BLOCK'S

DISINFECTION, STERILIZATION, *AND* PRESERVATION

SIXTH EDITION

BLOCK'S
DISINFECTION, STERILIZATION, *AND* PRESERVATION

SIXTH EDITION

GERALD McDONNELL, BSc, PhD

Senior Director, Microbiological Quality &
Sterility Assurance
Johnson & Johnson
Raritan, NJ

JOYCE M. HANSEN, BS, MBA

Vice President, Microbiological Quality &
Sterility Assurance
Johnson & Johnson
Raritan, NJ

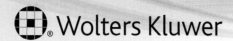

Philadelphia • Baltimore • New York • London
Buenos Aires • Hong Kong • Sydney • Tokyo

Acquisitions Editor: Nicole Dernoski
Development Editor: Ariel Winter
Editorial Coordinator: Tim Rinehart
Marketing Manager: Phyllis Hitner
Production Project Manager: David Saltzberg
Design Coordinator: Steve Druding
Art Director, Illustration: Jennifer Clements
Manufacturing Coordinator: Beth Welsh
Prepress Vendor: Absolute Service, Inc.

6th edition

Library of Congress Cataloging-in-Publication Data

Names: McDonnell, Gerald E., editor. | Hansen, Joyce M., editor.
Title: Block's disinfection, sterilization, and preservation / [edited by]
  Gerald McDonnell, Joyce M. Hansen.
Other titles: Disinfection, sterilization, and preservation
Description: Sixth edition. | Philadelphia : Wolters Kluwer, [2021] |
  Preceded by Disinfection, sterilization, and preservation / editor,
  Seymour S. Block. 5th ed. 2001. | Includes bibliographical references
  and index.
Identifiers: LCCN 2020015254 (print) | LCCN 2020015255 (ebook) | ISBN
  9781496381491 (hardcover) | ISBN 9781975153960 (ebook)
Subjects: MESH: Anti-Infective Agents, Local | Disinfectants |
  Sterilization
Classification: LCC RM409 (print) | LCC RM409 (ebook) | NLM QV 220 | DDC
  615.7/92--dc23
LC record available at https://lccn.loc.gov/2020015254
LC ebook record available at https://lccn.loc.gov/2020015255

CCS0720

Contents

PART IV: STERILIZATION BY ANTIMICROBIAL TYPES

PART V: PRESERVATION

PART VI: MEDICAL AND HEALTH-RELATED APPLICATIONS

Contributors

Donald G. Ahearn, PhD
Research Professor of Microbiology (Emeritus)
Applied and Environmental Microbiology Center
Department of Biology
Georgia State University
Atlanta, GA

James E. Akers Jr
Owner and Principal Consultant
Akers Kennedy and Associates LLC
Leawood, KS

James W. Arbogast, PhD
Vice President
Hygiene Science and Public Health Advancements
GOJO Industries Inc
Akron, OH

Richard Bancroft, BSc (Hons)
Science & Technical Director
STERIS Corporation
Leicester, United Kingdom

Allan Bennett, BSc (Hons), MSc
Scientific Lead
Biosafety, Air and Water Microbiology Group
National Infection Service, Public Health England
Salisbury, United Kingdom

Alan J. Beswick, PhD
Principal Scientist
Microbiology
Health and Safety Executive
Derbyshire, United Kingdom

Paul L. Bigliardi, MD
Professor of Dermatology
Department of Dermatology
University of Minnesota
Minneapolis, MN

Elaine Black, PhD
Senior Regulatory Manager
Regulatory Affairs
Ecolab
St. Paul, MN

Tajah L. Blackburn, PhD, MPH
Senior Scientist
Antimicrobials Division
United States Environmental Protection Agency
Washington, DC

Ernest R. Blatchley III
Lee A. Rieth Professor in Environmental Engineering
Lyles School of Civil Engineering and Division of
    Environmental and Ecological Engineering
Purdue University
West Lafayette, IN

Dirk P. Bockmühl, PhD
Professor
Faculty of Life Sciences
Rhine-Waal University of Applied Sciences
Kleve, Germany

Catherine Makison Booth, DProf
Senior Scientist
Microbiology
Health and Safety Executive
Derbyshire, United Kingdom

Gwen Borlaug, MPH, CIC, FAPIC
Infection Prevention Consultant
Peoria, AZ

Kelvin G.M. Brockbank
Chief Executive Officer
Tissue Testing Technologies, LLC
North Charleston, SC

Christopher L. Brown, BA
Senior Analyst
N&P Ltd
Charles Town, WV

Elizabeth Bruning, BSc (Hons), LLB
Senior R&D Manager
Research & Development
RB (Reckitt Benckiser)
Montvale, NJ

Trabue D. Bryans, BS, M(ASCP)
President
BryKor LLC
Marietta, GA

Andre G. Buret, MSc, PhD
Professor
Biological Sciences
University of Calgary
Calgary, Canada

Peter A. Burke, PhD
Founder and Principal Consultant
Executive Offices
Strategic Regulated R&D Consultants LLC
Concord, OH

Christine F. Carson, PhD
Research Fellow
School of Biomedical Sciences
The University of Western Australia
Perth, Australia

Marc Cataldo, PharmD
Director
Medical Communications & Strategy/Medical Affairs
Medical Affairs Department
Purdue Pharma L.P.
Stamford, CT

Zhao Chen, PhD
Postdoctoral Associate
Joint Institute for Food Safety and Applied Nutrition
University of Maryland
College Park, MD

Nicholas P. Cheremisinoff, PhD
Principal Consultant
N&P Ltd
Charles Town, WV

Lipika Gopal Chugh, BDS, MDS
Senior Lecturer
Department of Periodontology
Manav Rachna Dental College
Fazidabad, India

Elizabeth Claverie-Williams, MS
Assistant Director
Disinfection, Reprocessing and Personal Protection
Center for Devices and Radiologic Health, Food and
    Drug Administration
Silver Spring, MD

Thomas Patrick Coohill, PhD
Professor
Physics and Astronomy
Siena College
Loudonville, NY

Bruna de Oliveira Costa, MSc
Research Scientist
Department of Biotechnology
Universidade Católica Dom Bosco
Mato Grosso do Sul, Brazil

Brian Crook, BSc, PhD
Principal Scientist
Microbiology
Health and Safety Executive
Derbyshire, United Kingdom

Patrick J. Crowley, FRPhSGB
Visiting Professor
School of Pharmacy
King's College London
London, United Kingdom

Mark A. Czarneski, BS, MS
Director of Technology
ClorDiSys Solutions Inc
Branchburg, NJ

Elaine M. Daniell, BS, CISS-EO, CISS-RAD
President
Sterility Assurance Consulting
EDan-SA LLC
Oxford, GA

Kimbrell R. Darnell, MS, CISS-RAD, CISS-EO
Senior Manager of Laboratories
Becton, Dickinson, and Company
Covington, GA

Sarah de Szalay, BS, MS
Global Category R&D Manager
Research and Development, Reckitt Benckiser, Inc.
Montvale, NJ

Eric Dewhurst, BSc, FRSB
Technical Director
Shepherd Green Ltd
Cumbria, United Kingdom

John A. Diemer, BS, MS
Senior Research Scientist
Research and Development, Reckitt Benckiser, Inc.
Montvale, NJ

Lawrence G. Doucet, PE, DEE
Environmental Consultant and Engineer
Yorktown Heights, NY

Charles E. Edmiston Jr, MS, PhD, CIC
Emeritus Professor of Surgery
Department of Surgery, Division of Vascular Surgery
Medical College of Wisconsin
Milwaukee, WI

Maren Eggers, PhD
Head, Virology
Department of Virology
Labor Prof. Dr. G. Eders MVZ GbR
Stuttgart, Germany

David P. Elder, PhD
Consultant
David P. Elder Consultancy
Hertfordshire, United Kingdom

Steven Elliott, MS
Center for Devices and Radiologic Health, Food and
    Drug Administration
Silver Spring, MD

Randal W. Eveland, PhD
Senior Manager
Research and Development
STERIS Corp
Mentor, OH

Nancy A. Falk, PhD
Research Fellow
Cleaning Growth and Innovation Group
The Clorox Co
Pleasanton, CA

Eamonn S. Fitzpatrick, FIBMS, FRMS
Former Chief Technical Officer
School of Veterinary Medicine
University College Dublin
Dublin, Ireland

Dan B. Floyd, BS, CISS-EO
Microbiologist
Tyvek Healthcare
DuPont Safety
South Jordan, UT

Helen E. Forsdyke, BSc (Hons)
Senior Director, Regulatory Compliance, EMEA
Johnson & Johnson Medical Ltd
North Yorkshire, United Kingdom

Octávio Luiz Franco, PhD
Professor
Department of Biotechnology
Universidade Católica Dom Bosco
Mato Grosso do Sul, Brazil

Manal M. Gabriel, DDS, PhD
Fellow
Microbiology—Preclinical Development
Alcon
Johns Creek Parkway, GA

Philip A. Geis, PhD
Principal
Geis Microbiological Quality (affiliated with Advanced Testing
    Laboratory)
The Villages, FL

Kurt Giles, DPhil
Associate Professor
Institute for Neurodegenerative Diseases
University of California, San Francisco
San Francisco, CA

Brendan F. Gilmore, BSc, PhD
Professor
School of Pharmacy
Queen's University Belfast
Belfast, United Kingdom

Prerna Gopal, BDS, PhD
Senior Research Associate
Science & Research Institute
American Dental Association
Chicago, IL

Sean P. Gorman, PhD
Emeritus Professor
School of Pharmacy
Queen's University Belfast
Belfast, United Kingdom

Evan Goulet, PhD
Senior Project Manager
Lexa Med Ltd
Toledo, OH

Katherine Ann Hammer, PhD
Senior Lecturer
School of Biomedical Sciences
The University of Western Australia
Perth, Australia

Joyce M. Hansen, BS, MBA
Vice President, Microbiological Quality & Sterility Assurance
Johnson & Johnson
Raritan, NJ

Jacqueline L. Hardy
Lead Biologist
Antimicrobials Division
United States Environmental Protection Agency
Washington, DC

Philippe G. Hartemann, MD, PhD
Emeritus Professor
Department of Public Health
School of Medicine—Lorraine University
Vandœuvre-lès-Nancy, France

Michael S. Harvey, BS
President and Chief Executive Officer
Enviro Tech Chemical Services
Modesto, CA

David W. Hobson, PhD, DABT
Adjunct Professor
Nuclear Medical Technology
University of the Incarnate Word
San Antonio, TX

Marlitt Honisch, MSc
Research Associate
Faculty of Life Sciences
Rhine-Waal University of Applied Sciences
Kleve, Germany

Jonathan N. Howarth, PhD
Senior Vice President, Technology
Enviro Tech Chemical Services
Modesto, CA

Eamonn V. Hoxey, PhD, B.Pharm, FRPharmS
Director
E V Hoxey Ltd
Gloucestershire, United Kingdom

Christon J. Hurst, PhD
Cincinnati, OH
Universidad del Valle
Cali, Colombia

Mohammad Khalid Ijaz, DVM, MSc (Hons), PhD
Adjunct Associate Professor
Department of Biology
Medgar Evers College—The City University of New York
Brooklyn, NY

Nicola J. Irwin, MPharm, PhD
Lecturer, Pharmaceutical Materials Science
School of Pharmacy
Queen's University Belfast
Belfast, United Kingdom

Alyce Linthurst Jones, PhD
Virginia Beach, VA

James Jay Kaiser, BS
Sterilization Sciences Consultant
Rochester, NY

Günter Kampf, MD
Associate Professor
Institute for Hygiene and Environmental Medicine
University Medicine Greifswald
Greifswald, Germany

Ram Prakash Kapil, PhD
Executive Director
Clinical Pharmacology
Purdue Pharma L.P.
Stamford, CT

Amy Jo Karren, BS, RM/SM, NCRM
Microbiologist
W.L. Gore and Associates
Flagstaff, AZ

Stephen Anthony Kelly, PhD
Research Fellow
School of Pharmacy
Queen's University Belfast
Belfast, United Kingdom

Daniel Klein, MA
Senior Manager, Microbiology
Research Development
Steric Corp
St. Louis, MO

Kerry Roche Lentine, MS
Director, Technology Management
Process Solutions
MilliporeSigma
Burlington, MA

Finola C. Leonard, MVB, PhD, MRCVS
Associate Professor
School of Veterinary Medicine
University College Dublin
Dublin, Ireland

Richard V. Levy, PhD
Editor-in-Chief
PDA Journal of Pharmaceutical Science and Technology
Parenteral Drug Association
Bethesda, MD

Joey S. Lockhart, MSc
Graduate Student
Biological Sciences
University of Calgary
Alberta, Canada

John R. Logar, BA
Senior Director, Aseptic Processing and Terminal Sterilization
Microbiological Quality & Sterility Assurance
Johnson & Johnson
Raritan, NJ

Luyan Z. Ma, PhD
Professor
State Key Laboratory of Microbial Resources
Institute of Microbiology, Chinese Academy of Sciences
Beijing, China

Marisa Macnaughtan, PhD
Scientist II
Professional Products Division
The Clorox Co
Pleasanton, CA

Jean-Yves Maillard, BSc, PhD
Professor of Pharmaceutical Microbiology
School of Pharmacy and Pharmaceutical Sciences
Cardiff University
Wales, United Kingdom

Bryan K. Markey, MVB, PhD, DipStat, DipECVM, MRCVS
Associate Professor
School of Veterinary Medicine
University College Dublin
Dublin, Ireland

John J. Matta, PhD
Shoreview, MN

Elaine Mayhall, PhD
Center for Devices and Radiologic Health, Food and
    Drug Administration
Silver Spring, MD

Patrick J. McCormick, PhD
Research Fellow
Microbiology and Sterilization Sciences
Bausch + Lomb
Rochester, NY

William C. McCormick III, MS
Research Fellow
Global Stewardship
The Clorox Co
Pleasanton, CA

Colin P. McCoy, PhD
Professor of Biomaterials Chemistry
School of Pharmacy
Queen's University Belfast
Belfast, United Kingdom

Gerald McDonnell, BSc, PhD
Senior Director
Microbiology Quality & Sterility Assurance
Johnson & Johnson
Raritan, NJ

John J. Merianos, PhD
Senior Science Fellow
Research and Development, Sutton Laboratories
Chatham, NJ

Vinod P. Menon, PhD
Lead Research Specialist
Health Care Business Group
3M Company
St. Paul, MN

James H. Michel, MS
Technical Manager
Copper Development Association
McLean, VA

Corinne A. Michels, PhD
Distinguished Professor Emerita
Biology Department
Queens College—The City University of New York
Queens, NY

Harold T. Michels, PhD
Senior Vice President (Retired)
Technology and Technical Services
Copper Development Association Inc
McLean, VA

Chris H. Miller, PhD
Professor Emeritus of Oral Microbiology
Executive Associate Dean Emeritus
Associate Dean Emeritus for Academic Affairs
Indiana University School of Dentistry
Indianapolis, IN

Emily F. Mitzel, MS
Senior Manager
Technical Consulting
Nelson Laboratories
Salt Lake City, UT

Douglas W. Morck, DVM, PhD
Professor
Biological Sciences
University of Calgary
Alberta, Canada

Kristopher Douglas Murphy, PhD
Global Manager, Chemistry
Cantel Medical Corp
Plymouth, MN

Clarence Murray III
Center for Devices and Radiologic Health
Food and Drug Administration
Silver Spring, MD

David B. Opie, PhD
Senior Vice President
Research and Development
Noxilizer Inc
Baltimore, MD

Charles John Palenik, MS, PhD, MBA[†]
Infection Control Research & Services Indiana University
    School of Dentistry
Indianapolis, IN

Lionel Pineau, PhD
Scientific Director
Eurofins Biotech-Germande
Marseilles, France

Thomas Pottage, BSc (Hons)
Project Team Leader
Biosafety, Air and Water Microbiology Group
National Infection Service, Public Health England
Salisbury, United Kingdom

Daniel L. Price, PhD
Director
Microbiology Research and Development
Interface Inc
Atlanta, GA

Daniel L. Prince, PhD
Chief Executive Officer
Prince Sterilization Services
Fairfield, NJ

Derek J. Prince, PhD
President
Prince Sterilization Services
Pine Brook, NJ

Stanley B. Prusiner, MD
Director
Institute for Neurodegenerative Diseases
University of California, San Francisco
San Francisco, CA

Michael K. Pugsley, PhD, DSP
Director, Toxicology
Cytokinetics Inc
South San Francisco, CA

Patrick Joseph Quinn, MVB, PhD, MRCVS
Professor Emeritus
Former Professor of Veterinary Microbiology and Parasitology
School of Veterinary Medicine
University College Dublin
Dublin, Ireland

Md Ramim Tanver Rahman, MEng
Research Assistant
State Key Laboratory of Microbial Resources
Institute of Microbiology, Chinese Academy of Sciences
Beijing, China

Mohammad Shafiur Rahman, MSc, PhD
Professor
Food Science and Nutrition
Sultan Qaboos University
Muscat, Oman

José A. Ramirez, MS, PhD
Executive Vice President and Lead Science Advisor
Virox Animal Health
Ontario, Canada

Suzana Meira Ribeiro, PhD
Visiting Professor
Faculty of Health Sciences
Universidade Federal da Grande Dourados
Mato Grosso do Sul, Brazil

Alfredo C. Rodríguez, PhD
PQS Technologies LLC
Arlington Heights, IL

Tony A. Rook, BS
Associate R&D Director
Global Microbiology Resource Center
Sherwin-Williams
Cleveland, OH

Suranjan Roychowdhury, PhD
Vice President
Global Director and Development
Cantel Medical Corp
Plymouth, MN

Akikazu Sakudo, PhD
Associate Professor
Faculty of Veterinary Medicine
Okayama University of Science
Ehime, Japan

Michael J. Schoene, BS
Senior Research Scientist
Microbiology and Sterilization Sciences
Bausch + Lomb
Rochester, BY

Michael H. Scholla, PhD
Emeritus Medical Packaging Fellow
Medical and Pharma Protection
DuPont Safety
Wilmington, DE

Elizabeth A. Scott, PhD
Professor
Department of Biology
Simmons University
Boston, MA

Jane E. Severin, PhD, MBA, CPP
Vice President
Technical Solutions
Network Partners Northville, MI

Rizwan Sharnez, PhD
Founder and Senior Consultant
Cleaning Validation Solutions
Mead, CO

Manjunath Shet, PhD
Director
Department of Pharmacokinetics and Drug Metabolism
Imbrium Therapeutics
Stamford, CT

Mikhail Shifrin
Project Engineer
Absolute Ozone®
Research and Development
Edmonton, Canada

Hideharu Shintani, PhD
Guest Professor
Department of Science and Engineering
Chuo University
Tokyo, Japan

Osmar Nascimento Silva, PhD
Assistant professor
Department of Pharmacy
Centro Universitario de Anápolis (Unievangelica)
Goiás, Brazil

Maruti N. Sinha, PhD
Principal Engineer
Research and Development
Cantel Medical Corp
Plymouth, MN

Mark A. Smith, PhD, CHP
Managing Director
Ionaktis LLC
Charlotte, NC

Scott R. Steinagel, BS, MBA
Senior Manager
Microbiology Services
Ecolab
St. Paul, MN

Atefeh Taheri, PhD
Scientist II
Professional Products Division
The Clorox Co
Pleasanton, CA

Stephen F. Tomasino, PhD
Senior Scientist
Biological and Economic Analysis Division
United States Environmental Protection Agency
Washington, DC

Daniel J. Vukelich, Esq
President and CEO
Association of Medical Device Reprocessors
Washington, DC

Thierry Wagner, MS
Global Director
Regulations and Standards Healthcare
DuPont Safety & Construction
Luxembourg, France

Mark Wainwright, PhD
Professor of Antimicrobial Chemotherapy
School of Pharmacy and Biomolecular Sciences
Liverpool John Moores University
Liverpool, United Kingdom

Craig A. Wallace, BS
Senior Technical Specialist (Retired)
3M Infection Prevention Division
St. Paul, MN

Linda K. Weavers, PhD
John C. Geapel Endowed Professor
Civil, Environmental and Geodetic Engineering
The Ohio State University
Columbus, OH

G. B. Wickramanayake
Program Manager
Environmental Restoration Department,
   Battelle Memorial Institute
Columbus, OH

Martell Winters, BS
Director of Science
Lab Management
Nelson Laboratories LLC
Salt Lake, UT

Amanda L. Woerman, PhD
Assistant Professor
Institute for Neurodegenerative Diseases
University of California, San Francisco
San Francisco, CA

Matthew P. Wylie, PhD
Professor of Biomaterials Chemistry
School of Pharmacy
Queen's University Belfast
Northern Ireland, UK

Yoshihito Yagyu, PhD
Associate Professor
Department of Electrical and Electric Engineering
National Institute of Technology
Sasebo College
Nagasaki, Japan

Dedication

Professor Seymour S. Block, PhD (1918–2014)
Professor Emeritus of Bioengineering Department of Chemical Engineering University of Florida Gainesville, Florida

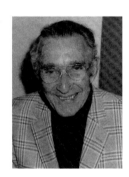

The sixth edition of *Disinfection, Sterilization, and Preservation* is dedicated to the memory of our good friend and colleague, Professor Seymour S. Block. He was the coeditor, with Carl A. Lawrence, of the first edition of this book in 1968 and the sole editor of the following four editions, with the fifth edition being published in 2001. He passed away in 2014 while still considering a sixth edition of this book. Over the years, *Disinfection, Sterilization, and Preservation* was for many the first introduction to the scientific principles and practices in this area and continues to be used as a key reference to this present day. Block graduated with a PhD from Penn State University in 1942, then the youngest person to earn a doctorate in the chemistry department and, after serving as a research chemist during World War II, came to the University of Florida for the remaining of his distinguished career. His initial work focused on larger fungi (mushrooms) but then studied preservation, disinfectant, and sterilizing agents. In addition to his teaching skills, he consulted with government and business and held many patents in the art. He was also a charter member of the Society for Industrial Microbiology and Biotechnology. In addition to his publications in science, he published works on Benjamin Franklin. He officially retired from the University in 1995 but remained active for many years after this. When he passed away at the age of 96, he was the longest serving professor in the State University System of Florida.

Preface

The first edition of *Disinfection, Sterilization, and Preservation* was published in 1968, edited by Drs. Carl A. Lawrence and Seymour S. Block. Since that time, there has been four further editions edited by Professor Block, with the fifth edition being published at the end of 2000. Sadly, in the interim, he passed away in 2014. Now 20 years since its last publication, it has been a great pleasure to bring together a new, sixth edition entitled *Block's Disinfection, Sterilization, and Preservation*. This edition is dedicated to Professor Block's memory, and we hope will continue to be a practical guide to the scientific principles and practices in this area.

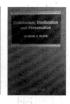

In planning for this edition, it has been useful to review the evolution of the book from its initial publication of approximately 800 pages in a compact book to the fifth edition with approximately 1 500 pages of larger size (and smaller font). The fifth edition included essential parts considered in the inaugural edition such as modes on modes of action, methods of testing, antiseptics and disinfectants, and sterilization. But the 2000 edition also focused on many important microbiological challenges of the day such as *Staphylococcus* and *Enterococcus* (with increased reports of antibiotic resistance), *Legionella* (due to notable outbreaks), human immunodeficiency virus (with debate at that time on the risks associated with infection prevention methods), and prions (soon after the height of the bovine spongiform encephalopathy outbreak in the United Kingdom and associated transmission to humans as variant Creutzfeldt-Jakob disease). Specific chapters on individual types of microorganisms have been reduced in the sixth edition, which returns to the initial outline of pre-

vious editions of the book. The new edition is collected into nine parts: introduction, fundamental principles of activity, disinfection, sterilization, preservation, medical and health applications, industrial and research applications, methods of testing, and miscellaneous topics. Following some introduction chapters are the fundamental chapters including consideration of microorganisms and the challenges to inactivation due to resistance mechanisms. There is a greater emphasis on the optimization of chemical and physical antimicrobial methods, such as by-product formulation and process exposure conditions. Consideration is also given to cleaning in many chapters, which can be effective not only in the physical removal of microorganisms but also as a prerequisite to disinfection/sterilization applications. This has been an area of scientific and regulatory attention in the last 20 years. The disinfection and sterilization parts consider the most commonly used physical and chemical methods, including newer chapters on the use of plant extractions, metals (copper and silver), proteins/peptides, and bacteriophages. The sterilization section also includes new chapters on gas methods such as those based on nitrogen dioxide, ozone, hydrogen peroxide, and gas plasmas. Part V has reestablished chapters on preservation methods, including a new chapter on sterile packaging as an essential component in maintaining the safety of products right up to the point of use. Part VI provides an update on medical and health applications, including antisepsis, environmental disinfection, and the reprocessing of single-use and reusable medical devices. Similarly, Part VII discusses industrial and research applications with updates on aseptic processing (as an alternative to terminal sterilization of sterile products), risks with water and foods, and control of microorganisms in laboratory and manufacturing environments. Part VIII on methods of testing has been consolidated to the widely used methods in testing antimicrobial method of microbicides but has been extended to include methods that support these including bioburden and the use of biological/chemical indicators. Finally, the last part provides a series of chapters on topics ranging from the risks with endotoxins and biofilms to regulations and standards and considers the increased focus in recent years on antimicrobial surfaces and nanotechnology.

It is important to recognize the knowledge and dedication of the various authors of the chapters in this book. Some have devoted their professional careers to this area, whereas others are the new generation of talent in the area. Our thanks to them in sharing their knowledge in this edition and for the late nights and weekends in completing chapters for this edition. We hope that a further generation of colleagues and friends will be inspired to contribute in future editions.

It is true to say that much has changed since the last edition. Primary to this is the challenge from microorganisms, with examples being the development of antibiotic-resistant bacteria (with the recent alarm from carbapenem-resistant *Enterobacteriaceae*), viral hemorrhagic fever viruses (eg, associated with Ebola virus disease and Lassa fever), influenza and corona virus pandemics (eg, Middle East respiratory syndrome, severe acute respiratory syndrome, swine flu, and COVID-19), and prion-associated diseases. Treatment of individuals infected or at risk from infection is a challenge requiring a revival in the identification of new anti-infectives, disease management methods, and more rapid immunization development. But greater emphasis has also been placed on preventing transmission and infection by using best practices of sterilization, disinfection, preservation, antisepsis, and asepsis methods described in this book. We have also learned that microorganisms can present with intrinsic and acquired mechanisms of tolerance to these methods if not applied correctly, although not to the same impact as observed with resistance to antibiotics and other anti-infectives. Despite this, many of these microbicides are dramatically less used today that in previous years, primarily due to other safety concerns. Fortunately, the correct application of microbiological quality controls can continue to ensure the provision of safe and effective products and services.

Despite the well-established impacts of disinfection, sterilization, and preservation methods on public health, we still observe how lapses in essential practices can lead to problems. Good examples include in the prevention of food or water contamination, failures in product preservation, and lapses in the reprocessing of reusable medical devices. These focus our attention not only on the efficient use of disinfection, sterilization, and preservation methods but also on the identification of risks that may be reduced before, during, and after the delivery of products and services. Balancing the requirements in the effective use of these methods to include environmental safety is also important to consider.

Medicine and surgery continue to make great advances, and microbicidal strategies and technologies need to continually evolve to meet these needs. The benefits of new treatment methods, reducing surgical intervention (eg, using endoscopic devices) or reducing human risks (or increasing surgical precision; eg, using robotics), are good examples. But these must be designed and handled appropriately to decrease risks of infection or other surgical complications. Many of these instruments are expected to become even more complicated and will increasingly be used in smaller clinic situations. Therefore, attention to ensuring adequate reprocessing and safe use in surgery is important to ensure patient safety. We continue to have more patients receiving various lifesaving or enhancing surgical procedures and implants such as pacemakers, mechanical joints, and other devices as well as transfers of whole living organs. Advances in artificial organs and three-dimensional printing technologies as well as combination devices (devices including drugs or tissues) will continue to challenge innovations to ensure products meet the microbiological quality necessary for their intended use.

It is a similar challenge with the development of chemicals (including drugs) or other products that are either used in the body, on the body surface (antiseptics), or in other applications. During the manufacturing and provision of large and small molecule drugs, it is imperative that products are provided to a defined microbiological quality as they are often used in those that are at their most vulnerable. In addition to the microbiological quality aspects of these products, the presence of biological associated toxins (some of which may or may not be inactivated by antimicrobial methods) can be a concern. An example is the focused attention in recent years on bacterial endotoxin. It is important not only that these products are provided on time to recipients but, that they are not the source of infections or other complications. Many of these technologies are themselves antiseptics and disinfectants, which are important in the provision of public health in many situations. As new therapeutic methods become more widely available, such as "vein-to-vein" chemotherapy (eg, chimeric antigen receptor cell therapy, Car-T), even greater attention on reducing infection risks and detection of those risks will be important.

Thankfully, we have a well-established armamentarium of antimicrobial technologies for our use with new and innovative products or applications. Many of these technologies are still used in similar ways to 50 years ago. This may not be so bad if these ways still meet our needs, but a new challenge is to develop from this foundation and to continue to adapt. Also consider that products and services will be different in the future, but by applying microbiological quality logic and best practices and continuing to innovate our processes, we can strike the right balance between man and microorganism.

Gerald McDonnell
Joyce M. Hansen

Historical Perspective

Eamonn V. Hoxey

The use of disinfection, preservation, and sterilization practices to kill microorganisms or to prevent or inhibit their growth is as old as human civilization or even older. The use of specific treatments to eliminate microorganisms and prevent deterioration or infection predates knowledge of the existence of living entities at a microscopic scale and has had a significant effect on health and welfare. Such treatments include those that have enabled development of animal husbandry and food preservation techniques to increase food production dramatically and create a safe food supply chain. Developments in public health and medical practices have decreased the occurrence and severity of infection, decreased morbidity and mortality, and improved the quality of life.

Developments in disinfection, preservation, and sterilization can be separated into three phases:

- Serendipitous—random actions prior to the discovery of microbes identified procedures that benefited human health, allowed food to be stored for longer, or improved animal welfare. Without understanding the reason for their effectiveness, these procedures became incorporated into routine practices that improved food supply and reduced illness and death.
- Empirical—knowledge of microorganisms and their link with spoilage and infection allowed observation and studies into the cause of deterioration and infection. Careful observation led to the definition of standard processes with demonstrable beneficial effect.
- Scientific—understanding the nature of inactivation of microorganisms, and the variables that influence it, allowed development of engineering control and monitoring of process variables. This has led to the development of optimized processes with risk-based, targeted outcomes.

▶ SERENDIPITOUS DEVELOPMENTS

Preservation of food by heating, drying, smoking, salting, fermenting, acidifying, adding sugar, and impregnating with spices and aromatics has been used by people throughout history. The Bible sets out instructions that soldiers returning from battle were required to disinfect their equipment and clothing with heat, either exposed to fire or boiling water.[1] Alexander the Great required his armies to boil their drinking water and bury feces. He is also reported to have ordered timber for bridge building to be covered with olive oil as a precaution against decay. This process was then followed in the Roman empire for all wooden construction that was exposed to severe moisture.[2] In Biblical and medieval times, fire was used to destroy clothes and corpses of diseased people. Historical reports from the Great Plagues mentioned the clothes of victims being burnt. Physicians who attended patients suffering from plague were careful to clothe themselves in protective garments comprising gloves, mask, hat, and long coat (Figure 1.1).

Alcohol has a long history of use for disinfection. Wine was used liberally throughout history, both externally and internally, to heal all kinds of ailments. Whereas the concentration of alcohol in wine provides little value as an antiseptic, distilled spirits provided a higher concentration of alcohol. Guy de Chauliac's *Inventarium sive Chirurgia Magna* (The Inventory, or the Great [work on] Surgery) reported the use of brandy for military dressings. The title of the book is often shortened to *Chirurgia Magna*; it was written in medieval Latin in 1363 and circulated in manuscript form before its first printing in 1478.[3] It was a compendium from previous authors with the addition of his own experience. There were 70 editions as it became the most influential surgical text for over 200 years, particularly in France.

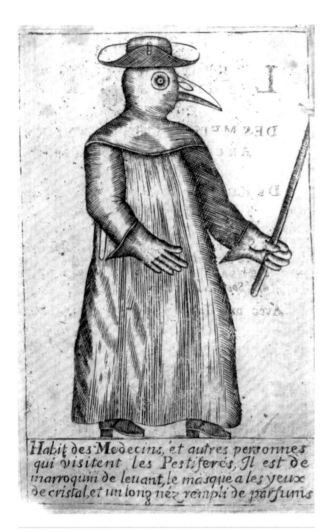

FIGURE 1.1   Plague physician's protective clothing, 17th century. From Father Maurice de Toulon, *Traite de la Peste*. Geneva, 1721. Courtesy of the Wellcome Collection.

▶ EMPIRICAL DEVELOPMENTS

The first true observations of the killing of microorganisms by chemicals dates from 1676. Antonie van Leeuwenhoek[4] (Figure 1.2) first observed viable organisms on a microscopic scale and reported that pepper and wine vinegar would kill microorganisms. Edmund King[5] followed up the work of van Leeuwenhoek by testing a number of substances including sulfuric acid, sodium tartrate, salt, sugar, wine, blood, and ink. He observed their effect on rate of kill, mobility, and shape of the organisms.

Methods of preservation of wood were standardized earlier than disease-preventive treatments for plants, animals, and humans. For example, the first patent for a wood preservative containing "the Oyle or Spirit of Tarr" was granted in 1716 for the protection of ship planking against decay and shipworm.[6] Coal-tar creosote, regarded

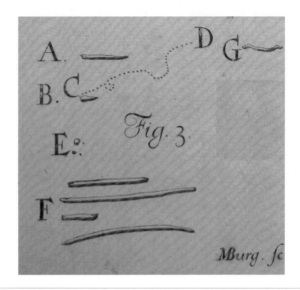

FIGURE 1.2   van Leeuwenhoek sketches of microorganisms, bacteria isolated from the teeth and sketched in 1684.

as the standard wood preservative, was patented in 1838 with the injection of creosote under pressure into wood.[7]

The cause of contagious fungal disease in plants and the means of its prevention by treatment with chemicals were discovered before disease in humans because the results of growth of fungal pathogens could be seen directly with the naked eye. Tillet[8] showed that chemicals in the form of saltpeter (potassium nitrate or other nitrogen-containing compounds) and lime (calcium oxide or calcium hydroxide) partially protected wheat seeds from infection by the bunt fungus. Prevost[9] used copper salts in field tests and demonstrated that they prevented the germination of fungal spores. Sulfur was used to prevent fungus disease of plants as early as 1802, and the effective lime-sulfur protective treatment was introduced in 1851.[10,11]

In 1718, Joblot[12] sterilized a hay infusion by boiling it for 15 minutes and then sealing the container. Appert[13] applied this procedure for preserving food to develop canning food by combining heat and closed containers. Spallanzani[14] noted that microorganisms in a liquid could be killed by heat and found that some organisms were more resistant than others; to kill resistant organisms, the liquid had to be boiled for 1 hour.

Semmelweis published his detailed observations[15] in 1847 and later compiled a seminal book, *Aetiologie*,[16] on his studies (Figure 1.3). He observed that when medical students came directly from the autopsy room and examined patients in the maternity ward, the rate of infection was greater than when students were not present. He noted odor from the autopsy room when students were present and insisted that they wash their hands with chloride of lime on leaving the autopsy room and before examining obstetric patients. The decrease in the death rate was spectacular.

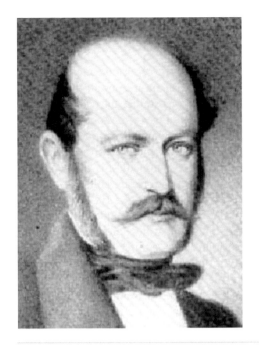 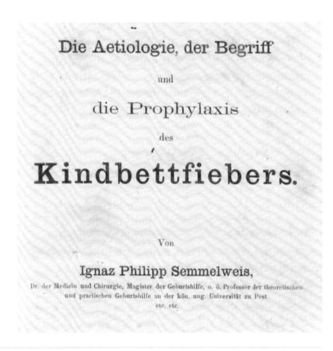

FIGURE 1.3   Ignaz Semmelweis (1818-1865) and the title page of his book on *Aetiologie* from 1861.

Louis Pasteur's experiments helped create the science of microbiology and inspired other scientists to investigate microbial diseases and the preservation of food and beverages. Pasteur (Figure 1.4) had to convince physicians that microorganisms cause disease. He advised surgeons to put their instruments through a flame before using them. He encouraged hospital personnel to heat sterilize bandages that were to be put on open wounds. He developed a process of heating wine briefly at 50°C to 60°C to prevent it being rejected because of off-flavors resulting from bacterial fermentations; a procedure now called pasteurization and still used for milk and other products.[17]

Lister[18] (see Figure 1.4) attributed the inflammation of wounds in compound fractures initially to microorganisms in the air but later recognized that microorganisms on surgeon's hands and dirty instruments were major causes of infection. He instituted a system of antiseptic surgery using phenol applied to the wound and to the floors and the walls of the operating rooms and wards. Lister commented that before antiseptic surgery, his wards were among the unhealthiest in the Glasgow hospital but, after the adoption of antiseptic treatment, the wards changed "so that during the last nine months not a single instance of pyemia, hospital gangrene, or erysipelas has

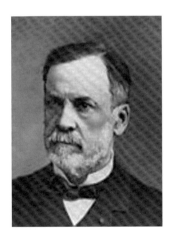 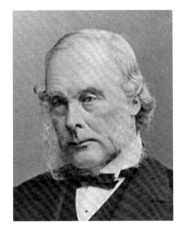 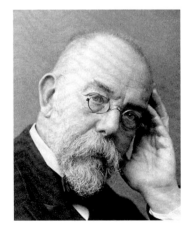

Louis Pasteur
(1822-1895)

Joseph Lister
(1827-1912)

Robert Koch
(1843-1910)

FIGURE 1.4   Pioneers in disinfection.

occurred in them."[18,19] Lister went to the United States in 1876 and lectured to the International Medical Congress. In the audience for his lectures was Robert Johnson, who started producing the gauze dressings soaked in phenol that Lister was using. This was the founding of Johnson & Johnson[20] as a provider of surgical dressings and sutures. In 1888, Fred B. Kilmer,[21] who had joined Johnson & Johnson, published a pamphlet and catalogue of products entitled *Modern Methods of Antiseptic Wound Treatment* with notes and suggestions from 10 eminent American physicians.

Robert Koch[22] (see Figure 1.4) introduced modern bacteriology with sterile technique, pure cultures, solid media, and antimicrobial test methodology. Using the achromatic microscope, Koch demonstrated that bacteria invaded tissues to produce disease. He wrote a comprehensive research paper titled *Uber Disinfektion* (or "On Disinfection")[22] that described the ability of over 70 chemicals at different concentrations and at different temperatures to kill *Bacillus anthracis* spores.

Kronig and Paul[23] established the basis of modern, scientific knowledge of the inactivation of microorganisms. They noted that

- Bacteria exposed to an inimical agent are not all killed at a fixed time but at a rate that depends on the concentration of the agent and the temperature.
- Inimical agents can be compared only when tested under controlled conditions, including challenge with a constant the number of microorganisms without interference from organic matter.
- Action of the inimical agent must be arrested promptly after a stated period.
- Surviving bacteria have to be transferred to the most favorable medium at optimal temperature.
- Results are determined by accurate count of survivors on plate cultures.

▶ SCIENTIFIC DEVELOPMENTS

The pioneering work of Kronig and Paul[23] established the scientific principles for standardization of tests for chemical disinfectants and the detailed investigation of the inactivation of a population of microorganisms. This investigation of microbial inactivation has been undertaken on innumerable occasions in academia, health institutions, research centers, and industry and has involved researchers in a variety of fields from health care to defense and space exploration to food science. These studies have led to an understanding of the nature of microbial inactivation and the influence of experimental variables on the effectiveness of disinfection, preservation, and sterilization. This, in turn, has led to the adoption of a risk-based measure to predicting the outcome of an applied process, with an emphasis on understanding and monitoring an optimized process rather than trying to measure process effectiveness by microbiological testing of resulting products.

As Kronig and Paul[23] reported, microorganisms exposed to an inimical agent are not all inactivated at the same instant. Numerous studies have shown that the inactivation of a pure culture of microorganisms by an inimical agent generally follows an exponential relationship between the number of microorganisms surviving and the extent of treatment applied. This relationship can be described by an inactivation rate constant or the extent of treatment needed to produce a 10-fold decrease in the number of microorganisms, termed the D_{10} value. After any given treatment, regardless of extent, there is always a finite probability that a microorganism will survive. This probability is determined by the initial number of microorganisms present, the inherent resistance of the test microorganisms, and the environment around them during treatment. Even when viable organisms cannot be detected, the probability of survival exists. The probability of a microorganism surviving decreases as the treatment is increased but never reaches zero.

Development of processes for disinfection, preservation, and sterilization has required the definition of test methods that allow the comparison of lethal processes against standardized challenges. The microorganism chosen, how it is grown, the number to be used, and the way that they are presented to the process under investigation all affect the outcome of the test. Once broad-spectrum antimicrobial activity has been demonstrated for a sterilization process, bacterial endospores have generally been used because of their relative resistance (see chapters 3 and 4), ease of presentation, and durability during storage. Standardized biological indicators are available for most methods of sterilization. The modern necessity of using biological indicators for routine monitoring of sterilization cycles, however, has been questioned as noted in the following text. There is greater variety of tests applied for disinfectants aimed at measuring the antimicrobial activity of a substance or preparation. Disinfectant tests can be considered at three levels: first, preliminary screening tests to establish antimicrobial activity of an agent; second, simulated tests to determine the conditions and concentration needed for a disinfection procedure; and, third, in situ tests to evaluate the disinfection procedure as it is to be used in practice.[24]

As understanding of the range of microorganisms and their inactivation has increased, so has the recognition of the different requirements for disinfection, reduction of the number of viable microorganisms to a level that is not harmful for health, and sterilization, attaining the absence of all viable microorganisms. In health care, Spaulding[25] proposed a system of classification that is still widely used around the world for identification of the need for disinfection and sterilization based on the associated risks. This classification system can be applied to surfaces and medical devices in the health care environment. It presents a ranking of the use of devices ranging from *critical* (presenting a high risk and requiring sterility) through *semicritical* to *noncritical* (presenting a low risk and often requiring disinfection or cleaning only). The use of sophisticated medical devices, such as flexible endoscopes, many of which had been classified as semicritical because they only contacted intact mucous membranes and being unable to withstand the rigorous processing necessary to achieve sterility at that time, led to the development of controlled disinfection processes with specified disinfectants and in automated equipment. The morbidity and mortality associated with hospital-acquired infection has led to greater attention to hygiene and the application of rational policies for disinfection in health care facilities,[26] including with flexible endoscopes.[27]

The food industry implemented a risk management approach termed Hazard Analysis Critical Control Point for the identification of process risks and the controls necessary at the critical steps to mitigate these risks. The basic requirement for the canning of food is the reduction of the chance of survival of spores of *Clostridium botulinum* by a sufficiently large factor.[28] The accepted magnitude of this factor is derived from Esty and Meyer's[29] studies, which proposed a 10^{12}-fold reduction of spore numbers to ensure an acceptable degree of safety of low-acid, thermally processed foods.

There was recognition by the National Academy of Sciences in 1958 that space exploration might lead to extraterrestrial bodies becoming contaminated with living terrestrial organisms.[30] The concern was, and remains, that contamination of planetary environments by terrestrial organisms could compromise investigations to identify indigenous life.[31] Historically, the approach used in establishing planetary protection requirements for spacecraft was that the probability of contamination with terrestrial microorganisms, that is, the probability that microorganisms would be introduced and then reproduce, is less than a threshold and the probability of contamination over multiple space launches would remain small. This overall probability was set to 10^{-3} by the Committee on Space Research (COSPAR), now the International Council for Science for all nations, with different nations then being allotted fractions of this probability.[32] The COSPAR[33] accepted "a sterilization level such that the probability of a single viable organism aboard any spacecraft intended for planetary landing or atmospheric penetration would be less than 1×10^{-4}, and a probability limit for accidental planetary impact by unsterilized flyby or orbiting spacecraft of 3×10^{-5} or less." National Aeronautics and Space Administration undertook a considerable body of research into the inactivation of microorganisms at the Scandia Laboratories in Albuquerque, New Mexico, in order to develop methods for meeting the sterilization requirements for space hardware.

Although Spaulding[25] classified the extent of processing required based on the use of medical devices, he did not propose criteria for sterility other than the absence of viable microorganisms. An approach of applying a fixed, minimum inactivation factor against a biological indicator of high nominal resistance to be delivered by a sterilization process was adopted initially in the food industry. A 10^{12} inactivation factor, described as an overkill approach, is still applied today for many sterilization processes. In 1970, however, an amendment to the Nordic Pharmacopoeia[34] (Figure 1.5) first included the notion that a maximal probability of survival of a single microorganism in or on a health care product after sterilization treatment of 1×10^{-6} should be required. It stated, "Sterile drugs must be prepared and sterilized under conditions that aim at such a result that in one million units there will be no more than one living microorganism." This was followed by similar concepts in statements in the United States Pharmacopeia XXI and the British Pharmacopoeia 1988.[35] The rationale for selection of this value has not been documented but corresponds with a general recognized level of risk considered "remote." The probability of

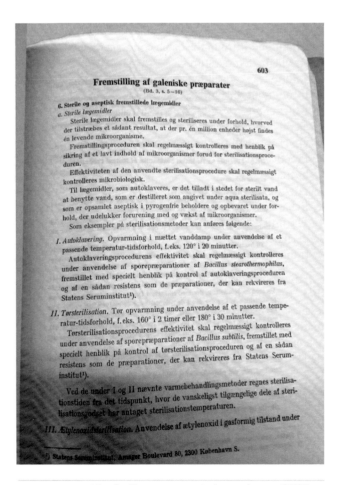

FIGURE 1.5 Nordic Pharmacopoeia Amendment (1970) stating "Sterile drugs must be prepared and sterilised under conditions that aim at such a result that in one million units there will be no more than one living microorganism."

survival of a single microorganism has been termed the *sterility assurance level* (SAL) and an acceptable maximal SAL of 10^{-6} for health care products labeled sterile has been stipulated regularly in pharmacopoeia and many other standards and guidance documents.

The UK Medical Research Council[36] investigated the use of steam sterilization and concluded "high vacuum sterilizers are fully instrumented and automatically controlled, and, once a sterilization procedure has been laid down and checked, the temperature record should provide an adequate assurance of sterility. Spore preparations should be used only for assessing new techniques or equipment, for research purposes, and for occasions when a rigorous full-dress inspection is needed for administrative or forensic reasons." This prompted a focus on the development of engineering controls and methods for independent monitoring of the sterilization process by measurements of the process variables, with the recognition of what has been termed *parametric release* of products following sterilization.

An incident at a hospital in the United Kingdom in 1971, in which use of a batch of 5% dextrose solution led to five deaths and at least two other patients affected, was investigated by a committee of inquiry.[37] The inquiry reported that

- About one-third of the batch concerned failed to attain sterilizing temperatures.
- Failure was caused by retention of air in the autoclave throughout the cycle.
- Instructions for operation of autoclaves were not sufficiently precisely worded.
- Operators had to interpret the instructions.
- Practices that were not included in the instructions had been allowed.
- Low-temperature recordings were habitually ignored.
- Reliance was placed on external autoclave instruments.
- The unit manager had "wholly inadequate" relevant experience and his superior did not ensure appropriate training was given.

The conclusions of the inquiry included the statement that "fundamental is human failings from simple carelessness to poor management of people and plant. Too many people believe that sterilization of fluids is easily achieved with simple plant operated by personnel of little skill under a minimum of supervision, a view of the task that is wrong in every respect." In a subsequent report on the prevention of microbial contamination of medicinal products, Rosenheim[38] added that the "correct way to control a sterilization process for which the physical requirements are known are by use of a sound method of physical measurement. The use of biological or chemical indicators are of secondary importance." These events and reports were influential globally in the implementation of good manufacturing practices (GMPs) for health care products in general and specific requirements for preparation of sterile products in particular. Emphasis was placed on engineering controls, preventive maintenance, independent control and monitoring, documentation of procedures, and requirements for competence of personnel.

The development of standardized and accurate methods of monitoring and control has also provided the opportunity for the optimization of processes to reduce the extent of treatment to achieve the defined SAL with a sterilization process while minimizing the detrimental effect on product.

- In moist heat treatment using steam at high pressure in the food and health care industries, the F_0-value is used as an alternative to defining the sterilization process as a minimum hold time at a given temperature. The lethality of a process includes the effects of the heating and cooling periods as well as the sterilization hold time. In a large fluid load, the heat-up and cool-down times can be long and have an appreciable microbicidal effect. The F_0-value expresses the lethality of the whole process as an equivalent hold time at 121°C, and its calculation has been extensively reviewed.[39-41] A similar concept is used for the application of thermal disinfection processes.[42]
- In radiation sterilization, methods of determining the radiation dose needed to achieve a defined SAL based on inactivation of the naturally occurring population of microorganisms as they occur on the product have been developed. The basis of these methods was first propounded by Tallentire et al.[43-45] Subsequently, standardized protocols were developed,[46,47] which have formed the basis of international standard procedures. The methods are based on a probability model for the inactivation of microbial populations. The model is applied to bioburden made up of a mixture of various microbial species and assumes that each such species has its own unique D_{10} value. In the model, the probability that an item will possess a surviving microorganism after exposure to a given dose of radiation is defined in terms of the initial number of microorganisms on the item prior to irradiation and the D_{10} values of the microorganisms. The methods involve performance of tests of sterility on product items that have received doses of radiation lower than the sterilization dose. The outcome of these tests is used to predict the dose needed to achieve a predetermined SAL. These same principles have also been used to develop a method (called method VD_{max}) for substantiating a selected sterilization dose achieving maximally an SAL of 10^{-6}, the selection of the dose being based on the number of microorganisms on product prior to sterilization.[48-50]
- In ethylene oxide sterilization, pressure to decrease levels of residuals of the sterilizing agent after processing have led the use of decreased concentration of ethylene oxide and developments of improved process control and monitoring include direct measurement of humidity and ethylene oxide concentration. This has allowed the acceptance of parametric release for ethylene oxide sterilization processes.

For a sterile health care product, achieving sterility is one thing, but sterility needs to be maintained until the point of use and the product has to be presented in a way that does not compromise sterility. Therefore, significant attention has to be paid to the way that the product is packaged and the materials used as well as how it is transported and stored so that the integrity of the package is maintained (see chapter 41). The environment in which the product is used and the clinical practice adopted by the user will also affect the risk of infection to which the patient is exposed.

Many health care products, particularly those containing water, have the capacity to support microbial growth. The stability of the product and the safety of the user can require specific measures to prevent survival and multiplication of microorganisms that might occur naturally in the product or enter it during storage or use. This could require the inclusion of one or more specific antimicrobial preservatives in the formulation. As the complex nature of the formulation of such products might influence the effectiveness of antimicrobial agents, the identification of a suitable preservative system requires careful evaluation (see chapter 6). Concerns over preservative toxicity by regulatory authorities means that the inclusion of preservatives has to be justified. These concerns have led to an almost complete transition to sterile single-use dosage forms with certain types of products, such as those for parenteral administration. Multidose containers for eye preparations, however, are still widely available and require preservative protection as the eye can be particularly susceptible to infection when damaged.[51] Other examples of the use of preservatives include application in cosmetics, water, foods, and industrial applications (see chapters 37 to 40).

As scientific knowledge has grown, methods of testing disinfectants, preservatives, and sterilizing agents have been codified in a variety of formats. In order to support regulations, these procedures have been defined as voluntary consensus standards, pharmacopoeia monographs, or professional codes of practice. In the health care field, for example, there has been significant alignment in expectations through the harmonization of pharmacopoeias and requirements for GMP, and the development of a portfolio of international standards for the development, validation, and routine control of sterilization processes. Antiseptic, disinfection, and preservative requirements can vary depending on regional regulatory requirements (see chapter 70).

Defining a process for disinfection, preservation, or sterilization remains a compromise between maximizing the microbicidal effect while minimizing damage to constituents of the product and potential toxicity to humans. Assurance of the effectiveness of disinfection, preservation, or sterilization comes from actions taken in all phases of development, validation, and routine control of the associated processes together with knowledge of the microbiological contamination on the item being processed and the surrounding environment. Typically, such actions include but are not limited to

- Defining an appropriate inimical agent
- Defining conditions that have adequate microbicidal effectiveness
- Selecting material combinations that can withstand exposure to the inimical agent
- Identifying the nature of the product to be treated and its presentation to the process
- Controlling the microbiological status of constituents of the product
- Validating and routinely controlling any cleaning and pretreatment procedures used
- Controlling the environment
- Controlling manufacturing equipment and processes
- Controlling personnel and their hygiene
- Controlling the manner in which a product is packaged
- Specifying the equipment that is needed to control the treatment conditions
- Showing that the defined process is effective and reproducible
- Demonstrating that the validated process has been delivered
- Maintaining the continued effectiveness of the process over time
- Controlling the conditions under which any product is stored.

◗ CONCLUSION

This chapter provides a glimpse of some of the highlights in the early developments of disinfection, sterilization, and preservation and the background to the foundations of modern practices. More detailed accounts of the early developments are found in previous editions of this book and the references to this chapter. The background to the individual treatments can be found in the specialized chapters in this edition.

◗ ACKNOWLEDGMENT

With thanks to A. Tallentire, PhD, Professor Emeritus, University of Manchester, United Kingdom, for the insights that have shaped my thinking on these topics and his feedback and helpful suggestions on this text.

REFERENCES

1. Numbers 31:21-24 (NIV).
2. Bulloch W. *The History of Bacteriology*. London, United Kingdom: Oxford University Press; 1938.
3. Ogden MS, ed. *Cyrurgie of Guy de Chauliac*. London, United Kingdom: Early English Text Society; 1971.

4. van Leeuwenhoek A. An abstract of a letter from Mr. Anthony Leeuwenhoek at Delft, dated Sept. 17, 1683, about some microscopical observations, about animals in the scurf of the teeth. *Philos Trans R Soc Lond B Biol Sci.* 1684;14:568-574.

5. King E. Several observations and experiments on the animalcula in pepper water, etc. *Philos Trans R Soc Lond B Biol Sci.* 1693;17(203):861-886.

6. Hunt GM, Garratt GA. *Wood Preservation.* 2nd ed. New York, NY: McGraw-Hill; 1953.

7. Bethell J. Dead oil of tar for treatment of wood. *British Patent 7751,* July 1838.

8. Tillet M. *Dissertation on the Cause of the Corruption and Smutting of the Kernels of Wheat in the Head and on the Means of Preventing These Untoward Circumstances.* Humphrey HG, trans-ed. Ithaca, NY: American Phytopathological Society; 1937.

9. Prevost I-B. *Memoir on the Immediate Cause of Bunt or Smut of Wheat, and of Several Other Diseases of Plants and on Preventives of Bunt.* Keitt GW, trans-ed. Menasha, WI: American Phytopathological Society; 1939.

10. McCallan SEA. History of fungicides. In: Torgeson DC, ed. *Fungicides.* New York, NY: Academic Press; 1967:1-29.

11. Keitt GW. History of plant pathology. In: Horsfall J, Dimond AE, eds. *Plant Pathology.* New York, NY: Academic Press; 1959:62-91.

12. Joblot L. *Descriptions and Use of Several New Microscopes.* Paris, France: Chez Jacques Collombat; 1718.

13. Appert N. *The Art of Preserving All Kinds of Animal and Vegetable Substances for Several Years.* New York, NY: D. Longworth; 1812.

14. Spallanzani L. Observations and experience about the animalcules of the infusion. In: *Writings on the Natural Animals and Vegetables of the Abbey Spallanzani.* Modena, Paris: 1776;3-221.

15. Semmelweis IP. Most important information on the etiology of puerperal fever in the birth delivery institution [in German]. *Zeitschrift der kaiserlich-Königlichen Gesellschaft der Aerzt zu Wien.* 1847; Jahrg. IV, 242; 1849, Jahrg. V, Bd. I,64.

16. Semmelweis IP. *The Etiology, Concept and Prophylaxis of Childbed Fever.* Pest, Vienna, and Leipzig: C.A. Hartleben's Verlag-Expedition; 1861.

17. Vallery-Radot R. *Pasteur.* New York, NY: Doubleday; 1923.

18. Lister J. On a new method of treating compound fracture, abscess, etc., with observations on the conditions of suppuration. *Lancet.* 1867;89(2274):387-389.

19. Lister J. On the antiseptic principle in the practice of surgery. *Lancet.* 1867;90(2299):353-356.

20. Johnson & Johnson. *History of Medical Product Sterilization.* New York, NY: Johnson & Johnson; 1998.

21. Kilmer FB. *Modern Methods of Antiseptic Wound Treatment.* New York, NY: Johnson & Johnson; 1888.

22. Koch R. On disinfection. *Mittheilungen aus dem Kaiserlichen Gesundheitsamte.* 1881;1:234-282.

23. Kronig B, Paul TL. The chemical foundations of the study of disinfection and of the action of poisons. *Zeitschrift für Hygiene.* 1897;25:1-112.

24. Reybrouk G. Evaluation of antibacterial and antifungal activity of disinfectants. In: Russell AD, Hugo WB, Ayliffe GAJ, eds. *Principles and Practice of Disinfection, Sterilization and Preservation.* 3rd ed. Oxford, United Kingdom: Blackwell Science; 1999:124-144.

25. Spaulding EH. Chemical disinfection and antisepsis in the hospital. *J Hosp Res.* 1957;9:5-31

26. Ayliffe GAJ, Babb JR. Decontamination of the environment and medical equipment in hospital. In: Russell AD, Hugo WB, Ayliffe GAJ, eds. *Principles and Practice of Disinfection, Preservation and Sterilization.* 3rd ed. Oxford, United Kingdom: Blackwell Science; 1999:395-415.

27. Kovaleva J, Peters FT, van der Mei HC, Degener JE. Transmission of infection by flexible gastrointestinal endoscopy and bronchoscopy. *Clin Microbiol Rev.* 2013;26:231-254.

28. Gould GW. Application of thermal processing in the food industry. In: Russell AD, Hugo WB, Ayliffe GAJ, eds. *Principles and Practice of Disinfection, Preservation and Sterilization.* 3rd ed. Oxford, United Kingdom: Blackwell Science; 1999:665-674.

29. Esty JR, Meyer KF. The heat resistance of the spores of *B. botulinus* and allied anaerobes XI. *J Infect Dis.* 1922;31:650-664.

30. Trauth CA Jr. A multi-stage decision model for mission non-contamination requirements. *Space Life Sci.* 1968;1:135-149.

31. National Research Council. *Preventing the Forward Contamination of Mars.* Washington, DC: The National Academies Press; 2006. doi:10.17226/11381

32. Committee on Space Research. *COSPAR Decision No. 16, COSPAR Information Bulletin.* Paris, France: Committee on Space Research; 1969.

33. Committee on Space Research. *COSPAR Resolution No. 26, COSPAR Information Bulletin.* Paris, France: Committee on Space Research; 1964.

34. Den danske Farmakopékommision. Fremstilling af galeniske praeparater. In *Pharmacopea Nordica Edico Danika Addendum.* Kobenhavn, Denmark: Nyt Nordisk Forlag Arnold Busk A/S; 1970.

35. Carson PA, Dent N. *Good Clinical, Laboratory and Manufacturing Practices: Techniques for the QA Professional.* Cambridge, United Kingdom: Royal Society of Chemistry; 2007.

36. Medical Research Council. Sterilisation by steam under increased pressure; a report to the Medical Research Council by the Working Party on pressure-steam sterilisers. *Lancet.* 1959;273:425-435.

37. Clothier CM. *Report of the Committee Appointed to Inquire into the Circumstances, Including the Production, which Led to the Use of Contaminated Infusion Fluids in the Devonport 37. Section of Plymouth General Hospital.* London, United Kingdom: Her Majesty's Stationery Office; 1972.

38. Rosenheim. *Report on the Prevention of Microbial Contamination of Medicinal Products.* London, United Kingdom: Her Majesty's Stationery Office; 1973.

39. Deindoerfer FH, Humphrey AE. Analytical method for calculating heat sterilization times. *Appl Microbiol.* 1959;7:256-264.

40. Stumbo CR. *Thermobacteriology in Food Processing.* 2nd ed. New York, NY: Academic Press; 1973.

41. De Santis P, Rudo VS. Validation of steam sterilization in autoclaves. In: Carleton FJ, Agalloco JP, eds. *Validation of Aseptic Pharmaceutical Processes.* New York, NY: Marcel Dekker; 1986:279-317.

42. McCormick PJ, Schoene MJ, Dehmler MA, McDonnell G. Moist heat disinfection and revisiting the A_0 concept. *Biomed Instrum Technol.* 2016;50:19-26.

43. Tallentire A, Dwyer J, Ley FJ. Microbiological quality control of sterilized products: evaluation of a model relating frequency of contaminated items with increasing radiation treatment. *J Appl Bacteriol.* 1971;34:521-534.

44. Tallentire A. Aspects of microbiological control of radiation sterilization. *J Rad Ster.* 1973;1:85-103.

45. Tallentire A, Khan AA. The sub-process dose in defining the degree of sterility assurance. In: Gaughran ERL, Goudie AJ, eds. *Sterilization by Ionizing Radiation.* Vol 2. Montreal, Canada: Multiscience Publications Ltd; 1978:65-80.

46. Davis KW, Strawderman WE, Masefield J, Whitby JL. DS gamma radiation dose setting and auditing strategies for sterilizing medical devices. In: Gaughran ERL, Morrissey RF, eds. *Sterilization of Medical Products.* Vol 2. Montreal, Canada: Multiscience Publications Ltd; 1981:34-102.

47. Davis KW, Strawderman WE, Whitby JL. The rationale and a computer evaluation of a gamma irradiation sterilization dose determination method for medical devices using a substerilization incremental dose sterility test protocol. *J Appl Bacteriol.* 1984;57:31-50.

48. Kowalski JB, Tallentire A. Substantiation of 25 kGy as a sterilization dose: a rational approach to establishing verification dose. *Radiat Phys Chem.* 1999;54:55-64.

49. Kowalski JB, Aoshuang Y, Tallentire A. Radiation sterilization—evaluation of a new approach for substantiation of 25 kGy. *Radiat Phys Chem.* 2000;58:77-86.

50. Kowalski JB, Tallentire A. Computer and field evaluations in support of the VD_{max} approach for selected sterilization doses greater than 25 kGy. *Radiat Phys Chem.* 2010;79:1005-1011.

51. Beveridge EG. Preservation of medicines and cosmetics. In: Russell AD, Hugo WB, Ayliffe GAJ, eds. *Principles and Practice of Disinfection, Preservation and Sterilization.* 3rd ed. Oxford, United Kingdom: Blackwell Science; 1999:457-484.

Definition of Terms

Gerald McDonnell

Words are meant to convey meaning, but we cannot be sure that any word will convey the same meaning to every person under every situation. People have different backgrounds and outlooks and derive different meanings from the same word. Furthermore, language is, in a sense, a living organism, and words can change their meaning with time. Consider the English language alone and the difference between reading a modern novel in comparison to the works of Shakespeare and Chaucer. In modern usage, the definition of words can make a difference to their general and legal use. In previous edition of this book,[1] as example was given with the word "whiskey" (or for those such inclined, "whisky"). Most people think they know what the term *whiskey* means, but they could be wrong, for it is a word with a legal as well as a popular meaning. Legally, whiskey is strictly a spirit distilled from a fermented mash of grain at less than 95% alcohol by volume (190 proof) having the taste, aroma, and characteristics generally attributed to whisky and bottled at not less than 40% alcohol by volume (80 proof). This term can be further subdivided into other subterms, such as Irish whiskey and Scotch whisky, that are related to spirits made in certain countries, according to laws of those specific countries. A product having the same color, odor, taste, and chemical composition might not satisfy the legal definition and its associated label claims.

Definitions are man-made and can therefore range considerably depending on different parts of the world and under different situations. Consider terms such as *disinfection*, *sterilization*, and *preservation*, which are often used in common practice but can have different legal requirements under different situations. Definitions attempt to make boundaries around terms, but these boundaries are often become vague and indistinct to accommodate different situations. Yet, we must work with them as best we can. A good example is trying to define what we mean when we use the term *dead*. We understand, no doubt, the term, but how do we define this? It is hard to be exact.

When is a person physically or legally dead? When they are no longer breathing? When he or she is brain dead? When all the cells in his or her body are dead? It is no different when we use terms such as *sterilization* and *sterile*. When is a product sterile? When all life in or on it has been killed, when it has been heated at x temperature for y minutes, or when its microbial population is reduced by a given number or scale? It is what we say it is, according to the way we construct our definition.

Definitions by lexicographers and lawyers serve the useful purpose of giving all people the opportunity of common understanding of what they mean when they use a word. When manufacturers label a product as an antiseptic, as disinfectant, or as "sterile," it is imperative that their product does or is what these terms imply. The legal implication of these terms became a focus in the 1920s in certain countries such as the United States. An initial judicial decision at this time in the United States stated that "language used in the label is to be given the meaning ordinarily conveyed by it to those to whom it was addressed." This was difficult to do if there was not clear and defined meanings (and expectations) for these various terms. Legal definitions therefore began to clarify their meanings. It was in 1925 that the US Bureau of Chemistry (now the US Food and Drug Administration [FDA]) deemed it necessary to give drug manufacturers a legal definition of the word *antiseptic* so that this class of drugs could be controlled by the government. Words such as *antiseptic*, *disinfectant*, and *sanitizer* were early examples of words that had loosely accepted meanings until they were more strictly defined during these times. Austin M. Patterson, a lexicographer of scientific terms, made a thorough study of many of these words in 1932, which served to further harmonize their meanings in the new era of antimicrobial controls.[2] Others such as those published by McCulloch,[3] Reddish,[4] Spaulding,[5] and earlier editions of this book, to name but a few, continued to evolve these growing series of definitions. In recent years, there has been much progress made on harmonizing many of the definitions that we use in the application of disinfection, sterilization, and preservation technologies internationally (eg, as defined in ISO 11139[6]). Despite that, different countries (or even regulatory agencies) can still use specific terms to represent legal requirements in their jurisdiction that can vary from their general or harmonized usage.

Overall, definitions are further discussed in this chapter. An initial consideration is given to four main terms, *disinfection, antisepsis* (as a specific type of disinfection application), *sterilization,* and *preservation,* with some discussion. This is followed by an alphabetic list of definitions that may be a useful reference during the reading of the subsequent chapters of this book. This list should not be considered strict or exclusive, and it is important to note that the general and, more importantly, legal requirements in the use of these terms for product labeling can vary from country (or area) to country.

▶ DISINFECTION

Disinfection is a process to inactivate viable microorganisms to a level previously specified as being appropriate for a defined purpose. It can be achieved using a variety of physical (eg, heat or radiation) and chemical methods or indeed a combination of both. Chemical disinfection, for example, can therefore be defined as the reduction of microorganisms achieved by the action of one or more chemicals. Note that processes such as cleaning and filtration can also physically remove viable microorganisms from surfaces or the air, others gases, or liquids but do not necessarily inactivate microorganisms. A *disinfectant* may be simply defined as the technology used for the purpose of disinfection. This can include the use of hot water, steam, or ultraviolet (UV) light, but the common use of the term *disinfectant* generally refers to a chemical or combination of chemicals used for disinfection. A harmonized term used is *disinfecting agent*, which refers to any physical or chemical agent used for disinfection.

The origin of the term is from the French *des-* and the verb *infecter*, to essentially mean the reversal of or to rid from infection. The word *disinfectant* was first recorded in writing in 1598, with the meaning of "to cure, to heal," but in 1658, it was used in the more modern sense, to remove infection. At this time, it was already appreciated that there was a benefit to burning the belongings used of those "that died of the pestilence to dis-infect them." In those days, it was believed that contagious diseases arose from effluvia, a flowing out of invisible particles from the diseased person or corpse, or from miasmas, which were noxious disease-bearing exhalations from putrefying organic matter emanating from damp, unhealthful places like malarial swamps. Miasmas were referred to in medical writing as early as 1665. But we can find earlier

evidence of the importance of disinfection methods in earlier times, such as in the use of chemical substances such as burning sulfur, the earliest reference for which can be at least traced back to the practice being described in Homer's *Odyssey* in approximately 800 BC, calling on his nurse to bring sulfur for fumigation following the massacre of suitors. The purifying effects of chemicals such as sulfur has been cited for many similar uses, such as in the 4th century for rooms used for surgery in India and during the Middle Ages in Europe during the plague epidemics. Because disease was associated with foul odors, disinfectants were expected to destroy or mask the odors to get rid of the infection.

The term became more widespread in its use during the 1800s in parallel with a greater understanding of microorganisms. Patterson[2] studied 143 definitions of *disinfectant* used from 1854 to 1930. Of these, 25, mostly of earlier date, made no mention of microorganisms. Of the rest, 95 defined disinfectants as germ destroyers. In this respect, the term *germ* refers to any microorganism. But the word *disinfectant* still carries with it much of its original connotation, namely, the cleaning of sickrooms, clothing, bedding, lavatories, stables, and so forth. Even the more legal definition[4] is similar but more detailed. It refers to an agent that frees from infection; usually a chemical agent that destroys disease germs or other harmful microorganisms or inactivates viruses. So, even at this time, the term was most commonly used to designate chemicals that kill the growing (or vegetative) forms of microorganisms but not necessarily the more resistant forms (such as the endospores of bacteria). Proper use of a disinfectant could therefore be contingent on the purpose for which it is used or the type of infectious (or contaminating) agent there is reason to suspect may (or is known) be present.

Block,[1] in a previous edition of this book, discussed in more detail the various medical, chemical, legal, and general definitions at the time. But the subsequent harmonization of the terms disinfection and disinfectant negates the need for further debate. But he also highlighted five elements in these definitions of disinfection. These were that a disinfectant (1) removes infection (or microbial contamination); (2) is ordinarily a chemical but can be a physical agent; (3) kills, not just inhibits, microorganisms in the vegetative stage; (4) does not necessarily kill spores (or other, more resistant forms of microbial life); and (5) is typically used only on inanimate objects, not on the human or animal body. These are useful in discussing disinfection further and other associated definitions.

As already discussed, a *disinfectant* in the past was often associated with ensuring the concept of being "free from infection" but should be more generally considered as any agent that destroys pathogenic (disease-causing) and other kinds of unwanted microorganisms by chemical or physical means. In many applications, disinfection is not only required to reduce pathogens but may also be just as concerned with other unwanted microorganisms (such as those leading to food or other product spoilage). We have also considered that this can encompass a wide range of chemical and/or physical methods, many of which are considered in greater detail in this book. But the types of microorganisms that are (or maybe) present can vary from situation to situation, ranging in their structures and levels of resistance to disinfectants. This is considered in detail in chapter 3, Microorganisms and Resistance, but a summary of their hierarchy of resistance (or sensitivity) to disinfectants is given in Figure 2.1.

This is important because a disinfectant may be capable of inactivating few or many types of microorganisms based on this hierarchy. From a labeling (and therefore legal) point of view, the disinfectant may be further defined based on the ability to inactivate different groups of microorganisms using specific terms. It is important to note that these terms can vary in their usage and requirements for the test methodology to be used to support such claims. This can vary from country to country, many of which require the demonstration (and often registration) of disinfectants or disinfection processes in different countries. Unfortunately, at the time of writing, there are no harmonized requirements for the claims and test methods used to support disinfectant efficacy internationally. The two most commonly cited systems are those based on disinfectant labeling requirements in the United States (eg, by the FDA, Environmental Protection Agency, and US Department of Agriculture, depending on the application) and the European Union (EU).[7] A common way is to refer to the specific ability to inactivate certain classes of microorganisms. Examples include the use of the suffix -cidal, such as in bactericidal (ability to kill vegetative bacteria), mycobactericidal (to kill mycobacteria, which are considered more difficult to kill than other types of bacteria), viricidal (to kill viruses), and sporicidal (the ability to kill spores, generally indicated by confirming efficacy against bacterial endospores). So, for example, a *sporicidal disinfectant* (which is some countries may be labeled a *liquid chemical sterilants*) is considered effective against bacterial spores and, when appropriate in some jurisdictions, may also be considered to be effective against other types of microorganisms given the hierarchy of resistance of microorganisms to disinfectants shown in Figure 2.1. But overall, the term *sporicidal* indicates the ability of a disinfectant or disinfection process to inactivate bacterial spores but does not directly indicate that all other forms of microorganisms are inactivated or that these products/processes can render a "sterile" situation (see the discussion on *sterilization* and *sterile* in the following text). It is important to understand the regulatory use of these terms to ensure the appropriate use of the disinfectant and the desired outcome. For example, in the United States, the term *germicide* is limited to the ability of the disinfectant to demonstrate bactericidal efficacy against certain vegetative bacteria (eg, *Staphylococcus aureus* and *Escherichia coli*). This does *not* ensure efficacy of the disinfectant against all germs, all bacteria (eg, mycobacteria are not included), or bacterial endospores (although the vegetative forms of spore-forming genus such as *Bacillus* would be included). Also, because the test methods used to verify such claims can vary from area to area, it is important to review the labeling and claims carefully to ensure the effectiveness of the disinfectant for any specific application.

A similar, yet distinct, designation using the suffix "-static" refers to the ability to inhibit the growth of a certain class of microorganisms (eg, fungistatic, bacteriostatic, and sporistatic). Note that strictly speaking, these terms would not meet the requirement of the definition of a disinfectant and may be considered more forms of *preservation* in some situations.

Another way is to define disinfectants based on their ability to inactivate a more general group of microorganisms based on their similar profile of resistance to inactivation. A commonly used system, as an example, defines disinfectants into three classes: low-level, intermediate-level, and high-level disinfectants (Table 2.1).

There is a range of other terms that may be considered to fall under the general definition of disinfection but in more specific ways. Many of these terms are often used interchangeable with disinfection or disinfectant. These include the following:

Sanitization is the removal or inactivation of microorganisms that pose a threat to public health, and therefore, sanitizers would be considered as types

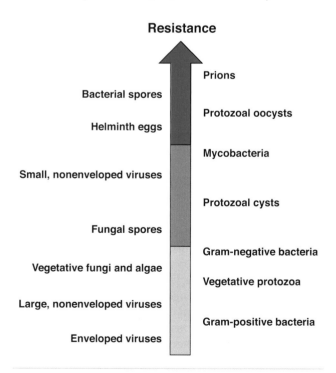

Resistance

Prions
Bacterial spores
Protozoal oocysts
Helminth eggs
Mycobacteria
Small, nonenveloped viruses
Protozoal cysts
Fungal spores
Gram-negative bacteria
Vegetative fungi and algae
Vegetative protozoa
Large, nonenveloped viruses
Gram-positive bacteria
Enveloped viruses

FIGURE 2.1 The estimated hierarchy of microorganism resistance to disinfection. The figure is given as a guide, and the specific resistance profile can vary depending on the disinfectant and the specific target microbial strain.

TABLE 2.1	A general classification of disinfection (and disinfectants), as defined by the US Food and Drug Administration[a]	
Disinfection	**Definition**	**Expected Efficacy**
Low level	A lethal process using an agent that kills vegetative forms of bacteria, some fungi, and lipid viruses	Bactericidal, virucidal (enveloped viruses)
Intermediate level	A lethal process using an agent that kills viruses, mycobacteria, fungi, and vegetative bacteria but no bacterial spores	Mycobactericidal, fungicidal, virucidal, bactericidal
High level	A lethal process using a sterilant under less than sterilizing conditions. The process kills all forms of microbial life except for large numbers of bacterial spores.	Sporicidal (but often over an extended period), mycobactericidal, fungicidal, virucidal, bactericidal

[a]From US Food and Drug Administration.[8]

of disinfectants. These terms are particular widely used in food and brewing industries for hard surface disinfection. The term *sanitizer* first appeared in the 1950s but became more widely used when published in the first edition of this book. Today, *sanitization* is a regulated term and is widely used in the United States to define disinfectants used to reduce, but not necessarily eliminate, microorganisms from the inanimate environment to levels considered safe as determined by public health codes or regulations. In this context, they can include a wide range of food-contacting surfaces and non–food-contacting surfaces as well as air sanitizers. The typical efficacy tests used to support such product claims are essentially bactericidal tests (eg, a specific hard surface carrier test demonstrating efficacy against a gram-positive and/or gram-negative bacteria, such as *S aureus* or *Salmonella enterica* [formerly *typhi*]). But the term is also often used in general terms, such as in the case of hand sanitizers, referring to liquids used to disinfect the hands (eg, alcohol-containing gels or solutions).

Fumigation may be defined as the delivery of an antimicrobial process (typically based on a liquid or gas) that is applied indirectly to an area for the purpose of disinfection. Although the typical use of disinfectant to a large area and its associated surfaces (such as in a room) is by a manual method (eg, spray and wiping), fumigation is achieved by applying the antimicrobial gas, liquid, or aerosol into the area for a given time for disinfection. The process may need to be followed by the active removal of residual disinfectant from the air/surface (or allowing the biocide to naturally degrade overtime) to allow for the safe entry into the area. Fogging or aerosolizing of disinfectants into an area is therefore considered methods of fumigation. Applications can include the use of disinfectants such as formaldehyde, hydrogen peroxide, or chlorine dioxide in high-risk areas to control pathogens; such as biosafety level 2, 3, or 4 laboratories; contaminated hospital wards; and controlled manufacturing environments.

Pasteurization is a very familiar term used to describe the antimicrobial reduction of microorganisms that can be harmful or cause product spoilage. The traditional and most common use of the term is in the heating of liquids, such as in treatment of foods and liquid (eg, milk and juices). The process was named after one of the founding fathers of modern microbiology, Louis Pasteur, based on his demonstration for the successful use of the use of heat in the prevention of beer and wine spoilage during the 19th century. It is important to note that the effects of heating of various liquid foodstuffs in preventing spoilage or extending shelf life had been described and used by many others for centuries before this time. Although the term is most widely used in food industry, it has often been used to describe the use of hot water (typically above 65°C or 149°F) for many surface disinfection purposes (eg, the disinfection of medical devices or manufacturing equipment).

Sterilant may be generically defined as an agent used to destroy microorganisms (ie, a disinfectant), but the term more specifically is used in the United States to define a liquid chemical sterilants as disinfectants that can destroy all forms of microbiological life, including high numbers of bacterial spores. This definition may appear to be similar to that of a high-level disinfectant, discussed earlier, but note that the FDA further defines a sterilant as a high-level disinfectant used under the same contact conditions except typically for a longer contact time. Therefore, such products can have a specified contact time for high-level disinfection but may have a much longer contact time for sterilant activity. The term *sterilant* begins to crossover to our understanding of our use of the term *sterilization* or rendering a surface "sterile," but note that although a sterilant has the ability to inactivate microorganisms, this does not necessarily mean that it achieves a sterile end point. A good example is the use of a liquid chemical sterilant to treat a surface, but then how is it removed following its use to ensure the surface is safe and without recontaminating the surface? Consider it this way: A sterilant on its own may have the ability to sterilize but only as part of a controlled process. This is discussed further under "sterilization."

Biocide (or more specifically *microbicide*) is a general term to describe any physical or (more commonly) chemical agent that inactivates a broad spectrum of microorganisms. It typically refers to the specific antimicrobial agent being used (eg, heat, hydrogen peroxide, or UV light) in comparison to "disinfectant" that can refer to the antimicrobial agent and the various product formulations that use the agent in combination with other ingredients (see following text for further definitions).

A further specific term is *antisepsis*. *Antisepsis* is defined as the destruction or inhibition of microorganisms in or on living tissue, for example, on the skin or mucous membranes. The word *antiseptic* is traditionally credited to John Pringle in his experiments published in the 1750s studying the effects of various substance to inhibit putrefaction. He was familiar with the word *septic*, first recorded in 1605, which means "putrefying." As a physician, he had written, "The miasma or septic ferment being received into the blood," and when he found chemicals (eg, salts, acids, and alkalis) that prevented putrefaction, the word *antiseptic* was generated.[9] In the EU, the term is specifically defined as application of an antiseptic on living tissues causing an action on the structure or metabolism of microorganisms to a level judged to be appropriate to prevent and/or limit and/or treat an infection of those tissues.[7] Therefore, antiseptics are types of products and antimicrobial agents (excluding antibiotics) that are used for that purpose. These include products such as preoperative preparations (used in the disinfection of skin prior to surgical intervention), surgical scrubs (used for the washing or treatment of hands prior to the donning of gloves by surgeons and other operating room staff), health care personal hand washes (used for routine disinfection of hands in health care facilities), and general or surgical hand disinfectants (or sanitizers defined earlier). Other terms such as *hygienic hand rubs* or *hand washes* are widely used in the EU. The regulatory (and labeling) requirements for products making such claims are controlled in many countries, including the United States, Canada, and the EU. Due to the sensitive nature of the target tissues in comparison to the air or hard surfaces, only a limited number of disinfectant types are used due to the balance of antimicrobial efficacy but in the absence of significant damage or irritation. These include biocides such as alcohols, iodine-releasing agents, chlorhexidine, and triclosan. An important consideration to note is the ability of many of these actives to be effective antimicrobials when initially applied to the skin (or other tissue) but then also to retain some (often bacteriostatic or even bactericidal) activity over time. This may be referred to as residual activity, persistence, or substantively. Biocides that include this attribute include chlorhexidine and other biguanides.

The word *antiseptic* is derived from the Greek language to mean "against putrefaction." The term was first used by Pringle in the 1750s to record the ability of substances to prevent the spoilage of organic matter such as egg and meat. After Lister's research in the use of antimicrobial agents in surgery, the term acquired a second meaning, that of a substance used to destroy pathogenic microorganisms. Patterson,[2] in his detailed review of definitions published in 1932, found some difference of opinion regarding the true meaning of the term—whether an antiseptic merely inhibited the growth of microorganisms, killed them, or both. Essentially, antiseptics can provide microbicidal and/or microbiostatic activity, depending on the target microorganisms, the biocide itself, and the product formulation. The mode of action will, of course, depend on such criteria as concentration used, time of contact, temperature, pH, and organic matter present. The antimicrobial efficacy of antiseptics is typically verified against bacteria but can also include fungi and viruses. Furthermore, the label efficacy claims associated with antiseptics are often controlled based on certain in vitro (and on skin) test criteria to ensure they meet the intended need. Although widely used in the EU, the use of term *disinfectant* for antimicrobial products used on the body, as in the case of "skin disinfectant," has traditionally been frowned on in the United States. The over-the-counter antimicrobial drug review panel[10] stated that *disinfection* properly referred to the use of such chemicals on inanimate objects and not on the human body. A hard distinction insofar as US governmental regulations is concerned is that disinfectants or antimicrobial chemicals labeled for use on inanimate objects ("hard surfaces") are considered economic poisons under the Federal Environmental Pesticide Control Act (7 USC §136), whereas agents such as antiseptics labeled for use on human or animal tissue are regulated as drugs under the Federal Food, Drug, and Cosmetic Act. The specific regulatory status in other countries or economic areas can also vary.

Overall, a disinfection process or disinfectant may have different antimicrobial designations depending on its application (eg, foods, food contact surfaces, devices, agricultural, veterinary). An example was given by Fraser[11] in writing about the antimicrobial properties of peracetic acid, although this could easily be applied to other chemical or physical disinfectants. The chemical product may be referred to as a "sanitizer" being particularly used in the food and brewing industries, "terminal disinfectants" in the dairy industry, as "biocides" in municipal water treatment, as "ovicides" in agricultural waste treatment, and as "high-level disinfectants" or "sterilants" in medical and pharmaceutical applications. Of course, a biocide such as peracetic acid may be bacteriostatic under certain (low concentration/temperature) conditions with short contact time, bactericidal at longer time, and sporicidal at even longer time. Each can be a proper designation for the conditions of use and its label. On the other hand, some industries may use terminology particular to that

industry with no regard to any properly accepted definitions. It would be desirable to have definitions accepted
internationally in all cases, but they are not; therefore,
there may be different interpretations of the terms as they
are used in different industries and countries.

▶ STERILE AND STERILIZATION

The term *sterile* (or also *sterility*) is simply defined as being
free from viable microorganisms. Theoretically speaking,
many technologies and practices can enable this end
point, depending on the chemical and/or physical process
used and the target microorganism(s). But legally, where
a product is labeled as being "sterile," there are two main
ways to demonstrate this end point. The first approach is
by *aseptic processing*, which is defined as the act of handling materials in a controlled environment, in which the
air supply, materials, equipment, and personnel are regulated to control microbial and particulate contamination
within acceptable levels. This is further discussed, in detail, in chapter 58. The other approach is by terminal sterilization, where *sterilization* is a defined process used to
render a surface or product free from viable microorganisms. *Sterilization*, as in "sterilization by heat or organic
liquids," was first found to be written in 1874, but the
word *sterile* did not appear widely used until after 1877.

Specifically, *terminal sterilization* is an active process
by which a product is sterilized within a *sterile barrier
system* that preserves the sterile state following the process (eg, during storage or transportation, essentially until
the product is used). A *sterile barrier system* is part of a
packaging system, specifically referring to the basic package that minimizes the risk of ingress of microorganisms
and allows aseptic presentation of the sterile product at
the point of use. The full packaging system is a combination of the sterile barrier system and any other protective
packaging. Sterilization is therefore an active process of
inactivating microorganisms to the level where no viable
microorganisms remain. Simple, yes? Well maybe not, on
further consideration. Even as far back as the 1930s, because of the misuse of this term, the Council on Pharmacy
and Chemistry of the American Medical Association[12]
officially went on record stating that sterilization was intended to convey an absolute meaning, not a relative one.
A product cannot be partially sterile. Nevertheless, the
word *sterile* is still used today in the partial sense. For example, in the case of some mechanically filtered solutions
called "sterile", although being free of bacteria and fungi
and their spores, they may contain active viruses that may
not be removed by the size of the filter (eg, 0.2- or 0.1-μm
filters; see chapter 30). Another example is in the treatment of human or animal tissues with certain types of
chemicals to reduce the risks of microbial contamination
but may not be able to absolutely confirm the total inactivation of all potential microorganisms (ISO 14160[13]).

But outside these unique examples, consider that it can
never be known with certainty whether all microorganisms of all types have been killed following a given antimicrobial process. First, we may not even be aware of
the existence of some species or have media suitable for
culturing all microorganisms to prove it. Second, we can
never prove the achievement of a negative absolute (eg,
even in zoology, lost species of animals once claimed to be
extinct occasionally turn up!). Therefore, it became more
practical, as pointed out by Bruch and Bruch,[14] to use a
process definition of sterilization. By this definition, sterilization is the process by which living microorganisms
are removed or killed to the extent that they are no longer
detectable in standard culture media in which they previously have been found to proliferate. According to this
definition, both the process used to achieve sterility and
the methods used to test for it are equally important.

But we have already mentioned that detecting the
presence (or absence) of all microorganisms would be difficult (if not impossible) to test, so what other options do
we have? This is where mathematics can help. First, we
do know (as shown in Figure 2.1) that microorganisms
range in their resistance to chemical and physical agents.
So, we can begin to study the effects of these agents on the
ability to kill the various types of microorganisms under
certain conditions of exposure (eg, time, temperature,
concentration, dose). This become the first prerequisite
for defining a sterilization process: evidence that supports that the process has the ability to kill various types
of microorganisms. Studies over many years have shown
this ability with the most widely used sterilization technologies, including heat, ionizing radiations, and certain
types of sporicidal gases such as ethylene oxide and hydrogen peroxide. Next, we can study the rate at which the
microorganisms are inactivated. Overall, when we study
this in the laboratory, we find that microorganisms typically demonstrate an exponential rate of kill on treatment
over time or dose. The rate of kill will be quicker with the
easier-to-kill microorganisms (eg, enveloped viruses) in
comparison to those that are harder to inactivate, such
as bacterial spores (see Figure 2.1). The rate of kill will
also vary with process conditions under test, for example, higher temperatures will inactivate microorganisms
quicker than lower temperatures. Therefore, if we know
the types and numbers of microorganisms that are present and we understand the rates of microbial inactivation,
then for a given process we can define the minimum exposure conditions to ensure they are all inactivated. A good
example of this is in studying the inactivation of the most
resistant forms of microorganisms to a given sterilization
method, as is the case with the use of *Geobacillus stearothermophilus* spores to test steam sterilization processes.
Hence, if we know we start with 100 bacterial spores and
we directly show we kill 100 bacterial spores under specified conditions, then is it "sterile"? Not so fast: We must
also remember that the term *sterile* implies an absolute,

and in practice, it becomes a matter of probability whether sterility has been achieved. So even when viable organisms cannot be detected, there is always a probability that a microorganism has survived. This probability can decrease with the longer or greater exposure conditions, which allows us to introduce another term in sterilization, the *sterility assurance level* (SAL). This term first became widely used during the 1970s in the United States.[15] An SAL is defined as the probability of a single viable microorganism occurring on an item after sterilization and is expressed as the negative exponent to the base 10 (eg, 10^{-3} or 10^{-6}). Remember that an SAL is a probability. A product may be sterile at an SAL of 10^{-2} or 10^{-22}, but the probability of a microorganism surviving at 10^{-22} is obviously much less. Historically, an SAL of 10^{-6} is the most widely used for terminal sterilization processes. But before we conclude this discussion, achieving a sterile product is not just the performance of a sterilization process. A further definition is warranted for the *assurance of sterility* as a qualitative concept comprising all activities that provide confidence that the product is sterile. This can include activities during the full manufacturing process (including sterilization) as well as the validation and routine monitoring of the various critical parts of that process that may impact microbiological quality. Examples will include monitoring microbiological contamination in raw materials or formed products, the manufacturing environment (including equipment, personnel, and environmental factors such as air and water), packaging systems and materials, the development and control of the sterilization process, and storage conditions following sterilization.

▶ PRESERVATION

Whereas the terms *disinfection* and *sterilization* specifically refer to the inactivation of microorganisms for various purposes, *preservation* refers to the control of the multiplication of microorganisms or preventing microbial contamination. For the purposes of discussion in this book, preservation can include any chemical or physical method to prevent microorganisms from deteriorating or even contaminating a product. The impact of natural preservation processes has been appreciated for millennium, such as in the use of heating, drying, and acidifying foods as well as the storage of liquids in silver- or copper-containing vessels that appeared to extend their shelf life (presumably through the leaching of these metals and their associated bacteriostatic activities). Modern preservation methods include the use of various antimicrobial chemicals to maintain, or in some cases reduce, the population of microorganisms that can be present in or introduced to a product over time. Examples include the treatment of water for drinking or other industrial purposes as well as various types of liquid or solid products such as skin creams, shampoos, paints, foods, and pharmaceutical preparations. The growth (or

overgrowth) of microorganisms, such as bacteria and fungi, in many of these situations have been implicated in the outbreaks of infection as well as leading to the spoilage of produce (often referred to as biodeterioration) and the obvious economic impacts. There is clearly a crossover to our discussion on disinfection earlier in this chapter, with the use of antimicrobial chemicals at bacteriostatic or fungistatic conditions. Bacteria and fungi are important in this regard because they can multiply over time in many of these products if given the opportunity unlike other microorganisms such as viruses. In some situations, these are referred to as *objectionable microorganisms*, which may be defined as microorganisms that can either cause illness or degrade a product, thus making the product less effective. This term was first widely used in the United States to define microbiological contaminants in drug products not required to be sterile and include microorganisms such as *S aureus*, *E coli*, many *Pseudomonas* species, *Burkholderia cepacia*, and *Candida albicans*. They may be detected from a variety of environmental sources, including the air, personnel, water, etc, and have even been detected as a concern in well-known antiseptic products, such as *Elizabethkingia meningoseptica* in povidone-iodine preoperative products and *Bacillus cereus* in alcohol products.[16] The impact of the overgrowth of pathogens in drinking water is another clear example and is actually an important illustration of the positive impact of preservation, sanitation, and disinfection on public health in modern years.[17]

Preservation can also include physical processes (or barriers) that prevent contamination over time, and the most obvious example of this is the use of packaging methods to prevent microbial contamination. These are essential barriers to contaminants during the storage or transportation of a product to its intended purpose, as highlighted earlier in this chapter during the terminal sterilization of products. But the classical demonstration of the impact of a physical preservation method was the torturous path experiment by Louis Pasteur in 1862 used to prove the germ theory of disease. The experiment was conducted to disprove the widely held theory at the time that microorganisms formed by spontaneous generation. Pasteur designed an experiment using a "swan-neck" or S-shaped flask (Figure 2.2); when culture media was added to the flask and heated, no growth was observed over time in the presence of the tortuous path in comparison to the absence of the swan neck. Modern microbial barrier packaging methods (or *sterile barrier systems*) are made of a variety of materials such as papers, textiles, and plastics (see chapter 41).

▶ GLOSSARY

The following definitions are given for general reference during the reading of this book. It is important to remember that, where possible, harmonized definitions are

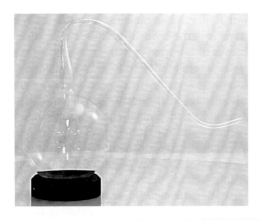

FIGURE 2.2 A representation of Pasteur's swan-shaped flask that provided the demonstration of a torturous path to prevent contamination of a growth media within the flask.

provided but that these can vary from country to country depending on their traditional or regulatory usages.

A_0: a measure of microbiological lethality delivered by a moist heat disinfection process. It is expressed as the equivalent time in seconds to microbial inactivation at 80°C (but in excess of 65°C) and with reference to a microorganism with a z-value of 10 K. The higher the A_0, the greater the level of disinfection is expected. It is calculated by the following equation:

$$A_0 = \Sigma\ 10^{(T-80)/z}\ \Delta t$$

where, t is the chosen time interval (in seconds) and T is the temperature in the load (in degrees Celsius).

Aeration: removal of chemical residuals to a predetermined level. Specifically, for gas sterilization processes, this is usually performed as part of (or following) the sterilization cycle during which the chemical sterilizing agent and/or its reaction products are removed from a load until predetermined levels (based on safety requirements) are reached.

Algicide: a substance that kills algae, and for the purpose of this book, algae are a diverse group of unicellular chlorophyll-containing organisms. Examples include *Chlamydomonas* (a green algae) and *Spirogyra*.

Antibiotic: a substance to kill or inhibit the growth of bacteria (but may include other microorganisms); used most often at low concentrations in the treatment of infectious diseases of humans, animals, and plants. It is usually used as a chemotherapeutic drug and must be low in toxicity while effective against target microorganisms.

Antimicrobial: the ability to kill or suppress the growth of microorganisms. The term is generally used to describe any chemical agent(s), products, or processes used for that purpose.

Antisepsis: destruction of inhibition of microorganisms in or on living tissues

Antiseptic: a chemical, product, or process used for antisepsis

Asepsis: prevention from contamination with microorganisms

Aseptic presentation: transfer of products, materials, etc, using conditions and procedures that minimize the risk of microbial contamination

Aseptic processing: a manufacturing term used to describe the handling of sterile product, materials, containers, devices, etc, in a controlled environment in which the air supply, materials, equipment, and personnel are regulated to maintain sterility

Aseptic technique: conditions and procedures used to minimize the risk of the introduction of microbial contamination

Assurance of sterility: qualitative concept comprising all activities that provide confidence that product is sterile (also used as *sterility assurance*)

Bactericidal: the ability to kill bacteria. This term may typically apply to any agent or product that can kill vegetative bacteria (both pathogenic and nonpathogenic) but not necessarily bacterial spores (see "sporicide"). Similar terms are specific to certain types of bacteria inactivated, such as mycobactericidal (against all mycobacteria) or tuberculocidal (against *Mycobacterium tuberculosis*).

Bacteriostatic: an agent, usually chemical, that prevents the growth of bacteria but that does not necessarily kill them. Sometimes the only difference as to whether a chemical is bacteriostatic or bactericidal depends on the conditions of application, such as time, concentration, temperature, or pH. Many bacteriostatic agents are also *sporistatic*, due to sensitivity of bacterial spores in the presence of these agents to prevent germination and/or outgrowth of these spores.

Bioburden: the population of viable (or detectable) microorganisms on or in a product or other material

Biocide: a chemical or physical agent that inactivates all living organisms. The term literally mean "life killing." *Microbicide* specifies an agent that kills microorganisms.

Biocompatibility: the condition of being compatible with living tissue or a living system by not being toxic, injurious, or causing an immunologic reaction

Biodecontamination: removal and/or reduction of biological contaminants to an acceptable level. Also see *decontamination*.

Biodeterioration: the deterioration of valuable materials due to biological activity. The causes are usually microbiological (eg, bacteria and fungi) but other examples can include insects, rodents, higher animals, or plants. Deterioration may be noted by the breakdown of the material, *biodegeneration*, as in natural decay of timber, or *aesthetic depreciation*, as in staining of works of art.

Biofilm: a community of microorganisms. Biofilms can consist of single or multiple types of microorganisms, either as actively multiplying, dormant, or generally associated with the biofilm structure. They can include "wet" (ie, associated with water) or "dry" biofilms and are typically developed on or associated with surfaces or interfaces (eg, water lines or storage systems).

Biological indicator (BI): test system containing viable microorganisms providing a defined resistance to a specified sterilization process. Common examples of BIs include standardized preparations of bacterial spores on or in a carrier and are widely used to test (or verify) the activity of sterilization processes such as those based on steam and gases. *Self-contained biological indicators* are specific designs that include the BI in a packaging system with an intrinsic incubation medium required for testing for growth of the indicator microorganisms but incubation.

Chemical indicator (CI): a test system widely used in disinfection and sterilization applications that reveals change in one or more predefined process variables based on a chemical or physical change resulting from exposure to a process (eg, by a color change)

Chemisterilant: a chemical agent or product used to kill all microorganisms, including spores

Chemitherapeutant: a chemical used inside the body that kills or suppresses microorganisms to control disease. Antibiotics are examples. The term may also apply to chemicals used to destroy malignant cells and tissues, such as cytotoxic drugs.

Clean: visually free of soil, or contaminant(s), and quantified as being below specified levels of analytes (eg, a specific contaminant such as protein)

Clean-in-place: cleaning of internal surfaces of parts of equipment or an entire process system, without or with minimal disassembly

Cleaning: removal of contaminants to the extent necessary for further processing or for intended use. Contaminants may include microorganisms, chemicals, extraneous materials, etc. Cleaning agents include detergents or other types of chemicals (eg, acids and alkalis) used during cleaning procedures.

Commensals: microorganisms living on or within another organism but not causing injury to the host under normal circumstances

Conditioning: in sterilization processes, refers to the treatment of product prior to the exposure (sterilization) phase to attain a specified temperature, relative humidity, or other process variable throughout the load.

Containment: combination of buildings, engineering functions, equipment, and work practices that allow safe handling of hazardous biological or chemical substances and prevent accidental release of these substances to the external environment

Contamination: to make impure or unsuitable by contact or mixture with something unwanted, such as microorganisms or chemicals. Contamination can be used as both a verb (to contaminate) and a noun (the contamination). Extrinsic contamination specifically refers to the ingress of viable or nonviable extraneous material during a manufacturing process, whereas intrinsic contamination is already present in the starting material (eg, raw material). Compare to the opposite of this term, which is *decontamination*.

Critical surface: surface that might come into direct contact with a product, including its containers or closures, or other material posing a risk of contamination

D-value, D_{10} value, or decimal reduction time: the time (or dose) required to achieve the inactivation of 90% of a population of microorganisms under stated conditions. A 90% reduction is equivalent to reducing the microbial population to one-tenth its starting population, that is, a one-logarithm ($1 \log_{10}$) reduction.

Death rate curve: See *survivor curve*.

Decontamination: the process of freeing a person or object from potentially harmful material. This material can be infectious microorganisms (biodecontamination), harmful insects (*disinfestation*), or toxic or radioactive chemicals (chemical decontamination). Decontamination can be achieved by chemical and/or physical means and is often used to describe a process to render a surface or item safe for use, handling, or disposal. Surface decontamination can include cleaning, disinfection, and/or sterilization as well as combinations thereof.

Deodorizer: any chemical, product, or process used to prevent or delay the growth of odor-producing microorganisms, or to mask, chemically destroy, or neutralize odors

Depyrogenation: the inactivation or removal of pyrogenic substances ("pyrogens")

Disinfectant: chemical or combination of chemicals used for disinfection

Disinfecting agent: physical or chemical agent used for disinfection

Disinfection: antimicrobial process to inactivate viable microorganisms to a level previously specified as being appropriate for a defined purpose (see discussion earlier).

Disinfestation: extermination or destruction of insects, rodents, or other animal forms that cause harm or transmit disease, which may be on a person or his or her belongings, clothing, or surroundings.

Dosimeter: a device having a reproducible, measurable response to radiation that can be used to measure the absorbed dose in a given system

Droplet nuclei: particles of 5 μm diameter or less that are formed by dehydration of airborne droplets and are capable of air dispersal

Endotoxin: types of toxins present in a microorganism and released on cell disintegration. Endotoxins are lipopolysaccharide component of the cell wall of gram-negative bacteria that are heat stable and can elicit a variety of inflammatory responses in animals and humans.

Environmental isolates: microorganisms cultured from processing or manufacturing environments

Excipient: chemical or biological component other than an active ingredient that is included in a *formulation*

Exotoxin: types of toxins produced and secreted from a microorganism. Examples include the botulinum toxin ("Botox") and enterotoxins from bacteria, and mycotoxins (eg, aflatoxins) from fungi.

F-value: measure of microbiological lethality delivered by a heat process expressed in terms of the equivalent time, in minutes, at a specified temperature with reference to microorganisms with a specified z-value. A commonly used F-value for a moist heat (steam) sterilization process is the F_0 that is equivalent time, in minutes, at a temperature of 121.1°C (or 250°F) with reference to microorganisms with a z-value of 10 K. Similarly, a dry heat sterilization process, the F_H, is the equivalent time, in minutes, at a temperature of 160°C (320°F) with reference to microorganisms with a z-value of 20 K. Overall, the F-value is a cumulative estimate of microbial lethality over multiple exposure temperatures/times expressed as an equivalent time to being exposed at one temperature (eg, 121°C or 160°C) and can be predicted based on our mathematical understanding of the lethal effects of temperature on microbial inactivation.

Fomites: inanimate objects or materials that may transmit infectious microorganisms (eg, toilet seats, toothbrushes, silverware)

Formulation: combination of chemical ingredients, includes active (eg, antimicrobial agents, enzymes) and other ingredients (eg, stabilizers, buffers, solvents, dyes) into a product for its intended use. Many antiseptic and disinfectant products are often known by their main active ingredients, such as "alcohols," "glutaraldehyde," and "chlorine" but are in fact often formulations. The term may also apply to liquid-formulated products, such as paints, shampoos, pharmaceuticals, that are preserved with low concentrations of water ("low water activity") or preservative chemicals to prevent microbial growth.

Fractional cycle: an equipment (eg, sterilizer or washing system) operating cycle in which the exposure (or defined antimicrobial reduction) phase is reduced compared with that specified for the normal cycle. A commonly used cycle is a "half cycle," which is a test cycle in which the holding time during the exposure period is only 50 % as compared with the operating cycle.

Fumigation: the delivery of an antimicrobial process that is applied indirectly to an area for the purpose of disinfection. The term may also be used for similar applications to control insects (using insecticidal agents) and vermin.

Fungicidal: an agent that kills fungi. This definition often assumes activity against both molds and yeasts, although terms like yeasticidal are also used. There is also the assumption that fungal spores are also killed or inactivated, although this may not always be the case.

Fungistatic: an agent that inhibits but does not necessarily kill fungi. The term typically applies to vegetative and spore forms of fungi.

Germicidal or germicide: an agent that destroys microorganisms and has been traditionally used in the past to refer to being effective against pathogenic microorganisms. The words *germ* (defined as a microorganism) and germicidal find extensive use in the technical as well as the popular literature. It refers to chemical agents, but the adjective *germicidal* may refer to physical agents, such as *germicidal* lamps. In some areas, the term is limited in its efficacy claim to be bactericidal against common bacterial pathogens such as vegetative bacteria (eg, *S aureus* and *E coli*). See discussion on *disinfection* earlier.

Germination: the initiation of vegetative growth in a dormant spore. Similar terms are used to describe the same event in other dormant forms of microorganisms, such as encystation of protozoal cysts.

Gowning or gowning procedure: defined actions for putting on protective clothing (including gowns, gloves, head or shoe covers, etc) to reduce the risks of contamination from people entering a defined area (eg, controlled areas such a cleanrooms)

Growth promotion: a type of test performed to demonstrate that a growth medium will support the growth of microorganisms

Health care–acquired infection (HCAI): an infection acquired by a patient during the course of receiving treatment for other conditions within a health care setting (eg, a hospital). Also see *nosocomial*.

Heat shock: sublethal heat treatment to induce spore germination and destroy vegetative microorganisms

High-level disinfectant: a disinfectant that is expected to kill all forms of microbial life except for large numbers of bacterial spores when used in sufficient concentration and under suitable exposure conditions. See Table 2.1 and discussion on *disinfection*.

Holding time: for an equipment (eg, sterilizer or washing system) operating cycle, the period during which process parameters are maintained, within their specified tolerances

Hydrophilic: ability to attract and absorb water. Literally, "water liking."

Hydrophobic: ability to repel and not absorb water. Literally, "water fearing."

Inactivation: to make inactive or no longer being able to grow or multiply

Infection: the invasion and multiplication of microorganisms in a host

Inoculated carrier: supporting material on, or in, which a defined number of viable test microorganisms has been deposited

Inorganic load: naturally occurring or artificial contamination containing inorganic contaminants, such as metal salts or hard water; used as a *soil* to challenge the efficacy of disinfection or sterilization products or processes

Intermediate-level disinfectant: an agent that destroys all vegetative bacteria, including tubercle bacilli, lipid and some nonlipid viruses, and fungus spores but not bacterial spores. See Table 2.1 and discussion on *disinfection*.

Isolator: a sealed enclosure capable of preventing the ingress of contaminants by means of physical separation of the interior from the exterior. Example of when isolators may be used include on the body (eg, during surgical procedures), laboratory procedures (eg, sterile testing), rearing germ-free animals, and during aseptic processing to prevent contamination by infective agents. An isolator may also be used to prevent invasion by microorganisms in sterility testing procedures or rearing germ-free animals.

Labeling: includes the label (affixed to a product), instructions for use, and any other information that is related to identification, technical description, intended purpose, and proper use of a product (but typically excludes shipping documents)

Laminar airflow: a system of parallel flows of air, horizontally or vertically, to reduce the opportunity for microbial contamination. The air is typically filtered to reduce contamination levels and force over an area, such as in a laminar flow cabinet, cleanroom, or surgical suite.

Lethal rate (L): measure of inactivation per unit time (eg, minutes) at the temperature, T, expressed in terms of a reference temperature (T_{ref}). The lethal rate at any temperature can be calculated using the equation:

$$L = 10 \, ([T - T_{ref}] / z)$$

where, T is the delivered temperature, T_{ref} is the reference temperature, and z is the change in temperature that produces a 10-fold change in D-value.

Load: the defined product, equipment, or materials to be processed together within an operating cycle. An example is shown in Figure 2.3. Note the alternative use of organic or inorganic *load*, being the presence of organic/inorganic material that may be present or interfere with the antimicrobial process.

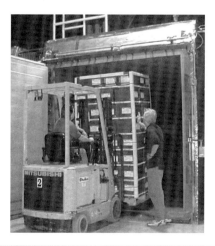

FIGURE 2.3   An example of a sterilizer load.

Low-level disinfectant: an agent that inactivates vegetative bacteria except mycobacteria; enveloped (lipid) viruses; fungi, but not necessarily fungal; or bacterial spores. See Table 2.1 and discussion on *disinfection*.

Master product: device or procedure set used to represent the most difficult to sterilize item in a product family or processing category

Microbial barrier: property of the sterile barrier system that minimizes the risk of ingress of microorganisms demonstrated under test conditions such as a sterilization process, handling, distribution, transport, and storage

Microbicide: See *biocide*.

Microbiostat: any chemical(s) that controls or prevents the growth of microorganisms

Minimum effective concentration (MIC): the lower concentration of a chemical or product, used in a specified disinfection or sterilization process, that achieves a claimed activity

Minimum recommended concentration (MRC): the lowest concentration of a chemical or product specified by use in a disinfection or sterilization process

Noncondensable gas: air and/or other gas that will not liquefy under the conditions of a saturated steam process

Nosocomial: acquired or occurring in a hospital. Nosocomial (or health care–acquired) infections are not present or incubating before admittance to the hospital but are obtained during the patient's stay in a health care facility. See *health care–acquired infection*.

Objectionable microorganism: microorganism that can either cause illness or degrade a product

Operating cycle: complete set of stages of a disinfection of sterilization process, carried out in a specified sequence

Organic load: naturally occurring or artificial contamination containing organic contaminants, such as blood or serum; used as a *soil* to challenge the efficacy of disinfection or sterilization products or processes

Ovicide: a substance that kills the eggs of very small infectious animals, such as the eggs of tapeworms

Packaging system: combination of a sterile barrier system and protective packaging

Parametric release: declaration that product has reached a desired state (eg, disinfected or sterile) based on records demonstrating that the process variables were delivered within specified tolerances

Pasteurization: a heat disinfection process (used with liquids, including milk, wine, or water) to 60°C to 100°C (or the equivalent) for a given time to reduce significantly or kill pathogenic and spoilage organisms

Pathogen: disease-producing microorganism

Planktonic: describes the growth of microorganism dispersed in solution, as in the case of free-swimming plankton

Preconditioning: treatment of product, prior to the operating cycle, to attain specified values, such as temperature, relative humidity, and/or other process variables

Preservation: the control of the multiplication of microorganisms or preventing microbial contamination

Preservative: an antimicrobial agent or mechanism used for preservation

Prions: transmissible agents composed entirely of protein material and do not appear to have unique associated nucleic acid. They are the causative agents in a unique group of diseases known as transmissible spongiform encephalopathies, including Creutzfeldt-Jakob disease, and scrapie.

Process challenge device (PCD): item providing a defined resistance to a cleaning, disinfection, or sterilization process and used to assess the performance of the process

Processing: activity to prepare a new or used health care product for its intended use. Typically refers to clinically used devices and can include cleaning, disinfection, and/or sterilization depending on the device and its risk to patients.

Product family: group or subgroup of product characterized by similar attributes determined to be equivalent for evaluation and processing purposes

Prophylactic: an agent that contributes to the prevention of infection and disease. This word is wide in scope, ranging from the use of biocides or antimicrobial drugs to the use of fresh air and a nutritious diet to ward off disease.

Protective packaging: configuration of materials designed to prevent damage to the sterile barrier system and its contents from the time of their assembly until the point of use

Pyrogen: a substance that causes a rise in body temperature ("fever producing"). An example are bacterial *endotoxins* from the outer membranes of gram-negative bacteria, composed of complex lipopolysaccharide molecules.

Qualification: activities undertaken to demonstrate that utilities, equipment, or methods are suitable for their intended use and perform properly. Equipment or process qualification typically includes three components: installation qualification (objective evidence that all key aspects of the installation comply with an approved specification), operational qualification (obtaining and documenting evidence that installed equipment operates within predetermined limits when used in accordance with its operational procedures), and performance qualification (establishing by objective evidence that the process, under anticipated conditions, consistently produces a product which meets all predetermined requirements).

Reference microorganism: a microbial strain obtained from a recognized culture collection

Reference standard: a standard, generally of the highest metrologic quality, from which measurements are derived

Reprocessing: See *processing*. Typically refers to the processing (eg, cleaning, disinfection, and/or sterilization) of used health care products following clinical use

Requalification: repetition of part or all of *validation* for the purpose of confirming the continued acceptability of a specified process

Resistance: the inability of an antimicrobial agent to be effective against a target microorganism

Resistometer: test equipment designed to create defined combinations of the physical and/or chemical parameters of a process (typically a sterilization process)

Reusable device: a device designated or intended by the manufacturer as suitable for processing and reuse

Safety data sheet: a document specifying the properties of a chemical product or substance, the potential hazardous effects for humans and the environment, and the precautions necessary to handle and dispose of the substance/product safely; used to be referred to as material safety data sheet

SAL: See *sterility assurance level*.

Sanitization: the removal or inactivation of microorganisms that pose a threat to public health

Sanitizer: an antimicrobial product or process used for the purpose of sanitization. See discussion on *disinfection*. Sanitizers are commonly applied to inanimate objects, particularly associated with the food industry.

Saturated steam: water vapor in a state of equilibrium between its liquid and gas phases

Self-contained biological indicator (SCBI): biological indicator presented such that the primary package, intended for incubation, contains the incubation medium required for incubation and recovery of the test organism

Sessile: the attachment and growth of microorganisms to a surface, not freely dispersed such as that described for *planktonic*

Single-use device: device designated or intended to be used on one individual, typically during a single procedure

Soil: natural or artificial contamination on a device or surface following its use or simulated use

Spores: the thick-walled resting cells produced by some bacteria and fungi that are capable of survival in unfavorable environments and are more resistant to antimicrobial agents than vegetative cells

Spore log reduction (SLR): negative exponent to the base 10, expressed as a logarithm, describing the decrease in the number of spores

Sporicide: an agent that inactivates microbial spores. The term is commonly used in reference to substances applied to inanimate objects.

Sporulation: the process of spore development in microorganisms. Spores are dormant forms of some types of microorganisms, including bacterial genus such as *Bacillus* and *Clostridium* (these are known as *endospores*), and fungi.

Standard distribution of resistances (SDR): a term typically used in radiation sterilization processes to describe a reference set of resistances of microorganisms and corresponding probabilities of occurrence

Sterilant: chemical or combination of chemicals used for disinfection or sterilization

Sterile: free from living microorganisms

Sterile barrier system (SBS): the minimum package that minimizes the risk of ingress of microorganisms and allows aseptic presentation of the sterile product at the point of use

Sterility: state of being free from viable microorganisms

Sterility assurance: See *assurance of sterility.*

Sterility assurance level (SAL): probability of a single viable microorganism occurring on an item after sterilization, expressed as the negative exponent to the base 10. See discussion on *sterilization.*

Sterilization: process used to render product free from viable microorganisms

Sterilization cycle: predetermined sequence of stages performed in a sterilizer or sterilization process to achieve product free of viable microorganisms

Sterilizer: equipment designed to achieve sterilization

Sterilizing agent: physical or chemical agent(s), or combination thereof, having sufficient microbicidal activity to achieve sterility under defined conditions

Surrogate: item designed to represent a product in process simulations and is comparable with the actual product

Survivor (or death rate) curve: the graphical representation of the microbial death rate kinetics for a specific antimicrobial product or process on a defined microbial population

Terminal process: final step of processing to render a medical device safe and ready for its intended use

Thermal death time: the time required to kill all spores at a specified temperature

Thermolabile: readily damaged by heat

Tolerance: a decreased effect of an antimicrobial agent against a target microorganism, requiring increased concentration or other modification to be effective

Toxicity: the quality of being toxic or poisonous

Tyndallization: a repeated process of heat treatment for killing microorganisms. The treated material is heated to given temperature (typically less than sterilization conditions) and then allowed to cool and stand to allow for the germination of any surviving spores. This process is then successively repeated for a defined number of times to destroy all vegetative forms and germinated spores.

Validation: confirmation process, through the provision of objective evidence that the requirements for a specific intended use or application have been fulfilled

Vegetative cells: microbial cells that are in the growth and reproductive phase of the growth cycle

Verification: the provision of objective evidence that specified requirements have been fulfilled

Viable: microorganisms alive and capable of reproduction under favorable circumstances

Viroids: virus-like infectious agents that produce diseases in higher plants. They differ from true viruses in that they are believed to contain no protein, only low-molecular-weight RNA.

Virucide: an agent that destroys or inactivates viruses to make them noninfective. The spelling *viricide* is also sometimes used.

z-value: change in temperature of a thermal sterilization or disinfection process that produces a 10-fold change in D-value for a particular microorganism. It may be considered the slope of the logarithm of the D-value against temperature and the number of degrees to change the D-value by a factor of 10. It is useful for comparing the death rate of bacterial spores with the destructive effect on the product over an equivalent temperature range.

REFERENCES

1. Block SS. Definition of terms. In: Block, SS ed. *Disinfection, Sterilization, and Preservation.* 5th ed. Philadelphia, PA: Lippincott Williams & Wilkins; 2001:19-30.
2. Patterson AM. Meaning of "antiseptic," "disinfectant" and related words. *Am J Public Health Nations Health.* 1932;22:465-472.
3. McCulloch EC. *Disinfection and Sterilization.* 2nd ed. Philadelphia, PA: Lea & Febiger; 1945:19-22.
4. Reddish GF. *Antiseptics, Disinfectants, Fungicides, and Chemical and Physical Sterilization.* 2nd ed. Philadelphia, PA: Lea & Febiger; 1957:23-29.
5. Spaulding EH. Chemical disinfection of medical and surgical materials. In: Lawrence CA, Block SS, eds. *Disinfection, Sterilization, and Preservation.* Philadelphia, PA: Lea & Febiger; 1968:517-531.
6. International Organization for Standardization. *ISO 11139: 2018: Sterilization of Heath Care Products—Vocabulary of Terms Used in Sterilization and Related Equipment and Process Standards.* Geneva, Switzerland: International Organization for Standardization; 2018.
7. British Standards Institution. *BS EN 14885:2015. Chemical Disinfectants and Antiseptics. Application of European Standards for Chemical Disinfectants and Antiseptics.* London, United Kingdom: British Standards Institution; 2015.
8. US Food and Drug Administration. *Reprocessing Medical Devices in Health Care Settings: Validation Methods and Labeling. Guidance for Industry and Food and Drug Administration Staff.* Washington, DC: US Government Printing Office; 2015.
9. Pringle J. Some experiments on substances resisting putrefaction. *R Soc Philos Trans.* 1750;46:480-488.
10. US Food and Drug Administration. Over the counter antimicrobial I drug review panel: over the counter topical antimicrobial products and drug and cosmetic products. *Fed Regist.* 1974;39(179):33102-33141.
11. Fraser JAL. Novel applications of peracetic acid in industrial disinfection. *Spec Chem.* 1987;7(3):178-186.
12. American Medical Association. Report of the Council on Pharmacy and Chemistry: use of the terms "sterile," "sterilize," and "sterilization." *JAMA.* 1936;107:38.
13. International Organization for Standardization. *ISO 14160:2011: Sterilization of Health Care Products—Liquid Chemical Sterilizing Agents for Single-Use Medical Devices Utilizing Animal Tissues and Their Derivatives—Requirements for Characterization, Development, Validation and Routine Control of a Sterilization Process for Medical Devices.* Geneva, Switzerland: International Organization for Standardization; 2011.
14. Bruch CW, Bruch MK. Sterilization. In: Martin EW, ed. *Husa's Pharmaceutical Dispensing.* Easton, PA: Mack; 1971:592-623.
15. Bruch CW. Factors determining choice of sterilizing procedure. In: GB Phillips, WS Miller, eds. *Industrial Sterilization.* Durham, NC: Duke University Press; 1973:119-124.
16. Sutton S, Jimenez L. A review of reported recalls involving microbiological control 2004-2011 with emphasis on FDA considerations of "objectionable organisms." *Am Pharm Rev.* 2012;15:42-57.
17. Mara D, Lane J, Scott B, Trouba D. Sanitation and health. *PLoS Med.* 2010;7(11):e1000363.

CHAPTER

3

Microorganisms and Resistance

Gerald McDonnell

Microbiology is the study of microorganisms. Microorganisms can be classified under eight major types based on their essential structures: prions, viruses, bacteria, archaea, fungi, algae, protozoa, and the helminths. They present a wide variety of structures and sizes, with known resistance profiles to inactivation (Table 3.1 and Figure 3.1).[1] Because these are the targets of the many types of preservation, disinfection, and sterilization, a basic understanding of their concerns to public health and commerce and their resistance to inactivation is a useful introduction. Prions and viruses are noncellular structures that depend on host cells for survival and replication. They are some of the smallest types of microorganisms, typically <0.4 μm, and for viruses, they consist of an essential nucleic acid (DNA or RNA structure) contained within a protein- (or lipid and protein) based structure. The essential protein-only structure (or infectivity component) of prions is even simpler than this and is still a matter of some investigation as to their true nature. Bacteria, archaea, fungi, algae, and protozoa are all unicellular organisms, but themselves range greatly in structure (from prokaryote to eukaryotic cell types) and size, typically from 0.1 μm to 200 μm (see Table 3.1). Our knowledge of many of these continues to develop, particularly in our understanding of archaea with remarkable abilities to survive extreme environments that would traditionally be considered adverse to life. Equally, it is often wrong to consider these unicellular microorganisms just as individual, free-living cells because they are often closely associated or even coexisting together in various environments. Communities of bacteria and fungi can grow to develop into colonial structures that are visible. But the advantageous and/or detrimental roles of these populations of microorganisms in the human body, animals, plants, or in the environment is an area of active research, such as in the study of biofilms (defined as a community of microorganisms; see chapter 67) and microbiomes (the combined genetic material of the microorganisms in an environment). The much larger, multicellular helminths (or microscopic worms) can be >1000 μm and are often directly visible to the human eye.

This diversity of life presents varying resistance profiles to the effects of the different types of physical and chemical antimicrobial processes used for disinfection, sterilization, and preservation. This chapter briefly considers the various types of microorganisms and particularly their resistance profiles to inactivation by physical and chemical biocidal mechanisms. Traditionally, certain types of microorganisms have been well studied in this area, such as bacteria and, to a much lesser effect, fungi. This is not only due to their ease of laboratory identification and manipulation (for many but not necessarily all of these) but also because they are common environmental contaminants and are frequently associated with negative impacts such as product spoilage, infection, or toxicity. Viruses have also been the subject of more recent investigations in the last 30 years, primarily due to their importance as pathogens and contaminants of mammalian biotechnology processes used for manufacturing protein therapeutics. But there has also been a greater focus on the investigation of other types of microorganisms such as prions, protozoa, and helminths, with the development of laboratory-based methodology to study their viability and a greater understanding of their impact on health and safety. Finally, a brief consideration will be given to the understanding on various toxins than can be produced from microorganisms, including when the vegetative organism is itself inactivated and its presence can continue to have potential negative health and product impacts.

▶ GENERAL HIERARCHY OF RESISTANCE

Microorganisms can be classified based on their innate resistance profiles to inactivation by chemical and physical microbicidal mechanisms.[1] A summary of this hierarchy

TABLE 3.1   The eight major types of microorganisms

Microorganism Type	Description	Examples
Prions 	Transmissible agents composed of protein and lacking any specific nucleic acid. They are associated with types of neurologic diseases known as transmissible spongiform encephalopathies.	PrP^{Sc} or PrP^{res} forms of proteins implicated in diseases such as scrapie, Creutzfeldt-Jakob disease, and chronic wasting disease
Viruses 	Consist of a virus-specific nucleic acid (DNA or RNA), surrounded by an external protein-based capsid. Some viruses are further surrounded by a lipid-based envelope. Enveloped viruses are relatively sensitive to inactivation, whereas nonenveloped viruses demonstrate greater resistance. They depend on host cells for multiplication, such as animal, plant, or bacterial cells depending on the virus type.	Enveloped viruses: human immuno-deficiency virus, hepatitis B virus, influenza virus, and herpes viruses. Nonenveloped viruses: parvoviruses, papillomaviruses, and poliovirus
Bacteria 	Bacteria (or eubacteria) are prokaryotic, single-celled microorganisms that can range from cell wall–free forms (mycoplasmas) and cell wall–containing types (traditionally classified based on the Gram stain and microscopic morphology). Some bacteria, such as *Bacillus* species and *Clostridium* species, can morph between vegetative cell and spore forms, the latter being particularly of high resistance to inactivation. They are ubiquitous and can multiply in various environments under desired growth conditions. Some forms are obligate intracellular bacteria, such as *Chlamydia* species and *Rickettsia* species.	Cell wall free: *Mycoplasma pneumoniae* Gram-positive: *Staphylococcus, Bacillus, Streptococcus* Acid-fast: *Mycobacterium* Gram-negative: *Escherichia, Klebsiella, Pseudomonas*
Archaea	Prokaryotic, single-celled microorganisms that are genetically distinct from bacteria. Often identified from "extreme" environments, so are often studied for their unique resistance to such conditions, such as heat and high salt; generally, not associated with being pathogenic or as routine environmental contaminants	*Thermococcus, Halobacterium, Methanococcus*

TABLE 3.1 The eight major types of microorganisms *(Continued)*

Microorganism Type	Description	Examples
Fungi	Eukaryotic, single-celled micro-organisms. The two major types include the molds (or filamentous fungi) that can grow as longer lines of cells and yeasts (unicellular growth forms). Fungi can also develop from vegetative forms of growth to dormant spores of various types, depending on the fungus type. These spores can also present varying resistance profiles to inactivation due to their structures. Fungi can be ubiquitous in the general environmental.	Molds: *Aspergillus, Penicillium, Trichophyton* Yeasts: *Candida, Saccharomyces*
Algae	Eukaryotic cells that can grow as filaments or single cells. Photosynthetic and frequently associated with water habitats, particularly when contaminated; can be a source of toxins that can lead to health risks	*Chlamydomonas, Gonyaulax*
Protozoa	Eukaryotic, cell wall–free cells that can develop into multiple forms during their life cycles, including dormant forms of cysts or oocysts. These latter structures can be highly resistant to chemical disinfectants; often associated with natural water supplies and as human or animal parasites	*Giardia, Cryptosporidium, Acanthamoeba*
Helminths	Multicellular eukaryotes that are often free-living (eg, in water) or as parasites in humans or animals (known as various types of microscopic "worms"). Many grow to such sizes as to be visible to the human eye. During their respective life cycles, they can form ova (or eggs) that present with high resistance to inactivation.	*Enterobius, Ascaris, Schistosoma*

Abbreviations: PrP^res, protease-resistant PrP; PrP^Sc, scrapie-type PrP.

and the relationship to the expectations of antimicrobial claims made with disinfectants is given in Figure 3.1.

Prions are well cited as being highly resistant to inactivation, and this should not be a surprise considering their nature as protein-only transmissible agents. It would be wrong to assume that the many types of physical and chemical antimicrobial methods would be effective against these proteins.[2] For example, methods such as those like radiation are known to target nucleic acids as their mechanisms of action and would not be expected,

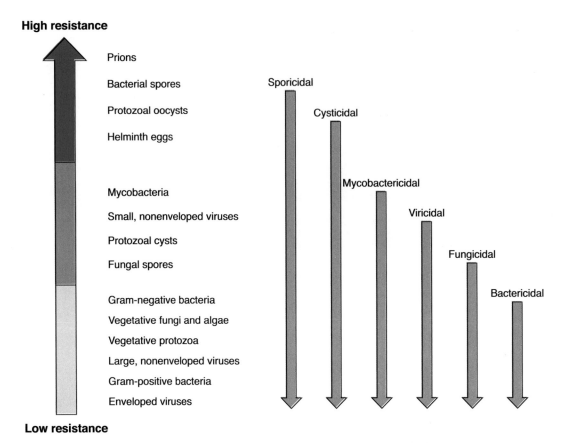

FIGURE 3.1   Hierarchy of the various types of microorganisms and their resistance profiles to inactivation. The various expectations from claims made with disinfectants are also shown (see chapter 2). The resistance profiles can vary depending on the specific antimicrobial method under investigation, and this profile is given as a guide. Specific claims of effectiveness against algae and helminths are less well defined and are given as estimates based on limited studies conducted with these microorganisms.

or have been shown, to have significant activity against prions due to the lack of specific DNA or RNA molecule in these agents. But equally, methods have been described as effective at neutralizing prion infectivity but may not be effective against other types of microorganisms (eg, proteases). Due to their unusual properties and unique risks of transmission, it is important to consider them as the most resistant forms of microorganisms to both physical and chemical methods.[2]

It is well established that many types of dormant forms of vegetative microorganisms such as bacterial endospores, protozoal oocysts, helminths, and, to a lesser extent, protozoal cyst forms and fungal spores classically demonstrate high resistance to inactivation.[1] By far the most studied in this group are bacterial spores such as those formed by *Bacillus atrophaeus* and *Geobacillus stearothermophilus*. They have been widely used to evaluate and test various types of sterilization processes, and the various stages of the development of spores from vegetative cells (sporulation) have been well described as well as detailed investigations at which stage the developing spores demonstrate increased resistance to various types

of biocidal processes (eg, earlier in the sporulation to ultraviolet [UV] and formaldehyde, whereas later to heat and glutaraldehyde). Much less yet more recent investigations have described the resistance profiles of protozoal cysts, or particularly oocysts, as well as helminth eggs. The dormant forms of protozoa have been a concern due to their unexpected resistance profiles to various types of antimicrobial chemistries used to treat water (eg, chlorine or bromine), thereby having the ability to survive water disinfection mechanisms and their association with waterborne illness (eg, dysentery). Fungal spores have been typically shown to be much less resistant than bacterial spores, but they should not be underestimated because they can be found within dried, tightly-packed, and protected bodies that resist the penetration of disinfectants and sterilants (eg, *Aspergillus* species ascospores and *Pyronema* species). Overall, the term *sporicidal* is generally confirmed using bacterial spores as being the most resistant to this group, and when demonstrated to be effective against these, they are often assumed to be effective against other types of dormant and vegetative forms of microorganisms, including fungal spores.

Viruses can also range dramatically in resistance profiles based on their structures.[1] They are typically classified into two major types—nonenveloped and enveloped—referring to the presence or absence of an external lipophilic envelope. The external envelope is derived from the modified cell membrane structure sourced from the host cell during infection and release of virus particles, consisting of host cell phospholipids and proteins as well some virus protein such as glycoproteins. Because the envelope structure is typically required to allow the virus to successfully infect target cells, damage to this relatively sensitive structure is often sufficient to render the virus nonviable and therefore particularly sensitive to biocidal physical and chemical effects. Notable enveloped viruses such as human immunodeficiency virus (HIV), hepatitis B virus (HBV), and the flu (or influenza) viruses are therefore considered relatively sensitive to inactivation to include drying, heat, and chemical biocidal treatments. Nonenveloped viruses are dramatically more resistant. They can be further subdivided into larger and smaller nonenveloped viruses, where larger viruses (such as adenoviruses) are considered more resistant than enveloped viruses but less resistant than smaller, nonenveloped viruses. Traditionally, the most studied virus in the smaller, nonenveloped class was poliovirus, which was widely used as the test virus for testing disinfectant efficacy (see chapters 62 and 63). But in recent years, there has been a greater understanding of the extremes of resistance in nonenveloped viruses from studies with pathogens such as noroviruses, coxsackieviruses, and parvoviruses. Parvoviruses particularly demonstrate higher levels of resistance to physical and chemical inactivation methods due to their unique, tightly packed protein-capsid structures.[3] Therefore, it is important to carefully inspect "virucidal" claims because efficacy against HIV or HBV will not be good indicators of efficacy against more resistant forms of viruses, and even then, the efficacy in certain types of nonenveloped viruses like poliovirus may not necessarily confirm efficacy against all nonenveloped viruses depending on the antimicrobial method under investigation.

Bacteria also range in resistance profiles. At a gross level, there has been three types of bacteria described as having increased levels of resistance to inactivation, from lower to higher being gram-positive bacteria, gram-negative bacteria, and mycobacteria. Such resistance profiles are due to their intrinsic cell wall structure differences, with gram-positive bacteria having a larger quantity of peptidoglycan in its cell wall, gram-negative bacteria with less peptidoglycan but containing an additional outer lipid-based membrane, and mycobacteria consisting of a tripartite structure of inner peptidoglycan, arabinogalactan, and outer lipid layer of mycolic acids. Mycobacteria have been traditionally found to have the highest level of resistance in the vegetative bacteria group to inactivation. Therefore, it is important to note that label claims or efficacy studies that often claim inactivation of bacteria (bactericidal; see

chapter 2) are typically restricted to testing representative gram-negative and gram-positive bacteria but not mycobacteria (claims against which are specifically referred to as mycobactericidal). Added to this complexity can be the ability of certain bacterial genera to develop into bacterial spores, as described earlier. But overall, such general statements of efficacy against bacteria can be an oversimplification due to the diversity of bacteria types described to date and their ability to adapt to various situations. Consider, for example, that mycoplasmas (eg, the pathogens *Mycoplasma pneumoniae* and *Mycoplasma genitalium*) are known as cell wall–free bacteria and for this reason were often assumed to be very sensitive to inactivation, but this may not always be the case due to the unique lipids in their cell membrane structures that provide greater rigidity and tolerance to microbicides.[4] Bacterial genera and species can vary in their tolerance levels to microbicides due to their structures, often depending on the chemical or physical antimicrobial method under investigation. For example, *Salmonella*, *Enterococcus*, and *Legionella* species have been described to have higher levels of tolerance to heat.[5,6] Bacteria can vary due to their ability to present various resistance mechanisms that can be both a natural ability in the bacteria type or due to their ability to mutate or acquire resistance mechanisms to survive adverse conditions, including the presence of preservatives, antiseptics, and disinfectants. Examples include innate stress responses, biofilm development, cell wall structural changes, and efflux of chemical microbicides out of the cell (see chapters 4 and 67). Acquired mechanisms can be due to mutations and the acquisition of transmissible genetic material that can encode resistance mechanisms (see chapter 4). These mechanisms of intrinsic and acquired tolerance to antimicrobials can allow bacteria to persist in harsh or hostile environments.

The archaea are notably missing from the resistance hierarchy in Figure 3.1. Due to their similarities (essentially as single-celled prokaryotes), they were traditionally classified as bacteria but are now considered to be phylogenetically distinct. But despite our expanding knowledge of archaea types, they are considered nonpathogenic, are not known to be associated with spoilage, and are typically associated with "extreme environments" such as extremes of heat. Unlike the other microorganisms described, the archaea are not typically targets for preservative, disinfection, and sterilization processes. But they are of interest to microbiologists due to their various unique structures and metabolism that allow them to survive extreme environments as vegetative microorganisms.

Although less studied, fungi and protozoa can present similar variability in their resistance profiles to biocidal mechanisms. Vegetative fungi (molds and yeast) and protozoa are traditionally considered midway in resistance between gram-positive and gram-negative bacteria, with their dormant forms of spores and cysts demonstrating higher resistance. But resistance profiles can vary significantly depending on their individual structures. As already noted earlier, *Aspergillus* and *Pyronema* species can demonstrate higher levels of resistance to some biocidal treatment methods. The ability of fungus to grow as masses of hyphal growth incorporating various types of spores can be a penetration barrier particularly to chemical microbicides. Protozoa, being more free-living, are considered more likely to be inactivated (such as in water) but can circumnavigate biocidal treatments by their association with bacterial biofilms. As described previously, the formation of dormant cyst forms can demonstrate resistance to chemical microbicides but generally not to physical methods such as heat inactivation. Helminths are much less studied, but their egg forms are known to be more resistant to inactivation than their adult worm forms.[1]

It is important to note that exceptions to these profiles are frequently cited in the literature. In considering these reports, it is important to look carefully at the test methods being use. Close inspection of many reports can show significant differences in the growth and isolation of test organisms and their presentation to an antimicrobial process for comparing their resistance profiles to inactivation. Important variables can include the ability of cells, dormant forms, or viruses to clump together; the presence of interfering factors (such as organic or inorganic materials that can compete or even neutralize the biocidal activity); and the presence of mixed populations of microorganisms or various forms. Despite these test methodology variances, there are reports of unique and dramatic resistance profiles to inactivation methods with specific types of microorganisms (Table 3.2).

TABLE 3.2   Examples of atypical resistance levels with microorganisms against biocidal mechanisms

Microorganism[a]	Biocidal Method(s)	Examples of Mechanisms of Resistance
Deinococcus radiodurans[7]	Ionizing and nonionizing radiation, including γ radiation in the 5-10 kGy range; can include cross-resistance to oxidizing agents and dehydration	Gram-positive, vegetative bacteria that can have multiple mechanisms of tolerance including DNA damage repair mechanisms, multiple copies of their genomes, presence of pigments that act as free-radical scavengers, and unusual (thicker) cell wall structure in comparison to other gram-positive bacteria. Other bacteria with high-level resistance include *Deinobacter*, *Rubrobacter*, and *Methylobacterium* species.
Pyronema domesticum[8]	Ethylene oxide	Fungi (molds) originally reported from cotton-containing products that survived typical ethylene oxide sterilization process, due to hyphal mass protection, tightly packed ascospore-containing fruiting bodies ("apothecia"), and desiccated ascospore protoplasm
Mycobacterium chelonae and *Mycobacterium massiliense*[9,10]	Glutaraldehyde and ortho-phthalaldehyde (OPA)	Certain strains of these acid-fast, nontuberculosis bacteria have demonstrated unique resistance to aldehyde disinfectants. Mechanisms may be related to the lack of available protein targets at the surface of their lipophilic cell wall surface.
Pseudomonas species[11]	Cross-resistance with antibiotics and certain types of microbicides such as triclosan, quaternary ammonium compounds, chlorhexidine, and metals (eg, copper)	Multiple efflux mechanisms that pump the antimicrobial out of the target cell and control of porin synthesis to allow for a greater level of tolerance to the microbicides, with consequences at preservative or lower levels. These mechanisms have been described in other gram-negative and gram-positive bacteria.
Staphylococcus species[12]	Quaternary ammonium compounds and cross-resistance with other microbicides and antibiotics	Efflux mechanisms that are hosted on plasmids and are known to be widespread in staphylococci
Escherichia coli[1,13]	Triclosan and cross-resistance to some antibiotics such as isoniazid	Mutations in genes expressing enoyl-(acyl-carrier-protein) reductases that prevent binding of the microbicide. These enzymes are involved in cellular fatty acid synthesis and have been described as important targets for triclosan; also identified in other bacteria. Efflux-associated mechanisms have also been described.
Cryptosporidium oocysts[14]	A wide variety of chemical disinfectants and sterilant depending on their formulation/exposure conditions	Thick-walled oocyst structure, consisting of a four-layered matrix of protein/carbohydrate/lipid. These structures were initially considered unique in their resistance profiles, but subsequent investigations of other protozoa (eg, *Acanthamoeba*[15]) have also demonstrated high-level resistance.

[a]Note that higher resistance levels have been described in some of the species listed but may not be a property of all strains in that species.

Prions

Although often considered a controversial topic, prions are well established as unique transmissible agents that are composed of protein and lacking any specific nucleic acid.[16] The specific source of the prion protein is PrP (or in its normal cellular form is known as PrP^c), a glycoprotein associated the cell membranes of human or animal cells and particularly in the neurons of neural tissues such as the brain and spinal cord. The protein is not considered essential for life, but it has been associated with various higher order functions including transport of copper, stress responses, central nervous system structure, and memory.[17] Like other proteins, PrP^c assumes a normal folded secondary and tertiary structure that is produced and broken down by normal protein metabolism processes. But in the disease process, a conformational change in its structure can occur to render the protein resistant to proteases and therefore to cellular degradation. This form of the protein, known as a prion, is referred to in the literature under a variety of similar names such as PrP^{res} (referring to "resistant"), PrP^{Sc} (denoting "scrapie"—a sheep prion disease), or PrP^{TSE} (for transmissible spongiform encephalopathies [TSEs] or prion diseases). The prion form acts to promote a conformational change in other PrP^c proteins. Because the prion form cannot be completely broken down by normal cellular processes, it accumulates in affected cells, can lead to cell damage/death, and can transfer to other cells. Over time, this cascade reaction has a significant impact on neural tissues, leading to gross damage and the pathologic implications typified in prion diseases such as loss of brain function and eventually death. It is firmly established that the PrP plays a central role in these diseases and is devoid of any unique nucleic acid typical for other transmissible diseases such as with viruses (see chapter 68). But there is some debate on the role of other cofactors in these diseases that may also be linked with disease infectivity, the prion conversion process, and "strain" diversity. These include various types of lipids and RNA fragments.[18,19]

The TSEs or prion diseases are fatal degenerative brain diseases of animals and humans.[20] Human diseases include Creutzfeldt-Jakob disease (CJD), kuru, and Gerstmann-Sträussler-Scheinker syndrome and are considered rare. For example, CJD is the most widely described and is reported to occur in about 1 to 3 cases in 1 million populations. Specific cases of disease transmission between humans has been reported with tissue transplantation, reusable medical devices, and, if often speculated (but not confirmed), blood transmission.[2] Zoonotic transmission has also been reported, most notably with the link between bovine spongiform encephalopathy (BSE or often referred to as mad cow disease) and a variant form of CJD (vCJD) in humans due to contaminated meat products.[21] Certain animal diseases are considered more widespread for reasons that are unknown, including scrapie (in sheep) and chronic wasting disease (CWD, in deer/elk).[20]

In addition to these specific TSEs, there is much speculation about the existence of prion-like mechanisms in other neurodegenerative diseases such as Parkinson disease and Alzheimer disease.[20] It is interesting to note that Alzheimer disease has been shown to be induced (by a protein-seeding mechanism) in certain animal models in mechanisms similar to those understood for prion diseases and suggesting the potential transmissibility of these diseases in contact with contaminated tissues.

Prions have noteworthy higher resistance profiles to most physical and chemical antimicrobial methods. A summary of processes known to be effective or ineffective against prions are given in Table 3.3. It is important to note that efficacy reports can vary widely and do depend on the methods used for evaluation (see chapter 68).[2] For example, many studies have focused on the investigation of tissues highly contaminated with prions under which conditions full efficacy against the target agents would not be expected, particularly if compared to investigations with other types of microorganisms. This is due to the interference of the tissue material in such investigations and the lack of penetration to the target agents. Despite this, some clear conclusions can be made from these studies. First, antimicrobial methods that specifically target nucleic acids as their primary modes of action are not effective. Despite this conclusion, there are some exceptions, such as in the case of certain unique phenolic-disinfectant formulations that were verified to be effective against prions.[22] Second, steam sterilization is considered effective, but dry heat methods are not. The effectiveness of steam can range depending on the material being inactivated (eg, whole tissue or contaminated surfaces with a cleaning step prior to steam treatment).[2,22] Incineration is considered effective, but even in this case, viable prions could be detected in some studies.[23] Third, processes that are effective at degrading protein structures are generally effective, especially aggressive chemical treatment based on alkalis (especially sodium hydroxide), some oxidizing agents (eg, sodium hypochlorite, gaseous hydrogen peroxide), and (in certain situations) with extended protease digestion. The reports of effectiveness can also range depending on the test method, product formulation or test conditions, and so forth.[2] For example, proteases may often appear effective in in vitro tests, but in infectivity (in vivo) tests, many of these methods were not found to be effective and this may be due to partial protein degradation.[2] Combinations of heat and chemical (eg, alkali) processes have been shown to be particularly effective, including for whole carcass degradation.

So overall, prions present a unique challenge for traditional disinfection and sterilization procedures. In many cases, control of prions and prion contamination, such as in the handling of animal tissues, is most often a risk reduction exercise. Examples include the sourcing of tissues used for human introduction from animals or human known to be at a low risk of prion disease, the

TABLE 3.3 A summary of antimicrobial processes known to be effective, potentially effective but requiring further investigation, and ineffective against prions[a]

Effective	Potential Effectiveness	Ineffective
Steam sterilization but typically under extended exposure time (eg, 121°C for 1 h and 134°C for 18 min) or, for surface contamination, when combined with a cleaning step prion to steam treatment	Oxidizing agents (such as liquid hydrogen peroxide, peracetic acid, or ozone) under certain formulation and/or process conditions	Aldehydes such as formaldehyde and glutaraldehyde
1 N sodium hydroxide for 1 h or with other alkaline-based chemistries or formulations	Some acids, depending on concentration, formulation, and temperature exposure	Alcohols
2% available chlorine for 1 h		Hot or boiling water
Incineration		Radiation (ionizing or nonionizing)
Hydrogen peroxide gas		Dry heat
Certain types of gas plasmas (eg, oxygen)		Ethylene oxide
Some phenolic formulations		Quaternary ammonium compounds
4 M guanidine hydrochloride ($\geq$1 h)		
Prolonged protease digestion		

[a]Reprinted from McDonnell.[2]

use of treatment that is known to inactivate or remove prion contamination (particularly alkaline and oxidizing agents), or the complete removal of prion risk by exclusion (eg, removing all materials that are of animal origin or disposal of any materials that contact tissues known to be contaminated). Despite this, specific inactivation methods for prions have been defined and this continues to be an area for further research and development. Further consideration of the unique nature and inactivation of prions is given in chapter 68.

Viruses

Viruses are a major group of pathogens and are therefore important targets for disinfection and sterilization applications. Unlike bacteria and fungi, they cannot grow or multiply in the environment without a specific host. Therefore, they are generally not targeted for preservative applications but are key targets for many purposes such as environmental disinfection (particularly in disease outbreak situations), treatment of foods or liquids for consumption, skin or mucous membrane infection treatments, mammalian biotechnology process systems, wastewater or material treatment, and device/tissue sterilization. Once viruses are in a host, they can lead to infections that are often serious and are responsible for significant rates of morbidity and mortality. Influenza outbreaks alone continue to be a significant cause of death during yearly flu seasons, but the different variants of influenza viruses do vary in virulence and have

been associated with pandemics. The most noteworthy was the Spanish influenza pandemic that is estimated to have led to about 50 million deaths in 1918 worldwide.[24] Previous editions of this book focused attention on viruses such as HIV and HBV due to serious concerns at that time on their risks of transmission and particularly in health care facilities.[25,26] In recent years, concerns with rotavirus, noroviruses, Zika virus, dengue, Ebola virus, and other emerging virus outbreaks, many with threats of pandemics, continue to highlight the risks of viruses as serious pathogens.[27] Even preventable diseases in first-world countries, such as measles, have reemerged as concerns and causes of death due to unfounded concerns with vaccinations.[28]

In such disease states, viruses have the ability to be disseminated, often at high levels, by many mechanisms such as through blood or other body fluids (eg, with HIV, HBV, and viral hemorrhagic fever viruses such as Ebola), diarrhea (eg, with noroviruses or rotaviruses), direct contact (eg, from warts such as with human papillomaviruses), and through the air or droplet routes (such as with smallpox, influenza, and rhinoviruses). Viruses are therefore often highly contagious or transmissible. Disinfection challenges can include the presentation of the virus (eg, often associated in blood or other body tissues/excretions), the viral load present (often high in cases such as active infections with Ebola or other hemorrhagic fever viruses estimated to be $\geq 10^6$ viruses per milliliter blood),[29] the ability of the virus to persist in the environment, and resistance of virus type to chemical and physical inactivation. Viruses can clump together, and this has often been linked as a tolerance factor to allow virus survival following disinfection.[1] Furthermore, they are often associated with various organic materials (such as patient's tissues or excretions that include proteins, carbohydrates, and lipids), which provide a penetration challenge to physical and chemical disinfectants. As with other microorganisms, the importance of cleaning (to remove extraneous materials) prior to disinfection or sterilization is important.[30] Even enveloped viruses that are considered relatively sensitive to environmental conditions, drying, and disinfection can show remarkable persistence profiles in the environment, depending on the specific virus protein structures[31] and the presence of nonviral extraneous materials.[32]

As introduced earlier in this chapter (see Table 3.1), viruses can present a wide resistance profile to disinfectants and disinfection processes due to their structures. The main determinants to resistance are the presence of an external envelope (therefore known as enveloped and nonenveloped viruses) and their size (large or small viruses). Traditionally, viruses were then classified into three types based on their innate resistance profiles to inactivation.[1,33] These include small nonenveloped viruses,

large nonenveloped viruses, and enveloped viruses. Enveloped viruses can range in size from approximately 40 to 400 nm, larger nonenveloped viruses are in the 50- to 100-nm range, and small nonenveloped viruses at 10 to 30 nm. Examples of pathogenic viruses in each of these types and their relationship to model or indicator viruses used for efficacy tests are given in Table 3.4.

In the past, viruses were much less studied in comparison to bacteria due to their unique and often difficult growth requirements for laboratory investigation. For most microbiology laboratories, a sensitive cell culture method needs to be available for the virus to multiply in, although animal-based infection models may also be used but are not preferred. Even with cell culture techniques, human pathogen surrogate viruses often need to be used that are considered equivalent to their human counterparts, such as in the case of earlier studies on the use of a duck hepatitis B model as a surrogate for human HBV[34] or the use of murine surrogates for human norovirus.[35] Another useful method to determine viricidal activity is with the use of bacteriophages (bacterial viruses) that are easier to manipulate in laboratory practice, are nonpathogenic to humans or animals, and also may present with a higher

TABLE 3.4 Examples of virus pathogens and surrogate viruses used to indicate disinfection effectiveness against viruses[a]

Viruses	Diseases	Examples of Indicator Viruses[b]
Group A: enveloped viruses		
HIV	AIDS	Duck hepatitis B virus
Ebola virus	Ebola virus disease, a viral hemorrhagic fever in humans and primates	Bovine viral diarrhea virus Influenza A virus
Influenza virus	Influenza or flu	Herpes simplex virus
Group B: large, nonenveloped viruses		
Adenoviruses	A wide range of symptoms similar to having a cold, sore throat, pneumonia, sometimes diarrhea, and conjunctivitis (commonly called "pink eye")	Adenovirus
Group C: small, nonenveloped viruses		
Poliovirus	Poliomyelitis or commonly called polio	
Human papilloma virus	Often asymptomatic but can lead to the development of skin or mucous membrane warts (eg, in the genital area) or precancerous lesions. Two types of viruses, HPV-16 and HPV-18, are associated with cervical cancer.	Feline calicivirus Poliovirus Parvovirus Murine norovirus Bovine Enterovirus
Parvovirus	Human (eg, fifth disease) and animal disease, particularly associated with the gastrointestinal tract and lymphatic system. Symptoms can include vomiting, diarrhea, immunosuppression, and infertility.	

[a]From Klein and DeForest.[33]

[b]Used as surrogate viruses for disinfection testing and can vary depending on geographical area (see chapters 62 and 63).

resistance profile to inactivation,[36] but they do vary in resistance depending on the bacteriophage type.[37] Mammalian indicator viruses became commonly used to establish antimicrobial claims against viruses (see Table 3.4). For example, claims against enveloped and nonenveloped viruses could be substantiated with disinfectants or sterilants and cleared by the US Food and Drug Administration by demonstrating efficacy against herpes simplex virus, adenovirus, and poliovirus (see chapters 62 and 71). Similar virus types are used in the European Union to make disinfection claims for various antiseptic or disinfectant applications by verifying efficacy with viruses such as bovine viral diarrhea virus and parvoviruses in defined test methods (see chapter 63). Although these approaches are widely accepted, there are often concerns over varying resistance profiles within these groups depending on the strain of virus and the disinfectant types under investigation.[3,31,38] Unexpected levels of resistance to heat and chemical disinfection methods have been reported with parvoviruses and other nonenveloped viruses in comparison to the poliovirus that had been widely used to demonstrate viricidal activity against these types of viruses.[3] Resistance profiles appear to be due to presence of inert surface protein-capsid structures and their tight, inaccessible structures.[39]

A final consideration with viruses is that they are essentially inert structures, unlike viable cells of bacteria, protozoa, and fungi. When such microbial cells are significantly disrupted in their structure and function, and this damage reaches a significant extent, they lose viability, die, and are incapable of further multiplication or infection. Viruses can be different. They can withstand a lot of damage, but once the viral components required for infection, such as the nucleic acid alone (in many nonenveloped viruses) and associated proteins (such as those associated with the envelope or capsid of enveloped viruses), are available or by reassociation, they may still lead to infection. This has been described in laboratory experiments and described as "multiplicity reactivation"[40]; although these results have not been reproduced or investigated in further detail, they do suggest that disrupted virus structures can still retain low-level infectivity capability.

Bacteria

Bacteria are by far the most widely studied and considered in disinfection, sterilization, and preservation applications. First, they are ubiquitous in nature and are often detectable (sometimes at high levels) in various environmental sources. For example, estimates of the total percentage biomass of the Earth suggest that the levels of bacteria far exceed that of animals and plants. An example of this is in the human body, where the number of bacteria living in the skin and mucous membranes or in the body (particularly the gut) are in excess of the total number of human cells in the body.[41] Second, they are both

noteworthy pathogens, as significant causes of disease, and are frequent sources of contamination or causes of product spoilage (Table 3.5). They are therefore important targets in preventing foods, liquid (including water), cosmetic, preserved products, and pharmaceuticals contamination as well as reducing the risks of acquired infections (eg, health care–acquired infections [HAIs]). The beneficial impact on public health with sanitization and pasteurization processes over the last 50 to 100 years is significant. Examples include the provision of safe drinking water; sewage disposal and treatment; milk or other liquid product pasteurization; and antiseptic, disinfection, and sterilization in high-risk situations such as during surgery or wound management.[42] Combined with other major controls such as immunization and availability of antibiotics, the impact has been significant on reducing the rates of once common bacterial infections and death such as cholera, dysentery, influenza, typhoid, and malaria (now replaced as leading causes of death by heart disease and cancer compared to estimates from 1900). But bacterial infections are still a major concern, especially in high-risk situations where certain populations such as the old, very young, or immunocompromised are at a greater risk of contracting bacterial diseases. For example, the top six causes of HAIs and associated with antimicrobial resistance are all bacteria, known as the ESKAPE pathogens.[43] This acronym refers to *Enterococcus faecium*, *Staphylococcus aureus*, *Klebsiella pneumoniae*, *Acinetobacter baumannii*, *Pseudomonas aeruginosa*, and *Enterobacter* species. Periodic outbreaks of community-acquired infections such as *Escherichia coli* or other Enterobacteriaceae and *Listeria monocytogenes* from food or water as well as the reemergence of diseases such as tuberculosis and malaria continue to be a concern. Furthermore, bacterial contamination is a constant cause of concern for manufacturers of preserved or aseptically manufactured products (see Part 5 and chapter 58).[44] The importance of the detection and risk reduction for the presence of certain bacterial pathogens, known as "objectionable" microorganisms, has become particularly important to nonsterile product manufacturers.[45] Examples can include *S aureus* and many gram-negative bacteria such as *A baumannii*, *P aeruginosa*, and *Burkholderia cepacia* complex. These examples highlight the third reason why bacteria are a concern in disinfection, sterilization, and preservation applications, having their ability to adapt to survive, multiply, and persist in unfavorable environments.

As previously stated, the major intrinsic mechanism of tolerance to inactivation in bacteria is their overall structures, particularly related to their outer or cell wall structure.[1] The most vulnerable are mycoplasmas because they do not contain an outer cell wall structure but do have a unique cell membrane structure that can present with higher levels of resistance to microbicides than animal or eukaryotic cells.[4] Next are gram-positive bacteria containing a larger outer component of peptidoglycan and then the gram-negative bacteria with a lower

TABLE 3.5	Examples of bacteria, Gram staining classifications, and frequent associated diseases	
Bacterial Genus	**Gram (or other) Stain Designation**	**Disease Examples**
Mycoplasma	Cell wall–free but stain as gram-negative	Pneumonia, bronchitis, and sexually transmitted infections; significant contaminants in cell cultures used in research laboratories
Chlamydia	Gram-negative, replicate intracellularly	Conjunctivitis, pneumonia, and urethritis
Bacillus	Gram-positive, aerobic, spore-forming	Food poisoning, keratitis, and anthrax; a common environmental contaminant in air and on surfaces
Clostridium	Gram-positive, anaerobic, spore-forming	Intestinal infection and intoxication
Staphylococcus	Gram-positive	Genus like *Staphylococcus epidermidis* are common flora of the skin. Along with other staphylococci, it is common environmental contaminants. *Staphylococcus aureus* is a major pathogen in cellulitis, impetigo, sepsis, wound infections, and other health care–acquired infections. Many strains, such as methicillin-resistant *S aureus* (MRSA) strains, are resistant to many antibiotics.
Streptococcus	Gram-positive	Meningitis, scarlet fever, pneumonia, bronchitis, rhinosinusitis, and dental caries
Escherichia	Gram-negative	Pneumonia, gastrointestinal infections, sepsis
Pseudomonas	Gram-negative	Conjunctivitis, keratitis, wound, and other health care–acquired infections commonly associated with water contamination, even in pure water systems
Klebsiella	Gram-negative	Opportunistic pathogens, particularly in health care–acquired infections such as urinary tract infections, pneumonia, surgical wound infections, and septicemia. Increasing rates of antibiotic resistant strains, such as carbapenem-resistant *Klebsiella pneumoniae*; widespread in nature but often associated with water or water system contamination
Mycobacterium	Gram-positive/variable, acid-fast	Tuberculosis, leprosy, and opportunistic infections. Many types are ubiquitous in soil and water environments.

component of peptidoglycan but an outer, lipid-based membrane. A further grouping of bacteria, notably including acid-fast mycobacteria and, to a lesser extent, bacteria that have a similar cell wall structure such as *Nocardia*, have a different tripartite structure external to the inner cell membrane that consists of peptidoglycan linked to an arabinogalactan polymer and outer lipid layer (in mycobacteria, containing long mycolic acids). The specific structure, depending on the bacterial genus, can limit the effects of heat and chemicals to affect the bacterial structure and therefore antimicrobial activity. The final group, already highlighted earlier, are bacteria spores produced by gram-positive bacterial genera such as *Bacillus*, *Geobacillus*, and *Clostridium* (Figure 3.2). Bacterial spores are considered some of the most resistant microorganisms to inactivation. These consist of an inner core structure (containing the essential DNA molecule and proteins), surrounded by various membranes, peptidoglycan-like layers, and outer spore coats (particularly consisting of proteins) that protect the spore from inactivation mechanisms (see chapter 3).[1]

Similar to other microorganisms, it is impossible to verify the effectiveness of each type of disinfectant or disinfection process to each species of bacteria, but key surrogates are used to verify efficacy based on these types of classification. Mycoplasmas are not widely studied, and there are no standardized test methods or recommended

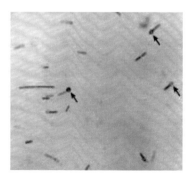

FIGURE 3.2 Gram-stained *Clostridium tetani* bacteria, showing the development of spores (indicated by *arrows*). For a color version of this art, please consult the eBook.

strains for disinfection efficacy claims to date, but strains of *M pneumoniae* and other genera have been used in some investigations.[4] Gram-positive bacteria surrogates include *S aureus* and *Enterococcus hirae*, whereas for gram-negative bacteria, these include *P aeruginosa*, *Salmonella enterica*, and *E coli*. In the past, *Mycobacterium tuberculosis* was widely used to indicate mycobactericidal activity, but due to risks of handling and requirements for long incubation times, other surrogates include *Mycobacterium terrae* and *Mycobacterium avium*. Finally, bacterial spores are widely used in standardized sporicidal disinfection and sterilization test methods, such as the AOAC sporicidal test[46] and EN 13704[47] with *Bacillus subtilis*, *Clostridium sporogenes*, and *Bacillus cereus* spores. Biological indicators (BIs), test systems containing viable microorganisms providing a defined resistance to a specified sterilization process, most commonly use bacterial spores to test, verify, and validate sterilization processes (see chapter 65). The types of spores used with BIs will depend on the known intrinsic resistance of those spores to specific sterilization methods, such as with *G stearothermophilus* spores in moist heat and hydrogen peroxide gas disinfection or sterilization and with *B atrophaeus* spores in ethylene oxide sterilization.

A subject that is not often considered in the use of these traditional, standardized test methods is the variety of mechanisms employed by certain types of bacteria to resist the activity of preservation, disinfection, and sterilization methodologies. These are summarized in Table 3.6 and are discussed in further detail in chapter 4. Bacteria can be very adaptable in different environments, particularly when under stress (as is in the case in the presence of chemical microbicides or biocidal processes). This is most frequently observed in the presence of low concentrations of microbicides (such as in the case of preserved products

or liquids), situations were bacteria are only subjected to periodic or sublethal disinfection (eg, in the periodic disinfection of water lines), or in the treatment of contaminated wastes that allow bacteria to escape inactivation or be injured and survive the antimicrobial process. These mechanisms can allow for the unexpected survival of bacteria in various environmental conditions, leading to cross-contamination, and can also lead to cases of cross-resistance to not only the microbicides being employed but also to antibiotics with further therapeutic ramifications. Examples of cross-resistance to antibiotics include in mycobacteria with high-level resistance to glutaraldehyde,[48] staphylococcal plasmids that are linked to efflux mechanisms of tolerance,[49] triclosan resistance mechanisms including efflux,[1] mutations in genes for protein associated with the mode of action of the microbicides,[1] cell wall changes causing exclusion of the microbicide/antibiotic,[1] and particularly the development of biofilms (see chapters 4 and 67).[1] Biofilms are a common mechanism found to allow for the bacteria to escape the activity of disinfection methods and are a natural, intrinsic mechanism of resistance and development in bacteria. These are discussed in more detail in chapters 4 and 67. Up to recent years, acquired resistance mechanisms (due to mutations and acquisition of transmissible genetic elements such as plasmids or transposons) were thought to only allow for marginal increases in the minimum inhibitory concentrations of microbicides such as chlorhexidine, quaternary ammonium compounds (QACs), and triclosan.[50] But the impact of increased cross-resistance to antibiotics cannot be underestimated, with the widespread, ubiquitous, and often unnecessary use of triclosan and maybe some other microbicides.[51] Further reports of more dramatic resistance mechanisms in certain bacteria leading to disinfection failure due to mutation or potentially plasmid

TABLE 3.6 Examples of intrinsic and acquired mechanisms of resistance

Intrinsic Resistance Mechanisms	Acquired Resistance Mechanisms
Cell wall structures, causing impermeability or lack of surface reactivity	Mutations in the structure and functions of the cell to include efflux mechanisms, cell wall surface changes, and modifications in the structures of certain cell targets (eg, with triclosan)
Sporulation in certain genera	Acquisition of plasmids or transposons that include genes conferring resistance determinants such as efflux mechanisms, microbicide inactivation, cell surface alterations, and sequestration
Production of enzymes and chemicals that neutralize chemical microbicides (eg, catalase against hydrogen peroxide) and protect against or repair damage to cell component during or following treatment	
Efflux, but the extrusion of chemical microbicides (eg, chlorhexidine, triclosan, or quaternary ammonium compounds) from the target cell	
Biofilm development	

acquisition (eg, with mycobacteria and glutaraldehyde) has been a cause of some concern.[1,9] It is important to note that most of these reports are related to the use of chemical disinfectants and not physical methods of inactivation, although examples of novel resistance determinants to heat and radiation that have evolved in certain types of bacteria and archaea are of interest to study due to their ability to allow for survival under extreme conditions (Tables 3.2 and 3.6). Overall, these reports highlight the importance of the correct use of disinfectants and monitoring their long-term effectiveness.

A final consideration is the production of different types of toxins in bacteria. These are important virulence factors because they can lead to various disease effects such as fever induction and tissue damage (see later in this chapter and chapter 66). They are generally classified into two groups—exotoxins and endotoxins. Exotoxins are actively produced by and released from bacteria during growth. They can be potent poisons to humans and animals including cholera, botulism, and toxic shock syndrome toxins with effects such as blocking neurotransmitters, cell damage/lysis, and inhibition of protein synthesis. These are generally a concern during active infection of hosts but are not normally considered as important contaminants on surfaces or products unless present at higher concentrations (such as in contaminated foods, where the bacteria have been actively multiplying). Endotoxins, which are an intrinsic part of the outer cell wall structure of gram-negative bacteria, are not normally released from the cell apart form on adjustments to environmental stress, cell damage, and cell death. When released, they can be resilient in the environment, surviving drying and inactivation methods, and persisting on contaminated surfaces or liquids. When these are introduced into the blood stream of animals or humans, they can lead to various immune reactions cascades including fever, which under some conditions can be fatal. Endotoxins are not readily inactivated by many chemical and physical disinfection or sterilization mechanisms, so control of these contaminants is often a matter of removing the source (ie, gram-negative bacteria) during manufacturing, water treatment processes, or other product-handling processes. Inactivation (or neutralization) methods can include extended dry heat sterilization (known as depyrogenation) and physical removal by filtration.[52]

Archaea

The archaea were once classified as bacteria (or "archaebacteria") because they are prokaryotic cells, but they are now known to be a diverse group of microorganisms phylogenetically distinct from bacteria.[53] As noted earlier in this chapter, little consideration of this group has been given in disinfection, sterilization, and preservation applications due to their lack of association with health,

environmental, or commercial (eg, food or product spoilage) risks. But it is interesting to note that there have been some concerns (but no direct evidence) over potential pathogenic risks[54] and the need for control of many archaea in the environment (eg, those that produce methane, a greenhouse gas) that have prompted some investigations (eg, with the use of antimicrobial peptides).[55] Probably of greater academic interest has been the detection of many archaea actively living and multiplying in what we, as humans, consider as extreme environments. These include extremes of temperature (even under boiling or steam sterilization conditions), saline conditions, and extremes of pH. Examples of these are given in Table 3.7, along with a summary of some of the tolerance mechanisms that have been identified that allow these microorganisms to survive under such conditions. Many of these examples, such as the thermophiles (or "hyperthermophiles," being resistant to temperatures in excess of 80°C), are not only found to be resistant to high temperatures but also to radiation. These include *Pyrococcus* species that can have optimal growth conditions at approximately 115°C and relatively higher levels of tolerance to gamma and other sources of radiation.[56] It may be speculated that the mechanisms of resistance would be similar to what was already described with certain bacteria, particularly those that develop highly resistant dormant forms (endospores), but this was not found to be the case in archaea (see Table 3.7).[1] The archaea had evolved (noting that they are often considered as ancient, earlier microorganisms) as vegetative prokaryotes that where actively able to metabolize and multiply under extreme conditions by an accumulation of tolerance mechanisms. These will vary depending on the exact environmental niches preferred by the specific genus and species of archaea but are remarkably similar. They include unique outer cell wall structures, such as the presence of external S-layer structures based on glycoproteins and the presence of certain types of lipids that given greater fluidity (eg, under cold conditions) or less sensitivity to breakdown (eg, under higher temperatures). Other mechanisms include unique protein structures (in cell structure and metabolism) that can perform their roles under such conditions, use of protective proteins (eg, that bind to protect the essential DNA molecules), efficient repair mechanisms that can restore damaged macromolecules, efflux or other cell wall–associated solute transportation mechanisms, and detoxification systems. It is tempting to speculate that if the accumulation of such mechanisms in vegetative prokaryotes is possible in archaea, they are also possible to evolve in other prokaryotes (ie, bacteria). Indeed, similar mechanisms of tolerance to chemical and physical methods of preservation and disinfection have been described in bacteria but have not been shown to lead to similar extremes of resistance (see chapter 4).[1] But there are some exceptions, such as those described in Table 3.2 and notably bacteria such as *Deinococcus radiodurans* that display high level resistance to radiation

TABLE 3.7   Examples of archaea, extreme growth conditions described, and some examples of mechanisms of resistance identified

Microorganism	Growth Conditions	Mechanisms of Resistance
Pyrococcus fumarii	Hyperthermophilic; have little growth at <85°C and optimal growth reported at 115°C; also display higher resistance to radiation	Unique cell membrane/wall structure Protective DNA-binding proteins Efficient DNA repair mechanisms Heat-resistant protein (structural and enzymes) and lipid structures Detoxification systems (eg, for reactive oxygen species)
Halobacterium species	Tolerate high-salt conditions, often up to 32% NaCl; also display higher resistance to radiation and other DNA-damaging agents	Cellular protection and detoxification from oxidative damage Repair mechanisms for cellular macromolecules Extracellular S-layer composed of glycoprotein Highly acidic protein structures (prevent precipitation) Osmotic stress control using efflux/influx mechanisms
Methanococcus species	Can survive just above freezing temperatures (2°C-3°C) and under high pressures (20-100 MPa); also display higher resistance to ultraviolet light	Unique protein and lipid structures that tolerate colder temperatures Increased cell membrane fluidity, reportedly due to the presence of unsaturated fatty acids Production of "cold-shock" protective proteins that bind to DNA or act as chaperones to control protein structures
Natronobacterium species	Survive under high alkaline conditions (eg, pH 10.5) and have high-saline tolerance	Control of membrane permeability and intracellular osmotic balance Cell wall structures Unique protein and other cell constituent structures

and other biocidal methods by a similar accumulation of cellular mechanisms in a vegetative microorganism. These included DNA damage repair mechanisms, multiple copies of their genomes, presence of pigments that act as free-radical scavengers, and unusual (thicker) cell wall structures in comparison to other gram-positive bacteria. There is an interesting link between radiation and thermotolerance in many thermophiles.[57]

Fungi

Fungi are eukaryotic microorganisms and have also been reasonably well studied in their resistance profiles to antimicrobial methods. Many are known pathogens in plants and animals, particularly as causes of opportunistic infection in immunocompromised patients, such as *Candida* species and *Aspergillus* species in humans or animals and *Magnaporthe oryzae* and *Botrytis cinerea* in plants. Other notable fungal pathogens include the various types of dermatophytes (eg, *Trichophyton* species) that can cause infections such as ringworm and athlete's foot and *Cryptococcus* species that can cause fungal pneumonia and meningitis. But due to their ubiquitous nature, they are widely known to be environmental contaminants and can be significant causes of food, drug, and product spoilage, particularly sourced from damp environments. Negative effects can include undesired changes in color, texture, and smell as well as product destruction. Examples of

such contaminants include species of *Penicillium* and *Aspergillus*. Many can lead to significant health effects, with an important example being *Stachybotrys* species (commonly known as "black mold") that is often associated with growth on water-damaged building materials and are linked to a range of health effects linked to the production of spores and toxins. For these reasons, fungi are important targets in a variety of disinfection and sterilization applications for contamination prevention or remediation. Fungi are also important targets in the use of preservatives in products, including building materials, foods, cosmetics, liquid pharmaceuticals, and other vulnerable products. But fungi have many commercial benefits such as in the production of breads, milk-based products (eg, cheese and yogurt), alcohol fermentation, and as sources of antibiotics (eg, penicillin).

Macroscopically and microscopically fungi have a wide range of structural types but are generally subdivided in two groups—unicellular (or yeasts) and filamentous fungi (molds) (see Table 3.1). Yeasts are similar to bacteria in how they grow as unicellular organisms yet are different in their eukaryotic cell structure organization and cell size (eg, in the 8-10 μm size compared to bacteria at 0.3-1 μm). Examples include *Candida albicans* and *Candida auris*; both are pathogens in humans, important causes of HAIs, and often cited as being resistant to antifungal therapeutic agents.[58] Other common yeasts include various species of *Saccharomyces* used in food production. Molds are different in that they tend to form

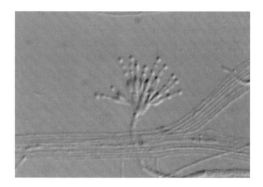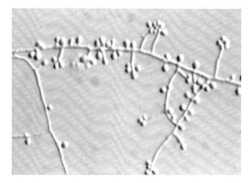

FIGURE 3.3 Examples of filamentous fungal growth showing hyphae, various fruiting bodies, and spores. For a color version of this art, please consult the eBook.

long filaments of cells (known as hyphae) because the cells do not separate following cell division (Figure 3.3). Depending on the various types of molds, the hyphal growth can specialize to produce spores (including sexual and asexual forms). Such structural arrangements have been traditionally used to identify mold genera.[59] The spores can be produced at the end of hyphal branches or contained within specialized structures known as fruiting bodies and are released into the environment. The production of spores and ease in their dissemination make fungi common sources of the environmental contamination both in the air and on surfaces.

Fungal structures can provide a variety of resistance factors to preservation, disinfection, and sterilization processes.[1] An important factor is the fungal cell wall structure, which is generally composed of an outer polysaccharide (glucans) and glycoprotein matrix that includes chitin or cellulose. In molds, the cell wall is often more rigid in structure and gives them a drier-looking macrostructure when observed on surfaces. Overall, the outer structure of molds, acting as a penetration barrier for water (eg, in thermal disinfection) and antimicrobial chemicals, is attributed to the higher level of resistance in comparison to most bacteria (see Figure 3.1). Molds are also considered more resistant than various types of yeasts. Another determinant of resistance is the overall protective nature of hyphal growth with molds that grow as clumps of cell (including spores forms) that can be difficult for chemicals to penetrate and allow for inactivation. Indeed, such populations may be considered as forms of fungal biofilms that allow for many protection effects from adverse environmental conditions, as discussed earlier with bacteria. But clearly a major resistance determinant in fungi is the development of spores, such as conidiospores, sporangiospores, ascospores, and basidiospores.[59,60] There are at least two protective mechanisms in place and their overall resistance will vary depending on the fungal genus or species. The first is the individual spore structure and the innermost structures are essential for life (eg, food reserves and, of course, DNA); have a low water content; and are surrounded by an outer, rigid,

and often dried spore coat that is composed primarily of polysaccharides but also including lipids and proteins. These are an excellent barrier, depending on the thickness of the spore coat; for example, sporangiospores (examples of asexual spores) have a thinner coat structure and are found to be more sensitive to microbicides in comparison to the more resistant ascospores (sexual spores). But many of these can be further protected in fruiting bodies. Such structures of genera including *Pyronema* (see Table 3.2) and *Aspergillus* are important examples because they often present with higher levels of resistance to chemical disinfection due to these structures. *Pyronema* species have been described as having greater tolerance to gaseous sterilization processes (eg, with humidified ethylene oxide processes; see chapter 31) due to hyphal mass protection, tightly packed ascospore-containing fruiting bodies ("apothecia"), and desiccated ascospore protoplasm.[8,61] Similarly, but less extreme, are *Aspergillus* species that have higher levels of tolerance to disinfection with heat, chemicals, and UV irradiation.[1,62] Although the mechanisms of resistance have not been studied in detail, the ascospores (usually eight per ascus) are included within an ascus structure and many of these are further protected within tightly packed masses of hypha within structures known as ascocarps. These structures add a significant challenge to inactivation of each individual and viable, ascospore.

Overall, these are the major known responses and mechanisms of resistance described for fungus to inactivation, but other minor intrinsic (and some acquired and mutational) mechanisms have been described and most of these are like those discussed for bacteria (see Table 3.6).[1] These include cell wall structure modifications and stress responses (eg, in yeast to tolerate the presence of high concentrations of ethanol during fermentation),[63] enzymatic degradation of microbicides (eg, a glutathione-dependent formaldehyde dehydrogenase in yeast *Saccharomyces cerevisiae* that neutralizes formaldehyde),[64] production of outer cell wall–associated capsules (eg, the polysaccharide [mannan]-based capsules in *Cryptococcus neoformans*),[65] and sequestration and/or efflux as

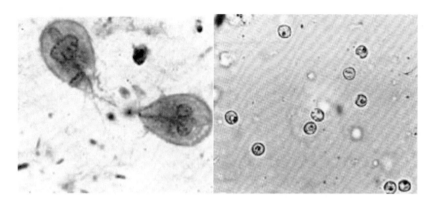

FIGURE 3.4 Examples of vegetative (left, *Giardia* trophozoite) and dormant (right, *Cryptosporidium* oocyst) forms of protozoa.

mechanisms of copper and other heavy metal tolerance in *Candida*[66] and *Aspergillus*.[67]

Different types of fungi have been used as indicator organisms for fungistatic and fungicidal activities. These include *C albicans*, *Trichophyton mentagrophytes*, *Aspergillus* species, and *Penicillium* species (see chapters 62 and 63). For example, preservative efficacy tests liquids or formulations include *C albicans* and *Aspergillus brasiliensis*, in addition to the bacteria *E coli*, *S aureus*, and *P aeruginosa* to evaluate microbicidal and microbiostatic activity over time within a prescribed set of experimental growth conditions.[68] The *T mentagrophytes* is still widely used in the United States to confirm the fungicidal activity of hard surface disinfectants,[69] whereas *A brasiliensis* and *C albicans* are used in the European Union.[70] *Aspergillus* species are often recommended because it is generally considered more resistant than other types of fungi to inactivation, but this can vary depending on the antimicrobial process. In certain applications, such as fungal contamination remediation or environmental disinfection in higher risk cleanrooms, the isolation, identification, and the use of specific fungal strains may be applicable.[71,72]

Protozoa

Protozoa are also single-celled eukaryotes and are widespread in the environment. But unlike fungi, they are not generally found in the air or as surface contaminants but are more generally waterborne, present in soil, and as parasites in humans or animals. Because many protozoa have specific mechanisms of mobility, they can be generally classified as being flagellates (ie, use flagella, such as *Giardia lamblia*), amoebas (moving by flowing cytoplasm, such as *Acanthamoeba*), ciliates (using cilia, such as *Paramecium* species), and those that have no specific mechanism (the sporozoans, such as *Cryptosporidium* and *Plasmodium* species). Although many types of protozoans are rarely implicated in diseases, there are some serious

life-threatening pathogens within this group. Examples include common causes of dysentery (*G lamblia* and *Cryptosporidium parvum*), eye infections (*Acanthamoeba castellanii*), and malaria (*Plasmodium* species).

Protozoa are also found to be present as both vegetative and dormant forms, depending on their specific life cycles (Figure 3.4). The vegetative forms, known as sporozoites or trophozoites, are classical eukaryotic structures but do not have a cell wall and are therefore not reported to present a high-resistance challenge to inactivation. But this will depend on the strain of protozoa and associated intrinsic defense mechanisms. Pathogens such as *Plasmodium* and *Leishmania* can tolerate living within host cells, escaping the cell and immune defense mechanisms.[73] Some of these evasive features will also aid in their tolerance to biocidal methods. Many tolerance mechanisms are similar to those described for bacteria and fungi (see Table 3.6), such as due to stress responses (eg, repair mechanisms and enzyme production), surface modifications, and efflux. Protozoa do not form their own biofilms but are found to be associated with and feed on bacterial biofilms,[74] which can protect them from various chemical or thermal disinfection methods (as described for bacteria earlier in this chapter). These environments can present some interesting survival dynamics and interactions between bacteria and protozoa, which in addition to environmental survival can also play a role in the development of persistence factors that allow for greater survival of pathogens in humans or animals.[74] An interesting indirect mechanism of resistance to microbicides associated with protozoa is the ability of bacteria and viruses to survive (and sometime multiply) within protozoa (in particular amoeba) both in their vegetative and dormant forms.[75] These include pathogens such as *Legionella*, *Mycobacterium*, *Acinetobacter*, and *Pseudomonas* species. This can allow bacterial and viral pathogens that are normally sensitive to chemical disinfection mechanisms to circumnavigate inactivation processes. There is also some interest in the use of amoeba as a cell culture technique to be able to identify new pathogens (eg, the giant viruses in amoeba)[76] and to facilitate the growth of fastidious bacteria.[75] As described for bacteria and fungi, protozoa also form resilient, dormant forms during their life cycle. The formation of cysts or oocysts, which are different in structure, are known to be particularly resistant to chemical inactivation (but less so to thermal or other radiation methods).[1] Their structures and disinfection tolerance profile can vary depending on the protozoa type. The cysts or *Acanthamoeba* species and oocysts of *Cryptosporidium species* are the most widely studied. *Acanthamoeba* cysts are not considered particularly tolerant to heat (typically requiring at least 55°C-65°C temperature range for inactivation) but do demonstrate higher levels of tolerance to chemical disinfection such as with glutaraldehyde and chlorine.[15] Specific strains, isolated from environmental sources, demonstrate greater resistance in comparison to those from culture collections, like prokaryotes in disinfection studies. The variability in resistance is believed to be due to the overall thickness of the cyst wall, consisting of two layers of an outermost polysaccharide-protein structure (exocyst) and an inner cellulose-based structure (endocyst).[1] *Cryptosporidium* oocysts have been described as highly tolerant to chemical disinfectants, including many used for high-level disinfection[77] and water sanitization.[78] Like *Acanthamoeba* cysts, the thickness of the oocyst walls has been correlated with higher tolerance levels to disinfection. The oocyst structure is different, consisting of four layers from the innermost polysaccharide layer, a protein layer, a lipid-based structure, and an outermost sugar-based glycocalyx.[1] The inner three layers that present a mixture of hydrophobic and hydrophilic structures are believed to provide a significant penetration challenge to chemical microbicides but not to the effects of thermal inactivation.[79]

Protozoa are not widely considered or tested in routine disinfection or sterilization applications. But reports of outbreaks of protozoal infections related to water contamination, such as in drinking water with *Giardia* and *Cryptosporidium* species (eg, dysentery)[80] or in cases of keratitis in contact lenses wearers (with *A castellanii*) due to inadequate disinfection or postdisinfection rinsing with contaminated water,[15] have seen an increase in the number of studies of protozoa disinfection/sterilization.

Helminths

The helminths are multicellular, parasitic eukaryotes, generally referred to as microscopic worms (see Table 3.1). Examples include the nematodes (roundworms), cestodes (tapeworms), and trematodes (the flukes). They can often be found in animals and human as asymptomatic parasites, and their benefits to human or animal health are a matter of some debate (such as in modulating immune responses).[81] But they can also lead to serious disease including pathogens such as *Wuchereria bancrofti* and

Ascaris lumbricoides that can lead to lymph/blood vessel or intestinal blockages, respectively. They are often sourced from contaminated water, foods, or from vectors such as mosquitoes or flies. Each type of helminth has a life cycle than can include adult worms and eggs (produced sexually), the eggs being predominantly persistent in different environments over time as the dormant forms of these microorganisms. The worms themselves can be relatively tolerant to the presence of chemical microbicides due to their overall structure (consisting of an external, rigid collagen-based cuticle) but die over time once outside of their respective hosts. Their eggs (or ova), consisting of multiple layers of protein and chitin that protect the inner core structure by exclusion,[1] are hardier to environmental conditions. Like protozoal cysts, they are typically inactivated at temperatures >65°C. They are therefore considered equivalent to protozoal cysts from a microbicides tolerance perspective (see Figure 3.1). Overall, helminths have not been well studied for their sensitivity to many disinfection and sterilization methods, but more recent studies have reemphasized the importance of understanding the risks associated with many of these pathogens including *Enterobius* (pinworms)[82] and *Ascaris*[83] in public and animal health situations.

Toxins

A very brief consideration of microbial toxins is given here, and they are considered in more detail in chapter 66. Toxins are toxic molecules, often protein or lipid based, produced by microorganisms that can cause many of the disease symptoms associated with microbial infections such as fever (a rise in body temperature), nausea, cell or tissue damage, nervous system disruption, and even death. Examples of different types of bacterial and fungal toxins are given in Table 3.8.

Microbial toxins can be classified in many ways, such as the target of their biological effects (eg, enterotoxins and neurotoxins), but for this review, they are subdivided in two broad types based on their production by microorganisms, exotoxins, and endotoxins. Exotoxins are produced and actively released by microorganisms during their normal growth. They are often produced in reaction to stressed conditions (as part of stationary phase growth of a microbial population), which can lead to significant health effects. Examples include the different types of staphylococcal or streptococcal toxins that elicit sepsis, fever, and significant tissue damage.[84] Another example in gram-negative bacteria is the production of shiga toxin from *E coli* O157:H7, which can lead to abdominal pain, colitis, diarrhea, and other effects, the toxin in this case being similar to toxins in *Shigella dysenteriae*. Fungal exotoxins (mycotoxins such as aflatoxins, ochratoxins, and the trichothecenes) can also lead to both chronic and acute health effects.[85] Toxins are potent virulence factors

TABLE 3.8   Examples of microbiological toxins and their effects on health

Toxin	Microorganism(s)	Toxicity
Clostridial neurotoxins	*Clostridium botulinum, Clostridium tetani*	Paralysis (or interference in different ways with the normal activity of neurons in animals or humans) in diseases such as tetanus (muscle spasms and other effects) and food poisoning (botulism). The botulinum toxin ("botox") is used for medical purposes as low concentrations such as in cosmetic surgery.
Anthrax toxin	*Bacillus anthracis*	Anthrax, a three-component toxin that can cause edema, disruption of cell functions, and can cause death
Diphtheria toxin	*Corynebacterium diphtheriae*	Diphtheria; fever and respiratory distress and other complications that can be fatal in approximately 5%-10% of cases
Endotoxin	Gram-negative bacteria, such as *Pseudomonas* and *Escherichia coli*	Fever, inflammation, and other immune response complications
Aflatoxins	*Aspergillus* species	Potent carcinogens (cancer promoting) and other health effects including liver damage
Trichothecene mycotoxins	*Stachybotrys chartarum*	Inflammation, nausea, respiratory distress, and other health effects
Microcystins	Cyanobacteria (blue-green algae)	Neurotoxins that attack nerve tissue and can affect the nervous systems in animals, fish, and humans

in both bacteria and fungi, but because they are typically protein-based structures, they can be neutralized by many different types of physical (eg, heat) and chemical (eg, oxidizing agent, aldehydes, and alcohols) microbicides. The presence of bacterial or fungal toxins in preserved or other commercial products (eg, parenteral injections and water) can lead to life-threatening health effects.

Endotoxins are an intrinsic part of gram-negative bacteria cell structures but can be released over time, particularly following cell damage or death, and may lead to toxic effects (see Table 3.8). They are released from the cell surface within outer membrane vesicles (OMVs) into their immediate environment. The OMVs are known to be involved in a diverse range of biological functions.[86] Therefore, although the microbial cells may be damaged or inactivated by antimicrobial methods, endotoxins can be released from these cells and remain resilient in various environments (such as in water, pharmaceutical products, and on surfaces) and may lead to adverse health effects. Endotoxins, also known as lipopolysaccharide (LPS), are specifically released from outer cell wall membrane. The specific LPS structure can vary from bacterial species to species but essentially consists of polysaccharides (the O-antigen and core polysaccharides) and lipids (lipid A), with the lipid portion being associated with its toxic effects in activating the immune system. Endotoxins are also referred to as microbial pyrogens, which can cause a temperature rise (fever) when introduced into the bloodstream of animals or humans. Pyrogenic substances can

be classified as microbial or nonmicrobial based on their origin, but endotoxins are the most frequently implicated sources of pyrogenic reactions in mammals. Other effects of endotoxins will depend on the specific immune reaction, such as septic shock, inflammation, and even death under extreme situations.[87] Therefore, the presence of gram-negative bacteria and their associated endotoxins can be a risk in many applications such as in the use of implantable medical devices or parenteral drugs. Sources of gram-negative bacteria can include plants, foods, animal or human tissues, raw materials, and water used for various purposes including water for injection, product manufacturing, cleaning, rinsing, and so forth.

The presence (or potential presence) of endotoxin can be controlled by exclusion of the sources (eg, gram-negative bacteria contamination) or using specific depyrogenation processes (see chapter 66).[87,88] These include physical removal (eg, by controlled distillation or membrane filtration) or by inactivation, with the most widely cited method being dry heat (eg, at 180°C-400°C, such as 250°C for 30 min) and a typical 3 log reduction of endotoxin demonstrated.[88] Such dry heat extremes are usually required because endotoxins are resilient in the environment and are not neutralized by many other widely used chemical and physical disinfection or sterilization methods, such as steam sterilization (noting that endotoxin can be transmitted in steam if the source water used for generating steam is contaminated). But reports of inactivation have included radiation methods, heated acids or alkaline-based treatments, hydrogen peroxide gas and liquid treatments, and other oxidizing agents.[87] Depyrogenation studies are typically performed using a standardized source of endotoxin, such as control standard endotoxin (CSE) derived from *E coli*, and tested for reactivity using limulus amebocyte lysate (LAL), amoebocyte lysate from the Atlantic horseshoe crab, or a suitable surrogate.[89]

▶ CONCLUSIONS

Overall, a good understanding of microbiology and the potential resiliency of microorganisms in harsh environments is important when considering the effective use of preservation, disinfection, and sterilization modalities. The eight major types of microorganisms can present a range of tolerance or resistance profiles that should be considered when developing or choosing such applications. Bacteria, fungi, and viruses have traditionally been more extensively investigated due to their widespread association with diseases and product spoilage, and in this group alone, a wide spectrum of resistance mechanisms have been described. Bacteria and fungi are known to have natural and/or intrinsic mechanisms, such as effective barriers to penetration in bacterial endospores and spore-containing ascocarps in *Aspergillus* species. Fungal hyphal growth and the development of biofilms (see chapter 67) are other important examples that allow these microorganisms (including those that can become protected within biofilms) to escape antimicrobial effects of chemical and physical antimicrobials. Bacteria, and to a certain extent fungi, although less studied, have shown the ability to mutate or acquire genetic material in the form of plasmids or transposons that can confer greater tolerance profiles to preservatives but have also been implicated in leading to ineffective disinfection or even sterilization situations (eg, with *Mycobacterium* and *Pyronema* species). Such instances are considered rare and may be overcome by optimization of processes or liquid product formulations but are still a cause of some concern. Investigations with archaea continue to impress in our minds on how microorganisms can adapt (or it may be more correct to state had evolved) to extremes of environmental growth conditions that we would have once considered impossible and using a combination of subtle mechanisms to survive. Other specific challenges in the inactivation of prions, protozoa, and helminths pose their own unique challenges and have required the development of newer test methods to allow further investigations of the effects of disinfection and sterilization methods on these pathogens. Overall, it is impossible (and unnecessary) to test all microorganisms to confirm the efficacy of preservation, disinfection, and sterilization modalities, but it is considered acceptable to use particular marker or surrogate microorganisms to verify effectiveness claims or expectation. A variety of compendial and standardized test methods have been described

and are widely used for this purpose, although in many cases, such as in the testing criteria for antiseptic and disinfectant efficacy, there are often no internationally recognized test methods that are used to establish label claims with such products. Different test methods can be used in different regulatory jurisdictions and may not often be considered equivalent. The expectations for sterilization are often more aligned, as defined in international standards that describe the minimum antimicrobial efficacy and process validation requirements.

REFERENCES

1. McDonnell G. *Antisepsis, Disinfection, and Sterilization: Types, Action, and Resistance.* Washington, DC: ASM Press; 2007.
2. McDonnell G. Decontamination of prions. In: JT Walker, ed. *Decontamination in Hospitals and Healthcare.* Cambridge, United Kingdom: Woodhead Publishing; 2014:346-369.
3. Eterpi M, McDonnell G, Thomas V. Disinfection efficacy against parvoviruses compared with reference viruses. *J Hosp Infect.* 2009; 73(1):64-70.
4. Eterpi M, McDonnell G, Thomas V. Decontamination efficacy against *Mycoplasma. Lett Appl Microbiol.* 2011;52(2):150-155.
5. Liu S, Tang J, Tadapaneni RK, Yang R, Zhu MJ. Exponentially increased thermal resistance of *Salmonella* spp. and *Enterococcus faecium* at reduced water activity. *Appl Environ Microbiol.* 2018;84(8):e02742-17.
6. Saby S, Vidal A, Suty H. Resistance of *Legionella* to disinfection in hot water distribution systems. *Water Sci Technol.* 2005;52(8):15-28.
7. Krisko A, Radman M. Biology of extreme radiation resistance: the way of *Deinococcus radiodurans. Cold Spring Harb Perspect Biol.* 2013;5(7):a012765.
8. Lampe CM, Hansen JM, Rymer TM, Sargent H. Sterilization of products contaminated with *Pyronema domesticum. Biomed Instrum Technol.* 2009;43(6):489-497.
9. Burgess W, Margolis A, Gibbs S, Duarte RS, Jackson M. Disinfectant susceptibility profiling of glutaraldehyde-resistant nontuberculous *Mycobacteria. Infect Control Hosp Epidemiol.* 2017;38(7):784-791.
10. Svetlíková Z, Skovierová H, Niederweis M, Gaillard JL, McDonnell G, Jackson M. Role of porins in the susceptibility of *Mycobacterium smegmatis* and *Mycobacterium chelonae* to aldehyde-based disinfectants and drugs. *Antimicrob Agents Chemother.* 2009;53(9):4015-4018.
11. Poole K. Efflux-mediated multiresistance in gram-negative bacteria. *Clin Microbiol Infect.* 2004;10(1):12-26.
12. Jang S. Multidrug efflux pumps in *Staphylococcus aureus* and their clinical implications. *J Microbiol.* 2016;54(1):1-8.
13. Saleh S, Haddadin RN, Baillie S, Collier PJ. Triclosan—an update. *Lett Appl Microbiol.* 2011;52(2):87-95.
14. Barbee SL, Weber DJ, Sobsey MD, Rutala WA. Inactivation of *Cryptosporidium parvum* oocyst infectivity by disinfection and sterilization processes. *Gastrointest Endosc.* 1999;49(5):605-611.
15. Coulon C, Collignon A, McDonnell G, Thomas V. Resistance of *Acanthamoeba* cysts to disinfection treatments used in health care settings. *J Clin Microbiol.* 2010;48(8):2689-2697.
16. Soto C, Pritzkow S. Protein misfolding, aggregation, and conformational strains in neurodegenerative diseases. *Nat Neurosci.* 2018;21(10):1332-1340.
17. Wulf MA, Senatore A, Aguzzi A. The biological function of the cellular prion protein: an update. *BMC Biol.* 2017;15(1):34.
18. Deleault NR, Walsh DJ, Piro JR, et al. Cofactor molecules maintain infectious conformation and restrict strain properties in purified prions. *Proc Natl Acad Sci U S A.* 2012;109(28):E1938-E1946.
19. Wang F, Wang X, Orrú C, et al. Self-propagating, protease-resistant, recombinant prion protein conformers with or without in vivo pathogenicity. *PLoS Pathog.* 2017;13(7):e1006491.

20. Scheckel C, Aguzzi A. Prions, prionoids and protein misfolding disorders. *Nat Rev Genet.* 2018;19(7):405-418.

21. Sanchez-Juan P, Cousens SN, Will RG, van Duijn CM. Source of variant Creutzfeldt-Jakob disease outside United Kingdom. *Emerg Infect Dis.* 2007;13(8):1166-1169.

22. Fichet G, Comoy E, Duval C, et al. Novel methods for disinfection of prion-contaminated medical devices. *Lancet.* 2004;364(9433): 521-526.

23. Brown P, Rau EH, Johnson BK, Bacote AE, Gibbs CJ Jr, Gajdusek DC. New studies on the heat resistance of hamster-adapted scrapie agent: threshold survival after ashing at 600 degrees C suggests an inorganic template of replication. *Proc Natl Acad Sci U S A.* 2000;97(7): 3418-3421.

24. Morens DM, Taubenberger JK, Harvey HA, Memoli MJ. The 1918 influenza pandemic: lessons for 2009 and the future. *Crit Care Med.* 2010;38(4 Suppl):e10-e20.

25. Thraenhart O. Measures for disinfection and control of viral hepatitis. In: SS Block, ed. *Disinfection, Sterilization, and Preservation.* Philadelphia, PA: Lea & Febiger; 1991.

26. Rubin J. Human immunodeficiency virus (HIV) disinfection and control. In: SS Block, ed. *Disinfection, Sterilization, and Preservation.* Philadelphia, PA: Lea & Febiger; 1991.

27. Howard CR, Fletcher NF. Emerging virus diseases: can we ever expect the unexpected? *Emerg Microbes Infect.* 2012;1(12):e46.

28. Bester JC. Measles and measles vaccination: a review. *JAMA Pediatr.* 2016;170(12):1209-1215.

29. Lanini S, Portella G, Vairo F, et al. Blood kinetics of Ebola virus in survivors and nonsurvivors. *J Clin Invest.* 2015;125(12):4692-4698.

30. Chaufour X, Deva AK, Vickery K, et al. Evaluation of disinfection and sterilization of reusable angioscopes with the duck hepatitis B model. *J Vasc Surg.* 1999;30(2):277-282.

31. Labadie T, Batéjat C, Manuguerra JC, Leclercq I. Influenza virus segment composition influences viral stability in the environment. *Front Microbiol.* 2018;9:1496.

32. Irwin CK, Yoon KJ, Wang C, et al. Using the systematic review methodology to evaluate factors that influence the persistence of influenza virus in environmental matrices. *Appl Environ Microbiol.* 2011;77(3):1049-1060.

33. Klein M, DeForest A. Principles of viral inactivation. In: Block SS, ed. *Disinfection, Sterilization, and Preservation.* 3rd ed. Philadelphia, PA: Lea & Febiger; 1983:422-434.

34. Sauerbrei A. Is hepatitis B-virucidal validation of biocides possible with the use of surrogates? *World J Gastroenterol.* 2014;20(2):436-444.

35. Brié A, Razafimahefa R, Loutreul J, et al. The effect of heat and free chlorine treatments on the surface properties of murine norovirus. *Food Environ Virol.* 2017;9(2):149-158.

36. EN 13610:2002. *Chemical Disinfectants. Quantitative Suspension Test for the Evaluation of Virucidal Activity Against Bacteriophages of Chemical Disinfectants Used in Food and Industrial Areas. Test Method and Requirements (Phase 2, Step 1).* Brussels, Belgium: European Committee for Standardization; 2002.

37. Gallandat K, Lantagne D. Selection of a biosafety level 1 (BSL-1) surrogate to evaluate surface disinfection efficacy in Ebola outbreaks: comparison of four bacteriophages. *PLoS One.* 2017;12(5):e0177943.

38. Rabenau HF, Steinmann J, Rapp I, Schwebke I, Eggers M. Evaluation of a virucidal quantitative carrier test for surface disinfectants. *PLoS One.* 2014;9(1):e86128.

39. McDonnell G, Burke P. Disinfection: is it time to reconsider Spaulding? *J Hosp Infect.* 2011;78(3):163-170.

40. Cairns HJ. Multiplicity reactivation of influenza virus. *J Immunol.* 1955;75(4):326-329.

41. Sender R, Fuchs S, Milo R. Revised estimates for the number of human and bacteria cells in the body. *PLoS Biol.* 2016;14(18):e1002533.

42. Centers for Disease Control and Prevention. Control of infectious diseases. *MMWR Morb Mortal Wkly Rep.* 1999;48(29):621-629.

43. Pendleton JN, Gorman SP, Gilmore BF. Clinical relevance of the ESKAPE pathogens. *Expert Rev Anti Infect Ther.* 2013;11(3):297-308.

44. Stewart SE, Parker MD, Amézquita A, Pitt TL. Microbiological risk assessment for personal care products. *Int J Cosmet Sci.* 2016;38(6): 634-645.

45. Sawant A, Cundell AM, Ahearn DG, et al. *Technical Report No. 67: Exclusion of Objectionable Microorganisms from Nonsterile Pharmaceuticals, Medical Devices, and Cosmetics.* Bethesda, MD: Parenteral Drug Association; 2014.

46. AOAC International. Method 966.04 sporicidal activity of disinfectants test—method II. In: *Official Methods of Analysis.* Gaithersburg, MD: AOAC International; 2006.

47. EN 13704:2018. *Quantitative Suspension Test For the Evaluation of Sporicidal Activity of Chemical Disinfectants Used in Food, Industrial, Domestic and Institutional Areas (Phase 2, Step 1).*

48. Duarte RS, Lourenço MC, Fonseca Lde S, et al. Epidemic of postsurgical infections caused by *Mycobacterium massiliense. J Clin Microbiol.* 2009;47(7):2149-2155.

49. Wassenaar TM, Ussery D, Nielsen LN, Ingmer H. Review and phylogenetic analysis of *qac* genes that reduce susceptibility to quaternary ammonium compounds in *Staphylococcus species. Eur J Microbiol Immunol (Bp).* 2015;5(1):44-61.

50. McDonnell G, Russell AD. Antiseptics and disinfectants: activity, action, and resistance. *Clin Microbiol Rev.* 1999;12(1):147-179.

51. Weatherly LM, Gosse JA. Triclosan exposure, transformation, and human health effects. *J Toxicol Environ Health B Crit Rev.* 2017;20(8):447-469.

52. Williams KL. *Endotoxins: pyrogens, LAL testing and depyrogenation.* 3rd ed. New York, NY: Informa Healthcare; 2007.

53. Adam PS, Borrel G, Brochier-Armanet C, Gribaldo S. The growing tree of archaea: new perspectives on their diversity, evolution and ecology. *ISME J.* 2017;11(11):2407-2425.

54. Aminov RI. Role of archaea in human disease. *Front Cell Infect Microbiol.* 2013;3:42.

55. Varnava KG, Ronimus RS, Sarojini V. A review on comparative mechanistic studies of antimicrobial peptides against archaea. *Biotechnol Bioeng.* 2017;114(11):2457-2473.

56. Jolivet E, Matsunaga F, Ishino Y, Forterre P, Prieur D, Myllykallio H. Physiological responses of the hyperthermophilic archaeon "*Pyrococcus abyssi*" to DNA damage caused by ionizing radiation. *J Bacteriol.* 2003;185(13):3958-3961.

57. Ranawat P, Rawat S. Radiation resistance in thermophiles: mechanisms and applications. *World J Microbiol Biotechnol.* 2017;33(6):112.

58. Colombo AL, Júnior JNA, Guinea J. Emerging multidrug-resistant *Candida* species. *Curr Opin Infect Dis.* 2017;30(6):528-538.

59. Guarro J, Gené J, Stchigel AM. Developments in fungal taxonomy. *Clin Microbiol Rev.* 1999;12(3):454-500.

60. Wyatt TT, Wösten HA, Dijksterhuis J. Fungal spores for dispersion in space and time. *Adv Appl Microbiol.* 2013;85:43-91.

61. Reeves F Jr. The fine structure of ascospore formation in *Pyronema domesticum. Mycologia.* 1967;59(6):1018-1033.

62. Dijksterhuis J, Meijer M, van Doorn T, Samson R, Rico-Munoz E. Inactivation of stress-resistant ascospores of *Eurotiales* by industrial sanitizers. *Int J Food Microbiol.* 2018;285:27-33.

63. Abreu-Cavalheiro A, Monteiro G. Solving ethanol production problems with genetically modified yeast strains. *Braz J Microbiol.* 2014;44(3):665-671.

64. Wehner EP, Rao E, Brendel M. Molecular structure and genetic regulation of SFA, a gene responsible for resistance to formaldehyde in *Saccharomyces cerevisiae*, and characterization of its protein product. *Mol Gen Genet.* 1993;237(3):351-358.

65. Chang AL, Doering TL. Maintenance of mitochondrial morphology in *Cryptococcus neoformans* is critical for stress resistance and virulence. *MBio.* 2018;9(6):e01375-18.

66. Ilyas S, Rehman A. Oxidative stress, glutathione level and antioxidant response to heavy metals in multi-resistant pathogen, *Candida tropicalis. Environ Monit Assess.* 2015;187(1):4115.

67. Antsotegi-Uskola M, Markina-Iñarrairaegui A, Ugalde U. Copper resistance in *Aspergillus nidulans* relies on the PI-type ATPase

CrpA, regulated by the transcription factor AceA. *Front Microbiol.* 2017;8:912.

68. United States Pharmacopeia. <51> Antimicrobial effectiveness testing. In: *United States Pharmacopeial Convention.* Rockville, MD: United States Pharmacopeia; 2011:52-54.

69. AOAC 955.17. *Fungicidal Activity of Disinfectants.* Rockville, MD. AOAC: 2006.

70. EN 1650: 2008. *Fungicidal Suspension Test for Disinfectants.*

71. ASTM D4445-10. *Standard Test Method for Fungicides for Controlling Sapstain and Mold on Unseasoned Lumber (Laboratory Method).*

72. ASTM E2614-15. *Standard Guide for Evaluation of Cleanroom Disinfectants.*

73. Zambrano-Villa S, Rosales-Borjas D, Carrero JC, Ortiz-Ortiz L. How protozoan parasites evade the immune response. *Trends Parasitol.* 2002;18(6):272-278.

74. Sun S, Noorian P, McDougald D. Dual role of mechanisms involved in resistance to predation by protozoa and virulence to humans. *Front Microbiol.* 2018;9:1017.

75. Thomas V, McDonnell G, Denyer SP, Maillard JY. Free-living amoebae and their intracellular pathogenic microorganisms: risks for water quality. *FEMS Microbiol Rev.* 2010;34(3):231-259.

76. Colson P, La Scola B, Raoult D. Giant viruses of amoebae: a journey through innovative research and paradigm changes. *Annu Rev Virol.* 2017;4(1):61-85.

77. Weir SC, Pokorny NJ, Carreno RA, Trevors JT, Lee H. Efficacy of common laboratory disinfectants on the infectivity of *Cryptosporidium parvum* oocysts in cell culture. *Appl Environ Microbiol.* 2002;68(5):2576-2579.

78. Pereira JT, Costa AO, de Oliveira Silva MB, et al. Comparing the efficacy of chlorine, chlorine dioxide, and ozone in the inactivation of *Cryptosporidium parvum* in water from Parana State, Southern Brazil. *Appl Biochem Biotechnol.* 2008;151(2-3):464-473.

79. Jenkins MB, Eaglesham BS, Anthony LC, Kachlany SC, Bowman DD, Ghiorse WC. Significance of wall structure, macromolecular composition, and surface polymers to the survival and transport of *Cryptosporidium parvum* oocysts. *Appl Environ Microbiol.* 2010;76(6):1926-1934.

80. Betancourt WQ, Rose JB. Drinking water treatment processes for removal of *Cryptosporidium* and *Giardia*. *Vet Parasitol.* 2004;126(1-2): 219-234.

81. Helmby H. Human helminth therapy to treat inflammatory disorders—where do we stand? *BMC Immunol.* 2015;16:12.

82. Rudko SP, Ruecker NJ, Ashbolt NJ, Neumann NF, Hanington PC. *Enterobius vermicularis* as a novel surrogate for the presence of helminth ova in tertiary wastewater treatment plants. *Appl Environ Microbiol.* 2017;83(11):e00547-17.

83. Strunz EC, Addiss DG, Stocks ME, Ogden S, Utzinger J, Freeman MC. Water, sanitation, hygiene, and soil-transmitted helminth infection: a systematic review and meta-analysis. *PLoS Med.* 2014;11(3):e1001620.

84. Ramachandran G. Gram-positive and gram-negative bacterial toxins in sepsis: a brief review. *Virulence.* 2014;5(1):213-218.

85. Pitt JI, Miller JD. A concise history of mycotoxin research. *J Agric Food Chem.* 2017;65(33):7021-7033.

86. Jan AT. Outer membrane vesicles (OMVs) of gram-negative bacteria: a perspective update. *Front Microbiol.* 2017;8:1053.

87. Magalhães PO, Lopes AM, Mazzola PG, Rangel-Yagui C, Penna TC, Pessoa A Jr. Methods of endotoxin removal from biological preparations: a review. *J Pharm Pharm Sci.* 2007;10(3):388-404.

88. US Department of Health and Human Services Food and Drug Administration. *Guidance for Industry Pyrogen and Endotoxins Testing: Questions and Answers.* Bethesda, MD: US Department of Health and Human Services Food and Drug Administration; 2012.

89. United States Pharmacopeia. <85> Bacterial endotoxins test. In: *United States Pharmacopeial Convention.* Rockville, MD: United States Pharmacopeia; 2011:1-5.

Bacterial Resistance to Biocides

Jean-Yves Maillard

Chemical biocides are heavily used as preservatives, disinfectants, or antiseptics[1] in an increasing number of industrial, health care, and domiciliary applications.[2] Biocides have a long usage history for preventing or controlling infection or controlling spoilage of water and foodstuff. Today, it is impossible to put a number to the quantities of chemical biocides that are being used on daily basis worldwide. It is, however, clear that their usage has dramatically increased during the last 15 years mainly for health care applications and in consumer products. Such increase in usage is causing concerns with issues such as environmental toxicity and emerging resistance in bacteria.[2] The number of active substances (ie, biocides) that can be used for different applications in Europe has been dramatically reduced.[3,4] The list of authorized biocides on the European market is currently being reviewed and amended, forcing manufacturers to change the composition of established formulations.[3,4] The revised European Biocidal Product Regulation[4] mentioned the need to demonstrate that a product will not induce bacterial resistance. The US Food and Drug Administration[5] recently enforced a rule that restricts the use of certain biocides, such as triclosan and triclocarban that have been linked to antimicrobial resistance (AMR) in bacteria, in antimicrobial soaps and similar products.

It is appropriate to question whether the widespread use of biocidal products today is justified. The increase usage of biocides not only in consumer products but also in health care may be due, at least in part, not only to a better education and awareness of consumers about microbial infections and contamination[6] but also to market pressures and opportunities. Important media coverage of poor hygiene and cleanliness in health care facilities also contributed to the demand for better, often biocide-based, solutions. A recent contributor for an increase usage of biocidal products has been the rise in AMR (specifically chemotherapeutic antibiotic) in bacteria. The AMR is a global issue with serious economical

and societal consequences.[7] Recommendations to tackle AMR include better hygiene and control of bacterial pathogens from surfaces in health care and veterinary settings.[7] Here, the conundrum is that although the use of biocidal products is important to control microbial pathogens, inappropriate applications might lead to an exacerbation of AMR.

One difficult issue about AMR is the definition of what resistance means particularly when biocides are concerned. The definition is usually linked to protocols that measure a change in susceptibility profile.[8-13] It is unfortunate that in many publications, the term *resistance* is only linked to an increase in the biocide minimum inhibitory concentration (MIC); MICs are often lower than the in-use concentration of a biocide or product, and the in-use concentration may still be effective.[8,14] Where MIC and minimum bactericidal concentration (MBC) may become more relevant is when the *during-use* concentration is considered. The during-use concentration is the lowest concentration of a biocide or product attained following product application; it encompasses, for example, residual concentration and dilution during use.[8,15,16] The use of the term *reduced susceptibility* when MIC or MBC are measured is more appropriate and is often expressed as a fold reduction in MIC or MBC. The practical significance of a *reduced susceptibility* remains, however, to be defined. Generally, the scientific community and regulators have no consensus on the definition of resistance,[2,8] owing the diversity of terms used, including *resistance*, *tolerance*, *decreased susceptibility*, *reduced susceptibility*, *insusceptibility*, and *acquired reduced susceptibility*. Today, with the diversity of products containing biocide(s) at various concentrations, a bacterium surviving in a product should be defined as resistant whatever the concentration of biocide is in that product.

This book chapter is exploring not only the evidence of bacterial resistance to biocides and products and the mechanisms of bacterial resistance but also the interaction between biocides and bacteria that would lead to the expression of *global* resistance mechanisms, putting in perspective the during-use concentration of a product and its effect.

▶ EVIDENCE OF BACTERIAL SURVIVAL IN BIOCIDAL PRODUCTS AND BIOCIDES

There are plenty of examples in the literature of bacteria-contaminating products containing a biocide that lead to an outbreak or pseudo-outbreak (Table 4.1). Bacteria-contaminating biocidal products have been described as early as 1958, with some references mentioning incident dating from the 1940s, and product contamination are still being reported today (see Table 4.1). Bacterial resistance to biocides is therefore not a new phenomenon.[2,8,9] Bacterial survival in a biocidal product can be driven by

1. Primarily a low concentration attained during product preparation and use (including phase separation for emulsion where the antimicrobial is retained in the oil phase)
2. The use of contaminated diluent during product preparation
3. Improper storage of biocidal products
4. The use of contaminated dispensers holding biocidal products
5. The use of contaminated disinfectant cloth to disinfect a sterile product

The nature of the biocides plays a role, and most examples provided in Table 4.1 concerned cationic biocides, mainly chlorhexidine and benzalkonium chloride solutions. If the nature of the biocide plays a role and less reactive membrane active agents may be a concern, bacterial resistance to highly reacting alkylating and oxidizing agents can also occur.[2,6] For example, failure of high-level disinfection during endoscope reprocessing has led to the isolation of resistant bacteria,[78-83] some of which have been suspected to be associated with outbreaks and pseudo-outbreaks.[67,84-86] The nature of the bacterial contaminant is also important to consider. Bacterial contaminants of biocidal products are predominantly gram-negative bacteria, particularly pseudomonads or *Burkholderia* species (see Table 4.1), reflecting the versatility of these bacterial genera.[87] For povidone-iodine, bacterial contaminants such as *Burkholderia cepacia* and pseudomonads are often considered intrinsically resistant to certain concentrations.[71-74,76] Likewise, contaminations of alcohol solutions with bacterial endospores of *Bacillus cereus*[18,19] reflect the innate resistance nature of the spores.

Biocides are overall very diverse[2] and often used in combination in biocidal products. Component of formulations that provide other functions, such as chelation and wettability, and pH may contribute to the overall antimicrobial activity of the product. Yet the efficacy of the full formulations is rarely investigated.[6,8,88,89] The use of biocidal products in the community or in health care settings on emerging bacterial resistance has not been widely studied, but the few published studies provide some interesting information. One of the main issues of such studies is the definition of bacterial resistance and by what measures it is defined. Thus, the comparison of the outcomes of these studies is difficult.[2] Investigations from Cole et al[90] failed to show any cross-resistance between the use of biocides and resistance to chemotherapeutic antibiotics. Likewise, two in situ studies did not observe any cross-resistance between triclosan or triclocarban used in over-the-counter antibacterial liquid hand and body cleansers and antibacterial bar soaps,[91] or triclosan used in consumer products,[92] and antibiotics. However, Carson et al[93] identified a correlation between elevated MIC to quaternary ammonium compounds (QACs) used in home consumer products and bacterial resistance to antibiotics.

The bulk of information regarding bacterial resistance to biocides remains from studies in vitro, which often lack consistency in their approach.[2,8] Overall, in vitro investigations looking at a change in bacterial susceptibility when exposed to a biocide can be divided into three categories:

1. Bacterial exposure to increasing concentration of a biocide in defined conditions of time, growth media, and temperature. Such protocols, often referred to as stepwise training of bacteria to biocide exposure, do not necessarily reflect conditions of exposure found in practice.[94-105]
2. The use of environmental isolates from health care, biocide manufacturing sites, slaughterhouses, etc, where biocidal products are commonly used. Bacterial isolates often show a reduced biocide susceptibility profile or resistance to specific biocides.[78,80,84,96,106-116]
3. Studies investigating biocidal product contamination that lead to an infectious outbreaks or pseudo-outbreaks (see Table 4.1)

The use of in vitro studies to understand bacterial behavior and survival when exposed to a specific biocide may suffer from unrealistic exposure such as excessive low concentrations of a biocide, unrealistic exposure to increasing concentrations, long contact time, absence of organic load, etc.[6,98] Biocides, however, are extensively used in a wide range of products for very diverse applications where inappropriate dilution (see Table 4.1) or exposure to a low concentration during use may occur.[2] Furthermore, some of these in vitro studies, such as stepwise training, contributed to a better knowledge of bacterial adaptation, albeit slow, to biocides, mainly through the expression of specific mechanisms such as changes in membrane permeability or increasing efflux capability.[94-100,117]

TABLE 4.1   Outbreaks and pseudo-outbreaks due to contaminated biocidal product[a]

Biocide	Contaminant(s)	Site(s) of Microbes	Mechanism of Contamination/Source	Year (Reference)
Alcohols				
Alcohols	Bacillus cereus	Automated radiometric blood culture system	Intrinsic contamination (spores)	1983 (Berger[17])
	B cereus	Blood (pseudobacteremia), pleural fluid	Intrinsic contamination (spores)	1999 (Hsueh et al[18])
	Burkholderia cepacia	Blood (catheter related)	Contaminated tap water used to dilute alcohol for skin antisepsis	2004 (Nasser et al[19])
Cationic biocides				
Chlorhexidine	Pseudomonas species	Not stated	Refilling contaminated bottles, washing used bottles using cold tap water, contaminated washing apparatus; low concentration (0.05%)	1967 (Burdon and Whitby[20])
	B cepacia	Blood, urinary, wounds	Not determined	1971 (Speller et al[21])
	Flavobacterium meningosepticum	Blood, CSF, wounds, skin	Not determined but possibly due to contaminated water and/or topping off of stock solution or low concentration (1:1000-1:5000)	1976 (Coyle-Gilchrist et al[22])
Chlorhexidine	Pseudomonas species, Serratia marcescens, Flavobacterium species	Not stated	Not determined, but authors speculate due to overdilution or refilling of contaminated bottles	1981 (Marrie and Costerton[23])
	Pseudomonas aeruginosa	Wounds	Tap water used to dilute stock solutions; low concentration (0.05%)	1982 (Anyiwo et al[24])
	B cepacia	Blood, wounds, urine, mouth, vagina	Metal pipe and rubber tubing in pharmacy through which deionized water passed during dilution of chlorhexidine; low concentration	1982 (Sobel et al[25])
	Ralstonia pickettii	Blood	Contaminated bidistilled water used to dilute chlorhexidine; low concentration (0.05%)	1983 (Kahan et al[26])
	R pickettii	Blood (pseudobacteremia)	Distilled water used to dilute chlorhexidine; low concentration (0.05%)	1985 (Verschraegen et al[27])
	R pickettii	Blood	Contaminated deionized water; low concentration (0.05%)	1987 (Poty et al[28])
	Achromobacter xylosoxidans	Blood, wounds	Atomizer (low concentration, 600 mg/L)	1998 (Vu-Thien et al[29])
	S marcescens	Blood, urine, wounds, sputum, others	Not determined, but use of nonsterile water for dilution to 2% and distribution in reusable nonsterile containers	1998 (Vigeant et al[30])
	R pickettii	Blood (pseudobacteremia)	Distilled water used to dilute chlorhexidine; low concentration (0.05%)	2000 (Maroye et al[31])

TABLE 4.1 Outbreaks and pseudo-outbreaks due to contaminated biocidal product[a] *(Continued)*

Biocide	Contaminant(s)	Site(s) of Microbes	Mechanism of Contamination/Source	Year (Reference)
Chlorhexidine	A xylosoxidans	Blood	Atomizer contamination	2005 (Tena et al[32])
	Burkholderia cenocepacia	Various patient specimen, blood, sputum, drainage, catheter	Chlorhexidine solution diluted with contaminated water	2013 (Lee et al[33])
	B cepacia	Blood	Intrinsic contamination, contaminated 0.5% chlorhexidine	2015 (Ko et al[34])
	S marcescens	Blood	Intrinsic contamination, 2% aqueous chlorhexidine antiseptic	2017 (de Frutos et al[35])
Chlorhexidine plus cetrimide	Pseudomonas multivorans	Wounds	Tap water used to prepare stock solutions; low concentrations (0.05% chlorhexidine and 0.5% cetrimide)	1970 (Bassett et al[36])
	Stenotrophomonas maltophilia	Urine, umbilical swabs, catheter tips, others	Deionized water used to prepare solutions; failure to disinfect contaminated bottles between use	1976 (Wishart and Riley[37])
Hexidine	S marcescens	Blood	Application of a contaminated solution to disinfect tunnelled catheters	2016 (Merino et al[38])
Benzalkonium chloride	Pseudomonas species	Blood	Storage of benzalkonium chloride (0.1%) with cotton/gauze	1958 (Plotkin and Austrian[39])
	P aeruginosa	Blood	Diluted solution of benzalkonium chloride	1959 (Shickman et al[40])
Benzalkonium chloride	Enterobacter aerogenes	Blood, sinus tract	Storage of benzalkonium chloride (0.13%) with cotton/gauze	1960 (Malizia et al[41])
	Pseudomonas-Achromobacteriaceae group	Blood, urine	Storage of benzalkonium chloride (0.1%) with cotton/gauze; dilution with nonsterile water	1961 (Lee and Fialkow[42])
	E aerogenes	Blood, sinus tract	Storage of benzalkonium chloride (0.1%) with cotton/gauze; dilution with nonsterile water	1961 (Lee and Fialkow[42])
	Pseudomonas kingii	Urine	Contamination (intrinsic) of antiseptic	1969 (Centers for Disease Control and Prevention[43])
	Pseudomonas EO-1	Urine	Contaminated (intrinsic) cleansing-germicide solution	1970 (Hardy et al[44])
	B cepacia, Enterobacter species	Blood (pseudobacteremia)	Storage of benzalkonium chloride with cotton/gauze, improper dilution, storage bottles infrequently sterilized	1976 (Kaslow et al[45])
	B cepacia	Bacteremia	Storage of benzalkonium chloride with rayon balls; failure to disinfect squeeze bottles	1976 (Frank and Schaffner[46])
	S marcescens	Intravenous catheters (dogs and cats), other sites	Storage of benzalkonium chloride (0.025%) with cotton/gauze	1981 (Fox et al[47])
	S marcescens	CSF	Contamination (extrinsic) of stock bottle	1984 (Sautter et al[48])

(continued)

TABLE 4.1   Outbreaks and pseudo-outbreaks due to contaminated biocidal product[a] *(Continued)*

Biocide	Contaminant(s)	Site(s) of Microbes	Mechanism of Contamination/Source	Year (Reference)
Benzalkonium chloride	*S marcescens*	Joint	Storage of benzalkonium chloride with cotton/gauze	1987 (Nakashima et al[49])
	S marcescens	Not specified	Multiple-dose medication vials contaminated with benzalkonium chloride–soaked cotton ball during disinfection	1987 (Nakashima et al[50])
	Mycobacterium chelonae	Skin abscesses	Storage of benzalkonium chloride with cotton/gauze; improper dilution	1990 (Georgia Division of Public Health[51])
	P aeruginosa	Corticosteroid injection multidose vial	Inoculation with pseudomonads via needle puncture after vial septa were wiped with contaminated disinfectant	1999 (Olson et al[52])
	Mycobacterium abscessus	Joint	Storage of benzalkonium chloride with cotton/gauze; dilution with probable contaminated tap water	2003 (Tiwari et al[53])
	B cepacia	Blood, catheter	1:1000 aqueous benzalkonium chloride solution	2008 (Lee et al[54])
Benzalkonium chloride/ picloxydine	*B cepacia*	Blood, urine, wound, sputum	Water used to dilute the antiseptic	1976 (Guinness and Levey[55])
	B cepacia	Blood	Water used to dilute the antiseptic	1976 (Morris et al[56])
Benzethonium chloride	*Pseudomonas* species	Blood (pseudobacteremia)	Contaminated (intrinsic solution; 0.2%)	1976 (Dixon et al[57])
Didecyldimethylammonium chloride	*Pseudomonas fluorescens*, *A xylosoxidans*	Blood	Contaminated dispenser—product used to decontaminate blood culture bottles	2007 (Siebor et al[58])
Didecyl diammonium chloride	*Achromobacter* species	Not specified	Hospital filtered tap water contaminating disinfectant atomizers and patients' rooms	2015 (Hugon et al[59])
QAC (not defined)	*S marcescens*	Not specified	Failure of hospital personnel to clean the disinfectant spray bottles before refilling	1980 (Ehrenkranz et al[60])
QAC (not defined)	*A xylosoxidans*	Blood, CSF, respiratory therapy devices	Detergent-disinfectant solution as the source of contamination	2002 (Lehours et al[61])
QAC (not defined)	*B cepacia*	Blood	Use of a contaminated disinfectant during quality controls in a university blood bank—QAC had been used in order to disinfect the rubber stopper of the blood culture bottle	2005 (Ebner et al[62])
Alkyldiaminoethylglycine hydrochloride solution	*B cepacia*, *P fluorescens*, *Alcaligenes xylosoxidans*, *P aeruginosa*, *Pseudomonas putida*	Not specified	Unwoven rayon cloths	2012 (Oie et al[63])
Glucoprotamin (surfactant)	*A xylosoxidans*	Blood	Suspected antiseptic reusable tissue dispensers	2016 (Günther et al[64])

TABLE 4.1	Outbreaks and pseudo-outbreaks due to contaminated biocidal product[a] *(Continued)*			
Biocide	**Contaminant(s)**	**Site(s) of Microbes**	**Mechanism of Contamination/Source**	**Year (Reference)**
Alkylating biocides				
Formaldehyde	*P aeruginosa*	Blood	Reused formaldehyde solution (low concentration present 0.0014% and 0.005%)	1992 (Vanholder et al[65])
Formaldehyde (with glyoxal and glutaral)	*Klebsiella oxytoca*	Blood	Intrinsic contamination to 0.25% formaldehyde	2000 (Reiss et al[66])
Glutaraldehyde	*M chelonae*	Automated endoscope washer disinfector	Biofilm formation	2001 (Kressel and Kidd[67])
	Methylobacterium mesophilicum	Automated endoscope washer disinfector	Biofilm formation	2001 (Kressel and Kidd[67])
Phenolics				
Chloroxylenol	*S marcescens*	Multiple sites	Contaminated (extrinsic) 1% chloroxylenol soap; sink	1997 (Archibald et al[68])
Triclosan	*S marcescens*	Conjunctiva	Intrinsic contamination	1995 (McNaughton et al[69])
Iodine				
Povidone-iodine	*B cepacia*	Blood (pseudobacteremia)	Intrinsic contamination 10% povidone-iodine (probable *B cepacia* proliferating on the deionizing resin in the water system)	1981 (Berkelman et al[70])
	B cepacia	Blood (pseudobacteremia)	Intrinsic contamination	1981 (Craven et al[71])
	B cepacia	Blood (pseudobacteremia), peritoneal fluid	Intrinsic contamination	1989 (Centers for Disease Control and Prevention[72])
	B cepacia	Blood (pseudobacteremia), peritoneal fluid	Intrinsic contamination	1991 (Jarvis[73])
	B cepacia	Blood (pseudobacteremia), peritoneal fluid	Intrinsic contamination	1992 (Panlilio et al[74])
	P putida	Blood, catheter tips	Not determined	2004 (Bouallègue et al[75])
Poloxamer-iodine	*P aeruginosa*	Peritoneal fluid, wound	Intrinsic contamination	1982 (Parrott et al[76])

Abbreviations: CSF, cerebrospinal fluid; QAC, quaternary ammonium compound.

[a]From Weber et al.[77] Reproduced with permission from American Society for Microbiology.

The choice of the bacterial isolate to study is important. A recent study, looking at hundreds of isolates of *Staphylococcus aureus*, reported clear differences in the genetic mutations occurring between isolates exposed to triclosan.[118] The investigation of environmental isolates is probably more realistic than the use of adapted standard culture collection strains to understand the ability of bacteria to adapt. Studies of environmental bacterial isolates that have been regularly exposed to biocides do not always show a decreased biocide susceptibility when compared to standard collection strains.[114,115,118,119]

There is a clear body of evidence that bacteria have a phenomenal ability to survive biocide exposure. Bacterial survival in biocidal products, at time at the in-use concentration, has been well reported (see Table 4.1). The artificial development of bacterial resistance, however, can be difficult to achieve using realistic in vitro protocols, reflecting, for example, high biocide concentrations or short contact time.[6,98] Nevertheless, it is now clear that bacteria can use an accumulation of mechanisms, ensuring their survival in biocides and certain biocidal products.

▶ MECHANISMS OF BACTERIAL RESISTANCE TO ANTIMICROBIAL BIOCIDES

Bacteria have a number of mechanisms that can be expressed to respond to an external stress and enable their survival. Overall, these mechanisms aim to reduce the damaging concentration of a stressor, such as a biocide, and allow repair to the bacterial cell. A short exposure to a biocide can lead to damages that are reversible (ie, damages can be effectively repaired), whereas a longer exposure often produces irreversible damages that will lead to cell death (Figure 4.1). Maintenance of the internal cytoplasmic pH appears to be key in the bacterial ability to survive.[120,121] Although this is quite a simplistic notion, reversible/irreversible damages will depend on the nature of the biocide, concentrations used, and time of exposure. Hence, highly reactive biocides such as alkylating and oxidizing agents are often considered to be more efficient

in killing bacteria when compared to cationic biocides.[8] With this in mind, examples of bacterial survival in a biocidal product often (but not exclusively) concern less reactive biocide chemistries such as cationics and phenolics, but resistance to alkylating agents such as glutaraldehyde have been reported (see Table 4.1).

Considering the importance of biocide concentration and exposure in the survival of bacteria, factors that negatively affect biocide/bacteria interactions need to be considered.[1,8] These factors can be divided into

1. Factors inherent to the biocide including concentration, formulation, mechanism(s) of action
2. Factors inherent to the bacteria including the type (ie, mycobacteria, gram-negative or gram-positive bacteria, bacterial endospores), metabolism (including presence of a biofilm), specific resistance mechanism (eg, overexpression of efflux pumps)
3. Factors inherent to product usage (ie, the during-use parameters), decreased concentration (ie, following dilution of stock solution or abundant rinsing with water, residual concentration), type and amount of organic load (soiling), effective exposure time, material/surface that is disinfected

The most important parameters to consider are those affecting products during use. These have been rarely considered during in vitro testing,[15,16] but these will clearly affect bacteria survival during disinfection/antisepsis and

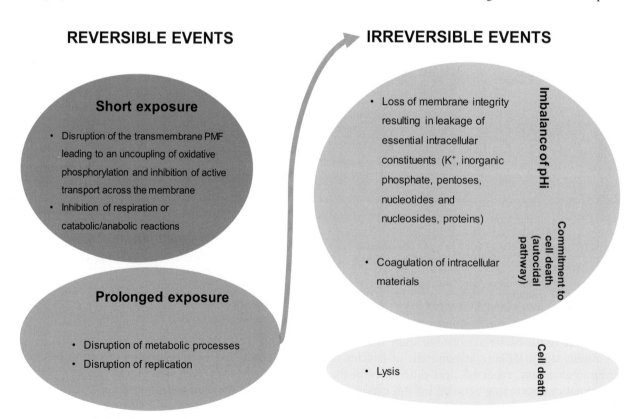

FIGURE 4.1 Levels of biocide interactions with a bacterial cell. Abbreviation: PMF, proton motive force.

account for bacterial survival in products (see Table 4.1). The concentration of a biocide in a product is key for its efficacy or for allowing bacterial survival.[122] Where the biocide concentration is close to the MBC, the product may allow bacterial survival and be prone to bacterial contamination.[123] During the use of a product, it is often difficult to predict what will be the target microorganisms to kill. In health care settings, outbreaks of *Clostridium difficile* will dictate the use of sporicides, which are considered the most effective disinfectant products.[124,125] However, despite claims from manufacturers, not all biocide chemistries are sporicidal and only oxidizing agents and alkylating agents have been shown to have efficacy against bacterial endospores.[124-126] Different microorganisms are recognized to have different susceptibility to biocides.[8] The main reason for being less susceptible to biocides is their intrinsic or natural properties, which are mainly structural including different cell envelope (eg, different membrane lipid composition, different outer membrane proteins [OMP]) or additional components (eg, efflux, glycocalyx). Bacterial endospores have all together a unique structure and are considered to be highly resistant to biocides (see following discussion). As such, they are often used as biological indicators for testing high-level disinfection of medical devices. Hence, a sporicidal product should be effective in killing vegetative microorganisms.[8] Apart from their intrinsic properties, a bacterium can acquire resistance to a biocide through gene transfer and mutations.[127] Whether the change in biocide susceptibility profile is transient or permanent, the mechanisms involved are often similar and initially result from the selective pressure exerted by the biocide or biocidal product in the first place.[15,128]

Mechanisms Leading to a Decrease in the Concentration of Biocides in Bacteria

Bacteria have several mechanisms at their disposal that enable to decrease a stressor (or biocide) concentration that would be detrimental to them. Bacterial *adaptation* to a stressor has been suggested from experiments in which bacterial growth curve in the presence of biocides resulted in an extended lag phase[129] before a normal exponential growth resumed. We now know that bacterial exposure to a biocide will trigger a stress response and lead to the expression of a number of mechanisms enabling survival (see following discussion). The mechanisms involved in bacterial response to a biocide exposure are principally global mechanisms such as changes in membrane composition and expression of efflux pumps, although specific mechanisms such as enzymatic expression and mutations have been reported. These mechanisms often work together to enable bacterial survival.[6,9,130-133] The use of protocols that informed on gene expressions following

a biocide exposure has shown that bacterial metabolism can be altered, leading to marked differences in decreased susceptibility to a specific biocide between susceptible and resistant isolates.[133-135]

Reducing Biocide Penetration

The impact of bacterial cell structure in decreasing the penetration of a biocide has been well described in the literature in vegetative bacteria, notably gram-negative bacteria and mycobacteria.[136,137] It is also a fundamental property of the bacterial endospore.[138] The lipopolysaccharide (LPS) layer in gram-negative bacteria has long been established as a barrier to biocide penetration, notably with cationic biocides such as biguanides and QAC. Evidence of the role of LPS comes from the use of permeabilizing agents such as ethylenediaminetetraacetic acid.[136,139,140] The role of the bacterial outer structure in reducing the effect of biocide exposure has also been demonstrated with the study of protoplasts.[141] Overall, the role of membrane-associated proteins in bacteria decreased susceptibility to a QAC and some antibiotics has been documented[142] together with the impact of reducing the expression of membrane porins.[97,130,143-146]

In mycobacteria, the mycolate layer associated with the arabinogalactan/arabinomannan cell wall and overall lipid-rich outer cell wall is responsible for preventing biocide and antibiotic penetration.[106,137,147-150] The reduced presentation of surface-associated porins has also been shown to play a role in reducing the activity of glutaraldehyde and ortho-phthalaldehyde.[151]

Changes to the bacterial cell envelope in response to biocide exposure have also been documented in a number of studies. Changes in membrane lipid composition,[130,152-157] membrane proteins,[97,130,158-161] membrane potential,[162] and membrane fluidity[104,105] have all been associated with decreased susceptibility to some biocides.

Efflux Pumps

The expression of efflux pumps allows bacteria to decrease the concentration of stressors that would eventually reach the cytoplasm. Five main efflux pumps have been described in bacteria: the drug/metabolite transporter superfamily, the major facilitator superfamily, the adenosine triphosphate (ATP)-binding cassette family, the resistance-nodulation-division (RND) family, and the multidrug and toxic compound extrusion family.[163-167] Carriage of efflux pump genes in environmental and hospital isolates has been particularly well documented in the last few years (Table 4.2). The correlation between decreased biocide susceptibility, antibiotic resistance, and efflux pump carriage in gram-positive and gram-negative bacteria food isolates has been reported in a number of studies.[172,173]

The role of efflux pumps in decreased bacterial susceptibility to QAC[166,171,174-186] and triclosan[94,133,181,187-193] has been well reported. Some publications reported that

TABLE 4.2 Examples of studies reporting carriage of efflux pump genes in environmental, food, and hospital isolates

Efflux Gene (% Carriage in Isolate)	Bacteria (Number of isolates)	Origin of Isolates	Biocides	Reference
qacA/B (83.0%) smr (77.4%) norA (49.0%) norB (28.8%)	High-level mupirocin-resistant, MRSA (53)	Health care	Chlorhexidine	Liu et al[110]
qacA/B (80%)	Staphylococcus epidermidis (25)	Health care	Chlorhexidine	Hijazi et al[111]
sepA (95.3%) mepA (89.4%) norA (86.4%) lmrS (60.8%) qacAB (40.5%) smr (3.7%)	MRSA (82) MSSA (219)	Health care	Chlorhexidine	Conceição et al[112]
acrB (96.29%) mdfA (85.18%) oxqA (37.03%) qacA/B (11.11%) qacE (7.40%)	Escherichia coli (27)	Food	Hexadecylpyridinium chloride (QAC)	Burgos et al[115]
qacA/B (83%) Smr (1.6%)	MRSA (60)	Health care	Benzalkonium chloride Benzethonium chloride Chlorhexidine	Shamsudin et al[168]
acrB (100%) AcrAB-TolC system (100%)	Gram-negative (29)	Food	Cetrimide Hexadecylpyridinium chloride Chlorhexidine Triclosan	Fuentes et al[169]
qacA (26% for HMRSA, 67% for VISA) qaC (5% for HMRSA, 4% for MSSA, 17% for VISA)	HMRSA (38) Community-acquired MRSA (25) VISA (6) MSSA (25)	Health care	QAC Chlorhexidine	Smith et al[170]
mdrL (33%) lde (42%)	Listeria monocytogenes (45)	Food	Benzalkonium chloride	Conficoni et al[171]

Abbreviations: HMRSA, hospital-acquired methicillin-resistant *Staphylococcus aureus*; MRSA, methicillin-resistant *Staphylococcus aureus*; MSSA, methicillin-sensitive *Staphylococcus aureus*; QAC, quaternary ammonium compound; VISA, vancomycin-insensitive *Staphylococcus aureus*.

the efflux pump gene expression is dependent on the concentration of the biocide.[171,182,183]

Efflux pump expression can be induced by some but not all biocides.[163,164,166] The overexpression of efflux pumps when bacteria are exposed to biocides or biocidal products is important to consider because it may impact on cross-resistance to antibiotics. For example, following triclosan exposure, a number of studies reported overexpression of efflux pumps such as AcrAB-TolC efflux system in *Salmonella* ser Typhimurium[133,191,194]; SmedEF in *Stenotrophomonas maltophilia*[195]; AcrAB in *Escherichia coli*[94,196]; TriABC,[181] MexCD-OprJ,[188] and MexJk[189] in *Pseudomonas aeruginosa*[181]; and CmeB in *Campylobacter jejuni*.[197] The overexpression of efflux pumps might be triggered by the expression of global regulatory genes such as *marA* and *soxS*[94,198] as a result of stress brought on by a biocide.

It is questionable that the sole expression of efflux can lead to bacterial survival in a high (in use) concentration of a biocide. Bacterial resistance to a high concentration of a biocides is more likely to arise from the expression of multiple mechanisms.[6,9,130-133]

Enzymatic Degradation

The degradation of active substances by microorganisms has been well documented for the biodeterioration and biodegradation of a wide range of pollutants. The main question as far as biocide and biocidal products are concerned is whether bacterial enzymatic activity is rapid enough for a bacterium to survive exposure to a biocide. There are plenty of examples of bacterial pathogens surviving in aquatic environments polluted with high concentration of heavy metals.[199,200] Questions arise as to whether heavy metal pollution in the environment plays a role in the maintenance or dissemination of biocide and antibiotic resistance genes.[201-204] Heavy metal pollution certainly contributes to the dissemination of a metal resistance genes.[205] Bacterial resistance to copper and silver can arise from a reduction to the metallic ions to the metal,[13,206] although resistance to copper and copper oxide nanoparticles also involves an expression of genes encoding for efflux (eg, RND family efflux, P-type ATPase efflux) and transporters (eg, cation diffusion facilitator transporters).[207-209]

The role of enzymatic degradation in enabling bacterial survival in biocide may be best illustrated with the degradation of alkylating agents such as formaldehyde and glutaraldehyde with aldehyde dehydrogenases[210] and with the degradation of oxidizing agents, notably hydrogen peroxide, with catalase, superoxide dismutase, and alkyl hydroperoxidases.[211,212] Catalase can react fast enough to quench the activity of oxidizing agents and is used as a neutralizer in standard efficacy tests, although bacterial resistance to the in-use concentration of oxidizing agents may not solely rely on enzymatic degradation.[213]

Physiological and Metabolic Changes

Biocide exposure on the bacterial cell has been observed to result in an extended lag phase in growth culture.[129,214-217] The assumption is that this extended lag phase enables bacteria to express (1) resistance mechanisms to decrease the damaging concentration of stressor and (2) repair mechanisms. According to Figure 4.1, initial damage caused by a biocide is reversible, but bacteria need time to repair it. It has also been recognized that high metabolic activity makes bacteria more susceptible to biocides.[129]

Following exposure to triclosan, Webber and colleagues[218] observed that *S* Typhimurium was able to modify its metabolic pathway as part of the expression "triclosan resistance network" to produce pyruvate and fatty acids; fatty acids synthesis is targeted by the bisphenol at a low concentration.[95,187,219] The induction of multiple pathways in *S* Typhimurium following exposure to biocides including triclosan, chlorhexidine, and benzalkonium chloride was also reported by Curiao and colleagues.[220]

Other studies looking at bacterial gene expression following biocide exposure identified changes in expression for genes responsible for various metabolic pathways.[135,156,221-225] In *E coli*, the σ^S (or RpoS) subunit of RNA polymerase plays a determinant role in general stress response and triggers changes in bacterial metabolism.[134] With that in mind, it may not be surprising that biocide as a stressor will eventually produce a change in metabolism in bacteria.

Biofilms

Bacteria are usually attached to or associated with surfaces in a community of microorganisms: a biofilm. Bacterial biofilms have been well documented to be highly resistant to antimicrobials whether antibiotics or biocides.[226,227] Additional biofilm mechanisms of resistance have been described in addition to the mechanisms of resistance present in a single bacterial cell (Table 4.3).[6,228-230] Newly adhered bacterial cells attached to surfaces already present decreased susceptibility to biocides.[231] It is now understood that the biofilm matrix that binds the microbial community together plays an important role in establishing the biofilms and their resistance to antimicrobials.[232] However, the matrix might not be responsible solely for the level of resistance to biocides. Martin and colleagues[80] isolated vegetative *Bacillus subtilis* from endoscope washer disinfector that was resistant to the in-use concentration of chlorine dioxide and hydrogen peroxide used in endoscope reprocessing, and they demonstrated that the matrix was not solely responsible for the resistance to these oxidizing agents.[213]

The presence of bacterial biofilms is an issue for the high-level disinfection of medical devices[80,230,233-236] and surface sanitizing in food handling environments.[237-240] The effect of biocide exposure on a mixed bacterial biofilm has been shown to contribute to a selection and clonal expansion of the least susceptible species.[241-245] This is not really surprising, and the consequence of such a selection has not been fully explored. What is more significant is the potential protection given from bacterial species highly resistant to a biocide to other susceptible bacteria within a biofilm.[246-250] In these studies, the matrix (ie, exopolysaccharides) was proposed to be responsible for the protection given by the resistant bacterial species.

Studies on bacterial biofilms refer in their majority to *wet* biofilms, where biofilms occur under wet conditions, for example, in a drain,[243] water pipes,[249] medical devices,[233] or tested in wet conditions.[241,244,245] Recently, *dry* biofilms occurring on dry surfaces have been identified.[251,252] These biofilms were particularly resistant to the in-use concentration of sodium hypochlorite (500 ppm)[252] and higher (20 000 ppm),[253] which questions the current infection control strategies in health care settings.[254]

Bacterial Endospores

Bacterial endospores have been well documented for their resistance to biocides and biocidal products.[255,256] Their multilayered structure, dehydration, and presence of small acid-soluble proteins in their core are responsible for such resistance.[255] It is not surprising that bacterial endospores are among the most difficult entities to kill.[8] Recently, the role of the spore cortex that exerts pressure on the spore cytoplasmic membrane has been shown to be an important

TABLE 4.3 Mechanisms of resistance of bacterial biofilms[a]

Resistance Mechanisms	Comments	Observation
Decreasing the effective concentration of a biocide	Establishing a reduced local biocide concentration following a diffusion gradient Nonspecific neutralizing interaction with cell constituents Lysed bacterial community offering mechanistic inactivation as a result of increased organic load	Depends on the nature of the matrix Highly reactive biocides (eg, oxidizing agents) more prone to react
Enhanced bacterial insusceptibility	Degradation of antimicrobials Efflux (more effective against lower concentrations) Change in membrane composition (proteins and lipids)	Biocides cause an early stress response and subsequent genes expression to specific *survival* mechanisms enhanced by effective cell-cell communication (quorum sensing) and gene transfer.
Slow growth/metabolism	A local chemical gradient (reduced nutrients/oxygen) can retard growth rate, mitigating against biocide injury. Presence of persisters	Persister cells have a specifically slow metabolism and are highly resistant to antimicrobials. They are scattered within the biofilm and thought to be responsible for biofilm survival and regrowth following antimicrobial exposure.
Acquisition of new resistance determinants	Increased genetic exchange	Effective communication between bacterial cells through quorum sensing and gene exchange

[a]Adapted from Maillard and Denyer.[6] Reprinted with permission of Tekno Scienze Srl.

mechanism to ensure the spore membrane is impermeable to any chemicals including water to some extent, and as such, the spore cortex adds some protection to the spore core.[257]

There are very few biocides that are sporicidal, and the review from Russell[258] in 1990 still holds true today. The efficacy testing for sporicidal activity relies heavily on neutralization of the biocide. Leggett and colleagues[125] reviewed a number of scenario where neutralizations of the biocide are suboptimal or absent. This question claims that amine-based disinfectants, as examples, are labeled as *sporicidal*[126] because failure of neutralization is likely to be responsible for any recorded activity.[124]

▶ BACTERIAL RESPONSE TO BIOCIDES LEADING TO A CHANGE IN ANTIMICROBIAL SUSCEPTIBILITY

Bacteria can express a number of mechanisms that make them less susceptible or resistant to biocides and biocidal products.[2] Biocides have multiple target sites at a high concentration, and the overall damage caused to the target sites and the type of target site damage will lead to an inhibitory, reversible effect of a lethal effect. If bacterial resistance to biocidal products has been documented and had an impact, for example, on patients, it has become clear that one needs to consider carefully the effect of biocide exposure at a low concentration on bacteria. Many biocides, and

notably cationic biocides such as the QAC and the biguanides, but also phenolics, might leave a low concentration residual following use on a disinfected surface. Likewise, the application of a product might require some important water dilution (rinsing) during or after use to render the surface safe for use. The during-use parameter has been recently mentioned to clearly define the concentration of a biocidal product and biocide that will effectively be in contact with the target microorganism during application.[8,15] Exposure to low concentrations that maybe subinhibitory is relevant to consider, not for a point of view of resistance to a product but for a realistic exposure of a biocide that will inevitably produce a stress response in the bacterial cell and the subsequent expression of a number of genes that will lead to a transient or permanent change in susceptibility profile to unrelated antimicrobials, including different classes of biocides and antibiotics.

Stress Response

Bacteria surviving in biocidal products displayed either intrinsic mechanisms of resistance or expressing mechanisms enabling their survival in a product.[195,259] Bacterial exposure to a low concentration of a biocidal product is realistic with the rise in consumer products containing a low concentration of biocide(s) and with the use of biocidal products, allowing a residual (low) concentration of biocides on surfaces during use or after use.[2,6,8]

It is now well recognized that biocide exposure produces a stress response in bacteria[260,261] (whether intrinsically resistant or not) that will lead to the expression of regulatory genes such as *fis*,[198] *marA*,[193,196,262-264] *soxRS*,[94,193,262-264] *rob*,[263] *oxyR*,[265] *ramA*,[94,193] and *sigB*,[266] triggering the expression of nonspecific resistance mechanisms such as efflux and changes in membrane permeability.[156,188,195,220,224,267-269] These mechanisms, when triggered, enable bacteria to survive the stressor. In *B subtilis*, exposure to a stressor enables the trigger of a cell envelope stress response, which regulates the production of both specific resistance determinants and general mechanisms to protect the bacterial envelope.[270]

A bacterial stress response may be indicated with a reduced bacterial growth rate,[101,214-216] which may result from the expression of mechanisms decreasing the concentration of the stressor to a level that enable growth to resume and/or effective repair mechanisms. To date, bacterial repair mechanisms as a mean to survive biocide exposure has received little consideration,[213,271-274] despite the knowledge that the initial interaction between a biocide and the bacterial cell is reversible (see Figure 4.1).

In the literature, this is often measured as an increased in MIC and/or MBC and a change in antibiotic susceptibility profile. Such response is usually transient while the stressor is present. The exposed bacteria are expected to revert to a *sensitive* susceptibility profile when the stressor is removed.[16,89,128,268,275] Thus, the concentration of biocide the bacteria is exposed to is paramount,[1,6,122,276,277] and in vitro studies using a nonlethal concentration become relevant because these concentrations would produce a bacterial stress response.

Mutations

Bacterial mutations occur naturally but can be driven by stress response mechanisms following exposure to antimicrobials. It is now well understood that the expression of SOS DNA-damage response, RpoS general stress response, and reactive-oxygen species regulators will drive the expression of low-fidelity DNA polymerases that allow for mutagenic break repair leading to mutations.[278] With the selective pressure exerted by a biocide, bacteria that can withstand this pressure will survive and the other will die.

Mutations resulting from a biocide exposure has been mainly investigated with triclosan.[94,95,118,187,229,279-284] Triclosan is so far unique as a biocide because at a low concentration it will interact specifically with enoyl acyl reductase inhibiting fatty acid synthesis.[95,187,219,280,285-287] A mutation in the gene responsible for this enzyme (eg, *fabI*, *inhA*) will result in bacterial survival to a somewhat higher concentration of the bisphenol in comparison to wild type strains. Ciusa and colleagues[118] identified different mutations in *sa-fabI* following *S aureus* strains exposure to triclosan. The mutations observed differed in their majority between those detected in clinical isolates and

those selected in vitro.[118] Furthermore, it was suggested that differences in MIC and MBC to triclosan between clinical isolates and strains selected in vitro that present the same *sa-fabI* mutation indicate accumulated compensating mutations that modify the phenotype of the clinical isolates.[118] This would also imply that for clinical isolates, the stressor (antibiotic or biocide) driving mutations might be difficult to ascertain.

A few studies have looked at other biocides and identified mutations such as *rpoA* and *ramA* following exposure to a QAC formulation, *fabI* and *gyrA*, following exposure to an oxidizing or amine-based formulation.[259] In *Serratia marcescens*, mutation in *sdeS*, a regulator gene likely to encode the repressor protein SdeS,[288] follows exposure to QAC[289] and is responsible for increased efflux and resistance to antimicrobials. In *Enterobacter* and *Klebsiella* species, mutation in *silS* gene accounted for phenotypic resistance to silver.[290,291]

Overexpression of some resistant gene determinants and mutations enabling survival in biocide might come as a fitness cost,[220,229,292] although this is not always the case.[293]

Cross-resistance to Unrelated Antimicrobials

Within the last few years, there have been plenty of examples of a bacterial isolate showing a change in susceptibility profile to both biocides and antibiotics, often resulting from an exposure to biocides (Table 4.4). Evidence of cross-resistance now include studies investigating different environments where biocides are used (eg, food industry, material industry [eg, paint]), although most evidence remain with studies looking at the food, veterinary, and health care environments. If some studies remain somewhat artificial in their protocol, for example, exposure to increasing concentration of a biocide,[103,104] a large number of recent publications studied clinical or environmental isolates with a change in susceptibility profile or resistance to antibiotics following exposure to biocide or biocidal products.[103-105,172,251,292,295,296,299] It is, however, clear that these isolates, which are often different bacterial genera, differ in their AMR profile, and publications refer to a percentage of total isolates resistant to specific antibiotics.[103,172,251,294-297] It is difficult to generalize that the exposure to a biocide will drive cross-resistance to antibiotics in all bacteria,[8] although there is enough documented evidence that biocide-driven cross-resistance occurs in situ in a large number of bacterial genera.

The mechanisms at the forefront of cross-resistance triggered by biocide exposure, or associated with increased biocide MIC, are (1) efflux,[8,115,143,163-166,182,185,188,196,197,300] as result of either efflux gene overexpression following a stress or SOS-type response; (2) mutation in regulatory genes; and (3) change in membrane permeability or composition (see Table 4.4).[130,143,151,156,165,198]

TABLE 4.4 Examples of cross-resistance between biocides and unrelated chemicals including antibiotics in the recent literature

Bacteria/Source of Isolates	Biocide Exposure	Resistance to Unrelated Biocides	Resistance to Antibiotics	Mechanisms	Reference
Burkholderia lata	CHG (0.005%) BZC (0.005%)	No significant change in MIC or MBC to CHG or BZC	Decrease in susceptibility to CAZ, CIP, IMP	Upregulation of outer membrane protein and ABC transporter	Knapp et al[128]
Staphylococcus aureus	TRI (0.0004%)	Increase in MIC and MBC to TRI	Resistance[a] to CIP, AMP	ND	Wesgate et al[15]
Escherichia coli	TRI (0.0004%)	Increase in MIC and MBC to TRI	Resistance[a] to AMP		
E coli	CHG (0.0004%)	No change in MIC or MBC to CHG	Resistance[a] to TOB, TIC, AMP		
S aureus	H₂O₂ (0.001%)	No change in MIC or MBC to H₂O₂	Resistance[a] to CIP, AMP		
E coli	H₂O₂ (0.001%)		Resistance[a] to AMP		
Clinical isolates of *S aureus*	In situ[b]	High MIC to CHG[c]	Resistance[a] CEF, RIF, TSX, CHL	Efflux: *qacAB*	Conceição et al[112]
Food isolates of *E coli*	In situ[b]	Increase in MIC to HDP[c]	Resistance[a] to AMP STR, TET, CHL, NA TSX	Efflux: *acrB*, *mdfA*, *oxqA*, *qacA/B*, *qacE*	Burgos et al[115]
Food isolates of *Pseudomonas* species	In situ[b]	Increase MIC to TRI, BZC, and CET[c] (remained sensitive to biocidal product)	Decrease in susceptibility to AMP, ERY, IMP, POL, SUL, STR	ND	Lerma et al[88]
Food isolates of *Leuconostoc pseudomesenteroides* and *Lactobacillus pentosus*[d]	TRI (0.1%) BZC (0.1%)	ND	Decrease in susceptibility to CHL, CIP, TET	SOS response not activated by biocide stress	Casado Muñoz Mdel et al[294]
Food isolates of gram-positive and gram-negative strains[d]	Stepwise exposure to BZC and HDP	Increase in MIC to BZC, HDP, TRI, and CHG	Resistance[a] to AMP, SXT, CTX, CAZ (following exposure to BZC)	Efflux: *acrB*, *sugE*, *norC*, *qacE*, *qacH* Increased membrane rigidity	Gadea et al[103]
Food isolates of gram-positive and gram-negative strains[d]	Stepwise exposure to CET	Increase in MIC to BZC, HDP, TRI, CHG, DDB, MT	Resistance[a] to CAZ, CTX, AMP, TET, STX, SMX	Changes in membrane fluidity	Gadea et al[104]
	Stepwise exposure to CHG	Increase in MIC to DDB, TRI, MT, CET, HDP, BZC	Resistance[a] to CTX, IMP, CAZ, SMX, NA		
Seafood isolates of gram-positive and gram-negative strains[d]	In situ[b]	Increase MIC to CHG, TRI[c] High MIC to copper sulfate and zinc chloride	Resistance[a] to AMP, CTX, IMP, CAZ, CHL, STR	Efflux: *qacE* delta Metal resistance genes *pcoA/copA*, *pcoR*, *chrB*	Romero et al[295]
E coli and *S aureus*	AgNPs	ND	Decrease in susceptibility to AMP, PEN, CHL, KAN	Promoting stress tolerance through induction of intracellular ROS	Kaweeteerawat et al[260]

TABLE 4.4 Examples of cross-resistance between biocides and unrelated chemicals including antibiotics in the recent literature *(Continued)*

Bacteria/Source of Isolates	Biocide Exposure	Resistance to Unrelated Biocides	Resistance to Antibiotics	Mechanisms	Reference
Dairy industry isolates of gram-positive and gram-negative strains[d]	In situ[b]	Increase in MIC to BZC, CET, HDP, TRI, HP, PHH[c]	Resistance[a] to AMP, CTX, CAZ, TSX, TET, STR	Efflux: *qacE* delta 1, *qacA/B*, *acrB*, *mdfA*	Márquez et al[172]
Food isolates of *Salmonella enterica Salmonella* species[d]	In situ[b]	Increase in MIC to BZC, CET, HDP, TRI, HP[c]	Resistance[a] to CHL, TET, STR, NA, CIP, TSX, NEL	Efflux: *acrB*, *oqxA*, *mdfA*, *qacA/B*, *qacE*	Márquez et al[296]
Organic food isolates of gram-positive and gram-negative strains[d]	In situ[b]	Increase in MIC to CET, HDP, TRI, CHG[c]	Cefuroxime, followed by amoxicillin and erythromycin	ND	Gadea et al[105]
Klebsiella pneumoniae	Repeated exposure to one-fourth MIC of CHG	Increase in MIC and MBC to CHG	Increase MIC to COL Change in MIC to AZM, TEC, FEP	Efflux: upregulation of *smvA* Change in membrane composition: upregulation of *pmrK*, mutation in PhoPQ	Wand et al[267]
Salmonella ser Typhimurium	Sublethal concentrations of Superkill (mixture of aldehydes and QAC) (0.0018%)	Increase in MIC to TRI	Increase in MIC to NA, CHL, TET	Efflux: de-repression of AcrAB-TolC	Webber et al[259]
	AQAS (QAC) (0.0018%)	ND	Increase in MIC to NA, CHL, TET	Efflux: de-repression of AcrAB-TolC Mutations in *rpoA*, *ramA*	
	Trigene (halogenated tertiary amine compound) (0.0005)	Increase in MIC to TRI	Increase in MIC to NA, CIP	Mutations in *fabI*, *gyrA*	
	Virkon (oxidative compound) (0.2%)	Increase in MIC to TRI	Increase in MIC to NA, CIP	Mutations in *fabI*, *gyrA*	
S aureus[d]	Exposure to sub-MIC of CHG	No change in CHG susceptibility Increase in MIC to plant extract	Resistance[a] to CIP, TET, GEN, AMK, FEP, MEM	ND	Wu et al[297]
	Plant extract (*Rhizoma coptidis*)	Increase MIC to plant extract	Resistance[a] to CIP, TET, GEN, AMK		

(continued)

TABLE 4.4   Examples of cross-resistance between biocides and unrelated chemicals including antibiotics in the recent literature *(Continued)*

Bacteria/Source of Isolates	Biocide Exposure	Resistance to Unrelated Biocides	Resistance to Antibiotics	Mechanisms	Reference
Enterococcus faecium *Enterococcus faecalis*	Exposure to one-fourth MIC of CHG (Hibiclens)	ND	ND (but assumed VAN resistance with expression of *vanA*)	Increased *vanH* promoter activity Increased expression of *VanA* Increased expression of *telA, xpaC, liaX, liaY* associated with daptomycin nonsusceptibility	Bhardwaj et al[298]
Dental plaques isolates[d]	Repeated exposure to CHG (0.0002%)	Increased MIC to CHG	Change in susceptibility to AMP, KAN, GEN, TET	Efflux (upregulation of expression of the HlyD-like periplasmic adaptor protein) Biofilm formation	Saleem et al[299]
Environmental isolates (biofilms)	During-use application of copper and zinc-based antifouling paint	Decreased susceptibility to copper and zinc	Decreased susceptibility to TET	Increase in abundance of metal and biocide resistance genes Increase in chromosomal RND efflux	Whiteley et al[251]
Acinetobacter baumannii[d]	CHG (4%)	Increased MIC to CHG	Resistance[a] to CIP, IMP, MEM, GEN, TOB, NEL, TET, DOX	Efflux: increased expression in *adeb, abeS, amvA* Porins: decreased expression in *ompA*	Fernández-Cuenca et al[143]
	BZC (0.1%)	Increased MIC to BZC	Resistance[a] to CIP, GEN, NEL, TET, DOX	Efflux: increased expression in *adeb, abeS* Porins: decreased expression in *ompA, carO*	
	Triclosan (Irgasan) (0.003%)	Increased MIC to Irgasan)	Resistance[a] to CIP, SUL, CAZ, IMP, MEM, GEN, TOB, AMK, NEL, TET	Efflux: increased expression in *adeJ*; decreased expression in *abeM, amvA* Expression in *ompA, carO, omp 33-36*	

Abbreviations: ABC, adenosine triphosphate-binding cassette; AgNPs, silver nanoparticles; AMK, amikacin; AMP, ampicillin; AZM, azithromycin; BZC, benzalkonium chloride; CAZ, ceftazidime; CEF, cefixime; CET, cetrimide; CHG, chlorhexidine digluconate; CHL, chloramphenicol; CIP, ciprofloxacin; COL, colistin; CTX, cefotaxime; DDB, didecyldimethylammonium bromide; DOX, doxycycline; ERY, erythromycin; FEP, cefepime; GEN, gentamicin; H_2O_2, hydrogen peroxide; HDP, hexadecylpyridinium chloride; HP, hexachlorophene; IMP, imipenem; KAN, kanamycin; MBC, minimum bactericidal concentration; MEM, meropenem; MIC, minimum inhibitory concentration; MT, methylenebis(3,4,6-trichlorophenol); NA, nalidixic acid; ND, not determined; NEL, netilmicin; PEN, penicillin; PHH, poly-(hexamethylene guanidinium) hydrochloride; POL, polymyxin B; QAC, quaternary ammonium compound; RIF, rifampin; RND, resistance-nodulation-division; ROS, reactive-oxygen species; SMX, sulfamethoxazole; STR, streptomycin; SUL, sulbactam; SXT, sulfamethoxazole; TEC, teicoplanin; TET, tetracycline; TIC, ticarcillin-clavulanic; TOB, tobramycin; TRI, triclosan; TSX, trimethoprim-sulfamethoxazole; VAN, vancomycin.

[a]Clinical resistance as defined by European Committee on Antimicrobial Susceptibility Testing, British Society for Antimicrobial Chemotherapy.

[b]Frequent exposure to biocidal products likely to have happened in situ.

[c]Increase in MIC compared to standard culture strains.

[d]Resistance to antibiotics and types of antibiotic depend on isolates.

Dissemination of Resistance

The effect of biocides and biocidal products on the maintenance and transfer of genes encoding for resistance is a concern that needs to be addressed.[301] There is also plenty of evidence that environmental isolates carry not only genes responsible for a nonspecific resistance mechanism such as efflux but also a battery of specific genes for antibiotic resistance.[111,112,115,171,172,200,250,295,302] A number of retrospective studies reported that genetic determinants encoding for biocide resistance (eg, *qacAB* and *smr*) are spreading not only in the clinical setting[118,303-306] but also in the food and veterinary environments.[295,307-309] The literature suggests that the selective pressure exerted by biocides can contribute to the selection of bacterial isolates carrying genes involved in cross-resistance or resistance to antibiotics.[250,302,303,307,310,311] There are plenty of examples where resistance genes to biocides and antibiotics are present on the same multidrug resistance plasmids,[312-314] enabling the coselection and transfer of these plasmids following biocide exposure.[118,204,209,295,312,315-318]

The role of biocide and biocidal product exposure in the maintenance of resistant genetic determinants to both biocides and antibiotics needs also to be considered.[307,319,320] By exerting a selective pressure, biocides, like other stressors including heavy metal pollution and antibiotics, are likely to contribute to the maintenance of resistant-determinant genes in bacteria. The full impact of such pressure on AMR has not been fully considered with biocides as of yet.

▶ CONCLUSION

Biocides and the application of biocidal products are essential to control microorganisms in different field of applications. It is probably appropriate to consider that bacteria exposure to a low concentration of some biocides during or after the application of a biocidal product is increasing, when one considers the increase in biocidal products (or biocides used in nonbiocidal products) commercially available today. With increased AMR and its health and economic consequences,[7] the quantity of biocides used routinely might need to be questioned. After all, one of the main causes responsible for the level of AMR currently reported is the use and abuse of chemotherapeutic antibiotics.[7,321] Are we heading in the same direction with biocides? The potential impact of biocide and biocidal products on emerging resistance bacteria is still being debated[2,321-323] and has driven some changes in the regulation of biocidal products.[4,5]

There is no doubt that bacteria have a phenomenal capacity to adapt and survive biocide exposure (see Table 4.1), and in doing so, bacteria can express a number of nonspecific mechanisms that can lead to cross-resistance to unrelated antimicrobials. However, based on the study of clinical and environmental isolates, not all bacteria have the same capacity to express resistance and cross-resistance mechanisms and to survive biocide exposure. There is also evidence that biocides are impacting on the maintenance and transfer of resistant genes in bacterial pathogens in environments where biocide exposure is common.

It is also evident from the literature that bacterial isolates showing an increase in a biocide MIC might nevertheless remain susceptible to a biocide at in-use concentration. Hence, not only the concentration of a biocide but also the exposure time to a biocide is paramount to ensure that target bacteria are destroyed. In addition, studies concerning biocidal products (a full formulation as oppose to just the biocide) remain scarce but tend to show that bacterial adaptation to a full formulation is more difficult.[15,16,109,324]

The question about how to define and measure bacterial resistance to biocides has not been resolved.[8] The introduction of the during-use concept,[8,15] where the concentration of a biocide in contact with the target bacteria is very low, is realistic and makes the use of MIC and MBC determination before and after exposure to a biocidal product practical,[15,16] although in this case, a change in susceptibility profile can be transient. Many in vitro studies have been based on exposing bacteria to repeated or increasing low concentrations of a biocide. These investigations have provided information on the impact of biocide exposure on bacterial mutations leading to a change in antimicrobial susceptibility profile, for example, linked to an overexpression of an efflux mechanism. The determination of MICs needs to be used as markers of change in the susceptibility profile[8,9,122] and not as a proof of bacterial resistance. The use of standard well-defined protocols to measure a change in bacterial susceptibility profile to chemotherapeutic antibiotics following biocide exposure should be followed because these provide a clinical interpretation based on set resistance breakpoints.[325,326] With regulatory pressure, the use of a predictive protocol to measure the risk associated with bacterial exposure to a biocidal product is needed. To date, a protocol relying on the strict control of the bacterial inoculum and the exposure to the during-use parameters (concentration of product, contact time, temperature, organic load) has been proposed[8] and evaluated.[15,16] This protocol measures a change in the susceptibility profile to the product (MIC and MBC) and relevant clinical antibiotics for the bacterial species investigated. It also measures the nature of the change whether it is transient or permanent, providing some useful information on the use of the product (eg, relying on residual activity post application).

The determination of the risk posed by emerging bacterial AMR and cross-resistance following exposure to biocidal product is important to consider for reassuring regulators, end users, and the public that the product will be safe to use.

REFERENCES

1. Maillard J-Y. Antimicrobial biocides in the healthcare environment: efficacy, policies, management and perceived problems. *Ther Clin Risk Manag.* 2005;(1):307-320.

2. Scientific Committee on Emerging and Newly Identified Health Risks. The antibiotic resistance effect of biocides. European Commission Web site. http://ec.europa.eu/health/ph_risk/committees/04_scenihr/docs/scenihr_o_021.pdf. Published 2009. Accessed May 2019.

3. Elsmore R, Wright S. The authorisation of biocidal products under the BPR. *Chimica Oggi.* 2016;34:51-54.

4. Biocidal Product Regulation. Regulation (EU) No 528/2012 of the European Parliament and of the Council. European Union Web site. http://eur-lex.europa.eu/legal-content/EN/TXT/PDF/?uri=CELEX:02012R0528-20140425&from=EN. Published 2013. Accessed May 2019.

5. US Food and Drug Administration. FDA issues final rule on safety and effectiveness of antibacterial soaps. http://www.fda.gov/NewsEvents/Newsroom/PressAnnouncements/ucm517478.htm. Published 2016. Accessed May 2019.

6. Maillard J-Y, Denyer SP. Emerging bacterial resistance following biocide exposure: should we be concerned? *Chimica Oggi.* 2009;27:26-28.

7. O'Neill J. *Tackling Drug-Resistant Infections Globally: Final Report and Recommendations. The Review on Antimicrobial Resistance.* London, United Kingdom: HM Government; 2016.

8. Maillard J-Y, Bloomfield S, Coelho JR, et al. Does microbicide use in consumer products promote antimicrobial resistance? A critical review and recommendations for a cohesive approach to risk assessment. *Microb Drug Resist.* 2013;19:344-354.

9. Maillard J-Y. Bacterial resistance to biocides in the healthcare environment: should it be of genuine concern? *J Hosp Infect.* 2007;65:60-72.

10. Chapman JS, Diehl MA, Fearnside KB. Preservative tolerance and resistance. *Int J Cosmet Sci.* 1998;20:31-39.

11. Hammond SA, Morgan JR, Russell AD. Comparative susceptibility of hospital isolates of gram-negative bacteria to antiseptics and disinfectants. *J Hosp Infect.* 1987;9:255-264.

12. Russell AD. Biocide use and antibiotic resistance: the relevance of laboratory findings to clinical environmental situations. *Lancet Infect Dis.* 2003;3:794-803.

13. Cloete TE. Resistance mechanisms of bacteria to antimicrobial compounds. *Int Biodeterior Biodegradation.* 2003;51:277-282.

14. Dettenkoffer M, Wenzler S, Amthor S, Antes G, Motschall E, Daschner FD. Does disinfection of environmental surfaces influence nosocomial infection rates? A systematic review. *Am J Infect Control.* 2004;32:84-89.

15. Wesgate R, Grascha P, Maillard J-Y. Use of a predictive protocol to measure the antimicrobial resistance risks associated with biocidal product usage. *Am J Infect Control.* 2016;44:458-464.

16. Knapp L, Amézquita A, McClure P, Stewart S, Maillard J-Y. Development of a protocol for predicting bacterial resistance to microbicides. *Appl Environ Microbiol.* 2015;81:2652-2659.

17. Berger SA. Pseudobacteremia due to contaminated alcohol swabs. *J Clin Microbiol.* 1983;18:974-975.

18. Hsueh P-R, Teng LG, Yang P-C, Pan H-L, Ho S-W, Luh K-T. Nosocomial pseudoepidemic caused by *Bacillus cereus* traced to contaminated ethyl alcohol from a liquor factory. *J Clin Microbiol.* 1999;37:2280-2284.

19. Nasser RM, Rahi AC, Haddad MF, Daoud Z, Irani-Hakime N, Almawi W. Outbreak of *Burkholderia cepacia* bacteremia traced to contaminated hospital water used for dilution of an alcohol skin antiseptic. *Infect Control Hosp Epidemiol.* 2004;25:231-239.

20. Burdon DW, Whitby JL. Contamination of hospital disinfectants with *Pseudomonas* species. *Br Med J.* 1967;2:153-155.

21. Speller DC, Stephens ME, Viant AC. Hospital infection by *Pseudomonas cepacia. Lancet.* 1971;1:798-799.

22. Coyle-Gilchrist MM, Crewe P, Roberts G. *Flavobacterium meningosepticum* in the hospital environment. *J Clin Pathol.* 1976;29:824-826.

23. Marrie TJ, Costerton JW. Prolonged survival of *Serratia marcescens* in chlorhexidine. *Appl Environ Microbiol.* 1981;42:1093-1102.

24. Anyiwo CE, Coker AO, Daniel SO. *Pseudomonas aeruginosa* in postoperative wounds from chlorhexidine solutions. *J Hosp Infect.* 1982;3:189-191.

25. Sobel JO, Hashman N, Reinherz G, Merzbach D. Nosocomial *Pseudomonas cepacia* infection associated with chlorhexidine contamination. *Am J Med.* 1982;73:183-186.

26. Kahan A, Philippon A, Paul G, et al. Nosocomial infections by chlorhexidine solution contaminated with *Pseudomonas pickettii* (biovar VA-1). *J Infect.* 1983;7:256-263.

27. Verschraegen G, Claeys G, Meeus G, Delanghe M. *Pseudomonas pickettii* as a cause of pseudobacteremia. *J Clin Microbiol.* 1985;21:278-279.

28. Poty F, Denis C, Baufine-Ducrocq H. Nosocomial *Pseudomonas pickettii* infection. Danger of the use of ion-exchange resins [in German]. *Presse Med.* 1987;20:1185-1187.

29. Vu-Thien H, Darbord JC, Moissenet D, et al. Investigation of an outbreak of wound infections due to *Alcaligenes xylosoxidans* transmitted by chlorhexidine in a burns unit. *Eur J Clin Microbiol Infect Dis.* 1998;17:724-726.

30. Vigeant P, Loo VG, Bertrand C, et al. An outbreak of *Serratia marcescens* infections related to contaminated chlorhexidine. *Infect Control Hosp Epidemiol.* 1998;19:791-794.

31. Maroye P, Doermann HP, Rogues AM, Gachie JP, Mégraud F. Investigation of an outbreak of *Ralsontia pickettii* in a paediatric hospital by RAPD. *J Hosp Infect.* 2000;44:267-272.

32. Tena D, Carranza R, Barberá JR, et al. Outbreak of long-term intravascular catheter-related bacteremia due to *Achromobacter xylosoxidans* subspecies xylosoxidans in a hemodialysis unit. *Eur J Clin Microbiol Infect Dis.* 2005;24:727-732.

33. Lee S, Han SW, Kim G, Song DY, Lee JC, Kwon KT. An outbreak of *Burkholderia cenocepacia* associated with contaminated chlorhexidine solutions prepared in the hospital. *Am J Infect Control.* 2013;41:93-96.

34. Ko S, An HS, Bang JH, Park SW. An outbreak of *Burkholderia cepacia* complex pseudobacteremia associated with intrinsically contaminated commercial 0.5% chlorhexidine solution. *Am J Infect Control.* 2015;43:266-268.

35. de Frutos M, López-Urrutia L, Domínguez-Gil M, et al. *Serratia marcescens* outbreak due to contaminated 2% aqueous chlorhexidine. *Enferm Infecc Microbiol Clin.* 2017;35:624-629.

36. Bassett DCJ, Stokes KJ, Thomas WRG. Wound infection with *Pseudomonas multivorans*: a water-borne contaminant of disinfection solutions. *Lancet.* 1970;295:1188-1191.

37. Wishart MM, Riley TV. Infection with *Pseudomonas maltophilia* hospital outbreak due to contaminated disinfectant. *Med J Aust.* 1976;2:710-712.

38. Merino JL, Bouarich H, Pita MJ, et al. *Serratia marcescens* bacteraemia outbreak in haemodialysis patients with tunnelled catheters due to colonisation of antiseptic solution. Experience at 4 hospitals [in Spanish]. *Nefrologia.* 2016;36:667-673.

39. Plotkin SA, Austrian R. Bacteremia caused by *Pseudomonas* sp. following the use of materials stored in solutions of a cationic surface-active agent. *Am J Med Sci.* 1958;235:621-627.

40. Shickman MD, Guze LB, Pearce ML. Bacteremia following cardiac catheterization: report of a case and studies on the source. *N Engl J Med.* 1959;260:1164-1166.

41. Malizia WF, Gangarosa EJ, Goley AF. Benzalkonium chloride as a source of infection. *N Engl J Med.* 1960;263:800-802.

42. Lee JC, Fialkow PJ. Benzalkonium chloride: source of hospital infection with gram-negative bacteria. *JAMA.* 1961;177:708-710.

43. Centers for Disease Control and Prevention. Food and Drug Administration warning—contaminated detergent solution. *Morb Mortal Wkly Rep.* 1969;18:366.

44. Hardy PC, Elderer GM, Matsen JM. Contamination of commercially packaged urinary catheter kits with *Pseudomonas* EO-1. *N Engl J Med.* 1970;282:33-35.

45. Kaslow RA, Mackel DC, Mallison GF. Nosocomial pseudobacteremia: positive blood cultures due to contaminated benzalkonium chloride. *JAMA.* 1976;236:2407-2409.

46. Frank MJ, Schaffner W. Contaminated aqueous benzalkonium chloride: an unnecessary hospital infection hazard. *JAMA.* 1976;236: 2418-2419.

47. Fox JG, Beaucage CM, Folta CA, Thornton GW. Nosocomial transmission of *Serratia marcescens* in a veterinary hospital due to contamination by benzalkonium chloride. *J Clin Microbiol.* 1981;14: 157-160.

48. Sautter RL, Mattman LH, Legaspi RC. *Serratia marcescens* meningitis associated with a contaminated benzalkonium chloride solution. *Infect Control.* 1984;5:223-225.

49. Nakashima AK, McCarthy MA, Martone WJ, Anderson RL. Epidemic septic arthritis caused by *Serratia marcescens* and associated with benzalkonium chloride antiseptic. *J Clin Microbiol.* 1987;25:1014-1018.

50. Nakashima AK, Highsmith AK, Martone WJ. Survival of *Serratia marcescens* in benzalkonium chloride and in multiple-dose medication vials: relationship to epidemic septic arthritis. *J Clin Microbiol.* 1987;25:1019-1021.

51. Georgia Division of Public Health. Abscesses in an allergy practice due to *Mycobacterium chelonae. Georgia Epidemiol Rep.* 1990;6:2.

52. Olson RK, Voorhees RE, Eitzen HE, Rolka H, Sewell CM. Cluster of postinjection abscesses related to corticosteroid injections and use of benzalkonium chloride. *West J Med.* 1999;170:143-147.

53. Tiwari TS, Ray B, Jost KC Jr, et al. Forty years of disinfectant failure: outbreak of postinjection *Mycobacterium abscessus* infection caused by contamination of benzalkonium chloride. *Clin Infect Dis.* 2003;36:954-962.

54. Lee C-S, Lee H-B, Cho Y-G, Park J-H, Lee H-S. Hospital-acquired *Burkholderia cepacia* infection related to contaminated benzalkonium chloride. *J Hosp Infect.* 2008;68:280-282.

55. Guinness M, Levey J. Contamination of aqueous dilutions of Resiguard disinfectant with *Pseudomonas. Med J Aust.* 1976;2:392.

56. Morris S, Gibbs M, Hansman D, Smyth N, Cosh D. Contamination of aqueous dilutions of Resiguard disinfectant with *Pseudomonas. Med J Aust.* 1976;2:110-111.

57. Dixon RE, Kaslow RA, Mackel DC, Fulkerson CC, Mallison GF. Aqueous quaternary ammonium antiseptics and disinfectants: use and misuse. *JAMA.* 1976;236:2415-2417.

58. Siebor E, Llanes C, Lafon I, et al. Presumed pseudobacteremia outbreak resulting from contamination of proportional disinfectant dispenser. *Eur J Clin Microbiol Infect Dis.* 2007;26:195-198.

59. Hugon E, Marchandin H, Poirée M, Fosdse T, Servent N. *Achromobacter* bacteraemia outbreak in a paediatric onco-haematology department related to strain with high surviving ability in contaminated disinfectant atomizers. *J Hosp Infect.* 2015;89:116-122.

60. Ehrenkranz NJ, Bolyard EA, Wiener M, Cleary TJ. Antibiotic-sensitive *Serratia marcescens* infections complicating cardiopulmonary operations: contaminated disinfectant as a reservoir. *Lancet.* 1980;316: 1289-1292.

61. Lehours P, Rogues AM, Occhialini A, Boulestreau H, Gachie JP, Megraud F. Investigation of an outbreak due to *Alcaligenes xylosoxydans* subspecies xylosoxydans by random polymorphic DNA analysis. *Eur J Clin Microbiol Infect Dis.* 2002;21:108-113.

62. Ebner W, Meyer E, Schulz-Huotari C, Scholz R, Zilow G, Daschner FD. Pseudocontamination of blood components with *Burkholderia cepacia* during quality controls. *Transfusion Med.* 2005;15:241-242.

63. Oie S, Arakawa J, Furukawa H, Matsumoto S, Matsuda N, Wakamatsu H. Microbial contamination of a disinfectant-soaked unwoven cleaning cloth. *J Hosp Infect.* 2012;82:61-63.

64. Günther F, Merle U, Frank U, Gaida MM, Mutters NT. Pseudobacteremia outbreak of biofilm-forming *Achromobacter xylosoxidans*: environmental transmission. *BMC Infect Dis.* 2016;16:584.

65. Vanholder R, Vanhaecke E, Ringoir S. *Pseudomonas* septicemia due to deficient disinfectant mixing during reuse. *Int J Artificial Organs.* 1992;15:19-24.

66. Reiss I, Borkhardt A, Fussle R, Sziegoleit A, Gortner L. Disinfectant contaminated with *Klebsiella oxytoca* as a source of sepsis in babies. *Lancet.* 2000;356:310.

67. Kressel AB, Kidd F. Pseudo-outbreak of *Mycobacterium chelonae* and *Methylobacterium mesophilicum* caused by contamination of an automated endoscopy washer. *Infect Control Hosp Epidemiol.* 2001;22:414-418.

68. Archibald LK, Corl A, Shah B, et al. *Serratia marcescens* outbreak associated with extrinsic contamination of 1% chloroxylenol soap. *Infect Control Hosp Epidemiol.* 1997;18:704-709.

69. McNaughton M, Mazinke N, Thomas E. Newborn conjunctivitis associated with 0.5% antiseptic intrinsically contaminated with *Serratia marcescens. Can J Infect Control.* 1995;10:7-8.

70. Berkelman RL, Lewin S, Allen JR, et al. Pseudobacteremia attributed to contamination of povidone-iodine with *Pseudomonas cepacia. Ann Intern Med.* 1981;95:32-36.

71. Craven DE, Moody B, Connolly MG, Kollisch NR, Stottmeier KD, McCabe WR. Pseudobacteremia caused by povidone-iodine solution contaminated with *Pseudomonas cepacia. N Engl J Med.* 1981; 305:621-623.

72. Centers for Disease Control and Prevention. Contaminated povidone-iodine solution—Texas. *Morb Mortal Wkly Rep.* 1989;38:133-134.

73. Jarvis WR. Nosocomial outbreaks: the Centers for Disease Control's Hospital Infections Program Experience, 1980–1990. *Am J Med.* 1991; 91(suppl 3B):101-106.

74. Panlilio AL, Beck-Sague CM, Siegel JD, et al. Infections and pseudoinfections due to povidone-iodine solution contaminated with *Pseudomonas cepacia. Clin Infect Dis.* 1992;14:1078-1083.

75. Bouallègue O, Mzoughi R, Weill FX, et al. Outbreak of *Pseudomonas putida* bacteraemia in a neonatal intensive care unit. *J Hosp Infect.* 2004;57:88-91.

76. Parrott PL, Whitworth EN, Terry PM, et al. *Pseudomonas aeruginosa* peritonitis associated with contaminated poloxamer-iodine solution. *Lancet.* 1982;320:683-685.

77. Weber DJ, Rutala WA, Sickbert-Bennett EE. Outbreaks associated with contaminated antiseptics and disinfectants. *Antimicrob Agents Chemother.* 2007;51:4217-4224.

78. Griffiths PA, Babb JR, Bradley CR, Fraise AP. Glutaraldehyde-resistant *Mycobacterium chelonae* from endoscope washer disinfectors. *J Appl Microbiol.* 1997;82:519-526.

79. van Klingeren B, Pullen W. Glutaraldehyde resistant mycobacteria from endoscope washers. *J Hosp Infect.* 1993;25:147-149.

80. Martin DJ, Denyer SP, McDonnell G, Maillard J-Y. Resistance and cross-resistance to oxidising agents of bacterial isolates from endoscope washer disinfectors. *J Hosp Infect.* 2008;69:377-383.

81. Fisher CW, Fiorello A, Shaffer D, Jackson M, McDonnell GE. Aldehyde-resistant mycobacteria bacteria associated with the use of endoscope reprocessing systems. *Am J Infect Control.* 2012;40:880-882.

82. Epstein L, Hunter JC, Arwady MA, et al. New Delhi metallo-β-lactamase–producing carbapenem-resistant *Escherichia coli* associated with exposure to duodenoscopes. *JAMA.* 2014;312:1447-1455.

83. Naryzhny I, Silas D, Chi K. Impact of ethylene oxide gas sterilization of duodenoscopes after a carbapenem-resistant Enterobacteriaceae outbreak. *Gastrointest Endosc.* 2016;84:259-262.

84. Duarte RS, Lourenco MCS, Fonseca LD, et al. Epidemic of postsurgical infections caused by *Mycobacterium massiliense. J Clin Microbiol.* 2009;47:2149-2155.

85. Guy M, Vanhems P, Dananché C, et al. Outbreak of pulmonary *Pseudomonas aeruginosa* and *Stenotrophomonas maltophilia* infections related to contaminated bronchoscope suction valves, Lyon, France, 2014. *Euro Surveill.* 2016;21:17-25.

86. Botana-Rial M, Leiro-Fernández V, Núñez-Delgado M, et al. A pseudo-outbreak of *Pseudomonas putida* and *Stenotrophomonas maltophilia* in a bronchoscopy unit. *Respiration.* 2016;4:274-278.

87. Rose H, Baldwin A, Dowson CG, Mahenthiralingam E. Biocide susceptibility of the *Burkholderia cepacia* complex. *J Antimicrob Chemother.* 2009;63:502-510.

88. Lerma LL, Benomar N, Casado Muñoz Mdel C, Gálvez A, Abriouel H. Correlation between antibiotic and biocide resistance in mesophilic and psychrotrophic *Pseudomonas* spp. isolated from slaughterhouse surfaces throughout meat chain production. *Food Microbiol.* 2015;51:33-44.

89. Cowley NL, Forbes S, Amézquita SA, McClure P, Humphreys GJ, McBain AJ. Effects of formulation on microbicide potency and mitigation of the development of bacterial insusceptibility. *Appl Environ Microbiol.* 2015;81:7330-7338.

90. Cole EC, Addison RM, Rubino JR, et al. Investigation of antibiotic and antibacterial agent cross-resistance in target bacteria from homes of antibacterial product users and nonusers. *J Appl Microbiol.* 2003;95:664-679.

91. Cole EC, Addison RM, Dulaney PD, Leese KE, Madanat HM, Guffey AM. Investigation of antibiotic and antibacterial susceptibility and resistance in *Staphylococcus* form the skin of users and non-users of antibacterial wash products in home environments. *Int J Microbiol Res.* 2011;3:90-96.

92. Aiello AE, Marshall B, Levy SB, Della-Latta P, Larson E. Relationship between triclosan and susceptibility of bacteria isolated from hands in the community. *Antimicrob Agents Chemother.* 2004;48: 2973-2979.

93. Carson RT, Larson E, Levy SB, Marshall B, Aiello AE. Use of antibacterial consumer products containing quaternary ammonium compounds and drug resistance in the community. *J Antimicrob Chemother.* 2008;62:1160-1162.

94. McMurry LM, Oethinger M, Levy SB. Overexpression of *marA*, *soxS*, or *acrAB* produces resistance to triclosan in laboratory and clinical strains of *Escherichia coli*. *FEMS Microbiol Lett.* 1998;166:305-309.

95. McMurry LM, McDermott PF, Levy SB. Genetic evidence that InhA of *Mycobacterium smegmatis* is a target for triclosan. *Antimicrob Agents Chemother.* 1999;43:711-713.

96. Cottell A, Denyer SP, Hanlon GW, Ochs D, Maillard J-Y. Triclosan-tolerant bacteria: changes in susceptibility to antibiotics. *J Hosp Infect.* 2009;72:71-76.

97. Winder CL, Al-Adham IS, Abdel Malek SM, Buultjens TE, Horrocks AJ, Collier PJ. Outer membrane protein shifts in biocide-resistant *Pseudomonas aeruginosa* PAO1. *J Appl Microbiol.* 2000;89:289-295.

98. Walsh SE, Maillard J-Y, Russell AD, Charbonneau DL, Bartolo RG, Catrenich C. Development of bacterial resistance to several biocides and effects on antibiotic susceptibility. *J Hosp Infect.* 2003;55:98-107.

99. Tattawasart U, Maillard J-Y, Furr JR, Russell AD. Development of resistance to chlorhexidine diacetate and cetylpyridinium chloride in *Pseudomonas stutzeri* and changes in antibiotic susceptibility. *J Hosp Infect.* 1999;42:219-229.

100. Thomas L, Maillard J-Y, Lambert RJ, Russell AD. Development of resistance to chlorhexidine diacetate in *Pseudomonas aeruginosa* and the effect of "residual" concentration. *J Hosp Infect.* 2000;46:297-303.

101. Thomas L, Russell AD, Maillard J-Y. Antimicrobial activity of chlorhexidine diacetate and benzalkonium chloride against *Pseudomonas aeruginosa* and its response to biocide residues. *J Appl Microbiol.* 2005;98:533-543.

102. Molina-González D, Alonso-Calleja C, Alonso-Hernando A, Capita R. Effect of sub-lethal concentrations of biocides on the susceptibility to antibiotics of multi-drug resistant *Salmonella enterica* strains. *Food Control.* 2014;40:329-334.

103. Gadea R, Fuentes MÁF, Pulido RP, Gálvez A, Ortega E. Effects of exposure to quaternary-ammonium-based biocides on antimicrobial susceptibility and tolerance to physical stresses in bacteria from organic foods. *Food Microbiol.* 2017;63:58-71.

104. Gadea R, Glibota N, Pulido RP, Gálvez A, Ortega E. Adaptation to biocides cetrimide and chlorhexidine in bacteria from organic foods: association with tolerance to other antimicrobials and physical stresses. *J Agric Food Chem.* 2017;65:1758-1770.

105. Gadea R, Fuentes MÁF, Pulido RP, Gálvez A, Ortega E. Adaptive tolerance to phenolic biocides in bacteria from organic foods: effects on antimicrobial susceptibility and tolerance to physical stresses. *Food Res Int.* 2016;85:131-143.

106. Manzoor SE, Lambert PA, Griffiths PA, Gill MJ, Fraise AP. Reduced glutaraldehyde susceptibility in *Mycobacterium chelonae* associated with altered cell wall polysaccharides. *J Antimicrob Chemother.* 1999;43:759-765.

107. Fraud S, Maillard J-Y, Russell AD. Comparison of the mycobactericidal activity of *ortho*-phthalaldehyde, glutaraldehyde and other dialdehydes by a quantitative suspension test. *J Hosp Infect.* 2001;48:214-221.

108. Wisplinghoff H, Schmitt R, Wöhrmann A, Stefanik D, Seifert H. Resistance to disinfectants in epidemiologically defined clinical isolates of *Acinetobacter baumannii*. *J Hosp Infect.* 2007;66:174-181.

109. Bock LJ, Wand ME, Sutton JM. Varying activity of chlorhexidine-based disinfectants against *Klebsiella pneumoniae* clinical isolates and adapted strains. *J Hosp Infect.* 2016;93:42-48.

110. Liu Q, Zhao H, Han L, Shu W, Wu Q, Ni Y. Frequency of biocide-resistant genes and susceptibility to chlorhexidine in high-level mupirocin-resistant, methicillin-resistant *Staphylococcus aureus* (MuH MRSA). *Diagn Microbiol Infect Dis.* 2015;82:278-283.

111. Hijazi K, Mukhopadhya I, Abbott F, et al. Susceptibility to chlorhexidine amongst multidrug-resistant clinical isolates of *Staphylococcus epidermidis* from bloodstream infections. *Int J Antimicrob Agents.* 2016;48:86-90.

112. Conceição T, Coelho C, de Lencastre H, Aires-de-Sousa M. High prevalence of biocide resistance determinants in *Staphylococcus aureus* isolates from three African countries. *Antimicrob Agents Chemother.* 2016;60:678-681.

113. Lear JC, Maillard J-Y, Dettmar P, Goddard PA, Russell AD. Chloroxylenol- and triclosan-tolerant bacteria from industrial sources. *J Ind Microbiol Biotechnol.* 2002;29:238-242.

114. Lavilla Lerma L, Benomar N, Gálvez A, Abriouel H. Prevalence of bacteria resistant to antibiotics and/or biocides on meat processing plant surfaces throughout meat chain production. *Int J Food Microbiol.* 2013;161:97-106.

115. Burgos MJG, Márquez FML, Pulido RP, Gálvez A, López RL. Virulence factors and antimicrobial resistance in *Escherichia coli* strains isolated from hen egg shells. *Int J Food Microbiol.* 2016;238:89-95.

116. Martínez-Suárez JV, Ortiz S, López-Alonso V. Potential impact of the resistance to quaternary ammonium disinfectants on the persistence of *Listeria monocytogenes* in food processing environments. *Front Microbiol.* 2016;7:638. doi:10.3389/fmicb.2016.00638.

117. Alonso-Calleja C, Guerrero-Ramos E, Alonso-Hernando A, Capita R. Adaptation and cross-adaptation of *Escherichia coli* ATCC 12806 to several food-grade biocides. *Food Control.* 2015;56:86-94.

118. Ciusa ML, Furi L, Knight D, et al. A novel resistance mechanism to triclosan that suggests horizontal gene transfer and demonstrates a potential selective pressure for reduced biocide susceptibility in clinical strains of *Staphylococcus aureus*. *Int J Antimicrob Agents.* 2012;40:210-220.

119. Lear JC, Maillard J-Y, Dettmar PW, Goddard PA, Russell AD. Chloroxylenol- and triclosan-tolerant bacteria from industrial sources—susceptibility to antibiotics and other biocides. *Int Biodeterior Biodegradation.* 2006;57:51-56.

120. Denyer SP, Stewart GSAB. Mechanisms of action of disinfectants. *Int Biodeterior Biodegradation.* 1998;41:261-268.

121. Maillard J-Y. Bacterial target sites for biocide action. *J Appl Microbiol.* 2002;92:16-27.

122. Russell AD, McDonnell G. Concentration: a major factor in studying biocidal action. *J Hosp Infect.* 2000;44:1-3.

123. Barry MA, Craven DE, Goularte TA, Lichtenberg DA. *Serratia marcescens* contamination of antiseptic soap containing triclosan: implications for nosocomial infection. *Infect Control.* 1984;5:427-430.

124. Wesgate R, Rauwell G, Criquelion J, Maillard J-Y. Impact of standard test protocols on sporicidal efficacy. *J Hosp Infect.* 2016;93:256-262.

125. Leggett MJ, Setlow P, Sattar SA, Maillard J-Y. Assessing the activity of microbicides against bacterial spores: knowledge and pitfalls. *J Appl Microbiol.* 2016;120:1174-1180.

126. Siani H, Cooper C, Maillard J-Y. Efficacy of "sporicidal" wipes against *Clostridium difficile*. *Am J Infect Control.* 2011;39:212-218.

127. Poole K. Mechanisms of bacterial biocide and antibiotic resistance. *J Appl Microbiol.* 2002;92:55-64.

128. Knapp L, Rushton L, Stapleton H, et al. The effect of cationic microbicide exposure against *Burkholderia cepacia* complex (Bcc); the use of *Burkholderia lata* strain 383 as a model bacterium. *J Appl Microbiol.* 2013;115:1117-1126.

129. Escalada MG, Russell AD, Maillard J-Y, Ochs D. Triclosan-bacteria interactions: single or multiple target sites? *Lett Appl Microbiol.* 2005;41:476-481.

130. Tattawasart U, Maillard J-Y, Furr JR, Russell AD. Outer membrane changes in *Pseudomonas stutzeri* strains resistant to chlorhexidine diacetate and cetylpyridinium chloride. *Int J Antimicrob Agents.* 2000;16:233-238.

131. Tattawasart U, Hann AC, Maillard J-Y, Furr JR, Russell AD. Cytological changes in chlorhexidine-resistant isolates of *Pseudomonas stutzeri. J Antimicrob Chemother.* 2000;45:145-152.

132. Braoudaki M, Hilton AC. Mechanisms of resistance in *Salmonella enterica* adapted to erythromycin, benzalkonium chloride and triclosan. *Int J Antimicrob Agents.* 2005;25:31-37.

133. Webber MA, Randall LP, Cooles S, Woodward MJ, Piddock LJ. Triclosan resistance in *Salmonella enterica* serovar Typhimurium. *J Antimicrob Chemother.* 2008;62:83-91.

134. Weber H, Polen T, Heuveling J, Wendisch VF, Hengge R. Genome-wide analysis of the general stress response network in *Escherichia coli*: σ^s-dependent genes, promoters, and sigma factor selectivity. *J Bacteriol.* 2005;187:1591-1603.

135. Condell O, Power KA, Händler K, et al. Comparative analysis of *Salmonella* susceptibility and tolerance to the biocide chlorhexidine identifies a complex cellular defense network. *Front Microbiol.* 2014;5:373. doi:10.3389/fmicb.2014.00373.

136. Denyer SP, Maillard J-Y. Cellular impermeability and uptake of biocides and antibiotics in gram-negative bacteria. *J Appl Microbiol.* 2002;92:35-45.

137. Lambert PA. Cellular impermeability and uptake of biocides and antibiotics in gram-positive bacteria and mycobacteria. *J Appl Microbiol.* 2002;92:46-54.

138. Leggett MJ, Schwarz JS, Burke PA, McDonnell G, Denyer SP, Maillard J-Y. Resistance to and killing by the sporicidal microbicide peracetic acid. *J Antimicrob Chemother.* 2015;70:773-779.

139. Champlin FR, Ellison ML, Bullard JW, Conrad RS. Effect of outer membrane permeabilisation on intrinsic resistance to low triclosan levels in *Pseudomonas aeruginosa. International J Antimicrob Agents.* 2005;26:159-164.

140. Ayres HM, Payne DN, Furr JR, Russell AD. Effect of permeabilizing agents on antibacterial activity against a simple *Pseudomonas aeruginosa* biofilm. *Lett Appl Microbiol.* 1998;27:79-82.

141. Munton TJ, Russell AD. Effect of glutaraldehyde on protoplasts of *Bacillus megaterium. J Gen Microbiol.* 1970;63:367-370.

142. Codling CE, Jones BV, Mahenthiralingam E, Russell AD, Maillard J-Y. Identification of genes involved in the resistance *Serratia marcescens* to polyquaternium-1. *J Antimicrob Chemother.* 2004;54:370-375.

143. Fernández-Cuenca F, Tomás M, Caballero-Moyano FJ, et al. Reduced susceptibility to biocides in *Acinetobacter baumannii*: association with resistance to antimicrobials, epidemiological behaviour, biological cost and effect on the expression of genes encoding porins and efflux pumps. *J Antimicrob Chemother.* 2015;70:3222-3229.

144. Pagès JM, James CE, Winterhalter M. The porin and the permeating antibiotic: a selective diffusion barrier in gram-negative bacteria. *Nat Rev Microbiol.* 2008;6:893-903.

145. Nikaido H. Molecular basis of bacterial outer membrane permeability revisited. *Microbiol Mol Biol Rev.* 2003;67:593-656.

146. Tabata A, Nagamune H, Maeda T, Murakami K, Miyake Y, Kourai H. Correlation between resistance of *Pseudomonas aeruginosa* to quaternary ammonium compounds and expression of outer membrane protein OprR. *Antimicrob Agents Chemother.* 2003;47:2093-2099.

147. Walsh SE, Maillard J-Y, Russell AD, Hann AC. Possible mechanisms for the relative efficacies of *ortho*-phthalaldehyde and glutaraldehyde against glutaraldehyde-resistant *Mycobacterium chelonae. J Appl Microbiol.* 2001;91:80-92.

148. McNeil MR, Brennan PJ. Structure, function and biogenesis of the cell envelope of mycobacteria in relation to bacterial physiology, pathogenesis and drug resistance; some thoughts and possibilities arising from recent structural information. *Res Microbiol.* 1991;142:451-463.

149. Broadley SJ, Jenkins PA, Furr JR, Russell AD. Potentiation of the effects of chlorhexidine diacetate and cetylpyridinium chloride on mycobacteria by ethambutol. *J Med Microbiol.* 1995;43:458-460.

150. Fraud S, Hann AC, Maillard J-Y, Russell AD. Effects of *ortho*-phthalaldehyde, glutaraldehyde and chlorhexidine diacetate on *Mycobacterium chelonae* and *Mycobacterium abscessus* strains with modified permeability. *J Antimicrob Chemother.* 2003;51:575-584.

151. Svetlíková Z, Škovierová H, Niederweis M, Gaillard J-L, McDonnell G, Jackson M. Role of porins in the susceptibility of *Mycobacterium smegmatis* and *Mycobacterium chelonae* to aldehyde-based disinfectants and drugs. *Antimicrob Agents Chemother.* 2009;53:4015-4018.

152. Jones MW, Herd TM, Christie HJ. Resistance of *Pseudomonas aeruginosa* to amphoteric and quaternary ammonium biocides. *Microbios.* 1989;58:49-61.

153. Méchin L, Dubois-Brissonnet F, Heyd B, Leveau JY. Adaptation of *Pseudomonas aeruginosa* ATCC 15442 to didecyldimethylammonium bromide induces changes in membrane fatty acid composition and in resistance of cells. *J Appl Microbiol.* 1999;86:859-866.

154. Guérin-Méchin L, Dubois-Brissonnet F, Heyd B, Leveau JY. Specific variations of fatty acid composition of *Pseudomonas aeruginosa* ATCC 15442 induced by quaternary ammonium compounds and relation with resistance to bactericidal activity. *J Appl Microbiol.* 1999;87:735-742.

155. Guérin-Méchin L, Dubois-Brissonnet F, Heyd B, Leveau JY. Quaternary ammonium compounds stresses induce specific variations in fatty acid composition of *Pseudomonas aeruginosa. Int J Food Microbiol.* 2000;55:157-159.

156. Tkachenko O, Shepard J, Aris VM, et al. A triclosan-ciprofloxacin cross-resistant mutant strain of *Staphylococcus aureus* displays an alteration in the expression of several cell membrane structural and functional genes. *Res Microbiol.* 2007;158:651-658.

157. Boeris PS, Domenech CE, Lucchesi GI. Modification of phospholipid composition in *Pseudomonas putida* A ATCC 12633 induced by contact with tetradecyltrimethylammonium. *J Appl Microbiol.* 2007;103:1048-1054.

158. Gandhi PA, Sawant AD, Wilson LA, Ahearn DG. Adaptation and growth of *Serratia marcescens* in contact lens disinfectant solution containing chlorhexidine gluconate. *Appl Environ Microbiol.* 1993;59:183-188.

159. Brözel VS, Cloete TE. Resistance of *Pseudomonas aeruginosa* to isothiazolone. *J Appl Bacteriol.* 1994;76:576-582.

160. Bore E, Hébraud M, Chafsey I, et al. Adapted tolerance to benzalkonium chloride in *Escherichia coli* K-12 studied by transcriptome and proteome analyses. *Microbiology.* 2007;153:935-946.

161. Karatzas KA, Randall LP, Webber M, et al. Phenotypic and proteomic characterization of multiply antibiotic-resistant variants of *Salmonella enterica* serovar Typhimurium selected following exposure to disinfectants. *Appl Environ Microbiol.* 2008;74:1508-1516.

162. Bruinsma GM, Rustema-Abbing M, van der Mei HC, Lakkis C, Busscher HJ. Resistance to a polyquaternium-1 lens care solution and isoelectric points of *Pseudomonas aeruginosa* strains. *J Antimicrob Chemother.* 2006;57:764-766.

163. Piddock LJ. Clinically relevant chromosomally encoded multidrug resistance efflux pump in bacteria. *Clin Microbiol Rev.* 2006;19:382-402.

164. Poole K. Efflux pumps as antimicrobial resistance mechanisms. *Ann Med.* 2007;39:162-176.

165. Poole K. Outer membranes and efflux: the path to multidrug resistance in gram-negative bacteria. *Curr Pharm Biotechnol.* 2002;3:77-98.

166. Buffet-Bataillon S, Tattevin P, Maillard J-Y, Bonnaure-Mallet M, Jolivet-Gougeon A. Efflux pump induction by quaternary ammonium compounds and fluoroquinolone resistance in bacteria. *Future Microbiol.* 2016;11:81-92.

167. Schindler BD, Kaatz GW. Multidrug efflux pumps of gram-positive bacteria. *Drug Res Updat.* 2016;27:1-13.

168. Shamsudin MN, Alreshidi MA, Hamat RA, Alshrari AS, Atshan SS, Neela V. High prevalence of qacA/B carriage among clinical isolates of meticillin-resistant *Staphylococcus aureus* in Malaysia. *J Hosp Infect.* 2012;81:206-208.

169. Fuentes MÁF, Morente EO, Abriouel H, Pulido RP, Gálvez A. Antimicrobial resistance determinants in antibiotic and biocide resistant gram-negative bacteria from organic foods. *Food Control*. 2014;37:9-14.

170. Smith K, Gemmell CG, Hunter IS. The association between biocide tolerance and the presence or absence of *qac* genes among hospital-acquired and community-acquired MRSA isolates. *J Antimicrob Chemother*. 2008;61:78-84.

171. Conficoni D, Losasso C, Cortini E, et al. Resistance to biocides in *Listeria monocytogenes* collected in meat-processing environments. *Front Microbiol*. 2016;7:1627. doi:10.3389/fmicb.2016.01627.

172. Márquez MLF, Burgos MJG, Aguayo MCL, Pulido RP, Gálvez A, Lucas RL. Characterization of biocide-tolerant bacteria isolated from cheese and dairy small-medium enterprises. *Food Microbiol*. 2017;62:77-81.

173. Márquez FML, Abriouel H, Morente EO, Pulido RP, Gálvez A. Genetic determinants of antimicrobial resistance in gram positive bacteria from organic foods. *Int J Food Microbiol*. 2014;172:49-56.

174. Mc Cay PH, Ocampo-Sosa AA, Fleming GT. Effect of subinhibitory concentrations of benzalkonium chloride on the competitiveness of *Pseudomonas aeruginosa* grown in continuous culture. *Microbiology*. 2010;156:30-38.

175. Tennent JM, Lyon BR, Midgley M, Jones IG, Purewal AS, Skurray RA. Physical and biochemical characterization of the *qacA* gene encoding antiseptic and disinfectant resistance in *Staphylococcus aureus*. *J Gen Microbiol*. 1989;135:1-10.

176. Littlejohn TG, Paulsen IT, Gillespie M, et al. Substrate specificity and energetics of antiseptic and disinfectant resistance in *Staphylococcus aureus*. *FEMS Microbiol Lett*. 1992;74:259-265.

177. Leelaporn A, Paulsen IT, Tennent JM, Littlejohn TG, Skurray RA. Multidrug resistance to antiseptics and disinfectants in coagulase-negative staphylococci. *J Med Microbiol*. 1994;40:214-220.

178. Heir E, Sundheim G, Holck AL. The *Staphylococcus qacH* gene product: a new member of the SMR family encoding multidrug resistance. *FEMS Microbiol Lett*. 1998;163:49-56.

179. Heir E, Sundheim G, Holck AL. The *qacG* gene on plasmid pST94 confers resistance to quaternary ammonium compounds in staphylococci isolated from the food industry. *J Appl Microbiol*. 1999;86:378-388.

180. Rouch DA, Cram DS, DiBernadino D, Littlejohn TG, Skurray RA. Efflux-mediated antiseptic resistance gene *qacA* in *Staphylococcus aureus*: common ancestry with tetracycline and sugar transport proteins. *Mol Microbiol*. 1990;4:2051-2062.

181. Ntreh AT, Weeks JW, Nickels LM, Zgurskaya HI. Opening the channel: the two functional interfaces of *Pseudomonas aeruginosa* OpmH with the triclosan efflux pump TriABC. *J Bacteriol*. 2016;198:3176-3185.

182. Romanova NA, Wolffs PFG, Brovko LY, Griffiths MW. Role of efflux pumps in adaptation and resistance of *Listeria monocytogenes* to benzalkonium chloride. *Appl Environ Microbiol*. 2006;72:3498-3503.

183. Tamburro M, Ripabelli G, Vitullo M, et al. Gene expression in *Listeria monocytogenes* exposed to sublethal concentration of benzalkonium chloride. *Comp Immunol Microbiol Infect Dis*. 2015;40:31-39.

184. Jaglic Z, Cervinkova D. Genetic basis of resistance to quaternary ammonium compounds—the *qac* genes and their role: a review. *Veter Med*. 2012;57:275-281.

185. Rushton L, Sass A, Baldwin A, Dowson CG, Donoghue D, Mahenthiralingam E. Key role for efflux in the preservative susceptibility and adaptive resistance of *Burkholderia cepacia* complex bacteria. *Antimicrob Agents Chemother*. 2013;57:2972-2980.

186. Ahn Y, Kim JM, Kweon O, et al. Intrinsic resistance of *Burkholderia cepacia* complex to benzalkonium chloride. *MBio*. 2016;7:e01716-16. doi:10.1128/mBio.01716-16.

187. McMurry LM, Oethinger M, Levy SB. Triclosan targets lipid synthesis. *Nature*. 1998;394:531-532.

188. Chuanchuen R, Beinlich K, Hoang TT, Becher A, Karkhoff-Schweizer RR, Schweizer HP. Cross-resistance between triclosan and antibiotics in *Pseudomonas aeruginosa* is mediated by multidrug efflux pumps: exposure of a susceptible mutant strain to triclosan selects *nxfB* mutants overexpressing MexCD-OprJ. *Antimicrob Agents Chemother*. 2001;45:428-432.

189. Chuanchuen R, Narasaki CT, Schweizer HP. The MexJK efflux pump of *Pseudomonas aeruginosa* requires OprM for antibiotic efflux but not for effect of triclosan. *J Bacteriol*. 2002;184:5036-5044.

190. Mima T, Joshi S, Gomez-Escalada M, Schweizer HP. Identification and characterization of TriABC-OpmH, a triclosan efflux pump of *Pseudomonas aeruginosa* requiring two membrane fusion proteins. *J Bacteriol*. 2007;189:7600-7609.

191. Randall LP, Cooles SW, Coldham NG, et al. Commonly used farm disinfectants can select for mutant *Salmonella enterica* serovar Typhimurium with decreased susceptibility to biocides and antibiotics without compromising virulence. *J Antimicrob Chemother*. 2007;60: 1273-1280.

192. Chuanchuen R, Karkhoff-Schweizer RR, Schweizer HP. High-level triclosan resistance in *Pseudomonas aeruginosa* is solely a result of efflux. *Am J Infect Control*. 2003;31:124-127.

193. Curiao T, Marchi E, Viti C, et al. Polymorphic variation in susceptibility and metabolism of triclosan-resistant mutants of *Escherichia coli* and *Klebsiella pneumoniae* clinical strains obtained after exposure to biocides and antibiotics. *Antimicrob Agents Chemother*. 2015;59: 3413-3423.

194. Buckley A, Webber MA, Cooles S, et al. The AcrAB-TolC efflux system of *Salmonella enterica* serovar Typhimurium plays a role in pathogenesis. *Cell Microbiol*. 2006;8:847-856.

195. Sánchez P, Moreno E, Martinez JL. The biocide triclosan selects *Stenotrophomonas maltophilia* mutants that overproduce the SmeDEF multidrug efflux pump. *Antimicrob Agents Chemother*. 2005;49:781-782.

196. Moken MC, McMurry LM, Levy SB. Selection of multiple-antibiotic-resistant (Mar) mutants of *Escherichia coli* by using the disinfectant pine oil: roles of the *mar* and *acrAB* loci. *Antimicrob Agents Chemother*. 1997;41:2770-2772.

197. Pumbwe L, Randall LP, Woodward MJ, Piddock LJ. Expression of the efflux pump genes *cmeB*, *cmeF* and the porin gene *porA* in multiple-antibiotic-resistant *Campylobacter jejuni*. *J Antimicrob Chemother*. 2005;54:341-347.

198. Bailey AM, Constantinidou C, Ivens AI, et al. Exposure of *Escherichia coli* and *Salmonella enterica* serovar Typhimurium to triclosan induces a species-specific response, including drug detoxification. *J Antimicrob Chemother*. 2009;64:973-985.

199. Gothwal R, Thatikonda S. Role of environmental pollution in prevalence of antibiotic resistant bacteria in aquatic environment of river: case of Musi river, South India. *Water Environ J*. 2017;31:456-462.

200. Laffite A, Kilunga PI, Kayembe JM, et al. Hospital effluents are one of several sources of metal, antibiotic resistance genes, and bacterial markers disseminated in sub-Saharan urban rivers. *Frontiers Microbiol*. 2016;7:1128. doi:10.3389/fmicb.2016.01128.

201. Östman M, Lindberg RH, Fick J, Björn E, Tysklind M. Screening of biocides, metals and antibiotics in Swedish sewage sludge and wastewater. *Water Res*. 2017;115:318-328.

202. Nayak SP, Ray P, Sahoo PK. Heavy metal tolerance and antibiotic profiling of bacterial isolates from hot springs of Odisha. *J Pure Appl Microbiol*. 2013;7:2301-2307.

203. Yamina B, Tahar B, Laure FM. Isolation and screening of heavy metal resistant bacteria from wastewater: a study of heavy metal co-resistance and antibiotics resistance. *Water Sci Technol*. 2012;66:2041-2048.

204. Chenia HY, Jacobs A. Antimicrobial resistance, heavy metal resistance and integron content in bacteria isolated from a South African tilapia aquaculture system. *Dis Aquat Org*. 2017;126:199-209.

205. Jie S, Li M, Gan M, Zhu J, Yin H, Liu X. Microbial functional genes enriched in the Xiangjiang river sediments with heavy metal contamination. *BMC Microbiol*. 2016;16:179. doi:10.1186/s12866-016-0800-x.

206. Argüello JM, Raimunda D, Padilla-Benavides T. Mechanisms of copper homeostasis in bacteria. *Front Cell Infect Microbiol*. 2013;3:73. doi:10.3389/fcimb.2013.00073.

207. Guo JH, Gao SH, Lu J, Bond PL, Verstraete W, Yuan ZG. Copper oxide nanoparticles induce lysogenic bacteriophage and metal-resistance genes in *Pseudomonas aeruginosa* PAO1. *ACS Appl Mat Inter*. 2017;9: 22298-22307.

208. Williams CL, Neu HM, Gilbreath JJ, Michel SL, Zurawski DV, Merrell DS. Copper resistance of the emerging pathogen *Acinetobacter baumannii*. *Appl Environ Microbiol*. 2016;82:6174-6188.

209. Staehlin BM, Gibbons JG, Rokas A, O'Halloran TV, Slot JC. Evolution of a heavy metal homeostasis/resistance island reflects increasing copper stress in enterobacteria. *Gen Biol Evol*. 2016;8:811-826.

210. Kümmerle N, Feucht HH, Kaulfers PM. Plasmid-mediated formaldehyde resistance in *Escherichia coli*: characterization of resistance gene. *Antimicrob Agents Chemother*. 1996;40:2276-2279.

211. Greenberg JT, Demple B. A global response induced in *Escherichia coli* by redox-cycling agents overlaps with that induced by peroxide stress. *J Bacteriol*. 1989;171:3933-3939.

212. Demple B. Redox signaling and gene control in the *Escherichia coli* *soxRS* oxidative stress regulon: a review. *Gene*. 1996;179:53-57.

213. Martin DJ, Wesgate R, Denyer SP, McDonnell G, Maillard J-Y. *Bacillus subtilis* vegetative isolate surviving chlorine dioxide exposure: an elusive mechanism of resistance. *J Appl Microbiol*. 2015;119:1541-1551.

214. Brown MR, William P. Influence of substrate limitation and growth-phase on sensitivity to antimicrobial agents. *J Antimicrob Chemother*. 1985;15:7-14.

215. Wright NE, Gilbert P. Influence of specific growth rate and nutrient limitation upon the sensitivity of *Escherichia coli* towards chlorhexidine diacetate. *J Appl Bacteriol*. 1987;62:309-314.

216. Gomez Escalada M, Harwood JL, Maillard J-Y, Ochs D. Triclosan inhibition of fatty acid synthesis and its effect on growth of *Escherichia coli* and *Pseudomas aeruginosa*. *J Antimicrob Chemother*. 2005;55:879-882.

217. Wu VC. A review of microbial injury and recovery methods in food. *Food Microbiol*. 2008;25:735-744.

218. Webber MA, Coldham NG, Woodward MJ, Piddock LJV. Proteomic analysis of triclosan resistance in *Salmonella enterica* serovar Typhimurium. *J Antimicrob Chemother*. 2008;62:92-97.

219. Levy CW, Roujeinikova A, Sedelnikova S, et al. Molecular basis of triclosan activity. *Nature*. 1999;398:383-384.

220. Curiao T, Marchi E, Grandgirard D, et al. Multiple adaptive routes of *Salmonella enterica* Typhimurium to biocide and antibiotic exposure. *BMC Genomics*. 2016;17:491.

221. Seaman P, Ochs D, Day MJ. Small-colony variants: a novel mechanism for triclosan resistance in methicillin-resistant *Staphylococcus aureus*. *J Antimicrob Chemother*. 2007;59:43-50.

222. Abdel Malek SM, Al-Adham IS, Winder CL, Buultjens TE, Gartland KM, Collier PJ. Antimicrobial susceptibility changes and T-OMP shifts in pythione-passaged planktonic cultures of *Pseudomonas aeruginosa* PAO1. *J Appl Microbiol*. 2002;92:729-736.

223. Wang S, Deng K, Zaremba S, et al. Transcriptomic response of *Escherichia coli* O157:H7 to oxidative stress. *Appl Environ Microbiol*. 2009;75:6110-6123.

224. Pi BR, Yu DL, Hua XT, Ruan Z, Yu YS. Genomic and transcriptome analysis of triclosan response of a multidrug-resistant *Acinetobacter baumannii* strain, MDR-ZJ06. *Arch Microbiol*. 2017;199:223-230.

225. Yan X, Budin-Verneuil A, Verneuil N, et al. Transcriptomic response of *Enterococcus faecalis* V583 to low hydrogen peroxide levels. *Curr Microbiol*. 2017;70:156-168.

226. Brown MR, Gilbert P. Sensitivity of biofilms to antimicrobial agents. *J Appl Bacteriol*. 1993;74:87S-97S.

227. Ashby MJ, Neale JE, Knott SJ, Critchley IA. Effect of antibiotics on non-growing planktonic cells and biofilms of *Escherichia coli*. *J Antimicrob Chemother*. 1994;33:443-452.

228. Fux CA, Costerton JW, Stewart PS, Stoodley P. Survival strategies of infectious biofilms. *Trends Microbiol*. 2005;13:34-40.

229. Donlan RM, Costerton JW. Biofilms: survival mechanisms of clinically relevant microorganisms. *Clin Microbiol Rev*. 2002;15:167-193.

230. Vickery K, Hu H, Jacombs AS, Bradshaw DA, Deva AK. A review of bacterial biofilms and their role in device-associated infection. *Health Infect*. 2013;18:61-66.

231. Das JR, Bhakoo M, Jones MV, Gilbert P. Changes in the biocide susceptibility of *Staphylococcus epidermidis* and *Escherichia coli* cells associated with rapid attachment to plastic surfaces. *J Appl Microbiol*. 1998;84:852-858.

232. Flemming HC, Wingender J, Szewzyk U, Steinberg P, Rice SA, Kjelleberg S. Biofilms: an emergent form of bacterial life. *Nat Rev Microbiol*. 2016;14:563-575.

233. Roberts C. The role of biofilms in reprocessing medical devices. *Am J Infect Control*. 2013;41:S77-S80.

234. Herrin A, Loyola M, Bocian S, et al. Standards of infection prevention in reprocessing flexible gastrointestinal endoscopes. *Gastroenterol Nurs*. 2016;39:404-418.

235. Pajkos A, Vickery K, Cossart Y. Is biofilm accumulation on endoscope tubing a contributor to the failure of cleaning and decontamination? *J Hosp Infect*. 2004;58:224-229.

236. Akinbobola AB, Sherry L, Mckay WG, Ramage G, Williams C. Tolerance of *Pseudomonas aeruginosa* in in-vitro biofilms to high-level peracetic acid disinfection. *J Hosp Infect*. 2017;97:162-168.

237. Pan Y, Breidt F Jr, Kathariou S. Resistance of *Listeria monocytogenes* biofilms to sanitizing agents in a simulated food processing environment. *Appl Environ Microbiol*. 2006;72:7711-7717.

238. Di Ciccio P, Vergara A, Festino A, et al. Biofilm formation by *Staphylococcus aureus* on food contact surfaces: relationship with temperature and cell surface hydrophobicity. *Food Control*. 2015;50:930-936.

239. Chmielewski RAN, Frank JF. Biofilm formation and control in food processing facilities. *Comp Rev Food Sci Food Safety*. 2003;2:22-32.

240. Kim CY, Ryu GJ, Park HY, Ryu K. Resistance of *Staphylococcus aureus* on food contact surfaces with different surface characteristics to chemical sanitizers. *J Food Safety*. 2017;4:e12354. doi:10.1111/jfs.12354.

241. Moore LE, Ledder RG, Gilbert P, McBain AJ. In vitro study of the effect of cationic biocides on bacterial population dynamics and susceptibility. *Appl Environ Microbiol*. 2008;74:4825-4834.

242. Kümmerer K, Al-Ahmad A, Henninger A. Use of chemotaxonomy to study the influence of benzalkonium chloride on bacterial populations in biodegradation testing. *Acta Hydroch Hydrobiol*. 2002;30:171-178.

243. McBain AJ, Bartolo RG, Catrenich CE, et al. Exposure of sink drain microcosms to triclosan: population dynamics and antimicrobial susceptibility. *Appl Environ Microbiol*. 2003;69:5433-5442.

244. Jones GL, Muller CT, O'Reilly M, Stickler DJ. Effect of triclosan on the development of bacterial biofilms by urinary tract pathogens on urinary catheters. *J Antimicrob Chemother*. 2006;57:266-272.

245. Forbes S, Cowley N, Humphreys G, Mistry H, Amézquita A, McBain AJ. Formulation of biocides increases antimicrobial potency and mitigates the enrichment of nonsusceptible bacteria in multispecies biofilms. *Appl Environ Microbiol*. 2017;83:e03054-16. doi:10.1128/AEM.03054-16.

246. Bridier A, Sanchez-Vizuete MDP, Le Coq D, et al. Biofilms of a *Bacillus subtilis* endoscope WD isolate that protect *Staphylococcus aureus* from peracetic acid. *PLoS One*. 2012;7:e44506.

247. Pang XY, Yang YS, Yuk HG. Biofilm formation and disinfectant resistance of *Salmonella* sp. in mono- and dual-species with *Pseudomonas aeruginosa*. *J Appl Microbiol*. 2017;123:651-660.

248. Sanchez-Vizuete P, Orgaz B, Aymerich S, Le Coq D, Briandet R. Pathogens protection against the action of disinfectants in multispecies biofilms. *Front Microbiol*. 2015;6:705. doi:10.3389/fmicb.2015.00705.

249. Lin HR, Zhu X, Wang YX, Yu X. Effect of sodium hypochlorite on typical biofilms formed in drinking water distribution systems. *J Water Health*. 2017;15:218-227.

250. Flach C-F, Pal C, Svensson CJ, et al. Does antifouling paint select for antibiotic resistance? *Sci Total Environ*. 2017;590-591:461-468.

251. Whiteley GS, Knight JL, Derry CW, Jensen SO, Vickery K, Gosbell IB. A pilot study into locating the bad bugs in a busy intensive care unit. *Am J Infect Control*. 2015;12:1270-1275.

252. Hu H, Johani K, Gosbell IB, et al. Intensive care unit environmental surfaces are contaminated by multidrug-resistant bacteria in biofilms: combined results of conventional culture, pyrosequencing, scanning electron microscopy, and confocal laser microscopy. *J Hosp Infect*. 2015;91:35-44.

253. Almatroudi A, Gosbell IB, Hu H, et al. *Staphylococcus aureus* dry-surface biofilms are not killed by sodium hypochlorite: implications for infection control. *J Hosp Infect*. 2016;93:263-270.

254. Otter JA, Vickery K, Walker JT, et al. Surface-attached cells, biofilms and biocide susceptibility: implications for hospital cleaning and disinfection. *J Hosp Infect*. 2015;89:16-27.

255. Leggett MJ, McDonnell G, Denyer SP, Setlow P, Maillard J-Y. Bacterial spore structures and their protective role in biocide resistance. *J Appl Microbiol*. 2012;113:495-498.

256. Maillard J-Y. Innate resistance to sporicides and potential failure to decontaminate. *J Hosp Infect*. 2010;77:204-209.

257. Cowan AE, Olivastro EM, Koppel DE, Loshon CA, Setlow B, Setlow P. Lipids in the inner membrane of dormant spores of *Bacillus* species are largely immobile. *Proc Natl Acad Sci U S A*. 2004;101:7733-7738.

258. Russell AD. Bacterial spores and chemical sporicidal agents. *Clin Microbiol Rev*. 1990;3:99-119.

259. Webber M, Whitehead RN, Mount M, Loman NJ, Pallen MJ, Piddock LJV. Parallel evolutionary pathways to antibiotic resistance selected by biocide exposure. *J Antimicrob Chemother*. 2015;70:2241-2248.

260. Kaweeteerawat C, Ubol PN, Sangmuang S, Aueviriyavit S, Maniratanachote R. Mechanisms of antibiotic resistance in bacteria mediated by silver nanoparticles. *J Toxicol Environ Health*. 2017;80: 1276-1289.

261. Greenway DL, England RR. The intrinsic resistance of *Escherichia coli* to various antimicrobial agents requires ppGpp and σ^s. *Lett Appl Microbiol*. 1999;29:323-326.

262. Pomposiello PJ, Bennik MH, Demple B. Genome-wide transcriptional profiling of the *Escherichia coli* responses to superoxide stress and sodium salicylate. *J Bacteriol*. 2001;183:3890-3902.

263. Pérez A, Poza M, Aranda J, et al. Effect of transcriptional activators SoxS, RobA, and RamA on expression of multidrug efflux pump AcrAB-TolC in *Enterobacter cloacae*. *Antimicrob Agents Chemother*. 2012;56:6256-6266.

264. Lawler AJ, Ricci V, Busby SJW, Piddock LJV. Genetic inactivation of *acrAB* or inhibition of efflux induces expression of *ramA*. *J Antimicrob Chemother*. 2013;68:1551-1557.

265. Dukan S, Touati D. Hypochlorous acid stress in *Escherichia coli*: resistance, DNA damage, and comparison with hydrogen peroxide stress. *J Bacteriol*. 1996;178:6145-6150.

266. Slany M, Oppelt J, Cincarova L. Formation of *Staphylococcus aureus* biofilm in the presence of sublethal concentrations of disinfectants studied via a transcriptomic analysis using transcriptome sequencing (RNA-seq). *Appl Environ Microbiol*. 2017;83:e01643-17.

267. Wand ME, Bock LJ, Bonney LC, Sutton JM. Mechanisms of increased resistance to chlorhexidine and cross-resistance to colistin following exposure of *Klebsiella pneumoniae* clinical isolates to chlorhexidine. *Antimicrob Chemother*. 2016;61:e01162-16. doi:10.1128/AAC.01162-16.

268. Sánchez MB, Decorosi F, Viti C, Oggioni MR, Martínez JL, Hernández A. Predictive studies suggest that the risk for the selection of antibiotic resistance by biocides is likely low in *Stenotrophomonas maltophilia*. *PLos One*. 2015;10:e0132816.

269. Karatzas KA, Webber MA, Jorgensen F, Woodward MJ, Piddock LJ, Humphrey TJ. Prolonged treatment of *Salmonella enterica* serovar Typhimurium with commercial disinfectants selects for multiple antibiotic resistance, increased efflux and reduced invasiveness. *J Antimicrob Chemother*. 2007;60:947-955.

270. Radeck J, Fritz G, Mascher T. The cell envelope stress response of *Bacillus subtilis*: from static signaling devices to dynamic regulatory network. *Curr Genet*. 2017;63:79-90.

271. Casado Muñoz Mdel C, Benomar N, Ennahar S, et al. Comparative proteomic analysis of a potentially probiotic *Lactobacillus pentosus* MP-10 for the identification of key proteins involved in antibiotic resistance and biocide tolerance. *Int J Food Microbiol*. 2016;222:8-15.

272. Motgatla RM, Gouws PA, Brözel VS. Mechanisms contributing to hypochlorous acid resistance of a *Salmonella* isolate from a poultry-processing plant. *J Appl Microbiol*. 2002;92:566-573.

273. Allen MJ, White GF, Morby AP. The response of *Escherichia coli* to exposure to the biocide polyhexamethylene biguanide. *Microbiology*. 2006;152:989-1000.

274. Slade D, Radman M. Oxidative stress resistance in *Deinococcus radiodurans*. *Microbiol Mol Biol Rev*. 2011;75:133-191.

275. Forbes S, Dobson CB, Humphreys GJ, McBain AJ. Transient and sustained bacterial adaptation following repeated sublethal exposure to microbicides and a novel human antimicrobial peptide. *Antimicrob Agents Chemother*. 2014;58:5809-5817.

276. McDonnell G, Russell AD. Antiseptics and disinfectants: activity, action and resistance. *Clin Microbiol Rev*. 1999;12:147-179.

277. Cerf O, Carpentier B, Sanders P. Tests for determining in-use concentrations of antibiotics and disinfectants are based on entirely different concepts: "resistance" has different meanings. *Int J Food Microbiol*. 2010;136:247-254.

278. Moore JM, Correa R, Rosenberg SM, Hastings PJ. Persistent damaged bases in DNA allow mutagenic break repair in *Escherichia coli*. *PLos Genet*. 2017;13:e1006733. doi:10.1371/journal.pgen.1006733.

279. Heath RJ, Yu YT, Shapiro MA, Olson E, Rock CO. Broad spectrum antimicrobial biocides target the FabI component of fatty acid synthesis. *J Biol Chem*. 1998;273:30316-30320.

280. Chen Y, Pi B, Zhou H, Yu Y, Li L. Triclosan resistance in clinical isolates of *Acinetobacter baumannii*. *J Med Microbiol*. 2009;58: 1086-1091.

281. Zhu L, Lin J, Ma J, Cronan JE, Wang H. Triclosan resistance of *Pseudomonas aeruginosa* PA01 is due to FabV, a triclosan-resistant enoyl-acyl carrier protein reductase. *Antimicrob Agents Chemother*. 2010;54: 689-698.

282. Heath RJ, Li J, Roland GE, Rock CO. Inhibition of the *Staphylococcus aureus* NADPH-dependent Enoyl-acyl carrier protein reductase by triclosan and hexachlorophene. *J Biol Biochem*. 2000;275:4654-4659.

283. Slater-Radosti C, Van Aller G, Greenwood R, et al. Biochemical and genetic characterization of the action of triclosan on *Staphylococcus aureus*. *J Antimicrob Chemother*. 2001;48:1-6.

284. Parikh SL, Xiao G, Tonge PJ. Inhibition of InhA, enoyl reductase from *Mycobacterium tuberculosis* by triclosan and isoniazid. *Biochemistry*. 2000;39:7645-7650.

285. Roujeinikova A, Levy CW, Rowsell S, et al. Crystallographic analysis of triclosan bound to enoyl reductase. *J Mol Biol*. 1999;294:527-535.

286. Stewart MJ, Parikh S, Xiao G, Tonge PJ, Kisker C. Structural basis and mechanisms of enoyl reductase inhibition by triclosan. *J Mol Biol*. 1999;290:859-865.

287. Heath RJ, Rubin JR, Holland DR, Zhang E, Snow ME, Rock CO. Mechanism of triclosan inhibition of bacterial fatty acid biosynthesis. *J Biol Chem*. 1999;274:11110-11114.

288. Maseda H, Hashida Y, Shirai A, Omasa T, Nakae T. Mutation in the *sdeS* gene promotes expression of the sdeAB efflux pump genes and multidrug resistance in *Serratia marcescens*. *Antimicrob Agents Chemother*. 2011;55:2922-2926.

289. Maseda H, Hashida Y, Konaka R, Shirai A, Kourai H. Mutational upregulation of a resistance-nodulation-cell division-type multidrug efflux pump, SdeAB, upon exposure to a biocide, cetylpyridinium chloride, and antibiotic resistance in *Serratia marcescens*. *Antimicrob Agents Chemother*. 2009;53:5230-5235.

290. Sütterlin S, Dahlö M, Tellgren-Roth C, Schaal W, Melhus Å. High frequency of silver resistance genes in invasive isolates of *Enterobacter* and *Klebsiella* species. *J Hosp Infect*. 2017;96:256-261.

291. Elkrewi E, Randall CP, Ooi N, Cottell JL, O'Neill AJ. Cryptic silver resistance is prevalent and readily activated in certain gram-negative pathogens. *J Antimicrob Chemother*. 2017;72:3043-3046.

292. Rensch U, Klein G, Kehrenberg C. Analysis of triclosan-selected *Salmonella enterica* mutants of eight serovars revealed increased aminoglycoside susceptibility and reduced growth rates. *PLos One*. 2013;8:e78310.

293. Furi L, Ciusa ML, Knight D, et al. Evaluation of reduced susceptibility to quaternary ammonium compounds and bisbiguanides in clinical isolates and laboratory-generated mutants of *Staphylococcus aureus*. *Antimicrob Agents Chemother*. 2013;57:3488-3497.

294. Casado Muñoz Mdel C, Benomar N, Lavilla Lerma L, Knapp CW, Gálvez A, Abriouel H. Biocide tolerance, phenotypic and molecular response of lactic acid bacteria isolated from naturally-fermented Alorena table to different physico-chemical stresses. *Food Microbiol*. 2016;60:1-12.

295. Romero JL, Burgos MJ, Pérez-Pulido R, Gálvez A, Lucas R. Resistance to antibiotics, biocides, preservatives and metals in bacteria isolated from seafoods: co-selection of strains resistant or tolerant to different classes of compounds. *Front Microbiol.* 2017;8:1650. doi:10.3389/fmicb.2017.01650.

296. Márquez MLF, Burgos MJ, Pulido RP, Gálvez A, López RL. Biocide tolerance and antibiotic resistance in *Salmonella* isolates from hen eggshells. *Foodborne Pathog Dis.* 2017;14:89-95.

297. Wu D, Lu R, Chen Y, Qiu J, Deng C, Tan Q. Study of cross-resistance mediated by antibiotics, chlorhexidine and *Rhizoma coptidis* in *Staphylococcus aureus. J Glob Antimicrob Resist.* 2016;7:61-66.

298. Bhardwaj P, Ziegler E, Palmer KL. Chlorhexidine induces VanA-type vancomycin resistance genes in enterococci. *Antimicrob Agents Chemother.* 2016;60:2209-2221.

299. Saleem HGM, Seers CA, Sabri AN, Reynolds EC. Dental plaque bacteria with reduced susceptibility to chlorhexidine are multidrug resistant. *BMC Microbiol.* 2016;16:214. doi:10.1186/s12866-016-0833-1.

300. Huet AA, Raygada JL, Mendiratta K, Seo SM, Kaatz GW. Multidrug efflux pump overexpression in *Staphylococcus aureus* after single and multiple in vitro exposures to biocides and dyes. *Microbiology.* 2008;154:3144-3153.

301. Scientific Committee on Emerging and Newly Identified Health Risks. Research strategy to address the knowledge gaps on the antimicrobial resistance effects of biocides. European Commission Web site. http://ec.europa.eu/health/scientific_committees/emerging/docs/scenihr_o_028.pdf. Published 2010. Accessed May 2019.

302. Pal C, Bengtsson-Palme J, Kristiansson E, Larsson JDG. Co-occurrence of resistance genes to antibiotics, biocides and metals reveals novel insights into their co-selection potential. *BMC Genomics.* 2015;16:964. doi:10.1186/s12864-015-2153-5.

303. Noguchi N, Suwa J, Narui K, et al. Susceptibilities to antiseptic agents and distribution of antiseptic-resistance genes *qacA/B* and *smr* of methicillin-resistant *Staphylococcus aureus* isolated in Asia during 1998 and 1999. *J Med Microbiol.* 2005;54:557-565.

304. Molina L, Udaondo Z, Duque E, et al. Antibiotic resistance determinants in a *Pseudomonas putida* strain isolated from a hospital. *PLos One.* 2014;9:e81604.

305. Pastrana-Carrasco J, Garza-Ramos JU, Barrios H, et al. *qacE* Delta 1 gene frequency and biocide resistance in extended-spectrum beta-lactamase producing Enterobacteriaceae clinical isolates [in Spanish]. *Rev Invest Clin.* 2012;64:535-540.

306. Zhang M, O'Donoghue MM, Ito T, Hiramatsu K, Boost MV. Prevalence of antiseptic-resistance genes in *Staphylococcus aureus* and coagulase-negative staphylococci colonising nurses and the general population in Hong Kong. *J Hosp Infect.* 2011;78:113-117.

307. Bjorland J, Sunde M, Waage S. Plasmid-borne *smr* gene causes resistance to quaternary ammonium compounds in bovine *Staphylococcus aureus. J Clin Microbiol.* 2001;39:3999-4004.

308. Couto N, Monchique C, Belas A, Marques C, Gama LT, Pomba C. Trends and molecular mechanisms of antimicrobial resistance in clinical staphylococci isolated from companion animals over a 16 year period. *J Antimicrob Chemother.* 2016;71:1479-1487.

309. Bjorland J, Steinum T, Sunde M, Waage S, Heir E. Novel plasmid-borne gene qacJ mediates resistance to quaternary ammonium compounds in equine *Staphylococcus aureus, Staphylococcus simulans,* and *Staphylococcus intermedius. Antimicrob Agents Chemother.* 2003;47:3046-3052.

310. Jennings MC, Minbiole KP, Wuest WM. Quaternary ammonium compounds: an antimicrobial mainstay and platform for innovation to address bacterial resistance. *ACS Infect Dis.* 2015;1:288-303.

311. Seier-Petersen MA, Jasni A, Aarestrup FM, et al. Effect of subinhibitory concentrations of four commonly used biocides on the conjugative transfer of Tn*916* in *Bacillus subtilis. J Antimicrob Chemother.* 2014;69:343-348.

312. Sidhu MS, Heir E, Leegaard T, Wiger K, Holck A. Frequency of disinfectant resistance genes and genetic linkage with beta-lactamase transposon Tn552 among clinical staphylococci. *Antimicrob Agents Chemother.* 2002;46:2797-2803.

313. Sidhu MS, Heir E, Sørum H, Holck A. Genetic linkage between resistance to quaternary ammonium compounds and beta-lactam antibiotics in food-related *Staphylococcus* spp. *Microb Drug Resist.* 2001;7:363-371.

314. Shearer JES, Wireman J, Hostetler J, et al. Major families of multiresistant plasmids from geographically and epidemiologically diverse staphylococci. *G3 (Bethesda).* 2011;1:581-591.

315. Gillings MR, Xuejun D, Hardwick SA, Holley MP, Stokes HW. Gene cassettes encoding resistance to quaternary ammonium compounds: a role in the origin of clinical class 1 integrons? *ISME J.* 2009;3:209-215.

316. Gaze WH, Zhang L, Abdouslam NA, et al. Impacts of anthropogenic activity on the ecology of class 1 integrons and integron-associated genes in the environment. *ISME J.* 2011;5:1253-1261.

317. Braga TM, Marujo PE, Pomba C, et al. Involvement, and dissemination, of the enterococcal small multidrug resistance transporter QacZ in resistance to quaternary ammonium compounds. *J Antimicrob Chemother.* 2011;66:283-286.

318. Poole K. At the nexus of antibiotics and metals: the impact of Cu and Zn on antibiotic activity and resistance. *Trends Microbiol.* 2017;25:820-832.

319. Peng ZX, Li MH, Wang W, et al. Genomic insights into the pathogenicity and environmental adaptability of *Enterococcus hirae* R17 isolated from pork offered for retail sale. *Microbiologyopen.* 2017;6:e00514.

320. Silveira E, Freitas AR, Antunes P, et al. Co-transfer of resistance to high concentrations of copper and first-line antibiotics among *Enterococcus* from different origins (humans, animals, the environment and foods) and clonal lineages. *J Antimicrob Chemother.* 2014;69:899-906.

321. Venter H, Henningsen ML, Begg SL. Antimicrobial resistance in healthcare, agriculture and the environment: the biochemistry behind the headlines. *Essays Biochem.* 2017;61:1-10.

322. Aiello AE, Marshall B, Levy SB, et al. Antibacterial cleaning products and drug resistance. *Emerg Infect Dis.* 2005;11:1565-1570.

323. Aiello AE, Larson EL, Levy SB. Consumer antibacterial soaps: effective or just risky? *Clin Infect Dis.* 2007;45:S137-S147.

324. Forbes S, Knight CG, Cowley NL, et al. Variable effects of exposure to formulated microbicides on antibiotic susceptibility in firmicutes and proteobacteria. *Appl Environ Microbiol.* 2016;82:3591-3598.

325. International Organization for Standardization. *ISO 20776-1:2006: Clinical Laboratory Testing and In Vitro Diagnostic Test Systems—Susceptibility Testing of Infectious Agents and Evaluation of Performance of Antimicrobial Susceptibility Test Devices—Part 1: Reference Method for Testing the In Vitro.* London, United Kingdom: International Organization for Standardization; 2006.

326. European Committee on Antimicrobial Susceptibility Testing. Breakpoint tables for interpretation of MICs and zone diameters. Version 4.0. European Committee on Antimicrobial Susceptibility Testing Web site. http://www.eucast.org/fileadmin/src/media/PDFs/EUCAST_files/Breakpoint_tables/v_9.0_Breakpoint_Tables.pdf. Accessed May 2019.

Principles of Antimicrobial Activity

Gerald McDonnell and Joyce M. Hansen

This chapter provides a general introduction to the central principles of antimicrobial activity and application as they apply to the different preservation, disinfection, and sterilization objectives discussed in this book. It starts with a general overview of the important balance between antimicrobial activity and safety in any application, with greater emphasis on environmental safety in the last 20 years. This chapter further considers central requirements in the development and practical application of preservation, disinfection, and sterilization technologies as well as an introduction into the antimicrobial mechanisms of action.

▶ GENERAL REQUIREMENTS

Antimicrobial technologies employed for preservation, disinfection, and sterilization are widely used for industrial and medical purposes in reducing or eliminating microorganisms. But in the development and application of these technologies, there are at least two major considerations: the desired antimicrobial effects (the most obvious reason behind employing these technologies) and safety requirements. Antimicrobial targets can range from preventing the growth of certain types of microorganisms such as bacteria and fungi (as in the goal in many types of preservation systems) to inactivating microorganisms, to either reduce the levels and types present (as is the goal in disinfection) or to completely eliminate all microorganisms to reach a sterile level (as with sterilization processes). Therefore, the objective of the desired end point with an antimicrobial process is important in its choice and application. This can range from the unique control of an individual type of microorganism (eg, in a biosafety or research laboratory that may only be used for a certain type of microorganism), to the control of a range of potential pathogenic or spoilage microorganisms (eg, in environmental disinfection requirements in food production,

research laboratory, general microbiology detection laboratories, and health care facilities), and to the complete eradication of all types of harmful or product degrading microorganisms in higher risk situation (as during the administration of injectable drugs or surgical intervention with devices). Safety requirements will also vary depending on the use of the antimicrobial technology. These can include material compatibility, safety to those using the technology, safety to the end consumer or patient, and safety for the environment. They will also vary depending on the application such as in the preparation of food/water for consumption, treatment of environmental surfaces, use on the skin, mucous membranes or in wounds, products to be placed or injected into the body or blood stream, or in other industrial situations such as during microelectronic manufacturing. Equally, the definition of these requirements and the risk-benefit balance in each situation are important to consider.

▶ ANTIMICROBIAL REQUIREMENTS

The desired antimicrobial end points will depend on a risk-benefit equation. If we consider preservation requirements, the goal is to prevent the multiplication of microorganisms. In many cases, the concern is the presence of environmental microorganisms in raw materials; during manufacturing or distribution; or from the use of the product, surface, or material over time. The greatest risks are bacteria and fungi because they can multiply under the right conditions (eg, water availability, presence of nutrients, temperature, time, etc.). Bacteria, particularly gram-negative bacteria, are equally a concern in water or water-based product systems, but other risks can come from the presence of alga and protozoa. These are often associated with the intrinsic microbiological quality of an environmental source (including the potential for cross-contamination with water used for hand washing or food preparation) or only seen as a concern under situations where they have the ability to survive and grow (eg, in contaminated drinking or recreational water with a ready supply of organic and inorganic nutrients). In many of these situations, preservation strategies may be appropriate to consider not only for during manufacturing or initial treatment but also for the intended use of the product. During product use it may be needed to ensure that any microorganisms it may contact from other sources (such as from water, air or human contact) are not allowed to proliferate to levels that can cause harm or product damage. An example was an outbreak of *Acanthamoeba* keratitis associated with use of a multipurpose contact lenses solution, which on investigation was not found to be due to microorganisms found during product manufacturing but was suggested to be due to the inability of the preservative system to control the presence of *Acanthamoeba* introduced during the use (or repeated use) of the product.[1] Equally important are measures taken to provide water for recreational use. Protozoal outbreaks are increasingly reported in recreational water, such as with *Cryptosporidium* and *Naegleria fowleri*. The Centers for Disease Control and Prevention[2] reported a 13% rise per year in reports of cryptosporidiosis in the United States from 2009 to 2017; although rarer, *N fowleri* outbreaks have been linked to nasal contamination from contaminated natural water sources (eg, hot springs, lakes, and rivers).[3] In other cases, microorganisms such as viruses and certain types of obligate intracellular bacteria can be present at low levels but may not have the opportunity to proliferate unless they are under unique environments such as in cell culture applications. Overall, the focus on preservation systems and applicable test methodologies to test preservative effectiveness predominantly focus on bacterial and fungal challenges in preserved products such as cosmetics and/or detection technologies (eg, in drinking water monitoring).[4]

For many other types of applications, it is not enough to prevent the growth of microorganisms, and their inactivation is a requirement or a specified goal, and this is the purpose of disinfection and sterilization. As already defined in chapter 2, disinfection is required to inactivate viable microorganisms to a level previously specified as being appropriate for a defined purpose, and sterilization is essentially the ultimate process that renders a surface or product free from viable microorganisms. In most practical cases, the objective is not limited to the inactivation of a specific, targeted microorganism, although this may be the case in certain situations such as in a research laboratory that may only be investigating a certain microbial strain or in a specific outbreak or contamination event (eg, with a known virus). It is more common that an attempt is made to reduce or control a range of microorganisms that may be present or are of a concern. In many cases, the exact types or strains of microorganisms present will not be known. Examples include environmental disinfec-

tion of surfaces in a food-handling facility or antiseptic hand washing or hand rinsing of staff that are employed in patient care. It would be impossible and impractical to test every type (genus, species, or even strain) of microorganisms that can be a concern; therefore, antimicrobial efficacy is usually demonstrated using indicator microorganisms that represent the different kinds of microbial life. These primarily include viruses, vegetative bacteria, fungi (molds and yeasts), mycobacteria, and bacterial spores as the major classes but may also include indicator protozoa, helminths, alga, and prions depending on the specific requirements (Table 5.1). If a disinfection application is shown to be effective against certain types of indicator organisms, this will imply activity against a wider range of microorganisms with similar structures or sensitivity to inactivation. This premise has led to the development and continued optimization of standardized antimicrobial test methods (see chapters 61-63). These test methods include requirements to meet regulatory claims and support product labeling associated with disinfection and/or sterilization as well as for testing specific antimicrobial applications such as the treatment of human/animal tissues (see chapter 50) or in the control of biofilms (see chapter 67). The differences in the intended use of disinfectants can lead to some confusion from users when considering the use of terms like *bactericidal*, *viricidal*, and *germicidal* (see chapter 2). It is important to remember that the suffix "-cidal" correctly implies the ability to kill a certain class or type of microorganisms. Therefore, "bactericidal" may be interpreted as killing all types of bacteria, but this may not be the case and is generally limited to many types of common vegetative bacteria; for example, this term may not apply to the inactivation of mycobacteria and spore forms of bacteria that are intrinsically more resistant (see chapter 3). "Viricidal" can be used to describe the inactivation of easier to kill enveloped viruses but not nonenveloped viruses, depending on the product, application, or associated labeled claims/validated test methods. Finally, "germicidal" may imply the ability to inactivate all germs (generally used to describe all microscopic microorganisms), but this is not the case such as in the United States, where this term is widely used but is only intended to indicate the ability to inactivate certain types of common vegetative bacteria (eg, *Staphylococcus aureus* and *Escherichia coli*). The original use of the term *germ* (from the 1600s, having its original from the Latin *germin* or French *germe* for the verb *to beget*), implies a small living substance capable of developing into some larger, which was essentially the basis of the germ theory in the 1800s and clearly focused on what was known at the time as the major types of germs, being types of vegetative bacteria. Although our knowledge of microbiology has certainly changed since that time, the use of these label claims needs to be closely considered to prevent misinterpretation.

Overall, the antimicrobial claims against indicator microorganisms in standardized test systems are the basis of

TABLE 5.1 Examples of microorganism types, commonly used indicator organisms of each group, and associated efficacy claims[a]

Microorganism Type	Indicator Organism Example	Associated Claim
Vegetative bacteria	Staphylococcus aureus Pseudomonas aeruginosa Salmonella choleraesuis Salmonella enterica Escherichia coli Klebsiella pneumoniae	Germicidal, bactericidal
Biofilm	Pseudomonas aeruginosa Staphylococcus aureus	N/A
Fungi	Trichophyton interdigitale (or mentagrophytes) Candida albicans Aspergillus niger	Fungicidal, yeasticidal, mildewicidal
Enveloped viruses	Hepatitis B virus HIV Herpes simplex Influenza	Viricidal
Nonenveloped viruses	Parvovirus Poliovirus Feline calicivirus	Viricidal
Mycobacteria	Mycobacterium bovis Mycobacterium terra	Mycobactericidal Tuberculocidal
Protozoa	Cryptosporidium parvum Giardia lamblia Acanthamoeba castellanii	Protozocidal, cysticidal
Algae	Oscillatoria	Algicidal
Helminths	Ascaris lumbricoides Enterobius vermicularis	Oocidal
Bacterial spores	Bacillus subtilis Bacillus cereus Clostridium sporogenes Clostridium difficile Geobacillus stearothermophilus	Sporicidal
Prions	Scrapie	Not applicable[b]

HIV, human immunodeficiency virus.

[a]Indicator microorganisms and claim structures can vary internationally and/or on the associated product or product application.

[b]No accepted claim to date but can be referred to as "reducing the risk of prion infectivity," "prion decontamination," or "prionocidal" as examples.

labeling requirements for disinfectants and disinfection processes internationally. The claims can range in their meaning and therefore specific label claims should be reviewed carefully to ensure expected efficacy. As we consider antimicrobial properties, it is important to remember that microorganisms range in their intrinsic resistance patterns to antimicrobial processes (see chapters 3 and 4). These can include types of pathogens that are relatively easier to inactivate by many different types of physical and/or chemical microbicidal technologies such as heat, radiation, and chemicals like aldehydes and oxidizing agents. Enveloped viruses and many (but not all types) of vegetative bacteria and fungi have been well described as being relatively susceptible to inactivation by many antimicrobial technologies (see chapter 3). But equally, types of mycobacteria (due to their unique tolerance profile to chemical disinfectants), nonenveloped viruses, protozoal (oo) cysts, and fungal and bacterial spores have much higher levels of tolerance and therefore create a more significant challenge (see chapters 3 and 4).[5] This known hierarchy of resistance is also the basis for the generalization of antimicrobial claims such as low-, intermediate-, or high-levels of disinfection that are widely used in many countries (see chapters 2 and 3).

So overall, with these claims and a close inspection of the hierarchy structure, we can expect the antimicrobial effectiveness against a wide range of microorganisms. For example, a low-level disinfection claim implies effectiveness against vegetative forms of bacteria (but not necessarily mycobacteria), some fungi, and enveloped (or lipid) viruses, whereas high-level disinfection can be considered effective against all of these, including a wider range of fungi and mycobacteria but also some activity against bacterial spores. Overall, this hierarchy can be challenged depending on the antimicrobial process or product under investigation or the intrinsic resistance of certain types of microorganisms that would be expected to be within these claims[5-7] (see chapters 3 and 4), but in general they apply. These terms are well established based on years of experience from industry and academic derived data proving antimicrobial efficacy against a wide range of microorganisms and, in most cases, the verification of such a claim based on regulatory requirements. Similarly, other disinfection requirements can be applied to specific applications such as for skin antisepsis (see chapters 42 and 43) and in the parametric control of moist heat treatments, as in thermal disinfection or pasteurization processes (see chapters 11 and 28). In the latter case, the ability of heat to reliably inactivate microorganisms above a given temperature (eg, 65°C-70°C) and then follow classical predictable profiles for kill in a temperature-time relationship allows for the demonstration of disinfection (and indeed sterilization) by simply confirming that the actual temperature is achieved over a given time. Disinfection can also be demonstrated by more traditional means, such as by applying the process/product and demonstrating that no viable microorganisms are detected or demonstrating that the quality of microorganisms have been reduced to a given level. This may seem to be a simple approach but can be laborious and difficult to control. Analysis is often hindered by the fact that only certain types of microorganisms (such as many bacteria and fungi) can be easily handled under laboratory conditions. Further, the risk of introduction of other microorganisms as contaminants can create misleading (false positive) results. This approach is still used to demonstrate the effectiveness of disinfection methods in high-risk or regulated environments or applications but is overall not considered practical or reliable if not performed with close attention to detail and best microbiological practices.

As noted previously, it is not always necessary to ensure the complete removal or inactivation of all microorganisms or essentially that a sterile condition is established and/or maintained. In situations like food or water consumption, industrial applications, or in the antimicrobial treatment of the skin or mucous membrane, many types of sterilization treatments (see Part IV) would not be appropriate due to limitations in application, costs, or deleterious effects on the application of these technologies such as changes in organoleptic properties on consumption, the presence of toxic by-products that cannot be tolerated, and damage to tissues or products. This is important to consider in the risk-benefit equation in considering requirements for antimicrobial applica-

tions. For these reasons, many gentler technologies may be practically used to reduce the presence of certain types of high-risk pathogens or spoilage microorganisms, such as vegetative bacteria and viruses in food, water or skin/mucous membranes, or many types of industrial products. These will be able to achieve relatively safe levels for human, animal, or plant situations but not at the expense of unacceptable safety risks or damage. There is also the growing consideration that the constant overexposure of antimicrobial technologies may themselves lead to unwanted effects, such as lack of fitness of the human or animal immune system and chemical-associated health risks linked to the direct or indirect use of antimicrobials.

But in certain situations, and more critical applications, sterilization is the expectation and can be readily achieved. Sterilization is essentially the ultimate disinfection process, being a process used to render product free from viable microorganisms. This definition is important in two aspects. First, it implies that the process should be well established or verified to inactivate all microorganisms that can be present (known or unknown) to render the target sterile and therefore free of living microorganisms. Therefore, all the requirements for disinfection discussed earlier will apply but will also need to encompass all types of microorganisms. Different methods to demonstrate and maintain these requirements are introduced later in this chapter as well as the antimicrobial properties of the limited types of technologies widely used for this purpose (see Part IV). But second, the definition also highlights that this is a controlled process. This will not only be in the act of applying the sterilization process itself but also will include the preparation before sterilization and the maintenance of sterility after the point of use. This concept is best considered as an "end-to-end" supply chain process to ensure microbiological quality, not just a focus on the terminal act of sterilizing (discussed later in this chapter). Both criteria and their ramifications essentially differentiate disinfection from sterilization, but although the end points and level of scrutiny may be different, the impact of both concepts to achieve the desired goal is essentially the same. For these reasons, in comparison to disinfection modalities (see Part III), there is a more restrictive list of technologies that are practically used to achieve sterilization such as heat, ionizing radiation, and certain types of chemical processes (see Part IV). To these we may also include filtration methods (although these generally do not provide antimicrobial processes but physically remove microorganisms) that can be used for liquids or gases (including air; see chapter 30) and the use of aseptic processing, based on the concept of ensuring the sterilization of various product components and keeping them under aseptic conditions during the manufacturing process to ensure a sterile product presentation (see chapter 58). In this latter case, the final product is not terminally sterilized (or subjected to a sterilization process in its final, manufactured state) but is essentially sterile based on best aseptic practices during the product manufacturing. The combined benefits of aseptic processing techniques and terminal sterilization can allow for unique applications for delivering new sterile products to continue to innovate rather than being considered as separate approaches.[8]

The requirements for the first or antimicrobial considerations for preservation, disinfection, and sterilization are further discussed in this chapter. These can be broadly considered based on the requirements for achieving desired end points. Similarly, the second requirement for safety will also be considered. Other chapters in this book discuss the different types of physical and chemical technologies used for microbial control and public health in further detail.

▶ SAFETY REQUIREMENTS

Preservation, disinfection, and sterilization technologies are used to control microorganisms, thereby reducing the risks of adverse impacts such as infection, toxicity, and spoilage. But there are other safety requirements that may need to be considered in using these technologies. These can be considered as relating to impacts on the target application (eg, surface, product, functionality, or material compatibility), safety to those applying the technology for a particular purpose, safety to the end consumer or patient, and safety for the environment. As an example of surface or material compatibility, types of construction metals and plastics can be damaged by heat, thereby restricting the types of antimicrobial processes that can be used in certain applications. As an example of an exception to this is with incineration or other treatments for waste disposal because materials in these cases are typically discarded (see chapter 54). An even more restrictive example is seen in the antimicrobial applications to living (eg, skin) or nonliving tissues and many pharmaceutical products. Food and water applications will also be affected by more subtle criteria such as organoleptic properties (eg, taste, smell) and consumer perception that may limit product acceptance (eg, visual appearance). So overall, the balance lies between obtaining the desired level of antimicrobial activity with the minimum acceptable level of deterioration or damage to the target application. For sterilization, this can be important in the choice of and application of sterilization processes that may damage certain types of materials of impede product functionality depending on the technology used.[9]

The next consideration is the risks associated with those using the technology, such as from burns (eg, due to handling and application of heat) to side effects from the use of various antimicrobial chemicals that are hazardous or toxic. It is important to remember that technologies that are designed to affect the growth or multiplication of microorganisms are likely to have similar effects on human, plant, or animal cells based on their more general mechanisms of action (see discussion later in this chapter). These requirements are especially important in understanding short- and long-term health impacts, which can range from those that may resolve quickly (eg, minor burns) to those that can be more dangerous to health over time (eg, carcinogenicity, mutagenicity, and, at an extreme, instant death). Many of these can be considered as occupational risks that should be minimized, such as those defined by regulatory agencies such as Occupational Safety and Health Administration in the United States, Control of Substances Hazardous to Health in the United Kingdom, and the International Labor Office.[10] Occupational risks may not only come from direct exposure to the antimicrobial process itself or by-products from that process but also due to accidents in the use or insufficient controls in using some of these technologies (eg, explosion accidents with ethylene oxide [EO] gas[11]). It is also important to consider that many widely used chemicals have been considered "safe" in the past but are now known to be of a higher risk, such as in the case of the historic use of mercury, types of organic solvents, and more recently with the ubiquitous use of microbicides such as hexachlorophene and triclosan.[12] Essentially, it may be simple to conclude that all microbicides by their nature will be expected to do harm as much as we expect them to have their effects on microbial targets, but also some technologies will be more of a concern than others.

The third consideration is an extension of the second, being safe to the patient or consumer. The associated risks can come from the presence of residual by-products from the use or application of the microbicidal technology. Obvious examples include the presence of residual levels of chemical disinfectants or sterilants. These will include low levels of chemical sterilants such as EO and hydrogen peroxide (see chapters 31 and 32). The EO, for example, is classified as a carcinogen and mutagen; therefore, it is prudent to ensure that the use of EO is controlled and even restricted in its use under some situations. As an antimicrobial, its most widespread use is in the sterilization of medical devices, although it is also used for other applications such as with some foodstuffs (see chapter 31). For medical device applications, regulatory and standard requirements restrict the levels of acceptable EO residues that can remain on devices prior to patient exposure.[13] These requirements include not only residuals of EO itself but also by-products on reaction with chlorine radicals (ethylene chlorohydrin) and water (ethylene glycol). As an example of a benefit-risk approach, the levels of acceptable residual levels can then be defined based on the expected patient contact, such as permanent contact, prolonged exposure, or limited exposure.[13] Another example of the health risks associated with chemicals is the use of chlorine for water disinfection (see chapter 15). Chlorine was introduced in the early 1900s as a widespread drinking water disinfectant with clear benefits in reducing the infection risk with water and foodborne pathogens (see chapters 37 and 56). But by 1974, it was reported that the chemical reaction of chlorine with organic and inorganic compounds in water can produce halogenated compounds associated with health risks (eg, chloroform and other trihalomethanes).[14] Disinfection by-products are associated with all types of chemical microbicides widely used for water disinfection, with health risks at different levels including genotoxicity and carcinogenicity; estimates of at least 600 by-products were reported from the use of chlorine in drinking water, with the trihalomethanes widely used as indicators for drinking water safety.[4,15] There is also a growing debate, often associated with conflicting data, on the effects of preservatives used in many consumer products that are used on the skin or mucous membrane, such as shampoos and cosmetics, or directly used in food. These can include effects on the immune system, complications in those with asthma, and at the extreme to include carcinogenicity risks.[16-18]

Central to the consideration of toxicity, particularly with chemical antimicrobials, is the concept of selective activity. Selective activity may be defined as injury to one kind of living organism without harming another that is intimately associated with it.[19] This principle is used in agriculture, pharmacology, and diagnostic microbiology, but its most dramatic application is the systemic chemotherapy of infectious disease (eg, antibiotic use in the prevention and treatment of bacterial infections). Selective action against microorganisms is based on differences in the cell physiology of the microorganism and the mammalian or other host. Despite the general similarity of nutritional requirements, enzyme composition, and nucleic acid structure among all forms of life, there are many differences between microbes and humans in structure and metabolism, especially in the processes of cell synthesis. Energy-yielding processes do not offer the same possibilities for selective toxicity. Chemicals that inhibit a specific step in a metabolic pathway that is vital to the microorganism, but that does not occur or is not accessible in the cells of the host, exhibit selective toxicity. The treatment of bacterial infections has traditionally been more successful than that of viral disease because viruses depend on many enzymes of the host cell for their replication. Overall, chemotherapeutic agents are therefore often limited in their target antimicrobial activity and, equally, due to the ability of microorganisms to adapt or mutate to their presence, are at a high risk of becoming less effective over time. This has been well established since the widespread introduction of antibiotics but with more alarming consequences recently with the lack of development of new anti-infectives and parallel emergence of multidrug-resistant bacteria such as carbapenem-resistant gram-negative bacteria.[20] The limitation for selective toxicity is different for surface disinfectants or sterilants that are used on inanimate surfaces or skin/wound antiseptics in comparison to systemic chemotherapeutic agents. A more limited range of chemicals can be practically used on the skin in comparison to a wider range used for work surface or product disinfection or sterilization. But in general, many of these chemicals demonstrate a broader range of antimicrobial effects with less specific, wider toxicity. Examples include the oxidizing agents that will target any microbial (or host) structure that can be oxidized to culminate in

inactivation or the effects of increased heat in disrupting the structure and function of the various macromolecules that make up life. It is also less likely for resistance to develop to such broad-spectrum antimicrobials over time in comparison to the chemotherapy agents with a high degree of selective toxicity that are associated with a narrow antimicrobial spectrum and the emergence of drug-resistant microorganisms. But in between these types of extremes, there are antimicrobials such as the bisphenol, quaternary ammonium compounds (QACs), and chlorhexidine that are in the midrange, with limited spectra of activity against microorganisms and variable degrees of selective toxicity between the microbial targets and hosts.

The final point is the impact to the environment. There has been a greater focus on the use of chemicals as microbicides and their impact on the environment, especially those that may not readily break down in the environment (or as highlighted earlier in this chapter, may breakdown or react with other chemicals to form by-products that can impact the environment and its associated life). An example is the harmonized data requirements for biocides under the European Union's *Biocidal Products Directive* (Directive 98/8/EC of the European Parliament[21]), which considers not only the toxicity risks on primary exposure to biocides (discussed earlier) but also the secondary risks through the environment.[22] The regulation defined four categories of biocides (disinfectants, preservatives, pest control, and other products, such as embalming fluids) and 23 product types (eg, for disinfectants based on their use for human or veterinary hygiene as well as food, public health, or water use). Registration requirements include toxicological studies, ecotoxicological studies, and data assessment. Similar requirements are also in place regarding other chemicals that can impact the formulation of antimicrobial products (see chapter 5) as defined under the European Union regulation *Registration, Evaluation, Authorisation and Restriction of Chemicals*.[23] The impact of these, and similar regulations in other countries and regional areas, has reduced the availability of many types of microbicides from practical use, particularly many chemicals known to be carcinogens, mutagens, and reprotoxic substances; endocrine disruptors; and those that are persistent and bioaccumulative.[24] Other examples of environmental safety considerations include the following:

- The safe disposal, including neutralization, of chemical disinfectants (eg, aldehydes) following their health care or industrial use into septic systems[25,26]
- The EO[27-29] and other gases released into the environment
- Incineration controls, often due to the release of toxic by-products from the incineration process[30] (see chapter 54)
- Handling and disposal of radioactive materials (see chapter 29)
- Energy sources for heat generation

It may be expected that further regulatory controls in different countries as well as international mandates regarding the short- and long-term risks to the environment will continue to impact the use of technologies for preservation, disinfection, and sterilization.

Overall, safety requirements can vary depending on the application. It is important to consider the risks and benefits in these situations to determine the best antimicrobial solution for a given situation, to include its safe, effective, and optimal use.

▶ REGULATORY REQUIREMENTS

The use of preservation, disinfection, and sterilization technologies will often be associated with legal requirements including international; regional; national; and area-specific (eg, state or province) regulations, standards, and guidelines (see chapter 70). These can include specific requirements in order to legally commercialize or use different technologies for various applications as well as determining the continued safety and effective use of antimicrobial methods under routine use in laboratory, medical, veterinary, food production/handling, public health, and industrial environments. These requirements can have different legal consequences with regulations having the greatest impact, being defined as a rule or directive made and maintained by an authority. Examples include the *Biocides Directive*[21] and *Registration, Evaluation, Authorisation and Restriction of Chemicals*[23] requirements in the European Union; US Food and Drug Administration (FDA) regulations regarding food,[31] medical devices[32] (FDA CFR 21-Part 807), and pharmaceuticals[33,34] (CFR 21 Parts 210 and 211); National Medical Products Administration (formerly China Food and Drug Administration or CFDA) regulations on medical devices[35] (Supervision and Regulation of Medical Devices, No. 680) and drugs (Drug Administration Law 2019)[36]; Indian regulations on medical devices[37]; and many other specific country regulations that are periodically subject to amendments or revisions that may impact antimicrobial applications.

The next level down from these are more specific standards that can also be international (International Organization for Standardization [ISO]), regional (European Standard [EN]), or country specific (eg, American National Standards Institute-Association for the Advancement of Medical Instrumentation, American Society for Testing and Materials International, or Association of Official Analytical Chemists [AOAC] in the United States; Canadian Standards Association in Canada; British Standards in the United Kingdom; Deutsches Institut für Normung in Germany; Australia/New Zealand standards in Australia-New Zealand; and the Guobiao (GB) standards in China). For pharmaceutical applications, including drug manufacturing or dispensing, many of these are published in various pharmacopeia such as the US pharmacopeia, European pharmacopoeia, and Japanese pharmacopoeia, with international efforts to ensure the standardization of these requirements. Standards can be harmonized internationally or regionally, where the same standard is applied (such as those developed by ISO or International Electrotechnical Commission [IEC]) or modified with exceptions for a specific country. They can also be considered as extensions of certain regulations when deemed appropriate or best practice. Many standards are more specific in their requirements, but some can be more general such as in the case of ISO 9001 quality management systems,[38] ISO 13485 for quality management systems in the manufacturing of medical devices,[39] and ISO/IEC 17025 for the competency of test and calibration laboratories.[40] Examples of specific standards in the area of disinfection and sterilization include those for washer disinfectors (ISO 15883 series), biological indicators (BIs) (ISO 11138 series), general sterilization processes (ISO 14937), specific sterilization processes such as steam (or moist heat sterilization under the ISO 17665 series), and radiation (ISO 11137 series).

Finally, there are different guidances published by many organizations that provide further information for specific applications such as in different health care situations, industrial manufacturing, food handling or manufacturing, and public health. Some are specific to those providing greater guidance of specific standards (eg, ISO/TS 11137-3 provides specific guidance on the parent ISO 11137-1 radiation sterilization standard), whereas others provide more general guidance on options for specific applications such as medical device reprocessing,[41,42] clinical practice (eg, surgical best practices[43-45]), biological safety,[46] water disinfection and preservation,[4] pharmaceutical manufacturing requirements,[47] and food safety.[48] Some of these guidances are based on detailed literature reviews (referred to as "evidenced based"), consensus building by expert committees, or developed by key opinion leaders for publication by industrial or public health organizations. Guidance documents can be useful in the development or application of best practices for many situations and in some cases may be expected to be employed as requirements by regulatory or auditing organizations. It is important to note that regulatory expectations are not only required, when defined, to allow for the safe and effective use of antimicrobials or antimicrobial processes in various situations but are also often subject to periodic verification of these requirements such as during announced and unannounced audits to ensure compliance to those requirements.

▶ MICROBICIDES AND ANTIMICROBIAL PROCESSES

Antimicrobial agents may be subdivided into either physical (eg, heat, radiation) or chemical (eg, halogens, oxidizing agents) types and in many cases are used in combination. Table 5.2 depicts some of the most common agents that are available and in widespread use. Chemotherapeutic agents are those that are used orally or systemically for the treatment of microbial infections of humans and animals.

TABLE 5.2 Major types of antimicrobial processes used for preservation, disinfection, and sterilization

Type of Process	Agent	Application[a]	Comments
Physical[b]	Dry heat (≥160°C)	Disinfection, sterilization	Less efficient than moist heat
	Moist heat (≥115°C)	Sterilization	Use of steam
	Moist heat (<100°C)	Disinfection	Inactivation of most pathogens over 70°C
	Cold/freezing	Preservation	Repeated freeze-thaw cycles can inactivate microbial cells.
	Ionizing radiation	Sterilization	Includes multiple sources (γ sources, x-ray, E-beam)
	Ultraviolet radiation	Disinfection	Requires direct light contact for optimal activity; may provide sterilization under some applications
	Other nonionizing radiation	Disinfection	Used as sources of heat
	Cell lysis methods such as those based on hydrostatic pressure changes or pulsed electrical field	Disinfection	Can inactivate microbial cells, with activity dependent on the application method, temperature, and in the presence of chemicals
Chemical (vapor phase)	Ethylene oxide	Sterilization	Most widely used chemical in sterilization processes
	Formaldehyde	Disinfection, sterilization	Laboratory room disinfection and limited use for sterilization
	Hydrogen peroxide, peracetic acid, chlorine dioxide, ozone	Disinfection, sterilization	Oxidizing agents for low-temperature disinfection and sterilization processes
	Gas plasma	Disinfection, sterilization	Can be generated from inert or antimicrobial gas(es)
Chemical (liquid phase)	Acids, alkali, and derivatives	Preservation, disinfection	Widely used for preservation, including foods
	Alcohols	Preservation, antisepsis, disinfection	Widely used in antiseptics and for surface cleaning/disinfection
	Aldehydes (glutaraldehyde, OPA)	Disinfection	Glutaraldehyde is used as a chemical sterilant.
	Halogens (including sources of chlorine, iodine and bromine)	Preservation, disinfection, sterilization	Widely used for surface disinfection and food applications
	Oxidizing agents (hydrogen peroxide, peracetic acid, chlorine dioxide, ozone)	Antisepsis, disinfection, sterilization	Increasing used as alternatives to aldehydes
	Antimicrobial metals including silver and copper	Antisepsis, disinfection	Often used in or as impregnated surfaces. Many other metals have been in traditional use such as mercury and tin.
	Phenolics	Antisepsis, disinfection	Skin applications and surface disinfectants
	Quaternary ammonium compounds	Antisepsis, disinfection	As surfactants, can be combined for cleaning applications
	Biguanides	Preservatives, antisepsis	Chlorhexidine is the most widely used, particularly as an antiseptic.
	Dyes	Preservatives, antisepsis	Examples include acridines and crystal violet.
	Essential oils	Preservatives, antisepsis, disinfection	Plant extracts, often consisting of multiple antimicrobials such as phenolics and aldehydes (eg, pine or tea tree oils)

(continued)

TABLE 5.2	Major types of antimicrobial processes used for preservation, disinfection, and sterilization *(Continued)*		
Type of Process	**Agent**	**Application**[a]	**Comments**
Other	Peptides, proteins, and enzymes Bacteriophages	Preservatives, antisepsis, disinfection	Often associated with limit spectrum of activity in comparison to other microbicides above

OPA, ortho-phthalaldehyde.

[a]Some of these methods can be applied for both disinfection and sterilization depending on their applications, but others are limited to disinfection due to their lack of practical antimicrobial activity against more resistant forms of microorganisms such as nonenveloped viruses, protozoal (oo)cysts, and bacterial spores (see chapters 3 and 4).

[b]Filtration methodologies used for disinfection and sterilization are generally excluded from this definition as they may be used for the same end points by physical removal but are not typically associated with antimicrobial activity (see chapter 30).

The most important agents are antibiotics, together with synthetic compounds that may be used for their antibacterial, antifungal, or antiviral properties. These are not considered further in this chapter.

Several physical processes such as moist heat, dry heat, and ionizing radiation under defined conditions can be relied on to kill all types of microorganisms, including more resistant forms such as bacterial spores, and thus are expected to achieve sterilization when correctly validated and maintained (see Part IV). These processes can be controlled even under sometimes difficult situations (such as in complex loads to be sterilized with features or materials that are difficult to ensure access of the antimicrobial process), and the assurance of such penetration capabilities has seen their widespread adoption as the major types of sterilization processes used today. Moist heat is not only a practical and relatively straight forward sterilization process to apply to heat-stable materials for traditional infectious agents but has also been shown to be effective against nontraditional infectious agents such as prions that are not readily inactivated by other methods such as radiation or dry heat (see chapter 68). Temperatures below 100°C (eg, as low as 50°C-60°C) can be of value in various thermal disinfection applications, including pasteurization (a widely used disinfection method in the preparation of and risk reduction in foods and many other materials or surfaces) and in the preparation of certain bacterial vaccines when the aim is to inactivate all the cells without affecting their antigenic identity. Moist heat is preferred over dry heat due to being more efficient as an antimicrobial process (a concept that is considered in more detail in chapters 11 and 28). At the opposite end of the heat spectrum, cold or even freezing temperatures are widely used as preservative methods. These are not generally appreciated to cause microbial death, although in some applications, freeze-thawing cycling can be associated with cell death and presumably due to the disruption of the membrane structure/function of cells. Ultraviolet (UV) radiation, as a nonionizing radiation source with less associated energy in comparison to ionizing radiation, is considered less effective as antimicrobial agent but still can have the ability to inactivate all microorganisms including bacterial and fungal spores; but due to limits in penetration capabilities and ensuring that all surfaces in a target applications have direct contact with UV light to enable antimicrobial activity, this technology has been more widely used for liquid, gas/air, and surface disinfection. Despite this, certain applications, such as in space with UV exposure, can be sustained, and high use of this technology for surface sterilization may be a practical reality.[49] Other physical methods have been identified for niche applications such as those based on hydrostatic pressure and pulsed electrical fields that target lysis of vegetative cells and may otherwise be limited in antimicrobial effectiveness (eg, against spores or viruses) and scope of applications (eg, in certain food or other industrial uses). Hydrostatic pressure, for example, is a method that uses the high pressures exerted by liquids on microorganisms, whereas pulsed electrical fields use an electric charge to cause disruption of cell walls in bacterial and fungi. Outside the scope of this section are physical methods used to preserve, disinfect, or sterilize by filtration mechanisms such as liquid or air filtration (see chapter 30) and the use of packaging materials for preservation or sterile presentation (see chapter 41) because these do not generally provide any intrinsic antimicrobial activity; their mechanism of action is simply by physical removal or exclusion of microorganisms.

A similar range of chemical agents and applications has been described. Like physical agents, they can range from those that are used to prevent the growth of or inactivate microorganisms. Chemicals can be limited not only in their antimicrobial activity but also in their ability to be safe for various applications. Preservatives, for example, need to be able to prevent the growth of many types of bacteria and fungi, and without reacting with or affecting the use of the product, they are used in either from a toxicity, effectiveness or, in many cases, aesthetic point of view. As discussed earlier, disinfection can be achieved with a wider range of chemical and physical methods. At the lower end are those microbicides that can be safely used on the skin or mucous membranes such as the bisphenol (eg, triclosan), chlorhexidine and other biguanides, alcohols, silver, and iodine, depending on their in-use concentration. Thermal methods are more restrictive as typically pain tolerance is in the 50°C to 55°C range, which only demonstrates limited antimicrobial activity. But these requirements become less of a concern with inanimate surfaces, applications to food and water, manufacturing equipment, etc. Therefore, in these cases, a wider variety of chemical (aldehydes, oxidizing agents, QACs, and phenolics) and physical (radiation sources and heat) methods can be used.

As a greater expectation of microbial inactivation is required, this list of choices becomes more limited to meet the needs for sterilization. A traditional and minimal requirement (or prerequisite) for this is often sporicidal activity due to their resistance profile to inactivation (see chapter 3). Physical methods (heat and radiation) are widely used but equally are certain types of chemicals (eg, aldehydes, oxidizing agents, and EO). Many types of chemical agents can also act as sporicides, such as glutaraldehyde (pentanedial), formaldehyde (methanal), hypochlorites, and EO gas. But their activity can often be slower against bacterial spores; however, this can be influenced by many factors such as the condition of the spores (present in liquid suspension or dried onto test objects), the presence of organic matter, the concentration and pH of the antimicrobial agent, presence of humidity, temperature, formulation, and state in which the chemical is in (eg, liquid or gas).[5,50,51] For example, optimal antimicrobial activity has been described under controlled humidity levels or, perhaps more accurately, the microenvironmental water content, for many sporicidal gases such as EO, formaldehyde, chlorine dioxide, and ozone. Methods of potentiating the activity of an agent are obviously important in antimicrobial product or process optimization. Formulation effects, defined as the combination of chemical ingredients such as microbicidal agents and antimicrobial agents and other ingredients (eg, stabilizers, buffers, solvents, chelating agents, etc), can have significant impacts in effectiveness (see chapter 6). pH can be important in optimizing antimicrobial activity and stability of the microbicide over time, with examples being in the use of chlorine (see chapter 15) and aldehydes (see chapter 23). Acids and bases can have intrinsic antimicrobial activity, but there can also be combined effects in increasing the activity of formulated microbicides. The activity of most compounds increases with an increase in temperature (see chapter 7),[50] but this will reach a limited dependent on the microbicide and may also increase the degradation of the antimicrobial to decrease its availability over time. The impact of other physical factors in the activity of microbicides is considered in further detail in chapter 7.

Combinations of antimicrobial agents may be used in disinfectant formulations. They offer the following advantages:

- Gaps in the range of action of a certain antimicrobial agent can be filled by a second agent. This helps to widen the range or have a broader spectrum of action. Some agents act preferentially against gram-positive bacteria, and others against gram-negative types. A third group may have preferable activity against molds and yeasts. Instead of increasing the concentration of an agent to get a broader spectrum of activity, it is often better to add a second agent of complementary activity. Only a small amount of the additional agent may be necessary.
- Lower toxic and ecologic risk. If a combination of two or more antimicrobial agents is used in a formulation, the concentration of each agent can be lower than in a formulation with only one of these agents. By reducing the concentration of an agent, the toxic effects are also reduced, if possible, below the threshold value (eg, for sensitization), which is becoming increasingly desirable.
- Solubility. If a saturated solution of a given agent of low solubility does not show sufficient efficiency, the required efficiency might be achieved by the addition of a second agent.
- Product or regulatory requirements. The choice of microbicides may be limited in some applications such as in the case of preservatives in cosmetics (see chapter 40) and on the skin (see chapters 42 and 43), where combinations are required to show product expectations. Commercial antiseptics and disinfectants may be subjected to official testing for registration purposes, and a variety of test method requirements may need to be fulfilled. A good example for this is the requirement of many test method or efficacy requirements in skin hygiene to show a substantiate (or residual) antimicrobial effect, which will be less likely with some microbicides (eg, alcohols) in comparison to others (see chapter 43), but the combination of these actives may provide some overall benefit.
- The risk of tolerance or resistance development against the antimicrobial(s) is lower when two or more antimicrobial agents are used.

In selecting antimicrobial agents, mutual effects on the action of the substances are of significance. Some substances have an inhibitory effect on each other, such as active chlorine compounds with an oxidative effect on aldehydes or phenols. Other combinations of active substances mutually enhance their actions, a fact well known from the patent literature. It is therefore the aim of those developing disinfectants (especially in liquid formulations) and sterilization processes to satisfy the demands on the product as far as possible by selecting suitable combinations of antimicrobial agents. Thus, the content of active substances in disinfectants may be reduced, which may even help to make production more economical.[52,53] Many studies have been published on the combined effects of two or more active substances, but it is important to consider that these effects may be considered as additive (when both microbicides contribute together to the antimicrobial effects), in synergism (where the they act together to give greater efficacy than either alone), or in antagonism (and therefore a negative overall impact).

These concepts not only apply to the various types of microbicides considered in this book but also to other chemotherapeutic agents. The effects can be best described graphically. In Figure 5.1, the full antimicrobial effect of two different substances, A and B, is displayed on the abscissa and the ordinate of a coordinate system at points M and N, respectively. This effect is achieved by substance A at concentration M and by substance B at concentration N, respectively. Assuming an increase up to the full effect has a linear character, the subdivision of the effect is supposed to be equivalent to the corresponding partial concentrations. There must be a series of partial concentrations of A and B giving the same effect in combination as the effective concentration of each substance alone. The simplest case would be the addition of the two partial effects corresponding to the respective partial concentrations. This may be shown graphically by drawing a straight line between N and M. All points on this line represent combinations giving identical effects (Figure 5.1A). The points M and N represent the inhibitory effects caused by the minimum inhibitory concentrations (MICs), M and N, of the two agents A and B. All points on the line between M and N represent the inhibitory effects caused by the different combinations of agents A and B. The combinations lying within the triangle of 0 (intersection of the X and Y axis), M and N (except those on the line MN) fail to give an inhibitory reaction. All the other combinations give positive results. This typical pattern is characteristic for additive effects. Synergism of antimicrobial combinations can be defined as the supra-additive effects of combined antimicrobials. Figure 5.1B shows an example of the synergistic action of two agents. Combinations of parts of the inhibitory concentrations of the two agents A and B reveal a higher activity than that expected on the basis of a purely additive effect. The curved line in Figure 5.1B indicates the limit of effectiveness.

A mathematical formula to describe these relationships can be given as:

$$\frac{x}{M} + \frac{y}{n} \leq 1$$

where x and y refer to the actual concentrations of the combination of the agents A and B, which exert the same antimicrobial effect as the MICs, M and N, of the two agents alone.[54] If the left side of this equation totals 1, we have a combination showing an additive effect. A result smaller than 1 indicates a synergistic effect of the combination.

These effects can also be demonstrated experimentally based on both microbiostatic and microbicidal test methods.[52,53] Examples include bacteriostatic tests such as MICs that are often employed in the testing of preservative considerations and bactericidal tests such a time-kill studies in the development and optimization of disinfectants (see chapter 61). The first step is the determination of the MIC of the two antimicrobial agents A and B alone. A series of successive dilutions of each agent is prepared in a liquid nutrient medium and then inoculated with the test bacteria (or fungi, if applicable) to be tested to give a known cell number (eg, 10^3-10^7/mL). After an incubation period (eg, for bacteria, 24-48 h), the tubes are examined for growth or no growth, where the lowest concentration observed for no growth is determined to indicate the MIC of each test agent. In a second step, the combination of A + B is tested in an analogous manner by using the MIC of the two agents and some higher and lower concentrations of this mixture. After inoculation and incubation, the MIC of the mixture is again determined. With the help of the formula in the earlier equation, it can be calculated whether the two components give an additive, a synergistic, or an antagonistic reaction. It is important to note in these cases that interference factors (eg, growth media) are present that can influence the activity of the microbicide(s).

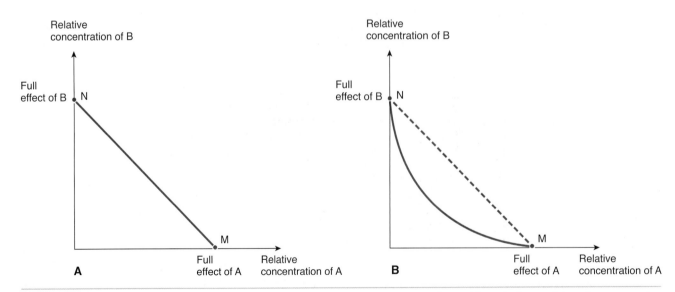

FIGURE 5.1   Combined effect of two antimicrobial agents A and B in the case of an additive behavior (A) and a synergistic behavior (B).

A good example would be attempting to demonstrate a true MIC with oxidizing agents (eg, chlorine, iodine, hydrogen peroxide) that will readily react with media components will clearly underestimate their true efficacy. In bactericidal tests, dilutions of the two disinfecting agents to be tested are also prepared separately and in combination, but in these cases, it is recommended for the test to be performed in water (or a similar noninterfering diluent) without any nutrient compounds. The dilutions are again inoculated with a known cell concentration (eg, 10^6-10^7/ mL). After exposures that can range from a few seconds to many hours (depending on the test microorganism and product requirements), samples are removed and analyzed for surviving cells (see chapter 61; note the importance of neutralization to ensure the antimicrobials under tests are immediately halted in their activity to give a true account of the extent of kill at each exposure time point). Microbial quantification can be done by two different methods, direct analysis of cell numbers remaining or end point analysis. In direct enumeration, the number of viable cells is determined by plating, indication, and counting, with the results plotted against time logarithmically (Figure 5.2). Synergism is shown by the combination of two agents showing a faster rate of killing than twice the concentration of either agent alone. Addition effects will show the rate of killing of the agents in combination is approximately that expected from simple algebraic summation of a single agent alone. Finally, antagonism will show a rate of killing of the combination lower than that of one or both of its components. In end point analysis, the samples are transferred into tubes containing liquid medium to allow the surviving cells to grow. After the desired incubation time, the tubes demonstrating growth/no growth are examined, and those with no growth indicate complete killing of the test population (end point). For each dilution, the time needed for complete inactivation can be determined, and again, addition effects will be indicated by the killing time of the combination being nearly the same as that needed by twice the concentration of either agent alone (ie, a mean value of the two killing times), and synergism where the combination is shorter, preferably by one-half or less, than that needed by twice the concentration of either agent alone. Many different iterations of these essential tests are useful in optimizing the benefits of formulation effects as well as combinations of actives (see chapters 6 and 61).

But it is worthwhile to have a note of caution at this stage in the identification and use of synergistic effects of two or more substances in disinfectants due to the potential inconsistency in the increase of effectiveness against different microorganisms. Many of the examples of synergism of two substances described in the literature and particularly in the patent literature concern a limited selection of test organisms. In some cases, improvement of action on one group of microorganisms may be accompanied by reduced effects on another group. For example, a combination of a QAC with the anionic agent undecylenic acid resulted in an antagonistic effect when *S aureus* was

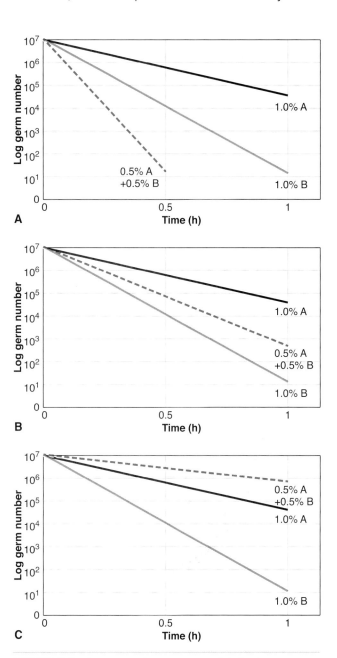

FIGURE 5.2 Interaction between two disinfecting agents A and B in a quantitative bactericidal test.[53] A, Synergism. B, Additivity. C, Antagonism.

used as the test organism but not with the fungus *Trichophyton mentagrophytes*.[55] Thus, some additive or synergistic combinations can be used only to compensate for a specific weakness against a single microbial species but may not apply to others.

It is outside of the scope of this chapter to provide further details of the many difficult combination of actives (including chemical-physical interactions) that can provide positive impact in antimicrobial activity, but some examples include the following[53]:

- Chelating agents (eg, ethylenediaminetetraacetic acid [EDTA]) with overall poor activity against bacteria is used at low concentrations to demonstrate greater bactericidal activity of bisphenol such as triclosan against gram-negative bacteria (where intrinsically gram-negative bacteria are more resistant than gram-positive bacteria).

- UV radiation (and indeed other energy sources such as temperature) potentiates the activity of hydrogen peroxide.[56]
- Hydrogen peroxide and peracetic acid have been shown to have synergistic activities in their subtly different modes of action against bacterial spores (see chapter 18).
- Combinations of QACs are widely used as broad-spectrum (against gram-positive and gram-negative bacteria, including in some situations mycobacteria) surface disinfectant formulations (see chapter 21).
- Reaction of two chemicals or microbicides that result in a more active product. For example, sodium iodide, a chemical without appreciable antimicrobial potency, may be oxidized by a reagent such as 2,2-dibromo-2-cyanoacetamide, a highly active disinfectant, giving free iodine, which provides an even higher antimicrobial activity than that of 2,2-dibromo-2-cyanoacetamide.[52] The microbicidal activity of peroxy compounds, such as hydrogen peroxide or sodium perborate, is enhanced by combination with a suitable catalyst, which accelerates the formation of oxygen radicals as the active principle of these compounds. Because of their high chemical reactivity, they have to be mixed just before application, giving a disinfectant solution with a short life span. This may be an advantage if only a short active period of disinfection is required, but similar and more stable combination products have also been described with greater benefits from a generational, stability, and safety points of view.
- Surfactants are often important constituents of disinfectants. They are used to achieve both uniform wetting of the surface to be treated and frequently for the additional cleaning effect they provide (see chapter 21). Particular attention should be given to this group of substances when formulating a disinfectant because there are many ways in which the two groups of compounds can interact (see chapter 6). For example, anionic surfactants promote the inactivation of cationic QACs, and nonionics (eg, Tween 80 or polyoxyethylene sorbitan monooleate) are capable of binding microbicides such as cetylpyridinium chloride, some phenols, and chlorhexidine (hence its use in neutralizing solutions[52,53]). In contrast, low surfactant concentrations of 0.1% or less are often accompanied by an improvement in the action of antimicrobial agents such as *p*-hydroxybenzoates preservatives.[57] Alkyl glucosides have shown synergistic activity in combination with biguanides, alcohols, and organic acids.[52] As another example, nisin is an antimicrobial peptide with antimicrobial properties that is produced by the gram-positive bacterium *Lactococcus lactis* subsp *lactis* particularly against gram-positive bacteria and has limited antimicrobial efficacy against gram-negative bacteria, yeasts, and mold; this can be significantly increased

in formulation with 30 to 300 ppm nisin, 20 mmol/L EDTA, and 0.1% to 1.0% Triton X-100.[58]

Overall, despite the individual or combinations of microbicides used, the response of microorganisms to adverse agents will depend on the type of target organism(s), the biocidal agent(s), and the intensity (eg, concentration of a chemical, temperature of exposure, radiation dose) and duration of exposure. In bacteriostasis or fungistasis, reversible inhibition of growth and multiplication can be achieved by restoring the organism to favorable conditions. Microorganisms injured but not killed by a particular process may be able to repair the damage inflicted on them, and such damaged cells should be considered in the design of procedures used for the validation of sterilization and disinfection processes, in their detection and enumeration, and as a health hazard in processed foods.[59] It may also be necessary to use an appropriate antagonist or neutralizing agent (inactivator, inactivating agent, neutralizer, antidote) to distinguish between a lethal effect and mere inhibition in cells exposed to disinfectants, antiseptics, or preservatives. The theoretic principles in using neutralizing agents is further discussed in chapter 61. Table 5.3 summarizes the uses of neutralizing agents. Moreover, in some instances (eg, mercury, silver, and thiol compounds), the chemical nature of the neutralizing agent may provide a clue as to the mechanism of action.

▶ PRESERVATION

The main goal of preservation is to prevent the growth of microorganisms in (or in the case of packaging systems, the ingress of microorganisms into) various products or applications. There are two main methods to achieve this goal: the physical exclusion of microorganisms and the use of antimicrobials or antimicrobial processes.

Physical exclusion as a concept for preservation was elegantly confirmed by Louis Pasteur in 1862 in the demonstration that a torturous path using a swan-neck shaped flask was sufficient to prevent the passage of microorganism to a culture media (see chapter 2, Figure 2.2). Similar designs (including food canning methods) and innovations in microbial barrier materials since that time are the basis of modern sterile barrier or exclusion systems used today (see chapter 41). Similarly, microbial retentive materials and methods are the basis for disinfection and sterile filtration technologies for air and liquid applications for products and environmental controls (see chapters 30 and 58-60). These are essentially based on the same exclusion processes such as providing a complex, torturous path to microorganisms or limiting their passage by size exclusion.

Historic methods of preservation were widely used in the past prior to any modern understanding of microbiology, including salting, drying, and use of heat. Salting and drying of food was found to allow foods to last for longer time periods without degradation by various bacteria and

TABLE 5.3   Examples of chemical agents that neutralize antimicrobial compounds[a]

Microbicide	Neutralizing Agent	Comment
Aldehydes	Dilution to subinhibitory level; glycine better	Sodium sulfite not recommended (may itself be toxic)
Phenolics	Dilution to subinhibitory level	Tween 80 is possible alternative.
Organic acids and their esters	Dilution to subinhibitory level	Tween 80 is possible alternative.
Hydrogen peroxide	Catalase, sodium thiosulfate	Rapid effect, but some bacteria can be inhibited by sodium thiosulfate
Peracetic acid	Sodium thiosulfate	Rapid effect, but some bacteria can be inhibited by sodium thiosulfate
Mercury compounds	Thiol compounds	Possible toxicity of sodium thioglycollate
Alcohols	Dilution to subinhibitory level	
Quaternary ammonium compounds, biguanides	Letheen broth (or agar); lecithin + Lubrol W	
Ethylenediaminetetraacetic acid and related chelating agents	Dilution	Mg^{2+} useful
Hypochlorites, iodine	Sodium thiosulfate	Rapid effect, but some bacteria can be inhibited by sodium thiosulfate
Silver compounds	Thiol compounds	As for mercury

[a]Note that membrane filtration may be alternative method, where the microbicide does not bind to the filter material.

fungi now known to be present. The use of other chemicals such as vinegar (as a mild acid) in pickling is another common example in more modern times, although the use of variety of chemicals was only directly shown to have effects on microorganisms (or "animalcules") by Antonie van Leeuwenhoek in the 1670s with the development of microscopy. Plants and plant extracts have a long traditional history of use in the treatment or even prevention of illness with examples from herbal remedies used in diverse worldwide cultures.[60] Although often controversial in modern scrutiny of therapeutic requirements, these extracts are known to have direct antibacterial requirements due to the presence of various natural antimicrobials such as aldehydes and phenolics. High heat mechanisms, including boiling and incineration have been historically appreciated for disinfection and preservation but only became fully understood since the 1800s and again with the development of methods such as pasteurization. Pasteurization is a disinfection method, but it is used to extend the shelf life of foods and liquids as a preservation method by reducing the numbers and therefore growth of microorganisms that lead to spoilage. Similar methods may be used to reduce the levels or types of microorganisms in raw materials used in a variety of manufacturing environments. Maintaining foods or tissues at cold or even freezing temperatures has the same impact as effective preservation methods. Similarly, product dehydration or drying is a useful way of preventing the growth of bacteria and fungi due to the reduced levels or even lack of available water for metabolism.

The earlier demonstration of the effects of chemicals as preservatives led to the development of modern chemi-cal preservation methods that continue to evolve today to meet product and regulatory requirements (see Part V). Examples include the use of chemical preservatives of products to prevent product spoilage (as in the case of cosmetics, paints, and natural products like those based on wood), decreased product acceptance by consumers (eg, organoleptic, being acceptance of a product due to taste, color, odor), or the overgrowth of microorganisms (such as in water or foods) that can lead to an unacceptable infection or associated toxicity risk in consumers. In most of these cases, the presence of a chemical preservative can be used not only to initially reduce the presence of microorganisms but also to prevent their potential growth over time during the manufacturing, storage, shipping, and even use of the product. For this reason, there is an emphasis on controlling bacterial and fungal contaminants due to their ubiquitous nature, their ability to be able to multiply even under sometimes unfavorable conditions, and the historical implications of such microorganisms in reported cases of product failure leading to spoilage, infections, or associated toxicity. In food preservation applications, these will include notable foodborne bacterial pathogens such as *Shigella*, *Escherichia*, and *Salmonella* (see chapters 37 and 56). But similarly, there is an increasing emphasis on viral and protozoal pathogens, with a focus on noroviruses and rotaviruses that have become prevalent in food and waterborne infections and outbreaks.[61,62] In cosmetic and non-sterile pharmaceutical applications, there is a much greater emphasis on certain pathogens that are known to be resilient or persistent in transmission situations such as those referred to as being objectionable or opportunistic microorganisms.[34,63,64] These terms has been become widely used in the United States in cosmetic and pharmaceutical applications. Microorganisms can be generally defined as being "objectionable" in view of the product's intended use and in general in relation to products not required to be sterile. But overall, the term may also be generally applied to any situations where the detection of a specific type of microorganism is considered a higher risk due to its known resilience and virulence based on previous experience. Many of these have been widely described in the past such as *Pseudomonas*, *Burkholderia*, and *Bacillus cereus* that once detected in a manufacturing environment are cause of an alert due to their known persistence and association with potential patient impacts including infection and toxicity.[63,64] Pseudomonads such as *Pseudomonas* and *Burkholderia* species are noteworthy given their propensity to persist in low nutrient availability conditions in even pure water conditions or the presence of low concentrations of biocides that are used for preservation conditions (eg, in cosmetics and drinking water situations); they are resilient due to many intrinsic and acquirement resistance mechanisms.[5] But in addition to their resilience, they can be pathogenic, are often associated with water contamination and biofilm formation, and are associated with product-associated outbreaks.[65,66] Other examples include bacteria such as *Aeromonas*, *Enterobacter*, *Klebsiella*, *Clostridium*, and *Staphylococcus* and fungi such as *Aspergillus* and *Penicillium*. As already stated, many of these microorganisms have been described as having known tolerance factors to antimicrobial processes such as spore formation, efflux mechanisms, cell surface alterations, and other innate and acquired tolerance of resistance factors that give them opportunities for survival in various industrial manufacturing and preservation technologies in comparison to other pathogens (see chapters 3 and 4). Therefore, these pathogens are often linked to product-associated outbreaks or contamination (eg, product spoilage) reports. It is important to note that microorganisms and their associated risks (eg, presence of toxin, enzymes, and chemicals) can lead to a variety of infection and toxic effects in consumers/patient depending on their quantitative levels, virulence, and host interactions.

Preservation requirements and technologies are further considered in chapters 38 to 40 for industrial, pharmaceutical, and cosmetic applications. Consideration is also given to the preservative requirements in food and water (see chapter 37) and for packaging, particularly sterile packaging, to maintain product integrity (see chapter 41).

▶ DISINFECTION

Disinfection, defined as a process to inactivate viable microorganisms to a level previously specified as being appropriate for a defined purpose, can encompass a wide range of applications and desired outcomes (see chapter 2). These include antiseptics, food or water disinfectants (including pasteurization), general or critical surface disinfection, area disinfection (fumigation), and medical/dental device applications. A variety of chemical and physical methods in their gaseous or liquid forms are used as summarized in Table 5.2. They vary in their antimicrobial effects and safety requirements. A good example of this is the restricted use of certain antimicrobials on the skin and mucous membranes due to their specific activity against certain microorganisms but also their minimal negative (including toxic) effects on those tissues. Other examples will include the direct use of antimicrobials on plants, foods, and in water. To these examples one can add the variety of filtration methods used to remove microorganisms depending on their sizes for a variety of liquids (including water) and gases (including air). The higher order of disinfection or filtration methods are associated with the complete inactivation or removal of microorganisms, which is further considered under the sterilization section in this chapter.

Before discussing the inactivation of microorganisms during disinfection, a brief consideration is given to filtration. Filtration is often considered separate to disinfection and sterilization methods as it generally does not encompass microbial inactivation, although in some cases, filtration can be combined with antimicrobial processes such as for filter disinfection/maintenance (eg, heat, UV light or periodic use of chemicals including chlorine, bromine, peracetic acid, and silver/copper) or where chemical antimicrobials are included into the structure of filter materials (eg, nanotechnology including silver or carbon, and natural products).[67] Microorganisms vary in size from larger cells such as yeasts, molds, and protozoa in the approximately 10 μm size down to smaller viruses to approximately 10- to 20-nm diameter range.[5] With this knowledge, filters can be designed to retain or prevent the passage of microorganisms by a knowledge of their exclusion size and demonstration of effectiveness by various test methods using physical tests (eg, the bubble-point test to determine the pressure at which a continuous stream of bubbles under pressure is observed passing through a wetted filter[68]), particulate tests (eg, testing the presence of particulates in air following filtration[69,70]), and indicator microorganisms (eg, the use of *Brevundimonas diminuta* or other challenge organisms[71,72]). Filters can be made of a variety of organic and inorganic materials including paper, glass, ceramics, metals, polysaccharides, and variety of polymers. For example, high-efficiency particulate air filters are widely used fiberglass filters that can be designed to remove particulates (including microorganisms) as low as 0.5 and 2.0 μm in diameter, such as those used in cleanrooms (see chapters 58 and 60) and microbiological cabinet designs (see chapter 59). Filters can be classified based on their size exclusion, with examples including course filtration methods (often used as prefilters to extend the lifetime of other more expensive, lower size exclusion filter types), microfiltration (generally including most bacteria and fungi to 0.1- or 0.2-μm diameter), and other methods such as nanofiltration or reverse osmosis methods that can be designed to ensure the removal of the smallest known viruses (eg, in the 10-20 nm range) as well as chemical contaminants such as metal ions. The latter methods can be considered sterile-grade filters because they can be validated to remove microbial contaminants to provide sterile products (see chapter 30).[73,74]

The hierarchy of resistance of microorganisms to inactivation as well as labeling or testing requirements to demonstrate the extent or indeed limits of various disinfectants and disinfection processes were introduced earlier. Antimicrobial claims can be specific to certain types of microorganisms (with claims such as bactericidal and viricidal) and broader claims defined by regulatory requirements in various countries/areas (eg, low-, intermediate-, or high-level disinfection; see chapter 2). The associated test methods used to demonstrate efficacy are useful to ensure these products/processes can be effective under recommended use conditions and are required to be verified (and/or validated) in many specific applications (eg, in industrial manufacturing, high-risk microbiological laboratories, or other regulated environments; see chapter 61). Best practices in disinfection (and sterilization) science dictate not only to demonstrate that a given microbicide, disinfectant formulation, or disinfection process can inactivate certain types of microorganisms but also to study the effects of these under various test conditions, including time and the presence of interfering factors. Microbiological survival curves, which are generally graphed as semilog plots of the ratio of the concentration of surviving organisms to the initial number versus time, are commonly used to present inactivation data and to interpret the inactivation kinetics of microorganisms. These curves can be useful in studying the kinetics of microbial inactivation, determining the predictability of the product/process in microbial inactivation, comparing the resistance of microorganisms to antimicrobial processes (eg, in D-valve estimations), and providing a more detailed analysis of what is occurring during the microbicidal application (see further specific details on the studies and impacts of this analysis in chapters 7, 11, 28, and 61). Typical curves, as shown in Figure 5.3, may be linear but are frequently nonlinear. Nonlinear curves can include sigmoidal, concave-upward, or concave-downward configurations. Several concepts, based on theoretic and mechanistic approaches, have been developed to explain the configurations of these curves.

A linear microbial survival curve demonstrates a predicable antimicrobial process against a uniform population of microorganisms, when the inactivation curve is well established (see the discussion later in this chapter on "Sterilization"). This can allow for the extrapolation of the continued antimicrobial activity over a longer time (or dose in the case of a radiation process), which is an important concept in the demonstration of a sterility assurance level (SAL) for

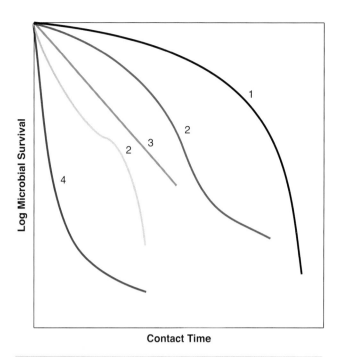

FIGURE 5.3 Representation of the configurations of microbial survival curves (showing $\log_{10}$ microbial reduction over time) on disinfection and sterilization process/product exposures: concave upward (1), sigmoidal (2), linear (exponential) (3), and concave downward (4).

sterilization processes discussed later. But other curve types can equally provide information about the target microbial population and/or the antimicrobial process/product being applied. An example was originally proposed in 1918 based on the assumption that the resistance of different individual cells in a population of apparently similar microorganisms may be different, and a vitalistic concept was used to explain the sigmoidal or upward-concave survival curves.[75] They suggested that organisms possessing an average degree of resistance to the antimicrobial process would be found in the majority of the population, whereas those possessing a maximum or minimum degree of resistance would be found in the minority. Consequently, the survival times were expected to be normally distributed, but no experimental evidence was available to verify this concept.[76] Others demonstrated that the logarithm of survival time for some organisms was normally distributed, and this indicated that the microorganisms resisting in a minimum degree are present in the greatest number, in contrast to the vitalistic concept.[77] In a comprehensive analysis of disinfection kinetics, several theoretic and practical drawbacks of the concept were discussed and indicated the need for further experimental evidence to substantiate the concept.[78]

The initial shoulder effect associated with many microbial survival curves (eg, curve 1, Figure 5.3) has been analyzed in different ways. The expressions developed from the multitarget[79] and multihit[80] phenomena were able to generate survival curves that were concave upward. The multitarget approach assumes that the microorganisms possess several vital sites, each of which must be hit once before inactivation. The multihit or series-event concept assumes that only one sensitive target requires several hits for inactivation. These approaches did not prove to be satisfactory in fitting data for some studies,[81] but they were successful in fitting data for others.[82] In another approach, it was considered that virus inactivation by iodine was first order and that the nonlinearity caused by the multihit effect was necessary to inactivate the organisms that remained as clumps.[83] Moreover, it was deduced that a typical lagging curve occurs if all the virions form clumps of approximately equal numbers of infectious particles. In contrast, survival curves for the chlorine inactivation of single virion preparations of poliovirus type 1 at low pH also resembled typical lagging curves.[84] Using the same organism and disinfectant at pH 6, others reported a similar curve configuration that was concave upward.[85] These curves are a typical example of how antimicrobial activity can vary depending on the exact antimicrobial being applied, including concentration, temperature, time, pH, etc. The inactivation of a suspension of clump-free protozoan cysts with ozone produced typical lagging curves.[86] Similar observations have been made in the inactivation of protozoan cysts by chlorine[87] and chlorine dioxide.[88] Thus, the existence of an initial lag in microbial inactivation may not be attributed solely to simple aggregation of particles.

The inactivation rate of a single-cell suspension of *Naegleria gruberi* cysts followed first-order kinetics when exposed to iodine, with a shoulder of survival curves proposed to be due to the aggregation of cysts.[89] A multi-Poisson distribution model was developed to explain cyst inactivation kinetics, assuming that the destruction of each individual of the clump was first order of kinetics. Two additional assumptions were made in the derivation of the distribution model: First, the rate of inactivation of clumped organisms is directly proportional to the concentration of clumps of a specific size, and second, the destruction of a clump is sequential, with only one individual inactivated at a time. Although no experimental evidence substantiated the last two assumptions, the multi-Poisson distribution model appeared successful in fitting their data.

It is evident that none of the various hypotheses can be considered entirely correct because they have not been subjected to adequate independent verifications. A common kinetic theory is difficult to apply universally because different microorganisms behave differently under similar experimental conditions, and the same microorganism may behave differently under various experimental or growth conditions. But kinetics based on empiric or mechanistic approaches can be used with reasonable confidence for engineering applications, such as designing full-scale treatment units or predicting the extent of inactivation under different hydraulic and mixing conditions. For example, using the multitarget and series-event kinetic parameters generated from batch data, the response of microorganisms to UV was successfully predicted for inactivation in flow-through reactors.[82]

Depending on the type of organism, the kinetics of the inactivation of relevant subcellular components such as DNA and RNA may also need to be established experimentally if the inactivation of those components is deemed necessary. Inactivation kinetics can be established for different viability endpoints as needed. For example, kinetic data can be established for the inactivation of the microorganism as well as the denaturation of its genetic materials if such treatments are deemed necessary based on the risk associated with microbial survival (eg, with some viruses). Such applications may be required in the treatment of infectious wastes and materials from bioprocessing facilities that contain genetically engineered organisms. Similar to microorganisms, inactivation kinetics can also be established for genetic elements ex vivo (eg, by investigating nucleic acid fragmentation). Once the kinetics is established, the extent of inactivation of biologic agents can be predicted for a variety of conditions such as different biocide concentrations, pH, and temperature.

Selection of an appropriate disinfection or sterilization process is determined by a number of criteria including:

- Effectiveness of the microbicide to inactivate microorganisms and, if necessary, the subcellular components
- Applicability of the method to different media (eg, air, wastewater, sludge, or surfaces)
- Availability of the antimicrobial process (eg, distribution of heat or chemical, presence of interfering factors, chemical demand, access to the microorganism, etc.)
- Detoxification requirements and lack of toxic by-product formation
- Hazards associated with the microbicide and treatment process
- Ease of handling and application
- Capital and operating costs, etc.

The effectiveness of different microbicides can also be evaluated by comparing the concentration-exposure time (C • t) data for the inactivation of microorganisms to a given level (eg, 99% inactivation). For a successful comparison, data should be generated under identical experimental conditions. For example, inactivation data need to be generated using the same suspension of organisms grown under similar conditions in a given medium (water or wastewater). Environmental conditions such as pH and temperature also should be the same. Finally, experiments should be conducted using appropriate reactors (eg, batch versus continuous flow) for which data will be applied. The C • t data can also be used to compare the relative resistance of different microorganisms to a given inactivation agent. This information is necessary, for example, when a waste stream contains several different microorganisms and subcellular components. In this case, inactivation data need to be obtained for each of the biologic agents of concern under identical environmental conditions.

A convenient way to evaluate C • t data is to compare the times required to inactivate 99% (2 log) of the organisms exposed to a certain concentration (eg, 1 ppm) of each of the microbicides. A unique concentration for all the inactivation agents does not seem to be feasible because of the significant variations in the effectiveness of the decontaminant and resistance of microorganisms. For example, when *E coli* was exposed to 0.07 mg/L of ozone at pH 7.2 and 1°C in a batch reactor, the time required to achieve 99% inactivation was only approximately 5 seconds.[90] In contrast, others reported that the time required to inactivate simian rotavirus by 10 mg/L chloramine at pH 8 and 5°C was more than 6 hours.[91] As a result of these wide variations, the C • t products for 99% inactivation were compared by several groups for a range of decontaminant concentrations.[92,93]

The C • t concept is based on an empiric logarithmic relationship[92] in the following form:

$$C^n \cdot t = k \qquad (1)$$

where C = concentration of biocide

n = coefficient of dilution

t = exposure time required to obtain a given level of inactivation (eg, 99%)

k = empiric parameter that varies with the disinfectant, microorganism, and extent of inactivation for a specific environmental condition

When $n = 1$, the C • t product is constant for a given range of values. When $n > 1$, the dominant factor that determines the extent of inactivation is concentration, and the C • t value decreases with increasing C. When $n < 1$, the dominant factor is contact time, and the C • t value increases with increasing C. The effects of various n values on C • t are presented in Figure 5.4.

A set of n values for different chemicals and microorganisms is given in Table 5.4. Reported n values range from 0.34 to 4.76. Data also indicate that n falls reasonably close to 1 in some cases. Under these conditions, C • t values can be used to compare either the efficiencies of different microbicides to inactivate the same organism or the resistance of different microorganisms to a given biocide. C • t data comparing the resistance of the protozoan cysts, *N gruberi* and *Giardia muris*, under various conditions of temperature, pH, ozone concentration, and contact time in a batch reactor are given in Table 5.5. The coefficient of dilution (n) for each organism was approximately 1. Comparison of C • t values for both organisms at pH 7 and 25°C shows that *N gruberi* has a C • t value approximately five times larger than *G muris*, indicating that *N gruberi* is approximately five times more resistant than *G muris*. Hence, the higher the C • t value, the more resistant the organism. C • t values can also be used to compare pH and temperature effects. For example, with an increase in temperature from 5°C to 15°C at pH 7, the resistance of *G muris* to inactivation by ozone was decreased approximately five times. In the case of *N gruberi*, the decrease in resistance under similar conditions was only by a factor of two.

The C • t values also can be used to compare the efficiency of different inactivation agents for the same

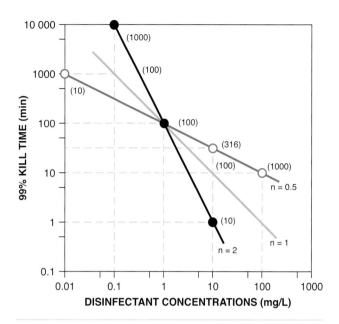

FIGURE 5.4 Effect of *n* value on concentration-exposure time (C • t) values at different disinfectant concentrations (C • t values given in parentheses).[93]

organism. Table 5.6 contains data comparing the efficacy of four chemical microbicides—ozone, chlorine dioxide, chlorine, and chloramines—against different microorganisms. In this case, the lower the C • t value, the higher the efficacy of the microbicide. Consequently, ozone appears to be the most effective of the four microbicides, with C • t values ranging from 0.006 to 2.0 mg-min/L. Chlorine dioxide and free chlorine are more or less comparable to each other in their disinfection efficiency. Chloramines are the least effective, with C • t values ranging from 95 to 6476 mg-min/L.

The C • t data for the inactivation of microorganisms may be presented as log-log plots of time versus concentration. An example used to compare the resistance of different organisms to inactivation by free available chlorine is given in Figure 5.5.[95] The inactivation lines for the most sensitive organisms fall closer to the origin of x- and y-axes, and the lines for resistant organisms fall further away from the origin. For example, *E coli* at pH 7 is the most sensitive, and *Bacillus anthracis* at pH 8.6 is the most resistant to chlorine inactivation at 20°C to 29°C.

A literature review on disinfection data compared the use of chlorine, chloramine, chlorine dioxide, and ozone in water.[93] One of the objectives of this study was to evaluate the applicability of the C • t concept in developing disinfection requirements for these chemical agents. It was concluded that the C • t values can be used to compare the efficacy of disinfectants against specific microorganisms and their relative resistance. The C • t values did vary depending on the microbicide when exposed to different concentrations at specific pH and temperature conditions, with some showing greater variability than others. But at the same time, the use of C • t values alone for defining

TABLE 5.4   Coefficient of dilution (n) for free chlorine, chlorine dioxide, and ozone[a]

Disinfectant	Organism	pH	Temperature (°C)	Range disinfectant concentration (mg/L)	n
Free chlorine	Naegleria gruberi	5.0	25	0.49-2.68	0.96
		7.0	25	0.78-3.44	1.19
		9.0	25	11.6-72.6	0.93
Free chlorine	Giardia muris	7.0	5	0.41-2.73	0.34
		7.0	5	11.1-78.5	1.52
		7.0	5	186-244	4.76
Free chlorine	G muris	5.0	25	4.9-13.0	1.35
		7.0	25	2.87-7.12	1.59
		9.0	25	15.5-84.1	0.90
Chlorine dioxide	Poliovirus type 1	7.0	5	0.4-1.0	1.05
		7.0	25	0.4-0.8	1.02
Chlorine dioxide	Escherichia coli	6.5	5	0.25-0.75	1.08
		6.5	10	0.25	1.18
		6.5	20	0.25	1.03
Chlorine dioxide	G muris	7.0	5	1.20	1.20
Chlorine dioxide	G muris	5.0	25	1.22	1.22
		7.0	25	1.30	1.30
		9.0	25	1.37	1.37
Chlorine dioxide	N gruberi	5.0	25	0.53-1.2	1.09
		7.0	25	0.41-1.3	0.93
		9.0	25	0.43-1.1	0.94
Ozone	N gruberi	5-9	25	0.21-1.05	1.0
		7	51-30	0.21-1.05	1.1
Ozone	G muris	5-9	25	0.02-0.19	1.2
		7	5-25	0.03-0.7	1.1

[a]From Hoff.[93]

disinfection application criteria had some problems including the following:

- Failure of disinfection to follow exponential rates described by the empirical C • t equation
- Differences in resistance between different isolates of the same species and between different species within groups (bacteria, viruses, cysts)
- Differences in the presentation of the microorganisms including aggregation, prior growth conditions, and protective effects
- Influence of practical experimental conditions (test configuration, mixing methodology, disinfectant, concentration variations, etc.)
- The relevance of laboratory data to in process conditions

Although the C • t concept was developed for measuring microbial inactivation by chemical agents, it can be applied to evaluate data for physical agents such as UV irradiation and heat. In the case of UV irradiation, the intensity (I) of the UV source falling on the treatment medium is given as power per unit area (eg, microwatts per square centimeter, $\mu W/cm^2$). The dose is given by the product of intensity and time, I • t (μW-sec/cm^2), and is similar to the C • t product used with chemical inactivation. As an example, Table 5.7 shows dose (I • t) data for 90% inactivation of test microorganism cultures. From this table, it appears that UV irradiation is effective in inactivating bacteria and viruses, whereas protozoan cysts and spore-forming bacteria are more resistant to inactivation by UV irradiation. In the case of heat, a temperature-time product (θ • t) can be used in place of the C • t product. Overall, the C • t values generated from laboratory or pilot

TABLE 5.5   Concentration-time (C · t) data for 99% inactivation of cysts with ozone[a,b]

Temperature (°C)	pH	Naegleria gruberi C (mg/L)	t (min)	C · t (mg-min/L)	Giardia muris C (mg/L)	t (min)	C · t (mg-min/L)
25	5	0.3-1.2	4.4-1.1	1.33	0.0-0.1	5.0-2.0	0.201
25	6	0.3-1.1	5.2-1.4	1.55	…	…	…
25	7	0.3-1.2	4.3-1.1	1.29	0.03-0.15	9-1.8	0.27
25	8	0.25-0.8	5.4-1.7	1.36	…	…	…
25	9	0.35-1.1	6.1-1.9	2.12	0.015-0.01	7.5-1.1	0.112
5	7	0.55-2.0	7.8-2.1	4.23	0.15-0.7	12.9-2.8	1.94
15	7	0.3-0.9	6.8-2.3	2.04	0.05-0.3	7.5-1.3	0.375
30	7	0.3-1.0	4-1.2	1.21	…	…	…

C, ozone concentration; t, time for 99% kill.

[a]C · t values are for average of three or more experiments. n values for N gruberi and C muris are 1.0-1.1 and 1.0-1.2, respectively.

[b]From Wickramanayake.[94]

scale experiments may be used to design full-scale treatment processes. Extrapolation of C • t values must be done with considerable caution and should be limited to the reported ranges of chemical concentrations, environmental conditions, and reactor types. Further discussion on studying the kinetic models for microbial inactivation are given in chapter 7 and in other chapters specifically to microbicide mechanisms (eg, heat disinfection and sterilization in chapters 11 and 28, respectively, or the effects of process variables in EO sterilization described in chapter 31).

▶ STERILIZATION

The term *sterile* is defined as being free from viable microorganisms, which as discussed earlier may be practically achieved by a variety of antimicrobial or physical removal technologies. But there are practical as well as regulatory implications in the use of this term. Practically, if the microbial content on or in a product or other material (the bioburden) is known and the activity of an antimicrobial process can reduce this by a known level, then this may be

TABLE 5.6   Summary of concentration-time value ranges (mg-min/L) for 99% inactivation of various microorganisms by chemical disinfectants at 5°C[a]

Microorganism	Disinfectant Free Chlorine pH 6-7	Preformed Chloramine pH 3-9	Chlorine Dioxide pH 6-7	Ozone pH 6-7
Escherichia coli	0.034-0.05	95-180	0.4-0.75	0.02
Poliovirus type 1	1.1-2.5	768-3740	0.2-6.7	0.1-0.2
Rotavirus	0.01-0.05	3806-6476	0.2-2.1	0.006-0.06
Phage f_2	0.08-0.18	…	…	…
Giardia lamblia cysts	47-150	…	…	0.5-0.6
Giardia muris cysts	30-630	…	7.2-18.5	1.3-2.0

[a]From Hoff.[93]

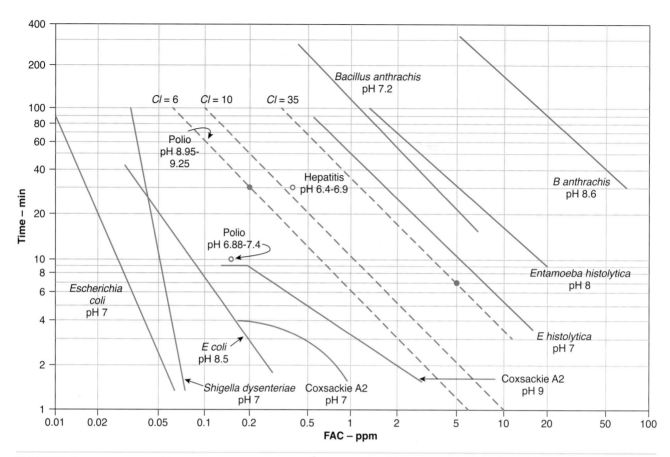

FIGURE 5.5   Inactivation of bacteria and viruses by free available chlorine at 20°C and 90°C.[95]

microbiologically considered to render the target material "sterile." But what happens if the bioburden changes, if the process being applied was not done correctly, and what about the maintenance of conditions over time? Would we have greater scientific confidence in the process if the level of antimicrobial activity could provide a greater level of assurance that sterility was indeed achieved consistently? Therefore, the regulatory implications come into our discussion on how the process of reaching a sterile state is achieved, documented, and maintained. As introduced earlier, there are two strategies that can be employed to ensure (and therefore label) a product "sterile":

- Aseptic processing, based on the concept of ensuring the sterilization (or sterile filtration) of various product components and keeping them under aseptic conditions during the manufacturing process and subsequent delivery to a point of use to ensure a sterile product presentation (see chapters 30 and 58)
- Terminal sterilization, a process used to render product free from viable microorganisms in the final product configuration and packaging

In both cases, the act of making a product sterile should not be considered as a single step in the overall manufacturing or processing process but can include multiple activities that provide confidence that at the end (or indeed

point of use) the product is sterile. This is a qualitative quality concept that may be defined as the assurance of sterility. This is clearly important during an aseptic manufacturing or handling, where the preparation and correct assembly of various components (raw materials, liquids, containers, manufacturing surfaces, subassemblies, air and water quality, etc.) need to be combined together to provide a sterile product and therefore scrupulously defined and controlled during the manufacturing process. But it is also important in the preparation of a product for terminal sterilization. An example includes providing a defined chemical or particulate cleanliness level of a product to ensure that the sterilization process can be effective because these residuals may hinder access of the antimicrobial effects to the target microorganisms. This may be important to ensure not only sterilization but also the overall safety of the product (because these materials may provide other risks such as toxicity, immune reactions, or other negative impacts in a patient or experimental situation). Another is that the sterilization process may only be defined to inactivate expected levels or even types of microorganisms. Equally, maintaining the sterile environment of the product over time needs to be considered to ensure, that following the manufacturing or processing strategies, the product is indeed sterile as intended for its point of use. Sterile packaging concepts are further considered in detail

TABLE 5.7	Reported microbial dose for 90% inactivation and kinetic inactivation constants resulting from ultraviolet irradiation[a]		
Group	**Microorganism**	**Dose Required for 90% Inactivation (mW · s/cm²)**	**First-Order Inactivation Constant (cm²/mW · s)**
Bacteria	*Aeromonas hydrophila*	1.54	1.50
	Bacillus anthracis	4.5	0.51
	B anthracis spores	54.5	0.0422
	Bacillus subtilis spores	12	0.19
	Campylobacter jejuni	1.05	2.19
	Clostridium tetani	12	0.19
	Corynebacterium diphtheriae	3.4	0.68
	Escherichia coli	1.33	1.73
	E coli	3.2	0.72
	E coli	3	0.77
	Klebsiella terrigena	2.61	0.882
	Legionella pneumophila	2.49	0.925
	L pneumophila	1	2.3
	L pneumophila	0.38	6.1
	Micrococcus radiodurans	20.5	0.112
	Mycobacterium tuberculosis	6	0.38
	Pseudomonas aeruginosa	5.5	0.42
	P aeruginosa	5.5	0.42
	Salmonella enteritidis	4	0.58
	S enteritidis	4	0.58
	Salmonella paratyphi	3.2	0.72
	Salmonella ser Typhi	2.26	1.02
	S Typhi	2.1	1.1
	S Typhi	2.5	0.92
	S Typhimurium	8	0.29
	Shigella dysenteriae	2.2	1.05
	S dysenteriae	0.885	2.60
	S dysenteriae	2.2	1.05
	Shigella flexneri	1.7	1.4
	Shigella paradysenteriae	1.7	1.4
	Shigella sonnei	3	0.77
	Staphylococcus aureus	5	0.46
	S aureus	4.5	0.51
	Streptococcus faecalis	4.4	0.52
	Streptococcus pyogenes	2.2	1.0
	Vibrio cholerae	0.651	3.54
	V cholerae	3.4	0.68
	Vibrio comma	6.5	0.35
	Yersinia enterocolitica	1.07	2.15

(continued)

TABLE 5.7 Reported microbial dose for 90% inactivation and kinetic inactivation constants resulting from ultraviolet irradiation[a] *(Continued)*

Group	Microorganism	Dose Required for 90% Inactivation (mW · s/cm²)	First-Order Inactivation Constant (cm²/mW · s)
Viruses	Coliphage	3.6	0.64
	Coliphage MS2	18.6	0.124
	F-specific bacteriophage	6.9	0.33
	Hepatitis A	7.3	0.32
	Hepatitis A	3.7	0.62
	Influenza virus	3.6	0.64
	Poliovirus	7.5	0.31
	Poliovirus 1	5	0.5
	Poliovirus type 1	7.7	0.30
	Rotavirus	11.3	0.204
	Rotavirus SA11	9.86	0.234
	Rotavirus SA11	8	0.3
Protozoa	*Giardia muris*	82	0.028
	Acanthamoeba castellanii	35	0.066

[a]From Water Environment Federation.[96]

in chapter 41. The routine maintenance of microbiological quality, including assurance of sterility, is considered later in this chapter.

Overall, the use of a terminal sterilization process is preferred and considered less of a risk in ensuring a sterile product is achieved. This is because the product is prepared in a manner to ensure microbiological consistency (eg, bioburden) and then subjected to a defined antimicrobial process in its final packaging orientation. Equally, it is an important step in the preparation of surfaces or materials used during an aseptic manufacturing process. For terminal sterilization, we can consider some essential requirements to ensure a sterile outcome that are like the concepts discussed in the previous section on "Disinfection" but are typically stricter.

- Sterilizing agent characterization. Broad-spectrum efficacy should be demonstrated against all types of microorganisms, under the conditions intended for use (eg, temperature, radiation dose, humidity, concentration, etc.). As highlighted previously, it is impossible and impractical to consider testing every type of microorganism known. But it is also unnecessary for the widely used technologies for sterilization (see Table 5.2) as they have been well established to inactivate the range of microorganisms known (by testing different indicator organisms within these groups; see Table 5.1) and have had a long history of successful sterilization applications. It is important to consider that the demon-

stration of broad-spectrum antimicrobial activity is not enough in the demonstration of a sterilization process because a more detailed knowledge is needed of how consistent the process is in predicting the reproducibility of antimicrobial activity over time (or dose). For this, a greater understanding of the mathematical kinetics of sterilization processes is needed (further discussed in the following text and in chapter 7). In addition, knowledge of the mechanisms of action of any sterilizing agent is useful to understand any risks of it not being effective against target microorganisms. Overall, newer sterilization processes (either based on the more traditional sterilization technologies in a new way or the use of alternative sterilizing agents) may be the subject of greater scrutiny to confirm microbicidal activity. But in addition to the microbicidal effectiveness, other safety requirements will need to be considered such as material compatibility, toxic residuals, and impact on the environment (as discussed earlier).

- Process and equipment characterization. The sterilizing agent will only be effective if the process controls defined earlier are reproducibility and reliably achieved. Therefore, the control of the process conditions and design of process equipment (sterilizers) is important. Examples include vacuum or pressure conditions, temperature provision and distribution, humidity controls, product loading patterns, conveyance of product to and from the sterilizing agent, etc. Specific requirements depend on the sterilization process defined during characterization and their applicable conditions (see Part IV chapters). In addition, the monitoring and recording equipment should be suitable for the sterilization environment (eg, the equipment should not be impaired by exposure to the sterilant and should have measurement accuracy needed for the process parameters. Safety requirements both in the initial and consistent use of the process/equipment over time will clearly be an important consideration given the impact to health and environment. Examples include the restricted access to radiation sources, pressure vessel standard compliance, and the safe abatement or neutralization of microbicidal gases or liquids.

- Product definition for exposure to the sterilization process. There are a number of key aspects to consider, which can also depend on the design of the sterilization process and associated equipment. The first can include the microbiological quality of the product prior to sterilization, defined as the bioburden (see chapter 64 and further discussed in the following text). Other product requirements have been previously discussed such as product cleanliness. But further considerations can be product design, packaging, and expected presentation for sterilization. A good example with product design and packaging is with a gas-based process, where the material should allow the penetration of the antimicrobial process conditions into the target product and associated parts of the product. But also, consideration may need to be given to the expansion or shrinking of the packaging material during extremes of process conditions during sterilization (eg, pressure change and rate of change, or temperature changes). Another example is when considering the difference between the sterilization of a single product in each sterilization cycle in comparison to thousands of products and how to ensure adequate access to each product reproducibility. Product loading patterns and load density can impact heat and radiation distribution. Product material and functionality tolerances to the sterilization process must be defined to ensure product safety on exposure to the process, and extremes in temperature, dose limitations, pressure changes, and gas concentration that may be observed. Overall, the product (including product design, packaging, and loading pattern) definition is important to ensure that the correct sterilization process can be defined and routinely maintained.

- Process definition and validation. Sterilization process definition includes the process conditions and tolerances to ensure consistent delivery of the desired endpoint. Process definition is confirmed during validation to demonstrate that the sterilization process conditions defined can be delivered reproducibly to a documented sterilization load, without compromising product and package functionality. It is not the purpose of this chapter to define validation requirements in detail as they will vary depending on the process and further consideration is given to this in the sterilizing agent-specific chapters (see Part IV) and associated standards (Table 5.8). But essentially, validation typically includes three essential stages: installation qualification, operational qualification, and performance qualification (PQ). Installation qualification protocols establish that the sterilization equipment (including ancillary equipment required for the process such as steam or gas generators, conveyors, abatement systems, etc.) are supplied and installed as intended to operate. This may also include the selection and calibration of measurement instrumentation (eg, instrumentation that measures temperature, pressure, dose, or speed of conveyance systems for a continuous sterilization process, etc.). OQ then confirms that the equipment and associated process functions correctly as defined and typically does not include product. The OQ protocols also typically include measurements that are used for comparison during future studies to demonstrate that the equipment maintains functionality over time. PQ is the ultimate test to demonstrate that the product when exposed to the process as defined confirms that the equipment can deliver the specified requirements, including provision of a sterile product. The approaches that can be used to demonstrate that the sterilization process is achieved during PQ testing is further discussed in the following text.

- Routine monitoring, release of product, and maintenance. It is logical that routine monitoring of the sterilization process (including parametric monitoring of process conditions, or indicators of process effectiveness such as biological and chemical indicators; see chapter 65) is essential to ensure a reliable sterilization process is achieved reproducibly over time. These can also used to ensure the safe release of a product load as being sterile and as part of an overall assurance of sterility quality process. This is important because it is not practical, or necessary, to ensure sterilization by randomly selecting and testing product for sterility following delivery of the defined process. There are several reasons for this (see chapter 64). Examples include that sterility testing is significantly limited in its ability to detect all types of microorganisms and there are risks of laboratory cross-contamination during the recovery and testing of products that can lead to false-positive results. But overall, the assurance of sterility concepts as part of a well-controlled quality system is necessary in the demonstration of a successful sterilization process. A final consideration with this is mind is process maintenance. Process maintenance starts with the control of the raw materials, manufacturing process and personnel impacts for environmental controls. The maintenance of the controls for industrial manufacturing are typically demonstrated by physical controls and measured by the product bioburden to demonstrate there is no change over time and/or that any changes do not impact the product bioburden. Process maintenance will also include (eg, calibration of sensors and

TABLE 5.8   Summary of international sterilization standards based on modality

Sterilization Technology	ISO Standard[a]	Title
All sterilization modalities	ISO 14937	Sterilization of health care products—general requirements for characterization of a sterilizing agent and the development, validation, and routine control of a sterilization process for medical devices
Radiation	ISO 11737-1	Sterilization of health care products—radiation—part 1: requirements for development, validation, and routine control of a sterilization process for medical devices
Ethylene oxide gas	ISO 11135	Sterilization of health care products—ethylene oxide—requirements for development, validation, and routine control of a sterilization process for medical devices
Moist heat	ISO 17665-1	Sterilization of health care products—moist heat—part 1: requirements for the development, validation, and routine control of a sterilization process for medical devices
Dry heat	ISO 20857	Sterilization of health care products—dry heat—requirements for the development, validation, and routine control of a sterilization process for medical devices
Liquid chemicals	ISO 14160	Sterilization of health care products—liquid chemical sterilizing agents for single-use medical devices utilizing animal tissues and their derivatives—requirements for characterization, development, validation, and routine control of a sterilization process for medical devices
Low temperature steam formaldehyde	ISO 25424	Sterilization of medical devices—low temperature steam and formaldehyde—requirements for development, validation, and routine control of a sterilization process for medical devices
Hydrogen peroxide gas	ISO 22441[b]	Sterilization of health care products—low temperature vaporized hydrogen peroxide—requirements for the development, validation, and routine control of a sterilization process for medical devices

[a]The most current version of these standards is defined by the date of publication and is purposefully omitted in this summary as each standard is subject to periodic review, modification, and voting for publication. There may also be different parts of the standard series, which are designated as ISO XXXX-1, etc, but only the parent standard for each series is shown.

[b]At the time of publication, this standard was under development.

servicing), requalification at defined intervals as initially validated (including repeating certain validation tests on equipment updates or significant servicing changes), and assessments of changes that can include equipment, process, load, or product manufacturing or design changes.

Due to the wealth of information with common sterilization processes, international standards have been developed that define these requirements for successful sterilization applications, including validation requirements (see Table 5.8).

For all sterilization processes, there is an expectation to demonstrate broad-spectrum antimicrobial activity as well as an understanding of the mathematical kinetics of inactivation with the defined process over time (or dose). Before we consider this further, there are some exceptions to this that are considered briefly. Examples include regulatory (or labeling) requirements in certain areas, product limitations, and microorganism limitations. The first relates to specific regulatory requirements

in certain countries or economic areas. Even though bacterial spores are considered some of the more resistant forms of microbial life, the demonstration of sporicidal activity is not enough to imply a sterilization end point. Sporicidal tests (see chapters 61-63) are widely used to demonstrate (and label for) the ability of an antimicrobial product or process to inactivate bacterial spores. Although these may show sporicidal activity (and likely to include other microorganisms), they may not always be used in a controlled, defined process to ensure sterility (eg, inactivate spores but not the maintenance of a sterile environment following treatment). In other cases, the application of a liquid sporicidal process may need to be followed by rinsing with water, which unless specifically controlled and validated may not preserve a sterile product or environment. In some areas, the demonstration of sporicidal activity (eg, using the stringent AOAC sporicidal test; see chapters 62, 71, and 72) can be used to support a claim of "sterilant" or even "sterilization" by certain regulatory agencies, but these may only imply a sporicidal disinfection process. It is therefore important to read and understand the associated labels with such products and processes.

Another exception is with product limitations that can be highlighted with living tissue sterilization applications (see chapter 50). Living (or associated) tissues and organs are essential to biomedical science and human health. Although many tissue-engineered products are currently under development, health care still depends on donations of tissues and organs from humans and animals. Given their cellular nature and the mechanisms of action of sterilization processes, it is not surprising that viable tissues will be damaged by such processes. To ensure their safety, a classical end-to-end microbiological quality approach has been adopted based on a risk assessment (see chapter 50). This includes detailed medical scrutiny of donors; screening for the presence of certain pathogens (eg, human immunodeficiency virus and hepatitis viruses); aseptic recovery; microbiological testing of recovered tissues; processing to include cleaning, disinfection, and/or liquid chemical sterilization of the tissue (eg, ISO 14160; see Table 5.8); microbiological testing following processing; and sterile packaging. In many of these cases, the liquid chemical disinfection or sterilization processing of the tissue may not be specifically effective against or penetrate to every potential type of microorganism that may be present, although there is a particular focus in these studies on bacteria or bacterial spores, and detectable bioburden reduction. In this case, it is common to conduct sterility tests on samples of the final product as a verification of the successful handling/treatment, similar to aseptically processed products.

A final example in sterilization science is limitations due to microorganism types, with a good example being transmissible proteinaceous agents, or prions (see chapters 3 and 68). Prions are not considered "living" but can be transmissible. Due to their unique structures, as uniquely folded peptides/proteins, they resist natural degradation and therefore form protein fibrils in the body. Prions in these forms are not found to be as sensitive to common disinfection and sterilization technologies as other classical microorganisms (bacteria, viruses, fungi, and protozoa[5,97]). Although in many cases further investigations are warranted, prions are known to persist in contaminated tissues subjected to many traditional sterilization methods such as those based on moist heat, radiation, and EO. Moist heat can be effective over time, but radiation and EO appear to have little impact from studies published to date. But at the same time, methods that have been shown to degrade protein structures, such as with chlorine, alkali, and hydrogen peroxide gas, have been shown to be effective.[97] Despite this, most of the sterilization standards specifically exclude consideration of prion inactivation and approaches to reducing risks associated with prion decontamination generally include detecting known or high-risk population and discarding materials that may contact associated high-risk tissues such as the brain or spinal cord.[98]

Widely used sterilization processes (see Table 5.8) have been well established to provide broad-spectrum antimicrobial activity, including against viruses, bacteria, fungi, and protozoa in their various vegetative and dormant states as applicable. In most of these cases, bacterial spores have been shown to be the most resistant microorganisms to inactivation. Exceptions to this rule have been described and are considered in chapter 3 (see Table 3.2) including certain types of vegetative bacteria that have varying and higher tolerance levels to radiation and the resistance of the fungus *Pyronema domesticum* to EO sterilization. In both of these cases, controls are recommended in the applicable radiation and EO sterilization standards to address these specific concerns and still apply a reliable sterilization process. As an example, with radiation sterilization, the product bioburden is characterized to understand the types as well as the number of microorganisms to determine a radiation dose acceptable to inactivate all microorganism with a wide range of radiation resistance profiles. Periodically the product bioburden resistance is verified by exposing manufactured product to a fractional dose of radiation in comparison to the sterilization dose ("dose verification"; see chapter 29). For other sterilization processes, bacterial spores have been widely used both in the process characterization (as representative resistant microorganisms) and their validation (such as in the use of spore-containing BIs; see chapter 65).

During the discussion on disinfection, we considered the importance of understanding the rate of microbial interaction over time on exposure to an antimicrobial process. Figure 5.3 provides an overview of typical inactivation kinetics on studying the microbicidal impact on a population of microorganisms over time. Essentially, the same concepts apply in understanding the microbicidal activity (characterization) of sterilization processes, particularly in studying bacterial spore inactivation kinetics. This concept is briefly discussed here and further considered in other chapters specific to sterilization (see Part IV). The first objective is to determine an accurate inactivation curve. The microbiological methods used are reasonably straightforward, by exposing the target microorganism (usually a population of bacterial spores) to the sterilization process conditions (or fractions thereof) to determine the level of microbial inactivation over time (or dose) with associated controls (see chapter 61). The most straightforward method is by direct enumeration, by serial dilutions and culturing of microorganisms present by plating on an applicable growth agar and incubation. The number of survivors can be directly counted and plotted (Figure 5.6).

To communicate these results visually, a survivor curve graph can be prepared in which the number of microorganisms surviving is plotted as a function of the length of time or dose of the sterilization process being tested.

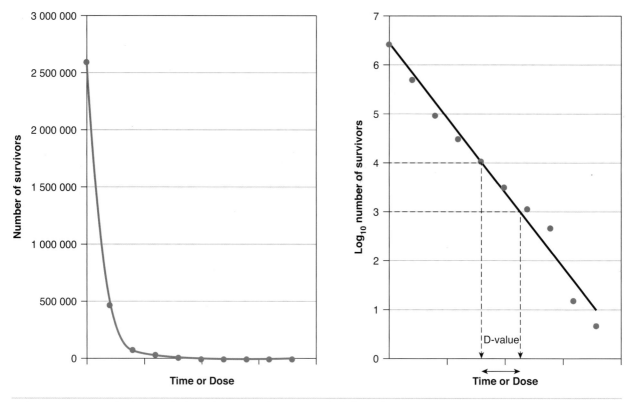

FIGURE 5.6 Microbial survival plotted on an arithmetic graph (left) and on a semilogarithmic graph (right). The estimation of the D-valve is demonstrated as the time (or dose) to give a 1 $\log_{10}$ reduction in the microbial population.

There are several ways to plot the data (see Figure 5.6). One is a survivor curve graph in which both the numbers of survivors and time are plotted on an arithmetic scale. In this case, the data forms an exponential decay-type curve. This is a nondistorted, visual perspective on the effect of a constant stress on a microbial population, but as the number of survivors approaches lower levels, this graph does not tell us much about the area of low levels of survival. But when we plot the number of surviving organisms on a logarithmic scale as a function of time/dose on an arithmetic scale, the y-axis is effectively expanded so we have equal readability at all survival levels. This is an appropriate way to treat microbial survivor data because in sterilization studies, we are interested in the rate of destruction of microorganisms as we approach zero survivors. But the direct enumeration method to detect low levels of survivors is limited and a greater sensitivity can be further determined using a most probable number (MPN) estimation by fraction-negative analysis (Figure 5.7).

This requires a different experimental design, where the number of surviving microorganisms is estimated based on a fraction of samples within a population. A typical example is in testing 10 samples inoculated with a known number of microorganisms (or 20 samples when using product with naturally existing bioburden for radiation) and exposing to a microbicidal process; as the levels of exposure to the process approaches a low level of (or to zero) survivors, a fraction of the 10 samples will show growth (therefore assumed to have at least one viable sur-

vivor) and others will have no growth (presumed to have no survivors). An example of the results from this experiment is shown in Figure 5.8.

This is the quantal or fraction-negative region of the survivor curve and allows the estimation of the survival of low levels of microorganisms. The estimation of the MPN is based on an equation described by Halvorson and Ziegler[99]:

$$N_u = \ln (n / r)$$

where, N_u = number of survivors in the quantal or fractional region of the survivor curve (see Figure 5.7)

n = number of units tested

r = number of units showing no growth

These valves can be added to the overall semilogarithmic graph of the survivor curve (see Figure 5.7). The points larger than 1×10^0 correspond to survival levels of more than one microorganism per unit. For a mean survival level less than 1×10^0, there is a fractional microbial survival level, where there may be 1 surviving organism in 10 units (0.1 or 10^{-1}), 1 in 100 units (0.01 or 10^{-2}), and so forth. The use of MPN and fraction-negative methods in the direct determination of D-values is considered in further detail in chapters 11 and 28.

Theoretically in this analysis, with a starting population of 10^6 microorganisms, a >6 $\log_{10}$ reduction is achieved over the time/dose indicated to provide a "sterile" product (where $\log_{10} 1 = 0$). If the number of starting

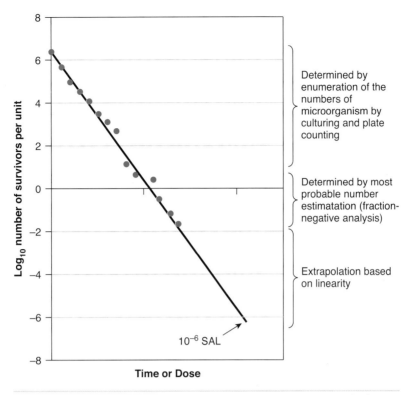

FIGURE 5.7 An ideal survivor curve showing the combined results from direct enumeration and fraction-negative (or quantal) measurement areas. From this combined analysis, a sterility assurance level (SAL) can be extrapolated giving confidence in the application of the sterilization process to provide sterility.

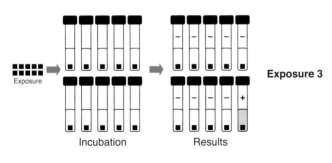

Exposure (Time/Dose)	n	r	n/r	$N_u{}^1$
1	10	1	10	2.30
2	10	5	2	0.69
3	10	9	1.1	0.09

$^1N_u = \ln (n/r)$

FIGURE 5.8 Examples of an most probable number (MPN) estimation of survivors by fraction negative analysis. In this example, 10 samples are exposed to a sterilization process over three exposure times (or doses), incubated, and assessed for growth (an example of the results for exposure 3 is shown above). The results and estimation of the MPN (N_u) is shown in the table.

microorganisms was less (eg, at 10^1 or 10^2), this end point would be achieved at a shorter time (or less dose). Theoretically, we can go further with this analysis, by continuing to expose the product to the process beyond the point of zero and therefore express the *probability* of a sterilization end point, such as the probability of one surviving organism per one thousand as 10^{-3} and one surviving organism per one million units as 10^{-6}. This is referred to as an SAL and is defined as the probability of a single viable microorganism occurring on an item after sterilization, expressed as the negative exponent to the base 10. The SAL is a quantitative probability assessment. Therefore, in the example given here, the product may be considered sterile at an SAL of 10^{-1} or 10^{-6}, but there is a greater assurance of sterility associated with a lesser SAL. It is important to use the correct nomenclature in referring to SALs, such as specifying the SAL as a maximum value and when comparing different SALs to refer to these being "less than" or "greater than" each other. The use of terms such as "higher" or "lower" SALs or that an SAL could be "better than" or "worse than" another can be misleading. Traditionally, an SAL of 10^{-6} has been accepted for sterilization processes internationally, but alternative SALs are acceptable based on a risk assessment and associated product need, with the overall goal being to provide a safe product for its intended purpose.[8,100]

It is useful at this stage to differentiate between the use of an SAL for a terminal sterilization process in comparison to estimation of the presence (or confirmation of the absence) of a nonsterile item following an aseptic process. Remember that an SAL is an extrapolation of an antimicrobial process that is known to occur over time or dose. In the case of an aseptic process, it is not possible to apply a sterility assurance level as there is the potential to have a non-sterile unit during the processing. In order to demonstrate that the risk of the presence of a non-sterile unit following asceptic processing has been systematically reduced, a sampling of a proportion of the units in an aseptically manufactured batch of product (or typically where the product is replaced with culture media, referred to as a "media fill") is often employed (see chapter 58). In this case sampling of, say, 1 in 10, 1 in 100, or 1 in 1000 for sterility testing can provide different levels of an assurance of sterility in the batch, but it would not be appropriate to refer to this as an SAL. A further term that is often used traditionally in these cases is the *probably of a nonsterile unit* (PNSU); a PNSU and SAL may have the same connotation but are often implied to different situations, where the SAL is the probably of sterility based on the extrapolation of an antimicrobial process, whereas the PNSU is most often used to the sampling of product for sterility testing following an aseptic process. But overall, in both cases, the aseptic manufacturing or terminal sterilization part of the treatment or manufacturing process is only part of the overall strategy of an assurance of sterility.[8,101]

To continue the discussion on the analysis of inactivation curves, these can be further studied for the impact on process variables to include temperature, humidity, dose, and chemical concentration depending on the sterilization process under investigation (see chapter 7). A good example of this is further considered for moist heat disinfection and sterilization processes (see chapters 11 and 28). By studying and determining the D-values at different temperature, a z-value can be determined by plotting the $\log_{10}$ D-valve over the test temperature and determining the slope of the resulting linear line to determine the average temperature required to change the D-value by a factor of 10. With both the D-value and associated z-value, the expected extent of the antimicrobial process can be determined over a range of temperatures. Similar effects can be determined by studying the different variables in other sterilization processes such as the effect of radiation dose (see chapter 29) and humidity, temperature, and concentration in EO processes (see chapter 31). These concepts can essentially apply to all sterilization methods, including alternative gas and liquid chemical sterilization processes.[102]

Finally, with this background, there are at least three approaches that can be used to demonstrate that the sterilization process is achieved during PQ testing (process definition).[103]

- Bioburden based, established on the inactivation of the microbial population on or in product in its natural state just prior to sterilization. This approach is based on a knowledge (both quantitative and qualitative) of the microbial population on representative product before sterilization (ie, the bioburden; see chapter 64). This is dependent on having a reasonably consistent manufacturing process, where the bioburden is relatively constant over time. Representative product is chosen and subjected to the sterilization process at increments of the expected exposure time, dose, or equivalent process variables for the process conditions. Following exposure, the product is tested for sterility to confirm antimicrobial activity (see chapter 64). The minimum sterilization process to ensure sterility can be defined based on the results of this test and extrapolating to apply an acceptable SAL. Such a method is widely used, or similarly applied, to the validation of radiation sterilization processes (see chapter 29).[104] It is important that not only the bioburden is periodically monitored to understand changes in numbers of microbial types but also that the susceptibility is routinely confirmed by a similar experimental design (eg, as defined for periodic dose verification testing for radiation sterilization processes; see chapter 29).

- Overkill, based on the inactivation of reference microorganisms. This is a more conservative approach and is probably the most widely used (eg, for heat and gas processes). It is particularly useful to employ if the microbiological challenge in or on the product (bioburden) is high, either in resistance or quantity, or variable. An example is during the reprocessing of reusable, critical medical devices where the bioburden is generally not known or routinely monitored (see chapter 47). The method is based on using an artificial challenge using test microorganisms (typically bacterial spores) at high levels (up to 10^6) with a known, high-level resistance to the sterilization process. Representative microorganisms include bacterial spore preparations of *Geobacillus stearothermophilus* (for steam sterilization processes) and *Bacillus atrophaeus* (for EO sterilization processes). The test microorganism is placed at specific or multiple locations within the product and/or associated load that are representative worst case for the sterilization process to access (usually determined based on knowledge of the process, product, and load being tested, and/or through experimental testing). The microbial challenge can be inoculated directly in or on the product, or more commonly using BIs that can be prepared in various designs (see chapter 65). The test product/load is then subjected to a fractional, defined sterilization process (fractionally less than the full, expected process for routine sterilization) and then the BIs or inoculated product recovered and tested to determine the extent of microbial inactivation. Examples include the use of a 10^6 spore inoculum or BI to test a sterilization process at one-half its exposure time or a 10^3 spore challenge to one-fourth sterilization cycle time. The effectiveness of the fractional sterilization process to inactivate a known population of microorganisms within a fractional time (or equivalent based on the sterilization process) can be used to extrapolate the time required to ensure sterility (including the desired SAL). The example earlier of a 6 $\log_{10}$ reduction of bacterial spores at a half sterilization cycle exposure time can be extrapolated to provide a theoretical 12 $\log_{10}$ reduction at the full cycle (therefore equivalent to an SAL of 10^{-6}). This approach is considered an "overkill" in most cases because the likely bioburden on the product for sterilization will be significantly lower than 10^6 (eg, <1000 colony-forming unit per product), and the bioburden is likely to be mixed population that has a significantly lower resistance to the sterilization process than the bacterial spores used in the test. In addition, mathematical calculations would indicate that total kill of BIs with a known population of 10^6 (if one were to use 10 BIs and observe ≤1/10 positive BIs following exposure to the half cycle) might demonstrate achievement of greater than a half-cycle kill (e.g., 10^{-1} SAL).

- A combined approach is based on the inactivation of reference microorganisms and knowledge of bioburden. This approach essentially uses a combination of the other two methods described. A knowledge of the bioburden (both initially and maintained over time) may be used to compare directly to the use of a test indicator microorganism at a defined population to verify and define a minimal process to achieve sterilization (with consideration of an acceptable SAL). The combined method and the bioburden-based approaches are typically applied when the product functionality is negatively impacted when using a longer exposure to the sterilant. Also, the combined or bioburden-based methods are beneficial to reduce demand on sterilization time or dose when there is a reduced capacity for sterilization (e.g., volume of medical device sterilization is larger than the sterilization throughput capacity available).

ASSURANCE OF MICROBIOLOGICAL QUALITY

The microbicidal processes described for preservation, disinfection, and sterilization are important in achieving safe products and other requirements (such as in laboratory, environmental, or public safety). But these processes should not be considered in isolation and are essentially part of an overall quality assurance process that considers an end-to-end philosophy (Figure 5.9). From a microbiological perspective, end-to-end refers to all stages of a supply process that should be considered as risks or critical control points in the development, manufacture, and delivery of a microbiologically controlled or sterile-labeled product to an end user or consumer. This objective not only applies to the manufacturer or supplier of products or utilities but also can be extended to the person or persons that are using such products themselves or with others (eg, health care providers, food distribution suppliers).

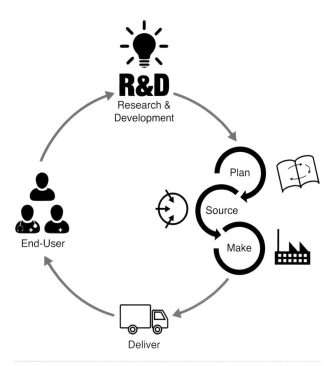

FIGURE 5.9 An example of an end-to-end product design and supply concept, where microbiological quality can play an essential role in each step of the process.

The impacts of not considering the importance of end-to-end microbiological controls can be highlighted by extreme excursions that led microbiological exposures, infections, and other negative impacts. In the cases where extreme excursions have been noted, the preservation, disinfection, or sterilization processes employed where not effective due to unforeseen errors in their application or subsequent use of products. Many are not reported in the peer-review literature as a retrospective on lessons learned but are often highlighted during periodic product recalls or infection outbreak reports worldwide. Examples include the following:

- The Cutter incident was reported as the transmission of polio virus from certain lots of inactivated-virus polio vaccine during the 1950s.[105] Due to incomplete inactivation of the virus during manufacturing, vaccine preparations were found to contain live virus that survived a formaldehyde treatment process. This was likely due not only to virion clumping but also to interference from the presence of other extraneous materials (from the virus preparation) that allow viruses to survive or be protected from the viricidal process used. Subsequent investigations of other formaldehyde-treated virus vaccines lead to the same conclusion and focused optimization of the treatment of virus preparations with disinfectants/sterilants.[106]

- There are frequent reports in the literature or associated product recalls that are associated with contaminated, preserved products. A review of FDA-associated recalls of cosmetics and personal care products highlighted many of the causes and sources.[107] These often include mold or gram-negative bacteria contamination that were isolated from the product and linked to their presence in associated manufacturing processes. A review of mold-associated contamination in preserved or aseptically manufactured products highlighted concerns with environmental monitoring, compliance to good manufacturing processes, and the isolation of molds with resistance to inefficient chemical or thermal disinfection methods.[108] Gram-negative bacteria (particularly pseudomonads) are common sources of contamination in liquid-preserved products due to their ability to adapt and multiply in low concentrations of preservatives and/or preservative types.[109] Some cases highlight concerns in the formulation or presentation of such products that allowed the chemical preservative activity to be separated from the contaminant and thereby allowing unexpected bacterial overgrowth or even biofilm development, despite the associated bacteria being confirmed to be sensitive to the preservation system.[110,111]

- Contaminated products due to lack of microbiological controls and adequate sterilization. Examples include prefilled syringes[112,113] and other pharmaceutical products due to lack of assurance of sterility practices[114] and cross-contamination prior to or at the point of use.[115] A common example of cross-contamination is from water at the point of use that can compromise product safety, such as in contact lenses hygiene.[116]

- Contaminated food products and water. It is not difficult to identify cases of infections or toxic effects due to the unexpected presence of microorganisms in water or food, and many are associated with insufficient manufacturing/treatment and delivery to the point of use (see chapter 56). Examples include virus-associated outbreak due to initial contamination and ineffective processes to control this risk,[117] cross-contamination at food processing facilities,[118] and inadequate transport or storage prior to consumption.[119] Uncontrolled water quality is an efficient source not only of microorganisms but also of their associated toxins, such as the implication of bacterial endotoxins in reports of toxic anterior segment syndrome.[120]

- Contamination of the environment due to failure of waste handling.[121,122] As an example, an outbreak of foot-and-mouth disease was suspected to be due to vehicles contaminated with the virus from a laboratory effluent system.[123]

- Infections related to the use of flexible endoscope. Flexible endoscopes are often cited as the most common medical devices associated with outbreaks of health care–associated infections.[124] Investigations of these outbreaks are most often related to lapses in best practices on reprocessing at health care facilities, including inadequate cleaning prior to disinfection or sterilization, control of water quality, disinfection controls, inadequate drying prior to storage, and more recently due to risks with the initial design of or damage to the devices over repeated clinical use.[125]

- Infections related to the use of surgical instrumentation following steam sterilization. Considering the multiple steps of cleaning, disinfection, and sterilization during reusable device reprocessing, including the reliability of steam sterilization processes, it is surprising that outbreaks are frequently reported with such devices. Examples include the failure of steam sterilization to inactivate *Pseudomonas aeruginosa* presumably due to the lack of adequate cleaning and/or drying of lumened devices[126] and the cross-contamination of devices following sterilization due to sterile packaged materials not being dried or maintained correctly prior to surgical use.[127]

- The presence of microorganisms with higher than expected resistance. A good example is with bacterial spore contaminant in alcohol-based disinfectants. Alcohols are broad-spectrum disinfectants but have little to no appreciable activity against bacterial spores (see chapter 19). Bacterial spore contamination of alcohol disinfectant can lead to environmental contamination in critical manufacturing environments and even patient infections. Reports of infections and pseudo-infections were sourced from alcohol prep pads (with 70% 2-propanol) contaminated with multiple *Bacillus* species, including the pathogen *B cereus*.[128] Another example is the persistence of protozoa cysts in drinking water due to inefficient controls in water treatment or cross-contamination.[129] A further example is the previously discussed presence of *P. domesticum* on cotton-based products sterilized with EO. The resistance of this organism to the sterilant was missed as the validation method did not test for the resistance of the naturally existing population against the BI resistance that was used to validate the sterilization process.

Therefore, it is not enough to depend on the intrinsic antimicrobial effects of preservation, disinfection, and sterilization to ensure public health and the safety of products/processes. An efficient end-to-end process requires an assurance of microbiological quality mindset, which can be defined as a qualitative concept comprising all activities that provide confidence that product is microbiologically safe according to its intended use. A good example of this is with assurance of sterility that should consider the various stages of a design, manufacturing, and delivery process to ensure the product is sterile at its point of use. Microbiological quality requirements should first align with overarching quality requirements such as those defined for medical devices, pharmaceutical products, laboratory, clinical practices, and food manufacturing (see chapter 70). But examples of assurance of microbiological quality at various stage of a product life cycle (see Figure 5.9) are discussed in the following text, where similar concepts may apply to any preservation, disinfection, or sterilization application.

- Research and development. This first step is the identification of the customer/patient/ consumer needs and the definition of the product to meet those needs. Microbiological requirements can be defined as essential design inputs, with examples being the products and services discussed in this chapter and associated chapters. Good examples are in the design of preservation, microbial reduction, and sterilization end points to ensure end user safety in the consumption of foods, cosmetics, pharmaceutical drugs, and/or devices. Many of these can be specified based on end user requirements, manufacturing capabilities, and regulatory (applicable regulations and standards) obligations (see Tables 5.8 and 5.9 for examples). Products or services can be designed to ensure microbiological quality early in the design process, with examples being the right types of chemical preservative are being used in liquid products, that defined levels of microbial or chemical reduction can be reproducibly attained (as in food disinfection and device cleaning processes), or products (including packaging systems) are compatible (and biocompatible) with or not adversely affected by a terminal sterilization process. Typically, in the product design phase is where the desired end point for product use should be defined (eg, sterile vs. non-sterile or microbiologically controlled) and the method of achieving the desired end point (eg, preservation or sterilization/aseptic processing) is selected. The requirements will clearly not only be impacted by microbial end points or controls but can include other safety and product-specific requirements, such as organoleptic properties, human factors considerations, usability, and shelf life. Once defined, these performance criteria can be tested and validated to meet expectations. For many healthcare products, the associated processes will need to be validated during this phase, and regulatory submissions are prepared and filed.

- Plan. In parallel and during R&D, manufacturing and supply chain organizations will plan where and how the product will be manufactured, which includes determining how to meet sourcing, production, and delivery requirements. Microbiological (and, when applicable, chemical and particulate contaminant) quality requirements can include, depending on the product type, raw material selection and specification; risks of contamination during product forming or assembly; the product and/or manufacturing equipment cleaning processes; environmental controls during manufacturing; housekeeping expectations for maintenance; and assembly, accessory equipment, and utilities (eg, water, compressed air, and environmental air specifications). A good example is when water quality may impact the stability of a preservative system. Another is in the design and use of environmental control or "clean" rooms to maintain particulate and microbiological levels during sensitive stages of the manufacturing process such as final product packaging or aseptic processing of sterile products. It may be necessary to consider manufacturing stages at different facilities, such as product development and collection

(eg, foods) or forming at one site, processing at another (eg, preparation for and final packaging), and sterilization at yet another site. During the planning stage, the selection of raw material specification (and sometimes the suppliers), the product and/or manufacturing equipment cleaning processes, environmental controls during manufacturing, housekeeping expectations for maintenance, and more depending on the product to be manufactured. As with all of the other stages, if the inputs or potential risks to impact microbiological quality are not evaluated there may be additional costly controls that need to be put in place once manufacturing has started. At this stage, it may also be necessary to include the need for indicators for process consistency over time, such as process monitoring, sampling, and testing (including trending analysis) as well as criteria for product testing (if required) and specifications for product release. Many of these requirements may be defined from associated regulations and standards (with examples given in Table 5.9).

Central to product development and manufacturing planning of microbiological-controlled products or processes is risk management.[8,130-133] Risk management should be an integral part of a quality management system and can be defined as a systematic application of management policies, procedures, and practices to the tasks of analyzing, evaluating, controlling, and monitoring risk. Microbiological risks are often considered in parallel with other contaminants such as chemicals and particulates. As the definition describes, there are at least four steps to consider:

- Identifying hazards (eg, raw material specifications, water and air quality, loading of product into a sterilization process)
- Estimating and evaluating associated risks
- Controlling these risks (eg, engineering controls such as water system design and maintenance and air quality and distribution in a controlled environment)
- Monitoring the effectiveness of controls (eg, bioburden, preservative concentration, detection of known foodborne pathogens)

It is outside of the scope here to consider risk assessment methods in detail because these will vary depending on the product or process under consideration. Methods used for risk assessment essentially have the same four steps, including Failure Modes and Effects Analysis, Hazard Analysis Critical Control Point (widely used in the food industry), Fault Tree Analysis, and Hazard and Operability Study.[134-137] For the purpose of this discussion, risk assessment can be considered in both the product development phase (product risk) and during the plan and manufacturing process (process risk). It is typical for the product risk assessment to be considered first because this can help in the identification of risks in the design and intended use of the product/service but also specify requirements for manufacturing (eg, labeling, including

TABLE 5.9   Examples of regulations, standards, and guidelines associated with microbiological quality in manufacturing[a]

Specification	Standard/Guideline	Title
Good manufacturing processes (GMPs)	EU GMP Annex 1 Revision	Manufacture of sterile medicinal products
Good manufacturing processes (GMPs)	US FDA GMPs 21 CFR 820	Quality System Regulation (QSRs)/Medical device good manufacturing practices
Compressed air	ISO 8573-1	Compressed air—part 1: contaminants and purity classes
Air quality in controlled environments particulates	ISO 14644-1	Cleanrooms and associated controlled environments—part 1: classification of air cleanliness by particle concentration
Controlled environments biocontamination controls	ISO 14698-1	Cleanrooms and associated controlled environments—biocontamination control—part 1: general principles and methods
Aseptic manufacturing equipment cleaning	PDA Technical Report No. 29, Revised 2012	Points to consider for cleaning validation
Pharmaceutical water systems	USP 1231	Water for pharmaceutical purposes
Reprocessing water quality	AAMI TIR34	Water for the reprocessing of medical devices
Steam quality/purity	EN 285	Sterilization—steam sterilizers—large sterilizers
Aseptic processing	ISO 13408-1	Aseptic processing of health care products—part 1: general requirements
Human or animal tissue handling	AATB guidance document	Microbiological process validation and surveillance program
Laboratory equipment	ISO 17025	General requirements for the competence of testing and calibration laboratories
Medical devices—bioburden	ISO 11737-1	Sterilization of health care products—microbiological methods—part 1: determination of a population of microorganisms on products
Drug product—bioburden	USP <1115>	Bioburden control of nonsterile drugs substances and products
Endotoxin	USP <85>	Bacterial endotoxin test

AAMI, Association for the Advancement of Medical Instrumentation; AATB, American Association of Tissue Banks; EN, European Standard; ISO, International Organization for Standardization; GMP, good manufacturing processes; PDA, Parenteral Drug Association; US FDA, Food and Drug Administration; USP, US Pharmacopeia.

[a]Note that examples of sterilization standards are summarized in Table 5.8.

instructions for use, levels of acceptable microbial levels or chemical cleanliness, and packaging tolerances). Manufacturing process risk assessment can then be useful to methodological-defined risks and associated procedures, equipment requirements, training, monitoring at critical-control points in the process, etc, to ensure product requirements. The combination of these risk analyses, considering the end-to-end concept, is important to reduce risk and ensure a quality process. Risk assessment can also be useful in minimizing the various source, manufacturing, and delivery steps to establish a lean supply chain and minimize associated costs.

• Source. This step includes the procurement of various materials and services to make sure that the sources for each process meet appropriate parameters for manufacturing. Typically, this is where suppliers of materials and services are audited and approved to provide the

items needed in both the quality and quantity desired for routine manufacturing (if not already completed during the product design phase. The source of raw materials and selection of suppliers is many times overlooked as a significant area of concern for microbiological quality. Examples of supply selections that have been found to be of concern have included water (either for direct use or to be provided into a process for further treatment), raw materials such as sugar and cotton, components washed prior to shipment for assembly, terminally sterilized components used for aseptic manufacturing, and the cleanliness of packaging materials. Other examples would include laboratory supplies or testing facilities, filters, cleaning agents, disinfectants, and indicators or equipment used to verify the effectiveness of sterilization processes. Not only is it critical to select the appropriate suppliers to meet the design specifications, but the route of shipment and the impact on raw materials might need to be considered if there is a food source that could support microbial growth. It is also useful at this stage to consider backup or secondary sources for key materials or services to ensuring business continuity. Connecting the dots between the source of materials and services, and applying the appropriate microbiological quality controls, can allow for the detection of problems early and prevent issues from occurring during routine manufacturing.

- Make. This step is the transformation of the raw materials and supplies into a final finished product. Greater attention is often placed on microbial quality during manufacturing, due to regulation and standard requirements (see Table 5.9; see chapter 70). These will include the various product and process specification that were identified in the development plan and source phases that will ensure a consistent and controlled microbiological quality supply. Typically, this includes assurance that the facility was designed appropriately with the right controls, the flow of materials and personnel are adequate, and that cleaning of the facility and environmental controls meet the design requirements for the product. This is the phase were routine monitoring and demonstration of consistency over time is necessary to demonstrate that processes will continue to be valid (e.g., product bioburden and equipment maintenance), and delivery of the desired endpoint is achieved (e.g., disinfection, aseptic techniques and sterilization). If contract terminal sterilization is employed, this step may occur following the make and transportation to the distribution systems for the next step in the manufacturing supply chain. These requirements will not only apply to products such as cosmetics, pharmaceuticals, devices, and foods but will also apply to the handling of wastes, laboratory supplies, and in clinical practice. These are further considered in more detail in other chapters of this book (see Parts V, VI, and VII).

- Delivery. The latter stage of the process is the delivery or shipment of the finished goods and services. Shipping and handling can subject a product to various extremes of environmental stresses such as physical stress (pressure differentials/rate of change), temperature, humidity, viable and non-viable particulates (eg, microorganisms, dust, and chemicals). Important microbiological quality considerations will include packaging design and tolerances (see chapter 41), shelf life (eg, for preserved or sterile products with known limitations), and conditions for storage defined in product labeling. In some cases, the product itself may provide the primary barrier to maintain the sterility of the contents (e.g., products with a tortuous pathway or container closure system to maintain integrity). Many preserved products, including chemical cleaners and disinfectants, can have limited shelf life due to expected (opening and reuse over a given time) or unexpected (eg, extremes in temperature) conditions. Others, such as in the case of sterile-packaged products, are essentially sterile until they are opened for use and exposed to a nonsterile environment. But there are at least two exceptions to this rule. The first is if the packaging has been compromised, with examples being due to physical damage or (in the case of many flexible packaging materials) wetness that compromises the sterile integrity of the packaging system (see chapter 41). The second is due to known limitations of the packaging system where the sterile integrity of the product may degrade (or otherwise compromised) over time, and in these cases, the product labeling should indicate a known limit in shelf life beyond which the product should not be used; these requirements are often specified by regulations and standards.

- End user. The microbiological integrity of any product and successful use of antimicrobial products/processes can be compromised at the point of use, with examples given earlier in this section. Common examples include the misuse of preserved products (eg, dilution in water, use of product after a claimed lifetime, or inadequate storage), disinfectants (inappropriate application, uncontrolled exposure conditions such as time or dilution, cross-contamination following disinfection), and with sterile products or sterilization processes (eg, bad water supply to steam sterilizers, cross-contamination of sterile product prior to surgical use, and inadequate storage). The risks associated with use should be considered during the research and development phase discussed earlier. An important aspect of this is an understanding of human factors that can be defined as a scientific discipline concerned with the understanding of interactions among humans and other elements of a system and the profession that applies theory, principles, data, and other methods to design in order to optimize human well-being and overall systems performance. Examples of microbiological quality considerations to reduce end-use error can include design criteria (eg, tamper-proof indications, robustness and ease of use of primary and secondary packaging, and sterilization end points), labeling (including instructions for use for inspection, reprocessing of medical devices, or preventing cross-contamination), and end user training (eg, aseptic technique). Examples of symbols used in labeling to indicate microbiological quality or risks are given in Table 5.10. But it is also important to note that an optimal end-to-end process is a closed loop (see Figure 5.9), where there is a constant feedback mechanism of performance and the ability to correct or improve on product design and process for continuous quality improvement. This is not only important in cases of specific complaints (eg, damaged product, toxicity, infection) dictated by regulatory processes internationally but also related to proactive preventative measures (eg, "near-misses" or suggested modifications to packaging or labeling) through the entire end-to-end process.

TABLE 5.10   Examples of microbiological quality–associated labeling or symbols[a]

Symbol	Description
	Biohazard, a biological substance (microorganisms or associated toxin) that poses a threat to the health of living organisms; often shown in yellow, red, or orange colors
	Toxic, substance poisonous, and harmful to people, animals, or the environment
	Use by date
	Do not use if package is damaged.
	Keep dry.
STERILE	Product subjected to a sterilization process
STERILE EO	Product subjected to an EO sterilization process
STERILE	Product subjected to a heat (moist or dry) sterilization process
STERILE R	Product subjected to radiation sterilization process
STERILE A	Aseptically manufactured, sterile product
②	Single-use product, do not use.
12m	Period after opening, identifying the useful lifetime of a cosmetic product after its package has been opened for the first time (in this case, 12 mo).

EO, ethylene oxide.

[a]Internationally harmonized symbols can be developed and changed over time; therefore, this table is given only as a guide.

▶ MECHANISMS OF ACTION

Chemotherapeutic agents, such as antibiotics, due to their selective toxicity generally have more specific mechanisms of action that have minimal direct effects on host cells or tissue structures. Studies over the last 50 to 70 years on the biochemical and molecular mechanisms of action of antibiotics highlight this conclusion.[5] Examples include the primary mechanisms of action of the aminoglycosides in the inhibition of protein synthesis by bind to bacterial ribosomal RNA and with β-lactams in binding to specific enzymes involved in the synthesis of peptidoglycan structures in bacterial cell walls. But it is not as easy to elucidate the exact mechanism of action of a microbicidal chemical agent or physical process.[138] The reason for this is that more than one cell or virus constituent are often affected, and consequently, the problem is to distinguish the primary effect from the secondary effects, which may all contribute to death. In general, the most useful information is obtained by studying the effects of low concentrations of a microbicide, or the effects of a low radiation dose or short exposure time at a defined temperature, on the organism being tested. For example, when heated at temperatures of 50°C to 60°C, S $aureus$ leaks amino acids, K^+, and 260-nm–absorbing material, whereas at much higher temperatures (>70°C), protein coagulation is a complicating issue with a clear impact in microbial structure and function.[139] Similarly, low (bacteriostatic) concentrations of chlorhexidine induces leakage of intracellular bacterial materials, but at high (bactericidal) concentrations, leakage is reduced as a result of intracellular precipitation.[139]

Over many years of investigation, different antimicrobial agents have been investigated for their mechanisms of action based on various methods. The majority of these studies have been performed with bacteria due to their ease of manipulation and associated tools in the laboratory, but these studies have also been substantiated by further investigations with other microorganisms such as fungi, protozoa, and noncellular forms such as viruses and prions in recent years. Examples of these methods may be summarized as follows[140]:

- Direct microscopic (including scanning and transmission electron microscopy) examinations to detect gross aberrations of microbial structures such as cell leakage, cell wall or viral capsid/structure disruption, and lysis
- Biocide treatment of cells under conditions of growth (eg, in broth) or nongrowth (use of washed suspensions) can indicate whether the test substance inhibits some biosynthetic process, in which case nongrowing cells are unaffected.
- The determination of the binding or uptake of an antimicrobial agent by microbial cells or their components. The basic principles are (1) the addition of the microbicide to the potential binding materials, (2) the separation of bound from unbound chemical, and (3) then assay of the free or bound quantities. These classical

approaches may use unlabeled as well as labeled (eg, radioactive) compounds. Initial studies were usually carried out with whole cells, but investigations of the interaction of certain compounds with cellular fractions were subsequently rewarding (eg, the interaction of acridines and triphenylmethane dyes with DNA).

- Experiments can determine whether the agent inhibits the synthesis or disrupt the function of specific cellular components or the assembly of virus particles such as in studies on bacterial cell wall synthesis or direct studies on specific macromolecules that make up cellular/viral structure such as proteins, lipids, RNA, or DNA. These include studies to show the cross-linking or coagulation of proteins, or indeed the specific breakdown of protein or lipid structures.
- Detection methods for the leakage of cell cytoplasmic (low-molecular-weight) materials either from the whole cell or cell wall–free forms that only have an exposed cytoplasm. In the latter context, studies on the proton flux across the cytoplasmic membrane has been an interesting experimental technique to investigate the activity of many microbicides on the function of the cell membrane.
- The effects of microbicides on the structure of microbial mutants that are known to lack certain microbial structures. A good example of these is with a series of bacterial spore mutants that lack or have modified spore structures that can affect their resistance profiles to antimicrobial.[141] Others have included bacterial cell envelope mutants, with defects in the lipopolysaccharide core and especially the protein components of the outer membrane of gram-negative bacteria.[142]
- Although less useful in studying most microbicides, other methods have been similar to those used in antibiotic research where the target microorganism is exposed to low concentration or exposure condition over time to allow for the development of mutants and then examined for the biochemical or molecular mechanisms of resistance. These studies have provided useful information in the identification of key microbial targets of antimicrobial agents. An example of this included the identification of primary mechanisms of action of the bisphenol triclosan, namely the binding to and inhibition of bacterial enoyl-acyl carrier protein reductases involved in the synthesis of fatty acids.[143]

Based on these studies, our knowledge of the structures of microorganisms and their associated functions (eg, metabolism, structure integrity, communication with their environment, protective mechanisms, pathogenic factors), and our general understanding of the impact of many antimicrobial methods on these structures, the modes of action of microbicides can be categorized into four groups[5]: oxidizing agents, transfer of energy, cross-linking agents, and a group of microbicides that bind to or specifically disrupt the structure of certain microbial structures (Table 5.11). Many of these effects have been well studied in bacteria

TABLE 5.11   General classification of microbicides based on their primary mechanisms of action

Classification	Example	Mechanism of Action
Oxidizing agents	Halogens such as chlorine, iodine, and bromine Hydrogen peroxide, ozone, peracetic acid, chlorine dioxide	Oxidation of various structural and functional macromolecules such as proteins, lipids, and nucleic acids
Cross-linking or coagulating agents	Aldehydes such as glutaraldehyde and formaldehyde Alkylating agents (eg, ethylene oxide) Phenolics Alcohols	Reaction and cross-reaction between macromolecules that disrupt structure and functions, particularly protein and nucleic acids. Many of these specifically cause cross-linking within and between target molecules that culminate in cell or viral death.
Energy transfer	Heat Radiation, including γ rays and UV light	Transfer of energy such as heat or radiation that lead to disruption of microbial structures and functions include specific effects on nucleic acids, protein, and liquid structures. The higher the energy sources (eg, heat transfer or radiation wavelength), the greater the impact. Lower energy sources such as UV light are sufficient to cause DNA damage that can cumulate in microbial death or with lower temperatures can retard growth but may not be sufficient to kill the target microorganism.
Specific structure disruption	Acridines	Target and intercalate into nucleic acids to disrupt their central role in microbial growth and survival
	Surfactants, including QACs Chlorhexidine	Disrupt the structure of microbial membranes (often internal to cellular cell walls and viral envelops) causing loss of structure and integrity
	Metals	Act as general cellular or structural poisons that interact with and disrupt the functions of proteins and nucleic acids in particular.

QACs, quaternary ammonium compounds; UV, ultraviolet.

(Table 5.12). This is the basis of their more broad-spectrum range of antimicrobial activity, for most microbicides in comparison to anti-infective drugs.[5]

It is important to remember that microorganisms are essentially composed of the same forms of macromolecules that make up human, animal, or plant life, although these structures and arrangements can be different and give us the variety of life that we understand today (see chapter 3). These are essentially protein, lipids, carbohydrates, and nucleic acids. Some of what we consider as the more "simpler" forms of life are proposed to be composed of one of these such as prions (protein only) and viroids (nucleic acid only), whereas other more "complex" forms present with a vast array of viral and cellular forms and organizations. In general, the more complex forms (as highlighted by eukaryotic cells), the more sensitive they are to microbicidal treatments, although some exceptions to this rule are the ability of some higher microbial forms to form dormant forms of their vegetative structures that can demonstrate higher tolerance levels of inactivation (eg, protozoa cysts or helminth eggs). These, like bacterial spores, demonstrate a lack of or slow penetration of microbicides into their inner structures as essential mechanisms of resistance (see chapters 3 and 4). The less complex forms are generally more resilient (such as nonenveloped viruses and prions), but this will also depend on the microbi-

cidal method under investigation, which can become clear in a better knowledge of their mechanisms of action.

Energy Transfer

Two of the most widely used methods of disinfection and sterilization are heat and radiation. Their antimicrobial effects are entirely based on attacking structures that are essential for microorganisms to metabolize, grow, replicate, and survive in different environments. This is well accepted in the study of bacteria and fungi that grow better under lower temperatures (psychrophiles), temperate environments (by human definitions, or mesophiles), or at higher temperatures (thermo- or even hyperthermophiles). The molecular structures can change dramatically by the addition or removal or energy sources in these balanced environments. The greater the energy applied, the greater the disruption that will culminate in death or the inability to replicate and cause disease or spoilage.

Ionizing radiation provides a process in which electrons are stripped from atoms of materials through which the radiation passes, whereas nonionizing radiation methods (such as UV) possesses insufficient energy to eject an electron and instead causes excitation of the

TABLE 5.12 Cellular targets of antimicrobial action[a]

Target	Agents	Effect
Cell wall	Lysozyme	Attacks peptidoglycan (β, 1-4 links)
	Aldehydes	Interaction with −NH$_2$ groups
	Anionic surfactants	Cell lysis
Outer membrane	EDTA (and similar chelating agents)	Chelates cations, induces release of up to 50% of lipopolysaccharide of outer membrane
	Polycations (eg, polylysine)	Displace cations
Cytoplasmic membrane	Moist heat, phenols, quaternary ammonium compounds, biguanides, parabens, hexachlorophene	Leakage of low-molecular-weight material and disruption of function
Nucleic acids	Acridines, dyes, alkylating agents, peroxygens, hypochlorites, ionizing and ultraviolet radiations	Binding, interacting, chelating, or disrupting structure (including fragmentation) of nucleic acids
Enzymes or proteins	Metal ions Alkylating agents, oxidizing agents, phenolics	−SH groups of enzymes, which may be membrane associated; also react with DNA or RNA

EDTA, ethylenediaminetetraacetic acid.

[a]From McDonnell[5] and McDonnell and Russell.[140]

atoms. Both types of radiation particularly damage DNA, although the nature of the damage is different.[144,145] Types of ionizing radiation are x-rays, γ-rays, high-speed electrons (β-rays), protons, and α-rays (positively charged helium atoms). In practice, β-rays and especially γ-rays (usually produced from a ^{60}Co source) are used; α-particles are charged and heavy and have little penetrating power. Bacterial and fungal spores are in general more resistant than other microorganisms to ionizing radiations. Among the clostridial and bacillus spores, *Clostridium botulinum* A and B and *Bacillus pumilus* E601, respectively, demonstrated higher resistance.[146] But one of the most resistant microorganisms found to date is the vegetative gram-positive coccus *Deinococcus radiodurans*, which possesses a number of resistant factors including efficient repair process for both ionizing and UV radiations (see chapter 3). Prions are even more resistant, which is proposed to be linked to the mode of action. The primary mechanism of action of ionizing radiation is believed to cause single- or double-strand breakages in DNA, the latter being more lethal.[147,148] But other effects can include disruption of structure and function of various other macromolecules such as proteins and lipids due to effects on covalent and noncovalent binds that make up these structures as well as leading to further cross-reactivity between these active molecules that can cause precipitation and microbial death.

These mechanisms of action are supported by observation on the mechanisms of resistance. For example, several reasons have been given for the comparatively high resistance in bacterial spores. These include the water content

of the spore-limiting reactivity and the ability of damaged cells to repair damage over time.[149] The DNA damage in spores has been shown to be repaired during postirradiation germination.[150] A highly radiation-resistant strain of *C botulinum* was also found to repair single-strand breaks in DNA under nonphysiologic conditions at 0°C and in the absence of germination.[151] With an exponential rate of microbial inactivation, it is presumed that a single "hit" on the sensitive target site (DNA) produces death, whereas multiple hits are necessary in cases where an initial shoulder is seen on the dose-response curve. Repair of injury can play an important role in this response. These investigations are likely the reason behind the lack of significant activity against prions with radiation because they have no proposed unique nucleic acid (although this is a conclusion that deserves further investigation given the other effects of radiation in biological systems). Furthermore, the mechanisms of resistance in *D radiodurans* (as well as other radiation-tolerant isolates such as *Methylobacterium* and *Kocuria* species) include not only the presence of efficient repair mechanisms but also the protective mechanisms (in cell wall structure and the production or pigments) as well as the presence of multiple (up to 4-10) copies of bacterial DNA molecules (see chapter 3).[5,152]

Similar conclusions can be made in the mode of action on nonionizing radiation sources such as UV. UV radiation has a wavelength range between approximately 328 and 210 nm, with maximal bactericidal activity near the wavelength (260 nm) of peak absorption of DNA. This is important given that DNA is the target of the action of UV radiation.[153] When nonspore forming bacteria are exposed to UV light, thymine dimers are formed between adjacent thymine molecules in the same strand of DNA. Other dimers may also be formed, such as uracil-thymine heterodimers. The induction of dimers is sufficient to explain the lethal nature of UV radiation. Some bacteria can repair this damage, a property that is highly developed in *D radiodurans* but is also a common feature in other bacteria.[153] For example the well-studied SOS response in *E coli* consists of a series of inducible genes that code for protective and repair mechanisms in cells, including DNA repair proteins that are activated following physiologic changes after UV radiation (or other DNA-damaging treatment) and controlled by RecA and LexA proteins.[5] These repair mechanisms include photoreactivation and excision repair. Bacterial spores have been found to have other mechanisms of resistance. For example, α- and β-type small, acid-soluble spore proteins (SASPs) interact with DNA in wild-type spores of *Bacillus subtilus* as a protective mechanism (see chapter 4). Spores (α^- β^-) lacking SASPs are significantly more sensitive to UV, even more so than vegetative cells.[141] Other, lower energy radiation processes such as infrared and microwave energy are believed to illicit any observed antimicrobial activity due to the generation of heat rather than direct impact on macromolecules themselves (see chapter 10).

The effects of heat-based processes on microbial life are easier to conclude based on the importance of temperature in the structure, growth, and survival or microorganisms. The impact of increased temperature alone on biological systems such as on enzymes is well established but so, too, is the separation of structures and function of proteins (causing unfolding and coagulation), separation and even fragmentation of double-stranded nucleic acids, and separation of lipid-based structures such as those that make up cell walls or viral envelopes. Overall, colder temperatures are less destructive and stall growth activity, but microorganisms remain viable and are therefore only considered preserved. This is considered briefly in the following text. But higher temperatures are more destructive due to a culmination of effective and reliable antimicrobial effects that are well established (see chapters 11 and 28).

Growth of microorganisms slows down and eventually stops if they are exposed to reduced temperatures. Some microorganisms can grow at temperatures approaching 0°C; these are termed *psychrophilic* and include important food-spoilage organisms.[154] Environmental factors such as nutrient status, pH, and water activity can alter the minimum growth temperature.[154,155] Modification of membrane lipid composition with temperature is also an important adaptation in some psychrophiles, whereas other psychrophiles show no membrane lipid alterations.[156] Microorganisms that can adapt to survive over a range of temperatures, including colder conditions, are known to be able to modify cell wall structure including cell membrane fluidity. Enzymes, being essential for metabolism in cells, are found to have a higher degree of structural flexibility due to the types of primary (amino acid) and higher order structures.[154]

'Cold shock' refers to a process in which microorganisms are suddenly chilled without freezing, and cell death has been shown to occur with gram-positive and gram-negative bacteria but not with yeasts.[157,158] Several factors influence the response of cells, particularly the age of culture, because exponential-phase (but not stationary-phase) cultures are more susceptible to cold shock. Likewise, the composition of the medium is an important factor, and various divalent cations protect the cells against chilling. Low-molecular-weight materials are released from chilled cells as a consequence of an increase in the permeability of the bacterial cell membrane, which in turn occurs because of a phase transition in membrane lipids.[158] A modification of this treatment is cold osmotic shock, in which bacteria are suspended in a hypertonic sucrose solution containing EDTA and are then resuspended in ice-cold magnesium chloride solution. This treatment does not cause death of the cells but does induce the release of periplasmic enzymes, including β-lactamases, from gram-negative bacteria. The procedure, with appropriate modifications, has also been used in preparing outer membranes of some gram-negative organisms.[159] Another option for microbial cell inactivation by low temperatures is the process of freezing and thawing. Membrane damage occurs, as evidenced by the leakage of intracellular materials and the increased penetrability into cells of certain compounds that are normally excluded. Damage to the outer membrane of the cell envelope has also been shown because frozen and thawed cells of *E coli* become sensitive to lysozyme. Comprehensive accounts of freezing/thawing and of repair of damage are provided elsewhere.[157,160] The effects against viruses is less clear. In some reports little to no effect of freezing and thawing (in studies testing the ability to be able to successfully store viruses at −80°C) was observed,[161] but more recent studies suggested the loss of viability of enveloped viruses and primarily due to envelope disruption.[162]

Although the precise manner how microorganisms are killed on exposure to water or steam at high temperatures is not fully elucidated, it is well established that heat will overall disrupt their structure and function. This can be shown by the effects on increasing temperatures on proteins (including enzymes), lipids and nucleic acids, and the various structures that make up cellular and viral structures.[5] These include protein unfolding, lipid bilayer separation, and double-stranded nucleic acid (eg, DNA) unravelling and fragmentation. Many studies with suspensions of nonspore forming bacteria being heated have shown several changes occurring in cells.[163] These include leakage of low-molecular-weight material, RNA and DNA breakdown, protein coagulation, and alterations in the appearance of the cell itself. In *S aureus*, Mg^{2+} is lost from cell wall teichoic acid, and a mutant lacking teichoic acid is more sensitive than the parent. In *E coli*, structural damage occurs to the outer membrane, and the cells become more sensitive to selective agents. Ribosomes from heat-injured cells of *Salmonella typhimurium* or *S aureus* have a sedimentation coefficient of 47S, with no 30S particles. Ribosomal RNA from heat-injured cells of *S typhimurium* suffers complete degradation of the 23S species. Single- and double-stranded breaks in DNA have been reported in *E coli* cells held at 52°C, similar to those induced by ionizing radiation. There is a link between the same repair processes being involved in the recovery from both types of damage.[164] *E coli* DNA repair-deficient mutants are more heat sensitive than the wild type. Cell revival appears to be related to repair of DNA breaks and is inhibited by inhibitors of DNA synthesis. Furthermore, mild heating causes an increase in mutation frequency. During heating, mesophilic bacteria and fungi can synthesize a number of proteins (heat shock proteins), which demonstrate the cells' capacity to express mechanisms that include repair to multitarget damage induced by moist heat and molecular stabilization of critical cellular components.[165] A considerable amount of evidence implicates the involvement of DNA in heat damage, probably a consequence of enzymatic action after thermal injury. Similar to the discussion at low temperatures, a range of bacteria and fungi can survive higher temperatures by modifications in their macromolecular structures that are adapted for heat tolerance. Examples include species of *Legionella* and *Enterococcus*, and extreme examples including vegetative bacteria and archaea hyperthermophiles (eg, *Thermococcus*, *Pyrococcus*) that can survive temperatures above 100°C (see chapter 3).[166] These types of microorganisms present with an array of resistance mechanisms that can allow for survival and even growth under these temperature extremes. These include fatty acid composition in the cell wall/membrane affecting fluidity/permeability and stability, higher guanine and cytosine content in double-stranded nucleic acids to improve thermostability, and modifications in the types of amino acids and secondary/tertiary structures of proteins, essentially opposite to those described for cold tolerance.

Bacterial spores, and to a lesser extent other dormant forms of fungi and protozoa (see chapter 3), have been traditionally studied for their unique resistance to higher temperatures. When bacterial spores are lethally heated, intracellular constituents are released, and there is a progressive loss of dipicolinic acid (DPA) and calcium, the rate of release being temperature dependent. Viability loss precedes DPA leakage, and consequently, leakage cannot be considered a primary effect. These effects reflect a breakdown in the various resistance mechanisms (including desiccation, presence of DPA, and unique proteins to protect the DNA molecule and impervious, multilayer spore layers) that are known to contribute to the overall resistance of spores to inactivation (see chapter 4).[165] The DPA is believed to play an important role in the resistance of bacterial spores to inactivation by moist heat. Higher growth temperatures enhance the thermal resistance of spores, and the ratio of total cation content to DPA content increases with increasing growth temperature. Heat resis-

tance of spores was found to be related directly to calcium content and inversely to their magnesium content.[167] In species with more than a 700-fold range in heat resistance, there was only a small range in DPA content. Thus, DPA does not appear to be directly involved in the heat resistance mechanism, although it might contribute by reducing or preventing thermally induced denaturation of proteins. The DPA is located in the spore core, as is almost all the spore calcium, magnesium, and manganese. The DPA-less mutants have varying resistance, with a mutant of *B cereus* demonstrating heat sensitivity and a mutant of *B subtilis* showing thermo-resistance as with the wild-type strain; but overall, there does appear to be a direct relationship between DPA content and spore resistance.[168]

The water content of the spore is likely to be a controlling factor in its sensitivity to moist heat. The water content of the protoplast is reduced by a mechanical contraction of the cortex about the protoplast (known as the "contractile cortex" theory).[169] In an alternative "expanded cortex" theory, an osmoregulatory hypothesis predicts that germinating spores heated in high concentrations of the nonpenetrating solute, sucrose, regain their heat resistance because of the decrease in water content of the cell. This theory also assumes a low water content of the spore core created initially during the sporulation process by osmotic dehydration by the mother cell, which is then maintained in the mature spore by electronegative peptidoglycan and positively charged counterions in the cortex.[170] Maintenance of the integrity of the cortex, by whatever means, is essential for the heat resistance of spores because removal of exosporium (if present) and of coats has no effect on heat resistance, whereas additional removal of cortex produces heat-sensitive protoplasts. Overall, the thermo-resistance of spores depends on several factors affecting the protoplast: (a) dehydration; (b) mineralization, with heat resistance decreasing if spores are demineralized and regained if re-mineralized; (c) thermal adaptation, because spores of a given species are most resistant when grown at maximum temperatures; and (d) protein thermotolerance. Calcium dipicolinate may be involved in the establishment and maintenance of dormancy.[170] Furthermore, SASPs found in the spore core may have a role to play. Spores lacking α-/β-type SASPs are more thermosensitive than wild-type spores,[141,171] but their impact is considered not to be a major determinant of thermal resistance.

The effects of dry heat on microorganisms are overall similar, although there are subtle differences in the mechanisms between moist and dry heat (see chapters 11 and 28). Overall, the presence of dry heat is a source of energy for the heating of water associated with cells, thereby having the same overall effects as moist heat. But heat in the absence of moisture is a much less efficient process than moist heat, and typically, higher temperatures for longer times must be used in practice. Much of this conclusion comes from studies with bacterial spores. Because desiccation (or the removal of water) is a mechanism of heat resistance in bacterial spores, thereby further water will be removed (or dried out) during heating up times with dry heat leading to greater resistance. Also, the overall heat penetration will be slower than that observed with moist heat, thereby delaying the heating mechanism. But overall, certain genus/species of bacterial spores show greater resistance to dry heat in comparison to moist heat, suggesting different protective mechanisms in both. Destruction of microorganisms by dry heat was originally considered to be primarily due to an oxidation process.[172] If this were true, bacterial spores heated in oxygen would be expected to be more sensitive to dry heat than when heated in the presence of other gases. But D-values (in minutes) of 1.40, 1.46, 1.47, 1.63, and 1.96 for *B subtilis* spores ranging from 1.40 to 1.96 minutes have been reported when heated in carbon dioxide, air, oxygen, helium, and nitrogen, respectively, indicate that this hypothesis may require further investigation.[173] Consequently, although oxidation may play an important part in the destruction of microorganisms, other possibilities must also be considered. An effect on DNA is one such possibility. Sublethal temperatures have been shown to induce mutants in *B subtilis* spores as a result of depurination, and it has been suggested that the dry heat sensitivity of spores could result from the genetically determined differences in the water content or the water-retaining capacity of the spores.[174] The water content of spores is, in fact, an important factor in determining their inactivation by dry heat. It is suggested that only a relatively small amount of water is needed to protect the heat-sensitive site in spores and that dry heat resistance depends mainly on the location of water rather than the amount, in the spore, together with the nature of its association with other molecules. Overall, the kinetics of heating between moist and dry heat is likely to be responsible for any differences, but once the right heat is achieved, the effects are likely similar.

It may be useful to mention at this stage the impact of heat on prions because they are rather resilient forms of transmissible agents and traditional methods of sterilization may not always be effective due to the unique nature of these agents (see chapter 3). It has been widely agreed that prions are heat tolerant, although many studies with prions are confounded by the fact that prion inactivation studies are conducted in the presence of gross amounts of related tissue (typically whole brain homogenates). In addition, moist heat sterilization can be effective but dry heat appeared to be less effective. Even though incineration is often recommended for waste removal (see chapter 68), residual prion infectivity was demonstrated following treatment at 360°C for 1 hour or on incineration at 600°C for 15 min).[175,176] It has been proposed that the effects of heat dry may be due to the presence of high lipid levels in the brain tissue material used in these studies that allow for heat transfer effects to the intrinsic prion molecules.[97] Moist heat (water heating) has been shown to have little effect, but higher temperature achieved by steam under pressure was very effective, which is the basis for the recommended prior sterilization cycle of 134°C for 18 minutes.[177] But, similar to dry heat, the data that support the reduction of prion infectivity following steam sterilization cycles show mixed results and is likely due to the difficulty in the delivery of uniform steam penetration to the infectious material embedded in contamination tissue. But when inoculated onto surfaces and subjected to cleaning and/or steam sterilization, prior inactivation can be reliably achieved if the correct cleaning process is used[178]; interestingly, the immersion of contaminated surfaces in water prior to and during the steam sterilization process alone was found to be an effective process, suggesting that a slower increase in temperature over time and up to 134°C was an effective process and did not require extended steam sterilization cycle conditions to be effective.

Oxidizing Agents

Oxidizing agents range considerably in antimicrobial activity depending on the microbicide, use in liquid or gas form, concentration, liquid formulation, temperature, etc. Therefore, reports in the literature on their effectiveness can often be misleading. Due to their mechanisms of action (oxidation of any material that can be oxidized), they can have broad-spectrum activity against all microorganisms; these effects will be less with certain types of microorganisms with greater resistance mechanisms such as limiting availability of reactive species (eg, requiring time to penetrate into cysts or spires), repair mechanisms, or limited, available structure-specific or accessible targets. Oxidizing agents include microbicides such as hydrogen peroxide, peracetic acid, ozone, and chlorine dioxide as well as the halogens chlorine and iodine. In addition to their direct roles as oxidizing agents, it is also postulated that the reaction and degradation of many of these microbicides will also lead to the generation of other reactive species that will also contribute to the antimicrobial effects. A simple, yet potent oxidizing agent like hydrogen peroxide is likely to generate a variety of free radicals (eg, the hydroxyl radical •OH) and other reactive species (eg, O_2•−, •OH, •OOH, •O, and •H) on degradation to water and oxygen, and reaction with microorganism component that will cause loss or viability. Similar effects have been reported for peracetic acid, ozone (in water) and chlorine dioxide, and particularly from bacteria or bacterial spore studies. Key targets for oxidizing agents are nucleic acids, where they can readily react with nucleotide bases and the sugar backbones in these molecules.[5] These effects can lead to fragmentation but also destabilize these structures for abnormal cross-reactivity that will culminate in loss of structure and function. Other effects include the impact on lipids, such as with shorter chained fatty acids and unsaturated fatty acid structures, which will also disrupt important cell structure components such as the cell membrane of bacteria, fungi, and enveloped viruses. Finally, the mechanisms of action against proteins and amino acids have also been studied, with similar effects to those noted earlier for nucleic acids. Certain types of amino acids, such as cysteine, are particularly sensitive, and due to the role of cysteine in the folding amino acid primary sequences into secondary and tertiary structures, these proteins can rapidly loose structure and therefore function.[140,179] Others include histidine and lysine.[180] The effects can also include cross-reactivity between oxidized side chains leading to cross-linking and breakage of peptide bonds that can cause protein fragmentation into peptides. Studies have suggested that the antimicrobial effects of oxidizing agents such as chlorine are primarily due to effects on proteins, followed by lipid peroxidation and nucleic acids.[181]

But there are subtle differences in the mechanisms of action of oxidizing agents. These effects may be important when considering the neutralization of nonviable structures such as prions or endotoxins or in the optimization of antimicrobial processes (eg, in the presence of residual soil). Examples of this have been shown with hydrogen peroxide and peracetic acid, depending on their formulation, temperature, and state (eg, in liquid or gas state). For example, hydrogen peroxide gas, some liquid peracetic acid formulations, chlorine dioxide, and chlorine have been shown to cause protein fragmentation by breaking peptide bonds.[182-185] Hydrogen peroxide gas was more reactive against amino acids than the liquid form, in addition to showing greater effects in protein fragmentation.[183,184] The reaction of hydrogen peroxide on the coats of bacterial spores facilitated the increased antimicrobial activity of peracetic acid, which appeared to be more destructive in activity to various spore structures,[186] although both oxidizing agents are effective against the internal spore DNA structure over time.[182,186,187] In studies of different formulations of peracetic acid in comparison to aldehyde-based disinfectants, it was shown that some formulations cause protein or biofilm degradation and increased cleaning effects, whereas others seemed to be potent cross-linking agents similar to the aldehydes (and thereby being less effective cleaning agents).[188,189] These differences suggested important effects in the formulation of oxidizing agent-based disinfectants to optimize their cleaning and associated antimicrobial activities. An important example of this is effectiveness of hydrogen peroxide gas to neutralize prion infectivity, but a limited effect when high concentrations of liquid hydrogen peroxide was tested.[97] High concentrations or formulations including liquid hypochlorites over time (eg, ≥2% available chlorine for 1 h) are well-established methods of prion inactivation due to structure degradation (see chapter 68).[97,190] It is likely that when used appropriately, the oxidizing agents will be effective against prions, but this class of microbicides requires further investigations to optimize and verify their activities for specific applications.

Cross-linking or Coagulating Agents

Cross-linking or coagulating agents are also widely used as microbicides including alcohols, phenols or cresols, alkylating agents (eg, EO), and the aldehydes (eg, glutaraldehyde and formaldehyde). These are general cellular or other microbial structure reactive agents as they bind to and can cause cross-reactivity between macromolecules, especially proteins and nucleic acids.

The mode of action of EO, as a typical alkylating agent, has been well described (see chapter 31). Alkylation is defined as the conversion:

$$H - X \rightarrow R - X$$

where R is an alkyl group.[191] Biologic activity of alkylating agents is indicated by reaction with nucleophilic groups. Epoxides, of which EO is one example, are known to interact with amino acids and proteins. The EO causes hydroxyethylation of amino acids, with the phosphate group of nucleic acids to form a triester and with guanine to give 7-(2′-hydroxyethyl) guanine.[5] The general antimicrobial activity of EO (CH_2CH_2O) and related substances parallels their activity as alkylating agents.[192] Thus, cyclopropane ($CH_2CH_2CH_2$), which is not an alkylating agent, has no antimicrobial action, whereas ethylene sulfide (CH_2CH_2S) has equal activity, and ethylene imine (CH_2CH_2NH) has greater activity.

The EO introduces alkyl groups (eg, ethyl groups) on reaction with nucleic acids (eg, DNA) and proteins. The DNA and RNA guanine (G) nucleotide residues are targeted form adducts that can disrupt their structure and function.[5,193] This not only can initiate a cascade of reactions including repair mechanisms in cells that can lead to further damage but also cause cross-linking between nucleotide bases that can inhibit their normal structure/function and culminate in cell death. These will include any microorganism with nucleic acids, so it is not surprising that EO demonstrates broad-spectrum antimicrobial activity (see chapter 31), including dormant forms such as bacterial spores, but is not known to be effective against prions.[97] Further reactions by alkylation have also been studied against amino acids (eg, cysteine, valine, histidine, and methionine) and lead to cross-linking of adjacent proteins.[194,195] Unique resistance mechanisms have been reported with certain fungi to EO, but these effects are primarily due to the desiccated nature of the associated fungal structures and lack of penetration of EO and humidity to elicit its optimal antimicrobial activity (see chapter 3). Similar mechanisms of action have been demonstrated in limited studies with other agents such as propylene oxide.

Aldehydes (including glutaraldehyde, formaldehyde and ortho-phthalaldehyde [OPA]) primarily elicit their antimicrobial effects by a similar mechanism, especially by reacting with proteins, but also nucleic acids to cause disruption and then cross-linking within and between adjacent proteins and nucleic acids.[5,196-199] The mechanisms of action against proteins have been particularly well studied over a number of years. Amino acids with free amine groups in their structures such as lysine, asparagine, glutamine, and arginine are particularly sensitive to reaction with aldehydes, which can then lead to cross-linking between adjacent amino acids within the same protein or adjacent proteins. This can lead to a cascade reaction leading to the formation of protein multimers that will break down microbial structure and function. Studies on the mechanisms of action of formaldehyde and glutaraldehyde on purified proteins and whole cells have also shown that surface proteins (or protein containing structures such as the cell wall and membrane) are early targets on exposure and alone can cause the shutdown of normal cellular function.[5] Increased rigidity or lack of normal functions of the cell wall/membrane continue, but further penetration into the cell structure will lead to further reactions with available proteins and associated nucleic acids that will culminate in cell death. The reaction of glutaraldehyde with nucleic acids follows pseudo first-order kinetics at high temperatures, but even at the higher temperatures, there is little evidence for the formation of intermolecular cross-links.[200] Glutaraldehyde inhibits synthesis of protein, RNA, and DNA in *E coli*, but this is believed to arise from an inhibition of precursor uptake as a consequence of aldehyde-protein interaction in the outer structures of the cell.[201] Equally, viral structures will lose the ability to infect cells and therefore their associated viability. But reports of greater resistance to bacterial spores, certain strains of mycobacteria, and nonenveloped viruses are most likely due to the lack of sensitive proteins on the surfaces or these microorganisms and antimicrobial activity dependent of the further penetration of the microbicide into these structures (see chapter 3). Equally, the ability of the aldehyde molecules to be able to cause cross-linking activity may explain the difference in activity of smaller molecular-sized aldehydes (formaldehyde and glutaraldehyde) to larger molecules (eg, OPA)[202] Interestingly, glutaraldehyde may be a more potent cross-linking agent but surface reactivity may prevent further penetration into microbial structures, whereas OPA is less reactive but allowing greater internal penetration (as described in some studies with mycobacteria)[203] Formaldehyde and glutaraldehyde are both effective against bacterial spores, but OPA has much slower activity depending on the spore species. Also, no appreciable activity against prions has been reported. Initial studies suggested that some effects could be observed, but this is more likely explained about the lack of availability of the prion material following exposure to cross-linking agents in the presence of encapsulated tissue, essentially preventing prion release.[97] Indeed, prion-contaminated tissue was found to allow the transmission of infection over years from a contaminated reusable device following alcohol and formaldehyde treatment likely to have caused the fixation of the transmissible agent to the device surface.[204]

The rest of the widely used microbicides in this group are more limited in their activity against dormant forms of microorganisms, but all demonstrated broad-spectrum antimicrobial activity against other forms. These include the alcohols and phenolics, and they can range in antimicrobial activity depending on their specific structures (eg, the bisphenols are more limited in activity than other broad-spectrum phenolics), their concentration, formulation, and application.[5] They both lead to reaction and interaction with proteins that lead to coagulation and loss of structure/function. The −OH groups of the alcohols react with hydrogen bonds to lead to protein denaturation and coagulation, but interestingly, the most optimal concentration for antimicrobial activity is in the 50% to 80% range so water is also considered to be required for efficacy (see chapter 19). In addition to protein, alcohols cause the disruption of cell membrane/walls by interaction with lipids and denature DNA/RNA molecules. They overall lack penetration into dormant forms of microorganisms such as bacteria spores but prevent the outgrowth of bacterial spores.[5] Phenolics are similar with reaction −OH groups and are also considered general cellular poisons when they have access to the reactive surface of internal structure essential for life. Even at low concentrations, they can be bacteriostatic/fungistatic due to cell surface interactions, but as the concentration is increased, so do the bactericidal/fungicidal effects that lead to breakdown of the cell wall/membrane (indicated by cytoplasmic leakage) and coagulation on cytoplasm components. For viruses, activity against the outer lipid and protein envelop leads to viricidal activity against enveloped viruses, but the effects against nonenveloped viruses can vary depending on the virus type (or availability of reactive surface proteins).[205,206]

It is useful to mention that phenolics do range in activity and their specific modes of activity, as shown in a range of studies interested in the specific modes of action and resistance to the bisphenols triclosan and hexachlorophene (see chapters 3 and 4).[207] Both microbicides were surprisingly found to specifically inhibit enoyl reductases in various bacteria. This has been studied in some detail, where triclosan interacts by hydrogen bonding, van der Waals forces, and other hydrophobic interactions with the enzyme's substrate binding site and its cofactor (NADH or NADPH). This inhibits the activity of the enzyme that is essential in the biosynthesis of fatty acids and inhibits growth/multiplication. This was significant because a similar mode of action was described for the antimycobacterial antibiotic isoniazid and changes in the access to or directly with the enzyme by mutation, overproduction, or efflux away from the site of action could lead to cross-resistance to both antimicrobials. But in the case of triclosan and hexachlorophene, as the concentration is increased, the other general effects of the phenolics are observed such the inhibition of other enzymes and cell membrane disruption. At this time, efficacy and particularly safety concerns have limited the practical application for triclosan and hexachlorophene, despite widespread use in the past.[208,209]

Specific Structure Disruption

It is beyond the scope of this chapter to consider the specific mechanisms of action of all microbicides that react with certain microbial structures, but a summary of some of the more important examples are given in Table 5.13. These vary in antimicrobial activity, ranging from those with limited bacteriostatic activity (eg, chelating agents), to chlorhexidine and QACs that are generally effective against most vegetative bacteria and fungi (but not typically mycobacteria, nonenveloped viruses, and bacterial spores) and metals such as copper and silver. Metals are often used for their microbiostatic activity but can be bactericidal and fungicidal depending on the concentrations used.

It makes sense that many of these chemical microbicides, as well as the oxidizing agents and cross-linking agents, will have an initial and often potent effect against microorganisms at their surfaces or interfaces with their environments. In all these cases, it is the accessibility of the microbicide to the surface and then internal structures of microorganisms that is the key to their antimicrobial activity and spectrum of activity. This is the essential basis of

microbial resistance to inactivation, where those microorganisms that are more accessible are more sensitive and those that are less accessible (eg, the mycobacteria, spores, cysts, or in the presence of a biofilm) are more or even completely resistant to the effects of the microbicide (see chapter 3). This has been particularly studied in bacteria (see chapter 4) and to a much less extent in fungi, viruses, and other microorganisms.

The basic bacteria prokaryotic cell consists of an inner cytoplasm (containing nucleic acids, protein, nutrients, salts, etc) surrounded by a cell membrane and a cell wall (see chapters 3 and 4). The basic unit of the bacterial cell wall, peptidoglycan (a polysaccharide), confers mechanical rigidity on the cell and protects the delicate, underlying cytoplasmic membrane. In gram-positive bacteria, the wall typically consists of a thicker layer of peptidoglycan interspersed with teichoic acid or another such acidic polymer. A typical gram-negative rod has a much thinner peptidoglycan layer closest to the cytoplasmic membrane, but external to the peptidoglycan is a periplasmic space (periplasm) and an outermost region known as the outer membrane. This complex outer membrane in gram-negative bacteria contains lipoprotein (covalently linked to the peptidoglycan layer), lipopolysaccharide, and phospholipids. Growth conditions in these bacteria are well known to cause changes in the cell wall structure

TABLE 5.13 Examples of microbicides with more specific mechanisms of action against microbial structures

Microbicide Group	Examples	Primary Mechanism[a]
Acridines	Proflavine, aminacrine	DNA, by intercalation between base pairs
Surfactants	Quaternary ammonium compounds (QACs), anionic surfactants	Cell or viral membranes, to disrupt lipid membrane structure/function and causing a breakdown in integrity (eg, cytoplasmic leakage)
Chelating agents	EDTA, EGTA	Removal of cations from microbial structures including proteins and cell membranes to disrupt their function, structure, or permeability rendering these structures sensitive to further damage or biocide penetration
Biguanides	Chlorhexidine	Disrupt the structure and function of cell membranes (by insertion into and interaction with lipids), when present and accessible to the microbicide. The loss of membrane integrity can also lead to further interaction and precipitation of cytoplasmic materials.
Acids and esters	Parabens, acetic acid, citric acid	Acidic pH can dramatically affect the metabolism of vegetative bacteria and fungi, limiting their growth. Specific effects include affinity for the cell to limit cell wall/membrane functions including energy generation, nutrient uptake, structure disruption, and enzyme inhibition.
Metals	Silver, copper	Affinity for cell surfaces disrupting activity (including energy generation) and integrity; binding to proteins (eg, cysteine sulfhydryl groups that play an important role in protein structure/function) and nucleic acids (causing pyrimidine dimers)

EDTA, ethylenediaminetetraacetic acid; EGTA, ethylene glycol tetraacetic acid.

[a]Other effects have been reported in some cases that overall disrupt cellular and some viral structures.[5]

and can impact their resistance to microbicides. Changes in outer membrane components of gram-negative bacteria can also take place, thereby modifying responses in disease and to biocides.[5,210] A good example of the effect of a microbicide at this level is EDTA and other chelating agents. They are known to cause destabilization of the outer cell wall and associated cell membranes (outer and inner membrane where present).[211] They are not powerful bactericides with some inhibitory effects against gram-negative, especially *P aeruginosa*, and gram-positive bacteria.[212] But they are well-known to potentiate the activity against bacteria with chemically unrelated antibacterial compounds. As chelating agents, they can combine with cations associated with the outer membrane of bacteria and especially gram-negative bacteria, with the release of large amounts of outer membrane lipopolysaccharide. The result is that the outer membrane is "opened up," permitting the entry into the cells of chemically unrelated molecules, including several antibiotics and biocides. These effects are less obvious with gram-positive bacteria.[213] Other useful permeabilizing agents include citric, malic, and gluconic acids.[214]

Several substances are known to disrupt the cytoplasmic membrane (Table 5.14). These cause the leakage of intracellular materials, although other effects are observed.[5] Phenolics have been found to particularly target the cell membrane and cause cell lysis, although they are also considered general cellular poisons because they react to proteins to cause precipitation. Chlorhexidine (as well as the QACs) in low concentrations demonstrate similar interactions at the cell wall/membrane level to induce cytoplasmic leakage, but at much higher drug concentrations, leakage is reduced as a consequence of the interaction of chlorhexidine with cytoplasmic protein and nucleic acid.[215] Chlorhexidine at bacteriostatic concentrations has also been found to inhibit membrane-bound enzymes such as adenosine triphosphatase (ATPase), and the QACs such as cetyltrimethylammonium bromide disrupt the cell wall/membrane proton-motive force, an electrochemical gradient across the wall that is used in the synthesis of adenosine triphosphate.[211] Chlorhexidine affects the outer membrane of gram-negative bacteria with the release of periplasmic enzymes and disturbs the functionality of the inner membrane.[211,216]

TABLE 5.14   Membrane-active antimicrobial agents

Antibacterial Agent(s)	Effect on Cell	Mechanism of Action
Phenol	Leakage; possible cell lysis; protein denaturation	Generalized membrane damage
Quaternary ammonium compounds	Leakage; protoplast lysis; interaction with membrane phospholipid; discharge of pH component of proton motive force (Δp)	Generalized membrane damage
Chlorhexidine	Leakage at low concentrations, interactions of high concentrations with cytoplasmic constituents; protoplast and spheroplast lysis (both also concentration-dependent); high concentrations inhibit membrane-bound adenosine triphosphatase	Concentration-dependent effect; low concentrations affect membrane integrity; higher ones congeal protoplasm
Hexachlorophene	Leakage, protoplast lysis (maximum at concentrations > bactericidal level); inhibits respiration	Membrane-bound electron transport chain
Phenoxyethanol	Leakage, low concentrations stimulate total oxygen uptake and uncouple oxidative phosphorylation; H^+ translocation and K^+ permeability are independent actions	Proton-conducting uncoupler
Fenticlor	Collapse of proton potential; prevents coupling of inward proton translation to active transport; relationship between bactericidal action and leakage; no leakage at bacteriostatic concentration	Uncoupler
Tetrachlorosalicylanilide	Inhibition of energy-dependent (not energy-independent) transport of phosphate and amino acids into *Staphylococcus aureus*; increase of oxygen uptake in presence of glucose; increased permeability to Cl^-	Uncoupler
Sorbic acid	Transport inhibition (conflicting results reported); inhibition of ΔpH across cytoplasmic membrane	Transport inhibitor (effect on PMF); possibly another unidentified mechanism
Parabens	Leakage of intracellular constituents; transport inhibition; selective inhibition; selective inhibition of ΔpH across membrane	Concentration-dependent effect; low concentrations inhibit transport; higher ones affect membrane integrity

PMF, proton motive force.

TABLE 5.15 Antimicrobial compounds and nucleic acids

Effect	Antimicrobial Compound	Comments
Intercalation to DNA	Acridines	DNA synthesis inhibited; binding to other macro-molecules observed
Alkylation	Ethylene oxide	Alkylation of phosphated guanine and other anti-microbial effects
DNA strand breakage	Hydrogen peroxide Peracetic acid	Has other effects on microbial structures

Similarly, detailed studies have been made on the interaction of a polymeric biguanide and polyhexamethylene biguanide.[217] In gram-negative bacteria, for example, it binds to negatively charged cell surface, impairs the outer membrane, and interacts with inner membrane phospholipids. K^+ loss occurs, and eventually, there is a complete loss of membrane function with precipitation of intracellular constituents.

Many microbicides will target nucleic acids (DNA or RNA) by different mechanisms (Table 5.15). The antibacterial activity of the acridines increases with the degree of ionization.[218] Ionization is, in fact, the most important factor governing their activity, but it must be cationic in nature. Acridine derivatives that are ionized to form anions or zwitterions are only poorly antibacterial by comparison. A considerable amount of research has been done on the mechanism of their antibacterial action.[219] They induce filamentous forms in gram-negative bacteria, inhibit DNA synthesis, and combine strongly to DNA, although binding to other sites, such as RNA, cell envelopes, and ribosomes, has also been reported. Binding to DNA has been studied extensively. The planar drug molecules become intercalated (sandwiched) between adjacent base pairs.[5,219] Thus, with proflavine, the compound is bound through the two primary amino groups, which are held in ionic linkage by two phosphoric acid residues of the Crick-Watson spiral, with the flat skeleton of the acridine ring resting on (and held by van der Waals forces to) the purine and pyrimidine molecules.

▶ CONCLUSION

The impact of the safe use of preservation, disinfection, and sterilization technologies has been well demonstrated from their impact on public health and safety over at least the last 100 years. In some cases, we can go further back in time to show their impact even if our knowledge of the reasons why at the time where unknown, such as best practices in food preservation. The optimal use of these technologies depends on balancing the desired antimicrobial end points while minimizing safety risks. These requirements have not dramatically changed in recent years. The challenge is the prudent use of these technologies at the right time, place, and under the right controls. We have at our disposal an armamentarium of well-described antimicrobial agents and processes but should continue to find new and novel ways to use these. Examples include a greater emphasis on environmental safety concerns, our understanding of microorganisms, optimization of technology use, and ensuring the safety of new product types.

There has clearly been a greater focus on understanding environmental safety risks in the last 20 years with examples highlighted in this chapter. These include new regulatory requirements (eg, in Europe with chemical safety), a better understanding of the environmental fate of chemicals, human risks on exposure to low levels of chemicals, and energy utilization. But we must be careful to ensure that the science to support conclusions on health risks is accurate and considers a risk-benefit analysis. Restrictions in the availability and use of certain (especially chemical) antimicrobial technologies can have a benefit in driving innovation. Examples include optimizing the use of different types of preservation chemicals or processes, development of liquid disinfectant formulations with increased activity despite the use of lower concentrations of microbicides, and innovations in sterilization practices for the prudent use of traditional and newer chemical sterilization methods. Combinations of best practices in microbiological quality (end-to-end), aseptic processing, and terminal sterilization methods have enabled new types of products/services such as drug or tissue-device combination products and three-dimensional printed devices or other materials.

Although it may be considered unlikely, we should not be complacent to think that our increasing knowledge of microorganisms and their risks to public health will not also challenge us. Examples such as the detection of microorganisms with unexpected resistance to chemical and physical microbicidal methods have taught us to be cautious, and we remain to learn more about the evolution of microorganisms under stressed conditions. The continued research into nonviable yet transmissible infectious agents such as viroids (naked nucleic acids) and prions (or transmissible protein structures) will no doubt indicate new risks previously not identified or considered. But there is also an opportunity to ensure that different (and in some cases the same) antimicrobial technologies can be employed to reduce the transmissibility of such agents. In all of these cases, applying microbiological quality best practices can ensure product or process safety and consistency and may also challenge us to deploy different strategies. A good example of this is with prions, where cleaning processes can be effective at reducing or eliminating the potential risk on contaminated surfaces rather than classical sterilization methods. The combination of these methods, as well as the prudent sourcing of materials used in or for manufacturing that do not contain high risk materials of an animal origin, are good examples. Equally, as stressed in this chapter, it is uncommon for the range of preservation, disinfection, and sterilization methods to fail, but when they do, the investigation of many of these cases present with opportunities to reduce risks by deploying best practices in microbiological quality through the full end-to-end process. This can be enabled with the use of rapid microbiological quality detection methodologies that can be employed to identify public health risks during these processes.

But it is also interesting to note that it is not our intention to eradicate the world from microbial life because microorganisms have often an underestimated benefit to health and well-being. In recent years, this has become an active area of research, such as in the influence of a healthy human immune system and impact of microbiome populations in health and disease states.[220] Consider, for example, the challenge of microbiological safety when the product is a microorganism or a population of microbes, which is not an unusual concept considering the development of vaccine technology since the inspiring work of pioneers in infection prevention and immunization such as Edward Jenner (1749-1823) and generations of microbiologists since that time. But new and more subtle ways of controlling the transmission of, or negative health impacts with, microorganisms are likely to be deployed. Examples include mixed populations of microorganism in affecting microbiome population shifts, subtle disruption of biofilms by quorum sensing or similar effects, and the use of microorganism-specific targets such as bacteriophages. These are good examples to challenge how we define microbiological safety in various situations.

Established principles, technologies, and practices of preservation, disinfection, and sterilization developed over the last 100 years should continue to be used and innovated. In some cases, this is reestablishing and evolving best practices in microbiological quality through a full end-to-end process to include product manufacturing/ delivery, water and food safety, waste handling and laboratory controls. It is important that we do not forget these best practices, if we can learn from errors in the past and encourage publication of lessons learned in the future. In other situations, it is innovating existing or developing new processes to allow for different applications and technologies that will enable new products and services.

A further consideration is in existing and developing regulations, standards, and guidance. In the interest of public health, it would be optimal to continue to move from an era of individual region or country requirements to more internationally harmonized practices that support the use of best practices around the world. These types of practices will also reduce the cost to public health and delivering safe and effective products. Efforts such as harmonization of European (EN) and international (ISO)

requirements for the development and validation of disinfection and sterilization processes should be encouraged because the overall risks from microorganisms are essentially the same and they do not recognize (or indeed respect) human borders. Other examples include harmonization of pharmacopeia requirements, antimicrobial test method development, and environmental safety standards. Close collaboration between regulators, users, and manufacturers is essential to this goal.

REFERENCES

1. Verani JR, Lorick SA, Yoder JS, et al; for Acanthamoeba Keratitis Investigation Team. National outbreak of *Acanthamoeba keratitis* associated with use of a contact lens solution, United States. *Emerg Infect Dis.* 2009;15:1236-1242.
2. Gharpure R, Perez A, Miller AD, Wikswo ME, Silver R, Hlavsa MC. Cryptosporidiosis Outbreaks—United States, 2009–2017. *MMWR Morb Mortal Wkly Rep.* 2019;68:568-572.
3. Yoder JS, Eddy BA, Visvesvara GS, Capewell L, Beach MJ. The epidemiology of primary amoebic meningoencephalitis in the USA, 1962–2008. *Epidemiol Infect.* 2010;138:968-975.
4. World Health Organization. Guidelines for drinking-water quality, 4th edition, incorporating the 1st addendum. World Health Organization Web site https://www.who.int/water_sanitation_health/publications/drinking-water-quality-guidelines-4-including-1st-addendum/en/. Accessed August 15, 2019.
5. McDonnell G. *Antisepsis, Disinfection, and Sterilization: Types, Action, and Resistance.* 2nd ed. Washington, DC: American Society for Microbiology Press; 2017.
6. McDonnell G, Burke P. Disinfection: is it time to reconsider Spaulding? *J Hosp Infect.* 2011;78:163-170.
7. Lewis T, Patel V, Ismail A, Fraise A. Sterilisation, disinfection and cleaning of theatre equipment: do we need to extend the Spaulding classification? *J Hosp Infect.* 2009;72:361-363.
8. International Organization for Standardization. *ISO/TS 19930:2017: Guidance on Aspects of a Risk-Based Approach to Assuring Sterility of Terminally Sterilized, Single-Use Health Care Product That Is Unable to Withstand Processing to Achieve Maximally a Sterility Assurance Level of 10^{-6}.* Geneva, Switzerland: International Organization for Standardization; 2017.
9. Association for the Advancement of Medical Instrumentation. *AAMI TIR17:2017. Compatibility of Materials Subject to Sterilization.* Arlington, VA: Association for the Advancement of Medical Instrumentation; 2017.
10. Alli BO. *Fundamental Principles of Occupational Health and Safety.* 2nd ed. Geneva, Switzerland: International Labour Organization; 2008.
11. American Chemistry Council's Ethylene Oxide/Ethylene Glycols Panel. *Ethylene Oxide Product Stewardship Guidance Manual.* 3rd ed. Washington, DC: American Chemistry Council; 2007. https://www.americanchemistry.com/ProductsTechnology/Ethylene-Oxide/EO-Product-Stewardship-Manual-3rd-edition/EO-Product-Stewardship-Manual-Hazards-of-Ethylene-Oxide.pdf. Accessed September 22, 2019.
12. Dann AB, Hontela A. Triclosan: environmental exposure, toxicity and mechanisms of action. *J Appl Toxicol.* 2011;31:285-311.
13. International Organization for Standardization. *ISO 10993-7:2008: Biological Evaluation of Medical Devices—Part 7: Ethylene Oxide Sterilization Residuals.* Geneva, Switzerland: International Organization for Standardization; 2008.
14. Morris RD, Audet AM, Angelillo IF, Chalmers TC, Mosteller F. Chlorination, chlorination by-products, and cancer: a meta-analysis. *Am J Public Health.* 1992;82:955-963.
15. Richardson SD, Plewa MJ, Wagner ED, Schoeny R, Demarini DM. Occurrence, genotoxicity, and carcinogenicity of regulated and emerging

disinfection by-products in drinking water: a review and roadmap for research. *Mutat Res.* 2007;636:178-242.

16. Kirchhof MG, de Gannes GC. The health controversies of parabens. *Skin Therapy Lett.* 2013;18:5-7.

17. Harvey PW, Darbre P. Endocrine disrupters and human health: could oestrogenic chemicals in body care cosmetics adversely affect breast cancer incidence in women? *J Appl Toxicol.* 2004;24:167-176.

18. Prabhakaran S, Abu-Hasan M, Hendeles L. Benzalkonium chloride: a bronchoconstricting preservative in continuous albuterol nebulizer solutions. *Pharmacotherapy.* 2017;37:607-610.

19. Albert A. Selectivity in the service of man. In: *Selective Toxicity.* 5th ed. London, United Kingdom: Methuen; 1973.

20. Logan LK, Weinstein RA. The epidemiology of carbapenem-resistant Enterobacteriaceae: the impact and evolution of a global menace. *J Infect Dis.* 2017;215 (suppl 1):S28-S36.

21. EUR-Lex. *Directive 98/8/EC of the European Parliament and of the Council Concerning the Placing of Biocidal Products on the Market.* Brussels, Belgium: European Union; 1998.

22. European Chemicals Agency. *Technical Guidance Document in Support of the Directive 98/8/EC Concerning the Placing of Biocidal Products on the Market: Guidance on Data Requirements for Active Substances and Biocidal Products.* Helsinki, Finland: European Chemicals Agency; 2008.

23. EUR-Lex. *Regulation (EC) No 1907/2006 of the European Parliament and of the Council of 18 December 2006 Concerning the Registration, Evaluation, Authorisation and Restriction of Chemicals (REACH), Establishing a European Chemicals Agency, Amending Directive 1999/45/EC and Repealing Council Regulation (EEC) No 793/93 and Commission Regulation (EC) No 1488/94 as well as Council Directive 76/769/EEC and Commission Directives 91/155/EEC, 93/67/EEC, 93/105/EC and 2000/21/EC.* Brussels, Belgium: European Union; 2006.

24. Hopkins JA. Legislation affecting disinfectant products in Europe: the biocidal products directive and the registration, evaluation and authorization of chemicals regulations. In: Fraise AP, Maillard JY, Sattar S, eds. *Russell, Hugo and Ayliffe's Principles and Practice of Disinfection, Preservation and Sterilization.* 5th ed. Chichester, United Kingdom: Wiley-Blackwell; 2013:255-261.

25. American National Standards Institute, Association for the Advancement of Medical Instrumentation. *ANSI/AAMI ST58:2013: Chemical Sterilization and High-Level Disinfection in Health Care facilities.* Washington, DC: AAMI; 2013/(R)2018.

26. Occupational Safety and Health Administration. *Best Practices for the Safe Use of Glutaraldehyde in Health Care.* Washington, DC: US Department of Labor, Occupational Safety and Health Administration; 2006.

27. Ethylene Oxide Sterilization Association (EOSA). *Flawed science and modeling by EPA result in inappropriate conclusions that could have disastrous adverse public health impacts.* https://www.eosa.org/sites/default/files/2018-09/EOSA%20Position%20Paper%20--%20Flawed%20Science%202018-09.pdf. Accessed December 2019.

28. Agency for Toxic Substances and Disease Registry. *Toxicological Profile for Ethylene Oxide.* Atlanta, GA: US Public Health Service, US Department of Health and Human Services; 1990. https://www.atsdr.cdc.gov/toxprofiles/tp137.pdf. Accessed August 15, 2019.

29. World Health Organization. *Ethylene Oxide.* Geneva, Switzerland: World Health Organization; 2003. https://www.who.int/ipcs/publications/cicad/en/cicad54.pdf. Accessed August 15, 2019.

30. Committee on Health Effects of Waste Incineration. *Waste Incineration & Public Health.* Washington, DC: National Academy Press; 2000.

31. Pub L No. 111-353, 124 Stat 3885.

32. US Food and Drug Administration. 21 CFR Part 807. Establishment registration and device listing for manufacturers and initial importers of devices. US Food and Drug Administration Web site. https://www.accessdata.fda.gov/scripts/cdrh/cfdocs/cfcfr/CFRSearch.cfm?CFRPart=807. Accessed August 2019.

33. US Food and Drug Administration. 21 CFR Part 210. Current good manufacturing practice in manufacturing, processing, packing, or holding of drugs; general. US Food and Drug Administration Web site. https://www.accessdata.fda.gov/scripts/cdrh/cfdocs/cfcfr/CFRSearch.cfm?CFRPart=210. Accessed August 15, 2019.

34. US Food and Drug Administration. 21 CFR Part 211. Current good manufacturing practice for finished pharmaceuticals. US Food and Drug Administration Web site. https://www.accessdata.fda.gov/scripts/cdrh/cfdocs/cfcfr/CFRSearch.cfm?CFRPart=211. Accessed August 15, 2019.

35. China State Council. *Supervision and Regulation of Medical Devices, No. 680.* Beijing, China: China State Council; 2017.

36. National People's Congress of the People's Republic of China. Drug Administration Law. 2019. National People's Congress Web site. http://www.npc.gov.cn/npc/c30834/201908/26a6b28dd83546d79d17f90c62e59461.shtml. Accessed August 15, 2019.

37. Ministry of Health and Family Welfare. *India Ministry of Health and Family Welfare Notification No. G.S.R, 78(E). Medical Devices Rules 2017.* New Delhi, India: Ministry of Health and Family Welfare; 2017.

38. International Organization for Standardization. *ISO 9000:2015: Quality Management Systems—Fundamentals and Vocabulary.* Geneva, Switzerland: International Organization for Standardization; 2015.

39. International Organization for Standardization. *ISO 13485:2016: Medical Devices—Quality Management Systems—Requirements for Regulatory Purposes.* Geneva, Switzerland: International Organization for Standardization; 2016.

40. International Organization for Standardization. *ISO/IEC 17025:2017: General Requirements for the Competence of Testing and Calibration Laboratories.* Geneva, Switzerland: International Organization for Standardization; 2017.

41. Association for the Advancement of Medical Instrumentation. *ANSI/AAMI ST79:2017: Comprehensive Guide to Steam Sterilization and Sterility Assurance in Health Care Facilities.* Arlington, VA: Association for the Advancement of Medical Instrumentation; 2017.

42. Department of Health and Social Care. Health Technical Memorandum (HTM) 01-01 series on the management and decontamination of surgical instruments (medical devices) used in acute care. UK Government Web site. https://www.gov.uk/government/publications/management-and-decontamination-of-surgical-instruments-used-in-acute-care. Accessed August 15, 2019.

43. Association of periOperative Registered Nurses. *Guidelines for Perioperative Practice.* Denver, CO: Association of periOperative Registered Nurses; 2019.

44. Berríos-Torres SI, Umscheid CA, Bratzler DW, et al; for Healthcare Infection Control Practices Advisory Committee. Centers for Disease Control and Prevention guideline for the prevention of surgical site infection, 2017. *JAMA Surg.* 2017;152:784-791.

45. World Health Organization. Global guidelines on the prevention of surgical site infection. 2016. World Health Organization Web site. https://www.who.int/gpsc/ssi-prevention-guidelines/en/. Accessed August 15, 2019.

46. World Health Organization. Laboratory biosafety manual—third edition. World Health Organization Web site. https://www.who.int/csr/resources/publications/biosafety/WHO_CDS_CSR_LYO_2004_11/en/. Accessed August 15, 2019.

47. World Health Organization. *WHO Good Manufacturing Practices for Sterile Pharmaceutical Products.* Geneva, Switzerland: World Health Organization; 2011. WHO Technical Report Series 961.

48. World Health Organization. *Exposure Assessment of Microbiological Hazards in Food.* Geneva, Switzerland: World Health Organization; 2008. https://www.who.int/foodsafety/publications/micro/MRA7.pdf. Accessed August 15, 2019.

49. Schuerger AC, Moores JE, Smith DJ, Reitz G. A lunar microbial survival model for predicting the forward contamination of the moon. *Astrobiology.* 2019;19:730-756.

50. Russell AD. Factors influencing the efficacy of antimicrobial agents. In: Russell AD, Hugo WB, Ayliffe GAJ, eds. *Principles and Practice of Disinfection, Preservation and Sterilization.* 3rd ed. Oxford, United Kingdom: Blackwell Scientific Publications; 1999:95-123.

51. Bloomfield SF. Bacterial sensitivity and resistance: C. resistance of bacterial spores to chemical agents. In: Russell AD, Hugo WB, Ayliffe GAJ, eds. *Principles and Practice of Disinfection, Preservation and Sterilization.* 3rd ed. Oxford, United Kingdom: Blackwell Scientific Publications; 1999:303-320.

52. Lehmann RH. Synergisms in disinfectant formulations. In: Payne KR, ed. *Industrial Biocides.* Chichester, United Kingdom: John Wiley & Sons; 1988:68-90.

53. Lehmann RH. Synergisms in disinfectant formulations. In: Block SS, ed. *Disinfection, Sterilization, and Preservation.* 5th ed. Philadelphia, PA: Lippincott, Williams & Wilkins; 2001:459-471.

54. Zipf HF. Practical points for experiments using combinations of two compounds. *Arzneimittelforschung.* 1953;3:398-403.

55. Kull FC, Eisman PC, Sylwestrowicz HD, Mayer RL. Mixtures of quaternary ammonium compounds and long-chain fatty acids as antifungal agents. *Appl Microbiol.* 1961;9:538-541.

56. Waites WM, Harding SE, Fowler DR, Jones SH, Shaw D, Martin M. The destruction of spores of *Bacillus subtilis* by the combined effects of hydrogen peroxide and ultraviolet light. *Lett Appl Microbiol.* 1988;7:139-140.

57. Allwood MC. Inhibition of *Staphylococcus aureus* by combinations of non-ionic surface active agents and antibacterial substances. *Microbios.* 1973;7:209-214.

58. Blackburn P, Polak J, Gusik SA, Rubino SD, inventors; Public Health Research Institute Of The City Of New York, assignee. Nisin compositions for use as enhanced, broad range bactericides. International Patent Application WO 1989012399. December 28, 1989.

59. Andrew MHE, Russell AD, eds. *The Revival of Injured Microbes.* London, United Kingdom: Academic Press; 1984. Society for Applied Bacteriology Symposium Series No. 12.

60. Grabley S, Thiericke R. *Drug Discovery from Nature.* London, United Kingdom: Springer; 1999:5-7.

61. Centers for Disease Control and Prevention. *Surveillance for Foodborne Disease Outbreaks United States, 2016: Annual Report.* Atlanta, GA: US Department of Health and Human Services, Centers for Disease Control and Prevention; 2018.

62. Moreira NA, Bondelind M. Safe drinking water and waterborne outbreaks. *J Water Health.* 2017;15:83-96.

63. Vu N, Lou JR, Kupiec TC. Quality control analytical methods: microbial limit tests for nonsterile pharmaceuticals, part 1. *Int J Pharm Compd.* 2014;18:213-221.

64. Vu N, Lou JR, Kupiec TC. Quality control: microbial limit tests for nonsterile pharmaceuticals, part 2. *Int J Pharm Compd.* 2014;18:305-310.

65. Lundov MD, Moesby L, Zachariae C, Johansen JD. Contamination versus preservation of cosmetics: a review on legislation, usage, infections, and contact allergy. *Contact Dermatitis.* 2009;60:70-78.

66. Eissa ME. Distribution of bacterial contamination in non-sterile pharmaceutical materials and assessment of its risk to the health of the final consumers quantitatively. *J Basic Appl Sci.* 2016;5:217-230.

67. Woo CG, Kang J-S, Kim H-J, Kim Y-J, Han B. Treatment of air filters using the antimicrobial natural products propolis and grapefruit seed extract for deactivation of bioaerosols. *Aerosol Sci Technol.* 2015;49:611-619.

68. American Society for Testing and Materials International. *ASTM F316 - 03(2011): Standard Test Methods for Pore Size Characteristics of Membrane Filters by Bubble Point and Mean Flow Pore Test.* West Conshohocken, PA: American Society for Testing and Materials International; 2011.

69. American Society of Heating, Refrigerating and Air-Conditioning Engineers. *ANSI/ASHRAE Standard 52.2-2012. Method of Testing General Ventilation Air-Cleaning Devices for Removal Efficiency by Particle Size.* Atlanta, GA: American Society of Heating, Refrigerating and Air-Conditioning Engineers 2015.

70. British Standards Institution. *BS. EN 1822-1:2009: High Efficiency Air Filters.* London, United Kingdom: British Standards Institution: 2009.

71. American Society for Testing and Materials International. *ASTM F838:2015: Standard Test Method for Determining Bacterial Retention of Membrane Filters Utilized for Liquid Filtration.* West Conshohocken, PA: American Society for Testing and Materials International; 2015.

72. American Society for Testing and Materials International. *ASTM D3862:13: Standard Test Method for Retention Characteristics of 0.2-µm Membrane Filters Used in Routine Filtration Procedures for the Evaluation of Microbiological Water Quality.* West Conshohocken, PA: 2013.

73. Antonsen HRK, Awafo V, Bender JL, et al; for Sterilizing Filtration of Liquids Task Force. Sterilizing filtration of liquids. Technical report no. 26 (revised 2008). *PDA J Pharm Sci Technol.* 2008;62(suppl 5, TR26):2-60.

74. Belgaid A, Benaji B, Aadil N, et al. Sterilisation of aseptic drug by sterile filtration: microbiology validation by microbiology challenge test. *J Chem Pharm Res.* 2014;6:760-770.

75. Lee RE, Gilbert CA. On the application of the mass law to the process of disinfection—being a contribution to the "mechanistic theory" as opposed to the "vitalistic theory." *J Phys Chem.* 1918;22:348-372.

76. Cerf O. A review: tailing of survival curves of bacterial spores. *J Appl Bacteriol.* 1977;42:1-19.

77. Withell ER. The significance of the variation in shape of time-survivor curves. *J Hyg (Lond).* 1942;42:124-183.

78. Koch AL. The logarithm in biology. II. Distributions simulating the log-normal. *J Theor Biol.* 1969;23:251-268.

79. Morris JC. Disinfectant chemistry and biocidal activities. In: *Proceedings of the National Specialty Conference on Disinfection.* New York, NY: American Society of Civil Engineering; 1970.

80. Oliver R, Shepstone BJ. Some practical considerations in determining the parameters for multi-target and multi-hit survival curves. *Phys Med Biol.* 1964;9:167.

81. Taylor DG, Johnson JD. Kinetics of viral inactivation by bromine. In: Rubin AJ, ed. *Chemistry of Water Supply, Treatment, and Distribution.* Ann Arbor, MI: Ann Arbor Science; 1974:369-408.

82. Severin BF, Suidan MT, Engelbrecht RS. Kinetic modeling of U.V. disinfection of water. *Water Res.* 1983;17:1669-1678.

83. Berg G, Chang SL, Harris EK. Devitalization of microorganisms by iodine. I. Dynamics of the devitalization of enteroviruses by elemental iodine. *Virology.* 1964;22:461-481.

84. Young DC, Sharp DG. Poliovirus aggregates and their survival in water. *Appl Environ Microbiol.* 1977;33:168-177.

85. Floyd R, Sharp DG, Johnson JD. Inactivation by chlorine of single poliovirus particles in water. *Environ Sci Technol.* 1979;13:438-442.

86. Wickramanayake GB, Rubin AJ, Sproul OJ. Inactivation of *Naegleria* and *Giardia* cysts in water by ozonation. *J Water Pollut Control Federation.* 1984;56:983-988.

87. Rubin AJ, Engle JP, Sproul OJ. Disinfection of amoebic cysts in water with free chlorine. *J Water Pollut Control Federation.* 1983;55:1174-1182.

88. Chen YSR, Sproul OJ, Rubin AJ. Inactivation of *Naegleria gruberi* cysts by chlorine dioxide. *Water Res.* 1985;19:783-789.

89. Wei JH, Chang SL. A multi-Poisson distribution model for treating disinfection data. In: Johnson JD, ed. *Disinfection: Water and Wastewater.* Ann Arbor, MI: Ann Arbor Science; 1975:11-48.

90. Katzenelson E, Kletter B, Shuval HI. Inactivation kinetics of viruses and bacteria in water by use of ozone. *J Am Water Works Assoc.* 1974;66:725-729.

91. Berman D, Hoff JC. Inactivation of simian rotavirus SA11 by chlorine, chlorine dioxide, and monochloramine. *Appl Environ Microbiol.* 1984;40:317-323.

92. Watson HE. A note on the variation of the rate of disinfection with change in the concentration of the disinfectant. *J Hyg (Lond).* 1908;8:536-592.

93. Hoff JC. *Inactivation of Microbial Agents by Chemical Disinfectants.* Cincinnati, OH: Water Engineering Research Laboratory, US Environmental Protection Agency; 1986. EPA-600/S2-86-067.

94. Wickramanayake GB. *Kinetics and Mechanism of Ozone Activation of Protozoan Cysts* [dissertation]. Columbus, OH: Department of Civil Engineering, The Ohio State University; 1984.

95. Baumann ER, Ludwig DD. Free available chlorine residuals for small nonpublic water supplies. *J Am Water Works Assoc.* 1962;54:1379-1388.

96. Water Environment Federation. *Wastewater Disinfection: Manual of Practice FD-10.* Alexandria, VA: Water Environment Federation; 1996.

97. McDonnell G. Decontamination of prions. In: Walker JT, ed. *Decontamination in Hospitals and Healthcare*. 2nd ed. England, United Kingdom: Woodhead Publishing; 2020.

98. Rutala WA, Weber DJ; for Society for Healthcare Epidemiology of America. Guideline for disinfection and sterilization of prion-contaminated medical instruments. *Infect Control Hosp Epidemiol*. 2010;31:107-117.

99. Halvorson HO, Ziegler NR. Application of statistics to problems in bacteriology. I. A means of determining bacterial population by the dilution method. *J Bacteriol*. 1933;25:101-121.

100. Association for the Advancement of Medical Instrumentation. *ANSI/AAMI-ST67:2019. Sterilization of Health Care Products—Requirements and Guidance for Selecting a Sterility Assurance Level (SAL) for Products Labeled "Sterile."* Arlington, VA: Association for the Advancement of Medical Instrumentation; 2019.

101. Association for the Advancement of Medical Instrumentation. *AAMI TIR100:2020. End-to-End Microbiological Quality and Assurance of Sterility. Draft Version 2020*. Arlington, VA: Association for the Advancement of Medical Instrumentation; 2020.

102. Justi C, Amato V, Antloga K, Harrington S, McDonnell G. Demonstration of a sterility assurance level for a liquid chemical sterilisation process. *Zentralsterilisation*. 2000;9:170-181.

103. International Organization for Standardization. *ISO 14937:2009: Sterilization of Health Care Products—General Requirements for Characterization of a Sterilizing Agent and the Development, Validation and Routine Control of a Sterilization Process for Medical Devices*. Geneva, Switzerland: International Organization for Standardization; 2009.

104. International Organization for Standardization. *ISO 11137-2:2013: Sterilization of Health Care Products—Radiation—Part 2: Establishing the Sterilization Dose*. Geneva, Switzerland: International Organization for Standardization; 2013.

105. Offit PA. The Cutter incident, 50 years later. *N Engl J Med*. 2005;352:1411-1412.

106. Brown F. Review of accidents caused by incomplete inactivation of viruses. *Dev Biol Stand*. 1993;81:103-107.

107. Janetos TM, Akintilo L, Xu S. Overview of high-risk Food and Drug Administration recalls for cosmetics and personal care products from 2002 to 2016. *J Cosmet Dermatol*. 2019;18:1361-1365.

108. Ahearn DG, Stulting RD. Moulds associated with contaminated ocular and injectable drugs: FDA recalls, epidemiology considerations, drug shortages, and aseptic processing. *Med Mycol*. 2018;56:389-394.

109. Cunningham-Oakes E, Weiser R, Pointon T, Mahenthiralingam E. Understanding the challenges of non-food industrial product contamination. *FEMS Microbiol Lett*. 2019;366(23):fnaa010.

110. Berkelman RL, Anderson RL, Davis BJ, et al. Intrinsic bacterial contamination of a commercial iodophor solution: investigation of the implicated manufacturing plant. *Appl Environ Microbiol*. 1984;47:752-756.

111. Anderson RL, Berkelman RL, Mackel DC, Davis BJ, Holland BW, Martone WJ. Investigations into the survival of *Pseudomonas aeruginosa* in poloxamer-iodine. *Appl Environ Microbiol*. 1984;47:757-762.

112. Brooks RB, Mitchell PK, Miller JR, et al; for Burkholderia cepacia Workgroup. Multistate outbreak of *Burkholderia cepacia* complex bloodstream infections after exposure to contaminated saline flush syringes: United States, 2016-2017. *Clin Infect Dis*. 2019;69:445-449.

113. Blossom D, Noble-Wang J, Su J, et al; for Serratia in Prefilled Syringes Investigation Team Group. Multistate outbreak of *Serratia marcescens* bloodstream infections caused by contamination of prefilled heparin and isotonic sodium chloride solution syringes. *Arch Intern Med*. 2009;169:1705-1711.

114. Jimenez L. Microbial diversity in pharmaceutical product recalls and environments. *PDA J Pharm Sci Technol*. 2007;61:383-399.

115. Patel PR, Larson AK, Castel AD, et al. Hepatitis C virus infections from a contaminated radiopharmaceutical used in myocardial perfusion studies. *JAMA*. 2006;296:2005-2011.

116. Seal D, Stapleton F, Dart J. Possible environmental sources of *Acanthamoeba* spp in contact lens wearers. *Br J Ophthalmol*. 1992;76:424-427.

117. Bozkurt H, Phan-Thien KY, van Ogtrop F, Bell T, McConchie R. Outbreaks, occurrence, and control of norovirus and hepatitis a virus contamination in berries: a review. *Crit Rev Food Sci Nutr*. 2020;3:1-23.

118. Wadamori Y, Gooneratne R, Hussain MA. Outbreaks and factors influencing microbiological contamination of fresh produce. *J Sci Food Agric*. 2017;97:1396-1403.

119. Li M, Baker CA, Danyluk MD, et al. Identification of biological hazards in produce consumed in industrialized countries: a review. *J Food Prot*. 2018;81:1171-1186.

120. Mamalis N, Edelhauser HF, Dawson DG, Chew J, LeBoyer RM, Werner L. Toxic anterior segment syndrome. *J Cataract Refract Surg*. 2006;32:324-323.

121. Eze CT, Nwagwe OR, Ogbuene EB, Eze HI. Investigating groundwater contamination following the disposal of hospital wastes in a government reserved area, Enugu, Nigeria. *Bull Environ Contam Toxicol*. 2017;98:218-225.

122. Devarajan N, Laffite A, Mulaji CK, et al. Occurrence of antibiotic resistance genes and bacterial markers in a tropical river receiving hospital and urban wastewaters. *PLoS One*. 2016;11:e0149211.

123. Auty H, Mellor D, Gunn G, Boden LA. The risk of foot and mouth disease transmission posed by public access to the countryside during an outbreak. *Front Vet Sci*. 2019;6:381.

124. Kovaleva J, Peters FT, van der Mei HC, Degener JE. Transmission of infection by flexible gastrointestinal endoscopy and bronchoscopy. *Clin Microbiol Rev*. 2013;26:231-254.

125. Rauwers AW, Troelstra A, Fluit AC, et al. Independent root-cause analysis of contributing factors, including dismantling of 2 duodenoscopes, to investigate an outbreak of multidrug-resistant *Klebsiella pneumoniae*. *Gastrointest Endosc*. 2019;90:793-804.

126. Tosh PK, Disbot M, Duffy JM, et al. Outbreak of *Pseudomonas aeruginosa* surgical site infections after arthroscopic procedures: Texas, 2009. *Infect Control Hosp Epidemiol*. 2011;32:1179-1186.

127. Dancer SJ, Stewart M, Coulombe C, Gregori A, Virdi M. Surgical site infections linked to contaminated surgical instruments. *J Hosp Infect*. 2012;81:231-238.

128. Centers for Disease Control and Prevention. Notes from the field: contamination of alcohol prep pads with *Bacillus cereus* group and *Bacillus species*—Colorado, 2010. *MMWR Morb Mortal Wkly Rep*. 2011;60:347.

129. Efstratiou A, Ongerth JE, Karanis P. Waterborne transmission of protozoan parasites: Review of worldwide outbreaks—an update 2011-2016. *Water Res*. 2017;114:14-22.

130. International Organization for Standardization. *ISO 31000:2018: Risk Management—Guidelines*. Geneva, Switzerland: International Organization for Standardization; 2018.

131. International Organization for Standardization. *ISO 14971:2019: Medical Devices—Application of Risk Management to Medical Devices*. Geneva, Switzerland: International Organization for Standardization; 2019.

132. International Organization for Standardization. *ISO 35001:2019: Biorisk Management for Laboratories and Other Related Organisations*. Geneva, Switzerland: International Organization for Standardization; 2019.

133. Food and Agriculture Organization/World Health Organization. Risk management and food safety; consultation report, 1997. Food and Agriculture Organization Web site. http://www.fao.org/3/W4982E/w4982e00.htm. Accessed December 15, 2019.

134. International Organization for Standardization. *IEC 31010:2019: Risk Management—Risk Assessment Techniques*. Geneva, Switzerland: International Organization for Standardization; 2019.

135. Food and Agriculture Organization. The use of Hazard Analysis Critical Control Point (HACCP) principles in food. Food and Agriculture Organization Web site. http://www.fao.org/3/w8088e/w8088e05.htm. Accessed December 15, 2019.

136. Sandle T. *Pharmaceutical Microbiology: Essentials for Quality Assurance and Quality Control*. Cambridge, United Kingdom: Woodhead Publishing; 2016.

137. Haas CN, Rose JB, Gerba CP. *Quantitative Microbial Risk Assessment*. New York, NY: Wiley & Sons; 1999.

138. Allwood MC, Russell AD. Mechanisms of thermal injury in nonsporing bacteria. *Adv Appl Microbiol.* 1970;12:89-119.

139. Hugo WB. Disinfection mechanisms. In: Russell AD, Hugo WB, Ayliffe GAJ, eds. *Principles and Practice of Disinfection, Preservation and Sterilization.* 3rd ed. Oxford, United Kingdom: Blackwell Scientific Publications; 1999:258-283.

140. McDonnell G, Russell AD. Antiseptics and disinfectants: activity, action, and resistance. *Clin Microbiol Rev.* 1999;12:147-179.

141. Leggett MJ, McDonnell G, Denyer SP, Setlow P, Maillard JY. Bacterial spore structures and their protective role in biocide resistance. *J Appl Microbiol.* 2012;113:485-498.

142. Nikaido H. Prevention of drug access to bacterial targets: permeability barriers and active efflux. *Science.* 1994;264:382-387.

143. Yazdankhah SP, Scheie AA, Høiby EA, et al. Triclosan and antimicrobial resistance in bacteria: an overview. *Microb Drug Resist.* 2006;12:83-90.

144. Russell AD. Radiation sterilization. A. Ionizing radiation. In: Russell AD, Hugo WB, Ayliffe GAJ, eds. *Principles and Practice of Disinfection, Preservation and Sterilization.* 3rd ed. Oxford, United Kingdom: Blackwell Scientific Publications; 1999:675-687.

145. Russell AD. Radiation sterilization. B. Ultraviolet radiation. In: Russell AD, Hugo WB, Ayliffe GAJ, eds. *Principles and Practice of Disinfection, Preservation and Sterilization.* 3rd ed. Oxford, United Kingdom: Blackwell Scientific Publications; 1999:688-702.

146. Russell AD. Microbial susceptibility and resistance to chemical and physical agents. In: Collier L, Balows A, Sussman M, eds. *Topley & Wilson's Microbiology and Microbial Infections.* 9th ed. London, United Kingdom: Edward Arnold; 1998:149-184. Balows A, Duerden BI, eds. *Systematic Bacteriology;* vol 2.

147. Farkas J. Tolerance of spores to ionizing radiation: mechanisms of inactivation, injury and repair. *Soc Appl Bacteriol Symp Ser.* 1994;23:81S-90S.

148. Moseley BEB. Ionizing radiation: action and repair. In: Gould GW, ed. *Mechanisms of Action of Food Preservation Procedures.* London, United Kingdom: Elsevier Applied Science; 1989:43-70.

149. Russell AD, Morris A, Allwood MC. Methods for assessing damage to bacteria induced by chemical and physical agents. In: Ribbons DW, Norris JR, eds. *Methods in Microbiology.* Vol 8. London, United Kingdom: Academic Press; 1973:95-182.

150. Terano H, Tanooka H, Kadota H. Repair of radiation damage to deoxyribonucleic acid in germinating spores of *Bacillus subtilis. J Bacteriol.* 1971;106:925-930.

151. Durban E, Grecz N, Farkas J. Direct enzymatic repair of deoxyribonucleic acid single-strand breaks in dormant spores. *J Bacteriol.* 1974;118:129-138.

152. Krisko A, Radman M. Biology of extreme radiation resistance: the way of *Deinococcus radiodurans. Cold Spring Harb Perspect Biol.* 2013;5:a012765.

153. Bridges BA. Survival of bacteria following exposure to ultraviolet and ionizing radiation. In: Gray TGR, Postgate JR, eds. *The Survival of Vegetative Microbes.* Cambridge, United Kingdom: Cambridge University Press; 1976:183-208. Society for General Microbiology Symposium No. 26.

154. De Maayer P, Anderson D, Cary C, Cowan DA. Some like it cold: understanding the survival strategies of psychrophiles. *EMBO Rep.* 2014;15:508-517.

155. Ingram M, Mackey BM. Inaction by cold. In: Skinner FA, Hugo WB, eds. *Inhibition and Inactivation of Vegetative Microbes.* London, United Kingdom: Academic Press; 1976:111-151. Society for Applied Bacteriology Symposium Series No. 5.

156. Herbert RA. Microbial growth at low temperatures. In: Gould GW, ed. *Mechanisms of Action of Food Preservation Procedures.* London, United Kingdom: Elsevier Applied Science; 1989:71-96.

157. MacLeod RA, Calcott PH. Cold shock and freezing damage to microbes. In: Gray TGR, Postgate JR, eds. *The Survival of Vegetative Microbes.* Cambridge, United Kingdom: Cambridge University Press; 1976:81-109. Society for General Microbiology Symposium No. 26.

158. Rose AH. Osmotic stress and microbial survival. In: Gray TGR, Postgate JR, eds. *The Survival of Vegetative Microbes.* Cambridge, United Kingdom: Cambridge University Press; 1976:135-182. Society for General Microbiology Symposium No. 26.

159. Neu HG, Heppel LA. The release of enzymes from *Escherichia coli* by osmotic shock and during the formation of spheroplasts. *J Biol Chem.* 1965;240:3685-3692.

160. Mackey BM. Lethal and sublethal effects of refrigeration, freezing and freeze-drying on microorganisms. In: Andrew MHE, Russell AD, eds. *The Revival of Injured Microbes.* London, United Kingdom: Academic Press; 1984:45-75. Society for Applied Bacteriology Symposium Series No. 12.

161. Estes MK, Graham DY, Smith EM, Gerba CP. Rotavirus stability and inactivation. *J Gen Virol.* 1979;43:403-409.

162. Hansen RK, Zhai S, Skepper JN, Johnston MD, Alpar HO, Slater NK. Mechanisms of inactivation of HSV-2 during storage in frozen and lyophilized forms. *Biotechnol Prog.* 2005;21:911-917.

163. Russell AD. Heat sterilization. B. Destruction of bacterial spores by thermal methods. In: Russell AD, Hugo WB, Ayliffe GAJ, eds. *Principles and Practice of Disinfection, Preservation and Sterilization.* 3rd ed. Oxford, United Kingdom: Blackwell Scientific Publications; 1999:640-656.

164. Ishino Y, Narumi I. DNA repair in hyperthermophilic and hyperradioresistant microorganisms. *Curr Opin Microbiol.* 2015;25:103-112.

165. Schumann W. Regulation of the heat shock response in bacteria. In: Kumar CMS, Mande SC, eds. *Prokaryotic Chaperonins: Multiple Copies and Multitude Functions.* Singapore, Singapore: Springer Nature Singapore; 2017:21-36. *Heat Shock Proteins;* vol 11.

166. Gould GW. Heat-induced injury and inactivation. In: Gould GW, ed. *Mechanisms of Action of Food Preservation Procedures.* London, United Kingdom: Elsevier Applied Science; 1989:11-42.

167. Mehta R, Singhal P, Singh H, Damle D, Sharma AK. Insight into thermophiles and their wide-spectrum applications. *3 Biotech.* 2016; 6:81.

168. Setlow P. I will survive: protecting and repairing spore DNA. *J Bacteriol.* 1992;174:2737-2741.

169. Murrell WG, Warth AD. Composition and heat resistance of bacterial spores. In: Campbell LL, Halvorson HO, eds. *Spores III.* Ann Arbor, MI: American Society for Microbiology; 1965:1-24.

170. Balassa G, Milhaud P, Raulet E, Silva MT, Sousa JC. A *Bacillus subtilis* mutant requiring dipicolinic acid for the development of heat-resistant spores. *J Gen Microbiol.* 1979;110:365-379.

171. Lewis JC, Snell NS, Burr HK. Water permeability of bacterial spores and the concept of a contractile cortex. *Science.* 1960;132:544-545.

172. Sykes G. *Disinfection and Sterilization.* 2nd ed. London, United Kingdom: F & N Spon; 1965.

173. Pheil CG, Pflug IJ, Nicholas RC, Augustin JAL. Effect of various gas atmospheres on destruction of microorganisms in dry heat. *Appl Microbiol.* 1967;15:120-124.

174. Molin G. Inherent genetic differences in dry heat resistance of some *Bacillus* spores. In: Barker AN, Wolf J, Ellar DJ, et al, eds. *Spore Research 1976.* New York, NY: Academic Press; 1976:487-500.

175. Brown P, Liberski PP, Wolff A, Gajdusek DC. Resistance of scrapie infectivity to steam autoclaving after formaldehyde fixation and limited survival after ashing at 360 °C: practical and theoretical implications. *J Infect Dis.* 1990;161:467-472.

176. Brown P, Rau EH, Johnson BJ, Bacote AE, Gibbs CJ Jr, Gajdusek DC. New studies on the heat resistance of hamster-adapted scrapie agent: threshold survival after ashing at 600°C suggests an inorganic template of replication. *Proc Natl Acad Sci U S A.* 2000;97:3418-3421.

177. World Health Organization. *WHO Infection Control Guidelines for Transmissible Spongiform Encephalopathies. Report of a WHO Consultation, Geneva, Switzerland, 23-26 March 1999. WHO/CDS/CSR/APH/2000/3.* Geneva, Switzerland: World Health Organization; 2000.

178. McDonnell G, Dehen C, Perrin A, et al. Cleaning, disinfection and sterilization of surface prion contamination. *J Hosp Infect.* 2013;85:268-273.

179. Cantoni O, Brandi G, Albano A, Cattabeni F. Action of cystine in the cytotoxic response of *Escherichia coli* cells exposed to hydrogen peroxide. *Free Radic Res.* 1995;22:275-283.

180. Choe JK, Richards DH, Wilson CJ, Mitch WA. Degradation of amino acids and structure in model proteins and bacteriophage MS2 by chlorine, bromine, and ozone. *Environ Sci Technol.* 2015;49:13331-13339.

181. Noguchi N, Nakada A, Itoh Y, Watanabe A, Niki E. Formation of active oxygen species and lipid peroxidation induced by hypochlorite. *Arch Biochem Biophys.* 2002;397:440-447.

182. Linley E, Denyer SP, McDonnell G, Simons C, Maillard JY. Use of hydrogen peroxide as a biocide: new consideration of its mechanisms of biocidal action. *J Antimicrob Chemother.* 2012;67:1589-1596.

183. Finnegan M, Linley E, Denyer SP, McDonnell G, Simons C, Maillard JY. Mode of action of hydrogen peroxide and other oxidizing agents: differences between liquid and gas forms. *J Antimicrob Chemother.* 2010;65:2108-2115.

184. McDonnell G. Peroxygens and other forms of oxygen: their use for effective cleaning, disinfection, and sterilization. In: Zhu PC. ed. *New Biocides Development: The Combined Approach of Chemistry and Microbiology.* New York, NY: Oxford University Press; 2006:292-308. ACS Symposium Series.

185. Ooi BG, Branning SA. Correlation of conformational changes and protein degradation with loss of lysozyme activity due to chlorine dioxide treatment. *Appl Biochem Biotechnol.* 2017;182:782-791.

186. Leggett MJ, Schwarz JS, Burke PA, McDonnell G, Denyer SP, Maillard JY. Mechanism of sporicidal activity for the synergistic combination of peracetic acid and hydrogen peroxide. *Appl Environ Microbiol.* 2015;82:1035-1039.

187. Shin S-Y, Calvisi EG, Beaman TC, Pankratz HS, Gerhardt P, Marquis RE. Microscopic and thermal characterization of hydrogen peroxide killing and lysis of spores and protection by transition metal ions, chelators, and antioxidants. *Appl Environ Microbiol.* 1994;60:3192-3197.

188. Kampf G, Fliss PM, Martiny H. Is peracetic acid suitable for the cleaning step of reprocessing flexible endoscopes? *World J Gastrointest Endosc.* 2014;6:390-406.

189. Kampf G, Bloss R, Martiny H. Surface fixation of dried blood by glutaraldehyde and peracetic acid. *J Hosp Infect.* 2004;57:139-143

190. McDonnell G, Fichet G, Antloga K, et al. Cleaning investigations to reduce the risk of prion contamination on manufacturing surfaces and materials. *Euro J Parent Pharmaceut Sci.* 2010;10:67-72.

191. Price CC. Fundamental mechanisms of alkylation. *Ann N Y Acad Sci.* 1958;68:663-668.

192. Albert A, Gibson MI, Rubbo SD. The influence of chemical constitution on antibacterial activity. VI. The bactericidal action of 8-hydroxyquinoline (oxine). *Br J Exp Pathol.* 1953;34:119-130.

193. Pottenger LH, Boysen G, Brown K, et al. Understanding the importance of low-molecular weight (ethylene oxide- and propylene oxide-induced) DNA adducts and mutations in risk assessment: insights from 15 years of research and collaborative discussions. *Environ Mol Mutagen.* 2019;60:100-121.

194. Windmueller HG, Ackerman CJ, Engel RW. Reaction of ethylene oxide with histidine, methionine, and cysteine. *J Biol Chem.* 1959;234:895-899.

195. Wu KY, Chiang SY, Shih WC, Huang CC, Chen MF, Swenberg JA. The application of mass spectrometry in molecular dosimetry: ethylene oxide as an example. *Mass Spectrom Rev.* 2011;30:733-756.

196. Power EGM. Aldehydes as biocides. *Prog Med Chem.* 1997;34:149-201.

197. Hoffman EA, Frey BL, Smith LM, Auble DT. Formaldehyde cross-linking: a tool for the study of chromatin complexes. *J Biol Chem.* 2015;290:26404-26411.

198. Wine Y, Cohen-Hadar N, Freeman A, Frolow F. Elucidation of the mechanism and end products of glutaraldehyde crosslinking reaction by x-ray structure analysis. *Biotechnol Bioeng.* 2007;98:711-718.

199. Migneault I, Dartiguenave C, Bertrand MJ, Waldron KC. Glutaraldehyde: behavior in aqueous solution, reaction with proteins, and application to enzyme crosslinking. *Biotechniques.* 2004;37:790-802.

200. Hopwood D. The reactions of glutaraldehyde with nucleic acids. *Histochem J.* 1975;7:267-276.

201. Gorman SP, Scott EM, Russell AD. Antimicrobial activity, uses and mechanism of action of glutaraldehyde. *J Appl Bacteriol.* 1980;48:161-190.

202. Simons C, Walsh SE, Maillard JY, Russell AD. A note: ortho-phthalaldehyde: proposed mechanism of action of a new antimicrobial agent. *Lett Appl Microbiol.* 2000;31:299-302.

203. Fraud S, Hann AC, Maillard JY, Russell AD. Effects of ortho-phthalaldehyde, glutaraldehyde and chlorhexidine diacetate on *Mycobacterium chelonae* and *Mycobacterium abscessus* strains with modified permeability. *J Antimicrob Chemother.* 2003;51:575-584.

204. Bernoulli C, Siegfried J, Baumgartner G, et al. Danger of accidental person-to-person transmission of Creutzfeldt-Jakob disease by surgery. *Lancet.* 1977;1(8009):478-479.

205. Eterpi M, McDonnell G, Thomas V. Disinfection efficacy against parvoviruses compared with reference viruses. *J Hosp Infect.* 2009;73:64-70.

206. Springthorpe S, Sattar SA. Chemical disinfection of virus-contaminated surfaces. *Crit Rev Environ Cont.* 1990;20:169-229.

207. Saleh S, Haddadin RN, Baillie S, Collier PJ. Triclosan—an update. *Lett Appl Microbiol.* 2011;52:87-95.

208. Weatherly LM, Gosse JA. Triclosan exposure, transformation, and human health effects. *J Toxicol Environ Health B Crit Rev.* 2017;20:447-469.

209. Dhillon GS, Kaur S, Pulicharla R, et al. Triclosan: current status, occurrence, environmental risks and bioaccumulation potential. *Int J Environ Res Public Health.* 2015;12:5657-5684.

210. Stickler DJ, King BJ. Bacterial sensitivity and resistance. A. Intrinsic resistance. In: Russell AD, Hugo WB, Ayliffe GAJ, eds. *Principles and Practice of Disinfection, Preservation and Sterilization.* 3rd ed. Oxford, United Kingdom: Blackwell Scientific Publications; 1999:284-296.

211. Russell AD, Chopra I. *Understanding Antibacterial Action and Resistance.* 2nd ed. Chichester, United Kingdom: Ellis Horwood; 1996.

212. Kraniak JM, Shelef LA. Effect of ethylenediaminetetraacetic acid (EDTA) and metal ions on growth of *Staphylococcus aureus* 196E in culture media. *J Food Sci.* 1988;53:910-913.

213. Russell AD, Furr JR. The antibacterial activity of a new chloroxylenol preparation containing ethylenediamine tetraacetic acid. *J Appl Bacteriol.* 1977;43:253-260.

214. Ayres HM, Payne DN, Furr JR, Russell AD. Use of the Malthus-AT system to assess the efficacy of permeabilizing agents on the activity of antibacterial agents against *Pseudomonas aeruginosa. Lett Appl Microbiol.* 1998;26:422-426.

215. Longworth AR. Chlorhexidine. In: Hugo WB, ed. *Inhibition and Destruction of the Microbial Cell.* London, United Kingdom: Academic Press; 1971:95-106.

216. Barrett-Bee K, Newboult L, Edwards S. The membrane destabilising action of the antibacterial agent chlorhexidine. *FEMS Microbiol Lett.* 1994;119:249-254.

217. Hübner NO, Kramer A. Review on the efficacy, safety and clinical applications of polihexanide, a modern wound antiseptic. *Skin Pharmacol Physiol.* 2010;23(suppl):17-27.

218. Albert A. Fourth Smissman Award Address. The long search for valid structure-action relationships in drugs. *J Med Chem.* 1982;25:1-5.

219. Foster JHS, Russell AD. Antibacterial dyes and nitrofurans. In: Hugo WB, ed. *Inhibition and Destruction of the Microbial Cell.* London, United Kingdom: Academic Press; 1971:185-208.

220. Sharma A, Gilbert JA. Microbial exposure and human health. *Curr Opin Microbiol.* 2018;44:79-87.

CHAPTER 6

The Impact of Formulary Components on Antimicrobial Products

Peter A. Burke and José A. Ramirez

Many applications of antimicrobials use the antimicrobial agent or precursor in its pure form (eg, ethylene oxide sterilization, chlorination of potable water) or incorporated into a suitable solvent or matrix at the point of use (eg, most preservatives and antimicrobials used in the impregnation of manufactured materials). However, most products used for topical applications or for the disinfection of environmental surfaces (which includes the US Environmental Protection Agency [EPA]-defined categories of sanitizer, disinfectant, and sterilant) are complex chemical mixtures designed to meet multiple product performance specifications demanded by the user. These include, besides the required biocidal efficacy levels, properties such as product toxicity (oral, ocular, dermal, inhalation, etc), cleaning efficacy, ease of use, cost in use, desired aesthetic characteristics (eg, foaming, scent, visual appearance), shelf life, etc. Many times, it is the nature of the chemical matrix into which an active antimicrobial is formulated—the formulation—that provides a manufacturer with certain competitive advantages over other participants in the marketplace.

In this chapter, references are made to a number of chemically functional materials that comprise a formulated antimicrobial product. The terms presented in Table 6.1 are used extensively in the following pages to describe such materials and are defined therein for clarity of discussion.

This chapter focuses on the formulation of antimicrobial actives into finished products. As alluded to earlier discussion, attention is drawn toward topical or environmental disinfection applications, with treatment limited to the more relevant antimicrobial actives for those applications as examples of the importance of formulation. Preservative application and formulation vary in complexity and are highly dependent on the desired product features and performance specifications. Preservation system selection and formulation have to not only meet the desired preservation specifications, but also not alter or negatively affect other important product properties such as appearance, color, odor, rheology, and other relevant mechanical, physical, chemical, or electrical properties inherent to the commercialized product or material. For an extended treatment on preservation systems, the reader is referred to the relevant chapters in this book.

▶ SYNERGISM, ANTAGONISM, AND ADDITIVE EFFECTS

Fundamental concepts in formulation science are those of synergism, antagonism, and additivity. Multiple references exist defining these, including in the specific context of antimicrobial and pharmaceutical formulations.[2-4] Limiting ourselves to the practical descriptions of the term as used in this context, a mixture is said to exhibit additive effects when its overall performance can be expressed as a linear combination of the individual effects of the components. In other words, the overall effect can be predicted by simple addition of the individual component effects (ie, additivity). On the other hand, a mixture is said to exhibit synergy when the observed effect is greater than the additive effect. Mathematically speaking, higher order (nonlinear) positive interactions between components contribute to an additional effect beyond the linear, additive one. In contrast, antagonism pertains to diminished overall effect from the mixture as compared to the individual components. This could be due to negative linear interactions between species, negative nonlinear (higher order) effects between components, or both. It is noted that these concepts apply not only to the combination of antimicrobial species but also to the combination of antimicrobial species with "inert" components. It is also important to note that the "effect" on which synergism, antagonism, or additivity is measured can not only be antimicrobial activity (eg, log reduction of viable organisms) but also irritation profile, shelf life/stability, odor, or any other relevant product feature.

TABLE 6.1 Definition of key formulation terms employed in this chapter[a]

Ingredient	Functionality	Examples
Biocide, antimicrobial	Destruction or prevention of microbial subsistence and/or reproduction	QACs, aldehydes, phenolics, alcohol, peroxygens, halogens, etc
Solvent	Organic molecules, for the most part polar in nature and mostly containing at least an oxygen atom; employed for dissolving hydrophobic substances in water; also used in some cases to improve detergency, streaking, or improve drying rates	Short-chain alcohols (eg, ethanol, isopropanol), alkylene glycols, glycol ethers
Surfactants/emulsifiers	Surface active agents typically comprising a hydrophobe-lipophobe pair structure; used to impart detergency, lower surface tension, emulsify insoluble species, impart or reduce foaming	Sodium lauryl sulfate, linear alkylbenzene sulfonates, ethoxylated alcohols, betaines
Thickeners	A substance used to increase the viscosity of a formulation	Polyethylene glycols, polysaccharides (eg, pectin, gums, alginates)
Chelating or sequestering agents	Compounds that bind dissolved metals (such as calcium, magnesium, iron, copper, etc); used for reducing ill effects of hardness in water on biocide and detergency action and reducing transition metal-aided decomposition of peroxygens and halogens	Ethylenediamine, EDTA, EGTA, MGDA, GLDA, HEDP
Alkali or acid	pH stabilization to desired specification for optimal performance	Alkalis (NaOH, KOH, silicates); acids (organic acids, H_2SO_4, H_3PO_4, HCl, etc)
Buffer	Maintaining pH over time and increasing alkalinity	Disodium phosphate
Corrosion inhibitor	Reducing the corrosion rates and protecting metal surfaces	Nitrates, phosphates, molybdates, triazoles

Abbreviations: EDTA, ethylenediaminetetraacetic acid; EGTA, ethylene glycol-bis(2-aminoethylether)-N,N,N′,N′-tetraacetic acid; GLDA, glutamate diacetate; H_2SO_4, sulfuric acid; H_3PO_4, phosphoric acid; HCl, hydrochloric acid; HEDP, 1-hydroxyethane 1,1-diphosphonic acid; KOH, potassium hydroxide; MGDA, N-(1-carboxylatoethyl)iminodiacetate, methylglycinediacetic acid; NaOH, sodium hydroxide; QACs, quaternary ammonium compounds.

[a]Adapted from McDonnell.[1]

With this in mind, some of the more relevant approaches to formulation with the key antimicrobial material types are discussed further in this chapter. Because it would be impossible to delve into the almost boundless field of formulation science in antimicrobial products, the material presented here is considered a starting point for formulators—the critical, need-to-know, basic principles that enable the reader to plan a formulation approach, devise a registration strategy, or gain a better understanding of the makeup of an existing product.

▶ HALOGENS

Various halogen compounds have been widely used for over a century and a half. The main classes of chemistries are chlorine, bromine, and iodine compounds that are very effective antimicrobials at low concentrations. For instance, iodophors have been used in household settings for the disinfection (or sanitization) of the toilet bowl water at concentrations in the part per billions to react biocidally with gram-negative bacteria in potable water like *Escherichia coli*.[5]

Chlorine is not normally distributed in nature but is found in a salt form as either sodium, potassium, calcium or magnesium. Iodine was first used in medical treatment of wounds as Lugol solution (USP XXIII) or tincture of iodine.[6] Bromine has been used in a solid released form from hydantoin compounds like 1-bromo-3-chloro-5,5 dimethylhydantoin forming active bromine and chlorine active species. These hydantoin compounds have been effectively used for years in swimming pool sanitization.[7]

Different approaches have been employed depending on the active selected (chlorine, bromine, or iodine) to formulate an effective industrial antimicrobial product with specific commercial end points as the product's goal. These approaches include the following methods:

- Direct liquid or gas injection
- Slow dissolving granular or tablet mixtures forms
- Two parts in situ formation of the active to maximize active stability
- Tincture of iodine solution for skin and wound treatment

The formulation is always specific to the intended use of the antimicrobial product. Uses are broad in this category because halogens are used for very diverse applications such as drinking water disinfection, sterilization, and wound treatment as well as medical devices, to list just a few examples. Thus, the formulation type coupled with packaging or method of application strategy is rigorously considered at project initiation depending on the market need and industry regulations to be served. The pharmaceutical and medical device applications have much stricter guidelines and antimicrobial requirements. This fact drives different consideration from a concentration perspective as well as toxicity (including ecotoxicity) profile relating to excipient ingredients. This section focuses on formulating halogen-based products for general and some specific applications.

Working with halogen compounds can be very challenging because they are naturally very reactive from a pure chemical perspective and many times are toxic in pure chemical form. Chlorine is a green gas that can react quickly with organic materials in an exothermic reaction that is hard to control. Additionally, this reactive nature makes these agents effective at low concentrations but leads to shorter stability profiles once the active ingredient is dosed into the area for disinfection. The finished formulated product must carefully define the best method of application to the point of antimicrobial action. Many chlorine, bromine, and iodine products are relatively unstable once placed in water or the environment requiring treatment. For instance, hypochlorous acid, a major active entity in many chlorination products used to disinfect swimming pool water, has a very rapid degradation profile once in the water, which is influenced by pH, salts, organic materials, and divalent cations. If the pH of the solution is maintained at 2 to 3, it provides a greater release of hypochlorous acid and longer period of activity. However, this pH is not appropriate for pool chlorination due to the irritancy potential to eye and skin to the humans using this water for exercise. Thus, the pH must be balanced against other important product requirements rather than just antimicrobial efficacy. The impact of pH effect on hypochlorous acid is depicted in Figure 6.1. Therefore, the specific concentration of the active needs to be adjusted to permit application at a suitable pH to achieve the goal. Nevertheless, because less than 1 ppm of hypochlorous acid is typically sufficient for disinfection of the water, there is a lot of potential formulation range to optimize the product to achieve the end point requirements.

To maximize the performance, many factors other than just pH need to be factored in the final formulation or delivery system. Antimicrobial efficacy needs to consider the calcium and magnesium concentrations found as hard water salts in water to prevent any effect of these divalent cations causing active reduction or neutralization. These factors, coupled with the concentrations of organic compounds in the water source, need to be accounted for to minimize the negatively catalyzing agents to hypochlorous acid.

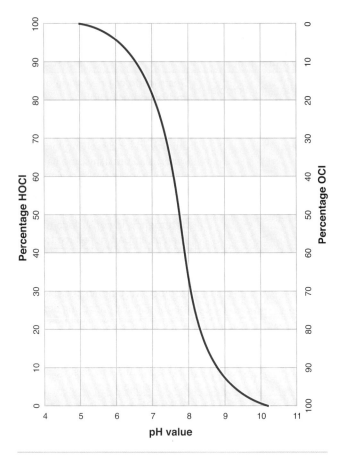

FIGURE 6.1   Relationship between hypochlorous acid (HOCl) and hypochlorite ion (OCl) concentration as a function of pH. Adapted from Baker.[8] Copyright © 1959 American Water Works Association. Reprinted by permission of John Wiley & Sons, Inc.

Bromine compounds and iodine in the form of iodophors (iodine-releasing polymers; see following discussion) all have stability challenges centering around the active nature of the antimicrobial agent in the environment resulting in shorter half-lives of the active in solution. Of course, iodine solutions or iodine-releasing compounds have a classic brownish color that needs to be dealt with from an end product perspective because it will discolor clothing, skin, etc, that contact these compounds.

In the case of solid or crystalline compounds releasing halogens, the products are formulated to maximize storage shelf life by mixing the powders under low humidity conditions and using binding agents that have limited chemical interactions with the hydantoin compounds. For example, ethylene oxide-propylene oxide (EO-PO) block copolymers permit very slow release of active ingredients into the application site.[5] Most of these products are in tablet form, being made using a Mainstay 10- to 20-ton tablet press after appropriate granularization by a Fitz Mill or equivalent to achieve the desired particle size and density. Iodophor liquid active agents have been incorporated using similar method of manufacture with some additional steps to reduce humidity.

Some halogen forms have superior stability, especially those that are in granular or powder form such as 1-bromo-3-chloro-5,5-dimethylhydantoin or calcium isocyanuric acid, which are presented in tablet form. These solid forms of chlorine-releasing compounds have excellent shelf life until at the point of use. The ability to present these products as solids permits a long-term stability profile. These types of products have been used in swimming pool sanitizers, toilet bowl sanitizers, medical device disinfectants, and general disinfecting agents for various water sources and are commercially sold in granular or tablet form. For instance, hydantoin tablets are commonly used for hot tub sanitization on a weekly basis due to the slow release technology.

Generally, for chlorine and bromine solution products, the first and most important stabilizing consideration is maintaining liquid formulations at higher pH. The maintenance of higher pH will reduce the rate of decomposition and loss of active agent. The formulation manufacturing needs to have high-quality water with rigid control of ionic contaminants. The presence of transition metals (such as iron, cobalt, and copper) and hardness factors (calcium, magnesium) will increase the rate of degradation of active.[9] Thus, chelating agents such as ethylenediaminetetraacetic acid (EDTA) or phosphonates incorporated as an additive in the formula will enhance the stability of the active agent as a function of time. For instance, hypochlorous acid will want to chemically react to form chloramines, chlorides, or chlorates. These compounds typically have lesser or no antimicrobial properties (see chapter 15).

Iodine is a very toxic compound if ingested or absorbed percutaneously, so it is formulated specifically to minimize these negative factors while maintaining its excellent antimicrobial activity. Iodophors are formed to achieve this goal, such as in the use of povidone-iodine complexes. The iodine is reacted by incorporation into a carrier molecule such as polyvinylpyrrolidone (PVP), which has very low toxicity profile. The PVP had been used in the past as a potential blood substitute, having neglectable toxicity.[10] This combination has been used for many years in wound healing formulations designed to either reduce or prevent infection by various skin microorganisms on abraded skin or burns. Povidone-iodine complexes have been used in the healing of burned skin for decades without any significant negative impact on the patient or users (see chapter 16).

There are a number of compounds with potential to contribute to the inherent properties of halogens, increasing antimicrobial efficacy while minimizing their negative oxidative properties. As mentioned earlier, pH, by itself, is a synergistic agent to halogens. Thus, the mere control of pH can dramatically improve antimicrobial activity under constant conditions. Agents that control the pH provide the active agent a more active efficacy per unit and greater stability profile presenting greater microbial reaction. This profile is seen most easily under difficult microbial conditions such as in the presence of bacterial endospores, which are intrinsically more resistant naturally to halogens than vegetative microorganisms. Various surfactants or other surface-active agents act as synergists with halogens as well. Anionic surfactants are most effective due to their low pH tolerance. Thus, alkylbenzene sulfonates, alkyl sulfates, and alkyl phosphonates are good formulary compounds that provide positive benefits to halogens in solution. Some nonionic surfactants can be used but are much more difficult to formulate with many side interactions that negatively impact the halogen antimicrobial effectiveness. Nevertheless, their ability to increase wettability and reduce the interfacial surface tension of solutions to be able to suspend soil particles at low concentrations impart important benefits for removal of soiled surface particles permitting greater antimicrobial activity because of the combination with cleaning activity.

Finally, cationic and amphoteric surfactants have also been used in formulated products; however, the superior effects observed with anionic surfactants makes the use of these alternative agents less likely in practice. Hence, most standard nonspecific application formulas usually contain an anionic or nonionic surfactant as a preferred cleaning agent.

Other common compounds found in halogen-containing formulations begin with high-quality water without ionic characteristics (ie, deionized water). Second, solvents are used as cosolvents as well for cleansing and solubility factors. Thus, other than water, common solvents include short-chain alcohols such as methanol, ethanol, and isopropanol. Other solvents used are glycol ethers for solubility and freezing point depression and benzyl alcohol to provide wettability and detergency properties. Examples of general formulations such as an iodine-based, toilet bowl-sanitizing tablet and a chlorine-releasing, extruded lavatory sanitizing block are provided in Table 6.2.

ALCOHOLS

Alcohols have been used for many years as antimicrobial agents and are perhaps the oldest biocidal active still in use. They are known to have been used as early as 131-201 AD as a wound treatment and cleaning aid. In the late 1870s, Koch studied these agents and suggested they were ineffective, at least with relevance to *Bacillus anthracis* spores. This finding, although correct, did not reflect the agent's action on vegetative cells on which it has been proven to be very efficacious. By 1888, Furbringer[12] was recommending alcohol as a hand disinfectant for surgeons, which has remained a potential use even today.

TABLE 6.2   Examples of halogen formulations

Ingredient	Concentration (%)
US 4,911,859[5]	
Calcium sulfate dihydrate	59.8
Calcium sulfate anhydrous	10.0
Fumed silica	4.0
Iodophor (Biopal NR-20)	8.5
Polyvinylpyrrolidone-iodine complex (povidone)	5.7
Dye (acid blue #9)	5.0
Polyethylene oxide polymer (Polyox 60K)	2.0
Polyethylene glycol (PEG 4500)	5.0
	100.0
US 5,449,473[11]	
Sodium dodecylbenzene sulfonate	52.0
Chloramine T	31.5
Neodol 91 (alcohol ethoxylate)	8.0
Polybutene	4.0
Perfume	0.5
Volatile silicone oil	4.0
	100.0

As a group, alcohols have played an active role over the years as either a disinfectant or an antiseptic. The broad-spectrum antimicrobial activity against both gram-positive and gram-negative bacteria, fungi, and viruses made the common alcohols of ethanol and isopropanol widely used agents for many years. The mode of action is thought to be a combination of protein degradation and cell membrane disruption (see chapter 19). Nevertheless, unlike antibiotics but like most chemical disinfectants, alcohols are considered nonspecific antimicrobials from a pure mechanistic perspective. Because they have been in use for many years in hospitals settings, it can be speculated if the microbial flora is becoming resistant to these agents and require reformulation with either other antimicrobial agents or compounds to prevent this effect. Studies to date do not show any marked resistance to alcohols especially at the use concentrations used for either disinfectants or antiseptics. Both Willie and Wigert[13] showed minimal resistance profiles and, more importantly, reversal of any developed resistance with termination of alcohol exposure.

Alcohols are typically used in concentrations of 70% to 80% to be effective, which can often limit their use for surface disinfection in comparison to other available antimicrobials. There are many factors such as toxicity, ecology, and general cleansing properties that often favor other formulations. The use of alcohols for submersion of a limited number of medical devices is still performed but is limited in scope. By submerging the device for 10 minutes in 70% to 80% alcohol, disinfection can be achieved. However, the use of alcohols for general environmental surface disinfection is often limited because these formulations are poor cleaners and evaporate rapidly, preventing sufficient contact time for biocidal activity. However, it should be noted that simple aqueous dilutions of alcohol are still used with great effectiveness against vegetative bacteria.

The high concentration requirement (more than 70% ethanol or isopropanol) is a potential cost disadvantage and leaves little room for synergistic compound incorporation or for improvement in the cleansing properties in surface disinfectant products. Simple alcohols diluted in water are widely used as a surface disinfectant without necessary formulation to gain effectiveness for this application and because they are not registered disinfectants no further improvement will occur. Despite this, examples can include combinations of alcohols and formulations with oxidizing agents (such as hydrogen peroxide or peracetic acid) (see chapter 19). In contrast, the majority of alcohol and alcohol formulations have been used significantly in wound healing, skin degerming, and antiseptic waterless hand washes. Alcohols have been very widely used in skin treatments for medical procedures. Therefore, the majority of this review focuses on the formulation of skin care products using alcohols as an antiseptic.

Skin has a normal microbial flora natural for each individual depending on the area of anatomical skin, which can harbor both transient and pathogenic organisms that can infect disrupted (abraded) skin (see chapters 42 and 43). Alcohol application to the skin limits these organisms from colonizing the skin by reducing the entire microbial population, part of which may include very low numbers of pathogenic organisms such as methicillin-resistant *Staphylococcus aureus*. The alcohol formulation itself has an optimal concentration of 95% for maximum effectiveness.[14] However, to balance cost, safety risks, and ultimate antimicrobial effectiveness, a 70% concentration has been found to be very efficacious with excellent results for many years in hospitals and other health care facilities.

The use of alcohols in hospitals as prophylactics against cross-contamination and infection has prompted the use of waterless agents every time a health care professional or visitor enters the patient area or tends to the patient. These measures have been effective in helping to prevent the spread of health care–acquired infections from one patient to another via the health care worker. Thus, the alcohol disinfection or washing of hands assists in the potential hand-to-hand contact resulting in limited but potentially dangerous cross-contamination of hospital pathogens among patients.[15]

To achieve effective formulations for this application, the alcohols have been incorporated into gels and foam products. A variety of polymers are used to achieve this gelling effect such as Carbopol®.[16] The use of this polymer permits the user to dispense and rub together their hands without alcohol loss from running off the skin surface to the floor presenting a hazard. This is important because the hands need to be vigorously rubbed together to entirely cover the skin surface of the hand. This treatment can result in improved antimicrobial efficacy, some claiming to be in excess of a 5 log reduction of bacteria under certain test conditions.[17]

In the United States, the US Food and Drug Administration (FDA) regulates these products from a regulatory perspective relative to toxicity and efficacy. These antiseptics were initially regulated under the tentative final monograph of 1976. However, this monograph has been under careful review by FDA to examine the toxicity requirement of these products for future use and registration with FDA for use in the United States. This review will take an extended period of time between government requirement and generation of industry-based data to depict the toxicity profile in modern toxicology methods. The criteria for acceptance of these products is thus still under flux regarding toxicity at the time of writing. These regulatory decisions will potentially have a significant impact relative to formulary practice.

One of the main concerns from health care professionals using these products multiple times per day is the irritancy and sensitization potential of the products. Hence, formulators have focused on this point to ensure the emollient nature of the product provide a less irritating formulation while not reducing the efficacy profile. Various humectant components have been incorporated into formulae to achieve a gentler product for multiple use applications. A basic moisturizing agent is a glycerin-like compound that provides this property to the alcohol-based formulation. The most simplistic formulary action can be the mere reduction in alcohol content from 60% to 70%, which reduces cost with minimal-if any-effect on antimicrobial efficacy. This formulary consideration affects efficacy by reduction of evaporation, providing while greater contact time of active. The added water provides very basic moisturizing benefits. Of course, there are many complex chemistries that can be used for these moisturizing purposes depending on the formula properties.

Finally, the regulations often require these antiseptics to have reduced microbial skin population (eg, after 10 successive hand washes), which retard microbial repopulation. Alcohols by themselves are not substantive in nature to skin, and hence, other formulary constitutions are often added to achieve this goal. This typically includes the addition of a low concentration of another biocide, such as chlorhexidine gluconate (CHG) or triclosan (Figure 6.2). The bisphenol triclosan is one of many ingredients that has shown to be substantive to skin at low concentration making this compound useful for this purpose. This compound has been found to be

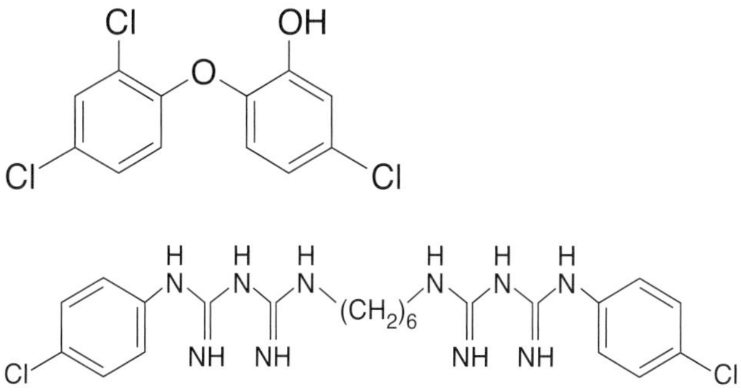

FIGURE 6.2 Example of biocides (top, triclosan, and bottom, chlorhexidine) used in combination with alcohols to provide substantivity to skin.

effective for this use due to not only its substantive properties but also its traditionally considered low toxicity and rare sensitization potential. These properties have led to the incorporation of this compound like others in medicated soap, hand antiseptic products, antiperspirants, deodorants, and dentifrices. The CHG is being used widely today in comparison to other compounds for residual effect due to both antimicrobial efficacy with excellent toxicity and environmental profile. However, recent evidence would suggest concerns on the safety of triclosan, particularly in nonessential applications such as routine handwashing in the general public.[18] These include human toxicity impacts, environmental bioaccumulation and persistence potential, effects on natural microbiomes, and development of bacterial tolerance mechanisms as well as cross-resistance to antibiotics.[19] In certain situations, this has led to banning the use of triclosan and indeed other similar antimicrobials in certain applications (such as antimicrobial soap–based products by the FDA).[17] For further reviews of this subject, see McDonnell.[1]

In conclusion, alcohol-containing waterless hand gels have been shown effective in reducing the potential for cross-contamination leading to hospital-acquired infections. Until safer and more effective agents are developed, alcohol-containing formulations will be used in hand washes to protect patients from cross-contamination in the hospital setting. The formulation of alcohol-containing antiseptics can be modified to improve efficacy, as well as to address any toxicity concerns to patients and health care workers, or ecology concerns to provide the desired efficacy but limiting environmental impact.

▶ PHENOLICS

Phenolics, in particular coal tar compounds, have been used as early as 1815 for antimicrobial purposes. The first medical application of phenol itself as an antimicrobial was by Lister[20] in 1867 as a wound dressing treatment and

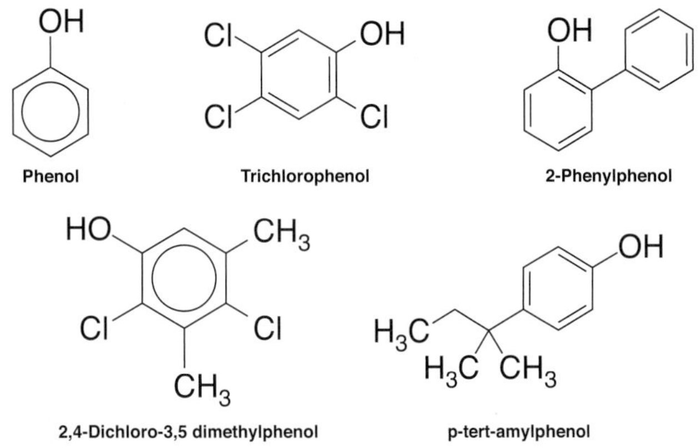

FIGURE 6.3 Examples of antimicrobial phenolic compounds.

surgical antiseptic solution. Most phenolic compounds today are synthetically derived as pure actives substances (see chapter 20). Alkylated phenol homologs are very effective agents, and generally, as the number of methylene groups increases in substitution, the antimicrobial potency increases likewise. A few phenolic compounds are presented in Figure 6.3 to demonstrate the variation in molecular structure.

Phenolic disinfectants compounds have been used since the early 19th century, and today, at least 10 million pounds of active are used in various biocidal applications.[21] The most common phenolic derivatives used in health care applications are ortho-phenylphenol (OPP) (2-phenylphenol); ortho-benzyl, para-chlorophenol (OBPCP); and 4-tert-amylphenol.

Several approaches are possible to formulate industrial or hospital-grade disinfectant products containing a phenolic compound or blended compounds as the active agents. The formulations are based on the use of the active against the organisms required to be eradicated by the location such as a hospital versus the use in industrial settings (such as in food or general housekeeping). Hence, many factors need to be considered when formulating the component parts with varying interaction with the phenolic compounds to either enhance or synergize activity. Phenolics are generally more effective in acidic solutions. Hence, the inclusion of soaps and emulsifiers is required to make the phenols more soluble while maintaining a balance of pH necessary for optimal efficacy. As the pH increases in solution, the phenol is converted to sodium or potassium phenate that is less active. Therefore, using the correct combination of soap and phenolic compound at a given pH can increase the antimicrobial potential. The phenates themselves can act as a solubilizing agent for the phenol. Fully formulated phenolic disinfectants take into consideration the use of cosolvents, pH adjustment, surface active agents, and chelation agents, which will maximize the efficacy potential when used in unison.

Most phenolic disinfectants concentrates are formulated for dilution to 400 to 1400 ppm at use. These formulations are used as broad-spectrum disinfectants that possess vegetative, viricidal, and tuberculocidal activity but are not sporicidal generally. Phenolic dispersions have been made in natural soaps, but this is not recommended due to the effect of hard water salts that readily precipitate calcium and magnesium soaps when diluted. Most modern synthetic soaps can be easily diluted in 400 ppm of hard water without any clarity issues while maintaining its antimicrobial activity. Surfactants are used to solubilize the active ingredient while providing cleansing properties as well as solvating the soils present in the environment for formula effectiveness.

Of the various classes of surfactant ingredients, only the anionic class is generally used in the formulation of phenolic disinfectant products. Wallhausser[22] has reported that alkane sulfonates as solubilizing agents are very effective solvents with phenolic compounds. Nonionic surfactants can inactivate the antimicrobial properties of phenolics. The use of cationic surfactants (such as quaternary ammonium compounds [QACs]) has been reported as being used in some specific applications but are generally considered incompatible with phenolic disinfectants. Synergy has been reported with certain quaternary compounds.[23] The theory is that the QAC reduces the surface tension to such a degree that solution falls below the critical micelle concentration permitting more phenol to interact at the cell membrane. Anionics are the mainstay for surfactants used for cleansing, wettability, and solubilization of phenolic compounds with agents such as dodecylbenzene sulfonates commonly used. This type of compound provides good solvent action while not affecting the antimicrobial potency of the phenolic compound when diluted to the use dilution during application.

Furthermore, other cosolvents are used to formulate the final phenolic disinfectant product such as alcohols, glycol ethers, and propylene glycol. These cosolvents permit greater incorporation of the agent at various pH's while maintaining the antimicrobial potency with limited decline of active. Hence, the use of various agents to aid in the incorporation of phenolics is critical for formulation maximization. The selection of detergents, builders, cosolvents, and appropriate chelating agents will greatly improve the formula.

Stability of phenolic disinfectants is generally good provided no interaction with incompatible ingredients incorporated in error. It is important to have a long-term stability profile of the phenolic agent as a function of time with a minimum of 1 year with a goal of 2 years of acceptable shelf life. Thus, negative interacting compounds such as nonionic surfactants should be carefully screened with the specific phenolic compound via assays to maintain long-term disinfectant stability (shelf life). Examples of a few phenolic formulation used commercially are shown in Table 6.3.

TABLE 6.3 Examples of formulated commercialized phenolic formulations[a]

Ingredient	F1	F2	F3	F4	F5	F6	F7	F8	F9	F10	F11
OPP	15	18	18	15	15	15	7.5	14	14	14	5
4-Chloro, cyclopentylphenol	6	7	—	5.9	6	—	2.9	—	—	—	—
4-Chloro, 2-benzylphenol	—	—	7	—	—	6.3	—	7.5	8.5	—	—
4-Tert-amylphenol				2.5		2.5	1.25	2.0	2.0		0.8
2,4-Dichloro, 3,5-dimethylphenol	—									12	4.7
Alkyldiphenyloxide disulfonate (45%)	7	8.5	8.5	4.5	6.5	4.5	4.5	8.1	6.8	6.8	4.5
Sodium lauryl sulfate	3				3.5	4.0	1.0		2.1	—	—
Dodecylbenzene sulfonate	—	1.5	1.5	2.0						2.0	
NTA	—									1.0	
EDTA	3.3	3.3	3.3	3.3	2.5	0.8	0.4	1.0	1.0		1.0
Sodium hydroxide	3.0	3.5	3.7	3.6	3.3	3.2	1.4	3.0	2.6	2.8	1.4
Isopropanol	10	10	10	5		10	10	10			5
Hexylene glycol	—						5.0		10		
Sodium sulfite	—	0.5	0.5	0.5	0.5	0.5	0.25	0.6	0.6	0.5	0.5
Sodium xylene sulfonate										4	
Perfume	—	0.3	0.4	0.3	0.3	0.3	0.2			0.2	
Dye	—	.002	.002	.001	.001	.001	.001			.001	

Abbreviations: EDTA, ethylenediaminetetraacetic acid; F, formula; NTA, nitrilotriacetic acid; OPP, ortho-phenylphenol.

[a]Data from Winicov and Schmidt.[24]

The use of phenolic disinfectants has come under greater regulatory security especially in Europe due to environmental impact and aquatic effects. It has been shown that certain phenolic agents exhibit higher toxicity and lower biodegrading in the environment.[25] The biodegradation of the compound is important and must be considered because the governmental regulatory agencies have critical standards for disinfectant formulations to achieve or exceed. This will play a greater role in the future years to come, particularly in Europe.

In conclusion, phenolic disinfectants are among the oldest synthetic chemical compounds used today as antimicrobial agents. Thus, they are an important class of compounds for use as disinfectants, antiseptics, and preservatives. Certain phenolics and other formulation excipients will come under greater regulatory pressure due to their oral and percutaneous toxicity as well as their environmental profiles. Nevertheless, these compounds will be effectively used in industrial, domestic, and medical applications for many years to come until more effective agents with superior toxicity and biodegradation profiles are developed.

▶ QUATERNARY AMMONIUM COMPOUNDS

The QACs are surface-active agents and have surfactant molecule structure in their most basic function. Surfactants all have a hydrophobic and hydrophilic sections of the molecule that provides their ability to disperse oil/soils in water. The basic structure of a QAC is shown in Figure 6.4.[26] This balance of solubility as well as the charge of the molecule are critical to function.

The QACs are cationic charged molecules unlike other surfactants that are anionic, nonionic, or amphoteric. A fundamental property of surface-active agents is

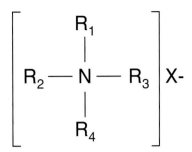

FIGURE 6.4 General structure of a quaternary ammonium compound.

the formation of micelles, which reduces the free energy of the system by decreasing the hydrophobic surface area exposed to the water. Micelles are the reservoir for surfactant molecules. The ability to reduce the interfacial surface tension and increase wettability is dependent on the critical micelle concentration, which is an important and distinct property unique to each surfactant molecule individually. Most surfactants are used as cosolvents, cleansers, wettability agents; however, the QACs are particularly used as antimicrobial agents (see chapter 21).

From Figure 6.4, it is seen that a QAC consists of a central nitrogen with four attached groups that vary in structure and size that creates different functional properties as well as antimicrobial profiles. The anion is usually either a chlorine or bromine element linked to the nitrogen to form the quaternary ammonium salt. Various R groups can be substituted dependent on requirements of the antimicrobial agent including the number of nitrogens, degree of saturation, linear or branched chains, and the use of aromatic groups. There are many structural molecules formed by different R group substitution. Examples include monoalkyl trimethyl ammonium salts, dialkyldimethylammonium salts, heteroaromatic ammonium salts, and polysubstituted quaternary ammonium salts. The QACs are further considered here as a general class of agents to provide an overview of basic formulary approaches dictated by antimicrobial requirements for industrial and health care use.

The antimicrobial activity of QACs varies depending on the selection of chemical agents and whether multiple compounds are formulated together to achieve a broader, more active formulation against a select microbial population. For instance, a hospital disinfectant may have different actives than a household disinfectant or sanitizer due to the flora required to be eradicated. Furthermore, due to the substantive nature of QACs, this can be an advantage in food preparation applications due to low toxicity, but this same property in certain pharmaceutical applications can be a concern due to requirements for residue-free surfaces.

Generally speaking, the sanitizing-disinfectant range of the QACs at use dilution is typically between 200 and 1200 ppm. The formulation is usually odorless, colorless, noncorrosive, and stable in formulation as well as at the use dilution. The QACs have good pH stability with a wide range of acceptable action, generally between pH 3 and 10.5. Other properties are good detergency, wettability, tolerance to organic materials, and low toxicity and irritancy as well as stability under increased temperatures. The QACs can be substantive to many surfaces leaving a bacteriostatic benefit following application, which can be used as a benefit in some applications, for instance, in food preparation. However, QACs do have antimicrobial limits because their effectiveness against gram-negative bacteria and certain viruses requires either greater contact times or concentration in comparison to other biocides. The QACs are not effective against spores, bacteriophages, and some viruses, in particular nonenveloped forms. They are also not effective against mycobacteria, although formulation with coactives and/or other excipients can yield mycobactericidal activity. These limitations can sometimes be resolved by formulary additives and modified inert materials.

From a formulary perspective, concerning concentrated products diluted on use, QACs are sensitive to hard water salts requiring a chelation agent such as EDTA to permit their successful use when diluted in hard water applications. The selection of nonionic surfactant is critical to maximize the QAC antimicrobial profile. Of course, anionic surfactants like alkylbenzene sulfonates will inactivate the cationic compound rapidly due to their negative charge and therefore must be avoided in formulation. Furthermore, the selection of QACs has a greater activity if the chain length of the active is C_{10} to C_{14}, with C_{10} and C_{12} demonstrating the most effective antimicrobial efficacy.[27] The ratio of nonionic to QAC has been found to be important, and this ratio should not exceed 4:1. The efficacy of 2:1 or 3:1 is considered superior due to the micellization. The cationic agents are found to be less bound in micelles and more reactive under these conditions. Finally, the moles of ethoxylation of the nonionic surfactant additive can be a negative contributor to the formulation and should be chosen at lower moles of ethoxylation while still achieving the cosolvency and solubility characteristics. Ethoxylation plays a role in solubility and micelle formation that can greatly affect the presentation of the active agent to the microorganism (P. Burke, written communication, November, 1976).

In conclusion, QACs will continue to be used because of the broad range of potential applications, residual bacteriostasis, low toxicity, and often a more favorable environmental fate profiles. In Europe, the regulatory requirements placed on all biocides but particularly phenolic compounds due to unfavorable biodegradation profile may make certain QACs viewed in a more favorable light. From a formulary perspective, QACs will be enhanced by inclusion of other charged molecules and superior new surfactants with less negative interactions.

◗ ALDEHYDES

Various aldehydes are powerful biocidal agents used in mostly the medical field with particular use for the disinfection of medical devices. The most well-known and first used with modern medical devices as either a high-level disinfectant (HLD) is glutaraldehyde (1,5-pentanedial). The molecule was first synthetized by Harries and Tank[28] in 1908. There are now three predominant aldehyde compounds widely used as disinfectant and/or sterilant formulations; namely, glutaraldehyde, ortho-phthaldehyde (OPA), and formaldehyde. The structures of these agents are given in Figure 6.5. Formaldehyde is in limited use and only used for special purposes today because of the toxicity profile by oral, dermal, or inhalation including carcinogenic potential (see chapter 36).

Aldehydic compounds predominantly react with proteins, causing cross-linking and inactivation of the enzymatic or structural functions of these molecules on or within microbiological structures. Furthermore, data shows these compounds also react with the RNA, DNA, and other macromolecules. The specific mode of action is believed to be due to alkylation with amino acids of the surface proteins. The agents are thought to react with amine and sulfhydryl groups forming intermolecular bridges that disrupt the catalytic activity of the protein.[29] Thus, cross-bridging action is confirmed by the fact that a higher concentration of biocidal action, meaning greater resistance, is required with *Mycobacterium* strains that have a waxy lipid layer external to the cell wall/membrane. The additional lipid barrier is believed to provide a greater resistance profile. Thus, for aldehyde formulations, all *Mycobacterium* species are more difficult to kill in comparison to other vegetative bacterial cells.

The rate of reaction with the protein (amino acids) is pH dependent and increases significantly over the pH ranges from 4 to 9.[30] The reaction product is a compound stable to acid hydrolysis with an absorption characteristic at 265 nm. The fact that it is acid hydrolysis–stable rules out Schiff base reaction formation.[29] It has been further reported that the aldehyde reacts with the primary amine (lysine) of the protein, and the condensation of the glutaraldehyde leads to formation of 1,3,4,5-substituted pyridinium salt analogues to the amino acid desmosine.[31]

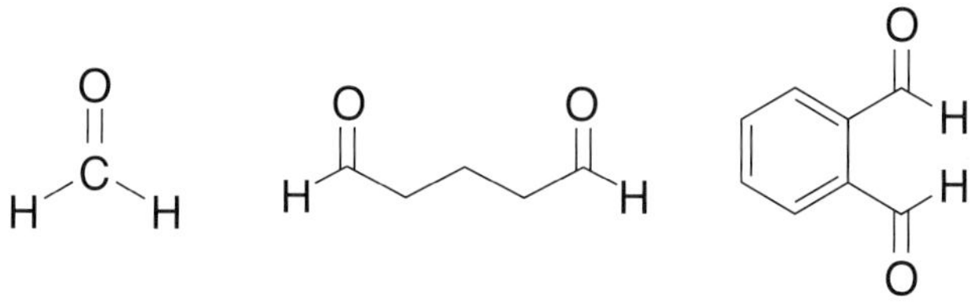

This confirms the observation of a peak absorption of light at 265 nm as proteins which are labile to alkaline hydrolysis, cross-linked. Thus, control of the pH in a tight range is critical to formulations containing aldehydes for achieving the most effective biocidal formula.

Glutaraldehyde and OPA formulations are widely used as low-temperature liquid disinfectants for medical devices as well as in limited applications for general surface disinfection. Formulations are particularly used for the high-level disinfection of semicritical devices, such as flexible endoscopes. In the United States, HLDs are regulated by the FDA after registration with the agency having met the toxicity and efficacy criteria. These criteria include demonstrated sporicidal activity. Although the products are used normally as a disinfectant, sporicidal potential must be shown even if for an extended period like overnight (8-12 h) contact. However, a typical product is used for 8 to 30 minutes at 25°C by submersion or processed within an automatic endoscope reprocessor. Formulations usually contain between 1.5% and 3.5% of glutaraldehyde under acidic conditions to maintain the shelf life stability prior to treatment of the endoscope at which point the solution is activated by being made alkaline with a pH around 8. By the use of additives, modern formulations are able to have a stable acidic stock solution that does not require activation during application. Single-component OPA formulations are available with the active ingredient incorporated at 0.55% at a pH of 7.5 for HLD treatment of heat-sensitive medical devices at 20°C. The use of an automatic endoscope reprocessor reduces the contact time greatly by controlling the temperature at 55°C, which concomitantly increases the rate of antimicrobial action. The OPA is slowly replacing glutaraldehyde because the latter has both inhalation toxicity and sensitization profiles that require health care facilities to closely monitor and control the environment. The OPA has a lower vapor pressure, which makes OPA odorless and overall less irritating to hospital staff. Another advantage of OPA is it has wider pH tolerance (3-9), has higher efficacy against mycobacteria, and does not autopolymerize under alkaline conditions. Both aldehydes have an advantage over other HLD products commercially because aldehydes are noncorrosive to medical devices, which is a potential negative factor for certain oxidizing agent products (eg, hydrogen peroxide and peracetic acid) sold as HLD treatment for endoscopes. However, the aldehyde products, both glutaraldehyde and OPA, can stain any hospital clothing, hard surfaces, and, in some cases, skin, all deemed undesirable.

The basic formulation for either glutaraldehyde or OPA contains buffering agents, corrosion inhibitors, chelating agents, and, sometimes, dye. The OPA formulations, for example, use these ingredients to balance the formulation from an ionic perspective and buffer the critical pH for maximum antimicrobial efficacy. Most formulas contain both dipotassium monophosphate and

FIGURE 6.5 Structures of the most common aldehyde compounds.

potassium dihydrophosphate to act as buffering agents for salts, which also aids in pH balance. Normally, a corrosion inhibitor is incorporated to protect the device from a long-term corrosion potential from the product. Benzotriazole is the most routinely used corrosion inhibitor for this purpose. Lastly, to prevent any hard water salt effect that can diminish antimicrobial efficacy or causes a precipitate, a chelation agent such as hydroxyethyl-ethylenediaminetriacetic acid is used in the formulation to prevent this potential interaction. The key factors are the control of pH in the use dilution while minimizing any precipitation effects that might reduce antimicrobial efficacy.

Surface active agents such as cationic compounds and nonionic surfactants like linear alcohol ethoxylates as well as anionic surfactants (eg, alkylbenzene sulfonates) have been incorporated to potentiate the antimicrobial efficacy. However, no significant benefit has been reported to be worthy of the expense and formulary considerations for medical device application from a commercial perspective. For hard surface applications, a much smaller commercial potential, some of these ingredients are used for cleansing, wettability, and solvent properties. Of course, sodium bicarbonates have been used because it has an immediate pH adjustment property, which enhances antimicrobial potential. Finally, the addition of a second antimicrobial agent such as phenol to provide a synergistic effect has been commercialized and has been reported to show positive effects.[32] Cationic agents were attempted without any significant benefit.[33]

In conclusion, aldehydes will continue to be used for medical device reprocessing, especially flexible endoscopes. The relative stability and ease of formulation of aldehydes in comparison to other agents such as peroxygens makes these agents desirable. The current OPA formulations marketed globally are effective and have a significant cost advantage over other HLD marketed products.

▶ PEROXYGEN COMPOUNDS

The two main classes of peroxides employed in the formulation of environmental antimicrobial products are hydrogen peroxide and peroxyacids (or peracids). Hydrogen peroxide is a ubiquitous industrial chemical available commercially in active concentrations ranging from 3% to 90% by weight. Several different peracids are also available commercially for diverse industrial use. The most common by far is peracetic acid, available in concentrations from 1% to 40% by weight in an equilibrium mixture that also contains hydrogen peroxide, acetic acid, and water. The salt form of peroxymonosulfuric acid (Caro acid) is also a commercial product. Other organic peroxides are sold in Europe for use in antimicrobial products, including

monoperphthalic acid[34] and ε-phthalimido perhexanoic acid.

Several approaches are possible for the formulation of environmental antimicrobial products with peroxygens, including:

- Single-phase liquids, aqueous, or anhydrous form
- One part granular or crystalline mixture
- Two part systems mixed on use
- Gas or vapor phase application

For the first three approaches, the formulation and packaging or application strategy are closely interrelated and are determined by market, manufacturing and logistics, and company-specific considerations.

Stability

In general, the shelf life of a formulated peroxygen product will be determined by the rate of the autodecomposition. Self-decomposition is accelerated by temperature and peroxygen concentration and is subject to catalysis by inorganic dissolved species. The catalytic effect of these dissolved species, typically transition metals, is dramatically enhanced with increasing pH.[35]

In complex formulated matrices, additional ingredients are present to impart certain desired characteristics to the final product. Examples are filling an efficacy spectrum gap or improving efficacy of claimed active(s), imparting detergency to the product, or delivering a desired color or scent. This introduces an additional variable to the stability problem—that is, the potential for degradation of the peroxygen by direct reaction with the added functional material(s). Additionally, the functional material may also introduce catalytic impurities carried over from their manufacturing, which can accelerate the decomposition of the peroxygen. In order to mitigate these effects, a variety of materials have been cited as stabilizers.[35] First and foremost for stabilizing, is formulation at an acid pH (less than 5). This reduces the rate of the peroxygen self-decomposition reaction. Second, use of high-quality water and formula ingredients that bring minimal dissolved ions into the mixture. In particular, the presence of transition metals (iron, copper, manganese, nickel, cobalt, especially), chlorides, and hardness (calcium, magnesium) needs to be minimized. Third, chelant species with high binding affinity for the aforementioned species can be added directly to the formulation or indirectly via stabilized peroxygen stock from the manufacturer. The more common stabilizers are phosphonic acids (eg, hydroxy ethylidene [1,1-diphosphonic acid], aminotris[methylene phosphonic acid], diethylenetriamine penta[methylene phosphonic acid]), stannates, and pyrophosphates.[35]

One of the main issues in the formulation with peracids in an aqueous matrix is the hydrolysis of the peracid back to the parent carboxylic acid and hydrogen peroxide. Thus, it is important to consider the equilibrium of the hydrolysis reaction:

$$R - CO_2H + H_2O_2 \overset{H^+}{\rlap{\raise2pt\hbox{$\longrightarrow$}}\lower2pt\hbox{$\longleftarrow$}} R - CO_3H + H_2O$$

A key consideration for the formulation of peracid products in liquid form is that the expected concentrations of peracid (R-CO$_3$H), water, parent acid (R-CO$_2$H), and hydrogen peroxide will not be the same as those obtained initially on addition of the peracid stock solution to the manufacturing batch (or dilution of the concentrate product on use for that matter). Thus, equilibration of the mixture will typically occur in the hours after product batching and/or packaging.[36]

Some peroxygens are so prone to self-decomposition in water that they are better formulated in dry, granular form. Examples are perborates, permonosulfuric acid, monoperphthalic acid, and ε-phthalimido perhexanoic acid. Hydrogen peroxide itself has also been commercialized in powdered form as an adduct of sodium carbonate, referred to as "sodium percarbonate," but it is typically not used on its own given stable liquid hydrogen peroxide solutions can be easily formulated and are more convenient to use. The peracids can be used in powdered or tableted formulations; however, perborate and monopersulfate salts find better application for in situ generation discussed briefly in the following text. Other peracids like monoperphthalic acid and ε-phthalimido perhexanoic acid have been commercialized in disinfection products in Europe[37] but may not have yet clearance in other jurisdictions (such as by the EPA in the United States).

The availability of crystalline forms enables a common approach to overcome stability issues in the liquid form; namely, the generation of the peracid in situ. The most common approach for disinfectants by far is the generation of peracetic acid by the combination of tetraacetylethylenediamine (TAED) with an oxygen donor such as a perborate or percarbonate salt. Diverse product presentations exist, ranging from a compacted tablet containing all ingredients to two parts solid-solid or solid-liquid (TAED needs to be in solid form given its susceptibility to hydrolysis). The main drawback with TAED-generated peracetic acid is the preparation process, time involved in dissolution of the TAED, the competing requirements of low pH for maximum efficacy versus high pH for hydrolysis reaction speed, and the short shelf life of the prepared solution.

Potassium monopersulfate (or Caro acid potassium salt—KHSO$_5$) is typically not employed by itself but as a precursor to generating hypochlorous acid by reaction in water with chloride ions (typically provided as sodium chloride):

$$HSO_5^- + Cl^- \rightarrow H^+ + OCl^- + SO_4^{2-}$$

as disclosed originally in 1960.[38] The hypochlorous acid and monopersulfuric acid mixture provides for a powerful oxidizing disinfectant.

Synergists

There are a number of compounds that potentiate a desired performance attribute inherent to the peroxide (such as efficacy or bleaching) and others that minimize undesirable effects (such as odor or irritation). As mentioned earlier, acidified peroxygen formulations exhibit a longer shelf life given the direct relation between pH and self-decomposition rate. However, pH itself is a synergistic factor with the peroxygen for all classes of organisms but in particular in the destruction of viruses, fungi, mycobacteria, and bacterial endospores. Thus, the majority of liquid peroxygen antimicrobial formulations exhibit pH's of 5 or below.

As with other antimicrobial actives, surfactants are another key synergist in peroxygen formulations. Anionic surfactants are particularly useful, given that many of them exhibit additive or synergistic behavior with peroxygens, especially at low pH. Particularly useful surfactants are the alkylbenzene sulfonates, alkyl sulfates, and alkyl phosphate esters. Nonionics are also incorporated into antimicrobial peroxygen mixtures and, in many cases, show a synergistic effect with the peroxygen. Their ability to reduce surface tension and suspend soil particles at relatively low in-use concentrations is important for formulation efficacy under "dirty" conditions. The most common combinations are alcohol ethoxylates, alkyl polyglycosides, and EO-PO block copolymers.

Cationic and amphoteric surfactants have been combined to a lesser extent with peroxygens but mostly because combinations with anionics give a better overall performance among other product functional features (eg, better cleaning, better peroxide stability, better environmental profile). A particularly useful class of surfactant that is widely used with peroxygens are amine oxides, especially in acid formulations. In amine oxides, that strictly speaking are considered nonionics, the nitrogen protonates in acid medium giving it a cationic character. They tend to provide good foaming, improve detergency and mildness, and have been reported to reduce odor in peracid formulations as well.[39] Betaines are by far the most widely used amphoteric in peroxygen formulations, especially where copious foaming and/or skin mildness are key performance requirements.

Another common synergistic material is solvents. Solvents are organic molecules, for the most part polar in nature, and mostly contain at least an oxygen atom. Some of these materials exhibit synergistic antimicrobial effects in peroxygen formulations while at the same time provide additional desirable characteristics such as hydrotroping, detergency against oily soils, reducing streaking, and accelerating drying times. Examples of such solvents

TABLE 6.4   Multidilution hydrogen peroxide concentrate detergent disinfectant[a]

Ingredient	F1	F2	F3
HEDP (60% active)	0.48		
ATMP (50% active)		0.58	
90% Sodium tripolyphosphate			0.32
C6 Diphenyl disulphonate (45%)	0.18	0.18	0.18
C6-C10, 3.5 moles EO alcohol ethoxylate	0.05	0.05	0.05
Hydrogen peroxide (50%)	1.10	1.10	1.10
DDBSA (98%)	0.18	0.18	0.18
Total	100	100	100

Abbreviations: ATMP, aminotris(methylenephosphonic acid); DDBSA, dodecyl benzene sulfonic acid; EO, ethylene oxide; F, formula; HEDP, hydroxyethylidene diphosphonic acid. All ingredients in water to 100%.

[a]Data from Ramirez and Rochon.[40]

TABLE 6.6   Two-part peracetic acid sterilization solution[a]

Ingredients	%
Part 1	
Sodium perborate monohydrate	20
Tetraacetylethylenediamine	15
Sodium triphosphate	40
Sodium carbonate	15
Alkylbenzene sulfonate	2
Sodium sulfate	8
Part 2	
Octane phosphonic acid	0.2
Fatty alcohol ethoxylate	0.4
Cumene sulfonate	0.4
Water	39
Phosphoric acid	60

[a]Data from Scoville and Novicova.[41]

are the short-chain alcohols (methanol, ethanol, isopropanol), cyclic alcohols (eg, benzyl alcohol), and glycol ethers. Other ingredients may be added to formulations for the purpose of minimizing corrosion to substrates from the peroxygen and acid conditions.

Examples of commercial formulations leveraging one or more of the tools described here are presented in Tables 6.4 to 6.6. These include a multidilution, concentrate detergent disinfectant (Table 6.4), a formulated peracetic acid for instrument sterilization (Table 6.5), and a two-part activated sterilization product based on peracetic acid (Table 6.6).

TABLE 6.5   Peracetic acid instrument sterilization solution[a]

Ingredient	%
1-Hydroxyethylene-1,1-diphosphonic acid	0.70
8-Hydroxyquinoline	0.0035
Peracetic acid	0.23
Propylene glycol	4.10
Nonylphenol surfactant	0.002
Hydrogen peroxide	7.3
1,2,3-Benzotriazole	1.00
Sodium nitrite	0.25
Sodium molybdate	0.25
Water Total	100

[a]Data from Scoville and Novicova.[41]

▶ NITROGEN COMPOUNDS

The types and classes of biocidal compounds containing nitrogen are quite extensive.[43] Formulation with specific classes such as QACs and the important halogen –(N-H) compounds (especially those based on chlorine and iodine) have been treated earlier in this chapter. Other classes of nitrogen-containing compounds are used extensively as preservatives in many consumer and industrial products such as cleaners, paints, glues, metal working fluids, paper, construction materials, textiles, etc, or for the control of algae, fungi, and slime-producing bacteria in cooling tower systems. These include formaldehyde-releasing products from the reaction of primary amines with formaldehyde or the methylolate derivations of nitroalkanes, halogenated nitriles, pyridines (used extensively as therapeutic agents and cosmetics, in particular the bispyridine octenidine hydrochloride used in Europe as an antiseptic), thiazoles, and nitrogenated phenols (eg, bronopol, 2-bromo-2-nitropropane-1,3-diol).

In this section, examples of nitrogen compound formulations intended for topical or surface sanitation or disinfection are considered. The QACs have already been considered in detail separately. The compounds of focus here exhibit the right combination of germicidal activity and low toxicity that permit their use in topical and environmental surface decontamination. These can be classified generally as amine derivatives and comprise principally the bisguanadines and alkylamines. Another class of materials used extensively in the past for antiseptic products are the anilides (eg, triclocarban), but

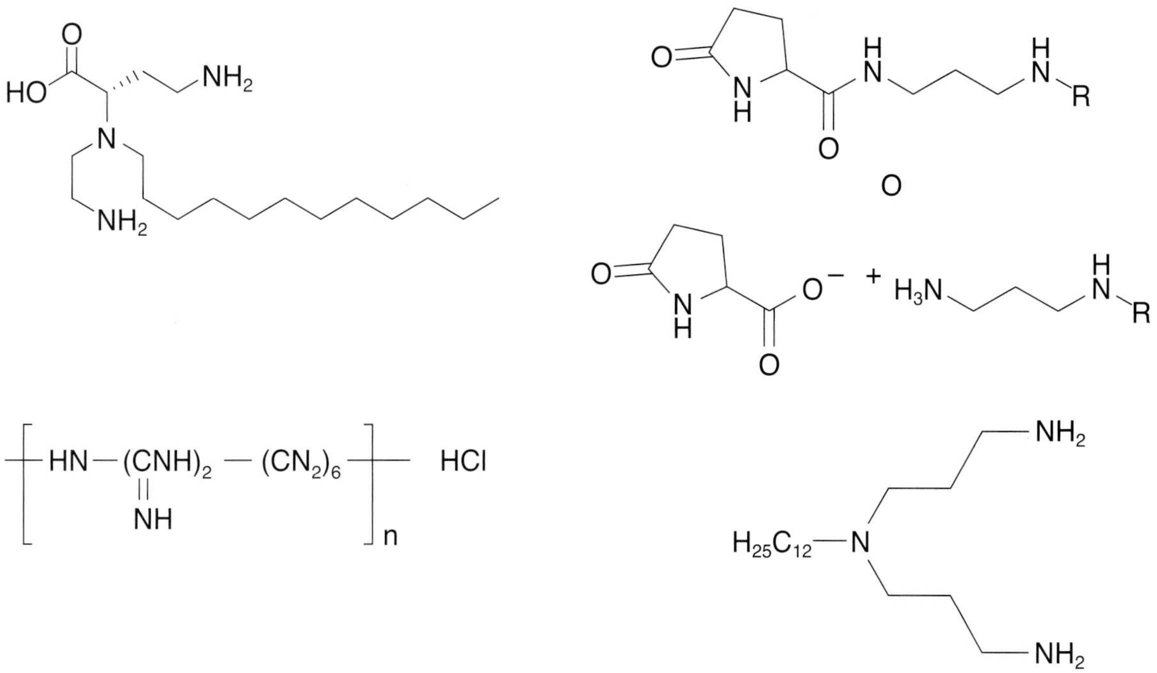

FIGURE 6.6 Common nitrogen-based compounds used in disinfectant formulation, clockwise beginning at top left, dodecyl di(aminoethyl) glycine, glucoprotamine, and N,N-bis-(3-aminopropyl)laurylamine, with poly-hexamethylene biguanide hydrochloride in the lower left.

rising concerns on their actual efficacy and toxicity has resulted in gradually less reliance on them by formulators. Of the biguanides, asides from chlorhexidine gluconate that is discussed in more detail later in this chapter, the most common compound is the quaternary polymer, polyhexamethylene biguanide hydrochloride (PHMB) (Figure 6.6).

Although PHMB has recently come under scrutiny in Europe as a suspected carcinogen (depending on its application, use has been limited to certain concentrations[44]), it is still useful in a variety of topical and hard surface formulations globally. Being a cationic material, it is not compatible with anionic surfactants and generally not stable in the presence of oxidizers (such as chlorine or peroxygens) or in highly alkaline media. It is of most interest because of its high activity against pseudomonads and other gram-negative bacteria; hence, it is frequently formulated in conjunction with QACs to cover their known weaknesses in that area. Additionally, because it is not considered surface active, it is preferred for applications where foaming needs to be limited or controlled.[45]

An exemplary formulation for a disinfectant-impregnated wipe is given in Table 6.7.[46] The composition employs an active content of PHMB of just over 350 ppm combined with a QAC at 300 ppm. Detergency is provided by either nonionic surfactants, an EO-PO block copolymer, or an alkyl polyglycoside. These specific choices exhibit low residue and streaking, thus are especially suited for use on reflective or transparent surfaces. Isopropanol is included in order to provide rapid

evaporation from the surface, particularly useful in no-rinse applications.

The alkylamines are much more popular outside of North America, and the principal compounds used in topical or hard surface disinfection are the amphoteric surfactants dodecyl di(aminoethyl) glycine and

TABLE 6.7 Disinfectant liquids based on PHMB for impregnated wipe[a]

Ingredient	F1	F2	F3
Deionized water	82.556	80.448	80.498
Alkyl polyglucoside (C8-C10), Glucopon 215	0.133	0.133	—
EO-PO block copolymer, Pluronic L64	—	—	0.083
DDABC quat, Carboquat H, 50%	0.060	0.060	0.060
Isopropyl alcohol, 99.5%	0.392	2.500	2.500
PHMB, Vantocil P, 20%	0.189	0.189	0.189
Suominen SX-145 polyester wipe substrate	16.670	16.670	16.670
Total	100	100	100

Abbreviations: DDABC, didecyldimethylammonium bicarbonate; EO-PO, ethylene oxide-propylene oxide; F, formula; PHMB, poly-hexamethylene biguanide hydrochloride.

[a]Data from Kloeppel et al.[46]

N,N-bis-(3-aminopropyl)laurylamine as well as the reaction product of cocopropylene 1,3-diamine and L-glutamic acid, glucoprotamine (see Figure 6.6).

The dodecyl di(aminoethyl) glycine is often formulated with other QACs and/or phenolics in the presence of a nonionic surfactant at slightly alkaline pH. The in-use active concentration of the material is in the order of 1000 to 2500 ppm, with concentrates of up to 15% active amine possible.[47] The main utility of these formulations is for mycobactericidal activity, particularly in Europe, where higher contact times are allowed by regulation and are more common in the marketplace. Similarly, the N,N-bis-(3-aminopropyl)laurylamine is typically combined with phenolics, or other aromatic alcohols, as well as short-chain alcohol and aldehydes. The pH of these formulations is slightly alkaline, and most contain one or more nonionic surfactants, although formulation with anionic surfactants is possible. Examples of synergistic formulations with phenoxyethanol are shown in Table 6.8.[48] These are concentrates that are diluted in water upon use at the rate of between 2% and 5%. A small amount of isopropyl alcohol is needed as a hydrotrope for the phenoxyethanol, the laurylamine is quite readily soluble in water. A nonionic surfactant such as an ethoxylated alcohol or an ethoxylated carboxylate can be used in order to impart some detergency and improve wetting.

The glucoprotamines can be formulated over a wide range of pH, but a slight decrease in activity is observed as the pH is made slightly more alkaline, with an optimum approaching pH of 9.[49] The material is highly soluble in water (440 g/L) and is quite compatible with nonionic and amphoteric surfactants. It is not very compatible with anionic surfactants. In fact, even the small presence of alkyl sulfonates or alkyl sulfates results in an antagonistic biocidal effect.[50] On the other hand, dramatic synergies have been reported with certain nonionic surfactants, in particular with alcohol ethoxylates with hydrophobe lengths between C_8 and C_{14}, and 2 to 4 moles ethoxylation, and with C_8 to C_{12} alkyl polyglucosides with 1.4 to 1.6 glucoside units.[50]

The material is also compatible with most solvents used in cleaning and detergent formulations as well as with most chelating agents and sequestrants.

▶ CHLORHEXIDINE

Although technically a nitrogen-based biocide, chlorhexidine is so widely used in formulations that it deserves treatment on its own. It is commercially available typically as a salt, commonly as gluconate, acetate, or hydrochloride salts. The most used form is the gluconate salt, given its higher solubility in both aqueous and nonaqueous solvents. Because of its characteristic germicidal spectrum (essentially effective against gram-positive and gram-negative bacteria as well as fungi/yeasts and enveloped viruses) and compatibility to skin, it is widely used in antiseptic products. Its limited solubility in water restricts its use mainly to ready-to-use formulated products (as opposed to concentrate-diluted at the point of use).

There are several key considerations in formulations with chlorhexidine gluconate:

- At pH above 8, the chlorhexidine begins to precipitate out of aqueous solution, whereas in acid conditions (pH lower than about 4), hydrolysis to p-chloroaniline causes a gradual loss of activity. The range of pH for optimal activity is reported widely as between 5 and 8.
- Because chlorhexidine is a cationic molecule, it is generally incompatible with anionic species, including inorganic anions (eg, sulfates or carbonate), organic anions such as anionic surfactants (carboxylates, sulfonates, sulfates, phosphate esters, etc), and many anionic dyes.
- Although compatible with other cationic species (such as QACs, other biguanides, other cationic surfactants), it may form complexes with the counterion of the cationic material that could cause precipitation or loss of activity due to complexation with said counterions.
- As with many active agents, chlorhexidine may be incorporated into nonionic micelles. This can be used to

TABLE 6.8 Examples of combined alkyl-amine/phenolic hard surface disinfectant formulations[a]

Ingredient	F1	F2	F3	F4
Phenoxyethanol	30.0	30.0	30.0	30.0
Lonzabac® 12	12.0	12.0	12.0	12.0
Isopropanol	15.0	10.0	10.0	10.0
Alkyl ethoxylate (11 EO)	20.0	—	—	—
Laureth-11-carboxylic acid	—	15.0	18.0	—
Laureth-5-carboxylic acid	—	—	—	18.0
Water	To 100	To 100	To 100	To 100

Abbreviations: EO, ethylene oxide; F, formula; PHMB, polyhexamethylene biguanide hydrochloride.

[a]Data from Eggensperger et al.[48]

an advantage, such as in increasing the availability or rate of transport into the target organism (and hence improving biocidal activity in formulation), but in most cases, this actually becomes a detriment to the formulator by reducing the available concentration of chlorhexidine for kill or impeding rates of absorption into target organisms.

In topical formulations, the traditionally required concentration is between 2% and 6% chlorhexidine gluconate, although formulations containing lower concentrations (such as 1% or 0.5%) have been described. Because chlorhexidine formulations are usually aimed at topical (skin) use, two important functional requirements of the formulation are low irritancy to skin and/or eye and suitable foaming and rinsability (or residue, tackiness, etc, for the case of leave-on products) profiles. In order to impart suitable foaming to the composition, high-foaming surfactants need to be incorporated into the formulation. However, given the incompatibilities mentioned earlier, high-foaming anionics are typically not an option. Most cationic surfactants available commercially do not exhibit acceptable foaming (or acceptable irritation profiles for that matter); hence, the most common options for the formulator are nonionic or amphoteric surfactants. As mentioned earlier, many of these seemingly acceptable options reduce the availability or transport rates of the chlorhexidine molecule, and hence, actual in vitro biocidal confirmatory testing must be part of the product development protocol.

A prototypical antiseptic formulation is presented in Table 6.9.[51] The combination of nonionic surfactants is usually necessary in order to get the right balance between foaming, detergency, and skin mildness while minimizing the deactivation of the chlorhexidine gluconate. Common nonionic surfactants such as carboxylates and linear or branched alcohol ethoxylates inactivate chlorhexidine to greater degree, and experimentation throughout the

years has narrowed the best options to compounds such as ethylene-propylene block copolymers, aromatic alcohol ethoxylates, certain low hydrophilic-lipophilic balance, linear and branched chain alcohol ethoxylates, and alkyl polyglycosides in combination with betaines and/or amine oxides. In the example formulation, a dye and a fragrance are formulated into the product with isopropyl alcohol as the carrier of choice. The pH is adjusted within the optimal pH of activity, typically requiring acidification, which is usually done with carboxylic acids such as acetic, glycolic, citric, or lactic acid.

Formulations will frequently include a viscosity modification agent in concentrations of up to 2% wt/wt; reliable candidates for chlorhexidine formulations are alkyl, hydroxyalkyl, or carboxyalkyl cellulose. Typical glycol emollients such as propylene or triethylene glycol can also be used in concentration of up to 10% wt/wt. It is possible to improve the efficacy and mildness by formulating at lower CHG active levels by using one or more coactives, for example, by increasing the level of a short-chain alcohol. Other formulations will be unique to particular applications, such as for mouth rinses, surgical preoperative preparations, and the treatment of wounds or mucous membranes (see chapter 22).

▶ ESSENTIAL OILS

The working definition of an essential oil applies to oily compounds, largely obtained from plant sources (leaves, buds, fruits, flowers, roots, seeds, barks, etc) and typically composed of complex mixtures of up to 60 components but where usually one to three components dominate the composition.[52] They are usually terpenoids that can be aromatic or not (see chapter 14). Common examples used in sanitizing and disinfecting products include pine, thyme, lemongrass, lemon, orange, anise, clove, rose, lavender, citronella, eucalyptus, peppermint,

TABLE 6.9 Example of a CHG-based antimicrobial hand wash[a]

Ingredient	Amount (% wt/wt)	Functionality
Chlorhexidine gluconate (20%)	20	Antimicrobial
Laurylaminedimethyl oxide	3.75	Nonionic surfactant (foaming)
Ethylene oxide-propylene oxide block copolymer (PEO_{67}-PPO_{39}-PEO_{67})	25	Nonionic surfactant (foaming and detergency)
Isopropyl alcohol	4	Solubilization of dye and fragrance
Dye (eg, red carmoisine dye)	0.005	Serve as indicator on treated area
Fragrance (eg, Herbacol 15.393/T)	0.1%	Fragrance
	Adjust to pH 5.5	

Abbreviation: CHG, chlorhexidine gluconate; PEO, polyethylene oxide; PPO, polypropylene oxide.

[a]Data from Billany et al.[51]

TABLE 6.10   Dilutable hard surface disinfectant based on thymol and origanum oils as actives[a]

Ingredient	Amount (% wt/wt)	Functionality
Thymol	18	Antimicrobial
Origanum oil	4	Antimicrobial
Sodium citrate	1	Sequestering agent for hardness and pH buffering (when diluted with tap water on use)
Propylene glycol methyl ether	18	Solubilization of essential oils
Sodium lauryl sulfate	12	Solubilization of essential oils, detergency, and foaming
Water	47	
	Resulting pH is 8.8.	Used at 1:100 dilution

[a]Data from Daigle et al.[55]

camphor, sandalwood, and cedar oils. Because of their hydrophobic nature, it is very difficult to formulate essential oils into aqueous matrices, and one typically requires the use of a solubilizing system.

There are several commercially viable ways to solubilize essential oils into a water-based product, but invariably, they involve the use of surfactants, water-soluble solvents, or both. The usual solvents employed in essential oil antimicrobial compositions are typically short-chain alcohols such as methanol, ethanol, or isopropanol; glycols such as propylene and hexylene glycol; or a variety of glycol ethers. Surfactants may also be used to aid solubilization but at the same time impart desired additional functional properties such as detergency, foaming, or viscosity. In this regard, surfactants used can be any of the type: anionic, nonionic, or amphoteric. In some cases, cationic surfactants can be used, but in this case, it usually involves a combination of a QAC with an essential oil to obtain additive or synergistic activity in the final formulation. In cases where the surfactant is relied on mostly for solubilization, well-known hydrotropes such as the toluene, cumene, or xylene sulfonates are good choices, whereas when nonionic surfactants are used, low hydrophilic-lipophilic balances typically higher than 12 to 13 are preferred. Synergistic solubilization systems based on mixtures of solvents and anionic-nonionic surfactants are possible, but the reader is referred to one of the many detergent formulation treatises available.[53,54]

An example of a dilutable composition with bactericidal activity based on a mixture of thymol and origanum oil is presented in Table 6.10.[55]

Another composition illustrating a slightly different solubilization system is presented in Table 6.11.[56]

In this case, a ready-to-use formulation has been shown to have bactericidal efficacy according to the AOAC use dilution method.[57] These compositions are typical of essential oil-based disinfectants where the required in-use concentration of the essential oil for efficacy is in the order of 2000 ppm. As can be inferred from comparing both formulations, the solubilization capacity of the short-chain alcohols is not as high as for glycol ethers; thus, there is a need to supplement the solubilizing package with the anionic surfactants. But as mentioned earlier, techniques for hydrotroping poorly water-soluble compounds are abundant in the detergent formulation literature.

The most prevalent natural oil used in environmental surface decontamination is pine oil. This natural oil extracted from pine trees has been used as an antimicrobial product for many years. α-Terpineol is the predominant compound accounting for the antimicrobial

TABLE 6.11   Hard surface disinfectant based on thymol[a]

Ingredient	Amount (% wt/wt)	Functionality
Thymol	0.15	Antimicrobial
Ethyl alcohol	15	Solubilizing agent
C12-C15 alcohol, ethoxylated, carboxylated	1.5	Solubilizing agent plus detergency and foaming
Dodecylbenzene sulfonate	0.25	Solubilizing agent and detergency and foaming
Water	83.10	
	Resulting pH is 2.9.	

[a]Data from McCue and Smialowickz.[56]

activity of the oil. Pine oil has a limited antimicrobial profile, largely restricted to gram-negative bacteria like coliforms (eg, *E coli*). The first such formulation was invented soon after the economic depression in the United States on 1929. The original product, Pine-Sol™, was a commercial product brand that has been sold for over 50 years for household cleaning and disinfecting. As formulated, it has a clear yellowish solution that becomes milky on dilution with water. The formulation combines the natural pine oil with anionic surfactants, builders, chelation agents, and alcohol cosolvents in a homogeneous product. It is noted that due to limited availability of pine oil stocks, some of these products have been recently reformulated, with a switch in antimicrobial active from pine oil to glycolic acid.[58] Other pine oil–based formulations with wide spectrum of activity incorporate a second biocide; namely, a QAC coupled with a nonionic surfactant to achieve proper solubility and increase the antimicrobial activity.[59]

▶ BIOCIDAL FORMULATION WITH METALS

The use of certain metals such as silver and copper as antimicrobials has seen a resurgence of interest in recent years. Prevalent applications include use of silver and copper in topical/therapeutical products, for the impregnation of materials (especially polymers and fabrics), and for the control of bacteria such as *Legionella* in water systems (whereby ions are generated by ion dissolution from energized electrodes). Formulated germicidal products for environmental surface disinfection have recently begun making some inroads commercially (although still not gaining significant traction in the marketplace at the time of writing) and is thus our focus here.

The most common metallic antimicrobial in use for environmental and medical device surfaces impregnation is silver.[60] Nonetheless, use of silver-based formulations for the decontamination of environmental surfaces is still not widespread. As a point of reference, in the United States alone, out of the more than 50 companies holding EPA registrations with silver as an active, there are only 3 that have formulated environmental surface germicides (most registrations are unformulated raw materials for use in manufacturing of impregnated materials or cartridges/ electrodes for electrolysis units for *Legionella* control). In registered environmental surface formulations, silver is typically coupled to another species (many times another antimicrobial) in order to preserve its stability. Another approach is to formulate as a two-part system, especially when the second part is a strong oxidizer that oxidizes the elemental silver from an oxidation state of (+1) to (+2) or (+3) where it is more effective but less stable. It is well-known that ionic silver solutions can be stabilized in a colloidal dispersion by combining them with

a dispersant, with PVP, polyethyleneimine, polyethylene glycol, lipoic acid, and citric acid being the most common.[61] One formulation coupled the silver ions with citric acid by generating the silver ions from an energized silver electrode in a solution of citric acid.[62] Another approach employs a similar technique, formulating an aqueous silver composition by dissolving a silver salt such as silver chloride, silver nitrate, silver sulfate, sodium-silver chloride, or commercial colloidal silver solution in a low pH (lower than pH 2), acidified by phosphoric acid, sulfuric or nitric acid, and citric or tartaric acid solution.[63] In this case, the end-use product is a mixture of the silver solution with hydrogen peroxide, presumably to provide an oxidative source to keep or restore the silver valence at higher than +1. Another example of a surface disinfectant product based on silver follows a similar approach, but in that case, the second part is a peracetic acid/ hydrogen peroxide solution. The difficulty of stabilizing the ionic silver in complex matrices and its relatively weak biocidal potential to meet stringent hard surface disinfection tests without the presence of an oxidizer have limited its application in formulated environmental sanitizers and disinfectants.

The major traditional uses of copper as an antimicrobial are by far as a fungicide or mildewcide where it is applied to plants and crops, a component incorporated in the manufacture of articles with impregnated copper as a form of inherent biocidal protection (such as paper fibers, cardboard, etc), and an algicide in water, cooling tower, and pool treatment. The use of dissolved copper/ silver as produced by dissolution from solid-state electrodes in an electrolysis unit has gained relatively wide acceptance in *Legionella* control applications in institutional and health care settings.[64] In the last 10 years, there has been an increased interest in the use of copper alloy surfaces and fixtures (eg, in health care facilities) due to several studies citing reduced microbiological levels on those surfaces.[65-67] However, no copper-based formulated germicidal environmental sanitizer or disinfectants are currently marketed, likely due to the fact that although effective, the stringent contact times and bioburden reduction levels cannot be met by formulated ionic copper solutions alone.[68]

In conclusion, it is expected that antimicrobial applications of metals will continue to be mostly focused on low-concentration/long-contact time scenarios; namely, water treatment (especially recirculation systems), preservation, and materials impregnation. Given the unfavorable relationship between required biocidal concentrations for disinfection and toxicity, public concerns about environmental persistence, and the difficulty of formulation in a homogeneous, multicomponent matrix, the use of metals in formulated topical or surface sanitizers and disinfectants will likely remain limited to few products.

REFERENCES

1. McDonnell GE. *Antisepsis, Disinfection, and Sterilization: Types, Action, and Resistance.* 2nd ed. Washington, DC: ASM Press; 2017.

2. Friese C, Lehmann R, Leinen H, inventors; Henkel AG and Co KGaA, assignee. Use of surfactants to boost the anti-microbial properties of a carboxylic acid amide. European patent 0783246B1. November 18, 1988.

3. Zipf HF. Practical points for experiments using combinations of two compounds. *Arzneimittelforschung.* 1953;3:398-403.

4. Loewe S. The problem of synergism and antagonism of combined drugs. *Arzneimittelforschung.* 1953;3(6):285-290.

5. Bunczk CJ, Burke PA, Camp WR, inventors; Kiwi Brands Inc, assignee. Toilet bowl cleaners containing iodophors. US patent 4,911,859. March 27, 1990.

6. Lugol JGA. Mémoire sur l'Emploi de l'Iode dans les maladies scrofuleuses. *Glasgow Med J.* 1832;5(17):83–92.

7. Putnan EV. Iodine vs. chlorine treatment of swimming pools. *Parks Recreations.* 1961;44:162.

8. Baker RJ. Types and significance of chlorine residuals. *J Am Water Works Assoc.* 1959;51(9):1185–1190.

9. Shere L. Some comparisons of the disinfecting properties of hypochlorite and quaternary ammonium compounds. *Milk Plant Monthly.* 1948;37:66-69.

10. Hunt JL, Sato R, Heck EL, Baxter CR. A critical evaluation of povidone-iodine absorption in thermally injured patients. *J Trauma.* 1980;20(2):127-129.

11. Bunczk CJ, Burke PA, Camp WR, Orehotsky JL, inventors; Kiwi Brands Inc, assignee. Lavatory cleansing and sanitizing blocks containing a halogen release bleach and a polybutene stabilizer. US patent 5,449,473. September 12, 1995.

12. Fürbringer P. *Untersuchungen und Vorschriften über die Desinfektion der Hande des Arztes nebst Bemerkungen über den Bakterilogischen Chakter des Nagleschmutzes.* Wiesbaden, Germany: J. F Bergmann; 1988.

13. Willie B. Praktische Laborversuche zur Resistenzentwicklung von Mikoorganismengenen Disinfektionsmittel. 1976;1:17-22.

14. Price PB. New studies in surgical bacteriology and surgical technique with special reference to disinfection of skin. *JAMA.* 2019;111(22):1993-1996.

15. Healthcare Infection Control Practices Advisory Committee (FDA); 2012.

16. Lins C, inventor; SC Johnson and Son Inc, assignee. High alcohol content aerosol antimicrobial mousse. US patent 5,167,950. December 1, 1992.

17. US Food and Drug Administration. FDA website announcement. https://www.fda.gov/NewsEvents/Newsroom/PressAnnoucements/ucm517478.htm. Accessed March, 5, 2018.

18. Weatherly LM, Gosse JA. Triclosan exposure, transformation, and human health effects. *J Toxicol Environ Health B Crit Rev.* 2017;20(8):447-469.

19. Levy SB. The challenge of antibiotic resistance. *Sci Am.* 1998;278(3):46-53.

20. Lister J. On the antiseptic principle in the practice of surgery. *Br Med J.* 1867;2(351):246-248.

21. Kline & Company. *Specialty Biocides of North America.* Little Falls, NJ: Kline & Company; 2000.

22. Wallhausser KH. Compatibility of surfactants with disinfectants. *Seifen Öle Fette Wachse.* 1980;111:106-107.

23. Davis B. Surfactants-biocide interactions. In: Porter MR, ed. *Recent Developments in the Technology of Surfactants (Critical Reports on Applied Chemistry).* Vol. 30. Dordrecht, Netherlands: Kluwer Academic; 1990:65-131.

24. Winicov MW, Schmidt W, inventors; West Laboratories Inc, assignee. Phenolic synthetic detergent-disinfectant. US patent 3,824,190. July 16, 1974.

25. Directive 98/9/EC of the European Parliament and of the Council of 16 February 1998 concerning the placing of biocidal products on the market. *Official Journal of the European Communities.* 1998;41(L123, 24.4.98):1-56.

26. McDonnell GE. QACs and other surfactants. In: *Antisepsis, Disinfection, and Sterilization.* Washington, DC: ASM Press; 2007:140-143.

27. Tomlinson E, Brown MR, Davis SS. Effect of colloidal association on the measured activity of alkylbenzyldimethylammonium chlorides against *Pseudomonas aeruginosa. J Med Chem.* 1977;20(10):1277-1282.

28. Harries HP, Tank L. Conversion of the cyclopentene into the mono- and dialdehyde of glutaric acid. *Berichte.* 1908;41:1701-1711.

29. Korn AH, Feairheller SH, Filachione EM. Glutaraldehyde: nature of the reagent. *J Mol Biol.* 1972;65(3):525-529.

30. Hoopwood D, Callen CR, McCabe M. The reactions between glutaraldehyde and various proteins. An investigation of their kinetics. *Histochem J.* 1970;2(2):137-150.

31. Hardy PM. The nature of the cross-linking of proteins by glutaraldehyde. *J Chem Soc Perkin Trans.* 1979;1:2282-2288.

32. Schattner RI, inventor. Buffered phenol-glutaraldehyde sterilizing compositions. US patent 4,103,001. July 25, 1978.

33. Gorman SP, Scott EM, Russell AD. Antimicrobial activity, uses and mechanism of action of glutaraldehyde. *J Appl Bacteriol.* 1980;48(2):161-190.

34. Baldry MG. The antimicrobial properties of magnesium monoperoxyphthalate hexahydrate. *J Appl Bacteriol.* 1984;57(3):499-503.

35. Schumb WC, Satterfield CN, Wentworth RL. *Hydrogen Peroxide.* New York, NY: Reinhold Publishing Corp; 1955.

36. Swern D. Organic peracids. *Chem Rev.* 1949;45(1):1-68.

37. Deutschen Gesellschaft für Mikrobiologie und Hygiene. *Approved List of Disinfectants.* Wiesbaden, Germany: mhp-Verlag GmbH; 2002.

38. Hinegardner WS, Stephanou SE, Lake DB, D'addieco AA, inventors; E I du Pont de Nemours and Co, assignee. A process for the production of Caro's acid and monopersulfates and monopersulfates containing salt mixtures. German patent application DE1080083B. March 29, 2019.

39. Smith KR, Hei R, inventors; Ecolab Inc, assignee. Peroxycarboxylic acid compositions with reduced odor. US patent 20,040,143,133. November 24, 2009.

40. Ramirez JA, Rochon MJ, inventors; Virox Technologies Inc, assignee. Hydrogen peroxide disinfectant with increased activity. US patent 6,803,057B2. October 12, 2004.

41. Scoville JR Jr, Novicova IA, inventors; Metrex Research LLC, assignee. Hydrogen peroxide disinfecting and sterilizing compositions. US patent 5,900,256. May 4, 1999.

42. Biering H, Bansemir K-P, Sorns J, inventors; Ecolab Inc, assignee. Process for disinfecting instruments. US patent 6,540,960. April 1, 2003.

43. Block S. *Disinfection, Sterilization, and Preservation.* 5th ed. Philadelphia, PA: Lippincott Williams & Wilkins; 2001.

44. Scientific Committee on Consumer Safety. Opinion on polyaminopropyl biguanide (PHMB)—submission III. https://ec.europa.eu/health/sites/health/files/scientific_committees/consumer_safety/docs/sccs_o_204.pdf. Accessed September 23, 2018.

45. Lonza Microbial Control. *Vantocil TG Antimicrobial.* Atlanta, GA: Lonza Corp; 2013.

46. Kloeppel A, Koehl D, Colurciello A, inventors; Lonza Inc, assignee. Food contact disinfecting/sanitizing formulation and wipe. US patent application 20,140,171,512. March 21, 2019.

47. Behrends S, Dettmann A, Mohr M, inventors. Tuberculocidal disinfectant. WIPO patent WO1999035912. March 2, 2000.

48. Eggensperger H, Bernd L, Mohr M, Goroncy-Bermes P, Beilfuss W, inventors; Schulke and Mayr GmbH, Eastman Kodak Co, assignees. Amine- and alcohol-based disinfectant concentrate and disinfectant and use thereof. US patent 5,393,789. February 28, 1995.

49. Disch K. Glucoprotamine—a new antimicrobial substance. *Zentralbl Hyg Umweltmed.* 1994;195(5-6):357-365.

50. Lehmann RH. Synergism in disinfectant formulation. In: Block SS, ed. *Disinfection, Sterilization, and Preservation.* 5th ed. Philadelphia, PA: Lippincott Williams & Wilkins; 2001:459-472.

51. Billany M, Longworth A, Shatwell J, inventors; Imperial Chemical Industries Ltd, assignee. Cleansing compositions. US patent 3,855,140. December 17, 1974.

52. Kalemba D, Kunicka A. Antibacterial and antifungal properties of essential oil. *Curr Med Chem.* 2003;10(10):813-829.

53. Mackay RA. Solubilization. In: Schick MJ, ed. *Nonionic Surfactants: Physical Chemistry.* Vol 23. New York, NY: Marcel Dekker; 1987:297-368.

54. Lange KR, ed. *Detergents and Cleaners: A Handbook for Formulators.* Cincinnati, OH: Hanser/Gardner Publications; 1994.

55. Daigle F, Lettelier A, Quessy S, inventors; Laboratoire M2, assignee. Disinfectant formulation. US patent 20,100,034,907. April 8, 2014.

56. McCue KA, Smialowickz DT, inventors; Eastman Kodak Co, Reckitt Benckiser LLC, assignees. Disinfectant and sanitizing compositions based on essential oils. US patent 5,403,587. April 4, 1995.

57. United States Environmental Protection Agency. *Standard Operating Procedure for AOAC Use Dilution Method for Testing Disinfectants.* Fort Meade, MD: United States Environmental Protection Agency; 2016.

58. United States Environmental Protection Agency. Registered products database. https://iaspub.epa.gov/. Accessed November 3, 2018.

59. Manske SD, McPherson MS, inventors; Clariant International Ltd, assignee. Pine oil cleaning composition. US patent 6,465,411. October 15, 2002.

60. Cloutier M, Mantovani D, Rosei F. Antibacterial coatings: challenges, perspectives, and opportunities. *Trends Biotechnol.* 2015;33(11):637-652.

61. Tejamaya M, Romër I, Merrifield RC, Lead JR. Stability of citrate, PVP, and PEG coated silver nanoparticles in ecotoxicology media. *Environ Sci Technol.* 2012;46(13):7011-7017.

62. Arata A, inventor; Pure Bioscience, assignee. Disinfectant and method of making. US patent 6,197,814. March 6, 2001.

63. Gömöri J, inventor; SANOSIL AG General Wille Strasse, Sanosil AG, assignees. Process for preparing a disinfectant. US patent 4,915,955. April 10, 1990.

64. Walraven N, Pool W, Chapman C. Efficacy of copper-silver ionisation in controlling *Legionella* in complex water distribution systems and a cooling tower: over 5 years of practical experience. *J Water Proc Eng.* 2017;13:196-205.

65. Mikolay A, Hugget S, Tikana L, Grass G, Braun J, Nies DH. Survival of bacteria on metallic copper surfaces in a hospital trial. *Appl Microbiol Biotechnol.* 2010;87(5):1875-1879.

66. Rai S, Hirsch B, Attaway H, et al. Evaluation of the antimicrobial properties of copper surfaces in an outpatient infectious disease practice. *Infect Control Hosp Epidemiol.* 2012;33(2):200-201.

67. Salgado C, Sepkowitz K, John J, et al. Copper surfaces reduce the rate of healthcare-acquired infections in the intensive care unit. *Infect Control Hosp Epidemiol.* 2013;34(5):479-486.

68. Health Protection Scotland. *Literature Review and Practice Recommendations: Existing and Emerging Technologies Used for Decontamination of the Healthcare Environment—Antimicrobial Copper Surfaces.* Glasgow, United Kingdom: Health Protection Scotland; 2017.

CHAPTER

7

Kinetics of the Inactivation of Microorganisms

Alfredo C. Rodríguez

This chapter considers the changes in the number of survivors (individual microorganisms capable of reproduction) with time. It is often applied to industrial disinfection, pasteurization, and sterilization (terminal or commercial sterilization) processes aimed at assuring safety, stability, and quality of pharmaceutical parenteral drugs and devices and of shelf-stable food products. These concepts can be studied using a variety of individual microorganism types or even mixed populations. But the emphasis of this chapter is focused on the inactivation of bacterial spores because they are highly resistant to antimicrobial agents and also have stability properties that support their use as biological indicators to verify the efficacy of sterilization processes (see chapter 65). Development, improvement, and troubleshooting of sterilization processes benefit from a good understanding of related inactivation kinetics.[1,2] When a validated mathematical model is available, the related tasks may be supported more efficiently than using a purely empirical trial-and-error approach because the time, money, and other resources are significantly reduced. Indeed, in the food industry, a simulation package is well accepted by the regulatory and process authorities for simulation of moist heat–based (F_0; see equation 10 and chapters 11 and 28) processes.

Bacterial spore structure, formation, and significant transformations are well understood[3] (see chapter 3). The significant transformations concerning sterilization are dormancy, activation, inactivation, clumping,[4] and injury. Figure 7.1 presents a system diagram that includes these transformations and the corresponding subpopulations. "D" is applied to the inactivation transformation of the different subpopulations, and the inverted triangles represent the inactivated individuals corresponding to the different subpopulations. System analysis from population dynamics is used here to work on the corresponding models at the conceptual and mathematical levels. Dormancy

is the transformation of the bacteria into its corresponding spore that renders it resistant to antimicrobial processes (see chapter 3), including moist heat, and microscopically birefringent. Activation is the transformation of dormant bacterial spores that enables them to potentially germinate into an actively dividing cell that can produce colony-forming units (CFUs) on culturing. Activated spores lose their high heat resistance and birefringence (looking opaque in the phase contrast microscope, discussed in the following text). Inactivation is a transformation of microorganisms that renders them unable to multiply and therefore produce CFUs. Clumping of bacterial spores (and other microorganisms) is where they form groups or clumps, but due to this affinity may only produce one CFU per clump of cells on cultivation. Finally, injury renders them initially incapable of producing a CFU, unless modified growth conditions (such as additional nutrients, lower incubation temperature, enzymatic treatments, extended incubation time, etc) are applied or occur. Other transformations have been conceptually described[5] but have not yet been described mathematically well enough for practical applications.

Survival curves, which are generally semilog plots of the ratio of the concentration of surviving organisms to the initial number versus time, are commonly used to present inactivation data and to interpret the inactivation kinetics of microorganisms. Typical curves may be linear but are frequently observed to be nonlinear. Figure 7.2 presents some microbial inactivation curve types that may be seen in practice due to the presence of the different subpopulations and transformations described earlier. For instance, activated spores or vegetative cells will lead to an initial sharp drop in survivors because activated spores have a significantly lower resistance to moist heat that is similar to the resistance of vegetative cells. In addition, the activation transformation leads to a negative exponential curve and will lead to a hump

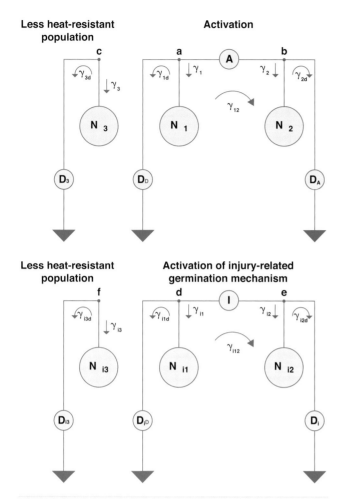

FIGURE 7.1 System diagram for bacterial spores undergoing sterilization. This system includes inactivation, activation, injury, and the presence of a less resistant subpopulation. The gamma (γ) symbols represent the rate for these subpopulations (undergoing a transformation ie, injury, activation, death, etc.); mathematically, they are the time derivatives of the density (individuals per unit volume or unit mass; colony-forming units per gram, etc.) of the corresponding subpopulation undergoing a transformation.

in the inactivation curve that may be significant at relatively lower temperatures and other conditions. These survivorship/inactivation curves may be described by the validated models available. Despite this, it is important to design products and processes that minimize the complexity of the description of the kinetics of inactivation without introducing significant error in practical terms. For instance, a more resistant subpopulation that may occur at occluded interfaces between glass and rubber stoppers may be eliminated by supersaturating the stoppers with water before sterilization, for example (see chapter 28). Figure 7.3 gives examples of how dormant bacterial spores change when viewed under phase-contrast microscopy. Dormant spores show birefringence

and are heat resistant, whereas bacterial spores that have broken dormancy look opaque and have lost their high heat resistance. The bacterial spore resistance properties were recently reviewed.[6]

Conceptually, the inactivation of microorganisms under the effect of a lethal agent follows well-defined patterns, with the rate of inactivation diminishing with time in a mostly ordered fashion. The exponential nature of inactivation prevents the goal of zero survivorship from being realistic (infinite time would be required). Thus, low levels of survivorship have been defined and validated practically as the goals of related industrial sterilization or disinfection (including pasteurization) processes, such as terminal sterilization for the medical device and pharmaceutical industry and commercial sterilization for the low acid–canned foods in the food industry. This chapter reviews procedures that can be used to assist in the efficient development and validation of such processes. The complexity and diversity of industrial sterilization processes precludes the selection of a single approach to describe mathematically the inactivation of microorganisms. In addition, different lethal agents may attack different components of the targeted microorganisms (see chapter 5). For instance, DNA, enzymes, or other subsystems required for germination and growth may be targeted and can affect the results. Finally, study of the kinetics of microbial inactivation caused by some lethal agents such as radiation may benefit from a non-homogeneous kinetic approach (see chapter 29). As an illustration, Figure 7.4 presents the damage caused by an electric field in a piece of wood. Clearly, if electroporation was intended as the lethal process, some regions would receive high-intensity treatments, whereas most of the material would receive negligible treatments. Therefore, the model used to describe the corresponding kinetics of inactivation should be the simplest model that describes the inactivation process properly. Models with corresponding degrees of complexity are further discussed in this chapter. Moist heat (including ultrahigh pressure), dry heat, chemical, and radiation sterilization processes are reviewed in detail, due to their practical importance. Application of mathematical models to such practical problems is currently enabled using mathematical software in various computer systems. Use of mathematical programs eliminates the need to use traditional procedures (eg, semilog paper). Examples presented here as illustrations correspond to worksheets developed using MathCAD versions 14 or 15 (MathSoft Engineering and Education Inc, Cambridge, MA). The worksheets presented have been carefully developed, but no warranty is given regarding their application. Computerized systems must be validated properly in each instance per the corresponding regulatory requirements or guidelines.

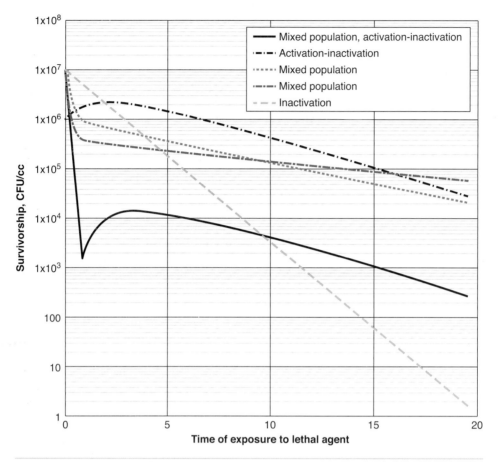

FIGURE 7.2 Examples of survivorship curves of bacterial spores undergoing sterilization that are commonly found in industrial practice.

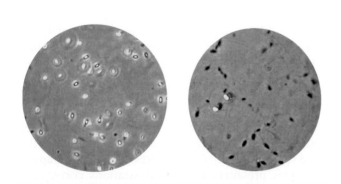

FIGURE 7.3 Bacterial spores seen through the phase-contrast microscope showing the birefringence of dormant spores (*left*) that coincides with high spore heat resistance, and opaque spores (*right*) that have germinated and lost their resistance to heat.

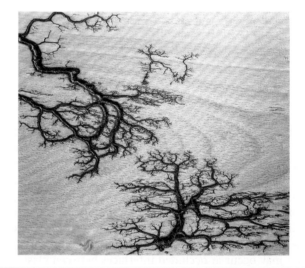

FIGURE 7.4 Fractal nature of high-voltage electric field into wood as an illustration of lethal agents where nonhomogeneous kinetics may be useful (ie, with radiation).

▶ MATHEMATICAL MODELING

In 1910, Chick[7] showed that microbial inactivation by moist heat resembled a first-order chemical reaction and that the temperature dependency of the corresponding rate constant was well described by Arrhenius law (note that "Acronyms and Abbreviations" section is provided at the end of this chapter for reference)

$$\frac{dN}{dt} = -kN \tag{1}$$

where, N is the concentration of microorganisms at time t, and k is the pseudo–first order inactivation rate constant, and t is time. The rate of inactivation (minus sign) was found to be proportional to the number of survivors (N). For isothermal lethal conditions, the solution is

$$ln[N(t)] = ln(No) - Kt \tag{2}$$

The last expression has the form of a straight line when the dependent variable is the logarithm of the number of viable spores. Using decimal logarithms equation (equation 2) is

$$log[No/N(t)] = t/D \tag{3}$$

The decimal reduction time (D) is the time required by the inactivation curve to go through an order of magnitude (for instance, from 1 000 000 to 100 000 CFUs/mL or a 1 log_{10} reduction of the population). Therefore, for isothermal conditions (square-wave heating), the time required to reach a desired reduction in the population of microorganisms can be estimated by multiplying the number of orders of magnitude by the decimal reduction time. The effect of temperature on the decimal reduction time is normally described using the parameter z, or the number of degrees of temperature required to change the decimal reduction time by a factor of 10. The Arrhenius law has been shown to be a better descriptor, but the temperature range of moist heat sterilization processes is small enough that both equations are expected to work reasonably well.[8] In addition, the decimal reduction time is often used to define the effect of the menstruum composition on the resistance of the test organisms. Figure 7.5 presents the application of the decimal reduction time obtained from corresponding thermal destruction time studies to define which of two solutions should be used as a master solution for routine qualification tests when z-values are significantly different.

In 1908, Chick[9] also explored chemical disinfection processes and found that the kinetics of inactivation could be described as a first-order chemical reaction and that the rate of inactivation was proportional to the number of survivors times the concentration to a power n. Thus, when the concentration of the lethal agent is to be considered, the model is

$$\frac{dN}{dt} = -kC^n N \tag{4}$$

Enter D_{250} and z data, and identify the corresponding solutions.

$z_1 := 10.09$ $z_2 := 12.31$ $D_1 := .54$ $D_2 := .45$

Solution 1 is: yyyyyyyy

Solution 2 is: xxxxxxxxxxx

The temperature at which the curves intersect each other in this case is:

intersetTemperature = 254.43   °F

n := 50   Number of points for the figure.
ORIGIN ≡ 1   i := 1.. n

Main formula to calculate D.   Temperature range.

$$D(T, D_{250}, z) := \frac{D_{250}}{\frac{T-250}{z}}$$ $T_1 := 230$ $T_2 := 260$

$$T_i := T_1 + \left(\frac{T_2 - T_1}{n}\right) \cdot (i - 7)$$ Temperatures for the graph.

Temperature := 250   First tentative value:
Solution block:
Given
D(Temperature, D_1, z_1) = D(Temperature, D_2, z_2)

Equation above will be satisfied at a temperature such that the values of D corresponding to different values for D at 250°F and z are equal.

intersetTemperature := Find(Temperature)

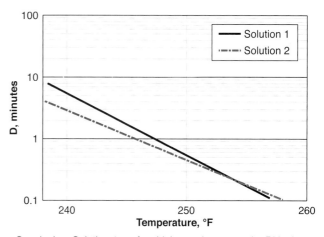

Conclusion: Solution 1 confers higher resistance to the BI in the temperature range of practical interest.

FIGURE 7.5   Use of the Bigelow (D_{250}, z) model to select a solution that imparts a higher resistance to bacterial spores within a temperature range for intended sterilization processes. This worksheet example performs the calculations to decide which solution will impart a higher heat resistance to a biological challenge (BI) when z-values differ significantly in the solutions (based on inspection of the decimal reduction time, D, and temperature curves). The data for D at 250°F and z-values for each solution are entered and analyzed between 245°F and 260°F (the temperature range of practical interest).

In this case, for instance for gas sterilization using ethylene oxide (EO), the decimal reduction time will include the kinetic constant k and the concentration to the power n.

The power n is often near one, and the rate of inactivation will be twice as fast if the concentration is doubled.

TABLE 7.1　Coefficient of dilution (n) for free chlorine, chlorine dioxide, and ozone[a]

Disinfectant	Organism	pH	Temperature (°C)	Range Disinfectant Concentration (mg/L)	n
Free chlorine	Naegleria gruberi	5.0	25	0.49-2.68	0.96
		7.0	25	0.78-3.44	1.19
		9.0	25	11.6-72.6	0.93
Free chlorine	Giardia muris	7.0	5	0.41-2.73	0.34
		7.0	5	11.1-78.5	1.52
		7.0	5	186-244	4.76
Free chlorine	G muris	5.0	25	4.9-13.0	1.35
		7.0	25	2.87-7.12	1.59
		9.0	25	15.5-84.1	0.90
Chlorine dioxide	Poliovirus type 1	7.0	5	0.4-1.0	1.05
		7.0	25	0.4-0.8	1.02
Chlorine dioxide	Escherichia coli	6.5	5	0.25-0.75	1.08
		6.5	10	0.25	1.18
		6.5	20	0.25	1.03
Chlorine dioxide	G muris	7.0	5	1.20	1.20
Chlorine dioxide	G muris	5.0	25	1.22	1.22
		7.0	25	1.30	1.30
		9.0	25	1.37	1.37
Chlorine dioxide	N gruberi	5.0	25	0.53-1.2	1.09
		7.0	25	0.41-1.3	0.93
		9.0	25	0.43-1.1	0.94
Ozone	N gruberi	5-9	25	0.21-1.05	1.0
		7	51-30		1.1
Ozone	G muris	5-9	25	0.02-0.19	1.2
		7	5-25	0.03-0.7	1.1

[a]From Hoff.[11]

There are cases such as the disinfection using phenolic compounds when n is near three.[10] This means that if the concentration is twice as large, the rate of inactivation will be 8 times faster. This theory may be limited within certain ranges of concentrations depending on the antimicrobial chemical under investigation and associated process conditions (eg, temperature, humidity, formulation, pH). Table 7.1 presents published values for exponent n corresponding to disinfection processes using chlorine, chlorine dioxide, or ozone as lethal agents.[11] Table 7.2 presents results of the application of these kinetic models to spore inactivation by EO in transient processes showing the accuracy of this approach and its potential usefulness to simulate practical applications[12] (see chapter 31 on EO sterilization).

TABLE 7.2　Comparison between calculated (using n = 1) and experimental numbers of survivors for transient ethylene oxide experiments[a]

Study	Target Concentration in mg/L	Microbial Enumeration = Average	Calculated Results
1	200	6.2×10^5	1.8×10^5
2	600	2.61×10^2	33
3	600	84	51
4	800	0	0.1

[a]From Rodriguez et al.[12]

In general, the decimal reduction time defines the rate of microbial inactivation.

There are a series of factors that have been found to have a significant effect on the value of the decimal reduction time such as temperature (T), water activity (Aw), pressure (P, at very high values), pH, radiation dose, etc. The decimal reduction time (D), or its natural logarithm [ln(D)] is therefore a function of a series of variables

$$\ln(D) = f(T, P, C, Aw, pH, dose, ...) \qquad (5)$$

Correspondingly, the spore log reduction (SLR) may be estimated for transient lethal treatments using the following formula:

$$SLR = \log\left(\frac{N_0}{N}\right) = \int_0^{time} \frac{dt}{D(T(t), C(t), P(t), pH, ...)} \qquad (6)$$

Use of this formula is illustrated in detail in Figure 7.6, as an example of the effect *of Aw* in a process.

The differential of the decimal reduction time as function of the mentioned series of variables is

$$d[\ln(D)] = \frac{\partial f}{\partial T}dT + \frac{df}{dP}dP + \frac{\partial f}{\partial C}dC + \frac{\partial f}{\partial A_w}dA_w$$
$$+ \frac{\partial f}{\partial pH}dpH + \frac{\partial f}{\partial dose}d\,dose + ... \qquad (7)$$

(Note: The notation is standard mathematical notation for partial derivatives of functions.)

Application of the Gauss law for the propagation of error enables us to define the corresponding variance

$$\sigma^2(\ln(D)) = \frac{\partial f}{\partial T}\sigma^2 T + \frac{df}{dP}\sigma^2 P + \frac{\partial f}{\partial C}\sigma^2 C$$
$$+ \frac{\partial f}{\partial A_w}\sigma^2 A_w + \frac{\partial f}{\partial pH}\sigma^2 pH + \frac{\partial f}{\partial dose}\sigma^2 dose + ... \qquad (8)$$

Therefore, the kinetic mathematical differential and its statistical variances are closely linked concepts.

Moist and Dry Heat

The ordered nature of the inactivation using thermal methods may be understood based on the idea that the corresponding molecular transformations require that the molecules surpass the energetic barrier represented by the activation energy. The Boltzmann distribution of the speed of the molecules for a certain molecular structure depends only on the absolute temperature. Figure 7.7 shows an example of the effect of absolute temperature on the shape of the corresponding frequency distribution curves for several absolute temperature values. Therefore, the fraction that will reach the energy needed to overcome the energetic barrier

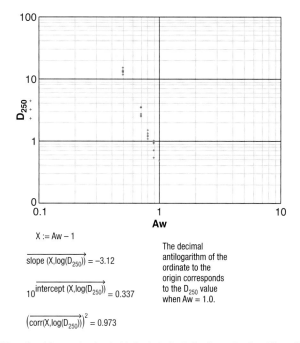

$X := Aw - 1$

$\overrightarrow{slope\ (X, \log(D_{250}))} = -3.12$

$10^{\overrightarrow{intercept\ (X, \log(D_{250}))}} = 0.337$

$\left(\overrightarrow{corr(X, \log(D_{250}))}\right)^2 = 0.973$

The decimal antilogarithm of the ordinate to the origin corresponds to the D_{250} value when Aw = 1.0.

Values of model parameters to calculate the decimal reduction time as function of Aw and T.

$D_0 := 0.4 \qquad m := -3.12 \qquad z := 11$

$$D(x) := D_0 \cdot 10^{m \cdot (Aw(x)-1)+\left(\frac{T_0 - T(x)}{z}\right)}$$

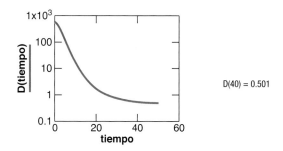

$D(40) = 0.501$

$$SLR(x) := \int_0^x \frac{1}{D(y)}\,dy$$

This function calculated the SLR. It uses the concentration and temperature regimes together with the kinetic parameters D0, m, and z.

FIGURE 7.6 Empirical description of the effect of water activity on the decimal reduction time. The function needed to calculate the spore log reduction corresponding to a sterilization process with variable Aw is included.

remains constant (for instance, 90%); thus, after D minutes, the inactivation transformation is expected to diminish the survivors by the same factor (for instance, 90%) and so on. In addition, the fraction that reaches the higher speed increases with temperature leading to a corresponding reduction in the value of the decimal reduction time. This interpretation has also been verified for condensed systems (eg, DNA suspensions).[13-15]

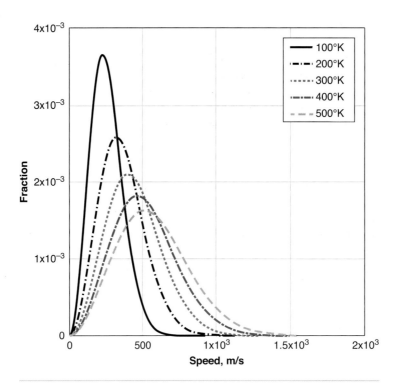

FIGURE 7.7 Distribution of the speed of molecules as a function of absolute temperature.

Estimation of the survivors to a moist or dry heat process may be performed using the following formula. The integration is to be performed numerically

$$N(t) = \frac{N_0}{10^{\left[\frac{1}{D_{250}}\int_0^t 10^{\frac{T(t)-250}{z}} dt\right]}} \quad (9)$$

Figure 7.8 presents the calculation of D_{250} (the D-value at 250°F) and z using survivorship data obtained with Stumbo method using the most probable number (MPN).[16]

Accumulated lethality is a very useful concept that enables comparison of sterilization processes performed using different temperature regimes [$T(t)$]. In particular, when the reference temperature is 250°F (121.1°C) and the z-value is 18°F (10°C), the F_0 is defined by the following formula:

$$Fo = \int_0^{time} 10^{\frac{T(t)-250}{18}} dt \quad (10)$$

Each minute of F_0 corresponds to the lethal effect of one minute at 250°F (121.1°C).

Thus, it enables comparison of diverse temperature regimes [$T(t)$]. For further discussion on thermal heat inactivation kinetics, see chapters 11 and 28.

Figure 7.9 presents an example of the determination of the kinetic parameters for Bigelow model (D_{250}, and z) using nonlinear regression. This is a powerful approach and it is sensitive to the initial values assumed for the parameters to be estimated. A graph of the temperature regime used is presented at the beginning of the worksheet and evidently not a perfect square wave. The sum of squares to be minimized consists of the accumulated differences between the estimated and the experimental values. The set of values for D_{250} and z selected will be the ones that minimize the sum of squares and therefore the difference between the experimental and estimated values for the survivors. This method enables the use of the actual temperature curves of the resistometer instead of the assumption of square wave heating or the use of empirical correction factors.

Chemical Inactivation (With Ethylene Oxide Gas)

Chemical inactivation kinetics has been particularly studied for EO sterilization (see chapter 31). The model described in the following text was validated for minimum moisture of 15%.[12] Chick model[9] applies

$$\frac{dN}{dt} = -kC^n N \quad (11)$$

$n := rows(time)$ Number of data pairs.

$p := degree + 1$ Number of parameter to be determined.

$i := 1..n$

$i := 1.. degree + 1$ Index variables

$a := 0.01$ Aliquot used

$MPN_i := \dfrac{1}{a} \cdot \ln\left(\dfrac{tubes_i}{negativeTubes_i}\right)$ Most probably number (MPN) of survivors calculated using Halvorson's Formula.

$N_0 := 6 \cdot 25600$ Initial number of survivors.

$D_i := \dfrac{time_i}{\log(N_0) - \log(MPN_i)}$

$X_{i,j} := (shiftedTemperature_i)^{j-1}$ Matrix X has the first column made of ones and the second column contains the shifted temperature data. This equation adjusts itself to the degree of the polynomial (in this case 1).

$Y_i := \log(D_i)$ Vector Y has the decimal logarithm of the decimal reduction times.

$b := (X^T \cdot X)^{-1} \cdot X^T \cdot Y$ Solve for coefficients b.

$b := \begin{pmatrix} 0.273 \\ -0.058 \end{pmatrix}$

$Y_{calculated}(x) := \sum_j \left(b_j \cdot x^{j-1}\right)$ This equation calculates the regression line. it adjusts itself to the degree of the polynomial (in this case 1).

A First-degree linear regression

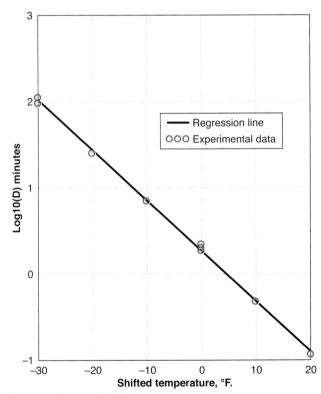

B Data and regression line

Analysis: Formulae for sums of squares and R^2 from Netter et al. 1990.

J is a matrix n by n made of ones: $J_{j,i} := 1$

Total sum of squares: $SSTO := Y^T \cdot Y - \dfrac{1}{n} \cdot Y^T \cdot J \cdot Y$

Error sum of squares: $SSE := Y^T \cdot Y - b^T \cdot X^T \cdot Y$

Regression sum of squares: $SSR := b^T \cdot X^T \cdot Y - \dfrac{1}{n} Y^T J \cdot Y$

Coefficient of multiple determination R^2: $R^2 := \dfrac{SSR}{SSTO}$ $R^2 = 0.999$

$MSE := \dfrac{SSE}{n-p}$ $MSR := \dfrac{SSR}{p-1}$

$F_{test} := \dfrac{MSR}{MSE}$ $F_{test} = 13261.104$

Compare F_{test} against $F_{critical}$ for $(1-\alpha)$ significance; and $p-1, n-p$ degrees of freedom:

$\alpha := 0.05$ level of significance.

$F_{critical} := qF(1-\alpha, p-1, n-p)$ $F_{critical} = 4.844$

The slope of the log-linear equation is b2. Thus, in this particular case, the mean z value in °F is

$z := \dfrac{-1}{b_2}$ $z := 17.152$

The mean value of D250 corresponds to a shifted temperature of zero:

$D_{250} := 10^{Y_{calculated}(0)}$ $D_{250} = 1.873$

In this section, we estimate the confidence intervals for z and D_{250}.

The estimated variance-covariance matrix $s^2\{b\}$ is

$$s_{squared} := MSE \cdot (X^T \cdot X)^{-1}$$

C Regression analysis

The confidence intervals for the elements of b are as follows:

$LowerCL_j := b_j - qt\left(1 - \dfrac{\alpha}{2}, n-p\right) \cdot \sqrt{s_{squared_{j,j}}}$

$UpperCL_j := b_j - qt\left(1 - \dfrac{\alpha}{2}, n-p\right) \cdot \sqrt{s_{squared_{j,j}}}$

qt(p,ν) is a MathCAD function that returns the inverse cumulative probability distribution for the student's t frequency distribution with p=(1−α/2) and n-p degrees of freedom.

We can calculate the corresponding confidence limits for z because of its relationship with the slope.

$LLD := \dfrac{-1}{LowerCL_2}$ $LLD = 16.761$

$ULD := \dfrac{-1}{UpperCL_2}$ $ULD = 17.562$

Therefor, we are $(1-\alpha) \cdot 100\%$ confident that the value of z is between LLD and ULD.

We shifted to the ordinates (temperature) by 250°F in order for the intercept of the curve to correspond to D_{250} and the formulae applied to element 1 of b enable us to calculate the confidence limits for D_{250}.

$LowerCL_1 = 0.246$ $10^{LowerCL_1} = 1.979$

$UpperCL_1 = 0.296$ $10^{UpperCL_1} = 1.979$

Upper and lower confidence limits for the decimal reduction time D.

D Estimation of confidence-level upper and lower values for D_{250} and z

FIGURE 7.8   Analysis of most probable number thermal death time results using the Stumbo procedure.[16]

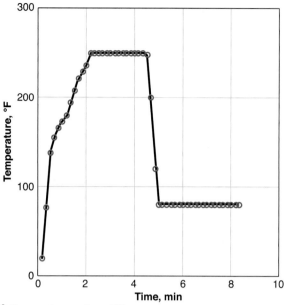

A Temperature regime - T(t)

$D_{250} := 0.55$ Tentative values for D_{250}, z, and the initial number of survivors.

$z := 20$

$Survs_0 := 3 \cdot 10^4$

$Temp(t) := interp(cs, time, T2, t)$ Temperature as a function of time using the cubic spline approximation.

$Temp(2.5) = 250$ Test.

$$Survs(t, D_{250}, z) := \frac{Survs_0}{\left[10^{\left[\frac{1}{D_{250}} \int_0^t \left[10^{\left(\frac{Temp(t) - 250}{z} \right)} \right] \right]} \right]}$$

Sum of squares to be minimized:

$$SSE(D_{250}, z) := \sum_k [\ln((testSurvs_k)) - \ln(Survs(testTime_k, D_{250}, z))]^2$$

Solution Block:

Given

$SSE(D_{250}, z) = 0$ $1 = 1$

$\begin{pmatrix} D_{250} \\ z \end{pmatrix} := Minerr(D_{250}, z)$

Here, the set of values for D_{250} and z that minimizes the difference between experimental and calculated data is determined using nonlinear regression.

$D_{250} = 0.7$ These are the values for D_{250} and z that minimize the error as previously defined.

$z = 11.295$

C Parameter determination (D_{250} and z) using nonlinear least squares

$$testTime := \begin{pmatrix} 1 \\ 1.5 \\ 2 \\ 2.5 \\ 3 \\ 3.5 \end{pmatrix} \qquad testSurvs := \begin{pmatrix} 22617 \\ 17883 \\ 11921 \\ 880 \\ 69 \\ 42 \end{pmatrix}$$

$$testTime := testTime + \frac{40}{60}$$

40 s added due to prevacuum time.

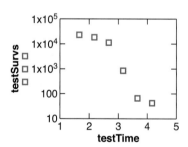

B Survivor experimental data

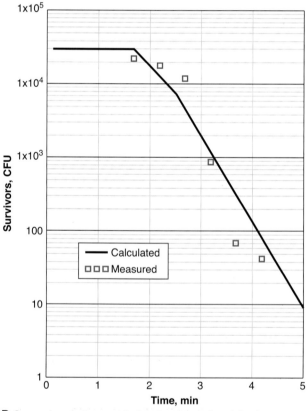

D Comparison between calculated and experimental values

FIGURE 7.9   Estimation of the decimal reduction time and z using nonlinear least squares regression.

As discussed previously, the coefficient of dilution n can vary depending on the antimicrobial and process conditions. The temperature and concentration are functions of time.

$$\frac{dN}{dt} = -k[T(t)]C(t)^n N \qquad (12)$$

Therefore, the logarithmic survivorship change is described by the following equation:

$$\ln\left(\frac{N_0}{N(t)}\right) = \int_0^{end} k[T(t)]C(t)^n \, dt \qquad (13)$$

The effect of temperature on the kinetic rate constant can be calculated using a Bigelow model

$$k[T(t)] = k_{T_r}10^{\frac{T-T_R}{z}} \qquad (14)$$

The survivors [CFUs; $N(t)$] can be calculated using the following equation:

$$N(t) = \frac{N_0}{\exp\left\{ k_{Tr} \int_0^{end} C(t)^n 10^{\frac{T-T_R}{z}} dt \right\}} \qquad (15)$$

And lethality (F) can be defined as follows:

$$F \equiv \frac{1}{kC^n} \ln\left(\frac{N_0}{N}\right) \qquad (16)$$

Equivalence between the decimal reduction time and the rate constant when concentration is relevant may be given by

$$D = \frac{ln(10)}{kC^n} \qquad (17)$$

And the formula for the accumulated lethality may be given by

$$F_{T_R, C_R, z} = \frac{1}{C_R^n} \int_0^t C^n(t) 10^{\frac{T(t)-T_R}{z}} dt \qquad (18)$$

Each minute corresponds to the lethal effect of 1 minute at the reference EO concentration and temperature. Thus, it should enable comparison of diverse concentration and temperature regimes. Figure 7.10 presents graphically the experimental and calculated data obtained using the earlier model to describe the inactivation of bacterial spores due to the lethal effect of EO.[12] The EO sterilization is further discussed in chapter 31.

Figure 7.11 presents the application of the kinetic model combined with the transport phenomena calculations

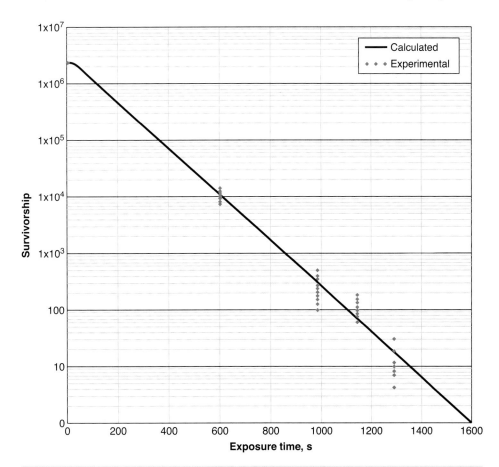

FIGURE 7.10   Comparison between measured and calculated Biological Indicator (BI) (spore) survivorship under an ethylene oxide sterilization cycle. The model applies when relative humidity is at least 15%.

Work sheet developed to calculate the mass transfer into the wall of a hollow cylinder.

This worksheet used MKS SI units.

Diffusivity (m²/s):   Internal radius (m): $a := \dfrac{0.00239}{2}$

$\alpha \equiv 2.35 \cdot 10^{-11}$ External radius (m): $b := \dfrac{0.00634}{2}$

$\text{radio} := \dfrac{0.00417}{2}$ Radius at the interface between the cap and the Luer, m.

Initial condition: $f(r) := 0$ The initial concentration of EO at the region of interest is zero.

Boundary condition:

$p(t) := 400$ BC at a.

$q(t) := 400$ BC at b.

Given

$\dfrac{1}{\alpha} \cdot u_t(r,t) - u_{rr}(r,t) - \dfrac{1}{r} \cdot u_r(r,t) = 0$

$u(r,0) = f(r)$

$u(a,t) = p(t) \qquad u(b,t) = q(t)$

$u := \text{Pdesolve}\left[u, r, \begin{pmatrix} a \\ b \end{pmatrix}, t, \begin{pmatrix} 0 \\ 10000 \end{pmatrix}, 50, 200\right]$ Solve for u(x,t) over the range r=a to b and t=0 to 10000

$r := a, (a + 0.00001) .. b \qquad t := 600$

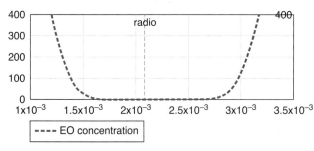

Figure showing that EO concentration reaches a minimum at the interface.

$t := 0, 10 .. 3000$

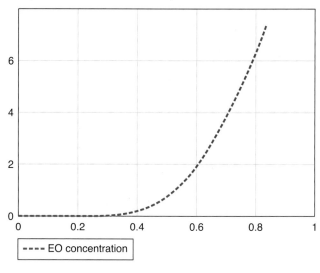

Figure showing the change in the EO concentration at the center with respect to the dimensionless time.

$T(x) := 120 \cdot \dfrac{9}{5} + 273.15 \qquad i := 1 .. (25 \cdot 60) \qquad t_i := i$

$C(x) := \dfrac{u(\text{radio}, x)}{1000}$

$k_R := \dfrac{2.303}{2.9 \cdot 60 \cdot \dfrac{600}{1000}} \qquad k_R = 0.022059$ Rate constant for D=2.9 min.

$N_0 := 1.6 \cdot 10^6$ Initial number of survivors.

$T_R := 54 + 273.15 \qquad T_R = 327.15 \qquad z := 29.4$ Reference temperature and z,K.

$N(x) := \dfrac{N_0}{e^{K_R \cdot 10 \int_0^x C(x) \cdot 10^{\frac{T(x) - T_R}{z}} dx}}$ This function calculates the survivors.

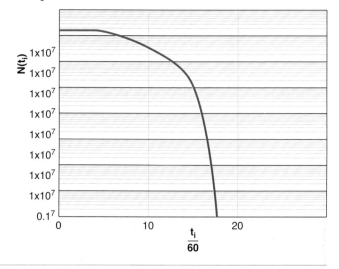

FIGURE 7.11   Estimation of the mass transfer of ethylene oxide gas in a hollow-cylinder configuration and of the corresponding lethal effect on survivorship of a biologic indicator.

required to estimate the mass transfer of EO through some plastic material configuration in the shape of a hollow cylinder. This configuration is very common in medical devices. This approach may be particularly used for occluded surfaces.

Initially, the mass transfer part is defined including the geometry, the initial condition, the boundary conditions, the diffusivity α, and the differential equation. Pdsolve is a numerical solver for partial differential equations provided by MathCAD versions 14 and 15. A graphical presentation of the change in EO concentration at the point of interest and the definition of inactivation is shown, in this case with an initial population of 1 million and a reference decimal reduction time of 2.9 minute. Finally, the spore inactivation is calculated using equation (15) and the numerical integration function provided by MathCAD. Other mathematical programs may be similarly used. Simulation of vented components is simpler because the mass transfer of EO does not need to be simulated using a convection approach.

Ultrahigh Pressure–High Temperature

The value of the kinetic constant in a moist heat sterilization process is determined by the composition of the menstruum, the physiological status of the spores, the temperature, and pressure. Under normal application conditions, the effect of pressure is negligible; however, when pressure reaches very high values, of the order of 680 MPa, there is a significant effect on the inactivation rate constant. For instance, in preliminary test of inactivation of *Geobacillus stearothermophilus* spores in a glucose solution, the process time required to achieve terminal sterilization in a large bag diminished from almost 2 hours for moist heat at 250°F to approximately 3 minutes using an ultrahigh-pressure system. In this system, the governing model remains as Chick defined in 1910:[7]

$$\frac{dN}{dt} = -kN \tag{19}$$

But the effect of pressure is added to the effect of temperature on the kinetic constant.[17] The differential of the logarithm of the kinetic rate constant has a pressure and a temperature component.

$$d\ln k \left(\frac{\partial \ln k}{\partial T}\right)_T dT + \left(\frac{\partial \ln k}{\partial P}\right)_P dP \tag{20}$$

The effect of temperature may be described using Arrhenius equation.

$$\left(\frac{\partial \ln k}{\partial T}\right)_P = \frac{Ea}{RT^2} \tag{21}$$

Where Ea is the activation energy, and R is the universal gas constant.

And the effect of pressure may be described using a similar activation volume equation.

$$\left(\frac{\partial \ln k}{\partial P}\right)_T = \frac{\Delta V^*}{RT} \tag{22}$$

Where ΔV^* is the activation volume.

Therefore, the combined model of the effects of temperature and pressure on the microbial inactivation rate constant is

$$k = k_o \exp\left\{-\left[\frac{\Delta V^*}{RT_0}(P - P_0) + \frac{Ea}{R}\left(\frac{1}{T} - \frac{1}{T_0}\right)\right]\right\} \tag{23}$$

And a corresponding equation for the survivorship is

$$N(t) = N_o \exp\left\langle -k_o \int_0^{processTime} \exp\left\{-\left[\frac{\Delta V^*}{RT_0}(P(t) - P_0)\right.\right.\right.$$
$$\left.\left.\left. + \frac{Ea}{R}\left(\frac{1}{T(t)} - \frac{1}{T_0}\right)\right]\right\}dt\right\rangle \tag{24}$$

Finally, the accumulated lethality equation can be

$$F_0 = \int_0^{processTime} \exp\left\{-\left[\frac{\Delta V^*}{RT_0}(P(t) - P_0)\right.\right.$$
$$\left.\left. + \frac{Ea}{R}\left(\frac{1}{T(t)} - \frac{1}{T_0}\right)\right]\right\}dt \tag{25}$$

Figure 7.12 presents the description of the inactivation of spores of *Clostridium botulinum* using the strain found at that time to be the most resistant bacterial spore to high-pressure inactivation.[18]

High pressure has also the effect of activating bacterial spores. Activated spores have broken dormancy and have lost most of their intrinsic resistance (resembling that of vegetative cells). Figure 7.13 presents the conceptual model including the activation, inactivation of activated spores, and the inactivation of dormant spores. The subpopulations are the dormant spores and the activated spores. Both subpopulations are undergoing the inactivation transformation (D), and the inverted triangles represent the inactivated spores corresponding to the two subpopulations. The corresponding formula for the survivors is

$$N_2[t] \to \frac{e^{-kdAt}(kA((-1 + e^{-(kA - kdA + kdD)t})}{\frac{N10 - N20) + (kdA - kdD)N20)}{-kA + kdA - kdD}} \tag{26}$$

where, $N_2(t)$ represents the CFUs. Figure 7.14 presents graphically the results of this activation-inactivation analysis compared to corresponding experimental results. The figure shows the activation hump expected whenever activation is a significant transformation.

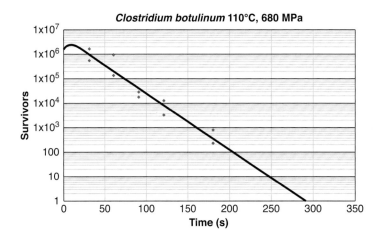

FIGURE 7.12   Model and verification for the inactivation of bacterial spores using ultrahigh pressure.

Radiation

The inactivation of microorganisms by lethal radiation follows also a well-ordered pattern similar to the one found for the effect of moist heat or other lethal agents. The main difference is that in the formula used to describe kinetics of inactivation due to radiation, the dose, instead of time, is used as the main independent variable (see chapter 29). Dose refers to the radiation energy delivered to a region. It is different from the radiation energy incident (fluence) because only a fraction of the radiation energy delivered to a region will be absorbed. The rate of change of the logarithm of the survivors with respect to dose can be given by

$$\frac{d \ln (N(Dose))}{dDose} = -a \qquad (27)$$

$$S(Dose) = \frac{N(Dose)}{N_0} = \exp(-a \times Dose) \qquad (28)$$

where S is the fraction of survivors to the radiation treatment.

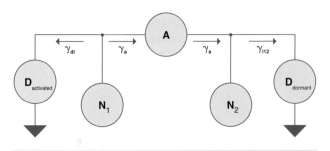

FIGURE 7.13   System diagram for bacterial spores undergoing sterilization. This system includes inactivation and activation and is applicable to ultrahigh-pressure processes. From Rodriguez et al.[17]

Equation 28 describes well the inactivation of many systems. For example, using data for the γ (^{60}Co) radiation inactivation of T1 phages,[19] the agreement with the model was excellent and enabled the calculation of the estimated mass of DNA present:

a = 0.0011 Gy^{-1}
Mean number of hits in the target region = a × Dose
E = mean energy transfer for primary ionization
E = 80 eV
1 eV = 1.602 × 10^{-19}J
1 Gy = 1J per kg
Mean energy per target region = a Dose E = D m
Mass (m) = E a = 1.4 × 10^{-17} kg

The actual mass of DNA double-strand molecule of the T1 phage was 5×10^{-17}, and this difference may be due to the fraction of inactive DNA. Overall, the model describes the lethal effect of radiation dose on the virus very well, but practical applications are more complicated. Lethality of radiation processes is primarily due to damage to the DNA (or other target nucleic acids). Radiation sterilization processes are more complicated due to the nonhomogeneous nature of the kinetics, to the potential of more than one copy of the chromosome in some microorganisms, and to the DNA repair mechanisms protecting the microorganisms. Thus, a bioburden-oriented approach to sterilization validation based on careful estimated measurement of the bioburden, determination of the lethal dose required using ISO standard reference tables, and dose distribution and verification provide the current practical solution to define the sterilization parameter required for safe radiation-sterilized products (see chapters 5, 29, and 64). Unfortunately, food products often have high bioburden values that require dose values that would render the corresponding radiation-sterilized food unacceptable (eg, due to malodor production).

Seed values and survivorship function:

$N_{10} := 10^6$

$N_{20} := 10^5$

$kdA := 1$

$kA := 0.01$

$kdD := 0.001$

$N_2(x,kdA,kA,kdD,N_{10},N_{20}) := \dfrac{\exp(-kdA \cdot x) \cdot [kA \cdot [[-1 + \exp[-(kA - kdA + kdD) \cdot x] \cdot N_{10} - N_{20}] + [(kdA - kdD) \cdot N_{20}]]]}{kdA - kA - kdD}$

A Response equations

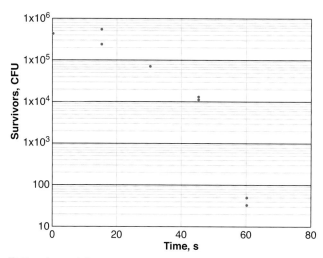

B Experimental data

$SSE(kdA,kA,kdD,N_{10},N_{20}) := \sum_k (\ln(testN_k) - \ln(N_2(testt_k,kdA,kA,kdD,N_{10},N_{20})))^2$

Given

$SSE(kdA,kA,kdD,N_{10},N_{20}) = 0$

$kdA > (kA,kdD)$

$N_{10} > 0$

$N_{20} > 0$

$\begin{pmatrix} kdA \\ kA \\ kdD \\ N_{10} \\ N_{20} \end{pmatrix} := Minerr(kdA,kA,kdD,N_{10},N_{20})$

$\begin{pmatrix} kdA \\ kA \\ kdD \\ N_{10} \\ N_{20} \end{pmatrix} = \begin{pmatrix} 0.186 \\ 0.071 \\ 0.109 \\ 3.005 \times 10^6 \\ 3.211 \times 10^6 \end{pmatrix}$

C Parameter determination

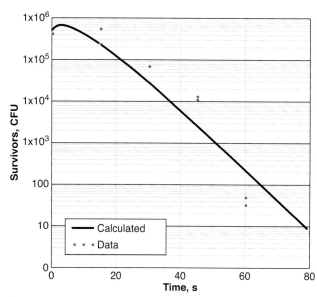

D Comparison between calculated and experimental values.

FIGURE 7.14 Description of spore (*Clostridium botulinum*) inactivation by ultrahigh-pressure and temperature using an activation-inactivation model.

◗ ANALYSIS OF CELL INACTIVATION DATA

Figure 7.15 presents data of microbial survivorship under lethal conditions, with the variability typical of industrial processes. Variability is originated by the microbiological agent under investigation, together with other sources such as the local conditions inside the production vessel, tolerances corresponding to the product components, etc. Currently, it is not practical to describe real-life industrial sterilization processes to the degree of detail that would include every source of variation. But this section deals with the task of estimating a process time that will lead to

a certain probability of a nonsterile unit (normally 10^{-6}) at a desired tolerance level (for instance, 95%-99%). One of the most powerful tools to do this includes least square regression; the other is distribution analysis of the results. Data analyzed may be a logarithmic-survivor curve in the form of CFUs or accumulate physical lethality (F_0). Least square regression will fit data to a linear combination of functions:

$$y(x) = b_0 + b_1\Phi_1(x) + b_2\Phi_2(x) + \ldots + b_n\Phi_n(x) \quad (29)$$

Not surprisingly, the most common such combination of functions for our purpose corresponds to polynomials

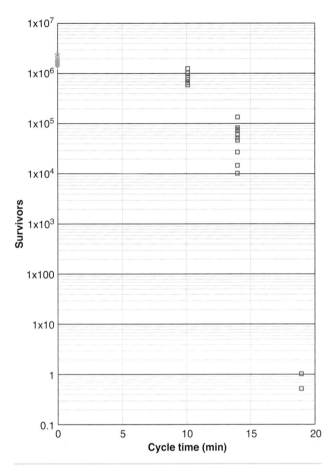

FIGURE 7.15 Typical bacterial spore inactivation behavior of inoculated product during an industrial sterilization cycle.

Distribution analysis allows for the normalization of the data with emphasis on the tails of the frequency distribution curves. This is important because in sterilization processes, the critical goal is to prevent process failure, and failure would occur at the worse-case tail regions. Thus, even if the normalization process shows some discrepancy in the areas closer to the mean, passing the included tests will enable the use of the normalized curves concerning the tails. Software used for this analysis (eg, Distribution Analyzer; Variation.com) has been validated by protocol for regulatory submissions such as to the US Food and Drug Administration in the United States. These software programs can enable the definition of the data and related parameters such as the upper specification (spec) limit, etc, and the data corresponds to a certain time in the process when the intended F_0-value was expected to have been reached. Figure 7.17 shows the results of the distribution analysis including the statement "with 99% confidence more than 99.9474% of the values are in spec.," which way be extremely useful to reach a conclusion regarding the efficacy of the sterilization process being developed, tested, or validated.

▶ MECHANISMS OF INACTIVATION AND RESISTANCE

Intrinsic and acquired resistance mechanisms in microorganisms can be important to consider in understanding the kinetics of microbial inactivation. Bacterial spores (particularly from *Bacillus subtilis*) are often cited and investigated as some of the more resistant forms of microorganisms to disinfection and sterilization processes (see chapters 3 and 4) and have been studied in some detail for their mechanisms of resistance and inactivation.[3,4,6] There are at least two main mechanisms of microbial inactivation: DNA damage (noting that injured organisms may lead to subsequent vegetative mutants) and damage to other structures required for activation and germination of the spores (see chapter 5). Damage to DNA is characteristic of inactivation using dry heat, ultraviolet light, γ radiation, EO, and other disinfectants such as nitrite, formaldehyde, desiccation, and, perhaps, antimicrobial plasmas. Wet heat and ultrahigh pressure affect other critical structures required for germination although the details are not completely understood. The lethal effect of chemical disinfectants may be further affected by the presence of detoxifying enzymes (including catalase in the case of hydrogen peroxide) and chemicals.[22] But the effect of ionizing radiation on fungal and vertebrate cells found that unrepaired DNA double-strand breaks are generally lethal.[23] The damage to DNA may be affected by DNA repair mechanisms present, particularly during germination and outgrowth. In addition, aqueous iodine was reported to elicit its antimicrobial activity by causing lysis after germination and not by causing DNA damage.[24] But bacterial

(expressions of more than two algebraic terms, especially the sum of several terms that can contain different powers of the same variable or variables), where powers of the independent variable are used. These are often expressed up to the first or second power. Polynomials are particularly useful, but the functions Φ may be very diverse including exponentials, trigonometric functions, etc. A great advantage of this approach is that the coefficients (b_i) of a linear combination of functions follow the F distribution[20] and the corresponding analysis leading to defining tolerance intervals, etc, are available.[21] For example, Figure 7.16 presents the regression and analysis of the survivorship data including the calculation of the exposure time needed to achieve the desired survivorship (or antimicrobial efficacy) at the agreed tolerance level (in this case, the upper 99%). It is important to use the extreme worse-case tolerance levels because failures due to the corresponding variability may occur within this interval; thus, the exposure time must account for the variability induced by the process, materials, test or target microorganism, etc, in order to achieve exposure process times that can be trusted.

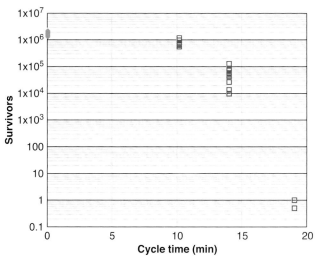

A Survivorship data of inoculated product during a production sterilization cycle

reducedData$_{q+rows(control),w}$:= data$_{(q),w}$ Data for regression include control data.

Regression

n := rows (reducedData)   n = 40   Number of experiments or observations used in calculations.

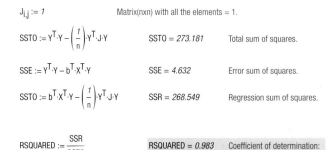

X$^{\langle 2 \rangle}$:= reducedData$^{\langle 1 \rangle}$ y := $\overline{log\left(reducedData^{\langle 2 \rangle}\right)}$ Y := y   Data values are presented in the last page.

degree := 2   Degree of Polynomial

i := 1.. n   j := 1.. n   l := 1 .. (degree + 1)   Index variables

X$_{i,l}$:= $(X_{i,2})^{l-1}$ Create columns of powers of X as required for selected polynomial degree. Elements of the first column of X matrix are equal to one as required by the least-square approach.

p := cols (X)   p = 3

k := p − 1   k = 2   Number of independent variables.

A := X^T·X   g := X^T·y

b := $\left(X^T \cdot X\right)^{-1}$·X^T·y

b = $\begin{pmatrix} 6.1888847097 \\ 0.3892220586 \\ -0.0379863099 \end{pmatrix}$ Coefficients for the quadratic model.

J$_{i,j}$:= 1   Matrix(nxn) with all the elements = 1.

SSTO := Y^T·Y − $\left(\frac{1}{n}\right)$·Y^T·J·Y   SSTO = 273.181   Total sum of squares.

SSE := Y^T·Y − b^T·X^T·Y   SSE = 4.632   Error sum of squares.

SSTO := b^T·X^T·Y − $\left(\frac{1}{n}\right)$·Y^T·J·Y   SSR = 268.549   Regression sum of squares.

RSQUARED := $\frac{SSR}{SSTO}$ RSQUARED = 0.983   Coefficient of determination:

B Least-square regression and analysis using a second degree polynomial

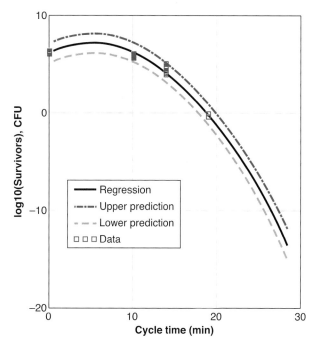

C Comparison of calculated and experimental values including corresponding 99% prediction-interval values

Calculate time required to reach logarithmic survivorship of −1 at the upper 99% prediction interval, spore log reduction (SLR) and probability of nonsterile unit (PNSU).

t := 40   Initial guess.

Given linterp (x$_o$, UP, t) = −1   timeNeeded99 := Find(t)

timeNeeded99 = 20.71

fracExposure99 := ceil(timeNeeded99 − exposureStart)

Results: Minutes of exposure required to reach 0.1 survivorship at the
Initial fracExposure99 = 11   up 99% tolerance level.

D Calculation of the required exposure time to reach 10^{-1} survivorship (or SLR >6) at the 99% upper prediction level

FIGURE 7.16 Estimation of the exposure time to a lethal agent needed to reach the desired spore logarithmic reduction (SLR) in a production sterilization cycle. Data correspond to representative inoculated product units placed randomly (or following an experimental design pattern) in the production load.

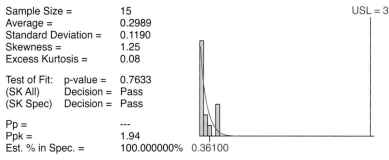

Minutes to reach 3 min. Fo (min) - Penetration
Beta Distribution (0.300343, 0.960209, 1.774071, 7.396485)

Sample Size =	15	
Average =	0.2989	
Standard Deviation =	0.1190	
Skewness =	1.25	
Excess Kurtosis =	0.08	
Test of Fit: p-value =	0.7633	
(SK All) Decision =	Pass	
(SK Spec) Decision =	Pass	
Pp =	---	
Ppk =	1.94	
Est. % in Spec. =	100.000000%	0.36100

USL = 3

With 99% confidence more than 99% of the values are below 1.66113
With 99% confidence more than 99.9474% of the values are in spec.

FIGURE 7.17   Using Distribution Analyzer (Variation.com) to establish that more than 99.9% of the accumulated F_0-values for a process are within specification at the 99% confidence interval.

spores are often not the only types of microorganisms that demonstrate extreme resistance mechanisms. A robust repair mechanism in *Deinococcus radiodurans*, as well as other resistance mechanisms, contributes to its extreme resistance to radiation.[25] *D radiodurans* can repair hundreds of radiation-induced double-strand break in the DNA molecule.[26] Further, *D radiodurans* is a polyploid organism enabling genomic protection to lethal agents that attack DNA, a luxury that is not present in other vegetative bacteria.[27] But at the same time, genes responsible for increased radiation resistance of *D radiodurans* can also transfer increased resistance into other bacteria such as *E coli* suggesting that many of these resistance factors can be induced in other bacteria.[28]

Microbial resistance can also be impacted by accessibility of the microbicidal process to the internal structures of the target microorganism. A good example has been described with the resistance *Pyronema domesticum* ascospores to physical and chemical (in particular EO) sterilization processes.[22] For example, the resistance of *P domesticum* ascospores to radiation was reported as D_{10} values of 2.83 kGy, which is higher than the D_{10} of 1.7 kGy used in the radiation sterilization (ISO 11137) standard.[29] On the other hand, others found that samples naturally contaminated with *P domesticum* had resistance levels no greater than that predicted by the bioburden-based resistance model (ie, population C) used for dose determination (method 1) described in ISO 11137 series of standards.[30] These results suggest variability in laboratory studies, which cannot be underestimated and should be read in detail.

A review of resistance mechanisms to radiation, recombination repair of DNA and chromosome organization if further considered elsewhere.[22,31] In addition, chapters 3, 4, and 5 discuss the mechanisms of action and resistance of lethal agents in greater detail.

▶ EFFECTS OF ENVIRONMENTAL CONDITIONS

Temperature

The effect of temperature on the kinetics of inactivation happens mostly through its effect on the value of the corresponding kinetic constant. This effect is described by the z parameter of the Bigelow model, the activation energy of the Arrhenius model, the activation enthalpy and entropy of Eyring model, etc. The temperature ranges used for sterilization or disinfection (including pasteurization) processes are relatively small, and any of the mentioned models describe the changes of the kinetic constant due to the temperature. In addition, many processes are performed using transient temperature regimes, where the temperature at the critical regions of the material(s) undergoing disinfection/sterilization is often far from a perfect isothermal regime. Therefore, a numerical integration of the contribution of many time increments needs to be performed. The formulas presented here may be implemented using available mathematical software, or even accounting worksheets. Figure 7.9 presents an example of the calculations needed to determine the parameters and to verify the accuracy of the corresponding estimated microbial inactivation. The effects of heat can be cumulative overtime, and this has been particularly shown in more heat-resistant microorganisms. For example, suboptimal moist heat treatment of *G stearothermophilus* spores that were subsequently stored under conditions that prevented their germination or outgrowth was shown to complete the lethal effect of the initial treatment.[32] Fungal ascospores, although less studied than bacterial spores, deserve some attention as they may be quite resistant to heat and radiation. Ascospores of *Neosartorya fischeri* were reported to survive heat treatment at 84°C for 120 minutes[33] and have been cited to have higher heat resistance than other fungal spores.[34] Concerning moist heat inactivation, others have explored the germination of *G stearothermophilus* using Raman spectroscopy and differential interference contrast microscopy.[35] Luu et al[36] studied the effects of heat activation on *Bacillus* spores with nutrients under high pressure.

Moisture

Kinetics of the inactivation of microorganisms is often strongly affected by the moisture content, often measured as relative humidity or *Aw*. For example, decimal reduction time of bacterial spores increases significantly (up to more than 20 times or more) when the Aw is below approximately 0.98. Therefore, occluded zones or other potential dry regions or conditions must be taken into consideration. Figure 7.6 shows the extremely significant effect and also illustrates the calculation of corresponding estimated survivor values. For many sterilization methods, humidification is an important variable to control to ensure an optimum inactivation process (eg, chemical disinfection or sterilization with EO, chapter 31, ozone in chapter 33, and chlorine dioxide in chapter 27).

pH

pH has a strongly significant effect on microbial inactivation kinetics in liquids. When applicable for the product, thermal-death-time tests are to be performed covering the intended pH range. An additional consideration is that pH and temperature interact and can be considered in the kinetics; for instance, the value of the decimal reduction time under different pH and temperature conditions benefits when the interaction terms are included into the corresponding analysis. Figure 7.18 presents the corresponding analysis of the effect of pH on the decimal reduction time for *C botulinum* spores undergoing moist heat sterilization. Earlier analysis showed that the percentage of variation in the decimal reduction time with respect to the mean value increased from 45% to 96% by including the temperature-pH interaction term into the analysis.[37] In addition, for food products, if the pH is lower than 4.6, the risk of botulin toxin formation through germination and growth of *C botulinum* becomes negligible. This fact leads to the classification of low acid–canned foods as the shelf-stable food products that require commercial sterility.[38]

Expected Chemical Demand

For many disinfectants, variables such as the environment in which the disinfectant is being applied and the presence of contaminating soils such as organic and inorganic

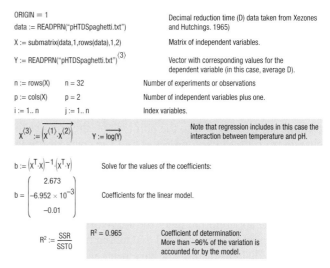

A Regression including interaction between pH and temperature

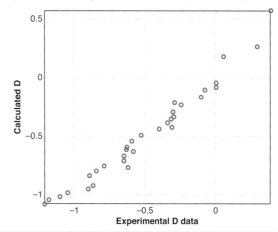

B Graph showing the correspondence between calculated and experimental values when the interaction between pH and temperature is considered. $r^2 > 0.96$.

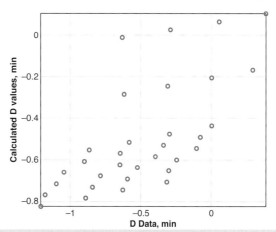

C Graph showing the correspondence between calculated and experimental values when pH and temperature are considered independently (no interaction). $r^2 > 0.45$.

FIGURE 7.18 Empirical description of the effect of pH on the value of the decimal reduction time (D) that benefits strongly in including a term to account for the interaction between pH and temperature.

materials can react with the lethal agent and reduce its availability for the intended process. A very relevant concern is that the kinetic models presented here to describe the kinetics of disinfection/sterilization assume that the availability of the lethal agent is not a limiting factor. If the demand for the disinfectant is high enough (for instance, after a long exposure time), the availability of the disinfectant may become low to the point where the kinetics to change from first to second order and the corresponding impact on the rate of inactivation is very significant. This was likely as a contributing factor to the development of the generation of kinetic models such as the Hom model[39] that include fractional powers of time as needed to fit the curve to the apparent tailing of the survivorship data. It is very important to keep in mind that tailing means that the intended lethal effect may not have been achieved or can be assumed, regardless of the circumstance that apparently good curve-fitting results may be obtained using fractional powers of time. Indeed, fractional powers of time would need further scientific justification in order to accept their use for rigorous industrial and scientific applications.

Accessibility of a Biocide to Targeted Organisms

Chemical disinfection processes depend strongly on the concentration of the lethal agent. If conditions are different from direct exposure to the biocide, and it must first go through a process of diffusion or convection in order to reach the regions intended for sterilization or disinfection, this transport process dominates the dynamics of the inactivation through the concentration terms in the appropriate formula. Some details of these transport phenomena are beyond the scope of this chapter; however, Figure 7.11 presents an example concerning sterilization using EO into an occluded area (a hollow cylinder), where the gas must diffuse through the cylinder to reach the master site or region of interest.[12] The corresponding calculation of the effect of the diffused gas on survivorship is also presented to illustrate the intimate linkage between transport phenomena and kinetics of inactivation in chemical sterilization or disinfection.

In addition, other processes can be affected by accessibility. Examples include:

- Presence or a biofilm (chapter 67) or other interfering factors
- Limit of radiation penetration or dose distribution (eg, with electron beam or ultraviolet light)
- Presence of air or other noncondensing gases in steam sterilization
- Cold spots in a load leading to longer come up times for dry heat or excessive condensation in steam leading to nonuniform cycles
- Break down of biocides on material contact (eg, with hydrogen peroxide into water oxygen due to presence of catalase or reactions with stainless steel)

◗ ADDITIONAL REFERENCES

The review by Ball and Olson[38] captures the most significant aspects of sterilization technology and science before the advent of computers systems. It includes the description of the Bigelow (D_{250}, z) model and of the Ball formula method currently used by the food industry to develop commercial sterilization cycles. Busta[40,41] presented the activation and injury transformations of bacterial spores; this is very relevant as it indicates the need to include other transformations besides the inactivation transformation to describe the sterilization processes. Wang et al[8] showed that both Bigelow model (D, z) and Arrhenius equation could be used to describe the parameters of inactivation kinetics using moist heat. The principles of thermal destruction are also described in some detail in previous editions of this book and further in chapters 11 and 28 of this edition. Finally, this author[13,42] describes in more detail the mathematical models and kinetic concepts presented here.

◗ ACRONYMS AND ABBREVIATIONS

ΔV^*:　activation volume

a:　proportionality constant in equations 27 and 28

Aw:　water activity or the relative humidity expressed as a fraction

b_i:　least square coefficients in equation 29

C:　concentration of the lethal agent

$C(t)$:　concentration of the lethal agent (eg, EO) as a function of time

C_R:　reference concentration of the lethal agent

D:　decimal reduction time

D_{250}:　decimal reduction time at 250°F

Ea:　activation energy

F:　time in minutes of exposure at T_R and C_R that would cause the same killing effect as the $T(t)$ and $C(t)$ regime

F_0:　time in minutes of exposure at *250°* and *z = 18°F* that would cause the same killing effect as the $T(t)$ regime

k:　rate constant

n:　Coefficient of dilution is an exponent that defines the effect of the concentration on the rate of inactivation. For instance, if n is 1 doubling the concentration will double the rate of inactivation (ie, EO), and if n is 3 (some phenolic compounds), doubling the concentration will increase the rate of inactivation by a factor of eight. Table 7.1 presents some published values corresponding to chlorine, chlorine dioxide, and ozone.

N:　number of survivors

$N(s)$:　number of survivors as function of dose in equations 27 and 28

$N(t)$:　number of survivors as function of time

N_0:　initial number of survivors

P: pressure
P_0: initial or reference pressure
R: universal gas constant
t: time
$T(t)$: temperature as a function of time
T_0: initial or reference temperature
T_R: reference temperature
z: number of degrees (°F) required to reduce the decimal reduction time by 90%
Φ: (Greek letter phi), function in equation 29

REFERENCES

1. US Food and Drug Administration. 21 CFR Part 113. Thermally processed low-acid foods packaged in hermetically sealed containers. US Food and Drug Administration Web site. https://www.accessdata.fda.gov/scripts/cdrh/cfdocs/cfcfr/CFRSearch.cfm?CFRPart=113. Accessed April 1, 2019.
2. US Food and Drug Administration. Compliance program guidance manual. Sterile drug process inspections. US Food and Drug Administration Web site. https://www.fda.gov/media/75174/download. Accessed April 1, 2019.
3. Gould GW, Hurst A. *The Bacterial Spore*. London, United Kingdom: Academic Press; 1969.
4. Aiba S, Toda K. Some analysis of thermal inactivation of bacterial-spore clump. *J Fermentation Tech*. 1966;44:301-304.
5. Andrew MHE, Russell AD. *The Revival of Injured Microbes*. London, United Kingdom: Academic Press; 1984.
6. Setlow P. Spore resistance properties. In: Driks A, Eichenberger P, eds. *The Bacterial Spore*. Washington, DC: ASM Press; 2016:201-215.
7. Chick H. The process of disinfection by chemical agencies and hot water. *J Hyg (Lond)*. 1910;10:237-286.
8. Wang DIC, Scharer J, Humphrey AE. Kinetics of death of bacterial spores at elevated temperatures. *Appl Microbiol*. 1964;12:451-454.
9. Chick H. An investigation of the laws of disinfection. *J Hyg (Lond)*. 1908;8:92-158.
10. Lambert RJW, Johnston MD, Hanlon GW, Denyer SP. Theory of antimicrobial combinations: biocide mixtures–synergy or addition? *J Appl Microbiol*. 2003;94:747-759.
11. Hoff JC. *Inactivation of Microbial Agents by Chemical Disinfectants*. Cincinnati, OH: Water Engineering Research Laboratory; 1986.
12. Rodriguez AC, Young W, Caulk K, Zelewski J, Kwasnica S, Aguirre S. Calculating accumulated lethality and survivorship in EtO sterilization processes. *Med Device Diagn Industry*. 2001;23:100-107.
13. Rodriguez AC. Modeling the inactivation of bacterial spores. In: Gomez M, Moldenhauer J, eds. *Biological Indicators for Sterilization Processes*. Bethesda, MD: Parenteral Drug Association; 2009:75-95.
14. Wang JC. Helical repeat of DNA in solution. *Proc Natl Acad Sci U S A*. 1979;76:200-203.
15. Depew RE, Wang JC. Conformational fluctuations of DNA helix. *Proc Natl Acad Sci U S A*. 1975;72:4275-4279.
16. Stumbo CR. *Thermobacteriology in Food Processing*. New York, NY: Academic Press; 1965.
17. Rodriguez AC, Larkin JW, Dunn J, et al. Model of the inactivation of bacterial spores by moist heat and high pressure. *J Food Sci*. 2006;69:E367-E373.
18. Margosch D, Ehrmann MA, Buckow R, Heinz V, Vogel RF, Gänzle MG. High-pressure-mediated survival of *Clostridium botulinum* and *Bacillus amyloliquefaciens* endospores at high temperature. *Appl Environ Microbiol*. 2006;72:3476-3481.
19. Kellerer AM. Models of cellular radiation action. In: Freeman RG, ed. *Kinetics of Nonhomogeneous Processes: A Practical Introduction for Chemists, Biologists, Physicists, and Materials Scientists*. New York, NY: John Wiley & Sons; 1987:305-375.
20. Neter J, Wasserman WW, Kutner MH, eds. *Applied Linear Statistical Models*. 3rd ed. Homewood, IL: Irwin; 1990.
21. Walpole RE, Meyers RH. *Probability and Statistics for Engineers and Scientists*. 6th ed. New York, NY: Macmillan Publishing Company; 1985.
22. McDonnell GE. *Antisepsis, Disinfection, and Sterilization: Types, Action, and Resistance*. 2nd ed. Washington, DC: ASM Press; 2017.
23. Resnick MA. Similar responses to ionizing radiation of fungal and vertebrate cells and the importance of DNA double-strand breaks. *J Theor Biol*. 1978;71:339-346.
24. Li Q, Korza G, Setlow P. Killing the spores of *Bacillus* species by molecular iodine. *J Appl Microbiol*. 2017;122:54-64.
25. Slade D, Lindner AB, Paul G, Radman M. Recombination and replication in DNA repair of heavily irradiated *Deinococcus radiodurans*. *Cell*. 2009;136:1044-1055.
26. Repar J, Cvjetan S, Slade D, Radman M, Zahradka D, Zahradka K. RecA protein assures fidelity of DNA repair and genome stability in *Deinococcus radiodurans*. *DNA Repair (Amst)*. 2010;9:1151-1161.
27. Ohtani N, Tomita M, Itaya M. An extreme thermophile, *Thermus thermophilus*, is a poliploid bacteria. *J Bacteriol*. 2010;192;5499-5505.
28. Gao G, Tian B, Liu L, Sheng D, Shen B, Hua Y. Expression of *Deinococcus radiodurans* Pprl enhances the radioresistance of *Escherichia coli*. *DNA Repair (Amst)*. 2003;2:1419-1427.
29. Richter SG, Barnard J. The radiation resistance of ascospores and sclerotia of *Pyronema domesticum*. *J Ind Microbiol Biotechnol*. 2002;29:51-54.
30. Lampe C, Hansen JM, Rymer TM, Sargent H. Sterilization of products contaminated with *Pyronema domesticum*. *Biomed Instrum Technol*. 2009;43:489-497.
31. Fletcher HL. Resistance to radiation, recombination repair of DNA and chromosome organisation. *Mutat Res*. 1981;80:75-89.
32. Mtimet N, Trunet C, Mathot AG, et al. Die another day: fate of heat-treated *Geobacillus stearothermophilus* ATCC 12980 spores during storage under growth-preventing conditions. *Food Microbiol*. 2016;56:87-95.
33. Conner DE, Beuchat LR. Heat resistance of ascospores of *Neosartorya fischeri* as affected by sporulation and heating medium. *Int J Food Microbiol*. 1987;4:303-312.
34. Zimmermann M, Miorelly S, Massager P, Aragao GM. Modeling the influence of water activity and ascospore age on the growth of *Neosartorya fischeri* in pineapple juice. *LWT Food Sci Tech*. 2011;44:239-243.
35. Zhou T, Dong Z, Setlow P, Li YQ. Kinetics of germination of individual spores of *Geobacillus stearothermophilus* as measured by Raman spectroscopy and differential interference contrast microscopy. *PLoS One*. 2013;8(9):e74987.
36. Luu S, Cruz-Mora J, Setlow B, Feeherry FE, Doona JD, Setlow P. The effects of heat activation on *Bacillus* spore germination, with nutrients or under high pressure, with or without various germination proteins. *Appl Environ Microbiol*. 2015;81:2927-2938.
37. Xezones H, Hutchings IJ. Thermal resistance of *Clostridium botulinum* (62A) spores as affected by fundamental food constituents. *Food Tech*. 1965;1003:113.
38. Ball CO, Olson FCW. *Sterilization in Food Technology: Theory, Practice, and Calculations*. New York, NY: McGraw-Hill; 1957.
39. Hom LW. Kinetics of chlorine disinfection of an ecosystem. *J Sanitary Eng Division*. 1972;2:183.
40. Busta FF. Introduction to injury and repair of microbial cells. In: Perlman D, ed. *Advances in Applied Microbiology*. New York, NY: Academic Press; 1978.
41. Busta FF, Ordal ZJ. Heat-activation kinetics of endospores of *Bacillus subtilis*. *J Food Sci*. 1964;29:345-353.
42. Rodriguez AC. Kinetics of the inactivation of bacterial spores in steam sterilization. In: Moldenhauer J, ed. *Steam Sterilization*. Bethesda, MD: Parenteral Drug Association; 2003:25-90.

Importance and Processes of Cleaning

Rizwan Sharnez

The purpose of cleaning a device or equipment is to render it suitable for further processing or for its intended use. From a regulatory and an end-user perspective, surfaces that are reusable should be free of visible residue, and microbial and chemical contaminants should be reduced to acceptable levels. The acceptable level of a contaminant depends on the purpose of the subsequent operation. For example, if cleaning is followed by disinfection or sterilization, it may be important for some applications that the bioburden (population of viable microorganisms) after cleaning should be less than the acceptable microbial load for the subsequent antimicrobial step. This criterion, an acceptance limit for postcleaning bioburden, is important in many environmental, manufacturing, and health care situations, such as in cleanrooms, pharmaceutical operations, food processing, and in health care facilities, where surface contamination with pathogens can pose an infection risk to humans. The ability of the cleaning operation to reduce contaminants to an acceptable level is also important in the preparation of newly manufactured and reusable medical devices prior to disinfection and sterilization. In addition to the requirements of the subsequent operation, storage conditions that affect microbial growth, such as time, temperature, moisture, and residual nutrients, are also important to consider when setting an acceptance limit for microbial contaminants.

Acceptance limits for chemical contaminants in many applications are derived from toxicological data. The data are used to derive an acceptable daily exposure (ADE) for the contaminant.[1-4] The ADE of a substance is the largest dose a subject can be exposed to per day for a lifetime by any route of administration without any observable adverse effects. The lower the ADE of the contaminant, the lower its acceptance limit, and therefore, the more sensitive the analytical method needs to be to verify that the contaminant is reduced to an acceptable level.

Initially, cleaning mechanisms, methods, processes, and equipment design considerations are discussed. The effect of cleaning parameters, clean hold time (CHT), and storage conditions on microbial growth and the formation of biofilms are then considered. Later in the chapter, cleaning practices for preventing corrosion and microbial contamination and a first principles approach for setting rational alert and action limits for postcleaning bioburden and chemical residues are described. The cleaning of reusable devices and clinical surfaces is further discussed in chapter 47.

▶ CLEANING METHODS, MECHANISMS, AND PROCESSES

The development and optimization of a cleaning process requires an understanding of cleaning methods and mechanisms, the interaction between chemical and transport processes, and the physicochemical properties of the soil and the surface. These elements of cleaning and cleaning process and equipment design considerations are discussed in this section.

Cleaning Methods and Processes

In industrial applications, cleaning methods and processes fall into two broad categories: *clean-in-place* and *clean-out-of-place*. Cleaning can also be categorized as *automated*, as in washer-disinfectors (see chapter 47) or *manual*, which typically involves wiping or scrubbing in a sink with the cleaning solution or solvent—hereafter referred to as the cleaning fluid.

Clean-in-place

Clean-in-place (CIP) is a widely used method of automated cleaning that is performed directly within manufacturing equipment with little or no equipment disassembly. It typically consists of a programmable cleaning cycle with multiple steps. In each step, a specific cleaning fluid (that may be a solvent such as water or a solution of various cleaning chemicals) is continuously circulated through the system at a controlled flow rate, temperature and cleaning agent concentration, and for a set duration. CIP is widely used in the food, dairy, beverage, brewing, pharmaceutical, and cosmetic industries to clean large fixed equipment, such as fermenters, bioreactors, centrifuges, heat exchangers, tanks, and piping. Vessels and other large equipment are cleaned by spraying the cleaning fluid on product contact surfaces, thereby creating a falling film of fluid on the surface. Piping and associated components, such as valves and pumps, are cleaned by flooding them with the cleaning fluid. Advantages of CIP systems include low labor requirement, fast equipment turnaround, and consistency. High initial investment and equipment maintenance costs and relatively high usage of water, chemicals, and energy are the main drawbacks.

Clean-out-of-place

Small vessels and parts that can be readily disassembled are typically cleaned out of place in a parts washer or a bath with a continuous circulation loop. Clean-out-of-place (COP) processes can be manual, semiautomated, or fully automated. COP systems are generally more customizable, require less initial investment and maintenance, and consume less water, chemicals, and energy than CIP systems. Labor requirements and equipment turnaround times, however, are generally higher for COP processes, especially for manual and semiautomated systems. Custom designed parts washers are generally more effective and efficient at removing tenacious deposits in localized "hot spots" that are deemed to be difficult to clean. This is because the nozzles in a parts washer can provide high fluid impingement and shear at specific locations. Examples of tenacious deposits are cell debris and denatured proteins that dry on heated surfaces in heat exchangers and autoclaves. Surfaces that are difficult to access, such as the insides of pumps, valves, and filling needles, can be cleaned effectively with sonication, typically at frequencies between 18 and 120 kHz. COP baths are also used to pre-soak and pre-clean parts to reduce cycle-time or facilitate the use of milder cleaning conditions for manual cleaning, such as a lower temperature and cleaning agent concentration, and the use of milder cleaning agents such as a weak alkali or acid.

Analytical Methods

Analytical methods that are widely used to quantitate chemical contaminants include conductivity, total organic carbon (TOC), chromatography, and ultraviolet and fluorescence spectroscopy. Additionally, sodium dodecyl sulfate polyacrylamide gel electrophoresis is used to assess fragmentation and aggregation of protein during cleaning.[5]

Conductivity is mainly used to verify clearance of ionic contaminants and cleaning chemicals such as alkali and acid cleaners. TOC is widely used to quantitate organic contaminants. It is also a useful method for detecting biological residues on reusable medical devices (see chapter 47).[6-8] The limit of quantitation (LOQ) of TOC is approximately 0.1 ppm, which is equivalent to approximately 5 μg/cm^2 for swab samples (R. Sharnez, unpublished data, 2019). In comparison, the visible residue limit of most process residues is between 1 and 4 μg/cm^2.[9] A drawback of TOC is that samples can become contaminated with organic solvents and disinfecting agents, such as alcohol, which in turn can result in apparent failures and complex investigations. Also, being a nonspecific method, TOC measures organic carbon in the *entire* residue, not just in the contaminant. Thus, *all* of the measured carbon in the residue is attributed to the contaminant, a worst-case assumption that can greatly overestimate the concentration of the contaminant. Another drawback of TOC is that the recovery is sometimes too low to accurately quantify the amount of *contaminant* in a sample.[10] Also, to accurately determine the recovery of a contaminant, the theoretical (ie, actual, not measured) carbon fraction of the contaminant in the residue is required. This information is seldom available for complex soils, such as human, plant and animal-based materials, proprietary culture media, and biological waste. These drawbacks are especially significant when the contaminant is composed of a relatively small fraction of the overall carbon in the residue. Product-specific assays, such as enzyme-linked immunosorbent assay and other immunoassays, overcome some of the limitations of TOC but can require more time and expertise to develop. They also have greater specificity and sensitivity; for example, the LOQ of most immunoassays is approximately 1 ppb.

Acceptance limits, when applicable, for bioburden and endotoxin, and alert and action limits for swab and rinse samples are discussed later in this chapter.

Cleaning Mechanisms

The effectiveness of a cleaning procedure is determined by numerous factors including the post-use equipment hold time, the type of soil, humidity, materials of construction, surface characteristics (defects, corrosion, and roughness), hydrodynamics (fluid shear), solubility, temperature, pH, cleaning chemistry, active and enabling ingredients in cleaning agents (surfactants, wetting chelating agents, and additives) and their concentrations, mechanical action (in manual cleaning), and the duration of each step in the cleaning process (time).[11] These factors are discussed in this section in the context of cleaning biological soils with aqueous cleaning solutions as an example.

Mechanisms Related to Soil and Surface Characteristics

The cleanability of a soil depends on several factors including composition, thickness of the deposit, surface defects and corrosion, affinity to the surface, and cohesive forces within the soil matrix; swelling, degradation, and denaturation of the soil during cleaning; and moisture content (dryness) and porosity (if the soil is sufficiently dry). Most soils become harder to clean as they lose moisture, but some soils can become easier to clean, and even slough off the surface, when they are sufficiently dry. Thus, the post-use hold time and drying rate can be critical in evaluating the cleanability of a soil. The drying rate is primarily determined by humidity, temperature, and circulation rate of the surrounding air. Because of their strong adhesive bond with most materials, proteins are likely to be the first soil constituent to attach to equipment surfaces, forming the framework for other constituents to attach. The adhesive bonds between proteins and some surfaces can be quite strong, especially if the deposit is formed on a hot surface as in a heat exchanger. Also, denaturation and aggregation of proteins increases with temperature and pH, which generally makes them harder to remove.

Mechanisms Related to the Cleaning Process

Most cleaning processes remove surface residues by mechanical means (fluid shear or scrubbing) and chemical diffusion (Figure 8.1). These mechanisms are facilitated by wetting, chemical reactions (hydrolysis), and solubilization. Cleaning processes for biological residues generally rely on both shear and diffusion to adequately remove them.

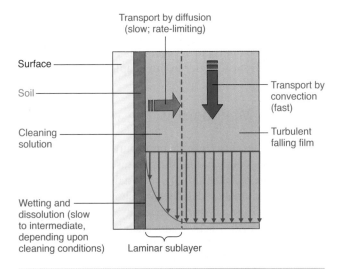

Transport by diffusion
(slow; rate-limiting)

Surface

Soil

Cleaning solution

Transport by convection (fast)

Turbulent falling film

Wetting and dissolution (slow to intermediate, depending upon cleaning conditions)

Laminar sublayer

FIGURE 8.1 Schematic representation of soil removal from a surface by diffusion-controlled mass transfer. Wetting and dissolution at the soil-cleaning fluid interface are followed by diffusion and convective transport.

Soil Removal by Fluid Shear

Fluid shear stress (τ_F) is the tangential force per unit of surface area exerted by the flowing cleaning fluid on the surface. For a given flow rate and configuration, τ_F increases with fluid viscosity. Also, viscosity decreases sharply with temperature; for example, the viscosity of water at 20°C (1 centipoise) is over 2.8 times greater than it is at 80°C (0.35 centipoise). Thus, at a given flow rate, τ_F decreases substantially with increasing temperature. For this reason, soil removal by fluid shear is more effective at a lower temperature.

Under optimum cleaning conditions, the shearing action of the fluid can remove over 90% of the soil. Depending on the type of soil and surface, and the drying conditions (post-use equipment hold time, temperature, and humidity), the minimum shear stress required to effectively remove process residues ($\tau_{F,MIN}$) is typically of the order of 1 N/m^2 (10 dynes/cm^2). For pipes and hoses, this corresponds to an average fluid velocity of approximately 5 ft/s and a Reynolds number (Re) of approximately 10,000. For dairy deposits, which are typically very difficult to remove, $\tau_{F,MIN}$ was reported to be between 0.75 and 2.5 N/m^2.[12] Fluid shear also aids in removing biofilms, especially those with structures that protrude beyond the laminar sublayer into the turbulent zone (see Figure 8.1).

Soil Removal by Diffusion

Diffusion is the movement of a chemical species A through a mixture of A and a medium B because of a concentration gradient of A. Ordinarily, this movement occurs from a region of higher concentration to a region of lower concentration. The rate of diffusion is determined by the magnitude of the concentration gradient of A in B, and the diffusivity of A in B (D_{AB}). For liquids, D_{AB} increases with temperature and decreases with viscosity and molecular weight (size) of A. Thus, for a given chemical contaminant (A) and cleaning fluid (B), the kinetics of cleaning by diffusion *increases* with temperature. Increasing the temperature generally also provides the additional advantages of higher solubility and faster rate of hydrolysis and other chemical reactions, such as those that break down proteins into peptides and other smaller fragments. Smaller fragments are generally more soluble and have higher diffusivities and are therefore more readily removed from the surface by diffusion.

Equipment and Design Considerations

Equipment should be designed and maintained to ensure adequate contact with cleaning fluids and proper drainage. Surfaces should be sloped at an angle of repose of at least 5 degrees to facilitate drainage. Dead ends should be avoided, but if they are necessary, the length-to-diameter ratio should be minimized and preferably should be less than two. Equipment should be fabricated with materials and surface finishes that resist corrosion under processing and cleaning conditions. Surfaces with high free surface energy, such as stainless steel and glass, are more hydrophilic and generally have greater bacterial attachment and biofilm formation rates than hydrophobic surfaces such as Teflon, Viton, ethylene propylene diene monomer, and silicone rubber.

Flow of cleaning fluids should be turbulent to provide sufficient fluid shear at the surface. Typically, this requires a Re greater than 4000 for pipes and hoses and a flow rate greater than 2.5 gpm per foot for a falling film. Also, the velocity of cleaning fluids should be sufficient to ensure flooding of pipes and hoses. Typically, this requires the average fluid velocity to be greater than 5 ft/s.

Another important consideration is the residence time or turnover rate of water in the system and its effect on microbial growth. For a given equipment configuration, the lower the fluid velocity, the longer the residence time. With longer residence times, disinfectants can become less effective and water temperatures can rise. These conditions generally favor microbial growth and the formation of biofilms. Increases in coliform contamination have been reported in distribution systems with longer residence times.[13] Additionally, at lower fluid velocities, particles are more likely to settle and thereby create new habitats for microbial growth. Residence time can be reduced by eliminating dead legs in pipes and periodic flushing of stagnant zones. Routine flushing and equipment maintenance can help identify mistakenly closed valves, dead legs, and other areas of poor circulation.

Cleaning Cycle

Based on the cleaning mechanisms and equipment design considerations discussed in previous sections, cleaning cycles in industrial processes often include the following steps.

Pre-rinse

The purpose of a pre-rinse is to wet the soil and physically remove it from the equipment. Wetting weakens the cohesive bonds between soil components, thereby facilitating their removal by fluid shear. It also opens up pathways for soil components to diffuse into the cleaning fluid, and for cleaning chemicals to diffuse into the soil matrix during subsequent chemical washes. As discussed earlier, because of the inverse relation between temperature and fluid shear, pre-rinses are generally more effective at a lower temperature. Pre-rinsing at a lower temperature also minimizes denaturation, aggregation, and subsequent redeposition of proteins and other biological macromolecules on equipment surfaces.

At sufficiently high fluid shear (typically of the order of 1 N/m^2), the pre-rinse can remove over 90% of the soil. Under these conditions, the optimum duration of the pre-rinse is generally between 1 and 5 minutes. A more precise estimate of the optimum duration of the pre-rinse can be obtained by monitoring the concentration of solids in the effluent rinse water by measuring optical density, for example, and noting the time it takes for the effluent to become clear.

Alkaline Wash

Alkaline cleaning chemicals such as sodium hydroxide (NaOH) can be very effective at removing proteins and other biological resides from device and equipment surfaces. Alkaline cleaning agents hydrolyze proteins into peptides and other fragments that are more soluble and therefore less likely to aggregate and redeposit on equipment surfaces. They can also enhance wetting and solubilization. These mechanisms are generally favored at higher NaOH concentration, that is, higher pH; however, most proteins denature and aggregate rapidly at NaOH concentrations above 1% and temperatures greater than 70°C (R. Sharnez, unpublished data, 2019). Because denatured protein aggregates are generally more difficult to clean, the optimum concentration and temperature of NaOH for cleaning proteinaceous soils is typically between 0.5% and 1% (pH approximately 12.5) and between 50°C and 70°C. Under optimum conditions, an alkaline wash can reduce most proteinaceous residues to visually undetectable levels within 5 to 10 minutes.

In some instances, the duration of the alkaline wash can be shortened or otherwise optimized by adding surfactants and wetting agents (as in formulated cleaning agents; see chapter 6). Nonionic wetting agents are good emulsifiers and can reduce foaming. Sequestrants, such as sodium phosphate derivatives, may be required to chelate minerals in hard water and prevent them from precipitating during the cleaning process. Chlorine compounds and peroxides, such as sodium hypochlorite (bleach) and hydrogen peroxide, can also enhance the effectiveness of alkaline cleaning agents; however, they can corrode stainless steel and other metals, especially at concentrations and temperatures above 1% and 50°C (R. Sharnez, unpublished data, 2019).

Intermediate Rinse

The alkaline wash is typically followed by an intermediate rinse to remove the cleaning agent and entrained particles.

Acid Wash

An acid wash is sometimes necessary to remove inorganic constituents and precipitated minerals. It is also used to passivate stainless steel and other metal surfaces.

Final Rinse

The purpose of the final rinse is to reduce residual cleaning chemicals and entrained particles to acceptable levels. The final rinse is performed with high purity water, such as water for injection (WFI), or distilled or deionized water.

The effectiveness of the earlier steps is determined by several equipment parameters such as contact between cleaning fluids and soiled surfaces (spray coverage), drainability of equipment surfaces, and effective control of critical process parameters (CPPs) such as flow rate and temperature and concentration of the cleaning fluids.[14-16] Spray coverage is evaluated at full scale with a dilute aqueous suspension of riboflavin. Bench-scale cleanability studies are used to optimize CPPs[12,17-19] and identify suitable master soils for developing and validating cleaning procedures at full scale.[20,21]

Various other cleaning formulations and processes can be used depending on the type of soil and the acceptable level of the contaminant. These can be as simple as using high purity water alone, particularly for residues that are highly soluble in water, but can also include the following:

- Organic solvents such as methanol for residues that are not water soluble
- Acid cleaners as described earlier for inorganic residues
- Formulated cleaners with additives that facilitate cleaning, such as surfactants, chelators, and wetting agents
- Enzyme-based cleaners that target specific types of biological macromolecules, such as proteases for proteins and lipases for lipids (see chapter 47)

▶ EFFECT OF CLEANING PARAMETERS ON GROWTH OF MICROORGANISMS

The effect of cleaning parameters and operating conditions on the growth rate of bacteria in clean equipment and the formation and propagation of biofilms and surface pitting are discussed in this section. The growth rate of bacteria serves as a good indicator of the growth of other microorganisms in the environment because conditions that limit the growth of bacteria generally also limit the growth of other environmental microorganisms.

The growth rate of microbes in clean equipment is determined primarily by the initial bioburden and concentration of nutrients (organic carbon) in the residual final rinse water. In sterile operations, the final rinse is typically performed with WFI, for which the specifications for bioburden and TOC are <10 colony-forming units (CFUs)/100 mL heterotrophic plate count (HPC) and <0.5 ppm organic carbon, respectively. Published data on the growth rates of bacteria under similar conditions is reviewed in the next section. The results are used to estimate microbial growth during storage and its potential impact on the effectiveness of subsequent operations.

Growth Rate of Bacteria in Water

The growth rate of bacteria in water has been investigated by several researchers. Their data are reviewed in this section and the results are used to determine acceptable postcleaning bioburden and storage times for process equipment.

Culture generation times for stock cultures of six enteric bacterial species in autoclaved river water samples were estimated to be between 33 and 90 hours at 30°C, and between 100 and 1000 hours at 20°C.[22] No growth was detected for three of the six species (*Proteus rettgeri*, *Salmonella* ser Senftenberg, and *Enterobacter aerogenes*) at 5°C; generation times for the other three species (*Escherichia coli*, *Arizona arizonae* [now *Salmonella enterica* subsp *arizonae*], and *Shigella flexneri*) ranged between 500 and 1000 hours at 5°C. The results are summarized in Table 8.1. Nutrient levels in these studies were of the order of 10 ppm (3.0 ppm ammonia nitrogen, 5.1 ppm protein, 2.8 ppm carbohydrates, and 3.2 ppm orthophosphates; pH 6.9). In water samples with approximately half the concentration of these nutrients, no growth was detected, suggesting that neither of these species were capable of significant growth at nutrient levels below 5 ppm under the test conditions. These results are consistent with those of others who observed generation times between 39 and 100 hours at 37°C for *E aerogenes* in media where the carbon source was rate limiting,[23,24] and bacterial growth rates between 0.008 and 0.049 per day in drinking water systems.[25] In other studies, the lag phase for bacteria in river water samples and water distribution systems was estimated to be about 24 hours.[28,29]

The earlier results are corroborated by studies on the kinetics of microbial growth in purified water.[29,30] In these studies, when bacterial counts were brought below the limit of detection (LOD) of the assay, it took approximately 72 hours for the counts to reach 10 CFUs/100 mL, the specification for WFI. Also, results from studies on the growth of heterotrophic bacteria in fresh drinking water from three surface water samples indicate that there was no measurable change in viable counts in all three samples for the first 7 days.[26] The TOC content of the three samples was 2.6, 3.1, and 3.7 ppm.

In studies of groundwater that was contaminated with treated waste, the growth rate (G) of planktonic bacteria was estimated to be between 0.001 and 0.047 per hour, which corresponds to doubling times ($\tau = \ln 2/G$) between 14.7 and 693 hours.[27] The samples were collected at different distances from the source of contamination and evaluated based on assimilation of tritium-labeled thymidine into bacterial nucleic acid. A more recent study investigated the survival and growth of total coliform,

TABLE 8.1 Culture generation times for stock cultures of six enteric bacterial species in autoclaved river water samples

Bacterial Species	Culture Generation or Doubling Time	Water Source or Nutrient Concentration (ppm)	Temperature (°C)	Comments
Hendricks[22]				
Escherichia coli	>500 hours	~10[a]	5	In water samples with approximately half the concentration of these nutrients, no growth was detected, suggesting that neither of these species were capable of significant growth at nutrient levels below 5 ppm.
Arizona arizonae	>500 hours	~10[a]	5	
Shigella flexneri	>500 hours	~10[a]	5	
Proteus rettgeri	NA (no growth detected)	~10[a]	5	
Salmonella ser Senftenberg		~10[a]	5	
Enterobacter aerogenes		~10[a]	5	
Postgate et al[23] and Postgate and Hunter[24]				
E aerogenes	39–100 hours	Carbon source was rate limiting.	37	
Boe-Hansen et al[25]				
Various	14–87 days	Drinking water	Ambient	Bacterial growth rates: 0.008-0.049 per day
Miettinen et al[26]				
Various heterotrophic bacteria	NA (no growth detected)	Three drinking water samples with the following TOC content: 2.6, 3.1, and 3.7 ppm C	Ambient	There was no measurable change in viable counts in any of the three samples for the first 7 days.
Harvey and George[27]				
Various planktonic bacteria	14–693 hours	Groundwater contaminated with treated waste	Ambient	

NA, not applicable.

[a]3.0 ppm ammonia nitrogen, 5.1 ppm protein, 2.8 ppm carbohydrates and 3.2 ppm orthophosphates; pH 6.9.

E coli and HPC bacteria in surface water and contaminated drinking water.[31] The water samples were spiked with monocultures of *E coli* and other HPC bacteria, and the viable counts were monitored over a period of 21 days. Their data are summarized in Table 8.2. The results indicate that at 25°C, the viable count of HPC bacteria increased by only 23% over the first 5 days and then decreased steadily over the next 16 days, and those of total coliforms decreased steadily from the start and dropped below LOD of the assay by the 10th day.

TABLE 8.2 Growth of detectable coliforms, *Escherichia coli*, and heterotrophic plate count bacteria in surface water and contaminated drinking water[a]

Species	Class	Change in Viable Counts (VC) Over 21 Days		
		15°C	**25°C**	**37°C**
HPC	Oligotrophic	Increased by 12% over first 4 days and then decreased over next 17 days	Increased by 23% over first 5 days and then decreased over next 16 days	Increased by 40% over first 5 days and then decreased over next 16 days
Coliforms	Copiotrophic	VC decreased from the start and fell below the limit of detection after 10 days.		
Escherichia coli				

HPC, heterotrophic plate count.

[a]From Sakyi and Asare.[31]

Relevance to Aseptic Operations

The growth rate of microbes in water increases with the concentration of nutrients. Also, TOC is a good indicator of nutrient levels in water. In most aseptic operations, TOC in the final rinse water is typically below 1 ppm organic carbon (OC) (R. Sharnez, unpublished data, 2019). The water used in the earlier studies had significantly higher levels of TOC, and yet, the observed growth rates of bacteria were insignificant. Thus, the much lower levels of nutrients in WFI and other high purity water would not support significant microbial growth. It follows that when essential nutrients in the final rinse are at sub-ppm levels, which is typical for cleaning processes in aseptic and other high-risk operations, the growth of microbes in the residual water after cleaning would not present a tangible risk to the efficacy of the subsequent disinfection and sterilization steps and, therefore, to microbial contamination of the product or device. But sub-ppm levels of nutrients are sufficient for some microorganisms to form biofilms. Also, trace levels of chloride and sulfate ions can lead to pitting and other types of corrosion in stainless steel and other metals. The importance of cleaning in preventing the formation and propagation of biofilms and corrosion is discussed later in this chapter.

▶ IMPLICATIONS FOR STORAGE AND CLEAN HOLD TIME

In this section, the growth rates of bacteria in water presented in the previous section are used to justify acceptance limits for bioburden and TOC in the context of storage following cleaning.

Clean Hold Time

Clean hold time (CHT) refers to the duration for which the device or equipment is stored following cleaning. It is the time interval between the end of cleaning and the start of the subsequent operation, typically disinfection (or sanitization), sterilization-in-place, steam sterilization (autoclaving), or batch processing.

Equipment that is stored in a wet state after cleaning is at risk of becoming contaminated. For this reason, validation of CHTs is a regulatory expectation for equipment that is used to manufacture pharmaceutical products and intermediates:

> There should be some evidence that routine cleaning and storage of equipment does not allow microbial proliferation. For example, equipment should be dried before storage, and under no circumstances should stagnant water be allowed to remain in equipment subsequent to cleaning operations.[32]
>
> The period and when appropriate, conditions of storage of equipment and the time between

cleaning and equipment reuse, should form part of the validation of cleaning procedures. This is to provide confidence that routine cleaning and storage of equipment does not allow microbial proliferation. In general, equipment should be stored dry, and under no circumstances should stagnant water be allowed to remain in equipment subsequent to cleaning operations.[33]

In both these references, the primary concern is microbial growth and proliferation during storage. Requirements for CHT validation studies are described elsewhere.[34,35] In these studies, the equipment or parts are held for the specified duration after cleaning and then rinsed with WFI, distilled water, or water of comparable quality. Rinse water samples are collected and tested for bioburden and endotoxin. Acceptance limits for these samples are typically set to compendial specifications, such as to the United States Pharmacopeia (USP) specifications for WFI at <10 CFUs/100 mL for bioburden and <0.25 EU/mL for endotoxin.

The variables that affect microbial growth during storage include the initial storage state (including initial bioburden, nutrient levels, and residual water), the time and temperature of storage, and protection from external recontamination. Studies on the growth of several enteric bacterial species in water indicate that at nutrient levels below 5 ppm OC growth slows down to undetectable levels (see previous section). Also, numerous studies on the growth of bacteria in river and drinking water samples indicate that in the context of CHTs less than a few days, microbial growth in water does not present a tangible risk of contamination at levels below 1 ppm OC. Nonetheless, organic carbon levels in the final rinse should be minimized and equipment hold times should be as short as possible to reduce the risk of forming a biofilm, especially in systems that are not disinfected or sterilized after cleaning.

Drying the equipment after cleaning is an effective way to prevent microbial growth during storage. Equipment, glassware, devices, and hoses can be stored for extended periods if they are dried and closed or sealed after cleaning to prevent the entry of microbes, water, or other extraneous matter. This criterion is based on the rationale that water is essential for the growth of microorganisms. With this approach, it is important to thoroughly inspect the equipment or part to make sure that it is dry before it is sealed and that it does not become wet during storage. The drying time can be reduced by improving drainage, using hot water for the final rinse, and adding an air blow or an alcohol wipe or rinse following the cleaning. If hot water is used for the final rinse, the equipment or part should not be closed or sealed until it reaches the storage temperature. This practice prevents moisture in the air from condensing on internal surfaces during storage.

For equipment that cannot be dried after cleaning, bioburden at the end of the CHT can be estimated from first principles and by making reasonable worst-case assumptions. For instance, assuming that the cells are in the exponential phase of growth during storage represents a worst-case scenario from the standpoint of microbial growth and the final bioburden (n). With this assumption, the growth of the cells can be modeled as

$$n = n_0\, e^{G\,(t - t_0)} \tag{1}$$

where n and n_0 are the final and initial number of viable cells, respectively (ie, the bioburden at time t and t_0), and G is the growth rate of the cells. The doubling time (τ) is obtained by setting n/n_0 to 2, thus

$$\tau = (\ln 2)\,/\,G \tag{2}$$

Based on data from studies on the growth rate of bacteria in water (see previous section), the average growth rate at ambient temperature (20°C-25°C) is estimated to be approximately 0.01 hr^{-1}, thus

$$\tau = \frac{\ln 2}{0.01/\mathrm{hr}} \sim 3\ \text{days} \tag{3}$$

Historical data for representative WFI rinse water samples indicate that the initial bioburden should typically be ≤1 CFUs/100 mL (R. Sharnez, unpublished data, 2019). Based on this initial bioburden (n_0) and a doubling time of approximately 3 days, the bioburden in the residual rinse water in the equipment can be estimated as a function of CHT (t) (Table 8.3). Thus, even with the worst-case assumption of exponential growth, it would take about 10 days for the bioburden to increase by 1 log (10-fold) under these conditions (ie, if the TOC of the final rinse water is approximately 1 ppm OC). A change in bioburden of this magnitude is well within the capability of most disinfection and sterilization processes because they are generally designed to reduce bioburden by several orders of magnitude. Note that this analysis is based on a relative change in bioburden, that is, it is independent of the initial bioburden; thus, the above conclusion

applies to cleaned equipment in general, regardless of the initial bioburden in the final rinse water. Additionally, for cleaning procedures with a process capability of about 1 CFU/100 mL for the final rinse, it would take approximately 10 days for the bioburden to exceed the USP specification for WFI, which is, 10 CFUs/100 mL. Based on this analysis, a CHT of less than 10 days should not typically present a tangible risk for closed systems if the TOC of the final rinse water is approximately 1 ppm OC.

Implications for Endotoxin in the Final Rinse

Bacterial growth and proliferation can result in elevated levels of endotoxin in residual rinse water. This is a concern for parenterals, for example, because endotoxin can be pyrogenic (see chapter 66). The implications of CHT on endotoxin levels in residual rinse water are assessed in this section for equipment that is rinsed with WFI. The USP specification for endotoxin for WFI is 0.25 EU/mL. Also, at least 500 bacterial cells are required to generate approximately 0.25 EU. The minimum time required to generate 0.25 EU in 1 mL of WFI can be estimated using Equation 1

$$n = n_0\, e^{G\,(t - t_0)}$$

Therefore, if we consider the worst-case substitutions of the final number of cells (n) = 500, the initial number of cells (n_0) = 10 CFUs/100 mL (the USP specification for bioburden for WFI), and G = 0.01 hr^{-1} (the growth rate of bacteria in water, discussed previously), then

$$\Delta t = \frac{\ln (500/0.1)}{0.01/\mathrm{hr}} = 852\ \text{hr} \tag{4}$$

where $\Delta t\,(t - t_0)$ is the *minimum* time required to generate 500 cells, and therefore 0.25 EU, in 1 mL of WFI. Thus, even under the most favorable conditions, it would take at least 852 hours or 35 days for the endotoxin concentration to increase by 0.25 EU/mL in WFI. Consequently, a CHT of a few days should be acceptable from the standpoint of endotoxin concentration in the final WFI rinse. This analysis illustrates the importance of cleaning and CHT in the context of disinfection and sterility assurance. It also provides a rational approach for deriving acceptance limits for post-cleaning bioburden and TOC.

▶ IMPLICATIONS FOR CORROSION AND FORMATION OF BIOFILMS

Nutrient-deficient conditions trigger phenotypic changes of planktonic (unattached) bacteria and their transition to the sessile (attached) state. Under these conditions, the attachment of bacteria to wet surfaces can occur within

TABLE 8.3 Estimated bioburden in residual rinse water from equipment at a doubling time of 3 days as a function of clean hold time

Clean Hold Time (Days)	Bioburden (CFUs/100 mL)
0	1
3	2
6	4
9	8
12	16

CFUs, colony-forming units.

a few minutes of making contact with the surface. Once attached, microorganisms can aggregate, grow into microcolonies, and form biofilms (see chapter 67). Other factors that influence biofilm formation are substrate composition, surface chemistry, topography,[13,36] and inadequate fluid shear during cleaning.[37] In most sterile operations, high-risk product contact surfaces are cleaned and disinfected daily; however, many environmental surfaces, such as storage tanks and pump exteriors, walls and ceilings are cleaned less frequently, which increases the risk of biofilms forming on wet surfaces.

Biofilm Formation

Improperly cleaned surfaces promote soil buildup and contribute to the development of biofilms. Recent studies have shown that biofilms can even develop under relatively dry conditions.[38] Microorganisms within biofilms can be pathogenic and can contaminate process fluids or the product either via direct contact with contaminated surfaces or indirectly through exposure to aerosols or condensate that originate from contaminated surfaces. Biofilms are difficult to remove because they have an insoluble layer of sticky extracellular polymeric substances (EPS) that protects them from cleaning and disinfecting agents. Therefore, effective control of biofilms relies on good equipment design, environment controls, and effective cleaning and disinfecting procedures to prevent their formation. The effectiveness of biofilm control can be monitored using analytical methods such as adenosine triphosphate bioluminescence for rapid nonspecific estimation of active biological residues or plate count methods for enumeration and identification of viable microbes.

The formation of a biofilm begins with the attachment of planktonic cells to the surface (see chapter 67 for a detailed description of the underlying mechanisms and kinetics of this phenomena). Adhesion of the cells to the surface is enabled by secretion of sticky EPS. Once attached, they continue to secrete EPS, forming a biofilm around them. The layers of EPS associated with biofilms form a protective barrier between the microorganisms inside the biofilm and the outside environment. Thus, microorganisms within biofilms are far more resistant to cleaning and disinfecting agents than planktonic microorganisms and, consequently, are more likely to survive and proliferate. The higher survival rate of the microbes increases the risk of contamination, reduced shelf life, and disease transmission. Additionally, EPS that are not removed during cleaning provide attachment sites for microorganisms newly introduced to the cleaned system. As they mature and propagate, biofilms can clog fluid handling systems, impede heat transfer, and corrode metal surfaces. Some microorganisms in biofilms catalyze chemical and biological reactions that can lead to pitting and other types of corrosion in stainless steel and other metals. The pits provide a protective habitat for microorganisms to grow and form biofilms, thereby increasing the possibility of microbial contamination.

Preventing the Formation of Biofilms

Methods used to prevent the formation of biofilms include mechanical and manual cleaning, chemical cleaning and disinfection; good equipment design and maintenance; periodic flushing for 5 to 30 minutes with hot water at 70°C to 80°C or superheated water at approximately 125°C at high fluid shear (of the order of 3 N/m^2). Equipment should be prerinsed with water at ambient temperature and high fluid shear before being flushed with hot cleaning fluids. The prerinse prevents biological macromolecules such as carbohydrates and proteins from "cooking" onto and attaching more firmly to hot surfaces. Also, the flushes should be sufficiently hot to prevent insoluble particles from redepositing on equipment surfaces. The application and effectiveness of the earlier methods has been discussed in the literature.[13,36,37] The importance of cleaning in preventing the formation and propagation of biofilms and pits is further discussed in this section.

Cleaning problems often occur at dead ends and at flange gasket interfaces. Such locations may not have sufficient exposure to cleaning and disinfecting chemicals to remove soil and kill microorganisms effectively. The surviving microorganisms can form a biofilm that resists subsequent cleaning and disinfection. An effective way to prevent the formation of biofilms is to steam critical surfaces after cleaning and disinfection. Biofilms are very unlikely to form in well-designed and operated equipment that is routinely and effectively steam-treated. Typically, biofilms form on external surfaces such as drains and walls. Also, aerosols containing viable microorganisms can form during cleaning. Aerosolization provides a means of dispersal of microorganisms present in biofilms. Aerosols are formed during the washing and spraying of surfaces and drains or when biofilms dry and release dust particles.

Once biofilms form, cleaning the surface becomes a lot more difficult because of the EPS matrix associated with the biofilm. An effective cleaning procedure must break up or dissolve the EPS matrix so that disinfecting agents can gain access to the colonizing cells. Chlorine is commonly applied as a disinfectant due to its oxidizing and disinfecting properties (see chapter 15). Its most toxic form, hypochlorous acid, is generated from hypochlorite ion at pH 4 to 7. Up to 15 to 20 ppm residual chlorine for 5 to 30 minutes may be required to control biofilm fouling.[39] Depending on its concentration, chlorine can be readily inactivated by organic compounds, so the presence of soil and biofilm can significantly reduce its effectiveness. Chlorine dioxide and chloramines are more effective as sanitizers and are widely used in the food industry (see chapters 15 and 27). Monochloramine was found to be more effective at penetrating bacterial biofilms than chlorine, but chloramines required longer contact time to be effective.[39-41] Alkali cleaners, especially with chelators such as ethylenediaminetetraacetic acid (EDTA), were found to be more effective than acidic cleaning agents in removing biofilms. Prolonged cleaning with alkali cleaners containing chelators is necessary to remove biofilms. Further, disinfectants may be required to inactivate microorganisms remaining on the surface after cleaning.

A well-designed and operated cleaning process can remove 90% or more of microorganisms associated with the surface but cannot be relied on to always reduce bioburden to an undetectable level. Surviving bacteria in particular can redeposit at locations that favor the formation of biofilms. Thus, including a disinfection step after cleaning to prevent the formation of biofilms may be necessary in some instances. Separate disinfecting steps following cleaning are not very common, particularly if the cleaning process involves the use of hot, alkaline cleaning solutions. They are more common in situations where the cleaning process involves a neutral pH cleaner at ambient temperature, as with manual cleaning of disassembled parts. In such cases, a disinfectant that is commonly used is 70% isopropanol or other alcohols (see chapter 19). In addition to being effective disinfectants, alcohols can also facilitate drying of the equipment, which reduces the possibility of biofilm formation.[35]

The major types of disinfectant used in the bioprocess industry are halogens, peroxygens, acids, and quaternary ammonium compounds. The effectiveness of chemical disinfectants is limited by the presence of soil, hardness of water, temperature, and their ability to physically contact the surviving microorganisms. Disinfectant selection may also be based on whether or not a biofilm is likely to be present, the organic load associated with the biofilm, and the ability of the disinfectant to physically remove contaminants as opposed to causing them to become more firmly attached to the surface (see chapter 67). The risk of biofilm formation and subsequent microbial proliferation can also be reduced by minimizing hold times and cleaning down to lower residue (nutrient) levels. Lower concentrations of nutrients on the surface generally result in a longer lag phase and lower microbial growth rate.

Corrosion of metals can influence the effectiveness of chlorine-based cleaning agents and disinfectants against microorganisms in biofilms, especially when they are used at lower concentrations. The corrosion products react with residual chlorine, preventing the active ingredients from penetrating the biofilm and gaining access to the microorganisms. Thus, the choice of pipe material and the accumulation of corrosion products can have a significant impact on the formation of biofilms. In addition to the level of generalized corrosion, localized pitting and other surface defects can provide a protective habitat for microorganisms to form biofilms or colonize existing ones. Chlorides and sulfates can increase pitting in some metals, especially at high concentrations, whereas phosphoric acid and phosphate-based corrosion inhibitors

can help reduce corrosion rates. In full-scale studies, phosphate-based corrosion inhibitors were found to reduce coliform levels in water purification systems.[42]

▶ ALERT AND ACTION LIMITS FOR BIOBURDEN AND TOTAL ORGANIC CARBON

The risk of microbial contamination in most systems increases with post-cleaning (initial) bioburden and the concentration of available nutrients. A good indicator of available nutrients is the TOC of the final rinse water. In this section, alert and action limits for bioburden and TOC in the final rinse water are set based on the data for bacterial growth in water presented in previous sections.

Total Organic Carbon

In previous sections, the doubling time of bacteria in water that contained approximately 5 ppm OC was estimated to be about 72 hours. Thus, an alert limit of 5 ppm OC provides assurance that bacterial growth during the growth phase, typically a few days, would be of the order of 1 log. This level of change in bioburden is not significant in the context of typical disinfection and sterilization operations. Additionally, most well-designed and operated cleaning processes are capable of reducing organic carbon levels in the final rinse water to that of the incoming water, which is typically below 1 ppm OC. Thus, an alert limit of 5 ppm OC is also reasonable from the standpoint of processes capability. If the process capability limit for TOC in the rinse water is greater than 5 ppm, the alert limit should be set to the process capability limit. Action limits for TOC should be set based on a risk assessment and analysis of historical data and trends. If such data are unavailable, it is recommended that the action limit be set to two times the alert limit.

Bioburden

Because of the potentially serious consequences of a microbial contamination, the alert limit for bioburden in the final rinse (B_{ALT}) should be set based on the capability of the cleaning process (B_{PCL}). Also, most well-designed and operated cleaning processes can physically remove or kill most detectable microorganisms (R. Sharnez, unpublished data, 2019). For such cleaning processes, B_{PCL}, the process capability limit for bioburden, would be virtually the same as that of the incoming water that is used for the final rinse (B_{IN}), that is, B_{PCL} is approximately equal to B_{IN}. In such instances, the alert limit for bioburden in the final rinse should be set based on B_{IN}. Action limits for bioburden should be set based on a risk assessment and analysis of historical data and trends. If such data are unavailable, it is recommended that the action limit be initially set to two times the alert limit.

REFERENCES

1. International Society for Pharmaceutical Engineering. *ISPE Baseline Guide. Risk-Based Manufacture of Pharmaceutical Products.* 2nd ed. North Bethesda, MD: International Society for Pharmaceutical Engineering; 2017.
2. Sharnez R, To A. Strategies for setting rational MAC-based limits part III: leveraging characterization and toxicological data. *J Validation Technol.* 2011;17:24-28.
3. Sharnez R, Horner M, Spencer A, Tholudur A. Biopharmaceutical cleaning validation: leveraging acceptable exposure of host-cell protein to set acceptance limits for inactivated product. *J Validation Technol.* 2012;18:38-44.
4. Sharnez R, Spencer A, To A, Tholudur A, Mytych D, Bussiere J. Biopharmaceutical cleaning validation: acceptance limits for inactivated product based on gelatin as a reference impurity. *J Validation Technol.* 2013;19:1.
5. Sharnez R, Spencer A, Romero J, et al. Methodology for assessing product inactivation during cleaning Part I: Experimental approach and analytical methods. *J Validation Technol.* 2012;18:42-45.
6. International Organization for Standardization. *ISO/DIS 15883-5:2019: Washer disinfectors—Part 5: Performance Requirements and Test Method Criteria for Demonstrating Cleaning Efficacy.* Geneva, Switzerland: International Organization for Standardization; 2019.
7. McDonnell G, Sheard D. *A Practical Guide to Decontamination in Healthcare.* Oxford, United Kingdom: Wiley-Blackwell; 2012.
8. US Food and Drug Administration. *Reprocessing Medical Devices in Health Care Settings: Validation Methods and Labeling; Guidance for Industry and Food and Drug Administration Staff.* Silver Spring, MD: US Food and Drug Administration; 2015.
9. Forsyth R. Ruggedness of visible residue limits for cleaning validation. *Pharm Technol.* 2009;33:102-111.
10. Sharnez R, To A. Recovery factors for cleaning validation Part I—Homogeneous solutions and suspensions. *J Validation Technol.* 2012;18:57-60.
11. Sharnez R, Klewer L. Strategies for developing a robust cleaning process part II: demonstrating cycle effectiveness. *Am Pharm Rev.* 2012;15:3.
12. Fan M. *Fundamental Understandings and Optimization Strategies of In-Place Cleaning* [dissertation]. Columbus: Ohio State University; 2018.
13. LeChevallier MW. Conditions favouring coliform and HPC bacterial growth in drinking water and on water contact surfaces. In: Bartram J, Cotruvo J, Exner M, Fricker C, Glasmacher A, eds. *Heterotrophic Plate Counts and Drinking-Water Safety: The Significance of HPCs for Water Quality and Human Health.* London, United Kingdom: IWA Publishing; 2003.
14. Sharnez R, VanTrieste M. Quality-by-design for cleaning validation. In: Pluta P, ed. *Cleaning and Cleaning Validation.* Vol 1. Bethesda, MD: Davis Healthcare; 2009; chap 6.
15. Sharnez R. Strategies for developing a robust cleaning process Part I: Application of quality by design to cleaning. *Am Pharm Rev.* 2010;13:77-80.
16. Sharnez R, Monk M. Strategies for enhancing the performance of cleaning processes Part I: A framework for assessing performance. *J Validation Technol.* 2011;17:36-39.
17. Sharnez R, Lathia J, Kahlenberg D, Prabhu S, Dekleva M. In situ monitoring of soil dissolution dynamics: A rapid and simple method for determining worst-case soils for cleaning validation. *PDA J Pharm Sci Technol.* 2004;58(4):203-214.
18. Sharnez R. Leveraging small-scale models to streamline validation. *J Validation Technol.* 2008;14:4.
19. Sharnez R, To A, Annapragada R. Experimental parameters for small-scale cleaning characterization. Part II: Effect of fluid velocity on the kinetics of cleaning. *J Validation Technol.* 2015;21:1.
20. Sharnez R. Streamline new product introductions with master soils. *J Validation Technol.* 2009;15:24-29.
21. Sharnez R. Master soils for cleaning cycle development and validation: a case study. In: Pluta P, ed. *Cleaning and Cleaning Validation.* Vol 2. Bethesda, MD: Davis Healthcare; 2009; chap 9.
22. Hendricks C. Enteric bacterial growth rates in river water. *Appl Microbiol.* 1972;24:168-174.
23. Postgate JR, Crumpton JE, Hunter JR. The measurement of bacterial viabilities by slide culture. *J Gen Microbiol.* 1961;24:15-24.
24. Postgate JR, Hunter JR. The survival of starved bacteria. *J Gen Microbiol.* 1962;29:233-263.
25. Boe-Hansen R, Albrechtsen HJ, Arvin E, Jørgensen C. Bulk water phase and biofilm growth in drinking water at low nutrient conditions. *Water Res.* 2002;36:4477-4486.
26. Miettinen IT, Vartiainen T, Martikainen PJ. Contamination of drinking water. *Nature.* 1996;381:654-655.
27. Harvey RW, George LH. Growth determination for unattached bacteria in a contaminated aquifer. *Appl Environ Microbiol.* 1987;53:2992-2996.
28. Adam O, Kott Y. Bacterial growth in water. *Toxicity Assess.* 1989;4:363-375.
29. Mittleman MW. Biological fouling of purified-water systems: Part III, Treatment. *Microcontamination.* 1986;4:30-40.
30. Dreeszen PH. *Biofilm: The Key to Understanding and Controlling Bacterial Growth in Automated Drinking Water Systems.* 2nd ed. Waterford, WI: Edstrom Industries; 2003.
31. Sakyi PA, Asare R. Impact of temperature on bacterial growth and survival in drinking-water pipes. *Res J Environ Earth Sci.* 2012;4:807-817.
32. US Food and Drug Administration. *Guide to Inspections of Validation of Cleaning Practices.* Washington, DC: US Government Printing Office; 1993.
33. Pharmaceutical Inspection Co-Operation Scheme. *Recommendations on Validation Master Plan, Installation and Operational Qualification, Non-Sterile Process Validation Cleaning Validation, Pharmaceutical Inspection Convention.* Geneva, Switzerland: Pharmaceutical Inspection Co-Operation Scheme; 2007. Document PI 006-3.
34. LeBlanc DA. Equipment cleaning validation: microbial control issues. *J Validation Technol.* 2002;8:40-46.
35. LeBlanc DA. Microbiological issues in process equipment cleaning validation, Part I: Basic issues. *Pharm Microbiol Forum Newsl.* 2007;15:10.
36. Chmielewski R, Frank JF. Biofilm formation and control in food processing facilities. *Compr Rev Food Sci Food Saf.* 2003;2:22-32.
37. Mittleman MW. Structure and functional characteristics of bacterial biofilms in fluid processing operations. *J Dairy Sci.* 1998;81:2760-2764.
38. Alfa MJ. Biofilms on instruments and environmental surfaces: do they interfere with instrument reprocessing and surface disinfection? Review of the literature. *Am J Infect Control.* 2019;47(suppl):A39-A45.
39. LeChevallier MW, Cawthon CD, Lee RG. Inactivation of biofilm bacteria. *Appl Environ Microbiol.* 1988;54:2492-2499.
40. LeChevallier MW, Lowry CD, Lee RG. Disinfecting biofilms in a model distribution system. *J Am Water Works Assoc.* 1990;82:87-99.
41. LeChevallier MW, Lowry CD, Lee RG, Gibbon DL. Examining the relationship between iron corrosion and the disinfection of biofilm bacteria. *J Am Water Works Assoc.* 1993;85:111-123.
42. LeChevallier MW, Welch NJ, Smith DB. Full-scale studies of factors related to coliform regrowth in drinking water. *Appl Environ Microbiol.* 1996;62:2201-2211.

CHAPTER

9

Ultraviolet Disinfection

Ernest R. Blatchley III and Thomas P. Coohill

Downes and Blunt[1-3] conducted a series of logical, ordered experiments to examine the behavior of bacteria and fungi when exposed to sunlight. Their experiments, which were conducted in the absence of many of the analytical tools that are common among academic and industrial laboratories today, demonstrated several interesting conclusions:

- (Sun)light is detrimental to the development of bacterial and fungal communities.
- The extent of exposure to sunlight appears to be related to the extent to which growth of these microbial communities is suppressed.
- The actinic (ie, ultraviolet [UV]) portion of the solar spectrum is primarily responsible for this behavior.

This classic work may be viewed as the first demonstration of the effects of UV radiation on microbial communities. In the time since these basic discoveries were reported, the effects of UV radiation on microorganisms and microbial communities have been elaborated in detail. Today, UV-based disinfection systems are commonly applied in many settings. Numerous important contributions to our current understanding of the mechanisms of action of UV radiation on microorganisms and critical biomolecules were presented in the 1950s and 1960s. Subsequent expressions of concern with common forms of disinfection, such as chlorination, promoted research to incorporate these findings with developments of fundamental photochemical reactor theory, which in turn facilitated rapid increases in the usage of UV radiation for disinfection of water after roughly 1980. Today, UV disinfection is among the most commonly applied disinfectants for water; it is also being used for disinfection and preservation of solids, surfaces, and air. The goal of this chapter is to describe the fundamental concepts that are needed to understand

the design, behavior, and validation of UV-based microbial inactivation systems used in water treatment. Similar principles apply with applications of UV disinfection to other media. Because the process relies on photochemistry, the basic principles of photochemistry are presented first, followed by a development of some of the practical issues related to UV-based microbial inactivation processes.

BASIC PRINCIPLES OF PHOTOCHEMISTRY

Photochemical processes are initiated by absorption of electromagnetic radiation. Two basic laws of photochemistry have been presented. The first law of photochemistry, also known as the Grotthus-Draper law, states that light (electromagnetic radiation) must be absorbed for a photochemical reaction to take place. The second law of photochemistry, also known as the Stark-Einstein law, states that for each photon of radiation absorbed, only one molecule will be excited. The second law also forms the basis for the concept of a quantum yield (Φ), which defines the ratio of molecules that react to photons absorbed. In turn, this allows for assignment of 1:1 equivalence between photons and molecules. The laws of photochemistry also indicate that two conditions must be met for a photochemical reaction to take place. First, a photon must be absorbed by a target molecule, or in some cases by a neighboring molecule, which may act as a photosensitizer. Second, the absorbed photon must have sufficient energy to break an existing bond or form a new one. If these two conditions are met, it is possible, although not certain, that a photochemical reaction may take place. If either condition is not met, a photochemical reaction will not take place.

Photon Energy

The German physicist Max Planck is credited with the development of the basic mathematical expression used to define photon energy:

$$E = h\frac{c}{\lambda} \tag{1}$$

Where:

E = photon energy
h = Planck constant
c = speed of light
λ = wavelength

Because reacting molecules and photons normally react on a 1:1 basis (as described by the Stark-Einstein law), it is often useful to express Planck law in an alternative form (note that 1 einstein is defined as being equal to Avogadro's number of photons):

$$Q_E = h\frac{c}{\lambda}A \tag{2}$$

Where: Q_E = energy per einstein
A = Avogadro's number

Much in the same way that molecules (or atoms) may be viewed as the smallest discrete units of a chemical compound, the photon may be viewed as the smallest discrete unit of radiation energy. Across the electromagnetic spectrum, there exists a wide range of wavelengths and corresponding photon energies (Figure 9.1). The focus of this chapter is on photochemical reactions that take place within biomolecules. It is impractical to develop a comprehensive summary of bond energies associated with all

moieties that are relevant in these molecules because of the dependence on molecular substituent groups and other factors. It is possible, however, to summarize representative values of the bond energies that characterize some of the common bonds in biological systems (see Figure 9.1). From this summary, it is evident that the bond energies of interest in microbial molecules are generally coincident with photon energies in the UV portion of the spectrum. Radiation with wavelengths less than approximately 320 nm is often sufficiently energetic to promote reactions in biomolecules. Radiation in the vacuum UV (VUV) portion of the spectrum is highly energetic but also tends to be absorbed strongly. Because of this, VUV radiation does not penetrate far into liquid or solid media; it is strongly absorbed by molecular oxygen (O_2), which limits its ability to be transmitted through gases. As such, most UV photoreactors are based on radiation in the UVB and UVC portions of the electromagnetic spectrum. UV radiation is defined as the portion of the electromagnetic spectrum that lies between visible light (ie, electromagnetic radiation that can be detected by a healthy human eye) and X-radiation. The UV spectrum is further subdivided into several subregions. Table 9.1 provides a summary of wavelength cutoffs for these regions (see Figure 9.1) as well as distinguishing features of each wavelength range.

Although the preceding arguments suggest that essentially all photons within the UV range should be capable of promoting photobiochemical reactions, photons at wavelengths of less than 320 nm tend to be the most effective for this purpose. Solar UV disinfection processes are strongly influenced by the effects of UVA radiation, largely by mechanisms that involve heat and the formation of O_2-based reactive intermediates. For some solar UV disinfection systems, incorporation of materials that allow for inclusion of UVB radiation can increase the rate of microbial inactivation; however, the vast majority of contemporary (nonsolar) UV disinfection systems employ "artificial" sources of UVC radiation to accomplish microbial inactivation.

Photochemical Kinetics

The rate of a photochemical reaction is directly related to the rate at which the target molecule absorbs incident radiation. For the case of monochromatic radiation, the rate of a photochemical process can be described as[4]:

$$r(\lambda) = -\frac{d[B]}{dt} = I_a(\lambda) \cdot \Phi(\lambda) \tag{3}$$

Where:

$r(\lambda)$ = rate of photochemical reaction
$[B]$ = molar concentration (activity) of absorbing (reacting) compound
t = time
$I_a(\lambda)$ = volumetric rate of photon (λ) absorption by the target molecule
$\Phi(\lambda)$ = quantum yield

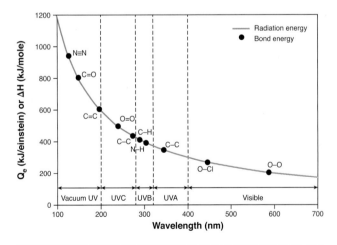

FIGURE 9.1   Photon energy (Q_E) as a function of wavelength. Superimposed on this figure are the wavelength ranges that define vacuum ultraviolet (UV), UVC, UVB, UVA, and visible radiation. Also included are typical bond energies (ΔH) for a number of bonds that are relevant to UV-based applications in water treatment and disinfection, as well as their corresponding wavelengths.

TABLE 9.1 Summary of wavelength regions within the ultraviolet spectrum and some corresponding characteristics

Type of Radiation	Nominal Wavelength Range (nm)	Characteristics
UVA	320-400	Comprises >99% of ambient solar UV radiation at sea level near mid-latitudes; promotes microbial inactivation through heat and formation of O_2-based reactive intermediates
UVB	280-320	Comprises roughly 1% of ambient solar radiation at sea level near mid-latitudes; promotes microbial inactivation through photochemical damage to nucleic acids; promotes skin cancer and damage to other external tissues
UVC	200-280	Absent from ambient solar spectrum at sea level near mid-latitudes because of absorption by stratospheric ozone; must be generated locally to the application; causes damage to nucleic acids, proteins, and other biomolecules
Vacuum UV	10-200	Strongly absorbed by gas-phase O_2 and to a lesser degree N_2; highly energetic radiation that can be used to photolyze H_2O and many other molecules that are normally stable

Abbreviations: H_2O, water; N_2, dinitrogen; O_2, molecular oxygen; UV, ultraviolet.

Parenthetical terms (λ) are included in equation (3) to emphasize that these attributes of photochemical reactions may display wavelength dependence. From this point forward, the parenthetical terms will be dropped in the interest of simplifying the resulting mathematical expressions.

The volumetric rate of photon absorbance depends on the geometry and optical characteristics of the reaction vessel in which the reaction takes place. For highly transparent conditions, or for the situation where we examine the rate of a photochemical reaction at a point in a system, equation (3) reduces to the following:

$$r = -\frac{d[B]}{dt} = \frac{2.303 \cdot E_0 \cdot \varepsilon \cdot [B]}{Q_E} \cdot \Phi \qquad (4)$$

Where:

E_0 = local fluence rate
ε = molar absorption coefficient
Q_E = energy per einstein

Equation (4) also indicates that the *local rate of a photochemical reaction* is proportional to the *local fluence rate*. As described in the following text, the fluence rate within a photochemical reactor often displays strong spatial gradients; as such, we observe equally strong spatial gradients in local photochemical reaction rates in these systems. Because photochemical reactions tend to be rapid, mixing behavior within photochemical reactors tends to have a strong influence on reactor performance.

In the case of UV disinfection, wherein the photochemical target is one or more biomolecules within a microbe, the physical interpretations of ε and $[B]$ become nebulous. Moreover, data to describe these parameters in a disinfection context are rarely available. Because of this, the common practice is to resort to a mathematical expression to describe microbial inactivation kinetics

(or UV dose-response behavior) based on the same logic that is used to describe the kinetics of purely photochemical reactions. Equation (5) illustrates the most basic form of a UV disinfection kinetic model:

$$\frac{dN}{dt} = -k \cdot E_0 \cdot N \qquad (5)$$

Where:

N = concentration of viable microbial target organisms
k = inactivation rate constant

In effect, the inactivation constant (k) is a combined parameter that accounts for efficiency of photon absorbance (analog of ε), the efficiency of absorbed photon use to inactivate the microbial target (analog of Φ), and the energy of an einstein of photons (analog of Q_E). This modeling approach implicitly assumes that a 1:1 correspondence exists between a photochemical event and inactivation of an individual microbial target. In other words, this model suggests that a single photochemical event leads to inactivation of the microbial target. This approach is valid for some simple organisms, over a limited range of conditions. As will be demonstrated later, this simple model fails to describe the intrinsic kinetics of all UV disinfection processes; however, it does provide a starting point for a discussion of this topic.

Because equations (4) and (5) describe photochemical reaction rates at any point in space, they are broadly applicable for description of the behavior of photochemical reactor systems. Their application requires detailed information regarding the spatial distribution of radiant energy (ie, the fluence rate field) within a photochemical reactor system; for many UV photoreactors, additional information is also required to develop quantitatively accurate predictions or reactor behavior.

SOURCES OF ULTRAVIOLET RADIATION

UV radiation can be generated from natural and manufactured sources. Although the source of radiation does not influence the effects of photons that it generates, it is useful to understand the basic physics of radiation generation by these sources as well as their corresponding output spectra.

The sun represents perhaps the most basic source of UV radiation.[5] The sun emits radiation as a result of incandescence, a process by which any hot object emits radiation. Planck's law can be used to simulate the spectrum of radiation emitted from a blackbody at any given temperature; blackbody emission represents the maximum possible emission spectrum for a surface at a given temperature. The spectrum of solar radiation received outside the earth's atmosphere has been measured by satellite-based instruments and high-altitude aircraft. The spectrum of solar radiation received at earth's surface is influenced by time of day, time of year, latitude, and altitude, as well as atmospheric composition. Numerical models have been developed to simulate these effects and to allow simulation of ambient solar spectra at essentially any time and location. One model that have been developed for this purpose is the Simple Model of the Atmospheric Radiative Transfer of Sunshine (SMARTS).[6]

Figure 9.2 provides a summary of several reference solar spectra. Included in this figure are two spectra that are used to describe solar radiation that is imposed on earth's atmosphere. The term *air mass zero* is used to de-scribe these spectra. Air mass describes the path length of light through earth's atmosphere relative to the path length that would be involved for radiation imposed at a zenith angle of zero (ie, perpendicular to earth's surface).[9] Therefore, air mass zero corresponds to solar radiation that has not yet encountered earth's atmosphere (ie, the spectrum of radiation imposed on earth's atmosphere). Another reference spectrum is included for air mass 1.5, which describes the spectrum of solar radiation imposed at an angle of 37 degrees. Also included in Figure 9.2 are spectra that were simulated using Planck's law for blackbodies at 5777 K and 6000 K. These two temperatures span the nominal estimates of the surface temperature on the sun.

Solar radiation received at earth's surface is substantially attenuated as compared to the air mass zero spectrum largely because of absorption by constituents of the atmosphere. Atmospheric ozone is a particularly strong absorber of UV radiation. The shortest wavelength of solar radiation received at near sea level elevations is roughly 290 nm. Earth's atmosphere is essentially opaque to radiation at wavelengths shorter than 290 nm. This means that ambient solar radiation received at earth's surface will include UVA and UVB radiation but essentially no UVC or VUV radiation. Although UVA and UVB radiation can be used to inactivate microbial pathogens, the most effective wavelengths for disinfection are found in the UVC range. Therefore, systems that employ UVC radiation for disinfection must rely on "artificial" sources of UV radiation. The most common artificial sources of UV radiation are mercury (Hg) lamps, of which there are two basic types: low pressure (LP) and medium pressure (MP).[10] Hg lamps operate by striking an electrical arc across a space that contains Hg and an inert carrier gas, usually argon. Collisions between electrons and the atoms (or molecules) that occupy the space between the lamp electrodes result in electronic excitation of those atoms; electronically excited argon can transfer some of its energy to a nearby Hg atom. Relaxation of electronically excited Hg atoms to lower energy states results in photon emission. In addition to conventional LP lamps, there are also lamps that are based on an Hg amalgam rather than pure metallic Hg. The Hg amalgam lamps are characterized by essentially the same output spectrum as conventional LP Hg lamps (Figure 9.3), but they can generate more power than their conventional LP Hg lamp analogs. For practical purposes, LP Hg lamps are often considered to be monochromatic ($\lambda = 253.7$ nm) sources of UV radiation; however, LP Hg lamps are also characterized by several other, smaller lines in their output spectra, including a line at 185 nm and a few lines in the visible range that are responsible for the pale blue color that is evident when these lamps are illuminated.

The output spectra of MP Hg lamps are considerably more complex than those of LP Hg lamps. The MP lamp output spectra are characterized by numerous discrete lines superimposed on a continuum. The MP lamps tend to be much less efficient than LP Hg lamps in terms of

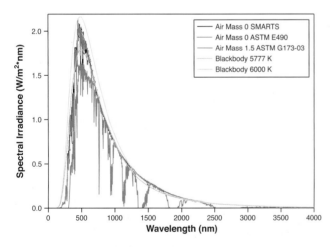

FIGURE 9.2 Reference solar spectra. Air mass zero spectra define radiation that is incident on the outside of earth's atmosphere.[7] The air mass 1.5 spectrum corresponds to solar radiation received at sea level imposed on earth's atmosphere at a zenith angle of 37 degrees.[8] The blackbody spectra are presented for temperature estimates that have been used to describe the surface of the sun. For a color version of this art, please consult the eBook.

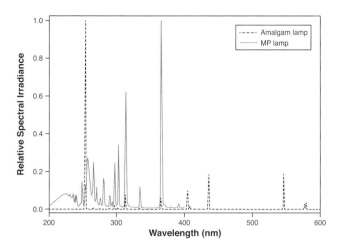

FIGURE 9.3 Normalized output spectra of Hg lamps. For both lamp types, spectra are normalized to the maximum value measured in the spectrum. Abbreviation: MP, medium pressure. Data courtesy of Trojan Technologies. For a color version of this art, please consult the eBook.

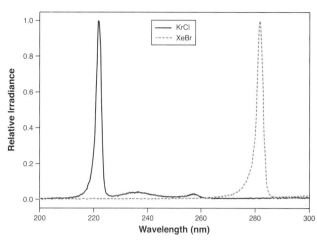

FIGURE 9.4 Normalized output spectra of krypton chloride (KrCl) and xenon bromide (XeBr) exciplex lamps. For a color version of this art, please consult the eBook.

conversion of electrical power (input) into UV photons (output). The MP lamps can be much more powerful than LP lamps, and as such, they can be used to develop systems that are characterized by a smaller footprint and less complexity than equivalent systems based on LP Hg lamp technology. A normalized MP lamp spectrum is included in Figure 9.3. The spectra presented for LP (amalgam) and MP Hg lamps were normalized against the maximum values that were measured for each lamp type. Normalization was applied because the output spectrum measured for any lamp will depend on the location of the measuring device relative to the source as well as the composition of the media located between the source and the measurement location.

Historically, Hg lamps have been viewed as the default option for generation of germicidal UV radiation. However, the inclusion of Hg in these devices presents safety risks that motivate the development of alternative sources of UV radiation. From the regulatory perspective, some pressure to develop alternatives to Hg lamps can be found in the *Minamata Convention on Mercury*,[11] an international treaty that was developed to protect human health and the environment from anthropogenic emissions of Hg. A similar piece of legislation in Europe has also resulted in restrictions on the use of Hg.[12] As with the *Minamata Convention*, Hg-based lamps for general lighting are allowed, but there are restrictions on the mass of Hg that can be included in these lamps.

Excilamps represent a family of UV and VUV sources that include excimers (*exci*ted di*mer*) and exiplexes (*exci*ted com*plex*). In both cases, a diatomic molecule or complex is electronically excited; relaxation back to a ground state results in photon emission at a characteristic wavelength. Excilamps are characterized by relatively narrow

emission spectra, typically in the range of 2 to 30 nm at half maximum.[10,13,14] Figure 9.4 illustrates the normalized spectral output of two common exciplex lamps: krypton chloride and xenon bromide. The output spectrum of an exciplex lamp can be adjusted through selection of the constituent gases that are used to form the exciplex. The most common configuration for these lamps is a so-called dielectric barrier discharge lamp,[15-17] which usually is manufactured with a cylindrical geometry. Many other geometric configurations are possible with these lamps, including flat-panel displays. This geometric flexibility may provide opportunities to improve the optical characteristics of UV photoreactors.

UV light-emitting diodes (LEDs) have emerged as important sources of antimicrobial UV radiation in recent years.[18-22] Diodes are semiconductor materials that have been doped with chemicals to alter their ability to carry electrical current. Doping materials are added to semiconductors, such as silicon, to allow formation of charge carriers. A so-called p-n (positive-negative) junction is established by bringing into contact materials that have been doped to promote formation of positive charge carriers (holes) and negative charge carriers (electrons). Holes and electrons naturally migrate toward each other because of electrostatic attraction, but their migration can be influenced by application of electrical current. When applied properly, this current promotes migration of holes and electrons toward each other, resulting in their recombination. In turn, this causes the electron to experience a drop in energy, yielding a photon that corresponds to the bandgap of the dopant materials. Visible and infrared LEDs are commonly applied in electronic devices, including cell phones, televisions, room lighting, etc. The production of UV LEDs is possible through the use of group III nitrides as doping materials, especially including the aluminum-gallium nitride doping system. The spectral

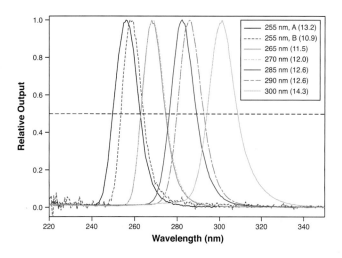

FIGURE 9.5 Normalized output spectra of ultraviolet light-emitting diodes as a function of aluminum-gallium composition (data from AquiSense Technologies). Parenthetical entries in the legend indicate peak width (nm) at half maximum. For a color version of this art, please consult the eBook.

output of these devices depends on the composition of the dopants. Figure 9.5 provides an illustration of the range of outputs observed among commercially available UV LEDs. Because of this, it is possible to select UV LEDs to have an output spectrum that is tailored to a given application.

UV LEDs have a number of other important advantages relative to conventional sources of UV radiation, such as Hg lamps. They contain no Hg, which is relevant in the context of the *Minamata Convention* and general public pressure. The UV LEDs are compact and durable and allow for instant on/off switching. Packaging of LEDs (including UV LEDs) allows for inclusion of optical elements that can provide for directional irradiation. As such, UV LEDs can function as nearly point sources of radiation, which offers considerable flexibility in reactor design. On the other hand, it is also important to recognize the drawbacks of UV LEDs. At present, the efficiency of these devices is lower than Hg lamps, and their costs are higher. Historic trends in LED development have indicated that as applications for these devices emerge, production processes improve to yield increasingly efficient and powerful LEDs.

▶ MICROBIAL INACTIVATION AND REPAIR

Mechanisms of Inactivation

The mechanisms of microbial inactivation depend on the range of wavelengths imposed on the microbes. As illus-

trated in Figures 9.2 to 9.5, the spectra of radiation from natural and artificial sources of UV radiation vary widely. Similarly, the mechanisms of inactivation that result from UV exposure also demonstrate considerable variability.

Exposure to solar UV radiation is governed by time of day, time of year, position of the target, materials that exist between the target and the radiation source (eg, shade), and numerous microenvironmental parameters; however, ambient solar radiation is limited to the UVA and UVB portions of the electromagnetic spectrum. UVA radiation causes microbial inactivation largely through the formation of reactive O_2 species (ROS), which then go on to react with microbial constituents.[23-26] UVB radiation is known to cause damage to nucleic acids, including DNA.[27] In general, the rates of microbial inactivation resulting from exposure to ambient solar UVA and UVB radiation are slow but can be relevant in some situations. Most UV disinfection systems employ artificial sources of UV radiation, usually in the UVC range. UVC radiation can alter nucleic acids, proteins, and even cellular structures like membranes, which are heavily involved in respiration. But DNA is the major target chromophore in much of the region where it absorbs most heavily, 240 to 310 nm, typically with a peak at 260 nm. The DNA also has the fewest copies of any major macromolecule and is the genetic material.[28,29]

Until the 1940s, most biologists believed that genetic material was protein, which UV radiation can alter. But in the 1920s, Gates[30-32] showed that the action spectra (see the following text) for both cell inactivation and mutation closely followed the absorption spectrum for nucleic acids in bacteria; his results were not readily accepted. Later, the photobiological community began to study UV effects on nucleic acids, predominantly DNA, and were surprised to discover that the genetic material was easily altered by UV radiation and then, even more surprisingly, that these alterations could sometimes be repaired. These studies helped form the basis for a new field of research known as molecular biology. DNA can be modified by absorption of UV photons in a variety of ways.[33] Individual bases can be altered by deamination, ring cleavage, or other direct effects. For example, adjacent bases can be covalently linked by UV into a cyclopyrimidine dimer (CPD). The CPDs are the major photoproduct near the DNA absorption peak (260 nm). Covalent bonds are stable at physiological temperatures. UV radiation can also form 6 to 4 pyrimidine photo-adducts (6-4 PPs, also referred to as 6-4 photoproducts) at a lower rate (about 30% of CPD formation). The 6-4 PPs have an absorption maximum near 320 nm.[34] DNA replication is altered by UV photoproducts; as few as one lesion in the form of a CPD or 6-4 PP can stop it.

The distribution of PPs varies with wavelength. In vegetative cells, dimers predominate in the UVC. After exposure to UVB, other PPs such as single strand breaks (SSBs) and DNA-protein cross-links begin to accumulate.

Although UV does not directly cause strand breaks in DNA, some of the mechanisms that repair UV PPs can. This damage is often overlooked but can have major effects on cell survival.[35] In the UVA, SSBs may be the predominant lesions.[33] UV radiation can also promote the formation of DNA photohydrates. If the cell contains certain photosensitizers, UVA and visible radiation can also produce indirect DNA effects where the photons are absorbed by other compounds which, in turn, damage DNA.[36] Unique PPs have been discovered in some studied cells. For example, the spores of *Bacillus subtilis* (and some other sporulating bacteria) produce a unique "spore PP" (5,6-dihydrothymine) and have a unique spore product photolyase for photoreactivation (PR, see the following text). In addition, the spore coat protein can act as an effective shield to UV. Dormant spores cannot readily repair UV damage, but vegetative cells can.[37] Whether the cell survives after germination to the vegetative form depends on how much UV damage it contains and whether the vegetative cell had enough time to repair that damage. Spores irradiated under wet conditions are several orders of magnitude more sensitive to UV than spores exposed to UV when dry.[38] As described previously, UVA is also associated with the production of ROS and damage to a variety of other endogenous chromophores.

Because DNA is closely associated with proteins in the chromatin structure of cells or in virus structures, it is not surprising that these close but separate moieties can cross-link after UV exposure. Some cells also contain pigments that can act in a similar manner. The replicating portion of DNA is most sensitive to UV-induced cross-linking with proteins. These cross-links cannot undergo PR but can be cleared by postreplication repair. In addition, Dewar valence isomers are formed by the photoisomerization of 6-4 PPs at wavelengths longer than 290 nm (peak production at 320 nm). They can be repaired by the (6-4 PP) photolyase.[34]

Physiological Responses Other Than Inactivation

Jagger[39] showed that irradiation of amoeba cytoplasm can damage cells. He further showed this was due mainly to PP formation in mitochondrial DNA. Singlet O_2 and free radicals can also be produced in some chromophores by UVA, and they can act as photosensitizers by destroying cellular components including membranes.[34] For many microbes, loss of viability or infectivity takes place at modest UV doses as compared to the doses of UVC radiation required to bring about other observable physiological changes. For example, Blatchley et al[40] observed roughly 6.8 $\log_{10}$ units of inactivation of *Escherichia coli* at a UV_{254} dose of 100 mJ/cm²; at the same dose, respiratory/metabolic activity was reduced by only 0.64 $\log_{10}$ units. Similar results were observed with *Streptococcus faecalis*. Redford

and Myers[41] reported inactivation of the algal species *Chlorella pyrenoidosa* to be approximately six times faster than reductions in photosynthesis as a result of UV_{254} exposure. Effective inactivation of the protozoan parasites *Cryptosporidium parvum* and *Giardia lamblia* (and related species) has been observed at remarkably low doses of UVC radiation, whereas interruption of other parts of their life cycle requires much larger UVC doses.[42-47] These observations suggest that UVC irradiation is effective for preventing replication of waterborne microbes, but actual death of the organisms will require UVC doses that are substantially larger than those needed to accomplish loss of the ability to reproduce or infect.

Disinfection Kinetics

As indicated by equation (5), the rate of photochemical damage to a molecule at a local level is first order with respect to the concentration of the target molecule and the local fluence rate. If it is assumed that a microorganism will be inactivated when it accumulates a single unit of photochemically induced damage, then the rate of microbial inactivation will also follow these same principles, as indicated previously in equation (5) (repeated here for clarity):

$$\frac{dN}{dt} = -k \cdot E_0 \cdot N \qquad (6)$$

Rearrangement of equation (6) to allow separation of variables, followed by integration yields the following form:

$$ln\left(\frac{N}{N_0}\right) = -k \int_0^\tau E_0 \cdot dt \qquad (7)$$

Where:

$$\tau = \text{period of exposure (s)}$$
$$\int_0^\tau E_{0,i} \cdot dt = \text{UV dose (mJ/cm}^2)$$

Equation (7) indicates that a plot of $ln\left(\frac{N}{N_0}\right)$ as a function of UV dose should yield a straight line with a slope of $-k$. In practice, it is common to present graphs of this nature in the form of $log_{10}\left(\frac{N}{N_0}\right)$ versus dose, probably because most people are more comfortable with base 10 logarithms than they are with natural logarithms. In either form, equation (7) implies a straight line that passes through the origin on a semilogarithmic plot. When data from an experiment are fit to equation (7), the slope of the best-fit line through the origin will have a value of $-\frac{k}{2.303}$.

Equations (6) and (7) describe the rate of inactivation for a microbe that is inactivated as a result of a single unit of damage, the so-called single-event model. Figure 9.6 illustrates the shape of the UV dose-response behavior that is predicted by the single-event model. Some simple organisms (eg, some viruses) follow dose-response behavior

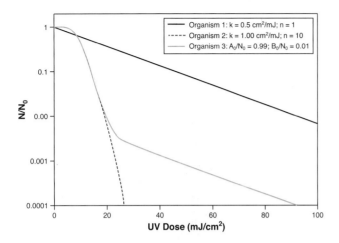

FIGURE 9.6   Illustration of common ultraviolet (UV) dose-response models. Model parameters are indicated in the legend. Organism 1 obeys single-event kinetics; organism 2 follows the series-event model, which includes a lag in inactivation, evident at relatively low doses; organism 3 comprises a population that demonstrates dose-response behavior that is a blend of those displayed by organisms 1 and 2. For a color version of this art, please consult the eBook.

that can be accurately simulated by the single-event model, at least for limited extents of microbial inactivation. Common deviations from single-event behavior have also been observed, including a shoulder in the limit of low doses and lag or tailing behavior that is often observed at large doses (see Figure 9.6). Models have been developed to account for these deviations. The series-event model[48,49] was developed based on the assumption that microbes within a population would accumulate damage in a serial manner, as follows:

$$M_0 \xrightarrow{h\nu} M_1 \xrightarrow{h\nu} M_2 \xrightarrow{h\nu} \cdots \xrightarrow{h\nu} M_{n-1} \xrightarrow{h\nu} M_n \xrightarrow{h\nu} \cdots \quad (8)$$

Where M_i represents a microorganism with i units of damage. An implicit assumption of the series-event model is that each unit of damage is caused by a discrete photochemical event, and that the reactions that are responsible for this damage have the same rate constant, k. Furthermore, it is assumed that microbes in this population will retain viability (ie, ability to reproduce and infect) until they accumulate damage beyond the threshold of n units of damage. All microbes with $n-1$ units of damage or less are assumed to be viable.

In the series-event model, a population of microorganisms will comprise individuals with many different levels of damage. The term N_i is used to define the concentration of microbes with i units of damage. Following this logic, it is then possible to define how the concentration of microbes at each level of damage will change because of UV exposure:

$$\frac{dN_i}{dt} = k \cdot E_0 \cdot N_{i-1} - k \cdot E_0 \cdot N_i \quad (9)$$

Equation (9) represents a series of differential equations that can be used to describe the entire population of microbes under the series-event model. If we recognize that the concentration of viable organisms (N) can be represented by the sum of the concentrations of all organisms with $n-1$ units of damage or less:

$$N = \Sigma_{i=0}^{n-1} N_i \quad (10)$$

then equations (9) and (10) can be combined to yield the overall prediction of the series-event model:

$$\frac{N}{N_0} = exp(-k \cdot E_0 \cdot t) \cdot \Sigma_{i=0}^{n-1} \frac{(k \cdot E_0 \cdot t)^i}{i!} \quad (11)$$

Organism 2 in Figure 9.6 provides an illustration of the series-event model. In practical terms, we observe that microbial inactivation does not start until a threshold dose has been surpassed, after which it follows roughly first-order inactivation behavior.

Another common deviation from the single-event model is the presence of tailing or reduced inactivation rate in the limit of large dose or large extent of inactivation. It is thought that this behavior may be attributable to shielding of microbes by ambient particles or to the existence of phenotypically advantaged microbial subpopulations. It is difficult to determine which of these aspects is responsible for tailing behavior; both processes can be simulated using the same mathematical approach. An example of a modeling approach that has been used to describe this behavior is the phenotypic persistence and external shielding (PPES) model.[50] The PPES model assumes that a microbial population can be described by two subpopulations: one that is sensitive to UV exposure and a second that is resistant. It is further assumed that each subpopulation can be simulated using an existing model, such as the single-event model and the series-event model. Equation (12) defines the application of the PPES model for a microbial population in which the majority of the population $\left(\frac{A_0}{N_0}\right)$ follows series-event behavior, with a small fraction of the population $\left(\frac{B_0}{N_0}\right)$ that follows slower inactivation that is described by the single-event model. Equation (12) is also illustrated in Figure 9.6 as the dose-response behavior of organism 3.

$$\frac{N}{N_0} = \frac{A_0}{N_0} \cdot exp(-k_A \cdot E_{0,i} \cdot t) \cdot \Sigma_{i=0}^{n-1} \frac{(k_A \cdot E_{0,i} \cdot t)^i}{i!}$$
$$+ \frac{B_0}{N_0} \cdot exp(-k_B \cdot E_{0,i} \cdot t) \quad (12)$$

Microbial Sensitivity to UV_{254nm} Radiation

Malayeri et al[51] compiled a summary of measured UV sensitivity of many waterborne microbes. Similar lists of microbial responses to UV exposure have been assembled,[38,52-55] which include quantitative descriptions of the sensitivities of a many bacterial cells, spores, and viruses to 254-nm radiation. Collectively, these and other summaries indicate that most vegetative protozoa and bacteria can be effectively inactivated (3-4 $\log_{10}$ units of change) by 254-nm radiation by a fluence (dose) as low as a few mJ/cm^2; other, more resistant microbes including some viruses and bacterial spores may require several hundred mJ/cm^2. All inactivation tables show a substantial variety in UV response within species among strains. Therefore, overlap and even reordering of any sequence listed here may be necessary from time to time. But a general estimate of UV sensitivity can be described as follows:

(From most sensitive to most resistant)
Protozoa > Bacteria > Viruses > Bacterial spores
≈ Yeast and other vegetative fungi > Fungal spores >
Adenoviruses > Algae > Some extremophiles > Prions

Adenoviruses are highly resistant to UV compared to other viruses (by a factor of 4), but the action spectrum (AS) (see the following text) for adenovirus inactivation[56] indicates that wavelengths shorter than approximately 240 nm are more effective than longer wavelengths for adenovirus inactivation, presumably due to photochemical damage to proteins. Protozoa, long believed to be highly resistant to UV, are actually among the most sensitive organisms when infectivity is used as the assay to quantify their responses to UV exposure.[42,43,45-47] Many studies report that enormous UV fluences are needed to "inactivate" prions; however, some recent results show that lower UV fluences may stop the pathogenic folding of the prion protein molecule.[57]

Biological Action Spectra

An action spectrum (AS) is a graphical depiction of a rate of a biological or physiological effect as a function of wavelength. When a measured AS for an effect matches the absorption spectrum of a molecule that can reasonably be considered to be causing that effect, this information is taken as evidence of identification of the target chromophore. In turn, this can point to the mechanism causing such important cellular responses as cell death.[30] The AS analysis discussed will be limited to the wavelength region that corresponds to the biologically active part of the UV spectrum (200-400 nm). Because electromagnetic radiation is absorbed as photons and a 200-nm photon has twice the energy of a 400-nm photon, it is proper to consider the number of photons at any given wavelength that can yield the same effect. For AS over the wide range of UV wavelengths, a quantum correction (QC, conversion of total energy to photon energy) generates a measurable difference in the final AS curve. For those AS limited to a narrow region of wavelengths, the differences between QC-corrected and uncorrected spectra are proportionately less.

It is common for a response at a given wavelength to be used as the basis for normalization of AS; common wavelengths used for this purpose include 254 nm (the dominant resonance emission line for Hg lamps) or

260 nm (the nominal absorption peak for DNA). The QC values for the effect plotted on the ordinate will increase at shorter wavelengths and decrease at longer wavelengths. The choices of scale are linear for the abscissa (wavelength) and for the ordinate either logarithmic, when trying to match the AS to an absorption spectrum for a suspected target (eg, DNA[30]) because that is the way absorption spectra are plotted to make them independent of concentration and thickness,[28] or linear, if one is just concerned with the fluence needed for a given effect. Employing a QC can be a simple matter of division. Unfortunately, even though it has been suggested for decades,[58-62] most authors have not followed this approach.

Action spectra in the ranges 230 to 297 nm were the first to show that bacterial cell inactivation and mutation are attributable to nucleic acids, not proteins.[30] A lack of understanding of AS hindered the acceptance of this fact until the 1940s. Several scientists then began to target nucleic acids (in particular DNA) by using an LP Hg "germicidal" lamp that emits the majority of its output at 254 nm, close to the absorption peak of DNA at about 260 nm. Cytoplasmic screening and absorption and scattering by endogenous pigments and organelles before the radiation reaches the target all are wavelength-dependent and can alter the amount and wavelengths that impinge on target molecules, such as DNA. These optical behaviors can also alter the response measured. These cellular screenings are minimal in small pathogens like viruses and unpigmented bacterial cells but become important in bacterial spores (due to shielding by the protein coat) and larger cells such as protozoa (due to cytoplasmic screening). Therefore, absorption within cells is not merely a summation of the absorption properties of their individual components but rather is influenced by their concentration and arrangement within the cell.

Figure 9.7 illustrates a quantum corrected composite AS derived from various data sets for inactivation of biological cells and viruses. The varying AS curve shapes are partly due to differences in the sensitivity of the various organisms and assay methods used.[29,56,58,59,62] The generalized AS presented in Figure 9.7 indicates that most of the damage occurs in the UVC range. The primary chromophores for damage at wavelengths between 240 nm and 280 nm are nucleic acids, usually DNA, because the absorption spectrum for these molecules peaks at around 260 nm. At the more energetic UVC wavelengths (200-240 nm), proteins, especially peptide bonds, become the dominant chromophore. The UVB (280-320 nm) portion of this AS shows a transition region where damage to DNA is still prevalent but the response begins to deviate from the absorption spectrum of DNA implying that other mechanisms in addition to direct DNA damage are occurring. Finally, organism responses to UVA radiation (320-400 nm) is greatly diminished relative to UVB and UVC and generally involves indirect processes, wherein UVA radiation leads to production of ROS that can damage important biological molecules, including lipids,

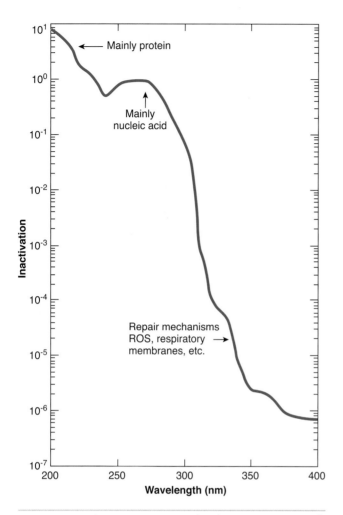

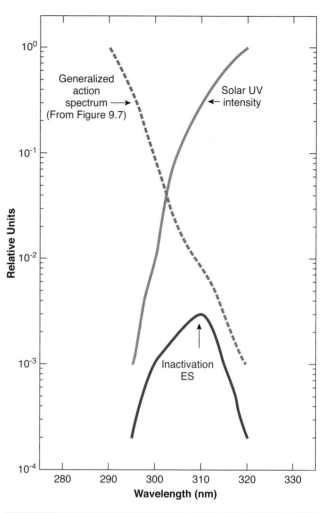

FIGURE 9.7 A composite generalized quantum corrected action spectrum for cell and virus inactivation throughout the biological ultraviolet range. Data compiled from a variety of sources,[56,58,62-63] some of which are composite data sets themselves. Abbreviation: ROS, reactive oxygen species.

FIGURE 9.8 An effectiveness spectrum (ES) that combines the action spectrum from Figure 9.7 with the available solar radiation reaching the earth's surface. The product of these two spectra gives an ES for cellular inactivation. The wavelength region selected (ultraviolet B [UVB]) was chosen to demonstrate the usefulness of such a plot.

enzymes, and even DNA (which is almost totally transparent to UVA). This damage, in turn, can affect membranes, respiration, and cellular repair mechanisms. Endogenous chromophores often absorb in this region and can either be damaged themselves or shield the organisms from further damage. The UVA fluences (doses) needed for microbial inactivation tend to be orders of magnitude higher than those of UVB or UVC radiation but can be of practical relevance in systems that involve solar UV radiation.

Cell inactivation and loss of infectivity are not the only types of physiological damage observed among microorganisms and higher organisms. Changes in respiration, membrane channels, abnormal cell growth (cancer), nitrogen uptake, and other biological effects are amenable to AS analysis. Early AS were the first to identify chlorophyll as the crucial molecule required for photosynthesis. Sometimes an AS cannot identify a single chromophore as the cause of an effect, but at a minimum, it does show the effect of separate

wavelengths on a biological response, and as such is of use for determining what will happen after UV exposure.

A related concept is that of the effectiveness spectrum (ES), which is a product of an AS and the QC-corrected output spectrum of the UV source used in the system (Figure 9.8). Sutherland[61] described the mathematical procedures for calculating the biological effects from exposing samples to polychromatic UV. The use of polychromatic UV sources (including solar radiation) sometimes allow the construction of a useful ES. For example, the generalized plant damage response to UV follows an AS that peaks in the UVC; however, UVC radiation is rarely relevant for plant tissues because it is absent from the solar spectrum received on earth. Typical ES for plant tissues peak in the UVB range.[58]

The AS for several important microbial pathogens, indicator organisms, and challenge organisms have been summarized, *C parvum, MS2, T1UV, Q Beta, T7, T7m,* and *Bacillus pumilus*.[56,62] All exhibited local maxima in the vicinity of 260 nm; however, for some microorganisms, a second maximum was observed at wavelengths between 210 and 240 nm, suggesting the involvement of proteins.

▶ REPAIR MECHANISMS

In most applications of UV disinfection, the doses of UV radiation applied to microorganisms do not cause death of the microbe but instead lead to damage that prevents their replication or their ability to infect a host cell. Depending on the extent of damage imposed, some microbes have developed repair mechanisms that allow viability or infectivity attributes to be restored. Basic attributes of these repair mechanisms are described in the following text.

Photorepair

Photorepair (PR) is the simplest method for correcting errors in DNA after exposure to UV. An enzyme (photolyase) directly binds to a CPD or 6-4 PP and splits it using the energy it absorbed from a UVA or blue light photon. Once the dimer is spilt, the enzyme detaches and the original bases are restored to their original configuration. Depending on the extent of UV-induced damage, PR can restore cell viability by anywhere from 20% to 100 %.[37] The CPD photolyases are common in many microorganisms; 6-4 PP photolyase, although not as common, can still repair 6-4 PPs by a similar method.[64] The PR also repairs mitochondrial DNA in the cytoplasm.[28] If the proper wavelengths of light are available, PR is often the first method that begins a chain of repair processes. The detection and distribution of photolyases across different species is currently unpredictable.

Dark Repair

Nucleotide excision repair (NER) is one of several repair processes that can occur in the absence of light. Lesions in DNA caused by UV-induced alteration of the bases often lead to distortion of the DNA structure. A DNA nuclease cuts out the distorted section, leaving a gap. The DNA polymerase then fills in the gap using a remaining undamaged strand as a template, and this is then closed by a DNA ligase. Hence, the original DNA sequence is restored using new bases.

In prokaryotes, only three proteins are needed for NER, although about 30 genes can be required in eukaryotes. This mechanism does not produce mutations; however, any process that involves substitution of new for damaged DNA bases can lead to an error, which may be caused by translesion synthesis wherein an incorrect DNA base is inserted into a gap or some other incorrect nucleotide is introduced. These errors are far more common during the repair of 6-4 PPs than for CPDs.[34]

Base excision repair (BER) was initially thought of as a constitutive system needed to repair small (single base) nonhelix distorting lesions in DNA caused by chemicals or ionizing radiation. BER was identified as common and helpful in preventing mutations for these DNA damaging events. But UVA can produce ROS that can also lead to similar individual base DNA damages, and BER can remove them.[34] Some of the UV-induced endonucleases required for BER were originally thought to be present only in highly UV-resistant cells; however, yeast cells and certain bacteriophages have similar enzymes and more UVA exposure studies may expand this list. Mutations in BER genes can lead to human cancer, as can the age-related decline in the production of BER proteins.[65]

Recombinational Repair

Recombinational repair is the most complicated repair process and can involve more than 20 gene products, which can lead to repair errors (mutations). Some of the mutations left behind by this repair can themselves lead to cell inactivation. Often ignored, recombinational repair is a major contributor to a cell's response to UV exposure.[33] Recombinational repair is not due to the cell's UV exposure, per se, but, rather from the repair of that UV damage. The UV exposure can cause the production of specific enzymes to complete recombinational repair. Basically, UV repair of DNA can sometimes leave gaps (strand breaks) that require a recombinational process to be repaired. Single strand breaks (SSBs) are easily repaired by DNA polymerase and DNA ligase. Double strand breaks (DSBs) occur when gaps form across from each other in double-stranded DNA while the DNA is undergoing repair. If these gaps are left unrepaired, DSBs can lead to cell inactivation and, in some cases, become the dominant cause of inactivation after UV exposure.[33] If PR occurs before other types of repair, then DNA breaks cannot form because PR itself removes the template for dark repair. Hence, the availability of other repair mechanisms, the extent and type of DNA damage, the position of the DNA replicating mechanism relative to the DNA damage (closer is worse), where the damage occurs, and the timing of the repair combine to determine which cells retain viability. For example, it has been known since 1949 that just "holding" cells in media that does not allow division promotes maintenance of viability.[39,66] This is called liquid holding recovery (LHR). The major reason why this allows cells to retain viability is that during this period of nongrowth, repair mechanisms have more time to remove the damage from DNA. Under common conditions used in municipal or industrial applications of UV disinfection, Bohrerova et al[66] showed that bacterial regrowth after UV is common and inactivated cells can provide a significant source of nutrients. These authors also suggested that concerns about extensive repair of UV damage may be overestimated.

SOS Repair

After studies showed DNA to be the genetic material and to harbor damaging PPs when exposed to UV, a repair system now labeled SOS (after the universal distress signal) was elucidated.[67] Several observations led to the conclusion that UV-irradiated cells are "primed" to repair DNA damage. This is demonstrated by an interesting example with UV-irradiated *E coli* being better than unirradiated cells at repairing and replicating UV-irradiated phage after cell infection using the cell's repair enzymes. This is called host cell repair. This SOS repair system uses more than 40 separate genes.

NER is an initial manifestation of SOS repair but is often not sufficient to fix all damage. Cells may remain in an arrested state but can accumulate damage such as SSBs. SOS repairs this damage but does so in a highly mutagenic fashion, such as translesion synthesis.[34] Although SOS demonstrates an almost "duct tape" response, where survival is worth the risk of faulty repair, current thinking suggests it plays an essential role in antibiotic resistance and evolution. Much of the initial success in elucidating DNA repair emerged from studies involving PR, NER, or recombinational repair. But this is still a very active field of research, and alternative repair mechanisms continue to be discovered. For example, studies with yeast have shown new repair endonucleases.[34,68] Cells can also protect their survival by check points that stop the cell from progressing to cell death much as the original growth delay observed with LHR.

Cells have a wide range of defense mechanisms to ameliorate UV (and other) damage. The governing repair mechanism will depend on the types of lesions produced, the microenvironment in which the cell lives, the stage in the cell cycle when the damage is inflicted, the timing of repair, and numerous other constraints.[38] A damaged cell that does not die after UV exposure could then recover later and start reproducing.[66] Hijnen et al[53] noted that bacteria in the natural environment often exhibit more UV resistance than laboratory-grown strains. This is not surprising because UV damage caused by sunlight is constantly "priming" cells to begin repair. But if sufficient damage is imposed on microbes by UV irradiation, they may be unable to repair this damage.

Ultraviolet-Resistant Microorganisms

Although extremely UV-resistant organisms are not always found at disinfection sites, their existence could point to different possible standards for microbial quality by cell inactivation and serve as examples of how, when challenged, some organisms evolved UV defense mechanisms. A few examples are described in the following text.

While attempting to sterilize spacecraft, the National Aeronautics and Space Administration Jet Propulsion Lab in the United States that has one of the most aseptic cleanrooms in existence, discovered *B pumilus* and other UV-resistant bacteria.[69] One isolate, SAFR-032

(*B pumilus*—WN669) produces a UV-resistant bacterial spore.[69,70] These spores are more than 300-fold more resistant to UVC exposure than the standard *B subtilis* spores strain WN667. When exposed to UVC radiation, *B pumilus* are able to form multilayered shields of cells that protect the cells in the core. After exposure, these protected cells can begin cell division. Even they would be totally inactivated (but still "intact") after one day's exposure on Mars unless they were covered by a coating of dust during common Mars storms. Genetic changes after UV are being studied among *B pumilus*.[18] The *B subtilis* wild-type spores themselves display high resistance to UV, partly due to their protective spore coat and their special photoproducts and repair capabilities.[37] It has been postulated that in their dormant state, spore-forming bacteria may be able to travel between planets, possibly even surviving the large UV and ionizing radiation doses inflicted during the journey.[71]

There are other microorganisms that also have extremely high UV resistance.[72] On Earth, extremophiles have been isolated from high-altitude lakes where the UVB flux can be as great as 170-fold higher than at sea level. These organisms often employ defenses to limit UV damage and can have efficient repair systems.[73] They have displaced *Deinococcus* (formally *Micrococcus*) *radiodurans* (itself 30-fold more resistant to UV than *E coli*) as one of the most UV-resistant organisms currently known. Accordingly, in some cases, they may serve as pathogen surrogates to set new standards. These resistant cells make excellent models for searching for novel strategies to control UV damage and for setting new limits for the UV inactivation of microorganisms, the details of which standards to set are beyond the scope of this chapter.

▶ PROCESS BEHAVIOR

Dose (or fluence) is the master variable in all photochemical processes. The dose of radiation delivered to a solution containing photochemical targets will determine the extent to which the photoreaction(s) of interest will proceed. Alternatively, the dose applied to a target will determine the likelihood that an individual target will undergo photochemical transformation. An important complicating feature of UV disinfection systems is the fact that essentially all contemporary photoreactor systems deliver a dose distribution.[74-76] As such, it is important to recognize the attributes of photoreactors that influence the dose distribution and the effects of this distribution on overall process behavior.

Fluence Rate Field

The UV disinfection systems that are used for treatment of fluids such as water or air are characterized by several common features. In general, the UV source (often one or more Hg lamps) is encased in a material that separates the lamp from the surrounding fluid while being highly transmissive of UV radiation. The most common materials used for this purpose are quartz and fused silica; when Hg lamps are used as the source, this barrier usually takes the form of a cylindrical sleeve. Lamp/sleeve assemblies are arranged in an array of fixed positions within a reactor. The fluid of interest, either water or air, is pumped through the array of ignited lamps to allow exposure of suspended microbial targets to UV radiation from these lamps.

As described previously, the local photochemical reaction rate within a reactor is directly proportional to the local fluence rate. Within virtually all contemporary photoreactors, strong spatial gradients in local fluence rate are evident. A number of factors influence the spatial distribution of radiation energy from the lamps within an array, including lamp output power, lamp spacing, absorption of emitted radiation by dissolved or suspended constituents in the fluid, reflection, refraction, and dissipation in space. Mathematical expressions have been developed to describe each of these phenomena, and these expressions have been incorporated into numerical models to allow simulations of the fluence rate field within UV photoreactors.

Perhaps the most basic of these models are discrete point source summation (PSS)[77] and the continuous analog known as line-source integration (LSI).[78] In these methods, a cylindrical lamp is simulated as a set of colinear point sources of radiation. A mathematical expression is developed to describe the effects of dissipation and absorption on the spatial distribution of radiant energy around a single point source. The fluence rate field around a lamp is then simulated by summing the contributions from all hypothetical point sources. The PSS and LSI models provide estimates of the fluence rate field that are in good agreement with measurements at locations that are far from the lamp itself; however, the difference between PSS/LSI model predictions and measurements increases as the distance from the source decreases. In part, the divergence between model simulation results and measurements is attributable to the fact that the PSS/LSI models do not account for the effects of reflection and refraction. Moreover, the PSS and LSI models imply a simplification of lamp geometry that becomes increasingly important as distance from the source decreases.

Figure 9.9 (left) illustrates the application of the PSS and LSI models for simulation of the fluence rate (E) field around an LP Hg lamp. Figure 9.9 (right) illustrates the

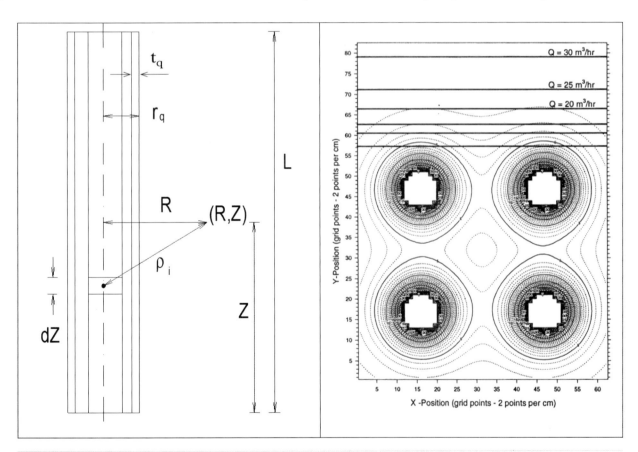

FIGURE 9.9   Left, Schematic illustration of single low-pressure mercury (Hg) lamp and the variables used to simulate the fluence rate (E) field in the vicinity of the lamp by the point source summation and line-source integration models. Variables include: r_q = radius of quartz sleeve; t_q = thickness of quartz sleeve; R = radial position of receptor site; z = longitudinal position of receptor site; rho_i = distance from i^{th} point source to receptor site; L = lamp length. Right, Two-dimensional cross-section of simulated fluence rate field in a four-lamp reactor system based on low-pressure Hg lamps. Dashed and solid lines in the figure illustrate lines of constant fluence rate. Horizontal lines at the top of the figure illustrate locations of the free surface for various flow rate conditions. Reprinted from Blatchley.[78] Copyright © 1997 Elsevier.

application of this same approach for simulation of the fluence rate field cross-section in a four-lamp, open channel reactor. Fluence rate is observed to fall off rapidly with distance from the lamps. In this open-channel system, the effects of free surface elevation are also evident. If this free surface is allowed to extend beyond the part of the channel cross-section where UV radiation is able to reach, then a substantial fraction of the fluid flowing through the system will be essentially unexposed to UV radiation. Under these circumstances, process performance will be very poor. Because of this, liquid level-control devices are crucial to the operation of open-channel systems. Many other fluence rate field models have been developed as improvements to the PSS/LSI approach. In general, these models include logic that is similar to the PSS model but may relax one or more of the assumptions used in the PSS/LSI approach, or include terms (eg, reflection or refraction) that are not accounted for by PSS/LSI.

Fluid Mechanics

As described earlier, many UV disinfection systems operate by pumping a fluid (usually water or air) through an array of lamps/jackets to allow exposure of dissolved or suspended constituents to UV radiation from these lamps. In virtually all practical applications of UV disinfection, flow through these lamp arrays is within the turbulent regime. In addition, the lamp/sleeve assemblies often impart aggressive mixing behavior on the fluid being treated. Collectively, these attributes of UV disinfection system design dictate that fluid mechanics are quite complicated.

Computational fluid dynamics (CFD) is a family of numerical methods that are used to simulate complex fluid flows. CFD models and computer hardware have advanced to the point that accurate simulations of fluid mechanics can be developed in relatively short periods of time for a wide range of engineering applications. CFD simulations involve numerical approximations to the equation of continuity and the equations of motion. For systems that operate in the turbulent regime, a turbulence closure model is also required. CFD simulations involve discretization of the computational domain, which will generally include the part of the system through which fluid flows, plus representative segments of the connecting pipes or ducts. Numerical methods are applied to converge on a solution to the governing equations that describes fluid flow within the system.

Computational Fluid Dynamics-I Field Simulations

Modeling of UV disinfection systems generally involves simulations that integrate the results of fluence rate field models with the output from a CFD simulation, so-called CFD-I models.[74-76,79-81] A common approach involves interrogation of CFD simulation results to allow simulations of individual particle trajectories through the system. In turn, the results of the fluence rate field simulation are then mapped on to each simulated trajectory to allow estimation of the dose received by a particle that follows such a trajectory.

Figure 9.10 illustrates the application of a CFD-I simulation to a simple UV disinfection system that involves a single lamp. The flow field approximation was developed for a fixed flow rate and the geometry of the reactor system, including inlet and outlet geometries. This flow field was then interrogated to allow simulation of particle trajectories following a "random walk" modeling approach. An LSI simulation was applied to the reactor (inset, lower right) based on the output characteristics of the lamp, the optical (absorbance) characteristics of the water being pumped through the reactor, and the geometry of the system. The fluence rate field was then mapped onto each particle trajectory to allow estimation of the dose received by each particle as it traverses the system. This calculation was repeated for a large number of particle trajectories, thereby allowing simulation of the dose distribution delivered by the reactor.

It is important to recognize that each particle trajectory through the reactor is unique, as is the dose delivered to a particle based on that trajectory. Variation in the dose distribution is influenced by differences in initial position for a particle as it enters the array. But even for two particles that start their trajectory at the same location, the turbulence characteristics of the flow field dictate that their trajectories and corresponding doses will be different.

Simulations of Disinfection Performance

The overall behavior of a UV disinfection system is governed by the combined effects of the dose distribution and the dose-response behavior of the target microbes. Mathematically, this is accounted for by application of the segregated-flow model:

$$\left(\frac{N}{N_0}\right)_{reactor} = \int_0^\infty \underbrace{\left(\frac{N}{N_0}\right)_{batch}}_{\substack{Dose-Response\\Behavior}} \cdot \underbrace{E(D) \cdot dD}_{\substack{Dose\\Distribution}} \quad (13)$$

The left side of equation (13) describes the fraction of organisms that retain viability after passing through the reactor. The first term in the integrand describes the dose-response behavior of the target microbe; this behavior is assigned using a dose-response model that fits the measured dose-response behavior of the target microbe. The second term in the integrand describes the dose distribution, which is a characteristic of the reactor system that can be simulated using the CFD-I approach. Equation (13) has been demonstrated to provide accurate, reliable predictions of reactor behavior, when the dose-response behavior of the target microbe and the dose distribution can be accurately described.[74-76]

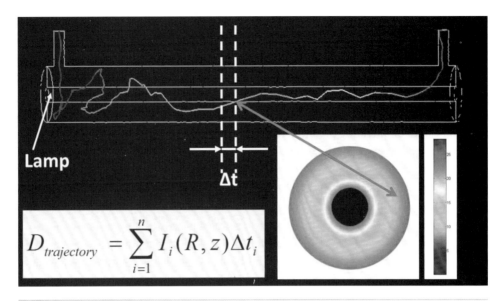

$$D_{trajectory} = \sum_{i=1}^{n} I_i(R, z) \Delta t_i$$

FIGURE 9.10 Illustration of the application of computational fluid dynamics (CFD)-I modeling for simulation of process behavior in a ultraviolet disinfection system. A CFD model was used to simulate the turbulent flow field in irradiated zone of the reactor. In turn, a random walk model was used to interrogate the simulated flow field so as to simulate individual particle trajectories through the reactor system, one of which is shown above. The simulated fluence rate field was then mapped onto each trajectory to allow estimation of the trajectory-specific dose ($D_{trajectory}$). By repeating this calculation for a large number of particles, it is possible to estimate the dose distribution delivered by the reactor. Integration of the dose distribution with a dose-response model for the target microbe via the segregated flow model allows estimation of the efficacy of the reactor system. For a color version of this art, please consult the eBook.

These simulations have taught that the most efficient UV disinfection systems tend to be characterized by a narrow dose distribution because most of the microorganisms that retain viability after passing through the system will have experienced a relatively small dose. By eliminating or reducing the number of organisms that receive low doses, fewer microbes are able to "survive" (ie, retain viability). Narrow dose distributions are achieved in systems where the fluence rate field shows relatively little spatial variation, and in systems where fluid flow lacks "dead zones" or patterns of flow that allow short-circuiting of the irradiated zone.

▶ REACTOR VALIDATION

UV irradiation is the disinfection process of choice for inactivation of the protozoan parasites *C parvum* and *G lamblia*; it is also effective for inactivation of a wide range of other microbes. As such, it has emerged as an important process for production of drinking water from surface water or groundwater sources, where opportunities for contamination by protozoan parasites and other microbial pathogens are likely to exist. The UV disinfection systems used in production of potable water for municipal applications are required to undergo validation

testing. The goal of validation testing is to demonstrate the ability of the system to achieve a desired extent of microbial inactivation based on attributes of the system and its operation that can be measured in real time. The default method for validation is called *biodosimetry*, which involves a series of linked experiments.

Biodosimetry is conducted by subjecting a challenge organism to UV exposure. Ideal characteristics for challenge organisms include ease of culture and assay, resistance to UV exposure, nonpathogenicity toward humans, and UV dose-response behavior that mimics that of the target organism for treatment. Examples of challenge organisms used in biodosimetric testing include coliphages MS2, Qβ, T1UV, and the spores of *B subtilis*. A suspension of the challenge organism is pumped through the reactor undergoing validation over a range of operating conditions. Operating variables included in biodosimetric testing generally include flow rate, UV transmittance, and lamp output power. For each operating condition applied in biodosimetric testing, the concentration of viable or infective challenge organism is measured in the influent and effluent at steady state. The same challenge organism suspension is also subjected to a range of well-defined UV doses under a collimated beam. The observed $\log_{10}$-transformed inactivation responses of the reactor being tested are then compared to the dose-response behavior for the challenge organism as a means of assigning a *reduction equivalent dose* (RED) to each condition. Nonlinear regression is then applied to develop a model to describe the RED as a function of operating conditions. In turn, this information can be programmed into the operating system of the reactor in an actual application, thereby allowing a target level of performance to be maintained in real time based on measured values of operating parameters.

Figure 9.11 illustrates an example of a biodosimetry data set for an actual reactor system. For this test, the challenge organism was coliphage MS2. The test itself was conducted over a period of several days. For each day of the test, a suspension of the challenge organism was prepared and pumped through the reactor, with influent and effluent samples being collected over a range of steady-state operating conditions to allow measurement of $\log_{10}$-transformed

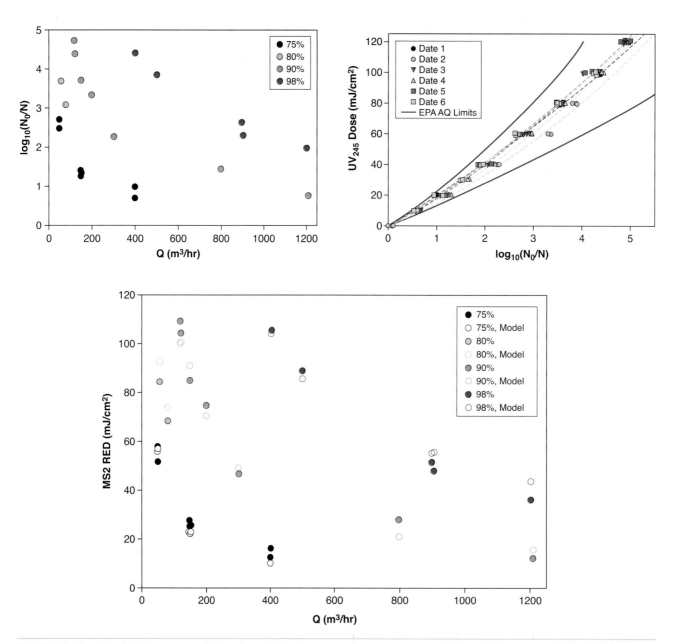

FIGURE 9.11   Graphical summary of data from biodosimetry experiments. Upper left panel illustrates measured values of $\log_{10}$-transformed MS2 inactivation fraction as a function of flow rate. For this experiment, data are shown only for the 100% power setting on the lamps. Separate data sets were developed for each of four values of ultraviolet (UV) transmittance. Upper right panel illustrates measured values of dose-response behavior for MS2 on each of 6 days of testing. A quadratic best-fit line is drawn through each data set to allow interpolation. The data from each test in the upper left panel is used to estimate a MS2 reduction equivalent dose (RED) value based on the interpolation functions that are defined in the upper right panel. The bottom panel illustrates MS2 RED as a function of flow rate for four values of UV transmittance. Data courtesy of HDR Engineering. For a color version of this art, please consult the eBook.

inactivation ratio, $\log_{10}(N_0/N)$ (Figure 9.11, top left). For each day of testing, the same suspension is subjected to a range of well-defined UV doses under a collimated beam to allow definition of the UV dose-response behavior of the challenge organism (Figure 9.11, top right). The observed values of $\log_{10}(N_0/N)$ from the test with the reactor being evaluated are then used to estimate the RED by interpolation of the dose-response data. This allows development of a function to illustration RED as a function of operating conditions for the reactor. Figure 9.11 (bottom) illustrates validated reactor RED as a function of flow rate for a range of UV transmittance values. In turn, these data can be used to assign inactivation credit for a given target microbe, such as *C parvum* or *G lamblia*, based on predefined tables that have been developed for this purpose. Furthermore, the results of this testing approach can be used to develop a control function for the validated reactor based on real-time measurements of operating parameters.

Several guidance documents have been developed to define this process in greater detail. The *UV Disinfection Guidance Manual* was developed by the US Environmental Protection Agency[82] to provide state and local regulators with guidance on validation of UV disinfection systems. The methods defined by this document allow a reactor to be operated to achieve a given level of inactivation of a target microbe, such as *C parvum, G lamblia,* or viruses. Similar documents have been developed in Austria and Germany to define the validation process.[83-85] The European standards call for validation to define operating conditions that will achieve a RED of 40 mJ/cm², which has been demonstrated to be effective for disinfection in most applications.

▶ SOLAR ULTRAVIOLET DISINFECTION

Access to safe, affordable water is a common problem in developing countries. In many cases, contamination by microbial pathogens is a cause of chronic illness; women and children are affected disproportionately by these problems in developing countries. Effective interventions to improve water potability in developing countries generally involve systems that are simple and inexpensive to operate and that employ locally available resources. Given that many developing countries are in near-equatorial areas, a common resource in these areas is solar radiation. As such, there has been considerable interest in the development of solar UV disinfection systems. At least three different classes of solar UV disinfections systems have been developed.

SODIS

SODIS is an abbreviation for *solar disinfection*.[86,87] In this process, water is typically placed in a polyethylene terephthalate (PET) plastic bottle and exposed to ambient solar radiation for a period of 6 hours. This exposure scenario has been demonstrated to be effective for inactivation of most microbial pathogens. Moreover, among communities who have adopted SODIS, the incidence of waterborne, communicable diseases has dropped significantly. SODIS relies largely on exposure of a water sample to ambient UVA radiation. UVA radiation is relatively ineffective at causing direct photochemical damage to microbes. But UVA radiation is known to promote the formation of several ROS, which in turn have the ability to inactivate microbes. Heating of water is also thought to contribute to disinfection in some settings.

SODIS is widely used for disinfection, with more than 2 million people from 28 countries applying the process on a regular basis. It is simple and inexpensive to apply and is effective. But SODIS suffers from two important disadvantages. First, it is a batch process. This limits production based on the number of containers that are available for this purpose. Second, it is generally conducted in a PET plastic bottle. PET is essentially opaque to UVB radiation, which represents the most germicidally active portion of the ambient solar spectrum at most locations.

Full-Spectrum Solar Disinfection

In this process, ambient solar radiation is amplified through the use of as simple device, such as a compound parabolic collector (CPC). A UV-transparent tube is placed in the focus of the CPC cross-section and water is pumped through the tube to allow exposure. Figure 9.12 illustrates a CPC-based system that was developed for this purpose.

The full-spectrum device allows direct solar disinfection based on the entire (amplified) ambient spectrum. The inclusion of UVB radiation in this method is crucial, in that it allows for direct photochemical damage to microbial DNA, as is observed with UVC radiation. Direct solar exposure has been demonstrated to be effective for inactivation of the microbial pathogens that are responsible for a large fraction of waterborne microbial illnesses, including *C. parvum* and surrogates for the bacteria that cause typhoid fever and cholera. Although the CPC-based system is designed as a continuous-flow device that includes UVB radiation, the flow rate that can be achieved through these systems is modest.

Indirect Solar Disinfection

SODIS and full-spectrum solar UV disinfection both depend on the antimicrobial characteristics of ambient solar radiation. As such, both of these systems are effective but quite slow. The ambient solar spectrum is dominated by radiation that is nongermicidal or poorly germicidal, including the entire visible spectrum. In indirect solar UV disinfection, ambient solar radiation is collected on solar panels. This energy is converted into electrical energy that is stored on batteries. In turn, this stored electrical energy

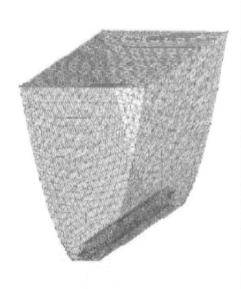
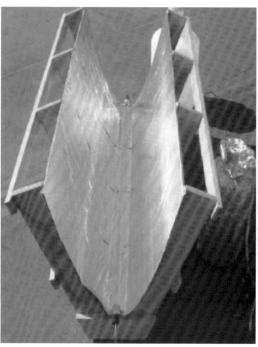

FIGURE 9.12 Left, Digitized image of compound parabolic collector (CPC). Note the ultraviolet-transparent transmission tube located in the focus of the CPC cross-section. Right, Photo of CPC used in field testing. For a color version of this art, please consult the eBook. Reprinted from Mbonimpa et al.[27] Copyright © 2012 Elsevier.

is used to power a small, commercially available UV reactor. As an illustration, there are commercially available reactors that are able to treat on the order of 5000 L of water per day at a power requirement of 10 to 12 W. When coupled with a system to accomplish physical separation of particles (ie, filter), these systems are able to provide safe water to communities of 500 people or more.

▶ EFFECTS OF ULTRAVIOLET RADIATION ON WATER CHEMISTRY

UV irradiation promotes a wide range of photochemical reactions. When applied to water, some of the most important reactions involve damage to nucleic acids and proteins, which in turn lead to microbial inactivation (ie, disinfection). It is important to recognize, however, that UV-induced photoreactions can also cause changes in the composition of dissolved chemical constituents. Some of these chemical changes can lead to improvements in water quality, whereas others lead to degradation of water quality.

Nitrate

Nitrate (NO_3^-) is a critical form of nitrogen within the nitrogen cycle and a common product of oxidation of organic and inorganic compounds that contain reduced nitrogen. As such, it is a common form of nitrogen in many water sources. NO_3^- strongly absorbs radiation at wavelengths less than approximately 240 nm; this radiation is used to cause photolysis of NO_3^- to yield a range of products, including nitrite (NO_2^-) and reactive intermediates, such as the nitric oxide radical (NO), O_2 radical ($O_2^-•$), and hydroxyl radical (HO•).[88] NO_3^- is a form of nitrogen that is readily assimilated by many plants, whereas NO_2^- causes methemoglobinemia. Limits on the acceptable concentrations of both forms of nitrogen have been defined for drinking water supplies; the limits based on NO_2^- are substantially lower than those based on NO_3^-.

The reactive intermediates that form from photolysis of NO_3^- are important to water quality in at least two ways. First, these radicals can react with other constituents in water to yield disinfection by-products (DBPs) that are potentially harmful to human health. As an example, photolysis of NO_3^- by the output of MP Hg lamps has been shown to promote the formation of halonitromethanes and haloacetonitriles.[89] Second, these reactive intermediates, especially HO•, can promote the degradation of contaminants that are present in water. It has been shown that trace pollutants can be degraded by HO• that is produced by photolysis of NO_3^-.[90]

Nitrogen-Chlorine Photolysis

In settings where reduced nitrogen (eg, amines, ammonia) and free chlorine are present, nitrogen-chlorine (N-Cl) bonds are readily formed. The N-Cl bond is quite photolabile and exposure to germicidal UV radiation leads to cleavage of the N-Cl bond, yielding a chlorine radical and an aminyl radical.[91] These radical products then go on to participate in further reactions. The copresence of amines and free chlorine is common in swimming pools, in water reuse settings, and in production of potable water. The reactions that are promoted by UV-induced cleavage of the N-Cl bond lead to a wide range of reaction products. For example, UV photolysis of mono-, di-, and trichloramine (NH_2Cl, $NHCl_2$, NCl_3) lead to formation of NO_2^-, NO_3^-, N_2O, and N_2.[91] Photolysis of chlorinated amine compounds, including amino acids and creatinine has been shown to promote the formation of several toxic DBPs, including cyanogen chloride (CNCl) and dichloracetonitrile.[92-94] The combined application of UV and free chlorine has also been demonstrated to be an effective strategy for oxidation of ammonia-N.[95] Similarly, chlorination followed by UV irradiation has been demonstrated to be effective for degradation and detoxification of the cyanotoxin microcystin-LR.[96]

Hydrogen Peroxide Photolysis

UVC radiation is able to photolyze the hydrogen peroxide (H_2O_2) molecule[97,98]:

$$H_2O_2 + hv \rightarrow 2HO \qquad (14)$$

This reaction is relatively inefficient because of the low molar absorptivity of the H_2O_2 molecule; however, the product of this reaction is the hydroxyl radical, which is a powerful oxidant. Like NO_3^- photolysis, UV/H_2O_2 represents an example of an advanced oxidation process, one in which highly reactive oxidizing intermediates, such as HO•, are generated. The UV/H_2O_2 process is used to oxidize highly recalcitrant contaminants in water supplies.

Hypochlorous Acid Photolysis

Similarly, hypochlorous acid (HOCl) can be photolyzed by exposure to UVC radiation[99-101]:

$$HOCl + hv \rightarrow HO\cdot + Cl \qquad (15)$$

This reaction is characterized by a slightly larger value of molar absorptivity than H_2O_2 for most UVC wavelengths, and as such, it is a more efficient generator of hydroxyl radicals than the UV/H_2O_2 process. It also leads to formation of a chlorine radical, which can open up reaction pathways that would not be involved in the UV/H_2O_2 process.

▶ CONCLUSIONS

UV irradiation is effective for control of pathogenic microorganisms in a broad range of applications. The ability

of UV irradiation to function over such a diverse set of applications is attributable to the basic characteristics of the process. Of critical importance is the fact that microbial inactivation is accomplished at relatively low doses of UV radiation, which allows the process to be applied in a cost-effective manner. In a general sense, the photochemical reactions that lead to microbial inactivation tend to be rapid, whereas other reactions that can lead to DBP formation tend to be slow. Collectively, these attributes lead to favorable results of treatment through the application of UV disinfection. There are some circumstances where adverse changes in water composition can result from UV irradiation, and these need to be accounted for in process design. The development of computational and experimental hardware for characterization of the fundamental physicochemical characteristics that govern process behavior in UV systems have made it possible to develop predictive mathematical models for these systems. These models have been demonstrated to be capable of providing accurate predictions of process performance and are likely to represent important tools in the design of UV-based disinfection systems in the future.

REFERENCES

1. Downes A, Blunt TP. On the influence of light upon protoplasm. *Proc R Soc London.* 1878;28:199-212.
2. Downes A, Blunt TP. The influence of light upon the development of bacteria. *Nature.* 1877;16:218-219.
3. Downes A, Blunt TP. Researchers upon the effect of light upon bacteria and other organisms. *Proc R Soc London.* 1877;26:488-500.
4. Stumm W, Morgan JJ. *Aquatic Chemistry: Chemical Equilibria and Rates in Natural Waters.* New York, NY: Wiley; 1995.
5. Iqbal M. *An Introduction to Solar Radiation.* Toronto, Ontario, Canada: Academic Press; 1983.
6. National Renewable Energy Laboratory. SMARTS: simple model of the atmospheric radiative transfer of sunshine 2013. National Renewable Energy Laboratory Web site. https://www.nrel.gov/grid/solar-resource/smarts.html. Accessed 2013.
7. American Society for Testing and Materials International. *E490: Standard Solar Constant and Zero Air Mass Solar Spectral Irradiance Tables.* West Conshohocken, PA: American Society for Testing and Materials International; 2014.
8. American Society for Testing and Materials International. *G173: Standard Tables for Reference Solar Spectral Irradiances: Direct Normal and Hemispherical on 37° Tilted Surface.* West Conshohocken, PA: American Society for Testing and Materials International; 2012.
9. Finlayson-Pitts BJ, Pitts J, James N. *Chemistry of the Upper and Lower Atmosphere: Theory, Experiments, and Applications.* San Diego, CA: Academic Press; 2000.
10. Phillips R. *Sources and Applications of Ultraviolet Radiation.* London, United Kingdom: Academic Press; 1983.
11. United Nations Environment Programme. *Minamata Convention on Mercury: Text and Annexes.* Nairobi, Kenya: United Nations Environment Programme; 2013.
12. European Union. Directive 2011/65/EU of the European Parliament and of the Council of 8 June 2011 on the restriction of the use of certain hazardous substances in electrical and electronic equipment. *Off J Eur.* 2011:L174/88-L/10.
13. Lomaev MI, Sosnin EA, Tarasenko VF. Excilamps and their applications. *Chem Eng Technol.* 2016;39(1):39-50.
14. Lomaev MI, Sosnin EA, Tarasenko VF. Excilamps and their applications. *Prog Quantum Electron.* 2012;36:51-97.

15. Kogelschatz U, ed. Collective phenomena in volume and surface barrier discharges. In: *25th Summer School and International Symposium on the Physics of Ionized Gases*. Donji Milanovac, Serbia: Symposium on the Physics of Ionized Gases; 2010.

16. Kogelschatz U. Dielectric-barrier discharges: their history, discharge physics, and industrial applications. *Plasma Chem Plasma Processing*. 2003;23:1-46.

17. Eliasson B, Kogelschatz U. UV excimer radiation from dielectric-barrier discharges. *Appl Phys B*. 1988;46:299-303.

18. Song K, Mohseni M, Taghipour F. Application of ultraviolet light-emitting diodes (UV-LEDs) for water disinfection: a review. *Water Res*. 2016;94:341-349.

19. Khan A, Balakrishnan K, Katona T. Ultraviolet light-emitting diodes based on group three nitrides. *Nat Photonics*. 2008;2:77-84.

20. Ding K, Avrutin V, Ozgur U, Morkoc H. Status of growth of group III-nitride heterostructures for deep ultraviolet light-emitting diodes. *Crystals*. 2017;7(10):300.

21. Orton JW, Foxon CT. Group III nitride semiconductors for short wavelength light-emitting devices. *Rep Prog Phys*. 1998;61:1-75.

22. Yoshida S, Misawa S, Gonda S. Properties of AlxGa1-xN Films prepared by reactive molecular-beam epitaxy. *J Appl Physics*. 1982;53:6844-6888.

23. Boehm AB, Yamahara KM, Love DC, Peterson BM, McNeill K, Nelson KL. Covariation and photoinactivation of traditional and novel indicator organisms and human viruses at a sewage-impacted marine beach. *Environ Sci Technol*. 2009;43:8046-8052.

24. Kohn T, Nelson KL. Sunlight-mediated inactivation of MS2 coliphage via exogenous singlet oxygen produced by sensitizers in natural waters. *Environ Sci Technol*. 2007;41:192-197.

25. Reed RH, Mani SK, Meyer V. Solar photo-oxidative disinfection of drinking water: preliminary field observations. *Lett Appl Microbiol*. 2000;30:432-436.

26. Read RH. Solar inactivation of faecal bacteria in water: the critical role of oxygen. *Lett Appl Microbiol*. 1997;24:276-280.

27. Mbonimpa EG, Vadheim B, Blatchley ER III. Continuous-flow solar UVB disinfection reactor for drinking water. *Water Res*. 2012;46:2344-2354.

28. Jagger J. *Introduction to Research in Ultra-Violet Photobiology*. Englewood Cliffs, NJ: Prentice-Hall; 1967.

29. Coohill TP. Exposure response curves action spectra and amplification factors. In: Biggs RH, Joyner MEB, eds. *Stratospheric Ozone Depletion/UV-B Radiation in the Biosphere*. Berlin, Germany: Springer; 1994:57-62.

30. Gates FL. A study of the bactericidal action of ultra violet light: III. The absorption of ultra violet light by bacteria. *J Gen Physiol*. 1930;14:31-42.

31. Gates FL. A study of the bactericidal action of ultra violet light: I. The reaction to monochromatic radiations. *J Gen Physiol*. 1929;13:231-248.

32. Gates FL. A study of the bactericidal action of ultra violet light: II. The effect of various environmental factors and conditions. *J Gen Physiol*. 1929;13:249-260.

33. Smith KC. Basic ultraviolet radiation photobiology. Photobiological Sciences Online Web site. http://photobiology.info/UVphoto.html. Accessed August 23, 2019.

34. Sinha RP, Häder DP. UV-induced DNA damage and repair: a review. *Photochem Photobiol Sci*. 2002;1:225-236.

35. Smith KC, Shetlar MD. DNA-protein crosslinks. Photobiological Sciences Online Web site. http://photobiology.info/Smith_Shetlar.html. Accessed August 23, 2019.

36. Friedberg EC, Walker GC, Siede W, Wood RD, Schultz RA, Ellenberger T. *DNA Repair and Mutagenesis*. Washington, DC: ASM Press; 2006.

37. Setlow P. Resistance of spores of *Bacillus* species to ultraviolet light. *Environ Mol Mutagen*. 2001;38(2-3):97-104.

38. Coohill TP, Sagripanti JL. Overview of the inactivation by 254 nm ultraviolet radiation of bacteria with particular relevance to biodefense. *Photochem Photobiol*. 2008;84:1084-1090.

39. Jagger J. *Solar-UV Actions on Living Cells*. New York, NY: Praeger Scientific; 1985.

40. Blatchley ER III, Dumoutier N, Halaby TN, Levi Y, Laîné JM. Bacterial responses to ultraviolet irradiation. *Water Sci Technol*. 2001;43:179-186.

41. Redford EL, Myers J. Some effects of ultraviolet radiations on the metabolism of *Chlorella*. *J Cell Comp Physiol*. 1951;38:217-243.

42. Clancy JL, Bukhari Z, Hargy TM, Bolton JR, Dussert BW, Marshall MM. Using UV to inactivate *Cryptosporidium*. *J Am Water Works Assoc*. 2000;92:97-104.

43. Clancy JL, Hargy TM, Marshall MM, Dyksen JE. UV light inactivation of *Cryptosporidium* oocysts. *J Am Water Works Assoc*. 1998;90:92-102.

44. Bukhari Z, Marshall MM, Korich DG, et al. Comparison of *Cryptosporidium parvum* viability and infectivity assays following ozone treatment of oocysts. *Appl Environ Microbiol*. 2000;66:2972-2980.

45. Craik SA, Weldon D, Finch GR, Bolton JR, Belosevic M. Inactivation of *Cryptosporidium parvum* oocysts using medium- and low-pressure ultraviolet radiation. *Water Res*. 2001;35:1387-1398.

46. Craik SA, Finch GR, Bolton JR, Belosevic M. Inactivation of *Giardia muris* cysts using medium-pressure ultraviolet radiation in filtered drinking water. *Water Res*. 2000;34:4325-4332.

47. Slifko TR, Huffman DE, Dussert B, et al. Comparison of tissue culture and animal models for assessment of *Cryptospridium parvum* infection. *Exp Parasitol*. 2002;101:97-106.

48. Severin BF, Suidan MT, Engelbrecht RS. Mixing effects in UV disinfection. *J Wat Pollut Control Fed*. 1984;56:881-888.

49. Severin BF, Suidan MT, Engelbrecht RS. Kinetic modeling of UV disinfection of water. *Water Res*. 1983;17:1669-1678.

50. Pennell KG, Aronson AI, Blatchley ER III. Phenotypic persistence and external shielding ultraviolet radiation inactivation kinetic model. *J Appl Microbiol*. 2008;104:1192-1202.

51. Malayeri AH, Mohseni M, Cairns B, Bolton JR, Chevrefils G, Caron E. *Fluence (UV Dose) Required to Achieve Incremental Log Inactivation of Bacteria, Protozoa, Viruses and Algae*. Chevy Chase, MD: IUVA News; 2016.

52. Kowalski WJ, Bahnfleth WP, Witham DL, Severin BF, Whittam TS. Mathematical modeling of ultraviolet germicidal irradiation for air disinfection. *Quant Microbiol*. 2000;2:249-270.

53. Hijnen WA, Beerendonk EF, Medema GJ. Inactivation credit of UV radiation for viruses, bacteria and protozoan (oo)cysts in water: a review. *Water Res*. 2006;40:3-22.

54. Coohill TP, Sagripanti JL. Bacterial inactivation by solar ultraviolet radiation compared with sensitivity to 254 nm radiation. *Photochem Photobiol*. 2009;85:1043-1052.

55. Lytle CD, Sagripanti JL. Predicted inactivation of viruses of relevance to biodefense by solar radiation. *J Virol*. 2005;79:14244-14252.

56. Beck SE, Rodriguez RA, Linden KG, Hargy TM, Larason TC, Wright HB. Wavelength dependent UV inactivation and DNA damage of adenovirus as measured by cell culture infectivity and long range quantitative PCR. *Environ Sci Technol*. 2014;48:591-598.

57. Bellinger-Kawahara C, Cleaver JE, Diener TO, Prusiner SB. Purified scrapie prions resist inactivation by UV irradiation. *J Virol*. 1987;61:159-166.

58. Coohill TP, Ghetti F. Action spectroscopy: ultraviolet radiation. In: Greisbeck A, Oelgemöller M, Ghetti F, eds. *CRC Handbook of Organic Photochemistry and Photobiology*. 3rd ed. Boca Raton, FL: CRC Press; 2012:1093-1103.

59. Coohill TP. UV action spectra for marine phytoplankton. *Photochem Photobiol*. 1997;65:259-260.

60. Bolton JR, Mayor-Smith I, Linden KG. Rethinking the concepts of fluence (UV dose) and fluence rate: the importance of photon-based units—a systemic review. *Photochem Photobiol*. 2015;91:1252-1262.

61. Sutherland JC. Biological effects of polychromatic light. *Photochem Photobiol*. 2002;76(2):164-170.

62. Beck SE, Wright HB, Hargy TM, Larason TC, Linden KG. Action spectra for validation of pathogen disinfection in medium-pressure ultraviolet (UV) systems. *Water Res*. 2015;70:27-37.

63. Coohill TP. Historical aspects of ultraviolet action spectroscopy. *Photochem Photobiol*. 1997;(suppl 65):123S-128S.

64. Jagger J. Photoreactivation. Photobiological Sciences Online Web site. http://photobiology.info/Jagger.html. Accessed August 23, 2019.

65. Cleaver JE. Nucleotide excision repair in human cells. Photobiological Sciences Online Web site. http://photobiology.info/CleaverNER.html. Accessed August 23, 2019.

66. Bohrerova Z, Rosenblum J, Linden KG. Importance of recovery of *E. coli* in water following ultraviolet light disinfection. *J Environ Eng.* 2015;141:6.

67. Janion C. Inducible SOS response system of DNA repair and mutagenesis in *Escherichia coli. Int J Biol Sci.* 2008;4(6):338-344.

68. Moeller R, Douki T, Cadet J, et al. UV-radiation-induced formation of DNA bipyrimidine photoproducts in *Bacillus subtilis* endospores and their repair during germination. *Int Microbiol.* 2007;10:39-46.

69. Link L, Sawyer J, Venkateswaran K, Nicholson W. Extreme spore UV resistance of *Bacillus pumilus* isolates obtained from an ultraclean spacecraft assembly facility. *Microb Ecol.* 2004;47:159-163.

70. Mahnert A, Vaishampayan P, Probst AJ, et al. Cleanroom maintenance significantly reduces abundance but not diversity of indoor microbiomes. *PLoS One.* 2015;10(8):e0134848.

71. Horneck G, Bucker H, Reitz G. Long-term survival of bacterial-spores in-space. *Adv Space Res.* 1994;14:41-45.

72. Onofri S, de Vera JP, Zucconi L, et al. Survival of Antarctic cryptoendolithic fungi in simulated Martian conditions on board the international space station. *Astrobiology.* 2015;15:1052-1059.

73. Albarracín VH, Gärtner W, Farías M. UV resistance and photoreactivation of extremophiles from high-altitude Andean lakes. Photobiological Sciences Online Web site. http://photobiology.info/Albarracin.html. Accessed August 23, 2019.

74. Lyn DA, Chiu K, Blatchley ER III. Numerical modeling of flow and disinfection in UV disinfection channels. *J Environ Eng-Asce.* 1999;125:17-26.

75. Chiu K, Lyn DA, Savoye P, Blatchley ER III. Integrated UV disinfection model based on particle tracking. *J Environ Eng-Asce.* 1999;125:7-16.

76. Chiu KP, Lyn DA, Savoye P, Blatchley ER III. Effect of UV system modifications on disinfection performance. *J Environ Eng-Asce.* 1999;125:459-469.

77. Jacob SM, Dranoff JS. Light intensity profiles in a perfectly mixed photoreactor. *AIChE J.* 1970;16:359-363.

78. Blatchley ER III. Numerical modelling of UV intensity: application to collimated-beam reactors and continuous-flow systems. *Water Res.* 1997;31:2205-2218.

79. Lyn DA, Blatchley ER III. Numerical computational fluid dynamics-based models of ultraviolet disinfection channels. *J Environ Eng-Asce.* 2005;131:838-849.

80. Liu D, Wu C, Linden K, Ducoste J. Numerical simulation of UV disinfection reactors: evaluation of alternative turbulence models. *Appl Math Model.* 2007;31:1753-1769.

81. Ducoste J, Linden K, Rokjer D, Liu D. Assessment of reduction equivalent fluence bias using computational fluid dynamics. *Environ Eng Sci.* 2005;22:615-628.

82. US Environmental Protection Agency. *Ultraviolet Disinfection Guidance Manual for the Final Long Term 2 Enhanced Surface Water Treatment Rule.* Washington, DC: US Environmental Protection Agency; 2006.

83. ÖNORM. *Plants for the Disinfection of Water Using Ultraviolet Radiation—Requirements and Testing—Part 2: Medium Pressure Mercury Lamp Plants.* Vienna, Austria: ÖNORM; 2003.

84. ÖNORM. *Plants for the Disinfection of Water Using Ultraviolet Radiation—Requirements and Testing—Part 1: Low Pressure Mercury Lamp Plants.* Vienna, Austria: ÖNORM; 2001.

85. Deutscher Verein des Gas- und Wasserfaches. *UV Disinfection Devices for Drinking Water Supply—Requirements and Testing.* Bonn, Germany: Deutscher Verein des Gas- und Wasserfaches; 2006.

86. Meierhofer R, Wegelin M. *Solar Water Disinfection—A Guide for the Application of SODIS.* Dubendorf, Switzerland: Swiss Federal Institute of Environmental Science and Technology: 2002.

87. Eawag. SODIS: safe drinking water for all 2018. SODIS Web site. http://www.sodis.ch/index_EN. Accessed March 13, 2019.

88. Mack J, Bolton JR. Photochemistry of nitrite and nitrate in aqueous solution: a review. *J Photochem Photobiol Chem.* 1999;128:1-13.

89. Shah AD, Dotson AD, Linden KG, Mitch WA. Impact of UV disinfection combined with chlorination/chloramination on the formation of halonitromethanes and haloacetonitriles in drinking water. *Environ Sci Technol.* 2011;45:3657-3664.

90. Keen OS, Love NG, Linden KG. The role of effluent nitrate in trace organic chemical oxidation during UV disinfection. *Water Res.* 2012;46:5224-5234.

91. Li J, Blatchley ER III. UV photodegradation of inorganic chloramines. *Environ Sci Technol.* 2009;43(1):60-65.

92. Weng SC, Li J, Wood KV, et al. UV-induced effects on chlorination of creatinine. *Water Res.* 2013;47(14):4948-4956.

93. Weng SC, Blatchley ER III. Ultraviolet-induced effects on chloramine and cyanogen chloride formation from chlorination of amino acids. *Environ Sci Technol.* 2013;47:4269-4276.

94. Weng S, Li J, Blatchley ER III. Effects of UV 254 irradiation on residual chlorine and DBPs in chlorination of model organic-N precursors in swimming pools. *Water Res.* 2012;46:2674-2682.

95. Zhang XR, Li W, Blatchley ER III, Wang X, Ren P. UV/chlorine process for ammonia removal and disinfection by-product reduction: comparison with chlorination. *Water Res.* 2015;68:804-811.

96. Zhang XR, Li J, Yang JY, et al. Chlorine/UV process for decomposition and detoxification of microcystin-LR. *Environ Sci Technol.* 2016;50:7671-7678.

97. Rivera-Utrilla J, Sánchez-Polo M, Ferro-García MÁ, Prados-Joya G, Ocampo-Pérez R. Pharmaceuticals as emerging contaminants and their removal from water. A review. *Chemosphere.* 2013;93:1268-1287.

98. Wols BA, Hofman-Caris CH. Review of photochemical reaction constants of organic micropollutants required for UV advanced oxidation processes in water. *Water Res.* 2012;46:2815-2827.

99. Sichel C, Garcia C, Andre K. Feasibility studies: UV/chlorine advanced oxidation treatment for the removal of emerging contaminants. *Water Res.* 2011;45(19):6371-6380.

100. Jin J, El-Din MG, Bolton JR. Assessment of the UV/chlorine process as an advanced oxidation process. *Water Res.* 2011;45:1890-1896.

101. Fang J, Fu Y, Shang C. The roles of reactive species in micropollutant degradation in the UV/free chlorine system. *Environ Sci Technol.* 2014;48:1859-1868.

Nonionizing Radiation: Microwave Radiation, Infrared Radiation, and Pulsed Light

Mark A. Smith

Electromagnetic radiation has proven to be effective for disinfection or sterilization for many applications. Effectiveness of such methods in various applications is generally a function of the energy, or wavelength, of the radiation and can vary widely. As described by Maxwell[1] in his original paper of 1865, electromagnetic radiation consists of a transverse wave, with electric and magnetic field oscillations perpendicular to each other and to the direction of propagation, which occurs at the speed of light in a vacuum. Figure 10.1 shows an electromagnetic wave schematically. Two parameters are of importance in discussing electromagnetic radiation, frequency, and wavelength.

The wavelength, as noted in Figure 10.1, is the physical distance over which a wave pattern repeats, depicted as the distance from a specific point on a given wave cycle to the corresponding point on the succeeding wave cycle. The frequency of oscillation is the number of repeating cycles over a given time period. The two terms are inversely related[1]:

$$c = \lambda v \qquad (1)$$

where c is the speed of light in a vacuum (299 792 458 m/s), λ is the radiant energy wavelength, and v is the wave frequency. The frequency of oscillation is proportional to the radiant energy, a relationship elucidated by Planck[2] in a seminal paper on quantum theory in 1900. Frequency and energy are connected by a proportionality constant:

$$E = hv \qquad (2)$$

where E is the radiation energy, h is Planck's constant (6.626×10^{-34} J · s or 4.136×10^{-15} eV · s), and v again represents the wave frequency.

Planck's equation formed the fundamental basis of quantum theory, stating that radiant energy in the electromagnetic spectrum is actually quantized or formed of discrete and separate bundles of energy. For electromagnetic radiation, these quanta are called photons. Characteristics of the interaction between electromagnetic radiation quanta and matter are largely dependent on the photon energy.

Maxwell's equations predicted, among other things, a spectrum of electromagnetic energy with an infinite number of frequencies, which led to the formulation of what has become known as the electromagnetic spectrum. The common depiction of this spectrum is arranged by one of the three parameters: wavelength, frequency, or energy (Figure 10.2). The electromagnetic spectrum is divided into bands or sections, each of which is named. In the lowest energy band, wavelengths are on the order of a kilometer or more. At the high-energy end of the spectrum, wavelengths are comparable in size to an atomic nucleus. Boundaries between bands on the spectrum are not clearly defined, with no precise demarcation from one type of radiation to another. Several boundaries overlap, such that a given energy radiation could be in more than one band. For example, a photon of 500 keV electromagnetic radiation could be either an X-ray or a gamma ray. The difference is one of origin and not energy, in that the X-ray is generated in the electron cloud of an atom, whereas the gamma ray arises from the nucleus.

Apart from the individual bands across the spectrum as shown in Figure 10.2, electromagnetic radiation is generally divided into two large categories, differentiated by the type of reaction that occurs between photons and the matter with which they interact. At wavelengths of several nanometers and shorter, corresponding to an energy of approximately 10 eV or higher, the photons have a sufficient energy to overcome atomic or molecular ionization energy, resulting in the ejection of an electron from atoms with which the photon interacts. Photons in this energy range are referred to as ionizing radiation, whereas those with longer wavelengths are considered

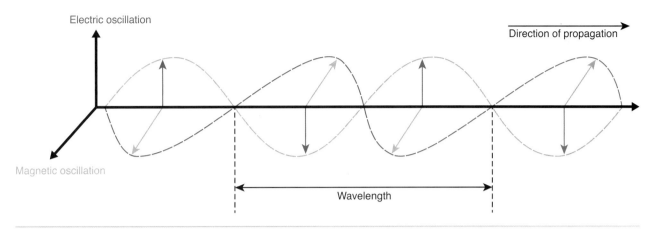

FIGURE 10.1   Diagram of electromagnetic radiation, consisting of electrical and magnetic oscillations in planes perpendicular to each other and to the direction in which the wave front is propagated. A wavelength is defined as the distance between successive waves, as measured from the same point in the oscillation cycle, for example, from one crest to the next crest.

nonionizing radiation. There is also no clear demarcation in terms of wavelength (or energy) between the two divisions. Instead, radiation is classified as one or the other on the basis of the reactions it creates. Ionizing radiation is generally considered to start within the ultraviolet (UV) range and extend to higher energies[3]; however, these are not definitive boundaries. For example, the photoelectric effect (ejection of an electron from an atom as a result of incident photon energy) can occur in some metals (eg, sodium) at wavelengths in the visible portion of the spectrum, even though visible light is considered nonionizing.

The distinction between ionizing and nonionizing radiation is important in considering the effect that the type of radiation has on organisms. Photochemical reactions may occur at energies that correspond to the visible light portion of the spectrum, for example, photosynthesis, with chemical reactions resulting from ion creation occurring at higher energy. At energies lower than the visible range, the energy deposited typically results in molecular vibration or oscillation of charge carriers. The macroscopic

effect of such reactions tends to be thermal as opposed to chemical. Most or all electromagnetic radiation reactions with matter can be used for disinfection or sterilization. This chapter concentrates on processes involving nonionizing radiation, with some inclusion of techniques using radiation in the UV range. Other chapters describe methods that employ ionizing radiation, from UV (see chapter 9) through X-rays and gamma rays (see chapter 29).

▶ MICROWAVE DISINFECTION AND STERILIZATION

In 1945, a patent application submitted by Percy L. Spencer[4] of Raytheon Manufacturing Company described a method for heating food that used electromagnetic energy with a wavelength of about 10 cm. This invention, the now near ubiquitous microwave oven for home use, grew out of radar technology and represented a new method for heating food.

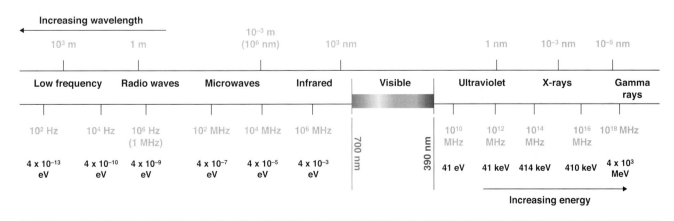

FIGURE 10.2   Diagram of the electromagnetic radiation spectrum, divided into bands according to wavelength, frequency, and energy.

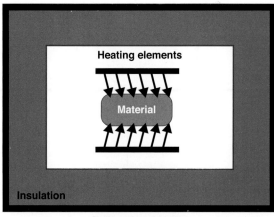
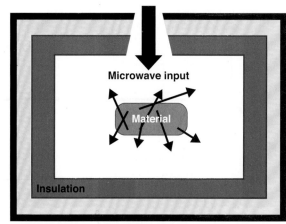

FIGURE 10.3   Depiction of microwave heating versus conventional radiant heating. On the left, the conventional heating system uses a heat source external to the material being treated, resulting in thermal effects beginning on the outside of the material, moving inward through conduction. On the right, microwaves penetrate the material being treated and thermal effects begin inside the material, moving both inward and outward through conduction.

Microwaves can also be used for heat treatment in an industrial setting. For disinfection or sterilization, the microbiological efficacy of the process is the same as for other processes that use heat to achieve the desired effect (see chapters 11 and 28). The difference is in the method whereby heat is generated. Various applications of microwave heating for disinfection in medical facilities are soft contact lenses, dental instruments, dentures, milk, and urinary catheters.[5]

In describing the relationship between microwaves and materials, it is convenient to divide all materials into three categories. They may be classified as conductors, insulators, or dielectrics. A conductor, which is a material in which electrons flow freely, allows for electricity flow in the material. Most common conductor materials are metals. When microwaves interact with conductors, the radiant energy tends to be reflected by the conductor. An insulator, conversely, is a material that inhibits the free flow of electrons and tends to not allow electricity to be conducted. Common insulator materials are plastics, ceramics, and glass. When microwaves interact with insulators, the radiant energy passes through the material and little interaction or energy deposition occurs. A dielectric material absorbs and stores energy without conducting it. In theory, it is a special class of insulator, in that the energy interacts with the material, but electricity is not conducted. The microwave heating process occurs with dielectric materials, principally as interactions involving the dipole properties of the material. Because microwaves have somewhat limited penetration into the materials, microwave heating of bulky or thick material also relies on conductive heating within the material, such that the heating occurs not necessarily from the center outwards but from a point within the material to other points within the material.[6]

Figure 10.3 shows a simple representation of a microwave heating process as compared to a conventional electrical heater. On the left, the conventional heater creates a temperature rise in the material by an externally applied heat source, creating the thermal effect beginning at the outer surface of the material. On the right, a microwave heating system bombards the material with radiant energy, and the heating process begins within the interior of the material.

Microwave Theory

Heat is generated within a material by microwaves in a process known as dielectric heating, a physical process whereby energy from electromagnetic radiation generates vibrational energy in molecules of the insulating material (dielectric) that causes a temperature increase within the material, a process originally described in 1954.[6] Other factors also contribute to the process, including uniformity of the radiation field and heat transfer driven by temperature gradients.

Because microwaves exist in the same general region of the electromagnetic spectrum as radio waves used for communications, industrial and consumer microwave equipment is general limited to specified wavelengths. In the United States, two frequencies are typically used in microwave heating processes: 915 and 2450 MHz. Both are used in commercial applications, but the latter is more commonly encountered in home-use microwave ovens. Outside of the United States, other frequencies are also used, specifically 433.92, 896, and 2375 MHz.[7]

Microwave heating occurs when the radiant energy interacts at a molecular level, generating friction by dipole rotation of polar solvents and migration of dissolved ions. Dipole rotation occurs with an alternating current electric field, where the field polarity varies at the wave frequency and the molecules continually attempt to align with the polarity. Friction from this process creates heat. In microwave ovens used for heating food, water is the dipole principally responsible for the heating effect. Migration of dissolved ions creates friction in a similar manner, where heat is generated as the ions realign with the field oscillations.[8] Therefore, microwave heating principally results from dipole rotation and ionic polarization. The volumetric heating rate (Q) of microwave is related to the electric field strength by

$$Q = 2\pi f \varepsilon_o \varepsilon'' E^2 \qquad (3)$$

where f is the frequency of microwaves, E the strength of electric field of the wave at that location, ε_o the permittivity of free space (a physical constant), and ε'' the dielectric loss factor (a material property called dielectric property) representing the material's ability to absorb that particular wavelength of electromagnetic radiation. The dielectric constant, ε'', also affects the strength of the electric field inside the object being irradiated with microwaves.[7]

Microwave Equipment

A simplified representation of equipment for microwave processing consists of a magnetron (a microwave cavity wherein materials are heated), waveguides that direct microwaves from the magnetron to the cavity, and a control system.[9] Microwaves are generated by the magnetron, which is composed of the two parts of a diode: a cathode and an anode. Both electrodes are cylindrical and concentric, with an anode resonant cavity surrounding the cathode, as shown in Figure 10.4. A magnetic field is created by a magnet placed around the anode. Heating the cathode generates electrons with negative charge that move toward the anode, which has a positive charge. The magnetic field perturbs the path of the electrons, causing them to deviate from a straight-line trajectory. As they pass the resonator cavity, the electrons oscillate at a high frequency. The frequency of the resultant microwave matches the oscillation frequency of the electrons in the resonator cavity. These oscillations are collected by an antenna and transmitted via a wave guide to the cavity wherein material heating occurs.[7]

Microwave Applications

Microwave technology serves as a heat source for disinfection or sterilization purposes. Therefore, the microbiological efficacy of the method is based on the heat

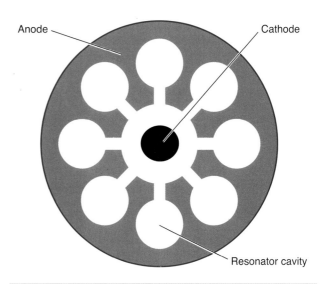

FIGURE 10.4 Cross-sectional diagram of a resonant cavity magnetron, which generates microwaves from interaction between electrons and a magnetic field while moving past a series of open metal cavities. Electrons passing the cavities generate radio wave oscillations, serving as a source of microwaves. Resonant frequencies are determined by the size and shape of the resonant cavities.

properties and is similar to other heat-based techniques. There have been studies that suggest microwaves could be a microbicide apart from the thermal effects, but this has been difficult to verify. Using a microwave oven designed similarly to a home kitchen appliance, studies showed inactivation of bacterial cultures, mycobacteria, viruses, and *Geobacillus stearothermophilus* spores, although the suggestion was that that water and higher power microwaves may be needed for sterilization.[10-15] One concern is that the microwave heaters that are available commercially may have uneven energy distribution limiting treatment applications with devices (ie, hot and cold spots on solid devices), which is difficult to characterize adequately to ensure that the entire device has sterilized or disinfected.[5]

Microwaves have been used in the food industry for several purposes including, tempering of frozen meat and poultry products; precooking of bacon for foodservice; sausage cooking; drying of various foods; baking of bread, biscuit, and confectionery; thawing of frozen products; blanching of vegetables; heating and sterilizing fast food, cooked meals, and cereals; and pasteurization and sterilization of various foods. For pasteurization and sterilization, the process using microwaves is dependent on thermal properties and heat generated during processing. In that way, the microbicidal effect is the same as any other heating method, a function of the temperature attained and the time the product is held at the higher temperature.[7] Commercialization of the microwave heating process for pasteurization or sterilization has proven to be problematic, with only limited success.[16]

In medical applications, microwaves have been studied and shown to be effective for disinfection of soft contact lenses, dental instruments, dentures, milk, and urinary catheters. For catheters, it was found that the microwave heating process tended to cause melting in certain plastics, making choice of materials a critical step. Although experience in home appliance microwave ovens suggests that disinfection of metal objects would be an issue due to arcing, with certain precautions in presentation of the objects (eg, immersed in water or controlling the application of microwave energy), it has been shown possible to use microwave heating for some metal objects.[17-23]

One use of microwaves related to medical applications is for disinfection of medical waste. This process again relies on the heating effects of microwaves to attain and maintain temperature adequate for disinfection. Medical waste is processed first by shredding the materials, depicted in Figure 10.5, which gives a more uniform and smaller particle size that does not require as high a temperature as would be required for intact materials. Shredded waste is moistened and passed through a series of microwave units for thermal processing, as shown in Figure 10.6. The small, uniform particle size and the water content ensure that microwaves heat the waste efficiently for microbial reduction, rendering it suitable for disposal as municipal solid waste in a sanitary landfill. Validation of the process can be difficult, but at least one study has been published in using biological indicators to monitor process effectiveness.[24]

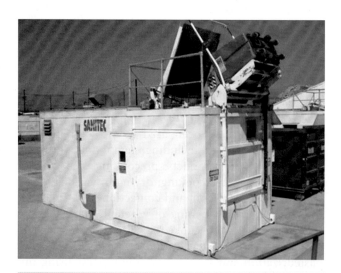

FIGURE 10.5   Commercial equipment for microwave disinfection of medical waste. Waste containers are emptied into the process via an automated handler and shredded into tiny particles in a system specifically designed for medical waste. Photograph courtesy of Sanitec Industries, Inc. For a color version of this art, please consult the eBook.

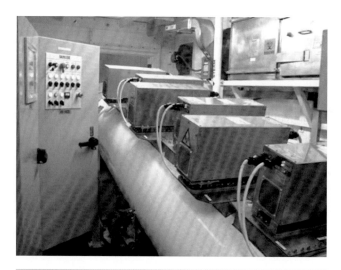

FIGURE 10.6   Commercial equipment for microwave disinfection of medical waste. Shredded waste consisting of small particles is moved on a stainless steel screw conveyor, moistened with steam, and passed by a series of microwave units. Thermal treatment of each individual waste particle occurs from the inside out, assuring thorough disinfection. Treatment is verified on a regular basis by challenge testing using spores of *Bacillus atrophaeus*. Photograph courtesy of Sanitec Industries, Inc. For a color version of this art, please consult the eBook.

▶ INFRARED DISINFECTION AND STERILIZATION

Moving higher in energy on the electromagnetic spectrum, just above the microwave range and below visible light is a region called the infrared. Infrared radiation was discovered more than half a century before James Clerk Maxwell[1] formulated the equations describing behavior of electromagnetic radiation. Frederick William Herschel,[25] a musician and composer as well as an astronomer in Great Britain, was testing filters to be used in observing sun spots when he discovered that a red filter caused a rise in temperature that was significantly larger than observed with unfiltered light. Although illumination of any surface with light will cause the object to become warm, Herschel[25] found that the temperature was surprisingly higher when he passed light through a prism and held a thermometer in the area just beyond the red end of the visible light spectrum. His theory was that there was a band of light beyond the visible spectrum that produced enhanced heating effects. This radiation he referred to as *calorific rays*, a term that was replaced by *infrared* in the late 19th century.[25,26]

Infrared Theory

Infrared is considered to be the range of wavelengths approximately from 700 nm to 1 mm, as shown in Figure 10.2. As with the other longer wavelength bands of the electromagnetic spectrum, infrared radiation creates rotational or vibrational energy in molecules, particularly as related to creating fluctuations in the dipole moment of the molecules, a process similar to what was discussed in regard to use of microwaves. The specific types of interactions occurring in infrared energy absorption are related to the wavelength of the incident radiation, encompassing changes to the vibrational state at shorter infrared wavelengths and changes in the rotational state at longer infrared wavelengths.[27]

The microbicidal effects of infrared radiation result from heating of the material being treated, similarly to the discussion with microwaves. Therefore, the efficacy of the process is dependent principally on those parameters that determine the efficiency and extent of thermal effects. Of particular importance are infrared power level, peak wavelength and bandwidth of the infrared source, sample size, temperature of the material, types of microorganisms and the state of growth phase, and the moisture content.[28]

The effect of power level is somewhat intuitive, in that greater infrared power means higher energy deposition and subsequently more energy absorbed by the material. The wavelength effect is related in that energy and wavelength are inversely related as shown in the equations at the beginning of this chapter. However, a less obvious wavelength effect also occurs, as was shown in 2006 when a study was conducted on inactivation of *Bacillus subtilis* when treated with differing wavelengths. Samples of an aqueous solution the bacterium were air-dried on a stainless steel petri dish and treated with three different infrared wavelengths: 950, 1100, and 1150 nm, corresponding to radiant energies 4.2, 3.7, and 3.2 μW/cm^2/nm, respectively. Each petri dish for the three samples was raised to a temperature of 100°C, but pathogen inactivation was greater for the shorter wavelength, presumably a result of the greater penetration depth of shorter wavelength infrared.[29]

In food products, for example, it has been shown that water molecules have the greatest effect from infrared radiation. Proteins, lipids, and carbohydrates containing polar groups (eg, $-NH_2$, $-CO$, $-OH$) also tend to show significant response to infrared. The microbicidal action from infrared heating, which is a primarily direct radiation thermal effect, may also include inactivation mechanisms similar to UV light, which can cause DNA damage and is discussed in a separate chapter, and induction heating similar to the process during microwave irradiation.[30]

Infrared Equipment

Conventional infrared heating systems are usually either gas-fired or electric heaters, with temperature ranges of 343°C to 1100°C for gas and electric, and 1100°C to 2200°C for electric only.[30] The wavelength of infrared radiation, or any electromagnetic radiation, is related to the temperature of the radiant energy through Wien's dis-

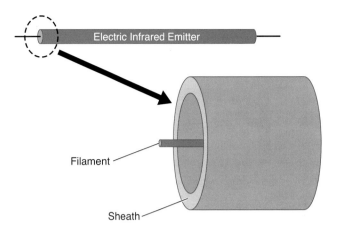

FIGURE 10.7 Diagram of an electric infrared source. Infrared radiation is generated by passing electric current through a resistor. Resistance to electron flow generates heat, transmitted in the form of infrared radiation.

placement law, most popularly in the form elucidated by Max Planck[2] some years after Wilhelm Wien first stated theories related to black body radiation.

For electric heaters, infrared radiation is generated by passing electric current through a resistor. Resistance to electron flow generates heat, transmitted in the form of infrared radiation. A typical tube emitter cross-section is shown in Figure 10.7. The more common electrical infrared sources appropriate for disinfection or sterilization purposes are metal sheath rods, first developed in the 1920s. A metal wire (conductor) is wrapped in a spiral around a ceramic body (insulator) and the wire heated by electrical current. Chromel wire, which is an alloy of chromium and nickel, has been used, in part because heating the wire to high temperature creates a chromium oxide layer on its outer surface, helping to protect against corrosion and burning[31]; however, a variety of metals may be used for different applications, as appropriate. The most common filament in current use if tungsten, electrical infrared sources may include ceramic heating elements, quartz lamps, quartz-tungsten lamps, or carbon fiber heating elements. The differences among these electrical sources are the range of wavelengths that are generated by the process, which is in turn related to the radiant energy temperature.[30]

Gas-fired infrared heaters consist of a plate that is heated on one side by a gas flame. The thermal effects on the plate, which is usually either metal or ceramic, result in emission of heat where the infrared wavelength involved is related to the temperature. Figure 10.6 shows a simplified diagram of a gas-fired infrared emitter. Radiant tube heaters, which are gas-fired infrared emitters, are more typically used in applications wherein large areas are heated. The more directed heat associated with disinfection or sterilization applications is the gas-fired emitter as represented in Figure 10.8.[32]

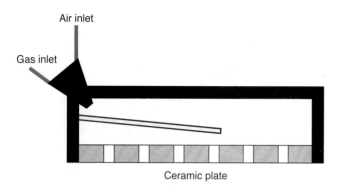

FIGURE 10.8 Diagram of a gas-fired infrared source, consisting of a plate heated by gas flame. The thermal effects on the plate result in emission infrared radiation, where the wavelength is related to the temperature.

Infrared Applications

Applications of direct application of infrared radiation, as opposed to general dry heat sterilization, is not common in health care facilities or medical equipment manufacturing and use. Studies have been done to show efficacy of sterilization using infrared,[33] but the process is largely used for sterilization of equipment in laboratories, including glassware. In food processing, infrared radiation has been used to inactivate bacteria, spores, yeast, and mold in both liquid and solid foods.[30] Various other applications include surface disinfection in bakeries as well as reducing mold formation on bread prior to packaging and bacterial disinfection of rice.[34]

▶ PULSED LIGHT DISINFECTION AND STERILIZATION

Extensive studies have shown the ability of continuous visible and UV light to inactivate cellular organisms. A technique has been in development and commercial application for some time that uses electrical energy to create intense pulses of light, which creates somewhat different bactericidal effects.[35] Because of the high peak power of the flash and its ability to provide high doses of broad-spectrum UV light in very short times, the process is much more effective than conventional UV sources.

Because chapter 9 in this book discusses UV light, this chapter focuses on the use of pulsed light for disinfection and sterilization. In particular, this chapter provides a discussion of two important applications: (1) the pulsed light treatment of water and (2) the use of pulsed light as a terminal sterilization process for aseptically manufactured pharmaceuticals. In the former application, pulsed light is used as a highly effective disinfection process; in the latter, pulsed light is used for sterilization.

Pulsed Light Theory

Pulsed light flashes are produced using pulsed power to convert alternating current line voltage to a high-voltage, direct current pulses for energizing a tubular lamp. In this process, electrical energy is stored and concentrated in a capacitor over a relatively long time (ie, tenths of a second) and then released as a high-power electrical pulse a few hundred millionths of a second in duration. This short-duration, high-voltage pulse is conducted through cables to a xenon flashlamp, a quartz or sapphire tube containing xenon gas and sealed at each end about an electrode. The electrical pulse ionizes the gas in the lamp to create a plasma that expands to fill the lamp. The wall of the lamp eventually confines the plasma, where it becomes superheated by further electrical energization. During thermal ionization of the gas, outer shell electrons are stripped away and an intense pulse of radiation is emitted.[35]

The light generation process is efficient in converting electrical to light energy. Approximately 50% to 75% of the electrical power energizing the lamp is converted to light emission. Because of power compression associated with the pulsed-power components of the system, average electrical requirements for routine operation are modest (<16 kW); however, peak electrical power into the lamp and power of the emitted flash are high, greater than approximately 4 MW.

The wavelengths of pulsed light in this context fall within the electromagnetic spectrum in the visible and UV ranges, which are considered nonionizing radiation. These wavelengths are absorbed only by specific resonant molecular bonding structures. The wavelengths of light in a pulsed light flash cannot, for example, interact with water molecules to produce hydroxyl radicals, which are produced by and represent an important lethal species during treatment of microorganisms with the more energetic photons from ionizing radiation sources. Instead, the wavelengths of light present in a pulsed light flash are quite specific in the types of molecular bonds with which they interact. The emitted pulsed light flash contains nonionizing wavelengths in the far UV (UVC), mid UV (UVB), near UV (UVA), visible, and infrared. Approximately 25% of the light is in the UV range. At shorter wavelengths, the emitted light is limited by the transmission properties of the lamp envelope to wavelengths greater than approximately 190 to 200 nm.

The only chemical structures of any consequence that absorb at wavelengths greater than approximately 200 nm are carbonyls ($C = O$), carboxyls ($O = COH$), sulfhydryls ($S-H$), nitrates ($O-N = O$), and the conjugated carbon-to-carbon double-bond systems present in unsaturated or aromatic molecules. For the wavelengths and photon energies present in the pulsed light flash, the unsaturated or aromatic bonds in polyaromatic hydrocarbons represent the primary and most important absorbing molecular structures. Most cells and biologic tissues are relatively colorless and absorb light poorly in the near UV at wavelengths above approximately 320 to 340 nm. Near UV is not significantly absorbed by proteins or nucleic acids. Absorption in the near UV is primarily restricted to highly aromatic, colored molecules, such as carotenes, isoprenes, pterins, flavins, cyanins, porphyrins, hemes, or chlorophylls, which are in general present in low concentration except in specialized cells or tissues. Thus, typical bacteria and spores are relatively transparent above approximately 320 nm, and it is wavelengths between this upper bound and the vacuum UV that are primarily responsible for the lethal effects of UV light.

The relative response of a system to light of different wavelengths is defined as its action spectrum. The peak of the action spectra for the killing and mutagenic effects of UV light on cells and biologic tissues lies in the far UV.[36] For most organisms, this lethal activity peaks at wavelengths between 250 and 275 nm and relates to nucleic acid absorption. For example, consider an *Escherichia coli* bacterium exposed to UV light. A typical cell from a logarithmic growth-phase culture contains approximately 80% water. Of the dry weight of the cell, approximately 70% is protein, 20% nucleic acids, and less than 10% carbohydrate and lipid. Sugars, starches, and saturated fats do not usually show absorption above approximately 200 nm. The amino bond loses absorption above approximately 220 nm. Thus, at wavelengths greater than approximately 220 nm, cellular absorption of UV light occurs primarily in polyaromatic bonds in nucleic acids. Nucleic acids absorb UV light strongly because all of the pyrimidine and purines bases are highly aromatic in structure. Absorption in proteins occurs in the aromatic amino acids (primarily tyrosine, tryptophan, and phenylalanine) and in the cystine disulfide bond. Absorption of UV by protein is less than that of nucleic acids because only approximately 10% of the amino acid residues of protein are aromatic. Nucleic acid absorption is 10 to 30 times greater per unit weight than that of protein through the wavelength range of 240 to 280 nm, so that even though *E coli* has much more protein than nucleic acid, its absorption of light in this region is very largely due to nucleic acids. Consequently, although nucleic acids in general represent less than approximately 1% of the total weight of a microorganism, they can be responsible for more than 70% of UV light absorption.

Continuous UV light treatment primarily affects DNA through mechanisms that are reversible under experimental conditions. Pulsed light treatment has been studied in the context of this repair mechanism, which has shown that the repair mechanism present with continuous treatment does not occur. Explanatory theories have included the idea that DNA damage from pulsed light treatment is too severe for repair to occur or that the DNA repair mechanism itself is inactivated from the pulsed light treatment.[35]

There are significant similarities between the spectrum of a typical pulsed light flash with that of sunlight. Both contain nonionizing wavelengths from the UV to the infrared. They also have similar emission peaks, with the peak spectral output of both occurring at approximately 425 to 450 nm. There are also significant differences between sunlight and pulsed light. Pulsed light is rich in UV at wavelengths less than 300 nm that are filtered by the earth's atmosphere and therefore not present in sunlight at the surface of the earth. Pulsed light is also much more intense. At an incident energy of 1 J/cm², the pulsed light flash is more than 20 000 times brighter than sunlight.[37] Normally, the pulsed light flash is shaped or concentrated on a treated product or surface by a reflector. It is often beneficial to use lamps in a reflective cavity to obtain the increased efficiency provided by entrapment and multiple reflections of the light. For sterilization purposes, pulsed light is usually used at incident light energies greater than approximately 2 J/cm² per flash.

Pulsed Light Equipment

An in-line, automated pulsed light treatment system usually includes four basic components:

1. A shielded tunnel (to protect operators from the intense light), including an integrated conveyor for receiving and treating the product directly from a manufacturing line
2. A pulse generation and control module that maintains and controls lamp operation and tunnel treatment
3. A data logger for verifying and recording electronic signals from photodetector assemblies designed to measure the light and monitor the critical parameters of every flash
4. A water system for lamp cooling. The lamp cooling system usually comprises a qualified water source for circulation through a jacket surrounding the lamp(s). This requirement is often met with a recirculating water source of purified water, such as deionized water. This recirculating water cooling the lamps may be thermally maintained by a heat exchanger coupled to a building water supply.

The pulsed light incident on a treated surface or plane is measured as energy per area, or fluence, in J/cm² or mJ/cm². Calorimetry is used to measure pulsed light and calibrate pulsed light measurement systems. Although several types of systems are available for pulsed light calorimetry, in general, surface-absorbing thermopile calorimeters offer a good compromise between sensitivity and ability to withstand high-peak-power treatments without damage.

A typical thermopile comprises a sensor head coupled to a signal measurement digital display. A small carbon disc in the thermopile head efficiently absorbs broadband light across the pulsed light spectrum. Just as an absorbing surface is warmed when exposed to the sun, a thermal gradient is produced across the carbon disc during exposure to a pulsed light flash. A temperature measurement device, in intimate thermal contact with the back surface of the carbon disc, generates an electrical signal proportional to the change in temperature produced by light absorption on the surface of the carbon disc. This signal is measured against background and the result displayed digitally.

In instances where finer mapping of the fluence distribution is required, it may be desirable to reduce the area of the calorimeter's absorbing surface. The manufacturer can achieve this by reducing the size of the carbon disc or by properly designed masking of the disc surface. In addition, a filter may be placed over the carbon disc to allow the unit to measure the energy contained in specific bandwidths of light passing the filter. For example, a 260-nm bandpass filter, with proper calibration, may be used to measure pulsed light intensity through a corresponding with peak biologic activity for many cells and tissues.

Online measurement systems capable of monitoring each flash for energy, spectral properties, or lamp operating parameters are available. One such system consists of a filter and silicon photodiode combination mounted to view the lamp directly or, alternatively, to monitor the light within a reflective treatment cavity. Because the UV content of the pulsed light flash is strongly affected by changes in lamp operating conditions, because flash content may change more dramatically than total light output, and because of the importance of wavelength to the production of biologic effects, it is essential to design the system to measure UV content such as by incorporating bandpass filtration in flash monitoring systems.

An alternative online pulsed light monitoring system comprises a digital spectrograph capable of capturing the intensity and spectral distribution of each flash. In such systems, a dispersion element is used to spread the incident light spectrum (in much the same way that a prism is able to spread the visible light spectrum of sunlight) onto a charge-coupled device for registering the energy in discrete portions of the incident light. Under some conditions, both of these online photodetector systems potentially can "drift," and periodic recalibration is required as a safeguard. One way this requirement can be met is through regular adjustment of the system using a standardized calorimeter.

A variety of electrical measurements that relate closely to the properties of the resulting flash are obtainable. For example, verification of the intensity, density, and duration of the electrical current energizing the lamp can provide further assurance of system performance. Similar assurances can be drawn using other parameters, such as the voltage and duration of the pulse energizing the lamp or the voltage and charge on the system's energy storage capacitor. Such electrical measurements of lamp operating parameters can provide further online verification of system performance because they are redundant to and therefore capable of reinforcing photoelectric flash measurements.[38]

Pulsed Light Applications

Pulsed light can be used as a sterilization method in situations and with products where light can access all of the surfaces and volume where contamination may occur. In addition, pulsed light treatment can be effectively applied through materials that are sufficiently transmissive in the range of wavelengths involved, such as many plastics, such that it may be used to treat products through a filled and sealed plastic container. Obviously, metal does not transmit light, and glass usually absorbs too strongly in the UV region to allow treatment through a glass container. Printing or labels on a container or package can obstruct treatment and should be applied after pulsed light processing.

Many solutions can be effectively treated to sufficient depth to allow the bulk treatment of a filled container. The primary limitation on depth of treatment relates to the degree of unsaturated aromatic compounds or color present in the molecular composition of the liquid. Because most colored compounds are, by definition, composed of molecules that interact strongly with light and are also often aromatic in molecular structure, it is quite natural that color should hinder transmission and pulsed light treatment. Some absorptive or colored materials, although not treatable at filled container depths, are treatable as thin or millimeter-thick layers and may then be aseptically filled. Because pulsed light is readily transmitted through air, water, saline, dextrose, ophthalmic, and many other pharmaceutical solutions, effective microbial inactivation and sterilization can be achieved.

Pulsed light treatment through both containers and solutions is determined and limited by the laws of light absorption, scatter, reflection, and refraction. As used in commercial pulsed light systems, light absorption is the most important of these factors in determining the ability to treat a particular container or product. The absorption of light in a material or solution is described by Beer–Lambert–Bouguer law, which in its traditional form is

$$T = P / P_0 = e^{-\varepsilon cl} = e^{-\alpha l} = \% \, T / 100 \qquad (4)$$

where the transmittance, T, is the ratio of the spectral radiant power, P, to that incident on the sample, P_0, e is the base of natural logarithms, ε is the molar (Napierian) absorption coefficient of the test material at the specific test wavelength, c is the concentration of the solute, l is the pathlength or penetration depth, α is the absorption coefficient and is the product of ε and c, and $\%T$ is the percent transmission. The absorption coefficient of a material is wavelength dependent and experimentally derived. It is often convenient to express these properties of light penetration in decadic form or in terms of absorbance:

$$T = P / P_0 = 10^{-\varepsilon cl} \qquad (5)$$

$$A = \log (P_0 / P) = \varepsilon cl = \alpha l = -\log T = 2 - \log \%T \quad (6)$$

where ε is in this instance the decadic molar absorption coefficient, A is the absorbance, and α is the decadic absorption coefficient. The depth of penetration is the inverse of the absorption coefficient $(1/\alpha)$ and in the decadic system is the distance at which the spectral radiant power decreases to one tenth of the incident value. If the Napierian absorption coefficient is used, the depth of penetration $(1/\alpha)$ is the distance at which the spectral radiant power decreases to $1/e$ of its incident value, which called the *e-fold penetration depth*. The absorption coefficients of biologic tissues are such that e-fold penetration depths for wavelengths of light in the UV range are on the order of tens of micrometers, hundreds of micrometers in the visible, and centimeters in the infrared.

It is seen from these equations that not only the absorption characteristics of a particular product or container material, but thickness plays a role in determining the ability of pulsed light effectively to treat the product and package combination. Using these relationships and a spectrophotometer, it is often possible to predict the suitability of a container or product for treatment with pulsed light. These absorption equations do not hold in the presence of significant light scatter, and prediction of pulsed light treatment suitability is sometimes more relevant for the product than container. The translucence of polyethylene and polypropylene containers is an indication of the degree of visible light scatter sometimes present in these materials. Similar scattering in the pulsed light wavelength range sometimes makes it more difficult to predict the degree of transmission that will be observed using a particular container. In such instances, the level of pulsed light treatment effectiveness to be expected is sometimes best demonstrated through biologic testing.

Food Disinfection by Pulsed Light

In microbial disinfection of food, pulsed light has an advantage over other techniques because it is a nonthermal process. Thermal treatment may cause undesirable changes to the food, particularly on minimally processed foods (ie, usually consumed without further washing or heating), that can be avoided or minimized using pulsed light as a disinfecting agent. Based on studies that have attempted to define factors that influence pulsed light treatment efficacy, the extent of microbial decontamination of food relies on the total fluence striking the cell surface, which is influenced by

- Number of applied light flashes
- The applied discharge voltage
- The distance between target and flash lamp
- The spectral range of the light flashes
- The sensitivity of various groups of microorganisms
- The extent and kind of contamination
- The impact of the surrounding matrix in which microorganisms are embedded[39]

In some studies, it was found that highly reflective surfaces and rough surfaces both resulted in lower microbial inactivation as compared to smooth and less reflective surfaces. A shadowing phenomenon is believed to be the cause in both situations. Rough surfaces create complex surface features that give rise to nonuniform adherence by bacteria to the surface, whereas highly reflective surfaces, particularly hydrophobic materials, tend to promote cell clustering. Both cause additional nontransmissive material to be interposed in the light path, giving rise to shadowing, a significant phenomenon in electromagnetic radiation with low penetration ability, such as visible and near-UV light.[39]

A variety of foods have been studied for efficacy of pulsed light disinfection as well as evaluated potential detrimental effects on the foods themselves.[39] These included produce meat and meat product, fish, beverages, and others. Overall, the observed antimicrobial efficacy depends on the product presentation (eg, surfaces and liquids) and design of the pulsed light exposure system. Negative effects, similar to those described for UV treatments, can include those related to the generation of free radicals on or within the food that can damage nutrients (eg, vitamins), changes in the sensorial properties (eg, of meat), textural properties (of fruit and vegetables), and some organoleptic (smell, taste) properties. These effects can be minimized based on exposure conditions, including temperature controls.[39] There is also an opportunity to combine pulsed light with other disinfection methods to enhance antimicrobial activity and minimize negative effects, such as combination with hydrogen peroxide, chlorine, and acids. In treatment of fruit juices, in particular, the combination of pulsed light with the nonchemical methods of pulsed electric field and thermosonication (ie, ultrasound combined with slight temperature increase) proved to be effective in microbial reduction, although some studies show degradation in organoleptic properties.[40]

Water Treatment With Pulsed Light

Chlorine chemistries have for many years been the public health mainstay of municipal drinking water systems. Recently, UV light has increasingly found use, in both municipal drinking water facilities and in high-quality pharmaceutical- or electronics-grade water systems, for the disinfection of water.[41] One drawback and public health issue associated with conventional water disinfection systems is their lack of effectiveness against protozoan dormant forms (see chapter 3), such as the chemical- and UV-resistant cysts or oocysts of *Cryptosporidium*, *Giardia*, *Cyclospora*, and others.[42] *Cryptosporidium parvum* oocysts are representative of the group. The *C parvum* is a protozoan parasite that has increasingly been implicated as a threat to water safety. Infectious epidemics of waterborne diarrhea and death have been associated with cryptosporidial contamination of drinking water systems at sites throughout the world. These outbreaks are usually associated with runoff or flooding leading to water supply contamination from livestock sources. The *C parvum* oocysts are notoriously resistant to disinfection, especially in the treatment of drinking water by chlorination.[43] Because of the threat this organism poses, preliminary tests were conducted to determine the potential for pulsed light to disinfect waterborne suspensions of *C parvum* oocysts. Initial results demonstrated that pulsed light treatment could effectively inactivate high concentration suspensions of *C parvum* oocysts when assayed using in vivo mouse infectivity assays. Subsequent tests using both in vivo and in vitro assays have confirmed the high degree of effectiveness of pulsed light against *C parvum* oocysts. Tests performed to titrate the effects of pulsed light at lower treatment levels have shown the method is highly effective against oocysts, even at relatively low doses.[44]

The high degree of effectiveness shown in these results provided impetus for the further development and testing of a pulsed light water treatment system. The design concept was a point-of-entry system capable of treating water at the inlet to a residence or restaurant anywhere in the world and producing high-quality water free of potential protozoan, bacterial, or viral pathogens. Pulsed light dose-response tests were conducted using multiple strains of a wide range of potentially pathogenic waterborne organisms, including *C parvum*, *E coli*, *Salmonella* species, *Klebsiella* species, and poliovirus to determine appropriate treatment conditions. These studies led to the design and fabrication of the 4 gal/min point-of-entry pulsed light water treatment unit shown in Figure 10.9. The unit contains a pulsed light lamp mounted in a 316-grade stainless steel treatment chamber, with associated valves, sensors, and control elements. Three separate units were tested using *Klebsiella terrigena*, *C parvum* oocysts, poliovirus type 1, rotavirus, and bacteriophages PRD-1 and MS-2.[40,44] Tests were performed both in "clean" and "dirty" water (clean water was dechlorinated municipal water; dirty water was 10 nephelometric turbidity unit water with 2.5 mg/L total organic carbon and 500 mg/L total dissolved solids). Even the "dirty" water results show the pulsed light unit provides greater than 7 log cycle reductions in *K terrigena* colony-forming units, more than 3.4 log cycle reductions in oocyst infectivity using in vivo mice infectivity or in vitro tissue

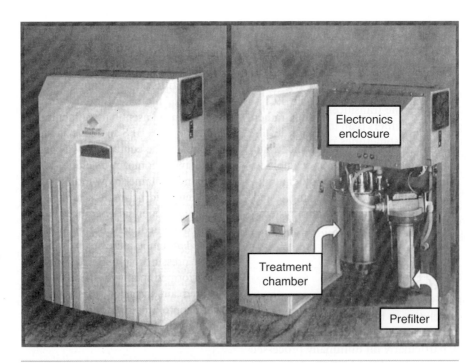

FIGURE 10.9 A pulsed light water treatment unit. The system shown is designed as a 4 gal/min point-of-entry water treatment unit to provide high levels of protozoan oocyst, bacterial, and viral inactivation. The face of the wall-mounted unit is 16″ × 30″, and it weighs approximately 75 lb. On the right, the unit is shown opened to reveal the key components.

TABLE 10.1	Microbiologic effectiveness of pulsed light water treatment system shown in Figure 10.9[a]		
Test Organism	**Count**		**Log Inactivation**
	Influent	Effluent	
Klebsiella terrigena	3.3×10^5	<0.01	>7.5
Cryptosporidium parvum oocysts	2.5×10^5	<10	>4.6
Poliovirus type 1	6.2×10^5	0.37	6.2
Simian rotavirus SA11	2.6×10^3	<0.04	>4.9
Bacteriophage PRD-1	2.5×10^5	<1	>5.4
Bacteriophage MS-2	2.0×10^4	<1	>4.3

[a]Results obtained during treatment of a standardized "dirty" water: absorbance 2601 nm 0.125/cm, total organic carbon 2.5 mg/L, total dissolved solids 500 mg/L, turbidity 10 nephelometric turbidity units.

culture assay procedures, and more than 4 to 6 log cycle reductions in viral tissue culture infectivity (Table 10.1).

Packaging Sterilization With Pulsed Light

In-line or in-process sterilization of packaging materials is advantageous in some circumstances to minimize contamination prior to final assembly of the product or to reduce the need for subsequent disinfection or sterilization of the entire package. Examples where packaging material may be sterilized with pulsed light include aseptic processing lines, plastic beverage bottles, contact lenses packed into sterile solutions, and simple medical tools, that is, without shadowed surfaces or grooves. It has also been suggested as a method for control of hospital acquired infections, defined as worker or patient infections that are acquired through unintended exposure.[45]

Pulsed light technology has been shown to be advantageous for sterilizing packaging materials and processing equipment in aseptic packaging, using wavelengths in the UV to the near-infrared region. Packaging materials are typically exposed to a series of 1 to 20 light-intensity pulses of approximately 1 millisecond to 0.1 second in duration. At a pulse rate of 1 to 10 per second, microbicidal effects have been shown to be efficient with a higher UV content spectrum providing more efficiency based on the increased total fluence. Comparison of antimicrobial effects of pulsed light as compared to continuous UV sources have shown higher inactivation levels for pulsed light.[46] Packaging materials compatible with pulsed light sterilization are those that will transmit light over the range of wavelengths used in the process. Several plastics have proven to be mostly transparent in this range, including linear low-density polyethylene, low-density polyethylene, nylon, fluoropolymer films such as Aclar, high-density polyethylene, and polypropylene. Light transmission is critical, such that the presence of shadowing negates the process efficacy.[46]

▶ SUMMARY

Three nonionizing radiation methods were discussed in this section, microwave radiation, infrared radiation, and pulsed light. Each of these techniques provides a variation on a different disinfection or sterilization method as discussed elsewhere in this book. For microwave and infrared radiation, the disinfection process is heating, such that antimicrobial mechanisms from those techniques are the same as discussed for other methods employing heat for microbial inactivation. For pulsed light, the antimicrobial mechanism may be a combination of heating effects or UV radiation. The unique aspect of these methods is in the manner in which the radiation is delivered to the microbes in order to achieve the desired effect.

▶ ACKNOWLEDGMENTS

Disinfection, Sterilization, and Preservation, 5th edition (SS Block [editor], 2000), chapter 39 was written by Joseph Dunn and was explicitly devoted to pulsed light as a disinfection or sterilization method for water treatment and for aseptic processing. In this edition, the chapter has been expanded to include other methods, but a large portion of the section on pulsed light was used from the fifth edition. Some sections were minimally edited and appear largely unchanged from the chapter prepared by Dr Dunn.

REFERENCES

1. Maxwell JC. A dynamical theory of the electromagnetic field. *Philos Trans R Soc Lond.* 1865;155:459-512.
2. Planck M. Über eine Verbesserung der Wienschen Spektralgleichung. *Verhandlungen der Deutschen Physikalischen Gesellschaft.* 1900;2:202-204. ter Haar D, trans-ed. On an improvement of Wien's equation for the spectrum. *The Old Quantum Theory.* Oxford, United Kingdom: Pergamon Press; 1967:79-81.

3. Johnson TE. *Introduction to Health Physics*. 5th ed. New York, NY: McGraw-Hill; 2017.

4. Spencer PL, inventor; Raytheon Manufacturing Co, assignee. Method of treating foodstuffs. US patent 2,495,429. January 24, 1950.

5. Rutala WA, Weber DJ; and Healthcare Infection Control Practices Advisory Committee. *Guideline for Disinfection and Sterilization in Healthcare Facilities*. Atlanta, GA: Centers for Disease Control and Prevention; 2008.

6. Von Hippel AR. *Dielectrics and Waves*. New York, NY: Wiley; 1954.

7. Ahmed J, Ramaswamy HS. Microwave pasteurization and sterilization of foods. In: *Handbook of Food Preservation*. 2nd ed. Boca Raton, FL: CRC Press; 2007:691-711.

8. Oliveira MEC, Franca AS. Microwave heating of foodstuffs. *J Food Eng*. 2002;53:347-359.

9. Tang J. Unlocking potentials of microwaves for food safety and quality. *J Food Sci*. 2015;80:E1776-E1793.

10. Najdovski L, Dragas AZ, Kotnik V. The killing activity of microwaves on some non-sporogenic and sporogenic medically important bacterial strains. *J Hosp Infect*. 1991;19:239-247.

11. Rosaspina S, Salvatorelli G, Anzanel D, Bovolenta R. Effect of microwave radiation on *Candida albicans*. *Microbios*. 1994;78:55-59.

12. Welt BA, Tong CH, Rossen JL, Lund DB. Effect of microwave radiation on inactivation of *Clostridium sporogenes* (PA 3679) spores. *Appl Environ Microbiol*. 1994;60:482-488.

13. Latimer JM, Matsen JM. Microwave oven irradiation as a method for bacterial decontamination in a clinical microbiology laboratory. *J Clin Microbiol*. 1977;6:340-342.

14. Sanborn MR, Wan SK, Bulard R. Microwave sterilization of plastic tissue culture vessels for reuse. *Appl Environ Microbiol*. 1982;44(4):960-964.

15. Rosaspina S, Salvatorelli G, Anzanel D. The bactericidal effect of microwaves on *Mycobacterium bovis* dried on scalpel blades. *J Hosp Infect*. 1994;26:45-50.

16. Tops R. Industrial implementation: microwave pasteurized and sterilized products. In: *Symposium on Microwave Sterilization*. Chicago, IL: Institute of Food Technologists; 2000.

17. Webb BC, Thomas CJ, Harty DW, Willcox MD. Effectiveness of two methods of denture sterilization. *J Oral Rehabil*. 1998;25:416-423.

18. Rohrer MD, Bulard RA. Microwave sterilization. *J Am Dent Assoc*. 1985;110:194-198.

19. Rohrer MD, Terry MA, Bulard RA, Graves DC, Taylor EM. Microwave sterilization of hydrophilic contact lenses. *Am J Ophthalmol*. 1986;101:49-57.

20. Douglas C, Burke B, Kessler DL, Cicmanec JF, Bracken RB. Microwave: practical cost-effective method for sterilizing urinary catheters in the home. *Urology*. 1990;35:219-222.

21. Kindle G, Busse A, Kampa D, Meyer-König U, Daschner FD. Killing activity of microwaves in milk. *J Hosp Infect*. 1996;33:273-278.

22. Harris MG, Rechberger J, Grant T, Holden BA. In-office microwave disinfection of soft contact lenses. *Optom Vis Sci*. 1990;67:129-132.

23. Mervine J, Temple R. Using a microwave oven to disinfect intermittent-use catheters. *Rehabil Nurs*. 1997;22:318-320.

24. Neto AG, de Carvalho JN, Costa da Fonseca JA, da Costa Carvalho AM, de Melo Vasconcelos Castro MM. Microwave medical waste disinfection: a procedure to monitor treatment quality. Paper presented at: 1999 SBMO/IEEE MTT-S International Microwave and Optoelectronics Conference; August 9-12, 1999; Rio de Janeiro, Brazil.

25. Herschel W. Experiments on the refrangibility of the invisible rays of the sun. *Philos Trans R Soc Lond*. 1800;90:284-292.

26. Rowan-Robinson M. *Night Vision: Exploring the Infrared Universe*. Cambridge, United Kingdom: Cambridge University Press; 2013.

27. Decareau RV. *Microwaves in the Food Processing Industry*. Orlando, FL: Academic Press; 1985.

28. Bhattacharya S, ed. *Conventional and Advanced Food Processing Technologies*. West Sussex, United Kingdom: John Wiley & Sons; 2005.

29. Hamanaka D, Uchino T, Furuse N, Han W, Tanaka S. Effect of the wavelength of infrared heaters on the inactivation of bacterial spores at various water activities. *Int J Food Microbiol*. 2006;108:281-285.

30. Krishnamurthy K, Khurana HK, Soojin J, Irudayaraj J, Demirci A. Infrared heating in food processing: an overview. *Compr Rev Food Sci Food Saf*. 2008;7:2-13.

31. Allphin W. *Primer of Lamps and Lighting*. 3rd ed. Boston, MA: Addison-Wesley Educational Publishers Inc; 1973.

32. Mujumdar AS, ed. *Handbook of Industrial Drying*. 3rd ed. Boca Raton, FL: CRC Press; 2006.

33. Mata-Portuguez VH, Pérez LS, Acosta-Gío E. Sterilization of heat-resistant instruments with infrared radiation. *Infect Control Hosp Epidemiol*. 2002;23:393-396.

34. Wang B, Khir R, Pan Z, et al. Effective disinfection of rough rice using infrared radiation heating. *J Food Prot*. 2014;77:1538-1545.

35. Elmnasser N, Guillou S, Leroi F, Orange N, Bakhrouf A, Federighi M. Pulsed-light system as a novel food decontamination technology: a review. *Can J Microbiol*. 2007;53:813-821.

36. Harm W. *Biological Effects of Ultraviolet Radiation*. London, United Kingdom: Cambridge University Press; 1980.

37. Gast PR. Solar irradiance. In: Valley SF, ed. *Handbook of Physics and Space Environments*. Bedford, MA: Air Force Cambridge Research Laboratories, Office of Aerospace Research, United States Air Force, Hanscom Field; 1948: Section 16-1.

38. Clark RW, Lierman JC, Lander D, Dunn JE, inventors; Sanwa Bank California, assignee. Parametric control in pulsed light sterilization of packages and their contents. US patent 5,925,885, July 20, 1999.

39. Kramer B, Wunderlich J, Muranyi P. Recent findings in pulsed light disinfection. *J Appl Microbiol*. 2017;122:830-856.

40. Bhavya ML, Umesh Hebbar H. Pulsed light processing of foods for microbial safety. *Food Qual Saf*. 2017;1(3):187-201.

41. Friedman-Huffman D. Pulse white light takes aim at conventional UV. *Water Condition Purificat*. 1998;40:66-68.

42. Wright MS, Collins PA. Waterborne transmission of *Cryptosporidium*, *Cyclospora*, and *Giardia*. *Clin Lab Sci*. 1997;10:287-290.

43. Fayer R. Effect of sodium hypochlorite exposure on infectivity of *Cryptosporidium parvum* oocysts for neonatal BALB/c mice. *Appl Environ Microbiol*. 1995;61:844-846.

44. Slifko TR, Friedman D, Griffin D, et al. *Cryptosporidium* viability and infectivity for the water industry. Paper presented at: American Water Works Association Annual Convention; June 15-19 1997; Atlanta, GA.

45. Wekhof A, Trompeter F-J, Franken O. Pulsed UV disintegration (PUVD): a new sterilisation mechanism for packaging and broad medical-hospital applications. In: Proceedings from the 1st International Conference on Ultraviolet Technologies; June 14-16, 2001; Washington, DC.

46. Ansari IA, Datta AK. An overview of sterilization methods for packaging materials used in aseptic packaging systems. *Food Bioprod Process*. 2003;81:57-65.

CHAPTER 11

Microbial Inactivation Kinetics and Heat Disinfection

Patrick J. McCormick, James J. Kaiser, and Michael J. Schoene

Any discussion of the kinetics of the thermal destruction of microorganisms must acknowledge the defining contributions of individuals such as Rahn,[1] Pflug,[2] Holcomb and Pflug,[3] Bigelow,[4] Stumbo,[5] Ball,[6] Halvorson and Zielger,[7] Russell,[8] and many others. Their work laid the foundation for the development and validation of effective heat sterilization and disinfection treatments. Although heat processing has been used for centuries to reduce or eliminate microbial contamination and render items and goods safe for use or consumption, much of our knowledge of the kinetics of the thermal destruction of microorganisms and control of heat processing treatments has been derived from studies initially performed in the food industry during the first half of the 20th century. Stumbo[5] describes how advances in canning, measurement, and processing technology developed concurrently and led to breakthroughs in our understanding of the kinetics of inactivation of microorganisms subjected to heat processing conditions. Many of the principles and concepts established during this time remain in widespread use today and have been incorporated into international pharmacopeias, disinfection, and sterilization standards.

Perhaps the greatest challenge in developing accurate models of the kinetics of heat inactivation is the microorganisms themselves. We can employ either homogenous populations of defined test organisms deposited on some form of carrier placed with or inoculated directly onto or within the product or goods being processed, or we can study the heterogeneous populations of microorganisms that are normally resident on the product (bioburden). The former approach is preferred when modeling heat inactivation kinetics because a hypothetical and homogenous population of microorganisms will respond in a more uniform manner to an applied heat stress as compared to a heterogonous population. Heterogeneous populations of microorganisms frequently consist of mixed genus and species in different states of growth or natural contamination with varying levels of heat resistance.

This can complicate data analysis and lead to an inconsistent response to the applied heat stress as can studying the microorganisms in a different matrix native for the population. Most studies of applied heat processes are performed with a homogenous population of test organisms such as spores of *Geobacillus stearothermophilus*, *Bacillus atrophaeus*, *Bacillus coagulans*, *Clostridium sporogenes*, or others, many of which are commercially available and used in the form of biological indicators (BIs). The BIs are generally well characterized for their homogeneity and heat resistance as compared to product bioburden and are important tools in the development and validation of heat treatment processes (see chapter 65). In most circumstances, the use of a defined sterilization challenge in the form of a BI will provide a greater level of resistance to a given heat treatment than the bioburden that is typically present on or in the product and thus provide an additional margin of safety.[9]

As noted by Schmidt,[10] "The only single practical criterion of the death of microorganisms is the failure to reproduce when, as far as is known, suitable conditions for reproduction are provided. This means that any organism which fails to show evidence of growth when placed under what is considered, in the light of our present knowledge of bacterial nutrition and growth requirements is considered as dead." This statement is as true today as it was in 1954, even though our knowledge of the many different types of microorganisms has improved (eg, viruses). It underscores the fact that our knowledge and effective control of heat treatment processes rely primarily on our ability to recover and accurately enumerate microorganisms following exposure to heat treatment. This is critical to the development of effective heat treatment processes capable of attaining the desired level of microbial inactivation on a reproducible basis. Unfortunately, as anyone who has worked with microorganisms well knows, the recovery and enumeration of microorganisms is often subject to considerable variability. Although physical measurement systems such as thermocouples, resistance temperature detectors, and pressure transducers can be calibrated to traceable standards with a high degree of accuracy, in most cases, this is not possible with viable microbiological systems. At best, the microbiological systems employed to document the efficacy of a given sterilization or disinfection process may be characterized as to their homogeneity and relative resistance to an applied heat treatment,[11-13] but they cannot be calibrated to traceable physical standards.[14] Thus, although calibrated physical measurement systems may be employed to accurately measure and control the critical parameters of an applied heat treatment process, the determination of the microbicidal efficacy of the process is often less precise. Studies regarding the thermal inactivation of microorganisms should therefore consider not only the inherent variability of the microorganisms themselves but also the variability associated with their enumeration and recovery. As discussed by Sutton,[15] when considering bacteria and fungi, a plate count method often employed for the enumeration of microorganisms is subject to significant limitations such as growth abilities of the microorganisms present, accuracy, reproducibility, and the countable range per plate, as examples. Alternate microbiological enumeration techniques that rely on sophisticated technologies to detect the presence of viable microorganisms may also exhibit limited analytical capability because their performance is ultimately correlated to conventional microbiological methods.[16,17] There also exists the specter of viable but nonculturable microorganisms that may not exhibit growth under the laboratory conditions tested but may remain capable of further reproduction when introduced into a suitable host.[18] Further compounding this situation is that many studies have documented a wide range of variables that may impact the recovery of heat-stressed microorganisms. These must be controlled to the greatest extent possible to generate reliable data. Ultimately, as noted by Sutton,[15] any quantitative measurement of microorganisms using conventional or alternative microbiological methods is at best an estimate of the true population of microorganisms that may be present in any given sample at any given time. On initial consideration, this would suggest that studies of the thermal inactivation of microorganisms could be fraught with error. A review of the literature indicates, however, that there are numerous studies documenting controlled and reproducible microbial inactivation kinetics across a broad range of conditions. Although these studies reflect the diligence of the investigators in controlling the many variables associated with microbiological testing and the recovery of injured microorganisms, they also reflect the fact that the raw data is frequently subject to logarithmic transformation based on the semilogarithmic model of the inactivation of microorganisms. Logarithmic transformation has the effect of both normalizing the distribution of errors in the data[19] and stabilizing the variance.[20] Indeed, the semilogarithmic model of microbial

inactivation is the cornerstone of contemporary sterilization processing as a plot of the logarithm of the number of surviving microorganisms versus the duration of exposure or applied dose frequently yields a straight line. The selected processing conditions can then be extrapolated to the desired level of probability of microbial recovery. This model requires an acceptable degree of correlation or "goodness of fit" between the applied treatment and the resulting microbiological data, although this may be difficult to rigorously define from a statistical perspective, and the microbiological data may only span a limited range.

▶ THE SEMILOGARITHMIC SURVIVOR CURVE MODEL

As can be seen in Figure 11.1, when microbial inactivation data are plotted on a linear scale versus the duration of treatment under constant conditions, the resulting curve is of an exponential nature with an asymptotic decrease in the number of surviving microorganisms as the duration of exposure increases. Although it is evident that a greater number of microorganisms are being inactivated the longer the duration of the applied treatment, the information generated is of limited utility. As the number of surviving microorganisms decreases with the duration of exposure, resolution is lost; thus, it is difficult to use this data to extrapolate to a level of probability of a surviving

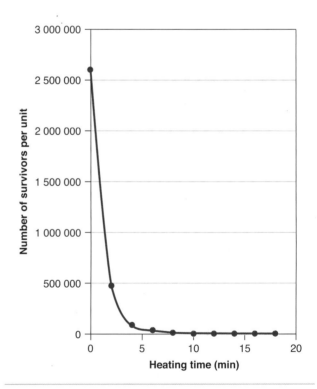

FIGURE 11.1 Microbial survivor curve data plotted on an arithmetic scale, number of survivors per unit versus heating time.

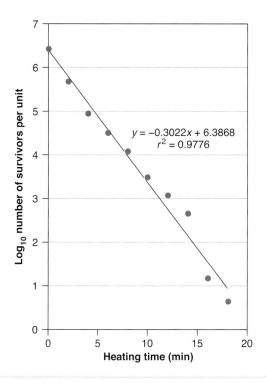

FIGURE 11.2 The same microbial survivor data as per Figure 11.1, plotted on a semilogarithmic scale, with the number of survivors per unit plotted on the log scale on the y-axis versus the heating time on the arithmetic scale on the x-axis.

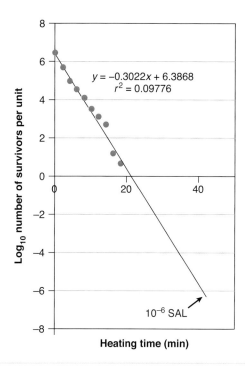

FIGURE 11.3 Extrapolation of the data of Figure 11.2 to a sterility assurance level (SAL) of 10^{-6} or a one-in-a-million probability of a surviving microorganism.

microorganism and thereby establish effective and reproducible treatment conditions. When the logarithm of the number of surviving microorganisms is plotted versus the duration of treatment under constant conditions, the effective population range that may be visualized is expanded and a linear relationship between the population of surviving microorganisms and the duration of treatment can become apparent (Figure 11.2). This information is far more useful as a linear relationship between microbial inactivation and the duration of the applied treatment or dose because it allows one to extrapolate to the desired probability of a surviving microorganism as appropriate to the intended application (Figure 11.3). This is of course an oversimplification because there are many factors involved in generating accurate and reproducible semilogarithmic inactivation curves of this nature, but it does serve to illustrate the primary attribute on which successful heat treatments for sterilization and disinfection are based; namely, the semilogarithmic nature of microbial inactivation.

The mathematical basis for the semilogarithmic inactivation of microorganisms follows from the work of Rahn.[1] Rahn[1] observed that, in contrast to multicellular organisms, bacteria exposed to lethal agents were inactivated at a nearly constant rate, whereas multicellular organisms exhibited an initial lag followed by concave downward survivor curves. When mosquito larvae were immersed in heptylic acid or tadpoles heated at 35.5°C, no effect was

apparent during the initial stages of treatment followed by an increase in the death rate to a maximum level, with a gradual decline in the rate of kill as the few remaining resistant organisms were killed off. With unicellular organisms, such as spores of *Bacillus anthracis* exposed to mercuric chloride or yeast of *Torula monosa* heated at 50°C, there was little or no lag apparent and inactivation occurred in a progressive geometric manner. For example, if one-half of the total population of bacteria or yeast were killed off in the first minute of exposure, one-half of the remaining population would be killed off in the second minute of exposure leaving one-fourth of the initial population alive at the second minute, etc. By plotting the logarithm of the surviving population of bacteria or yeast versus the time of exposure (or dose) of the lethal agent, a straight line was apparent. Based on the law of mass action, Rahn[1] attributed the logarithmic order of death of bacteria to the inactivation of a single critical molecule within the cell. This was analogous to the single hit theory of inactivation as proposed by Chick[21] for chemical disinfectants based on a first-order chemical reaction.

$$\frac{d[A]}{dt} = -K[A] \tag{1}$$

For sterilization and disinfection processes, the rate of this inactivation can be expressed as the following differential equation:

$$\frac{dN}{dt} = -KN \tag{2}$$

where N is the number of microorganisms surviving after treatment time (t) and K is a reaction-rate constant, which for thermal treatments is a function of temperature. A negative term is assigned to the right side of the equation to reflect the inactivation of microorganisms with continued treatment. Integrating this equation

$$\int \frac{dN}{N} = K \int dt \qquad (3)$$

$$\ln N = -Kt + C \qquad (4)$$

One can then evaluate the constant C using the boundary conditions. At time zero, C becomes the initial population, which is N_0. The equation thus becomes:

$$\ln N = -Kt + \ln N_0 \qquad (5)$$

Converting this equation from natural logarithms of base e to logarithms of base "10"

$$\log N = -kt + \log N_0 \qquad (6)$$

Note that in the base 10 system, the lower case term k is used to replace the term K; the two constants are related in that $k = 0.4343\ K$.

Now that the differential equation for first-order reaction kinetics has been converted to a form that is relatively user friendly, one must also consider the treatment of time in this process. As the rate of microbial inactivation is not necessarily related directly to the sterilizer clock time due to lag factors and other considerations, the term t is replaced with the term U, which is the equivalent minutes at the test temperature. The equation then becomes

$$\log N = -kU + \log N_0 \qquad (7)$$

We must now consider the D-value, or decimal reduction time, which is generally defined as the time or dose required to reduce a population of microorganisms by 1 log (90%) under a stated set of conditions. This is a useful measure of the resistance of a given population of microorganisms to a heat treatment process and is frequently employed to define a minimum acceptable level of sterilization such as a 12D reduction in a population of test organisms or bioburden.[22] Although a D-value (also known as a D_{10} value) can be determined in several ways, it is perhaps most easily visualized as the exposure time or dose required for the survivor curve to traverse 1 log cycle. From equation (7), we see that if $\log N$ is plotted versus the equivalent exposure time U, a straight line is obtained with slope $-k$ (Figure 11.4). By definition, the slope of a straight line is the tangent of the angle θ, which is expressed as ($\Delta\log N/\Delta U$). Examining the values of $\Delta\log N$ and ΔU in Figure 11.4, we find that the numerator in the slope equation

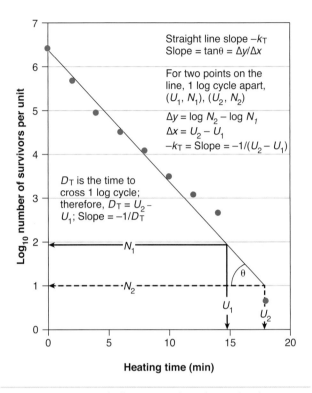

FIGURE 11.4 Graph illustrating the relationship between D-value and slope of the survivor curve on a semilogarithmic graph. Based on Pflug et al.[23]

($\Delta\log N/\Delta U$) when $\log N_2 - \log N_1$ are 1 log apart has a negative slope and is always -1. For example, $\log 10 - \log 100 = 1 - 2 = -1$. For the denominator in the slope equation for a 1-log change in N, the value of U is $U_2 - U_1$, which is ΔU. Therefore, for a 1-log change in N, the slope is $-1/\Delta U$.

$$\text{Slope} = -k_T = \tan\Theta = \frac{\Delta\log N}{\Delta U} = \frac{-1}{U_2 - U_1} = \frac{-1}{\Delta U} \qquad (8)$$

$$\Delta U = \frac{1}{k_T} \qquad (9)$$

Over time, the use of the reaction rate constant k was replaced with the use of the term D or D-value, which is the time at temperature T for the straight-line semilogarithmic survivor curve to traverse 1 log cycle (a 90% reduction in N) as discussed earlier. Because the rate of microbial inactivation will vary with the temperature of the heat stress applied, the D-value is usually denoted as the term D_T to denote exposure to constant temperature conditions (eg, $D_{121°C}$). Substituting the term D_T for the term kt in equation (7) based on the equivalency of these terms as expressed in equation (9), we have

$$\log N = \frac{-U}{D_T} + \log N_0 \qquad (10)$$

As can be seen from this equation, the D-value can also be defined as the negative reciprocal of the slope of the semilogarithmic survivor curve. Rearranging the terms of the earlier equation, a more useful equation for the determination of the D-value based on plate count data generated from a semilogarithmic survivor curve is

$$D_{\mathrm{T}} = U/\log N_0 - \log N \qquad (11)$$

One of the issues that is frequently encountered when modeling semilogarithmic inactivation kinetics is that even though most of the curve is of a linear nature, during the initial phases of exposure, shoulders that are concave either upward or downward may be apparent and/or tailing may occur, which can skew the fit of the model (Figure 11.5). Several factors can explain this departure from linearity, including multiple hit as opposed to single-hit inactivation kinetics,[24] cell clumping,[1] mixed populations of cells of varying ages,[1] spore dormancy,[25] variations in the applied heat treatment, poor control over experimental variables, presence of interfering factors, etc. Note that the linearity of the survivor curve is a function not only of the homogeneity of the population of microorganisms being tested but also of one's ability to control the applied heat treatment within a narrow temperature band. Where variations from linearity occur during the initial phases of heating such as those indicated

for curves B and D in Figure 11.5, it may be acceptable in some circumstances to ignore the N_0 data and construct a survivor curve based on the remainder of the data. A better means to reconcile the deviation from linearity during the initial phases of heating is to modify equation (10) by incorporating an intercept ratio (IR), which is defined as $\log Y_0/\log N_0$ where Y_0 is the intercept of the curve with the y-axis and N_0 is the initial population of microorganisms. The resulting equation will take the following form:

$$\log N = \frac{-U}{D_{\mathrm{T}}} + \log N_0 \, (IR) \qquad (12)$$

Thus, for survivor curves with an IR value >1.0, the curve will be concave downward (see Figure 11.5, curve B), whereas those with an IR value <1.0 will be concave upward (see Figure 11.5, curve C). Survivor curves with an IR value of 1.0 will obviously be straight lines through N_0 (see Figure 11.5, curve A). Holcomb et al[26] have also suggested the use of an intercept index defined as $\log$ (y-intercept at $U = 0 / N_0$) in order to address deviations from linearity in the initial phases of the semilogarithmic survivor curve. Although it is possible to use different mathematical approaches to assess the goodness of fit of the data, visual inspection of the survivor curve remains one of the easiest means to evaluate its linearity.

In addition to the shoulders that may be present in the survivor curve during the initial heating phase of the process, one must also consider how well the data from the linear portion of the curve fits the resulting model. A best fit estimate of the data can be readily determined using a graphing function or statistics package with a resulting coefficient of determination (r^2) of not less than 0.8 (eg, as defined for heat-based BIs in ISO 11138-1). Although this is acceptable for many applications, it is not necessarily the most rigorous approach because the range over which it is applied is not linked to a maximum degree of uncertainty. The least squares method of Draper and Smith[27] may also be employed to estimate the best fit of the data to a straight line as discussed by Pflug et al.[23] The least squares method makes the following assumptions: (1) the true model describing the relationship between the logarithm of the number of surviving organisms and heating time is a linear one, (2) the deviation in the log number of survivors from the straight line is a random variable with expected value of zero, (3) the expected deviation is the same for all heating times, and (4) the deviations for different heating times are uncorrelated. The following model is employed:

$$y_{\mathrm{u}} = \alpha + \beta U + \varepsilon \qquad (13)$$

where $y_{\mathrm{u}} = \log N_{\mathrm{U}}$ the logarithm of the number of survivors at time U; U = equivalent heating time at the test temperature; α = the y-intercept at $U = 0$; β = slope of the line; and ε = deviation component, a random variable with mean zero, constant variance equal to some value σ^2, and which is uncorrelated for different heating times.

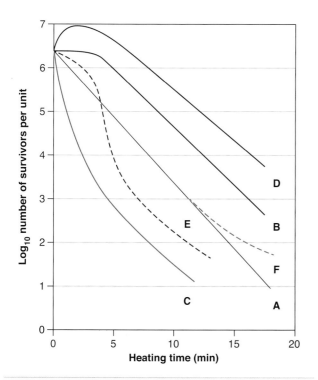

FIGURE 11.5 Shape of semilogarithmic survivor curves: straight line through the initial number, N_0 (curve A); concave downward (curve B); concave upward (curve C); activation effect (curve D); sigmoid (curve E); and a straight line with a tail (curve F). Based on Pflug et al.[23]

If n observations have been made at various heating times ($U_1, U_2, \ldots U_n$), not all necessarily distinct, we can derive estimates of α and β, which are denoted as $\hat{\alpha}$ and $\hat{\beta}$. This is done by choosing α and β to minimize the following sum of squared deviations:

$$S = \sum_{i=1}^{n} \varepsilon_i^2 = \sum_{i=1}^{n} [y_i - (\alpha + \beta U_i)]^2 \qquad (14)$$

By taking the partial derivatives $\partial S/\partial \alpha$ and $\partial S/\partial \beta$, we get two equations that, when set equal to zero and solved simultaneously for α and β, give

$$\hat{\beta} = \frac{\sum_{i=1}^{n} (U_i - \overline{U})(y_i - \overline{y})}{\sum_{i=1}^{n} (U_i + \overline{U})^2} \qquad (15)$$

$$\hat{\alpha} = \overline{y} - \hat{\beta}\overline{U} \qquad (16)$$

where

$$\overline{U} = \sum_{i=1}^{n} \frac{U_i}{n} \quad \text{and} \quad \overline{y} = \sum_{i=1}^{n} \frac{y_i}{n}$$

An unbiased estimate (s^2) of the variance σ^2 of the random variable ε is given by

$$s_\varepsilon^2 = \frac{\sum_{i=1}^{n} (y_i - \hat{\alpha} - \hat{\beta}U_i)^2}{n-2} \qquad (17)$$

Similarly, estimates of the standard errors of $\hat{\alpha}$ and $\hat{\beta}$ can be given using the result for s_ε^2.

$$S\hat{E}(\hat{\alpha}) = \left[\frac{\sum_{i=1}^{n} U_i^2}{n \sum_{i=1}^{n} (U_i - \overline{U})^2} \right]^{0.5} S\varepsilon \qquad (18)$$

$$S\hat{E}(\hat{\beta}) = \frac{S\varepsilon}{\left[\sum_{i=1}^{n} (U_i - \overline{U})^2 \right]^{0.5}} \qquad (19)$$

Equations (14) to (19) are defining equations and can be expanded and put into a simpler form for computation.

Because there are estimates of α and β and standard errors of those estimates, we can form confidence intervals (CIs) for the two parameters. The 95% CIs based on our experimental data would be

$$\hat{\alpha} \pm t_{.975} (n-2) \, S\hat{E}(\hat{\alpha}) \qquad (20)$$

and

$$\hat{\beta} \pm t_{.975} (n-2) \, S\hat{E}(\hat{\beta}) \qquad (21)$$

where $t_{.975} (n-2)$ is the 0.975 percentage point of the Student's t distribution with ($n-2$) degrees of freedom.

These CIs for the intercept and slope parameters have the following interpretation in our model: If an experiment is carried out many times in exactly the same way, then we would expect the CIs calculated from each set of data to cover the true values of α and β approximately 95% of the time.

An estimate for the parameter D, defined in equation (10), can be obtained from the following equation:

$$\hat{D} = -\frac{1}{\hat{\beta}} \qquad (22)$$

The estimate in equation (22) is called the quasi–least squares estimator of D because the minimization of the sum of squares in equation (14) was with respect to $\beta = -1/D$, and not D. McHugh and Sundararaj[28] described various methods for estimating D, including quasi–least squares and the weighted and unweighted least squares methods, and the method of maximum likelihood.

An approximate 95% CI for D is

$$\left[-\frac{1}{\hat{\beta}_1}, -\frac{1}{\hat{\beta}_2} \right] \qquad (23)$$

where $\hat{\beta}_1$ and $\hat{\beta}_2$ are the 95% confidence limits (CLs) of $\hat{\beta}_1$ (obtained from equation [21]).

▶ NONLINEAR SURVIVOR CURVES

The phenomenon of nonlinear survivor curves has been attributed to a number of potential causes including clumping of microorganisms, population heterogeneity, differences in heat resistance within the population,[29,30] increase in heat resistance during the heating process,[31] activation (germination) at high temperatures of a normally dormant spore population,[32] and various other causes. Although there has been much speculation regarding the potential causes, it should be remembered that nonlinear survivor curves may be simply caused by either poor control over the heat treatment process or issues associated with the laboratory analysis phase and the enumeration of surviving microorganisms. Nonlinear behavior can occur with any sterilization or disinfection process.[33] To address this, a number of alternative models to the classic first-order inactivation kinetics have been proposed for the heat inactivation of bacteria. For example, van Boekel[34] discussed the application of the Weibull distribution model to address the nonlinearity of observed semilogarithmic inactivation curves of vegetative cells subjected to heat treatment. As opposed to assuming that the inactivation of microorganisms is a consequence of a single lethal event, the Weibull approach considers lethal events as probabilistic events with the resulting survivor curve being a cumulative form of the individual inactivation time of each cell. As described by van Boekel[34] and Head and Cenkowski[35] in the Weibull model, the distribution of different individual inactivation times takes the following form:

$$\log \left(\frac{N}{N_0} \right) = -\frac{1}{2.303} \left(\frac{t}{\alpha} \right)^\beta \qquad (24)$$

Where: N = number of survivors at time t
N_0 = initial number of microorganisms
t = treatment time
α = scale parameter (typically minutes or seconds)
β = shape parameter (Weibull slope)

If the resulting semilogarithmic plot is linear, $\beta = 1.0$, whereas if $\beta > 1.0$, the curve is concave downward and concave upward if $\beta < 1.0$. The 90th percentile of the failure time distribution, t_R, which is also referred to as the reliable life in failure analysis (roughly analogous to the D-value when 1 log reduction is concerned), may be calculated as

$$t_R = \alpha(2.303)^{\frac{1}{\beta}} \qquad (25)$$

The Weibull model has been successfully employed by a number of investigators to address nonlinear inactivation kinetics in various systems including vegetative cells heated in various menstruum,[34] bacterial spores,[35-37] and heat-resistant fungi.[38-40] Other models include the shoulder/tail model discussed by Geeraerd et al[41] that incorporates an initial shoulder followed by an exponential inactivation phase and subsequent tailing phase, the Gompertz model that also addresses shoulders and tailing of the survivor curve,[42-44] and the biphasic model for which there are two different inactivation slopes (eg, assuming two distinct subpopulations of microorganisms[29,45]). Many of these models have been developed to address the kinetics of inactivation associated with the thermal treatment of foods and juices under low-temperature processing conditions as well as combination treatments.[46] Although these models are very useful and may indeed provide a better understanding of the behavior of a population of microorganisms when subjected to a particular stress or combination of stresses, it is likely that the semilogarithmic model will remain predominant for the foreseeable future due to its simplicity and ease of application.

▶ QUANTAL OR FRACTION-NEGATIVE ANALYSIS

As discussed earlier, the continued application of a controlled heat treatment to a homogenous population of microorganisms generally results in a predictable semilogarithmic order of inactivation that can be readily visualized by plotting the logarithm of surviving microorganisms versus the duration of heat treatment. This model is effective only to the limit of quantitation of plate count technology, which is approximately 25 to 250 colony-forming units (CFUs) for most microorganisms. As one would anticipate, counting error increases significantly the fewer the number of colonies present on a plate with an error of 20% as a percentage of the mean for 25 CFUs, 44.7% for 5 CFUs, and 100% for 1 CFU.[47] Due to the increase in counting error associated with the loss of countable colonies as

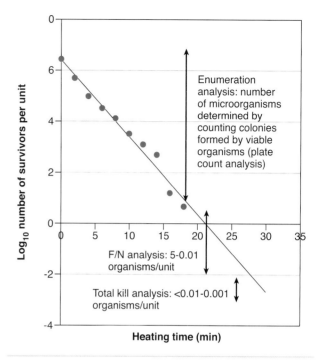

FIGURE 11.6 Survivor curve illustrating the enumeration, fraction-negative (F/N, or quantal) measurement areas, and region where there is essentially total kill.

the heat treatment progresses, we must therefore rely on quantal or fraction-negative analysis, which is capable of measurements in the range of 5 to 0.01 microorganisms per unit (Figure 11.6). In quantal or fraction-negative analysis, replicate samples of the challenge microorganism are subjected to graded exposures of treatment under constant conditions and the number of samples surviving treatment qualitatively determined (growth or no growth) for each exposure period. This typically takes the form of culturing each set of replicate samples processed for a given exposure time in individual tubes of growth medium and determining the fraction of tubes positive or negative for growth of the test organism based on visible turbidity following incubation for a defined period of time. Each set that is processed may exhibit complete recovery or growth of all samples tested, partial (dichotomous) recovery of the samples tested, or complete inactivation of all samples tested with increasing duration of heat treatment.

One of the earliest approaches to the analysis of quantal data was the thermal death time or end point analysis as described by Bigelow and Esty[48] and Townsend et al.[49] The thermal death time approach was initially employed in the canning industry to establish retort process times. This approach consisted of plotting the positive and negative results of replicate samples processed at various times and temperatures as a function of time on a logarithmic scale versus temperature (Figure 11.7). When any of the replicate units were positive, this was indicated with a plus sign. For those times when all replicates were negative, a zero was employed. The thermal death time for a given temperature was

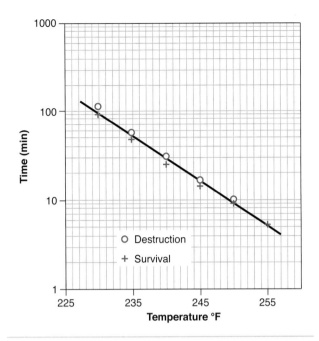

FIGURE 11.7 Thermal death time curve for spores of PA 3679 in beef and gravy in thermal time cans. F_0 = 9.5 min and z = 20°F. Based on Pflug.[2]

assumed to be between the longest heating time when a positive unit was obtained and the shortest heating time when all the units were negative. A shortcoming of this approach is that it does not consider the initial inoculum level (N_0) or the number of replicates per time point. Nevertheless, it was a reasonable if somewhat simplistic attempt at establishing effective process control based on the rate of inactivation of microorganisms under varying conditions. Today, the most common approach to the analysis of quantal data is to employ either the Stumbo-Murphy-Cochran method, which is based on most probable number (MPN) analysis, or the Holcomb-Spearman-Karber method, which is based on the mean time until sterility (U_{HSK}) as indicated in ISO 11138-1.[50]

The Stumbo-Murphy-Cochran method is a modification of the semilogarithmic model expressed in equation (10). This is easily rearranged to express the D-value as follows:

$$D_T = \frac{U_i}{\log N_0 - \log N} \quad (26)$$

Where: U_i = a specific heating time
N_0 = the initial number of microorganisms in each replicate unit
N = number of survivors at U_i

Stumbo et al[51] proposed that an estimate of N (the number of survivors in the quantal region) could be based on the MPN equation of Halvorson and Zeigler[7]:

$$N_U = \ln (n / r) \quad (27)$$

Where: n = number of units heated
r = number of units negative for growth

The MPN equation is essentially the probability of the "no survivors term" of the Poisson equation $P(0) = e^{-N}$. A dichotomous result in the quantal region occurs because of a probabilistic distribution of a few surviving microorganisms among replicate units. In fraction-negative testing when we have dichotomous results, the units that show no growth (the P[0] units) are the critical units in the analysis because only in these units do we truly know the number of surviving organisms (zero) per sample because we cannot determine by inspection the number of surviving microorganisms at a given exposure time in those units that are positive (turbid) for growth. Table 11.1 provides an estimate of the number of surviving microorganisms (N) per unit calculated by the MPN method from 1 to 99 units negative for growth based on processing 100 units per exposure interval. In this example, the use of the MPN equation (27) makes it possible to generate a survivor curve over approximately 2.5 log cycles between fractions negative of 1/100 to 99/100 or approximately 5 microorganisms per unit to 0.01 microorganisms per sample as noted earlier.

Substituting the MPN equation (27) into the D-value equation (26), we have

$$D_T = \frac{U_i}{\log N_0 - \log [2.303 \log (n / r)]} \quad (28)$$

Where: U_i = a specific heating time
N_0 = the initial number of microorganisms in each replicate unit
n = number of units heated
r = number of units negative for growth.

As can be seen from equation (28), the Stumbo-Murphy-Cochran method requires the initial number of microorganisms be known and at least one dichotomous result in the fraction-negative region. For each heating interval where quantal or fraction-negative data is recovered, a D-value may be calculated and the resulting D-values averaged together to provide an estimate of the D-value.

If $[n \times (r / n) \times (n - r / n)]$ is greater than or equal to 0.9 and 50 replicates have been tested at each exposure interval, then the upper and lower 95% CIs can be calculated about the D-value estimate as described in ISO 11138-1.[50]

$$D_{calc} = \frac{t}{\log_{10} N_0 - \log_{10} \left(\ln \frac{(1)}{a} \right)}$$

$$\text{where } a = \frac{r}{n} \pm 1.96 \sqrt{\frac{r}{n} \times \frac{1 - r / n}{n}} \quad (29)$$

For calculation of the upper CL, a value of -1.96 is employed for equation (29); for calculation of the lower CL, a value of $+1.96$ is employed.

Essentially, the Stumbo-Murphy-Cochran method is a two-point equation and assumes that the survivor curve is a straight line between N_0 and N_U. Although this assumption

TABLE 11.1 Estimation of the number of viable microorganisms per unit based on quantal data[a]

r (Number Negative Out of 100)	n / r	N (Estimated Number of Organisms per Unit)[b]	Log N
1	100.0	4.605	0.6632
5	20.0	2.996	0.4765
10	10.0	2.303	0.3622
15	6.667	1.897	0.2781
20	5.0	1.609	0.2067
25	4.0	1.386	0.1419
30	3.333	1.204	0.0806
35	2.857	1.050	0.0211
40	2.500	0.916	−0.0380
45	2.222	0.799	−0.0977
50	2.000	0.693	−0.1592
55	1.818	0.598	−0.2234
60	1.667	0.511	−0.2917
65	1.538	0.431	−0.3657
70	1.429	0.357	−0.4477
75	1.333	0.288	−0.5411
80	1.250	0.223	−0.6514
85	1.176	0.163	−0.7891
90	1.111	0.105	−0.9773
95	1.053	0.051	−1.2899
99	1.010	0.010	−1.9978

[a]Based on Pflug et al.[23]

[b]N is estimated using the equation of Halvorson and Zeigler[7]: $N = \ln n / r$.

holds in many applications, the user must be aware of potential variability in the method as the number of microorganisms at both time zero (N_0) and time U (N_u) are estimates and the resulting D_T value will vary with the variation in N_0 and N_U. As opposed to the Stumbo-Murphy-Cochran approach based on the use of MPN analysis to estimate the number of surviving microorganisms, the Holcomb-Spearman-Karber method is used to estimate the U_{HSK} value or mean time until sterility when a sample containing microorganisms becomes sterile. In very simplistic terms, the Stumbo-Murphy-Cochran estimates the number of surviving microorganisms on the y-axis of the survivor curve at time U when N_U is between 5 and 0.01 microorganisms per unit, whereas the Holcomb-Spearman-Karber method estimates the time (U_{HSK}) on the x-axis of the survivor curve at which there are no surviving microorganisms in a set of data in the quantal or fraction-negative region. Of the two methods, the Holcomb-Spearman-Karber method requires a more complete set of data in the quantal region,

with at least five successive heating intervals where all samples are positive for growth in the first (shortest) heating interval, at least two successive heating intervals with dichotomous results, and two successive heating intervals where all samples are negative for growth.[50] In contrast, the Stumbo-Murphy-Cochran can provide an estimate of the D-value based on one result in the quantal region if the initial population (N_0) is known.

Based on the semilogarithmic inactivation equation for estimating the number of surviving microorganisms at heating time U and assuming that the population of surviving microorganisms follows the Poisson distribution, Holcomb and Pflug derived the basic equation[3,52]:

$$U_{HSK} = \frac{\gamma + \ln N_0}{k} \qquad (30)$$

Where: U_{HSK} = mean time until sterility
Y = Euler's constant (0.5772)
k = reaction rate constant

Converting this to base 10 logarithms and replacing k with D_T (see discussion under equation [9]), we arrive at

$$D_T = \frac{U_{HSK}}{\log N_0 + 0.2507} \quad (31)$$

Using equation (31), if the U_{HSK} is known, in addition to the initial number of microorganisms (N_0) the D_T value can be estimated.

When r_i is the number of sterile replicates out of n; heated to a time U_i, then the HSK estimate of U_{HSK} is given by

$$U_{HSK} = \sum_{i=1}^{k-1} \left(\frac{U_{i+1} + U_i}{2} \right) \left(\frac{r_{i+1}}{n_{i+1}} - \frac{r_i}{n_i} \right) \quad (32)$$

where U_{HSK} = HSK heating time estimate (mean time until sterility)

  U_k = first heating time with all units negative

  U_i = ith heating time

  r_i = number of replicate units negative at U_i

  n_i = total number of replicate units heated at U_i

If successive times differ by a constant d and the same number of replicates n is heated at all times (this is known as the Limited Holcomb-Spearman-Karber method), we can write equation (32) as follows:

$$U_{HSK} = \frac{d}{2} - \frac{d}{n} \sum_{i=1}^{k-1} r_i \quad (33)$$

where U_{HSK} = HSK heating time estimate (mean time until sterility)

  U_k = first heating time with all units negative

  d = time between exposures (should be identical)

  n = number of replicates at each exposure interval (should be identical)

  $\sum_{i=1}^{k-1} r_i$ = the sum of negative cultures following the last heating time at which all cultures are positive for growth (U_2) and U_{k-1}

The estimated variance (V) of U_{HSK} assuming equal times between exposure periods and the same number of replicates per exposure period is given by

$$V = \frac{d^2}{n^2(n-1)} \times \sum_{i=1}^{k-1} r_i(n - r_i) \quad (34)$$

The 95% CI for the mean D-value is calculated from the variance of U_{HSK} as follows:

D lower CL:

$$= \frac{U_{HSK} - 2SD}{\log_{10} N_0 + 0.2507} \quad (35)$$

TABLE 11.2	Hypothetical fraction-negative data[a]	
Heating Interval (U_i)	No. of Samples Tested	No. of Samples Sterile
7 min	20	0
8 min	20	0
9 min	20	2
10 min	20	8
11 min	20	20
12 min	20	20

[a]Hypothetical inactivation data of a biological indicator (BI) inoculated with a population of 1.5×10^6 spores of *Geobacillus stearothermophilus* processed in a moist heat resistometer at 121°C.

D upper CL:

$$= \frac{U_{HSK} + 2SD}{\log_{10} N_0 + 0.2507} \quad (36)$$

Where: $SD = \sqrt{V}$

Based on the earlier discussion and the data in Table 11.2, it is a simple exercise to calculate the D-value for a hypothetical BI with a population of 1.5×10^6 spores per carrier processed at a temperature of 121°C using both the Stumbo-Murphy-Cochran and the Limited Holcomb-Spearman-Karber method as follows:

1. Stumbo-Murphy-Cochran method:

$$D_T = \frac{U_i}{\log N_0 - \log [2.303 \log (n/r)]} \quad (28)$$

Because there are two heating time intervals with fraction-negative results, a D_T value is calculated for each fraction-negative interval and averaged together as follows:

$$D_1 = \frac{t}{\log N_0 - \log [2.303 \log (n/r)]}$$

$$D_1 = \frac{9 \text{ min}}{\log (1.5 \times 10^5) - \log [2.303 \log (20/2)]}$$

$$D_1 = \frac{9 \text{ min}}{5.1761 - 0.3623}$$

$$D_1 = 1.87 \text{ min}$$

$$D_2 = \frac{t}{\log N_0 - \log [2.303 \log (n/r)]}$$

$$D_2 = \frac{10 \text{ min}}{\log (1.5 \times 10^5) - \log [2.303 \log (20/8)]}$$

$$D_2 = \frac{10 \text{ min}}{5.1761 - (-0.0379)}$$

$$D_2 = 1.92 \text{ min}$$

$$D_{avg.} = \frac{1.87 \text{ min} + 1.92 \text{ min}}{2}$$

$$D_{avg.} = 1.89 \text{ min}$$

2. Limited Holcomb-Spearman-Karber method

First designate the appropriate terms of the method as follows with respect to the data:

n = number of specimens per group (20)

d = the difference in minutes between adjacent exposure times (1 min)

U_1 = response of all specimens showing growth in the shortest exposure time adjacent to a dichotomous response (8 min)

U_k = response of all specimens showing no growth in the longest exposure time adjacent to a dichotomous response (11 min)

Where:

	exposure	(n) # samples	(r_1) # sterile	$(n - r_1)$	$f_i(n - r_1)$
	7 min	20	0	20	0
U_1	8 min	20	0	20	0
	9 min	20	2	18	36
U_{k-1}	10 min	20	8	12	96
U_k	11 min	20	20	0	0
	12 min	20	20	0	0

$$\sum_{i=1}^{k-1} U_i = 10$$

$$\sum_{i=1}^{k-1} U_i (n - f_i) = 132$$

Calculate the mean heating time until sterility (U_{HSK}) using equation (33):

$$U_{HSK} = U_k - d/2 - \left(d/n \times \sum_{i=1}^{k-1} U_i\right)$$

$$U_{HSK} = 11 \text{ min} - \frac{1 \text{ min}}{2} - \left(\frac{1 \text{ min}}{20} \times 10\right)$$

$$U_{HSK} = 11 \text{ min} - 0.5 \text{ min} - (0.5 \text{ min})$$

$$U_{HSK} = 10 \text{ min}$$

Calculate the D-value using equation (31):

$$D = \frac{U_{HSK}}{\log N_0 + 0.2507}$$

$$D = \frac{10 \text{ min}}{5.1761 + 0.2507}$$

$$D = 1.84 \text{ min}$$

Calculate the variance of U_{HSK} (V_T) as follows:

$$V_T = \frac{d^2}{n^2 (n-1)} \times \sum_{i=1}^{k-1} r_1 (n - r_1)$$

$$V_T = \frac{1^2}{400 (20-1)} \times (132)$$

$$V_T = \frac{1}{7600} \times (132)$$

$$V_T = 0.0174$$

Calculate the standard deviation:

$$SD = \sqrt{Vt}$$

$$SD = 0.1318$$

Calculate the lower and upper 95% CL for D:

$$CL_{lower} = \frac{T - 2SD}{\log N_0 + 0.2507}$$

$$= \frac{10 - 0.2636}{5.1761 + 0.2507}$$

$$= \frac{9.7364}{5.4268}$$

$$= 1.79 \text{ min}$$

$$CL_{upper} = \frac{T + 2s_T}{\log N_0 + 0.2507}$$

$$= \frac{10 + 0.2636}{5.1761 + 0.2507}$$

$$= \frac{10.2636}{5.4268}$$

$$= 1.89 \text{ min}$$

Although there may be sound reasons for selecting one form of quantal D-value analysis over another, depending on the application and nature of the data, experience suggests that under well-controlled conditions, the differences between D-values calculated using either the Stumbo-Murphy-Cochran or the Holcomb-Spearman-Karber method are not that significant when the data is suitable for calculation by both methods. A review of the D-values calculated for 30 lots of BIs processed in a moist heat resistometer using both methods suggests that there is little difference in the resulting D-values (<10%) regardless of the method of calculation employed (Table 11.3). Of the two methods, the Holcomb-Spearman-Karber method is generally assumed to be the most rigorous because one can estimate the mean time until sterility (U_{HSK}) and corresponding CIs based solely on the quantal data without knowledge of the initial population or shape of the survivor curve. This in turn can be used to compare the effect of various treatment variables, although calculation of the D_T value obviously requires that the initial population be known. Where data are limited, however, the Stumbo-Murphy-Cochran method can provide a reasonable estimation of the efficacy of the treatment conditions. For estimation of the D-value both the Stumbo-Murphy-Cochran and Holcomb-Spearman-Karber methods are subject to any errors associated with the determination of the initial population (N_0) or nonlinearity of the survivor curve. It is also assumed that for each exposure interval, the replicate samples are processed under identical conditions. When replicate samples are processed under ideal conditions in a resistometer (or essentially tightly controlled conditions) as in Table 11.3, these assumptions usually hold and the resulting errors are of a small magnitude such that either method (Stumbo-Murphy-Cochran or Holcomb-Spearman-Karber) will provide an acceptable result.

STERILITY ASSURANCE LEVEL

Thus far, we have presented an analysis of the semi-logarithmic model of the inactivation of microorganisms based on modeling performed in the direct

TABLE 11.3   Comparison of $D_{121°C}$-values of moist heat biological indicators calculated by both the Stumbo-Murphy-Cochran and Limited Holcomb-Spearman-Karber methods

BI type	Labeled $D_{121°C}$-Value	LL	UL	SMC $D_{121°C}$-Value	LHSK $D_{121°C}$-Value
Paper strip	1.7	1.36	2.04	1.9	1.9
Paper strip	2.0	1.6	2.4	1.9	1.8
Paper strip	2.1	1.68	2.52	1.8	1.8
Paper strip	1.9	1.52	2.28	1.7	1.7
Paper strip	1.8	1.44	2.16	1.6	1.6
Paper strip	1.9	1.52	2.28	1.6	1.6
Paper strip	2.4	1.92	2.88	2.4	2.4
Paper strip	1.5	1.2	1.8	1.8	1.8
Paper strip	2.2	1.76	2.64	1.9	1.9
Paper strip	1.7	1.36	2.04	1.9	1.9
Self-contained	2.1	1.68	2.52	2.1	2.1
Self-contained	2.1	1.68	2.52	2.3	2.3
Self-contained	1.9	1.52	2.28	2.2	2.2
Self-contained	2.1	1.68	2.52	2.1	2.1
Self-contained	2.1	1.68	2.52	2.1	2.1
Self-contained	1.7	1.36	2.04	1.8	1.7
Self-contained	1.7	1.36	2.04	1.8	1.8
Self-contained	2.0	1.6	2.4	1.9	2.0
Self-contained	1.8	1.44	2.16	1.8	1.9
Self-contained	1.7	1.36	2.04	1.5	1.5
Ampule	1.8	1.44	2.16	1.7	1.7
Ampule	1.7	1.36	2.04	1.8	1.8
Ampule	2.1	1.68	2.52	2.2	2.2
Ampule	2.0	1.6	2.4	2.3	2.3
Ampule	1.8	1.44	2.16	1.8	1.8
Ampule	1.9	1.52	2.28	1.9	1.7
Ampule	1.9	1.52	2.28	1.8	1.8
Ampule	1.9	1.52	2.28	1.9	1.9
Ampule	2.3	1.84	2.76	2.5	2.4
Ampule	1.7	1.36	2.04	1.5	1.5

Abbreviations: BI, biological indicator; LHSK, Limited Holcomb-Spearman-Karber method; LL, lower limit (labeled D-value −20%); SMC, Stumbo-Murphy-Cochran method; UL, upper limit (labeled D-value +20%).

enumeration (plate count) and quantal or fraction-negative regions of the survivor curve. From this data, we can then predict that region of the survivor curve where we would expect to recover less than 0.01 or 0.001 surviving microorganisms. This region (known as the total kill region—see Figure 11.6) represents the practical limit of measurement of the survivor curve using current methodology because the use of a significant number of replicates (ie, BIs or products inoculated with the test organism) is required. Confidence in and correlation of the data provided by total kill analysis coupled with the data generated in the direct enumeration and quantal or fraction-negative analysis regions of the survivor curve allows us to extend the processing time to a desired probability of a surviving microorganism or sterility assurance level (SAL), which is typically 12D or 10^{-6} for most sterilization applications (see Figure 11.3). This relationship is generally well established for most moist heat sterilization processing conditions over a temperature range of 110°C to 135°C and dry heat sterilization conditions of 160°C to 190°C and is recognized in many international pharmacopeias and standards as overkill or conservative processing conditions as described in Table 11.4. Note that there is nothing magical about an SAL of 10^{-6}. This is simply a level of probability (one-in-a-million) that provided a conservative level in risk assessments and was apparently established during the 1960s with the development of guidelines for animal safety testing.[55] Other SALs such as 10^{-3} may be perfectly acceptable depending on the application, such as in the past with products that contact intact skin or mucosa such as electrocardiogram electrodes or examination gloves. Overall, alternative SALs to demonstrate sterility may be acceptable when associated with a rigorous risk assessment.[56] If we have established the D-value of a suitable test organism (typically spores of *G stearothermophilus* for moist heat sterilization and spores of *B atrophaeus* for dry heat sterilization conditions) based on both the survivor curve method and quantal or fraction-negative method and demonstrated reasonably good agreement between the predicted D-values, one can determine the desired sterilization value (F_T) as follows:

$$F_T = (SLR)\,D_T \qquad (37)$$

Where: F_T = sterilization value at temperature T
   D_T = D-value at temperature T
   SLR = spore log reduction

Note that this term is also frequently referenced as F_{BIO}, where $F_{BIO} = D\,(\log N_0 - \log N)$. In those instances, where the D_T value predicted by the survivor curve method and quantal or fraction-negative method are different, prudence would suggest that the higher estimate would be employed to determine F_T or F_{BIO}.

Assuming one desires to attain an SAL of 10^{-6}, this would correlate to 12 log reduction of the appropriate test organism if considering a worst case starting population of 10^6. If we have documented a D-value of 1.5 minutes, the minimum exposure time or sterilization

TABLE 11.4 Typical overkill or conservative heat processing conditions

Conditions	Minimum BI D-Value (ISO)	Temperature	12D Hold Time[a]	Typical Cycles
Moist heat	1.5 min 121°C	121°C	18 min	Gravity displacement: 30 min[b]
		132°C	1.4 min[c]	Prevacuum: 4 min[b]
Dry heat	2.0 min 160°C	160°C	24 min	120 min[d]
		180°C	2.4 min	30 min[e]
		250°C	NA[f]	30 min (depyrogenation)[g]

[a]USP <1221>. Parenteral Drug Association (PDA) Technical Monograph No. 1 2007. Theoretical hold time based on 12D reduction. Actual sterilization exposure times should be determined by validation.

[b]Typical preprogrammed health care cycles that include allowance for lag time with standard loads.[53] Liquid loads may exhibit significant temperature lag depending on container configuration and volume (Joslyn, 1991).

[c]Estimated based on a z-value of 10°C. Actual hold time may vary depending on construction of biological indicator (BI) (Joslyn, 1991).

[d]Data from Joslyn.[58]

[e]Data from Hancock.[54]

[f]NA, not applicable. Validation based on 3 log reduction of endotoxin challenge.

[g] Data from Williams.[184]

value necessary to achieve an SAL of 10^{-6} is easily calculated as $F_T = (1.5 \text{ min}) (12) = 18$ minutes. Although this provides a sound theoretical basis for the initial sterilization process design, further work is necessary to confirm that the sterilization processing conditions within the product and load are within the desired range. It may also be necessary to establish the relationship between the resistance of the test organism employed for process development and validation and the resistance of the microorganisms present on or with the product (product bioburden). For most thermal processing conditions, it is usually accepted that the resistance of the reference test organism exceeds that of most common forms of product bioburden, but this assumption should be verified particularly for applications where product may have been exposed to microorganisms of unusually high number or heat resistance, such as prions. In these circumstances, further pretreatment or extended thermal processing conditions may be necessary to render the product or goods safe for use.

▶ THE TEMPERATURE COEFFICIENT MODEL OF MICROBIAL DESTRUCTION

In the earlier discussion, we have assumed that temperature has remained relatively constant. In reality, this is often not the case. As the astute reader well knows under most thermal processing conditions, the goods or items being processed may exhibit a significant temperature lag with the temperatures within the chamber because they are being heated to the desired exposure conditions. Further fluctuations of the temperature within the load will occur during the exposure phase of the process because the chamber temperatures fluctuate about the temperature set point with a further lag in load temperature at the end of the process as temperature of the chamber returns to ambient. Depending on the nature of the load and processing conditions, the variation in temperature between the load and the chamber may be significant. Thus, how is one to resolve the ideal processing conditions discussed earlier (exposure at a fixed temperature for a fixed time) with the realities of real-world processing conditions? Fortuitously, just as a linear relationship exists between exposure time and the inactivation of microorganisms under constant temperature conditions (the semilogarithmic model), a linear relationship also exists between the rate of inactivation of microorganisms (the D-value) and variation in temperature. This relationship (known as the temperature coefficient or z-value) is also of a semilogarithmic nature.[4] As seen in Figure 11.8, a plot of the logarithm of the D-value at various temperatures versus temperature on an arithmetic scale generally

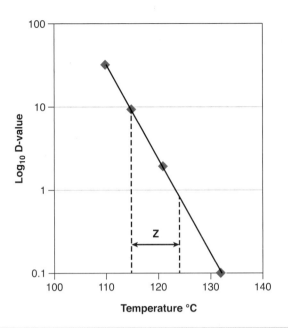

FIGURE 11.8   Plot of the z-value of a paper strip biological indicator processed in a moist heat resistometer over a temperature range of 115°C to 132°C. z = 8.9°C.

results in a straight line, the negative reciprocal of the slope of which is known as the z-value, or the change in temperature required for a 90% or 1-log change in the D-value. Note that this relationship holds regardless of whether one plots the logarithm of the D-value or the F-value (D [log N_0 − log N]) as both the thermal resistance curve (log D versus temperature) and thermal death time curve (log F versus temperature) parallel one another. An estimate of the z-value can be obtained as follows when data is available at two different temperatures:

$$z = (T_2 - T_1) / (\log D_1 - \log D_2) \qquad (38)$$

$$z = (T_2 - T_1) / (\log F_1 - \log F_2)$$

Generally, determination of the z-value should include measurements of the D-value or F-value made over at least three and preferably four different temperatures with the z-value determined by linear regression analysis of a plot of the log of the D- or F-value versus temperature. For moist heat applications, temperatures ranging from 110°C to 138°C are typical,[11] whereas temperatures of 150°C to 180°C are most often employed for dry heat applications.[12] The goodness of fit of the data can then be evaluated from determination of the coefficient of determination, r^2.[11] Pflug et al[23] have presented a detailed discussion of the correlation of the Bigelow z-value model with the Arrhenius model of reaction rate kinetics and shown that both methods of analysis are essentially equivalent with the Q_{10} value (the change in the reaction rate constant k for a 10°C change in temperature, typically a value of 2 for many chemical and biological reactions) being related to the z-value as follows:

$$z°C = \frac{10}{\log Q_{10}} \qquad (39)$$

For most calculations related to moist heat processing, a z-value of 10°C (18°F) based on the thermal resistance of bacterial spores is employed, although z-values reported in the literature have ranged from as low as 1°C to as high as 21°C for various microorganisms.[57] For dry heat processing conditions, a z-value of 20°C (38°F) is assumed as dry heat is less efficacious than moist heat regarding the inactivation of microorganisms at any given temperature. Some of the discrepancy in reported z-values may be attributed to variations in experimental conditions or other factors. Of particular importance is the menstruum in which the test organisms are suspended and also the construction of the test organism system. Whereas for moist heat sterilization, paper strip BIs consisting of paper strip carriers on which a suspension of spores of *G stearothermophilus* is deposited and packaged within a glassine envelope typically display consistent z-values in the range of 9°C to 11°C, self-contained BIs may exhibit different z-values due to the effect of thermal lag.[58] For most commercially available BIs employed for process development and validation, a minimum z-value of 6°C is required for application with moist heat sterilization[11] and a minimum z-value of 20°C is required for application with dry heat sterilization processes.[12] Note that BIs are best employed under the same conditions as which they have been qualified; otherwise, the results may be misleading.

▶ EQUIVALENT LETHALITY

As discussed earlier, the efficacy or lethality of a particular thermal process may be defined by the F-value, or the multiple of the D-value at a given temperature (D_T) and the desired level of log reduction of the designated test organism. Likewise, the change in the D-value of the test organism with temperature is generally linear and is known as the z-value. This makes it possible to account for the change in the rate of inactivation of the test organism as temperature varies during thermal processing by means of the lethal rate equation.

$$L = \Sigma\, 10^{(T - Tref)/z} \qquad (40)$$

Where: T = product temperature at time t
$Tref$ = reference temperature
z = z-value

For moist heat sterilization reference conditions of 121°C (250°F), a z-value of 10°C (18°F), and a $D_{121°C}$-value

of 1.0 minutes are typically employed, whereas for dry heat sterilization conditions reference conditions of 160°C (320°F), a z-value of 20°C (36°F), and a D_{160C}-value of 2.5 minutes are generally accepted. To determine the equivalent sterilization conditions for moist heat (F_0) or dry heat processing (F_H) conditions, it is a simple matter to multiply the lethal rate equation by the number of minutes at a given temperature T as follows:

$$F_0 \text{ or } F_H = \Delta t \times \Sigma\, 10^{(T - Tref)/z} \qquad (41)$$

Where: Δt = time in minutes at temperature T

For example, assume one is processing a product with a maximum moist heat temperature tolerance of 119°C. To allow for over temperature during processing, it has been decided to process the product at a set point temperature of 115°C. How long would the product need to be processed at 115°C to achieve the equivalent of 12 minutes processing at 121°C ($F_0 = 12$) assuming a $D_{121°C}$-value of 1.0 minutes?

$$\begin{aligned} L &= \Sigma\, 10^{(T - Tref)/z} \\ L &= \Sigma\, 10^{(115 - 121)/10} \\ L &= \Sigma\, 10^{-0.6} \\ L &= 0.2512 \end{aligned} \qquad (40)$$

Thus, under moist heat processing conditions, each 1 minute of exposure at 115°C is equivalent to 0.2512 minutes of exposure at 121°C and 48 minutes of exposure at 115°C would be necessary to realize conditions equivalent to 12 minutes exposure at 121°C. For cycle development and validation purposes, the temperatures within the load can be monitored continuously and the effects of varying temperature conditions throughout the cycle integrated via the lethal rate equation to realize the desired processing conditions.

$$L = \int 10^{(T - Tref)/z}\, dt \qquad (42)$$

A similar calculation may be performed for temperature-sensitive products processed under dry heat sterilization conditions using a z-value of 20°C. Assuming that one wishes to process a temperature-sensitive product under dry heat conditions at 120°C, how long would the product need to be processed in order to achieve the equivalent of a 12 $\log_{10}$ reduction of a test organism with a D_{160C}-value of 2.5 minutes ($F_H = 30$)?

$$\begin{aligned} L &= \Sigma\, 10^{(T - Tref)/z} \\ L &= \Sigma\, 10^{(120 - 160)/20} \\ L &= \Sigma\, 10^{-2} \\ L &= 0.01 \text{ min} \end{aligned} \qquad (40)$$

Thus, under dry heat processing conditions, 1-minute exposure at 120°C is equivalent to 0.01 minute exposure at 160°C and a minimum of 50 hours of exposure at 120°C would be necessary to realize conditions equivalent to

30 minutes exposure at 160°C. Note that in many applications, dry heat is employed not only to sterilize a given product but also to achieve depyrogenation; thus, a z-value (typically 50°C) based on the inactivation of endotoxin is employed as opposed to a z-value of 20°C (based on the inactivation of spores of *B atrophaeus*) when one is concerned with depyrogenation as well as sterilization of the product.[59]

PROCESS DEVELOPMENT AND VALIDATION

The development of a successful heat treatment process requires the consideration of many factors not the least of which is the tolerance of the product and packaging to the proposed heat processing conditions. The following discussion regarding process development and validation is of a limited nature. It is included solely to illustrate how the principles of thermal inactivation discussed earlier may be applied to the development and validation of heat processing treatments. The reader is advised to consult relevant international standards[60-62] and pharmacopeial guidelines on these topics as well as guidance provided by organizations such as the Parenteral Drug Association (PDA)[63,64] and the Association for the Advancement of Medical Instrumentation for further detail regarding sterilization process development and validation.

One of the key factors in designing a successful thermal treatment process is the extent to which one has control over the product and processing conditions. In industrial applications, one typically has a greater degree of control over the product and its bioburden as compared to health care applications where the product bioburden and the state of cleanliness of the product can vary widely.[65] Generally, sterilization process development falls into one of two general categories: Those under which the bioburden of the product is maintained in a state of control and those where the bioburden of the product is less controlled and processing parameters are selected with a worst-case scenario in mind. The former is generally regarded as bioburden-based processes and the latter as the conservative process or overkill approach. With bioburden-based (either bioburden or a combination BI/bioburden) methods, it is assumed that one can maintain the level of bioburden on a product within a desired range and that the bioburden itself does not present an unusual level of resistance to the applied thermal treatment. The advantage of this approach is that reduced heat processing conditions may be applied, which may be beneficial to the integrity of the product and packaging and allow for more rapid processing, although a higher degree of control and routine monitoring of bioburden is expected. With the overkill or conservative process approach, sterilization parameters are typically established based on the use of BIs inoculated with a high population

of bacterial spores resistant to the sterilization process as a worst-case model for the product bioburden. For products and processes that are under a high degree of control, parametric release of product based on the measurement and control of physical process parameters may be an option.[60,61,66]

For the bioburden-based approach, one can typically process replicate samples representative of actual product under fractional cycle conditions followed by sterility testing to estimate the D_T value of the bioburden on or in the product using either the plate-count or fraction-negative method of analysis as discussed earlier. In order to ensure reproducible data, this testing is best performed in a resistometer at the desired temperature conditions. Based on the bioburden present in the product and the determined product D_T value, the minimum processing conditions to achieve the desired bioburden reduction or SAL in/on the product can be determined as follows. Assume an in situ volume of 120 L and a bioburden of 50 CFUs/mL = 6 × 10^6 CFUs total bioburden, a bioburden $D_{121°C}$-value of 0.5 minutes and a desired SAL of 10^{-6}. Therefore,

$$F_T = (SLR) \, D_T \qquad (37)$$
$$F_T = (\log_{10} \text{bioburden} - \log_{10} \text{SAL}) \, D_T$$
$$F_T = (6.7781 + 6) \, 0.5 \text{ min}$$
$$F_T = (12.7781) \, 0.5 \text{ min}$$
$$F_T = 6.4 \text{ min}$$

Thus, a sterilization processing time of 6.4 minutes exposure at 121°C would be adequate to realize an SAL of 10^{-6} for a product bioburden level of 50 CFUs/mL and load size of 120 L, when the bioburden has a $D_{121°C}$-value of 0.5 minutes. Note that in equation (37), the total bioburden reduction is substituted for the spore log reduction (SLR) term. Obviously, these processing conditions would present less of a thermal insult to the product than a traditional overkill sterilization cycle such 30 minutes exposure to 121°C. Two important considerations to note, however, are that (1) one must ensure that the desired sterilization treatment (F-value) is delivered to the coolest location within the product and load and (2) not only should the bioburden of the product be routinely enumerated (eg, using ISO 11737-1)[67] but also the bioburden resistance should also be considered on a routine basis. For bioburden determination of the product, it may be advisable to incorporate a heat shock treatment such as 15 minutes at 80°C to 85°C as part of routine enumeration testing to rule out the presence of heat-resistant microorganisms within or on the product. Depending on the nature of the product and extent of control over the process, one may also wish to incorporate a margin of safety in the bioburden level employed for calculation of the heat processing time (ie, 500 CFUs/mL as opposed to 50 CFUs/mL) to allow for variation in bioburden population and resistance. Likewise, an additional safety factor may be added by assuming a bioburden $D_{121°C}$-value of

1.0 minute with a resulting processing time of 12.8 minutes (if this is tolerated by the product) in order to reduce the potential risk of spikes in bioburden population and/or resistance.

The combined bioburden/BI method of process validation likewise requires that the resistance and population of the product bioburden be known and is based on the principle that the resistance of the BI is typically well in excess of that of the product bioburden. With this approach, BIs with a reduced population of test organisms (a minimum of 10^3 spores per carrier) may be employed. This approach requires that process conditions be selected to inactivate the bioburden to the desired SAL, although not all BIs need to be inactivated when processed under reduced heat treatment conditions. A series of sublethal treatments are processed to verify that the resistance of the product bioburden is less than that of the BI. For example, assuming processing a device that can tolerate a maximum of 12 minutes exposure at 121°C:

Initial population of BI: 1×10^6 spores per carrier
$D_{121°C}$-value of BI: 1.5 minutes
$D_{121°C}$-value of bioburden: 0.4 minutes
Bioburden population: 10^2 CFUs per device

A cycle is processed at 121°C for 6 minutes, and the BIs are recovered and assayed via the plate count method, yielding an average of 10^2 spores per carrier for a total reduction of 4 logarithms. In turn, the bioburden would be reduced by a total of 15 logarithms following 6 minutes exposure. With an initial bioburden population of 10^2 CFUs per device, this would correspond to an SAL of 10^{-13} with respect to the bioburden (Figure 11.9).

Overkill heat sterilization processes are generally defined as capable of achieving a minimum 12 log reduction of a population of microorganisms having either a minimum $D_{121°C}$-value of 1.5 minutes[11] for moist heat sterilization conditions or a D_{160C}-value of 2.0 minutes[12] for dry heat sterilization conditions. The extent of treatment required to reproducibly inactivate 10^6 microorganisms is established and the resulting exposure time doubled for routine processing. The advantage of the overkill or conservative process definition based on the use of BIs is that a substantial safety margin is incorporated relative to the product bioburden[9] and the requirement for routine bioburden population and resistance determination diminished relative to the bioburden or BI/bioburden approach. Although there is some controversy regarding the definition of overkill sterilization,[68] it is generally agreed that an overkill process will result in a reduction of product bioburden substantially beyond a minimum SAL of 10^{-6}. In developing overkill sterilization processes, it is important to keep in mind that (1) establishing processing conditions based on the minimum D-value requirement for the BI may create complications during future revalidation because most commercially available BIs typically have D-values in excess of the

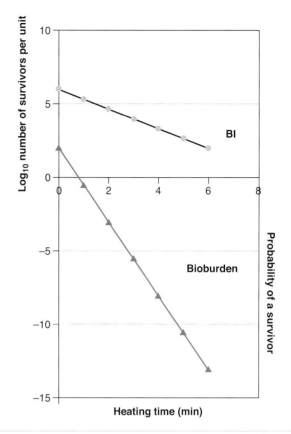

FIGURE 11.9 Combined biological indicator (BI)/bioburden method.

minimum required and (2) placement of the BI within product may lead to a substantial increase in the effective D-value of the BI (Figure 11.10) (see Sadowski[69] and Berger et al[70]). Validation of an overkill method can be realized using either a half-cycle or full cycle approach. With the half-cycle approach, BIs with a minimum population of 10^6 test organisms/carrier (complying with the minimum D-value requirement or an equivalent combination of population and D-value) and temperature sensors are placed at the worst-case locations within product throughout the load and processed for one-half of the normal processing time. Attainment of the desired log reduction of the BI population (typically 6 logarithms or no recovery) and minimum F-value (typically 6) is then demonstrated at the half-cycle.

For the full cycle approach, the nominal population of the BI should exceed by at least $0.5 \log_{10}$ of the population calculated from F_{BIO}[12] and the certified D-value for the BI where F_{BIO} is determined as follows:

$$F_{BIO} = D_T (\log N_0 - \log N) \qquad (37)$$

Where: D_T = the D-value of the BI at temperature T
N_0 = the initial population of the BI
N = postexposure population of the BI (eg, 10^{-6})

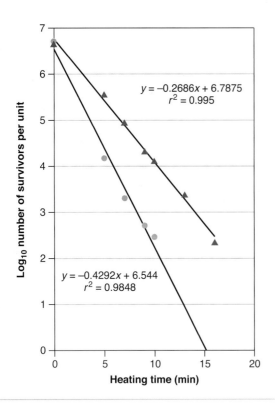

FIGURE 11.10 Comparative D-values *Geobacillus stea-rothermophilus* spores suspended in purified water for injection (●) $D_{121°C} = 2.3$ min and borate buffered saline (Δ) $D_{121°C} = 3.72$ min.

From the earlier discussion, it can be easily seen that 12 minutes exposure would be required to achieve an SAL of 10^{-6} for a BI with a $D_{121°C}$-value of 1.0 minutes. Assuming a moist heat BI with a $D_{121°C}$-value of 2.1 minutes, the BI population necessary to execute a full cycle validation (assuming a minimum F_0 of 12 minutes) can be calculated as follows:

$$N_0 = 10^{(F_0 / D_{121°C} + \log N)} \qquad (42)$$
$$N_0 = 10^{(12 / 2.1 + \log 1 \times 100)}$$
$$N_0 = 10^{(5.7143)}$$
$$N_0 = 517\,947$$
$$N_0 = 5.2 \times 10^5$$

In other words, a BI with a population of 5.2×10^5 and a $D_{121°C}$-value of 2.1 minutes ($F_{BIO} = 12$ min) would be equivalent in resistance to a BI with a (theoretical) population of 1.0×10^{12} and a $D_{121°C}$-value of 1.0 minutes ($F_{BIO} = 12$ min). The requirement of the full cycle validation approach for an additional 0.5 $\log_{10}$ of the population calculated from F_{BIO}^{12} and the certified D-value for the BI requirement is to account for issues in microbiological manipulations of the BI and provide for potential changes in the effective D-value of the BI due to placement in product, etc. Therefore, a BI with a population of $5.2 \times 10^5 + (0.5) = 5.7 \times 10^5$ would be necessary to comply with the full cycle validation approach

assuming a $D_{121°C}$-value of 2.1 minutes. Note that the advantage of the full cycle approach to validation of overkill sterilization processes is that many existing overkill cycles were established when the minimum $D_{121°C}$-value requirement for moist heat BIs were lower (1.0 min) than current requirements (1.5 min). Thus, for a 12D overkill cycle established with a BI with a $D_{121°C}$-value of 1 minute, there is a potential for the recovery of BIs positive for growth if the traditional half-cycle approach is employed using BIs with a minimum $D_{121°C}$-value of 1.5 minutes. It is difficult to consistently obtain commercially available BIs with a minimum $D_{121°C}$-value of 1.5 minutes because BI manufacturers must account for loss of potency during the expiration dating period of the BI; thus, most commercially available BIs have labeled D-values in excess of the minimum requirement of 1.5 minutes.

▶ MOIST HEAT TREATMENT

Moist heat (steam) sterilization is one of the oldest and most effective sterilization methods for those products and goods, which can withstand exposure to elevated temperatures and high moisture levels. In its simplest form, water is heated to temperatures in the typical range of 110°C to 140°C with a concomitant increase in pressure forming a saturated vapor that is introduced into a pressure vessel containing the goods to be sterilized (see chapter 28). Although water boils at 100°C under standard atmospheric conditions, to effectively regulate the sterilization process and achieve efficient sterilization, higher working pressures are often desired. Therefore, most modern autoclaves operate under pressure over a temperature range of 110°C to 135°C with the upper limit being determined by extremely conservative pressure vessel calculations. Although 1 kcal of energy is required to heat 1 kg (1 L) of water and increase the temperature by 1°C up to a temperature of 100°C, 540 kcal of energy is required at 100°C for a phase change from a liquid to a vapor state. This is known as the latent heat of vaporization. Additional energy is then required to raise the temperature of the steam to the desired temperature and pressure. When steam in the vapor state contacts a colder surface, it collapses and returns to a liquid state, releasing its latent heat energy that is highly effective at killing a broad range of microorganisms, primarily through the coagulation or disintegration of macromolecules within the cell or virus.[71,72] In addition to the high level of heat energy, which is released as the steam collapses back to a liquid state, a localized vacuum is formed that is rapidly replaced by more steam until the system reaches equilibrium. Thus, not only is steam a highly effective sterilant due to its high-energy level and the presence of moisture, but the dynamics of steam sterilization also provide an effective driving force for penetration of the products or goods being sterilized. In addition to the potential limitations of the high temperatures, pressures, and moisture content of steam sterilization on the products or goods being sterilized, slight variations in temperature along the saturated vapor curve (eg, superheat >5°C), the presence of residual air or noncondensable gasses (>3.5%), and poor steam quality (less than 95% dry, saturated steam) are generally recognized as having the potential to interfere with effective steam sterilization. Another concern is the purity or chemical composition of the steam, which is based on the quality of water used for steam generation.[73,74] For further discussion of steam sterilization see Hancock,[54] Young,[75] Agalloco,[76] PDA,[63] and Perkins[53] and see chapter 28.

▶ DRY HEAT TREATMENT

It is generally accepted that for any given temperature dry heat treatment is less effective than treatment with moist heat with regard to microbial inactivation. In order to achieve the same sterilization effect under dry heat conditions, one must typically employ higher temperatures and longer exposure times as reflected in the commonly accepted z-values of 10°C for moist heat sterilization processing and 20°C for dry heat sterilization conditions. Nevertheless, dry heat processing offers a number of advantages over moist heat processing, including the ability to process materials with a low water content such as heat-stable oils, ointments, powders, pharmaceutical ingredients, etc that may otherwise not be processed with moist heat or other forms of sterilization such as gamma irradiation or ethylene oxide. As dry heat processing frequently takes place under atmospheric conditions, the use of pressure-rated chambers or vessels is generally not required. Dry heat also has the significant advantage of being able to inactivate endotoxin over time, unlike moist heat, under high-temperature processing conditions for those heat-stable products that must not only be sterile but also comply with strict endotoxin limits or be pyrogen free.

Dry heat treatment can be realized by various means but almost always involves the transfer of heat energy to the goods or products being processed by means of either convection, conduction, radiation, or a combination of these methods. With a convective heat transfer processes, heat energy flows from one body to another due to the differences in temperature via a given medium or fluid. This typically takes the form of air as the working medium, which is heated and then passed over the load, thereby increasing its temperature. Once the heated air contacts the load, it then transfers heat energy to the load by means of conduction as the high-energy electrons of the heated air collide with the lower energy electrons of the load, thereby raising the molecular energy (temperature)

of the load. With some low-energy radiation methods, such as microwave or infrared heating (see chapter 10), high-energy photons are generated and transmitted to the load via electromagnetic waves. The high-energy photons collide with the goods being heated increasing their molecular energy and hence temperature. Depending on the situation and the product being processed, one form of dry heat processing may be preferred over the other, but from a microbiological perspective, the means whereby heat energy is transferred to the microorganisms is less critical than the temperatures that are realized.

As with moist heat, time and temperature are the most critical parameters associated with the dry heat destruction of microorganisms. The water activity (a_W) within target microbial cells is perhaps the next most critical factor. Water activity may be defined as follows:

$$a_W = (P_V) / (P_{VS}) \qquad (43)$$

Where: P_V = water vapor pressure in a system
P_{VS} = saturation water vapor pressure at the temperature of the system

Murrell and Scott[77] equilibrated six species of bacterial spores to differing a_W levels by storing them over different salt solutions for a period of several weeks followed by immediate heating to temperatures of 100°C to 120°C in a water or oil bath. Spores equilibrated to an intermediate moisture content of 0.2 to 0.4 a_W exhibited the greatest resistance to dry heat (Figure 11.11). Based on this and other studies, it is apparent that the rate of destruction of microorganisms under dry heat conditions is a function of the water content of the cell, which may vary depending on a number of factors including the water vapor pressure of the environment in which the cell is being heated. As described by Pflug,[2] the heating environment surrounding the microorganism can be considered as either a closed or open system with respect to the ability to gain or lose water from within the microbial cell. In a closed system, water movement into or out of the microbial cell from the heating environment is restricted, whereas in an open system, water can be readily gained or lost from the microbial cell via the heating environment. As one would anticipate, microorganisms heated in a dry open environment will rapidly lose water with a corresponding decrease in resistance. Studies by Doyle and Ernst[78] found a significant increase in resistance to dry heat with spores of *Bacillus subtilis* subsp *niger* encapsulated in calcium carbonate crystals (a closed system) in comparison to controls that were not encapsulated (an open system). Similar results have been reported for spores encapsulated in polymethylmethacrylate[79] and other materials.[80] The effect of different gas atmospheres on the resistance of spores processed under dry heat conditions has also been studied, although the results are somewhat confounded by the experimental conditions employed and whether testing was performed

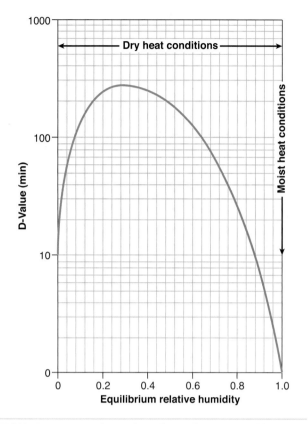

FIGURE 11.11   Relationship of D_T value and equilibrium relative humidity. Relative humidity is the ratio of the water vapor pressure to water vapor pressure if it were saturated at the same temperature (P/P_S). In theory, under equilibrium conditions, the relative humidity and water activity are equal. Based on Pflug et al.[23]

using an open or closed system. Using a closed system, Pheil et al[81] found little difference in the D-values of spores of *B subtilis* and *C sporogenes* with dry gasses of air, oxygen, helium, or nitrogen. Davis et al[82] reported lower survival of dry spores under a vacuum at 60°C as compared to atmospheric pressure, although little difference was noted at 25°C. Based on a review of this and other data, Pflug et al[23] concluded that the dry heat destruction rates appear to parallel the drying rates of the spores and that spore viability decreases because the spores are exposed to near-zero a_W conditions.

In keeping with the effect of a_W on the destruction of microorganisms by dry heat as discussed earlier, numerous studies have been performed on the effect of various added solutes on a_W and the destruction of microorganisms. In general, these studies suggest that when the a_W of a particular heating menstruum is decreased by the addition of solutes, there is an increase in heat resistance. This phenomenon has been observed for a wide variety of microorganisms: yeast,[83-88] mold spores,[89,90] vegetative cells of bacteria,[91-94] and bacterial spores.[95-100] This effect can vary with the type of solute

employed; however, because the extent of resistance conferred at a particular a_W varies with the solute employed, thus it is likely that other factors in such as cell shrinkage and plasmolysis may impact the heat resistance of a particular microorganism/solute combination.[101] Dry heat treatment is often used to process ointments and oils with low water content that otherwise cannot be processed with moist heat. Studies of the heat inactivation of microorganisms in a lipid environment were reviewed by Pflug et al[23] (Table 11.5). In general, it has been found that microorganisms are more resistant in lipids and oils than when they are heated in aqueous systems leading some to conclude that heating microorganisms in oil and lipids is equivalent to dry heat exposure conditions.[102] This supposition is supported to some extent by studies that have demonstrated that the addition of water to oil in which the microorganisms are suspended decreases their heat resistance.[103,104] Senhaji et al[105,106] demonstrated that when microorganisms in oil and water suspensions were agitated to increase the effective a_W, heat resistance was reduced significantly. Studies by Ababouch et al[32,107] likewise support the correlation between the reduced a_W and increased heat resistance of various spores suspended in oils.

The correlation between a_W and the heat resistance of microorganisms in low-moisture foods was recently reviewed by Syamaladevi et al.[108] Their review confirmed a_W as a critical factor in the heat processing of low-moisture foods and discussed a number of related product and process-related factors that influence heat resistance. They proposed the addition of a_W as a critical factor along with temperature to determine the heat resistance of pathogenic microorganisms in low moisture foods as follows:

$$D = f\,[\mathrm{T}, a_{\mathrm{w}(T, X_{\mathrm{w}})}] \tag{44}$$

Where: D = D-value
  T = temperature
  a_{W} = water activity
  X_{w} = mole fraction of water

On this basis, the effect of water activity on the temperature coefficient and lethal rate equations could also be considered, although further work would likely be necessary to fully develop this concept and establish its range of applicability.

▶ THERMAL DISINFECTION

Our discussion to this point has been focused on the application of moist and dry heat treatments at temperatures of 110°C and above that are intended to render products and goods sterile based on the semilogarithmic inactivation of highly heat-resistant bacterial spores. There are also many applications where moist heat treatments

TABLE 11.5 Summary of key reports in literature on heat resistance of bacteria in lipids[a]

Organism	Test Conditions		Finding or Results		Reference
Bacillus subtilis	100°C		Longest survival time (min)		Bartlett and Kline (1913)
	Glycerin		75		
	Oil		50		
	Water		3		
	~112°C				
	Glycerin		15		
	Oil		10		
Clostridium botulinum	121°C		Thermal death time (min)		Dickson et al (1925)
	Oil/broth mixture		15-23		
	Broth alone		3-5		
Streptococcus	*Condition*	*Temp (°C)*	*Kill time (min)*		Yesair et al (1944)
	Moist in broth	55	Moist heat 30-45		
	Dried in broth	55	30-45		
	Dried in moist fat	100	15-20		
	Dried	110	Dry heat 135-150		
	Dried in dry fat	100	135-150		
Bacillus cereus	*% Water added to soy oil*		*% Survival: 15 min at 121°C*		Molin and Snygg (1967)
	0		25.0		
	1		0.06		
	3		0.04		
	30		0.01		
Staphylococcus aureus	Peanut oil		$D_{121°C} = 9$ min; $z = 21°C$		Thuillot et al (1968)
	Peanut oil +0.3% water		$D_{65.5°C} = 15$ min; $z = 8°C$		
S aureus			*z-value (°C)*		Zaleski et al (1971)
	Soy oil		23		
	Soy oil + 0.1% water		15		
	Soy oil + 0.2% water		14		
	Soy oil + 0.3% water		13		
	Nutrient broth		6.5		
B subtilis	95°C		$D_{95°C}$ (min)		Senhaji (1977) Senhaji et al (1976) 137 7
	Soy oil		167		
	Soy oil + 2.5% water				
	Soy oil + 2.5% water				
	(agitated during heating)				
	Buffer		4.8		
B subtilis	95°C and 105°C		$D_{95°C}$ (min)	$D_{105°C}$ (min)	Senhaji and Loncin (1975 and 1977)
	Soy oil		142	71	
	33% oil in buffer, 2 phases		53	38	
	same, but shaken to emulsify		10	0.9	
	1-2 drops of oil on top of buffer		12	1.0	
	Buffer		7.3	0.6	

(continued)

TABLE 11.5   Summary of key reports in literature on heat resistance of bacteria in lipids[a] *(Continued)*

Organism	Test Conditions		Finding or Results	Reference
C botulinum	129.2°C			Ababouch and Busta (1987)
		Olive oil, commercial oil	D = 5.3 min; z = 28.5°C	
		(rapeseed + soy)	D_1 = 1.6 min; D_2 = 13 min	
	114°C			
		Buffer	D = 1.5 min; z = 11.2°C	
B subtilis	105°C			Ababouch et al (1995)
		Buffer	D = 17 min	
	130°C			
		Olive oil	D_1 = 7 min; D_2 = 39 min	
		Mineral oil/commercial oil	D_1 = 3 min; D_2 = 21 min	

[a]Reprinted from Pflug et al.[23]

below 100°C can be employed to reduce the number of vegetative microorganisms, viruses, and certain types of fungal spores on a product to a level considered safe for use or consumption as opposed to being sterile. Examples include the pasteurization of milk,[109] the heat treatment of vaccines,[110] viral disinfection,[111,112] bone marrow treatment,[113] the disinfection of health care equipment such as anesthesia apparatus and other respiratory therapy devices,[114-116] the heat treatment of high purity water systems,[117] the application of hot water to render surgical instruments safe for further processing,[116] etc. In these situations, it is either not necessary for the product or goods to be sterile based on their application or there may be no other practical means to process them such that they are safe for use. In many of these applications, heating at temperatures of 65°C to 95°C for various lengths of time are used to render the product or goods safe for use. Because one might anticipate, many of the principles discussed earlier regarding the semilogarithmic rate of microbial inactivation, D_T values, z-values, and integrated lethality also apply with regard to thermal disinfection. The kinetics of microbial inactivation under thermal disinfection conditions are very similar to those of sterilization with nearly identical methods employed to determine the D-value, temperature coefficient, and integrated lethality of a given microbiological system and process. The range of z-values associated with thermal disinfection is quite broad, with z-values as low as 3.7°C reported for *Aspergillus niger* in Pilsen beer[118] and as high as 21.1°C for hepatitis A virus in strawberry mash.[119] The variation in reported z-values for thermal disinfection is likely due to the impact of matrix effects on both heat transfer at the lower temperatures associated with thermal disinfection and the physiological state of the microorganisms being processed. For health care applications where surgical and

medical equipment is cleaned prior to thermal disinfection treatment, a z-value of 10°C is commonly assumed,[116] although this has been questioned by some.[120]

Not surprisingly, in health care applications, the classification of thermal disinfection mirrors that of chemical disinfection with low-, intermediate-, and high-level thermal disinfection categories based on the extent of contact of the device with intact tissue, mucous membranes, or compromised skin surfaces according to the Spaulding classification[121] (see chapter 47). The US Food and Drug Administration Guidance for washer-disinfectors,[115] for example, indicates that testing must be performed with various microorganisms suspended in an organic soil matrix in order to document attainment of a particular level of thermal disinfection. A low-level thermal disinfection claim must be substantiated by demonstrating a 6 $\log_{10}$ reduction of a mixture of vegetative bacteria such as *Pseudomonas aeruginosa*, *Staphylococcus aureus*, *Escherichia coli*, and representatives from the *Klebsiella-Enterobacter* group. Intermediate-level thermal disinfection requires the same 6 $\log_{10}$ reduction of vegetative microorganisms as low-level disinfection and a 3 $\log_{10}$ reduction of a thermophilic *Mycobacterium* species. High-level thermal disinfection requires the demonstration of a 6 $\log_{10}$ reduction of the indicated vegetative microorganisms and a 6 $\log_{10}$ reduction of a thermophilic *Mycobacterium* species. The ISO 15883-1 classification of thermal disinfection for washer-disinfectors is different in that classification as a low-, intermediate-, or high-level disinfection process is based on the minimum integrated lethality (A_0 values) attained by the process, where A_0 is defined as the "equivalent time in seconds at 80°C, delivered by the disinfection process, with reference to a microorganism with a z value of 10 K."[116] The A value expresses heat treatment in terms of the equivalent effect of a stated time at some

TABLE 11.6   Thermal disinfection classification

Final Processing	Instrument Categories	Recommended A_0 Value	Examples of Typical Time/Temperature Combinations
Sterilization	Critical instruments—items that contact the bloodstream or sterile areas of body	NA (sterilization required)	135°C for 3 min 121°C for 30 min
High-level disinfection	Semicritical instruments—items that contact intact mucous membranes or nonintact skin (but not sterile areas) that cannot tolerate sterilization	600-3000[a] Based on suspected contamination with heat-resistant viruses such as HIV, HBV, HCV	3000: 90°C for 5 min 80°C for 50 min 600: 90°C for 1 min
Intermediate-level disinfection	Semicritical instruments—items that contact intact mucous membranes or nonintact skin (but not sterile areas). These items *should* be further processed by sterilization if possible.	600 Based on suspected contamination with *Mycobacterium* Typically employed with anesthesia equipment and to render surgical instruments safe for further processing	90°C for 1 min 80°C for 10 min 70°C for 100 min
Low-level disinfection	Noncritical instrument—items that contact intact skin only. Further processing by sterilization *may* not be necessary.	60 For use with equipment or instruments that contact intact skin only Based on contamination with common bacteria and fungi	80°C for 1 min 70°C for 10 min

Abbreviations: HBV, hepatitis B virus; HCV, hepatitis C virus; NA, not applicable.

[a]Varies with regional requirements.

stated temperature for a particular z-value, that is, the A_0 value is the equivalent time in seconds at 80°C for an organism of specified z-value, the term being the equivalent of the lethal rate equation (40).

$$A_0 = \Sigma \, 10^{(T - 80)/z} \, \Delta t \qquad (45)$$

Where: $A_0 = A$ value when z is 10°C
t = chosen time interval, in seconds
T = temperature in the load, in degrees Celsius

Readers will recognize this equation as being similar to that employed to calculate F_0 values (equation [41]) for moist heat sterilization processes, the only differences being the reference temperature (80°C as opposed to 121°C) and time intervals of seconds as opposed to minutes. In calculating A_0 values, a lower temperature limit for the integration defined in the current version of the standard is set at 65°C; a higher minimum level may be specified based on unique thermal resistance of certain types of viruses.[112] At temperatures below 65°C, the z-value and D_T value of thermophilic organisms may change dramatically, and below 55°C, there are a number of organisms that will actively replicate. Typical time/temperature combinations for low-, intermediate-, and high-level thermal

disinfection treatments are provided in Table 11.6 (based on the ISO 15883 series of standards).

As noted by Röhm-Rodowlad et al,[122] there is not as large of a body of data regarding the experimental fundamentals of the A_0 concept as with the F_0 concept of moist heat sterilization. McCormick et al[123] evaluated the efficacy of thermal disinfection treatments at A_0 values of 60, 600, and 3000 with a range of different microorganisms (Table 11.7). The 0.2-mL aliquots of overnight cultures of the test organisms suspended in sterile saline to an approximate population of 10^6 CFUs/mL were added to thin wall polypropylene snap cap tubes and processed in thermocyclers[120] as indicated in Figure 11.12 for either 10 minutes at 70°C (A_0 = 60), 10 minutes at 80°C (A_0 = 600), or 5 minutes at 90°C (A_0 = 3000). A greater than 6 log reduction (no recovery [NR]) was realized for all organisms tested including a mixed culture biofilm of *S aureus*, *E coli*, and *Candida albicans*. Although this study did not consider the impact of different matrix constituents, it does demonstrate the efficacy of the applied thermal treatments with a range of different microorganisms.

A study by Almatroudi et al[124] compared the effect of dry and moist heat treatments on the recovery of dry-surface and hydrated biofilms of *S aureus*. Significant (>7 log) reductions were observed with dry-surface

TABLE 11.7   Antimicrobial efficacy of thermal disinfection[a,b]

Test Organism	Medium	N_0	A_0		
			60 (10 min × 70°C)	600 (10 min × 80°C)	3000 (5 min × 90°C)
Staphylococcus aureus ATCC 6538	TSA	1.4×10^7	≥6 (NR)	≥6 (NR)	≥6 (NR)
Pseudomonas aeruginosa ATCC 9027	TSA	3.1×10^7	≥6 (NR)	≥6 (NR)	≥6 (NR)
Escherichia coli ATCC 8739	TSA	1.4×10^7	≥6 (NR)	≥6 (NR)	≥6 (NR)
Candida albicans ATCC 10231	SDA	1.2×10^7	≥6 (NR)	≥6 (NR)	≥6 (NR)
Aspergillus brasiliensis ATCC 16404	SDA	1.0×10^7	≥6 (NR)	≥6 (NR)	≥6 (NR)
Fusarium solani ATCC 36031	SDA	6.6×10^6	≥6 (NR)	≥6 (NR)	≥6 (NR)
Serratia marescens ATCC 13880	TSA	7.6×10^6	≥6 (NR)	≥6 (NR)	≥6 (NR)
Staphylococcus epidermidis ATCC 17917	TSA	9.1×10^7	≥6 (NR)	≥6 (NR)	≥6 (NR)
Micrococcus luteus environmental isolate	TSA	5.6×10^6	≥2	≥6 (NR)	≥6 (NR)
Acinetobacter CC08077F3 clinical isolate	TSA	7.0×10^7	≥6 (NR)	≥6 (NR)	≥6 (NR)
MRSA CC08054 F11 clinical isolate	TSA	1.1×10^9	≥6 (NR)	≥6 (NR)	≥6 (NR)
MRSA CC08055 F11 clinical isolate	TSA	7.2×10^7	≥6 (NR)	≥6 (NR)	≥6 (NR)
MRSA CC08056 F11 clinical isolate	TSA	3.1×10^8	≥6 (NR)	≥6 (NR)	≥6 (NR)
Enterobacter aerogenes ATCC 13408	TSA	1.9×10^8	≥6 (NR)	≥6 (NR)	≥6 (NR)
Klebsiella pneumoniae ATCC 33495	TSA	1.2×10^8	≥6 (NR)	≥6 (NR)	≥6 (NR)
Enterococcus durans ATCC 6056	TSA	7.2×10^7	≥6 (NR)	≥6 (NR)	≥6 (NR)
Ralstonia insidiosa ATCC 49129	TSA	5.2×10^7	≥6 (NR)	≥6 (NR)	≥6 (NR)
Saccharomyces cerevisiae ATCC 27570	TSA	1.1×10^6	≥6 (NR)	≥6 (NR)	≥6 (NR)
Mycobacterium thermoresistibile ATCC 19529	BA	3.5×10^6	≥6 (NR)	≥6 (NR)	≥6 (NR)
Mixed population biofilm (containing *Staphylococcus aureus* ATCC 6538, *Escherichia coli* ATCC 8739 and *Candida albicans* ATCC 10231)	TSA	1.6×10^8	≥6 (NR)	≥6 (NR)	≥6 (NR)

Abbreviations: ATCC, American Type Culture Collection; BA, blood agar; MRSA, methicillin-resistant *Staphylococcus aureus*; N_0, initial population; NR, no recovery; SDA, Sabouraud dextrose agar; TSA, trypticase soy agar.

[a]Data presented as log reduction.

[b]Reprinted with permission from McCormick et al.[123] © Association for the Advancement of Medical Instrumentation.

and hydrated biofilms when processed with moist heat treatments ranging from 1 hour at 60°C to 4 minutes at 134°C. Similar results were observed with hydrated biofilm when processed with dry heat treatments ranging from 1 hour at 60°C to 20 minutes at 121°C, but less than a 2 log reduction was observed in the population of dry-surface biofilm processed under the same conditions. Interestingly, dry-surface biofilm subjected to autoclaving at 121°C for 30 minutes exhibited recovery and released planktonic cells on prolonged incubation. This study, in conjunction with the study by Doyle and Ernst[78] concerning the increased resistance to dry heat of spores of *B subtilis* subsp *niger* embedded in calcium

carbonate crystals, illustrates the significant impact that matrix effects and dehydration may have on the effective heat resistance of microorganisms and underscores the need for effective cleaning prior to disinfection and/or sterilization processing.

▶ OTHER HEAT TREATMENT METHODS

In addition to the classic moist heat (steam), dry heat, and thermal disinfection methods, there are many other heat treatment processes, such as subatmospheric steam

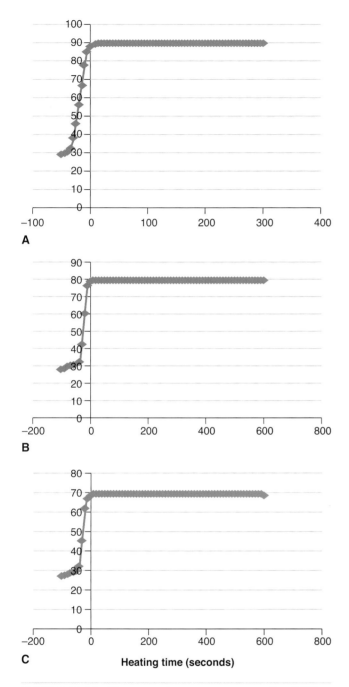

FIGURE 11.12 Thermocycler temperature profiles 90°C (A), 80°C (B), 70°C (C). Average of 12 runs.

sterilization,[125] low-temperature steam formaldehyde mixtures,[126] low-temperature steam combined with high hydrostatic pressure,[127] heating in the presence of a low-pH environment,[128] combined heating and cold storage methods,[129] etc, that have been successfully developed. Low-temperature steam refers to steam under vacuum conditions, in relation to the gas laws. Normally, when water is heated to a temperature of 100°C under standard atmospheric conditions, it undergoes a phase change from a liquid to a vapor state (see prior discussion

regarding the latent heat of vaporization). By reducing the pressure within the chamber below atmospheric levels, water will boil and form steam at lower temperatures, although with lower energy adequate for disinfection but not sterilization. Many of these processes were developed in the food and beverage industry and are intended for specific applications where conventional heat treatment methods may cause irreversible damage to the qualities of the goods being processed. Some of these processes may involve multiple methods of microbial inactivation that may complicate modeling of the inactivation kinetics. In many instances, these processes may successfully inactivate vegetative microorganisms but may not inactivate bacterial spores and thus are more realistically viewed as pasteurization or disinfection processes as opposed to sterilization processes. Each of these processes must be assessed based on their own merit and evaluated with regard to their effectiveness with the intended application. For medical devices, ISO 14937[130] provides useful guidance of those factors that must be considered when evaluating novel sterilization methods and combined treatments.

◗ FACTORS AFFECTING THE HEAT RESISTANCE OF MICROORGANISMS AND MICROBIOLOGICAL TEST SYSTEMS

As discussed earlier, one of the greatest challenges to developing reliable models of heat inactivation is the accurate enumeration of microorganisms. This is compounded by the variation in the response of different microorganisms to an applied heat stress. This response can be influenced by many factors both intrinsic and extrinsic to the microorganism. These factors have been commented on by authors including by Roberts,[131] Warth,[132] Davis et al,[133] Moldenhauer,[134] Pflug et al,[23] Coleman and Setlow,[135] Sadowski,[69] and others. These factors are associated with the growth and preparation of the microorganisms, their packaging and presentation to the applied heat treatment, the equipment employed to model the heat treatment process, and the recovery conditions following heat treatment. As noted by Pflug et al,[23] "The many variables introduced by the type of organism studies and the techniques used, and the unrecognized involvement of the many factors make a sound interpretation of previously reported data difficult."

One area where there seems to be general agreement regarding the use of microbiological test systems for the evaluation of heat treatment processes is the designation of spores of *G stearothermophilus* and *B atrophaeus* as the preferred test organisms for the evaluation of moist heat and dry heat sterilization treatments, respectively. Although other spore-forming microorganisms may also be employed to monitor heat treatment processes, these two microorganisms are the most frequently referenced in international pharmacopeias and sterilization standards. One of the most significant factors affecting the intrinsic heat resistance of BIs of *G stearothermophilus* and *B atrophaeus* is the sporulation medium and culture conditions (time and temperature) employed to prepare the spore crop from which the subsequent batch of BIs is manufactured. The sporulation medium may consist of either a solid or liquid medium but almost always includes supplemental divalent cations (typically calcium and/or magnesium) to both increase the heat resistance of the spore and yield of the spore crop. As demonstrated by the studies of Friesen and Andersen,[136] Marquis et al,[137] Beaman and Gerhardt,[138] Graham and Boris,[139] Penna et al,[140,141] Cazemier et al,[142] and others, the composition of the sporulation medium and presence of specific divalent cations within the medium play an important role in the heat resistance of the resulting spore crop. The factors affecting heat resistance and yield have been studied by the manufacturers of BIs for many years in order to develop optimal sporulation mediums and conditions. In addition to the presence of divalent cations in the sporulation medium, elevated incubation temperatures are also employed as a means to promote increased heat resistance. The intended outcome is to yield mature spores whose protoplasts have low-water content because this contributes to their heat resistance as discussed by Russell,[8] Gould,[143] and Lindsay et al.[144] Following sporulation, the spore crop is harvested and purified, typically by repeated centrifugation and resuspension in sterile water or buffer to concentrate the spore suspension and remove residual organic material and debris. Depending on the initial volume of sporulation medium, this may yield several hundred milliliters of a highly concentrated spore suspension. The solution employed to store the concentrated spore suspension is critical to its stability. Because the spore protoplast is subject to ion exchange when suspended in an aqueous media, the use of a dilute medium such as distilled water may lead to leaching of cations from the spore protoplast and subsequent loss of heat resistance. The loss of cations from the spore protoplast may be retarded by using a concentrated buffer and storage at low temperature to inhibit the extent of ion exchange that occurs. Following initial quality control checks for purity and yield, the spores are then inoculated onto the desired carrier and their heat resistance evaluated. The carrier may consist of a paper strip or other substrate depending on the design of the BI. Paper strip carriers have been employed for many years with paper strip and self-contained BIs, whereas BIs consisting of inoculated sutures, metal wires or discs, or other carriers are also available for specific applications. As one would anticipate, the microenvironment including the type of carrier employed and resulting BI design will influence the effective heat resistance of the BI. As previously noted, Doyle and Ernst[78] demonstrated

that occlusion of spores of *B subtilis* subsp *niger* within crystals of calcium carbonate significantly increased their resistance to both moist and dry heat. Finocchario[145] reported the influence of the paper carrier on the $D_{121°C}$-value of moist heat BIs, whereas Graham and Boris[139] compared the effect of different lots of glassine and kraft paper envelopes on the resistance of paper strip BIs subjected to both moist and dry heat processing. Spicher et al[146] found that paper carriers can exhibit superheating due to hygroscopic condensation and that storage conditions prior to exposure could influence the resistance of the BI to moist heat treatment. Pflug[147] demonstrated a difference in D-values when paper strip carriers were removed from their glassine envelopes and heated directly in growth medium. As discussed earlier, self-contained BIs for which the inoculated carrier is placed in close juxtaposition to an ampule of growth medium within the BI may result in a thermal lag effect because the indicator is heated and may influence the resulting D_T and z-values.[148] Similarly, the placement of BIs within process challenge devices may also impact the effective heat resistance of the BI. These studies underline the fact that when selecting BIs for an application, one must be aware of the many microenvironmental and design factors that may influence the overall heat resistance of the BI.

Another critical factor influencing the effective heat resistance of a BI is the recovery conditions employed to culture the BI after heat processing. The literature contains numerous references regarding the influence of different types of growth medium and incubation conditions on the overall heat resistance of BI test organisms. Davis et al[133] compared the recovery of *G stearothermophilus* BIs heated under moist heat conditions and *B atrophaeus* BIs heated under dry heat conditions in various commercially available recovery mediums and documented different D-values and z-values when BIs were incubated in different mediums and at different incubation temperatures. This was confirmed by Graham and Boris.[139] Roberts[131] reported the impact of various factors including the addition of sodium chloride, starch, and bicarbonate to the recovery medium on the recovery of heat-damaged spores; Mallidis and Scholefield[149] also noted that changes in the pH of the recovery medium and the addition of starch or charcoal led to statistically significant differences in the recovery of spores of *Bacillus stearothermophilus* processed with moist heat. Pflug et al[150] reported on the effect of different lots of Soybean Casein Digest Medium on the recovery of heat-treated spores of *G stearothermophilus*, noting that the performance of the recovery medium should be validated with heated spores as opposed to nonheated spores. Shintani et al[151] also noted the effect of different lots of commercially available Soybean Casein Digest Medium on the recovery of *G stearothermophilus* BIs processed in a moist heat resistometer. They identified significantly higher D-values determined by the survivor curve method in Soybean Casein Digest Agar as compared

TABLE 11.8 ISO 18472 Resistometer performance criteria

Parameter	Moist Heat	Dry Heat
Time	Selectable ±1 s	Selectable ±2 s
Temperature	110°C − 145°C ± 0.5°C	120°C − 200°C ± 2.5°C
Pressure	100 kPa − 420 kPa ± 3.5 kPa[a]	NA
Time to prevacuum	2 min	NA
Come-up period	11 s	1 min
Stabilization period	10 s (±1°C)	2 min (±4°C)
Come-down period	11 s	1 min

Abbreviation: NA, not applicable.

[a]Tolerance at 121°C.

to the D-values obtained by fraction-negative analysis using Soybean Casein Digest Broth. They attributed the difference in recovery to the different levels of available calcium ions and phosphate buffer (K_2HPO_4) in the mediums tested. Based on these and other studies, it is evident that the composition of the growth medium and methods employed for the recovery of heat-stressed BIs are indeed critical factors in determining the effective heat resistance of a BI. This is further complicated by the fact that most commonly used BI growth mediums such as Soybean Casein Digest Broth are composed primarily of crude extracts of animal and plant materials that makes it difficult to ensure that consistent recovery conditions are employed. Although this can be mitigated to some extent by purchasing large quantities of a particular lot of growth medium, this may not be practical in all circumstances. Self-contained BIs have an advantage over paper strip BIs in this regard because their design usually ensures that the same lot of growth medium is employed with each BI during initial validation and subsequent use throughout its shelf life. Of course, the medium must be both heat stable and capable of promoting the growth of heat-stressed test organisms following processing.[152]

In addition to the aforementioned list of factors that may impact the effective heat resistance of microorganisms, one must also consider the equipment employed to provide the desired heating conditions under which the heat resistance of the test organism is determined. Pflug et al[23] reviewed many of the different test apparatus employed to study the heat resistance of microorganisms. The variety of test equipment is considerable, ranging from simple capillary tubes placed in heating blocks[149] to computer-controlled resistometers.[153] Although the design of the equipment employed to evaluate the heat resistance of microorganisms has become increasingly sophisticated, much of the knowledge gained previously using less complex apparatus is still valid. Today, one of the most widely employed systems for determining the

heat resistance of microorganisms is a resistometer. The increased use of biological and chemical indicators in sterilization monitoring in health care and industry led to the need for the development of standardized test apparatus to characterize their heat resistance. As defined in ISO 18472,[154] a resistometer is a "test equipment designed to create defined combinations of the physical and/or chemical variables of a sterilization process." This is of necessity a rather broad definition, but the performance criteria for time to temperature, tolerances about the set point temperature, and time-to-ambient criteria listed in the standard are quite stringent and require sophisticated control technology (Table 11.8). Problems may arise, however, when one attempts to compare results of BI testing between laboratories using different types of resistometers. As reported by Oxborrow et al,[155] there was significant variability between laboratories using different models of moist heat resistometers when the same BI lots were tested with two different growth mediums. At that time, they concluded that a ±20% variability in D-values between laboratories as specified by the United States Pharmacopeia (USP) was not supportable. A review of this data by Mosly and Gillis[156] noted that much of the variability could be attributed to a combination of the operating limits of the resistometer and z-values of the BIs as well as unaccounted lag factors and nearly undetectable air leaks within the resistometers employed in testing. Pflug[157] also reviewed the data of Oxborrow et al[155] and also concluded that there was not only variability in the performance of resistometers between laboratories but that this was also further exacerbated by procedural differences between and within each laboratory. More recently, McCormick et al[158] in a study of commercially available moist heat BIs evaluated the operating precision of a moist heat resistometer using nonparametric process capability analysis and demonstrated an average Cnpk of 1.655863 over 30 cycles processed at a temperature of 121°C (Figure 11.13). This study found a high degree of correlation (within ±20%)

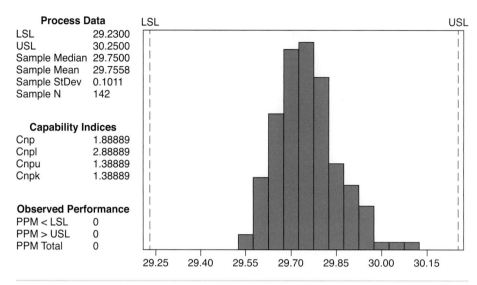

Process Data	
LSL	29.2300
USL	30.2500
Sample Median	29.7500
Sample Mean	29.7558
Sample StDev	0.1011
Sample N	142

Capability Indices	
Cnp	1.88889
Cnpl	2.88889
Cnpu	1.38889
Cnpk	1.38889

Observed Performance	
PPM < LSL	0
PPM > USL	0
PPM Total	0

FIGURE 11.13 Example of empirical process capability analysis of a moist heat resistometer. The process exhibits good capability relative to centering about the set point temperature of 121°C (29.7373 psia), but the data is skewed toward the upper specification limit. Abbreviations: Cnp, empirical process capability analysis for two-sided specification limit (LSL and USL) without regard for process centering; Cnpk, empirical process capability relative to the lower and upper specification limit accounting for process centering; Cnpl, empirical process capability relative to the lower specification limit; Cnpu, empirical process capability relative to the upper specification limit; LSL, lower specification limit; PPM, parts per million; USL, upper specification limit.

between the labeled D-value provided by the BI manufacturer and the D-value verified in the testing laboratory for self-contained BIs tested from 2008 to 2017, but this correlation was not as strong for paper strip BIs. Although it is evident that our understanding of those factors that can impact BI performance and resistometer design has improved considerably, the truism expressed by Pflug[157] that "in general, on a day-to-day basis, no two persons perform exactly the same and no two pieces of equipment operate exactly the same" remains valid.

▶ MOLECULAR MECHANISMS OF HEAT RESISTANCE

The impact of an applied heat stress on microorganisms varies with the nature of the heat stress (dry heat or moist heat), the magnitude and duration of the heat stress applied, the nature of the microorganism (spore form or vegetative form), the environment in which the microorganism is heated, the recovery conditions, and other factors. Although much has been learned about how microorganisms respond to an applied heat stress, there does not appear to be one single mechanism by which microorganisms are inactivated or a single mechanism by which they acquire heat resistance. This has been studied in some detail in various vegetative bacteria and archaea isolated from hot water sources, such as deep-sea hydrothermal vent environments. Some of these isolates,

such as *Pyrolobus fumarii* can survive at temperatures typically at 113°C and have many resistance factors including unique cell wall and protein structures.[70,159] Although this seems at odds with the single-hit theory of Chick discussed earlier in the chapter, Casolari[57] notes that the single-hit theory is quite limiting with regard to heat processing in view of the phenomenon of sublethal injury that may be inflicted on microorganisms by a various means including heat treatment. Rather, Casolari[57] suggests that microbial inactivation should be viewed as an end point of a progressively damaging process rather than a single event.

The primary damage that is inflicted on microorganisms by an applied heat stress is the cumulative disruption of the structure of macromolecules within the cell. This obviously has significant consequences with regard to the metabolic functioning, virus structure, cell wall-membrane integrity, and the reproductive potential of the cell. In most applications, the general order of resistance to heat treatment appears to be prions > bacterial spores > nonenveloped viruses > fungal spores > mycobacterium > vegetative bacteria and fungi > enveloped viruses with most microorganisms exhibiting less resistance to moist heat than dry heat and with quiescent cells exhibiting greater resistance to an applied heat stress than actively growing cells. At this date, little is known regarding the true mechanisms of resistance of prions to applied heat treatments (see chapter 68). Müller et al[160] has suggested that the reduction in prion effectivity with heat treatment proceeds in a stepwise manner, with an initial degradation in secondary structure and multimeric aggregation followed by subsequent backbone degradation (loss of primary structure). McDonnell et al[161] have cautioned, however, that although heat treatment can be effective against prions, some of the data is inconclusive due to assay variability, presence of contaminating materials, and the use of different test conditions. Clearly, further work in this area is necessary before the mechanism of heat inactivation of prions is fully understood.

In contrast to prions, the mechanism of heat resistance of bacterial spores to heat treatment is better understood, although there are differences depending on whether moist heat or dry heat is employed. Setlow[162] in reviewing the resistance of spores of *B subtilis* to heat treatment noted that spore resistance to moist heat is largely determined by the water content of the spore core, which is much lower than that of the vegetative cell protoplast. This correlates with the studies of Gerhardt and Marquis[163] who demonstrated an inverse relationship between the water content of the core and moist heat resistance. Other mechanisms that contribute to the wet heat resistance of spores is the binding of small acid-soluble proteins to the spore DNA[164] and the presence of large quantities of dipicolinic acid (DPA) in the spore core, which is postulated to play a role in both heat and radiation resistance of the spore.[165] Perhaps, not unexpectedly due to the difference in heating conditions and cellular structure, heat shock proteins induced by mild heat treatment that have been shown to enhance the survival of vegetative cells[166,167] do not appear to play a significant role in the resistance of spores to moist heat[168] but can influence the survival of vegetative bacteria to certain disinfection treatments. Dry heat treatment is believed to impact spores in a different manner than moist heat in that only dry heat treatment kills spores by DNA damage and mutagenesis.[169] This is supported by studies that demonstrate that spores that are deficient in DNA repair enzymes exhibit greater sensitivity to dry heat treatment than wild type spores.[162]

Damage to vegetative cells resulting from heat treatment appears to be of a broader spectrum as compared to spores with many potential targets including the cell membrane and cell wall,[170,171] ribosomes and RNA polymerase,[172] DNA damage,[173,174] protein denaturation and enzyme inactivation,[170,175] and other effects. In some cases, if the thermal treatment is not extensive, vegetative cells may be able to repair the damage induced by the applied heat treatment or make adaptive changes, but this is unlikely to occur with the majority of common microorganisms because temperatures are elevated significantly above their normal growth range.[72] In this context, one must also consider extremophiles that are capable of growth under extreme conditions of temperature, pressure, pH, salinity, etc. Extremophiles were previously classified as Archaebacteria and have now been classified as Archaea, a domain of single-celled microorganisms separate from prokaryotes and eukaryotes. Similar to prokaryotes in that they have no defined cell nucleus, Archaea apparently evolved along a separate evolutionary path and have significant biochemical differences. First described by Brock,[176] extremophiles have been shown to be capable of proliferating at temperatures as high as 122°C and pressures as high as 20 MPa.[177,178] Adaptations to extreme temperature conditions include significant differences in gene expression,[179] membrane structure,[180,181] DNA stabilization,[182] etc. Extremophiles have been isolated from a wide range of severe environments including the nutrient-limited conditions of cleanrooms.[183] Although it is unlikely that extremophiles present a significant concern from a health care perspective, they do demonstrate the astounding ability of microorganisms to adapt to severe environmental conditions. As more is learned regarding these amazing microorganisms, it will be interesting to determine whether their inactivation kinetics are congruent with our current understanding of the principles of the thermal destruction of microorganisms or whether new models of microbial inactivation kinetics will need to be developed.

◗ ACKNOWLEDGMENTS

The authors wish to thank and acknowledge Irving J Pflug, PhD, for his many valuable contributions to the study of sterilization science and for the original text of this chapter on which this revision is based.

REFERENCES

1. Rahn O. Injury and death of bacteria by chemical agents. In: Luyet BJ, ed. *Biodynamica Monograph No. 3*. Normandy, MO: Biodynamica; 1945:9-41.
2. Pflug IJ. Some observations regarding factors important to dry-heat sterilization. In: Sneath PNA, ed. *Sterilization Techniques for Instruments and Materials as Applied to Space Research*. Paris, France: Murray Print; 1968:51-58. COSPAR Technical Manual no. 4.
3. Holcomb RG, Pflug IJ. The Spearman–Karber method of analyzing quantal assay microbial destruction data. In: Pflug IJ, ed. *Selected Papers on the Microbiology and Engineering of Sterilization Processes*. Minneapolis, MN: Environmental Sterilization Laboratory, University of Minnesota; 1978:83-100.
4. Bigelow WD. The logarithmic nature of thermal death time curves. *J Infect Dis*. 1921;29:528-536.
5. Stumbo CR. *Thermobacteriology in Food Processing*. New York, NY: Academic Press; 1965.
6. Ball CO. Mathematical solution of problems on thermal processing of canned foods. *University California Public Health*. 1928;1:15-245.
7. Halvorson HO, Ziegler NR. Application of statistics in bacteriology: I. A means of determining bacterial population by the dilution method. *J Bacteriol*. 1933;25:101-121.
8. Russell AD, ed. *The Destruction of Bacterial Spores*. London, United Kingdom: Academic Press; 1982.
9. Agalloco J, Akers J, Madsen R. Moist heat sterilization—myths and realities. *PDA J Pharm Sci Technol*. 1998;52(6):346-350.
10. Schmidt CF. Thermal resistance of microorganisms. In: Reddish GF, ed. *Antiseptics, Disinfectants, Fungicides, and Sterilization*. Philadelphia, PA: Lea & Febiger; 1954:720-759.

11. International Organization for Standardization. *ISO 11138-3:2017: Sterilization of Health Care Products—Biological Indicators—Part 3: Biological Indicators for Moist Heat Sterilization Processes.* Geneva, Switzerland: International Organization for Standardization; 2017.

12. International Organization for Standardization. *ISO 11138-4:2017: Sterilization of Health Care Products—Biological Indicators—Part 4: Biological Indicators for Dry Heat Sterilization Processes.* Geneva, Switzerland: International Organization for Standardization; 2017.

13. International Organization for Standardization. *ISO 11138-5:2017: Sterilization of Health Care Products—Biological Indicators—Part 5: Biological Indicators for Low-Temperature Steam and Formaldehyde Processes.* Geneva, Switzerland: International Organization for Standardization; 2017.

14. Pflug IJ, Odlaug TE. Biological indicators in the pharmaceutical and medical device industry. *J Parenter Sci Technol.* 1986;40(5):242-248.

15. Sutton S. The limitations of CFU: compliance to CGMP requires good science. *J GXP Compliance.* 2012;16(1):74-80.

16. Parenteral Drug Association. Technical Report No 33. Evaluation, validation and implementation of new microbiological testing methods. *PDA J Pharmaceutical Sci Technology.* 2013;54(3): TR33.

17. United States Pharmacopeia. Validation of alternative microbiological methods. In: *United States Pharmacopeial Convention.* 40th ed. Rockville, MD: United States Pharmacopeia; 2017:1756-1770.

18. Li L, Mendis N, Trigui H, Oliver JD, Faucher SP. The importance of viable but non-culturable state in human bacterial pathogens. *Front Microbiol.* 2014;5:258.

19. Kilsby DC, Davies KW, McClure PJ, Adair C, Anderson WA. Bacterial thermal death kinetics based on probability distributions: the heat destruction of *Clostridium botulinum* and *Salmonella* Bedford. *J Food Prot.* 2000;63:1197-1203.

20. Ross T. Indices for performance evaluation of predictive models in food microbiology. *J Appl Bacteriol.* 1966;81:501-508.

21. Chick H. An investigation into the laws of disinfection. *J Hyg (Lond).* 1908;8:92-158.

22. United States Pharmacopeia. Sterilization and sterility assurance. In: *United States Pharmacopeial Convention.* 40th ed. Rockville, MD: United States Pharmacopeia. 2017;1744-1749.

23. Pflug IJ, Holcomb RG, Gomez M. Principles of the thermal destruction of microorganisms. In: Lawrence CA, Block SS, eds. *Disinfection, Sterilization, and Preservation.* Philadelphia, PA: Lea & Febiger; 2001:79-129.

24. Moats WA. Kinetics of thermal death of bacteria. *J Bacteriol.* 1971;105:165-171.

25. Corradini MG, Normand MD, Eisenberg M, Peleg M. Evaluation of a stochastic inactivation model for heat-activated spores of *Bacillus* spp. *Appl Environ Microbiol.* 2010;76(13):4402-4412.

26. Holcomb RG, Chapman P, Fischer D. Definition of intercept ratio. In: *Progress Report No. 9: Environmental Microbiology as Related to Planetary Quarantine.* Minneapolis, MN: University of Minnesota; 1972:55-59. National Aeronautics and Space Administration grant NGL 24-005-160.

27. Draper NR, Smith H. *Applied Regression Analysis.* 2nd ed. New York, NY: John Wiley & Sons; 1981.

28. McHugh RB, Sundararaj N. Decimal reduction time estimation in thermal microbial sterilization. In: *Progress Report No. 9: Environmental Microbiology as Related to Planetary Quarantine.* Minneapolis, MN: University of Minnesota; 1972:77-78. National Aeronautics and Space Administration grant NGL 24-005-160.

29. Cerf O. Tailing of survivor curves of bacterial spores. *J Appl Bacteriol.* 1977;42:1-19.

30. Sharpe K, Bektash RM. Heterogeneity and the modeling of bacterial spore death: the case of continuously decreasing death rate. *Can J Microbiol.* 1977;23:1501-1507.

31. Han YW, Zhang HI, Krochta JM. Death rates of bacterial spores: mathematical models. *Can J Microbiol.* 1976;22:295-300.

32. Ababouch LH, Grimit L, Eddafry R, Busta FF. Thermal inactivation kinetics of *Bacillus subtilis* spores suspended in buffer and in oils. *J Appl Bacteriol.* 1995;78:669-676.

33. Shintani H. Interpretation of tailing phenomenon of survivor curve and inactivation of virus by plasma exposure. *Pharmaceutica Analytica Acta.* 2012;3(6). doi:10.4712/2153-2435.1000181.

34. van Boekel MA. On the use of the Weibull model to describe thermal inactivation of microbial vegetative cells. *Int J Food Microbiol.* 2002;74:139-159.

35. Head D, Cenkowski S. Weibull model of inactivation of *Geobacillus stearothermophilus* spores in superheated steam. Paper presented at: CSBE/SCGAB 2009 Annual Conference; August 2009; Prince Edward Island, Canada. Paper No. CSBE01-301.

36. Collado J, Fernández A, Cunha LM, Ocio MJ, Martínez A. Improved model based on the Weibull distribution to describe the combined effect of pH and temperature on the heat resistance of *Bacillus cereus* in carrot juice 2003. *J Food Prot.* 2003;66(6):978-984.

37. Couvert O, Gaillard S, Savy N, Mafart P, Leguérinel, I. Survival curves of heated bacterial spores: effect of environmental factors on Weibull parameters. *Int J Food Microbiol.* 2005;101:73-81.

38. Sant'ana AS, Rosental A, Massaguer PR. Heat resistance and the effects of continuous pasteurization on the inactivation of *Byssochlamys fulva* ascospores in clarified apple juice. *J Appl Microbiol.* 2009;107:197-209.

39. Da Rocha Ferreira EH, Rosental A, Calado V, Saraiva J, Mendo S, De Massaguer PR. Thermal inactivation of *Byssochlamys nivea* in pineapple juice combined with preliminary high pressure treatments. In: Taoukis PS, Stoforos NG, Karanthanos VT, Saracacos GD, eds. In: *Food Process Engineering in a Changing World. Proceedings of the 11th International Congress on Engineering and Food (ICEF11).* Athens, Greece; 2011: 1879-1880.

40. Souza PBA, Poltronieri KF, Alvarenga VO, et al. Modeling of *Byssochamys nivea* and *Neosatorya fischeri* inactivation in papaya and pineapple juices as a function of temperature and solids content. *LWT.* 2017;82(1):90-95.

41. Geeraerd AH, Herremans CH, Van Impe JF. Structural model requirements to describe microbial inactivation during a mild heat treatment. *Int J Food Microbiol.* 2000;59(3):185-209.

42. Linton RH, Carter WH, Pierson MD, Hackney CR, Eifert JD. Use of a modified Gompertz equation to predict the effects of temperature, pH, and NaCl on the inactivation of *Listeria monocytogenes* Scott A heated in infant formula. *J Food Protect.* 1995;59(1):16-23.

43. Miller FA, Gil MM, Brandão TRS, Teixeira P, Silva CLM. Sigmoidal thermal inactivation kinetics of *Listeria innocua* in broth: influence of strain and growth phase. *Food Control.* 2009;20(12):1151-1157.

44. Gill MM, Miller FA, Brandao TRS, Silva CLM. Predictions of microbial thermal inactivation in solid foods: isothermal and non-isothermal conditions. *Procedia Food Sci.* 2016;7:154-157.

45. Geeraerd AH, Valdramidis VP, Van Impe JF. GinaFIT, a freeware tool to assess non-log-linear microbial survivor curves. *Int J Food Microbiol.* 2005;102(1):95-105.

46. Bevilacqua A, Speranza B, Sinigaglia M, Corbo MR. A focus on the death kinetics in predictive microbiology: benefits and limits of the most important models and some tools dealing with their application in foods. *Foods.* 2015;4:565-580.

47. United States Pharmacopeia. Validation of microbial recovery from pharmacopeial articles. In: *United States Pharmacopeial Convention.* 40th ed. Rockville, MD: United States Pharmacopeia. 2017;1787-1790.

48. Bigelow WD, Esty JR. Thermal death point in relation to time of typical thermophilic organisms. *J Infect Dis.* 1920;27:602-617.

49. Townsend CT, Esty JR, Baselt FC. Heat resistance studies on spores of putrefactive anaerobes in relation to determination of safe processes for canned foods. *Food Res.* 1938;3:323-346.

50. International Organization for Standardization. *ISO 11138-1:2017: Sterilization of Health Care Products—Biological Indicators—Part 1: General Requirements.* Geneva, Switzerland: International Organization for Standardization; 2017.

51. Stumbo CR, Murphy JR, Cochran J. Nature of thermal death time curves for P.A. 3679 and *Clostridium botulinum. Food Technol.* 1950;4: 321-326.

52. Pflug IJ, Holcomb RG. Principles of thermal destruction of microorganisms. In: Block SS, ed. *Disinfection, Sterilization, and Preservation.* 4th ed. Philadelphia, PA: Lea & Febiger; 1991:85-128.

53. Perkins JJ. *Principles and Methods of Sterilization in Health Sciences.* 2nd ed. Springfield, IL: Charles C. Thomas Publisher Ltd; 1983.

54. Hancock CO. Heat sterilization. In: Maillard JY, Fraise A, Sattar S, eds. *Principles and Practice of Disinfection, Preservation and Sterilization*. 5th ed. West Sussex, United Kingdom: Blackwell Publishing; 2013:277-293.

55. Hunter PR, Fewtrell L. Acceptable risk. In: *World Health Organization (WHO) Water Quality: Guidelines, Standards and Health*. London, United Kingdom: TWA Publishing; 2001.

56. International Organization for Standardization. *ISO/TS 19930:2017: Guidance on Aspects of a Risk-Based Approach to Assuring Sterility of Terminally Sterilized, Single-Use Health Care Product That Is Unable to Withstand Processing to Achieve Maximally a Sterility Assurance Level of 10^{-6}*. Geneva, Switzerland: International Organization for Standardization; 2017.

57. Casolari A. Microbial death. In: Bazin MJ, Prosser JI, eds. *Physiological Models in Microbiology*. Vol 2. Boca Raton, FL: CRC Press; 1988.

58. Joslyn L. Sterilization by heat. In: Block SS, ed. *Disinfection, Sterilization, and Preservation*. 4th ed. Philadelphia, PA: Lea & Febiger; 1991:515-516.

59. United States Pharmacopeia. Dry heat sterilization. In: *United States Pharmacopeial Convention*. 40th ed. Rockville, MD: United States Pharmacopeia; 2017:1840-1842.

60. International Organization for Standardization. *ISO 17665-1:2006: Sterilization of Health Care Products—Moist Heat—Part 1: Requirements for the Development, Validation and Routine Control of a Sterilization Process for Medical Devices*. Geneva, Switzerland: International Organization for Standardization; 2006.

61. International Organization for Standardization. *ISO 20857:2010: Sterilization of Health Care Products—Dry Heat—Requirements for the Development, Validation and Routine Control of a Sterilization Process for Medical Devices*. Geneva, Switzerland: International Organization for Standardization; 2015.

62. International Organization for Standardization. *ISO 14161:2009: Sterilization of Health Care Products—Biological Indicators—Guidance for the Selection, Use and Interpretation of Results*. Geneva, Switzerland: International Organization for Standardization; 2009.

63. Parenteral Drug Association. *Validation of Moist Heat Sterilization Processes Cycle Design, Development, Qualification and Ongoing Control*. Bethesda, MD: Parenteral Drug Association; 2007. Technical report no. 1.

64. Parenteral Drug Association. *Validation of Dry Heat Processes Used for Sterilization and Depyrogenation*. Bethesda, MD: Parenteral Drug Association; 2013. Technical Report No. 3.

65. Chu NS, McAlister D, Antonoplos PA. Natural bioburden levels detected on flexible gastrointestinal endoscopes after clinical use and manual cleaning. *Gastrointest Endosc*. 1998;48(2):137-142.

66. US Food and Drug Administration. Guidance for industry. In: *Submission of Documentation in Applications for Parametric Release of Human and Veterinary Drug Products Terminally Sterilized by Moist Heat Processes*. Silver Spring, MD: US Food and Drug Administration; 2010.

67. International Organization for Standardization. *ISO 11737-1:2018: Sterilization of Health Care Products—Microbiological Methods—Part 1: Determination of a Population of Microorganisms on Products*. Geneva, Switzerland: International Organization for Standardization; 2018.

68. Agalloco J. Understanding overkill sterilization: an end to the confusion. *Pharm Technol*. 2007;2007(suppl 2):60-67.

69. Sadowski M. The use of biological indicators in the development and qualification of moist heat sterilization processes. In: Gomez M, Moldenhauer J, eds. *Biological Indicators for Sterilization Processes*. Bethesda, MD: Parenteral Drug Association; 2009:219-269.

70. Berger TJ, Kiernan JT, Grillo JF. Influence of parenteral solutions and closure systems on biological indicator behavior. In: Gomez M, Moldenhauer J, eds. *Biological Indicators for Sterilization Processes*. Bethesda, MD: Parenteral Drug Association; 2009:117-160.

71. Russell AD. Theoretical aspects of microbial inactivation. In: Morrissey RF, Phillips GB, eds. *Sterilization Technology: A Practical Guide for Manufacturers and Users of Health Care Products*. New York, NY: Van Nostrand Reinhold; 1993:3-16.

72. McDonnell GE. Physical sterilization. In: McDonnell GE, ed. *Antisepsis, Disinfection, and Sterilization: Types, Action, and Resistance*. 2nd ed. Washington, DC: ASM Press; 2017:165-189.

73. British Standards Institution. *EN 285. Sterilization. Steam Sterilizers. Large Sterilizer*. London, United Kingdom: British Standards Institution; 2015.

74. Association for the Advancement of Medical Instrumentation. *AAMI TIR 34. Water for the Reprocessing Medical Devices*. Arlington, VA: Association for the Advancement of Medical Instrumentation; 2014.

75. Young JH. Sterilization with steam under pressure. In: Morrissey RF, Phillips GB, eds. *Sterilization Technology: A Practical Guide for Manufacturers and Users of Health Care Products*. New York, NY: Springer; 1993:120-151.

76. Agalloco J. Steam sterilization in-place technology and validation. In: Carleton F, Agalloco J, eds. *Validation of Pharmaceutical Processes: Sterile Products*. New York, NY: Marcel Dekker; 1998:451-482.

77. Murrell WG, Scott WJ. The heat resistance of bacterial spores at various water activities. *J Gen Microbiol*. 1966;43:411-425.

78. Doyle JE, Ernst RR. Resistance of *Bacillus subtilis* var. *niger* spores occluded in water-insoluble crystals to three sterilization agents. *Appl Microbiol*. 1967;15:726-730.

79. Angelotti R. Protective mechanisms affecting dry-heat sterilization. In: Sneath PNA, ed. *Sterilization Techniques for Instruments and Materials as Applied to Space Research:*. Paris, France: Murray Print; 1968:59-74. COSPAR technical manual no. 4.

80. Bruch CW, Koesterer MG, Bruch MK. Dry-heat sterilization: its development and application to components of exobiological space probes. *Dev Ind Microbiol*. 1963;4:334-342.

81. Pheil CG, Pflug IJ, Nicholas RC, Agustin JA. Effect of various gas atmospheres on the destruction of microorganisms in dry heat. *Appl Microbiol*. 1967;15:120-124.

82. Davis NS, Silverman GJ, Keller WH. Combined effects of ultrahigh vacuum and temperature on the viability of some spores and soil organisms. *Appl Microbiol*. 1963;11:202-210.

83. Gibson B. The effect of high sugar concentrations on the heat resistance of vegetative microorganisms. *J Appl Bacteriol*. 1973;36:365-376.

84. Beuchat LR. Combined effects of solutes and food preservatives on rates of inactivation and colony formation by heated spores and vegetative cells of molds. *Appl Environ Microbiol*. 1981;41:472-477.

85. Berger MA, Richard N, Cheftel JC. Influence de l'activité de l'eau sur la thermorésistance d'une levure osmophile: *Saccharomyces rouxii*, dans tin aliment a humidité intermédiaire. *Lebensmittel-Wissenschaft und Tecnologie*. 1982;15:83-88.

86. Put HMC. The heat resistance of ascospores of *Kluyveromyces* spp. isolated from spoiled heat processed fruit products. In: Dring GJ, Ellar DJ, Gould GW, eds. *Fundamental and Applied Aspects of Bacterial Spores*. London, United Kingdom: Academic Press; 1985:421-453.

87. Splittstoesser DF, Leasor SB, Swanson KMJ. Effect of food composition on the heat resistance of yeast ascospores. *J Food Sci*. 1986;51:1265-1267.

88. Jermini M, Schmidt-Lorenz W. Heat resistance of vegetative cells and asci of two *Zygosaccharomyces* yeasts in broth at different water activity values. *J Food Protect*. 1987;50:835-841.

89. Beuchat LR. Injury and repair of yeasts and moulds. In: Andrew MHE, Russell AD, eds. *The Revival of Injured Microbes*. London, United Kingdom: Academic Press; 1984:293-308.

90. Beuchat LR. Thermal tolerance of *Talaromyces flavus* ascospores as affected by growth medium and temperature, age and sugar content in the inactivation medium. *Transact British Mycologic Soc*. 1988;90:359-364.

91. Fay AC. The effect of hypertonic sugar solution on the thermal resistance of bacteria. *J Agr Res*. 1934;48:453-468.

92. Baumgartner JG. Heat sterilised reducing sugars and their effects on the thermal resistance of bacteria. *J Bacteriol*. 1938;36:369-382.

93. Corry JEL. The effect of sugars and polysols on the heat resistance of salmonellae. *J Appl Bacteriol*. 1974;37:31-43.

94. Corry JEL. The effect of sugars and polyols on the heat resistance and morphology of osmophilic yeasts. *J Appl Bacteriol*. 1976;40:269-276.

95. Weiss H. The heat resistance of spores with special reference to the spores of *B. botulinus*. *J Infect Dis*. 1921;28:70-92.

96. Rahn O. Incomplete sterilization of food products due to heavy syrups. *Canning Age*. 1928;8:705-706.

97. Von Angerer K, Küster E. Uber die Verzögerung des Hitzetodes von Bakterien und Sporen durch hochkonzentrierte als Funktion Medien des Tyndalleffectes. *Arch Hyg Bakterial*. 1939;122:57-97.

98. Braun OF, Hays GL, Benjamin HA. Use of dry sugar in sweetening foods canned in syrup: part II. Bacteriological aspects. Decrease in lethal value of sterilization process results from use of dry sugar in packing sweet potatoes. *Food Industry.* 1941;13:645.

99. Anderson EE, Esselen WB Jr, Fellers CR. Effect of acids, salt, sugar, and other food ingredients on thermal resistance of *Bacillus thermoacidurans. Food Res.* 1949;14:499-510.

100. Sugiyama H. Studies of factors affecting the heat resistance of spores of *Clostridium botulinum. J Bacteriol.* 1951;62:81-96.

101. Corry JEL. Sugar and polyol permeability of *Salmonella* and osmophilic yeast cell membranes measured by turbidimetry, and its relation to heat resistance. *J Appl Bacteriol.* 1976;40:277-284.

102. Yesair J, Bohrer CW, Cameron EJ. Effect of certain environmental factors on heat resistance of micrococci. *Food Res.* 1946;11:327-331.

103. Molin N, Snygg BG. Effect of lipid materials on heat resistance of bacterial spores. *Appl Microbiol.* 1967;15:1422-1426.

104. Zaleski S, Sobolewska-Ceronik K, Ceronik E. Influence de l'hydratation de l'huile de soja sur la résistance du staphylocoque enterotoxique a la chaleur. *Ann Inst Pasteur Lille.* 1971;22:263-267.

105. Senhaji AF, Loncin M. The protective effect of fat on the heat resistance of bacteria: I. *J Food Technol.* 1977;12:203-216.

106. Senhaji AF. The protective effect of fat on the heat resistance of bacteria: II. *J Food Technol.* 1977;12:217-230.

107. Ababouch LH, Busta FF. Effect of thermal treatments in oils on bacterial spore survival. *J Appl Bacteriol.* 1987;62:491-502.

108. Syamaladevi RM, Tang J, Villa-Rojas R, Sablani S, Carter B, Campbell G. Influence of water activity on thermal resistance of microorganisms in low-moisture foods: a review. *Comp Rev Food Sci Food Safety.* 2016;15:353-370.

109. Wilson GS. *The Pasteurization of Milk.* London, United Kingdom: Edward Arnold; 1942.

110. Pace JL, Rossi HA, Esposito VM, Frey SM, Tucker KD, Walker RI. Inactivated whole-cell bacterial vaccines: current status and novel strategies. *Vaccine.* 1998;16(16):1563-1574.

111. Uetera Y, Kawamura K, Kobayashi H, Saito Y, Yasuhara H, Saito R. Studies on viral disinfection: an evaluation of moist heat disinfection of HBV by using A0 concept defined in ISO 15883-washer-disinfectors. *PDA J Pharm Sci Technol.* 2010;64:327-336.

112. Eterpi M, McDonnell G, Thomas V. Disinfection efficacy against parvoviruses compared with reference viruses. *J Hosp Infect.* 2009;73(1):64-70.

113. Pruss A, Kao M, von Garrel T, et al. Virus inactivation in bone tissue transplants (femoral heads) by moist heat with the 'Marburg bone bank system.' *Biologicals.* 2003;31:75-82.

114. Association for the Advancement of Medical Instrumentation. *ANSI/AAMI ST79. Comprehensive Guide to Steam Sterilization and Sterility Assurance in Health Care Facilities.* Arlington, VA: Association for the Advancement of Medical Instrumentation; 2017.

115. US Food and Drug Administration. *Class II Special Controls Guidance Document: Medical Washers and Medical Washer-Disinfectors: Guidance for the Medical Device Industry and FDA Review Staff.* Silver Spring, MD: US Food and Drug Administration; 2002.

116. International Organization for Standardization. *ISO 15883-1:2006: Washer-Disinfectors—Part 1: General Requirements, Terms and Definitions and Tests.* Geneva, Switzerland: International Organization for Standardization; 2006.

117. United States Pharmacopeia. Water for pharmaceutical purposes. In: *United States Pharmacopeial Convention.* 40th ed. Rockville, MD: United States Pharmacopeia; 2017:1852-1858.

118. Reveron IM, Barreiro JA, Sandoval AJ. Thermal death characteristics of *Lactobacillus paracasei* and *Aspergillus niger* in Pilsen beer. *J Food Engineering.* 2005;66(2):239-243.

119. Deboosere N, Legeay O, Caudrelier Y, Lange M. Modelling effect of physical and chemical parameters on heat inactivation kinetics of hepatitis A virus in a fruit model system. *Int J Food Microbiol.* 2004;93:73-85.

120. Diab-Elschahawi M, Fürnkranz U, Blacky A, Bachhofner N, Koller W. Re-evaluation of current A0 value recommendations for thermal disinfection of reusable human waste containers based on new experimental data. *J Hosp Infect.* 2010;75:62-65.

121. Spaulding E. The role of chemical disinfection in the prevention of nosocomial infections. In: *Proceedings of the International Conference on Nosocomial Infections, 1970.* Chicago, IL: American Hospital Association; 1971:247-254.

122. Röhm-Rodowald E, Jakimiak B, Chojecka A, Wiercińska O, Ziemba B, Kanclerski K. Recommendations for thermal disinfection based on the A0 concept according to EN ISO 15883 [in Polish]. *Przegl Epidemiol.* 2013;67:687-690.

123. McCormick PJ, Schoene MJ, Dehmler MA, McDonnell G. Moist heat disinfection and revisiting the A0 concept. *Biomedic Instrum Technol.* 2016;50(suppl 3):19-26.

124. Almatroudi A, Tahir S, Hu H, et al. *Staphylococcus aureus* dry-surface biofilms are more resistant to heat treatment than traditional hydrated biofilms. *J Hosp Infect.* 2018;98(2):161-167.

125. Alder VG, Gillespie WA. Disinfection of woolen blankets in steam at subatmospheric pressure. *J Clin Pathol.* 1961;14:515-518.

126. Hoxey EV. Low temperature steam formaldehyde. In: Morrissey RF, Prokopenko YI, eds. *Sterilization of Medical Products.* Vol 5. Morin-Heights, Canada: Polyscience Publishers; 1991:359-364.

127. Barbosa-Canovas GV, Juliano P. Food sterilization by combining high pressure and thermal energy. In: Gutierrez-Lopez GF, Barbosa-Canovas GV, Welti-Chanes J, Parada-Arias E, eds. *Food Engineering: Integrated Approaches.* New York, NY: Springer; 2008:9-46.

128. Murphy RY, Hanson RE, Johnson NR, Chappa K, Berrang ME. Combining organic acid treatment with steam pasteurization to eliminate *Listeria monocytogenes* on fully cooked frankfurters. *J Food Prot.* 2006;69(1):47-52.

129. Mossel DAA, Struijk CB. Public health implication of refrigerated pasteurized ('sous-vide') foods. *Int J Food Microbiol.* 1991;13:187-296.

130. International Organization for Standardization. *ISO 14937:2009: Sterilization of Health Care Products—General Requirements for Characterization a Sterilizing Agent and the Development, Validation and Routine Control of a Sterilization Process for Medical Devices.* Geneva, Switzerland: International Organization for Standardization; 2009.

131. Roberts TA. Symposium on bacterial spores: VII. Recovering spores damaged by heat, ionizing radiation or ethylene oxide. *J Appl Bacteriol.* 1970;33:74-94.

132. Warth AD. Relationship between the heat resistance of spores and the optimum and maximum growth temperatures of *Bacillus* species. *J Bacteriol.* 1978;134:699-705.

133. Davis SB, Carls RA, Gillis JR. Recovery of sublethal sterilization damaged *Bacillus* spores in various culture media. In: Underkofler LA, Wulf ML, eds. *Developments in Industrial Microbiology.* Arlington, VA: Society for Industrial Microbiology; 1979:427-438.

134. Moldenhauer JE. Contributing factors to variability in biological indicator performance data. *PDA J Pharm Sci Technol.* 1999;53(4):157-162.

135. Coleman WH, Setlow P. Analysis of damage due to moist heat treatment of *Bacillus subtilis. J Appl Microbiol.* 2009;106(5):1600-1607.

136. Friesen WT, Andersen RA. Effects of sporulation conditions and cation-exchange treatment on the thermal resistance of *Bacillus stearothermophilus* spores. *Canadian J Pharmaceutical Sci.* 1974;9(2):50-53.

137. Marquis RE, Carstensen EL, Child SZ, Bender GR. Preparation and characterization of various salt forms of *Bacillus megaterium* spores. In: Levinson HS, Sonensheim AL, Tipper DJ, eds. *Sporulation and Germination.* Washington, DC: American Society for Microbiology; 1981:266-268.

138. Beaman TC, Gerhardt P. Heat resistance of bacterial spores correlated with protoplast dehydration, mineralization, and thermal adaptation. *Appl Environ Microbiol.* 1986;52:1242-1246.

139. Graham GS, Boris CA. Chemical and biological indicators. In: *Sterilization Technology: A Practical Guide for Manufacturers and Users of Health Care Products.* New York, NY: Van Nostrand Rheinhold; 1993:36-39.

140. Penna TCV, Machoshvili IA, Taqueda MES, Ferraz CAM. *Bacillus stearothermophilus* sporulation response to different composition media. *PDA J Pharm Sci Technol.* 1998;52(5):198-208.

141. Penna TCV, Machoshvili IA, Taqueda MES, Ishii M. The effect of media composition on the thermal resistance of *Bacillus stearothermophilus. PDA J Pharm Sci Technol.* 2000;54(5):398-412.

142. Cazemier AE, Wagenaars SFM, ter Steeg PF. Effect of sporulation and recovery medium on the heat resistance and amount of injury of spores from spoilage bacilli. *J Appl Microbiol.* 2001;90:761-770.

143. Gould GW. Modification of resistance and dormancy. In: Dring GJ, Ellar DJ, Gould GW, eds. *Fundamental and Applied Aspects of Bacterial Spores.* London, United Kingdom: Academic Press; 1985:371-382.

144. Lindsay JA, Murrell WG, Warth AD. Spore resistance and the basic mechanisms of spore heat resistance. In: Harris LE, ed. *Sterilization of Medical Products.* Vol 3. Sydney, Australia: Lindsay-Yates; 1985: 162-183.

145. Finocchario CJ. The use of biological indicators as an affirmation of sterilization process effectiveness. Part 2. *Pharm Eng.* 1993;13:42-44.

146. Spicher G, Peters J, Borchers U. Superheating of germ carriers falsifies the steam resistance of biological indicators [in German]. *Zentralbl Hyg Umweltmed.* 1993;194:369-370.

147. Pflug IJ. *Microbiology and Engineering of Sterilization Processes.* 10th ed. Minneapolis, MN: Environmental Sterilization Laboratory, University of Minnesota; 1999.

148. McCormick PJ. Biological indicators. *Infect Control Hosp Epidemiol.* 1988;9(11):504-507.

149. Mallidis CG, Scholefield J. Evaluation of recovery media for heated spores of *Bacillus stearothermophilus. J Appl Bacteriol.* 1986;61:517-523.

150. Pflug IJ, Smith GM, Christensen R. Effect of soybean casein digest agar lot on number of *Bacillus stearothermophilus* spores recovered. *Appl Environ Microbiol.* 1981;42(2):226-230.

151. Shintani H, Sasaki K, Kajiwara Y, Itoh J, Takahashi M, Kokubo M. Validation of D value by different SCD culture medium manufacturer and/or different SCD culture medium constituent. *PDA J Pharm Sci Technol.* 2000;54(1):6-12.

152. Kaiser JJ, inventor; Getinge/Castle, Inc, assignee. Culture medium containing glycerol that are pH and color stable when heat sterilized. US patent 5,968,807. October 19, 1999.

153. Agalloco J, McCauley K, Gillis JR. Innovation in biological indicator evaluator resistometer vessel technology. *Pharm Technol.* 2007;31: 58-65.

154. International Organization for Standardization. *ISO 18472:2006: Sterilization of Health Care Products—Biological and Chemical Indicators-Test Equipment.* Geneva, Switzerland: International Organization for Standardization; 2006.

155. Oxborrow GS, Twohy CW, Demetrius CA. Determining the variability of BIER Vessels. *Medical Device Diagnostic Industry.* 1990;12(5):78-83.

156. Mosley GA, Gillis JR. Operating precision of steam BIER vessels and the interactive effects of varying Z values on the reproducibility of listed D values. *PDA J Pharm Sci Technol.* 2002;56(6):318-331.

157. Pflug IJ. Variability in the data generated by laboratories measuring D-values of bacterial spores. *PDA J Pharm Sci Technol.* 2005;59(1):3-9.

158. McCormick PJ, Schoene MJ, Pedeville D, Kaiser JJ, Conyer J. Verification testing of biological indicators for moist heat sterilization. *Biomed Instrum Technol.* 2018;52:199-207.

159. Stetter KO. Extremophiles and their adaptation to hot environments. *FEBS Lett.* 1999;452(1-2):22-25.

160. Müller H, Stitz L, Wille H, Prusiner S, Riesner D. Influence of water, fat, and glycerol on the mechanism of thermal prion inactivation. *J Biol Chem.* 2007;282:35855-35867.

161. McDonnell GE, Dehen C, Perrin A, et al. Cleaning, disinfection and sterilization of surface prion contamination. *J Hosp Infect.* 2013;85(4):268-273.

162. Setlow P. Spores of *Bacillus subtilis*: their resistance to and killing by radiation, heat and chemicals. *J Appl Microbiol.* 2006;101:514-525.

163. Gerhardt P, Marquis RE. Spore thermoresistance mechanisms. In: Smith I, Slepecky RA, Setlow P, eds. *Regulation of Prokaryotic Development.* Washington, DC: American Society for Microbiology; 1989:43-63.

164. Setlow P. I will survive: protecting and repairing spore DNA. *J Bacteriol.* 1992;174(9):2737-2741.

165. Moeller R, Schuerger AC, Reitz G, Nicholson WL. Protective role of spore structural components in determining *Bacillus subtilis* spore resistance to simulated Mars surface conditions. *Appl Environ Microbiol.* 2012;78(24):8849-8853.

166. Lund PA. Microbial molecular chaperones. *Adv Microb Physiol.* 2001;44:93-140.

167. Maleki F, Khosravi A, Nasser A, Taghinejad H, Azizian M. Bacterial heat shock protein activity. *J Clin Diagn Res.* 2016;10(3):BE01-BE03.

168. Melly E, Setlow P. Heat shock proteins do not influence wet heat resistance of *Bacillus subtilis* spores. *J Bacteriol.* 2001;183(2):779-784.

169. del Carmen Huesca Espitia L, Caley C, Bagyan I, Setlow P. Base-change mutations induced by various treatments of *Bacillus subtilis* spores with and without protective small, acid-soluble spore proteins. *Mutat Res.* 2002;503(1-2):77-84.

170. Teixeira P, Castro H, Mohácsi-Farkas C, Kirby R. Identification of sites of injury in *Lactobacillus bulgaricus* during heat stress. *J Appl Microbiol.* 1997;83:219-226.

171. Markova N, Slavchev G, Michallova L, Jourdanova M. Survival of *Escherichia coli* under lethal heat stress by L-form conversion. *Int J Biol Sci.* 2010;6:303-315.

172. Nguyen HTT, Corry JEL, Miles CA. Heat resistance and mechanism of heat inactivation in thermophilic Campylobacters. *Appl Environ Microbiol.* 2006;72(1):908-913.

173. Kadota H, Uchida A, Sako Y, Harada K. Heat-induced DNA injury in spores and vegetative cells of *Bacillus subtilis.* In: Chamblis G, Vary JC, eds. *Spores III.* Washington, DC: American Society for Microbiology; 1978:27-50.

174. Andrews MHE, Greaves JP. Production of single strand breaks in the DNA of *Streptococcus faecalis* after mild heating. *J Gen Microbiol.* 1979;111:239-242.

175. Russell AD. Lethal effects of heat on bacterial physiology and structure. *Sci Prog.* 2003;86(pt 1-2):115-137.

176. Brock TD. Life at high temperatures. Evolutionary, ecological, and biochemical significance of organisms living in hot springs is discussed. *Science.* 1967;158(3804):1012-1019.

177. Lonsdale P. Clustering of suspension-feeding macrobenthos near abysmal hydrothermal vents at oceanic spreading centers. *Deep-Sea Res.* 1977;24(9):857-863.

178. Takai K, Nakamura K, Toki T, et al. Cell proliferation at 122°C and isotopically heavy CH_4 production by a hyperthermophilic methanogen under high-pressure cultivation. *Proc Natl Acad Sci U S A.* 2008;105(31):10949-10954.

179. Cusick KD, Lin B, Malanoski AP, et al. Molecular mechanisms contributing to the growth and physiology of an extremophile cultured with dielectric heating. *Appl Environ Microbiol.* 2016;82(20):6233-6246.

180. Koga Y. Thermal adaptation of the Archaeal and bacterial lipid membranes. Hindawi Web site. https://www.hindawi.com/journals/archaea/2012/789652/. Accessed December 20, 2017.

181. Oger PM, Cario A. Adaptation of the membrane in *Archaea. Biophys Chem.* 2013;183:42-56.

182. Nakasu S, Kikuchi A. Reverse gyrase; ATP-dependent type I topoisomerase from *Sulfolobus. EMBO J.* 1985;4:2705-2710.

183. La Duc MT, Dekas A, Osman S, Moissl C, Newcombe D, Venkateswaran K. Isolation and characterization of bacteria capable of tolerating the extreme conditions of clean room environments. *Appl Environ Microbiol.* 2007;73(8):2600-2611.

184. Williams KL. Depyrogenation validation, pyroburden, and endotoxin removal. In: Williams KL., ed. *Endotoxins: Pyrogens, LAL Testing and Depyrogenation.* 3rd ed. New York, NY: Informa Healthcare; 2007:301-303.

FURTHER READING

Abraham G, Debray E, Candau Y, Piar G. Mathematical model of thermal destruction of *Bacillus stearothermophilus* spores. *Appl Environ Microbiol.* 1990;56:3073-3080.

Adams DM. Heat injury of bacterial spores. *Adv Appl Microbiol.* 1978;23: 245-261.

Alderton G, Ito KA, Chen JK. Chemical manipulation of the heat resistance of *Clostridium botulinum* spores. *Appl Environ Microbiol.* 1976;31:492-498.

Alderton G, Snell N. Base exchange and heat resistance in bacterial spores. *Biochem Biophys Res Commun.* 1963;10:139-143.

Alderton G, Snell N. Bacterial spores: chemical sensitization to heat. *Science.* 1969;163:1212-1213.

Alderton G, Snell N. Chemical states of bacterial spores: dry-heat resistance. *Appl Microbiol.* 1969;17:745-749.

Alderton G, Snell N. Chemical states of bacterial spores: heat resistance and its kinetics at intermediate water activity. *Appl Microbiol.* 1970;19:565-572.

Alderton G, Thompson PA, Snell N. Heat adaptation and ion exchange in *Bacillus megaterium* spores. *Science.* 1964;143:141-143.

Alpin SJ, Hodges NA. Changes in heat resistance during storage of *Bacillus stearothermophilus* spores from complex and chemically defined media. *J Appl Bacteriol.* 1979;46:623-626.

Amaha M, Ordal ZJ. Effect of divalent cations in the sporulation medium on the thermal death rate of *Bacillus coagulans* var. *thermoacidurans*. *J Bacteriol.* 1957;74:596-604.

Amaha M, Sakaguchi K. Effects of carbohydrates, proteins, and bacterial cells in the heating media on the heat resistance of *Clostridium sporogenes. J Bacteriol.* 1954;68:338-345.

Andersen AA, Michener HD. Preservation of foods with antibiotics: 1. The complementary action of subtilin and mild heat. *Food Technol.* 1950;4:188-189.

Anderson EB, Meanwell U. Studies in bacteriology of low temperature pasteurization: part II. The heat resistance of a thermoduric streptococcus grown at different temperatures. *J Dairy Res.* 1936;7:182-191.

Anderson TE. *Some Factors Affecting the Thermal Resistance Values of Bacterial Spores as Determined With a Thermoresistometer* [master's thesis]. East Lansing, MI: Michigan State University; 1959.

Ando Y, Tsuzuki T. Mechanisms of chemical manipulation of the heat resistance of *Clostridium perfringens* spores. *J Appl Bacteriol.* 1983;54:197-202.

Anellis A, Lubas J, Rayman MM. Heat resistance in liquid eggs of some strains of the genus *Salmonella. Food Res.* 1954;19:377-395.

Angelotti R, Maryanski JH, Butler TF, Peeler JT, Campbell JE. Influence of spore moisture content on the dry-heat resistance of *Bacillus subtilis* var. *niger. Appl Microbiol.* 1968;16:735-745.

Aref H, Cruess WV. An investigation of thermal death point of *Saccharomyces ellipsoideus. J Bacteriol.* 1934;27:443-452.

Armitage P, Allen I. Methods of estimating LD 50 in quantal response data. *J Hyg (Lond).* 1950;48:298-322.

Augustin JAL. *Recovery Patterns of Putrefactive Anaerobe No. 3679 in Various Subculture Media Following Moist and Dry-heat Treatment* [dissertation]. East Lansing, MI: Michigan State University; 1964.

Ball CO. Thermal process time for canned food. *Bull Natl Res Counc.* 1923;7(pt 1, 37):1-76.

Ball CO, Olson FCW. *Sterilization in Food Technology.* New York, NY: McGraw-Hill; 1957.

Bartlett CJ, Kline F. Resistance of microorganisms suspended in glycerine or oil to the sterilizing action of heat. *Science.* 1913;38:372 (N.S.).

Beaman TC, Pankratz HS, Gerhardt P. Heat shock affects permeability and resistance of *Bacillus stearothermophilus* spores. *Appl Environ Microbiol.* 1988;54:2515-2520.

Beamer PR, Tanner FW. Heat resistance studies on selected yeasts. *Zentralblatt für Bakteriologie Parasitenk II.* 1939;100:202-211.

Bender GR, Marquis RE. Spore heat resistance and specific mineralization. *Appl Environ Microbiol.* 1985;50:1414-1421.

Bond WW, Favero MS, Korber MR. *Bacillus* sp. ATCC 27380: a spore with extreme resistance to dry heat. *Appl Microbiol.* 1973;26:614-616.

Bond WW, Favero MS, Petersen NJ, Marshall JH. Dry-heat inactivation kinetics of naturally occurring spore populations. *Appl Microbiol.* 1970;20:573-578.

Bond WW, Favero MS, Petersen NJ, Marshall JH. Relative frequency distribution of $D_{125\,C}$ values for spore isolates from the Mariner-Mars 1969 spacecraft. *Appl Microbiol.* 1971;21:832-836.

Brannen JP. A rational model for thermal sterilization of microorganisms. *Math Biosci.* 1968;2:165-170.

Brannen JP. On logarithmic extrapolation of microbial survivor curves for planetary quarantine requirements. *Space Life Sci.* 1968;1:150-152.

Brannen JP, Garst DM. Dry heat inactivation of *Bacillus subtilis* var. *niger* spores as a function of relative humidity. *Appl Microbiol.* 1972;23:1125-1130.

Bréand S, Fardel G, Flandrois JP, Rosso L, Tomassone R. Model of the influence of time and mild temperature on *Listeria monocytogenes* nonlinear survival curves. *Int J Food Microbiol.* 1998;40:185-195.

Brown B. Some properties of the Spearman estimator in bioassay. *Biometrika.* 1961;48(3/4):293-302.

Brown KL. Spore resistance and ultra heat treatment processes. *Soc Appl Bacteriol Symp Ser.* 1994;23:67S-80S.

Brown KL, Gaze JE, McClement RH, et al. Construction of a computer controlled thermoresistometer for the determination of the heat resistance of bacterial spores over the temperature range 100 to 150°C. *Int J Food Sci and Technol.* 1988;23:361-371.

Bruch CW. Dry-heat sterilization for planetary-impacting spacecraft. In: *Proceedings of the National Conference on Spacecraft Sterilization Technology.* Washington, DC: National Aeronautics and Space Administration; 1966:207-230.

Bruch MK, Smith FW. Dry heat resistance of spores of *Bacillus subtilis* var. *niger* on Kapton and Teflon film at high temperatures. *Appl Microbiol.* 1968;16:1841-1846.

Busta FF, Foegeding PM, Adams DM. Injury and resuscitation of germination and outgrowth of bacterial spores. In: Levinson HL, Sonenhein AL, Tipper DJ, eds. *Sporulation and Germination.* Washington, DC: American Society for Microbiology; 1981:261-265.

Cameron MS, Leonard SJ, Barrett EL. Effect of moderately acidic pH on heat resistance and recovery of *Clostridium sporogenes* spores in phosphate buffer and buffered pea puree. *Appl Environ Microbiol.* 1980;39:943-949.

Campbell JE. *Eighteenth Quarterly Report of Progress. Ecology and Thermal Inactivation of Microbes in and on Interplanetary Space Vehicle Components.* Washington, DC: National Aeronautics and Space Administration; 1969. National Aeronautics and Space Administration research project R-R-36-015-001.

Campbell JE. *Thirty-Seventh Quarterly Report of Progress. Ecology and Thermal Inactivation of Microbes in and on Interplanetary Space Vehicle Components.* Washington, DC: National Aeronautics and Space Administration; 1974. National Aeronautics and Space Administration order no. W-13411.

Campbell LL Jr, O'Brien RT. Antibiotics in food preservation. *Food Technol.* 1955;9:461.

Campbell LL Jr, Sniff EE. Effect of subtilin and nisin on the spores of *Bacillus coagulans. J Bacteriol.* 1959;77:766-770.

Casolari A. A model describing microbial inactivation and growth kinetics. *J Theor Biol.* 1981;88:1-34.

Cerf O, Davey KR, Sadoudi AK. Thermal inactivation of bacteria—a new predictive model for the combined effect of three environmental factors: temperature, pH and water activity. *Food Res Int.* 1996;29:219-226.

Chapman PA, Pflug IJ. Effect of the biological indicator envelope on the heat destruction rate of *Bacillus stearothermophilus* spores. *Bacteriol Proc.* 1973;73:E144.

Charm SE. The kinetics of bacterial inactivation by heat. *Food Technol.* 1958;12:4-8.

Cochran WG. Estimation of bacterial densities by means of the "the most probable number." *Biometrics.* 1950;6:105-116.

Cole MB, Davies KW, Munro G, et al. A vitalistic model to describe the thermal inactivation of *Listeria monocytogenes. J Industrial Microbiol.* 1993;12:232-239.

Cole MB, Jones MV. A submerged-coil heating apparatus for investigating thermal inactivation of micro-organisms. *Lett Appl Microbiol.* 1990;11:233-235.

Cook AM, Gilbert RJ. The effect of storage conditions on the heat resistance and heat activation response of *Bacillus stearothermophilus* spores. *J Pharm Pharmacol.* 1968;20:626-629.

Curran HR. The influence of some environmental factors upon thermal resistance of bacterial spores. *J Bacteriol.* 1934;27:26.

Curran HR. The influence of some environmental factors upon the thermal resistance of bacterial spores. *J Infect Dis.* 1935;56:196-202.

Czechowicz SM. *Effect of Storage Time on the Characteristics of Bacillus stearothermophilus Spores Suspended in Phosphate Buffers and Water* [master's thesis]. Minneapolis, MN: University of Minnesota; 1992.

Davey KR, Lin SH, Wood DG. The effect of pH on continuous high temperature/short time sterilization of liquid food. *Am Inst Chem Eng J.* 1978;24:537-540.

David J, Merson RL. Kinetic parameters for inactivation of *Bacillus stearothermophilus* at high temperatures. *J Food Science.* 1990;55:488-493, 515.

Delves-Broughton J. Nisin and its use as a food preservative. *Food Technol.* 1990;44:100-112.

Denny CB, Reed JM, Bohoer CW. Effect of tylosin and heat on spoilage bacteria in canned corn and canned mushrooms. *Food Technol.* 1961;15: 338-340.

Denny CB, Sharpe LE, Bohrer CW. Effect of tylosin and nisin on canned food spoilage bacteria. *Appl Microbiol.* 1961;9:108-110.

Dickson EC, Burke GS, Beck D, et al. Studies on thermal death time of spores of *Clostridium botulinum. J Infect Dis.* 1925;36:472-483.

Doyle MP, Marth EH. Thermal inactivation of conidia from *Aspergillus flavus* and *Aspergillus parasiticus. J Milk Food Technol.* 1975;38: 678-682.

Dring GJ, Ellar DJ, Gould GW, eds. *Fundamental and Applied Aspects of Bacterial Spores.* London, United Kingdom: Academic Press; 1985.

Drummond DW. *Effects of Humidity, Location, Surface Finish, and Separator Thickness on the Dry-heat Destruction of Bacillus subtilis var. niger Spores Located Between Mated Surfaces* [dissertation]. Minneapolis, MN: Division of Environmental Health, University of Minnesota; 1972.

Drummond DW, Pflug IJ. Dry-heat destruction of *Bacillus subtilis* spores on surfaces: effect of humidity in an open system. *Appl Microbiol.* 1970;20:805-809.

El-Bisi HM, Ordal ZJ. The effect of certain sporulation conditions on the thermal death rate of *Bacillus coagulans* var. *thermoacidurans. J Bacteriol.* 1956;71:1-9.

El-Bisi HM, Ordal ZJ. The effect of sporulation temperature on the thermal resistance of *Bacillus coagulans* var. *thermoacidurans. J Bacteriol.* 1956;71:10-16.

Ellicker PR, Frazier WC. Influence of time and temperature of incubation on heat resistance of *Escherichia coli. J Bacteriol.* 1938;36:83-98.

Esty JR, Meyer KF. The heat resistance of the spores of *B. botulinus* and allied anaerobes: XI. *J Infect Dis.* 1922;31:650-663.

Esty JR, Williams CC. Heat resistance of bacterial spores. *J Infect Dis.* 1924;34:518-528.

Eyring H. The activated complex and the absolute rate of chemical reactions. *Chem Rev.* 1935;17:65-77.

Farkas J. Tolerance of spores to ionizing radiation: mechanisms of inactivation, injury and repair. *Soc Appl Bacteriol Symp Ser.* 1994;23: 81S-90S.

Fernández PS, Ocio MJ, Rodrigo F, Rodrigo M, Martínez A. Mathematical model for the combined effect of temperature and pH on the thermal resistance of *Bacillus stearothermophilus* and *Clostridium sporogenes* spores. *Int J Food Microbiol.* 1996;32:225-233.

Fischer DA, Pflug IJ. Effect of combined heat and radiation on microbial destruction. *Appl Environ Microbiol.* 1977;33:1170-1176.

Foegeding PM, Ray B. Repair and detection of injured microorganisms. In: Vanderzant C, Splittstoesser DF, eds. *Compendium of Methods for the Microbiological Examination of Foods.* Washington, DC: American Public Health Association; 1992:121-134.

Fox K, Pflug IJ. Effect of temperature and gas velocity on the dry-heat destruction rate of bacterial spores. *Appl Microbiol.* 1968;16:343-348.

Frederickson AG. Stochastic models for sterilization. *Biotechnol Bioeng.* 1966;8:167-182.

Fujikawa H, Itoh T. Thermal inactivation analysis of mesophiles using the Arrhenius and z-value models. *J Food Prot.* 1998;61:910-912.

Garst DM, Lindell KF. *A Precisely Controlled, Low Range Humidity System.* Albuquerque, NM: Sandia Laboratories; 1970. National Aeronautics and Space Administration contract no. W-12853. Report SC-RR-70-775.

Gay FP, Atkins KN, Holden M. The resistance of dehydrated pneumococci to chemicals and heat. *J Bacteriol.* 1931;22:295-307.

Gerhardt P, Murrell WG. Basis and mechanism of spore resistance: a brief preview. In: Chambliss G, Vary JC, eds. *Spores VII.* Washington, DC: American Society for Microbiology; 1978:18-20.

Gibbs BM, Hurst A. Limitations of nisin as a preservative in non-dairy food. In: *Proceedings of the 4th International Symposium on Food Microbiology.* Göteburg, Sweden: Swedish Institute for Food and Biotechnology; 1964:151-165.

Gillespy TG. Studies on the mould *Byssochlamys fulva*: progress report. In: *Annual Report on Fruit and Vegetable Preservation Standards.* London, United Kingdom: Campden; 1937:68-75.

Gillespy TG. The heat resistance of the spores of thermophilic bacteria: II. Thermophilic anaerobes. In: *Annual Report on Fruit and Vegetable Preservation Standards.* London, United Kingdom: Campden; 1947:40-54.

Gillespy TG. The heat resistance of spores of thermophilic bacteria: III. Thermophilic anaerobes (con't). In: *Annual Report on Fruit and Vegetable Preservation Standards.* London, United Kingdom: Campden; 1948:34-43.

Görtzen S. Untersuchungen über die Widerstandsfähigkeit nativer anaerober Erdsporen gegen Siedehitze. *Zentralblatt für Bakteriologie Parasitenk 1 Orig.* 1937;138:227-241.

Gombas DE. Bacterial spore resistance to heat. *Food Technol.* 1983;37: 105-110.

Gould GW. Effect of food preservatives on the growth of bacteria from spores. In: *Proceedings of the 4th International Symposium on Food Microbiology.* Göteburg, Sweden: Swedish Institute for Food and Biotechnology; 1964:17-23.

Gould GW, Dring GJ. Heat resistance of bacterial endospores and concept of an expanded osmoregulatory cortex. *Nature.* 1975;258:402-405.

Gould GW, Russell AD, Stewart-Tull DES. Fundamental and applied aspects of bacterial spores. In: *The Society for Applied Bacteriology Symposium Series No. 23.* Oxford, United Kingdom: Blackwell Scientific Publications; 1994.

Greenberg RA, Silliker JH. The action of tylosin on spore-forming bacteria. *J Food Science.* 1962;27:64-68.

Greenberg RA, Silliker JH. Spoilage patterns in *Clostridium botulinum* inoculated canned foods treated with tylosin. In: *Proceedings of the 4th International Symposium on Food Microbiology.* Göteburg, Sweden: Swedish Institute for Food and Biotechnology; 1964:97-103.

Hansen NH, Reiman H. Factors affecting the heat resistance of nonsporing organisms. *J Appl Bacteriol.* 1963;26:314-333.

Härnulv BG, Snygg BG. Heat resistance of *Bacillus subtilis* spores at various water activities. *J Appl Bacteriol.* 1972;35:615-624.

Hawley HB. Nisin in food technology. *Food Manufacturing.* 1957;32: 370-373, 430-434.

Heinemann R, Stumbo CR, Scuolock A. Use of nisin in preparing beverage-quality sterile chocolate-flavored milk. *J Dairy Science.* 1964;47:8-12.

Hirsch A. Antibiotics in food preservation. *Proceedings Soc Appl Bacteriol.* 1953;16:100-106.

Hoffman RK, Gambill VM, Buchanan LM. Effect of cell moisture on the thermal inactivation rate of bacterial spores. *Appl Microbiol.* 1968;16:1240-1244.

Holdsworth SD. *Thermal Processing of Packaged Foods.* London, United Kingdom: Blackie Academic and Professional; 1997.

Hurst A. Injury. In: Hurst A, Gould GW, eds. *The Bacterial Spore 2.* London, United Kingdom: Academic Press; 1983:255-274.

Hurst A, Gould GW, eds. *The Bacterial Spore 2.* London, United Kingdom: Academic Press; 1983.

Ingram M. Sporeformers as food spoilage organisms. In: Gould GW, Hurst A, eds. *The Bacterial Spore.* London, United Kingdom: Academic Press; 1969.

Jacobson RL, Pflug IJ. Dry-heat destruction of bacterial spores: a study of destruction rates at low levels of water at 90, 110, and 125°C. In: *Progress Report No. 9: Environmental Microbiology as Related to Planetary Quarantine.* Minneapolis, MN: University of Minnesota; 1972:19-31.

Jaynes JAI, Pflug IJ, Harmon LG. Some factors affecting the heating and cooling lags of processed cheese in thermal death time cans. *J Dairy Science.* 1961;44:2171-2175.

Jensen LB. *Microbiology of Meat.* 3rd ed. Champaign, IL: Gerrard Press; 1954:273-274.

Johnson E, Brown B. The spearman estimator for serial dilution assays. *Biometrics.* 1961;17:79-88.

Jonsson UB, Snygg G, Harnulv G, et al. Testing two models for the temperature dependence of the heat inactivation rate of *Bacillus stearothermophilus* spores. *J Food Sci.* 1977;42:1251-1252.

Kaufmann OW, Andrews RH. The destruction rate of psychrophilic bacteria in skim milk. *J Dairy Sci.* 1954;37:317-327.

Koesterer MG. *Sterilization of Space Probe Components.* Washington, DC: National Aeronautics and Space Administration; 1962. Final report of contract NASr-31.

Koesterer MG. *Studies for Sterilization of Space Probe Components.* Rochester, NY: Wilmot Castle Co; 1965. National Aeronautics and Space Administration contract no. NASW-879.

Kooiman WJ, Geers JM. Simple and accurate technique for the determination of heat resistance of bacterial spores. *J Appl Bacteriol.* 1975;38: 185-189.

Lamanna C. Relation of maximum growth temperature to resistance to heat. *J Bacteriol.* 1942;44:29-35.

Lang OW. Thermal processes for canned marine products. *University of California Public Health.* 1935;2:1-175.

Lang OW, Dean SJ. Heat resistance of *Clostridium botulinum* in canned sea foods. *J Infect Dis.* 1934;55:39-59.

Lechowich RV, Ordal ZJ. The influence of the sporulation temperature on the heat resistance and chemical composition of bacterial spores. *Can J Microbiol.* 1962;8:287-295.

Levine AS, Fellers CR. Action of acetic acid on food spoilage microorganisms. *J Bacteriol.* 1940;39:499-515.

Levine M, Buchanan JH, Lease G. Effect of concentration and temperature on germicidal efficiency of sodium hydroxide. *Iowa State Coll J Sci.* 1927;1:379.

Lewis JC. The estimation of decimal reduction times. *Appl Microbiol.* 1956;4:211-221.

Lewis JC, Michener HD, Stumbo CR, et al. Additives accelerating death of spores by moist heat. *J Agri Food Chem.* 1954;2:298-302.

López M, González I, Condón S, Bernardo A. Effect on pH heating medium on the thermal resistance of *Bacillus stearothermophilus* spores. *Int J Food Microbiol.* 1996;28:405-410.

Mackey BM, Derrick CM. Changes in heat resistance of *Salmonella typhimurium* during heating at rising temperatures. *Lett Appl Microbiol.* 1987;4:13-16.

Mafart P, Leguerinel I. Modeling combined effects of temperature and pH on heat resistance of spores by a linear-Bigelow equation. *J Food Sci.* 1998;63:6-8.

Malin B, Greenberg RA. The effect of tylosin on spoilage patterns of inoculated and non-inoculated cream style corn. In: *Proceedings of the 4th International Symposium on Food Microbiology.* Göteburg, Sweden: Swedish Institute for Food and Biotechnology; 1964:87-95.

Marquis RE, Sim J, Shin SY. Molecular mechanisms of resistance to heat and oxidative damage. *Soc Appl Bacteriol Symp Ser.* 1994;23:40S-48S.

Marshall BJ, Murrell WG, Scott WJ. The effect of water activity, solutes, and temperature on the viability and heat resistance of freeze-dried bacterial spores. *J Gen Microbiol.* 1963;31:451-460.

Mayou JL, Jezeski H. Effect of sporulation media on the heat resistance of *Bacillus stearothermophilus* spores. *J Food Protect.* 1977;40:232-233.

Mazzotta A, Montville TJ. Characterization of fatty acid composition, spore germination, and thermal resistance in a nisin-resistant mutant of *Clostridium botulinum* 169B and in the wild-type strain. *Appl Environ Microbiol.* 1999;65:659-664.

Michels MJM, Visser FMW. Occurrence and thermoresistance of spores of psychrophilic and psychrotrophic aerobic sporeformers in soil and foods. *J Appl Bacteriol.* 1976;41:1-11.

Moats WA, Dabbadh R, Edwards WM. Interpretation of non-logarithmic survivor-curves of heated bacteria. *J Food Sci.* 1971;36:523-526.

Moore B, Pflug IJ, Haugen J. Dry-heat destruction rates of *B. subtilis* var. *niger* in a closed system. In: *Progress Report No. 3: Environmental Microbiology as Related to Planetary Quarantine.* Minneapolis, MN: University of Minnesota; 1969. National Aeronautics and Space Administration grant NGL 24-005-160.

Mudd S, Mudd EH. The penetration of bacteria through capillary spaces: IV. A kinetic mechanism in interfaces. *J Exp Med.* 1924;40:633-645.

Mullican CL, Hoffman RK. Dry heat or gaseous chemical resistance of *Bacillus subtilis* var. *niger* spores included within water-soluble crystals. *Appl Microbiol.* 1968;16:1110-1113.

Murrell WG, Scott WJ. Heat resistance of bacterial spores at various water activities. *Nature.* 1957;179:481-482.

Nank WK, Schmidt CF. The effect of the addition of manganese to a nutrient agar sporulation medium upon the resistance of thermophilic flat sour spore crops. *Bacteriol Proc.* 1958;42.

National Aeronautics and Space Administration. *NASA Standard Procedures for the Microbiological Examination of Space Hardware.* Washington, DC: Government Printing Office; 1968. National Aeronautics and Space Administration document no. NHB5340.1A.

National Aeronautics and Space Administration. *Planetary Quarantine Provisions for Unmanned Planetary Missions.* Washington, DC: Government Printing Office; 1969. National Aeronautics and Space Administration document no. NHB8020.12.

Nichols AA. The effect of variations in the fat percentage and in the reaction (pH) of milk media on the heat resistance of certain milk bacteria. *J Dairy Sci.* 1940;11:274-291.

Odlaug TE, Pflug IJ. Thermal destruction of *Clostridium botulinum* spores suspended in tomato juice in aluminum thermal death time tubes. *Appl Environ Microbiol.* 1977;34:23-29.

Palop A, Sala FJ, Condon S. Heat resistance of acid and demineralized spores of *Bacillus subtilis* sporulated at different temperatures. *Appl Environ Microbiol.* 1999;65:1316-1319.

Peeler JT, Reyes AL, Crawford RG. Thermal resistance of *Bacillus subtilis* var. *niger* in a closed system. *Appl Environ Microbiol.* 1977;33:52-57.

Pflug IJ. Dry-heat destruction rates for microorganisms on open surfaces, in mated surface areas and encapsulated in solids of spacecraft hardware. In: *Life Sciences and Space Research; VII.* Amsterdam, Netherlands: North-Holland Publishing; 1970:63-84.

Pflug IJ. Using the straight-line semilogarithmic microbial destruction model as an engineering design model for determining the F-value for heat processes. *J Food Protect.* 1987;50:342-346.

Pflug IJ. Collecting wet-heat microbial-destruction data using a miniature retort system: operation, temperature calibration, lag correction factors, and minimum heating times. In: Pflug IJ, ed. *Selected Papers on the Microbiology and Engineering of Sterilization Processes.* Minneapolis, MN: Environmental Sterilization Laboratory, University of Minnesota; 1988:125-142.

Pflug IJ. Biologically validating the sterilization process delivered to particles in a heat-hold-cool system. In: *Proceedings at the 1st International Congress on Aseptic Processing Technologies.* Lafayette, IN: Department of Food Science and Nutrition, Purdue University; 1989:88-104.

Pflug IJ. *Microbiology and Engineering of Sterilization Processes.* 8th ed. Minneapolis, MN: Environmental Sterilization Laboratory, University of Minnesota; 1995.

Pflug IJ. Discussion of the Z-value to use in calculating the F0-value for high-temperature sterilization processes. *PDA J Pharm Sci Technol.* 1996;50:51-54.

Pflug IJ, Augustin JAL. Dry-heat destruction of microorganisms. In: *Progress Report on Project 830.* East Lansing, MI: Food Science Department, Michigan State University; 1962.

Pflug IJ, Esselen WB. Development and application of apparatus for study of thermal resistance of bacterial spores and thiamine at temperatures above 250°F. *Food Technol.* 1953;7:237-241.

Pflug IJ, Esselen WB. Observations on the thermal resistance of putrefactive anaerobe no. 3679 spores in the temperature range of 250–300°F. *J Food Sci.* 1954;19:92-97.

Pflug IJ, Esselen WB. Heat transfer into open metal thermoresistometer cups. *Food Res.* 1955;20:237-246.

Pflug IJ, Gould GW. Heat treatment. In: Lund BM, Baird-Parker TC, Gould GW, eds. *The Microbiological Safety and Quality of Food.* Vol 1. Gaithersburg, MD: Aspen Publishers; 2000:36-64.

Pflug IJ, Holcomb RG. The use of bacterial spores as sterilization process monitoring devices: a discussion of what they can do and some of their limitations. In: *Proceedings of the 3rd PMA Seminar Program on Validation of Sterile Manufacturing Processes: Biological Indicators.* Washington, DC: Pharmaceutical Manufacturers Association; 1980:153-204.

Pflug IJ, Schmidt CF. Thermal destruction of microorganisms. In: Lawrence CA, Block SS, eds. *Disinfection, Sterilization, and Preservation.* Philadelphia, PA: Lea & Febiger; 1968:63-105.

Pflug IJ, Smith GM. Survivor curves of bacterial spores heated in parenteral solutions. In: Barker AN, Wolf J, Ellar DJ, et al, eds. *Spore Research.* Vol 2. London, United Kingdom: Academic Press; 1977:501-525.

Pflug IJ, Smith GM. The use of biological indicators for monitoring wet heat sterilization processes. In: Gaughran ERL, Kereluk K, eds. *Sterilization of Medical Products.* New Brunswick, NJ: Johnson & Johnson; 1977: 193-230.

Pheil CG, Pflug IJ. Effect of heating temperature on the thermal resistance of *Bacillus subtilis.* Paper presented at: *Institute of Food Technology Meeting Program;* May 1964; Washington, DC. Abstract 170.

Pilcher RW. *The Canned Food Reference Manual.* 3rd ed. New York, NY: American Can; 1947.

Poole G, Malin B. Some aspects of the action of tylosin on *Clostridium* species PA 3679. *J Food Science.* 1964;29:475-478.

Prokop A, Humphrey AE. Mechanism of thermal death of bacterial spores: electron-microscopic observations. *Folia Microbiol (Praha).* 1972;17:437-445.

Puleo JR, Favero MS, Oxborrow GS, Herring CM. Method for collecting naturally occurring airborne bacterial spores for determining their thermal resistance. *Appl Microbiol.* 1975;30:786-790.

Rahn O. Physical methods of sterilization of microorganisms. *Bacteriol Rev.* 1945;9:1-47.

Read RB Jr. Current status of instrumentation in milk and food research. *Am J Public Health Nations Health.* 1963;53:1579-1586.

Reed JM, Bohrer CW, Cameron EJ. Spore destruction rate studies on organisms of significance in the processing of canned foods. *Food Res.* 1951;16:383-408.

Reichart O. Modelling the destruction of *Escherichia coli* on the base of reaction kinetics. *Int J Food Microbiol.* 1994;23:449-465.

Reynolds H, Kaplan AM, Spencer FB, et al. Thermal destruction of Cameron's putrefactive anaerobe 3679 in food substrates. *Food Res.* 1952;17:153-167.

Robertson AH. Influence of age on the heat resistance of non-sporeforming bacteria. *J Bacteriol.* 1928;15:27.

Rodrigo M, Martinez A, Sanchez T, et al. Kinetics of *Clostridium sporogenes* PA3679 spore destruction using computer-controlled thermoresistometer. *J Food Sci.* 1993;58:649-652.

Sames T. Zur Kenntnis der bei höher Temperatur wachsenden Bakterien und Streptococcusarten. *Zeitschrift für Hyg Infektionsk.* 1900;33: 313-362.

Schalkowsky S, Wiederkehr R. Estimation of microbial survival in heat sterilization. In: Sneath PNA, ed. *Sterilization Techniques for Instruments and Materials as Applied to Space Research.* Paris, France: Murray Print; 1967:87-108. CO SPAR technical manual no. 4.

Schmidt CF. The effect of subculture media upon the apparent thermal resistance of spores of members of the genus *Bacillus. Bacteriol Proc.* 1955;40.

Schmidt CF. Thermal resistance of microorganisms. In: Reddish GF, ed. *Antiseptics, Disinfectants, Fungicides and Sterilization.* 2nd ed. Philadelphia, PA: Lea & Febiger; 1957:831-884.

Schmidt CF, Bock JH, Moberg JA. Thermal resistance determinations in steam using thermal death time retorts. *Food Res.* 1955;20:606-613.

Schmidt CF, Nank WK. Cultural factors influencing the thermal resistance of a strain of *Bacillus subtilis. Bacteriol Proc.* 1958;42:.

Segmiller JL, Xezones H, Hutchings U. The efficiency of nisin and tylosin lactate in selected heat sterilized products. *J Food Science.* 1965;30: 166-171.

Senhaji AF, Bimbenet JJ, LeMaguer M. Protection des microorganismes par les matiéres grasses au cours des traitements thermiques: 2 partie. *Industries Alimentaires et Agricoles.* 1976;93:13-20.

Senhaji AF, Loncin M. Protection des microorganismes par les matiéres grasses au cours des traitements thermiques: premiere partie. *Industries Alimentaires et Agricoles.* 1975;92:611-617.

Sherman JM, Albus WR. Physiological youth in bacteria. *J Bacteriol.* 1923;8:127-138.

Sherman JM, Cameron GM. Lethal environmental factors within the natural range of growth. *J Bacteriol.* 1934;27:341-348.

Shull JJ, Cargo GT, Ernst RR. Kinetics of heat activation and of thermal death of bacterial spores. *Appl Microbiol.* 1963;11:485-487.

Silverman GJ. *The Resistivity of Microorganisms to Inactivation by Dry Heat.* Cambridge, MA: Massachusetts Institute of Technology; 1968.

Simko GJ, Devlin JD, Wardle MD. Dry-heat resistance of *Bacillus subtilis* var. *niger* spores on mated surfaces. *Appl Microbiol.* 1971;22:491-495.

Skillinglaw CA, Levine M. Effects of acid and sugar on viability of *Escherichia coli* and *Eberthella typhosa. Food Res.* 1943;8:464-476.

Smith G, Kopelman M, Jones A, Pflug IJ. Effect of environmental conditions during heating on commercial spore strip performance. *Appl Environ Microbiol.* 1982;44:12-18.

Smith G, Pflug IJ, Gove R, et al. Survival of microbial spores under several temperature and humidity conditions. In: *Progress Report No. 6: Environmental Microbiology as Related to Planetary Quarantine.* Minneapolis, MN: University of Minnesota; 1971. National Aeronautics and Space Administration grant NGL 24-005-160.

Sobernheim G, Mündel O. Grundsätzliches zur Technik der Sterilisationsprüfung. *Zeitschrift für Hyg Infektionsk.* 1936;118:328-345.

Sobernheim G, Mündel O. Grundsätzliches zur Technik der Sterilisationsprüfung: II. Verhalten der Erdsporen bei der Dampfsterilisation. Ihre Eignung als Testsporen. *Zeitschrift für Hyg Infektionsk.* 1938;121:90-112.

Sognefest P, Benjamin HA. Heating lag in thermal death-time cans and tubes. *Food Res.* 1944;9:234-243.

Sognefest P, Hays GL, Wheaton E, et al. Effect of pH on thermal process requirements of canned food. *Food Res.* 1948;13:400-416.

Sommer EW. Heat resistance of the spores of *Clostridium botulinum. J Infect Dis.* 1930;46:85-114.

Stark CN, Stark P. The relative thermal death rates of young and mature bacterial cells. *J Bacteriol.* 1929;18:333-337.

Stern JA, Proctor BE. A micro-method and apparatus for the multiple determination of the rates of destruction of bacteria and bacterial spores subjected to heat. *Food Technol.* 1954;8:139-143.

Stevenson KE, Shafer BD. Bacterial spore resistance to hydrogen peroxide. *Food Technol.* 1983;37:111-114.

Stoforos N, Noronha J, Hendrickx M, Tobback P. A critical analysis of mathematical procedures for the evaluation and design of in-container thermal processes for foods. *Crit Rev Food Sci Nutr.* 1997;37:411-441.

Streips UN, Qoronfleh MW, Khoury PH, et al. Involvement of heat shock proteins in the heat resistance of *Bacillus subtilis* spores. In: *Program of Tenth International Spore Conference.* Woods Hole, MA: Marine Biological Laboratory; 1988:8.

Stumbo CR. A technique for studying resistance of bacterial spores to temperatures in the higher range. *Food Technol.* 1948;2:228-240.

Stumbo CR. Bacteriological considerations relating to process evaluation. *Food Technol.* 1948;2:115-132.

Stumbo CR, Gross CE, Viton C. Bacteriological studies relating to thermal processing of canned meats. *Food Res.* 1945;10:260.

Thuillot ML, Bossard J, Thomas G, et al. A propos de la thermorésistance de *S. aureus* dans l'huile. *Ann Inst Pasteur Lille.* 1968;19:153-157.

Townsend CT, Somers II, Lamb FC, et al. *A Laboratory Manual for the Canning Industry.* 2nd ed. Washington, DC: National Canners Association Research Laboratories; 1956:chap 4.

Townsend CT, Somers II, Lamb FC, et al. *A Laboratory Manual for the Canning Industry.* 2nd ed. Washington, DC: National Canners Association Research Laboratories; 1956:chap 6.

Townsend CT, Somers II, Lamb FC, et al. *A Laboratory Manual for the Canning Industry.* 2nd ed. Washington, DC: National Canners Association Research Laboratories; 1956:chap 7.

Townsend CT, Yee L, Mercer WA. Inhibition of the growth of *Clostridium botulinum* by acidification. *Food Res.* 1954;19:536-542.

Viljoen JA. Heat resistance studies: II. The protective effect of sodium chloride on bacterial spores heated in pea liquor. *J Infect Dis.* 1926;39:286-290.

Wang DI-C, Scharer J, Humphrey AE. Kinetics of death of bacterial spores at elevated temperatures. *Appl Microbiol.* 1964;12:451-454.

Weil R. Zur Biologie der Milzbrandbazillen. *Arch Hyg Bakteriol.* 1899;35: 355-408.

Wheaton E, Hays GL. Antibiotics and the control of spoilage in canned foods. *Food Technol.* 1964;18:549.

Wilder CJ, Nordan HC. A micromethod and apparatus for the determination of rates of destruction of bacterial spores subjected to heat and bactericidal agents. *Food Res.* 1957;22:462-467.

Williams CC, Merrill CM, Cameron EJ. Apparatus for determination of spore-destruction rates. *Food Res.* 1937;2:369.

Williams FT. Attempts to increase the heat resistance of bacterial spores. *J Bacteriol.* 1936;32:589-597.

Williams OB. The heat resistance of bacterial spores. *J Infect Dis.* 1929;44:421-465.

Withell ER. The significance of the variation in shape of time-survivor curves. *J Hyg (Lond).* 1942;42:124-132.

Xezones H, Hutchings U. Thermal resistance of *Clostridium botulinum* spores as affected by fundamental food components. *Food Technol.* 1965;19:113-115.

Yamazaki K, Kawai Y, Inoue N, Shinano H. Influence of sporulation medium and divalent ions on the heat resistance of *Alicyclobacillus acidoterrestris* spores. *Lett Appl Microbiol.* 1997;25:153-156.

Yesair J, Cameron EJ. Inhibitive effect of curing agents on anaerobic spores. *Canner.* 1942;94:89-92.

Yesair J, Cameron EJ, Bohrer CW. Comparative resistance of desiccated and wet micrococci heated under moist and dry conditions [abstract]. *J Bacteriol.* 1944;47:437-438.

Zakula R. Results on investigations of thermoresistance of some bacteria suspended in meat, lard, and tallow. In: *Proceedings of 15th European Meeting of Meat Research Workers.* Helsinki, Finland; 1969:226-232.

Zechman LG. *Heat Inactivation Kinetics of* Bacillus stearothermophilus *Spores* [dissertation]. Minneapolis, MN: University of Minnesota; 1989.

Zuccaro JB, Powers JJ, Morse RE, Mills WC. Thermal death times of yeast in oil and movement of yeast between the oil and water phases of French dressing. *Food Res.* 1951;16:30-38.

Acids and Alkalis

Md Ramim Tanver Rahman, Luyan Z. Ma, and Mohammad Shafiur Rahman

The word acid originates from the Latin word *acere* and essentially means to taste sour, associated with natural acidic solutions such as vinegar and lemon juice. A base, or alkali, is derived from Arabic *al-qali* that means roasting or ash because alkalis where originally sourced from burned plant material (eg, wood) ashes. In 1887, the Swedish scientist Svante Arrhenius claimed that in an aqueous (aq) solution, an acid produces hydrogen ions (H^+) (eg, $HCl[aq] \rightarrow H^+[aq] + Cl^-[aq]$) and a base produces hydroxide ions (OH^-) (eg, $NaOH[aq] \rightarrow Na^+[aq] + OH^-[aq]$). In 1923, the proton theory of acids and bases (ie, an acid is a proton, H^+ contributor, and a base is a proton, H^+ acceptor, eg, $HF + H_2O \leftrightarrow H_3O^+ + F^-$) was introduced by the Johannes Brønsted and Thomas Lowry. Gilbert Lewis, an American physical chemist, proposed the electron pair theory of *acids* and *bases*. He suggested that an acid accepts a pair of electrons, whereas a base donates a pair of electrons (eg, $NH_3 + H^+ \rightarrow NH_4^+$).

Figure 12.1 shows the effect of acid and base in water. Generally, acid reacts with metals, metal oxides, metal hydroxides, and metal carbonates, and a salt is produced. Acids also react with alkalis to form salts and water, otherwise called neutralization reactions. The pH scale measures the extent to which a substance is acidic or basic. The term *pH* is a measure of the hydrogen ion [H^+] concentration of a solution and is defined as the negative logarithm of ion concentration. Solutions with a high concentration of hydrogen ions have a low pH and are called *acidic solutions*; solutions with low concentrations of H^+ ions are considered as high pH and are called *alkaline* (also known as caustic or basic) solutions. The pH value varies from 0 (most acidic) to 14 (most basic), and 7 is considered as its neutral point (Figure 12.2). Although the pH range seems like a linear scale, it is important to remember that it is in the logarithm function. A 10-fold change in concentration of hydrogen ion happens when one pH unit is changed. Therefore, a pH of 11.0 is 10 times as basic as a pH of 10.0. This definition of pH was introduced in 1909

by the Danish biochemist Søren Peter Lauritz Sørensen. It is expressed mathematically as $pH = -\log[H^+]$, where [H^+] is hydrogen ion concentration in mol/L. In special cases, it is found that commercially available concentrated hydrochloric acid (HCl) solution (37% by mass) has $pH \approx -1.1$, whereas saturated sodium hydroxide solution has $pH \approx 15.0$, which indicates that more than 14 pH values and negative values exist.[1,2]

The value of pH is important for living system, for example, gastric (stomach) acid (pH 1.5-3.5), lysosomes (pH 4.5), urine (pH 6.0), cytosol (pH 7.2), blood (pH 7.34-7.45). The severity of periodontal (gum) disease is determined by the pH of saliva. All living cells are naturally maintaining pH balance homeostasis. Therefore, abnormality in pH balance (acidity and alkalinity) can be harmful to any organism. In a broad sense, pH can be used as a regulator for numerous applications, for example, agronomy, agriculture, medicine, biology, civil engineering, chemistry, forestry, food science, nutrition, environmental science, oceanography, chemical engineering, water treatment, and water purification. In many of those applications, pH can be used as a preservative as well as a disinfectant to control pathogens or other microorganisms.[3] Several factors can affect the general efficacy of extremes of pH as disinfectants, such as concentration, contact time, organic load, temperature, relative humidity, and microbial characteristics.[4,5] In this chapter, the modes of action of acids and alkalis (ie, pH in disinfection processes) are discussed.

◗ CRITICAL LIMITS FOR MICROBIAL GROWTH

Most bacteria are neutrophiles in nature. They develop optimally at a pH within one or two pH units of the neutral pH of 7 (Figure 12.3). Most common bacteria, like *Escherichia coli*, staphylococci, and *Salmonella* are neutrophiles

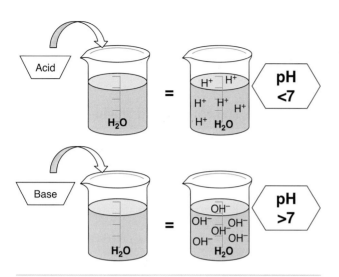

FIGURE 12.1   Acid and base in water. Abbreviations: H⁺, hydrogen ion; H₂O, water; OH⁻, hydroxide ion.

and do not proliferate under extremes of pH (eg, in the stomach's acidic pH). On the other hand, there are many pathogenic strains such as *E coli*, *Salmonella* ser Typhi, and other types of intestinal pathogens that are much more resistant to stomach acid. In comparison, fungi thrive at slightly acidic pH values of 5.0 to 6.0.

Helicobacter pylori is a primary cause of peptic ulcers and gastric cancer. Although its natural habitat is the acidic gastric mucosa, *H pylori* is a neutrophile (ie, thriving in a relatively neutral pH range). The bacterium can survive brief exposure to pHs of <4, but growth occurs only at the pH range of 5.5 to 8.0, with optimal growth at neutral pH.[6] Also, the composition of the gut bacteria community in the stomach and colon is distinctive, which is because of various physicochemical conditions such as pH value, nutrients, intestinal motility, and host secretions (eg, gastric acid, bile, digestive enzymes, and mucus). The organic acids affect bacterial growth in the colon by affecting colonic water absorption and decreasing fecal pH.[7,8] *S aureus* can colonize the human host over a range of pH. Examples include blood at pH 7.4, mouth at pH 5 to 7, nose at pH 6.5 to 7, lungs at 6.8 to 7.6, the vagina at pH 4.2 to 6.6, in abscesses at pH 6.2 to 7.3, urinary tract at pH 4.6 to 7, and the skin at pH 4.2 to 5.9.[9]

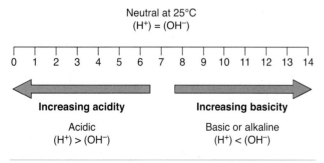

FIGURE 12.2   pH scale. Abbreviations: H⁺, hydrogen ion; OH⁻, hydroxide ion.

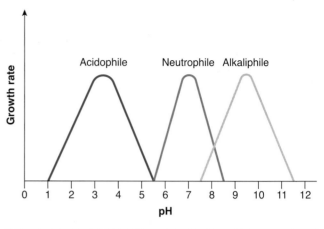

FIGURE 12.3   The curves show the approximate pH ranges for the growth of the different classes of pH-specific prokaryotes. Each curve has an optimal pH and extreme pH values at which growth is much reduced. Most bacteria are neutrophiles and grow best at near-neutral pH (center curve). Acidophiles have optimal growth at pH values near 3, and alkaliphiles have optimal growth at pH values above 9.

Microorganisms that grow optimally at pH <5.5 are called *acidophiles*. For example, the sulfur-oxidizing *Sulfolobus* species, isolated from hot springs in Yellowstone National Park and in sulfur mud fields, are extreme acidophiles. These archaea can survive at pH range of 2.5 to 3.5. Species of the Archaean genus *Ferroplasma* have been identified to grow in acid mine drainage at pH range of 0 to 2.9. An important bacterium of the normal microbiota of the vagina, *Lactobacillus*, can tolerate acidic environments at pH ranges 3.5 to 6.8 and participates in controlling the pH (acidity) of the vagina (pH of 4, except at the onset of menstruation) through their metabolic production of lactic acid. The acidity of the vagina plays a vital role in inhibiting other microbes that are not tolerable to acidity. Acidophilic microorganisms have been shown to have some critical adaptations to allow them to survive in strongly acidic environments. For example, proteins show increased negative surface charge that stabilizes them at low pH. Surface proton pumps in the cells actively expel H⁺ ions out of the cells. The changes in the composition of phospholipids in membrane probably reflect the need to maintain membrane fluidity at low pH level.[10]

At the opposite end of the range are the alkaliphiles, or microorganisms that grow best at pH range 8.0 to 10.5. *Vibrio cholerae*, the pathogenic agent of disease cholera, survives best at the slightly basic pH of 8.0. It can survive at pH of 11.0 but can be inactivated by the stomach acid. Extreme alkaliphiles have adapted to their harsh environment through modification of lipid and protein structure and compensatory mechanisms to maintain the proton motive force in an alkaline environment.[11] For example, the alkaliphile *Bacillus firmus* derives energy for transport reactions and motility from a Na⁺ ion gradient rather than

TABLE 12.1   pH tolerance of selected bacteria

Organism	Optimum pH	Extremes Reported	Reference
Campylobacter species	6.5-7.5	4.9	Doyle and Roman[13]; Doyle[14]
Clostridium botulinum	Proteolytic 4.6; nonproteolytic 5.0	pH ≤5 and ≥8.3	Fernandes[15]
Clostridium perfringens	6-7	N/A	Fernandes[15]
Escherichia coli O157	4.0-4.4	3.6-4.0	Fernandes[15]
Listeria species	5	4.3	Fernandes[15]
Salmonella species	6.5-7.5	3.8-9.5	Fernandes[15]
Staphylococcus aureus	7.0-7.5	4.2-9.3	Fernandes[15]
Yersinia species	7.0-8.0	<4.2 or >9.0	Fernandes[16]
Aeromonas species	5.5	4-10	Fernandes[16]
Vibrio cholerae	7.6	5-9.6	Fernandes[16]

a proton motive force.[12] Many enzymes from alkaliphiles showed a higher isoelectric point due to an increase in the number of basic amino acids as compared to homologous enzymes from neutrophiles. Table 12.1 shows the optimum pH tolerance of some foodborne bacteria.

TYPES OF ACIDS AND BASES

Acids such as acetic acid, benzoic acid, and the parabens and bases such as sodium hydroxide, potassium hydroxide, and sodium bicarbonate are used directly as preservatives and disinfectants. Note that stronger acids and bases have limited use due to safety concerns (eg, user safety and material compatibility). Acids are often considered unsafe and some (eg, concentrated sulfuric acid, nitric acid, HCl) are extremely destructive. But, many acids are commonly used in every day life, such as acetic acid (ethanoic acid) in vinegar, citric acid in fruits (ie, oranges and lemons), malic acid in apple, and folic acid in strawberries. Similarly, a large portion of concentrated alkali substances are considered poisonous, and some might be destructive (to hard surfaces, as well as human tissues such as the skin and eyes). Used at higher concentrations, temperatures, and contact times, they can even degrade full carcass. Mild alkalis, such as aluminium hydroxide or magnesium hydroxide, are used as oral drugs (as antacids in liquid or tablet form) or in toothpastes. Foods (for the purpose of preservation) can also be classified as being naturally high acidic, such as pickles, berries, and sauerkraut (pH 3.7 and lower), whereas low acidic foods include tomatoes and pears (pH 3.7-4.5), pumpkin and spinach (pH 4.6-5.3), milk, corn, and seafood (pH 5.4 and higher). The human stomach contains gastric juice that is acidic and aids in food digestion, whereas blood is slightly alkaline (ie, 7.35-7.45). Acidic or alkaline eating behavior is considered important for a

healthy life.[17] A list of common acids and alkalis are listed in Table 12.2. Many of these are more commonly known as food/beverage preservatives by their corresponding International Numbering System for Food Additives (INS), such as in the European Union by their "E" number, such as E-200 (sorbic acid) and E-270 (lactic acid). Note that it is typical for the INS number to be preceded by an E in the European Union, an A in Australia, and a U in the United States.

METHODS OF CONTROLLING pH

Acids and alkalis are considered either "strong" or "weak." For acids, this relates to the number of free hydrogen ions in solution for a given concentration. Thus, nitric acid is a strong acid because all of the acid molecules are dissociated into active H^+ and nitrate ions. Acetic acid is a weak acid; a solution of this acid of the same molar concentration as nitric acid would have a very different pH value because most of the acetic acid molecules do not separate into H^+ and acetate ions. Both nitric acid and acetic acid have the same total available acidity and, therefore, each requires the same amount of neutralizing base. Similarly, there are strong and weak bases. Sodium hydroxide is a strong base, whereas ammonia and sodium carbonate are weak bases. Equal molar concentrations of these bases possess the same capacity to neutralize a given quantity of acid. Thus, acids and bases are commonly used to control the pH of the cleaning and disinfectant solutions. Generally, the increment or decrement of pH can be achieved by two methods. The first one is a direct method, when the product is acidified or made more basic by adding one or more acids or bases respectfully. The second is an indirect method based on the use of microorganisms, such as that used in fermentation processes.[18,19]

TABLE 12.2 Examples of common types of acids and alkali

Name	Acid/Alkali	Remarks
Acetic acid	Acid	Found in vinegar, widely used in the pickling industry as a natural preservative. A 1% solution is considered an effective antiseptic.
Citric acid	Acid	Citric acid was originally extracted from lemons and limes, but it is now produced commercially by a fermentation process. Widely used for flavoring and as a preservative in food and beverages; used in effervescent salts, as a chelating agent, for surface passivation, and in cleaning solutions
Fumaric acid	Acid	It is manufactured synthetically from malic acid; widely used as a food/beverage additive for taste (sourness or vinegar) and as a preservative (eg, in tortillas)
Lactic acid	Acid	Lactic acid is widely used in the production of boiled sweets, pickled foods, and as a raw material in the manufacture of important emulsifiers for the baking industry intravenous fluids; widely used as a food preservative, flavoring agent, in cleaning formulations (for descaling), and as a surface disinfectant in the meat industry
Malic acid	Acid	Malic acid is found naturally in apples, pears, tomatoes, bananas and cherries; used for food flavoring and as a preservative
Phosphoric acid	Acid	Phosphoric acid is manufactured commercially from mined phosphate rock; used as an inorganic soil cleaning agent (eg, rust removal or descaling), cleaning/disinfectant excipient, food flavoring/preservative, and as a mild disinfectant
Tartaric acid	Acid	Tartaric acid is used in baking, in pharmaceuticals as effervescent salts, as a chelating agent, and in cleaning solutions
Sorbic acid	Acid	Sorbic acid and sodium and potassium sorbate are used to inhibit the growth of molds and yeasts in foods/beverages.
Formic acid	Acid	Used as a preservative and antibacterial agent in livestock feed and other food applications as well as in cleaning products (eg, for descaling or stain removal); can be an irritant at concentrations >2%
Benzoic acid	Acid	Benzoic acid, such as in the form of sodium benzoate, is widely used as a food preservative. Inhibits the growth of fungi and some bacteria. Typically used in the 0.05%-0.1% range in foods; also used as a topical antiseptic for the treatment of fungal skin infections such as athlete's foot
Propionic acid	Acid	It is found in Swiss cheese at concentrations of up to 1%. It is effective against molds and bacteria at concentrations of 0.1%-1%; widely used as a food preservative and for flavoring
Calcium hydroxide	Alkali	Commonly called *lime*, used to neutralize excess acid in soil. Widely used as a flocculant in water/sewage treatment and in clarifying foods/beverages; sometimes used as a viricide and surface cleaning agent (in formulation)
Sodium hydroxide	Alkali	Used in making soaps and detergents, as well as a viricide/bactericide and surface cleaning agent (in formulation), particularly for protein removal/degradation. Widely cited as being an effective cleaning and inactivation agent for prion decontamination; used for tissue and whole carcass digestion
Ammonia	Alkali	Used as a general purpose cleaner, as a preservative (eg, in foods), and as a disinfectant
Sodium bicarbonate	Alkali	Commonly known as baking soda, which is widely used in cooking. It is also considered a weak disinfectant (or preservative), being particularly used for odor control or activity against fungi; used as an antiseptic in toothpastes and mouthwashes as well as a mild cleaning agent

IMPORTANCE OF pH IN DISINFECTION METHODS

The pH is one of the major parameters that can affect the efficiency of disinfection in a wide range by diversified reactions. Husson[20] showed that pH and redox potential are individually and jointly major drivers of soil/plant/microorganism systems. The effectiveness of various antimicrobials is enhanced under different pH conditions. An environment-friendly, cost-effective disinfectant such as peracetic acid (an oxidizing agent) shows more effectiveness at lower pH <7.5, whereas hypochlorite (available chlorine) is more effective at lower pH due to dissociation.[21] The inactivation of *Tubifex tubifex* (an aquatic oligochaete) in drinking water by chlorine is affected by pH. Higher pH levels exhibited pronounced inactivation effectiveness, with decreased turbidity and chemical oxygen demand when potassium permanganate was used in chlorine inactivation studies.[22] The disinfection efficiency of free chlorine is increased at lower pH values, whereas chlorine dioxide efficacy is greater at alkaline pH levels. Chlorine (Cl_2) reaches an equilibrium in water to produce HClO (hypochlorous acid), H^+, Cl^-, and ClO^- (hypochlorite ion), with HClO having the greatest impact on antimicrobial activity (see chapter 15). If sodium is combined with hypochlorite to form sodium hypochlorite, the following responses would be initiated in water:

$$Cl_2 + H_2O \rightarrow HClO + H^+ + Cl^-$$

$$NaOCl + H_2O \rightarrow NaOH + HClO$$

$$HClO \rightleftharpoons H^+ + ClO^-$$

The dissociation of hypochlorous acid is dependent chiefly on pH and, to a much lesser extent, temperature, with almost 100% hypochlorous acid present at pH 5 and almost 100% hypochlorite ion present at pH 10.[23,24] A recent study showed that the pH of drinking water could also affect the composition and diversity of commensal bacteria in the gut. The invasion of pathogenic bacteria is believed to be prevented by the presence of commensal bacteria due to the reduction of the intestinal pH by the production of lactate and short-chain fatty acids (SCFAs).[7] Chlorination successfully inactivates viruses if the turbidity of the water is ≤1.0 nephelometric turbidity unit (NTU); it requires a free chlorine residual of ≥1.0 for 30 minutes and a pH of lower 8.0. Enteric viruses are generally more resistant to free chlorine than enteric bacteria, with CT (concentration and contact time, CT in mg-min/L) values for 99% inactivation, ranging from about 2 to more than 30 mg-min/L. White[25] suggested the CT guidelines for the 99% virus inactivation on pH range 7 to 9 at 0°C to 5°C and 10°C and shown the disinfection (2 log) of microorganisms by free available chlorine at various pH levels.

Various studies have shown that many biocides, such as glutaraldehyde, formaldehyde, phenols, and quaternary ammonium compounds are more effective at alkaline pH.[26] For example, the efficacies of aldehydes in formulation (eg, formaldehyde, glutaraldehyde) are dependent on pH, and their performance is generally better at a pH greater than 7. Quaternary ammonium compound formulations typically have the highest performance at pH of 9 to 10, for example, Roccal, Zephiran, DiQuat, and D-256. These are more active at neutral to slightly alkaline pH but lose their activity at pH less than 3.5. The activity of phenolics, hypochlorite, and iodine compounds can be affected by the pH.[27] Halogens, for example, chlorine or iodine compounds, lose efficacy over time, temperatures >110°F or at high pHs (>9). On the other hand, sodium hypochlorite and standard phenol showed high antimycotic efficacy under acidic pH than alkaline ones.[28] Biguanides (eg, chlorhexidine) in highly basic solution are detrimental to the negatively charged groups on cell membranes of microorganisms, which alters the permeability of membranes. Soaps and detergents can quickly inactivate the biguanides, and it shows good performance on a narrow pH range (5-7). The incremental decrease in pH reduced turbidity and stimulated other changes that play a vital role in disinfection process. In general, shifts in pH can enhance the rate of destruction of microbial growth by other microbicides (see chapter 6).

▶ OTHER CONSIDERATIONS

pH Effects on Viruses

Chemical disinfectants are considered important in stopping virus transmission and as an effective strategy for controlling their spread. Many commercially available disinfectants are commonly used in a variety of applications, including animal husbandry/breeding farms.[29,30] The type of target virus, presence of salts in solution (cation, anion, monovalent, divalent), and associated pH can be important in the aggregation and therefore survival of viruses in the environment.[31] pH plays a role on viruses not only as a disinfectant but also in affecting disease transmission. For example, an alkaline pH of 9.0 was found to enhance the binding and entry of the *Alpharetrovirus Helicoverpa armigera* stunt virus (HaSV).[32] The chikungunya virus is endocytosed into *Aedes albopictus* cells and requires membrane cholesterol as well as a low-pH environment for entry.[33] A study demonstrated the ability of low pH alone or in combination with pepsin digestion to inactivate enveloped viral contaminants in plasma.[34] Where duck plaque virus is noninfective above 42°C and structurally unstable above 65°C, changes in the presence of salts or pH was found to significantly decrease the stability of the virus.[35] Human noroviruses (NoVs) are recognized as one of the leading causes of foodborne or intestinal illnesses worldwide. Hydrogen peroxide, ethanol, sodium hypochlorite, quaternary ammonium compounds, and iodine showed little to no effectiveness on NoV GII.4 under the concentrations tested.[36,37] There is a need to develop optimized disinfection methods effective against norovirus on environmental surfaces, and in particular, fast-acting disinfectants are desired. A study suggested that the virus removal efficiency in wastewater treatment plant by coagulation could be improved by simply adjusting the pH.[38] Epigallocatechin gallate was found to be effective in reducing the titers of hepatitis A virus and murine norovirus in a dose-dependent manner at neutral and alkaline pH, but it was ineffective at pH 5.5.[39] These effects may not be specifically associated with gross viral structure disintegration but may have more subtle impacts. For example, during cell infection, the influenza virus coat undergoes a pH-induced rearrangement in endosomes specifically as the pH is reduced to <6 and leading to the release of the genome and the infectious cycle.[40] It is well established that proteins can undergo dynamic structural changes to elicit their functions and within a varied range of physical and chemical conditions of their microenvironments. The variations in these environments affect their activity unless certain mutations preserve their proper function under certain environmental conditions, such as pH. The pH effects on the stability of influenza A virus hemagglutinin has been of interest, and the sensitivity or stability of the protein to changes in pH is believed to impact the virus ability to cross species barriers.[41]

pH Effects on Biofilms

It is well known that biofilm formation is significant in pathogenesis (see chapter 67). Commercially available environmental disinfectants are often ineffective in killing all pathogens when harbored within biofilms. Biofilms are a major threat to human health and industrial productivity, to include water quality, the food processing industry, power generation efficiency, and dental carries.[42-47] Since the late 1970s, the detailed study of biofilms has received much attention when first brought to public attention by Costerton and coworkers[48] in 1978. Pathogens such as *H pylori*, *Legionella pneumophila*, and *Salmonella* ser Typhimurium have been shown to survive within biofilm structures. Microorganisms within biofilm, including pathogens, are widely known to be more resistant to disinfection than planktonic organisms.[49] For example, in *Salmonella* biofilm population densities, intrinsic cell disinfectant resistance and the presence of extracellular polymeric substances (EPS) greatly influenced resistance of biofilms against disinfection treatments.[50] Cellular EPS production is modulated by pH.[51,52] Changes in pH is considered as a stress factor for *Staphylococcus epidermidis* in biofilm formation, and it plays a possible role in the pathogenesis of biomaterial-related infections.[53]

The effect of alkaline pH on bacterial attachment can affect the development of biofilm. Therefore, in clinical settings (such as catheters or other indwelling medical devices) or in the food industry, alkaline formulations could be promising disinfectants to reduce biofilm development over time.[54] Alkaline formulations are also effective in the physical removal of organic-based soils from surfaces. For example, caustic soda (ie, sodium hydroxide) solutions are widely used for CIP (clean-in-place) processes, or techniques for cleaning the inside surfaces of channels, vessels, process equipment, channels, and related fittings, without dismantling. However, the effect of pH may vary depending on the bacteria present. For example, lower pH levels have been found to promote biofilm formation by a subset of hypervirulent ST-17 *Streptococcus agalactiae* strains.[55] In contrast, increased pH levels lead to a higher biofilm formation of *Pseudomonas aeruginosa*, *Klebsiella pneumoniae*, *V cholerae* non-O1, and *V cholerae* O1.[56] At pH 4.2, clinical strains were significantly more resistant than food isolates. *Listeria monocytogenes* survived and even grew at the high pHs.[57] Zhou et al[58] showed that alkali resistance of *P aeruginosa* biofilm formation was greater than that observed with acids. Chopp et al[59] found, based on a mathematical model, that the critical biofilm depth varied with the pH of the surrounding fluid, where increasing the pH effectively increased the critical biofilm depth and impact on quorum sensing. In cellular processes of a wound, pH is known to play a role, both directly and indirectly, to influence the healing process. Furthermore, the pH will also affect the antimicrobial efficacy of antiseptics used in at-risk or infected wounds.[60] At neutral pH (pH = 7), maximal adhesion of *E coli* 0157:H7 was noted, whereas no significant specific bacterial adhesion could be observed at pH 5.5. Biofilm formation by *Salmonella* ser Enteritidis on stainless steel over time was found to be independent of the pH value in the range 4.5 to 7.4; variations in pH lead to dissociation or protonation of the electrolytes, modulating electrostatic interactions between substratum and bacteria through changes in their surface charge.[61]

▶ MODES OF ACTION

The structure of all macromolecules will be affected by extremes of pH. As an example, hydrogen bonds, which hold together strands of DNA, are broken at higher pH. Lipids are also hydrolyzed by extremes in basic pH. More subtle effects on cellular structures and functions include the impact of pH on the cell surface proton motive force that is responsible for the production of adenosine triphosphate (ATP) in cellular respiration and essentially depends on the concentration gradient of H^+ across the plasma membrane. If H^+ ions are neutralized by hydroxide ions, the concentration gradient collapses and impairs energy production, which can lead to cell inhibition or even death. The cell component that is often cited as the most sensitive to pH are proteins, the workhorses of the cell. Fluctuations in pH modify the ionization of amino acid functional groups and disrupt hydrogen bonding, which in turn promote changes in the folding of the molecule, promoting denaturation and destroying structure and therefore function (Figure 12.4).[62-64] In summary, pH has been shown to (1) damage the cell wall (ie, by blocking the pathway of cell wall synthesis and degradation of cell wall components), (2) alter the membrane

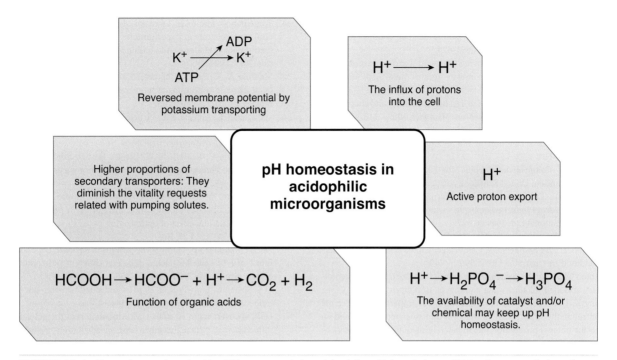

FIGURE 12.4 Procedures related with pH homeostasis in acidophiles. Abbreviations: ADP, adenosine diphosphate; ATP, adenosine triphosphate; CO_2, carbon dioxide; H^+, hydrogen ion; H_2, hydrogen; $HCOO^-$, methanoate; HCOOH, formic acid; H_2PO_4, dihydrogenphosphate ion; H_3PO_4, phosphoric acid. Reprinted from Baker-Austin and Dopson.[62] Copyright © 2007 Elsevier. With permission.

function (ie, bind and penetrate membrane lipids, loss of selective permeability resulting in leakage of cytoplasmic contents), (3) damage the proteins, (4) damage the nucleic acids, (5) act on energy metabolism, and (6) act on bacterial spores. The bonds of nucleic acids are destroyed, and proteins are precipitated by acidic disinfectants. Acids also change the pH of the environment making it detrimental to many microorganisms. The disinfection activities of acids (eg, acetic acid, citric acid) are highly pH dependent.

Additionally, the pH has broad effects on the cellular transcription of virulence genes and other accessory genes, which are presumably initiated through signaling elements and mediated through complex regulatory networks that controls the expression of all accessory genes.[65-67] An example has been shown in the effect of pH on *sae* expression (a key signaling locus, *sae* is involved in the regulation of the expression of many exoproteins in staphylococci); it has been shown that the transition in the *sae* transcription pattern occurred at pH 7.5 but not at pH 5.5, and the level of transcription is decreased at the lower pH.[9] The motility of *E coli* was also affected by low pH via the control of H-NS *flhDC* expression.[68] In *Pseudomonas mandelii*, levels of gene expression of *nirS* and *cnorB* at pH 5 were 539-fold and 6190-fold lower, respectively, in comparison to levels of gene expression for cells grown at pH 6, 7, and 8 between 4 and 8 hours. Cumulative denitrification levels were 28 μmol, 63 μmol, and 22 μmol at pH 6, 7, and 8, respectively, at 8 hours, whereas negligible denitrification was measured at pH 5.[69]

▶ ACKNOWLEDGEMENT

Authors would like to acknowledge the Sultan Qaboos University and University of Chinese Academy of Sciences for their supports to participate in this book project.

REFERENCES

1. Buck RP, Rondinini S, Covington AK, et al. Measurement of pH. Definition, standards, and procedures. *Pure Appl Chem.* 2002;74: 2169-2200.
2. Lim KF. Negative pH does exist. *J Chem Edu.* 2006;83:1465.
3. World Health Organization. *Laboratory Biosafety Manual.* 3rd ed. Geneva, Switzerland; 2004.
4. Maillard JY. Testing the effectiveness of disinfectants and sanitizers. In: Lelieveld H, Holah J, Gabrić D, eds. *Handbook of Hygiene Control in the Food Industry.* 2nd ed. Cambridge, United Kingdom: Woodhead; 2016:569-586.
5. Taylour J, Rosner D. Traceability of cleaning agents and disinfectants. In: Lelieveld H, Holah J, Gabrić D, eds. *Handbook of Hygiene Control in the Food Industry.* 2nd ed. Cambridge, United Kingdom: Woodhead Publishing; 2016:617-626.
6. Kusters JG, van Vliet AHM, Kuipers EJ. Pathogenesis of *Helicobacter pylori* infection. *Clin Microbiol Rev.* 2006;19:449-490.
7. Sofi MH, Gudi R, Karumuthil-Melethil S, Perez N, Johnson BM, Vasu C. pH of drinking water influences the composition of gut microbiome and type 1 diabetes incidence. *Diabetes.* 2014;63:632-644.
8. Zhang YJ, Li S, Gan RY, Zhou T, Xu DP, Li HB. Impacts of gut bacteria on human health and diseases. *Int J Mol Sci.* 2015;16:7493-7519.
9. Weinrick B, Dunman PM, McAleese F, et al. Effect of mild acid on gene expression in *Staphylococcus aureus*. *J Bacteriol.* 2004;186: 8407-8423.

10. Siliakus MF, van der Oost J, Kengen SWM. Adaptations of archaeal and bacterial membranes to variations in temperature, pH and pressure. *Extremophiles.* 2017;21:651-670.

11. Singh A, Barnard TG. Surviving the acid barrier: responses of pathogenic *Vibrio cholerae* to simulated gastric fluid. *Appl Microbiol Biotechnol.* 2016;100:815-824.

12. Fujinami S, Terahara N, Krulwich TA, Ito M. Motility and chemotaxis in alkaliphilic *Bacillus* species. *Future Microbiol.* 2009;4:1137-1149.

13. Doyle MP, Roman DJ. Growth and survival of *Campylobacter fetus* subsp. *jejuni* as a function of temperature and pH. *J Food Prot.* 1981;44:596-601.

14. Doyle MP. *Campylobacter jejuni.* In: Cliver DO, ed. *Foodborne Diseases.* London, United Kingdom: Academic Press; 1990:218-222.

15. Fernandes R. Pathogen profiles. In: Fernandes R, ed. *Microbiology Handbook: Meat Products.* Cambridge, United Kingdom: Leatherhead Food International Ltd; 2009:263-277.

16. Fernandes R. Pathogen profiles. In: Fernandes R, ed. *Microbiology Handbook: Fish and Seafood.* Cambridge, United Kingdom: Leatherhead Food International Ltd; 2009:225-240.

17. Fenton TR, Huang T. Systematic review of the association between dietary acid load, alkaline water and cancer. *BMJ Open.* 2016;6:010438.

18. Yang X, Tu M, Xie R, Adhikari S, Tong Z. A comparison of three pH control methods for revealing effects of undissociated butyric acid on specific butanol production rate in batch fermentation of *Clostridium acetobutylicum. AMB Express.* 2013;3:3.

19. Mohd-Zaki Z, Bastidas-Oyanedel JR, Lu Y, et al. Influence of pH regulation mode in glucose fermentation on product selection and process stability. *Microorganisms.* 2016;4:E2.

20. Husson O. Redox potential (Eh) and pH as drivers of soil/plant/microorganism systems: a transdisciplinary overview pointing to integrative opportunities for agronomy. *Plant and Soil.* 2013;362:389-417.

21. McFadden M, Loconsole J, Schockling AJ, Nerenberg R, Pavissich JP. Comparing peracetic acid and hypochlorite for disinfection of combined sewer overflows: effects of suspended-solids and pH. *Sci Total Environ.* 2017;599-600:533-539.

22. Nie XB, Li ZH, Long YN, He PP, Xu C. Chlorine inactivation of *Tubifex tubifex* in drinking water and the synergistic effect of sequential inactivation with UV irradiation and chlorine. *Chemosphere.* 2017;177:7-14.

23. McDonnell G, Russell AD. Antiseptics and disinfectants: activity, action, and resistance. *Clin Microbiol Rev.* 1999;12:147-179.

24. National Research Council. *Drinking Water and Health.* Washington, DC: National Academic Press; 1980.

25. White GC. *Handbook of Chlorination and Alternative Disinfectants.* 4th ed. New York, NY: John Wiley & Sons; 1999.

26. McDonnell GE. *Antisepsis, Disinfection, and Sterilization.* Washington, DC: ASM Press; 2007.

27. Ewart SL. Disinfectants and control of environmental contamination. In: Smith BP, ed. *Large Animal Internal Medicine: Diseases of Horses, Cattle, Sheep, and Goats.* 3rd ed. Warsaw, Poland: Elsevier Science Health Science Division; 2001:1371-1380.

28. Mohamed SAS. Studying effect of pH on the antimycotic performance of some disinfectants by using quantitative suspension test. *Ass Univ Bul Environ Res.* 2004;7:45-55.

29. Martin H, Le Potier MF, Maris P. Virucidal efficacy of nine commercial disinfectants against porcine circovirus type 2. *Vet J.* 2008;177:388-393.

30. Yamanaka T, Bannai H, Tsujimura K, et al. Comparison of the virucidal effects of disinfectant agents against equine influenza A virus. *J Equine Vet Sci.* 2014;34:715-718.

31. Gerba CP, Betancourt WQ. Viral aggregation: impact on virus behavior in the environment. *Environ Sci Technol.* 2017;51:7318-7325.

32. Penkler DL, Jiwaji M, Domitrovic T, Short JR, Johnson JE, Dorrington RA. Binding and entry of a non-enveloped T=4 insect RNA virus is triggered by alkaline pH. *Virology.* 2016;498:277-287.

33. Gay BE, Bernard M, Solignat N, Chazal N, Devaux C, Briant L. pH-dependent entry of chikungunya virus into *Aedes albopictus* cells. *Infect Genet Evol.* 2012;12:1275-1281.

34. Torgeman A, Mador N, Dorozko M, et al. Efficacy of inactivation of viral contaminants in hyperimmune horse plasma against botulinum toxin by low pH alone and combined with pepsin digestion. *Biologicals.* 2017;48:24-27.

35. Makhija A, Kumar S. Characterization of duck plague virus stability at extreme conditions of temperature, pH and salt concentration. *Biologicals.* 2017;45:102-105.

36. Whitehead K, McCue KA. Virucidal efficacy of disinfectant actives against feline calicivirus, a surrogate for norovirus, in a short contact time. *Am J Infect Control.* 2010;38:26-30.

37. Ha JH, Choi C, Lee HJ, Ju IS, Lee JS, Ha SD. Efficacy of chemical disinfectant compounds against human norovirus. *Food Control.* 2016;59:524-529.

38. Lee S, Ihara M, Yamashita N, Tanaka H. Improvement of virus removal by pilot-scale coagulation-ultrafiltration process for wastewater reclamation: effect of optimization of pH in secondary effluent. *Water Res.* 2017;114:23-30.

39. Falcó I, Randazzo W, Gómez-Mascaraque L, Aznar R, López-Rubio A. Effect of (−)-epigallocatechin gallate at different pH conditions on enteric viruses. *LWT.* 2017;81:250-257.

40. Li S, Sieben C, Ludwig K, et al. pH-Controlled two-step uncoating of influenza virus. *Biophys J.* 2014;106:1447-1456.

41. Lella SD, Herrmann A, Mair CM. Modulation of the pH stability of influenza virus hemagglutinin: a host cell adaptation strategy. *Biophys J.* 2016;110:2293-2301.

42. Garrett TR, Bhakoo M, Zhang Z. Bacterial adhesion and biofilms on surfaces. *Pro Nat Sci.* 2008;18:1049-1056.

43. Otto K. Biophysical approaches to study the dynamic process of bacterial adhesion. *Res Microbiol.* 2008;159:415-422.

44. Hori K, Matsumoto S. Bacterial adhesion: from mechanism to control. *Biochem Eng J.* 2010;48:424-434.

45. Liu Y, Zhang W, Sileika TR, Warta R, Cianciotto NP, Packman AI. Disinfection of bacterial biofilms in pilot-scale cooling tower systems. *Biofouling.* 2011;27:393-402.

46. Araújo P, Lemos M, Mergulhão F, Melo LF, Simões M. Antimicrobial resistance to disinfectants in biofilms. In: Méndez-Vilas A, ed. *Science Against Microbial Pathogens: Communicating Current Research and Technological Advances.* Badajoz, Spain: Formatex Research Center; 2011:826-834.

47. Otter JA, Vickery K, Walker JT, et al. Surface-attached cells, biofilms and biocide susceptibility: implications for hospital cleaning and disinfection. *J Hosp Infect.* 2015;89:16-27

48. Costerton JW, Geesey GG, Cheng KJ. How bacteria stick. *Sci Am.* 1978;238:86-95.

49. Rose LJ, Rice EW. Inactivation of bacterial biothreat agents in water, a review. *J Water Health.* 2014;12:618-633.

50. Pang X, Yang Y, Yuk HG. Biofilm formation and disinfectant resistance of *Salmonella* sp. in mono- and dual-species with *Pseudomonas aeruginosa. J Appl Microbiol.* 2017;123:651-660.

51. Dogsa I, Kriechbaum M, Stopar D, Laggner P. Structure of bacterial extracellular polymeric substances at different pH values as determined by SAXS. *Biophys J.* 2005;89:2711-2720.

52. Guibaud G, Bordas F, Saaid A, D'abzac P, Van Hullebusch E. Effect of pH on cadmium and lead binding by extracellular polymeric substances (EPS) extracted from environmental bacterial strains. *Colloids Surf B Biointerfaces.* 2008;63:48-54.

53. Chaieb K, Chehab O, Zmantar T, Rouabhia M, Mahdouani K, Bakhrouf A. *In vitro* effect of pH and ethanol on biofilm formation by clinical *ica*-positive *Staphylococcus epidermidis* strains. *Ann Microbiol.* 2007;57:431-437.

54. Nostro A, Cellini L, Di Giulio M, et al. Effect of alkaline pH on staphylococcal biofilm formation. *APMIS.* 2012;120:733-742.

55. D'Urzo N, Martinelli M, Pezzicoli A, et al. Acidic pH strongly enhances in vitro biofilm formation by a subset of hypervirulent ST-17 *Streptococcus agalactiae* strains. *App Environ Microbiol.* 2014;80:2176-2185.

56. Hoštacká A, Čižnár I, Štefkovičová M. Temperature and pH affect the production of bacterial biofilm. *Folia Microbiol (Praha).* 2010;55:75-78.

57. Borges SF, Silva JG, Teixeira PC. Survival and biofilm formation of *Listeria monocytogenes* in simulated vaginal fluid: influence of pH and strain origin. *FEMS Immunol Med Microbiol.* 2011;62:315-320.

58. Zhou L, Xia S, Zhang Z, et al. Effects of pH, temperature and salinity on extracellular polymeric substances of *Pseudomonas aeruginosa* biofilm with N-(3-oxooxtanoyl)-L-homoserine lactone addition. *J Water Sust.* 2014;2:91-100.

59. Chopp DL, Kirisits MJ, Moran B, Parsek MR. The dependence of quorum sensing on the depth of a growing biofilm. *Bull Math Biol.* 2003;65:1053-1079.

60. Jones EM, Cochrane CA, Percival SL. The effect of pH on the extracellular matrix and biofilms. *Adv Wound Care (New Rochelle).* 2015;4:431-439.

61. García-Gonzalo D, Pagán R. Influence of environmental factors on bacterial biofilm formation in the food industry: a review. *J Postdoc Res.* 2015;3(6):1-11.

62. Baker-Austin C, Dopson M. Life in acid: pH homeostasis in acidophiles. *Trends Microbiol.* 2007;15:165-171.

63. Maris P. Modes of action of disinfectants. *Rev Sci Tech.*1959;14:47-55.

64. Krulwich T, Sachs G, Padan E. Molecular aspects of bacterial pH sensing and homeostasis. *Nat Rev Microbiol.* 2011;9(5):330-343.

65. Olson ER. Influence of pH on bacterial gene expression. *Mol Microbiol.* 1993;8:5-14.

66. Bumke MA, Neri D, Elia G. Modulation of gene expression by extracellular pH variations in human fibroblasts: a transcriptomic and proteomic study. *Proteomics.* 2003;3:675-688.

67. Lager I, Andréasson O, Dunbar TL, Andreasson E, Escobar MA, Rasmusson AG. Changes in external pH rapidly alter plant gene expression and modulate auxin and elicitor responses. *Plant Cell Environ.* 2010;33:1513-1528.

68. Soutourina OA, Krin E, Laurent-Winter C, Hommais F, Danchin A, Bertin PN. Regulation of bacterial motility in response to low pH in *Escherichia coli*: the role of H-NS protein. *Microbiology.* 2002;148:1543-1551.

69. Saleh-Lakha S, Shannon KE, Henderson SL, et al. Effect of pH and temperature on denitrification gene expression and activity in *Pseudomonas mandelii. Appl Environ Microbiol.* 2009;75:3903-3911.

CHAPTER 13

Antimicrobial Dyes

Mark Wainwright

M an's need to color his environment, and often himself, has been felt since prehistoric times, as might be seen in ancient cave paintings and the tradition, particularly among druidic sects, of staining the skin with the indole pigment woad.[1] Whereas self-coloration, in terms of cosmetics, became increasingly popular from the middle ages, especially among women, the medical use of colorants is relatively recent and may be traced back to 19th century Europe and medico-scientists such as Gram, Koch, and Ehrlich who recognized the differential cell-staining potential of the then new aniline dyes when applied to microscopic samples.[2] This, in turn allowed Ehrlich's thesis regarding the medical use of related dyes, particularly in an antimicrobial capacity, with the eventual use of methylene blue (MB) as an antimalarial in 1890 and the introduction by Browning of antiseptic "flavine therapy" during World War I.[3] Further research, particularly in postwar Germany, produced new "colored antimicrobials," which led to the development of a range of conventional drugs against infectious and tropical disease that are still in use.[4] However, this productive era was rapidly sidelined, initially by the dye-derived sulfonamide antibacterials and then the penicillins, in the period 1935 to 1945.[5] The natural product nature of the original penicillins and streptomycin altered the drug discovery paradigm and further distanced previously useful dyes from the clinic. This situation lasted until perhaps the late 1980s, when conventional drug resistance became a significant clinical problem in Western medicine. At this time, the potential of photoactivated cationic dyes, such as MB, as antimicrobials ("photoantimicrobials") was revisited and, ironically, they now represent one of the few demonstrably effective methods of circumventing conventional drug resistance. This chapter deals with antimicrobial dyes, both as conventional and photoactivatable agents. Within the chapter, the term *dye* covers only organic colorants.

▶ DYE CLASSES AND ANTIMICROBIAL ACTION

Conventionally, dyes are synthesized in order to produce a colored effect on a given substrate—acid dyes on wool, for example. In this way, the desired results are coloration and fastness (ie, permanent adherence to the substrate), neither of which criteria is obviously associated with an antimicrobial effect. Dyes were discovered to have antimicrobial effects as a result, usually, of their chance testing—because, scientifically, this testing would be considered haphazard, rather than structurally systematic. Furthermore, very little scientific method was ever applied to investigating the modes of action of antimicrobial dyes, so that structure–activity relationships were uncommon in the past, the only real example being the sterling work of Albert et al on aminoacridine antibacterials and the establishment of bacterial DNA as a site of action.[6]

The outcome of almost 130 years of research, thus, does not allow anything approaching activity relationships by chemical class, that is, azoic, triphenylmethane, and so forth because logically, antimicrobial activity arises from direct interactions of chemical groups attached to the molecule—usually at its periphery—with groups or regions within the microbial target. Such groups, for example, quaternary ammonium $(-NR_3^+)$ or iminium $(=NR_2^+)$ moieties, are not usually unique to specific dye classes and are, indeed, often interchangeable or even ubiquitous among examples.

Obviously, dye structures vary with class, but the overall constitution is that of a larger, heteroaromatic chromophore (color-forming) portion, often with smaller pendant groups that can alter the chromophoric electron cloud via delocalization, therefore affecting the resulting light absorption profile. Such groups are thus termed *auxochromes*, a good example of which is the dimethylaminium group ($=NMe_2^+$) found in the phenothiazinium dye MB (as well as many others, including toluidine blue, acridine orange, and neutral red). As noted earlier, in addition to their contribution to molecular light absorption, these groups are often responsible for, at least, the initial interaction with microbial biomolecules such as the lipoteichoic acid in gram-positive bacterial cell wall exteriors.

How different dyes interact with microbial targets depends on several general factors: overall charge, molecular shape, and hydrophilic/lipophilic balance (effectively relative water/oil solubility). For conventional antimicrobial action, this does not of course differ from that of nondye molecules such as antibiotics or biocides. Similarly, how the same dye interacts with different cells can demonstrate morphologic variations, as is seen quite obviously with the triphenylmethane dye crystal (gentian) violet in the Gram stain, differentiating between the two main classes of bacteria by virtue of decreased dye interaction/penetration due to the presence of the outer membrane in gram-negative species.[7]

From the point of view of antimicrobial action, such variations in interaction with the target(s) are important because decreased interaction suggests weaker activity. It is important, therefore, to understand the processes involved so that activity can be maintained. Much of this understanding has emanated from the renaissance in photoantimicrobial research, which began in the early 1990s, and is based mostly on MB as a lead compound.[8] This work has demonstrated the importance of cationic nature for broad-spectrum activity (ie, against gram-positive and gram-negative bacteria) because anionic and electronically neutral dyes have little activity against gram-negative species. The idea of assisted uptake of cationic examples was suggested by Hamblin and Hasan,[9] describing the displacement by such dyes of stabilizing magnesium and calcium ions among the head groups in bacterial membranes, leading to membrane defects that allow increased dye ingress and subsequent internal damage.

Dye aggregation is a well-established phenomenon caused by the generally planar nature of such molecules, due to the extended nature of the conjugated pi/aromatic regions essential in dye structures. Aggregation can be envisaged as a kind of plate- or tray-stacking and is, indeed, essential in the visualization of cells by microscopy, that is, aggregation endows intensity of coloration in the cells being stained. Interestingly, dye aggregation is a *disadvantage* in the far more effective method of cell killing via photodynamic action (see in the following text).

The following sections have been arranged by chemical class because this allows a simpler approach to structure activity but are also discussed under "conventional" and "photoantimicrobial" headings because there are significant differences in levels of range and activity, and thus utility.

◗ CONVENTIONAL ANTIMICROBIALS

Azoic Dyes

Although of little current utility in terms of infection control, azo dyes have a considerable pedigree in terms of the development of conventional drugs and antiseptics. It was, after all, the azo dyes KL695 and prontosil that ushered in what is now considered to be the "antibiotic era" in the 1930s, as a result of a considerable chemical and microbiological effort at the Bayer company premises in Elberfeld.[10] The discovery that the azoic structure represented a prodrug, breaking down to sulfanilamide in the mammalian colon, gave rise to the sulfonamide class of antibacterial agents, and it is this class—not the penicillins—that furnished the commencement of useful clinical infection control.[10] The continued presence, although in diminishing import, of drugs such as sulfadiazine and sulfamethoxazole is entirely due to Domagk's screening of azoic dyes, but it is less well appreciated that other related drug classes were developed by him during World War II, such as the thiosemicarbazones with useful activity against mycobacterial infection.[11]

The demonstrable efficacy of the many sulfanilamide derivatives arising from Bayer's eventual disclosure of prontosil in 1935 belies the fact that several azoic dyes had been previously reported to have antibacterial activity that did not contain the azobenzenesulfonamide moiety (ie, would not produce sulfanilamide on breakdown).

Azo dyes had, in fact, been suggested and trialed in vitro as antiseptic agents as early as 1913. Excellent results had previously been reported for the simple dye chrysoidine by Eisenberg[12] and for pyridium and serenium by Ostromislensky.[13] The latter two were still in use as urinary antiseptics in the 1930s,[14] and pyridium remains in use.[15] Although such results were not observed in Bayer's animal testing,[16] the structural similarity to the prontosil rubrum molecule is obvious, but the lack of a sulfonamide residue (Figure 13.1) suggests that the mode of antibacterial action is different.

Triarylmethanes

It can be argued that the first major impact of dyes as antimicrobial agents was, in fact, the use of the triarylmethane derivative crystal (gentian) violet (Figure 13.2) in

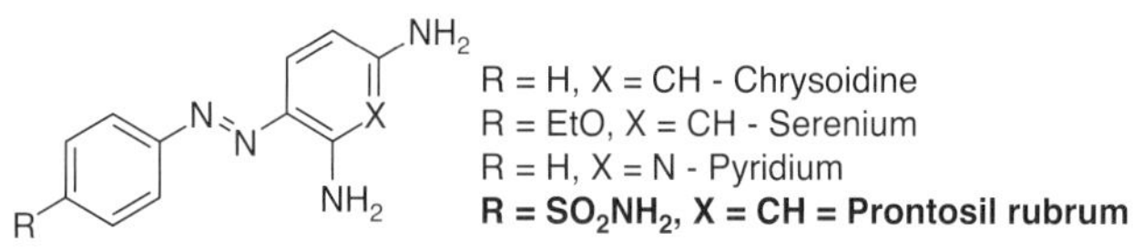

R = H, X = CH - Chrysoidine
R = EtO, X = CH - Serenium
R = H, X = N - Pyridium
R = SO₂NH₂, X = CH = Prontosil rubrum

FIGURE 13.1 Antiseptic (in vitro) azoic dyes and prontosil rubrum.

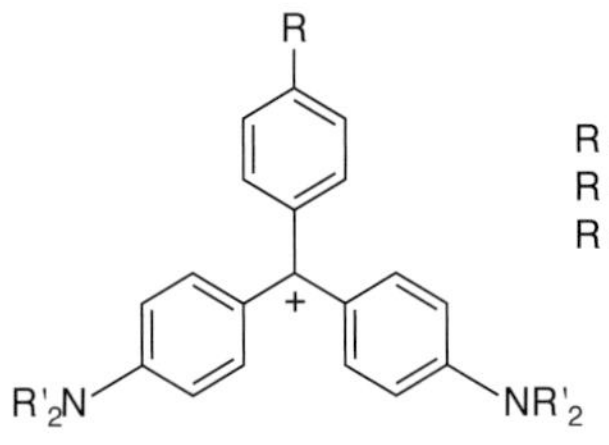

FIGURE 13.2 Simple antimicrobial triarylmethane dyes.

R = NMe2, R' = Me - Crystal violet
R = H, R' = Me - Malachite green
R = H, R' = Et - Brilliant green

Hans-Christian Gram's development of bacterial typing. Although this immensely valuable work was not aimed at bacterial killing, the demonstrated dye-cell interactions and selectivity underpinned the ensuing labors of scientists such as Koch and Ehrlich and led, ultimately, to the development of antimicrobial chemotherapy.[1] As noted earlier, "flavine therapy" was introduced by Browning and Gulbransen[3] during the second half of World War I, "flavines" referring generally to the dyes employed for wound disinfection, rather than being chemically specific. One of the principal dyes used here was brilliant green, a closely related analogue of crystal violet (see Figure 13.2). Similar work was carried out at the same time by others.[17-20]

Interestingly, Fung and Miller[21] examined the effects of a range of dyes—42 in all—from different classes and observed a distinct difference in activity along Gram classification lines, with very little activity shown against gram-negative bacteria but high activity by over half of the examples used against gram-positive bacteria. Little modern work has focused on this class of agents in terms of new and improved derivatives. Crystal violet was also found to be active against fungi and was used until relatively recently against skin infections such as ringworm.[22] In a parallel field, the dye was, until recently, added to donated blood by South American agencies to inactivate the parasite responsible for Chagas disease, *Trypanosoma cruzi*.[23] Additionally, crystal violet has proved to be highly effective in the treatment of patients infected with methicillin-resistant *Staphylococcus aureus* (MRSA).[24]

Acridines

The use of acridines as antimicrobial agents was first proposed[25] following the clinical introduction of proflavine and acriflavine as wound disinfectants[3] in 1917; several other derivatives were introduced during the World War II, mainly due to the work of Albert et al[26] and including the antimalarial drug mepacrine. Albert et al's efforts in this area allowed the development of structure-activity ideas, indicating that the microbial target was DNA and that active acridines intercalated into the structure. However, the interaction of quinolone antibacterials[27] and some acridine-based anticancer drugs[28] with DNA-managing enzymes such as gyrases and topoisomerases suggests that alternative/additional modes

of action are possible. Albert et al's experimentally derived criteria for antibacterial activity among the acridines, to include their cationic nature, high levels of ionization at physiological pH, and a planar molecular surface area ≥ 38 Å^2, led to the discovery that the heteroaromatic chromophore could be varied, or that a purely benzenoid structure was equally effective.[29] Thus, activity became predictable (or explainable) not only in the related azine dyes (phenazines, phenoxazines, phenothiazines, etc) but also in cationic anthracene derivatives.[29] Furthermore, nonlinear ring fusion (as in the phenanthridines) or bridged structures, where the bridge is part of the delocalized pi system of the molecule (eg, styryl and cyanine derivatives), also furnished active examples.

In terms of the clinical use of acridine derivatives, the principal entries are provided in Table 13.1.

In antiseptic and disinfection applications, the main acridine derivatives used have been proflavine, acriflavine/euflavine, and aminacrine, although local use of these agents was rapidly superseded by systemic β-lactam administration in the mid-1940s. Local application, for example, in wound disinfection, continued for a considerable time, both alone and in combination with sulfonamide derivatives.[31] In addition, acriflavine, the quaternary 10-methyl derivative of proflavine containing varying levels of proflavine hydrochloride, had been used as a systemic therapy in cases of trypanosomiasis (as trypaflavin) and gonorrhoea (as gonaflavin), the latter being administered intravenously at 0.1 g 3 times per week,[32] or in 10 doses of 40 to 80 mg at 2- to 3-day intervals.[33] The pure quaternary compound is euflavine (see Table 13.1).

The aqueous solubility of aminoacridine derivatives is obviously an important parameter in the proposed use of such compounds as injectable antibacterials, that is, for systemic use. The hydrophilic nature of the simple aminoacridines covered here furnishes correspondingly short half-lives in the bloodstream, and their use in the clinical treatment of bloodborne infection, for example, staphylococcal septicemia, has never been a realistic option as a consequence. For example, intravenous treatment of septicemia with argoflavin, a mixture of euflavine lactate and silver lactate, was not usually successful,[34] the concentration in the blood of administered acriflavine (200 mg) having decreased by 90% over 5 minutes and being undetectable at 30 minutes.[35] Aminacrine and rivanol exhibited similar pharmacokinetics.[36,37] Despite the absence of currently suitable injectables, there is a considerable patent literature, particularly concerning quaternized acridines, which emanated from earlier work on euflavine. However, simple aminoacridines were synthesized as blood antimicrobials, notably by IG Farben, for example, 3-amino-10-methyl-6-haloacridinium species.[38-40]

Further forays in this area might well use the antimalarial acridine mepacrine (quinacrine, atebrin) as a lead compound from a pharmacologic standpoint, with alterations to the much longer C-9 side chains, for example,

TABLE 13.1 Clinical antibacterial acridines[a]

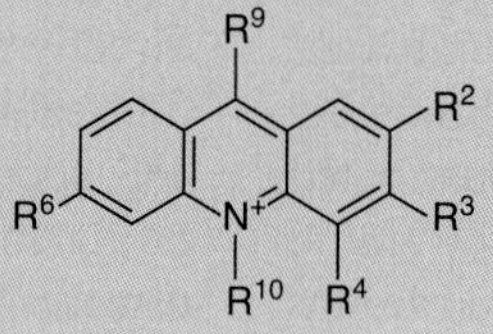

	R²	R³	R⁴	R⁶	R⁹	R¹⁰
Bases						
Aminacrine[b]	H	H	H	H	NH₂	H
Diflavine	NH₂	H	H	NH₂	H	H
Ethacridine[b]	EtO	H	H	NH₂	NH₂	H
Proflavine[b]	H	NH₂	H	NH₂	H	H
Salacrin[b]	H	H	Me	H	NH₂	H
Quaternary salts						
Euflavine[b,c]	H	NH₂	H	NH₂	H	Me
Flavicid	Me	NH₂	H	Me₂N	H	Me
Sinflavin	H	MeO	H	MeO	H	Me

[a]From Wainwright M et al.[30] Reproduced by permission of British Society for Antimicrobial Chemotherapy.

[b]Photobactericidal examples.

[c]Purified acriflavine.

with Nitroakridin 3582. This compound, [2,3-dimethoxy-6-nitro-9-(3′-diethylamino-2′-hydroxypropylamino) acridine], has been used in the treatment of clinical typhus.[41] The works of Steck et al[42] on antirickettsial acridines, based on Nitroakridin 3582, and of Elslager and Tendick[43] on acridine N-oxides represent the last major research efforts in systemic acridine antibacterials. Tabern's[44,45] "Phenacridane" series was intended as a topical anti-infective, and this has indeed been the major area of acridine-based antibacterial treatment since that time, mainly using proflavine or acriflavine.

The use of orally administered acridine drugs has been much more common, for example, euflavine pastilles employed for throat disinfection (Panflavine or Planacrine brands). Gonorrhoea was also treated via the oral route using acriflavine.[46] Ethacridine (2-ethoxy-6,9-diaminoacridine; see Table 13.1) has found long-term use in the oral treatment of enteric disease such as shigellosis due to low absorption and lower toxicity than acriflavine.[36,47]

Phenazines

Heteroatomic replacement of the C9 carbon of the acridine nucleus with nitrogen furnishes the phenazine analogue, responsible for biological stains such as neutral red and safranin, among others. Although a range of phenazines was included in Browning's examination of a range of

available dyes for antimicrobial activity in the post–World War I period,[48] no significant activity was reported. However, clofazimine, a phenazine-containing molecule, has formed part of the antimycobacterial effort since the 1950s. Clofazimine (Figure 13.3) was originally synthesized in the search for drugs against Hansen disease.[49]

Clofazimine is a purple- or damson-colored compound. Although, as noted, Barry's original drug target was Hansen bacillus (*Mycobacterium leprae*),[50] it is also active against *Mycobacterium avium*, one of the opportunistic pathogens associated with human immunodeficiency virus (HIV)-positive status.[51] Clofazimine has also found use in the treatment of Crohn disease[52] and in drug-resistant tuberculosis.[53]

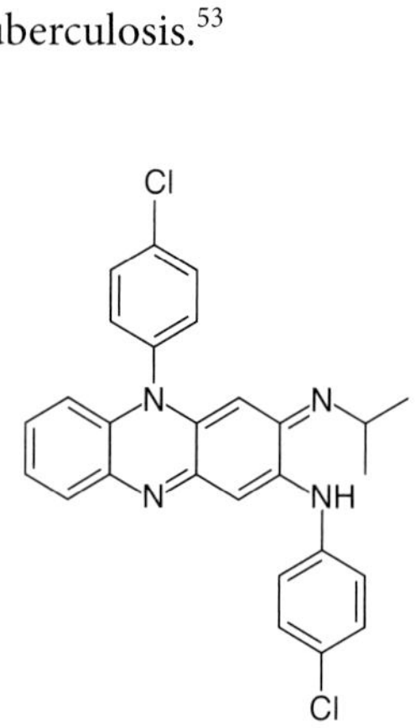

FIGURE 13.3 Clofazimine.

Cyanine and Styryl Dyes

Research in this area grew out of the success of flavine therapy during World War I and was due, in the most part, to Carl Browning, a one-time assistant of Paul Ehrlich.[54] Browning and his main chemical collaborator, Cohen, deconstructed the acridine chromophore and thus experimented on amino derivatives of pyridines and quinolines with olefinic groups attached in partial replacement of the fused benzene rings in acridine, producing both cyanine- and styryl-type molecules. As Browning was interested both in bacterial and trypanosomal infection, the resulting compounds were tested against both types of pathogen, producing a considerable body of work. In addition, styryl (aryl-CH=CH-aryl) and imino (aryl-CH=N-aryl) derivatives were examined.[48,55-59]

The activity of several of the derivatives was such that a clinical trial was run with compound 48S (Table 13.2) at the General Infirmary in Leeds, United Kingdom,[61] and included more than 2000 subjects. The 48S was employed in most areas requiring antisepsis/antiseptic dressings, local application, wound or infection site irrigation, and even intravenous administration in septicemia. Due to the instability of imino structures in acidic solution where

hydrolysis occurs, 48S was not administered by mouth. Generally, the activity of 48S in human subjects was sufficient to give cures in most cases where it was applied directly rather than systemically, although some successful treatments of septicemia were reported. In many ways, 48S appears to be similar in activity to acriflavine and proflavine, although these are not effective in blood-borne disease. That the clinical trial of the iminoquinoline was not extended cannot be due to lack of efficacy, and it was described as being bland and nonirritating to the tissues. As can be seen from Table 13.2, the variation in amino side chain length produced considerable differences in activity, longer chain derivatives generally being more active, in many cases more so than 48S itself. This may indicate a "lipophilic tail" influence due to interaction with outer/inner membrane structures in the bacterial target.

The strongly antibacterial nature of cyanines against gram-positive bacteria was shown in conjunction with low toxicity in the mouse.[62] Later work by Abd El-Aal and Younis[63] with more structurally complex examples exhibited activity against bacteria and fungi but at millimolar levels,[64] somewhat removed from the activity of the earlier Browning examples.

TABLE 13.2 Antibacterial activity of analogues of clinical compound 48, provided in μmol (10^{-6} M)[a]

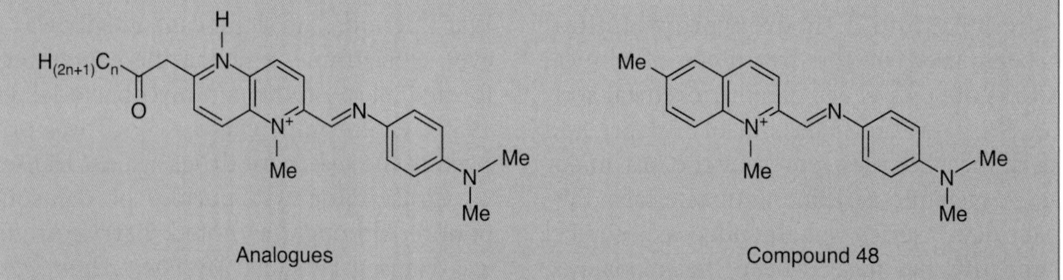

Analogues

Compound 48

n	MBC *Staphylococcus aureus* (μmol)	MBC *Escherichia coli* (μmol)
1	13	7
2	12	2
3	57	23
4	11	5
5	11	5
6	6	11
7	5	5
8	5	10
10	10	10
11	5	10
Compound 48	15	15
Acriflavine	19	38

Abbreviation: MBC, minimum bactericidal concentration.

[a]Data from Browning et al.[59,60]

Antimicrobial Textile Dyes

Textile dyes can be used for aesthetic purposes (eg, for dyeing) but can provide some antimicrobial activity (as a preservative or disinfectant). This is obviously a logical approach to fabric protection, but it should also be extended to the fight against health care–acquired infections, given that infection may be communicated via the environment—for example, soft furnishings, bedding, hospital scrubs. To this end, dyes having similar structural motifs to conventional biocidal agents have been produced, for example, quaternary ammonium salt derivatives (Figure 13.4; see chapter 21). Because the majority of textile dyes contain amino functionality, the synthesis of these biocidal analogues is relatively straightforward, as reported both for simple azoic.[65] Antibacterial cyanine dyes having overall cationic nature have also been reported (see Figure 13.4); because the positive charge in such cases is delocalized throughout the chromophore, molecular interactions with bacteria may be different from those of the point charges presented by the quaternary ammonium salt azoics mentioned earlier and most probably act via interference at the bacterial membrane.

One series of bisazo dyes, based on the pyrazole nucleus (see Figure 13.4), proved to be highly active against both bacteria and fungi, in some cases being more effective than the triazole drug fluconazole[66] and providing new leads for conventional drug discovery/development.

As noted earlier, the use of dyes as disinfectants was commonplace before the ingress of the sulfonamides and antibiotics into infection control in the 1930s and 1940s. The visible staining nature of dyes used conventionally has always been problematic for patients and clinicians—and presumably for environmentalists—and this has hindered any return to the fray for dyes, even in the face of frightening levels of conventional drug resistance in health care. However, the antimicrobial power of certain dyes and their derivatives used photodynamically provides some opportunities in 21st century disinfection applications.

▶ DYES ALLOWING PHOTODYNAMIC DISINFECTION

Unlike conventional dyes, photosensitizers are light-absorbing molecules that can populate the excited electronic triplet state significantly, therefore allowing electron transfer reactions or energy transfer involving oxygen in the environment. Cytotoxic photosensitization results from the generation of reactive oxygen species in situ. The superoxide anion, hydroxyl radical, and peroxides are produced via electron transfer and singlet oxygen via energy transfer (Figure 13.5). Photosensitizing dyes that are selectively taken up by microorganisms thus offer considerable potential for their eradication.

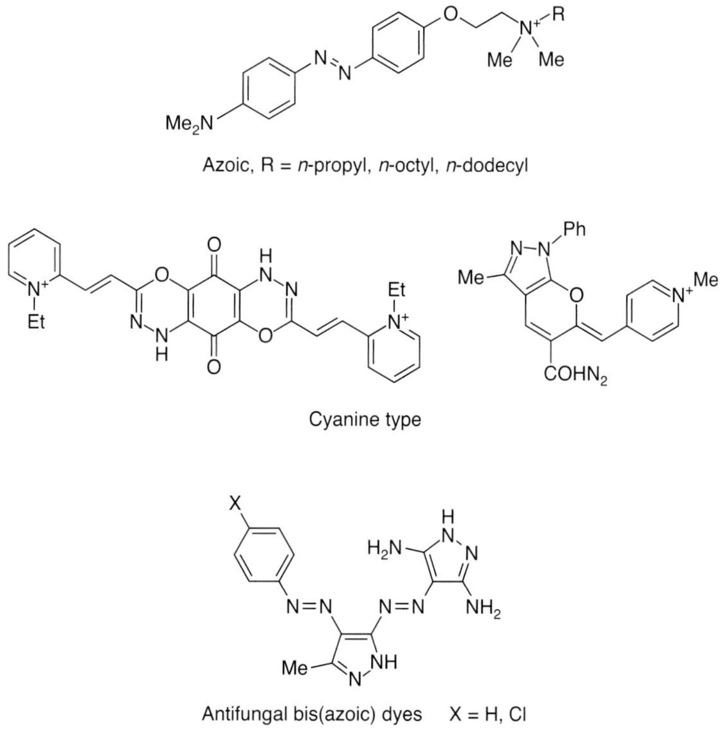

Azoic, R = *n*-propyl, *n*-octyl, *n*-dodecyl

Cyanine type

Antifungal bis(azoic) dyes   X = H, Cl

FIGURE 13.4 Antimicrobial textile dyes.

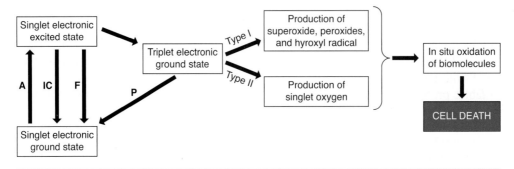

FIGURE 13.5 Pathways involved in photoantimicrobial action. Abbreviations: A, energy of absorbed photon, deactivation processes; F, fluorescence; IC, internal conversion; P, phosphorescence.

The mode of action of photosensitizing dyes illustrated is distinct to that of conventional anti-infective drugs or biocidal agents and, indeed, to the conventional, that is, non–light-activated action of the same photosensitizers. The intermediacy of reactive oxygen species ensures both varied and variable targeting and chemistry of interaction, thus making the development of resistance very difficult. Conversely, single-site/single-mode activity among conventional anti-infectives, such as antibiotics, encourages resistance.[67]

In terms of range of activity, reactive oxygen species theoretically can ensure efficient microbial cell inactivation over time, given suitable photosensitizer uptake by or association with the target microorganism. However, it should be noted that anionic dyes are significantly less effective against gram-negative bacteria due to poor interaction with the outer membrane in such organisms resulting from the preponderance of anionic head groups in this region. Conversely, the interaction is advantageous for cationic photosensitizers, which should be considered to be broad spectrum with regard to antibacterial activity.

A considerable research effort has been made in photoantimicrobial (= photodynamic + antimicrobial) discovery.[68] Although this conforms to the same design paradigm as conventional antimicrobial research in aiming for microbial selectivity, there are added requirements in both light absorption and efficiency of reactive oxygen species production.

Light absorption is required for activation of the photosensitizer so that the energy absorbed might be converted into reactive oxygen production, as shown earlier in Figure 13.5. Consequently, the light employed is determined by the chromophore involved, and this has an impact on the disinfection presentation (eg, on the skin). This is because of the presence, in some cases, of light-absorbing species in the environment, for example, heme pigments in blood and melanin in skin tissue. Clearly, for useful activation, the photoantimicrobials employed must absorb light in other regions of the electromagnetic spectrum. To avoid heme/melanin absorption of light, chromophores absorbing at long wavelengths of the visible

spectrum (normally ≥630 nm) are required, that is, far-red or near-infrared. Photoantimicrobials for use in surface disinfection (skin or environmental) are free of this restriction and can be blue or even ultraviolet absorbers.

Efficiency of reactive oxygen production can be improved by the inclusion of lower period atoms in a given lead-compound structure. This is known as the heavy-atom effect and is due to the stabilization of the triplet excited state by atoms such as sulfur, selenium, bromine, or iodine.[69] However, in terms of drug design, such inclusions usually increase the lipophilic character of the resulting molecule, which often alters solubility and cellular uptake behavior. Furthermore, reactive oxygen efficiency measured in vitro is not a guarantee of antimicrobial effects because there are other criteria contributing to this (such as the microbial cellular uptake mentioned earlier).

▶ PHOTOANTIMICROBIAL RATIONALE

The discovery of photoantimicrobial action was made,[70] reporting the photosensitizing action of acridine and the xanthene derivative eosin. The literature has various reports concerning the photoantimicrobial effects of synthetic dyes throughout the next 60 years, but it required the proper development of photodynamic therapy (PDT)[71] as a cancer treatment, beginning in the 1960s, to allow a renaissance in photoantimicrobial research. The PDT was—and is—firmly based on naturally occurring porphyrin derivatives, with synthetics constituting something of a lower class. This is also true in the related field of photodynamic antimicrobial chemotherapy[68] despite the fact that there is far less rationale for the use of anionic porphyrins used in cancer PDT as photoantimicrobials. Without PDT, photoantimicrobials would be firmly based on cationic dyes such as MB and the benzo[a]phenoxazine Nile blue.

The lead compounds used in the discovery of synthetic photoantimicrobials are, in the main, a subclass of established biological stains. The long-established phenothiazinium stain MB is premier among these, being first in class in terms of clinical use, but it is important to recognize that it is not the only choice, despite its many medical applications in the past.[72] Many candidate chromophores for novel photosensitizers can be found in the field of biological staining, the demonstrable selectivity for microbes offering a sound approach to drug discovery for photoantimicrobial agents. Given the requirement for cationic nature in producing broad-spectrum agents, several lead compounds are present in the tricyclic cationic class, for example, MB, Nile blue, and acriflavine. However, other classes such as the phthalocyanines and xanthenes have seen significant progress toward useful photoantimicrobial action.

It should be noted that the principal driver in moving the field of photoantimicrobial research to clinical use is largely governed by the potential for toxicity in the human or animal host. Consequently, there is a significant lobby for the use of compounds already licensed for use in medicine, albeit in other areas. As noted, MB is the principal example, having been employed clinically in various guises since the 1890s.[72] It is unfortunate that less effective anticancer PDT agents are suggested for clinical use in infection control via the same argument (viz, that they are already used in clinical PDT). This argument is fallacious on two counts. Although intended for use against tumors, there is invariably also some uptake of these photosensitizers by normal cells. This causes a small amount of collateral damage, which is acceptable in anticancer therapies but would not be in routine antimicrobial protocols. Furthermore, the photosensitizers in question, such as chlorins and hematoporphyrin derivatives, are lipophilic and anionic in nature and thus poorly active against gram-negative bacteria, for the reasons noted earlier.

The enormous difference in antimicrobial activity between dyes used in the conventional way, as covered in the initial section of this chapter, and photoantimicrobials means that there are many more examples of useful dyes used in this fashion, and with a far greater range. These are dealt with generally by chemical class in the following text.

Clinical Areas

As with anticancer PDT, the requirement for light activation means that localized, rather than systemic, infection is the logical presentation for photoantimicrobial use. However, it should not be surmised that only topical antisepsis or surface disinfection is achievable. The availability of fiber-optic light delivery offers the potential for treatment anywhere in—as well as on—the body. The mainstays of photoantimicrobial use since the noted renaissance around 1990 have been the application of MB to oral disease and in blood plasma disinfection. The former represents a relatively simple local application, typically into the gingival pocket, but exhibits broad-spectrum efficacy because infections here are often polymicrobial

(gram-positive or gram-negative bacteria and yeasts). The latter is single-unit disinfection, principally aimed at antiviral capability (since the advent of HIV) but also requiring antibacterial activity, typically against the gram-negative organisms *Pseudomonas fluorescens* and *Yersinia enterocolitica*.[73]

Toxicity

The desired combination of planar structure, surface area, and cationic charge of most of the photoantimicrobials covered here provides examples of potential nucleic acid intercalators, that is, molecules that, because of their geometry and charge, are able to fit between consecutive base pairs in the double helical structure of DNA. The relationship between sufficient molecular planar area/positive charge in this interaction as the mode of action of the aminoacridines was discussed earlier.[29] From the photodynamic perspective, such targeting of an essential biomolecule is highly appealing; however, this does not necessarily produce a magic bullet. For example, introducing MB into a solution of DNA leads to intercalation, which is observable via spectrophotometry. Subsequent red-light irradiation of the solution causes oxidative breakdown of the nucleic acid, which is again easily observable via HPLC of the resulting mixture, producing 8-hydroxyguanosine.[74] If the DNA target is contained in a eukaryotic cell nucleus, demonstrating the interaction and subsequent damage represents a much more difficult proposition, with the degree of difficulty being in proportion to cellular complexity. The DNA damage following photosensitization requires careful analysis because this event may occur indirectly after critical damage to the cell elsewhere, for example, in the lysosome, followed by relocalization as is the case for MB.[75]

The potential for cellular DNA damage by dyes is not a straightforward proposition and requires careful consideration. Dyes such as MB and acriflavine have been used in medicine and clinical laboratories since the late 19th century, but there have been no documented associated cases of cancer. A similar argument is possible for the photosensitizers discussed in the following text. Although it is imperative to carry out efficacy/safety testing on novel drugs, overall objectivity is also essential. The earlier mentioned MB, for example, is clearly safe for human use and, yet, produces a positive Ames (bacterial mutagenicity) test result in vitro.[76] Despite this, it should be noted that adverse effects have been reported following clinical photoantimicrobial activity. During the 1960s and 1970s, a significant number of cases of genital herpes were treated, usually with the acridine proflavine or the phenazine neutral red, given their reported efficacy against herpesviruses.[77] In a very small number of cases, posttreatment Bowen disease occurred. This may have been due to the use of ultraviolet light as the activating energy source, but

TABLE 13.3   Photoantimicrobial chemical classes and photoproperties

Photoantimicrobial Class	Typical Wavelength Range (nm)	Activating Light[a]
Acridine	400-450	Violet/blue
Phenazine	500	Green
Phenothiazinium	620-660	Red
Indocyanine green	800	Near-infrared
Xanthene	500-550	Green
Phthalocyanine	630-670	Red
Porphyrin	420-630	Blue/red

[a]Ultraviolet light may also be used but is not recommended for human clinical disinfection.

this was not established. The use of ultraviolet light with photoantimicrobials has not been recommended during the more recent renaissance in this field of research.

The principal classes of photosensitizer, exemplars of which are either clinically used photoantimicrobials or are approaching this status, are covered in Table 13.3 and the following sections. As with the dyes used as conventional antimicrobials, the photoantimicrobials are sectioned by chemical class.

Acridines

The parent molecule, acridine, was one of the dyes used in the initial laboratory demonstration of the photodynamic effect.[70] Little work has been carried out in developing useful photoantimicrobials from this chromophore and has been limited to the early derivatives proflavine and acriflavine. This is unusual, given that several members of the class have been used clinically (noted earlier) as conventional antimicrobials, without significant side effects. The in vitro antibacterial effects of a range of these agents

have been reported, and data concerning activities against *S aureus* and *Pseudomonas aeruginosa* are provided in Table 13.4. The associated dark (ie, conventional) toxicities occurred at much increased concentrations, in agreement with literature reports concerning bacterial DNA interference via an intercalative mechanism.[78] Given this mode of action, the increased activity of the acridines on photoactivation should be considered as the disastrous consequence of critically localized photosensitizers, where bacterial DNA intercalation leads to interference with cellular reproduction but is reversible on removal of the agent; photoactivation of the agent in situ leads to oxidation at various points, catastrophic breakdown, and is thus irreversible.

During their work on the structure-activity relationships of antibacterial examples, Albert and his coworkers[26] produced many simple aminoacridines,[79] of which only a handful have been examined as photoantimicrobials and are a potentially profitable area for drug discovery. The simple aminoacridines exhibit their most intense visible absorptions in the 400 to 500 nm light range (violet/blue). Practically speaking, because these compounds are

TABLE 13.4   Toxicity and phototoxicity of aminoacridines against bacteria[a]

Acridine	MBC (μmol)			
	Staphylococcus aureus		*Pseudomonas aeruginosa*	
	Dark	Light[b]	Dark	Light[b]
Ethacridine	10	5	100	25
Aminacrine	50	2.5	500	500
Salacrine	25	2.5	500	500
Acridine orange	25	1	500	100
Proflavine	25	2.5	250	10

Abbreviation: MBC, minimum bactericidal concentration.

[a]From Wainwright et al.[30] Reproduced by permission of British Society for Antimicrobial Chemotherapy.

[b]Fluence rate = 1.7 mW cm^{-2}; fluence = 6.3 J cm^{-2} (white light). See Table 13.1 for structural information.

aimed at photodynamic infection control, this might lead to problems with endogenous absorption. Despite this, it should be stated that riboflavin (vitamin B₂) has a strong absorption at 475 nm and yet retains its photoantimicrobial activity in the presence of red blood cells,[80] so it may be that there is potential for the aminoacridines. Conversely, as mentioned earlier, blue light photoactivation is proposed for surface decontamination. Proflavine was one of the photosensitizers employed in the clinical treatment of genital herpes in the 1970s.[81]

Phenazines

The phenazine dyes resemble the acridines closely, due to the fact that the acridine and phenazine chromophores differ due only to a single –CH= to −N= substitution in the central ring. Consequently, several examples of the phenazine class also have the capability for DNA intercalation.[82,83] The only derivatives concerning significant photoantimicrobial potential are neutral red and safranine T (Figure 13.6), and the former is certainly the major contributor, having also been used in the treatment of genital herpes in the 1960s and 1970s.[84]

As with the simple acridines, the planarity and structural simplicity of neutral red lead to significantly aggregated dyes in solution. Thus, in terms of singlet oxygen generation, the correct (monomeric) absorption band must be targeted on illumination ($\lambda_{max\ monomer}$ = 450 nm; $\lambda_{max\ aggregate}$ = 536 nm).[85] It should be remembered that neutral red is mainly employed in the histopathology laboratory as a live/dead stain for mammalian cells, and this may preclude its use as a clinical photoantimicrobial on the grounds of lack of selectivity, but this does not affect its potential for use in surface disinfection.

Phenothiaziniums

As mentioned earlier, MB has found use in a variety of clinical roles, in addition to providing a lead compound in antimalarial, antipsychotic, and antidepressant research.[1] Such is its importance in the photoantimicrobial field, the ubiquitous use of MB (Figure 13.7) has inhibited the clinical introduction of novel phenothiazinium

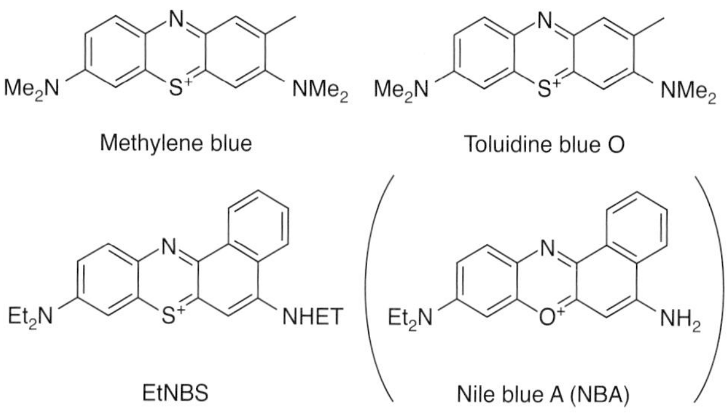

FIGURE 13.7 Phenothiazinium-based photoantimicrobials.

photosensitizers. The principal reason here is that MB is safe for human use, whereas any new chemical compound based on this structure would have to undergo extensive testing prior even to preclinical phases. There are many examples of new compounds based on MB that have far greater photoantimicrobial potential—MB itself is only a moderate example—but these face huge regulatory barriers, whereas MB is already licensed for use in blood product pathogen reduction,[73] oral and nasal photodisinfection,[86] and has been employed on a smaller scale against herpes lesions,[87] diabetic ulcers,[88] and onychomycosis.[89] In terms of initial-stage drug development, the synthesis of novel phenothiaziniums has seen higher productivity than any other potentially photoantimicrobial class.

Most reported series of MB derivatives have significantly greater photoantimicrobial activities than the parent. This has not necessarily been correlated to in vitro singlet oxygen yields; singlet oxygen measurement in vitro and cell killing in culture are two very different processes, particularly because the latter includes the cellular uptake and possible metabolism of the photosensitizer. This phenomenon is exemplified by the impressive pentacyclic derivative of MB, known as DO15. This derivative produces lower yields of singlet oxygen than the parent in vitro but is considerably more active as a photoantimicrobial under the same conditions (Table 13.5).[90] Additionally, its gram-negative efficacy is greater than usually seen with phenothiazinium photosensitizers and is due to lower aggregate formation, due to its bulkier molecular shape, and ability to alter outer membrane structure.[91]

The benzo[a]phenoxazine Nile blue became a lead compound in antitumor PDT during the late 20th century.[69] Resulting photosensitizers all contained "heavy" atoms (ie, lower chemical period) due to the poor conversion rates associated with the oxygen-containing chromophore (see Figure 13.7). More effective ring analogues with sulfur or selenium replacing oxygen have provided excellent scaffolds for photoantimicrobial development, and the principal compound in this group is Foley's EtNBS compound (see Figure 13.7).[92]

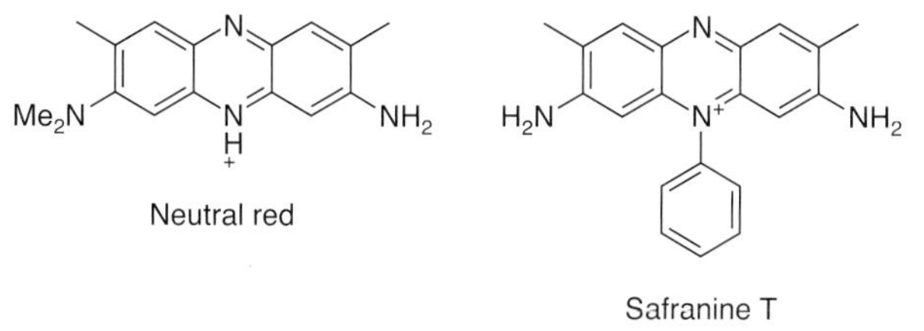

FIGURE 13.6 Phenazinium dyes.

TABLE 13.5 Properties and photoactivities of a series of methylene blue derivatives

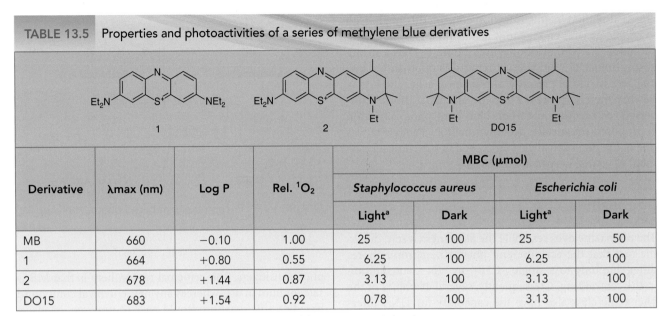

Derivative	λmax (nm)	Log P	Rel. ¹O₂	MBC (μmol)			
				Staphylococcus aureus		*Escherichia coli*	
				Light[a]	Dark	Light[a]	Dark
MB	660	−0.10	1.00	25	100	25	50
1	664	+0.80	0.55	6.25	100	6.25	100
2	678	+1.44	0.87	3.13	100	3.13	100
DO15	683	+1.54	0.92	0.78	100	3.13	100

Abbreviations: MB, methylene blue; MBC, minimum bactericidal concentration; Rel., relative.

[a]Fluence rate = 100 mW cm⁻²; fluence = 6.2 J cm⁻² (red light).

Cyanines

The sole realistic example in the cyanine class is that of indocyanine green (ICG), principally because it has been used in vital staining of cancer[93] and blood flow measurement.[94] Such clinical experience, in parallel with photodynamic research, has developed into the application of ICG in angiography and in the treatment of choroidal neovascularization in age-related macular degeneration.[95] As with other photosensitizers, this activity has also allowed development in the antimicrobial direction.

Long-wavelength absorption in cyanine dyes is gained from an extended polymethine (–CH=) pi system. In ICG,

this extends to seven methine units (see Figure 13.8) and results in a λmax around 800 nm. Such near-infrared absorption offers considerable potential in terms of the avoidance of endogenous absorption. Furthermore, although ICG was originally expected to act as a photosensitizer, and phototoxic effects have indeed been reported,[96] research suggests that these effects are often due to photothermal rather than type I/type II photosensitization pathways. The λmax allows excitation by a 808-nm diode laser, and the photoexcited molecule releases the excitational energy to its surroundings, causing thermal damage to cells.[97] Highly effective killing of periodontal and wound pathogens has been reported.[98,99]

Xanthenes

Indocyanine green

X	X'	R	R'	R"	λmax (nm)	Φ△	Common Name
H	H	Br	Br	Br	516	0.50	Eosin Y
H	H	I	I	I	526	0.63	Erythrosine
Cl	Cl	I	I	I	548	0.75	Rose bengal

FIGURE 13.8 Xanthene and indocyanine photoantimicrobials. Φ△, singlet oxygen efficiency (maximum = 1.00). Data from Pooler and Valenzeno.[100]

Xanthene Derivatives

Xanthene-based dyes containing heavy halogens are among the higher singlet oxygen–producing synthetic dyes. In addition, this class has been in constant use in humans either in medicine or as food colorants for over a century. In addition, eosin Y (Figure 13.8) was one of Raab's[70] "breakthrough" dyes in his experiments with paramecia.

These established dyes are less useful than might be expected, despite their high yields of singlet oxygen, because they are anionic in nature and in most cases the usual correlation of poor gram-negative bacteria efficacy.[21] Activities are, not surprisingly, very high against gram-positive bacteria and, for this reason, dyes such as rose bengal, erythrosine, and eosin Y have been suggested for oral disinfection, especially of the gingival pocket, given the preponderance of the gram-positive organism *Enterococcus faecalis* in this location.[101,102]

Phthalocyanines

As with porphyrins, of which they might be considered to be derivatives, there is no historical rationale for the use of phthalocyanines in infection control. From Figure 13.9, it can be seen that the latter have an extended aromatic network due to the four fused benzene rings around the outside of the structure, and this provides a much more intense long wavelength (red) absorption than the porphyrins, which is effective in terms of practical use where there is a possibility of endogenous absorption. The central atom usually has little effect on this absorption, but high yields of singlet oxygen are associated with phthalocyanines having a suitable central metal atom—greater than that of standard photosensitizers such as MB, for example,[103] and central atoms include aluminum, zinc, germanium, gallium, and silicon.[104] Conversely, derivatives having a central atom with an open "d" shell or paramagnetic metal ions such as V(II), Fe(II), Cr(II), Co(II),

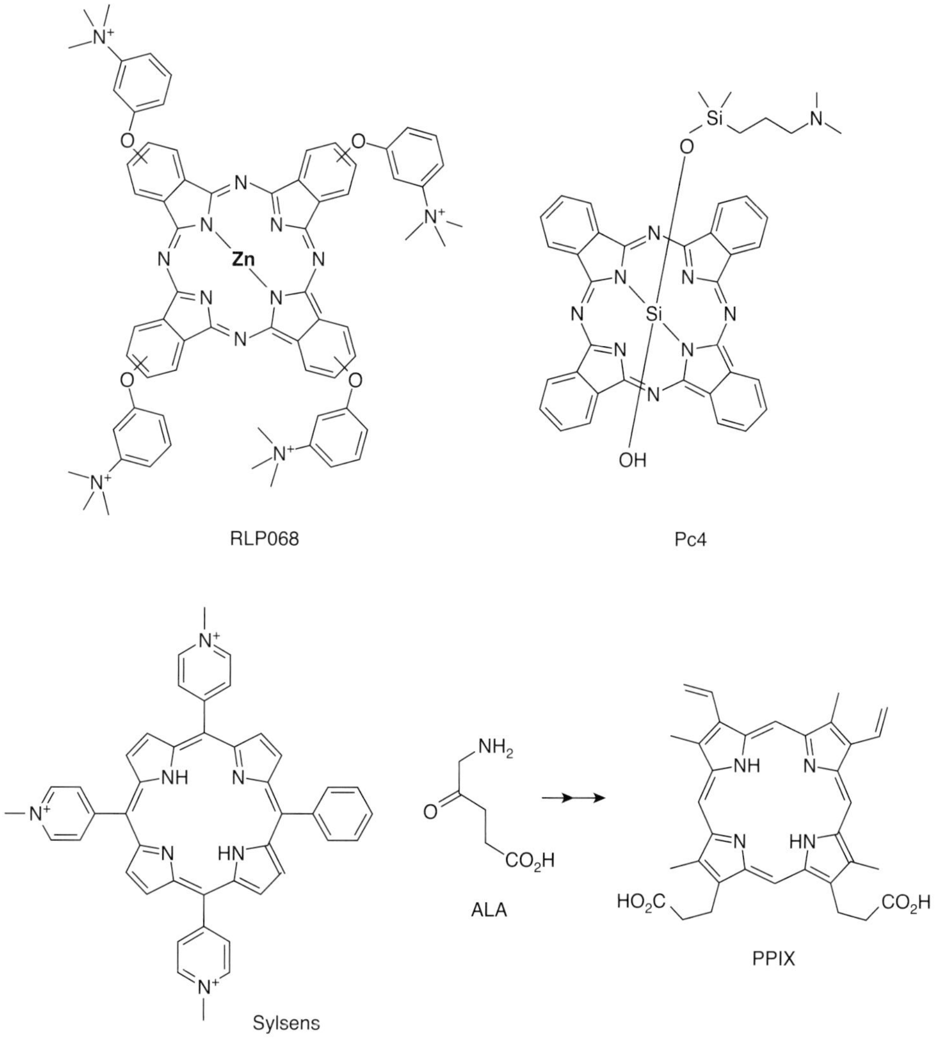

FIGURE 13.9 Phthalocyanine photoantimicrobials and protoporphyrin IX (PPIX).

Ni(II), and Cu(II) have short triplet lifetimes due to much more rapid reversion to the singlet ground state (see Figure 13.5) and are thus poor photosensitizers.[105]

There is a considerable photoantimicrobial literature associated with phthalocyanines, mainly due to the work concerning silicon phthalocyanines, carried out by Ben-Hur and coworkers in the 1990s, into their use in blood product disinfection protocols.[106,107] However, much work has also been reported subsequently by others concerning peripherally rather than axially functionalized derivatives, especially those of a cationic nature[108,109]; this has realized the clinically useful zinc phthalocyanine derivative, RLP068 (see Figure 13.9).[110]

One of the problems with phthalocyanine synthesis is the number of isomers formed when a nonsymmetrical starting material is used. This is obviously not a problem when the functionalization is added via the central atom, as is the case with the silicon phthalocyanines mentioned earlier. The intention with the derivative Pc4, for example, was to employ the intense long wavelength absorption to provide disinfection capability in red blood cell concentrates, that is, with very strong endogenous heme absorption typically against HIV-1 and HIV-2. This was extended to the requirement for blood disinfection protocols that both enveloped and nonenveloped viruses should be eradicated so that unknown viral contaminants would be removed by the same process. Enveloped viruses such as HIV and herpes simplex viruses (HSV) are generally susceptible to photoinactivation, whereas nonenveloped viruses are not, suggesting that the viral envelope is the primary target for phthalocyanine photosensitization.[111]

Thus, Pc4, with its cationic dialkylaminoalkylsilyloxy residue on the central silicon (see Figure 13.9), was not only active against cell-free HIV but also active against the actively replicating virus and latently infected red blood cells.[112] Although this activity profile against viruses is highly desirable, there remains the problem of collateral red blood cell damage, which requires the addition of an antioxidant.

Although the successful MB-plasma treatment has already been alluded to, the phthalocyanines have yet gained clinical approval in this area. However, the results of photoantiviral phthalocyanine testing have been impressive enough for several derivatives to been screened as anti-HIV agents per se. Thus, sulfonated copper, nickel, and vanadyl derivatives as well as the metal-free analogue have all been found to be inherently viricidal, suggesting their use, for example, in blocking the sexual transmission of HIV.[113] Viral contamination is obviously not the only factor in disease transmission through the transfusion of donated blood. Consequently, it has also been reported that blood-borne pathogens involved in parasitic tropical diseases can be photoinactivated using Pc4. For example, the malarial and trypanosomal parasites *Plasmodium falciparum* and *T cruzi*, respectively, important in many nontemperate parts of the world, are susceptible to this approach.[107]

Unsurprisingly, given the excellent performance of Pc4, the photobactericidal testing of various photodynamic phthalocyanine derivatives has also been carried out, in vitro. Several groups have screened derivatives aimed more at conventional bacterial and fungal infection (ie, intended for use in health care facility infection control). Thus, activity has been demonstrated for phthalocyanines against multidrug-resistant organisms[114] and bacteria in biofilms,[115] whereas photobactericidal materials have been produced from phthalocyanines incorporated into polymer films.[116] Testing of anionic, cationic, and neutral zinc phthalocyanines against both gram-positive and gram-negative bacteria again confirmed that only the positively charged phthalocyanine (a pyridinium salt) was active.[117] This is a similar effect to that observed with cationic *meso*-porphyrins (discussion in the following text).

Porphyrins

A considerable amount of research has been carried out in attempting to produce porphyrin-based photoantimicrobials, but, as mentioned previously, because most of the lead compounds used have been lipophilic, anionic examples, a poor profile has been obtained in most cases with respect to gram-negative bacteria. This has been remedied from two main angles: the provision of cationic examples and the use of a protoporphyrin precursor 5-aminolevulinic acid (ALA). Sylsens (see Figure 13.9) is a meso-tetrasubstituted porphyrin, having three cationic pyridinium pendant groups. This has exhibited considerable activity against both bacteria and fungi, being intended for use in onychomycosis and related conditions.[118]

The lack of uptake by gram-negative bacteria of anionic porphyrins can be circumvented by the use of ALA and its esters because these are converted into protoporphyrin IX in situ (see Figure 13.9), biochemistry that is essential to many bacteria. Consequently, gram-negative organisms are made highly susceptible to subsequent illumination.[119] However, the lack of cell selectivity in a clinical situation, noted previously, suggests that the potential for collateral damage (eg, at a wound site) would be too high to allow use in routine disinfection.

▶ CONCLUSION

In the 21st century, dyes are considered to be "old technology." Outside cosmetics, if the skin or other body surfaces are exposed to dyes, tissue staining normally results, and this is unpopular. Encouraging dye use in infection control is therefore quite a difficult proposition. However, the problem of increasing antimicrobial drug resistance means that the options available for conventional drug replacement are few. Furthermore, due to resistance epidemiology, any option must be useful across infection control, which means including veterinary as well as human applications. This is a considerable undertaking but one that has been promulgated by governments and infection control agencies alike.

The photodynamic use of cationic dyes (ie, photoantimicrobials) offers considerable scope for the improvement of the current situation, due to its multifactorial mode of action and lack of resistance development potential. Although there are established resistance mechanisms against some old classes of conventionally used dyes, these are usually circumvented on light activation and the generation of reactive oxygen species in situ. This should not only encourage the use of photoantimicrobials but should also provide impetus for the photodynamic investigation of other conventionally used dye disinfectants to the same end as well as the continued search for novel photoantimicrobial structures.

Looking forward, it is probably true that conventional anti-infective drugs and biocides will not be used in the same, sometimes wasteful, way as they have been in the past 80 years. Limits on prescription and clinical protocols are likely to be used in order to maintain the efficacy of the dwindling stock of actives. Topical and local photoantimicrobial dye use both in infection prophylaxis and the substitution—and thus conservation—of these actives should be a logical step, but it is one that will require considerable scientific persuasion, and the community should be prepared for this.

REFERENCES

1. Wainwright M. Dyes in the development of drugs and pharmaceuticals. *Dyes Pigments.* 2008;76:582-589.
2. Wainwright M. Dyes, flies, and sunny skies: photodynamic therapy and neglected tropical diseases. *Coloration Technol.* 2017;133:95-103.
3. Browning CH, Gulbransen R, Thornton LHD. The antiseptic properties of acriflavine and proflavine, and brilliant green: with special reference to suitability for wound therapy. *Br Med J.* 1917;2:70-75.
4. Wainwright M, Amaral L. Photobactericides—a local option against multi-drug resistant bacteria. *Antibiotics (Basel).* 2013;2:182-190.
5. Wainwright M. The problem of dyes in medicine. *Dyes Pigments.* 2017;146:402-407.
6. Lerman LS. Structural considerations in the interaction of DNA and acridines. *J Mol Biol.* 1961;3:18-30.
7. Page MGP. The role of the outer membrane of gram-negative bacteria in antibiotic resistance: Ajax' shield or Achilles' heel? *Handb Exp Pharmacol.* 2012;(211):67-86.
8. Wainwright M, McLean A. Rational design of phenothiazinium derivatives and photoantimicrobial drug discovery. *Dyes Pigments.* 2017;136:590-600.
9. Hamblin M, Hasan T. Photodynamic therapy: a new antimicrobial approach to infectious disease? *Photochem Photobiol Sci.* 2004;3: 436-450.
10. Wainwright M, Kristiansen JE. On the 75th anniversary of prontosil. *Dyes Pigments.* 2011;88:231-234.
11. Shane SJ, Riley C, Laurie JH, Boutilier M. Thiosemicarbazones in tuberculosis. *Can Med Assoc J.* 1951;64:289-293.
12. Eisenberg P. The action of dyes on bacteria and the effect of vital staining on growth of bacteria. *Zbl Bakteriol Parasiten Infektkr.* 1913;71:420.
13. Ostromislensky I. Note on bacteriostatic azo compounds. *J Am Chem Soc.* 1934;56:1713-1714.
14. Gillespie JB. Experiments on the antibacterial properties of pyridium and serenium. *Am J Dis Child.* 1933;45:254-270.
15. Gold NA, Bithoney WG. Methemoglobinemia due to ingestion of at most three pills of pyridium in a 2-year-old: case report and review. *J Emerg Med.* 2003;25:143-148.
16. Hörlein H. The chemotherapy of infectious diseases caused by protozoa and bacteria. *Proc R Soc Med.* 1936;29:313-24.
17. Churchman JW. The selective bactericidal action of gentian violet. *J Exp Med.* 1912;16:221-247.
18. Churchman JW. The selective bactericidal action of stains closely allied to gentian violet. *J Exp Med.* 1913;17:373-378.
19. Churchman JW, Michael WH. The selective action of gentian violet on closely related bacterial strains. *J Exp Med.* 1912;16:822-830.
20. Churchman JW. The selective bacteriostatic action of gentian violet and other dyes. *J Urol.* 1924;11:1-18.
21. Fung DYC, Miller RD. Effect of dyes on bacterial growth. *Appl Microbiol.* 1973;25:793-799.
22. Laube S. Skin infections and ageing. *Ageing Res Rev.* 2004;3:69-89.
23. Esteva M, Ruiz AM, Stoka AM. *Trypanosoma cruzi*: methoprene is a potent agent to sterilize blood infected with trypomastigotes. *Exp Parasitol.* 2002;100:248-251.
24. Saji M, Taguchi S, Uchiyama K, Osono E, Hayama N, Ohkuni H. Efficacy of gentian violet in the eradication of methicillin-resistant *Staphylococcus aureus* from skin lesions. *J Hosp Infect.* 1995;31:225-228.
25. Benda L. Über das 3.6-Diamino-acridin. *Chem Ber.* 1912;46:1787-1799.
26. Albert A, Rubbo SD, Goldacre RJ, Davey ME, Stone JD. The influence of chemical constitution on antibacterial activity. Part II: a general survey of the acridine series. *Br J Exp Pathol.* 1945;26:160-192.
27. Aldred KJ, Kerns RJ, Osheroff N. Mechanism of quinolone action and resistance. *Biochemistry.* 2014;53:1565-1574.
28. Goodell JR, Ougolkov AV, Hiasa H, et al. Acridine-based agents with topoisomerase II activity inhibit pancreatic cancer cell proliferation and induce apoptosis. *J Med Chem.* 2008;51:179-182.
29. Albert A, Rubbo SD, Burvill MI. The influence of chemical constitution on antibacterial activity. Part IV: a survey of heterocyclic bases, with special reference to benzquinolines, phenanthridines, benzacridines, quinolines and pyridines. *Brit J Exp Pathol.* 1949;30:159-175.
30. Wainwright M, Phoenix DA, Marland J, Wareing DRA, Bolton FJ. In-vitro photobactericidal activity of aminoacridines. *J Antimicrob Chemother.* 1997;40:587-589.
31. Mitchell GAG, Buttle GAH. Proflavine in closed wounds. *Lancet.* 1943;242:749.
32. Jauison H, Pecker A, Medioni G. Les accidents de l'acridinothérapie. Innocuite des doses usuelles. *Soc Med Hop Paris.* 1931;47:397-406.
33. Assinder EW. Acriflavine as a urinary antiseptic. *Lancet.* 1936;227: 304-305.
34. Sievers O, Stein B. In: Hörlein H, ed. *Medicine in Its Chemical Aspects.* Leverkusen, Germany: Bayer; 1963:60-63.
35. Bernstein F, Carrié C. Zu pharmakologie des trypaflavins. *Derm Zeit.* 1933;66:330-335.
36. Levrat M, Morelon F. Contribution à l'étude pharmacodynamique et toxicologique de la trypaflavine, du rivanol et d'autres dérivés de l'acridine. *Bull Sci Pharmacol.* 1933;40:582-592.
37. Keogh PP, Bentley GA. The pharmacology of monacrine. *Aust J Sci.* 1948;11:98-99.
38. IG Farben, assignee. Process for the manufacture of acridine derivatives. British Patent 367,037. February 1932.
39. IG Farben, assignee. Method for the production of 3-aminoacridine and its substitution products. German Patent 547,983. April 1932.
40. Mietzsch F, Mauss H, inventors; Winthrop Chemical Company, assignee. Salts of aminoacridines. US Patent 2,092,131. September 1937.
41. Miller CS, Wagner CA. 2,3-dimethoxy-6-nitro-9-(γ-diethylamino-β-hydroxypropylamino)acridine. *J Org Chem.* 1948;13:891-894.
42. Steck EA, Buck JS, Fletcher LT. Some 9-amino-3-nitroacridine derivatives. *J Am Chem Soc.* 1957;79:4414-4417.

43. Elslager EF, Tendick FH. 9-Amino-2,3-dimethoxy-6-nitroacridine 10-oxides. *J Med Pharm Chem*. 1962;5:1149-1153.

44. Tabern D, inventor; Abbott Laboratories, assignee. Antiseptic acridane compounds. US patent 2,645,594. July 1953.

45. Tabern D, inventor; Abbott Laboratories, assignee. Alkoxyphenyl-alkoxy-acridanes. US patent 2,684,367. July 1954.

46. Birch CA, Hanschell HM. Acute toxic hepatitis after acriflavine. *Lancet*. 1931;217:269-270.

47. Manson-Bahr P, ed. In: *Manson's Tropical Diseases*. 7th ed. London, United Kingdom: Cassell; 1940:516.

48. Browning CH, Cohen JB, Gaunt R, Gulbransen R. Relationships between antiseptic action and chemical constitution with special reference to compounds of the pyridine, quinoline, acridine and phenazine series. *Proc Roy Soc*. 1922;93B:329-366.

49. Barry VC, Belton JG, Conalty ML, et al. Anti-tubercular activity of oxidation products of substituted *o*-phenylenediamine. *Nature*. 1948;162:622-623.

50. Lockwood DNJ. Leprosy. *Medicine*. 2005;33:26-29.

51. Arbiser JL, Moschella SL. Clofazimine: a review of its medical uses and mechanisms of action. *J Am Acad Dermatol*. 1995;32:241-247.

52. Selby W, Pavli P, Crotty B, et al. Two-year combination antibiotic therapy with clarithromycin, rifabutin, and clofazimine for Crohn's disease. *Gastroenterology*. 2007;132:2313-2319.

53. Shah A, Bhagat R, Panchal N. Resistant tuberculosis: successful treatment with amikacin, ofloxacin, clofazimine, and PAS. *Tuber Lung Dis*. 1993;74:64-65.

54. Wainwright M, Kristiansen JE. Quinoline and cyanine dyes—putative anti-MRSA drugs. *Int J Antimicrob Agents*. 2003;22:479-486.

55. Browning CH, Cohen JB, Gulbransen R. Further observations on the relation between chemical constitution and antiseptic action. *J Path Bact*. 1921;24:127-128.

56. Browning CH, Cohen JB, Gulbransen R. The antiseptic properties of cyanine dyes. *Br Med J*. 1922;1:514-515.

57. Browning CH, Cohen JB, Ellingworth S, Gulbransen R. The antiseptic action of the styryl-pyridines and styryl-quinolines. *Br Med J*. 1923;2:326.

58. Browning CH, Cohen JB, Ellingworth S, Gulbransen R. The antiseptic action of anil-pyridines and anil-quinolines. *J Path Bact*. 1924;27:121-122.

59. Browning CH, Cohen JB, Ellingworth S, et al. Antiseptic properties of the amino derivatives of styryl and anilquinoline. *Proc Roy Soc*. 1926;100B:293-325.

60. Browning CH, Gulbransen R, Kennaway EL, Thornton LHD. Flavine and brilliant green, powerful antiseptics with low toxicity to the tissues: their use in the treatment of infected wounds. *Br Med J*. 1917;1:73-78.

61. Armitage G, Gordon J, Cohen JB, Ellingworth S, Dobson JF. The use of a new quinoline derivative in the treatment of infection. *Lancet*. 1929;214:968-971.

62. McKinstry DW. The antibacterial properties of cyanine. *J Am Pharm Assoc*. 1949;38:146-149.

63. Abd El-Aal RM, Younis M. Synthesis and antimicrobial activity of *meso*-substituted polymethine cyanine dyes. *Bioorg Chem*. 2004;32:193-210.

64. Chu WC, Bai PY, Yang ZQ, et al. Synthesis and antibacterial evaluation of novel cationic chalcone derivatives possessing broad spectrum antibacterial activity. *Eur J Med Chem*. 2018;143:905-921.

65. Liu S, Ma J, Zhao D. Synthesis and characterization of cationic monoazo dyes incorporating quaternary ammonium salts. *Dyes Pigments*. 2007;75:255-262.

66. Karcı F, Şener N, Yamaç M, Şenera I, Demirçalı A. The synthesis, antimicrobial activity and absorption characteristics of some novel heterocyclic disazo dyes. *Dyes Pigments*. 2009;80:47-52.

67. Wainwright M, Maisch T, Nonell S, et al. Photoantimicrobials—are we afraid of the light? *Lancet Infect Dis*. 2017;17:e49-e55.

68. Wainwright M. Photodynamic antimicrobial chemotherapy (PACT). *J Antimicrob Chemother*. 1998;42:13-28.

69. Cincotta L, Foley JW, Cincotta AH. Novel red absorbing benzo[*a*]phenoxazinium and benzo[*a*]phenothiazinium photosensitizers: in vitro evaluation. *Photochem Photobiol*. 1987;46:751-758.

70. Raab O. Uber die wirkung fluorescierenden stoffe auf infusorien. *Z Biol*. 1900;39:524-546.

71. Lipson RL, Baldes EJ. The photodynamic properties of a particular hematoporphyrin derivative. *Arch Dermatol*. 1960;82:508-516.

72. Wainwright M, Crossley KB. Methylene blue—a therapeutic dye for all seasons? *J Chemother*. 2002;14:431-443.

73. Wainwright M, Mohr H, Walker W. Phenothiazinium derivatives for pathogen inactivation in blood products. *J Photochem Photobiol B*. 2007;86:45-58.

74. Floyd RA, West MS, Eneff KL, Schneider J. Methylene blue plus light mediates 8-hydroxyguanine formation in DNA. *Arch Biochem Biophys*. 1989;15:106-111.

75. Mellish KJ, Cox RD, Vernon DI, Griffiths J, Brown SB. In vitro photodynamic activity of a series of methylene blue analogues. *Photochem Photobiol*. 2002;75:392-397.

76. Webb RB, Hass BS, Kubitschek HE. Photodynamic effects of dyes on bacteria. II. Genetic effects of broad-spectrum visible light in the presence of acridine dyes and methylene blue in chemostat cultures of *Escherichia coli*. *Mutat Res*. 1979;59:1-13.

77. Wainwright M. Photoinactivation of viruses. *Photochem Photobiol Sci*. 2004;3:406-411.

78. Albert A. *The Acridines*. 2nd ed. London, United Kingdom: Arnold; 1966.

79. Rubbo SD, Albert A, Maxwell M. The influence of chemical constitution on antiseptic activity. I: a study of the mono-aminoacridines. *B J Exp Pathol*. 1942;23:69-83.

80. Goodrich RP. The use of riboflavin for the inactivation of pathogens in blood products. *Vox Sang*. 2000;78:211-215.

81. Kaufman RH, Adam E, Mirkovic RR, et al. Treatment of genital herpes simplex virus infection with photodynamic inactivation. *Am J Obstet Gynecol*. 1978;132:861-869.

82. Li J, Wei YX, Wei YL, Dong C. Study on the spectral behavior of four fluorescent dyes and their interactions with nucleic acid by the luminescence method. *J Lum*. 2007;124:143-150.

83. Cao Y, He X. Studies of interaction between safranine T and double helix DNA by spectral methods. *Spectrochim Acta A Mol Biomol Spectrosc*. 1998;54:883-892.

84. Kaufman RH, Gardner HL, Brown D, Wallis C, Rawls WE, Melnick JL. Herpes genitalis treated by photodynamic inactivation of virus. *Am J Obstet Gynecol*. 1973;117:1144-1146.

85. Urrutia MN, Ortiz CS. Spectroscopic characterization and aggregation of azine compounds in different media. *Chem Phys*. 2013;142:41-50.

86. Andersen R, Loebel N, Hammond D, Wilson M. Treatment of periodontal disease by photodisinfection compared to scaling and root planing. *J Clin Dent*. 2007;18:34-38.

87. Tardivo JP, Wainwright M, Baptista MS. Local clinical phototreatment of herpes infection in São Paulo. *Photodiagnosis Photodyn Ther*. 2012;9:118-121.

88. Tardivo JP, Adami F, Correa JA, Pinhal MA, Baptista MS. A clinical trial testing the efficacy of PDT in preventing amputation in diabetic patients. *Photodiagnosis Photodyn Ther*. 2014;11:342-350.

89. Tardivo JP, Wainwright M, Baptista M. Small scale trial of photodynamic treatment of onychomycosis in São Paulo. *J Photochem Photobiol B*. 2015;150:66-68.

90. Wainwright M, Meegan K, Loughran C. Phenothiazinium photosensitisers IX. Tetra- and pentacyclic derivatives as photoantimicrobial agents. *Dyes Pigments*. 2011;91:1-5.

91. Bacellar IOL, Pavani C, Sales EM, Itri R, Wainwright M, Baptista MS. Membrane damage efficiency of phenothiazinium photosensitizers. *Photochem Photobiol*. 2014;90:801-813.

92. Foley JW, Song X, Demidova TN, Jilal F, Hamblin M. Synthesis and properties of benzo[*a*]phenoxazinium chalcogen analogues as novel broad-spectrum antimicrobial photosensitizers. *J Med Chem*. 2006;49:5291-5299.

93. Tagaya N, Yamazaki R, Nakagawa A, et al. Intraoperative identification of sentinel lymph nodes by near-infrared fluorescence imaging in patients with breast cancer. *Am J Surg.* 2008;195:850-853.

94. Unno N, Suzuki M, Yamamoto N, et al. Indocyanine green fluorescence angiography for intraoperative assessment of blood flow: a feasibility study. *Eur J Vasc Endovasc Surg.* 2008;35:205-207.

95. Gomi F, Ohji M, Sayanagi K, et al. One-year outcomes of photodynamic therapy in age-related macular degeneration and polypoidal choroidal vasculopathy in Japanese patients. *Ophthalmology.* 2008;115:141-146.

96. Mamoon AM, Gamal-Eldeen AM, Ruppel ME, Smith RJ, Tsang T, Miller LM. In vitro efficiency and mechanistic role of indocyanine green as photodynamic therapy agent for human melanoma. *Photodiagnosis Photodyn Ther.* 2009;6:105-116.

97. Chen WR, Adams RL, Bartels KE, Nordquist RE. Chromophore-enhanced in vivo tumor cell destruction using an 808-nm diode laser. *Cancer Lett.* 1995;94:125-131.

98. Boehm TK, Ciancio SG. Diode laser activated indocyanine green selectively kills bacteria. *J Int Acad Periodontol.* 2011;13:58-63.

99. Omar GS, Wilson M, Nair SP. Lethal photosensitization of wound-associated microbes using indocyanine green and near-infrared light. *BMC Microbiol.* 2008;8:111.

100. Pooler JP, Valenzeno DP. Physicochemical determinants of the sensitizing effectiveness for photooxidation of nerve membranes by fluorescein derivatives. *Photochem Photobiol.* 1979;30:491-498.

101. Wood S, Metcalf D, Devine D, Robinson C. Erythrosine is a potential photosensitizer for the photodynamic therapy of oral plaque biofilms. *J Antimicrob Chemother.* 2006;57:680-684.

102. Borba ASM, da Silva Pereira SM, Borba MCM, et al. Photodynamic therapy with high-power LED mediated by erythrosine eliminates *Enterococcus faecalis* in planktonic forms. *Photodiagnosis Photodyn Ther.* 2017;19:348-351.

103. Griffiths J, Schofield J, Wainwright M, Brown SB. Some observations on the synthesis of polysubstituted zinc phthalocyanine sensitisers for photodynamic therapy. *Dyes Pigments.* 1997;33:65-78.

104. Darwent JR, Douglas P, Harriman A, Porter G, Richoux M. Metal phthalocyanines and porphyrins as photosensitizers for reduction of water to hydrogen. *Coord Chem Rev.* 1982;44:83-126.

105. Chan VS, Marshall JF, Svensen R, Phillips D, Hart IR. Photosensitising activity of phthalocyanine dyes screened against tissue culture cells. *Photochem Photobiol.* 1987;45:757-761.

106. Zmudzka BZ, Strickland AG, Beer JZ, Ben-Hur E. Photosensitized decontamination of blood with the silicon phthalocyanine Pc 4: no activation of the human immunodeficiency virus promoter. *Photochem Photobiol.* 1997;65:461-464.

107. Zhao XJ, Lustigman S, Li YS, Kenney ME, Ben-Hur E. Structure-activity and mechanism studies on silicon phthalocyanines with *Plasmodium falciparum* in the dark and under red light. *Photochem Photobiol.* 1997;66:282-287.

108. Segalla A, Borsarelli CD, Braslavsky SE, et al. Photophysical, photochemical and antibacterial photosensitizing properties of a novel octacationic Zn(II)-phthalocyanine. *Photochem Photobiol Sci.* 2002;1:641-648.

109. Maisch T, Szeimies RM, Jori G, Abels C. Antibacterial photodynamic therapy in dermatology. *Photochem Photobiol Sci.* 2004;3:907-919.

110. Giuliani F, Martinelli M, Cocchi A, Arbia D, Fantetti L, Roncucci G. *In vitro* resistance selection studies of RLP068/Cl, a new Zn(II) phthalocyanine suitable for antimicrobial photodynamic therapy. *Antimicrob Agents Chemother.* 2010;54:637-642.

111. Ben-Hur E, Moor ACE, Margolis-Nunno H, et al. The photodecontamination of cellular blood components: mechanisms and use of photosensitization in transfusion medicine. *Transfus Med Rev.* 1996;10:15-22.

112. Margolis-Nunno H, Ben-Hur E, Gottlieb P, Robinson R, Oetjen J, Horowitz B. Inactivation by phthalocyanine photosensitization of multiple forms of human immunodeficiency virus in red cell concentrates. *Transfusion.* 1996;36:743-750.

113. Vzorov AN, Marzilli LG, Compans RW, Dixon DW. Prevention of HIV-1 infection by phthalocyanines. *Antiviral Res.* 2003;59:99-109.

114. Wilson M, Pratten J. Lethal photosensitisation of *Staphylococcus aureus* in vitro: effect of growth phase, serum, and pre-irradiation time. *Lasers Surg Med.* 1995;16:272-276.

115. Wilson M, Burns T, Pratten J. Killing of *Streptococcus sanguis* in biofilms using a light-activated antimicrobial agent. *J Antimicrob Chemother.* 1996;37:377-381.

116. Bonnett R, Buckley DG, Burrow T, et al. Photobactericidal materials based on porphyrins and phthalocyanines. *J Mat Chem.* 1993;3:323-324.

117. Minnock A, Vernon DI, Schofield J, Griffiths J, Parish JH, Brown ST. Photoinactivation of bacteria. Use of a cationic water-soluble zinc phthalocyanine to photoinactivate both gram-negative and gram-positive bacteria. *J Photochem Photobiol B.* 1996;32:159-164.

118. Smijs TG, Pavel S, Talebi M, Bouwstra JA. Preclinical studies with 5,10,15-tris(4-methylpyridinium)-20-phenyl-[21*H*,23*H*]-porphine trichloride for the photodynamic treatment of superficial mycoses caused by *Trichophyton rubrum. Photochem Photobiol.* 2009;85:733-739.

119. Nitzan Y, Salmon-Divon M, Shporen E, Malik Z. ALA induced photodynamic effects on gram positive and negative bacteria. *Photochem Photobiol Sci.* 2004;3:430-435.

Essential Oils

Katherine A. Hammer and Christine F. Carson

This chapter describes the use of essential oil products for antisepsis and disinfection. Essential oils are plant-derived, volatile, multicomponent liquids that are oily or lipid-like and are produced in many plant tissues. Many have a strong fragrance and have traditionally been extracted by steam or hydrodistillation.[1] There is a wealth of scientific data describing the antimicrobial activity of essential oils against many different microorganisms using standard in vitro susceptibility tests, which has been summarized elsewhere.[2] This type of data, including minimum inhibitory concentrations (MICs), zones of inhibition, or time kill data, are not discussed in detail in this chapter, where the focus instead is on data pertaining specifically to antisepsis and disinfection applications, including results generated by standard disinfection and antisepsis testing protocols, in-use studies, and in vivo clinical studies. This chapter is also limited to the description of antimicrobial activity relating to plant essential oils and does not include other types of plant extracts, such as hydrosols, preparations from desiccated plant material, or solvent extractions.

▶ CHEMISTRY AND COMPOSITION

Essential oils are typically distilled or pressed from fresh plant material, primarily leaves, and are not water miscible because they are composed largely of hydrocarbons and their oxygenated derivatives. They are generally regarded as secondary metabolites occurring in many, but not all, higher plants. As secondary metabolites, they are not essential for plant growth and often have no known function. Essential oils are complex mixtures, often containing more than 100 volatile, lipophilic, low-molecular-weight compounds that may be roughly divided into two chemical classes: terpenaceous and phenylpropanoid compounds.[1] In plants, they are produced via three major biosynthetic pathways. Terpenaceous compounds are produced in plants by the mevalonic or nonmevalonic acid pathways or a combination of both. The nonmevalonic acid pathway is also known as the methylerythritol phosphate pathway.[3] Phenylpropanoid compounds are produced by the shikimic acid pathway.[4]

Terpenaceous compounds arising from the mevalonic and nonmevalonic acid pathways may or may not contain oxygen. Sensu stricto, the term *terpene* refers to the hydrocarbon compounds from these pathways containing only carbon and hydrogen, whereas *terpenoid* refers to compounds that also contain oxygen. In practice, the terms are often used interchangeably.[1] The former is used in this chapter to refer collectively to terpene and terpenoid compounds. Historically, the word *terpene* comes to us from *turpentine*, the liquid originally derived from various *Pinus* species, although modern turpentine is a petroleum-based product. It was from the original, natural turpentine that the first members of the terpene class of compounds were isolated and characterized.

Terpenes are the largest group of natural compounds with more than 30 000 known structures, ranging from the smaller terpenes found in essential oils to higher terpenes such as beta carotene.[5] The basic biosynthetic building block for terpenes is an isoprene unit (C_5H_8) that is generally joined together in a head-to-tail fashion, although other combinations such as head-to-head do occur. The number of isoprene units from which a terpene is derived, with or without the subsequent loss or addition of carbon atoms, is used to classify the large number of compounds in this class into smaller groups. The terpenaceous compounds in essential oils are almost entirely limited to monoterpenes and sesquiterpenes with a few diterpenes.

Monoterpenes are the most common group of compounds found generally in essential oils.[1] In terms of the compounds present in essential oils used commercially in antisepsis and disinfection products, most fall into this chemical class. They are formed when two isoprene (C_5H_8) units combine yielding a compound with a molecular formula of $C_{10}H_{16}$. At first glance, the scope for variation on this theme may seem limited. However, through subsequent substitutions, cyclizations, and/or isomerizations, the derivatives fall into categories of alcohols, esters, phenols, ketones, lactones, aldehydes, and oxides, and about 1500 monoterpenes have been described,[6] although not all are found in essential oils.

Many cyclic monoterpenes contain a benzene ring[7] that has been shown to make a significant contribution to the antimicrobial activity of both the isolated compound and to essential oils that it occurs in. The antimicrobial activity of the benzene ring may be further enhanced by the attachment of a hydroxyl group to the ring, forming a phenol.[8-10] Phenolic monoterpenes rank among the most well-known and well-characterized antimicrobial essential oil compounds and include thymol and carvacrol.

Sesquiterpenes are the second most frequent group of compounds found generally in essential oils and arise from the combination of three isoprene units.[7] They are not highly prevalent among the oils or compounds used commercially for antisepsis or disinfectant products, although many are known to possess antimicrobial activity. Diterpenes are minor components of essential oils and are not purposefully exploited in commercial antisepsis or disinfectant products, although they may be present in oils that are.

Lastly, phenylpropanoids occur in plant oils much less consistently and generally less abundantly than terpenes but sometimes at high proportions.[1] They are derived from the shikimic acid pathway that occurs in microorganisms and plants but never in animals. They are a small group of compounds with only about 50 described. Among these are a few antimicrobial compounds that historically have enjoyed widespread use such as eugenol and anethole.

▶ SPECTRUM AND MODE OF ACTION OF ESSENTIAL OILS

The specific biological activity of an essential oil is a function of its composition. Different oil components inhibit or kill different microorganisms and by different means. Because the term *essential oil* applies to plant extracts containing a diverse array of antimicrobial components, the mechanism of action for each essential oil is not identical. That said, there are some mechanisms of action that are common to a number of different essential oils.

As a general rule, essential oils show concentration-dependent activity, with minor antimicrobial effects at lower or subinhibitory concentrations and gross effects including death at higher concentrations. Many of the commonly studied essential oils and components, such as oregano oil, thyme oil, and tea tree oil, show bactericidal activity rather than bacteriostatic activity.[1,11,12] Understandably, bacteriostatic essential oils would be of limited use for many disinfection applications.

A mechanism of action common to many essential oils and components is the disruption or damage of microbial membranes, which results in the loss of membrane barrier or metabolic function. Damage typically occurs in a concentration-dependent manner, with minor membrane changes occurring at lower concentrations and gross membrane damage occurring at higher concentrations.[13] This is often due to the oxygenated monoterpene components, examples of which are thymol, carvacrol, terpinen-4-ol, linalool, and 1,8-cineole. Examples of oils or components shown to elicit membrane damage include oregano oil,[14] carvacrol,[15,16] thymol,[17] 1,8-cineole,[18] tea tree oil, and terpinen-4-ol.[19] Additional mechanisms of action shown for some essential oils and components include inhibition of respiration by tea tree oil[20] and inhibition of cell division by cinnamaldehyde.[21]

Essential oils also vary in their spectrum of antimicrobial activity, which relates to both the chemical composition of the oil and microbial characteristics. As a generalization, essential oils rich in components with higher water solubility, such as the oxygenated monoterpene alcohols, will have higher antibacterial activity, whereas those rich in components with lower water solubility will have lower activity.[2] Most essential oils do not show large differences in levels of activity against gram-positive and gram-negative bacteria, although minor variations are common.[2] The effect of essential oils on bacterial endospores has not been extensively studied, and available data suggest that essential oils can have sporicidal activity and can also affect the germination and outgrowth of endospores.[2] Mycobacteria, which are known to be less susceptible to disinfectants compared to other bacteria, have been tested for susceptibility to essential oils.[22,23] Studies indicate that mycobacteria are inhibited by a range of essential oils; however, due to the growth requirements of mycobacteria, special testing conditions must be used, which means that susceptibility results are not directly comparable to those obtained for bacteria. Yeasts are largely susceptible to essential oils at concentrations similar to those affecting bacteria.[24] Other fungi, such as dermatophytes and molds, are also inhibited and killed, although the effects vary according to test conditions, concentration, and type of oil.[2,25] A number of different viruses have been tested for susceptibility to a range of essential oils, and antiviral activity has thus far been observed for enveloped viruses but not for nonenveloped viruses.[24,26,27]

▶ COMMERCIAL PRODUCTS CONTAINING VOLATILE OILS OR COMPONENTS

Several essential oil products have been commercially available for decades. These include disinfectants traditionally containing pine oil, such as Pine-O-Cleen® and Pine-Sol®. Pine-O-Cleen® was developed in Australia by

Len Hunter during World War II and now contains benzalkonium chloride as the active ingredient but historically contained pine oil.[28] Similarly, the disinfectant Pine-Sol®, developed in the United States in 1929, contained pine oil until recently when it was removed due to lack of availability.[29] Interestingly, many Pine-Sol® products contain limonene, among the other components. The product Listerine® was developed in 1879 in the United States.[30] Originally developed as a general disinfectant, it was aggressively marketed in the 1920s as a mouthwash, which is how we know it to be used today. Listerine® contains the essential oil components menthol, thymol, methyl salicylate (wintergreen), and eucalyptol. These days, a large number of disinfection and antiseptic products are commercially available that contain essential oils. These range from hand washes and hand gels, to surface disinfectants and sanitizers, to gel products for air conditioning systems. Many of these formulated products also contain other disinfectant ingredients as active components. The essential oil is often not included as an active component but rather as a fragrance or to enhance consumer appeal, particularly for those products marketed as "natural," "eco-friendly," or "green." In these products, the essential oil is likely to be present at concentrations that are too low to have any significant antimicrobial effect.

▶ OILS MOST FREQUENTLY USED IN DISINFECTION

Relatively few of the large number of essential oils produced worldwide in commercial quantities[31] are used for disinfection. The oils described in the following discussion include those most commonly included in cleaning, disinfectant, and antiseptic products as well as essential oils that have been investigated specifically for disinfection applications.

Citrus Oils

The two citrus oils most frequently found in disinfectant products are orange and lemon oils. The major citrus oil component limonene (synonymous with dipentene) is also used in some products.

Orange oil, also called *sweet orange oil* (to differentiate it from bitter orange oil), is obtained from the peel of *Citrus sinensis* (in the *Rutaceae*, or citrus tree, family) and contains at least 90% D-limonene.[32] Orange oil is the top essential oil produced in the world by volume[31] and is obtained largely as a by-product of orange juice production.[33] Brazil is the largest global producer of oranges[34] and as such also produces the largest quantities of orange oil.[31] Lemon oil is obtained from *Citrus limon* (also in the *Rutaceae*) and contains D-limonene (60% to 75%) and β-pinene.[32] Relatively large volumes of lemon oil are produced compared to many other essential oils, with most produced in Argentina.[31] Lemon oil is one of several products obtained from lemon processing, in addition to lemon juice.

Citrus oils are included in a range of "cleaner-disinfectant" type products but are generally not widely used in antisepsis. In addition, citrus oils are included in "degreaser" preparations due to the solvent properties of the essential oil components and the fact that they can be used instead of chlorinated solvents. These products may also be referred to as *terpene cleaner*.

Tea Tree Oil

Tea tree oil is produced largely from *Melaleuca alternifolia* (*Myrtaceae* family). The oil contains monoterpenes and related alcohols, and the most abundant component is terpinen-4-ol, which comprises about 40% of the oil.[35] The International Standard ISO 4730 stipulates acceptable ranges for 15 components,[36] and oils must meet the compositional criteria in order to be legally sold as "tea tree oil." Originally obtained from natural stands of trees, the oil is now produced from plantations of *M alternifolia* in several countries including Australia, Kenya, and China. The essential oil has historically been used as a topical antiseptic in Australia based on its documented broad-spectrum antimicrobial activity.[37] Tea tree oil is used primarily in hand hygiene and skin antisepsis products and, to a lesser extent, in products for surface cleaning or disinfection.

Eucalyptus Oil

Eucalyptus oil is produced from a number of Australian *Eucalyptus* and *Corymbia* tree species and falls into two broad categories. Oil produced from *Corymbia citriodora* (formerly *Eucalyptus citriodora*, also known as lemon-scented gum) is used largely in perfumery, whereas the oil used for medicinal or cleaning purposes is produced from a number of species including *Eucalyptus globulus*. This second oil type contains high levels of 1,8-cineole, also known as *eucalyptol*, and it is this oil type that is discussed further. The International Standard ISO 3065:2011 specifies that this type of eucalyptus oil must contain 80% to 85% 1,8-cineole.[38]

Eucalyptus oil in some instances was originally a by-product of timber production but is now a crop in its own right. The largest quantities of cineole-type eucalyptus oil are currently produced in China,[31] with other countries including Australia, Spain, Portugal, and Southern Africa producing smaller but still substantial quantities.[39] Eucalyptus oil was historically used in a manner similar to tea tree oil, which was as a general medicinal agent in the preantibiotic era. In terms of current commercial uses, it is used mainly in cleaning and disinfectant products and, to a lesser extent, as a medicinal or antiseptic agent.

Pine Oil

Pine oil is obtained by steam distillation from wood, stems, twigs, and leaves of several pine species, including *Pinus sylvestris*. It is not to be confused with turpentine oil, which is also derived from *Pinus* species but is distilled from resin harvested from live trees. Pine oils generally contain α-pinene, β-pinene, or α-terpineol as major components.[40,41] However, because there are several different types of pine oil, the composition varies. An additional product, pine needle oil, is obtained from the leaves and cones of several *Pinus* species including *P sylvestris*.[40] Pine oil has a long history as a component of disinfection and cleaning products, as discussed in the following text. Pine oil is not as commonly used now due to declining production and increased cost of the essential oil.[29]

Other Oils and Components

Essential oils, other than those described earlier, that have been identified in commercially available disinfectants include lavender oil, peppermint oil, lemon myrtle oil (from *Backhousia citriodora*), and lemongrass oil (from *Cymbopogon citratus*). Essential oil components have also been identified in disinfectants and antiseptics. These include thymol, a monoterpene and a component of thyme oil (*Thymus vulgaris*); carvacrol, which is a monoterpene component of both thyme and oregano oils; and eugenol, which is an allylbenzene and is a major component of clove oil. As previously mentioned, the components limonene (from citrus oils) and 1,8-cineole (from eucalyptus oils) are also present in many commercial products.

▶ ANTISEPSIS

Hand Hygiene

Commercial hand hygiene products that contain essential oils or components are increasingly common. Essential oils have been included in both surfactant-based and foaming hand wash products and in leave-on alcohol-based hand rubs. In many instances, the essential oil may be present at relatively low concentrations and as such may not provide any significant antimicrobial activity. At these low concentrations, the essential oil is likely to have been included in the formulation as a fragrance or to increase the general appeal of the product to consumers rather than to have an antiseptic effect.

A limited number of clinical studies have been published that investigate the clinical efficacy of certain hand wash formulations containing essential oils or components.[42-45] Of the four studies identified, two evaluated products containing tea tree oil, one investigated an oregano oil product, and the remaining study investigated a product containing farnesol.

The first of the tea tree oil hand hygiene studies assessed several different hand wash formulations, using volunteers and the hygienic hand wash standard protocol EN 1499.[42] The "in-house" products evaluated included a skin wash containing 5% tea tree oil, a skin wash containing both 5% tea tree oil and 10% alcohol, a solution of 5% tea tree oil in water, and a soft soap comparator containing no tea tree oil. Results showed that the skin wash containing both tea tree oil and alcohol, as well as the 5% tea tree oil solution, performed significantly better than the soft soap in reducing numbers of *Escherichia coli* on hands. Results for the 5% tea tree oil skin wash were not significantly different from soft soap.[42] This lack of antibacterial effect compared to soft soap may be due to insufficient contact time or partial inactivation of tea tree oil by other hand wash ingredients, as is mentioned in a subsequent section of this chapter. The second hand wash study evaluating a tea tree oil product, also using protocol based on EN 1499 on hands artificially contaminated with *E coli*, showed that two commercial hand wash products containing either 0.3% tea tree oil or 0.5% triclosan did not perform significantly better than nonmedicated soft soap hand wash, whereas soft soap hand wash followed by the use of 60% propan-2-ol performed significantly better than the nonmedicated tea tree oil and triclosan products.[45] A consideration for the outcomes of this last study is that the concentration of tea tree oil included in the commercial product is relatively low, and as such, it is unlikely to exert any profound antibacterial effect.

An experimental hand rub containing a combination of farnesol (a sesquiterpenoid, undisclosed concentration), benzethonium chloride, and polyhexamethylene biguanide was evaluated in human volunteers whose hands were artificially contaminated with *Serratia marcescens* using a method proposed by the US Food and Drug Administration Tentative Final Monograph protocol. Results showed a 3.2 log reduction in *S marcescens* count after 1 application of product and a 5.5 log reduction after 10 applications. The comparator commercial hand rub product resulted in log reductions of 3.6 after 1 application and 3.4 after 10 applications. The farnesol product also showed a residual antibacterial effect when tested on ex vivo porcine skin challenged with *Staphylococcus aureus* or *E coli*. However, the in vivo and ex vivo studies[43,44] did not assess the activity of the experimental hand rub without farnesol, or with farnesol alone, making it difficult to assess the true contribution of farnesol to the final result.

Lastly, a study examining the normal flora of the hands found that significantly fewer bacteria were recovered from hands washed with soap containing 0.5% oregano oil compared to washing with either water alone or with nonmedicated soap.[46] Results obtained after washing with the 0.5% oregano oil soap did not differ significantly from the commercial antibacterial soap, which was Dettol® antibacterial cream soap,[46] suggesting that the oregano oil was exerting an antibacterial effect similar to the commercial product.

General Skin Antisepsis

Essential oil products have the potential to be used for the reduction, or removal, of flora from body sites other than hands due to antimicrobial activity. Furthermore, several essential oils, including tea tree oil and eucalyptus oil, were historically used as topical antiseptic agents, indicating a historical precedent for this particular use.[37] However, little published data are available on the use of essential oils as topical antiseptics. A number of topical antiseptic or wound care products containing oils such as thyme, lemongrass, basil and rosemary,[47] *E citriodora* oil,[48] and tea tree oil[49] have been evaluated preclinically. No studies that evaluate products containing essential oils or components for pre- or postoperative infection prevention were identified, and no studies were identified evaluating the clinical effectiveness of topical antiseptic creams, gels, or ointments that contain essential oils. However, two studies evaluating essential oil products for the eradication of methicillin-resistant *S aureus* (MRSA) were identified, which both describe the use of tea tree oil.

A pilot study showed that 5 of 15 patients using 4% tea tree oil nasal ointment and 5% tea tree oil body wash were cleared of MRSA compared to 2 of 15 (13%) patients receiving standard therapy (2% mupirocin cream and triclosan body wash). However, due to low numbers of patients, the difference was not significant.[50] A larger study[51] showed that application of a 10% tea tree oil nasal ointment cleared 41% of patients of MRSA, but the standard treatment of 2% mupirocin cream was significantly more effective, with 78% of patients cleared. The use of body wash containing 5% tea tree oil or 4% chlorhexidine gluconate soap to eliminate MRSA carried at sites such as the axillae and groin was also evaluated. Clearance rates in the tea tree oil group were 57% and 80% for axilla and groin, respectively, whereas rates for axilla and groin were 50% and 29%, respectively, in the chlorhexidine group. Overall, the tea tree oil body wash product was considered superior to the chlorhexidine regimen for clearance of skin sites.[51] A later study evaluating the use of a 5% tea tree oil body wash to prevent MRSA colonization did not find any difference in rates compared to standard body wash.[52] This suggests that tea tree oil products may not actually prevent colonization but may assist in eradication if colonization has already occurred.

Oral Cavity

Antisepsis in the oral cavity includes the use of mouthrinses to reduce plaque and gingivitis, which are caused by the growth of bacteria in the mouth, and antiseptic solutions may also be used as irrigants during root canal or endodontic procedures (see chapters 45 and 51). Although essential oil–containing irrigants do not appear to be widely studied, a considerable number of studies have evaluated the clinical effectiveness of essential oil mouthrinses, usually as an adjunct to toothbrushing. A substantial number of these studies have particularly evaluated the product Listerine®, which contains menthol, thymol, methyl salicylate, and eucalyptol.[30] Overall, significant benefits associated with the use of essential oil mouthrinses have been reported.[53-56]

To summarize, for antiseptic applications, although some of the hand wash studies show promising results, at this stage, there are insufficient data to determine the usefulness of essential oils and components as antimicrobial additives to hand wash products. Little data are available to support the use of essential oils in skin antisepsis, whereas the use of essential oil mouthrinses is relatively well established. Additional studies are required for both hand hygiene and skin antisepsis to provide more basic data, to optimize the concentrations of essential oil required, and to further explore efficacy.

▶ DISINFECTION

Essential oil formulations have been evaluated for disinfection efficacy using a range of methods, both standard and nonstandard, including in vitro quantitative suspension tests, surface carrier tests, and the "in use" evaluation of products. In addition, rapid bactericidal activity has been shown for many essential oil-based formulations in standard time kill assays,[12,19,57] indicating that this type of activity is present.

Suspension Tests

Standard suspension test protocols have not been widely used to evaluate the activity of essential oils, as evidenced by the fact that only four publications at the time of writing were identified that use these methods.

Several formulations containing tea tree oil were evaluated using suspension test EN 1276,[58] with a number of the formulations achieving a >5 log reduction in viability after only 1-minute contact, whereas other formulations required the longer contact time of 5 minutes to achieve the same log reduction. These results may not be surprising, considering the impact of formulation on biocide efficacy (see chapter 6). Solutions of tea tree oil (5% to 10% vol/vol) were rapidly effective against *Pseudomonas aeruginosa* and *E coli* but did not achieve >5 log reductions against *Acinetobacter baumannii* or *S aureus* after 5-minute contact.[58] In a different study, evaluation of solutions of *Salvia officinalis* essential oil (containing β-thujone; 1,8-cineole; and camphor) using EN 1276 found >5 log reductions against a range of gram-positive and gram-negative pathogens after 5-minute contact time, at concentrations of 0.5% and 0.75% essential oil. Higher concentrations of oil (up to 2%) were required for the same log reduction values for fungi.[59] Orange essential oil, eugenol, and *Pituranthos chloranthus* essential oil (containing 30% terpinen-4-ol) were also evaluated using EN 1276, and whereas the *P chloranthus* oil and eugenol (both at 0.5% to 1.0% vol/vol) resulted in log reductions of >5 after 5-minute contact, the orange oil (1.0%) was less active with reductions of <10^5.[60] Lastly, an eco-friendly cleaner containing alcohol, sodium citrate, lactic acid, and limonene was tested at a final concentration of 1.2% (vol/vol) using EN 1276 and had little effect on MRSA or methicillin-sensitive *S aureus* after 5 minutes.[61] However, this product was tested at a relatively low concentration and was labeled as a cleaning product rather than a disinfectant and as such would not be expected to have substantial antibacterial activity.[61]

Surface Tests

Similar to suspension tests, only a handful of published studies have examined the activity of essential oil products using standard surface testing protocols. Several additional studies have investigated efficacy using modified or in-house surface testing protocols.

Formulations containing tea tree oil have been tested against bacteria dried onto stainless steel and glass carrier surfaces using EN 13697 and ASTM E2111 for each surface type, respectively.[62] The 5% tea tree oil product complied with EN 13697 requirements for bactericidal activity and achieved a >4 log reduction against *E coli* after 1-minute contact time, and for the remaining test organisms, which were *S aureus*, *A baumannii*, and *P aeruginosa*, the log reduction values after 5-minute contact ranged from 1 to 3. Similarly, for the glass carrier test, the 5% tea tree oil solution achieved a >4 log reduction after 5 minutes against *A baumannii* and *P aeruginosa*. The 5% tea tree oil showed little activity against *S aureus* on either carrier type.[62] Another study with tea tree oil tested solutions containing 0.2% tea tree oil to disinfect toothbrushes.[63] This study showed a decrease in *Streptococcus mutans* recovered from toothbrushes after the study period, and the decrease was significantly larger than that achieved with the distilled water control.[63]

A US Environmental Protection Agency (EPA) sanitizer test for inanimate surfaces (Disinfectant Technical Science Section [DIS/TSS-10]) was used to evaluate various formulations containing tea tree oil, vinegar, and borax for reducing loads of *E coli*, *Listeria*, and *Salmonella* on high-density polyethylene (HDPE), glass, and Formica (laminate) surfaces after 60-second contact time.[64] Formulations containing tea tree oil combined with borax or vinegar or both resulted in reductions ranging from 2 to 4 $\log_{10}$, depending on the surface and the test organism. The final concentration of tea tree oil in these formulations was relatively low and ranged from 0.007% to 0.03%. Tea tree oil alone, at a concentration of 100%, produced log reductions of >4 for all organisms on all surfaces after 60 seconds.[64]

Several natural cleaning products, one containing 0.05% thymol as an ingredient and a do-it-yourself ("DIY") recipe containing tea tree oil (approximately 0.021%), club soda, and vinegar, were evaluated using an in-house surface testing protocol.[65] Surface tests were conducted with stainless steel and ceramic coupons contaminated with bacteria. Product was sprayed onto the coupons, left for 30 minutes, and then bacteria were recovered. The product containing thymol achieved log reductions of approximately 6, on both surfaces, against both *S aureus* and *E coli*. The DIY product was less effective, achieving log reductions of 2.5 to 3 on ceramic surfaces and 1.5 to 4 on stainless steel. Also, the DIY product was less effective on stainless steel against *S aureus* compared to *E coli*. It should be noted that the DIY product contained a very low concentration of tea tree oil, so it is questionable whether there was enough essential oil present to have any effect. Also, it is possible that the commercial cleaner that contained thymol contained other ingredients that may have contributed to the antibacterial activity.[65]

A standard surface test (European Standard WI216028, which is now BS EN 13697:2015) was used to evaluate solutions of carvacrol (2 mM, equivalent to approximately 0.03% vol/vol), which were shown to decrease the viability of microbial populations predried onto stainless steel discs after 5-minute contact time.[66] The carvacrol solution was most effective against *Listeria monocytogenes* and *Salmonella* Typhimurium and was least effective against *S aureus*.

In one of the few studies investigating the widely used orange oil,[67] bacteria suspended in a solution containing 5% peptone were dried onto stainless steel and plastic cutting board surfaces, which were then immersed in solutions containing orange oil at several different concentrations, or a detergent solution for 1 minute. Contaminated surfaces were removed to a buffer solution, rubbed for 2 minutes to remove bacteria, and viable counts were performed. Log reductions of >5 were found for *Vibrio parahaemolyticus*, *Salmonella* Typhimurium, and *E coli*, but not for *S aureus*, at concentrations of orange oil as high as 10%. Higher activity was found on stainless steel compared to plastic. When the tests were conducted with bacteria suspended in whole-fat milk and then dried onto the surfaces, log reductions were about 4 for *V parahaemolyticus* and were less than 1 for the remaining three test organisms, for both the orange oil and the comparator detergents. This indicates that the proteins and fats present in the whole milk interfered with the activity of the orange oil.[67] Cleaning products containing orange oil were also evaluated for removing the indoor fungus *Stachybotrys chartarum* from artificially contaminated gypsum wallboard.[68] Although results varied according to the type of wallboard surface, such as whether it was unpainted or painted, the three cleaners containing orange oil yielded positive results in terms of reducing the regrowth of fungus after surface treatment.

Two studies have evaluated the antibacterial effects of cloths and wipes impregnated with essential oil solutions. In the first study, oregano oil was evaluated at several different concentrations in cleaning solutions that were used to soak cloths.[46] The study assessed whether cloths soaked with the solution exerted an antibacterial effect when artificially contaminated with bacteria and whether cloths soaked with the solution were effective for reducing bacteria dried onto stainless steel, wood, or plastic surfaces. Bacterial survival on cloths was significantly reduced after 2 minutes by the presence of 0.05% to 1.0% oregano oil. At 10% oregano, numbers of all four test organisms were reduced to below the limit of detection. Also, when cloths soaked in a solution containing 0.5% oregano oil were used to clean stainless steel, wood, or plastic surface, viable counts recovered were lower than those recovered using plain soap or water alone, suggesting an antibacterial effect. In the second study, wipes impregnated with 5% and 2% eucalyptus oil were evaluated[69] by wiping five times across discs onto which inocula of MRSA, *E coli*, and *Candida albicans* had been dried. Although all wipes resulted in decreases in microbial load, there were no significant differences between the reductions after wiping with the water (control) wipe and those containing eucalyptus oil.

These tests on surfaces show that tea tree oil, oregano oil, orange oil, carvacrol, and thymol can all reduce microbial loads on surfaces, whereas eucalyptus oil did not have any effect under the conditions used in the test. The studies also illustrate that results depend on both the concentration of oil present and formulation used, and also the target organism, with *S aureus* notably less susceptible in some studies.[67]

Biofilm on Food Contact Surfaces

The formation of microbial biofilm on food contact surfaces contributes to the persistence of both food spoilage and gastrointestinal pathogens in food preparation environments.[70] Eradication of biofilm is therefore an important factor in maintaining food freshness and safety. However, biofilm can be difficult to eradicate for several reasons; microbes within a biofilm are protected by the extracellular material surrounding them, which restricts the penetration of antimicrobial substances, and cells within a biofilm are also metabolically less active.[71] Although a number of studies have evaluated the effects of essential oils on microbial

biofilms formed on plastic or polystyrene,[2] this section focuses on biofilms formed on food contact surfaces such as stainless steel because this is of most relevance to the food industry. Essential oils (at various concentrations) shown to eradicate or reduce biofilms formed on stainless steel include oregano and carvacrol,[72] oils from *Cinnamomum cassia* and *S officinalis*,[73] peppermint (*Mentha piperita*),[74] lemongrass (*C citratus*),[74] and cinnamon.[75] These studies provide proof of concept that essential oils are capable of reducing biofilms formed on food contact surfaces. Contact time and essential oil concentrations are important variables affecting the outcome.

Reduction of Microbial Loads in Air

Essential oils may be dispersed in air as vapors based on their volatile nature or more likely as droplets that can be dispersed over wide areas and long distances using an aerosol-generating product or fogging device. Furthermore, application of oils in this manner may be used to reduce numbers of microbes in air or on surfaces after the oil settles out of the air. Although essential oil vapors have been shown to inhibit microbial growth in numerous laboratory studies,[76,77] there are relatively few published studies investigating the in situ application of essential oils via air for reducing microbial loads.

Three studies investigated the effects of essential oils on microbial counts in air, which were determined using air sampling devices. The first study investigated aerosolized oil from *S officinalis* (sage oil; containing 1,8-cineole, camphor, and β-thujone as major components) at a dose of 0.25 mL/m³ and showed reductions in total microbial air counts.[59] The second evaluated several components including eugenol, carvacrol, cinnamaldehyde, and perillaldehyde and showed that all components resulted in decreased total air counts compared to the control.[78] The third study evaluated peppermint and thyme oils for reducing bacterial loads in broiler housing.[79] In this study, a fogging machine was used to produce particles of less than 50 μM of essential oil solutions (1:500 dilution, equivalent to 0.2% vol/vol) and to disperse the particles throughout the selected room. Distilled water was used as a negative control. Air was sampled in addition to surfaces, including the straw litter, walls, and drinkers in the area. Results showed that microbial counts were reduced after essential oil fogging, although not to any large extent. This may be due to factors such as the relatively low concentration of essential oil used or to insufficient contact between the essential oil and pathogen. A later study by the same group evaluated fungal counts in air and showed a reduction in air counts after application of peppermint but not thyme oil.[25]

With regard to aerosolized essential oils to reduce microbial loads on surfaces, one study evaluated a vaporized mixture of essential oils in solution (0.02%) in addition to standard cleaning, in a tertiary care environment.[80]

Microbial loads were followed for 5 months and were monitored by sampling surfaces, including table and cabinet surfaces within patient rooms and handrail surfaces in a corridor. The microbial count in the air was not monitored. The data indicated that microbial counts were lower in essential oil–treated areas compared to control areas that received standard cleaning only,[80] suggesting that the vaporized essential oil had a beneficial effect.

To summarize, most of the studies investigating aerosolized essential oils for reduction of microbial loads found a positive effect, although in some instances, the effect was marginal.

Essential Oil Products as Sanitizers

Sanitizers are widely used in the food industry to reduce microbial contamination and extend the shelf life of food such as fresh fruit and vegetables, poultry and poultry products, fish, and meat. The essential oils evaluated as sanitizers tend to be those derived from plants that are used as food spices, such as thyme, oregano, cinnamon, and rosemary.[81] Studies with oils that are not typically used as food spices, such as orange oil, lemon oil, eucalyptus, or tea tree oil, were not found. In addition, essential oils have been evaluated for food preservation, either incorporated into the food itself, the food atmosphere, or the packaging (including edible films), as reviewed elsewhere.[82]

Thyme oil and the component thymol have been investigated for sanitizing a range of foods, examples of which include eggs,[83] chicken meat,[84] carrots,[85] and lettuce.[86] These studies showed that the application of the sanitizer resulted in reductions in microorganisms,[84,86] except for a study with eggs[83] that did not show significant reductions in bacterial counts after application of a spray containing 0.7% thyme oil. Similarly, oregano oil and the component carvacrol have been evaluated for sanitizing a range of foods including eggs,[87,88] apples,[89] spinach and lettuce,[90,91] and sprouts,[92] with all studies showing reductions in levels of pathogens present after washing or sanitization. Lastly, the component cinnamaldehyde has been evaluated for sanitizing apples,[89] lettuce,[93] and spinach,[94] with all studies showing reductions in numbers of contaminating microorganisms. Several other essential oils have been investigated[81] but not to any significant extent. The available data on the use of essential oils in sanitizers suggest that several different oils may be effective in reducing microbial loads on different food types. Whether these oils represent a feasible alternative to conventional sanitizers remains to be determined.

Sterilant Applications

Most, if not all, natural essential oils are inherently sterile due to their chemical composition and the absence of water and contain no viable microorganisms, including bacterial endospores. This is because neat essential oils are likely to be highly antimicrobial at 100% concentration, and also most (if not all) essential oils do not contain the components necessary to support the growth of microorganisms. A study evaluating eight essential oils for their capacity to support the growth of microorganisms showed that bacteria could survive for up to 6 hours in some neat oils, and *C albicans* could survive for up to 48 hours in ylang-ylang oil.[95] This indicates that neat oils may indeed have the capacity to act as sterilants, achieving complete microbial death given enough time. However, the use of essential oils as sterilants is likely to be limited by a number of practical considerations, several of which are described in the following text.

▶ PRACTICAL CONSIDERATIONS

There are a number of practical issues that must be considered before essential oils can be adopted for disinfection or even sterilization. First, although some essential oils may be able to achieve complete sterility over time by neutralizing all forms of bacteria, fungi, and viruses, the contact time required is likely to be long, the concentration of oil is likely to be very high, and large volumes of oil may be required depending on the item being treated. In addition, there are little data available to suggest that high concentrations of essential oils can achieve sterility against nonenveloped viruses and other hardy microorganisms, indicating that further research is required. Using high concentrations and large volumes may be expensive compared to other commercially available disinfectants and may also result in damage to the item being disinfected due to the solvent properties of many essential oils. Also, the essential oil would most likely need to be washed off at the end of the process, which would require both water and a detergent to emulsify the oil, both of which would contribute to overall costs. For example, when the feasibility of using oregano oil to disinfect household greywater was assessed, it was deemed to be impractical due to the relatively large volumes of oil required, land mass required to cultivate the oil-bearing plants, and overall costs.[96]

Essential oils have a number of chemical properties that also require consideration. Essential oils are volatile, which has the potential to cause issues with fumes or vapors if used in an enclosed environment. As mentioned previously, essential oils are generally water insoluble, meaning that surfactants or alcohol must be used to make solutions or emulsions in water. Many essential oils also have solvent-like properties and will interact with low-density polyethylene plastics or even HDPE.[97] These interactions result in the loss of essential oil as well as deformation of the plastic. Some of these issues are encountered at relatively high concentrations of oil and as such can be avoided by the use of lower concentrations of oil as long as efficacy is not compromised.

Factors Affecting Efficacy

The activity of many standard disinfectants and antiseptics is reduced or neutralized in the presence of extraneous material such as organic matter, soaps, or cations. The available data, summarized in the following text, suggest that the antimicrobial activity of several essential oils is also adversely affected by organic matter.

Assessment of tea tree oil solutions (5%) using EN 1276 under perfect, clean (0.3% albumin), and dirty (3% albumin) conditions showed a stepwise decrease in the effectiveness of tea tree oil in the presence of increasing quantities of albumin.[58] In contrast, a previous in vitro study of antimicrobial activity indicated that tea tree oil activity was not affected by organic matter or cations.[98] Assessment of orange oil against bacteria suspended in either whole-fat milk or a 5% peptone solution and then dried onto surfaces showed that bacteria in milk were largely unaffected by the orange oil, whereas the bacteria in 5% peptone solution were significantly affected.[67] Solutions of carvacrol and trans-cinnamaldehyde were evaluated for reducing numbers of *E coli* from apples in different conditions, and whereas carvacrol was not affected by the presence of 1% soil (organic matter), the activity of trans-cinnamaldehyde was reduced.[89] Essential oils from *P chloranthus*[60] and *S officinalis* (sage)[59] were determined to be effective disinfectants under dirty conditions. However, clean conditions were not tested in these studies; therefore, no comparison of activity is possible. Lastly, MIC studies with clove oil showed minor impairment of activity in the presence of rabbit serum, brewer's yeast, and bovine serum albumin,[99] and the addition of 0.25% lecithin reduced the activity of both thyme and oregano oils.[100]

It is also possible that other excipients present within disinfectant formulation may influence the antimicrobial activity of the essential oils (see chapter 6). These excipients may be included to ensure a homogenous solution or emulsion, and as such, their inclusion may be unavoidable. For example, emulsification of oregano, lavender, tea tree, and cinnamon with rhamnolipids actually increased bioactivity[101] compared to nonemulsified oils, whereas the surfactant Tween 80 diminished the activity of tea tree oil.[98] Although minimal data are available in this area, it is reasonable to assume that formulation may play an important role in the overall effectiveness of essential oil disinfectants.

The development of microbial resistance to essential oils is also an issue that must be considered. Similar to several disinfectants and antiseptics, many essential oils have a nonspecific mode of action, which involves disruption of the cell membrane and cell homeostasis. Based on this generalized and combined mode of action, it is hypothesized that true antimicrobial resistance is unlikely to develop.[102,103] Most studies examining the potential for bacteria to become truly resistant to essential oils have found little evidence, although minor changes in susceptibility, ascribed to microbial adaptive mechanisms, have been observed.[11,102-107]

Safety and Toxicity

Essential oils, like most, if not all, chemicals with disinfectant action, can have toxic side effects. Instances of irritancy and allergy to essential oils have been documented after skin[108] or occupational exposure,[109] and ingestion may result in systemic toxicity.[110] Therefore, precautions must be taken if working extensively with essential oils. In addition, the safe disposal of large volumes of essential oils or essential oil solutions would need to be managed. Evidence shows that terpenes in wastewater in activated sludge biodegrade into other compounds,[111] indicating that biodegradation does indeed occur. However, it has also been noted that although terpenes are considered biodegradable, they have a high biological or chemical oxygen demand,[112] and as such, it would be detrimental to release large volumes into wastewater. Similar to many industrial chemicals, the accidental release of large volumes of essential oil would likely result in harm to the local environment, and as such, measures must be taken to prevent this from occurring.

▶ SUMMARY

This chapter has summarized the available evidence describing the effectiveness of essential oils for a number of applications, including hand hygiene, skin and oral antisepsis, the disinfection or sanitization of surfaces, and potential use as a sterilant. Although the majority of studies found promising results, there was also major variation between the studies with regard to type of oil studied, concentration of oil used, and the protocol used to investigate effectiveness. As such, a clear picture of overall efficacy is not evident at this time.

There is no doubt that many essential oils have antimicrobial activity. This property is potentially useful for a broad range of applications, ranging from consumer to medicinal to industrial. Plant essential oils have not been widely adopted as medicinal agents and likewise have not been widely adopted in antisepsis and disinfection. That said, essential oils are included in a broad range of products for antisepsis, sanitization, and disinfection, and it appears that their use in this arena is relatively more widespread compared to medicine. The adoption of essential oils in antisepsis and disinfection is limited by a number of factors, including economic viability, efficacy, and feasibility. As it stands, it is unlikely that essential oils will be economically competitive substitutes for many of the commonly available commercial antiseptics and disinfectants. Although essential oils may be able to achieve equivalent activity, the concentrations required are likely to be higher than for standard disinfectants, and costs are likely to be substantially higher. Whether plant essential oils will transition from their current role as "eco-friendly fragrance" in antiseptics and disinfectants to more significant roles as bona fide active components remains to be seen.

REFERENCES

1. Carson CF, Hammer KA. Chemistry and bioactivity of essential oils. In: Thormar H, ed. *Lipids and Essential Oils as Antimicrobial Agents.* Chichester, United Kingdom: John Wiley & Sons; 2011:203-238.

2. Hammer KA, Carson CF. Antibacterial and antifungal activities of essential oils. In: Thormar H, ed. *Lipids and Essential Oils as Antimicrobial Agents.* Chichester, United Kingdom: John Wiley & Sons; 2011:256-306.

3. Singh B, Sharma RA. Plant terpenes: defense responses, phylogenetic analysis, regulation and clinical applications. *3 Biotech.* 2015;5:129-151.

4. Vogt T. Phenylpropanoid biosynthesis. *Mol Plant.* 2010;3:2-20.

5. Theis N, Lerdau M. The evolution of function in plant secondary metabolites. *Int J Plant Sci.* 2003;164:S93-S102.

6. Breitmaier E. *Terpenes: Flavors, Fragrances, Pharmaca, Pheromones.* Mörlenbach, Germany: Wiley-VCH; 2006.

7. Başer KHC, Demirci F. Chemistry of essential oils. In: Berger RG, ed. *Flavours and Fragrances: Chemistry, Bioprocessing and Sustainability.* Berlin, Germany: Springer; 2007:43-86.

8. Ultee A, Bennik MHJ, Moezelaar R. The phenolic hydroxyl group of carvacrol is essential for action against the food-borne pathogen *Bacillus cereus. Appl Environ Microbiol.* 2002;68:1561-1568.

9. Cristani M, D'Arrigo M, Mandalari G, et al. Interaction of four monoterpenes contained in essential oils with model membranes: implications for their antibacterial activity. *J Agric Food Chem.* 2007;55:6300-6308.

10. Liolios C, Gortzi O, Lalas S, Tsaknis J, Chinou I. Liposomal incorporation of carvacrol and thymol isolated from the essential oil of *Origanum dictamnus* L. and in vitro antimicrobial activity. *Food Chem.* 2009;112:77-83.

11. Melo ADB, Amaral AF, Schaefer G, et al. Antimicrobial effect against different bacterial strains and bacterial adaptation to essential oils used as feed additives. *Can J Vet Res.* 2015;79:285-289.

12. Zu Y, Yu H, Liang L, et al. Activities of ten essential oils towards *Propionibacterium acnes* and PC-3, A-549 and MCF-7 cancer cells. *Molecules.* 2010;15:3200-3210.

13. Hammer KA, Heel KA. Use of multiparameter flow cytometry to determine the effects of monoterpenoids and phenylpropanoids on membrane polarity and permeability in staphylococci and enterococci. *Int J Antimicrob Agents.* 2012;40:239-245.

14. de Souza EL, de Barros JC, de Oliveira CE, da Conceição ML. Influence of *Origanum vulgare* L. essential oil on enterotoxin production, membrane permeability and surface characteristics of *Staphylococcus aureus. Int J Food Microbiol.* 2010;137:308-311.

15. Khan I, Bahuguna A, Kumar P, Bajpai K, Kang S. Antimicrobial potential of carvacrol against uropathogenic *Escherichia coli* via membrane disruption, depolarization, and reactive oxygen species generation. *Front Microbiol.* 2017;8:2421.

16. Di Pasqua R, Hoskins N, Betts G, Mauriello G. Changes in membrane fatty acids composition of microbial cells induced by addiction of thymol, carvacrol, limonene, cinnamaldehyde, and eugenol in the growing media. *J Agric Food Chem.* 2006;54:2745-2749.

17. Chauhan AK, Kang SC. Thymol disrupts the membrane integrity of *Salmonella* ser. *typhimurium* in vitro and recovers infected macrophages from oxidative stress in an ex vivo model. *Res Microbiol.* 2014;165:559-565.

18. de Sousa JP, Torres RD, de Azerêdo GA, Figueiredo RC, Vasconcelos MA, de Souza EL. Carvacrol and 1,8-cineole alone or in combination at sublethal concentrations induce changes in the cell morphology and membrane permeability of *Pseudomonas fluorescens* in a vegetable-based broth. *Int J Food Microbiol.* 2012;158:9-13.

19. Carson CF, Mee BJ, Riley TV. Mechanism of action of *Melaleuca alternifolia* (tea tree) oil on *Staphylococcus aureus* determined by time-kill, lysis, leakage, and salt tolerance assays and electron microscopy. *Antimicrob Agents Chemother.* 2002;46:1914-1920.

20. Cox SD, Gustafson JE, Mann CM, et al. Tea tree oil causes K^+ leakage and inhibits respiration in *Escherichia coli. Lett Appl Microbiol.* 1998;26:355-358.

21. Li X, Sheng JZ, Huang GH, et al. Design, synthesis and antibacterial activity of cinnamaldehyde derivatives as inhibitors of the bacterial cell division protein FtsZ. *Eur J Med Chem.* 2015;97:32-41.

22. Nowotarska SW, Nowotarski K, Grant IR, Elliot CT, Friedman M, Situ C. Mechanisms of antimicrobial action of cinnamon and oregano oils, cinnamaldehyde, carvacrol, 2,5-dihydroxybenzaldehyde, and 2-hydroxy-5-methoxybenzaldehyde against *Mycobacterium avium* subsp. *paratuberculosis* (Map). *Foods.* 2017;6:E72.

23. Wong SY, Grant IR, Friedman M, Elliot CT, Situ C. Antibacterial activities of naturally occurring compounds against *Mycobacterium avium* subsp. *paratuberculosis. Appl Environ Microbiol.* 2008;74:5986-5990.

24. Reichling J, Schnitzler P, Suschke U, Saller R. Essential oils of aromatic plants with antibacterial, antifungal, antiviral, and cytotoxic properties—an overview. *Forsch Komplementmed.* 2009;16:79-90.

25. Witkowska D, Sowińska J, Żebrowska JP, Mituniewicz E. The antifungal properties of peppermint and thyme essential oils misted in broiler houses. *Braz J Poultry Sci.* 2016;18:629-637.

26. Sharifi-Rad J, Salehi B, Schnitzler P, et al. Susceptibility of herpes simplex virus type 1 to monoterpenes thymol, carvacrol, p-cymene and essential oils of *Sinapis arvensis* L., *Lallemantia royleana* Benth. and *Pulicaria vulgaris* Gaertn. *Cell Mol Biol.* 2017;63:42-47.

27. Schnitzler P, Astani A, Reichling J. Antiviral effects of plant-derived essential oils and pure oil components. In: Thormar H, ed. *Lipids and Essential Oils as Antimicrobial Agents.* Chichester, United Kingdom: John Wiley & Sons; 2011:239-254.

28. Hunter Industrials. The history of Hunter Industrials. Hunter Industrials Web site. http://huntind.com.au/about-us/. Accessed February 2, 2018.

29. Pine-Sol. 1221 Market Web site. https://1221market.com/collections/pinesol. Accessed February 2, 2018.

30. Fine DH. Listerine: past, present and future—a test of thyme. *J Dent.* 2010;38(suppl 1):S2-S5.

31. Lawrence BM. A preliminary report on the world production of some selected essential oils and countries. *Perfumer & Flavorist.* 2009;134:38-44.

32. Brayfield A, ed. *Martindale: The Complete Drug Reference.* 39th ed. London, United Kingdom: Pharmaceutical Press; 2017.

33. Hardin A, Crandall PG, Stankus T. Essential oils and antioxidants derived from citrus by-products in food protection and medicine: an introduction and review of recent literature. *J Agric Food Inf.* 2010;11:99-122.

34. Food and Agriculture Organization of the United Nations. *Citrus Fruit: Fresh and Processed.* Rome, Italy: Food and Agriculture Organization of the United Nations; 2017. Statistical Bulletin 2016.

35. Brophy JJ, Davies NW, Southwell IA, Stiff IA, Williams LR. Gas chromatographic quality control for oil of *Melaleuca* terpinen-4-ol type (Australian tea tree). *J Agric Food Chem.* 1989;37:1330-1335.

36. International Organization for Standardization. *ISO 4730:2017: Essential oil of Melaleuca, Terpinen-4-ol Type (Tea Tree Oil).* Geneva, Switzerland: International Organization for Standardization; 2017.

37. Carson CF, Hammer KA, Riley TV. *Melaleuca alternifolia* (tea tree) oil: a review of antimicrobial and other medicinal properties. *Clin Microbiol Rev.* 2006;19:50-62.

38. International Organization for Standardization. *ISO 3065:2011: Oil of Eucalyptus Australian Type, Containing a Volume Fraction of 80 % to*

85 % of 1,8-Cineole. Geneva, Switzerland: International Organization for Standardization; 2011.

39. Coppen JJW. *Flavours and Fragrances of Plant Origin.* Rome, Italy: Food and Agriculture Organization of the United Nations; 1995. *Non-wood Forest Products*; vol 1.

40. Kelkar VM, Geils BW, Becker DR, Overby ST, Neary DG. How to recover more value from small pine trees: essential oils and resins. *Biomass Bioenerg.* 2006;30:316-320.

41. Tisserand R, Young R. *Essential Oil Safety: A Guide for Health Care Professionals.* 2nd ed. London, United Kingdom: Elsevier Health Sciences; 2013.

42. Messager S, Hammer KA, Carson CF, Riley TV. Effectiveness of hand-cleansing formulations containing tea tree oil assessed ex vivo on human skin and in vivo with volunteers using European standard EN 1499. *J Hosp Infect.* 2005;59:220-228.

43. Shintre MS, Gaonkar TA, Modak SM. Efficacy of an alcohol-based healthcare hand rub containing synergistic combination of farnesol and benzethonium chloride. *Int J Hyg Environ Health.* 2006;209: 477-487.

44. Shintre MS, Gaonkar TA, Modak SM. Evaluation of an alcohol-based surgical hand disinfectant containing a synergistic combination of farnesol and benzethonium chloride for immediate and persistent activity against resident hand flora of volunteers and with a novel in vitro pig skin model. *Infect Control Hosp Epidemiol.* 2007;28:191-197.

45. Gnatta JR, Pinto FMG, Bruna CQ, Souza RQ, Graziano KU, Silva MJ. Comparison of hand hygiene antimicrobial efficacy: *Melaleuca alternifolia* essential oil versus triclosan. *Rev Lat Am Enfermagem.* 2013;21:1212-1219.

46. Rhoades J, Gialagkolidou K, Gogou M, et al. Oregano essential oil as an antimicrobial additive to detergent for hand washing and food contact surface cleaning. *J Appl Microbiol.* 2013;115:987-994.

47. Shukr MH, Metwally GF. Evaluation of topical gel bases formulated with various essential oils for antibacterial activity against methicillin-resistant *Staphylococcus aureus.* *Trop J Pharm Res.* 2013;12: 877-884.

48. Akhtar MM, Srivastava S, Sinha P, et al. Antimicrobial potential of topical formulation containing essential oil of *Eucalyptus citriodora* Hook. *Ann Phytomed.* 2014;3:37-42.

49. Han JI, Park SJ, Kim SG, Park HM. Antimicrobial effects of topical skin cream containing natural oil mixtures against *Staphylococcus pseudintermedius* and *Malassezia pachydermatis.* *Vet Med.* 2015;60:202-207.

50. Caelli M, Porteous J, Carson CF, Heller R, Riley TV. Tea tree oil as an alternative topical decolonization agent for methicillin-resistant *Staphylococcus aureus.* *J Hosp Infect.* 2000;46:236-237.

51. Dryden MS, Dailly S, Crouch M. A randomized, controlled trial of tea tree topical preparations versus a standard topical regimen for the clearance of MRSA colonization. *J Hosp Infect.* 2004;56:283-286.

52. Blackwood B, Thompson G, McMullan R, et al. Tea tree oil (5%) body wash versus standard care (Johnson's Baby Softwash) to prevent colonization with methicillin-resistant *Staphylococcus aureus* in critically ill adults: a randomized controlled trial. *J Antimicrob Chemother.* 2013;68:1193-1199.

53. Azad MF, Schwiertz A, Jentsch HF. Adjunctive use of essential oils following scaling and root planing—a randomized clinical trial. *BMC Complement Altern Med.* 2016;16:171.

54. Charles CA, McGuire JA, Qaqish J, Amini P. Increasing antiplaque/ antigingivitis efficacy of an essential oil mouthrinse over time: an in vivo study. *Gen Dent.* 2013;61:23-28.

55. Araujo MWB, Charles CA, Weinstein RB, et al. Meta-analysis of the effect of an essential oil-containing mouthrinse on gingivitis and plaque. *J Am Dent Assoc.* 2015;146:610-622.

56. Stoeken JE, Paraskevas S, van der Weijden GA. The long-term effect of a mouthrinse containing essential oils on dental plaque and gingivitis: a systematic review. *J Periodontol.* 2007;78:1218-1228.

57. Dunn LL, Davidson PM, Critzer FJ. Antimicrobial efficacy of an array of essential oils against lactic acid bacteria. *J Food Sci.* 2016;81: M438-M444.

58. Messager S, Hammer KA, Carson CF, Riley TV. Assessment of the antibacterial activity of tea tree oil using the European EN 1276 and EN 12054 standard suspension tests. *J Hosp Infect.* 2005;59:113-125.

59. Bouaziz M, Yangui T, Sayadi S, Dhouib A. Disinfectant properties of essential oils from *Salvia officinalis* L. cultivated in Tunisia. *Food Chem Toxicol.* 2009;47:2755-2760.

60. Yangui T, Bouaziz M, Dhouib A, Sayadi S. Potential use of Tunisian *Pituranthos chloranthus* essential oils as a natural disinfectant. *Lett Appl Microbiol.* 2009;48:112-117.

61. Adukwu EC, Allen SC, Phillips CA. A comparison of the sensitivity of four *Staphylococcus aureus* isolates to two chlorine-based disinfectants and an eco-friendly commercially available cleaning agent. *Int J Environ Health Res.* 2015;25:115-125.

62. Messager S, Hammer KA, Riley TV. *Assessing the In Situ Efficacy of Tea Tree Oil as a Topical Antiseptic.* Barton, Australia: Rural Industries Research and Development Corp; 2005.

63. Chandrdas D, Jayakumar HL, Chandra M, Katodia L, Sreedevi A. Evaluation of antimicrobial efficacy of garlic, tea tree oil, cetylpyridinium chloride, chlorhexidine, and ultraviolet sanitizing device in the decontamination of toothbrush. *Indian J Dent.* 2014;5:183-189.

64. Zekert AE. *Effect of Alternative Household Sanitizing Formulations Including: Tea Tree Oil, Borax, and Vinegar, to Inactivate Foodborne Pathogens on Food Contact Surfaces.* Blacksburg, VA: Virginia Polytechnic Institute and State University; 2009.

65. Goodyear N, Brouillette N, Tenaglia K, et al. The effectiveness of three home products in cleaning and disinfection of *Staphylococcus aureus* and *Escherichia coli* on home environmental surfaces. *J Appl Microbiol.* 2015;119:1245-1252.

66. Knowles J, Roller S. Efficacy of chitosan, carvacrol, and a hydrogen peroxide-based biocide against foodborne microorganisms in suspension and adhered to stainless steel. *J Food Prot.* 2001;64:1542-1548.

67. Lin CM, Sheu SR, Hsu SC, Tsai YH. Determination of bactericidal efficacy of essential oil extracted from orange peel on the food contact surfaces. *Food Control.* 2010;21:1710-1715.

68. Menetrez MY, Foarde KK, Webber TD, Dean TR, Betancourt DA. Testing antimicrobial cleaner efficacy on gypsum wallboard contaminated with *Stachybotrys chartarum.* *Environ Sci Pollut Res Int.* 2007;14:523-528.

69. Hendry E, Conway B, Worthington T. Antimicrobial efficacy of a novel eucalyptus oil, chlorhexidine digluconate and isopropyl alcohol biocide formulation. *Int J Mol Sci.* 2012;13:14016-14025.

70. Oliver SP, Jayarao BM, Almeida RA. Foodborne pathogens in milk and the dairy farm environment: food safety and public health implications. *Foodborne Pathog Dis.* 2005;2:115-129.

71. Jain A, Gupta Y, Agrawal R, Khare P, Jain S. Biofilms—a microbial life perspective: a critical review. *Crit Rev Ther Drug Carrier Syst.* 2007;4:393-443.

72. dos Santos Rodrigues JB, de Carvalho RJ, de Souza NT, et al. Effects of oregano essential oil and carvacrol on biofilms of *Staphylococcus aureus* from food-contact surfaces. *Food Control.* 2017;73:1237-1246.

73. Campana R, Casettari L, Fagioli L, Cespi M, Bonacucina G, Baffone W. Activity of essential oil-based microemulsions against *Staphylococcus aureus* biofilms developed on stainless steel surface in different culture media and growth conditions. *Int J Food Microbiol.* 2017;241:132-140.

74. Valeriano C, de Oliveira TLC, de Carvalho SM, das Graças Cardoso M, Alves E, Piccoli R. The sanitizing action of essential oil-based solutions against *Salmonella enterica* serotype Enteritidis S64 biofilm formation on AISI 304 stainless steel. *Food Control.* 2012;25:673-677.

75. de Oliveira MMM, Brugnera DF, do Nascimento JA, Batista NN, Piccoli RH. Cinnamon essential oil and cinnamaldehyde in the control of bacterial biofilms formed on stainless steel surfaces. *Eur Food Res Technol.* 2012;234:821-832.

76. Ács K, Bencsik T, Böszörményi A, Kocsis B, Horváth G. Essential oils and their vapors as potential antibacterial agents against respiratory tract pathogens. *Nat Prod Commun.* 2016;11:1709-1712.

77. Frankova A, Smid J, Kloucek P, Pulkrabek J. Enhanced antibacterial effectiveness of essential oils vapors in low pressure environment. *Food Control.* 2014;35:14-17.

78. Sato K, Krist S, Buchbauer G. Antimicrobial effect of trans-cinnamaldehyde, (-)-perillaldehyde, (-)-citronellal, citral, eugenol and carvacrol on airborne microbes using an airwasher. *Biol Pharm Bull.* 2006;29:2292-2294.

79. Witkowska D, Sowinska J. The effectiveness of peppermint and thyme essential oil mist in reducing bacterial contamination in broiler houses. *Poult Sci.* 2013;92:2834-2843.

80. Gelmini F, Belotti L, Vecchi S, Testa C, Beretta G. Air dispersed essential oils combined with standard sanitization procedures for environmental microbiota control in nosocomial hospitalization rooms. *Complement Ther Med.* 2016;25:113-119.

81. Patrignani F, Siroli L, Serrazanetti DI, Gardini F. Innovative strategies based on the use of essential oils and their components to improve safety, shelf-life and quality of minimally processed fruits and vegetables. *Trends Food Sci Technol.* 2015;46:311-319.

82. Burt S. Essential oils: their antibacterial properties and potential applications in foods—a review. *Int J Food Microbiol.* 2004;94:223-253.

83. Shahein EHA, Sedeek EK. Role of spraying hatching eggs with natural disinfectants on hatching characteristics and eggshell bacterial counts. *Egypt Poult Sci J.* 2014;34:213-230.

84. Lu Y, Wu C. Reductions of *Salmonella enterica* on chicken breast by thymol, acetic acid, sodium dodecyl sulfate or hydrogen peroxide combinations as compared to chlorine wash. *Int J Food Microbiol.* 2012;152:31-34.

85. Singh N, Singh RK, Bhunia AK, Stroshine RL. Efficacy of chlorine dioxide, ozone, and thyme essential oil or a sequential washing in killing *Escherichia coli* O157:H7 on lettuce and baby carrots. *LWT-Food Sci Technol.* 2002;35:720-729.

86. Ozturk I, Tornuk F, Caliskan-Aydogan O, et al. Decontamination of iceberg lettuce by some plant hydrosols. *LWT-Food Sci Technol.* 2016;74:48-54.

87. Copur G, Arslan M, Duru M, Baylan M. Use of oregano (*Origanum onites* L.) essential oil as hatching egg disinfectant. *Afr J Biotechnol.* 2010;9:2531-2538.

88. Zeweil HS, Rizk RE, Bekhet GM, Ahmed MR. Comparing the effectiveness of egg disinfectants against bacteria and mitotic indices of developing chick embryos. *J Basic Appl Zool.* 2015;70:1-15.

89. Baskaran SA, Upadhyay A, Kollanoor-Johny A, et al. Efficacy of plant-derived antimicrobials as antimicrobial wash treatments for reducing enterohemorrhagic *Escherichia coli* O157:H7 on apples. *J Food Sci.* 2013;78:M1399-M1404.

90. Poimenidou SV, Bikouli VC, Gardeli C, et al. Effect of single or combined chemical and natural antimicrobial interventions on *Escherichia coli* O157:H7, total microbiota and color of packaged spinach and lettuce. *Int J Food Microbiol.* 2016;220:6-18.

91. de Medeiros Barbosa I, da Costa Medeiros JA, de Oliveira KÁR, et al. Efficacy of the combined application of oregano and rosemary essential oils for the control of *Escherichia coli*, *Listeria monocytogenes* and *Salmonella enteritidis* in leafy vegetables. *Food Control.* 2016;59:468-477.

92. Landry KS, Komaiko J, Wong DE, Xu T, McClements DJ, McLandsborough L. Inactivation of *Salmonella* on sprouting seeds using a spontaneous carvacrol nanoemulsion acidified with organic acids. *J Food Prot.* 2016;79:1115-1126.

93. Yossa N, Patel J, Millner P, Ravishankar S, Lo Y. Antimicrobial activity of plant essential oils against *Escherichia coli* O157:H7 and *Salmonella* on lettuce. *Foodborne Pathog Dis.* 2013;10:87-96.

94. Yossa N, Patel J, Millner P, Lo YM. Essential oils reduce *Escherichia coli* O157:H7 and *Salmonella* on spinach leaves. *J Food Prot.* 2012;75: 488-496.

95. Maudsley F, Kerr KG. Microbiological safety of essential oils used in complementary therapies and the activity of these compounds against bacterial and fungal pathogens. *Support Care Cancer.* 1999;7: 100-102.

96. Winward GP, Avery LM, Stephenson T, Jefferson B. Essential oils for the disinfection of grey water. *Water Res.* 2008;42:2260-2268.

97. Chaliha M, Cusack A, Currie M, Sultanbawa Y, Smyth H. Effect of packaging materials and storage on major volatile compounds in three Australian native herbs. *J Agric Food Chem.* 2013;61:5738-5745.

98. Hammer KA, Carson CF, Riley TV. Influence of organic matter, cations and surfactants on the antimicrobial activity of *Melaleuca alternifolia* (tea tree) oil in vitro. *J Appl Microbiol.* 1999;86:446-452.

99. Nuñez L, Aquino M. Microbicide activity of clove essential oil (*Eugenia caryophyllata*). *Braz J Microbiol.* 2012;43:1255-1260.

100. Burt SA, Reinders RD. Antibacterial activity of selected plant essential oils against *Escherichia coli* O157:H7. *Lett Appl Microbiol.* 2003;36:162-167.

101. Haba E, Bouhdid S, Torrego-Solana N, et al. Rhamnolipids as emulsifying agents for essential oil formulations: antimicrobial effect against *Candida albicans* and methicillin-resistant *Staphylococcus aureus*. *Int J Pharm.* 2014;476:134-141.

102. Hammer KA, Carson CF, Riley TV. Frequencies of resistance to *Melaleuca alternifolia* (tea tree) oil and rifampicin in *Staphylococcus aureus*, *Staphylococcus epidermidis* and *Enterococcus faecalis*. *Int J Antimicrob Agents.* 2008;32:170-173.

103. Hammer KA, Carson CF, Riley TV. Effects of *Melaleuca alternifolia* (tea tree) essential oil and the major monoterpene component terpinen-4-ol on the development of single- and multistep antibiotic resistance and antimicrobial susceptibility. *Antimicrob Agents Chemother.* 2012;56:909-915.

104. Gustafson JE, Cox SD, Liew YC, Willie SG, Warmington JR. The bacterial multiple antibiotic resistant (Mar) phenotype leads to increased tolerance to tea tree oil. *Pathology.* 2001;33:211-215.

105. Hollander A, Kalily E, Shachar D, Yaron S, Danin-Poleg Y. Draft genome sequence of *Salmonella enterica* serovar Senftenberg 070885 and its linalool-adapted mutant. *Genome Announc.* 2017;5: e01036-17.

106. Kalily E, Hollander A, Korin B, Cymerman I, Yaron S. Adaptation of *Salmonella enterica* serovar Senftenberg to linalool and its association with antibiotic resistance and environmental persistence. *Appl Environ Microbiol.* 2017;83:e03398-16.

107. Kalily E, Hollander A, Korin B, Cymerman I, Yaron S. Mechanisms of resistance to linalool in *Salmonella* Senftenberg and their role in survival on basil. *Environ Microbiol.* 2016;18:3673-3688.

108. Sabroe RA, Holden CR, Gawkrodger DJ. Contact allergy to essential oils cannot always be predicted from allergy to fragrance markers in the baseline series. *Contact Dermatitis.* 2016;74:236-241.

109. Ackermann L, Aalto-Korte K, Jolanki R, Alanko K. Occupational allergic contact dermatitis from cinnamon including one case from airborne exposure. *Contact Dermatitis.* 2009;60:96-99.

110. Janes SE, Price CS, Thomas D. Essential oil poisoning: N-acetylcysteine for eugenol-induced hepatic failure and analysis of a national database. *Eur J Pediatr.* 2005;164:520-522.

111. Alvarez FR, Shaul GM, Krishnan ER, et al. Fate of terpene compounds in activated sludge wastewater treatment systems. *J Air Waste Manag Assoc.* 1999;49:734-739.

112. Silla E, Arnau A, Tuñón I. Fundamental principles governing solvents use. In: Wypych G, ed. *Handbook of Solvents.* New York, NY: ChemTech; 2000:7-63.

Chlorine and Chlorine Compounds

Nancy A. Falk, Marisa Macnaughtan, Atefeh Taheri, and William McCormick

Although chlorine is one of the most widely distributed elements on earth, it is not found in a free state in nature. Instead, it exists mostly as a salt, whereas chloride is the anion in combination with sodium, potassium, calcium, and magnesium cations. Elemental chlorine (Cl_2) can be synthesized in the laboratory and is a heavy, greenish-yellow gas with a characteristic irritating and penetrating odor. It is likely that chlorine and its compounds must have been known to alchemists for many centuries but only in 1809 did Sir Humphrey Davy conclude that chlorine gas (Cl_2) was an element.[1] Elemental chlorine is a highly reactive compound. It will react readily with oxygen-containing species to form a variety of chlorine oxides. Elemental chlorine will react reversibly with water to form hypochlorous acid (HOCl) and hydrochloric acid (HCl) (equation [1]).

$$Cl_2 \text{ (aq)} + H_2O \rightleftharpoons HOCl \text{ (aq)} + HCl \text{ (aq)} \quad (1)$$

Observations of the bleaching properties of chlorine gas in a water solution led to its first practical application in textile bleaching, with subsequent commercial production in 1785. Development of sodium and calcium hypochlorites (chloride of lime, chlorinated lime) for more convenient use followed shortly thereafter. The reactions to form these compounds from elemental chlorine are shown in equations (2) and (3).[2]

$$Cl_2 \text{ (aq)} + 2NaOH \text{ (aq)} \rightarrow NaOCl \text{ (aq)} + NaCl \text{ (aq)} + H_2O \quad (2)$$

$$2Cl_2 \text{ (g)} + 2\,Ca(OH)_2 \text{ (s)} \rightarrow Ca(OCl)_2 \times 2H_2O \text{ (s)} + CaCl_2 \text{ (s)} + Ca_3(OCl)_2(OH)_4 \text{ (s)} + Ca_3Cl_2(OH)_4 \text{ (s)} \quad (3)$$

In 1846, Semmelweis used chloride of lime to combat and control puerperal fever in his clinic in Vienna. As early as 1854, chlorinated lime was applied in the treatment of sewage in London. Finally, in 1881, a German bacteriologist, Koch, demonstrated under controlled laboratory conditions that pure cultures of bacteria may be destroyed using hypochlorites. Five years later, the American Public Health Association issued a favorable report on the use of hypochlorites as disinfectants.[3] Chloride of lime was first introduced to the North American continent by Johnson in 1908 for purification of water. Within a short time, many plants throughout the United States installed the chlorination process for water purification, alone or in combination with filtration, so that by 1911 an estimated 800 000 000 gallons of water were purified by the chlorination process.[4]

The number of waterborne diseases that have been prevented through public water disinfection in the United States and in Europe is enormous and the list of diseases is extensive. These diseases can be protozoan (amoebiasis, giardiasis, or microsporidiosis), bacterial (botulism, cholera, dysentery, typhoid fever), viral (hepatitis A, polyomavirus infections), or algal (*Desmodesmus* infections) in nature.[5-9] Today, it is rare to find municipal water that is not treated by some form of chlorination. The introduction of elemental chlorine as a commercial product supplemented existing hypochlorite processes for the treatment of water and sewage. The use of chlorine as a disinfectant gained wide acceptance later in other industries. It is important to note that following common practice in industrial applications, the words *chlorine* or *bleach* is often broadly used to signify "active chlorine compounds" and are used interchangeably. Generally, what is intended is an "aqueous solution of active chlorine compounds, consisting of a mixture of HOCl, OCl⁻, Cl_2, and other active chlorine compounds." Where *elemental chlorine* (Cl_2) is intended, it will be referred to as "chlorine gas" or "elemental chlorine." Note that in some cases, "bleach" or "nonchlorine bleach" may be used to refer to some hydrogen peroxide (H_2O_2)-based chemistries.

Wide use of bleach as an antiseptic began during World War I when Dakin[10] introduced a 0.45% to 0.50% sodium hypochlorite (NaOCl) solution for disinfection of open and infected wounds. Treatment of wounds with hypochlorite necessitated information regarding solvent action, irritation, and toxicity as well as the rate of reaction on the necrotic tissue. Various toxicity studies were reported.[11-14] More recent innovations in this field are discussed in this chapter.

▶ CHEMISTRY

Elemental Chlorine

One of the most important commercial preparations is elemental chlorine (Cl_2 gas). Today, over 65 million short tons of elemental chlorine are produced globally and 14 million short tons in the United States.[15] The main method of manufacture is through electrolysis of a salt solution (either sodium or potassium chloride), known as the chloralkali process. Useful by-products of the process include hydrogen gas and sodium hydroxide. Although elemental chlorine is a gas (approximately 2.5 times as heavy as air), it is supplied through compression and cooling as an amber liquid (1.5 times as heavy as water) and shipped in steel cylinders or tank cars. When released to atmospheric conditions, liquid chlorine reverts immediately to a gaseous form. The largest use of elemental chlorine is in the manufacturing of polyvinylchloride plastics and other major polymers such as polyurethanes, followed closely by the synthesis of solvents, and other organic and inorganic products. Approximately 5% of the elemental

chlorine production goes to the pulp and paper industry, whereas another 5% is used for water disinfection.[16] Elemental chlorine is highly reactive in the presence of moisture and possesses a great tendency to combine with organic compounds. Another characteristic of chlorine and chlorine compounds is their unique ability to displace bromine or iodine from their respective salts by metathesis. This chemical mechanism is frequently used in practice for the controlled release of iodine and bromine in solution. Both elemental chlorine and sodium hydroxide produced through electrolysis are used as raw materials in the manufacturing of sodium hypochlorite solutions.[2]

Hypochlorite Salts

The most common liquid form is hypochlorite, particularly in aqueous solution, first discovered by Berthollet[17] in 1789 by contacting chlorine gas with potash lye. Hypochlorite salts are the oldest and most widely used of the active chlorine compounds in the field of chemical disinfection. They are (1) proven and powerful antimicrobials controlling a wide spectrum of microorganisms, (2) deodorizers, (3) being nonpoisonous to humans at use concentrations, (4) free of poisonous residuals, (5) colorless and nonstaining, (6) easy to handle, and (7) economical to use.[18] Hypochlorite salts are available in solid or liquid form, with details shown in Table 15.1.

TABLE 15.1	Commercially produced chlorine compounds		
Chemical Name	**Active Ingredient Chemical Formula**	**% Average Cl_2**	**CAS Registry No.**
Inorganic			
Calcium hypochlorite dihydrate	$Ca(OCl)_2*2H_2O$	65%-70%	7778-54-3
		50%-52%	
Sodium hypochlorite	NaOCl	12%-15%	7681-52-9
		5.25%	
		5.25%-8.35%	
Chlorinated trisodium phosphate	$4(Na_3PO_4 *11H_2O)NaOCl$	3.25%	56802-99-4
Chlorine dioxide decahydrate	ClO_2*10H_2O	17%	10049-04-4
Lithium hypochlorite	LiOCl	30%-35%	13840-33-0
Potassium hypochlorite	KOCl	12%-14%	7778-66-7
Organic			
1,3-Dichloro-5,5-dimethylhydantoin	Figure 15.2, 3	66%	118-52-5
Trichloro-s-triazinetrione	Figure 15.2, 1	89%-90%	87-90-1
Sodium dichloroisocyanurate	Figure 15.2, 2	60%-63%	2893-78-9
Sodium dichloroisocyanurate dihydrate	Figure 15.2, 2	55%	51580-86-0
Potassium dichloroisocyanurate	Figure 15.2, potassium salt of 2	59%	2244-21-5
Trichloromelamine	Figure 15.2, 6	70%-129%	7673-09-8

Abbreviation: CAS, Chemical Abstracts Service.

Calcium hypochlorite, lithium hypochlorite, and sodium hypochlorite combined with hydrated trisodium phosphate (chlorinated TSP) make up the solid forms; however, sodium and potassium hypochlorite are sold in solution form. Calcium hypochlorite dihydrate is a powder, granulated material, or tablet with a strong chlorine odor.[19] It may be blended with compatible inorganic diluents to produce lower available chlorine compounds. Calcium hypochlorite products are soluble in water and fairly stable on prolonged storage. Lithium hypochlorite is a free-flowing, white, granulated material, also with a strong chlorine odor. It is readily soluble in water and is also stable. On exposure to air, powdered hypochlorites attract moisture and become less stable. The sodium hypochlorite solutions range in concentration, with lower available chlorine products used for domestic applications and stronger solutions sold for industrial uses. Sodium hypochlorite in water solutions are less stable, especially in products with higher chlorine concentrations. Potassium hypochlorites are available as liquids, with a higher available chlorine content than the sodium counterparts. Chlorinated TSP is a fine, white crystalline material. In addition to producing hypochlorite ion for sanitizing properties, it also contains alkaline phosphate for detergency; it finds usage in disinfecting equipment used for winemaking and brewing but is subject to phosphate regulations in applicable jurisdictions.

Because of their wide acceptance as disinfectants in many industries, hypochlorite solutions serve as standards for testing of other disinfectants. Today, hypochlorites are used as disinfectants in most households, hospitals, schools, and public buildings. They are also widely used for microbial control in restaurants, soda fountains, and other public eating places and for sanitizing food processing plants, dairies, canneries, breweries, wineries, and beverage bottling plants. Hypochlorites are sold for treatment of pool and drinking water, sewage, and wastewater effluents. In addition, hypochlorite can be combined with surfactants, salts, fragrances, colorants, and polymers to create products that disinfect with better cleaning efficacy and with improved use experience. Details on forms and choices are discussed later in this chapter.

Chlorine Dioxide

Chlorine dioxide has received more attention in recent years. This chlorinated compound is used with greater frequency for drinking water disinfection, for wastewater treatment, for slime control in cooling tower waters, and for disinfection of spaces containing a complex mixture of surfaces (also see chapter 27). It has a unique ability to break down phenolic compounds and remove phenolic tastes and odors from water. Another favorable feature is its lack of reaction with ammonia. Finally, chlorine dioxide does not form trihalomethanes or chlorophenols, a characteristic of great importance to humans and the environment especially in large-scale municipal water treatment plants. There are some health risks associated with its use. Chlorine dioxide and its inorganic reaction products, such as chlorite, may present a high risk of toxicity.[20] Recommended minimum exposure levels for chlorine dioxide gas are an Occupational Safety and Health Administration (OSHA) permissible exposure limit (PEL) of 0.3 mg/m^3 (0.1 ppm) as a time-weighted average (TWA) and the short-term exposure limit (STEL) is set at 0.9 mg/m^3 (0.3 ppm). For elemental chlorine gas, the OSHA PEL is 1.5 mg/m^3 (0.5 ppm) TWA and the STEL is 2.9 mg/m^3 (1 ppm), indicating that chlorine dioxide gas is more toxic to humans than chlorine gas.[21,22]

Chlorine dioxide is used in the chlorination of drinking water as well as in wastewater and for elimination of cyanides, sulfides, aldehydes, and mercaptans. The oxidation capacity of ClO$_2$ in terms of available chlorine to be approximately 2.5 times that of chlorine.[23] Its oxidation-reduction potential is close to that of chlorine. The analysis for chlorine dioxide is like that of chlorine but with some modification. As in the case of chlorine detection, chlorine dioxide can be continuously measured by chlorine dioxide analyzer and transmitter systems based on amperometric sensing devices. Chlorine dioxide at room temperature is soluble in water at 2.9 g/L at 30 mm Hg partial pressure. In aqueous solution, the product is decomposed by light. It undergoes a valence change of five in the reduction reaction to chloride and does not pass through a hypochlorous acid phase during this reduction but rather follows a different reaction path.

Chlorine dioxide activity is considered at least equal to that of chlorine.[24] Bactericidal efficiency was found to be unaffected at pH levels of 6 to 10. In further work, it was found that chlorine dioxide's bactericidal activity decreases with lowering of temperature.[25] In later work with spores, the authors demonstrated greater sporicidal activity for chlorine dioxide than for chlorine. The greater sporicidal activity of chlorine dioxide is explained by greater utilization of its oxidation capacity, involving a full change of five electrons. Vegetative bacteria do not activate this full oxidation potential.[26] Harakeh et al[27] evaluated solutions of chlorine dioxide against *Yersinia enterocolitica* and *Klebsiella pneumoniae*. The authors showed when these were grown in a natural aquatic environment of low temperature and lower nutrient contents that they were more resistant to chlorine dioxide than the same microorganisms grown under optimum laboratory conditions.[27] Berman and Hoff[28] showed good antiviral activity by chlorine dioxide at pH 10 in less than 15 seconds. It also has been shown to be very effective in inactivating *Cryptosporidium parvum* oocysts in drinking water.[29]

Chlorine dioxide is an extremely reactive compound and consequently cannot be manufactured and shipped in bulk but is prepared at the place of consumption. In practice, this consists of mixing a solution of chlorine with a solution of sodium chlorite; the product is then applied to a water supply. The chlorine dioxide is formed according to equation (4):

$$Cl_2 + 2NaClO_2 \rightarrow 2ClO_2 + 2NaCl \qquad (4)$$

Chlorine dioxide may also be produced by the following reactions: (1) acidification of chlorates with hydrochloric or sulfuric acid; (2) reduction of chlorates in acid medium; (3) reacting acids with chlorites; and (4) through electrolysis, using sodium chloride, sodium chlorite, and water. By combining separate solutions of sodium chlorite and acid, Alliger[30] developed a disinfectant composition that produces chlorine dioxide at the site of application. Chlorine dioxide decahydrate may be prepared commercially, but it must be kept refrigerated because it decomposes at room temperature and can be dangerously explosive under some conditions. de Guevara[31] prepared stable antiseptic solutions using inorganic boron compounds such as sodium tetraborate, boric acid, and sodium perborate to stabilize chlorine dioxide in aqueous solutions, forming a labile complex. When the stabilized Anthium Dioxcide® ClO₂ formula is generated, all traces of chlorine are removed by passage through a column of sodium carbonate peroxide. The final product contains 5% of stabilized ClO_2 complex. To make this material biologically active, it is necessary to release the ClO_2 in solution by either acidification or introduction of chlorine. The manufacturer's instructions for use recommend that an adjustment of pH be made with either acetic acid, citric acid, phosphoric acid, or by adding a provided activator a solution.[32] Today, this type of stabilized ClO_2 is used in the paper industry for removing slimes from paper mill white water systems. The use of chlorine dioxide has been extended to the food industry to provide sanitation for different food products under a variety of situations.[33-35]

Inorganic Chloramines

When ammonia combines with chlorine in an aqueous solution, it forms monochloramine (NH_2Cl), dichloramine ($NHCl_2$), nitrogen trichloride (NCl_3), or nitrogen (N_2). The residual amine tends to suppress the release of hypochlorous acid. In monochloramine, the chlorine is not sufficiently active to demonstrate any antimicrobial activity. It has a low hydrolysis constant, which is too low for hypochlorous acid to be released in sufficient amounts. The activity of chloramines depends on the pH of the solution (Figure 15.1). Because they are highly unstable, inorganic chloramines are not commercialized as such. The instability of $NHCl_2$ is important in breakpoint chlorination used for water and sewage treatment.[37]

Inorganic chloramine treatment of water supplies was used in the 1930s and early 1940s to improve tastes and odors of water. The most efficient ratio of chlorine

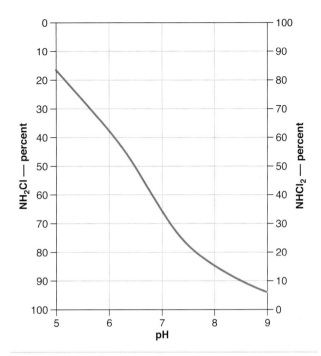

FIGURE 15.1 Relationships between monochloramine (NH_2Cl), dichloramine ($NHCl_2$), and pH. After Baker.[36] Copyright © 1959 American Water Works Association. Reprinted by permission of John Wiley & Sons, Inc.

to ammonia is 2:1 by weight.[4] Use of ammonia in water chlorination provided prolonged stability of chlorine in water distribution systems; however, inferior inactivation has been described when combined available chlorine was compared with free available chlorine.[38] It takes approximately 25 times as much chloramine as free available chlorine to effect a rapid bactericidal action; for chloramines, the contact time is approximately 100 times longer than that required for the same residual of free available chlorine to produce the same inactivation. Chloramines are being considered for chlorination of water to prevent trihalomethane formation and for inactivation of *Cryptosporidium*.[29,39] In addition, Kereluk and Borisenok,[40] working with 5 to 10 ppm monochloramine solutions, demonstrated antimicrobial activity against bacteria and fungi.

Organic Chloramines

Organic chloramines are produced by the equilibrium reaction of hypochlorous acid with an amine, amide, imine, or imide, as shown in equation (5).

$$HNR_2 + HOCl \rightleftharpoons ClNR_2 + H_2O \qquad (5)$$
$$R = \text{organic group}$$

The organic chloramines are the *N*-chloro derivatives of the following four groups: (1) sulfonamides: chloramine-T (Figure 15.2; 8, R = CH_3), dichloramine-T

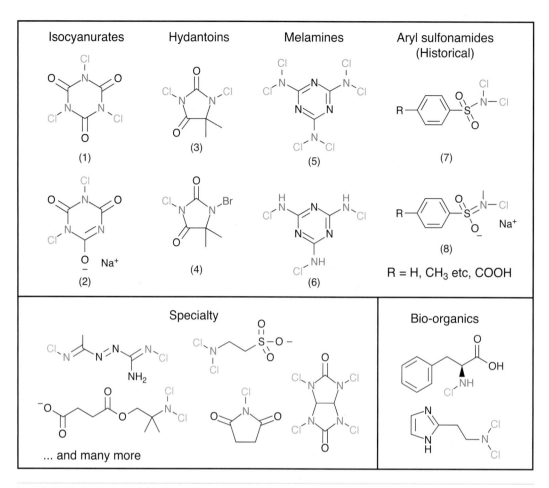

FIGURE 15.2   Selected *N*-chloramines and *N*-halamines.

(Figure 15.2; 7, R = CH₃), chloramine-B (Figure 15.2; 8, R = H), halazone (Figure 15.2; 7, R = COOH); (2) heterocyclic compounds with nitrogen in the ring: hydantoin, dichloroisocyanurate, trichloroisocyanurate, trichloromelamine (Figure 15.2; 3 and 4, 2, 1, and 6, respectively); (3) condensed amines from guanidine derivatives (chloroazodin; Figure 15.2; Specialty); and (4) anilides.[37] Once formed, some *N*-chloramine derivatives can be isolated as solids and are used as solid bleach precursors. When the *N*-chloramine is redissolved in water, the *N*-chloramine can undergo a hydrolysis reaction and release hypochlorous acid. Each *N*-chloramine will have unique properties depending on its water solubility and its hydrolysis constant. These two main factors control the amount of the timing of hypochlorous acid release. There are thousands of options for organic chloramines, and the wide variety of compounds also leads to a wide variety of properties such as solubility, chlorine release profile (hydrolysis constant), and toxicity.

Common uses for *N*-chloramine compounds include disinfection and cleaning in swimming pools and spas, toilets, laundry, dishwashing detergent, hard surface cleaning, textile bleaching, egg decontamination, water cooling system disinfection, pulp and paper bleaching, and wastewater treatment. The most common commercialized products today include sodium trichloroisocyanuric acid (trichloro-s-c), sodium dichloroisocyanurate, 1,3-dichloro-5,5-dimethylhydantoin, and 1-bromo-3-chloro-5,5-dimethylhydantoin (Figure 15.2; 1, 2, 3, and 4, respectively). Other *N*-halamines are available as specialty chemicals and therefore only manufactured in small quantities. Historically, *N*-halamines such as chloramine-T and others were commonly manufactured but no longer have active registration status in the United States.

PRINCIPLES, MECHANISMS, AND OTHER ASPECTS OF CHLORINE DISINFECTION

Definitions of Chemical Terms

Available chlorine may be defined as a measurement of oxidizing capacity and is expressed in terms of the equivalent amount of elemental chlorine. The concentration of hypochlorite (or any other oxidizing disinfectant) may be expressed as available chlorine by determining the electrochemical equivalent amount of Cl_2 to that compound. By equation (6), 1 mole of elemental chlorine is capable of reacting with two electrons to form inert chloride:

$$Cl_2 + 2e^- = 2Cl^- \tag{6}$$

From equation (7), it can also be noted that 1 mole of hypochlorite (OCl^-) may react with two electrons and two protons to form chloride and water:

$$OCl^- + 2e^- + 2H^+ = Cl^- + H_2O \tag{7}$$

Hence, 1 mole of hypochlorite is equivalent (electrochemically) to 1 mole of elemental chlorine and may be said to contain 70.91 g of available chlorine (identical to the molecular weight of Cl_2). Because calcium hypochlorite ($Ca[OCl]_2$) and NaOCl contain 2 and 1 moles of hypochlorite per mole of chemical, respectively, they also contain 141.8 g and 70.91 g available chlorine per mole. The molecular weights of $Ca(OCl)_2$ and NaOCl are, respectively, 143 and 74.5, so that pure preparations of the two compounds contain 99.2 and 95.8 weight percent available chlorine; hence, they are effective means of supplying chlorine for disinfection purposes.

Chlorine demand. In chlorination of water, a certain part of this chlorine is consumed by water impurities, and any unconsumed chlorine remains as residual available chlorine. The difference between the chlorine applied and the chlorine remaining in the water may be referred to as the *chlorine demand* of this water. Because of its electronic configuration, chlorine possesses a strong tendency to acquire extra electrons, changing to inorganic chloride ions. This affinity for electrons makes chlorine a strong oxidizing agent. Hence, chlorine in water reacts quickly with (1) inorganic-reducing substances, such as ferrous iron (Fe^{2+}), manganous manganese (Mn^{2+}), nitrites (NO_2-), and hydrogen sulfide (H_2S), and (2) organic materials (other than amines), wherein the chlorine atom loses its oxidizing properties by reduction to chloride and is lost as a disinfectant.[41] The reactions with the inorganic-reducing substances are quite rapid and stoichiometric, whereas those with organic material are in general slow and depend largely on the concentration of the free available chlorine.

Free and combined available chlorine. When chlorine survives the chlorine demand of the water, the chlorine measured may be reported as free, combined, or total residual chlorine depending on the analytic method used. The term *free* available chlorine is usually applied to three forms of chlorine that may be found in water: (1) elemental chlorine (Cl_2), (2) HOCl, and (3) hypochlorite ion (OCl^-).[41] These forms may be found in water, provided there is no ammonia or other nitrogenous compounds to form chloramines and there is enough chlorine to satisfy

the organic and inorganic water demands. During a chlorination process, a certain portion of chlorine combines with ammonia and other nitrogenous compounds present in natural water to form chloramines or *N*-chloro compounds. This combination of chlorine with ammonia or with other nitrogenous compounds is referred to as *combined* available chlorine. The free and combined available chlorine, when present in the water, are collectively described as *total residual* (available) *chlorine.*

Breakpoint chlorination refers to when a sufficient amount of chlorine is applied to satisfy the initial water demand, and an extra quantity of chlorine is added to provide a slight residual of free available chlorine. Before establishing this free residual, additions of chlorine (or hypochlorites) oxidize all the inorganic and organic material until at some so-called breakpoint, demand is fully satisfied. Any further additions of available chlorine result in a constant rise of free available chlorine in proportion to the dose (Figure 15.3). A detailed review of breakpoint chlorination and its application in water treatment is given by White.[43]

Marginal chlorination refers to the addition of chlorine to water sufficient just to overcome the chlorine demand consumption and to obtain an initial level of available chlorine regardless of the type of residual produced. *Superchlorination* is a further step in which chlorine is added beyond the level that is needed to yield an initial residual without regard to the type of residual produced. If too much chlorine is added, and a lower chlorine level is desired, a dechlorinating chemical (eg, sodium thiosulfate) may be added, and this process is referred to as *dechlorination.* The terms *prechlorination* and *postchlorination* generally relate to a position of chlorination before to or after filtration, respectively.[44]

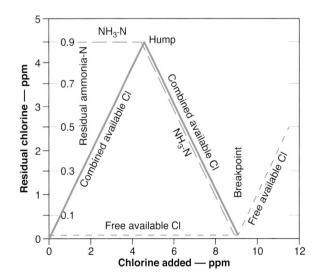

FIGURE 15.3   Ideal residual chlorine curve (ammonia solution). After Butterfield.[42] Copyright © 1948 American Water Works Association. Reprinted by permission of John Wiley & Sons, Inc.

Analysis of Available Chlorine

There are several methods to determine the available chlorine in solution or in products. In the iodometric method, the free chlorine liberates iodine in the acidified test solution containing potassium iodide (KI), and the liberated iodine is titrated with a standard sodium thiosulfate solution to a starch endpoint. In the sodium arsenite method, free chlorine is titrated with a standard sodium arsenite solution using KI-starch paper as the external indicator. In the orthotolidine (OT) method, when added to dilute chlorine solution (at the ppm level), the colorless OT reagent turns to yellow-orange-red depending on the chlorine concentration. The intensity of color determines the amount of available chlorine present and is compared with previously prepared color standards.[45] The Palin DPD method uses N,N-diethyl-p-phenylenediamine (DPD) reagent, and the dilute chlorine solution turns the reagent pink to red, depending on the concentration of chlorine (at the ppm level).[46] There are modifications in the OT and Palin methods to distinguish free available chlorine, total available chlorine, combined available chlorine, and chloramines. The DPD method is the basis for chlorine test strips used to quickly check chlorine levels in swimming pools and disinfectant solutions. The amperometric method consists of electrometric titration in which the current passes through a titration cell containing a dilute chlorine solution as the oxidizing agent and the standard phenylarsine oxide as titrating reducing agent. The volume of phenylarsine oxide consumed determines the free available chlorine (at the ppm level) in solution, and the endpoint is indicated electrically. This titrating detection unit is composed of an indicator electrode, a reference electrode, and a microammeter.[43]

Chlorine measurements can be accurately made using polarographic membrane techniques. The plastic probe contains an anode and electrolyte and is terminated by a membrane-covered noble metal cathode. When the probe is immersed in a chlorinated solution, the chlorine is reduced to chloride at the cathode; the generated current, linear with chlorine concentration, is displayed on the meter of the analyzer. The probe lead is the only connection between the analyzer and the sample being measured with no need for reagents of any kind. This probe can be installed in a pipeline or any other desirable location and requires virtually no maintenance. One of the more important features of probe analysis is the capability to distinguish between different forms of chlorine that may be present, thus yielding maximum efficiency at minimum cost. This application is widely accepted by various industries because of its safety, performance, and economy.[43]

Stability of Chlorine in Solution

The stability of free available chlorine in solution depends largely on the following factors: (1) chlorine concentration,

(2) presence and concentration of catalysts or reducing agents, (3) pH of the solution, (4) temperature of the solution, (5) presence of organic material, (6) ultraviolet irradiation, and (7) ionic strength. Any of these factors, alone or in combination, may greatly affect the stability of free available chlorine in solution. Iron and aluminum seem to have only a slight effect on the stability of chlorine in solution, whereas copper, nickel, and cobalt are powerful catalysts of decomposition. The most stable free available chlorine solutions are those having the following characteristics: (1) low chlorine concentration; (2) absence of copper, cobalt, nickel, or other catalysts; (3) high alkalinity; (4) low temperature; (5) absence of organic material; (6) storage in dark, closed containers (ie, shielded from ultraviolet light); and (7) low ionic strength. The stability of chlorine in solution or products may be rated by its half-life, which denotes the number of days required for the available chlorine content to be reduced to half its initial value.[47]

Organic chloramines are considerably more stable in solution than free chlorine compounds because they release chlorine rather slowly into solution, with delayed bactericidal action. Solutions of chloramine-T (see Figure 15.2; 8, R = CH$_3$) are quite stable, and a moderate exposure to high temperature, sunlight, or organic material does not seem to cause any appreciable decomposition.[48] To ensure free chlorine stability in solution, chlorine stabilizers are often used that combine with chlorine to form N-chloro compounds, prolonging the life of chlorine considerably but at the same time producing a slower germicidal effect.

Factors Affecting Chlorine Microbicidal Activity

A long history and wide use of chlorine compounds have yielded much laboratory and field evaluation data, mostly concerning hypochlorites, but with application to all active chlorine compounds to some extent. Disinfection effectiveness largely depends on the concentration of free, undissociated hypochlorous acid in water solution and the relationship between pH and the degree of dissociation of HOCl, as shown in Figure 15.4. In addition to pH, various other environmental factors, alone or in combination, determine the antimicrobial action of chlorine. A full understanding of these environmental factors and manipulation thereof enables the user of chlorine compounds to make proper adjustments for best results.

Effect of pH

The pH has perhaps the greatest influence on the antimicrobial activity of chlorine in solution. An increase in pH substantially decreases the biocidal activity of chlorine, and a decrease in pH increases this activity. Early works in 1921 and 1934 showed this pH dependency on hypochlorite effectiveness.[49,50] In 1937, Charlton and Levine,[51]

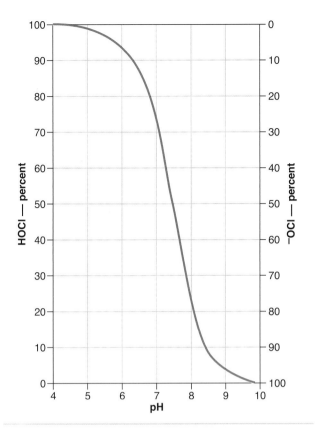

FIGURE 15.4 Relationships between hypochlorous acid (HOCl), hypochlorite (−OCl), and pH. After Baker.[36] Copyright © 1959 American Water Works Association. Reprinted by permission of John Wiley & Sons, Inc.

using *Bacillus metiens* and calcium hypochlorite solutions, showed that 100 ppm available chlorine at pH 8.2 exhibits approximately the same kill of spores as a 1000 ppm solution at pH 11.3, demonstrating the controlling effect of pH. Later, the effect of pH on 25 ppm available chlorine solution to produce 99% kill of *B metiens* spores was shown.[52] The results were 2.5 minutes for pH 6, 3.6 minutes for pH 7, 5 minutes for pH 8, 19.5 minutes for pH 9, 35.5 minutes for pH 9.35, 131 minutes for pH 10, and 465 minutes for pH 12.86. The authors attributed the striking changes in killing time to changes in concentrations of undissociated hypochlorous acid and concluded that the concentration of HOCl is closely related to the speed of inactivation by hypochlorites in solution.

Mercer and Somers,[53] using *Bacillus macerans* spores, showed that 15 ppm hypochlorite solution effected 99% reduction of organisms within 8.5 minutes at pH 6, and that approximately 42 minutes were required at pH 8 for the same reduction. They also found no significant difference in sporicidal activity with chlorine gas, sodium hypochlorite, and calcium hypochlorite.[53] Friberg and Hammarstrom,[54] in their work with bacteria and viruses, concluded that the viricidal effect of free available chlorine is affected by the pH in much the same manner as bactericidal action. Watkins et al[55] reported on the viricidal

activity of NaOCl solution, which at 12.5 ppm available chlorine completely inactivated phage of *Streptococcus cremoris* within a 30-second interval; as pH was lowered from 9 to 4.4, progressively faster phage destruction occurred. This increased activity at lower pH levels was somewhat similar to results obtained with hypochlorites against bacterial spores and non–spore-forming bacteria.

Bactericidal activity of chloramines is also influenced by pH. With a decrease in pH, there is a corresponding increase in dichloramine formation, which is a more effective bactericide than the monochloramine. Work using cysts of *Entamoeba histolytica* verified this point by showing that dichloramine was a considerably more powerful cyst-penetrating agent than monochloramine, attributed to faster penetrating power to one of the hydrolysis products of dichloramine (ie, HOCl).[56]

Effect of Concentration

It is logical to assume that an increase in concentration in available chlorine in a solution brings a corresponding increase in antibacterial activity. This supposition may hold true if other factors, such as pH, temperature, and organic content, are held constant. Experiments with *Staphylococcus aureus* at a constant pH value of 9 showed that by increasing the available chlorine in the hypochlorite solutions from 0.3 to 0.6, 1.2, to 2.0 ppm, the killing time was shortened or the bactericidal rate increased. The 2 ppm available chlorine produced complete kill in 5 minutes and 1.2 ppm in 10 minutes, whereas 0.3 ppm did not completely kill the organism even in 30 minutes.[57] Others tested hypochlorite solutions at concentrations of 25, 100, and 500 ppm of available chlorine at a constant pH of 10 and temperature of 20°C. The times required to provide the 99.9% kill of resistant *B metiens* spores were 31 minutes for 500 ppm, 63.5 minutes for 100 ppm, and 121 minutes for 25 ppm available chlorine solutions. It was concluded that a 4-fold increase in the concentration of hypochlorite solution results in a 50% reduction in killing time and a 2-fold increase in only a 30% reduction.[52,58]

Effect of Temperature

The effect of temperature was demonstrated with *Mycobacterium tuberculosis*; using 50 ppm available chlorine hypochlorite solution at pH 8.35, complete kill was obtained in 30 seconds at 60°C, in 60 seconds at 55°C, and in 2.5 minutes at 50°C.[59] Under the same test conditions, 200 ppm available chlorine solutions at pH 9 destroyed the organism in 60 seconds at 50°C and in 30 seconds at 55°C.

A temperature effect on the bactericidal activity of Ca(OCl)$_2$ solution was observed at 20°C, 30°C, 35°C, and 50°C. The 25 ppm hypochlorite solution at a constant pH of 10 killed in 121, 65, 38.7, and 9.3 minutes, respectively. A 60% to 65% reduction in killing time was observed with a 10°C rise in temperature.[52] Later, in work with hypochlorite solutions at 25 ppm available chlorine and three different pH levels (10, 7, 5), a rise of 10°C produced a reduction of 50% to 60% in killing time and that a drop of 10°C increased the necessary exposure time by approximately 2.1- to 2.3-fold. This work also revealed that temperature coefficients were only slightly affected by pH.[58] Work with *Pseudomonas fragi* showed that $Ca(OCl)_2$ at 3 ppm available chlorine produced a 99.99% kill in 4 minutes at 21°C, but in approximately 10 minutes at 4.4°C.[60] The effects of temperature on the bactericidal action of free available chlorine are especially evident at a pH higher than 8.5 and also when the chlorine residuals are low (0.02-0.03 ppm available chlorine).[61]

With respect to temperature effect on chloramines, it has been reported that 2.5-fold higher concentrations of chlorine and 9-fold longer exposure times are necessary to produce the same kill at 3°C as at 20°C.[41] From all this work, it is evident that an increase in temperature increases bactericidal activity.

Effect of Organic Material

Organic material in chlorine solution consumes available chlorine and reduces its capacity for bactericidal activity; this is evident especially in solutions with low levels of chlorine. It has been reported that hypochlorites are selective in their attack on various types of organic material. There seems to be a difference of opinion among various workers on this subject. Among different sugars, only levulose consumed chlorine and the chlorine loss with other nonnitrogenous substrates (lipids and alcohols) was negligible. Sodium hypochlorite was also more reactive with organic substrates than either chloramine-T or azochloramide.[62] Prucha[63] reported early on the effect of 1% to 5% skim milk on chlorine losses in solution. Loveless[64] studied the amount of available chlorine loss in hypochlorite solution in the presence of 1.5% whole milk at a temperature range of 21°C to 100°C for a period of 60 minutes, with all solutions showing some loss in available chlorine at 21°C and that the rate of loss increased with rising temperatures. The control solutions with no milk did not seem to lose any available chlorine during the 60 minutes, except for a small loss at 100°C. But the presence of milk in the tests with hypochlorite solutions did not seem adversely to affect the bactericidal action of chlorine.[65]

If the organic matter contains proteins, the chlorine reacts and forms chloramines, retaining some of its antibacterial activity even though the available chlorine levels are reduced considerably. This explains some questionable results in the early literature regarding the disappearance of anthrax spores from chlorinated tannery wastes in the absence of measurable free available chlorine, or that hypochlorite solution of 130 ppm of available chlorine completely killed *Salmonella pullorum* in the presence of 5% organic matter in the form of chicken manure.[66] Similar results were reported with *Salmonella typhosa* and human feces.[67]

Johns,[68] using a modification of glass slide technique and *Escherichia coli* and *S aureus* as test organisms, reported no evidence of germicidal reduction due to the presence of skim or whole milk in the freshly prepared hypochlorite solutions. This may be significant for the use of hypochlorites as sanitizers on milk farms and in dairy plants because minute amounts of milk may be encountered with no particular adverse effect on the activity of hypochlorites. However, Lasmanis and Spencer,[69] in their work with hypochlorite solutions using strains of staphylococci (coagulase positive and negative), found that with 3% of skim milk, they did not obtain complete kill of organisms, although smaller amounts of milk exhibited progressively lesser effects on the bactericidal action.

It appears that sugars and starches may affect the germicidal activity of chlorine. Shere[70] reported that 500 ppm of alkyl aryl sulfonate did not exhibit any slowing action on the germicidal effectiveness of the hypochlorite solutions. Other organic materials, such as tyrosine, tryptophan, cystine, egg albumin, peptone, body fluids, tissues, microbes, and vegetable matter, when present in a disinfecting solution, can consume chlorine to satisfy the organic water demand; in these cases, the chlorine may lose its function as a germicidal agent unless it forms chloramines or unless the chlorine dosage is adjusted to overcome this demand. This loss of chlorine due to organic matter may be significant in cases in which minute amounts of chlorine are used. Higher levels of chlorine tend to produce a safety reserve for performing the desired bactericidal action.

Effect of Hardness

Water hardness components such as Mg^{2+} and Ca^{2+} ions do not exhibit any impact on the antibacterial action of hypochlorite solution. In studies with 5 ppm available chlorine, sodium hypochlorite solution at 0 and 400 ppm hardness at 20°C, a complete kill of bacteria at two examined levels of hardness was obtained, indicating that raising the hardness from 0 to 400 ppm did not have any inhibitory action.[42]

Effect of Addition of Ammonia or Amino Compounds

The bactericidal activity of free chlorine is considerably diminished when chlorine is added to water containing ammonia or amino compounds and the concentration of chlorine is plotted against residual chlorine (see Figure 15.3). Chlorine can react immediately with ammonia to form monochloramines and dichloramines. As more chlorine is added to the ammonia solution, to a ratio of chlorine to ammonia of 5:1, formation of chloramines continues until all the ammonia has been converted. Up to this point, chlorine remains in the form of combined available chlorine. After the so-called "hump" has been obtained, added amounts of chlorine oxidize the chloramines, slowly reducing the residual chlorine and ammonia, until they both drop practically to zero. Increase of chlorine beyond this point (breakpoint) produces an increase in free available chlorine.[42] The available chlorine curves for different N-chloro compounds formed from amino acid or proteins vary because of variability of reactions and varying stabilities of the products of the reactions.

If ammonia concentrations are less than one-eighth of the total available chlorine added, the ammonia was found to be destroyed and the excess chlorine can remain as free available chlorine, exhibiting fast bactericidal action.[58] If the concentration of ammonia is greater than one-fourth that of free chlorine, the available chlorine will exist in the form of chloramines and thus will have slow bactericidal activity. Water temperature influences the antibacterial action of the ammonia-chlorine treatment, with efficiency decreasing with lower temperatures. An excess of ammonium salt in the presence of high levels of organic material enhanced the bactericidal effectiveness of hypochlorite solution.[71,72]

From the information available, it appears that the killing time of chlorine is extended considerably in chloramines or N-chloro compounds, and the higher the concentration of ammonia or nitrogenous compounds the greater the lag in bactericidal time.

Effect of Addition of Iodine or Bromine (Halogen Mixture)

There is considerable evidence that small additions of bromine or iodine to chlorine solutions greatly enhance the bactericidal activity of chlorine. Improvement of bactericidal results in solutions containing chlorine with a small amount of ammonia salt and bromide ions has been reported.[72] The addition of sodium bromide (NaBr) to hypochlorite solution resulted in a 33% to 1000% increase in bactericidal effectiveness against a variety of bacteria at pH 11.[73] Chlorine-bromine mixtures at various ratios increased the germicidal activity in purified and natural waters containing low and high amounts of nitrogenous growth-promoting material in a pH range of 5.4 to 8.6. Also chlorine reinforced by 5% to 10% bromide was effective in decreasing the number of chlorine- and bromine-resistant bacteria.[74] Kamlet,[75] using equimolecular mixtures of bromine and chlorine, obtained superior bactericidal effects against E coli compared with either chlorine or bromine alone. Others claimed an advantage in using germicidal mixtures of iodine and chlorine.[76]

Paterson[77] demonstrated that a halogen-substituted mixture, such as N-bromo-N-chlorodimethylhydantoin, exhibited bactericidal activity against test bacteria superior to that obtained for either N,N-dibromomethyl or N,N-dichlorodimethylhydantoin. Zsoldos[78] produced a germicidal mixture by introducing dichlorodimethylhydantoin and KI into aqueous solution, thereby generating a hypoiodous acid and chloramine combination. Table 15.2 summarizes the biocidal effect of free available chlorine for a number of microorganisms.

▶ MECHANISMS OF ANTIMICROBIAL ACTION

Hypochlorous Acid Formation in Cells

The HOCl is an example of a reactive oxygen species (ROS). The ROS are chemically reactive chemical species that assist mammals during host defense. During the process, macrophages and neutrophils produce high concentrations of H_2O_2, superoxide, and hypochlorous acid to kill invading microorganisms.[103] The buildup of ROS, a condition called oxidative stress, is suspected to be linked to the cause of different human diseases including Parkinson disease, Alzheimer disease, Huntington disease, and multiple sclerosis.[104] A series of reactions occur in the space between an ingested bacterium and the membrane of the phagosome and as a result the ingested bacteria within the phagosome are killed (shown in Figure 15.5). The NADPH oxidase system reduces molecular oxygen to the superoxide radical. The influx of protons (H^+) or other cations compensate the charge transfer. Nevertheless, the pH in the phagosome rises to about pH 8 that indicates that other cations such as potassium ions (K^+) may enter the phagosome instead of protons.[105] The protons are used to reduce superoxide to H_2O_2, which can be broken down to oxygen and water in a catalase-dependent reaction. Alternatively, H_2O_2 can combine with chloride to form HOCl in a reaction catalyzed by myeloperoxidase (MPO). Different peroxidases vary in their substrate specificity, and only MPO can generate HOCl.[106] Initial studies indicated that the halide requirement could be met by iodide, bromide, or chloride or by the pseudohalide, thiocyanate.[107-111] Additionally, it is shown nitrite might substitute halide in the MPO-mediated antimicrobial system in vitro[112,113]; however, it is not clear that nitrite is formed in sufficient amounts to contribute significantly to the microbicidal activity of the MPO system.[114]

MPO forms three different complexes on reaction with products of the respiratory burst of phagocytes: compounds I, II, and III.[114] H_2O_2 reacts rapidly with the iron of MPO (which is normally in the ferric form) to form a complex compound I, which has an oxygen bound by a double bond to the heme iron.[115] Compound I can also be formed by the reaction of MPO with HOCl. Compound I, the primary catalytic complex of MPO,

TABLE 15.2   Biocidal effect of free available chlorine on various microorganisms

Organism	pH	Temperature (°C)	Exposure Time	ppm Average Cl$_2$	Biocidal Results	References
Algae						
Chlorella variegata	7.8	22	NA	2.0	Growth controlled	Palmer and Maloney[79]
Gomphonema parvulum	8.2	22	NA	2.0	Growth controlled	Palmer and Maloney[79]
Microcystis aeruginosa	8.2	22	NA	2.0	Growth controlled	Palmer and Maloney[79]
Bacteria						
Achromobacter metalcaligenes	6	21	15 s	5	100%	Hays et al[80]
Bacillus anthracis	7.2	22	120 min	2.3-2.4	100%	Brazis et al[81,82]
Bacillus globigii	7.2	22	120 min	2.5-2.6	99.99%	Brazis et al[81,82]
Clostridium botulinum toxin type A	7	25	30 s	0.5	100%	Brazis et al[81,82]
Escherichia coli	7	20-25	1 min	0.055	100%	Butterfield et al[61]
Eberthella typhosa	8.5	20-25	1 min	0.1-0.29	100%	Butterfield et al[61]
Mycobacterium tuberculosis	8.4	50-60	30 s	50	100%	Costigan[59]
Listeria monocytogenes	9.5	20	30 s	100	99.999%	Lopes[83] and El-Kest and Marth[84]
Pseudomonas fluorescens IM	6	21	15 s	5	100%	Hays et al[80]
Shigella dysenteriae	7	20-25	3 min	0.046-0.055	100%	Butterfield et al[61]
Staphylococcus aureus	7.2	25	30 s	0.8	100%	Dychdala[85] and Bolton et al[86]
Streptococcus faecalis	7.5	20-25	2 min	0.5	100%	Stuart and Ortenzio[87]
All vegetative bacteria	9	25	30 s	0.2	100%	Snow[88]
Yersinia enterocolitica	9	20	5 min	100	99.99%	Orth and Mrozek[89]
Bacteriophage						
Streptococcus cremoris, phage stain 144F	6.9-8.2	25	15 s	25	100%	Hays and Elliker[90]
Fish						
Carassius auratus	7.9	Room	96 h	1	Killed	Davis[91]
Daphnia magna	7.9	Room	72 h	0.5	Killed	Davis[91]
Frogs						
Rana pipiens	8.3	21	4 d	10	100%	Kaplan[92]
Fungi						
Aspergillus niger	10-11	20	30-60 min	100	100%	Dychdala[93] and Costigan[94,95]
Rhodotorula flava	10-11	20	5 min	100	100%	Dychdala[93] and Costigan[94,95]
Nematodes						
Cheilobus quadrilabiatus	6.6-7.2	25	30 min	95-100	93%	Chang et al[96]
Diplogaster nudicapitatus	6.6-7.2	25	30 min	95-100	97%	Chang et al[96]

(continued)

TABLE 15.2 Biocidal effect of free available chlorine on various microorganisms *(Continued)*

Organism	pH	Temperature (°C)	Exposure Time	ppm Average Cl_2	Biocidal Results	References
Plants						
Cabomba caroliniana	6.3-7.7	Room	4 d	5	100%	Zimmerman and Berg[97]
Elodea canadensis	6.3-7.7	Room	4 d	5	100%	Zimmerman and Berg[97]
Protozoa						
Entamoeba histolytica cysts	7	25	150 min	0.08-0.12	99%-100%	Clarke et al[98]
Viruses						
Purified adenovirus 3	8.8-9	25	40-50 s	0.2	99.8%	Clarke et al[98]
Purified coxsackievirus A2	6.9-7.1	27-29	3 min	0.92-1	99.6%	Clarke and Chang[99] and Clarke and Kabler[100]
Purified coxsackievirus B1	7	25	2 min	0.31-0.4	99.9%	Clarke and Chang[99] and Clarke and Kabler[100]
Purified coxsackievirus B5	7	25-28	1 min	0.21-0.3	99.9%	Clarke and Chang[99] and Clarke and Kabler[100]
Infectious hepatitis	6.7-6.8	Room	30 min	3.25	Protected all 12 volunteers	Clarke and Chang[99] and Clarke and Kabler[100]
Purified poliovirus (Mahoney)	7	25-28	3 min	0.21-0.3	99.9%	Grabow et al[101]
Purified poliovirus (Lensen)	7.4-7.9	19-25	10 min	0.5-1	Protected all 164 inoculated mice	Clarke and Chang[99] and Clarke and Kabler[100]
Purified poliovirus III (Sankett)	7	25-28	2 min	0.11-0.2	99.9%	Clarke and Chang[99] and Clarke and Kabler[100]
Purified Theiler's Murine Encephalomyelitis virus	6.5-7	25-27	5 min	4-6	99%	Kelly and Sanderson[102]
Simian rotavirus	6	5	15 s	0.5	99.99%	Berman and Hoff[28]

Abbreviation: NA, not applicable.

reacts with a halide in a two-electron reduction to form the corresponding hypohalous acid and regenerating the native Fe^{3+}-MPO. The reaction of compound I with excess H_2O_2 results in the formation of compound II, which is inactive with respect to the oxidation of chloride. Compound II can be reduced to the active, native enzyme by oxygen radical anion or another reducing agent. Dioxygen radical anion can also react directly with native MPO to form compound III, an oxyperoxidase, which, like oxyhemoglobin, has oxygen attached to the heme iron. Compound III is unstable, decaying to native MPO with a half-decay time of several minutes at room temperature.

The current view is that in normal neutrophils, HOCl is primarily responsible for oxidative killing; however, deficiency of myeloperoxidase is a common condition and does not lead to obvious susceptibility to bacterial infections. This leads to the idea of existence of the backup systems to compensate for this deficiency.[105]

Hypochlorous Acid Reactivity

An ROS can be divided into two groups: one-electron (radicals) and two-electron (nonradical) oxidants such as H_2O_2 and HOCl.[116] The oxidizing strength of radicals can be ranked on the basis of one-electron reduction potential because the activation energy for radical reactions is low; therefore, thermodynamic drive is a good measure of reactivity. For two-electron oxidants, whereas the reduction potential determines the strength of the oxidant (thermodynamic drive), the kinetic aspect is more important in determining reactivity. This means that although H_2O_2 has a higher reduction potential than HOCl (E^o values of 1.776 and 1.482 for reduction to water and chloride, respectively), the reactions of H_2O_2 require higher activation energy and therefore rates are slower.

Generally, the reaction rates of peroxide with thiols, one of the very few biomolecules that H_2O_2 reacts is extremely slow ($k = 2.9 M^{-1}s^{-1}$ at pH 7.4-7.6).[117] HOCl reacts

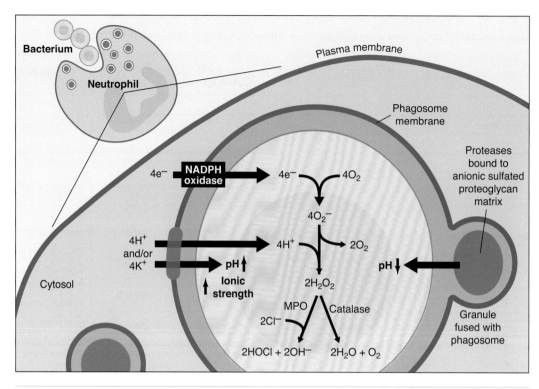

FIGURE 15.5   Chemical reaction schemes within phagocyte. From Roos and Winterbourn.[105] Reprinted with permission from AAAS.

with free cysteines about seven orders of magnitudes faster (k = 3.0 10^7 M^{-1}s^{-1} at pH 7.4) and shows high reaction rates with numerous other amino acid side chains.[118] These high rates of reaction will enable HOCl to oxidize residues that are buried and might be only transiently accessible for oxidative modifications. Interestingly, the reaction rate for chloramines that are produced upon reaction of HClO with nitrogen-containing compounds is about 300 to 700 M^{-1}s^{-1}.[119] It should be noted oxidants can have different effects depending on where they are generated.[120] It is possible to increase the possibility of an oxidant and a target by restraining them within the same cell compartment. For example, species like superoxide with low membrane permeability are largely restricted to reacting in the compartment in which they are generated.

Reaction of Products of Myeloperoxidase-Mediated Antimicrobial System

As HOCl has a pK$_a$ of 7.53, it exists as a mixture of the undissociated acid and the hypochlorite ion at physiologic pH levels. At lower pHs, HOCl predominates and can react with excess chloride to form molecular chlorine (Cl$_2$). All these products can react with any oxidizable group on the organism, for example, sulfhydryl groups, iron-sulfur centers, sulfur-ether groups, heme groups, unsaturated fatty acids, and be oxidized. As a consequence,

there may be a loss of microbial membrane transport, an interruption of the membrane electron transport chain, dissipation of adenylate energy reserves, and suppression of DNA synthesis with associated disruption of the interaction of the microbial cell membrane with the chromosomal origin of replication.[121-123] It seems that HOCl's damaging effects to bacteria during host defense and disinfection are likely due to its ability to cause protein unfolding and aggregation.[124] In vitro and in vivo data show that thermolabile proteins are particularly prone to HOCl-mediated oxidative unfolding and aggregation. Because these proteins are in rapid equilibrium with a partially unfolded conformation, bimolecular oxidation reactions that are fast enough to compete with the refolding reaction will cause protein unfolding and aggregation. Thermostable proteins, on the other hand, might be targeted predominantly on surface-exposed residues, which might not affect the activity or thermodynamic stability of the proteins.

In addition, HOCl reacts with nitrogen-containing compounds to form nitrogen-chlorine derivatives such as monochloramines and dichloramines, which can degrade to the corresponding aldehyde. Some of these compounds retain oxidizing activity. Taurine reacts with HOCl to form taurine chloramine, which is less toxic than HOCl, and this reaction has thus been implicated as a mechanism by which neutrophils are protected from HOCl released into the cytoplasm. Taurine chloramine can retain some biologic activity. The chloramines are long-lived, thus providing a mechanism for the prolongation of the oxidant activity of the peroxidase system and the penetration of MPO-derived oxidants into complex biological fluids, to be toxic at a distance under conditions in which the more reactive products are readily scavenged.

Additionally, it is proposed that MPO catalyzes the H_2O_2-dependent formation of HOCl, which reacts with dioxygen radical anion to form $\cdot$OH as follows:

$$H_2O_2 + Cl- \rightarrow HOCl + OH- \tag{8}$$

$$HOCl + O_2- \rightarrow \cdot OH + O2 + Cl- \tag{9}$$

Singlet oxygen has been detected as a product of the MPO-H_2O_2-chloride system with the following reactions:

$$H_2O_2 + 2Cl- \rightarrow 2HOCl + 2e- \rightleftharpoons \\ 2OCl- + 2H^+ + 2e- \tag{10}$$

$$HOCl + OCl- \rightarrow {}^1O_2 + H_2O + Cl- \tag{11}$$

Finally, it is proposed the oxidation of water by ${}^1O_2$ catalyzed by antibodies results in production of H_2O_2 and O_3; O_3 is also bactericidal.[125-128]

▶ FORMULATION OF PRODUCTS

Matching Compounds and Forms

The gaseous forms of chlorine and its compounds are elemental chlorine and chlorine dioxide. Where rapid, large-scale deployment is sought, for example, in fogging a large building or sparging gas into a large volume of liquid, these materials can be the most cost-efficient methods of rapid microbial control. These forms are very reactive, toxic at low exposure levels, and dissipate quickly. The differences between these two materials are discussed earlier. The choice of material depends on available equipment (eg, can chlorine gas be received, or chlorine dioxide be generated), the microbial species involved, and the operating conditions (eg, humidity, pH, level of organic matter).

While shelf-stable liquid solutions have been commercially available for over a century, particularly after the invention of the chloralkali process made chlorine and sodium hydroxide solutions easier to manufacture and therefore made hypochlorite solutions easier to manufacture,[129,130] innovations in formulation with fragrances,[131,132] surfactant,[133,134] thickeners, and polymers have enabled the formulation of sodium hypochlorite into trigger and aerosol sprays, foams, gels, and wipes.[135-138] These find applications as hard surface disinfecting cleaners, drain cleaners, and targeted soil and stain removers.

Solid chlorine-based compounds (hydantoins and chloramines) are used in laundry bleaches, pool and spa treatment chemicals, dishware detergents, and automatic toilet bowl and urinal cleaners. Fast-dissolving materials

(eg, sodium dichloroisocyanurate) are appropriate for shock treatment for pools and spas as well as for laundry bleaching and dishwashing. Slower dissolving materials (eg, trichloroisocyanuric acid and the chloro- and bromochlorohydantoins) are useful for continuous release of hypochlorite into solution, which is suitable for pool and spa maintenance as well as for automatic toilet and urinal cleaners. Often, these materials are tableted or granulated; the dissolution rate can also be controlled by tableting press conditions or granule particle size as well as the addition of processing aids.[139-141] Recent innovations in water-soluble films have yielded options for unit-dose bleaches for laundry and hard-surface disinfection applications, enabling faster dissolution than in a tablet form.[142-144]

Formulation Ingredients

When formulating with chlorine-based compounds, care must be taken to avoid incompatibilities with other ingredients. Incompatibilities reduce the efficacy of the chlorine-based compound due to its reaction with susceptible ingredients. These reactions in some cases are highly exothermic and can release by-products that can be harmful to human health. Packaging integrity may be compromised. Even in a dry state, chlorine-based materials can react with other components due to the presence of ambient moisture or water present in hydrated salts. In addition to the reaction chemistry information provided earlier in this chapter, useful guidance for choices of materials to formulate with chlorine-based materials comes from manufacturers through safety data sheets (SDS); those materials where the SDS indicates avoiding strong oxidizing agents are likely to react with chlorine-based disinfecting compounds. The SDS for the chlorine-based compound also gives guidance for personal protective equipment, handling, storage, and emergency procedures to be followed when working with chlorine-based compounds in the formulation laboratory and manufacturing facility.

Gaseous forms (chlorine and chlorine dioxide) are highly reactive and are unlikely to be formulated with other materials. Solid forms (dichloroisocyanurate, trichloroisocyanuric acid, halohydantoins) have been formulated with other ingredients, including salts, fragrances, and surfactants. The most commonly formulated chlorine-based compound is sodium hypochlorite, which finds use in products for laundry, hard-surface cleaning and disinfection, and mold control. Table 15.3 lists materials that have been used in cleaning and disinfecting products containing sodium hypochlorite.

Chemistry Considerations

Key incompatibilities when formulating with hypochlorite include unsaturated alkyl chains, primary or secondary alkyl amines, esters, amides, alcohols (or materials with terminal hydroxyl groups), thiols, and oxidizable metals. Compatibility is contingent on pH, with additional

TABLE 15.3	Materials used in formulations with sodium hypochlorite
Material Class	**Example Materials**
Surfactants	Alkyl and alkylaryl sulfates[145-147] Amine oxides[148-150] Alkyl trimethyl ammonium salts[150] Alkyl betaines[150] Fatty acid salts[150]
Thickeners (nonsurfactant)	Cross-linked polyacrylates[145] Alumina monohydrate[150] Clay[151,152]
Fragrances	Examples in reference [153] Proprietary lists of suitable materials used by fragrance houses
Polymers	Polyacrylates[145,150] Styrene/acrylate copolymer[150]
Other functional materials	Abrasives (silica, calcium carbonate)[145] Colorants[154] Corrosion inhibitors (silicates)[150]

hydroxide added where needed to improve stability by lowering the level of hypochlorous acid.[155]

When formulating with sodium hypochlorite, pH control during the process is essential to a stable formula and safety in manufacture. As discussed earlier, below pH 10, hypochlorous acid in notable concentrations is formed, and reacts more aggressively toward organic materials than does sodium hypochlorite. This reactivity lowers the efficacy of hypochlorite, breaks down functional ingredients, and in certain cases may generate hazardous by-products. Hypochlorous acid is also more corrosive to processing equipment than sodium hypochlorite. If possible, the hypochlorite is best added late in a formula, with the pH already adjusted to the desired final specification for the formula, and only minor ingredients added thereafter. When developing a new formulation, order of addition is thus an important consideration for stability. Scented bleaches are increasing in popularity. Two methods are used for scenting bleaches; they can be floated on top of the aqueous solution (recommended for diluted bleaches only), or they can be formulated into the bleach by use of surfactants (required for ready-to-use applications such as sprays or wipes).[155]

When working with hypochlorite solutions, it is noteworthy that a significant concentration of sodium chloride is present in the solution with sodium hypochlorite. When adjusting the hypochlorite level of a formula, the sodium chloride level is also being adjusted, providing an additional impact of electrolyte on various formula elements such as physical stability and rheology, especially for anionic and alkoxylated surfactants.[156] The sodium chloride content of a hypochlorite solution should be clearly stated on certificates of analysis.

Packaging Considerations

When selecting packaging for formulations of chlorine-based materials, several factors should be considered. First, the packaging materials (including cap liners and labels) should be compatible with the formula. Second, the packaging should not allow ultraviolet (UV) transmission into the formulation because this will decrease the stability of the formula. Third, the formulation should be evaluated to determine if a child resistant closure or the use of postconsumer recycled material is required. If the formulation will evolve gaseous by-product over its shelf life, the package should be vented to avoid pressure buildup that may result in package deformation or product leakage. The formulation should be tested for stability in the desired package for commercialization, and the package should be tested over the storage period to ensure that structural integrity is maintained.[157,158] Sodium hypochlorite solutions are typically sold in high-density polyethylene bottles, with the use of a child-resistant closure dependent on the formulation properties and regulatory requirements. Some flexible packaging options have emerged as well. For triggers and pumps, care in material selection, particularly with any metal parts in the dispenser, will improve product and package stability.

▶ PRACTICAL APPLICATIONS FOR DISINFECTION

Drinking Water Treatment

The chlorination practices for sanitizing drinking water to make it safe and palatable for human consumption have been established in North America since the early 20th century. Elemental chlorine or calcium hypochlorite has been used successfully to treat drinking water, with or without subsequent filtration; typically, 2 to 4 ppm suffices for controlling a wide range of microorganisms. Chlorine dioxide has been used as an alternative to chlorine for drinking water disinfection. At these concentrations, chlorine by itself may not completely control *Cryptosporidium* or *Giardia* oocysts. Although it has been reported that chlorine, when used sequentially with chloramines, can inactivate *Cryptosporidium*,[29] in practice, filtration is used to bring the levels of spore- or cyst-forming species to acceptable levels. Continuous chlorination of drinking water has been used to practically eliminate various waterborne pathogens, such as those responsible for cholera, dysentery, typhoid, and hepatitis A, thereby preventing epidemic due to drinking water. In the United States, drinking water quality and standards for impurity levels are mandated by the Safe Drinking Water Act, which is enforced by the US Environmental Protection Agency (EPA)[159]; in Europe, drinking water quality is regulated by the European Drinking Water Directive.[160] In addition, the World Health Organization (WHO) publishes guidelines for drinking-water quality.[161]

White[43] discusses in detail the "breakpoint phenomenon" as practiced in drinking water treatment with chlorine. By controlling pH, temperature, chlorine levels, and the chlorine/ammonia ratio, avoidance of undesirable by-products is achieved, resulting in potable water with better taste. The rate and equilibrium constants for the formation of mono-, di-, and trichloramine at varying chlorine and ammonia concentrations at different pH values create a complex modeling problem. For accurate modeling, the contribution from organic materials in the water, as well as side reactions from nitrate formation, needs to be considered. In the event of a malfunction of a public water supply or a natural disaster (eg, flood, typhoon, or hurricane), hypochlorite (either calcium or sodium) can be used to purify water for drinking, particularly where there are no facilities for boiling water; eight drops of 6% or 8% sodium hypochlorite bleach per gallon is recommended, followed by 30 minutes' time for disinfection of filtered tap water.[162]

Sewage and Wastewater Treatment

Chlorine or hypochlorites have been used effectively for sewage and wastewater treatment. Chlorination may be a continuous process or may be used intermittently or seasonally. The benefits of chlorination include (1) general disinfection, (2) control of odors, (3) reduction of biochemical oxygen demand, (4) chemical precipitation, (5) color reduction, and (6) cyanide treatment.[163,164] More recently, there has been some concern that chlorination of sewage and wastewater may result in the formation of toxic chlorinated organic compounds capable of contaminating drinking water. Therefore, the effluents from sewage plants and industrial plants, if not treated properly, can contribute to contamination of drinking water, bathing water, wells, rivers, lakes, and oceans, with adverse effects on animal and plant life. Dechlorination, using sulfur dioxide, sodium bisulfite, and sodium metabisulfite, is used to reduce chlorine levels before release to water systems.[165] Because of the public health hazard, sewage and wastewater disposal can be regulated by federal, state, and local water pollution control commissions.

Hard-Surface Cleaning and Disinfection

The most common chlorine-based compound used for hard-surface cleaning and disinfection is sodium hypochlorite, primarily because of its high stability in a liquid form. When used as a concentrated product, it is diluted to 1800 to 2400 ppm sodium hypochlorite for use; manufacturer instructions on dosage and contact time should be followed to ensure efficacy on the microorganisms of interest. Such solutions should be made just before use to ensure full potency of the hypochlorite; hypochlorite often degrades quickly in such solutions. To aid in cleaning, surfactants and polymers can be added to enhance penetration of soils for easier removal, yet still retain disinfection. Fast-dissolving solid bleaches, that is, sodium dichloroisocyanurate, can also be used for this purpose once diluted. Gaseous materials can be used, but the area being disinfected must be evacuated and sealed, limiting these materials to occasions where complete coverage is required for success.

Laundry Disinfection

Chlorine-based compounds, most commonly sodium hypochlorite, are used in sanitizing laundry in both commercial and household settings. Typically, 200 ppm hypochlorite is sufficient for disinfection in automatic washing machines. Laundry sanitization and disinfection claims are substantiated in the United States using ASTM International methods E2274 (for standard top load washing machines) or E2406 (for high-efficiency washing machines), adopted by the EPA.[166] In Europe, EN suspension and practice-oriented tests to validate antimicrobial laundry claims are delineated.[167] Not all fabrics and dyes are chlorine fast; patch testing of a dilution of hypochlorite (1 tsp per 1 cup water) can be done on fabrics prior to treatment if there is concern about compatibility of the dye or fabric with hypochlorite. Most notably, silk, wool, and nonwater fast fabrics should not be treated with hypochlorite.

Pool, Hot Tub, and Spa Maintenance

Swimming pools, hot tubs, and spas, both commercial and private, require water purification and disinfection of water handling systems as part of their maintenance. Use conditions and environmental factors contribute to the need for microbial control. Two types of chlorine products are used in purification of pool water. First, a recommended level of chlorine is maintained in the pool, tub, or spa during use. Sodium dichloroisocyanurate or trichloroisocyanuric acid are the most common materials for this purpose, as the cyanuric acid stabilizes chlorine in solution at a recommended level of 2 to 4 ppm,[168] particularly from UV light. Sodium hypochlorite solutions can also be used to boost chlorine levels. In addition, a "shock treatment" or superchlorination dosage of 5 and 6 ppm chlorine is recommended weekly when not in use to provide extra protection against algae and bacterial growth both in the water and in pumps, piping, and filters. Chlorination of water can cause formation of chloramines because of reactions between hypochlorite and protein contamination from swimmers, algae growth, and other environmental contamination, which result in a strong "chlorine" odor and user eye irritation. Following a recommended maintenance schedule, including careful filtration, chlorine monitoring, and pH control, helps mitigate these issues. For those who own or maintain pools, tubs, or spas, the Centers for Disease Control and Prevention's Model Aquatic Health Code[169] is a model regulation followed by many in the design and maintenance, including how to handle acute gross contamination incidents (eg, fecal, urine, or vomit). The chemicals used for maintenance, particularly trichloroisocyanuric acid, are highly concentrated oxidizers and should be protected from heat, humidity, and accidental access by children; use instructions should be followed carefully and proper personal protective equipment should be worn when handling. Users can refer to manufacturers' instructions or the SDS from the manufacturer for proper handling and storage instructions.

Food Processing and Food Service

In large-scale production operations, failure to control microbial contamination can have devastating consequences, including illness or even death of consumers, and significant financial impacts.[170] The owner of the Peanut Corporation of America was sentenced to 28 years in prison for his role in a deadly *Salmonella* outbreak.[171] Chlorine-based compounds find multiple uses in the food processing and food service industries to mitigate microbial contamination. First, chlorine-based compounds are often used to clean equipment as part of clean-in-place operations of food processing equipment. The US 40 CFR §180.940 states that hypochlorous acid and hypochlorite salts can be used in food contact sanitization provided the active concentration before use does not exceed 200 ppm available chlorine.[172] In addition, the Grade A Pasteurized Milk Ordinance[173] stipulates cleaning of dairy processing and storage equipment first, followed by sanitization, following manufacturer instructions for contact time and concentration. This ordinance allows for the use of electrolytic cell generation of hypochlorous acid in dairy processing operations.

The US Public Health Service/US Food and Drug Administration Food Code[174] specifies contact times and temperatures for chlorine solution for manual and mechanical ware washing, equipment, food contact surfaces, and utensils. For example, a contact time of at least 7 seconds is specified for a chlorine solution of 50 mg/L that has a pH of 10 or less and a temperature of at least 38°C (100°F) or a pH of 8 or less and a temperature of at least 24°C (75°F).[175] One manufacturer[176] indicates 200 ppm available chlorine with a 2-minute contact time, stressing the need to review manufacturer's instructions when using specific products.

Water used in process food preparation can be chlorinated as well. Plant chlorination of the water supply beyond the breakpoint level is referred to as in-plant chlorination. It is used in many food industry plants involved with canning, freezing, poultry dressing, and fish processing. Because it doesn't impact water pH or cause salt deposits, and due to its quick action, chlorine gas is the material of choice for in-plant chlorination[177]; hypochlorite can be used in limited amounts for small operations. Four to 7 ppm chlorine level was sufficient for normal operating conditions and that a higher chlorine level (10-20 ppm) was recommended for cleanup operations. In addition, a level of 5 ppm was shown to have negligible effect on flavor of a variety of canned foods. Even the 10 to 20 ppm levels did not show significant corrosion of processing equipment. In canneries and freezing plants, the bacteria, slimes, and foul odors are practically eliminated from plant premises because of in-plant chlorination. In poultry dressing plants, in-plant chlorination of water at a 18 to 30 ppm chlorine level postpicking, 20 to 23 ppm in evisceration, and 20 to 50 ppm in immersion chilling are recommended.[178]

Ice intended for human consumption or used in contact with water, food, food equipment, and utensils should be free of pathogenic organisms and should conform to local public health standards; ice should be made with drinking water if it contacts food or is consumed.[179] It is important that water handling equipment for ice making is disinfected regularly to avoid biofilm formation; mineral buildup from drinking water provides a surface for bacteria to grow if water systems are not properly cleaned and sanitized.

Fruits and vegetables may be decontaminated by washing in chlorine solution (4-5 ppm available chlorine) without damaging their quality.[180] Because eggs are contaminated by their environment and may be carriers of pathogens, they too are treated with chlorine compounds; 200 ppm hypochlorite is recommended after exterior cleaning.[176] Chlorination of food, when carefully controlled, checks the microbial population and makes the foods safer for consumption without adversely affecting the original nutritional value and palatability.

Disinfection to Prevent Diseases and Parasites in Agriculture

Purification of water and regular disinfection of equipment and buildings in agricultural operations can eliminate illnesses and parasites in livestock and crops, resulting in higher production and profit. The guidance described earlier is suitable for water purification and hard surface disinfection needs in agriculture, as part of biosecurity measures for the food supply.[181,182]

Disinfection as an Additional Benefit in Pulp Bleaching

Chlorine dioxide is the bleaching chemical of choice in Kraft paper operations, but a trend toward chlorine-free bleaching with more neutral pH operations and the open design of most pulp mills has resulted in increased microbial contamination including the formation of slimes.[183] In addition, the increased use of recycled material in food-contact paper products resulted in higher microbial counts.[184]

Medicine and Allied Sciences

As discussed earlier, hypochlorous acid is part of the body's response to injury or infection[185] and is now finding application in medical practice. Wang et al[186] demonstrated both wide antimicrobial activities with low animal toxicity for hypochlorous acid solutions in the pH range of 3.5 to 5.0. This combination indicates promise for soft tissue infection control, with minimum microbial control concentrations for 60 minutes at room temperature ranging from 0.17 μg/mL for *S aureus* to 86.6 μg/mL for *Aspergillus niger*. Hypochlorous acid can have two mechanisms in reducing infection and inflammation in periodontal applications.[187] Directly, hypochlorous acid exhibits antipathogen action, modulation of cytokine and growth factors, and lowering inflammation by affecting the nuclear factor κB and an activator protein in monocytes. Hypochlorous acid also reacts with taurine to create the anti-inflammatory and antimicrobial taurine chloramine.[188-190]

The original Dakin's solution was prepared by mixing chlorinated lime and sodium carbonate with boric acid. Because of the irritating properties then attributed to boric acid, the solution was modified to contain a mixture of sodium carbonate and sodium bicarbonate, replacing boric acid and sodium carbonate and resulting in greater stability of the hypochlorite and lesser irritation to open wounds. Up to 1963, Dakin's solution was a standard product in the *British Pharmacopoeia*[191] to disinfect open wound infections in the Carrel-Dakin surgical irrigation treatment. Hypochlorous acid was used in medical practice, both in soaking and application by gauze, for successful care of chronic wounds, particularly with diabetic patients.[192] The soaking and application methods provided a soft debridement not observed with Carrel-Dakin surgical irrigation. Krader[193] reports the use of stabilized 0.01% hypochlorous acid solution to clean lids, lashes, and periocular skin to manage blepharitis and prevent irritation and inflammation of the eyes. Approval was given in Brazil for hypochlorous acid-based products for acne, atopic dermatitis, scar treatment, and skin cleansing after laser skin resurfacing.[194] Hypochlorous acid has been reported to reduce skin inflammation and itching, but too much exposure can increase nerve factor growth and cause dermatitis.[195]

Chlorine dioxide has been used as a chemical disinfectant or sterilant for medical instruments that are not compatible with high heat, humidity, and pressure. It is not flammable, noncarcinogenic, and can work well at low temperatures (15°C to 40°C) at cycle times of about 2.5 hours, lending itself to use on medical devices with embedded batteries and electronics.[196] Hypochlorites find multiple uses in the medical field, hospitals, and dental and veterinary establishments for cleaning of environmental surfaces, disinfection of equipment, and in many applications for disinfecting the water used with modern instrumentation.[197]

Disaster, Outbreak, and Bioterrorism Response

Natural disasters, such as floods, tornadoes, hurricanes, wildfires, and earthquakes, can disrupt drinking water supplies and wastewater treatment. Hypochlorite is often used in such circumstances to purify drinking water, as mentioned earlier. It can also be used to remediate mold damage found in homes that have been flooded or have

damaged plumbing systems. During outbreaks of serious contagious illnesses, hypochlorite is often recommended to disinfect surfaces to prevent infections. It has aided efforts to control Ebola virus,[198,199] *Clostridium difficile*,[200,201] severe acute respiratory syndrome,[202] swine[203] (H1N1) and avian[204] flu outbreaks, methicillin-resistant *S aureus*,[205,206] norovirus,[207] and West Nile virus outbreaks.[208] Hypochlorite was used in disinfecting public spaces after a hepatitis A outbreak in San Diego, California.[209]

In September 2001, letters containing anthrax spores were mailed to two US senators and several media outlets in New York and Florida. As a result, five deaths and 17 additional hospitalizations with anthrax infections occurred.[210] Use of the mail to send the spores resulted in contamination of many buildings in which letters were processed. Ryan et al[211] present a comprehensive discussion of the approach and solutions used in the decontamination from this attack, which includes the use of a combination of hypochlorite disinfection and chlorine dioxide gas fumigation as effective and efficient treatments for spaces with complex surfaces.

◗ SURFACE COMPATIBILITY

Chlorine-based disinfectants are powerful oxidants. Because of this, certain surfaces may be oxidized on contact with these materials, particularly metals prone to oxidative corrosion and plastics with susceptible functional groups (particularly amides, unsubstituted amines, unsaturated hydrocarbons, and hydroxyl groups); damage may result. If in doubt about compatibility, the disinfectant can be patch tested on materials for the intended contact time. Lower concentrations and contact times can help to mitigate damage as well as thorough rinsing after disinfection. Resistant coatings can also help reduce damage to surfaces. Reducing agents, such as sodium thiosulfate, can also be used to neutralize oxidant disinfectants as a second step.[212] Ceramic, glass, and silica-based materials; titanium; baked-on enameled surfaces; and corrosion-resistant metals have good compatibility with chlorine-based materials. Tuthill et al[213] reviewed compatibility of various materials for chlorinated water. Plastics International has published a chart demonstrating the effect of exposure to chlorine and 15% hypochlorite to various plastic materials.[214] As mentioned earlier, chlorine dioxide has been used successfully as a chemical sterilant on surfaces that cannot tolerate heat or pressure extremes.

◗ RECENT INNOVATIONS

Electrolytic Cells

Chlorine gas is increasingly difficult to ship, particularly through populated areas, due to its inherent hazards. Thus, many patents have been granted globally for electrolytic cells that generate chlorine or hypochlorite at the point of use. The input is salt water; depending on the pH at the anode, the resulting product can be chlorine gas (pH below 5) or hypochlorous acid solution for disinfection (pH 5-7). At the cathode, the alkaline pH conditions yield a hypochlorite solution that can also be used for cleaning.

New devices for generating on-site sodium hypochlorite and hypochlorous acid are becoming more prevalent. These devices can do electrolysis of saline solutions on-site and the general term for the disinfecting or antiseptic solution is super-oxidized or electrolyzed water. Often, the main product of these devices is hypochlorous acid at a concentration of about 100 to 200 ppm at a pH of 5 to 6.5; however, the final concentration and pH is often dependent on the starting saline solution and any buffers or caustic that may be added to the starting solution and can occur in a wide range depending on the device manufacturer. Efficacy of the final solution will be strongly affected by the concentration of hypochlorous acid/sodium hypochlorite and the pH. Interestingly, there are products on market that range from 70 to 200 ppm bleach at pH 7 including Clorox® Anywhere®, CleanSmart™, and Puracyn®.[215] In some cases, the end result from the cell is the hypochlorous acid disinfecting solution[216-218]; in others, the electrolytic cell is part of another device that provides antimicrobial activity during the processing of the device, for example, a washing machine,[219,220] a bidet,[221] or an air disinfector.[222] The resulting hypochlorous acid solution has been studied for wound healing[223,224] as well as for surface disinfection.[225-227] The hypochlorous acid concentration in such solutions is typically 144 ppm, with some chlorine radicals present[228]; in general, the solutions have low toxicity and irritation potential to biological tissue and are less aggressive to sensitive surfaces. Regulatory approval has been granted to date for these materials to be used as disinfectants, as food-contact sanitizers, and for sanitizing food.[229-231]

Tissue Culture

The patent literature cites the use of hypochlorite as a key purification step for tissue culture for a wide variety of plant species, where maintaining purity of the cell culture is crucial for success. Weissman and Radaelli[232] sought to maintain dominance of *Nannochloropsis* in an algae cultivation system. Others used hypochlorite to decontaminate cuttings from mint plants with internodal segments prior to the culture process.[233]

Antimicrobial Surfaces

Technologies have been developed to coat a surface with a durable polymerized hydantoin coating. Upon exposure to hypochlorite, the resulting chlorohydantoin is antimicrobially active. Worley et al[234,235] developed a technology wherein a hydantoin is reacted with a silane to create a durable coating; this technology has been leveraged in medical scrubs, bedding, undergarments, and towels. Others covalently attached monomethylolhydantoin to a film made of castor oil and toluene diisocyanate.[236]

Other Processes Using Chlorine-Based Antimicrobials

Hypochlorite has been leveraged in recovery of polyhydroxyalkanoates from biological systems.[237,238] This biopolymer shows promise in replacing nonbiodegradable synthetic polymers. Hypochlorite, chlorine, and chlorine dioxide have been leveraged in enhanced oil recovery operations to kill bacteria that foul cooling water systems or form hydrogen sulfide; control of these bacteria means less corrosion and more efficient operations.[239-241]

▶ REGULATORY ASPECTS

United States Regulations

For the most part, disinfectant products are regulated as pesticides in the United States. The EPA oversees pesticide regulation under the Federal Insecticide, Fungicide, and Rodenticide Act (FIFRA). The FIFRA, as amended by the Food Quality Protection Act of 1996 and managed through the Office of Pesticide Programs, mandates the continuous review of existing pesticides. All pesticides distributed or sold in the United States generally must be registered by the EPA based on scientific data showing that they will not cause unreasonable risks to human health or to the environment when used as directed on product labeling. The agency reviews each registered pesticide every 15 years to determine whether it continues to meet the FIFRA standard for registration. The first such cycle that ended in 2008 was called the Reregistration Eligibility Decision (RED). The second 15-year cycle, called Registration Review, began in 2007 and will end in 2022. Each active ingredient will receive a final risk determination decision that allows the active to continue to be used as amended by the decision. The actions by EPA are recorded in individual dockets.[242] The registration review process consists of 5 stages[243]: (1) Open Docket (work plan review), (2) Data Call-In (DCI), (3) Preliminary Risk Assessment, (4) Final Risk Assessment and Proposed Decision, and (5) Final Decision. Public comment opportunities are available for stages 1, 2, and 4 in the process. The following is a short summary of the status of each active ingredient class for chlorine and chlorine-based disinfectants.

Chlorine Gas/Liquid

The registered uses of chlorine gas and aqueous chlorine includes disinfection of municipal drinking water. The EPA's

Office of Water has conducted a risk assessment for the use of chlorine in disinfection of municipal drinking water as well as disinfection by products resulting from the use of chlorine in municipal drinking water disinfection (Stage 1 Disinfectants and Disinfection Byproducts Rule [DBPR]: 63 FR 69390 -69476, December 16, 1998, Vol. 63, No. 241). Because of this assessment, a maximum residual disinfectant level of 4 mg/L for chlorine in municipal drinking water was determined as a safe level for human exposure (https://www.epa.gov/ground-water-and-drinking-water/national-primary-drinking-water-regulations#Disinfectants). Maximum contaminant levels of disinfection by-products were also established because of this assessment. Because the other registered uses of chlorine gas/aqueous chlorine are not likely to result in contamination of surface or groundwater and because the EPA's Office of Water has already assessed the drinking water use, the Office of Pesticide Programs does not anticipate conducting a drinking water assessment for chlorine gas/aqueous chlorine.

Chlorine Dioxide

The EPA first registered the aqueous form of chlorine dioxide for use as a disinfectant and a sanitizer in 1967. In 1988, EPA also registered chlorine dioxide gas as a sterilant. In 2013, EPA registered chlorine dioxide for use in potato storage facilities to fumigate against nonpathogenic spoilage organisms on potatoes. The recently added potato use will be reassessed, and the work plan revised, if necessary, as part of registration review.

Sodium Hypochlorite and Calcium Hypochlorite

Sodium hypochlorite and calcium hypochlorite were first registered in the United States in 1957. An RED was issued by the agency for sodium hypochlorite and calcium hypochlorite in 1992. There are no outstanding DCI requirements for these active ingredients. Products containing calcium hypochlorite and/or sodium hypochlorite are often referred to as bleach solutions. Sodium hypochlorite is a liquid chlorine product, whereas calcium hypochlorite is a solid. There are currently at least 457 EPA-registered sodium hypochlorite products. Registered uses for sodium hypochlorite include disinfectant, sanitizer, fungicide, and microbicide. Calcium hypochlorite currently has 129 EPA-registered products, with registered uses as a disinfectant, sanitizer, bactericide, algaecide, microbicide, fungicide, and viricide.

The most recent human health risk assessments for sodium hypochlorite and calcium hypochlorite were completed, in support of the 1992 RED. The RED determined that the products containing these active ingredients were eligible for reregistration, except the uses on sugar syrup and raw sugar (the processed commodity). In the Final Work Plan for the registration review of sodium hypochlorite and calcium hypochlorite, the agency decided

that additional data or updated risk assessments would not be necessary. The EPA believes that risks to human health from the use of sodium hypochlorite, calcium hypochlorite, and potassium hypochlorite are expected to be minimal when products are used according to directions for use and other labeling on product labels.

Chlorinated Isocyanurates

The chlorinated isocyanurates were first registered in the United States in 1958 for use as disinfectants, sanitizers, algicides, and fungicides. Sodium dichloro-s-triazinetrione was first registered in the United States in 1968; trichloro-s-triazinetrione was first registered in the United States in 1959; and sodium dichloroisocyanurate dihydrate was initially registered as a sanitizer in the United States on March 17, 1964. The agency completed an RED in 1992, which included a reregistration decision on all current uses except the material preservative uses, and all the existing uses at that time were found to be eligible for registration. The post-RED DCI was issued in May 1993.

Halohydantoins

The first pesticide product containing a halohydantoin was registered in October 1961. The registration review includes the four dihalodialkylhydantoins (PC Codes 006315, 006317, 028501, and 128826), which were evaluated in the 2007 RED for halodydantoins but also includes two dihalodialkylhydantoins (PC Codes 006322 and 128989) and a monohalodialkylhydantoin (PC Code 028500) that were registered after November 1, 1984. The agency combined several other halohydantoins into a single review. The sulfonylurea compounds mentioned in the last edition of this work (chloramine-T, chloramine-B, and halazone). Chloramine-T and chloramine-B remain active substances in the European Union.

European Union Regulations

In the European Union disinfectants are regulated as biocides under the Biocidal Product Regulation and are managed under the European Chemical Authority.[243] Biocides are divided into main groups and further delineated by product types. The main group disinfectants is broken down into five product types, shown in Table 15.4. Active substances are reviewed for each product type separately.[244,245]

▶ ACKNOWLEDGMENTS

The authors acknowledge the excellent foundational work of G. R. Dychdala (deceased), the author of "Chlorine and Chlorine Compounds" in past editions of *Block's Disinfection, Sterilization, and Preservation*. We also express our appreciation to The Clorox Company for supporting this work.

TABLE 15.4 Product types and usage approval status for main group 1: disinfectants, under the European Union Biocides Product Regulation relevant to chlorine and chlorine-based compounds

Number	Product Type	Usage and Approved/Evaluation Compounds
PT1	Human hygiene	For human hygiene purposes, applied on skin or scalp to disinfect skin or scalp Approved: sodium hypochlorite
PT2	Disinfectants and algaecides not intended for direct application to humans or animals	For disinfection of surfaces, materials, equipment, and furniture, which do not directly contact food or feeding stuffs For disinfection of air and water not used for human or animal consumption, chemical toilets, wastewater, hospital waste, and soil For algaecides for treatment of swimming pools, aquariums, and other waters and for remedial treatment of construction materials To be incorporated in textiles, tissues, masks, paints, and other articles or materials with the purpose of producing treated articles with disinfectant properties Approved: chlorine, chlorine dioxide, sodium hypochlorite, calcium hypochlorite Under evaluation: chlorinated isocyanurates, halohydantoins, chloramine-B and chloramine-T
PT3	Veterinary hygiene	For veterinary hygiene purposes such as disinfectants, disinfecting soaps, oral or corporal hygiene products, or with anti-microbial function To disinfect materials and surfaces associated with the housing or transportation of animals Approved: chlorine dioxide, sodium hypochlorite, calcium hypochlorite Under evaluation: chlorinated isocyanurates, chloramine-B and chloramine-T
PT4	Food and feed area	For the disinfection of equipment, containers, consumption utensils, surfaces, or pipework associated with the production, transport, storage, or consumption of food or feed (including drinking water) for humans and animals To impregnate materials that may come in contact with food Approved: chlorine dioxide, sodium hypochlorite, calcium hypochlorite Under evaluation: chlorinated isocyanurates, chloramine-B and chloramine-T
PT5	Drinking water	For the disinfection of drinking water for both humans and animals Approved: chlorine, chlorine dioxide, sodium hypochlorite, calcium hypochlorite Under evaluation: chlorinated isocyanurates, chloramine-B and chloramine-T
PT11	Preservatives for liquid cooling and processing systems	For the preservation of water or other liquids used in cooling and processing systems by the control of harmful organisms such as microbes, algae, and mussels; does not include products used for the disinfection of drinking water or of water for swimming pools Under evaluation: sodium hypochlorite, calcium hypochlorite, chlorinated isocyanurates, halohydantoins
PT12	Slimicides	For the prevention or control of slime growth on materials, equipment, and structures, used in industrial processes, for example, on wood and paper pulp, porous sand strata in oil extraction Under evaluation: sodium hypochlorite, chlorinated isocyanurates, halohydantoins

REFERENCES

1. Mellor JW. *A Comprehensive Treatise on Inorganic and Theoretical Chemistry*. New York, NY: Longmans Green; 1927:20.
2. Sconce JS. *Chlorine: Its Manufacture, Properties and Uses*. New York, NY: Huntington; 1962.
3. Hadfield WA. Chlorine and chlorine compounds. In: Reddish GF, ed. *Antiseptics, Disinfectants, Fungicides, Chemical and Physical Sterilization*. 2nd ed. Philadelphia, PA: Lea & Febiger; 1957:558-580.
4. Race J. *Chlorination of Water*. New York, NY: John Wiley & Sons; 1918:1-132.
5. Baker MN. *The Quest for Pure Water*. New York, NY; American Water Works Association; 1930.
6. Leal JL, Fuller GW, Johnson GA. *The Sterilization Plant of the Jersey City Water Supply Company at Boonton, NJ*. Milwaukee, WI: American Water Works Association; 1909:100-109.
7. Houston AC. *Studies in Water Supply*. London, United Kingdom; Macmillan & Co; 1913.
8. White CG. *The Handbook of Chlorination and Alternative Disinfectants*. 3rd ed. New York, NY: Van Nostrand Reinhold; 1992.
9. Horwood MP. *An Evaluation of the Factors Responsible for Public Health Progress in Boston*. Science. 1939;89:517-526.
10. Dakin HD. The antiseptic action of hypochlorites. *Br Med J*. 1915;2:809-810.
11. Taylor HD, Austin JH. The solvent action of antiseptics on necrotic tissue. *J Exp Med*. 1918;27:155-164.

12. Austin JH, Taylor HD. Behavior of hypochlorite and of chloramine-T solutions in contact with necrotic and normal tissues in vivo. *J Exp Med*. 1918;27:627-633.

13. Taylor HD, Austin JH. Toxicity of certain widely used antiseptics. *J Exp Med*. 1918;27:635-646.

14. Cullen GE, Taylor HD. Relative irritant properties of the chlorine group of antiseptics. *J Exp Med*. 1918;28:681-699.

15. The Chlorine Institute. Chlorine manufacture. The Chlorine Institute Web site. https://www.chlorineinstitute.org/stewardship/chlorine/chlorine-manufacture. Accessed October 15, 2017.

16. The Essential Chemical Industry. Chlorine. The Essential Chemical Industry Web site. http://www.essentialchemicalindustry.org/chemicals/chlorine.html. Accessed October 15, 2017.

17. Biography of Berthollet. *Sci Am*. 1853;8(26):202.

18. Lesser MA. Hypochlorites as sanitizers. *Soap Sanitary Chem*. 1949;25:119-125, 139.

19. Dychdala GR, inventor; Coastal Industries Inc, assignee. Calcium hypochlorite product and process for producing same. US patent 3,544,267. December 1, 1970.

20. Bull RJ. Health effects of alternative disinfectants and their reaction products. *J Am Water Works Assoc*. 1980;72:299-303.

21. The National Institute of Occupational Safety and Health. Chlorine. Centers for Disease Control and Prevention Web site. https://www.cdc.gov/niosh/npg/npgd0115.html. Accessed December 30, 2017.

22. The National Institute of Occupational Safety and Health. Chlorine dioxide. Centers for Disease Control and Prevention Web site. https://www.cdc.gov/niosh/npg/npgd0116.html. Accessed December 30, 2017.

23. Ingols RS, Ridenour GM. Chemical properties of chlorine dioxide in water treatment. *J Am Water Works Assoc*. 1948;40:1207-1227.

24. Ridenour GM, Ingols RS. Bactericidal properties of chlorine dioxide. *Water Sew Work*. 1947;39:561-567.

25. Ridenour GM, Armbruster EH. Bacterial effect of chlorine dioxide. *Water Sew Work*. 1949;41:537-550.

26. Ridenour GM, Ingots RS, Armbruster EH. Sporicidal properties of chlorine dioxide. *Water Sew Works*. 1949;96:279-283.

27. Harakeh MS, Berg JD, Hoff JC, et al. Susceptibility of chemostat-grown *Yersinia enterocolitica* and *Klebsiella pneumoniae* to chlorine dioxide. *Appl Environ Microbiol*. 1985;49:69-72.

28. Berman D, Hoff JC. Inactivation of simian rotavirus SA11 by chlorine, chlorine dioxide, and monochloramine. *Appl Environ Microbiol*. 1984;48:317-323.

29. Finch GR, Gyusek LL, Belosevic M. *The Effect of Chlorine on Waterborne* Cryptosporidium parvum. Edmonton, Canada: Department of Civil and Environmental Engineering, University of Alberta; 1996.

30. Alliger H, inventor. Germ killing composition and method. US patent 4,084,747. April 18, 1978.

31. de Guevara ML, inventor; van Buren C, Pearlman, Baldridge, Lyons, Browning, assignees. Aqueous chlorine dioxide antiseptic compositions and production thereof. US patent 2,701,781. February 8, 1955.

32. International Dioxcide, Inc. *Technical Properties of Anthium Dioxcide, a Chlorine Dioxide Complex. Bulletin 50*. Clark, NJ: International Dioxcide, Inc; 1966.

33. Masschelein WJ. *Chlorine Dioxide: Chemistry and Environmental Impact of Oxychlorine Compounds*. Ann Arbor, MI: Science Publishers; 1979.

34. Chlorine dioxide gains favor as effective sanitizer. *Food Eng*. 1977;49:143.

35. Olin Corporation. *Chlorine Dioxide: The Dioxolin Process and Food Processing. A Technical Bulletin from Olin Corporation*. Stanford, CT: Olin Corp; 1978.

36. Baker RJ. Types and significance of chlorine residuals. *J Am Water Works Assoc*. 1959;51:1185-1190.

37. Sheltmire WH. Chlorinated bleaches and sanitizing agents. In: Sconce JS, ed. *Chlorine: Its Manufacture, Properties and Uses*. New York, NY: Rheinhold; 1962:512-542.

38. Wattie E, Butterfield CT. Relative resistance of *Escherichia coli* and *Eberthella typhosa* to chlorine and chloramines. *Public Health Rep*. 1944;59:1661-1671.

39. Norman TS, Harms LL, Looyenga RW. The use of chloramines to prevent trihalomethane formation. *J Am Water Works Assoc*. 1980;72:176-180.

40. Kereluk K, Borisenok WS. The antimicrobial activity of monochloramine. *Dev Ind Microbiol*. 1983;24:24-31.

41. Weidenkopf SJ. Water chlorination. *U S Armed Forces Med J*. 1953;4:253-261.

42. Butterfield CT. Bactericidal properties of free and combined available chlorine. *J Am Water Works Assoc*. 1948;40:1305-1312.

43. White GC. *Handbook of Chlorination and Alternative Disinfectants*, 4th ed. New York, NY: John Wiley & Sons; 1999.

44. Griffin AE. Chlorination: a five-year review. *J N Eng Water Works Assoc*. 1944;58:322-332.

45. American Public Health Association. *Standard Methods for the Examination of Water and Wastewater*. 17th ed. Washington, DC: American Public Health Association; 1989.

46. Palin AT. Methods for the determination in water of free and combined available chlorine, chlorine dioxide, and chlorite, bromine, iodine, and ozone, using diethyl-*p*-phenylene diamine (DPD). *J Inst Water Eng*. 1967;21:537-547.

47. Chlorine bleach solutions. *Solvay Technical Engineering Service Bulletin*. 1957;14:6-7.

48. Dakin HD, Cohen JB. On chloramine antiseptics. *BMJ*. 1916;1:160-162.

49. Rideal EK, Evans UR. The effect of alkalinity on the use of hypochlorites. *J Soc Chem Ind*. 1921;40:64R-66R.

50. Johns CK. Germicidal power of sodium hypochlorite: effect of addition of alkali. *Ind Eng Chem*. 1934;26:787-788.

51. Charlton D, Levine M. *Germicidal Properties of Chlorine Compounds. Bulletin 132*. Ames, IA: Iowa Engineering Experiment Station; 1937.

52. Rudolph AS, Levine M. *Factors Affecting the Germicidal Efficiency of Hypochlorite Solutions. Bulletin 150* [dissertation]. Ames, IA: Iowa Engineering Experiment Station, Iowa State College; 1941.

53. Mercer WA, Somers II. Chlorine in food plant sanitation. *Adv Food Res*. 1957;7:129-160.

54. Friberg L, Hammarstrom E. The action of free available chlorine on bacteria and bacterial viruses. *Acta Pathol Microbiol Scand*. 1956;38:127-134.

55. Watkins SH, Hays H, Elliker PR. Virucidal activity of hypochlorites, quaternary ammonium compounds, and iodophors against bacteriophage of *Streptococcus cremoris*. *J Milk Food Tech*. 1957;20:84-87.

56. Chang SL. Destruction of micro-organisms. *J Am Water Works Assoc*. 1944;36:1192-1206.

57. Mallmann WL, Schalm O. *The Influence of the Hydroxyl Ion on the Germicidal Action of Chlorine in Dilute Solution. Bulletin 44*. Ann Arbor, MI: Michigan Engineering Experiments Station; 1932.

58. Weber GR, Levine M. Factors affecting germicidal efficiency of chlorine and chloramine. *Am J Public Health Nations Health*. 1944;34:719-728.

59. Costigan SM. Effectiveness of hot hypochlorites of low alkalinity in destroying *Mycobacterium tuberculosis*. *J Bacteriol*. 1936;32:57-63.

60. Collins EB. Factors involved in the control of gelatinous curd defects of cottage cheese: II. Influence of pH and temperature upon the bactericidal efficiency of chlorine. *J Milk Food Tech*. 1955;18:189-191.

61. Butterfield CT, Wattie E, Megregian S, et al. Influence of pH and temperature on the survival of coliforms and enteric pathogens when exposed to free chlorine. *Public Health Rep*. 1943;58:1837-1866.

62. Guiteras AF, Schmelkes FC. The comparative action of sodium hypochlorite, chloramine-T, and azochloramid on organic substrates. *J Biol Chem*. 1934;107:235-239.

63. Prucha MJ. Chemical sterilization in the dairy industry. *Proc Int Assoc Dairy Milk Inspectors*. 1927;16:319-328.

64. Loveless WG. *The Use of Chlorine Products as Germicides on Dairy Farms. Bulletin 369*. Burlington, VT: Free Press Printing, Vermont Agricultural Experimental Station; 1934.

65. Mudge CS, Smith FR. Relation of action of chlorine to bacterial death. *Am J Public Health Nations Health*. 1935;25:442-447.

66. Tilley FW, Chapin RM. Germicidal efficiency of chlorine and the *N*-chloro derivatives of ammonia, methylamine and glycine against anthrax spores. *J Bacteriol*. 1930;19:295-302.

67. McCulloch EC. *Disinfection and Sterilization*. 2nd ed. Philadelphia, PA: Lea & Febiger; 1945.

68. Johns CK. Influence of organic matter on the germicidal efficiency of quaternary ammonium and hypochlorite compounds. *Can J Res.* 1948;26(Sect F 2):91-104.

69. Lasmanis J, Spencer GR. The action of hypochlorite and other disinfectants on micrococci with and without milk. *Am J Vet Res.* 1953;14:514-516.

70. Shere L. Some comparisons of the disinfecting properties of hypochlorites and quaternary ammonium compounds. *Milk Plant Monthly.* 1948;37:66-69.

71. Geiger KH, Moloney PJ. Enhanced effectiveness of chlorination. *Can J Public Health.* 1952; 43:359-367.

72. Houghton GU. Bromide content of underground waters: II. Chlorination of water containing free ammonia and naturally occurring bromide. *J Soc Chem Ind.* 1946;65:304-328.

73. Kristoffersen T, Gould IA. Effect of sodium bromide on the bactericidal effectiveness of hypochlorite sanitizers of high alkalinity. *J Dairy Science.* 1958;41:950-955.

74. Farkas-Himsley H. Killing of chlorine-resistant bacteria by chlorine-bromine solutions. *Appl Microbiol.* 1964;12:1-6.

75. Kamlet J, inventor. Microbiocidal treatment of water with bromine chloride. US patent 2,662,855. December 15, 1953.

76. Darragh JL, House R, inventors; California Research LLC, assignee. Addition products of halogen and quaternary ammonium germicides and method for making the same. US patent 2,679,533. May 25, 1954.

77. Paterson LO, inventor. Process of disinfecting water. US patent 3,147,219. September 1, 1964.

78. Zsoldos FP Jr, inventor. Procedure for water treatment. US patent 3,161,588. December 15, 1964.

79. Palmer CM, Maloney TE. Preliminary screening for potential algicides. *Ohio J Sci.* 1955;55:1-8.

80. Hays H, Elliker PR, Sandine WE. Effect of acidification on stability and bactericidal activity of added chlorine in water supplies. *J Milk Food Tech.* 1963;26:147-149.

81. Brazis AR, Leslie JE, Kabler PW, et al. The inactivation of spores of *Bacillus globigii* and *Bacillus anthracis* by free available chlorine. *Appl Microbiol.* 1958;6:338-342.

82. Brazis AR, Bryant AR, Leslie JE, et al. Effectiveness of halogens or halogen compounds in detoxifying *Clostridium botulinum* toxins. *J Am Water Works Assoc.* 1959;51:902-912.

83. Lopes JA. Evaluation of dairy and food plant sanitizers against *Salmonella typhimurium* and Listeria monocytogenes. *J Dairy Sci.* 1986;69:2791-2796.

84. El-Kest SE, Marth EH. Inactivation of *Listeria monocytogenes* by chlorine. *J Food Prot.* 1988;51:520-524.

85. Dychdala GR. *Studies on Bactericidal Effectiveness of Calcium Hypochlorite Stabilizers for Swimming Pool Use.* Philadelphia, PA: Pennwalt Corp; 1960.

86. Bolton KJ, Dodd CER, Mead GC, et al. Chlorine resistance of strains of *Staphylococcus aureus* isolated from poultry processing plants. *Appl Microbiol.* 1988;6:31-34.

87. Stuart LS, Ortenzio LF. Swimming pool chlorine stabilizers. *Soap Chem Spec.* 1964;40:79-82,112-113.

88. Snow WB. Recommended chlorine residuals for military water supplies. *J Am Water Works Assoc.* 1956;48:1510-1514.

89. Orth R, Mrozek H. Is the control of *Listeria*, *Campylobacter* and *Yersinia* a disinfection problem? *Fleischwirtschaft.* 1989;69:1575-1576.

90. Hays H, Elliker PR. Virucidal activity of a new phosphoric acid-wetting agent sanitizer against bacteriophage of *Streptococcus cremoris.* *J Milk Food Tech.* 1959;22:109-111.

91. Davis HW. Discussion. *Trans Am Fisheries Soc.* 1934;64:1-280.

92. Kaplan HM. Toxicity of chlorine for frogs. *Proc Anim Care Panel.* 1962;12:259-262.

93. Dychdala GR. *Evaluation of Yeasts and Molds Against Different Fungicides.* Philadelphia, PA: Pennwalt Corp; 1961.

94. Costigan SM. *Germicidal Test of B-K Using* Aspergillus niger *as the Test Organism.* Philadelphia, PA: Pennwalt Corp; 1931.

95. Costigan SM. Fungicidal studies of some products commonly used in foot baths. Paper presented at: 59th Annual Convention of the Proprietary Association of America; May 12, 1941; New York, NY.

96. Chang SL, Berg G, Clarke NA, et al. Survival and protection against chlorination of human enteric pathogens in free-living nematodes isolated from water supplies. *Am J Trop Med Hyg.* 1960;9:136-142.

97. Zimmerman PW, Berg RO. Effects of chlorinated water on land plants, aquatic plants, and goldfish. *Contrib Boyce Thompson Inst.* 1934;6:39-49.

98. Clarke NA, Kabler PW, Stevenson RE. The inactivity of purified type 3 adenovirus in water by chlorine. *Am J Hyg.* 1956;64:314-319.

99. Clarke NA, Chang SL. Enteric viruses in water. *J Am Water Works Assoc.* 1959;51:1299-1317.

100. Clarke NA, Kabler PW. The inactivation of purified Coxsackie virus in water by chlorine. *Am J Hyg.* 1954;59:119-127.

101. Grabow WOK, Gauss-Müller V, Prozensky OW, et al. Inactivation of hepatitis A virus and indicator organisms in water by free chlorine residuals. *Appl Environ Microbiol.* 1983;46:619-624.

102. Kelly S, Sanderson W. The effect of chlorine in water on enteric viruses. *Am J Public Health Nations Health.* 1958;48:1323-1334.

103. Miller RA, Britigan BE. Role of oxidants in microbial pathophysiology. *Clin Microbiol Rev.* 1997;10:1-18.

104. Aliev G, Smith MA, Seyidov D, et al. The role of oxidative stress in the pathophysiology of cerebrovascular lesions in Alzheimer's disease. *Brain Pathol.* 2002;12:21-35.

105. Roos D, Winterbourn CC. Immunology. Lethal weapons. *Science.* 2002;296:669-671.

106. Klebanoff SJ. Oxygen metabolites from phagocytes. In: Gallin JI, Snyderman R, eds. *Inflammation: Basic Principles and Clinical Correlates.* 3rd ed. Philadelphia, PA: Lippincott Williams & Wilkins; 1999:721-727.

107. Klebanoff SJ. A peroxidase-mediated antimicrobial system in leukocytes. *J Clin Invest.* 1967;46:1078.

108. Klebanoff SJ. Iodination of bacteria: a bactericidal mechanism. *J Exp Med.* 1967;126:1063-1078.

109. Klebanoff SJ. Myeloperoxidase-halide-hydrogen peroxide antibacterial system. *J Bacteriol.* 1968;95:2131-2138.

110. Klebanoff SJ, Luebke RG. The antilactobacillus system of saliva. Role of salivary peroxidase. *Proc Soc Exp Biol Med.* 1965;118:483-486.

111. Klebanoff SJ, Clem WH, Luebke RG. The peroxidase-thiocyanate-hydrogen peroxide antimicrobial system. *Biochim Biophys Acta.* 1966;117:63-72.

112. Klebanoff SJ. Reactive nitrogen intermediates and antimicrobial activity: role of nitrite. *Free Radic Biol Med.* 1993;14:351-360.

113. Gaut JP, Byun J, Tran HD, et al. Myeloperoxidase produces nitrating oxidants in vivo. *J Clin Invest.* 2002;109:1311-1319.

114. Klebanoff SJ. Myeloperoxidase: friend and foe. *J Leukoc Biol.* 2005;77(5):598-625.

115. Odajima T, Yamazaki I. Myeloperoxidase of the leukocyte of normal blood. I. Reaction of myeloperoxidase with hydrogen peroxide. *Biochim Biophys Acta.* 1970;206:71-77.

116. Winterbourn CC. Reconciling the chemistry and biology of reactive oxygen species. *Nat Chem Biol.* 2008;4(5):278-276.

117. Winterbourn CC, Metodiewa D. Reactivity of biologically important thiol compounds with superoxide and hydrogen peroxide. *Free Radic Biol Med.* 1999;27:322-328.

118. Pattison DI, Davies MJ. Absolute rate constants for the reaction of hypochlorous acid with protein side chains and peptide bonds. *Chem Res Toxicol.* 2001;14:1453-1464.

119. Peskin AV, Winterbourn CC. Histamine chloramine reactivity with thiol compounds, ascorbate, and methionine and with intracellular glutathione. *Free Radic Biol Med.* 2003;35:1252-1260.

120. Wood ZA, Poole LB, Karplus PA. Peroxiredoxin evolution and the regulation of hydrogen peroxide signaling. *Science.* 2003;300:650-653.

121. Albrich JM, Gilbaugh JH III, Callahan KB, et al. Effects of the putative neutrophil-generated toxin, hypochlorous acid, on membrane permeability and transport systems of *Escherichia coli.* *J Clin Invest.* 1986;78:177-184.

122. Rakita RM, Michel BR, Rosen H. Differential inactivation of *Escherichia coli* membrane dehydrogenases by a myeloperoxidase-mediated antimicrobial system. *Biochemistry*. 1990;29:1075-1080.

123. Barrette WC Jr, Albrich JM, Hurst JK. Hypochlorous acid-promoted loss of metabolic energy in *Escherichia coli*. *Infect Immun*. 1987;55:2518-2525.

124. Winter J, Ilbert M, Graf PC, et al. Bleach activates a redox-regulated chaperone by oxidative protein unfolding. *Cell*. 2008;135(4):691-701.

125. Wentworth AD, Jones LH, Wentworth P Jr, et al. Antibodies have the intrinsic capacity to destroy antigens. *Proc Natl Acad Sci U S A*. 2000;97:10930-10935.

126. Wentworth P Jr, Jones LH, Wentworth AD, et al. Antibody catalysis of the oxidation of water. *Science*. 2001;293:1806-1811.

127. Wentworth P Jr, McDunn JE, Wentworth AD, et al. Evidence for antibody-catalyzed ozone formation in bacterial killing and inflammation. *Science*. 2002;298:2195-2199.

128. Wentworth P Jr, Wentworth AD, Zhu X, et al. Evidence for the production of trioxygen species during antibody-catalyzed chemical modification of antigens. *Proc Natl Acad Sci U S A*. 2003;100: 1490-1493.

129. O'Brien TF, Bommeraju TV, Hine F. *Handbook of Chlor-Alkali Technology, Volume 1: Fundamentals*. New York, NY: Springer Science and Business Media; 2005.

130. Baldwin RT. History of the chlorine industry. *J Chem Ed*. 1927;4:313.

131. Laufer RJ, Geiger JH Jr, inventors; International Flavors & Fragrances, Inc, assignee. Perfumed aqueous hypochlorite composition and method for preparation of same US patent 3,876,551. April 8, 1975.

132. DeSimone RS, inventor; Polak's Frutal Works, Inc, assignee. Bleach compositions containing perfume oils. US patent 4,113,645. September 12, 1978.

133. Hartman WL, O'Brien DA, Taylor TH, inventors; Procter and Gamble Co, assignee. Hypochlorite bleach containing surfactant and organic antifoamant. US patent 4,552,680. November 12, 1985.

134. Otten JG, Kinnaird MG, Greenough RE, et al, inventors; BASF Corp, assignee. Sterically hindered polyether polyols as chlorine bleach stable surfactants. US patent 4,913,833. April 3, 1990.

135. Bertacchi G, Scialla S, inventors; Procter and Gamble Co, assignee. Liquid bleaching compositions packaged in spray-type dispenser and a process for pretreating fabrics therewith. European patent EP0776966. September 11, 2002.

136. Abel D, Gurge RM, Trumbore MW, inventors; Collegium Pharmaceutical, Inc, assignee. Stable aerosol topical foams comprising a hypochlorite salt. US patent application 2011/0052506. April 3, 2011.

137. van Buskirk G, Adair M, Salwasser M, et al, inventors; Clorox Co, assignee. Method and device for delivery and confinement of surface cleaning composition. US patent 7,144,177. December 5, 2006.

138. Katsigras G, Bains S, Cheng L, et al, inventors; Clorox Co, assignee. Disinfecting article and cleaning composition with extended stability. US patent 7,008,600. March 7, 2006.

139. Keast RR, inventor; FMC Corporation, assignee. Preparation of stable, free-flowing mixtures of alkali metal dichloroisocyanurates and sodium tripolyphosphate. US patent 3,354,090. November 21, 1967.

140. Shuttlewood VC, Taylor RK, inventors; Chlor-Chem Ltd, assignee. Water treatment. US patent 4,728,442. March 1, 1988.

141. Dave PR, Jambekar GU, inventors; Conopco Inc, assignee. Biocide composition. US patent 8,889,183. November 18, 2014.

142. Vicari R, Hann BF, inventors; Sekisui Specialty Chemicals America LLC, assignee. Polyvinyl alcohol films with improved resistance to oxidizing chemicals. US patent 8,728,593. May 20, 2014.

143. Verrall AP, Goodrich SD, inventors; Mono-Sol Corp, assignee. Halogen-resistant composition. US patent 7,803,872. September 28, 2010.

144. Mizayaki H, inventor; Kuraray Co Ltd, assignee. Water-soluble film. European patent EP0884352. September 5, 2001.

145. Procter & Gamble. Product safety & compliance, document search. Procter & Gamble Web site. http://www.pgsdscpsia.com /productsafety/search_results.php?searchtext=All%20Product%20 Ingredients&category=ingredients&submit=Search&submit=Search. Accessed December 21, 2017.

146. Rosen MJ, Zhu ZH. The stability of sodium hypochlorite in the presence of surfactants. *JAOCS*. 1992;69:667-671.

147. Dow Chemical Company. Answer ID 1441; Dow answer center. Dow Chemical Company Web site. https://www.epa.gov/ground-water -and-drinking-water/national-primary-drinking-water-regulations #Disinfectants. Accessed October 30, 2019.

148. Reckitt Benckiser. Brands ingredient information. Reckitt Benckiser Web site. http://rbnainfo.com/brands.php. Accessed December 21, 2017.

149. S. C. Johnson & Son, Inc. Our ingredients. S. C. Johnson & Son, Inc Web site. http://www.whatsinsidescjohnson.com/us/en/ingredients. Accessed December 21, 2017.

150. The Clorox Company. Ingredients inside. The Clorox Company Web site. https://www.thecloroxcompany.com/brands/what-were-made-of /ingredients-inside/. Accessed December 21, 2017.

151. Julémont M, Marchal M, inventors; Colgate-Palmolive Co, assignee. Automatic dishwasher detergent compositions with chlorine bleach having thixotropic properties. US patent 4,740,327. April 26, 1988.

152. Zmoda BJ, inventor; Colgate-Palmolive Co, assignee. Thickened liquid bleach compositions. British patent application GB1237199. June 30, 1971.

153. Bolsen KA, inventor; Steris Corp, assignee. Daily air removal test for sterilizers. US patent 5,942,193. August 24, 1999.

154. Ahmed FU, Shevande M, inventors; Colgate-Palmolive Co, assignee. Linear viscoelastic aqueous liquid automatic dishwasher detergent composition having improved chlorine stability US patent 5,225,096. July 6, 1993.

155. Julémont M. Applications of hypochlorite. In: Broze G, ed. *Handbook of Detergents: Properties*. New York, NY: CRC Press; 1999:631-638.

156. Rosen MJ, Kunjappu JT. *Surfactants and Interfacial Phenomena*. 4th ed. New York, NY: Wiley; 2012.

157. The Association for Postconsumer Plastic Recyclers. HDPE bottle application test (HDPE-A-01). The Association for Postconsumer Plastic Recyclers Web site. https://www.plasticsrecycling.org/images /pdf/design-guide/test-methods/HDPE_Bottle_Application_Test _HDPE-A-01.pdf. Accessed December 21, 2017.

158. Clifford T. *All This Fun and a Paycheck, Too?* Bloomington, IN: Author House; 2013.

159. US Environmental Protection Agency. Safe Drinking Water Act (SDWA). US Environmental Protection Agency Web site. https:// www.epa.gov/sdwa. Accessed December 21, 2017.

160. European Commission. Environment: drinking water. European Commission Web site. http://ec.europa.eu/environment/water/water -drink/index_en.html. Accessed December 21, 2017.

161. World Health Organization. Guidelines for drinking water quality, 4th edition, incorporating the 1st addendum. World Health Organization Web site. http://www.who.int/water_sanitation_health/publications /drinking-water-quality-guidelines-4-including-1st-addendum/en/. Accessed December 21, 2017.

162. US Environmental Protection Agency. Emergency disinfection of drinking water. US Environmental Protection Agency Web site. https://www.epa.gov/ground-water-and-drinking-water/emergency -disinfection-drinking-water. Accessed November 30, 2017.

163. Laubusch EJ. State practices in sewage disinfection. *Sewage Ind Wastes*. 1958;30:1233-1240.

164. Laubusch EJ. Chlorination of waste-water. *Water Sewage Works*. 1958; 105:12-18.

165. US Environmental Protection Agency. Wastewater technology fact sheet: dechlorination. US Environmental Protection Agency Web site. https://www3.epa.gov/npdes/pubs/dechlorination.pdf. Accessed December 21, 2017.

166. US Environmental Protection Agency. Product performance test guidelines: OCSPP 810.2400: disinfectants and sanitizers for use on fabrics and textiles—efficacy data recommendations. US Environmental Protection Agency Web site. https://www.regulations.gov/document? D=EPA-HQ-OPPT-2009-0150-0024. Accessed December 21, 2017.

167. Bockmühl D. Hygiene aspects in domestic laundry. *Hyg Med*. 2011; 36:280-286.

168. American Chemistry Council. Pool treatment 101: introduction to chlorine sanitizing. American Chemistry Council Web site. https://chlorine.americanchemistry.com/Chlorine/Pool-Treatment-101/. Accessed December 21, 2017.

169. Centers for Disease Control and Prevention. The Model Aquatic Health Code (MAHC): an all-inclusive model public swimming pool and spa code. Centers for Disease Control and Prevention Web site. https://www.cdc.gov/mahc/index.html. Accessed December 21, 2017.

170. Mohr A. The 5 largest food recalls in history. Investopedia Web site. https://www.investopedia.com/financial-edge/0512/the-5-largest-food-recalls-in-history.aspx. Accessed November 30, 2017.

171. Associated Press. Executive gets 28 years in prison for food-poisoning case. New York Post Web site. https://nypost.com/2015/09/21/executive-gets-28-years-in-prison-in-food-poisoning-case/. Accessed December 21, 2017.

172. US Government Publishing Office. Tolerance exemptions for active and inert ingredients for use in antimicrobial formulations (food-contact surface sanitizing solutions). 40 CFR §180.940. https://www.ecfr.gov/cgi-bin/text-idx?tpl=/ecfrbrowse/Title40/40cfr180_main_02.tpl. Accessed December 21, 2017.

173. US Department of Health and Human Services, US Public Health Service, and US Food and Drug Administration. Grade "A" Pasteurized Milk Ordinance. US Food and Drug Administration Web site. https://www.fda.gov/downloads/food/guidanceregulation/guidancedocumentsregulatoryinformation/milk/ucm513508.pdf. Accessed December 21, 2017.

174. US Food and Drug Administration. 2013 Food Code §4-501.114. US Food and Drug Administration Web site. https://www.fda.gov/downloads/Food/GuidanceRegulation/RetailFoodProtection/FoodCode/UCM374510.pdf. Accessed December 21, 2017.

175. US Food and Drug Administration. 2013 Food Code §4-703.11. US Food and Drug Administration Web site. https://www.fda.gov/downloads/Food/GuidanceRegulation/RetailFoodProtection/FoodCode/UCM374510.pdf. Accessed December 21, 2017.

176. Spray Chem Chemical Company. MultiChlor product information. Spray Chem Chemical Company Web site. http://www.spraychem.com/page/multichlor.php. Accessed December 21, 2017.

177. Severn Trent Services. Chlorination in food processing plants. Severn Trent Services Web site. http://www.es2inc.com/wp-content/uploads/2011/07/Chlorination-in-Food-Processing-Plants.pdf. Accessed December 21, 2017.

178. Curtis P, Butler J. Controlling Salmonella in poultry plants. For the FSIS "How To" workshops. US Department of Agriculture Web site. https://www.fsis.usda.gov/wps/wcm/connect/f2dac782-69af-4bba-8bf1-719592ff6ce7/how_to_salmonella.ppt?MOD=AJPERES. Accessed December 21, 2017.

179. US Food and Drug Administration. 2013 Food Code §3-202.16. US Food and Drug Administration Web site. https://www.fda.gov/downloads/Food/GuidanceRegulation/RetailFoodProtection/FoodCode/UCM374510.pdf. Accessed December 21, 2017.

180. Somers II. Studies on in-plant chlorination. *Food Technol*. 1951;5:46-51.

181. Scotmas Group. Agriculture: purified water for unbeaten performance. Scotmas Group Web site. http://www.scotmas.com/industries/agriculture.aspx. Accessed December 21, 2017.

182. Manitoba Agriculture. Use of chlorine in the food industry. Government of Manitoba Web site. https://www.gov.mb.ca/agriculture/food-safety/at-the-food-processor/use-of-chlorine.html. Accessed December 21, 2017.

183. Flemming HC, Meier M, Schild T. Mini-review: microbial problems in paper production. *Biofouling*. 2013;29(6):683-696.

184. Hladíková Z, Kejlová K, Sosnovcová J, et al. Microbial contamination of paper-based food contact materials with different contents of recycled fiber. *Czech J Food Sci*. 2015;33(4): 308-312.

185. Kavros S. The use of hypochlorous acid solution in wound management. Foundation for Alternative and Integrative Medicine Web site. http://www.faim.org/the-use-of-hypochlorous-acid-solution-in-wound-management. Accessed December 8, 2017.

186. Wang L, Bassiri M, Najafi R, et al. Hypochlorous acid as a potential wound care agent: part I. Stabilized hypochlorous acid: a component of the inorganic armamentarium of innate immunity. *J Burns Wounds*. 2007;6:e5.

187. Sam CH, Lu HK. The role of hypochlorous acid as one of the reactive oxygen species in periodontal disease. *J Dent Sci*. 2009;4(2):45-54.

188. Gottardi W. Residual effects on the skin after application of disinfectants containing active halogen. *Hyg Med*. 1988;13:157-161.

189. Nagl M, Gottardi W. In-vitro experiments on the bactericidal action of N-chloro taurine. *Hyg Med*. 1992;17:431-439.

190. Nagl M, Gottardi W. Enhancement of the bactericidal efficacy of N-chlorotaurine by inflammation samples and selected N-H compounds. *Hyg Med*. 1996;21:597-605.

191. General Medical Council. *British Pharmacopoeia 1958*. London, United Kingdom: The Pharmaceutical Press: 1958.

192. Liden BA. Pearls for practice: hypochlorous acid: its multiple uses for wound care. *Ostomy Wound Management*. 2013;59(9):1-6.

193. Krader CG. Hypochlorous acid lid cleanser provides novel advantages. Ophthalmology Times Web site. http://ophthalmologytimes.modernmedicine.com/ophthalmologytimes/content/tags/advanced-i-lid-cleanser/hypochlorous-acid-lid-cleanser-provides-nove?page=full. Accessed December 21, 2017.

194. Sonoma Pharmaceuticals, Inc. Sonoma Pharmaceuticals receives Brazilian approvals to market multiple hypochlorous acid based dermatology products. GlobeNewswire Web site. https://globenewswire.com/news-release/2017/10/31/1169511/0/en/Sonoma-Pharmaceuticals-Receives-Brazilian-Approvals-to-Market-Multiple-Hypochlorous-Acid-Based-Dermatology-Products.html. Accessed December 21, 2017.

195. Pelgrift RY, Friedman AJ. Topical hypochlorous acid (HOCl) as a potential treatment of pruritus. *Curr Dermatol Rep*. 2013;2:181-190.

196. Consolidated Sterilizer Systems. Chlorine dioxide gas sterilizer. Consolidated Sterilizer Systems Web site. https://consteril.com/products/sterilizers/chlorine-dioxide-gas-sterilizer/. Accessed December 21, 2017.

197. Rutala WA, Weber DJ. Uses of inorganic hypochlorite (bleach) in health-care facilities. *Clin Micro Rev*. 1997;10(4):597-610.

198. Cook BWM, Cutts TA, Nikiforuk AM, et al. The disinfection characteristics of Ebola virus outbreak variants. *Sci Rep*. 2016;6:38293.

199. Centers for Disease Control and Prevention. Rationale and considerations for chlorine use in infection control for non-U.S. general health-care settings. Centers for Disease Control and Prevention Web site. https://www.cdc.gov/vhf/ebola/hcp/international/chlorine-solutions.html. Accessed December 8, 2017.

200. MacLeod-Glover C, Sadowski C. Efficacy of cleaning products for *C. difficile*: environmental strategies to reduce the spread of *Clostridium difficile*-associated diarrhea in geriatric rehabilitation *Can Fam Physician*. 2010;56(5):417-423.

201. Balsells E, Filipescu T, Kyaw MH, et al., Infection prevention and control of Clostridium difficile: a global review of guidelines, strategies, and recommendations. *J Glob Health*. 2016;6(2):020410.

202. Lai MYY, Cheng PK, Lim WW. Survival of severe acute respiratory syndrome coronavirus. *Clin Infect Dis*. 2005;41(7):e67-e71.

203. Centers for Disease Control and Prevention. Interim biosafety guidance for all individuals handling clinical specimens or isolates containing 2009-H1N1 influenza A virus (novel H1N1), including vaccine strains. Centers for Disease Control and Prevention Web site. https://www.cdc.gov/h1n1flu/guidelines_labworkers.htm. Accessed December 21, 2017.

204. World Health Organization. Collecting, preserving and shipping specimens for the diagnosis of avian influenza A(H5N1) virus infection. Guide for field operations. World Health Organization Web site. http://www.who.int/csr/resources/publications/surveillance/WHO_CDS_EPR_ARO_2006_1/en/. Accessed December 21, 2017.

205. Fisher RG, Chain RL, Hair PS, et al., Hypochlorite killing of community-associated methicillin-resistant *Staphylococcus aureus*. *Pediatr Infect Dis J*. 2008;27(10):934-935.

206. Blazek N. Hypochlorite solutions may be useful in managing CA-MRSA. Healio Web site. https://www.healio.com/pediatrics /emerging-diseases/news/print/infectious-diseases-in-children /{b07d99b2-7f3e-4183-a948-a2e6c2276b6a}/hypochlorite-solutions -may-be-useful-in-managing-ca-mrsa. Accessed December 21, 2017.

207. Hall AJ, Vinjé J, Lopman B, et al. Updated norovirus outbreak management and disease prevention guidelines. Centers for Disease Control and Prevention Web site. https://www.cdc.gov/mmwr/preview /mmwrhtml/rr6003a1.htm. Accessed December 21, 2017.

208. Spickler AR. Technical factsheets: West Nile virus infection. The Center for Food Security & Public Health, Iowa State University Web site. http://www.cfsph.iastate.edu/DiseaseInfo/factsheets.php. Accessed December 21, 2017.

209. Warth G. Power-washing is a dirty job, but could help contain hepatitis A outbreak. The San Diego Union-Tribune. Web site. https:// www.sandiegouniontribune.com/news/hepatitis-crisis/sd-me -power-washing-20170928-story.html. Accessed December 21, 2017.

210. National Public Radio. Timeline: how the anthrax terror unfolded. National Public Radio Web site. https://www.npr.org/2011 /02/15/93170200/timeline-how-the-anthrax-terror-unfolded. Accessed December 21. 2017.

211. Ryan SP, Calfee MW, Wood JP, et al. Research to support the decontamination of surfaces and buildings contaminated with biothreat agents. In: Rutala WA, ed. *Disinfection, Sterilization and Antisepsis: Principles, Practices, Current Issues, New Research, and New Technologies.* Washington, DC: APIC; 2010:260-306.

212. Dorr RT, Alberts DS, inventors; Mayne Pharma USA Inc, assignee. Method and composition for deactivating HIV infected blood and for deactivating and decolorizing anticancer drugs. US patent 5,811,113. September 22, 1998.

213. Tuthill AH, Lamb S, Kobrin G, et al. Effect of chlorine on common materials in fresh water. Paper presented at: CORROSION 98; March 22-27, 1998; San Diego, CA.

214. Plastics International. Chemical resistance chart. Plastics International Web site. http://www.plasticsintl.com/plastics_chemical _resistence_chart.html. Accessed December 20, 2017.

215. Gottardi W, Debabov D, Nagl M. *N*-chloramines, a promising class of well-tolerated topical anti-infectives. *Antimicrob Agents Chemother.* 2013;57(3):1107-1114.

216. Gram HF, Muller ME, Pendergrass AM, et al, inventors; Miox Corp, assignee. Electrolytic method and cell for sterilizing water. US patent 4,761,208. August 2, 1988.

217. Gardner SP, inventor; Ozo Innovations Ltd, applicant. Electrolyzed water composition. US patent application 20,170,267,553. September 21, 2017.

218. Durham CJ, Morgan RA, Pawlak MC, inventors; Zurex Pharmagra, assignee. Systems and methods for generating germicidal compositions. US patent 8,771,753. July 8, 2014.

219. Mallouki M, Hamiti AE, Archambeaud E, inventors; Ceram Hyd, assignee. Electrolytic cell for producing at least one chemical substance and washing machine. WIPO application 2016162327. October 13, 2016.

220. Bhuta HJ, Bhatt NR, inventors; XH20 Solutions Private Ltd, assignee. System and a method for washing, cleaning, disinfecting and sanitizing laundry using electrolytic cell having boron-doped diamond electrode. US patent application 2013/0125316. May 23 2013.

221. Morotomi Y, Matsushita K, Matsumoto S, et al, inventors; Toto Ltd, assignee. Sanitary washing apparatus. US patent 9,328,497. May 3, 2016.

222. Yamamoto T, Nishino S, Shimizu K, et al, inventors; Sanyo Electric, assignee. Air filtering apparatus. Japanese patent 5340856. November 13, 2013.

223. Rossi-Fedele G, Figueiredo JA, Steier L, et al. Evaluation of the antimicrobial effect of super-oxidized water (Sterilox®) and sodium hypochlorite against *Enterococcus faecalis* in a bovine root canal model. *J Appl Oral Sci.* 2010;18(5):498-502.

224. Eftekharizadeh F, Dehnavieh R, Hekmat SN, et al. Health technology assessment on super oxidized water for treatment of chronic wounds. *Med J Islam Rep Iran.* 2016;30:384.

225. Gunaydin M, Esen S, Karadag A, et al. In vitro antimicrobial activity of Medilox® super-oxidized water. *Ann Clin Microbiol Antimicrob.* 2014;13:29.

226. Tanaka H, Hirakata Y, Kaku M, et al. Antimicrobial activity of super-oxidized water. *J Hosp Infect.* 1996;34:43-49.

227. Selkon JB, Babb JR, Morris R. Evaluation of the antimicrobial activity of a new super-oxidized water, Sterilox, for the disinfection of endoscopes. *J Hosp Infect.* 1999;41:59-70.

228. Rutala WA, Weber DC. New disinfection and sterilization methods. *Emerg Infect Dis.* 2001;7(2):348-353.

229. Centers for Disease Control and Prevention. Chemical disinfectants. Centers for Disease Control and Prevention Web site. https://www .cdc.gov/infectioncontrol/guidelines/disinfection/disinfection -methods/chemical.html. Accessed December 21, 2017.

230. US Department of Agriculture, Food Safety and Inspection Service. Safe and suitable ingredients used in the production of meat, poultry, and egg products. Food Safety and Inspection Service. https://www.fsis .usda.gov/wps/wcm/connect/bab10e09-aefa-483b-8be8-809a1f051d4c /7120.1.pdf?MOD=AJPERES. Accessed December 29, 2017.

231. US Government Publishing Office. Food and drugs: subchapter B— food for human consumption. Electronic Code of Federal Regulations Web site. https://www.ecfr.gov/cgi-bin/text-idx?SID=e297 b78c5cfba6b87538f7d6f5d5bec4&mc=true&tpl=/ecfrbrowse/Title21 /21CIsubchapB.tpl. Accessed December 29, 2017.

232. Weissman J, Radaelli G, inventors; Aurora Algae, Inc, assignee. Systems and methods for maintaining the dominance of *Nannochloropsis* in an algae cultivation system. US patent 8,940,340. January 27, 2015.

233. Kumar S, Gupta SK, Bhat S, et al, inventors; Council of Scientific and Industrial Research (CSIR), assignee. Tissue culture process for producing a large number of viable mint plants in vitro from internodal segments. US patent 5,898,001. April 27, 1999.

234. Worley SD, Eknoian MW, Li Y, inventors; Auburn University, assignee. Surface active N-Halamine compounds. US patent 6,469,177. October 22, 2002.

235. Worley SD, Liang J, Chen Y, et al, inventors; Auburn University Office of Technology Transfer, assignee. Biocidal N-halamine epoxides. US patent 8,821,907. September 2, 2014.

236. Bisquera W Jr, Sumera F. Regenerable antimicrobial polyurethane coating based on N-hydroxymethylated hydantoin. *Philippine J Sci.* 2011;140(2):207-219.

237. Heinrich D, Madkour MH, Al-Ghamdi MA, et al. Large scale extraction of poly(3-hydroxybutyrate) from Ralstonia eutropha H16 using sodium hypochlorite. *AMB Express.* 2012;2:59.

238. Sayyed RZ, Gangurde NS, Chincholkar SB. Hypochlorite digestion method for efficient recovery of PHB from Alcaligenes faecalis. *Indian J Microbiol.* 2009;49(3):230-232.

239. Miox Ltd. Oil and gas management: enhanced oil recovery. Miox Web site. http://www.miox.com/industries/oil-gas-water/enhanced-oil -recovery/. Accessed December 12, 2017.

240. Scotmas Group. Enhanced oil recovery. Scotmas Group Web site. https://www.scotmas.com/industries/oil-gas/enhanced-oil-recovery .aspx. Accessed December 21, 2017.

241. Electrolytic Technologies. Applications: oil and gas water treatment. Electrolytic Technologies Web site. https://electrolytictech.com/oil -and-gas-water-treatment/. Accessed December 21, 2017.

242. US Environmental Protection Agency. eRulemaking project management office, US EPA docket references. eRulemaking Program Web site. https://www.regulations.gov. Accessed December 27, 2017.

243. Kyprianou R. Registration and reregistration review programs and DCIS—status and response issues. Paper presented at: CSPA Antimicrobials Workshop; March 10-11, 2015; Arlington, VA.

244. European Chemicals Agency. Information on biocides; biocidal active substances. European Chemicals Agency Web site.https://echa .europa.eu/information-on-chemicals/biocidal-active-substances. Accessed December 27, 2017.

245. European Chemicals Agency. Product-types. European Chemicals AgencyWebsite.https://echa.europa.eu/regulations/biocidal-products -regulation/product-types. Accessed December 27, 2017.

Iodine and Iodine-Containing Compounds

Paul L. Bigliardi, Maren Eggers, Marc Cataldo, Ram Kapil, Manjunath Shet, and Michael K. Pugsley

Iodine, a nonmetallic, essential element discovered in 1812 by the French scientist Bernard Courtois, was named by Joseph Louis Gay-Lussac in 1814 after the Greek word meaning "violet," which is the color of iodine vapor. It is not found in elemental form in nature but occurs sparingly in the form of iodides primarily in seawater, other brackish waters, in sea deposits, in Chilean saltpeter, and nitrate-bearing earth. Besides the single stable isotope, which is iodine 127 (^{127}I), there are more than 30 artificial isotopes with half-lives that range between 0.2 second and 1.57×10^7 years. Some of these isotopes have resulted from the dangerous fallout following nuclear accidents or attacks, whereas others are used in nuclear medicine (mainly iodine 131 [^{131}I] [8.04 d] and iodine 123 [^{123}I] [13.2 h]).

The first use of iodine in medical practice was as a remedy for bronchocele (a segment of a bronchus that is closed because of congestion).[1] Soon afterward, Lugol[2] treated scrofuloderma (tuberculous lesions of the skin) with an iodine/iodide solution bearing his name that is still in use today (known as *strong iodine solution*).[3] Iodine was officially recognized by the *United States Pharmacopeia* in 1830, specifically as *tinctura iodini* (tincture of iodine). Clinicians and microbiologists described a great quantity of experimental data and numerous clinical applications, which can be found in numerous reviews.[4-10]

Despite the successes that have been achieved with iodine, it was ascertained early that it also possesses properties, such as unpleasant odor, staining the skin, or reactivity with iron and other metals, that could make it unsuitable for some practical applications.[11] Furthermore, iodine solutions are not stable (under certain circumstances); it is well known that they can irritate tissue and may be a poison at certain doses or concentrations. The adverse side effects associated with acute iodine toxicity include vomiting, diarrhea, metabolic acidosis, seizure, stupor, delirium, and collapse.[12] High levels of iodine are also linked to disruption of thyroid hormone metabolism, the thyroid-pituitary axis, and the compensatory

mechanisms that exist to protect such metabolism against low or high levels of iodine intake[12] and associated with pain when administered as an iodine-alcohol solution on open wounds. Additionally, some risk of allergic reactions in the past 100 years led to the development of many iodine-based preparations that were designed to reduce these unwanted side effects without a significant loss of antimicrobial efficiency. This problem can be approached by using the appropriate concentration for different applications and developing formulations allowing controlled and regular release of active iodine for optimal antimicrobial activity. The iodophors (eg, povidone-iodine) were the first such compounds largely to achieve this goal. More recently, graphene-iodine nanocomposites have been developed, which can inhibit bacterial growth and have been found to be potentially biocompatible with human cells with very low cytotoxic effects for human cell cultures, although they have not yet been proven effective in clinical practice.[13]

▶ CHEMISTRY

Iodine is the halogen with the highest atomic weight (126.9 amu) of the common halogens. It is the weakest oxidizing agent of the group unlike its iodide anion, I^-, which is the strongest reducing agent of the halogens and forms grayish-black metallic scales that melt at 113.5°C to a black, mobile liquid. Iodine boils at 184.4°C (at atmospheric pressure) to produce the characteristic violet-colored vapor. Despite the high boiling point, it has an appreciable vapor pressure at room temperature (22°C) and sublimes before it melts if it is not heated too fast and with too high degree of heat.

Elemental iodine is only slightly soluble in water (ie, 1 g dissolves in 3450 mL at 20°C), forming a brown solution. Its solubility in water is increased with the addition of alkali iodides by which triiodide and higher polyiodides are formed (see equations [3], [5], and [6] in the following text). In polar organic solvents (such as alcohols, ketones, carbonic acids), iodine forms a brown solution whose color is explained by the formation of an electrostatic attraction between iodine and the solvent molecule that provides a stabilizing force for the molecular complex. This complex is known as an electron-donor-acceptor complex or charge transfer complex. In nonpolar solvents (such as carbon tetrachloride [CCl_4], benzene, hydrocarbons), iodine dissolves to a violet color that is explained by the presence of iodine in the free state (I_2), as in the gas phase.

Properties of Disinfecting Iodine Solutions

Iodine-based disinfectants can be divided into three main groups according to the solvent and substances interfering (by complexing) with the iodine species: (1) pure aqueous solutions, (2) alcoholic solutions, and (3) iodophoric preparations or combinations of two or three components. Each of them exhibits intrinsic differences in their chemical, antimicrobial, and toxic/irritant properties.

A reliable understanding of the processes occurring at disinfection, which includes not only killing of microorganisms but also interactions with the material or host tissue (eg, innate surfaces, living tissue, body fluids), is essential based on knowledge of the microbial mixture and the environment, the formulation, and the elimination of the active ingredient over time.

Aqueous Solution

For the iodine-water system, nine different equilibria (equations [1] to [9]) are specified[14] that produce at least 10 iodine species: I^-, I_2, I_3^-, I_5^-, I_6^{2-}, HOI, OI^-, HI_2O^-, I_2O^{2-}, H_2OI^+, and IO_3^-.

$$I_2 + H_2O \leftrightarrow HOI = I^- + H^+ \text{ (hydrolysis, } K_1) \quad (1)$$

$$HOI \leftrightarrow OI^- + H^+ \text{ (dissociation of HOI, } K_2) \quad (2)$$

$$I_2 + I^- \leftrightarrow I_3^- \text{ (triiodide formation, } K_3) \quad (3)$$

$$HOI + H^+ \leftrightarrow H_2OI^+ \text{ (protonation of HOI, } K_4) \quad (4)$$

$$I_3^- + I_2 \leftrightarrow I_5^- \text{ (pentaiodide formation, } K_5) \quad (5)$$

$$2I_3^- \leftrightarrow I_6^{2-} \text{ (dimerization of } I_3-, K_6) \quad (6)$$

$$OI^- + I^- + H_2O \leftrightarrow HI_2O^- + OH^-$$
$$\text{(iodination of } OI^-, K_7) \quad (7)$$

$$HI_2O^- \leftrightarrow I_2O^- + H^+ \text{ (dissociation of } HI_2O^-, K_8) \quad (8)$$

$$3HOI \leftrightarrow IO_3^- + 2I^- + 3H^+ \text{ (disproportionation) } \quad (9)$$

As noted earlier, this is a system of appreciable complexity, with several associated equilibria governed mainly by H^+ and I^- ions, which implies that pH and additional iodide influence equilibrium concentrations. Another important feature is the reaction rate; whereas the reactions in equations (1) to (8) are thought to occur instantaneously, disproportionation to iodate (equation [9]) proceeds comparatively slowly, with a rate highly influenced by pH and additional iodide, as can easily be deduced from the rate law[15]:

$$d\,[IO_3^-]\,/\,dt \approx 4 \times 10^{-38}\,[I_2]^3\,/\,[I^-]^3\,[H^+]^4 \quad (10)$$

where [ ] means equilibrium concentration of the bracketed species.

Because the reactions in equations (1) to (9) are well studied, with focus on the fate of radioiodine species that emerge in the course of nuclear accidents,[14] a calculation may represent the easiest way to approach equilibrium concentrations. It is difficult to determine all iodine species experimentally because for some species, limited analytical methods are available.[16] In natural water samples, concentrations of I^- and IO_3^- have been recently determined with a two-column high-performance liquid chromatography system; I^- was detected with amperometry, and IO_3^- was detected with spectrophotometry.[17]

Several investigations into the equilibrium concentrations of aqueous iodine solutions conducted differ mainly regarding the equilibria considered and the regulating parameters, pH, and additional iodide. One study investigated all the immediately established equilibria (equations [1] to [8]) and both regulating parameters.[18] It dealt with fresh iodine solutions not altered by disproportionation (iodate formation) and provided results about the equilibrium concentrations of the species I^-, I_2, I_3^-, I_5^-, I_6^{2-}, HOI, OI^-, HI_2O^-, IO_2^-, and H_2OI^-. The results for selected variations of total iodine and iodide, Lugol solution and its dilutions, and the rates of iodate formation (Figures 16.1 to 16.4) are the basis for most of the following conclusions:

- Additional iodide and pH have a marked influence on the individual equilibrium concentrations, and consequently, conditions can be indicated in which the number of species of importance is substantially reduced. In the most common case, only I^-, I_2, and I_3^- play a role for iodine in the presence of additional iodide at pH 6 or less (Figure 16.2).
- In such a system, HOI and all species derived from it (OI^-, HI_2O^-, I_2O^{2-}, H_2OI^+) and the higher polyiodides can be neglected without any noticeable loss of precision. In other words, in this case, only the triiodide equilibrium (equation [3]) is relevant and it is not influenced by pH. This has two consequences: (1) the distribution of the three species is the same at pH 6 or less, and (2) a sufficiently precise evaluation

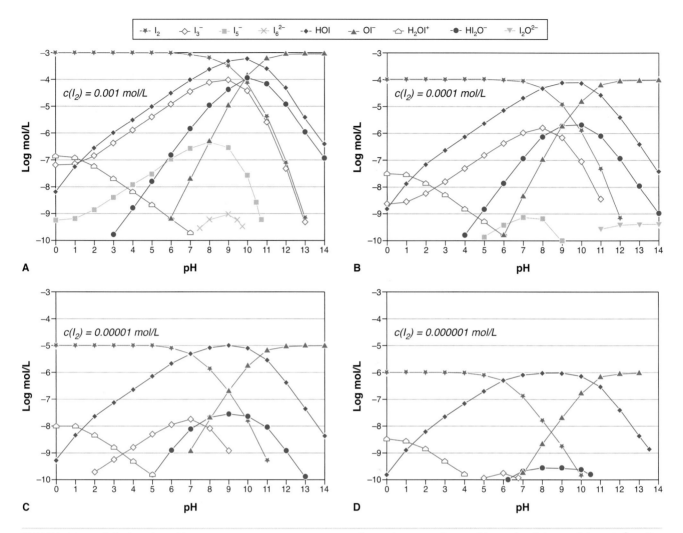

FIGURE 16.1 Calculated equilibrium concentrations in aqueous iodine solutions without additional iodide. A, $c[I_2] = 10^{-3}$ mol/L. B, $c[I_2] = 10^{-4}$ mol/L. C, $c[I_2] = 10^{-5}$ mol/L. D, $c[I_2] = 10^{-6}$ mol/L.

can be based solely on the determination of $[I_2]$ (eg, potentiometrically[19] or by dialysis[20]) and $[I^-]$ (iodide electrode), whereas triiodide is calculated from both; however, there are also methods that measure these species in a single operation.[16,21]

- Exceptions for the aforementioned quoted restriction to I^-, I_2, and I_3^- in presence of additional iodide are systems with very high iodide and iodine concentrations in which the equilibria in equations (5) and (6) are also important but are independent of pH as is the case with the equilibrium in equation (3). For example, in high-level Lugol solution, the species I_5^- and I_6^{2-} make up 8.2% of the oxidation capacity and should not be neglected (Figure 16.3A). On the other hand, in the absence of additional iodide, at pH 8 to 9 and at high dilution ($c[I_2] \leq 10^{-5}$ mol/L), HOI accounts for over 90% of the oxidation capacity (Figure 16.1C). Absence of iodide is also obligatory for the presence of the iodine cation H_2OI^+,[22] but because this is associated

with an extremely acid milieu, this has little relevance in practice.

- The problem of stability (ie, the rate of iodate formation) arising at pH above 7 can be reduced to the equilibrium concentration of HOI, which manifests in the simple rate law:

$$d[IO_3^-] / dt = 0.25 [HOI]^3 / [H^+]$$

which allows for an estimate of stability at weak alkaline conditions.[18] Figure 16.4 shows the initial rates of iodate formation (as a measure of stability) for iodine solutions (10^{-6} to 10^{-3} mol/L) without additional iodide and for a 0.001 mol/L iodine solution in the presence of additional iodide (10^{-4} to 10^{-1} mol/L).

The poor solubility of elemental iodine in water (338.3 ppm, 25°C, pH 5) can be increased by the addition of iodide, as first demonstrated by Lugol.[2] Lugol solution is

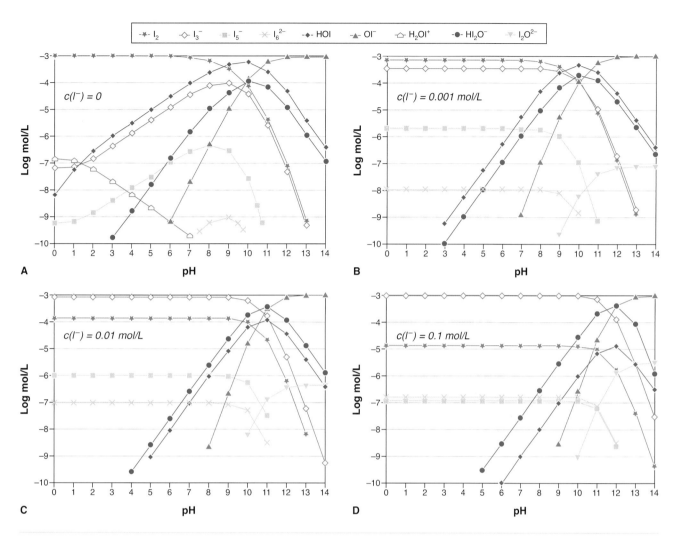

FIGURE 16.2 Calculated equilibrium concentrations in aqueous 10^{-3} mol/L iodine solutions in presence of additional iodide. A, No additional iodide. B, $c[I^-] = 10^{-3}$ mol/L. C, $c[I^-] = 10^{-2}$ mol/L. D, $c[I^-] = 10^{-1}$ mol/L.

a high-concentration iodine formulation with 5% (vol/vol) iodine (0.197 mol/L) and 10% (vol/vol) potassium iodide (KI) (0.6024 mol/L) and the following equilibrium concentrations: $6.129e^{-4}$ mol/L (155.6 ppm) free molecular iodine, 0.406 mol/L (51 650 ppm) iodide, 0.1803 mol/L (68 640 ppm) triiodide, 9.95×10^{-4} mol/L (631 ppm) pentaiodide, and 7.03×10^{-3} mol/L (5350 ppm) hexaiodide. Lugol solution, with a threefold molar excess of iodide, is completely soluble at any dilution. This applies to all iodine/iodide ratios at least down to a twofold excess of iodide. Less iodide results in a gap of solubility of free molecular iodine.

Alcoholic Solution

Iodine equilibrates with alcohols by undergoing "outer" and "inner" complexes that finally result in the formation of triiodide, a reaction that takes approximately 24 hours[23]

$$\text{ROH} + I_2 \leftrightarrow \underset{\text{"outer complex"}}{\text{ROH} \cdot I_2} \leftrightarrow \underset{\text{"inner complex"}}{\text{ROHI}^+I^-} \leftrightarrow \text{ROHI}^+I^-$$

$$I_2 + I^- \leftrightarrow I_3^-$$

$$I_3^- + \text{ROH} \leftrightarrow \text{ROH} \cdot I_3^-$$

Therefore, as in the aqueous system, we have several oxidizing iodine species: I_2, ROH $\cdot$ I_2, ROHI$^+$, I_3^-, and ROH $\cdot$ I_3^-. However, calculations concerning their distribution, even if possible, are of no use in a bactericidal context in a solvent that is itself a strong disinfectant.

Solutions of Iodophors

Iodophors are polymeric organic molecules (alcohols, amides, sugars) capable of complexing iodine species, resulting in reduced equilibrium concentrations of the species compared with those of pure aqueous solutions with the same total iodine and total iodide concentrations.

Because iodophoric preparations always contain appreciable iodide, the relevant species that must be considered

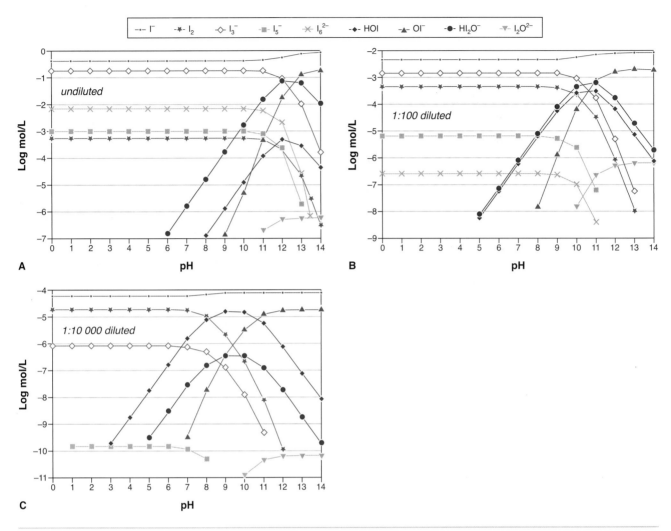

FIGURE 16.3   Calculated equilibrium concentrations in Lugol solution and its dilutions. A, Undiluted. B, 1:100. C, 1:10 000.

are restricted to I^-, I_2, and I_3^-, for which the following (simplified) complexing reactions can be written:

$$I_2 + R \leftrightarrow R \cdot I_2 \ldots K_{I2} \qquad (11)$$

$$I_3^- + R \leftrightarrow R \cdot I_3^- \ldots K_{I3} \qquad (12)$$

$$I^- + R \leftrightarrow R \cdot I^- \ldots K_{I-} \qquad (13)$$

where R = structural regions of the iodophor molecule that can form complexes by steric or electronic effects.

To the extent that the chemistry of aqueous disinfectant solutions containing iodophors is understood, both electronic and steric effects are thought to be responsible for these interactions.[24] Thus, taking as an analogy known interactions with oxygen compounds of low molecular weight, such as amides, esters, ketones, and ether,[25,26] it can be assumed that between molecular iodine and iodophor, molecules without exception contain such functional oxygen-containing groups (eg, povidone contains

a carbonyl oxygen of the amide function in the pyrrolidinone ring), donor-acceptor complexes are formed (see also equation [11]), and iodine plays the part of the acceptor:

$$\overset{\delta+ \quad \delta-}{>C=O} + I_2 \rightarrow \, >C=O \quad I-I$$

The iodophors, especially at high concentrations, are able to surround the iodine species in the manner of clathrates and withdraw it from equilibrium (equations [11] to [13]) because of the spatial arrangement of the dissolved polymer molecules that exists with near regions of helix-like structure.[20] This interaction must be important for the iodide ion and particularly for the large-mass triiodide ion, which cannot form a donor-acceptor complex because of their negative charge.

However, because no quantitative data (mass law constants) are available, an exact calculation for iodophoric preparations is not feasible. Nevertheless, qualitative investigations of the interactions with the iodophoric molecule polyvinylpyrrolidone (PVP) reveal that K_{I^-} is much less than K_{I2^-} and K_{I3^-}. With regard to the normal

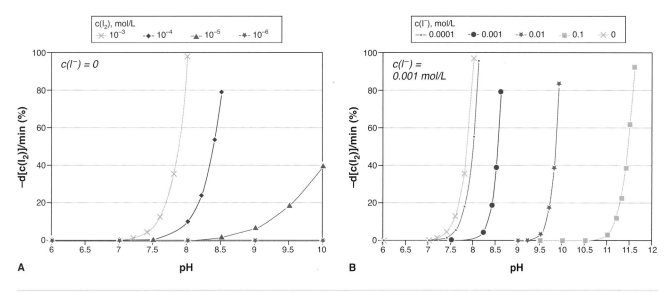

FIGURE 16.4 Initial rates of iodate formation expressed as percentage loss of initial oxidation capacity. A, $c[I_2] = 10^{-3}$, 10^{-4}, 10^{-5}, 10^{-6} mol/L; no additional iodide. B, $c[I_2] = 10^{-3}$ mol/L; $c[I^-] = 0$, 10^{-4}, 10^{-3}, 10^{-2}, 10^{-1} mol/L. From these curves, it can be determined that, for example, in a 10^{-4} mol/L iodine solution at pH 8, the initial rate of loss of oxidation capacity is approximately 10% of the initial concentration per minute.

conditions of use (ie, presence of appreciable iodide and pH <7), this has the following consequences[18]:

1. The HOI and the species derived from it (OI$^-$, HI$_2$O$^-$, I$_2$O^{2-}, and H$_2$OI$^+$) can be neglected.
2. Because the reactions in equations (11) to (13) reduce the equilibrium concentrations of I$_2$, I$_3^-$, and, to a certain degree, I$^-$, the species I$_5^-$ and I$_6^{2-}$ can be ignored as well.

Therefore, in iodophoric preparations, only the triiodide equilibrium (equation [3]) and the interactions of the iodophoric molecules with I$_2$, I$_3^-$, and I$^-$ are important, all of which are independent of pH. Because HOI is virtually absent, stability problems concern only interactions with oxidizable components but not disproportionation to iodate.

Influence of Temperature

Although not usually considered, temperature should not be overlooked. In a study dealing with 10 different povidone-iodine preparations, the results for the relative alteration of free iodine with temperature fitted to an exponential function of the form

$$\Delta\% \, [I_2]_{\Delta t} = 100 \, [10^{(0.023 \pm 0.0026)\Delta t} - 1]$$

which is valid from 10°C to 40°C.[27] Following this equation, [I$_2$] increases approximately 5.4% and 100% if the temperature rises 1.0°C and 13.1°C, respectively. This increase of [I$_2$] must be considered in the application of povidone-iodine preparations as disinfectants or antiseptics on living tissues. Because of their higher temperature

(30°C-36°C), povidone-iodine preparations used on living tissues exhibit a significantly higher [I$_2$] than they do at room temperature ($\Delta t = 10°C$-16°C; $\Delta\% \, [I_2] = 70\%$-130%).

In a clinical study examining the application of iodophoric preparations, no difference was found in the germicidal effectiveness of povidone-iodine (10% vol/vol) against *Staphylococcus aureus*, *Enterococci*, *Escherichia coli*, or group B *Streptococcus* that was warmed to 32°C versus povidone-iodine that was used at 25°C during application.[28]

Atypical Behavior of Iodophors at Dilution

If 10% povidone-iodine is diluted, the concentration of free molecular iodine unexpectedly increases and passes through a maximum in the 0.1% solution. As can be seen in Figure 16.5, the concentration of free iodine in a 10% povidone-iodine solution is approximately 2.0 mg and 8×10^{-6} mol/L and rises in a 1:100 dilution nearly 10-fold. On further dilution, after passing the maximum ([I$_2$] $\approx 10^{-4}$ mol/L), the free iodine behaves increasingly "normally"—that is, it decreases—and below 0.01%, the povidone-iodine solution can be regarded as a simple aqueous solution of iodine.

Because [I$_2$] depends not only on the concentration of povidone-iodine but also on total iodine (in general, 1%) and total iodide (iodine-iodide ratio; see Pinter et al[30]), and the presence of iodine-complexing pharmaceutical additives, it undergoes considerable variation. Figure 16.5 shows the typical course of [I$_2$] of a pure aqueous povidone-iodine at dilution. The ordinate of the maximum (and to a lesser degree, its abscissa) therefore is not a constant for different iodophors and preparations containing

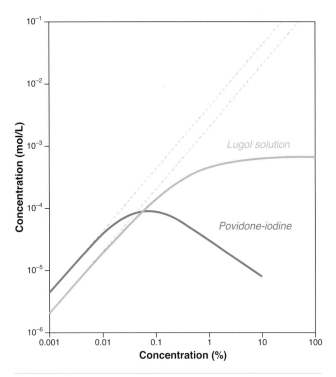

FIGURE 16.5   Total available (*dashed lines*) and free molecular (*solid lines*) iodine in aqueous povidone-iodine (determined potentiometrically) (Gottardi[19]) and in Lugol solution (calculated after Gottardi[29]).

iodophors. Figure 16.3 also shows the behavior of Lugol solution on dilution, which explains the drastic reduction of free iodine caused by the complexing properties of the povidone molecules.

This atypical behavior has been confirmed in a study that compared three distinct solutions of povidone-iodine, ranging in povidone-iodine concentrations from 7.5% (wt/vol) to 10% (wt/vol).[31] The maximum free iodine concentration after dilution ranged from 31 to 51 mg/L. All three solutions exhibited a similar trend in that the amount of free iodine increased with increasing dilution factor, up to a dilution factor of 1 and then began decreasing for the subsequent dilution factors of 10 and 100.

Individual Reactivity of Iodine Species

Iodide (I^-), as a nonoxidizing species, has no antiseptic activity. This is true for iodate (IO_3^-) as well, which acts as an oxidant only at acidic pH, as HIO_3 (pH <4).

Free iodine (I_2) is the only species with a proved correlation between equilibrium concentration and bactericidal activity. Its solvated forms, $I_2 \cdot H_2O$ or $I_2 \cdot ROH$, are thought to be the effective antimicrobial agents in aqueous and alcoholic solution. The term *free* serves to distinguish this I_2 from complex-bound I_2, as discussed later for iodophoric preparations, and refers to the solvated forms $I_2 \cdot H_2O$ and $I_2 \cdot ROH$.

Triiodide (I_3^-) probably has no antiseptic activity, which was deduced from the negative effect that increasing the iodide concentration has on inactivation of poliovirus.[32] On the other hand, triiodide represents the reservoir oxidation capacity in noniodophoric preparations (Lugol solution). It is the main species responsible for staining of tissue.[33]

The HOI is thought to contribute to bactericidal action, which is a plausible analogy with Cl_2/H_2O solutions, where HOCl is the true active species (see chapter 15). Chang[34] claimed differing behaviors of I_2 and HOI against certain microbes, reports on the bactericidal properties of HOI, and on attempts to establish a difference between I_2 and HOI. However, these observations should be treated cautiously.[18] It is possible to manipulate an aqueous iodine solution to exhibit greater than 90% of its oxidation capacity as HOI (pH ≈ 8.5, no additional iodide); such systems in general have no practical importance, mainly because of stability problems. On the other hand, given a similar reactivity of I_2 and HOI in highly diluted systems ($c[I_2] \leq 10^{-5}$ mol) without additional iodide (as is usual in drinking water disinfection) and in the pH range of 3 to 9, a more or less constant bactericidal activity of iodine in aqueous solution can generally be expected.[35]

Iodine cation (H_2OI^+) is thought to be a very potent iodinating agent. Many publications identify this species as being responsible for disinfection, which can be traced back to a comprehensive and often-cited study dealing with the halogens in disinfection.[32] However, exact calculations[18] show that the iodine cation has some importance, if any, only under very acidic conditions (pH <1) and in the total absence of additional iodide, where it amounts to only approximately 0.3% of the total iodine at high dilutions (Figure 16.2D). However, under conditions used in practice (ie, in the presence of iodide to regulate the concentration of free molecular iodine and improve stability), the iodine cation is virtually absent and therefore likely of no significance. For example, a solution with $c[I_2] = 0.001$ and $c[I^-] = 0.01$ mol/L generates $[I_2] = 1.31 \times 10^{-4}$ mol/L or 33.3 ppm at pH <8 (Figure 16.3C). The concentration of the iodine cation, however, is $[H_2OI^+] = 2.15 \times 10^{-13}$ mol/L (not shown in Figure 16.3C), which is approximately nine orders of magnitude less than $[I_2]$. Even if a higher reactivity is attributed to the iodine cation, which is thought to play an important role in certain substitutions, this is not likely able to explain any real contribution to a disinfecting process.

Virtual Impossibility of Discriminating Antimicrobial Activities of I_2 and HOI

The contribution of free molecular iodine, I_2, and HOI to the disinfection processes and differences in their bactericidal power has been previously discussed.[32] A solution containing predominantly I_2 requires a pH of less than 5 and absence of iodide, whereas a solution containing predominantly HOI needs a pH of approximately 8.4. A comparison of the killing effect of I_2 and HOI presupposes that the susceptibility of bacteria for interaction with these iodine species is the same in both pH ranges.

Stability of Iodine-Based Disinfectants

Iodine and other disinfectants based on halogens in the oxidation states 0 or +1, if they are not present as pure substances (ie, without a solvent), can gradually lose their antimicrobial properties (eg, during storage). This is due to (1) substitutions of covalent hydrogen (eg, O-H, N-H, C-H, as a result of reactions with solvent molecules and other formulation additives); (2) additions to olefinic double bonds; and (3) the disproportionation of hypohalous acid to halate in aqueous preparations (equation [9]), which has little to no antimicrobial properties. Although substitutions, which in the case of iodine are thought to be fewer than with chlorine and bromine, and additions can be avoided by an appropriate composition, the equilibria in equations (1) to (8) are established in any case if water is present, and iodate formation (equation [9]) can begin.

Based on calculated equilibrium concentrations, reaction times, and initial rates of iodate formation, the following conclusions have been drawn concerning the stability of iodine-containing disinfecting solutions[14,18,35]:

1. Below pH 6, a decrease in disinfection efficacy because of the formation of iodate can be excluded.
2. Above pH 7, the formation of iodate, the extent of which largely depends on the pH value as well as on the iodide concentration, must be taken into consideration. Raising the pH value lowers the stability (iodate formation increases), whereas raising the iodide concentration improves the stability (iodate formation is reduced).
3. Because of the stabilizing effect of the iodide ion, provided its concentration is sufficiently high, the opposing effect of the pH value can be overcompensated. As a result, iodine-based preparations can also exhibit sufficient stability for practice in the weak alkaline range (eg, Lugol solution, at pH <9).
4. In highly diluted iodine solutions (<10^{-5} mol/L, or 2.54 mg/L), which are used to disinfect potable water or swimming pool water, only a slow iodate formation can be expected even in absence of additional iodide and pH 8 or lower. In accordance with this, in iodine-based disinfection plants, no significant amounts of iodate have been detected.[36]
5. Atemnkeng et al[31] studied the dilution of three commercial povidone-iodine formulations (Braunol®, standardized Betadine®, and unstandardized iso-Betadine®). The pH values were found to increase as a function of the dilution ranging from 5.55 to 5.80 for unstandardized iso-Betadine®, whereas being higher (5.65-6.20) for Braunol® and standardized Betadine® solutions. The values remain constant with increase in

dilution factors. The observed pH for all three solutions is advantageous because their values approximate the pH of the skin at any dilution. The pH >5 in formulations is also important to control Dushman reaction, which could raise free iodine concentrations to an intolerable level for skin application.[31]

The Absence of N-iodo Compounds in Aqueous Solution

The well-known equilibria of halogen with N-H compounds is shown below:

$$X_2 + {>}N-H \leftrightarrow {>}N-X + H^+ + X^- \quad (14a)$$

$$HOX + {>}N-H \leftrightarrow {>}N-X + H_2O \quad (14b)$$

These lead to numerous N-chloro compounds that play an important role in chlorine-based disinfection practice; this, however, is not the case with iodine. Although N-iodo compounds can be synthesized in a nonaqueous system,[37,38] in contact with water, they immediately hydrolyze:

$${>}N-I + H_2O \rightarrow {>}N-H + HOI \quad (15)$$

This assertion complies with the pH range relevant for disinfection (pH 4-8) and not with alkaline conditions at 0°C, where N-iodo alkylamines can be synthesized even in aqueous solutions.[39]

The HOI immediately begins to disproportionate according to equation (9); iodide and protons develop, and a comproportionation or synproportionation chemical reaction in which each reactant, containing the same element but with different oxidation numbers, forms a product with the same oxidation number; and the reverse of reaction in equation (1) also takes place, forming molecular iodine. Within minutes, the reaction settles, and the ratio of resulting products, I_2 and IO_3^-, complies with the stoichiometry set forth in equation (16)[40]:

$$5{>}N-I + 3H_2O \rightarrow 5{>}N-H + 2I_2 + H^+ + IO_3^- \quad (16)$$

Because the equilibria of equations (15) and (16) are lying far on the right side, practically no N-iodo compound is present and the reverse reactions of equations (14a) and (14b) do not take place. N-iodo compounds, therefore, are virtually without any relevance for disinfection.

Reaction With Proteins: Antimicrobial Action and Consumption Effects

Halogens can react with both living and dead microorganisms and with dissolved proteins. In contrast to chlorine, where oxidizing (and antimicrobial) N-chloro compounds still emerge, reactions with compounds of iodine (consumption effects) are associated only with a loss of oxidation capacity (equations [16] to [18]) because *N*-iodo compounds are not formed (see earlier).

Interactions with thiol groups in proteins (S-H compounds) can result in formation of different compounds whereby oxidation to disulfides (equation [16a]) can occur on the one hand and to sulfur-oxygen acids (ie, sulfenic, sulfinic, and sulfonic acids; equation [16b]) on the other hand. Because these reactions occur with similar speed, the proportions of the diverse products are mainly governed by the mode of mixing. Equation (17) describes substitution at activated aromatic compounds (eg, the amino acids tyrosine, histidine, and the nucleosides cytosine and uracil), whereas equation (18) refers to the addition of I_2 to the olefinic function of unsaturated fatty acids

$$R - SH \xrightarrow[-2H^+, 2I^-]{+I_2, +R - SH} R - SS - R \qquad (16a)$$

$$R - SH \xrightarrow[-2H^+, 2I^-]{+I_2, H_2O} R - SOH \xrightarrow[-2H^+, 2I^-]{+I_2, H_2O}$$

$$R - SO_2H \xrightarrow[-2H^+, 2I^-]{+I_2, H_2O} R - SO_3H \qquad (16b)$$

$$= CH^- + I_2 \rightarrow = CI^- + H^+ + I^- \qquad (17)$$

$$-CH = CH^- + I_2 \rightarrow -CIH - CHI^- \qquad (18)$$

▶ PREPARATIONS CONTAINING OR RELEASING FREE IODINE

Solutions of Iodine and Iodide

To this group belongs a great variety of preparations containing elemental iodine and potassium (or sodium) iodide in water, ethyl alcohol, and glycerol, or in mixtures of these solvents. They rank with the oldest disinfectants and have survived more than 150 years owing to their efficacy, economy, and stability. The following are the official preparations according to the *United States Pharmacopeia and the National Formulary*[3]: (1) iodine topical solution, an aqueous solution containing 2.0% iodine and 2.4% sodium iodide; (2) strong iodine solution (Lugol solution), an aqueous solution containing 5% iodine and 10% KI; (3) iodine tincture, containing 2.0% iodine and 2.4% sodium iodide in aqueous ethanol (1:1); and (4) strong iodine tincture, containing 7% iodine and 5% KI in 95% ethanol. Because all these preparations contain large amounts of iodide (0.16-0.6 mol/L), only the triiodide equilibrium (equation [3]) becomes important. As a result, these solutions virtually contain only molecular iodine, iodide, and triiodide and are therefore very stable because there is no HOI present (see earlier).

Because of their high content of free molecular iodine (eg, Lugol solution [I_2] = 155.6 ppm), they are powerful disinfectants with the disadvantage of staining and a toxic potential that should not be underestimated.

Preparations Containing Organic Complexing Agents

In addition to preparations with complexing agents of low molecular weight, such as tetraglycine hydroperiodide,[10] the inclusion compound iodine-maltosylcyclodextrin[41] or quaternized chitosan with iodine,[42] this group includes the important *iodophors*, a term indicating in general the combination of iodine with a carrier (as these complexing agents usually are called) of high molecular weight. In aqueous solution, iodophors form comparable iodine species as pure aqueous iodine solutions (see earlier overview). However, the polymer carriers, because of their complexing properties, partly reduce the equilibrium concentrations of the iodine species and give the iodophor preparations properties that make them superior in some respects to solutions containing only iodine and iodide.

Iodophors

An iodophor is a complex of iodine with a carrier that has at least three functions: (1) to increase the solubility of iodine, (2) to provide a sustained-release reservoir of the halogen, and (3) to reduce the equilibrium concentration of free molecular iodine. The carriers are usually neutral polymers, such as PVP, nonylphenoxy polyethoxyethanol, polyether glycols, polyvinyl alcohols, polyacrylic acid, polyamides, polyoxyalkylenes, and polysaccharides.

In the solid state, iodophors form deep brown to black, crystalline powders that usually do not smell of iodine, indicating a tight bonding with the carrier molecules. The solubility of iodophors in water is good but depends on the chain length of the polymeric molecules. In the case of povidone-iodine, the solubility can vary between 5% (type 90/04, average molecular weight near 1 000 000) and more than 20% (type 17/12, average molecular weight near 10 000). The best known iodophor is povidone-iodine, a compound of l-vinyl-2-pyrrolidone polymer with iodine, which according to United States Pharmacopeia and National Formulary[3] contains no less than 9.0% and no more than 12.0% of available iodine when calculated on the dried basis. On the basis of spectroscopic investigations,[43] it was found that povidone-iodine (in the solid state) is an adduct not with molecular iodine (I_2) but with hydrotriiodic acid (HI_3), where the proton is fixed by a short hydrogen bond between two carbonyl groups of two pyrrolidone rings and the triiodide anion is bound ionically to this cation (Figure 16.6).

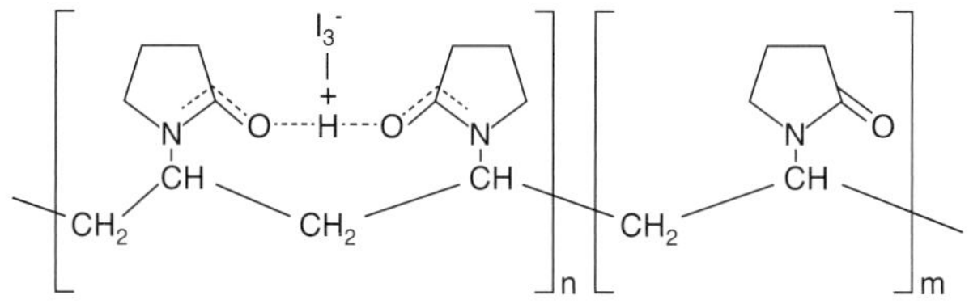

FIGURE 16.6 Structure of solid povidone-iodine. Reprinted from Schenck et al.[43] Copyright © 1979 Wiley-Liss, Inc., A Wiley Company. With permission.

A completely different situation occurs in solution, where this structure no longer exists and equilibria between I_2, I^-, I_3^-, and the polymeric organic molecules are established (equations [3] and [11] to [13]). The high concentration of carrier molecules (approximately 90 g/L) results in the content of free molecular iodine being greatly reduced in such preparations (10% aqueous solution of povidone-iodine: $c[I_2] \approx c[I^-] \approx 0.04$ mol/L, $[I_2] \approx 1 \times 10^{-5}$ mol/L or 2.54 ppm) compared with pure aqueous solutions with the same total iodine and total iodide content (aqueous iodine solution: $c[I_2] = c[I^-] = 0.04$ mol/L, pH 5: $[I_2] = 5.77 \times 10^{-3}$ mol/L or 1466 ppm). Note that this is a hypothetical value because the solubility of molecular iodine is 334 ppm (at 25°C), and an aqueous solution of this composition contains unquantifiable, undissolved iodine. The high content of free iodide (which varies between 10^{-3} and 10^{-1} mol/L, according to the preparation) also means that HOI can be disregarded and only I_2 is responsible for disinfection (see earlier).

Forms of Application

According to the USP 41-NF 36,[3] the following application forms of povidone-iodine are approved: povidone-iodine topical solution, povidone-iodine cleansing solution, povidone-iodine ointment, and povidone-iodine topical spray solution. Regarding available iodine, all must contain no less than 85% and no more than 120% of the labeled amount. In general, povidone-iodine preparations contain 1% to 10% povidone-iodine, which is equivalent to 0.1% to 1.0% available iodine; the cleansing solutions contain one or more surface-active agents.

Iodine Use on the Efficacy of Povidone-iodine Preparations

Because iodophoric preparations are mainly used as antiseptics, the influence of iodine-consuming body fluids is a very important feature regarding antimicrobial potency and rate. Mainly in presence of blood, which is characterized by numerous SH group functions, the reservoir of available iodine is substantially diminished and, because of the formed iodide, the triiodide equilibrium (equation [3]) is shifted to the right. Both effects

decrease the proportion of free molecular iodine (see earlier).

On the other hand, when povidone-iodine preparations are contaminated with liquid substrates, the dilution effect (see earlier) causes an increase in the equilibrium concentration of free molecular iodine (see Figure 16.5). The extent to which this effect compensates for the other two depends on the content of reducing substances. Thus, with whole blood, a large decrease in the concentration of free molecular iodine occurs, whereas in the presence of plasma or exudates, the concentration remains unchanged if the ratio of blood to povidone-iodine is not too high.[44]

Quantitative analysis of iodine (and other oxidizing substances) with blood has poor reproducibility due to the multiple different reactions of iodine with various SH groups (equations [16a] and [16b]). In practice, no substantial decrease in the bactericidal efficacy of 10% povidone-iodine preparations is likely with body fluids having a composition similar to plasma (volume substrate/volume 10% povidone-iodine ≤0.6). However, contamination by 25% or more of whole blood can significantly limit the observed antimicrobial activity.

Iodophoric Preparations and "Active Agents"

In the search for the ideal disinfectant, particularly antiseptics including the combination of immediate microbial kill with complete lack of unwanted side effects on host tissue, much work was done by microbiologists comparing various preparations and formulations containing different antimicrobials (eg, chlorine, iodine, aldehydes, peroxides, chlorhexidine, and quaternary ammonium compounds). The results of such studies usually are presented in such terms as, for example, "0.25% chlorhexidine and 0.025% benzalkonium chloride was more (or less) effective than 10% povidone-iodine." Such descriptions imply that povidone-iodine is an active agent; however, this is not the case. The basic requirements to designate a substance as an active agent are (1) a defined molecule and (2) a positive correlation between the concentration of these defined molecules and antimicrobial activity. Despite its extensive use, both criteria are not fulfilled when using povidone-iodine preparations and may lead to misleading results.

Regarding the nature of povidone-iodine and its disinfecting properties, the following points have been made[45]:

1. Although povidone-iodine in the solid state forms a crystalline powder with a delineated structure in which iodine is present in form of discrete HI_3 units (see Figure 16.6), it is not a uniform compound because the polymeric carrier molecules show a molecular weight distribution. In aqueous solution, however, there are no longer HI_3 molecules but an equilibrium between I^-, I_2, and I_3^-, which are complexed with the organic carrier molecules.

2. Povidone-iodine preparations with 10% povidone-iodine and 1% titratable iodine can easily be adjusted to contain a range of 0.1 to more than 20 ppm free molecular iodine (I_2). Indeed, in a comparison of 10 commercially available preparations, a range of 0.2 to 10 ppm free molecular iodine was found.[27]

3. Because of a possible range in [I_2] of approximately two orders of magnitude, preparations specified to contain 10% povidone-iodine will probably exhibit remarkable variations in bactericidal activity.

4. Because there is no direct and positive correlation between antimicrobial activity and the concentration of povidone-iodine (dose-action relation), it follows that povidone-iodine cannot be regarded as an active agent (like chlorhexidine) but rather as a pharmaceutical base material or additive.

5. As long as free molecular iodine (the most important species) is not specified, both quantitative killing results (log reductions) and evaluation of toxicity relate only to the *batch number X* of the *preparation Y* of the *manufacturer Z* and do not contribute to solution of basic issues of iodine and disinfection.

6. Results of comparisons of povidone-iodine with preparations with specified active agents (eg, 70% alcohol, 0.2% octenidine, 0.5% chlorhexidine) should not be generalized because they are misleading.

Although they have been published,[45] these assertions are not uniformly accepted; this also applies to the previously stated necessity to specify for iodine-based preparations, in addition to total (titratable) iodine, at least the free molecular iodine, which provides information about toxic effects as well as antimicrobial activity.

Solid Iodine-Based Antimicrobial Formulations

This group includes resins containing quaternary ammonium groups loaded with triiodide and higher polyiodide ions (eg, pentaiodide). In contrast to the "classic" disinfectants, which contain antimicrobial agents that are dispersed in a liquid (or gas) phase, these resins rank among the "nonclassic chemical disinfectants," which consist of active moieties attached to, associated with, or stored in (or a combination thereof) a solid phase.[46] Their mode of action is explained either by direct physical contact with their surface or by slow release of a disinfecting agent (in this case, iodine) into the bulk phase being disinfected. Because the residuals of total iodine washed out by the water flowing through the resin are very low, the resins seem to be ideally suited for application in point-of-use water purification units.[47]

Some et al[13] studied the antibacterial effects of the triiodide molecule onto a graphene (ie, an allotrope of carbon in the form of a honeycomb lattice) surface based on the number of oxygen-containing functional groups.

The antibacterial potency was increased with the number of oxygen-containing functional groups contained within the graphene derivatives due to the large surface area, which can undergo extensive iodine interactions via electrostatic interaction, thereby generating graphene-iodine composites.[13]

Preparations Producing Iodine In Situ

Preparations of this kind do not contain elemental iodine, but rather iodide (sodium iodide [NaI] or KI), and produce the former by an oxidation process ($2I^- \rightarrow I_2 + 2e^-$) that can be performed either chemically or by electrical current. The first (chemical) case generally deals with stable, dry powder concentrates that start to produce iodine only when they placed in contact with water. Examples of oxidants that were used to produce iodine in situ are chloramine-T, 1,3-dichloro-5,5-dimethylhydantoin,[48] and NH_2Cl.[49] A more recent development uses calcium peroxide as an oxidant and horseradish peroxidase as a catalyst.[33] The advantage of this concept, called *enzyme-based iodine* (EBI), is in the combination of a relatively high concentration of free molecular iodine (15 ppm) with a comparatively very low concentration of total iodine (≈ 30 ppm). This contrasts with, for example, iodophoric preparations, where the ratio is not 1:2 but rather 1:1000. In addition, the EBI system can reoxidize reduced iodine, which results in a constant level of active iodine during its use life. This feature was demonstrated in repeated cycles of use in disinfecting flexible fiber-optic endoscopic equipment[50]; despite this report, the use of such systems for device disinfection has not been further developed.

The production of iodine by anodic oxidation of an aqueous iodide solution is another possibility for supplying a diluted disinfecting solution in situ in the large volumes recommended for municipal drinking water supplies, cooling towers, and swimming pools.[51] In a closed disinfecting system, electric current can be used to reoxidize consumed (reduced) iodine for which potentiometric steering is possible.

Synopsis of Composition and Active Iodine Forms in Disinfectant Solutions

Table 16.1 summarizes preparations containing iodine and their applications. Besides the total concentration of iodine and iodide, the presumable active species and their calculated, measured, or estimated equilibrium concentrations are shown. Furthermore, a tentative description of the conditions in alcoholic solutions is given. In contrast to pure alcoholic solutions (containing only iodine and an alcohol), where iodine predominantly occurs in the solvated molecular form, $I_2 \cdot ROH$ (besides some triiodide; see Alcoholic Solution), alcoholic preparations used in practice (tincture and strong tincture of iodine)[3] also

TABLE 16.1 Composition and active iodine form in disinfectant solutions containing iodine

Components	Solvent	Examples	Total Iodine Content (Total Iodide Content)	Iodine Form Mainly Responsible for Antimicrobial Effect (Concentration Proportion of the Total Iodine Concentration)
I_2	Ethanol	Solution of iodine in alcohol	1%	$I_2 \cdot ROH$
	H_2O	Drinking water, swimming pool iodination	10^{-5} to 10^{-6} mol/L	$I_2 \cdot aq$, HOI ($[I_2] + [HOI]$: 0.25-2.5 ppm[a]; 98%-100%)
I_2, I^-	H_2O	Lugol solution	5% (10% KI)	$I_2 \cdot aq$ (155.6 ppm[a]; 0.31%)
I_2, I^-	H_2O	Enzyme-based iodine 30-40 ppm (110-130 ppm)		$I_2 \cdot aq$ (15 ppm; −50%)
	Ethanol/H_2O	Iodine tincture	2% (2.4% NaI)	$I_2 \cdot ROH$, $I_2 \cdot aq$
I_2, I^-, polymeric organic complexing agents,[b] additives[c]	H_2O	Mucosal disinfectant and washing concentrates based on iodophors	0.5%-1.0% (Iodide content varies greatly depending on the preparation.)	$I_2 \cdot aq$ (0.2-10 ppm[d]; 0.003%-0.1%)
	Propanol/H_2O	Skin disinfectants (sprays)	0.1% (0.05%)	$I_2 \cdot ROH$, $I_2 \cdot aq$

[a]Calculated (see Gottardi[18]).

[b]Povidone, polyoxyalkylenes, polyether glycols, and the like.

[c]Buffers, detergents, foam stabilizers, artificial colorings, and the like.

[d]Measured potentiometrically (see Gottardi[19]) in commercially available products.

contain iodide and water, with the result that the equilibria in equations (1) to (8) are also established. However, because of the iodide content, no HOI is present and only the solvated iodine molecules $I_2 \cdot ROH$ and $I_2 \cdot H_2O$—apart from the alcohol itself—appear to be responsible for disinfection. A differentiation between the two forms, regarding relative reactivity, should favor the hydrated complex because of the greater stability of the I_2-alcohol-solvate complex (the inductive effect of the alkyl group increases the electron-donating properties of the oxygen).

The HOI, as a virtual contributor to the antimicrobial process, may be expected only in iodine/water systems of high dilution and very low iodide concentration, as in the case with iodine disinfection of drinking and swimming pool water.

▶ ORGANIC IODINE COMPOUNDS

Compounds of this class contain iodine bound to a carbon atom, and they differ from the previously described disinfectants in that they contain no free iodine and are not oxidizing. Iodoform (triiodomethane), probably the oldest pharmaceutically used organoiodine compound, forms yellow crystals with a characteristic anesthetic odor. It came into extensive use as a dusting powder, especially as a local anti-infective agent to promote granulation and diminish infections of open wounds.[10] Because

of its toxicity (it has been reported to lead to sleeplessness, hallucinations, and spasms), it has been replaced by other preparations, especially those containing iodophors or other biocides/antibiotics, and it is no longer specified in the USP 41-NF 36.[3]

A special application still in use is the filling of cavities in dentistry and oral surgery with triiodomethane-containing pastes or triiodomethane-coated gauzes. Particularly, a calcium hydroxide–iodoform mixture was favored as a root filling material.[52] Filling of large cavities, however, should be avoided because O'Connor et al[53] reported on a severe iodoform toxicity with bismuth-iodoform-paraffin paste gauze after a total maxillectomy. With regard to its bactericidal mechanism, iodoform was thought to produce elemental iodine and formaldehyde in connection with water.[9] This assertion seems doubtful because it was impossible to detect any free iodine in an aqueous slurry of CHIS at 37°C and pH 7 with a method that is sensitive down to 2.5×10^{-8} mol/L.[54]

Iodine derivatives of quinoline exhibit protozoicidal and metazoicidal properties and have shown excellent results in prophylactic and therapeutic use.[10] Iodoquinol[3] (5,7-diiodo-8-quinolinol) and clioquinol[3] (5-chloro-7-iodo-8-quinolinol) are the best known active substances of this type and serve as the basis for creams, ointments, powders, and tablets. To this class of compounds also belong the iodine-containing X-ray contrast media. Examples are iocetamic acid and iopanoic acid, which are no longer included in the current USP 41-NF 36; however, iothalamic acid remains.[3] Each molecule contains a benzene ring system with three iodine atoms in the meta-position and are used as such. The radioactive compounds iodohippurate sodium ^{123}I and ^{131}I are used for nuclear medicine purposes.[3] Of only historical interest are the iodonium compounds, with the general formula $[R_2I^+]X^-$, where R is an organic radical and X^- an inorganic or organic anion (eg, diphenyliodonium chloride). The structure resembles that of the onium compounds (eg, quaternary ammonium), and the active part of these compounds is iodine in the oxidation state +3.[55]

▶ MODE OF ANTIMICROBIAL ACTION

Iodine, mainly in its molecular form, has been shown to penetrate the cell wall/membranes of microorganisms rapidly,[34] which can be deemed important in its activity. Although exact details about the nature of the killing of a living cell by the I_2 molecule (or one of the reaction products occurring in aqueous solution) are not known, it is plausible that microbial kill by iodine is based on the reactions outlined in equations (16) to (18), which could have the following consequences:

1. Oxidation of the SH group[32] of the amino acid cysteine results in loss of its ability to connect protein chains by disulfide (—S—S—) bridges, an important factor in the synthesis and activity of many proteins.
2. Iodination of the phenolic and imidazolic groups of the amino acids tyrosine and histidine, which easily form monoiodomono-iodo or diiododi-iodo derivatives, and iodination of the pyrimidine derivatives cytosine and uracil could increase the bulk of the molecules, leading to a form of steric hindrance in hydrogen bonds. As was postulated for the interaction with hypochlorous acid,[56] this could cause denaturation of DNA through dissociation of the double strand into single strands and disruption of protein structure/function. Because of the bulk of the large iodine atoms, this effect should be even more pronounced in case of an iodine-based disinfectant.
3. The addition of iodine to unsaturated fatty acids (equation [18]) is thought to lead to a change in the physical properties of the lipids and to cause membrane immobilization.[57] Electron microscopy and biochemical observations support the conclusion that iodine, by interacting with the double bonds of phospholipids, causes damage to the cell wall, which leads to a loss of intracellular material.[58]

Of the preceding points, the first might be the most important both because of the ubiquitous SH groups and the very fast and irreversible reaction with iodine. These effects are not only important in the antimicrobial activity against vegetative cells but are also applicable to the observed action against viruses and dormant forms of microorganisms over time, such as bacterial and fungal spores.

In in vitro experiments using peptone solutions, it was shown that iodine reacts with free proteins at least 3 times slower than chlorine and nearly 4 times slower than bromine.[59] In clinical practice, disinfection in the presence of dissolved proteins (blood, serum, sputum), iodine is much more efficient than chlorine (and bromine) because the share of the halogen concentration available for the actual antimicrobial reaction is considerably greater. The comparatively low reactivity with many of these proteins (no N-iodo compounds), which is sufficient to achieve high killing rates, is one of the reasons for the excellent antimicrobial properties of iodine.

However, there is a minor drawback with iodine that is not relevant for chlorine disinfection. As can be deduced from equations (16) to (18), consumption effects are always connected with the formation of iodide, which is the only iodine-derived reaction product in equations (16a) and (16b). Thus, according to the reactions in equation (16) to (18), not only is the reservoir of available iodine (oxidation capacity) diminished but also the triiodide equilibrium (equation [3]) is shifted to the right. This means that the antimicrobial power (which is a function of $[I_2]$) is diminished to a higher degree than would be estimated on the basis of the loss of total iodine. This disadvantage is avoided with formulations that can reoxidize the formed iodide, such as EBI,[33,50] or by removing gross soiling (cleaning) prior to surface disinfection with iodine formulations.

▶ RANGE OF ACTION

Iodine is an excellent, prompt, effective antimicrobial with a broad range of effects on almost all the disease-relevant microorganisms, such as vegetative bacteria, enveloped and nonenveloped viruses, bacteriophages, and protozoa, including some of their cyst forms.[60] Mycobacteria and bacterial spores can also be killed by iodine, depending on the formulation and contact time.[61] Furthermore, iodine also exhibits a fungicidal and trichomonicidal activity.[9] As is expected, varying amounts of iodine are necessary to achieve complete disinfection of the different classes of organisms. However, within the same class of organisms, published data have reported highly variable disinfecting effects of iodine. The published killing times for spores[61] and nonenveloped viruses[9] are widely disparate. One reason for this might be the nonuniform sensitivity of microorganisms to iodine, which applies not only to the type of organism but also to the growth conditions, nature of the cell wall, and environment (eg, protein, pH, temperature). Another aspect is the effects of extraneous materials such as growth media used in these disinfection studies, particularly with viruses.

In European Union (EU), as per European Biocidal Products Regulation (BPR, Regulation [EU] 528/2012), iodine including PVP-I has been approved as an active substance for use in biocidal products for product types: human hygiene (1), veterinary hygiene (3), food and feed area disinfectants (4), and embalming and taxidermist fluids (22). This illustrates its importance as a holistically active disinfectant due to the availability of data for its widespread use, with an acceptable toxicity and environmental profile.[62]

Efficacy of Povidone-iodine in Prevention of Infection

Povidone-iodine is commonly used in health care settings, and therefore, its range of efficacy has been investigated in multiple studies to demonstrate its impact in infection prevention and control. The accumulated data demonstrate that povidone-iodine can be efficient against various bacteria associated with health care–acquired infections, including methicillin-resistant strains of *S aureus* and *Staphylococcus epidermidis*[63-69] and vancomycin-resistant *Enterococcus*.[65] The activity extends to a broad range of microbes of importance in preventing health care–acquired infections, including gram-positive bacteria such as *Staphylococcus* species, *Streptococcus* species, *Micrococcus luteus*, and *Enterococcus* species including *Enterococcus faecalis*, and gram-negative bacteria such as *Acinetobacter anitratus*, *Acinetobacter baumannii*, *Enterobacter cloacae*, *E coli*, *Klebsiella* species, *Proteus mirabilis*, *Pseudomonas aeruginosa*, *Serratia marcescens*, *Bacteroides fragilis*, and *Haemophilus influenzae*; and *Candida* species.[63-66,70-72]

Povidone-iodine has shown persistent efficacy against strains of *P aeruginosa*, *Candida albicans*, and *S aureus*, with consistent concentration-time curves of iodine over a period of 1 to 1000 minutes.[73] Notably, these bacterial strains have documented higher level of tolerance to chlorhexidine, suggesting that povidone-iodine may be a suitable replacement for chlorhexidine under certain circumstances.[74] Although mechanisms of tolerance development to chlorhexidine (including mutations and plasmid transmission) have been described, these have not been reported for iodine, presumably due to its more wide-spectrum and nonspecific mechanisms of action. Diluting povidone-iodine may improve its efficacy in some circumstances; one study found that dilution had no effect on bactericidal activity against *P aeruginosa* and *E coli* but increased colony reductions against *S aureus* from <2.12 to >5 log.[70] However, such off-label use of antiseptics is not considered prudent.

Povidone-iodine has also been demonstrated to have broad antiviral activity. Human and avian influenza viruses,[75,76] Ebola viruses,[77] Middle East respiratory syndrome coronavirus,[78] and a model virus developed for testing in the EU called modified vaccinia virus Ankara[77,78] have all been effectively controlled with povidone-iodine. A comparative evaluation of povidone-iodine solution, povidone-iodine gargle, chlorhexidine gluconate, alkyldiaminoethylglycine hydrochloride, benzalkonium chloride, and benzethonium chloride found that only the povidone-iodine products had efficacy against all strains tested in parallel, including human immunodeficiency virus, measles, mumps, herpes virus, influenza virus, and rotavirus with full efficacy and adenovirus, rhinovirus, poliovirus, and rubella virus with some lesser efficacy.[79,80] The latter reflect the greater resistance of nonenveloped viruses to disinfection typical of other biocides (see chapter 3).

In vivo, povidone-iodine has shown immediate and persistent effects as a scrub for hands of medical personnel, conferring colony reductions on naturally contaminated hands[81-85] and on hands that had been experimentally contaminated with methicillin-resistant *S aureus*[86] or *A baumannii*.[87] As a preparation for presurgical skin, povidone-iodine has been demonstrated to achieve quick and sustained bacterial reductions at inguinal sites and abdominal sites,[63,64,88] and reductions were shown to be maintained after 6 hours in some studies.[63] Repeat applications have increased the bactericidal effect.[64,88,89]

The efficacy of a povidone-iodine formulation was superior to that of plain soap or a chlorhexidine soap tested against norovirus.[90] In this regard, Hartmann[91] found, by a special method, that the reduction of the total resident skin flora was significantly higher using povidone-iodine than with isopropanol. This is in contrast to the usual findings, mainly in testing preparations for surgical hand scrubs, which in general exhibit a better antiseptic activity of alcohols.[92]

Povidone-iodine solutions have also been shown to be effective against oral bacterial diseases.[93,94] In a study evaluating four gram-negative (two isolates each of *P aeruginosa* and *Klebsiella pneumoniae*) and three gram-positive bacteria (three isolates of *S aureus*), gargled povidone-iodine solution had more potent bactericidal activity when compared to chlorhexidine gluconate and cetylpyridinium chloride gargles tested.[93] Gargled povidone-iodine solution has also been shown to be more effective at killing *S aureus* and *P aeruginosa* when compared to benzethonium chloride and chlorhexidine gluconate products tested.[94] The observed effectiveness was maintained in the presence of oral organic matter. The effectiveness of povidone-iodine gargles at preventing respiratory illnesses has been tested; however, data are contradictory in terms of effectiveness because some studies have supported this hypothesis[95] and others have shown that a water gargle may be more effective at preventing respiratory illnesses.[96]

The use of gargled povidone-iodine solutions is not without drawbacks. These solutions have been linked to the development of hypothyroidism in people who gargle povidone-iodine solutions on a regular basis.[97] Indeed, gargling with povidone-iodine has been associated with higher serum inorganic iodine levels.[98] As such, it is recommended that people at higher risk of developing thyroid dysfunction, pregnant women, and breastfeeding women avoid gargling such solutions.[98]

Activity of Iodine in Water Disinfection

Pyle and McFeters[99] demonstrated that bacterial isolates (predominantly *Pseudomonas* species) from water systems disinfected by iodine showed differences of up to 4 log reduction in colony-forming units (CFUs) after contact with iodine (1 mg/L, pH 7, 1 min) if they were grown in brain-heart infusion or in phosphate buffer. A similar result was attained with *Legionella pneumophila*, which also showed a differing susceptibility to iodine with cultures grown in well water, on rich agar media, or attached to stainless steel (biofilm). Water cultures of legionellae associated with stainless steel surfaces were 135 times more resistant to iodination than were unattached legionellae and were 210 000 times more resistant to iodination than were agar-grown cultures.[100] Both studies indicate that growth conditions can dramatically affect the susceptibility to iodine (and other biocides) and must be considered when evaluating the efficacy of a disinfecting agent.

As mentioned by Hoehn,[60] the comparison of previously published references on the effectiveness of disinfection processes against different microorganisms is difficult because of the different environmental conditions under which experiments are conducted (eg, pH value, temperature, concentration and type of iodine preparation, time of exposure to the disinfectant, and amount and type of dissolved organic and inorganic substances). Another problem is the fact that, in general, most of these conditions are not described in detail, and an exact comparison of the antimicrobial effectiveness of iodine against different microorganisms, as well as a comparison with the other halogens, is therefore practically impossible. In spite of these difficulties, some authors have tried to summarize the disinfecting properties of iodine and the other halogens by reviewing the literature and analyzing the existing data. The most important conclusions are described in the following text.

A standard inactivation (ie, a 99.99% kill or a 5 log reduction in 10 min at 25°C) of enteric bacteria, amoebic cysts, and enteric viruses requires I_2 residuals of 0.2, 3.5, and 14.6 ppm, respectively[34]; however, on a weight basis, iodine can inactivate viruses more completely over a wide range of water quality than other halogens.[32] In the presence of organic and inorganic nitrogenous substances, iodine is often cited as the cysticide of choice because it does not produce side reactions that can interfere with its disinfecting properties.[32] Iodine requires the smallest dosage (in milligrams per liter) compared with chlorine or bromine to "break any water" to provide a free residual.[32] I_2 is 2 to 3 times as cysticidal and 6 times as sporicidal as

HOI, whereas HOI is at least 40 times as viricidal as I_2. This behavior is explained on the one hand by the higher diffusibility of molecular iodine through the cell walls of cysts and spores and on the other hand by the higher oxidizing power of HOI.[34] For some microorganisms, iodine tolerance also has been ascertained (eg, *Pseudomonas alcaligenes* and *Alcaligenes faecalis*), which can account for the bulk of the microbial flora in iodinated swimming pools.[101] This is due to the intrinsic resistance and persistence of such bacteria in situations such as biofilms. Other studies have shown that iodine does not induce tolerance in isolates of *Pseudomonas*, *Klebsiella*, *Enterobacteria*, *E coli*, and other species.[58,102] Indeed, different microorganisms are expected to have different susceptibilities to iodine.[12] On a spectrum of increasing susceptibility, certain protozoa (particularly oocyst forms) are the most resistant (least susceptible) to iodine disinfection, with vegetative bacteria being the least resistant (most susceptible) and viruses exhibiting intermediate resistance, depending on their structure. Variables that will affect the efficacy of iodine for disinfection include delivery, pH, and temperature (as described earlier). A summary of the disinfection capabilities for iodine solutions and iodine resins is provided in Table 16.2, which indicates that iodine solutions tested may not meet the World Health Organization minimum performance recommendations for point of use treatment products, whereas iodine resins (without filters) could achieve the minimum performance recommendations for two of the three pathogen classes (bacteria and viruses).[2]

Because iodine disinfection is a chemical reaction, the influence of temperature on reaction speed—as a rule of thumb, lowering the temperature approximately 10°C reduces the speed by one-half—must be considered for antimicrobial events in such a way that either the contact time or the concentration of the disinfectant is increased if cold water is to be treated. The lack of efficiency at low temperatures was demonstrated by Regunathan and Beauman,[103] who showed that some iodine preparations designed to purify canteen water worked well against *Giardia* at 20°C but not at 3°C, if used according to the instructions.

With regard to culture conditions, iodine (1500 times) exhibits a greater difference in CM · t values (concentration in molarity multiplied by time in minutes to achieve 99% decrease in viability) than chlorine (68 times) against water-cultured and agar-grown legionellae. Iodine was 50 times more effective than chlorine against agar-grown cultures but was only twice as effective when tested against water-grown legionellae cultures.[100]

▶ SAFETY AND TOXICITY

Toxicity comprises all unwanted side reactions that can be classified as primary effects, like irritation, which may range from simple skin erythema to cellular/tissue necrosis

TABLE 16.2 Water disinfection capabilities of iodine solutions and resins[a]

Parameter	Iodine Solutions	Iodine Resins
General	Cysts most resistant. Achieving *Giardia* cyst inactivation will ensure adequate bacteria and virus inactivation.	Cysts most resistant. Achieving *Giardia* cyst inactivation will ensure adequate bacteria and virus inactivation.
Bacteria	4 log inactivation at concentrations <10 mg-min/L[b]	Triiodide and pentaiodide resins can potentially provide a 6 log bacterial inactivation under most situations.
Viruses	2 log inactivation at concentrations of 15-75 mg-min/L[c]; reduction of 4 $\log_{10}$ for hepatitis A virus, poliovirus 1, and echovirus 1 by doses of 8 and 6 mg/L in 60 min or less, depending on water quality, pH, and temperature	Triiodide and pentaiodide resins can potentially provide a 4 log virus inactivation under most natural water quality conditions.
Giardia cysts	3 log inactivation at concentrations of 45-241 mg-min/L at >20°C. Provide additional contact time and higher disinfectant concentration multiplied by the exposure time (CT) at <20°C to achieve 3 log inactivation.	3 log reduction at 25°C and 4°C using pentaiodide resin compared with 0.2-0.4 log reduction with triiodide resin; additional contact time after passing through resin needed
Cryptosporidium oocysts	Not effective	Not effective
Effect of temperature	Major effect. Increase contact time and/or dose at colder temperatures; CTs up to 720 mg-min/L recommended for *Giardia* cyst inactivation in colder waters (<5°C)	Major effect. Increase contact time after passing through pentaiodide resin at colder temperatures; allow up to 40 min additional contact time for *Giardia* cysts inactivation in colder waters (<5°C)
Effect of pH	Minor effect; generally effective over typical pH levels for natural waters	Minor effect; generally effective over pH range typical for natural waters
Effect of turbidity	Affects disinfection capability; provide additional contact time and/or increase iodine dose in more turbid waters	Affects disinfection capability. Heavy organic matter loading can significantly reduce disinfection capability.

[a]Testing was carried out using iodinated resins only, with no filter applied. Although bacteria and viruses are not physically filtered by the resin, due to electrostatic interactions, *Giardia* cysts and *Cryptosporidium* oocysts are filtered by the resin bed. However, subsequent use of the resin leads to release or wash off of oocysts that could remain viable.

[b]Assuming a contact time of 20 min, a 0.5 mg/L iodine residual would be necessary to provide 4 log inactivation of *Escherichia coli* at near neutral pH at any temperature encountered in natural waters (20 min × 0.5 mg/L = 10 mg-min/L).

[c]2 log inactivation at near neutral to alkaline pH levels (6-10) and various water temperatures (5°C-30°C) at concentrations of 15-75 mg-min/L with the higher concentrations occurring at lower pH levels and colder water temperatures.

resulting in erosions or ulcerations of the epithelial tissue. Toxicity is directly related to the type of application (occlusion, alcoholic, or aqueous solution) and formulation/concentration. Secondary effects are the biological consequences of incorporation (eg, thyrotoxicity) and specific allergic reactions to the iodine itself or additives in the formulation. For all these effects, it is necessary to take into account (1) the composition of the preparation, that is, the equilibrium concentrations of the iodine species I_2, I^-, and I_3^-; (2) their specific contribution to toxic effects; (3) the nature and condition of the tissue coming in contact with the iodine system; and (4) the mode and time of application.

Irritation relates to a minor toxic effect of the active ingredient or additives on the host tissue—most commonly the epithelia—and is a result of iodinating or oxidizing reactions for which free molecular iodine is chiefly

responsible. Because these reactions are the same as those that cause microbial inactivation, in general, a positive correlation between both features can be expected. However, the surprisingly low toxicity of the low-level EBI disinfecting system[50] reveals that a high concentration of free molecular iodine (15 ppm) is well tolerated if total iodine (triiodide) is very low (30-40 ppm).

Staining is mainly caused by the triiodide ion and, only to a minor degree, by free molecular iodine.[33] The deep brownish color on skin or other surfaces is often misinterpreted as a kind of burn or damage. It is usually just a cosmetic problem.

For incorporation effects, two routes are possible: diffusion through the treated tissue and uptake as with drinking water. In the first case, uncharged molecular iodine plays the main role because it can diffuse through the skin. For the ionic species like I^- and I_3^-, however, intact skin acts as a barrier.[104] The triiodide ion, therefore, is retained in the outer, horny layers of the skin, where it causes staining that cannot be removed by washing. However, because of the equilibrium $I_3^- \leftrightarrow I_2 + I^-$, if staining is visible, molecular iodine is formed and diffuses into deeper regions of the skin, where its reduction causes an increase in serum iodide. On the other hand, there is also diffusion out of the skin, causing a remnant bactericidal action (see following discussion). Therefore, staining, although caused by the charged species I_3^-, also leads to real incorporation and should be viewed as a sign of toxicity. The contribution of iodide to incorporation is confined to ingestion (iodinated drinking water, iodide-containing foodstuffs) and resorption with disinfection of mucous membranes.

Although the symptoms are clear for both irritation and staining, the secondary effects (based on incorporation) have diverse manifestations. These can include elevated iodide levels in urine and serum and deviations (usually an increase) in serum levels of parameters connected with thyroid function, T_4 (thyroxine or tetraiodothyronine), T_3 (triiodothyronine), and thyrotropin (thyroid-stimulating hormone [TSH]). These hormones are critical in the maintenance of normal physiologic function of the metabolic and cardiovascular systems.

Topical Antiseptic Preparations

Iodine Tincture

High doses of free iodine, such as in the form of iodine tincture, are highly toxic if brought into body cavities and cause swelling and bleeding of mucous membranes. Consumption of 30 g of iodine tincture can be fatal.[105] As an antidote for such accidents, 10 to 20 g sodium thiosulfate (reduction of iodine to iodide) or starch (formation of inclusion compounds) orally is recommended.[106]

Lugol Solution

The high concentration of free iodine ($[I_2] = 155.6$ ppm) in Lugol solution makes it a powerful disinfectant but also a rather toxic solution, with strong staining properties grounded in the high triiodide concentration (0.18 mol/L). It should be used only externally on very small areas, where it can be recommended in emergencies (eg, at injuries by contaminated hypodermic needles).

Enzyme-Based Iodine

Toxicity tests, including oral toxicity, primary dermal irritation, acute inhalation, ocular toxicity, acute dermal irritation, and sensitization assays in test animals (rat, rabbit, and guinea pig), showed that except for slight irritation to the unwashed rabbit's eye and in the primary dermal test, there was no evidence of toxicity for EBI.[50] The authors attribute this low toxicity for external and internal surfaces of animals to the low level of total iodine (ie, triiodide) in the disinfectant

Povidone-iodine

Povidone-iodine preparations were introduced in the 1960s with the aim of preventing primary toxic effects, based on their low concentration of free molecular iodine. Their low toxic potential was inferred from the increase in serum iodide with their use, which is less than with iodine tincture or Lugol solution.[9] Because the carrier PVP was used as a blood substitute, toxicity can be considered a secondary problem.

The good tolerance to povidone-iodine is apparent in its successful application in healing burned skin, although iodine resorption remains a drawback. In vitro absorption studies using exposure chambers with skin samples clamped between them concluded that 10% povidone-iodine can be absorbed through the skin, and the degree of permeation is dependent on the time of contact.[107] Hunt et al[108] found that the amount of absorbed iodine was directly related to the size of a burn. A case of nephrotoxicity associated with an iodine level of 949 μg/L found that the amount of absorbed iodine was directly related to *P aeruginosa* infection of second- and third-degree burns that covered 26% of the body surface area has been reported.[109] Kuhn et al[110] stated that on treating burns with a povidone-iodine preparation, plasma iodine (ie, iodide) sharply increased from 6.4 ± 0.4 to 20.7 ± 4.7 μg/100 mL; however, the authors also state that thyroid function does not seem to be modified by plasma iodine overload. Glöbel et al[111] investigated iodine uptake after use of povidone-iodine preparations (Betaisodona®) as oral antiseptic, vaginal gel, and liquid soap in subjects with normal thyroid function. By measuring serum iodide, T_3, T_4, and TSH and the urinary iodide excretion (as an index of thyroid function), the authors observed an increase in the iodine supply of up to 2 mg daily but in no case the development of hyperthyroidism or hypothyroidism. The drastic test conditions (eg, hands and forearms were washed 10 times for 2.5 min with povidone-iodine liquid soap within 5 h) permit the conclusion that povidone-iodine preparations are nontoxic under normal label use, at least for healthy adults.

Povidone-iodine, not unexpectedly, has been reported to show cytotoxic effects in in vitro studies.[112] One evaluation found that exposure of sinonasal mucosal cells to povidone-iodine 5% or 10% led to decrease in the active area of a cell monolayers and to a reduction of ciliary beats.[113] However, Niedner[112] has noted that, in vivo, cytotoxic effects are typically seen only when povidone-iodine is used in conjunction with a detergent in open wounds. Cytotoxicity may be a particularly important consideration in the setting of burn dressings because cytotoxic effects might delay wound healing.[114]

Application of topical iodinated antiseptics in neonates (term and preterm) caused, besides a notable increase in urinary iodide excretion, significantly high levels of TSH that were interpreted as transient thyroid dysfunction.[115,116] In a large-scale study at an obstetric ward, it was found that iodine overload in the mothers, caused by skin disinfection before delivery using an iodophor preparation, induces a transient impairment of thyroid function in the infants, especially if they are breastfed. Because this situation is detrimental to screening for congenital hypothyroidism, iodophor preparations are not recommended in obstetrics.[117] When povidone-iodine 10% was applied to approximately 20% to 30% of the body surface area of 15 infants in preparation for cardiothoracic surgery, blood levels of iodine were found to increase by fourfold.[118] All four author groups recommend that caution be exercised in the use of iodine-containing antiseptics in neonates and that noniodinated substances with similar antibacterial efficacy should preferably be used. One study in neonates determined that application of povidone-iodine to an area corresponding to peripheral central line insertion on an upper limb showed no effect on the infants' thyroid function measured 5 days after delivery.[119]

Use of povidone-iodine as a preparation for cesarean delivery has been specifically investigated. One research team observed that use of povidone-iodine in preparation for cesarean delivery led to increased urinary iodine excretion in the mother and the neonate, but no adverse effect on the mothers or on the thyroid tests in the neonates were noted.[120] In another study of 153 cases of cesarean delivery preparation, the mean levels of TSH and T_4 in cord blood were within normal ranges, and there was a normal distribution among the cord blood samples.[121] However, 14.4% of the cord blood samples showed T_4 levels ≤ 7.3 μg/dL. Furthermore, in cases where T_4 level was <13 μg/dL, levels of T_4 levels and TSH showed a significant negative correlation ($r = -0.204$; $P = .014$), and each 1-unit reduction in T_4 was associated with an increase in TSH levels of 0.269 units. These observations led the authors to speculate that thyroid function tests could be affected by povidone-iodine use during skin preparation for cesarean delivery.

A prospective, controlled study found that transient hypothyroidism is not a common sequela of routine skin cleansing with povidone-iodine in premature neonates in North America, an iodine-sufficient area.[122] This result differs from the foregoing studies performed in Europe, which is generally considered an iodine-deficient area. Further potential dangers of pediatric exposure were highlighted in a series of 28 children who underwent strabismus surgery. Episodes of apnea at the time of preparation with povidone-iodine were noted in 54% of patients for periods of 20 to 262 seconds, and an additional two patients had durations of breath holding <20 seconds. No mechanistic basis for this effect was proposed but could include a reaction to temperature change or to a stinging sensation induced by the instilled solution, perhaps associated with the sevoflurane anesthesia employed in the surgery and/or the midazolam that was administered preoperatively.[123]

The irritation potential of povidone-iodine solutions was investigated by comparing subjective and objective assessment techniques with three similar formulations (all containing 10% povidone-iodine and variable amounts of potassium iodate: 0%, 0.03%, and 0.225%) that were applied for 1 to 8 hours to the skin.[124] The methods used, subjective assessment of erythema, objective measurement of skin color (erythema meter), and laser Doppler blood flow measurements, showed consistent results indicating a steady increase in cutaneous irritation, which in the preparation with the highest level of potassium iodate was essentially elevated. Because these experiments were conducted with the povidone-iodine specimen occluded by an aluminum chamber, the results should not be extrapolated to normal conditions in which the povidone-iodine solution dries on the skin, forming a protective film with greatly reduced free iodine.

After use of 10% povidone-iodine to prepare 146 surgical sites, there was no postoperative irritation at the incision or suture site[125]; however, Borrego et al[126] reported a series of 27 cases in which contact dermatitis developed away from the site of incision after presurgical povidone-iodine product use. This type of reaction is suspected to occur in areas of prolonged exposure, particularly where embedded medical devices are painted with povidone-iodine, where liquid may pool during surgery, or when medical draping or coverage with padding may interfere with drying. In most patients in this series, surgery was for >2 hours. An additional case report described erythema with blistering where povidone-iodine 10% (wt/wt) was suspected to have impregnated tourniquet padding.[127] In the Borrego et al[126] series of 27 cases, only one of the patients responded to patch testing with a sensitivity reaction to povidone-iodine 10%. An investigation in 16 patients who had experienced burning, stinging, and eyelid redness and swelling during intravitreal injections found that five patients had positive patch test results with povidone-iodine 10%.[128]

The potential that povidone-iodine can evoke fatal consequences if misapplied was shown in a case report on surgical debridement of a hip wound where a patient died 10 hours after continuous postoperative wound irrigation with Betadine®. Toxic manifestations of systemic iodine absorption appeared to be the cause of death.[129]

Regarding the toxicity of topical preparations, the following generalizations can be made:

1. Because the stratum corneum of intact skin is an effective barrier against electrolytes,[104] it is penetrated by iodine in the form of molecular iodine but not by iodide or triiodide.

2. In body cavities (eg, during treatment of mucous membranes, perineal wash) that are not protected

by a stratum corneum, the incorporation of iodide and triiodide also becomes important because iodine preparations always contain these species.

3. Depending on the chemical nature of the tissue—dry skin with a lower or surfaces of body cavities with a higher reducing potential—the penetrating iodine will be reduced more or less quickly to iodide.

4. The degree of irritation and the amount of total iodine absorbed by the body mainly depend on
   a. The composition and concentration of the applied solution and the concentrations of the main iodine species, I_2, I_3^-, and I^-
   b. The time (duration) of application
   c. The size of the treated area
   d. The nature of the treated area (horny skin, mucosa)
   e. The physical condition of the treated area (intact skin, open wounds)
   f. The type of application, for example, under semi-occlusive dressing or in ointment with occlusive effects or just solutions without this occlusive effect (particularly on skin)
   g. Skin location (more absorption occurs on facial than on back skin) and if mucous membranes are involved
   h. Overall, long-term applications (irrigation) on open wounds with concentrated formulations (eg, undiluted povidone-iodine preparations) should be avoided.

5. As long as it is not reduced, free iodine present on the skin diffuses not only into deeper regions but also back out of the skin, resulting in a certain period of residual bactericidal activity on the skin surface (see later). The reduced portion remains in the body for some time and gives rise to an increased level of serum iodide.

6. The incorporated iodine in the form of iodide and organically bound iodine (that comes to approximately 75% of the total resorbed iodine) leaves the body by urinary excretion and has a biological half-life of approximately 2 days.[111] This finding also suggests that the frequency of treatments (eg, in case of burned skin) needs to be considered because it can provoke an unexpected accumulation.

7. If the mode of application of an iodine preparation is expected to cause a measurable increase in serum iodide, a change to another disinfectant is indicated for neonates and patients with disturbed thyroid function.

Residual Effects of Iodine Preparations

The aforementioned back diffusion of the nonreduced portion of the absorbed iodine, which takes place much more slowly than uptake, was not initially recognized.[130] By means of a photometric method, this iodine flux (dim = mass / area × time) has been ascertained on the skin after application of Lugol solution and povidone-iodine preparations with various concentrations of free iodine.

The most important finding was that the intensity of the iodine flux is dependent on the amount of iodine absorbed by the skin, which increases with the concentration of free iodine of the applied solution and the time of application. Applying Lugol solution (155.6 ppm free iodine) for only 1 minute, the flux could be detected for approximately 24 hours (range: 50-0.005 μg I_2/cm^2/min), whereas after application of a povidone-iodine preparation (10 ppm free iodine) for 3 to 5 minutes, the flux was detectable for 0.5 to 1 hour (range: 0.2-0.005 mg I_2/cm^2/min). The latter result suggests that even the application of iodophor preparations could give rise to a persistent (residual) antimicrobial action. This has been proved by comparing the surviving CFUs of *M luteus* (applied to the skin by artificial contamination) on normal skin with those on skin that was treated for 5 minutes with a povidone-iodine preparation (10% povidone-iodine preparation [10 ppm free iodine]) immediately before contamination.[130] A log reduction rate of 0.4 was found, a result that confirmed the bactericidal action of the iodine diffusing out of the skin. As long as iodine diffuses out of the skin, active disinfection from the inner regions of the skin may occur, and an effective action on the residential pathogens can be expected, a feature that seems to be unique in the field of skin disinfection.

Ingestion of Iodinated Drinking Water

Although it has limited use in terrestrial applications (with the exception of emergency use), elemental iodine is considered to be an appropriate drinking water disinfectant in particular applications such as on extended space flights because it does not present other hazards (eg, chlorine gas or ozone generation) that are unacceptable in a confined space. It was used aboard the National Aeronautics and Space Administration (NASA) space shuttle and was also incorporated into the water recovery and distribution system for the international space station.[131-133] In view of the known potential risks associated with elevated intake of iodine—in particular, congenital goiter—the effects of iodine and iodide on thyroid function in humans were investigated.[134] The experiments failed to confirm the differential effect of I_2 on maintenance of serum T_4 concentrations relative to the effect of I^- that was observed in previous experiments in rats.[135] Based on elevations in TSH, the authors suggested some concern over the potential impact of chronic consumption of I_2 in drinking water.

▶ PRACTICAL APPLICATIONS

Human Medicine

The most important application of iodine in human medicine is in the disinfection of skin, which has been in use since the mid-19th century.[7] In addition to prophylaxis (eg, preoperative preparation of the skin, disinfection of hands, disinfection of the perineum), iodine preparations are used for therapeutic purposes (eg, treatment of infected and burned skin). The oldest account of the therapeutic use of iodine dates to 1829: *Mémoire sur l'emploi de l'iode dans les maladies scrofuleuses.*[2]

The high-level aqueous and alcoholic iodine preparations used up to the 1960s have all but been replaced by the iodophors because of fewer unwanted side reactions (see previous discussion). Among the investigated iodophors, povidone-iodine is usually considered the compound of choice.[9] Antimicrobial effects of povidone-iodine have been confirmed in clinical settings for antisepsis of hands[81,82,84] and surgical sites.[63,64,88] Successful clinical outcomes have been noted after use of povidone-iodine with or without alcohol to prepare sites for mixed surgery, ophthalmic surgery, cesarean and other abdominal surgeries, and for insertion of peripheral and central venous catheters.[89,125,136-140] It has been reported that allowing preoperative povidone-iodine to dry for at least 5 minutes rather than commencing surgery immediately after preparation increased the antibacterial effect.[141]

The initial enthusiasm for this compound was curtailed by observation of intrinsic bacterial contamination of a 10% povidone-iodine preparation (Pharmadine®) by *Pseudomonas cepacia*, leading to an outbreak of pseudobacteremia in a hospital.[142] Another surprising feature was the increased bactericidal activity of dilute povidone-iodine preparations.[143] These events initiated a thorough study of the physicochemical fundamentals of povidone-iodine[19,20] and the articulation of the importance of galenics in the antimicrobial efficacy of povidone-iodine solutions.[30] Attempts also were made to replace the povidone carrier with other macromolecules that might be even more harmless than povidone, which after all had been used as a blood substitute. In this connection, polymers constructed of sugar molecules (eg, polydextrose) are of great interest. When rigid aseptic precautions are required and no painful irritations are to be expected, iodine tincture is still used as the strongest iodine-based disinfectant. A detailed review of the use of iodine in human medicine is given by Knolle,[9] and a good historical account and description of aqueous solutions of iodine and tincture is provided by Reddish.[4] In 2017, the US Food and Drug Administration ruled that iodine tincture was no longer generally recognized as safe and effective as a topical antiseptic for health care professional use because there was insufficient safety and efficacy information available.[144]

Iodine has also been used for the disinfection of medical equipment, such as catgut suture materials, catheters, knife blades, ampules, plastic items, rubber goods, brushes, multidose vials, and thermometers.[10] Disinfection with iodine, however, is not appropriate for every sort of material. For example, many metal surfaces are not resistant to oxidation and can be altered. Furthermore, some plastics absorb elemental iodine, causing a brownish staining that fades very slowly, if at all.

Veterinary Medicine

Disinfection of the cow's udder with iodine before and after milking was a widely adopted application, which started in 1958 when it was found that dipping teats in 0.1%, 1%, and 2.5% tinctures of iodine markedly reduced the numbers of staphylococci that were recovered from milking machine liners.[145] Today, it is performed, in general, by using iodophoric preparations with 0.25% to 1.0% available iodine. This treatment is well tolerated and reduces the incidence of intramammary infections caused by *Streptococcus* and *Staphylococcus* pathogens common around dairies.[146,147] Regarding the possible contamination of milk with iodine, contamination would seem to be less likely with a preparation containing low concentrations of total iodine. An example is the animal drug IodoZyme®, an EBI powder concentrate that produces on dissolution 500 ppm total iodine with 150 ppm I_2.[148] The manufacturer claims that it is as effective as conventional 0.5% iodine teat dip (based on povidone-iodine) but contains only the 10th part of total iodine compared to the latter.

Disinfection of Water

Drinking Water

The first known field use of iodine in water treatment was in World War I by Vergnoux,[48] who reported rapid sterilization of water for troops. Since that time, several studies[48] have shown that iodination is suitable for the disinfection of drinking water, especially in emergency situations. Of considerable importance is the work of Chang and Morris,[149] which led to the development of the tetraglycine hydroperiodide tablets (Globuline) that have been successfully used to disinfect small or individual water supplies in the US army. This method of water purification (addition of iodine tablets or calcium hypochlorite to water, followed by a 25- or 30-minute disinfectant contact period before drinking) is still used by the US army. The Travelers Medical and Vaccination Center[150] claims that chemical disinfection using iodine is more reliable for water purification than chlorine or silver. Because the killing effect of iodine depends on temperature, they recommend the following standing times: 60, 30, and 15 minutes at 5°C, 15°C, and 30°C, respectively (typically at one iodine tablet for 1 L of water).

The use of iodine for water disinfection involves some potential health risks because the chemicals carrying out the disinfection are not removed during these procedures.[151] On the other hand, it was demonstrated in two prison water systems that iodine in doses up to 1.0 ppm is sufficient for disinfection; does not produce any discernible color, taste, or odor; and has no adverse effect on general health or thyroid function. Thomas et al[152] reported a 15-year pilot project in which they observed no instances of ill effects caused by use of iodine for water disinfection. The authors found that iodination is an effective and economic means of water purification, particularly in rural and underdeveloped countries. More recently, the iodine resins have been successfully used as a basis for purifier units that, as long as they are not exhausted, work well and demonstrate approximately 4 $\log_{10}$ reduction of bacteria. For emergencies and for travelers, "pocket purifiers" have been developed whose performance was officially approved through registration by the US Environmental Protection Agency.[103] A description of iodine-containing ion exchange resins for point-of-use water, including a new resin type that provides a more consistent and controllable level of iodine, was given by Osterhoudt.[47] For the disinfection of the drinking water supplies aboard spacecraft, iodine was chosen because of its low risk potential compared with ozone or chlorine. For the Skylab mission, it was furnished by a 30-g/L stock solution containing KI and I_2 in a 2:1 molar ratio, whereas for the Space Shuttle program, a new device for the controlled release of I_2 was introduced—the microbial check valve—consisting of a canister containing iodinated strong base ion exchange resin packed with polyiodide anions (I_3^-, I_5^-, I_7^-).[131]

Swimming Pool Water

Compared with chlorine, iodine has the advantage that it virtually does not react with ammonia or other nitrogenous compounds and therefore produces no compounds that are likely to contribute to swimmers' discomfort in the form of eye irritation or obnoxious odors.[153] The use of iodine in swimming pool disinfection has the following advantages[154]: (1) an approximately one-third savings on chemical cost, (2) no disagreeable odor or taste, (3) no irritation of the mucous membranes, (4) good disinfection of swimming pool water, (5) no danger in storage or use because the material is in crystalline form, (6) the residual is stable and does not fluctuate quickly, (7) the pH is stable after balance is reached, and (8) the swimmers' comfort is enhanced.

On the other hand, iodine is a notoriously poor algicide, and the control of algae growth requires additional measures. Probably the most serious flaw in the use of iodine is the difficulty in controlling the color of the pool water, particularly in the presence of a large amount of iodide, which generates a yellowish-brown color (generated by I_3^- ions). The problem of color control plus its inability to control algae all but eliminate iodine from use by the swimming pool industry.[48] Subsequently, no important contributions to this topic have been made.

Wastewater

Only a few reports deal with the use of iodine in the disinfection of water that, in contrast to drinking and swimming pool water, do not come in direct contact with humans (eg, wastewater and industrial water). Because these waters in general are highly charged with dissolved nitrogenous substances (proteins and their hydrolysis products), the use of iodine, which does not react with nitrogen compounds, should confer great advantages.

For applications that range in technical dimensions, the question of costs also must be considered, and because iodine can be nearly 3 times as expensive as chlorine per mole, the advantages and disadvantages of iodine must be weighed carefully. In a study of disinfection with a mixture of I^- and NH_2Cl that generates elemental iodine, Kinman and Layton[49] found that this system offers considerable potential for use in water disinfection for potable water, industrial water, and water that must be discharged to shellfish areas. Investigating alternatives to wastewater disinfection in pilot plant studies, Budde et al[155] compared the disinfectants chlorine, ozone, and iodine and found that for the same level of fecal coliform destruction, iodine was the most expensive under all conditions studied. Nevertheless, some recent innovations have been presented that are maintaining the use of iodine in this field. Besides an electrolytic approach,[51] a method using solid iodine as a source has been published.[156] In both cases, the resulting diluted iodine solution is recommended for disinfection of cooling tower water, sewage, and wastewater.

The suitability of iodine for the food processing industry, particularly as iodinated ice for fish and fish product preservation, is also claimed.[156] This contribution is the only one for iodine that relates to the field of preservation.

Disinfection of Air

Since Lombardo[157] first advocated the use of iodine as an aerial disinfectant, experiments on the disinfection of air have been carried out, mainly during World War II. Plesch[158] recommended the aerial disinfection of air raid shelters with iodine vapors as a prophylactic measure against influenza. White et al[159] reported iodine to be effective as an aerial disinfectant at concentrations much below its saturation vapor pressure, and Raymond[160] found a "relatively tolerable" concentration of 0.1 mg/ft^3 (3.5 mg/m^3) to be sufficient for a rapid kill of freshly sprayed salivary organisms. However, the danger that iodine vapors pose to the respiratory organs must be kept in mind, as documented by the fact that the maximum allowed concentration of iodine is 1.0 mg/m^3 (threshold limit value),[161] which is less than one-third of the concentration recommended by Raymond.[160] Despite this drawback, iodine-based procedures have been proposed recently (mainly in East Asia) that aim to disinfect air by iodine-containing wall coatings,[162] ceramics loaded with iodine,[163] and vaporizing solutions containing iodine, among other constituents.[164,165]

❯ ENVIRONMENTAL CONSIDERATIONS

Oceans represent a significant source of natural and bioavailable iodine. Iodine enters the atmosphere, largely from ocean water in the form of sea spray or gas. Once iodine compounds reach the atmosphere, they can combine with water or particulate matter that ultimately leads to the transfer of iodine to land surfaces via rain and aerosols. Iodine can then enter the soil or surface water, thus affecting animals and vegetation. When combined with organic matter found in the soil, iodine becomes stabilized and can remain in the soil for a significant amount of time, thus allowing for uptake by plants and eventually by animals. To complete the environmental cycle, water-based iodine reenters the atmosphere as iodine gases. Furthermore, iodine can enter the atmosphere via the burning of coal or oil, although the significance of these anthropogenic sources is relatively small compared to the amount of iodine that enters the atmosphere from ocean water.[12]

Given its environmental cycle, iodine affects all ecosystems and it is important to better understand the balance of iodine among different compartments of those ecosystems.[166] For example, the effect of iodine on plant material is generally positive up to a certain concentration, above which effects become more neutral and/or negative.[166] There have been some documented reports highlighting that iodine released into the environment can be toxic to some species. For example, the bluegill sunfish (*Lepomis macrochirus*) and the water flea (*Daphnia magna*) are susceptible to the toxic effects of iodine.[12] Furthermore, high concentrations of iodine in drinking water supplies may cause adverse health effects in susceptible individuals because of excessive iodine intake.[167]

Recent concerns have been raised by scientists where new measurements of iodine in the Arctic show that small levels of molecular iodine (I_2) in the air and iodide (I^-) in the Arctic snowpack can both contribute to depletion of ozone in the lower atmosphere.[168] This was the first study that reported on atmospheric concentration of molecular iodine and snowpack concentrations of iodide and as such, further measurements must be taken in order to fully understand the iodine environmental cycle and its effects on such atmospheric conditions.[168]

Relevance of Free Molecular Iodine to the Efficiency of Iodophor Preparations

As discussed earlier, the real antimicrobial agent is free molecular iodine because it is this species alone for which a correlation between concentration and bactericidal activity has been proven and not for the total iodine or iodophor concentration.[30,33,143,169] Various commercial preparations differ in the amount and kind of pharmaceutical additives present such as detergents and back-fatting agents, all of which usually have iodine-complexing properties as well as in the ratio of total iodine to total iodide.[30] This results in a significant difference in the concentration of free molecular iodine, although the actual iodophor concentration or the concentration of the total (titratable) iodine might be the same. These circumstances make it necessary to determine the free iodine, which can be measured by three different methods: (1) by extraction with a nonpolar solvent, such as heptane[170]; (2) by dialysis[20]; and (3) by a potentiometric method.[19] Free iodine is the yardstick for bactericidal potency (killing rate), whereas the total iodine, which follows from the specification or simply can be assayed by titration, points to the disinfection capacity. The latter comprises *all* oxidizing iodine species and therefore should not be confused with the free molecular iodine, which (except in highly diluted solutions; see Figure 16.5) amounts to only a small fraction of the total available iodine. For aqueous preparations, determination of free iodine is a reliable and simple means to predict bactericidal properties[169] and, as already pointed out, should be specified by the manufacturer.

Because the aforementioned methods for analyzing free iodine are established for aqueous systems, measurements in alcoholic solutions or water/alcohol mixtures not only need special calibrations but also do not give true correlations with the bactericidal potential because the solvent is itself bactericidal. Another restraint is that some pharmaceutical ingredients (eg, detergents) in commercially available iodophor preparations may influence the susceptibility of a living microorganism to iodine and disturb the correlation between bactericidal activity, in particular, and concentration of free iodine.

❯ ACKNOWLEDGMENTS

Authors are grateful for the previous work done on this chapter by Dr Waldemar Gottardi. Medical writing and editing support was provided by Dr Richa Attre who is a former employee of Purdue Pharma L.P. Ram Kapil and Manjunath Shet are employees of Imbrium Therapeutics L.P, a subsidiary of Purdue Pharma L.P. Michael Pugsley was an employee of Purdue Pharma L.P. during the update of this chapter.

REFERENCES

1. Halliday A. Observations on the use of the different preparations of iodine as a remedy for bronchocele, and in the treatment of scrofula. *Lond Med Repos.* 1821;16:199.
2. Lugol JGA. *Mémoire sur l'emploi de l'iode dans les maladies scrofuleuses.* Paris, France: 1829. Cited by: Horn H, Privora M, Weuffen W. *Handbuch der Desinfektions und Sterilisation.* Vol 1. Berlin, Germany: VEB Verlag Volk und Gesundheit; 1972.
3. United States Pharmacopeia. *USP 41-NF 36.* Rockville, MD: United States Pharmacopeial Convention; 2017. http://www.uspnf.com/. Accessed December 20, 2017.

4. Reddish GF, ed. *Antiseptics, Disinfectants, Fungicides, and Chemical and Physical Sterilization*. 2nd ed. Philadelphia, PA: Lea & Febiger; 1957:223-225.

5. Sykes G. *Disinfection and Sterilization*. 2nd ed. London, United Kingdom: Chapman and Hall; 1972.

6. Bolek S, Boleva V, Schwotzer H. Halogen und Halogenverbindungen. In: Horn H, Privora M, Weuffen W, eds. *Handbuch der Desinfektion and Sterilisation*. Vol 1. Berlin, Germany: VEB Verlag Volk und Gesundheit; 1972:132.

7. Horn H, Privora M, Weuffen W. Grundlagen der Desinfektions. In: Horn H, Privora M, Weuffen W, eds. *Handbuch der Desinfektions und Sterilisation*. Vol 1. Berlin, Germany: VEB Verlag Volk und Gesundheit; 1972.

8. Horn H, Privora M, Weuffen W. Grundlagen der Desinfektions. In: Horn H, Privora M, Weuffen W, eds. *Handbuch der Desinfektion und Sterilisation*. Vol 3. Berlin, Germany: VEB Verlag Volk und Gesundheit; 1974.

9. Knolle P. Alt und aktuell-Keime und Jod. *Hosp Hyg*. 1975;67:389-402.

10. Gershenfeld L. Iodine. In: Block SS, ed. *Disinfection, Sterilization, and Preservation*. 2nd ed. Philadelphia, PA: Lea & Febiger; 1977:196-218.

11. Goebel W. On the disinfecting properties of Lugol's solutions. *Zentralblatt für Bakteriologie*. 1906;42:86-176.

12. World Health Organization. Iodine as a drinking water disinfectant. World Health Organization Web site. http://www.who.int/water _sanitation_health/water-quality/guidelines/chemicals/iodine-draft -oct16-public-review2.pdf. Accessed December 19, 2017.

13. Some S, Sohn JS, Kim J, et al. Graphene-iodine nanocomposites: highly potent bacterial inhibitors that are bio-compatible with human cells. *Sci Rep*. 2016;6:20015.

14. Clough PN, Starke HC. A review of the aqueous chemistry and partitioning of inorganic iodine under LWR severe accident conditions. *Eur Appl Res Rep*. 1985;6:631-776.

15. Gottardi W. The formation of iodate as a reason for the decrease of efficiency of iodine containing disinfectants. *Zentralbl Bakteriol Orig B*. 1981;172(6):498-507.

16. Gottardi W. Redox-potentiometric/titrimetric analysis of aqueous iodine solutions. *Fresenius J Anal Chem*. 1998;362:263-269.

17. Takeda A, Tsukada H, Takaku Y, et al. Determination of iodide, iodate and total iodine in natural water samples by HPLC with amperometric and spectrophotometric detection, and off-line UV irradiation. *Anal Sci*. 2016;32(8):839-845.

18. Gottardi W. Iodine and disinfection: theoretical study on mode of action, efficiency, stability, and analytical aspects in the aqueous system. *Arch Pharm (Weinheim)*. 1999;332(5):151-157.

19. Gottardi W. Potentiometric evaluation of the equilibrium concentrations of free and complex bound iodine in aqueous solutions of polyvinylpyrrolidone-iodine (povidone-iodine). *Fresenius Z Anal Chem*. 1983;314:582-585.

20. Horn D, Ditter W. Physikalisch-chemische Grundlagen der mikrobiziden Wirkung wässriger POVIDONE-Iod-Lösungen. In: Hierholzer G, Görtz G, eds. *POVIDONE-Iod in der Operativen Medizin*. Berlin, Germany: Springer-Verlag; 1984.

21. Gottardi W, inventor. Determination of the equilibrium concentrations of the components halogen, halide, hypohalite, and/or hypohalous acids in aqueous solutions. Germany patent DE4440872. 1998. March 23, 1996.

22. Bell RP, Gelles E. The halogen cations in aqueous solution. *J Chem Soc*. 1951;73:2734-2740.

23. Bhattacharjee B, Varshney A, Bhat SN. Kinetics of transformation of outer charge-transfer complexes to inner complexes. *J Indian Chem Soc*. 1983;60:842-844.

24. Gottardi W. The influence of the chemical behaviour of iodine on the germicidal action of disinfectant solutions containing iodine. *J Hosp Infect*. 1985;6(suppl A):1-11.

25. Yamada H, Kozima K. The molecular complexes between iodine and various oxygen-containing organic compounds. *J Am Chem Soc*. 1960;82:1543.

26. Schmulbach CD, Drago RS. Molecular addition compounds of iodine: III. *J Am Chem Soc*. 1960;82:4484-4487.

27. Gottardi W, Koller W. The concentration of free iodine in aqueous povidone-iodine containing systems and its variation with temperature. *Monatshefte für Chemie*. 1986;117:1011-1020.

28. Leung MP, Bishop KD, Monga M. The effect of temperature on bactericidal properties of 10% povidone-iodine solution. *Am J Obstet Gynecol*. 2002;186(5):869-871.

29. Gottardi W. Redox-potentiometric/titrimetric analysis of aqueous iodine. *Zentralbl Bakt Hyg I Abt Orig B*. 1980;170:422-430.

30. Pinter E, Rackur H, Schubert R. Die Bedeutung der Galenik für die mikrobizide Wirksamkeit von Polyvidon-Iod-Lösungen. *Pharmazeutische Industrie*. 1983;46:3-8.

31. Atemnkeng MA, Plaizier-Vercammen J, Schuermans A. Comparison of free and bound iodine and iodide species as a function of the dilution of three commercial povidone-iodine formulations and their microbicidal activity. *Int J Pharm*. 2006;317(2):161-166.

32. Krusé WC, Hsu Y, Griffiths AC, Stringer R. Halogen action on bacteria, viruses and protozoan. In: Proceedings of the National Specialty Conference on Disinfection; July 8-10, 1970; Amherst, MA. Abstract.

33. Hickey J, Panicucci R, Duan Y, et al. Control of the amount of free molecular iodine in iodine germicides. *J Pharm Pharmacol*. 1997;49(12):1195-1199.

34. Chang SL. Modern concept of disinfection. *J Sanit Eng Div Proc ASCE*. 1971;97:689.

35. Gottardi W. Aqueous iodine solutions as disinfectants: composition, stability, comparison with chlorine and bromine solutions. *Zentralbl Bakteriol Orig B*. 1978;167(3):206-215.

36. Black AP, Thomas WC, Kinman RN, et al. Iodine for the disinfection of water. *J Am Water Works Assoc*. 1968;60:69-83.

37. Gottardi W. Diiodamine: acyl derivatives. *Monatshefte für Chemie*. 1974;105:611-620.

38. Gottardi W. The reaction of N-bromo-compounds with iodine: a convenient synthesis of N-iodo compounds. *Monatshefte für Chemie*. 1975;106:1019-1025.

39. Jander J, Knuth K, Renz W. Studies on nitrogen iodine compounds: VI. Preparation and infrared studies on N-iodomethylamines. *Z Anorg Allg Cheni*. 1972;392:143-158.

40. Gottardi W. On the usability of N-iodo-compounds as disinfectants. *Zentralbl Bakteriol Orig B*. 1978;167:216-223.

41. Kawakami M, Sakamoto M, Kumazawa T, inventors. Mouthwashes containing iodine–maltosylcyclodextrin inclusion compound as a microbicide with high water-solubility. Japan patent 297473. December 16, 1988.

42. Tang Y, Xie L, Sai M, Xu N, Ding D. Preparation and antibacterial activity of quaternized chitosan with iodine. *Mater Sci Eng C Mater Biol Appl*. 2015;48:1-4.

43. Schenck HU, Simak P, Haedicke E. Structure of polyvinylpyrrolidone-iodine (povidone-iodine). *J Pharm Sci*. 1979;68(12):1505-1509.

44. Gottardi W, Koller W. The influence of the consumption on the efficacy of povidone-iodine preparations. *Hyg Med*. 1987;12:150-154.

45. Gottardi W. Povidone-iodine: bactericidal agent or pharmaceutical base material. Reflections on the term active agent in disinfecting systems containing halogens. *Hyg Med*. 1991;16:346-351.

46. Kril MB, Fitzpatrick TW, Janauer GE. Toward a protocol for testing solid microbial compositions. Paper presented at: 3rd Conference on Progress in Chemical Disinfection; April 3-5, 1986; Binghamton, NY.

47. Osterhoudt LE. Iodinated resin and its use in water disinfection. *Spec Publ R Soc Chem*. 1997;196:227-234.

48. White GC. *Handbook of Chlorination*. New York, NY: Van Nostrand Reinhold; 1972.

49. Kinman RN, Layton RF. New method for water disinfection. *J Am Water Works Assoc*. 1976;68:298-302.

50. Duan Y, Dinehart K, Hickey J, Panicucci R, Kessler J, Gottardi W. Properties of an enzyme-based low-level iodine disinfectant. *J Hosp Infect*. 1999;43(3):219-229.

51. Sampson RL, Sampson AH, inventors; HT Acquisition Corp, Ecolab USA Inc, Halox Technologies Inc, assignees. Electrolytic process and apparatus for the controlled oxidation of inorganic and organic species in aqueous solutions. US patent 5,419,816. May 30, 1995.

52. Kubota K, Golden BE, Penugonda B. Root canal filling materials for primary teeth: a review of the literature. *ASDC J Dent Child.* 1992;59(3):225-227.

53. O'Connor AF, Freeland AP, Heal DJ, Rossouw DS. Iodoform toxicity following the use of B.I.P.P.: a potential hazard. *J Laryngol Otol.* 1977;91(10):903-907.

54. Gottardi W. Die potentiometrische Bestimmung von Jod und jodfreisetzenden Oxidationsmitteln. *Mikrochimica Acta.* 1982;1:371-386.

55. Gershenfeld L, Witlin B. Iodonium compounds and their antibacterial activity. *Am J Pharmacol.* 1948;12:158-169.

56. Prütz WA. Hypochlorous acid interactions with thiols, nucleotides, DNA, and other biological substrates. *Arch Biochem Biophys.* 1996;332(1):110-120.

57. Apostolov K. The effects of iodine on the biological activities of myxoviruses. *J Hyg(Lond).* 1980;84(3):381-388.

58. Reimer K, Schreier H, Erdos G, König B, König W, Fleischer W. Molecular effects of a microbicidal substance on relevant microorganisms: electron microscopic and biochemical studies on povidone-iodine. *Zentralbl Hyg Umweltmed.* 1998;200(5-6):423-434.

59. Gottardi W. On the reaction of chlorine, bromine, iodine and some N-chloro and N-bromo compounds with peptone in aqueous solution. *Zentralbl Bakteriol Orig B.* 1976;162:384-388.

60. Hoehn RC. Comparative disinfection methods. *J Am Water Works Assoc.* 1976;68:302-308.

61. Wallhäusser KH. *Sterilisation, Desinfektion, Konservierung.* Stuttgart, Germany: Georg Thieme; 1978.

62. European Commission. Commission implementing regulation (EU) No 94/2014. European Commission Web site. http://eur-lex.europa.eu/legal-content/EN/ALL/?uri=CELEX:32014R0094. Accessed December 20, 2017.

63. Jeng DK, Severin JE. Povidone iodine gel alcohol: a 30-second, one-time application preoperative skin preparation. *Am J Infect Control.* 1998;26(5):488-494.

64. Jeng DK. A new, water-resistant, film-forming, 30-second, one-step application iodophor preoperative skin preparation. *Am J Infect Control.* 2001;29(6):370-376.

65. Inoue Y, Hagi A, Nii T, Tsubotani Y, Nakata H, Iwata K. Novel antiseptic compound OPB-2045G shows potent bactericidal activity against methicillin-resistant *Staphylococcus aureus* and vancomycin-resistant *Enterococcus* both in vitro and in vivo: a pilot study in animals. *J Med Microbiol.* 2015;64(pt 1):32-36.

66. Kargupta R, Hull GJ, Rood KD, et al. Foaming Betadine Spray as a potential agent for non-labor-intensive preoperative surgical site preparation. *Ann Clin Microbiol Antimicrob.* 2015;14:20.

67. Espigares E, Moreno Roldan E, Espigares M, et al. Phenotypic resistance to disinfectants and antibiotics in methicillin-resistant *Staphylococcus aureus* strains isolated from pigs. *Zoonoses Public Health.* 2017;64(4):272-280.

68. Zisi AP, Exindari MK, Siska EK, Koliakos GG. Iodine-lithium-alpha-dextrin (ILαD) against *Staphylococcus aureus* skin infections: a comparative study of in-vitro bactericidal activity and cytotoxicity between ILαD and povidone-iodine. *J Hosp Infect.* 2018;98(2):134-140. doi:10.1016/j.jhin.2017.07.013.

69. Silas MR, Schroeder RM, Thomson RB, Myers WG. Optimizing the antisepsis protocol: effectiveness of 3 povidone-iodine 1.0% applications versus a single application of povidone-iodine 5.0. *J Cataract Refract Surg.* 2017;43(3):400-404.

70. Salvatico S, Feuillolay C, Mas Y, Verrière F, Roques C. Bactericidal activity of 3 cutaneous/mucosal antiseptic solutions in the presence of interfering substances: improvement of the NF EN 13727 European Standard? *Med Mal Infect.* 2015;45(3):89-94.

71. Hoekstra MJ, Westgate SJ, Mueller S. Povidone-iodine ointment demonstrates in vitro efficacy against biofilm formation. *Int Wound J.* 2017;14(1):172-179.

72. Lanjri S, Uwingabiye J, Frikh M, et al. In vitro evaluation of the susceptibility of *Acinetobacter baumannii* isolates to antiseptics and disinfectants: comparison between clinical and environmental isolates. *Antimicrob Resist Infect Control.* 2017;6:36.

73. Koburger T, Hübner NO, Braun M, Siebert J, Kramer A. Standardized comparison of antiseptic efficacy of triclosan, PVP-iodine, octenidine dihydrochloride, polyhexanide and chlorhexidine digluconate. *J Antimicrob Chemother.* 2010;65(8):1712-1719.

74. Kampf G, Kramer A. Epidemiologic background of hand hygiene and evaluation of the most important agents for scrubs and rubs. *Clin Microbiol Rev.* 2004;17(4):863-893.

75. Sriwilaijaroen N, Wilairat P, Hiramatsu H, et al. Mechanisms of the action of povidone-iodine against human and avian influenza A viruses: its effects on hemagglutination and sialidase activities. *Virol J.* 2009;6:124.

76. Ito H, Ito T, Hikida M, et al. Outbreak of highly pathogenic avian influenza in Japan and anti-influenza virus activity of povidone-iodine products. *Dermatology.* 2006;212(suppl 1):115-118.

77. Eggers M, Eickmann M, Kowalski K, Zorn J, Reimer K. Povidone-iodine hand wash and hand rub products demonstrated excellent in vitro virucidal efficacy against Ebola virus and modified vaccinia virus Ankara, the new European test virus for enveloped viruses. *BMC Infect Dis.* 2015;15:375.

78. Eggers M, Eickmann M, Zorn J. Rapid and effective virucidal activity of povidone-iodine products against Middle East respiratory syndrome coronavirus (MERS-CoV) and modified vaccinia virus Ankara (MVA). *Infect Dis Ther.* 2015;4(4):491-501.

79. Kawana R, Kitamura T, Nakagomi O, et al. Inactivation of human viruses by povidone-iodine in comparison with other antiseptics. *Dermatology.* 1997;195(suppl 2):29-35.

80. Eggers M, Koburger-Janssen T, Eickmann M, Zorn J. In vitro bactericidal and virucidal efficacy of povidone-iodine gargle/mouthwash against respiratory and oral tract pathogens. *Infect Dis Ther.* 2018;7(2):249-259. doi:10.1007/s40121-018-0200-7.

81. Paulson DS. Comparative evaluation of five surgical hand scrub preparations. *AORN J.* 1994;60(2):246-256.

82. Gupta C, Czubatyj AM, Briski LE, Malani AK. Comparison of two alcohol-based surgical scrub solutions with an iodine-based scrub brush for presurgical antiseptic effectiveness in a community hospital. *J Hosp Infect.* 2007;65:65-71.

83. Faoagali J, Fong J, George N, Mahoney P, O'Rourke V. Comparison of the immediate, residual, and cumulative antibacterial effects of Novaderm R,* Novascrub R,* Betadine Surgical Scrub, Hibiclens, and liquid soap. *Am J Infect Control.* 1995;23(6):337-343.

84. Seifi B, Sahbaei F, Zare MZ, Abdoli A, Heidari M. A comparative study between povidone-iodine and Manugel 85 on surgical scrub. *Mater Sociomed.* 2016;28(5):348-352.

85. Tsai JC, Lin YK, Huang YJ, et al. Antiseptic effect of conventional povidone-iodine scrub, chlorhexidine scrub, and waterless hand rub in a surgical room: a randomized controlled trial. *Infect Control Hosp Epidemiol.* 2017;38(4):417-422.

86. Guilhermetti M, Hernandes SE, Fukushigue Y, Garcia LB, Cardoso CL. Effectiveness of hand-cleansing agents for removing methicillin-resistant *Staphylococcus aureus* from contaminated hands. *Infect Control Hosp Epidemiol.* 2001;22(2):105-108.

87. Cardoso CL, Pereira HH, Zequim JC, Guilhermetti M. Effectiveness of hand-cleansing agents for removing *Acinetobacter baumannii* strain from contaminated hands. *Am J Infect Control.* 1999;27(4)327-331.

88. Shindo K. Antiseptic effect of povidone-iodine solution on abdominal skin during surgery and on thyroid-gland-related substances. *Dermatology.* 1997;195(suppl 2):78-84.

89. Traoré O, Allaert FA, Fournet-Fayard S, Verrière JL, Laveran H. Comparison of in-vivo antibacterial activity of two skin disinfection procedures for insertion of peripheral catheters: povidone iodine versus chlorhexidine. *J Hosp Infect.* 2000;44(2):147-150.

90. Eggers M, Koburger-Janssen T, Ward LS, Newby C, Müller S. Bactericidal and virucidal activity of povidone-iodine and chlorhexidine gluconate cleansers in an in vivo hand hygiene clinical simulation study. *Infect Dis Ther.* 2018;7(2):235-247. doi:10.1007/s40121-018-0202-5.

91. Hartmann AA. A comparison of the effect of povidone-iodine and 60% n-propanol on the resident flora using a new test method. *J Hosp Infect.* 1985;6(suppl A):73-78.

92. Rotter M. Procedures for hand hygiene in German-speaking countries. *Zentralbl Hyg Umweltmed.* 1996;199(2):334-349.

93. Shiraishi T, Nakagawa Y. Evaluation of the bactericidal activity of povidone-iodine and commercially available gargle preparations. *Dermatology.* 2002;204(suppl 1):37-41.

94. Yoneyama A, Shimizu M, Tabata M, Yashiro J, Takata T, Hikida M. In vitro short-time killing activity of povidone-iodine (Isodine Gargle) in the presence of oral organic matter. *Dermatology.* 2006;212(suppl 1):103-108.

95. Nagatake T, Ahmed K, Oishi K. Prevention of respiratory infections by povidone-iodine gargle. *Dermatology.* 2002;204(suppl 1):32-36.

96. Satomura K, Kitamura T, Kawamura T, et al; for Great Cold Investigators-I. Prevention of upper respiratory tract infections by gargling: a randomized trial. *Am J Prev Med.* 2005;29(4):302-307.

97. Sato K, Ohmori T, Shiratori K, et al. Povidone iodine-induced overt hypothyroidism in a patient with prolonged habitual gargling: urinary excretion of iodine after gargling in normal subjects. *Intern Med.* 2007;46(7):391-395.

98. Nobukuni K, Kawahara S. Thyroid function in nurses: the influence of povidone-iodine hand washing and gargling. *Dermatology.* 2002;204(suppl 1):99-102.

99. Pyle BH, McFeters GA. Iodine sensitivity of bacteria isolated from iodinated water systems. *Can J Microbiol.* 1989;35(4):520-523.

100. Cargill KL, Pyle BH, Sauer RL, McFeters GA. Effects of culture conditions and biofilm formation on the iodine susceptibility of *Legionella pneumophila. Can J Microbiol.* 1992;38(5):423-429.

101. Favero MS, Drake CH. Factors influencing the occurrence of high numbers of iodine-resistant bacteria in iodinated swimming pools. *Appl Microbiol.* 1966;14(4):627-635.

102. Hingst V, Klippel KM, Sonntag HG. Investigations concerning the epidemiology of microbicidal resistance to biocides. *Zbl Hyg.* 1995;197:232-251.

103. Regunathan P, Beauman WH. A comparison of point-of-use disinfection methods. Paper presented at: 3rd Conference on Progress in Chemical Disinfection; April 3-5, 1986; Binghamton, NY.

104. Goldsmith LA. *Biochemistry and Physiology of the Skin.* Oxford, United Kingdom: Oxford University Press; 1983.

105. Wirth W, Hecht G, Gloxhuber C. *Toxikologie-Fibel.* Stuttgart, Germany: Georg Thieme; 1967.

106. Kuschinsky G, Lüllmann H. *Kurzes Lehrbuch der Pharmakologie und Toxikologie.* 10th ed. Stuttgart, Germany: Georg Thieme; 1984.

107. Nesvadbova M, Crosera M, Maina G, Larese Filon F. Povidone iodine skin absorption: an ex-vivo study. *Toxicol Lett.* 2015;235(3):155-160.

108. Hunt JL, Sato R, Heck EL, Baxter CR. A critical evaluation of povidone-iodine absorption in thermally injured patients. *J Trauma.* 1980;20(2):127-129.

109. Aiba M, Ninomiya J, Furuya K, et al. Induction of a critical elevation of povidone-iodine absorption in the treatment of a burn patient: report of a case. *Surg Today.* 1999;29(2):157-159.

110. Kuhn JM, Rieu M, Wasserman D, et al. Thyroid function of burned patients: effect of iodine therapy. *Rev Med Interne.* 1987;8(1):21-26.

111. Glöbel B, Glöbel H, Andres C. Resorption von Iod aus PVP-Iod-Preparation nach Anwendung beim Menschen. *Dtsch Med Wochenschr.* 1984;109(37):1401-1404.

112. Niedner R. Cytotoxicity and sensitization of povidone-iodine and other frequently used anti-infective agents. *Dermatology.* 1997;195(suppl 2):89-92.

113. Kim JH, Rimmer J, Mrad N, Ahmadzada S, Harvey RJ. Betadine has a ciliotoxic effect on ciliated human respiratory cells. *J Laryngol Otol.* 2015;129(suppl 1):S45-S50.

114. Hajská M, Dragúňová J, Koller J. Cytotoxicity testing of burn wound dressings: first results. *Cell Tissue Bank.* 2017;18(2):143-151.

115. Vilain E, Bompard Y, Clément K, Laplanche S, de Kermadec S, Aufrant C. Application breve d'antiseptique iode en soins intentensifs neonatale: consequences sur la fonction thyroidienne. *Arch Pediatr.* 1994;1(9):795-800.

116. Linder N, Davidovitch N, Reichman B, et al. Topical iodine-containing antiseptics and subclinical hypothyroidism in preterm infants. *J Pediatr.* 1997;131(3):434-439.

117. Chanoine JP, Boulvain M, Bourdoux P, et al. Increased recall rate at screening for congenital hypothyroidism in breast fed infants born to iodine overloaded mothers. *Arch Dis Child.* 1988;63(10):1207-1210.

118. Mitchell IM, Pollock JC, Jamieson MP, Fitzpatrick KC, Logan RW. Transcutaneous iodine absorption in infants undergoing cardiac operation. *Ann Thorac Surg.* 1991;52(5):1138-1140.

119. Jeng MJ, Lin CY, Soong WJ, Hsiao KJ, Hwang B, Chiang SH. Neonatal thyroid function is unaffected by single treatment with different preparations of povidone-iodine on a wide skin surface. *Zhonghua Min Guo Xiao Er Ke Yi Xue Hui Za Zhi.* 1997;38(1):28-31.

120. Tahirović H, Toromanović A, Grbić S, Bogdanović G, Fatusić Z, Gnat D. Maternal and neonatal urinary iodine excretion and neonatal TSH in relation to use of antiseptic during caesarean section in an iodine sufficient area. *J Pediatr Endocrinol Metab.* 2009;22(12):1145-1149.

121. Nili F, Hantoushzadeh S, Alimohamadi A, Shariat M, Rezaeizadeh G. Iodine-containing disinfectants in preparation for caesarean section: impact on thyroid profile in cord blood. *Postgrad Med J.* 2015;91(1082):681-684.

122. Brown RS, Bloomfield S, Bednarek FJ, Mitchell ML, Braverman LE. Routine skin cleansing with povidone-iodine is not a common cause of transient neonatal hypothyroidism in North America: a prospective controlled study. *Thyroid.* 1997;7(3):395-400.

123. Emhardt JD, Haider KM, Plager DA, Grundhoefer DL. Intraoperative apnea in children after buffered 5% povidone-iodine site sterilization for strabismus surgery. *Paediatr Anaesth.* 2015;25(2):193-195.

124. Dykes PJ, Marks R. An evaluation of the irritancy potential of povidone iodine solutions: comparison of subjective and objective assessment techniques. *Clin Exp Dermatol.* 1992;17(4):246-249.

125. Georgiade GS, Georgiade NG, Grandy RP, Goldenheim PD. The effect of povidone-iodine solutions used as surgical preparations on the bacterial flora of the skin. *Adv Ther.* 1990;7(1):1-8.

126. Borrego L, Hernández N, Hernández Z, Peñate Y. Povidone-iodine induced post-surgical irritant contact dermatitis localized outside of the surgical incision area. Report of 27 cases and a literature review. *Int J Dermatol.* 2016;55(5):540-555.

127. Ellanti P, Hurson C. Tourniquet-associated povidone-iodine–induced chemical burns. *BMJ Case Rep.* 2015;2015.

128. Veramme J, de Zaeytijd J, Lambert J, Lapeere H. Contact dermatitis in patients undergoing serial intravitreal injections. *Contact Dermatitis.* 2016;74(1):18-21.

129. D'Auria J, Lipson S, Garfield JM. Fatal iodine toxicity following surgical debridement of a hip wound: case report. *J Trauma.* 1990;30(3):353-355.

130. Gottardi W. The uptake and release of molecular iodine by the skin: chemical and bactericidal evidence of residual effects caused by povidone-iodine preparations. *J Hosp Infect.* 1995;29(1):9-18.

131. Atwater JE, Sauer RL, Schultz JR. Numerical simulation of iodine speciation in relation to water disinfection aboard manned spacecraft I. Equilibria. *J Environ Sci Health A Environ Sci Eng Toxic Hazard Subst Control.* 1996;A31(8):1965-1979.

132. McCuaig K. Aseptic technique in microgravity. *Surg Gynecol Obstet.* 1992;175(5):466-476.

133. Gibbons RE, Schultz JR, Sauer RL. *Iodine Sorption Study on the Proposed Use of Viton A in a Shuttle Galley Water Accumulator.* Houston, TX: National Aeronautics and Space Administration; 1988. NASA technical memorandum 100 467.

134. Robison LM, Sylvester PW, Birkenfeld P, Lang JP, Bull RJ. Comparison of the effects of iodine and iodide on thyroid function in humans. *J Toxicol Environ Health A.* 1998;55(2):93-106.

135. Thrall KD, Sauer RL, Bull RJ. Evidence of thyroxine formation following iodine administration in Sprague-Dawley rats. *J Toxicol Environ Health.* 1992;37(4):535-548.

136. Nguyen CL, Oh LJ, Wong E, Francis IC. Povidone-iodine 3-minute exposure time is viable in preparation for cataract surgery. *Eur J Ophthalmol.* 2017;27(5):573-576.

137. Srinivas A, Kaman L, Raj P, et al. Comparison of the efficacy of chlorhexidine gluconate versus povidone iodine as preoperative skin preparation for the prevention of surgical site infections in clean-contaminated upper abdominal surgeries. *Surg Today.* 2015;45(11):1378-1384.

138. Kunkle CM, Marchan J, Safadi S, Whitman S, Chmait RH. Chlorhexidine gluconate versus povidone iodine at cesarean delivery: a randomized controlled trial. *J Matern Fetal Neonatal Med.* 2015;28(5):573-577.

139. Park HM, Han SS, Lee EC, et al. Randomized clinical trial of preoperative skin antisepsis with chlorhexidine gluconate or povidone-iodine. *Br J Surg.* 2017;104(2):e145-e150.

140. Springel EH, Wang XY, Sarfoh VM, Stetzer BP, Weight SA, Mercer BM. A randomized open-label controlled trial of chlorhexidine-alcohol vs povidone-iodine for cesarean antisepsis: the CAPICA trial. *Am J Obstet Gynecol.* 2017;217(4):463.e1-463.e8.

141. Yasuda T, Hasegawa T, Yamato Y, et al. Optimal timing of preoperative skin preparation with povidone-iodine for spine surgery: a prospective, randomized controlled study. *Asian Spine J.* 2015;9(3):423-426.

142. Craven DE, Moody B, Connolly MG, Kollisch NR, Stottmeier KD, McCabe WR. Pseudobacteremia caused by povidone-iodine solution contaminated with *Pseudomonas cepacia. N Engl J Med.* 1981;305(11):621-623.

143. Berkelman RL, Holland BW, Anderson RL. Increased bactericidal activity of dilute preparations of povidone-iodine solutions. *J Clin Microbiol.* 1982;15(4):635-639.

144. Safety and effectiveness of health care antiseptics; topical antimicrobial drug products for over-the-counter human use. *Fed Regist.* 2017;82(243):60474-60503. https://federalregister.gov/d/2017-27317. Accessed March 5, 2018.

145. Newbould FHS, Barnum DA. Effect of dipping cow's teats in a germicide after milking on the number of micrococci on the teat-cup liners. *J Milk Food Technol.* 1958;21:348.

146. Boddie RL, Nickerson SC. Evaluation of two iodophor teat germicides: activity against *Staphylococcus aureus* and *Streptococcus agalactiae. J Dairy Sci.* 1997;80(8):1846-1850.

147. Boddie RL, Nickerson SC, Adkinson RW. Efficacies of teat germicides containing 0.5% chlorhexidine and 1% iodine during experimental challenge with *Staphylococcus aureus* and *Streptococcus agalactiae. J Dairy Sci.* 1997;80(11):2809-2814.

148. West Agro, Inc. *IodoZyme.* Kansas City, MO: West Agro, Inc; 1995.

149. Chang SL, Morris JC. Elemental iodine as a disinfectant for drinking water. *Ind Eng Chem.* 1953;45:1009.

150. Travelers Medical and Vaccination Centre. Drinking and eating safely. Travel Medicine and Vaccination Centre Web site. http://www.tmvc.com.au/info3.html. Accessed 1999.

151. Schaub AS. Preventive medicine considerations for army individual soldier water purification. Paper presented at: 3rd Conference on Progress in Chemical Disinfection; April 3-5, 1986; Binghamton, NY.

152. Thomas WC Jr, Malagodi MH, Oates TW, McCourt JP. Effects of an iodinated water supply. *Trans Am Clin Climatol Assoc.* 1979;90:153-162.

153. Black AP. Swimming pool disinfection with iodine. *Water Sewage Works.* 1961;108:286-289.

154. Putnam EV. Iodine vs chlorine treatment of swimming pools. *Parks Recreations.* 1961;44:162.

155. Budde PE, Nehm P, Boyle WC. Alternatives to wastewater disinfection. *J Water Pollut Control Fed.* 1977;49(10):2144-2156.

156. Harvey WA, Mullins TF, MacDonald DJ, inventors. Method of disinfecting water and food stuff preservation with iodine species. WIPO (PCT) patent WO9855404. May 29, 1998.

157. Lombardo F. Vapori di soluzione iodoiodurata come profilassi e terapia dell'influenza. *Riforma Med.* 1926;42:1011-1012.

158. Plesch J. Methods of air disinfection. *Br Med J.* 1941;1(4194):798.

159. White LJ, Baker AH, Twort CC. Aerial disinfection. *Nature.* 1944;153:141-142.

160. Raymond WF. Iodine as an aerial disinfectant. *J Hyg (Lond).* 1946;44:359-361.

161. Lewis RJ, Sweet DV, eds. *Regulations, Recommendations and Assessments Extracted from the Registry of Toxic Effects of Chemical Substances.* Cincinnati, OH: National Institute for Safety and Health US Department of Health and Human Services; 1986.

162. Suzuki K, inventor. Antimicrobial wall coatings containing iodinated anion exchange resins. Japan patent JPH10317529. December 2, 1998.

163. Okubo T, inventor. Device for deodorization of air in closed space using ceramics loaded with disinfectant. Japan patent JP 09070427. February 24, 1998.

164. Na F, Fan S, inventors. Method and apparatus for air disinfection and deodorization. Patent CN 1091319. August 31, 1994.

165. Huang D, Zhu X, inventors. Indoor air disinfectants and their manufacture. Patent CN 1069414. March 3, 1993.

166. Medrano-Macías J, Leija-Martínez P, González-Morales S, Juárez-Maldonado A, Benavides-Mendoza A. Use of iodine to biofortify and promote growth and stress tolerance in crops. *Front Plant Sci.* 2016;7:1146.

167. US Army Public Health Center. Iodine disinfection in the use of individual water purification devices. Army Public Health Center Web site. https://phc.amedd.army.mil/PHC%20Resource%20Library/Iodine%20Disinfection%20in%20the%20Use%20of%20Individual%20Water%20Purification%20Devices.pdf. Accessed December 20, 2017.

168. Raso ARW, Custard KD, May NW, et al. Active molecular iodine photochemistry in the Arctic. *Proc Natl Acad Sci U S A.* 2017;114(38):10053-10058.

169. Gottardi W, Puritscher M. Germicidal experiments with aqueous PVP-iodine-containing disinfecting solutions: effect of the content of free iodine on the bactericidal action against *Staphylococcus aureus. Zentralbl Bakteriol Mikrobiol Hyg B.* 1986;182(4):372-380.

170. Pollack W, Iny O. A physico-chemical study of PVP-I solutions leading to the reformulation of 'Betadine' preparations (5% PVP-I). *J Hosp Infect.* 1985;6(suppl A):25-30.

Bromine and Bromine-Releasing Biocides

Jonathan N. Howarth and Michael S. Harvey

Bromine disinfectant products have widespread commercial use. This chapter will be dedicated to those compounds that contain or release bromine in the +1 oxidation state. These are known as oxidizing bromine biocides. Important nonoxidizing bromine biocides, such 2,2-dibromo-3-nitrilopropionamide, and nonoxidizing bromine preservatives, such as 2-bromo-2-nitro-1,3-propanerdiol and β-bromo-β-nitrostyrene, have been discussed in chapter 17 of the fourth edition.[1] Elemental bromine does not occur naturally, but its bromide salt precursors are distributed in trace quantities throughout the earth. Seawater, for example, has a bromide content of approximately 65 ppm. Note that this is much less than the chloride content of seawater at 20 000 ppm. Although bromine can be (and still is) produced from seawater, certain bodies of water and underground formations contain much higher concentrations of bromide and serve as the major source for the bromine and bromine-based products manufactured today. The Smackover brine formation in the south central United States (Arkansas) is a concentrated source of bromide ion (4000-5000 ppm). Other sources of bromide include deep wells in the Great Lakes region of the United States and the Dead Sea in the Middle East. The Dead Sea is a particularly rich source with concentrations ranging from 5000 to 6500 ppm.[2] The bromide ion is further enriched using evaporative ponds. In the 1950s, bromine extraction commenced in both Arkansas (United States) and Israel to take advantage of these abundant sources of bromide. In the late 1990s, bromine extraction from the Dead Sea also commenced in Jordan.

The production of bromine requires oxidation of the bromide-containing brine. This can be accomplished by several methods. Commercial quantities of bromine were first produced in the United States in 1846 and in Germany in 1865 using a combination of manganese dioxide and sulfuric acid. In 1890, Herbert M. Dow built a small plant in Canton, OH, that produced bromine by an electrolytic process. Today, the only oxidant of any commercial importance employs chlorine gas fed countercurrent to the flow of brine in a bromine extraction tower.[3] According to the Arkansas Geological Commission, US bromine production in 2001 was 212,000 metric tons, with Arkansas' output accounting for 97% of US production and about 40% of that worldwide.[4]

Although bromine was discovered almost 200 years ago, it is only within the last 35 years that bromine-based biocide technologies have achieved significant commercial use in water treatment. Elemental bromine itself has not been employed commercially to any significant extent for control of microorganisms due to hazardous management issues (it is a corrosive, fuming liquid). The hazards associated with elemental bromine have not posed a detriment to innovation but rather have led to the development of a wide variety of bromine-based delivery chemistries which are safer, less hazardous, and more convenient to use than the elemental form. Today, the water treatment community has many bromine-based biocide technologies to choose from—liquid two-component systems such as activated sodium bromide (NaBr) (effectively, in-situ generation of bromine), solid hydantoin-based technologies, and single-feed, liquid products such as sulfamic acid-stabilized bromine. Bartholomew[5] reviewed the use of bromine chemistry in cooling water systems and this was subsequently updated to reflect the current state of the technology.[6] The review chronicles the development of bromine-based disinfectants from the earliest inception to the state of the art, up to 2004.

An update of the commercial developments of bromine biocides used in cooling water systems will be provided in this chapter, in addition to reviewing other applications where they are used. These include

- recreational water (swimming pools and spas)
- municipal wastewater treatment
- food safety

Other relevant topics in this chapter include the analytical methods for measuring bromine residuals, bromine-containing disinfection by-products (DBPs), and an overview of the worldwide regulatory outlook for bromine biocides.

▶ WATER TREATMENT—EARLY STUDIES AND FUNDAMENTAL PRINCIPLES

Although elemental bromine itself finds little application in water treatment, its use was suggested as far back as 80 years ago. In 1935, Henderson[7] patented a process for treating water with bromine "to destroy any pathogenic organisms that may be present." Henderson data showed that the performance of just 0.25 to 0.5 ppm bromine with *Escherichia coli*–contaminated water was equivalent to 1.5 to 2.0 ppm chlorine. It was also claimed, with the amounts of bromine used (<5 ppm) in the water, that elemental bromine was expected to disappear due to the presence of organic matter present and any after-treatment was unnecessary. Concepts contained in the patent, improved effectiveness and rapid residual decay, still contribute to use of bromine chemistry today. Subsequent laboratory studies of bromine confirmed a broad range of activity over many types of microorganisms. Reports of its ability to deactivate *E coli*; to disinfect water; and to kill spore-forming bacteria, yeasts, and molds appeared in the 1930s and 1940s.[8-13]

The addition of bromine to water generates hypobromous acid (HOBr) and hydrobromic acid (HBr). Depending on the pH, HOBr can further convert to hypobromite (OBr^-). In 1938, Shilov and Gladtchikova[13] correctly measured a pK_a value of 8.7 for the $HOBr - OBr^-$ conversion.

$$Br_2 + H_2O = HOBr + HBr$$

$$HOBr + OH^- = OBr^- + H_2O \; pK_a = 8.7$$

A few years earlier, others accurately determined the pK_a for the analogous chlorine system as 7.5.[14]

$$Cl_2 + H_2O = HOCl + HCl$$

$$HOCl + OH^- = OCl^- + H_2O \; pK_a = 7.5$$

The relative amounts of the two hypohalous acids will therefore vary with the system pH. Above pH 7.5, the relative concentration of hypochlorous acid (HOCl) declines rapidly, although this decline does not occur until above pH 8.7 with HOBr. The importance of the differences in the acid dissociation constants will be discussed graphically in the section on cooling water treatment.

The impact of pH on the effectiveness of chlorine had actually been known for many years (see chapter 15). Workers as far back as 1921 noted that high pH decreased the microbiological activity of hypochlorite.[15,16] A striking example of this is the work by Rudolph and Levine[17]

on spores of *Bacillus metiens*. Time to produce a 99% kill with 25 ppm available chlorine varied from 2.5 minutes at pH 6 to 131 minutes at pH 10. There was a dramatic change in performance from pH 8 to pH 9, a pH range at which the majority of the cooling water treatment programs run at today. The authors concluded that the rate of kill of chlorine was directly related to the concentration of HOCl, which decreases rapidly at elevated pH. Many other studies over the years have pointed to a reduction in performance with chlorine at high pH levels.[18] Additional studies pointed to improved performance of chlorine and bromine mixtures in the presence of ammonia (NH_3) and other nitrogenous-containing materials.[19-21] The chemistry of chlorine and bromine differs significantly in the presence of excess NH_3. Chlorine forms predominately monochloramine, which is a relatively ineffective biocide—some 50 to 100 times less active than free chlorine.[22] Bromine, in contrast, produces a mixture of bromamines in rapid equilibria (mainly mono- and dibroamamine at pH 7 to 9), which are relatively effective biocides. Dibromamine, for example, is said to have the same activity as HOBr itself.[23] At pH 8.2 and a mole ratio of NH_3 to diatomic bromine (Br_2) of 10 (ie, 1.1 ppm NH_3 to 1.0 ppm Br_2), the mixture consists of a 50:50 mixture of mono- and dibromamine.[24] Improved microbiological effectiveness of bromamines versus chloramines was demonstrated against an *E coli* strain at pH 8.2.[25]

Another feature of bromamines is that they typically decay much faster in the environment than chloramines.[24] The following equations summarize the chemistry of the haloamines as formed from chlorine or bromine in excess NH_3.

$$NH_3 + HOCl = NH_2Cl + H_2O \text{ (fast reaction, chloramine decays slowly)}$$

$$NH_2Cl + HOCl = NHCl_2 + H_2O \text{ (slow reaction, chloramine decays slowly)}$$

$$NH_3 + HOBr = NH_2Br + H_2O \text{ (fast reaction, bromamine decays rapidly)}$$

$$NH_2Br + HOBr = NHBr_2 + H_2O \text{ (fast reaction, bromamine decays rapidly)}$$

In the mid-1980s, environmental concerns caused the shift from acid feeds with chromate to acid feeds with chromate/zinc and finally to totally chromate-free, alkaline-based cooling water treatment programs.[26] These alkaline-based programs relied on polyphosphates and, later, phosphonates and copolymers for corrosion and scale control.[27] It was clear that the chlorine-based technologies were less effective at the new higher pH environment that was now typically around pH 8.5 to 8.8, compared to the acid-assisted pH 6.0 to 7.0 employed with chromate-based programs. Figure 17.1 is a graphical representation of the pH/CO_2 solution equilibria.[28]

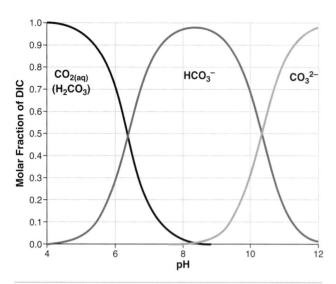

FIGURE 17.1 Carbon dioxide (CO₂) solution equilibria as a function of pH. Mole fraction of dissolved inorganic carbon (DIC). Abbreviations: H_2CO_3, carbonic acid; HCO_3^-, bicarbonate; CO_3^{2-}, carbonate.

It explains why discontinuation of acid causes pH to naturally rise into this range. As the hot water return cascades down the cooling tower fill, dissolved CO_2 is stripped out and escapes to the atmosphere along with the evaporated water. The CO_2 solution equilibria shift and stabilize around pH 8.5 to 8.8. When this occurs, the cooling water contains principally bicarbonate (HCO_3^-) alkalinity.

Increased energy costs also spurred the search for newer, more cost-effective technologies. It was realized that if system surfaces could be maintained under cleaner conditions, energy savings could outweigh the increased costs of biocidal treatment. Older cooling tower designs used plastic fiberglass or wood to break the water into smaller droplets of high surface area:volume ratios to facilitate heat transfer. High-efficiency film fill systems replaced these older splash fill designs. Film fill systems maximized

cooling tower performance but placed further demands on biocide programs.[29] It was essential that the thin gap between adjacent films had to be kept free of slime that could cause clogging and reduce cooling tower efficiency. In extreme cases, when biocontrol is lost, a film fill tower could even collapse under the weight of slime that accumulated.

Water recycling measures, especially those related to the use of municipal waste water as cooling water makeup, prompted intense industrial research into biocides effective in NH_3 and organic nitrogen rich environments. To accommodate the needs of this evolving landscape, it was clear that conventional chlorine programs could not meet these challenges. The spotlight fell front and center on bromine biocides. Due to volatility, handling difficulties, corrosivity, and expense, there had been little interest in elemental bromine as an industrial biocide up to then. Researchers focused on easy-to-handle, safer, nonvolatile, less corrosive, less expensive bromine-releasing biocidal products.

▶ BROMINE PRODUCTS AND BROMINE-RELEASING PRODUCTS

Halogenated Hydantoins

The first halogenated hydantoin introduced for water disinfection was 1-bromo-3-chloro-5,5-dimethylhydantoin (BCDMH). It was generally sold as 1″ 20 g tablets first for recreational water treatment and later for cooling water disinfection. Subsequently, 1,3-dibromo-5,5-dimethylhydantoin (DBDMH) was commercialized as the demand for product with a higher amount of free halogen was needed. Compared to BCDMH, the higher amount of bromine in DBDMH reduced its solubility and was therefore introduced as a high surface area granular product to ensure that sufficient bromine was released into the water being treated (Figure 17.2). A comparison of the properties of both hydantoins is provided in Table 17.1.

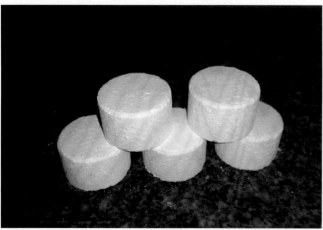
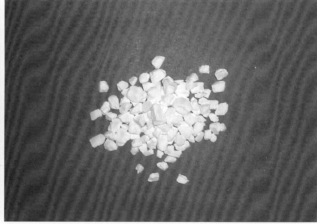

FIGURE 17.2 Solid forms of the halogenated hydantoins, 1-bromo-3-chloro-5,5-dimethylhydantoin (20 g tablets, left) and 1,3-dibromo-5,5-dimethylhydantoin (granules, right).

TABLE 17.1 Properties of halogenated hydantoins

Product	BCDMH	DBDMH
% Halogen (expressed as Cl_2)	54.4	49.4
Product form	One-inch diameter, 20 g tablets	Coarse granules ($-8 \times +14$ mesh)
Method of use	By-pass feeder	By-pass feeder
Molecular weight (g/mol)	241.4	285.9
pH saturated solution	3.5	6.6
Solubility	0.2% at 25°C (77°F)	0.1% at 25°C (77°F)
PMRA Reg. No.	19355	Not registered in Canada
US EPA Reg. No.	Various (eg, 63838-4)	3377-80

Abbreviations: BCDMH, 1-bromo-3-chloro-5,5-dimethylhydantoin; Cl_2, dichlorine; DBDMH, 1,3-dibromo-5,5-dimethylhydantoin; PMRA, Pest Management Regulatory Agency; US EPA, Environmental Protection Agency.

Another halogenated hydantoin product based on 1,3-chloro-5-ethyl-5-methyllhydantoin is available in the form of briquettes.[30] These require no binder in manufacturing. Due to its higher chlorine content, this product is more soluble (about 0.3%) than BCDMH alone. The 98% active product is formally registered as BCDMH (60.0%), 1,3-dichloro-5,5-dimethylhydantoin (27.4%), and 1,3-dichloro-5-ethyl-5-methylhydantoin (10.6%).

BCDMH is sparingly soluble in water. The chemistry of BCDMH can be described as a facile release of HOBr, followed by the sluggish oxidation of spent Br^- ion by monochloro DMH (Figure 17.3).

$$HOCl + Br^- = HOBr + Cl^-$$

Analysis of BCDMH in demand-free waters by the free and total the N,N-diethyl phenylenediamine (DPD) methods indicated that about half of the oxidant value analyzes as free halogen (ie, free HOBr) with the other half analyzing as combined halogen (ie, combined chlorine as chloro-DMH). Excess bromide ion and elevated water temperatures promote the hydrolysis of chloro-DMH with subsequent generation of HOBr. Cooling towers

having short Holding Time Index (HTI; residence times) waste chloro-DMH to the blowdown. Nevertheless, the combination of HOBr and combined chlorine chemistries are claimed to provide good penetration into and control of biofilms encountered in industrial water systems.[31] On the other hand, swimming pools have a near infinite residence time, losing water only to physical means (leaks, filter backwashing, bather drag out). These conditions allow full utilization of the halogen atoms of BCDMH into HOBr.

DBDMH is sparingly soluble in water. The product contains more available bromine activity than bromine itself—111% for DBDMH versus 100% for elemental bromine. Only one of the bromine moieties in Br_2 is manifest as HOBr in water, whereas DBDMH reacts with water to readily release two moles (Figure 17.4).

Virtually all of the halogen residual produced from DBDMH analyzes as being free, as determined by the DPD method, in contrast to other hydantoin products. In many applications, this property leads to lower relative product consumption than other hydantoin products and thus less product inventory and handling (Figure 17.5).

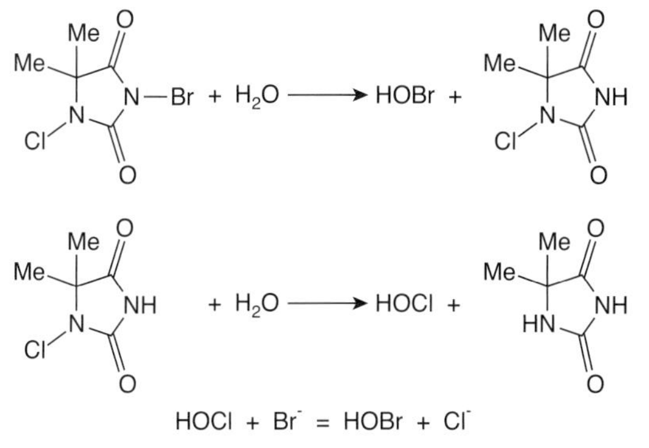

$$HOCl + Br^- = HOBr + Cl^-$$

FIGURE 17.3 Mechanism of 1-bromo-3-chloro-5,5-dimethylhydantoin hydrolysis to hypohalous acids in water.

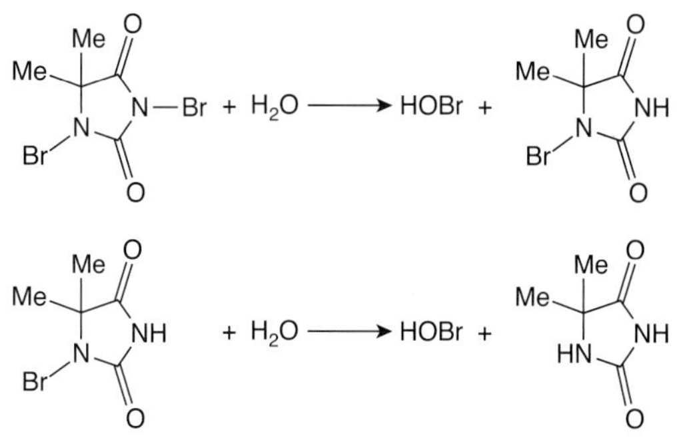

FIGURE 17.4 Mechanism of 1,3-dibromo-5,5-dimethylhydantoin hydrolysis to hypobromous acid in water.

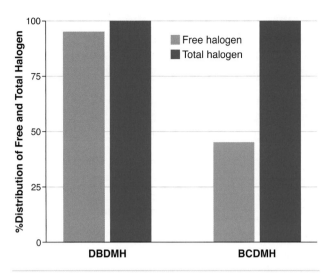

FIGURE 17.5   Relative distribution of free and total halogen residuals in demand-free water (using the N,N-diethyl phenylenediamine method). BCDMH, 1-bromo-3-chloro-5,5-dimethylhydantoin; DBDMH, 1,3-dibromo-5,5-dimethylhydantoin.

The DBDMH has lower water solubility than the BCDMH. Although a proprietary method was developed for making DBDMH tablets of excellent strength and structural integrity,[32] their low surface area meant insufficient bromine residual was released into the treated waters. Consequently, high surface area coarse granules were introduced to the market (see Figure 17.2). Many industrial water treaters elect to classify the microbiological quality of the treated water in terms of the amount of free-chlorine (DPD method) present. Because all the halogen in DBDMH reports as free-chlorine, whereas only half reports as free-chlorine for BCDMH, the former chemistry is often preferred, even though it is more expensive (because it contains twice the amount of bromine as BCDMH). Another property of DBDMH is the fact that saturated solutions are near-neutral in pH and low in halogen odor. This contrasts with other solid products available in the marketplace, which often yield acidic solutions with a strong irritating halogen odor.

Activated Sodium Bromide

The NaBr is a white, crystalline inorganic salt (Table 17.2). It is readily soluble in water and sold as a clear, pH-neutral solution containing 38 to 42 weight percent (wt%) product. Other sources of NaBr include NaOH-neutralized solutions of HBr vapors, which are the by-product of brominated flame-retardant manufacturing. The NaBr is not a biocide itself but must be used in conjunction with an activating agent such as chlorine gas, sodium hypochlorite (NaOCl) solutions (bleach), calcium hypochlorite, ozone (O_3), etc. The result of this dual feed approach is the generation of HOBr. Chemical activation examples are discussed in the cooling water uses section in this chapter.

Sulfamic Acid–Stabilized Bromine Products

To avoid the complexity of the two-component activated NaBr-oxidant system, research effort focused on single-feed liquid bromine products. The first products were based on perbromide (Br_3^-) salts that quell the vapor pressure of elemental bromine.[33,34] The products were wasteful in bromine because only one of the 3 bromine moieties in Br_3^- materializes as biocidal HOBr on hydrolysis in water. The highly acidic nature of these products further limited their appeal and the products were never US Environmental Protection Agency (EPA)-registered in the United States. STABR-EX was the first sulfamic acid–stabilized liquid bromine biocide that was commercialized; it was a breakthrough product of its era.[35] STABR-EX was manufactured by NaOCl oxidation of NaBr followed by stabilizing the mixture with sodium sulfamate. Unlike the acidic perbromide formulations, it was of high pH, possessed no headspace bromine vapors, and all the bromine values were exhibited as oxidizing bromine. Figure 17.6 compares the appearance of an acidic perbromide with that of a sulfamic acid–stabilized product.

TABLE 17.2   Properties of sodium bromide solutions

Product	Sodium bromide (NaBr) solutions
Concentration/wt%	38-42
Molecular Weight (NaBr) (g/mol)	102.9
Appearance	Clear, water white
pH 1-10 Dilution	7-9
Density (40% Solution)/g/ml (lb/gallons)	1.41 (11.8)
Freezing Point/°C (°F)	−25 (−13)
Activation Method	Requires source of chlorine, usually NaOCl
US EPA Reg. No.	Various (eg, 3377-25)

Abbreviations: NaOCl, sodium hypochlorite; US EPA, Environmental Protection Agency.

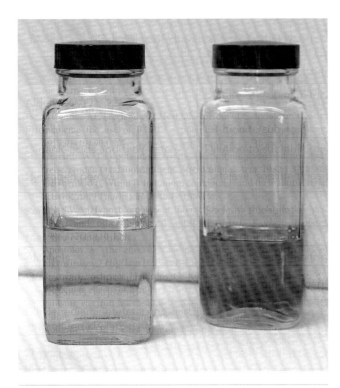

FIGURE 17.6 Comparative appearance of an alkaline sulfamic acid–stabilized product (left) and early generation acidic perbromide formulation (right). For a color version of this art, please consult the eBook.

There are four major sulfamic acid–stabilized bromine products commercially available. They are all single-feed liquids that require no external activation and were developed, in part, to overcome the complexities of dual feed activated NaBr, which requires the use of NaOCl or

dichlorine (Cl_2). As easily handled, preactivated liquids, these products are amenable to shock dosing, a feature not possible with the sparingly soluble halogenated hydantoins, which are generally administered through a by-pass feeder on a continuous or intermittent basis. The ease with which sulfamic acid-stabilized bromine products can be used, coupled with inexpensive shock dosing regimens, means they are rapidly gaining market share over solid bromine delivery systems. Sulfamic acid-stabilized bromine products are differentiated by their methods of manufacture and by their trade names: STABR-EX, STABROM 909, and BromMax 10.2 and 7.1 (Table 17.3). Compared to unstabilized NaOCl, these products typically have an excellent shelf-life greater than one year, even in hot climates (Figure 17.7).

As with NaOCl (or bleach) solutions, it is recommended to avoid contact of the concentrated materials with metals such as iron, copper, zinc, mild steel, and aluminum because these will be corroded over time. The transition metal ions released into solution could accelerate the deterioration of associated products. It is also recommended to avoid mixing with concentrated NaOCl solutions because this can give rise to exothermic decomposition. Finally, these products should be stored away from direct sunlight and other sources of heat to prevent degradation over time.

Sulfamic acid–stabilized bromine products can freeze at temperatures below 30°F (−1.1°C), so necessary precautions should be taken in cold climates. BromMax 10.2 is the exception. Because of the concentrated nature of this product, it crystallizes pure sodium N-bromosulfamate (Figure 17.8) above the freezing point of water. Therefore, this product should not be used if there is the possibility of exposure to cold weather. BromMax 10.2 is mostly sold into warmer climate countries. It contains

Product	STABR-EX	STABROM 909	BromMax 10.2	BromMax 7.1
TABLE 17.3 Properties of sulfamic acid–stabilized bromine products				
Active Ingredients	NaBr NaOCl	Sodium chloro and bromosulfamates	NaBr NaOCl	NaBr NaOCl
% Activity (expressed as Cl_2)	6.1	6.8	10.2	7.1
Method of Manufacture	NaBr + NaOCl	BrCl	TCCA + NaBr	Dilution BromMax 10.2
Physical Form	Yellow liquid	Yellow liquid	Yellow liquid	Yellow liquid
Density/g/mL (lb/gallons)	1.32 (11)	1.46 (12.2)	1.47 (12.3)	1.29 (10.8)
pH 1% Solution	12	12	12	12
Freezing Point/°C (°F)	−8 (17)	−8 (17)	6 (45)[a]	−8 (17)
US EPA Reg. No.	1706-179	3377-55	63838-3	63838-5
PMRA Reg. No.	25478	None	None	29408

Abbreviations: BrCl, bromine chloride; Cl_2, dichlorine; NaBr, sodium bromide; NaOCl, sodium hypochlorite; PMRA, Pest Management Regulatory Agency; TCCA, trichloroisocyanuric acid; US EPA, Environmental Protection Agency.

[a]Crystallization point.

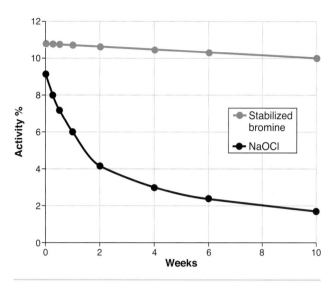

FIGURE 17.7 Long-term storage of a sulfamic acid–stabilized bromine product versus a bleach (sodium hypochlorite [NaOCl]) solution (dichlorine basis) at 40°C.

33% more active ingredient than other stabilized bromine products, and this higher activity has an economic advantage to contain overseas shipping costs. Far higher concentrations of bromine were possible through the use of trichloroisocyanuric acid (TCCA) as the oxidant.[36,37] The TCCA is a solid (91% available Cl_2) and does not dilute the product, as is the case for another stabilized bromine product where 12% NaOCl is used to affect the oxidation (see Table 17.3).

Subsequent to the commercialization of the four stabilized bromine products, another higher concentration (9.2% activity as Cl_2) product was introduced for larger industrial cooling water uses. It has the tradename MAXXIS and is a mixture of sodium chloro- and bromo-sulfamates. MAXXIS also has the same low temperature limitation as BromMax 10.2.

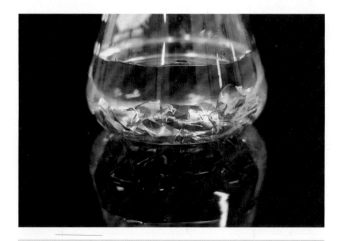

FIGURE 17.8 Hydrated crystals sodium N-bromosulfamate that can develop under cold conditions (6°C/45°F). For a color version of this art, please consult the eBook.

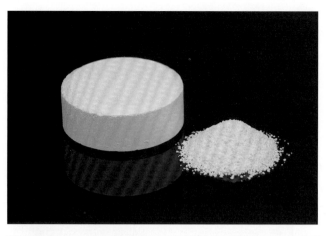

FIGURE 17.9 Trichloroisocyanuric acid/sodium bromide [NaBr] tablet and sodium dichlorisocyanurate/NaBr granules.

Bromine-Releasing Isocyanurate Compositions[38]

Bromine-releasing isocyanurate compositions include TCCA or sodium dichlorisocyanurate (SDIC) containing compositions mixed with a source of bromine (NaBr) (Figures 17.9 and 17.10). Examples of these products are summarized in Table 17.4. When either bromine-releasing isocyanurate composition is added to water, they effectively generate HOBr through the reaction of HOCl (liberated from the chlorinated isocyanurate) and NaBr. Because both compositions contain an excess of chlorine, the treated water will always contain mixed halogens. At elevated pH (>7) and at high dilution, the regeneration of the Br$^-$ ion into HOBr by the excess chlorinated isocyanurate is sluggish (J.N.H., unpublished data, 1990). The granules are often found to be too soluble to be used in any type of automatic feeding device and are only amenable by manual broadcast, usually for shock dosing (see Figure 17.9). On the other hand, the different solubilities of NaBr and TCCA mean that the NaBr preferentially leaches out of tablets over time. This causes the tablets to disintegrate into a high surface area mound of product, which accelerates dissolution even further (J.N.H., unpublished data, 1990). Thus, it may not be possible for the certain tablet formulations to deliver a controlled, meaningful dose of halogen to the water.

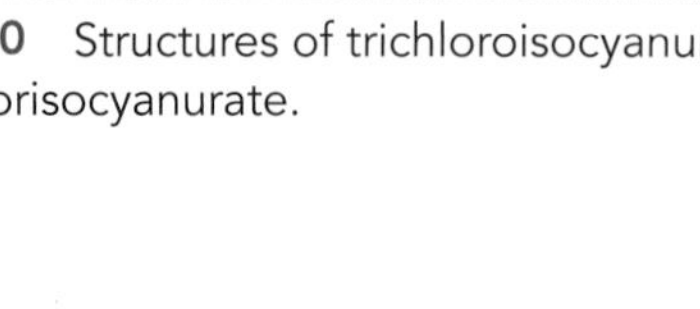

FIGURE 17.10 Structures of trichloroisocyanuric acid and sodium dichlorisocyanurate.

TABLE 17.4 Properties of bromine-releasing isocyanurate compositions

	TOWERBROM 90M	TOWERBROM 60M
Active Ingredients	92.9% TCCA + 6.9% NaBr	90% SDIC + 7.0% NaBr
% Expressed as Cl$_2$	84	57
Product Form	180 g and 14 g tablets	Free-flowing granules
Method of Use	Feeding, floating devices Hanging mesh bags	Manual broadcast
Bulk Density/ kg/m^3 (lb/ft^3)	1009.2 (63)	1009.2 (63)
pH 1% Solution	3	6
US EPA Reg. No.	939-72	939-71

Abbreviations: Cl$_2$, dichlorine; NaBr, sodium bromide; SDIC, sodium dichlorisocyanurate; TCCA, trichloroisocyanuric acid; US EPA, United States Environmental Protection Agency.

Bromine Chloride

Typical properties of bromine chloride (BrCl) are listed in Table 17.5.[39]

The BrCl has many of the hazardous properties commonly associated with elemental Br$_2$. But it does hydrolyze in water such that all available bromine materialize as HOBr (see the following text), whereas only about half will materialize with elemental Br$_2$.

$$BrCl + H_2O = HOBr + HCl$$

BrCl exists as an equilibrium mixture of Br$_2$ and Cl$_2$. It reacts rapidly with NH$_3$ to form bromamines,[24] which are much more effective bactericides and viricides compared to their chlorinated counterparts. Furthermore, the short environmental persistence of bromamines renders the treated effluent much less toxic to aquatic animals and plants and can even eliminate the need

TABLE 17.5 Properties of bromine chloride

Product	BrCl
Molecular Weight (BrCl) (g/mol)	115.4
% Available Br$_2$	138.5
Density (25°C)/g/mL (lb/gallon)	2.32 (19.3)
Flash Point	None
Fire Point	None
Boiling Point (760 mm)/°C (°F)	5 (41)
Vapor pressure (psig at 25°C)	34
Freezing Point/°C (°F)	−66 (−87)
Solubility in Water 20°C (68°F)	7.8 wt.%

Abbreviations: Br$_2$, diatomic bromine, BrCl, bromine chloride; Cl$_2$, dichlorine; NaBr, sodium bromide; SDIC, sodium dichlorisocyanurate; TCCA, trichloroisocyanuric acid; US EPA, United States Environmental Protection Agency.

for a dehalogenation (sulfite or metabisulfite) neutralization step. This is a costly and cumbersome practice often required to be employed before chlorinated effluent is discharged. Thus, BrCl has been effectively used for disinfection of municipal sewage. Unfortunately, the hazardous nature of BrCl, coupled with its high corrosivity, has led this product to be almost discontinued and it is no longer used for municipal wastewater treatment. More recently, the US Department of Homeland Security has placed BrCl on a restricted list of regulated chemicals due to other safety concerns.[40]

Electrobromination

Electrolysis of bromide ion-containing brines was first used in the early days of bromine recovery.[41] Borrowing from modern advances in chlor-alkali technology, in particular, the development of dimensionally stable anodes (DSAs) and membrane technology, the electrolysis of bromide ion solutions has come under renewed interest,[42] especially for disinfection purposes. The most widely practiced example of an electro bromination process is seawater electrolysis for microbiological control of ballast water onboard ocean-going vessels. The dominant anodic reaction is

$$2\,Cl^- + 2e^- = Cl_2 \qquad \text{Anodic reaction}$$

$$Cl_2 + H_2O = HOCl + HCl \qquad \text{Bulk solution}$$

In the bulk solution, the HOCl reacts with the 65 ppm bromide ion present in seawater to form HOBr. The cathodic reaction is reduction of water:

$$2\,H_2O - 2e^- = H_2 + 2\,OH^-$$

All seawater electrolysis systems are designed to safely manage the production of free hydrogen. The high localized pH in the vicinity of the cathode can cause precipitation of calcium scales that can impair the flow of current in such systems. A common feature is current reversal, where the polarity of the electrodes is switched so that scales formed on the cathodic cycle are dissolved on the anodic cycle. For this reason, electrodes are designed to possess dual anodic and cathodic properties; the most common configuration is platinized titanium. High volumetric flow rates through the cells also ensure that electrodes are swept free of current-blocking scale.

Direct Br^- ion electrolysis for disinfection of recreational water has been commercialized[43] but was later withdrawn from the market because photochemical bromate formation could not be adequately controlled. Direct electrolysis of a mixed NaCl/NaBr solution was reported to proceed with high efficiency and conversion of Br^- into a biocidal solution of HOBr. The patent assignee did not seek EPA regulatory approval for the product, so it has not been marketed to date (Howart et al[44]; R. Sergent, oral communication, June 1994).

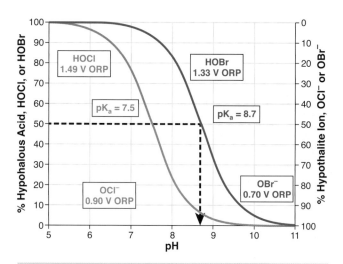

FIGURE 17.11 Hypochlorous acid (HOCl) and hypobromous acid dissociation curves. Both HOCl and hypochlorite (OCl^-) are considered "free available chlorine" or FAC. At pH 8.7, 50% of the bromine is in the most effective hypobromous acid (HOBr) form versus 5% for chlorine.

▶ COMMERCIAL USES OF BROMINE BIOCIDES

Cooling Water Treatment

Environmental concerns in the mid-1980s caused the shift from acid feed with chromate to acid feed with chromate/zinc and, finally, to alkaline-based water treatment programs for industrialized water treatment.[26] These alkaline-based programs relied on polyphosphates and, later, phosphonates and copolymers for corrosion and scale control.[27] Overall, traditional chlorine biocides were less effective in these new, higher pH environments that were now typically more like 8.5 versus the 6.0 to 7.0 employed with chromate-based programs (Figure 17.11). When pH control is discontinued, the pH of cooling water trends to pH 8.5 to 8.8. For example, at pH 8.7, 50% of HOBr is neutral and undissociated (the conjugate OBr^- ion is charged and is repelled away by the negative surface charge of microorganisms). Undissociated HOBr is not charged and suffers no repulsive forces. Compare this to the 5% HOCl present for chlorine treatment at the same pH. Thus, bromine treatment of cooling water has become mainstream, inspiring the development of the products discussed in this chapter.

One of the first applications of BCDMH to an industrial cooling system occurred in the late 1970s in a chemical plant located in El Dorado, AR (R. Sergent, oral communication, August 2003). In the 1980s, several patents were issued relating to the use of BCDMH in cooling systems.[45,46] Zhang and Matson[47] performed a thorough study of the disinfection effectiveness of BCDMH. Data showed that BCDMH was more effective than chlorine at pH 8.5 when dosed to the same residual against all bacteria tested—*E coli*, *Enterobacter aerogenes*, and *Pseudomonas*

aeruginosa. They also showed that BCDMH and other bromine biocides were effective in the presence of NH_3. Many studies have subsequently demonstrated that the effectiveness of BCDMH in the laboratory carries over to the field. A petrochemical plant with 90/10 copper/nickel alloy heat exchangers converted from gaseous chlorine to BCDMH.[48] The conversion resulted in lower overall biocide usage, consistent pH control, lower consumption of corrosion inhibitor (tolyltriazole), and overall lower corrosion rates on copper alloy. A 1-year field study in a refinery cooling system indicated that BCDMH use led to similar results with better control of both sessile and bulk water bacteria counts and lower corrosion rates on yellow metal compared to gaseous chlorine.[49]

Published case studies in 1993 compared the performance of BCDMH to chlorine gas in utility recirculating cooling systems.[50] In one system, BCDMH dosed to 0.4 ppm free residual chlorine (20 minutes feed time, once per day) provided improved microbiological control compared to the chlorine treatment regime (0.5 ppm free residual for 30 minutes per day). Bulk bacteria plate counts ranged from 10^5 to 10^7 CFU/mL under the chlorine/nonoxidizing biocide program compared with $<10^3$ CFU/mL under the BCDMH program. In addition, corrosion rates on 90/10 copper/nickel alloy decreased from 0.8 mpy (chlorine) to 0.1 to 0.4 mpy (BCDMH).

The hydrolysis chemistry of BCDMH was also studied and showed that it could be described as a facile release of HOBr, followed by a slow release of HOCl[47]:

$$BCDMH + H_2O = CDMH + HOBr \text{ fast}$$

$$CDMH + H_2O = DMH + HOCl \text{ slow}$$

Indeed, analysis of BCDMH in demand free waters by the free and total DPD methods indicate that about half of the oxidant value analyzes as free halogen (ie, free HOBr) with the other half analyzing as combined halogen (ie, combined chlorine as CDMH).[51] Excess bromide ion and warm water temperatures apparently aid the hydrolysis of the chlorine atom with generation of HOBr via the following reaction (see the following text). For example, it is common practice to preload a hot tub or spa on a BCDMH disinfection program with NaBr.[52] This suggests that under certain biocide application regimens, that is, shock dosing with short biocide residence time, both the halogens in BCDMH may not be fully used for microbiological control purposes.[5]

Older reports found that HOBr could be generated from an equimolar combination of NaBr and chlorine, as shown in the following text.[53,54]

$$HOCl + Br^- = HOBr + Cl^-$$

This reaction depends on the concentration of HOCl in solution and thus the rate decreases at higher pH.[55] Due to the instability of OBr^-, the solution must be used immediately. In the 1970s, it was realized that one could introduce NaBr and chlorine into a water system and thus generate bromine species in situ.[56] Proper mixing of bromide and oxidant is essential, particularly in the presence of NH_3 and other sources of contamination.[57]

Moore et al[58] replaced a combination of chlorine gas and a nonoxidizing biocide with activated NaBr in eight chemical plant cooling towers. The activated NaBr program provided effective biocontrol at low continuous residuals of 0.1 ppm and led to overall reductions in mild steel corrosion in 5 of the 8 towers in the study. In addition, the cooling tower discharge proved compatible with artificial marsh posttreatment, significantly reducing the amount of water disposed of using injection wells. Nalepa et al[59] compared activated NaBr to both high-dose and low-dose chlorine treatment regimens in an industrial cooling system operating between pH 8.2 to 8.4 using well water for makeup. Activated NaBr, fed continuously to an average residual of 0.11 free and 0.15 total (as Cl_2), provided effective microbiological control and led to a substantial decrease in general and pitting corrosion on mild steel. This was said to be due to the combination of chemical (less attack on passivated surfaces) and biological (better control of heterotrophic and sessile bacteria) factors.

Water treatment service companies have used a variety of ways of activating solutions of NaBr, including

- Addition of NaBr and NaOCl solutions to makeup or recirculating cooling water and then directing the solution to a residence chamber, where sufficient time is allowed for the activation to occur
- Addition of NaBr and NaOCl solutions together without any dilution water to an in-line static mixer then directing the mixture to the cooling water basin
- Addition of NaBr directly to the basin followed by separate addition an NaOCl to accomplish activation in the cooling water

The activation of NaBr with bleach has been reviewed.[60] The various means of introducing a source of NaBr and a source of bleach were compared on the basis of

- The time it took for the maximum bromine concentration to be attained
- The % conversion of Br^- ion in HOBr/OBr^-
- The % of total halogen recovered
- The stability of the activated solutions

Experimental data was compared to the model predicted by a landmark paper on the subject.[61] It was concluded that direct introduction of concentrated NaBr and NaOCl solutions into the opposite-end of a Tee-fitting in the absence of makeup/dilution water and then piping the mixture into the cooling water to be treated was the most efficient means of activating Br^- ion (Figure 17.12).

High conversion rates (85%) in such systems are immediately obtained. Although this type of activation occurs at an adversely high pH (12.86), the high concentration of the NaBr and NaOCl, reactants offsets any pH inefficiencies on the rate of the reaction. Use of a molar excess of NaOCl over the NaBr is advantageous in terms of cost because the excess hypochlorite serves to regenerate oxidizing bromine from the Br^- ion degradate of HOBr/OBr^-. This method benefits from ease of use in that no residence tanks are required. Furthermore, because it avoids the use of makeup or dilution water, calcium carbonate scaling problems in equipment and pipework caused by the high pH conditions of bleach solutions are eliminated.

The reaction of chlorine compounds with bromide still remains a widespread method of achieving the benefits of bromine chemistry in industrial water systems. It is the most inexpensive way of introducing bromine to water and is prevalent for large cooling systems at power plants, for example. Activated NaBr is the preferred bromine biocide for cooling water contaminated with NH_3 or urea (fertilizer plants), or if the NH_3 chiller systems are known to be leaking their contents. Cooling towers employing municipal wastewater as makeup water (rich in NH_3 and organic nitrogen) will also select activated NaBr as the biocide of choice.

As convenient single-feeds, sulfamic acid–stabilized products were widely embraced for use in industrial cooling water treatment. STABR-EX was the pioneering first product that was introduced.[62] The inventors sought to bolster the technology and a flurry of other US patents followed. These included widening the scope of suitable Br^- ion oxidants[62] and synergistic combinations with nonoxidizing biocides.[63] Since its introduction in 1997,

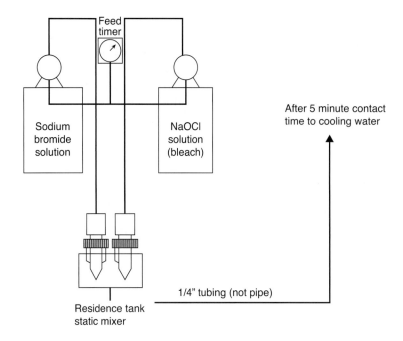

FIGURE 17.12 Depiction of the mixture method as a means of activating Br⁻ ions.

hundreds of billions of gallons of water have been treated with this product. McCoy et al[64] reviewed the advantages of a sulfamic acid–stabilized bromine product compared to traditional chlorine and bromine biocide technologies. These included 10 times higher thermal stability than NaOCl bleach, less aggressive than water treatment chemicals for scale and corrosion inhibitors, and an improved environmental toxicity profile. The success of STABR-EX spurred a competitive response[65-67] and a sulfamic acid–stabilized bromine product employing BrCl was introduced as Stabrom 909. Subsequent developments included methods for continuous processing,[68,69] biofilm removal,[70] and the use of Stabrom 909 for biocontrol in oil and gas environments such as hydraulic fracturing.[71]

With continued use of sulfamic acid–stabilized bromine products in cooling water systems, sulfamate ion can accumulate in treated water and give rise to a condition known as "overstabilization." This is manifest as reduced oxidation reduction potential measurements compared to the normal condition and diminished efficacy (higher planktonic plate counts, development of algae) despite maintaining target bromine residuals. It is generally associated with continuous dosing and high cycles of concentration. As the sulfamate accumulates in a cooling tower, Le Châtelier principle dictates that the bromine is less labile to release from the sulfamate moiety (Figure 17.13).

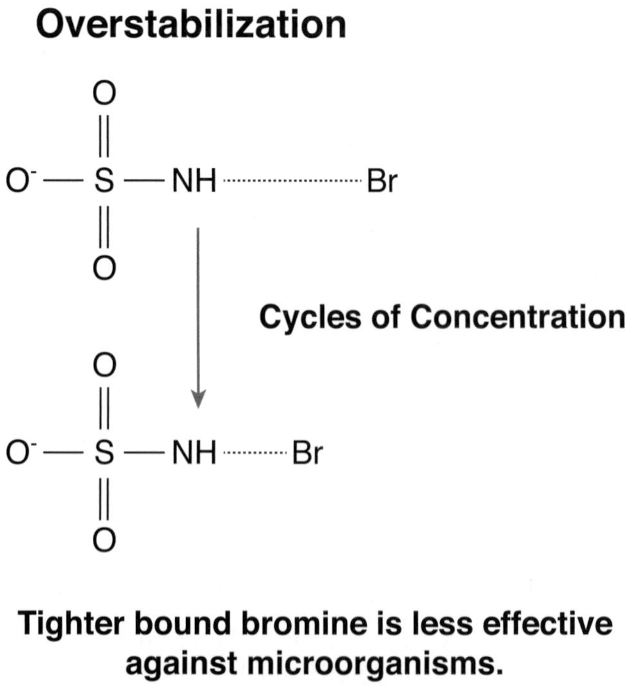

Overstabilization

$$O^- \!-\! S \!-\! NH \cdots\cdots\cdots Br$$

Cycles of Concentration

$$O^- \!-\! S \!-\! NH \cdots\cdots Br$$

Tighter bound bromine is less effective against microorganisms.

FIGURE 17.13 Depiction of the effects of overstabilization with sulfamic acid–stabilized bromine products.

A remediation measure to lower sulfamic acid residues is believed to exist. It involves the introduction of sodium nitrite, which reacts according to the following equation[72]:

$$NaNO_2 + HSO_3NH_2 = N_2 + NaHSO_4 + H_2O$$

A synthetic cooling water system designed to simulate treatment with stabilized bromine was prepared. The pH was adjusted to 8.8 to mirror that of typical cooling water and to deprotonate residual sulfamic acid. Sufficient $NaNO_2$ was introduced to react with 70 ppm of sulfamate ion. The treated sample was analyzed by ion chromatography (IC) for sulfamate ion. It was found that the nitrite treatment was ineffective in decreasing the amount of sulfamate ion present and 70 ppm was recovered quantitatively (M. Kondolf, oral communication, January 2019). It was concluded that $NaNO_2$ may only be reactive to sulfamic acid because it has no effect on its conjugate ion.

Unfortunately, there is no commercially available test kit for the water treater to determine the sulfamic acid level in the cooling water. Consequently, there is no way of knowing the amount of sodium nitrite to administer or if the remediation method has been effective at sulfamic acid removal/reduction. The only recognized cure for allegedly overstabilized water is to partially drain the system and refill with fresh water. This is not desirable as other water treatment products (eg, corrosion and scale inhibitors) are correspondingly diluted and must be replenished.

Sulfamic acid–stabilized bromine products are popular with water treatment service companies belonging to members of the Association of Water Technologies (AWT). These companies service the cooling water requirements of small evaporative condensers associated with heating, ventilation, and air conditioning (HVAC) and comfort cooling systems. The simplicity and convenience of these products permit efficient use of valuable time during service visits.

Finally, dry bromide/isocyanurate mixture commercial products for water treatment were introduced several years ago.[73,74] These products use a combination of SDIC or TCCA (see Figure 17.9) with NaBr to generate HOBr in situ in the water system. The mole ratio of NaBr to chlorine oxidant is less than one. This takes advantage of bromide buildup in recirculating water systems and promotes more efficient utilization of bromine values to optimize product economics.[75] Field studies indicate effective microbiological control at reduced consumption rates relative to other halogen donor systems, such as BCDMH and TCCA.

Recreational Water Treatment

A review on some aspects of bromine chemistry used for swimming pools was first published in the 1970s,[76] but it was not until the solid halogenated hydantoins were introduced in in the mid-1980s that their use for recreational water (swimming pools, spas) purposes gained momentum. Bather contamination, including urine, fecal matter, sweat, etc, means the properties of haloamines are exploited in the treatment of recreational water. Haloamines are formed as a result of the reaction of HOBr or HOCl with NH_3 and organic nitrogen. Bromamines and chloramines both have powerful lachrymator (eye irritation) properties. The main difference is that bromamines are very short-lived, whereas chloramines can persist for many days. What this translates to is

- Brominated water does not cause eye, skin, and respiratory discomfort that chlorinated pool water does.
- Brominated water does not require "breakpoint halogenation" (shocking) that chlorinated pool water does.
- Brominated recreational water does not give rise to odors and vapor phase corrosion that (indoor) chlorinated pool water does.

In addition, bromamines have potent biocidal properties, whereas chloramines diminish the efficacy of free chlorine. It is widely accepted in the recreational water industry that the bather experience in brominated water far surpasses that in chlorinated water. Why then does chlorination remain the overwhelming swimming pool sanitation practice? There are two main reasons for this. The first is cost. Bromine sanitizers such as BCDMH are 3 to 5 times more costly than inexpensive chlorinated sanitizers such as NaOCl in combination with hydrochloric acid (HCl) (also known as muriatic acid). The second is instability of bromine to sunlight. Chlorinated water can be stabilized to sunlight decomposition by introduction of cyanuric acid (CYA) (1,3,5-triazine-2,4,6-(1H,3H,5H)-trione) or its sodium salt.[77] The CYA forms a stable N-Cl chlorine complex that resists ultraviolet (UV) degradation. No such nitrogen additive exists for brominated products such as BCDMH. Of course, the relative strength of the N-Br bond (276 ± 21 kJmol^{-1}) compared to the N-Cl bond (334 ± 9.6 kJmol^{-1})[78] means the thermodynamics are not favorable. Regardless, it has been of some interest to find an additive that imparts UV stabilizing properties to brominated pool water. Such a quest has been met with spectacularly staggering failure to date (J.N.H., unpublished data, 1993). CYA imparts no UV stabilizing properties to brominated water. In fact, model experiments were subsequently conducted with a simple sunlamp in the laboratory to prove this and test a range of other potential stabilizer candidates possessing imide and amide functionality (J.N.H., unpublished data, 1991). The DMH alone enhanced UV stability of additive-free brominated water and DMH was patented for use with an electrobrominated pool water system.[79] An additional benefit was that DMH eliminated photochemical bromate formation. In general, high pK_a amides and imides such as DMH (pK_{a1} 9.1), succinimide (pK_a 9.6), and glutarimide (pK$_a$ 9.8) conveyed brominated water with superior UV stabilization properties over lower pK$_a$ materials such as CYA (pK$_{a1}$ 6.13).

For the reasons of cost and the inability to efficiently stabilize bromine from UV degradation, BCDMH has found use in small volume residential pools. Commonly, these pools are typically open for the relatively short summer season. The BCDMH is rarely used for commercial pools, such as those found at hotels, schools, and sports facilities. The volume of water requiring treatment is too large for bromination to be economical. One exception was the use of a BCDMH O$_3$ combination.[80] O$_3$ was used to regenerate HOBr from the spent Br$^-$ ion. Depending on the size of the O$_3$ generator employed, BCDMH consumption could be cut from 3 to 5 lb/10,000 gallon/week typically required for residential pools to a fraction of the amount. This system was employed on the competition pools at the 1996 Olympic Games in Atlanta, GA. Due to the high cost and unreliability of O$_3$ generators, the BCDMH/O$_3$ system is not offered today.

As indicated earlier in Figure 17.1, elevated temperatures and aeration drive off CO$_2$ and raise the pH of the water. Hence, bromination is the predominant sanitizer chemistry for spas and hot tubs because of the following properties that have been discussed earlier:

- Diminished efficacy of chlorine in the prevailing pH
- Reduced volatility of HOBr compared to HOCl[81]
- Higher bather inputs of NH$_3$ and organic nitrogen per volume of treated water compared to larger swimming pools

For routine maintenance, a few halogenated hydantoin tablets or granules can be introduced to the cartridge filter housing or used in small floating feeder devices. Halogenated hydantoins dissolve slowly due to their sparingly soluble nature. When a shock dose is required, such as just before or after a heavy bather load, the much more soluble SDIC/NaBr mixture is frequently administered. An alternative is to employ potassium peroxymonosulfate (2KHSO$_5$•KHSO$_4$•K$_2$SO$_4$; known by the tradename Oxone). This solubilizes rapidly and reoxidizes the Br$^-$ ion bank, which has accumulated in the water through routine use of brominated products.

Bromine is recognized to have superior algicidal properties in comparison to chlorine. This is because in the summer months, algae photosynthesize more dissolved CO$_2$ and drive the pool water pH upwards (see Figure 17.1). The acid dissociation curves shown Figure 17.11 explain the superior biocidal performance of bromine under conditions of elevated pH. When conventionally chlorinated pools developed algae problems, it was common practice to add a dose of NaBr to temporarily substitute the sanitizer chemistry to bromine to remediate the pool of algae. But this practice was accompanied by a large increase in consumption of the primary chlorine sanitizer in order to maintain normal halogen residuals. This was

because the CYA stabilization chemistry for chlorinated water conferred no such stabilization properties for brominated water. After a few days, the pool would revert to the normally stabilized condition. Clearly, the Br$^-$ ion has been depleted and irreversibly lost as highly stable BrO$_3^-$ ion, which is considered by EPA to be a possible human carcinogen. Once the fate of the Br$^-$ ion was understood, the suppliers of NaBr algaecides voluntarily withdrew their products from the market.

Sulfamic acid–stabilized bromine products are not registered as recreational water disinfectants. Preliminary testing indicated that these products could not pass the rigorous disinfection criteria that EPA requires. To qualify as a swimming pool sanitizer, the chemistry must perform the equivalent to 0.4 ppm residual chlorine against cultures of *E coli* and *Enterococcus faecium*.[82] Complete eradication must be demonstrated after 30 seconds for *E coli* and 2 minutes for *E faecium*.

Food Sanitation

The first use of a brominated product for food sanitation purposes was patented for DBDMH in the early 2000s.[83] A US Food and Drug Administration (FDA) food contact notification (FCN) was approved in 2003 as a sanitizer for use in poultry. During processing, poultry products are immersed in a cold water tank to reduce the temperature of the carcass and to arrest proliferation of disease-causing *Salmonella* and *Campylobacter* bacteria, which can be spread to people consuming contaminated chicken and turkeys. The chill tank represented an environment that depressed the activity of chlorinated products, namely high NH$_3$ and organic nitrogen loading from fecal and gastrointestinal releases into the water. The relatively higher volatility of chloramine,[84] coupled with its stability and powerful lachrymatory properties, caused discomfort to workers in the vicinity of the chill tank for these chlorine-based applications. Bromamines from DBDMH had no such negative properties. The DBDMH was also commercialized and patented for use on red meat (beef and pork).[85]

Although satisfied with the microbiological efficacy of DBDMH, the meat and poultry processing industries experienced difficulties due to its sparingly soluble nature. Solubilization of DBDMH granules proved troublesome. To obtain the required concentration, the water had to be directed through a series of chemical feeders housing the granules. Feeding was inconsistent because the height of the bed of granules was reduced as the granules dissolved. Moreover, the feeders required frequent, manpower-intensive refilling. Individuals charged with this task had to haul 50 lb (22 kg) pails of product into the chemical feeders, only to be confronted by risks of exposure to irritating dust as the granules were delivered. This prompted industry demand for an "all-liquid" HOBr product that was not limited by solubility issues and was capable of being dosed automatically. Shortly thereafter, an alternative system was offered meeting these needs.[86] Based on uncommercialized cooling water products developed earlier,[87] the product employed an aqueous solution of 24% aqueous HBr in conjunction with aqueous NaOCl bleach. Oxidation kinetics of Br^- to HOBr were virtually instantaneous and proceeded with 100% conversion unencumbered by the pH limitations of the reaction first reported by Kumar and Margerum[61] years earlier. It was reported that oxidation of Br^- by HOBr was 1.7×10^6 times faster than the reaction with OCl^-. In the oxidation of HBr by NaOCl, the reaction was accompanied by a dramatic color change as orange Br_2/Br_3^- (formed under acidic pH conditions) is hydrolyzed into a faint yellow HOBr solution as the pH swings from 1.6 to near neutral on NaOCl addition. This is depicted graphically in Figure 17.14 and represents the color changes observed as aliquots of NaOCl bleach are successively added to a dilute solution of HBr. In practice, the activation of HBr into HOBr is very rapid and can be accomplished continuously in a pipe with flow water flowing to the carcass wash or poultry chill tank. A simple sight glass and pH probe assures the operator proper activation has been achieved.

This trend is perfectly consistent with the phase diagram for bromine speciation during the activation event. The phase diagram in Figure 17.15 defines the thermodynamic speciation of bromine as a function of pH. At preactivation, the solution contains only HBr and is acidic. As the NaOCl is introduced, aqueous Br_2 predominates and the solution acquires a deep orange color. Continued addition of NaOCl oxidizes more Br^- ion and forces the pH to rise. Finally, when Br^- oxidation is complete, the pH is close to neutral and all of the bromine exists in the form of HOBr, which is nonchromophoric,

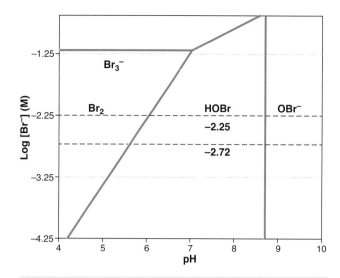

FIGURE 17.15 Principal species of bromine in equilibrium with the bromine and hydrogen ions at various pH values.[39]

hence the decrease in absorbance. The activated solution appears as a faint yellow coloration. The FDA has granted FCN when the safety and efficacy of food processing aids has been satisfactorily demonstrated. The FCNs 944 and 1036 allow solutions of HOBr to be used on meat at levels between 300 and 900 ppm (expressed as Br_2). The horizontal dotted lines at log $[Br^-]$ -2.25 and -2.72 define the boundary levels of Br^- ion activated into HOBr at the permitted levels.

Coupled with the more favorable economics of the 24% HBr/NaOCl system and the ease of use of all liquid products, this technology was rapidly adopted by the red meat industry where it was introduced to the carcass washing process.[88] As evidenced by the octanol/water partition coefficient,[86] the extreme lipophilicity of HOBr was particularly exploited by the beef processing industry. The exterior of beef carcasses is composed of 90% fat, and HOBr displays an affinity for the lipid phase. The success of the HOBr chemistries almost rendered the use of steam sterilization cabinets in certain applications obsolete because the beef processing industry sought to use an ambient temperature intervention step that did not cook the outside of the meat. When HOBr was introduced in early 2010, it was quickly adopted by a major meat packer at 6 of its 7 packing plants. Two other major meats packers also had processing plants using the 24% HBr/NaOCl system. In 2014, Japan permitted the reimportation of American beef and, at the time, the use of a bromine-based food processing aid was not permitted. There followed a lengthy approval period before industry interest was reawakened to this need in November 2018.[89]

The HOBr activity from both DBDMH and 24% HBr/NaOCl has been compared. Pieces of beef and pork were inoculated with field strain cultures of *E coli* O157:H7. 1 hour was allowed for surface attachment. Each piece

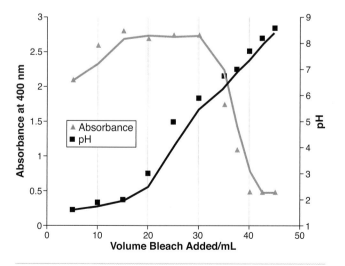

FIGURE 17.14 Absorbance versus pH of a solution of hydrobromic acid oxidizing to hypobromous acid as bleach is added. Reproduced from Howard et al.[87]

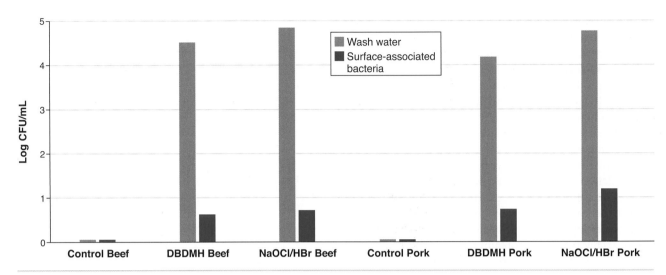

FIGURE 17.16 Log_{10} reduction of bacteria, both in wash water and surface associated, on beef and pork following 1,3-dibromo-5,5-dimethylhydantoin (DBDMH) or sodium hypochlorite (NaOCl)/hydrobromic acid (HBr) treatment.

was then sprayed for 30 seconds with 300 ppm as Br_2. The wash solutions were collected to determine the wash off, whereas any viable surface-associated bacteria remaining were dislodged into sterile water by vigorous agitation. The average results of triplicate analysis were compared to a city water control (Figure 17.16).

Both DBDMH and NaOCl/HBr treatments afford excellent reductions of bacteria present in the wash water; however, NaOCl/HBr displays a measurably greater efficacy than DBDMH. The same trend is apparent in reducing the surface-associated bacteria. The slightly better performance of the NaOCl/HBr system may be explained on the basis that it is unstabilized HOBr, whereas DBDMH confers stabilization properties rendering it less effective at short contact times representative of wash cabinets.

Animal carcasses are contaminated with bacteria during the hide removal process as the partially undressed hide contacts the inner food product. Hide-on carcass wash cabinets are employed to physically remove fecal matter with high-pressure water. The hide-on wash may be recycled carcass wash solution that has been replenished with HOBr by simple addition of NaOCl and inexpensive HCl. An in-plant trial was performed using NaOCl/HBr solutions as a hide-on wash. A concentration of 220 ppm as Br_2 afforded a 2.23 log_{10} reduction of *E coli* O157:H7 after a 15-second spray. Extending the spray time to 2 minutes reduced the number of hides with enumerable *Salmonella* by 80%.

Determination of Residual Bromine in Water

As discussed earlier, analytical methods for the determination of halogen concentrations in water frequently employ the indicator DPD, which is oxidized by halogens to yield a pink complex.[90] The color intensity is measured by photometric absorbance of the solution and is reflective of the amount of halogen initially present. Alternatively, a color comparator wheel is rotated until a match is made with the color that the sample develops on contact with the DPD indicator. Both methods are simple, inexpensive, and can be performed quickly with portable devices. The DPD procedure is accepted by the EPA for reporting halogen levels in wastewater.[91] The DPD method readily distinguishes free chlorine (eg, HOCl, OCl^-) from nitrogen bound chlorine (eg, NH_2Cl) via the free and total DPD reagents. The total chlorine DPD indicator contains buffer and solid potassium iodide (KI). Following a 3-minute development time, nitrogen-bound chlorine releases iodine which reacts with the DPD indicator to turn pink. Combined chlorine is then obtained by subtraction of free chlorine response from the total chlorine response.

In NH_3 and organic nitrogen rich environments, it is important to know how the chlorine is speciated because nitrogen-bound chlorine is much less efficacious to microorganisms than free chlorine. No method exists to distinguish free bromine (HOBr, OBr^-) from combined bromine. Indeed, a method is unnecessary because nitrogen-bound bromine is widely considered to be just as biocidal as the free bromine. Thus, the terms free bromine and combined bromine are synonymous. Residual bromine is a preferred description and embraces all active forms.

On the other hand, bromine-treated waters often contain chlorine used to activate or regenerate Br^- ion. NaBr/NaOCl, HBr/NaOCl, and BCDMH products represent the presence of mixed bromo-chloro-systems. Under these circumstances, it is critical to know how the halogens are speciated to confirm that effective use of the expensive Br moieties is accomplished. An elegant method is known as the glycine modification of the DPD method.[90]

It relies on the formation of N-chloroglycine when it is introduced with a mixed bromo-chloro-containing water. The chloroamino acid is unreactive to the DPD indicator and the free chlorine response is due solely to the presence of bromine. Addition of a few crystals of KI, or use of the total DPD reagent, reveals the total halogen content of the water. Subtraction of the free chlorine reading from the total chlorine reading affords the chlorine content of the water.

Other, less popular methods for determination of halogen in water have been described.[91] They include the iodometric titration method suitable for highly concentrated solutions and halogenated products. Test strips are popular with spa and hot tub owners because of their rapid response, simplicity of use, and low cost. In general, test strips are not as accurate or precise as the more sophisticated methods but are adequate in certain applications.

▶ BROMINATED DISINFECTION BY-PRODUCTS

A discussion of brominated DBPs is warranted because water treated with bromine may be discharged to natural bodies of water such as rivers and the sea or, more frequently, delivered to publicly owned treatment works. Here, the water is often subject to further oxidation (commonly chlorination but sometimes ozonation) for disinfection purposes prior to discharge to the environment. The oxidation of bromide ion into HOBr and how this interacts with other materials also present in the water can give rise to a series of DBPs of toxological and environmental concern. In general, there are two categories of brominated DBPs formed when waters containing bromide ion are further oxidized for disinfection purposes. The first category contains those in which the resulting HOBr reacts with natural organic matter (NOM) such as humic and fulvic substances present in the water and includes trihalomethanes (THMs) and haloacetic acids (HAAs). Those in the second category are those that result in the formation of bromate ion (BrO_3^-). Each category will be discussed separately.

Due to their potential to cause cancer, the EPA limits the amount of total THMs and HAA in drinking water to 80 and 60 μg/L, respectively. But brominated THMs and HAAs are considered more cytotoxic and genotoxic than their chlorinated counterparts. The formation and toxicity of brominated DBPs during chlorination and chloramination has been reviewed.[92] More than 500 DBPs (brominated and chlorinated) have been identified, but only 20 are currently regulated, a number that is likely to increase as further geno- and cytotoxicity studies are reported. Oxidation of waters containing naturally occurring sources of Br^- ion (eg, from seawater intrusion), as well as those from treatment of Br^- ions from use of bromine disinfectants (eg, cooling water blowdown),

is known to produce HOBr. This is a kinetically superior substitution agent to HOCl and reacts efficiently with NOM to produce brominated DBPs.[93] A number of other brominated DBPs have also been identified, including brominated phenols, brominated hydroxybenzoic acids, brominated hydroquinones, and brominated carboxylic acids,[94] but these have not come yet under regulatory scrutiny. Another study[95] reported the presence of 2,3,5-tribromopryrole in bromide ion–containing water treated with chlorine dioxide. This was reported to be many times more cytotoxic than dibromoacetic acid, 3-chlor-4-(dichlormethyl)-5-hydroxy-1-[5H]-furanone (more commonly referred to as MX), and potassium bromate with similar genotoxicity to that of MX. A review[96] identified over 100 DBPs found in indoor chlorinated (NaOCl) and brominated (BCDMH) swimming pool water. In fact, brominated DBPs were present in the chlorine-treated pool. This is hardly surprising because pool products containing Br^- ion are commonly introduced to chlorinated water for enhanced control of algae. Swimming pools represent a unique environment because the brominated DBP profile is governed by swimmer inputs including urine, fecal matter, sweat, cosmetics, skin, and hair. More brominated and chlorinated DBPs were found in these indoor pools than in previous outdoor pool studies, indicating that DBPs are volatilized and photolyzed in outdoor settings. The review concluded that the brominated and chlorinated indoor pools had different DBP profiles and bromoform was the prevalent THM in brominated water but possessed similar mutagenicity to that of typical chlorinated drinking water.

The hydrolytic stabilities of halogenated DBPs were reviewed[97] and followed the order haloketone > haloacetonitrile > haloacetaldehyde > haloacetic acid > trihalomethane for chlorinated and brominated species and increased with increasing number of halogen atoms with the DBP group. Similarly, the rate of hydrolysis increased in the order F < Cl < Br < I. Thus, although brominated THMs are considered to possess higher cyto- and geno-toxicities than their chlorinated counterparts, this is balanced by their shorter environmental persistence and faster break down in water.

The bromate ion (BrO_3^-) is considered to be a probable human carcinogen. The EPA limits its presence to 10 μg/L in drinking water. The most common source of bromate is ozonation of waters containing Br^- ion (Figure 17.17). The mechanism was first elucidated in the landmark paper of the subject.[98] The O_3 oxidizes Br^- ions at a moderate rate to OBr^- ions and HOBr (pK$_a$ HOBr 8.7). The O_3 reacts slowly with OBr^- ions to form BrO_3^-. Lower pH favors the formation of HOBr, which can be intercepted by organic matter and NH_3.[99] Notably, the rate of the reverse reaction (back to Br^- ion) is faster than the rate of bromate formation. Eventually, however, on prolonged ozonation, all of the Br^- ion would irreversibly be manifest as BrO_3^-. This work inspired a

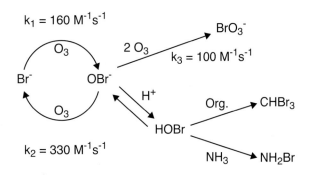

FIGURE 17.17   Schematic of mechanisms of the reactions of ozonation of water containing Br^- ions. Reprinted with permission from Haag and Hoigne.[98] Copyright © 1983 American Chemical Society.

later US patent[80] that covered the ozonation of BCDMH treated swimming pool water. It was shown that DMH in the ozonated water could intercept HOBr akin to NH_3 and suppress bromate formation.

Subsequent work[82,99-103] reported that BrO_3^- can also be formed by oxidation of Br^- through the intermediacy of $HOBr/OBr^-$ via a pure hydroxyl radical (OH^-) pathway in advanced oxidation processes (AOPs). In the presence of hydrogen peroxide (H_2O_2), BrO_3^- ceased because the production of OH radicals in the AOP was insufficient to overcome the rate of reduction of $HOBr/OBr^-$ by H_2O_2. Given that 10 μg/L BrO_3^- is allowed by EPA in drinking water, none of the methods are entirely satisfactory or economical. In fact, it might be argued that O_3 should not be considered as a drinking water disinfection option if the treated water contains any level of Br^- ion over 1 ppm.

Under the US Federal Insecticide, Fungicide, and Rodenticide Act (FIFRA) Section 6(a)(2) regulations, registrants of EPA-registered biocides are obligated to report factual information regarding unreasonable adverse effects on the environment through use of their pesticide. Oblivious to the known photolytic formation of bromate in chlorinated seawater,[104] registrants of certain recreational water bromine products have been compelled to report the formation of bromate under this regulation. Sometimes the copious amounts found have been many 100s of times the 10 μg/L permitted in drinking water.[105] Therefore, bromate formation in brominated swimming pool water has recently come to the attention of EPA. In response, a data call-in (DCI)[106] was issued to the registrants of brominated biocides used in recreational water treatment. The EPA has ordered the registrants of brominated hydantoins to perform a study on the formation of bromate. The results of the study are expected to be used as a risk assessment for human exposure, and, if necessary, set a limit on the amount of bromate that will be permitted. Unfortunately, bromate is a highly refractory ion and cannot be chemically reduced by any known practical means. Drainage and refill is the only recognized practice.

REGULATORY OUTLOOK

North America

Bromine biocides are pesticidal products promulgated by the EPA under the FIFRA regulation. Every 15 years, the EPA reviews the data on file for each and every pesticidal product. The EPA then decides whether the data on file is sufficient to reregister the product or whether there are data gaps that the EPA wishes to fill. Sometimes, data gaps are identified by the registrants themselves (see FIFRA 6(a)(2) in Brominated DBP section of this chapter). As a widely used halogenated product, brominated biocides are scrutinized. When concerns are identified, the EPA issues the registrants a DCI. This requires registrants to conduct studies deemed necessary. The agency allows the registrants a reasonable timeframe to fill the data gaps or to provide the agency with overwhelming technical arguments why such studies are unnecessary (submission of a waiver). Studies can range from something as simple as aquatic toxicity tests that might cost $5000 (in 2018) to be completed in 4 days, to 2-year carcinogenicity study costing $2.4 million. For budgetary reasons, registrants may pool resources and form a task force to obtain the necessary data. In addition, EPA requires that registrants pay annual maintenance fees of $3512 per registered product and state registration fees of around $100 to $400 are payable annually for biocides sold in those regions.

The Pesticide Management Regulatory Agency (PMRA) has regulatory oversight for biocides in Canada. Initial registration costs for a new pesticide not previously registered in Canada can be daunting. The agency requires registrants supply a suite of high-priced, lengthy (18-24 months) studies including oncogenicity, genotoxicity, prenatal development, and neurotoxicity. Certain sulfamic acid–stabilized products that feature NaOCl as an active ingredient (STABR-EX, BromMax 7.1) were exempt from these requirements and are registered in Canada, whereas the products employing a mixture of bromo- and chlorosulfamates (STABROM 909, MAXXIS) as active ingredients are not currently registered.

Europe

Historically, the regulation of biocidal products and the active substances that they contain has varied considerably across Member States within the EU, with some products being regulated and others not on a country by country basis. The complexities of the national regulatory systems were considered to be a barrier to free trade within the EU and new EU legislation, the Biocidal Products Directive (BPD), was proposed and finally adopted in 1998. Under the BPD, biocidal active substances that were already present on the market before May 14, 2000, could continue to be used in formulated products. The BPD was widely recognized to be difficult to implement. The inability to meet deadlines coupled with some confusion among the regulators, biocide suppliers, and consultants prompted a major revision in the form of a new regulation, the Biocidal Product Regulation (BPR).[107] The introduction of the BPR introduced new elements that were not included in the BPD, specifically Article 95 of the regulation. Under this article, suppliers had to submit to the European Chemicals Agency (ECHA) either an extensive data dossier or a letter of access to the data. The high costs involved in either approach meant that many companies elected not to pursue registration of their biocides in EU. Regrettably, if, and when, the BPR is fully implemented, EU countries will have a dwindling shorter list of biocide options from which to choose. It was originally planned to complete the evaluation of all active substances by 2010; this was then extended to 2014. Due to delays in achieving these targets, the current deadline for completion has been put back until December 31, 2014. Britain's exit from the EU ("Brexit") in 2019 is likely to foster further confusion; the country is one of the largest users of biocides in Europe. The regulatory outlook for bromine biocides in the EU paints an uncertain future.

Rest of the World

In contrast to North America and EU, the regulatory landscape for bromine biocides in most other countries (including Japan, Australia, Korea, and Latin America) is oftentimes very straightforward and streamlined. It is recognized that the use of brominated cooling water biocides has limited human health hazards. As long as the active ingredients are on the Toxic Substances Control Act (TSCA)-equivalent list, the biocide will be approved for use in that country. Usually the country will require submission of the product label, a Globally Harmonized System, Safety Data Sheet (SDS) and Technical Data Sheet.

The use of brominated biocides for direct use on food is different. Japan only allows products that are listed in the US Code of Federal Regulations (CFR) Title 21 Food and Drugs Parts 21 to 179. But as bromine-based biocides do not enjoy a CFR listing, there follows a lengthy approval process of up to 4 years by the Japanese Ministry of Health Labor and Welfare and Food Safety Commission before approval.[89] The Food Standards Australia New Zealand also has an arduous submission requirement but the review process may only take a year before approval.

Residential pools are not widely used outside certain countries, such as the United States and Australia. Outdoor commercial pools (eg, at hotels, sports clubs, schools and those open to the public) are almost universally treated with some form of chlorine, as the brominated hydantoins are too expensive to disinfect large bodies of water. Plus, as mentioned earlier, unlike with chlorine chemistry, bromine cannot be adequately stabilized to photolytic degradation by sunlight. Spas and hot tubs find residential use in many countries. Due to its enhanced efficacy at elevated

pH, in tandem with its low volatility, bromine represents the preferred disinfectant option. In order to obtain EPA approval, registrants of brominated hydantoins have undergone extensive testing (safety, efficacy, environmental fate, and toxicity) and are deemed safe for human exposure by the agency. Countries where brominated hydantoins are sold accept that these biocides represent little health or environmental hazards and often waive further requirements.

▶ ACKNOWLEDGMENTS

The authors would like to thank their colleague, Ms. Chrissa Easter MS for her invaluable assistance in preparation of the manuscript. Chris Nalepa PhD is thanked for his helpful review and comments.

REFERENCES

1. Rossmoore HW. Nitrogen compounds. In: Block SS, ed. *Disinfection, Sterilization, and Preservation*. 4th ed. Philadelphia, PA: Lea & Febiger; 1991:chap 17.
2. Grinbaum B, Freiberg M. Bromine. In: *Kirk-Othmer Encyclopedia of Chemical Technology*. 4th ed. New York, NY: John Wiley and Son; 2001:1-28.
3. Yaron F. Bromine manufacture: technology and economic aspects. In: Jolles ZE, ed. *Bromine and Its Compounds*. New York, NY: Academic Press, 1966:12-32.
4. Arkansas Geological Commission. Bromine brine. http://www.state.ar.us/agc/bromine.htm. Accessed January 8, 2018.
5. Bartholomew RD. *Bromine-Based Biocides for Cooling Water Systems: A Literature Review*. IWC 98-74. Pittsburgh, PA: Engineers' Society of Western Pennsylvania; 1998.
6. Nalepa CJ. *25 Years of Bromine Chemistry in Industrial Water Systems: A Review*. Houston, TX: NACE International; 2004.
7. Henderson CT, inventor; Henderson CT, assignee. Process of antisepticizing water. US patent 1,995,639. March 26, 1935.
8. Tanner FW, Pitner G. Germicidal action of bromine. *Proceedings Soc Exp Biol Med*. 1939;40:143-145.
9. Wood DR, Illing ET. The sterilisation of sea water by means of chlorine. *Analyst*. 1930;55:125.
10. Beckwith TD, Moser JR. Germicidal effectiveness of chlorine, bromine, and iodine. *J Am Water Works Assoc*. 1933;25:367-374.
11. McCarthy JA. Bromine and chlorine dioxide as water disinfectants. *J New England Water Works Assoc*. 1944;58:55-68.
12. Wyss O, Stockton RJ. The germicidal action of bromine. *Arch Biochem*. 1947;12:267-271.
13. Shilov EA, Gladtchikova JN. On the calculation of the dissociation constants of hypohalogenous acids from kinetic data. *J Am Chem Soc*. 1938;60:490-491.
14. Ingham JW, Morrison J. The dissociation constant of hypochlorous acid: glass-electrode potential determination. *J Chem Soc*. 1933:1200-1205.
15. Rideal EK, Evans UR. The effect of alkalinity on the use of hypochlorites. *J Soc Chem Ind*. 1921;40:64R-66R.
16. Johns CK. Germicidal power of sodium hypochlorite. *Ind Eng Chem*. 1934;26:787-788.
17. Rudolph AS, Levine M. Factors affecting the germicidal efficiency of hypochlorite solutions. *Bulletin 150*. Ames, IA: Iowa State College, Engineering Experimental Station; 1941:1-48.
18. Dychala GR. Chlorine and chlorine compounds. In: Block SS, ed. *Disinfection, Sterilization, and Preservation*. 4th ed. Philadelphia, PA: Lea & Febiger; 1991:135-136.

19. Houghton GU. Bromide content of underground waters. II. Chlorination of Water containing free ammonia and naturally occurring bromide. *J Soc Chem Ind*. 1946;65:324-328.

20. Farkas-Himsley H. Killing of chlorine-resistant bacteria by chlorine-bromine solutions. *Appl Microbiol*. 1964;12:1-6.

21. Kamlet J, inventor; Kamlet J, assignee. Microbiocidal treatment of water with bromine chloride. US patent 2,662,855. December 15, 1953.

22. Kabler PW. Relative resistance of coliform organisms and enteric pathogens of water with chlorine. *J Am Water Works Assoc*. 1953;43:553-560.

23. Johannesson JK. The bromination of swimming pools. *Am J Public Health Nations Health*. 1960;50:1731-1736.

24. Johnson JD, Sun W. Bromine disinfection of wastewater. In: Johnson JD, ed. *Disinfection Water and Wastewater*. Ann Arbor, MI: Ann Arbor Science; 1975:170-192.

25. Johannesson JK. Anomalous bactericidal action of bromamine. *Nature*. 1958;181:1799-1780.

26. Evolution of industrial water conditioning. In: *Betz Handbook of Industrial Water Treatment*. 7th ed. Trevose, United Kingdom: Betz Laboratories Inc; 1976:11-15.

27. Sullivan PJ, Hepburn BJ. *The Evolution of Phosphonate Technology for Corrosion Inhibition*. Houston, TX: NACE International; 1995.

28. Kemmer FN, ed. *The Nalco Water Handbook*. 2nd ed. New York, NY: McGraw-Hill Book Company; 1987.

29. Aull R, Krell T. Design features and their effect on high performance fill. Paper presented at: 2000 Cooling Technology Institute Annual Meeting; May 2000; Houston, TX.

30. Lonza Water Treatment. Dantobrom Briquettes & Granular. http://www.lonzawatertreatment.co.za/products/biocides/dantobrom-briquettes-and-granular.aspx. Accessed January 8, 2018.

31. Sergent RH. Enhanced water management using bromine chemistry. Paper presented at: 1986 Cooling Tower Institute Annual Meeting; January 1986; Houston, TX.

32. Howarth JN, Peters BC, inventors; Albermarle Corporation, assignee. Compacted forms of halogenated hydantoins. US patent 6,965,035B1. November 15, 2015.

33. Dadgar A, Howarth JN, Sergent RH, Favstritsky NA, McKeown JA, Borden DW, Sanders BM, Likens J, inventors; PABU Services Inc, assignee. Inorganic perbromide compositions and methods of use thereof. US patent 5,607,619. March 4, 1997.

34. Favstritsky NA, inventor; Great Lakes Chemical Corp, assignee. Water Soluble organic ammonium per halides. US patent 4,886,915. December 12, 1989.

35. Goodenough RD, Place J, Parks CF, inventors; ETHYL Corp 30 SOUTH FOURTH STREET RICHMOND VIRGINIA 23217 A CORP OF VA, assignee. Stable bromo-sulfamate composition. US patent 3,558,503. January 26, 1971.

36. Howarth JN, Harvey MS, inventors; Enviro Tech Chemical Services Inc, assignee. Methods for the preparation of concentrated aqueous bromine solutions and high activity bromine-containing solids. US patent 7,309,503B2. December 18, 2007.

37. Howarth JN, Harvey MS, inventors; Enviro Tech Chemical Services Inc, assignee. Highly concentrated bromine compositions and methods of preparation. US patent 7,455,859. November 25, 2008.

38. Occidental Chemical Corporations. *Towerbrom Microbicides by Oxychem* [pamphlet]. Dallas, TX: Occidental Chemical Corporations; 2016.

39. Ethyl Corporation. *Bromine Chloride (BrCl)* [pamphlet]. Ferndale, MI: Ethyl Corporation; 1975.

40. Department of Homeland Security: Chemical facility anti-terrorism standards chemicals of interest list. https://www.dhs.gov/publication/cfats-coi-list. Published. Accessed January 9, 2018.

41. Pletcher D, Walsh FC. *Industrial Electrochemistry*. London, United Kingdom: Blackie Academic & Professional; 1993.

42. Howarth JN, Dadgar A. Some modern applications of bromide ion electrolysis. Paper presented at: Fifth International Forum on Electrolysis; November 10-14, 1991; Fort Lauderdale, FL.

43. Williams RC, Kettle CD, Stebbins EE, McCullough LM, inventors; AD REM MANUFACTURING Inc A CORP OF FLORIDA, Ad rem Manufacturing Inc, assignee. Electrolytic cell assembly and process for production of bromine. US patent 5,254,226. October 19, 1993.

44. Howarth JN, Dadgar A, Sergent RH, inventors; PABU Services Inc, assignee. Recovery of bromine and preparation of hypobromous acid from bromide solution. US patent 5,385,650. January 31, 1995.

45. Macchiarolo NT, McGuire BG, Scalise JM, inventors; Great Lakes Chemical Corp, assignee. Method for the control of biofouling in recirculating water systems. US patent 4,297,224. October 27, 1981.

46. Puzig EH, inventor; Great Lakes Chemical Corporation, assignee. Biocidal composition. WO patent 1,989,010,696A1. November 16, 1989.

47. Zhang Z, Matson JV. Organic halogen stabilizers: mechanisms and disinfection efficiencies. Paper presented at: 1989 Cooling Tower Institute Annual Meeting; January 1989; Houston, TX.

48. Vanderpool D, Killoran M, Sergent R. *Improving the Corrosion Inhibitor Efficiency of Tolyltriazole in the Presence of Chlorine and Bromine*. Houston, TX: NACE International; 1987.

49. Spurrell C, Clavin JS. *Solid Halogen Donor Economically Answers the Challenge of SARA Title III and Corrosion Concerns*. Houston, TX: NACE International; 1993.

50. Smith, Breckenridge R, Clay V, Swidle D. *Bromine vs. Gaseous Chlorine: A Comprehensive Review of Case Histories*. Houston, TX: NACE International; 1993.

51. Nalepa CJ. *New Bromine-Releasing Granules for Microbiological Control of Cooling Water*. Houston, TX: NACE International; 2003.

52. Arch HTH Water Chemicals. http://www.hth-pro.com. Accessed January 10, 2018.

53. Job Clarens J. Préparation de l'hypobromite par le bromure pour le dosage de l'urée; Preparation of Hypobromite from a Bromide for the Estimation of Urea. *J Pharm Chim*. 1909;30(VI):100-101.

54. Meilliére G. Sur la préparation de l'hyporbomite par le bromure de potassium et l'eau de Javel; On the Preparation of Hypobromite from a potassium bromide and Javel water. *J Pharm Chim*. 1909;30(VI):211.

55. Lewin M, Avarahami M. The decomposition of hypochlorite-hypobromite mixtures in the pH range 7-10. *J Am Chem Soc*. 1955;77:4491-4497.

56. Mills JF. Interhalogens and halogen mixtures as disinfectants. In: Johnson JD, ed. *Disinfection: Water and Wastewater*. Ann Arbor, MI: Ann Arbor Science; 1975:113-143.

57. Zhang Z. *Disinfection Efficiency and Mechanisms of 1-Bromo-3-Chloro-5,5-Dimethylhydantoin* [doctoral dissertation]. Ann Arbor, MI: University Microfilms; 1988.

58. Moore RM, Lotz WC, Perry R. *Activated Sodium Bromide-Artificial Marsh Treatment: A Successful Plant-Wide Program*. paper IWC-95-61. Pittsburgh, PA: Engineers' Society of Western Pennsylvania; 1995.

59. Nalepa CJ, Moore RM, Golson GL, Wolfe TM, Puckorius RP. *Case Study: Minimization of Corrosion Using Activated Sodium Bromide in a Medium-Size Cooling Tower*. paper 485. Houston, TX: NACE International; 1996.

60. Howarth JN, Mesrobian C, Shaver T. A review of the cooling water methods for sodium hypochlorite activation of sodium bromine into a hypobromous acid-hypobromite biocide. Paper presented at: 72nd Annual International Water Conference; November 13-17, 2011; Orlando, FL.

61. Kumar K, Margerum DW. Kinetics and mechanism of general-acid-assisted oxidation of bromide by hypochlorite and hypochlorous acid. *Inorg Chem*. 1987;26(16):2706-2711.

62. Dallmier AW, McCoy WF, inventors; Ecolab USA Inc, assignee. Process to manufacture stabilized alkali or alkaline earth metal hypobromite and uses thereof in water treatment to control microbial fouling. US patent 5,683,654. November 4, 1997.

63. Cooper AJ, Dallmier AW, Kelly RF, McCoy WF, Ma X, inventors; Ecolab USA Inc, assignee. Compositions and method for controlling biological growth using stabilized sodium hypobromite in synergistic combinations. US patent 6,419,879. July 16, 2002.

64. McCoy WF, Allain EJ, Yang S, Dallmier AW. *Strategies Used in Nature for Microbial Fouling Control: Application for Industrial Water Treatment*. Houston, TX: NACE International; 1998.

65. Moore RM Jr, Nalepa CJ, inventors; Albemarle Corp, assignee. Concentrated aqueous bromine solutions and their preparation. US patent 6,068,861. May 30, 2000.

66. Nalepa CJ, Howarth JN, Moore RM. *A New Single-Feed Liquid Bromine Biocide for Treatment of Cooling Water.* McLean, VA: Association of Water Technologies; 1999.

67. Nalepa CJ, Howarth JN, Moore RM. *First Field Trials of a Single-Feed Liquid Bromine-Based Biocide for Cooling Towers.* paper TP00-09. Houston, TX: Cooling Technology Institute; 2000.

68. Torres JE, Moore RM Jr, Wilson RW Jr, Focht GD, inventors; Albemarle Corp, assignee. Continuous processes for preparing concentrated aqueous liquid biocidal composition. US patent 6,352,725B1. March 5, 2002.

69. Torres JE, Moore RM Jr, Wilson RW Jr, Focht GD, inventors; Albemarle Corp, assignee. Processes for preparing concentrated aqueous liquid biocidal compositions. US patent 6,348,219B1. February 19, 2002.

70. Nalepa CJ, inventor; Albemarle Corp, assignee. Control of biofilm. US patent 7,087,251B2. August 8, 2006.

71. Nalepa CJ, Carpenter JF, inventors; Albemarle Corp, assignee. Microbiological control in oil or gas field operations. US patent 7,578,968B1. August 25, 2009.

72. Brasted R. Reaction of sodium nitrite and sulfamic acid. *Analyt Chem.* 1952;24(7):1111-1114.

73. Kuechler TC. *Development of Monsanto's Towerbrom® Microbiocide, a New Bromine Microbiocide for Recirculating Systems.* McLean, VA: Association of Water Technologies; 1991.

74. Kuechler TC. *A Towerbrom® Progress Report.* McLean, VA: Association of Water Technologies; 1993.

75. Hight TVT, Matson JV, Rakestraw LF, Zhang Z, Kuechler TC, inventors; University of Houston, assignee. Biocidal methods and compositions for recirculating water systems. US patent 5,464,636. November 11, 1995.

76. Hanway JE. *Water Quality & Treatment. A Handbook of Public Water Supplies.* 3rd ed. New York, NY: McGraw Hill Book Company; 1971.

77. Harvey MS, Howarth JN, inventors; Enviro Tech Chemical Services Inc, assignee. Compositions for stabilizing chlorinated water to sunlight decomposition, and methods of preparation thereof. US patent 7,728,132B2. June 1, 2010.

78. Lide DR, ed. *CRC Handbook of Chemistry and Physics*, 83rd ed. Washington, DC.: CRC Press; 2002.

79. Nalepa C, inventor; Albemarle Corp, assignee. Efficient inhibition of bacterial and algicidal activity in aqueous media. US patent 6,086,746. July 11, 2000.

80. Howarth JN, McKeown JA, Sergent RH, inventors; Bio-Lab Services Inc, assignee. Methods for generating residual disinfectants during the ozonization of water. US patent 5,888,428. March 30, 1999.

81. McCoy WF, Blatchley ER III, Johnson RW. Hypohalous acid and haloamine flashoff in industrial evaporative cooling systems. Paper presented at: 1990 Cooling Tower Institute Annual Meeting; February 5-7; Houston, TX.

82. AOAC Official Method 965.13 Disinfectants (Water) for Swimming Pools. In: Horwitz W, Latimer GW, eds. *Official Methods of Analysis of AOAC International.* 18th ed. Gaithersburg, MD: AOAC International; 2005.

83. Howarth JN, inventor; Albermarle Corp, assignee. Microbiological control in poultry processing. US patent 6,908,636B2. June 21, 2005.

84. Schmidt JW, Wang R, Kalchayanand N, Wheeler TL, Koohmaraie M. Efficacy of hypobromous acid as a hide-on carcass antimicrobial intervention. *J Food Prot.* 2012;75(5):955-958

85. McNaughton JL, Liimatta EW, inventors; Albemarle Corp, assignee. Microbiocidal control in the processing of meat-producing four-legged animals. US patent 7,901,276. March 8, 2011.

86. Harvey MS, Howarth JN, Mesrobian CE, inventors; Enviro Tech Chemical Services Inc, Harvey MS, assignees. Methods and compositions for the reduction of pathogenic microorganisms from meat and poultry carcasses, trim and offal. US patent 2,011,020,068,8. August 18, 2011.

87. Howarth JN, Termine EJ, Yeoman AM, inventors; BioLab Services Inc, assignee. Halogen compositions for water treatment. US patent 5,641,520. June 24, 1997.

88. Bullard BR, Geornaras I, Delmore RJ, Woerner DR, Martin JN, Belk KE. Validation of antimicrobial interventions including the use of 1,3-dibromo-5,5-dimethylhydantoin applied in a final carcass wash in a commercial beef harvest operation. In: Proceedings from the 70th Reciprocal Meat Conference, American Meat Science Association; June 19-21, 2017; Texas A&M University-College Station, TX. Abstract No. 117.

89. Japan Food Chemical Research Foundation. Standards for use, according to use categories. https://www.ffcr.or.jp/en/upload/Standards%20for%20Use%202018%20Nov.%2030.pdf. Accessed January 9, 2018.

90. Palin AT. Analytical control of water disinfection with special reference to differential DPD methods for chlorine, chlorine dioxide, bromine, iodine and ozone. *J Inst Water Eng.* 1974;28:139.

91. Clesceri LS, Greenberg AE, Eaton AD, Franson MAH, eds. *Standard Methods for the Examination of Water and Wastewater.* 20th ed. Washington DC: American Public Health Association; 1998.

92. Sharma VK, Zboril R, McDonald TJ. Formation and toxicity of brominated disinfection byproducts during chlorination of water: a review. *J Environ Sci Health B.* 2014;49:212-228.

93. Heeb MB, Kristiana I, Trogolo D, Arey JS, von Guten U. Formation and reactivity of inorganic and organic chloramines and bromamines during oxidative water treatment. *Water Res.* 2017;110:91-101.

94. Hua G, Reckhow DA, Kim J. Effect of bromide and iodide ions on the formation and speciation of disinfection byproducts during chlorination. *Environ Sci Technol.* 2006;40:3050-3056.

95. Zhai H, Zhang X. Formation and decomposition of new and unknown polar brominated disinfection byproducts during chlorination. *Environ Sci Technol.* 2011;45:2194-2201.

96. Richardson SD, DeMarini DM, Kogevinas M, et al. What's in the pool? A comprehensive identification of disinfection by-products and assessment of mutagenicity of chlorinated and brominated swimming pool water. *Environ Health Perspect.* 2010;118:1523-1530.

97. Chen B. Hydrolytic stabilities of halogenated disinfection byproducts: review and rate constant quantitative structure—property relationship analysis. *Environ Eng Sci.* 2011;28:385-394.

98. Haag WR, Hoigne J. Ozonation of bromide-containing waters: kinetics of formation of hypobromous acid and bromate. *Environ Sci Technol.* 1983;17:261-267.

99. von Gunten U, Hoigne J. Bromate formation during ozonation of bromide-containing waters. Interaction of ozone and hydroxyl radical reactions. *Environ Sci Technol.* 1994;28:1234-1242.

100. Pinkernell U, Von Gunten U. Bromate minimization during ozonation: mechanistic considerations. *Environ Sci Technol.* 2001;35:2525-2531.

101. Kransner SW, Glaze WH, Weinberg S, Daniel PA, Najm IN. Formation and control of bromate during ozonation of waters containing bromide. *J Am Water Works Assoc.* 1993;85(1):73-81.

102. Galey C, Gatel G, Amy G, Cavard J. Comparative assessment of bromate control options. *Ozon Sci Eng.* 2008;22:267-278.

103. Lui Z, Cui J, Chen Z, Yan Z. The Control of bromate formation on ozonation of bromide-containing water. *Desal Water Treat.* 2014;52:4942-4946.

104. Macalady DL, Carpenter JH, Moore CA. Sunlight-induced bromate formation in chlorinated seawater. *Science.* 1977;25(195):1335-1337.

105. US Environmental Protection Agency. Ground water and drinking water: national primary drinking water regulations. https://www.epa.gov/ground-water-and-drinking-water/national-primary-drinking-water-regulations. Published. Accessed January 8, 2018.

106. Data Call In (DCI) No. GDCI-006315-1606. Enviro Tech Chemical Services Inc; 2017.

107. European Union. *EU Regulation no. 528/2012 of the European Parliament and of the Council of 22 May 2012 Concerning the Making Available on the Market and Use of Biocidal Products.* Brussels, Belgium: European Union; 2012.

CHAPTER
18
Peroxygen Compounds

John Matta, Maruti Sinha, Kris Murphy, and Suranjan Roychowdhury

Research efforts in chemical disinfection and sterilization research and development have taken many turns over the years. Recent advances and future guidelines seem clear: We will concentrate on chemicals that will be effective against microorganisms when highly diluted; will be low in toxicity to people, animals, aquatic life, etc; will not injure or have minimal impact on the environment; and will meet existing and developing regulatory requirements internationally. One such chemical, which will be considered in this chapter, was appraised many years ago by Dr. Samuel S. Wallian, in an address to the New York State Medical Society in 1892:

> One can hardly refer to the medical journals without finding enthusiastic recommendations of it as a disinfectant of rare efficiency, an antiseptic of recognized merit and a germicide of decided potency. . . . It is also a reliable sporicide, and at the same time it is nontoxic and noncorrosive qualities possessed by few if any of the other sporicides yet brought to notice.

The chemical Dr. Wallian referred to was then known as "oxidized water"; we know it as hydrogen peroxide (HP), which is the most common example of a peroxygen compound. Peroxygen compounds contain the functional group R-O-O-R, where R stands for either hydrogens or an organic group; it is the -O-O- functional structure that defines peroxides. Peroxide compounds are powerful oxidizing agents and are often thought of in terms of their bleaching power. But the peroxo group is also very reactive itself and in forming associated radicals and in attacking various organic compounds such as proteins, lipids, and nucleic acids. These effects can accumulate in potent antimicrobial activity. This chapter will address the use of peroxygen compounds, mainly HP and peracetic acid (PAA), in disinfection and sterilization. This chemistry has become very important because of the stability and ease of use of these compounds. Other similar chemicals are considered elsewhere in this book, such as chlorine dioxide (see chapter 27) and ozone (see chapter 33).

▶ HYDROGEN PEROXIDE

The HP has had a rocky road in its acceptance as a disinfectant; first popular, then unpopular, and more recently finding special application to serve functions of great value. Important early uses, in the preantibiotic world, were for wounds and for treating diphtheria. Eventually, its use expanded to general surface disinfection, treatment of skin infections, cleaning, air fumigation or disinfection, sterilization, and as an oral rinse or for direct use in the eye (at low concentrations). It is considered so safe under certain conditions that it was approved for use in foods in many countries.[1] One of the major applications in both liquid and gas form is in sterilizing containers for aseptically preserved foods like fresh milk and fruit juices. The HP can be easily destroyed by heat or by enzymes such as catalase and peroxidase to give the innocuous end products, oxygen and water.

The use of HP as a disinfectant can be traced back to the late 1800s.[2] First reported in the early 1800s by Louis-Jacques Thenard,[3] it was used primarily as a skin antiseptic. As industrial production and uses of HP developed through the 1800s, the wider application of peroxide in clinical and therapeutic uses was proposed by B. W. Richardson in 1891.[4] Although the germ theory of disease was still at a very early stage of understanding, it was noted that antimicrobial methods such as boiling water and the use of certain types of chemicals had a benefit in reducing the spread of disease or promoting healing. The antiseptic effects of HP solutions used on would infections is credited to Richardson in 1856.[1] Even at this early time in disinfection, there were reports of using peroxide as an aerosol or gas to refresh the air by DeSondalo (1842), in meeting places and mines.[2] The combination of developments in peroxide use for disinfection along with improved methods for bulk manufacture of HP led to its widespread use in therapeutic applications. These included infections of the skin, mucous membranes, wounds, and upper and lower respiratory tract. Marchand (1893), a leading supplier of "peroxide of hydrogen" preparations, used controlled demonstrations of the superiority of his bulk preparation of peroxide (purified and stabilized) to commercial grades available at the time.[2] These preparations were marketed for a variety of microbial illnesses and associated examples of clinical success.

The use of HP has had a checkered history, due to the range of concentrations (often unknown in many applications), preparations and temperatures used, as well as the interference from the presence of various soils that can react with and essentially neutralize the impact against target microorganisms. Many reports of tissue damage were due to the use of excessive concentrations of peroxide. Many failures of effectiveness were due to use of poorly stabilized preparations or inadequate temperatures for exposure or excessive amounts of contaminating soils. This was particularly true in the results of testing peroxide on bacterial spores.[2]

In wound application, low concentrations of unstable preparations of HP to tissues containing inactivating levels of catalase (present in blood) led to unfavorable results and general abandonment of this agent as an antiseptic; however, recent studies have begun to reevaluate the optimal use of HP in such applications as an alternative to antibiotics.[5] Examination of the early literature reveals that HP was satisfactory when used as a disinfectant for inanimate materials. For example, used in low concentrations, it was considered ideal for the preservation of milk and water[6] and for the sterilization of cocoa milk beverage.[7] By 1950, an electrochemical process had been developed that produced pure preparations in high concentrations that were stable even at elevated temperatures and that had long shelf lives.[1] Stabilization of peroxide with a small amount of acid provided a more reliable long-term concentration.

There has been an upsurge of interest in HP during the last 40 years. Yoshpe-Purer and Eylan[8] used low concentrations for the sterilization of drinking water. 0.1% HP at 54°C for 30 minutes was shown to reduce the total bacterial count in raw milk by 99.999%[9]; and the coliform, staphylococcal, salmonellae, and clostridial counts were reduced by 100%. Investigations of 3% HP to control contamination of hospital water sources, demonstrated that a final concentration of 0.03% in water killed 1 million colony-forming units (CFUs) per milliliter of seven bacterial strains overnight, with an 80% kill in 1 hour.[10] The rapid virucidal activity of HP against rhinovirus, tested both in suspension and on carriers, was demonstrated.[11]

In relatively high liquid concentrations (10%-25%), HP was also established as a sporicidal agent. D-values of 0.8 to 7.3 minutes at 24°C were reported with four aerobic

spore strains and one anaerobic spore strain.[12] Work in the Soviet Union indicated the practicability of this agent for sterilization of spacecraft; this view was supported by the studies in the United States.[13] These latter studies, reported using aerobic bacterial isolates from spacecraft and achieved a complete kill of spore suspensions at the level of 100 million CFUs per milliliter by a 10% concentration at 25°C in 60 minutes. A further understanding in the difference of antimicrobial efficacy between HP is liquid and gas form was developed, demonstrating that HP was particularly effective at lower concentrations in gas form leading to the development of area fumigation and low temperature gaseous sterilization processes (see chapter 32).[2] Gas and gas plasma forms became the focus on interest, particularly for single-use and reusable medical device sterilization applications (see chapter 32). Further developments focused on the optimization of HP antimicrobial activity and material compatibility by liquid formulation effects and in combination with other excipients and biocides (eg, alcohols),[14-16] and in PAA formulations) (see chapter 6).[2]

Pure HP is extremely stable. Discovery of factors that cause its decomposition led to the development of effective stabilizers that deactivate contaminating materials and do not act on HP itself.[1] Thus, the stability of concentrated HP can be retained when diluted to 3% if this step is carried out using clean equipment and a good grade of deionized water in clean bottles of inert material. Commercial grades of HP can contain chelants and sequestrants that minimize its decomposition. The common stabilizers include colloidal stannate and pyrophosphate, organophosphates, nitrate and phosphoric acid, and colloidal silicate.

A grade of HP (Super D®) used chiefly for the drug and cosmetic trade is highly stabilized. In the presence of added catalytic decomposing ions of aluminum, iron, copper, manganese, and chromium, a 6% solution retains 98% of its original active oxygen after being subjected to 100°C for 24 hours.[17] The ordinary in-use stability of 3% HP was checked, and there was no decrease in concentration when bottles (120 mL) were opened and 10 mL was discarded each day for 12 days. Seven randomly selected shelf samples of various brands were tested according to the USP XVIII, and all were found to meet the standards for nonvolatile residues, heavy metals, and HP concentration.

The stability of a 3% HP solution that had been heated also was examined in terms of biocidal activity. The time required for an unheated 3% HP solution to eliminate a 0^5/mL inoculum was compared with that of a solution that had previously been subjected for 8 hours daily to 45°C for a total of 7 days. There was no significant difference in the killing times between these two preparations for seven bacterial strains and one fungus.[18] Overall, commercial HP is available in a number of strengths, namely, 3%, 30%, 35%, 50%, 70%, and 90% (PeroxyChem Corp).

Special food-grade HP preparations in 35% and 50% strengths, which meet US Food and Drug Administration (FDA) safety regulations, are also available.

Peroxide is also available in dry forms, such as sodium percarbonate and sodium perborate, which release HP on contact with water. These types of formulation are used in bleaching, agricultural and environmental remediation applications (oxidizing soil and groundwater contaminants), and for generating peroxidated forms of organic acids (such as peracetic or perpropionic acid).

Mechanism of Action

The current status of the mechanism of action on the molecular level has been reviewed and summarized quite recently.[2,19] The mechanism of activity is usually attributed to its reactive nature (as an oxidizing agent) and the production of highly reactive radicals by peroxide. The production of short-lived radicals can also be catalyzed in target cells or in the environment by reaction of peroxide with available transition metal ions, such iron-II, in the classic Fenton reaction:

$$Fe^{2+} + H_2O_2 \rightarrow Fe^{3+} + OH + OH^-$$

It has been shown that the hydroxyl radical is a potent oxidizer of many cellular components (lipids, proteins, and nucleic acids),[20] so this mechanism is commonly cited. The evidence for this Fenton-like reaction includes that bacteria grown in iron-rich media (and thus having elevated iron concentrations) were more susceptible to peroxide. This effect could be inhibited by the addition of hydroxyl scavengers such as thiourea. The use of iron chelators that can penetrate cells can protect them against killing by peroxide.[21] Electron paramagnetic resonance (EPR) spin trapping of the bactericidal action of peroxides showed bactericidal activity was inhibited in the presence of antioxidants and indicated the hydroxyl radical to be part of the lethal species.[22] A strong inverse correlation was found between the concentration of the trapped radical signal and the relative strength of the peroxide concentration as a bactericide. It was concluded that strong bactericides produce radicals at a much faster rate than weak ones.

The hydroxyl radical is said to be among the strongest oxidants known,[1-3] and it is by this mechanism that HP is believed in part to elicit its antimicrobial activity. The hydroxyl radical, being highly reactive, can attack membrane lipids, DNA, and other essential cell or viral components. Transition metals, as described earlier, are believed to catalyze the formation of the hydroxyl radical; nontoxic quantity of iron, copper, chromium, cobalt, or manganese salts increased the activity of HP toward *Staphylococcus aureus* and *Escherichia coli* 100 times in one report.[23] It was also suggested that, in the case of water free of metal

ions, the bacteria themselves can provide the necessary metal ions.[8] In the absence of metal ions in the culture medium, or if these ions are chelated with ethylene diamine tetra-acetic acid, there was no bactericidal action on *E coli*.[24] Others suggested that the antimicrobial action of HP is particularly related to oxidation of sulfhydryl groups and double bonds in proteins, lipids, and surface membranes.[25] The hydroxyl radical is also thought to contribute most of the biologic damage done by other oxidizing agents and ionizing radiation (see chapter 29).

The study of the mechanism of peroxide action has focused on the damage to DNA because this is the genetic basis of the cell and many viruses. The DNA is composed of two strands of polynucleotide phosphates. The individual nucleotide phosphates of a strand are connected by the phosphate bond to form a long strand. These strands are linked together (in a pair of strands) by hydrogen bonds between specific pairs of nucleotides, one from each strand, to form a double-stranded structure. Increased peroxide levels are associated with increased single-stranded breaks in the phosphate bonds between nucleotides in a given strand.[2,19] This effect will, if unrepaired, prevent proper DNA replication or protein production. This effect has been observed for HP even at low concentrations. Cells can repair this damage, given time and nutrients. But if the damage is extensive, the result is cell death.

Observations of the exposure of bacterial cells to HP suggest two different categories of effects.[2,19] At low concentrations (<3 mM), surviving cells form filaments and some loss of intracellular components is seen (suggesting some damage to cell surfaces). The rate of bacterial killing requires active cellular metabolism. Notably, DNA-repair mutants were more sensitive to this mode of killing. At much higher concentrations of peroxide (>17 mM), the cells demonstrated a much greater loss of intracellular components and a noticeable decrease in cell volume. Cells exhibit a multihit dependence of peroxide concentration and exposure time. Notably, this mode of killing does not require active metabolism, and DNA-repair mutants are not especially susceptible. It was proposed that a first mode of antimicrobial activity (low peroxide concentration) was due to DNA damage, which occurs at a low, nonlethal level during aerobic growth. A second mode (at higher concentration of peroxide) appears to be due to multicomponent damage, similar to UV-damage (see chapter 9). Others have also observed these two modes of killing.[26,27] It was noted that free-radical scavengers (such as thiourea, ethanol) provided some protective effect against the higher concentration mode of killing. In addition, this could be augmented by intracellular iron content. They suggested that hydroxyl radicals are more involved high concentrations, but not lower concentrations, but this has not been confirmed. Copper-export deficient strains of *E coli* showed increased cellular copper inhibited antimicrobial activity and oxidative damage by peroxide.[28] The higher levels of copper were associated with both reduced activity and mutagenesis. Because copper is known to directly react with peroxide, this may be a dose-reducing phenomenon.

Direct in vitro demonstration of the damage to DNA by peroxide was shown using phage DNA incubated with ferrous sulphate and exposed to peroxide.[29] Single-stranded breaks in DNA were observed, which was dose-responsive at lower peroxide concentrations (<3 mM peroxide). Excess peroxide did not produce additional nicks in DNA. The damage was reduced by ethanol, a scavenger of hydroxyl radicals. The direct DNA oxidant in the low-concentration peroxide activity was not dependent on the production of free hydroxyl radicals, but rather free ferryl radical intermediates (from a Fenton-type reaction), possibly complexed to DNA. When iron chelators are added to cells (under nonbacteriostatic conditions), a decrease in sensitivity to peroxide was observed under low peroxide (<3 mM) exposures.[30] This reinforces the concept of the participation of a Fenton-like reaction under these conditions.

The DNA damage measurement in vivo was done by several groups by exposing bacteria to peroxide and measuring single-stranded breaks.[31-33] Breaks were found, dose-dependent on the peroxide exposure, and half to most could be repaired by incubating in medium at 37°C for a period. No studies have focused on the correlation of antimicrobial activity and DNA damage, and variations in exposure conditions, media, etc, make comparisons difficult. In addition, the presence of contaminating substances (eg, protein fragments or amino acids or other soils) can have a large impact on sensitivity to peroxide. Most studies used long exposures of peroxide at low concentrations (<2.5 mM), whereas in typical usage as a disinfectant, the exposures are shorter exposures at larger concentrations (eg, 3%).[19] It should also be noted that Fe^{2+} Fenton reaction-like damage will be less important in these applications because normally the peroxide is provided in a low iron medium. Therefore, it is anticipated that although peroxide does indeed cause damage to DNA, even at low concentrations, the killing observed in normal disinfection use must involve damage to other important macromolecules in the cell, notably proteins and membrane lipids.[2] Because viruses do not have such repair mechanisms, the damage from peroxide may not be recoverable in any concentration.

Peroxide is known to react with thiol amino acids cysteine[34-36] and methionine.[37] In addition, reactions with lysine, histidine, and glycine in solution have been demonstrated. The metal-catalyzed production of hydroxyl radicals, resulting in oxidation of amino acids in proteins, has also been demonstrated,[37] which can result in cleavage of the protein backbone as well as production of carbonyls. The *E coli* challenged with as little as 2 mM peroxide resulted in reduction in cell viability as well as an increase in protein carbonyl content.[38] Yeasts are also sensitive to this treatment, resulting in excessive protein oxidation.

These studies were done with low peroxide concentrations for a long exposure, so it is expected that exposure to a high concentration (eg, 3%) might cause similar damage.

Exposure of *E coli* to low concentrations of peroxide resulted in the expected effects as well as extensive cell filamentation.[39] At higher concentrations of 17.5 mM, this filamentation did not occur, but the cell volume decreased drastically. In addition, large increases in lactate dehydrogenase activity were seen that, coupled with the decreased cell volume, suggests membrane damage and loss of cell contents was a large factor in killing the bacteria. In other studies, cell membrane permeability was observed to markedly increase in various strains of bacteria at high peroxide concentrations.[40] Even in cyanobacteria exposed to peroxide, large increases in dissolved organic substances were observed as well as indicators of cell membrane damage.[41] The HP has substantial effects on membrane lipids even at low concentration.

Antimicrobial Activity of Hydrogen Peroxide

The HP is active against a wide range of organisms: bacteria, yeasts, fungi, viruses, and spores (Tables 18.1 to 18.3; Figures 18.1 to 18.3). Anaerobes are even more sensitive because they do not produce catalase to break down the peroxide. Twenty-five ppm or less was shown to prevent growth of vegetative bacteria (Table 18.4). A 3% solution of HP is rapidly bactericidal (see Table 18.3 and Figure 18.1). Even against bacteria in biofilms, it can be active at 0.5%.[43] In liquid form, it is less rapid in its action against yeasts, some viruses, and especially bacterial spores (see Tables 18.1 to 18.3); however, 6% (volume per volume [vol/vol]) HP was an effective sterilant in 6 hours.[52] In general, HP has greater activity against gram-negative than gram-positive bacteria. It is less affected by pH than are many other disinfectants, such as phenols and organic acids; little difference in antimicrobial activity was shown between pH 2 and 10.[53] As noted in Figures 18.2 and 18.3, an increase in concentration can have a marked effect on activity. Similar effects have been reported with gas phase HP (see chapter 32).[2]

Destruction of spores is greatly increased with both a rise in temperature and an increase in concentration, making HP an effective sporicide under these conditions. Under these conditions, the sporicidal activity of HP was unaffected by organic matter in the form of 25% fetal bovine serum or of salt as 3.4% sodium chloride (NaCl).[54] Comparing 10% HP with seven other disinfectants against 13 species of bacteria (Table 18.5), HP was favorable in observed antimicrobial activity.[55] In practical sporicidal applications with HP, high concentrations combined with high temperatures are used together to produce sterile conditions. In aseptic packaging, 35% HP at up to 80°C for 3 to 9 seconds has been used.

TABLE 18.1   Examples of antimicrobial activity of hydrogen peroxide toward bacteria, yeasts, and viruses[a]

Organism	Concentration (ppm)	Lethality (min)	Temperature (°C)	Reference
Bacteria				
Staphylococcus aureus	1000	60	—	Kunzmann[42]
S aureus	25.8 × 10⁴	0.2	24	Toledo et al[12]
S aureus biofilm	500	1	36	Lineback et al[43]
Escherichia coli	1000	60	—	Kunzmann[42]
E coli	500	10-30	37	Nambudripad et al[44]
Salmonella enterica (subsp. enterica)	1000	60	—	Kunzmann[42]
Enterobacter aerogenes	500	10-30	37	Nambudripad et al[44]
Sarcina species	500	150	37	Nambudripad et al[44]
Lactococcus lactis	500	150	37	Nambudripad et al[44]
Streptococcus liquefaceus	500	240	37	Nambudripad et al[44]
Micrococcus species	30	10	—	Wardle and Renninger[13]
Staphylococcus epidermidis	30	10	—	Wardle and Renninger[13]
Pseudomonas aeruginosa biofilm	500	1	21	Lineback et al[43]
Yeasts				
Torula species	500	180-210	37	Nambudripad and Lya[45]
Oidium species	500	180-210	37	Nambudripad and Lya[45]
Viruses				
Orthinosis virus	3.0 × 10¹	180	—	Nikolov and Popova[46]
Rhinovirus types 1A, 1B, 7	0.75 × 10¹	50-60	37	Mentel and Schmidt[11]
Rhinovirus types 1A, 1B, 7	1.5 × 10¹	18-20	37	Mentel and Schmidt[11]
Rhinovirus types 1A, 1B, 7	3.0 × 10¹	6-8	37	Mentel and Schmidt[11]
Poliovirus type 1	1.5 × 10¹	75	20	Kline and Hull[47]
Poliovirus type 1	3.0 × 10¹	75	20	Kline and Hull[47]

[a]Experiments were not conducted under the same conditions and may not be comparable.

Synergism With Hydrogen Peroxide

Overall, synergism between the antimicrobial activity of biocides can be difficult to demonstrate because the activity may not be specific due to a true synergistic activity between biocides but rather each biocide working independently in the mixture as antimicrobials.[56] Despite that, many reports in the literature suggest synergistic or combined antimicrobial effects with HP. The first, already suggested earlier, was reported in 1930,[23] where activity against E coli and S aureus was increased 100-fold when one part of cupric and ferric ions were added to 500 parts of HP. They knew that these ions promoted the free-radical oxidation of organic compounds with HP and concluded that the bactericidal action resulted from the same cause. The supposition that free radicals were responsible for this action was reinforced when it was observed that these metals with HP in a Fenton-type reaction produced mutations in bacteria, like those produced by radiation.[57]

When spores of *Clostridium bifermentans* were treated with 100 μM of copper sulfate or 0.28 M HP at 25°C, copper alone showed a minimal effect (95% colony formation) and peroxide alone was similar (87%).[58] When used together, the colony formation was significantly reduced (to 0.028%). Because HP is known to remove protein from spore coats, they tested it with dithiothreitol, which also possesses that property. Treatment with HP alone gave 93% colony formation and with dithiothreitol alone, 40%. Together, they gave 0.082%, a 500-fold reduction. It was proposed that dithiothreitol removes the protein in the spore coat that protects the spore from HP and that copper increases the rate of breakdown of HP and the rate of cleavage of peptide bonds by HP.

Studies with plasmid DNA showed that 10^{-2} M Cu^{+2} or 10^{-2} M HP alone did not significantly break the DNA, but a

TABLE 18.2 Sporicidal activity of hydrogen peroxide toward spore-forming bacteria and bacterial spores[a]

Organism	Concentration (ppm)	Lethality (min)	Temperature (°C)	pH	Comment[b]	Reference
Bacillus subtilis	500	420-1080	37	—	Mixed	Nambudripad et al[44]
Bacillus cereus	500	420-1080	37	—	Mixed	Nambudripad et al[44]
Bacillus megaterium	500	420-1080	37	—	Mixed	Nambudripad et al[44]
B subtilis ATCC 15411	3.0×10^1	1440	37	4.3	Spores on surface	Baldry[48]
B subtilis SA 22	25.8×10^4	7.3	24	3.8	Spores	Toledo et al[12]
Bacillus coagulans	25.8×10^4	1.8	24	3.8	Spores	Toledo et al[12]
Bacillus stearothermophilus	25.8×10^4	1.5	24	3.8	Spores	Toledo et al[12]
Clostridium sporogenes	25.8×10^4	0.8	24	3.8	Spores	Toledo et al[12]
B subtilis var *globigii*	25.8×10^4	2.0	24	3.8	Spores	Toledo et al[12]
B subtilis var *globigii*	35×10^4	1.5	24	3.8	Spores	Toledo et al[12]
B subtilis var *globigii*	41×10^4	0.75	24	3.8	Spores	Toledo et al[12]
B subtilis SA 22	17.7×10^4	9.4	20	—	Spores	Leaper[49]
B subtilis SA 22	17.7×10^4	0.53	45	—	Spores	Leaper[49]
B subtilis SA 22	29.5×10^4	3.6	20	—	Spores	Leaper[49]
B subtilis SA 22	29.5×10^4	0.35	45	—	Spores	Leaper[49]
B subtilis SA 22	35.4×10^4	2.3	20	—	Spores	Leaper[49]
B subtilis SA 22	35.4×10^4	0.19	45	—	Spores	Leaper[49]

[a]Experiments were not conducted under the same conditions and may not be comparable.

[b]Testing varied between studies. Mixed indicate a bacterial culture that may have contained vegetative and spore forms, spores indicate the use of a spore suspension, and all tests were done in suspension studies unless indicated on surfaces.

mixture of 10^{-6} Cu^{+2} with 10^{-5} M HP resulted in strand breaks and inactivated transforming ability.[59] The Cu^{+2} plus HP caused greater damage to the bases in DNA than Fe^{+3} plus HP.[60] Working with five representative viruses, it was found that the cupric and ferric ions alone were virucidal, but this action was greatly increased with HP, particularly for copper.[61] This effect extended for all of the viruses, and the investigators indicated that 0.05% Cu^{+2} plus 5% HP would have the virucidal activity equal to 2% glutaraldehyde. They stated that the Cu^{+2}-HP system was more efficient in their tests than glutaraldehyde and would inactivate most or all viruses that contaminate medical devices.

With the copper-HP system, the ID_{50} for *E coli* was 0.45 mg/L copper to 45 mg/L HP (1-100), whereas for glutaraldehyde, the ID_{50} was 4.6 mg/L.[62] For *Bacillus subtilis*, 2% glutaraldehyde gave a 1000-fold reduction in 35 minutes, equal to that of 0.2% copper plus 5% HP. A mix of 0.2% copper plus 10% HP gave a 1000-fold decrease in 15 minutes. Against the enveloped Junin virus (Argentinian mammarenavirus), the copper-HP mixture was reported to be 50 times more virucidal than glutaraldehyde. With 10 mg/L Cu^{+2} to 1000 mg/L HP in media containing 5% serum, the virus was inactivated about five times faster than with glutaraldehyde.

The addition of ascorbic acid to the copper-HP system caused a large increase in the DNA base damage, much greater than with the iron-HP ascorbic acid system.[60] They proposed that the copper ions bound to the DNA react with HP and ascorbic acid to generate hydroxyl radicals, which then immediately attack the DNA in a site-specific manner. With herpes simplex virus, the virucidal activity of copper was enhanced by reducing agents (HP can act as an oxidizing or reducing agent) in the following order: ascorbic acid $\gg$ HP $>$ cysteine.[63] Treatment of virus-infected cells with combinations of copper and ascorbate completely inhibited virus plaque formation to below 0.006% of the infectious virus input; it maintained 30% viability for the host mammalian cells. Other studies demonstrated the effectiveness of cupric ascorbate compared with other disinfectants, showing it to be equal or better in lower concentrations.[53,55,63]

The addition of other chemicals with biocidal properties to an HP solution has been shown to enhance its activity, particularly against aromatic hydrocarbons. As noted earlier, the activity can be enhanced with the addition of transition metals (although the lifetime of the reagent is short) to accelerate the production of hydroxyl radicals. Recent introduction of solutions of HP coupled with

| TABLE 18.3 | D-values with 3% hydrogen peroxide (H$_2$O$_2$) solution from lens disinfection studies |

Microorganism	Min	
	D-value[a]	Standard Error
Neisseria gonorrhoeae	[b]	—
Haemophilus influenzae	0.29	0.07
Pseudomonas aeruginosa	0.40	0.05
Bacillus subtilis	0.50	0.15
Escherichia coli	0.57	0.07
Proteus vulgaris	0.58	0.24
Bacillus cereus	1.04	0.12
Proteus mirabilis	1.12	0.33
Streptococcus pyogenes	1.50	0.25
Staphylococcus epidermidis	1.82	0.14
Staphylococcus aureus	2.35	0.18
Herpes simplex	2.42	0.71
Serratia marcescens	3.86	0.53
Candida albicans	3.99	0.54
Fusarium solani	4.92	0.54
Aspergillus niger	8.55	1.32
Candida parapsilosis	18.30	3.44

[a]Contamination level: 700 000 organisms per lens, 7 mL of H$_2$O$_2$ solution.

[b]Too rapid to measure.

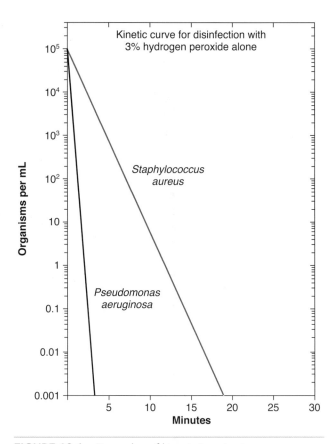

FIGURE 18.1 Examples of kinetic inactivation curves for disinfection with 3% hydrogen peroxide (in water) over time.

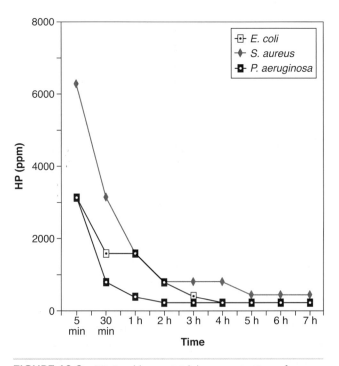

FIGURE 18.2 Minimal bactericidal concentration of hydrogen peroxide against time for water strains. Based on Alasri et al.[50]

alcohol, surfactants, and/or acids have shown enhanced antimicrobial activity and cleaning potential, particularly on surfaces.[64,65] The HP is also considered to play an active role in synergism with PAA both in liquid and gas form, particularly from mode of action studies.[66]

It already has been noted that heat sharply increases the activity of HP. One explanation is that HP makes spores more sensitive to heat, and so heat may be the actual true cause of death. The HP also acts synergistically with ultraviolet (UV) radiation 0.3% HP plus UV gave 2000 times greater increase of spore kill than radiation alone and 4000 times greater than HP alone.[67-69] Less than 1% HP in the presence of UV produced a synergistic kill, but the effect diminished, as the concentration increased. The absorption of UV by HP was postulated, as the cause for the loss of synergism. When high-intensity UV light (for 20 s) plus 2.5% HP was combined with heat up to 80°C for 60 seconds, a 5 log$_{10}$ inactivation of *B subtilis* was obtained. These researchers attributed the antimicrobial activity to the formation of hydroxyl radicals from HP within the spores, but they explained that at higher concentrations, the decrease in activity is due to reaction of breakdown products with HP molecules outside of the

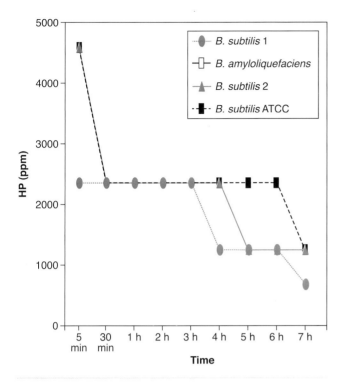

FIGURE 18.3 Minimal sporicidal concentration of hydrogen peroxide (HP) against time for *Bacillus* spores. Based on Alasri et al.[51]

spore. The major drawback of UV with peroxide, as with UV alone, is that UV is not particularly penetrating and is limited to surface action or to clear solutions that do not absorb UV (see chapter 9). The process for sterilization by a combination of UV and HP used sequentially was patented for the commercial sterilization of packaging before filling with ultrahigh-temperature processed foods.[70] A later development used a synchrotron radiation source to produce a narrow band of radiation, showing the greatest kill of *B subtilis* spores in the presence of HP with radiation close to 270 nm in wavelength.[71]

Another physical agent that has shown synergism with HP is ultrasonic energy. Experiments using ultrasonic waves in conjunction with HP found that sonication of *Candida albicans* and *Bacillus cereus* spores with 6% HP was lethal in 10 minutes, whereas the agents separately did not kill the organisms in 30 minutes' exposure at 35°C.[72] Ultrasonic energy was thought to disperse and agitate the cell aggregates, increasing surface contact with the disinfectants, increasing the permeability of the cell membrane to the disinfectant, and accelerating the rate between the disinfectant and the cell components.

Applications of Hydrogen Peroxide

Formerly used just as an antiseptic, HP now has many other applications for preservation, cleaning, disinfection, and sterilization. In swimming pools, for example, it is used in conjunction with other disinfectants such as Baquacil®, a polymeric biguanidine; it helps to prevent bacterial growth, control algae, and clean filters without producing eye irritation, harmful products, or unpleasant odors. It is used in ultrasonic disinfectant cleaning baths for dental and medical instruments. The HP is used for odor control in sewage and sewage sludges[73] and to treat landfill leachates to control microbial growth in waters that receive these discharges.[74,75] In the horticultural industry, it keeps capillary feed systems for nutrient supply to plants from being plugged by algae growths.[76]

As a sterilant, 6% HP over 6 hours in comparison to glutaraldehyde products, which took 8 and 10 hours in different tests[52]; 10% HP took 1 hour and 3% HP took 2.5 hours[13]. Six percent HP was also an effective high-level disinfectant for flexible endoscopes to be more effective than glutaraldehyde for killing or removing *B subtilis* in a 10-minute contact period.[77] In comparisons of 7.5% HP with 2% glutaraldehyde for disinfection of flexible endoscopes, HP needed half the exposure time of glutaraldehyde, 10 versus 20 minutes, and HP was highlighted as being less toxic to humans and the environment.[78] Formulations of HP for high-level disinfection have become widely used as alternatives to aldehydes (glutaraldehyde and ortho-phthalaldehyde (OPA); see chapter 23) for these reasons.[2,79]

At least two interesting papers reported on the production of HP in situ. Electroplated metal coatings produced HP when in contact with electrolytes.[80] It was proposed

TABLE 18.4 Effect of pH on the bacteriostatic activity of hydrogen peroxide (minimum inhibitory concentration in ppm)[a]

pH	*Pseudomonas aeruginosa* ATCC 15442	*Klebsiella pneumoniae* ATCC 4352	*Streptococcus faecalis* ATCC 10541	*Staphylococcus aureus* ATCC 6538
5.0	5	25	25	No growth
6.5	10	25	25	5
8.0	50	25	25	5

[a]Based on Baldry.[48]

360 **Part III** Disinfection by Antimicrobial Types

TABLE 18.5 Bacterial inactivation with hydrogen peroxide and peracetic acid compared to other biocidal agents[a,b]

Bacterium	Glutaraldehyde 2%	Formaldehyde 8%	Phenol 5%	Cupric Ascorbate 0.1%	Sodium Hypochlorite 0.05%	Hydrogen Peroxide 10%	Peracetic Acid 0.03%
Bacillus cereus	>5.0 (2)	>5.0 (2)	>5.0 (2)	>5.0 (2)	>5.0 (2)	>5.0 (2)	>5.0 (2)
Clostridium perfringens	>6.3 (2)	>6.3 (2)	>6.3 (2)	>6.3 (2)	0.14 ± 0.05 (2)	>6.3 (2)	4.1 ± 0.1 (2)
Escherichia coli	>6.9 (2)	>6.9 (2)	>6.9 (2)	6.3 ± 0.8 (2)	6.2 ± 0.9 (2)	>6.9 (2)	>6,9 (2)
Listeria monocytogenes	>6.1 (2)	>6.1 (1)	>6.1 (2)	>6.1 (1)	>6.1 (2)	>6.1 (2)	>6.1 (1)
Pseudomonas aeruginosa	3.8 ± 0.2 (2)	>6.1 (3)	5.8 ± 0.6 (3)	5.6 ± 0.9 (3)	1.3 ± 0.1 (2)	>6.1 (3)	5.0 ± 1.6 (3)
Salmonella ser Typhimurium	>6.4 (3)	>6.2 (3)	>6.4 (3)	>6.4 (3)	4.1 ± 1.3 (2)	>6.4 (3)	>6.4 (3)
Shigella sonnei	>6.3 (2)	>6.3 (2)	>6.3 (2)	>6.1 (1)	>6.3 (2)	>6.3 (2)	>6.3 (2)
Staphylococcus aureus	>6.5 (3)	>6.5 (3)	>6.5 (3)	5.5 ± 1.2 (3)	4.8 ± 1.8 (2)	5.6 ± 0.7 (3)	6.6 ± 0.3 (3)
Staphylococcus epidermidis	>6.3 (3)	5.9 ± 1.1 (3)	>6.3 (3)	5.1 ± 0.1 (2)	6.3 ± 0.4 (3)	>6.3 (3)	>6.3 (3)
Vibrio cholerae	>6.4 (2)	>6.4 (2)	>6.4 (2)	>6.4 (2)	>6.4 (2)	>6.4 (2)	>6.4 (2)
Vibrio parahaemolyticus	>6.2 (1)	>6.2 (2)	>6.2 (2)	>6.2 (2)	>6.2 (2)	>6.2 (2)	>6.2 (2)
Vibrio vulnificus	>6.3 (2)	>6.3 (2)	>6.3 (2)	>6.3 (2)	>6.3 (2)	>6.3 (2)	>6.3 (2)
Yersinia enterocolitica	>6.8 (2)	>6.8 (2)	>6.8 (2)	>6.8 (2)	>6.8 (2)	>6.8 (2)	>6.8 (2)

[a]Calculated as $-\log(T_d/T_w)$, where T_d is the titer of bacteria surviving 30 min exposure at 20°C to a given disinfectant and T_w is the titer of bacteria exposed under the same conditions to water. Results are expressed either as $x \pm s$ (n) where no surviving colonies were obtained or as $x \pm s$ (n) where n is the number of replicate experiments.

[b]Based on Sagripanti et al.[55]

that in the metal oxidation, the reactive O_2^* species is formed, which, with electrons from the metal, gives rise to the superoxide ion radical and this then to HP:

$$O_2^* + e^- \rightarrow O_2 \cdot^-$$

$$O_2 \cdot^- + e^- + 2H_2O \rightarrow H_2O_2 + 2OH^-$$

Electroplated metal coatings of cobalt; copper; and cobalt-containing alloys of nickel, zinc, and chromium inhibited the growth of pathogenic bacteria. This inhibition was shown not to be due to the metal ions themselves, and stainless steel without the coatings was found not to be inhibitory. It was suggested that these coatings could be used to reduce bacterial contamination in hospital facilities. Low-amperage electric current (DC) electric current was also used to produce HP on the surface of electrodes used as central venous catheters.[81] A zone of inhibition was demonstrated by inserting an anode and cathode into an agar plate inoculated with a lawn of bacteria. There was no zone under anaerobic conditions. The authors claimed that the electrode repels organisms from the electroconducting catheter, prevents intraluminal microbial migration, and is bactericidal to microorganisms attached to catheters, thus preventing the formation of biofilms on the electrodes.

The HP has been widely used in various forms for area disinfection (or fumigation). These include various misting systems and gas systems[82,83] that claim to use HP in a gas form (known as VHP®) or in a condensed gas form.[2] In these systems, liquid HP (with may include other chemicals in formulation such as silver, although the overall impact of these on antimicrobial activity is not clear) is either directly misted into the air/environment or generated into gas by heating. A typical process known as flash vaporization generates a gas by dropping a HP solution (at various concentrations between 3% and 55% in water) onto a hot surface. This forms a gas (or vapor) consisting of HP and water at the same proportion to the starting liquid). Both water and HP as vapors can readily condense into liquids (or if in a mist form go into a vapor/gas) under these conditions but dependent on the temperature in the area or on surfaces.[84] Under both conditions (gas or condensed gas), HP is an effective biocide in area fumigation or sterilization applications. Under gas conditions, HP has been shown to be an effective antimicrobial with greater efficacy at lower concentrations than liquid peroxide. But under condensed conditions, peroxide will condense preferably than water, depending on the surface temperature, to lead to a high concentration of HP initially; however, it is also logical that these systems can vary in material compatibility and safety due to the presence of condensed, concentrated peroxide on surfaces.[2,84] Such system applications have also been the basis for medical device or equipment disinfection[85] and sterilization (see chapter 32). The HP has also been widely

used in plasma sterilization systems (see chapter 32).[86,87] A plasma is essentially an ionized gas, generated by providing energy to any gas such as oxygen, nitrogen, or HP (see chapter 34). Initially, sterilization systems were described that used plasmas generated from HP gas within an exposure chamber, but such systems have not been commercially successful to date.[86] Despite this, many systems have been described that plasma as part of the sterilization process (see chapter 32).[2] These can include using plasma energy sources to generate peroxide gas from a liquid source (essentially as an alternative to heat) and the generation of a plasma following HP gas exposure to breakdown and remove peroxide residuals from the sterilization chamber and load. The impact of plasma in these cases to antimicrobial efficacy is not considered significant, as demonstrated in studies that compared efficacy of such systems in the presence or absence of the plasma phases.[88] But the overall impact to the safety of the sterilization process (in efficiency of peroxide residual removal) should not be underestimated. The use of HP in sterilization processes is further discussed on chapter 32.

The HP is widely used in food and food-contact surface disinfection. Advantages include no toxic residues, easily available and completely water soluble, and it readily degrades following application. It is used in milk and starch production, packaging, dried foods (such as eggs), and vinegars among others. Many such applications require regulatory approval, depending on the country or region. The HP is used in oral treatments (eg, in whitening and toothpaste). Although largely for the bleaching effect, it also provides antimicrobial capability. Dry sources of peroxide are also used. Examples include benzoyl peroxide, sodium percarbonate, perborate, and calcium peroxide.[89] A benefit of HP is its ability to be used on various types of living tissues, including the skin and mucous membranes. Clearly at higher concentrations, peroxide can be damaging to such tissues and has health hazards, but at lower concentrations (typically less than 3% in water), it can be used to reduce microbial levels but with minimal impact on the underlying tissue. The HP is used for the disinfection/sterilization of excised tissues and allografts, such as the Allowash® process using 3% HP in combination with surfactants, alcohol, and antibiotics in a defined antimicrobial process.[90,91] Certain applications have been described for use directly in the eye (at less than 1%), but overall, HP is an eye irritant and at higher concentrations can lead to irreversible eye tissue damage. The overall safety profile of HP has also seen it widely used as a preservative or cleaning/disinfection solutions/gels for contact lens and other devices that may contact the eye.[92,93]

But in such applications, the correct rinsing or neutralization of peroxide residuals is best practice to reduce eye irritation or damage.

The HP, as an effective oxidizing agent can be used to neutralize chemical contaminants. For example, it is used for treating pollutants (hydrocarbons, herbicide residuals, pesticide residuals) and as a deodorizer. It has also been used as an air scrubber, to control volatile organic compound (VOCs),[94] and for the neutralization of cytotoxic drug contamination in pharmacy dispensing cabinets.[95] The HP can also be used for treating wastewater systems,[96] typically using iron- or copper-based catalysts. It is useful form of wastewater disinfection and deodorization because bacteria are a common source of the problem.[2] It is also a major bleaching agent for wood pulp, paper, and paper products, where it is used more for its whitening capability than disinfectant properties but can be used for wood or other building material disinfection.[97]

▶ PERACETIC ACID

It would be desirable to have a chemical with the attributes of HP that has effective disinfection and sterilizing capabilities, no harmful decomposition products, and infinite water solubility but greater lipid solubility and freedom from deactivation by catalase and peroxidases. Such a compound exists. It is the peroxide of acetic acid, peroxyacetic acid, or PAA. As an effective biocide with essentially no toxic residuals, it has been the subject of considerable interest.[89,98,99] It is known as an ideal antimicrobial agent due to its high oxidizing potential and lack of deactivation by catalase and peroxidase, the enzymes that break down HP, with broad effectiveness against microorganisms.

The PAA is a more potent antimicrobial agent than HP,[48,100] being rapidly active at low concentration against a wide spectrum of microorganisms. It is sporicidal even at low concentrations and temperatures and can remain effective in the presence of organic matter, depending in the concentration and application process. As a weak acid, it is more active on the acid side but is antimicrobial at higher concentrations in the alkaline range, but the concentrations required are very high and the stability is lower. These effects can be optimized based on formulation and exposure process conditions. Like HP, it is useful both in solution (typically in formulation with other ingredients) and as a vapor (or gas). These properties make it a remarkably valuable compound. Sprossig[101] stated that it has advantages for disinfection and sterilization not found in any other agent.

Surprising as it may seem, the excellent bactericidal properties of PAA were first reported in 1902, highlighting "the excellent disinfecting and cold sterilization actions of PAA,"[102] but it was not until years later with the development of a commercial process for the production of 90% HP, necessary for PAA's manufacture, that it became generally available. In 1949, PAA was shown to be the most active of 23 germicides tested against spores of *Bacillus thermoacidurans*.[103] Others found it to be bactericidal at 0.001%, fungicidal at 0.003%, and sporicidal at 0.3%.[104] It found early application as a disinfecting agent in gnotobiotics, the production of germ-free animals at the Lobund Institute of the University of Notre Dame.[105] Developments in Europe and the United States followed, with applications include the treatment of waste materials, disinfection and sterilization of medical devices, and in the food processing industry because its residuals are only acetic acid, oxygen, water, HP, and dilute sulfuric acid.[89,99]

The PAA is normally synthesized by reaction of HP and acetic acid:

$$H_2O_2 + CH_3COOH \leftrightarrow CH_3COOOH + H_2O$$

This is an equilibrium, and the value of equilibrium constant depends not only on the concentrations but also on the temperature and, when applicable, the liquid product formulation. Most commercial PAA solutions are available as this equilibrium solution. This means that the PAA will normally be accompanied by peroxide and some amount of acetic acid. It is also possible to generate PAA on demand from other compounds. The most notable is tetraacetylethylenediamine (TAED). Reaction of TAED with peroxide will generate two molecules of PAA from every molecule of TAED.[106] This reaction is optimal under alkaline conditions and requires vigorous mixing. The result is initially a solution that has only PAA (not acetic acid) in water and a small amount of excess peroxide. Although not long-term stable, it can be used for on-demand PAA applications. It is commercially also used for pulp bleaching in some countries and is a component of some laundry detergents (as a nonchlorine bleaching additive).

Mechanism of Action

The PAA is well established as a broad-spectrum antimicrobial agent, including bactericidal, viricidal, mycobactericidal, sporicidal, fungicidal, and cystical activity depending on its application method (eg, concentration, gas or liquid, temperature, formulation). Clapp et al[22] initially used EPR spin trapping to examine the radical production of PAA and other peroxide compounds and to relate the radical formation with bacterial kill. They used 5,5-dimethyl-1-pyroline *N*-oxide (DMPO) as the trapping agent, which allowed them to detect carbon-centered and hydroxyl radicals produced at varying rates for the bacteria/peracid system studied. Employing *S aureus* and *E coli* with the peracid, they found that the inhibition of the bactericidal action by DMPO and two antioxidants indicated to them that radicals are the lethal species. A strong inverse correlation was found between the radical adduct signal and the strength of the bactericide. Of the peroxides tested, PAA was shown by this method to be the strongest bactericide, and that of the radicals formed, the hydroxyl radical is the lethal species. Added iron chelators gave evidence that iron species were involved.

Other reports investigated the sporicidal action of HP and PAA.[107,108] The HP was found to sensitize spores to heat damage and inactivated bacterial spores with 15% HP at elevated (60°C) but sublethal temperatures occurred without lysis, but prolonged exposure or higher concentrations of HP caused lysis with major damage to the coat, cortex, and protoplast. Spores were protected by oxidized transition metal cations. Vegetative cells were not protected by either oxidized or reduced metal ions and killing was enhanced (as discussed earlier). Metal chelators or free radical scavengers did not provide effective protection. But reducing agents such as sulfhydryl compounds and ascorbate were highly protective. The dependence of HP in liquid form on temperature for its sporicidal activity suggested that radicals are involved in the killing action. The protective effects of oxidized and reduced transition metal ions indicated that HP as a sporicide is different from its activity on vegetative cells killing. The PAA also aided hypochlorite and iodine in killing spores. As with HP, sulfhydryls and ascorbate protected spores against killing by PAA. Metal chelators were not protective of spores but did protect vegetative cells. Transition metal ions, especially the reduced forms, were highly protective. It was speculated that organic radicals formed from

$$\overset{O}{\underset{\|}{}} \qquad \overset{O}{\underset{\|}{}}$$

PAA, like $CH_3CO\bullet$ and $CH_3C\bullet$ because of their greater longevity than the hydroxyl radical, also may be involved in the sporicidal action. Whereas ions of reduced metal were highly protective of spores, in vegetative cells, the reduced transition metal ions sensitized the spores to killing by PAA. This was explained on the basis that the radical, by donating its unpaired electron or accepting another electron, can act either as a reducing or oxidizing agent. In the case of spores, which are said to be in the oxidized state,[109] they accept electrons and are reduced; thus, they are protected by reduced transition metal ions and other reducing agents. Vegetative cells, unlike spores, are metabolically active and can donate electrons from transition metals in the cell surface to the radicals, become oxidized, and are killed.[110]

Regarding the sensitization of spores to heat and to hypochlorite and iodine resulting from PAA treatment below lethal concentration, the importance of the small, acid-soluble proteins that coat the DNA was reported, and known to protect the DNA from HP (see chapter 3 on spore structure).[109] The PAA and HP may react with these proteins to leave the DNA unprotected and susceptible to attack by these agents. Subsequent studies with bacterial spore mutants that lack various components of the spores with PAA have shown that the resistance of spores to PAA is particularly due to the presence of the spore coats[111] and the mode of action of PAA was focused on damage to the inner membrane and, as for HP, the DNA molecule itself. The PAA and HP have shown synergistic antimicrobial activity against bacterial spores.[66] Spores were found to be sensitized to the sporicidal activity of PAA by pretreatment with HP even at low, nonlethal concentrations and

contact times, but the opposite was not true. The authors suggested that the HP effect was due to reaction with the outer spore layers including the spore membrane, which may be at least partially due to the removal or damage to proteins associated with the spore coat. But at the same time, direct activity of both biocides was also related to eventual damage to the inner core DNA as the ultimate source of spore viability. The direct effects of PAA on proteins, lipids, and nucleic acids has been shown,[112] although it is interesting to note that these effects can vary depending on the formulation, concentration, temperature, or even state (liquid or gas) of PAA. For example, some PAA-based formulations have been shown to cause protein cross-linking, whereas others do not.[113]

Maillard and Russell[114] investigated the action of a number of disinfectants, including PAA, on a virus. They tested PAA (1%), glutaraldehyde (1%), phenol (2%), chlorhexidine (1%), cetylpyridinium chloride (0.05%), ethanol (70% and 100%), and isopropanol (100%) against the nucleic acid of *Pseudomonas aeruginosa* PAO bacteriophage F116. It was considered that although the destruction of the proteins of the viral capsid and envelope would stop viral infection, only the breakdown of the nucleic acid would render the virus noninfectious and avoid reactivation. Of the disinfectants tested, only PAA significantly affected the phage genome, but it was not clear whether the nucleic acid was damaged inside the phage capsid or when the nucleic acid was released into the outside medium.

The disinfectant activity of PAA was hypothesized to be based on the release of active oxygen. It was thought that sensitive sulfhydryl and disulfide bonds in proteins are oxidized and reactions with double bonds were important.[115] It has been shown that PAA will oxidize small molecules containing double bonds, particularly when a sulfur is involved,[116] and PAA is well-known to epoxidate alkenes (the epoxide group will then quickly react further. The action of PAA (and other oxidants) on enzyme activity and individual amino acids was studied.[112] The PAA was found to oxidize cysteine, methionine, lysine, histidine, glycine and tryptophan. The PAA was found to be an efficient inhibitor of enzyme activity at 50 mM. Chang et al[117] studied the effect of 1 mM PAA on gene transcription of *Pseudomonas*. They found that the transcription of genes involved in metabolic pathways was repressed, and those genes that were associated with cellular protective processes (adaptation, DNA repair) were activated.

The specific action of PAA on *Pseudomonas* biofilms was observed by fluorescence imaging.[118] The PAA caused a uniform and linear loss of fluorescence (corresponding to leakage of the fluorophore out of the cells due to membrane permeabilization). This suggests that PAA was able to penetrate into the cells even though there was an extracellular matrix. But others have shown that mixed species in a biofilm showed increased resistance to PAA over time.[119] This phenomenon may due to many factors including PAA concentration, reactions with materials, clumping or accessibility of bacteria within the biofilm, etc. In certain cases, PAA has been used for biofilm removal, but this appears to be variable depending on the liquid formulation and application method for biofilm removal (as discussed earlier). Studies with PAA on *S aureus* and *Listeria monocytogenes* biofilms showed physical removal from stainless steel surfaces, but this was less efficient on polystyrene surfaces.[120]

In summary, PAA is known to react with many amino acids, particularly thiol-containing as well as peptide bonds. The inactivation of critical enzymes within the cell or virus structure has been demonstrated and the reaction with membrane proteins has also been observed. Reactions with membrane lipids are also likely. Although PAA can oxidize the nucleic acids of bacteria and viruses, it is likely that the damage caused by membrane permeabilization and loss of critical enzyme function will precede this and dictate the death of the cellular organisms. Overall, the accumulation of these general effects will cumulate to inactivate microorganisms both in vegetative and dormant forms.

Antimicrobial Activity of Peracetic Acid

The antimicrobial activity of PAA has been well established but, as highlighted earlier, can be dependent on the product or process application using PAA. Examples of efficacy against bacteria, yeasts, and fungi (Table 18.6; Figure 18.4),

TABLE 18.6   Antimicrobial activity of peracetic acid toward bacteria, yeasts, and fungi (pH = 7.0, temperature = 20°C)

Organisms	Concentration (ppm)	Lethality (min)	Comments	Reference
Bacteria				
Pseudomonas aeruginosa	50	—	Phosphate buffer	Greenspan and MacKellar[104]
P aeruginosa	250	—	Nutrient broth	Greenspan and MacKellar[104]
Escherichia coli	10	—	Phosphate buffer	Greenspan and MacKellar[104]
E coli	200	—	Nutrient broth	Greenspan and MacKellar[104]
Micrococcus pyogenes var *aureus*	10	—	Phosphate buffer	Greenspan and MacKellar[104]
M pyogenes var *aureus*	200	—	Nutrient broth	Greenspan and MacKellar[104]
E coli	10-15	5		Baldry et al[121]
Streptococcus faecalis	75-100	5		Baldry et al[121]
Staphylococcus aureus ATCC 6538	90	5		Orth and Mrozeck[122]
Enterococcus faecium DSM 2918	90	5		Orth and Mrozeck[122]
Listeria monocytogenes	90	5		Orth and Mrozeck[122]
Legionella pneumophila[a]	6	<5		Baldry and Fraser[76]
Mycobacterium chelonae (glut resistant)	800	10		Stanley[123]
Mycobacteria terrae	850	5	Phosphate buffer	Medivators (Cantel Medical)[124]
Yeasts				
Saccharomyces cerevisiae NCYC 762[b]	83	<5		Baldry[48]
S cerevisiae NCYC 1026[b]	42	<5		Baldry[48]
Zygosaccharomyces bailii NCYC 580[b]	25	<5		Baldry[48]
Fungi				
Aspergillus niger	50	—	Fungistatic, buffer	Greenspan and MacKellar[104]
A niger	500	—	Fungistatic, nutrient broth	Greenspan and MacKellar[104]
Penicillium roqueforti	50	—	Fungistatic, buffer	Greenspan and MacKellar[104]
P roqueforti	500	—	Fungistatic, nutrient broth	Greenspan and MacKellar[104]

[a]pH = 5.0, temperature = 25°C.

[b]pH = 6.5, temperature = 25°C.

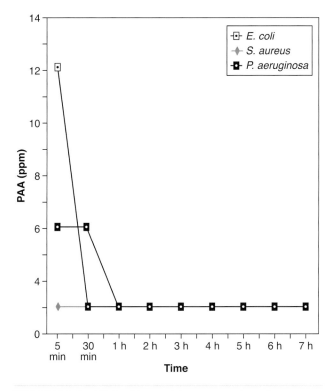

FIGURE 18.4 Minimal bacterial concentration of peracetic acid (PAA) against time for water strains. Based on Alasri et al.[50]

mycobacteria (Table 18.7), viruses (Table 18.8), and bacterial spores (Tables 18.9 to 18.12; Figures 18.5 to 18.9). All these tests confirmed the high activity of PAA against a broad spectrum of microorganisms and many PAA-based products are associated with antimicrobial efficacy claims, such as for high-level disinfection.[131] In addition, PAA has been shown to be effective against protozoa (vegetative and dormant, cyst, or oocyst forms), but efficacy varies depending on formulation and temperature of liquids tested.[132-134] The PAA liquid and gas systems have also been developed that demonstrate log-linear kinetics in the inactivation of spores, with *Geobacillus stearothermophilus* spores being the most resistant and demonstrating a sterility assurance level (SAL) of 10^{-6} in defined sterilization processes.[135-137]

As is well known, the test procedure affects the test results, and, as shown in Table 18.6, different media significantly changed the results with the same organism. In a comparison of the resistance of different bacteria to PAA, where the same test method and medium were employed, Table 18.5 shows that *P aeruginosa* was more resistant than the other bacteria tested. As shown in the tables, and comparing Figures 18.4 and 18.5, a much larger PAA concentration is required for sporicidal action than bactericidal and fungicidal action. Tables 18.9 and 18.11 demonstrate the effect of concentration on the sporicidal

TABLE 18.7 Mycobactericidal activity of 2% alkaline glutaraldehyde and Nu-Cidex® (0.35% peracetic acid).[a,b]

Test Organism	Log Initial Count	Log₁₀ Reduction in Test Organism (2% Glutaraldehyde [G]: Nu-Cidex [N]) (min)				
		1	4	10	20	60
Mycobacterium chelonae NCTC 946	G8.64	>5.64	>5.64	>5.64	>5.64	>5.64
	N8.76	>5.76	>5.76	>5.76	>5.76	>5.76
M chelonae WD 1	G8.43	0.24	0.30	0.35	0.51	0.64
	N8.06	4.06	>5.06	>5.06	>5.06	>5.06
M chelonae WD 2	G9.10	0	0.12	0.09	0.33	0.29
	N9.12	4.03	>6.12	>6.12	>6.12	>6.12
Mycobacterium tuberculosis H37Rv	G8.00	1.28	2.83	4.60	>5.00	>5.00
	N8.10	>5.10	>5.10	>5.10	>5.10	>5.10
Mycobacterium avium-intracellulare	G8.96	0.05	0.70	1.39	2.64	>5.96
	N9.87	2.08	5.24	>6.87	>6.87	>6.87
Mycobacterium kansasii WD 3	G8.56	2.44	3.96	>5.56	>5.56	>5.56
	N8.38	>5.38	>5.38	>5.38	>5.38	>5.38

Abbreviation: WD, endoscope-washer disinfector isolates 1, 2, and 3.

[a]The greater than symbol (>) denotes that the sensitivity of the recovery system does not allow reductions in log₁₀ counts of greater than the initial count less than 3 log₁₀ to be demonstrated.

[b]Based on Lynam et al[125] and Griffiths et al.[126]

TABLE 18.8   Inactivation of viruses by peracetic acid (temperature = 20°C)

Organisms	Concentration (ppm)	Lethality (min)	Comments	Reference
Poliovirus 1	400	5	7.5 log$_{10}$ reduction	Kline and Hull[47]
Coxsackievirus B-3	1280	5	5.5 log$_{10}$ reduction	Kline and Hull[47]
Coxsackievirus B-5	325	30	7.25 log$_{10}$ reduction	Kline and Hull[47]
Echovirus 10	1280	5	6.5 log$_{10}$ reduction	Kline and Hull[47]
Adenovirus 3,4,7	1280	5	4, 1.5, 3.5 log$_{10}$ reductions	Kline and Hull[47]
B virus	1280	5	7 log$_{10}$ reduction	Kline and Hull[47]
Herpes simplex	1280	5	3 log$_{10}$ reduction	Kline and Hull[47]
Enteric viruses	2000	10		Sprossig[101]
Enteric viruses	2000	30		Harakeh[127]
Human rotavirus	140	30		Harakeh[127]
Simian rotavirus	20	30		Harakeh[127]
Poliovirus 1	150-375	60	Water	Baldry et al[121]
	>750	30	Water	
	750-1500	15	Water	
	1500-2250	10	DM	
Coxsackievirus	100-375	60	DM	Baldry et al[121]
	250-500	15	DM	Baldry et al[121]
Echovirus	100-375	60	DM	Baldry et al[121]
Phage MS2	12-15	5	DM	Baldry et al[121]
Phi X 174	25-30	5	DM	Baldry et al[121]
Poliovirus 1	375-750,	60	YE	Baldry et al[121]
	750-1500,	30	YE	Baldry et al[121]
	1500-2250,	15	YE	Baldry et al[121]
	>2250	10	YE	Baldry et al[121]
Coxsackievirus	100-375,	60	YE	Baldry et al[121]
	500-1000	15	YE	Baldry et al[121]
Echovirus	100-375	60	YE	Baldry et al[121]
Phage MS2	75-94	5	YE	Baldry et al[121]
Phi X 174	94-113	5	YE	Baldry et al[121]
Vaccinia	850	10	>4 log$_{10}$ reduction in blood and BSA	Eterpi et al[128]
Adenovirus	850	10	>4 log$_{10}$ reduction in blood and BSA	Eterpi et al[128]
Poliovirus	850	10	>4 log$_{10}$ reduction in blood and BSA	Eterpi et al[128]
Porcine parvovirus	850	10	>4 log$_{10}$ reduction in blood and BSA	Eterpi et al[128]
Minute virus of mouse	850	10	1.9 log$_{10}$ reduction in blood and BSA	Eterpi et al[128]

Abbreviations: BSA, bovine serum albumin; DM, demineralized water; YE, yeast extract.

TABLE 18.9 Effect of concentration of peracetic acid on the survival of *Bacillus subtilis* (ATCC 9372) spores exposed for 30 min at 20°C and pH 3[a]

Concentration (%)	0.01	0.02	0.03	0.05	0.2
Log Reduction	<1	1	2	4	5

[a]Based on Sagripanti and Bonifacino.[53]

TABLE 18.10 Effect of pH on the survival of *Bacillus subtilis* (ATCC 9372) spores exposed to 0.03% peracetic acid at 30 min and 20°C[a]

pH	2	4	5	7	8
Log Reduction	4	3	2	1	<1

[a]Based on Sagripanti and Bonifacino.[53]

TABLE 18.11 Sporicidal activity of peracetic acid: effect of temperature and concentration

Temperature (°C)	Min for Lethality at Concentration (ppm)				Organism	Reference
	5000	10 000	20 000	30 000		
37	10	10	<0.5	<0.5	*Bacillus anthracis*	Hussaini and Ruby[129]
20	20	10	5	<0.5	*B anthracis*	Hussaini and Ruby[129]
4	>60	20	20	<0.5	*B anthracis*	Hussaini and Ruby[129]
0	—	—	—	1	*Bacillus subtilis* var *niger*	Jones et al[130]
−30	—	—	—	6	*B subtilis* var *niger*	Jones et al[130]
−40	—	—	—	600	*B subtilis* var *niger*	Jones et al[130]

TABLE 18.12 Minimum sporicidal concentration (ppm) of the antimicrobial agents tested for *Bacillus subtilis* ATCC 6633 spores[a]

Time	PAA	Combination of PAA + HP		HP	Chlorine	Formaldehyde
		PAA	HP			
5 min	1344	84	11 250	45 000	5376	3750
30 min	672	84	11 250	22 500	672	1875
1 h	336	42	5625	22 500	672	1875
2 h	168	42	5625	22 500	168	1875
3 h	168	42	5625	22 500	168	1875
4 h	168	21	2813	22 500	168	1875
5 h	168	21	2813	22 500	168	1875
6 h	168	21	2813	22 500	168	1875
7 h	168	21	2813	11 250	168	1875

Abbreviations: HP, hydrogen peroxide; PAA, peroxyacetic acid.

[a]Based on Alasri et al.[51]

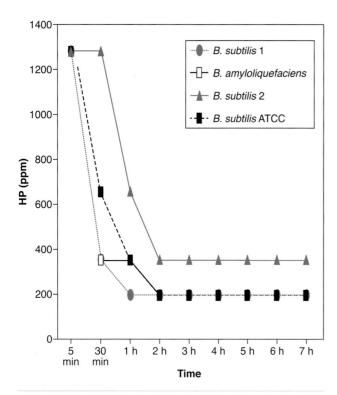

FIGURE 18.5   Minimal sporicidal concentration of per-acetic acid against time for *Bacillus* spores. HP, hydrogen peroxide. Based on Alasri et al.[51]

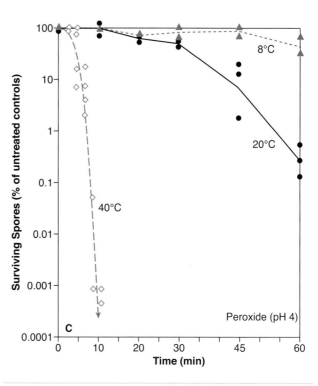

FIGURE 18.6   Sporicidal kinetics of 10% hydrogen peroxide, pH 4 at three different temperatures. Symbols represent the results of independent experiments.

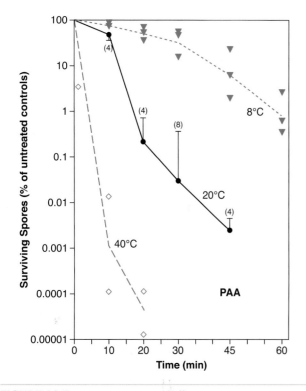

FIGURE 18.7   Spores surviving different time exposures to 0.03% peracetic acid (PAA). pH 3.4, at three temperatures. Symbols represent the results of independent experiments at 8°C or 40°C or averages ± standard deviations obtained from the parenthetically listed numbers of independent experiments at 20°C.

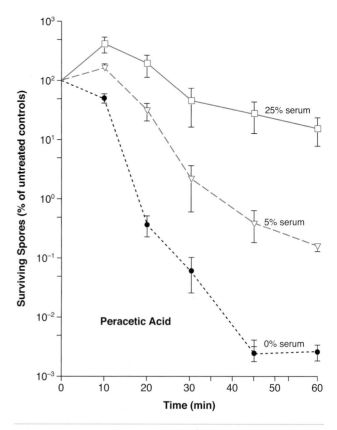

FIGURE 18.8   Kinetics of spore inactivation by peracetic acid in the presence of serum. Based on Sagripanti and Bonifacio.[54]

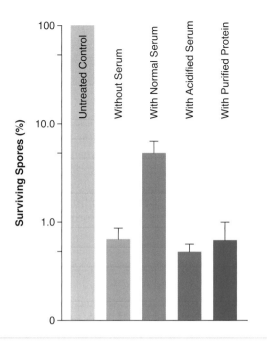

FIGURE 18.9 Kinetics of spore inactivation by peracetic acid in the presence of serum. Based on Sagripanti and Bonifacio.[54]

TABLE 18.14	Sporicidal activity of disinfectants to *Bacillus anthracis* spores with 4% horse serum at 20°C[a]	
Disinfectant	**ppm**	**Time (h)**
Peracetic acid	2500	0.5
Glutaraldehyde	20 000	2
Formaldehyde	40 000	2

Based on Lensing and Oei.[138]

concentration in 5 minutes at 20°C and 5°C. Alasri et al[50] tested PAA, HP, chlorine, and formaldehyde against 3 bacteria, PAA being bactericidal at much lower concentration than HP and formaldehyde, but against chlorine, it was approximately equal in 5 minutes, but after 3 hours, chlorine required only one-sixth the concentration of PAA against all the bacteria. Table 18.7 compares PAA with glutaraldehyde against 6 species of mycobacteria over a period of 60 minutes. With 5 of the 6 species, PAA acted more rapidly, and 2 species were resistant to glutaraldehyde after 60 minutes but not to PAA. In these tests, glutaraldehyde was used at 2% and PAA at 0.35%. The PAA was also confirmed to be effective against atypical mycobacteria strains (such as *Mycobacterium chelonae* and *Mycobacterium massiliense*) with known high-level resistance to glutaraldehyde disinfectants.[142,143]

Table 18.14 shows the results of tests of PAA, glutaraldehyde, and formaldehyde against spores of *Bacillus anthracis* in the presence of 4% horse serum. The PAA was sporicidal at lower concentration and shorter time. Table 18.12 presents the results over time of PAA, HP, chlorine, and formaldehyde against *Bacillus* spores. In 5 minutes, PAA was sporicidal at a lower concentration than the other disinfectants and continued so to HP and formaldehyde, but after 2 hours, chlorine was equally effective in these studies.[51]

Synergism With Peracetic Acid

Historical data (before 1999) seemed to support some synergy in antimicrobial activity with PAA and other biocides with spores, not with vegetative bacteria. But many problems exist with earlier data due to insufficient analytical chemical information on the composition of the solution reacting with the spores in the actual exposure vessel. Many studies do not report the levels of peroxide and acetic acid along with the PAA values. This is important because PAA usually exists (long term) in an equilibrium

TABLE 18.15	Bactericidal activity of disinfectants against test bacteria in 10 min by the use-dilution method—based on 100% active ingredient[a]				
		Bactericidal Concentration (ppm) Against			
Disinfectant	**Composition**	*Staphylococcus aureus*	*Escherichia coli*	*Proteus vulgaris*	*Pseudomonas aeruginosa*
Persteril	40% peracetic acid	1000	500	500	1000
Chloramine	25% available chlorine	2500	2500	2500	2500
Wescodyne	1.6% available iodine	1600	1600	1600	1600
Jodoseptan	1.9% available iodine	1520	950	1520	1900
Laurosept	25% laurylpyridinium bromide	2500	2500	2500	25 000
Sterinol	10% dimethyl-lauryl-benzyl ammonium bromide	8000	10 000	10 000	>10 000
Phenol	Phenol	20 000	15 000	15 000	15 000
Lysol	50% cresol	40 000	40 000	40 000	40 000
Septyl	7.5% o-phenylphenol + 3.2% p-tert, amyl phenol	2139	2139	2139	10 965
Formalin	37% formaldehyde	52 000	30 000	30 000	30 000
Alhydex	2% glutaraldehyde	6000	5000	5000	5000

[a]Based on Kryzywicka et al.[141]

with HP and acetic acid, and you can get the same level of PAA by pushing the equilibrium with peroxide or pushing with acetic acid. If you push with peroxide, you will have less acetic acid (hence, less potential of corrosion) but higher levels of peroxide that can obscure interpretation of synergy. Thus, it is very important to know the exact level of peroxide (and to a lesser extent the level of acetic acid) in the PAA solution being used in studies. In order to do a fair comparison of the biocidal activity of HP and PAA, controls of the individual components (PAA, peroxide, acetic acid), as well as any other components (eg, stabilizers) that may be present, are required in case they have some biocidal activity in their own right. Finally, the pH of the exposure solution is critical to the activity of PAA. The PAA is not as active as a biocide at alkaline pH. This is not a slow reaction, but it is a chemical protonation state that is a function of the existing pH of the solution.

The PAA may display synergism with other components in a given disinfectant formulation. Normally, PAA is available in an equilibrium solution at a given level of PAA, in equilibrium with peroxide and acetic acid. The exact position of the equilibrium depends mainly on the starting concentrations and on the temperature. Shifting of the equilibrium with time can happen if the concentration of any of the four components (eg, adding peroxide or diluting with water), but the shift is normally slow.[144] It can take hours to days to reach a new level. Similarly, changing the temperature can change the equilibrium, but slowly. Thus, raising the temperature may shift the equilibrium toward increasing peroxide and acetic acid, until the original temperature is restored. Thus, it is important to know that the exposure of the target microorganisms is at the same temperature as the evaluation of the test solution and that not too much time has elapsed before diluting the equilibrium solution to the testing level. Surprisingly, few studies provide this information.

The PAA, as well as HP, can display some synergism. As shown in Table 18.12, whereas 1344 ppm PAA or 45 000 ppm HP alone was required to kill *B subtilis* spores in 5 minutes, a combination of 84 ppm PAA with 11 250 ppm HP was equally effective.[51] A clear synergistic activity between HP and PAA was shown in mode of action studies, as described earlier in this chapter.[66] With vegetative bacteria, the effect was not so dramatic.[50] For example, with *S aureus*, 3 ppm PAA or 6250 ppm HP was lethal in 5 minutes; the combination of 3 ppm PAA with 390 ppm HP produced the same result. It appeared that the combination of PAA and peroxide did show some synergy. But the stock source of the PAA was a product that was known to have about the same amount of peroxide as PAA, and it was not clear how the final concentrations of each in the final biocide treatment solution (after dilution) were determined.

Leaper[49] reported the synergistic activity of PAA with alcohols. Using spores of *B subtilis* known to be resistant to PAA, he found a D-value of 0.08% PAA alone to be 47.2 minutes; combined with 9.9% of methanol, it was 17.3 minutes, with ethanol 4.7 minutes; and with *n*-propanol 1.6 minutes. Alcohols by themselves are known not to be sporicidal by themselves and have difficulty penetrating thick protein layers (see chapter 19). Synergistic responses were found for combinations of 0.04% PAA with up to approximately 20% ethanol, but higher concentrations of ethanol or PAA did not yield further sporicidal action. Because the stock source of the PAA was a stabilized PAA concentrate solution, it is likely that a fair amount of peroxide was also present. Details of the analytical values of the oxidizers in the exposure vessel were not given. Other studies tested soil spores with PAA in 70% ethanol and 60% isopropanol.[145] Without PAA, the alcohols were not sporicidal, but without the alcohols, 0.05% PAA was sporicidal in 48 hours. In combination, ethanol-PAA was sporicidal in two of three tests with 0.025% PAA and isopropanol-PAA were sporicidal in all tests at 0.0125%. The investigators recommended the combinations for the treatment of the skin and hands.

Synergism was reported for a combination of C_1 to C_4 peracids with C_6 to C_{18} peracids.[146] Thus, where PAA at 25 ppm against *E coli* had no observed log reduction and peroctanoic acid at 5 ppm had a log reduction of 0.1, a combination of the two of these concentrations had a log reduction of 3.8.

Leggett et al[66] exposed *B subtilis* spores to different combinations of PAA and HP. The analytical concentrations of each biocide were determined within the exposure vessel, so the accurate values at each concentration combination was known. Besides using wild type bacterial strains, they also used derivative strains that were most resistant to PAA. The study confirmed the synergistic activity of combinations of peroxide and PAA. The sporicidal activity was mostly due to the action PAA rather than the peroxide. But peroxide pretreatment of the spores for various times before exposure to PAA showed that the synergistic effect was dependent on initial reaction with the peroxide, allowing increased penetration by the PAA.

Applications

The powerful antimicrobial action of PAA at low temperatures along with the absence of toxic residuals led to a wide range of applications. It has been accepted worldwide in the food processing and beverage industries, which include meat and poultry processing plants, canneries, dairies, breweries, wineries, and soft drink plants, where it is said to be ideal for many clean-in-place (CIP) systems.[147] It is used as terminal disinfectant or sterilant for stainless steel and glass tanks, piping, tank trucks, and railroad tankers.[148] Its nonrinse feature—that is, its breakdown products in high dilution are not objectionable from the taste, odor, or toxicity standpoints—saves time and money in many of these applications, such as in water, beer, lemonade, and milk.[149] The virucidal effectiveness against bacteriophages specific for *Streptococcus lactis* and *Streptococcus cremoris* and the sporicidal effectiveness against *Clostridium tyrobutyricum* was confirmed.[150,151] The fungicidal effect of a PAA disinfectant was examined for its use as a room disinfectant in dairies.[152] In investigations of PAA for the beverage industry, all bacteria, yeasts, and fungi tested with 2500 ppm (0.25%) PAA were inactivated in 30 minutes and with 5000 ppm in 15 minutes.[153]

A preparation of PAA (known as P3-oxonia® active) was approved by the FDA in 1986, giving clearance for its ingredients as indirect food additives in sanitizing solutions. Subsequently, US Environmental Protection Agency (EPA) registration was issued and US Department of Agriculture (USDA) authorization granted.[147] In the food industry, plastic food containers were treated with a solution containing 0.1% PAA and 20% HP. They were sprayed on a conveyor belt using hot air to activate the solution and dry it off. Polyethylene strips with *B subtilis* spores were killed after treatment for 12 seconds at 65°C.[154]

The properties of PAA also have been recognized by the medical community. The US Centers for Disease Control listed it as a chemical sterilant and high-level disinfectant. The PAA-based formulations are now widely used for high-level disinfection and liquid chemical sterilization for reusable medical devices, including flexible endoscopes.[131] Application in the production and husbandry of germ-free animals, where sterility is paramount, came early.[155]

The use of PAA as an antiseptic in war-wound healing was investigated.[156] After selecting 35 patients with at least two similar wounds from the war in Croatia, wounds on one side of the body were treated with 0.2% PAA compresses, and those on the other side were treated with hypertonic NaCl solution. After 12 days, the PAA-treated wounds were significantly better cleansed, with fewer microorganisms than those conventionally treated.

In the preparation of pharmaceuticals, PAA permits the cold disinfection or sterilization of emulsions, hydrogels, ointments, and powders. An oil-in-water emulsion contaminated with *Aspergillus* was sterilized in 10 minutes with 0.1% PAA.[157] Skin preparations containing zinc oxide and talc were preserved with 0.05% to 0.2%, yielding the same microbicidal purity as hot air–sterilized products.[141] Zinc oxide lotions with 0.05% to 0.1% PAA were tested on 26 patients for 1 year and did not cause skin irritation.

In industrial application, PAA was been used in the disinfection of ion exchangers.[158] A 0.2% PAA solution was used for 1 hour to achieve complete disinfection and the capacity of the respective cation and anion exchangers was not changed under the conditions used (0.2%-1% PAA). The PAA is also used to disinfect reverse osmosis membranes,[159] removing a clinically significant biofilm. The PAA formulations have been used for biofilm prevention

and remediation of water systems (see chapter 67). Microorganisms are now recognized as causing many problems in industrial water systems. These include microbially induced corrosion, plugging, and fouling of heat exchangers, sprinklers, and cooling towers and disease caused by the *Legionella* bacteria. On-site trials for *Legionella* with 10 mg/L PAA on five cooling towers was reported,[76] with the organism eradicated in 20 minutes. Algae were controlled with 20 mg/L PAA disinfection performed twice a year, but a slug dose of 30 mg/L with 10 mg/L thereafter was better when there was heavy algae accumulation.

The PAA has many desirable attributes for wastewater disinfection, such as ease of implementation, broad activity, activity also against suspended organic matter, and absence of toxic by-products.[115] The known effectiveness of PAA against bacteria and viruses led to investigations of the use of PAA as a disinfectant for sewage and sewage effluents in laboratory and field trials.[160] The PAA was found to be an effective disinfectant for secondary effluent and stated that the ease of implementing PAA treatment without expensive equipment, the broad-spectrum activity even in the presence of organic matter, and the lack of environmentally undesirable by-products make PAA appear favorable for sewage treatment processes. Similar investigations studied the disinfection of sewage sludge.[76] Disinfection of sludge can eliminate it as a vehicle of transmission of infection to farm animals and also reducing the no-grazing interval of the land to which the sludge has been applied. Levels of 300 to 500 mg/L PAA reduced *Salmonella* levels below the limits of enumeration in all treated sludges. The PAA was effective against the cestode (tapeworm) oncosperes in sewage sludges producing lack of motion, dark coloration, granulation, and ovoid shrunken appearance.[161] In a digested sludge, 250 mg killed 99% of the embryos.

The breakdown products of PAA disinfection in wastewater are acetic acid, HP, oxygen, and water. At the pH of most wastewater, the spontaneous decomposition to acetic acid and oxygen dominate the products. Transition metals (eg, hard water, suspended iron, or copper) would accelerate the decomposition.[162] Some complicating factors are the increase in acetic acid from the decomposition, which may be broken down by bacteria. In addition, the production of oxygen (from the breakdown of both the PAA and any accompanying peroxide) will increase the oxygen content of the wastewater, and complicate chemical oxygen demand versus biological oxygen demand measurements.

The PAA is also used to disinfect membrane hollow fiber filters. For dialyzer reuse, automated systems fill hollow fiber hemodialyzers with disinfectant and allow the dialyzers to be reused 4 to 10 times.[163] The reuse with PAA was shown to not impact patient mortality[164] and have provided some improvements due to avoidance of first-use syndrome and improved biocompatibility.

The use of PAA in ultrafiltration membranes for water treatment was shown to be particularly efficient,[51] and the solution combination of PAA and HP was found to provide total disinfection of hollow fibers in 2 to 3 hours of contact time.

The PAA is widely used to disinfect reusable flexible endoscopes and other temperature-sensitive semicritical or critical devices at low temperatures (eg, 20°C-50°C) in short times (eg, approximately 5 min). When compared with other processes for disinfection of long narrow lumens, liquid PAA was found to be the most effective,[165] although these reports vary depending on the formulation and process control of the disinfectant application.[113] As liquid, PAA is often considered to aid in the cleaning (or physical removal of residual soil remaining after cleaning) as an alternative to cross-linking agents such as glutaraldehyde and OPA, this may not be taken for granted and can vary depending on the product formulation. Gas sterilization applications for medical devices (single use and reusable) have also been described but has not been widely used to date (see in the following text).[89]

Stability of Peracetic Acid

Peroxides in general are high-energy state compounds, and as such can be considered thermodynamically unstable. The PAA is considerably less stable than HP: 40% PAA loses 1% to 2% of its active ingredients per month compared with HP (30%-90%), which loses less than 1% per year. The decomposition products of PAA are acetic acid, HP, oxygen, and water. Dilute PAA solutions are even more unstable: A 1% solution loses half its strength through hydrolysis in 6 days.[155] The PAA is produced by the reaction of acetic acid or acetic anhydride with HP

in the presence of sulfuric acid, which acts as a catalyst, as shown:

$$CH_3C{\overset{O}{\underset{OH}{\vert\vert}}} + H_2O_2 \rightleftharpoons CH_3C{\overset{O}{\underset{OOH}{\vert\vert}}} + H_2O$$

To prevent the reverse reaction, the PAA solution is fortified with acetic acid and HP. In addition, a stabilizer is used. This may be a sequestering agent (hydroxyethylidene diphosphonate or sodium pyrophosphate) or a chelating agent (8-hydroxyquinoline) that removes trace metals, which accelerate the decomposition of peroxides.[1] Stabilization of the equilibrium mixture with a sequestrant/chelators has been shown to reduce the decomposition of PAA to almost immeasurable rates, even under alkaline conditions.[166] A patented process employing anionic surfactants with dilute PAA solutions shows not only greater stability but also greater antimicrobial activity.[167] Although a 1% PAA solution at pH 2.5 lost 13.4% PAA in 1 day, at pH 7.0 it lost 84% in 1 day.[155] On the other hand, a formulation of 1% PAA, 14.5% acetic acid, 5.0% HP, 78.5% water, and 1% sulfuric acid lost only 2.7% in 84 days. To maintain stability, solutions must be made up with especially pure chemicals and deionized water and kept free of dust and other contaminants. Commercial preparations with excellent stability are offered as shown in Table 18.16.

For stability, PAA should be stored at ordinary, preferably cool temperatures in original containers. It is unaffected by glass and most plastics, although if the equilibrium solution contains a high concentration of acetic acid (>17%), it may negatively affect the seams in plastic containers after >1 year. It may extract the plasticizer from some vinyl formulations used as gaskets and will attack natural and synthetic rubbers.[147] Pure aluminum,

---

TABLE 18.16 Examples of commercial peracetic acid equilibrium solution: approximate chemical composition (% by weight)

Ingredient	PeroxyChem LLC Philadelphia, PA	PeroxyChem LLC Philadelphia, PA	Solvay England	Ecolab St. Paul, MN	Cantel Medical Little Falls, NJ
	35% Peracetic Acid	15% Peracetic Acid	Proxitane 1507	P3 Oxonia Active	Minncare
Peracetic acid	35.5	15.0	15	5	5
H_2O_2	6.8	23.0	14	25	22
Acetic acid	39.3	16.0	28	6	9
H_2O	17.4	45.0	42	63	65
H_2SO_4	1.0	1.0	—	—	—
Stabilizer	0.05	0.05	<1.0	1.0	<0.5

Abbreviations: H_2O, water; H_2O_2; hydrogen peroxide; H_2SO_4, sulfuric acid.

stainless steel, and tin-plated iron are resistant to PAA, but plain steel, galvanized iron, copper, brass, and bronze are susceptible to reaction and corrosion.[149]

It is important to remember that the PAA/peroxide mixture is an equilibrium, and as such, it is subject to disturbances in the equilibrium that are not part of the decomposition of PAA. Thus, it should be noted that the position of the equilibrium mixture is dependent on the temperature (as well as initial concentration of reactants peroxide and acetic acid). Thus, at higher temperatures (eg, >50°C), the equilibrium slowly shifts toward the peroxide and acetic acid, and the PAA component appears to reduce. But if the solution is restored to the original temperature (eg, room temperature), and allowed to readjust for about 24 hours, the original level of PAA can be shown by analysis. Likewise, when the solution is diluted, it is important to remember that water is of the equilibrium equation (on the right, with PAA). Thus, dilution with water will drive the equilibrium equation to the left (toward peroxide and acetic acid). This is not the decomposition (destabilization) of PAA, but rather, it is the relaxation of the new equilibrium toward new levels of all components at the given temperature.

Peracetic Acid Vapor

The use of PAA in a vapor (or gas) form has seen more limited application in disinfection and sterilization. The PAA, in gas form, is considered a vapor because it readily condenses depending on the temperature of the area or surfaces it contacts. Similar to HP discussed previously, the correct control of such processes is important in the optimization of antimicrobial efficacy and safety. PAA vapor and aerosols have been used to disinfect devices, create germ-free isolators, and facilitate transfers of gnotobiotic specimens.[168] Vapor phase PAA (VPA) activity against spores was observed to be related to the relative humidity, implying that water plays an important component in the vapor activity.[169] Disinfection of laboratory animal rooms occurs more rapidly and across a larger area with vaporized PAA as compared to vaporized HP.[170] The PAA dry fogging is used to disinfect spaces like cleanrooms, biosafety cabinets, and animal care facilities.[171-174]

The PAA has been found to be effective in both the liquid and the vapor phase in room decontamination applications.[6] Vapor disinfection of hospital pharmacy isolators was found to be more rapid with a 3.5% PAA solution as compared to a 33% HP solution, occurring in 150 minutes with a standard load with VPA as compared to in 240 minutes with VHP.[175] The VPA was found to be effective against halophilic bacteria with complete kill of all test organisms observed after a 1-minute exposure.[176] Data indicates that 4000 ppm PAA vapor may have greater effectiveness at temperatures between 50°C and 60°C than HP vapor generated from a 35% HP solution under the

same sterilization conditions.[177] Equilibrium solutions of PAA benefit from the synergistic action of HP and PAA,[51,66] and it is expected that this synergy would be maintained under appropriate conditions in vapor phase PAA. The vapor phase permeability of PAA in narrow spaces and lumens likely occurs via a slip flow mechanism similar to that observed in gas permeability studies in porous sedimentary rocks, providing enhanced sterilant penetration capabilities compared to liquid phase PAA. Fluid dynamics considerations and control of condensation kinetics provide additional dimensions to the efficacy of VPA for disinfection and sterilization. When used for low temperature sterilization, VPA provides process efficiencies, a reduced exposure risk and compatibility with a variety of materials, including heat labile products and materials of biologic origin. With its short half-life on surfaces, it offers a safe, environmentally low temperature sterilization modality across a range of applications.

Limited data is available for the effects of vaporized peracetic sterilization on materials of construction. Directionally, materials compatibility can be crudely estimated by drawing conclusions based on a wider experience with VH_2O_2 sterilization (see chapter 32); however, due to the variation of process parameters and active chemical moieties between VH_2O_2 and VPA (sterilization modalities), a direct materials compatibility comparison between VH_2O_2 and VPA would be unreliable at best. A direct exposure of materials coupons is the best indicator of effects of a VPA gas or aerosol. A range of materials were exposed to both a 1-2 cycle process or to a >10 cycle sterilization process with VPA in a large-scale exposure system.[178] Materials compatibility was assessed based on changes in mass, sample dimensions, infrared spectral analysis, and degree of corrosion based on ASTM-G31-72.[179]

Aluminum compatibility to VPA depends greatly on the grade and need for anodizing. Aluminum 7075, 5056, 6061 display excellent compatibility with no notable corrosion as defined by ASTM-G31-72. Aluminum 1100 and 2024 displayed good to fair compatibility with apparent corrosion in 1-2x sterilization. In all cases, anodizing on aluminum was damaged by VPA sterilization. The VPA sterilization was seen to be compatible with stainless steel 304, 316, 430, and Hastelloy®. All of these were rated as excellent even after 30 sterilization cycles. Mild steels rated as fair compatibility, as corrosion was observed after 1-2 cycles of sterilization. Note that this is a difference from liquid PAA exposure, which is immediately deleterious to mild steel. Titanium grade 2 and the titanium alloy nitinol were rated as excellent after >30x and >10x sterilization respectively. Gold and nickel were rated excellent after >30x sterile. Chromium and silver were excellent up to 10x sterile with silver noting a color change around 10x sterile. Brass and copper were also tested at 10x sterile and rated at excellent; however, copper was noted to have dulled at after 10x sterile, which likely indicates the start of a corrosion process. Magnesium was rated as good after a 1-2x sterile and poor after 10x demonstrating significant corrosion.

According to data presented, most common thermoplastics display excellent compatibility at 30x sterile or less. This includes common plastics such as ABS, PTFE, PVF and PVDF, polycarbonate, polypropylene, and high- and low-density polyethylene. Polystyrene, PVC, polysulfone, and polyimides were also listed with excellent compatibility. Foamed plastic made of ethyl vinyl acetate were listed as "good" after 10 cycles due to a weight gain, which was indicated as an absorption of the sterilant into the materials.

Nonperoxide cured epoxies, and fluorinated versions thereof, were rated poor and good, respectively, and the literature suggested against their use if PAA sterilization is to be used. Common adhesive silicone, Loctite® 4061, and methacrylate were rated as excellent in their compatibility toward PAA sterilization. In general, the category of elastomers faired worst against VPA sterilization process. Butyl rubber, neoprene, FKM, viton, and natural rubber were all rated at fair to poor in their compatibility. Additionally, Pebax® and certain styrene copolymers fared poorly again a VPA sterilization process. The compatibility of elastomers with VPA will vary based on their individual molecular structures and processing history. Thus, like other classes of polymers, it is important to assess compatibility of elastomers on an application-specific basis.

Currently, it is proposed the liquid phase disinfection/sterilization processes using PAA derive their antimicrobial activity from a synergism between HP and PAA.[66] This PAA-HP synergism has yet to be described in the gas phase and to date, no detailed analysis of this synergy in the gas phase has been described, but it is suspected to exist.[180] But there is a described synergy between the PAA and water in gas phase sterilization processes.[169] For example, limited sporicidal activity was reported until relative humidity was greater than 40%, with the greatest activity being achieved when humidity was greater than 80%. Based on limited data,[181,182] it is hypothesized that the structure of PAA in an anhydrous (or low humidity) gas-phase environment is a 5-membered cyclic structure created with an intramolecular hydrogen bond between terminal hydrogen to the carbonyl oxygen of PAA:

Gas Phase PAA   Solution Phase PAA

In contrast, the aqueous solution phase structure is likely to be an open confirmation stabilized by numerous intermolecular hydrogen bonds to the available

bulk water. The cyclic, gas phase form of PAA allows the molecule to distribute electron density in a different manner as compared to its liquid phase structure.

Using a simple molecular mechanics calculation, it is possible to roughly estimate the energetic cost of rotating the -O-O- bond of gas phase PAA:

These calculations show PAA needs about 10 kcal/mol to achieve full bond rotation at the -O-O- bond. As a point of reference, a 3 to 4 kcal/mol difference would roughly equate to a 99:1 ratio of cyclic to open PAA structures. As such, a 10 kcal/mol difference means greater than 99% of the PAA in a low-humidity gas phase environment will be in the cyclic form. The subsequent lowing of microbicidal activity cause by this cyclic structure formation could be explained in two ways:

1. In low-humidity gas phase environments, PAA should take on a gas phase structure, as noted earlier. In a high-humidity gas phase environment, PAA would take on a structure like that of the solution phase PAA. This open structure of PAA does not allow for electron density to be distributed throughout the molecule and, therefore, may dramatically increase the reactivity of PAA. The difference in energy characteristics of the two molecules may be enough to affect sporicidal efficacy.

2. This cyclic confirmation may impede the ability of a "dry" PAA vapor to undergo the microcondensation process, which in a similar fashion to vaporized HP sterilization may be needed for microbial kill.[183-185] Increasing the humidity with PAA vapor will eventually lead to an adequate amount condensation in which PAA vapor can absorb/dissolve. Regardless of the mechanism, the described synergy between water and PAA has a marked effect on the efficacy of PAA vapor. Humidity levels greater than 60% at atmospheric pressure are needed for PAA to be usably efficacious in the gas phase.[169] The mechanistic reason for this synergy between PAA and water is still poorly understood but is not unusual in comparison to other gaseous sterilization processes. Additionally, further studies are needed to better define the interaction between HP and PAA during gas phase sterilization.

The mechanism of activity of PAA in the vapor phase has not been extensively investigated, but there are some published data that offer some insights. Vaporized PAA at room temperature and normal atmosphere was shown to inactivate viruses (reovirus 3, parvovirus minute virus of mice, and Avian polyomavirus) that had been evaluated as extremely stable to disinfectants.[174] In addition, the PAA vapor was shown to exhibit a $\log_{10}$ reduction value >4 on *G stearothermophilus* spores even when in difficult to access locations. The activity was connected to a high humidity level (>70% RH). Exposure of influenza viruses to PAA vapor under controlled box conditions[172] resulted in inactivation below detection levels within 5 minutes; activity versus other viruses varied, although the concentration of PAA used was lower than in.[174] In most cases, the RH was not kept above 70% for the whole disinfection run.

Physical chemical observations of PAA in the vapor phase were performed in the midinfrared region. Unusually strong hydroxide (OH) bending was observed,[181] which was attributed to intramolecular hydrogen bonding. Subsequently, the force constants were calculated.[186] The observed data was in agreement with an internal hydrogen bond, and it was noted to be unusually strong. The observed intramolecular hydrogen bond was characterized[182] and modeled to generate the force constants. These observations have been done on PAA vapor at very high concentrations and relatively little water vapor present. Because water is an excellent hydrogen bond donor, this may explain the effect of high relative humidity that has been observed[169,174] in increasing the antimicrobial effectiveness of vapor PAA.

The VPA has therefore been investigated for sterilization and disinfection purposes. Considering VPA as an alternative to formaldehyde, vaporized HP or gaseous chlorine dioxide, several notable products have been developed, for example, Minncare Dry Fog® and the Altrapure® fogging system for area disinfection applications, and the AbTox Plazlyte™ (discontinued), Revox® and STERIACE systems for terminal sterilization. Dry fogging system capability was investigated for its microbial activity and compatibility to electronics equipment.[187] Two different fogging systems were used, that is Mini Dry Fog® system (Mar Cor Purification, Skippack, PA) and a portable dry fog (Ikeuchi USA, West Chester, OH). For this study, liquid PAA, Minncare® Cold Sterilant was used, a registered disinfectant with the EPA. Composition percentages by weight of the sterilant are 4% to 6% PAA, 20% to 24% HP, and 8% to 10% acetic acid. To demonstrate its microbicidal activity, stainless steel coupons inoculated with various microbial agents (E coli, S aureus, Bacillus atrophaeus spores, vesicular stomatitis virus, and human adenovirus 5) were subjected to the dry fog. All five microbial agents were inactivated after exposure. A further area disinfection study inside an animal facility for antimicrobial and sporicidal character of VPA was reported.[170] This laboratory study consisting of four rooms ranging in area between 44.5 and 50.0 m^3, comparing the efficacy of PAA vapor to VHP. For this experiment, a dry fog unit (OZMIC-CJ-1, Oz Sangyo Co Ltd, Tokyo, Japan) was used. The PAA process inactivated the most resistant bacteria and mold spores tested within 15 minutes, with a total cycle time of 3 hours, in comparison to the VHP process that took 14 to 15 hours.

Others assessed the disinfection efficacy of VPA in an isolator, with a volume of approximately 0.8 m^3 and

equipped with an HEPA filtration and a vapor generator system.[180] The vapor generator maintained an air flow rate of 8 m^3/h and could measure time, temperature, and vapor flow. The PAA (generated from a 3.5% solution) and HP (from a 33% solution) vapor were tested in the isolator. It was observed that the time required to disinfect a standard load in the isolator required 150 minutes for VPA and 240 minutes for VHP. In conclusion, PAA vapor demonstrated better diffusion and requires a shorter contact time compared to HP.

Sporicidal activity of the PAA vapor has been demonstrated through various studies. The VPA was tested at varying relative humidity levels (20%, 40%, 60%, and 80% RH) and on different surfaces (paper and glass).[169] It was observed that the sporicidal action was faster on the paper than the glass. A possible explanation could be that spores in a drop of water easily spread over a large surface on porous materials. Therefore, they are not likely to pile up and provide a difficult penetration challenge as the liquid evaporates. On the contrary, microorganisms can pile up on impermeable surfaces and they create layers that can be relatively difficult to penetrate for VPA. The data shows spores on glass have a rapid initial death rate, but later, this kill rate slows down and ends up leveling off. The VPA reduced spore contamination on both porous and impermeable surfaces within approximately 10 minutes at RH ranging between 40% and 80%, but the inactivation rate was maximum at 80% RH and minimal at 20% RH. It was also concluded that level of microbial contamination and the cleanliness level of the surface is also important, in addition to the RH level. Overall, there is an opportunity for the further optimization of VPA processes for both disinfection and sterilization applications.

▶ OTHER PEROXYGEN COMPOUNDS

Performic and perpropionic acids are similar in antibacterial activity to PAA, but performic is volatile and unstable, and perpropionic is more costly.[188] Peroxyheptanoic and peroxynonanoic acids have been reported to have higher activity on a molar basis than PAA.[76] The perlauric acid has limited aqueous solubility but an antimicrobial spectrum somewhat like the quaternaries because of the long hydrocarbon chain. Monoperglutaric and diperglutaric acids and succinylperoxide are active, the latter having been marketed for disinfecting medical instruments. Derivatives of perbenzoic acid have been claimed in patents for sporicidal action. The magnesium salt of peroxyphthalate is a commercial product. It is a water-soluble, solid that is effective against bacteria, yeasts, and spores.[189] Its activity is increased in acid solution and with alcohol and with heat. It has been formulated as a sanitizer for bathrooms, kitchens, and diapers. As a powder with anionics, it has been proposed for use on walls and floors in health care facilities for environmental disinfection. Eggensberger[100] described peracid powder disinfectants made in situ by adding water to mixtures of organic acid reservoirs (anhydrides, amides, and esters) to HP reservoirs such as sodium peroxide. Products based on this procedure are on the market in Germany for treating dentures and general hospital disinfection. Benzoyl peroxide is in general use in skin formulations for treating acne, and *t*-butyl hydroperoxide with phenols has been suggested for preventing microbial attack on engine fuels, cutting oils, and timber.

Shin and Marquis[190] reported that *t*-butyl hydroperoxide was sporicidal and that its activity increased 10-fold for each 15°C temperature increase from 30°C to 70°C. Killing was thought to be due to the peroxyl radical (*t*-butylOO). Others were concerned about biofilm formation in hospital piping systems and evaluated peroxide solutions[191]; 1% HP was not effective against the test bacteria in 1 hour. A 1% solution of a mixture of 28% HP, 10% perglutaric acid, and 0.5% perbenzoic acid was highly effective. A 3% solution of 10% *t*-butyl hydroperoxide, 20% phenoxypropanols, and 48% dipropylene glycol gave a 5 log reduction in 3 hours.

Inorganic peroxides also have been used to combat microbes. Perborates have been used in toothpastes and powders. Permanganate is antibacterial, antifungal, and antiviral; it was used as an antiseptic, but its intense purple color is a disadvantage. It is said to be superior to copper sulfate as an algicide; 0.01% potassium permanganate kills algae in 4 to 6 hours in cooling towers.[192,193] A 1% solution of seven inorganic peroxygen compounds was evaluated for viricidal activity.[194] Permanganate was effective in 30 seconds with potassium peroxymonosulfate next in activity. Calcium peroxide is reported to protect seed from microbial inhibition during sprouting. The alkali metal perdisulphates are strong oxidants but demonstrate little antimicrobial activity. Monoperoxysulfuric acid is made from sulfuric acid and HP; partially neutralized with potassium hydroxide, it gives Caro's acid triple salt, which is used as a bleaching agent in toilet bowl and denture cleaners and as a swimming pool disinfectant. When investigated, it showed activity against bacteria and viruses but none toward yeasts and fungi.[195] With isopropanol, it was considered synergistic and active toward yeast. With chloride or bromide it generates the hypohalite useful for slime control, pool disinfection, and sanitation of baby diapers.[196]

ADVANCED OXIDATION SYSTEMS

Advanced oxidation systems include those where oxidizing radicals are generated, as for example with ozone (see chapters 10 and 33). In some cases, this action can be initiated by radiation. Solar UV on titanium dioxide (TiO_2) in aqueous systems generates the hydroxyl radical, which oxidizes many organic molecules and, as with peroxygen compounds, is strongly antimicrobial. The TiO_2 alone is inactive. Bacteria in the presence of solar UV and 0.01%

TiO_2 were killed in 5 minutes or less, whereas in sunlight alone, it took more than 1 hour.[197] In the disinfection of indoor air, UV photons and TiO_2 with 50% RH effectively destroyed bacteria and odors.[198,199] Addition of HP to ultraviolet A (UVA)/TiO_2 improves inactivation of *E coli*, presumably by weakening the cell wall due to OH attacks, allowing HP to diffuse into bacteria.[200] Addition of Fe^{+3} to the UV/TiO_2 decreases the disinfection time.[201]

TOXICITY AND HAZARDS OF PEROXYGEN COMPOUNDS

As peroxygen compounds are potent oxidizing agents, with known effects on various macromolecules essential to life, and are biocidal to microbial cells and viruses, they will also be hazardous overtime to humans and animals depending on the concentrations and forms (eg, liquid or gas) that they are exposed to. The HP is a clear, colorless liquid with a characteristic slightly acidic odor. It has low toxicity and is not a systemic poison because it is decomposed in the bowel before absorption.[202] Concentrated solutions are irritating to the skin, mucous membranes, and particularly to the eyes. The vapors can cause headache, dizziness, nausea, and vomiting; repeated exposure can cause inflammation of the respiratory tract and pulmonary edema. It is considered to be not classifiable as to its carcinogenicity to humans.[203] Rubber gloves, safety goggles, and protective clothing should be worn when handling concentrated HP, PAA, or any liquid peroxygen compound or solution. They should be washed off immediately using large quantities of water if splashed on the skin or in the eyes. If they are swallowed, milk or lukewarm water should be administered and a physician called. In a vapor HP sterilizing system using 30% HP, certain medical material polymers were cytotoxic after 12 hours aeration as a result of retained HP.[204] Peroxide condenses from the gas form at a higher rate than water, which can cause initial higher concentration of peroxide in the condensed liquid. This can lead to complications with using it for disinfection.[2] Under some conditions, peroxide can cause a severe burning sensation. In addition, surface materials can be damaged by the presence of the concentrated peroxide.

The PAA is a clear, colorless solution with a pungent odor that contains 40% or less of PAA. The 40% solution has a median lethal dose (LD_{50}) to rats of 1540 mg/kg.[205] The LD_{50} values for rats were reported at 315 for PAA and 263 for Wolfasteril®, a preparation containing 36% to 40% PAA.[206] For a 4% formulation (P3-oxonia® active), a value of 3.4 g/kg is given, which compares favorably to other common sanitizers.[147] The subchronic oral feeding studies with this formulation showed no change in growth of the animals in 8 weeks. The acute inhalation toxicity, LC 50, was 13 439 mg/m³. For the 35% PAA solution, the vapor is lachrymatory, and inhalation results in a stinging sensation in the nasal passages. The PAA solutions has

TABLE 18.17 Summary of Acute Exposure Guideline Levels for Hazardous Substance (AEGL) values for peracetic acid[a]

Classification	10 min	30 min	1 h	4 h	8 h	End Point/Reference
AEGL-1 (nondisabling)	0.52 mg/m^3 (0.17 ppm)	0.52 mg/m^3 (0.17 ppm)	0.52 mg/m^3 (0.17 ppm)	0.52 mg/m^3 (0.17 ppm)	0.52 mg/m^3 (0.17 ppm)	Threshold for irritation (Fraser and Thorbinson[211], McDonagh[212])
AEGL-2 (disabling)	1.6 mg/m^3 (0.5 ppm)	1.6 mg/m^3 (0.5 ppm)	1.6 mg/m^3 (0.5 ppm)	1.6 mg/m^3 (0.5 ppm)	1.6 mg/m^3 (0.5 ppm)	Mild irritation (Fraser and Thorbinson[211])
AEGL-3[b] (lethal)	60 mg/m^3	30 mg/m^3	15 mg/m^3	6.3 mg/m^3	4.1 mg/m^3	Highest concentration causing no deaths (Janssen[213])

[a]From National Research Council.[208] Adapted and reproduced with permission from the National Academy of Sciences. Courtesy of the National Academies Press, Washington, DC.

[b]AEGL-3 values are based on exposure to aerosol; therefore, concentrations are not converted to ppm.

been tested on skin and 0.4% to 0.8% PAA may be used directly as a body disinfectant for swine.[206]

Studies of acute mammalian toxicity did not reveal a clear dose-response that could be related to the PAA content or concentration alone.[207] The main effect of PAA is severe irritation and corrosion of skin, eyes, and mucous membranes, most obvious at higher concentrations. It causes irritation to the upper respiratory tract in humans after exposure to concentrations as low as 15.6 mg/m^3 (5 ppm).[208] At liquid concentrations of 0.2% or lower, PAA did not appear to cause skin irritation.[207] The skin sensitization potential of PAA appears to be low. In the vapor phase, a concentration of 4.6 mg PAA per m^3 was used for disinfection, with no deleterious symptoms.[209]

Using the Ames test, the mutagenicity of peroxygen compounds was studied.[210] The HP and PAA were not mutagenic, and neither was *m*-chloroperbenzoic acid. The only peroxygen compounds shown to be mutagenic were *t*-butylhydroperoxide and cumene hydroperoxide. The data for PAA do not raise immediate concern for carcinogenicity.[207] Genotoxicity studies with PAA have yielded some chromosomal and sperm anomalies in mice[208] but are insufficient for evaluation for humans.

Due to the continuous growing interest in PAA as an alternative modality for sterilization and disinfection, the US National Advisory Committee has established an Acute Exposure Guideline Levels for Hazardous Substance (AEGL Committee), falling under Federal Advisory Committee Act (FACA) Pub L No. 92-463 of 1972.[208] Three levels (AEGL-1, AEGL-2, and AEGL-3) have been created for each of five exposure periods, 10 minutes, 30 minutes, 1 hour, 4 hours, and 8 hours (Table 18.17). There is no current Occupational Safety and Health Administration guideline established for PAA yet.

By their chemical nature, the peroxygen compounds are powerful oxidizers. They appear to present no immediate danger from toxicity or other hazards when diluted in water to their effective concentration as disinfectants and sterilants but will do harm is not used in accordance with their instructions and safety precautions. In concentrated solution, they must be treated with caution, as is the case with any strong oxidant. They should be stored in a cool place, not over 30°C, in the original containers provided, with vents and flame resisters. The PAA is stable in linear PE containers but can slowly attack plastics after several years, especially with continuous heat. It can not only make plastic containers brittle but also degrade the seam lines of formed plastic containers. Spills or leaks of concentrated solutions should be treated carefully, evacuating and isolating the area. The spill should be approached from upwind (if possible), with adequate PPE. The spill should be contained, diluted, or mixed with an inert material (eg, sand or earth). Textiles or cellulose materials (eg, paper towels) are not recommended in these cases and consideration may need to be given to all local regulations for disposal.[207] Organic materials and heavy metals ions of copper, iron, and manganese should be avoided because they can cause decomposition so rapid as to cause ignition and produce fires.

ACKNOWLEDGMENTS

The authors are grateful for the excellent work done on the previous version of this chapter by Professor Seymour S. Block (deceased), University of Florida College of Engineering, Gainesville, Florida.

REFERENCES

1. Schumb WC, Satterfield CN, Wentworth RL. In: *Hydrogen Peroxide*. New York, NY: Van Nostrand Rheinhold; 1955:813-816.
2. McDonnell GE. The use of hydrogen peroxide for disinfection and sterilization applications. In: Marek I, ed. *Patai's Chemistry of Functional Groups*. Hoboken, NJ: John Wiley & Sons; 2014.
3. Schumb WC, Satterfield CN, Wentworth RL. *Report No. 42, Hydrogen Peroxide*. Cambridge, MA: Massachusetts Institute of Technology; 1953: 2ff.
4. Richardson BW. On peroxide of hydrogen, or ozone water, as a remedy. *Lancet*. 1891;1:707-709, 760-763.

5. Zhu G, Wang Q, Lu S, Niu Y. Hydrogen peroxide: a potential wound therapeutic target? *Med Princ Pract.* 2017;26(4):301-308.

6. Heinemann PG. The germicidal efficiency of commercial preparations of hydrogen peroxide. *JAMA.* 1913;60:1603-1606.

7. Wilson JB, Turner WR, Sale JW. Studies on bottled cocoa beverages. II. Efficiency of hydrogen peroxide in preserving cocoa-milk beverages. *Am Food J.* 1927;22:347-348.

8. Yoshpe-Purer Y, Eylan E. Disinfection of water by hydrogen peroxide. *Health Lab Sci.* 1968;5:233-238.

9. Naguib K, Hussein L. The effect of hydrogen peroxide on the bacteriological quality and nutritive value of milk. *Milchwessenschaft.* 1972;27:758-762.

10. Rosenzweig AL. Hydrogen peroxide in prevention of water contamination. *Lancet.* 1978;8070:944.

11. Mentel R, Schmidt J. Investigations on rhinovirus inactivation by hydrogen peroxide. *Acta Virol.* 1973;17:351-354.

12. Toledo RT, Escher FE, Ayres JC. Sporicidal properties of hydrogen peroxide against food spoilage organisms. *Appl Microbiol.* 1973;26: 592-597.

13. Wardle MD, Renninger GM. Bactericidal effect of hydrogen peroxide on spacecraft isolates. *Appl Microbiol.* 1975;30:710-711.

14. Ramirez JA, Omidbakhsh N, inventors; Virox Technologies Inc, assignee. Enhanced activity hydrogen peroxide disinfectant. US patent 8,637,085. January 28, 2014.

15. Rutala WA, Gergen MF, Weber DJ. Efficacy of improved hydrogen peroxide against important healthcare-associated pathogens. *Infect Control Hosp Epidemiol.* 2012;33(11):1159-1161.

16. Cosentino LC, Hnojewyj AM, Fischbach LJ, Jansen WB, Maltais JAB, inventors; Medivators Inc, assignee. Stable, shippable, peroxy-containing microbicide. US Patent 5,656,302. August 12, 1997.

17. Super D Hydrogen Peroxide, AOFARMA Hydrogen Peroxide, Peroxy-Chem, Philadelphia

18. Turner FJ. Hydrogen peroxide and other oxidant disinfectants. In: Block SS, ed. *Disinfection, Sterilization, and Preservation.* 3rd ed. Philadelphia, PA: Lea & Febiger; 1983:240-250.

19. Linley E, Denyer SP, McDonnell G, Simons C, Maillard J-Y. Use of hydrogen peroxide as a biocide: new consideration of its mechanisms of biocidal action. *J Antimicrob Chemother.* 2012;67(7):1589-1596.

20. Liochev SI. The mechanism of "Fenton-like" reactions and their importance for biological system. A biologist's view. *Metal Ions Biol Syst.* 1999;36:1-39.

21. Mello Filho AC, Hoffmann ME, Meneghini R. Cell killing and DNA damage by hydrogen peroxide are mediated by intracellular iron. *Biochem J.* 1984;218:273-275.

22. Clapp PA, Davies MJ, French MS, et al. The bactericidal action of peroxides; an E.P.R. spin-trapping study. *Free Radic Res.* 1994;21:147-167.

23. Dittmar HR, Baldwin IL, Miller SB. The influence of certain inorganic salts on the germicidal activity of hydrogen peroxide. *J Bacteriol.* 1930;19(3):203-211.

24. Colobert L. Mechanism of bactericidal activity of hydrogen peroxide and ascorbic acid on *Escherichia coli. Revue des Corps de Sante des Armees.* 1962;3(suppl):495-500.

25. Gould GW, Hitchins AD. Sensitization of bacterial spores to lysozyme and to hydrogen peroxide with reagents which rupture disulfide bonds. *J Gen Microbiol.* 1963;33:413-423.

26. Brandi G, Sestili P, Pedrini MA, Salvaggio L, Cattabeni F, Cantoni O. The effect of temperature or anoxia on *Escherichia coli* killing induced by hydrogen peroxide. *Mutat Res.* 1987;190:237-240.

27. Brandi G, Cattabeni F, Albano A, Cantoni O. Role of hydroxyl radicals in *Escherichia coli* killing induced by hydrogen peroxide. *Free Radic Res Commun.* 1989;6(1):47-55.

28. Macomber L, Rensing C, Imlay JA. Intracellular copper does not catalyze the formation of oxidative DNA damage in *Escherichia coli. J Bacteriol.* 2007;189:1616-1626.

29. Imlay JA, Chin SM, Linn S. Toxic DNA damage by hydrogen peroxide through the Fenton reaction in vivo and in vitro. *Science.* 1988; 240:640-642.

30. Luo Y, Han Z, Chin SM, Linn S. Three chemically distinct types of oxidants formed by iron-mediated Fenton reactions in the presence of DNA. *Proc Natl Acad Sci U S A.* 1994;91:12438-12442.

31. Ananthaswamy HN, Eisenstark A. Repair of hydrogen peroxide-induced single-stranded breaks in *Escherichia coli* deoxyribonucleic acid. *J Bacteriol.* 1977;130:187-191.

32. Hagensee ME, Moses RE. Repair response of *Escherichia coli* to hydrogen peroxide DNA damage. *J Bacteriol.* 1986;168:1059-1065.

33. Fernández JL, Cartelle M, Muriel L, et al. DNA fragmentation in microorganisms assessed in situ. *Appl Environ Microbiol.* 2008;74:5925-5933.

34. Luo D, Smith SW, Anderson BD. Kinetics and mechanism of the reaction of cysteine and hydrogen peroxide in aqueous solution. *J Pharm Sci.* 2005;94:304-316.

35. Ashby MT, Nagy P. Revisiting a proposed kinetic model for the reaction of cysteine residues and hydrogen peroxide via cysteine sulfenic acid. *Int J Chem Kinet.* 2007;39:32-82.

36. Kim JR, Yoon HW, Kwon KS, Lee S-R, Rhee SG. Identification of proteins containing cysteine residues that are sensitive to oxidation by hydrogen peroxide at neutral pH. *Anal Biochem.* 2000;283:214-221.

37. Dean RT, Fu S, Stocker R, Davies MJ. Biochemistry and pathology of radical-mediated protein oxidation. *Biochem J.* 1997;324:1-18.

38. Tamarit J, Cabiscol E, Ros J. Identification of the major oxidatively damaged proteins in *Escherichia coli* cells exposed to oxidative stress. *J Biol Chem.* 1998;273:3027-3032.

39. Brandi G, Salvaggio L, Cattabeni F, Cantoni O. Cytocidal and filamentous response of *Escherichia coli* cells exposed to low concentrations of hydrogen peroxide and hydroxyl radical scavengers. *Environ Mol Mutagen.* 1991;18(1):22-27.

40. Baatout S, De Boever P, Mergeay M. Physiological changes induced in four bacterial strains following oxidative stress. *Prikl Biokhim Mikrobiol.* 2006;42:418-427.

41. Peterson HG, Hrudey SE, Cantin IA, Perley TR, Kenefick SL. Physiological toxicity, cell membrane damage and the release of dissolved organic carbon and geosmin in *Aphanizomenon flos-aquae* after exposure to water treatment chemicals. *Water Res.* 1995;29(6):1515-1523.

42. Kunzmann T. Investigations on the disinfecting action of hydrogen peroxides. *Fortschr Med.* 1934;52:357-359.

43. Lineback CB, Nkemngong CA, Wu ST, Li X, Teska PJ, Oliver HF. Hydrogen peroxide and sodium hypochlorite disinfectants are more effective against *Staphylococcus aureus* and *Pseudomonas aeruginosa* biofilms than quaternary ammonium compounds. *Antimicrob Resist Infect Control.* 2018;7:154.

44. Nambudripad VKN, Laxminarayana II, Lya KK. Bactericidal efficiency of hydrogen peroxide. I. Influence of different concentrations on the rate and extent of destruction of bacteria of dairy importance. *Indian J Dairy Sci.* 1949;4:38-44.

45. Nambudripad VKN, Lya KK. Bactericidal efficiency of hydrogen peroxide. 2. Influence of different concentrations of peroxide on the rate and extent of destruction of additional bacteria of dairy importance. *Indian J Dairy Sci.* 1951;4:38-44.

46. Nikolov ZV, Popova OM. Action of chemical disinfectants on the orthinosis virus. *Kongr Bulg Mikrobiol Inst Sofia.* 1965:757-761.

47. Kline LB, Hull RN. The virucidal properties of peracetic acid. *Am J Clin Pathol.* 1960;33:30-33.

48. Baldry MGC. The bactericidal, fungicidal, and sporicidal properties of hydrogen peroxide and peracetic acid. *J Appl Bacteriol.* 1983;54:417-423.

49. Leaper S. Synergistic killing of spores of *Bacillus subtilis* by peracetic acid and alcohol. *J Food Technol.* 1984;19:355-360.

50. Alasri A, Roques C, Michel G, Cabassud C, Aptel P. Bactericidal properties of peracetic acid and hydrogen peroxide, alone and in combination, and chlorine and formaldehyde against bacterial water strains. *Can J Microbiol.* 1992;38:635-642.

51. Alasri A, Valverde M, Roques C, Michel G, Cabassud C, Aptel P. Sporicidal properties of peracetic acid and hydrogen peroxide, alone and in combination, in comparison with chlorine and formaldehyde for ultrafiltration membrane disinfection. *Can J Microbiol.* 1993;39:52-60.

52. Rutala WA, Gergen MF, Weber DJ. Sporicidal activity of chemical sterilants used in hospitals. *Infect Control Hosp Epidemiol.* 1993;14:713-718.

53. Sagripanti JL, Bonifacino A. Comparative sporicidal effects of liquid chemical agents. *Appl Environ Microbiol.* 1996;62:545-551.

54. Sagripanti JL, Bonifacino A. Effects of salt and serum on the sporicidal activity of liquid disinfectants. *J AOAC Int.* 1997;80:1198-1207.

55. Sagripanti JL, Eklund CA, Trost PA, et al. Comparative sensitivity of 13 species of pathogenic bacteria to seven chemical germicides. *Am J Infect Control.* 1997;25:335-339.

56. Lambert RJ, Johnston MD, Hanlon GW, Denyer SP. Theory of antimicrobial combinations: biocide mixtures—synergy or addition? *J Appl Microbiol.* 2003;94(4):747-759.

57. Demerec M, Bertani G, Flint J. A survey of chemicals for mutagenic action on *E. coli. Am Nat.* 1951;85:119-136.

58. Bayliss CE, Waites WM. The effect of hydrogen peroxide on spores of *Clostridium bifermentans. J Gen Microbiol.* 1976;96:401-407.

59. Sagripanti JL, Kraemer KH. Site-specific oxidative DNA damage at polyguanosines produced by copper plus hydrogen peroxide. *J Biol Chem.* 1989;264:1729-1734.

60. Aruoma OI, Halliwell B, Gajewski E, Dizdaroglu M. Copper-ion-dependent damage to the bases in DNA in the presence of hydrogen peroxide. *Biochem J.* 1991;273:601-604.

61. Sagripanti JL, Routson LB, Lytle CD. Virus inactivation by copper or iron ions alone and in the presence of peroxide. *Appl Environ Microbiol.* 1993;59:4374-4376.

62. Sagripanti JL. Metal-based formulations with high microbicidal activity. *Appl Environ Microbiol.* 1992;58:3157-3162.

63. Sagripanti JL, Routson LB, Bonifacino AC, Lytle CD. Mechanism of copper-mediated inactivation of herpes simplex virus. *Antimicrob Agents Chemother.* 1997;41:812-817.

64. Alfa MJ, Lo E, Wald A, Dueck C, DeGagne P, Harding GKM. Improved eradication of *Clostridium difficile* spores from toilets of hospitalized patients using an accelerated hydrogen peroxide as the cleaning agent. *BMC Infect Dis.* 2010;10:268.

65. Omidbakhsh N, Sattar SA. Broad-spectrum microbicidal activity, toxicologic assessment, and materials compatibility of a new generation of accelerated hydrogen peroxide-based environmental surface disinfectant. *Am J Infect Control.* 2006;34(5):251-257.

66. Leggett MJ, Schwarz JS, Burke PA, McDonnell G, Denyer SP, Maillard JY. Mechanism of sporicidal activity for the synergistic combination of peracetic acid and hydrogen peroxide. *Appl Environ Microbiol.* 2015;82(4):1035-1039.

67. Bayliss CE, Waites WM. The combined effect of hydrogen peroxide and ultraviolet irradiation on bacterial spores. *J Appl Bacteriol.* 1979;47:263-269.

68. Bayliss CE, Waites WM. The synergistic killing of spores of *Bacillus subtilis* by hydrogen peroxide and ultra-violet light irradiation. *FEMS Microbiol Lett.* 1979;5:331-333.

69. Bayliss CE, Waites WM. Effect of simultaneous high intensity ultraviolet irradiation and hydrogen peroxide on bacterial spores. *J Food Technol.* 1982;17:467-470.

70. Peel JL, Waites WM, inventors; BTG International Ltd, assignee. Improvement in methods of sterilization. US patent 4,289,728. September 15, 1981.

71. Waites WM, Harding SE, Fowler DR, Jones SH, Shaw D, Martin M. The destruction of spores of *Bacillus subtilis* by the combined effects of hydrogen peroxide and ultraviolet light. *Lett Appl Microbiol.* 1988;7:139-140.

72. Ahmed FIK, Russell C. Synergism between ultrasonic waves and hydrogen peroxide in the killing of microorganisms. *J Appl Bacteriol.* 1975;39:31-40.

73. Sims AFE. Industrial effluent treatment with hydrogen peroxide. *Chem Industries.* 1983;27:555-558.

74. Mather JD. Attenuation and control of landfill leachates. *Solid Wastes.* 1977;67:362-378.

75. Holmes R. The water balance method of estimating leachate production from landfill sites. *Solid Wastes.* 1980;70:20-33.

76. Baldry MGC, Fraser JAL. Disinfection with peroxygens. In: Payne KR, ed. *Industrial Biocides.* New York, NY: John Wiley & Sons; 1988:91-116.

77. Vesley D, Norlien KG, Nelson B, Ott B, Streifel AJ. Significant factors in the disinfection and sterilization of flexible endoscopes. *Am J Infect Control.* 1992;20:291-300.

78. Sattar SA, Taylor YE, Paquette M, Rubino J. In-hospital evaluation of 7.5% hydrogen peroxide as a disinfectant for flexible endoscopes. *Can J Infect Control.* 1996;11:51-54.

79. Arduino MJ, McDonnell G. Disinfection and sterilization. In: Carroll KC, Pfaller MA, Landry ML, et al, eds. *Manual of Clinical Microbiology.* 12th ed. Washington, DC: ASM Press; 2019:224-242.

80. Zhao Z-H, Sakagami Y, Osaka T. Toxicity of hydrogen peroxide produced by electroplated coatings to pathogenic bacteria. *Can J Microbiol.* 1998;44:441-447.

81. Liu W-K, Brown MRW, Elliot TSJ. Mechanisms of the bactericidal activity of low amperage electric current (DC). *J Antimicrob Chemother.* 1997;39:687-695.

82. Boyce JM. Modern technologies for improving cleaning and disinfection of environmental surfaces in hospitals. *Antimicrob Resist Infect Control.* 2016;5:10.

83. Han JH, Sullivan N, Leas BF, Pegues DA, Kaczmarek JL, Umscheid CA. Cleaning hospital room surfaces to prevent health care-associated infections: a technical brief. *Ann Intern Med.* 2015;163(8):598-607.

84. Hultman C, Hill A, McDonnell G. The physical chemistry of decontamination with gaseous hydrogen peroxide. *Pharm Eng.* 2007;27(1):22-32.

85. Rutala WA, Gergen MF, Sickbert-Bennett EE. Effectiveness of a hydrogen peroxide mist (Trophon) system in inactivating healthcare pathogens on surface and endocavity probes. *Infect Control Hosp Epidemiol.* 2016;37(5):613-614.

86. Jacobs PT, Lin SM, inventors; Ethicon Inc, assignee. Hydrogen peroxide plasma sterilization system. US patent 4,643,876. February 17, 1987.

87. Jacobs PT, Lin SM. Sterilization processes utilizing low-temperature plasma. In: Block SE, ed. *Disinfection, Sterilization and Preservation.* 5th ed. Philadelphia, PA: Lippincott Williams & Wilkins; 2001:747-763.

88. Krebs MC, Bécasse P, Verjat D, Darbord J. Gas-plasma sterilization: relative efficacy of the hydrogen peroxide phase compared with that of the plasma phase. *Int J Pharm.* 1998;160:75-81.

89. McDonnell GE. *Antisepsis, Disinfection, and Sterilization: Types, Action, and Resistance.* 2nd ed. Washington, DC: ASM Press; 2017.

90. McDonnell G. *American Association of Tissue Banks Guidance Document: Microbiological Process Validation & Surveillance Program.* McLean, VA: American Association of Tissue Banks; 2016.

91. Vangsness CT Jr, Garcia IA, Mills CR, Kainer MA, Roberts MR, Moore TM. Allograft transplantation in the knee: tissue regulation, procurement, processing, and sterilization. *Am J Sports Med.* 2003;31:474-481.

92. Nichols JJ, Chalmers RL, Dumbleton K, et al. The case for using hydrogen peroxide contact lens care solutions: a review. *Eye Contact Lens.* 2019;45(2):69-82.

93. Smith CA, Pepose JS. Disinfection of tonometers and contact lenses in the office setting: are current techniques adequate? *Am J Ophthalmol.* 1999;127(1):77-84.

94. Deo PV. The use of hydrogen peroxide for the control of air pollution. *Studies in Env Sci.* 1988;34:275-292.

95. Roberts S, Khammo N, McDonnell G, Sewell G. Studies on the decontamination of surfaces exposed to cytotoxic drugs in chemotherapy workstations. *J Oncol Pharm Pract.* 2006;12(2):95-104.

96. Perathoner S, Centi G. Wet hydrogen peroxide catalytic oxidation (WHPCO) of organic waste in agro-food and industrial streams. *Top Catal.* 2005;33:207-224.

97. Delgado DA, de Souza Sant'ana A, de Massaguer PR. Occurrence of molds on laminated paperboard for aseptic packaging, selection of the most hydrogen peroxide- and heat-resistant isolates and determination of their thermal death kinetics in sterile distilled water. *World J Microbiol Biotechnol.* 2012;28:2609-2614.

98. Block S. Peroxygen Compounds. In: Block SE, ed. *Disinfection, Sterilization and Preservation*. 5th ed. Philadelphia, PA: Lippincott Williams & Wilkins; 2001:185-204.

99. Malchesky PS. Medical applications of peracetic acid. In: Block SE, ed. *Disinfection, Sterilization and Preservation*. 5th ed. Philadelphia, PA: Lippincott Williams & Wilkins; 2001:979-996.

100. Eggensberger H. Disinfectants based on peracid splitting compounds [in Polish]. *Zentralbl Bakteriol B*. 1979;168:517-524.

101. Sprossig M. Peracetic acid and resistant microorganisms. In: Kedzia WB, ed. *Resistance of Microorganisms to Disinfectants: Second International Symposium*. Warsaw, Poland: Polish Academy of Sciences; 1975:89-91.

102. Freer PC, Novy FG. On the formation, decomposition and germicidal action of benzoylacetyl and diacetyl peroxides. *Am Chem J*. 1902;27:161-193.

103. Hutchings IJ, Xezones H. Comparative evaluation of the bactericidal efficiency of peracetic acid, quaternaries and chlorine containing compounds. In: Proceedings from the 49th Annual Meeting of the Society of American Bacteriology; May 17-20, 1949. Cincinnati, OH. Abstract 50B51.

104. Greenspan FP, MacKellar DG. The application of peracetic acid germicidal washes to mold control of tomatoes. *Food Technol*. 1951;5:95-97.

105. Reyniers JA. Germ-free life applied to nutrition studies. *Lobund Reports*. 1946;(1):87-120.

106. Davies DM, Deary ME. Kinetics of the hydrolysis and perhydrolysis of tetraacetylethylenediamine, a peroxide bleach activator. *J Chem Soc Perkin Trans*. 1991;1(2):1549-1552.

107. Shin SY, Calvisi EG, Beaman TC, Pankratz HS, Gerhardt P, Marquis RE. Microscopic and thermal characterization of hydrogen peroxide killing and lysis of spores and protection by transition metal ions, chelators, and antioxidants. *Appl Environ Microbiol*. 1994;60:3192-3197.

108. Marquis RE, Rutherford GC, Faraci MM, Shin SY. Sporicidal action of peracetic acid and protective effects of transition metal ions. *J Ind Microbiol*. 1995;15:486-492.

109. Setlow B, Setlow P. Binding of small, acid-soluble spore proteins to DNA plays a significant role in the resistance of *Bacillus subtilis* spores to hydrogen peroxide. *Appl Environ Microbiol*. 1993;59:3418-3423.

110. Rodriguez-Montelongo L, de la Cruz-Rodriguez LC, Farías RN, Massa EM. Membrane-associated redox cycling of copper mediates hydroperoxide toxicity in *Escherichia coli*. *Biochim Biophys Acta*. 1993;1144:77-84.

111. Leggett MJ, Schwarz JS, Burke PA, McDonnell G, Denyer SP, Maillard JY. Resistance to and killing by the sporicidal microbicide peracetic acid. *J Antimicrob Chemother*. 2015;70(3):773-779.

112. Finnegan M, Linley E, Denyer SP, McDonnell G, Simons C, Maillard J-Y. Mode of action of hydrogen peroxide and other oxidizing agents: differences between liquid and gas forms. *J Antimicrob Chemother*. 2010;65:2108-2115.

113. Kampf G, Bloss R, Martiny H. Surface fixation of dried blood by glutaraldehyde and peracetic acid. *J Hosp Infect*. 2004;57(2):139-143.

114. Maillard JY, Russell AD. Viricidal activity and mechanisms of action of biocides. *Sci Prog*. 1997;80:287-315.

115. Kitis M. Disinfection of wastewater with peracetic acid: a review. *Environ Int*. 2004;30:47-55.

116. Olojo R, Simoyi RH. Oxyhalogen-sulfur chemistry: kinetics and mechanism of the oxidation of thionicotinamide by peracetic acid. *J Phys Chem A*. 2004;108(6):1018-1023.

117. Chang W, Small DA, Toghrol F, Bentley WE. Microarray analysis of toxicogenomic effects of peracetic acid on *Pseudomonas aeruginosa*. *Environ Sci Technol*. 2005;39:5893-5899.

118. Bridier A, Dubois-Brissonnet F, Greub G, Thomas V, Briandet R. Dynamics of the action of biocides in *Pseudomonas aeruginosa* biofilms. *Antimicrob Agents Chemother*. 2011;55(6): 2648-2654.

119. van der Veen S, Abee T. Mixed species biofilms of *Listeria monocytogenes* and *Lactobacillus plantarum* show enhanced resistance to benzalkonium chloride and peracetic acid. *Int J Food Microbiol*. 2011;144:421-431.

120. Lee SHI, Cappato LP, Corassin CH, Cruz AG, Oliveira CAF. Effect of peracetic acid on biofilms formed by *Staphylococcus aureus* and *Listeria monocytogenes* isolated from dairy plants. *J Dairy Sci*. 2016;99:2384-2390.

121. Baldry MGC, French MS, Slater D. The activity of peracetic acid on sewage indicator bacteria and viruses. *Wat Sci Tech*. 1991;24(2):353-357.

122. Orth R, Mrozeck H. Is the control of *Listeria*, *Campylobacter*, and *Yersinia* a disinfection problem? *Fleischwirtsch*. 1989;69:1575-1576.

123. Stanley P. Efficacy of peroxygen compounds against glutaraldehyde-resistant mycobacteria. *Am J Infect Control*. 1999;27:339-343.

124. Mediavators (Cantel Medical). *High Level Disinfectant Rapicide PA, Safety, Efficacy, and Microbiological Considerations*. Minneapolis, MN: Medivators (Cantel Medical); 2011. Document 50096-959.

125. Lynam PA, Babb JR, Fraise AP. Comparison of the mycobactericidal activity of 2% alkaline glutaraldehyde and Nu Cidex (0.35% peracetic acid). *J Hosp Infect*. 1995;31:237-239.

126. Griffiths PA, Babb JR, Fraise AP. Mycobactericidal activity of selected disinfectants using a quantitative suspension test. *J Hosp Infect*. 1999;41:111-121.

127. Harakeh MS. Inactivation of enteroviruses, rotaviruses, and bacteriophages by peracetic acid in a municipal sewage effluent. *FEMS Microbiol Lett*. 1984;23:27-30.

128. Eterpi M, McDonnell G, Thomas V. Virucidal activity of disinfectants against parvoviruses and reference viruses. *Appl Biosafety*. 2010;15(4):165-171.

129. Hussaini SN, Ruby KR. Sporicidal activity of peracetic acid against B anthracis spores. *Vet Rec*. 1976;98:257-259.

130. Jones LA Jr, Hoffman RK, Phillips CR. Sporicidal activity of peracetic acid and beta-propiolactone at subzero temperatures. *Appl Microbiol*. 1967;15:357-362.

131. US Food and Drug Administration. FDA-cleared sterilants and high level disinfectants with general claims for processing reusable medical and dental devices—March 2015. US Food and Drug Administration Web site. https://www.fda.gov/medical-devices/reprocessing-reusable-medical-devices-information-manufacturers/fda-cleared-sterilants-and-high-level-disinfectants-general-claims-processing-reusable-medical-and. Accessed March 23, 2018.

132. Fouque E, Héchard Y, Hartemann P, Humeau P, Trouilhé MC. Sensitivity of *Vermamoeba (Hartmannella) vermiformis* cysts to conventional disinfectants and protease. *J Water Health*. 2015;13(2):302-310.

133. Coulon C, Collignon A, McDonnell G, Thomas V. Resistance of *Acanthamoeba* cysts to disinfection treatments used in health care settings. *J Clin Microbiol*. 2010;48(8):2689-2697.

134. Quilez J, Sanchez-Acedo C, Avendaño C, del Cacho E, Lopez-Bernad F. Efficacy of two peroxygen-based disinfectants for inactivation of *Cryptosporidium parvum* oocysts. *Appl Environ Microbiol*. 2005;71(5):2479-2483.

135. Wilson R. Evaluation of the Plazlyte sterilization system at the Richmond Hospital, Richmond, B.C. *J Healthc Mater Manage*. 1994;12(4):34, 37-40.

136. Moulton KA, Campbell BA, Caputo RA, inventors; DePuy Orthopaedics Inc, assignee. Plasma sterilizing process with pulsed antimicrobial agent treatment. US patent 5,084,239. January 28, 1992.

137. Justi C, Amato V, Antloga K, Harrington S, McDonnell G. Demonstration of a sterility assurance level for a liquid chemical sterilization process. *Zent Sterilis*. 2000;9:170-181.

138. Lensing HH, Oei HL. A study of the efficiency of disinfectants against anthrax spores. *Tijdschr Diergeneeskd*. 1984;109:557-563.

139. Evans DH, Stuart P, Roberts DH. Disinfection of animal viruses. *Br Vet J*. 1977;133:356-359.

140. Eterpi M, McDonnell G, Thomas V. Disinfection efficacy against parvoviruses compared with reference viruses. *J Hosp Infect*. 2009;73:64-70.

141. Kryzywicka H, Jaszczuk E, Janowska J. The range of antibacterial activity and the use concentrations of disinfectants. In: Kedzia WB, ed. *Resistance of Microorganisms to Disinfectants: Second International Symposium*. Warsaw, Poland: Polish Academy of Sciences; 1975:89-91.

142. Fisher CW, Fiorello A, Shaffer D, Jackson M, McDonnell GE. Aldehyde-resistant mycobacteria associated with the use of endoscope reprocessing systems. *Am J Infect Control.* 2012;40(9):880-882.

143. Burgess W, Margolis A, Gibbs S, Duarte RS, Jackson M. Disinfectant susceptibility profiling of glutaraldehyde-resistant nontuberculous mycobacteria. *Infect Control Hosp Epidemiol.* 2017;38(7):784-791.

144. Dul'neva LV, Moskvin AV. Kinetics of formation of peroxyacetic acid. *Russian J Gen Chem.* 2005;75(7):1125-1130.

145. Werner HP, Wewalka G. Destruction of spores in alcohol by peracetic acid [in Polish]. *Zentralbl Bakteriol Orig B.* 1973;157:387-391.

146. Oakes TR, Stanley PM, Keller J, inventors; Ecolab Inc, assignee. Peroxyacid antimicrobial composition. US patent 5,200,189. April 6, 1993.

147. Dychdala GR. New hydrogen peroxide-peroxyacetic acid disinfectant. In: Proceedings from the 4th Conference on Progress in Chemical Disinfection; April 11-13, 1988; Binghamtom, NY.

148. Blanchard AP, Bird MR, Wright SJL. Peroxygen disinfection of *Pseudomonas aeruginosa* biofilms on stainless steel discs. *Biofouling.* 1998;13:233-253.

149. Schroder W. *Peracetic Acid: Disinfectant for the Food Industry.* Nürnberg, Germany: Brauwelt International; 1984:115-120.

150. Teuber M. Testing of peracetic acid containing preparation "P-3 oxonia aktiv" on bacteriophage specifically for *Streptococcus lactis, S. cremonis,* and *S. lactis* subsp. *diacetilactis.* Kiel Institute for Microbiology and Dairy Investigations, Kiel, Germany; 1978:13:10.

151. Teuber M. Testing of the sporicidal properties the peracetic acid containing preparation "P-3 oxonia aktiv" and "P-3/VR 2828-20" against *Clostridium tyrobutyricum.* Kiel Institute for Microbiology and Dairy Investigations, Kiel, Germany; 1979:11:2.

152. Binder W, Foissy H. Test information on the fungicidal activity of "P3 oxonia aktiv." Institut für Milchwirtschaft und Mikrobiologie, Univers für Bodenkultur; 1979:26:2.

153. Jaeger P, Puespoek J. Peracetic acid as a disinfectant in breweries and soft drink factories. *Mitt Versuch Gaerung Wien.* 1980;34:32-36.

154. Dallyn H, inventor; Crown Packaging UK Ltd, assignee. Sterilization of articles. British patent GB1,570,492. July 2, 1980.

155. Greenspan FP, Johnsen MA, Trexler PC. Peracetic acid aerosols. In: Proceedings from the 42nd Annual Meeting of Chemical Special Manufacturers Association; May 1955.

156. Turcić J, Alfirević I, Cavcić J, Martinac P, Biocina B. Peroxyacetic acid effect on the bacteriologic status of war wound. *Acta Med Croatica.* 1997;51(3):159-162.

157. Kuehn H. Experiments with the antimicrobial treatment of dermatologic preparations containing peracetic acid. 2. *Pharmazie.* 1978;33:292-293.

158. von Ballmoos U, Soldavini H. Disinfection of ion exchangers with peracetic acid of special quality. IA. *Gass Wasser Abwaser.* 1979;59:487-488.

159. Molk DM, Karr-May CL, Trang ED, Sanders GE. Sanitization of an automatic reverse-osmosis watering system: removal of a clinically significant biofilm. *J Am Assoc Lab Anim Sci.* 2013;52(2):197-205.

160. Baldry MGC, French MS. Activity of peracetic acid against sewage indicator organisms. *Wat Sci Tech.* 1989;21:1747-1749.

161. Fraser JAL. Novel applications of peracetic acid in industrial disinfection. *Specialty Chem.* 1987;7:178-186.

162. Yuan Z, Ni Y, van Heiningen ARP. Kinetics of peracetic acid decomposition: part I: spontaneous decomposition at typical pulp bleaching conditions. *Can J Chem Eng.* 1997;75:37-41.

163. Francoeur R, Vas S, Uldall R. Dialyzer reuse: an automated system using peracetic acid. *Int J Artif Organs.* 1994;17(6):331-336.

164. Bond TC, Nissenson AR, Krishnan M, Wilson SM, Mayne T. Dialyzer reuse with peracetic acid does not impact patient mortality. *Clin J Am Soc Nephrol.* 2011;6(6):1368-1374.

165. Alfa M, DeGagne P, Olson N, Hizon R. Comparison of liquid chemical sterilization with peracetic acid and ethylene oxide sterilization for long narrow lumens. *Am J Infect Control.* 1998;26(5):469-477.

166. Koubek E, Haggett ML, Battaglia CJ, Ibne-Rasa KM, Pyun HY, Edwards JO. Kinetics and mechanism of the spontaneous decompositions of some peroxoacids, hydrogen peroxide and *t*-butyl hydroperoxide. *J Am Chem Soc.* 1963;85:2263-2268.

167. Bowing WG, Mrozek H, Schlussler HJ, Tinnefeld B, Vogele P, inventors; Ecolab Inc, assignee. Stable peroxy-containing microbicides. US patent 4,051,058. September 27, 1977.

168. Doll JP, Trexler PC, Reynolds LI, Bernard GR. The use of peracetic acid to obtain germfree invertebrate eggs for gnotobiotic studies. *Am Midl Nat.* 1963;69(1):231-239.

169. Portner DM, Hoffman RK. Sporicidal effect of peracetic acid vapor. *Appl Microbiol.* 1968;16(11):1782-1785.

170. Kimura T. Effective decontamination of laboratory animal rooms with vapour-phase ("vaporized") hydrogen peroxide and peracetic acid. *Scand J Lab Anim Sci.* 2012;30(1):17-23.

171. Mana TSC, Sitzlar B, Cadnum JL, Jencson AL, Koganti S, Donskey CJ. Evaluation of an automated room decontamination device using aerosolized peracetic acid. *Am J Infect Control.* 2016;45(3):327-329.

172. Knotzer S, Kindermann J, Modrof J, Kreil TR. Measuring the effectiveness of gaseous virus disinfectants. *Biologicals.* 2015;43:519-523.

173. Richter WR, Wood JP, Wendling MQS, Rogers JV. Inactivation of *Bacillus anthracis* spores to decontaminate subway railcar and related materials via the fogging of peracetic acid and hydrogen peroxide sporicidal liquids. *J Env Manage.* 2018;206:800-826.

174. Gregersen J-P, Roth B. Inactivation of stable viruses in cell culture facilities by peracetic acid fogging. *Biologicals.* 2012;40:282-287.

175. Bounoure F, Fiquet H, Arnaud P. Comparison of hydrogen peroxide and peracetic acid as isolator sterilization agents in a hospital pharmacy. *Am J Health Syst Pharm.* 2006;63:451-455.

176. Tasch P, Todd B. Halophilic bacteria susceptibility to peracetic acid vapor and ethylene oxide. *Appl Microbiol.* 1973;25(2):205-207.

177. Rovison JM Jr, Lymburner CJ, Abraham S, Thompson A, inventors; PeroxyChem LLC, assignee. Peracetic acid vapor sterilization of food and beverage containers. US patent 8,454,890. June 4, 2013.

178. Mar Cor Purification, Cantel Medical. *REVOX Materials Compatibility Guidance, Rev B.* New York, NY: Mar Cor Purification, Cantel Medical; 2015.

179. ASTM International. *ASTM-G31-72(2004) Standard Practice for Laboratory Immersion Corrosion Testing of Metals.* West Conshohocken, PA: ASTM International; 2004.

180. US Environmental Protection Agency. *EPA 600/R-14/332. Parametric Testing of Decontamination Chemistries to Guide Decontaminant Selection 1: Peracetic Acid.* Research Triangle Park, NC: US Environmental Protection Agency; 2014.

181. Giguere PA, Olmos A. Spectroscopic study of hydrogen bonding in performic acid and peracetic acid. *Can J Chem.* 1952;30:821-830.

182. Hazra MK, Kuang X, Sinha A. Influence of intramolecular hydrogen bonding on OH-stretching overtone intensities and band positions in peroxyacetic acid. *J Phys Chem A.* 2012;116:5784-5795.

183. Bentley K, Dove BK, Parks SR, Walker JT, Bennett AM. Hydrogen peroxide vapour decontamination of surfaces artificially contaminated with norovirus surrogate feline calicivirus. *J Hosp Infect.* 2012;80(2):116-121.

184. McAnoy AM, Sait M, Pantelidis S. *Establishment of a Vapourous Hydrogen Peroxide Bio-Decontamination Capability.* Victoria, Australia: Human Protection Performance Division DSTO; 2007. Report DSTO-TR-1994.

185. Dufresne S, Richards T. The first dual-sterilant low-temperature sterilization system. *Can J Inf Control.* 2016;31(3):169-174.

186. Cugley J, Gunthard H. Infrared spectra, force constants and thermodynamic functions of matrix isolated peroxyacetic acid. *Chem Phys,* 1976;54:281-292.

187. Krishnan J, Fey G, Stansfield C, et al. Evaluation of a dry fogging system for laboratory decontamination. *Appl Biosafety (Public Health Agency of Canada, Winnipeg, Manitoba, Canada).* 2012;17(3):132-141.

188. Greenspan FP. The convenient preparation of per acids. *J Am Chem Soc.* 1946;68:907.

189. Baldry MGC. The antimicrobial properties of magnesium monoperoxyphthalate hexahydrate. *J Appl Bacteriol.* 1984;57:499-503.

190. Shin SY, Marquis RE. Sporicidal activity of tertiary butyl hydroperoxide. *Arch Microbiol.* 1994;161:184-190.

191. Goroncy-Bermes P, Gerresheim S. Effectiveness of peroxide solutions against microorganisms in biofilms. *Zentralbl Hyg Umweltmed.* 1996;198:473-477.

192. Fitzgerald GP. Laboratory evaluation of potassium permanganate as an algicide in water reservoirs. *Southwest Water Works J.* 1964;45:16-17.

193. Fitzgerald GP. Evaluation of potassium permanganate as an algicide in water cooling towers. *Ind Eng Chem Prod Res Dev.* 1965;3:82-85.

194. Pieper K, Nehrkorn R, Steinmann J. Virucidal efficacy of inorganic per-compounds. *Zentral Hyg Umweltmed.* 1991;191(5-6):506-515.

195. Baldry MGC. A note on the biocidal properties of Caro's acid triple salt. *J Appl Bacteriol.* 1985;58:315-318.

196. Gaya H, Thirlwall J, Shaw EJ, Hassam Z. Evaluation of products for treating babies' napkins. *J Hyg (Lond).* 1979;82:463-471.

197. Block SS, Seng VP, Goswami DY. Chemically enhanced sunlight for killing bacteria. *J Sol Energy Eng.* 1997;119:85-91.

198. Goswami DY, Trivedi DM, Block SS. Photocatalytic disinfection of indoor air. *J Sol Energy Eng.* 1997;119:92-96.

199. Goswami TK, Hingorami SK, Greist H, et al. Photocatalytic system to destroy bioaerosols in air. *J Advanced Oxidation Technol.* 1999;4:185-188.

200. Pablos C, Marugán J, van Grieken R, Serrano E. Emerging micropollutant oxidation during disinfection processes using UV-C, UV-C/H_2O_2, UV-A/TiO_2 and UV-A/TiO_2/H_2O_2. *Water Res.* 2013;47:1237-1245.

201. Rincon A-G, Pulgarin C. Comparative evaluation of Fe^{3+} and TiO_2 photoassisted processes in solar photocatalytic disinfection of water. *Appl Catal B Environ.* 2006;63:222-231.

202. Gleason MN, Gosselin RE, Hodge HC, et al. *Clinical Toxicology of Commercial Products*, 3rd ed. Baltimore, MD: Williams & Wilkins; 1969:79.

203. World Health Organization International Agency for Research on Cancer. *IARC Monographs on the Evaluation of Carcinogenic Risks to Humans.* Lyon, France: World Health Organization International Agency for Research on Cancer; 1999. *Hydrogen Peroxide*; vol 71.

204. Ikarashi Y, Tsuchiya T, Nakamura A. Cytotoxicity of medical materials sterilized with vapour-phase hydrogen peroxide. *Biomaterials.* 1995;16:177-183.

205. National Institute of Safety and Health. *Toxic Substances List.* Rockville, MD: National Institute of Safety and Health; 1974.

206. Busch A, Werner F. Animal tolerance to peracetic acid. 1. Experimental results following the application of peracetic acid solutions on the skin of pigs. *Monatshefte für Veterinaermedizin.* 1974;29:494-498.

207. European Centre for Ecotoxicology and Toxicology of Chemicals. *Peracetic Acid (CAS No. 79-21-0) and Its Equilibrium Solutions.* Brussels, Belgium: European Centre for Ecotoxicology and Toxicology of Chemicals; 2001.

208. National Research Council. *Acute Exposure Guideline Levels for Selected Airborne Chemicals.* Washington, DC: National Academies Press; 2010. *Peracetic Acid*; vol 8.

209. Dworschak D, Linde J. Raumluftdesinfektion mit Peressigsäure (PES)-Aerosolen auf Intensivtherapiestationen und ihre Konsequenzen für die Behandlung des Hopitalismusproblems. *Dt Gesundh-Wesen.* 1976;31:1622.

210. Yaguchi T, Yamashita Y. Mutagenicity of hydroperoxides of fatty acids and some hydrocarbons. *Agri Biologic Chem.* 1980;44:1675-1678.

211. Fraser JAL, Thorbinson A. *Fogging Trials With Tenneco Organics Limited (30th June, 1986) at Collards Farm.* Warrington, United Kingdom: Solvay Interox; 1986.

212. McDonagh J. *Atmospheric Monitoring of Peracetic Acid on the Existing Caprolactone Plant Distillation Houses A and B. Assessment of Results.* Warrington, United Kingdom: Solvay Interox; 1997. Document No. EE9701992.M01. Memorandum to R.A. Haffenden et al from J. McDonagh.

213. Janssen PJM. *Acute Inhalation Toxicity Studies of Proxitane 1507 in Male Rats (I).* Weesp, The Netherlands: Duphar B.V. and Brussels, Belgium: Solvay; 1989. Report No. S. 8906, Int. Doc. No. 56645/25/89.

Alcohols

Günter Kampf and James W. Arbogast

Alcohol is perhaps the oldest of antiseptic agents being used for wound treatment as described by Claudius Galen (131-201 AD) and Guy de Chauliac (1363)[1] and as a hand disinfectant for surgeons in 1888 by Fürbringer.[2] Today, alcohols are used frequently for pathogen reduction on skin worldwide, and that is growing globally, especially in health care. Skin applications most frequently occur before blood draw, surgical procedures, and vascular catheter insertion as well as for routine hand hygiene with alcohol-based hand rubs (also known as "hand sanitizers" or "hygienic hand rubs") or prior to surgery (also known as surgical hand rubs). These products typically contain >60% ethanol, isopropanol, n-propanol, or mixtures thereof in a variety of formulation formats (rinses, gels, foams, and wipes).

Alcohols have also been used as hard surface (nonskin) disinfectants, including low-level disinfectants in health care settings as far back as the late 1800s.[3-5] Despite the lack of appreciable sporicidal effect that limits sterilization applications for alcohols, their general antimicrobial properties can be useful against surface-borne bacteria, including *Mycobacteria*, and other microorganisms. A variety of surface-disinfectant spray products claim effectiveness against bacteria, yeasts, fungi, and some viruses. Given the volatility and time-exposure requirements of alcohol, some of these claims are questionable. Seventy percent isopropanol is used as a surface spray in some food-handling situations in Europe as well as many other industrial disinfection applications. A recent review of alcohols as surface disinfectants in health care identified an effective solution with 29.4% ethanol[5]; however, the total formulation is important to the overall observed antimicrobial efficacy. Although alcohols are now nearly universally recognized as effective antimicrobial agents, the history of alcohol use for pathogen reduction and infection prevention involves controversy around the spectrum of antimicrobial activity, concentration levels, formulation impact, and dose/time of action.

For all types of application, it is critically important to consider experimental conditions and methods in detail when considering the antimicrobial performance of formulations based on alcohols.

As a group, the alcohols possess many features desirable for a disinfectant or antiseptic. They have excellent bactericidal efficacy as well as bacteriostatic action as a preservative, some virucidal efficacy (especially against enveloped viruses), and fungicidal efficacy. The low-molecular-weight alcohols evaporate readily and are therefore, under regular use conditions, not considered a risk for acquired microbial resistance (as compared to actives claiming persistent effect), are relatively inexpensive, are usually easily obtainable, are colorless but can be easily colored if needed, and are relatively nontoxic with topical (skin) application. Many alcohols can also have a surface cleaning action due to their lipid solvency and low surface tension.

▶ MODE OF ACTION

Alcohols have a nonspecific mode of action with a variety of toxic effects.[6,7] The main effect is often considered as the coagulation or denaturation of proteins.[6] This can occur in bacterial cells on the cell wall, on the cytoplasmic membrane, as well as on various cytoplasmic proteins or enzymes.[6] In 1939, it was already shown that both ethanol (2.5%-10%) and isopropanol (6.6%-20%) significantly reduced or abolished the dehydrogenase activity of *Escherichia coli*.[8] Coagulation of enzymes supports the loss of cellular activity. Enzymes for the production of bioethanol are also inactivated by ethanol in a concentration-dependent manner,[9] which supports the hypothesis of the unspecific nature of protein denaturation by alcohols. Specific cellular mechanisms, such as the inhibition or inactivation of cholinesterase activity, can additionally be influenced by the opening of the bacterial cell by ethanol.[10]

Protein denaturation is so nonspecific that basically all proteins and membrane components are coagulated by exposure to the alcohols. As early as 1921, Kamm[11] showed that both ethanol and *n*-propanol (1%-10%) can almost completely coagulate egg albumen in aqueous solution. Potato protein is also denatured by ethanol.[12] In addition, for ubiquitin, protein denaturation is triggered by pressure, temperature, and alcohols.[13] This nonspecific effect has been known for decades as a "protein deficit" in the efficacy testing of chemical disinfectants.[14] With alcohol-based disinfectants, the "protein deficit" occurs both in the determination of efficacy under protein load as well as during its application, for example, when high levels of protein are present on the hands or noncleaned surfaces in the sense of a pollution.[14] As a result, a higher concentration of active ingredient or a longer exposure time via higher doses are means to achieve equivalent antimicrobial efficacy when proteinaceous soil is present.

The penetration of the alcohols into the bacterial cell is explained by various mechanisms.[15] On the one hand, the alcohols can lower the surface tension of bacterial cells, which can lead to disruption of linkages in the cell membrane or membrane structure.[15] The alcohols ultimately penetrate into the hydrocarbon components of the bacterial membrane lipid bilayer, resulting in loss of function of the cell membrane and ultimately lysis of the cell.[16] Two factors of the cell membrane have proved to be relevant in yeast cells for tolerance to ethanol or isopropanol: strengthening the opposing potassium and proton electrochemical membrane gradients.[17] Whether these factors are of comparable relevance to bacterial cells is, according to current knowledge, unclear. In individual hospital isolates of *Enterococcus faecium*, a mutation (H486N/Y substitution in the rpoB gene) for increased tolerance to isopropanol at 23% was detected, possibly caused by exposure to rifampicin[16]; however, this mutation alone does not explain the increased tolerance of individual isolates to isopropanol, suggesting that isopropanol tolerance is a polygenic phenotype with multiple genetic changes across different loci.[16] This finding also suggests that there is no specific mode of action to explain the antimicrobial activity of the alcohols. Alcohols can also dissolve hydrogen bonds in the cell membrane.[15,18] In addition, it has been demonstrated in *E coli* that cell lysis can be explained by the weakening of hydrophobic interactions rather than from the intercalation of ethanol into membranes.[19]

Other nonspecific modes of action include the destruction of cytoplasmic integrity, lysis of the cell, and interference with cellular metabolism.[6] Lysis of the cells by alcohols has also been described in yeasts such as *Candida albicans*, *Torulopsis glabrata*, and *Saccharomyces cerevisiae*.[20] Depending on their concentration, ethanol and *n*-propanol can prolong the lag phase for bacterial multiplication, as demonstrated by *Aerobacter aerogenes*.[21] This effect is explained by a slowing of cell metabolism required for rapid cell division.[7] The halophilic bacterium *Halobacterium cutirubrum* has also been shown to increase envelope dissolution by 10% ethanol.[22] Similar effects can predict the effects on other types of microorganisms, such as the efficacy of alcohols against enveloped viruses due to their exposed lipid/protein surface in comparison to the greater resistance observed with nonenveloped viruses due to their unique protein exposed surfaces.[7]

◗ PHYSICAL CHEMICAL PROPERTIES

As the chain length and molecular weight of alcohol increases their specific gravity, boiling point, melting point, and lipophilicity generally increases, whereas solubility in water decreases. A nonlinear, branched carbon chain structure can improve the water solubility. These values are summarized for various alcohols in Table 19.1. Alcohols at higher chain lengths are solids at room temperature, which limits their applications as antimicrobial agents. The short-chain alcohols are inflammable liquids. The flash points for methanol, ethanol, propanols, and tert butanol are lower than 15°C. Therefore, caution should be exercised in handling these alcohols. Safety data for a range of alcohols are presented in Table 19.2.

The concentrations of alcohols are generally given in percentage by weight (gram per gram [g/g] or weight per weight [wt/wt]) or percentage in volume (milliliter per milliliter [mL/mL] or volume per volume [vol/vol]). Table 19.3 illustrates the percentages by volume and weight for ethanol, isopropanol, and *n*-propanol. Weight per weight has advantages of being easier to compare between products for end users and in manufacturing due to volume contraction on mixing. However, some parts of the world have regulations that specify vol/vol percentages to be specified on product labeling.[23]

◗ REGULATIONS AND GUIDELINES

European Regulations and Guidelines

In almost all countries within the European Union, products for hygienic and surgical hand disinfection are considered biocidal products (product type 1, intended for human hygiene). Products for surface disinfection belong to product type 2 (disinfectants and algaecides not intended for direct application to humans or animals) or product type 4 (food and feed area). Isopropanol has been approved in 2015 as an active biocidal agent for product types 1, 2, and 4.[24] *n*-Propanol has also been approved (November 2017) as an active biocidal agent for product types 1, 2, and 4.[25] Ethanol remains under review (June 2018) as an active biocidal agent for product types 1, 2, 4, and 6 (preservatives for products during storage).[26]

TABLE 19.1 Physical properties of alcohols								
Alcohol	Molecular Weight	Specific Gravity at 20°C	Boiling Point (°C)	Melting Point (°C)	Solubility in Water at 20°C (g/100 g Water)	Partition Coefficient (log P)[a]	Viscosity	
							(mPa · s)[b]	(°C)[b]
Methanol	32.04	0.791	64.7	−98	Unlimited	NA	0.52	20
Ethanol	46.07	0.789	78.4	−117	Unlimited	−0.58	1.22	20
Propan-1-ol[c]	60.10	0.805	97.2	−127	Unlimited	0.28	2.75	20
Propan-2-ol[d]	60.10	0.785	82.0	−89	Unlimited	−0.19	2.27	20
Butan-1-ol[e]	74.12	0.810	117.0	−89	7.7	0.89	2.95	20
Butan-2-ol[f]	74.12	0.808	99.8	−114	12.5	0.84	4.21	20
2-Methylpropan-1-ol[g]	74.12	0.802	108	−108	9.5	0.65	6.68	20
2-Methylpropan-2-ol[h]	74.12	0.779	82.9	24	Unlimited	0.34	3.30	30
Pentan-1-ol[i]	88.15	0.815	138	−79	2.7	NA	3.68	20
Pentan-2-ol[j]	88.15	0.808	119	−50	13.5	NA	NA	NA
3-Methylbutan-1-ol[k]	88.15	0.816	131	−117	2.5	NA	NA	NA
2-Methylbutan-1-ol[l]	88.15	0.816	128	70	3.6	NA	5.10	20
2-Methylbutan-2-ol[m]	88.15	0.800	102	−12	17.7 (30°C)	NA	3.70	25
Hexan-1-ol	102.20	0.814	157	−45	0.6	NA	0.45	24
Heptan-1-ol	116.21	0.824	175	−34	Slight	NA	NA	NA
Octan-1-ol	130.23	0.827	195	−16	Slight	NA	8.40	20
Benzyl alcohol	108.13	1.042	204.7	−15.3	3.5	NA	NA	NA

Abbreviation: NA, not available.

[a]System: diethyl ether/water.

[b]Centipoise.

[c]*n*-Propanol.

[d]Isopropanol.

[e]*n*-Butanol.

[f]sec-Butanol.

[g]Isobutanol.

[h]tert-Butanol.

[i]*n*-Amyl alcohol.

[j]sec-Amyl alcohol.

[k]Isoamyl alcohol.

[l]act-Amyl alcohol.

[m]tert-Amyl alcohol.

Skin antiseptics are commonly regulated as medicinal products. The efficacy requirements for a disinfectant depend on the intended use. In human medicine, a product for disinfection has to show at least bactericidal and yeasticidal activity. Additional claims such as fungicidal, tuberculocidal, mycobactericidal, virucidal (three levels of efficacy), and sporicidal activity are possible but not mandatory. The application of European efficacy standards is summarized in EN 14885.[27]

United States Regulations

In the United States the regulation of alcohols depends mostly on the product application. Skin antiseptics fall under the purview of the US Food and Drug Administration and are regulated as drugs, either as an over-the-counter under a drug monograph guideline or as a new drug approval, whereas alcohol-based antimicrobials for inanimate surface applications are regulated by the US Environmental Protection Agency.

World Health Organization Guidelines

Alcohol-based hand rubs are recommended as the first choice treatment for the decontamination of clean hands in health care since 2009.[28] In 2015, the World Health Organization (WHO) described alcohol-based hand rubs as essential medicines,[29] referencing the simple formulations using 80% ethanol or 75% isopropanol,[28] although they do not meet European efficacy requirements when applied

TABLE 19.2 Safety data of alcohols used for antiseptic purposes

Alcohol	Vapor Pressure at 20°C hPa	Vapor Density at 20°C	Flash Point[a] (°C)	Explosion Limits in Air (vol %)	Autoignition Temperature (°C)	Odor Threshold (ppm)
Methanol	128	1.1	11	6.0-36.0	385	5
Ethanol	59	1.6	13	3.3-19.0	363	10
Propan-1-ol	19	2.1	15	2.2-13.7	410	30
Propan-2-ol	43	2.1	12	2.0-12.7	399	40
Butan-1-ol	7	2.5	30	1.4-11.3	343	10
Butan-2-ol	17	2.6	23	1.7-9.8	405	0.6
Isobutanol	12	2.6	29	1.7-10.9	430	40
tert-Butanol	40	2.6	11	2.3-8.0	478	73
Pentan-1-ol	3	3.0	48	1.3-10.5	300	1
Pentan-2-ol	3	3.0	41	1.2-9.0	347	70
akt-Amyl alcohol	51[b]	NA	50	1.9-9.3	340	NA
tert-Amyl alcohol	13	3.0	20	1.3-9.6	425	2.3
Hexan-1-ol	1	3.5	63	2.1-7.7	292	5.2
Heptan-1-ol	0.5	4.0	70	NA	350	0.5
Octan-1-ol	0.3	4.5	81	0.8	270	NA
Benzyl alcohol	0.1	3.7	101	NA	436	NA

Abbreviation: NA, not available.

[a]For concentrated solutions.

[b]At 50°C.

Data from Hommel G. *Handbuch der Gefährlichen Güter.* 4th ed. Berlin, Germany: Springer; 1980, and Threon JF. *Alcohols, Industrial Hygiene and Toxicology.* 2nd ed. New York, NY: John Wiley & Sons; 1963. *Toxicology;* Vol 2.

with 3 mL for 30 seconds.[30] In 2016, WHO recommended the use of alcohol-chlorhexidine-skin-antiseptics for surgical site preparation in patients undergoing surgical procedures.[31] In the same guideline, "suitable" alcohol-based hand rubs are recommended next to surgical hand scrubs for the preoperative treatment of hands.[31]

Other National Guidelines

Other regions of the world may regulate alcohol use for antimicrobial purposes differently. Other national specific guidelines are not considered further in this review.

▶ ANTIMICROBIAL PROPERTIES OF ALCOHOLS

Measurement Methods

The spectrum of antimicrobial activity is usually determined in suspension tests or time kill tests. The test principle is the same. The disinfectant or antiseptic must demonstrate a minimum $\log_{10}$ reduction of culturable microorganisms or reduction of viral infectivity within a specific exposure time compared to a control (eg, pre-exposure or exposure to negative control).

In Europe, the spectrum of antimicrobial activity must include bactericidal activity according to EN 13727 and yeasticidal activity according to EN 13624. The same spectrum of antimicrobial activity is required in the United States, although the number of bacterial species to be investigated to determine bactericidal activity is much higher with at least 20 species compared to 4 species in EN 13727.[23] A mycobactericidal or virucidal activity is optional.[27] In veterinary medicine, the products must be at least bactericidal according to EN 13727.[27] Hygienic hand rub products used in food, industrial, domestic, and institutional areas have in Europe no specific minimum spectrum of antimicrobial activity. Tests are available to demonstrate bactericidal (EN 1276) and yeasticidal (EN 1650) activity.[27]

Spectrum of Bactericidal Activity

In the following sections, the alcohol concentrations are given as wt/wt unless otherwise indicated.

TABLE 19.3   Concentrations as percentages by weight and volume for aqueous ethanol, propan-2-ol, and propan-1-ol

Weight (% g/g)	Concentrations by Volume at 20°C (% mL/mL)		
Alcohol	Ethanol	Propan-2-ol	Propan-1-ol
40	47.4	47.0	46.5
50	57.8	57.0	56.5
60	67.7	67.2	66.2
70	76.9	76.5	76.1
80	85.4	85.0	84.5
90	93.2	93.8	93.5
95	96.7	97.5	97.2
100	100.0	100.0	100.0
Volume at 20°C (% mL/mL)	Weight (% g/g)		
40	33.4	33.5	34.0
50	42.6	43.0	43.4
60	52.1	53.7	53.9
70	62.6	62.8	63.5
80	73.4	73.5	74.5
90	85.8	86.0	86.0
95	92.5	92.8	93.0
100	100.0	100.0	100.0

Ethanol at 78% or more has comprehensive bactericidal activity within 30 seconds against *Acinetobacter baumannii*,[32] *Acinetobacter lwoffii*,[32] *Bacteroides fragilis*,[32] *Burkholderia cenocepacia*,[33] *Burkholderia cepacia*,[32] *Campylobacter jejuni*,[34] the vegetative cell form of *Clostridium difficile*,[32] *Corynebacterium jeikeium*,[35] *Enterobacter aerogenes*,[32] *Enterobacter cloacae*,[32] *Enterococcus faecalis*,[32,36] *E faecium*,[32,36] *Enterococcus hirae*,[37,38] *E coli*,[32,37,38] *Haemophilus influenzae*,[32] *Haemophilus parasuis*,[39] *Helicobacter pylori*,[40] *Klebsiella pneumoniae*,[32] *Klebsiella oxytoca*,[32] *Listeria monocytogenes*,[32] *Micrococcus luteus*,[32] *Proteus mirabilis*,[32] *Pseudomonas aeruginosa*,[32,37,38,41] *Serratia marcescens*,[32] *Staphylococcus aureus*,[32,37,38,41] *Staphylococcus epidermidis*,[32,35] *Staphylococcus haemolyticus*,[32] *Staphylococcus hominis*,[32] *Staphylococcus saprophyticus*,[32] *Streptococcus pneumoniae*,[32] *Streptococcus pyogenes*,[32] *Salmonella enteritidis*,[32] *Salmonella* Typhimurium,[32,42] and *Shigella sonnei*.[32] Lower concentration of ethanol may require longer exposure times to reach an equivalent efficacy, depending on the formulation.

Published data with isopropanol indicates a strong bactericidal activity of a 70% solution beginning after 15 seconds against *C jejuni*,[34] *Enterococcus* species,[43] *H parasuis*,[39] *S aureus*,[44] and *S epidermidis*.[45] Additional data with mixed propanols (eg, 45% isopropanol plus 30% *n*-propanol) indicate comprehensive bactericidal activity within 30 seconds.[37,46]

n-Propanol at 60% has a strong bactericidal activity beginning after 15 seconds against *A baumannii*,[47] *Enterococcus* species,[43] and *S aureus*.[48] Additional data with mixed propanols (eg, 30% *n*-propanol plus 45% isopropanol) indicate comprehensive bactericidal activity within 30 seconds.[37,46] The bactericidal activity of 60% *n*-propanol is considered to be equal to isopropanol at 70%, whereas lower concentrations such as 50% or 40% have a lower bactericidal activity.[49]

Spectrum of Fungicidal Activity

Ethanol is usually effective at 70% to 90% within 30 seconds to 5 minutes against fungi typically found in health care setting such as *C albicans*,[38,50] *Aspergillus niger*,[38] *Cryptococcus neoformans*,[50] or *Cryptococcus uniguttulatus*.[50] Food-related fungi such as ascospores,[51] conidia,[51] or yeasts[51,52] were often more resistant to ethanol with a variable efficacy of 70% ethanol in 10 minutes. In mixed suspensions of environmental isolates (*Rhodotorula rubra*, *C albicans*, *C uniguttulatus*) and clinical isolates (*R rubra*, *C albicans*, *C neoformans*), 70% ethanol is still fungicidal ($\log_{10}$ reduction ≥ 6) in 5 minutes, although the effect was somewhat less against the environmental mix.[50]

Isopropanol at 60% or 70% was mostly effective with 5 to 10 minutes against various types of yeasts including food-associated yeasts.[51,52] The efficacy of 70% isopropanol against food-associated fungal spores such as ascospores or conidia is low even at 10-minute exposure.[51]

Fourteen percent n-propanol has been described to inhibit multiplication of *C albicans* suggesting a levurostatic activity at that concentration.[53] At 89.5% (vol/vol), n-propanol is effective against *C albicans*.[54] A commercial product based on n-propanol (>30%) and isopropanol (15%-30%) has been investigated for yeasticidal activity against 25 strains isolated from food or food processing. Within 5 minutes, the product reduced the number of yeast cells by at least 4 $\log_{10}$ steps of 19 species; some species were less susceptible.[52]

Spectrum of Mycobactericidal Activity

Ethanol of 70% or more has sufficient activity against selected mycobacterial species such as *Mycobacterium chelonae*,[35] *Mycobacterium nonchromogenicum*,[35] *Mycobacterium smegmatis*,[35,55] *Mycobacterium terrae*,[38,56] and *Mycobacterium tuberculosis*[56,57] within 1 to 5 minutes. Only few data were found against aquatic nontuberculous mycobacteria. For example, *Mycobacterium marinum* was effectively reduced by ethanol at 50% and 70% in 1 minute.[58]

Early data from 1953 indicate a tuberculocidal activity of isopropanol at 50% to 70%.[59] In suspension tests, little has been published on the mycobactericidal activity of isopropanol. At 60%, it was mostly effective against both *M tuberculosis* and *M terrae* within 5 minutes.[56] Whether the tuberculocidal efficacy covers other mycobacterial species is not clear.

n-Propanol at 20% has been described to reduce *Mycobacterium avium* on frosted glass strips by >6 log in 20 minutes.[60] No other data were found to describe the efficacy of n-propanol against mycobacteria.

Spectrum of Virucidal Activity

Ethanol has been shown to be effective against various enveloped viruses.[61] Beginning at a concentration of 42.6%, ethanol was effective within 30 seconds against severe acute respiratory syndrome coronavirus[62]; Middle East respiratory syndrome coronavirus[63]; Ebola virus[63]; influenza A virus,[61,64,65] including the human type H3N2,[66] the avian type H3N8,[66] and human type H1N1[63]; influenza B virus[67]; human immunodeficiency virus (HIV)[38,68-71]; hepatitis B virus (HBV)[72,73]; vaccinia virus[61,64,74-78]; duck HBV[77]; togavirus[79]; pseudorabies virus[71]; Newcastle disease virus[80]; bovine viral diarrhea virus[71,78,81]; Zika virus[63]; herpes simplex viruses (HSVs)[66] types 1 and 2; and respiratory syncytial virus (RSV).[67] Ethanol is effective at 73.6% against hepatitis C virus (HCV) in 15 seconds[81] and 30 seconds[63] but not in 40%.[82]

Ethanol as a solution has mostly sufficient activity in 30 seconds against adenovirus type 5 (test virus of EN 14476) at concentrations between 45% (contains additional active ingredients) and 95%,[78,81,83,84] although one study indicates sufficient activity only in 1 minute with 77% ethanol.[85] Ethanol at 70% as a gel was sufficiently active in 2 minutes.[84] Adenovirus type 2 was less susceptible, requiring 2 minutes at 55%[67] and 85%.[38] In 30 seconds, 62.4% ethanol was not sufficiently effective[86] and at 50% required a 10-minute exposure time to be effective.[61] The combination of ethanol 73.6% and peracetic acid (0.2%) was effective in 30 seconds,[87] but this would be expected based on the potency of peracetic acid alone (see chapter 18). Data with other adenoviruses suggests that ethanol at 72.5% to 77% was effective in 60 seconds against adenovirus type 7 but not against adenovirus type 8.[88]

The effectiveness of ethanol on nonenveloped viruses has also been found to vary depending on the virus type. Gels based on 85% ethanol or the combination of 62.4% ethanol with additional citric acid were effective against rotavirus in 30 seconds[38,86] as well as a hand rub based on 55% ethanol, 0.7% phosphoric acid, and three other alcohols.[67] Today, murine norovirus (MNV), an enteric (gastrointestinal virus), is commonly used as a surrogate to assess activity of disinfectants and antiseptics against human noroviruses. Ethanol at concentrations between 62.4% and 85.8% is usually effective in 30 seconds[78,81,83,89-91] or 1 minute[91]; lower concentrations were less effective. A gel based on 53.2% ethanol was only effective in 1 hour.[92] Ethanol at 42.6% reduces MNV according to one study in 1 minute by 0.3 $\log_{10}$ and in 5 minutes by 0.4 $\log_{10}$.[91] In another study, 42.6% ethanol demonstrated approximately 3 $\log_{10}$ reduction in 30 seconds, whereas ethanol at 24.7% or 8% was ineffective within 3 minutes.[89] Feline calicivirus (FCV) has often been used in the past as a surrogate for human noroviruses, although it is not preferred because it is a respiratory tract virus and is highly sensitive to acidity.[93] The FCV is difficult to inactive by ethanol. Ethanol solutions at 42.5% and 62.4% were effective at 3 minutes, whereas 73.6% required 5 minutes.[94] Formulations with 72.5% ethanol did not reach a 4 $\log_{10}$ reduction in 60 seconds.[88] A solution based on 77% ethanol showed little activity against FCV in 60 seconds (<1 $\log_{10}$).[88] Even after 5 minutes, the efficacy was still insufficient (<2 $\log_{10}$).[85] A hand rub based on >85.8% ethanol was practically ineffective in 30 seconds (<1 $\log_{10}$).[78] Finally, ethanol at 42.6%, 62.4%, and 85.8% had insufficient efficacy in 5 minutes with the highest $\log_{10}$ reduction of 2.6.[91] Whenever different types of acid are added, ethanol in hand rubs has been described to be effective in 30 seconds at 45%,[78] 50.2%,[67,78] 55%,[95] 62.4%,[86] and 67.9%.[95] Malic acid at 0.35% has also been described to improve the efficacy of ethanol against FCV to some extent.[96] Data on the efficacy of ethanol against coxsackievirus are conflicting. Ethanol at 72.5% to 92.4% has been described to be effective against coxsackievirus B5 within 60 seconds[88,97] and also against coxsackievirus B1 within 10 minutes but not against coxsackievirus A7.[88] Higher ethanol concentrations (85%-90%) are effective against coxsackievirus B3 in 15 to 60 seconds.[98] The efficacy of ethanol against echoviruses is rather good. One study shows that ethanol at 92.4% is effective against echovirus 11 in 20 seconds.[99] Another study found a $\log_{10}$ reduction ≥ 3 within 1 minute for ethanol at 92.4% against the same virus, whereas ethanol at 67.9% was almost ineffective (<1 $\log_{10}$) at the same exposure time.[100] Against echovirus 6, ethanol was effective at 50% within 10 minutes.[61] With human enterovirus 71, ethanol had only little activity at 62.4% and 67.9% within 10 minutes (<1 $\log_{10}$). At 79.6%, a 3.2 $\log_{10}$ reduction was achieved in the same exposure time, and at 92.4%, this increased to 5.8 $\log_{10}$.[101]

Formulations with ethanol up to 80% and without acid were not sufficiently effective in up to 5 minutes against poliovirus type 1 when tested under standard conditions with 80% product proportion in the suspension. When the product proportion is increased in the suspension test to 97%, some formulations with 73.5% or 80% ethanol were effective within 1 minute. One formulation with 95% ethanol was effective in 30 seconds. Gels were mostly less effective compared to solutions. The addition of various types of acids can substantially improve the activity of ethanol against poliovirus type 1 so that the formulations are often sufficiently effective in 30 seconds.[102] Poliovirus type 2 is somewhat less susceptible to ethanol compared to poliovirus type 1.[103] A hand rub based on 55% ethanol, 0.7% phosphoric acid, and three other alcohols was effective in 30 seconds against rhinoviruses.[67]

A gel based on 54.2% ethanol showed no effect at all (0 $\log_{10}$) against hepatitis A virus (HAV) after 30 seconds.[86] Ethanol at 80% or 95% was not sufficiently effective within 2 minutes.[104] A hand rub based on 80% ethanol showed only little reduction of viral infectivity within 30 seconds (0.47) but increased efficacy on exposure at 2 minutes (≥ 2.2 $\log_{10}$).[71] When 0.7% phosphoric acid and three other alcohols are added to ethanol at 55%, the formulation was effective against HAV in 30 seconds.[67] Ethanol at 62.4% with additional 0.25% citric acid, however, was not sufficiently effective in 30 seconds with 1.75 $\log_{10}$.[86] The infectivity of the foot-and-mouth disease virus was insufficiently reduced by ethanol between 55.2% and 72.5% within 5 minutes.[105] Hand rubs with 70% to 75.2% ethanol and additional phosphoric acid (0.6%) or 50% ethanol and additional citric acid (0.5%) were effective within 30 seconds.[105]

Ethanol has little activity against polyomavirus SV40, an additional test virus that was chosen due to its resistance to alcohols by experts for the German test method to determine virucidal activity.[106] A gel based on 85% ethanol revealed sufficient activity in 15 minutes,[38] but a hand rub based on 78.2% ethanol had insufficient activity within 10 minutes (approximately 2 $\log_{10}$).[103] When 0.7% phosphoric acid and three other alcohols are added to ethanol at 55%, the formulation was able to reduce infectivity sufficiently in 60 seconds.[67] Ethanol at 73.6% in combination with 0.2% peracetic acid was effective in 30 seconds.[87] Ethanol has almost no virucidal activity against parvoviruses. At 80% ethanol, the infectivity of the canine parvovirus, as an example was reduced in 5 minutes only by 0.1 $\log_{10}$.[71]

Isopropanol at 40% is effective against the enveloped viruses duck HBV, vaccinia virus,[76] and the modified vaccinia virus Ankara.[77] At 75%, isopropanol is effective within 15 seconds against bovine viral diarrhea virus (a surrogate for HCV).[81] Seventy percent isopropanol was also shown to be effective against influenza A virus,[65] whereas 30% isopropanol was effective at a 10-minute exposure time.[61] The HIV can easily be inactivated by 70% isopropanol.[107] For inactivation of RSV, 35% isopropanol was effective within 1 minute.[108] The HSVs seem somewhat more resistant. The HSV types 1 and 2 were inactivated by 70% isopropanol in 5 minutes,[109] whereas another study indicated sufficient efficacy against HSV type 1 within 1 minute for isopropanol at 60% and 70%.[110] A concentration of 20% was still effective against HSV type 1 but required a 10-minute exposure.[61]

As for other alcohols, the results with other viruses vary depending on their structure. Isopropanol is considered to be ineffective against enteroviruses.[111] Against poliovirus type 1, human enterovirus 71, and coxsackieviruses B2 and B3, no efficacy was found at concentrations between 70% and 100% within 10 minutes.[61,98,101,112] The efficacy against echovirus[61,100,113] and astrovirus[113] is poor. Fifty percent isopropanol was, however, described as effective against adenovirus within 10 minutes.[61] The data with FCV, used as a surrogate for human noroviruses before the advent of MNV culture in vitro, are overall conflicting. The FCV was inactivated by isopropanol between 50% and 70% in 3 minutes, but at 80%, no sufficient efficacy was found after 5 minutes.[94] Another study indicated that isopropanol at 50%, 70%, and 90% for 5 minutes gave a maximum reduction of 0.8 $\log_{10}$.[91] The data with MNV are also not consistent. One study shows that isopropanol at 80% is effective against MNV in 30 seconds, whereas 50%, 60%, 70%, and 90% were not,[89] indicating that 80% may be the optimum concentration. Another study describes isopropanol at 70% in 5 minutes as effective ($\log_{10}$ reduction ≥ 2.6) and greater at 90% after 1 minute.[91] A third study shows that 60% isopropanol is effective against MNV in 60 seconds, but concentrations of 30% and 10% are not.[92] In contrast, rotaviruses have been found to be inactivated quite easily as shown with a mixture of 45% isopropanol and 30% n-propanol.[92]

Thirty percent and 60% n-propanol are effective within 1 minute against enveloped viruses such as HCV.[114] n-Propanol at 70% was described as effective against influenza A virus H1N1 within 1 minute.[65] A combination of 30% n-propanol and 45% isopropanol was effective within 15 seconds against various enveloped virus species.[66]

The FCV is inactivated within 30 seconds by *n*-propanol at 50% to 70%, but at 80%, an exposure time of 1 minute was necessary.[94] The MNV is also inactivated within 30 seconds by *n*-propanol at 50% to 90%.[89] The type 1 poliovirus is inactivated by *n*-propanol at 33% in 4 minutes by 3 $\log_{10}$.[115] The addition of 0.2% peracetic acid improved the efficacy resulting in a 4 $\log_{10}$ reduction within 1.5 minute.[115]

Spectrum of Sporicidal Activity

Bacterial spores are regarded to be resistant to ethanol,[116] isopropanol,[117] and *n*-propanol.

Activity Against Protozoans

Sixty-three percent and 80% isopropanol and ethanol at 5-minute contact have been shown to have some effects against cysts of *Giardia duodenalis* and *Entamoeba invadens* (a nonpathogenic model for *Entamoeba histolytica*), resulting in an almost complete collapse of the cyst wall of *Giardia*. Treatment with 80% isopropanol also prevented an oral infection of gerbils by 1000 *G duodenalis* cysts.[118]

▶ RESISTANCE

Acquired Bacterial or Fungal Resistance

In typical disinfectant applications, alcohols have an advantage of acting and evaporating rapidly and not leaving residue that allows time for bacteria to develop resistance. Apart from bacterial spores, no other bacteria with a notable resistance to *n*-propanol or propanol have been reported so far.[28,119,120] Conidia of *Penicillium chrysogenum*, *Penicillium digitatum*, and *Penicillium italicum* were shown to resist ethanol vapors under nonoptimal natural conditions probably caused by a reduced intracellular water activity of dry-harvested conidia,[121] but differences in the intrinsic resistance profiles of bacteria/fungi to alcohols may be demonstrated at low-level exposures.

Effect of Low-Level Exposure to Alcohols

Ethanol at 1.25% to 2.5% has been shown to significantly enhance *S aureus* biofilm formation by upregulation of some proteins with adhesive functions and others with cell maintenance functions and virulence factor EsxA.[122] Similar findings were reported with

L monocytogenes. When cells were exposed to 5% (vol/vol) ethanol for 60 minutes, they were significantly more difficult to kill by ethanol at 17.5%.[123] The adapted cells were also more difficult to kill by 0.1% hydrogen peroxide.[123] Attachment of cells can be significantly increased in some *L monocytogenes* strains when exposed to 2.5% ethanol, mostly at 10°C.[124] When the *Pseudomonas* species strain DJ-12 was exposed to 5% ethanol for 10 minutes, the cells were significantly more difficult to kill by 20% ethanol.[125] Cells treated with ethanol displayed irregular rod shapes with wrinkled surfaces.[125] Exposure of a *Pseudomonas putida* strain to toluene increased the tolerance to ethanol, which was explained by an inhibitory effect of ethanol on the biosynthesis of saturated fatty acids.[126] In *Bacillus subtilis* cells, the transfer of the mobile genetic element Tn916, a conjugative transposon, and the prototype of a large family of related elements was increased 5-fold by exposure to 4% ethanol for up to 2 hours. This may also result in a transfer of Tn916-like elements and any resistance genes they contain.[127]

The maximum ethanol tolerance of *S cerevisiae* has been described to be at 25% (vol/vol).[128] The presence of 2.5% ethanol was found to increase *S cerevisiae* colony growth by 20%, whereas 5% ethanol or more inhibited yeast colony growth.[129] When *S cerevisiae* cells were exposed for 30 minutes to sublethal concentrations of ethanol (8%, vol/vol), they became less susceptible to ethanol at a previously lethal concentration (14%, vol/vol).[130] Specific activities of glycolytic and alcohologenic enzymes within intact living cells remained high by the presence of sublethal ethanol.[128] Trehalose plays a role in ethanol tolerance at lethal ethanol concentrations but not at sublethal ethanol concentrations.[131] Using atomic force microscopy, it was shown that challenge of *S cerevisiae* with 9% ethanol (vol/vol) for 5 hours reduced the observed stiffness of glucose-grown yeast cells, suggesting that changes in the cell membrane due to the presence of ethanol could modify the biophysical properties of yeast cells.[132]

Less has been published on the effects of low-level exposure of isopropanol on microorganisms. One study indicated that attachment of cells can be significantly increased in some *L monocytogenes* strains when exposed to 2.5% isopropanol, mostly at 10°C.[124] Biofilm formation with 37 clinical icaADBC-positive *S epidermidis* isolates was investigated after exposure to isopropanol at 1%, 2%, 4%, or 6%. In 14 of the 37 strains, biofilm formation was inducible by isopropanol exposure.[133] With *C albicans*, it was described that 2% isopropanol inhibited to some extent biofilm development.[134] In *E coli*, it was shown that low-level exposure to isopropanol concentrations up to 2.7% for up to 24 days reduced the susceptibility of the six tested strains.[135]

n-Propanol at 0.2%, 1.5%, and 2% increased the attachment of marine *P aeruginosa* to polystyrene dishes and tissue culture dishes.[136] Biofilm formation with the same clinical *S epidermidis* isolates discussed earlier was investigated after exposure to *n*-propanol at 0.5%, 1%, 2%, and 4%. In 15 of the 37 strains, biofilm formation was also inducible by *n*-propanol exposure.[133] The *C albicans* biofilm development was similarly inhibited with 2% *n*-propanol.[134] In two food strains of *L monocytogenes*, the *n*-propanol minimum inhibitory concentration values remained unchanged after exposure to sublethal concentration of *n*-propanol.[137]

▶ ALCOHOLS FOR PRESERVATION

Ethanol, *n*-propanol, and isopropanol are traditionally the most frequently used aliphatic alcohols for preservation of cosmetic formulations and have been used as preservatives for many years.[138] Microbial growth is prevented in aqueous systems containing >20% by volume mass of absolute ethyl alcohol. However, lower alcohol levels (eg, 5%-20%) may have additive or synergistic activity when combined with other ingredients and physical/chemical factors (eg, pH).[139] The International Organization for Standardization guideline for cosmetic microbiology risk assessment recommends that products containing alcohol levels ≥20% by volume mass do not require microbiological testing (ie, challenge test and final product testing).[140] That guideline further suggests that data to support the conclusion that the microbiological risk is low for finished products with alcohol as the preservative may require well-designed experimental data or reviews of product history after launch. Short-chain alcohols as preservatives are generally universally allowed without regulatory restrictions.[141]

▶ ALCOHOLS FOR DISINFECTION ON HARD INANIMATE SURFACES

The use of ethanol and isopropanol for surface disinfection has been reviewed by Boyce[5] in 2018. *n*-Propanol is also used in quite a number of surface disinfectants.[142] Advantages include the fact that they are easy to use; are nonstaining; and have acceptable odor, rapid onset of action, and a broad spectrum of antimicrobial activity. Limitations include their slow action against nonenveloped viruses, lack of sporicidal activity, reduced activity in the presence of organic matter, limited detergent properties, flammability, and adverse effects on some types of equipment/materials. They may be used in health care for the disinfection of small noncritical items, vascular access devices, and environmental surfaces. Another application may be its use in flexible endoscopes after high-level disinfection (final flushing). The main aim is for disinfections when the water quality used for final rinsing cannot be assured.[143-145] Another advantage may be a faster drying after reprocessing.[146-148] Alcohols are also widely used in general and critical manufacturing environments such as cleanrooms.[149-151]

▶ ALCOHOLS FOR HYGIENIC HAND DISINFECTION

The bactericidal efficacy of ethanol-based hand rubs has been particularly evaluated on hands artificially contaminated with *E coli* according to EN 1500 with an application of 3 mL for 30 seconds (Table 19.4). Preparations with up to 70% ethanol mostly fail to meet the EN 1500 efficacy requirements, whereas solutions or gels with 80% or more are mostly effective. The application of larger volumes (eg, 6 mL) or smaller volumes (eg, 2 mL) can yield different results.[156,159-161] The application of volumes <3 mL is quite likely in clinical practice.[156,160] According to ASTM E2755, commercial preparations with volumes between 1.1 and 2 mL often reveal a between 2.0 and 3.3 $\log_{10}$ reduction on hands artificially contaminated with *S marcescens* (Table 19.5).

On artificially contaminated hands, ethanol is considered effective within 30 seconds against rotavirus but is inconsistent against MNV, human enterovirus, and FCV. Insufficient virucidal efficacy is also observed against poliovirus (Table 19.6). The addition of acids with ethanol-based formulations improves the virucidal efficacy to include adenovirus, poliovirus, and MNV but not HAV (Table 19.7).

Sixty percent (vol/vol) isopropanol was proposed in 1977 as a reference treatment for hygienic hand disinfection[171] and is the reference alcohol to determine the bactericidal efficacy of alcohol-based hand rubs for hygienic hand disinfection in EN 1500.[172] Numerous data exist for the reference treatment (2×3 mL for 2×30 s), which usually achieves a mean 4.6 $\log_{10}$ reduction on hands artificially contaminated with *E coli*.[173,174] The efficacy of hand rubs based on isopropanol has been mostly evaluated on hands artificially contaminated with *E coli* according to EN 1500 with an application of 3 mL for 30 seconds (Table 19.8). Hand rubs with an isopropanol concentration <75% may fail to meet these requirements depending on the entire composition. Longer application times or larger volumes may yield better results. The WHO has described hand rubs based on isopropanol at 75% (vol/vol) as essential medicines,[29] although they do not meet European efficacy requirements when applied with 3 mL for 30 seconds.[30]

On artificially contaminated hands, isopropanol can be considered to have insufficient efficacy within 30 seconds against FCV, human enterovirus, and poliovirus. The effect against MNV is unclear, but rotavirus is reduced substantially by isopropanol (Table 19.9).

TABLE 19.4 Efficacy of ethanol-based formulations for hygienic hand disinfection according to EN 1500[a,b]

Ethanol Concentration (wt/wt)	Viscosity (Type of Product)	Mean Log$_{10}$ Reduction Product	Mean Log$_{10}$ Reduction Reference Procedure	Reference(s)
45.5%[c]	Gel (C)	3.31[d]	4.28	Kramer et al[152]
49.3%[c]	Gel (C)	2.68[d]	3.78	Kramer et al[152]
52.1%[c]	Solution (S)	3.8[d]	4.2	Rotter[153]
52.1%[c]	Gel (C)	4.09[d]	5.07	Kramer et al[152]
52.1%[c]	Gel (C)	3.07[d]	4.12	Kramer et al[152]
54.1%[c]	Gel (C)	3.07[d]	4.10	Kramer et al[152]
62.4%[c]	Solution (S)	4.0	4.2	Rotter[153]
62.4%[c]	Gel (C)	5.25	5.11	Edmonds et al[154]
62.4%[c]	Foam (C)	5.06	5.11	Edmonds et al[154]
62.4%[c]	Gel (C)	5.17	4.80	Edmonds et al[154]
62.4%[c]	Gel (C)	3.33	3.87	do Prado et al[155]
62.4%[c]	Gel (C)	3.27	3.64	do Prado et al[155]
62.4%[c]	Gel (C)	2.91[d]	3.58	do Prado et al[155]
62.4%[c]	Gel (C)	3.49	3.71	do Prado et al[155]
62.4%[c]	Gel (C)	3.06[d]	3.68	do Prado et al[155]
62.4%[c]	Foam (C)	4.56	4.63	Macinga et al[156]
62.4%[c]	Gel (C)	2.13[d]	4.12	Kramer et al[152]
62.4%[c]	Gel (C)	3.36[d]	4.26	Kramer et al[152]
67.8%[c]	Solution (C)	4.78	4.78	Kramer et al[152]
70%	Solution (C)	3.95[d]	4.65	Kampf et al[84]
70%	Solution (C)	4.29[d]	5.00	Kampf et al[84]
70%	Solution (C)	4.04[d]	4.93	Kampf et al[84]
70%	Gel (C)	3.87[d]	4.62	Kampf et al[84]
70%	Gel (C)	4.38[d]	5.00	Kampf et al[84]
70%	Gel (C)	4.06[d]	4.99	Kampf et al[84]
70%	Gel (C)	3.63	3.62	do Prado et al[155]
70%	Gel (C)	3.27[d]	4.40	do Prado et al[155]
70%	Gel (C)	3.26[d]	3.81	do Prado et al[155]
70%	Gel (C)	3.25[d]	3.68	do Prado et al[155]
70%	Gel (C)	3.46[d]	4.35	do Prado et al[155]
70%	Gel (C)	3.40[d]	4.14	do Prado et al[155]
70%	Gel (C)	3.48[d]	4.00	do Prado et al[155]
70%	Solution (C)	3.32	3.62	do Prado et al[155]
73.5%[c]	Solution (S)	4.5	4.2	Rotter[153]
73.5%[c]	Solution (F)	3.59[d]	4.29	Suchomel et al[30]
73.5%[c]	Solution (C)	4.50	4.63	Macinga et al[156]
80%	Solution (F)	4.40	4.79	Suchomel et al[30]
85%	Gel (C)	3.30	3.50	Kampf et al[157]

TABLE 19.4 Efficacy of ethanol-based formulations for hygienic hand disinfection according to EN 1500[a,b] *(Continued)*

Ethanol Concentration (wt/wt)	Viscosity (Type of Product)	Mean Log$_{10}$ Reduction Product	Mean Log$_{10}$ Reduction Reference Procedure	Reference(s)
85%	Gel (C)	3.84	3.95	Kampf et al[38]
85%	Gel (C)	4.27	4.60	Kampf et al[38]
85%	Gel (C)	3.89	4.05	Kampf et al[38]
85%	Gel (C)	4.65	4.49	Kampf et al[38]
85%	Gel (C)	3.80	3.55	do Prado et al[155]
85%	Gel (C)	4.61	4.63	Macinga et al[156]

Abbreviations: C, commercial product; F, formulation with auxiliary agents or other active agents; S, ethanolic solution.

[a]All data sets with an application of 3 mL for 30 s.

[b]Adapted from Kampf.[158] Reprinted with permission from Günter Kampf, MD.

[c]Determined by calculation (originally described as vol/vol).

[d]Significantly less effective compared to reference procedure (EN 1500 efficacy requirement failed).

TABLE 19.5 Mean log$_{10}$ reduction of *Serratia marcescens* after application of ethanol-based hand disinfectants according to ASTM E2755[a]

Ethanol Concentration (wt/wt)	Viscosity (Type of Product)	Applied Volume	Mean Log$_{10}$ Reduction Product (Application 1)	Reference(s)
54.1%[b]	Gel (C)	0.75 mL	1.96	Macinga et al[162]
54.1%[b]	Gel (C)	1.5 mL	2.74	Macinga et al[162]
54.1%[b]	Gel (C)	1.5 mL	2.41	Macinga et al[162]
54.1%[b]	Gel (C)	3 mL	3.79	Macinga et al[162]
62.4%[b]	Gel (C)	1.1 mL	1.97	Kampf et al[163]
62.4%[b]	Foam (C)	1.1 mL	1.96	Kampf et al[163]
62.4%[b]	Foam (C)	1.5 mL	2.41	Macinga et al[162]
62.4%[b]	Gel (C)	2 mL	3.33	Edmonds-Wilson et al[164]
62.4%[b]	Foam (C)	Approx. 2 mL	3.29	Edmonds-Wilson et al[164]
85%	Gel (C)	1.5 mL	2.61	Macinga et al[162]
85%	Gel (C)	2 mL	2.90	Kampf et al[163]

Abbreviation: C, commercial product.

[a]Adapted from Kampf.[158] Reprinted with permission from Günter Kampf, MD.

[b]Determined by calculation (originally described as vol/vol).

1 Chapter 19 Alcohols

TABLE 19.6 Mean $\log_{10}$ reduction of viral infectivity (nonenveloped viruses) on hands or fingertips after application of ethanol-based hand rubs[a]

Virus	Ethanol Concentration (wt/wt)	Viscosity (Type of Product)	Application Time	Mean $\log_{10}$ Reduction	Reference(s)
Poliovirus type 1	80%	Solution (S)	30 s	0.42	Davies et al[165]
	80%	Solution (S)	10 min	2.2	Steinmann et al[166]
	96.8%	Solution (S)	10 min	3.2	Steinmann et al[166]
Murine norovirus	54.1%[b]	Gel (C)	20 s	2.8	Sattar et al[167]
	54.1%[b]	Gel (C)	30 s	3.5	Sattar et al[167]
	62.4%[b]	Solution (S)	30 s	4.69	Paulmann et al[89]
	67.8%[b]	Solution (S)	20 s	3.0	Sattar et al[167]
	67.8%[b]	Solution (S)	30 s	2.7	Sattar et al[167]
	68%[b]	Solution (S)	30 s	0.91	Macinga et al[86]
	73.5%[b]	Solution (S)	20 s	1.7	Sattar et al[167]
	>90%	Solution (C)	30 s	3.91	Steinmann et al[78]
Human enterovirus 71	68%[b]	Solution (S)	30 s	0.86	Chang et al[101]
	92.9%[b]	Solution (S)	30 s	4.06	Chang et al[101]
Rotavirus	70%[c]	Solution (S)	30 s	2.85	Bellamy et al[168]
Feline calicivirus	54.1%[b]	Gel (C)	20 s	1.4	Sattar et al[167]
	54.1%[b]	Gel (C)	30 s	2.1	Sattar et al[167]
	62%[c]	Solution (S)	30 s	0.50	Lages et al[169]
	62%[c]	Solution (S)	2 min	0.55	Lages et al[169]
	62.4%[b]	Solution (S)	30 s	3.78	Gehrke et al[94]
	62.4%[b]	Solution (S)	30 s	0.68	Kramer et al[67]
	67.8%[b]	Solution (S)	20 s	1.5	Sattar et al[167]
	67.8%[b]	Solution (S)	30 s	2.2	Sattar et al[167]
	70%	Solution (S)	30 s	2.66	Kampf et al[170]
	70%	Solution (S)	30 s	2.62	Kampf et al[170]
	70%	Solution (S)	30 s	1.18	Kampf et al[170]
	70%	Solution (S)	30 s	1.45	Kampf et al[170]
	70%	Solution (S)	30 s	1.33	Kampf et al[170]
	75.1%	Solution (C)	30 s	0.93	Kampf et al[170]
	80%	Solution (C)	30 s	1.34	Kampf et al[170]
	85.7%[b]	Solution (S)	30 s	2.84	Gehrke et al[94]
	95%	Solution (C)	30 s	1.90	Kampf et al[170]
	99.5%[c]	Solution (S)	30 s	1.00	Lages et al[169]
	99.5%[c]	Solution (S)	2 min	1.30	Lages et al[169]

Abbreviations: C, commercial product; S, ethanolic solution.

[a]Adapted from Kampf.[158] Reprinted with permission from Günter Kampf, MD.

[b]Determined by calculation (originally described as vol/vol).

[c]No information on vol/vol or wt/wt.

TABLE 19.7   Mean log$_{10}$ reduction of viral infectivity (nonenveloped viruses) on hands or fingertips after application of acid-containing ethanol-based hand rubs[a]

Virus	Ethanol Concentration (wt/wt)	Viscosity (Type of Product)	Application Time	Mean Log$_{10}$ Reduction	Reference(s)
Adenovirus type 5	62.4%[b]	Gel (C)[c]	15 s	≥3.16	Macinga et al[86]
			30 s	≥3.12	Macinga et al[86]
Poliovirus type 1	55%	Solution (C)[d]	30 s	3.04	Kramer et al[67]
			1 min	3.13	Kramer et al[67]
	62.4%[b]	Gel (C)[c]	30 s	2.98	Macinga et al[86]
Murine norovirus	45%	Solution (C)[d]	30 s	3.94	Steinmann et al[78]
	55%	Solution (C)[d]	30 s	3.91	Steinmann et al[78]
	62.4%[b]	Gel (C)[c]	30 s	2.48	Macinga et al[86]
Hepatitis A virus	62.4%[b]	Gel (C)[c]	30 s	1.32	Macinga et al[86]
Rotavirus	62.4%[b]	Gel (C)[c]	15 s	≥4.32	Macinga et al[86]
			30 s	≥3.84	Macinga et al[86]
Feline calicivirus	55%	Solution (C)[d]	30 s	2.38	Kramer et al[67]

Abbreviations: C, commercial product.

[a]Adapted from Kampf.[158] Reprinted with permission from Günter Kampf, MD.

[b]Determined by calculation (originally described as vol/vol).

[c]Contains citric acid.

[d]Contains phosphoric acid.

TABLE 19.8   Efficacy of isopropanol-based formulations for hygienic hand disinfection according to the test principle of EN 1500[a,b]

Isopropanol Concentration (wt/wt)	Viscosity (Type of Product)	Species	Application Time	Mean Log$_{10}$ Reduction	Reference(s)
53.7%[c]	Gel (C)	Escherichia coli	30 s	4.07[d]	Kramer et al[152]
53.7%[c]	Solution (S)		30 s	4.1	Herruzo et al[175]
53.7%[c]	Solution (S)		1 min	4.2	Rotter[153]
53.7%[c]	Solution (S)	Pseudomonas aeruginosa	15 s	6.05	Dharan et al[176]
53.7%[c]	Solution (S)		30 s	3.3	Herruzo et al[175]
53.7%[c]	Solution (S)		30 s	6.81	Dharan et al[176]
53.7%[c]	Solution (S)	Staphylococcus aureus	15 s	5.90	Dharan et al[176]
53.7%[c]	Solution (S)		30 s	6.36	Dharan et al[176]
53.7%[c]	Solution (S)		30 s	4.1	Herruzo et al[175]
53.7%[c]	Solution (S)	Enterococcus faecalis	15 s	5.03	Dharan et al[176]
53.7%[c]	Solution (S)		30 s	6.07	Dharan et al[176]
68.2%[c]	Solution (F)	E coli	30 s	3.57[d]	Suchomel et al[30]
75%	Solution (F)		30 s	4.36	Suchomel et al[30]

Abbreviations: C, commercial product; F, formulation with auxiliary agents or other active agents; S, propanolic solution.

[a]All data sets with an application of 3 mL.

[b]Adapted from Kampf.[177] Reprinted with permission from Günter Kampf, MD.

[c]Determined by calculation (originally described as vol/vol).

[d]Significantly less effective compared to reference procedure (EN 1500 efficacy requirement failed).

TABLE 19.9 Mean $\log_{10}$ reduction of viral infectivity (nonenveloped viruses) on hands or fingertips after application of isopropanol-based hand rubs[a]

Virus	Isopropanol Concentration (wt/wt)	Viscosity (Type of Product)	Application Time	Mean Log₁₀ Reduction	Reference(s)
Poliovirus type 1	53.7%[b]	Solution (S)	30 s	1.32	Kramer et al[67]
	53.7%[b]	Solution (S)	1 min	1.23	Kramer et al[67]
Murine norovirus	62.8%[b]	Solution (S)	30 s	2.24	Paulmann et al[89]
Human enterovirus 71	62.8%[b]	Solution (S)	30 s	0.53	Chang et al[101]
Feline calicivirus	62.8%[b]	Solution (S)	30 s	2.15	Gehrke et al[94]
	70%[c]	Solution (C)	30 s	0.67	Lages et al[169]
	70%[c]	Solution (C)	2 min	0.55	Lages et al[169]
	86%[c]	Solution (S)	30 s	0.76	Gehrke et al[94]
	91%[c]	Solution (C)	30 s	0.00	Lages et al[169]
	91%[c]	Solution (C)	2 min	0.43	Lages et al[169]
Rotavirus	70%[c]	Solution (S)	30 s	3.15	Bellamy et al[168]

Abbreviations: C, commercial product; S, propanolic solution.

[a]Adapted from Kampf.[177] Reprinted with permission from Günter Kampf, MD.

[b]Determined by calculation (originally described as vol/vol).

[c]No information on vol/vol or wt/wt.

Forty percent *n*-propanol was described as effective in 1 minute with a mean $\log_{10}$ reduction of 4.3, which was equivalent to the reference procedure with 4.2 $\log_{10}$.[153] Fifty percent *n*-propanol is very effective in 30 seconds (5.0 $\log_{10}$) and 1 minute (4.9 $\log_{10}$).[153,178] At 60%, it was reported to reach 5.5 $\log_{10}$.[153] The efficacy of *n*-propanol against *E coli* on artificially contaminated hands is considered to be at least as good as of isopropanol.[178]

On artificially contaminated hands, *n*-propanol can be considered to have insufficient efficacy against FCV within 30 seconds (Table 19.10).

TABLE 19.10 Mean $\log_{10}$ reduction of viral infectivity (nonenveloped viruses) on hands or fingertips after application of *n*-propanol–based hand rubs[a]

Virus	n-Propanol Concentration (wt/wt)	Viscosity (Type of Product)	Application Time	Mean Log₁₀ Reduction	Reference(s)
Feline calicivirus	63.5%[b]	Solution (S)	30 s	3.58	Gehrke et al[94]
	70%	Solution (S)	30 s	1.53[c] 1.56[c] 0.41[c] 0.95[c]	Kampf et al[170]
	70%	Solution (S)	30 s	0.99	Kampf et al[170]
	86%[b]	Solution (S)	30 s	1.38	Gehrke et al[94]

Abbreviation: S, propanolic solution.

[a]Adapted from Kampf.[179] Reprinted with permission from Günter Kampf, MD.

[b]Determined by calculation (originally described as vol/vol).

[c]Depending on the type of organic load.

For some activities, such as in patient care, it is recommended to wear medical gloves during the entire period of patient care, eg, in anesthetics, in patients with Ebola virus disease, in isolated patients (eg, infection with carbapenem-resistant Enterobacteriaceae), in patients with strong immunosuppression, or in emergency departments. Observational studies indicate that gloves are often worn in these situations, but hand disinfection is only performed very rarely once gloves are worn even if aseptic procedures are performed on the patient. In these situations or other long-term use of glove in critical environments, the disinfection of gloved hands can be considered as long as the gloves are not damaged and remain visibly clean because the efficacy of alcohol-based hand rubs can be used to significantly reduce microbial levels, and the microperforation rate does not increase for most glove-hand rub combinations.[180] The rate of health care–associated infections (HAIs) may even be affected in certain situations, as shown on a neonatal intensive care unit.[181] Whether this practice can be adopted to other areas such as room cleaning, cleanroom use, food processing, or food production is not clear.

ALCOHOLS FOR SURGICAL HAND DISINFECTION

Formulations with ethanol of less than 80% typically fail to meet the EN 12791 efficacy requirements even when applied for 5 minutes, but concentrations in the 80% to 85% range are usually effective (Table 19.11). According to ASTM E1115, the efficacy of ethanol-based preparations against the resident hand flora is poor (immediate efficacy, mean $\log_{10}$ reduction of 1.1) with 61% ethanol. Efficacies of 2.1 $\log_{10}$ and 3.1 $\log_{10}$ have been reported with formulations containing 70% or 80% ethanol (Table 19.12).

Formulations with isopropanol of at least 70% usually meet EN 12791 efficacy requirements when applied for 1.5 or 3 minutes (Table 19.13). Additional data with mixed propanols (eg, 45% isopropanol plus 30% n-propanol) indicate sufficient bactericidal efficacy for surgical hand disinfection within 1.5 minutes.[200-203]

In EN 12791, 60% vol/vol n-propanol is described as the reference alcohol for determination of the efficacy of products for surgical hand disinfection or surgical scrubbing.[204] Numerous data sets have been published

TABLE 19.11 Efficacy of ethanol-based hand rubs for surgical hand disinfection according to EN 12791[a]

Ethanol Concentration (wt/wt)	Viscosity (Type of Product)	Application Time	Mean Log$_{10}$ Reduction				Reference(s)
			Immediate Efficacy		3-h Efficacy		
			Product	Reference	Product	Reference	
61%	Emulsion (C)	3 min	1.82[b]	2.98	1.41[b]	2.56	Kampf and Ostermeyer[182]
73.5%[c]	Solution (F)	3 min	1.61[b]	2.38	0.76[b]	1.66	Suchomel et al[183]
		5 min	2.26[b]	3.06	0.95[b]	2.02	
73.5%[c]	Solution (F)	1.5 min	1.49[b]		0.87[b]		Kampf and Ostermeyer[184]
		3 min	1.50[b]	2.43	0.91[b]	2.22	
		5 min	1.41[b]		1.08[b]		
78.2%	Solution (C)	1.5 min	2.36[b]	2.92	1.69	1.91	Suchomel et al[185]
80%	Solution (C)	3 min	2.59	2.58	1.73	1.67	Kampf and Ostermeyer[182]
80%	Solution (F)	5 min	2.47	2.53	1.30[b]	2.03	Suchomel et al[183]
80%	Solution (F)	5 min	2.35	2.41	1.58	1.55	Suchomel et al[186]
80%	Solution (F)	5 min	2.37	2.41	2.04	1.55	Suchomel et al[186]
85%	Gel (C)	3 min	2.48	2.06	2.77	2.03	Kampf and Kapella[187]
85%	Gel (C)	3 min	2.13	2.23	2.18	1.44	Kampf and Kapella[187]

Abbreviations: C, commercial product; F, formulation with auxiliary agents or other active agents.

[a]Adapted from Kampf.[158] Reprinted with permission from Günter Kampf, MD.

[b]Significantly less effective compared to the reference procedure.

[c]Determined by calculation (originally described as vol/vol).

TABLE 19.12 Efficacy of ethanol-based hand rubs for surgical hand disinfection according to ASTM E1115 (only immediate effect)[a]

Ethanol Concentration (wt/wt)	Volume and Application Time	Immediate Effect Day 1	Immediate Effect Day 2	Immediate Effect Day 5	Reference(s)
61% (S)	3 × 2 mL until hands are dry	1.1	2.0	1.5	Mulberry et al[188]
70%[b] (C)	2 × 2 mL	2.3	2.9	3.2	Macinga et al[189]
70%[b] (C)	3 × 2 mL	3.1	3.4	3.0	Macinga et al[189]
80% (C)	Keep hands wet for 2 min (9.6 mL).	2.49	No data	2.53	Olson et al[190]
80% (C)	Keep hands wet for 2 min (8 mL).	2.1	2.4	2.4	Macinga et al[189]
80% (C)	Keep hands wet for 2 min (6-9 mL).	2.99	3.00	3.43	Kampf et al[191]

Abbreviations: C, commercial product; S, ethanolic solution.

[a]Adapted from Kampf.[158] Reprinted with permission from Günter Kampf, MD.

[b]Gel.

(Table 19.14). The reference alcohol has a rather weak bactericidal efficacy for surgical hand disinfection when applied for only 1 minute. Within the standard application time of 3 minutes, a mean $\log_{10}$ reduction between 2 and 3 is typically found immediately after application. The 3-hour value under the surgical glove is somewhat lower.[213] Additional data with mixed propanols (eg, 30% n-propanol plus 45% isopropanol) indicated sufficient bactericidal efficacy for surgical hand disinfection within 1.5 minutes.[196,201-203]

ALCOHOLS FOR SKIN ANTISEPSIS

Alcohols such as ethanol, isopropanol, or n-propanol are commonly used as skin antiseptics, not only before surgical procedures (often referred to as preoperative preparations) but also before the insertion of vascular catheters. For reducing the resident skin flora, n-propanol has been described as the most effective mono-alcohol.[214] Alcohols should not be used on the premature vulnerable skin of newborns.[31] The WHO has recommended since 2016 a combination of alcohols and chlorhexidine for skin antisepsis. The nonvolatile active ingredient is expected to yield a persistent efficacy in skin antisepsis. Octenidine dihydrochloride at 0.1% may be an alternative to chlorhexidine in addition to the alcohols.[215-217] The Centers for Disease Control and Prevention recommended in 2017 to use an alcohol-based antiseptic for the prevention of surgical site infections (category 1A).[218] The Robert Koch Institute in Germany recommended since 2018 the use of an alcohol-based skin antiseptic (category 1A). An additional active agent with a remnant efficacy can achieve

a long-lasting effect, although it is not clear which agent may be preferred (category 1B).[219]

THE IMPACTS OF ALCOHOLS FOR THE PREVENTION OF INFECTION

The use of alcohol-based hand rubs by health care workers according to specific indications has been shown in various studies to significantly reduce the rate of HAI. The impact on the infection rate depends largely on the compliance rate during patient care. In 2000, Pittet et al[220] were able to show that an increase of hand hygiene compliance from 48% to 66%, mainly by using the alcohol-based hand rub more frequently, was able to reduce the rate of HAI over 3 years significantly from 16.9% to 9.9%. Ever since, alcohol-based hand rubs are recommended for use in patient care according to the five moments for hand hygiene.[221] This includes the care for patients in hospitals, in practices, and in ambulant and domestic care. Its use at home can be recommended as an adjunct to hand-washing if infected persons or severely immunocompromised person are present.[222] Hand sanitizer products have also been tested in a variety of community settings in the United States, demonstrating that hand hygiene programs can reduce illness-related absenteeism and improve health outcomes.[223-225]

In 2010, it was shown that the application of a skin antiseptic based on 70% isopropanol in combination with 2% chlorhexidine resulted in a significantly lower rate of superficial (incidence rate: 4.2% versus 8.6%) and deep surgical site infections (incidence rate: 1.0% versus 3.0%) in abdominal, urologic, and gynecologic surgery

TABLE 19.13 Efficacy of isopropanol-based hand rubs for surgical hand disinfection according to EN 12791[a]

Isopropanol Concentration (wt/wt)	Viscosity (Type of Product)	Application Time	Immediate Efficacy	3-h Efficacy	Reference(s)
53.7%[b]	Solution (S)	5	1.65	1.04	Rotter et al[192]
62.8%[b]	Solution (S)	1	0.74	0.19	Suchomel et al[193]
62.8%[b]	Solution (S)	3	2.0[c]	0.7[c]	Rotter et al[194]
62.8%[b]	Solution (S)	3	2.1[c]	1.1[c]	Rotter et al[194]
62.8%[b]	Solution (S)	3	1.48	0.79	Suchomel et al[193]
62.8%[b]	Solution (S)	5	2.12	1.03	Suchomel et al[193]
68.2%[b]	Solution (F)	1.5	1.26[c]	1.13[c]	Kampf and Ostermeyer[184]
68.2%[b]	Solution (F)	3	1.43[c]	0.58[c]	Suchomel et al[183]
68.2%[b]	Solution (F)	3	1.74[c]	1.46[c]	Kampf and Ostermeyer[184]
68.2%[b]	Solution (F)	5	2.05[c]	1.00[c]	Kampf and Ostermeyer[184]
68.2%[b]	Solution (F)	5	1.46[c]	1.06[c]	Suchomel et al[183]
70%[d]	Solution (S)	0.5	1.50	1.24	Babb et al[195]
70%[d]	Solution (S)	2	1.65	1.58	Babb et al[195]
70%[d]	Solution (S)	2	0.82	1.21	Lowbury et al[196]
70%	Solution (F)	3	2.7[e]	1.7[e]	Rotter et al[197]
73.5%[b]	Solution (S)	3	2.3[e]	1.2[e]	Rotter et al[194]
73.5%[b]	Solution (S)	3	2.4[e]	1.4[e]	Rotter et al[194]
75%	Solution (S)	3	2.25	1.76	Suchomel et al[198]
75%	Solution (F)	3	2.09	1.32	Suchomel et al[198]
75%	Solution (F)	3	2.22	1.41	Suchomel et al[199]
75%	Solution (F)	3	2.53	2.08	Suchomel et al[199]
75%	Solution (F)	5	2.95[e]	2.04[e]	Suchomel et al[186]
75%	Solution (F)	5	2.41[e]	1.57[e]	Suchomel et al[186]
75%	Solution (F)	5	2.78[e]	1.36[c]	Suchomel et al[183]
75%	Solution (F)	5	2.65	1.74	Suchomel et al[199]
75%	Solution (F)	5	2.75	2.13	Suchomel et al[199]
86%[b]	Solution (S)	3	2.4[e]	1.4[e]	Rotter et al[194]
86%[b]	Solution (S)	3	2.6[e]	1.4[e]	Rotter et al[194]

Abbreviations: F, formulation with auxiliary agents or other active agents; S, propanolic solution.

[a]Adapted from Kampf.[177] Reprinted with permission from Günter Kampf, MD.

[b]Determined by calculation (originally described as vol/vol).

[c]Significantly less effective compared to the reference procedure (after 0 h, 3 h, or both).

[d]No information on vol/vol or wt/wt.

[e]Equivalent efficacy to EN 12791 reference procedure.

TABLE 19.14 Efficacy of 53.9% (wt/wt) *n*-propanol solution (reference alcohol) for surgical hand disinfection according to EN 12791[a]

Application Time (min)	Subjects (n)	Immediate Efficacy	3-h Efficacy	Reference(s)
1	21	1.05	0.45	Suchomel et al[193]
3	20	3.27	1.36	Suchomel and Rotter[205]
	24	3.1	2.2	Rotter et al[197]
	24	3.06	2.02	Suchomel et al[183]
	20	2.99	2.22	Kampf and Ostermeyer[202]
	20	2.98	2.56	Kampf and Ostermeyer[182]
	21	2.97	1.60	Suchomel et al[185]
	20	2.92	2.47	Kampf et al[191]
	21	2.92	1.91	Suchomel et al[185]
	20	2.87	2.50	Kampf et al[203]
	26	2.72	2.26	Kampf and Ostermeyer[184]
	200	2.70	2.20	Kampf and Ostermeyer[206]
	20	2.6	1.6	Rotter et al[194]
	20	2.58	1.67	Kampf and Ostermeyer[182]
	20	2.56	2.03	Suchomel et al[199]
	24	2.53	2.03	Suchomel et al[183]
	20	2.52	2.44	Kampf et al[201]
	40	2.52	2.05	Kampf et al[201]
	26	2.43	2.22	Kampf and Ostermeyer[184]
	25	2.41	1.55	Suchomel et al[186]
	20	2.4	1.0	Rotter et al[194]
	20	2.23	1.44	Kampf and Kapella[187]
	24	2.18	1.60	Suchomel et al[198]
	20	2.06	2.03	Kampf and Kapella[187]
	20	2.05	1.86	Hingst et al[207]
	21	2.03	1.01	Suchomel et al[193]
	19	2.01	1.63	Kampf et al[201]
	37	1.92	1.31	Kampf et al[201]
	20	1.86	1.50	Kampf et al[191]
	20	1.79	1.42	Hübner et al[208]
	23	1.63	1.72	Kampf[209]
	20	1.13	0.67	Barbut et al[210]
	20	0.83	0.50	Marchetti et al[211]
5	20	2.05	1.86	Hingst et al[207]
	21	2.30	1.60	Suchomel et al[193]
	20	2.49	1.78	Rotter and Koller[212]

[a]Adapted from Kampf.[179] Reprinted with permission from Günter Kampf, MD.

compared to the application of 10% povidone-iodine. No effect was found in organ/space surgical site infections.[226] Another study published in 2016 also yielded a significantly lower infection rate in 1147 patients undergoing cesarean section after a 3-minute use of a skin antiseptic based on 70% isopropanol and 2% chlorhexidine compared to the 3-minute application of a skin antiseptic based on 72.5% isopropanol and 8.3% povidone-iodine (incidence rate: 4.0% versus 7.3%).[227] The role of the different types of active ingredients on the preventive effect is still under controversial debate.[228-231]

A study from France among 1181 patients with 2457 vascular catheters on 11 intensive care units showed that the incidence of catheter-associated septicemia was 84% lower when 70% isopropanol in combination with 2% chlorhexidine was used compared to the application of 69% ethanol in combination with 5% povidone-iodine.[232] A similar study on 400 patients yielded a favorable but not significant result with a skin antiseptic based on 45% isopropanol, 30% *n*-propanol, and 0.1% octenidine compared to the application of a skin antiseptic based on 74% ethanol and 10% isopropanol.[216] Although the preventive effect cannot be clearly attributed to any of the active ingredients due to a lack of suitable controls, the alcohols are well recognized to have at least a very strong immediate effect that is substantial in skin antisepsis.

REFERENCES

1. Beck WC. Benefits of alcohol rediscovered. *AORN J.* 1984;40(2):172-176.
2. Fürbringer P. Zur Desinfection der Hände des Arztes. *Deutsche medizinische Wochenschrift (1946).* 1888;48:985-987.
3. Price PB. Ethyl alcohol as a germicide. *Arch Surg.* 1939;38:528-542.
4. Harrington C, Walker H. The germicidal action of alcohol. *Boston Med Surg J.* 1903;148(21):548-552.
5. Boyce JM. Alcohols as surface disinfectants in healthcare settings. *Infect Control Hosp Epidemiol.* 2018;39(3):323-328.
6. Ali Y, Dolan MJ, Fendler EJ, Larson EL. Alcohols. In: Block SS, ed. *Disinfection, Sterilization, and Preservation.* Philadelphia, PA: Lippincott Williams & Wilkins; 2001:229-253.
7. McDonnell G, Russell AD. Antiseptics and disinfectants: activity, action, resistance. *Clin Microbiol Rev.* 1999;12(1):147-179.
8. Sykes G. The influence of germicides on the dehydrogenases of Bact. coli: I. The succinic acid dehydrogenase of Bact. coli. *J Hyg (Lond).* 1939;39(4):463-469.
9. Skovgaard PA, Jørgensen H. Influence of high temperature and ethanol on thermostable lignocellulolytic enzymes. *J Ind Microbiol Biotechnol.* 2013;40(5):447-456.
10. Todrick A, Fellowes KP, Rutland JP. The effect of alcohols on cholinesterase. *Biochem J.* 1951;48(3):360-368.
11. Kamm O. The relation between structure and physiologic action of the alcohols. *J Am Pharmaceut Assoc.* 1921;10:87-92.
12. van Koningsveld GA, Gruppen H, de Jongh HH, et al. Effects of ethanol on structure and solubility of potato proteins and the effects of its presence during the preparation of a protein isolate. *J Agric Food Chem.* 2002;50(10):2947-2956.
13. Vajpai N, Nisius L, Wiktor M, Grzesiek S. High-pressure NMR reveals close similarity between cold and alcohol protein denaturation in ubiquitin. *Proc Natl Acad Sci U S A.* 2013;110(5):E368-E376.
14. Assadian O, Kramer A. *7.2.5.6 Eiweißfehler. Wallhäußers Praxis der Sterilisation, Desinfektion, Antiseptik und Konservierung.* Stuttgart: Georg Thieme Verlag; 2008.
15. Pethica B. Lysis by physical and chemical methods. *J Gen Microbiol.* 1958;15:166-168.
16. Pidot SJ, Gao W, Buultjens AH, et al. Increasing tolerance of hospital *Enterococcus faecium* to handwash alcohols. *Sci Transl Med.* 2018;10(452):eaar6115.
17. Lam FH, Ghaderi A, Fink GR, Stephanopoulos G. Biofuels. Engineering alcohol tolerance in yeast. *Science.* 2014;346(6205):71-75.
18. Ingram LO, Vreeland NS. Differential effects of ethanol and hexanol on the *Escherichia coli* cell envelope. *J Bacteriol.* 1980;144(2):481-488.
19. Ingram LO. Mechanism of lysis of *Escherichia coli* by ethanol and other chaotropic agents. *J Bacteriol.* 1981;146(1):331-336.
20. Brondz I, Olsen I, Sjöström M. Gas chromatographic assessment of alcoholyzed fatty acids from yeasts: a new chemotaxonomic method. *J Clin Microbiol.* 1989;27(12):2815-2819.
21. Dagley S, Dawes EA, Morrison GA. Inhibition of growth of *Aerobacter aerogenes*: the mode of action of phenols, alcohols, acetone, and ethyl acetate. *J Bacteriol.* 1950;60(4):369-379.
22. Onishi H, Kushner DJ. Mechanism of dissolution of envelopes of the extreme halophile *Halobacterium cutirubrum*. *J Bacteriol.* 1966;91(2):646-652.
23. US Department of Health and Human Services, US Food and Drug Administration. Tentative final monograph for health care antiseptic products; proposed rule. *Fed Reg.* 1994;59(116):31401-31452.
24. Juncker JC. Commission Implementing Regulation (EU) 2015/407 of 11 March 2015 approving propan-2-ol as an active substance for use in biocidal products for product-types 1, 2 and 4. *Off J Eur Union.* 2015;58(L 67):15-17.
25. Juncker JC. Commission Implementing Regulation (EU) 2017/2001 of 8 November 2017 approving propan-1-ol as an existing active substance for use in biocidal products of product-type 1, 2 and 4. *Off J Eur Union.* 2017;60(L 290):1-3.
26. European Chemicals Agency. Ethanol. Biocidal active substances. European Chemicals Agency Web site. https://echa.europa.eu/information-on-chemicals/biocidal-active-substances?p_p_id=echarevbiocides_WAR_echarevbiocidesportlet&p_p_lifecycle=1&p_p_state=normal&p_p_mode=view&p_p_col_id=column-1&p_p_col_pos=1&p_p_col_count=2&_echarevbiocides_WAR_echarevbiocidesportlet_javax.portlet.action=searchBiocidesAction). Accessed August 30, 2017.
27. European Committee for Standardization. *EN 14885:2015. Chemical Disinfectants and Antiseptics. Application of European Standards for Chemical Disinfectants and Antiseptics.* Brussels, Belgium: European Committee for Standardization; 2015.
28. World Health Organization. *WHO Guidelines on Hand Hygiene in Health Care. First Global Patient Safety Challenge Clean Care Is Safer Care.* Geneva, Switzerland: World Health Organization; 2009.
29. World Health Organization. WHO model list of essential medicines. http://www.who.int/medicines/publications/essentialmedicines/EML2015_8-May-15.pdf. Accessed August 30, 2017.
30. Suchomel M, Kundi M, Pittet D, Weinlich M, Rotter ML. Testing of the World Health Organization recommended formulations in their application as hygienic hand rubs and proposals for increased efficacy. *Am J Infect Control.* 2012;40(4):328-331.
31. World Health Organization. *Global Guidelines for the Prevention of Surgical Site Infections.* Geneva, Switzerland: World Health Organization; 2016.
32. Kampf G, Hollingsworth A. Comprehensive bactericidal activity of an ethanol-based hand gel in 15 seconds. *Ann Clin Microbiol Antimicrob.* 2008;7:2.
33. Peeters E, Nelis HJ, Coenye T. Evaluation of the efficacy of disinfection procedures against *Burkholderia cenocepacia* biofilms. *J Hosp Infect.* 2008;70(4):361-368.
34. Gutiérrez-Martín CB, Yubero S, Martínez S, Frandoloso R, Rodríguez-Ferri EF. Evaluation of efficacy of several disinfectants

against *Campylobacter jejuni* strains by a suspension test. *Res Vet Sci.* 2011;91(3):e44-e47.

35. Woo PC, Leung KW, Wong SS, Chong KT, Cheung EY, Yuen KY. Relatively alcohol-resistant mycobacteria are emerging pathogens in patients receiving acupuncture treatment. *J Clin Microbiol.* 2002;40:1219-1224.

36. Bradley CR, Fraise AP. Heat and chemical resistance of enterococci. *J Hosp Infect.* 1996;34:191-196.

37. Kampf G, Meyer B, Goroncy-Bermes P. Comparison of two test methods for the determination of sufficient antimicrobial efficacy of three different alcohol-based hand rubs for hygienic hand disinfection. *J Hosp Infect.* 2003;55(3):220-225.

38. Kampf G, Rudolf M, Labadie J-C, Barrett SP. Spectrum of antimicrobial activity and user acceptability of the hand disinfectant agent Sterillium Gel. *J Hosp Infect.* 2002;52(2):141-147.

39. Rodriguez Ferri EF, Martinez S, Frandoloso R, Yubero S, Gutierrez Martin CB. Comparative efficacy of several disinfectants in suspension and carrier tests against *Haemophilus parasuis* serovars 1 and 5. *Res Vet Sci.* 2010;88:385-389.

40. Akamatsu T, Tabata K, Hironga M, Kawakami H, Uyeda M. Transmission of *Helicobacter pylori* infection via flexible fiberoptic endoscopy. *Am J Infect Control.* 1996;24(5):396-401.

41. van Klingeren B. Disinfectant testing on surfaces. *J Hosp Infect.* 1995;(suppl 30):397-408.

42. Moretro T, Vestby LK, Nesse LL, Storheim SE, Kotlarz K, Langsrud S. Evaluation of efficacy of disinfectants against *Salmonella* from the feed industry. *J Appl Microbiol.* 2009;106:1005-1012.

43. Kampf G, Höfer M, Wendt C. Efficacy of hand disinfectants against vancomycin-resistant enterococci in vitro. *J Hosp Infect.* 1999;42(2):143-150.

44. Kampf G, Jarosch R, Rüden H. Limited effectiveness of chlorhexidine based hand disinfectants against methicillin-resistant *Staphylococcus aureus* (MRSA). *J Hosp Infect.* 1998;38(4):297-303.

45. Adams D, Quayum M, Worthington T, Lambert P, Elliott T. Evaluation of a 2% chlorhexidine gluconate in 70% isopropyl alcohol skin disinfectant. *J Hosp Infect.* 2005;61(4):287-290.

46. Kampf G, Hollingsworth A. Validity of the four European test strains of prEN 12054 for the determination of comprehensive bactericidal activity of an alcohol-based hand rub. *J Hosp Infect.* 2003;55(3):226-231.

47. Wisplinghoff H, Schmitt R, Wohrmann A, Stefanik D, Seifert H. Resistance to disinfectants in epidemiologically defined clinical isolates of *Acinetobacter baumannii*. *J Hosp Infect.* 2007;66:174-181.

48. Kampf G, Jarosch R, Rüden H. Wirksamkeit alkoholischer Händedesinfektionsmittel gegenüber Methicillin-resistenten *Staphylococcus aureus* (MRSA). *Der Chirurg.* 1997;68(3):264-270.

49. Rotter M, Koller W, Kundi M. Eignung dreier Alkohole für eine Standard-Desinfektionsmethode in der Wertbestimmung von Verfahren für die hygienische Händedesinfektion. *Zentralbl Bakteriol Hyg Orig B.* 1977;164:428-438.

50. Théraud M, Bédouin Y, Guiguen C, Gangneux JP. Efficacy of antiseptics and disinfectants on clinical and environmental yeast isolates in planktonic and biofilm conditions. *J Med Microbiol.* 2004;53(pt 10):1013-1018.

51. Bundgaard-Nielsen K, Nielsen PV. Fungicidal effect of 15 disinfectants against 25 fungal contaminants commonly found in bread and cheese manufacturing. *J Food Prot.* 1996;59(3):268-275.

52. Salo S, Wirtanen G. Disinfectant efficacy on foodborne spoilage yeast strains. *Food Bioprod Process.* 2005;83(4):288-296.

53. Lacroix J, Lacroix R, Reynouard F, Combescot C. In vitro anti-yeast activity of 1- and 2-propanols. Effect of the addition of polyethylene glycol 400 [in French]. *C R Seances Soc Biol Fil.* 1979;173(3):547-552.

54. Reichel M, Heisig P, Kampf G. Pitfalls in efficacy testing—how important is the validation of neutralization of chlorhexidine digluconate? *Ann Clin Microbiol Antimicrob.* 2008;7:20.

55. Best M, Sattar SA, Springthorpe VS, Kennedy ME. Comparative mycobactericidal efficacy of chemical disinfectants in suspension and carrier tests. *Appl Environ Microbiol.* 1988;54:2856-2858.

56. van Klingeren B, Pullen W. Comparative testing of disinfectants against *Mycobacterium tuberculosis* and *Mycobacterium terrae* in a quantitative suspension test. *J Hosp Infect.* 1987;10(3):292-298.

57. Best M, Sattar SA, Springthorpe VS, Kennedy ME. Efficacies of selected disinfectants against *Mycobacterium tuberculosis*. *J Clin Microbiol.* 1990;28(10):2234-2239.

58. Mainous ME, Smith SA. Efficacy of common disinfectants against *Mycobacterium marinum*. *J Aquat Anim Health.* 2005;17(3):284-288.

59. Frobisher M Jr, Sommermeyer L. A study of the effect of alcohols on tubercle bacilli and other bacteria in sputum. *Am Rev Tuberc.* 1953;68:419-424.

60. Beekes M, Lemmer K, Thomzig A, Joncic M, Tintelnot K, Mielke M. Fast, broad-range disinfection of bacteria, fungi, viruses, and prions. *J Gen Virol.* 2010;91(pt 2):580-589.

61. Klein M, Deforest A. Antiviral action of germicides. *Soap Chem Spec.* 1963;39:70-72.

62. Rabenau HF, Kampf G, Cinatl J, Doerr HW. Efficacy of various disinfectants against SARS coronavirus. *J Hosp Infect.* 2005;61:107-111.

63. Siddharta A, Pfaender S, Vielle NJ, et al. Virucidal activity of world health organization-recommended formulations against enveloped viruses, including Zika, ebola, and emerging coronaviruses. *J Infect Dis.* 2017;215:902-906.

64. Groupe V, Engle CC, Gaffney PE. Virucidal activity of representative antiinfective agents against influenza A and vaccinia virus. *Appl Microbiol.* 1955;3:333-336.

65. Jeong EK, Bae JE, Kim IS. Inactivation of influenza A virus H1N1 by disinfection process. *Am J Infect Control.* 2010;38(5):354-360.

66. Kampf G, Steinmann J, Rabenau H. Suitability of vaccinia virus and bovine viral diarrhea virus (BVDV) for determining activities of three commonly-used alcohol-based hand rubs against enveloped viruses. *BMC Infect Dis.* 2007;7:5.

67. Kramer A, Galabov AS, Sattar SA, et al. Virucidal activity of a new hand disinfectant with reduced ethanol content: comparison with other alcohol-based formulations. *J Hosp Infect.* 2006;62(1):98-106.

68. Martin LS, Meooougal JS, Loskoski SL. Disinfection and inactivation of the human T lymphotropic virus type III/lymphadenopathy associated virus. *J Infect Dis.* 1985;152:400-403.

69. Spire B, Barre-Sinoussi F, Montagnier L. Inactivation of lymphadenopathy associated virus by chemical disinfectants. *Lancet.* 1984;2:899-901.

70. van Bueren J, Simpson RA, Jacobs P, Cookson BD. Survival of human immunodeficiency virus in suspension and dried onto surfaces. *J Clin Microbiol.* 1994;32:571-574.

71. van Engelenburg FA, Terpstra FG, Schuitemaker H, Moorer WR. The virucidal spectrum of a high concentration alcohol mixture. *J Hosp Infect.* 2002;51(2):121-125.

72. Bond WV, Favero MS, Petersen NJ, Ebert JW. Inactivation of hepatitis B virus by intermediate to high-level disinfectant chemicals. *J Clin Microbiol.* 1983;18:535-538.

73. Kobayashi H, Tsuzuki M, Koshimizu K, et al. Susceptibility of hepatitis B virus to disinfectants or heat. *J Clin Microbiol.* 1984;20:214-216.

74. Bingel KF, Hermann C. Die experimentelle Desinfektion des Vakzinevirus als Grundlage für die klinische Pockenimpfung. *Med Welt.* 1966;2:76-82.

75. Grossgebauer K. Zur Desinfektion der mit Pocken kontaminierten Hand. *Gesundheitswes Desinfekt.* 1967;59:1-12.

76. Rabenau HF, Rapp I, Steinmann J. Can vaccinia virus be replaced by MVA virus for testing virucidal activity of chemical disinfectants? *BMC Infect Dis.* 2010;10:185.

77. Sauerbrei A, Schacke M, Glück B, Bust U, Rabenau HF, Wutzler P. Does limited virucidal activity of biocides include duck hepatitis B virucidal action? *BMC Infect Dis.* 2012;12:276.

78. Steinmann J, Paulmann D, Becker B, Bischoff B, Steinmann E, Steinmann J. Comparison of virucidal activity of alcohol-based hand sanitizers versus antimicrobial hand soaps in vitro and in vivo. *J Hosp Infect.* 2012;82(4):277-280.

79. Bucca MA. The effect of various chemical agents on eastern equine encephalomyelitis virus. *J Bacteriol.* 1956;71:491-492.

80. Cunningham CH. The effect of certain chemical agents on the virus of Newcastle disease of chicken. *Am J Vet Res.* 1948;9:195-197.

81. Steinmann J, Becker B, Bischoff B, et al. Virucidal activity of 2 alcohol-based formulations proposed as hand rubs by the World Health Organization. *Am J Infect Control.* 2010;38(1):66-68.

82. Ciesek S, Friesland M, Steinmann J, et al. How stable is the hepatitis C virus (HCV)? Environmental stability of HCV and its susceptibility to chemical biocides. *J Infect Dis.* 2010;201(12):1859-1866.

83. Steinmann J, Becker B, Bischoff B, Magulski T, Steinmann J, Steinmann E. Virucidal activity of formulation I of the World Health Organization's alcohol-based handrubs: impact of changes in key ingredient levels and test parameters. *Antimicrob Resist Infect Control.* 2013;2:34.

84. Kampf G, Ostermeyer C, Werner H-P, Suchomel M. Efficacy of hand rubs with a low alcohol concentration listed as effective by a national hospital hygiene society in Europe. *Antimicrob Resist Infect Control.* 2013;2:19.

85. Okunishi J, Okamoto K, Nishihara Y, et al. Investigation of in vitro and in vivo efficacy of a novel alcohol based hand rub, MR06B7. *Yakugaku zasshi.* 2010;130:747-754.

86. Macinga DR, Sattar SA, Jaykus LA, Arbogast JW. Improved inactivation of nonenveloped enteric viruses and their surrogates by a novel alcohol-based hand sanitizer. *Appl Environ Microbiol.* 2008;74:5047-5052.

87. Wutzler P, Sauerbrei A. Virucidal efficacy of a combination of 0.2% peracetic acid and 80% (v/v) ethanol (PAA-ethanol) as a potential hand disinfectant. *J Hosp Infect.* 2000;46:304-308.

88. Iwasawa A, Niwano Y, Kohno M, Ayaki M. Virucidal activity of alcohol-based hand rub disinfectants. *Biocontrol Sci.* 2012;17(1):45-49.

89. Paulmann D, Steinmann J, Becker B, Bischoff B, Steinmann E, Steinmann J. Virucidal activity of different alcohols against murine norovirus, a surrogate of human norovirus. *J Hosp Infect.* 2011;79(4):378-379.

90. Tung G, Macinga D, Arbogast J, Jaykus LA. Efficacy of commonly used disinfectants for inactivation of human noroviruses and their surrogates. *J Food Prot.* 2013;76:1210-1217.

91. Park GW, Barclay L, Macinga D, Charbonneau D, Pettigrew CA, Vinje J. Comparative efficacy of seven hand sanitizers against murine norovirus, feline calicivirus, and GII.4 norovirus. *J Food Prot.* 2010;73:2232-2238.

92. Belliot G, Lavaux A, Souihel D, Agnello D, Pothier P. Use of murine norovirus as a surrogate to evaluate resistance of human norovirus to disinfectants. *Appl Environ Microbiol.* 2008;74(10):3315-3318.

93. Cannon JL, Papafragkou E, Park GW, Osborne J, Jaykus LA, Vinje J. Surrogates for the study of norovirus stability and inactivation in the environment: a comparison of murine norovirus and feline calicivirus. *J Food Prot.* 2006;69:2761-2765.

94. Gehrke C, Steinmann J, Goroncy-Bermes P. Inactivation of feline calicivirus, a surrogate of norovirus (formerly Norwalk-like viruses), by different types of alcohol in vitro and in vivo. *J Hosp Infect.* 2004;56(1):49-55.

95. Shimizu-Onda Y, Akasaka T, Yagyu F, et al. The virucidal effect against murine norovirus and feline calicivirus as surrogates for human norovirus by ethanol-based sanitizers. *J Infect Chemother.* 2013;19:779-781.

96. Akasaka T, Shimizu-Onda Y, Hayakawa S, Ushijima H. The virucidal effects against murine norovirus and feline calicivirus F4 as surrogates for human norovirus by the different additive concentrations of ethanol-based sanitizers. *J Infect Chemother.* 2016;22:191-193.

97. Drulak M, Wallbank AM, Lebtag I, Werboski L, Poffenroth L. The relative effectiveness of commonly used disinfectants in inactivation of coxsackievirus B5. *J Hyg.* 1978;81:389-397.

98. Moldenhauer D. Quantitative evaluation of the effects of disinfectants against viruses in suspension experiments. *Zentralbl Bakteriol Mikrobiol Hyg B.* 1984;179(6):544-554.

99. Drulak M, Wallbank AM, Lebtag I. The relative effectiveness of commonly used disinfectants in inactivation of echovirus 11. *J Hyg (Lond).* 1978;81(1):77-87.

100. Kurtz JB. Virucidal effect of alcohols against echovirus 11. *Lancet.* 1979;1:496-497.

101. Chang SC, Li WC, Huang KY, et al. Efficacy of alcohols and alcohol-based hand disinfectants against human enterovirus 71. *J Hosp Infect.* 2013;83(4):288-293.

102. Kampf G. Efficacy of ethanol against viruses in hand disinfection. *J Hosp Infect.* 2018;98(4):331-338.

103. Schürmann W, Eggers HJ. Antiviral activity of an alcoholic hand disinfectant. Comparison of the in vitro suspension test with the in vivo experiments on hands, and on individual fingertips. *Antiviral Res.* 1983;3:25-41.

104. Wolff MH, Schmitt J, Rahaus M, König A. Hepatitis A virus: a test method for virucidal activity. *J Hosp Infect.* 2001;48:S18-S22.

105. Harada YU, Lekcharoensuk P, Furuta T, Taniguchi T. Inactivation of foot-and-mouth disease virus by commercially available disinfectants and cleaners. *Biocontrol Sci.* 2015;20(3):205-208.

106. Schwebke I, Eggers M, Gebel J, et al. Prüfung und Deklaration der Wirksamkeit von Desinfektionsmitteln gegen Viren zur Anwendung im humanmedizinischen Bereich: Stellungnahme des Arbeitskreises Viruzidie beim Robert Koch-Institut. *Bundesgesundheitsblatt.* 2017;60:353-363.

107. van Bueren J, Larkin DP, Simpson RA. Inactivation of human immunodeficiency virus type 1 by alcohols. *J Hosp Infect.* 1994;28(2):137-148.

108. Platt J, Bucknall RA. The disinfection of respiratory syncytial virus by isopropanol and a chlorhexidine-detergent handwash. *J Hosp Infect.* 1985;6:89-94.

109. Croughan WS, Behbehani AM. Comparative study of inactivation of herpes simplex virus types 1 and 2 by commonly used antiseptic agents. *J Clin Microbiol.* 1988;26(2):213-215.

110. Tyler R, Ayliffe GA. A surface test for virucidal activity of disinfectants: preliminary study with herpes virus. *J Hosp Infect.* 1987;9(1):22-29.

111. Eggers H-J. Experiments on antiviral activity of hand disinfectants. Some theoretical and practical considerations. *Zentralbl Bakteriol.* 1990;273:36-51.

112. Tuladhar E, Hazeleger WC, Koopmans M, Zwietering MH, Duizer E, Beumer RR. Reducing viral contamination from finger pads: handwashing is more effective than alcohol-based hand disinfectants. *J Hosp Infect.* 2015;90:226-234.

113. Kurtz JB, Lee TW, Parsons AJ. The action of alcohols on rotavirus, astrovirus and enterovirus. *J Hosp Infect.* 1980;1(4):321-325.

114. Doerrbecker J, Friesland M, Ciesek S, et al. Inactivation and survival of hepatitis C virus on inanimate surfaces. *J Infect Dis.* 2011;204:1830-1838.

115. Sproessig M, Muecke H. Increase in the virus-activating effect of peracetic acid by n-propyl alcohol [in German]. *Acta Boil Med Ger.* 1965;14:199-200.

116. Nerandzic MM, Sunkesula VC, C TS, Setlow P, Donskey CJ. Unlocking the sporicidal potential of ethanol: induced sporicidal activity of ethanol against *Clostridium difficile* and *Bacillus* spores under altered physical and chemical conditions. *PLoS One.* 2015;10:e0132805.

117. Powell UM. The antiseptic properties of isopropyl alcohol in relation to cold sterilization. *J Indiana State Med Assoc.* 1945;38:303-304.

118. Chatterjee A, Bandini G, Motari E, Samuelson J. Ethanol and isopropanol in concentrations present in hand sanitizers sharply reduce excystation of *Giardia* and *Entamoeba* and eliminate oral infectivity of *Giardia* cysts in gerbils. *Antimicrob Agents Chemother.* 2015;59(11):6749-6754.

119. Martro E, Hernandez A, Ariza J, et al. Assessment of *Acinetobacter baumannii* susceptibility to antiseptics and disinfectants. *J Hosp Infect.* 2003;55:39-46.

120. Ankarloo J, Wikman S, Nicholls IA. *Escherichia coli* mar and acrAB mutants display no tolerance to simple alcohols. *Int J Mol Sci.* 2010;11:1403-1412.

121. Dao T, Dantigny P. Preparation of fungal conidia impacts their susceptibility to inactivation by ethanol vapours. *Int J Food Microbiol.* 2009;135(3):268-273.

122. Cincarova L, Polansky O, Babak V, Kulich P, Kralik P. Changes in the expression of biofilm-associated surface proteins in *Staphylococcus*

aureus food-environmental isolates subjected to sublethal concentrations of disinfectants. *Biomed Res Int.* 2016;2016:4034517.

123. Lou Y, Yousef AE. Adaptation to sublethal environmental stresses protects *Listeria monocytogenes* against lethal preservation factors. *Appl Environ Microbiol.* 1997;63(4):1252-1255.

124. Gravesen A, Lekkas C, Knochel S. Surface attachment of *Listeria monocytogenes* is induced by sublethal concentrations of alcohol at low temperatures. *Appl Environ Microbiol.* 2005;71:5601-5603.

125. Park SH, Oh KH, Kim CK. Adaptive and cross-protective responses of *Pseudomonas* sp. DJ-12 to several aromatics and other stress shocks. *Curr Microbiol.* 2001;43(3):176-181.

126. Heipieper HJ, de Bont JA. Adaptation of *Pseudomonas putida* S12 to ethanol and toluene at the level of fatty acid composition of membranes. *Appl Environ Microbiol.* 1994;60(12):4440-4444.

127. Seier-Petersen MA, Jasni A, Aarestrup FM, et al. Effect of subinhibitory concentrations of four commonly used biocides on the conjugative transfer of Tn916 in *Bacillus subtilis. J Antimicrob Chemother.* 2014;69:343-348.

128. Wang M, Zhao J, Yang Z, Du Z, Yang Z. Electrochemical insights into the ethanol tolerance of *Saccharomyces cerevisiae. Bioelectrochemistry.* 2007;71(2):107-112.

129. Semchyshyn HM. Hormetic concentrations of hydrogen peroxide but not ethanol induce cross-adaptation to different stresses in budding yeast. *Int J Microbiol.* 2014;2014:485792.

130. Costa V, Reis E, Quintanilha A, Moradas-Ferreira P. Acquisition of ethanol tolerance in *Saccharomyces cerevisiae*: the key role of the mitochondrial superoxide dismutase. *Arch Biochem Biophys.* 1993;300:608-614.

131. Bandara A, Fraser S, Chambers PJ, Stanley GA. Trehalose promotes the survival of *Saccharomyces cerevisiae* during lethal ethanol stress, but does not influence growth under sublethal ethanol stress. *FEMS Yeast Res.* 2009;9(8):1208-1216.

132. Schiavone M, Formosa-Dague C, Elszetin C, et al. Evidence for a role for the plasma membrane in the nanomechanical properties of the cell wall as revealed by an atomic force microscopy study of the response of *Saccharomyces cerevisiae* to ethanol stress. *Appl Environ Microbiol.* 2016;82:4789-4801.

133. Knobloch JK, Horstkotte MA, Rohde H, Kaulfers PM, Mack D. Alcoholic ingredients in skin disinfectants increase biofilm expression of *Staphylococcus epidermidis. J Antimicrob Chemother.* 2002;49(4):683-687.

134. Chauhan NM, Shinde RB, Karuppayil SM. Effect of alcohols on filamentation, growth, viability and biofilm development in *Candida albicans. Brazilian J Microbiology.* 2013;44:1315-1320.

135. Horinouchi T, Sakai A, Kotani H, Tanabe K, Furusawa C. Improvement of isopropanol tolerance of *Escherichia coli* using adaptive laboratory evolution and omics technologies. *J Biotechnol.* 2017;255:47-56.

136. Fletcher M. The effects of methanol, ethanol, propanol and butanol on bacterial attachment to surfaces. *J Gen Microbiol.* 1983;129(3):633-641.

137. Aarnisalo K, Lundén J, Korkeala H, Wirtanen G. Susceptibility of *Listeria monocytogenes* strains to disinfectants and chlorinated alkaline cleaners at cold temperatures. *LWT Food Sci Technol.* 2007;40(6):1041-1048.

138. Bandelin FJ. Antibacterial and preservative properties of alcohols. *Cosmetic & Toiletries.* 1977;92:59-70.

139. Kabara JJ, Orth DS, eds. *Preservative-Free and Self-Preserving Cosmetics and Drugs: Principles and Practices.* New York, NY: Marcel Dekker; 1997.

140. International Organization for Standardization. *ISO 29621:2017. Cosmetics—Microbiology: Guidelines for the Risk Assessment and Identification of Microbiologically Low-Risk Products.* Vernier, Switzerland: International Organization for Standardization; 2017.

141. Steinberg DC. *Preservatives for Cosmetics.* 2nd ed. Carol Stream, IL: Allured; 2006.

142. Bloss R, Meyer S, Kampf G. Adsorption of active ingredients of surface disinfectants to different types of fabric used for surface treatment. *J Hosp Infect.* 2010;75:56-61.

143. Kovacs BJ, Chen YK, Kettering JD, Aprecio RM, Roy I. High-level disinfection of gastrointestinal endoscopes: are current guidelines adequate? *Am J Gastroenterol.* 1999;94(6):1546-1550.

144. Leiss O, Beilenhoff U, Bader L, Jung M, Exner M. Reprocessing of flexible endoscopes and endoscopic accessories—an international comparison of guidelines. *Z Gastroenterol.* 2002;40(7):531-542.

145. Kalenić S, Vukadinović MV, Janes-Poje V, Kotarski Z, Tripković V. Guidelines for cleaning and disinfection/sterilization of endoscopes. *Lic Vjesn.* 1999;121(7-8):221-226.

146. Kovaleva J. Endoscope drying and its pitfalls. *J Hosp Infect.* 2017;97(4):319-328.

147. Muscarella LF. Inconsistencies in endoscope-reprocessing and infection-control guidelines: the importance of endoscope drying. *Am J Gastroenterol.* 2006;101(9):2147-2154.

148. Rutala WA, Weber DJ. Reprocessing endoscopes: United States perspective. *J Hosp Infect.* 2004;56(suppl 2):S27-S39.

149. Salvage R, Hull CM, Kelly DE, Kelly SL. Use of 70% alcohol for the routine removal of microbial hard surface bioburden in life science cleanrooms. *Future Microbiol.* 2014;9(10):1123-1130.

150. Eaton T. Cleanroom airborne particulate limits and 70% isopropyl alcohol: a lingering problem for pharmaceutical manufacturing? *PDA J Pharm Sci Technol.* 2009;63(6):559-567.

151. Rubio S, McIver D, Behm N, Fisher M, Fleming W. Evaluation of the MicroWorks, Inc. Swab Sampling System (MSSSTM) for use in performing quantitative swab sampling. *PDA J Pharm Sci Technol.* 2010;64(2):167-181.

152. Kramer A, Rudolph P, Kampf G, Pittet D. Limited efficacy of alcohol-based hand gels. *Lancet.* 2002;359:1489-1490.

153. Rotter ML. Hygienic hand disinfection. *Infect Control.* 1984;5:18-22.

154. Edmonds SL, Macinga DR, Mays-Suko P, et al. Comparative efficacy of commercially available alcohol-based hand rubs and World Health Organization-recommended hand rubs: formulation matters. *Am J Infect Control.* 2012;40(6):521-525.

155. do Prado MF, Coelho AC, de Brito JP, et al. Antimicrobial efficacy of alcohol-based hand gels with a 30-s application. *Lett Appl Microbiol.* 2012;54:564-567.

156. Macinga DR, Shumaker DJ, Werner HP, et al. The relative influences of product volume, delivery format and alcohol concentration on dry-time and efficacy of alcohol-based hand rubs. *BMC Infect Dis.* 2014;14:511.

157. Kampf G, Shaffer M, Hunte C. Insufficient neutralization in testing a chlorhexidine-containing ethanol-based hand rub can result in a false positive efficacy assessment. *BMC Infect Dis.* 2005;5:48.

158. Kampf G. Ethanol. In: G Kampf, ed. *Kompendium Händehygiene.* Wiesbaden, Germany: mhp-Verlag; 2017:325-351.

159. Guilhermetti M, Marques Wiirzler LA, Castanheira Facio B, et al. Antimicrobial efficacy of alcohol-based hand gels. *J Hosp Infect.* 2010;74:219-224.

160. Kampf G, Marschall S, Eggerstedt S, Ostermeyer C. Efficacy of ethanol-based hand foams using clinically relevant amounts: a cross-over controlled study among healthy volunteers. *BMC Infect Dis.* 2010;10:78.

161. Goroncy-Bermes P, Koburger T, Meyer B. Impact of the amount of hand rub applied in hygienic hand disinfection on the reduction of microbial counts on hands. *J Hosp Infect.* 2010;74:212-218.

162. Macinga DR, Beausoleil CM, Campbell E, et al. Quest for a realistic in vivo test method for antimicrobial hand-rub agents: introduction of a low-volume hand contamination procedure. *Appl Environ Microbiol.* 2011;77(24):8588-8594.

163. Kampf G, Ruselack S, Eggerstedt S, Nowak N, Bashir M. Less and less-influence of volume on hand coverage and bactericidal efficacy in hand disinfection. *BMC Infect Dis.* 2013;13:472.

164. Edmonds-Wilson S, Campbell E, Fox K, Macinga D. Comparison of 3 in vivo methods for assessment of alcohol-based hand rubs. *Am J Infect Control.* 2015;43(5):506-509.

165. Davies JG, Babb JR, Bradley CR, Ayliffe GAJ. Preliminary study of test methods to assess the virucidal activity of skin disinfectants using poliovirus and bacteriophages. *J Hosp Infect.* 1993;25:125-131.

166. Steinmann J, Nehrkorn R, Meyer A, Becker K. Two in-vivo protocols for testing virucidal efficacy of handwashing and hand disinfection. *Zentralbl Hyg Umweltmed.* 1995;196:425-436.

167. Sattar S, Ali M, Tetro JA. In vivo comparison of two human norovirus surrogates for testing ethanol-based handrubs: the mouse chasing the cat! *PLoS One.* 2011;6(5):e17340.

168. Bellamy K, Alcock R, Babb JR, Davies JG, Ayliffe GA. A test for the assessment of 'hygienic' hand disinfection using rotavirus. *J Hosp Infect.* 1993;24:201-210.

169. Lages SL, Ramakrishnan MA, Goyal SM. In-vivo efficacy of hand sanitisers against feline calicivirus: a surrogate for norovirus. *J Hosp Infect.* 2008;68(2):159-163.

170. Kampf G, Grotheer D, Steinmann J. Efficacy of three ethanol-based hand rubs against feline calicivirus, a surrogate for norovirus. *J Hosp Infect.* 2005;60(2):144-149.

171. Wewalka G, Rotter M, Koller W, Stanek G. Wirkungsvergleich von 14 Verfahren zur hygienischen Händedesinfektion. *Zentralbl Bakteriol Orig B.* 1977;165:242-249.

172. European Committee for Standardization. *EN 1500:2013. Chemical Disinfectants and Antiseptics. Hygienic Hand Disinfection. Test Method and Requirement (Phase 2, Step 2).* Brussels, Belgium: European Committee for Standardization; 2013.

173. Kampf G, Ostermeyer C. Intra-laboratory reproducibility of the hand hygiene reference procedures of EN 1499 (hygienic hand wash) and EN 1500 (hygienic hand disinfection). *J Hosp Infect.* 2002;52(3):219-224.

174. Kampf G, Ostermeyer C. Inter-laboratory reproducibility of the hand disinfection reference procedure. *J Hosp Infect.* 2003;53(4):304-306.

175. Herruzo R, Vizcaino MJ, Herruzo I. In vitro-in vivo sequence studies as a method of selecting the most efficacious alcohol-based solution for hygienic hand disinfection. *Clin Microbiol Infect.* 2010;16:518-523.

176. Dharan S, Hugonnet S, Sax H, Pittet D. Comparison of waterless hand antisepsis agents at short application times: raising the flag of concern. *Infect Control Hosp Epidemiol.* 2003;24(3):160-164.

177. Kampf G, ed. Iso-propanol. In: *Kompendium Händehygiene.* Wiesbaden, Germany: mhp-Verlag; 2017:362-375.

178. Rotter ML, Koller W, Wewalka G, Werner HP, Ayliffe GAJ, Babb JR. Evaluation of procedures for hygienic hand disinfection: controlled parallel experiments on the Vienna test model. *J Hyg (Lond).* 1986;96:27-37.

179. Kampf G. *n*-Propanol. In: Kampf G, ed. *Kompendium Händehygiene.* Wiesbaden, Germany: mhp-Verlag; 2017:352-361.

180. Kampf G, Lemmen S. Disinfection of gloved hands for multiple activities with indicated glove use on the same patient. *J Hosp Infect.* 2017;97(1):3-10.

181. Ng PC, Wong HL, Lyon D, et al. Combined use of alcohol hand rub and gloves reduces the incidence of late onset infection in very low birthweight infants. *Arch Dis Child Fetal Neonatal Ed.* 2004;89:F336-F340.

182. Kampf G, Ostermeyer C. Efficacy of two distinct ethanol-based hand rubs for surgical hand disinfection—a controlled trial according to prEN 12791. *BMC Infect Dis.* 2005;5:17.

183. Suchomel M, Kundi M, Allegranzi B, Pittet D, Rotter ML. Testing of the World Health Organization-recommended formulations for surgical hand preparation and proposals for increased efficacy. *J Hosp Infect.* 2011;79(2):115-118.

184. Kampf G, Ostermeyer C. World Health Organization-recommended hand-rub formulations do not meet European efficacy requirements for surgical hand disinfection in five minutes. *J Hosp Infect.* 2011;78(2):123-127.

185. Suchomel M, Gnant G, Weinlich M, Rotter M. Surgical hand disinfection using alcohol: the effects of alcohol type, mode and duration of application. *J Hosp Infect.* 2009;71(3):228-233.

186. Suchomel M, Kundi M, Pittet D, Rotter ML. Modified World Health Organization hand rub formulations comply with European efficacy requirements for preoperative surgical hand preparations. *Infect Control Hosp Epidemiol.* 2013;34:245-250.

187. Kampf G, Kapella M. Suitability of Sterillium Gel for surgical hand disinfection. *J Hosp Infect.* 2003;54:222-225.

188. Mulberry G, Snyder AT, Heilman J, Pyrek J, Stahl J. Evaluation of a waterless, scrubless chlorhexidine gluconate/ethanol surgical scrub for antimicrobial efficacy. *Am J Infect Control.* 2001;29(12):377-382.

189. Macinga DR, Edmonds SL, Campbell E, McCormack RR. Comparative efficacy of alcohol-based surgical scrubs: the importance of formulation. *AORN J.* 2014;100(6):641-650.

190. Olson LK, Morse DJ, Duley C, Savell BK. Prospective, randomized in vivo comparison of a dual-active waterless antiseptic versus two alcohol-only waterless antiseptics for surgical hand antisepsis. *Am J Infect Control.* 2012;40(1):155-159.

191. Kampf G, Ostermeyer C, Heeg P, Paulson D. Evaluation of two methods of determining the efficacies of two alcohol-based hand rubs for surgical hand antisepsis. *Appl Environ Microbiol.* 2006;72(6):3856-3861.

192. Rotter M, Koller W, Wewalka G. Povidone-iodine and chlorhexidine gluconate-containing detergents for disinfection of hands. *J Hosp Infect.* 1980;1:149-158.

193. Suchomel M, Koller W, Kundi M, Rotter ML. Surgical hand rub: influence of duration of application on the immediate and 3-hours effects of *n*-propanol and isopropanol. *Am J Infect Control.* 2009;37:289-293.

194. Rotter ML, Simpson RA, Koller W. Surgical hand disinfection with alcohols at various concentrations: parallel experiments using the new proposed European standards methods. *Infect Control Hosp Epidemiol.* 1998;19(10):778-781.

195. Babb JR, Davies JG, Ayliffe GA. A test procedure for evaluating surgical hand disinfection. *J Hosp Infect.* 1991;18(suppl B):41-49.

196. Lowbury EJL, Lilly HA, Ayliffe GAJ. Preoperative disinfections of surgeons' hands: use of alcoholic solutions and effects of gloves on skin flora. *Br Med J.* 1974;4:369-372.

197. Rotter ML, Kampf G, Suchomel M, Kundi M. Population kinetics of the skin flora on gloved hands following surgical hand disinfection with 3 propanol-based hand rubs: a prospective, randomized, double-blind trial. *Infect Control Hosp Epidemiol.* 2007;28(3):346-350.

198. Suchomel M, Rotter M, Weinlich M, Kundi M. Glycerol significantly decreases the three hour efficacy of alcohol-based surgical hand rubs. *J Hosp Infect.* 2013;83:284-287.

199. Suchomel M, Weinlich M, Kundi M. Influence of glycerol and an alternative humectant on the immediate and 3-hours bactericidal efficacies of two isopropanol-based antiseptics in laboratory experiments in vivo according to EN 12791. *Antimicrob Resist Infect Control.* 2017;6:72.

200. Rotter ML, Kampf G, Suchomel M, Kundi M. Long-term effect of a 1.5 minute surgical hand rub with a propanol-based product on the resident hand flora. *J Hosp Infect.* 2007;66:84-85.

201. Kampf G, Ostermeyer C, Heeg P. Surgical hand disinfection with a propanol-based hand rub: equivalence of shorter application times. *J Hosp Infect.* 2005;59(4):304-310.

202. Kampf G, Ostermeyer C. A 1-minute hand wash does not impair the efficacy of a propanol-based hand rub in two consecutive surgical hand disinfection procedures. *Eur J Clin Microbiol Infect Dis.* 2009;28(11):1357-1362.

203. Kampf G, Ostermeyer C, Kohlmann T. Bacterial population kinetics on hands during 2 consecutive surgical hand disinfection procedures. *Am J Infect Control.* 2008;36(5):369-374.

204. European Committee for Standardization. *EN 12791:2015. Chemical Disinfectants and Antiseptics. Surgical Hand Disinfection. Test method and requirement (Phase 2, Step 2).* Brussels, Belgium: European Committee for Standardization; 2015.

205. Suchomel M, Rotter M. Ethanol in pre-surgical hand rubs: concentration and duration of application for achieving European Norm EN 12791. *J Hosp Infect.* 2011;77(3):263-266.

206. Kampf G, Ostermeyer C. Influence of applied volume on efficacy of 3-minute surgical reference disinfection method prEN 12791. *Appl Environ Microbiol.* 2004;70(12):7066-7069.

207. Hingst V, Juditzki I, Heeg P, Sonntag H-G. Evaluation of the efficacy of surgical hand disinfection following a reduced application time of 3 instead of 5 min. *J Hosp Infect.* 1992;20:79-86.

208. Hübner N-O, Kampf G, Kamp P, Kohlmann T, Kramer A. Does a preceding hand wash and drying time after surgical hand disinfection influence the efficacy of a propanol-based hand rub? *BMC Microbiol.* 2006;6:57.

209. Kampf G. Lack of antimicrobial efficacy of mecetronium etilsulfate in propanol-based hand rubs for surgical hand disinfection. *J Hosp Infect.* 2017;96(2):189-191.

210. Barbut F, Djamdjian L, Neyme D, Passot C, Petit JC. Efficacy of 2 alcohol-based gels and 1 alcohol-based rinse for surgical hand disinfection. *Infect Control Hosp Epidemiol.* 2007;28(8):1013-1015.

211. Marchetti MG, Kampf G, Finzi G, Salvatorelli G. Evaluation of the bactericidal effect of five products for surgical hand disinfection according to prEN 12054 and prEN 12791. *J Hosp Infect.* 2003;54(1):63-67.

212. Rotter ML, Koller W. Surgical hand disinfection: effect of sequential use of two chlorhexidine preparations. *J Hosp Infect.* 1990;16:161-166.

213. Kampf G, Ostermeyer C. Influence of applied volume on efficacy of 3-minute surgical reference disinfection method prEN 12791. *Appl Environ Microbiol.* 2004;70:7066-7069.

214. Reichel M, Heisig P, Kohlmann T, Kampf G. Alcohols for skin antisepsis at clinically relevant skin sites. *Antimicrob Agents Chemother.* 2009;53(11):4778-4782.

215. Lutz JT, Diener IV, Freiberg K, et al. Efficacy of two antiseptic regimens on skin colonization of insertion sites for two different catheter types: a randomized, clinical trial. *Infection.* 2016;44:707-712.

216. Dettenkofer M, Wilson C, Gratwohl A, et al. Skin disinfection with octenidine dihydrochloride for central venous catheter site care: a double-blind, randomized, controlled trial. *Clin Microbiol Infect.* 2010;16:600-606.

217. KRINKO am Robert Koch Institut. Prävention von Infektionen, die von Gefäßkathetern ausgehen. *Bundesgesundheitsblatt.* 2017;60:171-215.

218. Berríos-Torres SI, Umscheid CA, Bratzler DW, et al. Centers for Disease Control and Prevention guideline for the prevention of surgical site infection, 2017. *JAMA Surg.* 2017;152(8):784-791.

219. Commission for Hospital Hygiene and Infection Prevention at the Robert Koch Institute. Prävention postoperativer Wundinfektionen. *Bundesgesundheitsblatt.* 2018;61(4):448-473.

220. Pittet D, Hugonnet S, Harbarth S, et al. Effectiveness of a hospital-wide programme to improve compliance with hand hygiene. *Lancet.* 2000;356:1307-1312.

221. Sax H, Allegranzi B, Uçkay I, Larson E, Boyce J, Pittet D. 'My five moments for hand hygiene': a user-centred design approach to understand, train, monitor and report hand hygiene. *J Hosp Infect.* 2007;67(1):9-21.

222. Kampf G, Dettenkofer M. Desinfektionsmaßnahmen im häuslichen Umfeld—was macht wirklich Sinn? *Hyg Med.* 2011;36(1-2):8-11.

223. Guinan M, McGuckin M, Ali Y. The effect of a comprehensive hand-washing program on absenteeism in elementary schools. *Am J Infect Control.* 2002;30:217-220.

224. White C, Kolble R, Carlson R, Lipson N. The impact of a health campaign on hand hygiene and upper respiratory illness among college students living in residence halls. *J Am Coll Health.* 2005;53:175-181.

225. Arbogast JW, Moore-Schiltz L, Jarvis WR, Harpster-Hagen A, Hughes J, Parker A. Impact of a comprehensive workplace hand hygiene program on employer health care insurance claims and costs, absenteeism, and employee perceptions and practices. *J Occup Environ Med.* 2016;58(6):e231-e240.

226. Darouiche RO, Wall MJ Jr, Itani KM, et al. Chlorhexidine-alcohol versus povidone-iodine for surgical-site antisepsis. *N Engl J Med.* 2010;362(1):18-26.

227. Tuuli MG, Liu J, Stout MJ, et al. A randomized trial comparing skin antiseptic agents at cesarean delivery. *N Engl J Med.* 2016;374:647-655.

228. Maiwald M, Chan ES. The forgotten role of alcohol: a systematic review and meta-analysis of the clinical efficacy and perceived role of chlorhexidine in skin antisepsis. *PLoS One.* 2012;7:e44277.

229. Maiwald M, Widmer AF. WHO's recommendation for surgical skin antisepsis is premature. *Lancet Infect Dis.* 2017;17:1023-1024.

230. Allegranzi B, Egger M, Pittet D, Bischoff P, Nthumba P, Solomkin J. WHO's recommendation for surgical skin antisepsis is premature—authors' reply. *Lancet Infect Dis.* 2017;17:1024-1025.

231. Ngai IM, Van Arsdale A, Govindappagari S, et al. Skin preparation for prevention of surgical site infection after cesarean delivery: a randomized controlled trial. *Obstet Gynecol.* 2015;126:1251-1257.

232. Mimoz O, Lucet JC, Kerforne T, et al. Skin antisepsis with chlorhexidine-alcohol versus povidone iodine-alcohol, with and without skin scrubbing, for prevention of intravascular-catheter-related infection (CLEAN): an open-label, multicentre, randomised, controlled, two-by-two factorial trial. *Lancet.* 2015;386:2069-2077.

Phenolic Compounds

Sarah de Szalay and John A. Diemer

The first application of phenolic compounds as antimicrobial agents goes back as early as 1815 when coal tar was used as an antiseptic and disinfectant.[1] But it was not until Kuchenmeister in 1860 and Lister in 1867 used phenol (carbolic acid) as a dressing for wounds and in surgery, respectively, that the full potential of this type of agent began to be realized. Although phenol itself is no longer used as an antimicrobial agent, many of its derivatives are extremely important as the active component in numerous antiseptics, in institutional and commercial disinfectants, and in the preservation of various formulations and manufactured materials.[2]

Since the first use of phenol, hundreds of different phenol derivatives have been synthesized, isolated, and screened, with the aim of finding new compounds that are more effective, less toxic, and less irritating than the parent carbolic acid. Since the time of Kronig and Paul,[3] who first established test conditions and criteria for the evaluation of germicidal activity, numerous studies have been conducted that have provided a wealth of knowledge on the relationship between structure and germicidal activity of different phenolic derivative series. By understanding this relationship, an appreciation can be gained of why a certain derivative is used for a particular application.

Even though an understanding of the chemistry of phenolic agents is important, knowledge of how these compounds interact at the cellular and biochemical levels, and the physical chemistry of the interactions with various other formulation components, are also fundamental. This information provides insight into factors that control the rate and spectrum of microbicidal activity of a particular derivative. It is the summation of chemical, physical, and biologic data that allows the development of products or formulations that exhibit the desired efficacy and toxicologic properties necessary for commercial use. The structure and functional relationships of different

phenolic compounds were compiled by Suter[4] and offer an early comprehensive review, whereas Goddard and McCue[5] provided a more recent review. This chapter aims to provide a review of all these areas in order that the reader can gain an appreciation of why phenolics remain an important class of antimicrobial compounds.

▶ COAL-TAR DISINFECTANTS

Most phenolic antimicrobial agents are produced by efficient industrial-scale target-specific syntheses that supply extremely pure active substances.[6] For some applications in the United States, United Kingdom, and other countries, disinfectants based on coal, specifically coal-tar derivatives, are still used. Fractionation of coal tar obtained from the destructive distillation of coal leads to the production of a complex mixture of more than 50 phenolic substances,[7] which then can be broadly separated according to their boiling point with increased temperature. The initial substance to separate is phenol itself (boiling point 182°C), followed by the cresols (189°C-205°C), the xylenols (210°C-230°C), and the higher boiling point tar acids (230°C-310°C). The higher boiling point tar acids comprise a mixture of various higher alkyl homologs of phenol, such as the propylphenols, tetramethylphenols, diethylphenols, and the naphthols, to mention but a few.[7]

Whereas phenols and cresols are slightly soluble in water, the higher homologs obtained from coal-tar extraction display a decreasing solubility with the increasing weight of their substituting radicals. Solubility also depends on the structure of the substituent group, that is, whether it is a normal or a branched-chain alkyl radical or a cycloalkyl, aralkyl, aryl radical, and so on. Although solubility decreases, these higher homologs exhibit superior bactericidal activity and lower skin toxicity. The efficacy ratio against gram-negative to gram-positive bacteria remains fairly constant. The exception are the gram-negative pseudomonads, where activity decreases with decreasing water solubility. Finally, inactivation by organic soil also increases accordingly.

Two basic themes have been followed to overcome the poor solubility of these more active higher phenolic homologs and to allow their application in commercial disinfectant products. These are solubilization using a soap of natural origin and emulsification. Physically, products based on these two formulation methods can be distinguished following their dilution in distilled water. At low concentrations, the solubilized-type disinfectants produce practically clear solutions, whereas those based on emulsification give milky, turbid suspensions.

Historically, solubilized coal-tar disinfectants can be further divided into two groups: the *clear soluble phenolics* and the *black fluids*. The *clear soluble phenolics* comprise preparations containing low-molecular-weight cresols and xylenols as the active ingredients. Although these fluids are obsolete and no longer officially used in certain pharmacopeia, the "cresol and soap solution British Pharmacopoeia (BP)"[8] is an example of a mixture of cresols in soap prepared from linseed oil and potassium hydroxide. This mixture forms a clear solution and, upon dilution, has a wide spectrum of activity against vegetative bacteria, fungi, and some viruses. Unfortunately, this type of product retains some of its corrosive properties as a result of the phenolic fraction employed.[9]

The *black fluids*[10] are among the oldest type of phenolic disinfectant and are made from refined tar distillate dissolved in a carrier oil, such as castor oil, emulsified with a soap or surfactant. These products either give clear solutions or emulsions on dilution with water, but they retain their activity in the presence of large quantities of organic soil. They have a wide spectrum of activity, including bacteria and fungi. Unfortunately, they are corrosive to many materials, such as rubber and plastics, and should be handled with care.[9]

Products classified in the *emulsified* disinfectants contain, in addition to the phenolic constituents, varying proportions of coal-tar hydrocarbons and, in some instances, other constituents, such as neutral oils. They differ from the solubilized form in that the phenol fraction, rather than being dissolved in a soap base, is emulsified into a permanent concentrated suspension with the aid of gelatin, casein, or the carbohydrate extractable from Irish moss seaweed.[7,11] In the United Kingdom, this type of emulsified group are called the *white fluids*.[10] The neutral oils consist mostly of methyl and dimethyl naphthalenes, other hydrocarbons (acenaphthene), organic bases (quinoline, pyridine) and their alkyl derivatives, certain oxygenated compounds, and organic sulfur compounds. Neutral oil itself is practically free from phenol or phenol derivatives and hence has no inherent antimicrobial activity.[7] It is often used, however, because it acts as an adjuvant and gives the formulation greater stability.[11]

The emulsifiable-type disinfectant has a wide spectrum of activity and is again effective under heavy soiling conditions. This type of disinfectant, however, is still a potential skin irritant and is corrosive and hence should be handled with care.[9] Additionally, because emulsions are metastable systems, they are less stable in long-term storage conditions compared to the aforementioned black fluids. In more recent 2008 *British Pharmacopoeia*,[12] they have updated an emulsified formula for antiseptic use, with a mixture of chloroxylenol, a soap base (prepared from castor oil and potassium hydroxide), ethanol, and terpineol.

Historically, the bactericidal potency of coal-tar and related disinfectants has been assessed by using the *Salmonella ser typhi* phenol coefficient. The phenol coefficient compares the activity of different dilutions of the phenolic disinfectant after contact times of 5 and 10 minutes, with that obtained from a standard dilution series of phenol. The phenol coefficient is calculated by dividing the highest dilution of the phenolic disinfectant that shows growth on subculture at 5 minutes but not at 10 minutes by the standard dilution of phenol that shows the same response.

Hence, this method served as a cross-referencing cipher for many of the early papers written on phenolic compounds. However, phenol coefficients are no longer used for the most part because the conditions and organism types were chosen arbitrarily. Plus, the data generated from this test are not effective in evaluating disinfectants that are bacteriostatic, one is having a residual activity, or take into account microorganisms with an increased phenol resistance. The US Environmental Protection Agency (EPA) has ruled in 2001 the elimination of phenol testing (Pesticide Registration Notice 2001-4)[13] as part of its registration requirements; however, this test should be viewed historically because early work on phenolic compounds followed this procedure.

In the case of the lower homologs, such as the cresol and xylenol isomers, the phenol coefficient against *S typhi* gives a reasonable indication of the general germicidal potency against other microorganisms. This is borne out by the results obtained with three commercial *soluble* disinfectants of different germicidal strengths (cresol compound N.F. and cresylic disinfectants A and B).[14] With the higher phenol homologs used in *emulsifiable* disinfectants, the picture is entirely different. There appears to be no relationship between the *S typhi* phenol coefficients and those obtained with the other bacteria. Klarmann and Shternov[14] showed that for three disinfectants of the *soluble* group, the ratio of *S typhi* to *Staphylococcus aureus* phenol coefficients were between 1 and 2. For six commercial disinfectants, which used *emulsifiable* tar oils, the ratio varied between 8 to 1 and 20 to 1. Brewer and Ruehle[15] also concluded that the *S typhi* phenol coefficient was unable to describe adequately the germicidal potency of all coal-tar disinfectants. These authors showed that although certain products had comparatively high *S typhi* phenol coefficients, when tested against *Streptococcus pyogenes*, they were about 10 to 30 times less effective.

These findings indicate that the *S typhi* phenol coefficient alone should not be used to describe the activity of certain coal-tar disinfectants, as previously stated. In the case of the emulsifiable disinfectants, no quantitative relationship exists between the effect on *S typhi* and that on other microorganisms. Indeed, some disinfectants of this type, with high *S typhi* phenol coefficients, actually may be less effective against other pathogenic microorganisms than disinfectants with lower *S typhi* coefficients.

▶ SYNTHETIC PHENOL DERIVATIVES

Phenol itself and its derivatives are produced in large quantities through efficient synthetic processes. The structures of phenol and some of its important derivatives are shown in Figure 20.1. Extensive study over many years showed that introducing different substituents into the phenyl nucleus can influence the antimicrobial activity.

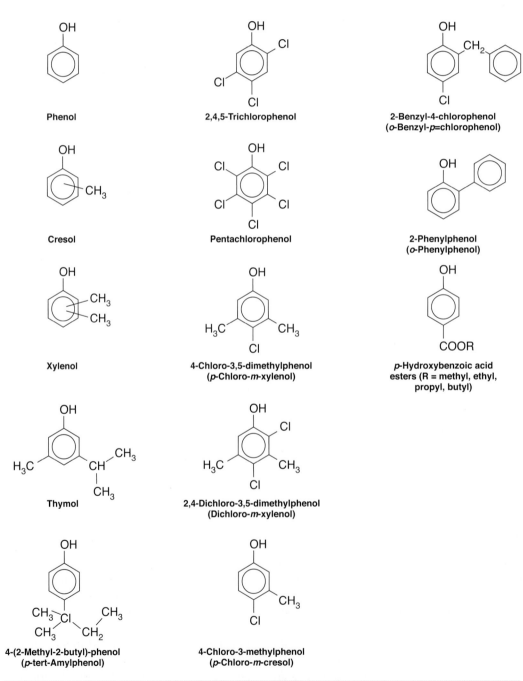

FIGURE 20.1   Structures of important phenolic compounds.

TABLE 20.1	Microbicidal action of phenol derivatives (phenol coefficients, 37°C)			
Name	*Salmonella typhi*	*Staphylococcus aureus*	*Mycobacterium tuberculosis*	*Candida albicans*
Phenol	1.0	1.0	1.0	1.0
2-Methyl-	2.3	2.3	2.0	2.0
3-Methyl-	2.3	2.3	2.0	2.0
4-Methyl-	2.3	2.3	2.0	2.0
4-Ethyl-	6.3	6.3	6.7	7.8
2,4-Dimethyl-	5.0	4.4	4.0	5.0
2,5-Dimethyl-	5.0	4.4	4.0	4.0
3,4-Dimethyl-	5.0	3.8	4.0	4.0
2,6-Dimethyl-	3.8	4.4	4.0	3.5
4-*n*-Propyl-	18.3	16.3	17.8	17.8
4-*n*-Butyl-	46.7	43.7	44.4	44.4
4-*n*-Amyl-	53.3	125.0	133.0	156.0
4-tert-Amyl-	30.0	93.8	111.1	100.0
4-*n*-Hexyl-	33.3	313.0	389.0	333.0
4-*n*-Heptyl-	16.7[a]	625.0	667.0	556.0

[a]Approximate.

Alkylated Phenol Derivatives

Table 20.1 gives the phenol coefficients of a series of simple alkylated phenol homologs against a range of organisms.[16] The germicidal potency increases as the number of methylene groups in the substituted alkyl group increases. After the *n*-amyl (C_5) derivative, a further increase in size of the alkyl chain produces an increase in activity against *S aureus*, *Mycobacterium tuberculosis*, and *Candida albicans*, but the effectiveness against *S typhi* declines. The three isomeric cresols (methylphenols) and the four isomers of xylenol (dimethylphenols) show increases in activity of up to 5 times that of phenol, but within each isomer series, there is no apparent difference in activity. These data again serve to indicate at the time that the phenol coefficient against *S typhi* cannot be used as a meaningful indicator of general antimicrobial activity. These results are in agreement with those of other workers.[17,18]

Suter[4] concluded that substitution in the 4-position of the phenolic ring of an alkyl chain of up to six carbons in length increases the antibacterial action of phenolics, presumably by increasing the surface activity and ability to orient at an interface. Activity falls off after this because of decreased water solubility. Because of the polarity enhancement of polar properties, straight-chain 4-position substitution confers greater activity than branched-chain substitution containing the same number of carbon atoms. Studies with the dermatophyte *Trichophyton*

mentagrophytes suggested that the optimum alkyl chain length may vary with the organism concerned. Etoh et al[19] showed that the lowest minimum inhibitory concentration (MIC) of a range of 4-*n*-alkyl substituted phenols was obtained with the nonyl (C_9) phenol. Introduction of bulky substituent groups in the 2-position of a phenol already substituted with an alkyl group in the 4-position dramatically reduced the antimicrobial activity against this fungus.

One simple alkylated phenol still in commercial use is 4-tert-amylphenol (*p*-tert-amylphenol; 4-[2-methyl-2-butyl]-phenol). This derivative is commonly used as an active ingredient in various disinfectant formulations, where it is combined with other phenols to give activity against pseudomonads. Paulus[6] reported the microbicidal concentration of this compound alone as 400 mg/L for *Salmonella choleraesuis* and 500 mg/L for *S aureus*.

Halogenated-Alkyl Phenol Derivatives

Halogenation of phenolic compounds, preferably by chlorination, leads to a potentiation of antibacterial effectiveness. The combination of alkylation and halogenation has produced a number of highly effective microbiocides. A systematic examination of the relationships between the chemical structure and the microbiocidal action of aliphatic and aromatic substitution derivatives of 2- and 4-chlorophenol was carried out

TABLE 20.2   Microbicidal action of 2-position alkyl derivatives of 4-chlorophenol (phenol coefficients, 37°C)

Name	Salmonella ser typhi	Salmonella schotmuelleri	Staphylococcus aureus	Streptococcus pyogenes	Mycobacterium tuberculosis	Trichophyton schoenleinii	Candida albicans
4-Chlorophenol	4.3	4.3	4.3	4.4	3.9	3.3	4.0
Methyl-	12.5	12.9	12.5	11.1	11.1	7.1	11.1
Ethyl-	28.6	28.6	34.4	31.1	27.8	25.0	32.5
n-Propyl-	93.3	714.0	93.8	77.8	66.7	714.0	100.0
n-Butyl-	141.0	114.0	257.0	250.0	178.0	156.0	178.0
n-Amyl-	156.0	100.0	500.0	556.0	389.0	278.0	389.0
sec-Amyl-	46.7	42.9	312.0	312.0	222.0	229.0	182.0
n-Hexyl-	23.2[a]	21.4[a]	1250.0	1333.0	333.0	357.0	556.0
Cyclohexyl-	<26.7	<14.3	438.0	361.0	278.0	222.0	300.0
n-Heptyl-	20.0	14.3[a]	1500.0	2222.0	>400.0	175.0	>363.0
n-Octyl-	NA	NA	1750.0	>312.0	NA	NA	NA

Abbreviation: NA, not available.

[a]Approximate.

by Klarmann et al.[16] Table 20.2 illustrates the situation found in the case of 2-position alkyl derivatives of 4-chlorophenol; Table 20.3 shows the effect of 4-position alkyl derivatives of 2-chlorophenol. The general trends are summarized as follows:

1. Halogen substitution intensifies the microbicidal potency of phenol derivatives; the presence of halogen in the 4-position to the hydroxyl group is more effective in this respect than in the 2-position.
2. Introduction of aliphatic or aromatic groups into the nucleus of halogen phenols increases the bactericidal potency even further (up to certain limits). The increase depends in the case of alkyl substitution on the number of carbon atoms present in the substituting group or groups.
3. As a rule, the intensifying effect on the bactericidal potency of a normal aliphatic chain with a given number of carbon atoms is greater than that of a branched-chain or of two alkyl groups with the same total of carbon atoms.
4. The 2-alkyl derivatives of 4-chlorophenol are more actively germicidal than 4-alkyl derivatives of 2-chlorophenol.

In addition to the homologous series of alkyl derivatives of 2- and 4-chlorophenol, a series of polyalkyl of 4-chlorophenol also was studied (Table 20.4). As with the

TABLE 20.3   Microbicidal action of 4-position alkyl derivatives of 2-chlorophenol (phenol coefficients, 37°C)

Name	Salmonella ser typhi	Salmonella schotmuelleri	Staphylococcus aureus	Streptococcus pyogenes	Mycobacterium tuberculosis	Candida albicans
2-Chlorophenol	2.5	2.1	2.9	2.0	2.2	2.2
Methyl-	6.3	5.4	7.5	5.6	5.6	8.3
Ethyl-	17.2	25.0	15.7	15.0	17.8	22.2
n-Propyl-	40.0	35.7	32.1	33.3	33.3	44.4
n-Butyl-	86.7	66.7	93.8	88.9	77.8	88.9
n-Amyl-	80.0	40.0	286.0	222.0	222.0	278.0
tert-Amyl-	32.1	21.4	125.0	122.0	111.0	100.0
n-Hexyl	23.3	NA	500.0	555.0	178.0	278.0
n-Heptyl-	16.7	NA	375.0	350.0	77.8	70.0

Abbreviation: NA, not available.

TABLE 20.4	Microbicidal action of polyalkyl derivatives of 4-chlorophenol (phenol coefficients, 37°C)			
Name	Salmonella ser typhi	Staphylococcus aureus	Mycobacterium tuberculosis	Candida albicans
4-Chlorophenol	4.3	4.3	4.4	3.9
3-Methyl-	10.7	11.3	11.3	11.1
3,5-Dimethyl-	30.0	25.7	27.5	28.1
6-Ethyl-3-methyl-	64.3	50.0	55.6	55.6
6-n-Propyl-3-methyl-	183.0	200.0	178.0	156.0
6-iso-Propyl-3-methyl-	107.0	150.0	138.0	138.0
2-Ethyl-3,5-dimethyl-	46.4	106.0	94.4	122.0
6-sec-Butyl-3-methyl-	50.0	500.0	361.0	389.0
2-iso-Propyl-3,5-dimethyl-	81.3	313.0	313.0	325.0
6-Diethylmethyl-3-methyl-	23.3	625.0	611.0	777.0
6-iso-Propyl-2-ethyl-3-methyl-	56.7	200.0	175.0	200.0
2-sec-Butyl-3,5-dimethyl-	28.6	563.0	556.0	556.0
2-sec-Amyl-3,5-dimethyl-	15.6[a]	750.0	889.0	700.0
2-Diethylmethyl-3,5-dimethyl-	<13.0	1143.0	1000.0	667.0
6-sec-Octyl-3-methyl-	21.4[a]	>89.0	122.0	>70.0

[a]Approximate.

monoalkyl series described previously (see Table 20.2), the number of methylene groups in the alkyl substitution group determines the degree of selective action against different microorganisms. With monoalkyl substitution, a compound with five carbon atoms (n-amyl) in the side groups gives maximum activity against S typhi. For the polyalkyl derivatives, maximum activity is reached when the compounds have a total of four substituting carbon atoms (6-n-propyl-3-methyl- and 6-isopropyl-3-methyl). Against the other test microorganisms, the greatest antimicrobial activity in these polyalkyl derivatives is seen when a total of seven carbon atoms are in the side groups (2-diethylmethyl-3,5-dimethyl).

Comparing the activity of the 4-chlorophenol derivatives with a total of four carbon atoms in the substituting groups against S typhi, it can be seen that substitution by one alkyl group (see Table 20.2; n-butyl) leads to a more effective compound than substitution by two groups (see Table 20.4; 6-n-propyl-3-methyl). This in turn is better than substitution by three groups (see Table 20.4; 2-ethyl-3,5-dimethyl) even though it contains the same total number of carbon atoms.

The halogenated alkyl phenolics commonly used today are 4-chloro-3,5-dimethylphenol (p-chloro-m-xylenol [PCMX]), 2,4-dichloro-3,5-dimethylphenol (dichloro-m-xylenol [DCMX]), 4-chloro-3-methylphenol (p-chloro-m-cresol [PCMC]), and 6-isopropyl-3-methyl-4-chlorophenol (chlorothymol) (see Figure 20.1).

Because of its strong microbicidal properties and low toxicity, PCMX is used today as a broad-spectrum antimicrobial in disinfectants, antiseptics, and soaps.[20] It also has been used as a fungicide for adhesives, paints, textiles, paper products, and polishes. It is reasonably soluble in water (0.33 g/L at 20°C), but it is more soluble in alkaline solution and organic solvents. The PCMX is not sporicidal and alone has some activity against mycobacteria. To improve its solubility and achieve its full antimicrobial potential, correct formulation of PCMX is essential. The impact of formulation on the activity and stability of antiseptics and disinfectants is considered in further detail later in this chapter and in chapter 6. But an example of a typical formulation containing a chloroxylenol solution containing soap, terpineol, and ethanol is still included in the 2008 British Pharmacopoeia[12] for application as an antiseptic.

The DCMX has similar properties and spectrum of activity as PCMX[6] and has been used in pine-type disinfectants and medicated soaps.[21] However, because of its lower aqueous solubility (0.2 g/L at 20°C) and its more distinctive phenolic odor, its use tends to be limited.

The aqueous solubility of PCMC is greater (3.85 g/L at 20°C) than that of other chlorophenols. Although it appears slightly less active against a range of microorganisms than PCMX,[6] it has gained considerable importance as an industrial preservative in protecting various functional fluids, such as thickeners, adhesives, and pigments as well as textiles and leather. This is principally because it remains active over a wide pH range (4-8), where, compared with other phenolic derivatives, only PCMC remains sufficiently soluble.

Chlorothymol makes a satisfactory antiseptic when applied in the form of a solution in alcohol and glycerin.[22] Monochloro and dichloro derivatives of carvacrol (5-isopropyl-2-methylphenol) were particularly effective against *S aureus*,[23] comparing favorably with the corresponding thymol derivatives. More recently, Paulus[6] reported that 4-chlorothymol is effective against fungi, less active against bacteria, and insufficient in its activity against *Pseudomonas*.

Among the aromatic halogenated substituted phenols, 2-benzyl-4-chlorophenol (*o*-benzyl-*p*-chlorophenol [OBPCP]; chlorophene) (see Figure 20.1) is still used today in combination with other phenolics in various institutional and domestic disinfectant formulations. It is almost insoluble in water (149 mg/L at 25°C), but this is improved in alkaline solution, in organic solvents, or with the aid of saturated vegetable oil soap, such as coconut oil or various anionic detergents. In a suitable formulation, chlorophene shows good broad-spectrum activity.[6] The formulation of disinfectants with benzylphenols and their halogen substitution products is the subject of a study by Carswell and Doubly.[24] A liquid soap properly formulated with chlorophene compared favorably with one containing the same proportion of hexachlorophene its effectiveness.[25] However, there are currently significant safety concerns for chlorophene and dichlorophen,[26] which eventually may place it under new regulatory classifications.

Phenylphenols

Phenylphenols, also referred to as *aryl phenols*, are compounds composed of a phenolic group connected directly to another aromatic ring. Two examples of these phenols are 2-phenylphenol (*o*-phenylphenol [OPP]) and 4-phenylphenol (*p*-phenylphenol [PPP]). Both compounds have similar broad-spectrum activity; however, PPP is not commercially used because of its poor solubility properties and cost.[6] OPP, on the other hand, is well known, is widely used, and has become one of the most important phenolic biocides for application in disinfectants and in industrial preservation.

The solubility of OPP (see Figure 20.1) in water is low (0.2 g/L at 20°C), but it has good solubility in various solvents. The MIC ranges from 50 to 500 mg/L for various bacteria, yeasts, and molds,[6,27] making it reasonably broad spectrum. Its activity against *Pseudomonas aeruginosa* is, however, less distinctive (MIC approximately 1500 mg/L).[6] The greatest use for OPP in its phenol form is in the formulation of general surface disinfectants. It is commonly used as the active ingredient in hospital-type disinfectants because of its strong activity against *M tuberculosis*. It may be formulated alone or in combination with other alkyl or halogenated phenolic derivatives. pH and the ratio/concentration of soap or detergents to OPP and the phenolic concentration are all critical factors in the germicidal potency of phenolic disinfectants. The sodium phenate form of OPP generally is used in preservation applications because of its high water solubility.[28] As a preservative, OPP is used to prevent the microbial degradation of industrial fluids, cosmetics, adhesives, paints, and textiles.

Bisphenols

Bisphenols are compounds that are composed of two phenolic groups connected either directly or by various linkages. Large numbers of this type of compound have been synthesized and have been described by Gump.[29] The compounds that exhibit the best activity are those that are separated by –CH$_2$– or –S– or –O– linkages. If a –CO–, –SO–, or –CH(OH)– group separates the phenyl groups, activity is low. Maximum activity is found with the hydroxyl groups at the 2,2-position of the bisphenol. Increased efficacy is also observed as the degree of halogenation of the phenol molecules increases; this is particularly the case against the gram-positive bacteria. When different members of a bisphenol series were tested in soaps against *S aureus*, the superiority of the highly chlorinated members was evident.[30] Gump[29] suggested that halogenation in the 4-position of each ring was the optimum position for activity against fungi. Increased halogenation, however, gave a decrease in activity against fungi, but this was considered to be due to a decrease in solubility. Unfortunately, increased halogenation is also accompanied by increased toxicity.[6] As a result of this, and other side effects, the practical use of many bisphenols has been abandoned.

All bisphenols have limited water solubility, but they are more soluble in organic solvents and dilute alkali solutions. Although certain of the bisphenols demonstrate high bacteriostatic or fungistatic properties, their bactericidal and fungicidal activity is low. Like many other phenolic agents, activity against *Pseudomonas* species is also low but may be improved by formulation effects (see chapter 6).

Beginning in 1937, halogenated bisphenols were studied intensively in the laboratories of the Givaudan Corporation. From a long series of compounds that were examined, two had important commercial applications. The first of these was 2,2′-dihydroxy-5,5′-dichlorodiphenyl-methane (alternatively 2,2′-methylene-bis[4-chlorophenol]; dichlorophen) (Figure 20.2). This was first prepared by Weiler et al[31] and later by the improved method of Gump and Luthy.[32] Although it exhibited reasonable activity against bacteria, its activity against fungi and yeast was relatively high.[6] Because of this and its low skin irritancy, it found application as a preservative for toiletries and as a treatment

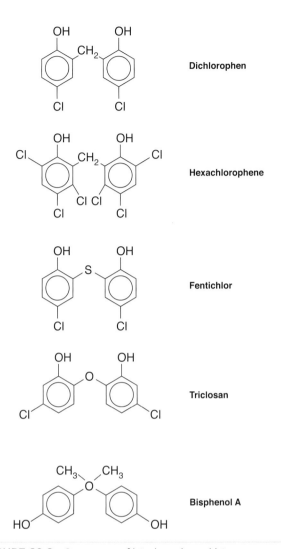

FIGURE 20.2 Structures of bisphenols and bis-(hydroxyphenyl) alkanes.

for athlete's foot.[7] Other applications include use as a fungicide and mildew-proofing agent for textiles, paper, cardboard, and adhesives; as a slimicide in paper manufacture; as preservative for lubricants and coolants; and to prevent microbial growth in water-cooling towers and humidifying plants. It also has been used in veterinary applications for its antiparasitic (anthelmintic and anti-protozoan, as a dewormer) activity, presumably due to its laxative activity.[33]

The other compound of commercial importance that was synthesized and described by Gump[29] was bis-(3,5,6-trichloro-2-hydroxyphenyl)-methane (alternatively, 2,2'-methylene-bis[3,4,6-trichlorophenol]; or hexachlorophene) (see Figure 20.2). Although it was essentially insoluble in water, the outstanding usefulness of this substance at that time was that it could be formulated into antiseptic soaps and detergents without a loss of activity. Like other bisphenols, it was also substantive to the skin, providing continuing bacteriostatic activity, especially against gram-positive bacteria.

Although hexachlorophene also has been used as a microbicide in cosmetics and textiles, its application in this area and as the active ingredient in consumer antimicrobial soap and detergent products has now been limited worldwide because of its potential for absorption through the skin and subsequent toxicity and neurotoxicity, particularly in neonates.[34] Another review by Evangelista de Duffard and Duffard[35] of chlorinated hydrocarbons, including hexachlorophene, showed it to cause motor dysfunction and developmental neurotoxicity.

A number of hydroxy-halogenated derivatives of diphenyl sulfide have been used as biocidal agents in a number of applications. One, 2,2'-dihydroxy-5,5'-dichlorodiphenyl-sulfide (alternatively, bis-[2-hydroxy-5-chlorophenyl]-sulfide; fentichlor) (see Figure 20.2), has good bacteriostatic activity against gram-positive bacteria and surprisingly good activity against fungi, yeast, and algae. As a result, it has been used as a preservative in lubricants and coolants to overcome the problem of fungal growth.[6] Hugo and Russell[7] reported that the chief application of fentichlor was originally in the treatment of dermatophytic conditions; however, this molecule is also a photosensitizer, and hence, its use in this application and as a preservative in cosmetics is now limited. The halogenated analogue of fentichlor, 2,2'-thiobis(2,4-dichlorophenol), which also found application in soaps and cosmetics,[36] also caused photosensitization and has been discontinued.

Although strictly a phenoxyphenol, 2,4,4'-trichloro-2'-hydroxydiphenyl ether, triclosan, is included in this section because of its structural similarity to the bisphenols (see Figure 20.2). Triclosan is sparingly soluble in water (10 mg/L at 20°C), but it is readily soluble in a range of solvents and dilute alkali.[37] In terms of its antimicrobial activity, triclosan is principally bacteriostatic with some fungistatic activity. Unlike the classic bisphenols, this inhibitory activity is reasonably broad, being equally effective against gram-positive and most gram-negative bacteria, good activity against *Candida* species and mycobacteria, and poor activity against filamentous fungi. Its activity is not affected by organic matter but can be inhibited by formulated surfactant micelles structures. However, its activity against *Serratia marcescens*, *Alcaligenes* species (MIC for both >100 mg/L), and *P aeruginosa* (MIC >1000 mg/L) is low.[38] A primary target for triclosan in bacteria is by inhibiting fatty acid synthesis via its binding to the enoyl-acyl carrier protein reductase (ENR) enzyme,[39] which is encoded by the gene *fabI*. This increases the enzyme's affinity for nicotinamide adenine dinucleotide (NAD^+) resulting in the formation of a stable complex of ENR-NAD^+-triclosan, making it unable to participate in fatty acid synthesis. These fatty acids are necessary for building and reproducing cell membranes in bacteria, and triclosan can specifically inhibit this biosynthesis.[40,41] Triclosan also has a persistent skin activity similar to chlorhexidine (see chapter 22), which can be affected pH, surfactants, and ionic nature of the formulation.

Triclosan has been incorporated into a large number of hospital and consumer products. This extensive use led to a number of questions related to the generation of triclosan-tolerant bacteria and its potential linkage to antibiotic resistance.[42] This was clearly a cause for concern. Currently, there is a plethora of evidence to indicate that products containing triclosan could lead to the generation of antibiotic-resistant bacteria, particularly under laboratory conditions. Bailey et al[43] observed differences in triclosan-dependent transcriptomes of *Escherichia coli* and *Salmonella ser typhimurium* with increased expression of efflux pump component genes. McBain et al[44] observed that sublethal concentrations of triclosan can decrease bacterial diversity and a limited decrease in susceptibility to portions of the population in environmental microcosms. For a review of bacterial resistance to triclosan and its implications with respect to antibiotics, the reader should refer to reviews by Carey and McNamara[45] and McDonnell.[46] The US Food and Drug Administration (FDA)[47] issued a ruling in 2016 relating to triclosan usage in over-the-counter consumer antiseptic wash products and recommended products containing triclosan should no longer be marketed. This ruling was based on a number of factors: first, lack of direct evidence that antibacterial washes were more effective at preventing the spread of germs than normal washing with soap and water; second, long-term exposure to triclosan could pose health risks, such as bacterial resistance; and/or hormonal effects were not satisfied or sufficient for the agency to find it safe.[47] However, it should be noted that triclosan's use in consumer hand sanitizers, wipes, or health care settings was left intact by the FDA ruling.

An analogue of triclosan, triclocarban (or 3-[4-chlorophenyl]-1-[3,4-dichlorophenyl]urea), is another compound that shares some features with bisphenols, such as its skin substantiveness. Although a trichlorocarbanilide, triclocarban is similar enough to bisphenols to be considered here. Triclocarban has found application in antimicrobial soaps, particularly bar soaps, lotions, deodorants, toothpaste, and plastics. Research has suggested triclocarban exerts its effect by inhibiting the activity of enoyl-acyl carrier protein (enoyl-ACP) reductase, widely distributed in bacteria, fungi, and plants. The ACP reductase catalyzes the last step in each cycle of fatty acid elongation in the type II fatty acid synthase systems. This is very similar to the inhibition effects of triclosan described earlier. As a result, this agent interrupts cell membrane synthesis and leads to bacterial growth inhibition.[48] As with triclosan, triclocarban is fairly broad spectrum with activity against gram-positive bacteria being greater than against gram-negative bacteria, good activity against *Candida* species, and poor activity against filamentous fungi. Its activity is not generally affected by the presence of organic matter.

The FDA[47] also issued a ruling in 2016 relating to triclocarban usage in consumer antiseptic wash products and recommended products containing triclocarban could no longer be marketed, similar to that described earlier with triclosan. Again, this ruling was based on two main factors: lack of direct evidence of the benefit over normal washing with soap and water and health risks. In fact, due to its use predominantly in bar soaps, a high percentage of the compound was found in wastewater biosolids,[49] which could provide a prime breeding ground for cross-resistance and promotion of antibiotic resistance via genetic exchange. Some recent evidence points to an altered antibiotic tolerance in biosolids containing triclocarban.[50]

Polyhydric (Resorcinol) Derivatives

Polyhydric phenols are identified as containing more than one hydroxyl group on the aromatic ring. The three dihydric phenols—catechol, resorcinol, and hydroquinone—and the two trihydric phenols—phloroglucinol and pyrogallol—are all reported as having comparatively low antibacterial activities.[11] Various derivatives of these phenols have been shown to have higher antibacterial potency.

Determination of the antibacterial properties of various resorcinol derivatives began with the studies of Johnson and coworkers.[51,52] Together, with additional data,[53-56] studies have indicated that optimum activity against *S typhi* activity occurs with the *n*-hexyl–substituted compound, whereas for *S aureus*, it continues to increase up to at least the 2-nonyl compound. Nevertheless, 4-*n*-hexyl resorcinol became an important antiseptic for topical use, particularly in medicated throat lozenges.

Hydroxycarboxylic Acids and Esters

Historically, various aromatic hydroxycarboxylic acids have found application as preservatives in the food, cosmetic, and pharmaceutical industries. Although they can be classified as "acid" preservatives, because of the appended hydroxyl group, they are considered here under the heading of phenolics.

Salicylic acid (ortho-hydroxybenzoic acid) is a weak acid with a dissociation constant of 1.07×10^{-3}. This compound was the subject of several early investigations, but its efficacy appeared to vary depending on the organism concerned. Cains et al[57] found that salicylic acid was less effective than phenol against *Yersinia pestis*, whereas Woodward et al[58] found it to have a phenol coefficient of 18.3. Since then, because of its low pK_a, salicylic acid has found application as a preservative in acidic products. Its optimum pH for antimicrobial activity lies between 4 and 6. Although it is directed primarily against yeast and mold,[59] its antibacterial activity is superior to that of benzoic acid. It is only in its undissociated state that it exhibits antimicrobial activity, but this significantly changes as the pH varies. At pH 2, 90% is undissociated; at pH 4, this value is 8.6%; and at pH 6, only 0.09% is in the active form.[27] The use of salicylic acid as a food preservative has now been abandoned principally because of its toxicity. It still finds application in topical skin care products, often in combination with benzoic acid, for the treatment of fungal infections or acne. This is in addition to its additional keratinolytic properties.[7] The European Union is assessing the toxicology of salicylic acid.[60]

The alkyl esters of *p*-hydroxybenzoic acid, or parabens as they are more commonly known, hold a position of considerable importance as antimicrobial agents, notably in the field of preservation. The parabens are relatively stable chemicals, being rapidly hydrolyzed only under extreme conditions, for example, at pH 10 or pH 1.[59] They are active over a wide pH range (pH 4-8) and have pK_a values between 8 and 8.5. From the antimicrobial results shown in Table 20.5, it is clear that the activity of the individual esters increases from methyl to butyl,[61] whereas their already low water solubility decreases further over the same series. This decrease in water solubility is mirrored by an increase in the lipid solubility.

Most of the data contributing to the understanding of the parabens activity have come from the early work of Sabalitschka and colleagues.[62-67] As early as 1939, the parabens were regarded as among the most useful preservatives available,[68] and this view is held today (see chapter 40).[59]

The parabens are generally more active against gram-positive bacteria, fungi, and yeast than against gram-negative bacteria, particularly *P aeruginosa*. Fukahori et al[69] investigated the relationship between paraben ester alkyl chain length and antimicrobial activity against *E coli*. Uptake into the bacterial cell and reduction in the minimum bactericidal concentration (MBC) were proportional to the number of carbon atoms in the alkyl chain. Interestingly, the actual level of paraben necessary to achieve the desired antibacterial effect decreased logarithmically because the alkyl chain length increased.

The parabens display a low order of acute and subacute toxicity.[70] Sokol[61] concluded that the parabens approximate the requirements of an "ideal" pharmaceutical preservative as formulated by Gershenfeld and Perlstein.[68] This was based on irritation, absorption, and excretion studies carried out in both animals and humans. These conclusions agree with those reached later by Matthews et al.[71] In addition, Paulus[59] indicated that they are broad spectrum, effective at low concentrations (0.05%-0.2%), stable, odorless, colorless, and effective over a wide range of temperature and pH.

Parabens have a long history in preservation from personal care products to food products. Over the last 10 years or so, the general media has created a myth about the safety and health risk parabens may pose, counter to the published research and global regulatory acceptability. Some of this myth came from a misunderstanding by the media

TABLE 20.5 Inhibition of bacteria and fungi by esters of *p*-hydroxybenzoic acid (percentages)

Name	Methyl	Ethyl	Propyl	Butyl
Salmonella ser typhi	0.2	0.1	0.1	0.1
Escherichia coli	0.4	0.1	0.1	0.4
Staphylococcus aureus	0.4	0.1	0.05	0.0125
Proteus vulgaris	0.2	0.1	0.05	0.05
Pseudomonas aeruginosa	0.4	0.4	0.8	0.8
Aspergillus niger	0.1	0.04	0.02	0.02
Rhizopus nigricans	0.05	0.025	0.0125	0.00625
Chaetomium globosum	0.05	0.025	0.00625	<0.003125
Trichophyton interdigitale	>0.008	0.008	0.004	0.002
Candida albicans	0.1	0.1	0.0125	0.0125
Saccharomyces cerevisiae	0.1	0.05	0.0125	0.00625
Molecular weight	152.2	166.2	180.2	194.2
Water solubility				
(g/100 g at 15°C)	0.16	0.08	0.023	0.005
(g/100 g at 25°C)	0.25	0.11	0.04	0.015
pK_a	8.5	NA	8.1	NA
Log P (octanol:water)	1.96	2.47	3.04	3.57

Abbreviation: NA, not available.

of a 2004 research study,[72] which mistakenly linked parabens to breast cancer. Parabens are normally broken down quite quickly in human body, metabolized, and harmlessly excreted, which seem to refute the aforementioned claim. A number of global organizations have stated acceptance of the use of parabens in personal care products. However, due to this toxicity profile, they were considered less favorable and their use in many applications was reduced. Currently, the FDA has limitations on the level of use of some parabens; however, these limits are based on the lack of human dermal and associated toxicity data required by this agency. Industry has argued that extensive animal studies should suffice and correlate to the human model, but this argument has been unsuccessful to fate.[73-77]

Other Phenolic Derivatives

Several other types of phenol derivatives have been evaluated for their antimicrobial properties. These include the nitrophenols, aminophenols, and naphthol and its derivatives. Although nitration increases the activity of the phenol against bacteria, it also increases systemic toxicity to higher species because of the specific biologic properties conferred on these molecules, allowing them to act as uncoupling agents and consequently interfere with oxidative phosphorylation. Of the other phenolic derivatives described earlier, most show limited antimicrobial activity; as a consequence, they have found little commercial application.

Natural Phenolic Derivatives

Natural phenolic ingredients from plants, which traditionally have been used in ancient times, are now being studied for incorporation into everyday products (see chapter 14). The use of natural plant products as medicines has grown significantly in the last decade, and its use in developing countries has also increased due to the low income of the general population.[78,79] Overall, this increase has been driven by traditional medicine uses, public awareness of chemical disinfection in the home environment (with recent studies indicating issues with the known chemicals used in home disinfection products), uses as additives in food products, and the growing resistance of bacteria to established antibiotics. Many natural plant products contain phenolic compounds as their principal constituent or as secondary constituents and possess antimicrobial properties.[80] Those compounds most commonly found are thymol, eugenol, quercetin, rutin, carvacrol, gallic acid, curcumin, phenol ethers, methyl eugenol ether, anethole, safrole, isosafrole, other polyphenols (flavonoids), and various terpene-type compounds. Because of their natural appeal and their common use as medicinal ingredients, natural plant products today are being reexamined for their preservative and antimicrobial value.[80-84]

Some of these natural products, such as thymol and pine oil, have already been brought to market in household disinfectants.

ANTIMICROBIAL ACTION OF PHENOLIC DERIVATIVES

It is the free hydroxyl group that constitutes the primary reactive entity of the phenol molecule. Introduction of the different substituents into the nucleus of phenol (and of polyphenols) modifies this reactivity in different respects. Thus, alkyl substitutions affect such things as the distribution ratio between the aqueous and the non-aqueous (including bacterial) phases, the capacity for reducing surface tension, and, in some instances, species selectivity, all of which determine the antibacterial action of a given phenol derivative. Halogen substitution probably has a similar effect; additionally, it affects the electrolytic dissociation of the phenol derivative, intensifying the acid character of the compound with the increase in the number of substituting halogen atoms.[85] It is the balance between the hydrophobic and polar groups that give the different phenol derivatives their membrane active properties and also contributes to their varying degrees of activity.

Factors Affecting Germicidal Action

In addition to differences attributable to chemical structure, germicidal action of phenolic antimicrobial agents is influenced by a number of other factors. Russell[86] provided a comprehensive review of these factors in relation to an entire range of antimicrobial agents. Following is a summary of those that relate specifically to the action of phenol and its derivatives.

All phenols act either bacteriostatically and/or bactericidally, depending on their concentration.[11] Most phenolic antimicrobial agents have relatively high concentration exponents (dilution coefficient) of between 4 and 6, whereas the parabens have a concentration exponent of 2 to 4.[86] This means that for a typical phenolic, dilution by one-half increases the length of time taken to kill a standard number of bacteria by between 2^4 and 2^6 times. From a practical point of view, the high concentration exponents for phenolics mean that they rapidly lose their bactericidal activity on dilution; however, they remain bacteriostatic even at extremely low concentrations.[11]

The number of bacteria to be killed and the environmental conditions will also determine the extent of bactericidal efficacy. Karabit[87] examined the effect of cell concentration on the rate of death of *S aureus* exposed to 0.5% phenol. The time required to produce a 1 $\log_{10}$ reduction in viable numbers, the D-value, was independent of cell concentration up to 10^6 organisms per milliliter

(2.25 h). Above this cell concentration, the D-values were significantly longer, such that at 10^8 organisms per milliliter, it was nearly 3 times as long (6.4 h). Presumably, this was due to the increased organic load and inaccessibility of the biocide resulting from the higher microbial concentration.

Bacteria on surfaces are known to be more resistant to the treatment of antimicrobial agents than those in suspension[88]; however, it has been reported that PCMX is more effective against *P aeruginosa* on surfaces than it is in suspension.[89] Das et al[90] showed that PCMX is equally effective against *Staphylococcus epidermidis* and *E coli* attached to surfaces as it was against those in suspension.

Phenolic antimicrobials act optimally under acidic and neutral conditions, that is, in their undissociated (unionized) state. Table 20.6 shows the pK_a values (pH at 50% undissociation) for a series of common phenolic derivatives. Clearly, the alkylated phenol derivatives have higher pK_a values than the simple halogenated phenols, and hence, the former group is more active under alkali conditions. Alkyl phenols have the ability to form alkali salts. These phenates dissolve readily in water but have lower antimicrobial activity. The benefit of phenates is that they are able to act as solubilizing agents for the free phenol.

Other environmental factors such as temperature and the presence of organic soil also affect germicidal efficacy. Phenols are always more effective as the temperature is increased. Russell[86] indicated that the Q_{10}, the change in activity for each 10-degree rise in temperature, for phenols and cresols is between 3 and 5. The presence of organic matter such as blood, serum, feces, and pus can reduce bactericidal activity. Although this reduction can be up to 90%,[11] the extent of this depends on the particular phenol concerned and the interfering soil.

TABLE 20.6	pK_a values of phenolic microbicidal agents[a]
Phenol Derivative	**pK_a**
3-Methyl-6-isopropylphenol (thymol)	10.6
2-Phenylphenol	11.6
Benzylphenol	11.6
2-Benzyl-4-chlorophenol	9.7
4-Chloro-3,5-dimethylphenol	9.7
4-Chloro-3-methylphenol	9.6
5,5'-Dichloro-2,2'-dihydroxy-diphenyl methane (dichlorophen)	8.7/12.6
2,4,6-Trichlorophenol	8.5
Pentachlorophenol	5.26

[a]Reprinted by permission from Paulus.[6] Copyright © 1993 Springer Science+Business Media Dordrecht.

Action Against Bacteria

Phenol and its derivatives exhibit several types of bactericidal action. At higher concentrations, the compounds act as a gross protoplasmic poison, penetrating and disrupting the cell wall and precipitating the cell proteins.[91,92] At lower concentrations, phenol and its derivatives exhibit more subtle effects.

Generally, gram-positive bacteria are more sensitive to phenolics than are gram-negative bacteria, which themselves are also more sensitive than mycobacteria. The sensitivity of mycobacteria is intermediate between that of the vegetative bacteria and the more resistant bacterial spores.[86] The increased resistance of the mycobacteria and bacterial spores probably relates to the higher lipid content of the cell walls and spore coats, respectively.[88] Table 20.7 shows the MIC of various phenolics against a range of bacteria, yeast, and fungi. Clearly, *Pseudomonas* species are particularly tolerant to the whole range of phenolics studied.

The initial reaction between a phenolic derivative and bacteria involves binding of the active to the cell surface. Bean and Das[94] studied the uptake of a range of phenols by *E coli*. Of the phenols studied, phenol itself, 2-chlorophenol, 3-methylphenol, PCMC, thymol (2-isopropyl-5-methylphenol), hexylresorcinol, and 5-chloro-2-hydroxyphenyl-methane all exhibited S-type uptake isotherms.[95] With this pattern, the initial linear portion of the curve indicates that uptake is proportional to the concentration in the bulk aqueous phase. At a concentration characteristic of each phenol, there was a sudden increase in uptake that corresponded to an increase in the opacity of the suspension. It was suggested that this was the result of precipitation and coagulation. Similar results were observed by Judis[96] for the uptake of 2,4-dinitrophenol and 2-tert-amylphenol in *E coli*, although in this case, uptake curves were interpreted as being of the C-type isotherms, suggesting constant partitioning of the active.[95] The only other phenolic agent examined by Bean and Das,[94] which is resorcinol, had an L-type uptake isotherm, which indicates that uptake is limited by the number of sites available on the cell surface.

Once the active has bound to the exterior of the cell, it needs to penetrate to its target site(s). Literature on penetration is sparse. Russell and Chopra[88] suggested that for gram-positive bacteria, biocides may often enter the cell by passive diffusion and partitioning. For gram-negative bacteria, it was proposed that hydrophobic actives, such as phenolics and parabens, use the hydrophobic lipid bilayer pathway. Greenberg and coworkers[97] studied the structure-active relationship of several phenolic compounds and how it relates to antimicrobial activity. They found that lipophilicity and steric effects are two key factors in determining bactericidal activity and appear to act as nonionic surface active compounds, which can disrupt the lipid-protein interface.

TABLE 20.7   Minimum inhibitory concentrations (MIC) of phenol derivatives in nutrient agar[a]

Organism	MIC (mg/L)						
	OPP	BP	OBPCP	PCMC	PCMX	DC	PCP
Aeromonas punctata	200	100	10	200	100	50	10
Bacillus subtilis	100	100	10	150	75	100	10
Escherichia coli	200	500	3500	250	200	100	500
Leuconostoc mesenteroides	100	100	10	200	100	5	35
Proteus vulgaris	200	200	100	200	200	50	100
Pseudomonas aeruginosa	1500	5000	5000	800	1000	>5000	500
Pseudomonas fluorescens	1500	5000	>5000	800	500	3500	500
Staphylococcus aureus	100	100	20	200	100	5	10
Desulfovibrio desulfuricans	50	100	50	35	50	20	35
Candida albicans	100	100	50	200	75	50	35
Torula rubra	100	100	50	50	100	50	100
Alternaria tenuis	100	75	20	200	75	50	1
Aspergillus flavus	85	200	75	100	100	50	100
Aspergillus niger	75	100	100	100	100	100	50
Aureobasidium pullulans	35	100	20	30	50	35	20
Chaetomium globosum	60	50	20	80	50	20	20
Cladosporium herbarum	60	200	100	200	100	200	50
Coniophora puteana	50	35	5	100	35	2	35
Lentinus tigrinus	100	75	20	3500	75	5	10
Paecilomyces variotii	100	100	50	200	100	50	50
Penicillium citrinum	35	100	75	100	50	50	50
Penicillium glaucum	80	100	50	100	35	50	50
Polyporus versicolor	65	100	50	5000	75	50	20
Rhizopus nigricans	50	100	50	100	100	35	15
Sclerophoma pityophila	100	100	20	100	75	20	10
Stachybotrys atra cords	50	35	20	100	35	15	15
Trichoderma viride	75	200	100	140	100	50	200
Trichophyton pedis	20	20	10	100	50	10	10

Abbreviations: BP, benzylphenol; DC, 5,5'-dichloro-2,2'-dihydroxy-diphenyl methane; OBPCP, 2-benzyl-4-chlorophenol; OPP, 2-phenylphenol; PCMC, 4-chloro-3-methylphenol; PCMX, 4-chloro-3,5-dimethylphenol; PCP, pentachlorophenol.

[a]From Paulus and Genth.[93] Reprinted by permission of Sheila Barry.

Pulvertaft and Lumb[98] studied the effect of certain antiseptic formulations on the lysis of bacterial cultures. They found that *E coli*, staphylococci, and streptococci underwent complete lysis at a phenol concentration of 0.032%, but at 0.54%, no lysis took place. Presumably, this was due to the precipitation and coagulation of the cell surfaces or contents at the higher phenol concentration. Srivastava and Thompson[99,100] reported that 0.5% phenol did cause lysis of *E coli* at the time of separation during division (mitosis), when the membrane was at its weakest.

The primary target site for the action of phenolic antimicrobial agents appears to be the cytoplasmic membrane. Damage to the cytoplasmic membrane can take several forms, depending on the concentration and the specific active employed. Although a particular agent may have one particular primary target site, because of the strong interdependency of cellular function, other sites will invariably be affected.[101] Jang et al[102] observed in *S aureus*, via microarray analysis, that OPP inhibits anabolism of amino acids and deregulates genes encoding enzymes involved in the diaminopimelate (DAP) pathway—essential for building up peptidoglycan cell walls. Nde et al,[103] via transcriptome analysis in *P aeruginosa* exposed to OPP, showed upregulation of genes encoding ribosomal, virulence, and membrane transport at treatment times of 20 and 60 minutes. Also at 20 minutes exposure, genes for anaerobic respiration and swarming motility were also upregulated. After 60 minutes, exposure increases synthesis of lipopolysaccharide, which could lead to cell wall modification.

One of the initial events to occur at the cytoplasmic membrane will be the inhibition of membrane-bound enzymes. This may even occur at subinhibitory concentrations of the phenolic. The manifestation of this activity may be the inhibition of the respiratory chain and energy transfer, inhibition of substrate oxidation, and inhibition of transport processes.[101] Frederick et al[104] showed that the primary site of action of hexachlorophene in *Bacillus megaterium* was the inhibition of the membrane-bound part of the electron-transport chain near the terminal electron acceptor. In *E coli*, subinhibitory concentrations of triclosan (1 μg/mL) have been shown to inhibit the uptake of the amino acids phenylalanine and uracil and other nutrients.[105]

At higher, but still subinhibitory phenolic concentrations, there may be a selective increase in the permeability of the cytoplasmic membrane to protons and other ions.[101] Within the bacterial cell, oxidative phosphorylation, adenosine triphosphate (ATP) synthesis, active transport, and maintenance of intracellular solute levels are all powered by a proton motive force (PMF) generated by ATP hydrolysis and other metabolic oxidation-reduction reactions. The PMF is expressed as a pH gradient across the cytoplasmic membrane, with the interior of the cell being more alkaline and negatively charged compared with the extracellular environment. Clearly, any agent that alters the permeability of the membrane to protons could result in the uncoupling of oxidative phosphorylation, inhibition of active transport, and loss of metabolites. Such effects have been observed with a number of different phenolic actives.

Commager and Judis[106] showed that low concentration (50% of the MIC level) of 4-chlorophenol, 2,4-dichlorophenol, 4-chloro-2-methylphenol, and 2,4-dinitrophenol stimulated oxygen uptake in *E coli* when glucose was used as the substrate presumably because of the uncoupling of oxidative phosphorylation. Hugo and Bowen[107] studied the effect of 4-ethylphenol on *E coli* and found that, among other things, uncoupling of oxidative phosphorylation also occurred. Fentichlor affects the metabolic activity of *E coli* and *S aureus*,[108] producing a selective increase in the permeability of the cytoplasmic membrane to protons. As a result, PMF was dissipated and oxidative phosphorylation uncoupled.[109] Other actives, such as various 4-*n*-alkyl phenols,[110] PCMC,[111] and the parabens[112,113] have similar effects.

The next level in damage to the cytoplasmic membrane is the loss of the membrane's ability to act as a permeability barrier. This is the result of a generalized loss in structural integrity and manifests itself as a leakage of intracellular material. Although these effects may begin to occur at bacteriostatic concentrations, if left to continue, autolytic processes will be initiated and death will follow.[101] Leakage of intracellular materials follows a defined pattern. The first index of membrane damage is the release of K+ ions,[114] followed by inorganic phosphates, pool amino acids, and then 260-nm absorbing material.[88] This latter material provides a nonspecific indication of the release of DNA, RNA, and, to some degree, protein.

Several authors examined the leakage of intracellular material on exposure to phenolic antimicrobial agents. Kroll and Anagnostopoulos[115] showed that there was a strong correlation between the kinetics of K+ leakage on exposure of *Serratia marcescens* to phenol and the loss of culture viability. Gale and Taylor[116] studied the leakage of amino acids from the bacterial cell on exposure to 1% phenol solution. They found that leakage of glutamic acid from *Streptococcus faecalis* was almost as intensive as that produced by boiling.

Judis[117] showed that exposure of prelabeled *E coli* to phenol, PCMX, PCMC, DCMX, 4-chloro-2-methylphenol, 2,4-dinitrophenol, and 2,4,6-trichlorophenol all caused leakage of 14C-glutamate from the bacteria. In detailed studies with phenol and PCMX, the extent of release was directly related to concentration of the active and appeared independent of pH over the range of 4.6 to 8.6. Initial release occurred at sub-MIC levels, where there was no detectable reduction in viability, suggesting that at low levels, the effects of the phenols were reversible. Subsequent work by Judis[118] using 14C-adenine and 32P-phosphate indicated that, although early leakage events in *E coli* were reversible, beyond a certain point leakage proceeded to cell death. Once this point has been passed, leakage of radiolabeled nucleic acid continued, even when the phenolic stress was removed. Subsequently, Commager and Judis[106] proposed that the primary site for the bactericidal action of phenolic antimicrobials was damage to the cytoplasmic membrane, which resulted in a loss of the permeability barrier. Because this occurred at concentrations of the phenolic that already inhibited the metabolic enzyme reaction responsible for repair, the bacteria were unable to recover and died.

Hugo and Bloomfield[108,119,120] found a close correlation between the bactericidal activity of fentichlor and the leakage of 260 nm of absorbing material from *E coli* and *S aureus*. At bacteriostatic concentrations, fentichlor did not cause the leakage of 260-nm absorbing material. Exposure of *E coli* B to bactericidal concentrations of triclosan results in rapid release of 260-nm absorbing material and cell death.[105] Similar observations were made by Joswick et al[121] who examined exposure of *B megaterium* to hexachlorophene and a number of other bisphenols. For hexachlorophene, release was dose dependent, achieving a maximum at 7 times the minimum lethal dose (10 μg/mg cell dry weight).

Interaction of phenolic antimicrobials with the cytoplasmic contents of bacteria is also an important event in the bactericidal activity. Effects can range from inhibition of certain enzymes to complete coagulation of the cytoplasmic contents. The degree of damage will depend on the concentration of the phenolic employed.

Bach and Lambert[122,123] studied the action of phenol on bacterial enzymes. A 1:1000 dilution of phenol acting for 30 minutes on *S aureus* destroyed the cell's ability to activate succinate, fumarate, pyruvate, and glutamate, whereas the lactate, glucose, formate, and butanol systems were only partially inactivated. According to Sykes,[124] the concentrations of phenol, 4-butylphenol, and hexylresorcinol required to inactivate the succinic dehydrogenase of *E coli* are slightly higher than the minimum killing concentration.

It has been reported that the primary target site for triclosan in *Escherichia coli*,[40] *Mycobacterium smegmatis*,[125] and other bacteria is an enoyl-reductase that is involved in fatty acid synthesis. These authors suggested that either upregulation of or a mutation in the gene responsible for encoding this enzyme resulted in an increased tolerance of these organisms to triclosan. The inhibitory effect of triclosan occurs at low concentrations because it mimics the natural substrate of the enzyme.[41] Although this may be the first target site that causes bacteriostasis, it is already known that this will not be the only target at higher bactericidal concentrations. Higher concentrations can also cause nonspecific damage to cytoplasmic membrane.[126] Genomic transcriptional analysis[102] shows effects on metabolism, downregulation of transcriptional genes for virulence, and energy metabolism while upregulating genes for multidrug resistance, coenzyme transport A, metabolism, and transcription. It could also downregulate transcription genes for major lipid metabolism enzymes (3-hydroxyacyl-CoA dehydrogenase, acetyl-CoA acetyltransferase, acetyl-CoA synthetase, and acetyl-CoA carboxylase). However, expression of the *fabL* gene was unchanged with the addition of 0.05 mM triclosan for 10 and 60 minutes. As reported earlier, Regös and Hitz[105] showed that bactericidal concentrations caused the rapid release of cellular components from *Escherichia coli*, resulting in cell death. Even at subinhibitory concentrations, triclosan also interfered with the uptake of essential nutrients. McDonnell and Russell[127] reported that in strains of *Escherichia coli* and *S aureus* with elevated MICs toward triclosan, although there were minor changes in fatty acid profiles, MBCs were unaffected. Escalada et al[128] observed during investigations on the effects of triclosan against *P aeruginosa*, *Escherichia coli*, and *Enterococcus hirae* at different population growth stages that the duration of the lag phase was increased in a concentration-dependent manner. Higher concentrations were bactericidal regardless of growth phase, although stationary phase and washed suspensions were more resilient to lethality. This, it was suggested, indicated that many other

target sites were involved and complex cellular interactions beyond metabolic pathways could be occurring at both low and high triclosan concentrations.

Hugo[95] described irreversible coagulation of cytoplasmic constituents occurring at high phenolic concentrations. Bancroft and Richter[129] observed coagulation of cell protein in *B megaterium* and *Klebsiella aerogenes* using ultraviolet microscopy. At concentrations of phenol higher than those that first caused lysis in *E coli*, Pulvertaft and Lumb[98] found that lysis was inhibited. The biphasic leakage response observed by Joswick et al[121] on exposure of *B megaterium* to high concentrations of hexachlorophene was thought to be due to coagulation effectively "sealing-in" the protoplasmic contents. These results were confirmed by Corner et al,[130] but it was concluded that these effects were secondary to the primary target, which was the inhibition of membrane-bound respiratory enzymes occurring at lower concentration.

As reported earlier, mycobacteria are generally more resistant to antimicrobial agents than other vegetative bacteria; however, phenol and phenolic compounds still are considered highly effective tuberculocidal agents. Tilley et al[131] found a 1:200 solution of OPP to be effective against *M tuberculosis* in the presence of organic matter. Klarmann et al[132] studied a series of homologous 4-chlorophenol derivatives and found them to be highly effective against several strains of mycobacteria. Using a modified phenol coefficient test, Wright and Shternov[133] showed that phenol and various combinations of phenolic derivatives demonstrated good tuberculocidal activity (Table 20.8). Hegna[134] found OPP with soap to be more effective than a mixture of PCMC and OBPCP in a detergent system against *M tuberculosis*. This work also showed that 1% and 2% OPP solutions with soap were

TABLE 20.8	Dilutions of phenolic combinations exhibiting tuberculocidal activity in 10 minutes

Phenolic Combinations	Dilutions
A, J	1:100
B, J	1:60
C, J, L	1:150
C, K	1:150
C, D, K	1:300
E, F, J	<1:20
G, H, I, J	<1:20

Abbreviations: A, coal-tar neutral oils and phenols; B, cresol; C, o-hydroxy-diphenyl; D, p-tert-amylphenol; E, o-benzyl-p-chlorophenol; F, sodium o-phenylphenate; G, potassium p-tert-amylphenate; H, potassium o-phenylphenate; I, potassium o-benzyl-p-chlorophenate; J, solubilized by soap; K, solubilized by potassium ricinoleate; L, cresylic acid.

more effective than a 3.5% solution with soap. It was concluded that the higher concentration of soap in the 3.5% solution reduced its tuberculocidal activity, probably by loss of the phenolic to the soap micelles.

Smith,[135] in a comprehensive study of disinfectants for tuberculosis hygiene, observed that mycobacteria were more difficult to kill than other bacteria. He concluded that phenolic disinfectants had great practical value. In a study of the disinfecting of clinical thermometers from a tuberculosis sanitarium, it was found that alcohol and phenolic disinfectants disinfected thermometers harboring *M tuberculosis*, whereas the quaternary ammonium compound (QAC) and the iodophor tested did not.[136] The mycobacterial cell wall consists of lipid-rich hydrophobic layers. It is the content of this cell wall that is probably responsible for the resistance of this organism to so many chemical disinfectants,[137] and a review of microbial resistance mechanisms by McDonnell[46] gives an excellent overall view. The ability of phenol and phenolic derivatives to dissolve this lipid material probably gives them their tuberculocidal capabilities. Rubin[138] and Russell[139] provided excellent reviews on the response of mycobacteria to various phenolics.

Phenolics are not sporicidal but are sporistatic, inhibiting germination and outgrowth.[86] Russell and Chopra[140] provided data showing that phenol and cresol are not sporicidal, even at concentrations much higher than those required for bactericidal activity; however, they are sporistatic at the same concentration at which they are bacteriostatic. These authors also presented data on the effect of phenol on spore germination. Inhibition of the germination of *Bacillus subtilis* spores by 0.15% phenol was reversible, under certain conditions (eg, by the use of membrane filtration). It was concluded that phenol binds loosely to sites on the spore surface to inhibit germination and/or outgrowth because additional washing of treated spores was sufficient to remove the phenol and allow for spore outgrowth. The increased resistance of bacterial spores is due to the more complex structure of the spore coat and cortex, which act as a permeability barrier preventing access to the underlying spore protoplast.[141]

A review of bacterial target sites of phenolics and other biocidal compounds was provided by Maillard.[142] An extensive review assessing the mechanistic investigations of plant phenolic antibacterial compounds and various survey system approaches to demonstrate the potential for identifying antibacterial mechanisms has been undertaken by Rempe et al.[143]

Action Against Fungi

Fungi and yeast are known to have a significantly higher resistance to biocidal compounds than the nonsporulating bacteria. In general, phenolic antimicrobials can be regarded as fungicidal or fungistatic, depending

	Exposure Time[a]		
Fungi	15 min	30 min	60 min
Candida albicans	−	−	−
Trichophyton rubrum	−	−	−
Trichophyton mentagrophytes	−	−	−
Epidermophyton floccosum	−	−	−
Microsporum canis	−	−	−
Microsporum gypseum	−	−	−
Scopulariopsis brevicaulis	±	−	−
Aspergillus niger	±	−	−
Aspergillus fumigatus	+	+	+
Mucor species	−	−	−
Fusarium species	−	−	−

TABLE 20.9 Survival and growth of fungi after 15, 30, and 60 minutes exposure to a 1:50 dilution of a phenolic disinfectant containing 15% 2-phenylphenol and 6.3% 4-tert-amylphenol

[a]−, no growth on three replicate agar slants; +, growth on three replicate agar slants; ±, growth on one of three replicate agar slants.

on their concentration. Many phenolics, notably the alkyl-halogenated forms, the bisphenols, and the parabens, exhibit good antifungal activity.[144] Karabit et al[145] studied the rate of kill (D-value) of 0.5% phenol against both bacteria and fungi and concluded that *Aspergillus niger* and *C albicans* were more resistant to phenol than *E coli*, *P aeruginosa*, and *S aureus*. A 2% dilution of a phenolic disinfectant exhibited fungicidal action over a wide spectrum of clinically important fungi (Table 20.9).[146] Hegna[147] showed that OPP in linseed oil and soya oil soap had greater fungicidal activity than did a combination of PCMC and OBPCP in a detergent system.

The parabens are commonly used as preservatives because of their good fungistatic activity. Comparing the results in Table 20.5 with those in Table 20.10 shows that the concentrations required to be fungicidal are considerably higher than those that are fungistatic. In both cases, the parabens show the classic response of increasing activity with increasing alkyl chain length of the homologous series from methyl to butyl ester.

Although a significant amount is known about the mode of action of phenolic antimicrobial agents on bacteria, little appears in the literature on their mode of action on yeast and fungi. The greater complexity of the eukaryotic physiology means that extrapolation of results from bacteria to fungi and yeast may be an oversimplification.[148]

TABLE 20.10 | Minimum lethal concentrations (percentages) of paraben esters against some common fungi[a]

Name	Methyl	Ethyl	Propyl	Butyl
Candida albicans	0.5	0.25	0.0625	0.0625
Penicillium chrysogenum	0.5	0.25	0.125	0.125
Aspergillus niger	0.5	0.5	0.25	0.125

[a]Derived from data in Wallhausser.[27]

Ansari et al[149] offer a good review of natural phenolic's modes of action against a number of different yeast and fungi.

As with bacteria, natural plant phenolics have also been investigated for their antimicrobial properties. Aziz et al[150] were able to show the antifungal properties of eight phenolic compounds, with complete inhibition against *Aspergillus flavus* and *Aspergillus parasiticus* by *p*-hydroxybenzoic acid and protocatechuic, syringic, and *p*-coumaric acids as well as quercetin. Zabka and Pavela[151] were able to show that efficacy of different natural phenolic compounds is dependent on the molecular structures and differing interspecies sensitivity against *Fusarium*, *Aspergillus*, and *Penicillium* species. Pizzolitto et al[152] demonstrated that antifungal activity of natural plant phenolics against *A parasiticus* was correlated to lipophilicity, reactivity, and steric aspects of the compounds. As far as potential mechanisms of action against *Candida* by phenolic agents, Teodoro et al[153] offered a number of possible pathways needing further investigation.

Action Against Viruses

In general, many viruses tend to be more resistant to phenolic antimicrobial agents than either the bacteria or fungi.[86] The susceptibility of viruses to phenolic biocides varies with the virus concerned. Viruses can be divided into three broad categories:

1. *Lipophilic viruses*, referred to as enveloped viruses, are surrounded by a lipid-containing envelope that combines readily with lipids.
2. *Hydrophilic viruses*, referred to as nonenveloped viruses, do not have a lipid envelope (ie, are naked viruses) and do not combine with lipids.
3. *Intermediate viruses* do not have a lipid envelope but do have some lipophilicity in the capsomere.[154]

Phenolic biocides show a greater ability to inactivate the lipophilic (enveloped) viruses than they do in any of the other types. Klein and Deforest[155] found that 5% phenol inactivated both hydrophilic and lipophilic viruses but that OPP was only effective against lipophilic viruses and not hydrophilic viruses. Moreover, OPP was approximately 10 times more active against these viruses than phenol (Table 20.11). The additional carbon atoms present in OPP makes the molecule more hydrophobic (lipophilic) than phenol. This greater lipophilicity accounts for its greater activity against lipophilic viruses and its low activity against hydrophilic viruses. In general, the more hydrophobic the phenolic active is, the greater the activity against enveloped viruses and the lower its activity against the nonenveloped viruses.

During the early 2000s, new emerging influenza and respiratory-type viruses, such as H1N1, severe acute respiratory syndrome (SARS), and Middle East respiratory syndrome-coronavirus (MERS-CoV), were discovered. These viruses are lipophilic by nature. As expected, phenolic disinfectants show a high degree of virucidal activity against them. Common household detergent-disinfectant (containing 4.8% PCMX) at 5% dilution produced a greater than 4 log reduction in virus within 10 minutes (unpublished data by Reckitt Benckiser, 2009, 2013, 2017). Today, numerous phenolic disinfectants are registered in the United States with EPA as virucidal agents.[156]

Wood and Payne[157] tested the liquid antiseptic Dettol™, which contains PCMX as the active ingredient, against a range of enveloped and nonenveloped viruses. At an

TABLE 20.11 | Lowest phenolic concentrations (percentage solution) exhibiting virucidal activity in 10 minutes

Virus	Classification	Phenol	2-Phenylphenol
Poliovirus type 1	Hydrophilic	5%	12% (no effect)
Coxsackievirus B-1	Hydrophilic	5%	12% (no effect)
Echovirus 6	Hydrophilic	5%	12% (no effect)
Adenovirus type 2	Intermediate	5%	0.12%
Herpes simplex virus	Lipophilic	1%	0.12%
Vaccinia virus	Lipophilic	2%	0.12%
Asian influenza	Lipophilic	2%	0.12%

in-test PCMX concentration of 0.24%, Dettol™ inactivated the enveloped viruses herpes simplex type 1 (HSV-1) and HIV type 1, even in the presence of significant amounts of organic load; however, the same antiseptic was less effective against the nonenveloped viruses: coxsackievirus, human adenovirus type 25, and poliovirus type 1. Surprisingly, the activity against the enveloped virus, human coronavirus, was variable, depending on the subtype.

Information about the extent of virucidal activity of different phenolics is limited because a full systematic study has yet to be performed.[158,159] These latter investigators reported that the activity of phenols is highly formulation dependent and affected by factors such as temperature, concentration, pH, and the presence of organic matter. For this reason, virucidal activity cannot be generalized, and formulated products must be tested against the specific virus to determine efficacy.

Although information about the spectrum of activity of certain phenolics against different virus types is available, the actual mode of action is poorly understood. Prince et al[154] suggested that inactivation by chemical biocides is exclusively the result of denaturation and chemical reaction with the surface structures on the viruses that are essential to attachment and penetration at the receptor site on the host cell. Maillard[158] provided an overview of viral structure and highlighted the likely target sites for antiviral activity. Russell and Chopra[88] proposed that phenols are likely to interact with the virus's envelope in a manner similar to their interaction with the bacterial membrane. Sattar and Springthorpe[159] concluded that the molecular mechanisms of disinfectant action on viruses probably do not differ from those that occur with bacteria. In an effort to elucidate the exact target site, Maillard and coworkers[160] used the *P aeruginosa* bacteriophage F116 as a model virus and found that a 2% phenol solution did not alter the nucleic acid within the capsid of F116 or the phage transduction properties.[161] Using the same phenol concentration, damage to the capsid structure and tail was evident, provided that a contact period of greater than 20 minutes may be needed.[162]

Chávez et al[163] evaluated the antiviral activity of synthetic plant phenolic compounds against the rabies virus and observed that the presence of free-hydroxyl and ether groups influences the antiviral behavior of the compound. Suárez et al[164] made both methanolic and acetonic extracts of apple pomace phenolics. Both extracts were able to inhibit both HSV-1 and herpes simplex type 2 (HSV-2) replication in Vero cells by more than 50% at noncytotoxic concentrations. Silva et al[165] observed that presence of rutin and quercetin in plant extracts displayed relevant antiviral activity against dengue virus.

In summary, one can expect phenolic derivatives to show virucidal action against lipophilic viruses, but activity against hydrophilic viruses is less certain and should be determined individually. The use of natural phenolic compounds as antiviral agents needs to be further explored.

▶ FORMULATION USING PHENOLICS

The fact that the more active phenol derivatives have limited solubility, and because the MICs (see Table 20.7) for many of the bacteria and fungi are relatively high, it is possible that bactericidal and fungicidal concentrations may not be that far removed from their saturated aqueous solubility.[166] Therefore, in an attempt to improve the microbicidal efficacy of phenolic preparations, various solubilization techniques have been used.

Simple Solubilization and Thermodynamic Activity

As discussed in the section on coal-tar phenol, the principal technique used to increase the solubilization of phenolic derivatives is the use of an anionic surfactant such as potassium laurate, a soap of natural origin, or a synthetic detergent such as an alkyl aryl sulfonate. This technique takes advantage of the fact that when surfactants are present as micelles above their critical micelle concentration (CMC), the hydrophobic core of the micelle has a high affinity for low water-soluble hydrophobic phenolic antimicrobial agents. Hence, these compounds readily dissolve in the micelles and essentially become solubilized in an aqueous environment.[167]

The nature of antibacterial action of these solubilized phenol systems has interested many workers over the years. Bean and Berry[168-170] examined the effect of increasing the amount in solution a phenolic antimicrobial and surfactant (potassium laurate), held at a fixed ratio. Initially, as the concentration was increased, there was an increase in antibacterial activity. This was higher than that obtained from the phenol alone and was attributed to potentiation of the bactericide by the undissociated soap molecule, probably through a reduction in interfacial surface tension at the bacterial cell surface, leading to a greater rate of adsorption of the phenolic antimicrobial onto the cell wall. Above the surfactant CMC, solubilization of the active began, and there was a decrease in bactericidal activity. Activity reached a minimum when the micelles attained their maximum size. This observation was attributed to a reduction in the relative amount of phenols per individual micelle. It was suggested that this was the result of the micelles growing more quickly than the phenol could be solubilized.

As the level of the phenol-surfactant mixture in the solution was increased further, bactericidal activity reappeared and increased almost back to its previous maximum level. Bean and Berry[168-170] attributed this to an increase in the total number of micelles rather than to an increase in the size of the existing micelles. They proposed that the lethal events were the result of adsorption of the micelles onto the bacterial cell surface, followed by passage of the biocide onto and into the bacteria. It was postulated that activity was a function of the phenol in the micelle and not the total concentration in solution. The reemergence in activity was attributed to the increased number of micelles being available to act as what were essentially delivery vehicles.

Alexander and Tomlinson[171] had a different interpretation for similar observations. These authors worked with a slightly different system, in which the concentration of phenol was kept constant at 1%, whereas the surfactant (sodium dihexyl sulfosuccinate) was varied. Although they concurred with the increase in activity below the surfactant CMC, they suggested that the reduction in activity above this was due to removal of the active from the aqueous phase into the micelle, decreasing the amount of phenol available to react with the cell. They proposed that under these circumstances, the activity of the system was solely a function of the concentration of the bactericide in the aqueous phase and not the total amount. At higher surfactant concentrations, when bactericidal effects returned, the detergent molecules were thought to be exhibiting bactericidal activity.

Allawala and Riegelman[172] showed that in accordance with the Ferguson principle, bactericidal activity of phenolic agents in water depended on the thermodynamic activity of the solutions. Different solutions were shown to be equitoxic to bacteria when the thermodynamic activity or degree of saturation of the solutions were the same and not when their actual concentrations of the active in those solutions were the same, that is, when all phases of a particular system were saturated.

An important conclusion was also drawn by Allawala and Riegelman[173] in their studies with iodine and hexachlorophene. Although simple aqueous saturated solutions have maximum thermodynamic activity, they are not of any practical value because the active agent dissolved in solution is rapidly depleted by interaction with the bacteria. The antimicrobial performance of a solution is therefore dependent not only on the intensity factor (immediate thermodynamic activity) but also on the capacity factor (reservoir activity). Solubilizing agents such as surfactants provide this reservoir potential so that antimicrobial activity can be maintained. This reservoir effect improved efficiency over simple aqueous solutions and is particularly important where active agents of low water solubility are being considered.[174]

The role of thermodynamic activity with respect to the efficacy of antimicrobial agents was thoroughly reviewed by Kostenbauder.[175]

Product Formulation

Many factors play a role in the performance of phenolic antimicrobial agents, and as a result, when formulating effective disinfectants, antiseptics, or preserved systems, a complete understanding of the interactions between these factors and the various formulation components is required.

Phenol and its derivatives act optimally in acidic and neutral media. Over this pH range, phenolics are in their undissociated or unionized state. Unfortunately, under these circumstances, the solubility of the phenolic is low. To increase the solubility, increasing the pH of the system and inclusion of soap or synthetic detergents can be used.

Increasing the pH results in the conversion of the phenol to its corresponding sodium or potassium phenate. These phenates are much more water soluble than the phenol from which they were derived, but they exhibit reduced bactericidal power. Indeed, increasing the pH may decrease the germicidal action to such an extent that efficacy may no longer be evident.[176,177] Under these circumstances, inclusion of the correct amount and kind of soap may allow a distinct germicidal effect to be produced at a pH and a concentration at which a simple phenol-alkali combination alone would show a limited degree of activity.[178,179] Another important feature of the phenates is that they also may act as a solubilizing agent for the free phenolics.

The effect of pH is particularly noticeable when phenols are solubilized with alkyl aryl sulfonates. Greater latitude in pH adjustment is possible because the alkyl aryl sulfonic acids have much greater water solubility than fatty acids. Highly active phenolic disinfectants can be made with high acidity (as low as pH 3). In some cases, activity against *S aureus* is greatly increased.[180,181]

As discussed earlier, a primary technique used in the formulation of phenolics in aqueous systems is the use of soap or synthetic detergents. The ratio of synthetic detergent to phenolic or natural soap to phenolic plays a significant role in the solubility and germicidal activity. As ratios and pH are changed, activity changes also, allowing the formulator to design the product to meet the desired germicidal criteria and solution properties.

Of the three general classes—anionic, nonionic, and cationic—only the anionic detergents are generally usable in formulating phenolic disinfectants. Nonionic detergents reduce or completely destroy the antimicrobial activity of the phenols. Cationic surfactants such as QACs are generally incompatible; however, Davis[182] indicated that various synergistic blends of phenolics with QACs can be produced for certain industrial applications. The synergy is thought to be due to the lowering of the interfacial surface tension by the QAC below its CMC, which is believed to allow greater permeation of the phenol into the cell membrane.

Another means of incorporating phenolics into aqueous systems is to solubilize the active in a concentrated form in a solvent such as alcohol, glycol ethers, or propylene glycol and then add this to the aqueous phase. Thoma et al[183] indicated that solvents of this type do not negatively impact the antibacterial activity of a number of phenols, including PCMX. This is also one of the methods recommended for the incorporation of the parabens into different formulations.[184] In an oil and water system, where the higher parabens will preferentially partition into the oil phase, incorporation of a solvent may help displace the equilibrium toward the aqueous phase.

Properly formulated phenolic disinfectants are essentially nonspecific with respect to their bactericidal and fungicidal action and are thereby qualified for use in disinfecting practice that is directed logically against pathogenic vegetative microorganisms in general rather than against any species or class in particular. In this connection, it is noteworthy that bacterial strains of staphylococci that have become resistant to antibiotics did not, at the same time, acquire a greater resistance to phenol or selected phenolic disinfectants.[185,186] Chuanchuen et al[187] observed that MexJK efflux pump of *P aeruginosa* does require OprM for antibiotic efflux but not for triclosan efflux. McDonnell and Russell[127] gave a general review of antiseptic/disinfectant resistance and possible mechanisms.

▶ SURVEY OF ANTIMICROBIAL APPLICATIONS FOR PHENOLICS

The practical application of phenolic compounds as antimicrobial agents began in the early part of the 19th century.[1] As history shows, many derivatives of phenol have been synthesized and used as antimicrobials, taking into consideration their varied properties for many applications. Today, phenolic biocides are still widely used throughout the world. A comprehensive evaluation of the US and Western Europe's specialty biocides market can be found in two recent reports produced by Kline & Company.[188,189] In 2016, the combined US and Western Europe consumption of specialty biocides was estimated to be 1580.2 million lb (718.7 million kg), with phenolics accounting for an estimated 23 million lb (10.45 million kg) or 1.5% of the total (Table 20.12). By application (Table 20.13), household, industrial, and institutional (HI&I) cleaning accounts for an estimated 3.1 million lb (1.35 × 10⁶ kg) of phenolic biocides or 12.8% of the total. The use of phenolics in cosmetics and toiletries has dropped significantly over the last 10 years from 9 million lb (4.09 million kg) to 573 000 lb (260 454 kg) due to regulatory changes. By far, the greatest use of phenolics remains in wood preservation, which is 69% of the total.[188,189]

Phenolic compounds are recognized and accepted as the antimicrobials of choice for many applications. They are used as the active ingredient in hard-surface disinfectants, antiseptics, germicidal soaps, and lotions and as preservatives in toiletries and household and institutional products. Although Steinberg[190] reviewed the maximum levels that may be included as preservatives in cosmetic and toiletry products in the European Union, these restrictions do not

TABLE 20.12	Estimated US and Europe biocides consumption by product type, 2016[a]	
Biocide Active Class	**Million Pounds**	**% of Total**
Halogenated	460.0	29.1
Nitrogen based	170.4	10.8
Organosulfur	30.7	1.9
Inorganic	162.3	10.3
Phenolics	23.9	1.5
Organometallic	3.8	0.2
Miscellaneous	716.5	45.3
All other	13.2	0.8
Grand total	1580.8	100.0

[a]With permission from Kline & Company.[189]

currently preclude their use at higher levels for purposes other than preservation, for example, as antiseptics.

The phenolic derivatives found in hospital, institutional, and household disinfectants in the United States today are OPP, OBPCP, and 4-tert-amylphenol. Their use in these applications is because they possess the following beneficial characteristics: They have broad-spectrum microbicidal activity against gram-negative and gram-positive bacteria, mycobacteria, fungi, and lipophilic viruses; they are tolerant of organic load and hard water; and they are biodegradable.

Phenolic disinfectants are considered low- to intermediate-level disinfectants. As such, they are appropriate for general disinfection of noncritical and semicritical areas, but they should not be used on semicritical medical equipment that comes into contact with mucous membrane or

TABLE 20.13	Estimated US and West Europe consumption of phenolic biocides by application, 2016[a]	
Application	**Million Pounds**	**% of Total**
Wood preservation	16.5	69.0
HI&I	3.1	12.8
Agriculture	0.5	2.0
Cosmetics and toiletries	0.6	2.4
Others[b]	3.3	13.8
Grand total	23.9	100.0

Abbreviation: HI&I, household, industrial, and institutional.

[a]With permission from Kline & Company.[189]

[b]Includes textiles, adhesives and sealants, hospital and medical antiseptics and sterilants, and metalworking fluids.

nonintact skin.[191] For general disinfection, levels of 400 to 1300 mg/L in the diluted formulation are typical. They are not sporicidal and should not be used when sterilization is required.

In the United States, the Federal Insecticide, Fungicide, and Rodenticide Act (FIFRA) of 1947, which has been amended several times, most recently in 2012 and 2018,[192] is the basic law covering the formal registration of disinfectant products. The FIFRA legislates the use of potential ecologic poisons to ensure effectiveness, safety, and no significant adverse effect on the environment. Enforcement now is the responsibility of the EPA.

Most of the earlier investigations used the Association of Official Analytical Chemists (AOAC) Phenol Coefficient Method as the standard to measure activity of different phenolic disinfectants. Because the use of phenol itself is no longer considered relevant, this method has been replaced by the AOAC Use-Dilution Method. All products with registered bactericidal claims must be supported by data using this method. Tuberculocidal, fungicidal, and virucidal claims are supported by AOAC or EPA methods, depending on the application.

Throughout the world, PCMX also has been widely used as the active antimicrobial ingredient in numerous disinfectant and antiseptic products. In formulation, it has proven effective against a wide range of bacteria and fungi and has gained acceptance as a safe active for use on the skin. Because of its low sensitization potential, PCMX is also commonly used in the nonsurgical antibacterial hand soap category.[193] It has been claimed that the resultant antimicrobial activity may even persist over a few hours.[20,194] PCMX also can be used as a preservative in household and institutional products and cosmetics. In the European Union, it can be incorporated up to a maximum of 0.5% in cosmetics and toiletries.[190] Of a total of 48 423 cosmetic products voluntarily registered with the FDA in 2014, 70 used PCMX as a preservative.[195]

Because of its broad spectrum of activity, triclosan historically found application in deodorant soaps, underarm deodorants, and liquid soaps. For years, it had become increasingly popular as an active ingredient in antibacterial soaps because of its long-lasting residual bacteriostatic properties.[20,193] Products containing up to 1% triclosan had been used to assist in the reduction of body odor.[194] In a more medical application, 0.3% to 2% triclosan-containing hand wash/bodywash products have been used successfully to reduce the incidence of methicillin-resistant *S aureus*.[196-199] However, despite its efficacy, new research came to light in recent years concerning its persistence in the environment and its endocrine-disrupting properties in animals. In December 2013, the FDA proposed a new ruling for consumer antiseptic wash products with the goal of updating the requirements for safety and effectiveness of actives in the monograph. In September of 2016, the new ruling was finalized and 19 actives, including triclosan and triclocarban, were removed from the monograph because

the requirements for updated safety and effectiveness data were not met. Products containing triclosan and triclocarban were mandated to be off the US market by September 2017. PCMX remains an allowable active, although the FDA has deferred a final decision on this and two other actives until safety and efficacy data have been submitted and reviewed.[200] In health care antiseptics, which were last reviewed in 2017, PCMX remains as an FDA-approved active for health care personnel hand wash and surgical hand scrubs.[201] As a preservative in cosmetics and toiletries, triclosan can still be used up to a maximum of 0.3% in Europe.[190]

Thymol formulations are used as disinfectants, antiseptics, in embalming fluid, and in mouthwash preparations. Indeed, one of the longest running mouthwash products, Listerine™, is a combination of thymol and eucalyptol mixed with menthol and methyl salicylate in a hydroalcoholic vehicle.[202] Chlorothymol, made by the action of sulfuryl chloride on thymol, also has been used as a preservative in cosmetics, antiseptic formulations, and mouthwash preparations. The optimal pH range for chlorothymol is 4 to 9.

Hexachlorophene, a bisphenol, was widely used in formulations of antimicrobial hand and bath soaps and skin antiseptics until the safety of the compound was questioned in the early 1970s.[34] As a result, FDA regulations now stipulate that the compound is available by prescription only. Use on broken skin and mucous membranes or for total-body bathing is also contraindicated.[203]

In addition to those phenolics described earlier, many others are used as preservatives for various applications. The parabens have been used for many years as preservatives in cosmetics, pharmaceuticals, foods, and even food packaging materials. With greater activity against fungi than against bacteria, there is also a tendency for the higher parabens to be more soluble in oils and organic solvents. Hence, in an effort to protect all phases of a particular product and to broaden the spectrum of activity, mixtures of different parabens esters are commonly used. Gottfried[204] reported that the main advantage of using paraben mixtures was that the solubilities of the individual esters were independent of each other; hence, higher total concentrations of the parabens can be used than would be possible if only one ester was used. Because of their high oil solubility, paraben mixtures also play an important role in the preservation of emulsions, creams, and lotions. The more water-soluble methyl ester protects the aqueous phase, and the more lipid-soluble propyl and butyl esters protect the oil phase.[205] In formulations, parabens are normally combined at concentrations according to their relative aqueous solubility. Therefore, for combinations of methyl and propyl, ratios of between 3:1 and 2:1 have been used. For methyl, ethyl, and propyl mixtures, the ratio is 5:3:1, whereas for methyl, ethyl, propyl, and butyl, a 7:1:1:1 mixture has been used successfully.[59]

The actual levels of parabens used depend on the end application. In the United States, as a food preservative, 0.1% paraben has been used to protect bakery products, pickles, and salad dressing from the growth of yeast and mold.[206] As a preservative in cosmetics and toiletries in Europe, it can be used up to 0.4% for one ester or 0.8% maximum for an ester mixture.[190] The frequency of paraben use in US cosmetic products is considerable. In 2014, methyl, ethyl, propyl, and butyl esters were used in 28.5%, 10.2%, 21.9%, and 10.4% of products, respectively.[195]

Pentachlorophenol, trichlorophenol, OPP, and their sodium or potassium salts are widely used preservatives for numerous industrial applications and processes. The chief application for pentachlorophenol is as a fungicide in wood preservation. Because of low water solubility and low volatility, it can be applied either by painting or by pressure treatment using solvents, after which it remains resistant to leaching. Other uses for pentachlorophenol have included paper and pulp (0.2%-1.0% by weight), recirculating water systems such as cooling towers (80 mg/L shock levels), leather (0.1%-3.0% by weight), and in enhanced oil recovery processes (various levels, depending on application). Trichlorophenol also has been used in enclosed water systems (50-100 mg/L), leather finishes and dressings (0.25%-0.5%), and enhanced oil recovery flooding water (10-50 mg/L).[28]

OPP is a particularly versatile antimicrobial. Because of its broad-spectrum antibacterial and antifungal activity, in addition to its use in disinfectant products, it has been used as a preservative, although infrequently. Other preservative applications include adhesives in which it is used at a concentration of 0.05% to 1.0%, metalworking fluids (0.1%-0.15%), and textiles (0.1%-0.75%).[28]

Of the other phenolic compounds used as preservatives in cosmetic products in Europe, PCMC and OBPCP both can be incorporated up to a maximum of 0.2%,[190,207] but their use is also infrequent.

TOXICITY AND ECOTOXICITY

For more than 100 years, a considerable amount of information has been gained on the physical and chemical factors that determine the antimicrobial effectiveness of different phenolic derivatives. Antimicrobial effectiveness, however, is not the only factor to be considered when choosing an appropriate agent for a particular application. The toxicity and ecotoxicity profiles of the particular derivative are also equally important. Because of the wealth of toxicity data available on the key commercial phenolic derivatives, no more than an overview can be provided in the space remaining in this chapter. For a review of the toxicity profiles of different phenolic compounds, the reader should refer to the comprehensive guide provided by Patnaik.[208]

Although a few phenolic agents exhibit high toxicity and low biodegradability, and as a result have been banned, many of those in common use possess toxicologic and ecotoxicologic profiles that allow them to be used safely. Although the oral LD_{50} for phenol itself is relatively low (LD_{50} = 317 mg/kg), the values for many other phenol derivatives are considerably higher.[209] For many of the compounds in commercial use, comprehensive toxicologic profiles are available in the literature. Those of particular interest include OPP,[210] OBPCP,[211] and PCMX.[212] Paulus and Genth[93] conducted a critical examination of several well-known phenolic microbicides with respect to their toxicity and ecotoxicity (Table 20.14). Of the derivatives examined, pentachlorophenol showed oral toxicity (LD_{50} = 150 mg/kg) and percutaneous toxicity (LD_{50} = 325 mg/kg), whereas PCMX and dichlorophen exhibited the least skin and mucosa irritation effects and

TABLE 20.14 Toxicologic data of phenol derivatives[a]

Phenol	LD$_{50}$ Oral (mg/kg Rat)	Irritation[b]		Percutaneous Toxicity
		Skin	Mucosa	
OPP	2700	+	++	−
BP	3360	++	++	NA
PCMC	1830	++	++	−
OBPCP	>5000	++	++	−
PCMX	3830	+	−	−
DC	3310	−	+	−
PCP	150	++	++	++[c]

Abbreviations: BP, benzylphenol; DC, 5,5′-dichloro-2,2′-dihydroxy-diphenyl methane; NA, not available; OBPCP, 2-benzyl-4-chlorophenol; OPP, 2-phenylphenol; PCMC, 4-chloro-3-methylphenol; PCMX, 4-chloro-3,5-dimethylphenol; PCP, pentachlorophenol.

[a]From Paulus and Genth.[93] Reprinted by permission of Sheila Barry.

[b]−, no effect; +, moderate effect; ++, strong effect.

[c]LD$_{50}$ = 325 mg/kg rat.

also possess a low order of oral toxicity (LD_{50} = 3830 mg/kg and 3310 mg/kg, respectively). The relevance of these toxicity data depends on the intended application of a particular phenolic derivative. For example, pentachlorophenol is clearly unsuitable for use as a disinfectant where the likelihood of skin contact may be high, whereas PCMX, on the other hand, has found considerable application globally as an antiseptic and ingredient in antimicrobial soaps.

Ecologic toxicity is also important when considering the use of phenolic microbicides in particular applications. Risk assessment of the effective concentration to which a particular system will be exposed is required to ensure that deleterious effects are not observed. It is therefore necessary to consider the scale of use, the likely dilution factor, and the extent of biodegradability of the phenolic derivative in the environment. Toxicity studies on fish and activated sludge-treatment organisms showed that different phenolic derivatives are tolerated to varying degrees (Table 20.15). Biodegradability studies (Figure 20.3) suggested that although some compounds, such as OPP and PCMC, are quickly and completely degraded, others, such as pentachlorophenol, are only broken down slowly. Clearly, with compounds of this latter type, the likely environmental levels need to be calculated, the degree of recalcitrance determined, and the associated risk assessment carried out. When these are high, restrictions on use can be applied to ensure that toxic levels are not routinely reached.

TABLE 20.15	Nontoxic concentration of phenol derivatives for fish (LC_0) and activated sludge organisms (tolerated concentration)[a]	
Phenol	**LC_0 (mg/L)**	**Tolerated Concentration (mg/L)**
OPP	5	100
BP	5-10	20
PCMC	2	70
OBPCP	2	25
PCMX	1	15
DC	0.5	25
PCP	0.2	15

Abbreviations: BP, benzylphenol; DC, 5,5'-dichloro-2,2-dihydroxy-diphenyl methane; OBPCP, 2-benzyl-4-chlorophenol; OPP, 2-phenylphenol; PCMC, 4-chloro-3-methylphenol; PCMX, 4-chloro-3,5-dimethylphenol; PCP, pentachlorophenol.

[a]From Paulus and Genth.[93] Reprinted by permission of Sheila Barry.

In recent years, a number of environmental studies have been conducted to look at the residual levels of microbicides in the environment including wastewater treatment influent/effluent, surface water, and ground water. Studies show that although these materials do biodegrade,

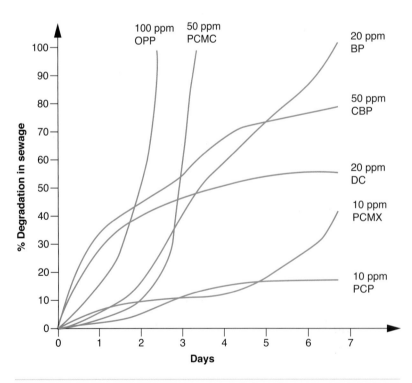

FIGURE 20.3 Decrease in concentration of phenols in activated sludge. Abbreviations: BP, benzylphenol; CBP, 4,4'-Bis(N-carbozolyl)-1,1'-biphenyl; DC, 5,5'-dichloro-2,2'-dihydroxy-diphenyl methane; OPP, 2-phenylphenol; PCMC, 4-chloro-3-methylphenol; PCMX, 4-chloro-3,5-dimethylphenol; PCP, pentachlorophenol. From Paulus and Genth.[93] Reprinted by permission of Sheila Barry.

trace amounts have been detected in a number of areas with the highest concentrations in wastewater influent and in sewage sludge. A study in the Hudson River Estuary by Wilson et al[213] recently detected triclosan at concentrations ranging from 1 ng/L in surface water to 9 ng/L near sediments. Another study in Savannah, Georgia, found triclosan in three rivers at levels of 1 to 10 ng/L in the dissolved phase and 2 to 16 ng/g in the sediment phase. Triclocarbon was also detected in three rivers at levels of 3 to 75 ng/L in the dissolved phase and 11 to 52 ng/g in the sediment phase. In wastewater treatment plants, the same study found triclosan in one treatment plant in influent (38 255 ng/L dissolved phase and 47 906 ng/g in the particulate phase), effluent (4760 ng/L dissolved phase and 13 ng/g particulate phase), and in sludge (0.3-1611 ng/g). Removal of triclocarban and triclosan was noted to be greater than 80%, depending on the treatment plant used.[214] Prior research has shown that activated sludge treatment removes an estimated 95% of triclosan present in waste streams with 80% to 90% of this being broken down by bacteria.[213] Incineration of wet sludge was noted to eliminate 99.99% of triclosan and triclocarban.[214]

Sampling techniques vary greatly in many of the recent studies conducted. As factors such as dilution of effluent into rivers, time of year, rainfall, and depth of water bodies may influence the concentrations found and the rate of degradation, more detailed studies are recommended to reliably quantify levels in the environment. This combined with more updated biodegradability studies will allow for better monitoring and assessment of environmental impact.

Regulatory agencies such as the EPA and FDA require substantial toxicity data to be provided as part of the registration of active agents and products containing these actives. Because potential exposures vary in different applications, the toxicologic data required for a particular application also differ. In 1994 and 2002, the EPA issued a "Data-Call In" notice requiring registrants of actives to submit subchronic and chronic toxicologic data to support the continued registration of these agents. As a result, the phenolic derivatives used as agricultural pesticides, industrial preservatives, and antimicrobial agents in disinfectants underwent extensive investigations and review of their toxicologic effects.

In Europe, the Biocidal Products Regulation (BPR) went into effect in September 2013 for the purpose of renewing the process for making available in the market and the use of biocidal products. The BPR now houses requirements for 22 different product types including those for human hygiene under product type 1 (PT1). Any active ingredients used in biocidal products must be approved for the target product type. Preservatives used must fall under the approved list for product type 6 (PT6).[215]

In terms of preservatives for cosmetics and toiletries, the EC Regulation No. 1223/2009,[216] plus subsequent amendments, contains Annex V, which lists preservatives that are allowed (part 1) or provisionally allowed (part 2). It also defines the maximum allowable concentration of the preservatives and specifies any limitations on use as well as any obligatory printed label warning. A similar situation exists in the United States, where preservatives used in drugs, foods, and cosmetics are controlled under the Federal Food, Drug, and Cosmetic Act, originally enacted in 1938.[207] The FDA carries out the implementation of this act.

◗ CONCLUDING REMARKS

Phenolic agents are some of the oldest chemical entities used for their antimicrobial properties and today still represent an important class of compounds used as the active ingredients in various commercial disinfectants, antiseptics, and preservatives. Because of their long history of use, a great deal of information is known about their structure-activity relationships, their bactericidal mode of action, and their formulation in commercial products. Although it is true that some phenolic compounds possess high oral and percutaneous toxicity and are difficult to degrade, others exhibit good toxicologic and ecotoxicologic profiles, and as a result, these compounds continue to be used in many different applications throughout the world. With the increased need for improved hygiene measures and the need to protect materials from spoilage, it is envisaged that chemical agents such as the phenolic compounds will continue to play an important role.

◗ ACKNOWLEDGMENTS

This chapter was previously authored by Paul Goddard and Karen McCue, whose basic text we humbly upgraded for this edition, and thanks to them for their extensive efforts in understanding phenolic compounds.

◗ ACRONYMS AND ABBREVIATIONS

AOAC	Association of Official Analytical Chemists
ATP	adenosine triphosphate
BACS	British Association of Chemical Specialities
BP	British Pharmacopoeia
CBP	4,4′-Bis(carazolyl)-1,1′-biphenyl
CIR	Cosmetic Ingredient Review
CMC	critical micelle concentration
DAP	diaminopimelate
DCMX	2,4-Dichloro-3,5-dimethylphenol
EC	European Commission
ECHA	European Chemical Agency
EU	European Union
EPA	US Environmental Protection Agency
FDA	US Food and Drug Administration
FIFRA	Federal Insecticide, Fungicide, and Rodenticide Act
HIV	human immunodeficiency virus

MBC	minimum bactericidal concentration
MIC	minimum inhibitory concentration
NAD$^+$	Nicotinamide adeneine dinucleotide
OBPCP	2-Benzyl-4-chlorophenol
OPP	2-Phenylphenol
PCMC	4-Chloro-3-methylphenol
PCMX	4-Chloro-3,5-dimethylphenol
PMF	proton motive force
PPP	4-Phenylphenol
QAC	quaternary ammonium compound
WHO	World Health Organization

REFERENCES

1. Hugo WB. Phenols: a review of their history and development as antimicrobial agents. *Microbios*. 1978;23:83-85.
2. Freney J. Composes phenoliques. In: Fleurette J, Frener J, Reverdy M-E, eds. *Antisepsie et Desinfection*. Paris, France: Editions ESKA; 1995:90-134.
3. Kronig B, Paul TH. Die Chemischen Grundlagen der Lehre von der Giftwirkung und Desinfektion. *Zentralbl Hyg Umweltmed*. 1897;25:1-112.
4. Suter CM. Relationships between the structure and bactericidal properties of phenols. *Chemical Reviews*. 1941;28:269-299.
5. Goddard PA, McCue KA. Phenolic compounds. In: Block SS, ed. *Disinfection, Sterilization, and Preservation*. 5th ed. Philadelphia, PA: Lippincott Williams & Wilkins; 2001:255-282.
6. Paulus W. Phenolics. In: *Microbicides for the Protection of Materials*. New York, NY: Chapman Hall; 1993:141-198.
7. Hugo WB, Russell AD. Types of antimicrobial agents. In: Russell AD, Hugo WB, Ayliffe GA, eds. *Principles and Practices of Disinfection, Preservation, and Sterilization*. 3rd ed. Oxford, United Kingdom: Blackwell Scientific; 1999:7-84.
8. Cresol and soap solution. In: *British Pharmacopoeia*. London, United Kingdom: Her Majesty's Stationery Office; 1968:258-259.
9. British Association of Chemical Specialities. *BACS Guide to the Choice of Disinfectants*. Harrogate, United Kingdom: British Association of Chemical Specialities; 1998.
10. Russell AD. Types of microbicidal and microbistatic agents. In: Russell AD, Hugo WB, Ayliffe GA, eds. *Principles and Practices of Disinfection, Preservation, and Sterilization*. 5th ed. Hoboken, NJ: Wiley-Blackwell; 2013:5-13.
11. Sykes G. Phenols, soaps, alcohols and related compounds. In: Bunbury HM, ed. *Disinfection and Sterilization*. London, United Kingdom: E.N. Spon; 1958:243-275.
12. Chloroxylenol solution. In: *British Pharmacopoeia*. Vol 3. London, United Kingdom: Her Majesty's Stationery Office; 2008:2525.
13. US Environmental Protection Agency. Pesticide registration (PR) notice 2001-4. Notice to manufacturers, producers, formulators, and registrants of pesticide products. US Environmental Protection Agency Web site. https://www.epa.gov/sites/production/files/2014-04/documents/pr2001-4.pdf. Accessed May 23, 2019.
14. Klarmann EG, Shternov VA. Bactericidal value of coal-tar disinfectants: limitations of the *B. typhosus* phenol coefficient as a measure. *Ind Eng Chem*. 1936;8:369-372.
15. Brewer CM, Ruehle GLA. Limitations of phenol coefficients of coal tar disinfectants. *Ind Eng Chem*. 1931;23:150-152.
16. Klarmann EG, Shternov VA, Gates LW. The alkyl derivatives of halogen phenols and their bactericidal action. I. Chlorophenols. *J Am Chem Soc*. 1933;55:2576-2589.
17. Coulthard CE, Marshall J, Pyman FL. The variation of phenol coefficients in homologous series of phenols. *J Chem Soc*. 1930;133:280-291.
18. Coulthard CE. The disinfectant and antiseptic properties of amyl-m-cresol. *Br J Exp Pathol*. 1931;12:331-336.
19. Etoh H, Ban N, Fujiyoshi J, et al. Quantitative analysis of the antimicrobial activity and membrane-perturbation potency of antifouling para-substituted alkylphenols. *Biosci Biotechnol Biochem*. 1994;58:467-469.
20. Bruch MK. Chloroxylenol: an old-new antimicrobial. In: Ascenzi JM, ed. *Handbook of Disinfectants and Antiseptics*. New York, NY: Marcel Dekker; 1996:265-294.
21. Blicke FF, Stockhaus RP. The germicidal action of 2-chloro-4-n-alkyl phenols. *J Am Pharm Assoc (Wash)*. 1933;22:1090-1092.
22. Beck AC. Chlorothymol as an antiseptic in obstetrics. *Am J Obstet Gynecol*. 1933;26:885-889.
23. Kuhn P. Über die Desinfektionswirkung von Thymol und Karvakrol-praparate. *Arch Hygiene*. 1931;105:18-28.
24. Carswell TS, Doubly JA. Germicidal action of formulation with sulphonated oil. *Ind Eng Chem*. 1936;28:1276-1278.
25. Bowers AG. Germicidal liquid soaps. *Soap Sanitary Chem*. 1950;26:36-38.
26. Yamarik TA. Safety assessment of dichlorophene and chlorophene. *Int J Toxicol*. 2004;(23, suppl 1):1-27.
27. Wallhausser KH. Antimicrobial preservatives used by the cosmetic industry. In: Kabara JJ, ed. *Cosmetic and Drug Preservation: Principles and Practice*. New York, NY: Marcel Dekker; 1984:605-745. *Cosmetic Science Technology Series*; vol 1.
28. Marouchoc SR. Classical phenol derivatives and their uses. *Developments in Indust Microbiol*. 1979;20:15-24.
29. Gump WS. The bis-phenols. In: Block SS, ed. *Disinfection, Sterilization, and Preservation*. 2nd ed. Philadelphia, PA: Lea & Febiger; 1977:252-281.
30. Kunz EC, Gump WS, inventors; Sindar Corp, assignee. Germicidal soaps containing halogenated dihydroxy diphenyl methanes. US patent 2,535,077. December 26, 1950.
31. Weiler M, Wenk B, Stotter H, inventors; IG Farbenindustrie AG, assignee. Condensation products from p-halogenated phenolic compounds and aldehydes. US patent 1,707,181. March 26, 1929.
32. Gump WS, Luthy M, inventors; BURTON T BUSH Inc, assignee. Process for making chlorinated phenol-aldehyde condensation products. US patent 2,334,408. November 16, 1943.
33. Schonfeld H, ed. Antiparasitic chemotherapy. In: *Antibiotic Chemotherapy*. Vol 30. Basel, Switzerland: Karger; 1981.
34. Kimbrough RD. Review of the toxicity of hexachlorophene, including its neurotoxicity. *J Clin Pharmacol*. 1973;13(11):439-444.
35. Evangelista de Duffard AM, Duffard R. Behavioral toxicology, risk assessment, and chlorinated hydrocarbons. *Environ Health Perspect*. 1996;104(suppl 2):353-360.
36. Schetty G, Stammbach W, inventors; JR Geigy AG, assignee. Bis(2-hydroxy-4, 5-dichlorophenyl) sulfide. US patent 2,760,988. August 28, 1956.
37. Savage CA. A new bacteriostat for skincare products. *Drug and Cosmetics Industry*. 1971;109:36-39, 161-163.
38. Vischer WA, Regös J. Antimicrobial spectrum of triclosan, a broad-spectrum antimicrobial agent for topical application. *Zentralbl Bakteriol Orig A*. 1974;226(3):376-389.
39. Ward WH, Holdgate GA, Rowsell S, et al. Kinetic and structural characteristics of the inhibition of enoyl (acyl carrier protein) reductase by triclosan. *Biochemistry*. 1999;38:12514-12525.
40. McMurry LA, Oethginger M, Levy SB. Triclosan targets lipid synthesis. *Nature (London)*. 1998;394:531-532.
41. Levy CW, Roujeinikova A, Sedelnikova S, et al. Molecular basis of triclosan activity. *Nature (London)*. 1999;398:383-384.
42. Levy SB. The challenge of antibiotic resistance. *Sci Am*. 1998;278:46-53.
43. Bailey AM, Constantinidou C, Ivens A, et al. Exposure of *Escherichia coli* and *Salmonella enterica* serovar *Typhimurium* to triclosan induces a species-specific response, including drug detoxification. *J Antimicrob Chemother*. 2009;64(5):973-985.
44. McBain AJ, Bartolo RG, Catrenich CE, et al. Exposure of sink drain microcosms to triclosan: population dynamics and antimicrobial susceptibility. *Appl Environ Microbiol*. 2003;69(9):5433-5442.
45. Carey DE, McNamara PJ. The impact of triclosan on the spread of antibiotic resistance in the environment. *Front Microbiol*. 2015;5:780.
46. McDonnell GE. *Antisepsis, Disinfection, and Sterilization: Types, Action, and Resistance*. 2nd ed. Washington, DC: ASM Press; 2017:143-154.

47. US Food and Drug Administration ruling on triclosan, TCC: safety and effectiveness of health care antiseptics: topical antimicrobial drug products for over the counter human use. *Fed Regist.* 2017;2(43):60474-60503. To be codified at 21 CFR §310.

48. Heath RJ, Rubin JR, Holland DR, Zhang E, Snow ME, Rock CO. Mechanism of triclosan inhibition of bacterial fatty acid synthesis. *J Biol Chem.* 1999;274(16):11110-11114.

49. McClellan K, Halden RU. Pharmaceuticals and personal care products in archived U.S. biosolids from the 2001 EPA National Sewage Sludge Survey. *Water Res.* 2010;44(2):658-668.

50. Carey DE, McNamara PJ. Altered antibiotic tolerance in anaerobic digesters acclimated to triclosan or triclocarban. *Chemosphere.* 2016;163:22-26.

51. Johnson TB, Hodge WW. A new method of synthesizing the higher phenols. *J Am Chem Soc.* 1913;35:1014-1023.

52. Johnson TB, Lane FW. The preparation of some alkyl derivatives of resorcinol and the relation of their structure to antiseptic properties. *J Am Chem Soc.* 1921;43:348-360.

53. Dohme ARL, Cox CH, Miller E. The preparation of aryl and alkyl derivatives of resorcinol. *J Am Chem Soc.* 1926;48:1688-1693.

54. Schaffer JM, Tilley FW. Further investigations of the relation between the chemical constitution and the germicidal activity of alcohols and phenols. *J Bacteriol.* 1927;14:259-273.

55. Hampil B. Bactericidal properties of the aryl and alkyl derivatives of resorcinol. *J Infect Dis.* 1928;43:25-40.

56. Rettger LF, Valley G, Plastridge WN. Disinfectant properties of certain alkyl phenols: I. Butyl resorcinol. *Centr Bakt Parasitenk, I Abt.* 1929;110:80-92.

57. Cains JF, Naidu BPB, Jang SJ. The bactericidal action of the common phenols and some of their derivatives on *B. pestis. Indian J Med Res.* 1928;15:117-134.

58. Woodward GJ, Kingery LB, Williams RJ. The fungicidal power of phenol derivatives. I. The effect of alkyl groups and halogens. *J Lab Clin Med.* 1934;19:1216-1223.

59. Paulus W. Acids. In: *Microbicides for the Protection of Materials.* New York, NY: Chapman Hall; 1993:199-226.

60. European Chemicals Agency. CLH report for salicylic acid 2014. European Chemicals Agency Web site. https://echa.europa.eu/documents/10162/9159532f-8623-453e-a4a2-625355b53608. Accessed June 18, 2018.

61. Sokol H. Recent developments in the preservation of pharmaceuticals. *Drug Stand.* 1952;20:89-106.

62. Sabalitschka T. Chemische konstitution und konservierungsvermogen. *Pharmazeutische Monatschefte.* 1924;5:235-237.

63. Sabalitschka T. Chemische konstitution und konservierungsvermogen. *Zeitschrift fürAngewandte Chemie.* 1924;37:811.

64. Sabalitschka T. Preservatives for pharmaceuticals and cosmetics. *Manufact Chemists.* 1931;2:5-7.

65. Sabalitschka T. Die konservierende Wirkung einiger Paraoxybenzoesaureester. *Pharmazeutische Monatschefte.* 1932;13:225-228.

66. Sabalitschka T, Tiedge KH. Synthetische studien über die Beziehung zwischen chemischer konstitution und antimikrober Wirkung. XII. 3-Nitro and 3-amino-4-hydroxylierte oder oxalkylierte Benzoesauren und deren Ester. *Archiv der Pharmazie.* 1934;272:383-394.

67. Sabalitschka T, Tietz H. Synthetische Studien über die Beziehung zwischen chemischer Konstitution und antimikrober Wirkung. XI. Zwei und derifach hydroxylierte oder oxyalkylierte Benzoesauren und deren Ester. *Archiv der Pharmazie.* 1931;269:545-566.

68. Gershenfeld L, Perlstein D. Preservatives for preparations containing gelatin. *Am J Pharm.* 1939;111:227-287.

69. Fukahori M, Akatsu S, Sato H, Yotsuyanagi T. Relationship between uptake of p-hydroxybenzoic acid esters by *Escherichia coli* and antibacterial activity. *Chem Pharm Bull (Tokyo).* 1996;44(8):1567-1570.

70. O'Connor DO, Rubino JR. Phenolic compounds. In: Block SS, ed. *Disinfection, Sterilization, and Preservation.* 4th ed. Philadelphia, PA: Lea & Febiger; 1991:204-224.

71. Matthews C, Davidson J, Bauer E, Morrison JL, Richardson AP. P-hydroxybenzoic acid esters as preservatives. II. Acute and chronic toxicity in dogs, rats, and mice. *J Am Pharm Assoc Am Pharm Assoc.* 1956;45:260-267.

72. Darbre PD, Aljarrah A, Miller WR, Coldham NG, Sauer MJ, Pope GS. Concentrations of parabens in human breast tumours. *J Appl Toxicol.* 2004;24(1):5-13.

73. Cosmetic Ingredient Review Expert Panel. CIR Expert Panel reaffirmed the safety of parabens used in cosmetics and personal care products—preservation vital to safety, 2012. Cosmetic Ingredient Review Web site. http://www.cir-safety.org/sites/default/files/paraben_build.pdf. Accessed December 1, 2017.

74. Scientific Committee on Consumer Safety. Opinion on parabens, SCCS/1348/10, 12/14/2010. European Commission Web site. http://ec.europa.eu/health/scientific_committees/consumer_safety/docs/sccs_o_041.pdf. Accessed December 1, 2017.

75. Scientific Committee on Consumer Safety. Clarification on opinion on parabens SCCS/1348/10 in the light of the Danish cause of safeguard banning the use of parabens in cosmetic products intended for children under three years of age. European Commission Web site. http://ec.europa.eu/health/scientific_committees/consumer_safety/docs/sccs_o_069.pdf. Accessed December 1, 2017.

76. Scientific Committee on Consumer Safety. Opinion on parabens. COLIPA no. P82. SCCS/1514/13. European Commission Web site. https://ec.europa.eu/health/sites/health/files/scientific_committees/consumer_safety/docs/sccs_o_132.pdf. Accessed December 1, 2017.

77. US Food and Drug Administration. Parabens in cosmetics 2017. US Food and Drug Administration Web site. http://www.fda.gov/cosmetics/productsingredients/ingredients/ucm128042.htm. Accessed December 1, 2017.

78. World Health Organization. WHO traditional medicine strategy 2002-2005. World Health Organization Web site. http://www.wpro.who.int/health_technology/book_who_traditional_medicine_strategy_2002_2005.pdf. Accessed November 28, 2017.

79. World Health Organization. WHO traditional medicine strategy: 2014-2023. World Health Organization Web site. http://www.who.int/medicines/publications/traditional/trm_strategy14_23/en/. Accessed November 28, 2017.

80. Gyawali R, Ibrahim SA. Natural products as antimicrobial agents. *Food Control.* 2014;46:412-429.

81. Lambert RJ, Skandamis PN, Coote PJ, Nychas GJ. A study of the minimum inhibitory concentration and mode of action of oregano essential oil, thymol and carvacrol. *J Appl Microbiol.* 2001;91(3):453-462.

82. Larrainzar MG, Rua J, Caro I, et al. Evaluation of antimicrobial and antioxidant activities of natural phenolic compounds against foodborne pathogens and spoilage bacteria. *Food Control.* 2012;26(2):555-563.

83. Cetin-Karaca H, Newman MC. Antimicrobial efficacy of natural phenolic compounds against gram positive foodborne pathogens. *J Food Research.* 2015;4(6):14-27.

84. Macé S, Hansen LT, Rupasinghe HPV. Anti-bacterial activity of phenolic compounds against *Streptococcus pyogenes. Medicines (Basel).* 2017;4(2):25.

85. Klarmann EG, Shternov VA, Von Wowern J. The germicidal action of halogen derivatives of phenol and resorcinol and its impairment by organic matter. *J Bacteriol.* 1929;17(16):423-442.

86. Russell AD. Factors influencing the efficacy of antimicrobial agents. In: Russell AD, Hugo WB, Ayliffe GA, eds. *Principles and Practice of Disinfection, Preservation, and Sterilization.* 3rd ed. Oxford, United Kingdom: Blackwell Scientific; 1999:95-123.

87. Karabit MS. Studies on the evaluation of preservative efficacy. V. Effect of concentration of microorganisms on the antimicrobial activity of phenol. *International J Pharmaceutics.* 1990;60:147-150.

88. Russell AD, Chopra I. Antiseptics, disinfectants and preservatives: their properties, mechanism of action and uptake into bacteria. In: *Understanding Antibacterial Action and Resistance.* 2nd ed. London, United Kingdom: Ellis Horwood; 1996:96-149.

89. Bloomfield SF, Arthjur M, Begun K, et al. Comparative testing of disinfectants using proposed European surface test methods. *Lett Appl Microbiol.* 1993;17:119-125.

90. Das JR, Bhakoo M, Jones MV, Gilbert P. Changes in the biocide susceptibility of *Staphylococcus epidermidis* and *Escherichia coli* cells associated with rapid attachment to plastic surfaces. *J Appl Microbiol.* 1998;84(5):852-858.

91. Cooper EA. The bactericidal action of cresols and allied compounds. *BMJ.* 1912;1:1234, 1293, 1359.

92. Cooper EA. Relations of phenols and their derivatives to proteins. *Biochem J.* 1913;7:175-185.

93. Paulus W, Genth H. Microbicidal phenolic compounds: a critical examination. *Biodet.* 1983;5:701-712.

94. Bean HS, Das A. The absorption by *Escherichia coli* of phenols and their bactericidal activity. *J Pharm Pharmacol.* 1966;18(suppl 1):107S-113S.

95. Hugo WB. Disinfection mechanisms. In: Russell AD, Hugo WB, Ayliffe GA, eds. *Principles and Practices of Disinfection, Preservation, and Sterilization.* 3rd ed. Oxford, United Kingdom: Blackwell Scientific; 1999:258-283.

96. Judis J. Mechanism of action of phenolic disinfectants. III. Uptake of phenol-C-14, 2,4-dichlorophenol-C-14, and p-tert-amylphenol-C-14 by *Escherichia coli. J Pharm Sci.* 1964;53:196-201.

97. Greenberg M, Dodds M, Tian M. Naturally occurring phenolic antibacterial compounds show effectiveness against oral bacteria by a quantitative structure-activity relationship study. *J Agric Food Chem.* 2008;56(23):11151-11156.

98. Pulvertaft RJ, Lumb GD. Bacterial lysis and antiseptics. *J Hyg (Lond).* 1948;46:62-64.

99. Srivastava RB, Thompson RE. Influence of bacterial cell age on phenol action. *Nature.* 1965;206(980):216.

100. Srivastava RB, Thompson RE. Studies on the mechanism of action of phenol in *Escherichia coli* cells. *Brit J Experimental Pathol.* 1966;67:315-323.

101. Denyer SP. Mechanisms of action of biocides. *Int Biodeterioration.* 1990;26:89-100.

102. Jang HJ, Nde C, Toghrol F, Bentley WE. Microarray analysis of toxicogenomic effects of ortho-phenylphenol in *Staphylococcus aureus. BMC Genomics.* 2008;9:411.

103. Nde CW, Jang HJ, Toghrol F, Bentley WE. Toxicogenomic response of *Pseudomonas aeruginosa* to ortho-phenylphenol. *BMC Genomics.* 2008;9:473.

104. Frederick JJ, Corner TR, Gerhardt P. Antimicrobial actions of hexachlorophene: inhibition of respiration in *Bacillus megaterium. Antimicrob Agents Chemother.* 1974;6(6):712-721.

105. Regös J, Hitz HR. Investigations on the mode of action of triclosan, a broad spectrum antimicrobial agent. *Zentralbl Bakteriol Orig A.* 1974;226(3):390-401.

106. Commager H, Judis J. Mechanism of action of phenolic disinfectants. VI. Effects on glucose and succinate metabolism of *Escherichia coli. J Pharm Sci.* 1965;54:1436-1439.

107. Hugo WB, Bowen JG. Studies on the mode of action of 4-ethylphenol on *Escherichia coli. Microbios.* 1973;8(31):189-197.

108. Hugo WB, Bloomfield SF. Studies on the mode of action of the phenolic antibacterial agent fentichlor against *Staphylococcus aureus* and *Escherichia coli.* III. The effect of fentichlor on the metabolic activities of *Staphylococcus aureus* and *Escherichia coli. J Appl Bacteriol.* 1971;34(3):579-591.

109. Bloomfield SF. The effect of the phenolic antibacterial agent fentichlor on energy coupling in *Staphylococcus aureus. J Appl Bacteriol.* 1974;37:117-131.

110. Denyer SP, Hugo WB, Witham RF. The antibacterial action of a series of 4-*n*-alkyl phenols. *J Pharm Pharmacol.* 1980;32:27P.

111. Denyer SP, Hugo WB, Harding VD. The biochemical basis of synergy between the antibacterial agent chlorocresol and 2-phenylethanol. *Int J Pharmacol.* 1986;29:29-36.

112. Eklund T. Inhibition of growth and uptake processes in bacteria by some chemical food preservatives. *J Appl Bacteriol.* 1980;48:423-432.

113. Eklund T. The effect of sorbic acid and esters of p-hydroxybenzoic acid on the proton motive force in *Escherichia coli* membrane vesicles. *J Gen Microbiol.* 1985;131(1):73-76.

114. Lambert PA, Hammond SM. Potassium fluxes, first indications of membrane damage in micro-organisms. *Biochem Biophys Res Commun.* 1973;54(2):796-799.

115. Kroll RG, Anagnostopoulos GD. Potassium leakage as a lethality index of phenol and the effect of solute and water activity. *J Appl Bacteriol.* 1981;50:139-147.

116. Gale EF, Taylor ES. Action of tyrocidine and some detergent substances in releasing amino acids from the internal environment of *Streptococcus faecalis. J Gen Microbiol.* 1947;1:77-84.

117. Judis J. Studies on the mechanism of action of phenolic disinfectants. I. Release of radioactivity from carbon-14-labeled *Escherichia coli. J Pharm Sci.* 1962;51:261-265.

118. Judis J. Studies on the mechanism of action of phenolic disinfectants. II. Patterns of release of radioactivity from *Escherichia coli* labeled by growth on various compounds. *J Pharm Sci.* 1963;52:126-131.

119. Hugo WB, Bloomfield SF. Studies on the mode of action of the phenolic antibacterial agent fentichlor against *Staphylococcus aureus* and *Escherichia coli.* I. The adsorption of fentichlor by the bacterial cell and its antibacterial activity. *J Appl Bacteriol.* 1971;34(3):557-567.

120. Hugo WB, Bloomfield SF. Studies on the mode of action of the phenolic antibacterial agent fentichlor against *Staphylococcus aureus* and *Escherichia coli.* II. The effects of fentichlor on the bacterial membrane and the cytoplasmic constituents of the cell. *J Appl Bacteriol.* 1971;34(3):569-578.

121. Joswick HL, Corner TR, Silvernale JN, Gerhardt P. Antimicrobial actions of hexachlorophene: release of cytoplasmic materials. *J Bacteriol.* 1971;108:492-500.

122. Bach D, Lambert J. Action de quelques antiseptiques sur la lacticodeshydrogenase du staphylocoque dore. *Compt Rend Soc Biol (Paris).* 1937;126:298-300.

123. Bach D, Lambert J. Action de quelques antiseptiques sur les deshydrogenase du staphylocoque dore; systemes activants le glucose, l'acide formique et un certain nombre d'autres substrates. *Compt Rend Soc Biol (Paris).* 1937;126:300-302.

124. Sykes G. Influence of germicides on dehydrogenase of *Bacterium coli*: succinic acid dehydrogenase of *Bacterium coli. J Hyg.* 1939;59:463-469.

125. McMurry LM, McDermott PF, Levy SB. Genetic evidence that InhA of *Mycobacterium smegmatis* is a target for triclosan. *Antimicrob Agents Chemother.* 1999;43:711-713.

126. Suller MT, Russell AD. Triclosan and antibiotic resistance in *Staphylococcus aureus. J Antimicrob Chemother.* 2000;46:11-18.

127. McDonnell G, Russell AD. Antiseptics and disinfectants: activity, action, and resistance. *Clin Microbiol Rev.* 1999;12:147-179.

128. Escalada MG, Russell AD, Maillard JY, Ochs D. Triclosan-bacteria interactions: single or multiple target sites? *Lett Appl Microbiol.* 2005;41(6):476-481.

129. Bancroft WD, Richter GH. The chemistry of disinfection. *J Phys Chem.* 1931;35:511-530.

130. Corner TR, Joswick HL, Silvernale JN, Gerhardt P. Antimicrobial actions of hexachlorophene: lysis and fixation of bacterial protoplasts. *J Bacteriol.* 1971;108:501-507.

131. Tilley FW, McDonald AD, Schaffer JM. Germicidal efficiency of o-phenylphenol against *Mycobacterium tuberculosis. J Agric Res.* 1931;42:653-656.

132. Klarmann EG, Shternov VA, Gates LW. The bactericidal and fungicidal action of homologous halogen phenol derivatives and its "quasi-specific" character. *J Lab Clin Med.* 1934;19:835-851.

133. Wright ES, Shternov VA. An adaption of the phenol coefficient method to *Mycobacterium tuberculosis. Proc Chem Soc Manufact Assoc.* 1958;95-99.

134. Hegna IK. An examination of the effect of three phenolic disinfectants on *Mycobacterium tuberculosis. J Appl Bacteriol.* 1977;43(2):183-187.

135. Smith CR. Disinfectants for tuberculosis hygiene. *Soap Sanitary Chem.* 1951;27:130-134.

136. Wright ES, Mundy RA. Studies on disinfection of clinical thermometers. II. Oral thermometers from a tuberculosis sanatorium. *Appl Microbiol.* 1961;9:508-510.

137. Russell AD. Mechanisms of bacterial resistance to biocide. *Int Biodeterioration Biodegradation.* 1995;36:247-265.

138. Rubin J. Mycobactericidal disinfection and control. In: Block SS, ed. *Disinfection, Sterilization, and Preservation.* 4th ed. Philadelphia, PA: Lea & Febiger; 1991:377-384.

139. Russell AD. Mycobactericidal agents. In: Russell AD, Hugo WB, Ayliffe GA, eds. *Principles and Practices of Disinfection, Preservation, and Sterilization.* 3rd ed. Oxford, United Kingdom: Blackwell Scientific; 1999:321-322.

140. Russell AD, Chopra I. Sporistatic and sporicidal agents: their properties and mechanism of action. In: *Understanding Antibacterial Action and Resistance.* 2nd ed. London, United Kingdom: Ellis Horwood; 1996:150-171.

141. Bloomfield SF, Arthur M. Mechanisms of inactivation and resistance of spores to chemical biocides. *Soc Appl Bacteriol Symp Ser.* 1994;23:91S-104S.

142. Maillard JY. Bacterial target sites for biocide action. *J Appl Microbiol.* 2002;92(suppl):16S-27S.

143. Rempe CS, Burris KP, Lenaghan SC, Stewart CN Jr. The potential of systems biology to discover antibacterial mechanisms of plant phenolics. *Front Microbiol.* 2017;8:422. https://www.frontiersin.org/articles/10.3389/fmicb.2017.00422/full.

144. Russell AD. Antifungal activity of biocide. In: Russell AD, Hugo, WB, Ayliffe GA, eds. *Principles and Practices of Disinfection, Preservation, and Sterilization.* 3rd ed. Oxford, United Kingdom: Blackwell Scientific; 1999:149-167.

145. Karabit MS, Juneskans OT, Lundgren P. Studies on the evaluation of preservative efficacy. I. The determination of antimicrobial characteristics of phenol. *Acta Pharm Suec.* 1985;22:281-290.

146. Terleckyj B, Axler DA. Quantitative neutralization assay of fungicidal activity of disinfectants. *Antimicrob Agents Chemother.* 1987;31:794-798.

147. Hegna IK. A comparative investigation of the bactericidal and fungicidal effect of three phenolic disinfectants. *J Appl Bacteriol.* 1977;43:179-181.

148. Russell AD, Furr JR. Biocides: mechanisms of antifungal action and fungal resistance. *Sci Prog.* 1996;79(pt 1):27-48.

149. Ansari SB, Anurag A, Fatima Z, Hameed S. Natural phenolic compounds: a potential anti-fungal agent. *Formatex.* 2013;1189-1195.

150. Aziz NH, Farag SE, Mousa LA, Abo-Zaid MA. Comparative antibacterial and antifungal effects of some phenolic compounds. *Microbios.* 1998;93(374):43-54.

151. Zabka M, Pavela R. Antifungal efficacy of some natural phenolic compounds against significant pathogenic and toxicogenic filamentous fungi. *Chemosphere.* 2013;93(6):1051-1056.

152. Pizzolitto RP, Barberis CL, Dambolena JS, et al. Inhibitory effect of natural phenolic compounds on *Aspergillus parasiticus* growth. *J Chemistry.* 2015;2015:1-7.

153. Teodoro GR, Ellepola K, Seneviratne CJ, Koga-Ito CY. Potential use of phenolic acids as anti-candida agents: a review. *Front Microbiol.* 2015;6:1420.

154. Prince HN, Prince DL, Prince RN. Principles of viral control and transmission. In: Block SS, ed. *Disinfection, Sterilization, and Preservation.* 4th ed. Philadelphia, PA: Lea & Febiger; 1991:411-444.

155. Klein M, Deforest A. The inactivation of viruses by germicides. *Proc Chem Soc Manufact Assoc.* 1963;49:116-118.

156. US Environmental Protection Agency. EPA pesticide registration (PR) notice 2001-4. Environmental Protection Agency Web site. https://www.epa.gov/sites/production/files/2014-04/documents/pr2001-4.pdf. Accessed December 1, 2017.

157. Wood A, Payne D. The action of three antiseptics/disinfectants against enveloped and non-enveloped viruses. *J Hosp Infect.* 1998;38(4):283-295.

158. Maillard J-Y. Viricidal activity of biocides. D. Mechanism of virucidal action. In: Russell AD, Hugo WB, Ayliffe GA, eds. *Principles and Practices of Disinfection, Preservation, and Sterilization.* 3rd ed. Oxford, United Kingdom: Blackwell Scientific; 1999:207-221.

159. Sattar AS, Springthorpe S. Virucidal activity of biocides. A. Activity against human viruses. In: Russell AD, Hugo WB, Ayliffe GA, eds. *Principles and Practices of Disinfection, Preservation, and Sterilization.* 3rd ed. Oxford, United Kingdom: Blackwell Scientific; 1999:168-186.

160. Maillard J-Y, Beggs TS, Day MJ, Hudson RA, Russell AD. Damage to *Pseudomonas aeruginosa* PAO1 bacteriophage F116 DNA by biocides. *J Appl Bacteriol.* 1996;80(5):540-544.

161. Maillard J-Y, Beggs TS, Day MJ, Hudson RA, Russell AD. The effects of biocides on the transduction of *Pseudomonas aeruginosa* PAO by F116 bacteriophage. *Lett Appl Microbiol.* 1995;21:215-218.

162. Maillard J-Y, Hann AC, Beggs TS, Day MJ, Hudson RA, Russell AD. Electron microscopic investigation of the effects of biocides on *Pseudomonas aeruginosa* PAO bacteriophage F116. *J Med Microbiol.* 1995;42(6):415-420.

163. Chávez JH, Leal PC, Yunes RA, et al. Evaluation of antiviral activity of phenolic compounds and derivatives against rabies virus. *Vet Microbiol.* 2006;116(1-3):53-59.

164. Suárez B, Álvarez ÁL, García YD, Del Barrio G, Lobo AP, Parra F. Phenolic profiles, antioxidant activity and *in vitro* antiviral properties of apple pomace. *Food Chem.* 2010;120:339-342.

165. Silva ARA, Morais SM, Marques MMM, et al. Antiviral activities of extracts and phenolic components of two *Spondias* species against dengue virus. *J Venom Anim Toxins Incl Trop Dis.* 2011;17(4):406-413.

166. Rapps NF. The bactericidal efficiency of chlorocresol and chloroxylenol. *J Soc Chemical Industry.* 1933;52:175T-176T.

167. Evans WP, Dunbar SE. Effect of surfactants on germicides and preservatives. In: *Surface Activity and the Microbial Cell.* London, United Kingdom: Society of Chemical Industries; 1965:169-192.

168. Bean HS, Berry H. The bactericidal activity of phenols in aqueous solutions of soap; the solubility of a water-insoluble phenol in aqueous solutions of soap. *J Pharm Pharmacol.* 1950;2:484-490.

169. Bean HS, Berry H. The bactericidal activity of phenols in aqueous solutions of soap. II. The bactericidal activity of benzylchlorophenol in aqueous solutions of potassium laurate. *J Pharm Pharmacol.* 1951;3(10):639-655.

170. Bean HS, Berry H. The bactericidal activity of phenols in aqueous solutions of soap. III. The bactericidal activity of chloroxylenol in aqueous solutions of potassium laurate. *J Pharm Pharmacol.* 1953;5:632-639.

171. Alexander AE, Tomlinson AJ. *Surface Chemistry.* Butterworth, London: Interscience Publishers; 1949:317.

172. Allawala NA, Riegelman S. Phenol coefficients and the Ferguson principle. *J Am Pharm Assoc Am Pharm Assoc.* 1954;43(2):93-97.

173. Allawala NA, Riegelman S. The release of antimicrobial agents from solutions of surface-active agents. *J Am Pharm Assoc Am Pharm Assoc.* 1953;42(5):267-275.

174. Wedderburn DL. Preservation of emulsions against microbial attack. In: Bean H, Beckett A, Carless J, eds. *Advances in Pharmaceutical Sciences.* Vol 1. New York, NY: Academic Press; 1964:195-268.

175. Kostenbauder HB. Physical factors influencing the activity of antimicrobial agents. In: Block SS, ed. *Disinfection, Sterilization, and Preservation.* 4th ed. Philadelphia, PA: Lea & Febiger; 1991:59-71.

176. Lundy HW. The effect of salts upon the germicidal action of phenol and sec-amyltricresol. *J Bacteriol.* 1938;35(6):633-639.

177. Ordal EJ, Wilson JL, Borg AF. Studies on the action of wetting agents on microorganisms. I. The effect of pH and wetting agents on the germicidal action of phenolic compounds. *J Bacteriol.* 1941;42(1):117-126.

178. Cade AR. Germicidal detergents—the synergistic action of soaps on the germicidal efficiency of phenols. *Soap.* 1935;11:27-30, 115-117.

179. Ortenzio LF, Opalsky CD, Stuart LS. Factors affecting the activity of phenolic disinfectants. *Appl Microbiol.* 1961;9:562-566.

180. Prindle RF. Practical aspects of interaction of surfactants and disinfectants. *Soap Chem Spec.* 1959;34:81-89.

181. Roesin M, Pilz I, Olerin G. The synergism between disinfectants and surface-active substances. *Farmatsiia.* 1960;8:629-631.

182. Davis B. Surfactant-biocide interactions. In: Porter MR, ed. *Recent Developments in the Technology of Surfactants: Critical Reports in Applied Chemistry.* Vol 30. Dordrecht, Netherlands: Elsevier Applied Science; 1990:65-131.

183. Thoma K, Ullmann E, Fickel O. Influence of auxiliary materials on pharmaceuticals. 23. Depreciating interactions of disinfectants and preservatives with non-ionogenic surfactants I: the antibacterial activity of phenols in the presence of polyoxyethylene sterates and polyethylene glycols. *Arch Pharm (Weinheim).* 1970;303:289-296.

184. Haag TE, Loncrini DF. Esters of para-hydroxybenzoic acid. In: Kabara JJ, ed. *Cosmetic and Drug Preservation: Principles and Practice.* New York, NY: Marcel Dekker; 1984:63-77. *Cosmetic Science Technology Series*; vol 1.

185. Klarmann EG. Environmental disinfection; a factor in the control of staphylococcal hospital sepsis. *Am J Pharm Sci Support Public Health.* 1957;129(2):42-52.

186. Rutala WA, Stiegel MM, Sarubbi FA, Weber DJ. Susceptibility of antibiotic-susceptible and antibiotic-resistant hospital bacteria to disinfectants. *Infect Control Hosp Epidemiol.* 1997;18(6):417-421.

187. Chuanchuen R, Narasaki CT, Schweizer HP. The MexJK efflux pump of *Pseudomonas aeruginosa* requires OprM for antibiotic efflux but not for efflux of triclosan. *J Bacteriol.* 2002;184(18):5036-5044.

188. Kline & Company. *Personal Care Ingredients: Global Market Analysis.* Parsippany, NJ: Kline & Company; 2015.

189. Kline & Company. *Specialty Biocides: Regional Market Analysis.* Parsippany, NJ: Kline & Company; 2016.

190. Steinberg DC. *Preservatives for Cosmetics.* 3rd ed. Carol Stream, IL: Allured Books; 2012.

191. Rutala WA. APIC guideline for selection and use of disinfectants. *Am J Infect Control.* 1990;18:99-117.

192. Federal Insecticide, Fungicide, and Rodenticide Act as amended, 540/09-89-012, revised Sept 2012.

193. Marzulli FN, Maibach HI. Antimicrobials: experimental contact sensitization in man. *J Soc Cosmet Chemists.* 1973;24:399A21.

194. Larson EL. APIC guideline for handwashing and hand antisepsis in health care settings. *Am J Infect Control.* 1995;23(4):251-269.

195. Steinberg DC. Frequency of use preservative use update through 2014. *Cosmetics and Toiletries.* 2014;131:56-60.

196. Brady LM, Thomson M, Palmer MA, Harkness JL. Successful control of endemic MRSA in a cardiothoracic surgical unit. *Med J Aust.* 1990;152(5):240-245.

197. Tuffnell DJ, Croton RS, Hemingway DM, Hartley MN, Wake PN, Garvey RJ. Methicillin resistant *Staphylococcus aureus*; the role of antisepsis in the control of an outbreak. *J Hosp Infect.* 1987;10(3):255-259.

198. Webster J. Handwashing in a neonatal intensive care nursery: product acceptability and effectiveness of chlorhexidine gluconate 4% and triclosan 1%. *J Hosp Infect.* 1992;21(2):137-141.

199. Zafar AB, Butler RC, Reese DJ, Gaydos LA, Mennonna PA. Use of 0.3% triclosan (Bacti-Stat) to eradicate an outbreak of methicillin-resistant *Staphylococcus aureus* in a neonatal nursery. *Am J Infect Control.* 1995;23(3):200-208.

200. FDA issues final rule on safety and effectiveness of antibacterial soaps [press release]. Silver Spring, MD: FDA Anonymous; September 2, 2016.

201. US Department of Health and Human Services, US Food and Drug Administration. Safety and effectiveness of health care antiseptics; topical antimicrobial drug products for over-the-counter human use; final rule. *Fed Regist.* 2017;82(242):60474-60503.

202. Mandel ID. Chemotherapeutic agents for controlling plaque and gingivitis. *J Clin Periodontol.* 1988;15(8):488-498.

203. Lockhart JD. Hexachlorophene and the Food and Drug Administration. *J Clin Pharmacol.* 1973;13(11):445-450.

204. Gottfried N. Alkyl p-hydroxybenzoate esters as pharmaceutical preservatives: a review of the parabens. *Am J Hosp Pharm.* 1962;19:310-314.

205. O'Neill JJ, Peelor P, Peterson AF, et al. Selection of parabens as preservatives for cosmetics and toiletries. *J Soc Cosmet Chem.* 1979;30:25-39.

206. Jay JM. Antimicrobial food preservatives. In: Rossmoore HW, ed. *Handbook of Biocide and Preservative Use.* New York, NY: Blackie Academic & Professional; 1995:334-348.

207. Hill G. Preservation of cosmetics and toiletries. In: Rossmoore HW, ed. *Handbook of Biocides and Preservative Use.* New York, NY: Blackie Academic & Professional; 1995:349-416.

208. Patnaik P. Phenols. In: *A Comprehensive Guide to the Hazardous Properties of Chemical Substances.* New York, NY: Van Nostrand Reinhold; 1992:582-592.

209. Registry of Toxic Effects of Chemical Substances. Tomes Micromedix; 1999. https://www.cdc.gov/niosh/rtecs/RTECSaccess.html.

210. Stouten H. Toxicological profile for *o*-phenylphenol and its sodium salt. *J Appl Toxicol.* 1998;18(4):261-270.

211. Stouten H, Bessems JG. Toxicological profile for *o*-benzyl-p-chlorophenol. *J Appl Toxicol.* 1998;18(4):271-279.

212. Anon. Final report on the safety assessment of chloroxylenol. *J Am Coll Toxicol.* 1985;4:147-169.

213. Wilson B, Chen R, Cantwell M, Gontz A, Zhu J, Olsen C. The partitioning of triclosan between aqueous and particulate bound phases in the Hudson River Estuary. *Mar Pollut Bull.* 2009;59(4-7):207-212.

214. Kumar KS, Priya SM, Peck AM, Sajwan KS. Mass loadings of triclosan and triclocarban from four wastewater treatment plants to three rivers and landfill in Savannah, Georgia, USA. *Arch Environ Contam Toxicol.* 2010;58(2):275-285.

215. Regulation (EU) No 528/2012 of the European Parliament and of the Council of 22 May 2012 concerning the making available on the market and the use of biocidal products. https://eur-lex.europa.eu/legal-content/EN/TXT/?uri=CELEX%3A32012R0528. Accessed April 2018.

216. Regulation (EC) No 1223/2009 of the European Parliament and of the Council of 30 November 2009 on cosmetic products. https://ec.europa.eu/health/sites/health/files/endocrine_disruptors/docs/cosmetic_1223_2009_regulation_en.pdf. Accessed April 2018.

Surface-Active Agents

John J. Merianos and Gerald McDonnell

Surface-active agents (*surfactants*) are amphiphilic compounds, which means one portion of the molecule is *hydrophilic*, or "water-loving," and the other portion of the molecule is *lipophilic*, or "oil-loving." The origin of the term *amphiphile* comes from the Greek word *amphi*, meaning that all surfactant molecules consist of at least two parts: one hydrophilic and one lipophilic. Chemically, the hydrophilic moiety of the molecule may be a carboxylate, sulfate, sulfonate, phosphate, or some other polar group. The lipophilic portion of the molecule is a nonpolar group, usually of a hydrocarbon nature. A schematic presentation of surfactant molecules is given in Figure 21.1, which illustrates the hydrophilic head group with a hydrophobic tail. The different surfactant molecules are typically classified based on the overall charge at their hydrophilic (polar) head groups: nonionic having no overall charge, cationic with a positive charge, anionic a negative charge, and amphoteric (or zwitterionic) with two oppositely charged groups. Figure 21.1 also shows how surfactants form micelles (or aggregates of surfactant molecule) and can be used to solubilize drugs or other insoluble molecules in various formulations as well as to aid in the removal of materials (eg, lipids on surfaces) in liquids such as water. By far, surfactants' most valuable application to the pharmaceutical and agricultural industries is their ability to solubilize drugs as a result of their amphiphilic nature, but they are also widely used as cleaning and disinfection agents.

▶ PHYSICAL PROPERTIES

The fundamental property of surfactants is their tendency to accumulate at interfaces, such as solid-liquid (*suspension*), liquid-liquid (*emulsion*), or liquid-vapor (*foam*).[1] Surface-active agents possess both water-soluble and oil-soluble characteristics. The dual solubility of the surfactants makes them able to exhibit unique properties.

If a compound is completely water soluble or completely oil soluble, it will not collect at the interface; instead, it will dissolve in the medium in which it is soluble. It is the nonpolar group that allows the compound to be partially oil soluble and the polar group that allows the compound to be partially water soluble.

Another important characteristic of surfactants is their capacity to lower surface or interfacial tension. Surface tension of a liquid is the force that opposes the expansion of the surface area of that liquid. Interfacial tension is similar to surface tension; however, one important difference is the location at which the tension occurs. Interfacial tension takes place at the interface of the two immiscible liquids, whereas surface tension takes place between the liquid surface and the air. Electrostatic or molecular forces are responsible for surface and interfacial tension. These forces are the reason for the mutual attraction of molecules for one another. Many molecules, although electrically neutral, have an uneven distribution of electrical charge, thus giving them polarity, or a negative or positive center of electricity. These negative and positive centers of electricity create the electrostatic forces within molecules.

The molecules in a liquid possess electrostatic forces, giving rise to intermolecular attraction. This attraction between "like" molecules is caused by *cohesive forces*. *Adhesional forces* occur because of the molecular attraction between the liquid's surface and the liquid molecules. The net result of the adhesional forces and the cohesive forces at the interface of two immiscible liquids is known as *interfacial tension*. If the cohesive forces, which tend to hold the liquid molecules together, are stronger than the adhesional forces, which tend to pull the surface of the molecules apart, the interfacial tension will be high and the two liquids will not mix. To lower the interfacial tension between two immiscible liquids, the interface between the two liquids must be altered by some means. This may be accomplished by adding a substance that is

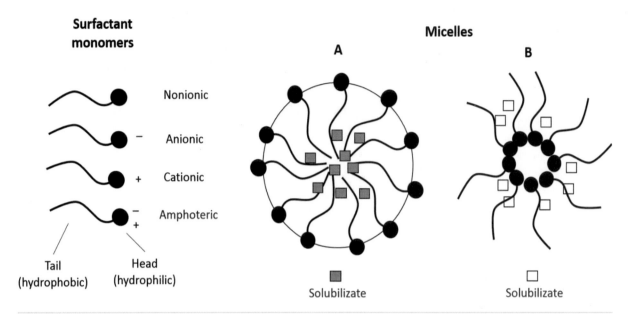

FIGURE 21.1   A representation of the structure of surfactant monomers and associated classification based on their overall charge (nonionic, anionic, cationic, and amphoteric). Also shown (right) are examples of micelles or aggregates of surfactants and the locations of solubilizates in spherical micelles. A, Ionic surfactant (solubilized molecules in this case have no hydrophilic groups). B, Nonionic surfactant (with polar solubilizate). Based on Zografi et al[1] and Harvey.[2]

capable of orienting itself between the liquid layers. On collection of a surface-active substance at the interface, there is a reduction of interfacial tension. These surface-active compounds are called *emulsified agents*, which help to hold together two immiscible liquids, forming a water-in-oil or an oil-in-water emulsion.

Stearic acid is an example of a surface-active compound. When stearic acid is placed in water, the molecules will collect at the surface. The molecules cannot go beyond the surface because the hydrophobic (or lipophilic groups) are insoluble in the water. Because of the dual-solubility characteristics of stearic acid molecules, they are adsorbed on the surface of the liquid and then are able to lower the surface tension of water. When the water and petrolatum are mixed, they have an interfacial tension of 57 dynes/cm. With the addition of a drop of stearic acid to water alone, the acid collects at the surface, with its polar groups projected in the water and its nonpolar groups oriented in an outward direction. The interfacial tension between the stearic acid and the water is 15 dynes/cm. When liquid petrolatum is added to the water-stearic acid mixture, the interfacial tension still remains at 15 dynes/cm. The monomolecular layer of the stearic acid between the liquid interface serves to lower the interfacial tension from 57 dynes/cm to 15 dynes/cm.

Another fundamental property of the surface-active agents is that in solution, they tend to form micelles or aggregates (see Figure 21.1). The different types of micelles formed by surfactants are shown in Figure 21.2. Micelle formation, or *micellization*, reduces the free energy of

the system by decreasing the hydrophobic surface area exposed to water. The surfactant molecules behave differently when present in micelles compared with free monomers in solution. Micelles are a reservoir for surfactant molecules, usually in their *monomer* (single molecule) form. The ability of the surfactant molecules to lower surface interfacial tension and dynamic phenomena, such as wetting and foaming, is governed by the concentration of free monomers in solution. Micelles are generated at low surfactant concentration in water. The concentration at which micelles start to form is called the *critical micelle concentration* (CMC) and is an important characteristic for each surfactant. Table 21.1 lists the CMC and micellar aggregation numbers for the three most common types of surfactants: anionic, cationic, and nonionic (with the values recorded in water at room temperature).

The global surfactants market was estimated to be approximately $43 million in 2017 and is projected to rise to approximately $66 million by 2025. The classification of surfactants is typically made on the basis of the charge of the hydrophilic (polar) group. There are four major classes of surfactants (in order of decreasing, estimated volume demand):

A. Anionics (approximately 40%)
B. Nonionics (approximately 30%)
C. Cationics (approximately 20%)
D. Amphoterics or zwitterions (<10%)

The anionic group, which consists of alkaline salts of fatty acids, is by far the largest group used by consumers

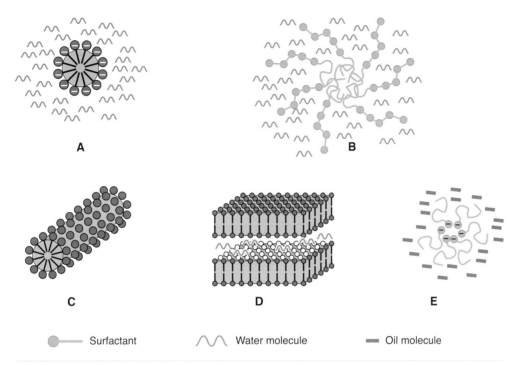

FIGURE 21.2 Examples of different types of micelles. A, Spherical micelle of an anionic surfactant. B, Spherical micelle of a nonionic surfactant. C, Cylindrical micelle. D, Lamellar micelle. E, Reverse micelle of an anionic surfactant in oil. Based on Zografi et al[1] and Harvey.[2]

in the form of soaps. Commercially, soaps are prepared by saponification of animal fats, vegetable oil, coconut oil, palm oil, or natural fatty acid glycerides in caustic solution. The soaps, in addition to their cleaning and detergent characteristics, are used in the pharmaceutical industry for their ability to solubilize compounds. They also act as wetting agent for solid dosage forms and emulsifying agent in emulsion formation. Monovalent soaps (Na^+, K^+) will give oil-in-water emulsions. Divalent soaps (Ca^{2+}, Mg^{2+}), due to their poor water solubility, will produce water-in-oil emulsions. The triethanolamine salts of fatty acids will give an oil-in-water emulsion. The synthetic anionic surfactants of commercial importance in this category include the following: alkyl sulfate, alkyl ether sulfate, alkyl benzenesulfonate, alkyl xylenesulfonate, dialkyl sulfosuccinate, alkyl phosphate, alkyl ether phosphate, alkyl ether carboxylate, and others.

The nonionic group is a major class of surfactants used widely throughout the pharmaceutical industry as a result of its low toxicity, good compatibility, and excellent stability in biologic systems. The most widely used compounds are the polyoxyethylene sorbitan fatty acid esters, which are found in both internal and external pharmaceutical formulations. The polar group in this category is a polyether or polyhydroxy oxyethylene unit attached to a fatty alcohol, fatty acid, or fatty amide moiety. These compounds can be water insoluble or quite water soluble, depending on the degree of ethoxylation. Ethoxylated surfactants can be tailor-made with regard to the average

number of oxyethylene units added to a specific fatty alcohol. Representative commercially available nonionic surfactants include fatty alcohol ethoxylate, fatty acid ethoxylate, fatty amide ethoxylate, fatty amine ethoxylate, alkyl glucoside, sorbitan alkanoate (Span™), ethoxylated sorbitan alkanoate (Tween™), alkylphenol ethoxylate (Igepal™ CO, Nonoxynol-9 or -11). The ethers offer an advantage over the esters in that they are quite resistant to alkaline or acidic hydrolysis. Nonionic surfactants are compatible with all other classes of surfactants and have been used as stabilizers, wetting agents, dispersants, detergents, and emulsifiers.

The interfacial properties of nonionics are greatly influenced by the polarity or nonpolarity of the system. As a result of the importance of polarity, a system was developed to assign a hydrophilic-lipophilic balance (HLB) number to each surfactant. The HLB value is the percentage weight of the hydrophilic group divided by 5 to reduce the range of values. On a molar basis, a 100% hydrophilic molecule (polyethylene glycol) would have a value of 20. The Atlas Powder Company[3] devised the HLB number system for nonionic surfactants used as emulsifying agents (Table 21.2). Griffin[4] developed an HLB scale, which is a numeric scale that extends from 1 to approximately 50. There is a relationship between the different applications of surfactants and the HLB range (Table 21.3), and there are methods available to calculate the HLB value of new surface-active agents. Table 21.4 provides examples of how to calculate the HLB value of

TABLE 21.1 Critical micelle concentrations (CMCs) and micellar aggregation numbers of various surfactants in water at room temperature

Structure	Name	CMC, mM/L	Surfactant Molecules/Micelle
Anionic			
$n\text{-}C_{11}H_{23}COOK$	Potassium laurate	24	50
$n\text{-}C_8H_{17}SO_3Na$	Sodium octant sulfonate	150	28
$n\text{-}C_{10}H_{21}SO_3Na$	Sodium decane sulfonate	40	40
$n\text{-}C_{12}H_{25}SO_3Na$	Sodium dodecane sulfonate	9	54
$n\text{-}C_{12}H_{25}OSO_3Na$	Sodium lauryl sulfate	8	62
$n\text{-}C_{12}H_{25}OSO_3Na$	Sodium lauryl sulfates	1	96
	Sodium di-2-ethylhexyl sulfosuccinate	5	48
Cationic			
$n\text{-}C_{10}H_{21}N(CH_3)_3Br$	Decyltrimethylammonium bromide	63	36
$n\text{-}C_{12}H_{25}N(CH_3)_3Br$	Dodecyltrimethylammonium bromide	14	50
$n\text{-}C_{14}H_{29}N(CH_3)_3Br$	Tetradecyltrimethylammonium bromide	3	75
$n\text{-}C_{14}H_{29}N(CH_3)_3Cl$	Tetradecyltrimethylammonium chloride	3	64
$n\text{-}C_{12}H_{25}NH_3Cl$	Dodecylammonium chloride	13	55
Nonionic			
$n\text{-}C_{12}H_{25}O(CH_2CH_2O)_8H$	Octaoxyethylene glycol monododecyl ether	0.13	132
$n\text{-}C_{12}H_{25}O(CH_2CH_2O)_8H^a$		0.10	301
$n\text{-}C_{12}H_{25}O(CH_2CH_2O)_{12}H$	Dodecaoxyethylene glycol monododecyl ether	0.14	78
$n\text{-}C_{12}H_{25}O(CH_2CH_2O)_{12}H^b$		0.091	116
$t\text{-}C_8H_{17}\text{-}C_6H_4\text{-}O$	Decaoxyethylene glycol mono-p,t-octylphenyl	0.27	100
$(CN_2CH_2O)_{9.7}N$	ether (octoxynol 9)		

[a]Interpolated for physiologic saline, 0.154 M NaCl.

[b]At 55°C instead of 20°C.

nonionic emulsifying blends to form an oil-in-water or a water-in-oil emulsion and thus to assign an HLB number. The hydrophilic groups on the surfactant molecule make a positive contribution to the HLB number, and the lipophilic groups exert a negative effect. There are several members of this class of surfactants, like nonoxynol-9, with spermaticidal and some disinfecting activity (eg, against human immunodeficiency virus [HIV] and some bacteria associated with sexually transmitted diseases).[5] Nonionic nonoxynol-9 can stabilize quaternary ammonium compound (QAC; types of cationic surfactant) formulations because nonionics are not sensitive to hard water. The hard-surface disinfecting activity of QACs is potentiated by the nonionics, such as nonoxynol-9. It is well documented that ethoxylated surfactants do support bacterial growth and deactivate preservatives,[6] such as the parabens. Although they are predominantly used for cleaning applications, they are not widely used as disinfecting agents. They can demonstrate some bactericidal activity and are sometimes used in combination with

other biocides as preservatives, demonstrating some bacteriostatic, fungistatic, and sporistatic activities. Further discussion of nonionic surfactants are outside the scope of this chapter.

Cationic surfactants arise due to a cationic charge on the nitrogen atom. Although phosphonium and sulfonium cationic surfactants exist,[7] this chapter primarily addresses the QACs with antimicrobial activity. This class of surfactants is hydrolytically stable and shows higher aquatic toxicity than most other classes; however, newer "soft" QACs, which were considered more environmentally friendly, have replaced dialkyl QACs as textile softening agents. They contain an ester or amide moiety in their hydrocarbon chain. Devinsky and coworkers,[8] using quantitative structure–activity relationships (QSAR) methods, give a good correlation of biologic activity (minimum inhibitory concentration or MIC) and lipophilicity, which is characterized by CMC and the length of the alkyl chain (Table 21.5). This topic is discussed later in this chapter. Several molecules in this class of soft

TABLE 21.2 Approximate hydrophilic-lipophilic balance (HLB) values for emulsifying agents

Generic or Chemical Name	HLB
Sorbitan trioleate	1.8
Sorbitan tristearate	2.1
Propylene glycol monostearate	3.4
Sorbitan sesquioleate	3.7
Glycerol monostearate (non–self-emulsifying)	3.8
Sorbitan monooleate	4.3
Propylene glycol monolaurate	4.5
Sorbitan monostearate	4.7
Glyceryl monostearate (self-emulsifying)	5.5
Sorbitan monopalmitate	6.7
Sorbitan monolaurate	8.6
Polyoxyethylene-4-lauryl ether	9.5
Polyethylene glycol 400 monostearate	11.6
Polyoxyethylene-4-sorbitan monolaurate	13.3
Polyoxyethylene-20-sorbitan monooleate	15.0
Polyoxyethylene-20-sorbitan monopalmitate	15.6
Polyoxyethylene-20-sorbitan monolaurate	16.7
Polyoxyethylene-40-stearate	16.9
Sodium oleate	18.0
Sodium lauryl sulfate	40.0

TABLE 21.4 Hydrophilic-lipophilic balance group numbers

Group	Group No.
Hydrophilic groups	
$-SO_4^-Na^+$	38.7
$-COO^-K^+$	21.1
$-COO^-Na^+$	19.1
N (tertiary amine)	9.4
Ester (sorbitan ring)	6.8
Ester (free)	2.4
$-COOH$	2.1
Hydroxyl (free)	1.9
$-O-$	1.3
Hydroxyl (sorbitan ring)	0.5
Lipophilic groups	
$-CH-$	
$-CH_2-$	
CH_3-	−0.475
$=CH-$	
Derived groups	
$-(CH_2-CH_2-O)-$	+0.33
$-(CH_2-CH_2-CH_2-O)-$	−0.15

TABLE 21.3 Relationship between HLB range and surfactant application

HLB Range	Use
0-3	Antifoaming agents
4-6	W/O emulsifying agents
7-9	Wetting agents
8-18	O/W emulsifying agents
13-15	Detergents
10-18	Solubilizing agents

Abbreviations: HLB, hydrophilic-lipophilic balance; O/W, oil-in-water emulsion; W/O, water-in-oil emulsion.

QACs have good antimicrobial activity and low systemic toxicity. Compared with "hard" counterpart benzalkonium bromide (dimethyldodecylbenzylammonium bromide, with an oral median lethal dose [LD$_{50}$] 410 mg/kg), the amides and the esters differ significantly (eg, LD$_{50}$ for compound no. 4 = 976 mg/kg, whereas compound no. 15 = 1450 mg/kg orally in mice) (see Table 21.5). It was concluded that "soft" QACs are two to three times less toxic than benzalkonium bromide based on LD$_{50}$ comparison. When the ester or the amide groups within a "soft" QACs are hydrolyzed, the surface activity of the QAC is lost, and so is its antimicrobial efficacy. As a result, the biodegradation order was proposed as ester, QAC >> amide >>>> benzalkonium bromide (the most resistant to biodeterioration); however, the "soft" QACs had limited application as commercial antimicrobials. Instead, they are mostly used as hair- and skin-conditioning agents in personal care industries and as fabric softeners in textile and paper industries.

The amphoteric (or zwitterionic) surfactants contain both an anionic and a cationic charge on the same molecule. An amphoteric surfactant is pH dependent and can therefore be either cationic, zwitterionic, or anionic. A change in pH of an amphoteric surfactant will change its charge and naturally affects its properties like detergency, wetting, and foaming. At the isoelectric point, the physiochemical properties of these amphoterics resemble that of nonionic surfactants. Above and below the isoelectric point, there is a gradual shift toward anionic and cationic character, respectively. The amphoterics have excellent dermatologic properties and show low eye and skin irritation.

TABLE 21.5	Antimicrobial activity and critical micelle concentrations of quats

$C_{11}H_{23}CO\text{-}X\text{-}(CH_2)_2\text{-}N^+(CH_3)_2C_mH_{2m+1}Br^-$						
				MIC $\times$ 10^6 (mol/dm^3)		
Comp	X	m	$-\log C_k{}^a$ (mol/dm^3)	Staphylococcus aureus	Escherichia coli	Candida albicans
1	NH	2	2.0044	105.4	1581.3^c	527.1
2	NH	4	2.1805	24.5	245.4	171.8
3	NH	6	2.3850	9.2	68.9	18.4
4	NH	8	2.9586	2.2	21.6	2.2
5	NH	10	3.5376	12.2	406.8	4.1
6	NH	12	3.8239	38.5	9620.9	57.7
7	NH	14	4.4089	2555.9	20 081.8	1277.9
8	0	1	1.9890	16.4	272.9	136.5
9	0	2	2.1192	15.8	210.3	157.7
10	0	3	2.2441	10.1	101.4	126.8
11	0	4	2.5528	9.8	73.4	73.4
12	0	5	2.6576	7.1	94.7	21.3
13	0	6	2.7969	1.1	68.7	18.3
14	0	7	3.1805	1.3	88.8	11.1
15	0	8	3.2879	6.5	86.1	21.5
16	0	9	3.5850	12.5	125.4	20.9
17	0	10	3.6383	18.3	151.8	81.2
18	0	11	3.7153	21.8	>1973.8^c	138.2
19	0	12	4.0000	96.0	>1920.5^c	576.2
20	0	13	4.2076	130.9	>1870.2^c	1309.1
Benzalkonium^b			2.0969	26.0	260.0	26.0

Abbreviations: MIC, minimum inhibitory concentration; NH, nitrogen-hydrogen.

^{a}From conductivity measurements.

^{b}Benzyldodecyldimethylammonium bromide.

^{c}Not included into calculations of regression equations.

These properties are well suited for use in shampoos and other personal care products. They are compatible with all other classes of surfactants, and they are stable in acidic and basic environments. Under strong alkaline conditions, betaines retain their surfactant properties. The most common commercial representatives of amphoteric surfactants are betaine (alkyldimethyl ammonium acetate from chloroacetic acid and alkyldimethylamine), alkyldimethylamine oxide (made by reaction of alkyldimetylamine with hydrogen peroxide), amidobetaine (made from fatty acid reaction with N,N-dimethylpropane-1,3 diamine, followed by reaction with chloroacetic acid), and alkyl imidazoline (synthesized by reaction of a fatty acid with aminoethanolamine, followed by treatment with chloroacetic acid). By far, the most widely used betaine is cocoamidopropyl betaine (under many trade names). It is used by many surfactant manufacturers, such as betaine C (TEGO™; Evonik Goldschmidt Chemical Co, Mapleton, Illinois), cocamidopropyl betaine (Lexaine™ C, Inolex, Philadelphia, Pennsylvania; Amphosol™ CA, Stepan, Northfield, Illinois; Mirataine™ BET C-30, Rhône-Poulenc, Collegeville, Pennsylvania; Empigen™ BS, Albright & Wilson, Oldbury, United Kingdom; Caltaine™ C-35, Pilot Chemical Co, Houston, Texas; Mackam™ 35-HP, McIntyre Group Ltd, University Park, Illinois), and oleamidopropyl betaine (Lonzaine™ C; Lonza, Walkersville, Maryland).

The amphoteric surfactants are also widely used in formulations due to their surfactancy and often low associated irritation, such as a foam booster, antistatic agents, and as shampoos, but also are reported to have some antimicrobial activity. They are both used for preservative (bacteriostatic and fungistatic) and disinfectant activity (bactericidal and fungicidal) at low concentrations,[9] including the yeast *Pityrosporum ovale* (associated with dandruff and formulations used for dandruff treatment).[10]

▶ QUATERNARY AMMONIUM ANTIMICROBIAL COMPOUNDS

The quaternary nitrogen moiety is an essential component for many biologically active compounds. The QACs play an important role in the living process. From vitamins (vitamin B complex and thiamine) to carboxylase enzymes, which participate in the carbohydrate metabolism, to choline, which is involved in the transmethylation reaction of fat metabolism, and to acetylcholine, a mediator in the transmission of nerve impulses all play a fundamental function. There are at least four types of physiologic actions[11] associated with QACs: (1) curare-like (curaremimetic or curareform) action, a muscular paralysis with no involvement of central nervous system or heart, produced by D-tubocurarine chloride used to induce muscular relaxation during surgery; (2) muscarinic-nicotinic action, which is a direct stimulation of smooth muscles and is a primary transient stimulation and secondary persistent depression of sympathetic and parasympathetic ganglia; (3) ganglia-blocking action; and (4) neuromuscular blockade. Table 21.6 illustrates the chemical structures of representative compounds responsible for these physiologic actions.

Medicinal chemists, using the principle of structure-activity relationships (SARs), have synthesized many QACs that will mimic certain biologic effects.[12] Thus, a complex structure of D-tubocurarine chloride can be reduced to a much simpler decamethonium structure, a neuromuscular-blocking agent. Hexamethonium acts as a ganglionic blocker by preventing the receptor from responding to acetylcholine. The decamethonium is too long to fit the ganglionic receptor but acts as a neuromuscular blocker by preventing the binding of acetylcholine to muscle endplate receptors. When the number of carbon atoms separating the quaternary nitrogens is increased above 12 carbons, the autonomic nervous activity disappears and the compounds become surface active and antimicrobial; however, there are exceptions to this rule, as discussed later in the case of bis-quaternary and polymeric QACs, where two and four carbon atoms separate the quaternary nitrogen, and the products have antimicrobial properties.

TABLE 21.6   Examples of quaternary structures with physiological actions

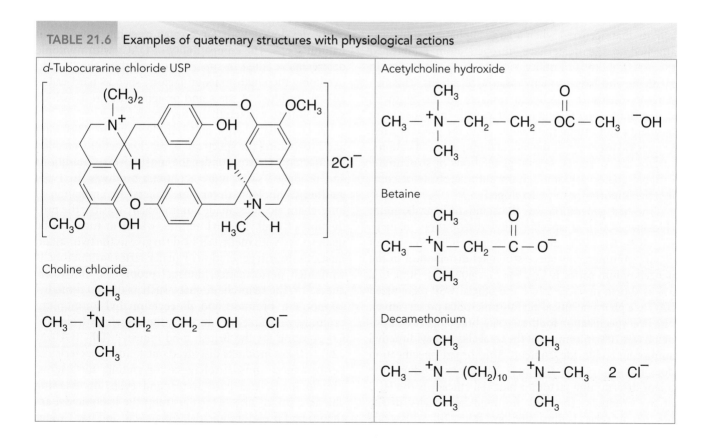

Although there are many stages in the historical development of quaternary ammonium antimicrobials, there is general agreement on at least two truly historical milestones. The first is the work of Jacobs and coworkers, which examined structure, preparation, and antimicrobial activity.[13] A number of papers published in 1915 described the preparation of various different series of the quaternary ammonium salts of hexamethylenetetramine.[14-20] In 1916, the antimicrobial activity of many of these synthesized QACs and additional derivatives were described.[13,21,22] In these publications, they related structure to antimicrobial activity. Although some reviews have challenged this work as the earliest investigations of QACs, their preeminence is assured by their quality, quantity, and treatment, which included antimicrobial activity and correlation between structure and antimicrobial activity. The only valid criticism may be the fact that some of the antimicrobial activity observed may be due to the release of formaldehyde from hexamethylenetetramine. Methenamine mandelate United States Pharmacopeia (USP) is still used as an antibiotic for urinary tract infection, acting by releasing formaldehyde in an acid medium.[2]

During the 1920s, additional information was published on the bacterial activity of quaternary derivatives of pyridine, quinoline, and other ring structures[23-25] as well as QACs of acylated alkylene diamines.[26] By 1935, with the demonstration of the antibacterial activity of long-chain quaternary ammonium salts, the second and most important milestone in the development of antimicrobial QACs took place.[27] The improved bactericidal activity that occurred when a large aliphatic residue was attached to the quaternary nitrogen atom established the practicability and utility of these compounds, first in medicine and later in many other applications. This important disclosure stimulated research in the synthesis and antimicrobial testing of QACs, with the consequent frequent publications and patents up to the present. After Domagk's discovery of the biocidal properties of cationic surface-active agents, several generations of structurally variable quaternary ammonium antimicrobials of commercial importance were developed.

The first generation was the standard benzalkonium chloride (BAC) of specific alkyl distribution, namely, C_{12}, 40%; C_{14}, 50%; and C_{16}, 10%. Another version of equally commercially successful alkyl distribution in the benzalkonium series is C_{12}, 5%; C_{14}, 60%; C_{16}, 30%; C_{18}, 5% as shown in Table 21.7. The official USP recognized BAC as a pharmaceutical aid (antimicrobial preservative). The USP specification for the C_{12}/C_{14} homologues components was 70% minimum of the total alkylbenzyldimethyl ammonium chloride content. This broad specification does not always give the most efficacious product. The major determining factor for biocidal efficacy is the HLB of the products. The peak for biocidal activity of the homologue series is illustrated on Table 21.8, with a carbon chain of 14 offering the best activity.[28-33]

Modifications in the first-generation QACs by substitution of the aromatic ring hydrogen with chlorine, methyl, and ethyl groups resulted in the second generation of the substituted benzalkonium compounds. Of this group, the product with commercial significance was the alkyldimethylethylbenzyl ammonium chloride under the trade name BTC 471 with alkyl distribution C_{12}, 50%; C_{14}, 30%; C_{16}, 17%; and C_{18}, 3%. Another product with antimicrobial activity in this group was alkyldimethyl-3,4-dichlorobenzyl ammonium chloride under the trade names of Tetrosan 3,4D and Riseptin with same alky distribution as previously described.

But by far, the greatest commercial significance was with third generation of QACs, the dual quats, initially developed in 1955 under the trade name BTC 2125M. This product was a mixture of equal proportions of alkyldimethylbenzyl ammonium and alkyldimethylethylbenzyl ammonium chlorides of specific alkyl distribution, as shown in Table 21.7. This combination of BAC with alkyl distribution (C_{12}, 5%; C_{14}, 60%; C_{16}, 30%; C_{18}, 5%) and alkyldimethylethylbenzyl ammonium chloride with alkyl distribution (C_{12}, 68%; C_{14}, 32%) is BTC 2125M, with claimed antimicrobial performance against vegetative bacteria. This synergistic combination of the third generation of quaternaries not only had an increased biocidal activity but also reduced the acute oral LD_{50} from 0.3 g/kg of BAC to an acute oral LD_{50} of 0.750 g/kg for BTC 2125M. The third generation of dual QACs offered improved biocidal activity, stronger detergency, and a relatively lower level of toxicity. In the early 1950s, the nonionic detergents were being developed with far greater cleaning power than natural soaps. The compatibility of QACs with nonionic detergents resulted in superior formulations that helped overcome the environmental factors, such as hard water, anionic residues of soap, and proteinaceous soils, which were found to weaken their effectiveness.[34]

A continual change and improvement in advancing and broadening the spectrum of biocidal activity enabled disinfectants to work under the most adverse conditions and produced safer, more economic products. In 1965, another technologic development, catalytic amination of long-chain alcohols, made commercially feasible the production of dialkylmethyl amines, which in turn can be quaternized with methyl chloride to give us the twin-chain quats, the fourth generation of quaternaries antimicrobials with high performance, unusual properties, and tolerances.[35,36] The twin-chain quats, such as dioctyl dimethyl ammonium bromide and didecyldimethyl ammonium bromide, were first introduced by the British Hydrological Corporation for the British food industry (DECIQUAM 222).[37] These products displayed outstanding bactericidal performance, unusual tolerance for anionic surfactants, protein loads, and hard water, and even low-foaming characteristics. Table 21.9 illustrates the bactericidal activities and pseudomonicidal, fungicidal, and hard-water tolerance (HWT) of five of the most active twin-chain

TABLE 21.7 Commercial antimicrobial quaternary ammonium compounds

Chemical Structure	Trade Names	Manufacturer Examples
Benzalkonium chlorides		
$R_1 = C_{12}$, 40%; C_{14}, 50%; C_{16}, 10% $R_1 = C_{12}$, 5%; C_{14}, 60%; C_{16}, 30%; C_{18}, 5%	BTC 835, BTC 824	Stepan
	BTC 50 USP	Lonza
	Barquat MB-50	Sherex
	Variquat 50 MC	Winthrop
	Zephiran chloride	Lonza
	Hyamine 3500	
Substituted benzalkonium chlorides		
$R_2 = C_{12}$, 50%; C_{14}, 30%; C_{16}, 17%; C_{18}, 3% $R_2 = C_{12}$, 68%; C_{14}, 32%	BTC 471	Stepan
	BTC 2125M	Lonza
	Barquat 4250	
Thin-chain quaternaries		
Dioctyl 25%, didecyl 25%, octyldecyl 50%	BTC 818, BTC 812	Stepan
	BTC 1010	Lonza
	Bardac 2050	
	Bardac 205M	
	Bardac 2250	
Cetylpyridinium chloride		
	Cepacol chloride	Merrell labs
	Ceepryn chloride	
N-(3-chloroallyl) hexaminium chloride		
	Dowicide Q	Dow
	Dowicil 200-	
	Dowicil 75	

(continued)

TABLE 21.7 Commercial antimicrobial quaternary ammonium compounds *(Continued)*

Chemical Structure	Trade Names	Manufacturer Examples
Domiphen bromide		
	Bradosol	Procter & Gamble
	Modic	CIBA
	Modicare	
Benzethonium chloride		
	Phemerol chloride	Park-Davis
	Hyamine 1622	Rohm and Haas
		Lonza
Methylbenzethonium chloride		
	Diaparene chloride	Rohm and Haas
	Hyamine 10×	

quats of 20 as measured by the official Association of Official Analytical Chemists (AOAC) procedure.[36] The product of choice in this series was C_8/C_{12}DMAC because of its superior water solubility and bactericidal activity; however, the odd number chain C_9/C_{11}DMAC is an equally active product, although its commercial feasibility was not explored at that time because of high cost of the odd carbon chain alcohols. Several odd carbon chain alcohols have been offered in commercial quantities. The concept of synergistic combination in the dual quats has been applied to twin-chain quats dialkyldimethyl ammonium chlorides (dioctyl, 25%; didecyl, 25%; octyldecyl, 50%)

TABLE 21.8 Effect of length of carbon chain on bactericidal activity: bactericidal test[a]

Long-Chain Length	*Staphylococcus aureus* #6538	*Salmonella typhosa* #6539	*Pseudomonas aeruginosa* #15 442
8	3000	4500	6000
9	800	1400	2500
10	450	300	1200
11	160	130	400
12	45	40	120
13	25	20	50
14	15	12	40
15	25	20	70
16	30	25	200
17	170	15	360
18	450	60	1000
19	330	90	1300

[a]Minimum concentration that kills in 10 min but not in 5 min in ppm.

TABLE 21.9 Antimicrobial activity of twin-chain quaternary ammonium compounds

Compounds	ppm		
	Pseudomonicidal	Fungicidal	HWT
$C_{10}/C_{10}DMAC$	500	210	1100
$C_8/C_{12}DMAC$	500	200	1200
$C_9/C_{11}DMAC$	500	190	1400
$C_9/C_{12}DMAC$	550	235	1300
$C_{10}/C_{11}DMAC$	550	210	1300

Abbreviation: HWT, hard-water tolerance.

was combined with BACs (R = C_{12}, 40%; C_{14}, 50%; C_{16}, 10%). A 60:40 blend of the previously mentioned quaternaries proved superior to the individual components tested by the AOAC use-dilution test (*Official Methods of Analysis of the AOAC*, 1984).[38] This newer blend of quaternaries represents the fifth generation of QACs. The blend remained active under the most hostile conditions, was less toxic and less costly, and provided more convenient disinfectants.

In the 1980s, the toxicity of QACs underwent scrutiny by the US Environmental Protection Agency (EPA) and other US regulatory agencies. The safety of the biocides in general received a greater priority over efficacy. A new class of biocides, the polymeric quaternaries, has emerged; these are less toxic than the standard BACs and less powerful than the dual quats or twin-chain quats. The polymeric quaternaries are milder and have found applications in pharmaceuticals as preservatives.[39,40] The polymeric quaternary ammoniums are polyelectrolytes, representing the sixth generation of QACs. They are generally considered milder and safer than all other classes based on LD_{50} and cytotoxicity.[39] More recently, other synergistic combinations, considered the seventh generation of quaternary, consisted of blends of bis-quats and polymeric quaternary (polyionenes). These offered excellent antimicrobial activity against oral flora bacteria, namely *Bacteroides gingivalis*, *Actinomyces viscosus*, and *Streptococcus mutans* at 1 to 5 ppm in pharmaceutically accepted polymer formulations.[40] These results required further testing to confirm safety and true synergism in this series of polymeric quaternaries with bis-quats blends, and a subsequent series of patents claiming antimicrobial, low-toxicity, blend composition of bis-QACs and polyvinylpyrrolidone.[40,41]

▶ CHEMISTRY

The QACs are the products of a nucleophilic substitution reaction of alkyl halides with tertiary amines. Chemically,

they have four carbon atoms linked directly to the nitrogen atom through covalent bonds; the anion in the original alkylating agent becomes linked to the nitrogen by an electrovalent bond. The general formula for the QACs is represented as follows:

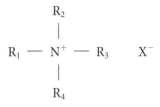

R1, R2, R3, and R4 are alkyl groups that may be alike or different, substituted or unsubstituted, saturated or unsaturated, branched or unbranched, and cyclic or acyclic and that may contain ether or ester or amide linkages; they may be aromatic or substituted aromatic groups. The nitrogen atom plus the attached alkyl groups forms the positively charged cation portion, which is the functional part of the molecule. The portion attached to the nitrogen by an electrovalent bond may be any anion but is usually chloride or bromide to form the salt. Depending on the nature of the R groups, the anion, and the number of quaternary nitrogen atoms present, the antimicrobial QACs may be classified in different salt groups as described in the following text.

Monoalkyltrimethyl Ammonium Salts

In these, one R group is a long-chain alkyl group, and the remaining R groups are short-chain alkyl groups, such as methyl or ethyl groups. All the compounds in this group are prepared from the reaction of a tertiary amine with an alkyl halide.[27,42,43] The tertiary amine may be the long-chain alkyldimethylamine or the short-chain trimethylamine, which react with methyl halide or with the long-chain alkyl halide, respectively. Examples of commercially available products in this group are cetyltrimethylammonium bromide as CTAB; alkyltrimethyl ammonium chloride as Arquad™ 16; alkylaryltrimethyl ammonium chloride as Gloquat™ C; and cetyldimethylethylammonium bromide as Cycloton™ D256B, Ammonyx™ DME, and Bretol™.

Monoalkyldimethylbenzyl Ammonium Salts

In this group, one R is a long-chain alkyl group, a second R is a benzyl radical, and the two remaining R groups are short-chain alkyl groups, such as methyl or ethyl groups. These compounds are prepared by the reaction of a long-chain alkyldimethylamine with the benzyl halide.[44-46] Examples of commercially available products in this group are alkyldimethylbenzyl ammonium chlorides as

BTC™ 824, Hyamine™ 3500, Cyncal™ Type 14, and Catigene™. In addition, there are substituted benzyl QACs such as dodecyldimethyl-3,4-dichlorobenzyl ammonium chloride, sold under the trade name of Riseptin™. There are also mixtures of alkyldimethylbenzyl and alkyldimethyl substituted benzyl (ethylbenzyl) ammonium chlorides, such as BTC 2125M and Barquat™ 4250.

Dialkyldimethyl Ammonium Salts

In this instance, two R groups are long-chain alkyl groups, and the remaining R groups are short-chain alkyl groups, such as methyl groups. These compounds are prepared by the reaction of the long-chain alkyldimethylamine with a long-chain alkyl halide or dialkylmethylamine with methyl halide.[47-50] Examples of commercially available products in this group are didecyldimethyl ammonium halides, such as Deciquam™ 222 and Bardac™ 22, and octyldodecyldimethyl ammonium chloride, such as BTC™ 812.

Heteroaromatic Ammonium Salts

In this group, one R chain is a long alkyl group, and the remaining three R groups are provided by some aromatic system. Thus, the quaternary nitrogen to which these three R groups are attached is part of an aromatic system such as pyridine, quinoline, or isoquinoline. These compounds are prepared by reaction of the aromatic amine with a long-chain alkyl halide.[42,51] Examples of commercially available products in this group are cetylpyridinium halide (CPC™ and Ceepryn™), reaction product of hexamethylenetetramine with 1,3-dichloropropene to give cis-isomer 1-[3-chloroallyl]-3,5,7-triaza-1-azoniaadamantane (Dowicil 200), alkyl-isoquinolinium bromide (Isothan™ Q), and alkyldimethylnaphthylmethyl ammonium chloride (BTC™ 1100).

Polysubstituted Quaternary Ammonium Salts

In this group, the cation portion of the molecule is the same as that described for any of the aforementioned groups; however, the anion portion is not a small inorganic ion as previously described, but a large, high-molecular-weight organic ion. These compounds are prepared by reaction of the quaternary ammonium halides with the sodium, potassium, or calcium salt of a high-molecular-weight organic moiety, so that an exchange of the anions is effected.[52,53] Examples of commercially available products in this group are alkyldimethylbenzyl ammonium saccharinate (Onyxide™ 3300 and Loroquat™ QA 100) and alkyldimethylethylbenzyl ammonium cyclohexylsulfamate (Onyxide 172).

Bis-Quaternary Ammonium Salts

In this group of compounds, there are two symmetric quaternary ammonium moieties arranged in the general formula:

$$R_1 - \underset{\underset{R_3}{|}}{\overset{\overset{R_2}{|}}{N^+}} - (Z) - \underset{\underset{R_6}{|}}{\overset{\overset{R_4}{|}}{N^+}} - R_5\ 2X^-$$

Here, the R groups are as described for any of the aforementioned groups, Z is a carbon-hydrogen attached to each quaternary nitrogen via an electrovalent bond. These compounds are prepared by reaction of a bis-tertiary amine with alkyl halide or of a di-halo compound with a tertiary amine.[54-56] An example of a commercially available product in this group is 1, 10-bis(2-methyl-4-aminoquinolinium chloride)-decane, sold under the trade name of Dequadin™ or Sorot™. Another example of bis-quat is 1,6-bis [1-methyl-3-(2,2,6-trimethyl cyclohexyl)-propyldimethyl-ammonium chloride] hexane or triclobisonium chloride sold by trade name Triburon™. Another commercially available bis-quat is CDQ™, used for industrial water treatment for controlling sulfate-reducing bacteria (*Desulfovibrio* species). The CDQ™ is prepared by reaction of alkyl[C_{12}, 40%; C_{14}, 50%; C_{16}, 10%] dimethylamine with dichloroethyl ether. Also, reaction of 1,4-dichloro-2-butene with 2 mol of alkyldimethylamines or hexamethylenetetramine offers another example of bis-quats with broad spectrums of biocidal activity.

Polymeric Quaternary Ammonium Salts

Many different types of polymeric quaternary ammonium salts have been reported to have antimicrobial activity.[57-62] The methods of preparation of these polymers are also many, from free radical polymerization of monomers containing quaternized nitrogen, to cationic, anionic polymerization, polycondensation of diamines with dihalides, or polycondensation of haloamines. The last method was used for the preparation of ionenes, which are polyelectrolytes with positively charged nitrogen atoms located in the backbone of polymeric chain. This type of polycation was first reported in 1941 and is formed by the Menshutkin reaction from ditertiary amines and dihalides.[62] Although a number of patents were published since 1941 concerning the applications of ionene polymers, little information was available on the mechanism and kinetics of their formation or their solution properties. The polymerization conditions for the formation of ionenes involve a total concentration of 3.0 mol (1.5 mol of each monomer) in a mixture of dimethylformamide/methanol solvent (1:1 or 4:1) and 5 to 7 days of reaction time at room temperature to give polyionenes with molecular weight (MW) of about 65 000. In condensation polymerization, the purity of the condensing species and stoichiometry are critical in obtaining high-molecular-weight polymer. Polyionenes exhibit bactericidal action, formation of insoluble complexes with DNA and heparin, neuromuscular-blocking action, cell lysis and aggregation, and cell adhesion.[62] The antimicrobial and antifungal properties of ionenes were studied by the zone of inhibition method against *Staphylococcus aureus, Escherichia coli, Pseudomonas aeruginosa, Bacillus subtilis, Candida sporogenes, Salmonella* Typhimurium, *Mycobacterium smegmatis, Pseudomonas mirabilis, Pseudomonas vulgaris, Candida globosum, M. verrucaris, Fusarium oxysporum,* and *Alternaria* species. The MIC for five of the most active ionenes bromides against *S aureus* and *E coli* are listed in Table 21.10.

The 6,10 ionene bromide was found to be the most active in these series and, at concentrations up to 4 ppm, stimulated the growth of normal cells. This range showed inhibition and death of the transformed human cells W138, possibly by electrostatic cytotoxic interaction.[63] It has been suggested that malignant cells are more electronegative than normal cells. If so, malignant cells should demonstrate a greater affinity for the electropositive ionene polymer. This hypothesis has been supported by experimental work; however, this preliminary study appears to warrant more extensive studies to evaluate this class of polymers as chemotherapeutic agents. Polyionenes and their low-molecular-weight analogues constitute a unique model system for a molecular probe of the living cell machinery because their structure, their positive-charge densities, their counterions, and their MWs can be varied systematically. These considerations apply not only to the study of toxicity or antimicrobial activity but also to the understanding of the interaction of the polyionenes with DNA or as molecular probes to elucidate the properties of cell membranes.

The high-charge density of polyionenes is responsible for their bactericidal and fungicidal activities, for the prolonged duration of the curarizing action, and for the formation of complexes with DNA and heparin. The differences in the biologic properties or stability of the complexes may be explained on the basis of electrostatic association between the negative and the positive moieties of the interacting molecules.

Because the normal and neoplastic cells show an array of different surface properties, including an increase in anodic mobility after transformation, some polyionenes (eg, 6,10 ionene bromide) may preferentially bind to cancer cells and inactivate them. This differential binding and toxicity to transformed cells conforms with topologic changes of membrane-binding sites in the transformed cells. All four products in Table 21.11 are ionenes that contain the quaternary nitrogen atom on the backbone of the polymer chain. The main difference is the MW, which is due to reactivity of the alkylating monomer, reaction time, solvent, temperature, and method of preparation. The WSCP™ or Busan™ 77 from Buckman Laboratories, which is chemically identified as poly[oxyethylene (dimethyliminio)-ethylene (dimethyliminio)-ethylene dichloride], was made by condensation of N,N,N′,N′-tetramethylethylenediamine with dichloroethyl ether in water to give an MW of 2000 to 3000. An MIC at 10- to 50-ppm levels indicated broad-spectrum antimicrobial activity, with dual functionality as polymer clarifiers for swimming pools or algicides. The presence of WSCP at only 2 ppm can reduce by 80% or more the chlorine needed to kill bacteria, where it enhances the activity of all oxidizers used in swimming pools. In addition, it was used as a cooling water treatment biocide for algae, bacteria, and fungi at 20 to 40 ppm.

Another polymeric QAC was the product Mirapol™ A-15, which is chemically identified as poly[N-3-dimethylammonio)propyl]N-[3-ethylneoxyethylenedimethylammonio)propyl]urea dichloride] or polyquaternium-2. This product is made by reacting a symmetrically substituted urea ditertiary amine with dichloroethylether in water to give an MW of 2000 to 3000. Initial uses were in hair-care products, with inhibitory levels of 100 ppm against *P ovale, S aureus,* and *E coli.* By a time/kill water treatment screening procedure, the product demonstrates a high-percentage kill of *P aeruginosa* and *Enterobacter aerogenes* at 10, 15, and 20 ppm of active product following a 30-minute contact period; however, these reports were debated,[64] and its primary use has been as a hair-conditioning agent in shampoos.

The last structure on Table 21.11 of the polymeric QACs is chemically identified as α-4-[1-tris(2-hydroxyethyl) ammonium chloride-2-butenyl] poly [1-dimethyl ammonium chloride-2-butenyl]-ω-tris(2-hydroxyethyl)ammonium chloride or Onamer™ M or Polyquat™ or with the name polyquaternium-1. The Onamer M is made by reacting 1,4-bis[dimethylamino]-2-butene (0.9 mol),

TABLE 21.10			Minimum inhibitory concentration (MIC) of polyionenes	
			MIC (ppm)	
			Staphylococcus aureus	*Escherichia coli*
3,3	Ionene	Bromide	>128	>128
6,6	Ionene	Bromide	16	16
6,10	Ionene	Bromide	4	4
2,10	Ionene	Bromide	4	8
6,16	Ionene	Bromide	4	32

TABLE 21.11　Polymeric polyquaternary ammonium compounds

A. Ionenes A. Rembaum applied polymer symposium No. 22 299-317 (1973)

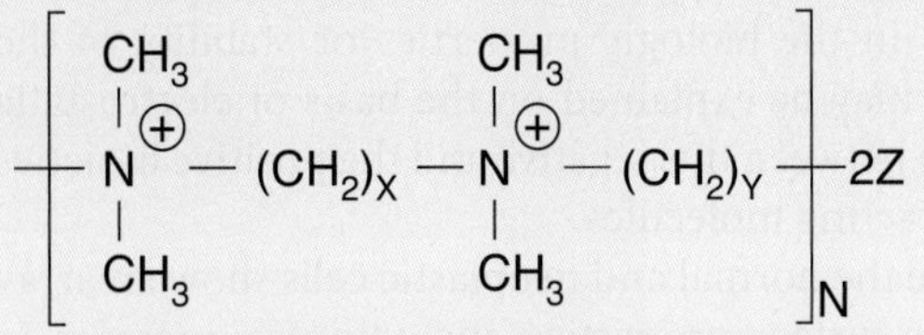

$$\left[\begin{array}{c} CH_3 \\ | \\ N^{\oplus} - (CH_2)_X - N^{\oplus} - (CH_2)_Y \\ | \\ CH_3 \end{array} \right]_N \cdot 2Z$$

B. Poly[oxyethylene(dimethyliminio)ethylene(dimethyliminio)ethylene dichloride] (WSCP or Busan 77)

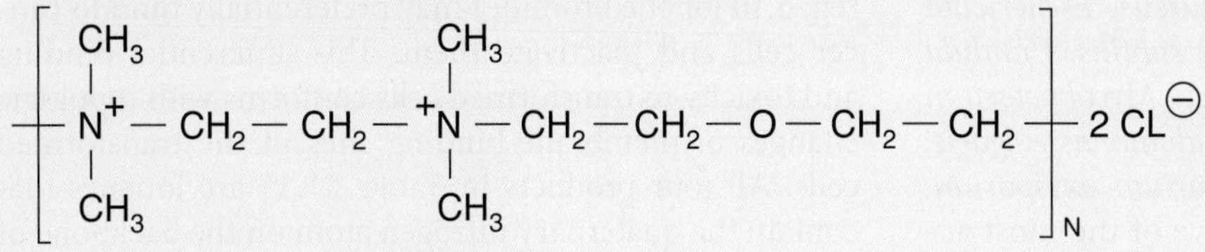

$$\left[\begin{array}{c} CH_3 \\ | \\ N^+ - CH_2 - CH_2 - {}^+N - CH_2 - CH_2 - O - CH_2 - CH_2 \\ | \\ CH_3 \end{array} \right]_N \cdot 2\,CL^{\ominus}$$

C. Polyquaternium-2 (Mirapol-A15)

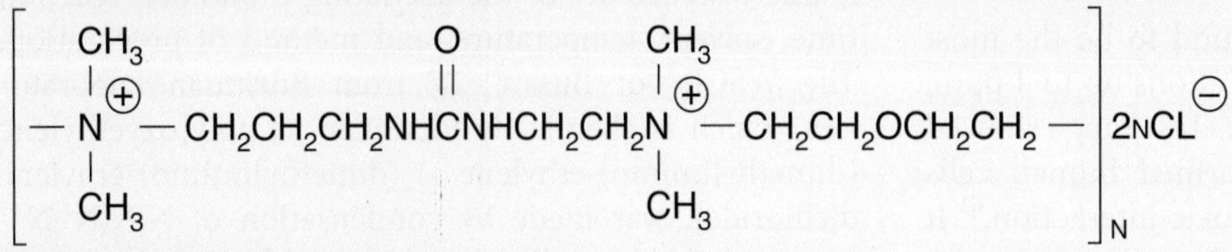

$$\left[\begin{array}{c} CH_3 \qquad\qquad O \qquad\qquad CH_3 \\ | \qquad\qquad || \qquad\qquad | \\ -N^{\oplus} - CH_2CH_2CH_2NHCNHCH_2CH_2N^{\oplus} - CH_2CH_2OCH_2CH_2 - \\ | \qquad\qquad\qquad\qquad\qquad | \\ CH_3 \qquad\qquad\qquad\qquad CH_3 \end{array} \right]_N 2NCL^{\ominus}$$

D. Polyquaternium-1 (Onamer M)

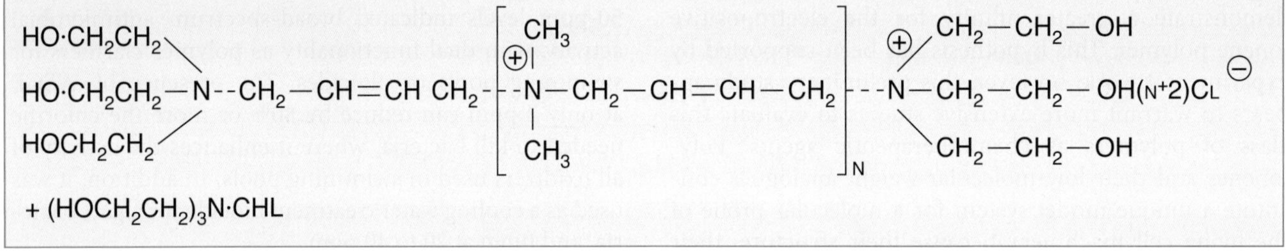

HO·CH₂CH₂
HO·CH₂CH₂—N--CH₂—CH=CH CH₂ $\left[\begin{array}{c} CH_3 \\ \oplus| \\ -N-CH_2-CH=CH-CH_2 \\ | \\ CH_3 \end{array} \right]_N$ $\begin{array}{c} CH_2-CH_2-OH \\ \oplus \diagup \\ --N-CH_2-CH_2-OH \\ \diagdown \\ CH_2-CH_2-OH \end{array}$ (N+2)CL$^{\ominus}$
HOCH₂CH₂

+ (HOCH₂CH₂)₃N·CHL

---

triethanolamine (0.2 mol), and 1,4-dichloro-2-butene (1.0 mol) in water to give an average MW of 5000 to 10 000.[65,66] The purpose of the triethanolamine in the preparation was randomly to terminate the polymeric chain so that we obtained a low-molecular-weight product by design. The 1,4-dichloro-2-butene alkylating agent is extremely reactive and gave a 98% conversion of organic chloride to ionic within 6 to 8 hours in water. Polyquaternium-1 was used for hair-conditioning applications but with demonstrated antimicrobial activity combined with excellent toxicologic data emerged as a preservative candidate for ophthalmic preparations.[39,67] Examples of the use of this preservative included contact lenses solutions such as Opti-Tears™, Opti-Clean™, Opti-Soft™, Opti-Free™, and Polyflex Tears-Naturale™ II (all are trade names of Alcon). Table 21.12 compares the cytotoxic response of Onamer™ M at various concentrations and other solutions by in vitro testing of mouse L929 cells.[39] The most common ophthalmic preservatives at this time were thimerosal, BAC, and chlorhexidine. These compounds can

be toxic to the eye and may cause corneal erosion and corneal ulceration, resulting in pain. This problem is particularly severe with QACs that are concentrated more than 400 times by hydrophilic lenses. Chlorhexidine is concentrated as much as 100-fold by hydrophilic contact lenses, which results in the potential for injury to the eye. The comparative cellular toxicity of soft contact lenses soaked in Onamer M at various concentrations and other solutions was determined by in vitro testing. The results from Table 21.12 showed that Onamer™ M was not cytotoxic. This cytotoxic response may be related to the acute oral LD_{50} of these compounds (Table 21.13). Earlier and more recent studies determined that the product was bacteriostatic against a range of bacterial pathogens such as S aureus, E coli, P aeruginosa, and Streptococcus faecalis at 50 ppm and bactericidal/yeasticidal in formulations.[68,69]

At least two characteristics are common to the WSCP and Onamer™ M polymeric quaternaries, making them uniquely different from other QACs. One is

TABLE 21.12 Comparative cytotoxicity of soft contact lenses soaked in preserved solutions on mouse L929 cells

Lens Soaked	Cytotoxic Response		Cytotoxicity Conclusion[a]
	Cell Lysis	Zone of Cell Death (mm)	
Saline	−	0	None
0.1% Onamer M	−	0	None
0.3% Onamer M	−	0	None
1.0% Onamer M	+	31	Moderate
Alkyltriethanol ammonium[b]			
Chloride (0.03%) + thimerosal (0.002%)[b]	+	16	Minimal
Chlorhexidine (0.005%) + thimerosal (0.001%)[b]	+	25	Moderate
Thimerosal (0.001%)[a]	+	10	Minimal
Sorbic acid (0.1%)[b]	+	16	Minimal
0.01% Benzalkonium chloride	+	48	Severe
0.01% Benzalkonium chloride	+	64	Severe

[a]Cytotoxicity was rated as follows: minimal when zone of decoloration was 20 mm. Moderate zone of decoloration was 20-40 mm. Severe zone of decoloration was 40 mm.

[b]Commercially available marketed solutions.

the absence of foaming, even at high aqueous concentrations. The other is the remarkably lower toxicity shared by these polymeric quaternary products. As an example, for Onamer M at 30% active material, primary abraded and intact skin irritation scores were zero for all observation periods. Draize eye irritation

TABLE 21.13 Acute oral LD_{50}: commercial antimicrobial quaternary ammonium compounds

Compounds	LD_{50}
Cetylpyridinium chloride	0.20 g/kg
Benzalkonium chloride	0.30 g/kg
Domiphen bromide	0.32 g/kg
Methylbenzethonium chloride	0.35 g/kg
Benzethonium chloride	0.42 g/kg
Didecyldimethylammonium chloride	0.53 g/kg
Octyldodecyldimethylammonium chloride	0.72 g/kg
BTC™ 2125 M	0.75 g/kg
Dowicil™ 200	2.20 g/kg
6,10–ionene bromide	1.00 g/kg
WSCP™ or Busan™ 77	2.77 g/kg
Mirapol™ A-15 (not sold as antimicrobial)	2.85 g/kg
Onamer™ M or Polyquat® or polyquaternium–1	4.47 g/kg

Abbreviation: LD_{50}, median lethal dose.

studies recorded a mild conjunctival irritation with scores of 2 or 4 in each rabbit, which cleared on the second day of observation. The acute oral LD_{50} in rats was determined to be 4470 mg/kg. The product was described as nonmutagenic by the mouse lymphoma forward mutation assay and by the sex-linked recessive lethal test in *Drosophila melanogaster*. In addition, it was not considered carcinogenic by the in vitro transformation of Balb/3T3 cells assay.

For reasons of structure, size, foaming, and toxicity, these polymeric quaternary compounds have encouraged the synthesis and evaluation of similar compounds for consideration. Besides the polyionene quaternary polymers, there are other classes of antimicrobial polymers in which the quaternary nitrogen is pendant away from the backbone chain of the polymer (Table 21.14). A number of quaternary monomers, homopolymers, and copolymers of N-vinyl-pyrrolidone and 2-methacryloxyethyl-N,N,N-triethyl ammonium bromide and iodide have been described to have antimicrobial activity.[60] This activity increases as the content of quaternary ammonium moiety increases. The quaternary nitrogen is pendant away from backbone chain and requires the proper lipophilic groups and proper charge density of the quaternary nitrogen for biocidal activity. None of these polymers are used as antimicrobials, but they are commercially available as hair-conditioning agents for shampoos and other industrial applications such as coagulating and flocculating agents. Examples are Gafquat™ (polyquaternium-11) and Merquat™ (polyquaternium-7). These products are made by the

TABLE 21.14   Free radical polymeric quaternary ammonium compounds

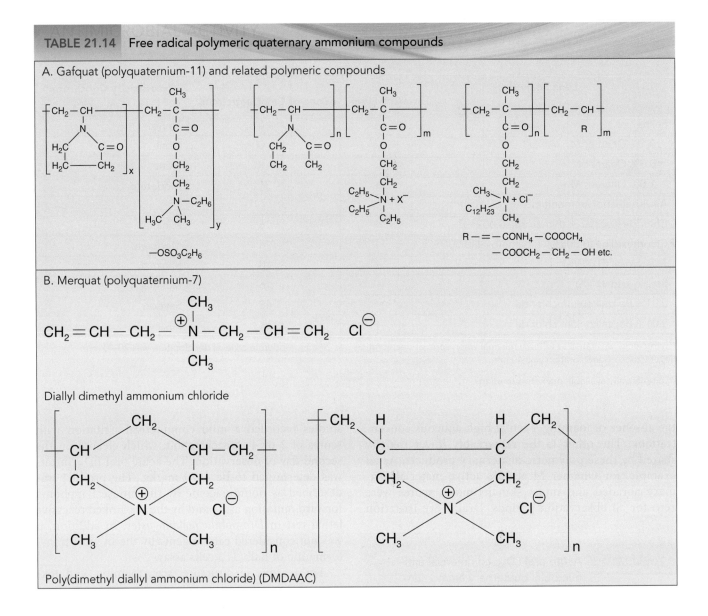

A. Gafquat (polyquaternium-11) and related polymeric compounds

B. Merquat (polyquaternium-7)

Diallyl dimethyl ammonium chloride

Poly(dimethyl diallyl ammonium chloride) (DMDAAC)

free radical polymerization of diallyl quaternary monomer, and their MW is greater than 100 000. But some related terpolymers, with MW 10 000 to 20 000, were reported to have antimicrobial activity such as against *Candida albicans* at 0.1% when used as a preservative for soft contact lenses.[70]

The antimicrobial activities (determined by MICs) of poly[trialkyl(vinylbenzyl)ammonium chloride] type of polycations against bacteria and fungi were considered more active than the corresponding monomers[71,72]; however, the absolute activity is low compared with commercially used quaternaries. The antibacterial assessment was based only on the conventional spread plate method, which has been widely used to evaluate the antibacterial activity of antibiotics and preservatives. But this method is subject to some variability, where the compound interacted with media negatively charged species (such as sodium caseinate of the agar plate) and produced an insoluble complex leading to inactivation of the polymer. Overall, the antibacterial activity of poly[dodecyldimethyl{vinylbenzyl} ammonium chloride] against *S aureus* at 0.5 ppm was effective within 30 minutes of contact, whereas the corresponding monomer was inactive. Compounds with the longest alkyl chain studied (dodecyl) exhibited high activity, which was ascribed to the contribution of the increased hydrophobicity of the compounds to the activity. In conclusion, the most significant finding was that the polymers are more active than the corresponding monomers, particularly against gram-positive bacteria. The higher activity of the polymers was interpreted as being due to favored adsorption onto the bacterial cell surface and the cytoplasmic membrane with subsequent disruption of its integrity, although they have the disadvantage of diffusing through the cell wall, especially with the gram-negative bacteria. Antimicrobial polymeric QACs with repeated vinyl-benzylammonium units have been described for preserving ophthalmic solutions.[73]

An optimal MW region of 14 300 for the 6,6-ionene bromide was shown to have antibacterial activity with a minimum bactericidal concentrations (MBC) of 6.6 ppm to 10 ppm against *S aureus*.[59] Polymeric biguanides of MW 11 900 and poly{alkyl[C_2-C_{12}] dimethyl[vinylbenzyl] ammonium chloride} of similar MW also exhibit better bactericidal action against gram-positive than gram-negative bacteria. The poly(dodecyldimethyl[vinylbenzyl] ammonium chloride) was the most active with 0.5 ppm against *S aureus*, which suggests that hydrophobicity plays an important role in bactericidal action. In conclusion, in all three types of polymers reported, there is a clear MW dependence of the biocidal activity; that is, polymers with low MW as well as high MW exhibit lower bactericidal activity, and there exists an optimal MW region for the biocidal action. This is a fine balance between the polymeric biocides between MW, biocidal activity (cytotoxicity), and (toxicity) acute oral LD_{50}.

ANALYSIS

The chemical structure of QACs permits a variety of quantitative procedures to determine their concentration. Various analytic methods have been reported for the determination of BACs by high-performance liquid chromatography (HPLC)[74] and gas chromatography.[75] Chemical ionization mass spectroscopy has been used to identify and determine the proportions of various alkyl chain lengths in commercial mixtures of BACs.[30] At least two methods for determining low concentration of Onamer™ M or polyquaternium-1 antimicrobial preservative in ophthalmic solutions have been reported.[66,76] A direct titration technique for the accurate, quantitative determination of cationic and anionic polyelectrolytes was reported.[77] The technique is based on a direct neutralization reaction between cationic and anionic forms of the polymers. Modification of poly[vinylsulfuric acid] potassium salt method was used for determination of high concentration of Onamer™ M.[78] The cationic polyelectrolytes show a light blue color in the presence of toluidine blue O dye, and the blue color turns to bluish purple when the titration end point is reached. With the many methods available, the method of choice is usually dictated by the level of QAC anticipated in the sample. For solutions estimated to contain 0.5% or more QAC, the chemist may use a diphasic or direct titration procedure.

STRUCTURE-ACTIVITY RELATIONSHIPS

Jacobs and Heidelberger[79] were the first to report the correlation between chemical structure and antimicrobial activity of benzyl and substituted benzyl hexamethylenetetrammonium salts. Forty substances tested against the bacillus typhosus (*Salmonella* Typhi) demonstrated the existence of direct relationships between chemical constitution and bactericidal action within the series. The degree of the bactericidal action was determined by the position, character, and number of groups substituted in the benzene nucleus. By introduction of the methyl, chlorine, bromine, iodine, cyano, and nitro groups into the benzene nucleus of the parent benzylhexamethylenetetrammonium salt, the bactericidal power of this compound was notably enhanced. The substitution of these groups in the ortho position almost invariably resulted in substances that were more active than their meta or para isomers; the introduction of the methoxy group was without marked effect.

Several substances in which two hexamethylenetetrammonium groups on the same aromatic nucleus (namely bis-quats 1,2-xylylenebis[hexamethylenetetrammonium chloride and mesitylenebis[hexamethylenetetrammonium chloride]) were the most active of the substances of this series when tested.[79] Comparative tests with other bacterial types demonstrated that these compounds possessed a marked degree of specificity. The bactericidal character is directly attributable to the presence of the hexamethylenetetramine nucleus.

The same general principle of increased antimicrobial activity was observed with benzalkonium and substituted BACs, as illustrated in Table 21.15. The AOAC germicidal and detergent sanitizer tests was used with *E coli*, and the HWT (ppm as $CaCO_3$) was measured. A 99.999% reduction in 30 seconds is required with quaternary level of 200 ppm to pass. A synergistic blend of alkyl[C_{12}:C_{14}; 70:30] 2,4,6-trimethylbenzyldimethyl ammonium chloride (C) has the highest HWT of 1300 ppm, with the 2,4,5 isomer (D) having the next best tolerance of 1200 ppm, which is twice as high as the corresponding BAC (A). The mesitylenyl and pseudocuminyl quaternary compounds are highly crystalline nonhygroscopic materials with excellent microbicidal properties; however, economics favors alkyl[C_{12}:C_{14}; 70:30] ethyl[15% ortho, 85% para]benzyldimethylammonium chloride(B). Synergistic blends of microbicidal QACs with dodecyl to tetradecyl proportion 85:15 to 55:45 are listed in Table 21.16.

A summary of the QSARs of antimicrobial N-lauryl-pyridinium iodides was summarized in Table 21.17.[80,81] The antimicrobial activities of N-laurylpyridinium iodides (19 compounds) having various substituents (methyl, ethyl, propyl, amino, carboxyl, and carbamoyl groups)

TABLE 21.15 Association of Official Analytical Chemists germicidal and detergent sanitizers test method with *Escherichia coli* at 200 ppm quaternary ammonium compound to give 99.999% reduction in 30 s

	Hard-Water Tolerance (ppm) CaCO$_3$			
Alkyl	**A**	**B**	**C**	**D**
R$_{12}$	100	400	900	1250
R$_{14}$	700	700	1000	700
R$_{16}$	400	400	600	500
R$_{18}$	100	300	550	350
R$_{12 (70)/14 (30)}$	650	1000	1300	1200

on the pyridine nuclei were studied against *E coli* K12, *B subtilis* var *niger*, *Aspergillus niger*, and *Candida utilis* with respect to their chemical structures. The N-lauryl-2,4,6-trimethylpyridinium iodide had the highest antimicrobial activity, whereas N-lauryl-2-carboxylpyridinium iodide had the lowest activity. In general, the electron-releasing groups on the pyridine nucleus such as amino or methyl group markedly enhanced the activities, and the electron-attracting groups such as carboxyl or carbamoyl group highly reduced them. There was a clearly linear relationship between the antimicrobial activities and the acidic dissociation constant (pK$_a$) for the corresponding pyridines, and the same relationships exist between the pK$_a$ and both bacteriolytic and bactericidal activities. The findings obtained suggest that the antimicrobial activities of the N-laurylpyridinium iodides are linearly dependent on the electron density of the ammonium moiety. The only widely commercialized pyridinium quaternary is cetylpyridinium chloride, as the active ingredient in mouthwashes/lozenges and in preservatives in pharmaceutical and other preparations. Economic considerations had initially prevented the commercialization of the substituted N-laurylpyridinium iodide quaternaries, but these are now widely used for a variety of medical and industrial applications.[82]

The relationship between hydrophobicity of bacterial cell surface and drug susceptibility to alkylpyridinium iodides has been investigated with different types of

bacteria.[83] The value of bactericidal activity of quaternary iodides having long alkyl chains (hexyl, octyl, decyl, dodecyl, tetradecyl, hexadecyl, octadecyl) was regarded as the drug susceptibility. The partition coefficient of bacterial cells between *n*-hexadecane and physiologic saline was regarded as representing their hydrophobicity of the cell surface. The logarithm of the coefficient was employed as a measure of hydrophobicity at 37°C. The hydrophobicity of the gram-negative bacteria was always higher than that of the gram-positive bacteria. The susceptibility of the bacteria to each of the alkylpyridinium iodides was analyzed by use of hydrophobicity, and a quantitative relationship between the susceptibility and their hydrophobicity was found. These findings led to the conclusion that the first step of the antimicrobial action of the iodides is a hydrophobic interaction at the cell surface and that the magnitude of the drug susceptibility of the bacteria depends on the hydrophobicity of the cell surface. The relationship between physicochemical properties and antimicrobial activity of a homologous series of alkyldimethylbenzyl ammonium chlorides against a variety of microorganisms was investigated to test if BAC mixtures could be improved as antimicrobial agents through a more rational choice of alkyl chain length composition.[29,30] The MICs of various members of the homologous series of alkyldimethylbenzyl ammonium chlorides were determined against 12 strains of microorganisms, representative of gram-positive and gram-negative bacteria, yeast,

TABLE 21.16 AOAC germicidal and detergent sanitizers test with *Escherichia coli* at 200 ppm active quaternary ammonium compound to give 99.999% reduction in 30 s

R		Hard-Water Tolerance (ppm)	
C_{12}	C_{14}	Calculated	Determined
100	0	400	400
95	5	415	500
90	10	430	750
85	15	445	1000
82.5	17.5	453	1050
80	20	460	1110
77.5	22.5	468	1000
75	25	475	1050
70	30	490	1000
65	35	505	1000
60	40	520	900
55	45	535	1000
50	50	550	900
45	55	565	1000
40	60	580	900
35	65	595	800
30	70	610	750
25	75	625	800
20	80	640	800
10	90	670	800
5	95	685	600
0	100	700	700

and fungi. The CMCs and octanol-water partition coefficient (P) were measured and calculated as the ratio of the concentration in the aqueous and oil (alcohol) phases expressed as the means of the replicate determination. Physicochemical data such as log P and log 1/MIC were subjected to multiple regression analysis to produce quadratic equations of the general form:

$$\log 1 / \text{MIC} = a + b \log P + C \left[\log P\right]^2$$

The log P values were plotted against biologic activity for a series of compounds, and a parabolic relationship was obtained. Log P_0 would in this instance be the value of log P for compounds with optimal biologic activity. This value of log P_0 will vary between different types of organisms. Many such parabolic relationships have been demonstrated, including several for QACs.[31,84] The levels of antimicrobial activity were observed to be parabolically related to the alkyl chain length, and thereby to log P. The chain lengths with optimal activity varied from organism to organism, reflecting differences in their cell wall structures. The lower chain lengths [C_{10}-C_{12}] were more active against yeast and fungi, whereas gram-negative bacteria were most susceptible toward the more lipophilic C_{16} compounds. This was probably a consequence of the lipophilic nature of the gram-negative

TABLE 21.17   Minimum inhibitory concentration (MIC) of N-laurylpyridinium iodides against *Escherichia coli* K12, *Bacillus subtilis, Candida utilis,* and *Aspergillus niger*

$$\left[\overset{3 \quad 2}{\underset{5 \quad 6}{\bigcirc}} N^+ - C_{12}H_{25} \right] I^-$$

No.	2	3	4	5	6	Abbreviation	MICs (M)[a]			
							E coli K12	B subtilis var niger	C utilis	A niger
1.	H	H	H	H	H	Py	53	5.6	61	85
2.	CH₃	H	H	H	H	2-Me-Py	21	3.6	26	26
3.	H	CH₃	H	H	H	3-Me-Py	51	4.9	59	82
4.	H	H	CH₃	H	H	4-Me-Py	31	4.6	45	72
5.	CH₃	H	CH₃	H	H	2,4-Me-Py	20	4.0	32	35
6.	CH₃	H	H	H	CH₃	2,6-Me-Py	20	5.0	30	40
7.	H	CH₃	CH₃	H	H	3,4-Me-Py	40	2.7	20	35
8.	H	CH₃	H	CH₃	H	3,5-Me-Py	74	5.5	17	69
9.	CH₃	H	CH₃	H	CH₃	2,4,6-Me-Py	2.6	0.39	0.49	29
10.	H	CONH₂	H	H	H	3-CONH₂-Py	71	20	210	67
11.	H	H	CONH₂	H	H	4-CONH₂-Py	84	24	220	77
12.	COOH	H	H	H	H	2-COOH-Py	1100	380	640	460
13.	H	COOH	H	H	H	3-COOH-Py	780	280	430	400
14.	H	H	COOH	H	H	4-COOH-Py	1000	350	700	460
15.	NH₂	H	H	H	H	2-NH₂-Py	44	10	13	23
16.	H	NH₂	H	H	H	3-NH₂-Py	29	1.8	3.8	35
17.	H	H	NH₂	H	H	4-NH₂-Py	10	1.6	7.0	23
18.	C₂H₅	H	H	H	H	2-C₂H₃-Py	45	12	160	130
19.	C₃H₇	H	H	H	H	2-C₂H₃-Py	24	6.3	53	120

[a]MICs against bacteria and yeast were measured by a Hitachi Recording Incubator and MICs against mold by the test tube dilution method.

cell wall and of the difficulties often encountered by hydrophilic molecules to traversing it. As a result, gram-negative microorganisms were the least sensitive toward all the homologues, MIC values being approximately 10 times greater than those toward the gram-positive organisms and the fungi.

The possibility of dual binding sites has experimental support from studies with cetyltrimethyl ammonium bromide, which binds in two stages, representing high- and low-affinity binding sites.[85] Such a mechanism implies potential synergy in combinations of BACs and might influence the choice of alkyl chain components for preservative mixture. Differences in the biologic activity of chemically related antimicrobials, acting at similar sites within the cell, also suggest their relative ease of penetration through the various liquid barriers of the cells and their ability to react at that site.[32,84] The outer components of the cells were considered as a series of aqueous and lipophilic layers. Substances of low water solubility would be unable to penetrate these aqueous layers and would accumulate within the lipid regions; similarly, those with low oil solubility would be unable to cross the lipophilic barriers. Compounds between these two extremes must exist that possess the optimum balance between hydrophilicity and lipophilicity for traversing the cell barriers. In summary, the antimicrobial activity of these compounds was found to be a parabolic function of their lipophilicity and maximized with *n*-alkyl chain length of between C_{12} and C_{16}.

Generally, yeast and fungi were most sensitive toward C_{12}, gram-positive bacteria toward C_{14}, and gram-negative bacteria toward C_{16}. The gram-negative bacteria were the most resistant toward all the compounds; gram-positive bacteria, the least.

The effect of colloidal associations on the activity of alkyldimethyl benzylammonium chlorides (ADBAC) homologous series C_8 to C_{18} have been reported with *P aeruginosa*.[86] The CMC is an important factor in the study of antimicrobial activity of QACs; at high concentrations of ADBAC, the formation of a micellar state of the salt interferes with the antibacterial action. These results questioned the normally accepted parabolic relationship reported to exist between the lipophilicity of many QACs and their antibacterial activities. The high concentration of nutrient salts, which are used in screening, would alter the concentration of monomeric quaternary ammonium salt. This may be responsible for some of the parabolic relationships rather than the intrinsic antibacterial activity of the compounds. As early as the 1950s, it was reported that for the homologous series of cationic surface-active agents, a parabolic relationship could exist between their antibacterial properties and their hydrophobic character. Thus, there is a linear relationship between activity and alkyl chain length with increased carbon number up to a maximum of between C_{12} and C_{14}, at which region there is observed decrease in activity. In Table 21.8, with broth dilution tests, a peak activity against various microorganisms could be observed at an alkyl chain length of 14 carbon atoms.[28] The turndown in activity probably is related to more than one physical property of the compounds: (1) the longer the chain, the greater the tendency for the molecule to be adsorbed at the surface of a bacterium; (2) there is a reduction of aqueous solubility of the molecule as the carbon number is increased. But the relevance of micellization to the thermodynamic state of the ADBAC molecule may be underestimated in the test system used. Salt additives are known to increase the tendency of ionic surface-active agents to micellize in water. In some instances, the micellar MWs (see Table 21.5) can increase, indicating a change in micellar type. In conclusion, the antibacterial activities of ADBAC homologous by the MIC procedure and by disinfection kinetics tests were studied in deionized water. There was a log-linear relationship between activity measured by kinetics test and carbon number. With the MIC method, there was a log-linear relationship up to C_{14} and then there was a turndown in activity. So consideration of the colloidal association of ADBAC in deionized water and in a simple salts growth media suggested that use of high concentrations of nutrient salts in MIC tests will lower the effective concentration of the surface-active agents. This change may be responsible for the turndown in activity observed in MIC tests, and in such circumstances, MIC tests do not give a true reflection of the intrinsic activity of these (and other) compounds.

The effects of the presence of organic materials on the bactericidal activity of BAC at various alkyl chain lengths during short contact times (10 s, 30 s, 1 min, 10 min) were investigated (Table 21.18).[87] The effect of human serum and dried yeast on the bactericidal activity of ADBAC standard blend OSN alkyl[C_{12}, 59%-63%; C_{14}, 29%-34%, C_{16}, 6.8-7.2%] dimethylbenzyl ammonium chloride and pure C_{12}BAC, C_{14}BAC, and C_{16}BAC was compared against 13 strains of bacteria. It was concluded that C_{12}BAC was the most effective component of the homologues series in the presence of organic materials. The bactericidal activity of BAC was inhibited by both dried yeast and human serum, with inhibition stronger by 2.5% dried yeast than by 10% human serum. As the carbon chain was increased, the inhibition increased. The C_{12}BAC was bactericidal against *Pseudomonas cepacia*, *P aeruginosa*, *Achromobacter guttatus*, *Alcaligenes faecalis*, and *Serratia marcescens* at 5000 ppm in a suspension of 2.5% dried yeast and at 2500 ppm in a 10% solution human serum at 1 minute of contact, but C_{14}BAC and C_{16}BAC was not effective at 10 000 ppm at 10 minutes. Many factors might be affected by the alkyl carbon length of BAC, producing changes in the bactericidal activity; for example, aqueous solubility, aqueous CMC, lipophilicity, and cell surface characteristics of the microorganisms used. The C_{12}BAC and C_{14}BAC were effectively bactericidal with all bacteria tested, even at a short contact time (30 s-1 min). The inhibition of bactericidal activity by organic materials was least for the C_{12}BAC (see Table 21.18). To clarify the relationship between inhibition of bactericidal activity of BAC by organic materials and binding of BAC to them, the authors assayed unbound C_{12}BAC and C_{14}BAC in a solution of bovine serum albumin by HPLC. As the carbon chain was lengthened, aqueous solubility decreased.

When the carbon chain is longer than C_{14}, the solubility and the CMC of BAC are extremely low. The binding to bovine serum albumin is increased with increase in the carbon chain; the C_{14}BAC bound to bovine serum albumin 2.5 to 3.7 times more than C_{12}BAC did. The bactericidal activity of BAC in a solution of bovine serum albumin depended on the amount of unbound BAC. The results showed that other factors in human serum may also inhibit antimicrobial activity. Interestingly, human serum tended to stimulate bactericidal activity against *S aureus* and *P cepacia* when the contact time was shorter. Human serum may make the surface of some bacteria more sensitive to BAC. These results suggest that C_{12}BAC is the most effective component of the homologous series of BAC in the presence of organic materials. The greater the content of C_{12}BAC in the blends, the more effective the mixture will be as a disinfectant from the practical point of view.

TABLE 21.18   Effect of human serum and dried yeast on bactericidal activity of homologues of the long-chain alkyl benzalkonium chlorides

Organism		Bactericidal Concentration (×10³ µg/mL)[a]															
		OSN				C₁₂BAC				C₁₄BAC				C₁₆BAC			
		10 s	30 s	1 min	10 min	10 s	30 s	1 min	10 min	10 s	30 s	1 min	10 min	10 s	30 s	1 min	10 min
Staphylococcus aureus FDA 209P	DW	0.5	0.5	0.2	0.05	5	1	0.5	0.1	1	0.4	0.1	0.025	0.4	0.2	0.025	0.01
	HS	1	0.5	0.5	0.5	1	1	0.5	0.5	5	1	0.5	0.5	0.5	0.5	0.5	0.5
	DY	5	5	2.5	2.5	5	5	2.5	2.5	5	5	2.5	2.5	>10	2.5	2.5	2.5
Staphylococcus epidermidis IFO 3762	DW	0.2	0.1	0.0125	0.006	1	0.4	0.4	0.025	0.8	0.025	0.025	0.006	0.05	0.006	<0.006	<0.006
	HS	0.5	0.5	0.5	0.5	2.5	1	0.5	0.5	0.5	0.5	0.5	0.5	2.5	0.5	0.5	0.5
	DY	2.5	2.5	2.5	2.5	2.5	2.5	2.5	2.5	2.5	2.5	2.5	2.5	2.5	2.5	2.5	1
Pseudomonas cepacia ATCC 17774	DW	5	1	1	0.4	1	0.8	0.5	0.5	>10	0.5	0.2	0.1	>10	>10	0.2	0.05
	HS	2.5	0.5	0.5	0.5	2.5	1	0.5	0.5	>10	5	2.5	0.5	>10	>10	>10	2.5
	DY	10	5	5	2.5	5	5	5	2.5	>10	>10	10	5	>10	>10	>10	>10
Pseudomonas aeruginosa H130	DW	5	5	0.2	0.1	5	5	1	0.5	10	5	5	0.2	>10	>10	>10	2.5
	HS	5	1	0.5	0.5	5	1	1	0.5	5	5	2.5	1	>10	>10	>10	5
	DY	>10	5	5	2.5	10	5	5	5	>10	>10	>10	10	>10	>10	>10	>10
P aeruginosa IFO 13736	DW	0.05	0.05	0.025	0.01	0.1	0.1	0.05	0.025	0.05	0.05	0.025	0.001	0.1	0.025	0.025	0.01
	HS	2.5	1	0.5	0.5	10	5	0.5	0.5	10	5	2.5	1	>10	>10	5	1
	DY	10	10	5	5	10	5	5	5	>10	>10	10	5	>10	>10	10	5
Proteus mirabilis 82-2-32	DW	0.1	0.1	0.025	0.01	0.2	0.1	0.1	0.025	0.2	0.2	0.025	0.01	10	0.1	0.05	0.01
	HS	2.5	2.5	0.5	0.5	5	5	2.5	1	10	5	2.5	1	5	5	0.5	0.5
	DY	>10	10	10	10	10	5	5	5	>10	>10	10	10	>10	>10	>10	>10

Organism	Medium																	
P mirabilis ATCC 21100	DW	0.2	0.05	0.05	0.05	0.2	0.4	0.05	0.2	0.01	0.01	0.05	0.05	0.05	0.1	0.05	0.05	0.01
	HS	5	2.5	0.5	0.5	1	5	1	10	0.5	1	2.5	5	5	>10	5	5	1
	DY	>10	5	2.5	2.5	5	10	5	>10	2.5	5	10	>10	>10	>10	>10	>10	10
P mirabilis 82-1-4	DW	5	0.2	0.1	0.01	1	1	0.2	1	0.2	0.05	0.1	0.05	0.05	>10	0.02	0.05	0.025
	HS	5	1	0.5	0.5	2.5	5	1	10	2.5	1	2.5	2.5	2.5	>10	>10	2.5	0.5
	DY	>10	5	5	5	10	10	5	>10	5	5	10	>10	10	>10	>10	>10	10
P morganii 82-2-11	DW	0.5	0.2	0.1	0.05	0.2	0.2	0.05	1	0.05	0.05	0.05	0.01	0.05	1	0.05	0.05	0.025
	HS	2.5	1	0.5	0.5	5	5	0.5	10	0.5	1	5	1	1	>10	>10	5	1
	DY	5	5	5	5	5	10	5	10	5	5	10	5	5	>10	>10	>10	10
Serratia marcescens 82-2-52	DW	5	0.4	0.2	0.05	0.4	0.4	0.025	>10	0.025	0.2	0.4	0.025	0.2	>10	0.025	0.025	0.025
	HS	5	2.5	1	0.5	5	5	0.5	>10	0.5	5	>10	2.5	5	>10	>10	>10	2.5
	DY	>10	>10	5	5	5	10	5	>10	5	>10	>10	10	10	>10	>10	>10	10
Havabacterium spp. 82-1-98	DW	0.1	0.05	0.05	0.025	0.2	0.2	0.05	0.2	0.25	0.05	0.05	0.025	0.05	0.2	0.025	0.025	0.01
	HS	2.5	0.5	0.5	0.5	1	5	0.5	5	0.5	1	1	2.5	1	10	5	2.5	0.1
	DY	2.5	2.5	2.5	2.5	5	5	2.5	10	1	2.5	5	5	5	10	5	5	2.5
Alcaligenes spp. A-39	DW	5	5	1	0.2	1	>10	0.2	>10	1	1	0.2	1	10	>10	>10	>10	0.5
	HS	5	5	1	0.5	5	5	0.5	>10	1	5	1	1	>10	>10	>10	>10	>10
	DY	>10	>10	>10	2.5	>10	>10	5	>10	5	>10	5	5	>10	>10	>10	>10	>10
Alcaligenes faecalis 572	DW	1	1	0.2	0.1	0.4	1	0.2	>10	0.2	0.2	0.4	0.2	0.2	>10	0.2	0.2	0.2
	HS	10	2.5	1	0.5	5	5	2.5	>10	2.5	5	5	10	10	>10	>10	>10	10
	DY	>10	>10	10	5	10	>10	5	>10	5	>10	10	>10	>10	>10	>10	>10	>10

Abbreviations: BAC, benzalkonium chloride; DW, deionized water; DY, 2.5% dried yeast; HS, 10% human serum; OSN, alkyl[C$_{12}$, 59%-63%; C$_{14}$, 29%-34%; C$_{16}$, 6.8%-7.2%] dimethylbenzylammonium chloride.

[a]Killed from 10^6 to <10^4 colony-forming units (CFUs)/mL at 25°C.

▶ ANTIMICROBIAL ACTIVITY

In the past, reports on the assessment of the antimicrobial activity of the QACs have often been misleading. On one hand, reports that by selecting the proper test method these compounds may appear as good disinfectants,[88] that efficacy is greater with suspension tests compared to inoculated carrier tests,[89] or that tests with QACs only demonstrate bacteriostatic instead of bactericidal activity[90] can be misleading. Unfortunately, a large amount of original work of the middle 1930s did indicate a wider spectrum of antimicrobial activity, including sporicidal and tuberculocidal activity at extremely low concentrations of QACs; there is little doubt that this was a result of inadequate neutralization of the test material carried over to the subculture medium, so that a static condition produced in the subculture was mistaken for destructive activity (see chapter 61). It must be remembered that the entire area of neutralization to prevent such carryover was inadequately dealt with at the time. A firm distinction between the biostatic and biocidal activities of an antimicrobial was not always determined. The necessity to obviate microbiostatic activity from the subculture medium was not always demanded as a requisite of antimicrobial testing, and the neutralization with specific chemical moieties used for individual classes of antimicrobials was not always insisted to be done. Any neutralization that occurred used dilution of the carryover antimicrobial from the aliquot sample to the volume of subculture medium to obtain a less than static concentration of the antimicrobial in the subculture medium.

The successful identification of discrete chemicals as specific QAC neutralizers, which may be incorporated into subculture media or into diluents, has made it mandatory that antimicrobial testing be performed only in the presence of such neutralizers (see chapter 61). Consequently, newer experimental results with QACs cannot be discredited as being purely static instead of destructive.

Also, the statement that the QACs may be made to look good by the proper test selection may be applied to any antimicrobial chemical. Certainly, a manipulation of the various test parameters, such as type and amount of soil, selection of test organisms, and many others, will bias any result, so that any chemical product will appear as a good or poor antimicrobial agent. The dynamics of testing carriers prepared with dried films of microorganisms can provide a more severe test than the liquid inoculum (suspension) test systems. This feature of carrier-type tests led to the development and use of such tests in the United States and the European Union to measure bactericidal, sporicidal, tuberculocidal, and viricidal activity (see chapters 62 and 63). In the United States, the regulation of antimicrobials intended for treatment of inanimate surfaces was formerly exercised by the US Department of Agriculture and currently by the EPA (see chapter 72). It includes deliberate scrutiny of a product for antimicrobial efficacy and toxicologic and chemical properties in compliance with the product-label claims and other attendant information, all prior to the initial sale of the product. Furthermore, the agency is required to monitor future production obtained on a periodic inspection schedule. The recent introduction of prescribed test methods by other agencies and in other countries is a most salutary development to eliminate the confusing conclusions developed here from many different kinds of experimental studies (see chapter 61).

In addition to the direct antimicrobial effects, QAC and other surfactant-based formulations are widely used for cleaning or combined cleaning-disinfection applications. Due to their surfactant abilities, they are often associated with increasing the physical removal of microbial contaminants from surfaces and particularly in the presence of contaminating soils such as foods and animals or human tissues. These physical removal capabilities may also allow for the greater penetration of the QACs or other associated biocides to intrinsic microorganisms and increased effectiveness of the cleaning/disinfection process. But in many cases, these effects may not be due to the direct antimicrobial activity of QACs against the target microorganisms.

The QACs have been tested by a multitude of different procedures, which may be generally classified as (1) in vitro static or minimum inhibitory level tests, usually as broth dilution tests; (2) in vitro or killing dilution tests, with suspensions tests such as the phenol coefficient test as an example; (3) simulated use-dilution tests, including inoculated carriers of representative surfaces such as stainless steel, porcelain, and fabric; and (4) in-use tests, which use the product in the actual environment. The results of such testing with QACs may be summarized as follows, but note that they can vary depending on the specific QAC and or associated formulations (see chapter 6): The active QACs sold as items of commerce are generally algistatic, bacteriostatic, tuberculostatic, sporostatic, and fungistatic at low concentration levels of 0.5 to 5 ppm[91,92]; they are algicidal, bactericidal, fungicidal, and virucidal against lipophilic viruses at medium concentration levels of 10 to 50 ppm[36,93]; they are generally not tuberculocidal, sporicidal, or virucidal against hydrophilic viruses at high concentration levels, but their activity can be enhanced in formulation with other excipient/biocides.[93-95] For example, although QACs are not considered effective against bacterial spores due to the lack of significant penetration into the spore structure, their presence will inhibit the outgrowth of spores following germination and in combination with germinants can render spores more susceptible to inactivation.[96,97] The activity of QACs against enveloped viruses such as HIV and hepatitis B virus may be expected due to the presence of a lipid envelop on these external structure of these viruses (see chapter 3) but not against nonenveloped viruses that have a protein-based external capsid structure.[98] There are mixed reports in the literature on the effectiveness of QACs against some nonenveloped viruses such as norovirus and caliciviruses,[92] but these studies may reflect the impact of formulation effects or physical effects on virus removal. They are bactericidal to both gram-positive and gram-negative bacteria, with some evidence for greater activity against the gram-positive bacteria.[97] In this regard, it should be remembered that the gram-negative

bacteria as a group, especially pseudomonad species, are typically more resistant to antimicrobial compounds (see chapters 3 and 4).

The QACs are bactericidal agents in acid and alkaline environments, with some evidence for greater activity in the alkaline range.[99] The following descriptions of antimicrobial results are considered as representative data for all QACs. The bacteriostatic, fungistatic, and algistatic activities of fatty nitrogen compounds, including QACs, were previously described[91] and are summarized in Table 21.19. The bactericidal dilutions for some widely used QACs after a 10-minute contact period at 20°C (using the phenol coefficient method against

TABLE 21.19 Inhibiting concentrations (in ppm) of fatty nitrogen compounds for some bacteria, fungi, and algae

Compound	Bacteria			
	Escherichia coli	*Pseudomonas fluorescens*	*Bacillus subtilis*	*Staphylococcus aureus*
Benzethonium chloride	1000	300	3	3
Benzalkonium chloride	200	300	3	4
Dodecyltrimethyl ammonium chloride	500	500	5	5
Dodocylbenzyldimethyl ammonium chloride	750	750	2	2
Cocobenzyldimethyl ammonium chloride	225	225	2	2
Didecyldimethyl ammonium chloride	225	750	0.7	7

Compound	Fungi			
	Aspergillus niger	*Chaetomium globosum*	*Myrothecium verrucaria*	*Trichoderma viridae*
Benzethonium chloride	300	30	300	200
Benzalkonium chloride	60	10	40	80
Dodecyltrimethyl ammonium chloride	500	50	500	500
Dodocylbenzyldimethyl ammonium chloride	75	7	150	75
Cocobenzyldimethyl ammonium chloride	20	7	20	20
Didecyldimethyl ammonium chloride	75	7	20	20

Compound	Algae			
	Chlorella vulgaris	*Stigeoclonium species*	*Anabena cylindrica*	*Oscillatoria tenuis*
Benzethonium chloride	3	1	1	1
Benzalkonium chloride	1	0.7	1	0.6
Dodecyltrimethyl ammonium chloride	50	5	5	0.5
Dodocylbenzyldimethyl ammonium chloride	0.2	0.2	0.2	0.2
Cocobenzyldimethyl ammonium chloride	2	0.5	2	0.7
Didecyldimethyl ammonium chloride	2	0.7	0.2	0.7

TABLE 21.20 Antimicrobial dilutions of commercially available quaternary ammonium germicide for 10-min contact periods at 20°C from phenol coefficients in manufacturers' brochures

Chemical	Antimicrobial Dilutions Versus	
	Staphylococcus aureus	*Salmonella typhosa*
Di-isobutylphenoxyethoxyethyl dimethyl benzyl ammonium chloride	1/25 000	1/25 000
40% Methyldodecylbenzyl trimethyl ammonium chloride, 10% methyldodecylxylylene bis(trimethyl ammonium chloride)	1/24 000	1/22 500
n-Alkyl[C_{12}, 40%; C_{14}, 50%; C_{16}, 10%] dimethyl benzyl ammonium chlorides	1/45 000	1/45 000
Benzyldimethyltetradecyl ammonium chloride	1/42 800	1/67 500
n-Alkyl[C_{12}, 5%; C_{15}, 60%; C_{16}, 30%; C_{18}, 5%] dimethylbenzyl ammonium chlorides	1/44 000	1/39 600
25% n-alkyl[C_{12}, 68%; C_{14}, 32%] dimethylethylbenzyl ammonium chlorides	1/55 500	1/54 300
n-Alkyl[C_{12}, 98%; C_{14}, 2%] dimethyl 1-naphthylmethyl ammonium chlorides	1/60 000	1/58 500
n-Alkyl[C_{12}, 50%; C_{14}, 30%; C_{16}, 17%; C_{18}, 3%] isoquinolinium bromides	1/38 000	1/40 000
Octyldodecyldimethyl ammonium chlorides	1/61 800	1/57 500
Alkyl[C_{12}, 40%; C_{14}, 50%; C_{16}, 10%] dimethylbenzyl ammonium saccharinates	1/43 500	1/40 500
Didecyldimethyl ammonium chlorides	1/63 000	1/84 000

S aureus and *Salmonella typhosa*) are also summarized in Table 21.20. These are at high dilutions for both organisms, and they are at significantly different dilutions depending on the specific chemical structure of the quaternary compound. The effect of the size of the quaternary molecule on the antimicrobial activity of a homologous series of alkyldimethylbenzyl ammonium chlorides was previously well documented,[28] who demonstrated a maximum activity as the highest 10-minute killing dilution against *S aureus* and *S typhosa* and *P aeruginosa* for the C_{14} member compound tested (see Table 21.8).

Additional evidence for the structure and antimicrobial activity relationship was published[34] and evaluated the interference of hard water with the sanitizing activity against *E coli* of a group of dialkyldimethyl ammonium chloride compounds of varying long-chain lengths. This comparison of HWTs, which are defined as the maximum concentrations of synthetic hard water (as $CaCO_3$) that 200 ppm of active quaternary compound will continue to disinfect (at 5 $\log_{10}$ reduction) a suspension of *E coli* after a 30-second contact period, is summarized in Table 21.21.

TABLE 21.21 Hard-water tolerances (ppm $CaCO_3$) of dialkyldimethyl quaternary ammonium compounds with long carbon chains ($R_1 + R_2$) that total 19 to 22 carbons

Totals Carbons ($R_1 + R_2$[a])	Hard-Water Tolerance (ppm $CaCO_3$)						
19	700	800	500	550			
20	500	900	1200	1400	1100		
21	300	700	900	1300	1300		
22	400	550	750	900	800	650	
	6	7	8	9	10	11	R_1 carbon length

[a]R_2 carbon chain length obtained by subtracting R_1 carbon chain length from the $R_1 + R_2$ total carbon chain length.

TABLE 21.22	Bactericidal activity of cetyl pyridinium chloride aqueous solution	
Organism	No. of Strains Tested	Average Critical Killing Dilution in Terms of Active Ingredients at 37°C
		No Serum
Staphylococcus aureus	5	1:83 000
Staphylococcus albus	1	1:73 000
Streptococcus viridans	1	1:42 500
Streptococcus hemolyticus	2	1:127 500
Neisseria catarrhalis	2	1:84 000
Diplococcus pneumoniae I	1	1:95 000
Pseudomonas aeruginosa	2	1:5800
Klebsiella pneumoniae	2	1:49 000
Corynebacterium diphtheriae	1	1:64 000
Mycobacterium phlei	1	1:1500
Eberthella typhosa	5	1:48 000
Escherichia coli	2	1:66 000
Proteus vulgaris	2	1:34 000
Shigella dysenteriae	1	1:60 000
Shigella paradysenteriae (Flexner)	2	1:52 000
Shigella paradysenteriae (Hiss)	1	1:49 000

Early investigations with cetyl pyridinium chloride illustrated several characteristics of QACs, such as the greater activity for gram-positive bacteria over gram-negative bacteria (Table 21.22), the positive effect of temperature, and the negative effect of organic matter on antimicrobial activity (Table 21.23).[100] Lawrence[101] also described the effect of pH on the antibacterial activity of an alkyldimethylbenzyl ammonium chloride at 5-, 10-, and 15-minute contact periods against S aureus (Table 21.24). The fungicidal activity of many QACs was initially investigated with Trichophyton interdigitale, demonstrating a higher resistance than bacteria (Table 21.25). Similar results have been shown with a

wider range of fungi, such as with a bis-QACS.[102] There are limited studies on the effects against protozoa,[92] but vegetative forms would be considered to be sensitive due to their structure and dormant forms (such as cysts and oocyst) are generally resistant (see chapter 3).

A final consideration is the numerous reports in the literature on the development of tolerance mechanisms to QACs in bacteria (see chapter 4).[92,103] As already mentioned, gram-negative bacteria are generally less sensitive to QACs due to their cell wall structure, but many types of bacterial and fungal structures including the mycobacterial cell wall and the outer surfaces of bacterial spores provide natural resistance mechanisms to the antimicrobial

TABLE 21.23	Effect of temperature and serum on germicidal activity of cetyl pyridinium chloride: critical killing dilutions expressed in terms of active ingredients			
Organisms	37°C 10% Bovine		20°C 10% Bovine	
	No Serum	Serum	No Serum	Serum
Staphylococcus aureus	1:110 000	1:11 500	1:67 500	1:6750
Salmonella Typhi	1:83 500	1; 1400	1:62 500	1:1300

TABLE 21.24   Effects of pH on the antiseptic efficiency of a quaternary ammonium germicide against *Staphylococcus aureus*

Quaternary Ammonium Compound Concentration	Exposure Acid or Alkali per 100 mL	Bacterial Growth After Minutes			
		pH	5	10	15
1:15 000	0.10 mL N/10 HCl	4.3	−	−	−
1:15 000	0.25 mL N/10 HCl	3.8	−	−	−
1:15 000	0.50 mL N/10 HCl	3.5	+	+	+
1:15 000	1.00 mL N/10 HCl	3.2	+	+	+
Control (no quaternary ammonium compound)	1.00 mL N/10 HCl	3.2	+	+	+
1:25 000	0	6.7	+	+	+
1:25 000	0.10 mL N/10 NaOH	9.4	+	+	+
1:25 000	0.25 mL N/10 NaOH	10.0	+	+	−
1:25 000	0.50 mL N/10 NaOH	10.2	+	+	−
1:25 000	1.00 mL N/10 NaOH	10.5	+	−	−
1:25 000	1.25 mL N/10 NaOH	10.6	+	−	−

effects of QAC (see chapters 3 and 4).[103] But there are many other acquired mechanisms of resistance in bacteria that have been described (with examples in Table 21.26) and proposed parallel mechanisms in other vegetative microorganisms such as fungi. These include additional cell wall modification, efflux mechanisms (where bacteria actively pump the biocides out of the inner cell surfaces across the cell wall), and enzymatic degradation of QACs. These mechanisms can increase dramatically the overall tolerance of bacteria to various QACs but may be overcome by various disinfectant formulation effects including multiple biocides and the presence of other excipients that may aid in biocide penetration and overwhelm

the cells resistance mechanisms. But these tolerance risks can be particularly important in the presence of lower levels of QACs (eg, being used for preservative purposes or in wastewater) and the cross-resistance to antibiotics with greater clinical consequences.[103,114] Some of these mechanisms (particularly associated with efflux) can be transmitted between bacteria by transmissible genetic elements (eg, plasmids), highlighting the risks of the broad use of such biocides to the developing concerns on antibiotic resistance. Overall, these concerns have led to the call for the appropriate and prudent use of biocides, including QACs, to reduce these and other potential toxicologic risks.[115,116]

TABLE 21.25   Critical killing dilution (10-min contact period) required for aqueous dilutions of quaternary compounds to kill spores of *Trichophyton interdigitale*[a]

Chemical Structure	Average Killing Dilution
40% methyldodecylbenzyltrimethyl ammonium chloride, 10% methyldodecylxylylene bis (trimethyl ammonium chloride)	1/2000
25% n-alkyl[C_{12}, 5%; C_{14}, 60%; C_{16}, 30%; C_{18}, 5%] dimethylbenzyl ammonium chloride, 25% n-alkyl[C_{12}, 68%; C_{14}, 32%] dimethylethylbenzyl ammonium chlorides	1/800
Octyldodecyldimethyl ammonium bromide	1/5000
Didecyldimethyl ammonium chloride	1/4750

[a]Dilutions are based on anhydrous germicide.

TABLE 21.26	Examples of tolerance or resistance mechanisms to quaternary ammonium compounds described in bacteria		
Mechanism	**Bacteria**	**Intrinsic or Acquired**	**References**
Modification of cell wall surface	*Pseudomonas aeruginosa*	Intrinsic and acquired, due to changes in surface protein, lipids, or other surface changes; exclusion from the mycobacterial and bacterial spore surface	McDonnell,[103] Tabata et al,[104] Guérin-Méchin et al,[105] and Bruinsma et al[106]
Efflux	*Serratia marcescens, Staphylococcus aureus* (*qacA-C* containing plasmids), *P aeruginosa* MexAB-OprM and MexXY-OprM (intrinsic) MexCD-OprJ, MexEF-OprN and MexJK-OprM (acquired), *Escherichia coli* AcrAB-TolC, EmrE	Intrinsic and acquired, including plasmids and mutational upregulation	Maseda et al,[107] Wassenaar et al,[108] Schweizer,[109] Weston et al,[110] and Poole[111]
Enzymatic degradation	*Pseudomonas, Burkholderia*	Intrinsic and acquired, including upregulation	Ahn et al[112] and Takenaka et al[113]

▶ TOXICOLOGY

The QACs are one of the mostly widely used preservative and disinfectant biocides worldwide due to their low associated toxicity,[92] but there has been a recent emphasis on investigating their toxicity to users and the environment.[116] In 1987, the EPA issued a "Data Call-In Notice" requiring all registrants of antimicrobial active ingredients to submit subchronic and chronic toxicologic data to support the continued registration of their products. Risk was evaluated by acquiring exposure and toxicity data under a three-tiered approach:

A. The first-tier studies: (1) 90-day dermal, (2) 90-day inhalation, (3) teratogenicity first, and (4) mutagenicity
B. The second-tier studies: (1) subchronic feeding, (2) teratogenicity second, (3) dermal absorption, (4) and 90-day neurotoxicity
C. The third-tier studies: (1) chronic feeding, two species; (2) oncogenicity, two species; (3) reproduction; (4) and metabolism to clarify issues concerning SARs

At this time, QACs were grouped into four groups so that toxicity studies would be facilitated by selecting one member from each group for testing:

Group I: The straight-chain alkyl or hydroxyalkyl quaternaries; the most common product in this group is the twin-chain quats; a full set of subchronic and chronic toxicity studies on didecyldimethyl ammonium chloride and teratology studies on alkyltrimethyl ammonium chloride
Group II: The nonhalogenated substituted benzyl and ADBACs, namely, BACs; a full set of subchronic and chronic studies on alkyl[C_{12}, 5%; C_{14}, 90%; C_{16}, 10%] dimethylbenzyl ammonium chloride

Group III: The alkyl[di- and tri-chlorobenzyl] dimethyl ammonium compounds; a full set of subchronic and chronic studies on alkyl[C_{12}, 5%; C_{14}, 90%; C_{16}, 5%] dimethyl 3,4-dichlorobenzyl ammonium chloride
Group IV: The heterocyclic ammonium compounds with unusual substituents. Each chemical in this category was expected to be tested separately unless otherwise justified. Representative compounds in group IV are (1) alkyl[C_{12}/C_{16}] substituted picolinium compounds, (2) alkyl[C_8/C_{18}] imidazolinium compounds, (3) alkyl[C_{14}/C_{18}] N-ethyl-morpholinium compounds, and (4) alkyl[C_{12}/C_{18}] isoquinolinium compounds and other heterogeneous structures.

Most of the resulting studies have not been published, but the QACs and their associated disinfectants remain in widespread use today, and specific toxicologic data is provided with their safety data sheets. A knowledge of the toxicologic properties of QACs is important so that the safety, health, and well-being of man and animals are not compromised by contact with these chemicals as they are manufactured, shipped, compounded, or used. Although these specific investigations are not germane, the studies to characterize the general toxicologic properties of antimicrobial QACs and the studies of the harmful consequences of these chemicals at concentrations simulating their use patterns are of primary importance. Toxicologic effect is measured at three levels: (1) at the amount necessary to bring about the response with 100% of the experimental animals, LD_{100}; (2) at the amount that will cause the response with 50% of the animals, LD_{50}; and (3) at the amount that does not produce the response with any of the animals, LD_0. The LD_{50} level is most frequently used to characterize toxicity. In addition, the methods of administering the chemical also are identified using descriptions such as oral, subcutaneous, intraperitoneal, intravenous, and dermal. Also, the toxicity is determined as an acute response following a single administration of the chemical; as a short-term or subacute response following a multiple, periodic administration of the chemical over a short period such as 30 or 90 days; and finally as a chronic response following a multiple, periodic administration over a long period, such as the animal's life span. The LD_{50} amounts of QAC depend on the route of administration. A notable example was with myristyl γ picolinium chloride, with a reported LD_{50} of 250 mg/kg by oral administration, 200 mg/kg for subcutaneous injection, 7.5 mg/kg for intraperitoneal injection, and 30 mg/kg for intravenous injection.[117] Using the acute oral LD_{50}, which is the toxicologic characteristic most frequently described, the toxicities of different quaternary compounds can be compared. For example, acute oral LD_{50} values in white rats were reported with 445 mg/kg for alkyldimethylbenzyl ammonium chloride, 500 mg/kg for alkenyldimethylethyl ammonium bromide, 730 mg/kg for alkyldimethyl 3,4-dichlorobenzyl ammonium chloride, 420 mg/kg for diisobutylphenoxyethoxyethyldimethylbenzyl ammonium chloride, and 389 mg/kg for alkyltolymethyltrimethyl ammonium chloride.[118,119] These and similar data obtained from studies in humans and in laboratory animals led to the generalized conclusion that the antimicrobial QACs examined to date exhibit similar toxicologic and pharmacologic properties.

Dermal toxicity also was examined and reported from animal and human testing that 0.1% was the maximum concentration of the aforementioned compounds that would not produce primary irritation on intact skin or act as a sensitizer.[118,119] The conjunctival mucous membrane obviously requires special consideration, which was undertaken by a number of investigators. A 1:3000 (333 ppm) solution of myristyl γ picolinium chloride produced a slight irritation of the conjunctival mucosa of rabbits.[117] A 1:1000 dilution (1000 ppm) of alkyldimethylbenzyl ammonium chloride instilled into the eyes of human subjects produced burning and stinging reactions, whereas a 1:5000 dilution (200 ppm) produced no unpleasant sensations.[120] The maximum nonirritating concentrations of alkyldimethylbenzyl ammonium chloride and cetylpyridimium chloride in the eyes of rabbits were reported to be 1:3000 (333 ppm) and 1:2000 (500 ppm), respectively.[121] Others observed comparable irritation levels for diisobutylphenoxyethoxyethyldimethyl ammonium chloride.[119]

An important toxicologic consideration arising from the widely encountered application area of sanitizing food contact surfaces is the cumulative effect in animals and humans with the ingestion of food contacted by the small residues QAC-based disinfectants. A laboratory study simulating this situation is conducted by the daily oral administration of QACs in the food or drinking water of test animals over a considerable period of time, including the normal life span of the animal. For example, myristyl γ picolinium chloride at 0.1% in the diet of rats did not interfere with their normal growth rate, but this concentration produced death when administered as a sole source of fluid and required reduction to 0.05% to permit a normal growth rate of the test animal.[117] Results of a 2-year chronic feeding study of rats on a diet containing 0.5, 0.25, 0.125, or 0.063% alkyldimethylbenzyl chloride found that all the quaternary compound concentrations were toxic to rats, as evidenced by lower growth rates over an untreated control group and as determined by the histopathologic lesions present in the treated animals.[122] But subsequent studies using a significantly larger number of experimental animals and a more randomized statistical design demonstrated that alkyldimethylbenzyl ammonium chloride at 0.25% in the diet of rats over a 2-year feeding period did not demonstrably affect the growth, food consumption, blood picture, or histopathology of the treated animals.[123] Dogs fed over a 15-week period a diet containing 0.12% or less quaternary compound demonstrated similar nontoxic effects. Similarly, a minimal toxicologic effect was observed, evidenced by weight loss, a depressed growth rate, and an abnormal blood or histopathology, for dogs that were allowed a 1:5000 aqueous dilution of either alkyldimethylbenzyl ammonium chloride, alkenyldimethylethyl ammonium bromide, laurylisoquinolinium bromide, or alkyldimethyl 3,4-dichlorobenzyl ammonium chloride as their sole source of drinking water over a 6-month period, for guinea pigs administered 25, 12.5, or 5 mg/kg of the aforementioned QACs daily for a 1-year period and for rats similarly treated daily over a 2-year period.[118] A concentration of 2500 ppm of alkyltolylmethyltrimethyl ammonium chloride or diisobutylphenoxyethoxyethyldimethyl benzyl ammonium chloride in the diet of rats produced minimal deleterious toxicologic effects over a 2-year period, whereas a concentration of 1000 ppm produced no undesirable toxicologic effects over the same period.[119]

In some cases, concerns over the adulteration of food, especially of milk, with residues from QAC disinfectants led to label statements for these products requiring a water rinse following use of the disinfectant and reuse of the food equipment. But in other cases, analysis of chronic feeding studies concluded that rinsing may not be necessary if the disinfectant solution did not exceed 200 to 400 ppm of quaternary compound and if the quaternary compound solution contains equal amounts of n-alkyl[C_{12}-C_{18}] benzyldimethyl ammonium chloride and n-alkyl[C_{12}-C_{14}] dimethylethylbenzyl ammonium chloride having an average MW of 384.[124,125]

A short time later, the same statement was made for an aqueous solution containing n-alkyl[C_{12}-C_{18}] benzyldimethyl ammonium chloride having an average MW of between 351 and 380 and consisting principally of alkyl groups with 12 to 16 carbon atoms with or without, but not over, 1% each of groups with 8 and 10 carbon atoms.[124]

Lower levels have been recommended in the European Union for food-contacting QACs such as didecyldimethylammonium chloride and BAC.[126]

In 1969, it was summarized that at least 10 human fatalities implicating QACs were medically recorded at that time as resulting from alkyldimethylbenzyl ammonium chloride solutions of 10% or 15% introduced into the victims via oral ingestion, intramuscular or intravenous administration, or intrauterine instillation.[127] In particular, the ingestion of concentrated solution leads to immediate burning pain in the mouth, throat, and abdomen. The toxicologic information can be summarized as follows. The QAC disinfectants as concentrated solutions of 10% or more are toxic, causing death if taken internally and severe irritation to the skin and conjunctival mucosa when applied externally. With normal precautions and operating procedures, the probability of such contact is extremely remote because the effective use-dilutions of these materials are well below the concentrated level causing death and severe injury. In addition, oral ingestion, the most likely route of accidental internal administration, is self-limiting for concentrated quaternary ammonium solutions because the immediate burning in the mouth and throat acts as a signal. At the dilute solutions of the use levels of QAC disinfectants, which range from several to about 1000 ppm, only the most deliberate distortions of normal operating procedures could offer acute toxicity problems. Finally, chronic toxicity, as from the cumulative effect of food adulterated with QAC germicides via residues from dilute disinfectant solutions used on food-processing equipment, is not considered a significant problem.

The ototoxic effects of QACs benzethonium chloride and BAC, which are frequently used for skin disinfection, have been studied.[128] The disinfectant QACs, at concentrations of 0.1% in water solution or in 70% alcohol, were introduced into the tympanic cavity (middle ear) of guinea pigs for exposure times of 10, 30, or 60 minutes. The animals were killed 2 or 9 weeks after the exposure, and the organ of Corti and vestibular neuroepithelia were studied as surface preparations with phase-contrast microscopy. Most of the ears exposed to the disinfectants had suffered damage, affecting both the vestibulum and the perilymphatic and endolymphatic spaces of the cochlea of the inner ear. The extent of the damage was related both to the duration of exposure and to the length of the animal's survival after the exposure. Furthermore, the tympanic cavity and the perilymphatic spaces of vestibulum and cochlea were pathologically changed. Furthermore, a report on the safety assessment of benzethonium chloride and methylbenzethonium chloride concluded that both compounds are safe at concentrations of 0.5% in cosmetics applied to the skin.[129] A maximum concentration of 0.02% was considered safe for cosmetics used in the eye area. Chronic and subchronic feeding studies indicated little or no toxic effects for both ingredients.

In clinical studies, benzethonium chloride produced mild skin irritation at 5% but not at lower concentrations. Neither ingredient was considered to be a sensitizer, but this may vary depending on the QAC or surfactant type (eg, quaternium-15 is a common cause of allergic contact dermatitis).[130]

There has also been a lot of interest in studying the environmental stability QACs and other surfactants in the environment.[116,131,132] They are detected in waste treatment plants, sewage, and sludge. They are considered biodegradable, including by microbial degradation, but overall, this can vary depending on their structures and availability. Many, under certain situations, can persist, and some can be toxic to aquatic organisms including fish.

APPLICATIONS

With the development of first- and second-generation QACs in the 1920-1930s, many application areas were developed for the QACs. Initially, they were used as an adjunct to surgery, such as in preoperative patient skin treatment, antisepsis of the hands of the surgical team preoperatively, and disinfection of surgical instruments. The superiority of 0.1% alkyldimethylbenzyl ammonium chloride in comparison to 60% alcohol for treatment of the surgeon's hands prior to surgery was demonstrated in a series of reports.[133-135] In 1938, alkyldimethylbenzyl ammonium chloride was also described as a skin preparation for a patient prior to surgery reduced the incidence of wound infection.[120,136] A comparison of the activity of cetylpyridinium chloride and alkydimethylbenzyl ammonium chloride with that of mercurials as skin preparation prior to surgery also found the quaternary compounds superior.[137] Some suggested that these effects were due to quaternary compounds applied to the skin forming a continuous residual sheet, beneath which bacteria actually survived.[138,139] It was proposed that the film is formed as an oriented adsorption of the quaternary compound on an organophilic surface, with the nontoxic ends directed toward the skin and the bactericidal active ends directed toward the outside, which explained the favorable results obtained for quaternary compounds in many studies. Others rejected the film concept and proposed instead that treatment with the quaternary compounds altered the charge of the skin to being positive, which attracted and held negatively charged bacteria, leading to the favorable, if inaccurate, results in wash studies with quaternary compounds.[140] In the same publication, they speculated that phospholipids present on the surface of the skin inhibited the antimicrobial activity of the quaternary compound. Overall, these negative comments and the widespread popular use of hexachlorophene-based products at the time (and since then discontinued due to toxicity concerns with hexachlorophene) lead to a decrease in the use of QACs to approximately 37% in 1965.[141] Combination products with alcohols, such as the use of mechanical soap hand scrubbing followed by application of a mixture of isopropyl alcohol, alkyldimethylbenzyl ammonium chloride, and cetyl alcohol were also described.[134] QACs are still used today for a variety of antiseptic applications, such as cetrimide and BAC in skin and mucous membrane (eg, mouth) washes but are not as widely used a routine skin disinfectants or as surgical scrubs (see chapters 42 and 43), with the exception of some formulations in combination with biocides such as chlorhexidine or alcohols (see chapters 19 and 22).[142] The most widely used are the alkyl BACs, and some newer formulations have been developed as alternatives to the now widely used alcohol-based hand rubs (see chapter 42).[143,144] In the United States, BAC and benzethonium chloride are currently under review by the FDA for safety and efficacy as over-the-counter health care antiseptic products.[145]

In the 1930s and 1940s, alkyldimethylbenzyl ammonium chloride and formulations thereof (to improve material compatibility) were recommended for the disinfection of surgical instruments.[120,146,147] Most early investigators, with few exceptions, did indeed subscribe to the idea of a total spectrum of microbicidal activity for the quaternary compounds, but clarity of the spectrum of efficacy was provided overtime. Early reports confirmed that QACs may not kill bacterial spores.[148] Similar studies with tubercle bacilli on simulate contaminated thermometers demonstrated that aqueous solutions of both alkyldimethylbenzyl ammonium chloride and cetylpyridinium chloride at high concentrations did not kill the organism after a 10-minute contact period, whereas tinctures of the same compounds (50% alcoholic) did in fact kill the organism.[149] The subsequent use of specific quaternary compound neutralizers as a requisite for testing prevented additional instances of residual bacteriostasis that were interpreted as bactericidal activity, as in the case of tuberculocidal and sporicidal testing. The inability of quaternary compounds to kill the tubercle bacillus or bacterial spores did limit their use as surgical instrument disinfection or sterilization, but they have continued to be widely used for noncritical device applications that are typically subjected to low or intermediate chemical disinfection (see chapter 47). Indeed, their combined cleaning and disinfection properties have seen their widespread use for such applications including on noncritical devices and environmental surfaces. Applications include concentrated products (requiring dilution prior to use), ready-to-use liquid formulations, and antimicrobial wipes.[92,103]

The widespread use of QACs for environmental disinfection of floors, walls, and equipment surfaces in hospitals, nursing homes, public places, and gymnasia required the development of a detergent compatible with the quaternary compounds that would permit the combination of the two operations of cleaning and disinfection. As early

example combined cetyldimethylethyl ammonium bromide with the nonionic wetting agent alkylated aryl polyether alcohol and inorganic salts.[150] The concentrated formulation was diluted as 1 oz/gal of aqueous solution and used to test disinfectant efficacy on cleaned glass slides contaminated with heavy artificial soil inoculated with bacteria. When the contact period of the slide and diluted formulation was extended to 10 minutes, all the bacteria on the soiled slides were killed, as demonstrated by negative broth subcultures of the slides and by zero-count agar plates prepared from the broth subcultures. This concept of a one-step operation to produce cleaning and antimicrobial activity, which made the treatment of large surface areas practical, met with success and furthered research to the present time toward the development of quaternary nonionic formulations with optimum cleaning and antimicrobial properties.[34] Both in vitro laboratory tests and of field tests under actual conditions attest to the utility of these products. Treatment of large areas of environmental surface is typically accomplished by a mop-and-bucket operation, by mechanical flooding and vacuum pickup, by sponge or cloth hand wipe operation, and by liquid spray. As an additional treatment procedure for disinfection of surfaces, QAC disinfectant formulations were developed in pressurized containers as an aerosol spray.[151] The treatment of area surfaces via a mist of QAC disinfectant generated from commercial fogging devices have been described.[152,153] These produced droplets of approximately 50 μm in diameter by the shearing action of air pressure on the liquid disinfectant solution, with 0.2% active aqueous solution of a 50:50 mixture of alkyldimethylbenzyl ammonium chloride and alkyldimethylethylbenzyl ammonium chloride. This procedure was suggested as an adjunct for terminal disinfection of hospital or other industrial areas in the 1960s, as area of particular resurgent interest in health care and animal husbandry applications.[154,155]

Treatment of food contact surfaces, that is, those found on equipment in the food processing industries and on food and beverage utensils in eating and drinking establishments, to obtain sanitary conditions that will prevent transmission of disease through the food, is defined in the United States as a sanitizing treatment or as sanitation of such surfaces. Practicable sanitizing requires that any treatment residual will not in itself be harmful; it does not require a destruction of all the bacteria present on the treated surface. The use of QACs to sanitize such surfaces was suggested by Krog and Marshall,[156,157] who experimentally contaminated the rims of glass drinking tumblers, allowed them to air-dry, and treated them with a 1:5000 aqueous dilution of alkyldimethylbenzyl ammonium chloride for various contact periods before swabbing and plating procedures were employed to enumerate the viable bacteria present; this demonstrated a reduction to less than 100 bacteria per rim after only a 1-minute contact period. Similarly, the use of alkyldimethylbenzyl ammonium chloride at a 1:6000 dilution in a dairy pasteurizing plant caused a 60% to 98% reduction of the bacteria count on the milk handling and processing equipment.[157] Subsequently, many other investigators confirmed the use of QACs as disinfectants for the dairy farm and dairy plant as well as other food-processing industries.[92]

The treatment of large amounts of water to destroy and prevent the proliferation of disease-producing microorganisms, of industrial process-interfering microorganisms, and finally of noxious, esthetically undesirable microorganisms is an important application area for QACs. The demonstration of the inactivation of bacteria and some protozoal cysts (*Entamoeba histolytica*) suggested that QACs could be useful for the emergency disinfection of drinking water.[158,159] Although QACs have not been widely used for the preparation of potable water, there are recent examples of their effective use as antimicrobial coatings attached to common filter media such as sand and zeolite. These have been used in the preliminary treatment of surface water for the removal of course particulate and to reduce microbial (particularly bacteria and virus) levels prior to further purification or treatment.[160] It is important to note that other reports suggest that "slow" sand filtration systems alone can reduce the levels of bacteria, viruses, and protozoa,[161] but the combination with QACs seems to offer an additional benefit to traditional sand filtration alone. These reports highlight the benefits of new ways to improve the activity of existing biocides, including QACs, including delivery to the point of use such as an antimicrobial surfaces (see chapter 73) or as nanotechnology (see chapter 74).

The general bactericidal, fungicidal, and algicidal (or associated static) activity of QACs have seen their effective use for many industrial, municipal, and other water treatment applications, such as in cooling systems and swimming pool water treatment. A product containing 0.5% of Hyamine 1622 was an example of the effective disinfectant of new water mains and in the preparation of joints on the mains.[162] The QACs were first recommended for treating process water in paper mills in the 1950s and 1960s to prevent the proliferation of microorganisms on the surface of equipment contacting the pulp solution.[163,164] These proliferations can form microbial slimes (biofilms; see chapter 67) that become detached and are carried along to become spots in the paper, often causing paper breaks during the manufacturing process that result in expensive, time-delaying machine shutdowns. The QACs were also recommended for use in cooling water systems to prevent proliferation of bacteria in the circulating cooling water system that would form microbial slimes that may reach the heat exchange units and impair their operational efficiency,[165,166] although the use of other biocides such as bromine are more widely used (see chapter 17). Dicocodimethyl ammonium chloride was recommended to prevent the proliferation of bacteria

in injection water or brine used in secondary oil recovery operations.[167] The injection water is pumped under pressure into injection wells drilled around the producing well, so that as it spreads through the subterranean sand structures containing residual oil, it will displace the residual oil in the direction of the producing well and increase the productivity of the well. If there is a proliferation of microorganisms in the injection waters, the subterranean sand structures will become plugged, requiring greater pressures to be applied to the injection waters until the operation cannot function. An example of this was described with the ability of *n*-alkyl crude tar base QACs to inhibit the proliferation of *Desulfovibrio desulfuricans*, a pseudomonad species primarily involved in plugging the sand formation.[168] Outdoor swimming pools are regularly treated with QACs to prohibit growth of algae, an aesthetic rather than a public health problem. The QACs at low concentrations (eg, 2-7 ppm) were found to be algicidal, algistatic, bacteriostatic, and/or bactericidal depending the concentration and formulation of QACs used.[169-171] For example, alkyldimethylisopropylbenzyl ammonium chloride at 7 ppm was found to be effective against *E coli* and *S faecalis* at a 30-second contact time by the AOAC test method prescribed for swimming pool bactericides at that time in the United States.[171]

The positively charged functional portion of the quaternary molecule is attracted to and substantive to negatively charged fabric; it may be applied to the fabric from a quaternary solution by rinsing, padding, or spraying. Taking advantage of this phenomenon, Benson et al[172,173] proposed that reusable diapers could be treated with [methylbenzethonium chloride]p-diisobutylcresoxyethoxyethyldimethylbenzyl ammonium chloride monohydrate in the final rinse of the laundry cycle. Treated diapers were proposed to prevent the formation of ammonia from urine by the action of ammonia-producing bacteria found in the infant's feces; thus, ammonia dermatitis leading to diaper rash could be prevented. The QACs were then soon recommended as alternatives to hot water for disinfection purposes in laundries. These applications make further practice sense considering the dual roles of QACs/surfactants for cleaning and disinfection, as described previously. Alkyldimethylbenzyl ammonium chloride was shown to be effective at reducing bacterial levels in laundry cycles at 1:5000 (200 ppm) or 1:10 000 (100 ppm) dilution, in these studies reducing bacteria to below detectable levels.[101] Similar studies confirmed these results under hot and cold water conditions.[174] Using the AOAC antimicrobial laundry additive test procedure, a simulated use test, others demonstrated fabric disinfection during the laundry cycle following addition of a 50:50 mixture of alkyldimethylbenzyl ammonium chloride and alkyldimethylethylbenzyl ammonium chloride at a 200 ppm level based on the weight of dry laundry fabric.[175] In addition, fabric treated similarly and allowed to air-dry demonstrated residual bacteriostatic activity against *S aureus*, *E coli*, and *Brevibacterium ammoniagenes* and also demonstrated residual self-disinfecting activity against *S aureus* and *E coli*. Since that time, QACs in various different formulations have been successfully used for laundry applications (see chapter 46).

Some of the miscellaneous applications for QACs are as preservatives. A large number of chemicals as preservatives for ophthalmic solution was reviewed in the 1950s and BAC at 1:5000 and 1:10 000 was highlighted as being superior.[101] Similarly, Stark[39] used polymeric QACs (namely Polyquat) for disinfecting and preserving solution for contact lenses, ointments, and other ocular medicaments. The polyquaterium-1 (Onamer™ M) was approved by the FDA as a preservative in several brands of contact lenses soaking solutions at 0.01% to 0.001% (Opti-Soft™, Opti-Clean™, Opti-Tears™, Opti-Free™, and Tears-Natural™ II). This product has almost replaced other QACs, such as BAC, and thimerosal in these many preparations. Water-soluble cationic polymers (Busan™ 77, WSCP™, Onyxsperse™ 12S, Onamer™ M), when formulated in an aqueous medium with one or more nonionic surfactants, provided stable, isotropic liquid laundry detergent and sanitizer compositions that have good detergency and bactericidal properties and, in addition, are less irritating to the eye and practically nonirritating to the skin.[176]

The QAC compounds, including a 50:50 mixture of alkyldimethylbenzyl ammonium and alkyldimethylethylbenzyl ammonium chlorides, were also investigated as preservatives for cosmetic oil-in-water systems using amine oxides as emulsifiers.[177] At 1000 or 2000 ppm, the QACs reduced the microbial count of the cosmetic system inoculated with bacteria and fungal spores from an initial count of several million per milliliter to less than 10/mL over an 8-week incubation period, including a reinoculation after 4 weeks of incubation. In another instance, as a fungistat for exterior latex paint films, alkyldimethyl ethylbenzylammonium cyclohexylsulfamate at about a 1% level in exterior latex paints was demonstrated to produce a paint film resistant to attack by fungi.[178] Other examples include their use in wood and natural materials such as wool fabric. The use of wood preservatives has been well described in patents, both in various QAC formulation or in combination with other actives such as essential oils.[179,180] Tricaprylylmethyl ammonium chloride (at 0.15%-0.4%) was found to be superior to all other QACs tested for the treatment of wool fabric from the black carpet beetle and the webbing clothes moth larvae.[181]

Finally, in addition to water disinfection/preservation treatments and for general food surface applications described earlier, QACs have also been described for use at low concentrations in water for use as rinsing agents for fruit and vegetables, and as alternatives to other biocides such as chlorine (see chapter 15). The QACs have been shown to be effective at reducing the levels of *S aureus*

and *E coli* in water used for irrigation of fresh produce.[182] Studies confirmed that gram-positive bacteria were more sensitive to the QACs used compared to gram-negative bacteria but also that the efficacy could be increased by QAC formulations; examples include mixtures of QACs, such as in combination with isothiazolinones or essential oils.[183]

▶ MODE OF ACTION

The earliest accounts of the QACs related antimicrobial activity to chemical structure by using homologous series of quaternary compounds and noting the effect on antimicrobial activity offered by variations in structure.[13] This method of collecting information on the antimicrobial attributes of a quaternary compound is constantly used to determine the most effective structure that may be used as an item of commerce. Beyond this purpose, this method contributes little to our understanding of the basic mechanism of QACs as antimicrobial agents. Although the mode of action has not been completely or definitively described in detail, there are well defined and accepted steps explaining the mode of action of cationic disinfectants or antiseptics.[59,103,184] Many techniques have been used in elucidating the mode of action of QACs. The most important site of adsorption is the cytoplasmic membrane, leading to disruption of its structure/function. Spheroplasts, or protoplasts lacking the outer cell wall layers, are known to bind the cationic biocides and may be lysed or damaged. Direct adsorption by isolated cell membranes has also been demonstrated.

The extent of bacterial death is governed by five principal factors: (1) concentration of biocide, (2) nature of bacterial cells and density, (3) time of contact, (4) temperature of medium, (5) pH and/or other formulation effects (when present), and (6) presence of foreign matter. The adsorption of a given amount of the compound per cell leads to the killing of a definite fraction of the bacterial population in the chosen time interval. The lowest concentration of QACs that induces bacterial death also brings about leakage of cytoplasmic constituents of low MW. The most immediately observed effect is loss of K^+ ions. The increased permeability is a sign of changes in the membrane that are initially reversible but become irreversible on prolonged treatment. The necessary characteristic of a QAC is its bactericidal action, but there is often a low and rather narrow concentration range in which its effect is bacteriostatic. At this low concentration, certain biochemical functions associated with the bacterial membrane may be inhibited. In the presence of a higher concentration of QAC and after prolonged treatment, the compound usually penetrates the cell and brings about extensive ill-defined disruption of normal cellular functions. The primary effect of QACs on the cytoplasmic membrane is thus established beyond doubt, but secondary actions on the cytoplasmic processes are less defined and may vary from one compound to another.

A review of the most reliable evidence on the mode of action of QACs suggests the following generalizations:

1. Adsorption of compound on the bacterial cell surface
2. Diffusion through the cell wall
3. Binding to the cytoplasmic membrane
4. Disruption of the cytoplasmic membrane
5. Release of K^+ ions and other cytoplasmic constituents
6. Precipitation of cell contents and the death of the cells

It is well known that the bacterial cell surfaces are usually negatively charged and that adsorption of polycations onto the negatively charged cell surfaces (process 1) is expected to be enhanced with increasing MW of the polymer due to the increasing charge density of the polycations. The binding of polymers to the cytoplasmic membranes and its disruption are expected to be facilitated by increasing the MW of the polymer and by increasing the amount of the bound polymers to the bacteria cells. To examine this hypothesis, Ikeda and Tazuke[59] studied the effect of polymer MW on lysis of protoplasts, which are bacteria cells freed entirely of cell walls, so that the interaction processes 1 (adsorption) and 2 (diffusion) of the polymer with the protoplasts can be left out of consideration. The amount of cytoplasmic constituents released from protoplasts and from intact cells of *B subtilis* was measured at 260 nm after exposure to fractionated samples of polymers of various MWs. Lysis of protoplasts was clearly enhanced with increases in MW of polymer[poly{*n*-butyldimethyl[vinylbenzyl]-ammonium chloride}]. A bell-shaped curve relationship of the activity to the MW of fractionated polymer was observed in the case of intact cells of *B subtilis*. Because separate experiments have shown that release of cytoplasmic constituents from intact cells correlates well with the death of the cells, these results support the concept that the mode of action of the polymeric biocides is disorganization of cytoplasmic membrane followed by rupture of membrane, leading to the death of the bacteria.[184]

The optimal MW region of 14 300 was reported for the 6,6-ionene bromide with antibacterial activity, with MBC of 6.6 to 10 ppm against *S aureus*.[59] The same workers reported that polymeric biguanides of MW 11 900 and poly{alkyl[C_2-C_{12}] dimethyl[vinylbenzyl]ammonium chloride} of similar MW exhibit better bactericidal action against gram-positive than gram-negative bacteria. The poly(dodecyldimethyl[vinylbenzyl]-ammonium chloride) was the most active at 0.5 ppm against *S aureus*, which suggests that hydrophobicity plays an important role in bactericidal action.

A primary consideration in examining the mode of action is the characterization of quaternary compounds as surface-active agents or surfactants. James[185] adequately defines these as compounds with a structural balance between one or more water-attracting (hydrophilic) groups; depending on the nature of the charge or absence of ionization of the hydrophilic group, they may be classified as anionic, cationic, or nonionic. The QACs are cationic surface agents and possess such properties as a reduction of the surface tension at interfaces on absorption; a ready attraction to an absorption on surfaces possessing a negative charge such as wool, glass, protein, and bacteria; the formation of ionic aggregates or micelles with attendant changes in electrical conductivity, surface tension, and solubility; a precipitation, complex formation, and denaturing effect on proteins; and an inhibiting or stimulating effect on enzymatic activity. With these demonstrable properties for cationic surfactants, it was natural to attribute the antimicrobial activity of QACs entirely to the presence and amount of surface activity. This obvious explanation has been refuted on initial and further studies.[186,187]

Hugo[187] provided an excellent overview on the mode of action of cationic surface-active agents on microbial cells. The concepts concerning the mode of action of surface-active agents on microorganisms was divided into five broad categories:

1. *Effects on protein*: The QACs are surface-active agents and will denature proteins[188] or cause the disruption of enzyme structure/function.[49] This effect is usually caused at concentrations much higher than those that are lethal to the microbial cells, and it is unlikely that this effect is the primary cause of the antibacterial activity of surface-active disinfectants except at high concentration.

2. *Effects on metabolic reactions*: Reported effects include the aerobic and anaerobic respiration of glucose by a variety of bacteria[189] and on the oxidation of lactate by *E coli* and *S aureus*.[190] Attempts have been made to relate inhibition of metabolism with inhibition of growth. Such a correlation has been observed at high concentration, and almost any degree of agreement or disagreement may be demonstrated, depending on the enzyme system chosen and the test organism. It can be expected that enzymes located in the cytoplasmic membrane will be the first to be affected. Penetration of the cell will follow, and cytoplasmic enzymes then will be inhibited. The enzyme inhibition is not the primary or main lesion caused by these compounds. A specific detergent-sensitive enzyme does not exist or has not been discovered.

3. *Effects on cell permeability*: These include cytolytic damage and phosphorus loss[191] as well as membrane damage and loss of potassium.[192] The cytoplasmic membrane is probably the organelle most sensitive to surface-active agents within the cell of bacteria and yeasts, and the alteration in the semipermeable properties of this structure can lead to leakage of metabolites and coenzymes and the disturbance of the

delicate balance of metabolite concentrations within the cell. This lesion may be a major contribution to the death of a cell and may cause an apparent loss of enzymatic activity due to the loss or dilution of coenzymes or substrates. There is a well-established relationship between cytolytic action and surface tension, which lends support to the idea that cytolytic damage may in fact be the primary lesion caused by surface-active substances. Direct damage to the structure/function of the viral membrane is also known to effect on the viability of enveloped viruses.[193]

4. *Stimulatory effect of the glycolysis reaction*: Has been suggested by a number of investigators.[194,195] This reaction is of interest, but because the effect is elicited at concentrations well below those that are antibacterial, it is not considered significant for the antibacterial action of surface-active agents.

5. *Effect on an enzymatically maintained dynamic membrane*: This is offered as a speculative theory by Newton.[196] Results to support this interesting hypothesis are awaited. This concept of the dynamic cell membrane enzymatically maintained could well be the detergent-sensitive enzyme, which, as it was stated before, may not exist.

Denyer and Hugo[197] selected the effect on the cytoplasmic membrane controlling the cell permeability as the mode of action for QACs. Overall, this is most consistent with the data presented to date, and it is well accepted. The metabolic imbalance that follows biocidal and other stresses is believed to lead to free radical production and self-destruction of the organism.[198] Four strategies were also proposed to enhance the mechanism of action of QACs and other biocides[198,199]:

1. Enhanced interaction
2. Accumulation at target site (intracellular biocide delivery)
3. Optimization of synergistic biocidal combination (biophysical and biochemical synergy)
4. Autocidal effect (engaging the bacterium in partnership with the biocide to invoke autocidal processes

The antibacterial action of such biocidal compounds then manifested final damage on the cells in at least six ways:

1. Disruption of the transmembrane proton motive force leading to an uncoupling of oxidative phosphorylation and inhibition of active transport across the membrane
2. Inhibition of respiration of catabolic or anabolic reactions
3. Disruption of replication
4. Loss of membrane integrity resulting in leakage of essential intracellular constituents
5. Lysis, the self-destructive event initiated by a biocide
6. Coagulation of intracellular materials

REFERENCES

1. Zografi G, Schott H, Swarbrick J. Disperse systems. In: Gennaro AR, ed. *Remington's Pharmaceutical Sciences*. 18th ed. Easton, PA: Mack; 1990:257-309.
2. Harvey S. Antimicrobial drugs. In: Gennaro AR, ed. *Remington's Pharmaceutical Sciences*. 18th ed. Easton, PA: Mack; 1990:269-305, 1167-1172.
3. Atlas Powder Company. *Atlas Surface Active Agents: Their Characteristics, the HLB System of Selection*. Senter, Michigan: Industrial Chemicals Department, Atlas Powder Company; 1950.
4. Griffin WC. HLB values of nonionics. *J Soc Cosmet Chem*. 1949;1:311.
5. Gupta G. Microbicidal spermicide or spermicidal microbicide? *Eur J Contracept Reprod Health Care*. 2005;10:212-218.
6. Evans WP. The solubilization and inactivation of preservatives by non-ionic detergents. *J Pharm Pharmacol*. 1964;16:323-331.
7. Kanazawa A, Ikeda T, Endo T. A novel approach to mode of action of cationic biocides: morphological effect on antibacterial activity. *J Appl Bacteriol*. 1995;78:55-60.
8. Devinsky F, Masarova L, Lacko I, Mlynarcik D. Structure-activity relationships of "soft" quaternary ammonium amphiphiles. *J Biopharm Sci*. 1992;2:1-10.
9. Vieira OV, Hartmann DO, Cardoso CM, et al. Surfactants as microbicides and contraceptive agents: a systematic in vitro study. *PLoS One*. 2008;3(8):e2913.
10. Fishlock-Lomax EG, inventor; Amphoterics International Ltd, assignee. Amphoteric surfactants for use in antimicrobial cleaning compositions. US patent 4,769,169. September 6, 1988.
11. Wolff ME. *Burger's Medicinal Chemistry and Drug Discovery*. Vol 1. 5th ed. New York, NY: Wiley-Interscience; 1995.
12. Goldstein A, Aronow L, Kalman SM. Principles of drug action: the basis of pharmacology. New York, NY: Wiley, 1974.
13. Jacobs WA. The bactericidal properties of the quaternary salts of hexamethylenetetramine. I: the problem of the chemotherapy of experimental bacterial infections. *J Exp Med*. 1916;23:563-568.
14. Jacobs WA, Heidelberger M. The quaternary salts of hexamethylenetetramine. I: substituted benzyl halides and the hexamethylenetetrammonium salts derived therefrom. *J Biol Chem*. 1915;20:659-683.
15. Jacobs WA, Heidelberger M. The quaternary salts of hexamethylenetetramine. II. Monohalogenacetylbenzylamines and their hexamethylenetetraminium salts. *J Biol Chem*. 1915;20:685-694.
16. Jacobs WA, Heidelberger M. The quaternary salts of hexamethylenetetramine. III. Monohalogenacylated aromatic amines and their hexamethylenetetraminium salts. *J Biol Chem*. 1915;21:103-143.
17. Jacobs WA, Heidelberger M. The quaternary salts of hexamethylenetetramine. IV. Monohalogenated simple amines, ureas, urethanes, and the hexamethylenetetraminium salts derived therefrom. *J Biol Chem*. 1915;21:145-152.
18. Jacobs WA, Heidelberger M. The quaternary salts of hexamethylenetetramine. V. Monohalogenacetyl derivatives of amino-alcohols and the hexamethylenetetraminium salts derived therefrom. *J Biol Chem*. 1915;21:403-437.
19. Jacobs WA, Heidelberger M. The quaternary ammonium salts of hexamethylenetetramine. VI. Halogenethyl esters and ethers and their hexamethylenetetraminium salts. *J Biol Chem*. 1915;21:439-453.
20. Jacobs WA, Heidelberger M. The quaternary salts of hexamethylenetetramine. VII. Halogen derivatives of aliphatic aromatic ketones and their hexamethylenetetraminium salts. *J Biol Chem*. 1915;21:455-464.
21. Jacobs WA, Heidelberger M, Amoss HL. The bactericidal properties of the quaternary salts of hexamethylenetetramine: II. The relation between constitution and bacterial action in the substituted benzyl-hexamethylenetetraminium salts. *J Exp Med*. 1916;23:569-576.
22. Jacobs WA, Heidelberger M, Bull CG. The bactericidal properties of the quaternary salts of hexamethylenetetramine: III. The relation between constitution and bactericidal action in the quaternary salts obtained from halogenacetyl compounds. *J Exp Med*. 1916;23:577-599.

23. Browning CH. Summary: experimental studies in tuberculosis. *BMJ*. 1926;1:73.

24. Browning CH, Cohen JB, Gaunt R, Gullbransen R. Relationship between antiseptic action and chemical constitution with special reference to compounds of the pyridine, quinoline, acridine and phenazine series. *Proc R Soc Med*. 1922;93B:329-366.

25. Browning CH, Cohen JB, Ellingsworth S, Gullbransen R. Antiseptic properties of the amino derivatives of styrl and anil quinoline. *Proc R Soc Med*. 1926;100B:293-325.

26. Hartmann M, Kagi H. Saure seifen. *Z Agnew Chem*. 1928;41:127-130.

27. Domagk G. A new class of disinfectants. *Dtsch Med Wochenschr*. 1935;61:829-832.

28. Cutler RA, Cimijotti EB, Okolwich TJ, Wetterau WF. Alkylbenzyldimethylammonium chlorides—a comparative study of the odd and even chain homologues. In: *Proceedings of the 53rd Chemical Specialties Manufacturers Association Annual Meeting*; May 15-18, 1966; Chicago, IL.

29. Daoud NN, Dickinson NA, Gilbert P. Antimicrobial activity and physico-chemical properties of some alkyldimethylbenzylammonium chlorides. *Microbios*. 1983;37:73-85.

30. Daoud NN, Crooks PA, Speak R, Gilbert P. Determination of benzalkonium chloride by chemical ionization mass spectroscopy. *J Pharm Sci*. 1983;72:290-292.

31. Hansch C, Clayton JM. Lipophilic character and biological activity of drugs II. The parabolic case. *J Pharm Sci*. 1973;62:1-21.

32. Lien EJ, Hanch C, Anderson SM. Structure-activity correlations for antibacterial agents on gram-positive and gram-negative cells. *J Med Chem*. 1968;11:430-441.

33. Lien EJ, Perrin JH. Effect of chain length upon critical micelle formation and protein binding of quaternary ammonium compounds. *J Med Chem*. 1976;19:849-850.

34. Greene DF, Petrocci AN. Formulating quaternary cleaner disinfectants to meet EPA requirements. *Soap Cosmet Chem Spec*. 1980;8:33-35, 61.

35. Ditoro RD. New generation of biologically active quaternaries. *Soap Chemical Specialties*. 1969;47:52, 86-88, 91-92.

36. Petrocci AN, Green HA, Merianos JJ, Like B. The properties of dialkyldimethyl quaternary ammonium compounds. In: *Proceedings of the 60th Chemical Specialties Manufacturers Association Annual Meeting*; May 12-15, 1974; Chicago, IL.

37. British Hydrological Corp. *Deciquam 22. Bochure*. London, United Kingdom: British Hydrological Corp; 1968.

38. Schaeufele PJ. Advances in quaternary ammonium biocides. *J Assoc OCS*. 1984;61:387-389.

39. Stark RL, inventor; Alcon Manufacturing Ltd, assignee. Aqueous antimicrobial ophthalmic solutions. US patent 4,525,346. June 25, 1985.

40. Merianos JJ. Structure activity relationships in quaternary ammonium antimicrobial compounds. Abstracts. *SIM NEWS Suppl*. 1988;38(4):S-63.

41. Merianos JJ, inventor; ISP Capital Inc, assignee. Antimicrobial, low toxicity, non-irritating composition comprising a blend of bis-quaternary ammonium compounds coprecipitated with a copolymer of vinylpyrrolidone and an acrylamido or vinyl quaternary ammonium monomer. US patent 5,242,684. September 7, 1993.

42. Shelton RS, van Campen MG, Tilford CH, et al. Quaternary ammonium salts as germicides. I. Non-acylated quaternary ammonium salts derived from aliphatic amines. *J Am Chem Soc*. 1946;68:753-755.

43. Hartmann M, Johann K, inventors; Novartis AG, assignee. Quaternary ammonium compound and process of making same. US patent 1,737,458. November 26,1929.

44. Wakeman RL, Tesoro GC, inventors; Onyx Oil and Chemical Co, assignee. Ethylbenzyl, lauryl, dimethyl ammonium salts. US patent 2,676,986. April 27, 1954.

45. Domagk G, inventor. Preserving and disinfecting media. US patent 2,108,765. February 15, 1938.

46. Dunn CC. A mixture of high molecular alkyldimethylbenzylammonium chlorides as an antiseptic. *Proc Soc Exp Biol Med*. 1936;35:427-429.

47. Kirby AHM, Frick EL. Greenhouse evaluation of chemicals for control of powdery mildews. *Ann Appl Biol*. 1963;52:45-54.

48. Tonaka F. Invert soaps as disinfectants. IX. Relationship between bactericidal actions and molecular weight. *J Pharmacol Soc Japan*. 1944;64:35-36.

49. Kuhn R, Dann O. Uber Invertseifen II; butyl-octyl-lauryl-, and cetyldimethyl sulfonium iodide. *Ber Dtsch Chem Ges*. 1940;73:1092.

50. Kuhn R, Jerchel D, Westphal O. Uber Invertseifen. III. Dialkylmethylbenzyl-ammonium-chlorid. *Ber Dtsch Chem Ges*. 1940;73:1095-1100.

51. Mosher HH, Howard FL, inventors; Onyx Oil and Chemical Co, assignee. Cationic isoquinoline pesticide. US patent 2,435,458. February 3, 1948.

52. Wakeman RL, Coates JF, inventors; Stepan Co, assignee. Quaternary ammonium compounds having a branched chain aliphatic acid anion. US patent 3,565,927. February 23, 1971.

53. Shibe WJ Jr, Cohen S, Frant MS, inventors; Gallowhur Chemical Corp, assignee. Quaternary ammonium saccharinates and process for preparing the same. US patent 2,725,326. November 29, 1955.

54. Hwa JCH, inventor; Rohm and Hass Co, assignee. Bis-quaternary ammonium compounds. US patent 3,079,436. February 26, 1963.

55. DeBenneville PL, Bock LH, inventors; Rohm and Haas Co, assignee. 1,4-but-2-yne bis-quaternary ammonium halides. US patent 2,525,778. October 17, 1950.

56. Babbs M, Collier HO, Austin WC, Potter MD, Taylor EP. Salts of decamethylene-bis-4-aminoquinaldinium (dequadin); a new antimicrobial agent. *J Pharm Pharmacol*. 1956;8:110-119.

57. Ghosh M. Effect of various parameters on the biological activities of polymeric drugs. *Polymer Mater Sci Eng ACS*. 1986;55:755-757.

58. Ghosh M. Synthetic macromolecules as potential chemotherapeutic agents. *Polymer News*. 1988;13:71-77.

59. Ikeda T, Tazuke S. Biocidal polycations. *Polymer Prep*. 1985;26:226-227.

60. Samour CM. Polymer drugs. *Chemtech*. 1978:494-501.

61. Rembaum A, Senyei AE, Rajaraman R. Interaction of living cells with polyionenes and polyionene-coated surfaces. *J Biomed Mater Res*. 1977;11:101-110.

62. Rembaum A. Biological activity of ionene polymers. In: *Proceedings of the Conference on Polymeric Materials for Unusual Service Conditions*; November 29-December 1, 1972; Moffett Field, CA.

63. Rembaum A, Sélégny E. *Polyelectrolytes and Their Applications*. Boston, MA: Reidel; 1975:131-144.

64. Petrocci AN, Prodo KW, Shay EG, Wakerman RL, inventors; Stepan Co, assignee. Synergistic blends of microbiocidal quaternary ammonium compounds. US patent 3,472,939. October 14, 1969.

65. Green HA, Merianos JJ, Petrocci AN, inventors; Stepan Co, assignee. Anti-microbial, cosmetic and water-treating ionene polymeric compounds. US patent 4,325,940. April 20, 1982.

66. Good RM Jr, Liao LC, Hook JM, Punko CL. Colorimetric determination of a polymeric quaternary ammonium antimicrobial preservative in an ophthalmic solution. *J Assoc Off Anal Chem*. 1987;70:979-980.

67. Rolando M, Crider JY, Kahook MY. Ophthalmic preservatives: focus on polyquaternium-1. *Expert Opin Drug Deliv*. 2011;8:1425-1438.

68. Petrocci AN, Clarke P, Merianos J, Green H. Quaternary ammonium antimicrobial compounds: old and new. *Dev Indust Microbiol*. 1979;20:11-14.

69. Lui AC, Netto AL, Silva CB, et al. Antimicrobial efficacy assessment of multi-use solution to disinfect hydrophilic contact lens, in vitro. *Arq Bras Oftalmol*. 2009;72:626-630.

70. Andrews JK, Howes JG, Selway RA, inventors; Chauvin Pharmaceuticals Ltd, assignee. Quaternary ammonium terpolymers. US patent 4,304,894. December 8, 1981.

71. Ikeda T, Tazuke S. Biologically active polycations: antimicrobial activities of poly[trialkylvinylbenzylammonium chlorides] type polycations. *Macromol Chem Rapid Commun*. 1983;4:459-461.

72. Ikeda T, Hirayama H, Yamaguchi H, Tazuke S, Watanabe M. Polycationic biocides with pendant active groups: molecular weight dependence of antibacterial activity. *Antimicrob Agents Chemother*. 1986;30:132-136.

73. Sheldon BG, Wingard RE Jr, Weinshenker NM, Dawson DJ, inventors; Novartis Corp, assignee. Quaternary ammonium group-containing polymers having antimicrobial activity. US patent 4,532,128. July 30, 1985.

74. Sato S, Tanaka S. Determination of benzalkonium chlorides by high-performance liquid chromatography. *Bunseki Kagaku.* 1984;33: 338-342.

75. Suzuki S, Nakamura Y, Kaneko M, Mori K, Watanabe Y. Analysis of benzalkonium chlorides by gas chromatography. *J Chromatogr.* 1989;463:188-191.

76. Stevens LE, Eckardt JI. Spectrophotometric determination of polyquaternium-1 with trypan blue by a difference procedure. *Analyst.* 1987;112:1619-1621.

77. Wang LK, Shuster WW. Polyelectrolyte determination at low concentration. *Indu Eng Chem Prod Res Dev.* 1975;14:312-314.

78. Merianos JJ, Smith LR, Weinstein M. Onamer M—a new cosmetic ingredient. *SCC Spec.* 1977;12:54-74.

79. Jacobs WA, Heidelberger M. The quaternary salts of hexamethylenetetramine. VIII. Miscellaneous substances containing aliphatically bound halogen and the hexamethylenetetraminium salts derived therefrom. *J Biol Chem.* 1915;21:465-475.

80. Kourai H, Takechi H, Horie T, Takeichi K, Shibasaki I. The antimicrobial characteristics of quaternary ammonium salts. Part XI: quantitative structure-activity relationship of antimicrobial n-laurylpyridinium iodides. *J Antibact Antifung Agents.*1985;13:245-253.

81. Kourai H, Takechi H, Horie T, Uchiwa N, Takeichi K, Shibasaki I. The antimicrobial characteristics of quaternary ammonium salts. Part X. Antimicrobial characteristics and a mode of action of N-alkylpyridinium iodides against *Escherichia coli* K12. *J Antibact Antifung Agents.* 1985;13:3-10.

82. Madaan P, Tyagi VK. Quaternary pyridinium salts: a review. *J Oleo Sci.* 2008;57(4):197-215.

83. Kourai H, Takechi H, Muramatsu K, Shibasaki I. The antimicrobial characteristics of quaternary ammonium salts. Part XIV. Relationship between hydrophobicity of bacterial cell surface and drug-susceptibility to alkylpyridinium iodides. *J Antibact Antifung Agents.* 1989;17:119-128.

84. Hansch C, Fujita T. A method of the correlation of biological activity and chemical structure. *J Am Chem Soc.* 1964;86:1616-1626.

85. Salt WG, Wiseman D. The uptake of cetyltrimethylammonium bromide by *Escherichia coli. J Pharm Pharmacol.* 1968;20:14-17.

86. Tomlinson E, Brown MRW, Davis SS. Effect of colloidal association on the measured activity of alkyldimethylbenzylammonium chlorides against *Pseudomonas aeruginosa. J Med Chem.* 1977;20:1277-1282.

87. Jono K, Takayama T, Kuno M, Higashide E. Effect of alkyl chain length of benzalkonium chloride on the bactericidal activity and binding to organic materials. *Chem Pharm Bull (Tokyo).* 1986;34:4215-4224.

88. Mailman WL, Kivela EW, Turner G. Sanitizing dishes. *Soap Sanit Chem.* 1946;22:130-133.

89. Stuart LJ, Ortenzio LF, Freidl JL. Use dilution confirmation test for results obtained by phenol coefficient methods. *J Assoc Off Anal Chem.* 1953;36:466-480.

90. Klarmann EG, Wright ES. An inquiry into the germicidal performance of quaternary ammonium disinfectants. *Soap Sanit Chem.* 1946;22:125-137.

91. Heuck HJ, Adema DMM, Weigmann JR. Bacteriostatic, fungistatic, and algistatic activity of fatty nitrogen compounds. *Appl Microbiol.* 1966;14:308-319.

92. Gerba CP. Quaternary ammonium biocides: efficacy in application. *Appl Environ Microbiol.* 2015;81:464-469.

93. Klein M, Deforest A. Antiviral action of germicides. *Soap Sanit.* 1963;39:70.

94. Smith CR, Nishihara H, Golden F, Hoyt A, Guss CO, Kloetzel MC. The bactericidal effect of surface-active agents on tubercle bacilli. *Public Health Rep.* 1950;65(48):1588-1600.

95. Davies GE. Quaternary ammonium compounds. A new technique for the study of their bactericidal action and the results obtained with Cetavlon (cetyltrimethylammonium bromide). *J Hyg (Lond).* 1949;47:271.

96. Nerandzic MM, Donskey CJ. A quaternary ammonium disinfectant containing germinants reduces *Clostridium difficile* spores on surfaces by inducing susceptibility to environmental stressors. *Open Forum Infect Dis.* 2016;3:196.

97. Kohler LJ, Quirk AV, Welkos SL, Cote CK. Incorporating germination-induction into decontamination strategies for bacterial spores. *J Appl Microbiol.* 2018;24:2-14.

98. Eterpi M, McDonnell G, Thomas V. Disinfection efficacy against parvoviruses compared with reference viruses. *J Hosp Infect.* 2009;73:64-70.

99. Gershenfeld L, Perlstein D. Significance of hydrogen ion concentration in the evaluation of the bactericidal efficiency of surface tension depressants. *Am J Pharmacol.* 1941;113:306.

100. Quisno R, Foter MJ. Cetyl pyridinium chloride; germicidal properties. *J Bacteriol.* 1946;52:111-117.

101. Lawrence CA. Mechanism of action and neutralizing agents for surface-active materials upon microorganisms. *Ann NY Acad Sci.* 1950;53:66-75.

102. Okazaki K, Yoshida M, Mayama M, et al. Antifungal characteristics of N,N′-hexamethylenebis (4-carbamoyl-1-decylpyridinium bromide). *Biocontrol Sci.* 2006;11:37-42.

103. McDonnell G. *Antisepsis, Disinfection, and Sterilization. Types, Action, and Resistance.* 2nd ed. Washington, DC: ASM Press; 2017.

104. Tabata A, Nagamune H, Maeda T, Murakami K, Miyake Y, Kourai H. Correlation between resistance of *Pseudomonas aeruginosa* to quaternary ammonium compounds and expression of outer membrane protein OprR. *Antimicrob Agents Chemother.* 2003;47:2093-2099.

105. Guérin-Méchin L, Dubois-Brissonnet F, Heyd B, Leveau JY. Specific variations of fatty acid composition of *Pseudomonas aeruginosa* ATCC 15442 induced by quaternary ammonium compounds and relation with resistance to bactericidal activity. *J Appl Microbiol.* 1999;87:735-742.

106. Bruinsma GM, Rustema-Abbing M, van der Mei HC, Lakkis C, Busscher HJ. Resistance to a polyquaternium-1 lens care solution and isoelectric points of *Pseudomonas aeruginosa* strains. *J Antimicrob Chemother.* 2006;57:764-766.

107. Maseda H, Hashida Y, Konaka R, Shirai A, Kourai H. Mutational upregulation of a resistance-nodulation-cell division-type multidrug efflux pump, SdeAB, upon exposure to a biocide, cetylpyridinium chloride, and antibiotic resistance in *Serratia marcescens. Antimicrob Agents Chemother.* 2009;53:5230-5235.

108. Wassenaar TM, Ussery D, Nielsen LN, Ingmer H. Review and phylogenetic analysis of *qac* genes that reduce susceptibility to quaternary ammonium compounds in *Staphylococcus* species. *Eur J Microbiol Immunol.* 2015;5:44-61.

109. Schweizer HP. Efflux as a mechanism of resistance to antimicrobials in *Pseudomonas aeruginosa* and related bacteria: unanswered questions. *Genet Mol Res.* 2003;2:48-62.

110. Weston N, Sharma P, Ricci V, Piddock LJV. Regulation of the AcrAB-TolC efflux pump in Enterobacteriaceae. *Res Microbiol.* 2018;169:425-431.

111. Poole K. Efflux pumps as antimicrobial resistance mechanisms. *Ann Med.* 2007;39:162-176.

112. Ahn Y, Kim JM, Kweon O, et al. Intrinsic resistance of *Burkholderia cepacia* complex to benzalkonium chloride. *MBio.* 2016;7(6):e01716-16.

113. Takenaka S, Tonoki T, Taira K, Murakami S, Aoki K. Adaptation of *Pseudomonas* sp. strain 7-6 to quaternary ammonium compounds and their degradation via dual pathways. *Appl Environ Microbiol.* 2007;73:1797-1802.

114. Scientific Committee on Emerging and Newly Identified Health Risks. *Assessment of the Antibiotic Resistance Effects of Biocides.* Brussels, Belgium: European Commission; 2009.

115. European Parliament, Council of the European Union. *Directive 98/8/EC Concerning the Placing of Biocidal Products on the Market.* Brussels, Belgium: European Parliament, Council of the European Union; 1998.

116. Zhang C, Cui F, Zeng GM, et al. Quaternary ammonium compounds (QACs): a review on occurrence, fate and toxicity in the environment. *Sci Total Environ.* 2015;518-519:352-362.

117. Nelson JW, Lyster SC. The toxicity of myristyl-gamma-picolinium chloride. *J Am Pharm Assoc Am Pharm Assoc.* 1946;35:89-94.

118. Shelanski HA. Toxicity of quaternaries. *Soap Sanit Chem.* 1949;25:125-129,153.

119. Finnegan JK, Dienna JB. Toxicity of quaternaries. *Soap Sanit Chem.* 1954;30:147-153, 157, 173, 175.

120. Walter CW. The use of a mixture of coconut oil derivatives as a bactericide in the operating room. *Surg Gynecol Obstet.* 1938;67:683-688.

121. Whitehill AR. Evaluation of some liquid antiseptics. *J Am Pharm Assoc (Wash).* 1945;34:219-221.

122. Fitzhugh OG, Nelson AA. Chronic oral toxicities of surface-active agents. *J Am Pharm Assoc Am Pharm Assoc.* 1948;37:29-32.

123. Alfredson BV, Stiefel JR, Thorp F Jr, Batten WD, Gray ML. Toxicity studies on alkyldimethyl-benzylammonium chloride in rats and dogs. *J Am Pharm Assoc.* 1951;40:263-267.

124. *Federal Register.* Part 121—food additives; subpart F—food additives resulting from contact with containers or equipment and food additives otherwise affecting food. 11/26/1969; *Federal Register* 34/117;18556. 12/13/1969; *Federal Register* 34/239;19655. 8/9 1974; *Federal Register* 39/155;28627.

125. US Environmental Protection Agency. *40 CFR 180.940. Tolerance exemptions for active and inert ingredients for use in antimicrobial formulations (Food-contact surface sanitizing solutions).* Washington, DC: US EPA; 2011.

126. European Food Safety Authority. Reasoned opinion on the dietary risk assessment for proposed temporary maximum residue levels (MRLs) of didecyldimethylammonium chloride (DDAC) and benzalkonium chloride (BAC). *EFSA Journal.* 2014;12(4):3675.

127. Gleason MN, Gosselin RE, Hodge HC, Smith RP. *Clinical Toxicology of Commercial Products: Acute Poisoning. 3rd ed.* Baltimore, MD: Williams & Wilkins; 1969.

128. Aursnes J. Ototoxic effects of quaternary ammonium compounds. *Acta Otolaryngol.* 1982;93:421-433.

129. Cosmetic, Toiletry, and Fragrance Association. The final report on the safety assessment of benzethonium chloride and methylbenzethonium chloride. *J Am Coll Toxicol.* 1985;4:65-106.

130. Cahill J, Nixon R. Allergic contact dermatitis to quaternium 15 in a moisturizing lotion. *Australas J Dermatol.* 2005;46:284-285.

131. Tezel U, Pavlostathis SG. Quaternary ammonium disinfectants: microbial adaptation, degradation and ecology. *Curr Opin Biotechnol.* 2015;33:296-304.

132. Ying GG. Fate, behavior and effects of surfactants and their degradation products in the environment. *Environ Int.* 2006;32:417-431.

133. Wetzel U. Handedisinfektionsversuche mit Zephirol. *Arch Hyg Bakteriology.* 1935;114:1.

134. Walter CW. Disinfection of hands. *Am J Surg.* 1965;109:691-693.

135. Swan H, Gonzalez RI, Harris A, Couslon C, Hopwood ML. Use of a quaternary ammonium compound for the surgical scrub. *Am J Surg.* 1949;77:24-37.

136. White CS, Collins JL, Newman HE. The clinical use of alkyldimethyl-benzylammonium chloride (Zephiran): a preliminary report. *Am J Surg.* 1938;39:607-609.

137. Hagan HH, Maguire CH, Miller WH. Cetyl pyridinium chloride as a cutaneous germicide in major surgery; a comparative study. *Arch Surg.* 1946;52:149-159.

138. Miller BF, Abrams R, Huber DA, Klein M. Formation of invisible, non-perceptible films on hands by cationic soaps. *Proc Soc Exp Biol Med.* 1943;54:174-176.

139. Rahn C. Protection of dry bacteria against cationic detergents. *Proc Soc Exp Biol Med.* 1946;62:2-4.

140. Blank IH, Coolidge MH. Degerming the cutaneous surface. I. Quaternary ammonium compounds. *J Invest Dermatol.* 1950;15:249-256.

141. King TC, Zimmerman JM. Skin degerming practices: chaos and confusion. *Am J Surg.* 1965;109:695-698.

142. World Health Organization. *WHO Guidelines on Hand Hygiene in Health Care.* Geneva, Switzerland: World Health Organization; 2009.

143. Dyer DL, Gerenraich KB, Wadhams PS. Testing a new alcohol-free hand sanitizer to combat infection. *AORN J.* 1998;68:239-241, 243-244, 247-251.

144. la Fleur P, Jones S. *Non-Alcohol Based Hand Rubs: A Review of Clinical Effectiveness and Guidelines.* Ottawa, Canada: Canadian Agency for Drugs and Technologies in Health; 2017.

145. US Food and Drug Administration. *21 CFR Part 310. Safety and Effectiveness of Health Care Antiseptics; Topical Antimicrobial Drug Products for Over-the-Counter Human Use.* Silver Spring, MD: US Food and Drug Administration; 2017.

146. Caesar F. Erfahrungen mit Zephirol. *Fortschritte der Ther.* 1935;4:249-250.

147. Post MH. Dust-borne infection in ophthalmic surgery. *Am J Ophthalmol.* 1946;29:1435-1443.

148. Zeissler J, Gunther O. Kann durch Kochen in Zephirol: quartamon-Losungen sterilisiert werden? *Zentralbl Bakteriol.* 1939;144:402-407.

149. Sommermeyer L, Frobisher M Jr. Laboratory studies on disinfection of oral thermometers. *Nurs Res.* 1952;1:32-35.

150. Guiteras AF, Shapiro RL. A bactericidal detergent for eating utensils. *J Bacteriol.* 1946;52:635-638.

151. Taylor GF, Prindle RF, inventors; STWB Inc, assignee. Surface disinfectant and space deodorant aerosol spray composition. US patent 3,287,214. November 22, 1966.

152. Friedman H, Volin E, Laumann D. Terminal disinfection in hospitals with quaternary ammonium compounds by use of a spray-fog technique. *Appl Microbiol.* 1968;16:223-227.

153. Hauser PH, Crawford RH, Clarke PH. Germicidal fogging of sick rooms. *Soap Chem Spec.* 1963;39:80-110.

154. Rutala WA, Weber DJ. Disinfectants used for environmental disinfection and new room decontamination technology. *Am J Infect Control.* 2013;41:S36-S41.

155. Jiang L, Li M, Tang J, et al. Effect of different disinfectants on bacterial aerosol diversity in poultry houses. *Front Microbiol.* 2018;9:2113.

156. Krog AJ, Marshall CG. Alkyl-dimethylbenzyl-ammonium chloride for sanitization of eating and drinking utensils. *Am J Public Health.* 1940;30:341-347.

157. Krog AJ, Marshall CG. Rocca in the dairy pasteurizing plant. *J Milk Technol.* 1942;5:343-347.

158. Fair GM, Chang SL, Taylor MP, Wineman MA. Destruction of waterborne cysts of *Entamoeba histolytica* by synthetic detergents. *Am J Public Health.* 1945;35:228-232.

159. Kessel JF, Moon FJ. Emergency sterilization of drinking water with heteropolar cationic antiseptics. I: effectiveness against cysts of *Entamoeba histolytica. Am J Trop Med Hyg.* 1946;26:345-350.

160. Torkelson AA, da Silva AK, Love DC, et al. Investigation of quaternary ammonium silane-coated sand filter for the removal of bacteria and viruses from drinking water. *J Appl Microbiol.* 2012;113:1196-1207.

161. Jenkins MW, Tiwari SK, Darby J. Bacterial, viral and turbidity removal by intermittent slow sand filtration for household use in developing countries: experimental investigation and modeling. *Water Res.* 2011;45:6227-6239.

162. Sotier AL, Ward HW. Quaternary ammonium germicidal treatment for jute-packed water mains. *J Am Water Works Assoc.* 1947;39:1038-1045.

163. Erskine AM, Gorin MH, Rosenstein L, Chesbro RM, inventors. Organic ammonium salts of lignin acids. US patent 2,850,492. September 2, 1958.

164. Shema BF, inventor; Suez WTS USA Inc, assignee. Slimicidal composition and method. US patent 3,231,509. January 25, 1966.

165. Darragh JL, Stayner RD. Quaternary ammonium compounds from dodecylbenzene algae control in industrial cooling systems. *Ind Eng Chem.* 1954;46:254-257.

166. Berenschot DJ, King EG, Stubbs RK, Bobalik GR, inventors; Armour Pharmaceutical Co, assignee. Quaternary ammonium germicide. US patent 3,140,976. July 14, 1964.

167. Prusick JH, Gregory VP, inventors; Armour and Co, assignee. Chemical treatment of flood waters used in secondary oil recovery. US patent 2,733,206. January 31, 1956.

168. Steinberger S, inventor; Onyx Chemical Corp, assignee Chemical treatment of flood waters used in secondary oil recovery. US patent 3,111,492. November 19, 1963.

169. Palmer CM, Maloney TC. Preliminary screening for potential algicides. *Ohio J Sci.* 1955;55:1-8.

170. Antonides JH, Tanner WS. Algicidal and sanitizing properties of Armazide. *Appl Microbiol.* 1961;9:572-580.

171. Shay EG, Clarke PH, Crawford R. An evaluation of some experimental chemicals for swimming-pool disinfection. In: *Proceedings of the 51st Chemical Specialties Manufacturers Association Annual Meeting*; May 18-20, 1964; Atlantic City, NJ.

172. Benson RA, Slobody LB, Lillick L, Maffia A, Sullivan N. A new treatment for diaper rash. *J Pediatr.* 1947;31:369-374.

173. Benson RA, Slobody LB, Lillick L, Maffia A, Sullivan N. The treatment of ammonia dermatitis with diaparene: report on 500 cases. *J Pediatr.* 1949;34:49.

174. McNeil E, Choper EA. Disinfectants in home laundering. *Soap Chem Spec.* 1962;38:51-54, 94, 97-100.

175. Petrocci AN, Clarke P. Proposed test method for antimicrobial laundry additives. *J Assoc Off Anal Chem.* 1969;52:836-842.

176. Bernarducci E, Harrison KA, inventors; STWB Inc, Reckitt Benckiser LLC, assignees. Isotropic laundry detergents containing polymeric quaternary ammonium salts. US patent 4,755,327. July 5, 1988.

177. Like B, Sorrentino R, Petrocci A. Utility of amine oxides in oil/water cosmetic systems. *J Soc Cosmet Chem.* 1975;26:155-168.

178. Ramp JA, Mancuso CG, Huig JG. *Dimethyl Alkyl Ammonium Cyclohexylsulfamate—A New Paint Mildewcide. VIII Congres FATIPEC.* Weinbeim, Bergstrasse: Verlag Chemie, GMBH; 1966.

179. Lichtenberg F, Fritschi J, Ranft V, inventors; Lonza Ltd, assignee. Wood preservatives. Canada patent 2,250,986. December 27, 2005.

180. Modak SM, Shintre MS, Gaonkar T, Caraos L, inventors; Columbia University of New York, assignee. Antimicrobial compositions containing synergistic combinations of quaternary ammonium compounds and essential oils and/or constituents thereof. US patent 7,871,649. January 18, 2011.

181. Tolgyesi E, Schwartz AM, Rader CA, et al. Mothproofing with ammonium quats. *Chemical Technology.* 1971;1:27-30.

182. Chaidez C, Lopez J, Castro-del Campo N. Quaternary ammonium compounds: an alternative disinfection method for fresh produce wash water. *J Water Health.* 2007;5:329-333.

183. Pablos C, Romero A, de Diego A, et al. Novel antimicrobial agents as alternative to chlorine with potential applications in the fruit and vegetable processing industry. *Int J Food Microbiol.* 2018;285:92-97.

184. Franklin TJ, Snow GA. *Biochemistry of Antimicrobial Action.* 4th ed. London, United Kingdom: Chapman & Hall; 1989.

185. James AN. Surface activity and the microbial cell. *SCI Monograph No. 19. Surface-Active Agents in Microbiology.* London, United Kingdom: Society of Chemical Industry; 1965:3-23.

186. Hotchkiss RD. The nature of the bactericidal action of surface-active agents. *Ann NY Acad Sci.* 1946;46:478-483.

187. Hugo WB. Some aspects of the action of cationic surface-active agents on microbial cells with special reference to their action on enzymes. In: *Surface Activity and the Microbial Cell.* New York, NY: Gordon and Breach Science; 1965:67-80.

188. Putnam FW. The interaction of protein and synthetic detergents. *Adv Protein Chem.* 1948;4:79.

189. Baker Z, Harrison RW, Miller BF. Action of synthetic detergents on the metabolism of bacteria. *J Exp Med.* 1941;73:249-271.

190. Ordal EJ, Borg AF. Effect of surface-active agents on oxidations of lactate by bacteria. *Proc Soc Exp Biol Med.* 1942;50:332-336.

191. Armstrong WM. Surface-active agents and cellular metabolism. I. The effects of cationic detergents on the production of acid and of carbon dioxide by bakers yeast. *Arch Biochem.* 1957;71:137.

192. Scharff TG, Maupin WC. Correlation of the metabolic effects of benzalkonium chloride with its membrane effects in yeast. *Biochem Pharmacol.* 1960;5:79.

193. Tsao IF, Wang HY, Shipman C Jr. Interaction of infectious viral particles with a quaternary ammonium chloride (QAC) surface. *Biotechnol Bioeng.* 1989;34:639-646.

194. Stickland LM. The Pasteur effect in normal yeast and its inhibition by various agents. *Biochem J.* 1956;64:503.

195. Bihler I, Rothstein A, Bihler L. The mechanism of stimulation of aerobic fermentation in yeast by a quaternary ammonium detergent. *Biochem Pharmacol.* 1961;8:289.

196. Newton BA. The mechanism of the bactericidal action of surface-active compounds: a summary. *J Appl Bacteriol.* 1960;23:345-349.

197. Denyer SP, Hugo WB. Biocide-induced damage to the bacterial cytoplasmic membrane. In: *Mechanism of Action of Chemical Biocides: Their Study and Exploitation.* Oxford, United Kingdom: Blackwell Scientific; 1991:171-187.

198. Denyer SP, Stewart GSAB. Mechanism of action of disinfectants. *Int Biodeterior Biodegradation.* 1998;41:261-268.

199. Denyer SP, Hugo WB. Intracellular delivery of biocides. *Mechanism of Action of Chemical Biocides: Their Study and Exploitation.* Oxford, United Kingdom: Blackwell Scientific; 1991: 263-270.

CHAPTER 22

Chlorhexidine

Vinod P. Menon

Chlorhexidine was first synthesized in 1950 in the laboratories of Imperial Chemical Industries Ltd (London, United Kingdom) during antimicrobial research into synthetic antimalarial agents of the proguanil type. It was found to possess a high level of antibacterial activity, low mammalian toxicity, and a strong affinity for binding to skin and mucous membranes. These properties led to the development of chlorhexidine principally as a topical antiseptic for application to such areas as skin, wounds, and mucous membranes and for dental use.[1] It is used as a surgical hand scrub or rub, for preoperative bathing, nursery neonatal umbilical stump care, surgical site disinfection, and oropharyngeal decontamination in ventilator patients. It is widely used for skin antisepsis before placement of epidural, arterial, and central venous catheters (CVCs). Chlorhexidine has also been impregnated into medical materials, including vascular cannulas and dressings for both vascular and epidural catheters. It has been used for decades by dentists and oral surgeons to control gingivitis and periodontitis. In addition, chlorhexidine has been used as a pharmaceutical preservative, particularly in ophthalmic and surgical irrigation solutions, and as a disinfectant for items such as inanimate surfaces and instruments.[2]

Chlorhexidine can also be found in dressings, ointments, suppositories, and contraceptive gels, and it is available as an over-the-counter solution for disinfection of minor cuts and wounds. It acts as preservative agent in various liquid soaps, shower foams, cosmetics, toothpaste, lubricants, and medical ointments because it prevents bacterial growth.[3] It is included as an antiseptic in the World Health Organization Essential Medicines list.

CHEMISTRY

Chlorhexidine is 1,6-di(4-chlorophenyl-diguanido) hexane, a bisbiguanide of the following formula:

Various resonance structures are assigned to the biguanide molecule. Although the biguanide structure shown previously—containing two iminic C=NH groups—is traditionally used for chlorhexidine and other biguanide structures, computational[4] analyses have suggested that the most stable conformer is better represented by the structure without iminic C=NH groups but containing two C-NH$_2$ primary amine sites.

Differences in the chemistry between the iminic groups of the nominal structure and the amine functionality may play an important role in understanding the degradation reactions of chlorhexidine.

Study of the related group of bisbiguanides has demonstrated that this compound, with a single chlorine substituent in each phenol ring, is the most active.[5] Chlorhexidine itself is a strong base, practically insoluble in water (0.008% wt/vol at 20°C), that reacts with acids to form salts of the RX_2 type. The water solubility of the different salts varies widely. Chlorhexidine was first made commercially available as the poorly soluble hydrochloride salt and subsequently as the moderately soluble acetate salt. The freely soluble gluconate salt was introduced in 1957 and is currently the favored form of chlorhexidine in disinfectant formulations.

Soluble chlorhexidine gluconate (CHG) cannot be easily isolated as a solid and is manufactured as a 20% wt/vol aqueous solution (eg, United States Pharmacopeia [USP] Chlorhexidine Gluconate Solution), higher concentrations being too viscous for convenient use. The diacetate salt has a solubility of 1.9% wt/vol (20°C), whereas the dihydrochloride and other inorganic salts are relatively insoluble (Table 22.1). The low solubility of the inorganic salts may cause problems of precipitation if a water-soluble salt such as the digluconate is formulated with, or diluted in, a solution containing inorganic anions such as chloride, sulfate, or nitrate. The aqueous gluconate salt solution is miscible with glacial acetic acid and with water and miscible with three times its volume of acetone and five times its volume of dehydrated alcohol; further addition of acetone or dehydrated alcohol yields a white turbidity.[6] The CHG solution should not be added directly to neat alcohol because precipitation may occur. In addition to water, the gluconate salt is soluble in methanol.[7] The gluconate salt is also soluble in hydrophobic vehicles with a hydrophilic-lipophilic balance (HLB) value less than 10, where the hydrophobic vehicles have two proximate hydrogen bonding groups with at least one group being a hydrogen donor. Examples include monoacylglycerides and higher alkanediols.[8]

Solutions and powders of chlorhexidine are colorless, or almost colorless, and usually odorless, although formulations prepared from the diacetate salt occasionally have an odor of acetic acid. Solutions prepared from all salts have an extremely bitter taste that must be masked in formulations intended for oral use. The taste quality–altering effects of chlorhexidine in humans were studied by analyzing confusions among taste stimuli in an identification task. Treatment with chlorhexidine was found to produce a profound and lengthy alteration of the salty taste of all salty compounds. It reduced the bitter taste of a subset of bitter compounds but had little effect on sweet and sour tastes.[9]

Chlorhexidine is moderately surface active and forms micelles in solution; the critical micellar concentration of the acetate is 0.01% wt/vol at 25°C.[10] The unusually high solubility of the gluconate salt has been attributed to self-association and formation of large aggregates.[11] Aqueous solutions of chlorhexidine are most stable within the pH range 5 to 8. Above pH 8.0, chlorhexidine base is precipitated, and in more acid conditions, there is gradual deterioration of activity because the compound is less stable. Hydrolysis yields para-chloroaniline; the amount is insignificant at room temperature, but it is increased by heating above 100°C, especially at alkaline pH.[12]

Chemical analysis of chlorhexidine, its degradation products, and its impurities can be performed using a variety of different methods. Qualitative assays for identification of the various chlorhexidine reagents are reported in the respective USP and European Pharmacopoeia monographs.[13,14] These may include infrared (IR) and melting point analyses. Quantitative analyses can generally be performed by several nonseparation methods including UV absorbance, acid titrimetry, and gravimetric determination of insoluble copper complexes in pharmaceutical products with chlorhexidine. High-performance liquid chromatography (HPLC) is the method most used to analyze this antiseptic; solid-phase extraction with UV spectrophotometry, gas-liquid chromatography, liquid chromatography, capillary electrophoresis, flow injection extraction-spectrophotometry, and voltammetry also are used to assess it.[15] Some induced colorimetric determinations of biguanides have been suggested.[16] Thin-layer chromatography methods have been used to evaluate CHG solutions, but although rapid, these lack the quantitative rigor and resolving power of HPLC. Para-chloroaniline in its free base form can be analyzed by gas chromatography (GC) methods; however, care must be exercised to avoid artificial increases in its concentration through thermal degradation of chlorhexidine during the GC injection process. Prolonged exposure to light should also be avoided.

Chlorhexidine Impurities and Degradants

Despite the widespread use of chlorhexidine in products, relatively little has been published with respect to the nature and characterization of the impurities present in chlorhexidine preparations. This dearth of data exists

TABLE 22.1	Solubility of chlorhexidine base and salts in water at 20°C (% wt/vol)	
Chlorhexidine Compound	**Aqueous Solubility (% wt/vol)**
Chlorhexidine base	0.008
Diacetate	1.9
Dihydrobromide	0.07
Dihydrochloride	0.06
Dinitrate	0.03
Sulfate	0.01
Carbonate	0.02

despite well-known issues with the degradation of chlorhexidine accelerated by thermal, acid/base, and photolytic processes. The most extensive characterization of the impurities and degradation products of chlorhexidine was published by Revelle et al from the US Food and Drug Administration (FDA).[17,18] The Revelle group identified, and confirmed by synthesis, 11 common impurities. The group encountered general retro-ene degradation of biguanide groups to guanide products, and aqueous acid catalyzed conversion of guanide groups to ureas, then to carbamates, and finally to amines. Although thermal and acidic stresses degraded chlorhexidine to similar products, dechlorinated degradation products were uniquely obtained through photolytic reactions. Ha and Cheung[19] identified the same products formed by an alternate hydrolytic chemical approach. The European Pharmacopoeia[14] identifies 12 impurities without further attribution or explanation.

Classes of chlorhexidine-related impurities and degradation products found in aged CHG-containing products tend to arise from three major sources or mechanisms:

1. *Manufacturing impurities*: Side products from the manufacture of the chlorhexidine-free base form are carried over into the subsequent chlorhexidine salts. These include species such as the mono-ortho-chloro isomer resulting from low-level ortho-chloroaniline impurities in the para-chloroaniline synthetic reagents. The levels of these species do not generally change significantly with sample aging.

2. *Chlorhexidine degradation reactions*: Chlorhexidine and its salts can degrade by various homogeneous and heterogeneous reactions. In general, the rates of these degradation reactions are significantly higher in solution than in solid reagent forms. These degradation reactions proceed primarily through three mechanisms: retro-ene reactions, hydrolysis reactions, and reactions with the counterion in the chlorhexidine salt.

3. *Side reactions with formulation reagents or sterilization byproducts*: Reactions of biguanide species with aldehydes, such as acetaldehyde, present at low levels in formulations including CHG can lead to systematic patterns of new impurities, which grow slowly with time. Free radical generators, including gamma irradiation used to treat such products, can result in formation of dechlorination products.

▶ PHARMACEUTICAL ASPECTS

Compatibility

Chlorhexidine is a cationic molecule in its salt forms and is thus generally compatible with other cationic materials, such as quaternary ammonium compounds (eg, cetrimide, benzalkonium chloride), although compatibility will depend on the nature and relative concentration of the second cationic species. It is, however, possible for a reaction to occur between chlorhexidine and the counterion of a cationic molecule, resulting in the formulation of a less soluble chlorhexidine salt, which may then precipitate.

Nonionic substances, although not directly incompatible with chlorhexidine salts, may inactivate the antiseptic to varying degrees, according to the chemical type and concentration used. In many cases, a suitable ratio of chlorhexidine to excipient can be chosen to give the required degree of bioavailability and hence activity, and this should be confirmed by suitable microbiologic tests. Chlorhexidine salts are compatible with most cationic and nonionic surfactants, but at higher concentrations of surfactant, chlorhexidine activity can be substantially reduced owing to micellar binding. In hard water, insoluble salts may form owing to interaction with calcium and magnesium salts; aqueous dilution is preferably carried out with deionized water. Solubility may be enhanced by the inclusion of surfactants such as cetrimide.[20]

Chlorhexidine is incompatible with inorganic anions in all but extremely dilute solutions (see Table 22.1). This incompatibility sometimes may be overcome by adding a suitable solubilizing agent in formulations in which this is acceptable. Residual antimicrobial activity of chlorhexidine on the skin can be reduced after a saline rinse or soak.[21] Chlorhexidine is also incompatible with organic anions, such as soaps, sodium lauryl sulfate, sodium carboxymethyl cellulose, alginates, and many pharmaceutical dyes. Commonly used synthetic anionic thickening agents in hydroalcoholic hand sanitizers, like carbomer and acrylates/C10-30 alkyl acrylate crosspolymer, have also been shown to have a significant negative impact on the persistent activity of chlorhexidine on the skin.[22] In certain instances, there will be no visible signs of incompatibility, but the antimicrobial activity may be significantly reduced because of the chlorhexidine being incorporated into micelles. Chlorhexidine forms inclusion complexes with β-cyclodextrins that can modulate both its efficacy and mammalian cytotoxicity.[23]

Effect of pH on Activity

The antimicrobial activity of chlorhexidine is pH dependent; the optimum range of 5.5 to 7.0 corresponds to the pH of the body surfaces and tissues. Within the pH range 5 to 8, antibacterial activity will vary with the microorganism and the type of buffer used. The pH in chronic wounds most commonly has a range of 6.5 to 8.5.[24] Notably, in vitro testing of activity against *Staphylococcus aureus* and *Pseudomonas aeruginosa*, among the most prominent bacteria in wound infections, showed pH independence in the range of 5.0 to 9.0.[25]

Isotonicity

Dilution of chlorhexidine in physiologic saline to render it isotonic with plasma should be regarded with caution because of the low solubility of chlorhexidine hydrochloride (<1 mg/100 mL). Although solutions may be free of precipitate on preparation, the solutions (normally containing at least 0.02% chlorhexidine) will be supersaturated, and precipitation of the hydrochloride salt is likely to occur on standing.

Sodium acetate may be used to adjust the tonicity of chlorhexidine solutions without the problem of precipitation; however, the pH of the required solution (2.1% wt/vol sodium acetate, European Pharmacopoeia) may be as high as 8.0 and should not, therefore, be stored for prolonged periods.

Coloring Agents

Only a limited number of approved dyes can be used to color chlorhexidine solutions, and even these are anionic in nature and therefore may not be fully compatible. They usually can be added at low concentrations to tint chlorhexidine solutions for identification purposes but are likely to form a precipitate when used at the higher concentrations necessary to give good skin-staining properties. For example, carmoisine (E122) at a concentration of 0.0005% provides sufficient coloring for identification purposes and will remain stable for long periods. At a concentration of 0.05%, it has good skin-staining properties but is usually given a shelf life of 7 days after preparation. On the other hand, there are commercial shelf-stable hydroalcoholic CHG skin preparation compositions with skin-staining properties for visualization of the prepped field that are tinted with approved dyes.[26] The stability of the tinted active is thus dependent on the solution composition as well as the identity, composition, and concentration of the individual tints. Solution tinting prevents inadvertently confusing the clear antiseptic with other clear medical solutions such as an injectable active drug solution. Such confusion can lead to tragic results.[27] Additionally, selection of the appropriate tint is important in applications such as preoperative skin preparations, where skin pigmentation can influence visibility. Failure to determine the field of prepared skin adequately could lead to an increased risk of surgical site infection (SSI). The tint enables surgeons to visualize the preparation of the skin adequately, which is a crucial component of anti-infection precautions.[28]

Packaging

The nature and quality of containers for concentrates and use dilutions are important. Glass, high-density polypropylene, and high-density polyethylene are usually suitable. Low-density polyethylene may be unsuitable because of excessive adsorption, and other packaging materials may interact with the antiseptic. Cork stoppers or cap linings never should be used because water-soluble tannins present may inactivate chlorhexidine.[29] Solutions of chlorhexidine should also be protected from prolonged exposure to light.

Sterilization

Dilute solutions of chlorhexidine (<1.0% wt/vol) may be sterilized by steam at 115°C for 30 minutes or at 121°C to 123°C for 15 minutes. Autoclaving of solutions greater than 1.0% can result in the formation of insoluble residues and is therefore unsuitable. Following autoclaving of a 0.02% wt/vol CHG solution at pH 9 for 30 minutes at 120°C, it was found that 1.56% wt/wt of the original chlorhexidine content had been converted into para-chloroaniline; for solutions at pH 6.3 and 4.7, the para-chloroaniline content was 0.27% wt/wt and 0.13% wt/wt, respectively, of the original gluconate content.[30] If sterile solutions are required at such high concentrations, filtration through a 0.22 μm membrane filter is recommended; however, the first 10 mL should be discarded because adsorption to the filter can occur in the initial stage; fibrous and porcelain filters are unsuitable.

Chlorhexidine hydrochloride powder is stable to dry-heat sterilization at 150°C. The solid salts are stable to sterilizing doses of gamma radiation, but chlorhexidine in solution is decomposed. Electron beam sterilization of a CHG/ethanol disinfectant combination results in more than 20% of the chlorhexidine content being altered by irradiation at the sterilization dose.[31]

Unsterilized aqueous chlorhexidine solutions or devices can be inadvertently contaminated by certain tolerant bacilli such as the *Burkholderia cepacia complex* or *Serratia marcescens*, which can lead to the antiseptic itself becoming the nidus of an infection outbreak.[32] Medical devices impregnated with chlorhexidine are routinely safely sterilized using the ethylene oxide modality without altering the activity of the drug or introducing harmful levels of residuals.[33-35]

Storage

Dilute chlorhexidine solutions may be stored at room temperature, and a shelf life of at least 1 year can be expected, provided preparation and packaging are adequate. Prolonged exposure to high temperature or light is to be avoided because this can adversely affect stability; chlorhexidine solutions exposed to light become discolored due to the polymerization of para-chloroaniline.[12,36] All dilute solutions to be stored should be either heat-treated (sterilized or pasteurized) or chemically preserved

(4% isopropanol or 7% ethanol) to eliminate the possibility of microbial contamination. For autoclaved solutions, the choice of container material is important, the best results being achieved by using neutral glass or polypropylene. Guidelines on the storage of locally prepared aqueous solutions are as follows, but care should be taken to review the antiseptic formulation instructions for use and safety sheets:

Untreated solutions: Prepare and use within 24 hours. Do not store.
Chemically preserved solutions: Store unopened for a maximum of 3 months. When opened, use within 7 days.
Sterilized solutions: Store unopened for a maximum of 12 months. When opened, use within 24 hours.

Chlorhexidine and Laundering

Chlorhexidine is absorbed onto the fibers of certain fabrics, particularly cotton, and resists removal by washing. If a hypochlorite (chlorine-releasing) bleach is used during the washing procedure, a fast brown stain may develop because of a chemical reaction between the chlorhexidine and hypochlorite causing precipitate formation.

There has been considerable debate about the composition of the precipitate, with different analytical techniques showing contradictory results and some indicating the presence of para-chloroaniline.[37] A decisive study employing a variety of techniques including high-performance, thin-layer, and GC techniques, proton nuclear magnetic resonance (^{1}H NMR), IR spectroscopy, and GC/mass spectroscopy (MS) showed that para-chloroaniline was not typically present in the precipitate.[38] Chlorophenylurea has been proposed as one of the components of the precipitate.[39] This problem of staining can be avoided by eliminating the use of bleach or replacing the chlorine-releasing bleach with one that is peroxide based, such as sodium perborate. Pretreatment of the fabrics with a dilute acidic detergent reduces or eliminates staining when a chlorine bleach is subsequently used.[40]

◗ MICROBIOLOGY

The antimicrobial activity of chlorhexidine is directed mainly toward vegetative gram-positive and gram-negative bacteria; it is inactive against bacterial spores except at elevated temperatures, and acid-fast bacilli are inhibited but not killed by aqueous solutions. The infectivity of some lipophilic viruses (eg, influenza virus, herpes virus, human immunodeficiency virus [HIV]) is rapidly inactivated by chlorhexidine, although aqueous solutions are not active against the small nonlipid viruses. Yeasts (including *Candida albicans*) and dermatophytes are usually sensitive, although chlorhexidine's fungicidal action in general is subject to species variation, as is observed with other biocides.

Mechanisms of Antibacterial Action

The mechanism of action of chlorhexidine and related biguanides was reviewed by Woodcock.[41] At relatively low concentrations, the action of chlorhexidine is bacteriostatic, and at higher concentrations, it is rapidly bactericidal, with the actual levels varying somewhat from species to species.

The lethal process consists of a series of related cytologic and physiologic changes, some of which are reversible, that culminate in the death of the cell. The sequence is thought to be as follows: (1) rapid attraction toward the bacterial cell; (2) specific and strong adsorption to certain phosphate-containing compounds on the bacterial surface; (3) overcoming the bacterial cell wall exclusion mechanisms; (4) attraction toward the cytoplasmic membrane; (5) leakage of low-molecular-weight cytoplasmic components, such as potassium ions, and inhibition of certain membrane-bound enzymes, such as adenosyl triphosphatase; and (6) precipitation of the cytoplasm by the formation of complexes with phosphated entities, such as adenosine triphosphate and nucleic acids.

Characteristically, a bacterial cell is negatively charged, and the nature of the ionogenic groups varies with bacterial species. It has been shown that given sufficient chlorhexidine, the surface charge of the bacterial cell is rapidly neutralized and then reversed. The degree of charge reversal is proportional to the chlorhexidine concentration and was found to reach a stable equilibrium within 5 minutes. The rapid electrostatic attraction of the cationic chlorhexidine molecules and the negatively charged bacterial cell undoubtedly contributes to the rapid rate of kill associated with chlorhexidine, although surface charge reversal is secondary to cell death. Electron microscopy and assays for characteristic outer membrane components, such as 2-keto-3-deoxyoctonate (KDO), demonstrate that sublethal concentrations of chlorhexidine bring about changes in the outer membrane integrity of gram-negative cells. An efflux of divalent cations, especially calcium ions, occurs prior to or during such outer-membrane changes. Chlorhexidine molecules are thought to compete for the negative sites on the peptidoglycan, thereby displacing metallic cations. Being 6 carbons long, rather than 12 to 16 carbons, the hydrophobic inner functionality of the chlorhexidine molecule is somewhat inflexible and incapable of folding sufficiently to interdigitate into the cell bilayer. Chlorhexidine therefore bridges between pairs of adjacent phospholipid head groups each being bound to a biguanide moiety and displaces the associated divalent cations. Interestingly, the distance between phospholipid headgroups in a closely packed monolayer is roughly equivalent to the length of a hexamethylene grouping.

A bisbiguanide would therefore be capable of binding to two adjacent phospholipid head groups. Such binding is critical for the bisbiguanides as activity is reduced significantly if the polymethylene bridge is made longer or shorter than six carbons. Although the action of multidrug efflux pumps is able to moderate the efficacy of quaternary ammonium compounds at low concentrations, they have relatively little effect[42] on the action of bisbiguanides. This is presumably because the bisbiguanides do not become solubilized within the membrane core.[43]

In terms of the lethal sequence, the bacterial cytoplasmic membrane appears to be the important site of action. Several changes indicative of damage to the cytoplasmic membrane have been observed in bacterial populations treated with bacteriostatic and bactericidal levels of chlorhexidine. Leakage of cytoplasmic contents

is a classic indication of damage to the cytoplasmic membrane, starting with low-molecular-weight molecules typified by potassium ions. Electron micrographs of these sublethally treated cells (Figure 22.1) show a shrinkage or plasmolysis of the protoplast.[44] Cells treated with bacteriostatic levels of compound can recover viability despite having lost up to 50% of their K$^+$. This is particularly true if the excess chlorhexidine is removed by a neutralizing agent, as happens in many in vitro testing situations.

As the chlorhexidine concentration is increased, higher molecular weight cell contents, such as nucleotides, appear in the supernatant fluid around the cell. Bacterial cells showing more than a 15% increase in nucleotide leakage have been found to be damaged irreversibly; levels of chlorhexidine producing this effect are therefore

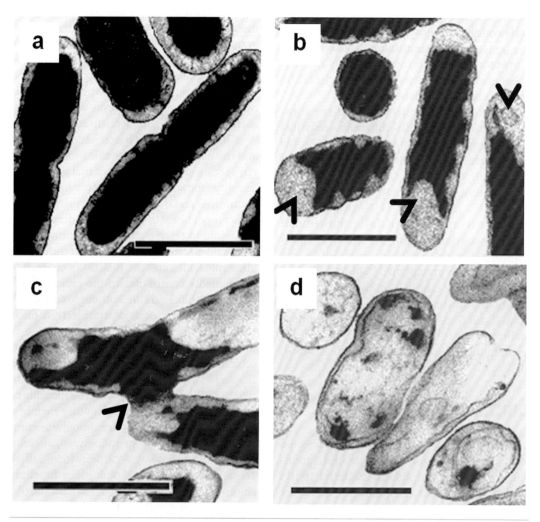

FIGURE 22.1 Cytological changes of *Escherichia coli* after treatment with chlorhexidine. Control cells possess intact cell membrane, cell wall, and complete cell content (A). After 4 h of incubation with 0.75 mg/L chlorhexidine, the treated *E coli* cells showed detached cytoplasmic membrane from the cell wall at both poles and cylindrical part of the cells (see *arrows* in B), leakage of cell content (see *arrow* in C), and formation of ghost cells (D). Magnification in all cases = ×20 500. Bar = 1 μm. Reproduced from Cheung et al.[44]

considered bactericidal. The rate of membrane disruption and cell leakage increases with chlorhexidine concentration up to a maximum and then falls back, and at concentrations that are rapidly bactericidal (100-500 mg/L), release of cell components does not occur. Electron microscopy shows the cytoplasm of these cells to be chemically precipitated—this precipitation having been caused by an interaction between the chlorhexidine and phosphated entities within the cytoplasm, such as adenosine triphosphate and nucleic acids.[44]

Antimicrobial Spectrum

Although numerous publications refer to the bacteriostatic and bactericidal properties of chlorhexidine against particular microorganisms, the methods used vary, and it is often difficult to compare results. A series of studies were therefore performed to provide a comprehensive spectrum of activity for chlorhexidine using both microbiostatic and microbicidal methods. The strains of organisms tested include clinical isolates, laboratory strains, and standard culture collection types. Each strain was tested to determine the minimum inhibitory concentration (MIC) of chlorhexidine and its susceptibility to the bactericidal action of 0.05% aqueous CHG using a rate-of-kill method.

Minimum Inhibitory Concentration Method

Twofold dilutions of CHG were prepared in Iso-Sensitest Agar, the surface of which was inoculated with a suspension of each test organism. After incubation at 37°C for 24 hours, the agar was examined for distinct growth. The MIC was recorded as the lowest chlorhexidine concentration that prevented growth.

Molds and yeasts were tested on Sabouraud agar incubated at 30°C for 24 to 72 hours. Anaerobes were incubated anaerobically for 2 to 3 days on agar containing 5% lysed blood. Fastidious organisms were incubated in carbon dioxide for 2 to 3 days (Tables 22.2 and 22.3).

Rate-of-Kill Test

The in vitro bactericidal and fungicidal activity of 0.05% CHG was determined using a procedure based on BS EN 1276:2009.[45] One milliliter of a 24-hour broth culture of the test organism was added to 10 mL of aqueous 0.05% wt/vol CHG solution, which was maintained at ambient temperature (18°C-21°C). One-milliliter aliquots of the mixture were removed after 20 seconds, 1 minute, and 10 minutes and transferred to inactivator broth containing 1.5% soya lecithin and 10% polysorbate 80. A viable count was performed on appropriate further dilutions,

and by comparison with an untreated control, a 10 log reduction factor was calculated (Tables 22.4 and 22.5).

Bacterial Susceptibility

The susceptibility of individual bacterial strains to chlorhexidine varies widely; however, few have been found to be capable of surviving concentrations of the antiseptic encountered in use.[46,47] It has been suggested that prolonged use of the antiseptic may lead to reduced susceptibility and to the development of resistant bacteria; however, this is not supported by the work of Martin[48] and Simpson et al,[49] who found that bacterial strains encountered in areas of prolonged and extensive use of the antiseptic have similar susceptibilities to strains of the same species encountered in areas where there is little or no chlorhexidine.

There is also no good evidence that the plasmid-mediated antibiotic resistance common among gram-negative bacteria is associated with resistance to chlorhexidine. Michel-Briand et al,[50] Ahonkhai et al,[51] and Sykes and Matthew[52] were unable to find any increase in chlorhexidine-resistance among antibiotic-resistant strains of *Escherichia coli*, *P aeruginosa*, *S marcescens*, or *Proteus mirabilis*.

Early studies with strains of methicillin-resistant *S aureus* (MRSA) using bacteriostatic MIC test procedures demonstrated a degree of reduced sensitivity to chlorhexidine compared to methicillin-sensitive strains of this organism (methicillin-sensitive *S aureus* [MSSA])[53,54]; however, this is considered of little clinical relevance because the highest MIC value for chlorhexidine quoted in these studies is 4 mg/L, and therefore, all strains of *S aureus*, including MRSA, can be regarded as sensitive to user concentrations of chlorhexidine. Both Haley et al[55] and Cookson et al[56] found the bactericidal activity of a 4% chlorhexidine hand wash to be similar for strains of MRSA and MSSA. A number of clinical reports also support the use of chlorhexidine preparations as part of programs for the control of outbreaks with MRSA[57-59]; however, Kampf et al[60] found a chlorhexidine in alcohol hand rub to be more effective than a chlorhexidine-based hand wash against MRSA and recommend this form of hand disinfection by staff treating MRSA patients.

Several outbreaks associated with contaminated CHG solutions have been reported,[61] indicating the ability of microorganisms to adapt to CHG. One mechanism of CHG resistance is through the cellular expression of efflux pumps, which can pump out of the bacterial cell various types of antibiotics and biocidal agents including CHG.[62] An indication of their ability can be gleaned through the study of 114 effluxing *S aureus* isolates where CHG was effluxed in 96% of the strains.[63] Other mechanisms of resistance can include the inactivation of the active ingredient or changes in the cell wall structure.[64]

TABLE 22.2   Bacteriostatic activity of chlorhexidine gluconate

Test Organism	MIC (mg/L)			Test Organism	MIC (mg/L)		
	(No. of Strains)	Mean	Range		(No. of Strains)	Mean	Range
Gram-positive cocci				Gram-negative bacilli *(continued)*			
Micrococcus flavus	1	0.5	NA	Bacteroides fragilis	11	34	8-64
Micrococcus lutea	1	0.5	NA	Campylobacter pyloridis	5	17	8-32
Staphylococcus aureus	16	1.6	1-4	Citrobacter freundii	10	18	4-32
Staphylococcus epidermidis	41	1.8	0.25-8	Enterobacter cloacae	12	45	16-64
Streptococcus faecalis	5	38	32-64	Escherichia coli	14	4	2-32
Streptococcus mutans	2	2.5	NA	Gardnerella vaginalis	1	8	NA
Streptococcus pneumoniae	5	11	8-16	Haemophilus influenza	10	5	2-8
Streptococcus pyogenes	9	3	1-8	Klebsiella aerogenes	5	25	16-64
Streptococcus sanguis	3	9	4-16	Klebsiella oxytoca	2	32	NA
Streptococcus viridans	5	25	2-32	Klebsiella pneumoniae	5	64	82-128
Gram-positive bacilli				Proteus mirabilis	5	120	64->128
Bacillus cereus	1	8	NA	Proteus morganii	5	73	16-128
Bacillus subtilis	2	1	NA	Proteus vulgaris	5	57	32-128
Clostridium difficile	7	16	8-32	Providencia stuartii	5	102	64-128
Clostridium welchii	5	14	4-32	Pseudomonas aeruginosa	15	20	16-32
Corynebacterium species	8	1.6	0.5-8	Pseudomonas cepacia	1	16	NA
Lactobacillus casei	1	128	NA	Pseudomonas fluorescens	1	4	NA
Listeria monocytogenes	1	4	NA	Salmonella ser Bredeney	1	16	NA
Propionibacterium acne	2	8	NA	Salmonella ser Dublin	1	4	NA
Gram-negative bacilli				Salmonella ser Gallinarum	1	8	NA
Acinetobacter anitratus	3	32	16-64	Salmonella ser Montevideo	1	8	NA
Acinetobacter lwoffi	2	0.5	NA	Salmonella ser Typhimurium	4	13	8-16
Alcaligenes faecalis	1	64	NA	Salmonella ser Virchow	1	8	NA
Bacteroides distasonis	4	16	NA	Serratia marcescens	10	30	16-64

Abbreviations: MIC, minimum inhibitory concentration; NA, not available.

The MIC and minimum bactericidal concentration (MBC) are commonly used to detect reduced susceptibility to chlorhexidine. However, there is neither a defined standardized method nor a consensus on the meaning of resistance to this agent.[65] Recently, Morrissey et al[66] attempted to define break points for chlorhexidine on the basis of normal distribution of MICs for a given bacterial species, known as the epidemiologic cutoff value. This value is described as the upper limit of the normal MIC distribution for chlorhexidine for a specific species and not the likelihood of treatment failure. In general, the advised dose of chlorhexidine usage is several times higher than the MBC; yet, if chlorhexidine concentration reaches sublethal levels over time,[67] those isolates with reduced susceptibility to chlorhexidine will remain viable, survive, and possibly persist. A more recent study[68] identifies the characteristics of lineages of S aureus with reduced susceptibility to chlorhexidine. The conclusion from this study is that clinical isolates with reduced susceptibility to chlorhexidine consist of strains that are genetically heterogeneous in their possession of biocide resistance genes. In order to reduce selection pressure in nosocomial pathogens, it has been suggested that the use of CHG be restricted to those indications with a clear patient benefit and to eliminate it from applications with a doubtful benefit.[69] Still, the overall risk for an acquired resistance to CHG is considered to be small as long as the antiseptics are used correctly.

TABLE 22.3	Fungistatic activity of chlorhexidine				
Organism	(No. of Strains)	Mean MIC (mg/L)	Organism	(No. of Strains)	Mean MIC (mg/L)
Mold fungi			Yeasts (continued)		
Aspergillus flavus	1	64	Saccharomyces cerevisiae	1	1
Aspergillus fumigatus	1	32	Torulopsis glabrata	1	6
Aspergillus niger	1	16	Dermatophytes		
Penicillium notatum	1	16	Epidermophyton floccosum	1	4
Rhizopus species	1	8	Microsporum canis	2	4
Scopulariopsis species	1	8	Microsporum fulvum	1	6
Yeasts			Microsporum gypseum	1	6
Candida albicans	2	9	Trichophyton equinum	1	4
Candida guilliermondii	1	4	Trichophyton interdigitale	2	3
Candida parapsilosis	2	4	Trichophyton mentagrophytes	1	3
Candida pseudotropicalis	1	3	Trichophyton quinkeanum	1	3
Cryptococcus neoformans	1	1	Trichophyton rubrum	2	3
Prototheca zopfii	1	6	Trichophyton tonsurans	1	3

Abbreviation: MIC, minimum inhibitory concentration.

Virulence Suppression

Whereas killing potentially pathogenic bacteria certainly will prevent them from causing infection, certain types of sublethal chemical treatment might also alter or damage bacterial cells in such a way as to reduce their ability to initiate the disease process. Thus, the bacteria could still be viable but less pathogenic. The ability of chlorhexidine to produce such a "depathogenizing" effect was first investigated by Holloway et al[70] using a peritonitis model in mice. Pathogenic strains of E coli and Klebsiella aerogenes were treated with sublethal concentrations of chlorhexidine after which the antiseptic was neutralized and the test suspension injected into susceptible animals. The results of these studies demonstrated that the pathogenicity of bacteria surviving treatment with chlorhexidine was reduced by more than 90%. This was confirmed by Rotter et al,[71] who could not demonstrate a similar effect with alcohol. This effect of chlorhexidine must be considered secondary to the direct bactericidal activity of the antiseptic; however, it is believed to be an additional, clinically relevant property that is not evident in conventional in vitro studies concerned with viability alone.

Sporicidal Activity

Chlorhexidine will inhibit the growth of the vegetative cells of spore-forming bacteria at relatively low concentrations (see Table 22.2) and also will inhibit spore germination/outgrowth. It is generally recognized, however,

that chlorhexidine has little direct sporicidal activity except at elevated temperatures. Shaker et al[72] investigated the sporicidal activity of an aqueous solution of CHG (25 mg/L) against Bacillus subtilis spores at various temperatures. At 20°C, 30°C, and 37°C, the antiseptic had little effect on spore viability, even after 120 minutes exposure. At a temperature of 70°C, however, the antiseptic reduced the number of spores by 5 logarithms. Physical and chemical conditions that alter the protective barriers of Clostridium difficile spores convey sporicidal activity to chlorhexidine. The C difficile spores became susceptible to heat killing at 80°C within 15 minutes in the presence of chlorhexidine, as opposed to spores suspended in water, which remained viable. The extent to which the spores were reduced was directly proportional to the concentration of chlorhexidine in solution, with no viable spores recovered after 15 minutes of incubation in 0.04% to 0.0004% wt/vol chlorhexidine solutions at 80°C. Reduction of spores exposed to 4% wt/vol chlorhexidine solutions at moderate temperatures (37°C and 55°C) was enhanced by the presence of 70% ethanol. However, complete elimination of spores was not achieved until 3 hours of incubation at 55°C. Elevating the pH to 9.5 significantly enhanced the killing of spores in either aqueous or alcoholic chlorhexidine solutions.[73]

Virucidal Activity

Chlorhexidine has good activity against viruses with a lipid component in their coats or with an outer envelope.

TABLE 22.4	Bactericidal activity of 0.05% chlorhexidine gluconate								

Test Organism	(No. of Strains)	Mean Log₁₀ Reduction After			Test Organism	(No. of Strains)	Mean Log₁₀ Reduction After		
		20 sec	1 min	10 min			20 sec	1 min	10 min
Gram-positive cocci					Gram-negative bacilli (continued)				
Micrococcus flavus	(1)	0.1	0.4	2.1	Bacteroides fragilis	(11)	3.0	4.2	5.2
Micrococcus lutea	(1)	0.2	0.7	2.9	Campylobacter pyloridis	(5)	NT	2.8	>4.0
Staphylococcus aureus	(16)	0.4	0.7	2.5	Citrobacter freundii	(10)	3.4	4.9	>6.0
Staphylococcus epidermidis	(41)	2.2	3.4	>5.1	Enterobacter cloacae	(12)	3.5	4.5	>6.3
Streptococcus faecalis	(5)	0.4	0.4	1.1	Escherichia coli	(14)	3.2	5.0	>6.4
Streptococcus mutans	(2)	0.8	>4.6	5.8	Gardnerella vaginalis	(1)	2.3	3.3	>5.8
Streptococcus pneumoniae	(5)	0.8	1.5	>3.5	Haemophilus influenza	(10)	>4.1	>4.1	>4.1
Streptococcus pyogenes	(9)	1.2	1.8	>3.7	Klebsiella aerogenes	(5)	2.7	3.9	>5.9
Streptococcus sanguis	(3)	1.1	2.2	>3.9	Klebsiella oxytoca	(2)	3.2	5.2	>6.4
Streptococcus viridans	(5)	0.4	0.8	2.3	Klebsiella pneumoniae	(5)	3.0	4.8	>6.2
Gram-positive bacilli					Proteus mirabilis	(5)	0.8	0.9	2.9
Bacillus cereus	(1)	2.0	2.0	4.7	Proteus morganii	(5)	1.0	1.5	4.2
Bacillus subtilis	(2)	0.5	0.5	0.3	Proteus vulgaris	(5)	0.8	1.0	4.1
Clostridium difficile	(7)	0.2	0.3	0.3	Providencia stuartii	(5)	0.6	0.9	1.8
Clostridium welchii	(5)	2.1	3.1	>4.8	Pseudomonas aeruginosa	(15)	1.7	2.7	4.9
Corynebacterium species	(8)	1.1	1.4	3.7	Pseudomonas cepacia	(1)	1.1	1.3	>4.6
Lactobacillus casei	(1)	0.2	0.2	4.1	Pseudomonas fluorescens	(1)	3.8	5.0	>6.7
Listeria monocytogenes	(1)	0.6	2.2	4.8	Salmonella ser Bredeney	(1)	1.6	3.4	>6.4
Propionibacterium acne	(2)	0.7	1.8	3.6	Salmonella ser Dublin	(1)	1.5	2.9	3.2
Gram-negative bacilli					Salmonella ser Gallinarum	(1)	2.5	4.0	>6.2
Acinetobacter anitratus	(3)	1.4	2.6	>5.3	Salmonella ser Montevideo	(1)	2.4	3.8	>6.3
Acinetobacter lwoffi	(2)	>4.0	>4.3	>4.8	Salmonella ser Typhimurium	(4)	2.0	3.7	>6.0
Alcaligenes faecalis	(1)	1.5	2.7	4.1	Salmonella ser Virchow	(1)	1.9	3.9	>6.2
Bacteroides distasonis	(4)	0.9	2.7	>4.9	Serratia marcescens	(10)	1.5	3.7	>5.9

Abbreviation: NT, not tested.

These include many respiratory viruses, herpes, and cytomegalovirus. The in vitro bactericidal and virucidal activity of throat lozenges containing CHG in relation to the main microorganisms responsible for upper respiratory tract infections, including the H1N1 influenza virus, was evaluated after short (5 min) and long (3 h) contact times. Antiviral activity inducing a 2 log (99%) destruction of the H1N1 virus after a 5-minute contact time at high CHG concentration was noted.[74]

In common with many other antiseptics, however, aqueous solutions of chlorhexidine do not have any significant activity against the small nonenveloped viruses, which include many of the enteric viruses, poliomyelitis, and papilloma (warts) virus.[75]

The HIV, the organism responsible for acquired immunodeficiency syndrome (AIDS), is known to be one of the enveloped viruses and can, therefore, be predicted to be sensitive to the action of chlorhexidine. This was confirmed in a series of in vitro studies. A 4% chlorhexidine hand wash preparation and 0.5% chlorhexidine in 70% alcohol were both found to be 100% effective against HIV type I after a 15-second contact. Aqueous solutions of chlorhexidine down to a final test concentration of 0.05% were 100% effective within 1 minute.[76] In a separate series of studies, chlorhexidine at 1 mg/mL (0.1%) was 80% to 100% effective.[77] A study in 2001 showed that intrapartum chlorhexidine lavage is not effective at preventing mother-to-child HIV transmission when used intravaginally

TABLE 22.5	Fungicidal activity of 0.05% chlorhexidine gluconate			
Test Organism	(No. of Strains)	Mean Log$_{10}$ Reduction After		
		20 sec	1 min	10 min
Mold fungi				
Aspergillus flavus	1	0.4	0.8	1.7
Aspergillus fumigatus	1	0.7	1.2	2.4
Aspergillus niger	1	0.7	1.2	3.0
Penicillium notatum	1	0.6	2.0	3.5
Rhizopus species	1	0.4	0.4	0.5
Scopulariopsis species	1	0.6	1.1	2.3
Yeasts				
Candida albicans	2	2.8	>4.1	>4.2
Candida guilliermondii	1	3.5	>4.3	>4.3
Candida parapsilosis	2	2.1	3.4	>4.2
Candida pseudotropicalis	1	3.6	>4.4	>4.4
Cryptococcus neoformans	1	4.0	>4.2	>4.2
Prototheca zopfii	1	3.3	>3.6	>3.6
Saccharomyces cerevisiae	1	3.7	>3.7	>3.7
Torulopsis glabrata	1	1.3	2.2	>4.4
Dermatophytes				
Epidermophyton floccosum	1	0.7	0.5	>1.8
Microsporum canis	2	0.4	1.0	>2.0
Microsporum fulvum	1	0.2	0.6	>2.4
Microsporum gypseum	1	0.1	0.3	2.0
Trichophyton equinum	1	0.5	1.1	>2.1
Trichophyton interdigitale	2	0.4	0.9	>2.4
Trichophyton mentagrophytes	1	1.3	>2.1	>2.1
Trichophyton quinkeanum	1	0.2	0.9	>2.8
Trichophyton rubrum	2	0.3	0.6	>2.4
Trichophyton tonsurans	1	0.4	0.3	1.6

during delivery. However, lavage with 0.4% chlorhexidine solely before rupture of the membranes tended toward lower transmission rates.[78] Published data on the activity of chlorhexidine against a wide range of viral agents are summarized in Table 22.6.[75,79-88]

CLINICAL APPLICATIONS AND EFFICACY

Oropharyngeal Disinfection: Ventilator-Associated Pneumonia

Ventilator-associated pneumonia (VAP) is a preventable secondary consequence of intubation and mechanical ventilation, which develops after 48 hours or more of mechanical ventilator support.[89] The VAP is the second most common nosocomial infection in intensive care units (ICUs). The condition is associated with increases in length of hospitalization and ICU stay, morbidity, mortality, and health care costs.[90] The VAP is considered a polymicrobial infection. Intubated patients are unable to swallow effectively due to incomplete glottis closure. Saliva and microorganisms reside in the mouth of intubated patients at a larger rate than normal.[91] Gram-positive streptococci typically predominate in the normal flora in the oropharynx. These can convert to gram-negative bacteria that can be more pathogenic. Additionally, stagnation of saliva promotes proliferation of such bacteria. If overgrowth of bacteria occurs in the oral cavity, then an immune response is initiated and the individual can become infected.[91] Gram-negative bacteria also accumulate along the endotracheal tube and can be propelled into the distal airways by inspiratory airflow from mechanical ventilation and endotracheal tube manipulation[92] or through microaspiration.[93] In recent years, many regimens of oral care with chlorhexidine have been used on mechanically ventilated patients to prevent the development of VAP. Oshodi and Bench[94] reviewed the available scientific evidence on the use of chlorhexidine in the prevention of VAP. Tantipong et al[95] investigated the effects of using a 2% chlorhexidine solution (n = 102) compared with using normal saline solution (n = 105) four times a day on 207 mechanically ventilated patients in ICUs and general medical wards. The incidence of VAP was 4.9% in the chlorhexidine group and 11.4% in the normal saline group, and the mean number of cases of VAP was 7 episodes per 1000 ventilator-days in the chlorhexidine group and 21 episodes per 1000 ventilator-days in the normal saline group. Although gram-negative bacilli were present at admission in 63 (61.8%) of the chlorhexidine group and 71 (67.6%) of the normal saline group, 19.1% of 63 patients in the chlorhexidine group, compared with none of the normal saline group, converted from being colonized with gram-negative bacilli to not being colonized. This study concluded that oral decontamination with a 2% chlorhexidine solution was effective in preventing VAP. Results from a recent systematic review and meta-analysis indicate that oral care with chlorhexidine is effective in reducing VAP incidence only in the adult population and if administered at a 2% concentration and/or four times daily.[96] A 2016 Cochrane Review included high-quality evidence from 18 randomized control

TABLE 22.6   Virucidal activity of chlorhexidine gluconate

Virus	Viral Family	Activity	Concentration (%)	References
Respiratory syncytial virus	Paramyxovirus	+	0.25	Platt and Bucknall[79]
Herpes hominis/simplex	Herpesvirus	+	0.02	Bailey and Longson [75]
Polio virus type 2	Enterovirus	−	0.02	Bailey and Longson[75]
Adenovirus type 2	Adenovirus	−	0.02	Bailey and Longson[75]
Equine infectious anaemia virus	Retrovirus	+	2.0	Shen et al[80]
Variola virus (smallpox)	Poxvirus	+	2.0	Tanabe and Hotta[81]
Herpes simplex types 1 and 2	Herpesvirus	+	0.02	Shinkai[82]
Equine influenza virus	Orthomyxovirus	+	0.001	Eppley et al[83]
Hog cholera virus	Togavirus	+	0.001	Eppley et al[83]
Bovine viral diarrhoea	Togavirus	+	0.001	Eppley et al[83]
Parainfluenza virus	Paramyxovirus	+	0.001	Eppley et al[83]
Transmissible gastroenteritis virus	Coronavirus	+	0.001	Eppley et al[83]
Rabies virus	Rhabdovirus	+	0.001	Eppley et al[83]
Canine distemper virus	Paramyxovirus	+	0.01	Eppley et al[83]
Infectious bronchitis virus	Coronavirus	+	0.01	Eppley et al[83]
Newcastle virus	Paramyxovirus	+	0.01	Eppley et al[83]
Pseudorabies virus	Herpesvirus	+	0.01	Matisheck[84]
Cytomegalovirus	Herpesvirus	+	0.1	Faix[85]
Coxsackie virus	Picornavirus	−	0.4	Narang and Codd[86]
Echo virus	Picornavirus	−	0.4	Narang and Codd[86]
Human rotavirus	Reovirus	−	1.5	Springthorpe et al[87]
Human immunodeficiency virus type I	Retrovirus	+	0.2	Harbison and Hammer[88]

Abbreviations: +, active in vitro at the concentration stated; −, not active in vitro at the concentration stated.

trials (RCTs) (2451 participants, 86% adults). It showed that chlorhexidine mouth rinse or gel, as part of oral hygiene care, reduced the risk of VAP compared to placebo or usual care from 24% to about 18% (relative risk [RR], 0.75; 95% confidence interval. 0.62-0.91; $P = .004$; I2 = 35%). This is equivalent to indicating that for every 17 ventilated patients in intensive care receiving oral health care including chlorhexidine, one outcome of VAP would be prevented.[97] The concentration of CHG used in these studies ranged from 0.12% to 2%, with the majority using concentrations of 0.12% to 0.2%.

Skin Disinfection

Chlorhexidine formulated in a detergent base is used extensively for disinfection of the hands of surgeons and nurses and for whole body skin disinfection of patients undergoing surgery. Alcohol-based chlorhexidine solutions with emollients also are used by surgeons and nurses for hand disinfection. Alcohol-based chlorhexidine solutions are particularly suitable for final-stage skin preparation of the operation site; the area should be kept wet for at least 2 minutes to achieve the maximal effect. The immediate bactericidal action of chlorhexidine typically surpasses that of similar preparations containing povidone-iodine, triclosan, hexachlorophene, or para-chloro-meta-xylenol (PCMX). Its valuable persistent (residual) effect, which prevents regrowth of organisms on the skin, is comparable to that of hexachlorophene or triclosan, although chlorhexidine has a broader spectrum of activity, particularly against gram-negative bacteria.

The evidence for efficacy is derived from extensive laboratory testing on volunteers and hospital staff and is generally supported by clinical experience now extending over more than 50 years. Some of this evidence is discussed, although differences such as experimental method inevitably make it difficult to compare data produced by different authors. Furthermore, because the efficacy of any formulation is significantly affected by the excipients present, trials demonstrating activity of one formulation cannot be used as evidence for the efficacy of another.

When assessing the effectiveness of an agent for skin disinfection, several properties of the product must be taken into consideration: immediate bactericidal action against both the resident and transient flora, persistence of action preventing regrowth of skin microorganisms, and a cumulative effect resulting from regular use. The product also must retain its activity in the presence of blood and have good cosmetic acceptability for the user. The relative importance of these individual properties varies to some degree according to the particular application of the antiseptic.

Surgical Hand Disinfection

The objective of surgical hand disinfection is to reduce the level of bacteria on the hands, thus preventing the escape of microorganisms into the operation wound through the punctures in surgical gloves, which occurs frequently during operation.[98] The procedure must particularly reduce many transient microorganisms that are likely to be present on the skin and reduce the resident flora to as low a level as possible. The agent should remain persistent on the skin to maintain the number of survivors at this low level throughout the course of the operation (see chapters 42 and 43).

In one of the first in-use studies involving a 4% chlorhexidine hand wash, Smylie et al[99] found this antiseptic to be at least as effective as hexachlorophane in reducing the numbers of bacteria on the hands of the surgical team and in maintaining these low numbers for several hours under gloves. A povidone-iodine hand wash was less effective initially and allowed the numbers of survivors on the hands to increase dramatically during the course of an operation. The chlorhexidine hand wash used was more acceptable to users than the other hand washes, undesirable side effects occurring most frequently with the povidone-iodine preparation.

In a large volunteer study using the official FDA guidelines for assessing surgical hand scrubs at the time, Peterson et al[100] found that a chlorhexidine hand wash produced significantly greater reductions in numbers of resident bacteria than either hexachlorophane or povidone-iodine preparations and maintained these low numbers for up to 6 hours under gloves. Povidone-iodine was not persistent, allowing a significant increase in bacterial numbers with time. This particular chlorhexidine hand wash (Hibiclens) was also the first surgical hand scrub to be approved as safe and effective by the Topical Antimicrobials Committee of the FDA.

Aly and Maibach[101] examined the effectiveness of sponge brushes impregnated with either chlorhexidine or povidone-iodine hand washes in a volunteer surgical hand disinfection study. The immediate and persistent effects of the agents and the effect of blood were assessed. Chlorhexidine proved to be significantly more effective than povidone-iodine in both the presence and absence of blood; this confirmed an earlier study by Lowbury and Lilly,[102] who found that blood significantly reduced the effectiveness of povidone-iodine but not of chlorhexidine.

Pereira et al[103] evaluated several procedures for surgical hand disinfection with detergent hand scrubs and alcohol-based hand rubs. The most effective treatments were a 5-minute scrub with 4% chlorhexidine detergent solution and combination treatments consisting of an initial 2-minute scrub with 4% chlorhexidine detergent solution, followed by a 30-second hand rub with chlorhexidine in alcohol solution. The authors considered the alcohol-based hand rubs to be as effective as the detergent-based hand scrub solution and no more damaging to the skin.

In an evaluation of duration of surgical scrub techniques, Okubo et al[104] found that a 3-minute "scrub" with chlorhexidine detergent solution without brushes was as effective as 3- or 6-minute scrubs with brushes, and there was much less risk of injury to the skin.

The Centers for Disease Control and Prevention (CDC) recommends 2 to 5 minutes of surgical scrub of hands and forearms up to the elbow, although the antiseptic of choice is not mentioned.[105] In a multicenter RCT, Parienti et al[106] demonstrated that hand rubbing with aqueous alcoholic solution, preceded by a 1-minute nonantiseptic hand wash was as effective as traditional hand scrubbing with antiseptic soap (4% povidone-iodine or 4% CHG) in preventing SSIs. However, no direct comparisons were performed between CHG and povidone-iodine and alcohol. In a meta-analysis of 14 clinical trials, Tanner et al[107] showed that CHG scrubs may reduce the number of bacterial colony-forming units (CFUs) on hands compared with povidone-iodine scrubs; however, it failed to show significant reduction in the rates of SSI. Also, they concluded that alcohol rubs with additional antiseptic ingredients like CHG may reduce bacterial CFUs compared with aqueous scrubs.

Olson et al[108] studied the benefit of the value of adding an active level of CHG to an alcohol-based surgical hand antiseptic in a prospective, randomized in vivo comparison against two alcohol-only waterless antiseptics for surgical hand antisepsis. The $\log_{10}$ reduction from baseline at the immediate and 6-hour time points on days 1 and 5 was compared between the alcohol plus CHG product and the individual alcohol-only products. The three brushless, waterless surgical hand antiseptics evaluated in this study showed similar efficacy immediately after use; however, the alcohol plus CHG product demonstrated superior persistent activity to both alcohol-only products after 6 hours of glove wear.

The surgical hand scrub has its obvious merits, but it is not without drawbacks as well. Many health care workers develop significant skin damage and allergies, and scrubbing can increase skin shedding 18-fold.[109] There is some evidence that alcohol-based surgical hand rubs cause less skin damage[106] and are preferred by health care personnel.[110] Some commercial brushless, waterless products are formulated with a lotion base to assist in preventing dry and cracked hands, thereby maintaining skin barrier integrity.[111] Similarly, the brushless CHG/ethanol emollient hand preparation was associated with less drying of the skin than the 4% CHG treatment as assessed by moisture content and was associated with significantly better skin condition scores for appearance, intactness, moisture content, and sensation scores in a 2001 study.[112] Because it is better tolerated and quicker to apply, in one of the largest studies comparing a surgical scrub with a brushless technique, Parienti et al[106] found that compliance was better with the brushless technique. Finally, the appropriate selection of inactive formulation excipients such as moisturizers and skin conditioning agents can provide products that encourage hand hygiene compliance through improved hand health outcomes for health care workers.[113]

Hygienic Hand Disinfection

The major source of infectious microorganisms within the hospital is the infected or heavily colonized patient, and the principal route of transmission is via the hands of hospital personnel (see chapter 42). Hand washing or disinfection is therefore considered to be the single most important measure to prevent nosocomial infection. The primary objective of hygienic hand disinfection is to eliminate the transient organisms that have been acquired on the hands, thus preventing their transfer between patients. The agent must act rapidly because busy hospital staff wash for only a short time. Persistence of antibacterial action on the skin is considered desirable to help prevent colonization with hospital pathogens and reduce the level of contaminants acquired between hand washes. User acceptability of a formulation is important in the ward situation, where frequent hand washing is often necessary. Factors such as soreness and dryness of the hands can have more influence on the use of a hand wash product than its antimicrobial efficacy.[114]

Rapidity of action of chlorhexidine against transient contaminants artificially applied to the skin was demonstrated by La Rocca et al.[115] In a study designed to mimic a ward hand wash, the hands of subjects were repeatedly contaminated with S marcescens and washed with chlorhexidine skin cleanser for 15 seconds. A 99.9% reduction of the contaminants was demonstrated after a single 15-second wash with chlorhexidine. Progressively greater reductions were obtained following repeated washing, owing to the cumulative activity of residual chlorhexidine.

Larson et al[114] compared the microbiologic and physiologic changes to skin brought about by frequent hand washing (15-s wash, 24 times daily). A chlorhexidine hand wash significantly reduced the bacterial hand flora compared with all other agents tested and produced no more skin trauma than nonmedicated soap.

Maki et al[116] compared the effectiveness of chlorhexidine skin cleanser with other hand wash preparations in a controlled trial with nurses in a neurosurgical unit. Following a single 15-second wash, chlorhexidine significantly reduced both the total skin flora and gram-negative organisms acquired naturally during patient contact. No significant reductions in bacterial counts were found following washing with unmedicated soap or an iodophor-containing preparation. The effect of regular use of the agents also was investigated. Each agent was used exclusively on the unit for 4 weeks, during which period repeated hand samples were taken. Regular use of chlorhexidine produced the lowest total bacterial counts and lowest mean numbers of gram-negative bacilli and S aureus. This finding confirmed the marked effectiveness of chlorhexidine skin cleanser in a single brief hand washing and demonstrates its persistent effect between repeated hand washes.

In a later study, Maki and Hecht[117] investigated the effect of different hand wash preparations on the incidence of nosocomial infection in a large ICU. Lower rates of infection were obtained with both chlorhexidine and povidone-iodine hand wash preparations than with unmedicated soap; however, chlorhexidine was better tolerated and was considered more acceptable for routine use. Stanley et al[118] also demonstrated that the rate of infection in an ICU was significantly lower when hands were washed with a 4% chlorhexidine preparation than when liquid soap and an alcohol rinse were used.

Barriers to appropriate hand hygiene among health care professionals have been reported to include (1) inaccessibility of hand hygiene supplies, (2) skin irritation from hand hygiene agents, and (3) an inadequate amount of time for hand hygiene. The introduction of alcohol-based hand rubs has helped improve hand hygiene compliance due to the accessibility and time savings of hand sanitizer application versus hand washing with soap and water.[119,120] Therefore, recent guidelines promote the use of alcohol-based hand rubs that are easily accessible.[121] Persistence, however, is a very important virtue in an antiseptic and one that most alcohol formulations lack, although bacteria appear to grow more slowly on the hands after alcohol use. The addition of 0.5% or 1% CHG to alcohol preparations can produce an antiseptic with excellent persistence. A comparative study showed that a 61% ethanol preparation did not achieve adequate persistent activity at 6 hours after use.[112] The same study showed that using 1% chlorhexidine with 61% ethanol without scrubbing or using water produced significantly greater microbial reduction on the hands of volunteers than using 4% chlorhexidine with a scrub brush in 2- to 3-minute surgical scrubs. The introduction of alcohol/chlorhexidine hand hygiene solution combined with education and motivation programs can improve hand hygiene compliance and reduce total nosocomial infections.[122,123] Frequent use of alcohol-based formulations for hand antisepsis can cause drying of the skin unless emollients or humectants are added to the formulations.

The drying effect of alcohol can be reduced or eliminated by adding skin-conditioning agents.[112]

Preoperative Skin Antisepsis

The SSI rates in the month following "clean" surgery can vary from 0.6% (knee prosthesis) to 5% (limb amputation).[124] The costs of these SSIs can be considerable in financial and social terms due to the large number of clean surgical procedures conducted annually. Preoperative skin antisepsis using antiseptics is performed to reduce the risk of SSIs by removing soil and transient organisms from the skin where a surgical incision will be made. Transient pathogenic skin flora present at the time of incision can be easily removed by a number of antiseptic agents. The iodophors (eg, povidone-iodine), alcohol-containing products, and chlorhexidine are the most commonly used agents for surgical skin preparation.[105] Although CHG is the preferred agent to prevent catheter-related infection,[125] the preferred antiseptic agent for surgical site preparation is less obvious. Alcohol is readily available, inexpensive, and has the fastest onset of action, whereas chlorhexidine has the greatest residual antimicrobial activity.[126] Studies have shown the superiority of CHG preparations in decreasing the bacterial load compared to iodine-based products.[127] In a single trial comparing 0.5% chlorhexidine in methylated spirit with povidone-iodine paint in alcohol, Berry et al[128] randomized 542 participants undergoing elective clean surgery. They found that there was a statistically significant difference in the number of SSIs in the chlorhexidine group (18/286; 6.3%) compared with the povidone-iodine paint treatment group (34/256; 13%). Thus, over the duration of follow-up there was a 53% reduction in the risk of getting an SSI in the chlorhexidine group compared to the povidone-iodine in alcohol paint group. In a separate multicenter, prospective, randomized clinical trial[129] comparing 10% povidone-iodine with 2% CHG and 70% isopropyl alcohol in clean-contaminated surgical cases, investigators found that the overall rate of SSI was significantly lower in the CHG/alcohol group compared with povidone-iodine group (9.5% versus 16.1%, respectively). The CHG/alcohol combination was superior to the povidone-iodine group in reducing the risk of both superficial incisional (4.2% versus 8.6%, respectively) and deep incisional (1% versus 3%, respectively) SSIs. On the other hand, surgical investigators at the University of Virginia conducted a single institution study[130] in general surgical patients (N = 3209 operations) looking at clinical outcomes associated with three separate skin-prepping regimens using a sequential (6 mo) implementation design. These included regimen A, 10% povidone-iodine scrub combination with an isopropyl alcohol application between steps; regimen B, 2% CHG / 70% isopropyl alcohol; and regimen C, 0.7% iodine povacrylex / 74% isopropyl alcohol. Patients were followed for 30 days postoperatively as part of an ongoing American College of Surgeons National Quality Improvement Program initiative. The primary outcome was overall rate of SSIs by 6 months performed in an intent-to-treat manner. The results were highly provocative with the lowest infection rate observed in regimen C, 3.9%, compared with 7.1% for regimen B. The authors suggest that iodine povacrylex in isopropyl alcohol solution may provide longer lasting antisepsis than other iodophor-based products because, when placed on skin, it dries to a film of disinfectant. It was suggested that this film may resist being washed away by fluids and blood and thus may provide potential for longer term protection than traditional povidone-iodine formulations.[130]

The preponderance of surrogate and clinical studies suggests that a CHG + alcohol combination is a very effective skin antiseptic agent for reducing the risk of surgical sites.[131] The addition of an alcohol base lends an enhanced component to the broad-spectrum activity of CHG, further augmented by documented residual activity of CHG on the surface of the skin. One cautionary comment has been provided by the authors: Any skin antiseptic agent containing alcohol, including CHG, must be allowed to dry prior to draping to reduce the likelihood of a fire occurring during electrocautery. For this reason, the FDA recommends a 3-minute wait period after applying a preoperative skin antiseptic agent containing high levels of ethanol or isopropanol.

Preoperative Whole Body Disinfection

A significant proportion of postoperative wound infections is caused by microorganisms from the patient's own skin, which may be derived from sites remote from that of the operation. Reducing the level of the skin microflora over the whole body is, therefore, thought to be of benefit in reducing the incidence of infection from these sources.

Brandberg and Anderson[132] demonstrated a significant reduction in total skin flora following a shower bath with a 4% chlorhexidine skin cleanser and found that this reduction was maintained for up to 1 week, emphasizing the persistent properties of the antiseptic. These results were confirmed by Kaiser et al,[133] who also demonstrated a beneficial cumulative effect with repeated application of chlorhexidine.

Following earlier microbiologic studies, Brandberg et al[134] performed a clinical investigation to determine the effect of preoperative showering with chlorhexidine skin cleanser on infection rates in patients undergoing vascular surgery. On admission, patients bathed daily with the antiseptic (three to eight baths, depending on the length of preoperative stay). Immediately prior to surgery, the operative site was washed with this same solution and finally prepared using 0.5% chlorhexidine in 70% alcohol. A control group of patients did not perform daily bathing but received the same operation-site preparation.

The infection rate was reduced from 17.5% in the control group to 8% in the patients who showered preoperatively with chlorhexidine.

In a closely monitored clinical study involving more than 2000 surgical patients, Hayek et al[135] demonstrated a significant reduction in the infection rate in patients who bathed with chlorhexidine skin cleanser on two occasions in the 24 hours prior to surgery. The overall infection rate was 9% for patients who bathed with chlorhexidine compared with 12.5% for those using unmedicated bar soap.

In addition to reducing patient morbidity, this infection control measure was considered to confer significant health economic benefits to the hospital in terms of improved bed use and cost-effectiveness. Hayek and Emerson[136] reported that the reduction in infection rate achieved by preoperative bathing with chlorhexidine would save 22 bed days per 100 patients, allowing almost 3% more patients to be admitted for elective surgery.

Other workers investigated the effect of both preoperative and postoperative bathing with chlorhexidine. Randall and coworkers reported the results of two prospective studies in men undergoing vasectomy. In the first of these,[137] preoperative bathing with chlorhexidine skin cleanser was microbiologically effective, but it did not reduce the postoperative infection rate, which was in excess of 30%. In the second study,[138] preoperative bathing with chlorhexidine was retained, and the effect of additional postoperative bathing on the days following operation was examined. This procedure, which involved both preoperative and postoperative bathing, reduced the infection rate from 37.8% to 6.7%. Wound infection in this group of patients was considered largely a secondary phenomenon occurring after the patient left the hospital.

Some trials failed to demonstrate a clinical benefit, although these either have not followed the recommended skin disinfection method or have included too few patients to show statistical significance. In a review of all studies on the use of chlorhexidine for whole body disinfection, Brandberg[139] concluded that the procedure is a valuable adjunct to existing antiseptic and aseptic measures that will contribute toward a reduction in infections caused by organisms derived from the patient's own skin.

Preoperative baths are now widely encouraged in clinical practice. Although it is expected that decreasing general skin contamination in preoperative patients will decrease the number of SSIs, a clear cause-and-effect relationship has not been established to date. Recent Cochrane systematic reviews identified RCTs of full-body bathing or showering with chlorhexidine, compared with placebo or regular soap, and found no clear evidence that preoperative bathing with chlorhexidine was more effective at reducing SSI.[140,141] Some of these studies entailed full-body rinsing after application of chlorhexidine, and this may have impacted chlorhexidine's antiseptic activity, so conclusions about preoperative bathing should be interpreted with caution. Two sets of guidelines support use of CHG

for preoperative cleansing to prevent SSI[142] and daily bathing in the ICU to prevent healthcare-associated infection (HAI).[143] The modality of whole body disinfection may also play an important role. Preoperative showering with 4% CHG soap resulted in effective antimicrobial coverage on most skin sites, but gaps in antiseptic coverage were noted at selective sites even after repeated application. Use of a 2% CHG-impregnated polyester cloth wipe resulted in considerably higher skin concentrations with no gaps in antiseptic coverage.[144]

Catheter Site Protection

Vascular access devices enable health care professionals to administer medications, nutritional support, blood products, and other therapies to patients. These invasive devices may also put patients at risk for local and systemic infections, including catheter-related bloodstream infections (CRBSIs). Most microorganisms responsible for short-term CRBSIs originate from the insertion site.[145] Among the strategies found to be successful in reducing CRBSI, the use of chlorhexidine as a skin antiseptic for site preparation has been included in the top five performance indicators for reducing CRBSI recommended by the CDC.[146] Chaiyakunapruk et al[147] conducted a systematic review that evaluated chlorhexidine against povidone-iodine in all vascular catheters, including arterial and central and peripheral venous catheters and showed that antiseptic solutions containing chlorhexidine reduced CRBSI on average by 49% compared with povidone-iodine. Although the use of CHG with isopropyl alcohol for antisepsis of the skin prior to catheter insertion provides substantial protection, viable bacteria may still remain on the skin, and regrowth occurs over time. A 2009 study of chlorhexidine-impregnated polyurethane foam disks in intravascular catheter dressings demonstrated a reduced risk of infection even when background infection rates were low.[148] More recently, other antimicrobial dressings have been developed, including a transparent intravenous (IV) dressing incorporating 2% (wt/wt) CHG in an aqueous gel pad.[149] The use of the transparent dressing containing CHG gel has likewise been associated with a reduction in catheter-related sepsis.[150] Chlorhexidine-impregnated dressings with an FDA-cleared label that specifies a clinical indication for reducing CRBSI or catheter-associated blood stream infection (CABSI) are now recommended by the CDC to protect the insertion site of short-term, nontunneled CVCs. This recommendation for patients aged 18 years and older was a 2017 update to the 2011 guidelines.[125] Transparent CHG-impregnated dressings are considered advantageous[151] when visualization of the catheter site is desired, as shown in Figure 22.2.

The CVCs are essential devices for giving fluids, medications, IV nutrition, and cancer treatment to patients. Compared to peripheral catheters (ie, tubes inserted via

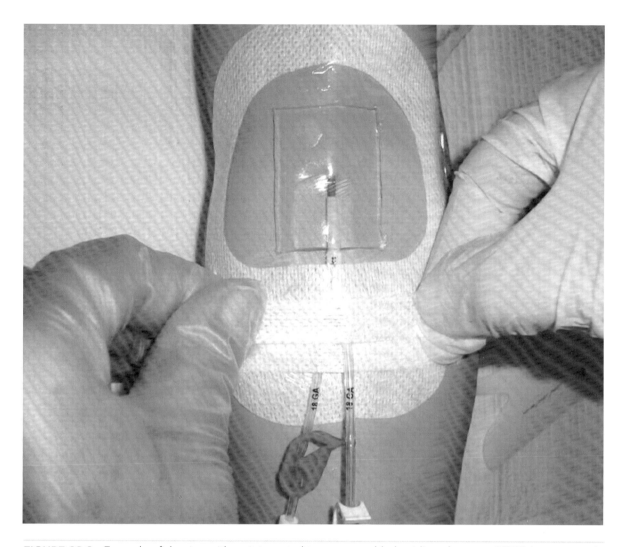

FIGURE 22.2   Example of draping with an integrated transparent chlorhexidine gluconate (CHG)-impregnated gel pad dressing on a peripherally inserted catheter in clinical practice. For a color version of this art, please consult the eBook. Reproduced from Pfaff et al[151] © 2012 by the American Association of Critical-Care Nurses. All rights reserved. Reprinted with permission.

veins in the limbs that are designed for short-term use), CVCs are longer and reach deeper into the major veins of the body, providing a more secure and durable IV access. However, infections, especially of the bloodstream, are common in patients with CVCs. It has been speculated that this is due, at least in part, to the placement technique where peripheral catheters are "tunneled" and CVCs enter the vessel directly. Several measures have been developed to reduce such infections, including coating or impregnation of CVCs with antiseptics or antibiotics. Of the various forms of antiseptic catheter impregnation that have been introduced since the late 1980s, chlorhexidine-silver sulfadiazine (CH-SS) impregnation is one of the most commonly used and studied. In a systematic review of 15 studies of catheters coated externally with CH-SS, Ramritu et al[152] found that pooling results demonstrates a significant reduction in risk of CRBSI associated with CH-SS relative to uncoated catheters.

In the same review, two RCTs of a second-generation CVC coated both internally and externally with CH-SS found a similar reduction in risk of CRBSI with a greater relative reduction in risk for the study with a longer insertion time.[153]

Urology

Numerous reports have described the effectiveness of chlorhexidine preparations in preventing urinary tract infections. A solution of 0.05% chlorhexidine in either glycerine[154] or ethylene glycol[155] was used successfully as a combined urethral antiseptic and lubricant. Intermittent bladder irrigation with 0.02% aqueous solution of chlorhexidine was effective in reducing the incidence of bacteria in catheterized patients.[156-158] Solutions used in the urinary tract should be prepared from compendial CHG solutions, which contain no additives. The inadvertent use of solutions containing surfactants causes hematuria in some patients.

Obstetrics and Gynecology

In one of the earliest reports involving chlorhexidine, Calman and Murray[159] reported on the suitability of several antiseptics for use in obstetrics. They considered that the most exacting test, and the one most relevant to practical obstetrics was a 2.5-minute bactericidal test in the presence of fresh blood. By this standard, only chlorhexidine achieved a complete kill of all microorganisms at its recommended user dilution of 1 in 2000 (0.05%). On the basis of this work and on the experience of 2.5 years of clinical use, chlorhexidine was considered the most satisfactory antiseptic available for use in midwifery.

Byatt and Henderson[160] compared the ability of different antiseptics to disinfect the perineum. The most effective aqueous preparation was a 4% chlorhexidine detergent preparation both undiluted and at a dilution of 1:80, which brought about reductions in recoverable bacteria of 98% and 82%, respectively. An equivalent concentration of chlorhexidine without added cleansing agents was less effective, suggesting that the mucus secretions and fatty acid exudates present in this situation prevented penetration of antiseptics to the bacteria.

Christensen et al[161] investigated the effectiveness of vaginal washing with a 0.2% chlorhexidine solution for the prevention of neonatal colonization with group B streptococci. A significant reduction in colonization with this organism was noted in the infants of treated mothers, and the investigators concluded that this procedure might prevent serious infection in the early neonatal period. Taha et al[162] reported that neonatal admissions and mortality due to sepsis were reduced when a sterile aqueous solution of chlorhexidine 0.25% was used to cleanse and disinfect the birth canal.

In a retrospective study of women undergoing laparotomy for gynecologic surgery, skin preparation with 2% CHG followed by 70% isopropyl alcohol resulted in a significant decrease in SSI compared with the use of 10% povidone-iodine scrub followed by 10% povidone-iodine paint with 65% alcohol.[163] To avoid irritation, CHG with high concentrations of alcohol should not be used in the vagina. Solutions that contain lower concentrations, such as the commonly used 4% CHG soap containing 4% alcohol, are usually well tolerated. One randomized trial compared the efficacy of 4% CHG with 4% isopropyl alcohol to a 10% povidone-iodine solution for vaginal preparation.[164] Fifty women who underwent vaginal hysterectomy were randomized to a preoperative vaginal scrub with one solution, and serial vaginal culture specimens were obtained to assess bacterial contamination throughout surgery. No cases of vaginal irritation occurred. Thirty minutes after the vaginal preparation, those in the iodine group were more than six times more likely to have contaminated cultures compared with the CHG group.

There is significant evidence to suggest that topical application of chlorhexidine to the umbilical cord reduces neonatal mortality in community and primary care settings in developing countries.[165]

Wounds and Burns

Platt and Bucknall,[166] using a wound model in guinea pigs, demonstrated that irrigation with 0.05% chlorhexidine was highly effective in preventing wound sepsis. This finding was confirmed in the clinical situation by Colombo et al,[167] who demonstrated a significant reduction in postoperative infection in patients whose wounds were sprayed with 0.05% chlorhexidine during suturing. Groups of workers in France also have found irrigation with chlorhexidine to be effective for controlling existing wound infection.[168,169] A recent review of the evidence on use of chlorhexidine in wound care[170] indicates that research on its effectiveness in reducing bacterial burden is limited to preparations of 1% or less concentration and has primarily been conducted in laboratory settings. Although effectiveness in eradicating bacteria has been tested in vitro and in animal studies, the limited research in clinical settings fails to demonstrate an associated improvement in the rate of wound healing. At the same time, there is no strong clinical evidence that chlorhexidine at low concentrations significantly impedes wound healing either.[171,172]

Chlorhexidine preparations have been used extensively in the management of burns for cleansing and antisepsis. In addition, several groups of workers have used the antiseptic for balneotherapy of major burns. The patients were immersed in baths containing aqueous solutions of CHG at concentrations ranging from 0.01% to 0.05%. This treatment was considered a valuable adjunct to the existing infection control measures.[173,174]

Oral Disease

The role of chlorhexidine as an effective agent for the prevention and treatment of oral disease has been widely recognized for a number of years. With the exception of fluoride, no chemical agent for use in the mouth has been so extensively studied. The effectiveness of chlorhexidine stems from its ability to adsorb to negatively charged surfaces in the mouth (eg, tooth, mucosa, pellicle, restorative materials), maintaining prolonged antimicrobial activity for many hours.[175] Retention studies with radiolabeled chlorhexidine show that approximately one-third of the dose is retained after a 60-second mouth rinse with 10 mL of a 0.2% solution.[176] Clinical studies demonstrated that this treatment, applied twice daily, produces optimum uptake and retention in the mouth.[177,178]

Gingivitis is a reversible condition when gums become red and swollen and can bleed easily. Gingivitis is also very common—studies suggest that as many as 50% to 90% of adults in the United Kingdom and United States suffer from it. The application of chlorhexidine varnishes seems to have beneficial effects in patients with chronic gingivitis, improving their plaque accumulation and bleeding levels and reducing their gingival index.[179] It is possible to maintain this beneficial effect for prolonged periods of time, although this requires reapplications of the varnish.

Plaque formation is a continual process, and an agent showing persistent activity offers an advantage over an agent with only a limited duration of effect. Chlorhexidine remains the agent of choice for supragingival plaque control.[180,181] Treatment with chlorhexidine mouthwash or gel reduces the duration of and discomfort from minor aphthous ulceration and increases the total number of ulcer-free days.[182,183] A recent review of 12 trials analyzing 950 participants showed a large positive effect of plaque reduction in favor of chlorhexidine rinse.[184]

Preoperative and postoperative use of chlorhexidine mouthwash reduces the oral microflora and the incidence of postextraction bacteremia.[185,186] Postoperative gingival healing is enhanced by the use of chlorhexidine applied as either a mouthwash or a gel. A recent RCT[187] on the efficacy of chlorhexidine prophylaxis on posttooth extraction bacteremia concluded that a 0.2% chlorhexidine mouthwash (10 mL for 1 min) significantly reduced the duration (at 15 min) of bacteremia secondary to tooth extraction under local anesthesia. Subgingival irrigation with a more potent 1% chlorhexidine did not increase the efficacy of the mouthwash. The antiseptic is thought to achieve this by reducing the level of microbial contamination of the wound.[188,189]

Oral hygiene can prove difficult to maintain in certain compromised groups. Persons who have mental or physical disabilities may be unable either to understand or perform adequate control measures. Immunocompromised patients are particularly susceptible to oral infections, especially with *Candida* species, and the same is true of denture wearers. Chlorhexidine mouthwash, gel, and spray have been effective in helping maintain the oral hygiene of mentally and physically handicapped groups[190,191]; the mouthwash and gel have been used successfully in immunocompromised patients to control candidiasis and mucositis.[192-194]

Soaking dentures in chlorhexidine is effective in reducing colonization with *Candida* species.[195,196] It is suggested that the antiseptic exerts both antifungal and antiadhesive effects, which may last for several days.[197]

Persons who have an increased caries risk can be identified from the high salivary levels of *Streptococcus mutans*. Use of chlorhexidine gel[198] or chlorhexidine fluoride mouthwash,[199] along with other preventive measures such as fluoride treatment and diet control, has been shown to reduce significantly the incidence of caries in these patients. Radiation-associated caries also can be controlled by a chlorhexidine/fluoride mouthwash.[200] Featherstone et al[201] reported an RCT where the primary study factor was caries management by means of chlorhexidine (antibacterial) and fluoride therapy guided by the patients' risk for caries. The authors concluded that chlorhexidine (antibacterial) and fluoride therapy based on salivary microbial and fluoride levels favorably altered the balance between pathologic and protective caries risk factors.

The most common side effect associated with oral use of chlorhexidine is extrinsic tooth staining, which seems to be an unavoidable consequence of having clinically effective chlorhexidine available at the tooth surface. The highly reactive molecule combines with dietary chromogens, which then are precipitated onto the tooth surface[202]; it is this chlorhexidine/chromogen complex that forms the characteristic stain. Maximum staining occurs in vitro at 0.1% chlorhexidine[203]; however, reducing the concentration to limit staining requires a corresponding increase in volume to maintain clinical efficacy. Thus, clinically equivalent doses of chlorhexidine have equivalent levels of stain. The stain is extremely variable from individual to individual and may be minimized by prior toothbrushing with a dentifrice.[181] Although tooth staining limits the long-term oral use of chlorhexidine, for some patient groups, the benefits outweigh the disadvantages. Indeed, for the physically and mentally handicapped, chlorhexidine may be the only option for effective oral hygiene.[204]

⬤ SAFETY

Chlorhexidine has been in use throughout the world for more than 50 years in a wide range of clinical situations; during this period, reports of adverse reactions have been relatively few. Extensive studies involving experimental animals and human volunteers as well as observations of hospital staff and patients have been carried out to determine the nature and probability of untoward reactions that may be associated with the varied applications of chlorhexidine to living tissues. These range from disinfection of intact adult skin to delicate mucous membranes (eg, bladder and eye) and traumatic or surgical wounds. Systemic (oral, intramuscular, IV) and topical routes of administration have been investigated for short- and long-term adverse effects.

Acute effects of accidental ingestion or injection have been rarely reported and are associated only with high doses of chlorhexidine. Long-term effects of animal feeding and topical (human) use showed that absorption from the alimentary tract or through the skin is negligible or absent. There is no evidence of carcinogenicity. The incidence of skin irritation and hypersensitivity is low when chlorhexidine is applied at its recommended concentrations. There is no deleterious effect on healing of wounds or grafting of burns. As with most disinfectants, a high probability of total deafness rules out the use of chlorhexidine during surgery on the inner or middle ear.[205] Chlorhexidine is toxic to nerve tissue, and therefore, contact with the brain and meninges must be avoided. Strong solutions of chlorhexidine and preparations that are formulated with other excipients, such as alcohols and surfactants, also should be kept away from the eyes.

Acute Toxicity

Systemic administration of formulations of chlorhexidine by oral, IV, and subcutaneous (SC) routes has been performed in rats and mice. Oral median lethal dose (LD_{50}) values are high because chlorhexidine is poorly absorbed from the gut and is excreted mainly unchanged in the feces. Administration by the IV route results in greater toxicity than by either the oral or SC routes because of a stromalytic effect on red blood cells resulting from its surfactant activity. Acute lethal doses of CHG are reported as follows[206]:

- LD_{50} (mouse, oral): 1220 to 2215 mg/kg
- LD_{50} (mouse, SC): 1140 mg/kg
- LD_{50} (mouse, IV): 13 mg/kg
- LD_{50} (rat, oral): 2000 to 2430 mg/kg
- LD_{50} (rat, SC): 3320 mg/kg
- LD_{50} (rat, IV): 24 mg/kg
- LD_{50} (rabbit, dermal): >2000 mg/kg (highest dose tested; no animal deaths)

Subacute and Chronic Toxicity

Slight toxic effects (details not provided) were reported in a review by Willis[207] in rats given a 20% CHG solution daily by gavage for 7 days at dose levels between 1000 and 15 000 mg/kg. Also mentioned was a report wherein no toxic effects were seen in rats given 20 000 mg/kg orally for 14 days.

In a subchronic oral study (up to 3 mo), there was a dose-related decrease in body weight of the animals that corresponded with a decrease in consumption of drinking water that the authors stated was likely from the unpalatable taste of CHG. The only adverse response noted in rats receiving 50, 100, or 200 mg/kg CHG daily in their drinking water for 60 days was evidence of reactive histiocytosis in the mesenteric lymph nodes. Because this response is known to occur naturally in aging rats, this effect was questioned as to whether it was drug related. The change was not neoplastic, and phagocytic function was normal. In longer-term tests of up to 2 years, the effect on the mesenteric lymph nodes was nonprogressive.

The effect of CHG at doses of 5 and 50 mg/kg daily on the reproductive performance of male and female rats also was studied. Mating performance, pregnancy rate, duration of gestation, litter parameters, and the condition of the dams at terminal necropsy were unaffected by the treatment.

Butler and Iswaran[208] reported on a 1-year oral study with dogs in which CHG was given in drinking water at various dose levels (specific intake levels not given). The only possible toxic effect found was an increase in salivation in a few animals.

In a 2-year oral dosing study with rats, Case[209] administered CHG to the animals via their drinking water at concentrations of 5, 25, or 50 mg/L. Water consumption was significantly reduced at the highest concentration. No drug-related changes were observed in any hematology parameter or in clinical chemistries. No effects were noted in either the macroscopic or microscopic pathology.

The effect of CHG at doses of 5 and 50 mg/kg daily on the reproductive performance of male and female rats also was studied. Mating performance, pregnancy rate, duration of gestation, litter parameters, and the condition of the dams at terminal necropsy were unaffected by the treatment.

Oncogenicity/Mutagenicity

Carcinogenicity studies have been performed in both rats and mice given oral chlorhexidine plus artificially increased levels of its degradation product para-chloroaniline. No evidence of carcinogenicity was found in rats after 2 years of up to 40 mg/kg of chlorhexidine plus 0.6 mg/kg/day para-chloroaniline daily.

Several reports of mutagenicity tests with CHG have been done based on modifications of the microbiologic Ames test procedure. This type of microbiologic test is considered to be fundamentally inappropriate for use with known antimicrobial agents because it is difficult to separate the legitimate lethal action of the drug on the bacterial cell from any toxicologic activity the drug may possess. However, Sakagami et al[210] were able to demonstrate that CHG was not genotoxic in both the presence and the absence of metabolic enzymes in an *umu* gene induction assay with *Salmonella* ser Typhimurium strain 1535/pSK1002. Sakagami et al[211] also evaluated the genotoxicity of CHG using the *rec*-assay with *B subtilis* (M-45[*rec*−] and H-17[*rec*+]). The CHG gave equivocal results in this assay system.[212]

In a chromosomal aberration test with cultured Chinese hamster ovary cells, CHG gave negative results both in the presence and absence of metabolic enzymes.[213] Withrow et al[213] evaluated the genotoxic effect of CHG using an in vitro cell culture assay system. In this study, CHG was negative for genotoxicity at the thymidine kinase locus of mouse lymphoma cells (L5178Y $TK^{+/-}$).

The CHG was tested for mutagenicity in an in vivo micronucleus assay with mice.[207] Ten animals per dose were used. Dose levels in this study were 10, 20, and 30 mg/kg. The CHG also produced a negative response in this test system. In another in vivo study, Ribeiro et al[214] treated groups of 10 Wistar rats orally with 0.5 mL of a 0.12% CHG solution twice daily for 8 days. At the end of this exposure period, oral mucosal cells were harvested using a wooden spatula; peripheral leukocytes and reticulocytes were isolated from blood samples. The DNA damage was tested using the comet assay and as micronuclei in blood reticulocytes. A significantly higher amount of DNA damage was observed in the oral mucosal cells and in the peripheral leukocytes compared to the controls. In contrast, no increase in the frequency of micronucleated reticulocytes was observed in the CHG-treated animals.

Dermal Absorption

All the available information on chlorhexidine suggests that the antiseptic is absorbed through skin to an extremely small degree, if at all. Case[215] reported on a series of studies to detect percutaneous absorption of chlorhexidine following application to the skin of volunteers. Radiolabeled chlorhexidine formulated as a 4% hand wash or 5% aqueous solution was applied to forearm skin and left in contact for 3 hours. Levels ranging from 96% to 98% of the radioactivity subsequently were recovered from the skin; no radioactivity was detected in blood or urine. The equivalent of 0.007% of the administered dose was detected in only one of the fecal samples. In a further study, subjects followed an exaggerated surgical scrub schedule using a 4% chlorhexidine hand wash five times daily for three 5-day weeks. Each treatment lasted 6 minutes and included 3 minutes of brush scrubbing. Blood samples were taken throughout the test period and analyzed for chlorhexidine using a gas liquid chromatography method with a sensitivity of 0.01 to 0.05 mg/L. No detectable blood levels were found in any of the volunteers at any time. Blood samples also were taken from hospital staff members who had been regular users of 4% chlorhexidine for surgical hand disinfection for at least 6 months. No detectable levels of chlorhexidine were found in any of the subjects.

Blumer et al,[216] who used 4% chlorhexidine hand wash for bathing infants, were unable to detect skin absorption of chlorhexidine on each of the 3 days following bathing. Cowen et al,[217] who also bathed infants with this preparation, did find significant levels of chlorhexidine in the blood when samples were taken by heel prick, but this was thought to be due to contamination from the treated skin. Samples of venous blood taken, in an attempt to avoid contamination, showed extremely low levels of chlorhexidine in some infants and no detectable levels in others.

Gongwer et al[218] bathed neonatal rhesus monkeys for 90 days with an experimental hand wash formulation containing 8% CHG. No adverse effects on the brain or other tissues were found. Minimal amounts of chlorhexidine were detected in a few tissues and in the feces, and it was suggested that the antiseptic had entered the body by oral ingestion following grooming.

Skin permeation studies have been performed on full-thickness excised human skin.[219] Overall, following 2- and 30-minute exposures, the skin penetration of CHG from both aqueous and alcoholic solutions was limited. At skin depths of >300 μm, the concentration of CHG detected from both solutions was negligible. In addition, CHG did not completely permeate through the full thickness of the human skin model. The concentration of CHG recovered within the top 100 μm skin sections was significantly less following a 2-minute exposure to alcoholic CHG than that following similar exposure to aqueous CHG. Following a 30-minute exposure, there was no significant difference in the skin penetration of the CHG from alcoholic and aqueous solutions within the model.

From the results of all the studies listed, it is clear that percutaneous absorption of chlorhexidine, if it occurs at all, is minimal. There is no evidence that any chlorhexidine absorbed would be toxic.

Skin Irritation and Sensitization

Primary dermal irritancy studies with aqueous CHG solutions (20%, 0.5%) or a 4% chlorhexidine hand wash were performed in rabbits using the Draize test method.[220] The results showed that none of the formulations was a primary skin irritant. A repeated-application dermal toxicity study was performed in rabbits with aqueous CHG (20%) applied once daily, 5 days a week for 3 weeks. The concentrated solution caused damage to both intact and abraded skin, which healed within 2 weeks of stopping treatment.

Chlorhexidine can induce allergic contact dermatitis at the site of application. The first case of well-described chlorhexidine contact dermatitis was reported in 1972.[221] Although allergy to chlorhexidine has been reported in the literature,[222] life-threatening anaphylactic shock is rare.[223] Life-threatening anaphylaxis is commonly associated with mucosal and parenteral exposure, when it occurs.[224] Although professional exposure may represent an important source of chlorhexidine sensitization among health care workers, the risk of sensitization and allergy to chlorhexidine in health care workers is not well established. The issue is further complicated by the fact that chlorhexidine is frequently formulated with excipients such as dyes, surfactants, and emollients that could be responsible for triggering contact allergies.[225,226] The FDA identified 52 cases of anaphylaxis, a severe form of allergic reaction, with the use of CHG products applied to the skin. In the 46 years between January 1969 and early June 2015, the FDA received reports of 43 cases worldwide. The serious allergic reaction cases reported outcomes that required emergency department visits or hospitalizations to receive drug and other medical treatments. These allergic reactions unfortunately resulted in two deaths. Eight additional cases of anaphylaxis were published in the medical literature between 1971 and 2015. This has prompted the FDA to encourage manufacturers of over-the-counter antiseptic products containing CHG to add a warning about the rare but serious allergic reactions risk to labeling.

Considered against the extensive use of the antiseptic over more than 50 years, the incidence of such side effects must be considered extremely low.

Wound Healing

Saatmann et al[227] assessed the effects of 0.05% and 4% CHG solutions on the healing of surgically induced wounds in guinea pigs. The wounds were irrigated after surgery and daily thereafter until necropsy. Daily progress of the wound appeared normal in all treatment groups, with no gross evidence of treatment effects. On histopathologic evaluation, the treated animals exhibited a slight delay in healing compared with saline-treated animals on days 3, 6, and 9; however, by days 14 and 21, no differences were detectable.

Hirst et al[228] investigated the effect of chlorhexidine on gingival wound healing in dogs. Biopsy sites were treated with 20% chlorhexidine or saline for 42 days, after which the sites were graded for inflammatory response. Sites exposed to chlorhexidine had less evidence of inflammation than the control sites, and healing was judged as complete.

Histologic findings indicate toxicity of chlorhexidine to proliferating skin.[229] It has been reported that chlorhexidine is cytotoxic to exposed fibroblasts when assessed in vitro using tissue culture methods; data from one study[230] found that chlorhexidine was cytotoxic to human dermal fibroblasts at concentrations of 5 to 2400 times below those used in clinical practice. Evidence from in vitro studies suggests that fibroblasts and keratinocytes exposed to 0.05% chlorhexidine for 15 minutes are nonviable within 24 hours.[229] Another in vitro study found that after 96 hours of exposure to chlorhexidine at a concentration of 0.0032%, there was a significant reduction in fibroblast proliferation. However, chlorhexidine at a concentration of 0.0004% was associated with a significant increase in fibroblast proliferation.[231] Sanchez et al[232] observed that the cytotoxicity observed in vitro did not correlate with in vivo data. Using an infected wound model, they found that chlorhexidine actually accelerated the rate of healing compared with saline-treated controls.

One histologic study showed that after 6 weeks of treatment with 5% CHG, chronic leg ulcers exhibited a decrease in microvessels, neutrophils, fibroblasts, and dendrocytes compared to ulcers treated with normal saline.[233] Expert opinion suggested that the decrease in microvessels might not be a significant issue because there was an excessive increase in vasculature related to lipodermatosclerosis in the ulcer bed; that is, although some microvessels may not survive exposure to 5% CHG, this only reduces microvessels from a pathogenically high level to a "normal" level.

The effect of chlorhexidine on human articular cartilage has been of particular concern, with a number of cases of marked chondrolysis and subsequent joint damage being reported. An in vitro study demonstrated that exposure of nonarthritic human cartilage to chlorhexidine for 1 minute reduced cell metabolic activity by 14%, which was not significant, but exposure for 1 hour had a marked effect—86% reduction. In arthritic cartilage even exposure of 1 minute had a significant impact on metabolic activity (43% reduction).[171] Chlorhexidine has a damaging effect on the articular cartilage of the knee and should not be used, even in low concentrations, to irrigate exposed articular cartilage.

Ototoxicity

Sensorineural deafness was found to occur in patients who had undergone vascular myringoplasty operations; the common factor was the use of 0.05% chlorhexidine in 70% alcohol for perioperative disinfection of the middle ear. It was thought that the solution had penetrated the membrane of the round window, entering the inner ear and causing damage to the cochlea, which resulted in permanent hearing loss.[234] This has since been extensively investigated using animal models. Severe vestibular and cochlear damage has been found to occur, the extent of which is related to concentration and duration of exposure.[235,236] In addition, the extent of damage was also shown to be related to the time lapse after exposure; that is, the injury had progressed in the 4-week period following exposure.[237] Other antiseptics have been similarly ototoxic when administered in this way. Toxicity is significantly enhanced in the presence of high levels of alcohol or detergent.[238] In a further study to examine the ototoxicity of chlorhexidine in an animal model, an electrophysiologic approach was employed. Perez and colleagues[239] demonstrated damage to the vestibular nerve and cochlear structures with the loss of vestibular and auditory evoked potentials when chlorhexidine was applied to the middle ear. On the contrary, povidone-iodine did not affect vestibular evoked potentials and had only a small effect on the auditory brainstem response.

Neurotoxicity

Limited information is available on the risk of neurotoxicity with chlorhexidine. In 1955, Weston-Hurst[240] reported that the neurotoxic concentration of aqueous chlorhexidine when injected into the cerebrospinal fluid of monkeys appeared to be in the region of 0.05%. In 1984, Henschen and Olsen[241] showed that injection of just 5 µL of 0.05% aqueous chlorhexidine into the anterior chamber of the eye produced adrenergic nerve degeneration in rats, and the authors postulated that the thin unmyelinated nerves of the central nervous system might be equally affected. More recently, Doan et al[242] found that chlorhexidine was neurotoxic at a concentration of 0.01% (the lowest concentration tested) when applied directly to neurons. However, in a rat model using a radioactive tracer, the same authors estimated mathematically that provided the antiseptic is allowed to dry fully, the concentration of antiseptic that could be delivered to the neuraxis would be extremely low.[242] It has been suggested that alcohol, which constitutes the main component of chlorhexidine solutions, might be the actual causative neurotoxic agent.[243]

Ocular Toxicity

Although dilute solutions of pure chlorhexidine have been used for eye irrigation (0.05%) and as a preservative for such preparations as eye drops (0.01%), higher concentrations and preparations containing other excipients may cause eye tissue damage.

If chlorhexidine inadvertently comes into contact with the ocular surface, progressive corneal damage can occur in a dose-dependent fashion.[244,245] At lower concentrations, chlorhexidine can cause toxic effects on the epithelial layers of the cornea and conjunctiva, which can cause transient epithelial disruption and abrasion. Typically, full recovery without lasting visual sequelae is possible.[244] However, at higher concentrations, irreversible injury occurs to the corneal endothelial monolayer, which in humans lacks the ability to regenerate.[244,245] With sufficient loss of endothelial cells, corneal edema ensues, and the cornea loses its transparency; the resultant visual loss can be severe. Although lesser degrees of corneal endothelial injury may heal over a period of weeks to months, severe corneal endothelial injury results in irreversible corneal edema and accompanying visual loss that can be treated only by corneal transplantation. The histopathologic findings in the cornea have been described in such cases; they include epithelial edema with bullous changes, marked loss of keratocytes, thickening of Descemet membrane, and an attenuated disrupted cell layer.[246] Care should be taken during preoperative skin preparation to keep chlorhexidine out of the eye and to flush copiously with sterile saline solution or sterile water if contact accidentally occurs.

Chlorhexidine has also been accidentally irrigated into the anterior chamber of the eye, instead of balanced salt solution, during cataract surgery.[247] Later in the operation, a decrease in corneal clarity was noted, and an epithelial abrasion had to be performed. The inadvertent use of chlorhexidine in this patient resulted in reduced endothelial function and loss of corneal clarity. Progressive ulcerative keratitis related to the use of CHG 0.02% eye drops has been reported.[248]

Isolated reports of injury resulting from accidental introduction into the eye of an antiseptic hand wash containing 4% chlorhexidine in a detergent base have been received. Accidental splashes entering the eye during normal hand washing caused irritation, which was resolved completely following prompt and thorough washing of the affected eye with water. Irreversible corneal damage occurred following more prolonged ocular exposure as a result of misuse of the antiseptic hand wash on anesthetized patients for skin preparation of the periorbital area and eyelids. The product had pooled on the eye surface and remained there for up to 1 hour.[249,250] From the information available, it would appear that the excipients present in the hand wash formulation, or possibly a combined effect of the excipients and chlorhexidine, are a more likely cause of permanent ocular damage than the chlorhexidine alone.

Accidental use of chlorhexidine solutions (1:666 and 1:1000) as irrigation during cataract surgery resulted in immediate corneal edema, which resulted in a bullous keratopathy.[251] Liu et al[252] described a case of a patient who underwent resection of gingival cancer with inadvertent ocular exposure to chlorhexidine skin preparation, which led to persistent corneal edema that eventually required corneal transplantation. Bever et al[253] recently reported two neurosurgical patients who experienced severe corneal toxicity and visual loss as a result of presumed inadvertent topical ocular exposure to the chlorhexidine skin preparation.

Phototoxicity

Chlorhexidine was tested for phototoxicity in the course of a European Union/European Cosmetic, Toiletry and Perfumery Association (EU/COLIPA) validation study of in vitro phototoxicity assays in the 3T3 neutral red uptake phototoxicity assay.[254] Chlorhexidine was cytotoxic with an IC_{50} of 61.5 µg/mL. The IC_{50} of CHG in the presence of UV-A irradiation was 74.4 µg/mL, which was not significantly different indicating that this chemical was not phototoxic. In another nonstandard in vitro assay for phototoxicity, CHG also gave no evidence of phototoxicity.[255]

Mucosal Exposure

The aqueous concentration of CHG normally recommended for contact with mucous surfaces is 0.05% (wt/vol). At this concentration, there is no irritant effect on soft tissues, nor is healing delayed. Harvey et al[256] investigated the effect of CHG on mucous membranes using hamster cheek pouch mucosa. The cheek pouch mucosae of groups of five male Syrian hamsters were treated with 0.2% or 2% aqueous solutions of CHG or with saline daily for 3 weeks. Thereafter, the animals were sacrificed and the cheek mucosa excised and examined histologically. In addition, the permeability of the cheek pouch mucosa was determined using a standard diffusion chamber with radiolabeled water. The high concentration of CHG caused the formation of discrete white hyperplastic areas with inflammation accompanying a significant increase in epithelial thickness. The high concentration also resulted in a significant reduction of mucosal permeability. The lower concentration had no adverse effect on either mucosa morphology or permeability.

The effects of CHG on the mucous membrane of the tongue were evaluated by Sonis et al.[257] In this study, groups of 10 to 12 male Lewis rats were given CHG via their drinking water at a concentration of 0.02% or 0.2% for 14 days. One additional group was given 0.2% CHG in the drinking water for 30 days. Three other animals each received 0.02% or 0.2% CHG in the drinking water for 14 days and were then maintained without exposure for another 16 days and sacrificed on day 30. All other animals were sacrificed at the end of their exposure time. The tongues were excised and prepared for histologic examination. The administration of 0.2% CHG in the drinking water caused the formation of hyperkeratotic plaques on the tongues in most animals within 14 days. Some ulceration was also noted. Microscopically, a generalized dysplasia and hyperkeratosis of the tongue mucosa was seen in these animals. These plaques disappeared within 30 days of exposure. At 0.02% CHG, hyperkeratotic plaques were seen only in a few animals. Animals in this group also showed generalized dysplasia, hyperkeratosis, and parakeratosis of the tongue mucosa but at a much lower severity than those of the high-dose group.

The effect of CHG on gingival wound healing was evaluated in six Labrador dogs. Biopsy sites in the facial gingival tissue were treated with 2% CHG or saline for 1 minute each day for 42 days, after which the sites were graded histologically for inflammatory response. The sites exposed to CHG exhibited less evidence of inflammation than did the control sites, and healing was judged to be markedly improved as compared to the control group.[228]

Topical chlorhexidine may cause anaphylaxis when applied on mucosal surfaces. Among 50 cases of adverse reactions to chlorhexidine due to mucosal application, 9 cases of anaphylactic shock were reported by the Japanese Ministry of Welfare between 1967 and 1984.[258] Vaginal instillation of chlorhexidine solution or chlorhexidine-containing gel application while placing an intrauterine device or during cervix conization can result in an anaphylactic shock.[259,260]

Concurrent Application of Chlorhexidine Gluconate and Povidone-Iodine

In clinical practice, no single antiseptic containing both chlorhexidine and povidone-iodine is currently available. However, many surgeons use a combination of chlorhexidine and povidone-iodine preparations in sequence. Their simultaneous application was once thought to form a less effective cocktail. This belief has recently been challenged in vitro, with evidence in fact for a potential synergistic effect.[261] A separate study showed that using a combination of chlorhexidine with povidone-iodine is safe and effective for skin antisepsis and preoperative surgical skin area scrubbing with chlorhexidine for 3 minutes, followed by cleaning once with povidone-iodine, could be enough for reducing skin bacterial flora before neurosurgical intervention.[262] Langgartner et al[263] compared three skin disinfection regimens prior to the insertion of a CVC and found that using sequential application of chlorhexidine/alcohol and povidone-iodine was superior to either of the disinfectants alone in reducing skin colonization rates at the insertion site. A recent systematic review and meta-analysis of preoperative antisepsis with a combination of chlorhexidine and povidone-iodine indicated that bacterial decontamination at the operative site is more effective when the combination is used.[264] These studies assume additional importance because several clinicians use iodine-impregnated surgical incise drapes to afford an additional level of antimicrobial protection in challenging surgeries[265] while simultaneously employing chlorhexidine-based preparations as the primary skin disinfection modality. Mechanistically, there is good reason to believe combination chlorhexidine and povidone-iodine would be of benefit. Although both have a broad spectrum of antibacterial activity, povidone-iodine can also target viruses, fungi, and bacterial spores, and chlorhexidine can target yeast. Additionally, the action of povidone iodine is intracellular, and therefore, the action of chlorhexidine, which disrupts cell membranes, would theoretically augment its potency.

▶ ACRONYMS AND ABBREVIATIONS

MIC	minimum inhibitory concentration
MRSA	methicillin-resistant *Staphylococcus aureus*
MSSA	methicillin-susceptible *Staphylococcus aureus*
CHG	chlorhexidine gluconate
VAP	ventilator-associated pneumonia
ICU	intensive care unit
FDA	US Food and Drug Administration
CDC	Centers for Disease Control and Prevention
SSI	surgical site infection
CFUs	colony-forming units
CVC	central venous catheter

REFERENCES

1. Milstone AM, Passaretti CL, Perl TM. Chlorhexidine: expanding the armamentarium for infection control and prevention. *Clin Infect Dis.* 2008;46:274-281.
2. Knox RW, Demons ST, Cunningham CW. A novel method to decontaminate surgical instruments for operational and austere environments. *Wilderness Environ Med.* 2015;26(4):509-513.
3. Lim KS, Kam PC. Chlorhexidine—pharmacology and clinical applications. *Anaesth Intensive Care.* 2008;36:502-512.
4. Bharatam PV, Patel DS, Iqbal P. Pharmacophoric features of biguanide derivatives: an electronic and structural analysis. *J Med Chem.* 2005;48(24):7615-7622.
5. Davies GE, Francis J, Martin AR, Rose FL, Swain G. 1:6-Di-4′-chlorophenyldiguanidohexane ("Hibitane"). Laboratory investigation of a new antibacterial agent of high potency. *Br J Pharmacol Chemother.* 1954;9:192-196.

6. United States Pharmacopeia, National Formulary. *Description and Relative Solubility/Reference Tables*. Rockville, MD: United States Pharmacopeial Convention; 2014.

7. Wibaux AM, Van de Pol V, inventors; Avery Dennison Corp, assignee. Chlorhexidine gluconate containing solvent adhesive. US patent 9,764,059. September 19, 2017.

8. Menon VP, Rule JD, Ross RB, Conrad-Vlasak DM, Wlaschin KF, inventors; 3M Innovative Properties Co, assignee. Chlorhexidine gluconate compositions, resin systems and articles. US patent 9,713,659. July 25, 2017.

9. Gent JF, Frank ME, Hettinger TP. Taste confusions following chlorhexidine treatment. *Chem Senses*. 2002;27(1):73-80.

10. Heard DD, Ashworth RW. The colloidal properties of chlorhexidine and its interaction with some macromolecules. *J Pharm Pharmacol*. 1968;20:505-512.

11. Zeng P, Zhang G, Rao A, Bowles W, Wiedmann TS. Concentration dependent aggregation properties of chlorhexidine salts. *Int J Pharm*. 2009;367(1-2):73-78.

12. Goodall RR, Goldman J, Woods J. Stability of chlorhexidine in solutions. *Pharm J*. 1968;200:33-34.

13. United States Pharmacopeial Convention. *United States Pharmacopeia National Formulary: USP 40-NF 35*. Rockville, MD: United States Pharmacopeial Convention; 2014:3364-3373.

14. European Pharmacopoeia Commission, Council of Europe. In: *European Pharmacopoeia*. 8th ed. Strasbourg, France: Council of Europe; 2013:1850-1854.

15. Fiorentino FAM, Corrêa MA, Salgado HRN. Analytical methods for the determination of chlorhexidine: a review. *Crit Rev Anal Chem*. 2010;40:89-101.

16. Goizman MS, Sarkisyan SO, Sarkisyan AA, Persianova IV. Differential spectrophotometric determination of biguanide derivatives. *Pharm Chem J*. 1985;19:503-508.

17. Doub WH, Ruhl DD, Hart B, Mehelic PR, Revelle LK. Gradient liquid chromatographic method for determination of chlorhexidine and its degradation products in bulk material. *J AOAC Int*. 1996;79(3):636-639.

18. Revelle LK, Doub WH, Wilson RT, Harris MH, Rutter AM. Identification and isolation of chlorhexidine digluconate impurities. *Pharm Res*. 1993;10(12):1777-1784.

19. Ha Y, Cheung AP. New stability-indicating high performance liquid chromatography assay and proposed hydrolytic pathways of chlorhexidine. *J Pharm Biomed Anal*. 1996;14(8-10):1327-1334.

20. Peltonen L. Chlorhexidine. In: Sheskey PJ, Quinn ME, Rowe RC, eds. *Handbook of Pharmaceutical Excipients*. 6th ed. London, United Kingdom: Pharmaceutical Press; 2009:162-166.

21. Stahl JB, Morse D, Parks PJ. Resistance of antimicrobial skin preparations to saline rinse using a seeded bacteria model. *Am J Infect Control*. 2007;35(6):367-373.

22. Kaiser N, Klein D, Karanja P, Greten Z, Newman J. Inactivation of chlorhexidine gluconate on skin by incompatible alcohol hand sanitizing gels. *Am J Infect Control*. 2009;37(7):569-573.

23. Teixeira KI, Denadai AM, Sinisterra RD, Cortés ME. Cyclodextrin modulates the cytotoxic effects of chlorhexidine on microrganisms and cells in vitro. *Drug Deliv*. 2015;22(3):444-453.

24. Dissemond J, Witthoff M, Brauns TC, Haberer D, Goos M. pH-Wert des Milieus chronischer Wunden. *Hautarzt*. 2003;54:959-965.

25. Wiegand C, Abel M, Ruth P, Elsner P, Hipler UC. pH influence on antibacterial efficacy of common antiseptic substances. *Skin Pharmacol Physiol*. 2015;28(3):147-158.

26. Kieser TM, Rose MS, Aluthman U, Montgomery M, Louie T, Belenkie I. Toward zero: deep sternal wound infection after 1001 consecutive coronary artery bypass procedures using arterial grafts: implications for diabetic patients. *J Thorac Cardiovasc Surg*. 2014;148:1887-1895.

27. O'Connor M. Responsiveness to the chlorhexidine epidural tragedy: a mental block? *J Law Med*. 2012;19(3):436-443.

28. McDaniel CM, Churchill RW, Argintar E. Visibility of tinted chlorhexidine gluconate skin preparation on varied skin pigmentations. *Orthopedics*. 2017;40(1):e44-e48.

29. Linton KB, George E. Inactivation of chlorhexidine ("Hibitane") by bark corks. *Lancet*. 1966;1(7451):1353-1355.

30. Jaminet F, Delattre L, Delporte JP, Moes A. Effect of temperature of sterilization and of pH on stability of chlorhexidine in solution [in French]. *Pharm Acta Helv*. 1970;45(1):60-63.

31. Yamaguchi T. Electron beam sterilization of chlorhexidine gluconate/ethanol disinfectant [in Japanese]. *J Antibacterial Antifungal Agents*. 2013;41(9):469-474.

32. Ko S, An HS, Bang JH, Park SW. An outbreak of *Burkholderia cepacia complex* pseudobacteremia associated with intrinsically contaminated commercial 0.5% chlorhexidine solution. *Am J Infect Control*. 2015;43(3):266-268.

33. US Food and Drug Administration. 3M Tegaderm CHG chlorhexidine gluconate I.V. port dressing 510(k) premarket notification. US Food and Drug Administration Web site. https://www.accessdata.fda.gov/cdrh_docs/pdf12/K123679.pdf. Accessed January 21, 2018.

34. US Food and Drug Administration. ARROW FlexBlock continuous peripheral nerve block kit/set 510(k) premarket notification. US Food and Drug Administration Web site. https://www.accessdata.fda.gov/cdrh_docs/pdf15/K153652.pdf. Accessed January 21, 2018.

35. US Food and Drug Administration. Biopatch antimicrobial dressing 510(k) premarket notification. US Food and Drug Administration Web site. http://www.accessdata.fda.gov/scripts/cdrh/cfdocs/cfpmn/pmn.cfm?ID=K003229. Accessed January 21, 2018.

36. Myers JA. Hospital infections caused by contaminated fluids. *Lancet*. 1972;2(7771):282.

37. Kolosowski KP, Sodhi RN, Kishen A, Basrani BR. Qualitative analysis of precipitate formation on the surface and in the tubules of dentin irrigated with sodium hypochlorite and a final rinse of chlorhexidine or QMiX. *J Endod*. 2014;40(12):2036-2040.

38. Orhan EO, Irmak Ö, Hür D, Yaman BC, Karabucak B. Does para-chloroaniline really form after mixing sodium hypochlorite and chlorhexidine? *J Endod*. 2016;42(3):455-459.

39. Nowicki JB, Sem DS. An in vitro spectroscopic analysis to determine the chemical composition of the precipitate formed by mixing sodium hypochlorite and chlorhexidine. *J Endod*. 2011;37(7):983-988.

40. Wilker C, McCormick SD, Lyle JM, inventors; Washing Systems, LLC, assignee. Reduction or removal of chlorhexidine and/or avobenzone from fabric materials. US patent 9,133,419. September 15, 2015.

41. Woodcock PM. Biguanides as industrial biocides. In: Payne KR, ed. *Industrial Biocides*. Chichester, United Kingdom: Wiley; 1988:19-36.

42. Poole K. Efflux-mediated antimicrobial resistance. *J Antimicrob Chemother*. 2005;56(1):20-51.

43. Gilbert P, Moore LE. Cationic antiseptics: diversity of action under a common epithet. *J Appl Microbiol*. 2005;99(4):703-715.

44. Cheung HY, Wong MM, Cheung SH, Liang LY, Lam YW, Chiu SK. Differential actions of chlorhexidine on the cell wall of *Bacillus subtilis* and *Escherichia coli*. *PLoS One*. 2012;7(5):e36659.

45. British Standards Institution. *Chemical Disinfectants and Antiseptics. Quantitative Suspension Test for the Evaluation of Bactericidal Activity of Chemical Disinfectants and Antiseptics Used in Food, Industrial, Domestic and Institutional Areas. Test Method and Requirements (Phase 2, Step 1)*. London, United Kingdom: British Standards Institution; 2009. BS EN 1276:2009.

46. Pitt TL, Gaston MA, Hoffman PN. In vitro susceptibility of hospital isolates of various bacterial genera to chlorhexidine. *J Hosp Infect*. 1983;4:173-176.

47. Hammond SA, Morgan JR, Russell AD. Comparative susceptibility of hospital isolates of gram-negative bacteria to antiseptics and disinfectants. *J Hosp Infect*. 1987;9:255-264.

48. Martin TDM. Sensitivity of the genus *Proteus* to chlorhexidine. *J Med Microbiol*. 1969;2:101-108.

49. Simpson RA, Hawkey PM, Woodcock PM. Antibiotic resistance and chlorhexidine susceptibility of gram negative bacteria in the hospital and community. Paper presented at: 29th Interscience Conference on Antimicrobial Agents and Chemotherapy; September 17-20, 1989; Houston, TX.

50. Michel-Briand Y, Laporte JM, Bassignot A, Plesiat P. Antibiotic resistance plasmids and bactericidal effect of chlorhexidine on *Enterobacteriaceae. Lett Appl Microbiol.* 1986;3:65-68.

51. Ahonkhai I, Pugh WJ, Russell AD. Sensitivity to antimicrobial agents of some mercury-sensitive and mercury-resistant strains of gram-negative bacteria. *Curr Microbiol.* 1984;11:183-185.

52. Sykes RB, Matthew M. The β-lactamases of gram-negative bacteria and their role in resistance to β-lactam antibiotics. *J Antimicrob Chemother.* 1976;2:115-157.

53. Brumfitt W, Dixson S, Hamilton-Miller JMT. Resistance to antiseptics in methicillin and gentamicin resistant *Staphylococcus aureus. Lancet.* 1985;1:1442-1443.

54. Mycock G. Methicillin/antiseptic-resistant *Staphylococcus aureus. Lancet.* 1985;2:945-950.

55. Haley CE, Marling-Cason M, Smith JW, Luby JP, Mackowiak PA. Bactericidal activity of antiseptics against methicillin-resistant *Staphylococcus aureus. J Clin Microbiol.* 1985;21:991-992.

56. Cookson BD, Bolton M, Platt J. Chlorhexidine resistance in methicillin-resistant *Staphylococcus aureus* or just an elevated MIC? An in vitro and in vivo assessment. Paper presented at: 4th European Congress of Clinical Microbiology; April 17-20, 1989; Nice, France.

57. Rumbak M, Cancio M. Significant decrease in MRSA nosocomial pneumonia following institution of an MRSA prevention protocol. *Crit Care Med.* 1994;22:A90.

58. Jones MR, Martin DR. Outbreak of methicillin-resistant *Staphylococcus aureus* infection in a New Zealand hospital. *N Z Med J.* 1987;100:369-373.

59. Lejeune B, Buzit-Losquin F, Simitzis-Le Flohic AM, Le Bras MP, Alix D. Outbreak of gentamicin-methicillin-resistant *Staphylococcus aureus* infection in an intensive care unit for children. *J Hosp Infect.* 1986;7:21-25.

60. Kampf G, Jarosch R, Rüden H. Limited effectiveness of chlorhexidine based hand disinfectants against methicillin-resistant *Staphylococcus aureus* (MRSA). *J Hosp Infect.* 1998;38:297-303.

61. Weber DJ, Rutala WA, Sickbert-Bennett EE. Outbreaks associated with contaminated antiseptics and disinfectants. *Antimicrob Agents Chemother.* 2007;51:4217-4224.

62. Levy SB. Active efflux, a common mechanism for biocide and antibiotic resistance. *J Appl Microbiol.* 2002;92(suppl):65S-71S.

63. DeMarco CE, Cushing LA, Frempong-Manso E, Seo SM, Jaravaza TA, Kaatz GW. Efflux-related resistance to norfloxacin, dyes, and biocides in bloodstream isolates of *Staphylococcus aureus. Antimicrob Agents Chemother.* 2007;51:3235-3239.

64. Kaulfers PM. Epidemiologie und Ursachen mikrobieller Biozidresistenzen. *Zentralbl Hygiene Umweltmed.* 1995;197:252-259.

65. Horner C, Mawer D, Wilcox M. Reduced susceptibility to chlorhexidine in staphylococci: is it increasing and does it matter? *J Antimicrob Chemother.* 2012;67(11):2547-2559.

66. Morrissey I, Oggioni MR, Knight D, et al; and BIOHYPO Consortium. Evaluation of epidemiological cut-off values indicates that biocide resistant subpopulations are uncommon in natural isolates of clinically-relevant microorganisms. *PLoS One.* 2014;9(1):e86669.

67. Bloomfield SF. Significance of biocide usage and antimicrobial resistance in domiciliary environments. *J Appl Microbiol.* 2002;92(suppl): 144S-157S.

68. Vali L, Dashti AA, Mathew F, Udo EE. Characterization of heterogeneous MRSA and MSSA with reduced susceptibility to chlorhexidine in Kuwaiti hospitals. *Front Microbiol.* 2017;8:1359.

69. Kampf G. Acquired resistance to chlorhexidine: is it time to establish an 'antiseptic stewardship' initiative? *J Antimicrob Chemother.* 2012;67(11):2547-2559.

70. Holloway PM, Bucknall RA, Denton GW. The effects of sub-lethal concentrations of chlorhexidine on bacterial pathogenicity. *J Hosp Infect.* 1986;8:39-46.

71. Rotter ML, Hirschl AM, Koller W. Effect of chlorhexidine-containing detergent, non-medicated soap or isopropanol and the influence of neutralizer on bacterial pathogenicity. *J Hosp Infect.* 1988;11:220-225.

72. Shaker LA, Russell AD, Furr JR. Aspects of the action of chlorhexidine on bacterial spores. *Int J Pharm.* 1986;34:51-56.

73. Nerandzic MM, Donskey CJ. Induced sporicidal activity of chlorhexidine against *Clostridium difficile* spores under altered physical and chemical conditions. *PLoS One.* 2015;10(4):e0123809.

74. Michel C, Salvatico S, Belkhelfa H, Haddioui L, Roques C. Activity of Drill® lozenges on the main microorganisms responsible for upper respiratory tract infections. *Eur Ann Otorhinolaryngol Head Neck Dis.* 2013;130(4):189-193.

75. Bailey A, Longson M. Virucidal activity of chlorhexidine on strains of *Herpesvirus hominis*, poliovirus, and adenovirus. *J Clin Pathol.* 1972;25:76-78.

76. Montefiori DC, Robinson WE Jr, Modliszewski A, Mitchell WM. Effective inactivation of human immunodeficiency virus with chlorhexidine antiseptics containing detergents and alcohol. *J Hosp Infect.* 1990;15:279-282.

77. Harrison C, Chantler E. The effect of nonoxynol-9 and chlorhexidine on HIV and sperm in vitro. *Int J STD AIDS.* 1998;9:92-97.

78. Gaillard P, Mwanyumba F, Verhofstede C, et al. Vaginal lavage with chlorhexidine during labour to reduce mother-to-child HIV transmission: clinical trial in Mombasa, Kenya. *AIDS.* 2001;15(3):389-396.

79. Platt J, Bucknall RA. The disinfection of respiratory syncytial virus by isopropanol and a chlorhexidine-detergent handwash. *J Hosp Infect.* 1985;6:89-94.

80. Shen DT, Crawford TB, Gorham JR, McGuire TC. Inactivation of equine infectious anemia virus by chemical disinfectants. *Am J Vet Res.* 1977;38:1217-1219.

81. Tanabe I, Hotta S. Effect of disinfectants on *Variola virus* in cell culture. *Appl Environ Microbiol.* 1976;32:209-212.

82. Shinkai K. Different sensitivities of type 1 and 2 herpes simplex virus to sodium p-chloromercuribenzoate and chlorhexidine gluconate. *Proc Soc Exp Biol Med.* 1974;147:201-204.

83. Eppley JR, Hayes BM, Kucera CJ. "Nolvasan"—a virucide. *Bio Chem Rev.* 1968;33:9-13.

84. Matisheck P. In vitro activity of chlorhexidine diacetate against pseudorabies virus. *Vet Med Small Anim Clin.* 1978;73:796-799.

85. Faix RG. Comparative efficacy of handwashing agents against Cytomegalovirus. *Infect Control.* 1987;8:158-162.

86. Narang HK, Codd AA. Action of commonly used disinfectants against enteroviruses. *J Hosp Infect.* 1983;4:209-212.

87. Springthorpe VS, Grenier JL, Lloyd-Evans N, Sattar SA. Chemical disinfection of human rotaviruses: efficacy of commercially-available products in suspension tests. *J Hyg (Lond).* 1986;97:139-161.

88. Harbison MA, Hammer SM. Inactivation of human immunodeficiency virus by Betadine products and chlorhexidine. *J Acquir Immune Defic Syndr.* 1989;2:16-20.

89. Fields LB. Oral care intervention to reduce incidence of ventilator-associated pneumonia in the neurologic intensive care unit. *J Neurosci Nurs.* 2008;40(5):291-298.

90. Melsen WG, Rovers MM, Groenwold RH, et al. Attributable mortality of ventilator-associated pneumonia: a meta-analysis of individual patient data from randomised prevention studies. *Lancet Infect Dis.* 2013;13(8):665-671.

91. O'Neal PV, Brown N, Munro C. Physiologic factors contributing to a transition in oral immunity among mechanically ventilated adults. *Biol Res Nurs.* 2002;3(3):132-139.

92. Estes RJ, Meduri GU. The pathogenesis of ventilator-associated pneumonia: I. Mechanisms of bacterial transcolonization and airway inoculation. *Intensive Care Med.* 1995;21(4):365-383.

93. Palmer LB. Ventilator-associated infection. *Curr Opin Pulm Med.* 2009;15(3):230-235.

94. Oshodi TO, Bench S. Ventilator-associated pneumonia, liver disease and oral chlorhexidine. *Br J Nurs.* 2013;22(13):751-758.

95. Tantipong H, Morkchareonpong C, Jaiyindee S, Thamlikitkul V. Randomized controlled trial and meta-analysis of oral decontamination with 2% chlorhexidine solution for the prevention of ventilator-associated pneumonia. *Infect Control Hosp Epidemiol.* 2008;29(2):131-136.

96. Villar CC, Pannuti CM, Nery DM, Morillo CM, Carmona MJ, Romito GA. Effectiveness of intraoral chlorhexidine protocols in the prevention of ventilator-associated pneumonia: meta-analysis and systematic review. *Respir Care.* 2016;61(9):1245-1259.

97. Hua F, Xie H, Worthington HV, Furness S, Zhang Q, Li C. Oral hygiene care for critically ill patients to prevent ventilator-associated pneumonia. *Cochrane Database Syst Rev.* 2016;(10):CD008367.

98. O'Connor AG. Glove puncture during operation. *Nurs Times.* 1984;80(40 suppl):5-6.

99. Smylie HG, Logie JRC, Smith G. From pHisoHex to Hibiscrub. *Br Med J.* 1973;4:586-589.

100. Peterson AF, Rosenberg A, Alatary SD. Comparative evaluation of surgical scrub preparations. *Surg Gynecol Obstet.* 1978;146:63-65.

101. Aly R, Maibach HI. Comparative evaluation of chlorhexidine gluconate (Hibiclens) and povidone-iodine (E-Z Scrub) sponge/brushes for presurgical hand scrubbing. *Curr Ther Res Clin Exp.* 1983;34: 740-745.

102. Lowbury EJL, Lilly HA. The effect of blood on disinfection of surgeon's hands. *Br J Surg.* 1974;61:19-21.

103. Pereira LJ, Lee GM, Wade KJ. An evaluation of five protocols for surgical handwashing in relation to skin condition and microbial counts. *J Hosp Infect.* 1997;36:49-65.

104. Okubo T, Kobayashi H, Ikeda T, et al. Study on short-term surgical scrubs without brushes. Paper presented at: 3rd International Conference of Hospital Infection Society; September 4-8, 1994; London, United Kingdom.

105. Mangram AJ, Horan TC, Pearson ML, Silver LC, Jarvis WR. Guideline for prevention of surgical site infection, 1999. Centers for Disease Control and Prevention (CDC) Hospital Infection Control Practices Advisory Committee. *Am J Infect Control.* 1999;27:97-132.

106. Parienti JJ, Thibon P, Heller R, et al. Hand-rubbing with an aqueous alcoholic solution vs traditional surgical hand-scrubbing and 30-day surgical site infection rates: a randomized equivalence study. *JAMA.* 2002;288:722-727.

107. Tanner J, Dumville JC, Norman G, Fortnam M. Surgical hand antisepsis to reduce surgical site infection. *Cochrane Database Syst Rev.* 2016;(1):CD004288.

108. Olson LK, Morse DJ, Duley C, Savell BK. Prospective, randomized in vivo comparison of a dual-active waterless antiseptic versus two alcohol-only waterless antiseptics for surgical hand antisepsis. *Am J Infect Control.* 2012;40(2):155-159.

109. Meers PD, Yeo FA. Shedding of bacteria and skin squames after handwashing. *J Hyg (Lond).* 1978;81:99-105.

110. Larson EL, Butz AM, Gullette DL, Laughon BA. Alcohol for surgical scrubbing? *Infect Control Hosp Epidemiol.* 1990;11:139-143.

111. Weight CJ, Lee MC, Palmer JS. Avagard hand antisepsis vs. traditional scrub in 3600 pediatric urologic procedures. *Urology.* 2010;76(1):15-17.

112. Mulberrry G, Snyder AT, Heilman J, Pyrek J, Stahl J. Evaluation of a waterless, scrubless chlorhexidine gluconate/ethanol surgical scrub for antimicrobial efficacy. *Am J Infect Control.* 2001;29(6): 377-382.

113. Kaiser EN, Newman JL. Formulation technology as a key component in improving hand hygiene practices. *Am J Infect Control.* 2006;34(10):S82-S97.

114. Larson E, Leyden JJ, McGinley KJ, Grove GL, Talbot GH. Physiologic and microbiologic changes in skin related to frequent handwashing. *Infect Control.* 1986;7:59-63.

115. La Rocca MAK, La Rocca PT, La Rocca R. Comparative study of three handwash preparations for efficacy against experimental bacterial contamination of human skin. *Adv Ther.* 1985;2:269-274.

116. Maki DG, Zilz MA, Alvarado CI. Evaluation of the antibacterial efficacy of four agents for handwashing. *Curr Chemother Infect Dis.* 1979;11:1089-1090.

117. Maki DG, Hecht JA. Comparative study of handwashing with chlorhexidine, povidone-iodine, and non-germicidal soap for prevention of nosocomial infection. *Clin Res.* 1982;30:303A.

118. Stanley G, Sheetz C, Pfaffer M, Wenzel R. The comparative effect of alternative handwashing agents on nosocomial infection rates. Paper presented at: 29th Interscience Conference on Antimicrobial Agents and Chemotherapy; September 17-20, 1989; Houston, TX.

119. Bischoff WE, Reynolds TM, Sessler CT, Edmond MB, Wenzel RP. Handwashing compliance by health care workers: the impact of introducing an accessible, alcohol-based hand antiseptic. *Arch Intern Med.* 2000;160:1017-1021.

120. Maury E, Alzieu M, Baudel JL, et al. Availability of an alcohol solution can improve hand disinfection compliance in an intensive care unit. *Am J Respir Crit Care Med.* 2000;162:324-327.

121. Boyce JM, Pittet D. Guideline for hand hygiene in health-care settings. Recommendations of the Healthcare Infection Control Practices Advisory Committee and the HICPAC/SHEA/APIC/IDSA Hand Hygiene Task Force. Society for Healthcare Epidemiology of America/ Association for Professionals in Infection Control/Infectious Diseases Society of America. *MMWR Recomm Rep.* 2002;51(RR-16):1-45.

122. Pittet D, Hugonnet S, Harbarth S, et al. Effectiveness of a hospital-wide programme to improve compliance with hand hygiene. Infection Control Programme. *Lancet.* 2000;356:1307-1312.

123. Johnson PD, Martin R, Burrell LJ, et al. Efficacy of an alcohol/ chlorhexidine hand hygiene program in a hospital with high rates of nosocomial methicillin-resistant *Staphylococcus aureus* (MRSA) infection. *Med J Aust.* 2005;183(10):509-514.

124. Dumville JC, McFarlane E, Edwards P, Lipp A, Holmes A. Preoperative skin antiseptics for preventing surgical wound infections after clean surgery. *Cochrane Database Syst Rev.* 2013;(3):CD003949.

125. O'Grady NP, Alexander M, Burns LA, et al; and Healthcare Infection Control Practices Advisory Committee. Guidelines for the prevention of intravascular catheter-related infections. *Am J Infect Control.* 2011;39(4)(suppl 1):S1-S34.

126. Larson E. Guideline for use of topical antimicrobial agents. *Am J Infect Control.* 1988;16:253-266.

127. Sistla SC, Prabhu G, Sistla S, Sadasivan J. Minimizing wound contamination in a 'clean' surgery: comparison of chlorhexidine-ethanol and povidone-iodine. *Chemotherapy.* 2010;56:261-267.

128. Berry A, Watt B, Goldacre M, Thomson J, McNair T. A comparison of the use of povidone-iodine and chlorhexidine in the prophylaxis. *J Hosp Infect.* 1982;3(1):55-63.

129. Darouiche RO, Wall MJ Jr, Itani KM, et al. Chlorhexidine-alcohol versus povidone-iodine for surgical-site antisepsis. *N Engl J Med.* 2010;362:18-26.

130. Swenson BR, Hedrick TL, Metzger R, Bonatti H, Pruett TL, Sawyer RG. Effect of preoperative skin preparation on postoperative wound infection rates: a prospective study of 3 skin prepping protocols. *Infect Control Hosp Epidemiol.* 2009;30:964-971.

131. Edmiston CE Jr, Bruden B, Rucinski MC, Henen C, Graham MB, Lewis BL. Reducing the risk of surgical site infections: does chlorhexidine gluconate provide a risk reduction benefit? *Am J Infect Control.* 2013;41(suppl 5):S49-S55.

132. Brandberg A, Anderson I. Whole-body disinfection by shower-bath with chlorhexidine soap. In: Newson SWB, Caldwell ADS, eds. *Problems in the Control of Hospital Infection.* London, United Kingdom: Royal Society of Medicine/Academic Press; 1980:65-70.

133. Kaiser AB, Kernodle DE, Barg NLB, Petracek MR. Influence of preoperative showers on staphylococcal skin colonization: a comparative trial of antiseptic skin cleansers. *Ann Thorac Surg.* 1988;45:35-38.

134. Brandberg A, Holm J, Hammarsten J, et al. Postoperative wound disinfection by shower bath with chlorhexidine soap. In: Newsom SWB, Caldwell ADS, eds. *Problems in the Control of Hospital Infection.* London, United Kingdom: Royal Society of Medicine/Academic Press; 1980:71-75.

135. Hayek LJ, Emerson JM, Gardner AMN. Clinical trial of "Hibiscrub" whole-body disinfection in elective surgery. *J Hosp Infect.* 1987;10: 165-172.

136. Hayek LJ, Emerson JM. Preoperative whole body disinfection— a controlled study. *J Hosp Infect.* 1988;11(suppl B):15-19.

137. Randall PE, Ganguli L, Marcuson RW. Wound infection following vasectomy ("Hibiscrub"). *Br J Urol.* 1983;55:564-567.

138. Randall PE, Ganguli LA, Keaney MG, Marcuson RW. Prevention of wound infection following vasectomy (chlorhexidine gluconate). *Br J Urol.* 1985;57:227-229.

139. Brandberg A. Preoperative whole body disinfection (viewpoint Sweden). *J Chemother.* 1989;1(suppl 1):19-24.

140. Webster J, Osborne S. Preoperative bathing or showering with skin antiseptics to prevent surgical site infection. *Cochrane Database Syst Rev.* 2007;(2):CD004985.

141. Webster J, Osborne S. Preoperative bathing or showering with skin antiseptics to prevent surgical site infection. *Cochrane Database Syst Rev.* 2015;(2): CD004985.

142. Institute for Healthcare Improvement. *How-to Guide: Prevent Surgical Site Infection for Hip and Knee Arthroplasty.* Cambridge, MA: Institute for Healthcare Improvement; 2012.

143. REDUCE MRSA Trial Working Group. *Universal ICU Decolonization: An Enhanced Protocol.* Rockville, MD: Agency for Healthcare Research and Quality; 2013. AHRQ publication no. 13-0052-EF.

144. Edmiston CE Jr, Krepel CJ, Seabrook GR, Lewis BD, Brown KR, Towne JB. Preoperative shower revisited: can high topical antiseptic levels be achieved on the skin surface before surgical admission? *J Am Coll Surg.* 2008;207(2):233-239.

145. Mermel LA. What is the predominant source of intravascular catheter infections? *Clin Infect Dis.* 2011;52:211-212.

146. O'Grady NP, Alexander M, Burns LA, et al. Summary of recommendations: guidelines for the prevention of intravascular catheter-related infections. *Clin Infect Dis.* 2011;52(9):1087-1099.

147. Chaiyakunapruk N, Veenstra DL, Lipsky BA, Saint S. Chlorhexidine compared with povidone-iodine solution for vascular catheter-site care: a meta-analysis. *Ann Intern Med.* 2002;136(11):792-801.

148. Timsit JF, Schwebel C, Bouadma L, et al. Chlorhexidine-impregnated sponges and less frequent dressing changes for prevention of catheter-related infections in critically ill adults: a randomized controlled trial. *JAMA.* 2009;301(12):1231-1241.

149. Jeanes A, Bitmead J. Reducing bloodstream infection with a chlorhexidine gel IV dressing. *Br J Nurs.* 2015;24(suppl 19):S14-S19.

150. Timsit JF, Mimoz O, Mourvillier B, et al. Randomized controlled trial of chlorhexidine dressing and highly adhesive dressing for preventing catheter-related infections in critically ill adults. *Am J Respir Crit Care Med.* 2012;186(12):1272-1278.

151. Pfaff B, Heithaus T, Emanuelsen M. Use of a 1-piece chlorhexidine gluconate transparent dressing on critically ill patients. *Crit Care Nurs.* 2012;32(4):35-40.

152. Ramritu P, Halton K, Collignon P, et al. A systematic review comparing the relative effectiveness of antimicrobial-coated catheters in intensive care units. *Am J Infect Control.* 2008;36:104-117.

153. Brun-Buisson C, Doyon F, Sollet J-P, Cochard J-F, Cohen Y, Nitenberg G. Prevention of intravascular catheter-related infection with newer chlorhexidine-silver sulfadiazine-coated catheters: a randomized controlled trial. *Intensive Care Med.* 2004;30:837-843.

154. Miller A, Gillespie WA, Linton KB, Slade N, Mitchell JP. Prevention of urinary tract infection after prostatectomy. *Lancet.* 1960;2:886-888.

155. Gillespie WA. Progress in the control of hospital cross-infection. *Public Health.* 1962;77:44-52.

156. Ball AJ, Carr TW, Gillespie WA, Kelly M, Simpson RA, Smith P. Bladder irrigation with chlorhexidine for the prevention of urinary infection after transurethral operations: a prospective controlled study. *J Urol.* 1987;138:491-494.

157. Kirk D, Dunn M, Bullock DW, Mitchell JP, Hobbs SJ. Hibitane bladder irrigation in the prevention of catheter-associated urinary infection. *Br J Urol.* 1979;51:528-531.

158. Bruun JN, Digranes A. Bladder irrigation in patients with indwelling catheters. *Scand J Infect Dis.* 1978;10:71-74.

159. Calman RM, Murray J. Antiseptics in midwifery. *Br Med J.* 1956;2:200-204.

160. Byatt ME, Henderson A. Pre-operative sterilization of the perineum: a comparison of six antiseptics. *J Clin Pathol.* 1973;26:921-924.

161. Christensen KK, Christensen P, Dykes AK, Kahlmeter G. Chlorhexidine for prevention of neonatal colonization with group B streptococci. III. Effect of vaginal washing with chlorhexidine before rupture of the membranes. *Eur J Obstet Gynecol Reprod Biol.* 1985;19:231-236.

162. Taha TE, Biggar RJ, Broadhead RL, et al. Effect of cleansing the birth canal with antiseptic solution on maternal and newborn morbidity and mortality in Malawi: clinical trial. *BMJ.* 1997;315:216-219.

163. Levin I, Amer-Alshiek J, Avni A, Lessing JB, Satel A, Almog B. Chlorhexidine and alcohol versus povidone-iodine for antisepsis in gynecological surgery. *J Womens Health.* 2011;20:321-324.

164. Culligan PJ, Kubik K, Murphy M, Blackwell L, Snyder J. A randomized trial that compared povidone iodine and chlorhexidine as antiseptics for vaginal hysterectomy. *Am J Obstet Gynecol.* 2005;192:422-425.

165. Imdad A, Bautista RM, Senen KA, Uy ME, Mantaring JB III, Bhutta ZA. Umbilical cord antiseptics for preventing sepsis and death among newborns. *Cochrane Database Syst Rev.* 2013;(5):CD008635.

166. Platt J, Bucknall RA. An experimental evaluation of antiseptic wound irrigation. *J Hosp Infect.* 1984;5:181-188.

167. Colombo AA, Perrotti F, Boriolo P, et al. Chlorhexidine in the prophylaxis of surgical wound infections. *Minerva Chir.* 1987;42:1999-2002.

168. Carrier-Clerambault R, Praud Y, Bruno G. Traitement des infections chirurgicales et urologiques par la chlorhexidine. *Mediterrannee Medicale.* 1978;164:61-63.

169. Gerard Y, Thirion Y, Schernberg F, et al. Utilisation de la chlorhexidine dans le traitement des infections osseuses et articulaires. *Ann Med Nancy.* 1979;18:1385-1389.

170. Wound Healing and Management Node Group. Evidence summary: wound management—chlorhexidine. *Wound Prac Res.* 2017;25(1):49-51.

171. Best A, Nixon M, Taylor G. Brief exposure of 0.05% chlorhexidine does not impair non-osteoarthritic human cartilage metabolism. *J Hosp Infect.* 2007;67:67-71.

172. Drosou A, Falabella A, Kirsner RS. Antiseptics on wounds: an area of controversy. *Wounds.* 2003;15(5):149-166.

173. Collier F, de Laet MH, Deconinck PG. Anti-infection prophylaxis of infantile burns. *Acta Chir Belg.* 1978;77:365-369.

174. Jouglard JP, Manelli JC, Palayret D. La place de la balneotherapie dans le traitement des grands brules. *Mediterranee Med.* 1979;192:75-77.

175. Gjermo P, Bonesvoll P, Rolla G. Relationship between plaque inhibiting effect and retention of chlorhexidine in the human oral cavity. *Arch Oral Biol.* 1974;19:1031-1034.

176. Bonesvoll P. Oral pharmacology of chlorhexidine. *J Clin Periodontol.* 1977;4(5):49-65.

177. Cancro LP, Paulovich DB, Bolton S, Picozzi A. Dose response of chlorhexidine gluconate in a model in vivo plaque system. *J Dent Res.* 1974;53:765.

178. Agerbaek N, Melsen B, Rölla G. Application of chlorhexidine by oral irrigation systems. *Scand J Dent Res.* 1975;83:284-287.

179. Puig Silla M, Montiel Company JM, Almerich Silla JM. Use of chlorhexidine varnishes in preventing and treating periodontal disease. A review of the literature. *Med Oral Patol Oral Cir Bucal.* 2008;13(4):E257-E260.

180. Addy M. Chlorhexidine compared with other locally delivered antimicrobials: a short review. *J Clin Periodontol.* 1986;13:957-964.

181. Kornman KS. The role of supragingival plaque in the prevention and treatment of periodontal diseases: a review of current concepts. *J Periodontal Res.* 1986;21(suppl):5-22.

182. Hunter L, Addy M. Chlorhexidine gluconate mouthwash in the management of minor aphthous ulceration: a double-blind, placebo controlled cross-over trial. *Br Dent J.* 1987;162:106-110.

183. Addy M, Carpenter R, Roberts WR. Management of recurrent aphthous ulceration: a trial of chlorhexidine gluconate gel. *Br Dent J.* 1976;141:118-120.

184. James P, Worthington HV, Parnell C, et al. Chlorhexidine mouthrinse as an adjunctive treatment for gingival health. *Cochrane Database Syst Rev.* 2017;(3):CD008676.

185. Martin MV, Nind D. Use of chlorhexidine gluconate for pre-operative disinfection of apicectomy sites. *Br Dent J.* 1987;162:459-461.

186. Field EA, Nind D, Varga E, Martin MV. The effect of chlorhexidine irrigation on the incidence of dry socket: a pilot study. *Br J Oral Maxillofac Surg.* 1988;26:395-401.

187. Barbosa M, Prada-López I, Álvarez M, Amaral B, de los Angeles CD, Tomás I. Post-tooth extraction bacteraemia: a randomized clinical trial on the efficacy of chlorhexidine prophylaxis. *PLoS One.* 2015;10(5):e0124249.

188. Langebaek J, Bay L. The effect of chlorhexidine mouthrinse on healing after gingivectomy. *Scand J Dent Res.* 1976;84:224-228.

189. Bakaeen GS, Strahan JD. Effects of a 1% chlorhexidine gel during the healing phase after inverse level mucogingival flap surgery. *J Clin Periodontol.* 1980;7:20-25.

190. Francis JR, Addy M, Hunter B. A comparison of three delivery methods of chlorhexidine in handicapped children. 1: effects on plaque, gingivitis and tooth staining. *J Periodontol.* 1987;58:451-455.

191. Usher PJ. Oral hygiene in mentally handicapped children. A pilot study of the use of chlorhexidine gel. *Br Dent J.* 1975;138:217-221.

192. Ferretti GA, Hansen IA, Whittenburg K, Brown AT, Lillich TT, Ash RC. Therapeutic use of chlorhexidine in bone marrow transplant patients: case studies. *Oral Surg Oral Med Oral Pathol.* 1987;63:683-687.

193. Jacobsen S, Brynhni I-L, Gjermo P. Oral candidosis-frequency, treatment and relapse tendency in a group of psychiatric inpatients. *Acta Odontol Scand.* 1979;37:353-361.

194. Ellepola AN, Samaranayake LP. Adjunctive use of chlorhexidine in oral candidoses: a review. *Oral Dis.* 2001;7:11-17.

195. Olsen I. Denture stomatitis. The clinical effects of chlorhexidine and amphotericin B. *Acta Odontolog Scand.* 1975;33:47-52.

196. Budtz-Jorgensen E. Hibitane in the treatment of oral candidiasis. *J Clin Periodontol.* 1977;4:117-128.

197. McCourtie J, MacFarlane TW, Samaranayake LP. A comparison of the effects of chlorhexidine gluconate, amphotericin B, and nystatin on the adherence of *Candida* species to denture acrylic. *J Antimicrob Chemother.* 1986;17:575-583.

198. Zickert I, Emilson CG, Krasse B. Effect of caries preventative measures in children highly infected with the bacterium *Streptococcus mutans. Arch Oral Biol.* 1982;27:861-868.

199. Luoma H, Murtomaa H, Nuuja T, et al. A simultaneous reduction of caries and gingivitis in a group of school children receiving chlorhexidine-fluoride applications: results after 2 years. *Caries Res.* 1978;12:290-298.

200. Katz S. The use of fluoride and chlorhexidine for the prevention of radiation caries. *J Am Dent Assoc.* 1982;104:164-170.

201. Featherstone JDB, White JM, Hoover CI, et al. A randomized clinical trial of anticaries therapies targeted according to risk assessment (caries management by risk assessment). *Caries Res.* 2012;46(2):118-129.

202. Addy M, Moran J, Griffiths AA, Wills-Wood NJ. Extrinsic tooth discoloration by metals and chlorhexidine. I. Surface protein denaturation or dietary precipitation? *Br Dent J.* 1985;159:281-285.

203. Prayitno S, Addy M. An in vitro study of factors affecting the development of staining associated with the use of chlorhexidine. *J Periodontol Res.* 1979;14:397-402.

204. Storhaug R. Hibitane in oral disease in handicapped patients. *J Clin Periodontol.* 1977;4:102-107.

205. Lai P, Coulson C, Pothier DD, Rutka J. Chlorhexidine ototoxicity in ear surgery, part 1: review of the literature. *J Otolaryngol Head Neck Surg.* 2011;40(6):437-440.

206. Registry of Toxic Effects of Chemical Substances number DU1950000. Canadian Centre for Occupational Health and Safety Web site. http://ccinfoweb2.ccohs.ca/rtecs/records/DU1950000.html. Accessed May 21, 2019.

207. Willis L. Final report on the safety assessment of chlorhexidine/chlorhexidine diacetate/chlorhexidine dihydrochloride/chlorhexidine digluconate. *J Am Coll Toxicol.* 1993;12:201-223.

208. Butler WH, Iswaran TJ. Chlorhexidine: safety evaluation in problems in the control of hospital infection. *Roy Soc Med Intl Congr Symp.* 1980;23:45-48.

209. Case DE. Safety of Hibitane. I. Laboratory experiments. *J Clin Periodontol.* 1977;4:66-72.

210. Sakagami Y, Yamazaki H, Ogasawara N, Yokeyama H, Ose Y, Sato T. The evaluation of disinfectants and their metabolites by umu test. *Mutat Res.* 1988;209(3-4):155-160.

211. Sakagami Y, Yamazaki H, Ogasawara N, Yokeyama H, Ose Y, Sato T. DNA repair test of disinfectants by liquid rec-assay. *Mutat Res.* 1988;193:21-30.

212. Ackermann-Schmidt B, Suessmuth R, Lingens F. Effects of 1,1′-hexamethylene-bis [(5-*p*-chlorophenyl)-biguanide] on the genome and on the synthesis of nucleic acids and proteins in the bacterial cells. *Chem Biol Interact.* 1982;40:85-96.

213. Withrow TJ, Brown NT, Hitchins VM, Strickland AG. Cytotoxicity and mutagenicity of ophthalmic solution preservatives and UVA radiation in L5178Y cells. *Photochem Photobiol.* 1989;50:385-389.

214. Ribeiro DA, Bazo AP, da Silva Franchi CA, Marques ME, Salvadori DM. Chlorhexidine induces DNA damage in rat peripheral leukocytes and oral mucosal cells. *J Periodontal Res.* 2004;39(5):358-361.

215. Case DE. Chlorhexidine. Attempts to detect percutaneous absorption in man. In: Newsom SWB, Caldwell ADS, eds. *Problems in the Control of Hospital Infection.* London, United Kingdom: Royal Society of Medicine/Academic Press; 1980:39-43.

216. Blumer JL, Husak MP, Wiltshire J, Fanaroff AA, Speck WT. Antibacterial efficacy and safety of neonatal bathing with Hibiclens. *Pediatr Res.* 1982;16(4 II):148A.

217. Cowen J, Ellis SH, McAinsh J. Absorption of chlorhexidine from the intact skin of newborn infants. *Arch Dis Child.* 1979;54:378-383.

218. Gongwer LE, Hubben K, Lenkiewicz RS, Hart ER, Cockrell BY. The effects of daily bathing of neonatal rhesus monkeys with an antimicrobial skin cleanser containing chlorhexidine gluconate. *Toxicol Appl Pharmacol.* 1980;52:255-261.

219. Karpanen TJ, Worthington T, Conway BR, Hilton AC, Elliott TSJ, Lambert PA. Permeation of chlorhexidine from alcoholic and aqueous solutions within excised human skin. *Antimicrob Agents Chemother.* 2009;53(4):1717-1719.

220. Organisation for Economic Co-operation and Development. *Test No. 405: Acute Eye Irritation/Corrosion.* Paris, France: OECD Publishing; 2017.

221. Ljunggren B, Möller H. Eczematous contact allergy to chlorhexidine. *Acta Derm Venereol.* 1972;52:308-310.

222. Lauerma AI. Simultaneous immediate and delayed hypersensitivity to chlorhexidine digluconate. *Contact Dermatitis.* 2001;44:59.

223. Stephens R, Mythen M, Kallis P, Davies DWL, Egner W, Rickards A. Two episodes of life-threatening anaphylaxis in the same patient to a chlorhexidine-sulphadiazine-coated central venous catheter. *Br J Anaesth.* 2001;87(2):306-308.

224. Ebo DG, Bridts CH, Stevens WJ. IgE-mediated anaphylaxis from chlorhexidine: diagnostic possibilities. *Contact Dermatitis.* 2006;55:301-302.

225. Calogiuri GF, Di Leo E, Trautmann A, Nettis E, Ferrannini A, Vacca A. Chlorhexidine hypersensitivity: a critical and updated review. *J Allergy Ther.* 2013;14:141.

226. Opstrup MS, Johansen JD, Zachariae C, Garvey LH. Contact allergy to chlorhexidine in a tertiary dermatology clinic in Denmark. *Contact Dermatitis.* 2016;74(1):29-36.

227. Saatmann RA, Carlton WW, Hubben K, Streett CS, Tuckosh JR, DeBaecke PJ. A wound healing study of chlorhexidine digluconate in guinea pigs. *Fundam Appl Toxicol.* 1986;6:1-6.

228. Hirst RC, Egelberg J, Hornbuckle GC, Oliver RC, Rathbun WE. Microscopic evaluation of topically applied chlorhexidine gluconate on gingival wound healing in dogs. *J South Calif Dent Assoc.* 1973;41(4):311-317.

229. Main R. Should chlorhexidine gluconate be used in wound cleansing? *J Wound Care.* 2008;17(3):112-114.

230. Hidalgo E, Dominguez C. Mechanisms underlying chlorhexidine-induced cytotoxicity. *Toxicol In Vitro.* 2001;15:271-276.

231. Thomas G, Rael L, Bar-Or R, et al. Mechanisms of delayed wound healing by commonly used antiseptics. *J Trauma.* 2009;66(1):82-90.

232. Sanchez I, Swaim SF, Nusbaum KE, Hale AS, Henderson RA, McGuire JA. Effects of chlorhexidine-diacetate and povidone-iodine on wound healing in dogs. *Vet Surg*. 1988;17:291-295.

233. Fumal I, Braham C, Paquet P, Pierard-Franchimont C, Pierard G. The beneficial toxicity paradox of antimicrobials in leg ulcer healing impaired by a polymicrobial flora; a proof-of-concept study. *Dermatology*. 2002;204:70-74.

234. Bicknell PG. Sensorineural deafness following myringoplasty operations. *J Laryngol Otol*. 1971;85:957-961.

235. Morizono T, Johnstone BM, Hadjar E. The ototoxicity of antiseptics (preliminary report). *J Otolaryngol Soc Aust*. 1973;3:550-553.

236. Igarashi Y, Suzuki JI. Cochlear ototoxicity of chlorhexidine gluconate in cats. *Arch Otorhinolaryngol*. 1985;242:167-176.

237. Willoughby K. Chlorhexidine and ototoxicity in cats. *Vet Rec*. 1989;124(20):547.

238. Morizono T, Johnstone BM, Entjep H. Sensorineural deafness caused by preoperative antiseptics. *Otologia Fukuoka*. 1974;20:97-99.

239. Perez R, Freeman S, Sohmer H, Sichel JY. Vestibular and cochlear ototoxicity of topical antiseptics assessed by evoked potentials. *Laryngoscope*. 2000;110:1522-1527.

240. Weston-Hurst E. Adhesive arachnoiditis and vascular blockage caused by detergents and other chemical irritants: an experimental study. *J Pathol Bacteriol*. 1955;38:167-178.

241. Henschen A, Olson L. Chlorhexidine-induced degeneration of adrenergic nerves. *Acta Neuropathol*. 1984;63:18-23.

242. Doan L, Piskoun B, Rosenberg AD, Blanck TJJ, Phillips MS, Xu F. In vitro antiseptic effects on viability of neuronal and Schwann cells. *Reg Anesth Pain Med*. 2012;37:131-138.

243. Patle V. Arachnoiditis: alcohol or chlorhexidine? *Anaesthesia*. 2013; 68:425.

244. Green K, Livingston V, Bowman K, Hull DS. Chlorhexidine effects on corneal epithelium and endothelium. *Arch Ophthalmol*. 1980;98: 1273-1278.

245. Mac Rae SM, Brown B, Edelhauser HF. The corneal toxicity of presurgical skin antiseptics. *Am J Ophthalmol*. 1984;97:221-232.

246. Varley GA, Meisler DM, Benes SC, McMahon JT, Zakov ZN, Fryczkowski A. Hibiclens keratopathy. A clinicopathologic case report. *Cornea*. 1990;9(4):341-346.

247. Klebe S, Anders N, Wollensak J. Inadvertent use of chlorhexidine as intraocular irrigation solution. *J Cataract Refract Surg*. 1998;24(6): 729-730.

248. Murthy S, Hawksworth NR, Cree I. Progressive ulcerative keratitis related to the use of topical chlorhexidine gluconate (0.02%). *Cornea*. 2002;21(2):237-239.

249. Hamed LM, Ellis FD, Boudreault G, Wilson FM II, Helveston EM. Hibiclens keratitis. *Am J Ophthalmol*. 1987;104:50-56.

250. Phinney RB, Mondino BJ, Hofbauer JD, et al. Corneal edema related to accidental Hibiclens exposure. *Am J Ophthalmol*. 1988;106:210-215.

251. van Rij G, Beekhuis WH, Eggink CA, Geerards AJ, Remeijer L, Pels EL. Toxic keratopathy due to the accidental use of chlorhexidine, cetrimide and cialit. *Doc Ophthalmol*. 1995;90(1):7-14.

252. Liu HY, Yeh PT, Kuo KT, Huang JY, Lin CP, Hou YC. Toxic keratopathy following the use of alcohol-containing antiseptics in nonocular surgery. *JAMA Ophthalmol*. 2016;134:449.

253. Bever GJ, Brodie FL, Hwang DG. Corneal injury from presurgical chlorhexidine skin preparation. *World Neurosurg*. 2016;96:610.e1-610.e4.

254. Spielmann H, Balls M, Dupuis J, et al. The international EU/COLIPA in vitro phototoxicity validation study: results of phase II (blind trial), part 1: the 3T3 NRU phototoxicity test. *Toxicology In Vitro*. 1998;12:305-327.

255. Spielmann H, Lovell WW, Holzle E, et al. In vitro phototoxicity testing. The report and recommendations of ECVAM workshop 2. *ATLA*. 1994;22:314-348.

256. Harvey BV, Squier CA, Hall BK. Effects of chlorhexidine on the structure and permeability of hamster cheek pouch mucosa. *J Periodontol*. 1984;55:608-614.

257. Sonis ST, Clark WB, Shklar G. Chlorhexidine-induced lingual keratosis and dysplasia in rats. *J Periodontol*. 1978;49:585-591.

258. Okano M, Nomura M, Hata S, et al. Anaphylactic symptoms due to chlorhexidine gluconate. *Arch Dermatol*. 1989;125(1):50-52.

259. Knudsen BB, Avnstorp C. Chlorhexidine gluconate and acetate in patch testing. *Contact Dermatitis*. 1991;24(1):45-49.

260. Porter BJ, Acharya U, Ormerod AD, Herriot R. Latex/chlorhexidine-induced anaphylaxis in pregnancy. *Allergy*. 1998;53(4):455-457.

261. Anderson MJ, Horn ME, Lin YC, Parks PJ, Peterson ML. Efficacy of concurrent application of chlorhexidine gluconate and povidone iodine against six nosocomial pathogens. *Am J Infect Control*. 2010;38:826-831.

262. Guzel A, Ozekinci T, Ozkan U, Celik Y, Ceviz A, Belen D. Evaluation of the skin flora after chlorhexidine and povidone-iodine preparation in neurosurgical practice. *Surg Neurol*. 2009;71:207-210.

263. Langgartner J, Linde HJ, Lehn N, Reng M, Scholmerich J, Gluck T. Combined skin disinfection with chlorhexidine/propanol and aqueous povidone-iodine reduces bacterial colonization of central venous catheters. *Intensive Care Med*. 2004;30:1081-1088.

264. Davies BM, Patel HC. Systematic review and meta-analysis of preoperative antisepsis with combination chlorhexidine and povidone-iodine. *Surg J*. 2016;2:e70-e77.

265. Casey AL, Karpanen TJ, Nightingale P, Conway BR, Elliott TS. Antimicrobial activity and skin permeation of iodine present in an iodine-impregnated surgical incise drape. *J Antimicrob Chemother*. 2015;70(8):2255-2260.

Aldehydes

Stephen A. Kelly, Sean P. Gorman, and Brendan F. Gilmore

Aldehydes (from the Latin *alcohol dehydrogenatum*, alcohol deprived of hydrogen) are compounds containing the functional group—CHO formed as a result of oxidation of primary alcohols, where the carbonyl group is bonded to at least one hydrogen atom. The general formula for an aldehyde and the structures of the aldehyde microbicides in widespread use are shown in Figure 23.1. Currently, only three aldehyde compounds are of widespread practical use as disinfectant biocides, namely glutaraldehyde, formaldehyde, and ortho-phthalaldehyde (OPA) despite the demonstration that many other aldehydes possess good antimicrobial activity. Glutaraldehyde is one of the most commonly used biocides worldwide across a diverse range of applications, and as such is considered the archetypal compound in this biocide class and is the primary focus of this chapter. Other aldehyde biocides such as acrolein (2-propenal, acrylaldehyde) whose applications are primarily as a biocide in agriculture and industrial water supply systems (and considered a high priority air and water toxicant by the US Environmental Protection Agency [EPA]) are not considered further in this chapter.

Glutaraldehyde (pentanedial; see Figure 23.1) possesses high microbicidal activity against both bacteria and bacterial spores, fungi and their spores, and viruses. Additionally, glutaraldehyde is an effective mycobactericidal agent. Glutaraldehyde is a highly reactive saturated five-carbon dialdehyde, which interacts strongly with the bacterial cell wall, although mode of action is most likely due to interaction with proteins and enzymes (which increases with increased pH). The rate of antimicrobial activity of glutaraldehyde is pH dependent, with glutaraldehyde usually commercially obtained as an acidic solution (2%, 25%, or 50%) with 2% solutions used for disinfectant applications. Before use, the glutaraldehyde solution is "activated" (made alkaline) before use, although stable formulations that do not require activation are also available. Glutaraldehyde has a broad spectrum of activity, with rapid microbicidal action and is noncorrosive to rubber, metals, and lenses; however, its toxicity is a matter for some concern, with its use restricted or banned in some countries.

Formaldehyde (methanal; see Figure 23.1), as well as formaldehyde release agents, can be used as a preservative, as a disinfectant either in liquid or vapor form, although use is primarily as a sterilant or fumigant in the vapor phase. The UK Health and Safety Executive has indicated that inhalation of formaldehyde vapor should be presumed to be a carcinogenic risk to humans. Formaldehyde has a broad spectrum of antimicrobial activity, exhibiting lethality to bacteria and bacterial spores (although the sporicidal activity of glutaraldehyde is more rapid), fungi, and many viruses. Formaldehyde rapidly combines with proteins, and as a result, its activity may be significantly and rapidly diminished in the presence of organic matter.

The OPA (benzene-1,2-dicarboxaldehyde; see Figure 23.1), an aromatic dialdehyde biocide, is the most recently introduced aldehyde biocide in widespread use, having received clearance by the US Food and Drug Administration (FDA) in October 1999. The OPA is a high-level disinfectant with excellent, broad-spectrum antimicrobial activity including superior mycobacterial activity compared with glutaraldehyde. Due to concerns over glutaraldehyde toxicity and resistance development, OPA (0.55%) has been proposed as a glutaraldehyde replacement in high-level disinfection (a disinfection process, which kills all microorganisms except bacterial spores; see chapter 47). The OPA has numerous advantages over glutaraldehyde including low volatility and high stability over a wide pH range (pH 3-9), being virtually odorless, has good material compatibility, and is nonirritant to eyes and nasal passages. Furthermore, OPA does not require activation prior to use and glutaraldehyde-resistant bacterial strains appear not to have acquired cross-resistance. The OPA, from the studies reported to date, has excellent activity against vegetative bacteria, superior to that of glutaraldehyde, but lower activity against bacterial spores.

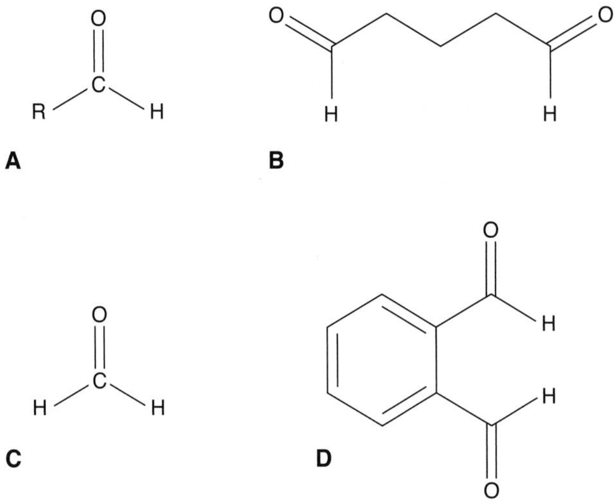

FIGURE 23.1 Chemical structures of aldehyde biocides: A, Aldehyde general structure. B, Glutaraldehyde. C, Formaldehyde. D, Ortho-phthalaldehyde.

▶ GLUTARALDEHYDE

Glutaraldehyde is a powerful biocidal agent with established reputation for the chemosterilization of equipment that cannot be sterilized by traditional physical or gaseous chemical methods (see Part IV). The first indications of its antimicrobial potential came from a survey of saturated dialdehydes in a search for an efficient substitute for formaldehyde.[1] In the following year, Stonehill et al[2] advocated that a suitably alkalinated solution of glutaraldehyde was rapidly sporicidal, and toward the end of 1963, a glutaraldehyde formulation was marketed for use as a chemosterilizer. The continuing interest in the compound is reflected in the numerous publications, even in recent years, on such basic aspects as its activity and mechanism of action. Emphasis is currently being applied to the toxicology of glutaraldehyde exposure, whereas much attention continues to be focused on increasing the range of applications and improvements in the activity of the compound.

Chemical Properties

Structure

Glutaraldehyde (1,5-pentanedial) appears in the official monographs of the United States Pharmacopeia and British Pharmacopoeia as glutaral concentrate and strong glutaraldehyde solution, respectively. Other synonyms used are glutaric dialdehyde and glutardialdehyde. It is usually supplied as an amber-colored liquid at an acidic pH. The saturated 5-carbon dialdehyde was first synthetized in 1908.[3] As with other aldehydes, the two aldehyde groups react

readily under suitable conditions, particularly with proteins.[4,5] A single absorption maximum at 280 nm is exhibited by pure glutaraldehyde, although a second maximum at 235 nm is normally observed in commercial solutions because of the presence of impurities of polymers.[6,7] The impurity may be removed by several methods.[6,8-11] Appearance of the 235-nm absorbing polymer in pure solutions depends on storage temperature,[12,13] and the rate of the polymerization depends on temperature and pH.[14,15]

The ratio of monomer to polymer and type of polymer present have been the subjects of numerous publications.[16] Essentially, it is considered that the presence of free aldehyde groups is a prerequisite for good biocidal activity. Schemes depicting glutaraldehyde polymerization in both acid and alkaline aqueous solution are outlined in Figures 23.2 and 23.3.[17] At acid pH, glutaraldehyde is in equilibrium with its cyclic hemiacetal and polymers of the cyclic hemiacetal, as proposed by Hardy et al.[7,18] Increase in temperature produces more free aldehyde in acid solution, whereas in alkaline solution loss of reactive aldehyde groups is possible. When pH is raised to the neutral or basic range, the dialdehyde undergoes an aldol condensation with itself followed by dehydration

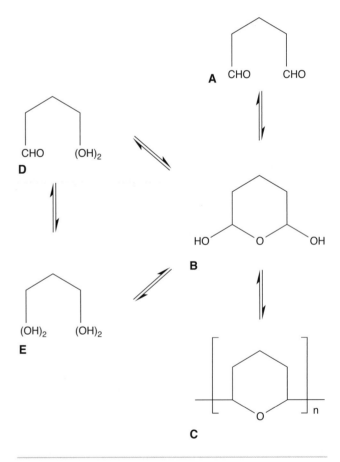

FIGURE 23.2 Glutaraldehyde polymerization in aqueous acid media. A, Monomer. B, Cyclic hemiacetal. C, Acetal-like polymer. D, Monohydrate. E, Dihydrate.

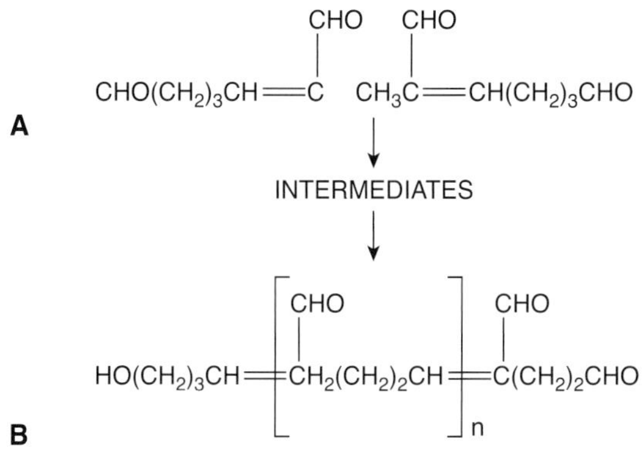

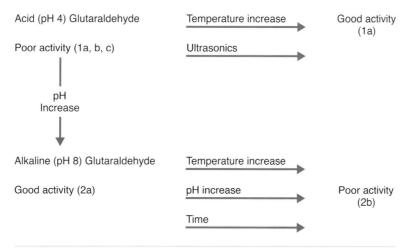

A

CHO(CH₂)₃CH═C   CH₃C═CH(CH₂)₃CHO

CHO   CHO

↓

INTERMEDIATES

↓

B

HO(CH₂)₃CH═CH₂(CH₂)₂CH═C(CH₂)₂CHO

CHO   CHO

FIGURE 23.3 Glutaraldehyde polymerization in aqueous alkaline media. Aldol-type polymer (A) progresses to a higher polymeric form (B) with time and increase pH.

to generate α,β-unsaturated aldehyde polymers. Progression to the higher polymeric form can also occur with increased time and pH. As the pH is raised, n increases (see Figure 23.3) in value until the polymer precipitates from solution. Loss of reactive aldehyde groups could therefore be responsible for the rapid loss of biocidal activity of alkaline solutions on storage. A study into the structure of the solid aldol condensation product showed that polymerization of glutaraldehyde under basic conditions results in the formation of water-soluble and water-insoluble polymers and that these polymers contain unconjugated aldehyde, conjugated aldehyde, hydroxyl, and carboxyl groups.[19] A number of other studies investigated the several products formed in the aldol condensation of glutaraldehyde and concluded that these new oligomers were glutaraldehyde trimer, pentamer, and heptamer having a 1,3,5-trioxane skeleton.[20-24] The glutaraldehyde trimer,

2,4,6-tris(4-oxobutyl)-1,3,5-trioxane, was named "paraglutaraldehyde," and this was proposed as being responsible for the precipitation observed occasionally during chemosterilization with alkaline glutaraldehyde.

Increased activity in acid solution through application of heat or ultrasonics[25] can be explained by displacement of equilibrium toward the monomer (see Figure 23.2). A scheme relating these various factors to biocidal activity is described in Figure 23.4.

Analysis

Various methods have been used to determine glutaraldehyde concentration. Measurement of the complex absorbances resulting from glutaraldehyde reaction with 2,4-dinitrophenylhydrazine[26] or 3-methyl-2-benzothiazolone hydrazone[27] were early reported methods. A relationship between concentration and osmolality of glutaraldehyde solutions has also been employed.[9,28] A number of methods involving measurement of the 235-nm and 280-nm absorption maxima have also been reported. The purification index (PI), defined as A_{235}/A_{280}, where A_{280} is the ultraviolet (UV) absorbance of monomeric glutaraldehyde at its λ_{max} 280 nm, and A_{235} is that of polymeric glutaraldehyde at its λ_{max} 235 nm, has been widely employed to grade glutaraldehyde products. Lower PI values represent higher purity. But care must be taken in the application of this index.[21,22] A commercial glutaraldehyde product was discovered to contain an impurity that exhibits absorption at 280 nm but not at 235 nm, indicating the unreliability of the PI value. Others used a 235-nm absorbance to concentration relationship.[29]

A 280-nm absorbance maximum was also reported,[6,13] although it was suggested that for routine laboratory use, a chemical titration method would be most suitable.[6,30] Titration methods have also been studied in the reaction of

Acid (pH 4) Glutaraldehyde → Temperature increase → Good activity (1a)

Poor activity (1a, b, c) → Ultrasonics →

↓ pH Increase

Alkaline (pH 8) Glutaraldehyde → Temperature increase →

Good activity (2a) → pH increase → Poor activity (2b)

→ Time →

FIGURE 23.4 Influence of time, temperature, and pH on the biocidal activity of acid and alkaline glutaraldehyde solutions: 1a,b,c and 2a,b relate to state of the molecule as described in Figures 23.2 and 23.3.

glutaraldehyde with hydroxylamine, hydrazine, and methylamine and found that a characteristic change in absorbance occurred.[31] From this, a spectrophotometric method was developed for the determination of low concentrations of the aldehyde in the presence of substrates absorbing in the same wavelength region. A microplate photometric method based on N-methylbenzo-thiazol-(2)-hydrazone and 4-amino-3-hydrazino-5-mercapto-1,2,4-triazole has been developed to measure various aldehydes, including glutaraldehyde, in disinfectant solutions.[32] Other methods of analysis have been developed for specific reasons such as the determination of glutaraldehyde at low levels in hospital air.[33] Chromatographic methods have also been described. These gas chromatographic[34,35] and high-performance liquid chromatographic (HPLC) methods[22] have compared favorably with UV methods. It is advised that the chromatographic methods should be used in preference to the UV-absorption (235/280 nm) or UV spectrophotometric method (hydroxylamine).[23,36] A HPLC method for glutaraldehyde determination was defined and validated by derivatization using 2,4-dinitrophenylhydrazine. The method was validated for concentration ranging from 1.25 mg/L with a detection limit of 0.2 mg/L.[37]

Reaction With Proteins

It is likely that several reactions occur between glutaraldehyde and proteins, giving rise to several products. Several studies of glutaraldehyde interaction with proteins in vitro have been published,[38-40] shedding some light on this subject. The composition/purity of the glutaraldehyde solution is known to dictate the type of reaction products formed with amino acids.[41] The rate of reaction with protein is pH dependent and increases considerably over the pH 4 to 9 range,[5] and it is known that the reaction gives rise to a product (or products) that is stable to acid hydrolysis and a chromophore with an absorption maximum at 265 nm. The stability of the cross-linkages to acid hydrolysis rules out Schiff base formation.[42] Aldol-type polymers formed in alkaline solution react with amino groups to give an imino bond stabilized by resonance with the ethylenic double bond (Figure 23.5), and it was proposed that glutaraldehyde does not react with proteins in its free form but as an unsaturated polymer.[43] On the other hand, the tanning actions of aqueous solutions of purified and unpurified glutaraldehyde are almost identical,[18,44-46] indicating that a possible cross-linking reaction does not depend on the initial presence of unsaturated compounds.

In a study of the mechanism of cross-linking of proteins employing bovine pericardium, it is suggested that glutaraldehyde fixes primarily the surface of the fibers and creates a polymeric network that hinders the further cross-linking of the interstitium of the fiber.[47]

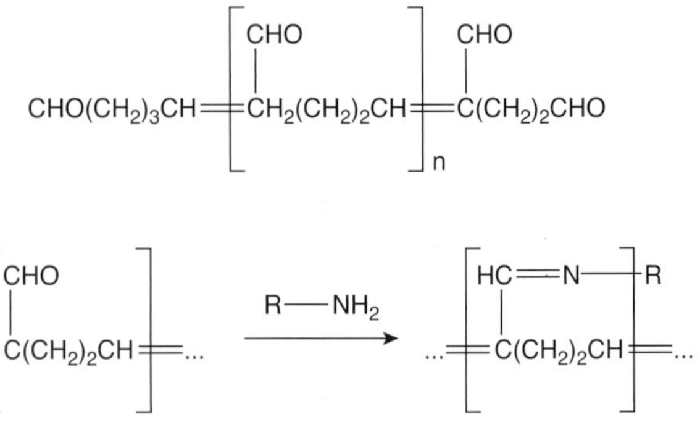

FIGURE 23.5   Reaction of aldol-type polymers of glutaraldehyde with amino acids.

Proteins are composed of amino acids, some of which contain free amino groups that readily react with glutaraldehyde. In particular, lysine possesses an ε-amino group that is the principal side chain of the molecule and therefore accessible to glutaraldehyde.[48] A further mechanism was proposed to explain the nature of glutaraldehyde-protein cross-links.[46] The reaction of free aldehyde with a primary amine of the protein is followed by condensation of additional free glutaraldehyde and leads to the formation of a 1, 3, 4, 5 substituted pyridinium salt analogous to the amino acid desmosine (Figure 23.6). This mechanism ties in with the observation of a new absorption peak at 265 nm as proteins are cross-linked, and the lability of pyridinium type cross-links to alkaline hydrolysis is similar to protein-glutaraldehyde cross-links treated in the same manner.[49] The pyridinium linkage is not the only type of cross-link in glutaraldehyde-treated proteins, but it most likely represents a significant portion of these, with other possibilities existing. The reaction of glutaraldehyde with adenosine, cytidine, and guanosine and with the equivalent deoxyribonucleosides has been investigated.[50] Multiple products were seen in HPLC for adenine and guanine nucleosides. In each nucleoside, the site of reaction was shown to be the exocyclic amino group. Chemically, the bonds were thought to be Schiff bases.

Although the interactions of glutaraldehyde with proteins are well studied over several decades, a number of more recent reviews have compiled current knowledge in this area.[51,52]

Antimicrobial Properties

Glutaraldehyde displays a broad spectrum of activity and rapid rate of kill against the majority of microorganisms (Table 23.1). Glutaraldehyde as a chemical sterilant is capable of destroying all forms of microbial life including bacterial and fungal spores, tubercle bacilli, and viruses. Similarly, it has been classified as a high-level disinfectant capable of producing sterility if the exposure was long enough.[54]

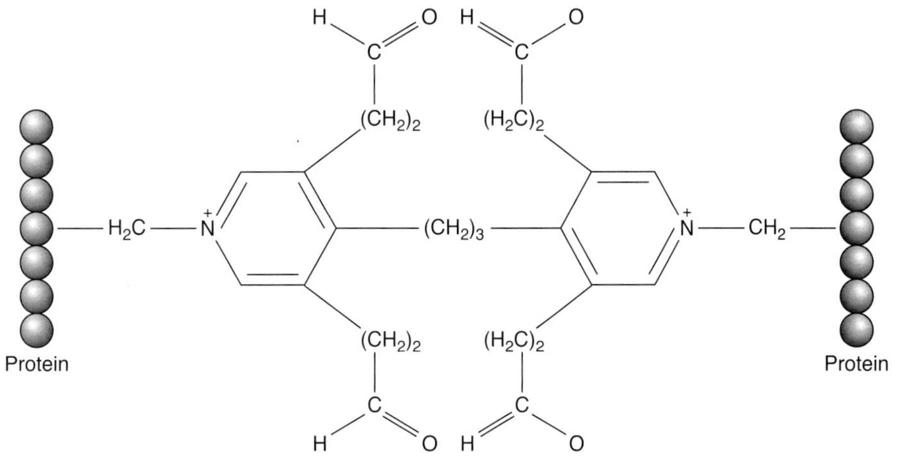

FIGURE 23.6 A protein-pyridinium cross-link resulting from glutaraldehyde reaction with protein.

TABLE 23.1 Lethal effects of aqueous 2% alkaline glutaraldehyde solutions[a]

Type of Microorganism	Specific Organism(s)	Killing Time
Vegetative bacteria	Staphylococcus aureus	<1 min
	Streptococcus pyogenes	
	Streptococcus pneumoniae	
	Escherichia coli	
	Pseudomonas aeruginosa	
	Serratia marcescens	
	Proteus vulgaris	
	Klebsiella pneumoniae	
	Micrococcus lysodeikticus	
Tubercle bacillus	Mycobacterium tuberculosis H37Rv	<10 min
Bacterial spores	Bacillus subtilis	<3 h
	Bacillus megaterium	
	Bacillus globigii	
	Clostridium tetani	
	Clostridium perfringens	
Viruses	Poli types I and II	<10 min
	Echo type 6\coxsackie B-1	
	Herpes simplex	
	Vaccinia	
	Influenza A-2 (Asian)	
	Adeno type 2	
	Mouse hepatitis (MHV3)	

[a]From Borick.[53]

TABLE 23.2   Comparative sporicidal activities of some aldehydes

Aldehyde	Chemical Structure	Sporicidal Activity
Formaldehyde (methanal)	HCHO	Good
Glyoxal (ethanedial)	CHO • CHO	Good
Malonaldehyde (propanedial)	CHO • CH$_2$CHO	Slightly active
Succinaldehyde (butanedial)	CHO • (CH$_2$)$_2$CHO	Slightly active
Glutaraldehyde (pentanedial)	CHO • (CH$_2$)$_1$CHO[a]	Excellent
Adipaldehyde (hexanedial)	CHO • (CH$_2$)$_4$CHO	Slightly active

[a]In simplest form: see text also.

Bacterial Spores

The ability of glutaraldehyde to kill bacterial spores is, perhaps, its most important property. Useful sporicidal activity is a relatively rarer property of chemical disinfectants, which are often bactericidal only (see chapter 5). Glutaraldehyde is the only aldehyde to exhibit excellent sporicidal activity (Table 23.2), an activated 2% solution having a greater effect than 8% formaldehyde against a range of bacterial spores (Table 23.3). Increasing attention has been focused on the development of alternative disinfectants having useful sporicidal activity. But difficulties remained in balancing useful activity with inherent disadvantages such as corrosivity, inactivation by organic matter and toxicity, which are all too often present. A comparative study into the sporicidal activity of several glutaraldehyde, sodium dichloroisocyanurate, and peroxygen disinfectants typified the situation.[55] Bacillus subtilis NCTC 10073 spores were rapidly eliminated (<1 h) in the absence of blood by the various chlorine-containing compounds (ranging from 1200 ppm to 5750 ppm Cl2). But presence of blood effectively negated this activity. Peroxygen disinfectants were variable in their activity, but the peracetic acid disinfectant tested proved effective in the presence and absence of blood at the concentrations tested. A glutaraldehyde-phenate and a "long-life" glutaraldehyde disinfectant were also

examined. These were tested at 30 days and 28 days, respectively, and found to much slower in action (>1 h) than the other disinfectants tested but did retain their activity in the presence of blood.

The time required for sterilant process by a chemical agent is based on the killing time achieved by the agent against a reasonable challenge of resistant spores. At the common use-dilution of 2%, a glutaraldehyde formulation was capable of killing spores of Bacillus and Clostridium in 3 hours.[2,56] Others reported a 99.99% kill of spores of Bacillus anthracis and Clostridium tetani in 15 and 30 minutes, respectively.[57] It was apparent from these results that not all species were equally susceptible, and of those organisms tested, Bacillus pumilis was the most resistant. Studies of the sporicidal activity of 2% glutaraldehyde against B subtilis var globigii, Geobacillus stearothermophilus, and Clostridium difficile found that the aerobic species, normally chosen for test purposes, survived for 2 hours, but C difficile was killed in under 10 minutes.[58] Overall, B subtilis spores are found to be the most resistant to treatment with glutaraldehyde.[59] Using the Association of Official Analytical Chemist (AOAC) sporicidal test and vacuum-dried spores, 10 hours was necessary for complete kill. In an investigation including nine glutaraldehyde formulations, it was reported that all were effective against a spore suspension of B subtilis var

TABLE 23.3   Comparison of the sporicidal activity of formaldehyde and glutaraldehyde[a]

Spores	Time (h) Required to Kill	
	2% Activated Glutaraldehyde[b]	8% Formaldehyde[b]
Bacillus globigii	2-3	>3
Bacillus subtilis	2	>3
Clostridium tetani	<2	>3
Clostridium perfringens	2-3	>3

[a]From Stonehill et al.[2]

[b]Age of solutions: 18 h.

globigii in 3 hours or less.[60] A similar result was obtained with a challenge of 10^6 spores dried onto aluminum foil. A 3-hour exposure was recommended at that time to be sufficient for practical purposes, particularly as spores are infrequent on clean medical equipment. Other work, using similar time-survivor measurements and aqueous suspensions of *B subtilis* spores, indicated that a 3-hour period gave approximately a 6 log drop in viable count.[61-64]

Glutaraldehyde was found to have a significant advantage over other compounds for which claims of sporicidal activity have been made, although some agent combinations, such as mixtures of hypochlorite and alcohol[65-68] and buffered hypochlorite solutions[60] are more powerful.

Antibacterial Activity

Vegetative bacteria are readily susceptible to the action of glutaraldehyde. As shown in Table 23.4, a 0.02% aqueous alkaline solution was rapidly effective against gram-positive and gram-negative species, and a 2% solution was capable of killing any vegetative species, including *Staphylococcus aureus*, *Proteus vulgaris*, *Escherichia coli*, and *Pseudomonas aeruginosa* within 2 minutes.[2] Complete kill in 10 minutes of *E coli* suspensions (2×10^8 cells/mL) by 100 µg/mL alkaline glutaraldehyde was reported, compared with a 45% kill produced by acid solution.[69] Glutaraldehyde preparations passed the Kelsey-Sykes capacity test with and without yeast, using *P aeruginosa* as the test organism, compared with hypochlorite under the concentrations tested, which failed the test when yeast was added.[60] Using stainless steel penicylinders, neoprene "O" rings, and polyvinyl tubing as carriers for a range of organisms including *P aeruginosa* and *Mycobacterium smegmatis* to simulate in-use conditions for the sterilization of instruments, catheter tubing, and anaesthetic equipment, a glutaraldehyde preparation was more effective on all three carriers than a cetrimide/chlorhexidine gluconate disinfectant, which was only partially effective.[70]

Mycobacteria

The tubercle bacillus is more resistant to chemical disinfectants than other nonsporing bacteria (see chapter 3). Because glutaraldehyde is widely used for the cold disinfection of respiratory equipment that may be contaminated with tubercle bacilli, it must have good activity against these organisms. Earlier reports of glutaraldehyde activity against mycobacteria have been conflicting, with some claiming good mycobactericidal activity.[2,56,64,71] Others have shown a slow action against *Mycobacterium tuberculosis*,[57] being less effective than formaldehyde or iodine[72] or hypochlorite.[73] Two percent glutaraldehyde formulations for 10 to 30 minutes were recommended for the chemical disinfection of fiberoptic endoscopes, where an iodophor formulation was less effective against the tubercle bacillus.[74] The use of glutaraldehyde as an alternative to other disinfectants in tuberculosis laboratory discard jars was investigated.[75] A 5 log reduction in viability of clinical isolates of *M tuberculosis* was obtained within 10 to 30 minutes at 25°C using alkaline glutaraldehyde, even in the presence of neutralizing materials such as swab sticks and sputum. A possible explanation for these varying conclusions was suggested, which found the official AOAC test procedure to be non-quantitative and to lack precision and accuracy.[76] It was concluded that use of carriers increased variability of results and suggested a new test method for mycobacterial efficacy. But another interpretation is that the cross-linking of mycobacterial cells onto the surface in the presence of extraneous materials (contaminating protein) may protect the cells from inactivation and, although still viable, are unable to grow unless physically dislodged (see chapter 61). The importance of accurate temperature control was also highlighted.[77] A significant change in rate of kill of *Mycobacterium bovis* bacille Calmette-Guérin by glutaraldehyde was observed as temperature was increased from 20°C to 25°C. Clumping of bacilli was proposed as another cause of erroneous results.

The choice of organism for use in mycobactericidal tests is also controversial. Investigators have often used *M smegmatis* in suspension and a variety of carriers in the presence of sputum to assess mycobactericidal activity of disinfectants.[78] In these tests, glutaraldehyde produced in excess of a 6 log reduction in viable count after 1 minute of contact; however, others suggested *M smegmatis* is more susceptible to disinfectants than *M tuberculosis*, and therefore, its use as a test organism is not appropriate.[79] These authors suggested using *Mycobacterium terrae*,

TABLE 23.4 Susceptibilities of nonsporing bacteria to 0.02% aqueous alkaline glutaraldehyde[a]

Organism	Inactivation Factor After Exposure (min)			
	5	**10**	**15**	**20**
Staphylococcus aureus	10^1	10^2	10^4	10^4
Escherichia coli	10^1	10^1	$>10^5$	$>10^6$
Pseudomonas aeruginosa	$<10^1$	10^1	10^1	10^4

[a]From Rubbo et al.[57]

TABLE 23.5 Mycobacterial activity of glutaraldehyde

Species	Time for Inactivation (min) With Organic Load		Treatment Conditions	Reference
	Present	Absent		
Mycobacterium avium			2% Glutaraldehyde	
Mycobacterium chelonae	10		Log$_{10}$ kill >5	Shetty et al[82]
Mycobacterium xenopi			Organic load—5% horse serum	
Mycobacterium smegmatis				
Mycobacterium tuberculosis	10	20	2% Glutaraldehyde	
Mycobacterium avium-intracellulare (clinical isolate)	10	60	Log$_{10}$ kill >5	
Mycobacterium fortuitum	1	1	Organic load—1% horse serum	Griffiths et al[83]
M chelonae (type strain)	1	1		
M chelonae (isolate)	>60	>60		
Mycobacterium tuberculosis (clinical isolate)	10	20	2% Glutaraldehyde	
M avium-intracellulare (clinical isolate)	11	60	Log$_{10}$ kill >5	Griffiths et al[84]
Mycobacterium terrae	10	60	Organic load—1% horse serum	
Mycobacterium gordonae		10	2% Glutaraldehyde	
		10	3.2% Glutaraldehyde	Jackson et al[85]
			Bronchoscope contaminated with 10^8 colony-forming units/mL	

which produced results more closely related to *M tuberculosis* in the suspension test employed. Once again, a glutaraldehyde formulation was found to be rapidly mycobactericidal. Variation in resistance to glutaraldehyde was shown by different strains of mycobacteria, with strains of *Mycobacterium avium* and *Mycobacterium intracellulare* requiring over 20 and 40 minutes, respectively, to achieve a 99% kill.[80] Differences in sensitivity to glutaraldehyde between laboratory strains and clinical isolates had been observed previously.[81] The antimycobacterial activity of glutaraldehyde is summarized in Table 23.5. But it is interesting to note increasing reports of high-level resistance to glutaraldehyde in atypical mycobacteria strains (*Mycobacterium chelonae*, *Mycobacterium massiliense*) that have been isolated from environmental conditions (eg, water and equipment) and from patient infections.[79,86-89] Some of these strains were also reported to be cross-resistant to other aldehydes (OPA) and demonstrated increased virulence in animal studies.[89-91] The resistance mechanisms have been studied and is most likely to be due to the lack of appreciable or sensitive protein molecules at the surface of the mycobacterial cell wall in these strains, thereby limiting the activity or penetrability of glutaraldehyde.[92]

In conclusion, claims of glutaraldehyde activity against mycobacteria must be regarded with caution,

taking into account the method and temperature used in the assessment and the criteria employed to measure success or failure of disinfection. All reports indicate activity of glutaraldehyde against these organisms; it is the rate of kill that is affected by method and conditions used. The practical implications of these reports are that adequate time for decontamination of equipment must be allowed.

Antifungal Activity

Glutaraldehyde has been shown to exhibit potent activity against a range of fungi, including the dermatophytes *Trichophyton interdigitale* and *Microsporium gypseum*, the yeasts *Candida albicans* and *Saccharomyces cerevisiae*, the common spoilage molds *Mucor hiemalis*, *Rhizopus stolonifer*, and *Penicillium chrysogenum*, and the resistant fruit spoilage mold *Byssochlamys fulva*.[93-96] Fungicidal activity of a 0.5% glutaraldehyde solution is illustrated in Figure 23.7 against spores of *Aspergillus niger*. This fungus was found to be more resistant than other fungi to glutaraldehyde,[57,96] presumably due to its greater intrinsic tolerance to microbiocides than other fungi (see chapter 3).[92] But in common with a range of other fungal species, both mycelial growth and sporulation are inhibited by 0.5% alkaline glutaraldehyde, whereas spore swelling is entirely halted by a 0.5% solution. *A niger* and

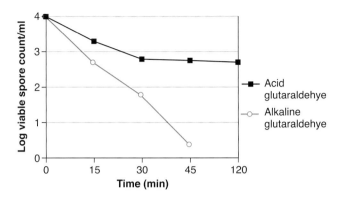

FIGURE 23.7 Effect of 0.5% acid or alkaline glutaraldehyde formulation on spores of *Aspergillus niger*. From Gorman and Scott.[96]

Aspergillus fumigatus were found to be the most resistant fungi encountered in a comparative study of fungicidal activity of disinfectants.[97] Sonacide® (an acid-based glutaraldehyde formulation) was effective against both fungi; however, a glutaraldehyde-phenate mixture (Sporicidin®) was not effective, even after 90 minutes of contact.

Antiviral Activity

Reliable scientific evidence of viricidal activity of disinfectants became increasingly necessary during the 1980s and 1990s because more information becomes available implicating direct contact with infected material as a significant means of transmission of infection. Two publications, while developing a test method to determine viricidal activity of disinfectants, have confirmed the antiviral activity of glutaraldehyde. When using an ultrafiltration dilution technique to separate disinfectant from virus, it was demonstrated that 2% glutaraldehyde was rapidly viricidal to poliovirus type 1.[98] A surface test in which a standard challenge of 3×10^7 plaque-forming units of herpes simplex was allowed to dry onto coverslips before exposure to a range of disinfectants was also investigated[99]; no viable virus was recovered after 1 minute of contact with 2% alkaline glutaraldehyde, and overall glutaraldehyde and ethanol or isopropanol were the most active of all the agents tested. A number of earlier reports showed that glutaraldehyde was effective against a range of viruses,[100-103] even in the presence of high levels of organic matter.[104,105] Enveloped lipophilic viruses usually show significantly less resistance than the nonlipid viruses (see chapter 3). The nonlipid enteroviruses—polio, echo, and coxsackie—showed greater resistance to disinfection with glutaraldehyde than other virus groups.[106] A potentiated acid glutaraldehyde formulation was also shown to have weak activity against coxsackievirus B5 and echovirus 11 in studies[107,108] and to be less effective than ethanol or a chlorine-based disinfectant against reovirus 3.[109]

Many studies concentrated on hepatitis B virus (HBV) and human immunodeficiency virus (HIV). The HBV infection continues to be a major health hazard, especially among health care professionals. Because of the risks to personnel and initial lack of data relating to disinfectant activity toward HBV, infection-prevention guidelines tended to recommend only strong disinfectants such as glutaraldehyde or high concentrations of hypochlorites for the treatment of HBV-contaminated material. These recommendations are supported by evidence that glutaraldehyde is capable of inactivating HBV antigen[110] and destroying HBV infectivity.[111,112] Glutaraldehyde was shown to produce a time and concentration-dependent reduction in hepatitis A viral titer and a decrease in antigenicity.[113] Further studies with HIV continued to support the efficacy of glutaraldehyde against the virus, displaying sensitivity to chemical disinfection similar to that of other enveloped viruses.[114] Reverse transcriptase was used as an indicator of viral inactivation, and although this assay was demonstrated to be less sensitive than measurement of infectious virus titer, it was also concluded that HIV behaved similarly to other enveloped viruses.[115]

Rotaviruses are responsible for numerous outbreaks of acute gastroenteritis in young children. The possible risk of transmission of these viruses by contaminated hand or fomite contact could be reduced by good disinfection practice. In an evaluation of disinfectant activity against human rotaviruses, 2% alkaline glutaraldehyde solution in the presence of an organic load produced at least a 3 log reduction in virus plaque titer within 1 minute in a suspension test[116] and using virus-contaminated inanimate surfaces.[117] Rotaviruses, similar to polioviruses, represent the nonenveloped viruses that generally have a greater resistance to microbicide inactivation. In this case, these viruses can demonstrate variable viricidal activity with glutaraldehyde due to their external protein capsid structure that may or may not react with glutaraldehyde (see chapter 3). Parvoviruses, for example, show variable activity with both glutaraldehyde and OPA but over time do show variable activity.[118] Recently, investigations claiming the unusual lack of activity again human papilloma viruses[119] have not been substantiated and are likely due to test method aberrations rather than lack of antiviral activity (Yarwood, personal communication, September 2019).

Resistance

Reports in the literature of resistance of microorganisms to glutaraldehyde resulting in contamination and occasionally infection may be attributed to two factors. First, where reference is made to outbreak of infection or spread of contamination through use of glutaraldehyde,[120-122] the agent was invariably employed as a disinfectant rather than as a sterilizing agent. The short time available between patients on, for example, endoscopy lists, has necessitated a reduction in contact time for decontamination in many instances, and this has inevitably led to the reported cases. Indeed, 45 minutes of glutaraldehyde contact was necessary to achieve sterilization of heavily contaminated flexible-fiber bronchoscopes.[123] It is also likely that in many of these cases, the disinfectant was not used appropriately or indeed cross-contamination following disinfection due to the use of tap water (which is often contaminated with pathogens are low levels at the point of use).

A second factor that must also be considered is intrinsic microorganism resistance. The TM strains of *M chelonae* survived 60 minutes of exposure to 2% alkaline glutaraldehyde, although no survivors of ATCC strains of *M chelonae* or *Mycobacterium fortuitum* were detected in fluids assayed at 2 minutes of contact time.[81] With 0.2% glutaraldehyde, both TM and ATCC strains showed survivors at 96 hours of exposure time. *M chelonae* organisms have been reported as intrinsic contaminants of porcine prosthetic heart-valve tissues treated and stored, respectively, in 1% and 0.2% glutaraldehyde solutions.[124]

Disinfectant solutions used to treat materials and equipment for patient use must therefore be carefully evaluated in terms of their potential for harboring rather than eliminating contaminants. Glutaraldehyde-resistant nontuberculous mycobacteria are becoming increasingly problematic for health care organizations. More than 2000 cases of infection from a single strain of glutaraldehyde-resistant *Mycobacterium abscessus* subsp *massiliense* (BRA100) were reported in Brazil between 2004 and 2008.[87,125] In a subsequent study, clinical BRA100 isolates were recovered following postsurgical infection. These strains once again proved highly resistant, with minimum inhibitory concentration (MIC) values of 8% glutaraldehyde. These isolates were susceptible to both OPA and peracetic acid, suggesting glutaraldehyde should be replaced with OPA or other solutions for high-level disinfection.[126] Nosocomial infections have also been traced to endoscopes, bronchoscopes, and dialyzers in the Netherlands, Japan, the United Kingdom, and the United States, with glutaraldehyde-resistant *M chelonae* and *M abscessus* isolates identified as the causative organisms.[88,89,127,128] As discussed earlier, changes in the protein availability on the surfaces of these strains appear to be the major mechanism of resistance to glutaraldehyde, and in some cases was also cross-resistant to OPA.[88,92] Others recently reported the emergence of glutaraldehyde-resistant *P aeruginosa* in a health care setting. Two strains of glutaraldehyde-resistant *P aeruginosa* were found in the rinsing water and drain of an endoscope reprocessor. A number of patients with lower respiratory tract and bloodstream infections were identified as having possible epidemiologic links to the resistant *P aeruginosa* strains.[129]

Efflux mechanisms have been shown to contribute to glutaraldehyde resistance in both *Pseudomonas fluorescens* and *P aeruginosa* biofilms. Transcriptomic analysis revealed genes involved in multidrug efflux were induced in the presence of sublethal concentrations of glutaraldehyde. Furthermore, glutaraldehyde activity was potentiated by the addition of efflux pump inhibitors (EPIs), resulting in significant improvements in biofilm inactivation,[130] but this mechanism of resistance is difficult to understand considering the mode of action of glutaraldehyde as a microbicide. The *P fluorescens* was also used as a model organism to investigate the genetic response elucidating tolerance to glutaraldehyde in reused wastewater (produced water). The altered resistance profile of microorganisms to glutaraldehyde was determined to be due to increased salinity of the produced water, with genes involved in osmotic stress, energy production and conversion, membrane integrity, and protein transport found to facilitate bacterial survival following biocide treatment.[131]

As with resistance to similar antimicrobial compounds, resistance to glutaraldehyde is considered multifactorial. Outer membrane structure and composition as well as the presence of integrons and modulators of biofilm formation all appear to play a role in resistance development.[130,132,133] Although examples of glutaraldehyde resistance are increasing, accepted breakpoint values to determine resistance do not currently exist. An MIC value of >4000 mg/L (0.4%) has been suggested for *Bacillus* strains, which may be suitable for other species to describe resistance.[134]

Sporicidal results[66] have shown that a spore population of *B subtilis* treated with alkaline glutaraldehyde, and presumed dead, can be revived in defined germination medium following removal of the outer coat layers of the spore with selective agents and by application of ultrasonic energy (Table 23.6). A small proportion may be recovered after 3 to 10 hours of contact with 2% glutaraldehyde solutions by application of ultrasonic energy, lysozyme, and protein-denaturing agents such as dithiothreitol and urea-mercaptoethanol. This revival may be considered academic in nature, but it has implications in practice, especially in view of the differences in resistance exhibited by natural and subcultured populations as suggested earlier. It is likely that viable spores have been protected from complete inactivation due to cross-linking and entrapment within contaminated surfaces. Furthermore, there is a risk attached to the use of sublethal concentrations of glutaraldehyde (ie, less than 2%) for disinfection or sterilizing purposes under soiled conditions. Such concentration levels may arise not only from in-use dilution but also from polymerization of alkaline solutions of glutaraldehyde and presence of organic matter.[135] The presence of various types and amounts of organic and inorganic materials, as well as changes in pH, may lead to adsorption, alteration, or inactivation of the disinfectant, significantly reducing recommended effective concentrations. Also, substandard preparation of the "activated" disinfectant, contamination of solutions,

TABLE 23.6 Revival of alkaline glutaraldehyde-treated *Bacillus subtilis* spores after coat removal and resuscitation[a]

Treatment Sequence	% Survivors After Dilution and Incubation in:		
	25% vol/vol Ringer	GM	GM + Lysozyme
Glutaraldehyde 2% (3 h)	0.0006	0.0006	0.0004
UDS	0	0	0.038
Sonication 10 min	0	0	0.046
Sonication 10 min	0	0	0.032
Glutaraldehyde 2% (10 h)	0	0	0
UDS	0	0	0.004
Sonication 10 min	0	0	0.006
Sonication 10 min	0	0	0.0015
Glutaraldehyde 1% (10 h)	0.27	0.26	0.26
UDS	0.035	0.075	0.75
Sonication 10 min	0.016	0.013	2.20
Sonication 10 min	0.018	0.031	1.05

[a]From Gorman et al.[67]

Abbreviations: GM, germination medium; UDS, urea/dithiothreitol/sodium dodecyl sulphate.

failure to replace solutions that have deteriorated on standing, or even dilution of residual glutaraldehyde solution may all modify the outcome of disinfection. Illustrating this point, the "reuse" of glutaraldehyde solutions has been investigated.[136] Samples of the disinfectant were collected from baths over the recommended 14 day reuse period, analyzed, and assessed for activity against *M bovis* and hepatitis A virus. Glutaraldehyde levels dropped to approximately 1% (from 2.25% initial) by 14 days. Due attention should therefore be exercised in the use of glutaraldehyde, as with any disinfectant, to avoid such an occurrence especially in view of the resurgence of pathogens such as mycobacteria, viruses, and antibiotic-resistant bacteria.

Initial viable spore count: 2×10^7 colony-forming units/mL

Exceptional resistance to sterilization and disinfection is exhibited by the causative agent of scrapie and other prion agents (see chapter 68).[137,138] Scrapie agent was shown to be more resistant than other organisms to glutaraldehyde and was not fully inactivated by 12.5% glutaraldehyde in 16 hours at 4°C.[138] In a more recent study, scrapie infectivity survived exposure to 12.5% unbuffered glutaraldehyde (pH 4.5) for 16 hours.[139] Furthermore, the causative agent for Creutzfeldt-Jakob disease (CJD) was not inactivated following 14-day exposure to 5% glutaraldehyde at pH 7.3.[140] Results are not unexpected due to the proteinaceous nature of prions and their associated structures (see chapter 68).

Microbial biofilm formation on medical devices is an acknowledged problem in respect to antimicrobial agent resistance. Whereas glutaraldehyde 2% has been shown to eradicate laboratory-grown biofilm cells of *P aeruginosa* within 1 minute,[141] concerns justifiably exist as to efficacy against biofilm formed on flexible endoscopes in automatic machines. Griffiths et al[86] examined glutaraldehyde 2% against *M chelonae* isolates from automatic machines and which had been exposed to selective pressure of disinfectant usage. These isolates were extremely resistant to glutaraldehyde. It was concluded that strict attention must be placed on sessional and regular cleaning of the machines to prevent biofilm formation. The effect of glutaraldehyde disinfection on microbial biofilms from a range of species was recently investigated.[142] Glutaraldehyde was not capable of preventing the survival of bacteria in biofilms of *Salmonella* ser Typhimurium, *E coli*, *Streptococcus mutans*, or *Bacteroides fragilis*. In a recent study on glutaraldehyde disinfection of *S aureus* and *P aeruginosa* biofilms from endoscopes, cells in residual biofilm remained viable after treatment with 2% glutaraldehyde.[143] Environmental issues surrounding glutaraldehyde use also remains a concern. Environmental partitioning studies suggest glutaraldehyde tends to remain in the aquatic compartment in wastewater, with little tendency to bioaccumulate. This exposes aquatic microorganisms to sublethal concentrations of glutaraldehyde, which may result in the proliferation of tolerant or resistant microbes.[144,145]

Mechanism of Action

Interactions With Bacterial Cell Constituents

Glutaraldehyde-protein interactions, as described earlier, indicate an effect of the dialdehyde initially on the surface of bacterial cells. Conclusions from a range of mode-of-action studies indicate a powerful binding of the aldehyde to the outer cell layers. Earlier studies found that the dialdehyde reacted with 30% to 50% of the ε-amino groups in isolated peptidoglycan, and it was proposed that two tripeptide side chains could be joined when free ε-amino groups are available.[146] Treatment of *E coli* whole cells and isolated walls with alkaline glutaraldehyde greatly reduced, or completely prevented, lysis by 2% sodium lauryl sulphate at 35°C to 40°C,[69] and pretreatment of *S aureus* and *P aeruginosa* cells with glutaraldehyde reduces subsequent lysis by lysostaphin and EDTA-lysozyme.[147,148] Strengthening of the outer layers of spheroplasts and protoplasts by glutaraldehyde has also been reported.[149,150] Cell agglutination, shown to occur on addition of glutaraldehyde to various microorganisms, was suggested to be due to the formation of intercellular bonds, thus confirming the hypothesis of a preferential action of glutaraldehyde on the outer layers of the cells.[151] But the biocidal effect of glutaraldehyde is unlikely to be due to a sealing of the cell envelope alone.[152,153] Transport of a low-molecular-weight amino acid, α-amino-isobutyric-acid-1-^{14}C (14 C-AIB), was compared in glutaraldehyde-treated and untreated cells of *E coli* and found to be reduced by only 50% in treated cells.

The reaction of glutaraldehyde with cytoplasmic constituents has received less attention. The inhibitory effect of the aldehyde on RNA, DNA, and protein syntheses in *E coli* is practically complete within 10 minutes of adding the disinfectant and is due to inhibition of precursor uptake as a consequence of a glutaraldehyde-protein reaction in the outer structures of the cell.[69] The reaction of the aldehyde with nucleic acids follows pseudo-first-order kinetics at high temperatures, but there is little evidence for the formation of intermolecular cross-links, even at the higher temperatures.[154] Comparatively few studies have examined the effects of glutaraldehyde on cell enzyme activity. Dehydrogenase activity is inhibited by concentrations that have little effect on cell viability.[150] This is possibly because the compound strengthens the outer cell surface and prevents ready access of substrate to enzyme. Glutaraldehyde was found to prevent the selective release of certain enzymes from the cytoplasmic membrane of *Micrococcus lysodeikticus*.[155] Direct effects on various intracellular proteins is expected given the cross-linking mode of action.[92] Various concentrations of glutaraldehyde were reported to directly inactivate several periplasmic enzymes,[156,157] including ATPase.[152,158] Glutaraldehyde fixation was shown to cause a shift of ATPase from the periplasmic space to the cell surface.[159] Thus, in addition to a sealing effect on the outer layer, glutaraldehyde also inactivates cell enzymes to achieve its rapid bactericidal effect.[152]

Interaction With Bacterial Spores

The importance attached to the interaction of glutaraldehyde with bacterial spores is observed in the continuing interest shown by researchers in this area. Low concentrations of glutaraldehyde (0.1% wt/vol) were shown to inhibit germination of spores of *B subtilis* and *Bacillus pumilus*, whereas much higher concentrations (2% wt/vol) are sporicidal.[160] The aldehyde, at acid and alkaline pH, appears to interact to a considerable extent with the outer layers of bacterial spores. This interaction reduces the release of dipicolinic acid (DPA) from *B pumilus* and peroxide-induced lysis of spores subsequently treated with thioglycolic acid; however, the small differences in results obtained with acid and alkaline glutaraldehyde in respect of interaction with the spore coat did not correlate with the much greater sporicidal effect of the aldehyde at alkaline pH. The data indicated that acid glutaraldehyde could interact at the spore surface and remain there, whereas alkaline glutaraldehyde may have a greater penetration into the spore.

A study found that spores of *Bacillus cereus* became heat-sensitive in the presence of high concentrations of salts.[161] The authors postulated that the cations interact with the loosely cross-linked and electronegative spore peptidoglycan to cause collapse of the cortex. Replacement of mobile counterions and a consequent fall in the osmotic dehydration of the spore core leads to a reduction in resistance. In this respect, replacement of the alkalinating agent or "activator salt" (eg, sodium bicarbonate) in glutaraldehyde solutions by, especially, divalent metal chlorides, retains a marked sporicidal effect in the absence of alkaline pH.[15] This may indicate a role for the alkalinating agent or other cation addition in facilitating penetration and interaction of glutaraldehyde with components of the spore cortex or core. An investigation into the resistance of ion-exchange and coat-defective spores of *B subtilis* to glutaraldehyde has also indicated the importance of the protective role of the spore coat.[162] This was further examined with normal and chemically altered (calcium-form and hydrogen-form) spores of *B subtilis* (Table 23.7).[163] The calcium (Ca)-form was more sensitive to glutaraldehyde (pH 4.0 and 7.9) than the normal or hydrogen (H)-form, whereas removal of the spore coat, or coat protein, dramatically increased sensitivity of the spore to glutaraldehyde. Spore protoplasts were also shown to provide no resistance to glutaraldehyde but pretreatment of coat-defective spores with glutaraldehyde (pH 7.9) reduced the rate of lysis by lysozyme and by sodium nitrite, thereby protecting the cortex.[163] Glutaraldehyde at pH 4.0 had little effect.

Further experimental observations found that the uptake of acid glutaraldehyde by isolated spore coats follows a similar pattern to the uptake by intact spores; however,

2% Glutaraldehyde	Time (min) to Kill 90% of Initial Spore Population[b]				
	Normal	H-form	Ca-form	UME	UDS
pH 7.9	85 (123)	95 (126)	30 (61)	47	<1
pH 4.0	190	220	97	85	16

TABLE 23.7 Effect of acid and alkaline glutaraldehyde on ion-exchange and coat-defective spore forms of *Bacillus subtilis* at 20°C[a]

[a]From Gorman et al.[163]

[b]Initial spore count: 1.5×10^7 colony-forming units/mL. The times (D-values) in parentheses are for spores produced in a defined liquid medium; otherwise, spores were produced on solid medium.

Abbreviations: Ca-form, calcium form (ion-exchange spore forms); H-form, hydrogen form; UDS, urea/dithiothreitol/sodium dodecyl sulphate (spore coatless forms); UME, urea/mercaptoethanol.

isolated spore coats take up alkaline glutaraldehyde at a faster rate than intact spores. These uptake patterns suggest that alkaline glutaraldehyde may penetrate beyond the coats in the intact spore, whereas acid glutaraldehyde may be confined to the spore coat layers. These results coupled with the possibility of revival of glutaraldehyde-treated spores[67] serve as strong evidence for a strictly glutaraldehyde—spore surface layer(s) reaction.

The emergence and development of resistance to alkaline glutaraldehyde has been investigated in sporulating cells of *B subtilis*.[163] Growth and sporulation were followed by electron microscopy and resistance assigned to specific stages in relation to phase brightness, calcium 45 (^{15}Ca), and DPA accumulation in the maturing spore. A sequential development of resistance was observed with thermal resistance appearing first at early stage V of sporulation, corresponding to maturation of cortex and deposition of rudimentary spore coat material. Resistance to glutaraldehyde developed within the range t_5 to t_6 (ie, 5-6 h after exponential development), coinciding with late stage V of the sporulation process. Similar findings were later reported by others.[164] This development of resistance is in agreement with the observations stated earlier[67,163] in respect of spore coat protection.

Interaction With Fungi and Viruses

Inhibition of germination, spore swelling, mycelial growth, and sporulation in fungal species at varying concentrations has been demonstrated.[96] The principal structural wall component of many moulds and yeasts is chitin, which resembles the peptidoglycan of bacteria and is thus a potentially reactive site for glutaraldehyde action. Other active sites could include the polysaccharide-protein complexes, found in yeast cells, and in which cystine residues,-S-S-bonds, are abundant. The formation of intercellular bonds in yeast causing agglutination of the cells is likely to be a contributing factor in microorganism death.[151]

Few studies relate to mechanism of viral inactivation by glutaraldehyde. Studies with foot-and-mouth-disease virus found that glutaraldehyde-treated virus particles had a smaller sedimentation coefficient than normal particles.[165] This was in contrast to the effect observed on treated poliovirus when no change occurred.[166] Considerable alterations in the arrangement of the RNA and protein subunits were reported.[165] The overall structural integrity of the virus particle was not maintained. Prolonged exposure of poliovirus to the aldehyde increased its buoyant density and permeability to phosphotungstic acid.[167] It was suggested by that interaction between glutaraldehyde and lysine residues on the surface of hepatitis A virus may occur because this amino acid was present on the most exposed structural protein of the virus.[113] Work with HBV indicated that glutaraldehyde did not cause virus disruption, but results indicated that a "fixing" reaction occurred in a manner analogous to that seen for bacteria.[110] These results correlate well with the mode of action of glutaraldehyde, particularly against surface or available proteins.

Effect of Alkalination

Because the degree of biocidal activity observed in glutaraldehyde solutions is so markedly dependent on the pH of the solution, it seems appropriate to deal with this effect from a mechanistic viewpoint. The enhanced biocidal activity of glutaraldehyde in alkaline solution is thought to be due to an effect on the glutaraldehyde molecule in relation to polymerization, the outer layers of the microbial cell, or a combination of both. Effect of pH on the glutaraldehyde molecule has been discussed in detail earlier. The requirement that free aldehyde groups be present for optimum activity is well established.[57,168] The presence of free aldehyde groups in glutaraldehyde allows formation of an aldol-type polymer at alkaline pH.[151] A similar biocidal effect may be obtained with substantially higher glutaraldehyde concentrations at acid pH.

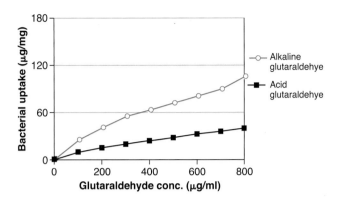

FIGURE 23.8   Effect of glutaraldehyde concentration on uptake by *Escherichia coli* under acid or alkaline formulations. From Gorman and Scott.[135]

A further interesting study found that acid glutaraldehyde did not react immediately with the outer cell layers or to the same overall extent as an alkaline solution.[169] This feature was considered to be compatible with the structure of the aldehyde at acid and alkaline pH.[151] Subsequent data obtained on bacterial uptake of glutaraldehyde have supported these views.[96] Uptake isotherms obtained from both acid and alkaline solutions are of the basic Langmuir (L) type, the acid solution having the further classification of L subgroup 2 and the alkaline, L subgroup 4, as illustrated in Figure 23.8. The second rise observed in the alkaline glutaraldehyde L-curve can be attributed to the development of fresh sites due to further penetration of the aldehyde and bicarbonate. The long plateau obtained for the acid solution indicates that a high-energy barrier must be overcome before additional absorption can occur on new sites. This observation correlates with the increased biocidal activity obtained on heating acid glutaraldehyde solutions.

The effect of sodium bicarbonate and other alkalinating salts is likely to be on the bacterial cell rather than on the aldehyde molecule.[29] Support for this hypothesis of bicarbonate was obtained from cell leakage data[170] and proton magnetic resonance studies.[171] The loosely bound outer layer of the gram-negative cell can be removed by washing with 0.5 M sodium chloride or sodium bicarbonate.[152] The alkalinating agent appears also to aid penetration of the glutaraldehyde molecule, as shown by its effect on the periplasmic-located enzyme, alkaline phosphatase.[152] This enzyme is equally inhibited by acid and alkaline glutaraldehyde in sodium chloride-washed cells of *E coli*, in contrast with the greater inhibitory action of alkaline glutaraldehyde on enzyme activity in whole cells. The possibility of a bicarbonate effect on the glutaraldehyde molecule was also investigated by estimating the degree of polymerization in acid and alkaline solutions.[170] The degree of polymerization is extensive at alkaline pH but negligible in acid solution. This polymerization, leading to an extensive loss of aldehyde groups, was measured

in weeks rather than in the short periods (minutes or hours) in which biocidal activity of alkaline glutaraldehyde is observed. An immediate effect is not, therefore, apparent on the glutaraldehyde molecule, and consequently, the primary effect of sodium bicarbonate must be on the bacterial cell. A further study showed that sodium bicarbonate at a concentration of 0.3%, which may conveniently be employed to alkalinate glutaraldehyde, inhibits bacterial spore germination.[172] This inhibitory effect was found to be due to HCO_3^- ion interaction with the dissociated protein from the carboxyl group of acidic amino acid residues on spore protein. This was postulated to cause degradative structural alterations within the spore.

Factors Influencing Efficacy and Evaluation of Activity

The antimicrobial activity of any compound cannot be looked at in isolation but must be described with reference to, for example, pH, temperature, organic challenge, and in-use dilution. Such factors significantly influence the usefulness of the preparation and how it is used. Reference has previously been made to the dramatic increase in biocidal activity of glutaraldehyde at alkaline pH. The difference in sporicidal activity of acid and alkaline solutions is illustrated in Figure 23.9. As temperature is increased, this difference in activity is reduced until at 70°C

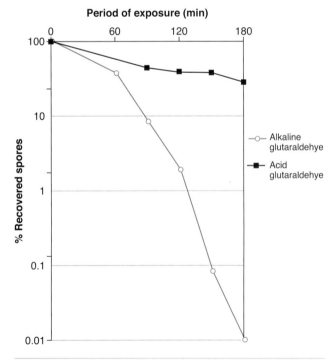

FIGURE 23.9   Effect of acid and alkaline glutaraldehyde (2%) on washed suspensions of *Bacillus subtilis* spores (3 × 10⁷/mL). Alkaline solution: sodium bicarbonate 0.3% activator, pH 7.9; acid solution, pH 4.0.

both are equally effective producing a complete kill of *B subtilis* spores (10^7/mL) within 5 minute.[61] Unfortunately, alkaline solutions have poor stability, and a loss of antimicrobial activity is observed in such solutions on storage (Table 23.8). This is related to a decrease in concentration of free aldehyde, which appears to be essential for biocidal activity. An estimate of the decrease in glutaraldehyde that can occur was reported.[53] A decrease from 2.1% (pH 8.5) to 1.3% (pH 7.4) was measured over a period of 28 days at ambient temperatures. These values have been confirmed by others, who also showed that glutaraldehyde concentrations in solutions of pH 7.3 and lower were not affected by storage.[64] As outlined earlier, several successful formulation exercises have resulted in much improved stability of alkaline glutaraldehyde solutions. Other preparations are formulated at a lower pH, some with other potentiators included to increase the otherwise low level of activity observed.

At one stage, glutaraldehyde-based disinfectants were generally available as 2% solutions to which an "activator" was added to bring the solution to alkaline pH. This activated solution has a limited shelf life, on the order of 14 days. The problem of in-use dilution of glutaraldehyde solutions is of concern especially about stabilized formulations designed for longer use. A long period of use would inevitably result in dilution of the sterilizing solution, which may be accompanied by pH changes and contamination by organic matter and contribute to loss of activity. But overall, repeated use of a solution, even if stable, for more than 7 to 14 days was undesirable.[174] In use conditions for disinfection and sterilization inevitably imply the presence of organic matter such as blood and pus. Ideally, therefore, a chemical agent should remain unaffected by organic matter. Many reports indicate a high resistance of glutaraldehyde to neutralization by organic matter, a surprising fact considering the reactivity of glutaraldehyde with protein. The presence of 20% blood serum[56] or 1% whole blood[71] did not appear to adversely affect activity of glutaraldehyde. In a study using a specially devised test method, the concentration (% wt/vol) of sterile baker's yeast (called the soil neutralization number) that a disinfectant could tolerate and still be able to kill bacteria in 10 minutes at 25°C was reported.[175] It was found that 2% alkaline glutaraldehyde had a maximum neutralization number of 50% against *S aureus* and *P aeruginosa*. This was explained based on the uptake pattern exhibited by glutaraldehyde, which is of the L (Langmuir) type. It was proposed that alkaline glutaraldehyde would react with a limited number of adsorption sites, either cell surfaces or other proteinaceous material, and would therefore remain relatively unaffected by a high content of organic matter.

One of the problems associated with determinations of the MIC has been the reactivity of glutaraldehyde with constituents of the growth medium (see chapter 61). For example, a darkening of nutrient broth in the presence of glutaraldehyde in these tests was proposed to explain the poor bacteriostatic results obtained.[57] Furthermore, a 60% decrease in free aldehyde concentration occurs when alkaline glutaraldehyde is added to malt extract broth,[135] although this is a fairly slow reaction over a 6-hour period at 37°C. Intentional neutralization of glutaraldehyde during time kill tests has been approached in a number of ways. In some reports, no inactivator has been used; however, in such cases, the results are only valid if dilutions were performed to subinhibitory levels. In a search for a suitable inactivator for glutaraldehyde, we found 1% glycine to be effective and nontoxic to the microorganism employed, *E coli*.[176]

In a report on bactericidal activity of 40 potential disinfectant inactivators, glycine was found to be nontoxic to *S aureus* and *P aeruginosa*.[177,178] Most of the other chemical inactivators used for glutaraldehyde inactivation have proven unsatisfactory.[29,72] Some methods of glutaraldehyde neutralization do not require the presence of an additional chemical inactivator; these include centrifuging the glutaraldehyde/cell mixture, followed by washing[63,73] and filtering with washing.[64]

TABLE 23.8 Effect of storage on the sporicidal activity[a] of 2% acid and alkaline glutaraldehyde[b]

Storage Time (wk)	Acid		Alkaline	
	Time (min) for 99.9% Kill	Glutaraldehyde Concentration (%)	Time (min) for 99.9% Kill	Glutaraldehyde Concentration (%)
0	>300	2.0	40	2.0
2	>300	1.9	120-180	1.6
6	>300	1.5	>300	0.7
12	>300	1.5	>300	0.6
24	>300	1.5	>300	0.3

[a]Activity determined at 18°C against *Bacillus subtilis* (initial spore count at 10^8/mL).

[b]From Gorman and Scott.[15,173]

The methods and problems of biocidal testing require consideration because they may influence claims for glutaraldehyde activity. The AOAC sporicidal test, as an example is well controlled and established as a standard procedure, although in the past this method has given variable results[179]; this may be partly due to the presence of high concentrations of interfering, organic soils in this test that may not allow for adequate glutaraldehyde penetration and antimicrobial activity. Survival curves of treated spore suspensions provide more information on the kinetics of sporicidal action but are also subject to wide variation. Many of the variables in such tests with glutaraldehyde were investigated for improvements.[63] The problems of spore resistance as affected by method of preparation and recovery of spores after treatment would appear to warrant more attention. This aspect was illustrated using chemically defined and complex media for the production of *B subtilis* spores.[180] The spore crops thus obtained differed in their resistance to glutaraldehyde. Table 23.7 provides examples of glutaraldehyde (pH 7.9) sporicidal activity against spores and spore forms produced on solid medium and defined liquid medium; significant differences in activity are observed.[163] A progressive development of resistance to glutaraldehyde also occurs on prolonged incubation of sporulating *B subtilis* in sporulation medium.[181] A time of 72 minutes was required for 2% glutaraldehyde to provide a 90% kill of 1-day *B subtilis* spores, compared to 94 minutes required for 14-day spores.

Formulations

Although glutaraldehyde has many advantages as a widely used disinfectant and sterilant, particularly for the heat-sensitive applications, it has disadvantages including stability, and being an irritant and sensitizer. Novel approaches to glutaraldehyde disinfectant formulation can aid in optimizing the activity, stability, and surface compatibility of the microbicide but at the same time limiting any disadvantages including toxicity (see chapter 6). Since the expiration of the original patent on the sterilizing action of alkalinated glutaraldehyde, many new products have been introduced, having equivalent activity and stability to the original patented product.[182] In addition, to improve the stability of activated glutaraldehyde, some preparations were formulated at lower alkaline pH values or at acid pH. This has the effect of reducing the rate of polymerization of glutaraldehyde and thus prolonging shelf life. Microbiologic activity was maintained usually by the inclusion of a surfactant in the formulation. Indeed, surfactants have been shown to engender synergistic disinfection efficacy with glutaraldehyde, with the cationic surfactants alkyl dimethyl benzyl ammonium bromide or alkyl dimethyl benzyl ammonium chloride. Complete killing of 10^6 *B subtilis* var *niger* spores was achieved in

2 hours with 2% glutaraldehyde in combination with either of the surfactants, versus 4 hours with glutaraldehyde alone. Similarly, these synergistic activities also resulted in complete killing of the same spore suspension with 1% glutaraldehyde in 4 hours instead of 2%.[183] The decrease in required glutaraldehyde concentration could prove beneficial in a health care setting, reducing occupational exposure of workers to glutaraldehyde and its associated implications for health. Another example is a formulation included 3.5% glutaraldehyde with 20% wt/wt isopropanol and 8% potassium acetate with improved efficacy to mycobacteria and spore-forming bacteria.[184] A glutaraldehyde composition containing an activator system that does not precipitate salts when diluted with hard water has been described.[185] This makes it possible to formulate solutions with an increased concentration of active glutaraldehyde to be diluted at the point of use without the attendant possibility of precipitate being deposited on medical instruments. Formulation can dramatically affect antimicrobial activity. In a comparison of nine glutaraldehyde products, all were effective against bacterial spores in suspension in 3 hours or less, but the acid glutaraldehyde preparations tested were less effective than alkaline ones, particularly against dried spores, and these formulation also tended to be more corrosive on surfaces.[60]

Numerous attempts have been made to potentiate the antimicrobial activity of glutaraldehyde solutions. These have frequently involved addition of surface active agents: cationic,[186] nonionic,[187,188] nonionic ethoxylates of isomeric linear alcohols,[59] amphoteric,[189] and anionic.[15] Addition of inorganic monovalent and divalent cations will further increase glutaraldehyde activity,[173] and therefore, it is perhaps not surprising that increased concentrations of sodium chloride and sodium bicarbonate also increase activity.[190] The application of ultrasonic energy to glutaraldehyde solutions has been used to good effect.[61] Addition of a second antimicrobial agent to provide a synergistic effect has also been reported. In this respect, addition of phenol to glutaraldehyde has proved to be beneficial.[191,192] Reports on other novel glutaraldehyde formulations have been reviewed elsewhere.[16] A different direction in formulation is to aim for increased effectiveness over time. A 3.2% alkaline glutaraldehyde solution has been evaluated in an automatic machine for disinfection of fiberoptic endoscopes.[193] The glutaraldehyde concentration in the solution remained higher than 2% even after 102 consecutive wash cycles and 28 days use. A variety of materials were tested in contact with this higher glutaraldehyde concentration and were not damaged.

Toxicology

The use of glutaraldehyde for the chemical disinfection of heat-sensitive equipment or other surfaces is widespread in clinical, industrial, and laboratory applications.

This type of specialized use brings possible risks of toxic reactions occurring (1) to the individual handling the equipment during the disinfecting or sterilizing process and (2) to the patient exposed to equipment treated with glutaraldehyde—in some cases, this may involve contact with the blood stream. With regard to individuals being exposed to glutaraldehyde during handling of equipment, investigators using results of a questionnaire reported that 37% of endoscopy units using glutaraldehyde for disinfection reported health problems among their staff that were attributed to glutaraldehyde use.[194] Other reports of occupational toxicity refer to small numbers of individuals.[195-198] Provocation testing was used to determine allergic reactions in nurses who reported respiratory symptoms that they attributed to exposure to glutaraldehyde.[199] Two of the four patients investigated had a confirmed reaction to glutaraldehyde. Estimates of percutaneous penetration of topically applied glutaraldehyde (10% aqueous solution) indicated that although no penetration of thick stratum corneum could be detected, approximately 3% penetrated epidermis and 3% to 13.8% penetration of thin stratum corneum occurred.[200] Irritation and one case of sensitization also resulted from application of glutaraldehyde to areas of thin stratum corneum. Evidence for a dose-dependent contact hypersensitivity response to glutaraldehyde was demonstrated in guinea pigs and mice.[201] Inhalation is severely toxic when high-aldehyde concentrations are allowed to evaporate in a closed system. Single inhalations of concentrated vapors (25% and 50% glutaraldehyde) by rats for 6 to 8 hours did not kill any of the exposed animals.[202] A number of more recent studies have shown glutaraldehyde causes damage to the upper respiratory tract in animals.[203-205] It is practical to state that safer use of liquid solutions, such as with adequate ventilation, etc, can reduce these risks significantly.[206]

It is important to reduce the risks of glutaraldehyde toxicity to staff by using clearly defined handling procedures such as wearing of rubber gloves (provided they are resistant to organic chemicals) and safety goggles. Siting of equipment in hoods or cabinets with exhaust is also necessary to prevent vapor inhalation. A patch-test was used to determine sensitivity levels to glutaraldehyde and found an increased level of sensitization (9.9% versus 2.6%) among health care workers.[207] A review of glutaraldehyde exposure and its impact in the health care environment suggested workplace exposure reduction could be achieved through maintenance of adequate ventilation levels where glutaraldehyde is in use, as well as rigid adherence to personal protective equipment guidelines, and banning unnecessary practices such as glutaraldehyde fogging.[208]

A number of publications have considered the risk to the patient from using glutaraldehyde-treated equipment. Approximately 10% of glutaraldehyde absorbed by rubber or plastic parts was found to be released slowly in 24 hours.[209] A useful and comprehensive report studied the residual glutaraldehyde in plastics and rubbers after exposure to alkaline glutaraldehyde solution.[210] The degree of absorption of glutaraldehyde into various materials correlated with time of contact between material and solution. The absorbed glutaraldehyde was confined to the surface of the exposed material, and a single 2-minute rinse procedure significantly reduced glutaraldehyde levels. Further rinsing had little effect, although an extended immersion in rinsing solution did cause considerable desorption. On repeated exposure to glutaraldehyde, as would occur in practice, a buildup in glutaraldehyde levels was apparent only in latex rubber. Therefore, for this material, extended soaking and rinsing procedures were recommended. In a report on the use of glutaraldehyde to process tissue heart valves, a glutaraldehyde concentration of greater than 10 to 25 ppm was reported to cause toxic effects on cells of any type.[49] A protocol of three separate rinses in 500 mL of sterile normal saline for 2 minute each with gentle agitation was recommended. This gave glutaraldehyde concentrations in the final rinse of less than 1 ppm. Glutaraldehyde release from bioprostheses can induce cytotoxic reactions.[49,211,212] Various rinsing procedures have been recommended to reduce aldehyde levels, including rinsing followed by storage in glutaraldehyde-free solutions.[211] There have been numerous reports of colitis resulting from glutaraldehyde contact with the gastrointestinal tract. This has been linked to the inadequate rinsing of flexible endoscope, including internal channels enabled glutaraldehyde to be introduced to the tissue.[213,214] In many of these cases, the instructions of use with glutaraldehyde disinfectant solutions may not be adequately followed to include the method of rinsing (eg, full immersion in water) and number of recommended rinses that can vary considerably depending on the disinfectant formulation and registered labeling.[182,215]

The LD$_{50}$ value of glutaraldehyde was estimated to be 15 mg/kg in mice and 9.8 mg/kg in rats.[2] These values correlated with other findings that damage to leucocytes was apparent only above a 100 μg/mL glutaraldehyde level.[210] In addition, no erythrocyte damage occurred at the glutaraldehyde concentrations used. From these observations, it was concluded that even in extremely adverse circumstances, there was little risk of damage to blood cells due to the use of glutaraldehyde-treated apparatus. A potentiated acid glutaraldehyde was judged not to be teratogenic to mice in spite of using relatively high doses.[216] Glutaraldehyde was not found to be mutagenic in the Ames test[217] and in four in-vitro systems involving microbial and mammalian-cell indicator tests.[218] A review by Zeiger et al[219] of the genetic toxicity and carcinogenicity of glutaraldehyde revealed that bone marrow hyperplasia and low levels of leukemia were seen in one chronic drinking water study in rats, but this was not observed in three other chronic inhalation studies with either rats or mice.

A study examined differences in toxicity between acid and alkaline glutaraldehyde.[220] Some differences were observed, for example, acute peroral LD_{50} values for rats were 3.45 g/kg (acid) and 4.16 g/kg (alkaline) with signs and gross pathology similar. No systemic effect following 24-hour cutaneous application was seen with acid glutaraldehyde and only a few with alkaline (unsteady gait, sluggishness, rapid breathing). Local skin irritation and corneal injury were also more marked with the alkaline solution. In a final report on the safety assessment of glutaraldehyde, the problems inherent with its use in cosmetic products was summarized.[221] No embryotoxic, fetotoxic, or teratogenic effects were observed at concentrations that did not cause severe maternal toxicity. The no-observable adverse effects level for reproduction toxicity was >1000 ppm. Bacterial mutagenesis tests produced mixed results as expected for a preservative. Further dermal carcinogenicity studies were required to complete the safety assessment of glutaraldehyde for use in "leave-on" products. Following the publication of this report, newly available studies were analyzed in terms of concentration and frequency of use. The panel determined not to reopen this safety assessment and confirmed the conclusions of the original report.[222,223] It was concluded that if glutaraldehyde did not exceed 0.5%, it could be used in "rinse-off" products for brief and discontinuous use, but because of its respiratory irritation, it should not be used in aerosolized cosmetic products. It was noted, however, that glutaraldehyde is currently being used in an aerosol product and in "leave-on" products.[224]

Concern as to the accuracy of testing (bias, precision, overall uncertainty) between European laboratories for aldehyde levels in workplace air has been addressed in a comprehensive study.[225] Thirty one laboratories from European Union member states participated in the study, which showed that glutaraldehyde testing complied with the standard EN 482 with an overall uncertainty of 30%.[226]

▶ APPLICATIONS

Glutaraldehyde is used extensively in several major nonmicrobiological areas, including the leather tanning industry and tissue fixation for electron microscopy. In a microbiologic context, glutaraldehyde has mainly been employed for the liquid chemical disinfectant (including sterilant activity) of medical and surgical material that cannot be sterilized by heat or irradiation.

Several advantages provide the basis for glutaraldehyde's use as a chemosterilizer:

1. Broad spectrum of activity, including sporicidal activity and rapidity of action
2. Activity in the presence of organic matter
3. Noncorrosive action toward metals, rubber, lenses, and most materials (although some formulations may not fulfill these criteria)[122]

But the increase in number of reports of occupational sensitivity reactions and mycobacterial resistance profiles has resulted in growing concern about glutaraldehyde use, and adequate safety precautions are required to minimize risk of toxicity among operators. In many areas, this has led to an increased use of alternative disinfectant types including OPA and oxidizing agents (see chapter 47). Disinfection of endoscopy equipment and other semicritical devices has become one of the main uses of glutaraldehyde. These instruments must be free of pathogens such as hepatitis B, HIV, and *M tuberculosis* to prevent transmission of infection between patients. The traditional heating methods of disinfection or sterilization are unsuitable because they damage the instruments, and although ethylene oxide is recommended, it is not always available and is a time-consuming process. The requirement for a rapid turnover of equipment necessitated rapid high-level liquid disinfection, and glutaraldehyde was regarded since the 1950s as the agent of choice.[227,228] A 30-minute immersion was recommended following use of an endoscope on a patient or carrier of hepatitis B or AIDS, and a 1-hour immersion following use in a tuberculosis patient.[228] In later work, glutaraldehyde was recommended as a first-line disinfectant and a 4-minute soak was proposed to be sufficient for the inactivation of vegetative bacteria and viruses, including HIV and HBV.[229] Many additional references have been made to the use of glutaraldehyde for rapid and safe disinfection of gastrointestinal endoscopy equipment.[230-233]

Early recommendations also suggested the use of glutaraldehyde for cold disinfection of hemostats, cystoscopes, food containers, and anaesthetic equipment.[234] The success of this practice was confirmed by several authors.[235,236] It has also proved useful for disinfection of urologic instruments[237] and gynecologic laparoscopy equipment.[238] Occasionally, adverse effects of glutaraldehyde on medical equipment are observed.[239] Glutaraldehyde was also widely used for disinfecting dental surgical instruments and working surfaces where the hepatitis B surface antigen may be present.[240] Peroxygen disinfectant, as alternatives, were also less practical in these situations due to material compatibility and costs. Glutaraldehyde-moistened sponges were shown to be suitable for disinfecting dental equipment that could not be heat sterilized or immersed in a fluid bath because of large size, fixed position, or destructible parts, although attention to detail on the careful rinsing of this equipment to prevent cross-contamination or toxicity (as with any liquid disinfectant/sterilant) is important to consider.[241] Also in the dental field, a low-concentration, stable glutaraldehyde disinfectant/cleaner was shown to be effective for aspirator care.[242] Dental unit waterlines are a problem in relation to infection spread to patients. Microbial biofilm formation on these can be inherently resistant to antimicrobial agents (see chapter 67). The efficacy of a number of agents in this situation was found glutaraldehyde to be effective in reducing the bacterial count but did not destroy the biofilm matrix allowing bacterial recurrence.[243] Other have reported concerns on the cross-linking of extraneous materials onto surfaces when using glutaraldehyde (particularly when surfaces have not be cleaned effectively), which can promote the development of biofilms and resistant bacteria.[92,244]

The effectiveness of vapor-phase glutaraldehyde for surface disinfection against vegetative bacteria and spores was reported, when in spite of its low volatility, it was more effective than formaldehyde on an added amount basis.[245] Others found glutaraldehyde to have good disinfectant activity in the aerosol state and recommended it for disinfection of surfaces.[246] In a related study, the effectiveness of glutaraldehyde in reducing surface contamination of packaged medical devices was investigated.[247] Glutaraldehyde was able to penetrate several types of packaging material, although not polyethylene film. Despite these initial reports, the use of glutaraldehyde in vapor or aerosol form has not seen widespread use, primarily due to safety risks.

The treatment of viral warts with glutaraldehyde has been reported on several occasions.[248-250] A 73.5% cure rate with 227 patients with viral warts treated with aqueous ethanol and collodion-based preparations of glutaraldehyde was demonstrated.[251] A 10% solution (pH 4.2) in aqueous ethanol was found to be most convenient. Similar results are claimed for glutaraldehyde (10%) as a semisolid aqueous-based gel for the treatment of plantar warts.[252] Aqueous solutions of glutaraldehyde have been used to treat hyperhydrosis,[253] and topically applied glutaraldehyde has been effective in the treatment of onychomycosis.[254] Several dental applications have been described, including anticaries formulations.[255,256] A glutaraldehyde-calcium hydroxide combination was shown to be an effective pulp dressing for dental work.[257]

Frequently in immunochemical work, the need arises to link proteins to particles, to polymerize proteins, or to form covalent conjugates of proteins and smaller peptides.[42] Glutaraldehyde is one of the few reagents that have been successfully used for all the earlier applications while also preserving the native antigenicity of the material under study. In the immunologic field, glutaraldehyde has been used in the preparation of vaccines such as tetanus[258-260] and pertussis.[261] In a study of detoxification of tetanus toxin, glutaraldehyde proved to be most favorable compared to the activity of formaldehyde or β-propiolactone.[262] The use of the agent in radioimmune assays for a specific antigen has been reported,[263] and the preparation of vaccines by the action of glutaraldehyde on toxins, bacteria, viruses, allergens, and cells has been reviewed elsewhere.[264]

The antimicrobial properties of glutaraldehyde have also been applied in other areas. In the poultry industry, glutaraldehyde has been employed as a disinfectant in the immersion chilling of poultry.[265] A 10-minute prechill in 0.5% glutaraldehyde (pH 8.6) extended shelf life of boiler

carcasses at 2°C approximately 6 days beyond controls[266]; salmonella transfer was also prevented. In the cosmetic industry, glutaraldehyde has been recommended for disinfection of production equipment[267] and as a preservative.[202,268] The sterilization of fermentation media has been reported in the patent literature.[269] Glutaraldehyde also has certain advantages over formaldehyde as the preservative employed in the ancient art of embalming.[270] In the veterinary field,[271] the introduction of glutaraldehyde as a teat-skin disinfectant for control of mastitis has been successful. Glutaraldehyde was shown to be more effective than iodine in preventing new intramammary infection, and no evidence of teat skin irritation was observed.

Glutaraldehyde has been applied in combating microbial contamination, particularly sulphate-reducing bacteria, in oil-field water injection systems.[272] It has been used as a gelling agent (hydroxypropylmethyl cellulose) for packaging agent and minimizing the hazards to personnel and materials during shipping of explanted medical devices for analysis.[273] The use of glutaraldehyde as a cross-linking agent for bioprostheses such as heart valves, vascular grafts, elastic cartilages, tendon xenografts, and artificial skin has been reviewed.[274] This includes its use for fixing of cells and its increasingly important application in controlled drug delivery systems whereby its ability to cross-link proteins and polysaccharides is employed to useful effect. Medical devices of many types are being increasing employed with the attendant risk of infection being transmitted to the patient. Glutaraldehyde is a very valuable agent in preventing this risk[275] with needleless or jet injector use for bone marrow aspirations, lumbar punctures, and cutaneous and intraoral injections.

In 2015, the European Commission approved glutaraldehyde as an active biocidal agent for various disinfection purposes, under the newer requirements defined in the Biocides Directive. These included hard surface disinfection in hospitals, poultry, and pig farm disinfection; food vessel and machinery disinfection; and food processing surface disinfection.[276] In 2017, the EPA in the United States re-registered glutaraldehyde as an active ingredient in pesticides.[277] Glutaraldehyde continues to find new applications, in particular in enzyme immobilization for biocatalysis[278-280] and cross-linking, such as with chitosan, for applications including drug delivery and antimicrobial activity.[281-283]

Formaldehyde

Formaldehyde (systematic name methanal) exists as a freely water-soluble gas. Unlike glutaraldehyde, which has two aldehyde functional groups, formaldehyde is a monoaldehyde. Formaldehyde has a similar mechanism of action to glutaraldehyde. Formaldehyde inactivates microorganisms by acting as an alkylating agent, causing protein cross-linking by reacting with the amino and sulfhydryl groups of proteins, as well as reacting with purine bases of DNA and RNA. For the purposes of disinfection, formaldehyde is normally used as a water-based solution known as formalin, which contains 37% formaldehyde by weight.

As with glutaraldehyde, formaldehyde can be bactericidal, sporicidal, fungicidal, and virucidal. Formaldehyde inactivated 10^4 M tuberculosis in 2 minutes with a 4% solution, and a 2.5% solution inactivated 10^7 Salmonella ser Typhi in 10 minutes in the presence of organic matter. A number of viruses were inactivated by 2% formalin, and 8% formalin solution inactivated poliovirus in 10 minutes. Although formaldehyde destroys a wide range of microorganisms, it has a slower sporicidal activity than glutaraldehyde, with a 4% formaldehyde solution requiring a 2-hour contact time with B subtilis spores to achieve an inactivation factor of 10^4, compared with 15 minutes for 2% glutaraldehyde.[284]

Specific MIC breakpoint values for formaldehyde have yet to be defined but are likely to be underestimated or difficult to define due to the direct reaction of the microbicide with the growth media constituents (see chapter 61). The susceptibility of a number of microorganisms to formaldehyde was investigated in a recent study, with MIC values determined for the following species: Bacillus stearothermophilus (0.03%), B subtilis (0.02%), Acinetobacter calcoaceticus (0.01%), Enterobacter cloacae (0.01%), E coli (0.02%), Serratia marcescens (0.01%), and S aureus (0.02%).[285] In a study by the same group, the decimal reduction time (D-value) was determined for B subtilis (11.8 min), B stearothermophilus (10.9 min), and A calcoaceticus (5.2 min), using a solution of 0.5% formaldehyde as disinfectant.[286] In a separate study, the susceptibility of 442 bacterial isolates from livestock in Denmark to formaldehyde was assessed, with MIC values ranging from 0.0008% to 0.0125%, with most isolates in the range 0.003% to 0.006%. In this study, development of resistance to formaldehyde was not apparent.[287] Resistance mechanisms to formaldehyde has been reported elsewhere.[92] For example, a formaldehyde-resistant strain of E coli (MIC = 0.07%) was reported, and the gene responsible was identified, which was subsequently found in other resistant E coli strains.[288-290] The formaldehyde resistance mechanisms in the formaldehyde-resistant strain E coli VU3695 were investigated. A large (4.6 kb) plasmid DNA fragment encompassing the formaldehyde resistance gene was sequenced. A single 1107-bp open reading frame encoding a glutathione-and NAD-dependent formaldehyde dehydrogenase was identified and sequenced, and the enzyme was expressed in an in vitro assay and purified. Amino acid sequence homology studies showed 62.4% to 63.2% identity with class III alcohol dehydrogenases isolated from horse, human, and rat livers. We demonstrated that the resistance mechanism in the formaldehyde-resistant strain E coli VU3695 and in other formaldehyde-resistant members of the family

Enterobacteriaceae is based on the enzymatic degradation of formaldehyde by a formaldehyde dehydrogenase. As with glutaraldehyde, nosocomial outbreaks caused by formaldehyde-resistant mycobacteria have been reported. Slow-growing species such as M avium, M intracellulare, and Mycobacterium gordonae were capable of surviving 2% formaldehyde for more than 10 minutes, with water-adapted strains of the faster growing Mycobacterium mucogenicum surviving for 24 hours, and even in 10% concentrations for shorter periods.[291] Several disease outbreaks have been associated with formaldehyde resistance, including the use of reusable hemodialysis equipment.[292] Formaldehyde resistance has also been due to cell surface modifications (including during spore development) and due to viral clumping.[92] Such mechanisms are not dissimilar to those described for glutaraldehyde.

Historically, formaldehyde was used in a health care setting to sterilize surgical instruments, especially when mixed with ethanol and/or in a humidified gas process. Gas processes have been traditionally used for area fumigation (especially in research laboratory applications) and for medical device sterilization (for further discussion, see chapter 36). Formaldehyde is also used in the production of viral vaccines, as an embalming agent, and as a disinfectant in hemodialysis equipment.[284] Use in the latter has experienced a considerable decline. A 2005 report surveying dialysis-associated disease in the United States showed the percentage of centers using formaldehyde to reprocess dialyzers had dropped from 94% to 20% in the preceding two decades.[293] Overall, equipment, device, or area/room applications with formaldehyde have seen a significant decline in use due to not only increased concerns on safety but also the availability of alternative technologies (especially with hydrogen peroxide disinfection and sterilization systems; see chapters 18 and 32).

Formaldehyde has also found widespread use as a disinfectant in poultry farms, although reports on its efficacy for removal of Salmonella species from poultry houses using a 1% vol/vol solution vary. A number of studies report formaldehyde having a greater efficacy at this concentration compared with glutaraldehyde, as well as proving more efficacious in field conditions, although total Salmonella elimination was not guaranteed.[294-298] Formalin is also one of the most used disinfectants in aquaculture, although the margin between effectively eliminating the infectious water-borne agent and avoiding damage to fish can be small. This can result in damage to gills and alterations in mucous cells as well as negative effects on water quality.[299] Further to its use as a disinfectant and preservative (especially formaldehyde-releasing agents; see chapters 38-40), formaldehyde is also used in the production of resins and binders for wood products and in the production of plastics, coatings, and flooring materials.[300]

The use of formaldehyde in disinfection has reduced significantly in recent decades, due largely to the detrimental health impacts following formaldehyde exposure, in particular long-term exposure via inhalation. Adverse health effects of formaldehyde have long been known, with irritation of the eyes and upper airways reported following formaldehyde exposure in prefabricated houses as early as the 1960s.[300] The International Agency for Research on Cancer has classified formaldehyde as "carcinogenic to humans (Group 1)," on the basis that formaldehyde may cause nasopharyngeal cancer and leukemia. The most recent reviews by the National Toxicology Program and the EPA have also classified formaldehyde as known human carcinogens, based also on epidemiologic evidence that formaldehyde exposure causes both of these cancers.[301-305] A recent meta-analysis revealed that current formaldehyde exposure concentrations are relatively safe in terms of cancer risk.[306] Airborne formaldehyde does, however, continue to cause eye irritation, with a concentration of less than 0.001 mg/m^3 required in order to be considered safe.[306] Formaldehyde exposure has also been linked to the development of asthma in children, as well as work-related asthma with health care professionals, although systematic reviews in this area suggest much more robust and wide-ranging studies are required to generate a more definitive evidence base.[307-309]

The use of formaldehyde for sterilization has been associated with a number of additional drawbacks, with infective agents for scrapie, CJD, and transmissible mink encephalopathy (TME) remaining viable following treatment with formaldehyde.[310,311] In fact, it has been suggested that the fixative properties of formaldehyde may have been responsible for the survival of these agents, fixing the agents to medical devices and enabling further iatrogenic transmission of diseases overtime such as CJD.[312] Formaldehyde has also been implicated in the development of Alzheimer disease, with formaldehyde shown to reduce lysine acetylation of cytosolic histones, compromising histone content in chromatin, a conserved feature of aging across different domains of life.[313]

Ortho-phthalaldehyde

The widespread application of glutaraldehyde as a high-level disinfectant and sterilant has been accompanied by the emergence of resistance[86,88] and reported health problems associated with glutaraldehyde use (including dermatitis and occupational asthma).[314-317] These concerns stimulated efforts to discover or design novel biocidal agents and associated formulations. These have included formulations based on oxidizing agents and alternative aldehydes, such as OPA. The OPA (systematic name 1,2-benzenedicarboxaldehyde) is the most recently approved aldehyde biocide to enter widespread use as a high-level disinfectant, having received approval from the FDA in October 1999. The OPA exhibits broad-spectrum bactericidal[318-320] but relatively slower sporicidal activity.[321]

Unlike glutaraldehyde formulations, OPA can be readily formulated to not require activation and exhibits excellent stability across a wide pH range (pH 3-9).[320] Due to its demonstrated excellent antimicrobial activity and apparent lack of toxicity to the eyes and nasal mucosa, lack of perceptible odor, low volatility, and excellent material compatibility, OPA has been promoted as a safe and effective replacement for glutaraldehyde for high-level disinfection, especially for dental and medical equipment including endoscopes. However, recent toxicity studies and clinical case studies challenge the initial claims of safety and further work to establish safe exposure concentration limits is certainly required.

The OPA is a soluble and stable aromatic dialdehyde, which in solution forms a clear, pale blue liquid (pH 7.5). Typical in-use concentrations for high-level disinfection of heat-sensitive medical devices and surfaces are 0.55%. It is sensitive to UV and oxidation in air. The mechanism of action of OPA is similar to that of glutaraldehyde, but OPA exhibits much less potent cross-linking activity. The OPA is more lipophilic, which may contribute to increased accumulation and uptake in mycobacteria and gram-negative bacteria.[322] A proposed mechanism for cross-linking primary amines in the peptide chain by the aromatic dialdehyde OPA is given in Figure 23.10.[322] The peptide-OPA-peptide complex formed as a result of modification of both aldehyde groups is expected to be energetically unfavorable due to steric hindrance; thus, monosubstituted OPA-peptide complex are likely to be preferable and accounting for a lower cross-linking capacity when compared to the flexible, aliphatic glutaraldehyde.

The OPA has excellent microbicidal activity, across a range of microorganisms.[318,320,323,324] It exhibits superior mycobacterial activity when compared with glutaraldehyde. In one study, the mean time to achieve a 6 log$_{10}$ reduction of *M bovis* using 0.21% OPA was 6 minutes, compared to 32 minutes for glutaraldehyde at 1.5% (Table 23.9).[325] The OPA has excellent microbicidal activity against pseudomonads,[324,326] *C albicans*,[327] and the intestinal parasite *Cryptosporidium parvum*.[328] In a number of studies using *P fluorescens*, the mechanism of action of OPA have been studied and reveal a multitarget mode of action.[324,326] The OPA binds membrane receptors due to cross-linkage, facilitates biocide entry to the cell by impairment of membrane function (alters cell surface hydrophobicity but not outer membrane protein expression), and interacts with intracellular molecules including RNA and DNA (the latter observed only at high concentrations of OPA.[324] Bovine serum albumin noticeably impaired the action of OPA at pH 9.[324] Aldehyde biocides also have fixative properties, which could potentially lead to the accumulation of organic material at surfaces, thus reducing their biocidal efficacy at surfaces.[329]

Initially, OPA was shown to be effective against strains of glutaraldehyde-resistant mycobacteria and *B subtilis*

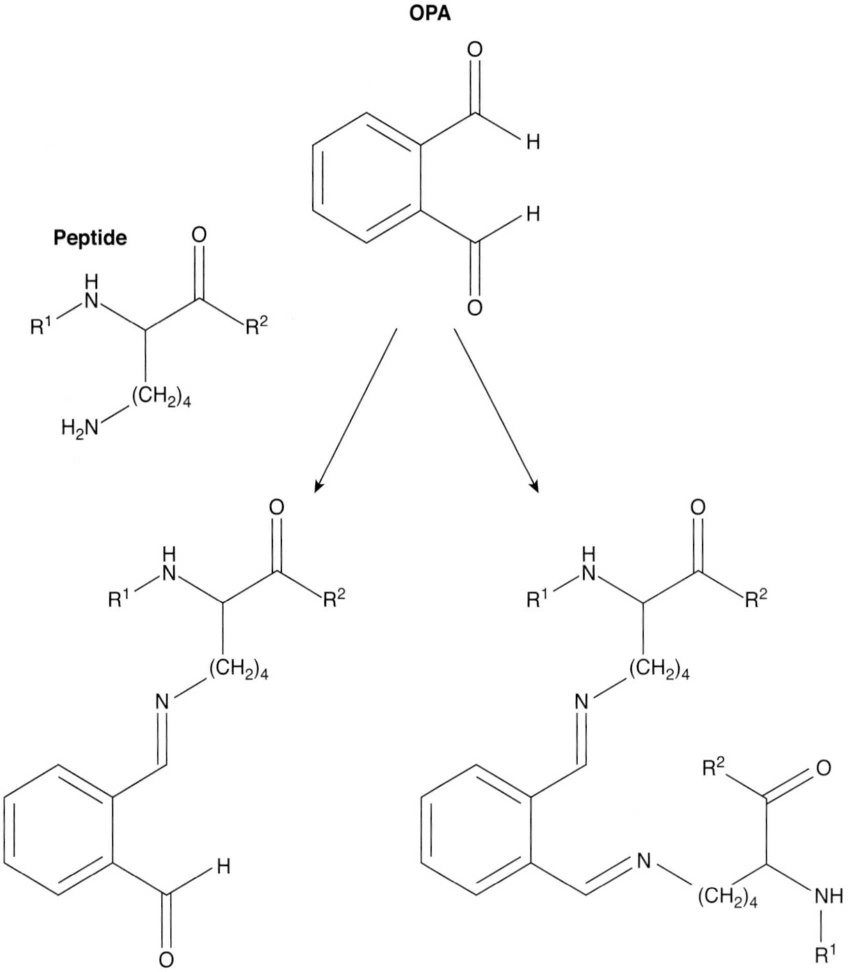

FIGURE 23.10 Two potential scenarios for cross-linking of ortho-phthalaldehyde (OPA) via reaction with primary amines on peptides and proteins: OPA-peptide cross-linking via a single aldehyde group (A) or peptide-OPA-peptide complex formed via cross-linking through both aldehyde functional groups with primary amines of two peptides (B). The reaction of both aldehydes is expected to produce an energetically unfavorable complex due to steric hindrance.[322]

spores,[321] indicating a lack of emergence cross-resistance between glutaraldehyde and OPA. A number of recent studies have indicated that cross-resistance to OPA may be an emerging risk and should be considered in longer term use of the biocide. *P aeruginosa* strains, which were resistant or multiresistant to antibiotics, have a decreased susceptibility to OPA, whereas at the same time, resistant and multiresistant *P aeruginosa* exhibit increased OPA sensitivity following laboratory adaptation.[330] In a follow-up study, the authors demonstrated an association with *P aeruginosa* antibiotic resistance and OPA susceptibility, indicating the importance of evaluating resistant

TABLE 23.9 Activity of glutaraldehyde and ortho-phthalaldehyde against *Mycobacterium bovis*

Disinfectant	Time for 6 Log_{10} Reduction
1.5% Glutaraldehyde	28-36 min
2.5% Glutaraldehyde	14-18 min
0.21% Ortho-phthalaldehyde	4.8-6.3 min

Range of values from two different laboratories.[320]

and multiresistant strains in routine disinfectant efficacy testing of OPA.[331] The isolation of mycobacteria (*M avium* and *M chelonae/M abscessus*) from automated endoscope reprocessing systems following OPA disinfection, which exhibited resistance to OPA at high-level disinfection in-use concentrations has recently been reported,[88] giving rise not only to concerns associated with transmission of infection via reprocessed endoscopic equipment and other medical devices but also to the emergence of stable resistance to OPA.

The OPA is a weakly sporicidal biocide,[320,321] and glutaraldehyde exhibits superior sporicidal activity.[321] As with glutaraldehyde, vegetative cells are much more sensitive to OPA than spores.[321,332] Although it was assumed that mechanisms of action and spore resistance are similar to those of glutaraldehyde, Cabrera-Martinez and coworkers[333] conducted detailed studies into the mechanism of spore inactivation by OPA and the development of resistance in *B subtilis* spores. In agreement with an earlier study, OPA (10 g/L) at pH 7.8 resulted in sporicidal activity, which was much less effective when the concentration of OPA was reduced to 5 g/L (a concentration that produced greater than 4 $\log_{10}$ reduction in vegetative bacteria within 5 min at room temperature [RT]). *B subtilis* spores were not sensitive to OPA at RT, but increasing the temperature to 37°C or 50°C increased spore sensitivity to OPA. In agreement with earlier work, the spore coat was found to be an important determinant of *B subtilis* spore sensitivity to OPA because spore decoating or mutation to *cotE* (which disrupts spore coat assembly) significantly increased sporicidal activity. Importantly, OPA-treated spores were found not to germinate and could not be recovered by exogenous germinants. Taken together, spore resistance to OPA appears to be related to the presence of spore coats, and sporicidal activity is not by DNA damage, with death possibly due to cross-linking of key membrane proteins by OPA.[333] A more recent study on *B anthracis* spores demonstrated that at typical in-use concentrations, glutaraldehyde exhibited significantly higher sporicidal (4 $\log_{10}$ reduction times) kill (19.2-34.46 min) compared to OPA (109.2-157.5 min) for a range of *B anthracis* strains,[334] supporting the earlier findings.[321]

To date, aside from manufacturer-reported studies, there is limited available data on the virucidal activity of OPA in the scientific literature. A number of reports indicate that OPA exhibits reasonable viricidal activity against a range of viruses. An initial report was on the activity of a range of disinfectants, including OPA, against adenovirus type 8.[335] In these studies, with an efficacy criterion of a 3 $\log_{10}$ reduction after 1-minute exposure, OPA (0.55%) achieved a >3 $\log_{10}$ reduction. The viricidal activity of OPA has also been reported against hepatitis B and C viruses (using surrogate viruses duck hepatitis B virus [DHBV] and bovine viral diarrhea virus [BVDV]). In this study, EPA guidelines for efficacy criterion of minimum

3 $\log_{10}$ reduction in surrogate virus beyond the cytotoxic level and at least 4 $\log_{10}$ reduction of the recovered dried virus control were adopted.[336] The OPA solutions (0.5%) at 20°C for 5 minutes gave a greater than 4 $\log_{10}$ reduction in BVDV titre on an inanimate surface, whereas 0.3% OPA was effective at against DHBV dried on an inanimate surface (4.4 $\log_{10}$ reduction after 5 min).[336] In an evaluation of 11 chemical biocides, formulated and unformulated, against a panel of enveloped and nonenveloped viruses dried on inanimate surfaces (5- and 10-min contact times), OPA (0.55%) at 10-minute exposure times gave a >5 $\log_{10}$ reduction of porcine parvovirus (PPV), whereas a 5-minute exposure was ineffective. Furthermore, 5-minute exposure of OPA (0.55%) proved effective against minute virus of mice, poliovirus strain Sabin, adenovirus type 5, and vaccinia virus with greater than 4 $\log_{10}$ reduction observed in each case.[118] When evaluated against two surrogate coronaviruses (mouse hepatitis virus [MHV] and transmissible gastroenteritis virus [TGEV]) using the quantitative carrier method on stainless steel coupons, OPA (0.55%) contact time 1 minute, achieved a $\log_{10}$ reduction factor of 2.3 and 1.7 for TGEV and MHV, respectively, indicating that contact time is a crucial consideration when OPA is employed for the disinfection of virally contaminated surfaces.[337] Currently, biocidal agents that have the potential to cross-link proteins (including OPA) should not be employed in the disinfection and decontamination of prion infected surfaces,[338] with OPA (0.55%) having been shown to be ineffective (≤ 3 $\log_{10}$ reduction within 1 h) in the inactivation of prions.[339]

The OPA has been promoted as a safer alternative to glutaraldehyde because its introduction into widespread use as a high-level disinfectant, despite the paucity of evidence available to either support or rebut such claims.[317] A recent review of the literature and manufacturer's toxicity data of a range of high-level disinfectant agents revealed that although all agents had the potential to act as dermal irritants, OPA is a potential dermal and respiratory sensitizer.[317] A summary of comparison of dermal and respiratory toxicity data for glutaraldehyde and OPA at concentrations approximating in-use conditions is given in Table 23.10. From the few toxicity studies available in the literature, OPA certainly appears to be chemical irritant and sensitizer and may act as an adjuvant for other allergens.[340,341] A 3-day inhalation exposure study found that OPA exposure leads to respiratory sensitization in mice.[342] In recent years, a number of clinical case reports have challenged the safety of glutaraldehyde substitution for OPA, these include the first reported cases of occupational asthma in health care workers following exposure to OPA, in each case as a result of exposure during disinfection of endoscopes and other medical devices.[343,344] More recently, the respiratory tract toxicity of OPA was studied in Harlan Sprague-Dawley rats and B6C3F1/N mice. In this study, experimental animals

TABLE 23.10 Summary of comparison of dermal and respiratory toxicity data for glutaraldehyde and ortho-phthalaldehyde at concentrations approximating in-use conditions[a]

	Glutaraldehyde	Ortho-phthalaldehyde
In-use concentration	2%-4%	0.55%
Cytotoxicity	Cytotoxic (2.5%)	Cytotoxic (0.6%)
Dermal sensitization	Allergic contact dermatitis/ skin sensitization (0.25%-5%)	Nonsensitizing
Skin/eye irritation	Skin irritant (1%-2%)	Nonirritating to skin; moderate eye irritant; corrosive
	Irreversible eye irritant (2.4%)	Skin, eye and mucous membrane irritant; nonallergic dermatitis (0.55%-0.56%)
Respiratory sensitization	Respiratory sensitization/ occupational asthmas (2%)	No known studies of respiratory sensitization
Respiratory irritation	Respiratory irritation (2%)	Respiratory irritation; aggravation of existing respiratory conditions (0.55%)

[a]From Rideout et al.[317]

were exposed to OPA by whole-body inhalation for 3 months at concentrations of 0.44 to 7.0 ppm. All animals presented exhibited a spectrum of lesions throughout the respiratory tract (nose, larynx, trachea, and lungs), as well as on the skin and eyes, which were consistent with a severe irritant response. Interestingly, this compared to an earlier study on glutaraldehyde toxicity, OPA exposure led to greater incidence and severity of nasal tract toxicity at similar exposure concentrations.[345] In a separate study, the authors also reported a significant reduction in survival and histopathologic lesions in the testes and epididymitis of male rats and mice in a 13-week OPA inhalation exposure study, which was limited to the two highest exposure concentrations tested (3.5 and 7.0 ppm).[346]

According to manufacturer guidance and Centers for Disease Control and Prevention–published guidance, OPA must be handled with care in appropriately ventilated areas and using appropriate personal protective equipment (gloves, eye protection),[284,347] due to potential contemporary concerns regarding respiratory tract toxicity, and OPA-mediated staining of proteins (including the skin) grey.[284,318] Following disinfection, endoscopes and other devices should be rinsed thoroughly with water (in accordance with manufacturer's instructions that can vary depending on the formulation) to reduce chemical residue to levels that would not induce an irritant, anaphylactic, or allergic response (<1 ppm).[348] Taken together, initial claims of limited or nontoxicity of OPA at in-use conditions and the replacement of glutaraldehyde by OPA for high-level disinfection based on superior toxicity profile appear to require closer scrutiny; further detailed and appropriately powered toxicity studies to determine actual safety profile and appropriate occupational exposure limits are required.

REFERENCES

1. Pepper R, Lieberman E, inventors; Ethicon Inc, assignee. Dialdehyde alcoholic sporicidal compositions. US patent 3,016,328. January 9, 1962.
2. Stonehill A, Krop S, Borick P. Buffered glutaraldehyde—a new chemical sterilizing solution. *Am J Hosp Pharm.* 1963;20:458-465.
3. Harries C, Tank L. Conversion of cyclopentene into the mono- and di-aldehyde of glutaric acid. *Berichte.* 1908;41:1701-1711.
4. Bowes J, Carter C. The reaction of glutaraldehyde with proteins and other biological materials. *J R Microsc Soc.* 1966;85:193-200.
5. Hopwood D, Allen C, McCabe C. The reaction between glutaraldehyde and various proteins: an investigation of their kinetics. *Histochem J.* 1970;2:137-150.
6. Anderson P. Purification and quantification of glutaraldehyde and its effect on several enzyme activities in skeletal muscle. *J Histochem Cytochem.* 1967;15:652-661.
7. Hardy P, Nicholls A, Rydon H. The nature of glutaraldehyde in aqueous solution. *J Chem Soc D.* 1969;1969:565-566.
8. Pease D. *Histological Techniques for Electron Microscopy.* 2nd ed. Amsterdam, Netherlands: Elsevier; 1964.
9. Fahimi H, Drochmans P. Essais de standardisation de la fixation au glutaraldehyde. *J Microsc.* 1965;4:725-736.
10. Hopwood D. Theoretical and practical aspects of glutaraldehyde fixation. *Histochem J.* 1972;4:267-303.
11. Dijk F, Oosterbaan J, Hulstaert C. A rapid method for obtaining monomeric glutaraldehyde. *Histochemistry.* 1985;83:573-574.
12. Gillett R, Gull K. Glutaraldehyde—its purity and stability. *Histochemie.* 1972;30:162-167.
13. Stibenz V. About the spectralphotometric analysis and the index of purification E235/E280 of glutaraldehyde. *Acta Histochem.* 1973;47:83-88.
14. Rasmussen K, Albrechtsen J. Glutaraldehyde. The influence of pH, temperature, and buffering on the polymerization rate. *Histochemistry.* 1974;38:19-26.
15. Gorman S, Scott E. Potentiation and stabilization of glutaraldehyde biocidal activity utilizing surfactant-divalent cation combinations. *Int J Pharm.* 1979;4:57-65.
16. Gorman S, Scott E, Russell A. Antimicrobial activity, uses and mechanism of action of glutaraldehyde. *J Appl Bacteriol.* 1980;48:161-190.
17. Gorman S, Scott E. The state of glutaraldehyde molecule in relation to its biocidal activity. *J Pharm Pharmacol.* 1980;32:131-132.

18. Hardy P, Hughes G, Rydon H. Formation of quaternary pyridinium compounds by the action of glutaraldehyde on proteins. *J Chem Soc Chem Commun.* 1976;5:157-158.

19. Margel S, Rembaum A. Synthesis and characterization of poly(glutaraldehyde). A potential reagent for protein immobilization and cell separation. *Macromolecules.* 1980;13:19-24.

20. Hashimoto K, Masada Y, Sumida Y, Tashima T, Satoh N. Studies of aqueous solutions of glutaraldehyde by gas chromatography-mass spectrometry. *Int J Mass Spectrom Ion Phys.* 1983;48:125-128.

21. Tashima T, Kawakami U, Harada M, et al. Isolation and identification of new oligomers in aqueous solution of glutaraldehyde. *Chem Pharm Bull.* 1987;35:4169-4180.

22. Tashima T, Kawakami U, Satoh N, Nakagawa T, Tanaka H. Detection of impurities in aqueous solutions of glutaraldehyde by high performance liquid chromatography with a multichannel diode array UV detector. *J Electron Microsc (Tokyo).* 1987;36:136-138.

23. Tashima T, Kawakami U, Harada M, Satoh N, Nakagawa T, Tanaka H. Relationship between precipitation in aqueous solution of glutaraldehyde for chemosterilization and impurities detected by gas chromatography. *Int J Pharm.* 1988;42:61-67.

24. Tashima T, Kawakami U, Harada M, et al. Polymerization reaction in aqueous solution of glutaraldehyde containing trioxane-type oligomers under sterilizing conditions. *Chem Pharm Bull.* 1989;37:377-382.

25. Boucher R. On biocidal mechanisms in the aldehyde series. *Can J Pharm Sci.* 1975;10:1-7.

26. Jones L, Hancock C. Spectrophotometric studies of some 2, 4-dinitrophenyl-hydrazones. *J Am Chem Chem Soc.* 1960;82:105-107.

27. Paz M, Blumenfeld O, Rojkind M, Henson E, Furfine C, Gallop P. Determination of carbonyl compounds with N-methyl-benzothiazolone hydrazone. *Arch Biochem Biophys.* 1965;109:548-559.

28. Smith R, Farquhar M. Lysosome function in the regulation of the secretory process in cells of the anterior pituitary gland. *J Cell Biol.* 1966;31:319-348.

29. Munton T, Russell A. Aspects of the action of glutaraldehyde on *Escherichia coli. J Appl Bacteriol.* 1970;33:410-419.

30. Frigerio N, Shaw M. A simple method for determination of glutaraldehyde. *J Histochem Cytochem.* 1969;17:176-181.

31. Hajdu J, Friedrich P. Reaction of glutaraldehyde with NH2 compounds. A spectrophotometric method for the determination of glutaraldehyde concentration. *Anal Biochem.* 1975;65:273-280.

32. Zurek G, Karst U. Microplate photometric determination of aldehydes in disinfectant solutions. *Anal Chim Acta.* 1997;351:247-257.

33. Wliszczak W, Meisinger F, Kainz G. Gaschromatographische bestimmung de disinfektionsmittels glutaraldehyd in der luft von Krankenhausern. *Mikrochim Acta.* 1977;2:139-148.

34. Lyman G, Johnson R, Kho B. Gas chromatographic determination of glutaraldehyde. *J Chromatogr.* 1978;156:285-292.

35. Harke H, Pust U. Quantitative determination of glutaraldehyde in disinfectants. *Zentralblatt für Bakteriol Mikrobiol und Hyg B.* 1978;167:87-89.

36. Millership J. A report on an initial comparative study of two methods for the determination of glutaraldehyde. *J Clin Pharm Ther.* 1987;12:33-38.

37. Menet M, Gueylard D, Fievet M, Thuillier A. Fast specific separation and sensitive quantification of bactericidal and sporicidal aldehyde by high-performance liquid chromatography: example of glutaraldehyde determination. *J Chromatogr B Biomed Sci Appl.* 1997;692:79-86.

38. Habeeb A, Hiramoto R. Reactions of proteins with glutaraldehyde. *Arch Biochem Biophys.* 1968;126:16-26.

39. Blass J, Verriest C, Leau A, Weis M. Monomeric glutaraldehyde as an effective cross-linking reagent for proteins. *J Am Leather Chem Assoc.* 1976;74:121-131.

40. Kirkeby S, Moe D. Studies on the actions of glutaraldehyde, formaldehyde, and mixtures of glutaraldehyde and formaldehyde on tissue protein. *Acta Histochem.* 1986;79:115-121.

41. Kirkeby S, Jacobsen P, Moe D. Glutaraldehyde—"pure and impure." A spectroscopic investigation of two commercial glutaraldehyde solutions and their reaction products with amino acids. *Anal Lett.* 1987;20:303-315.

42. Reichlin M. Use of glutaraldehyde as a coupling agent for proteins and peptides. *Methods Enzymol.* 1980;70:159-165.

43. Monsan P, Puzo G, Mazarguil H. Etude du mechanisme d'etablissement des liaisons glutaraldehyde-proteines. *Biochimie.* 1975;57: 1281-1292.

44. Hardy P, Nicholls A, Rydon H. The nature of the cross-linking of proteins by glutaraldehyde. Part I. Interaction of glutaraldehyde with the amino-groups of 6-aminohexanoic acid and of α-N-acetyl-lysine. *J Chem Soc Perkin 1.* 1976;1:958-962.

45. Hardy P, Hughes G, Rydon H. Identification of a 3-(2-piperidyl) pyridinium derivative ('anabilysine') as a cross-linking entity in a glutaraldehyde-treated protein. *J Chem Soc Chem Commun.* 1977;21:759-760.

46. Hardy P, Hughes G, Rydon H. The nature of the cross-linking of proteins by glutaraldehyde. Part 2. The formation of quaternary pyridinium compounds by the action of glutaraldehyde on proteins and the identification of a 3-(2-piperidyl)-pyridinium derivative, anabilysine, as a cross-linking entity. *J Chem Soc Perkin Trans.* 1979;1:2282-2288.

47. Cheung D, Perelman N, Ko E, Nimni M. Mechanism of crosslinking of proteins by glutaraldehyde III. Reaction with collagen in tissues. *Connect Tissue Res.* 1985;13:109-115.

48. Korn A, Feairheller S, Filachione E. Glutaraldehyde: nature of the reagent. *J Mol Biol.* 1972;65:525-529.

49. Woodroof E. Use of glutaraldehyde and formaldehyde to process tissue heart valves. *J Bioeng.* 1978;2:1-9.

50. Hemminki K, Suni R. Sites of reaction of glutaraldehyde and acetaldehyde with nucleosides. *Arch Toxicol.* 1984;55:186-190.

51. Kuznetsova NP, Mishaeva RN, Gudkin LR, Panarin EF. Reactions of glutaraldehyde with dipolar ions of amino acids and proteins. *Russ Chem Bull.* 2013;62(4):918-927.

52. Migneault I, Dartiguenave C, Bertrand MJ, Waldron KC. Glutaraldehyde: behavior in aqueous solution, reaction with proteins, and application to enzyme crosslinking. *Biotechniques.* 2004;37(5):790-802.

53. Borick P. Chemical sterilizers (chemosterilizers). *Adv Appl Microbiol.* 1968;10:291-312.

54. Spaulding E, Cundy K, Turner F. Chemical disinfection of medical and surgical materials. In: Block S, ed. *Disinfection, Sterilization and Preservation.* 2nd ed. Philadelphia, PA: Lea & Febiger; 1977:654-684.

55. Coates D. Sporicidal activity of sodium dichloroisocyanurate, peroxygen and glutaraldehyde disinfectants against *Bacillus subtilis. J Hosp Infect.* 1996;32:283-294.

56. Borick P, Dondershine F, Chandler V. Alkalinized glutaraldehyde, a new antimicrobial agent. *J Pharm Sci.* 1964;53:1273-1275.

57. Rubbo S, Gardner J, Webb R. Biocidal activities of glutaraldehyde and related compounds. *J Appl Bacteriol.* 1967;30:78-87.

58. Dyas A, Das B. The activity of glutaraldehyde against *Clostridium difficile. J Hosp Infect.* 1985;6:41-45.

59. Boucher R, inventor; Wave Energy Systems Inc, assignee. Method and sporicidal compositions for synergistic disinfection or sterilization. US patent 15,523,371. June 21, 1971.

60. Babb J, Bradley C, Ayliffe G. Sporicidal activity of glutaraldehydes and hypochlorites and other factors influencing their selection for the treatment of medical equipment. *J Hosp Infect.* 1980;1:63-75.

61. Sierra G, Boucher R. Ultrasonic synergistic effects in liquid-phase chemical sterilization. *Appl Microbiol.* 1971;22:160-164.

62. Kelsey J, Mackinnon I, Maurer I. Sporicidal activity of hospital disinfectants. *J Clin Pathol.* 1974;27:632-638.

63. Forsyth M. A rate of kill test for measuring sporicidal properties of liquid sterilisers. *Dev Ind Microbiol.* 1975;16:37-47.

64. Miner N, McDowell J, Willcockson G, Bruckner N, Stark R, Whitmore E. Antimicrobial and other properties of a new stabilized alkaline glutaraldehyde disinfectant sterilizer. *Am J Hosp Pharm.* 1977;34:376-382.

65. Coates D, Death J. Sporicidal activity of mixtures of alcohol and hypochlorite. *J Clin Pathol.* 1978;31:148-152.

66. Gorman S, Scott E, Hutchinson E. The effect of sodium hypochlorite-methanol combinations on spores and spore forms of *Bacillus subtilis. Int J Pharm.* 1983;17:291-298.

67. Gorman S, Hutchinson E, Scott E, McDermott L. Death, injury and revival of chemically treated *Bacillus subtilis* spores. *J Appl Bacteriol*. 1983;54:9-99.

68. Gorman S, Scott E, Hutchinson E. Hypochlorite effects on spores and spore forms of *Bacillus subtilis* and on a spore lytic enzyme. *J Appl Bacteriol*. 1984;56:295-303.

69. McGucken P, Woodside W. Studies on the mode of action of glutaraldehyde on *Escherichia coli*. *J Appl Bacteriol*. 1973;36:419-426.

70. Leers W, McAllister J, MacPherson L. A comparative study of Cidex and Savlon. *Can J Hosp Pharm*. 1974;17-18.

71. Snyder R, Cheatle E. Alkaline glutaraldehyde—an effective disinfectant. *Am J Hosp Pharm*. 1965;22:321-327.

72. Bergan T, Lystad A. Antitubercular action of disinfectants. *J Appl Bacteriol*. 1971;34:751-756.

73. Relyveld E. Etude du pourvoir bactericide du glutaraldehyde. *Ann Microbiol*. 1977;128B:495-505.

74. Leers W. Disinfecting fibreoptic endoscopes: how not to transmit *Mycobacterium tuberculosis* by bronchoscopy. *Can Med Assoc J*. 1980;123:275-283.

75. Collins J. The use of glutaraldehyde in tuberculosis laboratory discard jars. *Lett Appl Microbiol*. 1986;2:103-105.

76. Ascenzi J, Ezzell R, Wendt T. Evaluation of carriers used in the test methods of the Association of Official Analytical Chemists. *Appl Environ Microbiol*. 1986;51:91-94.

77. Collins F. Kinetics of the tuberculocidal response by alkaline glutaraldehyde in solution and on an inert surface. *J Appl Bacteriol*. 1986;61:87-93.

78. Best M, Sattar S, Springthorpe V, Kennedy M. Comparative mycobactericidal efficacy of chemical disinfectants in suspension and carrier tests. *Appl Environ Microbiol*. 1988;54:2856-2858.

79. van Klingeren B, Pullen W. Comparative testing of disinfectants against *Mycobacterium tuberculosis* and *Mycobacterium terrae* in a quantitative suspension test. *J Hosp Infect*. 1987;10:292-298.

80. Collins F. Bactericidal activity of alkaline glutaraldehyde solution against a number of atypical mycobacterial species. *J Appl Bacteriol*. 1986;61:247-251.

81. Carson L, Petersen N, Favero M, Aguero S. Growth characteristics of atypical mycobacteria in water and their comparative resistance to disinfectants. *Appl Environ Microbiol*. 1978;36:839-846.

82. Shetty N, Srinivasan S, Holton J, Ridgway G. Evaluation of microbicidal activity of a new disinfectant: Sterilox 2500 against *Clostridium difficile* spores, *Helicobacter pylori*, vancomycin resistant *Enterococcus* species, *Candida albicans* and several *Mycobacterium* species. *J Hosp Infect*. 1999;41:101-105.

83. Griffiths P, Babb J, Fraise A. Mycobacterial activity of selected disinfectants using a quantitative suspension test. *J Hosp Infect*. 1999;41:111-121.

84. Griffiths P, Babb J, Fraise A. *Mycobacterium terrae*: a potential surrogate for *Mycobacterium tuberculosis* in a standard disinfectant test. *J Hosp Infect*. 1998;38:183-192.

85. Jackson J, Leggett J, Wilson D, Gilbert D. *Mycobacterium gordonae* in fiberoptic bronchoscopes. *Am J Infect Control*. 1996;24:19-23.

86. Griffiths P, Babb J, Bradley C, Fraise A. Glutaraldehyde-resistant *Mycobacterium chelonae* from endoscope washer disinfectors. *J Appl Microbiol*. 1997;82:519-526.

87. Duarte RS, Lourenço MCS, Fonseca LDS, et al. Epidemic of postsurgical infections caused by *Mycobacterium massiliense*. *J Clin Microbiol*. 2009;47(7):2149-2155.

88. Fisher CW, Fiorello A, Shaffer D, Jackson M, McDonnell GE. Aldehyde-resistant mycobacteria bacteria associated with the use of endoscope reprocessing systems. *Am J Infect Control*. 2012;40:880-882.

89. De Groote MA, Gibbs S, De Moura VCN, et al. Analysis of a panel of rapidly growing mycobacteria for resistance to aldehyde-based disinfectants. *Am J Infect Control*. 2014;42:932-934.

90. Svetlíková S, Kovierová H, Niederweis M, Gaillard J, McDonnell G, Jackson M. Role of porins in the susceptibility of *Mycobacterium smegmatis* and *Mycobacterium chelonae* to aldehyde-based disinfectants and drugs. *Antimicrob Agents Chemother*. 2009;53:4015-408.

91. Shang S, Gibbs S, Henao-Tamayo M, et al. Increased virulence of an epidemic strain of *Mycobacterium massiliense* in mice. *PLoS One*. 2011;6:e24726.

92. McDonnell G. *Antisepsis, Disinfection, and Sterilization: Types, Action, and Resistance*. Washington, DC: ASM Press; 2017.

93. Dabrowa N, Landau J, Newcomer V. Antifungal activity of glutaraldehyde in vitro. *Arch Dermatol*. 1972;105:555-557.

94. Gorman S, Scott E. An assessment of the antifungal activity of glutaraldehyde. *J Pharm Pharmacol*. 1976;28:48.

95. Tadeusiak B. Fungicidal activity of glutaraldehyde. *Roc Panstw Zakl Hig*. 1976;27:689-695.

96. Gorman S, Scott E. A quantitative evaluation of the antifungal properties of glutaraldehyde. *J Appl Bacteriol*. 1977;43:83-89.

97. Terleckyj B, Axler D. Quantitative neutralization assay of fungicidal activity of disinfectants. *Antimicrob Agents Chemother*. 1987;31: 794-798.

98. Boudouma M, Enjalbert L, Didier J. A simple method for the evaluation of antiseptic and disinfectant virucidal activity. *J Virol Methods*. 1984;9:271-276.

99. Tyler R, Ayliffe G. A surface test for virucidal activity of disinfectants: preliminary study with herpes virus. *J Hosp Infect*. 1987;9:22-29.

100. Blough H. Selective inactivation of biological activity of myxoviruses by glutaraldehyde. *J Bacteriol*. 1966;92:266-268.

101. Graham J, Jaeger R. Inactivation of yellow fever virus by glutaraldehyde. *Appl Microbiol*. 1968;16:177.

102. Schümann K, Grossgebauer K. Experiments on disinfection of vaccinia virus embedded in scabs and/or at the hand. *Zentralbl Bakteriol Orig B*. 1977;164:45-63.

103. Shen D, Crawford T, Gorham J, McGuire T. Inactivation of equine infectious anaemia virus by chemical disinfectants. *Am J Vet Res*. 1977;38:1217-1219.

104. Saitanu K, Lund E. Inactivation of entero virus by glutaraldehyde. *Appl Microbiol*. 1975;29:571-574.

105. Evans D, Stuart P, Roberts D. Disinfection of animal viruses. *Br Vet J*. 1977;133:356-359.

106. Klein M, Deforest A. The inactivation of viruses by germicides. In: *Proceedings of the 49th Meeting of Chemical Specialities Manufacturers' Association*. New York, NY: Chemical Specialties Manufacturers Association; 1963:116-118.

107. Drulak M, Wallbank A, Lebtag I, Werboski L, Poffenroth L. The relative effectiveness of commonly used disinfectants in inactivation of coxsackievirus B5. *J Hyg London*. 1978;81:389-397.

108. Drulak M, Wallbank A, Lebtag I. The relative effectiveness of commonly used disinfectants in inactivation of echovirus 11. *J Hyg (Lond)*. 1978;81:77-87.

109. Drulak M, Wallbank A, Lebtag I. The effectiveness of six disinfectants in inactivation of reovirus 3. *Microbios*. 1984;41:31-38.

110. Adler-Storthz K, Sehulster L, Dreesman G, Hollinger F, Melnick L. Effect of alkaline glutaraldehyde on hepatitis B virus antigen. *Eur J Clin Microbiol*. 1983;2:316-320.

111. Bond W, Favero M, Petersen N, Ebert J. Inactivation of hepatitis B virus by intermediate-to-high-level disinfectant chemicals. *J Clin Microbiol*. 1983;18:535-538.

112. Kobayashi H, Tsuzuki M, Koshimizu K, et al. Susceptibility of hepatitis B virus to disinfectants or heat. *J Clin Microbiol*. 1984;20:214-216.

113. Passagot J, Crance J, Biziagos E, Laveran H, Agbalika F, Deloince R. Effect of glutaraldehyde on the antigenicity and infectivity of hepatitis A virus. *J Virol Methods*. 1987;16:21-28.

114. Spire B, Barré-Sinoussi F, Montagnier L, Chermann J. Inactivation of lymphadenopathy associated virus by chemical disinfectants. *Lancet*. 1984;2:899-901.

115. Resnick L, Veren K, Salahuddin S, Tondreau S, Markham P. Stability and inactivation of HTLV-III/LAV under clinical and laboratory environments. *JAMA*. 1986;255:1887-1891.

116. Springthorpe V, Grenier J, Lloyd-Evans N, Sattar S. Chemical disinfection of human rotaviruses: efficacy of commercially-available products in suspension tests. *J Hyg (Lond)*. 1986;97:139-161.

117. Lloyd-Evans N, Springthorpe V, Sattar S. Chemical disinfection of human rotavirus-contaminated inanimate surfaces. *J Hyg (Lond)*. 1986;97:163-173.

118. Eterpi M, McDonnell G, Thomas V. Disinfection efficacy against parvoviruses compared with reference viruses. *J Hosp Infect*. 2009;73:64-70.

119. Meyers J, Ryndock E, Conway M, Meyers C, Robison R. Susceptibility of high-risk human papillomavirus type 16 to clinical disinfectants. *J Antimicrob Chemother*. 2014;69:1546-1550.

120. Ringrose R, McKown B, Felton F, Barclay B, Muchmore H, Rhoades E. A hospital outbreak of *Serratia marcescens* associated with ultrasonic nebulizers. *Ann Intern Med*. 1968;69:719-729.

121. Bassett D. Common-source outbreaks. *Proc R Soc Med*. 1971;64:18-24.

122. Ayliffe G, Deverill C. Decontamination of gastroscopes. *Heal Soc Serv J*. 1979:538-540.

123. Scheidt A. Persistent contamination of the flexible fiberbronchoscope following disinfection in aqueous glutaraldehyde. *Chest*. 1980;78:352-353.

124. Laskowski L, Marr J, Spernoga J, et al. Fastidious mycobacteria grown from porcine prosthetic-heart-valve cultures. *N Engl J Med*. 1977;297:101-102.

125. Leão S, Viana-Niero C, Matsumoto C, et al. Epidemic of surgical-site infections by a single clone of rapidly growing mycobacteria in Brazil. *Future Microbiol*. 2010;6:971-980.

126. de Oliveira Loreno NS, Bettini M, Ii P, et al. Experimental surgical infections *Mycobacterium massiliense* BRA100 strain recovered from postsurgical infections: resistance to high concentrations of glutaraldehyde and alternative solutions for high level disinfection. *Exp Surg Infect*. 2010;25:455-459.

127. Burgess W, Margolis A, Gibbs S, Duarte RS, Jackson M. Disinfectant susceptibility profiling of glutaraldehyde-resistant nontuberculous mycobacteria. *Infect Control Hosp Epidemiol*. 2017;38:784-791.

128. Nomura K, Ogawa M, Miyamoto H, Muratani T, Taniguchi H. Antibiotic susceptibility of glutaraldehyde-tolerant *Mycobacterium chelonae* from bronchoscope washing machines. *Am J Infect Control*. 2004;32:185-188.

129. Tschudin-Sutter S, Frei R, Kampf G, et al. Emergence of glutaraldehyde-resistant *Pseudomonas aeruginosa*. *Infect Control Hosp Epidemiol*. 2011;32:1173-1178.

130. Vikram A, Bomberger JM, Bibby KJ. Efflux as a glutaraldehyde resistance mechanism in *Pseudomonas fluorescens* and *Pseudomonas aeruginosa* biofilms. *Antimicrob Agents Chemother*. 2015;59:3433-3440.

131. Vikram A, Lipus D, Bibby K. Produced water exposure alters bacterial response to biocides. *Environ Sci Technol*. 2014;48:13001-13009.

132. Kadry AA, Serry FM, El-Ganiny AM, El-Baz AM. Integron occurrence is linked to reduced biocide susceptibility in multidrug resistant *Pseudomonas aeruginosa*. *Br J Biomed Sci*. 2017;74:78-84.

133. Azachi M, Henis Y, Shapira R, Oren A. The role of the outer membrane in formaldehyde tolerance in *Escherichia coli* VU3695 and Halomonas sp. MAC. *Microbiology*. 1996;142:1249-1254.

134. Serry FME, Kadry AA, Abdelrahman AA. Potential biological indicators for glutaraldehyde and formaldehyde sterilization processes. *J Ind Microbiol Biotechnol*. 2003;30:135-140.

135. Gorman S, Scott E. Uptake and media reactivity of glutaraldehyde solutions related to structure and biocidal activity. *Microbios Lett*. 1977;5:163-169.

136. Mbithi J, Springthorpe V, Sattar S, Pacquette M. Bactericidal, virucidal, and mycobactericidal activities of reused glutaraldehyde in an endoscopy unit. *J Clin Microbiol*. 1993;31:2988-2995.

137. McDonnell G. Decontamination of prions. In: Walker J, ed. *Decontamination in Hospitals and Healthcare*. Cambridge, United Kingdom: Woodhead Publishing; 2013:346-369.

138. McDonnell G. Transmissible spongiform encephalopathies and decontamination. In: Fraise A, Lambert PA, Maillard JY, eds. *Principles and Practice of Disinfection, Preservation and Sterilization*. Oxford, United Kingdom: Blackwell Publishing; 2013:208-228.

139. Taylor DM, Fernie K, Steele PJ, McConnell I, Somerville RA. Thermostability of mouse-passaged BSE and scrapie is independent of host PrP genotype: implications for the nature of the causal agents. *J Gen Virol*. 2002;83:3199-3204.

140. Amyx H. Some physical and chemical characteristics of a strain of Creutzfeld-Jakob disease in mice. In: *Abstracts of the Twelfth World Congress of Neurology*. Dallas, TX: World Federation of Neurology; 1981:255.

141. Takeo Y, Oie S, Kamiya A, Konishi H, Nakazawa T. Efficacy of disinfectants against biofilm cells of *Pseudomonas aeruginosa*. *Microbios*. 1994;79:19-26.

142. Vieira CD, Farias LM, Diniz CG, Alvarez-Leite ME, Camargo ER, Carvalho MA. New methods in the evaluation of chemical disinfectants used in health care services. *Am J Infect Control*. 2005;33:162-169.

143. Neves MS, Da Silva MG, Ventura GM, Côrtes PB, Duarte RS, de Souza HS. Effectiveness of current disinfection procedures against biofilm on contaminated GI endoscopes. *Gastrointest Endosc*. 2016;83:944-953.

144. Leung HW. Ecotoxicology of glutaraldehyde: review of environmental fate and effects studies. *Ecotoxicol Environ Saf*. 2001;49:26-39.

145. Kampf G. Glutaraldehyde. In: *Antiseptic Stewardship: Biocide Resistance and Clinical Implications*. Switzerland: Springer; 2018:131-160.

146. Hughes R, Thurman P. Cross-linking of bacterial cell walls with glutaraldehyde. *Biochem J*. 1970;119:925-926.

147. Russell A, Haque H. Inhibition of EDTA-lysozyme lysis of *Pseudomonas aeruginosa* by glutaraldehyde. *Microbios*. 1975;13:151-153.

148. Russell A, Vernon G. Inhibition of glutaraldehyde of lysostaphin-induced lysis of *Staphylococcus aureus*. *Microbios*. 1975;13:147-149.

149. Munton T, Russell A. Effects of glutaraldehyde on protoplasts of *Bacillus megaterium*. *J Gen Microbiol*. 1970;63:367-370.

150. Munton T, Russell A. Effect of glutaraldehyde on cell viability, triphenyl tetrazolium reduction, oxygen uptake and β-galactosidase activity in *Escherichia coli*. *Appl Microbiol*. 1973;26:508-511.

151. Navarro J, Monsan P. Etude du mechanisme d'interaction du glutaraldehyde avec les micro-organismes. *Ann Microbiol (Paris)*. 1976;127B:295-307.

152. Gorman S, Scott E. Transport capacity, alkaline phosphatase activity and protein content of glutaraldehyde-treated cell forms of *Escherichia coli*. *Microbios*. 1977;19:205-212.

153. Gorman S, Scott E. Preparation and stability of mureinoplasts of *Escherichia coli*. *Microbios*. 1977;18:123-130.

154. Hopwood D. Reactions of glutaraldehyde with nucleic acids. *Histochem J*. 1975;7:267-276.

155. Ellar D, Muñoz E, Salton M. The effect of low concentrations of glutaraldehyde on *Micrococcus lysodeikticus* membranes. *Biochim Biophys Acta*. 1971;225:140-150.

156. Done J, Shorey C, Locke J, Pollak J. The cytochemical localization of alkaline phosphatase in *Escherichia coli* at the electron microscope level. *Biochem J*. 1965;96:27c-28c.

157. Wang H, Tu J. Modification of glycogen phosphorylase B by glutaraldehyde. Preparation and isolation of enzyme derivatives with enhanced stability. *Biochemistry*. 1969;8:4403-4410.

158. Wetzel B, Spicer S, Dvorak H, Heppel L. Cytochemical localization of certain phosphatases in *Escherichia coli*. *J Bacteriol*. 1970;104:529-542.

159. Cheng K, Ingram J, Costerton J. Alkaline phosphatase localization and spheroplast formation of *Pseudomonas aeruginosa*. *Can J Microbiol*. 1970;16:1319-1324.

160. Thomas S, Russell A. Studies on the mechanism of the sporicidal action of glutaraldehyde. *J Appl Bacteriol*. 1974;37:83-92.

161. Gould G, Dring G. Heat resistance of bacterial endospores and concept of an expanded osmoregulatory cortex. *Nature*. 1975;258:402-405.

162. McErlean E, Gorman S, Scott E. Physical and chemical resistance of ion-exchange and coat defective spores of *Bacillus subtilis*. *J Pharm Pharmacol*. 1980;32:32.

163. Gorman S, Scott E, Hutchinson E. Interaction of the *Bacillus subtilis* spore protoplast, cortex, ion-exchange and coatless forms with glutaraldehyde. *J Appl Bacteriol*. 1984;56:95-102.

164. Power E, Dancer B, Russell A. Emergence of resistance to glutaraldehyde in spores of *Bacillus subtilis* 168. *FEMS Microbiol Lett.* 1988;50:223-226.

165. Sangar D, Rowlands D, Smale C, Brown F. Reaction of glutaraldehyde with foot and mouth disease virus. *J Gen Virol.* 1973;21:399-406.

166. Baltimore D, Huang A. Isopycnic separation of subcellular components from poliovirus-infected and normal HeLa cells. *Science.* 1968;162:572-574.

167. Wouters M, Miller A, Fenwick M. Distortion of poliovirus particles by fixation with formaldehyde. *J Gen Virol.* 1973;18:211-214.

168. Boucher R. Biochemical mechanisms of saturated dialdehydes and their potentiation by ultrasound. *Proc West Pharmacol Soc.* 1973;16:282-288.

169. Munton T, Russell A. Interaction of glutaraldehyde with spheroplasts of *Escherichia coli. J Appl Bacteriol.* 1973;36:211-217.

170. Gorman S, Scott E. Effect of alkalination on the bacterial cell and glutaraldehyde molecule. *Microbios Lett.* 1977;6:39-44.

171. King J, McGucken P, Woodside W. Relationship between pH and antibacterial activity of glutaraldehyde. *J Pharm Sci.* 1974;63:804-805.

172. Cheung H, So C, Sun S. Interfering mechanism of sodium bicarbonate on spore germination of *Bacillus stearothermophilus. J Appl Microbiol.* 1998;84:619-626.

173. Gorman S, Scott E. Effect of inorganic cations on the biocidal and cellular activity of glutaraldehyde. *J Appl Bacteriol.* 1979;47:463-468.

174. Ayliffe G, Collins B, Babb J. Disinfection with glutaraldehyde. *Br Med J.* 1979;1:1019.

175. Miner N, Whitmore E, McBee M. A quantitative organic soil neutralization test for disinfectants. In: *Developments in Industrial Microbiology.* Port Jervis, NY: Lubrecht & Cramer; 1975:23-50.

176. Gorman S, Scott E. An evaluation of potential inactivators of glutaraldehyde in disinfection studies with *Escherichia coli. Microbios Lett.* 1976;1:197-204.

177. Reybrouk G. Bactericidal activity of 40 potential disinfectant inactivators. *Zentralblatt für Bakteriol Mikrobiol und Hyg B.* 1978;167:528-534.

178. Cheung H, Brown M. Evaluation of glycine as an inactivator of glutaraldehyde. *J Pharm Pharmacol.* 1982;34:211-214.

179. Starke R, Ferguson D, Garza P, Miner N. An evaluation of the Association of Official Analytical Chemists sporicidal test methods. *Dev Ind Microbiol.* 1975;16:31-36.

180. Hodges N, Melling J, Parker S. A comparison of chemically defined and complex media for the production of *Bacillus subtilis* spores having reproducible resistance and germination characteristics. *J Pharm Pharmacol.* 1980;32:126-130.

181. Gorman S, Scott E, Hutchinson E. Emergence and development of resistance to antimicrobial chemicals and heat in spores of *Bacillus subtilis. J Appl Bacteriol.* 1984;57:153-163.

182. US Food and Drug Administration. *FDA-Cleared Sterilants and High Level Disinfectants with General Claims for Processing Reusable Medical and Dental Devices.* Silver Spring, MD: US Food and Drug Administration; 2015. https://www.fda.gov/medical-devices /reprocessing-reusable-medical-devices-information-manufacturers /fda-cleared-sterilants-and-high-level-disinfectants-general-claims -processing-reusable-medical-and. Accessed March 18, 2019.

183. Shen W, Ge Y, Su Y. Increasing disinfection efficacy of glutaraldehyde via chemical and physical enhancement. In: Zhu P, ed. *New Biocides Development.* Washington, DC: American Chemical Society; 2007:348-361.

184. Miner N, Harris V, Cao T, Ebron T, Lukomski N. Aldahol high-level disinfectant. *Am J Infect Control.* 2010;38:205-211.

185. Jacobs P, inventor; Ethicon Inc, assignee. Buffered glutaraldehyde sterilizing and disinfecting compositions. European patent EP0184297. June 11, 1986.

186. Adam S, inventor; Ethicon Inc, assignee. Sporicidal compositions comprising a saturated dialdehyde and a cationic surfactant. US patent 3,282,775. November 1, 1966.

187. Sidwell R, Westbrook L, Dixon G, Happich W. Potentially infectious agents associated with shearling bedpads. I. Effect of laundering with detergent-disinfectant combinations on polio and vaccinia viruses. *Appl Microbiol.* 1970;19:53-59.

188. Wilkoff L, Dixon G, Westbrook L, Happich W. Potentially infectious agents associated with shearling bedpads: effect of laundering with detergent-disinfectant combinations on *Staphylococcus aureus* and *Pseudomonas aeruginosa. Appl Microbiol.* 1971;21:647-652.

189. Dick P, Rombi M, inventors. New sterilizing compositions. French patent 2,313,081. 1977.

190. Sagripanti J, Bonifacino A. Effects of salt and serum on the sporicidal activity of liquid disinfectants. *J AOAC Int.* 1997;80:1198-1207.

191. Schattner R, inventor. Buffered phenol-glutaraldehyde sterilizing compositions. US patent 4,103,001. July 25, 1978.

192. Leach E. A new synergized glutaraldehyde-phenate sterilizing solution and concentrated disinfectant. *Infect Control.* 1981;2:26-30.

193. Akamatsu T, Tabata K, Hironaga M, Uyeda M. Evaluation of the efficacy of a 3.2% glutaraldehyde product for disinfection of fibreoptic endoscopes with an automatic machine. *J Hosp Infect.* 1997;35:47-57.

194. Axon A, Banks J, Cockel R, Deverill C, Newmann C. Disinfection in upper digestive tract endoscopy in Britain. *Lancet.* 1981;1:1093-1094.

195. Sanderson K, Cronin E. Glutaraldehyde and contact dermatitis. *Br Med J.* 1968;3:802-805.

196. Lyon T. Allergic contact dermatitis due to Cidax. Report of a case. *Oral Surg.* 1971;32:895-898.

197. Hansen K. Glutaraldehyde occupational dermatitis. *Contact Dermatitis.* 1983;9:81-82.

198. Benson W. Exposure to glutaraldehyde. *Occup Med.* 1984;34:63-64.

199. Corrado O, Osman J, Davies R. Asthma and rhinitis after exposure to glutaraldehyde in endoscopy units. *Hum Toxicol.* 1986;5:325-327.

200. Reifenrath W, Prystowsky S, Nonomura J, Robinson P. Topical glutaraldehyde-percutaneous penetration and skin irritation. *Arch Dermatol Res.* 1985;277:242-244.

201. Stern M, Holsapple M, McCay J, Munson A. Contact hypersensitivity response to glutaraldehyde in guinea pigs and mice. *Toxicol Ind Health.* 1989;5:31-43.

202. Meltzer N, Henkin H. Glutaraldehyde—a preservative for cosmetics. *Cosmet Toilet.* 1977;92:95-98.

203. Ballantyne B, Myers R. The acute toxicity and primary irritancy of glutaraldehyde solutions. *Vet Hum Toxicol.* 2001;43:193-202.

204. Halatek T, Opalska B, Swiercz R, et al. Glutaraldehyde inhalation exposure of rats: effects on lung morphology, Clara-cell protein, and hyaluronic acid levels in BAL. *Inhal Toxicol.* 2003;15:85-97.

205. van Birgelen AP, Chou BJ, Renne RA, et al. Effects of glutaraldehyde in a 2-year inhalation study in rats and mice. *Toxicol Sci.* 2000;55: 195-205.

206. Association for the Advancement of Medical Instrumentation. *Technical Information Report: AAMI TIR67: 2018 Promoting Safe Practices Pertaining to the Use of Sterilant and Disinfectant Chemicals in Health Care Facilities.* Arlington, VA: Association for the Advancement of Medical Instrumentation; 2018.

207. Schnuch A, Uter W, Geier J, Frosch P, Rustemeyer T. Contact allergies in healthcare workers. Results from the IVDK. *Acta Derm Venereol.* 1998;78:358-363.

208. Smith DR, Wang RS. Glutaraldehyde exposure and its occupational impact in the health care environment. *Environ Health Prev Med.* 2006;11:3-10.

209. Varpela E, Otterström S, Hackman R. Liberation of alkalinized glutaraldehyde by respirators after cold sterilization. *Acta Anaesthesiol Scand.* 1971;15:291-298.

210. Osterberg B. Residual glutaraldehyde in plastics and rubbers after exposure to alkalinized glutaraldehyde solution and its importance on blood cell toxicity. *Arch Pharm Chemi Sci Ed.* 1978;6:241-248.

211. Gendler E, Gendler S, Nimni M. Toxic reactions evoked by glutaraldehyde-fixed pericardium and cardiac valve bioprosthesis. *J Biomed Mater Res.* 1984;18:727-736.

212. Wiebe D, Megerman J, L'Italien G, Abbott W. Glutaraldehyde release from vascular prostheses of biologic origin. *Surgery.* 1988;104:26-33.

213. West A, Kuan S, Bennick M, Lagarde S. Glutaraldehyde colitis following endoscopy: clinical and pathological features and investigation of an outbreak. *Gastroenterology.* 1995;108:1250-1255.

214. Dolcé P, Gourdeau M, April N, Bernard P. Outbreak of glutaraldehyde-induced proctocolitis. *Am J Infect Control.* 1995;23:34-39.

215. Ahishali E, Uygur-Bayramiçli O, Dolapçioğlu C, et al. Chemical colitis due to glutaraldehyde: case series and review of the literature. *Dig Dis Sci.* 2009;54:2541-2545.

216. Marks T, Worthy W, Staples R. Influence of formaldehyde and sonacide (potentiated acid glutaraldehyde) on embryo and fetal development in mice. *Teratology.* 1980;22:51-58.

217. Sasaki Y, Endo R. Mutagenicity of aldehydes in *Salmonella. Mutat Res.* 1978;54:251-252.

218. Slesinski R, Hengler W, Guzzie P, Wagner K. Mutagenicity evaluation of glutaraldehyde in a battery of in vitro bacterial and mammalian test systems. *Food Chem Toxicol.* 1983;21:621-629.

219. Zeiger E, Gollapudi B, Spencer P. Genetic toxicity and carcinogenicity studies of glutaraldehyde—review. *Mutat Res.* 2005;589:136-151.

220. Ballantyne B, Myers R, Blaszcak D. The influence of alkalinization of glutaraldehyde biocidal solutions on acute toxicity, primary irritancy, and skin sensitivity. *Vet Hum Toxicol.* 1997;39:340-346.

221. Andersen F. Final report on the safety of glutaral. *J Am Coll Toxicol.* 1996;15:98-139.

222. US Food and Drug Administration. *Frequency of Use of Cosmetic Ingredients.* Silver Spring, MD: US Food and Drug Administration; 2011.

223. Personal Care Products Council. *Update Concentration of Use by FDA Product Category: Glutaral.* Washington, DC: Personal Care Products Council; 2011.

224. Burnett CL, Heldreth B. Glutaral. *Int J Toxicol.* 2017;36:28S-30S.

225. Goelen E, Lambrechts M, Geyskens F. Sampling intercomparisons for aldehydes in simulated workplace air. *Analyst.* 1997;122:411-419.

226. European Committee for Standardization. *EN 482: Workplace Exposure—General Requirements for the Performance of Procedures for the Measurement of Chemical Agents.* Brussels, Belgium: European Committee for Standardization; 2012.

227. O'Connor H, Axon A. Gastrointestinal endoscopy: infection and disinfection. *Gut.* 1983;24:1067-1077.

228. Ayliffe G, Babb J, Bradley C. Disinfection of endoscopes. *J Hosp Infect.* 1986;7:295-309.

229. Weller I, Williams C, Jeffries D, et al. Cleaning and disinfection of equipment for gastrointestinal flexible endoscopy: interim recommendations of a Working Party of the British Society of Gastroenterology. *Gut.* 1988;29:1134-1151.

230. Axon A, Phillips I, Cotton P, Avery S. Disinfection of gastrointestinal fibre endoscopes. *Lancet.* 1974;1:656-658.

231. Tolon M, Thofern E, Miederer S. Disinfection procedures for fiberscopes in endoscopy departments. *Endoscopy.* 1976;8:24-29.

232. Carr-Locke D, Clayton P. Disinfection of upper gastrointestinal fibreoptic endoscopy equipment: an evaluation of a cetrimide, chlorhexidine solution and glutaraldehyde. *Gut.* 1978;19:916-922.

233. Noy M, Harrison L, Holmes G, Cockel R. The significance of bacterial contamination of fibreoptic endoscopes. *J Hosp Infect.* 1980;1:53-61.

234. Rittenbury M, Hench M. Preliminary evaluation of an activated glutaraldehyde solution for cold disinfection. *Ann Surg.* 1965;161:127-130.

235. George R. A critical look at chemical disinfection of anaesthetic apparatus. *Br J Anaesth.* 1975;47:719-722.

236. Lin K, Park M, Baker H, Sidorowicz A. Disinfection of anaesthesia and respiratory therapy equipment with acid glutaraldehyde solution. *Respir Care.* 1979;24:321-327.

237. Mitchell J, Alder V. The disinfection of urological endoscopes. *Br J Urol.* 1975;47:571-576.

238. Loffer F. Disinfection vs. sterilization of gynecological laparoscopy equipment. *J Reprod Med.* 1980;25:263-266.

239. Mostafa S. Adverse effects of buffered glutaraldehyde on the Heidbrink expiratory valve. *Br J Anaesth.* 1980;52:223-227.

240. Expert group on hepatitis in dentistry. *Report to the Chief Medical and Dental Officers of the Health Department of Great Britain.* London, United Kingdom: Her Majesty's Stationery Office; 1978.

241. Association for the Advancement of Medical Instrumentation. *ANSI/AAMI ST58: 2013 Chemical Sterilization and High-Level Disinfection in Health Care Facilities.* Arlington, VA: Association for the Advancement of Medical Instrumentation; 2013.

242. Gorman S, Scott E. A comparative evaluation of dental aspirator cleansing and disinfectant solutions. *Br Dent J.* 1985;158:402-405.

243. Meiller T, Depaola L, Kelley JI, Bacqui A, Turng B, Falkler W. Dental unit waterlines: biofilm, disinfection and recurrence. *J Am Dent Assoc.* 1999;130:65-72.

244. da Costa L, Olson N, DeGagne P, Franca R, Tipple A, Alfa M. A new buildup biofilm model that mimics accumulation of material in flexible endoscope channels. *J Microbiol Methods.* 2016;127:224-229.

245. Bovallius A, Anäs P. Surface-decontaminating action of glutaraldehyde in the gas-aerosol phase. *Appl Environ Microbiol.* 1977;34:129-134.

246. Nicklas W, Böhm K, Richter B. Studies on the corrosive action of some disinfectants suitable for the aerosol-disinfection. *Zentralbl Bakteriol Mikrobiol Hyg B.* 1981;173:365-373.

247. Eskenazi S, Bychkowski O, Smith M, Macmillan J. Evaluation of glutaraldehyde and hydrogen peroxide for sanitizing packaging materials of medical devices in sterility testing. *J Assoc Off Anal Chem.* 1982;65:1155-1161.

248. London I. Buffered glutaraldehyde solutions for warts. *Arch Dermatol.* 1971;104:440.

249. Bunney M, Nolan M, Williams D. An assessment of methods of treating viral warts by comparative treatment of trials based on a standard design. *Br J Dermatol.* 1976;94:667-679.

250. Bunney M. The treatment of viral warts. *Drugs.* 1977;13:445-451.

251. Allenby C. The treatment of viral warts with glutaraldehyde. *Br J Clin Pract.* 1977;31:12-13.

252. Scott K. Glutaraldehyde gel for warts. *Practitioner.* 1982;226:1342-1343.

253. Juhlin H, Hansson H. Topical glutaraldehyde for plantar hyperhidrosis. *Arch Dermatol.* 1968;97:327-330.

254. Suringa D. Treatment of superficial onychomycosis with topically applied glutaraldehyde. *Arch Dermatol.* 1970;102:163-167.

255. Eigen E, inventor; Colgate Palmolive Co, assignee. Oral compositions containing non-toxic, non-volatile aliphatic aldehydes. US patent 3,497,590. February 24, 1970.

256. Litchfield J, Vely V; inventors; Wm Wrigley Jr Co; assignee. Dialdehyde-containing anti-caries chewing gum compositions. US patent 3,679,792. July 25, 1972.

257. Hannah D. Glutaraldehyde and calcium hydroxide. A pulp dressing material. *Br Dent J.* 1972;132:227-231.

258. Relyveld E, Girard O, Désormeau-Bedot J. Procede de fabrication de vaccins a l'aide du glutaraldehyde. *Ann Immunol Hung.* 1973;17:22-31.

259. Relyveld E. Preparation de vaccins antitoxique et antimicrobiens a l'aide de glutaraldehyde. *C R Acad Sci Hebd Seances Acad Sci D.* 1973;227:613-616.

260. Relyveld E. Preparation de vaccins tetanique a l'aide du glutaraldehyde. In: Proceedings on the 4th International Conference on Tetanus; April 1975; Dakar, Sénégal.

261. Gupta R, Saxena S, Sharma S, Ahuja S. Studies on the optimal conditions for inactivation of *Bordetella pertussis* organisms with glutaraldehyde for preparation of a safe and potent pertussis vaccine. *Vaccine.* 1988;6:491-496.

262. Künzel W, Meissner C. Studies into detoxification of tetanus toxin. *Arch Exp Veterinarmed.* 1978;32:823-830.

263. Whei-Yang Kao W, Guzman N, Prockop D. Use of glutaraldehyde-fixed *Escherichia coli* cells as a convenient solid support for radioimmune assays. *Anal Biochem.* 1977;81:209-219.

264. Relyveld E, Ben-Efraim S. Preparation of vaccines by the action of glutaraldehyde on toxins, bacteria, viruses, allergens and cells. In: Wu R, ed. *Methods in Enzymology.* Amsterdam, Netherlands: Elsevier; 1983:24-60.

265. Mast M, MacNeil J. Use of glutaraldehyde as a disinfectant in immersion chilling of poultry. *Poult Sci.* 1978;57:681-684.

266. Thomson J, Cox N, Bailey J. Control of Salmonella and extension of shelf-life of broiler carcasses with a glutaraldehyde product. *J Food Sci.* 1977;42:1353-1355.

267. Janik D, Hall C, De Navarre M. Glutaraldehyde—a sanitizing agent for the equipment used in the manufacture of cosmetics. *Cosmet Toilet.* 1977;92:99-100.

268. Meltzer N, Henkin H. Glutaraldehyde—a new preservative for cosmetics. Paper presented at: 6th Congress of International Federation of Societies of Cosmetic Chemists; 1970; Barcelona, Spain.

269. Creamer CE, inventor; Union Carbide Chemicals Corporation, assignee. Sterilization process for fermentation media. Canadian patent CA1102725A. June 9, 1981.

270. Union Carbide Chemicals Corporation. Dialdehyde based fluids improve embalming process. *Chemical Progress.* February 1962.

271. Meaney W. Effective new teat disinfectant for dairy cows. *Farm Food Res.* 1981;12:13-15.

272. Stott J, Herbert B. The effect of pressure and temperature on sulphate-reducing bacteria and the action of biocides in oilfield water injection systems. *J Appl Bacteriol.* 1986;60:57-66.

273. Matchette L, Vegella T. Glutaraldehyde retains its disinfectant properties in presence of hydroxypropylmethyl cellulose (HPMC) gel. *J Biomed Mater Res.* 1996;33:101-105.

274. Jayakrishnan A, Jameela S. Glutaraldehyde as a fixative in bioprostheses and drug delivery matrices. *Biomaterials.* 1996;17:471-484.

275. Weintraub A, Ponce de Leon M. Potential for cross-contamination from use of a needless injector. *Am J Infect Control.* 1998;26:442-445.

276. Juncker J. Commission Implementing Regulation (EU) 2015/1759 of 28 September 2015 approving glutaraldehyde as an existing active substance for use in biocidal products for product-types 2, 3, 4, 6, 11 and 12. *Off J Eur Union.* 2015;257(1303):19-26.

277. US Environmental Protection Agency. *Reregistration Eligibility Decision for Glutaraldehyde.* Washington, DC: US Environmental Protection Agency; 2007. https://www3.epa.gov/pesticides/chem_search/reg_actions/reregistration/red_PC-043901_28-Sep-07.pdf. Accessed April 10, 2019.

278. Barbosa O, Ortiz C, Berenguer-Murcia Á, Torres R, Rodrigues RC, Fernandez-Lafuente R. Glutaraldehyde in bio-catalysts design: a useful crosslinker and a versatile tool in enzyme immobilization. *RSC Adv.* 2014;4:1583-600.

279. Pawar SV, Yadav GD. PVA/chitosan-glutaraldehyde cross-linked nitrile hydratase as reusable biocatalyst for conversion of nitriles to amides. *J Mol Catal B Enzym.* 2014;101:115-121.

280. López-Gallego F, Betancor L, Hidalgo A, et al. Preparation of a robust biocatalyst of D-amino acid oxidase on sepabeads supports using the glutaraldehyde crosslinking method. *Enzyme Microb Technol.* 2005;37:750-756.

281. Li B, Shan CL, Zhou Q, et al. Synthesis, characterization, and antibacterial activity of cross-linked chitosan-glutaraldehyde. *Mar Drugs.* 2013;11:1534-1552.

282. Mirzaei B, Ramazani S, Shafiee M, Danaei M. Studies on glutaraldehyde crosslinked chitosan hydrogel properties for drug delivery systems. *Int J Polym Mater Polym Biomater.* 2012;62:605-611.

283. Tahtat D, Mahlous M, Benamer S, Khodja AN, Oussedik-Oumehdi H, Laraba-Djebari F. Oral delivery of insulin from alginate/chitosan crosslinked by glutaraldehyde. *Int J Biol Macromol.* 2013;58:160-168.

284. Rutala W, Weber D; and Healthcare Infection Control Practices Advisory Committee. *Guideline for Disinfection and Sterilization in Healthcare Facilities, 2008.* Atlanta, GA: Centers for Disease Control and Prevention; 2019. https://www.cdc.gov/infectioncontrol/guidelines/disinfection. Accessed August 14, 2019.

285. Mazzola P, Jozala A, de Lencastre Novaes L, Moriel P, Penna T. Minimal inhibitory concentration (MIC) determination of disinfectant and/or sterilizing agents. *Braz J Pharm Sci.* 2009;45:241-248.

286. Mazzola PG, Penna TCV, Martins AM. Determination of decimal reduction time (D value) of chemical agents used in hospitals for disinfection purposes. *BMC Infect Dis.* 2003;3:24.

287. Aarestrup FM, Hasman H. Susceptibility of different bacterial species isolated from food animals to copper sulphate, zinc chloride and antimicrobial substances used for disinfection. *Vet Microbiol.* 2004;100:83-89.

288. Kümmerle N, Feucht HH, Kaulfers PM. Plasmid-mediated formaldehyde resistance in *Escherichia coli*: characterization of resistance gene. *Antimicrob Agents Chemother.* 1996;40:2276-2279.

289. Wollmann A, Kaulfers P. Formaldehyde-resistance in *Enterobacteriaceae* and *Pseudomonas aeruginosa*: identification of resistance genes by DNA-hybridization. *Zentralbl Hyg Umweltmed.* 1991;191:449-456.

290. Kaulfers PM, Brandt D. Isolation of a conjugative plasmid in *Escherichia coli* determining formaldehyde resistance. *FEMS Microbiol Lett.* 1987;43:161-163.

291. Wallace RJ, Brown BA, Griffith DE. Nosocomial outbreaks/pseudo outbreaks caused by nontuberculous mycobacteria. *Annu Rev Microbiol.* 1998;52:453-490.

292. Bolan G, Reingold AL, Carson LA, et al. Infections with *Mycobacterium chelonei* in patients receiving dialysis and using processed hemodialyzers. *J Infect Dis.* 1985;152:1013-1019.

293. Finelli L, Miller JT, Tokars JI, Alter MJ, Arduino MJ. National surveillance of dialysis-associated diseases in the United States, 2002. *Semin Dial.* 2005;18:52-61.

294. Marin C, Hernandiz A, Lainez M. Biofilm development capacity of Salmonella strains isolated in poultry risk factors and their resistance against disinfectants. *Poult Sci.* 2009;88:424-431.

295. Davies R, Wray C. Observations on disinfection regimens used on *Salmonella enteritidis* infected poultry units. *Poult Sci.* 1995;74:638-647.

296. Davies R, Breslin M, Corry JE, Hudson W, Allen VM. Observations on the distribution and control of Salmonella species in two integrated broiler companies. *Vet Rec.* 2001;149:227-232.

297. Davies R, Breslin M. Observations on Salmonella contamination of commercial laying farms before and after cleaning and disinfection. *Vet Rec.* 2003;152:283-287.

298. Gradel KO, Jørgensen JC, Andersen JS, Corry JEL. Monitoring the efficacy of steam and formaldehyde treatment of naturally Salmonella-infected layer houses. *J Appl Microbiol.* 2004;96:613-622.

299. Leal JF, Neves MGPMS, Santos EBH, Esteves VI. Use of formalin in intensive aquaculture: properties, application and effects on fish and water quality. *Rev Aquac.* 2018;10:281-295.

300. Salthammer T, Mentese S, Marutzky R. Formaldehyde in the indoor environment. *Chem Rev.* 2010;110:2536-2572.

301. Mundt KA, Gentry PR, Dell LD, Rodricks JV, Boffetta P. Six years after the NRC review of EPA's draft IRIS toxicological review of formaldehyde: regulatory implications of new science in evaluating formaldehyde leukemogenicity. *Regul Toxicol Pharmacol.* 2018;92:472-490.

302. International Agency for Research on Cancer. Formaldehyde. In: *IARC Monographs on the Evaluation of Carcinogenic Risks to Humans.* Lyon, France: International Agency for Research on Cancer; 2012.

303. Nielsen GD, Larsen ST, Wolkoff P. Re-evaluation of the WHO (2010) formaldehyde indoor air quality guideline for cancer risk assessment. *Arch Toxicol.* 2017;91:35-61.

304. Environmental Protection Agency. *Toxicological Review of Formaldehyde—Inhalation Assessment.* Washington, DC: Environmental Protection Agency; 2010.

305. National Toxicology Program. NTP 12th report on carcinogens. *Rep Carcinog.* 2011;12:iii-499.

306. Vazquez-Ferreiro P, Carrera Hueso F, Alvarez Lopez B, Diaz-Rey M, Martinez-Casal X, Ramón Barrios M. Evaluation of formaldehyde as an ocular irritant: a systematic review and meta-analysis. *Cutan Ocul Toxicol.* 2019;38:169-175.

307. McGwin G Jr, Lienert J, Kennedy JI Jr. Formaldehyde exposure and asthma in children: a systematic review. *Environ Health Perspect.* 2010;118:313-317.

308. Arif AA, Delclos GL. Association between cleaning-related chemicals and work-related asthma and asthma symptoms among healthcare professionals. *Occup Environ Med.* 2012;69:35-40.

309. Nurmatov UB, Tagiyeva N, Semple S, Devereux G, Sheikh A. Volatile organic compounds and risk of asthma and allergy: a systematic review. *Eur Respir Rev.* 2015;24:92-101.

310. Tateishi J. Properties of the transmissible agent derived from chronic spongiform encephalopathy. *Ann Neurol.* 1980;7:390-391.

311. Burger D, Gorham J. Observation of the remarkable stability of transmissible mink encephalopathy virus. *Res Vet Sci.* 1977;22:131-132.

312. Bernoulli C, Siegfried J, Baumgartner G, et al. Danger of accidental person-to-person transmission of Creutzfeldt-Jakob disease by surgery. *Lancet.* 1977;1:478-479.

313. Wang F, Chen D, Wu P, Klein C, Jin C. Formaldehyde, epigenetics, and Alzheimer's disease. *Chem Res Toxicol.* 2019;32:820-830.

314. Gannon P, Bright P, Campbell M, O'Hickey S, Burge P. Occupational asthma due to glutaraldehyde and formaldehyde in endoscopy and x ray departments. *Thorax.* 1995;50:156-159.

315. Di Stefano F, Siriruttanapruk S, McCoach J, Burge P. Glutaraldehyde: an occupational hazard in the hospital setting. *Allergy.* 1999;54:1105-1109.

316. Shaffer M, Belsito D. Allergic contact dermatitis from glutaraldehyde in health-care workers. *Contact Dermatitis.* 2000;43:150-156.

317. Rideout K, Teschke K, Dimisch-Ward H, Kennedy S. Considering risks to healthcare workers from glutaraldehyde alternatives in high-level disinfection. *J Hosp Infect.* 2005;59:4-11.

318. Rutala W, Weber D. Disinfection of endoscopes: review of new chemical sterilants used for high-level disinfections. *Infect Control Hosp Epidemiol.* 1999;20:69-76.

319. McDonnell G, Russell AD. Antiseptics and disinfectants: activity, action, and resistance. *Clin Microbiol Rev.* 1999;12:147-179.

320. Rutala W, Weber D. New disinfection and sterilization methods. *Emerg Infect Dis.* 2001;7:348-353.

321. Walsh S, Maillard J, Russell A. Ortho-phthalaldehyde: a possible alternative to glutaraldehyde for high level disinfection. *J Appl Microbiol.* 1999;86:1039-1046.

322. Simons C, Walsh S, Maillard J, Russell A. A note: ortho-phthalaldehyde: proposed mechanism of action of a new antimicrobial agent. *Lett Appl Microbiol.* 2000;31:299-302.

323. Alfa M, Sitter D. In-hospital evaluation of orthophthalaldehyde as a high level disinfectant for flexible endoscopes. *J Hosp Infect.* 1994;26:15-26.

324. Simões M, Simões LC, Cleto S, Machado I, Pereira MO, Vieira MJ. Antimicrobial mechanisms of ortho-phthalaldehyde action. *J Basic Microbiol.* 2007;47:230-242.

325. Gregory A, Schaalje G, Smart J, Robison R. The mycobactericidal efficacy of ortho-phthalaldehyde and the comparative resistances of *Mycobacterium bovis, Mycobacterium terrae,* and *Mycobacterium chelonae. Infect Control Hosp Epidemiol.* 1999;20:324-330.

326. Simões M, Pereira M, Machado I, Simões L, Vieira M. Comparative antibacterial potential of selected aldehyde-based biocides and surfactants against planktonic *Pseudomonas fluorescens. J Ind Microbiol Biotechnol.* 2006;33:741-749.

327. Seo H, Lee D, Yoon E, et al. Comparison of the efficacy of disinfectants in automated endoscope reprocessors for colonoscopies: tertiary amine compounds (Sencron2®) versus ortho-phthalaldehyde (Cidex®OPA). *Intest Res.* 2016;14:178-182.

328. Barbee S, Weber D, Sobsey M, Rutala W. Inactivation of *Cryptosporidium parvum* oocyst infectivity by disinfection and sterilization processes. *Gastrointest Endosc.* 1999;49:605-611.

329. Pineau L, Desbuquois C, Marchetti B, Luu Duc D. Comparison of the fixative properties of five disinfectant solutions. *J Hosp Infect.* 2008;68:171-177.

330. Herruzo-Cabrera R, Vizcaino-Alcaide M, Fernández-Aceñero M. The influence of laboratory adaptation on test strains, such as *Pseudomonas aeruginosa,* in the evaluation of the antimicrobial efficacy of ortho-phthalaldehyde. *J Hosp Infect.* 2004;57:217-222.

331. Herruzo R, Vizcaíno M, Herruzo I. An exception to the rule "no association between antibiotic resistance and decreased disinfectant microbicidal efficacy": orthophthalaldehyde (OPA) and *Pseudomonas aeruginosa* isolated from ICU and paraplegic patients. *J Prev Med Hyg.* 2017;58:42-47.

332. Walsh S, Maillard J, Simons C, Russell A. Studies on the mechanisms of the antibacterial action of ortho-phthalaldehyde. *J Appl Microbiol.* 1999;87:702-710.

333. Cabrera-Martinez R, Setlow B, Setlow P. Studies on the mechanisms of the sporicidal action of ortho-phthalaldehyde. *J Appl Microbiol.* 2002;92:675-680.

334. March J, Pratt M, Cohen M, Lindsey J, et al. The differential susceptibility of spores from virulent and attenuated *Bacillus anthracis* strains to aldehyde-and hypochlorite-based disinfectants. *Microbiologyopen.* 2012;1:407-414.

335. Rutala W, Peacock J, Gergen M, Sobsey M, Weber D. Efficacy of hospital germicides against adenovirus 8, a common cause of epidemic keratoconjunctivitis in health care facilities. *Antimicrob Agents Chemother.* 2006;50:1419-1424.

336. Roberts C, Chan-Myers H, Favero M. Virucidal activity of ortho-phthalaldehyde solutions against hepatitis B and C viruses. *Am J Infect Control.* 2008;36:223-226.

337. Hulkower R, Casanova L, Rutala W, Weber D, Sobsey M. Inactivation of surrogate coronaviruses on hard surfaces by health care germicides. *Am J Infect Control.* 2011;39:401-407.

338. McDonnell G, Burke P. The challenge of prion decontamination. *Clin Infect Dis.* 2003;36:1152-1154.

339. Rutala W, Weber D. Guideline for disinfection and sterilization of prion-contaminated medical instruments. *Infect Control Hosp Epidemiol.* 2010;31:107-117.

340. Anderson S, Umbright C, Sellamuthu R, et al. Irritancy and allergic responses induced by topical application of ortho-phthalaldehyde. *Toxicol Sci.* 2010;115:435-443.

341. Hasegawa G, Morinaga T, Ishihara Y. Ortho-phthalaldehyde enhances allergen-specific IgE production without allergen-specific IgG in ovalbumin-sensitized mice. *Toxicol Lett.* 2009;185:45-50.

342. Johnson V, Reynolds J, Wang W, Fluharty K, Yucesoy B. Inhalation of ortho-phthalaldehyde vapor causes respiratory sensitization in mice. *J Allergy (Cairo).* 2011;2011:751052.

343. Franchi A, Franco G. Evidence-based decision making in an endoscopy nurse with respiratory symptoms exposed to the new ortho-phthalaldehyde (OPA) disinfectant. *Occup Med.* 2005;55:575-578.

344. Robitaille C, Boulet L. Occupational asthma after exposure to ortho-phthalaldehyde (OPA). *Occup Environ Med.* 2015;72:381.

345. Catlin N, Wilson C, Stout M, Kissling G, et al. Evaluation of the respiratory tract toxicity of ortho-phthalaldehyde, a proposed alternative for the chemical disinfectant glutaraldehyde. *Inhal Toxicol.* 2017;29:414-427.

346. Catlin N, Wilson C, Creasy D, et al. Differentiating between testicular toxicity and sexual immaturity in ortho-phthalaldehyde inhalation toxicity studies in rats and mice. *Toxicol Pathol.* 2018;46:753-765.

347. Psaltikidis E, Loeschner Leichsenring M, Nakamura M, Bustorff-Silva J, Passeri L, Venâncio S. High-level disinfectants alternative to glutaraldehyde for processing flexible endoscopes. *Cogitare Enferm.* 2014;19:423-432.

348. Streckenbach S, Alston T. Perioral stains after ortho-phthalaldehyde disinfection of echo probes. *Anesthesiology.* 2003;99:1032.

24

Copper Alloy Surfaces Kill Bacteria and Reduce Infections

James H. Michel, Harold T. Michels, and Corinne A. Michels

Disinfection and sterilization, as well as ordinary cleaning, are necessary for infection control. Beyond the situations where surgical instruments and medical devices touch sterile surfaces within the human body, there are many opportunities to transmit infections in hospitals. These include interactions involving touching between patients, patient and visitor, and patient and health care worker as well as touching environmental surfaces by patient, visitor, and health care worker. It is well known that infection control and prevention is a serious problem not only in hospitals but also in other health care facilities, schools, public transportation systems, food production facilities, restaurants, public and office buildings, and cruise ships. According to a report from the Centers for Disease Control and Prevention, 1.7 million patients were infected (in 2002) while in a US hospital causing approximately 100 000 deaths and resulting in $35.7 to $45 billion in additional treatment costs.[1] Bacteria commonly reside in health care facilities and continue to cause health care–associated or health care–acquired infections. This together with emergence of new antibiotic-resistant strains complicates an already difficult situation. The ability of microbes to survive on surfaces for prolonged periods increases the probability that they will be transferred to patients and others. In addition, a variety of staph strains, sometimes including aggressively infectious strains, are found on the skin of most people and are easily transferred between patients, from visitors, from health care workers, and to objects. These objects are sources that transfer contaminants to others who touch them. Thus, it is not surprising that the microbial burden of frequently touched surfaces in health care facilities play a significant role in infection causality.[2]

Microbes are everywhere, not just in hospitals. You can become infected anywhere, just by going to work, at an event at your child's school, or having a night out at the movies. Mass transit systems are particularly problematic. A recent study conducted in the subway system of New York City identified 1688 bacterial, viral, archaea, and eukaryotic taxa in public areas.[3] Because this included disease-causing organisms, it is suggested that it is prudent to minimize touching of surfaces in transit systems and to wash or use hand sanitizers as soon as possible upon exiting. Then there are numerous school closings due to outbreaks of H1N1 influenza and even methicillin-resistant *Staphylococcus aureus* (MRSA) infections reported among school athletes; norovirus episodes on cruise ships that sometimes cause the vessels to return to port early[4]; as well as outbreaks of *Escherichia coli* O157:H7 related to ingesting contaminated food from major national restaurant chains, distributors of ground beef and poultry products, and tainted supermarket-prepared foods.

Aggressive sanitation procedures, like handwashing and regular cleaning and disinfecting, are the first line of defense. However, this alone has not solved the problem. In this chapter, the benefits of adding antimicrobial copper touch surfaces to help in the fight against infections are described and discussed. Antimicrobial copper should be viewed as an addition to and not a substitute for good sanitization and disinfection procedures. Keep in mind that antimicrobial copper surfaces, unlike other methods, require neither staff training nor behavioral changes to be effective. Antimicrobial copper alloys are continuously active, 24 hours a day, 7 days a week, without any human intervention. They are our newest weapon in the fight against infections.

▶ CHEMICAL COMPOSITION OF COPPER ALLOYS

Copper is listed in the periodic table of elements as a metal. Metals are usually solid at room temperature; have a luster; are hard, ductile, and malleable; and are good conductors of electricity and heat. Alloys are made by combining one metal with one or more other elements, typically metals, to create improved properties such as strength, hardness, and corrosion resistance. For example, C26000, a brass alloy, consists of 70% copper and 30% zinc. In this case, zinc is added to increase strength and decrease cost. Other attributes of brass include an attractive yellow gold-like appearance and acoustical properties desirable for musical instruments. Even C10200, which contains a minimum of 99.95% copper, is classified as an alloy. Modern metallurgy continues to develop alloys for specific uses and over 800 copper alloys of a variety of compositions and properties are available today. Of these, 500 are registered with the US Environmental Protection Agency as having significant antimicrobial activity. Table 24.1 lists the composition of a few examples of copper alloys.

▶ COPPER ALLOYS IN ANCIENT TIMES

Copper, as a metal, has been used by man since prehistoric times. It was one of the first metals to be used by humans,[6] most likely because it was found as "native copper," a natural uncombined metallic form of copper.

The earliest copper artifacts are from the Neolithic period. Early uses include jewelry, figurines, tools, bells, vessels, coinage, and weapons. The discovery of the 5300-year-old mummified body of the "Ice Man," in the Swiss Alps in 1991 was widely reported. He was found with a copper axe. This is just one indication of how copper was used in ancient times. Two periods in history are named after the metal, the Copper Age and the Bronze Age. Bronze is an alloy of copper and tin. Because bronze is strong and can hold a sharp edge, it was widely used in weapons until the introduction of iron.

▶ ANTIMICROBIAL COPPER IN ANCIENT TIMES

Thousands of years before the discovery of bacteria by Louis Pasteur, the ancients were aware of the sanitizing properties of copper.[7] The bible suggests that water stored in copper or bronze vessels was free of disease-causing agents. Ancient Hindu tradition recommends storing household water in copper vessels for improved health. It was confirmed in a recent study that overnight storage

TABLE 24.1   Copper alloy composition[a,b]

Alloy Number	Cu	Zn	Ni	Al	Sn	Mn	Fe	P	Si
High copper alloys									
C10200	99.95								
C11000	99.90								
Brasses									
C24000	80	20							
C26000	70	30							
C28000	60	40							
Bronzes									
C51000	95				5			0.2	
C61500	90		2	8					
C63800	95			3					2
C65500	97					1			2
Copper-nickel alloys									
C70600	89		10				1		
C71000	80		20						
C71500	69		30				1		
Copper-nickel-zinc alloys									
C73500	72	10	18						
C75200	65	17	18						

Abbreviations: Al, aluminum; Cu, copper; Fe, iron; Mn, manganese; Ni, nickel; P, phosphorus; Si, silicon; Sn, tin; Zn, zinc.

[a]The composition is in weight percentage. Intentional small additions of less than 1% are shown when required in their specifications.

[b]Reproduced with permission from Michels and Michels.[5]

of contaminated water in copper vessels kills bacteria, making the water safe to drink.[8]

An ancient medical text, written in Egypt circa 2400 BCE, was purchased in 1862 by a book dealer named Smith. Now commonly referred to as the *Smith Papyrus*, this text provides insight into the use of copper in medicine. It describes how to treat infected chest wounds and promote healing with copper. The *Papyrus* speaks of a "green pigment" that is believed to be a copper compound such as malachite (copper carbonate hydroxide mineral). It was also written in another ancient text, the *Ebers Papyrus* circa 1500 BCE, that metallic copper splinters and shavings, copper salts and oxides, can treat burns and promote healing of infected wounds. Similarly, the *Hippocratic Collection* (written, in part, by the Greek physician in 460-380 BCE) indicates that leg wounds can be treated with a poultice that includes verdigris, the natural patina formed when copper is exposed to air or seawater, and red copper oxide among other oxides and natural products, all dissolved in wine.

Hippocrates also recommended the use of bronze for medical instrumentation due its propensity to promote healing. The famous Roman surgeon Galen (130-200 CE) fabricated and used bronze instruments, which were found in Pompeii and Herculaneum. Many examples of early bronze surgical instrumentation survive until today.[9]

Even when the germ theory of infections was known, reports of the benefits of copper continued to be recorded. During two Paris cholera epidemics (1865 and 1866), the French physician Victor Burq determined, by statistical analysis, that only 16 deaths occurred among 30 000 workers in the copper industry, whereas the death rate was 10 to 40 times higher among similar noncopper workers. During World War I, it was found in a few cases that, when fragments from copper-containing projectiles were not removed from a wound, the wound healed surprisingly well and infection free.[7]

▶ COPPER ALLOYS IN THE MODERN ERA

Copper, which is highly recyclable, continues to be used in large quantities today in electrical applications (65%), construction (25%), transportation (7%), and elsewhere (3%). Some specific applications include industrial and home electrical wiring, potable water plumbing tube, electronic connectors, heat exchanger tubing in steam power plants, circuitry wiring and electrical contacts, tubing for natural gas, magnetrons on microwave ovens, seawater lines, welding electrodes, irrigation systems, medical gas distribution systems, printed circuit boards, locks and door hardware, wiring for glass defrosting systems, hydraulic lines, electromagnets, electrical motor windings, sleeve bearings (bronze), ship propellers, heat sinks in electronic devices, fittings, fasteners, screws, plumbing faucets, architectural roofing, statues, transformers, and the subject of this chapter, antimicrobial touch surfaces.

▶ ANTIMICROBIAL COPPER ALLOYS IN THE MODERN ERA AND THEIR SPECTRUM OF EFFICACY

As described in the following text, copper alloys have strong efficacy against a wide range of both gram-negative and gram-positive bacteria. Copper alloys are also effective against fungi and inactivate viruses.

In 1983, Kuhn[10] published a study of bacterial levels found on brass (C26000: 70% copper, 30% zinc) and stainless steel (S304000: 18% chromium, 8% nickel) doorknobs in a hospital in Erie, Pennsylvania. Whereas stainless steel doorknobs were heavily contaminated, the brass doorknobs contained only a few isolates of strep and staph bacteria. Almost 20 years later, this paper came to the attention of H. Michels, a coauthor of this chapter. It was decided to confirm the antimicrobial activity of copper alloys using *E coli* O157:H7, a toxin-producing bacterium responsible for numerous food recalls, that leads to hemorrhagic diarrhea and kidney failure.

As reported by Wilks et al,[11] a concentrated suspension of this microorganism was spread over the surface of coupons of several compositions of copper alloys in a sterile environment at room temperature and ambient relative humidity. At specified time intervals, the microorganisms were removed from the coupon surface and survival determined, with stainless steel as the experimental control. More than a 7.5 log (<99.99999%) in bacterial levels was observed at 45 minutes on two 99.9% copper containing alloys (C10200 and C11000), and only a few, if any, survivors were observed by 100 minutes of exposure. The other alloys showed similar but less dramatic results in proportion to their copper contents.

A few years later, Hong et al[12] observed similar results in a study using a standard laboratory *E coli* strain. The initial inoculum contained about 10^9 colony-forming units (CFUs), and at 45 minutes, a 9-log drop was measured indicating that all were killed, as can be seen in Figure 24.1. An approximately 1-log decrease was observed at 15 minutes, the time required for the sample to dry on the coupon surface, and more rapid killing occurred between 15 and 45 minutes. Again, no significant decrease in live bacteria was observed on the stainless steel. In regard to specific alloys, Hong et al[12] compared a series of copper alloys ranging from nearly 99.9% copper (C11000) to 60% copper (C28000). They found that the extent of initial killing at 15 and 30 minutes correlated with the copper content of the alloy (see Figure 24.1). However, complete killing was observed in all of the alloys at 45 minutes, ranging in copper content down to 60%. Several others achieved similar results and showed a strong correlation between the copper content of the alloy and killing efficacy, when challenged by *E coli*.[13-16]

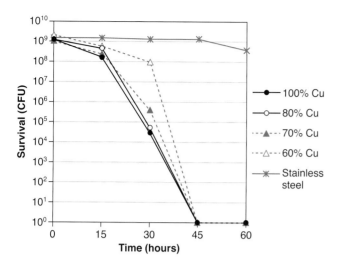

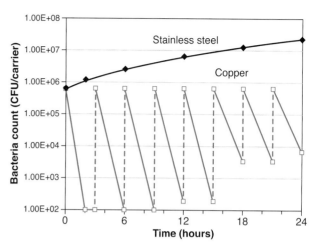

FIGURE 24.1 *Escherichia coli* survival on copper-zinc alloy surfaces containing different copper concentrations. *E coli* strain ATCC 23724 was grown in Luria Broth to mid-log phase (OD_{600} about 0.3), harvested by centrifugation from 100 mL of culture, and resuspended in 0.85% sodium chloride (NaCl) to a final volume of 500 μL. The 100 μL of concentrated cells were spread over the surface of metal coupons of 304 stainless steel (S30400); 99.90% copper (C11000); and copper-zinc alloys C24000, C26000, and C28000 containing 80%, 70%, and 60% copper, respectively (alloy compositions are listed in Table 24.1). Following the indicated time of exposure, the cells were washed from the coupon surface with 100 μL of 0.85% NaCl and samples taken to titer survival. The results represent at least two independent trials. Abbreviations: CFU, colony-forming unit; Cu, copper. From Hong et al.[12] Reproduced with permission from American Society for Microbiology. Copyright © 2012 American Society for Microbiology.

FIGURE 24.2 Methicillin-resistant *Staphylococcus aureus* (MRSA) survival on copper (C11000) and stainless steel (S30400) following multiple inoculations. *S aureus* (MRSA) samples spread over the surface of metal coupons of 304 stainless steel (filled diamonds) and nearly 100% copper (open squares). Following the indicated time of exposure, the cells were washed from the coupon surface and samples taken to titer survival. Reprinted with permission from Anderson and Michels.[13]

The "dry inoculation method" that uses a smaller inoculum was developed by Espírito Santo et al[17] to better simulate how environmental surfaces become contaminated. By limiting the sample volume, this method favors very rapid drying. When this "dry inoculum method" was used, it was observed that bacterial killing initiated immediately. When alloy C11000 (99.9% copper) was challenged with *E coli* O157:H7, a 9-log drop was observed in only 1 minute.[17] The dry inoculum method was also used to test a copper-nickel-zinc alloy (C75200, 65% copper) and a brass (C28000, 60% copper). The result was over 9 logs of killing of *E coli* on both alloys within 15 minutes. These findings suggest that the killing times reported by Wilks et al[11] and Hong et al[12] were a result of the time required for the larger sample applied to dry, thus effectively delaying direct contact between the microorganism and the alloy surface.

Approximately 126 000 hospitalizations each year in the United States are caused by the "super bug" MRSA.[18] The efficacy of copper alloys against MRSA has been repeatedly confirmed in independent studies.[15,16,19-21] The power of copper alloys is its ability not only to kill bacteria after its surface is initially contaminated but also to keep on

killing after being repeatedly recontaminated, without any intermittent cleaning. As illustrated in Figure 24.2, C11000, containing 99.9% copper, maintains efficacy after a total of 8 inoculations without cleaning between inoculations over 24 hours.[13] Although a fall-off in efficacy is seen in C11000 between 12 and 24 hours, this will decrease if the reinoculation time is extended. In contrast, the quantity of MRSA increases after each inoculation on the stainless steel.

Three out of five clinically important MRSA strains tested on pure copper were killed within 60 minutes, and the remaining two strains were killed within 80 to 100 minutes, as reported by Gould et al.[16] A series of copper alloys, including brass and bronze, were challenged by MRSA inoculations as high as 10^5 to 10^8 CFUs per coupon, and greater than 99.9% kill was observed within 2 hours, as reported by Anderson and Michels.[13] Noyce et al[15] found that lowering the initial bacterial load resulted in a shorter time for pure copper to kill MRSA, from 60 minutes at 10^7 CFUs per coupon to 15 minutes at 10^3 CFUs per coupon. The lower level is more representative of the amount of contamination found on surfaces in hospitals.

One-third of enterococcal infections that occur in intensive care units (ICUs) in the United States are caused by vancomycin-resistant enterococci (VRE).[22] It is primarily transferred from environmental surfaces to patients and health care workers by touch.[23] Strains of vancomycin-resistant *Enterococcus faecalis* and *Enterococcus faecium* were killed in less than an hour by copper alloys containing at least 90% copper, but in contrast, they survived for several weeks on stainless steel, as reported by Warnes et al.[22] Gould et al[16] also reported similar results. The aforementioned studies imply that the use of copper alloy surfaces in hospitals should help fight VRE infections in ICUs.

Clostridium difficile is hard to kill. Its spores survive under extreme conditions, including up to 5 months on dry inanimate surfaces.[24] They are also not killed by all hospital-grade disinfectants, including those containing quaternary ammonium. Patients taking broad-spectrum antibiotics or who are otherwise immunocompromised are quite susceptible to *C difficile*, and it is very hard to cure. Weaver et al[25] reported that *C difficile* vegetative cells are highly sensitive to exposure to copper alloys, but *C difficile* spores are relatively resistant. Copper alloys ranging from 65% to 100% copper killed 10^5 *C difficile* spores in between 24 and 48 hours, a rather prolonged period. However, no loss in viability was seen on stainless steel. Wheeldon et al[26] reported that, after inducing *C difficile* spore germination, greater than 99% reduction from 10^6 CFUs/cm^2 was observed within 3 hours of exposure to a pure copper surface. Another spore-forming *Bacillus* species displayed similar results, in that the vegetative cells were highly sensitive to copper alloys, whereas the spore form was resistant.[27,28] It was also reported that a sporulation-defective strain of *Bacillus subtilis* was rapidly killed on copper alloy surfaces containing 60% to 100% copper, but a sporulation-competent strain exhibited only 1 log of killing, according to San et al.[28] These findings suggest that the addition of germinant to cleaning formulations could enhance the antimicrobial efficacy of copper alloys against spore-forming bacteria.

Viruses must invade other organisms to reproduce. However, copper alloy samples were found to permanently inactivate 75% of influenza A (H1N1) in 1 hour and almost 100% after 6 hours, according to Noyce et al.[29] Norovirus can ruin a cruise ship vacation. It is insidious because it can be transferred by hand-to-hand contact, touching environmental surfaces, and even ingesting contaminated food. Presently, the only method available to control norovirus outbreaks is to thoroughly clean and disinfect surfaces with bleach. Neither a vaccine nor an effective treatment exists. It is also hard to study because human norovirus cannot be cultured in the laboratory. However, murine norovirus, MNV-1, has been identified as a close surrogate. In one study, murine norovirus was found to be no longer infectious after as little as 30 minutes of exposure to copper (99.9% copper) and 60 minutes of exposure to copper-nickel (90% copper) surfaces, but the viral particles remained infectious when exposed to stainless steel for even longer times, according to Warnes and Keevil.[30] When using the "dry inoculum method," the inactivation rates were found to be 5 minutes for both copper (99.9% copper) and copper-nickel (90% copper) surfaces. In a subsequent study, Warnes et al[31] observed that capsid integrity was compromised upon coming in contact with copper alloys. These findings suggest that copper alloy railings in hallways and stairs, elevator buttons, and door hardware on cruise ships should help control and prevent norovirus outbreaks.

There is significant variability in the sensitivity of fungal species to copper alloy surface exposure.[32,33] Quaranta et al[33] found that *Candida albicans* and *Saccharomyces cerevisiae* vegetative cells were both extremely sensitive to copper alloy surface exposure when tested using either the wet or dry inoculums. However, when Weaver et al[32] tested a number of spore-forming species including *Aspergillus niger*, *Aspergillus flavus*, *Aspergillus fumigatus*, *Penicillium chrysogenum*, *Fusarium culmorum*, *Fusarium oxysporum*, and *Fusarium solani* on copper and aluminum coupons, it was observed that spores of all of these species were extremely resistant to copper surface exposure. Note that Weaver et al[32] choose aluminum rather than stainless steel as the control material because their study was aimed at air conditioning systems where mold is a problem. Aluminum is commonly used as fins on tubes to facilitate heat (and cold) transfer. Aluminum, like stainless steel, has no antimicrobial efficacy. *P chrysogenum* and the *Fusarium* species were found to not survive on copper after 24 hours. In contrast, the spores exposed to the aluminum surface showed no decrease in viability over the same time period. It required 4 to 10 days of exposure to copper for complete killing of the spores of *A flavus* and *A fumigatus*. Amazingly, *A niger* spores were still viable and showed no evidence of killing even after 10 days of exposure to copper. However, when *A niger* was in the vegetative state, its hyphae were unable to grow over a copper coupon, demonstrating significant inhibition, but were able to readily grow over the surface of the aluminum coupon. Thus, growth and survival of vegetative cells of these fungal species appears to be sensitive to copper alloy surface exposure, but spores are extremely resistant.

▶ SPECTRUM OF EFFICACY OF MICROORGANISMS SUSCEPTIBLE TO COPPER ALLOY SURFACE KILLING

The publication of the paper by Wilks et al[11] and the Public Health registration of over 500 copper alloys as antimicrobial materials by the US Environmental Protection Agency, after having demonstrated antimicrobial activity against six different bacteria under government-approved protocols,[13] made others aware of the antimicrobial properties of copper alloys. This stimulated other researchers to conduct additional investigations that lead to many additional published papers on the efficacy of copper alloys. Several microorganisms, including a variety of bacteria, plus viruses and fungi have been shown to be susceptible to copper alloy surfaces killing as discussed earlier in this chapter. Copper alloy surfaces have demonstrated antimicrobial efficacy against a wide range of additional microorganisms including prokaryotes, viruses, and fungi, many of which are listed in Table 24.2. Although extensive tabulations have been published,[54] no

TABLE 24.2	Spectrum of microorganisms shown to exhibit sensitivity to copper alloy surfaces[a]

Microorganism	Reference
Bacterial species	
Acinetobacter species (MDR and other strains)	[19], [34], [35], [36]
Bacillus anthrax, Bacillus cereus, Bacillus subtilis (vegetative cells, not spores)	[17], [27], [28]
Brachybacterium conglomeratum	[17]
Brucella melitensis	[27]
Burkholderia species	[27], [37], [38]
Campylobacter jejuni	[39]
Clostridium difficile (vegetative cells, not spores)	[25], [26]
Deinococcus radiodurans	[17]
Enterobacter species	[13], [34], [40]
Enterococci species (vancomycin-resistant, other strains)	[16], [22], [41], [42], [43]
Escherichia coli (various strains)	[11], [12], [13], [14], [15], [16], [17]
Francisella tularensis	[27]
Klebsiella pneumonia	[19], [34], [44]
Legionella pneumophila	[32], [45], [46]
Listeria monocytogenes	[47], [48]
Mycobacterium tuberculosis	[19]
Pantoea stewartii	[36]
Pseudomonas species	[13], [16], [34], [35], [36]
Salmonella enterica	[39], [44], [49]
Staphylococcus aureus (MRSA, other strains); *Streptococcus pneumoniae*, other species	[13], [15], [16], [19], [20], [35], [50]
Yersinia pestis	[27]
Viruses	
Coronavirus 229E (human)	[51]
Influenza A	[15], [29]
Norovirus (murine, human)	[30], [31], [52]
T2 bacteriophage	[53]
Vaccinia, Monkeypox	[27]
Fungi	
Aspergillus species	[32]
Candida albicans	[19], [32], [33]
Fusarium species	[32]
Penicillium chrysogenum	[32]
Saccharomyces cerevisiae	[33]

Abbreviations: MDR, multi-drug resistant; MRSA, methicillin-resistant *Staphylococcus aureus*.

[a]Reproduced with permission from Michels and Michels.[5]

such list should be considered definitive or complete because other organisms are continuing to be evaluated. As the referenced articles used different protocols, detailed comparisons between studies are tenuous at best. That being said, some generalizations can be made. First, all the species of bacteria listed in Table 24.2, which includes both gram-negative and gram-positive, have shown significant sensitivity to copper alloy surface exposure (except for the spore forms of *C difficile* and *Bacillus anthracis*). Second, killing rate increases as the copper content of the alloys increases.[11,12,25,28] Third, spore formation, which is a survival mechanism that fungi and a few bacteria can resort to when stressed, provides significant protection against copper alloy surface killing.[25,27] Fourth, because there have been only a few studies of viral sensitivity to copper alloy surfaces and those viruses studied to date have very different capsid type, additional studies are needed on a larger group of related viruses using a single protocol.

▶ MODE OF ACTION

It is not an overstatement to say that the ability of bacteria to mutate and thus become resistant to multiple antibiotics is a serious issue. However, as discussed in the following text, bacteria do not appear to be able to develop resistance against copper alloy surfaces. Thus, the emergence of mutated strains displaying resistance to copper alloy surfaces is unlikely. Copper ions, Cu^+ and Cu^{++}, initially form[14,17,36,43,55,56] when bacterial cells come in contact with copper alloy surfaces. The ability of copper to transition between these two oxidation states allows it to act as a catalyst in several biological processes not only in bacteria but also in humans.[57,58] Thus, copper is an essential micronutrient. Nonetheless, it is toxic at high intracellular concentrations and also can disrupt membrane integrity when presented to the outside surface of the cell.[59-64] Understanding the mechanism of copper alloy surface killing allows us to understand why resistant mutant strains have not been observed.

Our current understanding of copper's role in homeostasis is based on bacterial, yeast, and mammalian models.[57,58,60,65-70] Species have evolved tightly regulated mechanisms for copper homeostasis to allow a small amount to enter the cell as a micronutrient but not large amounts to avoid toxicity. The possibility of overwhelming this control mechanism was considered as a mechanism of copper alloy surface killing because intracellular copper level were observed to increase soon after exposure to copper alloy surfaces.[14,17,42,43,50] However, extensive evidence from a large number of studies by Grass and colleagues[14,17,61] strongly support that the primary site of attack is at the cell surface membrane.

It is known that transition metals such as copper (and iron) are capable of catalyzing the formation of reactive oxygen species (ROS), particularly hydroxyl radicals (•OH), via the Fenton reaction shown in the following text.[71-74]

$$Cu^+ + H_2O_2 \longrightarrow Cu^{++} + \bullet OH + OH^-$$

The unpaired electron of the hydroxyl radical is highly reactive and capable of causing oxidative damage to cellular macromolecules including lipids, proteins, and nucleic acids. The possibility that peroxidation of the unsaturated fatty acids of membrane phospholipids is the initiating event in killing by copper alloy surfaces was investigated by Hong et al.[12] *E coli* cells were exposed to the surfaces of a series of copper-zinc alloys, specifically C24000, C2600, and C2800, and a high copper alloy, C11000 (see Table 24.1) and monitored the kinetics of killing and lipid peroxidation. They found a correlation between higher copper concentration of the alloy and more rapid killing and a faster rate of lipid peroxidation. In addition, the loss in membrane integrity coincided with the timing of cell death and peak lipid peroxidation. To test this correlation, Hong et al[12] used a mutant strain of *E coli* having an increased ratio of unsaturated to saturated fatty acids. They observed that the rate of lipid peroxidation increased in the mutant strain when compared to that observed in the parent strain, and the mutant strain was significantly more sensitive to copper alloy surface killing.

As initially hypothesized by Hong et al,[12] these results clearly implicate the peroxidation of unsaturated fatty acids in the *E coli* membrane as the cause of the rapid, efficient, and catastrophic cell death observed in cells exposed to dry metallic copper alloy surfaces. San et al[28] conducted a similar investigation of the gram-positive *B subtilis*. Because *B subtilis* spores were resistant to copper alloy surface exposure, they used a sporulation-defective mutant strain to demonstrate that lipid peroxidation correlated with cell death. It is believed that the loss of membrane integrity is the primary step in the killing mechanism. This damage to the membrane so severely compromises its integrity that death occurs so rapidly that the cell is unable to mount an effective repair response or mutate to a copper-resistant form.

▶ ANTIMICROBIAL COPPER ALLOYS IN A HOSPITAL CLINICAL TRIAL

A clinical trial was conducted in three major US hospitals by a US team of infectious disease specialists, microbiologists, metallurgical engineers, and statisticians and is described here in detail. The clinical trial was designed to answer the following key questions. Do the surfaces of components made from standard materials, such as stainless steel, plastics, and wood, harbor bacteria, and if so, in what quantity? Similarly, do the surfaces of components made from copper alloys harbor bacteria in the clinical environment, and if so, in what quantity? Will a quantifiable reduction in bacterial levels be observed on the surfaces made from copper alloys versus the components made from standard materials? Finally, and most importantly, will any observed reduction in bacteria on the components made from copper alloys translate into a reduction in infections by patients in these copper rooms versus patients in standard rooms?

The medical ICU was selected to conduct a clinical trial because its patients often have compromised immunity and are thus more susceptible to acquiring infections. The major premise was that if copper alloys were found to be antimicrobial in the clinical setting, their introduction would provide meaningful and measurable benefit in the ICU setting. The following three hospitals were selected to participate in the clinical trial:

- Memorial Sloan Kettering Cancer Center, in New York City, NY
- Medical University of South Carolina, in Charleston, SC
- Ralph H. Johnson Veterans Administration Medical Center, also Charleston, SC

The trial was designed in three phases, to be conducted sequentially:

- Phase 1 measured the baseline microbial burden on existing components in the "standard rooms" made from conventional or standard materials.
- Phase 2 installed a suite of components made with copper alloy surfaces in random patient rooms, identified as "copper rooms." Following several weeks of adaptation to the ICU environment, the microbial burden was measured on the suite of component surfaces in the "copper rooms" and compared to the measurements on the suite of components in the "standard rooms."
- Phase 3 measured infection rates of patients in "standard rooms" and compared these with the infection rates measured in "copper rooms."

On the basis of the microbial burdens found on a variety of components in phase 1, the following six components were found to be the most contaminated:

- Bed rails
- Nurses' call button
- Arms of the visitor's chair
- Over-the-bed patient tray table
- Intravenous (IV) pole
- Data input device, which varied by hospital (mouse, laptop, or the bezel on a touch screen patient monitor)

It was not a coincidence that these were the components positioned closest to the patient. It was decided that the same six components would be fabricated in copper alloys and installed in random ICU rooms, identified as "copper rooms" in phases 2 and 3.

Phase 1: The techniques used to collect samples of bacteria were developed and refined to optimize the quantity of bacteria removed from the surfaces of the components

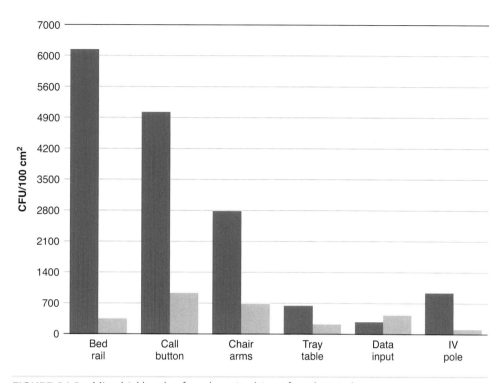

FIGURE 24.3 Microbial burden found on six objects from hospital intensive care unit (ICU) rooms. Samples were taken from the standard noncopper ICU rooms (dark blue bars) and from the copper component ICU rooms (light blue bars). Abbreviations: CFU, colony-forming unit; IV, intravenous. From Schmidt et al.[76] Reproduced with permission from American Society for Microbiology. Copyright © 2012 American Society for Microbiology.

in single-patient ICU rooms and subsequently released for culturing. For additional detail on the sampling protocol, refer to Attaway et al.[75] The nursing staff was only informed on the day that sampling would occur. Samples were collected randomly on a weekly basis. Surfaces that were sampled on the existing standard components were made of conventional materials including plastics, wood, coated steel, aluminum, and stainless steel but not copper alloys. The surfaces of selected standard components in the "standard rooms" were used as experimental controls in phases 2 and 3.

Phase 2: Those components, whose surfaces were the most highly contaminated in phase 1, were selected to be reproduced in copper alloys. A set of the six copper components listed earlier were placed in random ICU rooms, identified as "copper rooms." Eight "copper rooms" and 8 "standard rooms" were deployed over the three hospitals, for a total of 16 rooms. Patients were assigned to the first available room to achieve randomness. Trial personnel had no influence in timing, frequency, or method of cleaning, although hand hygiene was monitored. Sampling was performed weekly at random. The noncopper or standard foot rail of the bed was sampled in all 16 rooms to monitor cleaning on both the "standard rooms" and the "copper rooms" without informing the cleaning and health care teams. For additional detail regarding efforts to achieve maximum randomness and minimize bias, refer to Schmidt et al.[76]

Experts in the field of microbial burden generally accept below 250 CFUs/cm^2 as benign.[76-81] As shown in Figure 24.3,[76] the contaminated levels measured on all six items in the "standard rooms" exceeded the aforementioned benign level of 250 CFUs/cm^2, with the bed rail showing the most contamination. This is both alarming and significant because the bed rail is a major area of interaction between the patient, health care workers, and visitors. The contamination levels measured on the other five items in the "standard rooms" decrease in this order: the call button, chair arms, IV pole, tray table, and data input device. The average contamination level in the standard room was 2674 CFUs/cm^2 but only 465 CFUs/cm^2 in the copper rooms, which translates into a reduction of 83%. In addition to the much lower contamination levels on the components in "copper rooms," there were also relatively small differences in contamination levels found on the six components in those rooms. As shown in Figure 24.3, the call button in the "copper rooms" had the highest level followed by the chair arms, data input device, bed rail, tray table, and IV pole.

Phase 3: Hospital-acquired infections (HAIs) were determined by clinicians at each hospital according to National Healthcare Safety Network definitions, after examining relevant clinical information. However, patient identity and room type (either "standard" or "copper") were not disclosed in the records provided to the clinicians.

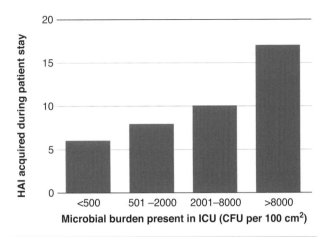

FIGURE 24.4 Distribution of health care–associated infection as a function of microbial burden. The number of hospital-acquired infections (HAIs) acquired during the patient stay is plotted versus the microbial burden of the intensive care unit (ICU) rooms during the patient stay. Standardized procedures were used to swab and titer the level of bacterial contamination on the surface of various components from standard (noncopper) and copper medical ICU patient rooms. Reproduced with permission from Salgado et al.[82]

Patients in both types of rooms had comparable clinical characteristics and demographics. The copper components were in the ICU rooms for 9 months prior to beginning the collection of infection rate data. Thus, health care workers became accustomed to seeing the copper surfaces every day. In addition, the ICU staff was not told that measurement of infection rates, phase 3, had started. As reported by Salgado et al,[82] 26 out of 320 patients, or 8.1%, were infected in the standard rooms, whereas 10 out of 320 patients, or 3.4%, displayed infection in the copper rooms. Thus, the infection rate displayed a measurable reduction, by introducing only six copper components into random ICU rooms. This translates into a 58% reduction with a *P* value of .013, which is an indication of high statistical significance.

High microbial burden correlates with greater infection, as shown in Figure 24.4.[82] Figure 24.4 includes all the data from both the standard and copper rooms and is statistically significant as indicated by its *P* value of .038. Only 17% of the total 4 450 545 CFUs of bacteria identified from all rooms were recovered from the copper surfaces, whereas the remaining 83% were found on the standard surfaces. Thus, the cleaner surfaces, meaning lower bacterial burden, favor the lower infection rates observed in the copper rooms.

The Salgado et al[82] trial was the first study that demonstrated that an active antimicrobial environmental surface could reduce HAIs. Therefore, as in all scientific research, additional studies are needed to confirm and verify the findings reported by Salgado et al.[82]

ANTIMICROBIAL COPPER ALLOYS IN PUBLIC SPACES

A short study was conducted over 10 weeks in Grand Central Terminal in New York city by measuring contamination levels on existing brass railings versus wood, marble and stainless railings, brass shelves versus marble ticket counters, and brass door pulls and push bars versus adjacent glass and wood surfaces. The brass rails showed a 97% reduction in bacteria, the brass shelves a 94% reduction, and the door hardware an 84% reduction when compared to the standard materials. This study indicated that copper alloy surfaces retain the efficacy for decades, even when they are not cleaned as frequently as in hospitals.

ANTIMICROBIAL COPPER ALLOYS AND TOXICITY

Copper is an essential nutrient for all forms of life, including humans. The US Food and Nutrition Board of the National Academies of Sciences, Engineering, and Medicine recommends copper intake of 0.9 mg/d in adults. Good sources of dietary copper include oysters, nuts, seeds, dark chocolate, whole grains, and liver. The ingestion of large amounts of copper as compounds can be toxic. They can damage the nervous system, leading to liver and kidney failure and even death. Those afflicted with Wilson disease, a rare recessive hereditary ailment, are unable to eliminate copper from the body. They are particular at risk of reaching toxic levels. That being said, there is no known harmful effect to humans from touching copper alloy surfaces. Unlike the membranes of bacteria, the skin of humans provides a high degree of protection against copper entering the body. Centuries of use of copper coinage, copper jewelry, and copper architectural materials is sufficient evidence of the high standard of safety of copper alloys used by humans.

ANTIMICROBIAL COPPER ALLOYS AND THE FUTURE

As stated previously, the ability of bacteria to mutate and thus become resistant to multiple antibiotics is a serious issue. The widespread overuse, misuse, and abuse, by humans and in raising poultry and other animals for human consumption, is contributing to the emergence of antibiotic-resistant strains of bacteria, according to the Centers for Disease Control and Prevention. Stimulating growth of these animals with subclinical doses of antibiotics has also made them hosts for antibiotic-resistant bacteria.[83] The use of copper surfaces in raising animals for food production could reduce the need for antibiotics in animal husbandry. Copper alloys could also reduce the transmission of antibiotic-resistant organisms, such as *E coli* O157:H7, if used in food processing facilities. Thus, copper could help prevent the emergence of other antibiotic resistance strains such an MRSA, which evolved in the hospital setting.

The first commercial antimicrobial components were produced in 2011. As of 2018, over 300 facilities have installed products made from antimicrobial copper that were manufactured by US suppliers. These installations are located in 37 states and 13 countries and include health care facilities, schools including universities, airports, office buildings, physical fitness facilities, laboratories, and restaurants. As the benefits of antimicrobial copper become better known, its use should increase. This will not only help reduce infections but also contribute to the decrease in the emergence of additional antibiotic-resistant infectious strains because of its ability to rapidly and completely kill bacteria.

▶ ACKNOWLEDGMENTS

We would like to thank Adam Estelle of the Copper Development Association, Inc. for his assistance and input in this review. We wish to also thank all the investigators we have interacted with over the years, especially Professors C. W. Keevil of the University of Southampton and Michael G. Schmidt of the Medical University of South Carolina. We also are grateful to the members and management of the International Copper Association, Ltd. and Copper Development Association, Inc. for their financial support, as well as the U.S. Army Materials Command that provided funding for the clinical trial.

REFERENCES

1. Scott RD. *The Direct Medical Cost of Healthcare-Associated Infections in U.S. Hospitals and the Benefits of Prevention*. Atlanta, GA: Centers for Disease Control and Prevention; 2009.
2. Boyce JM. Environmental contamination makes an important contribution to hospital infection. *J Hosp Infect*. 2007;65(suppl 2):50-54.
3. Afshinnekoo E, Meydan C, Chowdhury S, et al. Geospatial resolution of human and bacterial diversity with city-scale metagenomics. *Cell Syst*. 2015;1:72-87.
4. Centers for Disease Control and Prevention. Norovirus. https://www.cdc.gov/norovirus/trends-outbreaks.html. Accessed June 8, 2019.
5. Michels HT, Michels CA. Copper alloys—the new 'old' weapon in the fight against infectious disease. *Curr Trends Microbiol*. 2016;10:23-45.
6. Langner BE. *Understanding Copper: Technologies, Markets, Business*. Lunebürg, Germany: Druckerei Wulf; 2011.
7. Dollwet HHA, Sorenson JRJ. Historic uses of copper compounds in medicine. *Trace Elem Med*. 1985;2(2):80-87.
8. Sudha VBP, Ganesan S, Pazhani GP, Ramamurthy T, Nair GB, Venkatasubramanian P. Storing drinking-water in copper pots kills contaminating diarrhoeagenic bacteria. *J Health Popul Nutr*. 2012;30(1):17-21.
9. Milne JS. *Surgical Instruments in Greek and Roman Times*. Oxford, United Kingdom: Clarendon Press; 1907.
10. Kuhn PJ. Doorknobs: a source of nosocomial infection? *Diag Med*. 1983;6(8):62-63. https://www.antimicrobialcopper.org/sites/default/files/upload/media-library/files/pdfs/uk/scientific_literature/kuhn-doorknob.pdf. Accessed June 8, 2019.
11. Wilks SA, Michels HT, Keevil CW. The survival of *Escherichia coli* O157 on a range of metal surfaces. *Int J Food Microbiol*. 2005;105(3):445-454.
12. Hong R, Kang TY, Michels CA, Gadura N. Membrane lipid peroxidation in copper alloy-mediated contact killing of *Escherichia coli*. *Appl Environ Microbiol*. 2012;78(6):1776-1784.
13. Anderson DG, Michels HT. Antimicrobial regulatory efficacy testing of solid copper alloy surfaces in the USA. In: Collery P, Maymard I, Thephanides T, Khassanova, L, Collery T, eds. *Metal Ions in Biology and Medicine*. Vol 10. Montrouge, France: John Libbey Eurotext; 2008:185-190.
14. Espírito Santo C, Taudte N, Nies DH, Grass G. Contribution of copper ion resistance to survival of *Escherichia coli* on metallic copper surfaces. *Appl Environ Microbiol*. 2008;74(4):977-986.
15. Noyce JO, Michels HT, Keevil CW. Potential use of copper surfaces to reduce survival of epidemic meticillin-resistant *Staphylococcus aureus* in the healthcare environment. *J Hosp Infect*. 2006;63(3):289-297.
16. Gould SWJ, Fielder MD, Kelly AF, Morgan M, Kenny J, Naughton DP. The antimicrobial properties of copper surfaces against a range of important nosocomial pathogens. *Ann Microbiol*. 2009;59(1):151-156.
17. Espírito Santo C, Lam EW, Elowsky CG, et al. Bacterial killing by dry metallic copper surfaces. *Appl Environ Microbiol*. 2011;77(3):794-802.
18. Kuehnert MJ, Hill HA, Kupronis BA, Tokars JI, Solomon SL, Jernigan DB. Methicillin-resistant–*Staphylococcus aureus* hospitalizations, United States. *Emerg Infect Dis*. 2005;11(6):868-872.
19. Mehtar S, Wiid I, Todorov SD. The antimicrobial activity of copper and copper alloys against nosocomial pathogens and *Mycobacterium tuberculosis* isolated from healthcare facilities in the Western Cape: an in-vitro study. *J Hosp Infect*. 2008;68(1):45-51.
20. Michels HT, Noyce JO, Keevil CW. Effects of temperature and humidity on the efficacy of methicillin-resistant *Staphylococcus aureus* challenged antimicrobial materials containing silver and copper. *Lett Appl Microbiol*. 2009;49(2):191-195.
21. Weaver L, Noyce JO, Michels HT, Keevil CW. Potential action of copper surfaces on meticillin-resistant *Staphylococcus aureus*. *J Appl Microbiol*. 2010;109(6):2200-2205.
22. Warnes SL, Green SM, Michels HT, Keevil CW. Biocidal efficacy of copper alloys against pathogenic enterococci involves degradation of genomic and plasmid DNAs. *Appl Environ Microbiol*. 2010;76(16):5390-5401.
23. Drees M, Snydman DR, Schmid CH, et al. Prior environmental contamination increases the risk of acquisition of vancomycin-resistant enterococci. *Clin Infect Dis*. 2008;46(5):678-685.
24. Kramer A, Schwebke I, Kampf G. How long do nosocomial pathogens persist on inanimate surfaces? A systematic review. *BMC Infect Dis*. 2006;6:130.
25. Weaver L, Michels HT, Keevil CW. Survival of *Clostridium difficile* on copper and steel: futuristic options for hospital hygiene. *J Hosp Infect*. 2008;68(2):145-151.
26. Wheeldon LJ, Worthington T, Lambert PA, Hilton AC, Lowden CJ, Elliott TSJ. Antimicrobial efficacy of copper surfaces against spores and vegetative cells of *Clostridium difficile*: the germination theory. *J Antimicrob Chemother*. 2008;62(3):522.
27. Bleichert P, Espírito Santo C, Hanczaruk M, Meyer H, Grass G. Inactivation of bacterial and viral biothreat agents on metallic copper surfaces. *Biometals*. 2014;27(6):1179-1189.
28. San K, Long J, Michels CA, Gadura N. Antimicrobial copper alloy surfaces are effective against vegetative but not sporulated cells of gram-positive *Bacillus subtilis*. *Microbiologyopen*. 2015;4(5):753-763.
29. Noyce JO, Michels HT, Keevil CW. Inactivation of influenza A virus on copper versus stainless steel surfaces. *Appl Environ Microbiol*. 2007;73(8):2748-2750.
30. Warnes SL, Keevil CW. Inactivation of norovirus on dry copper alloy surfaces. *PLoS One*. 2013;8(9):e75017.
31. Warnes SL, Summersgill EN, Keevil CW. Inactivation of murine norovirus on a range of copper alloy surfaces is accompanied by loss of capsid integrity. *Appl Environ Microbiol*. 2015;81(3):1085-1091.
32. Weaver L, Michels HT, Keevil CW. Potential for preventing spread of fungi in air-conditioning systems constructed using copper instead of aluminium. *Lett Appl Microbiol*. 2010;50(1):18-23.
33. Quaranta D, Krans T, Espírito Santo C, et al. Mechanisms of contact-mediated killing of yeast cells on dry metallic copper surfaces. *Appl Environ Microbiol*. 2011;77(2):416-426.

34. Souli M, Galani I, Plachouras D, et al. Antimicrobial activity of copper surfaces against carbapenemase-producing contemporary gram-negative clinical isolates. *J Antimicrob Chemother*. 2013;68(4):852-857.

35. Eser OK, Ergin A, Hascelik G. Antimicrobial activity of copper alloys against invasive multidrug-resistant nosocomial pathogens. *Curr Microbiol*. 2015;71(2):291-295.

36. Santo CE, Morais PV, Grass G. Isolation and characterization of bacteria resistant to metallic copper surfaces. *Appl Environ Microbiol*. 2010;76(5):1341-1348.

37. Cui Z, Ibrahim M, Yang C, et al. Susceptibility of opportunistic *Burkholderia glumae* to copper surfaces following wet or dry surface contact. *Molecules*. 2014;19(7):9975-9985.

38. Ibrahim M, Wang F, Lou M, et al. Copper as an antibacterial agent for human pathogenic multidrug resistant *Burkholderia cepacia* complex bacteria. *J Biosci Bioeng*. 2011;112(6):570-576.

39. Faúndez G, Troncoso M, Navarrete P, Figueroa G. Antimicrobial activity of copper surfaces against suspensions of *Salmonella enterica* and *Campylobacter jejuni*. *BMC Microbiol*. 2004;4:19.

40. Tian WX, Yu S, Ibrahim M, et al. Copper as an antimicrobial agent against opportunistic pathogenic and multidrug resistant *Enterobacter* bacteria. *J Microbiol*. 2012;50(4):586-593.

41. Warnes SL, Keevil CW. Mechanism of copper surface toxicity in vancomycin-resistant enterococci following wet or dry surface contact. *Appl Environ Microbiol*. 2011;77:6049-6059.

42. Elguindi, J, Wagner J, Rensing C. Genes involved in copper resistance influence survival of *Pseudomonas aeruginosa* on copper surfaces. *J Appl Microbiol*. 2009;106:1448-1455.

43. Molteni C, Abicht HK, Solioz M. Killing of bacteria by copper surfaces involves dissolved copper. *Appl Environ Microbiol*. 2010;76(12):4099-4101.

44. Warnes SL, Highmore CJ, Keevil CW. Horizontal transfer of antibiotic resistance genes on abiotic touch surfaces: implications for public health. *MBio*. 2012;3(6):e00489-e00512.

45. Gião MS, Wilks SA, Keevil CW. Influence of copper surfaces on biofilm formation by *Legionella pneumophila* in potable water. *Biometals*. 2015;28(2):329-339.

46. Rogers J, Dowsett AB, Dennis PJ, Lee JV, Keevil CW. Influence of plumbing materials on biofilm formation and growth of *Legionella pneumophila* in potable water systems. *Appl Environ Microbiol*. 1994;60(6):1842-1851.

47. Abushelaibi A. *Antimicrobial Effects of Copper and Brass Ions on the Growth of Listeria monocytogenes at Temperatures, pH and Nutrients* [dissertation]. Baton Rouge, LA: Louisiana State University; 2005.

48. Wilks SA, Michels HT, Keevil CW. Survival of *Listeria monocytogenes* Scott A on metal surfaces: implications for cross-contamination. *Int J Food Microbiol*. 2006;111(2):93-98.

49. Zhu L, Elguindi J, Rensing C, Ravishankar S. Antimicrobial activity of different copper alloy surfaces against copper resistant and sensitive *Salmonella enterica*. *Food Microbiol*. 2012;30(1):303-310.

50. Santo CE, Quaranta D, Grass G. Antimicrobial metallic copper surfaces kill *Staphylococcus haemolyticus* via membrane damage. *Microbiologyopen*. 2012;1(1):46-52.

51. Warnes SL, Little ZR, Keevil CW. Human coronavirus 229E remains infectious on common touch surface materials. *MBio*. 2015;6(6):e01697-e01715.

52. Manuel CS, Moore MD, Jaykus LA. Destruction of the capsid and genome of GII.4 human norovirus occurs during exposure to metal alloys containing copper. *Appl Environ Microbiol*. 2015;81(15):4940-4946.

53. Li J, Dennehy JJ. Differential bacteriophage mortality on exposure to copper. *Appl Environ Microbiol*. 2011;77(19):6878-6883.

54. Borkow G. Using copper to fight microorganisms. *Curr Chem Biol*. 2012;6(2):93-103.

55. Elguindi J, Moffitt S, Hasman H, Andrade C, Raghavan S, Rensing C. Metallic copper corrosion rates, moisture content, and growth medium influence survival of copper ion-resistant bacteria. *Appl Microbiol Biotechnol*. 2011;89(6):1963-1970.

56. Zeiger M, Solioz M, Edongué H, Arzt E, Schneider AS. Surface structure influences contact killing of bacteria by copper. *Microbiologyopen*. 2014;3(3):327-332.

57. Hordyjewska A, Popiołek Ł, Kocot J. The many "faces" of copper in medicine and treatment. *Biometals*. 2014;27(4):611-621.

58. Ladomersky E, Petris MJ. Copper tolerance and virulence in bacteria. *Metallomics*. 2015;7(6):957-958.

59. Catalá A. An overview of lipid peroxidation with emphasis in outer segments of photoreceptors and the chemiluminescence assay. *Int J Biochem Cell Biol*. 2006;38(9):1482-1495.

60. Cervantes C, Gutierrez-Corona F. Copper resistance mechanisms in bacteria and fungi. *FEMS Microbiol Rev*. 1994;14(2):121-137.

61. Grass G, Rensing C, Solioz M. Metallic copper as an antimicrobial surface. *Appl Environ Microbiol*. 2011;77(5):1541-1547.

62. Macomber L, Imlay JA. The iron-sulfur clusters of dehydratases are primary intracellular targets of copper toxicity. *Proc Natl Acad Sci U S A*. 2009;106(20):8344-8349.

63. Ohsumi Y, Kitamoto K, Anraku Y. Changes induced in the permeability barrier of the yeast plasma membrane by cupric ion. *J Bacteriol*. 1988;170(6):2676-2682.

64. Grass G, Rensing C. Genes involved in copper homeostasis in *Escherichia coli*. *J Bacteriol*. 2001;183(6):2145-2147.

65. Kim BE, Nevitt T, Thiele DJ. Mechanisms for copper acquisition, distribution and regulation. *Nat Chem Biol*. 2008;4(3):176-185.

66. Brown NL, Rouch DA, Lee BT. Copper resistance determinants in bacteria. *Plasmid*. 1992;27(1):41-51.

67. Bondarczuk K, Piotrowska-Seget Z. Molecular basis of active copper resistance mechanisms in gram-negative bacteria. *Cell Biol Toxicol*. 2013;29(6):397-405.

68. Cooksey DA. Copper uptake and resistance in bacteria. *Mol Microbiol*. 1993;7(1):1-5.

69. Rademacher C, Masepohl B. Copper-responsive gene regulation in bacteria. *Microbiol*. 2012;158:2451-2464.

70. Argüello JM, Raimunda D, Padilla-Benavides T. Mechanisms of copper homeostasis in bacteria. *Front Cell Infect Microbiol*. 2013;3:73.

71. Kehrer JP. The Haber-Weiss reaction and mechanisms of toxicity. *Toxicology*. 2000;149(1):43-50.

72. Valko M, Morris H, Cronin MTD. Metals, toxicity and oxidative stress. *Curr Med Chem*. 2005;12(10):1161-1208.

73. Lemire JA, Harrison JJ, Turner RJ. Antimicrobial activity of metals: mechanisms, molecular targets and applications. *Nat Rev Microbiol*. 201;11(6):371-384.

74. Hans M, Mathews S, Mücklich F, Solioz M. Physicochemical properties of copper important for its antibacterial activity and development of a unified model. *Biointerphases*. 2015;11(1):018902.

75. Attaway HH III, Fairey S, Steed LL, Salgado CD, Michels HT, Schmidt MG. Intrinsic bacterial burden associated with intensive care unit hospital beds: effects of disinfection on population recovery and mitigation of potential infection risk. *Am J Infect Control*. 2012;40(10):907-912.

76. Schmidt MG, Attaway HH, Sharpe PA, et al. Sustained reduction of microbial burden on common hospital surfaces through introduction of copper. *J Clin Microbiol*. 2012;50(7):2217-2223.

77. Dancer SJ. How do we assess hospital cleaning? A proposal for microbiological standards for surface hygiene in hospitals. *J Hosp Infect*. 2004;56(1):10-15.

78. Lewis T, Griffith C, Gallo M, Weinbren M. A modified ATP benchmark for evaluating the cleaning of some hospital environmental surfaces. *J Hosp Infect*. 2008;69(2):156-163.

79. Malik RE, Cooper RA, Griffith CJ. Use of audit tools to evaluate the efficacy of cleaning systems in hospitals. *Am J Infect Control*. 2003;31(3):181-187.

80. Mulvey D, Redding P, Robertson C, et al. Finding a benchmark for monitoring hospital cleanliness. *J Hosp Infect*. 2011;77(1):25-30.

81. White LF, Dancer SJ, Robertson C, McDonald J. Are hygiene standards useful in assessing infection risk? *Am J Infect Control*. 2008;36(5):381-384.

82. Salgado CD, Sepkowitz KA, John JF, et al. Copper surfaces reduce the rate of healthcare-acquired infections in the intensive care unit. *Infect Control Hosp Epidemiol*. 2013;34(5):479-486.

83. Levy SB, Marshall B. Antibacterial resistance worldwide: causes, challenges and responses. *Nat Med*. 2004;10(suppl 12):S122-S129.

Silver and Silver Nanoparticles

Jean-Yves Maillard and Philippe Hartemann

KEYWORDS: silver, nanoparticles, mechanisms, efficacy, toxicity, resistance

Silver has been the most used metallic salt for its antimicrobial properties over centuries.[1-3] There are different forms of silver that can be incorporated in products, including metallic silver (Ag^0), silver ions (most common Ag^{1+}, Ag^{2+}, or Ag^{3+}), and silver nanoparticles (nanosilver; AgNPs) for this chapter, ionic silver will be abbreviated to Ag. An AgNP is defined as particulate matter, aggregate, or agglomerate for which 50% or more of the particles in the number size distribution are in the range 1 to 100 nm. The AgNPs can be used in a wide range of matrices and formulations including composites, colloids, fibers, gels, coatings, membranes, and thin films.[4-8] The form of silver and concentration, formulations, and matrices can impact antimicrobial efficacy and overall toxicity. The Ag and AgNPs are widely used today for their antimicrobial properties in a wide range of applications including consumer home products, health care industry, clothing and fabric industry, food industry, and construction industry (Table 25.1).[8-16] The number of clothing items (eg, cleaning textiles, sportswear, gloves, socks, underwear, helmet lining) incorporating Ag/AgNPs as an antimicrobial, notably to control malodors,[16-18] has rapidly increased in recent years. There are now thousands of products containing silver (AgNPs) for the consumer home and other markets. The AgNPs might be the most commonly used nanomaterials in consumer products (eg, see https://www.nanotech project.org). It is clear from these diverse applications that the majority of Ag- and AgNP-containing products are used in a dry condition as opposed to immersion in liquids (see Table 25.1). This is an important consideration, which will be discussed later. The use of AgNPs in the food industry can be categorized in different stages of food production such as crop harvest (use of Ag/AgNPs-based agricultural disinfectants), food processing (food

preparation equipment), and storage (sprays, refrigerators, storage containers).[19] In the European Union, no nanomaterials are admitted for use in plastics that come into contact with food unless authorized. The regulation of silver nanoparticles in products is complex and depends on the application.[3] In the United States, in contrast, the use of AgNPs in food containers is possible but has to be registered.[20] The US Food and Drug Administration (FDA) has issued guidance on the regulation of nanomaterials (https://www.fda.gov/scienceresearch/specialtopics/nano technology/ucm301114.htm). An important use of Ag/AgNPs is in the construction industry notably in paint products, sealants, etc, and incorporated onto various plastics. The AgNPs are also used for disinfection of drinking water, cooling towers, and recreational water applications.[2,21]

The Ag and AgNPs used for biomedical applications have recently been reviewed.[11] Applications include wound dressings, bandages,[1,8,12,22-24] medical devices such as catheters,[25-30] bone scaffolds,[31,32] and potentially ocular devices.[33] The combination of low concentrations of silver ion with hydrogen peroxide (5%) in an aerosol (dry mist) is also used for the disinfection of wards, medical equipments, and ambulances.[34,35]

The incorporation Ag/AgNPs in medical dressings was introduced in the 20th century with silver foil dressing[9,36,37] and then with silver nitrate (0.5%) in compresses for the treatment of burn wounds and particularly for the control of *Pseudomonas aeruginosa*.[38] The development of bacterial resistance to silver nitrate forced a change in formulations with combining actives, notably Ag-sulfonamide (silver sulfadiazine).[39-41] A number of additional combinations have been used such as silver sulfadiazine with chlorhexidine,[42] silver sulfadiazine, and cerium nitrate (Flammacerium).[43,44] The combination of Ag or AgNPs with other antimicrobials and various polymers in a dressing aims to improve antimicrobial efficacy with the effective release of Ag/AgNPs, decrease

TABLE 25.1	Examples of some Ag and AgNPs applications
Healthcare	Wounds dressings, antiseptics, hospital beds and furniture, water distribution networks (Cu-Ag)
Home consumer products	Fabric conditioners, baby bottles, food storage containers and salad bowls, kitchen cutting boards, bed mattress, vacuum cleaner, disposable curtains and blinds, tableware, independent living aids—bathroom products, furniture (chairs), kitchen gadgets and bath accessories, dishwashers, refrigerators and washing machines, toilet tank levers to sink stoppers, toilet seat, pillows and mattresses, food storers, containers, ice trays and other plastic kitchenware, hair brush, hair straightener, combs, brushes, rollers, shower caps
	Toothpaste, cosmetic deodorants, toothbrushes, tissue paper, epilator, electric shaver
	Pet shampoos, feeders and waters, litter pans, pet bedding and shelter, paper, pens and pencils, ATM buttons, remote control, handrails (buses), computer keyboards, hand dryers, wireless voice communicators with badge and the sleeves, yoga mat, coatings for use on laptop computers, calculators, sheet protectors, name badges and holders, shop ticket holders, media storage products, laminating film, report covers and project folders, photo holders, memory book, office accessories, transparency film, collapsible coolers
Clothing and fabrics	Baby clothes, underwear, socks, footwear, various fabrics and vinyls, bath towels, quilts, sleeping bags, bed linens, pillows, quilts, mattress protectors, and towels
Food	Packaging, nanobiotic poultry production
Construction	Powder coating (door knobs), wall paints, air conditioning, epoxy resin floor, PVC wall cladding, antimicrobial flooring, metal suspended ceiling systems, window blinds and shading systems, shelving systems, decorative wood laminates, electrical wiring accessories, no tile panels (alternative to standard tiling), hygienic laminated surfaces, wallpaper, borders and murals, carpet and carpet underlay, seals (door for cooler doors and freezer cells, tank lids, mixers and kneading machines, hospital doors, for vibrating screens/vibrosieves in the pharmaceutical industry)
Disinfectants	Agricultural disinfectants, industrial disinfectants, aquaculture disinfectants, pool disinfectants

Abbreviations: Ag, silver; AgNPs, silver nanoparticles; ATM, automated teller machine; Cu-Ag, copper-silver; PVC, polyvinyl chloride.

overall toxicity, and overall improve wound healing.[45-51] The use of antimicrobial (including Ag/AgNPs) dressing is recommended for infected acute and chronic wounds (eg, burns, traumatic wounds, and diabetic ulcers)[2] to reduce microbial bioburden that can prevent healing and for the prevention of infection and reinfection. A number of Ag/AgNP-based wound dressings have been authorized on the US market by the FDA.[7]

In dentistry, Ag has been used in amalgams[52,53] but is now replaced with more modern materials. Clinical evidence, in vitro and in vivo, originally indicated that Ag can prevent and stop caries in the primary and permanent dentition, although its use can be associated with tooth discoloration and pulp irritation.[53] Incorporation of AgNPs in dental materials (polymeric filling materials, cements, denture base materials, artificial teeth, etc) enhances the antimicrobial activity of the material, whereas staining can be reduced with reduced AgNP size for dental and other applications.[54-64]

The extent of Ag/AgNPs use in so many applications has highlighted it as an effective antimicrobial.[65]

ANTIMICROBIAL EFFICACY

Ionic silver and AgNPs have been shown to have broad spectrum of activity.[4,6,66-73] Gram-negative bacteria are generally more susceptible to Ag than gram-positive bacteria.[74,75] The activity of silver resides in ionic silver at a concentration of 10^{-9} to 10^{-6} mol/L while Ag^0 is inactive. Exopolysaccharide might reduce the concentration or penetration of ionic silver[76] and as such Ag activity against microbial biofilm may be limited. The AgNPs overall has been shown to have a better bactericidal efficacy (ng/L concentrations) than ionic silver (μg/L concentrations).[4,66,68-79] The AgNPs have also been reported to have some activity in the presence of bacterial biofilms.[78-81] The antimicrobial efficacy of Ag and AgNPs depends on their bioavailability.[82] Bioavailability can be reduced by complexation, sorption, and precipitation, for example, in the presence of chloride, sulfide and phosphate, and generally organic matter.[83] For this reason, the use of Ag in wounds has limitation both in terms of penetration and reduced bioavailability because of organic matter. The maximum concentration of available ionic silver attainable in wounds has been estimated not to exceed 1 μg/mL.[46] Likewise, activity of AgNPs against biofilm is hampered probably because of aggregation and retarded biosorption.[84]

An Ag/AgNPs needs to be in contact with the targeted microorganisms to exert an antimicrobial effect.[85] The level of hydration will significantly impact Ag efficacy. In dressings, the release of ionic silver is linked to the level of hydration.[86] For dry-surface applications, such as in many consumer products (see Table 25.1), the absence of hydration/moisture would prevent the release of ionic silver and its bioavailability. This unfortunately is not reflected in efficacy test protocols. The most common and accepted antimicrobial surface test is ISO 22196,[87] which is based on immersing the test surface in a bacterial test suspension for 24 hours. Such a test condition (100% humidity) maximizes the release and diffusion of ionic silver or other antimicrobial ionic metals or actives and ultimately antimicrobial activity. This test has been criticized for its lack of in situ correlation with surfaces that are not immersed in liquid and kept at a temperature of 37°C.[88,89] Further evidence of the lack of AgNPs diffusion from surfaces is given in studies on food packaging. The use of AgNPs in food packaging is considered to be safe[15] because AgNPs are not released to the food.[90,91] Williams et al[92] showed some release of AgNPs from food packaging under high moisture conditions (agar diffusion) or acidic conditions, although the AgNPs released had limited antimicrobial effect only delaying the growth of *Salmonella* ser Typhimurium. Other efficacy tests include diffusion of Ag/AgNPs either from a disk or material placed on a seeded agar plate or direct diffusion from a well in a seeded agar plate.[17,93] These inaccurate and limited methods rely on the diffusion of the antimicrobial active in a moist environment. These methods indicate that Ag/AgNPs/reactive oxygen species (ROS) can diffuse in the agar and inhibit the growth of the target microorganisms, but they do not provide information on the microbicidal activity of Ag/AgNPs products and importantly may not provide any valuable information on the efficacy of Ag/AgNPs in a dry environment.

The concentration exponent of silver nitrate is 1 and as such Ag efficacy will be retained on small dilutions.[94] Temperature and pH have little effect on Ag, although an increase in pH will increase efficacy.[46] Water hardness will affect Ag efficacy for the reasons described earlier, although the impact on efficacy against gram-positive and gram-negative bacteria might be different.[95] The AgNPs efficacy will be affected by size and morphology.[27,66,72,96,97] The reported superior efficacy of AgNPs over Ag is partially due to an increased surface area of the particle enhancing contact with target microorganisms. In addition, AgNPs might have the ability to generate more ionic silver,[1,98] although it is believed that the size, shape, surface coating, and surface charge of the nanoparticles will affect the rate, location, and/or timing of ionic silver release.[73,99] Pal et al[96] showed that truncated triangular nanoplates,

with a high number of {111} facets, were highly reactive compared to other shapes.

To increase antimicrobial efficacy of Ag or AgNPs, combinations with other actives and/or polymers have been used.[61,62,82,100] In dressings, ionic silver has been combined with antibiotics (eg, sulfonamide, silver sulfadiazine), chlorhexidine (Silvazine™), and cerium nitrate (Flammacerium). The type and nature of polymers used in combination of Ag/AgNPs will impact on the amount and release rate of ionic silver.[78,101] In the textile industry, the type of material fiber used impacts the release of ionic silver.[17]

▶ MECHANISMS OF ACTION

Ionic silver and AgNPs like many biocides have a multiple target sites in microorganisms. Although their interactions have been primarily studied against bacteria,[11,85,102,103] information against viruses[104,105] and fungi[106,107] has emerged. An AgNPs antimicrobial effect is believed to result from a combination to, or alteration of, microbial proteins, leading eventually to metabolic disruption and structural damage.[45,85,102] Some studies have mentioned membrane lipids has a potential target site for Ag action.[66,108-110] The interaction of Ag against bacterial cells is probably more pronounced at the cytoplasmic membrane, where Ag has been shown not only to inhibit the proton motive force and not surprisingly the respiratory electron transport chain but also to alter membrane permeability resulting in cell death.[67,85,102,111,112] The generation of damaging ROS by the bacterial cells following exposure to AgNPs has also been reported.[112-119] It has been reported that ROS can be generated not only at the cytoplasmic membrane but also within the bacterial cytoplasm following penetration of Ag/AgNPs.[85,120,121] The combination of Ag/AgNPs with hydrogen peroxide or povidone-iodine has been shown result in the production of free radicals causing damage to cytoplasmic membrane and cytoplasm constituents.[100,114,122]

Several studies demonstrated the importance of ionic silver for the antimicrobial activity of AgNPs.[70,123-126] The mechanism of lethality of AgNPs against bacteria has been linked to direct membrane damage, the release of ionic silver promoting the formation of ROS, and the modulation and modification of microbial signal-transduction pathways,[29,66,85,112,127-129] although studies have questioned the release of ionic silver as the bactericidal mechanism of action when AgNPs are immobilized on surfaces or matrices.[112,127] The mechanism of bactericidal action of AgNPs is mainly related to membrane disruption, although AgNPs (80 nm) have been identified in bacterial cytoplasm.[130,131] The efficacy of AgNPs with a 20- to 80-nm size has been linked to the release of ionic silver, whereas smaller nanoparticles (10 nm) efficacy leads to more surface interaction and higher intracellular penetration.[85] It is unclear if AgNPs accumulation in the cytoplasm followed cytoplasmic membrane damage. The scientific evidence points to the accumulation of AgNPs at the cytoplasmic membrane causing membrane disruption, pore formation, and cytoplasmic leakage.[66,85,96,128,129,131-135] When in the cytoplasm, AgNPs can interact with sulfur-containing proteins and enzymes and nucleic acids.[96,136,137] There are also indications that AgNPs might affect quorum sensing in gram-negative bacteria.[138]

▶ BACTERIAL RESISTANCE

Occurrence of Bacterial Resistance

Bacterial resistance to ionic silver has been well documented over the years.[2,139,140] Clinically, most information is related to the use of ionic silver and silver combinations with other antimicrobials in wound dressings. The clinical use of silver nitrate in dressings was followed rapidly by reports of *P aeruginosa* resistance.[74,141] Analysis of these studies[74,141] also showed that ionic silver was selectively active against *P aeruginosa*, allowing other bacterial species to grow, notably coliform bacilli. Conversely exposure of a microbiota to a sublethal concentration of AgNPs selected for *Bacillus* species, which became the dominant species.[142] Bacterial clinical resistance to silver sulfadiazine has also been reported for a number of bacterial species including *Enterobacter cloacae*,[143-145] *Providencia stuartii*,[146] *P aeruginosa*,[147] and *Salmonella* Typhimurium,[148] although resistance developed mainly because of the antibiotic component.[149] There have been a couple of clinical studies about the use of Ag dressings to combat bacterial infection in chronic leg ulcers. In an early study following 30 patients, all bacterial isolates remain susceptible to silver nitrate (170 mg/L) except one isolate of *E cloacae*.[150] In another study, however, a silver dressing was shown to have little activity over a 3-week period against wound isolates and one silver-resistant *E cloacae* (minimal inhibitory concentration [MIC] >512 mg/L) isolate was identified.[151]

If the clinical evidence of Ag bacterial resistance remains scarce, additional information is provided from in vitro studies. It has been suggested that Ag is contributing to selecting intrinsically resistant bacteria to Ag.[144,146,152-154] The Ag resistance has also been described in a number of environmental isolates including Enterobacteriaceae[155-158] and in *Acinetobacter baumannii*.[159] It is also possible to produce high resistance to silver (>1024 mg/L) in *Escherichia coli* experimentally following a stepwise training approach, whereby bacteria is gradually exposed to increasing concentrations of Ag.[160] Bacterial resistance to AgNPs has also been described even if the use of AgNPs is more recent than that of ionic silver.[110,117,118,161-163]

Bacterial Resistance Mechanisms

Bacterial mechanisms of resistance to Ag aim to reduce the concentration of ionic silver detrimental to the microorganism. These include reducing Ag uptake, accumulation, and transforming ionic silver into the inactive Ag[0], decrease in Ag/AgNPs binding and accumulation following a change in transporter,[164] bacterial membrane composition[110,118,156-158,165] including outer membrane proteins.[160,161,163] Increased efflux mechanisms that reduce Ag accumulation has been described.[154,166] A number of mechanisms aiming to reduce the effective Ag concentration have been described including the inactivation of ionic silver through chelation by the sulfhydryl groups of metal-binding proteins,[167] the decreased expression of succinate dehydrogenase,[156] and the transformation/neutralization of ionic silver to inactive metallic form.[164,168] Reduction in oxidative stress damage following exposure to AgNPs has also been described and resulted from an upregulation of antioxidant protective mechanisms.[169] Preexposure to sublethal concentrations of AgNPs followed with a recovery period led to the accumulation of ATP,[118] although exposure to higher AgNPs concentration resulted in the collapse of membrane potential and the depletion of ATP.[66,117]

If bacterial resistance mechanisms have been defined, these follow bacterial gene expression following exposure to Ag/AgNPs. The interaction of ionic silver with the bacterial cell membrane will produce a stress response and associated transcriptomic expression.[66,117,169] One study suggested that AgNPs can act as a mutagen causing a high rate of frameshift mutations similar to exposure to ultraviolet irradiation and oxidizing agents.[118] The impact of AgNPs ($\geq$20-80 μg/mL) exposure against bacterial cell can result in an extended lag phase followed with increased growth rate, indicating bacterial adaptation to AgNPs.[170] Proteomic analysis of *E coli* showed the induction of envelope proteins (OmpA, OmpC, OmpF, OppA, and MetQ) following exposure to AgNPs (10 nm).[66]

Possibly of a concern is the reported induction of antibiotic resistance following exposure to AgNPs. In *P aeruginosa*, exposure to AgNPs resulted in higher MICs to ampicillin, chloramphenicol, kanamycin, and tetracycline possibly following the upregulation of a number of mechanisms including efflux transporters and antioxidant system.[171] Such a decrease in antibiotic susceptibility was also observed by Kaweeteerawat et al[118] in *Staphylococcus aureus* and *E coli* possibly following adaptation to stress. Graves et al[172] observed an increase in *E coli* fitness following exposure to Ag/AgNPs.

Genetic Basis of Ionic Silver Resistance in Bacteria and Dissemination of Resistance

The genetic basis of bacterial resistance to silver has been well described in the literature. Bacterial resistance to ionic silver has often been found on plasmids in many gram-negative species,[9,144,173,174] although there is also evidence of chromosomal resistance.[173,175,176] In enteric bacterial isolates, the occurrence of silver-encoded resistance was found to exceed 10%.[154]

In *E coli* and *Salmonella* species, the role of the *sil* operon located on plasmid pGM101 has been linked to Ag/AgNPs resistance.[154,166] In *Salmonella* species, *silCBA* encodes a resistance nodulation division efflux pump.[154] SilA is an inner membrane cation pump protein, whereas SilC is an outer membrane[9] not dissimilar to the AcrAB efflux system in *E coli*. Carriage of silver-resistant genes in methicillin-resistant *S aureus* and methicillin-resistant coagulase-negative *S aureus* isolates from wounds and nasal cavities in human and animals may be low[177] and confined to *silE*. *silE* encodes for a periplasmic silver-binding protein.[9] Isolates harboring *silE* have been shown to remain susceptible to a silver-containing hydrofiber wound dressing.[177] Likewise, in *E cloacae* human and equine isolates *sil* operon carriage may be low.[174] When present, *sil* genes conferred an increased MIC to the isolates (>5 mg/L MIC), which however remained susceptible to a silver-containing product.[174] Silver-resistant (MIC >512 mg/L) *E cloacae* isolates from wounds treated with silver-based dressings, harbored the *silE*, *silS*, and *silP* determinants.[151]

One concern of plasmid encoding silver resistance is the dissemination of silver resistance and the cotransfer and expression of associated genes conferring new phenotypes including antibiotic resistance.[85,140,178] Deshpande and Chopade[159] demonstrated that in *A baumannii*, efflux-based resistance to Ag was encoded on a 54 kb plasmid, which could be easily transferred by conjugation.

◗ TOXICITY

With the increase number of consumer products containing silver, all nonrecycled waste will end up in the environment and silver compounds in textiles and cosmetics will end up in wastewater treatment plants. Demand for silver is increasing globally (https://www.silverinstitute.org/silver-industrial-demand-rebounded-2017-mine-supply-recorded-second-consecutive-loss/). Understanding the transformation of nanosilver in the environment is important. Following dissolution of silver is likely to form stable combination with chloride and sulfide that will impact on silver bioavailability and toxicity in the environment, although these silver complexes are less toxic than free silver ions. In slurry studies, AgNPs has been shown to decrease microbial species diversity.[179] Similar findings were reported about the impact of AgNPs in microbiota in a wastewater treatment plant.[180]

The best-described adverse effect in humans of chronic exposure to silver is argyria, a permanent bluish-gray discoloration of the skin or eyes.[181] Most familiar human exposure to Ag was from dental amalgams that contain 35% Ag^0 and 50% Hg^0.[182] Early studies on

the use of Ag/AgNPs in wound dressings has been associated with a number of side effects including cytotoxicity, staining, methemoglobinemia and electrolyte disturbance, longer slough separation time, retardation of wound healing, and the possible inactivation of enzyme-debriding agents.[183] These side effects have been decreased with the development of new dressings controlling the release of Ag/AgNPs and fluid handling.[24,46,184] A more recent study based on the study of fibroblasts has shown a positive effect of AgNPs on healing based on reduced inflammatory cytokine levels.[185] Conversely, the cytotoxicity of Ag against human fibroblasts is concentration dependent.[186]

The generation of oxidative stress as part of the mechanisms of action of AgNPs might also account for cell toxicity.[187] As with antimicrobial efficacy, the size and shape of nanoparticles can affect toxicity.[188,189]

◗ CONCLUSIONS

The commercial demand for the use of ionic silver and nanosilver continues to increase, including of Ag/AgNPs as antimicrobials for the use of domestic products including textile, plastic, and cosmetic. The majority of Ag/AgNPs usage as antimicrobials is in materials in a dry state that would not be continuously immersed in liquid. Conversely, the most common test protocols used to measure Ag/AgNPs efficacy are based on 100% humidity, high temperature (37°C), and long contact time (24 hr). With these parameters in mind, Ag/AgNPs showed high efficacy as ionic silver is able to diffuse and exert its potent antimicrobial activity. The question is when the Ag/AgNPs are not bioavailable, is the surface/textile still antimicrobial to microorganisms deposited on the surface? The answer to that question is likely to be negative. This is an issue for manufacturers, consumers, and regulators. In the absence of an appropriate surface or textile test protocol reflecting dry conditions, the value and benefit of incorporating Ag/AgNPs as antimicrobials in materials cannot be appropriately evaluated.

The AgNPs are more efficacious than ionic silver. Advances in AgNPs synthesis and combination with polymers and materials have renewed the interest in using silver as an antimicrobial for an increasing number of applications. The current market for AgNPs material is buoyant and will continue to grow. Academically, progress in understanding on the impact the shape, size, type of AgNPs particles, and combination with materials on bioavailability and efficacy has been made. With the increasing usage of AgNPs in personal care product, notably cosmetic and textile, long-term exposure effect studies are needed on the most common nanoparticles used. The number of silver-containing items discarded that will end up in the environment will increase. The bioavailability of AgNPs in the environment remains paramount to understand potential environmental toxicity.

REFERENCES

1. Wijnhoven SWP, Peijnenburg WJGM, Herbert CA, et al. Nanosilver—a review of available data and knowledge gaps in human and environmental risk assessment. *Nanotoxicol.* 2009;3:109-138.

2. Maillard J-Y, Hartemann P. Silver as an antimicrobial: facts and gaps in knowledge. *Crit Rev Microbiol.* 2013;39:373-383.

3. Schneider G. Antimicrobial silver nanoparticles—regulatory situation in the European Union. *Mat Today.* 2017;4:S200-S207.

4. Rhim J-W, Hong S-I, Park H-M, Ng PKW. Preparation and characterization of chitosan-based nanocomposite films with antimicrobial activity. *J Agric Food Chem.* 2006;54:5814-5822.

5. Porel S, Ramakrishna D, Hariprasad E, Gupta AD, Radhakrishnan TP. Polymer thin film with in situ synthesized silver nanoparticles as a potent reusable bactericide. *Curr Sci.* 2011;101:927-934.

6. Zewde B, Ambaye A, Stubbs J III, Raghavan D. A review of stabilized silver nanoparticles—synthesis, biological properties, characterization, and potential areas of applications. *JSM Nanotechnol Nanomed.* 2016;4:1043.

7. Verma J, Kanoujia J, Parashar P, Tripathi CB, Saraf SA. Wound healing applications of sericin/chitosan-capped silver nanoparticles incorporated hydrogel. *Drug Deliv Transl Res.* 2017;7:77-88.

8. Negut I, Grumezescu V, Grumezescu AM. Treatment strategies for infected wounds. *Molecules.* 2018;23:E2392.

9. Silver S, Phung le LT, Silver G. Silver as biocides in burn and wound dressings and bacterial resistance to silver compounds. *J Ind Microbiol Biotechnol.* 2006;33:627-634.

10. Gottschalk F, Sonderer T, Scholz RW, Nowack B. Possibilities and limitations of modeling environmental exposure to engineered nanomaterials by probabilistic material flow analysis. *Environ Toxicol Chem.* 2010;29:1036-1048.

11. Burduşel AC, Gherasim O, Grumezescu AM, Mogoǎnta L, Ficai A, Andronescu E. Biomedical applications of silver nanoparticles: an up-to-date overview. *Nanomaterials.* 2018;8:E681.

12. Zhou Y, Chen R, He T, et al. Biomedical potential of ultrafine Ag/AgCl nanoparticles coated on graphene with special reference to antimicrobial performances and burn wound healing. *ACS Appl Mater Interfaces.* 2016;8:15067-15075.

13. Zhou Y, Tang RC. Facile and eco-friendly fabrication of AgNPs coated silk for antibacterial and antioxidant textiles using honeysuckle extract. *J Photochem Photobiol B.* 2018;178:463-471.

14. Gupta SD, Agarwal A, Pradhan S. Phytostimulatory effect of silver nanoparticles (AgNPs) on rice seedling growth: an insight from antioxidative enzyme activities and gene expression patterns. *Ecotoxicol Environ Saf.* 2018;161:624-633.

15. Huang YK, Mei L, Chen XG, Wang Q. Recent developments in food packaging based on nanomaterials. *Nanomaterials.* 2018;8:E830.

16. Kumar S, Shukla A, Baul PP, Mitra A, Halder D. Biodegradable hybrid nanocomposites of chitosan/gelatin and silver nanoparticles for active food packaging applications. *Food Packag Shelf.* 2018;16:178-184.

17. Tan LY, Sin LT, Bee ST, et al. A review of antimicrobial fabric containing nanostructures metal-based compound. *J Vinyl Add Technol.* 2019;25(suppl 1):E3-E27.

18. Mokhena TC, Luyt AS. Electrospun alginate nanofibres impregnated with silver nanoparticles: preparation, morphology and antibacterial properties. *Carbohydr Polym.* 2017;165:304-312.

19. Bouwmeester H, Dekkers S, Noordam MY, et al. Review of health safety aspects of nanotechnologies in food production. *Regul Toxicol Pharmacol.* 2009;53:52-62.

20. von Goetz N, Lorenz C, Windler L, Nowack B, Heuberger M, Hungerbühler K. Migration of Ag- and TiO₂-(nano)particles from textiles into artificial sweat under physical stress: experiments and exposure modeling. *Environ Sci Technol.* 2013;47:9979-9987.

21. Silvestry-Rodriguez N, Sicairos-Ruelas EE, Gerba CP, Bright KR. Silver as a disinfectant. *Rev Environ Contam Toxicol.* 2007;191:23-45.

22. Toy LW, Macera L. Evidence-based review of silver dressing use on chronic wounds. *J Am Acad Nurse Pract.* 2011;23:183-192.

23. Kaba SI, Egorova EM. In vitro studies of the toxic effects of silver nanoparticles on HeLa and U937 cells. *Nanotechnol Sci Appl.* 2015;8:19-29.

24. Nam G, Rangasamy S, Purushothaman B, Song JM. The application of bactericidal silver nanoparticles in wound treatment. *Nanomater Nanotechnol.* 2015;5:23-37.

25. Stevens KNJ, Croes S, Boersma RS, et al. Hydrophilic surface coatings with embedded biocidal silver nanoparticles and sodium heparin for central venous catheters. *Biomaterials.* 2011;32:1264-1269.

26. Antonelli M, De Pascale G, Ranieri VM, et al. Comparison of triple-lumen central venous catheters impregnated with silver nanoparticles (AgTive®) vs conventional catheters in intensive care unit patients. *J Hosp Infect.* 2012;82:101-107.

27. Pollini M, Paladini F, Catalano M, et al. Antibacterial coatings on haemodialysis catheters by photochemical deposition of silver nanoparticles. *J Mater Sci Mater Med.* 2011;22:2005-2012.

28. Ballo MK, Rtimi S, Pulgarin C, et al. In vitro and in vivo effectiveness of an innovative silver-copper nanoparticle coating of catheters to prevent methicillin-resistant *Staphylococcus aureus* infection. *Antimicrob Agents Chemother.* 2016;60:5349-5356.

29. Thomas R, Soumya KR, Mathew J, Radhakrishnan EK. Inhibitory effect of silver nanoparticle fabricated urinary catheter on colonization efficiency of coagulase negative staphylococci. *J Photochem Photobiol B.* 2015;149:68-77.

30. Thomas R, Mathew S, Nayana AR, Mathews J, Radhakrishnan EK. Microbially and phytofabricated AgNPs with different mode of bactericidal action were identified to have comparable potential for surface fabrication of central venous catheters to combat *Staphylococcus aureus* biofilm. *J Photochem Photobiol B.* 2017;171:96-103.

31. Ciobanu CS, Iconaru SL, Pasuk I, et al. Structural properties of silver doped hydroxyapatite and their biocompatibility. *Mater Sci Eng C Mater Biol Appl.* 2013;33:1395-1402.

32. Zhou K, Dong C, Zhang X, et al. Preparation and characterization of nanosilver-doped porous hydroxyapatite scaffolds. *Ceram Int.* 2015;41:1671-1676.

33. Rizzello L, Pompa PP. Nanosilver-based antibacterial drugs and devices: mechanisms, methodological drawbacks, and guidelines. *Chem Soc Rev.* 2014;43:1501-1518.

34. Shapey S, Machin K, Levi K, Boswell TC. Activity of a dry mist hydrogen peroxide system against environmental *Clostridium difficile* contamination in elderly care wards. *J Hosp Infect.* 2008;70:136-141.

35. Andersen BM, Rasch M, Hochlin K, Jensen FH, Wismar P, Fredriksen JE. Decontamination of rooms, medical equipment and ambulances using an aerosol of hydrogen peroxide disinfectant. *J Hosp Infect.* 2006;62:149-155.

36. Konop M, Damps T, Misicka A, Rudnicka L. Certain aspects of silver and silver nanoparticles in wound care: a minireview. *J Nanomater.* 2016;76:14753.

37. Yang Y, Hu H. A review on antimicrobial silver absorbent wound dressings applied to exuding wounds. *J Microb Biochem Technol.* 2015;7:228-233.

38. Moyer CA, Brentano L, Gravens DL, Margraf H, Monafo WW Jr. Treatment of large human burns with 0.5% silver nitrate solution. *Arch Surg.* 1965;90:812-867.

39. Fox CL Jr. Silver sulfadiazine—a new topical therapy for *Pseudomonas* in burns. Therapy of *Pseudomonas* infection in burns. *Arch Surg.* 1968;96:184-188.

40. Fox CL Jr, Modak SM. Mechanism of silver sulfadiazine action on burn wound infections. *Antimicrob Agents Chemother.* 1974;5:582-588.

41. Modak SM, Sampath L, Fox CL Jr. Combined topical use of silver sulfadiazine and antibiotics as a possible solution to bacterial resistance in burn wounds. *J Burn Care Rehabil.* 1988;9:359-363.

42. Fraser JF, Cuttle L, Kempf M, Kimble RM. Cytotoxicity of topical antimicrobial agents used in burn wounds in Australasia. *ANZ J Surg.* 2014;74:139-142.

43. Garner JP, Heppell PS. The use of Flammacerium in British burns units. *Burns.* 2005;31:379-382.

44. Garner JP, Heppell PS. Cerium nitrate in the management of burns. *Burns.* 2005;31:539-547.

45. Maillard J-Y, Denyer SP. Focus on silver. In: *European Wound Management Association (EWMA) Position Document: The Role of Topical Antimicrobials in Managing Wound Infection.* London, United Kingdom: MEP; 2006.

46. Maillard J-Y, Denyer SP. Demystifying silver. In: *European Wound Management Association (EWMA) Position Document: The Role of Topical Antimicrobials in Managing Wound Infection.* London, United Kingdom: MEP; 2006.

47. El-Naggar MY, Gohar YM, Sorour MA, Waheeb MG. Hydrogel dressing with a nano-formula against methicillin-resistant *Staphylococcus aureus* and *Pseudomonas aeruginosa* diabetic foot bacteria. *J Microbiol Biotechnol.* 2016;26:408-420.

48. Hanif M, Juluri RR, Fojan P, Popok VN. Polymer films with size-selected silver nanoparticles as plasmon resonance-based transducers for protein sensing. *Biointerface Res Appl Chem.* 2016;6:1564-1568.

49. Jaiswal M, Koul V, Dinda AK. *In vitro* and *in vivo* investigational studies of a nanocomposite-hydrogel-based dressing with a silver-coated chitosan wafer for full-thickness skin wounds. *J Appl Polym Sci.* 2016;133:43472.

50. Higa AM, Mambrini GP, Hausen M, Strixino FT, Leite FL. Ag-nanoparticle-based nano-immunosensor for anti-glutathione S-transferase detection. *Biointerface Res Appl Chem.* 2016;6:1053-1058.

51. Nešović K, Kojić V, Rhee KY, Mišković-Stanković V. Electrochemical synthesis and characterization of silver doped poly(vinyl alcohol)/chitosan hydrogels. *Corrosion.* 2017;73:1437-1447.

52. Noronha VT, Paula AJ, Durán G, et al. Silver nanoparticles in dentistry. *Dent Mater.* 2017;33:1110-1126.

53. Peng JJ, Botelho MG, Matinlinna JP. Silver compounds used in dentistry for caries management: a review. *J Dent.* 2012;40:531-541.

54. Cheng L, Zhang K, Weir MD, Melo MA, Zhou X, Xu HH. Nanotechnology strategies for antibacterial and remineralizing composites and adhesives to tackle dental caries. *Nanomedicine.* 2015;10:627-641.

55. Elias Santos V, Targino A, Pelagio Flores MA, de Luna Freire Pessoa H, Galembeck A, Rosenblatt A. Antimicrobial activity of silver nanoparticles in treating dental caries. *RFO.* 2014;18:312-315.

56. Chambers C, Stewart SB, Su B, Jenkinson HF, Sandy JR, Ireland AJ. Silver doped titanium dioxide nanoparticles as antimicrobial additives to dental polymers. *Dent Mater.* 2017;33:e115-e123.

57. Kaur P, Luthra R. Silver nanoparticles in dentistry: an emerging trend. *SRMJ Res Dent Sci.* 2016;7:162-165.

58. Geng Z, Wang R, Zhuo X, et al. Incorporation of silver and strontium in hydroxyapatite coating on titanium surface for enhanced antibacterial and biological properties. *Mater Sci Eng C.* 2017;71:852-861.

59. Mirzaee M, Vaezi M, Palizdar Y. Synthesis and characterization of silver doped hydroxyapatite nanocomposite coatings and evaluation of their antibacterial and corrosion resistance properties in simulated body fluid. *Mater Sci Eng C.* 2016;69:675-684.

60. Zhang X, Chaimayo W, Yang C, Yao J, Miller BL, Yates MZ. Silver-hydroxyapatite composite coatings with enhanced antimicrobial activities through heat treatment. *Surf Coat Technol.* 2017;325:39-45.

61. Divakar DD, Jastaniyah NT, Altamimi HG, et al. Enhanced antimicrobial activity of naturally derived bioactive molecule chitosan conjugated silver nanoparticle against dental implant pathogens. *Int J Biol Macromol.* 2018;108:790-797.

62. Lee D, Lee SJ, Moon J-H, et al. Preparation of antibacterial chitosan membranes containing silver nanoparticles for dental barrier membrane applications. *J Ind Eng Chem.* 2018;66:196-202.

63. Yu W-Z, Zhang Y, Liu X, Xiang Y, Li Z, Wu S. Synergistic antibacterial activity of multi components in lysozyme/chitosan/silver/hydroxyapatite hybrid coating. *Mater Des.* 2018;139:351-362.

64. Bapat RA, Chaubal TV, Joshi CP, et al. An overview of application of silver nanoparticles for biomaterials in dentistry. *Mater Sci Eng C.* 2018;91:881-898.

65. Turner RJ. Is silver the ultimate antimicrobial bullet? *Antibiotics.* 2018;7:112-113.

66. Lok C-N, Ho C-M, Chen R, et al. Proteomic analysis of the mode of antibacterial action of silver nanoparticles. *J Proteome Res.* 2006;5:916-924.

67. Edwards-Jones V. The benefits of silver in hygiene, personal care and healthcare. *Lett Appl Microbiol.* 2009;49:147-152.

68. Fernández A, Picouet P, Lloret E. Cellulose-silver nanoparticle hybrid materials to control spoilage-related microflora in absorbent pads located in trays of fresh-cut melon. *Int J Food Microbiol.* 2010;142:222-228.

69. Fernández A, Soriano E, Hernández-Muñoz P, Gavara R. Migration of antimicrobial silver from composites of polylactide with silver zeolites. *J Food Sci.* 2010;75:E186-E193.

70. Marambio-Jones C, Hoek EMV. A review of the antibacterial effects of silver nanomaterials and potential implications for human health and the environment. *J Nanopart Res.* 2010;12:1531-1551.

71. Percival SL, Slone W, Linton S, Okel T, Corum L, Thomas JG. The antimicrobial efficacy of a silver alginate dressing against a broad spectrum of clinically relevant wound isolates. *Int Wound J.* 2011;8:237-243.

72. Dakal TC, Kumar A, Majumdar RS, Yadav V. Mechanistic basis of antimicrobial actions of silver nanoparticles. *Front Microbiol.* 2016;7:1831.

73. Slavin YN, Asnis J, Häfeli UO, Bach H. Metal nanoparticles: understanding the mechanisms behind antibacterial activity. *J Nanobiotechnol.* 2017;15:65.

74. Cason JS, Jackson DM, Lowbury EJ, Ricketts CR. Antiseptic and aseptic prophylaxis for burns: use of silver nitrate and of isolators. *Br Med J.* 1966;2:1288-1294.

75. Spacciapoli P, Buxton DK, Rothstein DM, Friden P. Antimicrobial activity of silver nitrate against periodontal pathogens. *J Periodontal Res.* 2001;36:108-113.

76. Miao A-J, Schwehr KA, Xu C, et al. The algal toxicity of silver engineered nanoparticles and detoxification by exopolymeric substances. *Environ Pollut.* 2009;157:3034-3041.

77. Agnihotri S, Mukherji S, Mukherji S. Immobilized silver nanoparticles enhance contact killing and show highest efficacy: elucidation of the mechanism of bactericidal action of silver. *Nanoscale.* 2013;5:7328-7340.

78. Kostenko V, Lyczak J, Turner K, Martinuzzi RJ. Impact of silver-containing wound dressings on bacterial biofilm viability and susceptibility to antibiotics during prolonged treatment. *Antimicrob Agents Chemother.* 2010;54:5120-5131.

79. Huang L, Dai T, Xuan Y, Tegos GP, Hamblin MR. Synergistic combination of chitosan acetate with nanoparticle silver as a topical antimicrobial: efficacy against bacterial burn infections. *Antimicrob Agents Chemother.* 2011;55:3432-3438.

80. Lu H, Liu Y, Guo J, Wu H, Wang J, Wu G. Biomaterials with antibacterial and osteoinductive properties to repair infected bone defects. *Int J Mol Sci.* 2016;17:334.

81. Mi GJ, Shi D, Wang M, Webster TJ. Reducing bacterial infections and biofilm formation using nanoparticles and nanostructured antibacterial surfaces. *Adv Health Mat.* 2018;7:1800103.

82. Anjum S, Gupta B. Bioengineering of functional nanosilver nanogels for smart healthcare systems. *Global Challenges.* 2018;2:1800044.

83. Gupta A, Maynes M, Silver S. The effects of halides on plasmid-mediated silver resistance in *Escherichia coli. Appl Environ Microbiol.* 1999;64:5042-5045.

84. Choi O, Deng KK, Kim NJ, Ross L Jr, Surampalli RY, Hu Z. The inhibitory effects of silver nanoparticles, silver ions, and silver chloride colloids on microbial growth. *Water Res.* 2008;42:3066-3074.

85. Durán N, Durán M, de Jesus MB, Seabra AB, Fávaro WJ, Nakazato G. Silver nanoparticles: a new view on mechanistic aspects on antimicrobial activity. *Nanomedicine.* 2016;12:789-799.

86. Lansdown AB, Williams A, Chandler S, Benfield S. Silver absorption and antibacterial efficacy of silver dressings. *J Wound Care.* 2005;14:155-160.

87. International Organization for Standardization. *ISO 22196:2011: Measurement of Antibacterial Activity on Plastics and Other Non-Porous Surfaces.* Geneva, Switzerland: International Organization for Standardization; 2011.

88. Michels HT, Noyce JO, Keevil CW. Effects of temperature and humidity on the efficacy of methicillin-resistant *Staphylococcus aureus* challenged antimicrobial materials containing silver and copper. *Lett Appl Microbiol*. 2009;49:191-195.

89. Ojeil M, Jermann C, Holah J, Denyer S, Maillard J-Y. Evaluation of new in vitro efficacy test for antimicrobial surface activity reflecting UK hospital conditions. *J Hosp Infect*. 2013;85:274-281.

90. Gallocchio F, Cibin V, Biancotto G, et al. Testing nano-silver food packaging to evaluate silver migration and food spoilage bacteria on chicken meat. *Food Addit Contam Part A Chem Anal Control Expo Risk Assess*. 2016;33:1063-1071.

91. Tiimob BJ, Mwinyelle G, Abdela W, Samuel T, Jeelani S, Rangari VK. Nanoengineered eggshell-silver tailored copolyester polymer blend film with antimicrobial properties. *J Agric Food Chem*. 2017;65:1967-1976.

92. Williams K, Valencia L, Gokulan K, Trbojevich P, Khare S. Assessment of antimicrobial effects of food contact materials containing silver on growth of *Salmonella* Typhimurium. *Food Chem Toxicol*. 2017;100:197-206.

93. Farrokhi Z, Ayati A, Kanvisi M, Sillanpää M. Recent advance in antibacterial activity of nanoparticles contained polyurethane. *J Appl Polymer Sci*. 2019;136:46997.

94. Denyer SP, Stewart GSAB. Mechanisms of action of disinfectants. *Int Biodeter Biodegrad*. 1998;41:261-268.

95. Jin X, Li MH, Wang JW, et al. High-throughput screening of silver nanoparticle stability and bacterial inactivation in aquatic media: influence of specific ions. *Environ Sci Technol*. 2010;44:7321-7328.

96. Pal S, Tak YK, Song JM. Does the antibacterial activity of silver nanoparticles depend on the shape of the nanoparticle? A study of the gram-negative bacterium *Escherichia coli*. *Appl Environ Microbiol*. 2007;73:1712-1720.

97. Samberg ME, Orndorff PE, Monteiro-Riviere NA. Antibacterial efficacy of silver nanoparticles of different sizes, surface conditions and synthesis methods. *Nanotoxicology*. 2011;5:244-253.

98. Zawadzka K, Kądziola K, Felczak A, et al. Surface area or diameter—which factor really determines the antibacterial activity of silver nanoparticles grown on TiO_2 coatings? *New J Chem*. 2014;38:3275-3281.

99. Abbaszadegan A, Ghahramani Y, Gholami A, et al. The effect of charge at the surface of silver nanoparticles on antimicrobial activity against gram-positive and gram-negative bacteria: a preliminary study. *J Nanomater*. 2015;16:720654.

100. Banerjee M, Mallick S, Paul A, Chattopadhyay A, Ghosh SS. Heightened reactive oxygen species generation in the antimicrobial activity of a three component iodinated chitosan-silver nanoparticle composite. *Langmuir*. 2010;26:5901-5908.

101. Monteiro DR, Gorup LF, Takamiya AS, Ruvollo-Filho AC, de Camargo ER, Barbosa DB. The growing importance of materials that prevent microbial adhesion: antimicrobial effect of medical devices containing silver. *Int J Antimicrob Agents*. 2009;34:103-110.

102. Durán N, Marcato PD, De Conti R, Alves OL, Costa FTM, Brocchi M. Potential use of silver nanoparticles on pathogenic bacteria, their toxicity and possible mechanisms of action. *J Braz Chem Soc*. 2010;21:949-959.

103. Alshareef A, Laird K, Cross RBM. Shape-dependent antibacterial activity of silver nanoparticles on *Escherichia coli* and *Enterococcus faecium* bacterium. *Appl Surf Sci*. 2017;424:310-315.

104. Etemadzade M, Ghamarypour A, Zabihollahi R, et al. Synthesis and evaluation of antiviral activities of novel sonochemical silver nanorods against HIV and HSV viruses. *Asian Pac J Trop Dis*. 2016;6:854-858.

105. Tamilselvan S, Ashokkumar T, Govindaraju K. Microscopy based studies on the interaction of bio-based silver nanoparticles with *Bombyx mori* nuclear polyhedrosis virus. *J Virol Methods*. 2017;242:58-66.

106. Dojčilović R, Pajović J, Božanić D, et al. Interaction of amino acid-functionalized silver nanoparticles and *Candida albicans* polymorphs: a deep-UV fluorescence imaging study. *Colloids Surf B Biointerfaces*. 2017;155:341-348.

107. Kalaivani R, Maruthupandy M, Muneeswaran T, et al. Synthesis of chitosan mediated silver nanoparticles (Ag NPs) for potential antimicrobial applications. *Front Lab Med*. 2018;2:30-35.

108. Dibrov P, Dzioba J, Gosink KK, Häse CC. Chemiosmotic mechanism of antimicrobial activity of Ag+ in *Vibrio cholerae*. *Antimicrob Agents Chemother*. 2002;46:2668-2670.

109. Anas A, Jiya J, Rameez MJ, Anand PB, Anantharaman MR, Nair S. Sequential interactions of silver-silica nanocomposite (Ag-SiO$_2$ NC) with cell wall, metabolism and genetic stability of *Pseudomonas aeruginosa*, a multiple antibiotic-resistant bacterium. *Lett Appl Microbiol*. 2013;56:57-62.

110. Hachicho N, Hoffmann P, Ahlert K, Heipieper HJ. Effect of silver nanoparticles and silver ions on growth and adaptive response mechanisms of *Pseudomonas putida* mt-2. *FEMS Microbiol Lett*. 2014;355:71-77.

111. Percival SL, Bowler PG, Russell D. Bacterial resistance to silver in wound care. *J Hosp Infect*. 2005;60:1-7.

112. Su HL, Chou CG, Hung DJ, et al. The disruption of bacterial membrane integrity through ROS generation induced by nanohybrids of silver and clay. *Biomaterials*. 2009;30:5979-5987.

113. Kim S-H, Lee H-S, Ryu D-S, Choi S-J, Lee D-S. Antibacterial activity of silver-nanoparticles against *Staphylococcus aureus* and *Escherichia coli*. *Korean J Microbiol Biotechnol*. 2011;39:77-85.

114. Xu H, Qu F, Xu H, et al. Role of reactive oxygen species in the antibacterial mechanism of silver nanoparticles on *Escherichia coli* O157:H7. *Biometals*. 2012;25:45-53.

115. Kon K, Rai M. Metallic nanoparticles: mechanism of antibacterial action and influencing factors. *J Comp Clin Path Res*. 2013;1:160-174.

116. Rai MK, Deshmukh SD, Ingle AP, Gade AK. Silver nanoparticles: the powerful nanoweapon against multidrug-resistant bacteria. *J Appl Microbiol*. 2012;112:841-852.

117. Lee WK, Kim J, Lee DG. A novel mechanism for the antibacterial effect of silver nanoparticles on *Escherichia coli*. *Biometals*. 2014;27:1191-1201.

118. Kaweeteerawat C, Ubol PN, Sangmuang S, Aueviriyavit S, Maniratanachote R. Mechanisms of antibiotic resistance in bacteria mediated by silver nanoparticles. *J Toxicol Environ Health A*. 2017;80:1276-1289.

119. Yuan Y-G, Peng Q-L, Gurunathan S. Effects of silver nanoparticles on multiple drug-resistant strains of *Staphylococcus aureus* and *Pseudomonas aeruginosa* from mastitis-infected goats: an alternative approach for antimicrobial therapy. *Int J Mol Sci*. 2017;18:E569.

120. Belluco S, Losasso C, Patuzzi I, et al. Silver as antibacterial toward *Listeria monocytogenes*. *Front Microbiol*. 2016;7:307.

121. Kim JS, Kuk E, Yu KN, et al. Antimicrobial effects of silver nanoparticles. *Nanomedicine*. 2007;3:95-101.

122. Hartemann P, Goeffert M, Blech MF. Efficacité bactéricide du peroxide d'hydrogène sur *Escherichia coli*. *Ann Med Nancy*. 1995;34:85-88.

123. Reidy B, Haase A, Luch A, Dawson KA, Lynch I. Mechanisms of silver nanoparticle release, transformation and toxicity: a critical review of current knowledge and recommendations for future studies and applications. *Materials*. 2013;6:2295-2350.

124. Manke A, Wang L, Rojanasakul Y. Mechanisms of nanoparticle induced oxidative stress and toxicity. *BioMed Res Int*. 2013;94:2916.

125. Rajeshkumar S, Malarkodi C. In vitro antibacterial activity and mechanism of silver nanoparticles against foodborne pathogens. *Bioinorg Chem Appl*. 2014;58:1890.

126. Dos Santos CA, Seckler MM, Ingle AP, et al. Silver nanoparticles: therapeutical uses, toxicity, and safety issues. *J Pharm Sci*. 2014;103:1931-1944.

127. Miyoshi H, Ohno H, Sakai K, Okamura N, Kourai H. Characterization and photochemical and antibacterial properties of highly stable silver nanoparticles prepared on montmorillonite clay in n-hexanol. *J Colloid Interface Sci*. 2010;345:433-441.

128. Akter M, Sikder MT, Rahman MM, et al. A systematic review on silver nanoparticles-induced cytotoxicity: physicochemical properties and perspectives. *J Adv Res*. 2018;9:1-16.

129. Zheng K, Setyawati MI, Leong DT, Xie J. Antimicrobial silver nanomaterials. *Coord Chem Rev*. 2018;357:1-17.

130. Xu X, Brownlow W, Kyriacou S, Wan Q, Viola J. Real-time probing of membrane transport in living microbial cells using single nanoparticle optics and living cell imaging. *Biochemistry*. 2004;43:10400-10413.

131. Taglietti A, Diaz Fernandez YA, Amato E, et al. Antibacterial activity of glutathione-coated silver nanoparticles against gram positive and gram negative bacteria. *Langmuir.* 2012;28:8140-8148.

132. Sondi I, Salopek-Sondi B. Silver nanoparticles as antimicrobial agent: a case study on *E. coli* as a model for gram-negative bacteria. *J Colloid Interface Sci.* 2004;275:177-182.

133. Ansari MA, Khan HM, Khan AA, et al. Interaction of silver nanoparticles with *Escherichia coli* and their cell envelope biomolecules. *J Basic Microbiol.* 2014;54:905-915.

134. Li WR, Xie XB, Shi QS, Zeng HY, Ou-Yang YS, Chen YB. Antibacterial activity and mechanism of silver nanoparticles on *Escherichia coli.* *Appl Microbiol Biotechnol.* 2010;85:1115-1122.

135. Gogoi SK, Gopinath P, Paul A, Ramesh A, Ghosh SS, Chattopadhyay A. Green fluorescent protein-expressing *Escherichia coli* as a model system for investigating the antimicrobial activities of silver nanoparticles. *Langmuir.* 2006;22:9322-9328.

136. Bondarenko O, Ivask A, Käkinen A, Kurvet I, Kahru A. Particle-cell contact enhances antibacterial activity of silver nanoparticles. *PLoS One.* 2013;8:e64060.

137. Yuan Z, Li J, Cui L, Xu B, Zhang H, Yu C-P. Interaction of silver nanoparticles with pure nitrifying bacteria. *Chemosphere.* 2013;90:1404-1411.

138. Hayat S, Muzammil S, Shabana, et al. Quorum quenching: role of nanoparticles as signal jammers in gram-negative bacteria. *Future Microbiol.* 2019;14:61-72.

139. Silver S, Gupta A, Matsui K, Lo JF. Resistance to Ag+ cations in bacteria: environments, genes and proteins. *Met Based Drugs.* 1999;6:315-320.

140. Mijnendonckx K, Leys N, Mahillon J, Silver S, Von Houdt R. Antimicrobial silver: uses, toxicity and potential for resistance. *Biometals.* 2013;26:609-621.

141. Cason JS, Lowbury EJL. Mortality and infection in extensively burned patients treated with silver-nitrate compresses. *Lancet.* 1968;1:651-654.

142. Gunawan C, Teoh WY, Marquis CP, Amal R. Induced adaptation of *Bacillus* sp. to antimicrobial nanosilver. *Small.* 2013;9:3554-3560.

143. Gayle WE, Mayhall CG, Lamb VA, Apollo E, Haynes BW Jr. Resistant *Enterobacter cloacae* in a burn center: the ineffectiveness of silver sulfadiazine. *J Trauma.* 1978;18:317-323.

144. Davis IJ, Richards H, Mullany P. Isolation of silver- and antibiotic-resistant *Enterobacter cloacae* from teeth. *Oral Microbiol Immunol.* 2005;20:191-194.

145. Kremer AN, Hoffmann HJ. Subtractive hybridization yields a silver resistance determinant unique to nosocomial pathogens in the *Enterobacter cloacae* complex. *J Clin Microbiol.* 2012;50:3249-3257.

146. Wenzel RP, Hunting KJ, Osterman CA, Sande MA. *Providencia stuartii,* a hospital pathogen: potential factors for its emergence and transmission. *Am J Epidemiol.* 1976;104:170-180.

147. Bridges K, Kidson A, Lowbury EJL, Wilkins MD. Gentamicin- and silver-resistant *Pseudomonas* in a burns unit. *Br Med J.* 1979;1:446-449.

148. McHugh GL, Moellering RC, Hopkins CC, Swartz MN. *Salmonella typhimurium* resistant to silver nitrate, chloramphenicol, and ampicillin. *Lancet.* 1975;1:235-240.

149. Klasen HJ. A historical review of the use of silver in the treatment of burns. II. Renewed interest for silver. *Burns.* 2000;26:131-138.

150. Lansdown ABG, Williams A. Bacterial resistance to silver in wound care and medical devices. *J Wound Care.* 2007;16:15-19.

151. Sütterlin S, Tano E, Bergsten A, Tallberg AB, Melhus A. Effects of silver-based wound dressings on the bacterial flora in chronic leg ulcers and its susceptibility in vitro to silver. *Acta Derm Venereol.* 2012;92:34-39.

152. Bridges K, Lowburry EJL. Drug resistance in relation to use of silver sulphadiazine cream in a burns unit. *J Clin Pathol.* 1977;30:160-164.

153. Haefeli C, Franklin C, Hardy K. Plasmid-determined silver resistance in *Pseudomonas stutzeri* isolated from a silver mine. *J Bacteriol.* 1984;158:389-392.

154. Silver S. Bacterial silver resistance: molecular biology and uses and misuses of silver compounds. *FEMS Microbiol Rev.* 2003;27:341-353.

155. Hendry AR, Stewart IO. Silver-resistant *Enterobacteriaceae* from hospital patients. *Can J Microbiol.* 1979;25:915-921.

156. Kaur P, Vadehra DV. Mechanism of resistance to silver ions in *Klebsiella pneumoniae. Antimicrob Agents Chemother.* 1986;29:165-167.

157. Starodub ME, Trevors JT. Silver resistance in *Escherichia coli* R1. *J Med Microbiol.* 1989;29:101-110.

158. Starodub ME, Trevors JT. Mobilization of *Escherichia coli* R1 silver-resistance plasmid pJT1 by Tn5-Mob into *Escherichia coli* C600. *Biol Met.* 1990;3:24-27.

159. Deshpande LM, Chopade BA. Plasmid mediated silver resistance *in Acinetobacter baumannii. Biometals.* 1984;7:49-56.

160. Li XZ, Nikaido H, Williams KE. Silver-resistant mutants of *Escherichia coli* display active efflux of Ag+ and are deficient in porins. *J Bacteriol.* 1997;179:6127-6132.

161. Lok CN, Ho CM, Chen R, et al. Silver nanoparticles: partial oxidation and antibacterial activities. *J Biol Inorg Chem.* 2007;12:527-534.

162. Hsu SH, Tseng HJ, Lin YC. The biocompatibility and antibacterial properties of waterborne polyurethane-silver nanocomposites. *Biomaterials.* 2010;31:6796-6808.

163. Radzig MA, Nadtochenko VA, Koksharova OA, Kiwi J, Lipasova VA, Khmela IA. Antibacterial effects of silver nanoparticles on gram-negative bacteria: influence on the growth and biofilms formation, mechanisms of action. *Colloids Surf B Biointerfaces.* 2013;102:300-306.

164. Nies DH. Microbial heavy-metal resistance. *Appl Microbiol Biotech.* 1999;51:730-750.

165. Ramalingam B, Parandhaman T, Das SK. Antibacterial effects of biosynthesized silver nanoparticles on surface ultrastructure and nanomechanical properties of gram-negative bacteria viz. *Escherichia coli* and *Pseudomonas aeruginosa. ACS Appl Mater Interfaces.* 2016;8:4963-4976.

166. Staehlin BM, Gibbons JG, Rokas A, O'Halloran TV, Slot JC. Evolution of a heavy metal homeostasis/resistance island reflects increasing copper stress in enterobacteria. *Gen Biol Evol.* 2016;8:811-826.

167. Liau SY, Read DC, Pugh WJ, Furr JR, Russell AD. Interaction of silver nitrate with readily identifiable groups: relationship to the antibacterial action of silver ions. *Lett Appl Microbiol.* 1997;25:279-283.

168. Simon-Deckers A, Loo S, Mayne-L'Hermite M, et al. Size-, composition-, and shape-dependent toxicological impact of metal oxide nanoparticles and carbon nanotubes toward bacteria. *Environ Sci Technol.* 2009;43:8423-8429.

169. McQuillan JS, Shaw AM. Differential gene regulation in the Ag nanoparticle and Ag(+)-induced silver stress response in *Escherichia coli*: a full transcriptomic profile. *Nanotoxicology.* 2014;8:177-184.

170. Schacht VJ, Neumann LV, Sandhi SK, et al. Effects of silver nanoparticles on microbial growth dynamics. *J Appl Microbiol.* 2013;114:25-35.

171. Yang Y, Mathieu JM, Chattopadhyay S, et al. Defense mechanisms of *Pseudomonas aeruginosa* PAO1 against quantum dots and their released heavy metals. *ACS Nano.* 2012;6:6091-6098.

172. Graves JL Jr, Tajkarimi M, Cunningham Q, et al. Rapid evolution of silver nanoparticle resistance in *Escherichia coli. Front Genet.* 2015;6:42.

173. Gupta A, Phung LT, Taylor DE, Silver S. Diversity of silver resistance genes in IncH incompatibility group plasmids. *Microbiology.* 2001;147:3393-3402.

174. Woods EJ, Cochrane CA, Percival SL. Prevalence of silver resistance genes in bacteria isolated from human and horse wounds. *Veter Microbiol.* 2009;138:325-329.

175. Silver S, Phung LT. Bacterial heavy metal resistance: new surprises. *Ann Rev Microbiol.* 1996;50:753-789.

176. Silver S, Phung LT. A bacterial view of the periodic table: genes and proteins for toxic inorganic ions. *J Ind Microbiol Biotechnol.* 2005;32:587-605.

177. Loh JV, Percival SL, Woods EJ, Williams NJ, Cochrane CA. Silver resistance in MRSA isolated from wound and nasal sources in humans and animals. *Int Wound J.* 2009;6:32-38.

178. Aminov RI. Horizontal gene exchange in environmental microbiota. *Front Microbiol.* 2011;2:158.

179. Colman BP, Arnaout CL, Anciaux S, et al. Low concentrations of silver nanoparticles in biosolids cause adverse ecosystem responses under realistic field scenario. *PLoS One.* 2013;8:e57189.

180. Durenkamp M, Pawlett M, Ritz K, Harris JA, Neal AL, McGrath SP. Nanoparticles within WWTP sludges have minimal impact on

leachate quality and soil microbial community structure and function. *Environ Poll.* 2016;211:399-405.

181. Temple RM, Farooqi AA. An elderly, slate-grey woman. *Practitioner.* 1985;229:1053-1054.

182. Dunne SM, Gainsford ID, Wilson NH. Current materials and techniques for direct restorations in posterior teeth. Part 1: silver amalgam. *Int Dental J.* 1997;47:123-136.

183. Hollinger MA. Toxicological aspects of topical silver pharmaceuticals. *Crit Rev Toxicol.* 1996;26:255-260.

184. Yang Y, Qin Z, Zeng W, et al. Toxicity assessment of nanoparticles in various systems and organs. *Nanotechnol Rev.* 2017;6:279-289.

185. Franková J, Pivodová V, Vágnerová H, Juránová J, Ulrichová J. Effects of silver nanoparticles on primary cell cultures of fibroblasts and keratinocytes in a wound-healing model. *J Appl Biomater Funct Mater.* 2016;14:137-142.

186. Anisha BS, Biswas R, Chennazhi KP, Jayakumar R. Chitosan-hyaluronic acid/nano silver composite sponges for drug resistant bacteria infected diabetic wounds. *Int J Biol Macromol.* 2013;62:310-320.

187. Kim S, Choi JE, Choi J, et al. Oxidative stress-dependent toxicity of silver nanoparticles in human hepatoma cells. *Toxicol In Vitro.* 2009;23:1076-1084.

188. Kim TH, Kim M, Park HS, Shin US, Gong MS, Kim HW. Size-dependent cellular toxicity of silver nanoparticles. *J Biomed Mater Res A.* 2012;100(A):1033-1043.

189. Liu W, Wu Y, Wang C, et al. Impact of silver nanoparticles on human cells: effect of particle size. *Nanotoxicology.* 2010;4:319-330.

CHAPTER 26

Peptides, Enzymes, and Bacteriophages

Suzana Meira Ribeiro, Osmar Nascimento Silva, Bruna de Oliveira Costa, and Octávio Luiz Franco

Resistance to anti-infective drugs is considered a worldwide threat.[1] The ability to overcome the action of antimicrobial drugs can be achieved through conditions related to an individual bacterial cell (eg, change the antimicrobial bacteria target, antibiotic deactivation, block entrance, and efflux of the antibiotic) and/or may be related to bacterial life in the form of a community, known as biofilm.[2,3] Bacteria in biofilm can show resistance to antimicrobial agents, even if individual bacteria within biofilm present susceptibility to antimicrobials. In this context, where there are specific microorganisms that are resistant to antibiotics, such as extended-spectrum β-lactamases (ESBL) and carbapenemases, biofilm formation can further amplify the resistance phenotype.[4]

Resistant microorganisms can impact the economy in different fields such as public health, agriculture, livestock, food industries, and water distribution systems.[5,6] In public health, difficulty in combatting bacterial infections caused by resistant planktonic bacteria and biofilms can prolong the stay of patients in hospitals, leading to reduced quality of life and raising costs due to hospitalization.[7] In agriculture, difficulties in bacterial control can increase the yield losses of plant and animal inputs.[8,9] In the production chains of food industries, microbial biofilms, for example, can favor the contamination and consequent spoilage of foods.[10] Some pathogens that contaminate food can synthetize toxins or cause infections in humans or animals.[11] This microbial organization can also develop in systems of water distribution, affecting the water quality and contributing to the corrosion process of pipes.[12] In addition, biofilms in water systems can serve as a contamination source of infectious bacteria.[12,13]

In order to minimize the issues occasioned by microorganisms in many of these scenarios, sterilization and disinfection techniques can be used.[14] Sterilization allows the elimination of all forms of microorganism life, including spores.[14] Disinfection consists of a process that eliminates most microorganisms, except their spores.[15]

The term *disinfectant* is commonly employed for chemical agents used on inanimate surfaces, whereas the term *antiseptic* is used for disinfectants applied on living tissues and skin.[16] Antiseptics and disinfectants can minimize or prevent economic losses related to the presence of undesirable microorganisms in a particular context.

Many marketed disinfectant and antiseptic agents have become inefficient in combatting resistant microorganisms and their biofilms.[17] A wide variety of proposals have been presented to overcome these concerns, such as peptides, other proteinaceous compounds (eg, enzymes), and bacteriophages.[18-20] Peptides have been isolated from different classes of living organisms. They can be promiscuous in their activity, showing, for example, antimicrobial, antibiofilm, and immunomodulatory effects (Figure 26.1).[21,22] These activities could be useful to disinfect a contaminated surface, such as skin, and additionally improve the immune response against invader pathogens.[21,22] Some enzymes have shown efficiency in disinfecting medical devices and in removing biofilms in food.[23,24] Bacteriophages (bacterial viruses) have also shown potential to be used in multiple situations in inanimate and live surfaces. Because their targets are bacterial cells, the advantage of bacteriophages are not only their lytic activity against bacterial cells but also their ability to replicate in bacteria and increase their dose, yet minimally interfering with the normal flora (when narrow-spectrum phages are used) and the absence of cross-resistance with normal flora.[25]

An interesting use of peptides, enzymes, and bacteriophages involves their application in biomolecular engineering.[26-28] This approach allows antimicrobial compounds to be manufactured with increased antimicrobial properties and with nonexistent or minimal toxicity and/or potential to cause hazardous waste.[26-28] Thus, in the era where antibiotics become a limited resource to combat harmful bacteria, the use of innovative approaches could prevent infections or issues caused by microorganisms

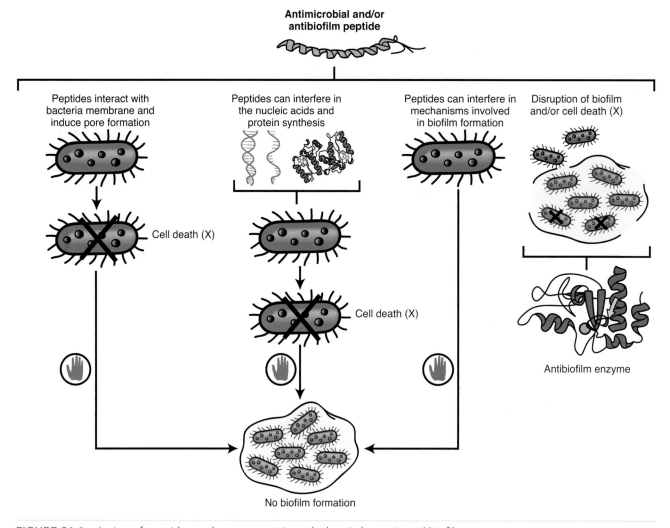

FIGURE 26.1　Action of peptides and enzymes against planktonic bacteria and biofilms.

in industrial sectors, the environment, and agriculture. Peptides, enzymes, and bacteriophages are interesting strategies to combat bacteria. This chapter sheds light on their potential use for the prevention and eradication of unwanted microorganisms and discusses the biotechnological approaches to improve the use of these agents in different contexts.

▶ PEPTIDES AND ENZYMES FOR DISINFECTION AND ANTISEPSIS OF SURFACES

Numerous peptides and proteins, such as enzymes, with antimicrobial properties have been isolated from different classes of organisms.[29] Alternatively, they can be used as a template for the development of compounds with improved antimicrobial and antibiofilm action.[30,31] In this context, peptides and enzymes could be used as for disinfectant or antiseptic applications.

For disinfection, peptides have been used alone or in combination to eradicate planktonic microorganisms and their biofilms.[27,28] Most studies have focused on the elimination of human or veterinary infectious disease. In dentistry, peptides are the potential active components in some products (eg, mouth rinse, root canal sealers, and composite resins) or can be promising candidates for the treatment of oral infections.[18] This strategy can be exemplified by the synthetic antibiofilm peptide 1018, which in developed studies showed potent activity against oral multispecies biofilms, thus being a promising candidate as an antibiofilm agent that is nontoxic and effective for antisepsis of bacterial plaques in clinical dentistry.[18] This peptide has also shown effectiveness in reducing biofilm on wounds[22] and therefore could be used as potential antiseptic agent.

Many peptides have emerged as potential candidates for development as antimicrobial drugs, such as magainin, a potent peptide that reached to phase III clinical trials. Some peptides are already commercially exploited, such as with nisin and aprotinin.[32,33] In food applications, nisin is a peptide produced by the bacterium *Lactococcus lactis* and has been used as a preservative.[28,32] Nisin can combat bacteria associated with food spoilage and human infections.[28,32] Aprotinin, an antifibrinolytic molecule, has been primarily explored for use in surgery to reduce bleeding[33]; however, studies have shown its potential as a direct antimicrobial and as a protease inhibitor (inhibiting surface-related proteases that are important virulence factors in certain bacteria).[34,35]

Another approach in antisepsis is to combine peptides with other agents, such as commercial antiseptics.[20] This approach is designed to prevent the emergence of resistant organisms, to expand the spectrum of target microorganisms, and to decrease toxicity, allowing the use of lower doses of both agents.[36] For example, the combination of the synthetic peptide 1018 with the commercial antiseptic chlorhexidine increased the antibiofilm activity of each compound compared to when they were used alone to combat infections caused by oral multispecies biofilms.[18]

Peptide mechanisms of action against planktonic bacteria involves electrostatic interaction between peptides and bacterial membranes, which then leads to increased cell membrane permeability, loss of barrier function, and leakage of cytoplasmic components, culminating in cell death (see Figure 26.1).[37] They also can prevent the cell-wall, protein, and nucleic acid synthesis (see Figure 26.1),[30] whereas the antibiofilm action has been related to the interference with a universal compound, known as (p)ppGpp (guanosine tetra- and penta-phosphates) (see Figure 26.1). This molecule seems to play an important role in the response to stress in bacteria and consequently in the development of biofilm in multiple bacterial species.[38]

Enzymes have been commonly used in cleaning formulations, used as prerequisites to disinfection of reusable medical devices or surfaces.[39] In particular, proteases have been employed to aid in the removal of bacterial biofilms from the various surfaces of medical devices, such as endoscopes, colonoscopes, and contact lenses. In the food processing industry, enzymatic detergents are also used to aid in the removals of foodborne pathogens[40] that contaminate equipment surfaces and the infrastructure, including thawing rooms, conveyor belts, shredders, commercial kitchens, and packaging materials.[41]

The mechanisms of action of antibiofilm enzymes consist in the degradation of polysaccharides, DNA, and proteins that compose the biofilm matrix.[42,43] They can also lead to cell lysis and affect cell signaling, thus interfering mechanisms associated with biofilm formation and maintenance.[23] Lysostaphin (an endopeptidase), for example, is able to disrupt biofilms formed by *Staphylococcus aureus* that grows on plastic and glass surfaces.[44] In addition, this enzyme has the ability to kill the bacterial cells present in biofilm.[44,45] An advantage of lysostaphin is its antimicrobial activity against nondividing as well as dividing cells.[46] The activity against nondividing cells could be explored against dormant cells in biofilms, a bacterial state resistant

to antimicrobials.[47] But overall, the antimicrobial activity is limited to certain staphylococci, particularly *S aureus*.

One potential enzyme that could be used as an antiseptic is α-amylase from *Bacillus subtilis*.[48] This enzyme was able to inhibit the biofilm of methicillin-resistant *S aureus* (MRSA) and *Pseudomonas aeruginosa*, bacteria commonly associated with wound infections.[49] Another strategy in this context would be the combination of enzymes with commercial antiseptic agents for a more effective antisepsis. In this situation, enzymes can degrade the biofilm matrix and thus facilitate the access of the antiseptics to the adhered bacteria in the living tissue or skin.[42]

A combination of enzymes and peptides also has been proved to be a potential strategy to inhibit pathogens. A combination of the antimicrobial peptide ranalexin with the enzyme lysostaphin reduced MRSA infection on human skin ex vivo to a greater extent than any of the individually tested compounds.[20]

As presented, there are many approaches to enable the disinfection of surfaces. Examples of antimicrobial and/or antibiofilm peptides and enzymes that have been used to combat pathogens are summarized in Table 26.1. These include various health and food industry applications for the use of these biomolecules.

▶ BACTERIOPHAGES AND ANTIMICROBIAL APPROACHES

Bacteriophages, viruses that infect bacteria, are considered ubiquitous microorganisms. There are more than 6000 phages described that infect bacteria or archaea.[50] These are classified based on their morphology, genetic content (DNA or RNA),[51,52] habitats (eg, soil, marine, or human gut bacteriophages),[53-55] particular hosts (eg, *Klebsiella* and *Pseudomonas* phages),[56,57] and their life cycle (lytic or lysogenic).[58] Because such organisms have the potential to destroy specific pathogenic bacteria and their biofilms,[59] and self-replicate, causing minimal or no effect on bacterial microflora of treated organisms (eg, animals infected with pathogenic bacteria),[60] they can potentially be used in different scenarios, such as clinical (medical and veterinary), industrial, and environmental (eg, treatment of contaminated water).[59,61]

In the early 20th century, bacteriophages were recognized as a potential antimicrobial to treat human bacterial infections.[59] However, after the introduction of antibiotics in 1940 and their success in combating infections caused by bacteria, interest in bacteriophages was reduced.[50] In addition, the Council on Pharmacy and Chemistry of the American Medical Association concluded that the antimicrobial properties of bacteriophages was uncertain and thus required more experiments to prove their efficacy.[59] Due to the rapid emergence of antibiotic-resistant bacteria, there has been a resurgent interest in bacteriophages

TABLE 26.1   Marketed antimicrobial and/or antibiofilm peptides and enzymes

Compound	Company	Use
Peptide		
C16G2	Chengdu Sen Nuo Wei Biotechnology Co	Dental caries
DPK-060	DermaGen AB	Atopic dermatitis
		Otitis externa
Dusquetide	Inimex Pharmaceuticals Inc	Melioidosis
Lactoferrin	DermaGen AB	Postsurgical adhesions
LL-37	Pergamum AB	Leg ulcer
LTX-109	Lytix Biopharma AS	Impetigo
		Staphylococcus aureus infections
MBI-226	Cadence Pharmaceuticals Inc	Acne vulgaris, genital warts, rosacea
MDL-63397	Durata Therapeutics Inc	Osteomyelitis, pneumonia
MK-4261	Cubist Pharmaceuticals Inc	*Clostridium difficile* infections
MSI-78	Dipexium Pharmaceuticals Inc	Diabetic foot ulcer, skin and soft tissue infections
NP108	NovaBiotics Ltd	Bovine mastitis
NP213	NovaBiotics Ltd	Onychomycosis
NP339	NovaBiotics Ltd	Cystic fibrosis, invasive fungal disease, oropharyngeal candidiasis
NP432	NovaBiotics Ltd	*C difficile*, MRSA, and *Pseudomonas aeruginosa* infections
NVB302	Novacta Biosystems Ltd	*C difficile* infections
POL7080	Polyphor Ltd	*P aeruginosa* infections
		Gram-negative infections
TD-1792	GlaxoSmithKline Co	Gram-positive infections
		Skin and soft tissue infections
TD-6424	Clinigen Group plc	Broad-spectrum antibiotic
Protein		
Alcalase	Novozymes A/S	Washing detergents
Durazym	Novozymes A/S	Washing detergents
Esperase	Novozymes A/S	Washing detergents
Everlase	Novozymes A/S	Washing detergents
Kannase	Novozymes A/S	Washing detergents
Lipex	Novozymes A/S	Washing detergents
Liquanase Ultra	Novozymes A/S	Washing detergents
Liquanase	Novozymes A/S	Washing detergents
Lysostaphin	Ruhof Co	*S aureus* infections
Neutrase	Novozymes A/S	Washing detergents
Ovozyme	Novozymes A/S	Washing detergents
Polarzyme	Novozymes A/S	Washing detergents
Primase	Novozymes A/S	Washing detergents
Properase	Medisafe International Co	Contact lens cleaners
		Washing detergents

TABLE 26.1   Marketed antimicrobial and/or antibiofilm peptides and enzymes *(Continued)*

Compound	Company	Use
Savinase	Medisafe International Co	Contact lens cleaners
		Washing detergents
Savinase Ultra	Novozymes A/S	Washing detergents
Savinase	Novozymes A/S	Washing detergents
Stainzyme	Novozymes A/S	Washing detergents
Subtilisin	Johnson & Johnson	Contact lens cleaners
		Washing detergents
		Skin infections
Termamyl	Novozymes A/S	Washing detergents

Abbreviation: MRSA, methicillin-resistant *Staphylococcus aureus.*

as alternatives to control pathogenic bacteria.[50,62,63] In 2006, the US Food and Drug Administration (FDA) and US Department of Agriculture (USDA) approved the use of a six-bacteriophage cocktail named MP-102 (Intralytix) for treating meat products to combat the bacteria *Listeria monocytogenes.*[64] Currently, there is a growing diversity of products and applications based on bacteriophages for different applications (Table 26.2).

The antimicrobial potential for the use of bacteriophages could be based on the lytic process alone. In this process, the viral genome becomes part of the bacterial genome and, after that, the virus genetic material induces the bacterium to replicate the components for new viral particles (Figure 26.2).[65] Cell lysis is mediated by enzymes produced by the viral genome, such as holins and endolysins. Holins have the ability to form pores in the plasma membrane.[65] This allows the endolysins to reach the peptidoglycan and break it down, favoring bacterial cell cytoplasm leakage (see Figure 26.2).[66] The diversity of endolysins and holins in nature can be further explored for antimicrobial purposes.[67,68] Besides, it is possible to modify their sequence to improve their antimicrobial potency. In this direction, some studies have developed chimeric endolysins with improved bacteriolytic activity.[69]

The selectivity of bacteriophages can vary. Some bacteriophages tend to have narrow-spectrum activity, killing only a subset of bacterial species or intraspecies.[70] For example, a study showed that different bacteriophages isolated from certain capsular types of *Klebsiella pneumoniae* showed selectivity against other types of *K pneumoniae.*[71] The bacteriophages KpV41, KpV475, and KpV71 presented lytic activity against mainly *K pneumoniae* of capsular type K1, whereas bacteriophages KpV74 and KpV763 presented lytic activity against K2 capsular types.[71] Phages KpV766 and KpV48 presented nonspecific capsular lytic activity.[71] An advantage of narrow-spectrum bacteriophages is preserving the microflora resident on a live surface, in the case of their use for an antiseptic purpose.

Other bacteriophages can present broad-spectrum activity against a broader range of bacterial types. A study showed that each one of four bacteriophages isolated from Lake Michigan was able to lyse *P aeruginosa* (*Proteobacteria*), *Arthrobacter* (*Actinobacteria*), *Chryseobacterium* (*Bacteroidetes*) and *Microbacterium* (*Actinobacteria*).[72] Broad-spectrum bacteriophages could be used to eliminate multiple harmful bacteria in a context of polymicrobial contamination. Another strategy for disinfection could be using a cocktail of different bacteriophages.[73] This last approach could minimize the probability of selecting resistant bacterial strains; however, the use of a multiple-phage cocktail could face complex pharmacological and regulatory issues because the quantities and quality of each phage should be characterized before and after exposure in a context of antimicrobial therapy.[27,63]

In order to improve bacteriophage efficacy against bacteria, re-engineering of bacteriophages has been investigated.[27] In a general way, different strategies can be used for bacteriophage bioengineering for antimicrobial application, such as homologous recombination, bacteriophage recombineering of electroporated DNA (BRED), and CRISPR-Cas-mediated genome engineering.[74] In the homologous recombination process, the viral injected DNA recombines with regions of a bacterial donor plasmid (that carries a gene or genes that will be introduced in the phage genome) resulting in recombinant phages. Pouillot et al,[75] for example, used homologous recombination to carry out an insertion of mutated genes, to develop a bank of T4 phages able to infect different bacterial species.

In BRED, purified phage DNA and the substrate (double-stranded DNA, single-stranded DNA containing a deletion, or a point mutation) are inserted in a bacterial cell by electroporation.[76] This process allows the recombination between homologous regions of both DNA parts, so that the desired mutant can later be selected.[55] Nobrega et al[77] employed BRED to construct phages resistant to the pH of the gastrointestinal tract of animals. This could

TABLE 26.2 Marketed antimicrobial bacteriophages

Product Name	Company	Condition Treated	Route of Administration (Probably)
Phage—human diseases			
Phagestaph	Biochimpharm Co	Treatment and prevention of diseases caused by *Staphylococcus aureus*	Oral and rectal
Phagyo	Biochimpharm Co	Treatment and prevention of purulent inflammatory diseases caused by *Streptococcus*, *Staphylococcus*, *Escherichia coli*, *Pseudomonas aeruginosa*, *Proteus*, and their combinations	Oral, local, and external
Septaphage	Biochimpharm Co	Treatment and prevention of diseases caused by *Shigella* species, *Salmonella* species, *E coli*, *Proteus* species, *Staphylococcus* species, *Pseudomonas* species, and *Enterococcus* species	Oral and rectal
Bioseptum	Biofarm-L	Treatment of intestinal infections	Oral
Pyobacteriophagum Liquidum	Biofarm-L	Treatment and prevention of inflammatory and enteric diseases caused by staphylococci, streptococci, *Proteus* species, *P aeruginosa*, and *E coli*	Oral and local
Artilysin	LISANDO GmbH	Treatment of systemic infections by gram-negative bacteria infections	Oral, local, and external
Medolysin	LISANDO GmbH	Broad spectrum antibacterial	Local and external
Complex pyobacteriophage	Microgen Co	Specifically lyse staphylococci, streptococci, enterococci, *Proteus* species, *Klebsiella pneumoniae* and *Klebsiella oxytoca*, *P aeruginosa*, and *E coli*	Oral, local, and external
Dysentery polyvalent bacteriophage	Microgen Co	Treatment and prevention of bacterial dysentery caused by *Shigella flexneri* of 1, 2, 3, 4, 6 serovariants and *Shigella sonnei*	Oral, local, and external
E coli bacteriophage	Microgen Co	Treatment and prevention of diseases caused by *E coli*	Oral, local, and external
E coli–Proteus bacteriophage	Microgen Co	Treatment and prevention of purulent inflammatory and enteric diseases, dysbacteriosis caused by bacteria *Proteus* species, and enterotoxigenic *E coli*	Oral, local, and external
Intesti-bacteriophage	Microgen Co	Treatment and prevention of diseases of the gastrointestinal tract caused by bacteria of dysentery, *Salmonella* species, *E coli*, *Proteus* species, enterococci, staphylococci, *P aeruginosa*, or a combination thereof	Oral and rectal
Klebsiella purified polyvalent bacteriophage	Microgen Co	Treatment and prevention of diseases caused by *K pneumoniae*, *Klebsiella ozaenae*, and *Klebsiella rhinoscleromatis*	Oral, local, and external
Sextaphag polyvalent pyobacteriophage	Microgen Co	Treatment and prevention of inflammatory and enteric diseases caused by staphylococci, streptococci, *Proteus* species, *Klebsiella* species, *P aeruginosa*, and *E coli*	Oral, local, and external
Streptococcus bacteriophage	Microgen Co	Treatment and prevention of diseases caused by *Streptococcus*	Oral, local, and external
Phagobioderm	Neopharm	Treatment and prevention of inflammatory and diseases caused by *P aeruginosa*, *E coli*, *Staphylococcus* species, *Streptococcus* species, *Proteus* species	Oral, local, and external
Otofag	MicroMir	Normalize the microflora and prevent purulent inflammatory diseases of the bacterial etiology of the ear, throat, and nose	Oral, local, and external

TABLE 26.2	Marketed antimicrobial bacteriophages *(Continued)*		
Product Name	**Company**	**Condition Treated**	**Route of Administration (Probably)**
Fagodent	MicroMir	Treatment of the bacterial inflammation of the oral cavity	Oral and local
Fagoderm	MicroMir	Normalize microflora and prevent bacterial infections of the skin	External
Fagonin	MicroMir	Normalize microflora and prevent bacterial infections of organs of the intimate sphere	External and rectal
Phage–food industry and animal health			
Staphage Lysate (SPL)	Delmont Laboratories, Inc	Treatment of recurrent canine pyoderma and related staphylococcal hypersensitivity or polymicrobial skin infections with a staphylococcal component	Local and external
Ecolicide	Intralytix	Targets *E coli* O157:H7 contamination in pet food	—
EcoShield	Intralytix	Controlling the foodborne bacterial pathogen *E coli* O157:H7	—
ListPhage	Intralytix	Targets *Listeria monocytogenes* contamination in pet food	—
ListShield	Intralytix	Controlling the foodborne bacterial pathogen *L monocytogenes*	—
SalmoFresh	Intralytix	Controlling the foodborne bacterial pathogen *Salmonella enterica*	—
SalmoLyse	Intralytix	Targets *Salmonella* species contamination in pet food	—
ShigaShield	Intralytix	Controlling the foodborne bacterial pathogen *Shigella* species	—
Artilysin	LISANDO GmbH	Broad spectrum antibacterial	Local and external
Listex P100	PhageGuard	Controlling the foodborne bacterial pathogen *L monocytogenes*	—
Salmonelex	PhageGuard	Controlling the foodborne bacterial pathogen *S enterica*	—
AgriPhage	Phagelux	Biological control for bacterial spot and bacterial speck on tomatoes and peppers	—
AgriPhage-Cmm	Phagelux	Biological control for bacterial canker disease on tomato	—
Lexia	Phagelux	Treatment of acute hepatopancreatic necrosis disease (AHPND) and early mortality syndrome (EMS) in shrimp	—
Bronchophagus	MicroMir	Prevention and treatment of the lower respiratory tract, including in complex therapy for the treatment of chronic obstructive bronchitis and chronic obstructive pulmonary disease in horses	Oral and local
Vetagin	MicroMir	Treatment of purulent, purulent catarrhal, catarrhal, fibrinous and other endometritis, caused or complicated by a bacterial infection	Oral and local
Fagovet	MicroMir	Prevention of bacterial infections and strengthening the immunity of birds	Oral
Phage—preharvest interventions			
Ecolicide PX	Intralytix	Targets *E coli* O157:H7 contamination on hides of live animals	—

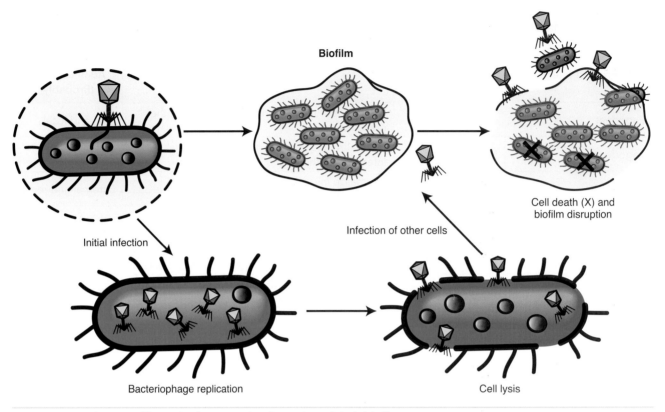

FIGURE 26.2 Activity of bacteriophages against bacteria and their biofilms.

be useful to improve antimicrobial phage therapy by oral administration.[78] Phages that are resistant to other environmental conditions could be developed and used for disinfection purposes.

Bacteriophage engineering has also been used in biotechnology to deliver the CRISPR system, a genome editing technology. CRISPR consists of a family of DNA sequences present in bacteria.[74] These sequences harbor fragments of DNA virus that were previously attached to the bacteria. This allows the bacteria to recognize and destroy the DNA of a similar virus that may later attack them. The CRISPR system is constituted of Cas protein that recognizes and cuts the foreign DNA and the CRISPR locus that guides Cas against the target DNA specified by the guide RNA.[53] In an antimicrobial context, for example, the CRISPR system was used to destroy antibiotic resistance genes present in plasmids of S aureus.[78] In addition, this system was able to kill S aureus in a mouse skin colonization model.[78] Elimination of resistance genes could prevent the spread of resistance between bacteria. Such bacteriophages could be used as antimicrobial topical therapy as well as an antiseptic.

Initially, the studies with bacteriophages were focused on clinical antimicrobial therapy. Currently, bacteriophage applications go beyond the treatment and prevention of infectious diseases.[79]

Among these are their uses as bactericidal agents in food, as a preservative tool, both of vegetable and animal

origin.[80] Studies have shown the potential to combat bacteria that commonly contaminate foods, such as *L monocytogenes*.[81] One of the advantages of using phages in the food industry is that they are a nonthermal intervention and can be used both in the elimination of bacteria from meats and cheeses and in the hygiene of whole and cut fruits, thus extending the useful life of food in addition to preventing bacterial food poisoning.[82]

Another potential use of bacteriophages is in water or waste treatment, such as direct use in sewage treatment. Bacteriophages have been shown to be effective against *Shigella* and *Escherichia coli*, both waterborne and foodborne pathogens.[61] Bacteriophages can also be used in the petroleum industry to combat bacteria associated with fouling and corrosion of pipelines. Samples of pipes with corrosion in a petroleum pipeline station revealed the presence of the bacteria *Stenotrophomonas maltophilia* and associated phages.[83] The lytic phage of this bacteria found in this study was related to the Siphoviridae family.[83] In this context, bacteriophages could reduce production costs and generate less environmental impact than the chemical agents used for the same purpose.[84,85]

There are thousands of bacteriophages described, and it is believed that millions will be isolated and characterized in the future. In spite of their potential, the number of formulations marketed using phages is relatively low. With advances in biotechnology for screening microbial biodiversity and to improve bacteriophage properties against unwanted microorganisms, bacteriophages can be better explored and used for commercial purposes, both for disinfecting live and inanimate surfaces.

MARKET PROSPECTS FOR PROTEINS, PEPTIDES, AND BACTERIOPHAGES

In recent decades, a significant concern in the incidence of bacterial infections has been reported, which has triggered an increase in attention to antiseptic agents and disinfectants. Concomitant to this, we have experienced a period where life expectancy has exceeded historical levels, accompanied by an increase in the incidence of chronic diseases, surgical procedures, and a greater concern with the hygiene of the body and the environment.[86] In 2016, the market for disinfectants and antiseptics was worth about USD $6.55 billion, and by 2017, it is estimated that this market grew by about 7% to reach a value of USD $7.1 billion, according to reports from companies and brands. Today, the United States alone accounts for approximately 40% of the worldwide market for antiseptics and disinfectants. The European Union represents another 34% of the total market. The predictions for the growth of this market are encouraging because emerging economies such as Brazil, Russia, India, China, and South Africa (the BRICS) have grown substantially, which directly contributes to the growth of the antiseptic and disinfectant market. It is estimated that the global antiseptic and disinfectant market will reach USD $9.1 billion in 2022, with an annual average growth between 5% and 7%.

One of the current challenges of this industry is the replacement of chemical compounds with more natural compounds. Among the strategies to be used are peptides, proteins, and enzymes (see Table 26.1), and bacteriophages (see Table 26.2) because the organic components present in these agents can be readily degraded in the environment. With the advance in biotechnology, these agents can be engineered to develop approaches with improved antimicrobial, antivirulent and/or antibiofilm properties. Enzymes, for examples, have been widely used as components of cleaning formulations and as accessories for disinfection processes, especially in the cleaning of medical and dental instruments. Enzymes have been chosen for medical use because they have the ability to cleave large, hard-to-remove molecules, and, particularly in the use of proteases, there is a high protein content in body fluids (such as blood and tissue fragments) that are not easily removed with conventional detergents/surfactants.[39] Further enhancements and use of these compounds can open possibilities for new applications.

However, despite all the benefits presented by bacteriophages and proteins/peptides, some limitations need to be taken into account in the commercial use of these bioproducts. A major limitation in comparison to traditional disinfectants is often the limited spectrum of activity (particularly with bacteriophages and antimicrobial peptides), but the more specific mechanisms of action against key target bacteria may be a benefit in some applications so as not to disrupt the local microbiome (eg, in the oral or gut cavities). A major challenge for the commercial use of bacteriophages in many countries is the adaptation of the regulatory frameworks to adequately reflect the new mode of action of these antimicrobials because they are self-replicating and self-limiting. Despite this, bacteriophage-based products have been widely marketed in some Eastern European countries. As for proteinaceous compounds, there are a number of limitations, including thermostability, narrow substrate scope and/or erroneous stereotype and/or region selectivity in the case of the enzymes, and the proteolytic degradation in the case of the peptides. But in overcoming these challenges for certain applications, there can be a diversity of compounds with future potential.

CONCLUSION

Advances in biotechnology present new opportunities to combat undesirable microorganisms using peptides, proteins, and bacteriophages. In the context of antimicrobial resistance, this possibility provides an effective and promising resource for disinfecting inanimate and alive surfaces. Prospection of these compounds in nature and development of these agents with improved activity can help different sectors of society in combating undesirable microorganisms. Although such compounds have emerged as new antimicrobial and antibiofilm agents, questions about safety need to be addressed before the world can benefit from peptides, enzymes, and bacteriophages in the arduous fight against microbial resistance. A combination of these agents with other compounds could increase success in the disinfection of surfaces and draw more attention to the use of peptides and enzymes in multiple situations, such as in pharmaceutical, industrial, and environmental fields.

REFERENCES

1. Roca I, Akova M, Baquero F, et al. The global threat of antimicrobial resistance: science for intervention. *New Microbes New Infect.* 2015;6:22-29.
2. Blair JMA, Webber MA, Baylay AJ, Ogbolu DO, Piddock LJV. Molecular mechanisms of antibiotic resistance. *Nat Rev Microbiol.* 2015;13:42-51.
3. Singh S, Singh SK, Chowdhury I, Singh R. Understanding the mechanism of bacterial biofilms resistance to antimicrobial agents. *Open Microbiol J.* 2017;11:53-62.
4. Chung PY. The emerging problems of *Klebsiella pneumoniae* infections: carbapenem resistance and biofilm formation. *FEMS Microbiol Lett.* 2016;363(20):fnw219.
5. Luepke KH, Suda KJ, Boucher H, et al. Past, present, and future of antibacterial economics: increasing bacterial resistance, limited antibiotic pipeline, and societal implications. *Pharmacotherapy.* 2017;37:71-84.

6. Boltz JP, Smets BF, Rittmann BE, van Loosdrecht MCM, Morgenroth E, Daigger GT. From biofilm ecology to reactors: a focused review. *Water Sci Techno.* 2017;75:1753-1760. doi:10.2166/wst.2017.061.

7. Wood TK. Strategies for combating persister cell and biofilm infections. *Microb Biotechnol.* 2017;10(5):1054-1056. doi:10.1111/1751-7915.12774.

8. Economou V, Gousia P. Agriculture and food animals as a source of antimicrobial-resistant bacteria. *Infect Drug Resist.* 2015;8:49-61. doi:10.2147/IDR.S55778.

9. Kim BS, French E, Caldwell D, Harrington E, Iyer-Pascuzzi AS. Bacterial wilt disease: host resistance and pathogen virulence mechanisms. *Physiol Mol Plant Pathol.* 2016;95:37-43. doi:10.1016/j.pmpp.2016.02.007.

10. Zhao X, Lin CW, Wang J, Oh DH. Advances in rapid detection methods for foodborne pathogens. *J Microbiol Biotechnol.* 2014;24:297-312.

11. Lerner A, Matthias T. Possible association between celiac disease and bacterial transglutaminase in food processing: a hypothesis. *Nutr Rev.* 2015;73:544-552. doi:10.1093/nutrit/nuv011.

12. Mahapatra A, Padhi N, Mahapatra D, et al. Study of biofilm in bacteria from water pipelines. *J Clin Diagn Res.* 2015;9(3):DC09-DC11. doi:10.7860/JCDR/2015/12415.5715.

13. Decker BK, Palmore TN. Hospital water and opportunities for infection prevention. *Curr Infect Dis Rep.* 2014;16:432. doi:10.1007/s11908-014-0432-y.

14. Rutala WA, Weber DJ. Disinfection, sterilization, and antisepsis: an overview. *Am J Infect Control.* 2016;44:e1-e6. doi:10.1016/j.ajic.2015.10.038.

15. Rutala WA, Weber DJ. Disinfection and sterilization: an overview. *Am J Infect Control.* 2013;41:S2-S5. doi:10.1016/j.ajic.2012.11.005.

16. McDonnell GE. *Antisepsis, Disinfection, and Sterilization: Types, Action, and Resistance.* Washington, DC: American Society for Microbiology; 2007.

17. Harbarth S, Tuan Soh S, Horner C, Wilcox MH. Is reduced susceptibility to disinfectants and antiseptics a risk in healthcare settings? A point/counterpoint review. *J Hosp Infect.* 2014;87:194-202. doi:10.1016/j.jhin.2014.04.012.

18. Wang Z, de la Fuente-Núñez C, Shen Y, Haapasalo M, Hancock RE. Treatment of oral multispecies biofilms by an anti-biofilm peptide. *PLoS One.* 2015;10:e0132512. doi:10.1371/journal.pone.0132512.

19. Aminov R, Caplin J, Chanishvili N, et al. Application of bacteriophages. *Microbiol Aust.* 2017;38:63-66. doi:10.1071/MA17029.

20. Desbois AP, Lang S, Gemmell CG, Coote PJ. Surface disinfection properties of the combination of an antimicrobial peptide, ranalexin, with an endopeptidase, lysostaphin, against methicillin-resistant *Staphylococcus aureus* (MRSA). *J Appl Microbiol.* 2010;108:723-730. doi:10.1111/j.1365-2672.2009.04472.x.

21. Mansour SC, de la Fuente-Núñez C, Hancock RE. Peptide IDR-1018: modulating the immune system and targeting bacterial biofilms to treat antibiotic-resistant bacterial infections. *J Pept Sci.* 2015;21:323-329. doi:10.1002/psc.2708.

22. Steinstraesser L, Hirsch T, Schulte M, et al. Innate defense regulator peptide 1018 in wound healing and wound infection. *PLoS One.* 2012;7:e39373. doi:10.1371/journal.pone.0039373.

23. Meireles A, Borges A, Giaouris E, Simões M. The current knowledge on the application of anti-biofilm enzymes in the food industry. *Food Res Int.* 2016;86:140-146. doi:10.1016/j.foodres.2016.06.006.

24. Stiefel P, Mauerhofer S, Schneider J, Maniura-Weber K, Rosenberg U, Ren Q. Enzymes enhance biofilm removal efficiency of cleaners. *Antimicrob Agents Chemother.* 2016;60:3647-3652. doi:10.1128/AAC.00400-16.

25. Loc-Carrillo C, Abedon ST. Pros and cons of phage therapy. *Bacteriophage.* 2011;1:111-114. doi:10.4161/bact.1.2.14590.

26. Thallinger B, Prasetyo EN, Nyanhongo GS, Guebitz GM. Antimicrobial enzymes: an emerging strategy to fight microbes and microbial biofilms. *Biotechnol J.* 2013;8:97-109. doi:10.1002/biot.201200313.

27. Brown R, Lengeling A, Wang B. Phage engineering: how advances in molecular biology and synthetic biology are being utilized to enhance the therapeutic potential of bacteriophages. *Quant Biol.* 2017;5:42-54. doi:10.1007/s40484-017-0094-5.

28. Wang G. *Antimicrobial Peptides: Discovery, Design and Novel Therapeutic Strategies.* 2nd ed. Oxfordshire, United Kingdom: CABI; 2017.

29. Zhao X, Wu H, Lu H, Li G, Huang Q. LAMP: a database linking antimicrobial peptides. *PLoS One.* 2013;8:e66557. doi:10.1371/journal.pone.0066557.

30. de la Fuente-Núñez C, Cardoso MH, de Souza Cândido E, Franco OL, Hancock RE. Synthetic antibiofilm peptides. *Biochim Biophys Acta.* 2016;1858:1061-1069. doi:10.1016/j.bbamem.2015.12.015.

31. Vaikundamoorthy R, Rajendran R, Selvaraju A, Moorthy K, Perumal S. Development of thermostable amylase enzyme from *Bacillus cereus* for potential antibiofilm activity. *Bioorg Chem.* 2018;77:494-506. doi:10.1016/j.bioorg.2018.02.014.

32. Gharsallaoui A, Oulahal N, Joly C, Degraeve P. Nisin as a food preservative: part 1: physicochemical properties. antimicrobial activity, and main uses. *Crit Rev Food Sci Nutr.* 2016;56:1262-1274. doi:10.1080/10408398.2013.763765.

33. Luque A, Junqueira SM, Cabra HA, Andrade PC, Oliveira FM. Aprotinin free hemostatic sealant to reduce blood loss in surgical patients: a systematic review. *Value Health.* 2015;18:A293. doi:10.1016/j.jval.2015.03.1707.

34. Brannon JR, Burk DL, Leclerc JM, et al. Inhibition of outer membrane proteases of the omptin family by aprotinin. *Infect Immun.* 2015;83(6):2300-2301. doi:10.1128/IAI.00136-15.

35. Pellegrini A, Thomas U, von Fellenberg R, Wild P. Bactericidal activities of lysozyme and aprotinin against gram-negative and gram-positive bacteria related to their basic character. *J Appl Bacteriol.* 1992;72:180-187.

36. Graham S, Coote PJ. Potent, synergistic inhibition of *Staphylococcus aureus* upon exposure to a combination of the endopeptidase lysostaphin and the cationic peptide ranalexin. *J Antimicrob Chemother.* 2007;59:759-762. doi:10.1093/jac/dkl539.

37. Yazici H, O'Neill MB, Kacar T, et al. Engineered chimeric peptides as antimicrobial surface coating agents toward infection-free implants. *ACS Appl Mater Interfaces.* 2016;8:5070-5081. doi:10.1021/acsami.5b03697.

38. de la Fuente-Núñez C, Reffuveille F, Haney EF, Straus SK, Hancock RE. Broad-spectrum anti-biofilm peptide that targets a cellular stress response. *PLoS Pathog.* 2014;10:e1004152. doi:10.1371/journal.ppat.1004152.

39. Augustin M, Ali-Vehmas T, Atroshi F. Assessment of enzymatic cleaning agents and disinfectants against bacterial biofilms. *J Pharm Pharm Sci.* 2004;7:55-64.

40. Singh R, Kumar M, Mittal A, Mehta PK. Microbial enzymes: industrial progress in 21st century. *3 Biotech.* 2016;6:174. doi:10.1007/s13205-016-0485-8.

41. Solanki K, Grover N, Downs P, et al. Enzyme-based listericidal nanocomposites. *Sci Rep.* 2013;3:1584. doi:10.1038/srep01584.

42. Lefebvre E, Vighetto C, Di Martino P, Larreta Garde V, Seyer D. Synergistic antibiofilm efficacy of various commercial antiseptics, enzymes and EDTA: a study of *Pseudomonas aeruginosa* and *Staphylococcus aureus* biofilms. *Int J Antimicrob Agents.* 2016;48:181-188. doi:10.1016/j.ijantimicag.2016.05.008.

43. Kaplan JB, LoVetri K, Cardona ST, et al. Recombinant human DNase I decreases biofilm and increases antimicrobial susceptibility in staphylococci. *J Antibiot (Tokyo).* 2012;65:73-77. doi:10.1038/ja.2011.113.

44. Belyansky I, Tsirline VB, Montero PN, et al. Lysostaphin-coated mesh prevents staphylococcal infection and significantly improves survival in a contaminated surgical field. *Am Surg.* 2011;77:1025-1031.

45. Craigen B, Dashiff A, Kadouri DE. The use of commercially available alpha-amylase compounds to inhibit and remove *Staphylococcus aureus* biofilms. *Open Microbiol J.* 2011;5:21-31. doi:10.2174/1874285801105010021.

46. Bastos MD, Coutinho BG, Coelho ML. Lysostaphin: a staphylococcal bacteriolysin with potential clinical applications. *Pharmaceuticals (Basel).* 2010;3:1139-1161. doi:10.3390/ph3041139.

47. Kester JC, Fortune SM. Persisters and beyond: mechanisms of phenotypic drug resistance and drug tolerance in bacteria. *Crit Rev Biochem Mol Biol.* 2014;49:91-101. doi:10.3109/10409238.2013.869543.

48. Kalpana BJ, Aarthy S, Pandian SK. Antibiofilm activity of α-amylase from *Bacillus subtilis* S8-18 against biofilm forming human bacterial pathogens. *Appl Biochem Biotechnol.* 2012;167:1778-1794. doi:10.1007/s12010-011-9526-2.

49. Serra R, Grande R, Butrico L, et al. Chronic wound infections: the role of *Pseudomonas aeruginosa* and *Staphylococcus aureus. Expert Rev Anti Infect Ther.* 2015;13:605-613. doi:10.1586/14787210.2015.1023291.

50. Wittebole X, De Roock S, Opal SM. A historical overview of bacteriophage therapy as an alternative to antibiotics for the treatment of bacterial pathogens. *Virulence.* 2014;5:226-235. doi:10.4161/viru.25991.

51. Koonin EV, Krupovic M, Yutin N. Evolution of double-stranded DNA viruses of eukaryotes: from bacteriophages to transposons to giant viruses. *Ann N Y Acad Sci.* 2015;1341:10-24. doi:10.1111/nyas.12728.

52. Krishnamurthy SR, Janowski AB, Zhao G, Barouch D, Wang D. Hyperexpansion of RNA bacteriophage diversity. *PLoS Biol.* 2016;14:e1002409. doi:10.1371/journal.pbio.1002409.

53. Han LL, Yu DT, Zhang LM, Shen JP, He JZ. Genetic and functional diversity of ubiquitous DNA viruses in selected Chinese agricultural soils. *Sci Rep.* 2017;7:45142. doi:10.1038/srep45142.

54. Lal TM, Sano M, Ransangan J. Isolation and characterization of large marine bacteriophage (*Myoviridae*), VhKM4 infecting *Vibrio harveyi. J Aquat Anim Health.* 2017;29:26-30. doi:10.1080/08997659.2016.1249578.

55. Yutin N, Makarova KS, Gussow AB, et al. Discovery of an expansive bacteriophage family that includes the most abundant viruses from the human gut. *Nat Microbiol.* 2018;3:38-46. doi:10.1038/s41564-017-0053-y.

56. Koberg S, Brinks E, Fiedler G, et al. Genome sequence of *Klebsiella pneumoniae* bacteriophage PMBT1 isolated from raw sewage. *Genome Announc.* 2017;5:e00914-e00916. doi:10.1128/genomeA.00914-16.

57. Krylov VN. Bacteriophages of *Pseudomonas aeruginosa*: long-term prospects for use in phage therapy. *Adv Virus Res.* 2014;88:227-278. doi:10.1016/B978-0-12-800098-4.00005-2.

58. Du Toit A. Viral infection: the language of phages. *Nat Rev Microbiol.* 2017;15:134-135. doi:10.1038/nrmicro.2017.8.

59. Salmond GP, Fineran PC. A century of the phage: past, present and future. *Nat Rev Microbiol.* 2015;13:777-786. doi:10.1038/nrmicro3564.

60. Mai V, Ukhanova M, Reinhard MK, Li M, Sulakvelidze A. Bacteriophage administration significantly reduces *Shigella* colonization and shedding by *Shigella*-challenged mice without deleterious side effects and distortions in the gut microbiota. *Bacteriophage.* 2015;5:e1088124. doi:10.1080/21597081.2015.1088124.

61. Jun JW, Giri SS, Kim HJ, et al. Bacteriophage application to control the contaminated water with *Shigella. Sci Rep.* 2016;6:22636. doi:10.1038/srep22636.

62. Yosef I, Manor M, Kiro R, Qimron U. Temperate and lytic bacteriophages programmed to sensitize and kill antibiotic-resistant bacteria. *Proc Natl Acad Sci U S A.* 2015;112:7267-7272. doi:10.1073/pnas.1500107112.

63. Nilsson AS. Phage therapy—constraints and possibilities. *Ups J Med Sci.* 2014;119:192-198. doi:10.3109/03009734.2014.902878.

64. Sharma M. Lytic bacteriophages. *Bacteriophage.* 2013;3:e25518. doi:10.4161/bact.25518.

65. Saier MH Jr, Reddy BL. Holins in bacteria, eukaryotes, and archaea: multifunctional xenologues with potential biotechnological and biomedical applications. *J Bacteriol.* 2015;197:7-17. doi:10.1128/JB.02046-14.

66. Young R. Phage lysis: three steps, three choices, one outcome. *J Microbiol.* 2014;52:243-258. doi:10.1007/s12275-014-4087-z.

67. Schmelcher M, Donovan DM, Loessner MJ. Bacteriophage endolysins as novel antimicrobials. *Future Microbiol.* 2012;7:1147-1171. doi:10.2217/fmb.12.97.

68. Catalão MJ, Gil F, Moniz-Pereira J, São-José C, Pimentel M. Diversity in bacterial lysis systems: bacteriophages show the way. *FEMS Microbiol Rev.* 2013;37:554-571. doi:10.1111/1574-6976.12006.

69. Mao J, Schmelcher M, Harty WJ, Foster-Frey J, Donovan DM. Chimeric Ply187 endolysin kills *Staphylococcus aureus* more effectively than the parental enzyme. *FEMS Microbiol Lett.* 2013;342:3036. doi:10.1111/1574-6968.12104.

70. Koskella B, Meaden S. Understanding bacteriophage specificity in natural microbial communities. *Viruses.* 2013;5:806-823. doi:10.3390/v5030806.

71. Solovieva EV, Myakinina VP, Kislichkina AA, et al. Comparative genome analysis of novel podoviruses lytic for hypermucoviscous *Klebsiella pneumoniae* of K1, K2, and K57 capsular types. *Virus Res.* 2018;243:10-18. doi:10.1016/j.virusres.2017.09.026.

72. Malki K, Kula A, Bruder K, et al. Bacteriophages isolated from Lake Michigan demonstrate broad host-range across several bacterial phyla. *Virol J.* 2015;12:164. doi:10.1186/s12985-015-0395-0.

73. Ando H, Lemire S, Pires DP, Lu TK. Engineering modular viral scaffolds for targeted bacterial population editing. *Cell Syst.* 2015;1:187-196. doi:10.1016/j.cels.2015.08.013.

74. Pires DP, Cleto S, Sillankorva S, Azeredo J, Lu TK. Genetically engineered phages: a review of advances over the last decade. *Microbiol Mol Biol Rev.* 2016;80:523-543. doi:10.1128/MMBR.00069-15.

75. Pouillot F, Blois H, Iris F. Genetically engineered virulent phage banks in the detection and control of emergent pathogenic bacteria. *Biosecur Bioterror.* 2010;8:155-169. doi:10.1089/bsp.2009.0057.

76. Marinelli LJ, Hatfull GF, Piuri M. Recombineering: a powerful tool for modification of bacteriophage genomes. *Bacteriophage.* 2012;2:5-14. doi:10.4161/bact.18778.

77. Nobrega F, Costa AR, Santos JF, et al. Genetically manipulated phages with improved pH resistance for oral administration in veterinary medicine. *Sci Rep.* 2016;6:39235. doi:10.1038/srep39235.

78. Bikard D, Euler CW, Jiang W, et al. Exploiting CRISPR-Cas nucleases to produce sequence-specific antimicrobials. *Nat Biotechnol.* 2014;32:1146-1150. doi:10.1038/nbt.3043.

79. Lin DM, Koskella B, Lin HC. Phage therapy: an alternative to antibiotics in the age of multi-drug resistance. *World J Gastrointest Pharmacol Ther.* 2017;8:162-173. doi:10.4292/wjgpt.v8.i3.162.

80. Sillankorva SM, Oliveira H, Azeredo J. Bacteriophages and their role in food safety. *Int J Microbiol.* 2012;2012:863945. doi:10.1155/2012/863945.

81. Oliveira M, Viñas I, Colàs P, Anguera M, Usall J, Abadias M. Effectiveness of a bacteriophage in reducing *Listeria monocytogenes* on fresh-cut fruits and fruit juices. *Food Microbiol.* 2014;38:137-142. doi:10.1016/j.fm.2013.08.018.

82. Goodridge LD, Bisha B. Phage-based biocontrol strategies to reduce foodborne pathogens in foods. *Bacteriophage.* 2011;1:130-137. doi:10.4161/bact.1.3.17629.

83. Pedramfar A, Beheshti Maal K, Mirdamadian SH. Phage therapy of corrosion-producing bacterium *Stenotrophomonas maltophilia* using isolated lytic bacteriophages. *Anti-Corros Methods Mater.* 2017;64:607-612. doi:10.1108/ACMM-02-2017-1755.

84. Haq IU, Chaudhry WN, Akhtar MN, Andleeb S, Qadri I. Bacteriophages and their implications on future biotechnology: a review. *Virol J.* 2012;9:9. doi:10.1186/1743-422X-9-9.

85. Rosenberg E, Bittan-Banin G, Sharon G, et al. The phage-driven microbial loop in petroleum bioremediation. *Microb Biotechnol.* 2010;3:467-472. doi:10.1111/j.1751-7915.2010.00182.x.

86. Lachenmeier DW. Antiseptic drugs and disinfectants. In: Ray SD, ed. *Side Effects of Drugs Annual.* Vol 36. Amsterdam, Netherlands: Elsevier; 2015:273-279. doi:10.1016/bs.seda.2015.06.005.

Chlorine Dioxide

Zhao Chen and Mark A. Czarneski

▶ CHEMICAL AND PHYSICAL PROPERTIES

Chlorine dioxide is a yellow-green gas that was first prepared by Chenevix in 1802.[1] Humphrey Davy independently prepared this compound in 1811, elucidated its composition, and proposed the name of euchlorine.[2] Although chlorine dioxide is the most widely accepted English name for this compound, the names chlorine oxide, anthium dioxide, chlorine(IV) oxide, chlorine peroxide, chloroperoxyl, and chloryl radical also have been used. The Chemical Abstracts Service Compound Registry Number (CAS RN) for chlorine dioxide is 10049-04-4.

Structural Properties

Chlorine dioxide contains one atom of chlorine and two atoms of oxygen and exists entirely or almost entirely as a free radical monomer (Figure 27.1).[3,4] Microwave spectra of chlorine dioxide in the gaseous phase have given chlorine-oxygen distances of about 0.147 nm; electronic diffraction indicates 0.149 nm. This chlorine-oxygen distance is approximately that of an average chlorine-oxygen double bond. The angle formed by the oxygen-chlorine-oxygen bonds is in the range of $117.7 + 1.7$ degrees.[4,5] Chlorine dioxide has considerable unsaturated bond character,[6] but, in solution, there is no evidence of dimerization or polymerization,[7] and at neutral pH, it does not hydrolyze.[8] Crystalline hydrates of chlorine dioxide have been reported, including a hexahydrate, an octahydrate, and a decahydrate.[4,9-11]

Chlorine dioxide is one member of a series of oxides that also includes chlorine monoxide (Cl_2O); chlorine peroxide [$Cl(O_2)$], which has the same molecular formula as chlorine dioxide but a different structure; chlorine trioxide (ClO_3); chlorine tetroxide (ClO_4); chlorine heptoxide (Cl_2O_7); as well as dimers and mixtures of these oxides. Although all are sometimes called chlorine oxide, each has distinctly different properties from chlorine dioxide.

Spectral Properties

The ultraviolet adsorption spectrum of chlorine dioxide dissolved in carbon tetrachloride shows maxima at 375 and 355 nm with a minimum at 263 nm.[8] The absorption spectrum in aqueous solution has a broad band near 360 nm.[4] The molar extinction coefficient is frequently reported as 1150 M/cm^{-1},[12] but when using high-resolution, narrow bandwidth spectrophotometers, it has been determined to be 1250 M/cm^{-1}.[11,13] The extinction coefficient is temperature, acid, and ionic strength independent from 25°C to 50°C, 0.2 to 4 N, and 2 to 4 M, respectively,[4,11] and is unaffected by chloride concentration up to 0.3 M.[11,14] The chlorine dioxide gas-phase spectrum is the same as that in aqueous solution,[4,11] providing a convenient method for monitoring concentration in various processes.

In the infrared, the fundamental vibrational frequencies of chlorine dioxide in the gaseous phase, measured as wave numbers, are 946 cm^{-1}, 448 cm^{-1}, and 1110 cm^{-1}, corresponding to the symmetric stretch, bend, and asymmetric stretch, respectively.[5]

Physical Properties

Under standard pressure, chlorine dioxide freezes at a temperature of −59°C and boils at 11°C.[15] Thus, it is a true gas at room temperature, where its density is about 1.6 g/cm^3.[16] The gas has an odor similar to that of chlorine.

Chlorine dioxide is soluble in water, and a formula has been developed to predict solubility under various conditions.[12,17] Solubilities at 0°C, 15°C, and 30°C were demonstrated to be linear,[15] and extrapolated solubility

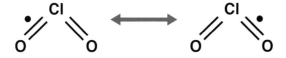

FIGURE 27.1 Structure of chlorine dioxide, indicating its radical character.

curves have been published.[8] At 20°C, chlorine dioxide gas present at a concentration of 4% by volume has a solubility of about 4 g/L. The partition coefficient of chlorine dioxide between water and the gaseous phase is expressed as:

$$L = \frac{C_{ClO2\ (aq)}}{C_{ClO2\ (g)}}$$

and is equal to 70 ± 0.7 at 0°C, 45 at 15°C, and 26.5 + 0.8 at 35°C.[8]

Chlorine dioxide in the gas phase is stable in concentrations of less than 10% in air at atmospheric pressure. The gas tends to be unstable at higher concentrations and can be destabilized further by contact with light or with substances that catalyze its decomposition. When decomposition occurs, the volume increase is relatively small, and the resulting explosion has sometimes been described as a "puff." Using chlorine dioxide in gas form for area disinfection/sterilization, the concentrations are typically 0.04% to 0.18% (1-5 mg/L). These concentrations are far below the "puffing" threshold for chlorine dioxide. Detonation has never been observed, even at much higher concentrations at temperatures less than 42°C.[18] Attempts to store chlorine dioxide in a compressed form, with or without other gases, have been unsuccessful[12] until recently when CDG Environmental obtained US Department of Transportation permission to ship 3000 ppm solutions (CDG Solution 3000 liquid concentrate). Recent studies have confirmed the lower limit for explosive decomposition at 9.5% (chlorine dioxide/air).[19] Thus, when the concentration of chlorine dioxide gas in air is below 9.5%, there is no explosion hazard.

METHODS OF PREPARATION

Because chlorine dioxide is not sufficiently stable to be stored, it is typically produced at the site of use. Many methods exist for the preparation of chlorine dioxide, and the method chosen for a specific application will depend on the amount required, the amount of side products that can be tolerated, and whether the gas is required in solution or the gaseous form. The large-scale commercial production of chlorine dioxide, as is required in the bleaching of paper, generally involves the reduction of sodium chlorate by a suitable acid.[4] Several alternative processes use this method, and the details can be found in the extensive compilation of Masschelein and Rice.[8]

Sterilization and disinfection applications are smaller scale processes in which production quantities do not exceed 2000 kg/d. For such processes, sodium chlorite is the preferred starting material.[11] In potable water–treatment facilities, all the chlorine dioxide used is generated from sodium chlorite.[12] As pointed out by Gordon et al,[4] the advantages of using chlorite in the generation of chlorine dioxide are its ease of use and the purity of chlorine dioxide that is produced. In some methods, acid is added to the chlorite/hypochlorite mixture.[20] Chlorine dioxide also has been generated by oxidation of chlorite with nitrogen trichloride.[4] Today, most small generators use an oxidative process in which chlorine (either as a gas or in solution) is mixed with sodium chlorite solution (either as a solid or in solution).[12] This reaction is rapid, readily goes to completion, and proceeds with following stoichiometry:

$$2NaClO_2 + Cl_2 \rightarrow 2ClO_2 + 2NaCl$$

A convenient application of this method of production consists of passing diluted chlorine gas through a column or tower of sodium chlorite to yield uncontaminated chlorine dioxide.[21] Chlorine dioxide generated by this method can be used immediately or dissolved in a solvent (typically water) for temporary storage. This method also can be used to remove traces of chlorine from a stream of chlorine dioxide gas prepared using another method.[4]

Numerous alternative methods for generating chlorine dioxide for smaller scale applications have been reported. Some examples include the electrolysis of chlorite solutions,[4,8] by passing nitrogen dioxide, obtained from the effluent gasses of an electric arc machine, through a column of sodium chlorite.[22] For the preparation of small quantities of chlorine-free chlorine dioxide, the oxidation of chlorite with persulfate, as illustrated by the following reaction, has been used[4,8]:

$$2NaClO_2 + Na_2S_2O_8 \rightarrow 2ClO_2 + 2Na_2SO_4$$

CHEMICAL REACTIONS OF CHLORINE DIOXIDE

Chlorine dioxide is a strong oxidizing agent and, in contrast to chlorine, does not tend to react with organic materials to form chlorinated species or with ammonia to form chloramine. The inorganic chemistry and reactions of chlorine dioxide with organic matter have been well studied and can be found in the comprehensive references written by Gordon et al,[4] Masschelein and Rice,[8] and Aieta and Roberts.[23]

Decomposition

As a free radical species, chlorine dioxide is not stable for long periods in storage and can decompose. Whereas the gas can be stable in concentrations of less than 10% by volume in air, decomposition is facilitated at higher concentrations. Although its instability precludes storage of chlorine dioxide in compressed form,[12] it is sufficiently stable to permit its routine use, and studies have been done to elucidate the factors that influence its stability.

The decomposition reaction of high concentration of chlorine dioxide has been studied in depth.[24-27] For concentrated chlorine dioxide gas (15%-30% by volume), the ignition temperatures are approximately 130°C; the presence of light, dust, petroleum-based lubricants, and sulfur all lower the decomposition temperature.[28] Further, chlorine dioxide can undergo autocatalytic decomposition, which may or may not involve explosion, and the ratios of products formed during decomposition depend on the concentration of water vapor and temperature.[24] Surface area can accelerate the decomposition of chlorine dioxide, but sufficiently large surface areas appear to inhibit catalytic decomposition by adsorption of the intermediates.

Exposure to light leads to decomposition of chlorine dioxide,[8,25] and in the gas phase, the primary photochemical reaction is the homolytic fission of the chlorine-oxygen bond to form $ClO^{\bullet}$ and $O^{\bullet}$.[8] The reaction mechanism for the light catalyzed decomposition of gaseous, dry chlorine dioxide is postulated as:

$$ClO_2 + h\nu \rightarrow ClO^{\bullet} + O^{\bullet}$$

$$ClO_2 + O^{\bullet} \rightarrow ClO_3$$

$$2ClO^{\bullet} \rightarrow Cl_2 + O_2$$

Interestingly, when moisture is present along with gaseous chlorine dioxide, exposure to light may induce the formation of a visible mist that does not contain chlorine but rather consists of a complex mixture of acids.[25] The following mechanism has been proposed for the photolytic decomposition of chlorine dioxide in the presence of moisture[7]:

$$ClO_2 + h\nu \rightarrow ClO^{\bullet} + O^{\bullet}$$

$$ClO_2 + O^{\bullet} \rightarrow ClO_3$$

$$2ClO_3 \rightarrow Cl_2O_6$$

$$ClO^{\bullet} + ClO_2 \rightarrow Cl_2O_3$$

$$Cl_2O_6 + H_2O \rightarrow HClO_3 + HClO_4$$

$$Cl_2O_3 + H_2O \rightarrow 2\ HClO_2$$

$$2\ HClO_2 \rightarrow HClO + HClO_3$$

In solution at neutral pH, in the absence of light, and at room temperatures (18°C-25°C) or cooler, chlorine dioxide is quite stable. The primary decomposition process, when it occurs, is hydrolysis and disproportionation of chlorine dioxide into chlorite and chlorate ions:

$$2ClO_2 + 2OH^- \rightarrow ClO_2- + ClO_3- + H_2O$$

The rate of hydrolysis is impacted by temperature and pH, increasing rapidly at elevated temperature and at pH values above 10, and is more rapid in the presence of chlorine and hypochlorite, producing chlorate and hydrochloric acid.[11]

In reducing environments, chlorine dioxide may undergo single electron transfer processes, which ultimately result in the formation of chloride. The standard potential (E°) for chlorine dioxide is 1.511 V,[29] although in solution, the electron potential is dependent on the pH and the number of electrons transferred.

Reactions With Organic Compounds

Chlorine dioxide is a selective yet versatile oxidant for many organic compounds. It does not act via chlorination, and thus, trihalomethane formation does not occur.[12] The chemistry and mechanisms of reactions of chlorine dioxide with organic compounds have been reviewed extensively,[8,30,31] and a compilation of kinetic data is also available.[32] The oxidation of amines with chlorine dioxide was studied in detail by Rosenblatt et al[33,34] and Hull et al[35,36] who found that, in aqueous solutions, primary and secondary amines react slowly or not at all with chlorine dioxide but that tertiary amines were readily oxidized, producing a secondary amine and an aldehyde.

Chlorine dioxide does not react with saturated aliphatic hydrocarbons, whereas alcohols, aldehydes, and ketones are oxidized to form carboxylic acids.[11] Chlorine dioxide reacts with carbohydrates, such as glucose, to oxidize the primary hydroxyl groups, first to aldehydes and then to carboxylic acids.[8] The reaction with lipids is mainly an oxidation at the double bond. Although most amino acids do not react readily with chlorine dioxide, tyrosine, tryptophan, and cysteine are exceptions.[31,37] Peptides and proteins are subject to oxidation, substitution, and addition reactions.[38] Chlorine dioxide solutions have been shown to denature proteins,[39] and the gas phase has been shown as an effective way of inactivating β-lactams from old production facilities.[40] Additionally, chlorine dioxide can cause destruction of lysozyme function via protein denaturation and degradation.[41]

Chlorine dioxide rapidly oxidizes phenolic compounds[42] and has been used to oxidize chlorinated phenolic compounds to reduce their toxicity.[11] Occasional chlorination of aromatic or unsaturated aliphatic hydrocarbons has been reported,[43] but no trihalomethanes were formed. Because chlorine dioxide does not tend to form dioxins or trihalomethanes or react with ammonia to form chloramines, it has great appeal for the treatment of water and wastewater.

▶ BIOCIDAL PROPERTIES

The antimicrobial properties of chlorine dioxide solutions were documented in the 1930s by Schaufler[44] and Kovtunovitch and Chemaya.[45] Later, Ridenour and Ingols[46] reported on the addition of chlorine dioxide along with chlorine to commercial water supplies to produce better tasting water, a practice that continues today. Numerous studies have been carried out since then to validate the biocidal properties of chlorine dioxide in an aqueous environment and have demonstrated broad-spectrum biocidal properties. Chlorine dioxide has several registered uses in water treatment, disinfection, and sterilization in both dissolved in water and applied as a gas.

Biocidal Activities

Studies have proved the efficacy of aqueous and gaseous chlorine dioxide on a wide variety of microorganisms, including bacteria, fungi, spores, viruses, and protozoa. The effect of chlorine dioxide has been proved in laboratory conditions on major bacterial pathogens responsible for principal outbreaks, such as *Escherichia coli* O157:H7, *Listeria monocytogenes*, and *Salmonella enterica*.[47] Meanwhile, some early studies have shown that chlorine dioxide is capable of inactivating enteroviruses, polioviruses, rotavirus, and human immunodeficiency virus (HIV).[48-55] The increasing interest in the potential biocidal uses of chlorine dioxide has also stimulated studies into the activity of this agent against various protozoal, fungal, and algal species, such as *Cryptosporidium parvum* oocysts, *Streptomyces griseus*, and yeasts.[56-59]

With the current concerns about prions and prion-associated diseases, it is not surprising that studies into the inactivation of these agents by chlorine dioxide have been undertaken. Brown et al[60-62] studied the inactivation of prions by chlorine dioxide and other disinfectants. Sodium hypochlorite produced consistently marked inactivation (3-4 log within 15 minutes), whereas chlorine dioxide (50 ppm) exhibited moderate to substantial inactivation. It was suggested that doubling or tripling the concentration of chlorine dioxide would be more effective in inactivating the agent of Creutzfeldt-Jakob disease.

Microorganisms differ greatly in the sensitivity to chlorine dioxide (Figure 27.2).[47] One of the most distinct features of some bacteria is the ability to produce stress-resistant spores. Because of sporulation, resistance to heat, radiation, desiccation, extreme pH, chemicals, enzymes, and high pressure are largely increased.[63] This resistance enables the bacteria to survive many antisepsis and disinfection (eg, pasteurization) processes. As noted in the previous sections, the broad-spectrum activity of chlorine dioxide in solution was well established in the 1940s and the years following; however, the sporicidal activity of gaseous chlorine dioxide and, thus, its efficacy as

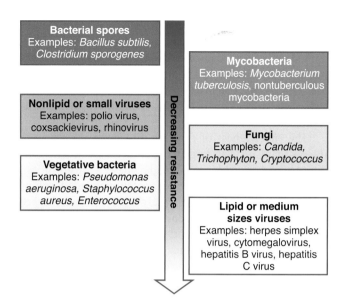

FIGURE 27.2 Typical resistance of microorganisms to chlorine dioxide.

a gas sterilant were not demonstrated until the 1980s. The lethal activity of chlorine dioxide gas on spores of *Bacillus subtilis* was first reported by Rosenblatt et al[64] in their patent of the use of chlorine dioxide as a gas sterilant. Sporicidal activity was present at concentrations as low as 11 mg/L. In a work reported subsequently, it was found that, analogous to ethylene oxide, adequate hydration of the spores was required for optimal activity.[65] Activity was also demonstrated against the anaerobic spore former *Clostridium sporogenes*.[66] In 1988, chlorine dioxide gas was registered as a sterilizing agent by the US Environmental Protection Agency (EPA) under the Federal Insecticide, Fungicide, and Rodenticide Act (FIFRA). Work by Jeng and Woodworth[67] confirmed the sporicidal activity of chlorine dioxide and provided further information about the conditions required for its effective use.

Biofilm can be defined as a community of microorganisms, generally associated with or attached to abiotic or biological surfaces (see chapter 67).[69] These cells are frequently embedded in exopolymeric substances. The tolerance of vegetative bacterial cells in biofilms to environmental stresses, such as routinely used disinfectants, can be profoundly increased than planktonic bacteria. The exopolysaccharide (EPS) matrix restricts the access of antimicrobial substances to cells within the biofilm by reducing diffusion and by maintaining cells at slow growth rate. For example, the survival of *Pseudomonas fluorescens* M2 cells after exposure to a chlorine dioxide solution was apparently enhanced by the presence of *P fluorescens* DL5 in binary biofilms.[70] Vaid et al[71] reported that a 10-minute treatment of 0.3 mg/L gaseous chlorine dioxide and 7 mg/L of aqueous chlorine dioxide resulted in reductions of 3.21 and 3.74 log CFUs/cm^2 of *L monocytogenes* within a biofilm matrix on stainless steel coupon, respectively.

Interestingly, Martin et al[72] isolated a *B subtilis* strain from a washer-disinfector whose vegetative form demonstrated unique resistance to 0.03% chlorine dioxide. It has been postulated that additional efficient intracellular mechanisms may be involved to explain its significant resistance to in-use concentrations of commonly used high-level disinfectants.

The effectiveness of chlorine dioxide on inactivating microorganisms also largely depends on treatment conditions, such as chlorine dioxide phase, concentration, contact time, temperature, pH, total suspended solids, and organic matter.[73] The efficacy increases at higher concentrations and treatment times but decreases with a decrease in temperature and pH. Concerning total suspended solids, their presence promotes pathogen aggregation and interferes with the disinfection performance of chlorine dioxide.[74] Nonetheless, when compared to chlorine, chlorine dioxide is a more effective biocide in the presence of high levels of organic matter, depending on the concentration.

Another factor associated with treatment conditions is the phase of chlorine dioxide. Studies have demonstrated that the application of chlorine dioxide in a gaseous form is more effective in inactivating microorganisms compared with its aqueous form, presumably due to its higher penetrability.[47]

Biocidal Mechanism

The possible modes of action of chlorine dioxide over microorganisms have been widely studied (see Figure 27.2). Research into the mechanism of the biocidal action of chlorine dioxide has involved the identification of specific chemical reactions between chlorine dioxide and biomolecules and evaluation of the effect of chlorine dioxide on physiological functions. The most widely reported mechanism is the disruption of cell protein synthesis primarily due to the oxidations of cell surface membrane proteins[12,75] and free fatty acids[76] and the increase in the permeability of the microbial cell.[77] Cho et al[78] reported that chlorine dioxide caused some levels of both surface damage and inner component degradation in *E coli*. Furthermore, Cho et al[78] explained that only after a certain level of surface damage, intracellular components were attacked because the initial lag phase in enzyme degradation was noticeable and was related to the time required for chlorine dioxide to penetrate the cell.

Chlorine dioxide has also been related to membrane damage on bacterial spores.[79,80] Chlorine dioxide caused damage to the inner cell membrane, change in cell permeability, and interruption of the complete germination of *B subtilis* spores.[79] In *Bacillus cereus*, chlorine dioxide caused surface roughness, indentations, and elongation of cells that resulted in the inhibition of division and associated metabolic damage of bacterial cells.[79] With respect

to viruses, chlorine dioxide inactivated poliovirus by altering viral capsid proteins and reacting with RNA separated from the capsids, which impaired RNA synthesis.[48] Li et al[81] reported that the inactivation mechanism of hepatitis A virus (HAV) by chlorine dioxide was due to the loss of the 5′ nontranslated regions (5′NTR) (the sequence from bp 1 to 671) and/or destruction of the antigenicity, which is different from that of chlorine.

However, most of the published studies have been focused on the inactivation mechanisms of chlorine dioxide on bacteria and viruses. And there are very few studies on the fungicidal mechanisms of chlorine dioxide. Zhu et al[82] has showed that the metal ion leakage, the inhibition of enzyme activities, and the alteration of cell structure were critical events in *Saccharomyces cerevisiae* inactivation by chlorine dioxide.

▶ TOXICOLOGY AND SAFETY

Chlorine dioxide is used in large quantities, and experience has demonstrated that it can be used safely. Because it is a chemical disinfectant and sterilizing agent, however, it is toxic to living systems. Its application, therefore, should be carefully managed, and steps should be taken to prevent unacceptable exposure. Smith and Willhite[83] indicated that although there are concerns about chlorine dioxide's acute toxicity, they concluded that the human experience with chlorine dioxide in both prospective studies and in actual use situations has failed to reveal adverse long-term health effects.

The threshold limit value (TLV) time-weighted average (TWA) signifying the level at which a human can be safely exposed for up to 8 hours has been established as 0.1 ppm for gaseous chlorine dioxide, and the short-term exposure level (STEL) has been set as 0.3 ppm, as required by the Occupational Safety and Health Administration (OSHA). The STEL is the 15-minute exposure safety level. This TWA concentration is also the most frequently cited odor threshold, which means that exposure to this gas is self-warning.[84]

Chlorine dioxide is considered a mucous membrane irritant, and inhalation of excessive amounts can lead to pulmonary edema.[85] Meggs et al[86,87] describe the nasal pathology of persistent rhinitis with chemical sensitivity after chlorine dioxide exposure.

Because chlorine dioxide is used for water treatment and in the food industry, most of the toxicity studies that have been done have involved ingestion of chlorine dioxide or its metabolites. Whereas most of these studies involved animals, some human studies have been reported. A few studies involving topical application[88,89] also have been done.

When ingested, chlorine dioxide is metabolized and excreted as chloride and chlorite.[90,91] It is difficult to separate effects attributable solely to chlorine dioxide from those of its metabolic products; therefore, many of these studies compared the effects of the administration of chlorine dioxide and chlorite.

Studies in rats and mice on the ingestion of chlorine dioxide in water[92-94] found little other than a transient increase in serum glutathione. By contrast, studies involving chlorite ingestion[92,95] found methemoglobinemia, decreases in glucose-6-phosphate dehydrogenase (G6PD) activity, and increased erythrocyte fragility. At the highest dose, a few deaths and significant erythrocyte abnormalities were observed in animals. Studies on the ingestion of chlorine dioxide conducted with rats,[96] monkeys,[97] and pigeons[98] all demonstrated decreases in thyroid function. In their work, Bercz et al[97] found that the effect was reversible on withdrawal of chlorine dioxide.

Animal studies to delineate the teratogenic potential of chlorine dioxide and chlorite showed no significant association,[99-101] except for the study on chlorine dioxide by Suh et al.[102] The evidence for mutagenicity of either chlorine dioxide or chlorite is contradictory.[68,103,104] Available data support that chlorite is not considered carcinogenic.[103] There appears to be no published research on the carcinogenicity, if any, of chlorine dioxide.

Studies with human subjects have not detected any serious toxicities associated with the acute or chronic ingestion of chlorine dioxide and chlorite. A wide-ranging, EPA-sponsored study determined the effect of administering discrete doses of increasing concentration of chlorine disinfectants, including chlorine dioxide, to normal healthy volunteers.[105-107] The impact on normal human subjects of daily ingestion of the disinfectants at concentrations of 5 mg/L over 12 weeks also was studied. Lastly, chlorite, at a concentration of 5 mg/L, was administered daily to G6PD-deficient subjects. The physiologic impact was assessed by a large battery of qualitative and quantitative tests. The study affirmed the relative safety and tolerance of normal, healthy, adult males and normal, healthy, adult male G6PD-deficient individuals to daily 12-week ingestion of 500 mL of chlorine dioxide at a concentration of 5 mg/L.[107,108]

Michael et al[109] studied the population of a village that converted to chlorine dioxide as a potable water disinfectant during the summer months to avoid taste and odor problems. One person, identified as being G6PD deficient, displayed a reduction of hemoglobin concentration, hematocrit, and red blood cell count. No other significant differences were observed in any subjects.

In 1982, Tuthill et al[110] published a retrospective study of neonates from Chicopee, Massachusetts, in the time frame of 1945-1950, when the town used chlorine dioxide (about 0.5 ppm) in water posttreatment. The data were compared, for the same time, with neonates from Holyoke, Massachusetts (a community with similar demographics but using chlorination). The rates of jaundice, birth defects, and fetal and neonatal mortality did not differ significantly between the communities. A statistically significant positive association was found between prematurity and the chlorine dioxide–treated water. Of the roughly 1000 births examined in each community, Chicopee showed 7.8% premature births, and Holyoke experienced a 5.8% rate. This finding was not statistically significant when the age of the mother was controlled.[111]

In 2004, Ouhoummane et al[112] compared thyroid function of newborns from 11 municipalities where chlorine dioxide disinfection was used with 15 municipalities that used chlorine disinfection. They found no evidence of suppressed thyroid function in newborns exposed to drinking water treated with chlorine dioxide. There was no statistical difference in thyroid-stimulating hormone (TSH) or prevalence of congenital hypothyroidism between those exposed to chlorine dioxide disinfection and those exposed to other disinfection. These results were compiled from 32 978 newborns over the period 1993-1999 in Quebec, Canada, for neonatal screening for congenital hypothyroidism.

Akamatsu et al[113] showed low levels of exposure (0.05 and 0.1 ppm of gas) to rats for 24 hours a day, 7 days a week, for a total time of 6 months and no chlorine dioxide gas–related toxicity was found. No weight gain, food or water consumption, or relative organ weight was observed. No biochemistry and hematology examinations changes occurred, and in the respiratory organs, no chlorine dioxide gas–related toxicity was observed.

Chlorine dioxide and sodium chlorite have gone through an EPA's Reregistration Eligibility Decision (RED) for Chlorine Dioxide and Sodium Chlorite (Case 4023) in 2006. Sodium chlorite is used as a precursor in the generation of chlorine dioxide, so the EPA combined the results of both because they have the same toxicologic end points. The RED compiled data and papers and summed up the safety aspects for chlorine dioxide. The Food Quality Protection Act (FQPA) Safety Factor (as required by FQPA) is intended to provide a 10-fold safety factor (10X), for the protection of infants and children in relation to pesticide residues in food, drinking water, or residential exposures. After the RED was completed, the FQPA Safety Factor has been removed (ie, reduced to 1X). This was based on a complete database for developmental and reproductive toxicity; the risk assessment does not underestimate the potential exposure for infants and children, and the end point selected for assessment of risk from dietary and nondietary exposure to chlorine dioxide is protective of potentially susceptible populations including children.

Also in the RED, the acute toxicity of chlorine dioxide was found to be moderate by the oral route and was assigned a toxicity category II. Toxicity category I is considered *danger*, toxicity category II is *warning*, toxicity category III requires *caution*, and toxicity category IV is safe. For skin, the acute toxicity of chlorine dioxide using sodium chlorite as the test material is considered minimal with a toxicity category of III and for inhalation using sodium chlorite as the test material, chlorine dioxide was moderately toxic category II. For eye irritation, chlorine dioxide was a mild irritant with a toxicity category of III. For primary dermal irritation, sodium chlorite was a primary irritant with a toxicity category of II. The EPA considers chlorine dioxide and sodium chlorite as essentially the same.

▶ APPLICATIONS

The list of applications and potential applications for chlorine dioxide continues to develop. A search of the recent patent literature disclosed hundreds of filings related to chlorine dioxide. Several of these are quite novel and involve applications employing small amounts of chlorine dioxide generated in situ for disinfection or deodorizing. An example of one such application is a novel plastic packaging film that releases chlorine dioxide over time.[114]

Potable Water

Chlorination has, for many years, been the standard for water disinfection in the United States. There are, however, problems associated with its use in this application. Some raw water supplies contain phenols, other organic compounds, and certain heavy metal ions, which, after chlorination, result in undesirable tastes and odors in the treated water. Furthermore, chlorination of certain waters results in the production of a variety of chlorinated species, including trihalomethanes and dioxins, in the finished water. The presence of these compounds with their associated toxicity raised serious concerns and led to the search for alternatives to chlorine.

The water industry was introduced to chlorine dioxide in 1940 when the Mathieson Chemical Company made available the first commercial quantities of sodium chlorite. This dry, flaked or powdered material dissolved readily in water, where it reacted with chlorine to liberate chlorine dioxide. The potential of generating chlorine dioxide from a water solution of this compound by simply passing chlorine through it had great appeal, especially because early studies indicated that chlorine dioxide was capable of treating water without producing a disagreeable odor or taste.

In 1944, a water-treatment plant in Niagara Falls, New York, was the first in the United States to adopt chlorine dioxide to their water purification process.[85] Used primarily for the control of odors and taste, it eliminated phenolic odors and the unpleasant taste caused by chlorination of dissolved ferrous ion. Cyanides, sulfides, aldehydes, and mercaptans also were oxidized, and pesticides and herbicides, particularly aldrin, methoxychlor, paraquat, and diquat, were reported to be "removed." Because of the higher cost of chlorine dioxide, its use was initially restricted to specialty applications.

In Europe, chlorine dioxide was used more widely in various water-treatment applications. As early as 1940, chlorine dioxide was, and still is, used in various stages of water processing. It is used in raw, presettled water or prior to filtration for disinfection, taste, and odor control where it is applied at levels of 0.1 to 5 mg/L. Today in Europe, several thousand utilities use chlorine dioxide in their water distribution systems.

In 1977, 103 facilities in the United States were identified to be using chlorine dioxide. Estimates place the number of US utilities with chlorine dioxide treatment equipment at 300 to 400, and rapid growth is projected for the next decade.[12]

Today, sodium chlorite remains the preferred raw material for the generation of chlorine dioxide in water treatment and disinfection applications.[11] Although in situ generation processes in which aqueous sodium chlorite is treated with chlorine or acid (HCl or H_2SO_4) and sodium hypochlorite remain the major methodology for water treatment, concerns have arisen about chlorite and chlorate residuals in the finished water. A promising alternative method involves the direct injection of gaseous chlorine dioxide produced from dry sodium chlorite and chlorine gas in a separate reactor into the water stream, thereby eliminating the problem of the contribution of the unreacted chlorite and side product chlorate.[115]

Antibiotic Inactivation

Many people have an allergy to β-lactams, an important class of antibiotics. Some of these allergies can be severe, and as such, pharmaceutical manufacturers must take precautions to avoid cross-contamination. The issue can be severe, and as such, there are regulations surrounding this issue (eg, in the United States, under 21 CFR 211.176):

> If a reasonable possibility exists that a non-penicillin drug product has been exposed to cross-contamination with penicillin, the non-penicillin drug product shall be tested for the presence of penicillin. Such drug product shall not be marketed if detectable levels are found when tested according to procedures specified in "Procedures for Detecting and Measuring Penicillin Contamination in Drugs."

Chlorine dioxide gas is an oxidizer, and as such, it was thought that this reaction will inactivate β-lactams. In one study, β-lactams from the penicillin, cephalosporin, and carbapenem groups were tested.[40] Specifically, penicillin G, penicillin V, ampicillin, and amoxicillin from the penicillin group; cefadroxil, cefazolin, and cephalexin from the cephalosporin group; and imipenem from the carbapenem group. A cocktail of these β-lactams were inoculated on three different carriers (stainless steel, aluminum, and Lexan) and tested at various concentrations and dosages. It was found that a dosage of 7240 ppm-h achieved a 3 log reduction of all the β-lactams. Based on this study, many old penicillin production facilities have been cleaned successfully with data submitted to US Food and Drug Administration (FDA) and other worldwide regulatory bodies.[116]

Chemical Weapon Decontamination

Chlorine dioxide gas, as an oxidizing agent, will oxidize items that it encounters, including many chemical agents. Gordon et al[117] at Public Health Agency in Canada showed gaseous chlorine dioxide as effective in inactivating anthrax toxins lethal factor and protective antigen within a short amount of time. When Snyder[118] performed studies for the EPA, chlorine dioxide fumigation achieved >99% inactivation of chemical nerve agent VX. But chlorine dioxide was found to be ineffective or only partially effective for thickened soman and sarin, which may be related to lack of penetration by the gas to the chemical tested.

Food Industry

Chlorine dioxide has found many applications in the food industry; it has been used for disinfecting both equipment and materials and raw and finished products. In solution, it is used to disinfect fruits and vegetables and, in poultry, chiller and process water to control contamination.[119] Chlorine dioxide is also used to bleach and mature flour.[8] At levels of 10 to 40 ppm, it oxidizes and decolorizes the carotenoid pigments and accelerates aging to produce flour that will make an elastic dough. It is used to bleach certain fats and fatty oils by oxidation of pigments to colorless forms.[8] Other applications include disinfection of spices, removal of the medicinal odor from cooked shrimp, and extension of the shelf life of tomatoes.[8] Reina et al[120] found that the cooling water for pickling cucumbers reached relatively high populations of bacteria during a typical day's operation, and these could be optimally controlled by the addition of 1.3 ppm chlorine dioxide.

Chlorine dioxide is legally permitted in at least the United States and China for sanitizing fruits and vegetables in water.[121,122] In the United States, the application of chlorine dioxide in the food industry is regulated by the FDA and the EPA. The FDA states the specific conditions in using chlorine dioxide as a food additive for human consumption and allows the use of chlorine dioxide as a disinfectant agent in water at a concentration not exceeding 3 mg/L residual to wash whole fruits and vegetables. Treatment of produce with chlorine dioxide is followed by a potable water rinse or by blanching, cooking, or canning.[121] However, the use of liquid chlorine dioxide to disinfect fresh-cut fruits and vegetables and the direct application of chlorine dioxide gas on fresh fruits and vegetables cannot be established in the regulations. Of note,

there are over 20 Food Contact Notifications (FCNs) issued by the FDA with the use of aqueous and gaseous chlorine dioxide (FCN 644, 645, 1400, 1421, 1804 to specify a few). Food contact notices or substances can be defined as "any substance intended for use as a component of materials used in manufacturing, packing, packaging, transporting, or holding food if such use is not intended to have a technical effect in such food" based on the Food, Drug, and Cosmetic Act. Chlorine dioxide is also allowed to be used in the production of organic foods according to 7 CFR §205.601, which specifies synthetic substances allowed for use in organic crop production. In the European Union (EU), there are no regulations concerning the use of chlorine dioxide for surface washing of fresh produce.

Numerous studies have proven that chlorine dioxide is effective in reducing some major foodborne pathogens in foods, such as *E coli* O157:H7, *Salmonella* species, *L monocytogenes*, as well as food spoilage microorganisms.[47] Overall, the disinfection level achieved through gaseous chlorine dioxide treatment is higher than those with aqueous washing, and a greater than 8 log reduction has been reported. But results can be greatly dependent on several factors, such as experimental design, sample type, and treatment scale.

Han et al[123] determined the reductions of *L monocytogenes* on injured and noninjured green pepper surfaces by both aqueous and gaseous chlorine dioxide. Gaseous chlorine dioxide showed significantly higher log reduction than aqueous chlorine dioxide treatment for both injured and uninjured food surfaces. The main advantage of gaseous chlorine dioxide over aqueous form is that gas has more powerful ability to penetrate. Gaseous chlorine dioxide could reach microorganisms present in foods, which are protected by surface irregularities, biofilms, and so on. The efficacy of gaseous chlorine dioxide in reducing *E coli* O157:H7 and *L monocytogenes* on strawberries was also determined using batch and continuous flow chlorine dioxide gas treatment systems.[124] A batch treatment of strawberries with 4 mg/L gaseous chlorine dioxide for 30 minutes and continuous treatment with 3 mg/L gaseous chlorine dioxide for 10 minutes achieved greater than a 5 log reduction for both *E coli* O157:H7 and *L monocytogenes*.

Due to the high populations of natural microflora in foods, microorganisms should be carefully controlled especially during storage because foods may contain some weakened or damaged points that can become niches for microbial contamination. It has been widely documented that gaseous chlorine dioxide is effective against natural microflora in foods. Gómez-López et al[125] found that after gaseous chlorine dioxide treatment, the disinfection levels of mesophilic aerobic bacteria, psychrotrophs, and yeasts in grated carrots achieved were 1.88, 1.71, 2.60, and 0.66 log CFUs/g, respectively. A lag phase of at least 2 days was observed for mesophilic aerobic bacteria, psychrotrophs, and lactic acid bacteria in treated samples, whereas mesophilic aerobic bacteria and psychrotrophs increased in parallel. Mahmoud and Linton[126] found lower levels of psychrotrophic bacteria, yeasts, and molds on shredded lettuce after gaseous chlorine dioxide treatment, which stayed lower compared to the untreated samples during storage at 4°C for 7 days. Apart from laboratory-scale tests, pilot studies have also been previously conducted. In a pilot study of Popa et al,[127] five separate half-pint plastic clamshell containers each containing 100 g of blueberries were placed on a metal rack inside a sealed 20-L bucket and exposed to gaseous chlorine dioxide. Significant reductions of 2.33, 1.47, 1.63, and 0.48 log CFUs/g were observed for mesophilic aerobic bacteria, coliforms, yeasts, and molds, respectively.

Aqueous chlorine dioxide has also been proved efficient to eliminate pathogens in foods, although no complete elimination has been observed. The early study of Zhang and Farber[128] showed only a 1.1 log reduction of *L monocytogenes*, when 5 mg/L aqueous chlorine dioxide was applied to shredded lettuce or cabbage for 10 minutes. Reductions as high as 5 log CFUs/mL have been lately reported by other authors. Rodgers et al[129] reported that 5 mg/L aqueous chlorine dioxide could achieve over 5 log reductions of *L monocytogenes* and *E coli* O157:H7 on apples, lettuce, and cantaloupe. The data obtained in the study of Pao et al[130] revealed significant reductions (5 log CFUs/cm^2) of *S enterica* and *Erwinia carotovora* after 20 mg/L chlorine dioxide treatment on tomato only when the fruit was freshly inoculated. When antimicrobial ice preparations containing chlorine dioxide was applied to mackerel skin for 120 minutes, total reductions of *E coli* O157:H7, *Salmonella* ser Typhimurium, and *L monocytogenes* were 4.8, 2.6, and 3.3 log, respectively.[131]

Studies on the disinfection of aqueous chlorine dioxide on the natural microflora in foods have indicated various results, ranging from no significant inactivation to higher reductions. An early study by Costilow et al[132] revealed that washing cucumbers in water with even high concentrations 100 mg/L chlorine dioxide failed to significantly reduce populations of yeasts, molds, and lactic acid bacteria. In contrast, some studies on the effect of aqueous chlorine dioxide on the spoilage microbiota of foods have yielded generally satisfactory results. Aqueous chlorine dioxide has been reported to significantly reduce the levels of aerobic mesophilic bacteria, aerobic psychrotrophic bacteria, yeasts and molds, and lactic acid bacteria in fresh-cut asparagus, lettuce, and mulberries.[133,134] In the study of Hong et al,[135] 100 mg/L aqueous chlorine dioxide treatment reduced the populations of total aerobic bacteria, yeast and mold, and coliforms in chicken legs by 0.93, 1.15, and 0.94 log CFUs/g, respectively. Researchers have also developed methods that implemented aqueous chlorine dioxide as one additional hurdle combined with other interventions to achieve effective control of spoilage microorganisms. Chen and Zhu[136] effectively inactivated aerobic mesophilic bacteria, aerobic psychrotrophic

bacteria, yeasts and molds, and lactic acid bacteria in plums using a combination of aqueous chlorine dioxide and ultrasound.

The effects of chlorine dioxide treatment in both its liquid and gaseous forms on the shelf life of foods have been thoroughly studied. On fruits and vegetables, chlorine dioxide is effective in controlling postharvest spoilage. Gómez-López et al[125] prolonged the shelf life of grated carrots stored at 7°C by 1 day using gaseous chlorine dioxide treatment. The treatment with 100 mg/L aqueous chlorine dioxide for 20 minutes could prolong the shelf life of fresh-cut asparagus lettuce stored at 4°C to 14 days, compared to 4 days for the control.[133] Chen et al[134] reported that aqueous chlorine dioxide treatment of 60 mg/L for 15 minutes prolonged the shelf life of mulberries to 14 days compared to 8 days for the control. Treatment of beef trimmings before grinding with 200 mg/L aqueous chlorine dioxide for 3 minutes could also extend the patty shelf life at 2°C.[137]

Chemical residues after both aqueous and gaseous chlorine dioxide treatments have been investigated. With respect to chlorine dioxide in the gaseous phase, Tsai et al[138] could not detect any residues of chlorine dioxide, chlorite, or chlorate in potatoes stored in an atmosphere with gaseous chlorine dioxide. As for Roma tomatoes, a 10 mg/L aqueous chlorine dioxide treatment for 3 minutes left residues of chlorine dioxide, chlorate, and chlorite but not chloride, although they were not detectable after 1 day.[139] Trinetta et al[140] evaluated the residues of chlorine dioxide, chlorite, chlorate, and chloride on tomatoes, oranges, apples, strawberries, lettuce, alfalfa sprouts, and cantaloupes after treatment with 5 mg/L gaseous chlorine dioxide for 10 minutes followed by a subsequent water rinse. The treatment may leave detectable residual levels on lettuce and sprouts, whereas treated tomatoes, oranges, apples, strawberries, and cantaloupes were all found to have very low residuals compared to the EPA acceptable levels for drinking water. The application of aqueous chlorine dioxide to mulberries and plums did not leave residues of chlorine dioxide, chlorite, or chlorate.[134,136] This could be attributed to the fact that the treatment was followed by a water rinse according to the FDA,[120] which was designed to remove chemical residues.

Food Facility Treatment

Gaseous or liquid chlorine dioxide is also used for the treatment of the food production facilities rooms and equipment. *E coli*, *Salmonella*, *Listeria* are a few organisms that are known pathogen concerns for facilities. These contaminations have been known to survive for years in facilities and are difficult to clean.[141] They last for years because many areas of a production facility are hard to or impossible to clean. Many facilities are old and were not designed with current cleaning practices in mind.

This can lead to ineffective decontamination, cleaning, and disinfection processes. The use of chlorine dioxide in its gas form has allowed these facilities to reduce these risks. Chlorine dioxide as a gas has a greater opportunity to get to all areas and allow for greater disinfection assurance because the gas molecule is small and can reach hard to reach areas. In the past, it was incumbent on the user to get the disinfecting agent, typically liquids, to all surfaces. When using chlorine dioxide in its true form (as a gas), it can reach all surfaces to provide a thorough kill independent of the users' actions.

Odor Control

Chlorine dioxide has been used for years in odor control in both the residential and industrial markets. In the industrial market, chlorine dioxide has been used in scrubbing systems to prevent emission of noxious odors. Chlorine dioxide scrubbers have been used to eliminate the odors associated with sulfur compounds as well as the difficult-to-control odors produced by fat-rendering works and fish reduction plants.[5,8]

In the residential market, there are hundreds of products that can produce small amounts of chlorine dioxide for use in deodorizing everything from refrigerators to garbage cans. As an example, NosGUARD SG (Fort Lauderdale, Florida) is used to eliminate foul odors caused by mold, mildew, pets, food, smoke, and more. Other companies have services based around odor control using chlorine dioxide solutions and gas.

Sanitization and Disinfection

In addition to the applications mentioned previously, solutions containing chlorine have been used for an additional variety of sanitization and disinfection applications. In these applications, the in situ generation of chlorine dioxide is most often used. The products used in these applications are advertised as "stabilized" chlorine dioxide and contain chlorite along with other proprietary ingredients. Chlorine dioxide is generated by the addition of an "activator," which may be provided by combination with or addition of another chemical or electrolytically. Gutman and Marzouk[142] disclosed solid compositions that, when dissolved in water, release chlorine dioxide quickly and almost quantitatively. These can be used in a variety of applications ranging from industrial and water-treatment installations to antiseptic and sanitizing preparations. Aseptrol (Engelhard Corp, Iselin, New Jersey) dissolvable capsules[143] are commercially advertised for application as hard-surface sanitizers. Aseptrol is solid sodium chlorite and a proprietary activator contained in a capsule. When placed in water, a chlorine dioxide solution results.

Yi et al[144] demonstrated the effective use of chlorine dioxide gas to disinfect gastrointestinal endoscopes.

Treatment with 4 mg/L chlorine dioxide gas for 30 minutes and 75% relative humidity (RH) resulted in complete inactivation of *Bacillus atrophaeus* spores and demonstrated the use of chlorine dioxide gas as an effective sterilant.

Chlorine dioxide generating preparations with sporicidal activity have been applied with hand sprayers to disinfect isolators used for the containment of gnotobiotic animals.[145] Novartis (formerly the Sandoz Corp) validated an isolated filling line that uses chlorine dioxide solution for sanitization,[145] although no data on sporicidal efficacy were published.

The Alcide Corp markets a line of products based on a technology in which chlorine dioxide is generated in situ when sodium chlorite and lactic acid are mixed. These products are intended for several different applications. One such application is the control of infectious diseases in aquaculture and for the treatment of surfaces, media, or animals directly to remove bacterial, viral, fungal, and protozoan parasites.[146] Two additional applications propose the treatment of blood to reduce the infectivity of HIV in blood and blood products and to reduce the risk of disease transmission through transplantation of optical sclera and corneas.[147,148]

Another patent addresses a method for inactivating viruses in blood using an unspecified two component method for chlorine dioxide generation and a process involving a closed, controlled-communication container.[149] Allergan Inc has patented some technologies for the use of stabilized or electrolytically prepared chlorine dioxide as a contact lenses disinfectant.[150-152]

Tristel Solutions Ltd produces a series of high-level and sporicidal liquid disinfectant products that harness the biocidal power of chlorine dioxide. The Tristel products based on the liquid formulation technologies contribute significantly to the prevention of hospital-acquired infections (HAIs) and can play an important role in managing cross-contamination and eliminating outbreaks.

Insect and Pest Fumigation

Chlorine dioxide has primary been shown as an antimicrobial agent. Czarra et al[152] have shown that chlorine dioxide gas can be effective against insects. In life science research, mice and rats have been widely used. When working with rodents, pinworms are typically nonpathogenic, but with immunocompromised rodents, they can have adverse effects on behavior, growth, intestinal physiology, and immunology, which may affect research. Rodents are typically treated with a special diet to eliminate the worms, but the environment still contains pinworm eggs, which typically leads to reinfection. In the lab, chlorine dioxide gas has been shown to completely render pinworm eggs (*Syphacia ova*) nonviable with a 1440 ppm-h cycle. Cole and Czarneski[153] demonstrated the complete pinworm egg inactivation in the field in a medical research animal facility in Australia and completely eradicated the infestation and remained pinworm free 18 months later.

Bedbugs (*Cimex lectularius* and *Cimex hemipterus*) have had a resurgence in recent years. These insects have proven themselves as hardy organisms with the capability of surviving for several months without an available food source. As such, they can be difficult to remove from the environment. Typically, the manual cleaning process is used to eliminate them. Gibbs et al[154] have shown that gaseous chlorine dioxide can achieve a 100% mortality rate after exposure to various concentrations (1, 2, and 3 mg/L) at various dosages (519, 1029, 1132, and 3024 ppm-h).

Gas Disinfection and Sterilization Applications

As noted previously, although the potent antimicrobial activity of chlorine dioxide in solution was known since 1947, it was not until 1985 that its sporicidal activity in the gas phase was recognized.[64,65] Subsequent development of disinfection and sterilization processes has opened new areas of application for this versatile agent and has been used in varied applications.

Chlorine dioxide gas has been shown to be effective at large-scale facility decontamination when new facilities were disinfected prior to the start of research. RIKEN, Japan's largest comprehensive research institution, disinfected a new facility, which houses approximately 20 000 mice and 3000 rats.[155] Czarneski[156] reported the use of chlorine dioxide gas to decontaminate a new 180 000 ft³ (5097 m³), 65-room facility, which included some new and used equipment. The whole facility disinfection process allowed the equipment to be treated in place, which reduced the probability of cross-contamination from old equipment to new equipment. Luftman et al[157] also demonstrated the successful disinfection of a *Salmonella*-contaminated facility at very low concentrations of 0.3 mg/L over time. In addition to entire facility disinfection, Girouard and Czarneski[158] demonstrated the disinfection of a three-room suite (approximately 4077 ft³ [115 m³]) in 3.5 hours total cycle time including aeration at low concentrations of 1 mg/L. Sensitive equipment such as computers and other lab equipment were disinfected in place during multiple validation exposures to demonstrate the relative good material compatibility of the gas phase. One computer underwent 35 exposures and continued to function normally. Likewise, Leo et al[159] showed the repeated disinfection of a pharmaceutical Blow-Fill-Seal machine at 1 mg/L chlorine dioxide concentrations and predicted a $\log_{10}$ spore reduction of a predicted minimum of 16.65 based on three different disinfection cycles with a summary of four 24-minute quarterly results. Sherman et al[160] showed good material compatibility by disinfecting a cryoelectron microscope with minimal impact on the equipment. Lowe et al[161-163] validated hospital rooms,

ambulances, and suites or rooms with various organisms and locations also showing material compatibility. Chlorine dioxide has also been validated in isolators from various manufacturers,[164-166] processing vessels and tanks,[167,168] and biological safety cabinets.[169,170] Isolator cycle times were as short as 83 minutes for small transfer isolator and 115 minutes for a train of isolators at 5 mg/L concentrations.[166] Eylath et al[164] observed kill under half suit armpits with the arms in the down position at 5 and 7.5 mg/L concentrations. They also showed no residuals after gas exposure by rinsing 304 stainless steel coupons with water for injection (WFI) and measured no residual as measured using a high-performance liquid chromatography (HPLC) method for detection of chloride.

In a study of the sterilization of overwrapped foil suture packages, Kowalski[171] demonstrated the practical utility of gas-phase chlorine dioxide sterilization. They found that excellent kill of spores could be achieved routinely at concentrations of as low as 10 mg/L of chlorine dioxide. Jeng and Woodworth[68] showed that blood oxygenators, devices that present a particularly rigorous challenge, could be sterilized with chlorine dioxide gas.

In 2001, ClorDiSys Solutions, Inc, acquired the rights to gaseous chlorine dioxide sterilization technology from Johnson & Johnson, the original developer of an automated dry gas technology. Since this acquisition, efforts directed toward further developing commercial markets (life science, health care, pharmaceutical, research, and food) for this process, and various types of generators have been developed for different markets. The life science market uses chlorine dioxide in research areas, where clean environments are needed in barrier facilities to keep research clean or to protect research animals or people. In research labs, such as biosafety level 3 or 4 labs, disinfection is critical because users in these labs regularly work with deadly infectious agents. In the health care industry, hospitals are becoming more important as more information is becoming known of HAI and the risks of environmental contamination in-patient isolation rooms or wings. In the pharmaceutical industry, isolators and clean rooms have routinely been disinfected with chlorine dioxide gas and in an increasing number of biologic facilities. These facilities are critical because any contamination can cause entire batches to be disposed of, often because of a small-level biological contamination. In recent years, the FDA Food Safety Modernization Act (FSMA) of 2011 has required facilities to be proactive instead of reactive. This has led to chlorine dioxide gas to be used on significantly large facilities (over 1 million ft³ [28 000 m³]) in the food industry, particularly in the dairy, dry processing and wet processing facilities.

A schematic diagram of a typical chlorine dioxide generator is shown in Figure 27.3.

The availability of small, production-scale chlorine dioxide disinfecting units or sterilizers has allowed detailed investigation of the applicability of chlorine dioxide sterilization to selected products. One such study involved

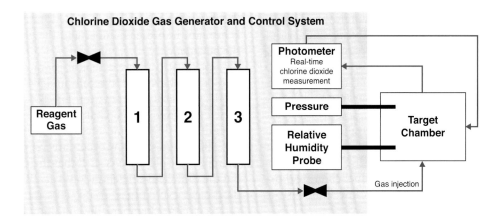

FIGURE 27.3 Typical dry gas chlorine dioxide generator. The reagent gas (2% chlorine/ 98% nitrogen) flows through sodium chlorite and generates >99% pure chlorine dioxide gas + sodium chloride. The chlorine dioxide/nitrogen mixture is delivered to the target chamber and the sodium chloride is left in the consumable cartridges (1-2-3). The relative humidity is measured, and the control system raises it to the typical target set point of 65%. The control system then injects and controls the concentration to reach a target set point of 0.5-20 mg/L depending on the application. The pressure is measured in some applications to ensure high pressure is released to protect the chamber.

polymethylmethacrylate intraocular lenses and was reported by Kowalski.[171] In this instance, humidification of product to be sterilized was conducted in the sterilization chamber itself. A representative process diagram for this study is shown in Figure 27.4.

The results of the intraocular lens study, as well as others, indicated the potential of chlorine dioxide as an alternative to ethylene oxide for selected applications. Chlorine dioxide offers some significant advantages over ethylene oxide for selected sterilization applications.[171] It is effective

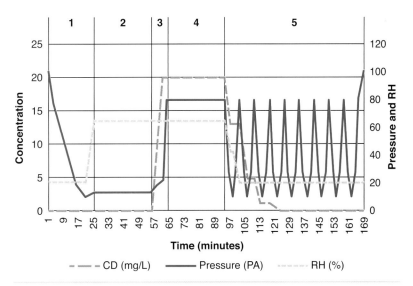

FIGURE 27.4 Typical vacuum sterilization cycle. Step 1—precondition: This step lowers the vacuum to set point (10 kPa) and adds relative humidity to set point (65%). Step 2—condition: This step holds the relative humidity at set point for typically 30 minutes. Step 3—charge: This step raises the chlorine dioxide gas concentration to set point (20 mg/L) and then backfills the chamber with filtered air to 80 kPa. Step 4—exposure: This step holds the chlorine dioxide gas concentration at 20 mg/L for 30 minutes. If the concentration drops for any reason, the gas is returned to the target set point. Step 5—aeration: This step removes the chlorine dioxide gas from the chamber by pulling vacuum and breaking with filtered air. Typically, eight vacuum/break cycles are required to remove the gas to safe levels. Abbreviations: CD, chlorine dioxide; PA, pascals; RH, relative humidity.

in comparatively low concentrations at atmospheric pressure or below. At the concentrations used, it is not explosive and does not require expensive, damaging limiting construction. Additionally, the light-absorbing properties of chlorine dioxide allow for convenient, real-time, spectrophotometric measurement of gas concentration during sterilization. Coupled with complete process control, the sterilization process is amenable to the validation of parametric release of sterilized product. Additionally, chlorine dioxide does not possess the "solvent-like" properties of ethylene oxide, and consequently, residual chlorine dioxide remaining in sterilized products is low and does not require extensive aeration.[171]

The demonstrated efficacy of chlorine dioxide at low concentrations and atmospheric pressure has established many applications for this agent. Figure 27.5 shows a typical isolator or small chamber cycle. Small isolators can have total cycle times under 90 minutes including the aeration time. The cycle consists of five phases or steps. The first step is precondition, which raises the relative humidity from ambient to 65%. This 65% is then maintained for 30 minutes in the condition step. Once the conditioning is completed, the cycle advances to the charge step, which injects chlorine dioxide gas to the target concentration. Once the concentration is reached and verified by photometric measurement, the cycle advances to the exposure step, which typically is 30 minutes at 5 mg/L for small chambers. When this time has elapsed,

the final step of aeration is started. In this step, fresh air is brought into the chamber and the gas is exhausted to the outside.

Figure 27.6 shows a typical room disinfection cycle. These cycles have times typically under 4 hours. Some large rooms or suites of rooms can have cycles under 8-hour total cycle time. Large chambers (20 000 ft[3] [566 m[3]]) typically use lower concentrations of 0.5 mg/L and hold for 240 minutes. Room cycles are very similar to small chamber or isolator runs such that the steps are identical, but the times and concentrations vary. Because of this and the longer cycle times, some steps were combined. For rooms or large chambers, the condition time is shortened. Because the chambers are large, the charge step is long and the conditioning time can be combined with the charge step. This allows the cycle times to be optimized.

To further shorten cycle times, the charge time and exposure time can be combined. This is done by using a dosage counter compared to an exposure timer. To do this, the concentration is measured as soon as it starts injecting and the ppm-h are accumulated. The value of 720 ppm/h is based on current published knowledge; for example, a minimum of 5 log$_{10}$ reduction of spores was demonstrated at 400 ppm/h by Luftman et al[157] inside a large animal hospital disinfection cycle, and a 6 log$_{10}$ reduction was demonstrated by Czarneski and Lorcheim[166] in an isolator at 900 ppm/h. Eylath et al[164] showed several cycles in isolators and processing vessels applications

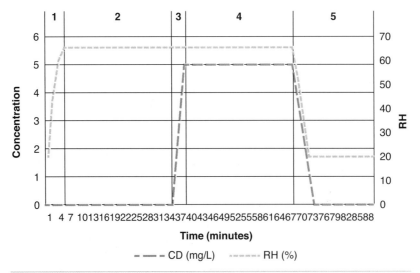

FIGURE 27.5 Typical ambient isolator decontamination cycle. Step 1—precondition: This step raises the relative humidity to set point (65%). Step 2—condition: This step holds the relative humidity at set point for typically 30 minutes. Step 3—charge: This step raises the chlorine dioxide gas concentration to set point (5 mg/L). Step 4—exposure: This step holds the chlorine dioxide gas concentration at 5 mg/L for 30 minutes. If the concentration drops for any reason, the gas is returned to the target set point. Step 5—aeration: This step removes the chlorine dioxide gas from the chamber by using house exhaust to remove the gas. Typically, 12-15 air exchanges are required to remove the gas to safe levels. Abbreviations: CD, chlorine dioxide; RH, relative humidity.

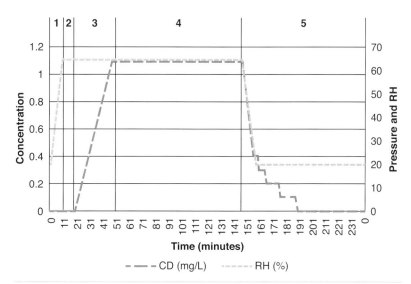

FIGURE 27.6 Typical ambient room decontamination cycle.
Step 1—precondition: This step raises the relative humidity to set point
(65%). Step 2—condition: This step holds the relative humidity at set point
for typically 10 minutes. Step 3—charge: This step raises the chlorine dioxide gas concentration to set point (1 mg/L). Step 4—exposure: This step
holds the chlorine dioxide gas concentration at 1 mg/L for 120 minutes.
If the concentration drops for any reason, the gas is returned to the target
set point. Step 5—aeration: This step removes the chlorine dioxide gas
from the chamber by using house exhaust to remove the gas. Typically,
12-15 air exchanges are required to remove the gas to safe levels.

that demonstrated 6 $\log_{10}$ reduction of spores. The tests
were run at various contact time ranging from 540 to
600 ppm/h as well as 900 ppm/h. In isolators, Eylath et
al[168] demonstrated 6 $\log_{10}$ reductions in exposures of 675
to 1800 ppm/h. A 4 $\log_{10}$ reduction was demonstrated by
Leo et al[159] at a low exposure of 180 ppm/h (1 mg/L for
30 minutes) and Czarneski[156] demonstrated a 6 $\log_{10}$ reduction at 820 ppm/h.

To follow up on all the various doses, Lorcheim and
Melgaard[172] performed studies with a constant dosage
(720 ppm/h) and varied the concentrations (0.3, 0.5, 1, 5,
10, and 20 mg/L) and found that the dosage of 720 ppm/h
provided a 6 $\log_{10}$ reduction of spores regardless of concentration. This indicates that dosage or contact time is
the more critical parameter compared to exposure time.
The dosage that is required for good cycles typically is
720 ppm/h. This dosage is the accumulation of concentration over time or labeled as ppm/h.

To calculate chlorine dioxide ppm from mg/L, the
below calculations can be used:

ppm calculation for 1 mg/L chlorine dioxide concentration
ppm = (mg/m³) (24.45) / molecular weight = (mg/L)
(1000) (24.45) / molecular weight
Chlorine dioxide ppm = (1 mg/L) (1000 L/m³) (24.45) /
67.5 = 362.2
Exposure contact time = 362 ppm × 2 h = 724 ppm/h

The number 24.45 in the equations is the volume
(liters) of a mole (gram molecular weight) of a gas at
1 atmosphere and at 25°C.

So, the overall dosage or contact time starts when gas
is being injected and the accumulation starts. This has the
effect of combining the exposure time and charge time
and shortening the overall cycle time.

CONCLUSIONS

Chlorine dioxide has a broad-spectrum biocidal activity
against a variety of bacteria, viruses, yeasts, mycobacteria, and bacterial spores. Because chlorine dioxide is an
oxidizing agent, the primary mode of action is via electron exchange within the microbial molecular structure.
Chlorine dioxide is favored over nonoxidizing disinfectants due to its greater efficacy. Although all oxidizing
agents are capable, at suitable concentrations, of providing
biocidal disinfection, they have several drawbacks when
compared to chlorine dioxide. Unlike chlorine, chlorine
dioxide does not readily form halogenated by-products
due to the nature of the molecular bonding. Chlorine
dioxide is known to be compatible with most of the materials commonly found in medical and pharmaceutical
equipment and environments and has an excellent health
and safety record when used at recommended levels.

Chlorine dioxide has been widely applied in medical and pharmaceutical environments. It has also been used in various applications such as drinking water treatment and the washing and treatment of foods. As with all choices among alternative approaches that provide solutions to a given problem, an informed choice based on current evaluation and understanding of pertinent existing data is the best one that can be made. It is the authors' intent that this overview of chlorine dioxide should aid in making an informed choice regarding its application.

REFERENCES

1. Sidgwick NV. Halogen oxides. In: *The Chemical Elements and Their Compounds*. Vol 2. Oxford, United Kingdom: Oxford University Press; 1951:1202-1218.
2. Davy H. On a combination of oxymuriatic gas and oxygen gas. *Philos Trans*. 1811;101:155-161.
3. Taylor NW, Lewis GN. The paramagnetism of "odd molecules." *Proc Natl Acad Sci U S A*. 1925;11:456-457.
4. Gordon G, Keiffer RG, Rosenblatt DH. The chemistry of chlorine dioxide. In: Lippaer SJ, ed. *Progress in Inorganic Chemistry*. Vol 15. New York, NY: John Wiley & Sons; 1972:201-287.
5. Vaida V, Simone JD. The photoreactivity of chlorine dioxide. *Science*. 1995;268:1443-1448.
6. Leonesi D, Piantoni G. Dissociation constant and spectrum of chlorous acid. *Annali di Chimica (Rome)*. 1965;55:668-675.
7. Nielson AH, Woltz PJH. The infrared spectrum of chlorine dioxide. *J Phys Chem*. 1952;20:1879-1883.
8. Masschelein WJ, Rice RG. *Chlorine Dioxide: Chemistry and Environmental Impact of Oxychlorine Compounds*. Ann Arbor, MI: Ann Arbor Science; 1979:111-145.
9. Bigorgne M. A new rapid method for the determination of the formula of certain hydrates. *C R Hebd Seances Acad Sci*. 1953;236:1966-1968.
10. Williamson HV, Hample CA, inventors; Cardox Corp, assignee. Nonexplosive chlorine dioxide hydrate composition and process for producing same. US patent 2,683,651. July 13, 1954.
11. Kaczur JJ, Cawfield DW. Chlorine oxygen acids and salts. In: *Kirk-Othmer Encyclopedia of Chemical Technology*. Vol 5. 4th ed. New York, NY: John Wiley & Sons; 1991:968-997.
12. Aieta EM, Berg JD. A review of chlorine dioxide in drinking water treatment. *J Am Water Works Assoc*. 1986;78:62-72.
13. Hong CC, Rapson WH. Kinetics of disproportionation of chlorous acid. *Can J Chem*. 1968;46:2053-2060.
14. Kieffer RG, Gordon G. Disproportionation of chlorous acid II. Kinetics. *Inorg Chem*. 1968;7:235-239.
15. Windholz M, ed. *Merck Index*. 10th ed. Rahway, NJ: Merck; 1983.
16. Cheesman GH. Parachor of chlorine dioxide. *J Chem Soc*. 1930;35-37.
17. Young CL. Sulfur dioxide, chlorine, fluorine, and chlorine oxides. In: Young CL, ed. *IUPAC Solubility Data Series*. Vol 12. Oxford, United Kingdom: Pergamon Press; 1988:xi-xvii, 454-456.
18. Cowley G. Safety in the design of chlorine dioxide plants. *Loss Prev*. 1993;113:1-12.
19. Jin R, Hu S, Zhang Y, et al. Concentration-dependence of the explosion characteristics of chlorine dioxide gas. *J Hazard Mater*. 2009;166:842-847.
20. Ward WJ, Gasper L, Gasper KE, inventors; Olin Corp, assignee. Chlorine dioxide generation. US patent 4,013,761. March 22, 1977.
21. Grubitsch H, Suppan E. Zur kenntnis der dampfdruckkurve von chlordioxid. *Monatsh Chem*. 1962;93:246-251.
22. Hutchinson WS, Derby RI. Improved flour bleaching process using chlorine dioxide produced by an electric arc method. *Cereal Chem*. 1947;24:372-376.
23. Aieta EM, Roberts PV. The chemistry of oxy-chlorine compounds relevant to chlorine dioxide generation. In: Jolley RL, ed. *Water Chlorination: Environmental Impact and Health Effects*. Vol 5. Chelsea, MI: Lewis; 1985:783-794.
24. McHale ET, von Elbe G. The explosive decomposition of chlorine dioxide. *J Phys Chem*. 1968;72:1849-1856.
25. Spinks JWT, Porter JM. Photodecomposition of chlorine dioxide. *J Am Chem Soc*. 1934;56:264-270.
26. Crawford RA, DeWitt B. Decomposition rate studies in the gaseous chlorine dioxide-water system. *Tappi J*. 1968;50:226-230.
27. Gray P, Ip JK. Spontaneous ignition supported by chlorine dioxide. *Combust Flame*. 1972;18:361-371.
28. Haller JF, Northgraves WW. Chlorine dioxide and safety. *Tappi J*. 1955;38:199-202.
29. Flis IE. The oxidation potentials of chlorite and chlorine dioxide solutions. *Zhurnal Fiziko Khimic*. 1958;32:573-579.
30. Noss CI, Hauchman FS, Olivieri VP. Chlorine dioxide reactivity with proteins. *Water Res*. 1986;20:351-356.
31. Hoigné J, Bader H. Kinetics of typical reactions of chlorine dioxide with substances in water. *Vom Wasser*. 1982;59:253-267.
32. Neta P, Huie RE, Ross AB, Alberta B. Rate constants for reactions of inorganic radicals in solution. *J Phys Chem Ref Data*. 1988;17:1027.
33. Rosenblatt DH, Hayes AJ Jr, Harrison BR, Streaty RA, Moore KA. The reaction of chlorine dioxide with triethylamine in aqueous solution. *J Org Chem*. 1963;28:2790-2794.
34. Rosenblatt DH, Hull LA, DeLuca DC, Davis GT. Oxidations with amines. II. Substituent effects in chlorine dioxide oxidations. *J Am Chem Soc*. 1967;89:1158-1163.
35. Hull LA, Davis GT, Rosenblatt DH. Oxidation of amines. 9. Correlation of rate constants for reversible one-electron transfer in amine oxidation with reactant potentials. *J Am Chem Soc*. 1969;91:6247-6250.
36. Hull LA, Davis GT, Rosenblatt DH, et al. Oxidation of amines III. duality of mechanism in the reaction of amines with chlorine dioxide. *J Am Chem Soc*. 1967;89:1163-1170.
37. Noss CI, Dennis WH, Olivieri VP. Reactivity of chlorine dioxide with nucleic acids and proteins. In: Jolley RL, ed. *Water Chlorination: Chemistry, Environmental Impact and Health Effects*. Vol 5. Chelsea, MI: Lewis; 1985:1077-1086.
38. Jolley RL, Jones G, Pitt WW, et al. Chlorination of organics in cooling water and process effluents. In: Jolley RL, ed. *Water Chlorination: Environmental Impact and Health Effects*. Vol 1. Ann Arbor, MI: Ann Arbor Science; 1977:105-138.
39. Ogata N. Denaturation of protein by chlorine dioxide: oxidative modification of tryptophan and tyrosine residues. *Biochemistry*. 2007;46:4898-4911.
40. Lorcheim K. Chlorine dioxide gas inactivation of beta-lactams. *Appl Biosaf*. 2011;16:34-43.
41. Ooi BG, Branning SA. Correlation of conformational changes and protein degradation with loss of lysozyme activity due to chlorine dioxide treatment. *Appl Biochem Biotechnol*. 2017;182:782-791.
42. Grimley E, Gordon G. The kinetics and mechanism of the reaction between chlorine dioxide and phenol in aqueous solution. *J Inorg Nucl Chem*. 1973;35:2383-2392.
43. Ghanbari HA, Wheeler WB, Kirk JR. Reactions of aqueous chlorine and chlorine dioxide with lipids: chlorine incorporation. *J Food Sci*. 1982;147:482-485.
44. Schaufler C. Antiseptic effect of chlorine solutions from interactions of potassium chlorate and hydrochloric acid. *Zentralbl Chir*. 1933;60:2497-2500.
45. Kovtunovitch GP, Chemaya LA. Bactericidal effects of chlorine solutions from interaction of potassium chlorate and hydrochloric acid. *Sovetskaya Khirurgiya*. 1936;2:214-221.
46. Ridenour GM, Ingols RS. Bactericidal properties of chlorine dioxide. *J Am Water Works Assoc*. 1947;39:561-567.
47. Gómez-López VM, Rajkovic A, Ragaert P, Smigic N, Devlieghere F. Chlorine dioxide for minimally processed produce preservation: a review. *Trends Food Sci Technol*. 2009;20:17-26.

48. Alvarez ME, O'Brien RT. Mechanisms of inactivation of poliovirus by chlorine dioxide and iodine. *Appl Environ Microbiol.* 1982;44: 1064-1071.

49. Sansebastiano G, Mori G, Tanzi ML, et al. Chlorine dioxide: methods of analysis and kinetics of inactivation of poliovirus type 1. *Ig Mod.* 1983;79:61-91.

50. Berman D, Hoff JC. Inactivation of simian rotavirus SA 11 by chlorine, chlorine dioxide, and monochloramine. *Appl Environ Microbiol.* 1984;48:317-323.

51. Harakeh MS, Butler M. Inactivation of human rotavirus, SA11 and other enteric viruses in effluent by disinfectants. 1984. *J Hyg.* 1984;93: 157-163.

52. Olivieri VP, Hauchman FS, Noss CI, et al. Mode of action of chlorine dioxide on selected viruses. In: Jolley RL, ed. *Water Chlorination: Chemistry Environmental Impact and Health Effects.* Vol 5. Chelsea, MI: Lewis; 1985:619-634.

53. Sansebastiano G, Cesari C, Bellelli E. Further investigations on water disinfection by chlorine dioxide. *Ig Mod.* 1986;85:358-380.

54. Chen YS, Vaughn JM. Inactivation of human and simian rotaviruses by chlorine dioxide. *Appl Environ Microbiol.* 1990;56:1363-1366.

55. Farr RW, Walton C. Inactivation of human immunodeficiency virus by a medical waste disposal process using chlorine dioxide. *Infect Control Hosp Epidemiol.* 1993;14:527-529.

56. Korich DG, Mead JR, Madore MS, Sinclair NA, Sterling CR. Effects of ozone, chlorine dioxide, chlorine, and monochloramine on *Cryptosporidium parvum* oocyst viability. *Appl Environ Microbiol.* 1990;56: 1423-1428.

57. Whitmore TN, Denny S. The effect of disinfectants on a geosmin-producing strain of *Streptomyces griseus. J Appl Bacteriol.* 1992;72: 160-165.

58. Wang Y, Jiang Z. Studies on bactericidal and algaecidal ability of chlorine dioxide. *Water Treat.* 1995;10:347-352.

59. Bundgaard-Nielsen K, Nielsen PV. Fungicidal effect of 15 disinfectants against 25 fungal contaminants commonly found in bread and cheese manufacturing. *J Food Prot.* 1996;59:268-275.

60. Brown P, Rohrer RG, Moreau-Dubois MC, Green EM, Gajdusek DC. Use of the golden Syrian hamster in the study of scrapie virus. *Adv Exp Med Biol.* 1981;134:365-373.

61. Brown P, Rohrer RG, Green EM, Gajdusek DC. Effect of chemicals, heat and histopathologic processing on the high-infectivity hamster-adapted scrapie virus. *J Infect Dis.* 1982;145:683-687.

62. Brown P, Gibbs CJ Jr, Amyx HL, et al. Chemical disinfection of Creutzfeld-Jakob disease virus. *N Engl J Med.* 1982;306:1279-1282.

63. Ryu JH, Beuchat LR. Biofilm formation and sporulation by *Bacillus cereus* on a stainless steel surface and subsequent resistance of vegetative cells and spores to chlorine, chlorine dioxide, and a peroxyacetic acid-based sanitizer. *J Food Prot.* 2005;68:2614-2622.

64. Rosenblatt DH, Rosenblatt AA, Knapp JE, inventors; Johnson and Johnson, assignee. Use of chlorine dioxide gas as a chemosterilizing agent. US patent 4,504,442. March 12, 1985.

65. Rosenblatt DH, Rosenblatt AA, Knapp JE, inventors; Johnson and Johnson, assignee. Use of chlorine dioxide gas as a chemosterilizing agent. US patent 4,681,739. July 21, 1987.

66. Rosenblatt AA, Knapp JE. Chlorine dioxide gas sterilization. Paper presented at: Health Industry Manufacturers Association Conference; October 31, 1988; Washington, D.C.

67. Jeng DK, Woodworth AG. Chlorine dioxide gas sterilization under square-wave conditions. *Appl Environ Microbiol.* 1990;56:514-519.

68. Jeng DK, Woodworth AG. Chlorine dioxide gas sterilization of oxygenators in an industrial scale sterilizer: a successful model. *Artif Organs.* 1990;14:361-368.

69. Donlan RM, Costerton JW. Biofilms: survival mechanisms of clinically relevant microorganisms. *Clin Microbiol Rev.* 2002;15:167-193.

70. Lindsay D, Brözel VS, Mostert JF, von Holy A. Differential efficacy of a chlorine dioxide-containing sanitizer against single species and binary biofilms of a dairy-associated *Bacillus cereus* and a *Pseudomonas fluorescens* isolate. *J Appl Microbiol.* 2002;92:352-361.

71. Vaid R, Linton RH, Morgan MT. Comparison of inactivation of *Listeria monocytogenes* within a biofilm matrix using chlorine dioxide gas, aqueous chlorine dioxide and sodium hypochlorite treatments. *Food Microbiol.* 2010;27:979-984.

72. Martin DJ, Wesgate RL, Denyer SP, McDonell G, Maillard Y. *Bacillus subtilis* vegetative isolate surviving chlorine dioxide exposure: an elusive mechanism of resistance. *J Appl Microbiol.* 2015;119:1541-1551.

73. Ayyildiz O, Ileri B, Sanik S. Impacts of water organic load on chlorine dioxide disinfection efficacy. *J Hazard Mater.* 2009;168:1092-1097.

74. US Environmental Protection Agency. *Alternative Disinfectants and Oxidants Guidance Manual.* Washington, DC: US Environmental Protection Agency; 1999.

75. Roller SD, Olivieri VP, Kawata K. Mode of bacterial inactivation by chlorine dioxide. *Water Res.* 1980;14:635-642.

76. Fukayama MY, Tan H, Wheeler WB, Wei CL. Reactions of aqueous chlorine and chlorine dioxide with model food compounds. *Environ Health Perspect.* 1986;69:267-274.

77. Berg JD, Roberts PV, Matin A. Effect of chlorine dioxide on selected membrane functions of *Escherichia coli. J Appl Bacteriol.* 1986;60: 213-220.

78. Cho M, Kim J, Kim JY, Yoon J, Kim JH. Mechanisms of *Escherichia coli* inactivation by several disinfectants. *Water Res.* 2010;44:3410-3418.

79. Young SB, Setlow P. Mechanisms of killing of *Bacillus subtilis* spores by hypochlorite and chlorine dioxide. *J Appl Microbiol.* 2003;95:54-67.

80. Peta ME, Lindsay D, Brözel VS, Von Holy A. Susceptibility of food spoilage *Bacillus* species to chlorine dioxide and other sanitizers. *S Afr J Sci.* 2003;99:375-380.

81. Li JW, Xin ZT, Wang XW, Zheng JL, Chao FH. Mechanisms of inactivation of hepatitis A virus in water by chlorine dioxide. *Water Res.* 2004;38:1514-1519.

82. Zhu C, Chen Z, Yu G. Fungicidal mechanism of chlorine dioxide on *Saccharomyces cerevisiae. Ann Microbiol.* 2013;63:495-502.

83. Smith RP, Willhite CC. Chlorine dioxide and hemodialysis. *Regul Toxicol Pharmacol.* 1990;11:42-62.

84. American Conference of Governmental Industrial Hygienists. *Industrial Hygiene Guide.* Cincinnati, OH: American Conference of Governmental Industrial Hygienists; 1990.

85. White GC. *Handbook of Chlorination.* New York, NY: Reinhold; 1972.

86. Meggs W, Elsheikh T, Metzger W, et al. Nasal pathology and ultrastructure in persistent rhinitis with chemical sensitivity after chlorine dioxide (ClO$_2$) exposure. *J Toxicol Clin Toxicol.* 1995;33:525.

87. Meggs WJ, Elsheikh T, Metzger WJ, et al. Nasal pathology of persistent rhinitis after chlorine dioxide exposure. *J Allergy Clin Immunol.* 1995;95:260.

88. Robinson GM, Bull RJ, Schamer M, Long RE. Epidermal hyperplasia of mouse skin following treatment with alternative drinking water disinfectants. *Environ Health Perspect.* 1986;69:293-300.

89. Abdel-Rahman MS, Skowronski GA, Turkall RM, Gerges SE, Kadry AR, Abu-Hadeed AH. Subchronic dermal toxicity studies of alcide allay gel and liquid in rabbits. *J Appl Toxicol.* 1987;7:327-333.

90. Abdel-Rahman MS, Couri D, Bull RJ. Metabolism and pharmacokinetics of alternate drinking water disinfectants. *Environ Health Perspect.* 1982;46:19-23.

91. Scatina J, Abdel-Rahman MS, Gerges SE, Alliger H. Pharmacokinetics of Alcide®, a germicidal compound in rats. *J Appl Toxicol.* 1983;3: 150-153.

92. Moore GS, Calabrese EJ. Toxicological effects of chlorite in the mouse. *Environ Health Perspect.* 1982;46:31-37.

93. Abdel-Rahman MS, Couri D, Bull RJ. Toxicity of chlorine dioxide in drinking water. *Int J Toxicol.* 1984;3:277-284.

94. Abdel-Rahman MS, Couri D, Bull RJ. The kinetics of chlorite and chlorate in rats. *J Environ Pathol Toxicol Oncol.* 1985;6:97-103.

95. Harrington RM, Romano RR, Gates D, Ridgway P. Subchronic toxicity of sodium chlorite in the rat. *J Am Coll Toxicol.* 1995;14:21-33.

96. Orme J, Taylor DH, Laurie RD, Bull RJ. Effects of chlorine dioxide on thyroid function in neonatal rats. *J Toxicol Environ Health.* 1985;15:315-322.

97. Bercz JP, Jones L, Garner L, Murray D, Ludwig DA, Boston J. Subchronic toxicity of chlorine dioxide and related compounds in drinking water in the nonhuman primate. *Environ Health Perspect.* 1982;46:47-55.

98. Revis NM, McCauley P, Bull R, Holdsworth G. Relationship of drinking water disinfectants to plasma cholesterol and thyroid hormones levels in experimental studies. *Proc Natl Acad Sci U S A.* 1986;83:1485-1489.

99. Couri D, Miller CH Jr, Bull RJ, Delphia JM, Ammar EM. Assessment of maternal toxicity, embryotoxicity and teratogenic potential of sodium chlorite in Sprague-Dawley rats. *Environ Health Perspect.* 1982;46:25-29.

100. Carlton BD, Basaran AH, Mezza LE, George EL, Smith MK. Reproductive effects in Long-Evans rats exposed to chlorine dioxide. *Environ Res.* 1991;56:170-177.

101. Skowronski GA, Abdel-Rahman MS, Gerges SE, Klein KM. Teratologic evaluation of Alcide liquid in rats and mice. I. *J Appl Toxicol.* 1985;5:97-103.

102. Suh DH, Abdel-Rahman MS, Bull RJ. Effect of chlorine dioxide and its metabolites in drinking water on fetal development in rats. *J Appl Toxicol.* 1983;3:75-79.

103. Ishidate M Jr, Sofuni T, Yoshikawa K, et al. Primary mutagenicity screening of food additives currently used in Japan. *Food Chem Toxicol.* 1984;22:623-636.

104. Hayashi M, Kishi M, Sofuni T, Ishidate M Jr. Micronucleus tests in mice on 39 food additives and eight miscellaneous chemicals. *Food Chem Toxicol.* 1988;26:487-500.

105. Bianchine JR, Lubbers JR, Chauhan S, Miller J. *Study of Chlorine Dioxide and Its Metabolites in Man.* Cincinnati, OH: US Environmental Protection Agency Health Effects Laboratory; 1981. EPA-600/1-81-068 (PB82-109356).

106. Lubbers JR, Chauhan S, Bianchine JR. Controlled clinical evaluations of chlorine dioxide, chlorite and chlorate in man. *Environ Health Perspect.* 1982;46:57-62.

107. Lubbers JR, Chauhan S, Miller JK, Bianchine JR. The effects of chronic administration of chlorine dioxide, chlorite and chlorate to normal healthy adult male volunteers. *J Environ Pathol Toxicol Oncol.* 1984;5:229-238.

108. Lubbers JR, Chauhan S, Miller JK, Bianchine JR. The effects of chronic administration of chlorite to glucose-6-phosphate dehydrogenase deficient healthy adult male volunteers. *J Environ Pathol Toxicol Oncol.* 1984;5:239-242.

109. Michael GE, Miday RK, Bercz JP, et al. Chlorine dioxide water disinfection: a prospective epidemiology study. *Arch Environ Health.* 1981;36:19-27.

110. Tuthill RW, Giusti RA, Moore GS, Calabrese EJ. Health effects among newborns after prenatal exposure to ClO$_2$-disinfected drinking water. *Environ Health Perspect.* 1982;46:39-45.

111. Condie LW. Toxicological problems associated with chlorine dioxide. *J Am Water Works Assoc.* 1986;78:73-78.

112. Ouhoummane N, Levallois P, Gingras S. Thyroid function of newborns and exposure to chlorine dioxide by-products. *Arch Environ Health.* 2004;59:582-587.

113. Akamatsu A, Lee C, Morino H, Miura T, Ogata N, Shibata T. Six-month low level chlorine dioxide gas inhalation toxicity study with two-week recovery period in rats. *J Occup Med Toxicol.* 2012;7:2.

114. Wellinghoff ST, inventor; Southwest Research Institute, assignee. Chlorine dioxide generating polymer packaging films. US patent 5,360,609. November 1, 1994.

115. Gordon G, Rosenblatt AA. Gaseous, chlorine-free chlorine dioxide for drinking water. Paper presented at: American Water Works Association Water Quality Technology Conference; November 12-15, 1995; New Orleans, LA.

116. Cole B. *Site Remediation of a Penicillin Production Facility Using Chlorine Dioxide Gas as Sterilant.* Beaumaris, Australia: Association of Biosafety for Australia & New Zealand; 2016.

117. Gordon D, Krishnan J, Theriault S. Inactivation studies of lipopolysaccharide and anthrax toxins using gaseous decontamination methods. Paper presented at: Canadian Biosafety Symposium; May 31-June 2, 2009; Halifax, Canada.

118. Snyder E. *Systematic Decontamination of Chemical Warfare Agents and Toxic Industrial Chemicals: Report on the 2008 Workshop on Decontamination Research and Associated Issues for Sites Contaminated with Chemical, Biological, or Radiological Materials.* Washington, DC: US Environmental Protection Agency; 2009. EPA/600/R-09/035.

119. Engelhard Corp. *Chlorine Dioxide from Engelhard.* Iselin, NJ: Engelhard Corp; 1997. Product bulletin EC7097.

120. Reina LD, Fleming HP, Humphries EG. Microbiological control of cucumber hydrocooling water with chlorine dioxide. *J Food Prot.* 1995;58:541-546.

121. US Food and Drug Administration. *Code of Federal Regulations 21 CFR 173.300: Secondary Direct Food Additives Permitted in Food for Human Consumption: Chlorine Dioxide.* Silver Spring, MD: US Food and Drug Administration; 2017.

122. National Health and Family Planning Commission of the People's Republic of China. *Hygienic Standards for Use of Food Additives.* Beijing, China: National Health and Family Planning Commission of the People's Republic of China; 2017.

123. Han Y, Linton RH, Nielsen SS, Nelson PE. Reduction of *Listeria monocytogenes* on green peppers (*Capsicum annuum* L.) by gaseous and aqueous chlorine dioxide and water washing and its growth at 7 degrees C. *J Food Prot.* 2001;64:1730-1738.

124. Han Y, Selby T, Schultze K, Nelson P, Linton H. Decontamination of strawberries using batch and continuous chlorine dioxide gas treatments. *J Food Prot.* 2004;67:2450-2455.

125. Gómez-López VM, Devlieghere F, Ragaert P, Debevere J. Shelf-life extension of minimally processed carrots by gaseous chlorine dioxide. *Int J Food Microbiol.* 2007;116:221-227.

126. Mahmoud BSM, Linton RH. Inactivation kinetics of inoculated *Escherichia coli* O157:H7 and *Salmonella enterica* on lettuce by chlorine dioxide gas. *Food Microbiol.* 2008;25:244-252.

127. Popa I, Hanson EJ, Todd EC, Schilder AC, Ryser ET. Efficacy of chlorine dioxide gas sachets for enhancing the microbiological quality and safety of blueberries. *J Food Prot.* 2007;70:2084-2088.

128. Zhang S, Farber JM. The effects of various disinfectants against *Listeria monocytogenes* on fresh-cut vegetables. *Food Microbiol.* 1996;13:311-321.

129. Rodgers SL, Cash JN, Siddiq M, Ryser E. A comparison of different chemical sanitizers for inactivating *Escherichia coli* O157:H7 and *Listeria monocytogenes* in solution and on apples, lettuce, strawberries, and cantaloupe. *J Food Prot.* 2004;67:721-731.

130. Pao S, Kelsey DF, Khalid MF, Ettinger MR. Using aqueous chlorine dioxide to prevent contamination of tomatoes with *Salmonella enterica* and *Erwinia carotovora* during fruit washing. *J Food Prot.* 2007;70:629-634.

131. Shin JH, Chang S, Kang DH. Application of antimicrobial ice for reduction of foodborne pathogens (*Escherichia coli* O157: H7, *Salmonella* Typhimurium, *Listeria monocytogenes*) on the surface of fish. *J Appl Microbiol.* 2004;97:916-922.

132. Costilow RN, Uebersax MA, Ward PJ. Use of chlorine dioxide for controlling microorganisms during the handling and storage of fresh cucumbers. *J Food Sci.* 1984;49:396-401.

133. Chen Z, Zhu C, Zhang Y, Niu D, Du J. Effects of aqueous chlorine dioxide treatment on enzymatic browning and shelf-life of fresh-cut asparagus lettuce (*Lactuca sativa* L.). *Postharvest Biol Technol.* 2010;58:232-238.

134. Chen Z, Zhu C, Han Z. Effects of aqueous chlorine dioxide treatment on nutritional components and shelf-life of mulberry fruit (*Morus alba* L.). *J Biosci Bioeng.* 2011;111:675-681.

135. Hong YH, Ku GJ, Kim MK, et al. Inactivation of *Listeria monocytogenes* and *Campylobacter jejuni* in chicken by aqueous chlorine dioxide treatment. *J Food Sci Nutr.* 2007;12:279-283.

136. Chen Z, Zhu C. Combined effects of aqueous chlorine dioxide and ultrasonic treatments on postharvest storage quality of plum fruit (*Prunus salicina* L.). *Postharvest Biol Technol.* 2011;61:117-123.

137. Jimenez-Villarreal JR, Pohlman FW, Johnson ZB, Brown AH Jr. Effects of chlorine dioxide, cetylpyridinium chloride, lactic acid and trisodium phosphate on physical, chemical and sensory properties of ground beef. *Meat Sci.* 2003;65:1055-1062.

138. Tsai LS, Huxsoll CC, Robertson G. Prevention of potato spoilage during storage by chlorine dioxide. *J Food Sci.* 2001;66:472-477.

139. Trinetta V, Morgan M, Linton R. Use of high-concentration-short-time chlorine dioxide treatments for the inactivation of *Salmonella enterica* spp. inoculated onto Roma tomatoes. *Food Microbiol.* 2010;27:1009-1015.

140. Trinetta V, Vaidya N, Linton R, Morgan M. Evaluation of chlorine dioxide gas residues on selected food produce. *J Food Sci.* 2011;76:T11-T15.

141. Carpentier B, Cerf O. Review—persistence of *Listeria monocytogenes* in food industry equipment and premises. *Int J Food Microbiol.* 2011;145:1-8.

142. Gutman Y, Marzouk Y, inventors; Marzouk Y, Abic Ltd, assignee. Solid composition releasing chlorine dioxide. US patent 5,399,288. March 21, 1995.

143. Engelhard Corp. *Controlled Sustained Release.* Iselin, NJ: Engelhard Corp; 1997. Product bulletin EC7098.

144. Yi Y, Hao L, Ma S, et al. A pilot study on using chlorine dioxide gas for disinfection of gastrointestinal endoscopes. *J Zhejiang Univ Sci B.* 2016;17:526-536.

145. Rickloff JR, Edwards LM. Modern trends in isolator sterilization. In: Wagner CM, Akers JM, eds. *Isolator Technology Applications in the Pharmaceutical and Biotechnology Industries.* Buffalo Grove, IL: Interpharm Press; 1995:151-152.

146. Kross AD, inventor; Treatment or prevention of microbial infections in mammals. PCT patent WO 9,523,511. 1995.

147. Rubenstein AI, inventor. Novel method to treat blood. US patent 4,944,920. July 31, 1990.

148. Rubenstein AI, inventor; International Medical Technologies Corp, assignee. Novel method for disinfecting red blood cells, blood platelets, blood plasma, and optical corneas and sclerae. US patent 4,971,760. November, 20, 1990.

149. Carmen R, Chong C, inventors; Miles Inc, assignee. Method for inactivating viruses in blood using chlorine dioxide. US patent 5,240,829. August 31, 1993.

150. Dziabo AJ, Ripley PS, inventors; Allergan Inc, assignee. Methods to disinfect contact lenses. US patent 5,320,806. June 14, 1994.

151. Dziabo AJ, Ripley PS, inventors; Allergan Inc, assignee. Aqueous ophthalmic formulations and methods for preserving same. US patent 5,424,078. June 13, 1995.

152. Czarra JA, Adams JK, Carter CL, Hill WA, Coan PN. Exposure to chlorine dioxide gas for 4 hours renders *Syphacia* ova nonviable. *J Am Assoc Lab Anim Sci.* 2014;53:364-367.

153. Cole B, Czarneski MA. A multiple-staged site remediation of a medical research animal facility affected by a rodent pinworm infestation. Paper presented at: Association of Biosafety for Australia & New Zealand 5th Annual Conference; November 9-13, 2015; Canberra, Australia.

154. Gibbs SG, Lowe JJ, Smith PW, Hewlwtt AL. Gaseous chlorine dioxide as an alternative for bedbug control. *Infect Control Hosp Epidemiol.* 2012;33:495-499.

155. Takahashi E, Czarneski MA, Sugiura A. Japan's RIKEN BSI: whole facility chlorine dioxide gas decontamination approach for a barrier facility—a case study. *Appl Biosaf.* 2014;19:201-210.

156. Czarneski MA. Microbial decontamination of a 65-room new pharmaceutical research facility. *Appl Biosaf.* 2009;14:81-88.

157. Luftman HS, Michael A, Regits MA, et al. Chlorine dioxide gas decontamination of large animal hospital intensive and neonatal care units. *Appl Biosaf.* 2006;11:144-154.

158. Girouard DJ Jr, Czarneski MA. Room, suite scale, class III biological safety cabinet, and sensitive equipment decontamination and validation using gaseous chlorine dioxide. *App Biosaf.* 2016;21:34-44.

159. Leo F, Poisson P, Sinclair CS, Tallentire A. Design, development and qualification of a microbiological challenge facility to assess the effectiveness of BFS aseptic processing. *PDA J Pharm Sci Technol.* 2005;59:33-48.

160. Sherman MB, Trujilloe J, Leahy I, et al. Construction and organization of a BSL-3 cryo-electron microscopy laboratory at UTMB. *J Struct Biol.* 2013;181:223-233.

161. Lowe JJ, Gibbs SG, Iwen PC, Smith PW. A case study on decontamination of a biosafety level-3 laboratory and associated ductwork within an operational building using gaseous chlorine dioxide. *J Occup Environ Hyg.* 2012;9:D196-D205.

162. Lowe JJ, Gibbs SG, Iwen PC, Smith PW, Hewlett AL. Impact of chlorine dioxide gas sterilization on nosocomial organism viability in a hospital room. *Int J Environ Res Public Health.* 2013;10:2596-2605.

163. Lowe JJ, Hewlett AL, Iwen PC, Smith PW, Gibbs SG. Evaluation of ambulance decontamination using gaseous chlorine dioxide. *Prehosp Emerg Care.* 2013;17:401-408.

164. Eylath AS, Wilson D, Thatcher D, Pankau A. Successful sterilization using chlorine dioxide gas: part one-sanitizing an aseptic fill isolator. *BioProcess Int.* 2003;7:52-56.

165. Barbu N, Zwick R. Isolators selection, design, decontamination, and validation. *Pharm Eng.* 2014;6-14.

166. Czarneski MA, Lorcheim P. Isolator decontamination using chlorine dioxide gas. *Pharma Technol.* 2005;4:124-133.

167. Han Y, Guentert AM, Smith RS, Linton RH. Efficacy of chlorine dioxide gas as a sanitizer for tanks used for aseptic juice storage. *Food Microbiol.* 1999;16:53-61.

168. Eylath AS, Madhogarhia ER, Lorcheim P, Czarneski M. Successful sterilization using chlorine dioxide gas: part two-cleaning process vessels. *BioProcess Int.* 2003;8:54-56.

169. Luftman HS, Regits MA, Lorcheim P, et al. Validation study for the use of chlorine dioxide gas as a decontaminant for biological safety cabinets. *Appl Biosaf.* 2008;13:199-212.

170. National Science Foundation. *Biosafety Cabinetry: Design, Construction, Performance, and Field Certification.* Alexandria, VA: National Science Foundation; 2008.

171. Kowalski JB. Sterilization of medical devices, pharmaceutical components, and barrier isolation systems with gaseous chlorine dioxide. In: Morrissey RF, Kowalski JB, eds. *Sterilization of Medical Products.* Vol 7. Champlain, NY: Polyscience; 1998:313-323.

172. Lorcheim K, Melgaard E. Linearity of the relationship between concentration and contact time for sterilization with chlorine dioxide gas. Paper presented at: American Biological Safety Association 58th Annual Biological Safety Conference; October 9-14, 2015; Providence, RI.

CHAPTER

28

Sterilization and Depyrogenation by Heat

Daniel L. Prince and Derek J. Prince

In the strictest sense of the word, "sterilization" implies the complete destruction of all viable microorganisms in order to deem an object "sterile." We note that sterilization is an absolute term meaning a product is either "sterile" or "nonsterile." The oldest and most effective sterilization procedure still used to this day is fire. Indeed, pharmaceutical and medical research laboratories alike use flames without issue to sterilize reusable inoculating loops, scalpels, hemostats, and other instruments as well as to disinfect the necks and caps of bottles. Similarly, incineration as a method of sterilization is commonly employed to kill harmful microorganisms from contaminated materials when destruction of the material is of no concern (see chapter 54). Of course, the use of fire/incineration as a sterilization method is often inadequate or useless because the entire destruction of all viable organisms is of no importance if the product of concern no longer exists or functions as intended. These same fundamentals still exist today as certain product types/materials are incompatible with certain sterilization modalities. Fortunately, the field of sterilization science has progressed to include several well-accepted modalities. The most commonly employed and well understood include ethylene oxide, gamma irradiation, and moist heat (steam) and dry heat. This chapter offers the reader an overview of moist heat (steam) and dry heat sterilization practices. Both processes use the lethal effect of heat to destroy all forms of life. The main distinction is that in the former heat energy is primarily delivered through saturated steam and in the latter through dry air. Sterilization by heat is a proven process used to effectively kill all microbial forms of life and can inactivate toxins such as endotoxin, the fever-producing substance from gram-negative bacteria (see chapters 3 and 66). A brief historic overview of moist heat steam sterilization is introduced, followed by a discussion on the kinetics of the lethal effects of heat and the important moist heat and dry heat sterilization and depyrogenation concepts.

▶ HISTORICAL OVERVIEW

Current practices and knowledge about sterilization of pharmaceuticals, medical devices, and other related products flow from thousands of years of discovery. Steam sterilization began during the renaissance when Denis Pavan invented the "digester" or pressure cooker.[1] It was found that heating water in a sealed vessel heated the air, causing it to expand. The pressure generated from this closed system caused the boiling point of water to increase from 100°C to 121°C at 15 psi, allowing food to cook more quickly. Later embodiments of this invention, which include microprocessor controls of temperature-pressure ranges, air removal, and pharmaceutical clean steam, have led to the present day commercial moist heat steam sterilizer.

In 1683, microbes became visible to the naked eye for the first time as Antonie van Leeuwenhoek improved on a primitive microscope that proved the existence of microorganisms. From 1860 to 1864, the French biologist Louis Pasteur convincingly demonstrated the germ theory of disease, namely that disease was caused by microorganisms and not by spontaneous generation. Pasteur demonstrated that processing by heat (ie, pasteurization) of wine and beer eliminated unwanted microbes. He recognized the importance of moist and dry heat as sterilization techniques. Charles Chamberlain, working in Pasteur's laboratory, improved on the digester design and, in 1879, invented the autoclave sterilization process wherein time and sterilization temperature was controlled and monitored. By the late 1800s, governments began to enact legislation to protect the quality of food. The US canning industry adopted a very conservative heat treatment, known as the "12D" process that reduces the probability of survival of heat-resistant *Clostridium botulinum* spores to one in a billion by causing a theoretical reduction of the initial population by 12 logarithms.[2] This is the historical thread that links today's 10^{-6} sterility assurance level (SAL) approach used for the heat processing of medical devices, instruments, and pharmaceuticals to food microbiology safety (see chapter 1).

In the 21st century, heat processing is a critical component throughout a broad spectrum of industries. Moist heat steam sterilization is perhaps the most well-known and most practiced form of sterilization because an "autoclave" can essentially be found in every university, hospital, research center, dental office, tattoo shop, testing laboratory, and health care manufacturing facility still to this day. Dry heat processes are also used for a variety of applications. In the pages that follow, we begin with the modes used to explain the lethal effect of heat on microorganisms followed by the theoretical foundation and practical applications of processing by moist steam heat and dry heat. Both processes have many favorable attributes that benefit many applications such as in product manufacturing of pharmaceuticals and medical devices, equipment sterilization, and waste disposal.

▶ MODELS USED TO DESCRIBE THE LETHAL EFFECT OF HEAT ON MICROORGANISMS

The theoretical framework for heat sterilization comes from research on the effects of time and temperature on bacterial spores such as from *Geobacillus* and *Bacillus* species (see chapters 7 and 11). Sterilization by steam or dry heat are lethal processes that destroy microbes by heat. Specifically, lethality is attributed to the transfer of steam or dry heat energy to its surroundings. This energy transfer acts directly on any contaminating microorganism's structure, replication, or metabolic process that is necessary to provide viability for survival.

The basis of the models used to explain lethality comes from the work of many investigators. They sometimes encountered results that were complex and difficult to extrapolate into a model. It was observed that exposure to a heat process was a lethal event and that the rate of death varied because the sensitivity of bacteria to heat was variable. Many factors were identified to explain the variation. For example, one was that two populations of the same species may be present in a sample and these two populations may have markedly different susceptibility to heat processing. One population may be much more resistant to the lethal process than the other. It is well understood that deviation from the linear logarithmic nature of the survival curve is usually due to two basic factors. The first is the presence of a hump or "lag" in the initial portion of the survival curve of a heat-resistant population of spores, due to Anand's "heat stimulation" or what is understood as "heat activation."[3-8] The second, the tailing of the final portion, is doubtless due to more than one thermoresistant variant in the population. Because of this, when the rate of death observed as a function of heat was graphed, nonlinear curves were often observed. In addition, many other factors are now known that significantly impact the rate at which a population of microorganisms are killed by heat processes. These factors are summarized in Table 28.1. Determining heat resistance for a specific microorganism can be a difficult task because many environmental and physiologic factors play a role.

Investigations of microbial inactivation in plant soil (or earth) have demonstrated many of these variables. Dry heat destruction characteristics of the microflora associated with soil particles suggest the following:

1. The population of microorganisms found in soil results in a dichotomous survival curve upon dry heat processing.
2. Resistance of cultured "hardy organisms" was variable,[36,37] and $D_{125°C}$ values[38] (the D-value at 125°C; see chapter 2) ranged from 5 to 139 hours. *Bacillus xerothermodurans* was found to have a $D_{125°C}$-value of 139 hours.[39]
3. Moderately resistant organisms such as *Bacillus atrophaeus* can be very resistant to dry heat when encapsulated in particles. Spores encapsulated in salt crystals can have increased dry heat resistance more than 10-fold.[40,41] In many soil particles, crystals with large waters of hydration may cause organisms normally of low dry heat resistance to become super-resistant spores. It seems probable that through soil wetting and drying cycles, spores can be completely encapsulated in soil particles, which could greatly increase dry heat resistance.
4. The relative number of resistant spores is small. It was estimated that 1 spore in 10^3 to 10^5 survives a dry heat treatment of approximately 30 hours at 110°C.[42]

In summary, bacterial spores are known to survive for long periods in harsh environmental conditions. This can be influenced by the spore structure itself, the presence of external protective factors, and water retention. These factors can allow some species of bacterial spores to survive even harsh sterilization processes.[43]

In experiments evaluating the effect of heat stress on a microbial population, aliquots of a suspension of microorganisms are subjected to heat for several different periods and then the number of survivors for each heating time determined. In addition, the number of microorganisms in the unheated control is determined as the starting point. To communicate these results visually (the change in the number of surviving microorganisms with increased heat stress), a survivor curve graph is prepared in which the number of survivors is plotted as a function of the length of heating time at temperature T. There are several ways to plot the data. When plotting microbial survivor data on a graph with an arithmetic scale on both the x- and the y-axes, the data form an exponential decay-type curve. This is a nondistorted, visual perspective on the effect of a constant stress on a microbial population.

TABLE 28.1	Factors affecting the heat resistance of microorganisms
Resistance Factor	**Rationale**
Water content	Destruction rate of microbial cells is a function of water content, which is determined by the relative humidity of the atmosphere surrounding the cells or the water activity of the environment in which the cells are suspended. Spores are more resistant to heat because they have a very low water content. Their water activity is much lower than vegetative bacteria. There is a free exchange of water between the spore and its environment, and the water activity is expected to change in relation to the suspending medium or the atmospheric environment.[9] The presence of humidity can raise the water activity of the spore making it susceptible to inactivation processes.
Growth phase	Vegetative microbial cells show differing degrees of susceptibility to adverse influences at various stages of the growth cycle.[10,11] Young cells are more susceptible to heat destruction than older and more mature cells.[12,13] Increased resistance of thermoduric streptococci to heat destruction was observed during the early logarithmic phase,[14] and greater heat resistance is exhibited during the stationary phase than during exponential growth.[15,16]
Growth temperature	Spores produced at higher temperatures were more resistant than spores produced at lower temperatures.[17-26] Spores of thermophilic organisms are inherently more resistant than those of mesophilic or psychrophilic species. The spores of a given species grown at a maximum temperature are in general more resistant than those grown at optimum or minimum temperature.[27]
Sublethal heating	Organisms, to a limited extent, have an adaptive response to protect themselves from the lethal effect of a heat process. Enhancement of resistance to lethal heating may result from prior sublethal heating of dormant spores, which reportedly can sometimes induce an increase in dormancy. Sporulation in the presence of cadmium, known to induce stress shock proteins, resulted in spores with increased resistance to heat. A mutant lacking the ability to produce heat shock proteins was more temperature sensitive.[28] The induction of increased heat resistance by sublethal heating has also been observed in vegetative cells. Heat resistance is increased not only by prior sublethal heating but also during the process of heating the cells to lethal temperature, with the extent of increase depending on the slowness of the rise in temperature.[29]
Nutrient conditions	Extensive studies of the effect of nutrient conditions and other factors on the resistance of spores of a strain of *Bacillus atrophaeus* have been performed.[19] Nutrient conditions can either increase or decrease the resistance compared with a standard nutrient condition. Different brands of peptone resulted in a change in resistance, although resistance appeared to be independent of concentration with any one peptone. Various digest media resulted in spores of low resistance, except casein digest, which enhanced resistance. Spores of high resistance were obtained using media prepared from vegetable extracts as well as isoelectric gelatin. The addition of either phosphate or magnesium to the standard peptone medium increased resistance. The addition of available carbohydrates, organic acids, or amino acids in some cases increased resistance. The increases in resistance obtained with varying nutrient conditions were reflected only in the specially produced spores; transfer to a standard medium restored the original resistance.
pH	The influence of pH on heat resistance of microorganisms depends on different factors, such as the strain investigated, suspending medium, water activity, and test temperature. Thus, because of the strong influence of the type of substrate on the effect of pH on heat resistance, resistance calculations based on one set of experimental conditions (pH, substrate, and temperature, among others) are not necessarily applicable to other experimental conditions.[30,31]
Physical environmental conditions	"Enclosure effect" on heat resistance, when *Geobacillus stearothermophilus* spores were dried on filter paper discs and placed in nonhermetic paper or foil envelopes, which in turn were heated in saturated steam, survival times were shorter than when no envelope was used.[32-34] Speculated that the envelope effect may occur because the spores are at an elevated temperature in an envelope at ambient temperature before they become saturated with water unlike "naked" exposed spores.[35] This is considered the result of a difference in the level of stabilization of critical molecules in the spore.

At longer heating times, the number of surviving organisms approaches zero, but because the y-axis scale is arithmetic 1, it does not identify with precision survival numbers smaller than approximately 2000; therefore, this graph does not tell us much about the area of low levels of survival. Learning from this, it came to be known that the lethal effect of heat is more clearly demonstrated in graphs when the number of microorganisms is expressed as $\log_{10}$. The number of organisms that survive (N_T) exposure to the heat process is plotted on the y-axis, and the time of exposure to the heat process is plotted on the arithmetic x-axis. Semilogarithmic graphs are optimal for this purpose because the magnitude of the initial target population (N_0) is very large (eg, 1 million colony-forming units [CFUs]). Using the semilogarithmic curve, it is possible to see with accuracy when there are only a small number of surviving organisms (chapters 7 and 11).

The Bigelow[44] or the z-value model is the temperature coefficient model that is used worldwide in designing and monitoring heat sterilization processes. It is also derived from experimental data on the effect of heat on the survival of microorganisms and is portrayed graphically. Bigelow observed that when the logarithm of the destruction time was plotted on the y-axis against temperature on an arithmetic scale on the x-axis, the resultant shape of the survivor curve over the range of temperatures studied was a straight line. The time at a given temperature that causes a 1 log reduction (ie, 90%) in the specific target microbial population is referred to as D-value. The graph of log D versus temperature is called the thermal resistance (TR) curve and from it, one learns the change in temperature that causes a 10-fold change in the D, known as the z-value. Thus, D- and z-values are measures of the destruction of microorganisms caused by the lethality of a heat process. These were recommended for the analysis of microbial survival data generated from a heat process.[45,46] Thus, since that time, survivor curves are typically plotted on semilogarithmic scales.

Today, commercially available biological indicators (BIs) are widely used as biological reference standards for sterilization processes and are manufactured according to US Food and Drug Administration, International Organization for Standardization 11138, or other current good manufacturing practices. The BIs are challenge devices that contain biological spores (as the most resistant microorganisms to heat inactivation processes) at a known count and resistance (see chapter 65). The BIs are often used to develop, validate, and monitor the effectiveness of the heat process. They can also verify the process parameters relied on for the parametric release of sterile products. As a challenge device, they are manufactured to contain higher numbers of resistant bacterial spores than the organisms expected to be found in manufacturing facilities or on surfaces. A certificate of quality is provided with each shipment certifying the population per BI (N_0) and its resistance to the heat process (D-value). Thus, BIs can be used to biologically verify and/or validate the lethality of heat processes.

Lethality is also referred to as an F-value in moist heat steam (F_0) and dry heat processes ($F_{D\ or\ H}$). The F_0-value is the equivalent exposure time in a moist heat steam process related to the temperature of 121°C and to z = 10 (see chapter 2). A standard moist heat steam process is defined as 121°C for 15 minutes, whereas a standard dry heat sterilization process is defined at a minimum of 160°C for at least 120 minutes.[47] Accordingly, commercial cycles used by the pharmaceutical and medical device industries are designed to be very conservative such that after the heat

process, there is a very high probability that the product sterilized is sterile.

In summary, the international experimental approach to validate the lethality of a sterilization heat process is appropriate for heat-stable materials. It is conservatively based on experiments with typical starting populations of millions of heat-resistant spores. The results are plotted semilogarithmically as described earlier, and the resultant survivor curve will typically be a straight line. Its slope is used to extrapolate the exposure time needed to achieve a theoretical reduction greater than the starting spore population log N_0, for example, a 12 log reduction of N_0. The attainment of a theoretical log reduction greater than what can be empirically measured (because there are no surviving organisms) is known as an SAL. For heat-sensitive materials, the SAL can be obtained by substituting the highly resistant spores with the relevant bioburden typically found on the surfaces being sterilized as discussed later. For further analysis of the mathematical theories behind thermal survivor curves, see chapter 10 and previous editions of this book.[48,49]

Moist Heat Steam Sterilization

Sterilization by steam is perhaps the most common and frequently used sterilization modality. This is carried out using sterilization equipment designs that operate at high levels of pressure and temperature. Steam is an ideal form of sterilization except for materials that are compromised by high heat, high pressures, and moisture. Sterilization exposures inside the typical steam sterilization temperature range from 110°C to 135°C and are optimal to achieve microbial lethality with a high degree of confidence. Due to the mass heat transfer generated as the steam condenses to liquid, steam sterilization is more effective than most other sterilization processes at destroying resistant bacterial spores in relatively short periods of exposure. In addition, steam sterilization is also considered one of the most economically friendly sterilization modalities. The main principle of a steam sterilizer design is the vaporization of water by raising its temperature in a closed vessel, producing pressurized saturated steam. The exact control of this process will depend on the specific cycle parameter design to be able to accommodate the load being sterilized and to attain the minimum requirements for sterilization (in these cases, temperature over time). Pure saturated steam is recommended to be made from highly purified water to provide the optimal physical (eg, lack of appreciable levels of air or other noncondensable gases) and chemical (noncontaminated) characteristics of steam.

Saturated Steam

Pure steam (clean steam or high-purity steam) is steam condensate that complies with a defined water specification (eg, water for injection [WFI], as defined by

TABLE 28.2	Recommended levels of contaminants in condensate from steam[a]
Determinant	**Acceptable Levels in Steam Condensate**
Silicate	≤0.1 mg/L
Iron	≤0.1 mg/L
Cadmium	≤0.005 mg/L
Lead	≤0.05 mg/L
Other heavy metals (except iron, cadmium, lead)	≤0.1 mg/L
Chloride	≤0.1 mg/L
Phosphate	≤0.1 mg/L
Conductivity (at 20°C)	≤4.3 µS/cm
pH (20°C)	~5-7
Appearance	Colorless, no sediment
Hardness	≤0.02 mmol/L

[a]Reprinted with permission from British Standards Institution.[50]

TABLE 28.3	Advantageous properties of saturated steam as a sterilant
Property	**Advantage**
Rapid, even heating through latent heat transfer	Improved product quality and productivity
Pressure can control temperature.	Temperature can be quickly and precisely established.
High heat transfer coefficient	Smaller required heat transfer surface area, enabling reduced initial equipment outlay
Originates from water	Safe, clean, and low cost

pharmaceutical monographs or in associated standards such as EN 285:2015 for steam sterilizers[50]) (Table 28.2).

To have optimal pure steam for sterilization, it is important to ensure that saturated steam (water vapor in a state of equilibrium between its liquid and gas phases) is free from noncondensable gases and superheat. Both factors have the potential to adversely affect sterilization lethality, especially for loads containing porous/hard goods. Noncondensable gases such as air, nitrogen, and carbon dioxide (CO_2) can change steam from a pure state to a mixture of steam and gas, thereby limiting the effectiveness of steam to reliably condense onto desired surfaces. "Super-heated" steam occurs when the liquid/gas equilibrium no longer exists, and steam is in excess relative to water, therefore taking on drier and less efficacious state because it is less likely to efficiently condense on desired surfaces. It is important to monitor that the cycle is free from these effects because it is pure, saturated steam that is most effective at achieving sterilization.

Saturated steam has many properties that make it an excellent heat source, particularly at temperatures of 100°C (212°F) and higher (Table 28.3). When discussing the use of steam as a sterilant, it is important to note the differences between water and steam because it relates to pressure and temperature relationships. According to Boyle law and the Gay-Lussac pressure temperature law, for a fixed mass of gas, the product of pressure and volume is constant, and the temperature is directly proportional to pressure:

$$\text{Pressure} \times \text{Volume} = \text{Constant}$$

$$\text{Pressure} \propto \text{Temperature}$$

In water's liquid form, hydrogen bonding pulls water molecules together. Because it exists below its boiling point and therefore steam is absent, this form of water is referred to as unsaturated water (water in its most recognizable state) and has a relatively compact, dense, and stable structure. Saturated water, on the other hand, occurs at a given temperature-pressure combination where both liquid water and water vapor (ie, steam) are present in equilibrium. Thus, water exists in different phases based on the temperature and pressure of the environment it is present in. The temperature at which water boils changes with ambient pressure, such that a low pressure corresponds to a low boiling point temperature and a high pressure corresponds to an increased boiling point temperature. When a saturation condition is reached, the liquid phase and the vapor phase are in equilibrium with one another, that is, both phases exist simultaneously. If a small amount of energy is added to saturated liquid, it turns into vapor at constant temperature. Likewise, if a small amount of energy is removed from saturated vapor, it will condense to liquid at constant temperature. The transference of heat energy to the microbe from the change of phase from steam to water is the major lethal event that causes sterilization.

For most medical devices and pharmaceutical applications, the most relevant conditions for sterilization are shown in Figure 28.1. In the optimal region of the temperature-pressure curve, steam and liquid water exist in equilibrium with each other. It is a biphasic mixture of water in its gas and liquid phases that are in thermal equilibrium. Saturated steam can exist at a variety of temperature and pressure combinations. As indicated by the curved line, the optimal conditions for steam sterilization exist at the temperature and pressure where steam is in equilibrium with water. As the process begins to drift to the left (liquid phase) and away from the curved line, steam is considered too "wet," and as it drifts to the right and away from the curved line (gas), the steam is considered too "dry." With respect to a moist heat steam

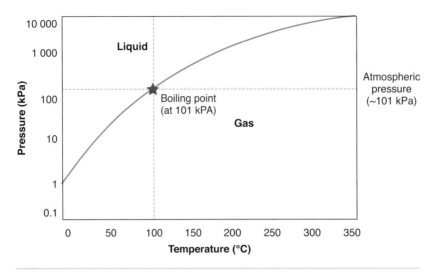

FIGURE 28.1   Phase diagram of water at various temperature and pressure conditions.

sterilizer, temperature and pressure are carefully controlled and monitored to introduce saturated steam to achieve lethality.

When the saturated steam molecules condense from steam to liquid, thermal energy is released and transferred to the materials as well as any organisms present in the load causing the exposed materials to be sterilized. As indicated in Figure 28.1, saturated steam can occur over a wide range of temperatures and pressures where steam (gas) and water (liquid) can coexist. It occurs when the rate of water vaporization is equal to the rate of condensation. In many applications, the parameters of temperature and pressure used for saturated moist steam heat sterilization are in the range of 115°C to 134°C and 1.1 bar (15.9 psia) to 1.89 bar (27.4 psia), respectively. Where the liquid-vapor boundary terminates is the critical temperature (T_c) and critical pressure (p_c) (ie, critical point) at which the liquid and gas phases of water are indistinguishable from each other. In water, the critical point occurs at around 647 K (374°C; 705°F) and 22 MPa (220.6 bar). If steam is heated above the saturation point, it becomes superheated steam. Although some degree of superheat can be tolerated, higher degrees result in a loss of sterilizing efficiency.[51] Superheated steam can arise from several sources. For one, the sterilization chamber jacket heat can be heated above the sterilizing temperature produces heating of materials with high emissivity characteristics by radiant heat transfer to the surface of materials in the sterilizing chamber. As steam is admitted to the sterilizing environment and passes through the material, it picks up heat from both the chamber walls and the material, resulting in superheat in a surface layer of the material. In the presence of water, the superheated steam loses its additional heat energy when it contacts the water or any surface at a temperature below the superheated steam temperature. Savage[52] found that as the deviation from the saturation phase boundary

increased, the rate of spore destruction decreased phenomenally. These data indicate that at temperatures above 132°C, superheat was not efficacious; however, this is an area that requires more investigation using appropriately designed test equipment. Rates of reaction are so fast at temperatures above 121°C that the accuracy of test results must be considered questionable for any of the test methods reported to date. In general, based on the bacteriologic results obtained at lower temperatures, superheat below 5°C (approximately 85% RH) should not be objectionable.

As mentioned earlier, condensation of steam causes a tremendous transfer of heat energy from the steam to the contact surface, including the presence of microorganisms. As an example, at 100°C, the steam molecules will transfer approximately 2676 kJ/kg of steam when condensed, heating the microorganisms to a lethal temperature. Condensation will continue to occur so long because the temperature of the condensing surface is less than that of steam. This allows for rapid heating of surfaces, penetration of dense materials, denaturation of proteins and other macromolecules essential for life, and subsequent sterilization of microorganisms including more resistant forms such as nonenveloped viruses and spores (see chapter 3). Even at 80°C, there is still substantial lethality via heat transfer upon condensation, only differing 3% from that of the calculated lethality at 134°C (Table 28.4). The direct transfer of energy from steam to the contaminating microorganism is not the only mechanism of sterilization by heat. In fact, the United States Pharmacopeia (USP) recognizes this and divides steam sterilization into two general informational subchapters: steam sterilization by direct contact[53] and aqueous liquids.[54] This is because the sterilization parameters where steam comes into direct contact with the target is substantially different than from when steam is simply used as a heating agent with

TABLE 28.4	Specific enthalpy of saturated steam at various temperatures
Temperature (°C)	**Specific Enthalpy (kJ/kg)**
134	2726
120	2707
100	2676
80	2643

no direct contact on the material to be sterilized. Thus, unlike direct contact, sterilization by steam of liquids in filled containers, for example, is not a result of direct contact chamber supplied steam contact or penetration. In general, the theories and validation principles behind the two methods of steam sterilization are shared; however, certain challenges such as determination of the TR for the BI within the liquid and container mapping to identify internal cold spots are unique to the validation where chamber-supplied steam does not come into direct contact with the load. Although potentially difficult to assess (eg, blow-fill-seal systems), these concepts are important in understanding how the thermal conditions applied to the external components of the load target affect the internal portion intended to be sterile. These latter assessments may not be used by many moist heat sterilization practitioners; however, they have proven to be extremely useful for terminal sterilization of pharmaceutical products such as liquids in sealed glass vials or syringes and blow-fill-seal containers.

Although often considered the most common and eco-friendly method of sterilization, heat sterilization of health care products are often avoided due to material incompatibility with temperature and time profiles. But, with correct cycle development considerations, it has been estimated that as many as 30% of aseptically manufactured products may in fact be compatible with terminal sterilization by steam.[55] The reasoning behind the avoidance of developing a terminal sterilization cycle is most likely attributed to the abuse of the "overkill" mentality most commonly used and referenced when validating a steam and dry heat sterilization processes. This type of cycle validation uses extremely exaggerated and often unrealistic "worst case" assumptions to validate the cycle, resulting in lengthy cycle times at high temperatures. Whereas this type of validation approach is conservative and useful for heat-stable materials, other case-specific optimization approaches should be used for the terminal sterilization of products desirous of being sterilized by heat. Strict reliance on heat process parameters designed to kill 12 logs of resistant spores will limit the application of terminal sterilization by such methods.[56] For this reason, method development cycles on products in their final container shall

be performed to assess the efficacy of steam sterilization at alternative time and temperature combinations so that an appropriate SAL can be achieved. According to the European Medicines Evaluation Agency, if a decision is made to not use terminal sterilization (thereby electing to use aseptic processing alternatives; see chapter 58), a scientific justification must be included within the applicable regulatory dossier.[57]

An outcome with a validated cycle that achieves a defined F_0 provides greater sterilization assurance than aseptic manufacturing on its own. In fact, this thinking has long been discussed in Japan, where the use of an F_0 >2 was discussed for products prepared via aseptic processing, such as filtered products.[58]

Steam Sterilizer Designs

The typical construction of a steam sterilizer (commonly known as an autoclave) is shown in the longitudinal cross-section of Figure 28.2. The basic system consists of a pressure vessel, steel shell equipped with a sealable door on one end (or both ends) and a permanent closure (back-head) on the other end. A thermostatically trapped steam jacket surrounds the autoclave on all sides (except the back-head, when present, and the door). Both the main shell and the jacket are fed with steam through control valves, and both are equipped with pressure gauges and safety relief valves. A chamber temperature indicator/controller probe is usually located in the chamber drain vent line. Well-designed steam sterilization equipment delivers steam in a controlled process to the load. The major problems during this process are air removal, superheat, load wetness, and material damage. To minimize these problems, common design elements of the sterilizer are the baffle, water separator, and splash pan for optimal process controls (eg, removal of water during the process or steam delivery or from condensation during the process). Underpowered steam boilers, inadequate traps, and undersized piping may contribute to steam wetness and rouging (surface rusting or residual buildup) of a chamber.

Most modern sterilizers are often rectangular vessels to minimize floor space and maximize loading volume. The design of such vessels are important to ensure water drainage; for example, flat-bottomed vessels are not adequately sloped for water to exit the drain vent, therefore, low spots retain condensate in the chamber (Figure 28.3). After sterilization, rapid venting of the sterilizing chamber can result in violent ebullition of the water on the hot floor of the autoclave chamber. This can propel water up onto materials being processed and can cause spot wetting on the bottom of wrapped materials. Such gross wetting is not always dried during the drying process. To prevent this wetting, some manufacturers provide a splash pan (see Figure 28.2).

There are four critical parameters in any steam sterilization process: steam, pressure, temperature, and time.

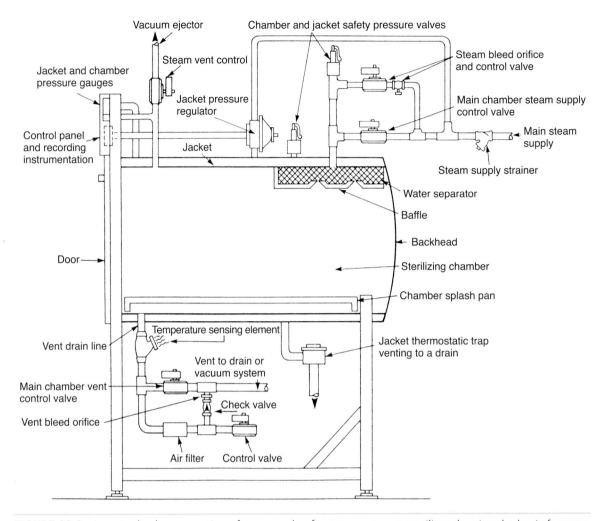

FIGURE 28.2   Longitudinal cross-section of an example of a steam pressure sterilizer showing the basic features. From Joslyn.[48(p704)]

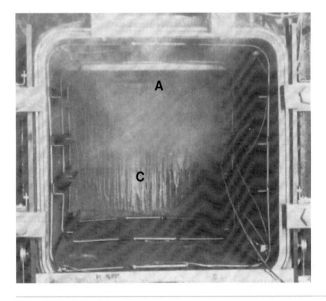
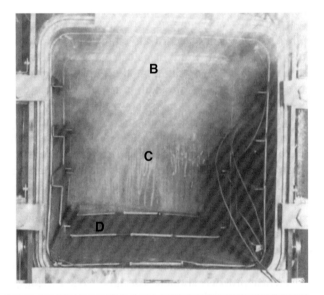

FIGURE 28.3   Chamber water separator and baffle design for a gravity displacement–based steam sterilizer. A, Improper design results in mixing of air and steam. B, Proper design results in a smooth cloud layer that acts as a piston to displace air from the chamber. C, Entrained water from the steam supply is separated and runs down to the backhead to the drain. D, Accumulation of water on the chamber floor. From Joslyn.[48(p706)]

The operation of a sterilizer is programmed and follows a sequence of steps designed to optimally achieve the desired level of assurance. In summary, the steps of the sequence in a prevacuum, or forced air removal, steam sterilizer design are as follows:

1. Begin the vacuum pump to evacuate air from the chamber. Air is an insulator that, if present, does not conduct heat very well and interferes with the uniform delivery of steam to or within the load (see the following discussion).
2. Steam is bled into the chamber. After the first evacuation, there will still be some residual air present. At this step, the load begins to heat but the temperature effect at this part of the sequence is not counted as part of the specified exposure time.
3. Steps 1 and 2 may be repeated for a total of 3 to 5 times as appropriate, to various vacuum or positive pressure levels.
4. Steam is charged into the chamber and the temperature monitored by a sensor. When the sterilization temperature is reached, the steam valve is closed and a timer is initiated to hold the temperature for the specified time. This step is often referred to as the "hold time" or "plateau period phase."
5. Controls in the chamber monitor the temperature, and steam is bled into the chamber as necessary to maintain the chamber at the specified sterilization temperature.
6. At the conclusion of the hold time, the steam supply is turned off and the vacuum pump is signaled to turn on to evacuate the steam from the chamber.
7. A drying cycle is performed by the delivery of sterile air that circulates in the hot chamber under controlled pressure conditions.

Many other cycle variables can be programmed or controlled depending on the load being sterilized, such as simple venting systems and air pressurization cycles.[59]

Importance of Air Removal

The injection of steam and achievement of the appropriate steam conditions are of minimal effect if the appropriate preconditioning steps are not carefully carried out. The first and most important step in this process is the removal and replacement of residual air from within the chamber with steam. Alternatives can include the equal distribution of air and steam within the sterilization chamber/load, under specific cycle development conditions. Due to the higher density of air, residual air can form blankets that can inhibit the ability of steam to contact the load. Similarly, air is an insulator and therefore not an efficient conductor of heat/moisture. For these reasons, it is of critical importance to ensure the removal of air from within the chamber prior to initiating the cycle. The most common techniques used for air removal are by gravity displacement or high vacuum ("prevacuum"), although

other methods can include dilution by mass flow, dilution by pressure pulsing, and pressure pulsing in combination with gravity displacement.[48]

Gravity displacement. A common form of sterilization by steam is the gravity displacement cycle where steam is injected into the chamber and displaces the colder air simply by pushing it to the bottom toward the drain and steam trap. This cycle is best used with items with a low potential of trapping air, such as unwrapped metal components, glassware, and nonporous materials. The higher density steam eventually mass displaces the air downward faster than the air can diffuse into the constantly renewed supply of pure steam. This effect ultimately pushes the air to the bottom of the chamber where it can exit through the drain. Gravity displacement steam sterilizers are equipped with a water separator and a steam baffle located at the steam entry point. This is to aid in the removal of atomized water particles and the raw entrained water trapped within high-velocity steam in order to produce the highest quality steam (98% or better) possible. Similarly, these components help reduce the velocity of steam entering the chamber. This is important because steam entering the chamber at a high velocity poses the risk of mixing with the unwanted air instead of pushing it out. Efficient gravity displacement cycles should reduce steam velocity to approximately 1 ft/s.[60] Baffles located along the side of the chamber that do not extend to the chamber top were found to be less effective at avoiding air steam mixing. It's also important to ensure proper sizing of the drain vent. If properly sized, the chamber pressure should not exceed 1 to 2 psig when steam is admitted to the chamber. During sterilization exposure, removal of condensate and residual air is maintained via a thermostatic trap strategically located at the bottom of the chamber drain. Air removal and time to reach sterilization conditions usually takes longer when a gravity displacement cycle is employed relative to mechanical air removal processes. These points all help to ensure that the most effective gravity displacement cycle is being performed.

Prevacuum. A common drawback of the gravity displacement cycle is that it is not effective at removing air from porous loads, partially vented containers, and materials with tubing or other components where removal of residual air may be difficult. For these types of materials, a prevacuum cycle can be employed, where mechanically assisted vacuum/pressure pulses aid in the removal of air from the chamber and load items to increase the penetration/circulation of steam. The number of pulses can vary depending on the complexity of the material and load configuration and is typically determined during development studies. Although more effective and faster at accomplishing the removal of residual air from the chamber and material, aggressive vacuum and pressure pulsing may result in unwanted stressing of the materials being sterilized (eg, packaging systems). In principle, pressure pulsing reduces the concentration of air in a sterilizing environment by pressurization with a diluent gas (steam) and evacuating or venting the resulting mixture of air and steam. This is repeated until the air concentration is reduced to below a predetermined acceptable concentration. Assuming each vacuum pulse occurs at 0.1 atmosphere, each pulse will reduce the air in the sterilizer by approximately 90%.[61] Therefore, a cycle containing three vacuum pulls can effectively remove 99.9% of air within the chamber. Assuming uniform mixing of air and steam, a mathematical model showing the approximate partial pressure of air after each pulse is given by

$$A_n = P_2 (A_{n-1}) / P_1$$

where A_n is the partial pressure of air in the sterilizing chamber after each pressure pulse (n), A_{n-1} is the partial pressure of air in the sterilizing chamber before each pressure pulse, P_2 is the final absolute chamber pressure on evacuation, and P_1 is the final absolute chamber pressure during pressurization. Analysis of this equation shows that an increased partial pressure of steam (P_1 increases) and lower vacuum levels (P_2 decreases) result in an increase in the rate of air removal. In practice, the calculated number of pulses required for removal of air to a partial pressure less than 5 mm Hg results in a load temperature that generally follows the temperature and pressure of saturated steam in the chamber (no thermal lag). Figure 28.4 shows the heating

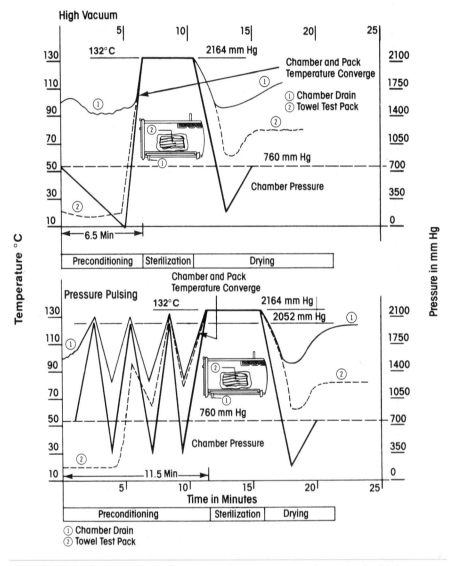

FIGURE 28.4   A comparison of steam sterilization cycles using a single, high-vacuum preconditioning phase in comparison to a pressure-pulsing air removal process. Note atmospheric pressure (760 mm Hg) is indicated as a horizontal dashed line and chamber pressure indicated by the solid black line. The temperature measured in the chamber drain (1) and in a towel test pack (42-towel double-muslin-wrapped test packs) (2) are shown. When the partial pressure of air in the chamber is below 5 mm Hg, heating in the load usually follows the chamber steam temperature, as shown. From Joslyn.[48]

character of a pressure-pulsing system versus a single high vacuum to remove air for uniform heating of a single towel pack. With deeper vacuum levels, air removal is efficient and fewer pulses are required to reduce the concentration of air to acceptable levels for efficient steam heating. When the vacuum is less than 250 mm Hg, the air removal characteristics are more like those of a high-vacuum system.

An interesting characteristic of pressure-pulsing systems is that air can be removed more efficiently from dense, porous loads than from the sterilizing chamber. This is because pressurization of the system compresses air into a spherical ball in the load. At the depth at which steam does penetrate, it condenses and heats the material. When the chamber pressure is reduced, the air expands into the heated region and the steam revaporizes because of the lower pressure. This drives the air out of the load. Thus, the relative inefficiency of the pressure-pulsing system is the result of the remaining chamber air being re-entrained in the load during repressurization. This infers that in comparing the sterilization parameters used, for example, for the reprocessing of medical instruments in their sterilization tray that a minimally loaded chamber may be more of a challenge than the same tray system maximally loaded in the chamber.[62]

Caution should be employed to ensure that this type of conditioning step will not harm the materials, including packaging systems. Along with helping remove air from the chamber prior to injecting steam to initiate a cycle, vacuum pulses can also be used at the end of cycle to help remove residual steam and condensate to facilitate drying of the load items.

Airtightness of the Sterilizer Chamber

Regardless of the chosen preconditioning technique, proper conditioning of the load before exposure at a given temperature is vital. Under normal conditions, the process should ensure that the entire load is exposed for a sufficient period of time at a high enough temperature to be acceptably sterilized. Common causes of air remaining within the chamber of vacuum sterilizers are air leaks through mechanical components such as valves and door gaskets or fatigue cracks in piping. Even with diligent equipment checkout efforts, the sterilizer may develop an air leak between tests or exhibit intermittent leak problems that compromise proper sterilization.

For this reason, there are several tests that can be used to periodically test for air removal in a sterilizer.[50] Traditionally, the most common is the Bowie-Dick test. This test simulates a porous load, consisting of a chemical indicator placed within the center of a test pack; the chemical indicator is designed to change color on exposure to the correct steam conditions following penetration of the porous materials. Another is the hollow load test that also uses a similar chemical indicator placed at the end of a dead-end lumen to check for the air removal/ steam penetration in a worst-case location.

Importance of Drying

In a wet state, sterilized packaged materials are more susceptible to recontamination. It has been known for some time now that bacteria can pass through wet or damp wrapping materials.[63,64] To ameliorate the problem of wetness, most steam sterilization processes typically provide a drying phase or specific drying of loads may be required following a steam sterilization process. For example, in many cases in the past, following a steam sterilization cycle, the sterilizer door would be opened partially so that steam vented out of the chamber while radiant and convective heat from the sterilizing chamber provide the heat energy to dry the load; this is not a preferred method because unsterile air contacts the load at a vulnerable time. A more reliable method uses a system (eg, an aspirator) to pull steam out of the sterilizing chamber while admitting air through a bioretentive filter until the load is sufficiently dried. It is important to remove the steam through the top of the chamber while admitting air in the bottom (the reverse of gravity displacement) until the sterilizer door is opened. This is because steam accumulates at the top of the chamber and would not be totally removed. This is also a safety risk, as operators frequently have reported burns from steam after opening an autoclave door and reaching for panel controls, which are often located above the door. Steam causes severe burns with only a moment's contact.

When applicable, drying can also be optimized using the same vacuum pump system that assists with air removal. For example, after sterilization, the chamber can evacuate to between 100 and 40 mm Hg absolute to revaporize a percentage of the condensate and thereby drying the load. Drying in vacuum sterilizers usually produces acceptably dry loads under validated cycle conditions in accordance with the manufacturer's instructions. The presence of "wet" loads in such situations typically indicates problems with the sterilizer load (eg, overloading or not positioning materials to drain during the cycle) or steam quality (eg, "wet" steam, see the following discussion).

Steam Quality

There are several types of steam that can be used for moist heat sterilization. These include plant steam, process steam, and pure steam. Although the primary focus in the following discussion is on pure steam, an understanding of the other steam types may be useful. The quality of steam is the weight of dry steam present in a mixture of dry saturated steam and entrained water. If the steam quality is 97%, the wet steam mixture consists of 3 parts by weight of saturated water and 97 parts by weight of saturated steam. Ideal steam for sterilization is 100% saturated steam. Factors such as boiler priming, poorly trapped steam supplies, and normal pipe wall condensation entrained by high-velocity steam flow all contribute to produce a steam quality that is less than 100%. Steam that is not saturated is less efficacious and will potentially cause other problems as described earlier.

Steam quality for steam sterilization can be controlled at the point of use (in the autoclave chamber) by using a well-designed steam separator and baffling system. These design elements can reduce the risks of an autoclave not performing consistently regardless of the steam quality delivered to the autoclave. When pure steam (that is required to be pyrogen free) is required, it is required to made from a high-purity water source and by using a steam separator design. The steam separator is designed to direct the clean steam in a rigorous path where any impurities or remaining moisture are reduced and lead to a drain. The resultant condensed steam will typically need to meet the WFI water quality standards[50,65] as listed in the following text when condensed and tested properly:

- Total organic carbon of <500 ppb (suggested alert level of >250 ppb and action level >350 ppb)
- Conductivity (online) to meet USP WFI requirements adjusted for temperature (nominal conductivity <1.3 μS/cm at 25°C to pass stage 1 requirements)
- Endotoxin levels ≤0.25 EU/mL (suggested alert level ≥0.06 EU/mL and action level ≥0.12 EU/mL)
- Heterotrophic plate count ≤10 CFUs/100 mL (alert ≥5 CFUs/100 mL, action ≥10 CFUs/100 mL)

Alternatively, the sterilizer can be equipped with a dedicated electric clean steam generator that is provided with the required water quality. Electric clean steam generators are equipped with an approved pressure vessel typically constructed from 316 L stainless steel. All connections on the vessel including the heating elements are also sanitary and sloped to drain. Three-phase voltage can typically assure faster heat up times. Such designs are often equipped with an automatic timed blow-down system that carries any impurities that may have built up in the system to the drain. If pure steam is required, as described earlier, a steam separator may also be added to the outlet of the evaporator.

Steam quality affects the degree of sterilization and dryness of processed materials. When materials such as dressings, linens, and outer wrappings are sterilized, the fabrics can become saturated with moisture. Excessive wetting of the materials hinders diffusion of air from the load. When the material is dry, air can pass more freely. When the material is wet, the diffusivity of air through the material decreases. This trapped air can significantly reduce the rate at which a dense, porous load heats. After sterilization, grossly wetted materials are not easily dried. Penikett et al[66] reported that materials are noticeably damp that contain up to 6% water by weight. Figure 28.5 shows the typical moisture gain of a test towel pack, with various percentages of initial pack moisture after sterilization in 99% saturated steam. High initial pack

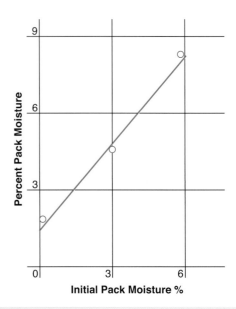

FIGURE 28.5   Percentage of moisture in a towel pack (12 lb) with various initial moisture contents after high-vacuum sterilization with approximately 99% saturated steam at 132°C. From Joslyn.[48(p712)]

moisture results in increased moisture gain. Figure 28.6 shows the increase in moisture gain relative to steam quality for a towel pack with an initial pack moisture level of 3%. The moisture gain increases as the steam quality decreases. Steam quality can be more important depending on the steam sterilizer and cycle designs used to eliminate air from the system. For this reason, drying parameters and acceptance criteria for dryness should be included in sterilization protocols. The attainment of finished product sterility without consideration of the impact of drying is not acceptable, although drying for some loads may not be applicable (eg, for the sterilization of liquid loads).

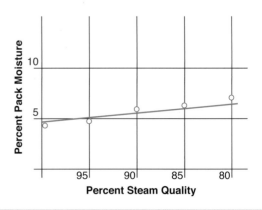

FIGURE 28.6   The effect of steam quality on moisture gain for a towel pack (912 lb) with 3% initial moisture content after high vacuum sterilization at 132°C. From Joslyn.[48(p712)]

▶ DRY HEAT PROCESSING

The two major applications of dry heat processing are for sterilization and depyrogenation. Dry heat sterilization serves as an alternative to moist heat, especially for moisture-sensitive materials, and depyrogenation acts to inactivate endotoxins.

Hot air sterilizers are usually heated electrically and can be designed with heaters underneath a perforated bottom plate to provide natural convection currents. As the heated air rises and contacts the colder load, the air cools around the load. This air moves in a downward direction, and the air in contact with the heaters again moves upward, setting up convection currents. This type of sterilizer is a *gravity convection* type. On the other hand, *mechanical convection* sterilizers are fitted with a motor-driven fan, which assists in air circulation and increasing heat transfer by convection.

Dry heat should be used only for those materials that cannot be sterilized by steam, where the moisture would either damage the materials or they would be impermeable to it. Such materials include petrolatum, oils, powders, sharp instruments, and glassware. It is necessary not to overload a dry heat sterilizer with materials; overloading delays heat convection either by circulation or by heat absorption. Enough space should be left between materials for good circulation. Wrappings and other barriers should be kept to a minimum. A heavy load can require an abnormally long time to heat, and residual organic matter on surfaces will tend to char and bake onto them.

Dry heat is an effective tool for the sterilization of glassware, many types of supplies, and other critical materials and equipment that cannot be sterilized by steam. Compared with moist heat sterilization, dry heat processing is relatively slower, requiring higher temperatures and longer heating times. Sterilization by dry heat uses hot air that contains little or no moisture. Therefore, unlike steam sterilization, moisture plays a minimal or no role in the process of sterilization by dry heat. Within the pharmaceutical and health care industries, it is used to sterilize heat-stable items such as glass, stainless steel, nonaqueous liquids, powders, and petrolatums and when items must be maintained dry. The exterior of the exposed material first absorbs the heat before passing it from the exterior to the interior portion of the material, inactivating microorganisms by oxidation and protein coagulation. The typical parameters for dry heat sterilization are 160°C to 190°C,[67-69] and once the temperature is uniform within the load, these processes can range in contact time from 120 to 60 minutes, respectively. These processes, in comparison to steam sterilization at lower temperatures, take longer to achieve sterilization because dry heat is based on the use of air as a medium for the transference of heat energy to the load items rather than water (steam). Air is much less efficient in the release of thermal energy when compared to the phase change of steam to water.

But similar to steam, the higher the temperature, the shorter the exposure time needed to achieve the desired SAL. Sterilization lethality (F_H) is defined as the amount of time necessary for the load to receive the equivalent to 160°C using a z-value of 20°C. When the entire sterilization cycle is considered from heating up to cooling down, the F_H accumulates over the range of temperatures present. By using this approach, the sterilization cycle can be defined by a designated lethality target rather than by a time at a given temperature such as 160°C.

Because dry heat sterilization is typically used for heat-stable items, practitioners routinely validate dry heat processes using the overkill method. This process is like that previously discussed in the moist heat steam validation section and also includes equipment qualification, empty chamber temperature distribution, component mapping, load mapping, and heat penetration and, when appropriate, BIs. Heat penetration data is collected in parallel to microbial challenge data to certify the load's effectiveness at achieving the appropriate lethality. Whereas *Geobacillus stearothermophilus* is used to validate moist heat steam cycles, *B atrophaeus*, a thermophilic spore-former, is used for testing dry heat as it demonstrates higher resistance.

The second major use of dry heat is for depyrogenation, specifically the inactivation of endotoxins. For some industries and product types, such as containers intended to contain liquid parenteral injectables, more stringent levels of sterilization are applied to inactivate not only all viable microorganisms but also all biological material. It is important to note that although a product is labeled as sterile, it may still be pyrogenic. Endotoxins are a type of pyrogen that are present in microorganisms and released upon cell disintegration (see chapter 66). Specifically, endotoxins are lipopolysaccharide substances located within the outer membrane of gram-negative bacterial cell walls. In pharmaceutical manufacturing, water sources are a common cause of endotoxin due to contamination from gram-negative bacteria such as *Escherichia coli* and *Pseudomonas* species. When this contamination persists in parenteral or other implantable products, the patient can experience a strong immune response and a febrile reaction. These substances are heat stable and will not be destroyed in a standard moist heat steam autoclave cycle. Depyrogenation is referred to a method that will remove/destroy a minimum of 3 logs of endotoxin challenged at 1000 or more USP international units (IU).[69] Processes to achieve this are typically limited to include some cleaning processes and the use of extreme dry heat temperatures. Depyrogenation is commonly performed as a dry heat process at 250°C or higher for a defined period.[40] When compared to dry heat sterilization, depyrogenation is performed at higher temperatures and often for longer exposure times.

In terms of inactivation activity by heat, the F_D is used as the measurement of depyrogenation comparable to F_0

TABLE 28.5 Depyrogenation temperature versus time relationships to accomplish 3 log reduction of endotoxin (at a Z = 50C and D = 5 minutes)

Temperature	3 Log Reduction of Endotoxin
250°C	15 min
300°C	90 s
343°C	9 s

used for steam and F_H used for dry heat. An F_D of 1 is defined as the depyrogenation effect achieved by 1 minute at 250°C. The z-value for the depyrogenation process is usually given as 50°C. Depyrogenation in tunnels or mechanical forced air dry heat ovens are typically performed for 30 minutes at 250°C, but for heat-labile materials, lower temperatures may need be considered with proper development and validation (eg, ≥180°C).[69] As shown in the Table 28.5, higher temperatures lead to shorter exposure times needed to accomplish depyrogenation.

Like the lethality caused by moist heat steam, destruction of bacterial spores by dry heat sterilization is also a first-order reaction wherein a linear death curve is observed by plotting spore survival in a population over time on a semilogarithmic graph; however, the destruction of endotoxin by dry heat is a second-order reaction depending on both temperature and time.[70] The shape of the depyrogenation curve is therefore biphasic (Figure 28.7), where initially, the rate of depyrogenation is very rapid and subsequently the rate slows down considerably (k2).

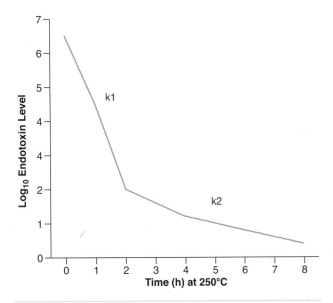

FIGURE 28.7 Depyrogenation is a biphasic reaction. Note the rapid destruction of endotoxin in the first phase (indicated as k1), followed by a slow rate of destruction (k2).

The depyrogenation process is typically validated by the demonstrated attainment of a 3 $\log_{10}$ reduction of endotoxin following analysis with a validated bacterial endotoxin test (chapter 66). The heat lethality F_D delivered by the dry heat depyrogenation process provides a large margin of safety with regard to also assuring sterilization because the reference dry heat–resistant organism used for validating dry heat sterilization, namely, *B atrophaeus* spores has a D-value of only a *few seconds* at the temperature used for depyrogenation. Therefore, one can anticipate an excess of microbial reduction and process lethality can be defined solely on the basis of endotoxin inactivation.

The principal advantages of using dry heat is its lack of water that makes it less corrosive than steam for metals and glass and the ability to achieve depyrogenation and sterilization within one process. The primary disadvantages are that the extreme temperatures limit its use with a broad spectrum of materials and devices and that heat penetration and microbial inactivation is much slower when compared to steam.

Validation of a Heat Sterilization Process

The validation of a steam or dry heat sterilization process begins well before a routine sterilization cycle is conducted. A typical validation plan for a specific good manufacturing practice (GMP) facility comprises four main phases such as design qualification (DQ), installation qualification (IQ), operational qualification (OQ), and performance qualification (PQ). For some processes, such as for health care steam sterilizers, the qualification steps can be standardized by the manufacturer to meet the labeling and/or registration requirements with the sterilizer (eg, to meet steam sterilizer design criteria as defined in standards such as EN 285:2015[50] and American National Standards Institute [ANSI]/Association for the Advancement of Medical Instrumentation [AAMI] ST8[71]). The PQ components of a typical sterilization validation is discussed, which serves to confirm the physical and microbiological performance of the selected sterilization cycle for specific loads. This phase should involve the preparation and performance of a development cycle to gather important preliminary data prior to the design and execution of the official PQ or performance validation. Although the following text discusses important considerations when validating a process for heat sterilization, it includes specific emphasis on validation of moist heat steam processes.

Once the appropriate sterilization modality (ie, steam or dry heat) and type of cycle (ie, gravity displacement or vacuum) has been identified, it's important to next consider the type of sterilization validation method to be carried out during the PQ. With respect to steam and dry heat, three methods are commonly employed and are briefly defined in the following text.

Overkill Method

Where sensitivity to the heat process is of no concern to the load items, an overkill method should be employed. This is the safest and most conservative sterilization method as a high and unrealistic population (eg, $\geq 10^6$) of heat-resistant ($D_{121°C}$-value ≥ 1 min) microorganisms (most often endospores of *G stearothermophilus* or *B atrophaeus*) are used to define the process. This all but guarantees that the same process would be capable of reducing any contaminant that would be introduced during normal manufacturing and handling of the material. It is often preferred when no heat sensitivity exists or when the actual bioburden of the material to be sterilized cannot be easily determined or is variable. Similarly, this method is preferred because it would not typically require the practitioner to perform routine monitoring of facility and material bioburden. If limitations exist with package and product integrity, a terminal sterilization cycle at a lower time and temperature should be investigated and implemented whenever possible.

Bioburden/Biological Indicator

The second approach is known as the bioburden/BI combination method. In this method, the identification of the actual bioburden present on the materials to be sterilized is used to select an appropriate BI with a known higher resistance to the sterilization process. Based on the cycle's ability to destroy a modest population of the more resistant BI, it can be calculated that the same method would reliably destroy the natural and less resistant bioburden present on the materials to be sterilized. Because this method is also dependent on knowing the product bioburden and its resistance to heat sterilization, these variables are also required to be controlled and monitored.

Bioburden Method

When an overkill approach is not suitable, the bioburden approach can be considered because it allows for the attainment of an SAL to be applied to a broader range of products including heat-labile solutions and materials. In this method, the actual microbial load of the product is identified and characterized. Identification and characterization refer to the number and heat resistance of the bioburden. A moist heat process is then developed whereby the process will render the product free of those specific microbial contaminants with a defined SAL (eg, 10^{-6}). In this approach, the experimental design allows for a reduction in sterilization temperature and or time when compared to temperature and time combinations typically used in an overkill approach. Although the process impact on materials is lower when this method is implemented, continuous process monitoring with respect to environmental monitoring and product bioburden data are needed to ensure this type of reduced heat

cycle remains adequate for future loads. Therefore, routine monitoring of the product bioburden and its resistance to the sterilization method is required. Development studies using this strategy can be performed prior to disqualifying a device or drug product for terminal sterilization. If the device, drug product, and packaging system function as intended after terminal sterilization exposure, a cycle achieving an F_0 of ≥ 2 should be performed because it offers more safety when compared to using the same drug or device that may not be exposed to a terminal sterilization process.[58]

Once the appropriate sterilization validation approach is chosen, a development and subsequent performance validation cycle can be performed. At this stage, physical and, if appropriate, microbiological data, will be collected in order to support the routine usage of the cycle. Physical data includes heat distribution data on empty and loaded chambers, the use of thermocouples to monitor temperature profiles, and heat penetration studies among other important measurements. Microbiological data most typically involves the use of BIs containing heat-resistant spore-forming organisms to further confirm lethality as well as bioburden determinations when applicable as discussed earlier. Although BIs can serve an important role in validating the performance of a sterilization cycle, their use should not take the place of physical measurements. Instead, they should be used to support the physical measurement data and complement it whenever appropriate. For example, when using a steam sterilization cycle to sterilize a container system outfitted with complex tubing, physical measurements may not always capture the ability of steam to adequately penetrate the unique load item(s). But, this can be verified during cycle development by placing a BI at the location identified as most difficult for steam penetration, the physical air removal and steam penetration data previously gathered can be further supported with that of the growth results of the BIs following exposure to a partial sterilization process. When used in physical and microbiological performance validations, it's important to ensure that BIs or other indicators are placed throughout the load, adjacent to thermocouples, at "cold spots" and slowest to heat/most difficult to penetrate locations previously identified during empty or loaded chamber assessment cycles. In addition to the empty chamber cycle, performance validations should include three cycles per load configuration (ie, three independent cycles for a maximum load and three independent cycles for a minimum load) to ensure reproducibility. Once the cycle has been validated, routine production can be carried out with or without the use of BIs for product release, where release can be based solely on that of the cycle physical data.

It is important to note that widely used steam sterilization cycles typically expose products to excessive and unnecessary levels of sterilization; however, for heat-labile solutions and heat-sensitive materials, terminal sterilization is still preferable to not performing terminal sterilization. The F_0 concept and bioburden-based design approach address this concern by allowing practitioners to assess microbial lethality at temperatures other than 121°C.

▶ UNDERSTANDING F_0 AND ITS PRACTICAL USAGE

In the European Pharmacopoeia, a prescribed steam sterilization cycle is 15 minutes at 121°C.[47] This is a widely cited steam sterilization overkill cycle based on a 12 $\log_{10}$ reduction of *G stearothermophilus* spores (with a $D_{121°C}$ of 1 min, therefore 12 × 1 min = a 12-min cycle and a further overkill of 3 min is added for additional assurance, resulting in a total cycle time of 15 min). This cycle is clearly an overkill cycle, but in many cases, it is preferable to use a sterilization exposure temperature other than 121°C. When moist heat steam sterilization is performed at specific temperature (T) (other than the generally recognized reference temperature of 121°C), then at T, the lethality can be equivalent to that of the process performed at 121°C. The time required at T to accomplish the same lethality as would be obtained at 121°C is known as the F_0-value (or $F_{121°C}$). Therefore, the F_0-value is defined in time and can be calculated prior to cycle initiation in order to determine how long of a cycle is required for a temperature other than 121°C or after the cycle to calculate total accumulated lethality (explained in more detail in the following text). Both cases require the use of a temperature coefficient model in order to calculate the expected lethality. In Europe, for example, a minimum F_0 is recommended at 8 minutes and the lowest acceptable temperature for any moist heat steam process is 110°C[47]; however, it is not necessary to define a minimum F_0 of 8, as any F_0 with an appropriate validated and well-defined terminal sterilization can be acceptable.[58] To fully understand F_0, it is important to understand its related values, the D-value, z-value, and SAL. As briefly defined earlier, the *D- (decimal or decay) value* is the time required, at a specified temperature (in the case of heat sterilization), to reduce the microbial population by one logarithmic value (ie, by a factor of 10) from the initial value. For example, the D-value for a given bacterial spore preparation at 121°C would be given as $D_{121°C}$ = 1 minute. The *z-value* is the temperature coefficient of microbial destruction, being the change in temperature required to alter the D-value by a factor of 10. The z-value for a population of bacterial spores subjected to steam sterilization is often assumed or tested to be approximately 10°C. Finally, the *SAL* is the probability of a single viable microorganism occurring on an item after sterilization, expressed as the negative exponent to the base 10. Because it is not possible to confirm directly if a process was capable of destroying all organisms and rendering all product sterile, the probability of

survival of an individual microorganism can never be zero but can be reduced to a low level. An effective sterilization process has a low SAL (higher negative exponent). It is important to remember that the SAL is a probability, not an estimate of how many items are sterile or not. An example is given with a glass vial manufacturer. The bioburden of each glass vial in this case is 100 CFUs per unit and, therefore, a 2 $\log_{10}$ (or 100 CFUs) reduction would be theoretically required to render the vials "sterile." If a moist heat steam sterilization process, by definition, causes a 1 log reduction (D-value) after a 1-minute exposure at 121°C, then at least 2 minutes of exposure would be required to reduce the 100 CFUs to zero. But, if the bioburden varied, for example, to 101 or 110 CFUs, it would also be assumed that a proportion of those vials would not be considered sterile. As the exposure time of the sterilization process increases, the probability of sterility increases, and there is less probability of the survival of a single microorganism. Today, the most widely used SAL is 10^{-6}, which in this example would equate to a minimum 8-minute exposure time (2 min to reduce the known, theoretical population on each vial of 100 and a further 6 min to give an SAL of 10^{-6}). Therefore, a theoretical 8-min cycle at 121°C in a controlled steam process would be an acceptable sterilization process for these vials.

As mentioned and with respect to steam, the F_0-value is the equivalent exposure time at 121°C and z-value of 10°C. An example of an overkill cycle would be a process providing an F_0 = 12 minutes, essentially assuming a starting bioburden of 10^6, a 6 $\log_{10}$ reduction of the population, and a further 6 log 10 reduction to give an SAL of 10^{-6}. As the temperature goes below 121°C, the predicted lethality will decrease because it takes longer for the population to be inactivated, and as it increases above 121°C, the lethality will increase (Figure 28.8). The typical phases of a heat sterilization cycle involve (1) heating up, (2) exposure/holding, and (3) cooling down (Figure 28.9). In a standard cycle, it is only when the sterilization exposure set point parameters are reached that the contact time begins and sterilization assurance is calculated. Within this context, the F_0 can be used to calculate what's referred to as accumulated lethality during the whole exposure cycle. This concept calculates the lethality achieved at temperatures other than 121°C that are recorded during the heating up and cooling down phases of a cycle. The summation of lethality calculated from this step can then be added to the known lethality achieved during the exposure time to determine the total lethality that the product was subjected to.

Thus, in combination with the depth of knowledge surrounding the lethality of heat, the concept of F_0 allows the user to take into consideration the heating up and cooling down phases of a sterilization cycle. Because heat-resistant spores typically begin to die at temperatures of approximately 110°C, conservative F_0 cycles typically do not include temperatures lower than that value because

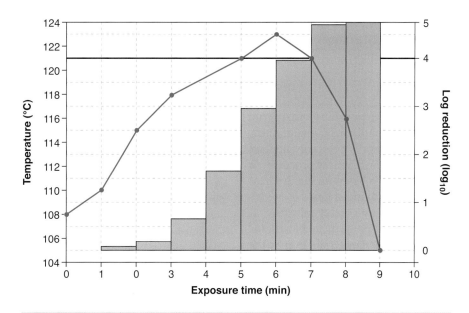

FIGURE 28.8 Cumulative lethality (log reduction) of *Geobacillus stearothermophilus* spores exposed to a sterilization cycle with a set exposure time of ≥121°C (solid horizontal line) for 2 min. The temperature profile is plotted, and lethality shown as a bar graph (cumulating to approximately 5 log reduction). There is little to no appreciable log reduction below 110°C, but this increases as the temperature increases to above 121°C.

it is safe to assume minimal spore reductions are occurring. Note that when using bioburden-based monitoring of a load, microbial death may be calculated at temperatures lower than 110°C depending on the contaminating microorganism's resistance to heat.

In addition to using F_0 to calculate accumulated lethality, this type of calculation can also be used to calculate total lethality at temperatures other than the standard reference temperature of 121°C. An F_0 of 12 minutes means the product was exposed to the equivalent of 12 minutes at 121°C but as described earlier does not require a dwell time of exactly 12 minutes at 121°C. In the equation for F_0,

it is shown that lethality accumulates over the course of the process:

$$F_0 = \Delta t \sum 10^{T - 121 / z}$$

Where: Δt = time interval between two next measurements of T
T = temperature of the sterilized product at time t
Z = temperature coefficient, assumed to be equal to 10°C

When using this equation to assess a sterilization cycle lasting 15 minutes at a constant temperature of 121°C, as expected from the definition of F_0, the result is 15 minutes.

$F_0 = 15 \times 10^{121 - 121 / 10} = 15 \times 10^0 = 15 \times 1 = 15$ minutes

However, if we keep the same 15-minute sterilization cycle but change the temperature by 10°C to 111°C, we instead obtain:

$F_0 = 15 \times 10^{111 - 121 / 10} = 15 \times 10^{-10 / 10} = 15^{-1} = 1.5$ minutes

It can be seen that a steam sterilization cycle lasting 15 minutes at 111°C is equivalent, in terms of lethal effect, to 1.5 minutes at 121°C. Therefore, if a practitioner wanted to achieve the same lethality of a 15-minute cycle

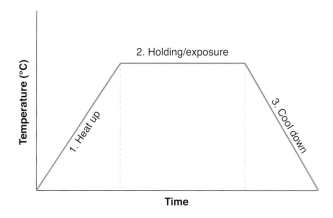

FIGURE 28.9 Typical autoclave processing phases (heat up, hold/sterilization, and cooling).

at 121°C at a temperature of 111°C, they would need to sterilize the load for approximately 10 times the amount of time or 150 minutes in this example:

$$F_0 = 150 \times 10^{111 - 121/10} = 150 \times 10^{-10/10} = 15 \text{ minutes}$$

It should be noted that these relationships remain true only if exposure to moist-heat conditions is maintained, and for this reason, the F_0 concept is primarily applied to moist heat steam processes. For dry heat processes, a similar concept of F_H is used and is based on the dry heat resistance profiles in comparison to moist heat.

Steam sterilization can therefore be successfully used as a terminal step for a wide range of products and loads, including more sensitive pharmaceutical materials. Even in the absence of an "overkill" cycle, sterilization with a high probability of assurance can still be obtained by the appropriate selection of alternative sterilization parameters. One approach, as discussed earlier, is the bioburden method, where the sterilization temperature and exposure time are based on the products' actual bioburden count and heat resistance.

In many manufacturing facilities, the environment and subsequently the bioburden of the product being subjected to sterilization can be controlled. In many cases, the bioburden may consist of vegetative bacteria shed from personnel (such as *Staphylococcus* species), and if this is found to be consistently low (eg, $\leq$100 CFUs) and to have a $D_{121°C}$ at 100 times less than that of *G stearothermophilus* spores, the challenge is much lower for sterilization. Therefore, a much shorter exposure to the sterilization temperature is necessary to achieve a 10^{-6} SAL. As seen in the following example using realistic bioburden data, the product would only need to be subjected to moist heat steam conditions for 0.16 minutes at 121°C in order to reduce the bioburden by 8 logs (from a starting population up to 100 CFUs/product) and achieve an SAL of 10^{-6}.

If $n = 100$ or $\log_{10} = 2$ and $D = 0.02$

The total log reduction (TLR) necessary for a 10^{-6} SAL = $2 + 6 = 8$ logs

10^{-6} SAL = TLR $\times$ D = 8×0.02 is only 0.16 minutes at 121°C

When applying this same realistic bioburden data to a steam sterilization cycle at 121°C with an F_0 target of 12, the calculation of the SAL is

$$\text{Log } N_u = (-F) / D + \text{Log } N_0$$

$$N_u = \text{SAL}$$

D = D-value of the natural bioburden, 0.02 minutes

F = F-value of the process (lethality)

N_0 = bioburden population per container = 100 CFUs

$$\text{Log } N_u = (-12) / 0.02 + 2 = -598$$

$$\text{SAL} = 10^{-598}$$

Such a process would provide a significant (and unnecessarily conservative) SAL, and a lower temperature and time combination could be used to achieve the objective of a 10^{-6} or lesser SAL and reduce negative risks such as impact to product and package integrity. Product potency can often be a limiting step for the attainment of terminal sterilization of heat-labile products. By lowering the sterilization exposure temperature from 121.1°C to 111.1°C, for example, the D-valve will become 0.2 minutes when using the accepted z-value of 10°C. However, note that the estimated D-values depicted here for non–spore-forming bacterial species, such as *Staphylococcus aureus*, are conservative. The D-values for several vegetative bacterial pathogens were recently reinvestigated and estimated at higher temperatures based on a conservative z-value of 10°C (Table 28.6).[72] Therefore, with a knowledge of the bioburden, the extent of overkill present in heat sterilization process can be significant and can be used to optimize terminal sterilization processes for product applications that may have been traditionally considered damaging to products and manufactured by aseptic processing (see chapter 58).[54]

Parametric Release

An important concept regarding validation of a heat process is the use of physical parameter monitoring for the parametric release of sterilized product loads.[73] Parametric release is the acceptance of the attainment of sterility in a sterilization load, without the use of BIs or end-product sterility testing to verify microbial inactivation. This type of verification mechanism requires that the sterilization cycle first be designed and validated to achieve the desired SAL. Batches or lots of terminally sterilized products can then be released according to the critical parameters defined during validation. A few examples of critical operating parameters may include dwell time limits, minimum and maximum limits for process peak dwell temperature, and average peak dwell temperature. When time and temperature relationships are well characterized, it is acceptable to also use F_0 as a critical parameter. Note that although the inclusion of a BI is not necessary in routine loads to be released by a parametric process, they may be included during initial cycle validation as an effort to complement or verify the physical parameters. It is important to ensure product release is based on well-supported scientific rationale as well as documented validation data because use of a parametric release program often requires prior regulatory approval.[74] When parametric release programs are based on sterilization methods other than that of an overkill method (eg, bioburden based as described earlier), it is necessary to have microbiological control programs in place to ensure the manufacturing facilities

TABLE 28.6	D-valves for vegetative bacteria, estimated D-valves at different temperatures, assuming a z-valve of 10°C and $N_0 = 100$ CFU ($\log_{10} = 2$), and estimated sterility assurance levels[a]						
	Reported Value (min)	Estimated Values[b] (min)			TLR for 10^{-6} SAL	Minutes at 121°C Needed for 10^{-6} SAL[c]	$F_0 = 1$ Estimated SAL[d]
	$D_{60°C}$	$D_{80°C}$	$D_{100°C}$	$D_{121°C}$			
Escherichia coli	2.0	0.02	0.0002	0.000002		0.00002	$10^{-500\,000}$
Salmonella species	2.5	0.03	0.0003	0.000003		0.000024	$10^{-333\,330}$
Staphylococcus aureus	3.0	0.03	0.0003	0.000003	8	0.000024	$10^{-333\,330}$
Listeria monocytogenes	16.7	0.2	0.001	0.00002		0.0002	$10^{-50\,000}$

Abbreviations: CFU, colony-forming unit; SAL, sterility assurance level.

[a]From Pflug.[72]

[b]Based on $D_{60°C}$[72] and z-value of 10°C.

[c]SAL 10^{-6} = total log reduction (TLR) × D-valve.

[d]Estimated SAL based on an $F_0 = 1$; Log $N_u = (-F) / D + $ Log N_0.

state of microbial control remains similar to how it was during validation. This means gathering environmental data from the manufacturing site itself as well as periodically confirming product bioburden prior to sterilization. Any identification of new contaminants that have a higher count or resistance to the organisms used to previously validate the sterilization process would trigger the need to reassess the cycle and possibly revalidate (Table 28.6).

REFERENCES

1. Hugo WB. A brief history of heat and chemical preservation and disinfection. *J Appl Bacteriol.* 1991;71(1):9-18.
2. Berry MR, Pflug IJ. Canning. In: Caballero B, Finglas P, Toldra F, eds. *Encyclopedia of Food Sciences and Nutrition.* 2nd ed. Academic Press; 2003:817.
3. Busta FF, Ordal ZJ. Heat-inactivation kinetics of endospores of *Bacillus subtilis. J Food Sci.* 1964;29:345-353.
4. Curran HR, Evans FR. Heat inactivation inducing germination in the spores of thermotolerant and thermophilic aerobic bacteria. *J Bacteriol.* 1945;49:335-346.
5. Curran HR, Evans FR. The viability of heat-activatable spores in nutrient and nonnutrient substrates as influenced by prestorage and post-storage heating. *J Bacteriol.* 1946;51:567-568.
6. Curran HR, Evans FR. The viability of heat-activatable spores in nutrient and nonnutrient substrates as influenced by pre-storage and post-storage heating and other factors. *J Bacteriol.* 1947;53:103-113.
7. Evans FR, Curran HR. The accelerating effect of sublethal heat on spore germination in mesophilic aerobic bacteria. *J Bacteriol.* 1943;46:513-523.
8. Shull JJ, Ernst RR. Graphical procedure for comparing thermal death of *Bacillus stearothermophilus* spores in saturated and superheated steam. *Appl Microbiol.* 1962;10:452-457.
9. Angelotti R. Protective mechanisms affecting dry-heat sterilization. In: Sneath PNA, ed. *Sterilization Techniques for Instruments and Materials as Applied to Space Research.* Paris, France: Muray-Print; 1968:59-74. COSPAR technical manual no. 4.
10. Sherman JM, Albus WR. Physiological youth in bacteria. *J Bacteriol.* 1923;8:127-138.
11. Sherman JM, Cameron GM. Lethal environmental factors within the natural range of growth. *J Bacteriol.* 1934;27:341-348.
12. Robertson AH. Influence of age on the heat resistance of non-spore forming bacteria. *J Bacteriol.* 1928;15:28.
13. Stark CN, Stark P. The relative thermal death rates of young and mature bacterial cells. *J Bacteriol.* 1929;18:333-337.
14. Anderson EB, Meanwell U. Studies in bacteriology of low temperature pasteurization: part II. The heat resistance of a thermoduric *Streptococcus* grown at different temperatures. *J Dairy Res.* 1936;7:182-191.
15. Ellicker PR, Frazier WC. Influence of time and temperature of incubation on heat resistance of *Escherichia coli. J Bacteriol.* 1938;36:83-98.
16. Bréand S, Fardel G, Flandrois JP, Rosso L, Tomassone R. Model of the influence of time and mild temperature on *Listeria monocytogenes* nonlinear survival curves. *Int J Food Microbiol.* 1998;40:185-195.
17. Weil R. Zur biologie der milzbrandbazillen. *Arch Hyg Bakteriol.* 1899;35:355-408.
18. Sames T. Zur Kenntnis der bei höher Temperature wachsenden Bakterien und Streptococcusarten. *Zeitschrift für Hyg Infektionsk.* 1900;33:313-362.
19. Williams OB. The heat resistance of bacterial spores. *J Infect Dis.* 1929;44:421-465.
20. Curran HR. The influence of some environmental factors upon thermal resistance of bacterial spores. *J Bacteriol.* 1934;27:28.
21. Sobernheim G, Mündel O. Grundsatzliches zue technick der sterilisations prufing: II. Verhalten der erdsporen bei der dampfsterilisation. Ihre ignung als sporen test. *Z Hyg Infectionskrankh.* 1938;121:90-112.
22. Lamanna C. Relation of maximum growth temperature to resistance to heat. *J Bacteriol.* 1942;44:29-35.
23. Sugiyama H. Studies on factors affecting the heat resistance of spores of *Clostridium botulinum. J Bacteriol.* 1951;62:81-96.
24. El-Bisi HM, Ordal ZJ. The effect of certain sporulation conditions on the thermal death rate of *Bacillus coagulans* var. thermoacidurans. *J Bacteriol.* 1956;71:1-9.
25. Nank WK, Schmidt CF. The effect of the addition of manganese to a nutrient agar sporulation medium upon the resistance of thermophilic flat sour spore crops. *Bacteriol Proc.* 1958;42.
26. Lechowich RV, Ordal ZJ. The influence of the sporulation temperature on the heat resistance and chemical composition of bacterial spores. *Can J Microbiol.* 1962;8:287-295.
27. Gerhardt P, Marquis RE. Spore thermoresistance mechanisms. In: Smith I, Slepecky RA, Setlow P, eds. *Regulation of Procariotic Development.* Washington, DC: American Society for Microbiology; 1989:43-63.
28. Streips UN, Qoronfleh MW, Khoury PH, et al. Involvement of heat shock proteins in the heat resistance of *Bacillus subtilis* spores. In: *Program of Tenth International Spore Conference.* Woods Hole, MA: Marine Biological Laboratory; 1988:8.

29. Mackey BM, Derrick CM. Changes in heat resistance of *Salmonella typhimurium* during heating at rising temperatures. *Lett Appl Microbiol.* 1987;4:13-16.

30. Cameron MS, Leonard SJ, Barrett EL. Effect of moderately acidic pH on heat resistance and recovery of *Clostridium sporogenes* spores in phosphate buffer and buffered pea puree. *Appl Environ Microbiol.* 1980;5:943-949.

31. Fernández PS, Ocio MJ, Rodrigo F, Rodrigo M, Martínez A. Mathematical model for the combined effect of temperature and pH on the thermal resistance of *Bacillus stearothermophilus* and *Clostridium sporogenes* spores. *Int J Food Microbiol.* 1996;32:225-233.

32. Chapman PA, Pflug IJ. Effect of the biological indicator envelope on the heat destruction rate of *Bacillus stearothermophilus* spores. *Bacteriol Proc.* 1973;73:E144.

33. Pflug IJ, Smith GM. The use of biological indicators for monitoring wet heat sterilization processes. In: Gaughran ERL, Kereluk K, eds. *Sterilization of Medical Products.* New Brunswick, NJ: Johnson & Johnson; 1977:193-230.

34. Smith G, Kopelman M, Jones A, et al. Effect of environmental conditions during heating on commercial spore strip performance. *Appl Environ Microbiol.* 1982;44:12-18.

35. Pflug IJ. *Microbiology and Engineering of Sterilization Processes.* 10th ed. Minneapolis, MN: Environmental Sterilization Laboratory, University of Minnesota; 1999.

36. Koesterer MG. *Studies for Sterilization of Space Probe Components.* Rochester, NY: Wilmot Castle Co; 1965. National Aeronautics and Space Administration contract no. NASW-879.

37. Bond WW, Favero MS, Petersen NJ, Marshall JH. Relative frequency distribution of $D_{125°C}$ values for spore isolates from the Mariner-Mars 1969 spacecraft. *Appl Microbiol.* 1971;21:832-836.

38. Campbell JE. *Ecology and thermal inactivation of microbes in and on interplanetary space vehicle components. 37th Quarterly Report of Progress.* Washington, DC: National Aeronautics and Space Administration: 1974. National Aeronautics and Space Administration order no. W-13411.

39. Bond WW, Favero MS, Korber MR. *Bacillus* sp. ATCC 27380: a spore with extreme resistance to dry heat. *Appl Microbiol.* 1973;26:614-616.

40. Doyle JE, Ernst RR. Resistance of *Bacillus subtilis* var. *niger* spores occluded in water-insoluble crystals to three sterilization agents. *Appl Microbiol.* 1967;15:726-730.

41. Mullican CL, Hoffman RK. Dry heat or gaseous chemical resistance of *Bacillus subtilis* var. *niger* spores included within water-soluble crystals. *Appl Microbiol.* 1968;16:1110-1113.

42. Puleo JR, Favero MS, Oxborrow GS, Herring CM. Method for collecting naturally occurring airborne bacterial spores for determining their thermal resistance. *Appl Microbiol.* 1975;30:786-790.

43. Friedline AW, Zachariah MM, Middaugh AN, Garimella R, Vaishampayan PA, Rice CV. Sterilization resistance of bacterial spores explained with water chemistry. *J Phys Chem B.* 2015;119(44):14033-14044.

44. Bigelow WD. The logarithmic nature of thermal death time curves. *J Infect Dis.* 1921;29:528-536.

45. Pflug IJ. Discussion of the Z-value to use in calculating the F0-value for high temperature sterilization processes. *PDA J Pharm Sci Technol.* 1996;50:51-54.

46. Stoforos N, Noronha J, Hendrickx M, et al. A critical analysis of mathematical procedures for the evaluation and design of in-container thermal processes for foods. *Crit Rev Food Sci Nutr.* 1997;37:411-441.

47. European Pharmacopoeia. *Ph Eur 9.2, 5.1.1. Methods of Preparation of Sterile Products.* Strasbourg, France: European Pharmacopoeia; 2017.

48. Joslyn LJ. Sterilization by heat. In: Block SS, ed. *Disinfection, Sterilization, and Preservation.* 5th ed. Philadelphia, PA: Lippincott Williams & Wilkins; 2001:695-728

49. Pflug IJ, Holcomb RG, Gomez MM. Principles of the thermal destruction of microorganisms. In: Block SS, ed. *Disinfection, Sterilization, and Preservation.* Philadelphia, PA: Lippincott William & Wilkins; 2001:79-129.

50. British Standards Institution. *EN 285:2015. Sterilization—Steam Sterilizers—Large Sterilizers.* London, United Kingdom: British Standards Institution; 2016.

51. Walter CW. Sterilization. *Surg Clin North Am.* 1948;28:350.

52. Savage RHM. Experiments on the sterilizing effects of mixtures of air and steam, and of superheated steam. *Q J Pharmacol.* 1937;10:451-462.

53. United States Pharmacopeia. *42-NF 37, General Chapter <1229.1> Steam Sterilization by Direct Contact.* Bethesda, MD: United States Pharmacopeia; 2019.

54. United States Pharmacopeia. *42-NF 37, General Chapter <1229.2> Moist Heat Sterilization of Aqueous Liquids.* Bethesda, MD: United States Pharmacopeia; 2019.

55. Cundell AM. Justification for the aseptic filling for sterile injectable products. *PDA J Pharm Sci Technol.* 2014;68(4):323-332.

56. Agalloco JP. Increasing patient safety by closing the sterile production gap-part 1. Introduction. *PDA J Pharm Sci Technol.* 2017;71(4):261-268.

57. European Agency for the Evaluation of Medicinal Products. *Note for Guidance on Manufacture of the Finished Dosage Form.* London, United Kingdom: European Agency for the Evaluation of Medicinal Products; 1996.

58. Sasaki T. Parametric release for moist heated pharmaceutical products in Japan. *PDA Journal of GMP and Validation in Japan.* 2002;4(1).

59. International Organization for Standardization. *ISO 17665-1:2006: Sterilization of Health Care Products—Moist Heat—Part 1: Requirements for the Development, Validation and Routine Control of a Sterilization Process for Medical Devices.* Geneva, Switzerland: International Organization for Standardization; 2006.

60. Joslyn LJ. *Empirical Determination of Steam Flow Rates for Maximum Gravity Displacement Efficiency. Research Project.* Macedon, NY: Joslyn Valve Co; 1976.

61. Parental Drug Association. *Validation of Moist Heat Sterilization Processes: Cycle Design, Development, Qualification and Ongoing Control.* Bethesda, MD: Parental Drug Association; 2007. PDA technical report no. 1.

62. Prince DL, Mastej J, Easton D, Hoverman I, Chatterjee R. *Case Study: Moist Heat Sterilization of Reusable Device and Tray System.* Chagrin Falls, OH: Bonezone; 2013.

63. Beck WC, Collette TS. False faith in the surgeon's gown and surgical drape. *Am J Surg.* 1952;83:125.

64. Probst HD. The effect of bacterial agents on the sterility of surgical linen. *Am J Surg.* 1953;86:301-308.

65. United States Pharmacopeia. *42-NF 37, General Chapter <1231> Water for Pharmaceutical Purposes.* Bethesda, MD: United States Pharmacopeia; 2019.

66. Penikett EJK, Rowe TWG, Robinson E. Vacuum drying of steam sterilized dressings. *J Appl Microbiol.* 1959;71:282-290.

67. United States Pharmacopoeia. *42-NF 37, General Chapter <1229.8> Dry heat sterilization.* Bethesda, MD: United States Pharmacopeia; 2019.

68. Parental Drug Association. *Validation of Dry Heat Processes Used for Depyrogenation and Sterilization.* Bethesda, MD: Parental Drug Association; 2013. PDA technical report no. 3.

69. International Organization for Standardization. *ISO 20857:2013: Sterilization of Health Care Products—Dry Heat—Requirements for the Development, Validation, and Routine Control of a Sterilization Process for Medical Devices.* Geneva, Switzerland: International Organization for Standardization; 2013.

70. Tsuji K, Harrison S. Dry-heat destruction of lipopolysaccharide: dry-heat destruction kinetics. *Appl Environ Microbiol.* 1978;36(5):710-714.

71. American National Standards Institute, Association for the Advancement of Medical Instrumentation. *ANSI/AAMI ST8:2013. Hospital Steam Sterilizers.* Arlington, VA: Association for the Advancement of Medical Instrumentation.

72. Pflug I. *Microbiology and Engineering of Sterilization Processes.* 14th ed. Otterbein, IN: Environmental Sterilization Laboratory; 2010.

73. United States Pharmacopeia. *42-NF 37, General Chapter <1222> Terminally Sterilized Pharmaceutical Products-Parametric Release.* Bethesda, MD: United States Pharmacopeia; 2019.

74. US Food and Drug Administration. *Guidance for Industry: Submission of Documentation in Applications for Parametric Release of Human and Veterinary Drug Products Terminally Sterilized by Moist Heat Processes.* Silver Spring, MD: US Food and Drug Administration; 2010.

Sterilization and Preservation by Radiation

John R. Logar and Elaine Daniell

The use of radiation for industrial application requires a multidisciplinary approach. There is a materials related component regarding the determination of the radiation effect (ie, cross-linking or degradation) of the product and/or packaging materials; a physics-related component regarding the determination of the absorbed-dose distribution throughout the product loading configuration used in the irradiation process; and, for sterile products, there is a microbiology-related component regarding the determination of the radiation resistance of the microbiological population on the product. The three main industrial applications of ionizing radiation are the sterilization of health care products, modification of materials, and the preservation of food. The industrial application of radiation for the sterilization of health care products is widespread, and its application is well established because it has been proven to be economical and reliable. Sterilization is used for the elimination of microorganisms on health care products to greatly reduce and/or eliminate the potential for patient infection from the sterilized product. Radiation sterilization uses energy from a radiation source to pass through the material to deactivate the microorganisms present. By contrast, the industrial application of radiation for both the preservation and enhanced microbial quality of food has experienced limited application due to consumer confidence in the process (benefit versus impact) even though the process is very similar to food pasteurization (the reduction and elimination of certain pathogenic microorganisms such as *Listeria*, *Escherichia coli*, and *Salmonella*). The third application of ionizing radiation is focused on the modification of materials by scission or cross-linking chemical bonds to deliver a predetermined effect and create an alternate form of the material (eg, cross-linked polyethylene, wire coating). For this chapter, we primarily focus on the use of ionizing radiation for the sterilization of health care products and the modification of materials used in health care products.

The history of processing with radiation in the health care industry began in the early 1950s. The first attempts were with electron beam irradiation, but due to the unreliability of the equipment available at the time, this method was abandoned. It was not until the advent of the use of cobalt 60 (^{60}Co) isotope in the early 1960s that routine processing with radiation truly began. From the 1960s to today, there have been continual advances in the design and reliability of the irradiation equipment and thus the continued expansion in the use of both gamma and electron beam radiation applications. Additionally, in the late 1990s, with the development of high energy, high-current electron beam technology, the radiation processing industry renewed its interest in the use of electron beam and X-ray irradiation. That interest and expansion continues today. As a result, there are many types of irradiator designs and applications available to the health care industry that enables the selection of the most effective and efficient process for products and applications.

SOURCES OF RADIATION ENERGY

In general, radiation may be classified into two groups, electromagnetic and particle radiation. For the various types of radiation in the electromagnetic spectrum, they produce antimicrobial effects by transferring the energy of an electron or photon into characteristic ionizations in or near a biological target. In addition to creating pairs of positive and negative electrons, ions can also produce free radicals and activated molecules. These effects, which are produced without any appreciable rise (compared to other sterilization modalities) in temperature, have been termed *cold sterilization* because it relates to the destruction of microorganisms.

Electromagnetic Radiation

Of the types of electromagnetic radiation used for the destruction of microorganisms, microwave, ultraviolet, gamma, and X-rays, only the latter two are dealt within this chapter (for others, see chapters 9 and 10). The X-ray and gamma radiation, although nearly identical in nature, have different origins. The emission of an X-ray from an atom occurs when there is a transition of an electron from an outer shell to a vacancy in an inner shell; this is produced by bombarding a heavy metal target (eg, tantalum) with high-energy electrons from an electron beam accelerator. Gamma radiation is the result of a transition of an atomic nucleus from an excited state to a ground state, as seen in most radioactive materials, yielding electromagnetic radiation. The difference between gamma rays and X-rays are the wavelength frequency and energy spectrum of the emitted photons. X-rays and gamma rays have essentially the similar penetrating power because they carry no charge; however, the maximum energy of the electrons used to create the X-rays creates a subset of higher energy photons that will result in greater penetration.

The radioisotopes that are typically used for gamma processing are ^{60}Co and cesium 137 (^{137}Cs). The ^{60}Co is produced as an intentional by-product of nuclear reactors used to produce electricity. It is formed when naturally occurring ^{59}Co absorbs an additional neutron, creating the radioisotope ^{60}Co. This radioisotope has a half-life of 5.27 years and decays with the emission of two high-energy gamma rays (1.17 and 1.33 MeV) and a lower energy (0.318 MeV) β particle to become the nonradioactive element nickel 60 (^{60}Ni). Because of an isotope's decay, it is necessary to periodically replenish the isotope to maintain a desired throughput capacity. The ^{60}Co is the radioisotope most commonly used for industrial radiation sterilization due to its availability and effectiveness in delivering the intended effect.

The ^{137}Cs is also produced as a nuclear reactor by-product. It is formed during the separation of chemicals from other nuclear wastes and is then encapsulated. The ^{137}Cs exists as cesium chloride, which is readily soluble in water. This radioisotope has a half-life of 30 years and decays with the emission of two β particles (0.51 and 1.17 MeV) and one gamma ray (0.66 MeV) to become barium 137 (^{137}Ba). The lower energy gamma ray produced as ^{137}Cs decays results in a reduction in penetrating power compared with ^{60}Co. Typically, the capsules for storage of ^{137}Cs are intended for dry storage, due to the repeated thermo-quenching required with wet storage and the increased risk of encapsulation failures. Therefore, this isotope is not currently used for the industrial radiation processing applications. Other radioisotopes have been investigated for industrial application but have not been developed further because of high production costs, limited commercial availability, low penetrating power, or short half-life.

Particle Radiation

Particles usually considered of importance in radiation biology are the α, β, neutron, meson, positron, and neutrino. The only particle currently applicable to sterilization is the β particle or electron. The α particles, although capable of causing dense ionizations, have limited penetrating ability; neutrons, which are uncharged, have great penetrating power but are unacceptable because they can induce radioactivity. Mesons and protons are produced only by expensive, high-energy machines and are therefore not used for industrial application. The β radiation, arising from the decay of an isotope source, consists of electrons with a single negative charge, a low mass and low energy; because of their low energy, these electrons cannot penetrate materials deeply.

Electrons produced by machines can be emitted or accelerated to a predetermined energy. The higher the energy electron produced, the greater the penetration into materials, products, and packages. Machines that are used in the acceleration of electrons vary in both their design and output with regard to energy and power. This flexibility enables the user to customize the machine to the application. The range of machine energy and power, and examples of their applications, are provided in Table 29.1. Electron beam emitters produce low-energy electrons in the range of 80 to 300 kV and machine-accelerated electrons fall into low-, medium-, and high-energy categories; 100 keV to 25 MeV. For machine-accelerated electrons, the accelerating field

TABLE 29.1   Machine classification, design, and application

Classification	Machine Type	Energy Range (MeV)	Power Upper Limit (kW)	Application Examples
Low	DC	<1	300	Treat web stock to obtain a chemical reaction (cross-linking, surface modification).
Medium	DC	1-5	200	Sterilize health care products.
High	Radiofrequency Microwave AC	>5	150	Sterilize health care products and pasteurize food.

Abbreviations: AC, alternating current; DC, direct current.

TABLE 29.2 Units and conversion factors in radiation	
Units of Measure for Sterilization or Pasteurization	**Units of Measure for Personnel Safety**
1 Gy = 1 J/kg	1 Sv = 1 J/kg
1 Gy = 10^2 rad	1 Sv = 100 rem
1 kGy = 10^5 rad	1 mSv = 100 mrem
1 Mrad = 10^6 rad	
1 kGy = 0.1 Mrad	

is generated using direct current, radiofrequency or microwave energy. Once the electrons are accelerated to the desired energy, the beam can then be managed by magnetic fields to achieve such results as increasing its size, changing its shape, or scanning over a predetermined area.

Radiation Units

The fundamental measurement parameter in radiation processing is the amount of energy deposited per unit mass, which is referred to as *absorbed dose*. The unit of absorbed dose is the gray (Gy), where 1 Gy is equivalent to absorption of 1 J/kg (Table 29.2). Dose measurements are typically related to the amount of absorbed dose in water. This relationship is used because most of the products (health care products) that undergo radiation processing are focused on delivering a dose to microbiological flora and thus the targeted density is similar to water. The dose equivalent is used to express the quantity of dose used in radiation protection; it expresses all radiation on a common scale for calculating the effective absorbed dose. The units of dose equivalent are the sievert and rem. The radiation dose used for sterilization is typically expressed in the kGy unit of measure.

▶ EFFECTS OF IONIZING RADIATION

The primary effect of the absorption of high-energy radiation is ionization in matter. Ionization is the product of either direct interaction of charged particles with matter that dislodges both ions and individual atomic particles or an indirect interaction of a photon with atoms that causes electrons to be ejected. Ionization is the transformation of individual atoms or molecules from an uncharged or stable state to a charged or excited state. It is the formation of these excited state particles and their interactions that alter materials exposed to radiation.

At any given time, all portions of a material are not equally subjected to the energy of ionizing radiation. Ionizing radiation is by nature discrete, and in passage through a material, the photons or electrons produce a number of localized events along their passage or track. Certain portions of the material exposed to radiation may experience a slight alteration, whereas an adjacent area is subjected to intense energy. Along a track, photons of energy ionize the material and can produce free radicals and excited atoms. Secondary electrons, if they possess sufficient energy, ionize or excite additional adjacent atoms, forming a spur of delta rays (Figure 29.1). The sequence of events along a track is therefore localized and intense, and the alterations in affected molecules can be severe. Examples of ionization include the radiolysis of water or the formation of oxygen radicals. This breaking of chemical bonds and formation of free radicals results in changes to the structures of both materials and microorganisms.

Effects on Material

Polymers are typically described as chain-like molecules that contain either a carbon or silicone backbone structure. In general, the longer the chain, the greater the strength of the polymer. Exposure to radiation causes breakage of this backbone structure, and subsequently one of three reactions can occur. The first type of reaction that might occur is simply a recombination of the structure that does not result in a physical change. The second type of reaction is cross-linking, which is the combination of multiple chains to produce even longer chains with greater interaction between chains. This type of reaction can result in a physical change toward greater strength and consequently a decrease in the elongation properties of the polymer. The third type of reaction is chain scission, where the broken chain is terminated by something other than the original backbone molecule. The free radicals that are produced by the irradiation process often terminate this structure, and this results in a physical change characterized by a decrease in strength and elongation. Other types of radiation-induced changes to polymers can include color changes and odor inducement. In the manufacture of health care products that are composed of polymers, either a radiation-resistant polymer can be used or antioxidants can be added to the polymer base to minimize the effects of radiation processing.[1] The effects of radiation on metals are typically very small, especially at the doses necessary for sterilization.

The interaction of radiation with food also produces changes. At the doses required for food irradiation

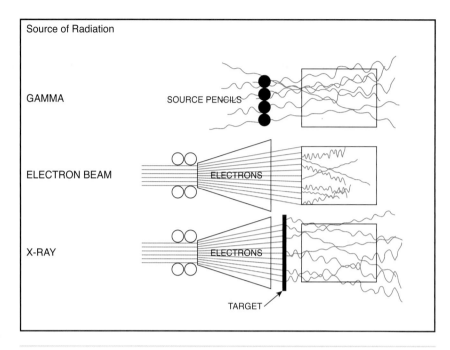

FIGURE 29.1   Interaction of gamma rays and electrons with matter.

(0.4-8 kGy), the changes are usually limited to nutritional quality, odor, taste, and color; however, the degree of change(s) is mostly related to the overall dose delivered (either no change up to significant change). The interaction with biological liquids, tissues, or drug components can also produce changes. At the doses used in the sterilization process, changes may occur that cause a degradation of the drug content or functional aspects of the biological liquids or tissue such as protein-based substances (eg, collagen, human or recombinant albumin, tissue). Radiation may modify these by breaking of the protein chains and disrupting the ability of the amino acid to combine with other polymers, which can change the function of the material. Fluids may undergo changes when exposed to radiation, the type and degree of which are based on the chemical makeup of the fluid, the dose, and the dose rate of the radiation process. As with all other materials, free radicals are produced that combine to result in a change in the fluid. The most observed and easiest to quantitate change is that of pH. Reactions in fluids are completed in less time than those in solid materials, thus resulting in less additional change over time.

▶ LETHAL EFFECTS OF RADIATION ON MICROORGANISMS

Intracellular Effects

Radiation can cause a wide variety of physical and biochemical effects in microorganisms. It is most likely that the primary cellular target governing loss of viability is the DNA molecule.[2] The radiation sensitivity of 79 organisms, ranging from viruses to higher plants and animals, was correlated with their nucleic acid volume.[3] The larger the nucleic acid volume, the more sensitive the microorganism was to radiation. It also appears that appreciable differences in radiation sensitivity may be the result of an ability to repair DNA damage or cellular protective properties such as the spore coats rather than an inherent radiation resistance of the DNA target.[4-7] Such protective and repair mechanisms are known to be important in microorganisms with higher resistance to radiation inactivation.[8] The damage to the DNA molecule by the radiation energy renders the microorganism unable to replicate, thereby eliminating the ability of the cell to remain viable.

For the purpose of this discussion, microbial survival is defined as the ability of a microorganism either to reproduce significantly in nutrient broth or to produce a colony-forming units (CFUs) on a recovery medium after exposure to radiation.

Survival Curves

The destruction or inactivation of microorganisms by radiation occurs in geometric progression. In other words, the same fraction of microorganisms is inactivated with application of successive increments of radiation; therefore, the radiation effect is cumulative. Graphing the logarithm of the surviving organisms against the amount of radiation dose can best plot this relationship. Some representative types of curves are shown in Figure 29.2. Curve 1 represents the exponential relationship previously described.[9] Curve 2 is representative of organisms

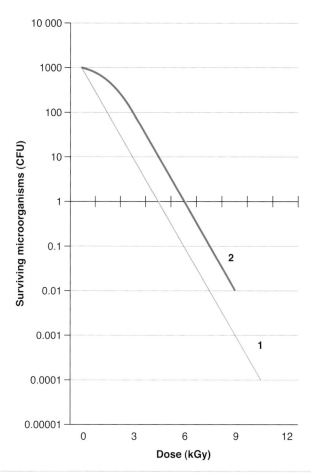

FIGURE 29.2 Schematic diagram of survival curves. The initial number, N_0, of microorganisms was 1000 colony-forming units. Curve 1 represents an exponential relationship, and curve 2 shows a shoulder effect before the exponential relationship is achieved.

that exhibit a shoulder effect before exponential inactivation, which may be due to repair mechanisms. Examples of these organisms are *Deinococcus* (originally *Micrococcus*) *radiodurans*[10] and radiation-resistant mutants of *Salmonella* ser Typhimurium.[4] These curves are indicative of typical homogeneous populations.

The number and types of microorganisms found on products before sterilization is typically referred to as the *bioburden*. Bioburden typically consists of a heterogeneous population of microorganisms, with a mixture of minimally to highly resistant microorganisms based on microorganism type and product environment (see the following text and chapter 64). The number of each type of microorganism varies based on raw materials, control of the manufacturing environment, type of manufacturing process (manual or automated), and geographic location of the manufacturing site. The resistance of a heterogeneous population is typically evaluated by eliminating the minimally resistant population of microorganisms using a low radiation dose and then characterizing the radiation resistance of the remaining population of

highly resistant microorganisms. For populations of microorganisms that have a radiation resistance similar to curve 1 in Figure 29.2, the D_{10} value can be obtained from any portion of the straight line. The D_{10} value in this case is defined as the radiation dose required to kill 90% of a homogeneous microbial population, where it is assumed that the death of microorganisms follows first-order kinetics. For populations of microorganisms that have a radiation resistance similar to curve 2, the D_{10} value can be best obtained from the straight-line portion. To determine the extent of radiation treatment, the shoulder effect may need to be considered.

The primary method for determining a D_{10} value is that of Stumbo et al. (1950).[11] This method adapted the most probable number (MPN) technique for obtaining the D_{10} value and derived an equation capable of describing either inoculated or indigenous microorganisms. From the MPN equation,[12]

$$\bar{x} = 2.303 \log\left(\frac{n}{q}\right) \quad (1)$$

where $\bar{x}$ is the MPN of surviving organisms per unit tested, n is the number of units irradiated, and q is the number of units rendered sterile. The D_{10} value is derived by using the equation

$$D_{10} = \frac{\text{dose}}{(\log \text{bioburden} - \log \bar{x})} \quad (2)$$

This model assumes exponential inactivation.

Radiation Resistance

The radiation resistance of microorganisms can be altered, either increased or decreased, by altering the environment that exists during irradiation. Representative factors that alter the radiation resistance are presented in Table 29.3. For example, if the radiation conditions are such that the supply of oxygen is not limited, the resistance of the organism can be decreased. In other words, if the supply of oxygen is limited for an aerobic organism or an anaerobic environment exists, the resistance of the aerobic organism may be increased.

Although many external factors may influence the radiation resistance of various microorganisms, in general, microorganisms can be grouped based on their relative resistance (Table 29.4). Bacterial spores, with few exceptions, are generally the most resistant to radiation, gram-negative rods are the least resistant, and yeast and fungi have an intermediate resistance. There are specific organisms that have been found to show resistance to radiation such as *Roseomonas mucosa* and *D radiodurans*.[8] In some cases, the manufacturing environment may lead to increased resistance such as a harsh dry environment or freezing of product may increase resistance of spore-forming organisms and a bacterial biofilm in water sources or liquid vessels

TABLE 29.3　Factors that modify radiation resistance

Modifier	Examples	Effect on Resistance	Conditions That Influence Modifier
Atmosphere	Oxygen	Decrease	Reducing agents
			Protectors
			Anaerobiosis by microbial metabolism or by dose
Protectors	Sulfhydryl-containing compounds	Increase	Oxygen
	Reducing agents		pH
	Alcohols		Temperature
	Glycerol		
	Dimethyl sulfoxide		
	Proteins		
	Carbohydrates		
Sensitizers	N-Ethylmaleimide	Decrease	Oxygen
	Quinones		pH
	Iodoacetic acid		Temperature
	p-Chloromercuribenzoic acid		Protectors
	Nitrous oxide		Catalase
	Dimethyl sulfoxide		Superoxide dismutase
	Halides		OH scavengers
	Nitrites		Spore or vegetative cell
	Nitrates		
	Radiation products		
	H_2O_2		
Temperature	Freezing	Increase	
	Elevated	Decrease	
Water content of cell	Desiccation of cell	Increase—vegetative	Relative humidity
		Decrease—spore or yeasts	Oxygen
Recovery technique	Incubation temperature	Variable	
	Composition of medium		
	Salts		
	Diluent		
	Oxygen		
Age of microorganism		Variable	Dependent on stage in organism life cycle
Dose rate	High-dose rate	Increase	Oxygen

Abbreviations: H_2O_2, hydrogen peroxide; OH, hydroxide.

may increase organism resistance due to repeated contact with chemical disinfectants. This increased resistance may require a radiation pretreatment of raw materials or components to mitigate resistance developed by the microbial flora. Alternatively, another sterilization method might be selected for pretreatment of raw materials or components, depending on the microorganism observed and the root cause of the increased radiation resistance.

MICROBIAL VALIDATION AND ESTABLISHMENT OF DOSE

Typically, the product radiation sterilization dose is validated using the published methods by International Organization for Standardization (ISO)[28,29] along with other technical publications.[30,31] The method chosen for establishing the sterilization dose may be based on the natural

TABLE 29.4	Radiation resistance of microorganisms and other biological units			
Species	D_{10}[a]	Presence of a Shoulder (kGy)	Menstruum Used for Irradiation	References
Anaerobic spore formers				
Clostridium botulinum				
Type A 36	3.3	4.0	Buffer	Grecz[13]
Type B	1.1-3.3	4.0-10.0	Buffer	Grecz[13] and Roberts and Ingram[14]
Type D	2.2	2.5-3.5	Water	Roberts and Ingram[14]
Type E beluga	0.8	2.5-3.5	Water	Roberts and Ingram[14]
Type F	2.5	2.5-3.5	Water	Roberts and Ingram[14]
Types A, B	3.4-4.2		Beef	Krieger et al[15]
Clostridium sporogenes	1.6-2.2	2.5-3.5	Water	Roberts and Ingram[14]
Clostridium perfringens	1.2-2.0	2.5-3.5	Water	Roberts and Ingram[14]
Clostridium tetani	2.4	2.5-3.5	Water	Roberts and Ingram[14]
Aerobic spore formers				
Bacillus subtilis	0.6		Saline + 5% gelatin	Lawrence et al[16]
Bacillus pumilus E601	1.7	11.0	Water	Van Winkle et al[17]
B pumilus E601	3.0		Dried	Van Winkle et al[17]
B pumilus ATCC 27142	1.4-4.0		Dried	Prince and Rubino[18]
Bacillus sphaericus C_1A	10.0		Dried, organic	Gaughran and Goudie[19]
Vegetative bacteria and fungi				
Salmonella ser Typhimurium	0.2		PO_4 buffer	Thornley[20]
S Typhimurium R6008	1.3	4.0	PO_4 buffer	Davies and Sinskey[4]
S Typhimurium	0.8		Egg yolk magma	Brogle et al[21]
Salmonella ser Senftenberg	0.9		Egg yolk magma	Brogle et al[21]
Pseudomonas species	0.06		PO_4 buffer	Thornley[20]
Lactobacillus brevis NCDO 110	1.2	0.2-0.5	PO_4 buffer	Prince and Rubino[18]
Staphylococcus aureus	0.2		PO_4 buffer	Krieger et al[15]
Streptococcus faecium	2.8		Dried	Christensen[22]
Deinococcus radiodurans	2.2	12.0	PO_4 buffer	Duggan et al[23]
Moraxella osloensis	5.8		Ice	Welch and Maxcy[24]
Acinetobacter radioresistens	1.3-2.2		PO_4 buffer	Nishimura et al[25]
Aspergillus niger	0.5		Saline + 5% gelatin	Lawrence et al[16]
Saccharomyces cerevisiae	0.5		Saline + 5% gelatin	Lawrence et al[16]
Viruses				
Foot and mouth	13.0		Frozen at $-60°C$	McCrea and Horton[26]
Coxsackievirus	4.5		Eagle + 2% bovine serum albumin	Sullivan et al[27]

Abbreviation: PO_4, phosphate.

[a]Dose required to reduce the initial population by 1 log.

bioburden population count or bioburden resistance. Method 1 and VD_{max} are both based on the bioburden count that fall within the microorganism standard distribution of resistance (SDR). The SDR specifies resistances of microorganisms in terms of D_{10} values and the probability of occurrence of values in the total population.[29] For families of products where the product microbial resistance is less than or equal to the SDR, method 1 may be used to validate a lower sterilization dose; however, if groups of products need to run together at a standardized dose or products are of high value (eg, implants), then the VD_{max} method that requires less samples may be more favorable. If the product microbial resistance is not less than or equal to the SDR, then the method must be based on the determination of microbial resistance, which would require the use of method 2. The method of choice may also be governed by the functional dose limitations of the product due to material compatibility that would require a dose establishment method capable of qualifying a lower sterilization dose such as method 1 or method 2.

For all establishment methods, it is important to understand the microbial flora that makes up the product natural bioburden. The determination of the minimum sterilization dose typically starts with the determination of the level of bioburden, or the number of microorganisms, on the product before sterilization. Regardless of the method used for validating the sterilization dose, the periodic monitoring and understanding of the microbial flora is required for the establishment and maintenance of the substantiation of the established dose. Test methods for performing this estimation of bioburden on health care products may be found in ISO standards.[32] Examples of bioburden magnitude are presented in Table 29.5.[33-35] The bioburden type and magnitude can be influenced by the source and types of raw materials used as the basis for the product; product design and size; and the manufacturing process (manual or automated), manufacturing and packaging environment, and geographic location.

TABLE 29.5	Examples of typical bioburden levels on health care products[a]
Type of Material or Product	**Average Colony-Forming Units/Product**
Biological tissue patch—raw material	10^7-10^9
Nonwoven drape	10^5-10^7
Dressing	10^5
Water-based gels	10^2
Multicomponent kits	10^2-10^3
Heparin Na	830/g
Solution containers	50
Sutures	20
Orthopedic implant	10
Pacemaker	5
Syringe	0.5
Aprotinin solution	0.1/mL
Needles	0.01

Abbreviation: Na, sodium.

[a]Levels can vary depending on the manufacturing process and environment.

Once the product is manufactured and placed in primary packages before sterilization, its bioburden may change over time. For those products that contain no microbial growth support medium, typically, the vegetative organisms can die over time and bacterial spores remain constant.[36] For those products that contain a microbial growth support medium, the bioburden magnitude may have to be evaluated between the time of manufacture and sterilization to understand the potential impact on microbial validation as required by published standards.[29] Some microbial supporting substances may see a significant increase of microbial organisms over a period of time prior to sterilization. As an example, several organisms were tested for viability at 6 and 24 hours after inoculation into water and saline. In most cases, a 1- or 2-log decline was seen within the first 6 hours for vegetative organisms. The saline provided greater viability for gram-negative and gram-positive microorganisms than did distilled water.[18]

It is important to understand the product raw materials, supplier handling and storage environments, the product manufacturing environment, the manufacturing processes, and personnel practices contribute to the overall level of microbial bioburden on the finished packaged product being presented to the validated sterilization process. Because the radiation validation methods are bioburden based, the impact to the sterilization validation must be evaluated in conjunction with product bioburden monitoring data.

Because radiation sterilization validation is based on product natural bioburden, the use of biological indicators for validation and process monitoring is not recommended for radiation sterilization of health care products and is not necessary to demonstrate the sterility assurance level (SAL) demonstrated with the validation methods. Many organisms have been found to have a higher resistance to radiation than the traditional biological indicator consisting of spores of *Bacillus pumilus*. These organisms can have a naturally higher resistance to radiation or, when irradiated under certain circumstances, can become more resistant to radiation (see Table 29.3).[8,37] This raises the question as to why a radiation-resistant biological indicator was not developed. Primarily, the validation methods that have been developed better address the sterilization effectiveness for the level and resistance of the natural microbial flora associated with the medical products and manufacturing environment. In addition, if a radiation-resistant biological indicator were to be used, the minimum sterilization dose required to achieve the desired SAL could exceed the dose allowed for materials degradation, and this would inhibit the use of radiation as a sterilization process.

Therefore, the minimum sterilization dose for health care products is best established using bioburden-based validation methods outlined in ISO standards,[29] such as methods 1, 2, and VD_{max}. These methods are based on ideas first propounded by Tallentire and others[38-41] and further developed by Whitby and Gelda[42] and Davis et al.[43,44] Variations of these methods have been developed and outlined in technical industry publications[4] that may be used; however, the basic principles behind the methods are consistent.

The methods 1, 2, and VD_{max} outlined in ISO standards and other technical publications are based on a probability model for survival of microbial populations. The probability model, as applied to a bioburden comprising a heterogeneous population of microorganisms, assumes each species has its own unique D_{10} value. In the model, the probability that a product unit will be sterile after exposure to a given dose of irradiation is defined in terms of the average initial number of organisms on the product unit before irradiation and their respective resistance or D_{10}, values. The methods involve testing products for sterility after exposure to a dose of radiation that is considerably less than the full sterilization dose. A summary of the device industry's experience using these methods has been considered separately.[37,45-47]

Method 1 is based on experimental verification that the radiation resistance of the product bioburden is less than or equal to that of a microbial population having an SDR. The first step is the determination of the average bioburden level for the product. Next, this average bioburden number is used to identify a target verification dose from a lookup table in the ISO standard.[29] The target verification dose is intended to demonstrate an SAL of 10^{-2}, which represents the dose that will reduce the microbial population with a standard distribution of radiation resistance to a level that gives a 1 in 100 chance of occurrence of a nonsterile product unit for the selected product. A sample size of 100 product units is exposed to the selected target verification dose and each product

is tested individually for sterility.[48] If there are no more than 2 positive tests of the 100 tests, the product bioburden is considered less than or equal to the SDRs, and the sterilization dose can be calculated or obtained from the lookup table to achieve the desired SAL in the routine process. This method of dose determination for the health care industry is simple to apply, to obtain the verification dose during establishment and the final sterilization dose. An example of how the probability of a nonsterile unit for an SDR is calculated for a bioburden population of 1000 CFUs exposed to a delivered dose of 11.0 kGy is shown in Table 29.6. Given the probability of occurrence for a D_{10} value population (based on 1000 CFUs) and the corresponding log reduction in the population based on a radiation dose of 11 kGy, the probability of samples testing positive for the number of samples tested following this dose is 9.79×10^{-3} or an SAL of $10^{-2.0}$ (1 in 100).[49]

Another method based on the radiation resistance of the product bioburden with a microbial population less than or equal to the SDR is the VD_{max} method.[41] Components of the SDR of high resistance that have significant effect on the attainment of an SAL of 10^{-6} have been used to define the maximal resistances on which this substantiation method is based. In carrying out substantiation, the method verifies that bioburden present on product prior to sterilization is less resistant to radiation than a microbial population of maximal resistance consistent with the attainment of an SAL of 10^{-6} at the selected sterilization dose; verification of this is conducted. This approach involves the calculation of a maximal acceptable verification dose (VD_{max}) for a given bioburden and provides a direct link between the outcome of the verification dose experiment and the attainment of an SAL of 10^{-6} at a defined sterilization dose. A sample of product units is exposed to the VD_{max} dose and each product is tested individually

TABLE 29.6	Average bioburden of 1000 colony-forming units/product exposed to a radiation dose of 11.0 kGy[a,b]									
D_{10} **Value (kGy)**	1.0	1.5	2	2.5	2.8	3.1	3.4	3.7	4.0	4.2
Population (%)	65.487	22.493	6.302	3.179	1.213	0.786	0.350	0.111	0.072	0.007
No. of Organisms / 1000	654.87	224.93	63.02	31.79	12.13	7.86	3.5	1.11	0.72	0.07
Log Reduction	11.00	7.33	5.50	4.40	3.93	3.55	3.24	2.97	2.75	2.62
Remaining CFUs	6.55E-09	1.04E-05	1.99E-04	1.27E-03	1.43E-03	2.22E-03	2.04E-03	1.18E-03	1.28E-03	1.68E-04
Total Remaining CFUs	9.79E-03									
SAL	$10^{-2.0}$									

Abbreviations: CFUs, colony-forming units; SAL, sterility assurance level.

[a]Where log reduction = dose / D_{10} value; remaining CFUs = number of microorganisms / $10^{(log\ reduction)}$; total remaining CFUs = summation of remaining CFUs for each D_{10} value population of organisms; SAL = $\log_{10}$ (total remaining CFUs)

[b]Reprinted from Logar.[49]

for sterility.[48] If there are no more than the acceptable number of positive tests, the product bioburden radiation resistance is considered less than or equal to the VD_{max}, and the sterilization dose is substantiated.

The validation by the VD_{max} method is similar in approach as with method 1 in that the product bioburden is determined and then the average bioburden level is used to obtain the verification dose from the tables within the ISO standard and associated technical publications depending on the VD_{max} sterilization dose being substantiated. A bioburden level less than or equal to 1000 CFUs is required for substantiation of a 25-kGy sterilization dose and a bioburden level less than or equal to 1.5 CFUs is required for substantiation of a 15-kGy sterilization dose.[29] Alternate doses may be substantiated that allow other levels of maximum bioburden.[30] A sample size of 10 product units is exposed to the selected verification dose indicated on applicable tables for the VD_{max} dose selected that represents the SAL of 10^{-1} dose and each product item is tested individually for sterility.[48] If there is no more than one positive test of sterility in the 10 tests, the preselected dose of 15-kGy, 25-kGy, or other alternate sterilization dose is substantiated. In addition, other applications of VD_{max} for sample number and selected SAL to obtain the verification dose, which substantiates a selected sterilization dose has been developed as part of an electronic calculation tool.[50]

Although method 2 does not require the determination of the product bioburden and does not use the SDRs to determine the sterilization dose, it is a good practice to conduct product bioburden testing as part of the validation process to assist in demonstrating maintenance of the sterilization dose over time. To determine the sterilization dose, this method uses information about the radiation resistance of microorganisms as they occur on the product. Product units are exposed to incremental amounts of radiation and these units are tested individually for sterility. The method uses this information to calculate an estimated verification dose to achieve a 10^{-2} SAL. A sample of 100 product units is exposed to the estimated verification dose and each product is tested individually for sterility.[48] The microorganisms surviving exposure to such a dose should have a more homogeneous D_{10} value than the initial bioburden. From the verification dose experiment, an estimate of the D_{10} value is calculated, and this estimate is used for extrapolation to determine the sterilization dose needed to achieve the SAL desired. This method of dose determination is not routinely used in the health care industry because it is more difficult to apply, requires significantly more time for completion, and requires a large number of product units for test. This method of dose determination is typically used when the product natural bioburden has a radiation resistance outside the SDR as indicated when method 1 or VD_{max} fails or if the product bioburden is very low, and a lower dose can be attained to achieve the desired SAL and meet maximum dose limitations for product functional acceptance.

The method chosen for establishing the sterilization dose may not only depend on the bioburden population and/or resistance but may also depend on the selected SAL to be achieved. Examples of the sterilization doses determined for health care products are provided in Table 29.7. Methods 1 and 2 provide for the selection of the SAL based on the intended use of the product. The VD_{max} method is primarily for substantiation of a sterilization dose to achieve the SAL of 10^{-6} for the product. Essentially, there are two major SALs that are routinely used for medical products, 10^{-3} and 10^{-6}. A 10^{-6} SAL is used for products that have contact with compromised tissues, and a 10^{-3} SAL can be used for products that do not come into contact with compromised tissue or are used for diagnostic applications. Guidance for the determination and selection of the appropriate SAL may be found in US industry standards[52]; however, other international standards and guidance's may need to be considered.[53] Historically, the selection of an SAL was very restrictive in what was required for supporting the use of SALs other than 10^{-6}. More updated approaches in some standards allows manufacturers to select an alternate SAL, such as 10^{-5} or 10^{-4}, for those types of products that are sensitive to 10^{-6} sterilization processes. The revised standard requires the use of the most rigorous SAL that the product can withstand as well as a risk assessment in order to select an alternate SAL. This focus on risk assessment also aligns with other regulatory documents.[54]

TABLE 29.7	Examples of sterilization doses for health care products			
Type	**Sterility Assurance Level**	**Method Used**	**Dose (kGy)**	**References**
Heparin	10^{-6}	Method 1	24.7	Dám et al[34]
Aprotinin solution	10^{-6}	Method 1	11.0	Dám et al[34]
Variety of medical devices	10^{-6}	Method 1, 2, or VD_{max}	11.0-35	Hansen and Whitby[37] Kowalski et al[51]
Variety of medical devices	10^{-3}	Method 1 or 2	5.2-25.0	Hansen and Whitby[37]

Dosimetry

Dosimetry systems are used in radiation sterilization to quantify the dose absorbed in a material. A dosimetry system consists of dosimeters and any associated packaging and all related measurement instrumentation. There are two types of dosimeters: type I dosimeters and type II dosimeters (see ISO/ASTM 52626).[55] Type I dosimeters are defined as dosimeter of high metrological quality, the response of which is affected by individual influence quantities in a well-defined way that can be expressed in terms of independent correction factors. Type II dosimeters are defined as dosimeters where the response of which is affected by influence quantities in a complex way that cannot practically be expressed in terms of independent correction factors. These two types of dosimeters can be used in either a reference standard dosimetry system, transfer standard dosimetry system, or a routine dosimetry system. All systems are traceable to a primary standard that are maintained at national standards institutes such as the National Institute of Standards and Technology in the United States or the National Physical Laboratory in the United Kingdom. Reference standard dosimetry systems typically use type I dosimeters that are calibrated to a primary standard and meet well-established criteria for accuracy, precision, and stability and are maintained in defined quality systems. A reference standard dosimetry system can be used to transfer absorbed dose measurements for the calibration of routine dosimeters at the irradiation facility.

Routine dosimetry systems, which include the dosimeter and all ancillary measurement equipment, must be rugged enough to withstand normal irradiation processing procedures. Each batch of dosimeters used for routinely monitoring dose must be calibrated before use. In addition, all ancillary measurement equipment (eg, a spectrophotometer or spectrometer) must also be included in the calibration program and calibrated at the same frequency (ie, must be calibrated together as a system).

In the operating ranges used for health care product sterilization, the three main routine dosimetry systems are dyed polymethyl methacrylate (PMMA), radiochromic film, and alanine pellets or films. All of these systems infer the amount of absorbed dose through the measurement of the change in optical density of radiation-sensitive dyes, for PMMA and radiochromic film, or the change in number of free radicals, for alanine. All three types of routine dosimetry systems can be used for gamma and X-ray radiation processes; however, only radiochromic films and alanine films are used for electron beam processing due to the influence of mass and thickness of PMMA and alanine pellets on the stopping power of the electrons. Acceptability of a dosimetry system must be user defined and depends on the range of use, sensitivity of the dosimeter response, and the overall uncertainty for the application.[56]

Products that have been irradiated in a validated process are typically released based on dosimetry results. Dosimeters that have been irradiated with the product or at a point of reference are analyzed and an absorbed dose is determined (referred to as *dosimetric release*). If the absorbed dose for the process is within the specified minimum and maximum dose for the process, the product can be released. If the absorbed dose is not within the specified minimum and maximum dose for the process, the product must be reviewed for disposition.

▶ GAMMA PROCESSING

Industrial gamma radiation facilities have several similar features: a radiation shield, an isotope source, a storage for the isotope when not in use, and a means of transporting or conveying product through the radiation process. The radiation shield is usually made of concrete or lead and provides protection for the personnel operating the facility. The radiation shield typically consists of 6- to 8-ft-thick concrete walls and ceiling (referred to as the *radiation cell*). The isotope is placed into double-encapsulated stainless steel pencils, and these pencils are then placed into a source rack, which is typically stored in water when the isotope is not in use for radiation processing (Figure 29.3). Product is conveyed through the

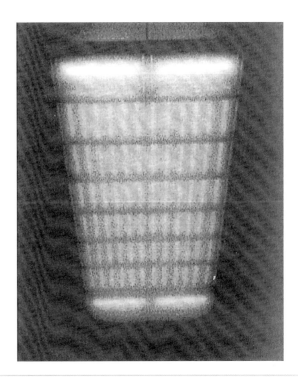

FIGURE 29.3 Gamma isotope pencils placed in a rack in a storage position.

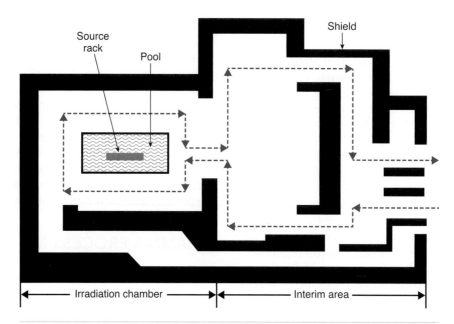

FIGURE 29.4   Overview of a typical gamma facility layout. The arrows depict the travel of the product through the irradiation facility and around the isotope source rack.

facility (Figure 29.4) in an irradiation container, which may consist of individual cardboard boxes, totes, carriers, or pallets containing multiple boxes in a specified or defined configuration. Each conveyance system has advantages and disadvantages, and each system is chosen to best suit the processing needs. All conveyance systems are similar in that they expose the product, in single or multiple passes, to the radiation field such that a nearly uniform dose of radiation is delivered throughout the product in the product loading configuration chosen. The movement of the conveyance system is typically referred to as "shuffle and dwell" because the irradiation container moves through the facility and stops for a predetermined amount of time at each of the designated positions around the source rack. In the use of individual boxes, totes, and carriers, the product is typically conveyed around the source in a symmetric fashion such that two sides are directly exposed to the radiation field for an equal amount of time. When processing using a pallet irradiator, typically the pallet is conveyed around the source such that either two sides or in some cases, all four sides of the pallet are directly exposed to the radiation field for an equal amount of time depending on the dose uniformity required.

Use of the radiation field is different for each of these facilities depending on the arrangement of isotope and the height of the conveyance system (Figure 29.5). The configuration that best uses the radiation field is an arrangement of isotope such that the product being conveyed is taller than the source rack containing the isotope (referred to as *product overlap*). This configuration is typically used for individual boxes and totes and requires that

the conveyance system move around the isotope in the manner previously described and at multiple levels. The second configuration is an arrangement of isotope such that the isotope configuration is taller than the product being conveyed (referred to as *source overlap*). This configuration is typically used for carriers and pallets and is highly dependent on the configuration of the isotope in the source rack to deliver the desired dose uniformity to the product loading configuration.

There are generally two types of processing, batch and continuous. In batch irradiators, the irradiation containers are loaded outside the radiation shield and are moved as a batch into the irradiation cell while the source rack is in a shielded position. The irradiation cell is then cleared, the safety systems are set, and the source rack is raised out of its shielded position. The irradiation containers are then moved through the irradiation process in a shuffle-and-dwell pattern through each of the positions around the source. After all irradiation containers have dwelled at each position for the predetermined amount of time, the source rack is lowered into its shielded position, and the irradiation containers are removed from the cell as a batch. This type of processing provides great flexibility and is typically used for processing small amounts of product volume or for simultaneously processing a large variety of products with different density and dose requirements. In continuous irradiators, the irradiation containers are loaded outside the radiation shield and then continuously shuffled through the irradiation cell (as one comes out of the cell, one goes in the cell) while the source rack is raised out of storage. The irradiation containers will dwell at a defined position

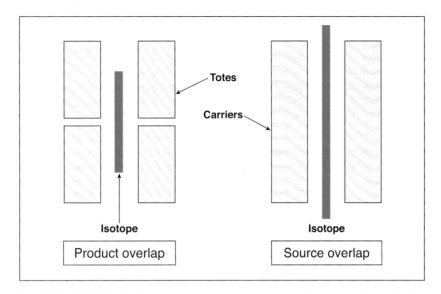

FIGURE 29.5 A representation of two types of gamma facilities. A product overlap system is used when totes are used to transport the product through the irradiation facility. A source overlap system is used when carriers are used to transport the product through the irradiation facility.

for a predetermined amount of time and then shuffle, one at a time to each position in the irradiation cell. After dwelling at each position, the fully processed container of product exits the cell and an unirradiated container of product then enters the cell. This type of processing is performed using any of the four types of irradiation containers. Figure 29.6 depicts a typical continuous irradiator that uses a tote irradiation container for product overlap. Continuous irradiators are generally less flexible than a batch irradiator and are typically used for processing large volumes of product having similar densities and dose ranges.

Routine gamma radiation processing has primarily one parameter to control, time. The length of time that the product is exposed to the radiation field is determined by the amount of isotope in the facility, the means of transportation of the product through the facility (irradiation container), density of the product, the product loading configuration, and the minimum dose required for sterilization or intended effect. The typical exposure time for a given product is 1 to several minutes at each dwell position in the irradiation cell. The exposure time for a terminally sterilized batch of product usually takes between 3 and 12 hours depending on the batch size.

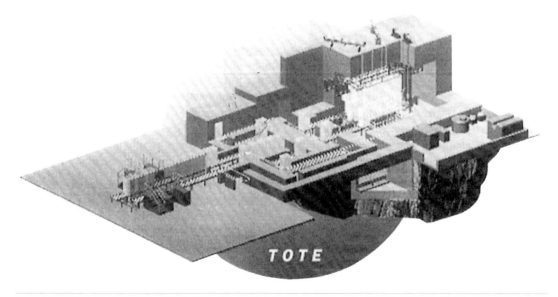

FIGURE 29.6 Typical product overlap that uses totes to process product through the gamma facility.

The amount of ^{60}Co isotope in the facility is measured in curies, a measure of the number of nuclear transformations per unit time; 1 Ci equals 3.7×10^{10} nuclear transformations per second. The amount of curies in an isotope decays over time in a predictable manner, and this time is referred to as the isotope *half-life*. The amount of ^{60}Co isotope determines the amount of energy produced per unit of time and therefore the amount of product that can be processed. Thus, as the ^{60}Co isotope decays, additional ^{60}Co isotope must be added to the source rack to maintain the throughput capacity over time.

Gamma rays or photons from ^{60}Co, have no mass and therefore have greater penetration capabilities than the electrons, which have mass, from an electron beam. Thus, the bulk density and product loading configuration are the two primary product characteristic that must be controlled. The bulk density should be consistent for a given product and package and the way it is loaded into the irradiation container should be defined. These characteristics in addition to the minimum dose required are used to determine the length of time the irradiation container dwells at each position in the irradiation cell.

Dose distributions (mappings) are determined for each product to determine the locations or zones of delivered minimum and maximum dose, the dose uniformity, and irradiation processing times.[57] Products with like bulk densities and product loading configurations can be dose mapped as a group because the distribution of dose within these like bulk densities should be the same. Any changes to the product bulk density or product loading configuration, requires an evaluation of the effect of that change on the dose distribution, including, if necessary, a new dose mapping. In addition, any changes to the irradiation, for example, a change to the isotope in the source rack (through the addition or removal of isotope pencils or rearrangement of isotope) or installation of new irradiation containers, the impact on process qualification and product dose distribution needs to be evaluated.

▶ ELECTRON BEAM PROCESSING

Electron beam processing consists of two main properties, the generation and output of the electron beam and the conveyance of the product through the beam; a typical facility layout is presented in Figure 29.7. Because it is directional, electron beam irradiation enables a more direct application of radiation as compared to either gamma or X-ray processing. This unique feature has resulted in many customized applications.

Electron beam irradiator designs used in the sterilization of health care products are typically either an emitter

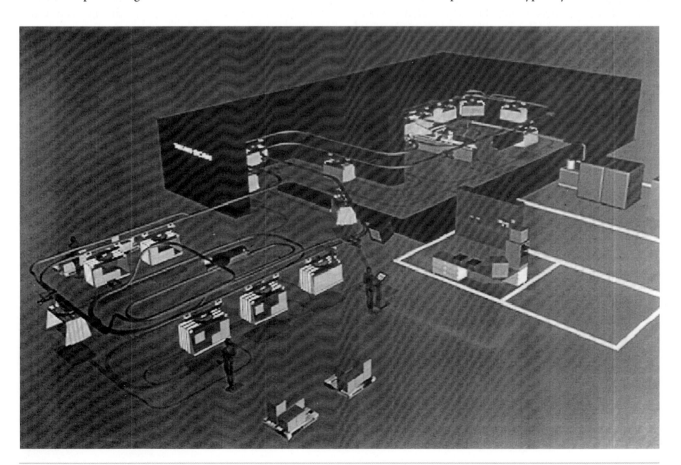

FIGURE 29.7 Typical horizontal electron beam facility.

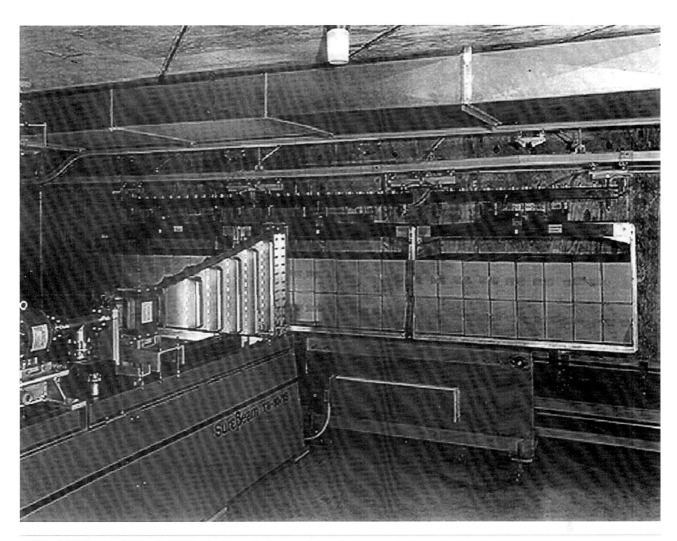

FIGURE 29.8 Product in front of a horizontal electron beam for processing.

technology or accelerator technology. Each design produces electrons at a desired energy (under vacuum) and then the electrons are delivered to the product through a beam window. For the emitter technology, the electrons leave the window at their defined energy in a unidirectional cloud. For the accelerator technology, prior to the beam window is a scan horn, which defines the maximum width of the delivered electron beam. The scan horn magnet directs the beam of electrons (coming from the accelerator) in a sweeping motion across the scan horn at a defined width. This is referred to as the scan width. The result is a narrow curtain of electrons that leave the beam window at the desired target energy. The scan horn can be placed in either a vertical (perpendicular to the ground) or horizontal (parallel to the ground) position. In either design, the scan width is controlled to ensure that the entire product is irradiated. If double-sided irradiation is necessary, the product must be flipped over 180 degrees and irradiated a second time.

The conveyance mechanisms in the irradiators are quite different for either the horizontal or the vertical scan horn position. In a horizontal scanning position, the most commonly used conveyor system is a roller conveyor, where the product is placed flat on the conveyor and transported under the beam. In a vertical scan horn position, the product is either placed into a carrier or placed on a roller conveyor and is then conveyed in front of the beam (Figure 29.8). In either design, penetration of electrons into the product depends on the energy of the electrons. The depth of penetration is also be greatly influenced by the density of the material being irradiated (Figure 29.9). Figure 29.10 depicts a typical depth-dose curve for 10-MeV electrons. These depth-dose curves are for single-sided irradiation. For products that are either rotated or turned over to accomplish double-sided irradiation, the resulting depth-dose curves would be a summation of the two single-sided curves (see Figure 29.10). Processing large metal items using the electron beam may pose some unique challenges associated with the ability to reach all surfaces of the device (due to the density of the material and penetration energy of the electrons), whereas gamma or X-rays may be able to pass through the device.

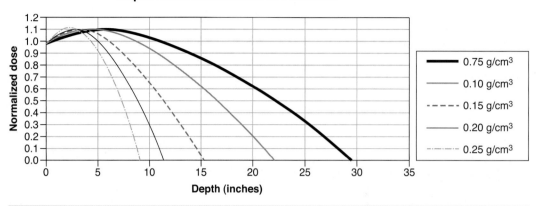

FIGURE 29.9 Depth-dose distributions in products with various densities (g/cm³) for a 10-MeV electron beam.

These depth-dose curves are applicable only if the material being processed is homogeneous, such as sheets of Styrofoam™, corrugate, or plastic. If the product is not homogeneous but heterogeneous, such as plastic tubing with multiple connectors, syringes, or practically any product made up of multiple components, the product must be dose mapped to determine the dose distribution characteristics. Electrons have both charge and mass, and thus, the distribution of dose within the product will be greatly influenced by the type of material and its orientation to the electron beam. The results of the product dose mapping are used to determine the optimum product loading configuration and routine processing parameters, such as conveyance speed and scan width. If the product is changed, the effect of that change on the dose distribution needs to be evaluated, and most likely, the dose mapping performed again. In addition, if the delivery of the beam or the beam energy is changed or any change to the carriers or the product loading configuration, the impact on the process qualification and product dose distribution needs to be evaluated, and if necessary, a new dose mapping should be performed.[57]

Due to the high dose rate achieved in industrial electron beam irradiators, the typical processing time for a given product in an electron beam irradiator is only seconds. The typical processing time for a batch of product is a few minutes up to an hour or 2. The actual throughput is determined based on the size of the batch of product and power of the electron beam irradiator. The power of the system (kW) is based on the energy of the electrons (ie, electron volts) and the current (the number of electrons accelerated per unit time).

For electron beam processing, there are three parameters that can be varied—current, speed, and scan width. Some systems are enabled to allow for these parameters to be changed very rapidly; therefore, the ability to change from one product to another requiring different parameters can be accomplished in seconds, thus allowing for a true first-in–first-out system and resulting in lower inventories for the manufacturer.

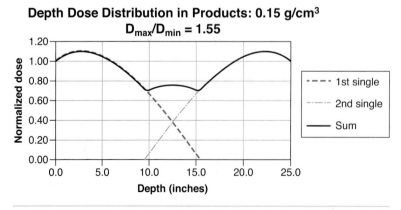

FIGURE 29.10 Depth-dose distribution for a 10-MeV electron beam in a product with a density of 0.15 g/cm³ and a maximum-to-minimum dose ratio of 1.55.

X-RAY PROCESSING

X-ray irradiators used in health care sterilization typically have three main properties in their design: an electron beam accelerator, a target (to convert the electrons to photons), and a conveyance system (Figure 29.11). The electron beam accelerator will determine the maximum energy of the photons produced and the amount of throughput (ie, product that can be processed per unit time). The electron energy is typically limited to <7.5 MeV due to the potential for activation of processed materials and the converted photon energies are a range from very low (approximately 100 keV) to the maximum accelerated electron energy (ie, 7.5 MeV). The amount of throughput is a fraction of the potential electron beam accelerator throughput because the conversion of electrons to X-rays is inefficient, and much of the energy is lost in the form of heat in the target used to generate the X-rays. Thus, an accelerator that can produce high energy along and high current is desirable to maximize the throughput and efficiency of the irradiator. Designs for X-ray facilities typically use a conveyance mechanism that can transport large totes or full pallet loads in front of the X-ray target in a manner very similar to electron beam processes; however, several passes, product manipulations, and product rotations may be required to deliver the desired dose uniformity ratio.

The depth-dose curves achieved with X-rays are similar to those that can be obtained with gamma processing. But the overall penetration is typically better than gamma due to the subset of higher energy photons (>1.3 MeV) that are produced from the high-energy electrons being converted. Changes to the X-ray target or beam energy, as well as changes to the carrier or product loading configuration, which may affect the process qualification, should be evaluated and, if necessary, requalified.[57]

The typical processing time for a given product in an X-ray irradiator is several minutes, in each of multiple passes, because of the moderate dose rate achieved in industrial X-ray facilities. The processing time for a batch of product is typically 1 to several hours depending on the batch size and product manipulations. An overall comparison of the relative properties of gamma rays, electron beams, and X-rays is provided in Table 29.8.

PROCESS ACCEPTANCE

Typically, products that have undergone radiation processing are released based on dosimetry results as it pertains to delivery of dose to a product. But in radiation processing, the more reliable estimate is determining acceptance of a process and to rely on a parametric release process that uses dosimetry as a means of verifying the process as being in a state of control.

Parametric release requires that the design of the irradiation process and the control system must include redundant, independent monitoring systems on all critical control points. Parametric release for radiation processing

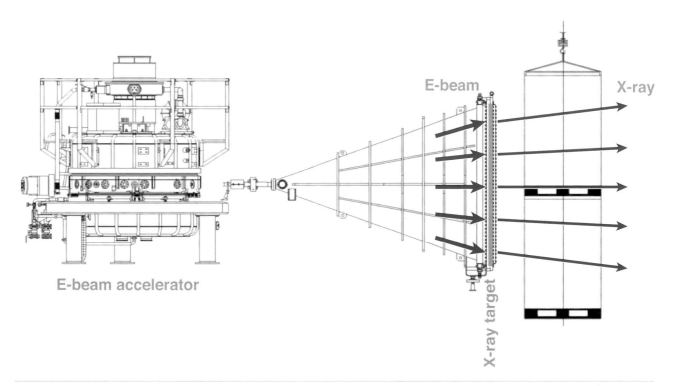

FIGURE 29.11 Schematic of an X-ray irradiator using a hanging tote conveyance system. The X-rays are generated by bombarding a heavy metal target with high-energy electrons from an electron beam accelerator.

TABLE 29.8   Comparison of gamma, electron beam, and X-ray[a]

Comparison Area	Gamma	Electron Beam (<5 MeV)	Electron Beam (>5 MeV)	X-ray
Dose rate	Low	High	High	Medium
Material effects	High	Low	Low	Medium
Penetration	High	Low	Medium	High
Processing time	Hours	Seconds	Seconds	Minutes
Replenishment or replacement part costs	High	Low	Low	Low
Licensing and installation	Hard	Easy	Easy	Easy

[a]This comparison is relative, not absolute.

is done by reviewing the critical control points within the process to determine that the process was within an acceptable state of control throughout the entire process and, if required, using dosimeters only to confirm a delivery of the dose at a predetermined target and magnitude. As a result of determining a process is under a state of control, the process can be deemed acceptable and thus, the products validated within this process are also deemed to have met their acceptable dose specifications. Establishing and defining a process is under a state of control enables the user to support the disposition of routing processing errors such as a misplaced or missing dosimeter, dosimeter reading error, or damaged dosimeter. The measurement is one of the critical parameters used in assessing the process delivered its intended effect; however, when a measurement is not obtained, the other critical parameters can be used to determine whether the process was in a state of control and calculations can be made from acceptable measurement to determine the best estimate for the missing values. Conversely, when a process goes out of control (eg, process interruption), the dosimeter measurements can be used to determine the extent that the process went out of control.

Another part of process acceptance is the continued acceptance of the established minimum sterilization dose by the performance of periodic dose audits at the original verification dose estimate to substantiate the validated sterilization dose. The dose audit for a specific sterilization product family are typically performed on a quarterly basis; however, other frequencies are allowed or required for special circumstances and conditions as outlined in approved standards.[2] As part of the dose audit, the product bioburden is determined to monitor the state of control of the product being presented routinely to the sterilization process. The bioburden and dose audit provide the data to demonstrate that the microbial flora remain in a state of control within the conditions of the original dose determination for continued acceptance of the measured sterilization dose by dosimetry during routine release.

CHANGE CONTROL

With radiation sterilization processing, it is very important to understand the inputs of the manufacturing environment and processes, materials, suppliers, and packaging configuration so that changes can be evaluated for impact to the validated sterilization process. Because radiation dose determination methods are based on the bioburden population and/or resistance of the product and the dose mapping qualification establishes the achieved dose distribution across the product load with a specified orientation and density, even minor changes to the product, manufacturing processes, or environment or packaging may have an impact on the product being presented to the validated sterilization process. Changes should be evaluated and documented through a formal change control process to ensure there has been no shift to the product bioburden or impact to the dose distribution across the product loading within the routine sterilization process.

EXCURSIONS AND DEVIATIONS

With routine monitoring of the manufacturing environment through periodic bioburden and dose audit testing, it is also important to understand the meaning and actions to be taken when a bioburden excursion or dose audit result deviation is encountered. Bioburden excursions can be the result of a shift in the microbial flora in the manufacturing; however, typical manufacturing can have periodic bioburden spikes that may not indicate a meaningful shift (see chapter 64). The routine bioburden monitoring data should be used to determine alert and action levels based on statistical calculations to provide documented responses to be taken with excursions or deviations. The response to an excursion or deviation is based on the extent of the excursion and the results of the investigation.

For an excursion to a bioburden alert or action level, one must understand that the results obtained from the bioburden sample lot selected to represent a family of products is representative of all product lots within the family for the monitoring time period. The bioburden and/or dose audit result on a specific batch does not only impact the batch tested but the entire family of products represented by the selected batch. Any actions taken based on a result from a specific batch must also be applied to all batches within the family for the monitoring period. In the case of a bioburden alert level excursion, the result only indicates a possible shift and not necessarily a sustained event or change in the manufacturing that would impact the sterilization dose. For this reason, it is important to perform the periodic dose audit on the same lot that is being monitored for bioburden.

In the case of a bioburden excursion, the acceptable results of the dose audit provide confirmation that the bioburden excursion does not impact the substantiation of the sterilization dose; therefore, the routine sterilization dose remains valid. If the dose audit results in a number of samples showing growth outside the acceptable number for the method, then the dose must be augmented accordingly,[29] and an investigation initiated for the bioburden excursion and dose audit result.

The bioburden excursion and/or dose audit failure should require an investigation that includes but is not limited to the following:

1. Characterization and identification (where possible) of the predominate bioburden organisms and dose audit samples demonstrating growth
2. Sample representation of routine manufacturing and handling
3. Laboratory investigation of testing materials, environment, and technique
4. Manufacturing environment and personnel practices
5. Change control of any product material, supplier, or manufacturing process

Based on the investigation, if the bioburden excursion or the dose audit failure is a direct result of the samples being handled improperly or the verification dose being applied incorrectly, the bioburden and/or dose audit may be repeated to confirm if there is a true shift. If the investigation results in a determination of a root cause for the shift, corrective action may be performed, and additional testing performed to confirm effectiveness of the corrective action to return to the state of control represented by the original dose establishment and bioburden levels. During the investigational period, the routine sterilization dose should remain augmented until corrective action is complete to indicate a return to the original validated dose or the dose is reestablished.

For radiation routine processing deviations, the routine processing where the product does not meet the minimum sterilization dose may have an incremental irradiation dose added to the product or "topped off" to meet the minimum sterilization dose with the cumulative total exposure. For routine processing deviations where products exceeded the established maximum allowed dose, the product would require material evaluation for product and package fit/form/function. If a processing deviation occurs in the loading pattern or dosimeter placement, a dose mapping may be required to confirm the minimum and maximum dose distribution and dosimeter correlation factors associated with the erroneous loading configuration or dosimeter placement to complete the risk impact to the product.[57]

▶ RADIATION SAFETY

This section discusses the level of radiation exposure or radiation safety limits and puts into perspective the doses allowed for safety and the doses required for sterilization or pasteurization. Everyone is exposed to radiation from the sun, earth, and space in different levels based on their geographic location. This exposure is typically referred to as *background* radiation and averages from 10 to 200 mrem per year. In contrast, the maximum permissible occupational exposure for radiation workers is 5000 mrem per year or 0.0005 kGy per year. On average, people who work with industrial irradiators receive a dose slightly higher than background but is far below the permissible levels. All personnel who work around industrial irradiators should be monitored with personal dosimeters to determine the amount of radiation exposure as part of the radiation safety program.

The safety systems in industrial irradiators protect workers and surrounding areas from the radiation produced in the facility.[58] The primary mechanism for this protection is a biological shield, which is constructed of concrete or metal. The thickness of the shield is determined by the type of radiation and the amount of the isotope or the power and energy of the electron beam. In addition to the biological shield, there are systems to ensure that the workers do not inadvertently enter the irradiator while it is in operation.

Ionization radiation produces ozone in the environment. Ozone is considered to be an irritant to the mucosal membranes (see chapter 33). Irradiators are constructed with ventilation systems to exhaust the ozone to minimize worker exposure to this irritant. The need to treat the exhaust depends on the levels produced and the local environmental restrictions. Gamma radiation facilities produce a higher amount of ozone than electron beam or X-ray radiation facilities.

Radiation facilities are audited and regulated through governmental regulatory agencies, and reviews of the implementation of safety systems are performed regardless of the licensing agency.

REFERENCES

1. Association for the Advancement of Medical Instrumentation. *AAMI TIR17:2017. Compatibility of Materials Subject to Sterilization.* Arlington, VA: Association for the Advancement of Medical Instrumentation; 2017.

2. Ginoza W. The effects of ionizing radiation on nucleic acids of bacteriophages and bacterial cells. *Annu Rev Microbiol.* 1967;21:325-368.

3. Sparrow AH, Underbrink AG, Sparrow RC. Chromosomes and cellular radiosensitivity: I. The relationship of D_{10} to chromosome volume and complexity in seventy-nine different organisms. *Radiat Res.* 1967;32:915-945.

4. Davies R, Sinskey AJ. Radiation-resistant mutants of *Salmonella typhimurium* LT2: development and characterization. *J Bacteriol.* 1973;113:133-144.

5. Davies R, Sinskey AJ, Botstein D. Deoxyribonucleic acid repair in a highly radiation-resistant strain of *Salmonella typhimurium.* *J Bacteriol.* 1973;114:357-366.

6. Matsuyama A. Present status of food irradiation research in Japan with special reference to microbiological and entomological aspects. In: *Radiation Preservation of Food.* Vienna, Austria: International Atomic Energy Agency; 1973:261-278.

7. Town CD, Smith KC, Kaplan HS. Production and repair of radiochemical damage in *Escherichia coli* deoxyribonucleic acid; its modification by culture conditions and relation to survival. *J Bacteriol.* 1971;105:127-135.

8. Jung KW, Lim S, Bahn YS. Microbial radiation-resistance mechanisms. *J Microbiol.* 2017;55(7):499-507.

9. Lea OE. *Actions of Radiations on Living Cells.* London, United Kingdom: Cambridge University Press; 1956.

10. Anderson AW, Nordan HC, Cain RF, Parrish G, Duggan D. Studies on a radio-resistant micrococcus: I. Isolation morphology, cultural characteristics, and resistance to gamma radiation. *Food Technol.* 1956;10:575-577.

11. Stumbo CR, Murphy JR, Cochran J. Nature of thermal death time curves for PA 3679 and *Clostridium botulinum.* *Food Technol.* 1950; 4(8):321-326.

12. Halvorson HO, Ziegler NR. Application of statistics to problems in bacteriology: I. a means of determining bacterial population by the dilution method. *J Bacteriol.* 1933;25:101-121.

13. Grecz N. Biophysical aspects of *Clostridia.* *J Appl Bacteriol.* 1965; 28:17-35.

14. Roberts TA, Ingram M. Radiation resistance of spores of *Clostridium* species in aqueous suspension. *J Food Sci.* 1965;30:879-885.

15. Krieger RA, Snyder OP, Pflug IJ. *Clostridium botulinum* ionizing radiation D-value determination using a micro food sample system. *J Food Sci.* 1983;48:141-145.

16. Lawrence CA, Brownell LE, Graikoski JT. Effect of cobalt-60 gamma radiation on microorganisms. *Nucleonics.* 1953;11:9-11.

17. Van Winkle W, Borick PM, Fogarty M. Destruction of radiation-resistant microorganisms on surgical sutures by ^{60}Co-irradiation under manufacturing conditions. In: *Radiosterilization of Medical Products.* Vienna, Austria: International Atomic Energy Agency; 1967.

18. Prince HN, Rubino JR. Bioburden dynamics: the viability of microorganisms on devices before and after sterilization. *Med Dev Diagn Industry.* 1984;6:47

19. Gaughran ERL, Goudie AJ. *Sterilization of Medical Products by Ionizing Radiation.* Montreal, Canada: Multiscience; 1978.

20. Thornley MJ. *Microbiological Aspects of the Use of Irradiation for the Elimination of Salmonellae from Foods and Feeding Stuffs.* Vienna, Austria: International Atomic Energy Agency; 1963. Technical report series 22.

21. Brogle RC, Nickerson JTR, Proctor BE, et al. Use of high-voltage cathode rays to destroy bacteria of the *Salmonella* group in whole egg solids, egg yolk solids, and frozen egg yolk. *J Food Sci.* 1957;22: 572-589.

22. Christensen EA. Radiation resistance of enterococci dried in air. *Acta Pathol Microbiol Scand.* 1964;61:483-486.

23. Duggan DE, Anderson AW, Elliker PR. Inactivation of the radiation-resistant spoilage bacterium *Micrococcus radiodurans.* I. Radiation inactivation rates in three meat substrates and in buffer. *Appl Microbiol.* 1963;11:398-403.

24. Welch AB, Maxcy RB. Characterization of radiation-resistant vegetative bacteria in beef. *Appl Microbiol.* 1975;30:242-250.

25. Nishimura Y, Ino T, Iizuka H. *Acinetobacter radioresistens* isolated from cotton and soil. *Int J Syst Bacteriol.* 1988;38:209-211.

26. McCrea JF, Horton RF. *Literature Survey of Viruses and Rickettsiae in Foods.* Natick, MA: Q.M. Research and Engineering Center; 1962. Contract DA19-129-QM-1810, report no. 4 final.

27. Sullivan R, Fassolitis AC, Larkin EP, Read RB Jr, Peeler JT. Inactivation of thirty viruses by gamma radiation. *Appl Microbiol.* 1971;22:61-65.

28. International Organization for Standardization. *ISO 11137-1:2006: Sterilization of Healthcare Products—Radiation—Part 1: Requirements for the Development, Validation and Routine Control of a Sterilization Process for Medical Devices.* Geneva, Switzerland: International Organization for Standardization; 2006.

29. International Organization for Standardization. *ISO 11137-2:2013: Sterilization of Healthcare Products—Radiation—Part 2: Establishing the Sterilization Dose.* Geneva, Switzerland: International Organization for Standardization; 2013.

30. Association for the Advancement of Medical Instrumentation. *ANSI/AAMI/ISO TIR13004:2013. Sterilization of Health Care Products—Radiation—Substantiation of a Selected Sterilization Dose: Method VD_{max}^{SD}.* Arlington, VA: Association for the Advancement of Medical Instrumentation; 2013.

31. Association for the Advancement of Medical Instrumentation. *AAMI TIR40:2018. Sterilization of Health Care Products—Radiation—Guidance on Dose Setting Utilizing a Modified Method 2.* Arlington, VA: Association for the Advancement of Medical Instrumentation; 2018.

32. International Organization for Standardization. *ISO 11737-1:2018: Sterilization of Health Care Products—Microbiological Methods—Part 1: Determination of the Population of Microorganisms on Product.* Geneva, Switzerland: International Organization for Standardization; 2018.

33. Anger CB. Radiation sterilization validation for dosimetric release. *Med Dev Diagn Industry.* 1981;3(9):47-50.

34. Dám AM, Gazsó LG, Kaewpila S, et al. Radiation sterilization dose calculation for heparin and aprotinin based on ISO method 1. *Int J Pharm.* 1995;121:245-248.

35. Hoxey EV. Validation of methods for bioburden estimation. In: *Sterilization of Medical Products: Proceedings of the International Kilmer Memorial Conference on the Sterilization of Medical Products.* Montreal, Canada: Polyscience Publications; 1993:297-304.

36. Christensen EA, Emborg C, Holm NW. *Microbiological Control of Radiation Sterilization of Medical Supplies: II. Number of Microorganisms on Medical Products Prior to Sterilization as a Function of the Storage Time Between Production and Microbiological Control.* Roskilde, Denmark: Danish Atomic Energy Commission; 1969. RISÖ report no. 194.

37. Hansen JM, Whitby J. Gamma radiation sterilization practice in the U.S. device industry. *Med Dev Diagn Industry;* July 1994.

38. Tallentire A. Aspects of microbiological control of radiation sterilization. *J Radiat Steril.* 1973;1:85-103.

39. Tallentire A, Dwyer J, Ley FJ. Microbiological quality control of sterilized products: evaluation of a model relating frequency of contaminated items with increasing radiation treatment. *J Appl Bacteriol.* 1971;34:521-534.

40. Tallentire A, Khan AA. The sub-process dose in defining the degree of sterility assurance. In: Gaughran ERL, Goudie AJ, eds. *Sterilization by Ionizing Radiation.* Vol 2. Montreal, Canada: Multiscience Publications; 1978:65-80.

41. Kowalski JB, Tallentire A. Substantiation of 25 kGy as a sterilization dose: a rational approach to establishing verification dose. *Radiat Phys Chem.* 1999;54(1):55-64.

42. Whitby JL, Gelda AK. Use of incremental doses of cobalt 60 radiation as a means to determine radiation sterilization dose. *J Parenter Drug Assoc.* 1979;33:144-155.

43. Davis KW, Strawderman WE, Masefield J, et al. DS gamma radiation dose setting and auditing strategies for sterilizing medical devices. In: *Sterilization of Medical Products: Proceedings of the International Kilmer Memorial Conference on the Sterilization of Medical Products.* Montreal, Canada: Multiscience Publications; 1981:51-81.

44. Davis KW, Strawderman WE, Whitby JL. The rationale and a computer evaluation of a gamma irradiation sterilization dose determination method for medical devices using a substerilization incremental dose sterility test protocol. *J Appl Bacteriol.* 1984;57:31-50.

45. Hansen JM. AAMI dose setting: ten years' experience. In: *Sterilization of Medical Products: Proceedings of the International Kilmer Memorial Conference on the Sterilization of Medical Products.* Montreal, Canada: Polyscience Publications; 1993:449-459.

46. Kowalski JB, Herring C, Baryschpolec L, et al. Field evaluations of the VDmax approach for substantiation of a 25kGy sterilization dose and its application to other preselected doses. *Radiat Phys Chem.* 2002;64:411-416.

47. Hansen J, Bryans T. Radiation dose setting method 2 and modified method 2: use and experience. *Biomed Instrum Technol.* 2019;53:38-42.

48. International Organization for Standardization. *ISO 11737-2:2009: Sterilization of Medical Devices—Microbiological Methods—Part 2: Tests of Sterility Performed in the Definition, Validation and Maintenance of a Sterilization Process.* Geneva, Switzerland: International Organization for Standardization; 2009.

49. Logar JR. Exploring the probability of a device being nonsterile following irradiation. *Biomed Instrum Technol.* 2019;53:43-48.

50. Kowalski JB. Setting standards: extending the VD_{max} approach: AAMI TIR76 and its web-based calculation tool. *Biomed Instrum Technol.* 2019;53:232-236.

51. Kowalski J, Aoshuang Y, Tallentire A. Radiation sterilization—evaluation of a new method for substantiation of 25 kGy. *Radiat Phys Chem.* 2000;58:77-86.

52. Association for the Advancement of Medical Instrumentation. *ANSI/AAMI ST67:2011/(R)2017. Sterilization of Health Care Products—Requirements and Guidance for Selecting a Sterility Assurance Level (SAL) for Products Labeled "Sterile."* Arlington, VA: Association for the Advancement of Medical Instrumentation; 2017.

53. International Organization for Standardization. *ISO/TS 19930:2017: Guidance on Aspects of a Risk-Based Approach to Assuring Sterility of Terminally Sterilized, Single-Use Health Care Product That Is Unable to Withstand Processing to Achieve Maximally a Sterility Assurance Level of 10-6.* Geneva, Switzerland: International Organization for Standardization; 2017.

54. International Organization for Standardization. *ISO 13485:2016: Medical Devices—Quality Management Systems—Requirements for Regulatory Purposes.* Geneva, Switzerland: International Organization for Standardization; 2016.

55. International Organization for Standardization. *ISO/ASTM 52628:2013: Standard Practice for Dosimetry in Radiation Processing.* Geneva, Switzerland: International Organization for Standardization; 2013.

56. International Organization for Standardization. *ISO/ASTM 51707:2015: Guide for Estimation of Measurement Uncertainty in Dosimetry for Radiation Processing.* Geneva, Switzerland: International Organization for Standardization; 2015.

57. International Organization for Standardization. *ISO 11137-3:2017: Sterilization of Health Care Products—Radiation—Part 3: Guidance on Dosimetric Aspects of Development, Validation and Routine Control.* Geneva, Switzerland: International Organization for Standardization; 2017.

58. International Atomic Energy Agency. *Radiation Safety of Gamma and Electron Irradiation Facilities.* Vienna, Austria: International Atomic Energy Agency; 1992. IAEA safety series 107.

CHAPTER 30

Sterile Filtration of Liquids and Gases

Kerry Roche Lentine and Richard V. Levy

Sterile filtration is used successfully in a variety of applications at a variety of scales. Medical practitioners employ sterilizing grade syringe filters or in-line large volume parenteral filters as an extra measure of safety for their patients at the 1 mL to 1 to 2 L range. Laboratory scientists employ sterilizing grade filters to safeguard media and reagents to ensure robust and consistent experimental results. These laboratory scale processes can range from self-contained, disposable vacuum-driven filtration devices in the 50 to 500 mL range to pressure-driven filter capsules that can process several liters of feed. In pharmaceutical manufacturing for plasma, vaccines, biotherapeutics, and small molecule drugs, sterile filtration is the portion of a process that includes the installation, sterilization, system preparation, integrity testing, and filtering of a liquid or gas through a sterilizing-grade filter with the intention of removing microorganisms. Sterilizing grade filters are used at multiple points throughout the pharmaceutical manufacturing process from media and gas filtration for bioreactor protection to process intermediate and bulk drug substance bioburden reduction to final sterile drug product filtration at scales from 10 L to greater than 10 000 L.

From a regulatory standpoint, sterile filtration is defined as the complete removal of microorganisms and particles within a specific size range from liquids or gases to produce a drug product that meets the current aseptic processing guidelines set by each country such as the US Food and Drug Administration (FDA)[1] or the European Medicines Agency (EMA).[2,3] In the spirit of harmonization, sterile filtration may also be defined by other organizations, including the Pharmaceutical Inspection Co-operation Scheme (PIC/S),[4] World Health Organization (WHO),[5] the International Organization for Standardization (ISO),[6] or by a compendium such as the United States Pharmacopeia (USP).[7]

The intent of this chapter is to provide the reader a general overview of sterile filtration of liquids and gases with an emphasis on their application in the pharmaceutical industry.

◗ CONTAMINATION AND THE ROLE OF FILTRATION

Types of Contaminants

Three broad classes of contaminants are found in biological and pharmaceutical solutions: (1) dissolved impurities, (2) suspended particulate matter, and (3) suspended microorganisms.

Water is a major source of dissolved impurities. Dissolved contaminants can be subdivided into inorganic (ionic) and organic impurities. Inorganic salts find their way into water supplies from soil, rocks, tanks, pipes, and other sources. Organic compounds include lignins, tannins, detergents, polysaccharides, proteins, and other biodecomposition products that are commonly associated with surface water supplies. Suspended particulate matter includes colloidal solids, metal, cotton, dust, lint, and an endless variety of other solid contaminants. When used generically, the term is assumed to include microorganisms.

Microorganisms can be a problem whether alive or dead. Alive, they can multiply at logarithmic rates, overburden prefilters and final filters, and overpower preservative systems. Dead, they are a cause of premature filter plugging and the source of certain types of endotoxins, which may prove to be pyrogenic when introduced with drugs into humans and animals.[8] Because of the low absorption characteristics of many membrane filters, pyrogens in solution are not removed by simple size exclusion alone. There are filters that supplement sieving removal with charge (usually cationic) to capture endotoxin. These must be carefully validated because removal by charge is in general less robust. Pyrogenic activity may be attributed to the presence of bacterial cells. Intact cells may be removed quantitatively, but no assurance can be given that cell lysis, and thus release of the soluble pyrogenic constituents into the solution, has not taken place.

Controlling Exogenous Contamination

Some of the major exogenous contamination sources that need to be recognized and addressed are related to the design of the work area, raw materials entering the facility, equipment used for processing intermediates, drug substance, and final drug product as well as the people associated with the process. Specifically, the following are points of consideration when performing a sterile filtration:

1. The manufacturing area, including its physical layout, location, traffic patterns, and use, influences the particulate burden in the air. Most airborne microscopic contaminants are associated with dust or other particles that are dispersed by the movement of people.

2. Raw materials: All raw materials pose a risk of contaminating the drug manufacturing process such as cell culture media, buffer salts, surfactants, solvents, and excipients are potential sources of contaminating debris, dissolved impurities, and microorganisms. Dead bacteria and mycotic spores left over from sterilization processes such as autoclaving or ultraviolet radiation remains a source of particles and pyrogens. Chemical incompatibility of raw materials with processing equipment may lead to insoluble precipitates, which fail to go entirely into solution.

3. Equipment, piping, vessels, tubing, and nearly every surface to which the fluid is exposed can contribute contaminants. Particles are inevitable wherever there are moving parts, valves, bungs, O-ring seals, threaded connectors, tubing, or any surface subject to abrasion or wear, as in even the best-designed filling machines and apparatus. Furthermore, improper cleaning can result in formation of biofilm (see chapter 67). Biofilms can be attached to internal surfaces of process systems or detached and suspended within the fluid to be filtered. Bacteria are the most common type of organism present in biofilm or bioburden in fluid system being sterile filtered. Although prefiltration systems are designed to remove physically intact bacteria and parts of bacteria cells, microbial by-products produce many compounds that can cause immune responses. For further understanding of both biofilm and bioburden in this context, consult Parenteral Drug Association (PDA) Technical Report 69, entitled *Bioburden and Biofilm Management in Pharmaceutical Manufacturing Operations.*[8]

4. People are a well-known source of both microbial contamination as well as fomites that contaminate the pharmaceutical environment such as skin cells, hair, clothing fibers, and sputum.

5. Postfinal filtration particle generation from containers and closure systems is another concern. Both glass and elastomeric particles are shed when a stopper is inserted into a bottle or a plunger is inserted into a syringe.[9] Glass vial delamination can occur from vial handling or product container interactions.[10] When detected, this type of contamination can result in discarding the drug product batch or in product recalls. A recall in 2018 described a sterile injectable drug contaminated with particulate matter believed to be from the manufacturing process. The recall discussed concern that particles, even sterile particles may be harmful to the patient. "In the absence of in-line filtration, these particles may cause local vein irritation, inflammatory reaction, aggravation of preexisting infections, allergic reactions, phlebitis, pulmonary emboli, pulmonary granulomas, immune system dysfunction, pulmonary dysfunction, pulmonary infarction, and systemic embolization."[11] Although there is some debate concerning the clinical impact of particle contamination in injectables, point of use sterile filtration in the form of syringe filters or in-line infusion filters can provide the patient an extra measure of safety.[12]

▶ HISTORY OF STERILIZING FILTRATION

Filtration is used as a means of stabilizing pharmaceutical and biological fluids. The Pasteur-Chamberlin filter was one of the first filters designed for the removal of bacteria from solutions and was patented in 1894.[13] These porous unglazed porcelain tubes were originally designed to purify drinking water. Also, in the 1890s Theobald Seitz, seeking to remove spoilage microorganisms in wine, developed a fibrous filter structure. In 1909, he filed a patent in the United States where he described the layering of asbestos, cellulose, and/or cotton fibers in a graded density to remove successively finer particles from a liquid stream. This patent also described the use of support materials to strengthen the structure of the filter material.[14] In 1918, his brother Georg Seitz and Friedrich Schmitthenner[15] were awarded a patent for a depth filter specifically designed to sterilize liquids. This filter material combined diatomaceous earth or clay with asbestos, cotton, and flax fibers for higher throughput in a presterilized, easy to replace format that eliminated filter cleaning. Although asbestos was a highly effective filter material, in 1973 the FDA proposed that parenteral manufacturers eliminate asbestos or other fiber-releasing filters from their manufacturing process.[16]

Retention of bacteria by these media depends on absorption to the inner filter structure and random entrapment throughout the filter matrix. Starting in 1919, Zsigmondy and Buchmann[17,18] patented true membrane filters for the removal of bacteria from solutions that were larger than the pore size at or near their surface. These membranes were screen-like cellulose ester-based media produced by phase inversion—a technique still used for most of microporous membranes to this day. In 1927, Membranefiltergesellschaft m.b.n. was founded with Zsigmondy and Wilhelm Sartorius of Sartorius-Werke A. G. among group of owners and produced these membranes with laboratory scale operations until the 1960s.[19] The primary use of this technology in Germany during World War II was to determine the degree of bacterial contamination of potable water supplies. After the war, Goetz, under contract with the US military, acquired the membrane technology and worked from 1947 to 1950 with the California Institute of Technology to refine these membranes to increase porosity and uniformity while eliminating the need to boil filters prior to use.[20] These developments led to the analytical membrane filters for bacterial recovery and enumeration referenced in industry standards today.[21] In 1950, the Lovell Chemical Company won a contract to further develop Goetz's work for large-scale membrane manufacturing. In 1954, Jack Bush acquired the rights to this membrane technology and founded the Millipore Filter Company to expand the applications for these membranes.

Many of the mid-century cellulosic microporous membrane applications focused on laboratory scale bacterial recovery for enumeration; however, as researchers began to use polymers such as polyamides, polyvinylidene fluoride (PVDF), polyethersulfone, and polytetrafluoroethylene, they developed more robust membrane filters for particle removal, bioburden reduction, and sterilization of gas, liquids, water, and certain types of drug products.[22-27] These removal applications required more surface area than that used in laboratory settings resulting in the development of various sanitary filtration device formats such as tube filters, stacked disks, and pleated cartridge filters.[28-33]

Because many sterile filter applications in a pharmaceutical process are for aqueous fluids and most of the membrane polymers used in these applications are natively hydrophobic, surface modification methods such as grafting of hydrophilic coatings, radiation polymerization, and other techniques are employed to hydrophilize these membranes. Surface modification can also be designed to reduce nonspecific protein binding.[34]

During the 1960s, 0.45-μm rated membrane was quickly applied to the removal of bacteria, yeast, and molds from biological and pharmaceutical fluids as well as for sterility testing of drug products.[35,36] But in the late 1960s, a pseudomonad-like organism, now known as *Brevundimonas diminuta*, associated with a proteinaceous solution, was isolated, which could pass through that membrane during the filtration process.[37] Membranes with a "tighter" pore size rating of 0.2 (or 0.22-μm) were then introduced for critical sterilizing filtration applications.

Although filter media are used to affect separations such as solid/liquid, chromatographic, electrophoretic, and molecular separations, this chapter is limited to the removal of microorganisms other than viruses, which have been considered elsewhere and, in general, are not expected to be removed to any degree by sterilizing-grade filters.[38] In addition to many other commercial and scientific applications, sterile filtration is used extensively in the production of sterile and particle-free biopharmaceutical fluids that cannot be sterilized by any other means. Because terminal sterilization methods (eg, autoclaving, ionizing radiation) are preferred by worldwide regulatory agencies, pharmaceutical manufacturers must demonstrate that terminal sterilization cannot be used. The filters then must be validated to ensure that they perform effectively under process conditions. Adherence to rigid Good Manufacturing Practice (GMP) performance criteria imposed on filtration media and filtration systems, particularly those used to produce parenteral drug products, is required and enforced by regulatory inspection.[39,40] Even higher standards for sterile filtration are being established as the complexity and duration of processing has increased. Simultaneously, there has been an increase in the physicochemical and biological complexity of the drugs themselves, further complicating the filtration equation.

▶ FILTER TYPES

The filtration process consists of passing a mixture of fluid and solids through a porous medium that retains the solids on the surface, entraps them in the matrix, or both. Filters may be broadly categorized as primarily depth, surface, or screen filters, depending on their composition and construction characteristics, particle-fluid-filter interactions, and mechanisms of filtration. The distinction between depth, surface (prefilters), and screen filters is of considerable importance, particularly to pharmaceutical process filtration.

Filtration devices and systems typically operate by two different modes: normal flow (also known as dead ended) and tangential flow (also known as cross flow). Normal flow filtration (NFF) occurs when the flow of the feedstock is driven perpendicular to the filter medium with the objective of filtering all the feed through the filter. Tangential flow filtration (TFF) occurs when the feed material flows parallel to the filter medium and a portion of the feedstream permeates through the filter medium by the effect of transmembrane pressure and the bulk of the feedstream moves across the membrane and is recirculated for multiple passes to accomplish the separation. In TFF devices, the cross flow provided by a feed pump helps in reducing buildup of the retained products on the filter surface. This chapter focuses on NFF as it relates to sterile filtration. The topic of TFF in biopharmaceutical processing has been comprehensively reviewed by Lutz.[41]

When used independently, no one type of filter is cost-effective for most high-volume pharmaceutical filtration applications that require complete removal of microorganisms and particles down to a specific size. High-volume microfiltration usually calls for removing particles in a precise, definable way and at an optimal cost. The most effective way to accomplish this is to capitalize on the complementary properties of depth, surface (prefilters), and screen filters. Depth and surface filtration are the most economical ways to remove the bulk of the particulate burden from a fluid.[42] Prefilters can be depth, surface, or screen filters depending on the application and are necessary for most sterilizing applications. The optimum choice of filters involves a careful weighing of two factors: filtration efficiency and particle and colloid loading capacity. These are discussed later in this chapter.

Depth Filters

Depth Filters in Liquid Applications

Depth filters are used in bioprocessing for the clarification of centrate or direct harvest from the bioreactor to remove large particles and colloids as well as host cell proteins. In plasma processes, they can be used for clarification of plasma fractions and precipitate removal. In small molecule processes, depth filters can be used for color and haze removal, catalyst recovery, as well as removal of carbon fines and undissolved intermediates and excipients. Depth filters can be combined with prefilters and sterilizing-grade filters for economical process trains, which are discussed later in this chapter.

A depth filter consists of fibrous, granular, or sintered materials pressed, wound, fired, or otherwise bonded into a tortuous maze of flow channels. Particles in a fluid that pass through the irregular channels defined by the tortuous orientation are principally retained by a combination of mechanical entrapment and adsorption that occur throughout the depth of the filter matrix. The depth of the filter bed can range from 3 to 30 mm providing longer residence time for the capture of smaller particles through adsorptive mechanisms. Figure 30.1 illustrates the role of small particle adsorption inherent with depth filters. Materials commonly selected for pharmaceutical processes include cellulose, cellulose esters, polymeric fibers such as polypropylene, and inorganic fibers and may include filter aids such as diatomaceous earth and carbon. Surface modification, such as a cationic treatment, can be used to remove negative species. These filters are typically used in lenticular pads installed in stainless steel housings or in enclosed single-use pods or capsules.

Because there are many permutations of materials and fabrication methods, depth filters cannot realistically be assigned an absolute particle retention rating. Instead, they are assigned a nominal rating, that is, some particle

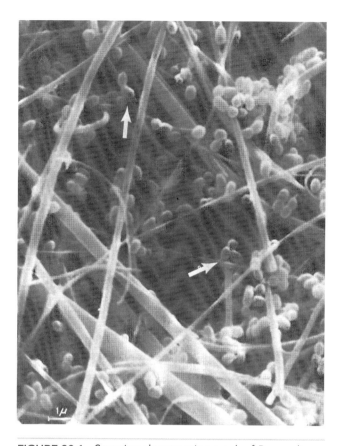

FIGURE 30.1 Scanning electron micrograph of *Brevundimonas diminuta* ATCC 19146 on a glass fiber depth filter. *Arrows* indicate examples of bacterial cells adsorbed to fibers.

size above, which a certain percentage of contaminants is retained. The nominal rating can be determined experimentally after fabrication by passing a test fluid through the depth filter. This fluid, having a known concentration of suspended particles and a known size distribution, is assayed with membrane filters (screen-type filters) before and after filtration. Particle size counts are made on the pre- and postfiltration assay filters, and the percentage retained (in various size ranges) by the depth filter is calculated. The nominal rating of a depth filter is valid only under a strictly defined set of conditions (flow, temperature, pressure, and viscosity). Changes in any one of these parameters may affect the retention mechanisms and may have an important bearing on critical filtration. For instance, when a solid contaminant in a fluid moves through a depth filter, it follows the path of least resistance until it becomes trapped or is adsorbed. As the pressure differential increases, which often results from filter plugging or an increase in operating pressure, particles and microorganisms are driven deeper into the matrix, eventually "breaking through" to enter the downstream process.

Depth Filters in Air and Gas Applications

Of the two types of filter classifications (depth and membrane) used in air and gas filtration, the fibrous depth type is the most common when very large volumes of air must be handled. Glass fibers are commonly used for this application such as those used in high-efficiency particulate air (HEPA) filters for cleanroom air. The gas passing through the matrix of such filters follows a tortuous path, and the microorganisms present are trapped both on the surface and in the depth of the filter.

Advantages of Depth Filters

The advantages of depth filters may be summarized as follows: (1) Depth filters normally exhibit a highest particle capacity (because depth filters can collect contaminants throughout their thicknesses and because they have relatively large spaces between the interstices compared with surface or screen filters) and (2) depth filters retain a substantial percentage of contaminants smaller than their normal size rating because of adsorption.

Disadvantages of Depth Filters

The following are considered disadvantages of depth filters:

1. Media migration, or the tendency of the filter media (filter fragments) to slough off during filtration, is a severe drawback peculiar to all depth filters. Although continuous throughout the life of the filter, media migration becomes more pronounced when a hydraulic surge or continuous flexing of the filter matrix takes place.
2. Release of microorganisms initially trapped in the matrix downstream also presents a problem, particularly during long filtration runs. If adsorption has played a role in the removal of certain particles, even minute changes in the fluid-particle-filter matrix interactions may trigger a release of those particles. Under certain conditions, microorganisms may reproduce within the filter matrix, penetrate deeper into the matrix, and emerge on the downstream side to contaminate the filtrate.[43] This phenomenon is often called *grow-through*.
3. Because they have no meaningful pore size, depth filters impose no definite limitation on the size of particles that may pass through the filter bed.
4. The relatively large amount of liquid retained by depth filters (holdup volume) can be a serious shortcoming with valuable feedstreams.

Selection of Depth Filters in Pharmaceutical Processing

Selection of depth filters requires (1) clearly defining objectives of the filtration step such as product quality, yield, and impurity removal; (2) specifying batch size; (3) identifying the desired process endpoint such as turbidity, pressure, or process time; (4) understanding the properties of the feed material, including feed lot to lot variability; (5) understanding how material from this filtration step can affect subsequent steps in the purification process; and

(6) describing any microbiological needs for the filtrate such as low bioburden or low endotoxins, which would necessitate pre-use sterilization or sanitization of the filter and system. Finally, establishment of the desired capacity and surface area to achieve the processing goals of this step requires bench-scale testing.

Surface Filters

A surface filter, in the context of pharmaceutical filtration, is composed of multiple layers of nonwoven media, usually glass or polymeric microfibers, or web-supported cellulosic membranes. When a fluid is passed through a surface filter, particles larger than the interstices in the microfiber matrix are retained on the surface, whereas smaller particles may be trapped within the matrix, giving a surface filter the advantages of both depth filters and screen filters.

Surface filters can be constructed of microfibers of glass, cellulose, or a variety of polymers or nonwoven supported cellulose membranes. These materials can be used singly or combined to create the filter structure. In addition to traditional fiber laid processes, polymeric microfibers can be melt blown to develop an integral structure that does not require binders. Surface filters are often rolled or pleated and supported by nonwoven base materials for incorporation into a variety of device formats.

Selection of Prefilters in Pharmaceutical Processing

Prefiltration is an effective method to reduce production costs by extending the throughput of downstream membrane filters. Selection of the appropriate prefilter requires (1) clear definition of the objectives of the filtration step, including the objectives of the other filters in the train; (2) specifying batch size; (3) specification of the desired process endpoint such as pressure rise or process time; (4) determination of compatibility with the feedstream, cleaning, sanitizing, or sterilization agents such as steam or gamma radiation; (5) understanding of extractable and leachable contributions; and (6) assessment of impact of protein, preservative, or formulation binding. As with depth filters, establishment of the desired capacity and surface area to achieve the processing goals of this step requires bench-scale testing, which is discussed later in this chapter.

Prefilter Applications

Typical applications that use prefilters include filtration of IVs and small volume parenterals (SVP), ophthalmics, topicals, oral liquids, rinse water such as for vial and stopper washers, solvents, and excipients as well as prefiltration of buffers, cell culture media, and serum.

Screen Filters

Screen filters or sieve filters are used to achieve controlled and predictable particle removal, particularly for final filtration applications that produce a sterile effluent. A screen filter is a highly uniform, rigid, and continuous structure with regularly spaced uniform meshes or irregularly formed spaces or pores. When a fluid is passed through a screen filter, all particles and microorganisms larger than the pore size are retained predominantly on its surface. Particles that penetrate the surface are captured if they are large enough to be retained by the pores within the filter matrix. Examples of screen filters are stainless steel; polymeric mesh; and microporous, polymeric membrane filters, which are the focus of this chapter.

Advantages of Microporous Membrane Filters

The following may be considered advantages of using microporous membrane filters:

1. Filter efficiency is independent of flow rate and pressure differential for particles larger than the pore size.
2. There is no media migration with membrane filters because of their homogeneous structure or do such filters permit passage of particles or organisms larger than the most open pore size, even at very high-pressure differentials. For example, hyaluronic acid filtration can reach pressure differentials approaching 500 psid. Because sterilizing filter cartridge construction does not withstand these excessive pressures, this type of filtration is conducted with large areas of flat sheets in specialized high-pressure housings.
3. Large, inflexible particles tend to form a filter cake on the membrane filter surface. Although interfering little with flow, this porous mat acts as a depth filter by retaining particles smaller than the membrane pore size, thereby increasing the efficiency of the membrane filter.
4. Membrane filters are thin ($<$150-μm), and because there is little void volume within the filter structure, there is minimal feedstream loss.

Disadvantages of Membrane Filters

There are two main disadvantages to using microporous membrane filters. First, because of their surface-retention mechanism, membrane filters have a relatively low capacity, particularly if the particles approximate the pore size of the filter surface. Such particles can plug the pores and prevent fluid flow. Second, not all particles smaller than its pore size pass through the membrane filter. Some of these particles are collected on the membrane surface, and some are trapped in the tortuous interstices themselves. If there are enough of these smaller particles, a rapid buildup in pressure will occur.

▶ RETENTION MECHANISMS

Retention Mechanisms in Air and Gas Filtration

The interstices or pores within a gas filter may be large compared with the size of the particles or microorganisms being trapped, but the mechanism of filtration is such that efficiency in removing small particles is high. A filter having an effective diameter on the order of 5 to 100-μm removes more than 99% of submicron particles.[44] One of the primary ways of increasing the efficiency of a fibrous filter is to reduce the spacing among the fibers. Filters constructed of fine rather than coarse fibers tend to decrease the gap. The removal of particles or microorganisms from air and other gases may be attributed to the following five basic mechanisms.[44] Figure 30.2 schematically depicts these mechanisms.

Interception

Interception is the contact of the surface of the microorganism or particle with the surface of the filter. An assumption is made and can be readily demonstrated that particles adhere to the filter surface once they make contact. Interception would be favored, then, by a small fiber diameter of the filter matrix.

Sedimentation

The sedimentation mechanism is of secondary practical importance because the settling rate of microorganisms is low. If a stream of gas is flowing through a filter matrix, eventually, the microorganisms settle on the surfaces of the filter fibers.

Impaction

The momentum of microorganisms traveling in a gas stream does not allow them to make sharp changes of direction, so they impact on the fiber surface. The efficiency of impaction is favored by a higher gas velocity through the filter and by the small fiber diameter of the filter matrix, which gives rise to a more abrupt change in the flow path of the gas.

Diffusion

Low velocities of air or gas through the filter matrix favor diffusion. Bacteria undergo Brownian movement to some extent and can diffuse to the surfaces of the fiber matrix where van der Waals forces contribute to particle capture.

Electrostatic Attraction

Gas flowing through a filter matrix causes a triboelectric effect, resulting in the charging of the filter fibers. The charge

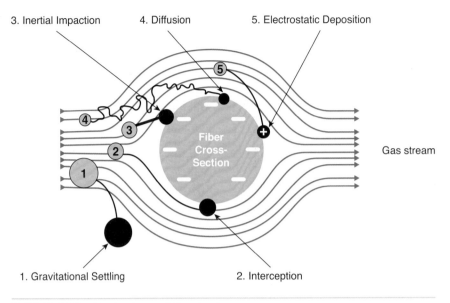

FIGURE 30.2   Mechanisms of filtration in gas streams.

acquired depends on the nature of the fiber. Microorganisms carrying a charge become attracted to the surfaces of the filter. Coating the fibers of a filter with a good electrical insulator was shown to increase the efficiency of the filter.[45] In a sterile filtration application, the filters should not become moist or the retention effect caused by the electrostatic charge could dissipate. Thus, hydrophobicity is an important characteristic of air filters.

These particle-capture mechanisms lead to a most penetrating particle size and dictate construction of a filter with a surface area as large as is practical. The most penetrating particles for fibrous filter media and for membrane filters have been measured to be 0.15- and 0.05-μm, respectively.[46] Retention ratings for HEPA fiberglass filters have been determined to be 99.99%, and for typical membrane filter, 99.9999999%. These mechanisms dictate that it is desirable to construct a filter with a surface area as large as is practical. A large surface area maintains a low differential pressure across the filter and maintains filter efficiency by decreasing the translational velocity of the gas. The large surface areas of HEPA filters in use today are obtained by pleating the filter material back and forth around fluted separator plates.

Retention Mechanisms in Liquid Streams

Size Exclusion

The primary filtration mechanism of a microporous membrane filter in liquids is physical sieving or size exclusion, whereby all particles larger than the surface opening or pore size are retained at or near its surface (Figure 30.3). Uniformity of pore size permits well-defined limits of particle retention to be determined by appropriate testing

(ie, high bacterial challenge levels at a defined number of microorganisms per square centimeter of effective filtration area equals no passage detected).

Adsorption

Adsorption is also a contributing factor in the capture of particles smaller than the pores they encounter. Charge differentials between sites on a particle and within the membrane structure is one of many adsorptive mechanisms. Process conditions and physicochemical properties of the feedstream can affect both size exclusion and adsorption mechanisms. The physicochemical properties of the feedstream could overcome adsorptive forces and allow

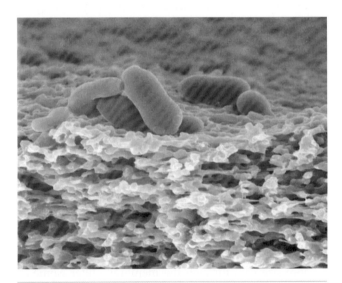

FIGURE 30.3   Cross-sectional scanning electron micrograph of a microporous membrane filter with microorganisms retained on the membrane surface. The cross section highlights the irregular torturous nature of the membrane.

particles to be released into the downstream. Deformable particles retained by size exclusion could be forced through the filter structure by high pressure or flow rates, whereas feedstream properties such as pH or a high salt concentration could decrease the size of microorganisms retained by size exclusion allowing them to be released into the downstream. This is one reason that process-specific bacterial challenge testing of sterilizing-grade membranes is required for critical applications.

❱ FILTER RATINGS

Filter pore ratings can be a confusing topic in pharmaceutical filtration. In theory, pore size relates to a filter's ability to retain particles, including microorganisms, larger than the rated pore size. In practice, the pore rating may have very little to do with the actual relevant performance of the filter. For example, a 0.2-μm rated, sterilizing-grade filter will allow passage of 0.2-μm particles into the effluent, this grade of filter is characterized for the removal of standard bacteria, not for the removal of 0.2-μm particles. The special case of sterilizing-grade filters is discussed in detail later.

Another confusion arises from the use of *absolute* and *nominal* pore ratings. *Nominal* is intended to mean that the filter will remove a certain amount, but not all particles, whereas the term *absolute* is intended to indicate that all particles above a specified size will be removed by the filter. These are both functional terms based on the particle challenge test used. Without information on the test parameters, one might assume that an absolute filter will remove everything "absolutely." The method used by one manufacturer to determine the pore rating and provide an absolute claim can be very different than the method and claim used by another, particularly among different filter structures. Even though manufacturers establish their removal claims under well-controlled laboratory conditions, particle removal in an end user's process will be impacted by feed quality and process conditions; these need to be carefully understood prior to implementation.

Additionally, filters from various manufacturers with the same pore size rating and same polymer components may structurally be very different. This could lead an end user to assume that the filters are equivalent or that one filter will perform better than another based solely on the filter rating. Therefore, pore size rating alone is unreliable selection criterion because these ratings vary from manufacturer to manufacturer and from product to product. The responsibility squarely rests with the user to understand the manufacturer's filter claims to select the appropriate filter for the intended use.

Approaches to Filter Ratings

Approaches to establish pore ratings are varied and depend on the filter type (depth, surface, or screen) and whether it will be used for a liquid or gas application. Methods include gas-liquid or liquid-liquid intrusion tests, flow rate, particle challenge tests, aerosolized oil tests, and microscopy.

Microscopy

In scanning electron microscopy, a sample of membrane is evaluated, using appropriate imaging software to determine pore size and distribution. Track etched membranes can be reasonably sized using this technique owing to their flat surface punctuated by cylindrical pores.

Gas-Liquid or Liquid-Liquid Intrusion Tests

Porosimetry is a physical method where liquid is forced into the membrane under pressure from a gas or other liquid and the penetration profile is analyzed mathematically to determine pore size, porosity, and pore distribution. Porosimetry is based on the assumption that the pores are straight cylindrical pores and flow is directed vertically from upstream to downstream. Microporous membrane filters are complex structures with irregular torturous pathways that move multidirectionally and even dead-end throughout the structure. Correction factors are employed to account for this.

Bubble point is simple method for determining the largest pores in a membrane structure. When the pores of a microporous membrane are full of a wetting liquid (eg, water in a hydrophilic membrane), a gas (eg, air) only displaces the liquid from the pores if the gas pressure is high enough to overcome the local liquid surface tension–induced capillary forces. This method is not practical for depth filters where interstices are so large that the force required to displace liquid is too low be impractical. For membrane filters, the bubble point test can be used for membrane characterization as well as a nondestructive in-process test for filter system integrity during pharmaceutical processing. The principles of the bubble point test are discussed in detail later.

Particle Challenges

Manufacturers use a variety of particles of defined sizes to determine the minimum size that can be retained by the filter. The choice of challenge conditions is dependent on the filter type, desired claims and application and is often used for filters claimed to have a nominal pore size rating.

A filter efficiency rating should indicate the particle size or the microorganism being used for the test and is calculated as described in equation 1 (Particle Removal Efficiency):

$$E_{ps} = 1 - \left(\frac{C_u}{C_d}\right) \times 100\% \qquad (1)$$

Where

E_{ps} = particle removal efficiency at a specified test particle size

C_u = downstream particle count

C_d = upstream particle count

A pore rating for a filter can be helpful as a high-level classification. Regardless of the claimed particle removal efficiency, in actual use, particle removal can be different than product claims due to the interactions of the filter material and structure with the infinite permutations of end user feed compositions and processing conditions.

Sterilizing-Grade Membrane Filter Ratings

Sterile filtration is the process of removing microorganisms from a fluid stream without adversely affecting the feedstream. A sterilizing-grade designation is not pore size dependent despite the common industry use of the 0.2-μm descriptor. It is a functional definition whereby membrane filter demonstrates removal of a standard test organism *B diminuta* (formerly classified in the genus *Pseudomonas*) at a minimum challenge concentration of 1×10^7 colony-forming units (CFUs)/cm^2 under a specific flow rate or pressure. Those filters carrying a sterilizing-grade claim will have data to support that claim. If the manufacturer of a 0.2-μm does not provide a sterilizing-grade filter claim or data to support such a claim, the filter cannot be considered sterilizing grade. To be qualified as sterilizing grade, filter manufacturers will typically perform studies based on American Society for Testing and Materials (ASTM) F838-15a.[47] In addition to membrane filter qualification, manufacturers also perform lot release bacterial challenge tests on samples of membrane and devices.

Functionality of sterilizing-grade membrane filter performance is further demonstrated by the end user for critical operations such as aseptically processed final drug products. It is a regulatory requirement for the end user to conduct process-specific bacterial challenge test validation using the actual drug product under actual (downscaled) processing conditions.[1-6] The PDA Technical Reports 26 and 40 provide the end user guidance on best practices related to filter validation of liquids and gases.[48,49]

▶ FILTRATION APPLICATIONS OF LIQUIDS AND GAS IN PHARMACEUTICAL APPLICATIONS

Filter Sterilization of Liquids

Sterilizing-grade filters are used throughout pharmaceutical and biopharmaceutical processes where either bioburden reduction or sterilizing performance is needed, particularly for feedstreams that cannot be terminally sterilized by heat. Common applications include media and feed filtration into bioreactors, buffer filtration, chromatography column protection, process intermediates, aggregate removal prior to virus filtration, bulk drug substance as well as critical final formulated drug product in both terminal sterilized, and aseptically processed applications.

End users should define the objectives of each filtration step to establish the process claims and determine the data needed from the manufacturer, the type of testing required to justify the filter selection, and any in-process testing to demonstrate fitness for use. For example, a user states the objective for a 0.2-μm filter used for aseptic processing of a heat labile drug product into vials is that the filtrate will be sterile. The manufacturer of a 0.2-μm filter with a sterilizing claim will need to supply data supporting the sterilizing claim. The user will need to meet regulatory expectations and validate that the filter will exhibit sterilizing performance in their product under their usage conditions and will need to perform integrity after use to demonstrate the filter is fit for use. In certain countries, there may also be a regulatory requirement to conduct a pre-use integrity test. On the other hand, a user may select the same 0.2-μm filter for protection of a chromatography column and describes the objective of the filtration as controlling bioburden. In this less critical application, the end user could perform a risk assessment to determine what type of testing is appropriate to indicate the filter is suitable for use.

Filter Sterilization of Air and Other Gasses

Filters are by far the most commonly used devices for the sterilization of air and other gases. The relative ease of handling, the low cost per unit volume of air sterilized, and the efficiency in removing not only microorganisms but also other submicron particles all account for the extensive use of filters. Filtration is the method used for the sterilization of both small and large volumes of air and gas. The mechanics are such that large volumes may be processed economically. For efficient and economic operation, however, the aerosol content of the gas to be filtered must be low; otherwise, a prefilter may be necessary. This is of importance with microporous membrane filters in use today for the removal of bacteria, yeasts, and molds.

Microorganisms, particles, or droplets of liquid dispersed in a gas are referred to as aerosols. The behavior of aerosols is of concern in many scientific and industrial applications. Dwyer[43] reports that particles suspended in a gaseous medium behave according to the classic laws of mechanics. Complications are involved, however, because the mass of these particles is so small that they have an extremely small inertia but high viscous drag properties. Dwyer points out that this is not surprising given that for a spherical particle, inertial effects are a function of the cube of the radius, whereas the viscous drag effects are a manifestation of surface area and are a function of the square of the radius. It is expected, then, that as particle size decreases, the viscous effects become predominant.

Many viable microorganisms exist in aerosols. In fact, the air around us serves as the vehicle for many species of bacteria, molds, yeasts, and their spores. The constant presence of microorganisms is of concern to the food and beverage processing industries, the pharmaceutical industry, hospitals, and the many smaller laboratories requiring sterile environments.

Selection of the appropriate filter for critical gas-sterilizing applications is important. Due to the varied retention mechanisms operating in gas filtration, microorganisms smaller than the specified pore size are retained. A filter having an average pore diameter of 0.8-μm was demonstrated to retain particulate material as small as 0.05-μm.[50] Electrostatic charge plays a greater role in removal than any other mechanism in gas streams.

Hydrophobic membrane filters are ideally adaptable to the filtration of sterile air of venting air for sterile tanks or containers from which sterile pharmaceuticals are being filled, stored, or withdrawn. Sparging for bioreactor applications is ideally suited to membrane filtration because an entire filtration element may be sterilized in place. Vents on fermenters protect not only the influent into the tank but also the environment from the exhaust material. Sterile air filters protect the environment in a blow-fill-seal filling area, and parison support air provides robust and reliable sterility assurance. Autoclave and lyophilizer vacuum breaks require sterilizing-grade hydrophobic filters to ensure the contents remain sterile. In these cases, vent filter material should be hydrophobic; otherwise, moisture droplets, often found in pressurized gas systems, would wet a hydrophilic membrane, essentially reducing the effective filtration area (EFA) by blocking the pores to bulk flow of gas to the extent that a pressure above the bubble point (described later) of the membrane would be required to force air through. In addition, wetting of an air filter may decrease its retention efficiency.

Unlike conventional depth-type filter, hydrophobic microporous membranes (if properly qualified) will not allow bacterial passage when challenged with copious amounts of moisture that may arise in certain applications such as hot water-for-injection (WFI) tanks and fermenter/bioreactor vent applications; however, the addition of coalescing prefilters prior to the sterilizing filter, jacketed filter housings, and proper system design can mitigate the deleterious effects of filter wetting.

▶ FILTER INTEGRITY TESTING OF STERILIZING FILTERS

Filter Integrity Tests

A key feature of an integrity test is its ability to predict membrane performance. In sterilizing filtration, the removal of microorganisms to high levels of efficiency is the most critical performance characteristic. Sterilizing filters must perform to total removal levels of 10^{10} to 10^{11} total microorganisms. Expressed in percentage of efficiency (equation 1), the removal ability equates to greater than 99.999999999%, a high level indeed. This high efficiency is needed because even one organism emerging from a sterilizing filter renders the filtrate nonsterile.

The process of sterilization is often characterized by both physical and biological parameters. For example, the physical measurement of a moist heat process such as steam-in-place (SIP) or autoclaving includes the time/temperature profile of the sterilization cycle (see chapter 28). Examples of physical measurement on sterilizing filters include gas-liquid integrity tests such as diffusional flow or bubble point. These physical parameters are used during each sterilization process to monitor and assess performance. A biological parameter would use a biological indicator (BI) as a measure, expressed in quantitative terms, of the microbial kill for a moist heat process or microbial removal for a filtration process. A BI is a standardized preparation of a specific microorganism at a specific concentration that is relevant to the sterilization process. For example, *Geobacillus stearothermophilus* spores are used as BIs for moist heat processes because the spores are resistant to heat. But these spores would be too large to pass through a 0.2-μm sterilizing-grade filter. *B diminuta*, described in the next section, is the analogous BI for sterilizing filtration.

Biological parameters are used during characterization and validation of the sterilization process and are not employed during routine processing; therefore, a relationship or correlation between the physical and biological parameters is a critical feature. The physical measurement should predict the biological performance of the sterilization process. In an analogous manner, the most useful integrity test of filtration is one that provides information on its ability to remove microorganisms.

Bubble Point

An important advantage of a membrane filter is its ability to be nondestructively tested for integrity before and after filtration. Commonly used integrity tests are the bubble point, diffusive airflow, and pressure hold tests. Test theory has been thoroughly reviewed by others.[51-53]

When the pores of a membrane filter structure are full of a wetting liquid (eg, water in a hydrophilic membrane), a gas (eg, air) displaces the liquid from the pores only if the gas pressure is high enough to overcome the local liquid surface tension–induced capillary forces. The critical pressure at which this occurs is controlled by the size of the pores and the surface tension of the wetting liquid (Figure 30.4) (equation 2, Bubble Point):

$$BP = \frac{4K\gamma\cos\theta}{d} \qquad (2)$$

Where:
BP = bubble point pressure
K = shape correlation factor
γ = surface tension
θ is the liquid-solid contact angle
d is the pore diameter

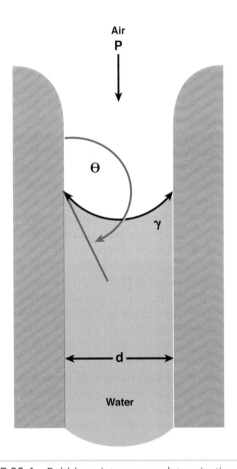

FIGURE 30.4 Bubble point pressure determination. Schematic of a pore cross section. γ is the surface tension, θ is the liquid-solid contact angle, and d is the pore diameter as shown in equation 2. As the pore diameter increases, the force required to overcome the capillary forces decreases resulting in a lower bubble point value. The surface tension of the wetting fluid will also impact the bubble point value. Using a lower surface tension fluid than water, such as alcohol, will reduce the liquid-solid contact angle. In this case, less force will be required to displace the liquid in the pore resulting in a lower bubble point value than for the identical filter tested with water as the wetting fluid.

The bubble point pressure is determined experimentally by observing the pressure at which gas bubbles flow from the downstream side of the membrane or filter, hence the name *bubble point pressure* (Figure 30.5). The relationship between the bubble point pressure and the pore size is an inverse one (ie, the bubble point is higher for smaller pores), and thus, a large membrane defect is identified by a bubble point value below the manufacturer's bubble point specification.

Diffusional Flow Testing

Another valid integrity test that is especially useful for large-area filters is the diffusion flow test (also known as the forward flow test). In this test, the rate for flow of a gas is measured as it diffuses through the water in a wetted integral filter or convectively flows through defects in a nonintegral filter.

Diffusive flow through an integral membrane consists of a three-step process: (1) solution of the test gas in the liquid on the high-pressure upstream side of the membrane, (2) migration of individual gas molecules through the liquid (described mathematically by Fick's law of diffusion), and (3) evaporation of the gas molecules on the low-pressure downstream side of the membrane. The overall rate at which this occurs depends on (1) the solubility of the gas in the liquid, (2) the diffusivity of the gas through the liquid, (3) the pressure difference between the upstream and downstream sides, (4) the temperature, (5) the membrane thickness and porosity, and (6) the total frontal area of the membrane in the filter.

If a diffusion test pressure is selected appropriately by the filter manufacturer (typically near 80% of the bubble point pressure specification), defective filters can be identified as those for which measured gas flow rates are higher than the manufacturer's specification for acceptable flow rates (see Figure 30.5).

Due to the dependence of the overall diffusion rate on the membrane area, the amount of diffusion that is experienced by small-area filters (eg, those with areas less than approximately 2000 cm^2) is not enough to obscure the identification of the bubble point. Instead, the difference observed visually between the effluents at pressures below and above the bubble point is quite dramatic. (For small-area devices, little or no flow is observed below the bubble point, whereas very large flow rates are observed at pressures above the bubble point.) The larger diffusive flows experienced by large-area devices result in a much less dramatic difference in what is observed immediately below and above the bubble point, which in turn makes identification of bubble point much more difficult. Analysts performing manual integrity tests should be trained and certified to perform these tests and the end user should understand the degree of subjectivity that is involved in a manual test. Automated filter integrity test

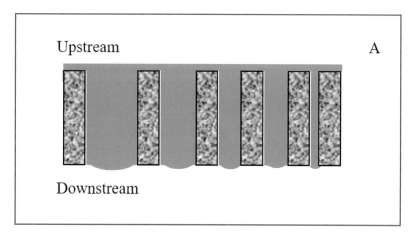

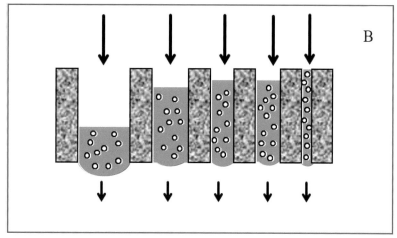

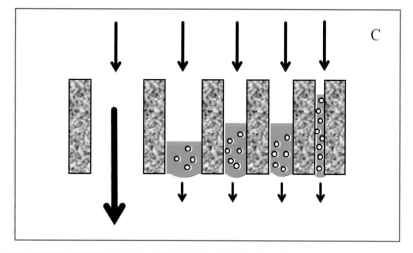

FIGURE 30.5 Diffusion and bubble point. This schematic is a highly simplified depiction of bubble point and diffusion concepts. The pores of membrane filter are highly torturous flow paths, not the straight top to bottom capillaries depicted here. A, A cross section of a filter with different pore sizes. *Blue* indicates water held in the pores by capillary forces. The pressure is equal on the upstream and the downstream of the filter. B, The upstream pressure is higher than the downstream pressure. Air dissolves in the water and diffuses into the downstream; however, pressure is not yet sufficient to overcome the capillary forces holding the water in the pores. For the diffusion test, the upstream air pressure is increased to 80% of the bubble point test pressure. This test pressure is not sufficient to overcome the capillary forces holding the water in the pores. The pressure is held for a defined time, and the flow rate of the diffusing gas is measured. C, For the bubble point test, the upstream pressure is not held at the diffusion test pressure. Instead, the upstream pressure is steadily and continuously increased to a point where the force of this pressure overcomes the capillary forces of the largest pores in the filter resulting in bulk flow of air. The measurement of this pressure is called the bubble point.

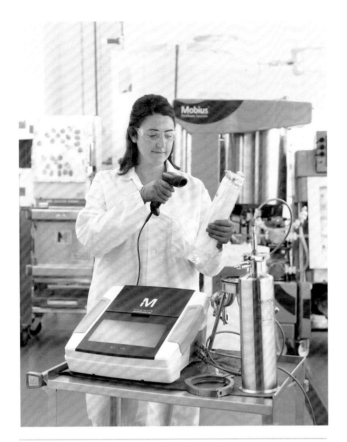

FIGURE 30.6   Example of a portable, automated integrity test device for measuring bubble point and diffusional air flow. For a color version of this art, please consult the eBook. MERCK Image materials/images reproduced with permission of Merck Sharp & Dohme Corp., a subsidiary of Merck & Co., Inc., Kenilworth, New Jersey, USA. All rights reserved.

instruments are commercially available to perform both the diffusion and bubble-point tests (Figure 30.6).

These instruments have greater precision and reproducibility, reduce the degree of test error, and provide documented evidence of the test results in either electronic or printed form. Automatic integrity test instruments should be qualified during installation and the instrument performance should be recorded and analyzed during use with the actual fluids being tested.[54] By following the manufacturer's recommendations for the appropriate test and test conditions for the filter in question, users can obtain quantitative results that, when compared with the manufacturer's specifications, determine the integrity of the filter.

Minimum Production Integrity Test Value in Filter Validation

Manufacturers of sterilizing-grade membrane filters often provide data on the comparison between their suggested integrity test and bacterial retention. In addition, they can provide guidance on performing and interpreting integrity tests obtained from the wide variety of fluids that are sterilized by filtration. For performing a microbial retention validation, it is recommended that at least one of the filters tested have a minimum integrity test value at or near the minimum production limit or specification.[48] The definition of the term *at or near* is defined by regulatory reviewers on a case-by-case basis. Within 10% of the minimum integrity value is considered a good rule of thumb.

Integrity Testing of Critical Sterilizing Filters

Filter integrity tests are important for indicating whether a filter assembly is fit for the intended use. Filter manufacturers will provide integrity test specifications such as bubble point or diffusion for their products. These specifications will indicate the test temperature, test gas such as air or nitrogen, and the wetting liquid such as water or an alcohol-water solution. Validation is discussed later in this chapter.

Post-use Integrity Testing

Post-use integrity testing is a regulatory requirement for final sterile-filtered aseptically processed drug products that cannot be sterilized in their final container. The objective is to document that the filter was integral, thereby indicating the effluent was sterilized. It is important to establish the conditions for the post-use integrity test. In some cases, a post-use water flush step may be conducted to remove residual drug product prior to conducting the integrity test. In other cases, an end user may choose not to flush the filter and to develop a correction factor to establish a drug product–based integrity test value.

Pre-use Integrity Tests

Pre-use integrity tests can be conducted prior to sterilization to understand whether the filter was damaged by the shipping, warehousing, or assembly process prior to carrying out the sterilization operation. Pre-use poststerilization integrity tests (PUPSIT) can be conducted after the sterilization process to understand whether the sterilization process caused the filter device to be unseated from its housing or if the process damaged the filter device structure. Unlike the post-use test, regulatory expectations for conducting pre-use tests vary and typically focus on the concern of the impact of SIP and autoclave process on filter integrity. An EU GMPs explicitly require PUPSIT for the final sterile-filtered aseptically processed products that cannot be sterilized in their final container.[55] In many countries, a PUPSIT is suggested but not required. In this case, the decision not to conduct a PUPSIT should be based on a risk assessment. In these cases, the risk often centers around how to maintain sterility of the system during and after a pre-use test, for example, how to maintain downstream sterility if the system was not designed for in situ testing. If a redundant filtration setup is used, both the interstitial space between the filters and the downstream need to maintain sterility.

A system design has been described to maintain sterility as well as manage gas and liquid flow during integrity testing for a redundant filter system.[56]

Integrity Testing of Gas and Vent Filters

Compressed gas filters and tank vent filters are used throughout a pharmaceutical facility, often in place for months and may experience multiple sterilization cycles. Therefore, assessment of the filtration objective, process location, degree of contact with the drug product, among other risk parameters will dictate the frequency of filter integrity testing for these filters. For example, the EMA differentiates the frequency of integrity testing of gas and vent filters by criticality; recommending critical sterile gas and vent filters to be integrity tested after use while recognizing noncritical air or gas vent filters should be integrity tested "at appropriate intervals."[55]

▸ CHARACTERIZING MICROBIAL REMOVAL PROPERTIES OF STERILIZING-GRADE FILTERS

Microbial Challenge Tests

Elford[57] presented the earliest report of a microbial (bacterial) retention test being used to predict the performance properties of membrane filters. Although his studies emphasized membrane formation, he investigated several biological applications for his filters. Using three different genera of bacteria, he showed that retention of microorganisms by filters of various pore sizes depended on the size of microorganisms used in the test. These tests were performed on membranes composed of nitrocellulose. Studies were carried out at low-pressure drops across the filter, and little attention was given to the culturing of the test microorganisms.

The basis of the modern microbial retention testing was described by Bowman et al[37] who had isolated an unusual microorganism contaminating a protein solution. They described it as a small pseudomonad that, when present in high concentrations, consistently passed through a 0.45-μm membrane filter; they used this as their test microorganism. Realizing the need for a standardized test microorganism, they deposited it with the ATCC. Subsequently, the organism was identified as *Pseudomonas diminuta* and given the accession number of 19146. This bacterium was reclassified to the genus *Brevundimonas* in 1994 based on DNA homology.[58]

Rogers and Rossmoore[59] later proposed a procedure for determining the biologically defined pore size of membrane filters. Their intent was to develop a pore-size characterization for microporous membranes using microbiological

methods as a supplement to physical measurements. While also using *B diminuta* for sterilizing-grade membranes, they could examine larger pore sizes by using microbes of greater dimensions.

Standard Challenge Microorganism

B diminuta ATCC 19146 has emerged as the challenge test microorganism of choice in sterilizing filtration performance and is recognized by such organizations as the FDA,[1] ASTM International,[47] and the PDA.[48,49] These methods are compared in Table 30.1. Choosing *B diminuta* as a "biological indicator" to characterize the performance of membrane filters follows the same logic used in choosing *G stearothermophilus* for moist heat sterilization and *Bacillus atrophaeus* for ethylene oxide sterilization. When considering physiochemical agents such as moist heat and ethylene oxide, the most logical choice for a test organism is one that has been shown to be resistant to the agent to be applied, as have the two spore-forming organisms just mentioned. Similarly, certain smaller bacteria rigorously challenge the ability of a filtration system to physically remove bacteria. *B diminuta* is a natural candidate for a test organism for several reasons. It was originally isolated from contaminated solutions after filtration. Under properly controlled cultivation conditions, the cells can be induced to be small coccobacilli (0.2- to 0.9-μm) with a length-to-width ratio of 2:1 and monodispersed (nonaggregated). The organism is easily maintained and can be grown to high cell densities in a short time (18 to 24 h). It is considered nonpathogenic to healthy populations and is therefore lower risk to use at high concentrations in large volumes of liquid under the high-pressure conditions used during bacterial challenge studies.

B diminuta, is a small, rod-shaped, asporogenous, nonfermenting, gram-negative bacterium. It possesses a single polar flagellum that has a uniquely short wavelength (0.6-μm). *B diminuta* forms small colonies 1 to 2 mm in diameter on soybean casein digest agar after 48 hours of incubation at 30°C. The colonies exhibit a light tan pigment and are round and slightly convex, with entire edges. Morphologically, *B diminuta* is difficult to differentiate from other gram-negative nonfermenting rods. Ballard et al[60] provide a comprehensive review of the taxonomy and physiology of this organism.

Microbial Size

Just as the heat resistance of *G stearothermophilus* spores is a principal factor in moist heat sterilization validation, the size of the test microbe is critical for the determination of retention characteristics of membranes. In much the same way that D-values (a measure of resistance) can fluctuate for a particular lot of *G stearothermophilus* spores, the size of bacteria, for instance, can vary with

TABLE 30.1   A comparison of guidelines for performing microbial retention testing of sterilizing grade filters

Bacterial Challenge Test Parameters	ASTM F838-15a[a]	FDA Aseptic Processing Guideline[b]	PDA Technical Report 26 for Liquids[c] and Technical Report 40 for Gases[d]
Test organism	Brevundimonas diminuta ATCC 19146	B diminuta ATCC 19146	B diminuta ATCC 19146 or relevant bioburden
Challenge level of the effective frontal surface area	10^7 CFUs/cm^2	$\geq 10^7$ CFUs/cm^2	$\geq 10^7$ CFUs/cm^2
Culturing method	Saline lactose broth frozen cell paste or an equivalent method	Properly grown, harvested, and used	Saline lactose broth frozen cell paste or an equivalent method
Challenge volume	Not considered	Not considered	Simulate an actual process
Challenge ΔP across the test membrane	30 psid (206 kPa)	Simulate an actual process	Simulate an actual process
Challenge flow rate	2 to 4 × 10^{-3} L/min/cm^2	Simulate an actual process	Meet or exceed actual process conditions
Challenge vehicle	Saline lactose broth or sterile saline	Simulate an actual process	Actual product or surrogate if bactericidal effects impact the culture
Methods for detecting test organism passage	0.45-μm analytical membrane filter	Not considered	0.45- or 0.2-μm analytical membrane filter
Integrity test	Perform post-use test	Correlate to filter performance	Must correlate to bacterial retention

[a]From ASTM International.[47]

[b]From US Food and Drug Administration.[1]

[c]From Parenteral Drug Association.[48]

[d]From Parenteral Drug Association.[49]

different physiologic states and with different cultivation media. Size is controlled by two factors: the organism's environment and its genetics. The environmental influences that affect size include changes in the growth phase of an organism, nutrient content of culture medium, the concentration of dissolved oxygen, and, of renewed interest, the concentration of dissolved ions and other excipients and active pharmaceutical ingredients.

Also, fundamental to producing an appropriate challenge for the current microbial retention test is the distribution of cell sizes and shapes of a microorganism as it goes through the various growth phases. Figure 30.7 provides an example of a bacterial growth curve. The curve is obtained by plotting either log of bacterial mass (a measure of size) or log of bacterial numbers versus time of incubation. In the late 1920s, Henrici[61] observed that freshly inoculated cells show a size increase during the lag phase while the organism adjusts to a new environment. In so doing, the cell increases its intracellular components (ribosomes, messenger RNA, enzymes) and thus prepares for the increase in the cellular division rate that is to follow. After this preparation, the organism enters the exponential growth phase, a time of rapid growth. During the

transition from the exponential to the stationary phase, cells again become smaller because they divide faster than they grow. Although the extracellular concentration of nutrients is depleted, the organism is still capable of maintaining a growth rate (ie, continuation of division) by using intracellular reserves. As the cell depletes the intracellular reserves, its size decreases, and the population enters the stationary phase of growth. The stationary phase is that period of growth during which the number of cells no longer increases, that is, during which there is essentially a zero growth rate. Once into stationary phase, although there is no net increase in bacterial numbers, the population is still in a dynamic state. Although some cells continue to divide at a basal rate, others die because of the severity of the environment (lack of nutrients and accumulation of waste products). Cultures from late stationary phases may have a level of viable cells equivalent to that of early stationary-phase cultures, but they may also contain many dead cells and much autolytic cellular debris.

The entire effective frontal surface area of a membrane filter must be challenged with viable bacterial cells for the retention test to be rigorous. If significant portions of the membrane being tested become plugged

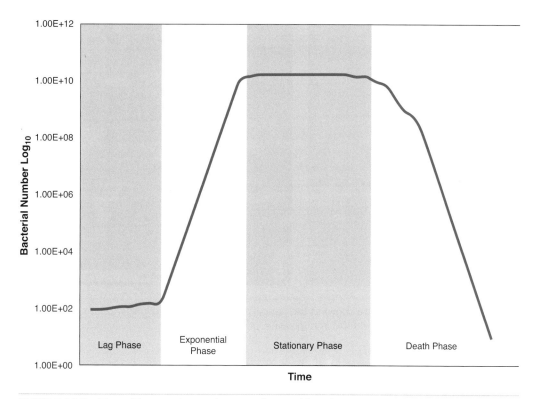

FIGURE 30.7 Typical bacterial growth curve obtained by plotting either log of bacterial mass (a measure of size) or log of bacterial numbers versus time of incubation.

with debris, the viable cells cannot effectively challenge that portion of the membrane. The particulate debris and viable cells in this case must compete for test sites on the membrane surface; thus, results of retention tests may be a false negative. Early stationary phase cultures are clearly the most appropriate for bacterial retention testing of membrane filters because they are small, are still capable of further division, and have few dead and dying cells in the population. Choice of the growth phase requires a thorough understanding of the population dynamics of the test organism under defined conditions of cultivation.

The cultivation medium can also have a profound effect on both cell size and cell arrangement. Schaechter et al[62] working with another gram-negative bacterium, *Salmonella* Typhimurium, observed profound effects caused by different cultivation media on cell size and composition (RNA and DNA). They concluded that size and composition depended on the growth rate afforded by the medium, with an increase in growth rate resulting in an increase in cell size. Other researchers have found substantial increases in cell size and mass under conditions of progressively faster growth rates.[63,64]

Leahy and Sullivan[65] studied the effect of different culturing conditions on *B diminuta* cultivated in nutrient rich soybean casein digest broth (SCDB) and comparatively nutrient-depleted saline lactose broth (SLB). This response is illustrated in the scanning electron micrographs in Figure 30.8. The *B diminuta* cultivated in SCDB are large, forming cells that are distinctly rod shaped (aspect ratios

approximately 4:1) as shown in Figure 30.8A. Production of exopolysaccharides favors aggregation in the form of multiple cell clusters (rosettes) as well as pellicle formation at the air-liquid interface. The rosettes are commonly composed of 10 to 15 cells each. Wet mount and stain preparations show extensive aggregation and debris. These bacterial aggregates result in particles whose effective filtration size is at least five times that of a single cell in SLB. Figure 30.8B shows *B diminuta* grown in SLB, a medium widely used in the cultivation of challenge microorganisms for filter retention testing. The formula for SLB is 7.6 g NaCl, 970.0 mL reagent-grade water, and 30.0 mL lactose broth (1.3 g dehydrated lactose broth per 100 mL reagent-grade water). In the Leahy and Sullivan SLB cultivation method, an aliquot from a 30°C 18- to 24-hour SCDB culture of *B diminuta* was transferred into SLB for incubation at 30°C. *B diminuta* exhibited a generation time of 2.6 hours in SLB and reached cell densities 10^7 organisms/mL in 18 to 22 hours of incubation. The comparatively lower nutrient conditions of the SLB culture produced a predominantly monodispersed suspension of small coccobacillary cells. Comparatively little detrital material is seen with light microscopic viewing of wet mount or stained preparations.

Other methods of cultivation of *B diminuta* for bacterial retention tests such as the frozen paste method are also acceptable. The SLB method and the frozen paste method of preparation of *B diminuta* were described in the 1982 Health Industry Manufacturers Association (HIMA) guidelines on which the ASTM F838-15a standard is

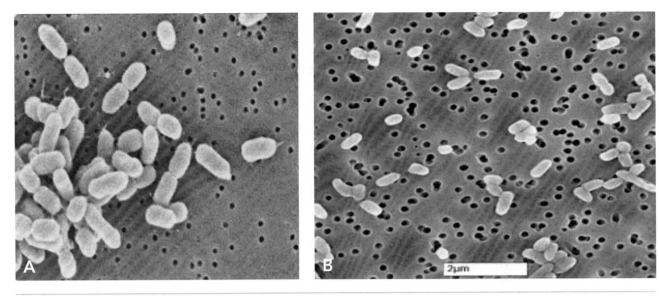

FIGURE 30.8 Scanning electron micrograph showing the typical morphology of *Brevundimonas diminuta* ATCC 19146 when cultivated in soybean casein digest broth (A) and in saline lactose broth (B).

heavily based and subsequently replaced the HIMA guideline in the 1990s.[47,66] Subsequently, detailed advances have been made in the SLB cultivation method and the frozen paste method.[67,68]

Detection Assay

The sensitivity of any test for bacterial retention depends on the efficient detection of any organism that may traverse the filter. Because the presence of even one organism in the filtrate is significant, recovery methods for the test organism should be as sensitive as possible. Maximum sensitivity may be achieved by examining the entire filtrate for sterility. Aliquot sampling of the filtrate (ie, testing only a portion of the filtrate rather than all of it) can miss detecting organisms when they are in low concentrations (less than one organism per 100 mL). The membrane filter method is widely used to analyze large fluid volumes for the presence or absence of bacteria in sterility testing.[36,69] Leahy and Sullivan[65] described a modification of the USP method that allows quantitation of bacterial passage instead of merely growth/no-growth results. Furthermore, Carter[70] conducted studies to demonstrate the continued suitability of using of 0.45-μm analytical membranes as recovery filters in sterilizing-filter bacterial challenge tests.

Challenge Test System Considerations

The test apparatus design for conducting a bacterial challenge test is dependent on (1) the filter format tested such as a 47-mm membrane disc or a cartridge in a stainless steel holder or single-use capsule, (2) the number of filters tested simultaneously (eg, 3 to 4 filters or 20 filters), and (3) whether the system is pressure driven with compressed air or flow driven via a pump. Independent of the test system design, the standard bacterial retention test for claiming sterilizing-grade filter performance will exhibit (1) consistent and well-documented cultivation of *B diminuta*, (2) a minimum concentration of *B diminuta* per unit area of the filter, (3) the use of sensitive bacterial recovery methods, (4) standard process conditions (eg, differential pressure, flow rate), and (5) a common suspending vehicle for the challenge bacteria.

Quantifying Sterilizing Performance

As mentioned previously, the quantification of microbial kill or removal is an essential element in the characterization of any sterilization process. For such sterilization methods as those using moist heat or ethylene oxide, the rate of kill is described as the D-value. The D-value, expressed in minutes, is the amount of exposure time to the conditions of sterilization that results in a 1 log reduction in bacterial numbers. It is the relationship between microbial kill and physical measurements of the sterilization system such as time and temperature that allows prediction of sterilization performance.

The quantification of bacterial retention by membrane filters is determined experimentally. The test filter is challenged with defined concentration of microorganisms. The filtrate is assayed to determine the total number of microorganisms that have passed through the filter. Investigators have proposed the term *beta ratio* to express the microbial removal efficiency of filters.[65,71] The beta ratio was defined as the number of organisms challenging the filter divided by the number that pass

TABLE 30.2 Hypothetical log reduction value in the context of membrane surface area and bacterial passage

Surface Area Tested (cm²)	EFA Challenge (CFUs/cm²)	Upstream Challenge (CFUs/filter)	Downstream Bacterial Passage (CFUs)	Log Reduction Value (LRV)
14	1×10^7	1.4×10^8	0[a]	>8.15
7000	1×10^7	7.0×10^{10}	0[a]	>10.85
14	1×10^7	1.4×10^8	10	7.15
7000	1×10^7	7.0×10^{10}	10	9.85

Abbreviations: CFUs, colony-forming units; EFA, effective filtration area.

[a]For absence of bacteria, a "1" is used in the denominator of the LRV calculation and the result is reported with a greater than symbol (>).

through the filter (equation 3, Beta Ratio). In a later study, the term *titer reduction* was proposed, which is synonymous with the beta ratio[72]:

$$\beta = \left(\frac{C_u}{C_d} \right) \quad (3)$$

Where:
C_u = upstream bacterial challenge concentration
C_d = downstream bacterial count

To standardize terminology, HIMA adopted the term *log reduction value* (LRV) in 1982 as an expression of the microbial removal efficiency by filters (equation 4).[66] The $\log_{10}$ of the beta ratio is the LRV. This calculation is useful for filters that exhibit high levels of retention efficiency. For example, a filter with an LRV of 8 can reduce the number of test microorganisms by eight orders of magnitude. If this retention efficiency was expressed as a percentage, the value would be 99.999999%. Sterilizing filters do not commonly exhibit passage of test organisms; such filters, therefore, express LRVs as "greater than" the log to of the total challenge level.

Log Reduction Value

$$LRV = \text{Log}_{10} \left(\frac{C_u}{C_d} \right) \quad (4)$$

Where:
LRV = log reduction value
C_u = total upstream bacterial challenge concentration
C_d = total downstream bacterial challenge concentration

When C_d is zero, the term "1" is used in the calculation and the results reported as greater than ">."

The upstream challenge concentration in CFUs/filter is used in the LRV calculation. The EFA challenge equation is used to determine whether the challenge test met the minimum acceptance criterion of 1×10^7 CFUs/cm² (equation 5).

$$\text{EFA challenge} = \frac{\beta}{A} \quad (5)$$

Where;
β = beta ratio in CFUs (colony-forming units)
A = filter effective frontal surface area

When reviewing LRV results, it is important to understand the total challenge in CFUs/filter, concentration, and the effective frontal surface area in addition to the EFA Challenge concentration LRV to put the results in context.

Table 30.2 provides an example of a single 0.2-μm filter type with two different surface areas challenged with *B diminuta*. Each device met the minimum acceptance criterion was 1×10^7 CFUs/cm². In the first case, both devices exhibited no bacterial passage downstream. The LRVs were >8.15 and >10.85. If the surface area was not provided, one could conclude that the filter that achieved the higher LRV was superior than the other. In the second case, if the LRVs of 7.15 and 9.85 were provided without indicating the surface or the degree of passage, one might assume that both devices were retentive because the LRVs were greater than 7 when in fact, both exhibited bacterial passage. As in the first case, the LRV difference for the same degree of bacterial passage are an artifact of the need to adjust the upstream challenge concentration to account for the surface area.

Relationship of Integrity Test Value to Microbial Retention

In the 1970s, researchers used *B diminuta* to show the relationship between integrity tests and bacterial retention.[71,72] Because bacterial retention tests are destructive tests, meaning that the filter would not be used in a pharmaceutical production process after such a test, nondestructive filter integrity tests were implemented to both facilitate membrane characterization and lot release testing of membrane filters by the manufacturer and later, to demonstrate the filter is fit-for-use in the process by the end user. One approach to establishing a relationship between a filter integrity test and the bacterial retention test is during sterilizing-grade membrane development and validation. In this approach, a series of membranes with increasing bubble point values is produced. Replicate samples are pre-use bubble point tested then challenged with bacteria using a method such as ASTM F838-15a.[47]

Figure 30.9 demonstrates how the experimental data can be represented. In this hypothetical example, a series of membranes with increasing bubble points are challenged in a standard bacterial retention test. The bacterial counts in the filtrate are transformed to the log of the count. When the log of the count is less than 1, a portion of the tests will have a sterile filtrate, and the remaining portion of tests will have very low bacterial counts. For simplicity, Figure 30.9 depicts an extrapolation to a bubble point value that delivers a certain degree of confidence. In this example, where the log of the count is −3, the retention confidence would translate to 99.9% at a bubble point value of 57 psig. In actual practice, a variety of statistical techniques would be applied to the data to establish the bubble point with high retention confidence and a high safety margin.

The bubble point specification can then be used in quality release tests.[73,74] After a membrane has been developed and validated, that membrane can then incorporate into the filter device development process where the bacterial retention will be verified as part of the device validation and the device integrity tests claims verified. During routine membrane production, membrane manufacturers perform bacterial retention tests and integrity tests on samples from the lot as part of release testing. For device testing, in process integrity tests can be performed on the entire lot of devices, whereas samples from the lot can be tested for bacterial retention.

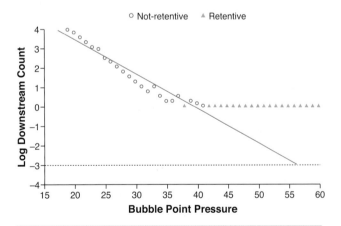

FIGURE 30.9 Bubble point versus log of the count. A series of membranes with increasing bubble points are challenged in a standard bacterial retention test. Open circles represent nonretentive filters. Solid triangles represent retentive (or sterilizing performance) filters. In this hypothetical example, where the log of the count is −3, the retention confidence would translate to 99.9% for a bubble point of 57 psi.

Sterilizing-grade filters are provided with integrity test specifications such as a minimum bubble point value or a maximum diffusion value. In an end user's environment, the integrity test can be considered a fit-for-use test to indicate either pre-use or post-use whether the filter device experienced damage or unseating from the housing. If the device meets the acceptance criterion for the specified integrity test, the end user can have a high degree of assurance that the device will exhibit sterilizing-grade performance.

Variables Affecting of Sterilizing Performance

As discussed, membrane manufacturers use standard bacterial retention tests to develop and characterize sterilizing grade filters; however, end users will have different feedstream properties and processing conditions, which could affect the removal of *B diminuta* by these same filters. It is important to understand these factors to select and validate the appropriate sterilizing grade filter for a process.

Adsorptive Effects

Several researchers have sought to understand the role of adsorption versus size exclusion on the retentive properties of membrane filters ranging from the impact of filter layering to the impact of the challenge suspension liquid properties such as divalent cations and surfactants in bacterial retention.[75-78]

Robertson and DeVisser[79] studied *B diminuta* retention using liquids that varied in surface tension, ionic strength, and viscosity. In both studies, bacterial retention was not affected, that is, the sterilizing filters under study remained completely retentive. Leahy[80] provided a comprehensive examination of chemical attributes of the liquid vehicle on filter performance. Further refining this work, Levy used *B diminuta* as a test microorganism to study the effects of solution chemistry (pH, viscosity), surfactant (Triton X-100), and divalent ($MgCl_2$) and trivalent ($AlCl_3$) cations on the retention of these bacteria by PVDF membranes. Retention was independent of solution attributes and pressure of filtration (30 to 50 psid).[81] Summaries of the literature regarding the role of adsorption in sterilizing filtration are published elsewhere.[82,83]

Challenge Concentration

Clearly, the number of organisms that challenge a filter per unit area of the filter is an important test variable. Elford[84] observed that passage of microorganisms through membranes with even larger pore sizes (>0.5-μm) depended on the number of organisms present. Wallhäusser[77] obtained a similar result in his testing of filter cartridges. This phenomenon is illustrated by the data

TABLE 30.3	Effect of bacterial challenge level on passage of *Brevundimonas diminuta* through a 0.45-μm membrane filter	
	Total No. of Organisms Challenging Filter	**Total No. of Organisms Passing Through Filter**
Retention threshold	10^2	0
	10^4	0
	10^6	10^0
	10^8	10^2
	10^{10}	10^4

TABLE 30.4	Bacterial retention test performed by recirculation of continually inoculated liquid through a 0.2-μm pore size membrane filter		
Replicate	**Microbial Challenge per cm^2 of Filter Area**	**Total Microbial Challenge**	**Log Reduction Value**
1	1.6×10^7	7.6×10^9	>9.88
2	1.3×10^7	6.0×10^9	>9.78
3	1.9×10^7	8.9×10^9	>9.95
4	1.4×10^7	6.6×10^9	>9.82

[a]Test organism: *Brevundimonas diminuta*; test duration: 16 hours.

shown in Table 30.3. Under standard conditions, passage of *B diminuta* through a 0.45-μm filter does not occur until some threshold concentration is exceeded. Below that threshold, the filtrate is sterile. Although the bioburden of liquids that are sterilized by filtration are often known, reliable sterilization procedures should consider an unexpected increase of bioburden and should also provide some margin of safety to obtain sterile filtrates. In this way, sterilizing filters are commonly challenged at relatively high concentrations of microorganisms to validate their performance. The industry standard minimum concentration of 10^7 organisms/cm^2 of effective filtration area will adequately challenge a filtration element.[1]

Test Duration

Time is another factor that can influence the performance of bacterial filtration. Although most sterilizing filtrations are limited to short processing times (<8 h), extended filtration duration may allow microorganisms to replicate to the point of membrane passage. Howard and Duberstein[85] showed that filters that were constantly fed well water show passage of microorganisms as a function of time. In general, passage did not occur until after 24 hours and increased with time.

Leahy et al[86] demonstrated that sterilizing-grade filters were completely retentive to daily challenges of 10^6 of a variety of microorganisms. Experiments were run for 28 days under simulated conditions of continuous ambulatory peritoneal dialysis. It appears that the impact of time includes a subset of variables that affect retention. Examples of these are (1) numbers and types of microorganisms in liquid stream, (2) physiochemical makeup of liquid stream (eg, temperature, pH, ionic strength), and (3) nutritional makeup of liquid stream (ie, stimulatory or inhibitory to microbial growth).

Table 30.4 provides data on *B diminuta* retention using a test system that recirculates fluid containing a constant feed of organisms for 16 hours. The experimental conditions

were designed to simulate pharmaceutical-type filtrations. Sterilizing filters (0.2-μm) successfully retained all organisms throughout the test period. The factor of time must be considered when determining the useful life of a filtration element.

Pressure

Another key factor in bacterial retention is the pressure drop across the filter element. Leahy and Sullivan,[65] Tanny et al,[75] and Reti et al[76] have shown the dependence of transmembrane pressure on bacterial retention. These studies used filters with pore sizes larger than those recommended for sterilization. This effect is illustrated by the data in Table 30.5.

At pressure drops that differ by an order of magnitude, there is a corresponding order-of-magnitude change in the rate of bacterial passage. The efficiency of retention decreases with increasing pressure drop. Sterilizing filters (0.2-μm pore size) are independent of pressure (ie, no passage is detected at any of the test pressures). Performance tests should be run at relatively high transmembrane pressures (eg, 30 psid) to maximize the likelihood of detecting bacterial passage if it occurs.

TABLE 30.5	Impact of differential pressure (ΔP) on retention of *Brevundimonas diminuta*	
Pore size of Membrane Filter (μm)	**Log Reduction Value**	
	5 psi ΔP	**50 psi ΔP**
0.22	>10^{10}	>10^{10}
0.45	8.65	7.60
0.65	4.61	3.14
0.80	2.00	1.32

Summary

Sterilizing filtration has been applied successfully to a wide variety of liquids that differ in their physical (including pressure and duration) and chemical attributes (including pH, ionic strength, polarity, surface tension, and viscosity). But it is impossible to design any one bacterial retention test procedure that considers all these variables. A standard method under controlled conditions affords the manufacturer a consistent way to develop and trend performance of their products and produce product claims; the end user can then compare sterilizing-grade filter claims among filter manufacturers to aid in the selection process. Product- and process-specific bacterial retention filter validation is required for critical filtration processes to assess the impact of the variables specific to an end user's products and processes.

▶ STERILIZING FILTER SELECTION AND SYSTEM DESIGN CONSIDERATIONS

Selecting a Sterilizing Membrane

Choosing Between 0.2-μm Versus 0.1-μm Rated Filters for Final Drug Product Applications

Since the early 1970s, 0.2-μm rated filters with sterilizing-grade claims have been the standard for sterilizing filtration and have been used successfully to sterilize billions of doses of parenteral drug products. (R. Wilkins, oral communication, January 15, 2018). On occasion, microorganisms smaller than *B diminuta* (such as *Ralstonia pickettii*, strains of *Leptospira*, and strains from the *Mollicutes* class such as of the genus *Mycoplasma*) have been reported to penetrate some 0.2-μm and 0.1-μm membrane.[85,87-92] Although bacteria can pass through 0.2-μm filters, it is an uncommon occurrence in pharmaceutical processes. There are few published studies where the root cause for contamination of commercial aseptically processed drug products was shown to be bacterial penetration through the filter. In 1985, Anderson et al[87] demonstrated that *R pickettii* (formerly of the genus *Pseudomonas*), found in a sodium chloride solution used in respiratory therapy, could pass reproducibly through one manufacturer's sterilizing-grade filter. In 1998, another filter-sterilized sodium chloride solution was recalled due to isolates of *R pickettii* in the respiratory tract cultures of 13 patients.[93] Sundaram reports on many cases of bacterial penetration through 0.2-μm filters, many of the cases cited are laboratory studies in nonpharmaceutical applications such as estuary water and sea water and in laboratory cell culture applications. Some relevant studies cited relate to extended duration sterile filtration well in excess of

8 hours.[91] In 1997, Leo et al[94] reported that under specific conditions, a bioburden microorganism penetrated a certain 0.2-μm rated filter.

Safety Margin

Because there could be a process risk, understanding, characterizing, and controlling bioburden is essential for aseptically processed drug products. In well-controlled processes, the bioburden levels reaching the sterilizing filter are significantly lower than the validated challenge level greater than 1×10^7 CFUs/cm^2 used to claim sterilizing-grade performance suitable for use in the process. For example, if the bioburden count for the feed preceding a sterilizing filter was 10 CFUs/100 mL and a 10 000 L batch was filtered through a single filtration device with 6000 cm^2 of effective frontal membrane surface area, the challenge per unit area would be 1.7×10^2 CFUs/cm^2, illustrating the margin of safety provided by a properly designed, validated, operated, and maintained sterile filtration process.

Challenge Microorganism

Although *B diminuta* is widely recognized as the sterilizing-grade challenge standard, relevant bioburden isolates found to be smaller than *B diminuta* in process bioburden should be considered for product- and process-specific bacterial challenge validation studies. The decision to use alternate test microorganisms should be based on a thorough risk assessment and sound understanding of the bioburden history and profile. There are cases, during product- and process-specific challenge tests where product attributes such as high salts, pH, viscosity, osmolarity and process attributes such as test duration, flow rate, or pressure where bacterial penetration have been observed. In these cases, 0.1-μm rated filter may then be the appropriate choice for validation and implementation. For most cases, a sterilizing grade 0.2-μm will provide the appropriate level of safety in the process.

The 0.2-μm Versus 0.1-μm Rated Filters for Media and Cell Culture Applications

In cell culture–derived processes, *Mollicutes* (*Mycoplasma*, *Acholeplasma*, *Spiroplasma*) contamination of cell banks and cell culture media was typically associated with animal-derived components such as trypsin or serum. As the industry moved to remove animal-derived components from cell culture media, it was thought that 0.2-μm filtration was sufficient for these serum-free media formulations. In 2005, 0.2-μm filtered SCDB used in a process simulation was found to be contaminated with *Acholeplasma laidlawii*.[95] This case moved the industry to either autoclave SCDB for process simulations, or if filtered, to use preirradiated raw materials. It also created awareness in the biopharmaceutical industry of the risk of *Mollicutes* contamination of plant-based hydrolysate components of cell culture media.[96,97] The following example illustrates potential sources of *Mollicutes* contamination in raw materials. The starting material for plant hydrolysates is obtained from farms where they are exposed to a variety of environmental conditions, animals, animal waste, and insects. The production processes are industrial, not pharmaceutical, and some processes might use animal-derived enzymes or be produced in facilities that also manufacture materials derived from animal tissues.

The end user must understand the origin of raw materials to determine the risk to their process. While risk to patient from the bioreactor unit operation, so far upstream from the final drug product, *Mollicutes* contamination will result in discarding the batch, intensive investigation for root cause, facility and equipment decontamination, sterilization, and documentation. This type of investigation and implementation of corrective and preventative actions can take weeks to months to resolve with the potential to impact final drug product supply to the patient. Therefore, it is now common to select 0.1-μm filters in cell culture media applications.

Summary

Ultimately, the selection of a 0.2- or 0.1-μm filter will depend on the application (bioreactor medium, chromatography buffer, final drug product), bioburden (concentration, profile), feedstream attributes, processing conditions, and process endpoints (filtration time, volumetric throughput, differential pressure limit). A data-driven analysis and risk assessment will support the correct approach for the application.

Filtration System Sizing Considerations

Filtration systems generally consist of a series of filters in series called a filter train, where each filter in the series extending the life of the next filter in series. Performance is defined by answering two questions: How fast can the feedstream be filtered (flow rate) and how much can be filtered (capacity).

Flow rate (volume filtered per unit of time) is a function of filtration area, differential pressure, and fluid viscosity. The resistance to flow offered by the filter medium is related to both pore size and porosity in addition to the quantity, size distribution, and composition of particles in the feedstream. Capacity is the maximum volumetric throughput (volume per effective frontal surface area) of a given feed for a given filter or filter train. Practically speaking, the filter is considered plugged when the pressure

differential across the filter reaches the practical limits of the system or when flow has decreased to the point at which it becomes impractical to continue. In practice, end users typically define process endpoints related to duration, pressure rise, or flow-rate decline.

Particles plug filters by a variety of mechanisms such as cake formation, complete pore plugging and gradual pore plugging. Figure 30.10 illustrates different plugging models in terms of differential pressure versus volumetric throughput. Cake formation occurs with nondeformable particles larger than the pore sizes in the filter. These particles build up on the surface forming cake-like structure. In cake formation, resistance to flow increases linearly with cake thickness. Complete pore plugging occurs with deformable particles that are slightly larger than the pore size distribution of the filter. During processing, pressure forces these particles to completely block the pore resulting in a rapid buildup in pressure. This can occur in the absence of proper prefiltration. Gradual pore plugging occurs when particles build up within the pore opening slowly blocking the pore. This type of plugging is most common with biological feedstreams.

As seen in Figure 30.10, both gradual pore plugging and complete pore plugging do not have a linear relationship between differential pressure and capacity

Certain feedstreams such as buffers or water exhibit predictable filtration behavior; as such, filter selection and sizing can often be determined from manufacturer performance data such as flow rate versus pressure curves. Other feedstreams such as hydrolysate rich cell culture media, bulk drug substance, or a formulated drug product are typically complex fluids composed of many components with different particle profiles. In these cases, laboratory studies are necessary.

When small-scale laboratory studies are conducted to determine filter sizing it is important to use the actual feed material to effectively estimate the amount of filtration

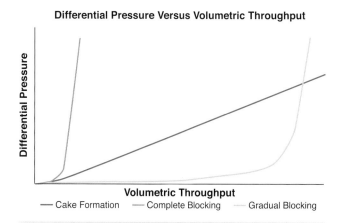

Differential Pressure Versus Volumetric Throughput

Differential Pressure (y-axis)

Volumetric Throughput (x-axis)

— Cake Formation — Complete Blocking — Gradual Blocking

FIGURE 30.10 Three different filter plugging models: cake, complete, and gradual pore plugging. Gradual pore plugging effects are commonly seen in feeds with biological or other complex components.

area needed for larger scale filtration systems. Key factors in proper scale up include membrane pore size, porosity, filtration device construction, equipment design, and feed properties. Lot to lot variation of the feed material is important to understand and control, particularly for biological feedstreams. For practical reasons, there can be a significant gap in time between obtaining feed samples and performing filter sizing studies that necessitate storage. Storage temperature and time or freeze/thaw cycles can negatively impact test sample feed quality resulting in filter sizing data that leads to unnecessary oversizing of the filtration system.

Mok et al[98] provides guidance for sizing filters in relatively clean feedstreams such as water or buffers, and Raghunath et al[99] discusses best practices for sizing filters using the Vmax technique for feedstreams that generally follow a gradual pore plugging model such as cell culture media, centrate, sera, complex buffers, and process intermediates. Safety factors are an important consideration in sizing filtration systems where a balance between process efficiency and process economy is needed. Additionally, Lutz[100] presents a comprehensive analysis for applying safety factors in filter sizing.

Prefilter/Final Filter Combinations: An Economic Consideration

Because depth and surface filters retain large amounts of fine particulates, they find wide use as prefilters for membrane filters. Materials used as the prefilter medium usually are low in cost compared with membrane filters. It is important, then, that they remove the larger share of particulate contamination so that the life of the membrane filter is extended as far as possible, acting as an insurance policy by removing all particles and microorganisms to a high level of efficiency.

To maximize the effective life of a membrane filter, a prefilter must have the proper retention efficiency and the optimum filtration area. The membrane filter pore size determines the retention efficiency required of the prefilter, that is, the prefilter must remove most of the particulates that approximate the pore size rating of the membrane filter. For example, if product considerations dictate the use of a 0.2-μm pore–sized membrane filter, the nominal rating of the prefilter must be more open than that of the final filter. With the proper filtration area, a prefilter that has the required retention efficiency will make the most efficient and economic use of the membrane filter.

Figure 30.11 illustrates the impact of prefiltration in terms of efficiency and capacity. In these hypothetical examples, the feedstream is being filtered at a constant flow rate through a series of two filters, the first a surface type prefilter and the second a microporous membrane final filter.

As particles in the feed accumulate in and on the filters, both flow resistance and differential pressure increase. Figure 30.11A depicts very low volumetric throughput for a final filter used in the absence of prefilter. The life of the filter is drastically shortened without prefiltration. In Figure 30.11B, a final filter is protected by a prefilter that has a very open filter structure where the particles are not being captured efficiently by the prefilter. The differential pressure as a function of volume is shown for each filter separately, then as a function of both filers combined in series. The prefilter is not providing enough retention efficiency to protect the final filter because there is little pressure buildup across the prefilter. As a result, the poorly protected final filter plugs rapidly, and maximum pressure is exceeded, with most of the batch still to be processed. The situation is different in Figure 30.11C. Here, a much tighter prefilter has been used. In this case, the prefilter has more than adequate retention efficiency but insufficient capacity. This time, it is the prefilter that plugs prematurely. Figure 30.11D depicts an optimized prefilter and final filter combination. The prefilter has just the right retention efficiency and capacity for the final filter. The properties of the two filters are properly matched, and the capacity for the process has been significantly improved. In this example, at the end of the run, both filters have exhausted almost all their dirt-handling capacity.

Serial, Redundant, and Bioburden Reduction Filtration Strategies

Serial filtration is a filter train with two or more filters in a series, typically the same filter type such as a 0.2-μm followed by a 0.2-μm filter. In some cases, one of the filters may be tighter than the other such as a 0.2-μm followed by a 0.1-μm. There are several different process objectives for developing a serial filtration process such as (case a) managing the bioburden or particulate load before the final sterile filter or (case b) as a filter failure backup strategy commonly called "redundant filtration" or (case c) both filters together provide the sterilizing performance.

For critical sterile filtration of aseptically processed drug products, the way the objective for the sterilizing performance in combination with regulatory expectations is defined will dictate the integrity testing approach. For case a where a single filter was validated as providing sterilizing performance and two of these filters are used in series with one being claimed as a bioburden reduction filter and the second one is claimed for sterilizing performance, then only the one that is claimed as sterilizing is integrity tested. If it fails the integrity test, the bioburden filter is not tested as a backup. For redundant filtration, case b, where a single filter was validated as providing sterilizing performance and two of these filters are used in series with one being a backup for the other, the integrity

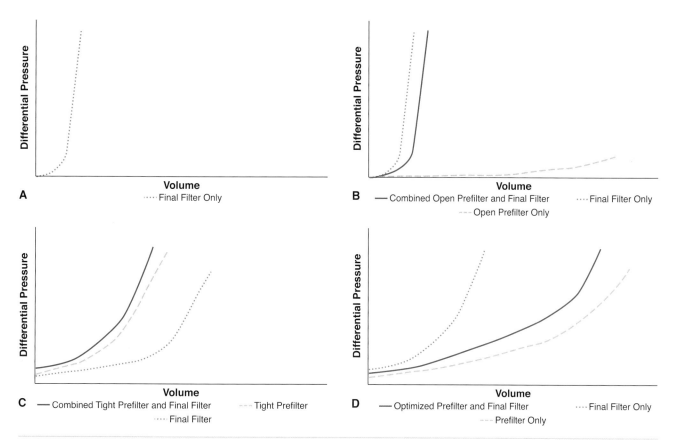

FIGURE 30.11 Optimization of prefilter and filter will improve volumetric throughput. A single microporous membrane filter. Without prefiltration, the microporous membrane filter quickly plugs, resulting in insufficient throughput (A). Microporous membrane filter protected by relatively coarse prefilter. Inadequate prefiltration has resulted in premature plugging the microporous membrane filter (B). Microporous membrane filter protected by prefilter with insufficient capacity, leading to premature plugging of prefilter (C). Properly matched prefilters and microporous membrane filter, resulting in full use of both filter capacities and complete filtration of batch (D).

test needs to be performed on one of the filters only. If that filter fails the integrity test, then the backup filter will be tested and if it passes the filtration is considered to have met the acceptance criterion. For the rare occurrence of case c, if both filters must be in series to achieve sterilizing performance and have been validated as such, both filters must be individually integrity tested and both must pass the integrity test.

Meltzer et al[53] reviewed the theory of filter efficiencies and how that theory can assist the filter user to decide the merits of implementing redundant filtration. The authors discussed one method of evaluating the relative efficiencies of redundant filters (eg, 0.2-μm) versus a single filter of tighter pore distribution (eg, 0.1-μm). In any case, empiric determinations of filter efficiencies are preferred and required for validation of the filters. For further consideration, others offer practical advice for designing single-use filter assemblies and filter-cartridges in stainless steel systems as well as considerations for implementing redundant filtration and strategies for integrity testing redundant filtration systems.[98,101]

VALIDATION OF STERILIZING-GRADE FILTERS

Manufacturers of sterilizing-grade filters conduct process and product validation studies to demonstrate that the products they have developed perform as designed. Process monitoring, in-process testing, and lot release testing are employed to confirm that the products are in a state of control and meet established claims. Data trending is used to monitor and understand process behavior. Although filter manufacturers design and validate their products to operate under a wide variety of conditions, they cannot account for the infinite number of variables encountered when installed in an end user's process. It is the end user's responsibility to understand the impact of their feed and processing conditions on the selected filtration system. It is also the end user's responsibility to operate within the claims established by the manufacturer.

Relevant regulations, guidelines, standard methods, and industry best practices are available to guide the end user in conducting filter validation studies. Risk assessment exercises will help define the types of testing necessary for a consistent and robust filtration step appropriate to the unit operation. The strategy for which filter validation constituents are necessary may be different in an upstream process than for an aseptically processed final drug product. For example, one end user might determine his or her bioreactor media filtration step is at minimal risk for contamination and choose not to conduct the bacterial retention studies, another user might determine his or her bioreactor media filtration step is at elevated risk for contamination and opt to conduct bacterial retention studies. In contrast, the bacterial retention component of filter validation is required in applications where filters are used to sterilize sterile drug products.

Filter validation studies document that the filters are fit for their intended use and that the filter does not affect the safety, efficacy, potency, or quality of the final drug product. They also provide supporting data for the effective range in which the process reproducibly operates. Whereas filter validation is the responsibility of the end user, the filter manufacturer plays a key role in suppling performance data on how the filter performs under a set of standard conditions. Some of these data can be used directly by the end user as part of a paper exercise to document suitability for the selection of a filter. Other data must be generated empirically by the end user to establish performance in their process under their operating conditions with their feedstream. Some of these data, such as bacterial retention studies, can be outsourced to qualified external laboratories.

The validation of sterilizing-grade filters has been reviewed in detail in PDA Technical Report 26 and by McGrath and Levy.[48,102] Table 30.6 outlines the responsibilities of filter manufacturers and filter users for critical sterile filtration applications. These responsibilities make up the basic elements of filter selection and filter validation studies. Essential constituents of filter validation include feed and process compatibility, binding (adsorption), sterilization, integrity, extractables, and leachables as well as bacterial retention. These elements can be addressed in a sterilizing filter validation master plan (SFVMP). An SFVMP is a document that will provide justification and supporting data for the intended use of the selected filter(s) in a process. The SFVMP typically includes a description of the operating parameters for the process and information on the fluid to be filtered. It will also outline the test criteria and the justification for why a test was selected, a description of the test parameters, the acceptance criteria, and possibly deviation handling criteria. There may be a test method summary, or the SFVMP may reference a separate document that covers the details and actual test data for that test.

Key Constituents of a Sterilizing Filter Validation

Compatibility

Compatibility studies demonstrate the feed does not adversely impact the filtration device. The need for a comparability study and the type of study will be based on the process step. The approach could be different for a buffer versus final drug product. The filter manufacturer's compatibility tables and material qualification documentation as well as published literature, historical data, and the end user's previous experience will also inform the type of testing required. Compatibility studies should account for the entire device. In certain situations, it may be more practical to test individual components. The studies should address process parameters for the filtration such as temperature, duration, and feed properties (solvents, surfactants, stabilizers, biological components) as well as filtration device sterilization conditions.

Binding or Adsorption

Binding studies will document that the filter does not intentionally remove feed components such as protein, surfactants, or preservatives. If binding is unavoidable, the binding study can document a mitigation strategy that effectively addresses binding. For example, if a preservative in a final drug product is found to bind to the membrane, the mitigation procedure could be to prime the filter housing with the product and hold for a specified time followed by flushing product until a steady state of preservative in the effluent is established. This procedure would be covered in the binding study to demonstrate that the procedure consistently produces effluent that meets the designated preservative target range. An understanding of the effect of filtration device sterilization should also be included as well as consideration for any planned process interruptions during the filtration process.

Sterilization

Filtration devices can be provided either presterilized by the manufacturer or are sterilized by the end user. The objective of filter sterilization qualification is to document that the sterilization method is effective and does not compromise the filter. Presterilized filtration devices and assemblies are predominantly sterilized by gamma radiation (see chapter 29). The end user should review the filter sterilization qualification data supplied by the manufacturer and use this documentation in the SFVMP to demonstrate the sterilization process is effective and meets the manufacturer's claims. Filtration devices and assemblies prepared and sterilized by the end user will require assessment using the actual devices, sterilization equipment, and conditions that

TABLE 30.6 Responsibilities of manufacturers and end users for validation of sterilizing-grade filters in critical applications such as final-drug product filtrations

Filter Performance Elements	Filter Manufacturer	Filter User
Filtration objective	NA	Paper exercise: Establish and define the purpose of the filter for the defined process step.
Chemical compatibility	Disclose materials of construction.	Paper exercise: Document compatibility. Perform studies.
Extractables/leachables	Develop methods. Provide data under standard conditions.	Review manufacturer's data. Perform studies.
Binding/adsorption	NA	Perform studies.
Bacterial retention	Provide bacterial retention claims. Provide validation data. Provide correlation of retention with the integrity test. Offer validation services.	Perform studies: for critical sterile filtration using product and process-specific microbial retention studies (typically using an outside laboratory). Paper exercise: Ensure correlation to bacterial retention exists.
Filer integrity	Provide integrity test specifications. Provide validation data. Provide test procedures. Provide test correlation with bacterial retention.	Develop flush procedures for post-use integrity tests or develop product-specific integrity test values. Ensure correlation to bacterial retention exists. Ensure operators are qualified to perform integrity tests.
Filter reproducibility	Validate the filter claims and the manufacturing process.	Review the validation data and conduct audit of the manufacturer.
Drug activity and stability	NA	Verify no conformational changes or activity losses. Perform stability studies.
Endotoxins	Perform analysis on a per lot basis.	Verify low endotoxin levels from filters. Ensure process operation does not contribute endotoxins.
Animal origin	Provide animal origin statement.	Paper exercise: Review manufacturer's documentation.
Operation	Provide limits for operating, temperature, and temperature.	Review filtration objectives to ensure manufacturer's product meets the objectives. Design process to not exceed manufacturer's specifications.
Particulates and nonfiber-releasing properties	Provide test data.	Paper exercise: Review manufacturer's documentation.
Product reproducibility	Provide validation data.	Paper exercise: Review manufacturer's data.
Sterilization	Provide recommended procedures with limits for time, temperature, and number of cycles. Provide test data.	Ensure process conditions do not exceed manufacturer's specifications. Validate sterilization process.
Toxicity	Perform testing and provide results such as (USP class VI plastics, cytotoxicity).	Paper exercise: Obtain and include filter data with clinical trials or perform toxicologic review.
Flow rate and pressure drop	Provide test data for flow rate and pressure drop.	Paper exercise: Use manufacturer data to aid in the filter selection process.
TOC and conductivity	Provide test data. Provide flushing test methods.	Use manufacturer information as guidance to establish appropriate pre-use flushing procedures.

TOC, total organic carbon; USP, United States Pharmacopeia.

will be used in process; scaled down devices or systems will not appropriately capture performance effects of sterilization. Depending on the sterilization method chosen, appropriate documentation of acceptable sterilization processing (eg, biological/chemical indicators and/or process parameters) as well as filter integrity tests can be used to document suitability of the sterilization process.

In SIP and autoclaving applications, if the filtration device is wetted prior to use, it is important to understand the risk of possible filter damage if the filter is sterilized wet. These applications subject filtration systems to fluctuating differential pressures and temperatures that could approach the softening point of some polymers; therefore, it may be advisable to "blow down" the filter prior to sterilization. This can be accomplished by applying pressurized air at a greater pressure than the specified bubble point to drive liquid out of the pores. The pressure and the duration of the blow down should be determined experimentally. If it is not practical to blow down the filtration device, care must be in designing the sterilization cycle. Water-wet filters will require a longer time to reach the designated sterilization temperature and will produce additional condensate that should be managed as part of the system design. Thermocouples should be augmented with BIs to profile the sterilization dynamics within the filter. For autoclaving, the cycle should be designed with gradual ramp up and exhaust parameters such as provided in a liquid goods or slow exhaust cycle. For SIP, gradual ramp-up will minimize the stress on a wet filter.

Integrity Testing

Integrity testing is a critical in-process test that documents that a filtration device is appropriately installed in the system and confirms the bacterial retention capabilities of the filter. End users need to validate the integrity test equipment used. Operators must be trained and qualified to conduct integrity tests and interpret the test results to verify the validity of the results. Depending on the regulatory requirements, these critical filters may only need to be tested after use, but there may be a requirement to test both pre-use and post-use.

The manufacturer should provide instructions on how to wet the filter so that all the pores are filled with liquid prior to testing. It is important to assess the impact of the feed material on integrity test values, typically in the form of false integrity test failures. Feed components such as detergents or alcohols or process artifacts such as antiscaling agents, cleaning residues, oils, or tubing plasticizers can impact surface tension negatively affecting integrity test results as compared to suppliers' (typically water based) specifications in the form of false failures. Contaminants must be controlled by removal from the process. In the case of feed components, a flushing procedure can be established to remove feed residuals from the filter or a product-specific integrity test can be experimentally determined.

The end user should provide justification for when the integrity test will be performed (pre-use, pre-use poststerilization, and final integrity test) and where the test will be performed. While in-line testing is preferred, there may be cases where the filtration device must be removed from the process for off-line testing. During the qualification, the filtration flush parameters can be confirmed. If a PUPSIT is necessary, the qualification should document that the system of flushing, flush waste removal, gas introduction, venting, and valve sequencing are operating as intended and that PUPSIT procedure does not introduce contamination into the system.

Extractables and Leachables

The objectives of extractables and leachable studies are to identify, quantify, and assess the impact of compounds that migrate from the filtration device into the process stream. Extractables are compounds extracted from plastic or elastomeric materials in solvents under aggressive conditions or worst-case conditions. Leachables are compounds that leach from the plastic or elastomeric materials into actual drug product under normal processing and/or storage conditions. An easy way to remember the difference is "extractables are 'extreme' and leachables are 'life-like.'"

In filtration device qualification, extractable and leachable studies have different objectives. Extractable studies should be designed to identify and quantify as many compounds as possible that have the potential to become leachable. Leachable studies should be designed to identify and quantify as many compounds as possible that migrate from the filtration process or storage systems into the actual drug product. Leachable evaluation starts with data from a well-defined extractables study. Data from extractable and leachable studies can then be used to calculate patient risk and to establish mitigation strategies should they be necessary.

Bacterial Retention

As discussed earlier, manufacturers of sterilizing grade membranes use standard bacterial challenge test methodologies during development and support sterilizing grade membrane claims during validation and lot release; however, the unique conditions of an end user's product and process could affect the size and morphology of the microorganisms present, affect the structure or integrity of the filtration device, or a combination of both. For this reason, in final drug product filtration, the end user must conduct customer drug product and process-specific validation studies to demonstrate that the filter will reproducibly remove viable microorganisms, to produce a sterile effluent.

Factors that can affect bacterial retention include (1) drug product properties such as pH, viscosity, conductivity, surface tension, and osmolarity; (2) drug product formulation components such as the active ingredient, presence of surfactants, oils, adjuvants, or interactions with other excipients; and (3) process properties such as pressure, flow rate, temperature, and maximum process duration. These factors need to be considered and simulated as much as possible in the bacterial retention qualification study.

As part of the planning for a bacterial retention study, it is important to understand the process bioburden. The bioburden level should be quantified and identified to the species level and assessed to justify and document the use of the standard test microorganism *B diminuta*. If the assessment indicates that a bioburden isolate would be more penetrating than *B diminuta*, it should be considered for use in the bacterial retention study.

Bacterial retention studies are conducted at small scale with membrane discs (approximately 14 cm^2 effective frontal surface area) or small devices. The challenge test microorganism is cultivated under standard conditions, as described earlier in this chapter, then inoculated into the drug product to achieve a minimum challenge concentration of 1×10^7 CFUs/cm^2. The test filters are integrity tested before use and then the challenge suspension is delivered to the test filters under scaled down process conditions, the full effluent volume for each test filter is separately collected and assayed. The test filters are integrity tested after use. Mitigation strategies are available if the components in the drug product negatively affect the challenge bacteria and are explained in the PDA Technical Report 26. This technical report also provides best practices for on designing and conducting product- and process-specific bacterial retention studies.[48]

▶ CONCLUSION

For more than 50 years, membrane filtration has been an accepted and reliable method for both liquid and gas sterilization in aseptic processing. In many cases, it is the only practical method for ensuring that a variety of products reach the end user in a sterile form. Because the applications are so varied, selecting the optimum sterilizing grade membrane and filtration system is a significant and demanding exercise. To remove all bacteria, the membrane pore size distribution must be smaller than the bioburden size distribution. The filter device itself must be manufactured in a reliable manner to ensure integrity and strength, and when installed into a processing system, must be properly sealed to prevent bypass and allow sterilization of the filter and filtration system before use. Filter choice, system size, and design depend on many factors such as the process contamination risk, feed material profile, and processing conditions.

Manufacturer and users of sterilizing grade filters share responsibilities for ensuring sterilizing filters perform as expected. The manufacturer is responsible for designing, developing, and validating that a sterilizing grade

filter will perform as intended. The manufacturer will employ standard test methods under controlled conditions to develop and trend performance of their products and to produce product claims. The end user will assess the manufacturer's claims to aid in the selection process. The accountability for demonstrating that a sterilizing grade filter is fit for use in the end user's process rests solely on the end user owing to the unique variables in the end users feed material, equipment, and processing conditions. This will require empirical testing often in the actual feed material under actual or downscaled conditions. Regardless of the intended application, sterilizing filtration is expected to produce a sterile product as introduced into the final container.

REFERENCES

1. US Food and Drug Administration. *Guidance for Industry Sterile Drug Products Produced by Aseptic Processing—Current Good Manufacturing Practice*. 2004. Retrieved (or Downloaded) from https://www.fda.gov/regulatory-information/search-fda-guidance-documents/sterile-drug-products-produced-aseptic-processing-current-good-manufacturing-practice. Accessed April 9, 2019.

2. European Medicines Agency. *Guideline on the Sterilisation of the Medicinal Product, Active Substance, Excipient and Primary Container*. Amsterdam, The Netherlands: European Medicines Agency; 2019.

3. European Medicines Agency. *Guideline on Manufacture of the Finished Dosage Form*. Amsterdam, The Netherlands: European Medicines Agency; 2017.

4. Pharmaceutical Inspection Co-operation Scheme. *Guide to Good Manufacturing Practice for Medicinal Products 2018; PE 009-13: Annex 2*. Geneva, Switzerland: Pharmaceutical Inspection Convention Co-operation Scheme.

5. World Health Organization. *Annex 6: WHO Good Manufacturing Practices for Sterile Pharmaceutical Products*. Geneva, Switzerland: World Health Organization; 2011.

6. International Organization for Standardization. *ISO 13408-2:2018: Aseptic Processing of Health Care Products—Part 2: Sterilizing Filtration*. Geneva, Switzerland: International Organization for Standardization; 2018.

7. United States Pharmacopeia. Sterilizing filtration of liquids. In: *United States Pharmacopeial Convention*. 40th ed. Rockville, MD: United States Pharmacopeia; 2017.

8. Parenteral Drug Association. *Bioburden and Biofilm Management in Pharmaceutical Manufacturing Operations*. Bethesda, MD: Parenteral Drug Association; 2015. Technical report no. 6.

9. Shearer GL. Taking a closer look at parenteral contaminants. *Pharm Technol*. 2016;40:34-38.

10. Rayaprolu BM, Strawser JJ. Glass delamination in parenterals: a brief overview. *J Pharmacovigil*. 2017;5:4.

11. American Pharmaceutical Review. *Baxter expands voluntary nationwide recall to include second lot of Nexterone injection*. American Pharmaceutical Review Web site. http://www.americanpharmaceuticalreview.com/1315-News/346332-Baxter-Expands-Voluntary-Nationwide-Recall-to-Include-Second-Lot-of-Nexterone-Injection/. Accessed April 15, 2019.

12. Langille SE. Particulate matter in injectable drug products. *PDA J Pharma Sci Technol*. 2013;67:186-200.

13. Chamberland CE, inventor, assignee. Filter. US patent 519,664. May 8, 1984.

14. Seitz TF, inventor, assignee. Filter. US patent 956,832. May 3, 1910.

15. Seitz GH, Schmitthenner F, inventors; Firm of Seitz-Werke, Theo. & Geo. Seitz, of Kreuznach. A. D. Vahe, Germany, assignees. Filter-body. US patent 1,256,171. February 12, 1918.

16. National Archives and Records Administration. Federal Register: 38 Fed. Reg. 27039. *Fed Regist.* 1973;38. https://www.loc.gov/item/fr038188/.

17. Zsigmondy R, Bachmann F, inventors; Zsigmondy R, Bachmann F, assignees. Process for the preparation of membrane filters or ultrafilters of specific pore size (translated from German). German patent DE 329060 C. November 12, 1920.

18. Zsigmondy R, Bachmann W, inventors; Zsigmondy R and Bachmann W, assignees. Filter and method of producing same. US patent 1421341. June 27, 1922.

19. Sartorius AG. *Evolving from a University Mechanician to a Global Player: Sartorius Chronicle from 1870 to 2005.* Göttingen, Germany; 2006.

20. Goetz A, Tsuneishi N, Kabler PW, Streicher L, Neumann HG. Application of molecular filter membranes to the bacteriological analysis of water. *J Am Water Works Assoc.* 1951;43(12):943-984.

21. American Public Health Association, American Water Works Association, Water Environment Federation. 9215 heterotrophic plate count (2017). In: *Standard Methods for the Examination of Water and Wastewater.* https://doi.org/10.2105/SMWW.2882.188.

22. Lovell SP, Bush JH, inventors; Millipore Filter Corp, assignee. Microporous nylon film. US patent 2,783,894. March 3, 1957.

23. Yamazaki E, inventor; Gore Enterprise Holdings, Inc, assignee. Production of porous sintered PTFE products. US patent 4,110,392. August 29, 1978.

24. Grandine JD II, inventor; Millipore Investment Holdings Ltd, assignee. Processes of making a porous membrane material from polyvinylidene fluoride, and products. US patent 4,203,848. May 20, 1980.

25. Pall DB, inventor; Pall Corp, assignee. Process for preparing hydrophilic polyamide membrane filter media and product. US patent 4,340,479. July 20, 1982.

26. Kraus M, Heisler M, Katsnelson I, Velazques D, inventors; Pall Corp, Bank One Michigan NA, assignees. Filtration membranes and method of making the same. US patent 5,108,607. April 28, 1992.

27. Bowser JJ, Hyde CT, inventors; Gore W L and Associates Inc, assignees. Irradiated expanded polytetrafluoroethylene composites, and devices using them, and processes for making them. US patent 5,019,140. May 28, 1991.

28. Porter DB, Paine RA, inventors; EMD Millipore Corp, assignee. Method of applying a microporous plastic membrane filter on a support. US patent 3,198,865. August 3, 1965.

29. Pall DB, Keedwell C, inventors; Pall Corp, assignee. Process for preparing filters having a microporous layer attached thereto. US patent 3,407,252. October 22, 1968.

30. Bush JH, Weyand JE, inventors; EMD Millipore Corp, assignee. Filter cartridge for filtering liquids. US patent 3,406,831. October 22, 1968.

31. Pall DB, Estates R, Jasaitis TK, inventors. Cylindrical filter elements with improved side seam seal. US patent 3,865,919. February 11, 1975.

32. Ganzi GC, Paul CT, inventors; Millipore Corp, assignee. Method and structure for sealing tubular filter elements. US patent 4,512,892. April 23, 1985.

33. Reulecke F, inventor; Sartorius GmbH, assignee. Filter element for the filtration of fluids. Germany patent DE 3145552. November 17, 1981.

34. Steuck MJ, inventor; Millipore Investment Holdings Ltd, assignee. Porous membrane having hydrophilic surface and process. US patent 4,618,533. October 21, 1986.

35. United States Pharmacopeia. Microbiological examination of nonsterile products: microbial enumeration tests. In: *United States Pharmacopeial Convention.* 40th ed. Rockville, MD: United States Pharmacopeia; 2017.

36. United States Pharmacopeia. Sterility tests. In: *United States Pharmacopeial Convention.* 40th ed. Rockville, MD: United States Pharmacopeia; 2017.

37. Bowman FW, Calhoun MP, White M. Microbiological methods for quality control of membrane filters. *J Pharm Sci.* 1967;56:222-225.

38. Parenteral Drug Association. Technical Report No. 41 (revised 2008): virus filtration. *PDA J Pharma Sci Technol.* 2008;62:1-65.

39. US Federal Register. Current good manufacturing practice for finished pharmaceuticals 21 CFR part 211.

40. US Food and Drug Administration. Drug quality assurance sterile drug process inspections. In: *Compliance Program Guidance Manual.* Washington, DC: Center for Drugs and Biologics, Office of Regulatory Affairs; 2015.

41. Lutz H. *Ultrafiltration for Bioprocessing.* Cambridge, United Kingdom: Elsevier; 2015.

42. Meltzer TH. Filtration: the practice of pre-filtration and its related considerations. *Ultrapure Water.* 1989;6:24-34.

43. Dwyer JL. The technology of absolute microfiltration. *Technol Quarterly Master Brewers Assoc Am.* 1968;5:246G.

44. Dwyer JL. *Contamination Analysis and Control.* New York, NY: Reinhold; 1966.

45. Rossano AT Jr, Silverman L. Electrostatic effects in fiber filters for aerosols. *Heating Ventilating.* 1954;51:101.

46. Accomazzo MA, Grant DC. Mechanisms and devices for filtration of critical process gases. In: Raber RR, ed. *Fluid Filtration: Gas.* Vol 1. Philadelphia, PA: ASTM International; 1986.

47. ASTM International. *ASTM F838-15a: Determining the Bacterial Retention of Membrane Filters Utilized for Liquid Filtration.* West Conshohocken, PA: ASTM International; 2015. doi:10.1520/F0838-15A.

48. Parenteral Drug Association. Technical Report No. 26: sterilizing filtration of liquids. *PDA J Pharma Sci Technol.* 2008;52:1-62.

49. Parenteral Drug Association. Technical Report No. 40: sterilizing filtration of gases. *PDA J Pharma Sci Technol.* 2005;58:1-44.

50. Megaw WJ, Wiffen RD. The efficiency of membrane filters. *Air Water Pollut.* 1963;7:501-509.

51. Meltzer TH. Filtration: a critical review of filter integrity testing. Part I: the bubble point method: assessing filter compatibility—initial and final testing. *Ultrapure Water.* 1989;6:40-51.

52. Meltzer TH. Filtration: a critical review of filter integrity testing. Part II: the diffusive air flow and pressure-hold methods: assessing filter compatibility—initial and final testing. *Ultrapure Water.* 1989;6:44-56.

53. Meltzer TH, Madsen RE, Jornitz MW. Considerations for diffusive airflow integrity testing. *PDA J Pharm Sci Technol.* 1999;53:56-59.

54. Lee JY. Validating an automated filter integrity test instrument. *Pharm Technol.* 1989;13:48-56.

55. European Commission. EudraLex—Volume 4—Good Manufacturing Practice (GMP) guidelines. European Commission. https://ec.europa.eu/health/documents/eudralex/vol-4_en. Accessed April 9, 2017.

56. Mok Y, Besnard L, Love T, et al. Best practices for critical sterile filter operation, a case study. *Bioprocess Int.* 2016;14:28-33.

57. Elford WJ. A new series of graded collodion membranes suitable for general bacteriological use, especially in filterable virus studies. *J Pathology Bacteriol.* 1931;34:505-521.

58. Segers P, Vancanneyt M, Pot B, et al. Classification of *Pseudomonas diminuta* Leifson and Hugh 1954 and *Pseudomonas vesicularis* Büsing, Döll, and Fretag 1953 in *Brevundimonas* gen. nov. as *Brevundimonas diminuta* comb. nov. and *Brevundimonas vesicularis* comb. nov., respectively. *Int J Syst Bacteriol.* 1994;44:499-510.

59. Rogers BG, Rossmoore HW. Determination of membrane filter porosity of microbiological methods. *Developments in Industrial Microbiology.* 1970;2:453-459.

60. Ballard RW, Doudoroff M, Stanier RY. Taxonomy of the aerobic pseudomonads: *Pseudomonas diminuta* and *P. vesiculare. J Gen Microbiol.* 1968;53:349-361.

61. Henrici AT. *Morphologic Variation and the Rate of Growth of Bacteria.* London, United Kingdom: Bailliere, Tindall and Cox; 1928.

62. Schaechter M, Maaloe O, Kjeldgaard NO. Dependency on medium and temperature of cell size and chemical composition during balanced growth of *Salmonella typhimurium. J Gen Microbiol.* 1958;19: 595-605.

63. Herbert D. Some principles of continuous culture. In: Tunevall G, ed. *Recent Progress in Microbiology.* Springfield, IL: Charles C Thomas; 1958:381-402.

64. Maaloe O, Kjeldgaard NO. *Control of Macromolecular Synthesis.* New York, NY: Benjamin: 1966.

65. Leahy TJ, Sullivan MJ. Validation of bacterial retention capabilities of membrane filters. *Pharm Technol.* 1978;2:65-75.

66. Health Industry Manufacturers Association. *Microbiological Evaluation of Filters for Sterilizing Liquids.* Washington, DC: Health Industry Manufacturers Association; 1982.

67. Carter J, Levy RV. Microbial retention testing in the validation of sterilizing filtration. In: Meltzer TH, Jornitz MW, eds. *Filtration and the Biopharmaceutical Industry.* New York, NY: Marcel Dekker; 1998:577-604.

68. Fennington GJ Jr, Howard G Jr. Preparation and evaluation of bacterial stocks for filter validation. *PDA J Pharm Sci Technol.* 1997;51:153-155.

69. International Council for Harmonisation. *Q4B Evaluation and Recommendation of Pharmacopoeial Texts for Use in the ICH Regions: Annex 8 (R1) : Sterility Test General Chapter.* Retrieved (or Downloaded) from https://www.fda.gov/regulatory-information/search-fda-guidance-documents/q4b-annex-8-sterility-test-general-chapter. Accessed April 12, 2019.

70. Carter J. Evaluation of recovery filters for use in bacterial retention testing of sterilizing-grade filters. *PDA J Pharma Sci Technol.* 1996;50(3):147-153.

71. Reti AR. An assessment of test criteria for evaluating the performance and integrity of sterilizing filters. *Bull Parenter Drug Assoc.* 1977;31:187-194.

72. Pall DB, Kirnbauer EA. Bacteria removal production in membrane filters. Paper presented at: The 52nd Colloid and Surface Science Symposium, American Chemical Society; June 1978; Knoxville, TN.

73. Blanchard MM. Quantifying sterilizing membrane retention performance. *BioProcess International.* 2007;5:44-51.

74. Blanchard MM. Ensuring aseptic processing through quality by design. *BioProcess Int.* 2012;10:52-56.

75. Tanny GB, Strong DK, Presswood WG, Meltzer TH. Adsorptive retention of *Pseudomonas diminuta* by membrane filters. *J Parenter Drug Assoc.* 1979;33:40-91.

76. Reti AR, Leahy TT, Meier PM. The retention mechanism of sterilizing and other submicron high efficiency filter structures. In: Uplands Press. *Second World Filtration Congress.* London, United Kingdom; 1979:427-435.

77. Wallhäusser KH. Is the removal of microorganisms by filtration really a sterilization method? *J Parent Drug Assoc.* 1979;33:156-170.

78. Wallhäusser KH. Recent studies on sterile filtration. *Pharm Industry.* 1979;41:475-481.

79. Robertson JH, DeVisser A. Microbiological qualification and validation of sterilizing membrane filters. Paper presented at: Interphex Annual Meeting; September 1980; New York, NY.

80. Leahy TJ. *Validation of bacterial retention by membrane filtration: a proposed approach for determining sterility assurance* [dissertation]. Amherst: University of Massachusetts; 1983.

81. Levy RV. The effect of pH, viscosity and additives on the bacterial retention of membrane filters challenged with *Pseudomonas diminuta*. In: Johnston PR, Schroeder HG, eds. *Fluid Filtration: Liquid.* Vol II. Philadelphia, PA: American Society for Testing Materials; 1987:80-89.

82. Levy RV. The mechanisms and reliability of sterilizing filtrations with microporous membranes. Paper presented at: The Pharmaceutical Technology Conference '87; September 22-24,1987; East Rutherford, NJ.

83. Meltzer TH. *Filtration in the Pharmaceutical Industry.* New York, NY: Marcel Dekker; 1987:1091.

84. Elford WJ. The principles of ultrafiltration as applied in biological studies. *Proc R Soc.* 1933;112B:384-406.

85. Howard G Jr, Duberstein R. A case of penetration of 0.2-micrometer rated membrane filters by bacteria. *J Parenter Drug Assoc.* 1980;34:95-102.

86. Leahy TJ, Sullivan MJ, Slingeneyer A, Mion C. The efficiency of microbial retention by peritoneal dialysis filters. *Trans Am Soc Artif Intern Organs.* 1980;26:225-230.

87. Anderson RL, Bland LA, Favero MS, et al. Factors associated with *Pseudomonas pickettii* intrinsic contamination of commercial respiratory therapy solutions marketed as sterile. *Appl Environ Microbiol.* 1985;50:1343-1348.

88. Morowitz HJ, Tourtellotte ME, Pollack ME. Use of porous cellulose ester membranes in the primary isolation and size determination of pleuropneumonia-like organisms. *J Bacteriol.* 1963;85:134-136.

89. Tully JG. Cloning and filtration techniques for mycoplasmas. In: Razin S, Tully JG, eds. *Methods in Mycoplasmology.* Vol 1. New York, NY: Academic Press; 1983:173-177.

90. Roche KL, Levy RV. Methods used to validate microporous membranes for the removal of mycoplasma. *BioPharm.* 1992;5:22-33.

91. Sundaram S, Eisenhuth J, Howard G Jr, Brandwein H. Method for qualifying microbial removal performance of 0.1 micron rated filters. Part I: characterization of water isolates for potential use as standard challenge organisms to qualify 0.1 micron rated filters. *PDA J Pharm Sci Technol.* 2001;55:346-372.

92. Chen J, Bergevin J, Kiss R, et al. Case study: a novel bacterial contamination in cell culture production—*Leptospira licerasiae. PDA J Pharm Sci Technol.* 2012;66:580-591.

93. Centers for Disease Control and Prevention. Nosocomial *Ralstonia pickettii* colonization associated with intrinsically contaminated saline solution—Los Angeles, California, 1998. *MMWR Morb Mortal Wkly Rep.* 1998;47:285-286.

94. Leo F, Auriemma M, Ball P, et al. Application of 0.1 µm filtration for enhanced sterility assurance in pharmaceutical filling operations. *BFS News.* 1997:15-24.

95. US Food and Drug Administration. Questions and answers on current good manufacturing practices—production and process controls. US Food and Drug Administration Web site. https://www.fda.gov/Drugs/GuidanceComplianceRegulatoryInformation/Guidances/ucm124782.htm#3. Accessed April 9, 2019.

96. Parenteral Drug Association. *Proceedings from the PDA Workshop on Mycoplasma Contamination by Plant Peptones.* Bethesda, MD: Parenteral Drug Association; 2007.

97. Windsor HM, Windsor GD, Noordergraaf JH. The growth and long term survival of *Acholeplasma laidlawii* in media products used in biopharmaceutical manufacturing *Biologicals.* 2010;38:204-210.

98. Mok Y, Besnard L, Pattnaik P, Raghunath B. Sterilizing-grade filter sizing based on permeability: a quick reference tool for buffer filtration. *Bioprocess Int.* 2012;10:58-63.

99. Raghunath B, Pailhes M, Mistretta T. Predicting filter size using Vmax testing. *BioProcessing J.* 2006;5:38-40.

100. Lutz H. Rationally defined safety factors for filter sizing. *J Membr Sci.* 2009;341:268-278.

101. Felo M, Oulundsen G, Patil R. Single-use redundant filtration. *BioPharm Int.* 2012;25:38-41.

102. McGrath J, Levy R. Validation of sterilizing-grade filters. In: Carleton FJ, Agalloco JP, eds. *Validation of Pharmaceutical Processes: Sterile Products.* 2nd ed. New York, NY: Marcel Dekker; 1999:555-583.

CHAPTER 31

Ethylene Oxide Sterilization

Craig A. Wallace

Ethylene oxide (EO), also known as epoxyethane or EO, is a colorless gas that is used as a fumigant to treat food products such as spices and as a chemical sterilant for medical devices and other health care products. For many years, EO sterilization was the primary low-temperature process used by hospitals for sterilization of medical devices that were not compatible with the elevated temperature and high humidity of steam sterilization (Figure 31.1). The EO is still used in hospitals around the world, although vaporized hydrogen peroxide–based processes have replaced EO in many facilities because of faster cycle times and control of personnel safety requirements. The EO is used extensively in industrial sterilization of medical devices that are not compatible with radiation or steam sterilization (Figure 31.2). EO is an excellent sterilant because EO molecules exhibit an ability to permeate through most polymeric materials while retaining molecular integrity and producing only negligible changes in the wide variety of materials used in medical devices (Figure 31.3).[1] The physical properties of EO are provided in Table 31.1.

The EO was discovered in 1859, but its biocidal properties were not recognized until the 1920s and then primarily as an insecticide.[2] The ability of EO to kill microorganisms was first noted in the 1940s and was first applied as a treatment for spices and gums. This antimicrobial property was expanded for use as a sterilant for heat and moisture sensitive medical devices in the 1950s.[3] The development of medical devices made of heat-sensitive thermoplastic materials drove the need for the further development and optimization of EO sterilization processes.

▶ BIOCIDAL MECHANISM AND EFFICACY

The primary biocidal mechanism for EO is alkylation or the replacement of a hydrogen atom with an alkyl group.[4,5] The primary targets of the alkylation process are sulfhydryl, amino, carboxyl, phenolic, and hydroxyl groups contained in cellular macromolecules such as nucleic acids and proteins.[3] The alkylation of nucleic acids was confirmed in studies on *Salmonella*[6] and *Clostridium*.[7] Alkylation of these critical macromolecules disrupts cellular replication.

The EO has been shown in many studies to be a highly efficacious biocide, having a broad spectrum of activity against vegetative bacteria, bacterial spores, and viruses.[4,8-19] One study indicated that *Pyronema domesticum*, a type of fungus, had a higher than expected resistance to EO.[20] EO is used as a chemical sterilant and, like all chemical sterilants, requires direct contact with the microorganism to inactivate it. Studies have demonstrated that the presence of organic soil (10% fetal bovine serum) and 0.65% salt reduces the effectiveness of EO on exposed surfaces and inside lumens, with similar effects noted for other chemical sterilants such as vaporized hydrogen peroxide and vaporized peracetic acid.[21] In another lumen study, a liquid chemical sterilant system was more effective than gaseous EO in tests involving organic soil and salt. But EO was found to be effective in inoculated lumen testing where the soil challenge included only fetal bovine serum but no salt.[22] EO was not found to be efficacious in the sterilization of dental handpieces where the internal surfaces of the devices were inadequately cleaned.[23] Another study demonstrated greater EO efficacy in lumen challenge testing when compared to one vaporized hydrogen peroxide system, whereas EO was equivalent in performance to a second vaporized hydrogen peroxide system.[17]

The high diffusivity of the EO molecule enables penetration through many polymers and into narrow lumens. Studies have confirmed the ability of EO to penetrate lumens[24] and to penetrate some tissue matrices used for human tissue allografts.[25] A number of carbapenem-resistant Enterobacteriaceae infections and outbreaks related to use of contaminated duodenoscopes

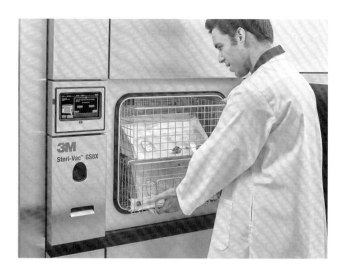

FIGURE 31.1 Small chamber ethylene oxide sterilizer for hospital and industrial use. For a color version of this art, please consult the eBook. Photo courtesy of 3M.

in endoscopic retrograde cholangiopancreatography procedures have been reported in the literature. These endoscopes contain long narrow lumens and are typically reprocessed by high-level disinfection. Several health care facilities reported that implementation of EO sterilization of their endoscopes halted the outbreaks.[26-30]

$$H_2C - CH_2$$
$$\diagdown O \diagup$$
Ethylene Oxide

FIGURE 31.3 Ethylene oxide molecule. From Block.[1(p580)]

▶ STERILIZATION FORMULATIONS

Medical device sterilization processes have used EO in pure form (100% EO) as well as in gas mixtures with EO combined with inert gases such as fluorocarbons, hydrofluorocarbons, and carbon dioxide (CO_2).[31,32] The mixtures are used to improve safety by reducing explosion and fire risk. Mixture processes operate at higher pressures than typically used for 100% EO systems, which allows processing of some packaged devices that cannot withstand the low pressures (vacuum) used in the 100% EO systems.[3] The commonly used mixture of 12% EO and 88% chlorofluorocarbon (CFC) was phased out in the mid-1990s when the CFC gases themselves were phased out because of environmental concerns and regulations. Hydrochlorofluorocarbon (HCFC) replacements were used until similar environmental regulations stopped

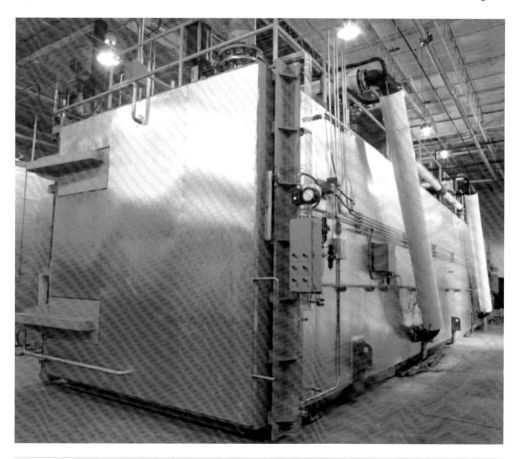

FIGURE 31.2 Industrial large chamber ethylene oxide sterilizers.

TABLE 31.1   Physical properties of ethylene oxide[a]

Liquid	
Molecular weight	44.05
Apparent specific gravity at 20°C/20°C (68°C/68°F)	0.8711
ΔSp. gr./Δt at 20°C-30°C (68°F–86°F)	0.00140
Coefficient of expansion at 20°C (68°F)	0.00161
Water solubility	Complete
Heat of vaporization at 1 atm	6.1 kcal/g-mole
Surface tension	28.0 dynes per cm
Viscosity at 10°C (50°F)	0.28 cps
Vapor pressure at 20°C (68°F)	1095 mm Hg
Boiling point at 760 mm	10.4°C (50.7°F)
at 300 mm	−11.0°C (−12.2°F)
at 10 mm	−66°C (−86.8°F)
ΔBP/ΔP at 740-760 mm Hg	0.033°C per mm
Freezing point	−122.6°C (−170.7°F)
Refractive index, n_o at 7°C (44.6°F)	1.3597
Heat of fusion	1.236 kcal/g-mole
Specific heat at 20°C (68°F)	0.44 cal per g per °C
Explosive limits in air at 760 mm Hg	
Upper	100% by volume
Lower	3% by volume
Flash point, tag open cup (ASTM Method D 1310)	< −18°C (<0°F)
Vapor	
Critical temperature	196.0°C (384.8°F)
Critical pressure	1043 psia
Autoignition temperature in air at 1 atm	429°C (804°F)
Decomposition temperature of pure vapor at 1 atm	560°C (1040°F)
Heat of combustion of gas, gross	312.15 kcal/g-mole
Heat of formation	12.2 kcal/g-mole

Abbreviation: ASTM, American Society for Testing and Materials.

[a]Data from Block,[1] Table 33.1, p 581.

their production in 2014 in the United States.[33,34] Common EO and CO_2 (EO/CO_2) mixtures consist of 8.5% EO and 91.5% CO_2 or 20% EO and 80% CO_2.[35]

STERILIZATION PROCESS VARIABLES

Process variables are defined as conditions within a sterilization process, changes in which alter microbicidal effectiveness.[36] The primary process variables for EO sterilization are temperature, EO gas concentration, relative humidity (RH), and exposure time.[3,5,32,33,37-41] Exposure time

is determined based on the temperature, EO concentration and RH selected. One international standard also lists pressure as a sterilization process variable.[42]

Temperature

Typical EO sterilization process temperatures range from 37°C to 63°C. Inactivation of *Bacillus atrophaeus* spores at various temperatures are shown in Figure 31.4.[43] The Q_{10} value for this data is approximately 1.9. This corresponds to the reported values of 1.8 for *B atrophaeus*[44] and 2.18 for *Bacillus subtilis* (ATCC 9524).[45] A Q_{10} value of 1.55 to 1.64

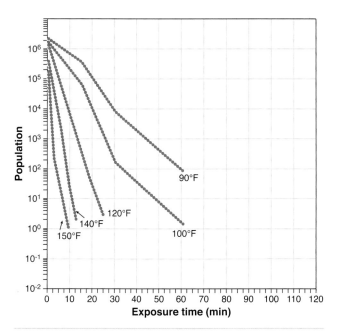

FIGURE 31.4 Inactivation of *Bacillus atrophaeus* spores at different temperatures at 500 mg/L ethylene oxide and 40% relative humidity. From Block,[1(p586)] Figure 33.2.

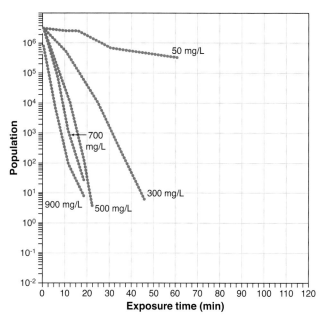

FIGURE 31.5 Inactivation of *Bacillus atrophaeus* spores at different ethylene oxide concentrations at 117.5°F and 40% relative humidity. From Block,[1(p586)] Figure 33.1.

has been reported for spores of *Bacillus coagulans*[46] and a Q_{10} of 1.7 to 2.2 for spores of *Clostridium botulinum*.[47] These data indicate that, in general, for every 10°C change in temperature, the inactivation rate for spores will double when the EO concentration is not limiting.[3] This value has been corroborated in other summary publications.[5]

Concentration

Typical EO concentrations in sterilization processes are reported to range from 450 to 1200 mg/L.

Survivor curves for the inactivation of *B atrophaeus* spores at different EO concentrations are shown in Figure 31.5.[43] As the gas concentration increases from 50 to 500 mg/L, the inactivation rate increases significantly. At gas concentrations greater than 500 mg/L, there is no significant increase in the rate of spore inactivation. For *B atrophaeus* spores, at gas concentrations of 200 to 1200 mg/L, the most dramatic decrease in resistance occurs when the given concentration is increased from 200 to 400 mg/L at 54.4°C.[3,8] More recent investigations using more precisely controlled test equipment have shown that inactivation of *B atrophaeus* followed second-order kinetics over EO concentrations of 100 to 1200 mg/L and temperatures of 22°C to 60°C.[93]

It is expected that the lethality of 100% EO and EO blends would be equivalent when the concentration of EO in the processes are equivalent.[1] A more recent publication that compared the effect of 100% EO to an EO/HCFC gas blend on *B atrophaeus*–based EO biological indicators found that 100% EO had greater lethality at equivalent EO concentrations. The authors speculate that when using an HCFC blend

gas, the HCFC competes with the EO molecules for access to the critical binding sites on the spores. With HCFC present in the exposure chamber and blocking EO access to the critical binding sites, the result is fewer alkylation reactions and thus decreased lethal impact on the spores.[34]

Relative Humidity

The RH has long been recognized as a critical factor in EO sterilization. Studies demonstrated that at RH between 30% and 75%, the inactivation curves were linear, whereas below 30%, nonlinearity exists (Figure 31.6 and 31.7).[43] Others have demonstrated the need for RH of at least 30% for effective EO sterilization.[48] The requirement for the presence of water for EO sterilization is not surprising because water will react with EO to open the epoxide ring.[3,49] A commonly accepted range of RH for EO sterilization processes is 30% to 90%[5,39] with most processes setting the minimum RH at least 35% as a safety margin.[32] The range minimum (30%-35%) is driven by efficacy of the process because of the significant reduction in process lethality below this level. The upper end of the range (at or below 90%) is driven by the desire to avoid condensation in the chamber during the process.

▶ STERILIZATION PROCESSES

EO sterilization cycles typically have six phases: preconditioning, conditioning, air removal, gas exposure, gas removal, and aeration. In some processes, certain phases may

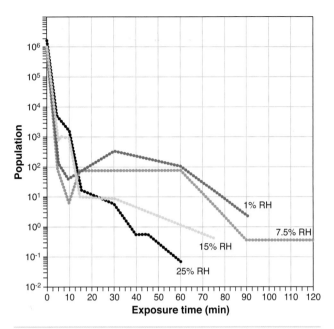

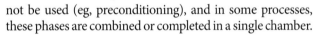

FIGURE 31.6 Inactivation of *Bacillus atrophaeus* spores at relative humidity (RH) levels ranging from 1% to 25% at 500 mg/L ethylene oxide and 117.5°F. From Block,[1(p584)] Figure 33.3.

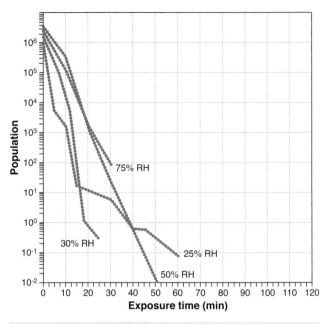

FIGURE 31.7 Inactivation of *Bacillus atrophaeus* spores at relative humidity (RH) levels of 25% to 75% at 500 mg/L ethylene oxide and 117.5°F. From Block,[1(p587)] Figure 33.4.

not be used (eg, preconditioning), and in some processes, these phases are combined or completed in a single chamber.

Preconditioning: Preconditioning is the treatment of product, prior to the sterilization cycle, in a room or chamber to attain specified conditions for temperature and RH.[42] Preconditioning is typically performed using environmental conditions of higher temperature and RH (eg, 100°F and 80% RH) and an exposure time based on the size and density of the load. The objective of preconditioning is to bring the product load close to the target process temperature and RH, to improve efficacy and reduce the amount of time required for in-chamber conditioning, thereby reducing costs.

Conditioning: Conditioning is the continued process to bring the product load to target temperature and RH conditions but performed inside the sterilization chamber as part of the sterilization process. The time required for this process is dependent on the effectiveness of the preconditioning stage. This stage is often accomplished using a dynamic environment using multiple steam pulses.

Air removal: The significance of effective air removal is often overlooked in gaseous chemical sterilization processes, even though it has a major influence on the speed and reliability of the process. Air inhibits sterilant penetration in gaseous processes the same way it inhibits steam penetration in steam sterilization processes. For systems that do not pull a deep vacuum, in the order of 1 Torr or less, a sequence of flushes and pulses with subatmospheric steam or subatmospheric

steam and sterilant might be used to complete the air removal by dilution.[1]

Gas exposure: The exposure phase commences after the injection of the EO gas as well as any carriers or diluents (eg, CO_2, nitrogen). International standards differentiate EO injection time from the exposure time, where the exposure time is defined as the period for which the process parameters are maintained within their specified tolerances, and for calculation of cycle lethality is essentially the period between the end of EO injection and the beginning of EO removal.[42] Exposure time is a key variable optimized in cycle development and validation.

Gas removal: The primary objective of this step is removal of gas from the headspace of the chamber for operator safety (if the chamber door is opened before aeration is completed), and to lower the head space concentration to facilitate the start of aeration process. The EO is removed from the head space of the sterilizer chamber by drawing a vacuum in the chamber. This may be followed by pressurization of the sterilizing chamber with air and repeating a chamber evacuation. This sequence may be repeated several times to remove EO by dilution.[1]

Aeration: Aeration is defined as part of the sterilization process during which EO and/or its reaction products desorb from the processed medical devices until predetermined residual levels are reached. This can be performed within the sterilizer and/or in a separate chamber or room.[42] The EO that has permeated out of the sterilized materials diffuses into an air stream that will be vented from the chamber. The rate of diffusion into the air stream can increase significantly with increased temperature. Aeration rate can be affected by the type and thickness of packaging materials, the loading configuration, and air temperature and flow rate. Aeration on the industrial scale is often performed in a separate chamber or room; however, handling materials during a transfer from the sterilizing chamber to an aerator may result in higher potential worker exposure to the sterilizing agent that can be mitigated by use of personal protective equipment. In many current applications, materials are aerated in the sterilizing chamber to minimize potential worker exposure.[1,50]

Improvements in aeration removal time are achieved by evacuating and pressurizing the sterilizer chamber with air, sometimes referred to as *air washes*, to help remove air from inside the chamber and load. Newer approaches to facilitate faster and more effective aeration include use of microwave radiation[51,52] and steam with high pressure nitrogen washes.[53] There are also developments in using technology such as green fluorescent protein as a monitor for dissipation of EO residues.[54] Optimization of the cycle allowing reduction of the exposure time and gas concentration and more effective gas removal processes can result in lower amounts of residual EO in the devices and shorter aeration times required to reach the target residual levels.[31]

Process Development and Validation

The fundamentals of process development and validation for EO sterilization processes are the same as for other terminal sterilization processes, with specific accommodations for the unique properties of EO (eg, aeration). Key factors to be considered for preconditioning, the sterilization cycle, and aeration include[3,42]

1. product design and materials
2. product bioburden
3. packaging, chamber loading, and load mass
4. preconditioning time and conditions
5. gas exposure time
6. gas concentration
7. temperature
8. RH
9. evacuation rates
10. depth of vacuum

Process validation is composed of Installation, Operational, and Performance Qualification. Installation Qualification (IQ) is the process of obtaining and documenting evidence that equipment has been provided and installed in accordance with its specification.[36] This step verifies that the sterilizer and any critical ancillary equipment have been installed according to the manufacturer's specifications,

including utilities and the physical environment. The IQ also verifies that proper documentation is completed, including use instructions. Operational Qualification (OQ) is the process of obtaining and documenting evidence that installed equipment operates within predetermined limits when used in accordance with its operational procedures.[36] The OQ is designed to demonstrate that the sterilizer operates as intended in its design specifications. Verification of sensor calibration is a requirement in OQ as well as testing with independent sensors to ensure that the selected process parameters are delivered by the equipment. The OQ testing is typically done in an empty chamber but may be done with selected test materials and loads. Performance Qualification (PQ) is the process of obtaining and documenting evidence that the equipment, as installed and operated in accordance with documented procedures, consistently performs in accordance with predetermined criteria and thereby yields product meeting its specification.[36] The PQ is composed of the Physical Performance Qualification, in which physical parameters of the process (eg, temperature, RH, EO concentration) are measured and validated throughout the process and the product load. In the Microbiological Performance Qualification (MPQ), the biocidal effectiveness of the process is evaluated and validated throughout the process and the product load. There are two approaches used for the MPQ. The first, the biological indicator/bioburden approach, combines knowledge of the resistance of a biological indicator to a given sterilization process with knowledge of the product/load bioburden population and resistance to establish the sterilization process parameters (sterilization cycle exposure time). Use of this method requires that product bioburden levels shall be demonstrated to be relatively consistent over time, and the resistance of the bioburden be shown to be equal to or less resistant than the resistance of the biological indicator.[42] The second, the overkill approach, assumes that the product bioburden level consists of less than or equal to 10^6 organisms that have a resistance that is less than or at least equal to that of the biological indicator.[42] It also assumes that the challenge can be reduced to 10^0 at one-half the normal exposure (Figure 31.8). Although little information regarding product bioburden is required, the assumptions must be confirmed. The inactivation of the biological indicator, on which the gas exposure time will be based, must occur at the most difficult-to-sterilize location within or on the product.[3]

Sterilization in Health Care Facilities

Health care facilities are typically unable to complete process validations for their EO sterilization processes because of lack of validation expertise, budget, and equipment. They will instead rely on information on proper processing provided in the instructions for use from both the sterilizer manufacturer and the medical

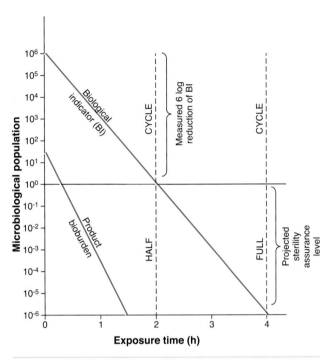

FIGURE 31.8 Overkill approach to cycle development. From Block,[1(p591)] Figure 33.12.

device manufacturer. In the United States, the Food and Drug Administration (FDA) regulates the sale of sterilizers used in health care facilities and provides guidance to manufacturers on the information and data that must be submitted to the FDA as part of the regulatory clearance process. This information will include validation of biocidal efficacy, confirmation of effects of the sterilization process on devices and materials, and labeling requirements.[55] The Association for the Advancement of Medical Instrumentation provides guidance for health care facilities regarding facility design; personnel training; device preparation and packaging; process quality testing; and sterilizer design, installation, and maintenance.[56]

◗ EFFECTS ON MATERIALS AND DEVICES

The EO can sterilize most heat or moisture-sensitive medical devices without adverse effects on the polymers or other materials used in the medical devices.[5,33] The EO sterilization processes operate at relatively low temperatures (below 60°C) that are tolerated by most common medical device polymers, optics, and electronics. The EO processes do not generate free radicals or other oxidative moieties that can damage some materials.[57]

Several studies on the effects of EO sterilization on various medical device and specialty polymers and materials have been published. These studies often compared the effects of EO sterilization to the effects of other sterilization processes such as moist heat, dry heat, or radiation on new and complex polymers and biomaterials. Several studies on complex polymers and proteins for drug delivery and therapeutic applications found that EO changed the physical properties of the materials.[58-62] Other studies found no measurable effects or superior performance of EO compared to other sterilization modalities for medical materials including specialty polymers,[63-67] specialty fibers,[68-70] and other specialized materials.[71-74] A study on the effects of EO on polylactic acid and polyglycolic acid polymers used for treatment of hard and soft tissue wounds indicated that EO is an appropriate method for sterilization if the materials are properly aerated.[75]

◗ SAFETY

The EO sterilization carries certain risks for sterilizer operators and patients. If not properly handled, EO's flammability and explosive properties present risks to sterilizer operators, and its toxic and carcinogenic properties can present risks to operators, patients, and the environment. Appropriate facility and equipment design, installation, and maintenance and staff training on safe handling procedures of the EO gas itself and the sterilized devices (pre-aeration), are effectively used to mitigate these risks.

Sterilizer Operator Safety—Flammability

The EO is flammable and explosive in air in concentrations from 3% to 100% by volume.[1,3,76] Operators of large chamber EO sterilizers such as contract sterilizers and large-scale medical device manufacturers have used engineering controls such as specialized ventilation systems and careful selection of pumps and ancillary equipment to mitigate these risks. Large chamber 100% EO sterilizers will typically add nitrogen gas to the chamber with the EO to reduce the risk of fire or explosion.[3,42] Small chamber EO sterilizers (less than 10 ft³) use single-dose cartridges of 100% EO (less than 200 g). The smaller chamber and smaller EO containers pose less risk and are not required to conform, for example, to the National Fire Protection Association (NFPA) regulations that cover larger containers and chambers.[77-79]

Sterilizer Operator Safety—Exposure

The EO is an effective biocidal agent and carries with it hazardous properties that must be addressed in its handling and application. The EO is categorized as a carcinogen and a mutagen, is directly toxic in certain concentrations.[33,76,80] The Occupational Health and Safety Administration has established a permissible exposure limit of 1 ppm for an 8-hour time-weighted average (TWA), and a short-term exposure limit (STEL) (15 min) of 5 ppm. The 8-hour TWA integrates the exposure to which an operator can be exposed in an 8-hour period and also provides an average exposure level during that period.[1,33,81,82] Operators of large chamber EO sterilizers use engineering controls such as specialized ventilation to reduce the risk of operator exposure. In addition, staff training (including training for facility staff not directly involved with the EO sterilization equipment), airborne monitoring, and use of personal protective equipment such as respirators are used to reduce risks of worker exposure to EO.[1,80,83]

The safety of workers using small chamber EO sterilizers in health care facilities or medical device manufacturing is also addressed with sterilizer engineering controls and worker training and appropriate monitoring.[1,82,84,85] Processes in small chamber sterilizers using 100% EO operate at subatmospheric pressures, to eliminate the chance of a chamber leak resulting in release of EO to the environment (Figure 31.9). Risks are also reduced with the use of small, single-cycle containers rather than large cylinders or tanks of EO (Figure 31.10). The US Environmental Protection Agency requirement for aeration to be completed in the sterilizer chamber, thus eliminating any potential exposure occurring during transfer of the load from sterilizer to aerator, also reduces the risk of worker exposure.[80]

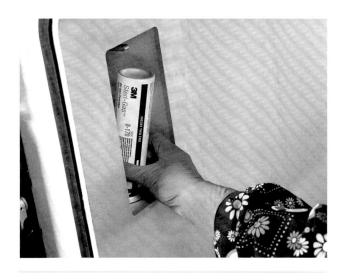

FIGURE 31.10 Single-use ethylene oxide cartridges for small chamber sterilizers. For a color version of this art, please consult the eBook. Photo courtesy of 3M.

Patient Safety—Ethylene Oxide Residuals

Most polymeric medical device materials will retain varying levels of EO at the completion of the exposure phase of the sterilization cycle. In addition, there may also be residues of the EO by-products ethylene chlorohydrin and ethylene glycol. Ethylene chlorohydrin can be formed if the device materials present a chlorine source.[5,76,86]

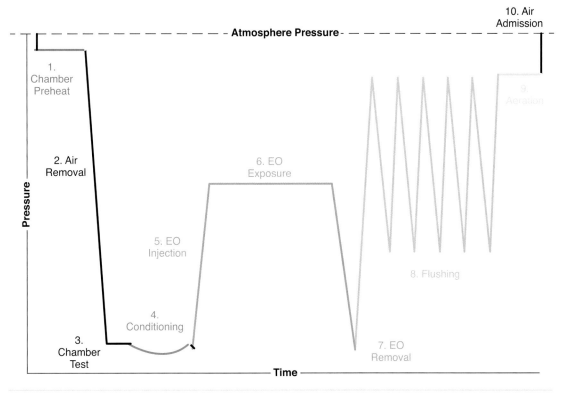

FIGURE 31.9 Subatmospheric 100% ethylene oxide (EO) sterilization cycle.

Ethylene glycol and ethylene chlorohydrin are more difficult to remove from the device postprocess than EO residues. These residues can cause burns and skin reactions on patients if not reduced to safe levels.[87,88] Removal of these chemical residues from the medical devices begins during the gas removal phase of the process that is also used to reduce the EO levels in the head space of the chamber for operator safety. Reduction of residuals is the primary objective of the aeration process.

Acceptable levels of residual EO and ethylene chlorohydrin in medical devices have been established and published by the International Organization for Standardization. There are no limits specified for ethylene glycol because it is less toxic than the other residues and the calculated allowable levels are not likely to occur in a medical device.[89] The requirements are categorized based on the expected contact time of the medical device with the patient tissue and include the categories limited exposure, prolonged exposure, and permanent contact. There are also requirements for some specific types of devices (eg, blood oxygenators). The standard also provides information on chemical extraction and analysis methodologies. The EO residual levels are part of the sterilization process validation criteria used by medical device manufacturers.[42]

Environmental Safety

Environmental emissions of EO are regulated at the national and local levels in the United States, with allowable emission levels varying by location. Emission reduction technologies can be used to meet the required emission levels for both large chamber and small chamber sterilizers. The EO scrubbers convert EO to ethylene glycol by acid hydrolysis, and the ethylene glycol can then be used in other applications. Large chamber EO sterilizers can also use reclamation processes to condense the EO to a liquid state and subsequently reuse it as a sterilant. Catalytic conversion to CO_2 and water vapor uses heat and a catalytic bed in the presence of oxygen. For catalytic systems the sterilizer effluent will typically require dilution with air because of limitations on the EO concentration that can be processed by these systems.[1,3,90-92]

▶ CONCLUSIONS

The EO will continue to play a very important role in medical device sterilization and other applications well into the future. Manufacturers rely on EO for devices and materials that are not compatible with heat or radiation methods. Most of the active research related to EO sterilization in recent years has focused on the effects of different sterilization processes on new medical device polymers and biomaterials, and these studies show that EO is, in most cases, the best option for terminal sterilization of these complex materials. Others have described the optimization of this process to gain efficiency and reduce safety concerns.[93] Although the volume of goods sterilized with EO in health care facilities has diminished, there continues to be a role for EO in this area as well, for devices that are not suited to steam or vaporized hydrogen peroxide. There has been frequent misinformation in this area that EO is being banned or discontinued (perhaps confusion related to the phase out of CFC and HCFC carrier gases) as well as an ongoing emphasis about the risks associated with EO without reasonable clarity about the benefits of EO and how the risks are mitigated. The novel properties of EO, efficacy, high penetrability, and materials compatibility, will continue to have applications in the field of sterilization in the years ahead as medical devices and materials continue to evolve in complexity and applications.

REFERENCES

1. Parisi AN, Young WE. Sterilization with ethylene oxide and other gases. In Block SS, ed. *Disinfection, Sterilization, and Preservation*. 4th ed. Philadelphia, PA: Lea & Febiger; 1991:580-596.
2. Joslyn LJ. Gaseous chemical sterilization. In Block SS, ed. *Disinfection, Sterilization, and Preservation*. 5th ed. Philadelphia, PA: Lippincott Williams & Wilkins; 2001:337-359.
3. Cotton RT, Rourke, RC. Ethylene oxide as a fumigant. *Eng Chem*. 1928;20:805.
4. Bruch CW. Gaseous sterilization. *Ann Rev Microbiol*. 1961;15:245-262.
5. Mendes GC, Brandão TR, Silva CL. Ethylene oxide sterilization of medical devices: a review. *Am J Infect Control*. 2007;35:574-581.
6. Michael GT, Stumbo CR. Ethylene oxide sterilization of *Salmonella* Senftenberg and *Escherichia coli*: death kinetics and mode of action. *J Food Sci*. 1970;35:631-634.
7. Winarno FG, Stumbo CR. Mode of action of ethylene oxide on spores of *Clostridium botulinum* 62A. *J Food Sci* 1971;36:892-895.
8. Kereluk K, Gammon RA, Lloyd RS. Microbiological aspects of ethylene oxide sterilization. II. Microbial resistance to ethylene oxide. *Appl Microbiol*. 1970;19(1):152-156.
9. Sidwell RW, Dixon GJ, Westbrook L, Dulmadge EA. Procedure for the evaluation of the virucidal effectiveness of an ethylene oxide gas sterilizer. *Appl Microbiol*. 1969;17(6):790-796.
10. Alfa M, DeGagne P, Olson N. Bacterial killing ability of 10% ethylene oxide plus 90% hydrofluorocarbon sterilizing gas. *Infect Control Hosp Epidemiol*. 1997;18(9):641-645.
11. Klarenbeek A, van Tongeren HAE. Virucidal action of ethylene oxide gas. *J Hyg (Lond)*. 1954;52:525-528.
12. Tomkins GJ, Cantwell GE. The use of ethylene oxide to inactivate insect viruses in insectaries. *J Invertebr Pathol*. 1975;25:139-140.
13. Savan M. The sterilizing action of gaseous ethylene oxide on foot-and-mouth disease virus; a preliminary report. *Am J Vet Res*. 1955;16:158-159.
14. Mathews J, Hofstad MS. The inactivation of certain animal viruses by ethylene oxide (carboxide). *Cornell Vet*. 1953;43:452-461.
15. Hartman FW, Kelly AR, LoGrippo GA. Four-year study concerning the inactivation of viruses in blood and plasma. *Gastroenterology*. 1955;28:244-264.
16. Dadd AH, Daley GM. Resistance of micro-organisms to inactivation by gaseous ethylene oxide. *J Appl Bacteriol*. 1980;49:89-101.
17. Rutala WA, Gergen MF, Weber DJ. Comparative evaluation of the sporicidal activity of new low-temperature sterilization technologies: ethylene oxide, 2 plasma sterilization systems, and liquid peracetic acid. *Am J Infect Control*. 1998;26:393-398.

18. Ries MD, Weaver K, Beals N. Safety and efficacy of ethylene oxide sterilized polyethylene in total knee arthroplasty. *Clin Orthop Relat Res.* 1996;(331):159-163.

19. Dekker A. Inactivation of foot-and-mouth disease virus by heat, formaldehyde, ethylene oxide and γ radiation. *Vet Rec.* 1998;143:168-169.

20. Lampe CM, Hansen JM, Rymer TM, Sargent H. Sterilization of products contaminated with *Pyronema domesticum. Biomed Instrum Technol.* 2009;43(6):489-497.

21. Alfa MJ, DeGagne P, Olson N, Puchalski T. Comparison of ion plasma, vaporized hydrogen peroxide, and 100% ethylene oxide sterilizers to the 12/88 ethylene oxide gas sterilizer. *Infect Control Hosp Epidemiol.* 1996;17:92-100.

22. Alfa MJ, DeGagne P, Olson N, Hizon R. Comparison of liquid chemical sterilization with peracetic acid and ethylene oxide sterilization for long narrow lumens. *Am J Infect Control.* 1998;26:469-477.

23. Parker HH IV, Johnson RB. Effectiveness of ethylene oxide for sterilization of dental handpieces. *J Dent.* 1995;23(2):113-115.

24. Kanemitsu K, Imasaka T, Ishikawa S, et al. A comparative study of ethylene oxide gas, hydrogen peroxide gas plasma, and low-temperature steam formaldehyde sterilization. *Infect Control Hosp Epidemiol.* 2005;26(5):486-489.

25. Kearney JN, Franklin UC, Aguirregoicoa V, Holland KT. Evaluation of ethylene oxide sterilization of tissue implants. *J Hosp Infect.* 1989;13:71-80.

26. Chang CL, Su LH, Lu CM, Tai FT, Huang YC, Chang KK. Outbreak of ertapenem-resistant *Enterobacter cloacae* urinary tract infections due to a contaminated ureteroscope. *J Hosp Infect.* 2013;85(2):118-124.

27. McCool S, Muto CA, Querry A, et al. High level disinfection (HLD) failure in gastrointestinal scopes with elevator channels: is it time to switch to ethylene oxide (ETO) sterilization? Poster presented at: IDWeek 2014; October 8-12, 2014; Philadelphia, PA.

28. Epstein L, Hunter JC, Arwady MA, et al. New Delhi metallo-β-lactamase-producing carbapenem-resistant *Escherichia coli* associated with exposure to duodenoscopes. *JAMA.* 2014;312(14):1447-1455.

29. Smith ZL, Oh YS, Saeian K, et al. Transmission of carbapenem-resistant Enterobacteriaceae during ERCP: time to revisit the current reprocessing guidelines. *Gastrointest Endosc.* 2015;81(4):1041-1045.

30. Naryzhny I, Silas D, Chi K. Impact of ethylene oxide gas sterilization of duodenoscopes after a carbapenem-resistant Enterobacteriaceae outbreak. *Gastrointest Endosc.* 2016;84(2):259-262.

31. Strain P, Young WT. Ethylene-oxide sterilisation aids speed to market. *Med Device Technol.* 2004;15:18-19.

32. Burgess DJ, Reich RR. Ethylene oxide sterilization: scientific principles. In Reichert M, Young JH, ed. *Sterilization Technology for the Health Care Facility.* 2nd ed. Gaithersburg, MD: Aspen; 1997:178-184.

33. Rutala WA, Weber DJ; for Healthcare Infection Control Practices Advisory Committee. *Guideline for Disinfection and Sterilization in Health Care Facilities, 2008.* Atlanta, GA: Center for Disease Control and Prevention; 2008.

34. Krushefski G, Piotrkowski A, Wallace C, Matzinger, K. Effects of 100% ethylene oxide test gas on the resistance of ethylene oxide biological indicators. *Pharm Technol.* 2014;38(12).

35. Association for the Advancement of Medical Instrumentation. *AAMI TIR15:2016. Physical Aspects of Ethylene Oxide Sterilization.* Arlington, VA: Association for the Advancement of Medical Instrumentation; 2016.

36. International Organization for Standardization. *ISO/TS 11139:2006: Sterilization of Health Care Products—Vocabulary.* Geneva, Switzerland: International Organization for Standardization; 2006.

37. Ernst RR, Doyle JE. Sterilization with gaseous ethylene oxide: a review of chemical and physical factors. *Biotech Bioeng.* 1968;10:1-31.

38. Phillips CR. The sterilizing action of gaseous ethylene oxide; sterilization of contaminated objects with ethylene oxide and related compounds; time, concentration and temperature relationships. *Am J Hyg.* 1949;50(3):280-288.

39. Mosley GA, Gillis JR, Whitbourne JE. Calculating equivalent time for use in determining the lethality of EtO sterilization processes. *Medical Device and Diagnostics Industry Magazine.* February 2002.

40. Heider D, Gomann J, Junghann BU, Kaiser U. Kill kinetics study of *Bacillus subtilis* spores in ethylene oxide sterilization processes. *Zentr Steril.* 2002;10:158-167.

41. Rutala WA, Weber DJ. Infection control: the role of disinfection and sterilization. *J Hosp Infect.* 1999;(suppl 43):S43-S55.

42. International Organization for Standardization. *ISO/TS 11135:2014: Sterilization of Health Care Products—Ethylene Oxide—Requirements for Development, Validation and Routine Control of a Sterilization Process for Medical Devices.* Geneva, Switzerland: International Organization for Standardization; 2014.

43. Caputo RA, Rohn KJ, Mascoli CC. Biological validation of an ethylene oxide sterilization process. In: *Developments in Industrial Microbiology.* Fairfax, VA: Society for Industrial Microbiology; 1980:22.

44. Ernst RR, Shull JJ. Ethylene oxide gaseous sterilization. I. Concentration and temperature effects. *Appl Microbiol.* 1962;10:337-341.

45. Liu TS, Howard GL, Stumbo CR. Dichlorodifluoromethane-ethylene oxide mixture as a sterilant at elevated temperatures. *Food Technol.* 1968;22:86-89.

46. Blake DF, Stumbo CR. Ethylene oxide resistance of microorganisms important in food spoilage of acid and high acid foods. *J Food Sci.* 1970;35:26-29.

47. Kuzminski LN, Howard GL, Stumbo CR. Thermochemical factors influencing the death kinetics of spores of *Clostridium botulinum* 62A. *J Food Sci.* 1969;34:561-567.

48. Kaye S, Phillips CR. The sterilizing action of gaseous ethylene oxide; the effect of moisture. *Am J Hyg.* 1949;50(3):296-306.

49. Politzer P, Estes VM, Baughman M. Epoxide nucleophile interactions: acid catalyzed reaction of ethylene oxide with water. *Int J Quantum Chem Quantum Biol Symposium.* 1978;5:291-299.

50. Cyr HW, Glaser Z, Jacobs ME. A CDRH risk assessment of ethylene oxide residues on medical devices. In: *Sterilization in the 1990s.* Washington, DC: Health Industry Manufacturers Association; 1989: 269-279. Report 89-1.

51. Samuel AH, Matthews IP, Gibson C. Microwave desorption: a combined sterilizer/aerator for the accelerated elimination of ethylene oxide residues from sterilized supplies. *Med Instrum.* 1988;22(1): 39-44.

52. Matthews IP, Gibson C, Samuel AH. Enhancement of the kinetics of the aeration of ethylene oxide sterilized polymers using microwave radiation. *J Biomed Mater Res.* 1989;23:143-156.

53. McClaren J. A design of experiments approach to ethylene oxide sterilization cycle optimization—aeration. Poster presented at: Association for the Advancement of Medical Instrumentation—Technical Poster Session; October 2015; Silver Spring, MD.

54. Dias FN, Ishii M, Nogaroto SL, Piccini B, Penna TC. Sterilization of medical devices by ethylene oxide, determination of the dissipation of residues, and use of green fluorescent protein as an indicator of process control. *J Biomed Mater Res B Appl Biomater.* 2009;91: 626-630.

55. US Food and Drug Administration. *Guidance for Premarket Notification [(510)k] for Sterilizers Intended for Use in Health Care Facilities.* Silver Spring, MD: US Food and Drug Administration; 1993.

56. Association for the Advancement of Medical Instrumentation. *ANSI/AAMI ST41:2008. Ethylene Oxide Sterilization in Health Care Facilities: Safety and Effectiveness.* Arlington, VA: Association for the Advancement of Medical Instrumentation; 2008.

57. Association for the Advancement of Medical Instrumentation. *AAMI TIR17:2008. Compatibility of Materials Subject to Sterilization.* Arlington, VA: Association for the Advancement of Medical Instrumentation; 2008.

58. Chen L, Sloey C, Zhang Z, et al. Chemical modifications of therapeutic proteins induced by residual ethylene oxide. *J Pharm Sci.* 2015;104:731-739.

59. Ah YC, Choi Y, Kim SY, Kim SH, Lee KS, Byun Y. Effects of ethylene oxide gas sterilization on physical properties of poly(L-lactide)-poly (ethylene glycol)-poly(L-lactide) microspheres. *J Biomater Sci Polym Ed.* 2001;12(7):783-799.

60. Edlund U, Albertsson AC, Singh SK, Fogelberg I, Lundgren BO. Sterilization, storage stability and in vivo biocompatibility of poly(trimethylene carbonate)/poly(adipic anhydride) blends. *Biomaterials.* 2000;21:945-955.

61. Kiminami H, Krueger AB, Abe Y, Yoshino K, Carpenter JF. Impact of sterilization method on protein aggregation and particle formation in polymer-based syringes. *J Pharm Sci.* 2017;106:1001-1007.

62. Phillip E Jr, Murthy NS, Bolikal D, et al. Ethylene oxide's role as a reactive agent during sterilization: effects of polymer composition and device architecture. *J Biomed Mater Res B Appl Biomater.* 2013;101(4):532-540.

63. Simmons AJ, Hyvarinen J, Poole-Warren L. The effect of sterilisation on a poly(dimethylsiloxane)/poly(hexamethylene oxide) mixed macrodiol-based polyurethane elastomer. *Biomaterials.* 2006;27(25):4484-4497.

64. Collier JP, Sutula LC, Currier BH, et al. Overview of polyethylene as a bearing material: comparison of sterilization methods. *Clin Orthop Relat Res.* 1996;(333):76-86.

65. Pietrzak, WS. Effects of ethylene oxide sterilization on 82:18 PLLA/PGA copolymer craniofacial fixation plates. *J Craniofac Surg.* 2010;21(1):177-181.

66. Fray ME, Bartkowiak A, Prowans P, Slonecki J. Physical and mechanical behavior of electron-beam irradiated and ethylene oxide sterilized multiblock polyester. *J Mater Sci Mater Med.* 2000;11:757-762.

67. Holl K, Seul T. Changes in the mechanical properties of laser-welded polymer specimens of polypropylene and polycarbonate through different sterilization procedures. *Polymer Eng Sci.* 2016;:536-540.

68. Stolov AA, Slyman BE, Burgess DT, Hokansson AS, Li J, Allen RS. Effects of sterilization methods on key properties of specialty optical fibers used in medical devices. *Proc SPIE.* 2013;8576:857606.

69. Zhao Y, Xiaoli Y, Ding F, Yang Y, Gu X. The effects of different sterilization methods on silk fibroin. *J Biomed Sci Eng.* 2011;4:397-402.

70. Nuutinen JP, Clerc C, Virta T, Törmälä P. Effect of gamma, ethylene oxide, electron beam, and plasma sterilization on the behaviour of SR-PLLA fibres in vitro. *J Biomater Sci Polym Ed.* 2002;13(12):1325-1336.

71. Seitz JM, Collier K, Wulf E, et al. The effect of different sterilization methods on the mechanical strength of magnesium based implant materials. *Adv Eng Mat.* 2011;13(12):1146-1151.

72. França A, Pelaz B, Moros M, et al. Sterilization matters: consequences of different sterilization techniques on gold nanoparticles. *Small.* 2010;6(1):89-95.

73. Halpern JM, Gormley CA, Keech MA, von Recum HA. Thermomechanical properties, antibiotic release, and bioactivity of a sterilized cyclodextrin drug delivery system. *J Mater Chem B.* 2014;2:2764-2772.

74. Holtan JR, Olin PS, Rudney JD. Dimensional stability of a polyvinylsiloxane impression material following ethylene oxide and steam autoclave sterilization. *J Prosthet Dent.* 1991;65(4):519-525.

75. Zislis T, Martin SA, Cerbas E, Heath JR III, Mansfield JL, Hollinger JO. A scanning electron microscope study of in vitro toxicity of ethylene-oxide-sterilized bone repair materials. *J Oral Implantol.* 1989;15(1):41-46.

76. Shintani H. Ethylene oxide gas sterilization of medical devices. *Biocontrol Sci.* 2017;22(1):1-16.

77. National Fire Protection Association. *Standard for the Storage, Handling, and Use of Ethylene Oxide for Sterilization and Fumigation.* Quincy, MA: National Fire Protection Association; 2007. NFPA 560.

78. National Fire Protection Association. *Standard for the Storage, Use, and Handling of Compressed Gases and Cryogenic Fluids in Portable and Stationary Containers, Cylinders, and Tanks.* Quincy, MA: National Fire Protection Association; 2013. NFPA 55.

79. Conviser SA, Woltz C. Ethylene oxide sterilization: sterilant alternatives. In Reichert M, Young JH, ed. *Sterilization Technology for the Health Care Facility.* 2nd ed. Gaithersburg, MD: Aspen; 1997:187-198.

80. US Environmental Protection Agency. *Reregistration Eligibility Decision for Ethylene Oxide.* Washington, DC: US Environmental Protection Agency; 2008.

81. Occupational Health and Safety Administration. Occupational health and safety standards, toxic and hazardous substances: ethylene oxide. 29 CFR §1910.1047. https://www.osha.gov/laws-regs/regulations/standardnumber/1910/1910.1047. Accessed October 7, 2019.

82. Schneider PM. Ethylene oxide sterilization: employee monitoring. In Reichert M, Young JH, ed. *Sterilization Technology for the Health Care Facility.* 2nd ed. Gaithersburg, MD: Aspen; 1997:220-225.

83. Desai PR, Buonicore AJ. Engineering controls to minimize worker exposure to ethylene oxide at sterilization facilities. *Plant/Operations Prog.* 1990;9(2):103-107.

84. Wallace CA, Pearson R, Walt M, Murphy M, Pederson J. Operator safety studies—breathing zone analyses when using a small chamber ethylene oxide sterilizer. Poster presented at: Association for the Advancement of Medical Instrumentation—Technical Poster Session; October 2015; Silver Spring, MD.

85. Elliott L, Mortimer V, Ringenburg V, Kercher S, O'Brien D. Effect of engineering controls and work practices in reducing ethylene-oxide exposure during the sterilization of hospital supplies. *Scand J Work Environ Health.* 1988;14(suppl 1):40-42.

86. Whitbourne J, Page BFJ, Centola DT. Ethylene oxide sterilization: ethylene oxide residues. In Reichert M, Young JH, ed. *Sterilization Technology for the Health Care Facility.* 2nd ed. Gaithersburg, MD: Aspen; 1997:200-206.

87. Cárdenas-Camarena L. Ethylene oxide burns from improperly sterilized mammary implants. *Ann Plast Surg.* 1998;41:361-369.

88. Karacalar A, Karacalar SA. Chemical burns due to blood pressure cuff sterilized with ethylene oxide. *Burns.* 2000;26(8):760-763.

89. International Organization for Standardization. *ISO 10993-7:2008: Biological Evaluation of Medical Devices—Part 7: Ethylene Oxide Sterilization Residuals.* Geneva, Switzerland: International Organization for Standardization; 2008.

90. Young JH. Ethylene oxide: current status and future prospects. In: *Proceedings from the International Kilmer Memorial Conference on the Sterilization of Medical Products*; Moscow, Union of Soviet Socialist Republics; 1991; September 11-15, 1989.

91. Klobucar JM. *Safely Controlling Ethylene Oxide Emissions Using Thermal Oxidation.* San Diego, CA: Air and Waste Management Association; 1998.

92. Santello L. Controlling ethylene oxide and chlorofluorocarbon emissions at sterilization facilities. In: *Sterilization in the 1990s.* Washington, DC: Health Industry Manufacturer's Association; 1989. Report 89-1.

93. Mitchel G, Pricer K. Effects of EO concentration and temperature on inactivation of *B. atrophaeus.* In: *Industrial Sterilization—Research from the Field.* Arlington, VA: Association for the Advancement of Medical Instrumentation; 2013:31-36.

Disinfection and Sterilization With Hydrogen Peroxide

Randal W. Eveland

Hydrogen peroxide was first isolated by Louis Jacques Thénard in 1818 from the reaction of barium peroxide with nitric acid. The first proposed disinfectant use was in 1858 by the English physician B. W. Richardson. Since that first report, hydrogen peroxide has become one of the most widely used microbiocides for antiseptic, disinfectant, and sterilization applications, with well-established effectiveness against a wide range of microorganisms.

The use of hydrogen peroxide, in liquid formulation or particularly in gas (or vapor) form, for disinfection and sterilization has continued to increase for a number of reasons. Within health care facilities, steam sterilization has been the sterilization method of choice for well over 100 years, but many electronic devices and instruments with heat- and moisture-sensitive materials cannot withstand the process conditions. Ethylene oxide gas was widely used in hospitals as a low-temperature method, but its use has decreased due to long process time (in particular for aeration or removal of toxic residues), the health hazards associated with its use (eg, carcinogenic potential of both the sterilant and its decomposition products), and government regulations. Hydrogen peroxide sterilization technologies have become popular in these cases. Similarly, gas or liquid phase sterilization processes have found applications as alternatives in various industrial processes, including medical device or component sterilization. Furthermore, gas or aerosolized peroxide processes are widely used for area disinfection (fumigation) applications (eg, pharmaceutical, animal research, production spaces, and infection outbreak remediation) due to undesired use of formaldehyde due to the chemicals' known carcinogenicity and the long process time (see chapter 36).

Gaseous hydrogen peroxide processes can offer broad-spectrum activity, short cycle times, and good material compatibility and are environmentally friendly. Hydrogen peroxide decomposition into environmentally safe and nontoxic byproducts (water and oxygen) is a major force driving the effort to use hydrogen peroxide for disinfection and sterilization applications.

▶ PHYSICAL PROPERTIES

The chemical formula for hydrogen peroxide is H_2O_2. In its pure form, it is a pale blue liquid, whereas hydrogen peroxide solutions with water are clear and colorless. Hydrogen peroxide can be mixed with water at any concentration. The chemistry of hydrogen peroxide is characterized by the reactivity of the peroxide (double oxygen) bond. This oxygen-oxygen bond is weak and will disassociate to a powerful oxidizing agent. Hydrogen peroxide decomposes into water and oxygen upon heating or in the presence of numerous chemicals, particularly transition metal salts of metals such as iron, copper, manganese, nickel, or chromium that may catalytically decompose the peroxide.

Commercial grades of liquid hydrogen peroxide typically contain stabilizers to prevent decomposition and provide stability during storage and transport. Typical stabilizers include chelants and sequestrants, with stannates and phosphates being commonly used. Stabilizers are not known to have an effect on disinfection or sterilization processes, but they are a consideration for the equipment manufacturers.

Hydrogen peroxide is a strong oxidizing agent with a standard reduction potential (E°) of 1.78 V. In comparison to hydrogen peroxide (with a larger reduction potential indicating a stronger oxidizer), ozone is a stronger oxidizer (E° = 2.07 V), peracetic acid is similar in oxidizing capability (E° = 1.81 V), whereas chlorine is a weaker oxidizer (E° = 1.36 V).[1,2] The hydroxyl radical, key to efficacy, has a standard reduction potential of 2.80 V.[1]

The terms *gas* or *vapor* are used interchangeably when discussing vaporized hydrogen peroxide processes, and both terms refer to the same physical state of matter.

All vapors are gases, but not all gases are vapors. For a vapor, changes in pressure or temperature can allow the vapor to change to a liquid (condense). Distinctly different from a gas or vapor, an aerosol is a fine dispersion of liquid droplets. For hydrogen peroxide disinfection and sterilization processes, the control of temperature, pressure, sterilant delivery, and vaporization method is critical to ensure the gaseous hydrogen peroxide is delivered and maintained as intended (eg, at or below the condensation point) for an efficacious process.

A wide variety of hydrogen peroxide concentration solutions (with the balance as water) are used. A 3% hydrogen peroxide solution is used over-the-counter as a topical antiseptic, with a maximum of 8% hydrogen peroxide concentration recommended for home use. Various concentrations may also be used in liquid-based formulations, such as in combination with peracetic acid and under acidified formulations (see chapter 18). For disinfection and sterilization applications, hydrogen peroxide concentrations from 30% to 59% are commonly used to generate the gas under various conditions, for example, under- or oversaturated (to allow for gas condensation on target surfaces). Hydrogen peroxide concentrations from 60% to 100% are considered more dangerous to transport, for example, being classified by the US Department of Transportation (DOT) as "Packing Group 1," the same classification used for transporting hydrogen peroxide rocket fuel. The DOT classification helps explain why concentrations at or above 60% are not routinely used as a source of hydrogen peroxide in liquid or gas disinfection or sterilization applications.

▶ SAFETY AND TOXICITY

The hazards and properties of hydrogen peroxide are well established in the scientific literature.[3] Hydrogen peroxide is a natural constituent of the body; it is present in exhaled breath at levels of 300 to 1000 $\mu g/m^3$ and in food at levels of 3 to 7 ppm.[4] The human liver, one organ that generates hydrogen peroxide, produces an estimated 3.8 g/kg of liver per day.[5] In an adult man with a liver weighing 1800 g, this amounts to 6.8 g/d or 97 mg/kg of body weight per day. As the body readily produces hydrogen peroxide, the in vivo toxicity is moderated by the presence of enzymes such as catalase (an enzymatic, highly effective, catalytic decomposer of hydrogen peroxide) and metal ion sequestration that limits hydroxyl radical production.

The primary exposure routes to hydrogen peroxide are via inhalation, ingestion, skin, and/or eye contact. Hydrogen peroxide solutions of 35% and greater are severely irritating to corrosive and may result in irreversible eye damage including blindness. Hydrogen peroxide can be harmful if inhaled or swallowed. The potential for a toxic effect will vary greatly depending on the hydrogen peroxide concentration and the route of exposure.

Hydrogen peroxide is not a sensitizing agent.[3] There are no known effects of hydrogen peroxide to reproduction/development.[3] Although there is limited evidence of hydrogen peroxide carcinogenicity with animal studies, the relevance and significance of this information for humans is unclear and therefore inadequate to characterize hydrogen peroxide as a carcinogen to humans.[3] In vitro studies have shown hydrogen peroxide can have mutagenic, genotoxic, and cytotoxic effects; however, the relevance to in vivo systems is questionable due to natural mechanisms (as stated earlier) present to mitigate hydrogen peroxide.[3]

Although hydrogen peroxide is classified as odorless, some users have identified a nasal irritation response (likely via chemosensitive trigeminal nerve response versus an olfactory nerve interaction)[6] and characterized the odor as slightly pungent or acidic. Hydrogen peroxide irritation has been identified to occur at 150 mg/m^3 (108 ppm),[7] but it should be noted that odor thresholds and sensory thresholds are often highly variable because methodology and individual sensitivity will vary.

▶ MECHANISM OF ACTION

Oxidizing agents are widely used for various antimicrobial medical, dental, industrial, and agricultural applications (see chapter 18). Oxidizing agents, such as hydrogen peroxide, can be powerful antimicrobial agents due to their ability to remove electrons from other substances such as proteins, lipids, and nucleic acids.[8]

The mechanism of action is believed to be based on the formation and subsequent reaction of hydroxyl radicals via the superoxide ($O_2^{\cdot 2}$) and hydrogen peroxide as first proposed by Haber and Weiss.[9] The reaction to form the radicals is believed to be catalyzed in vivo by transition metal ions via the Fenton reaction. The first step in the process is the reduction of iron(III) to iron(II) (equation 1). Iron(II) can then react with hydrogen peroxide to generate the hydroxyl radical ($\cdot OH$) (equation 2). The net reaction to form hydroxyl radical is shown in equation 3.

$$Fe^{3+} + \cdot O_2^- \rightarrow Fe^{2+} + O_2 \qquad (1)$$

$$Fe^{2+} + H_2O_2 \rightarrow Fe^{3+} + OH^- + \cdot OH \qquad (2)$$

$$\cdot O_2^- + H_2O_2 \rightarrow \cdot OH + OH^- + O_2 \qquad (3)$$

The hydroxyl radical ($\cdot OH$) is a potent oxidizer to cellular components, nucleic acids, and proteins. It is the oxidation and subsequent loss in viability and function that inactivates microorganisms to provide the antimicrobial effect. The process begins on the outer surfaces and can progress, as structure damage progresses, to intercellular components.[8] The oxidation (or loss of an electron by a molecule, an atom, or an ion) and damage to these molecules will have dramatic effects on their structure and function, which culminate to give biocidal activity. Oxidation reactions with biocides have been shown to cause macromolecular unfolding, fragmentation, and cross-reaction with oxidized groups.[8] Proteins, carbohydrates, and lipids on the surface of microorganisms are particularly accessible targets, followed by various intercellular components, including proteins and nucleic acids, as the structure of the microorganism disintegrates.

The effects of hydrogen peroxide on nucleic acids have been well described as hydrogen peroxide, and other reactive oxygenated species (including the short-lived but extremely reactive superoxide ions and hydroxyl radicals) are formed during cellular respiration and can have detrimental effects in eukaryotic cell components; indeed, these effects have been linked to cell aging and mutagenesis.[10] For example, hydrogen peroxide has a dramatic effect on DNA and RNA structures, attacking both the nucleotide bases and the sugar-phosphate backbone of these structures.[11] The oxidation of these groups will lead to strand breakage and cross-reactions between converted bases/sugars, which will affect the replication, transcription, translation, and other roles of these essential structures. With respect to proteins and amino acids, a difference has been reported in the specific reactivity and modes of action between hydrogen peroxide in liquid or gas form.[12,13]

Overall, oxidizing agents such as hydrogen peroxide have multiple effects on proteins, lipids, carbohydrates, and nucleic acids, which leads to loss of their structure and, hence, function. Specific effects include changes in structure, breakdown of these macromolecules into smaller constituents, and transformation of structural and functional groups as well as some effects leading to cross-linking within and between these molecules under some conditions. These effects will result in the loss of viability of the microbial target. The effects are clearly significant on vegetative and actively metabolizing microorganisms, including bacteria and fungi. The overall damage to the structures of spores, cysts, and viruses also appears to cause a loss in viability presumably due to specific effects not only on surface proteins and lipids but also on penetration to the nucleic acid.

▶ BROAD-SPECTRUM ACTIVITY

As an oxidizing chemistry, hydrogen peroxide in various forms and concentrations has demonstrated broad-spectrum activity against a wide variety of microorganisms. Considering pathogens, E. H. Spaulding taught that certain classes of microorganisms can be generally classified as being more resistant to disinfection and biocides than others.[14] This classification is shown in Table 32.1 and includes a summary of those microorganisms that have

been shown to be inactivated by gaseous hydrogen peroxide. The list of organisms is not exclusive but provides an understanding of the potential and likelihood for hydrogen peroxide to disinfect/sterilize microorganisms in the same classification group. The most resistant organism to gaseous hydrogen peroxide is generally recognized as *Geobacillus stearothermophilus* spores, although spores of *Bacillus atrophaeus* (*Bacillus subtilis* var *globigii*) have been reported to be more resistant to liquid formulations.[53] Bacterial spores are much more resistant to hydrogen peroxide than the vegetative form of the organism. The list of organisms within the resistance spectrum, from least to most resistant, is meant as a general guide. The resistance of organisms, even within the same classification, can vary greatly depending on experimental methods. Experimental conditions such as exposure time, concentration, and test system play a significant role in defining resistance, but other factors such as culture purity and the presence of organic or inorganic soil will also affect the observed resistance.

Efficacy has also been demonstrated against the mycoplasma *Acholeplasma laidlawii*, against *Cryptosporidium parvum* oocyst,[54] and helminths (parasitic worms, eg, tapeworm or nematode) *Caenorhabditis elegans* and *Syphacia muris*.[55] For *S muris*, there is research suggesting that effectivity may vary when considered in vivo versus in vitro.[46]

Prion disease–causing agents, for example, those associated with the diseases scrapie, Creutzfeldt-Jakob disease, and chronic wasting disease, are not strictly considered as living microorganisms because they are believed to consist solely of protein with no associated nucleic acids (see chapter 68). Although not viable, prions are transmissible and can be a significant contamination concern in the presence of high-risk tissues (eg, contaminated brain tissue). Prions are considered difficult to inactivate and are therefore ranked as more resistant than bacterial spores in Table 32.1. Inactivation of prions on contaminated surfaces has been documented for subatmospheric pressure sterilizers using 59% hydrogen peroxide gas,[15] but certain subatmospheric pressure sterilizers that used plasma required precleaning with alkaline formulations prior to being effective or a process to increase gas-phase hydrogen peroxide concentration to approximately 90% to 95% for repeatable effectivity.[56]

When similar concentrations are considered, disinfection and sterilization processes with liquid hydrogen peroxide solutions are not nearly as rapid as those with gaseous hydrogen peroxide. The formation and subsequent reaction of hydroxyl radicals occur more readily in the gas phase because water can stabilize hydrogen peroxide in solution via hydrogen bonding. The rate of reaction differences between liquid and gaseous hydrogen peroxide has been evaluated experimentally and compared via a difference in D-value. The D-value refers to the time required to reduce the population of a microorganism by 90% (or 1 $\log_{10}$).

TABLE 32.1   Classification of microorganism resistance and identification of microorganisms for which gaseous hydrogen peroxide efficacy has been demonstrated

Spaulding Classification		Efficacy Demonstrated With Gaseous Hydrogen Peroxide
More Resistant ⬆	Prions	Scrapie 263K strain,[15] bovine spongiform encephalopathy (BSE) 6PB1 strain[15]
	Bacterial spores	*Bacillus anthracis*,[16-18] *Bacillus atrophaeus* (formerly *Bacillus subtilis*),[16,18-22] *Bacillus cereus*,[19,20] *Bacillus circulans*,[19] *Bacillus firmus*,[21] *Bacillus megaterium*,[21] *Bacillus pumilus*,[20,21] *Bacillus thuringiensis*,[18] *Clostridium botulinum*,[23] *Clostridium difficile*,[20,24-26] *Clostridium perfringens*,[20] *Clostridium sporogenes*,[22] *Clostridium tetani*,[20] *Geobacillus stearothermophilus*[a] (formerly *Bacillus stearothermophilus*)[16,18-20,25-28]
	Mycobacteria	*Mycobacterium avium*,[29] *Mycobacterium bovis*,[20] *Mycobacterium chelonae*,[20] *Mycobacterium smegmatis*,[22] *Mycobacterium terrae*,[29] *Mycobacterium tuberculosis*,[20,30,31] *Mycobacterium fortuitum*[32]
	Small nonenveloped viruses	*Calciviridae* (feline calicivirus, *Murine norovirus*, vesicular exanthema of swine virus),[33-37] *Flaviviridae* (hog cholera virus),[34] *Paramyxoviridae* (Newcastle disease virus),[34] *Parvoviridae* (mouse and porcine parvovirus),[33,38] *Picornaviridae* (polio type 1, foot-and-mouth disease virus, swine vesicular virus),[20,33,34] *Reoviridae* (bluetongue virus),[34] *Rhabdoviridae* (vesicular stomatitis virus)[34]
	Gram-negative bacteria	*Acinetobacter baumannii*,[25,26,28,39,40] *Acinetobacter calcoaceticus*,[20] *Bacteroides fragilis*,[20] *Brucella suis*,[41,42] *Burkholderia cepacia*,[26] *Burkholderia mallei*,[43] *Burkholderia pseudomallei*,[41] *Enterobacter cloacae*,[40] *Escherichia coli*,[20,22,26] *Francisella tularensis*,[41,42] *Klebsiella pneumoniae* (*Legionella* species),[22,26] *Moraxella osloensis*,[20] *Pseudomonas aeruginosa*,[20,21,26] *Pseudomonas cepacia*,[20] *Salmonella choleraesuis*,[22] *Serratia marcescens*,[20,44] *Xanthomonas maltophilia*,[20] *Yersinia pestis*[41,42,45]
	Fungi	*Alternaria* species,[46] *Aspergillus brasiliensis* (formerly *Aspergillus niger*),[20,46] *Blastomyces dermatitidis*,[47] *Candida albicans*,[20,46] *Candida parapsilosis*,[20,46] *Coccidioides immitis*,[47] *Histoplasma capsulatum*,[46] *Penicillium* species,[46] *Trichophyton mentagrophytes*[19,20]
	Large, nonenveloped viruses	*Adenoviridae* (adenovirus),[33,35,48] *Parvoviridae* (parvovirus)[38]
	Gram-positive bacteria	*Deinococcus radiodurans*,[20] *Enterococcus faecium*/*Enterococcus faecalis* (VRE),[20,26,39,49,50] *Enterococcus hirae*,[46] *Listeria monocytogenes*,[20,22] *Staphylococcus aureus* (MRSA),[20,26,28,39,51] *Staphylococcus epidermidis*,[20,51] *Streptococcus pneumoniae*[26]
Less Resistant	Enveloped viruses	*Orthomyxoviridae* (avian influenza virus, influenza A[H1N1]),[34,35,52] *Herpesviridae* (pseudorabies virus),[20,34] *Poxviridae* (Vaccinia)[32,33]

Abbreviations: MRSA, methicillin-resistant *Staphylococcus aureus*; VRE, vancomycin-resistant enterococci.

[a]Most resistant organism to vaporized hydrogen peroxide.

As shown in Table 32.2, the D-value for three spore species was evaluated at different hydrogen peroxide liquid and vapor concentrations (250 000 and 1.5 mg/L, respectively). Even at the concentration of 1.5 mg/L hydrogen peroxide, the gaseous sterilant has a faster D-value than aqueous hydrogen peroxide at 250 000 mg/L.

It has been suggested that the differences in reactivity observed for liquid and gaseous hydrogen peroxide may be due to mechanistic differences between the liquid and gas forms.[13] Hydrogen peroxide in the gas form may be able to better penetrate and interact with protein structure in ways, minus enhancements via formulation, that are not possible with liquid peroxide.

The role of humidity for gaseous hydrogen peroxide systems appears to be less critical than for other gas processes in that humidification does not seem to be required as for other agents such as ozone, chlorine dioxide, formaldehyde, and ethylene oxide where >60% humidity is typically required. Gaseous hydrogen peroxide has been shown effective at both high and low humidity, with many health care subatmospheric sterilization processes using no humidification beyond that provided with water from the vaporized sterilant solution.

Processed materials may also have an impact on disinfection process efficacy. It was noted that absorptive, porous materials (such as polyurethane, Viton, and paper) present a greater challenge to the disinfection process, requiring a longer exposure time to achieve a 6 $\log_{10}$ reduction of *G stearothermophilus* spores.[19]

TABLE 32.2	Sporicidal efficacy comparison of aqueous and gaseous hydrogen peroxide (H_2O_2)[a]

Spore	D-Value (min)[b]	
	H_2O_2 Aqueous Concentration: 250 000 mg/L	H_2O_2 Gas Concentration: 1.5 mg/L
Geobacillus stearothermophilus	2	1.5
Bacillus atrophaeus	5	0.7
Clostridium sporogenes	1	0.5

[a]Data from McDonnell.[8]

[b]The D-value refers to the time required to reduce the population of a microorganism by 90% (or 1 log).

▶ MATERIAL COMPATIBILITY

Hydrogen peroxide is a widely used chemical, and the compatibility of hydrogen peroxide aqueous solutions is well understood. The general compatibility knowledge can be broadly applied to material performance in disinfection and sterilization applications; however, the specific conditions within each process will also contribute to the compatibility profile of processed materials and, as appropriate, the enclosure area. Gaseous hydrogen peroxide concentration as well as exposure time, temperature, humidity, and risk of condensation as well as the material properties themselves will all have an effect on material compatibility. Hence, any material compatibility discussions or comparisons between processes must take into account the process-specific conditions and their potential impact on compatibility.

Hydrogen peroxide demonstrates good compatibility with a wide array of plastics. Color stability should be understood as oxidizing chemistries like hydrogen peroxide may cause color bleaching depending on the dyes used. Plastics that have oxidable functional groups, some nylons for example, will be oxidized and may show loss of functionality after repeated sterilization. Metals in general have good compatibility with hydrogen peroxide. Colored anodized aluminum surfaces may also have the colorant oxidized from the surface and fade. Adhesives are compatible to varying degrees depending on the formulation, and adhesive suitability to gaseous hydrogen peroxide processes may be affected by its location and application on a device.[57]

Cellulosic materials are not compatible with hydrogen peroxide and should be avoided. Furthermore, exposed fabrics can pose a fire hazard because during exposure, the water can preferentially evaporate from the fabric leaving behind highly concentrated hydrogen peroxide, which

can react with organic material and autoignite. Liquids cannot be sterilized with gaseous hydrogen peroxide, but the surfaces of sealed liquid-containing containers can be.

A benefit to aid in understanding the compatibility of hydrogen peroxide is that the chemical has such a long history of use and its potential for reaction with many materials is understood. Failure to appreciate or take this knowledge into account could lead to negative material interactions and, in the case of medical devices, potentially negative results for the device and the patient it is used on. One such example of this indirect material compatibility effect is based on the known reaction of hydrogen peroxide with the dry lubricant molybdenum sulfide (MoS_2) to form sulfuric acid (H_2SO_4).[58] Following a range of outbreaks with multiantibiotic-resistant bacteria involving gastrointestinal (GI)-flexible endoscopes (specifically duodenoscopes),[59] many have advocated for the sterilization of these GI devices between patient use. Some have advocated to use gaseous hydrogen peroxide processes with these devices, even though GI-flexible endoscopes are known to use molybdenum sulfide as a dry lubricant inside the medical device. Once formed inside a GI device, sulfuric acid is known to decompose the elastomeric materials in the endoscope insertion tube from the inside, eventually exposing the exterior of the device, and potentially patients, to sulfuric acid.[60]

▶ LIQUID APPLICATIONS

Liquid hydrogen peroxide in solution with water only or in formulation has been shown to be effective against bacteria, yeasts, fungi, viruses, and spores is well described.[61] Although a 6% solution was shown to be an effective sterilant in 6 hours,[62] it is in formulation with other chemicals that hydrogen peroxide is most used as a disinfectant and sterilant. In particular, its extensive use with peracetic acid and under acidified formulations (see chapter 18) have the most applicability in disinfection. Higher concentrations of liquid hydrogen peroxide (eg, at 30%-35%) have been used under controlled temperature conditions (up to 80°C) for the disinfection and sterilization of containers used in high-speed filling applications.[63]

▶ ATMOSPHERIC PROCESSES

Atmospheric vaporized hydrogen peroxide processes can be developed and have been widely used to include for the disinfection and sterilization of packaged medical items, area disinfection, isolator and laminar flow cabinet disinfection, and production line sterilization processes. The quick microbial kill of gaseous or condensed hydrogen peroxide and the nontoxic nature of the decomposition products are key factors as to where and how it is used. Hydrogen peroxide solutions at 30% to 35% concentration in water are typical, but lower concentrations in the 3% to 6% range and up to 59% solutions can also be used to generate the gas or aerosols.

Hydrogen peroxide can be generated into an area via one of three methods: (1) as an aerosol, (2) as a gas, or (3) as a condensed gas. The most commonly used processes are either as a gas or condensed gas. Equipment designed for these processes typically include systems with preset cycles and operator-controllable cycles that allow the user to establish appropriate parameters for their application (Figure 32.1). Various systems and accessories are offered that allow scaling of systems for the area to be disinfected, such as biosafety cabinets to large rooms. In these systems, the hydrogen peroxide solution is typically flash vaporized across a heated surface or nebulized to create hydrogen peroxide gas or aerosol.

In the "dry" or gas process, the gas concentration and humidity (depending on the area temperature) can be controlled to prevent condensation within the treatment area when hydrogen peroxide is introduced.[64] The dry process allows for the maintenance of a stable hydrogen peroxide gas concentration within the treatment area over the disinfection cycle. In an alternative process, the peroxide solution in nebulized and released into the area, where it can be present as a gas over time and depending on the concentration, humidity, and temperature of the area. In condensed gas processes, the concentration of gaseous peroxide in the air is purposely increased above the saturation point to form a "microcondensation" layer of hydrogen peroxide and water onto surfaces.[65] As hydrogen peroxide has been shown to be more corrosive in the presence of water, a lower concentration is often used overtime to ensure material compatibility. The differences in approach are evident in the application instructions for United States Environmental Protection Agency claims.

During decontamination, one manufacturer instructs to maintain hydrogen peroxide concentration at 250 ppm for 90 minutes or at 400 ppm for 30 minutes, whereas another manufacturer directs to apply 35% hydrogen peroxide solution at a rate of 3.1 g/min for 55 minutes and then hold for 3 hours or to apply at a rate of 10 g/min for 2.5 hours and then hold for 15 minutes.

The critical parameters for atmospheric vaporized hydrogen peroxide applications are peroxide concentration, temperature, relative humidity, and contact time. A defined hydrogen peroxide gas concentration, to include both the starting solution concentration (eg, 35% wt/wt) and application rate, is used to ensure the required process concentrations can be achieved. The starting peroxide liquid concentration is typically 30% to 59% (wt/wt) hydrogen peroxide to achieve process concentrations from approximately 0.3 to 2.5 mg/L hydrogen peroxide (approximately 200-1800 ppm hydrogen peroxide). Temperature is important to the process to maintain the required hydrogen peroxide concentration in the gas phase. Typical temperatures are from 25°C to 40°C, with process temperatures as low as 4°C possible.[66] Relative humidity control can allow for process optimization and management, in particular of whether the process is "dry" or if sterilant is microcondensed onto all surfaces. During a typical, controlled atmospheric process, the initial relative humidity may range from 10% to 60% before the introduction of the gas. With the addition of vaporized hydrogen peroxide and water into the area, the relative humidity can typically vary from 40% to 90%.

Atmospheric vaporized hydrogen peroxide applications can include the general process steps of preconditioning, conditioning, decontamination, and aeration as shown in Figure 32.2, but these processes can range in application. During the preconditioning phase, the application area is prepared for introduction of vaporized hydrogen peroxide. Requirements for temperature, humidity, and air flow within the area can be established during this phase. The hydrogen peroxide gas generation system is readied for use. During the conditioning phase,

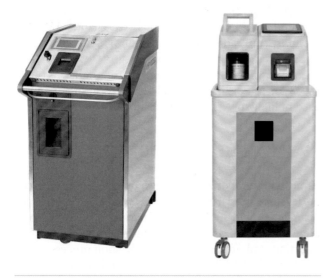

FIGURE 32.1 Examples of hydrogen peroxide gas generator systems for atmospheric applications. For a color version of this art, please consult the eBook.

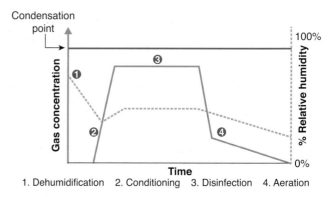

FIGURE 32.2 Example of an atmospheric decontamination process maintained below the condensation point.

vaporized hydrogen peroxide is introduced into the exposure area to achieve the required concentration in the area. The decontamination (or disinfection) phase begins once appropriate conditions are met and lasts as long as required based on efficacy of the process at the exposure conditions. For the aeration phase, vaporized hydrogen peroxide is removed from the exposure area and hydrogen peroxide residual is reduced to a safe level (typically <1 ppm).

Atmospheric applications have mainly included disinfection (including sporicidal disinfection) of spaces as small as a biological safety cabinet or into areas as large as 28 000 m^3 (performed in sections as large as 7000 m^3) for the 2001 Federal Government building anthrax remediation.[17] Applications only included not only for antimicrobial purposes but also in the neutralization of chemical contaminants such as chemical weapons and cytotoxic drugs.[67,68] Integration into room and building systems designed for compatibility with the vaporized hydrogen peroxide process is increasing. Sterilization applications have also been validated for certain industrial processes.

▶ SUBATMOSPHERIC (VACUUM) PROCESSES

Hydrogen peroxide gas exposure under vacuum is used to sterilize a variety of product applications such as reusable medical devices (eg, in a health care or clinical setting) to sterilize single-use medical devices or to sterilize drug product packaging (health care products). The advantages to using hydrogen peroxide in low-pressure, controlled applications include air removal, increased rate of sterilant diffusion into a load, and an increase in the relative concentration of hydrogen peroxide at the point of contact. For example, at 25°C and 1 atm (101.3 kPa, 760 mm Hg, or 760 Torr), a 1 mg/L hydrogen peroxide concentration is best case approximately 720 ppm, whereas at 50°C and 0.0013 atm (0.13 kPa, 1 mm Hg, or 1 Torr), a 9 mg/L hydrogen peroxide concentration is possible for >6400 ppm.

Health Care Reusable Device Sterilization

In the United States, there are two major types of hydrogen peroxide gas, low-temperature sterilization system products used in the hospital environment: those that use plasma and those that do not (Figure 32.3). Both types of sterilizers offer users unalterable cycles based on device characteristics and claims established by the manufacturer. Total cycle times vary from approximately 17 to 70 minutes depending on the cycle and, to a certain extent, the device load. Liquid hydrogen peroxide (typically at 59% concentration in water) is used to generate the gas adjacent to or directly within the sterilization chamber. Once vaporized, the hydrogen peroxide is then diffused into the load for antimicrobial action. In all cases, the load is exposed to the gas, which can be introduced over multiple "pulses" of gas introduction, exposure, and removal

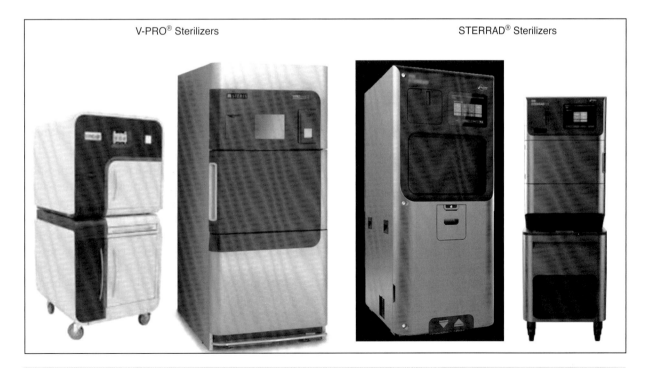

FIGURE 32.3 Examples of hospital sterilizers that use hydrogen peroxide gas (V-PRO®) sterilizers and use hydrogen peroxide gas-plasma (STERRAD®) sterilizers. For a color version of this art, please consult the eBook.

as defined by the sterilization process. Both systems, with or without plasma, break down hydrogen peroxide to acceptable levels via catalytic conversion of all chamber effluent and venting from the chamber to atmosphere.

Relative humidity, although critical for effective repeatable sterilization with other sterilization methods, does not seem to be a critical factor for subatmospheric hydrogen peroxide gas sterilization. Rather than humidification, the first step in the sterilization process is to reduce pressure and remove all gaseous water present in the chamber. Any water present on the prepared load may also be removed during the chamber evacuation, depending on the cycle design. From this point, water is only introduced by the sterilizer into the chamber in two specific ways during the sterilization cycle: (1) with (or on breakdown of) the gaseous sterilant or (2) from atmospheric humidity during the transition to near atmospheric/atmospheric conditions in the sterilizer cycle.

Temperature in low-pressure hydrogen peroxide gas sterilization plays a different role than it would in other sterilization methods, for example, steam. For steam sterilization, it is important to heat the entire load to the sterilization temperature to ensure conditions are met for sterilization (see chapter 28). For hydrogen peroxide gas sterilizers, the role of the chamber wall temperature (approximately 50°C is common) is to help maintain the sterilant in the gaseous state not to heat the load. For gaseous hydrogen peroxide sterilization under vacuum, there is no good mechanism to transfer heat to the loads. The exception is sterilizers with plasma because the high energy provided to the chamber from radiofrequency (RF) coils can heat the load depending on the process design. This is evidenced by device temperature poststerilization because a device load in a hospital hydrogen peroxide gas sterilizer can typically have increased temperature from room temperature (approximately 20°C) to approximately 25°C to 40°C, whereas a hydrogen peroxide gas-plasma sterilizer load will be less than or equal to 55°C.[20,69]

As shown in the pressure versus time graph in Figure 32.4, hydrogen peroxide gas sterilizers typically have three general phases: condition, sterilize, and aeration. For the condition phase, air is removed from the sterilizer and is loaded to a pressure set point. The sterilizer also prepares sterilant for injection and may perform other conditioning checks, such as evaluating the load for moisture content. The sterilize phase can vary depending on the sterilizer and process type, but typically during this phase, two to four sterilization pulses may be used with a set quantity of hydrogen peroxide used for each pulse. For the sterilization pulse, liquid sterilant is vaporized at low pressure and enters the chamber. The pressure within the chamber is held for a set time while sterilant diffuses into the load. Filtered air can then be introduced into the chamber and held for a set time. This transition step (transitioning the chamber to a higher pressure) has been shown to move sterilant within the load. Next, chamber pressure is reduced in preparation for the next sterilization

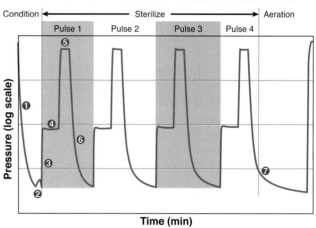

V-PRO® maX 2 Sterilizer Pressure Versus Time

1. Evacuate chamber
2. Moisture check
3. Preparation for injection, inject
4. Post injection hold
5. Transition to 500 Torr, hold
6. Evacuate (remove H$_2$O$_2$), prepare for next pulse
7. Evacuate chamber to aerate

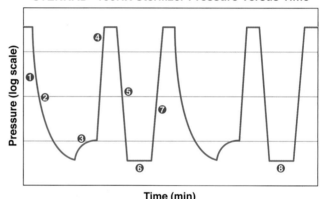

STERRAD® 100NX Sterilizer Pressure Versus Time

1. Sterilant injection
2. Sterilant concentration
3. Transfer sterilant
4. Diffusion, transition to atm
5. Evacuate (remove H$_2$O$_2$)
6. Plasma
7. Ventilate, prepare for next pulse
8. Evacuate chamber, plasma and vent to atmospheric

FIGURE 32.4 Example of pressure versus time graphs for hydrogen peroxide sterilizers with and without plasma.

pulse, or after the last sterilization pulse, in preparation for the aeration phase. For the aeration phase, the chamber is evacuated for a set time to essentially remove residual hydrogen peroxide from the load and chamber.

As shown in Figure 32.4, hydrogen peroxide gas-plasma sterilizers operate similarly. There is an initial condition phase where air is removed from the chamber to a pressure set point, followed in some sterilizers with the generation of an air plasma to heat the load and assist to remove any moisture present. Also during the condition phase for some sterilizers, sterilant is concentrated in a separative vessel from approximately 59% to approximately 90% to 95% hydrogen peroxide concentration, with the water removed based on differences in the vapor pressure between water and hydrogen peroxide. Following the condition phase, chamber pressure is reduced for the sterilize phase, where sterilant is transferred to the chamber and allowed to diffuse through the load. Filtered air can be introduced into the chamber (a similar transition step to that discussed earlier), and chamber pressure held for a set time. Sterilant and air is removed from the chamber as the chamber pressure is again reduced. A plasma is then initiated within the chamber by RF energy provided to a plasma coil. Following the plasma phase, the cycle can either vent to atmospheric pressure then evacuate the chamber to the sterilant injection pressure or proceed directly to the sterilant injection for the next sterilization pulse. The plasma exposure in the final sterilization pulse serves as aeration for the cycle. Plasma is used under vacuum during this phase to reduce process residuals.

One significant process difference between the sterilizers in Figure 32.3 is whether the sterilizer uses plasma or not. The use of hydrogen peroxide based on gas-plasma sterilizer during the sterilization phase makes sense conceptually as a method to create reactive species (such as hydroxyl radicals) for a more effective process. In simplest terms, plasma is an ionized gas created when sufficient energy is applied to a gas to cause electron removal from an atom, thus creating ionized particles (see chapter 34). The plasma state in the hydrogen peroxide gas sterilizer is created using an RF coil located inside of the chamber. Although plasmas are used for their antimicrobial properties, with antimicrobial activity attributed to the various ions, electrons, radicals, or UV light present, the plasma in these hydrogen peroxide–based sterilizers may not have a significant contribution to microbicidal activity.[70] Instead, plasma can be used in these sterilizers for other purposes such as during conditioning and aeration as a source of heat or as a mechanism to volatilize adsorbed/absorbed hydrogen peroxide residuals in the chamber or on the load.

Beyond plasma, multiple strategies have been introduced into the hydrogen peroxide gas sterilizer cycle designs to improve device penetration capabilities, such as improved lumened device claims. As an example, liquid hydrogen peroxide–filled adapters (known as "boosters") can be applied to a device lumen to allow for longer lumen sterilization during a cycle. The adapters allow for the direct application of liquid hydrogen peroxide within a lumened device. Concentrating sterilant from 59% to 80% to 95% is also a part of some sterilizers because the higher hydrogen peroxide concentration could theoretically allow increased penetration of hydrogen peroxide sterilant into difficult to penetrate areas of the load, such as lumens, without water (as a breakdown product from hydrogen peroxide) interference. As with other sterilization systems, increases in sterilant exposure time can also lead to increased efficacy claims. Multiple exposures (sterilization pulses) may also be used to increase sterilant exposure time or a priming injection of sterilant (introduction of sterilant to the chamber while the chamber is evacuated by vacuum) may be used to condition the chamber and load. Furthermore,

exposure times may be varied depending on the type of devices intended for the sterilization cycle, for example, surface sterilization versus sterilization within a lumen. Some processes have also developed alternative hydrogen peroxide delivery systems in combination with ozone gas during the exposure process, but the overall benefit of the ozone under such conditions has not been defined.[57]

Each of the strategies applied by the sterilizer manufacturers is essential and required for their respective sterilization cycles; however, the relative importance of each strategy would have to be evaluated in terms of the claims made by each sterilizer cycle. Beyond the potential contributions to sterilizer cycle efficacy, the impact the processes have on material compatibility should be considered. As an example, plasma can negatively affect material compatibility because plasma is known to generate secondary reactions that can be detrimental to outer layers of sterilized devices.[20] The plasma effect is most pronounced on surfaces of nonmetallic materials such as soft plastics, for example, the insertion tube of flexible endoscopes. The increased load temperature achieved due to plasma in combination with a higher sterilant concentration will likely contribute to an increase in the reactions of hydrogen peroxide with oxidable materials (eg, for every 10°C increase in temperature, the reaction rate doubles). All other elements in a cycle being equal, longer sterilant exposure times will increase the exposure times of materials to the sterilant and can affect compatibility of materials susceptible to oxidation.

Commercially available chemical indicators (CIs) and biological indicators (BIs) are available to monitor the cycle performance. Improvements have been made to BIs for hydrogen peroxide sterilizers resulting in significantly reduced incubation times, with BIs now available with incubation times from 20 to 30 minutes. Figure 32.5 shows examples from several manufactures with the BIs and their validated read time. These BIs are typically qualified with a specific incubator/reader to provide the quick detection of viable test microorganisms.

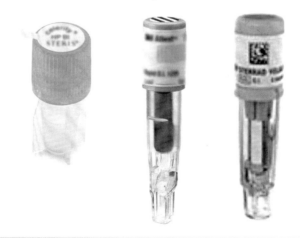

FIGURE 32.5 Examples of biological indicators for VH_2O_2 with fast read times. For a color version of this art, please consult the eBook.

Packaging for hydrogen peroxide gas sterilizers in hospitals is typically (1) sterilization wrap, (2) Tyvek/plastic pouches, or (3) rigid reusable sterilization containers. Importantly, paper or cellulosic materials should not be used because hydrogen peroxide can condense within these materials, potentially leading to autoignition and fire as well as reducing the concentration of peroxide within the exposure chamber.

A key benefit to the use of hydrogen peroxide gas for reusable medical devices is that the process does not leave residual water on devices, which is particularly important when sterilizing moisture-sensitive devices such as electronics, cameras, and devices with electronic components. The processes are designed such that the concentration of water and sterilant within the chamber (which helps maintain the sterilant in the gas phase) will not condense onto surfaces. Due to the fast kill kinetic (D-value) of gas phase reactions in comparison to liquid phase reactions, the microbicidal efficacy is generally described as resulting from gas phase interactions. This, however, can vary in sterilizer process design.

Despite this, devices must be thoroughly dried before processing in subatmospheric gaseous hydrogen peroxide processes. Some sterilizer designs have mechanisms to identify the presence of moisture in the load but only to a certain extent. Because evaporation is an endothermic process, moisture will evaporate under vacuum and cool the local environment. Depending on the quantity of water and the thermal conductivity of its surroundings, water could freeze and subsequently condense hydrogen peroxide. Upon warming, this liquid water with hydrogen peroxide may remain on the device and pose a safety hazard on subsequent handling and patient use.

The potential for terminally sterilized, packaged loads to be processed within approximately 20 to 30 minutes and that these loads required no additional aeration or cooldown postprocessing will offer new options for health care departments currently using immediate-use sterilization. Coupled with a BI read within 20 to 30 minutes, many of the risks users face when deciding to use immediate-use sterilization can be eliminated using a hydrogen peroxide gas sterilizer (as an alternative to steam sterilization) when devices must be sterilized quickly.

Industrial Gas Sterilization Applications

Hydrogen peroxide gas sterilizers to sterilize single-use medical devices and components or to sterilize drug product packaging follow the same general processes as described earlier. These sterilizers offer users greater control for cycle parameter optimization, and users are responsible to validate the specific sterilization process for their product and load criteria.

Hydrogen peroxide gas sterilization can be used as an alternative to other heat and low-temperature sterilization processes but particularly for devices with sensitive components that cannot be sterilized with steam, gamma radiation, or ethylene oxide. These have included plastic orthopedic implants, prefilled syringes, drug delivery systems, and biological drug packages.[71] The sterilization processes typically operate in the range of 28°C to 40°C (with lower temperatures possible) and therefore provide a near-room temperature method to sterilize heat-sensitive devices. In prefilled pharmaceutical drug applications, the process and packaging should be designed to ensure that the hydrogen peroxide sterilant does not interact with the drug, and the sterilization process is used to sterilize the packaging and external surfaces of the device.

Hydrogen peroxide sterilant (typically from 35% to 59%) is used to generate the gas adjacent to or directly within the sterilization chamber. Process conditions can include use of plasma (inside or immediately outside the sterilization chamber) and low-temperature steam depending on the system used. A very general cycle description is provided in Figure 32.6. Cycles will also typically feature three phases: preconditioning, sterile (vaporized hydrogen peroxide exposure), and aeration (postconditioning). The cycles operate similarly to those used in health care sterilizers. The preconditioning phase is used to control the chamber environment and prepare the load for sterilization, removing air and moisture, and, for some processes, controlling the load temperature prior to hydrogen peroxide introduction. For the sterile (vaporized hydrogen peroxide exposure) phase, pressure is reduced in the chamber, and hydrogen peroxide is introduced and allowed to diffuse through the load. Unlike the reusable device sterilizers described earlier, the amount of hydrogen peroxide introduced is not set as a single injection for some systems. The sterilizer controller may monitor process parameters and add additional sterilant during a sterilization pulse based on process design requirements. At the end of the sterilization pulse, the sterilizer may either progress into the aeration phase or execute additional sterilization pulses. Figure 32.6 shows a cycle with two sterilization pulses, but sterilizers may use one, two, or more sterilization pulses depending on the sterilant exposure required for a user to validate sterilization of their

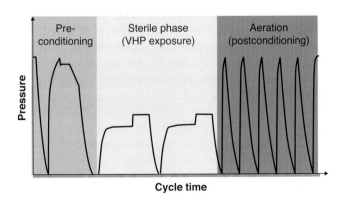

FIGURE 32.6 Health care product sterilizer cycle example. Abbreviation: VHP, vapor hydrogen peroxide.

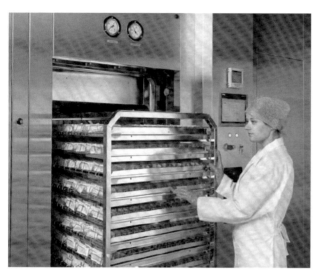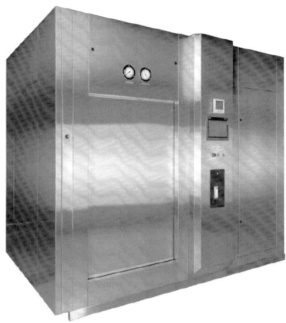

FIGURE 32.7 An industrial hydrogen peroxide sterilizer (the STERIS LTS-V Low Temperature Sterilizer). For a color version of this art, please consult the eBook.

load. Following the sterilize phase, the aeration phase is used to remove sterilant from the chamber and the load. Typically, a series of air flushes is used to reduce sterilant concentration within a chamber, but other aeration approaches can be used.

Device packaging can affect the hydrogen peroxide gas sterilization process. From compatible materials, hard nonporous plastics are usually chosen for medical device and device packaging. Although hydrogen peroxide is not known to penetrate materials, it can adsorb/absorb onto surfaces. A nonabsorptive material will allow for shorter aeration time and a shorter sterilization process. A typical device packaging for sterilization would be a device inside a plastic tray, with the tray covered in a gas-permeable material such as Tyvek (sometimes called a blister pack). The packaging must be designed to allow for sterilant contact on all surfaces and for sterilant removal during the aeration process. Figure 32.7 shows product loaded onto a cart for sterilization. Available systems, such as the STERIS LTS-V sterilizer shown, have sterilizer volumes from 2 to 8 m^3 (70-283 ft^3). Due to the incompatibility of hydrogen peroxide with cellulosic materials (eg, wood, cardboard, and paper) and the need to ensure sterilant delivery to the device, medical devices cannot be sterilized within shipping packaging.

REFERENCES

1. Parsons SA, Williams M. Introduction. In: Parsons SA, ed. *Advanced Oxidation Processes for Water and Wastewater Treatment.* London, United Kingdom: International Water Association; 2004:1-5.
2. Rahman MS. *Handbook of Food Preservation.* 2nd ed. Boca Raton, FL: CRC Press; 2007.
3. Munn S, Allanou R, Aschberger K, et al, eds. *European Union Risk Assessment Report. Hydrogen Peroxide.* Luxembourg, Luxembourg: Publications Office of the European Union; 2003. CAS no. 7722-84-1. EINECS no. 231-765-0.
4. Weiner ML, Freeman C, Trochimowicz H, et al. 13-week drinking water toxicity study of hydrogen peroxide with 6-week recovery period in catalase-deficient mice. *Food Chem Toxicol.* 2000;38: 607-615.
5. DeSesso JM, Lavin AL, Hsia SM, Mavis RD. Assessment of the carcinogenicity associated with oral exposures to hydrogen peroxide. *Food Chem Toxicol.* 2000;38:1021-1041.
6. Meredith M. Trigeminal response to odors. In: Adelman, ed. *Sensory Systems II: Senses Other Than Vision (Readings from the Encyclopedia of Neuroscience).* Boston, MA: Birkhäuser Boston; 1988:139.
7. Ruth JH. Odor thresholds and irritation levels of several chemical substances: a review. *Am Ind Hyg Assoc J.* 1986;47:142-151.
8. McDonnell G. *Antisepsis, Disinfection, and Sterilization: Types, Action, and Resistance.* 2nd ed. Washington, DC: ASM Press; 2007.
9. Haber F, Weiss J. The catalytic decomposition of hydrogen peroxide by iron salts. *Proc R Soc London.* 1934;147(861):332-351.
10. Cabiscol E, Tamarit J, Ros J. Oxidative stress in bacteria and protein damage by reactive oxygen species. *Int Microbiol.* 2000;3:3-8.
11. Linley E, Denyer SP, McDonnell G, Simons C, Maillard JY. Use of hydrogen peroxide as a biocide: new consideration of its mechanisms of biocidal action. *J Antimicrob Chemother.* 2012;67: 1589-1596.
12. McDonnell G. The use of hydrogen peroxide for disinfection and sterilization applications. In: Marek I, ed. *Patai's Chemistry of Functional Groups.* Hoboken, NJ: Wiley; 2014.
13. Finnegan M, Linley E, Denyer SP, McDonnell G, Simons C, Maillard JY. Mode of action of hydrogen peroxide and other oxidizing agents: differences between liquid and gas forms. *J Antimicrob Chemother.* 2010;65:2108-2115.
14. Spaulding EH. Chemical disinfection and antisepsis in the hospitals. *J Hosp Res.* 1972;9:5-31.
15. Fichet G, Antloga K, Comoy E, Deslys JP, McDonnell G. Prion inactivation using a new gaseous hydrogen peroxide sterilisation process. *J Hosp Infect.* 2007;67(3):278-286.

16. Rogers JV, Sabourin CL, Choi YW, et al. Decontamination assessment of *Bacillus anthracis*, *Bacillus subtilis*, and *Geobacillus stearothermophilus* spores on indoor surfaces using a hydrogen peroxide gas generator. *J Appl Microbiol.* 2005;99:739-748.

17. Rogers JV, Richter WR, Shaw MQ, Shesky AM. Large-scale inactivation of *Bacillus anthracis Ames, Vollum,* and *Sterne* spores using vaporous hydrogen peroxide. *Appl Biosafety.* 2009;14:127-134.

18. United States Environmental Protection Agency. *Compilation of Available Data on Building Decontamination Alternatives.* Washington, DC: United States Environmental Protection Agency; 2005.

19. Meszaros JE, Antloga K, Justi C, Plesnicher C, McDonnell G. Area fumigation with hydrogen peroxide vapor. *Appl Biosafety.* 2005;10(2):91-100.

20. Smith D. *STERRAD® NX Sterilization System.* Irvine, CA: Advanced Sterilization Products; 2004.

21. Kokubo M, Inoue T, Akers J. Resistance of common environmental spores of the genus *Bacillus* to vapor hydrogen peroxide. *PDA J Pharm Sci Technol.* 1998;52:228-231.

22. McDonnell G, Grignol G, Antloga K. Vapour phase hydrogen peroxide decontamination of food contact surfaces. *Dairy Food Environ Sanitat.* 2002;22:868-873.

23. Johnston MD, Lawson S, Otter JA. Evaluation of hydrogen peroxide vapour as a method for the decontamination of surfaces contaminated with *Clostridium botulinum* spores. *J Microbiol Methods.* 2005;60(3):403-411.

24. Boyce JM, Havill NL, Otter JA, et al. Impact of hydrogen peroxide vapor room decontamination on *Clostridium difficile* environmental contamination and transmission in a healthcare setting. *Infect Control Hosp Epidemiol.* 2008;29:723-729.

25. Otter JA, French GL. Survival of nosocomial bacteria and spores on surfaces and inactivation by hydrogen peroxide vapor. *J Clin Microbiol.* 2009;47:205-207.

26. McDonnell G, Antloga K, Azad S, Robinson N. Amsco V-PRO 1: a new low temperature sterilization system. *Zentral Sterilization.* 2009;17:101-113.

27. Rickloff JR, Orelski PA. Resistance of various micro-organisms to vaporized hydrogen peroxide in a prototype tabletop sterilizer. Paper presented at: 89th General Meeting of the American Society for Microbiology; May 14-18, 1989; New Orleans, LO.

28. Fu TY, Gent P, Kumar V. Efficacy, efficiency and safety aspects of hydrogen peroxide vapour and aerosolized hydrogen peroxide room disinfection systems. *J Hosp Infect.* 2012;80(3):199-205.

29. Moy A, Speight S. *Assessment of the Efficacy of Vapour Phase Hydrogen Peroxide Generated by the Bioquell Q10 Against* Mycobacterium avium *and* Mycobacterium terrae. Horsham, PA: Bioquell; 2014. PHE report no. 14/006.

30. Kahnert A, Seiler P, Stein M, Aze B, McDonnell G, Kaufmann SHE. Decontamination with vaporized hydrogen peroxide is effective against *Mycobacterium tuberculosis. Lett Appl Microbiol.* 2005;40:448-452.

31. Hall L, Otter JA, Chewins J, Wengenack NL. Use of hydrogen peroxide vapor for deactivation of *Mycobacterium tuberculosis* in a biological safety cabinet and a room. *J Clin Microbiol.* 2007;45(3):810-815.

32. Beswick AJ, Farrant J, Makison C, et al. Comparison of multiple systems for laboratory whole room fumigation. *Appl Biosafety.* 2011;16:139-157.

33. Eterpi M, McDonnell G, Thomas V. Virucidal activity of disinfectants against parvoviruses and reference viruses. *Appl Biosafety.* 2010;15(4):165-171.

34. Heckert RA, Best M, Jordan LT, Dulac GC, Eddington DL, Sterritt WG. Efficacy of vaporized hydrogen peroxide against exotic animal viruses. *Appl Environ Microbiol.* 1997;63(10):3916-3918.

35. Goyal SM, Chander Y, Yezli S, Otter JA. Evaluating the virucidal efficacy of hydrogen peroxide vapour. *J Hosp Infect.* 2014;86:255-259.

36. Bentley K, Dove BK, Parks SR, Walker JT, Bennett AM. Hydrogen peroxide vapour decontamination of surfaces artificially contaminated with norovirus surrogate feline calicivirus. *J Hosp Infect.* 2012;80(2):116-121.

37. Holmdahl T, Walder M, Uzcategui N, et al. Hydrogen peroxide vapor decontamination in a patient room using feline calicivirus and *Murine norovirus* as surrogate markers for human norovirus. *Infect Control Hosp Epidemiol.* 2016;37(5):561-566.

38. McDonnell G, Belete B, Fritz C, Hartling J. Room decontamination with vapor hydrogen peroxide VHP for environmental control of parvovirus. Paper presented at: 52nd Annual Meeting of the American Association for Laboratory Animal Science; October 2001; Baltimore, MD.

39. Lemmen S, Scheithauer S, Häfner H, Yezli S, Mohr M, Otter JA. Evaluation of hydrogen peroxide vapor for the inactivation of nosocomial pathogens on porous and nonporous surfaces. *Am J Infect Control.* 2015;43(1):82-85.

40. Otter JA, Yezli S, Schouten MA, van Zanten AR, Houmes-Zielman G, Nohlmans-Paulssen M. Hydrogen peroxide vapor decontamination of an intensive care unit to remove environmental reservoirs of multidrug-resistant gram-negative rods during an outbreak. *Am J Infect Control.* 2010;38(9):754-756.

41. Rogers J, Richter W, Wendling M, Shesky A. Inactivation of *Brucella suis, Burkholderia pseudomallei, Francisella tularensis,* and *Yersinia pestis* using vaporous hydrogen peroxide. *Appl Biosafety.* 2010;15(1):25-31.

42. United States Environmental Protection Agency. *Persistence Testing and Evaluation of Fumigation Technologies for Decontamination of Building Materials Contaminated with Biological Agents.* Washington, DC: United States Environmental Protection Agency; 2010.

43. Rogers J, Lastivka A, Richter W. Persistence and inactivation of *Burkholderia mallei* China 7 deposited on nonporous laboratory materials. *Appl Biosafety.* 2016;21(2):66-70.

44. Bates CJ, Pearse R. Use of hydrogen peroxide vapour for environmental control during a *Serratia* outbreak in a neonatal intensive care unit. *J Hosp Infect.* 2005;61(4):364-366.

45. Rogers JV, Richter WR, Shaw MQ, Choi YW. Vapour-phase hydrogen peroxide inactivates *Yersinia pestis* dried on polymers, steel, and glass surfaces. *Lett Appl Microbiol.* 2008;47:279-285.

46. Bioquell. *Hydrogen Peroxide Vapor Biological Efficacy.* Horsham, PA: Bioquell; 2017.

47. Hall L, Otter JA, Chewins J, Wengenack NL. Deactivation of the dimorphic fungi *Histoplasma capsulatum, Blastomyces dermatitidis* and *Coccidioides immitis* using hydrogen peroxide vapor. *Med Mycol.* 2008;46(2):189-191.

48. Berrie E, Andrews L, Yezli S, Otter JA. Hydrogen peroxide vapour (HPV) inactivation of adenovirus. *Lett Appl Microbiol.* 2011;52(5):555-558.

49. Otter JA, Cummins M, Ahmad F, van Tonder C, Drabu YJ. Assessing the biological efficacy and rate of recontamination following hydrogen peroxide vapour decontamination. *J Hosp Infect.* 2007;67(2):182-188.

50. Fisher D, Pang L, Salmon S, et al. A successful vancomycin-resistant enterococci reduction bundle at a Singapore hospital. *Infect Control Hosp Epidemiol.* 2016;37(1):107-109.

51. Health Protection Agency. *Determination of the Effectiveness of VPHP Against Methicillin-Resistant Staphylococcus aureus, Staphylococcus epidermidis and Bacillus stearothermophilus.* Porton Down, United Kingdom; 2001.

52. Rudnick SN, McDevitt JJ, First MW, Spengler JD. Inactivating influenza viruses on surfaces using hydrogen peroxide or triethylene glycol at low vapor concentrations. *Am J Infect Control.* 2009;37(10):813-819.

53. Toledo RT, Escher FE, Ayres JC. Sporicidal properties of hydrogen peroxide against food spoilage organisms. *Appl Microbiol.* 1973;26(4):592-597.

54. Barbee SL, Weber DJ, Sobsey MD, Rutala WA. Inactivation of *Cryptosporidium parvum* oocyst infectivity by disinfection and sterilization processes. *Gastrointest Endosc.* 1999;49(5):605-611.

55. Gustin EJ, McDonnell GE, Mullen G, Gordon BE. The efficacy of vapor phase hydrogen peroxide against nematode infestation: the *Caenorhabditis elegans* model. Paper presented at: 53rd Annual Meeting of the American Association for Laboratory Animal Science; October 27-31, 2002; San Antonio, TX.

56. Rogez-Kreuz C, Yousfi R, Soufflet C, et al. Inactivation of animal and human prions by hydrogen peroxide gas plasma sterilization. *Infect Control Hosp Epidemiol.* 2009;30(8):769-777.

57. Association for the Advancement of Medical Instrumentation. *AAMI TIR17: 2017: Compatibility of Materials Subject to Sterilization.* Arlington, VA: Association for the Advancement of Medical Instrumentation; 2018.

58. Schumb W, Satterfield CN, Wentworth RL. *Hydrogen Peroxide.* New York, NY: Reinhold Publishing Corp; 1955.

59. US Food and Drug Administration. *Executive Summary. Effective Reprocessing of Endoscopes used in Endoscopic Retrograde Cholangiopancreatography (ERCP) Procedures.* Silver Spring, MD: US Food and Drug Administration; 2015.

60. Hui H, Feldman LA, Nguyen HP, Timm D, Albers R, inventors; Ethicon Inc, Johnson & Johnson, assignee. Medical instrument and method for lubrication and sterilization thereof. US patent 5,716,322. February 10, 1998.

61. Block SS, ed. Peroxygen compounds. In: *Disinfection, Sterilization and Preservation.* 5th ed. Philadelphia, PA: Lippincott Williams & Wilkins; 2001:185-204.

62. Rutala WA, Gergen MF, Weber DJ. Sporicidal activity of chemical sterilants used in hospitals. *Infect Control Hosp Epidemiol.* 1993;14: 713-718.

63. Ansari IA, Datta AK. An overview of sterilization methods for packaging materials used in aseptic packaging systems. *Trans IChemE.* 2003;81(C):57-65.

64. Hultman C, Hill A, McDonnell G. The physical chemistry of decontamination with gaseous hydrogen peroxide. *Pharm Eng.* 2007;27(1): 22-32.

65. Watling D, Ryle C, Parks M, Christopher M. Theoretical analysis of the condensation of hydrogen peroxide gas and water vapour as used in surface decontamination. *PDA J Pharm Sci Technol.* 2002;56(6): 291-299.

66. Klapes NA, Vesley D. Vapor-phase hydrogen peroxide as a surface decontaminant and sterilant. *Appl Environ Microbiol.* 1990;56(2): 503-506.

67. McVey I, Schwartz LI, Centanni MA, Wagner GW, inventors; US Secretary of Army, STERIS Inc, assignee. Activated vapor treatment for neutralizing warfare agents. US patent 7,651,667. January 26, 2010.

68. Roberts S, Khammo N, McDonnell G, Sewell GJ. Studies on the decontamination of surfaces exposed to cytotoxic drugs in chemotherapy workstations. *J Oncol Pharm Pract.* 2006;12(2): 95-104.

69. STERIS. *V-PRO maX 2 Low Temperature Sterilization System.* Mentor, OH: STERIS; 2018.

70. Krebs MC, Bécasse P, Verjat D, Darbord JC. Gas-plasma sterilization: relative efficacy of the hydrogen peroxide phase compared with that of the plasma phase. *Int J Pharm.* 1998;160:75-81.

71. Vogel DB. Bringing sterilization inside. *Med Design Technol.* 2004: 24-27.

CHAPTER
33

Disinfection and Sterilization Using Ozone

Linda K. Weavers, G. B. Wickramanayake, Mikhail Shifrin, and Gerald McDonnell

Ozone (O_3), an unstable three-atom allotrope of oxygen, is formed by the excitation of molecular oxygen (O_2) into atomic oxygen (O) in an energizing environment that allows the recombination of atoms into O_3, which is a powerful oxidizing agent with a standard reduction potential of $+2.07$ V (O_3/O_2).[1] Pure O_3 melts at a temperature of $-192.5°C \pm 0.4°C$ and boils at $-111.9°C \pm 0.3°C$.[2] At ambient temperatures, O_3 is a blue-colored gas, but this color is not noticeable at the low concentrations typically used for disinfection purposes.[3] The O_3 was first introduced as a chemical disinfectant in drinking water treatment in 1893 at Oudshoorn, Netherlands,[4] but has subsequently been described and used for a variety of disinfection and sterilization applications. Ozone is used in its gas form, as well as when dissolved in liquids such as water, for antimicrobial purposes.

BENEFITS OF AND CHALLENGES WITH OZONE IMPLEMENTATION

For practical applications, it is important to note that ozone is potentially the strongest and fastest acting oxidizer/disinfectant commercially available today based on its chemical properties, depending on how it is applied. That puts ozone in the position to be theoretically applied in any applications where other widely used oxidizing biocides such as chlorine or chlorine-releasing products (see chapter 15), chlorine dioxide (see chapter 27), hydrogen peroxide, and peracetic acid (see chapter 18) are used but typically more effectively and economically. In addition to ozone being considered more ecologically safer unlike many other biocides, it is produced from a raw product (air, or specifically the oxygen in air) that is free, and this makes ozone in most applications more economically attractive than other alternative oxidizers that are not typically produced on site. There are few applications where ozone cannot be practically used for antimicrobial

purposes, and at worst, these are only considered to be slower in practice due to some external factors. Examples include the presence of extraneous materials (eg, organic soils or in the presence of biofilms; see chapter 67) that can react with to neutralize ozone and make it less available for antimicrobial activity, other restrictions in the access of ozone to target microorganisms, and other factors such as temperature. At lower temperatures in water, ozone was effective in inactivating *Escherichia coli* at lower temperatures and in the absence of contaminating (in this case, rumen content or feces-contaminated water).[5] Ozone was found to inactivate *E coli* in water at an estimated concentration of 22 to 24 ppm ozone at 5°C, but efficacy was dramatically reduced in the presence of soil. Others found that the antimicrobial activity of ozone in water was greater at lower pH (pH 6 compared to 8) and at higher temperatures (35°C compared to 15°C), suggesting that optimal conditions can be applied depending on the exposure conditions and concentration of ozone applied.[6] But equally, the stability of ozone will increase as the temperature increases. For water applications, typical ozone concentrations used are in the 0.2 to 0.4 mg/L range at a pH of 6 to 7, but higher concentrations (eg, 5 mg/L) are recommended in the presence of organic materials (eg, in wastewater) due to the increased neutralization of ozone. The process does not necessarily become more expensive even at lower temperature conditions because half-life of ozone in cold water is significantly longer and less ozone is therefore needed to be dissolved to achieve the desired antimicrobial concentration.

A further economic advantage, with the installation of a good quality ozone generating system, is limited operating costs other than a small electric consumption. In many cases, ozone is generated directly for air (approximately 20% oxygen), from which it is naturally made on exposure to ultraviolet (UV) light in the atmosphere. In general, no other consumables are regularly required, such as in the case of the use of chlorine systems or UV light installations. But higher capacity ozone generators (eg, at 50-400mg/L) have also been developed that can generate ozone from oxygen (oxygen concentrators, liquid oxygen (LOX) or bottled oxygen), such as by passing through corona discharge or dielectric barrier discharge. Other methods such as with UV light and electrolytic generating cells are used for smaller applications, as they often have lower efficiency and higher associated costs.

Although ozone itself can be toxic to health at antimicrobial concentrations, the implementation of ozone is often considered a safer option than the use of most chemical oxidizers. Ozone has been reported to be mutagenic, causes reproductive damage, and inhalation leads to irritation of the lungs and upper respiratory tract.[7,8] Higher exposure can cause headache, vomiting, and pain. Inhalation can cause tightness of the chest, including coughing, shortness of breath, and sensitivity to allergens. Repeated high exposure can cause lead to further lung damage and a fluid buildup in the lungs (pulmonary edema). At the same time, ozone has a relatively sharp odor that can be detected at low concentrations (approximately 0.01 to 0.005 ppm). The recommended occupational exposure limits in air (based on an 8-hour time weighted average) is at 0.1 ppm (at 25°C and 760 mm Hg) and 5 ppm as a ceiling or immediately dangerous to life or health.[7,8] The rapid and reactive nature of ozone with contaminants allows it to be used effectively at often low concentrations and in a safe manner while limiting significant negative effects on human health. In many cases, such as in drinking water disinfection, swimming pool water treatment, life support systems, etc, that require higher concentrations of chemicals for proper disinfection, there is often direct and indirect harmful effect to people and other species from the use of chemical oxidizers, including by-products of their use such as trihalomethanes in the case of chlorine that are considered potentially harmful.[8-10] Water disinfection by-products may also formed with ozone, but the safety in the use of ozone in comparison to chlorine continues to be a matter of debate.[11,12] Ozone may also reduce problems associated with the risks of using other chemicals, such as chlorine. Ozone can be easily produced on site eliminating any need for chemical storage, transportation, and stringent personal training where injuries and death from accidents related to chemical handling have been reported.

The practical implementation of ozone in disinfection and sterilization applications is not without its challenges, where many reports in the literature can be misleading on the successful application, advantages, and disadvantages of the technologies. But there has been an increased focus in the area to understand ozone technology and demonstrate successful implementation. These include

- Drinking water and waste water disinfection[13,14]
- Water handling system sanitization, such as heat and cooling water and high purity water distribution systems[15-18]
- Marine aquaria and ponds[19,20]

- Food surface (eg, fruit, vegetables, and fish), packaging, and food-handling surface disinfection[21,22]
- Laundry disinfection[23,24]
- Air, air-handling systems, and area deodorization and disinfection[15,25]
- Medical and dental device disinfection[21,26,27] and sterilization.[28,29] Over the last 20 to 30 years, there have been such systems patented and developed, but all have had little commercial success. This has been particularly due to material compatibility with devices, including metals, polymers, and adhesives that have limited repeated applications with ozone at higher concentrations to be able to meet disinfection and sterilization expectations for regulatory approval, such as sporicidal activity in the presence of high levels of organic and inorganic contaminants.[29-31] Systems that claim to combine hydrogen peroxide and ozone gas for sterilization claim to have much greater material compatibility profiles than ozone alone, primarily due to the lower concentrations of ozone used in these sterilization systems.
- In addition, there are reports on the therapeutic use of ozone, such as with skin diseases, wound healing, dentistry, periodontics, and other applications.[32-36] This is an area of active research and further evidence is required to substantiate the safe and effective use of ozone for many of these applications in infection prevention and control.

▶ OZONE GENERATION

Ozone generation is more efficient at low temperatures because of thermal decomposition at high temperatures and it is therefore important to remove as much heat from the discharge chamber (ozone cell) as possible. Ozone is typically generated for commercial applications by the same essential methods for 30 to 40 years, although advances have been made in the efficiencies of these systems (Figure 33.1). The most widely used methods use dielectric barrier discharge cells, also known as corona discharge cells (where a metallic mesh is used as an electrode material and plasma created around the wires of the mesh appears like a corona).

Ozone-generating cells are nothing more than an electric capacitor with two metal electrodes separated by quartz glass or ceramic dielectric material, through which dry air or oxygen is passed through to generate ozone (Figure 33.2). Just like any electric capacitor ozone-generating cell could be flat or cylindrical in geometry. Modern developments have included improvements in the density of electric discharge that creates more ozone per unit surface of an electrode, to the gas gap/electrode geometry to optimize and assist in improvement of power density, and to improvements in the materials, configurations, or cooling systems that facilitate efficient heat control inside the ozone cell created from the generation process.

The ozone produced can be used directly for air-based systems or in liquids bubbled or otherwise directly

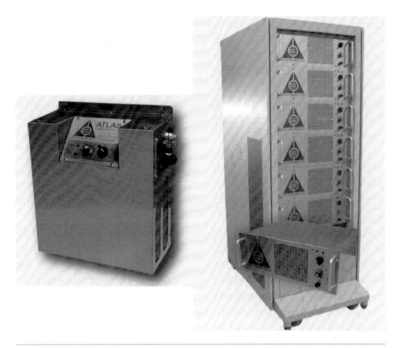

FIGURE 33.1   Examples of ozone generation systems. Courtesy of Absolute Ozone®, Edmonton, Canada.

injected into the water or other liquid. In these generation systems, ozone concentrations ranging from 1% to 3% can be produced if the feed gas is air and higher concentrations (eg, 3% to 24%) if the feed gas is oxygen. For water applications, due to low dissolved efficiency of ozone in water at low concentrations, dry air fed systems are considerably more expensive per gram of ozone dissolved than oxygen fed ones in water treatment applications. Although now less common than these discharge methods due to high power consumption and high operating cost, ozone may be generated by photochemical (eg, use of UV lights), electrolytic, and radiochemical means. The electrolytic methods can be cost-effective and convenient for certain low-volume applications, such as in laboratory or research work, where ozone can be produced already dissolved in the water. More specific details on ozone generation have been reviewed in detail by others.[37-39] The focus on recent research has been on the design of more

efficient ozone generators, to include the generation of higher ozone concentrations, high-pressure delivery systems for dissolution, decreased energy demand, and less oxygen consumption (when applicable).

STABILITY OF OZONE

The instability of gaseous and aqueous O_3 prevents the prior generation and storage of ozone for later applications. Consequently, O_3 needs to be generated on-site as needed for disinfection and sterilization purposes. Ozone is more stable in the gas phase than in the aqueous phase. For example, the half-life of gaseous O_3 in ambient atmosphere is approximately 12 hours, but this can also vary depending on the other variables such as the temperature, quality of air, and presence of various contact surfaces.[40,41] As shown in Table 33.1 the half-life of aqueous O_3 varies

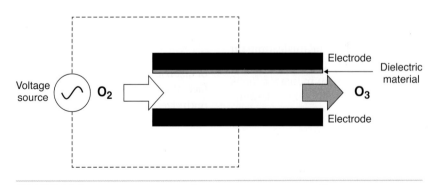

FIGURE 33.2   A representation of an ozone-generating cell.

TABLE 33.1	Estimated half-lives ($t_{1/2}$) of ozone in air and different water qualities[a]
Conditions	**Estimated Half-life ($t_{1/2}$)**
Air at −25°C	8 d
Air at 20°C	3 d
Air at 120°C	1.5 h
Water at pH 7 and 20°C	20 min
Water at pH 7 and 30°C	12 min
Water at pH 7 and 40°C	<4 min
Water at pH 7.5 and 15°C	15 min
Water at pH 8.5 and 15°C	10 min
Water at pH 9.5 and 15°C	5 min
Water at pH 10.5 and 15°C	<30 s
Distilled water	6 h
Tap water	30 min
Filtered lake water	10 min

[a]From McClurkin and Maier DE,[40] Weschler,[41] Staehelin and Hoigne,[42] Batakliev et al,[43] and Gardoni et al.[44]

from hours to seconds, depending on water conditions, such as temperature, pH, water contaminants, O_3 concentration, and concentration of promoters (that can speed up the decay rate) or radical scavengers (eg, carbonate ions that can inhibit the degradation rate).[42-44]

Gurol and Singer[45] developed the following empirical equation to incorporate some of these parameters to express the rate of decrease of O_3 concentration in the pH range of 2 to 9.5:

$$-\frac{D[O_3]}{dt} = k[O_3][OH^-]^{-0.55}$$

where $[O_3]$ and $[OH^-]$ are O_3 and hydroxide ion concentrations, respectively, and k is the rate constant, which is a function of temperature.

▶ ANALYTIC METHODS

Determination of residual O_3 concentrations in aqueous solutions is rather difficult because of its rapid decomposition rates, its volatility from solution, and its reactivity with many organic and inorganic chemicals. It is important to note that most methods of measuring O_3, which are often modifications of chlorine residual methods, are based on the determination of total oxidants in solution. Most of the O_3 disinfection and sterilization data reported in the literature are collected using analytic techniques such as iodometric methods, which do not necessarily measure the O_3 alone. For example, ozonation of olefins produces oxidizing species such as peroxides, hydro alkyl

peroxides, and peroxy acids that interfere with iodometric and many other analytic techniques. Therefore, O_3 disinfection data should be interpreted carefully, especially when different analytical techniques are used during the generation of inactivation data.

There are a wide variety of analytical methods used to determine dissolved ozone concentrations (Table 33.2).[46] Overall, the most widely used, practical, and specific method is by UV adsorption, but other specific methods include the indigo method, amperometric method, and the stripping and gas phase detection method.[47] The UV method is based on the absorption at 254 nm wavelength (provided from a mercury lamp at this wavelength in the UV spectrum), which is preferably absorbed by ozone.[47] Although this method is more straightforward in most water applications, the effects of temperature and pressure in the sample chamber should be considered for air applications. The indigo method is the recommended standard method for measuring ozone residuals.[48,49] In the indigo method, ozone adds across the carbon-carbon double bond of sulfonated indigo dye and decolorizes it. The change in absorbance is determined spectrophotometrically.[49,50] The indigo method is generally considered to be subject to fewer interferences than most of the alternative colorimetric methods and all iodometric procedures that may be used.[46,47] Overall, for dissolved ozone concentrations, the most accurate and widely used is the UV-based method, but these can often be more costly than alternative electrochemical methods.

Accurate measurement of gas-phase ozone is important in the determination of cost, efficiency, safety, and improvement in the design and construction of O_3 generators that produce ozone at much higher concentrations.[46,51] Accurate measurement of dissolved ozone is important for determining cost, efficiency, and effectiveness of water-dissolving devices as Venturi injectors or diffusers for water and wastewater disinfection as well as for establishing ozone demand and ozone system sizing. Therefore, precise and accurate analytic methods are necessary to measure O_3 in the gas phase and dissolved in water. The most commonly used gas-phase analytic methods include iodometry, UV absorption, and chemiluminescence.[46,51] Another method that can be used for O_3 analysis includes gas-phase titration with excess nitric oxide and O_3.[52] The most widely used gas-phase O_3 analytic techniques are listed in Table 33.3. Based on available information, the UV spectrophotometric method remains to be the most recommended for accurate determination of gas-phase ozone.[46,47,51] Overall, most industrial applications use ozone analyzers for measuring ozone concentration in gases and dissolved in liquids, and the most common are based on photometric UV absorption or alternative electrochemical measurement methods. Recent focus has been placed on the use of small, potable, and personal monitoring technologies for better monitoring of personal safety exposures to ozone and other gases.[53,54]

TABLE 33.2   Analytical methods for ozone in aqueous solutions[a]

Analytical Method	Detection Limit (mg/L)	Working Range (mg/L)	Expected Accuracy (%)	Expected Precision (%)	Interferences	pH Range	Current Status
Ideal	0.01	0.01-10	0.5	0.1	None	Independent	Recommended
Iodometric	0.002	0.5-100	1-35	1-2	All ozone byproducts and oxidants	<2	Not widely used
Arsenic back titration	0.002	0.5-65	1-5	1-2	Oxidizing species	6.8	Continued study
FACTS syringaldazine	0.02	0.5-5	5-20	1-5	Oxidizing species	6.6	NR
DPD	0.1	0.2-2	5-20	5	Oxidizing species	6.4	NR
Indigo spectrophotometric	0.001	0.01-0.1	1	0.5	Cl_2, Mn ions, Br_2, I_2	2	Recommended
	0.006	0.05-0.5	1	0.5	Cl_2, Mn ions, Br_2, I_2	2	Recommended
	0.1	>0.3	1	0.5	Cl_2, Mn ions, Br_2, I_2	2	Recommended
	0.01	0.01-0.1	5	5	Cl_2, Mn ions, Br_2, I_2	2	Recommended
		>0.1	5	5	Cl_2, Mn ions, Br_2, I_2	2	Recommended
GDFIA	0.03	0.03-0.4 Other ranges possible	1	0.5	Cl_2 at >1 mg/L	2	Comparison studies needed
LCV	0.005	NR	NR	NR	S^{2-}, SO_3^{-}, Cr^{4-}	2	Continued study
ACVK	0.25	0.05-1	NR	NR	Mn >1 mg/L Cl_2 >10 mg/L	2	Continued study
o-Tolidine	*Not quantitative*		NR	NR	Metal ions, NO^{2-}	2	Abandon
Bisterpyridine	0.004	0.05-20	2.7	2.1	Cl_2	<7	Recommended (lab test)
Carmine indigo	<0.5	NR	NR	NR	NR	2	Continued study
Electrochemical amperometric	~1	NR	5	5	Oxidizing species	2	Relative monitoring
Amperometric iodometric	~0.5	NR	5	5	Oxidizing species	4-4.5	NR
Bare electrode	0.2	NF	5	5	NR	NR	Continued study
Membrane electrode	0.062	NF	5	5	NR	NR	Continued study
Differential pulse dropping mercury	NR	NR	NR	NR	NR	NR	Research lab
Differential pulse polarography	0.003	NR	NR	NR	NR	4	Continued study
Potentiometric	NR	NR	NR	NR	NR	NR	Continued study
Ultraviolet	0.02	>0.02	0.5	0.5	Other absorber	Independent	Establish molar absorptivity
Isothermal pressure change	4×10^{-3}	4×10^{-3} to 10	0.5	0.5	None	Independent	Comparison study

Abbreviations: ACVK, acid chrome violet potassium; DPD, N-N-diethyl-p-phenylenediamine; FACTS, free available chlorine test with syringaldazine ; GDFIA, gas diffusion flow injection analysis; LCV, leuco crystal violet; NR, not reported; NF, not found.

[a]From Gordon et al.[46] Copyright © 1988 American Water Works Association. Reprinted by permission of John Wiley & Sons, Inc.

TABLE 33.3 Analytical methods for ozone in gas phase[a]

Analytical Method	Detection Limit (mg/L)	Working Range (mg/L)	Expected Accuracy (%)	Expected Precision (%)	Interferences	pH Range	Current Status
Ideal	1	1-50 000	1	1	None	Independent	Recommended
Ultraviolet	0.5	0.5-50 000	2	2.5	None	NA	Recommended
Stripping absorption iodometry	0.002	0.5-100	1-35	1-2	SO$_2$, NO$_2$	NA	Not widely used
Chemiluminescence	0.005	0.005-1	7	5	None	NA	Recommended
Gas-phase titration	0.005	0.005-30	8	8.5	None	NA	NR
Rhodamine B gallic acid	0.001	NR	NR	5	NR	NA	NR
Amperometry	NR	NR	NR	NR	NR	NA	NR

Abbreviations: NA, not applicable; NR, not reported.

[a]Based on a previous report[46] but some of the indicated ranges are debated.

From Gordon et al.[46] Reprinted by permission of John Wiley & Sons, Inc.

IMPLEMENTING OZONE IN WATER TREATMENT APPLICATIONS

One of the biggest problems that stands on the way of successful ozone implementation in water treatment is often a misunderstanding of Henry's law of dissolving gases in liquids; a popular misconception often promoted in the literature suggests the larger the surface contact between source gas (bubbles) and target liquid, the more gas will be dissolved. Henry's law states that, at a given temperature, the amount of gas dissolved in a liquid is proportional to the partial pressure of that gas to the liquid. Therefore, in considering the efficiency of ozone dissolution in water applications, the efficiency of dissolution is actually relatively low, with typical reports of <10% dissolved ozone efficiency with microbubble diffusers and about 5% dissolved ozone efficiency when regular diffusers are used. Ozone dissolution can be increased by increasing the concentration of ozone in the gas, increasing the gas (oxygen pressure), and reducing the temperature and pH of the water. As an alternative to simpler diffusers, an inexpensive Venturi-type injector (using the reduction in pressure that results from the flow through a constricted section of a pipe) can deliver 70% to 90% or higher dissolved ozone efficiency when the ozone concentration injected is 6% weight per volume and higher. An example of dissolved ozone concentrations in shallow water is given in Figure 33.3.

Reports suggest that dissolved ozone efficiency will improve somewhat in other deeper water applications, but overall, such applications of the gas are considered more efficient than the use of bubble diffusers.[55,56] This is supported by Henry's law as there is no consideration of the size of the interface surface, only pressure, temperature, and gas concentration. In diffuser systems, for available ozone to dissolve in water, it needs energy and most of this comes

from the speed of the bubble moving up in the liquid; the application of smaller bubbles to offer greater contact surface will actually move much slower and there is therefore less energy to allow for dissolution. Inside Venturi injectors, the gas is injected in to a vacuum area behind the restrictor and from that moment onward the pressure of the system grows to allow for greater dissolution until the liquid pressure is equalized with the system pressure. Overall, the greater the ozone dissolution achieved, the greater the disinfection efficacy can be for most practical applications.

INACTIVATION OF MICROORGANISMS

Bacteria

Ozone, as a potent oxidizing agent, has been well established as an effective disinfectant for bacteria.[57] Reports in the literature can vary considerably due to various different test systems, including ozone generation methods (including inaccurate methods of determining ozone concentrations over exposure time), presence of interfering substances (which can rapidly react with ozone to neutralize its activity), and other factors previously discussed, such as concentration, temperature, and pH. Although such studies are rare, a useful comparison of the antimicrobial efficacy of ozone against a range of bacteria, viruses, and yeasts was useful to determine the response and relative resistance of these organisms to ozonation.[58] The organisms tested include *Mycobacterium fortuitum*, *E coli*, *Salmonella* Typhimurium, poliovirus type 1 (Mahoney), and the yeast *Candida parapsilosis*. The experiments were conducted on two different test systems at pH 7.0 and 24°C. The first experiment was performed in deionized

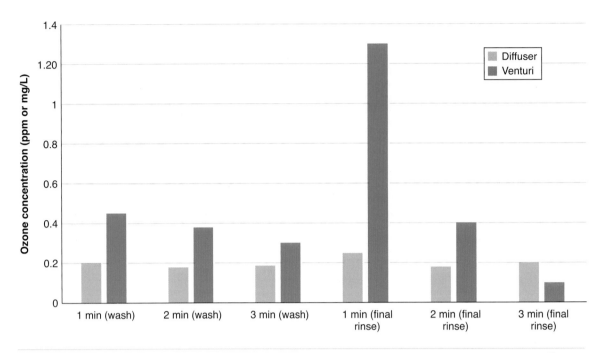

FIGURE 33.3   The efficiency of an ozone dissolution using a Venturi injector compared to a bubble diffuser. Testing was conducted in a laundry washer during a washing phase (that was affected by the presence of a higher pH detergent) in comparison to a final water rinse phase (M. E. Moore, written communication, March 2019).

water with O_3 residual levels maintained between 0.23 and 0.26 mg/L. The second experiment was performed on an activated sludge effluent with the O_3 residual levels maintained between 0.29 and 0.36 mg/L. Contact time for both systems was approximately 1.7 minutes. The resistance of these organisms to inactivation was in the following order for both systems: *M fortuitum* > poliovirus type 1 > *C parapsilosis* > *E coli* > *Salmonella* Typhi (Tables 33.4 to 33.6). This profile is roughly as expected in comparison to other physical and chemical antimicrobial methods (see chapter 3).[57] Table 33.4 compares the results from these studies with others against bacteria. For example, ozone concentrations of 0.1 to 0.63 mg/L were studied with *Legionella pneumophila* and demonstrated 4.6 to 5.2 $\log_{10}$ reductions at a contact time of 20 minutes.[59] A similar study with *E coli* and fecal streptococci studied contact times ranging from 2.7 to 19 minutes with applied O_3 concentrations from 0.45 to 4 mg/L. Under the conditions tested, the most effective levels of bactericidal activity in wastewater ranged from 2.2 to 4.0 mg/L for a 19-minute contact time. This gave an approximately 3 $\log_{10}$ reduction (99.9%) and leaving residual ozone concentrations of 0.06 to 0.35 mg/L.

Since these studies, many more reports verifying the efficacy of ozone against a wide range of bacteria including *Pseudomonas aeruginosa* and methicillin-resistant *Staphylococcus aureus* at concentrations as low as 0.1 to 0.4 mg/L in water,[66] *E coli* O157:H7 and *Salmonella* on the surface of raspberries and strawberries,[67] and as an alternative method for root canal treatment in periodontitis, including

efficacy against a wide range of bacteria such as *Streptococcus* species.[68] Dissolved ozone at 1.5 to 2.0 ppm successfully passed US Environmental Protection Agency Disinfectant Technical Science Section AOAC antimicrobial tests (see chapters 61 and 62) in various studies with *Salmonella choleraesuis, S aureus, P aeruginosa, Campylobacter jejuni,* and *Listeria monocytogenes* as well as with the test fungi *Aspergillus flavus* and *Trichophyton mentagrophytes.* In addition, ozone has been shown to be an effective sporicidal biocide against a range of bacterial spores including *Bacillus subtilis, Geobacillus stearothermophilus,* and *Bacillus cereus.*[21] In these studies, 11 mg/L aqueous ozone showed the greatest efficacy against *B cereus* (approximately 6 $\log_{10}$ reduction) and *G stearothermophilus* the greatest resistance (approximately 0.3 $\log_{10}$ reduction). Similar studies confirmed the effectiveness against *Bacillus* (aerobic) and *Clostridium* (anaerobic) spore-forming bacteria, even in the presence of extraneous soils and dependent on the concentration and exposure times.[69] *G stearothermophilus* has been well established as the most resistant organism to ozone and is used for the validation and routine monitoring of ozone (and other) sterilization processes.[28,29] Log-linear kinetics have been described as the basis of the development of sterilization processes using ozone alone, such as a vacuum-based, humidified process at a starting concentration of 85 mg/L ozone for 15 minutes at approximately 35°C.[29,57] Investigations of the structure of spores by electron microscopy following ozone treatment suggested the outer spore coat layers had significant surface damage, which is therefore an important sporicidal site of action of ozone.[21]

TABLE 33.4 Inactivation of bacteria by ozone

Organism	Percentage Reduction	Time (min)	Concentration[a] (mg/L)	pH	Temperature (°C)	Medium	Reactor Type	Comments	Reference
Escherichia coli	99.99	1.67	0.23-0.26	7	24	Ozone demand free water	Completely mixed continuous flow-through		Farooq and Akhlaque[58]
Legionella pneumophila	>99.997	20	0.32	7	24	Sterile distilled water	Batch		Edelstein et al[59]
	>99.999	20	0.47	7	24	Sterile distilled water	Batch		Edelstein et al[59]
Mycobacterium fortuitum	90	1.67	0.23-0.26	7	24	Ozone demand free water	Completely mixed continuous flow-through		Farooq and Akhlaque[58]
Salmonella Typhimurium	99.995	1.67	0.23-0.26	7	24	Ozone demand free water	Completely mixed flow-through		Farooq and Akhlaque[58]
	17	19	0.85 (0)	7.5	16	Raw wastewater	Continuous flow-through	TSS 85 mg/L COD 100 mg/L	Joret et al[60]
E coli	97	19	1.4 (0)	7.5	16	Raw wastewater	Continuous flow-through	TSS 85 mg/L COD 100 mg/L	Joret et al[60]
	99.9	19	2.2 (0.06)	7.5	16	Raw wastewater	Continuous flow-through	TSS 85 mg/L COD 100 mg/L	Joret et al[60]
	17	19	0.85 (0)	7.5	16	Raw wastewater	Continuous flow-through	TSS 85 mg/L COD 100 mg/L	Joret et al[60]
Fecal streptococci	93	19	1.4 (0)	7.5	16	Raw wastewater	Continuous flow-through	TSS 85 mg/L COD 100 mg/L	Joret et al[60]
	99.6	19	2.2 (0.06)	7.5	16	Raw wastewater	Continuous flow-through	TSS 85 mg/L COD 100 mg/L	Joret et al[60]
	99.9998	0.16	0.51	7.0	20	Water	Continuous flow-through		Boyce et al[61]
E coli	99.9995	0.16	0.18	7.0	20	Water	Continuous flow-through		Boyce et al[61]
	99	0.33	0.065	7.2	1	Water	Batch		Katzenelson et al[62]

Abbreviations: COD, chemical oxygen demand; TSS, total suspended solids.

[a]Some concentrations are reported as initial concentration with the residual levels in parentheses.

TABLE 33.5 Inactivation of viruses by ozone

Organism	Percentage Reduction	Time (min)	Concentration[a] (mg/L)	pH	Temperature (°C)	Medium	Reactor Type	Comments	Reference
Poliovirus type 1 (Mahoney)	99.7	1.67	0.23-0.26	7	24	Ozone demand free water	Completely mixed continuous flow-through		Farooq and Akhlaque[58]
	90	4.9	0.18	7.2	20	Activated sludge reactor effluent	Batch	TSS 12.5 mg/L	Harakeh and Butler[63]
Coxsackievirus B5	0	10	0.1				Batch	NH₃ 1.55 mg/L BOD₃ 10.6 mg/L COD 37.2 mg/L	
	99	5.5	0.25				Batch		
	99	2.0	0.32				Batch		
	99.99	2.5	0.40				Batch		
Poliovirus type 1	90	5	0.2	7.2	20	Activated sludge reactor effluent	Batch	TSS 12.5 mg/L	Harakeh and Butler[63]
	99	5	0.25				Batch	NH₃ 1.55 mg/L BOD₃ 10.6 mg/L COD 37.2 mg/L	
	99	10	0.2				Batch		
Poliovirus type 1 (Mahoney)	90	0.53	0.51	7.2	20	Water	Completely mixed continuous flow-through		Roy et al[64]
	90	0.50	0.32	7.2	22	Water			
	90	0.75	0.32	4.3	NR	Water			
Enteric virus	92	19	1.4 (0)	7.5	16	Raw wastewater	Continuous flow-through	TSS 85 mg/L COD 100 mg/L	Joret et al[60]
Enteric virus	92	19	2.2 (0.06)	7.5	16	Raw wastewater	Continuous flow-through	TSS 85 mg/L COD 100 mg/L	Joret et al[60]
Enteric virus	>98	19	4.10 (0.02)	7.8	18	Raw wastewater	Continuous flow-through	TSS 103 mg/L COD 231 mg/L	Joret et al[60]
Echovirus type 1	99	10	0.26	7.2	20	Activated sludge effluent	Batch	TSS 12.5 mg/L NH₃ 1.55 mg/L BOD₃ 10.6 mg/L COD 37.2 mg/L	Harakeh and Butler[63]
Bacteriophage f₂	80	10	0.1	7.2	20	Activated sludge effluent	Batch	TSS 12.5 mg/L NH₃ 1.55 mg/L BOD₃ 10.6 mg/L COD 37.2 mg/L	Harakeh and Butler[63]

TABLE 33.5 Inactivation of viruses by ozone (Continued)

Organism	Percentage Reduction	Time (min)	Concentration[a] (mg/L)	pH	Temperature (°C)	Medium	Reactor Type	Comments	Reference
Simian rotavirus SA11	96	10	0.26	7.2	20	Activated sludge effluent	Batch	TSS 12.5 mg/L NH₃ 1.55 mg/L BOD₃ 10.6 mg/L COD 37.2 mg/L	Harakeh and Butler[63]
Human rotavirus	80	10	0.31	7.2	20	Activated sludge effluent	Batch	TSS 12.5 mg/L NH₃ 1.55 mg/L BOD₃ 10.6 mg/L COD 37.2 mg/L	Harakeh and Butler[63]
	99	9	0.2	4	20	Activated sludge effluent	Batch	TSS 12.5 mg/L	Harakeh and Butler[63]
Poliovirus type 1	75	10	0.2	7.2	20		Batch	NH₃ 1.55 mg/L BOD₃ 10.6 mg/L	
	80	10	0.2	9	20		Batch	COD 37.2 mg/L	
Poliovirus type 1 Sabin	>96	0.16	0.21	7.0	20	Water	Continuous flow-through	1 TU, bentonite	Boyce et al[61]
	>97	0.16	0.21	7.0	20	Water	Continuous flow-through	5 TU, bentonite	Boyce et al[61]
Coxsackievirus A9	>98	0.16	0.144	7.0	20	Water	Continuous flow-through	5 TU, bentonite	Boyce et al[61]
	>98	0.15	0.035	7.0	20	Water	Continuous flow-through	5 TU, bentonite	Boyce et al[61]
Bacteriophage, f₂	>99.97	0.16	0.40	7.0	20	Water	Continuous flow-through	5 TU, bentonite	Boyce et al[61]
	>99.995	0.16	0.41	7.0	20	Water	Continuous flow-through	5 TU, bentonite	

Abbreviations: BOD₃, biochemical oxygen demand (at 3 days); COD, chemical oxygen demand; NH₃, ammonia; NR, not reported; TSS, total suspended solids; TU, turbidity units of bentonite clay.

[a]Some concentrations are reported as initial concentration with the residual levels in parentheses.

TABLE 33.6 Inactivation of yeasts by ozone

Organism	Percentage Reduction	Time (min)	Concentration (mg/L)	pH	Temperature (°C)	Medium	Reactor Type	Reference
Candida parapsilosis	99.8	1.67	0.23-0.26	7	24	Demand-free water	Completely mixed continuous flow-through	Farooq and Akhlaque[58]
Candida tropicalis	99	0.30	0.02	7.2	20	Demand-free water	Completely mixed continuous flow-through	Kawamura et al[65]
		0.08	1.0					

Viruses

Ozone is also well established as an effective virucide.[58,60-62,63,64,70] As shown in Table 33.5, only relatively low concentrations and contact times are necessary for the inactivation of certain viruses. For example, exposure of poliovirus type 1 (Mahoney) to 0.25 mg/L of ozone for 5 minutes at pH 7.2 and 20°C caused 99% inactivation.[63] Exposure of the same organisms to 0.4 mg/L of chlorine for 15 minutes in more favorable environmental conditions at pH 6 and temperature 25°C resulted in only 38% inactivation.[70] The concentration and time product, concentration × time (C · t) value, for 4 log inactivation of coxsackievirus B5 at neutral pH and room temperature is estimated to be only 1 mg-min/L (see Table 33.5). As the concentration increases, the observed log reduction of viruses also increased (Figure 33.4). Under similar environmental conditions and C · t values, poliovirus inactivation was only 1 log. These results indicate that significant variation in levels of resistance to O_3 inactivation exists among viruses, similar to what has been observed

with other viruses.[64,70,71] Enveloped viruses, due to their sensitive enveloped structures, are more sensitive than nonenveloped viruses in general (see chapter 3).[57,71] The presence of extraneous soils often present with viruses (as they are sourced from cells or cell cultures) and their ability to form clumps will also present with some practical variability. As may be expected from previous discussions, ozone-driven inactivation of microorganisms in wastewaters required longer contact times and larger doses than inactivation of microorganisms in demand-free systems. A comparison of data in Table 33.5 shows the effects of suspended solids and organic matter on the virucidal effectiveness of ozone.[60,63] As with chlorine and other oxidants, a portion of the applied O_3 will react with any oxidizable materials present in the medium. The fraction of O_3, or any disinfectant, that does not inactivate microorganisms often is difficult to predict for these systems.

More recent studies have continued to optimize the effectiveness of ozone against viruses for a variety of applications including food surfaces,[72] wastewater treatment,[73] and drinking water[74] with both enveloped and nonenveloped viruses.

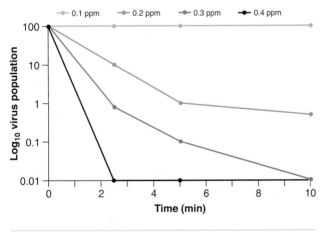

FIGURE 33.4 The effect of ozone concentration on the inactivation of virus (coxsackievirus B5) in activated sludge effluent at pH 7.2, 20°C. From Harakeh and Butler.[63] Reprinted by permission of Taylor & Francis Ltd. http://www.tandfonline.com.

Prions

Prions are atypical transmissible agents being composed only of protein but responsible for accumulation in neural tissues that lead to disease states such as animal (scrapie and bovine spongiform encephalopathy) and human diseases (such as Creutzfeldt-Jakob disease [CJD] and variant CJD) (see chapters 3 and 68). Although these diseases are rare, they are 100% fatal and are a particular concern as contaminants from materials of animal or human origin as they present with unusual resistance profiles to inactivation by disinfection and sterilization methods (see chapter 3 and 68).[57,75] The antimicrobial activity with ozone was of some interest to investigate, given the known effects of other oxidizing agents, including chlorine and hydrogen peroxide in the neutralization of prions (or loss of infectivity) due to protein/peptide degradation.[75] Initial studies have shown that ozone may be effective at inactivating prion infectivity, as indicated by prion (brain homogenate infected with the prion disease scrapie strain 263K) degradation by detection using a traditional Western blot analysis or an alternative protein misfolding cycle amplification (PCMA) that is indicative of the transmissible nature of prions.[76] The most optimal conditions were at >13 mg/L ozone at pH 4.4 and 20°C. Overall, the lower pH conditions tested (pH 4.4 compared to pH 6.0 or 8.0) were more effective, as were higher concentrations and temperatures (20°C compared to 4°C). These results considered the significant presence of contaminating materials (in the brain homogenate tested) that would have limited penetration to the prion proteins under investigation. Indeed, greater efficacy was observed in similar studies, conducted in infected brain homogenate that was further diluted in saline, and proposed to be more applicable for applications such as wastewater treatment.[77,78] Although the methods used, particularly the PCMA method, are useful indicators of effectiveness against prions, the gold standard still requires the demonstration of infectivity reduction in animal studies and generally with two strains of prions, as there is some suggestion the strain can vary considerably in prion inactivation profiles (see chapter 68).[75]

Fungi and Yeasts

Similar to the studies with bacteria discussed earlier, ozone is also effective against fungi including molds and yeasts. The effect of ozone on *Candida tropicalis* was tested at pH 7.2 and 20°C with 99% kill times ranging from 18 seconds at 0.02 mg/L O_3 to approximately 5 seconds at 1 mg/L O_3 (see Table 33.6).[65] *C tropicalis* was 10 or more times as resistant to O_3 inactivation as *E coli*, *S* Typhi, and *S aureus*, but it was approximately 15 times less resistant than the spores of *Bacillus* species. As with most other microorganisms, O_3 appears to be an effective fungicide but with midrange activity between vegetative bacteria and bacterial spores (see chapter 3). Specific investigations have included the use of ozone to reduce the contamination rates of footwear with the fungus (dermatophyte) species *Trichophyton rubrum* and *T mentagrophytes* in the control of onychomycosis and tinea pedis,[79] and of various fungal contaminants on dried aromatic plants.[80] Again, as for bacterial studies, optimization of ozone process depends on the process conditions and application targets for consideration of optimized fungicidal activity.

Protozoa and Helminths

Ozone inactivation data for protozoan vegetative and cyst (or dormant forms) has increased substantially since the early 1990s due to reports of outbreaks of protozoan cysts

or oocysts in drinking water treatment plants and detection in a large number of surface waters.[81] Inactivation data generated from selected studies are summarized in Table 33.7. Early studies investigated the ozone inactivation of three different organisms under different pH and temperatures: cysts of the nonpathogenic soil and water amoeba (*Naegleria gruberi*), the mice parasite *Giardia muris*, and the human pathogen *Giardia lamblia*.[82] Based on linear C · t data, *Naegleria* was the most resistant to O_3 inactivation, and *G lamblia* was slightly less resistant than *G muris*. This study was the initial source of the O_3 inactivation criteria in the US Surface Water Treatment Rule aspect of the Safe Drinking Water Act.[86] But subsequent studies showed that Table 33.7 shows that *Cryptosporidium parvum* oocysts are many times more resistant to ozone than *Giardia* species cyst (see Table 33.7), similar to studies with other chemical antimicrobials (see chapter 3); however, significant variation exists among various studies because of the lack of reliable and completely reproducible tests for oocyst viability as well as known variability in the innate resistance of protozoal cysts to inactivation and cyst purification techniques.[87-89]

Due to the overall oxidation effects, more recent studies have continued to demonstrate the efficacy of ozone against the vegetative and dormant forms of protozoa, including pathogens such as *Acanthamoeba* species (at 500 mg/h O_3 in dental water lines)[26] and *Toxoplasma gondii* (6 mg/L over a 12-min contact time).[90] Efficacy has also been confirmed against helminth eggs, which are much larger in structure.[50,91] As expected from earlier studies, efficacy against protozoal and helminth dormant forms varies depending on the concentration of ozone and test conditions (eg, pH, temperature, and presence of interfering substances), supporting the conclusion that optimal exposure conditions will depend on the specific application. This is not unexpected, as in comparison with other biocidal treatments. For example, Table 33.8 compares the effectiveness of ozone, chlorine dioxide, chlorine, and monochloramine in the inactivation of *C parvum*.[92] Based on linear C · t values, O_3 was found to be the most effective disinfection agent, followed by chlorine dioxide and chlorine. Monochloramine was the least effective disinfection agent in this specific study. Generally, and depending on the test conditions used, O_3 is known to be a more effective microbicide than either chlorine, chlorine dioxide, or monochloramine for water applications.[93,94]

Mode of Action

Ozone, and its ability to generate other short-lived and reactive oxidizing agents such as the hydroxyl radicals (˙OH), causes oxidation of both organic and inorganic compounds.[93,94] This will include the variety of microbial cellular and structural components. Initially, this will lead to outer surface damage such as at the cell wall/membrane

TABLE 33.7 Inactivation of protozoan cysts by ozone

Organism	Percentage Reduction	Time (min)	Concentration (mg/L)	pH	Temperature (°C)	Medium	Reactor Type	C · t (mg-min/L)	Reference
Naegleria gruberi	99	7.8	0.55	7	5	0.01 M demand-free phosphate buffer	Semibatch	4.23	Wickramanayake et al[82]
	99	2.1	2.0	7	5			4.23	
	99	4.3	0.3	7	25			1.29	
	99	1.1	1.2	7	25			1.29	
Giardia muris	99	12.9	0.15	7	5	0.01 M demand-free phosphate buffer	Semibatch	1.94	Wickramanayake et al[82]
	99	2.8	0.7	7	5			1.94	
	99	9.0	0.03	7	25			0.27	
	99	1.8	0.15	7	25			0.27	
Giardia muris	99.994	5	0.52	6.70	22	0.05 M demand-free phosphate buffer	Batch	2.6	Finch et al[83]
	99.92	5	0.18	6.70	22			0.9	
Giardia lamblia	99	5.3	0.1	7	5	0.01 M demand-free phosphate buffer	Semibatch	0.53	Wickramanayake et al[82]
	99	1.1	0.5	7	5			0.53	
	99	5.5	0.03	7	25			0.17	
	99	1.2	0.15	7	25			0.17	
Giardia lamblia	99.97	5	1.44	6.85	22	0.05 M demand-free phosphate buffer	Batch	7.2	Finch et al[83]
	99.5	2	0.79	6.85	22			1.58	
	99	12.5	0.5	6.9	7			6.3	
Cryptosporidium parvum	99	7.6	1.0	6.9	7	0.05 M demand-free phosphate buffer	Batch	7.6	Finch et al[84]
	99	5.2	0.5	6.9	22			2.6	
	99	4.0	1.0	6.9	22			4.0	
Cryptosporidium parvum	99	6	0.77	NR	Room	Deionized water	Batch	4.6	Peeters et al[85]
	99	8	0.51		Room			4	

TABLE 33.8 Comparison of *Cryptosporidium parvum* inactivation by disinfectants[a]

Disinfectant	Inactivation (%)	Time (min)	Concentration (mg/L)	C · t (mg-min/L)
Ozone	99	5-10	1	5-10
Chlorine dioxide	90	60	1.3	78
Chlorine	99	90	80	7200
Monochloramine	90	90	80	7200

[a]From Korich et al.[92]

of bacteria and outer structures of viruses and then inner components such as enzymes and nucleic acids.[57] For example, in studies with *Vibrio parahaemolyticus*, lower concentrations of ozone (0.125 mg/L) were adequately neutralized and tolerated by the test bacteria, but in higher concentrations (>1 mg/L), damage was observed to the cell wall/membrane leading to leakage of intracellular cytoplasmic components.[95] This was followed by direct inactivation of intracellular enzymes and specific degradation of nucleic acids (DNA and RNA), which culminated in cell death. Although these effects are likely to be due to the direct oxidization of ozone alone, the generation of radicals (including hydroxyl radicals) are thought to play a particular role under alkaline pH conditions.

Ozone is known to target certain types of amino acids such as lysine, histidine, and tyrosine, which will disrupt structural and enzymatic proteins. Similarly, lipid double bonds and the DNA backbone structure are particularly sensitive to oxidation damage. Although this type of damage can be repaired in cellular microorganisms, the culmination of damage can culminate in cell death and loss of virus viability.[57] The accumulation of such damage is also responsible for the loss of viability of dormant forms of microorganisms such as bacterial spores, with a particular emphasis on damage to the inner spore membranes and the nucleic acid that has been described for oxidizing agents.[96] Similar degradation effects on virus, including lipid, protein, and nucleic acids have been described in both liquid and gas form.[97-99] When poliovirus type 1 (Mahoney) was exposed to O_3, it was observed that the damage to the viral nucleic acid is the major cause of the inactivation of organism.[64] The RNA was observed to be damaged by ozone concentrations less than 0.3 mg/L within 2 minutes of contact times. Also, O_3 altered two of the four polypeptide chains present in the viral protein coat. In studies on the kinetics and mechanism of O_3 inactivation of bacteriophage f_2, it was also reported that the RNA enclosed in the phage coat was inactivated less by ozone than were whole phages but was inactivated more than naked RNA.[100] Important results of this study include the fact that subcellular components of a microorganism can be more resistant than the whole organism

and that the inactivation of a microorganism does not necessarily denature the genetic materials in it, which may be required for full virus inactivation (loss of viability).

OZONE STERILIZATION APPLICATIONS

With optimization of generation methods, broad spectrum antimicrobial efficacy, and the benefit of breaking down into innocuous residuals (oxygen), it is not surprising that ozone has been investigated for sterilization applications. Methods have included the use of ozone in liquid and gaseous forms. These have been described in food processing and medical situations, and most often, where surface materials are defined and the microbial bioburden levels known.[101-103] A recent example was for sterilization of silicone hydrogels, which investigated the use of ozone, steam, and γ radiation.[103] The ozone process was shown to be preferred to the other sterilization processes, depending on the defined process to provide the required log reduction for sterilization but minimizing any negative impact on the compatibility with the hydrogel material. Other examples include the liquid sterilization of dialyzers[104] and foods with nonporous outer surfaces.[105] Such optimization of applications may assist in the development of ozone as an alternative sterilization method for specific applications that are often limited due to the classical requirements of, and regulatory pathways for, sterilization processes.[106,107]

But in other to meet the classical requirements for sterilization processes (eg, in the sterilization of a load of medical devices or other products either following manufacturing or for reusable use in health care facility), ozone has had little commercial success to date. This is due to the higher levels of controlled, sustained ozone levels often required to be maintained to meet the regulatory requirements internationally for such sterilization processes and the negative effects on ozone at these concentrations and exposure conditions on surface or materials such as metals, polymers, and elastomers with used in devices.[28-31] There are several ozone sterilization methods described in the literature, including patents on such a such processes.[57,105,108,109] Ozone itself can provide the necessary sterilization activity under defined conditions, but some of these processes have been described that combine ozone with other oxidizing agents such as hydrogen peroxide.[29,31,110] The role of ozone itself or any synergistic activity with other oxidizing agents in these cases are unknown and may be debated. A significant problem in the investigation of ozone for disinfection and sterilization applications has been on underdosing (therefore not achieving the desired antimicrobial effects) or overdosing of ozone (thereby leading to surface or product damage/incompatibility), overall not producing desired results. An example would be the investigation of the use of ozone in gaseous form under atmospheric conditions to disinfect porous substrates or tissues (eg, for mold remediation or dentistry applications); however, it would be well understood that gases do not have the necessary capillary characteristics to penetrate to the target microorganisms present in various pores or locations within such applications (eg, due to competition with air that will be intrinsically present and be difficult to displace with ozone alone). If possible, the ozone to be used is dissolved in water at a sufficiently high concentration and then forced into such areas (eg, by flushing or extracting through the material) to provide the required antimicrobial activity effective disinfectant. An easier application has been to remove the competing air in a similar fashion to that employed in steam and other gaseous sterilization methods, such as by applying a vacuum or series or positive/negative pressure pulses to remove the air and replace with the antimicrobial gas (see chapters 28, 31, and 32). Vacuum conditions, for example, create a situation where not only the air is removed but also when gaseous ozone is applied to the sterilization load, it can rapidly get to various areas of the load and illicit its antimicrobial effects. In cases where a vacuum or series of pressure pulses cannot be applied, ozone dissolved in water or a liquid formulation may be an effective alternative method. As mentioned earlier, for certain practical applications if the number and types of microorganisms (or bioburden; see chapter 64) are known, then the ozone concentration and conditions required to achieve sterilization (based on the concentration-time, CT, factors that are available from many sources or as demonstrated for an application) can be applied. In these cases, the ozone demand can be theoretically calculated for an application and the design of ozone system needed for an effective process.

Vacuum-based ozone systems for the low-temperature sterilization of reusable medical devices have been previously commercialized.[105,108,109] These systems have all been based on similar processes consisting of placing the load in a sealed chamber, pulling a deep vacuum (to remove air), humidifying the load (typically at 75%-95% relative humidity), exposure to ozone gas at 20°C to 30°C, and finally aeration by removing residual ozone from the chamber/ load (by pulling a single or series of vacuum pulses). These process conditions are not unlike those described for other oxidizing agent-based sterilization process (eg, hydrogen peroxide; see chapter 32). A series of such sterilizers, partially commercialized as STER-O3-Zone designs, described the use of defined chambers that could directly couple to the humidity/ozone source and then subsequently used for sterile device storage following the process. The process consisted of humidification at 75% to 95% relative humidity and ozone exposure for 40 to 60 minutes at ambient temperatures (25°C to 30°C). A further system (commercialized as the 125L ozone sterilizer) was described for use with various reusable devices.[28] The sterilizer consisted of an exposure chamber, a humidifier, an ozone generator, and a vacuum pump but also required water (for humidification) and medical grade oxygen (for ozone generation). The sterilization process had three phases, conditioning, sterilization, and ventilation. During conditioning, the load was humidified at approximately 85% to 100% relative humidity but claimed to prevent water (or subsequent ozone) condensation. During sterilization under low pressure, ozone gas (generated from oxygen exposed to a corona discharge system) was introduced into an evacuated chamber up to approximately 85 mg/L ozone under the same humidified conditions and approximately 30°C to 36°C for 15 minutes and then repeated for a further exposure time. The chamber was then simply aerated by evacuating the gas (through a catalytic converter) and released to atmospheric pressure, for an overall cycle time of 4.5 hours. Although these systems had many benefits, including having low operating costs, the higher ozone concentrations used for sterilization were found to be incompatible with many types of materials used in reusable device manufacturing such as metals (aluminum, brass) and polymers (polyurethanes, rubber). More recent sterilizer designs use combinations of hydrogen peroxide and a lower dose of ozone for sterilization.[110,111] The method is like those described earlier but without the need for controlled humidification. During the cycle, the load is evacuated to a deep vacuum, exposed to hydrogen peroxide gas at 20°C to 26°C (using a dynamic injection system until the pressure to reach 19 Torr), introduction of 2 mg/L of ozone, and then exposed for 5 minutes; this is repeated twice to achieve sterilization and then aerated by evacuation and ventilation to allow access to the load. The introduction of ozone during the cycle is claimed to enhance antimicrobial activity by reaction with hydrogen peroxide to form hydroxyl radicals.

ACKNOWLEDGMENT

The chapter has been updated based on the previous fifth edition and owes substantially to the contributions of Linda K. Weavers and G. B. Wickramanayake.

REFERENCES

1. Latimer WM. *The Oxidation States of the Elements and Their Potentials in Aqueous Solutions.* 2nd ed. Englewood Cliffs, NJ: Prentice-Hall; 1952.

2. Kroschwitz JL, Howe-Grant M, eds. *Encyclopedia of Chemical Technology.* Vol 17. 4th ed. New York, NY: John Wiley & Sons; 1996:953-994.

3. Rice RG. Application of ozone in water and wastewater treatment. In: Rice RG, ed. *Analytical Aspects of Ozone: Treatment of Water and Wastewater.* Chelsea, MI: Lewis; 1986:7-26.

4. Rice RG, Robson CM, Miller GW, et al. Uses of ozone in drinking water treatment. *J Am Water Works Assoc.* 1981;73:44-57.

5. Zhao T, Zhao P, West JW, Bernard JK, Cross HG, Doyle MP. Inactivation of enterohemorrhagic *Escherichia coli* in rumen content- or feces-contaminated drinking water for cattle. *Appl Environ Microbiol.* 2006;72:3268-3273.

6. Association for the Advancement of Medical Instrumentation. *ANSI/AAMI TIR67. Promoting Safe Practices Pertaining to the Use of Sterilant and Disinfectant Chemicals in Health Care Facilities.* Arlington, VA: Association for the Advancement of Medical Instrumentation; 2016.

7. US Department of Health and Human Services, National Institute for Occupational Safety and Health. *Occupational Health Guideline for Ozone.* Washington, DC: US Department of Health and Human Services; 1978.

8. Chang EE, Chiang PC, Chuang CL. Assessment of mutagenic potency of source water treated by ozone and adsorption processes. *Toxicolog Environ Chem.* 1999;68:321-333.

9. Komulainen H. Experimental cancer studies of chlorinated by-products. *Toxicology.* 2004;198:239-248.

10. Centers for Disease Control and Prevention. Disinfection by-products. Centers for Disease Control and Prevention Web site. https://www.cdc.gov/safewater/chlorination-byproducts.html. Accessed December 2, 2016.

11. Richardson SD, Plewa MJ, Wagner ED, Schoeny R, Demarini DM. Occurrence, genotoxicity, and carcinogenicity of regulated and emerging disinfection by-products in drinking water: a review and roadmap for research. *Mutat Res.* 2007;636:178-242.

12. Krasner SW. The formation and control of emerging disinfection by-products of health concern. *Philos Trans A Math Phys Eng Sci.* 2009;367:4077-4095.

13. US Environmental Protection Agency. *Wastewater Technology Fact Sheet: Ozone Disinfection.* Washington, DC: US Environmental Protection Agency; 1999.

14. Ngwenya N, Ncube EJ, Parsons J. Recent advances in drinking water disinfection: successes and challenges. *Rev Environ Contam Toxicol.* 2013;222:111-170.

15. Martinelli M, Giovannangeli F, Rotunno S, Trombetta CM, Montomoli E. Water and air ozone treatment as an alternative sanitizing technology. *J Prev Med Hyg.* 2017;58:E48-E52.

16. Rice RG, Netzer A, eds. *Handbook of Ozone Technology and Applications.* Vol 1. Ann Arbor, MI: Ann Arbor Science; 1982.

17. Cohan N. Understanding dissolved ozone and its use in pharmaceutical water systems. *Pharm Eng.* 2013;5:1-4.

18. Edwards HB. Treatment of cooling tower water with ozone in lieu of chemicals. In: Rice RG, ed. *Ozone Treatment of Water for Cooling Applications.* Norwalk, CT: International Ozone Association; 1981:21-30.

19. Rice RG. Ozone in the United States of America—state-of-the-art. *Ozone Sci Eng.* 1999;21:99-118.

20. Ramos NG, Ring JF. The practical use of ozone in large marine aquaria. *Ozone Sci Eng.* 1980;2:225-228.

21. Khadre MA, Yousef AE. Sporicidal action of ozone and hydrogen peroxide: a comparative study. *Int J Food Microbiol.* 2001;71:131-138.

22. Brodowska AJ, Nowak A, Śmigielski K. Ozone in the food industry: principles of ozone treatment, mechanisms of action, and applications: an overview. *Crit Rev Food Sci Nutr.* 2018;58:2176-2201.

23. Cardoso CC, Fiorini JE, Ferriera LR, Gurjão JW, Amaral LA. Disinfection of hospital laundry using ozone: microbiological evaluation. *Infect Control Hosp Epidemiol.* 2000;21:248.

24. Rice RG, DeBrum M, Cardis D, Tapp C. The ozone laundry handbook: a comprehensive guide for the proper application of ozone in the commercial laundry industry. *J Internat Ozone Assoc.* 2009;31:339-347.

25. Boeniger MF. Use of ozone generating devices to improve indoor air quality. *Am Ind Hyg Assoc J.* 1995;56:590-598.

26. Hikal W, Zaki B, Sabry H. Evaluation of ozone application in dental unit water lines contaminated with pathogenic *Acanthamoeba. Iran J Parasitol.* 2015;10:410-419.

27. Bhatt S, Mehta P, Chen C, et al. Efficacy of low-temperature plasma-activated gas disinfection against biofilm on contaminated GI endoscope channels. *Gastrointest Endosc.* 2019;89:105-114.

28. Murphy L. Ozone—the latest advance in sterilization of medical devices. *Can Oper Room Nurs J.* 2006;24:28, 30-32, 37-38.

29. Association for the Advancement of Medical Instrumentation. *ANSI/AAMI ST58:2013/(R)2018. Chemical Sterilization and High-Level Disinfection in Health Care Facilities.* Arlington, VA: Association for the Advancement of Medical Instrumentation; 2018.

30. Association for the Advancement of Medical Instrumentation. *AAMI TIR17:2008. Compatibility of Materials Subject to Sterilization.* Arlington, VA: Association for the Advancement of Medical Instrumentation; 2008.

31. Association for the Advancement of Medical Instrumentation. *AAMI TIR17:2017. Compatibility of Materials Subject to Sterilization.* Arlington, VA: Association for the Advancement of Medical Instrumentation; 2017.

32. Zeng J, Lu J. Mechanisms of action involved in ozone-therapy in skin diseases. *Int Immunopharmacol.* 2018;56:235-241.

33. Borges GÁ, Elias ST, da Silva SM, et al. In vitro evaluation of wound healing and antimicrobial potential of ozone therapy. *J Craniomaxillofac Surg.* 2017;45:364-370.

34. Gupta G, Mansi B. Ozone therapy in periodontics. *J Med Life.* 2012;5:59-67.

35. Nogales CG, Ferrari PH, Kantorovich EO, Lage-Marques JL. Ozone therapy in medicine and dentistry. *J Contemp Dent Pract.* 2008;9:75-84.

36. Maslennikov OV, Kontorshchikova CN, Gribkova IA. *Ozone Therapy in Practice: Health Manual.* Nizhny Novgorod, Russia: Ministry of Health Service of the Russian Federation; 2008.

37. Kogelschatz U, Eliasson B, Hirth M. Ozone generation from oxygen and air: discharge physics and reaction mechanisms. *Ozone Sci Eng.* 1988;10:367-377.

38. Langlais B, Reckow DA, Brink DR, eds. *Ozone in Water Treatment: Application and Engineering.* Washington, DC: Lewis; 1991.

39. Masschelein WJ, ed. *Ozonization Manual for Water and Wastewater Treatment.* New York, NY: John Wiley & Sons; 1982.

40. McClurkin JD, Maier DE. Half-life time of ozone as a function of air conditions and movement. Paper presented at: 10th International Working Conference on Stored Product Protection; June 27 to July 2, 2010; Estoril, Portugal.

41. Weschler CJ. Ozone in indoor environments: concentration and chemistry. *Indoor Air.* 2000;10:269-288.

42. Staehelin J, Hoigne J. Decomposition of ozone in water: rate of initiation by hydroxide ions and hydrogen peroxide. *Environ Sci Technol.* 1982;16:676-681.

43. Batakliev T, Georgiev V, Anachkov M, Rakovsky S, Zaikov GE. Ozone decomposition. *Interdiscip Toxicol.* 2014;7(2):47-59.

44. Gardoni D, Vailati A, Canziani R. Decay of ozone in water: a review. *Ozone Sci Eng.* 2012;34:233-242.

45. Gurol MD, Singer PC. Kinetics of ozone decomposition: a dynamic approach. *Environ Sci Technol.* 1982;16:377-383.

46. Gordon G, Cooper WJ, Rice RG, Pacey GE. Methods of measuring disinfectant residuals. *J Am Water Works Assoc.* 1988;80:94-108.

47. Majewski J. Methods for measuring ozone concentration in ozone-treated water. *Przegląd Elektrotechniczny.* 2012;88:253-255.

48. Rice EW, Baird RB, Eaton AD. *Standard Methods for the Examination of Water and Wastewater*. 23rd ed. Washington, DC: American Water Works Association; 2018.

49. Bader H. Determination of ozone in water by the indigo method: a submitted standard method. *Ozone Sci Eng*. 1982;4:169-176.

50. Bader H, Hoigné J. Determination of ozone in water by the indigo method. *Water Research*. 1981;15:449-456.

51. Rakness K, Gordon G, Langlais B, et al. Guideline for measurement of ozone concentration in the process gas from an ozone generator. *Ozone Sci Eng*. 1996;18:209-229.

52. Rehme KA, Puzak JC, Beard ME, Smith CF, Paur RJ. *Evaluation of Ozone Calibration Procedures. Project Summary, EPA-600/S4-80-050*. Washington, DC: US Environmental Protection Agency; 1981.

53. McKercher GR, Salmond JA, Vanos JK. Characteristics and applications of small, portable gaseous air pollution monitors. *Environ Pollut*. 2017;223:102-110.

54. Sagona JA, Weisel C, Meng Q. Accuracy and practicality of a portable ozone monitor for personal exposure estimates. *Atmos Environ*. 2018;175:120-126.

55. Barnes RA, inventor. Venturi injector with self-adjusting port. US patent 6,192,911. February 27, 2001.

56. Schulz CR, inventor; ITT Manufacturing Enterprises Inc, assignee. Apparatus and method for disinfection of water by ozone injection. US patent 5,273,664. December 28, 1993.

57. McDonnell, GE. *Antisepsis, Disinfection, and Sterilization: Types, Action, and Resistance*. 2nd ed. Washington, DC: ASM Press; 2017.

58. Farooq S, Akhlaque S. Comparative response of mixed cultures of bacteria and virus to ozonation. *Water Research*. 1983;17:809-812.

59. Edelstein PH, Whittaker RE, Kreiling RL, Howell CL. Efficacy of ozone in eradication of *Legionella pneumophila* from hospital plumbing fixtures. *Appl Environ Microbiol*. 1982;44:1330-1333.

60. Joret JC, Block JC, Richard Y. Wastewater disinfection: elimination of fecal bacteria and enteric viruses by ozone. *Ozone Sci Eng*. 1982;4:91-99.

61. Boyce DS, Sproul OJ, Buck CE. The effect of bentonite clay on ozone disinfection of bacteria and viruses in water. *Water Res*. 1981;15:759-767.

62. Katzenelson E, Kletter B, Shuval HI. Inactivation kinetics of viruses and bacteria in water by use of ozone. *J Am Water Works Assoc*. 1974;66:725-729.

63. Harakeh MS, Butler M. Factors increasing the ozone inactivation of enteric viruses in effluent. *Ozone Sci Eng*. 1984;6:235-243.

64. Roy D, Wong PKY, Engelbrecht RS, Chian ES. Mechanism of enteroviral inactivation by ozone. *Appl Environ Microbiol*. 1981;41:718-723.

65. Kawamura K, Kaneko M, Hirata T, Taguchi K. Microbial indicators for the efficiency of disinfection processes. *Water Sci Tech*. 1986;18:175-184.

66. Choudhury B, Portugal S, Mastanaiah N, Johnson JA, Roy S. Inactivation of *Pseudomonas aeruginosa* and methicillin-resistant *Staphylococcus aureus* in an open water system with ozone generated by a compact, atmospheric DBD plasma reactor. *Sci Rep*. 2018;8:17573.

67. Bialka KL, Demirci A. Utilization of gaseous ozone for the decontamination of *Escherichia coli* O157:H7 and *Salmonella* on raspberries and strawberries. *J Food Prot*. 2007;70:1093-1098.

68. Kist S, Kollmuss M, Jung J, Schubert S, Hickel R, Huth KC. Comparison of ozone gas and sodium hypochlorite/chlorhexidine two-visit disinfection protocols in treating apical periodontitis: a randomized controlled clinical trial. *Clin Oral Investig*. 2017;21:995-1005.

69. Rickloff JR. An evaluation of the sporicidal activity of ozone. *Appl Environ Microbiol*. 1987;53:683-686.

70. Alvarez ME, O'Brien RT. Effects of chlorine concentration on the structure of poliovirus. *Appl Environ Microbiol*. 1982;43:237-239.

71. Eterpi M, McDonnell G, Thomas V. Disinfection efficacy against parvoviruses compared with reference viruses. *J Hosp Infect*. 2009;73:64-70.

72. Wang Q, Markland S, Kniel KE. Inactivation of human norovirus and its surrogates on alfalfa seeds by aqueous ozone. *J Food Prot*. 2015;78:1586-1591.

73. Tondera K, Klaer K, Gebhardt J, et al. Reducing pathogens in combined sewer overflows using ozonation or UV irradiation. *J Int J Hyg Environ Health*. 2015;218:731-741.

74. Lénès D, Deboosere N, Ménard-Szczebara F, et al. Assessment of the removal and inactivation of influenza viruses H5N1 and H1N1 by drinking water treatment. *Water Res*. 2010;44:2473-2486.

75. McDonnell G, Comoy E. Decontamination of prions. In: Walker J, ed. *Decontamination in Hospitals and Healthcare*. 2nd ed. Cambridge, United Kingdom: Woodhead; 2019.

76. Ding N, Neumann NF, Price LM, et al. Inactivation of template-directed misfolding of infectious prion protein by ozone. *Appl Environ Microbiol*. 2012;78:613-620.

77. Ding N, Neumann NF, Price LM, et al. Kinetics of ozone inactivation of infectious prion protein. *Appl Environ Microbiol*. 2013;79:2721-2730.

78. Ding N, Neumann NF, Price LM, et al. Ozone inactivation of infectious prions in rendering plant and municipal wastewaters. *Sci Total Environ*. 2014;470-471:717-725.

79. Gupta AK, Brintnell WC. Sanitization of contaminated footwear from onychomycosis patients using ozone gas: a novel adjunct therapy for treating onychomycosis and tinea pedis? *J Cutan Med Surg*. 2013;17:243-249.

80. Kazi M, Parlapani FF, Boziaris IS, Vellios EK, Lykas C. Effect of ozone on the microbiological status of five dried aromatic plants. *J Sci Food Agric*. 2018;98:1369-1373.

81. LeChevallier MW, Norton WD. *Giardia* and *Cryptosporidium* in raw and finished water. *J Am Water Works Assoc*. 1995;87:54-68.

82. Wickramanayake GB, Rubin AJ, Sproul OJ. Inactivation of *Naegleria* and *Giardia* cysts in water by ozonation. *J Water Pollut Control Federation*. 1984;56:983-988.

83. Finch GR, Black EK, Labatiuk CW, Gyürék L, Belosevic M. Comparison of *Giardia lamblia* and *Giardia muris* cyst inactivation by ozone. *Appl Environ Microbiol*. 1993;59:3674-3680.

84. Finch GR, Black EK, Gyürék L, Belosevic M. Ozone inactivation of *Cryptosporidium parvum* in demand-free phosphate buffer determined by in vitro excystation and animal infectivity. *Appl Environ Microbiol*. 1993;59:4203-4210.

85. Peeters JE, Mazas EA, Masschelein WJ, Villacorta Martiez de Maturana I, Debacker E. Effect of disinfection of drinking water with ozone or chlorine dioxide on survival of *Cryptosporidium parvum* oocysts. *Appl Environ Microbiol*. 1989;55:1519-1522.

86. US Environmental Protection Agency. National primary drinking water regulations; filtration, disinfection; turbidity, *Giardia lamblia*, viruses, *Legionella*, and heterotrophic bacteria: final rule. *Fed Regist*. 1989;54:27486.

87. Jenkins MB, Eaglesham BS, Anthony LC, Kachlany SC, Bowman DD, Ghiorse WC. Significance of wall structure, macromolecular composition, and surface polymers to the survival and transport of *Cryptosporidium parvum* oocysts. *Appl Environ Microbiol*. 2010;76:1926-1934.

88. Coulon C, Collignon A, McDonnell G, Thomas V. Resistance of *Acanthamoeba* cysts to disinfection treatments used in health care settings. *J Clin Microbiol*. 2010;48:2689-2697.

89. Rennecker JL, Marinas BJ, Owens JH, Rice EW. Inactivation of *Cryptosporidium parvum* oocysts with ozone. *Water Research*. 1999;33:2481-2488.

90. Wainwright KE, Miller MA, Barr BC, et al. Chemical inactivation of *Toxoplasma gondii* oocysts in water. *J Parasitol*. 2007;93(4):925-931.

91. Mun S, Cho SH, Kim TS, Oh BT, Yoon J. Inactivation of *Ascaris* eggs in soil by microwave treatment compared to UV and ozone treatment. *Chemosphere*. 2009;77:285-290.

92. Korich DG, Mead JR, Madore MS, Sinclair NA, Sterling CR. Effects of ozone, chlorine dioxide, chlorine, and monochloramine on *Cryptosporidium parvum* oocyst viability. *Appl Environ Microbiol*. 1990;56:1423-1428.

93. von Gunten U. Ozonation of drinking water: part I. Oxidation kinetics and product formation. *Water Res*. 2003;37:1443-1467.

94. von Gunten U. Ozonation of drinking water: part II. Disinfection and by-product formation in presence of bromide, iodide or chlorine. *Water Res*. 2003;37:1469-1487.

95. Feng L, Zhang K, Gao M, et al. Inactivation of *Vibrio parahaemolyticus* by aqueous ozone. *J Microbiol Biotechnol*. 2018;28:1233-1246.

96. Cortezzo DE, Koziol-Dube K, Setlow B, Setlow P. Treatment with oxidizing agents damages the inner membrane of spores of *Bacillus subtilis* and sensitizes spores to subsequent stress. *J Appl Microbiol*. 2004;97:838-852.

97. Predmore A, Sanglay G, Li J, Lee K. Control of human norovirus surrogates in fresh foods by gaseous ozone and a proposed mechanism of inactivation. *Food Microbiol*. 2015;50:118-125.

98. Murray BK, Ohmine S, Tomer DP, et al. Virion disruption by ozone-mediated reactive oxygen species. *J Virol Methods*. 2008;153:74-77.

99. Thurston-Enriquez JA, Haas CN, Jacangelo J, Gerba CP. Inactivation of enteric adenovirus and feline calicivirus by ozone. *Water Res*. 2005;39:3650-3656.

100. Kim CK, Gentile DM, Sproul OJ. Mechanism of ozone inactivation of bacteriophage f$_2$. *Appl Environ Microbiol*. 1980;39:210-218.

101. Horvitz S, Cantalejo MJ. Application of ozone for the postharvest treatment of fruits and vegetables. *Crit Rev Food Sci Nutr*. 2014;54:312-339.

102. Guillard V, Mauricio-Iglesias M, Gontard N. Effect of novel food processing methods on packaging: structure, composition, and migration properties. *Crit Rev Food Sci Nutr*. 2010;50:969-988.

103. Galante R, Ghisleni D, Paradiso P, et al. Sterilization of silicone-based hydrogels for biomedical application using ozone gas: comparison with conventional techniques. *Mater Sci Eng C Mater Biol Appl*. 2017;78:389-397.

104. Blakeman R, Pearse TW, inventors; Medaco International Health, LLC, assignee. Sterilizing using ozone. US patent 10,258,704. April 16, 2019.

105. Mielnik TJ, Burke PA, inventors; Steris, Inc, assignee. System for decontaminating food articles having a porous outer surface. US patent 9,968,105. May 15, 2018.

106. International Organization for Standardization. *ISO 14937:2009: Sterilization of Health Care Products—General Requirements for Characterization of a Sterilizing Agent and the Development, Validation and Routine Control of a Sterilization Process for Medical Devices*. Geneva, Switzerland: International Organization for Standardization; 2009.

107. International Organization for Standardization. *ISO/TS 19930:2017: Guidance on Aspects of a Risk-Based Approach to Assuring Sterility of Terminally Sterilized, Single-Use Health Care Product That Is Unable to Withstand Processing to Achieve Maximally a Sterility Assurance Level of 10^{-6}*. Geneva, Switzerland: International Organization for Standardization; 2017.

108. Taggart DS, McKelvie JI, Steppan JJ, Hinklin TR, Boxley CJ, inventors; SteriO3, LLC, assignee. Sterilization device and methods. US patent 10,039,850. August 7, 2018.

109. Turcot R, Robitaille S, Dufresne S, inventors; Technologies of Sterilization with Ozone TSO3 Inc, assignee. Method and apparatus for ozone sterilization. US patent 7,588,720. September 15, 2009.

110. Robitaille S, Dufresne S, Vallieres JM, et al, inventors; TSO3 Inc Technologies of Sterilization with Ozone TSO3 Inc, assignee. Sterilization method and apparatus. US patent 9,101,679. August 11, 2015.

111. TSO$_3$ Inc. Sterizone: Technical monograph. TSO$_3$ Web site. https://www.tso3.com/wp-content/uploads/2018/06/MA-200-045_r3_VP4-Technical-Monograph_US_en.pdf. Accessed April 9, 2019.

Plasma Sterilization

Akikazu Sakudo, Hideharu Shintani, and Yagyu Yoshihito

The term *plasma*, referring to ionized gas, was first coined by Irving Langmuir in 1927 and was so named because it reminded him of blood plasma.[1,2] Since the 1970s, different types of plasmas have been recognized to inactivate microorganisms. In the early 1990s, commercial instruments that use plasma during sterilization of medical devices became available. For more than a decade, plasma medicine, which refers to the application of plasma for biological decontamination as well as for therapeutic purposes, has undergone rapid development. These applications include the "plasma" treatment of blood plasma, such as argon plasma coagulation (APC).[3] This terminology for "plasma" might cause confusion, which is why "gas plasma" is often used instead. In this chapter, because we do not deal with the treatment of blood, the term *plasma* is used throughout to refer to an ionized gas.

Diverse applications of plasma disinfection have recently been reported in the fields of medicine,[4] dentistry,[5,6] agricultural,[7,8] and environmental science[9-11] (Figure 34.1). Indeed, numerous scientific papers and patents over the past 20 years cite the microbicidal effect of plasma. Commercialized patents of plasma sterilization describe the use of oxidizing agent gases such as hydrogen peroxide[12] and peracetic acid[13] as well as ozone (O_3) and chlorine dioxide (ClO_2).[14] However, it should be noted that these instruments are not true plasma sterilizers because the sterilization factor is the oxidizing agent gases rather than the plasma. In the case of the widely used hydrogen peroxide gas plasma sterilizers STERRAD (Advanced Sterilization Products, Irvine, California), common cycle conditions clearly show that the plasma is only generated following exposure and removal of the gas by a vacuum.[15] In addition there was little or no contributory microbicidal activity in the presence and absence of plasma.[16] The D-value (decimal reduction time: the time required for killing 90% [1 log] of the exposed microorganisms) for 1 mg/L of hydrogen peroxide gas against *Geobacillus stearothermophilus* was about 1 minute, whereas the estimated D-value in the presence of plasma at 300 W at the same concentration was 5 minutes.[17] Therefore, the observed antimicrobial effect of STERRAD is due to the hydrogen peroxide gas and not the plasma. However, in such processes, the plasma is important because it may be involved as a heating mechanism and can aid in the removal of hydrogen peroxide (gas and liquid) residues from the sterilizer load, thereby making the contents safe. Furthermore, US Food and Drug Administration (FDA) issued a toxicity safety alert for hospital devices using a different plasma-based system, which involved peracetic acid gas exposure followed by plasma generation.[18,19] Although this system has proven microbicidal activity, there were potential problems associated with compatibility of the device as well as toxicity issues.[20]

Interestingly, the authors' studies have revealed that performance comparison of endotoxin inactivation showed that plasma of nitrogen (N_2) gas (Figure 34.2) was superior to hydrogen peroxide gas plasma using STERRAD (Table 34.1).[22] These findings prompted the authors to further study the potential use of this technology to ascertain whether it could elicit a broad spectrum of microbicidal activity against bacteria (including bacterial spores), viruses (enveloped and nonenveloped viruses), and fungi as well as the inactivation of prions and toxins (endotoxins, bacterial toxins, and fungal toxins). Our findings clearly showed that plasma sources could be suitable for these applications. Thus, plasma-based technologies can be applied not only for disinfection/sterilization but also for cleaning.[23] In addition some recalcitrant forms of bacteria in the environment, including biofilms, could be inactivated by the plasma. As well as N_2, plasma may be generated from a range of different gases including oxygen (O_2); carbon dioxide (CO_2); mock air (mixture of 20% O_2 and 80% N_2); and noble gases such as argon (Ar), helium (He), neon (Ne), krypton (Kr), and xenon (Xe) and mixtures thereof. The plasma generated from these gases caused inactivation of microorganisms, although the efficiency is dependent on the type of gas used.[24]

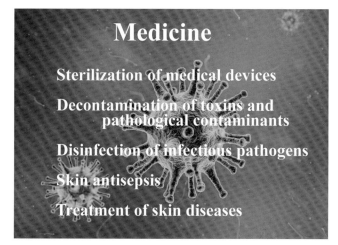
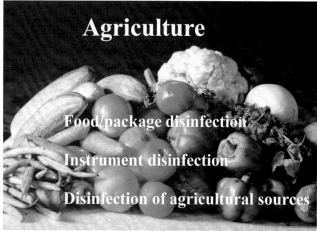
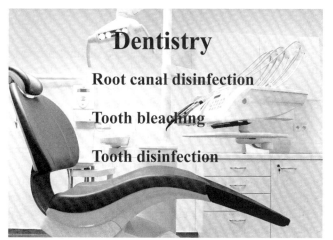
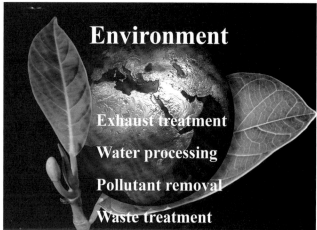

FIGURE 34.1 Recent applications of plasma technology for disinfection and decontamination. For a color version of this art, please consult the eBook.

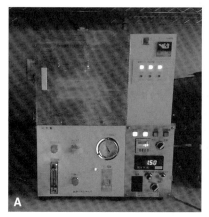
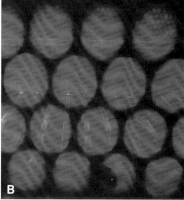

FIGURE 34.2 A representative nitrogen gas plasma instrument, BLP-TES (Bi-polar and Low-pressure Plasma-Triple Effects Sterilization) device. A, Photograph of the nitrogen gas plasma instrument (BLP-TES device; NGK Insulators, Ltd, Komaki, Japan). The BLP-TES device produces nitrogen gas plasma using a fast high-voltage pulse applied by a static induction (SI) thyristor power supply at 1.5 kpps and 0.5 atm. B, Photograph of the blue luminescence observed upon operation of the BLP-TES device. For a color version of this art, please consult the eBook. Reprinted from Sakudo et al.[21] Copyright © 2016 Elsevier. With permission.

TABLE 34.1	Performance of inactivation efficiency compared between hydrogen gas plasma and nitrogen gas plasma against endotoxin[a,b]	
	D-Value at 60°C	**Endotoxin Inactivation Level**
Hydrogen gas plasma	2.47 min	1 log reduction
Nitrogen gas plasma	Less than 1.3 min	More than 5 log reduction

[a]STERRAD (Advanced Sterilization Products, Irvine, California) was used as the hydrogen gas plasma instrument, whereas BLP-TES device was used as nitrogen gas plasma instrument. Endotoxin is derived from *Escherichia coli*.

[b]From Shintani et al[22] with permission from the Society for Antibacterial and Antifungal Agents, Japan.

Overall, plasma disinfection/sterilization can be used in three ways: (1) plasma is directly generated at the site of application (direct treatment of plasma), (2) plasma is generated at a remote site and transferred to the target site (indirect treatment of plasma by afterglow), and (3) plasma-treated solutions are used for disinfection/sterilization (solutions used as disinfectants are often referred to as "plasma-activated water [PAW]"[25] or "plasma-treated water [PTW])."[26,27] Plasma-treated solutions known as "plasma-activated medium (PAM),"[28] "plasma-stimulated medium (PSM),"[29] "plasma-treated phosphate-buffered saline (pPBS),"[30] or "nonthermal plasma-conditioned media (NTP media)"[31] have been reported to inactivate cancer cells but not healthy cells under certain test conditions. These solutions may also be used for therapeutic tests in the laboratory. In addition several cold plasma sources were certified as medical devices and have been used for the treatment of chronic wounds as well as other skin diseases.[32-34] Several groups have developed devices for such clinical purposes including kINPen,[32-35] Plasma-Derm,[36] and MicroPlaSter.[37] Because this book focuses on disinfection/sterilization, we would not deal with these plasma therapies in any further detail. If readers are interested in this issue, they should refer to some recent excellent reviews.[38-40]

In this chapter, we summarize the fundamentals of plasma and focus on plasma disinfection/sterilization of various microorganisms using nonoxidizing agent (or essentially inert) gases such as air, N_2, O_2, or noble gases.

▶ PROPERTIES OF PLASMA

Plasma is known as the fourth state of matter and comprises a gas containing electrons and charged particles.[41] When energy is applied, matter changes state from solid to liquid and then from liquid to gas. When additional thermal energy is applied to the gaseous matter, the constituent molecules (or atoms in the case of a noble gas) collide with greater frequency and kinetic energy, resulting in a loss of electrons and the formation of an ionized state. This ionized gas is called plasma. The number of charged particles and the number of electrons are nearly equal in a plasma because positive ions and electrons are always generated in a pair during ionization, and a plasma is in an electrically quasi-neutral state, at least from a macroscopic perspective. Plasma has a distinct property in which physical, chemical, and electrical actions are mixed and interact in a composite manner. First, plasma is a gas that contains charged particles and therefore exhibits conductivity. Second, there is chemical activity, which makes the plasma highly reactive. Third, plasma glows and therefore can be used as a light source. Final, plasma has a high temperature, and the particles possess significant kinetic energy. Of particular relevance, plasma sterilization takes advantage of the plasma property in which plasma is able to generate highly reactive chemical species at a low temperature. Generally, using electrical energy is simpler and more efficient than using thermal energy. Acceleration in an electric field is made possible because the electrons are negatively charged. Plasma can be generated from ionizing neutral particles by providing kinetic energy that is greater than the ionization potential.

Aside from electrons and positive ions, other species including atoms, molecules, and neutral particles without charge, such as radicals, exist within the gas in a plasma state.[42] A characteristic indicator of plasma is the degree of ionization β. Assuming an electron density n_e, ion density n_i, and neutral particle density n_n, these indicators are defined as shown in equation (1).

$$\beta = \frac{n_e}{n_e + n_n} \tag{1}$$

A plasma with 100% degree of ionization is called a completely ionized plasma; ionization of several percentage or higher is called strongly ionized plasma; and a degree of ionization (0.1% or below) where neutral particles occupy the majority of space is called weakly ionized plasma. The properties of plasma are greatly dependent on the pressure. Because the area near the atmospheric pressure is highly dense, intense collisions between electrons, ions, and neutral particles take place and kinetic energy of the particles are exchanged. The kinetic energy of a gas is determined by absolute temperature only. If the temperatures of electrons, ions, and neutral particles are Te, Ti, and Tn, respectively, then Te ≒ Ti ≒ Tn in an atmospheric plasma. A state in which each temperature is equal is called thermal equilibrium plasma, or simply, thermal plasma. However, plasma generated under a low pressure (less than a few hundred Pascal) has a low density of particles, and Te ≫ Ti ≒ Tn because electrons do not lose kinetic energy through collisions. Plasma in a thermally nonequilibrium state is referred to as nonthermal equilibrium plasma or low-temperature plasma.

Recent research in the field of medicine and bioscience involving the application of plasma technology has resulted in the development of pulse power sources that do not heat up under atmospheric pressure as well as atmospheric pressure plasma jets that use alternating current high-voltage discharge of several kilohertz and several kilovolts in an He gas.[43]

❱ GENERATION OF PLASMA

In the air, there are ions of particles and electrons generated under the influence of radiation from cosmic rays and from the natural world. These electrons are known as accidental electrons (initial electrons) and play an important role in initiating the generation of plasma.[44] If voltage is applied between electrodes to generate plasma, accidental electrons (initial electrons) that accidentally existed between the electrodes are accelerated by the electric field, generating new ions and electrons through collisions with other particles. Similarly, newly liberated electrons generated by ionization are also accelerated by the effect of the electric field leading to further ionization events, creating a phenomenon known as an electron avalanche, which in turn maintains the plasma state. Properties of plasma that differ from those of neutral particles including conductivity, luminescence, and chemical activation are derived from the collision between electrons in the plasma and gas molecules.[42]

This section explains the ionization process for the atoms. When an electron e collides with atom X, the elastic collision takes place if the collision energy is small and the kinetic energy of the electrons (electron temperature) does not significantly change. Outer shell electrons may be stripped away from the atomic nucleus resulting in ionization as described in equation (2). This occurs when electrons collide with atoms with kinetic energy greater than that of the ionizing voltage. Ions with two or greater valence are sometimes generated when the electron energy is high.

An electron collision with an atom does not necessarily result in ionization. Excitation may take place where the bound electrons within the atom absorb energy during the collision and are promoted to a higher energy orbit (equation [3]). Excitation state of atom X is denoted as X*. Because the excited atom is unstable, it returns to the ground state in a very short period of time ($<10^{-8}$ s). As shown in equation (4), excess energy is released at this point as photon energy hv. A collision in which excitation takes place during the first electron collision and ionization takes place during the second electron collision is referred to as a cumulative collision, expressed by equations (5) and (6). When the energy of the ordered stable state X* of atom X is higher than the ionization voltage of atom Y, atom Y ionizes through its collision with X*. This phenomenon is known as the Penning effect in which atom Y can be ionized at almost 100% probability resulting in highly effective ionization, leading to efficient generation of plasma. Although ionization may also occur via collision of ions (equation [8]), collision of neutral particles (equation [9]), or by interaction with light (equation [10]), these processes are less likely to occur than ionization by collision of electrons and, as such, can effectively be ignored in normal weak ionization plasma.

$$X + e \rightarrow X^+ + e + e \qquad (2)$$

$$X + e \rightarrow X^* + e \qquad (3)$$

$$X^* \rightarrow X + hv \qquad (4)$$

$$X + e \rightarrow X^* + e \qquad (5)$$

$$X^* + e \rightarrow X^+ + e + e \qquad (6)$$

$$X^* + Y \rightarrow X + Y^+ + e \qquad (7)$$

$$X^+ + Y \rightarrow X^+ + Y^+ + e \qquad (8)$$

$$X + Y \rightarrow X + Y^+ + e \qquad (9)$$

$$X + hv \rightarrow X^+ + e \qquad (10)$$

Another process occurs in which positive ions and electrons collide and recouple back into neutral particles. Recoupling of positive ions and electrons occur via a three-body collision of positive ion-electron-electron (equation [11]) and positive ion-electron-neutral particles (equation [12]). If the electrons have a high temperature, the main process is radiating recoupling in which excess energy is released as light (equation [13]).

$$A^+ + e + e \rightarrow A + e \qquad (11)$$

$$A^+ + e + B \rightarrow A + B \qquad (12)$$

$$A^+ + e \rightarrow A + hv \qquad (13)$$

Next, the process of collision between a molecule and an electron is explained. A process similar to the collision of an atom and an electron occurs, and molecule XY may be ionized directly through collision with an electron (equation [14]) or become excited (equation [15]). The colliding particles may result in promotion of electrons in an atom to a higher energy orbit. If the electron gains sufficient energy to overcome the Coulombic force that maintains its association with the positively charged nucleus, the electron is ejected and the atom ionizes to a positively charged ion. Molecules in an excited state where the total sum of internal energy of the particle changed before and after an inelastic collision is called an excited molecule, denoted by the symbol XY*. An electron shifted to the orbit of an excited state will subsequently drop back to the ground state after a short period of time, and this excess energy is released as a photon resulting in a glowing plasma.

A dissociation process in which a molecule dissociates into several molecules and atoms by collision with an electron may also occur. Through collision with an electron, molecule XY dissociates into X and Y, generating radicals with unpaired electrons. Neutral radicals generated during the dissociation process, as shown in equations (16), (17), and (18), increase the chemical reactivity of the plasma. Dissociation into X and Y by electron collision does not take place at the ground state but occurs spontaneously after the molecule is excited by collision with electrons. When an electron of low energy collides with a molecule, the molecule transiently becomes an anion (equation [19]) with an electron dissociating from the molecule (equation [20]).

$$XY + e \rightarrow XY^+ + e + e \tag{14}$$

$$XY + e \rightarrow XY^* + e \tag{15}$$

$$AB + e \rightarrow A + B + e \tag{16}$$

$$XY + e \rightarrow X^+ + Y + e + e \tag{17}$$

$$XY + e \rightarrow X + Y^+ + e + e \tag{18}$$

$$XY + e \rightarrow XY^- \tag{19}$$

$$XY + e \rightarrow X^- + Y \tag{20}$$

▶ GAS DISCHARGE PLASMA

Atmospheric gas is a very good insulator that does not conduct electricity.[45] As an insulator, gas ionizes and generates plasma when a high voltage is applied between an anode and a cathode. At this point, a dielectric breakdown (discharge) takes place when the conductivity of the gas rises rapidly. Dielectric breakdown occurs when accidental electrons that exist between electrodes serve as an initiator for the generation of plasma. Accidental electrons accelerated by the work of the electric field cause ionization as they collide with neutral molecules and atoms between the electrodes. Electrons produced through this ionization process are also accelerated by the electric field, causing further ionization. The chain of

events increases the density of charged particles between the electrodes, eventually leading to a dielectric breakdown in the gas. This ionization phenomenon in the gas phase is described by Townsend theory.[46]

According to the Townsend theory, weak current (undercurrent) I prior to the start of a discharge is proportional to the initial electron current I_0 and increases exponentially with the distance between electrodes d.

$$I = I_0 \ \exp(\alpha d) \tag{21}$$

If we suppose the number of collisions and ionizations caused over a unit length by a single electron under the force of an electric field is called α (first Townsend coefficient, otherwise known as α coefficient), this collision-ionization process is referred to as α action. The α coefficient depends on pressure p and electric field $E = \dfrac{V}{d}$ and can be expressed by the following equation. A and B are constants determined by the type of gas between the electrodes.

$$\frac{\alpha}{p} = A \exp\left(-\frac{B}{\dfrac{E}{p}}\right) \tag{22}$$

These equations describe a process known as an electron avalanche, in which initial electrons that serve as a trigger to the start of the discharge are accelerated by an electric field, collide, and ionize neutral particles. The number of electrons then multiplies in a manner reminiscent to that of an avalanche. An increase in current I depends on the presence of the initial electron current I_0. In the absence of I_0, the electron avalanche stops and exponential growth of charged particles does not occur, and a plasma is not generated.

Positive ions generated in a pair with electrons by α action accelerate toward the cathode by an electric field and collide with the cathode. Given that secondary electrons are released from a surface of a solid when high-energy ions and photons collide with the solid, Townsend named this release of secondary electrons from the cathode surface as γ action and the number of electrons released per colliding positive ion as γ coefficient. Note that β action is a phenomenon in which ionization takes place as ions collide with gas molecules, but, in reality, ion energy is insufficient to cause ionization. We calculate the discharged current that flows to the electrodes by taking α and γ actions into account. An increase in electron current is expressed as $I_0\exp(\alpha d) - I_0$, and assuming a monovalent positive ion was generated from ionization by α action, then the increase in electron current is equal to the number of positive ions. The positive ions are also influenced by the electric field but, in this case, accelerate in the cathode direction, releasing secondary electrons by γ action upon collision with the cathode. The secondary electron current at the cathode is $\gamma I_0\{\exp(\alpha d) - 1\}$.

Secondary electrons released by γ action are accelerated in the anode direction by the electric field as was the case for the initial electrons, and collisions and ionization events take place due to α action. When the secondary electron reaches the anode, electron current increases to $\gamma I_0\{\exp(\alpha d) - 1\}\exp(\alpha d)$. The α and γ actions are then repeated through this process. Addition of all the electron current that reaches the anode yields the following equation.

$$I = I_0\exp(\alpha d) + \gamma I_0\{\exp(\alpha d) - 1\}\exp(\alpha d) + \gamma I_0\{\exp(\alpha d) - 1\}\exp(\alpha d) + \cdots$$

$$= I_0 \frac{\exp(\alpha d)}{1 - \gamma\{\exp(\alpha d) - 1\}} \qquad (23)$$

When the denominator of equation 23 is zero, I becomes infinite and shows an electrically shorted state. Therefore, plasma is generated between the electrodes and a breakdown has taken place. In light of the earlier discussion, Townsend expressed the condition for the start of the discharge as follows, which is called the Townsend breakdown criterion.

$$\gamma\{\exp(\alpha d) - 1\} = 1 \qquad (24)$$

With regard to the relationship between the voltage and the start of a discharge (spark voltage) and gas pressure (p) as well as the length of the gap between electrodes (d), this voltage is determined by the product of p and d and has a minimum value. This relationship is known as Paschen law, and a graph of the relationship between voltage at the start of discharge V_s and the product of p and d (or pd) is known as Paschen curve.

Experimentally derived Paschen law can also be derived theoretically from Townsend spark condition equation (24). Equation (24) is rewritten as ad equation as follows.

$$ad = \ln\left(\frac{1}{\gamma} + 1\right) \qquad (25)$$

Multiplying both sides of equation (22) with pd and inserting equation (25) results in:

$$ad = Apd \exp\left(-\frac{B}{\frac{E}{p}}\right) = \ln\left(\frac{1}{\gamma} + 1\right) \qquad (26)$$

where voltage between electrodes Ed is equal to voltage V_s at the start of the discharge, and calculating spark voltage from equations (22) and (26) yields:

$$V_s = \frac{Bpd}{\ln\left\{\dfrac{A}{\ln\left(\dfrac{1}{\gamma} + 1\right)}\right\} + \ln(pd)} = \frac{Bpd}{C + \ln(pd)} \qquad (27)$$

where C is the constant determined by the gas and cathode material. From equation (27), small product of pd results in a greater value of voltage V_s at the start of discharge,

but as the product of pd becomes greater, V_s gradually increases after reaching a minimum value.

METHOD OF PLASMA GENERATION

Depending on the maintenance mechanism of plasma, forms of plasma are categorized into arc discharge, corona discharge, and glow discharge. As for the method of generating plasma, its categorization includes those that depend on the frequency of the power source, such as direct current discharge and high-frequency discharge; those that depend on ambient gas pressure, such as low-pressure and atmospheric pressure plasma; and those that depend on the electrode shape and form of discharge.[4,47] Among them, for the purposes of medical and bio-applications, several discharge methods for generating plasmas have been used including corona, glow, dielectric barrier, pulse, and high frequency. This section focuses on plasma generation methods that are most frequently used in plasma medical and bio-applications.

Corona Discharge

A corona discharge occurs when an electric field is concentrated at the tip of a needle. The electrodes are structured so that the electric field surrounding the electrode is uneven (such as a combination of a needle and a plate electrode) and a voltage is then applied. At this point, neutral gas near the tip of the needle ionizes by the concentrated electric field and generates plasma. A discharge caused by a local dielectric breakdown through concentration of the electric field is called a corona discharge. As discussed next, there are several modes of corona discharge. The tip of the needle electrode glows weakly as a result of a current running between electrodes at a few microamperes, forming a state of plasma known as glow corona. Raising the voltage further, the plasma at the needle tip extends along the plate electrode and becomes a state known as brush corona generated from an electric current with a pulse of approximately 1 μs. Raising the voltage even further, the plasma extended from the tip of the needle electrode connects to the plate electrode, forming a stringlike state known as streamer corona. Streamer corona is generated in a high-pressure region (700 Pa · m), and its mechanism of formation cannot be explained by the Townsend theory. This discharge phenomenon occurs over a very short period of time of less than 10^{-7} seconds and is not influenced by ions. As such, the discharge does not require γ action. In the streamer theory, α action on initial electrons causes an electron avalanche, and its intense spatially charged electric field accelerates electrons formed by photoionization and creates a smaller electron avalanche. A streamer is generated when this secondary electron avalanche enters the plasma pillar formed by the primary avalanche.

Glow Discharge

Glow discharge is a sustainable discharge phenomenon that typically occurs when 100 V to several kV of direct voltage is applied to a gas with a low pressure of approximately 100 Pa. Plasma generated by glow discharge is a nonthermal equilibrium plasma where energy of electrons is greater than the ion energy. The ability of the plasma generated by glow discharge to process at a low temperature gives it a wide range of potential applications. Atmospheric glow discharge can generate plasma under atmospheric pressure, leading to the generation of plasma using various gases such as He and Ar, air, and N_2. Compared to other forms of discharge, glow discharge is spatially highly homogeneous and is capable of generating plasma at low temperature and in a large volume. These properties make the plasma useful for applications in the field of medicine and the biosciences. An example of a discharge plasma is an atmospheric pressure plasma jet, which uses a mixture of He and Ar gas. Atmospheric pressure plasma jet is generally obtained by sending gas into an insulator tube of several millimeters in diameter and applying a high voltage of several kilovolts to several tens of kilovolts to the tube. A typical use is of an afterglow discharge type in which high-temperature plasma generated inside the tube, made of either glass or ceramic, is pushed out of the tube as it is cooled.

Dielectric Barrier Discharge

Barrier discharge is a form of discharge that is used frequently because it can be generated relatively easily under atmospheric pressure. This approach generates streamer discharge over a large area by placing a dielectric that does not conduct electricity on either side or both sides of electrodes to prevent arc discharge and by applying an alternating high voltage ranging from 10 Hz to several kilohertz. The temperature of the ions and neutral particles does not increase because the discharge takes place over a very short period of time. Aside from being called a dielectric barrier discharge (DBD), the discharge is also known as a silent discharge. The gap between the electrodes is the plasma-processing region, known as the gap length, that is generally in the range of several millimeters to several centimeters, which is quite narrow. To improve on the arrangement, another type of discharge, known as floating electrode DBD (FE-DBD), has been developed where one of the electrodes is replaced with a floating electrode.

Pulse Discharge

Although the method of generating plasma by atmospheric discharge is very attractive for applications in biological and medical sciences, it nonetheless transitions easily into an arc discharge, and the generation of a stable plasma in a large area is difficult to achieve. By applying voltages in the form of short pulses, electrons are accelerated but heavy ions are not, creating a stable discharge even under atmospheric pressure. Because voltages with a very short duration are applied, the transition into an arc discharge can also be suppressed. With the development of magnetic pulse compression circuit technology, a short-pulsed, highly repetitive, small-scale, high-voltage power source may be feasible.

High-Frequency Plasma

This plasma is typically generated with radiofrequency (RF) electromagnetic radiation of 13.56 MHz. Electrodes are not necessarily needed, and plasma can be generated using antennas. Highly dense plasma with a large volume can be generated under low atmospheric pressure, and its low temperature tends to prevent objects from being damaged. Discharge can be maintained without secondary electron emission (γ action) from the cathode. Depending on the shape of the antenna, this plasma is classified into capacitively coupled plasma (CCP) and inductively coupled plasma (ICP).

▶ INACTIVATION OF MICROORGANISMS BY PLASMA

Plasma has been shown to display broad-spectrum microbicidal activity as well as the ability to eliminate toxins associated with microorganisms.[17,48,49] As such, plasma is a useful means of disinfection/sterilization. In the next section, we introduce current knowledge on the inactivation of microorganisms by plasma, together with an introduction to the authors' own studies in this field. Generally, microbes exhibit a wide variation in intrinsic resistance to disinfectants (Figure 34.3). To date, plasma disinfection covers almost all the microbiological hierarchy from the most susceptible, enveloped viruses, to the most resistant pathogens, prions.

Bacteria

Recently, extensive research has been performed on the use of plasma to inactivate various bacteria. *Escherichia coli*, *Bacillus* species, *Salmonella* species, *Staphylococcus aureus*, and *Enterococcus faecalis*, in addition to bacterial spores such as *G stearothermophilus*, have been shown to be efficiently inactivated by plasma treatment,[50-53] indicating that this technology is highly effective as a means of disinfection.

There are numerous recent reviews covering a range of different topics concerned with disinfection/sterilization using plasma. Moisan et al[54] describes inactivation of several bacterial species including *E coli*, *S aureus*, and *Bacillus*

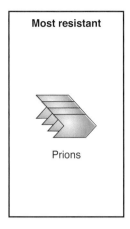

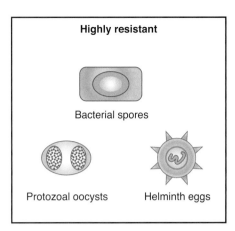

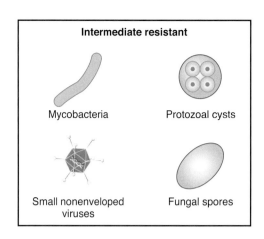

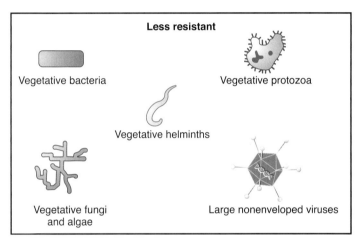

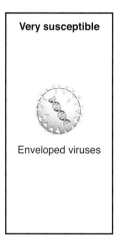

FIGURE 34.3 Resistance hierarchy of microorganisms.

subtilis spores using discharge of microwaves and DBD and various gases (air; Ar; O_2; CO_2; and mixtures of N_2, O_2, and Ar), which are compared and discussed. Ehlbeck et al[55] summarizes the inactivation efficiency of various plasma sources including discharge of corona, microwaves, as well as DBD and plasma jet against about 20 different microorganisms including gram-positive and gram-negative bacteria. A comparison of the inactivation of various bacteria was performed by Scholtz et al.[56,57] These studies showed that the sensitivity of all vegetative bacteria was comparable, whereas *Candida* and *Geobacillus* spores[56] or yeast[57] are more resistant to plasma than vegetative bacteria.

A most promising application of plasma disinfection is the eradication of antibiotic-resistant bacteria. Recently, the growing risk of disease from drug-resistant pathogens has caused considerable public health concern. Indeed, the danger of antibiotic-resistant bacteria was recently prioritized by both the World Health Organization (WHO)[58] and the Centers for Disease Control and Prevention (CDC).[59] The extensive and indiscriminate use of antibiotics has been recognized to alter the environmental microbiome, contributing to the emergence of drug-resistant bacteria.[60] Thus, innovative methods for inactivating multidrug-resistant bacteria are sought. The plasma method is especially useful

for eliminating multidrug-resistant bacteria that are otherwise difficult to neutralize.[61,62] This is because the mechanisms of action of the plasma are unlikely to differ between multidrug-resistant and susceptible bacteria.

Nonetheless, there is a paucity of published studies devoted to identifying potential mechanisms of plasma-induced bacterial inactivation. Our research group analyzed the bactericidal/disinfecting effect of N_2 gas plasma on *Salmonella* and its influence on components of the bacterial cell as well as which factors constitute the main mechanism of disinfection by N_2 gas plasma from a BLP-TES (Bi-polar and Low-pressure Plasma-Triple Effects Sterilization) device,[63] where a fast high-voltage pulse applied by a static induction (SI) thyristor power supply was used for plasma generation (see Figure 34.2). Our biochemical analyses demonstrated that *Salmonella* exposed to N_2 gas plasma have altered cell surface *O*-antigens and DNA, whereas the plasma treatment did not influence the lipopolysaccharide (LPS) component located in the inner region of the cell wall (Figure 34.4). The lack of LPS changes may be due to low penetration of the plasma. Images obtained from scanning electron microscope (SEM) highlighted changes at the bacterial cell surface. These alterations to the outer region of *Salmonella* may be related to the mechanisms

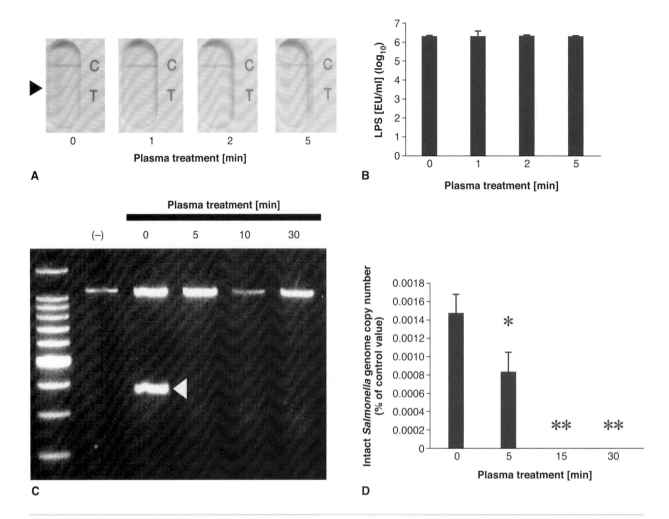

FIGURE 34.4 Nitrogen gas plasma treatment induces biochemical changes in *Salmonella*. A, After nitrogen gas plasma treatment with BLP-TES device, the *Salmonella* samples were subjected to immunochromatography for the *O*-antigen (Singlepath *Salmonella*; Merck Group, Darmstadt, Germany). The bands for *Salmonella* *O*-antigen are indicated by an arrowhead. C, control line; T, test line. B, The plasma-treated *Salmonella* samples were subjected to the chromogenic Limulus test for lipopolysaccharide (LPS) (Limulus-Color KY Series; Wako Pure Chemical Industries, Ltd, Osaka, Japan). The LPS concentration is shown in terms of endotoxin units per milliliter (EU/mL). C, The plasma-treated *Salmonella* samples were subjected to polymerase chain reaction (PCR) analysis using *Salmonella* One-Shot PCR (Takara Bio Inc, Kusatsu, Japan) for the *invA* gene. Negative control (−), which lacks DNA, is also shown. D, Real-time PCR assay by CycleavePCR *Salmonella* Detection Kit Ver. 2.0 (Takara Bio Inc, Kusatsu, Japan) using nitrogen gas plasma–treated *Salmonella*. Differences where $P < .05$ (*asterisk*) and $P < .01$ (*double asterisks*) versus control (0 min) were considered significant. For a color version of this art, please consult the eBook. Reprinted from Maeda et al.[63] Copyright © 2014 Elsevier. With permission.

by which N_2 gas plasma inactivates the bacteria. However, further biochemical analyses of cell components using both gram-negative and gram-positive bacteria as well as alternative plasma sources are needed to fully elucidate whether the mechanism of inactivation is common among various bacterial species and different forms of plasma.

Bacterial Spores

Except for prions, bacterial spores are generally considered to be the most resistant microorganisms to inactivate. Indeed, bacterial spores are often used as an index

for the demonstration of sterilization effectiveness.[64] By contrast, vegetative bacteria are generally susceptible to disinfection/sterilization treatment.[65] Next, we introduce a selection of representative papers related to inactivation of bacterial spores by plasma.

Lerouge et al[66] used low-temperature plasma generated from several different gases to inactivate *B subtilis* spores. Potential etching of spores upon treatment with various gas plasmas was compared to that induced by O_2 gas plasmas. Plasmas of Ar, hydrogen (H_2), CO_2, and tetrafluoromethane (CF_4) gases did not present any etching phenomenon. Etching resistance was discussed in terms of spore morphology and spore complex coating structure. The D-value of O_2/CF_4

was 1.5 minutes, whereas that of pure O_2 was 3.8 minutes. These observations indicate O_2/CF_4 was more efficient at spore inactivation with reduced levels of etching, which enhances functional/material compatibility while maintaining a sterility assurance level (SAL) of 10^{-6}.

Lassen et al[67] optimized the inactivation of *G stearothermophilus* ATCC 7953 endospores using RF-generated CF_4/O_2 gas plasma in terms of several factors such as power, flow rate, exposure time, and RF system type. Specifically, the dependency of the sporicidal effect on spores inoculated in the chamber of the RF system was studied based on survival curves and D-values. Their results indicated that the power value of the RF excitation source was the only parameter to influence inactivation of endospore.

Lassen et al[68] also evaluated the sporicidal effect of different RF plasma processes produced by combining various gas mixtures. Sporicidal effects of O_2-containing gas plasma were found to be dependent on the power. In the absence of O_2, no power dependency was observed. Survival curves obtained with the use of plasma generated from Ar/H_2 indicated a straight line from the initial population that may be used to extrapolate on SAL of 10^{-6} and less etching. The CF_4/O_2 caused more damage to the material by etching than Ar/H_2, indicating that the sporicidal and etching phenomenon do not always coincide. The CF_4/O_2 gas mixture may be appropriate for inactivation efficiency but inappropriate in attaining functional and material compatibility due to etching by O_2 gas. Inactivation through etching by O_2 gas was a highly power-dependent phenomenon. The authors concluded that an inactivation mechanism might combine a sporicidal effect with substrate damage by etching of the endospore with O_2 gas, whereas the effect of the presence of ultraviolet (UV) radiation is negligible.

Hury et al[69] studied the inactivation of *Bacillus* spores in O_2-based plasma. The study clearly shows O_2, H_2O_2, and CO_2 plasmas to be more efficient in eliminating *B subtilis* spores than Ar plasma.

Takamatsu et al[24] suggest the reactive species responsible for the inactivation of endospores in CO_2 plasma is singlet O_2 ($^1O_2$) and that of N_2 gas plasma is the hydroxyl ($\cdot$OH) radical. Variation in bacterial density on the carrier material leads to significant differences in the inactivation efficiency of spores when using CO_2 plasma. This observation is due to the shallow penetration depth of reactive species of CO_2 gas plasma ($^1O_2$, 10-40 nm). If the vegetative cells form multiple layers, such as in a biofilm, the killing efficiency is drastically reduced.

Winter et al[70] reported the Ar gas plasma inactivation of *B subtilis* endospores. The authors investigated the plasma-specific response of *B subtilis* toward Ar as well as air-generated plasmas. Cellular responses, such as DNA damage and oxidative stress, were observed due to the synergistic effect of Ar and air plasma treatment. A variety of gas-dependent cellular responses such as growth retardation and morphologic changes, including shrinkage by O_2 gas in air, were also observed.

Fungi

Compared to vegetative bacteria, studies on plasma-treated fungi are limited. Nonetheless, it is clear that fungi are more resistant to plasma than vegetative bacteria because they require a longer exposure time to achieve an equivalent level of inactivation. We showed that N_2 gas plasma generated from a BLP-TES device inactivated *Aspergillus brasiliensis*, which belongs to the same genus as the aflatoxin B_1 (AFB1)-producing fungi.[21] However, the viable cell number of *A brasiliensis* was unchanged after 5-minute treatment,[21] whereas *Salmonella* was completely inactivated after an identical exposure time.[63] Nonetheless, the viable cell count of *Aspergillus* significantly decreased following treatment with N_2 gas plasma for 15 minutes or more. Therefore, the N_2 gas plasma treatment inactivates molds but needs a longer time for inactivation compared to bacteria.

Similarly, Souškova et al reported no significant differences in susceptibility against plasma generated by corona discharge among bacteria including *E coli* and *Staphylococcus epidermidis*, but the susceptibility of fungi is different between species including *Aspergillus oryzae*, *Cladosporium sphaerospermum*, and *Penicillium crustosum*.[71-73] Intriguingly, of these fungi, *Aspergillus* displayed the greatest resistance to plasma inactivation.

Taken together, these studies suggest complete inactivation of vegetative bacteria is achieved after only a short exposure to plasma of about 5 minutes, although this may vary depending on the plasma source and precise operating conditions. By contrast, however, a longer exposure time of more than 15 minutes is required to fully inactivate fungi. This is possibly due to the presence of spores in the fungi but not in the vegetative bacteria. Spores appear to enhance the resistance of fungi to plasma.

Viruses

Recently, extensive research has been carried out to assess the potential application of plasma for inactivation of viruses. These studies include N_2 plasma inactivation of influenza virus,[74,75] respiratory syncytial virus (RSV),[76] and adenovirus,[77] as well as air plasma inactivation of adenovirus,[78] O_2 plasma inactivation of human parainfluenza virus type 3 and influenza virus A (H5N2).[79] It should be noted that the inactivation of feline calicivirus (FCV) by plasma was confirmed using various gases such as Ar and mixtures of O_2 and air.[80,81] In addition, bacteriophage can be inactivated by plasma jet in a flowing gas mixture of O_2 and He.[82] However, at the time of writing, no studies on the inactivation of plant viruses by plasma have been reported in the literature.

Most viruses are inactivated after a short exposure to plasma. According to the US Environmental Protection Agency (EPA)[83] *Guide Standard and Protocol for Testing Microbiological Water Purifiers*, the minimum performance standards of inactivation efficiency are a 6 log reduction/inactivation of bacteria and 4 log reduction/inactivation of viruses. The N_2 gas plasma generated by a high-voltage pulse using an SI thyristor power supply shows a 4 log reduction of virus titer of adenovirus within 4 minutes,[77] more than a 4 log reduction of RSV within 5 minutes, and about a 2 log reduction of influenza virus titer after 1 minute,[75] whereas Ar plasma caused more than a 5 log reduction within 2 minutes.[80] The O_2 plasma also reduced the titer of human parainfluenza virus type 3, RSV, and influenza virus A (H5N2) by approximately 4 to 6 log at a flow velocity of 0.9 m/s and reaction time of 0.44 second.[79] Air plasma achieved >5 log reduction in FCV titer within a treatment time of 3 minutes.[81] These findings suggest that plasma treatment against all virus types for 5 minutes or more meets the aforementioned performance standard of EPA.

Taken together, these studies demonstrate that plasma treatment is a potentially useful method for the rapid inactivation of viruses. Analysis of inactivation mechanisms suggests that the reactive chemical products produced in the plasma may induce damage to the viral genome (DNA or RNA) and other viral components such as proteins and lipids.[76,77] Therefore, optimization of each plasma system to generate increased levels of reactive chemical products is expected to improve the virucidal efficiency of these procedures.

Toxins

Bacteria and fungi sometimes produce toxins, which act as causative agents for diseases. For example, Shiga toxin (Stx)-producing *E coli* (STEC) leads to food poisoning by causing hemorrhagic colitis and hemolytic uremic syndrome. Aflatoxins are a group of toxic metabolites produced by fungal species belonging to the genus *Aspergillus*, such as *Aspergillus flavus* and *Aspergillus parasiticus*, that display potent mutagenic and carcinogenic properties. We and others have recently demonstrated that plasma can be used to inactivate not only bacteria and fungi but also toxins.

We applied an N_2 gas plasma apparatus to the inactivation of Stxs[84] and an aflatoxin[70] (Figure 34.5). Samples

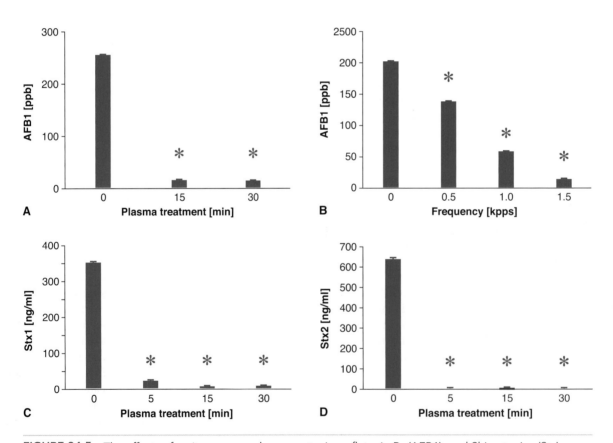

FIGURE 34.5   The effects of a nitrogen gas plasma on toxins, aflatoxin B_1 (AFB1), and Shiga toxins (Stx). Quantitative measurement of AFB1 (A and B), Stx1 (C), and Stx2 (D) after nitrogen gas plasma treatment with BLP-TES device at 1.5 kpps for the indicated times (A, C, and D) and at 0-1.5 kpps for 15 minutes (B) was performed by an enzyme-linked immunosorbent assay (ELISA) using MycoJudge Total Aflatoxin Kit (NH Foods Ltd, Osaka, Japan) and RIDASCREEN Verotoxin kit (R-Biopharm AG, Darmstadt, Germany). Differences where $P < .01$ (*asterisk*) versus control (0 min) were considered significant. A and B reprinted from Sakudo et al.[21] Copyright © 2016 Elsevier. With permission. C and D is cited from Sakudo and Imanishi.[84] https://creativecommons.org/licenses/by/4.0/.

of Stx1 and Stx2 as well as AFB1 were treated with an N_2 gas plasma generated by a plasma device using BLP-TES device. Quantification by enzyme-linked immunosorbent assay (ELISA) showed that both toxins were efficiently degraded to less than one-tenth of their original concentration within 5 minutes of treatment. Moreover, an assay using human epithelial cell (HEp-2) as an index of cytotoxicity showed that plasma treatment reduced the toxic activity of Stx. The ELISA also demonstrated that 200 ppb solution of AFB1 was efficiently degraded to less than 20 ppb ($<1/10$) within 15 minutes. The FDA guidelines to maintain a safe level of aflatoxin contaminants in human food sets 20 ppb as the safe maximum concentration of AFB1.[85] Thus, N_2 plasma technology could decrease AFB1 to safe levels. Moreover, a cell-based assay using human liver cancer cells (HepG2) as an index to measure the cell growth–promoting properties of AFB1 showed that plasma treatment reduced the biological activity of the mycotoxin.

When we consider possible inactivation mechanisms, a previous observation suggested that conformational changes in a protein induced by the N_2 gas plasma, but not a result of direct heating, may be responsible.[86] Thus, conformational changes or degradation of Stx1 and Stx2 proteins by the plasma may play an important role in their inactivation. In the case of AFB1, as the amount of heat and UV radiation is insufficient to inactivate the toxin, the reactive chemical products may contribute to the degradation of AFB1; however, further studies are required to fully understand the inactivation mechanisms of the toxins.

Studies have also analyzed the inactivation of LPS, which acts as an endotoxin, using a different technology for producing plasma.[22,87] Takamatsu et al[88] has also demonstrated plasma-induced decomposition of tetrodotoxin using various gas sources. Tetrodotoxin is generally known as fugu toxin and is also an alkaloid produced by some eubacteria such as *Vibrio* and *Pseudomonas*. The authors used a multigas plasma jet operated at 16 kHz and 9 kV provided by an alternating current power supply[89] and showed that N_2 plasma exhibited the optimal capability for tetrodotoxin decomposition, followed by O_2, Ar, and CO_2 plasmas. In this system, the tetrodotoxin concentration decreased to 1/100th its original level by N_2 plasma treatment within 10 minutes.

Microcystin-LR (MC-LR) is one of the most commonly encountered microcystins, which are a class of toxins produced by certain freshwater cyanobacteria that display potential hepatotoxicity in humans. Zhang et al[90] succeeded in degrading MC-LR following exposure to glow discharge plasma using a direct current power supply. In this system, plasma was generated at the gas-solution interface in an Ar atmosphere. Therefore, this arrangement enables the efficient inactivation of toxins in aqueous solution. These studies suggest that plasma may be a promising method for water treatment to help maintain water quality by removing toxins in both freshwater and wastewater.

Biofilms

Plasma inactivation of biofilms or biofilm-forming microorganisms is also an innovative means of reducing the incidence of nosocomial infections and iatrogenic diseases.[73,91-100]

Bacterial biofilms are responsible for disease, prostheses colonization, biofouling, damage to equipment, and pipe plugging.[91] Biofilms are more resistant than free-living vegetative cells against plasma exposure. Therefore, it is necessary to develop appropriate procedures to efficiently remove these biofilms. The use of gas charge plasmas is a good inactivation procedure because plasmas contain a mixture of reactive species that can inactivate microorganisms. Studies on plasma inactivation of biofilms have been reported in the literature.

Pseudomonas aeruginosa biofilms were inactivated after plasma exposure.[91] The adhesiveness and thickness of *Pseudomonas* species biofilms were significantly reduced by etching using an O_2 gas plasma. Morphologic changes and loss of viability upon gas plasma treatment were determined. Plasma-mediated inactivation of *P aeruginosa* biofilms was observed using a culture system. Both biofilm structure and cell culturability were influenced by the gas plasma treatment. The effect of plasma treatment on vegetative cells ranged from minimal modification to major structural changes with an associated loss of viability. The changes in biofilm structure leading to the loss of culturability and viability are related to a decrease in adhesiveness.

Salmonella species can form chemical-resistant biofilms that are difficult to remove from the attached surface.[92] Treatment with cold plasma reduced the thickness of *Salmonella* species biofilms. The D-value of *Salmonella* species biofilms was 7 seconds. The use of cold plasma is particularly suited to antimicrobial processes that need to be biocompatible such as in the medical, pharmaceutical, or food industries.

In other studies, O_2 gas plasma gave the best antibiofilm activity due to its significant etching properties, although this resulted in poor biocompatibility when O_2 was abundant.[96] The DNA on the regenerated surface after removal of biofilms did not have a negative impact on tissue cell surfaces. The results indicated that the application of a restricted percentage of O_2 gas plasma gave promising antibiofilm activity as well as biomaterial compatibility.

Furthermore, the same group reported that discharge O_2 inactivation gave high levels of antibiofilm activity due to its strong etching effects, although this damaged the underlying material.[97] Discharge N_2 and Ar maintained excellent antibacterial ability and antibiofilm activity but had negligible etching effects. An effective inactivation procedure using discharge Ar and N_2 was established in which bacteria could be inactivated in situ and the biofilms removed from the contaminated biomaterials without degradation of the material itself. Moreover, the procedures were found to be applicable to biomedical devices in an in vivo and clinical trial setting.

In addition, discharge gases from O_2, N_2, and Ar demonstrated almost the same antibiofilm activity.[101] Bacteria and biofilm regrowth from discharge gas–treated biofilms was not observed. These observations provide a clue to the mechanism of action of the plasma, which involves severe damage to the cell membranes of the bacteria in the biofilms resulting loss of viability.

An in-depth analysis of the mechanism of plasma action showed that the different reactive species mediated specific antibacterial and/or antibiofilm activity and the etching effect could be manipulated.[102] No bacteria or biofilm regrowth from Ar or N_2 discharge gas–treated biofilms was observed. The inactivation activity of plasmas for the treatment of biofilm-related contamination on materials was also confirmed. The D-value of a *S aureus* biofilm was reported as 3.3 minutes.

Another group reported removal of a *Candida albicans* biofilm following plasma treatment when O_2 gas was added to the Ar gas discharge, whereas Ar gas plasma alone was insufficient for biofilm removal.[94] Plasma etching may be the major factor in biofilm removal because O_2 gas plasma showed a significant etching phenomenon in contrast to Ar gas plasma. A 10- to 20-μm thick *C albicans* biofilm was removed within 5 minutes using an O_2/Ar discharge.

Recently, treatment using an Ar jet plasma with an O_2 gas mixture on a biofilm resulted in effective cleaning of the surface of a tooth due to extensive removal of proteins.[103] Protein removal was confirmed by the decrease of carbon and N_2 detected by X-ray photoelectron spectroscopy (XPS) analysis.

A study to quantify the inactivation of a plasma system on clinically relevant biofilms has also been performed.[93] Clinical isolates of *S epidermidis* and methicillin-resistant *S aureus* (MRSA) were grown as biofilms. The strains produced a biofilm and colony counts were 10^9 colony-forming units (CFUs)/cm^2. Colony-forming units were almost halved ($10^{4.5}$ CFUs/cm^2) after 1 hour of plasma exposure, and the calculated D-value was 13.3 minutes (60 min/4.5). Biofilm samples were placed in medical device bags, and almost identical D-values were obtained against the produced biofilm.

However, bacteria in deeper biofilms are more resistant to nonthermal Ar gas plasma treatment.[104] This is because the penetration depth of Ar gas species is shallow (10-40 nm) and biofilms comprising multilayers of vegetative cells or endospores have a thickness of >10 to 20 μm.[94] Nonetheless, the study showed that nonthermal Ar gas plasma displayed considerable efficiency in eliminating pathogenic bacteria from biofilms and wound surfaces. The role of reactive species in this process remains

unclear because abundant nonionized Ar gas is not bactericidal. The D-value of a *Streptococcus pyogenes* biofilm was reported as 2.8 minutes.

The influence of an atmospheric pressure nonthermal plasma jet in an He and O_2 gas mixture under ambient pressure was evaluated against biofilms of *Bacillus cereus* (gram-positive, endospore), *S aureus* (gram-positive, vegetative cell), *E coli* (gram-negative, vegetative cell), and *P aeruginosa* (gram-negative, vegetative cell).[105] The complete eradication of the two gram-positive bacterial biofilms was achieved. By contrast, gram-negative biofilms required longer plasma treatment than gram-positive biofilms because of the difference in surface morphology. This study provides clues to understanding the mechanism of plasma treatment for the inactivation of biofilms and the differential tolerance of gram-positive and gram-negative bacteria against plasma. Nonetheless, it is difficult to rationalize why gram-positive spore-forming *B cereus* is more susceptible to plasma than gram-negative vegetative cells. All microorganisms tested in this study were in biofilms.

Nutritive components inhibit the penetration of reactive O_2 species (ROS) into bacteria cells, resulting in reduced cell death.[106] These findings can be used to optimize decontamination of meat using atmospheric cold plasma technology. The D-value of atmospheric cold plasma with high O_2 levels using *E coli*, *Listeria monocytogenes*, and *S aureus* was 3.3 minutes, whereas air or a high-N_2 atmosphere yielded lower antimicrobial activities.

In addition, deterioration of functional and material compatibility was not observed in atmospheric He/O_2 plasmas despite displaying effective bacterial inactivation.[107] However, the results depend on the precise concentration of O_2 gas because of its etching phenomenon.

A mixture of He/O_2 cold atmospheric pressure plasma (CAPP) has been known to enhance the wear performance of ultrahigh-molecular-weight polyethylene without affecting the cytocompatibility of the material.[108] Exposure to a CAPP results in a higher level of crosslinking of the polyethylene chains. The higher degree of cross-linking leads to greater stiffness in the treated polymer. The He/O_2 plasma afterglow was shown to effectively inactivate the biofilm and improve material compatibility due to increased hydrophobicity.[98,107,108] Detailed analysis of the system reveals that the primary role in inactivation by plasma exposure is played by ROS (eg, atomic O_2 and •OH radicals) with a subsidiary effect from UV photons, charged particles, heat, and electric fields.[109-113]

A recent article by Puligundla and Mok[114] reviews the inactivation mediated by nonthermal plasma and suggests the technology has great potential for the control of biofilms. Several aspects related to the inactivation of biofilm-associated vegetative cells with different types of nonthermal plasmas under in vitro conditions are presented. The review summarizes methods for biofilm inactivation as well as the characteristics of plasma reactive species and their inactivating mechanisms. The significance of nonthermal plasma inactivation of biofilm-associated bacteria, especially those of medical importance such as pathogenic bacteria and bacteria associated with implants, is described.

Prions

Prions are proteinaceous infectious particles that are the causative agents of transmissible spongiform encephalopathy.[115] The animal prion diseases include bovine spongiform encephalopathy (BSE) in cattle, chronic wasting disease (CWD) in cervids, feline spongiform encephalopathy (FSE) in cats, exotic ungulate encephalopathy (EUE) in zoo animals (eg, kudu, nyala, gemsbok, eland, and oryx), and scrapie in goats and sheep as well as transmissible mink encephalopathy (TME) in mink. Human prion diseases include Creutzfeldt-Jakob disease (CJD), fatal familial insomnia (FFI), Gerstmann-Sträussler-Scheinker syndrome (GSS), and kuru. Although the transmissible agent is the most resistant of all pathogens, it is reported to be inactivated by plasma treatment.

Baxter et al[116] reported decontamination of prion from a metal surface using RF plasma generated from an Ar/O_2 gas mixture. In these experiments, stainless steel spheres were contaminated with scrapie prion and then treated with the RF plasma for 1 hour. The treated and untreated spheres were subjected to intraperitoneal inoculation into hamsters. The results indicated that hamsters inoculated with untreated spheres showed clinical signs at 92 days, whereas hamsters inoculated with plasma-treated spheres survived more than 466 days, suggesting that Ar/O_2 RF plasma successfully decontaminated scrapie prions.

The European project BIODECON[117] reported studies on prion treatment using low-pressure ICP of Ar and Ar mixed with various other gases. The results of animal bioassays using mice and hamsters showed that Ar plasma treatment decreased the transmission rate of prions, but the addition of N_2 to Ar increased the transmission rate compared to 100% for Ar, suggesting that Ar plasma efficiently inactivated prions compared to Ar/N_2. In addition, cell infectivity assays showed decreased transmission of prions following plasma treatment. Taken together, these studies demonstrate successful inactivation of prions by exposure to plasma generated using various methods and gas mixtures.

Julák et al[118] investigated plasma-treated scrapie prions by cell infectivity assay and Western blot analysis, indicating that treatment with plasma generated by corona discharge in open air decreased both PrP^{Sc} (abnormal isoform of prion protein, which is the main component of prions) and PrP^C (cellular isoform of prion protein, which is expressed in healthy cells).

We have carried out preliminary studies of prion inactivation using N_2 gas plasma. Scrapie prion on cover glass was treated with N_2 gas plasma using BLP-TES device and subjected to mouse inoculation via an intracerebral route. The results demonstrate efficient inactivation of the prion by N_2 gas plasma (A. S., unpublished data, 2019).

Taken together, the aforementioned reports suggest that prions can be inactivated by plasma with various plasma sources and gases. However, when the plasma disinfection/sterilization is applied to medical devices, it should be noted that the contaminated prion is derived from humans in a clinic or hospital setting. The previously described reports all use animal prions, which may behave differently from human prions in terms of susceptibility to plasma. Further studies into the effect of plasma exposure on human prion are required before this technology can be used in the clinic.

Moreover, recent studies have suggested misfolded proteins in neurodegenerative diseases such as Alzheimer disease, Parkinson disease, Huntington disease, amyotrophic lateral sclerosis (ALS), frontotemporal dementia, corticobasal degeneration, and progressive supranuclear palsy act as prions or share prion-like mechanisms[119] with transmissible properties. Thus, it would be interesting to establish whether plasma can inactivate these potential agents in order to develop methods to reduce the risk of contamination.

Other Microorganisms

Plasma is also known to be effective for the inactivation of other microorganisms besides those mentioned earlier. For example, cold atmospheric plasma inactivation of *Prototheca zopfii*, a yeast-like algae, has been reported.[120] In this study, 20 strains of *P zopfii* isolated from the milk of cows with clinical and subclinical mastitis were found to be highly susceptible to plasma treatment. In contrast, *C albicans*, which is the most common fungal species isolated from biofilms, either formed on implanted medical devices or on human tissues, was more difficult to inactivate using plasma.[121,122]

A recent paper reported that the waterborne helminth *Schistosoma japonicum* could be inactivated by atmospheric DBD plasma.[123] As shown in Figure 34.3, helminth eggs are generally known to be highly resistant microorganisms. In this system, plasmas generated in O_2 and air gas discharges were more effective in killing *S japonicum* than that generated in He. In addition, similar results were obtained using a gliding arc discharge plasma jet generated in air.

Studies of plasma inactivation on almost all of the microorganisms categorized in Figure 34.3 have already been performed. However, to date, no studies on the plasma treatment of protozoa, including protozoal oocysts and cysts, have been reported. Investigation of the effect of plasma on these microorganisms would contribute to a better understanding of the applicability of this technology.

▶ MECHANISMS OF PLASMA STERILIZATION

Several factors are considered to contribute to the antimicrobial effects of plasma. These factors include various types of ions, electrons, radicals, UV radiation, electric fields, and metastable species. It is important to note that these active species may differ depending on the types of gas used for plasma formation and the methods employed to generate the plasma. In addition, sterilization mechanisms may depend on target microorganisms. These considerations are further discussed in the following text, based on the various types of gases commonly used. It should be noted that most of these discussions of inactivation mechanisms are derived from experiments using bacterial spores.

Oxygen

The most popular gas investigated to date for plasma sterilization is O_2. The O_2 produces •O, •OH, and •OOH radicals and a mixture of other radicals that contribute to the sterilization effect.[82,96,124-129] Among them, the •OH radical is often considered the most efficient for microbial inactivation, despite its short lifetime (10^{-6} s = 1 μs).

The percentage of O_2 gas in the He carrier gas was found to positively correlate with the rate of virucidal activity, indicating ROS play a major role in the virucidal phenomenon.[82] Virucidal rate increased with increasing O_2 concentration, and the D-value was 1.3 minutes under the conditions of H_2/O_2 (99.25/0.75), which was the most appropriate for virucidal activity.

Low-temperature plasma was shown to be effective for the inactivation of bacterial spores.[127] Moreover, the penetrating (etching) effect of charged particles and the oxygenation effect of ROS are thought to play a dominant role in plasma-induced bacterial spore inactivation.

The CAPP with different gas compositions, He with or without N_2 or O_2, was used to inactivate bacteria.[130] Results indicated that CAPP induced a bactericidal phenomenon with He plasma containing O_2 gas giving the most pronounced effect. The *E coli* exposed to the plasma were found to have undergone morphologic changes resulting in membrane leakage. Biochemical analysis of bacterial macromolecules, namely proteins, indicated substantial intracellular protein oxidation. The ROS and reactive N_2 species (RNS) are involved in the inactivation of *E coli*, and the bactericidal mechanism is believed to involve various O_2 radicals, which have an etching effect.[54,66,68,94,131]

Three gases (O_2, N_2, and Ar) for low-power gas discharge plasma were tested and, of these, O_2 displayed the greatest antibiofilm activity because of its excellent inactivating effect of bacteria in biofilms and deeper penetration ability due to etching.[96] However, as described earlier, although O_2 gas may display a powerful bactericidal activity and efficiently remove biofilms, its etching effect may alter the surface chemistry of the underlying biomaterial and adversely affect biocompatibility and biofunctionality. Based on SEM observations of bacterial endospores, the length of exposure to O_2 plasma positively correlates with the degree of observed shrinking of the spores.[132] Moreover, there was a significant relationship between the degree of shrinking and spore death (ie, coefficient of relationship of the regression line was 0.949). By contrast, exposure of spores to N_2 gas plasma did not result in any detectable shrinkage.[133,134] The difference in the mechanisms of O_2 and N_2 gases has yet to be clarified. These findings should be carefully considered in terms of antimicrobial and material/product compatibility.

Tamazawa et al[135] reported that O_2 gas plasma combined with H_2O produced a significant sterilization effect and that sterilization using a mixture of O_2 and H_2O was superior to O_2 alone. These results are consistent with those reported elsewhere.[128,136-138]

Wu et al[139] reported that waterborne viruses showed various levels of damage to both surface proteins and RNA after exposure to atmospheric pressure cold plasma (APCP), leading to a loss in viability and infectivity. The ROS, such as atomic O in APCP, was detected with Ar-O_2 and He-O_2 gas carriers.

Brun et al[140] reported that thymine dimers did not form after exposure to O_2 gas plasma, suggesting the effect of shortwave UV radiation (UV-C) (200-280 nm) was negligible. However, increased expression of 8-hydroxy-2'-deoxyguanosine (8-OHdG) was detected in ocular cells.

Hury et al[69] reported that O_2 gas plasma was much superior to other gas plasmas, such as CO_2, H_2O_2, Ar, or He, for the sterilization of spore formers. Spore surfaces displayed significant disorder when treated with CO_2 gas plasma. However, contrary to the observations of other reports, O_2 gas plasmas did not show significant etching. Given that these results contradict all other reports on this point, the observations need to be reexamined.

Kim et al[141] compared air and N_2 gases in DBD plasma for the inactivation of *Campylobacter jejuni*. Plasma treatment with N_2 gas alone did not reduce the number of CFUs. However, a 0.8 log reduction in CFUs, namely to 0.8 *D-value*, was observed when N_2 gas was supplied with 2% air, equivalent to the addition of 0.4% O_2. The use of air alone (20% O_2) or air supplied with 2% N_2 (almost 20% O_2) or O_2 alone (100% O_2) caused a further decrease in CFUs by 0.7 to 1.7 *D-value*. These results show that O_2 gas in plasma generation is critically important for the increased inactivation due to the etching effect induced by O_2 gas plasma. The SEM analysis showed the presence of cell debris after treatment with air plasma, whereas no cell debris was detected following exposure to N_2 gas plasma, presumably due to reduced levels of etching. The *C jejuni* cells treated with air plasma had truncated flagella with sharp edges, whereas cells treated with N_2 gas plasma were morphologically normal. These observations suggest that air plasma, mostly O_2 gas plasma, damaged the cellular membrane, whereas N_2 gas plasma did not. The degree of damage to the membrane was consistent with the reduced CFUs. However, prolonged exposure to N_2 gas plasma extensively damaged the cellular membranes, although the underlying mechanism remains unclear. Kim et al[141] suggested that air, in particular the O_2 component, was more effective than N_2 gas at inactivating *C jejuni* and that membrane damage may be the major mechanism for the observed bactericidal effect.

Another study used low-pressure inductive discharge for the plasma inactivation process.[142] The O_2 and a mixture of O_2 and H_2O_2 were used as plasma source gases. *Bacillus atrophaeus* ATCC 9372 spore former was used to evaluate the efficacy of the plasma processes. D-values were estimated using survivor curves. D-values between 3 and 8 minutes were obtained depending on the process conditions. The best result, with a D-value of 3 minutes, was achieved at a high-power level using pure O_2 gas due to its significant etching effect.

According to Yong et al,[143] various treatment conditions may affect the inactivation efficiency of *E coli*. The optimum condition was determined by the incorporation of O_2 gas into the N_2 gas flow. The greater the initial CFUs, the greater the observed reduction of viable cell count, probably due to clumping at higher cell densities. Therefore, the initial decrease in CFUs caused by surface destruction was more significant than cell death at deeper regions within the clumps. This phenomenon was not observed if no clumping was present.

Lerouge et al[66] investigated mechanisms of inactivation of spores mediated by low-temperature plasma and compared this with the etching of *B subtilis*, which was exposed to different plasma gas compositions (O_2, O_2/Ar, O_2/H_2, CO_2, and O_2/CF_4). Except for CO_2, these gases are known to cause an etching phenomenon due to the presence of O_2 gas. The O_2/CF_4 plasma exhibited the highest efficacy among all the gases tested. The D-value of *B subtilis* exposed with O_2/CF_4 was less than 1.5 minutes compared to over 4 minutes with O_2 gas alone. It is not known why CO_2 exhibited the etching phenomenon. However, the mechanism of sterilization for the CO_2 gas is thought to be due to the presence of $^1O_2$ species,[24] and examination of SEM images confirmed that the spores were significantly etched. Moreover, the etching rate coincided with the observed death rate.[49]

Nitrogen

Because the N_2 molecule contains a triple bond, its dissociation energy into a plasma is high (Table 34.2). The dissociation energy for N_2 is 9.91 eV, whereas for O_2, it is 5.21 eV. Thus, N_2 gas is resistant to ionization. Consequently, reactive species generated in plasma from N_2 will

Gas	Dissociation Energy (V)
N_2	9.91
O_2	5.21
H_2O	5.11
NO	6.50
SO_2	5.60
N_2O	4.93
CO_2	5.52
O_3	1.05
H_2O_2	2.21

TABLE 34.2 Dissociation energy of several source gases

Abbreviations: CO_2, carbon dioxide; H_2O, water; H_2O_2, hydrogen peroxide; N_2, nitrogen; N_2O, nitrous oxide; NO, nitric oxide; O_2, oxygen; O_3, ozone; SO_2, sulfur dioxide.

Data from Shintani et al[22] with permission from the Society for Antibacterial and Antifungal Agents, Japan.

possess high energy, leading to rapid inactivation of microorganisms. Indeed, N_2 gas plasma has high efficiency and broad spectrum against microorganisms.

Interestingly, Rossi et al[133,134] demonstrated that N_2 gas plasma generated active species, which had no or insufficient ability to shrink bacterial endospores, suggesting a different mechanism of action from O_2. From this, it can be speculated that N^+ ion or •N radicals are difficult to obtain in comparison with O_2. However, it is not known which active species are present to cause the inactivation effect observed with N_2 gas plasmas. The UV-C may be generated but in amounts that are considered to be too low to elicit the observed biological effects.[22,109,144] Vacuum UV radiation (VUV, 10-200 nm) has, however, been confirmed.[145]

If we consider the effects observed with pulsed plasma processes, the direct or contributory effects of the pulsed voltage may lead to direct structural changes in spores, where cracks are evident on microscopic analysis.[22] Overall, whether such physical species significantly contribute to these effects is difficult to assess, and further research is needed to elucidate the true antimicrobial effects and active species involved in N_2 gas plasmas. Although the mechanism of action of the N_2 gas plasma has not been identified, it is well known that N_2 gas plasma is superior in terms of material and functional compatibility.[146] Our group[86] has reported that N_2 gas plasma induced secondary structural changes in the protein bovine serum albumin (BSA). Specifically, exposure to N_2 gas plasma induced an increase in α-helix and decrease in β-sheet content. Nonetheless, the exact mechanism that leads to these changes is still not known. Importantly, however, the plasma-induced effects were different from heat denaturation of BSA, which results in decreased α-helix and increased β-sheet content.

Our group has also reported that the N_2 gas plasma caused DNA and RNA oxidation and protein denaturation after N_2 gas plasma inactivation.[74,147] The DNA oxidation produces 8-OHdG.[147] Roth et al[148] also reported the identical phenomenon of DNA damage and protein inactivation. They speculated that DNA might be the primary target for spore inactivation as a result of UV-C radiation emitted by the N_2/O_2 gas plasma.

Han et al[149] studied an atmospheric cold plasma process for bactericidal activity by examining cell membrane integrity and damage to DNA. The bacteria used were *E coli* and *L monocytogenes*. Working gas mixtures used were air, N_2/O_2 (4/1), N_2/O_2 (9/1), and $O_2/CO_2/N_2$ (13/6/1). Enhanced bactericidal results were observed using working gas mixtures with a higher O_2 content. Cell leakage was assessed by measuring absorbance at 254 nm, and damage to DNA was also monitored. Exposure to plasma compromised membrane integrity and damaged the DNA. The authors speculated that these effects were due to etching mediated by O_2 gas.

Takamatsu et al[24] studied the effect of various gas atmospheric nonthermal plasmas on microbial suspensions. The CO_2 and N_2 gas plasma had high inactivation effects. The CO_2 plasma, which generated the greatest amount of $^1O_2$, inactivated vegetative cells. The N_2 plasma, which generated the largest amount of •OH radicals, inactivated vegetative cells and spore formers with a D-value ranging from 10 seconds to 2.5 minutes. The authors identified the reactive species responsible for the bactericidal effect as being $^1O_2$ and •OH radicals.

The penetration depth of reactive species (ions and radicals) in the case of N_2 gas appears to be approximately 10 to 40 nm from the surface of spores, as observed by atomic force microscopy.[22] This conclusion was consistent with results obtained by Takamatsu et al[24] and Shintani et al,[136] where the major species from RNS were •OH, •NO, and •OONO radicals and those from ROS were $^1O_2$ and •OH radicals. The lifetime of these reactive species is very short.

In our study,[22] the penetration depth of N_2 gas plasma was predicted to be more than 40 nm, whereas O_2 gas plasma had a penetration depth of more than 1 μm.[133,134] Thus, O_2 gas plasma penetrates more than 10 to 100 times deeper than N_2 gas plasma.

Rare or Noble Gases Such as Helium, Neon, Argon, Krypton, and Xenon

There are only a limited number of published reports using Ne, Kr, or Xe gas plasma in contrast to the plethora of papers using He or Ar gas plasma. Plasmas generated from rare gases of He or Ar have been studied in some detail.[61,68,70,94,96,109,128,131,133,150-159]

Pignata et al[150] reported D-values of 8.6 minutes against *A brasiliensis* with the use of Ar alone or O_2 alone. These observations indicated Ar alone and O_2 alone have identical inactivation capacities, which is difficult to reconcile. The authors also reported a D-value of 1 minute with a mixture of Ar/O_2 (10/1). A D-value of 15 or 8 seconds against *E coli* (vegetative cells) was observed with Ar or O_2, respectively, indicating fungi are more tolerant to plasma than vegetative cells. The Ar/O_2 mixture was superior to Ar or O_2 alone because of the enforced plasma inactivation capability due to ROS addition.

Lee et al[131] studied APCP using He/O_2. The authors found the observed result was not due to UV, but ROS. A D-value for the *B subtilis* spore former was 14 minutes compared with a few seconds to a few minutes for vegetative cells. The SEM observations indicated that vegetative cells suffered serious cell damage, evidenced by a shrunken morphology, with an SAL of 10^{-6} and functional/material compatibility.

Yu et al[154] studied the bactericidal effect mediated by Ar gas plasma. Two types of bacteria, *E coli* and *Micrococcus luteus*, were exposed to Ar gas plasma and the survivability was studied. The Ar atmospheric plasma is very effective in the destruction of bacterial cells. The D-value of *E coli* was 0.7 minute and that of *M luteus* was 0.5 minute. The effect of plasma treatment on the bacterial cell was examined by SEM, which revealed significant structural alterations following exposure to the plasma.

Lassen et al[68] studied the sporicidal effect using RF plasma. Experiments using *G stearothermophilus* exposed to plasma generated from Ar/H_2 (3/17) gave a straight-line survivor response, and the D-value was less than 2 minutes. Exposure to CF_4/O_2 plasma caused more damage to the substrate than the Ar/H_2 (3/17) plasma due to the etching effect of O_2. Results indicated that cell inactivation due to UV radiation was insignificant, whereas inactivation through etching by O_2 gas plasma was thought to be a major factor in the observed sporicidal effect. Thus, a sterilization process was realized that combines a sporicidal effect with low substrate damage, due to a low amount of O_2 gas, thereby achieving functional and material compatibility.

Hesby et al[160] indicated that Ar RF glow discharge caused simultaneous inactivation and improvement of surface hydrophilicity of materials. Changes in surface hydrophilicity were determined by contact angle measurements. Enhanced hydrophilicity and wettability were indicated by a lower contact angle and improved biocompatibility.

Park et al[61] investigated two inactivation methodologies—nanosecond pulsed plasma (NPP) and an Ar gas-feeding DBD (Ar-DBD). The experiments were carried out using *S aureus* (wild-type) and multidrug-resistant *S aureus* (penicillin-resistant, methicillin-resistant, and gentamicin-resistant *S aureus*). Both plasma sources can inactivate several types of *S aureus*. Following exposure to the plasma, the authors observed a change in the surface morphology, gene expression, and β-lactamase activity.

Functional groups of the peptidoglycan after plasma exposure were identified, which is indicative of degradation. The observed fragmentation of peptidoglycan was mostly ascribed to the action of ROS such as •OH, •O, as well as •OOH.

Tseng et al[155] reported that there was no detectable fragmentation of the DNA when spores were treated with RF atmospheric He plasma for up to 20 minutes (ie, 10 *D-value* times). The authors reported release of the spore core dipicolinic acid (DPA) almost immediately after the He plasma treatment, indicating rapid and severe damage to the spore envelope resulting in the liberation of spore components.[161]

Rossi et al[133] suggested that direct effects of Ar on exposed spores were similar to those observed following N_2 gas plasma treatment. Similar results were observed using He gas plasma, as shown in other publications.[109,153] Experiments conducted on spores exposed to He gas plasma showed evidence of spore cracking, suggesting He and N_2 share a common mechanism of action.[22,109]

Kim and Kim[153] used an APCP generated using an He/O_2 mixture. Plasma from He/O_2 generates low levels of UV but significant amounts of ROS. Exposure to this plasma resulted in damage to proteins and DNA.

Deng et al[109] studied the mechanisms of cold atmospheric plasma with *B subtilis*. The flow gas was He alone or an He/O_2 mixture. The mechanism of action mainly involved ROS (eg, atomic O_2 and •OH radicals) with a minor contribution from UV. An He/O_2 mixture was superior to He alone due to the etching effect of O_2 gas and more abundant ROS.

Hury et al[69] indicated that O_2, H_2O_2, and CO_2 gas plasma were more efficient for the inactivation of bacterial spores than Ar plasma due to etching by O_2 gas and more abundant ROS. The CO_2 plasma produced abundant •OH radicals. The CO_2 plasma also produced $^1O_2$ species.[24]

A study using Ar plasma was carried out by Nishioka et al,[162] which indicated that exposure to the plasma can damage both the cell membrane and DNA. Contributors responsible for the inactivation of cells remained unidentified, although minor effects due to heat and O_3 were noted. According to their data, the survivor curve gave a significant tailing, that is, a decrease in viable cell number of 3.9 log after 5-minute treatment (D-value 1.28 minutes) and 6.6 log after 40-minute treatment (D-value 6.06 min).

Hosseinzadeh Colagar et al[163] reported that exposure of *E coli* to Ar plasma results in the formation of inactivation zones where DNA and malondialdehyde levels were significantly increased. Banding patterns of total protein were altered, and the amino acid concentration increased due to degradation of proteins from the cell surface.

Hertwig et al[164] reported that plasma generated by Ar alone resulted in negligible emission of UV and atomic O_2, although VUV was detected. Plasma generated with Ar plus trace amounts of O_2 and N_2 as feed gas emitted the highest level of UV-C and considerable amounts of ROS and RNS. Plasma generated with Ar plus a trace amount of O_2 gave the highest emission of ROS, although UV-C levels were negligible. The maximum inactivation of *B subtilis* was achieved using a three-feed gas composition (Ar, O_2, N_2) due to the synergistic effect of UV-C, ROS, and RNS. Taken together, these findings indicate UV-C, VUV, ROS, and RNS play a role in the inactivation of *B subtilis* endospores.

Because rare gases are difficult to ionize, it is unlikely that ions, electrons, radicals, or even UV contribute as active species in the observed plasma sterilization process.[109] Direct comparison to UV exposure alone did not show any sporicidal effects.[109,140]

Tyczkowska-Sieroń and Markiewicz[165] reported that the inhibition zone of *C albicans* ATCC 10231 increased with exposure time to He plasma. This study confirmed that a variety of inactivating species generated in the cold atmospheric plasma, such as UV, radicals, ions, and energetic electrons, play a role in the observed inactivation. Several reports have confirmed the effect of VUV.[145,166,167] Indeed, direct research on the effects of exposure to VUV (174-nm emission using an Ekishima UV apparatus from Iwasaki Electric Co, Ltd, Tokyo, Japan) was conducted, which confirmed the previous observations.[145]

The active species during O_2 gas plasma exposure that are responsible for the observed activity are •O, •OH, and •OOH radicals. However, the active species present in N_2 and rare gas plasmas are more difficult to predict. The O_2 gas plasmas tested to date induce a deterioration in materials due to an etching phenomenon, which is incompatible with many sterilization applications. By contrast, inert gases such as N_2 or rare gases inactivate spores by a different mechanism and are thus more desirable because they can achieve both an SAL of 10^{-6} together with material and functional compatibility required for sterilization validation. The application of these plasmas may prove to be a useful alternative to conventional sterilization methods, such as humidified ethylene oxide gas, gamma ray, electron beam, moist heat sterilization, and dry heat.

Virard et al[168] reported the effects on cell behavior upon exposure to a cold plasma device generating ionization carried by He. This cold plasma treatment induces a predominantly necrotic cell death. Death is not triggered by a direct interaction of the cold plasma with cells but rather via a transient modification in the microenvironment. Thus, necrosis seems to be an active response to an environmental trigger.

Winter et al[70] studied the interaction between *B subtilis* and Ar plasma. The authors investigated the plasma-specific stress response of *B subtilis* toward not only Ar but also air plasma. Cellular responses were observed due to the synergistic effect of Ar and air plasma treatment, which included DNA damage and oxidative stress. A variety of gas-dependent cellular responses, such as growth retardation and morphologic changes, were observed, mostly due to the etching effect by O_2 gas in the air plasma.

Brun et al[140] tested APCP combined with He gas flow effects on *P aeruginosa*, *E coli*, *S aureus*, *C albicans*, *Aspergillus fumigatus*, and herpes simplex virus type 1. A reduction of microbial viability was observed following exposure to APCP. Increased levels of intracellular ROS in exposed microorganisms and cells were detected. Immunoassays demonstrated no induction of thymine dimers (ie, absence of UV-C irradiation) in cell cultures. Transient increased expression of 8-OHdG and genes and proteins related to oxidative stress was detected in ocular cells exposed to plasma.

Hong et al[125] studied an electrical discharge plasma at an RF. The discharge gas was He with 0% to 2% O_2. For the plasma treatment, *E coli* or *B subtilis* endospores were exposed to O_2 downstream in an He atmosphere. The inactivation effect of the RF plasma was highest with 0.2% O_2, corresponding to the maximum production of O_2 radicals.

According to Yu et al,[154] Ar atmospheric plasma was effective in the inactivation of *E coli* (gram-negative vegetative cells) and *M luteus* (gram-positive vegetative cells). D-values of *E coli* and that of *M luteus* were 0.7 and 0.5 minutes, respectively. The SEM observations indicated that the cellular structures of both organisms were damaged after plasma treatment.

Speculated Mechanisms of Action of Plasma

The mechanisms of action of plasma are clearly an area for further research. It has been suggested that they are related to various oxidation and reduction effects on the macromolecules that make up microbial structures (such as protein, lipids, and nucleic acids).[169] None of the studies published to date have directly demonstrated or clarified the mechanisms of plasma action. Furthermore, differences in the mechanisms of action have been reported between O_2-based plasmas in comparison to other inert gases, such as N_2, He, and Ar.

The external and internal structure of a bacterial endospore vary depending on the bacterial species and growth conditions. A useful description for the purpose of this discussion is given.[170] The inner spore membranes are relatively rigid structures, where only molecules of less than 200 Da are capable of passing through. These membranes are important because they contain receptors for various germinants that promote germination and outgrowth of the spore.[171] Despite their importance, if the inner membrane is damaged, DPA leaks out (as a clear indicator of both structural spore damage and initial germination) and germination is subsequently prevented.[155] According to Roth et al,[148] treatment of *B subtilis* with N_2/O_2 gas plasma damages DNA, proteins, and the spore membrane. Moreover, inactivation of catalase activity

and the leakage of DPA were observed. Small acid soluble proteins (SASPs) were particularly sensitive to plasma treatment. The UV-C appears to be the most effective agent in plasma, although this may vary depending on the source gases or plasma production procedures. Access to spore membranes is limited due to the various spore coats at the outermost part of the spore structure. Extensive damage/penetration is required for the inner membrane to be exposed. The inner core of the spore itself has various protection mechanisms, including the SASPs that are tightly associated with DNA and protect it from physical/chemical attacks. Thus, DNA damage is an important factor to consider. Inert gases are inactive, but excited inert gas (metastable gas) atoms and radicals are thought to be capable of penetrating into the interior of the spore, without interfering with charged proteins and lipids surrounding the inner membrane and core. Excited atoms and radicals may therefore pass through the inner membrane in order to attack the DNA at the core. In this sense, cations, anions, and electrons are not thought to be candidates for damaging the interior of the spore. Whether the inner membrane is damaged or not can be clarified by observation using phase-contrast microscopy or SEM.[172] The DPA release can be monitored in the culture medium in the vicinity of the spores.[161] The reader should refer to Setlow[173] for an insightful discussion on this topic, even though the experiments do not use plasma.

Sporicidal effects are predominantly observed at the spore surface, leading to etching and shrinkage. These effects may initially cause spore surface damage (by oxidation-reduction reactions), but the affected proteins and other macromolecules are then cross-linked to each other, resulting in the loss of spore viability.

▶ CONCLUSION

To minimize the risk of microbial hazards, plasma technology may provide an innovative disinfection/sterilization method with numerous potential applications in the field of medicine, dentistry, agriculture, and environmental science. However, further studies are necessary before this technology can be put into practical use.

First, safety aspects of the application must be established. This can be achieved by implementing existing engineering designs and safety standards as well as considerations in applicable regulations and standards. Plasma exposure of aqueous solution results in the generation of ROS and RNS, which may react to form further toxic compounds.[174,175] Therefore, the levels of these harmful by-products generated during plasma treatment should be investigated. In addition, the choice of gases or their mixed composition is important for optimization and safety of the procedure. This is because source gases of plasma are a major determinant in generating reactive species.

Second, information concerning the effect of plasma treatment on bacteria is accumulating, although data on other microorganisms and toxins remain limited. In particular, there is a lack of data on the effect of plasma treatment on plant viruses and protozoa. Moreover, susceptibility of microorganisms to plasma may be different depending on the derived species. For example, in the case of prions, susceptibility of scrapie prion to plasma may differ from that of human prion. Therefore, further studies using matched species are required.

Third, at present, most plasma instruments use a sample box for gas injection to control atmospheric pressure. Thus, the application/target space is limited, which in turn restricts sample size and current range of applications. If the plasma can be generated in the open air, it will remove this size limitation. Thus, the development of an instrument enabling an open air system would be advantageous in processing both large objects and high numbers of samples, which would considerably enhance the scale of the instrumentation. An alternative approach is to generate plasma at a remote site and then transfer it to a small target (eg, a plasma jet). In this case, to enlarge the target site, an array setup of plasma jets or a fundamental modification of plasma generation will be required.

Fourth, we need to better understand the mechanism of action of the plasma. Information on the mechanisms by which each pathogen is inactivated remains rather limited. The disinfection mechanisms may depend on the plasma instrument and gas inlet as well as the microorganisms being treated. In particular, the energy used for gas ionization by discharge brings about significant differences in disinfection properties.[176-178] Furthermore, it should be noted that recent studies have shown that the relative humidity (RH) during plasma generation significantly influences the efficacy of microorganism inactivation, possibly due to the change of ROS generation and their species caused by different RH levels.[138,179] Therefore, RH levels may be a critical control parameter in practical use. Therefore, detailed analysis of inactivation mechanisms using various plasma sources and gases as well as various microorganisms is required. Additional understanding will undoubtedly contribute to the optimization of disinfection efficiency. Optimization of the plasma-generating conditions, such as using mixtures of gases and controlling RH levels, may facilitate the development of a highly efficient equipment.

REFERENCES

1. Mott-Smith HM. History of "plasmas." *Nature.* 1971;233(5316):219.
2. Langmuir I. Oscillations in ionized gases. *Proc Natl Acad Sci U S A.* 1928;14(8):627-637.
3. Raiser J, Zenker M. Argon plasma coagulation for open surgical and endoscopic applications: state of the art. *J Phys D Appl Phys.* 2006;39:3520-3523.
4. Laroussi M, Kong MG, Morfill G, Stolz W. *Plasma Medicine: Applications of Low-Temperature Gas Plasmas in Medicine and Biology.* London, United Kingdom: Cambridge University Press; 2012.
5. Hoffmann C, Berganza C, Zhang J. Cold atmospheric plasma: methods of production and application in dentistry and oncology. *Med Gas Res.* 2013;3(1):21.
6. Cha S, Park YS. Plasma in dentistry. *Clin Plasma Med.* 2014;2(1):4-10.
7. Cullen PJ, Lalor J, Scally L, et al. Translation of plasma technology from the lab to the food industry. *Plasma Process Polym.* 2018;15(2):e1700085.
8. Ito M, Oh JS, Ohta T, Shiratani M, Hori M. Current status and future prospects of agricultural applications using atmospheric-pressure plasma technologies. *Plasma Process Polym.* 2018;15(2):e1700073.
9. Hashim SA, Samsudin FN, Wong CS, Abu Bakar K, Yap SL, Mohd Zin MF. Non-thermal plasma for air and water remediation. *Arch Biochem Biophys.* 2016;605:34-40.
10. Bansode AS, More SE, Siddiqui EA, et al. Effective degradation of organic water pollutants by atmospheric non-thermal plasma torch and analysis of degradation process. *Chemosphere.* 2017;167:396-405.
11. Magureanu M, Piroi D, Mandache NB, et al. Degradation of antibiotics in water by non-thermal plasma treatment. *Water Res.* 2011;45(11): 3407-3416.
12. Jacobs PT, Lin SM, inventors; Ethicon Inc, assignee. Hydrogen peroxide plasma sterilization system. US patent 4,643,876. February 17, 1987.
13. Moulton KA, Campbell BA, Caputo RA, inventors; DePuy Orthopaedics Inc, assignee. Plasma sterilizing process with pulsed antimicrobial agent treatment. US patent 5,084,239. January 28, 1992.
14. Finnegan M, Linley E, Denyer SP, McDonnell G, Simons C, Maillard JY. Mode of action of hydrogen peroxide and other oxidizing agents: differences between liquid and gas forms. *J Antimicrob Chemother.* 2010;65(10):2108-2115.
15. Jacobs PT, Lin SM, inventors; Ethicon Inc, assignee. Hydrogen peroxide plasma sterilization system. US patent 4,756,882. July 12, 1988.
16. Krebs MC, Bécasse P, Verjat D, Darbord JC. Gas plasma sterilization: relative efficacy of the hydrogen peroxide phase compared with that of the plasma phase. *Int J Pharm.* 1998;160:75-81.
17. Sakudo A, Shintani H. *Nova Medical: Sterilization and Disinfection by Plasma: Sterilization Mechanisms, Biological and Medical Applications (Medical Devices and Equipment).* New York, NY: Nova Science; 2010.
18. U.S. Food and Drug Administration (FDA). FDA Talk paper No. T98-17, April 2, 1998.
19. Gibbs J, Matthees S. Lessons learned from the AbTox ruling. MDDI Web site. https://www.mddionline.com/lessons-learned-abtox-ruling. Accessed May 28, 2019.
20. Furuhata S, Nishimura C, Furuhashi N, et al. Effectiveness test of low temperature plasma sterilization method using peracetic acid and hydrogen peroxide [in Japanese]. *Jpn J Assoc Operative Med.* 2000;21:140-144.
21. Sakudo A, Toyokawa Y, Misawa T, Imanishi Y. Degradation and detoxification of aflatoxin B_1 using nitrogen gas plasma generated by a static induction thyristor as a pulsed power supply. *Food Control.* 2017;73:619-626.
22. Shintani H, Shimizu N, Imanishi Y, et al. Inactivation of microorganisms and endotoxins by low temperature nitrogen gas plasma exposure. *Biocontrol Sci.* 2007;12(4):131-143.
23. McCombs GB, Darby ML. New discoveries and directions for medical, dental and dental hygiene research: low temperature atmospheric pressure plasma. *Int J Dent Hyg.* 2010;8(1):10-15.
24. Takamatsu T, Uehara K, Sasaki Y, et al. Microbial inactivation in the liquid phase induced by multigas plasma jet. *PLoS One.* 2015;10(7):e0132381.
25. Kamgang-Youbi G, Herry JM, Meylheuc T, et al. Microbial inactivation using plasma-activated water obtained by gliding electric discharges. *Lett Appl Microbiol.* 2009;48(1):13-18.
26. Park JY, Park S, Choe W, Yong HI, Jo C, Kim K. Plasma-functionalized solution: a potent antimicrobial agent for biomedical applications from antibacterial therapeutics to biomaterial surface engineering. *ACS Appl Mater Interfaces.* 2017;9:43470-43477.
27. Ikawa S, Tani A, Nakashima Y, Kitano K. Physicochemical properties of bactericidal plasma-treated water. *J Phys D Appl Phys.* 2016;49: 425401.
28. Duan J, Lu X, He G. The selective effect of plasma activated medium in an in vitro co-culture of liver cancer and normal cells. *J Appl Phys.* 2017;121:013302.

29. Yan D, Talbot A, Nourmohammadi N, et al. Principles of using cold atmospheric plasma stimulated media for cancer treatment. *Sci Rep.* 2015;5:18339.

30. Van Boxem W, Van der Paal J, Gorbanev Y, et al. Anti-cancer capacity of plasma-treated PBS: effect of chemical composition on cancer cell cytotoxicity. *Sci Rep.* 2017;7:16478.

31. Liedtke KR, Bekeschus S, Kaeding A, et al. Non-thermal plasma-treated solution demonstrates antitumor activity against pancreatic cancer cells in vitro and in vivo. *Sci Rep.* 2017;7:8319.

32. Bekeschus S, Schmidt A, Weltmann KD, von Woedtke T. The plasma jet kINPen—a powerful tool for wound healing. *Clin Plasma Med.* 2016;4:19-28.

33. Isbary G, Zimmermann JL, Shimizu T, et al. Non-thermal plasma—more than five years of clinical experience. *Clin Plasma Med.* 2013;1:19-23.

34. Daeschlein G, Napp M, von Podewils S, et al. In vitro susceptibility of multidrug resistant skin and wound pathogens against low temperature atmospheric pressure plasma jet (APPJ) and dielectric barrier discharge plasma (DBD). *Plasma Process Polym.* 2014;11:175-183.

35. Kluge S, Bekeschus S, Bender C, et al. Investigating the mutagenicity of a cold argon-plasma jet in an HET-MN model. *PLoS One.* 2016;11(9):e0160667.

36. Brehmer F, Haenssle HA, Daeschlein G, et al. Alleviation of chronic venous leg ulcers with a hand-held dielectric barrier discharge plasma generator (PlasmaDerm® VU-2010): results of a monocentric, two-armed, open, prospective, randomized and controlled trial (NCT01415622). *J Eur Acad Dermatol Venereol.* 2015;29(1):148-155.

37. Isbary G, Morfill G, Schmidt HU, et al. A first prospective randomized controlled trial to decrease bacterial load using cold atmospheric argon plasma on chronic wounds in patients. *Br J Dermatol.* 2010;163(1):78-82.

38. Weltmann KD, von Woedtke T. Plasma medicine—current state of research and medical application. *Plasma Phys Control Fusion.* 2017;59:014031.

39. Yan D, Sherman JH, Keidar M. Cold atmospheric plasma, a novel promising anti-cancer treatment modality. *Oncotarget.* 2017;8(9):15977-15995.

40. Tanaka H, Mizuno M, Toyokuni S, et al. Cancer therapy using non-thermal atmospheric pressure plasma with ultra-high electron density. *Phys Plasmas.* 2015;22:122004.

41. Nandkumar N. Plasma—the fourth state of matter. *Int J Sci Tech Res.* 2014;3(9):49-52.

42. Fridman A. *Plasma Chemistry.* Cambridge, United Kingdom: Cambridge University Press; 2012.

43. Teschke M, Kedzierski J, Finantu-Dinu EG, Korzec D, Engemann J. High-speed photographs of a dielectric barrier atmospheric pressure plasma jet. *IEEE Trans Plasma Sci.* 2005;33:310-311.

44. Conrads H, Schmidt M. Plasma generation and plasma sources. *Plasma Sources Sci Technol.* 2000;9:441-454.

45. Xiao D, ed. Fundamentals of gas discharge. In: *Gas Discharge and Gas Insulation. Energy and Environment Research in China.* Vol 6. Berlin, Germany: Springer; 2016:19-45.

46. Xiao D, ed. Fundamental theory of Townsend discharge. In: *Gas Discharge and Gas Insulation. Energy and Environment Research in China.* Vol 6. Berlin, Germany: Springer; 2016:47-88.

47. Fridman A, Friedman G. *Plasma Medicine.* Oxford, United Kingdom: Wiley-Blackwell; 2013.

48. Shintani H, Sakudo A. *Gas Plasma Sterilization in Microbiology: Theory, Applications, Pitfalls and New Perspectives.* London, United Kingdom: Caister Academic Press; 2016.

49. Shintani H, Sakudo A, Burke P, McDonnell G. Gas plasma sterilization of microorganisms and mechanisms of action. *Exp Ther Med.* 2010;1(5):731-738.

50. Niemira BA. Cold plasma reduction of *Salmonella* and *Escherichia coli* O157:H7 on almonds using ambient pressure gases. *J Food Sci.* 2012;77(3):M171-M175.

51. Klampfl TG, Isbary G, Shimizu T, et al. Cold atmospheric air plasma sterilization against spores and other microorganisms of clinical interest. *Appl Environ Microbiol.* 2012;78(15):5077-5082.

52. Sung SJ, Huh JB, Yun MJ, Chang BM, Jeong CM, Jeon YC. Sterilization effect of atmospheric pressure non-thermal air plasma on dental instruments. *J Adv Prosthodont.* 2013;5(1):2-8.

53. Tian Y, Sun P, Wu H, et al. Inactivation of *Staphylococcus aureus* and *Enterococcus faecalis* by a direct-current, cold atmospheric-pressure air plasma microjet. *J Biomed Res.* 2010;24(4):264-269.

54. Moisan M, Barbeau J, Moreau S, Pelletier J, Tabrizian M, Yahia LH. Low-temperature sterilization using gas plasmas: a review of the experiments and an analysis of the inactivation mechanisms. *Int J Pharm.* 2001;226(1-2):1-21.

55. Ehlbeck J, Schnabel U, Polak M, et al. Low temperature atmospheric pressure plasma sources for microbial decontamination. *J Phys D Appl Phys.* 2011;44:013002.

56. Scholtz V, Julák J, Kříha V. The microbicidal effect of low-temperature plasma generated by corona discharge: comparison of various microorganisms on an agar surface or in aqueous suspension. *Plasma Process Polym.* 2010;7:237-243.

57. Scholtz V, Kommová L, Julák J. The influence of parameters of stabilized corona discharge on its microbicidal effect. *Acta Phys Polon A.* 2011;119:803-806.

58. World Health Organization. Antimicrobial resistance. World Health Organization Web site. http://www.who.int/mediacentre/factsheets/fs194/en/. Accessed May 28, 2019.

59. Centers for Disease Control and Prevention. National Antimicrobial Resistance Monitoring System for Enteric Bacteria (NARMS). Centers for Disease Control and Prevention Web site. https://www.cdc.gov/narms/index.html/. Accessed May 28, 2019.

60. Krauland MG, Marsh JW, Paterson DL, Harrison LH. Integron-mediated multidrug resistance in a global collection of nontyphoidal *Salmonella enterica* isolates. *Emerg Infect Dis.* 2009;15(3):388-396.

61. Park JH, Kumar N, Park DH, et al. A comparative study for the inactivation of multidrug resistance bacteria using dielectric barrier discharge and nano-second pulsed plasma. *Sci Rep.* 2015;5:13849.

62. Kvam E, Davis B, Mondello F, Garner AL. Nonthermal atmospheric plasma rapidly disinfects multidrug-resistant microbes by inducing cell surface damage. *Antimicrob Agents Chemother.* 2012;56(4):2028-2036.

63. Maeda K, Toyokawa Y, Shimizu N, Imanishi Y, Sakudo A. Inactivation of *Salmonella* by nitrogen gas plasma generated by a static induction thyristor as a pulsed power supply. *Food Control.* 2015;52:54-59.

64. International Standards Organization. *Sterilization of Health Care Products—General Requirements for Characterization of a Sterilizing Agent and the Development, Validation, and Routine Control of a Sterilization Process for Medical Devices.* Geneva, Switzerland: International Standards Organization; 2009.

65. Rutala WA, Weber DJ; for Healthcare Infection Control Practices Advisory Committee. Guideline for disinfection and sterilization in healthcare facilities, 2008. Centers for Disease Control and Prevention Web site. https://www.cdc.gov/infectioncontrol/guidelines/disinfection/. Accessed May 28, 2019.

66. Lerouge S, Wertheimer MR, Marchand R, Tabrizian M, Yahia L. Effect of gas composition on spore mortality and etching during low-pressure plasma sterilization. *J Biomed Mater Res.* 2000;51(1):128-135.

67. Lassen KS, Nordby B, Grun R. Optimization of a RF-generated CF_4/O_2 gas plasma sterilization process. *J Biomed Mater Res B Appl Biomater.* 2003;65(2):239-244.

68. Lassen KS, Nordby B, Grun R. The dependence of the sporicidal effects on the power and pressure of RF-generated plasma processes. *J Biomed Mater Res B Appl Biomater.* 2005;74(1):553-559.

69. Hury S, Vidal DR, Desor F, Pelletier J, Lagarde T. A parametric study of the destruction efficiency of *Bacillus* spores in low pressure oxygen-based plasmas. *Lett Appl Microbiol.* 1998;26(6):417-421.

70. Winter T, Bernhardt J, Winter J, et al. Common versus noble *Bacillus subtilis* differentially responds to air and argon gas plasma. *Proteomics.* 2013;13(17):2608-2621.

71. Soušková H, Scholtz V, Julak J, Kommová L, Savická D, Pazlarová J. The survival of micromycetes and yeasts under the low-temperature plasma generated in electrical discharge. *Folia Microbiol (Praha).* 2011;56(1):77-79.

72. Soušková H, Scholtz V, Julák J, Savická D. The fungal spores survival under the low-temperature plasma. In: Machala Z, Hensel K, Akishev Y, eds. *Plasma for Bio-Decontamination, Medicine and Food Security* (NATO Science for Peace and Security Series A: Chemistry and Biology). New York, NY: Springer; 2012:57-66.

73. Scholtz V, Pazlarova J, Soušková H, Khun J, Julak J. Nonthermal plasma—a tool for decontamination and disinfection. *Biotechnol Adv.* 2015;33(6, pt 2):1108-1119.

74. Sakudo A, Misawa T, Shimizu N, Imanishi Y. N_2 gas plasma inactivates influenza virus mediated by oxidative stress. *Front Biosci (Elite Ed).* 2014;6:69-79.

75. Sakudo A, Shimizu N, Imanishi Y, Ikuta K. N_2 gas plasma inactivates influenza virus by inducing changes in viral surface morphology, protein, and genomic RNA. *Biomed Res Int.* 2013;2013:694269.

76. Sakudo A, Toyokawa Y, Imanishi Y, Murakami T. Crucial roles of reactive chemical species in modification of respiratory syncytial virus by nitrogen gas plasma. *Mater Sci Eng C Mater Biol Appl.* 2017;74: 131-136.

77. Sakudo A, Toyokawa Y, Imanishi Y. Nitrogen gas plasma generated by a static induction thyristor as a pulsed power supply inactivates adenovirus. *PLoS One.* 2016;11(6):e0157922.

78. Zimmermann JL, Dumler K, Shimizu T, et al. Effects of cold atmospheric plasmas on adenoviruses in solution. *J Phys D Appl Phys.* 2011;44:505201.

79. Terrier O, Essere B, Yver M, et al. Cold oxygen plasma technology efficiency against different airborne respiratory viruses. *J Clin Virol.* 2009;45(2):119-124.

80. Aboubakr HA, Williams P, Gangal U, et al. Virucidal effect of cold atmospheric gaseous plasma on feline calicivirus, a surrogate for human norovirus. *Appl Environ Microbiol.* 2015;81(11):3612-3622.

81. Nayak G, Aboubakr HA, Goyal SM, Bruggeman PJ. Reactive species responsible for the inactivation of feline calicivirus by a two-dimensional array of integrated coaxial microhollow dielectric barrier discharges in air. *Plasma Process Polym.* In press.

82. Alshraiedeh NH, Alkawareek MY, Gorman SP, Graham WG, Gilmore BF. Atmospheric pressure, nonthermal plasma inactivation of MS2 bacteriophage: effect of oxygen concentration on virucidal activity. *J Appl Microbiol.* 2013;115(6):1420-1426.

83. US Environmental Protection Agency. *Guide Standard and Protocol for Testing Microbiological Water Purifiers.* Washington, DC: US Environmental Protection Agency; 1987.

84. Sakudo A, Imanishi Y. Degradation and inactivation of Shiga toxins by nitrogen gas plasma. *AMB Express.* 2017;7(1):77.

85. US Food and Drug Administration. Sec. 683.100 Action levels for aflatoxin in animal feeds. Compliance policy guide. Guidance for FDA staff. US Food and Drug Administration Web site. http://www.fda.gov/ICECI/ComplianceManuals/CompliancePolicyGuidanceManual/ucm074703.htm. Updated March 2019. Accessed 28 May, 2019.

86. Sakudo A, Higa M, Maeda K, Shimizu N, Imanishi Y, Shintani H. Sterilization mechanism of nitrogen gas plasma: induction of secondary structural change in protein. *Microbiol Immunol.* 2013;57(7):536-542.

87. Park BJ, Takatori K, Sugita-Konishi Y, et al. Degradation of mycotoxins using microwave-induced argon plasma at atmospheric pressure. *Surf Coat Tech.* 2017;201:5733-5737.

88. Takamatsu T, Hirai H, Sasaki R, Miyahara H, Okino A. Surface hydrophilization of polyimide films using atmospheric damage-free multigas plasma jet source. *IEEE Trans Plasma Sci.* 2013;41:119-125.

89. Takamatsu T, Miyahara H, Azuma T, Okino A. Decomposition of tetrodotoxin using multi-gas plasma jet. *J Toxicol Sci.* 2014;39(2): 281-284.

90. Zhang H, Huang Q, Ke Z, Yang L, Wang X, Yu Z. Degradation of microcystin-LR in water by glow discharge plasma oxidation at the gas-solution interface and its safety evaluation. *Water Res.* 2012;46(19):6554-6562.

91. Vandervoort KG, Brelles-Marino G. Plasma-mediated inactivation of *Pseudomonas aeruginosa* biofilms grown on borosilicate surfaces under continuous culture system. *PLoS One.* 2014;9(10):e108512.

92. Niemira BA, Boyd G, Sites J. Cold plasma rapid decontamination of food contact surfaces contaminated with *Salmonella* biofilms. *J Food Sci.* 2014;79(5):M917-M922.

93. Cotter JJ, Maguire P, Soberon F, Daniels S, O'Gara JP, Casey E. Disinfection of meticillin-resistant *Staphylococcus aureus* and *Staphylococcus epidermidis* biofilms using a remote non-thermal gas plasma. *J Hosp Infect.* 2011;78(3):204-207.

94. Fricke K, Koban I, Tresp H, et al. Atmospheric pressure plasma: a high-performance tool for the efficient removal of biofilms. *PLoS One.* 2012;7(8):e42539.

95. Liu D, Xiong Z, Du T, Zhou X, Cao Y, Lu X. Bacterial-killing effect of atmospheric pressure non-equilibrium plasma jet and oral mucosa response. *J Huazhong Univ Sci Technolog Med Sci.* 2011;31(6):852-856.

96. Traba C, Chen L, Liang JF. Low power gas discharge plasma mediated inactivation and removal of biofilms formed on biomaterials. *Curr Appl Phys.* 2013;13(suppl 1):S12-S18.

97. Traba C, Chen L, Liang D, Azzam R, Liang JF. Insights into discharge argon-mediated biofilm inactivation. *Biofouling.* 2013;29(10): 1205-1213.

98. Joaquin JC, Kwan C, Abramzon N, Vandervoort K, Brelles-Mariño G. Is gas-discharge plasma a new solution to the old problem of biofilm inactivation? *Microbiology.* 2009;155(pt 3):724-732.

99. Ojano-Dirain C, Antonelli PJ. *Pseudomonas* biofilm formation after *Haemophilus* infection. *Otolaryngol Head Neck Surg.* 2011;145(3): 470-475.

100. Ayliffe G; for Minimal Access Therapy Decontamination Working Group. Decontamination of minimally invasive surgical endoscopes and accessories. *J Hosp Infect.* 2000;45(4):263-277.

101. Traba C, Liang JF. Susceptibility of *Staphylococcus aureus* biofilms to reactive discharge gases. *Biofouling.* 2011;27(7):763-772.

102. Traba C, Liang JF. The inactivation of *Staphylococcus aureus* biofilms using low-power argon plasma in a layer-by-layer approach. *Biofouling.* 2015;31(1):39-48.

103. Jablonowski L, Fricke K, Matthes R, et al. Removal of naturally grown human biofilm with an atmospheric pressure plasma jet: an in-vitro study. *J Biophotonics.* 2017;10(5):718-726.

104. Ermolaeva SA, Varfolomeev AF, Chernukha MY, et al. Bactericidal effects of non-thermal argon plasma in vitro, in biofilms and in the animal model of infected wounds. *J Med Microbiol.* 2011;60(pt 1):75-83.

105. Alkawareek MY, Algwari QT, Gorman SP, Graham WG, O'Connell D, Gilmore BF. Application of atmospheric pressure nonthermal plasma for the in vitro eradication of bacterial biofilms. *FEMS Immunol Med Microbiol.* 2012;65(2):381-384.

106. Han L, Ziuzina D, Heslin C, et al. Controlling microbial safety challenges of meat using high voltage atmospheric cold plasma. *Front Microbiol.* 2016;7:977.

107. Vleugels M, Shama G, Deng XT, et al. Atmospheric plasma inactivation of biofilm-forming bacteria for food safety control. *IEEE Trans Plasma Sci.* 2005;33:824-828.

108. Perni S, Kong MG, Prokopovich P. Cold atmospheric pressure gas plasma enhances the wear performance of ultra-high molecular weight polyethylene. *Acta Biomater.* 2012;8(3):1357-1365.

109. Deng X, Shi J, Kong MG. Physical mechanisms of inactivation of *Bacillus subtilis* spores using cold atmospheric plasmas. *IEEE Trans Plasma Sci.* 2006;34:1310-1316.

110. Perni S, Shama G, Hobman JL, et al. Probing bactericidal mechanisms induced by cold atmospheric plasmas with *Escherichia coli* mutants. *Appl Physics Lett.* 2007;90:073902.

111. Shi J, Liu D, Kong M. Effects of dielectric barriers in radio frequency atmospheric glow discharges. *IEEE Trans Plasma Sci.* 2007;35:137-142.

112. Walsh JL, Kong MG. Sharp bursts of high-flux reactive species in sub-microsecond atmospheric pressure glow discharges. *Appl Phys Lett.* 2006;89:231503.

113. Walsh JL, Shi JJ, Kong MG. Contrasting characteristics of pulsed and sinusoidal cold atmospheric plasma jets. *Appl Phys Lett.* 2006;88:171501.

114. Puligundla P, Mok C. Potential applications of nonthermal plasmas against biofilm-associated micro-organisms in vitro. *J Appl Microbiol.* 2017;122(5):1134-1148.

115. Sakudo A, Onodera T. *Prions: Current Progress in Advanced Research.* Poole, United Kingdom: Caister Academic Press; 2013.

116. Baxter HC, Campbell GA, Whittaker AG, et al. Elimination of transmissible spongiform encephalopathy infectivity and decontamination of surgical instruments by using radio-frequency gas-plasma treatment. *J Gen Virol.* 2005;86(pt 8):2393-2399.

117. Keudell A, Awakowicz P, Benedikt J, et al. Inactivation of bacteria and biomolecules by low-pressure plasma discharges. *Plasma Process Polym.* 2010;7:327-352.

118. Julák J, Janoušková O, Scholtz V, Holada K. Inactivation of prions using electrical DC discharges at atmospheric pressure and ambient temperature. *Plasma Process Polym.* 2011;8:316-323.

119. Prusiner SB. Biology and genetics of prions causing neurodegeneration. *Annu Rev Genet.* 2013;47:601-623.

120. Tyczkowska-Sieron E, Markiewicz J, Grzesiak B, Krukowski H, Glowacka A, Tyczkowski J. Short communication: cold atmospheric plasma inactivation of *Prototheca zopfii* isolated from bovine milk. *J Dairy Sci.* 2018;101:118-122.

121. Kumamoto CA. *Candida* biofilms. *Curr Opin Microbiol.* 2002;5(6):608-611.

122. Donlan RM. Biofilm formation: a clinically relevant microbiological process. *Clin Infect Dis.* 2001;33(8):1387-1392.

123. Wang XQ, Wang FP, Chen W, Huang J, Bazaka K, Ostrikov KK. Non-equilibrium plasma prevention of *Schistosoma japonicum* transmission. *Sci Rep.* 2016;6:35353.

124. Jacobs PT, Lin SM. Sterilization processes utilizing low temperature plasma. In: Block SM, ed. *Disinfection, Sterilization, and Preservation.* 5th ed. Philadelphia, PA: Lippincott Williams & Wilkins; 2001:747-764.

125. Hong YF, Kang JG, Lee HY, Uhm HS, Moon E, Park YH. Sterilization effect of atmospheric plasma on *Escherichia coli* and *Bacillus subtilis* endospores. *Lett Appl Microbiol.* 2009;48(1):33-37.

126. Thiyagarajan M, Sarani A, Gonzales XF. Characterization of an atmospheric pressure plasma jet and its applications for disinfection and cancer treatment. *Stud Health Technol Inform.* 2013;184:443-449.

127. Shi XM, Zhang GJ, Yuan YK, Ma Y, Xu GM, Gu N. Inactivation of bacterial spores using low-temperature plasma. *Nan Fang Yi Ke Da Xue Xue Bao.* 2009;29(10):2033-2036.

128. Purevdorj D, Igura N, Ariyada O, Hayakawa I. Effect of feed gas composition of gas discharge plasmas on *Bacillus pumilus* spore mortality. *Lett Appl Microbiol.* 2003;37(1):31-34.

129. Halliwell B, Gutteridge JMC. *Free Radicals in Biology and Medicine.* 4th ed. Oxford, United Kingdom: Oxford University Press; 2007.

130. Dezest M, Bulteau AL, Quinton D, et al. Oxidative modification and electrochemical inactivation of *Escherichia coli* upon cold atmospheric pressure plasma exposure. *PLoS One.* 2017;12(3):e0173618.

131. Lee K, Paek KH, Ju WT, Lee Y. Sterilization of bacteria, yeast, and bacterial endospores by atmospheric-pressure cold plasma using helium and oxygen. *J Microbiol.* 2006;44(3):269-275.

132. Kylian O, Sasaki T, Rossi F. Plasma sterilization of *Geobacillus stearothermophilus* by O_2:N_2 RF inductively coupled plasma. *Eur Phys J Appl Phys.* 2006;34:139-142.

133. Rossi F, Kylian O, Hasiwa M. Decontamination of surfaces by low pressure plasma discharges. *Plasma Process Polym.* 2006;3:431-442.

134. Rossi F, Kylian O, Hasiwa M. Mechanisms of sterilization and decontamination of surfaces by low-pressure plasma. In: D'Agostino R, Favia P, Kawai Y, et al, eds. *Advanced Plasma Technology.* Weinheim, Germany: Wiley-VCH Verlag GmbH & Co; 2008:319-340.

135. Tamazawa K, Shintani H, Tamazawa Y, Shimauchi H. Sterilization effect of wet oxygen plasma in the bubbling method. *Biocontrol Sci.* 2015;20(4):255-261.

136. Shintani H, Shimizu N, Tange S, et al. Efficiency of atmospheric pressure nitrogen gas remote plasma sterilization and the clarification of sterilization major factors. *Int J Clin Pharm Toxicol.* 2015;2:150-160.

137. Stephan KD, McLean RJ, DeLeon G, Melnikov V. Effect of feed-gas humidity on nitrogen atmospheric-pressure plasma jet for biological applications. *Technol Health Care.* 2016;24(6):943-948.

138. Muranyi P, Wunderlich J, Heise M. Influence of relative gas humidity on the inactivation efficiency of a low temperature gas plasma. *J Appl Microbiol.* 2008;104(6):1659-1666.

139. Wu Y, Liang Y, Wei K, et al. MS2 virus inactivation by atmospheric-pressure cold plasma using different gas carriers and power levels. *Appl Environ Microbiol.* 2015;81(3):996-1002.

140. Brun P, Brun P, Vono M, et al. Disinfection of ocular cells and tissues by atmospheric-pressure cold plasma. *PLoS One.* 2012;7(3):e33245.

141. Kim JS, Lee EJ, Kim YJ. Inactivation of *Campylobacter jejuni* with dielectric barrier discharge plasma using air and nitrogen gases. *Foodborne Pathog Dis.* 2014;11(8):645-651.

142. Boscariol MR, Moreira AJ, Mansano RD, Kikuchi IS, Pinto TJ. Sterilization by pure oxygen plasma and by oxygen-hydrogen peroxide plasma: an efficacy study. *Int J Pharm.* 2008;353(1-2):170-175.

143. Yong HI, Kim HJ, Park S, Choe W, Oh MW, Jo C. Evaluation of the treatment of both sides of raw chicken breasts with an atmospheric pressure plasma jet for the inactivation of *Escherichia coli.* *Foodborne Pathog Dis.* 2014;11(8):652-657.

144. Kawamura K, Sakuma A, Nakamura Y, Oguri T, Sato N, Kido N. Evaluation of bactericidal effects of low-temperature nitrogen gas plasma towards application to short-time sterilization. *Microbiol Immunol.* 2012;56(7):431-440.

145. Kinoshita S. Examination of UV and VUV effect on sterilization. *J Antibact Antifung Agent.* 2010;38:521-526.

146. Wiegand C, Fink S, Beier O, et al. Dose- and time-dependent cellular effects of cold atmospheric pressure plasma evaluated in 3D skin models. *Skin Pharmacol Physiol.* 2016;29(5):257-265.

147. Sakudo A, Toyokawa Y, Nakamura T, Yagyu Y, Imanishi Y. Nitrogen gas plasma treatment of bacterial spores induces oxidative stress that damages the genomic DNA. *Mol Med Rep.* 2017;15(1):396-402.

148. Roth S, Feichtinger J, Hertel C. Characterization of *Bacillus subtilis* spore inactivation in low-pressure, low-temperature gas plasma sterilization processes. *J Appl Microbiol.* 2010;108(2):521-531.

149. Han L, Patil S, Keener KM, Cullen PJ, Bourke P. Bacterial inactivation by high-voltage atmospheric cold plasma: influence of process parameters and effects on cell leakage and DNA. *J Appl Microbiol.* 2014;116(4):784-794.

150. Pignata C, D'Angelo D, Basso D, et al. Low-temperature, low-pressure gas plasma application on *Aspergillus brasiliensis*, *Escherichia coli* and pistachios. *J Appl Microbiol.* 2014;116(5):1137-1148.

151. Justan I, Cernohorska L, Dvorak Z, Slavicek P. Plasma discharge and time-dependence of its effect to bacteria. *Folia Microbiol (Praha).* 2014;59(4):315-320.

152. Hauser J, Esenwein SA, Awakowicz P, Steinau HU, Köller M, Halfmann H. Sterilization of heat-sensitive silicone implant material by low-pressure gas plasma. *Biomed Instrum Technol.* 2011;45(1):75-79.

153. Kim SM, Kim JI. Decomposition of biological macromolecules by plasma generated with helium and oxygen. *J Microbiol.* 2006;44(4):466-471.

154. Yu QS, Huang C, Hsieh FH, Huff H, Duan Y. Bacterial inactivation using a low-temperature atmospheric plasma brush sustained with argon gas. *J Biomed Mater Res B Appl Biomater.* 2007;80(1):211-219.

155. Tseng S, Abramzon N, Jackson JO, Lin WJ. Gas discharge plasmas are effective in inactivating *Bacillus* and *Clostridium* spores. *Appl Microbiol Biotechnol.* 2012;93(6):2563-2570.

156. Rosani U, Tarricone E, Venier P, et al. Atmospheric-pressure cold plasma induces transcriptional changes in *ex vivo* human corneas. *PLoS One.* 2015;10(7):e0133173.

157. Liao WT, Lee WJ, Chen CY, Shih M. Decomposition of ethylene oxide in the RF plasma environment. *Environ Technol*. 2001;22(2):165-173.

158. Whittaker AG, Graham EM, Baxter RL, et al. Plasma cleaning of dental instruments. *J Hosp Infect*. 2004;56(1):37-41.

159. Meding JB, Keating EM, Davis KE. Acetabular UHMWPE survival and wear changes with different manufacturing techniques. *Clin Orthop Relat Res*. 2011;469(2):405-411.

160. Hesby RM, Haganman CR, Stanford CM. Effects of radiofrequency glow discharge on impression material surface wettability. *J Prosthet Dent*. 1997;77(4):414-422.

161. Shintani H. Role of metastable and spore hydration to sterilize spores by nitrogen gas plasma exposure and DPA analysis by HPLC and UV. *J Pharm Sci Drug Des*. 2014;1:1-4.

162. Nishioka T, Takai Y, Mishima T, et al. Low-pressure plasma application for the inactivation of the seed-borne pathogen *Xanthomonas campestris*. *Biocontrol Sci*. 2016;21(1):37-43.

163. Hosseinzadeh Colagar A, Memariani H, Sohbatzadeh F, Valinataj Omran A. Nonthermal atmospheric argon plasma jet effects on *Escherichia coli* biomacromolecules. *Appl Biochem Biotechnol*. 2013;171(7):1617-1629.

164. Hertwig C, Steins V, Reineke K, et al. Impact of surface structure and feed gas composition on *Bacillus subtilis* endospore inactivation during direct plasma treatment. *Front Microbiol*. 2015;6:774.

165. Tyczkowska-Sieroń E, Markiewicz J. Inactivation of *Candida* species using cold atmospheric plasma on the way to a new method of eradication of superficial fungal infections. *Med Dosw Mikrobiol*. 2014;66(2):121-129.

166. Halfmann H, Bibinov N, Wunderlich J, Awakowicz P. Correlation between VUV radiation and sterilization efficiency in a double inductively coupled plasma. Paper presented at: 28th International Conference on Phenomena in Ionized Gases; July 15-20, 2007; Prague, Czech Republic.

167. Lerouge S, Fozza AC, Wertheimer MR, Marchand R, Yahia L'H. Sterilization by low-pressure plasma: the role of vacuum-ultraviolet radiation. *Plasma Polymers*. 2000;5:31-46.

168. Virard F, Cousty S, Cambus JP, Valentin A, Kémoun P, Clément F. Cold atmospheric plasma induces a predominantly necrotic cell death via the microenvironment. *PLoS One*. 2015;10(8):e0133120.

169. McDonnell G. Peroxygens and other forms of oxygen: their use for effective cleaning, disinfection, and sterilization. In: Zhu PC, ed. *New Biocides Development: The Combined Approach of Chemistry and Microbiology*. Oxford, United Kingdom: Oxford University Press; 2006:292-308.

170. McDonnell G. Gas plasma sterilization. In: Adam PF, Jean-Yves M, Syed AS, eds. *Principles and Practice of Disinfection, Preservation and Sterilization*. 5th ed. Hoboken, NJ: Wiley; 2013:333-342.

171. Russell AD, ed. The bacterial spore. In: *The Destruction of Bacterial Spore*. London, United Kingdom: Academic Press; 1982:1-29.

172. Cortezzo DE, Koziol-Dube K, Setlow B, Setlow P. Treatment with oxidizing agents damages the inner membrane of spores of *Bacillus subtilis* and sensitizes spores to subsequent stress. *J Appl Microbiol*. 2004;97(4):838-852.

173. Setlow P. Spores of *Bacillus subtilis*: their resistance to and killing by radiation, heat and chemicals. *J Appl Microbiol*. 2006;101(3):514-525.

174. Naïtali M, Kamgang-Youbi G, Herry JM, Bellon-Fontaine MN, Brisset JL. Combined effects of long-living chemical species during microbial inactivation using atmospheric plasma-treated water. *Appl Environ Microbiol*. 2010;76(22):7662-7664.

175. Traylor MJ, Pavlovich MJ, Karim S, et al. Long-term antibacterial efficacy of air plasma-activated water. *J Phys D Appl Phys*. 2011;44:472001.

176. Pankaj SK, Bueno-Ferrer C, Misra NN, et al. Applications of cold plasma technology in food packaging. *Trend Food Sci Technol*. 2014;35:5-17.

177. Bárdos L, Baránková H. Cold atmospheric plasma: sources, processes, and applications. *Thin Solid Films*. 2010;518:6705-6713.

178. Afshari R, Hosseini H. Nonthermal plasma as a new food preservation method: its present and future prospect. *J Paramed Sci*. 2014;5:2008-4978.

179. Matsui K, Ikenaga N, Sakudo N. Effects of humidity on sterilization of *Geobacillus stearothermophilus* spores with plasma-excited neutral gas. *Jpn J Appl Phys*. 2015;54:06GD02.

Nitrogen Dioxide

David Opie and Evan Goulet

Nitrogen dioxide (NO_2) is an antimicrobial gas with many beneficial properties. In 2016, NO_2 was registered as a sterilant with the US Environmental Protection Agency (EPA) under the Federal Insecticide, Fungicide, and Rodenticide Act.[1] The EPA registration required the demonstration that NO_2 is a sterilant, capable of destroying or eliminating all forms of microbial life; this included representative forms of vegetative bacteria, bacterial spores, fungi, fungal spores, and viruses. This registration covered uses that are not specifically applied to medical devices. The use of NO_2 for the sterilization of medical devices follows International Organization for Standardization (ISO) 14937:2009 as the general sterilization standard for methods that inactivate microorganisms by any physical or chemical means and is recognized by many regulatory agencies.[2] The NO_2 sterilization has also been recognized by the US Food and Drug Administration (FDA) with the 510(k) clearance of a medical device sterilized by NO_2 gas.[3]

The properties and use of NO_2 as a sterilant are detailed in this chapter. The mechanism of action for the sterilant is described and is shown to act in the same way as the natural in vivo processes by which animals control pathogens. To understand the mechanism of action, the surface chemistry must be considered because only referring to the gas phase concentration of the sterilant cannot lead to a sufficient analytical interpretation of the sterilization process. This may have implications in the study of other sterilization processes. Finally, this chapter discusses material compatibility and examples of applications with the NO_2 process.

▶ HISTORICAL REVIEW OF NITROGEN DIOXIDE REFERENCES IN MICROBIOLOGY AND HEALTH CARE

In the environment, NO_2 is known as a persistent gaseous component in air pollution. In industry, NO_2 is used in a variety of industrial applications, such as bleaching flour and as a polymerization inhibitor in acrylates.[4,5] Although the use of NO_2 as a sterilant is a relatively recent development, there is long a history of studying NO_2 as a pollutant, in medical applications, and as a biological contributor to reactive nitrogen species (RNS).

The NO_2 is found in ambient air at varying concentrations. Nitric oxide (NO) and NO_2 are produced by internal combustion engines and natural processes such as forest fires, lightning, and fermentation. NO_2 is the by-product of NO oxidation. Due to anthropogenic sources, any large city with a high density of internal combustion engines and fossil fuel power plants will have more NO_2 in the ambient air than will regions without such sources. In and near these cities, the ambient NO_2 concentration measured in 2017 ranged between 20 and 60 ppb.[6] Across the United States, the average daily maximum value (from a 1-hr average) has dropped 30% from 2001 to 2010. This drop reflects a long-term trend of NO_2 reduction, where the average daily maximum was 110 ppb in 1980 to 43 ppb in 2016.[6,7] Historically, and before air quality standards began to improve air quality, this value could range as high as 1300 ppb (1.3 ppm), as recorded in the Los Angeles area in 1964.[8] Given the prevalence of NO_2 in the environment, and the large contribution from man-made sources, NO_2 has been thoroughly studied. Studies have evaluated the sources of NO_2, links to acid rain, and the impact of NO_2 on materials and living things. This wealth of information facilitates the evaluation of health and safety issues associated with using NO_2 as a sterilant gas and provides a technical understanding for the detailed chemical reactions in a typical NO_2 sterilization chamber.

One of the earliest mentions of NO_2 used in health care–related applications is the use of high concentrations of NO_2 for making oxidized cellulose, also called oxycellulose.[9] Since the 1940s, manufacturers have exposed cellulose preparations (initially, cotton gauze) to a high concentration of NO_2, resulting in its oxidized form.

The oxidized cellulose is used as a bioabsorbable and hemostatic wound dressing (eg, the Surgicel® absorbable hemostatic wound dressing). Additional beneficial properties of this type of wound dressing have been identified, such as antimicrobial and osteogenic properties.[10,11] Oxidized cellulose products are still used today.

In 1962, researchers in Poltava, Ukraine, exposed *Bacillus anthracis* spores to very high concentrations of NO_2.[12] Although these researchers believed they observed microbicidal inactivation of the spores and other microorganisms, repeated studies showed efficacy was due to the bacteriostatic properties of the oxidized cotton gauze inoculated in the wound dressing products studied, rather than direct NO_2-mediated lethality of the spores.[13] In another example of the microbicidal evaluation of NO_2, researchers measured the effect of NO_2 on airborne microorganisms. Atmospheric test chambers, under controlled temperature and humidity conditions, were used to simulate atmospheric conditions with gaseous atmospheric pollutants. In one test, researchers used *Rhizobium meliloti* as the test organism and found that at 50% relative humidity (RH) and 3 ppm NO_2 concentration, a 2 log_{10} reduction was observed over a 3-hour exposure period.[14] A similar study observed more than 1 log_{10} reduction in the population of airborne Venezuelan equine encephalomyelitis (VEE) virus using a 10-ppm NO_2 concentration and 85% RH.[8] In both studies, *Bacillus subtilis* spores were used as controls because they were not damaged by exposure to NO_2 under these conditions. Therefore, the population of the test organisms, either *R meliloti* or VEE, was quantified in proportion to *B subtilis* spores. Under these exposure conditions, NO_2 did not exhibit sterilant properties because the control organism (*B subtilis*) was not inactivated. The reason that *B subtilis* spores survived these exposure conditions is a result of the relatively low NO_2 concentration and the short exposure time used in these tests.

Another study of airborne NO and NO_2 tested cultured Chinese hamster cells (V79 cells) for DNA degradation after exposure to either NO or NO_2.[15] The V79 cells were exposed to NO and NO_2 in varying concentrations, from 0 ppm to 500 ppm and over varying periods (from 5 to 30 min). It was found that NO_2 led to a dose- and time-dependent increase of the rate of single-strand breaks in V79 cellular DNA. However, NO treatment did not result in any detectable DNA damage. The lowest observable effective concentration of NO_2, which was statistically different from control values, was 10-ppm exposure for 20 minutes. The lack of DNA degradation with NO exposure can be understood by examining the Henry's law coefficient of NO compared to NO_2, as discussed in the following text.[16]

The DNA single strand-breaks were also observed using conditions appropriate for sterilization and area disinfection applications.[17] Purified DNA and *B subtilis* spores were tested at 2.85 mg/L NO_2 and 75% RH, with varying exposure time. After exposure, the purified DNA and DNA extracted from the intact spores was evaluated using gel electrophoresis, with both denaturing and nondenaturing gel. The NO_2 was found to cause increasing DNA single-strand breaks, with breakages occurring after only 2 minutes of exposure. Complete DNA degradation was observed after 16 minutes under these conditions. The mechanism by which NO_2 can cause such damage is discussed later in this chapter.

Although there has been an interesting history of NO_2 for use in health care–related applications and in studies of microbicidal behavior of NO_2, the work to evaluate and develop NO_2 as a sterilant did not start until 2004. This work was motivated, in part, in response to the great interest in NO, which is one of the several RNS recognized as contributing to many biological processes.[18,19] The NO is released by neutrophils and macrophages in response to inflammation and infection and thus plays a role in the immune response in vivo. Also, NO is a vasodilator used in treating cardiac and pulmonary diseases.[20,21] In vivo, NO will autoxidize to form NO_2, and from the point of having both intercellular and intracellular NO and NO_2, subsequent chemical reactions lead to species that will cause microorganism apoptosis.[22,23]

Given this remarkable span of biological activity associated with NO, the exogenous application of NO was tested for antimicrobial properties that might be useful for sterilization and disinfection.[17] These investigations revealed that the NO cycle of in vivo chemical reactions can be reproduced in vitro. However, it was further recognized that NO_2 provides a more direct route to initiate the microbicidal chemical reactions involving RNS. Once again, the Henry's law constant for the gases involved helps to explain the advantages of using NO_2 instead of NO as the sterilant gas.

By now, NO_2 has been thoroughly tested for its ability to inactivate microorganisms. To be registered as a sterilant with the EPA, a chemical agent must destroy or eliminate representative forms of microbial life in the inanimate environment.[24] Recommended microorganisms for testing the microbicidal activity of a sterilant are listed in regulatory documents and international standards, such as ISO 14937:2009.[2] The organisms tested with the NO_2 process included those listed in Table 35.1.[25] For these tests, a known population of each microorganism was inoculated onto a carrier surface and allowed to dry. These were exposed to NO_2 sterilization cycles with increasing exposure time and with the concentration and RH for the cycles held constant at 2.75 mg/L NO_2 concentration (2000 ppm at 600 mm Hg) and 70% to 80% RH. The D-values for each microorganism were calculated using the fraction negative technique (single point, Stumbo-Murphy-Cochran [SMC]; see chapter 11) and based on the first exposure time where partial exposed inoculated carriers were sterile. Whereas most microorganisms exhibited rapid lethality upon exposure to NO_2, spores of *Geobacillus stearothermophilus* exhibited the greatest resistance to the

TABLE 35.1   List of estimated D-values observed with selected microorganisms

Organism Type	Reference Organism	D-value (min)
Bacterial spores	*Bacillus atrophaeus* (ATCC 9372)	0.34
	Bacillus pumilus (ATCC 27142)	0.63
	Clostridium sporogenes (ATCC 3584)	<0.28
	Bacillus subtilis var niger (ATCC 49278)	0.34
	Geobacillus stearothermophilus (ATCC 7953)	1.27
Vegetative spores	*Pseudomonas aeruginosa* (ATCC 27559)	0.28
	Salmonella enterica ser Typhimurium (ATCC 14028)	0.30
	Staphylococcus aureus (ATCC 6538)	<0.28
Mycobacteria	*Mycobacterium terrae* (ATCC 15755)	0.33
Fungi	*Trichophyton mentagrophytes* (ATCC 18748)	0.39
	Candida albicans (ATCC 10231)	0.54
Nonlipid viruses	*Porcine parvovirus*	<1.2
Lipid viruses	Herpes simplex virus type 1	<1.2

NO_2 process. Table 35.1 shows that the D-value observed for the *G stearothermophilus* was 1.3 minutes, under the conditions used for this evaluation.

Aside from demonstrating that NO_2 can kill all forms of microbial life, screening a wide range of microorganisms permits the identification of microorganisms that have higher resistance to the NO_2 process. The indicator organism in a biological indicator (BI) must be a highly resistant microorganism (typically, a spore-forming organism) that is appropriate for used in a BI.[26] The indicator organism should be more resistant than the bioburden found on medical devices or surfaces to be decontaminated. The BI consists of a known population of highly resistant spores that are inoculated onto a suitable carrier (see chapter 65). The inoculated carrier can be placed in a permeable barrier package (eg, a small Tyvek pouch), built into a self-contained BI (SCBI), or used in a process challenge device (PCD). The PCD can provide some additional and controllable protection to the BI so that the PCD resistance to the NO_2 process is adjusted to represent the resistance of the load to be sterilized.

▶ INACTIVATION KINETICS WITH NITROGEN DIOXIDE

The BIs, consisting of spores of *G stearothermophilus*, exhibit log-linear inactivation kinetics with increasing NO_2 process exposure time. The log-linear response with increasing exposure duration is expected and is typically observed with other sterilization processes.[27] Like with other sterilization processes, analysis tools like Holcomb-Spearman-Karber (HSK), survivor curve method, and others can be used to evaluate the D-value of the indicator

organism population (see chapter 11). As with all sterilization methods, but especially when using NO_2, hydrogen peroxide (H_2O_2), and other gaseous sterilants, some mathematical tools like HSK, SMC, and most probable number are not valid when tailing occurs or when the survivor curve does not agree with the fraction negative methods.[27]

Figure 35.1 illustrates the log-linear progression of population reduction as a function of exposure time to the NO_2 process. The data represented in Figure 35.1 was determined by the direct enumeration of the surviving viable spore population on each BI and with a fraction negative method. The BIs used to measure these data were composed of *G stearothermophilus* spores inoculated onto 6-mm diameter stainless steel discs. Once the inoculum is dried, the BI discs were packaged in Tyvek/Mylar

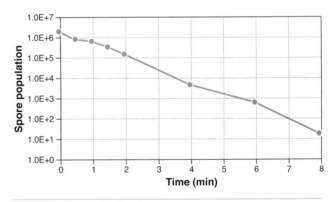

FIGURE 35.1   The spore population surviving the nitrogen dioxide (NO_2) exposure process is shown to decrease with increasing exposure time. The sterilant concentration (2.0 mg/L NO_2) and relative humidity (70%-80%) were constant for the exposure cycles.

pouches, placed into a test chamber, and exposed to 2.0 mg/L of NO_2 with 70% to 80% RH. The D-value calculated by direct enumeration was found to be 26 seconds. The D-value value calculated with the fraction negative method (HSK) was 35 seconds. A log-linear response to exposure time shown in Figure 35.1 provides a predictable model for inactivation. These results show that NO_2 can be a sterilant under the conditions tested. Predictable inactivation kinetics permit the use of the conservative overkill approach, as described in Annex D of ISO 14937:2009.[2]

▶ CHEMICAL AND PHYSICAL PROPERTIES

This section reviews some general physical and chemical properties of NO_2 that are important for using NO_2 as a sterilant. A more detailed discussion of chemical reactions, mechanism of microorganism lethality, and material compatibility are described later in this chapter.

Some selected and noteworthy chemical properties of NO_2 include:

- The NO_2 boils at 21.2°C (294 K) at sea level to form a yellow-brown gas.[28]
- The NO_2 freezes at −9°C (264 K) to form a colorless solid of the dimer dinitrogen tetroxide (N_2O_4).[28]
- The NO_2 has one unpaired electron, which means that this molecule is a free radical, and sometimes the formula for nitrogen dioxide is written as $NO_2^•$, with the dot indicating the radical.
- Due to the weakness of the single N–O bond, NO_2 is an oxidizer, but a relatively weak oxidizer compared to other common oxidizers (Table 35.2).[29,30]

The Lewis dot representation of the principle oxides of nitrogen are shown in Figure 35.2. As shown, there is an unpaired electron on the nitrogen with both NO and NO_2. Therefore, NO and NO_2 are radicals. However, these unpaired electrons are paired in the reactions forming dinitrogen trioxide (N_2O_3) and N_2O_4. Therefore, N_2O_3 and N_2O_4 are not radicals.

TABLE 35.2 Oxidation potential for selected gases[a]

Oxidation Potential of Selected Gases	
Oxidant	**Oxidation Potential (V)**
Fluorine	3.0
Hydroxyl radical	2.8
Ozone	2.1
Hydrogen peroxide	1.8
Noxilizer's sterilant, NO_2	−0.8

Abbreviation: NO_2, nitrogen dioxide.

[a]From Vanýsek[29] and *Standard Electrode Reduction and Oxidation Potential Values.*[30]

▶ COMMON CHEMICAL REACTIONS

Nitrogen dioxide found in the environment is formed in most combustion processes where the temperature is high enough to cause a reaction between the N_2 and O_2 molecules. The formation of NO is shown in equation (1):

$$O_2 + N_2 \rightarrow 2\,NO \tag{1}$$

The NO is a precursor to NO_2, and nitrogen dioxide is formed by the oxidation of NO. This reaction occurs in the air and in biological systems,[22] following the formula in equation (2):

$$NO + O_2 \rightarrow 2\,NO_2 \tag{2}$$

The hydrolysis of NO_2 results in nitrous acid (HNO_2) and nitric acid (HNO_3):

$$2NO_2 \,(or\, N_2O_4) + H_2O \rightarrow HNO_2 + HNO_3 \tag{3}$$

or

$$2NO_2 \,(or\, N_2O_4) + H_2O \rightarrow HONO + HNO_3 \tag{4}$$

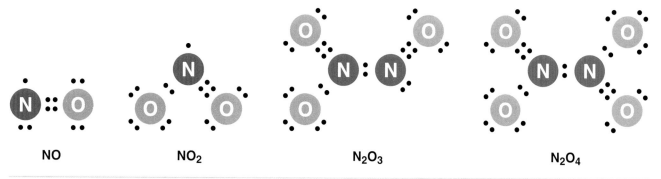

FIGURE 35.2 Lewis dot diagrams of the principle oxides of nitrogen involved in the nitrogen dioxide (NO_2) sterilization process. Abbreviations: NO, nitric oxide; N_2O_3, dinitrogen trioxide; N_2O_4, dinitrogen tetroxide.

This reaction is one step in the Ostwald process used in the industrial production of HNO_3 from ammonia.[31] The two isomers of nitrous acid are HONO (nitrous acid) and HNO_2 (nitryl hydride or isonitrous acid). The HNO_2 will ionize in water, like an acid, whereas HONO is more stable, will be found as a gas, and is the source of reactive OH in air pollution.[32]

The HNO_3 decomposes to nitrogen dioxide, water and oxygen, as shown in equation (5).

$$4\ HNO_3 \rightarrow 4\ NO_2 + 2\ H_2O + O_2 \qquad (5)$$

This decomposition occurs during evaporation and within the liquid phase of HNO_3. The NO_2 gives the characteristic yellow color of HNO_3 and HNO_3 fumes. The reactions involving NO_2 will be described in the discussion of the detailed physical and chemical reactions that comprise the NO_2 process.

When two sterilization molecules of NO_2 collide, either in the gas or liquid phase, there is a probability that these two molecules may bond together, forming the dimer N_2O_4. This is described by equation (6):

$$N_2O_4 \rightleftharpoons 2\ NO_2 \qquad (6)$$

The NO_2 is a radical, with one unpaired electron on the nitrogen. In molecular collisions that result in a molecular bond, these unpaired electrons form a single covalent bond between the nitrogen atoms. However, this bond is relatively weak, and at room temperature, the N_2O_4 will dissociate due to ambient thermal energy. The lifetime of an N_2O_4 molecule is short, with the half-life of the N_2O_4 being less than 10 µs at 25°C (298.15 K).[33] Therefore, an equilibrium state is described for NO_2 where molecules of NO_2 are constantly forming dimer molecules and then dissociating to return the monomer form.

When referring to a gas composed of both NO_2 and N_2O_4, the relative amounts of NO_2 and N_2O_4 are not typically mentioned because this can be readily calculated. Instead, a mixture of NO_2 and N_2O_4 is simply referred to as "NO_2 gas," and it should be assumed that there will be some fraction of the NO_2 molecules momentarily bound in the dimer form. It is convenient to refer to the total NO_2, which includes both monomer and dimer forms of NO_2. For any quantity of gas containing NO_2, the total number of moles of NO_2 is n_{total}, which is the sum of the monomer NO_2 moles, $n\ (NO_2)$, plus two times the dimer moles, $2n\ (N_2O_4)$, as shown in Equation (7).

$$n_{total} = n(NO_2) + 2n(N_2O_4) \qquad (7)$$

The ratio of monomer to dimer is described by the temperature-dependent equilibrium constant, K_p, shown in Equation (8).[33]

$$K_p = p^2(NO_2)\ /\ p(N_2O_4) \qquad (8)$$

In equation (8), $p(NO_2)$ and $p(N_2O_4)$ are the partial pressures of the nitrogen dioxide and dinitrogen tetroxide, respectively. The temperature-dependent fraction of dimer and monomer can be calculated from the temperature dependence of the equilibrium constant.

The equilibrium constant K_p is calculated from the thermochemical properties:

$$K_p = \exp(\Delta G° / RT) \approx \exp(21.13 - 6880 / T) \qquad (9)$$

In equation (9), $\Delta G°$ is the Gibbs free energy change per mole of reaction for unmixed reactants and products at standard conditions, R is the universal gas constant, and T is the absolute temperature of the gas.[33] At a single temperature, equation (8) shows that the square of the NO_2 partial pressure divided by the partial pressure of N_2O_4 will be constant. The temperature dependence of K_p shows that for a given number of moles of NO_2, the number of N_2O_4 molecules will increase as the temperature decreases. The calculated temperature-dependent relationship between NO_2 and N_2O_4 is shown in Figure 35.3. From this graph, it is clear that the partial pressure of N_2O_4 will increase exponentially with a decrease in temperature.

Another observation from the inspection of equations (7) and (8) is that the relative concentration of N_2O_4 will increase as the total amount of NO_2 increases. This concentration-dependent relationship between NO_2 and N_2O_4 is shown in Figure 35.4. The rate of collisions causing N_2O_4 formation increases as the concentration of NO_2 increases, whereas the dissociation rate is only dependent on temperature and is independent of the NO_2 concentration. Therefore, as the concentration of total NO_2 increases, the partial pressure of N_2O_4 will increase more rapidly than the total NO_2 concentration.

Referring to Figures 35.3 and 35.4 and their underlying equations, consider a liter of gas that is composed of dry air with a total NO_2 concentration ($NO_2 + N_2O_4$) of 10 mg/L. At 288.3 K (15°C), this 1 L of gas has 8.77 mg/L (191 µmol)

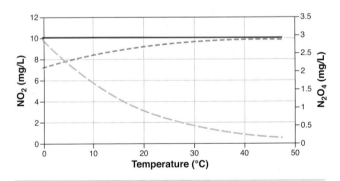

FIGURE 35.3   Graph of the temperature dependence of the nitrogen dioxide (NO_2) and dinitrogen tetroxide (N_2O_4) concentration in a gas with 10 mg/L of total NO_2. The total NO_2 concentration is shown with the solid line, the NO_2 monomer concentration is shown as the dotted line, and the N_2O_4 concentration is shown as the dashed line.

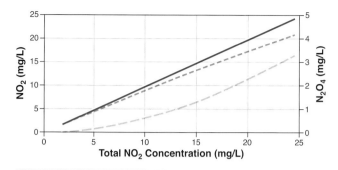

FIGURE 35.4 Graph of the concentration dependence of the nitrogen dioxide (NO_2) and dinitrogen tetroxide (N_2O_4) concentration in a gas at 25°C. The total NO_2 concentration is shown with the solid line, the NO_2 monomer concentration is shown as the dotted line, and the N_2O_4 concentration is shown as the dashed line.

of monomer NO_2 and 1.23 mg/L (13.4 μmol) of N_2O_4. At 298.3 K (25°C), the same 1 L of dry air with 10 mg/L of total NO_2 will have 9.36 mg/L (203 μmol) of NO_2 and 0.65 mg/L (7.1 μmol) of N_2O_4. From this example, as the temperature increases from 15°C to 25°C, the equilibrium has shifted to have less dimer. Also, the pressure of the gas increases as the temperature increases from 15°C to 25°C due to both increased kinetic energy of the molecules and the increased number of gas molecules (as more N_2O_4 dissociates into NO_2). Due to the increased NO_2 partial pressure caused by dissociation of the dimer, a gas containing NO_2 cannot be considered an ideal gas. As another example, consider an increase of NO_2 concentration while the temperature remains unchanged. As described earlier, at 298.3 K (25°C), 1 L of dry air with 10 mg/L of total NO_2 will have 9.36 mg/L (203 μmol) of NO_2 and 0.65 mg/L (7.1 μmol) of N_2O_4. When the total NO_2 concentration in this 1 L of dry air is doubled to 20 mg/L NO_2 (at 25°C), this liter of gas will have 17.69 mg/L (385 μmol) of NO_2 and 2.33 mg/L (25.3 μmol) moles of N_2O_4. This is shown in Figure 35.4. Notice that doubling the total NO_2 concentration, from 10 mg/L to 20 mg/L, more than triples the dimer concentration from 7.1 μmol to 25.3 μmol. Whereas these nonlinear examples illustrate the nonideal nature of NO_2 gas, these examples also show that the exact concentration for various conditions can be readily calculated.

DETECTION METHODS AND SPECTRAL PROPERTIES

Measuring the gas concentration in a chamber is easily done using a gas sampling circuit, where a small pump circulates a small amount of gas from the sterilization chamber, through the measurement system, and returns the gas back to the chamber. The type of sensor used for the measurement of NO_2 and other gas constituents will depend on the concentration of the gas being measured. For example, at very low concentrations of NO_2 (from

0 to 200 ppb), chemiluminescence is a common measurement method. Chemiluminescence is often used in environmental monitoring because ambient NO_2 levels are typically between 0 and 200 ppb. For NO_2 concentration ranges from 0 to 100 ppm, the electrochemical cells (EC cells) and solid-state detectors are appropriate. These types of detectors are relatively inexpensive, are available for many different types of gases (NO, NO_2, H_2O_2, etc), sold by multiple vendors, and are appropriate for monitoring the environment around the NO_2 processing equipment.

For higher concentration levels (from 100 ppm to 100 000 ppm), spectral measurement methods are appropriate using a gas cell with a short beam path. The absorption spectrum of NO_2 consists of many absorbance bands facilitating the measurements of NO_2 using standard laboratory equipment, like Fourier Transform-Infrared (FTIR) spectroscopy systems, visible light spectrophotometry systems, and photometric analyzer in the ultraviolet (UV) and visible (VIS) bands. The measurements in the infrared (IR), VIS, or UV bands will follow Beer's law, simplifying interpretation of the measured absorbance. The NO_2 absorbance bands include the visual violet, blue and green regions, between 300 and 600 nm, as shown in Figure 35.5. There is much less absorbance at wavelengths longer than 600 nm, resulting in the characteristic orange-red appearance of the gaseous NO_2.[34]

The N_2O_4 gas will not contribute to the measured absorbance at wavelengths longer than 400 nm, so that absorbance between 400 and 600 nm can be attributed to the NO_2 monomer. Regardless, the amount of dimer component of the total NO_2 must be considered. Heating the measurement gas cell greatly reduces the amount of dimer NO_2, as indicated in the graph shown in Figure 35.3. When 10 mg/L of total NO_2 is added to a chamber, heating the gas from 25°C to 50°C reduces the amount of N_2O_4 from 3.38% to 0.67% of the total amount of NO_2.

The choice of spectroscopic method may depend on other capabilities of the instruments and properties of the spectral bands. For example, being able to measure multiple gas constituents with the same instrument is helpful. The FTIR can measure NO_2, NO, and humidity in the chamber dosed with NO_2. The UV-VIS measurements will not measure water but lend themselves to simplified detector systems, such as using filtered light in the blue region of the visual spectrum.

USE OF NITROGEN DIOXIDE AS A STERILANT

When using NO_2 as a sterilant for disinfection or sterilization applications, there are three process variables that directly affect the lethal action of NO_2: sterilant concentration, exposure time, and RH. These process variables constitute the principle cycle parameters necessary for establishing the antimicrobial environment. For example,

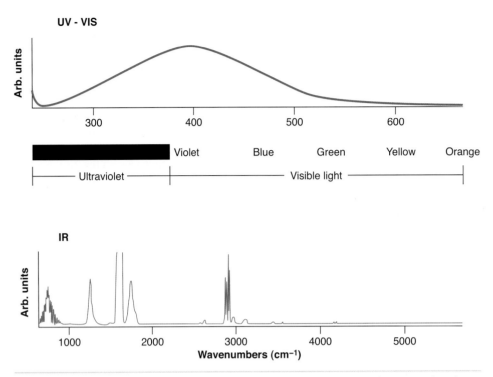

FIGURE 35.5   Nitrogen dioxide (NO_2) has a broad absorbance band in the UV-VIS band, absorbing violet and blue light. In the IR band, NO_2 molecule has discrete absorbance bands.

the process parameters might be 10 mg/L NO_2 concentration, 75% RH, and 10 minutes of exposure time. However, these parameters can be changed depending on the load configuration. Loads composed of simple packages and simple device geometry might require less sterilant and a shorter exposure time. Complex device configurations or very large and dense loads may require longer exposure times. The use of NO_2 permits a wide range of sterilant concentrations. Values as low as 200 ppm and with a 3-hour dwell have been successfully tested with BIs. The maximum NO_2 concentration tested is over 20 000 ppm. This range offers ample opportunity to balance cycle time, cycle cost, and material compatibility.

Beyond the principle cycle parameters (exposure time, NO_2 concentration, and RH), there are other cycle variables that can be viewed as secondary parameters. These secondary parameters are those that can be manipulated to overcome the challenges associated with specific loads. Factors like packaging, device geometry, materials, and other impedances that hinder the homogeneous achievement of the principle cycle conditions at every location within the chamber and load. These secondary cycle parameters are factors like vacuum depth and the number of sterilant exposure dwell phases, to name a few. These secondary cycle parameters are manipulated to deliver the principle cycle parameter conditions to the hardest-to-reach locations, throughout the load.

Temperature is important, but it is not as critical for the NO_2 sterilization process as it is with other sterilization processes. The NO_2 process has no liquid-to-gas

phase transition near the operating parameter set points. For example, the H_2O_2 sterilization process relies on the saturated vapor pressure of H_2O_2, which is highly dependent on temperature. When generating an H_2O_2 sterilant environment, the goal is to maximize the amount of H_2O_2 in the chamber. Operating at (and often, above) the saturation point of H_2O_2 applies a high sensitivity of the H_2O_2 process to temperature fluctuations. The NO_2 process does not work near the vapor-phase transition, where a dose of 10 mg/L NO_2 represents approximately 0.5% of the saturated vapor pressure of NO_2 at 21°C; however, the temperature of the sterilization chamber should be controlled within a specific temperature range (chiefly for maintaining a consistent RH). Process temperatures from 10°C to 35°C have been tested and shown to provide good sterilization efficacy. Additionally, as will be shown in the following text, large temperature changes can result in relatively small changes in the D-value, compared to the temperature-dependent D-value sensitivity observed with other sterilization methods (Arrhenius temperature dependence).

Humidity is known to play a critical role in many gas sterilization processes, and this remains true for the NO_2 process. With H_2O_2 sterilization, increasing humidity at certain temperatures has been shown to reduce observed D-values by increasing condensation (so-called microcondensation) of the H_2O_2 onto surfaces.[35] With ethylene oxide, increasing humidity is proposed to increase the water content of the spore coat, thereby increasing permeability of the spore coat to the sterilant molecules.[36,37]

Similarly, humidity plays an important role in the use of NO$_2$ sterilant. With the NO$_2$ process, the influence of humidity relies on both of these previously identified mechanisms. Furthermore, RH in the sterilizing chamber creates the conditions where specific heterogeneous chemical reactions (reactions on surfaces) can occur that contribute to the sterilization process. The details of these heterogeneous chemical reactions are described in the following text.

The D-value measured at different humidity levels demonstrates that the D-value decreases as the humidity increases.[38] For example, at 40% RH and 4 mg/L, a lot of BIs is found to have a 2.4-minute D-value. At 50% RH and 4 mg/L, this same lot of BIs is found to have a 0.4-minute D-value. At very low humidity levels (below 30% RH), the measurement of BI D-values with the NO$_2$ process is confounded by inconsistent results. Whereas at humidity levels above 70% RH, NO$_2$ has a rapid microbicidal action. The mechanism by which the RH level alters the chemistry of the NO$_2$ process is explained later in this chapter.

Different types of cycles are possible with NO$_2$ as the sterilant. Generally, NO$_2$ cycles can be divided into two categories: cycles with a vacuum step and cycles without a vacuum step (completed at or near ambient pressure). The use of vacuum during the sterilization cycle can facilitate rapid distribution of the sterilant and humidity throughout the load, and vacuum rinses at the end of the cycle facilitate rapid aeration. A cycle that includes a vacuum step requires that the chamber being used is compatible with low pressures, for example, an autoclave-style sterilization chamber. Conversely, an NO$_2$ sterilization or disinfection process that does not include an evacuation step has no such requirements on the structure of the enclosure being treated with the NO$_2$ process. For example, a cycle without a vacuum step is appropriate for disinfecting isolators and material transfer airlocks. Sterilant gas uniformity and aeration are largely dependent on air circulation patterns and air circulation velocity. The time required for distribution of the gas throughout the chamber and the time required for aeration may be much longer when no vacuum is used because air circulation and diffusion are the main mechanisms for the gas distribution processes.

Vacuum Nitrogen Dioxide Cycles

Figure 35.6 illustrates the essential design of a sterilization system configured for vacuum cycles using the NO$_2$. A graph of the chamber pressure versus time for a vacuum cycle is shown in Figure 35.7. In this graph, the pressure within the sterilization chamber is graphed as a function of elapsed time. The first step is the evacuation of the chamber to remove the atmosphere in the chamber. Next, the prechamber is filled to the appropriate pressure of sterilant gas. Then, the prechamber is opened to the evacuated sterilization chamber allowing the NO$_2$ to flow into the sterilization chamber. Pressure transducers, recording the pressure rise associated with the sterilant gas addition, or optical NO$_2$ detectors can be used to confirm delivery of the sterilant to the sterilization chamber. After the sterilant is added to the chamber, humidified air may be added to the sterilization chamber until the target RH is achieved, and dry air may be added until the target pressure for the exposure dwell is reached. The chamber pressure during the exposure dwell is typically between 500 mm Hg and 600 mm Hg (roughly between 65 and 80 kPa). These steps can be repeated, as needed, to achieve the intended sterilization process. Figure 35.7 shows two exposure dwells, representing the first half cycle and second half cycle of an overkill approach, described in

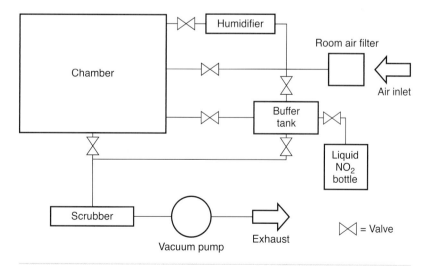

FIGURE 35.6 Block diagram of a nitrogen dioxide (NO$_2$) sterilization system configured for vacuum cycles. When using a scrubber, the air pumped from the chamber can be safely vented.

Phases of the Cycle

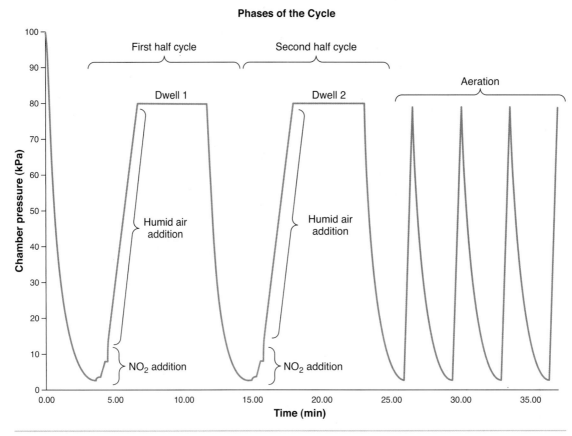

FIGURE 35.7   Pressure versus time for a typical nitrogen dioxide (NO₂) cycle with vacuum. The sterilant exposure phase has an evacuation step, a gas filling step, and an exposure dwell. These phases can be repeated as needed to complete the sterilization cycle. The exposure phases are followed by an aeration phase.

Annex D of ISO 14937:2009.[2] After the final exposure dwell is completed, the sterilant gas is removed from the sterilization chamber, and the load therein, using repeated evacuation and rinsing with air or inert gas (eg, nitrogen).

The sterilant in the chamber exhaust can be scrubbed by chemical means. The scrubbing process removes unsafe levels of NO₂ from the exhaust. The chemical removal of sterilant from the air stream may use a solid chemical scrubber material (eg, sodium permanganate) or water scrubber systems. The sodium permanganate (solid media) scrubber material neutralizes and captures the NO₂ in a nonhazardous, solid material. The spent scrubber material may be disposed of as nonhazardous solid waste with no special handling measures required. With water-based scrubber systems (appropriate for larger volume systems), the NO₂ is captured in water and neutralized before draining.

Nonvacuum Nitrogen Dioxide Cycles

Cycles that do not have a vacuum step are appropriate for vacuum-sensitive loads and for structures that are not designed for internal pressures that are significantly below ambient pressure. For example, the disinfection of isolators and material transfer airlocks, or the surface sterilization of packaged, prefilled syringes are cases in which a nonvacuum cycle may be appropriate. The system configuration for a nonvacuum cycle is illustrated in Figure 35.8. Note that in this case, and throughout the rest of this document, the word "chamber" is used to refer to isolators, airlocks, sterilization chambers, and any other volume to be exposed to the process. This nonvacuum chamber is a closed-loop system for the humidity introduction, sterilant addition, and dwell phases of the process. Humidity is added to the chamber first by recirculating the gas through the humidifier path until it reaches the target level. The NO₂ sterilant is added by recirculating the humidified air through the buffer tank until the specified NO₂ concentration is reached. The order of gas additions (humidification prior to NO₂) is essential to prevent the humidification system from becoming fouled with NO₂. The NO₂ buffer tank is easily returned to a dry state after the cycle using a small vacuum pump. The dwell time begins after the NO₂ addition phase is completed and closed-loop recirculation continues to mix the gases in the chamber. The aeration phase is open-loop with the exhaust gas, has the NO₂ removed by the

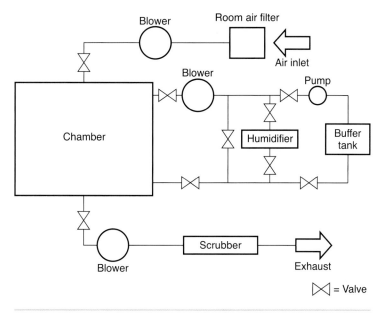

FIGURE 35.8 Diagram of nonvacuum system.

scrubber, and where inlet and outlet blowers can be used for pressure regulation. An example of the NO_2 and humidity concentration profiles measured in a nonvacuum cycle is shown in Figure 35.9. Note that when the NO_2 gas is added to the humidified chamber, the concentrations of both NO_2 and humidity decrease. This is a key phenomenon in NO_2 processes because both species are deposited and react heterogeneously on surfaces. This phenomenon and how it pertains to the mechanism of inactivation will be considered later in the chapter.

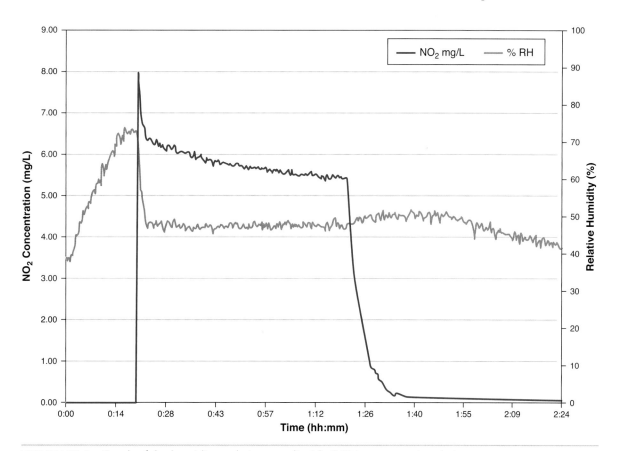

FIGURE 35.9 Graph of the humidity and nitrogen dioxide (NO_2) concentration during a nonvacuum process. Abbreviation: RH, relative humidity.

In both vacuum and nonvacuum cycles, an important part of the NO_2 process is measuring and applying the NO_2 dose to a chamber. The dose is often set as the number of grams of NO_2 applied to a specific load in a chamber. One method for preparing the dose uses a small auxiliary vacuum chamber (often called a prechamber or buffer tank) for preparing and measuring the NO_2 dose, as shown in Figure 35.6 and Figure 35.8. With this method, the buffer tank, which is connected by valves to a vacuum pump and a source of NO_2, is first evacuated and then filled with the sterilant dose. The sterilant dose is metered by measuring the pressure rise in the buffer tank due to the addition of the NO_2 gas. The calculated pressure rise for a specific dose NO_2 must account for the relative concentration of the dimer and the monomer. After filling the buffer tank with the correct dose of NO_2, the sterilant is flushed into the chamber.

► NITROGEN DIOXIDE STERILANT SOURCES

There are several methods for storing, delivering, or generating NO_2. For any given application, the most suitable method of providing NO_2 depends on several factors. These include the amount of sterilant needed per cycle, the frequency of sterilant usage, transportation considerations, convenience, and single-dose or multiple-dose containers. In consideration of these factors, several methods of providing sterilant to the target chamber have been used successfully. Some of these methods are the following:

1. Delivering NO to a chamber with an ambient amount of oxygen. In the presence of ambient air, which contains about 20% oxygen, the NO will oxidize to form NO_2, as shown in equation (2). This reaction is sufficiently fast that only a few minutes are needed to have a high fraction of the NO converted to NO_2.

   The NO can be compressed in a cylinder to a high pressure. A 44-L compressed gas cylinder of NO pressurized to 130 atm holds 1900 g NO. This amount of NO is sufficient to fill a 1000-L volume chamber 290 times with a dose that produces 10 mg/L NO_2. This method has been thoroughly tested and provides sterilization results that are not significantly different from using NO_2 gas as the sterilant source.[17]

2. The NO_2 sterilant can be generated at the time of use using a chemical reaction. For example, combining HNO_3 with copper metal generates NO_2 gas. This method has been developed and tested using a gas generating module that held a small amount of HNO_3 an excess of copper metal, such that the reaction resulted in the liberation of a target number of grams of NO_2 gas. This method is best suited for generating a single dose of sterilant gas at the point of use.[39,40]

3. Using a chemical reaction to make NO and adding this to a chamber with an ambient concentration of oxygen.

There are many chemical reactions that will generate NO gas. For example, the first stage of the Ostwald process (in which ammonia is converted to HNO_3) produces NO.[31] In the first stage of this process, ammonia is oxidized by heating with oxygen in the presence of a catalyst such as platinum with 10% rhodium, to form NO, as shown in equation (10).

$$4\,NH_3\,(g) + 5\,O_2\,(g) \rightarrow 4\,NO\,(g) + 6\,H_2O\,(g) \quad (10)$$

Another reaction that can be used for generating NO is the use of a diazeniumdiolate.[41] The NO-releasing compositions, such as the carbon-based diazeniumdiolates, release NO spontaneously under physiologic (aqueous) conditions or mixed with an acid.[41]

4. Another sources of NO_2 are compressed gas cylinders in which NO_2 gas is in a mixture of 10% NO_2 and balance nitrogen. The limitation with these is that the cylinders can only hold an NO_2 partial pressure of 0.5 atm. Above this concentration, there is a risk of condensing some of the NO_2 into liquid, thereby disturbing the expected stoichiometry of a measure of gas taken from the cylinder. Therefore, the nitrogen serves as a carrier gas for the NO_2 in the cylinder.

5. Because NO_2 boils at room temperature, the NO_2 sterilant can be stored and transported as a liquid. The cylinder used for storage and transportation does not need to be rated for high pressure because the vapor pressure of NO_2 is 1 atm at 21.2°C. As a liquid, this is the densest form of the sterilant and is very convenient. Dosing from a cylinder of liquid NO_2 is accomplished by evaporating gas from the surface of the liquid into an evacuated buffer tank. The pressure rise in the buffer tank can be directly correlated to moles of NO_2 added to the tank, when equilibrium conditions are considered. Therefore, it is important to know the temperature of the gas in the buffer tank. Once the dose is prepared in the buffer tank, the sterilant can be flushed into the sterilization chamber.

6. Generating NO_2 at the point of use with a plasma source is a novel method. The plasma is used to react with air, which is about 80% nitrogen and 20% oxygen, to yield NO_2.[42,43] This is accomplished by focusing a high-strength electric field from a microwave source on the stream of filtered air that causes the N_2 and O_2 molecules to dissociate. As the gas of dissociated air molecules flows away from the high-field strength region, atoms combine to form molecules, and a fraction of these molecules will result in NO_2 formation.

   A microwave source can be used to generate an oscillating electromagnetic field. Using a specific configuration of waveguide, a standing wave is established so that the highest amplitude electric fields oscillate in one specific location. By placing a metal electrode in this location, the electrode acts as an antenna to couple the electric field to the gas, igniting the plasma. At the highest electric field amplitude, dielectric breakdown occurs, and electrons leave the metal surface, accelerating in the electric field. The electron collisions with the oxygen and nitrogen molecules results in the formation of plasma of nitrogen and oxygen ions and radicals.

$$O_2 + e^- \rightarrow O + O^- \qquad (11)$$

$$N_2 + e^- \rightarrow 2N^{\bullet} + e^- \qquad (12)$$

Once the dissociation of the N_2 and O_2 begins, many other chemical reactions occur, only some of which are shown here:

$$N^{\bullet} + O_2 \rightarrow NO^{\bullet} + O^{\bullet} \qquad (13)$$

$$O^{\bullet} + N_2 \rightarrow NO^{\bullet} + N^{\bullet} \qquad (14)$$

$$O_2 + O^{\bullet} \rightarrow O_3 \qquad (15)$$

$$N_2 + 2O_3 \rightarrow 2NO^{\bullet} + O_2 \qquad (16)$$

$$NO^{\bullet} + O_2 \rightarrow NO_2^{\bullet} + O^{\bullet} \qquad (17)$$

$$NO^{\bullet} + O_3 \rightarrow NO_2^{\bullet} + O_2 \qquad (18)$$

As is apparent from equations (16) to (18), there are many atomic and molecular species that are formed in the plasma.[44] Ozone, nitrous oxide, and other species are formed. However, after a short time, the only stable and persistent chemical species are O_2, N_2, and NO_2, and other gaseous species are reduced to negligible levels through chemical reaction.[43,44] The rate of NO_2 generation can be accelerated by mixing O_2 with the air, approaching a stoichiometric ratio closer to the final NO_2 composition.

These methods of storing, delivering, or generating NO_2 gas allow for the optimization of economical and convenient methods for applying NO_2 to a wide range of scenarios.

▶ CHEMICAL REACTIONS AND MECHANISM OF ACTION

The NO_2 process occurs in a chamber in which a controlled amount of NO_2 sterilant is combined with humidified air. Although there are chemical reactions that occur in the gas phase, the rate of these gas-phase reactions between NO_2 and water (humidity) is relatively slow[45] and does not contribute to the sterilizing chemical reactions. However, the rate of the reactions on the surfaces exposed to the sterilant gas and RH is much faster. Also, it is worth noting that the microorganisms that will be sterilized are on the surfaces where these chemical reactions occur. Therefore, the impact of the surface chemistry should be evaluated. To understand the chemical reactions that lead to microbial lethality, it is helpful to recall the many

biological roles of NO. It was stated before that NO is produced by neutrophils and macrophages in response to inflammation and infection in vivo.[19] In vivo, the process by which one cell can cause another cell's death, extrinsic apoptosis, has several steps. These steps are summarized as follows: NO generated by a cell auto-oxidizes to form NO_2; NO and NO_2 combine to form N_2O_3; the N_2O_3 reacts with DNA through the nitrosation of nucleosides cytosine and guanine.[46] Excluding the cytosine and guanine reactions, these steps can occur either in the extracellular region, within the cell membrane, or within the microorganism.[23] It is interesting to note that the oxidation of NO and rate of reactions producing N_2O_3 can be 30 times faster in the hydrophobic lipid bilayer (as in the cell or spore membrane) than the same reactions in the extracellular, aqueous environment.[23] The NO_2 sterilization processes in vitro follow this same chemical reaction cycle found in vivo, leading to the degradation of a microorganism's DNA. There are three scenarios where oxides of nitrogen interact with the microorganism, and these are shown in Figure 35.10. The first scenario is the known in vivo reaction described earlier, where macrophages produce NO, causing extrinsic apoptosis of target microorganisms (Figure 35.10, Reaction A). The second scenario to consider is the direct interaction of microorganisms (eg, spores) with the humidified sterilant gas (see Figure 35.10, Reaction B). The third scenario is the interaction of the microorganisms with the chemical environment that develops on the surfaces exposed to the NO_2 process (see Figure 35.10, Reaction C).

The first scenario, in vivo, as mentioned earlier is well described in the literature.[46] The second scenario is more directly related to sterilization, when one considers the interaction of the humidified microorganisms with the gases in the sterilization chamber. The spore coat (or cell membrane) will become hydrated with the RH in the air. The humidity greatly increases the size of the spores, the water content of the spore coat, and the permeability of the spore to gases.[37,47] The NO gas is generated as a product of the water film interactions (see the following text). The gas constituents (NO_2, N_2O_4, NO, etc) enter the water-containing spore coat. Thereafter, the reactions continue as with the in vivo reactions of the RNS with the internal nucleic acid. In this scenario, the extrinsic apoptosis process in vivo is triggered by in vitro sources of NO_2.

The third scenario describes the reactions that occur in the water film that forms on all surfaces in the chamber exposed to the humidified air. These water film reactions result in new molecular nitrogen species. Some of these molecules remain in the water film; others leave the water film as gaseous products from the water film reactions. Gaseous reaction products like HONO and NO molecules supplement the NO_2 monomer and dimer gases in the chamber. The dissolved molecules remaining in the water film can interact directly with the cell membrane or spore coat of the microorganisms in contact with the water film. Figure 35.10 shows these as Reaction C. For additional clarity, these reactions within the water film

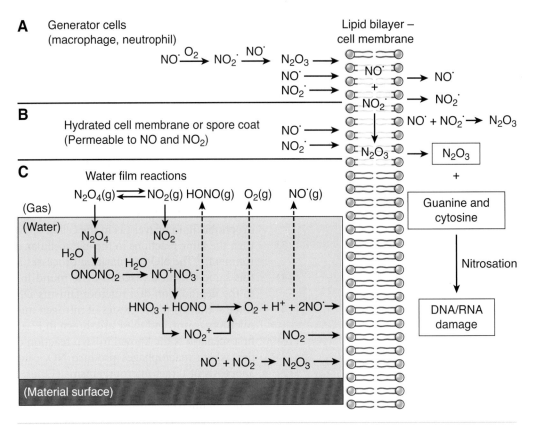

FIGURE 35.10   Diagram showing the chemical reactions that lead to the cellular microbicidal properties of reactive nitrogen species (RNS). Abbreviations: H_2O, water; HONO, nitrous acid; NO, nitric oxide; NO_2, nitrogen dioxide; NO_3^-, nitrate; N_2O_3, dinitrogen trioxide; N_2O_4, dinitrogen tetroxide; O_2, oxygen; $ONONO_2$, nitrosonitrate.

are outlined in Table 35.3 have been found in the literature, determined by calculation, and directly measured in NO_2 sterilization chambers. The analysis in the following text develops an analytical form of the temperature-dependent D-value for NO_2 sterilization processes. From this, the process shown as Reaction B in Figure 35.10 is the dominant lethal mechanism for isolated microorganisms. This would be the case for spores widely distributed in a BI surface or bioburden on a medical device. Furthermore, it is found that the temperature-dependent D-value for spores in clumps on the BI surface require the strong temperature dependence that can only arrive from the water film chemistry described in Reaction C.

In Table 35.3, step 1 consists of the dimerization of NO_2 to form N_2O_4, as is described earlier in discussions of the equilibrium between the monomer NO_2 and the dimer N_2O_4. This is a well-known behavior for NO_2. The NO_2 molecules that collide will momentarily bond and then return to the monomer state. The dissociation of the N_2O_4 is quite fast, with a half-life of less than 10 μs (at 25°C).[33] Therefore, whenever NO_2 gas is present, some fraction of the NO_2 will be momentarily bound in the dimer form. Step 2 refers to the formation of a water film on surfaces in the sterilization chamber. The NO_2 sterilization process occurs in a humidified environment. The microorganisms, spores, and all the surfaces (surfaces of the chamber, sur-

faces of the items to be sterilized, etc) will adsorb water in these conditions,[47-49] forming a surface. In most applications of the NO_2 sterilization process, a chamber will have roughly ambient temperature and RH below 90%.

The interactions of water films and NO_2 was first reported in atmospheric test chambers, in which scientists would recreate atmospheric conditions that include air, humidity, and atmospheric pollutants like NO_2.[46,50] Where the homogeneous (gas phase) reaction rate between NO_2 and H_2O is known to be slow, in the atmospheric test chambers researchers would observe that the hydrolysis of NO_2 in these chambers and the formation of reaction products was much faster than expected.[45] It was determined that the fast reactions occur in the water films that form on the surfaces of the chamber (heterogeneous reactions), and not in the gas-phase reactions.[50] The thickness of the water film on a surface depends on the surface material and is measured in monolayers of water.[48,49,51] In the literature, estimates of the thickness of a single monolayer of water range from 1.9 Å (0.19 nm)[49] to 2.7 Å (0.27 nm).[45] The thickness of the water film on a material surface will be some multiple of a water monolayer and is dependent on the surface material and the partial pressure of water at the surface (RH).[49] The water film thickness will vary from 1 to 3 monolayers at 20% RH and increases to more than 60 monolayers of water at RH values above 75% RH.[49]

TABLE 35.3 Chemical reactions that occur in water films on surfaces and that contribute to the nitrogen dioxide sterilization process

Step Number	Reaction	Reaction Type	Reference	Evidence
1	Gas phase dimerization of NO_2 to N_2O_4	Dimerization of the NO_2, forming N_2O_4	Leenson[33]	Observation of pre-chamber gas pressures (number of moles) compared to sterilization chamber concentration
2	Humidity forms water films on surfaces. Films of water do not react like bulk water.	Adhesion of water onto surfaces	Ewing[48]; Liebe et al[49]	Humidity drops in chamber due to heterogeneous reaction with NO_2.
3	N_2O_4 and NO_2 enter water film following Henry's law. Because of water-film chemistry, NO_2 hydrolysis (forming HNO_2 and HNO_3) is not the dominant reaction.	Solubilization of gas into liquid	Sander[16]; Finlayson-Pitts et al[45]	Measured concentration of NO_2 is lower than dose introduced into the chamber. Nitrate on surface is measured as residual.
4	$N_2O_4 \rightarrow NO^\bullet + NO_2^\bullet$	Surface reaction where N_2O_4 isomerizes to form $ONONO_2$, HONO, and NO are products	Möller et al[23]; Caulfield et al[46]	HONO and NO are measured in the chamber during sterilization process.
	$2NO^\bullet + O_2 \rightarrow 2NO_2^\bullet$	Auto-oxidation of NO	Lonkar and Dedon[19]; Caulfield et al[46]	
	$NO^\bullet + NO_2^\bullet \rightarrow N_2O_3$	Reaction of NO and NO_2	Nguyen et al[22]; Möller et al[23]; Caulfield et al[46]	
5	N_2O_3 reaction with DNA (cytosine and guanine)	Nitrosation of nucleosides	Lonkar and Dedon[19]; Nguyen et al[22]; Möller et al[23]; Caulfield et al[46]	DNA SSBs measured by noxilizer and others

Abbreviations: HNO_2, isonitrous acid; HNO_3, nitric acid; HONO, nitrous acid; NO, nitric oxide; NO_2, nitrogen dioxide; N_2O_3, dinitrogen trioxide; N_2O_4, dinitrogen tetroxide; O_2, oxygen; $ONONO_2$, nitrosonitrate; SSBs, single strand breaks.

Table 35.3, step 3 describes the interaction between the water film, the NO_2 sterilant gas, and the other gases in the sterilization chamber.[51] A gas will dissolve into water until the concentration in the water reaches equilibrium with the gas phase concentration. This phenomenon is called Henry's law, which states that the equilibrium concentration of a gas dissolved into a liquid is C_{aq}, and is given by

$$C_{aq} = P_g H_{CP} \qquad (19)$$

In equation (19), P_g is the partial pressure of the gas at the water/gas interface and H_{CP} is the Henry's law constant.[16] In thin films of water, this equilibrium is established very quickly. Table 35.4 lists the Henry's law constants, at 25°C, for the prominent gases found in the NO_2 sterilization process. The value for CO_2 is included as a reference and because of general familiarity with carbonated beverages. Table 35.4 also includes values for H_2O_2 and ethylene oxide (C_2H_4O), suggesting that this fundamental principle

TABLE 35.4 Henry's law coefficients and enthalpy of dissolution for selected gases

Henry's Law Coefficients and Constants	N_2O_4	NO_2	NO	HONO	CO_2	H_2O_2	C_2H_4O
H_{cp}^{θ} (M/atm)	1.4	0.012	0.0019	49	0.0034	0.074	0.0017
$\Delta_{sol}H$ (J/mol^{-1})	3500	2400	1600	4900	2400	7000	3500

Abbreviations: C_2H_4O, ethylene oxide; CO_2, carbon dioxide; H_2O_2, hydrogen peroxide; HONO, nitrous acid; NO, nitric oxide; NO_2, nitrogen dioxide; N_2O_4, dinitrogen tetroxide.

may be used to interpret the mechanisms associated with other sterilant gases. Step 4 describes the chemical reactions that occur on the surfaces and in the water film. The properties of this water film vary with the thickness of the water film. From the measurement of several physical and chemical properties, water films do not behave as bulk, aqueous water until the water film is several monolayers thick.[51] Even with the thicker water film, surface reactions of NO_2 are different from the bulk water reactions.

A large fraction of the NO_2 and water in the chamber are involved in these surface reactions. For example, the significance of the NO_2 (and N_2O_4) interactions with the water film is illustrated in Figure 35.10. During the NO_2 sterilization process, where the chamber is humidified prior to the addition of NO_2, the RH has an initial value of 75%. Before the NO_2 addition to the chamber, the humidity is in equilibrium with the water film formed on all surfaces. Once the NO_2 is added, the measured RH value drops from 75% to 50%, and the NO_2 gas concentration decreases sharply as well. Therefore, the addition of the NO_2 gas quickly shifts the equilibrium between the humidity and water film in the chamber and increases the amounts of water and NO_2 that reside in the water film. The N_2O_4 and NO_2 that dissolves into the water can form several chemical species, including $NO^{\bullet}$, $NO_2^{\bullet}$, NO_2^-, nitrate (NO_3^-), HONO, and HNO_3 (see Figure 35.10).[45,51] The most reactive species on the water film surface is the asymmetric form of N_2O_4, nitrosonitrate ($ONONO_2$), which results from the water-induced isomerization of symmetric N_2O_4.[52] The asymmetric $ONONO_2$ has two reaction pathways: it auto-ionizes to generate $NO^+NO_3^-$ or it has a back reaction with gas phase NO_2 to form symmetric N_2O_4 (this reaction step is not shown in Figure 35.10).[51] The $NO^+NO_3^-$ complex reacts with water to generate HNO_3 and HONO. Some of the HONO escapes from the water surface into the gas phase. The HNO_3 on the surface generates NO_2^+, a well-known reaction in concentrated solutions of HNO_3. The NO is generated by the reaction of HONO with NO_2^+.

Given all these chemical reactions, the literature suggests that gaseous NO and HONO will be formed. The formation of the NO and HONO was confirmed in NO_2

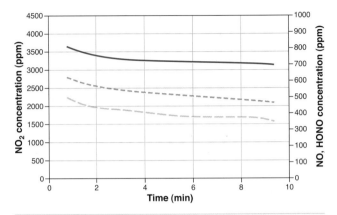

FIGURE 35.11 The gas concentration measured during the sterilant exposure dwell shows nitric oxide (NO) and nitrous acid (HONO) are formed. The solid black line is the nitrogen dioxide (NO_2) concentration, HONO concentration is represented by the dashed line, and NO is represented by the dotted line.

sterilization chambers using FT-IR spectroscopy. A measurement of the HONO and NO formed in the sterilization chamber is shown in Figure 35.11. The data were acquired during a cycle consisting of 10 mg/L NO_2 dose added to a chamber that had been humidified to 75% RH. After 6 minutes, the amount of HONO was found to be approximately 390 ppm and the amount of NO in gas was 502 ppm.

Table 35.3, step 5 is the reaction between the NO and NO_2 to form the N_2O_3. The NO, NO_2, and N_2O_3 can enter and cause critical damage to a microorganism.[23] The N_2O_3 reacts with the cytosine and guanine to damage DNA and RNA.[23,46] As previously described, DNA degradation within *B subtilis* spores was observed to proceed rapidly upon exposure to the NO_2 process.[19] Therefore, it may be concluded that the principle oxide of nitrogen associated with microorganism lethality is N_2O_3.[15,22,23,46] This reaction is the same reaction that is part of the human body's response to infection.

The measured partial pressures of gaseous RNS, shown in Table 35.5, correspond to NO_2 gas concentration values. In this table, the indicated concentration of 6 mg/L,

TABLE 35.5 Gas phase partial pressure and water film concentration for the main nitrogen species in the sterilization chamber

Nitrogen Species	6 mg/L Total NO₂ Gas Concentration		1 mg/L Total NO₂ Gas Concentration	
	Partial Pressure (atm)	Concentration in the Water Film (μM)	Partial Pressure (atm)	Concentration in the Water Film (μM)
NO_2	3.2×10^{-3}	3700	5.3×10^{-4}	640
N_2O_4	6.6×10^{-5}	9400	2.0×10^{-6}	280
NO	5.0×10^{-4}	63	3.3×10^{-5}	4.4
HONO	3.9×10^{-4}	6200	1.3×10^{-5}	440

Abbreviations: HONO, nitrous acid; NO, nitric oxide; NO_2, nitrogen dioxide; N_2O_4, dihydrogen tetroxide.

which would be the typical value measured during sterilization cycles, and 1 mg/L NO_2, which is a sterilant level that would be typically measured during BI D-value characterization. From these values and using the Henry's law constants from Table 35.4, the water film concentrations of the RNS can be calculated. At a chamber concentration of just 1 mg/L NO_2, the concentration of NO in the water film is 4.4 μM. This is a biologically relevant level. In biological systems, the NO concentration near stimulated generator cells is up to 0.5 μM, and this level will cause cell apoptosis[19] through deamination and cross-linking of DNA and single-strand breaks.[15,23,46]

TEMPERATURE DEPENDENCE OF THE NITROGEN DIOXIDE PROCESS

For the chemistry on the surface and in the water film, there are three temperature-dependent factors to consider. These factors are the following: first, the gas phase N_2O_4/NO_2 equilibrium constant, K_p, from equation (8); second, the Henry's law constant; and third, the Arrhenius temperature dependence of the chemical reaction rate. These factors can be combined to determine the overall reaction rate that includes changes in the temperature and NO_2 concentration.

With regard to the first factor, it has been shown that Kp decreases with decreasing temperature (equation [9]). This shifts the equilibrium to favor the formation of N_2O_4, thereby creating an inverse temperature dependence of N_2O_4 in the gas phase (see Figure 35.3). The second factor is the temperature-dependent Henry's law constant for NO_2 and N_2O_4. The Henry's law constant shown in equation (19) will increase with decreasing temperature. The temperature-dependent $H_{cp}(T)$ is given by

$$H_{cp}(T) = H_{cp}^{\theta} \times \exp[(\Delta_{sol}H / R) \times (1/T - 1/T^{\theta})] \quad (20)$$

where H_{cp}^{θ} is the Henry's law constant at 25°C, $\Delta_{sol}H$ is the enthalpy of dissolution, R is the gas constant and is equal to 0.082057 L atm mol^{-1} K^{-1}, and T^{θ} is the temperature at which H^{θ} is measured 25°C.[17] The values of H_{cp}^{θ} and $\Delta_{sol}H$ for some sterilization process–related gases are shown in Table 35.4. This table shows that N_2O_4 has a much greater solubility in water than does NO_2. This is an important point in understanding the water film chemistry involved with using NO_2 as the sterilant gas.

Combining these first two temperature-dependent factors, Kp and $H_{cp}(T)$, the concentration in the water film of NO_2 and N_2O_4 can be calculated as a function of temperature. The estimated water film concentration of total NO_2 is shown in Figures 35.12 and 35.13, for 6 and 1 mg/L NO_2 gas concentration, respectively. When a dose of 10 mg/L is added to the sterilization chamber and most of the species have diffused into the water

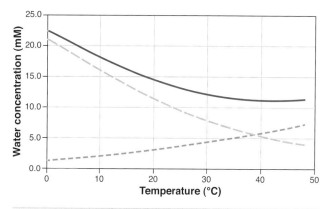

FIGURE 35.12 Graph of the equilibrium concentration in water as a function of temperature for nitrogen dioxide (NO_2) (dotted line), dinitrogen tetroxide (N_2O_4) (dashed line), and the sum of NO_2 and N_2O_4 (solid line) for a 6 mg/L concentration of NO_2 gas in the sterilization chamber.

film, the measured NO_2 concentration is about 6 mg/L (see Figure 35.8). Therefore, 6 mg/L was used for this calculation, as shown in Figure 35.12. For comparison, two additional NO_2 concentration values were analyzed, 1 and 3 mg/L, and these values are summarized in Table 35.6. The graph for water film total NO_2 concentration for 1 mg/L gas phase NO_2 is shown in Figure 35.13.

The water film concentration of the gas is proportional to the gas concentration. However, the gas partial pressure is not constant. For a fixed gas concentration, for example, 6 mg/L, the partial pressure will increase in proportion to the temperature increase (following Gay-Lussac's Law). At 15°C and with 1.0 mg/L of NO_2, the partial pressure of NO_2 in the gas is 0.51 mbar. At 35°C with 1.0 mg/L of NO_2, the partial pressure of NO_2 in the gas is 0.55 mbar. This temperature-dependent increase in the partial pressure is due to the increase kinetic energy of the gas. This is most clearly seen in Table 35.6, with 1 mg/L NO_2 gas concentration, where the water film concentration increases

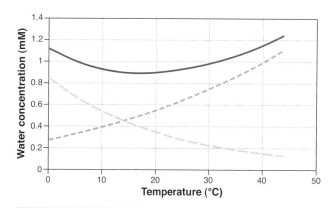

FIGURE 35.13 Graph of the equilibrium concentration in water as a function of temperature for nitrogen dioxide (NO_2) (dotted line), dinitrogen tetroxide (N_2O_4) (dashed line), and the sum of NO_2 and N_2O_4 (solid line) for a 1.0 mg/L concentration of NO_2 gas in the sterilization chamber.

TABLE 35.6	Tabulated values of total nitrogen dioxide (NO_2) concentration in the water film		
Temperature (°C)	Total NO_2 in Water Film (mM) at 1 mg/L NO_2 Gas Concentration	Total NO_2 in Water Film (mM) at 3 mg/L NO_2 Gas Concentration	Total NO_2 in Water Film (mM) at 6 mg/L NO_2 Gas Concentration
15	0.90	5.0	16.1
25	0.92	4.3	13.1
35	1.05	4.2	11.5

slightly going from 25°C to 35°C. For higher NO_2 concentration values, the increase in pressure from kinetic energy is obscured by the inverse temperature dependence of the N_2O_4 concentration. Overall, some important observations from Table 35.6 and Figures 35.12 and 35.13 include the following:

- The total sterilant dissolved in the water film is not linear with the measured NO_2 gas concentration.
- The total NO_2 concentration in the water film is temperature dependent.
- The slope of the temperature dependence of the dissolved total NO_2 in the water film changes sign between 1 and 3 mg/L, as the dimer concentration has a greater influence at the higher NO_2 gas concentration.

The third temperature-dependent factor of the NO_2 process comes from the Arrhenius equation, which provides the temperature dependence of chemical reaction rates. In general, the rate of a first-order chemical reaction follows the exponential time-dependence function, given as

$$P(t) = P_o \exp(-kt) \qquad (21)$$

In this equation, P is the concentration of the reaction products, P_o is the initial concentration of the reactant, k is the rate constant for the reaction, and t is the reaction time. The temperature dependence of the chemical reaction rate constant, k, is given by the Arrhenius equation:

$$k = A \exp(-E_a / RT) \qquad (22)$$

where k is the rate constant for the reaction, T is the absolute temperature (in Kelvin), A is a factor that is unique for a chemical reaction and describes the rate of the chemical interactions (units are sec^{-1}, like the frequency of collisions that might result in the chemical reaction), E_a is the activation energy of the reaction (L atm mol^{-1}), and R is the universal gas constant. The values of A and E_a can be found by fitting the log linear inactivation of P versus t at a single temperature, like 25°C. When P(t) is considered as the time-dependent population of viable spores on a BI carrier, and P_o is the initial population of spores on the carrier, then this equation yields the familiar log-linear graph of spore inactivation kinetics, like that

shown in Figure 35.1. Additionally, this assumes that this simplified reaction is a first order and depends on the concentration of only one reactant, the spore population; however, there is a reaction rate dependence on the sterilant concentration. In order to include the concentration dependence and the temperature-dependent changes in the NO_2 concentration, the rate constant needs to include the concentration using the pseudo first-order rate constant. For this, a new rate constant, k', is used, where

$$k' = k [C]^\alpha \qquad (23)$$

In equation (23), k' is the product of k from equation (22) and a term representing the concentration, [C] is the concentration of sterilant, and α is the exponent describing the order of the reaction. The sterilant concentration [C] is referring to the concentration of total dissolved NO_2 in the water film. The chemical reactions that will cause microbicidal reactions depend on the reaction products that occur in the water film. The pseudo first-order interpretation is appropriate because the rate during the reaction does not directly cause a measureable reduction in the sterilant concentration. The pseudo first-order assumption is implied when citing the observation of first-order microbial inactivation kinetics during a sterilization process. Using equations (21), (22), and (23), the rate of spore inactivation is given by the rate equation:

$$dP / dt = -k [C]^\alpha P(t) \qquad (24)$$

Here, P is the population of spores from equation (21). Substituting equation (23) into equation (22) gives the temperature-dependent rate constant:

$$k' = [C]^\alpha A' \exp(-E_a / RT) \qquad (25)$$

The combined factor, $[C]^\alpha A'$, can be interpreted as a concentration-dependent collision frequency. In equation (25), $[C]^\alpha$ modifies the factor A from equation (22), and A' changes with α so that the units of the term $[C]^\alpha$ A' remain sec^{-1}. To determine the factors A', E_a and α, requires D-value data. E_a and A' are determined by fitting the data at a single temperature. The exponent α is determined by fitting the data over a range of temperature. In the case where $\alpha = 0$, then k' = k. Often, complex

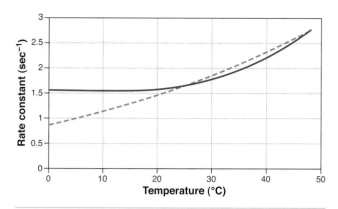

FIGURE 35.14 Graph of the rate constant for the Arrhenius temperature dependence (dotted line) and the calculated rate constant that includes the temperature-dependent total nitrogen dioxide (NO_2) concentration in the water film (solid line), with $\alpha = 1$.

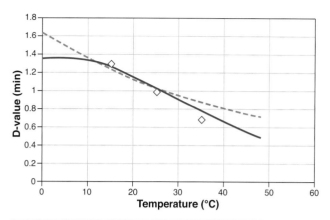

FIGURE 35.15 Comparison of the measured D-value versus temperature and the calculated temperature dependence. The calculated D-value with the water film chemistry ($\alpha = 1$) is shown with the solid line. The Arrhenius temperature dependence is shown with the dashed line ($\alpha = 0$). The measured D-value data is shown with the diamond symbols at 15°C, 25°C, and 35°C, measured with nitrogen dioxide (NO_2) dose = 1.5 mg/L. The biological indicators (BIs) used for the D-value measurement were glass filter carriers with 2.6×10^6 spores per BI.

chemical reactions, with intermediate reaction steps, have noninteger orders of reactions and α can be between -1 and 1 or greater than 1.[53]

Figure 35.14 shows the rate constant, k', for the total NO_2 concentration in the gas equal to 3.0 mg/L, and with $\alpha = 1$ (solid line). This curve is compared to the Arrhenius temperature dependence, k (dotted line). This graph shows that below 30°C, the concentration-dependent rate constant has a weak temperature dependence when compared to the Arrhenius (concentration independent) rate constant. At 45°C, the slope of the Arrhenius temperature dependence is slightly less than that of the water film temperature dependence. This is because the sterilant gas will be measured by absolute concentration, like mg/L or mmol/L.[54] However, the rate at which the sterilant gas enters the water film is dependent on the gas partial pressure of the sterilant, not the absolute concentration. For example, with the concentration held constant in units of mg/L, the partial pressure of the sterilant will increase with temperature, according to Gay-Lussac's Law.

Equation (25) has the three temperature-dependent factors included in the reaction rate constant k'. This rate constant can be used to directly calculate the temperature-dependent D-value, D(T), for the NO_2 process. Writing the equation for the D-value in terms of equation (21) and using k' from equation (25):

$$D(T) = t/[(\log (P_o) - \log (P_o \exp (-k't)] \quad (26)$$

Like with equation (21), the variable P_o is the original population of spores on the BI carrier, and t is the exposure time of the BI to the NO_2 process.

In order to evaluate the temperature-dependent D-value calculations, two types of BIs were selected for testing. The first type of BIs used a glass filter media as the carrier, and the second type used a stainless steel disc carrier. A comparison of the measured and calculated D-values versus temperature for the first type of BIs

(on glass filter media carriers) is shown in Figure 35.15. The BIs used for the measurement consisted of 6-mm diameter discs of glass filter media as the carrier, with 2.6×10^6 spores per carriers. These BIs were packaged in Tyvek/Mylar pouches during the NO_2 exposure process, at a dose of 1.5 mg/L NO_2. The variables A and E_a were determined at 25°C, and then the coefficient, α, was adjusted to find a fit with the data. The temperature dependence from equation (26) is shown as the solid line, and where $\alpha = 1$, which suggests the influence of the water film chemistry. The Arrhenius (concentration independent) temperature dependence for the D-value is shown as the dotted line (equation [26] with $\alpha = 0$). For most of the temperature range shown in Figure 35.15 (from 10°C to 35°C), there is reasonable agreement between the data and both curves. Without testing the D-value at higher and lower temperature values, it is not possible to determine the degree to which the temperature dependence of the water film chemistry (illustrated in Figure 35.13) contributes to the measured lethality rate. Regardless, the unique temperature dependence of the total NO_2 concentration in the water film is not required to represent the data measured with the BIs on the glass filter media.

Using the second type of BIs, the temperature-dependent D-value is shown in Figure 35.16, with the concentration-independent case. These BIs were 7.2-mm diameter stainless steel carrier discs, with 1.4×10^6 spores per carriers, and packaged in Tyvek/Mylar pouches. In Figure 35.16, the Arrhenius temperature dependence ($\alpha = 0$) is shown with the dotted line and the calculated temperature dependence from equation (26). The calculated D-value that depends on the water film chemistry is shown with a solid line. The NO_2 concentration was 3 mg/L

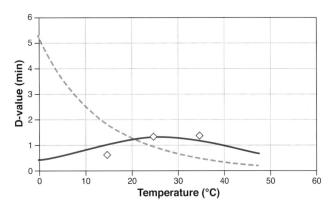

FIGURE 35.16   Comparison of the measured D-value versus temperature and the calculated temperature dependence. The calculated D-value with the water film chemistry is shown with the solid line. The Arrhenius temperature dependence is shown with the dashed line ($\alpha = 0$). The measured D-value data is shown with the diamond symbols at 15°C, 25°C, and 35°C, measured with nitrogen dioxide (NO$_2$) dose = 3.0 mg/L. The biological indicators (BIs) used for the D-value measurements were 7.2-mm diameter stainless steel carriers with 1.44×10^6 spores, packaged in small Tyvek pouches.

for these exposure cycles. The temperature dependence from equation (26) is shown as the solid line, and where $\alpha = 4$. The variables A and Ea were determined at 25°C, and then the coefficient, α, was adjusted to find a fit with the data. The calculated Arrhenius temperature dependence for the D-value has a slope that is contrary to the measured temperature dependence.

An analysis of these results provides insight into the NO$_2$ sterilization process, the use of BIs, and the interpretation of the measured BI D-value behavior as a function of temperature. One observation from Figures 35.15 and 35.16 is that BI quality influences the observed temperature dependence of the D-values. Another observation is that the simple Arrhenius temperature dependence (equation [22]) cannot completely represent the measured D-value results for the two types of BIs. The BIs with the stainless steel carriers have a higher resistance to the NO$_2$ process than the BIs on glass filter media. Both BI types were made using the same lot of spores; however, there is a significant difference in the resistance of two types of BIs. The difference in resistance is highlighted, first, by the different doses of NO$_2$ sterilant required to measure the D-values for the two types of BIs. For the stainless steel carriers, an NO$_2$ dose of 3 mg/L was used. For the glass filter carrier BIs, the NO$_2$ dose was 1.5 mg/L. Also, the population measured for the two types of BIs confirmed that the stainless steel BIs had fewer spores. The stainless steel carriers averaged 1.4×10^6 spores per carrier BIs versus an average of 2.6×10^6 spores per carrier with the glass filter carrier BIs. The measured resistance of a BI is known to increase with the number of spores on a carrier.[52] In spite of the difference, the magnitude of the

measured D-values are similar for both types of BIs, about 1 minute for both types, because the concentration used compensated for the difference in observed resistance. Therefore, we can conclude that the stainless steel carrier BIs have an inherently higher resistance than the glass filter carrier BIs. The reason for the difference in resistance with the two types of BIs may be the distribution of the spores on the different types of carriers. As the inoculum dries on the stainless steel carriers, the water dries from the edge of the droplet, and as the water (or other inoculation medium) evaporates from the edges, there is a flow of liquid from the center of the droplet to the edges.[55] This flow of liquid carries the suspended spores and any dissolved matter (like salts, proteins, and debris) to the out edge of the droplet. The result is an agglomeration of the spores at the edge, forming a ring of dried spores that can be many spore-layers deep. The agglomeration of spores (at the droplet edge or wherever it occurs) can be referred to as clumping.[56,57] Spore clumping is common with BIs using a stainless steel carrier and can be seen under microscopy.[27]

During a sterilization process, spores on the BI can be protected by clumping. The driving mechanisms of lethal process required to kill such protected spores can be temperature-dependent factors like liquid film sterilant concentration, diffusion, rate of forming reaction products, and others. Because diffusion and rate of forming reaction products are also functions of concentration, it is appropriate to use α in equation (25) to represent this higher order concentration dependence. Therefore, the temperature dependence of the D-value, from equations (25) and (26), is fit better to the temperature dependence in Figure 35.16 with $\alpha = 3$ or 4. This implies that the water film chemistry is strongly important to the lethality of the most protected spores. Conversely, spores that are at the surface are directly exposed to the sterilizing environment and should be sterilized with only the spore's intrinsic resistance to the process.[56] With the glass filter media carriers, the spores have three dimensions over which they can distribute themselves (eg, see Figure 40.1, page 797 of Block[27]). During the deposition of the aqueous inoculum on the glass filter carriers, the liquid wicks into the filter, carrying the spores a short distance. During the drying of the inoculum, the spores on the glass filter media are deposited on the individual fibers of the filter and do not travel to the drying front of the inoculum, as they would during the drying of the inoculum on the surface of a stainless steel carrier. This gives the spores on the glass filter media a better opportunity to remain as unclumped spores. These spores respond more directly to the sterilizing gas environment ($\alpha = 1$, as in Figure 35.15). With $\alpha = 1$, the liquid phase contribution to the D-value is relatively weak. This implies that the liquid phase is not a strong contributor to the temperature dependence of the D-value.

Recognizing these conclusions, the tailing of the inactivation kinetics may be understood. A fraction of the total spore population is not protected by clumping and is exposed directly to the gas process, as described with $\alpha = 0$ or $\alpha = 1$. Another fraction of the spores are protected by the clumping of spores on the BI and have a greater measured resistance because of this protection. Therefore, clumping contributes to tailing and lethality of spores in the clumps require highly concentration-dependent factors like diffusion and chemical reaction product generation.[58] Furthermore, tailing causes disagreement between the results of BI characterization methods like SMC, HSK, survival-kill method, and overall survivor curve. Conversely, characterization of the BIs with minimal clumping has shown improved agreement between various characterization methods, when compared to BIs with more clumping.[59,60]

These results with the NO_2 process shows the impact of BI quality on the observed BI response, where BI clumping can result in unexpected temperature dependence of the D-value. This is not only an aspect of the NO_2 sterilization process. Testing has been completed where the same lot of BIs was used for testing in both NO_2 and vapor H_2O_2 processes. From these results, both processes have similar requirements for BI performance. Both the NO_2 and H_2O_2 processes are sensitive to the clumping of the spores, which can be observed as tailing during fraction negative investigations. Furthermore, the shape of the temperature dependence of the D-value curve shown in Figure 35.16 (solid line) has been measured with the H_2O_2 process as well.[61] When testing H_2O_2 sterilization, researchers found that the measured D-value as a function of temperature had a maximum value at 35°C, where increasing or decreasing the temperature away from this temperature resulted in a reduction of the D-value. Also, as described with the stainless steel BIs in this report, photographs of the inoculum exhibit a ring of greater density spores[61] and tailing of the inactivation curves.[61] Therefore, the distribution of spores on the BI carrier greatly changes the observed inactivation kinetics. Furthermore, with BIs that exhibit tailing, the measured gas concentration may be insufficient to describe the rate of microbial inactivation, and factors that influence the surface chemistry can play a dominant role.

Other observations and conclusions from this analysis include the following:

- Relating the D-value to chemical reaction factors like activation energy (Ea), the frequency factor (A), and the reaction rate constant provides appropriate degrees of freedom for the modeling of the inactivation kinetics.
- Spores (and microorganisms) presented to the NO_2 process in a monolayer will more closely follow the traditionally expected temperature dependence (Arrhenius equation).
  - Bioburden on devices to be sterilized is not normally found in clumps and will follow the results represented with the temperature dependence shown in Figure 35.16.
  - For reusable instruments, device cleaning is important, and this importance is underscored by the higher sterilant concentrations often recommended to sterilize devices with the potential of soils remaining on the device surfaces (see chapter 47). These soils have the potential to produce the contrary temperature dependence seen in Figure 35.16.
- The temperature dependence on the molecular concentration of total NO_2 in the water film can cause temperature-dependent changes in the compatibility of very sensitive materials.

▶ STERILANT RESIDUALS

The water film chemistry, described earlier, produces several molecular species on the NO_2-sterilized surfaces. These molecular species include NO, NO_2, N_2O_3, HONO, HNO_2, and HNO_3. Most of the sterilant residues are removed during aeration, with a small amount of HNO_3 and HNO_2 remaining, barring any underlying reaction with the material. Any molecular nitrogen species that remain are identified as the residues of the process. The remaining residues have been characterized on many medical devices and different types of materials and can be shown not to cause known biocompatibility issues. The quantification of residues on devices uses standard assays.

The mechanisms to cause residual molecules to leave the water films and surfaces in a sterilization chamber depend on the temperature of the system, the inverse of the Henry's law constant, and the chemical reactions that result in molecular products that more easily enter the gas phase. The amount of water that adsorbs on surfaces, and the amount of molecular nitrogen species formed on a surface, depends on the material properties.[62] A material with molecular binding sites on the surface can have an affinity for water and residues. This binding slows the rate of residue removal. During aeration, the vapor pressures of the gaseous molecular nitrogen species are reduced, and the molecules dissolved in the water film leave the surface (Henry's law). The NO, NO_2, N_2O_4, and HONO molecules are removed following this mechanism. The N_2O_3 dissociates to NO and NO_2 gas when it leaves the surface.[63] Chemical reactions that decompose HNO_2, HONO, and HNO_3 form gaseous products are shown in equations (27) and (28).[64]

$$2\,HNO_2 + 3\,H_2O + NO \rightarrow \\ NO_{2(g)} + N_2O_{4(surface)} + 4\,H_2O_{(L)} \tag{27}$$

$$HNO_{3(surface)} + HONO_{(surface)} \rightarrow \\ N_2O_{4(surface/gas)} + H_2O_{(L)} \tag{28}$$

Despite these mechanisms, some undissociated HNO_3 and HNO_2 (and its isomer, HONO) can remain attached to binding sights on the material surface.[64] Therefore, the expectation is that the residue of the sterilant will be mostly HNO_3 and HNO_2. Measurements of the residues recovered from medical devices and material samples confirm that the residue from the NO_2 process is more than 90% NO_3^- and less than 10% nitrite (NO_2^-). Typically, NO_3^- extracted from processed surfaces ranges from <1 to 100 $\mu g/cm^2$. This agrees with the literature, where the residuals are measured spectroscopically as principally consisting of undissociated HNO_3.[52] The hazards posed by these residuals are considered low. The RNS, $NO^{\bullet}$, and $NO_2^{\bullet}$ are reacted during the process and only the less reactive species persist. Both nitrite and NO_3^- were tested for DNA-damaging activity. It was found that exposing cells to a 1-mM concentration caused no observed DNA damage.[15] Additionally, other trace residues were not cytotoxic.[65] From all the testing completed as part of sterilization testing, exposure to the NO_2 process does not change the cytotoxicity of materials.

Two analytical methods available for testing residues are ion chromatography and the Griess reagent assay. Ion chromatography is available from many test laboratories. The Griess reagent assay is commonly used to measure NO_3^- anions in drinking water. Generally, the Griess reagent assay is more sensitive than ion chromatography. For these test methods, extraction of the residuals and residues from the surface is necessary. An extraction technique that works well is to immerse the samples in purified water (eg, American Society for Testing and Materials [ASTM] type 1 water) at a specified temperature for a specified period of time. The international standard regarding extract preparation, ISO 10993-12:2012,[66] is appropriate for use with medical devices. The extract is then assayed for the residues, measured as NO_3^- or NO_2^- using either ion chromatography or the Griess reagent assay.

At present, no international standard exists to determine the acceptability of NO_2 sterilant residuals. The level of residuals measured by the assay is not "high" or "low" because this value measured is not a measure of "unsafe" or "safe." Rather, after characterizing the level of residuals on a medical device that passes biocompatibility testing and device functionality testing, then the level of residues measured is established to be a safe level.

▶ SAFETY

The safety of using NO_2 as a sterilant was thoroughly reviewed in the application to the EPA for registration of NO_2 as a sterilant (approved and registered in January 2016).[1] The health risks associated with NO_2 sterilization include patients exposed to sterilant residuals on device surfaces and those from operator exposure. Device residues are not yet considered to pose a significant risk as discussed earlier. The primary operator exposure risk is an acute inhalation risk. This can result in irritation of mucosal membranes and the lungs. Inhalation of high concentrations of NO_2 can lead to pulmonary edema. The Occupational Safety and Health Administration (OSHA) permissible exposure limit (PEL) for NO_2 is 5 ppm, whereas the National Institute for Occupational Safety and Health (NIOSH) recommended exposure limit (REL) is 1 ppm. The OSHA PEL is a ceiling value that should not be exceeded at any time, whereas the NIOSH REL value is a time-weighted average (TWA) over a 10-hour workday (in a 40-hr work week). These values are compared to other chemical sterilants, in Table 35.7.[67]

TABLE 35.7	Characteristics and relative safety of sterilant gases					
Sterilant	NIOSH REL (ppm)	OSHA PEL (ppm)	IDLH (ppm)	Odor Threshold (ppm)	Odor Threshold Below PEL?	Typical Use Concentration (ppm)
NO_2	1[a]	5[b]	20	0.1	Yes	500-10 000
ClO_2	0.1[c]	0.1	5	0.1	No	360
Ethylene oxide	0.1[d]	1[e]	800	500	No	500 000
H_2O_2	1	1	75	None	No	1000-3000
Ozone	0.1[b]	0.1	5	<0.1	Yes	200-20 000

Abbreviations: IDLH, immediately dangerous to life and health; NIOSH, National Institute for Occupational Safety and Health; OSHA, Occupational Safety and Health Administration; PEL, permissible exposure limit; REL, recommended exposure limit.

[a]NIOSH short-term REL, 15-min time-weighted average (TWA), not to be exceeded in any one workday.

[b]Ceiling REL/PEL, must not be exceeded at any time during the workday.

[c]NIOSH short-term REL of 0.3 ppm, 15-min TWA, not to be exceeded in any one workday.

[d]NIOSH ceiling REL is 5 ppm, over 10 min per workday.

[e]OSHA PEL allows an excursion to 5 ppm for 15 min per workday.

The relative safety of sterilant gases is compared for informational purposes only. Odor thresholds are given to call attention to whether an operator can discern a potential hazard by nose prior to exposure conditions reaching a nonpermissible level.

There are two significant differences in the safety of NO_2 sterilant versus other gas and vapor sterilants. First, NO_2 is visible due to the reddish-brown color of the gas. Second, the odor threshold of NO_2 is 0.1 ppm, which is well below the PELs of 1.0 ppm.[68] Neither ethylene oxide nor H_2O_2 can be detected by odor at safe levels.[69,70] Therefore, based on color and odor, NO_2 can be more easily detected by operators than other gas and vapor sterilants.[71,72]

The NO_2 is considered noncarcinogenic, whereas some other sterilant gases such as ethylene oxide and formaldehyde are considered carcinogenic in humans (group 1) by the International Agency for Research on Cancer (IARC).[73,74] The H_2O_2 is classified as an animal carcinogen (with unknown relevance to humans) by the IARC[75]; however, it is not classified as to its carcinogenicity in humans (group 3).

As with all applications of sterilants, manufacturers have developed systems and practices that minimize operator exposure to sterilant used. The NO_2 chambers, whether for sterilization or decontamination applications, are designed to minimize operator risk. This means that compatible materials of construction are used throughout. As with any sterilization process, calibration and preventive maintenance are also key components to the safe operation of the system. As was mentioned previously, electrochemical cells for NO_2 detection are commercially available. Cells that measure in the range of 0 to 10 ppm are appropriate for monitoring the work environment and alerting operators to potential hazardous conditions. They may be stationary units or portable, handheld units. Stationary units can be hardwired into a plant monitoring system to send a general alert when a hazardous condition is measured.

▶ MATERIAL COMPATIBILITY

As with other sterilization processes, including liquid chemical sterilants, radiation, gas sterilants, or heat sterilization, the development and validation of a sterilization or disinfection process requires an understanding the compatibility of the materials in the products or equipment being subjected to the process. Each sterilization process has its own set of materials compatibility limitations, depending on their application. Judging compatibility of materials, particularly polymers, requires testing the material formulation to be used in the device or equipment. Additionally, accelerated aging or real-time aging should be included in a material evaluation program. Many widely used materials are compatible with the NO_2 process; however, much of this discussion is devoted to materials that are not compatible or may be compatible within a limited set of applications. These general guidelines of material compatibility with NO_2 include suggestions for alternative materials and the application of protective coatings to minimize the impact of NO_2 on materials that are subject to reaction with the gas. Polymers are generally not used in their native state. Additives are included in the polymer formulations, improving the performance of the polymer with the additional of colorants, antioxidants, mold release agents, plasticizers, etc. Therefore, beyond the chemical compatibility of the native polymer with a sterilization process, the polymer compatibility along with the additives must be considered.

Materials are considered compatible with a sterilization process when no chemical reactions occur between the materials, the sterilization process is demonstrated to be effective on the material surface, and the material maintains its functional properties after the sterilization cycle. Several aspects of chemical compatibility include chemical changes, color changes, and the degree of change during a single sterilization cycle. Some materials may experience a slight discoloration (eg, yellowing). But, as with some other sterilization processes, the slight discoloration does not signal incompatibility of a material. Furthermore, there are materials that perform well after a single exposure but are not suited for multiple exposures to the process. These materials would be appropriate for single-use medical devices. Materials that perform well after multiple exposures would be appropriate for both single-use and reusable devices as well as isolators and airlocks that undergo repeated disinfection cycles. The reactions between the material and the sterilant gas compete with the reactions that result in the inactivation of microbes on the material surface. This results in increased apparent resistance to the sterilization process on these surfaces. For example, with soft polyvinyl chloride (PVC) materials, D-value of bacterial spores on soft PVC can be four times longer than the same spores placed on hard PVC or stainless steel surfaces.[76,77] This is true with both NO_2 and H_2O_2 sterilization and disinfection processes.

It is not practical to list all materials that are generally compatible with NO_2 gas in this document, but a few relevant materials are contained in Table 35.8. These materials are common in medical devices, parenteral drug containers, and the aseptic processing equipment. The fact that a material is listed as generally compatible does not obviate the need for testing the material compatibility or biocompatibility of the actual device or equipment being sterilized.

Polyamides and Polyurethanes

The NO_2 process chemistry will react with polyamides and polyurethanes.[78-80] The primary reaction pathways have been described in the literature,[81] and they result in scission of the amide and urethane bonds. Degradation due to NO_2 is inhibited when the amide or urethane bonds undergo hydrogen bonding with either neighboring polymer chains or chemical additives. The hydrogen bonds serve to protect these vulnerable groups from attack. When investigating material interactions with NO_2

TABLE 35.8   A list of common medical device and equipment-related materials that are compatible with nitrogen dioxide

Metals and Alloys	
Stainless steel: 304, 304L, 316, 316L	Platinum and Pt/Ir alloys
Gold	Titanium alloys
Silver	ASTM F-75 Co/Cr alloy

Ceramics	
Glass	Alumina
Quartz	Zirconia

Polymers	
Polyethylene (PE, LDPE, HDPE)	Acrylonitrile butadiene styrene (ABS)
Polypropylene (PP)	Polymethyl methacrylate (PMMA)
Polystyrene (PS)	Polyetherimide (PEI, Ultem®)
Polyesters (PET, PETE, PETG, APET)	Methyl methacrylate butadiene styrene (MABS, Zylar®)
Polyether ether ketone (PEEK)	Styrene methyl methacrylate (SMMA, NAS®)
Cyclic olefins (COC, COP)	Styrene acrylonitrile (SAN, Lustran®)
Fluoropolymers (PTFE, PFA, FEP)	Polysulfone (PSU, Udel®)
Polycarbonate (PC, Lexan®)	Polyphenylsulfone (PPSU, Radel®)
Rigid polyvinyl chloride (PVC)	Polyar", etherketone (PAEK)

Elastomers	
Fluoroelastomers (FKM, FFKM, Viton®, Kalrez®)	Halobutyl rubbers (Chloro-, Bromo-)[a]
Silicone (PDMS)	Styrene butadiene rubber (SBR)[a]
Chlorosulfonated polyethylene (CSPE, Hypalon®)	Nitrile rubber (BUNA, NBR)[a]

[a]Materials recommended for single-use devices or with limited exposure.

sterilization, it is important to look at both short-term (immediately after sterilization) and long-term (accelerated or real-time aging) effects.

Whereas some reactions are expected, some polyamide and polyurethane material formulations have been successfully tested for NO$_2$ process exposure. These tests were typical for limited exposure scenarios (eg, single-use devices). With long-term exposure or repeated sterilization cycles, chemical reactions can alter the surface properties of the material, often resulting in a glossy, tacky surface due to the scission of the polymeric chains. In nylon materials, the surface effects are partially reversible and may dissipate over time, indicating a reorganization of the polymeric chains at the surface.[82] With polyurethane materials, the material changes appear irreversible.[83] Urethanes also tend to go undergo discoloration upon exposure to NO$_2$ gas. Some urethane-based adhesives are also not recommended for NO$_2$ sterilization because they will undergo similar reactions, and the resulting low-molecular-weight products can result in adverse reactions with the bonded polymeric materials.

Other materials can be considered in place of polyamides or polyurethanes. Depending on the application, materials such as polypropylene, polysulfone, high-density polyethylene (HDPE), acrylonitrile butadiene styrene, or silicone may be appropriate. In the case of adhesives, acrylic- or silicone-based adhesives could be considered in place of urethane-based formulations.

Peptide-Based Materials

Peptide bonds are similar in nature to urethane and amide bonds in their susceptibility to attack by NO$_2$. Proteins such as collagen, often used in tissue scaffolds, or fibroin, the primary component of silk fibers, can undergo reaction with NO$_2$ that results in a loss of mechanical properties.

Polyacetal

Polyacetal is also known as acetal, polyformaldehyde, and polyoxymethylene. It is often referred to by trade names such as Delrin®, Celcon®, and Hostaform®. It is commonly used in applications where its lubricious properties are advantageous, such as gears in medical devices or rollers in filling lines. The polymeric structure reacts with the NO_2 process.[84] Attenuated total reflectance (ATR) FT-IR spectroscopy of the material in the postexposure condition indicated an increasing concentration of carboxyl bonds at the surface of the material. This is consistent with the scission of the C-O-C bond that serves as the backbone of the polyacetal structure.[82]

The degradation of the polyacetal results in the formation of friable particles of paraformaldehyde and the release of formaldehyde, the odor of which is readily detectable in polyacetal materials that have been exposed to NO_2. Both of these species are cytotoxic and carcinogenic, which renders this material incompatible with NO_2 sterilization. Design alternatives, such as polyetherimide (Ultem®), HDPE, polysulfone, and polyphenylsulfone (Radel®) should be considered.

Polyvinylchloride

Whereas the base polymer has been shown to be generally compatible with NO_2 gas sterilization, some formulations of PVC are not recommended for use with NO_2 sterilization. The PVC used for flexible tubing or sheets may contain up to 40% of plasticizer. Even some more rigid PVC will contain small percentages of plasticizer. A common plasticizer currently used in the industry is di(2-ethlyhexyl) phthalate (DEHP). However, DEHP is being replaced by alternative materials, based on guidance from regulatory agencies and concerns over DEHP causing adverse health effects.[85,86] Polymers that contain DEHP may exhibit surface blooming of DEHP. Also, there may be a loss of mechanical properties of the bulk material. Alternative plasticizers like trioctyl trimellitate may serve as suitable alternatives.

Hydrogels

Whereas some special process parameters have been developed for specific hydrogel materials, materials that are very hygroscopic and form hydrogels require special care in the development of the NO_2 sterilization process. Because the hydrogel materials will absorb water from the sterilization environment, this can result in the acidification of the material upon absorption of NO_2 as well as discoloration. These changes can alter the performance of the device.

Cellulose

Cellulosic materials are generally not compatible with the NO_2 sterilization process. Cellulose will react with NO_2 and the acids that form in the water film on the surface.

The reactions will result in oxidation and nitration of the cellulose material.[87,88] The primary effects of these reactions are discoloration of the material and embrittlement. Additionally, the reaction between the cellulose and the NO_2 serves to increase the apparent resistance of microorganisms on the cellulosic material. In the case of cellulose-based polymers, such as cellulose acetate or cellulose propionate, material alternatives to be considered are polycarbonate, copolyesters, and cyclic polyolefins.

Stainless Steel

The 300 series of stainless steels, especially 316, 316L, 304 and 304L have demonstrated excellent compatibility with the NO_2 sterilization and disinfection process. As evidence, the sterilization chambers and other accessories used for NO_2 gas are manufactured from the low-carbon, "L", version of one or both alloys. The martensitic 400 series of stainless steels, which are commonly used in cutting and load-bearing applications, will exhibit corrosion upon exposure to the NO_2 sterilization process. However, corrosion of these alloys is not limited to NO_2 sterilization, as corrosion has been observed in steam-sterilized devices as well.[89]

Aluminum

In air, bare aluminum will oxidize, forming a protective layer. Upon exposure to the NO_2 sterilization process, this protective layer is preserved. Some aluminum alloys (eg, 6063 T6, 6061 T6) has been tested and shown to be satisfactory for repeated exposure to the NO_2 disinfection process. Anodized aluminum can perform well in both single-use and reusable applications. For parenteral drug product containers such as vial or cartridges, aluminum crimp caps should be coated with an enamel to protect against cosmetic levels of corrosion. As with other materials, adding color to the enamel can mask any slight discoloration that the clear enamel may undergo.

Other Metal Alloys and Circuit Boards

Copper-containing alloys can be subject to corrosion upon exposure to the NO_2 sterilization process. This includes base alloys such as brass, as well as alloys used for brazing or soldering applications. Care should be taken to investigate the composition of alloys used in joining applications as even "silver solder" may contain a fraction of copper. The corrosion may not be evident immediately after exposure, and it may require several weeks to be visibly noticeable. Controlling humidity to a lower level (eg, 40% RH) may result in reduced corrosion of the copper and other alloys. Consider stainless steel alloys 316 and 304 are alternatives to brass materials in medical devices to be sterilized by NO_2.

For certain applications, such as printed circuit boards, motors, and other wiring, a conformal coating process will improve compatibility by virtually eliminating corrosion concerns. An example of a conformal coating material would be Parylene®, which has been shown to protect electric motors from corrosion over multiple NO_2 exposure cycles. Gold coating or plating of electrical contacts is generally not sufficient to eliminate corrosion concerns. Metallic coatings that are deposited via electrochemical methods often have microscopic defects such as pinholes. Whereas the gold will not corrode, these pinholes can permit the underlying metal to corrode, and potentially disturbing the gold plating. There are coating technologies that can protect these pinholes and reduce the potential for corrosion of the underlying metal.

Parenteral Drug Containers

The NO_2 sterilization process is well suited for parenteral drug container applications such as prefilled syringes or cartridge-based drug delivery devices where the external, gas-accessible surfaces are required to be sterile. It can be applied to parenteral products as an adjunct, batch sterilization process using minimal vacuum (depending on device geometry) and low temperature (10°C-30°C), with total processing times typically less than 4 hours, depending on chamber volume. These conditions can allow for the processing of sensitive parenteral biologic and pharmaceutical products with minimal impact to the time-temperature budget compare to other sterilization processes that operate at temperature ranges that typically exceed 30°C.

One measure of compatibility with parenteral containers is the measurement of sterilant ingress into the container. It is known that sterilant gases (eg, ethylene oxide) will permeate through the elastomer and contaminate the container contents. For syringes, a common configuration is staked-needle syringes composed of ASTM type 1 glass and cyclic olefin copolymer, tip caps, plunger rods, and pistons composed of pharmaceutical rubbers with and without fluoropolymer coatings. These types of syringes have been thoroughly studied with the NO_2 sterilization process. The syringes were filled with ASTM type 1 water, exposed in sterilization pouches to a cycle like that shown in Figure 35.8: 70% RH to 80% RH, 10 mg/L NO_2, 60-minute dwell, and 90-minute aeration. Upon completion of the cycle, the syringes were tested for NO_2 ingress into the water. The water from the syringes was tested via a colorimetric, Greiss-reagent assay for NO_3^- and nitrite anions, to confirm if any penetrating NO_2 would be present as HNO_3 or HNO_2. In all cases, the results of testing have indicated that the NO_3^- levels in the syringes were below the limit of detection (LOD) for the test (0.025 ppm NO_3^-).[90,91] And in all cases, the absorbance measured at the characteristic wavelength for the NO_3^- chromophore was similar for the unexposed controls and exposed samples. The LOD for the test was four times lower than the maximum level of NO_3^- allowed in water for injections (WFI) by the European Pharmacopoeia,[92] which is 0.2 ppm. This indicated that many existing parenteral container materials should provide an adequate barrier to NO_2 ingress to preserve the product integrity when the external surfaces of the container are sterilized with NO_2 gas.

Packaging Materials

Due to the general incompatibility of paper-based products, it is recommended that NO_2 sterilization be carried out on products in the primary, sterile-barrier packaging. As with other gas sterilization technologies, the primary package must include a means for sterilant gas ingress and egress. The NO_2 is compatible with many polymeric packaging materials that are currently in use including spunbonded or melt-blown olefin fibers, like Tyvek®, which allows for ready penetration of the NO_2 gas into the sterilization pouch or tray. All grades of Tyvek® provide adequate gas access for the NO_2 to both enter and leave the package. Unless adhesive is required for a tray sealing operation, uncoated Tyvek® is preferred.

Adhesives used for packaging should be validated for use with NO_2. It has been demonstrated that NO_2 sterilization may be used with flood-coated, water-based adhesives. Some hot-melt adhesives may react with NO_2 and undergo discoloration. This reaction can also provide a greater challenge to the sterilization process than will the water-based adhesives. Zone coating of adhesives on Tyvek® lid stock is also option, although it is mainly done for cosmetic reasons. Blue-tinted adhesives may help to mask any slight discoloration that the adhesive undergoes upon exposure to NO_2 gas.

For sterilization pouches with a clear film layer, the film should consist of coextruded polyester and polyethylene. Polypropylene may also be appropriate as a backing layer to the polyester. The clear film should not include an amide-based tie layer because this will discolor during the NO_2 process.

Standard tray materials such as polyester (PETG, APET, or PET), polystyrene, polyethylene, and copolyester (eg, Eastman Tritan®) are appropriate for use. Materials containing nylon, even when incorporated as an inner layer of laminated foil, should be avoided. As with any sterilization technology, the specific materials should be validated for use with the defined process. Trays that include nylon or polyurethane inserts or layers are not appropriate.

Given the general incompatibility of cellulosic materials, polymer-based label stock should be selected for use with NO_2 sterilization. Polystyrene or polyester stock is preferred because both perform well. The ink on the printed labels may be made more color fast, using a clear polyester (Mylar®) laminate.

▶ APPLICATION EXAMPLES

Medical Device Sterilization

In April 2016, a 510(k) application for a stainless steel, surgical ruler sterilized with NO_2 gas was cleared by the FDA for distribution as a medical device.[2] The vacuum-based NO_2 sterilization process was validated per ISO 14937:2009, using an overkill approach. The device was presented to the sterilization process in a Tyvek® pouch, and an SCBI containing more than 1.0×10^6 colony-forming units (CFUs) *G stearothermophilus* spores was placed inside of the pouch as an internal process challenge device (iPCD). The geometry of the SCBI provided a significant challenge to the process as compared to that of the relatively simple geometry of the stainless steel surface. A summary of the sterilization validation process is given here as a case study.

The challenge presented by the iPCD was compared directly to that presented by the native bioburden present. The bioburden was evaluated and found to be less than 20 CFUs/unit of aerobic bacteria and fungi, during process definition. A series of fractional cycles were carried out with NO_2 dose as the process variable. The vacuum level employed was 20 mm Hg (± 2 mm Hg) and humidified air was added to 590 mm Hg (± 59 mm Hg) after NO_2 dosing, which equated to 70% RH ($\pm 10\%$RH). A single exposure pulse with a dwell time of 5 minutes (± 10 s) was used, and aeration was affected through a series of evacuation air exchanges, from 20 to 590 mm Hg, with room air filtered through a 0.2-μm filter. The results are shown in Table 35.9. The results from the 2.0 mg/L NO_2 fractional cycle established that the iPCD was more resistant to the process than the native bioburden, whereas the complete inactivation of the iPCD in the 3.0 mg/L NO_2 fractional cycle established that more than 6 log reduction in indicator organism population was achieved.[93] Based on these initial results, a conservative half-cycle sterilization process was specified using an NO_2 dose at 10.0 mg/L ($\pm 10\%$), and the number of exposure pulses was doubled to yield two 5-minute long (± 10 s) dwells. The specified

vacuum was 20 mm Hg (± 2 mm Hg), the specified humidified air addition was 590 mm Hg (± 59 mm Hg), and the specified number of evacuative air exchanges was 12. A reduced half cycle with NO_2 set to 9.0 mg/L ($\pm 10\%$), humid air set to 531 mm Hg (± 59 mm Hg), and a dwell time of 4 minutes and 50 seconds (± 10 s) was repeated three consecutive times. In each half cycle, all five iPCDs were negative, and the half cycle was qualified.[94]

In order to quantify residuals from the process and demonstrate the biocompatibility of the ruler, samples were exposed to two times the full-cycle process (four exposure pulses) with parameters set to the upper bounds of the tolerance limits: NO_2 was 11.0 mg/L ($\pm 10\%$), humid air was 649 mm Hg (± 59 mm Hg), and the dwell time of each exposure pulse was 5 minutes and 10 seconds (± 10 s). After two consecutive exposures, extractions of ruler samples were carried out per ISO 10993-12:2012.[67] The NO_2 residuals were measured as extracted NO_3^- and nitrite via ion chromatography, using purified water as an extraction medium. Biocompatibility testing followed the guidance in ISO 10993-1:2009 for a short-duration, skin-contacting device and consisted of sensitization (Kligman maximization test), irritation (intracutaneous injection test), and cytotoxicity (MEM elution assay with L929 mouse fibroblast cells).[95] The results of these tests are shown in Table 35.10.[96] The 2X sterilization condition was chosen to allow for the potential resterilization of product after an interrupted cycle during the manufacturing process.

Sterilization of Filled and Packaged Syringes

The NO_2 sterilization has been shown to be a rapid and effective adjunct process for sterilization of the external, gas-accessible surfaces packaged, prefilled syringes. Many prefilled products are indicated for use in the sterile field, either in surgical site or ophthalmic indications. In 2004 guidance to industry, the FDA acknowledged that temperature-sensitive biologics and active ingredients

---

TABLE 35.9 NO_2 sterilization microbiological results for process definition

NO_2 Dose ($\pm 10\%$) (mg/L)	iPCD Results (Fraction Negative)	Product Test of Sterility Results (Fraction Negative)
2.0	20%	100%
3.0	100%	100%
5.0	100%	100%

Abbreviation: iPCDs, internal process challenge devices.

The microbiological results of process definition for a stainless steel ruler sterilized with nitrogen dioxide (NO_2) gas are shown. The load size was 22 rulers, and five each of iPCDs and products for tests of sterility were distributed throughout the load.

TABLE 35.10   The results of nitrogen dioxide (NO_2) residuals testing along with biocompatibility testing for a ruler sterilized two times with NO_2 gas

Test	Description	Result	Pass/Fail
Ion chromatography	Nitrate residuals	0.29 µg/cm^2	Pass
Ion chromatography	Nitrite residuals	None detected	Pass
pH measurement	pH of extract	7.19	Pass
Sensitization	Kligman maximization test	Grade 1	Pass[a]
Irritation	Intracutaneous injection test	No significant reaction observed	Pass
Cytotoxicity	MEM elution assay with L929 mouse fibroblast cells	Grade 0	Pass

[a]The grade 1 result was the difference between a 0.33 control score and a 0.67 test score.

may prevent terminal sterilization of the aseptically filled product via traditional methods. As means of mitigating risk to the patient, they recommended that manufacturers employ an adjunct sterilization process to mitigate risk.[97] The NO_2 sterilization can be applied to products with minimal vacuum and at temperatures in the range of 10°C to 30°C, providing less impact on the time-temperature stability budget of sensitive products.

As an analog for product-filled syringes, a process was developed for prefilled syringes containing WFI. The intent of the study was to develop a batch-release sterilization process for the external, gas-accessible surfaces of syringes intended for clinical trials or other situations where a process has not yet been validated. An ASTM type 1 glass syringe with a bromobutyl rubber plunger and a staked needle covered by a bromobutyl needle shield were selected. Using a load of 300 syringes, which might represent a clinical trial batch size, a nonvacuum half cycle was defined following an overkill cycle.[3] For half-cycle testing, 10 BIs (in the syringe barrel, external to the plunger) and 20 syringes were cultured in tests of sterility (external surfaces). Following the half cycle, a full cycle was performed with 10 BIs serving as microbiological challenges. The prefilled syringes were exposed to a total of one and a half cycles. As a result, the entire batch of syringes was exposed to temperature range of 20°C to 25°C for approximately 7 hours, which included the chamber loading and unloading time.[91]

The cycle parameters and microbiological data are shown in Table 35.11, and all BIs and product tests of sterility were negative.[91] After exposure to the one-and-a-half-cycle process, three syringes were tested for NO_2 ingress via the Griess reagent colorimetric assay for NO_3^-/nitrite residuals. The three exposed syringes, along with three unexposed controls, were found to be below the LOD for the test, 0.025 ppm NO_3^-.[91] This LOD was eight times lower than the limit for NO_3^- in WFI per the European Pharmacopoeia,[92] which indicated that the bromobutyl plungers and tip caps were a sufficient barrier to the NO_2 gas. This further indicated that the product contents of a prefilled syringe would be minimally impacted by the application of an adjunct NO_2 process. Similar NO_2 ingress results have been obtained for a 2X application of the full cycle shown in Table 35.11.[90]

Disinfection of Material Transfer Airlocks

For the purpose of introducing work materials into a controlled space, disinfected airlocks are used. Methods for transferring work materials include manual wiping, gas processes, and radiation. An example of using NO_2 sterilant for disinfection is the airlock system design for introducing packages into the filling

TABLE 35.11   The cycle parameters and microbiological results of the batch-release process

Cycle	Vacuum (mm Hg)	Rel. Hum. (%RH)	NO$_2$ Dose (mg/L)	Dwell Time (mm:ss)	Aeration Time (mm:ss)	BI Result (Neg. / Total)	Product Test of Sterility Result (Neg. / Total)
Half	700	75	10	30:00	90:00	10 / 10	20 / 20
Full	700	75	10	60:00	90:00	10 / 10	NA

Abbreviations: BI, biological indicator; Neg., negative; NO_2, nitrogen dioxide; Rel. Hum., relative humidity.

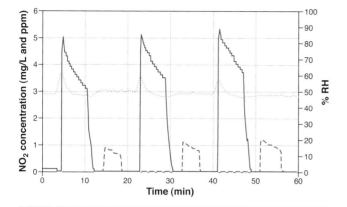

FIGURE 35.17 Graph of the humidity and nitrogen dioxide (NO_2) in the biodecontamination airlock during normal operation. The graph shows the humidity (dotted line), NO_2 concentration in mg/L during the process (solid line), and the NO_2 concentration during aeration (dashed line). Abbreviation: RH, relative humidity.

line isolator. This airlock is designed for decontaminating packages (tubs) that contain sterile, clean, and ready-to-fill syringes. The objective of this disinfection process is to complete all steps of the cycle within 20 minutes, including loading, disinfection, unloading, and returning the cart to the loading side of the airlock. Airlocks for other products have been built and put into service.

For airlocks, the disinfection process begins with humidification of the chamber, followed by the addition of sterilant. The parameters for the process are 80% to 85% RH and 10 mg/L NO_2 concentration. The dwell time for the process is 6 minutes. After the dwell, aeration begins and continues until the sterilant concentration in the chamber is below 1 ppm, as measured by an electrochemical cell detector. The measured humidity and sterilant for consecutive cycles is shown in Figure 35.17. The aeration phase of the process takes between 6 minutes and 7 minutes to reach 1 ppm of NO_2 in the chamber. This type of disinfection process can be used for a variety of work materials that are moving to a zone that has a higher classification. As the process does not include a vacuum phase, many types of packages can be used.

Material compatibility considerations for this application are limited to compatibility of the materials with the process and the impact that the process may have on the primary containers (syringes) that will be filled. Compatibility means that the package materials must permit the rapid disinfection of the package surfaces. For the syringes, sterilant residues must not cause interactions with the syringes after filling. Whereas the level of residuals can be measured with extraction and assay methods, compatibility needs to be evaluated with stability testing of the filled syringe.

REFERENCES

1. US Environmental Protection Agency. *Notice of Pesticide Registration.* Washington, DC: US Environmental Protection Agency. EPA reg. number 89265-1. https://www3.epa.gov/pesticides/chem_search/ppls /089265-00001-20160415.pdf. Accessed July 10, 2018.
2. International Organization for Standardization. *ISO 14937:2009: Sterilization of Health Care Products—General Requirements for Characterization of a Sterilizing Agent and the Development, Validation and Routine Control of a Sterilization Process for Medical Devices.* Geneva, Switzerland; International Organization for Standardization; 2009.
3. US Department of Health and Human Services. *Noxilizer Surgical Ruler, US FDA 510(k) Clearance Number: K160501.* Baltimore, MD: US Department of Health and Human Services; 2016.
4. Ladd EF, Bassett HP. Bleaching of flour. *J Biol Chem.* 1909;6:75-86.
5. Watson JM, inventor; Cosden Technology Inc, assignee. NO_2 polymerization inhibitor for vinyl aromatic compound distillation. US patent 3,964,978. June 22, 1976.
6. US Environmental Protection Agency. Nitrogen dioxide trends. US Environmental Agency Web site. https://www.epa.gov/air-trends/nitrogen -dioxide-trends. Accessed February 1, 2018.
7. Lamsal LN, Duncan B, Yoshida Y, et al. U.S. NO_2 trends (2005–2013): EPA Air Quality System (AQS) data versus improved observations from the Ozone Monitoring Instrument (OMI). *Atmos Environ.* 2015;110: 130-143.
8. Ehrlich R, Miller S. Effect of NO_2 on airborne Venezuelan equine encephalomyelitis virus. *Applied Microbiol.* 1972;23:481-484.
9. Kenyon RL, Hasek RH, Davy LG, Broadbooks KJ. Oxidation of cellulose. *Ind Eng Chem.* 1949;41(1):2-8.
10. Dineen P. Antibacterial activity of oxidized regenerated cellulose. *Surg Gynecol Obstrect.* 1976;142(4):481-486.
11. Spangler D, Rothenburger S, Nguyen K, Jampani H, Weiss S, Bhende S. In vitro antimicrobial activity of oxidized regenerated cellulose against antibiotic-resistant microorganisms. *Surg Infect (Larchmt).* 2003;4(3):255-262.
12. Poliakov AA, Trazhetsetska TA, Arbuzov KN, Akhumova AA, Chepurov KP. Bactericidal action of nitrogen dioxide on the vegetative and sporous forms of *Bacillus anthracis* [in Ukrainian]. *Mikrobiol Zh.* 1962;24:43-45.
13. Opie DB, Goulet EM. *Evaluation of the Method for Employing Nitrogen Dioxide, as Described by Polyakov 2010.* Noxilizer internal report: NR.0072.
14. Won WD, Ross H. Reaction of airborne *Rhizobium meliloti* to some environmental factors. *Appl Microbiol.* 1969;18:555-557.
15. Görsdorf S, Appel KE, Engeholm C, Obe G. Nitrogen dioxide induces DNA single-strand breaks in cultured Chinese hamster cells. *Carcinogenesis.* 1990;11:37-41.
16. Sander R. Compilation of Henry's law constants for water as solvent. *Atmos Chem Phys.* 2015;15:4399-4981.
17. Kulla J, Reich R, Broedel S Jr. *Sterilizing Combination Products Using Oxides of Nitrogen.* Minneapolis, MN: MDDI; 2009.
18. SoRelle R. Nobel prize awarded to scientists for nitric oxide discoveries. *Circulation.* 1998;98(22):2365-2366.
19. Lonkar P, Dedon PC. Reactive species and DNA damage in chronic inflammation: reconciling chemical mechanisms and biological fates. *Int J Cancer.* 2011;128:1999-2009.
20. Archer SL, Huang JMC, Hampl V, Nelson DP, Shultz PJ, Weir EK. Nitric oxide and cGMP cause vasorelaxation by activation of a charybdotoxin-sensitive K channel by cGMP-dependent protein kinase. *Proc Natl Acad Sci U S A.* 1994;91:7583-7587.
21. Ichinose F, Roberts JD Jr, Zapol WM. Inhaled nitric oxide: a selective pulmonary vasodilator: current uses and therapeutic potential. *Circulation.* 2004;109:3106-3111.
22. Nguyen T, Brunson D, Crespi CL, Penman BW, Wishnok JS, Tannenbaum SR. DNA damage and mutation in human cells exposed to nitric oxide in vitro. *Proc Natl Acad Sci U S A.* 1992;89: 3030-3034.

23. Möller MN, Li Q, Vitturi DA, Robinson JM, Lancaster JR Jr, Denicola A. Membrane "lens" effect: focusing the formation of reactive nitrogen oxides from the •NO/O$_2$ reaction. *Chem Res Toxicol*. 2007;20:709-714.

24. Pesticide Registration Manual. *Chapter 4—Additional Considerations for Antimicrobial Products*. https://www.epa.gov/pesticide-registration /pesticide-registration-manual-chapter-4-additional-considerations. Accessed June 27, 2018.

25. Opie DB. Sterilization and decontamination with nitrogen dioxide gas. In: Moldenhauer J, ed. *Environmental Monitoring—A Comprehensive Handbook*. Vol 7. Bethesda, MD: PDA/DHI; 2014:127-151.

26. International Organization for Standardization. *ISO 11138-1:2017: Sterilization of Health Care Products—Biological Indicators—Part 1: General Requirements*. Geneva, Switzerland: International Organization for Standardization; 2017.

27. Block SS, ed. *Disinfection, Sterilization, and Preservation*. 5th ed. Philadelphia, PA: Lippincott Williams & Wilkins; 2001.

28. Lewis RJ Sr. *Hawley's Condensed Chemical Dictionary*. 15th ed. New York, NY: John Wiley & Sons; 2007:896.

29. Vanýsek P. Electrochemical series. In: Haynes WM, ed. *CRC Handbook of Chemistry and Physics*. 91st ed. Boca Raton, FL: Taylor & Francis; 2010:8-26-8-28.

30. *Standard Electrode Reduction and Oxidation Potential Values*. https:// rsteyn.files.wordpress.com/2010/07/reduction-and-oxidation -potential.pdf. Accessed October 28, 2019.

31. Ostwald W, inventor. Improvements in the manufacture of nitric acid and nitrogen oxides. European patent no. GB190200698. March 20, 1902.

32. Astrayan R, Bozzelli JW, Simmie JM. Thermochemistry for enthalpies and reaction paths of nitrous acid isomers. *Int J Chem Kinet*. 2007;39:378-398.

33. Leenson IA. Approaching equilibrium in the N$_2$O$_4$-NO$_2$ system: a common mistake in textbooks. *J Chem Educ*. 2000;77:1652-1659.

34. Harris L. The absorption spectrum of nitrogen dioxide. *Chemistry*. 1928;14:690-694.

35. Unger-Bimczok B, Kottke V, Hertel C, Rauschnabel J. The influence of humidity, hydrogen peroxide concentration, and condensation on the inactivation of *Geobacillus stearothermophilus* spores with hydrogen peroxide vapor. *Pharm Innov*. 2008;3:123.

36. Oxborrrow GS, Placencia AM, Danielson JW. Effects of temperature and relative humidity on biological indicators used for ethylene oxide sterilization. *Appl Environ Microbiol*. 1983;45:546-549.

37. Westphal AJ, Price PB, Leighton TJ, Wheeler KE. Kinetics of size changes of individual *Bacillus thuringiensis* spores in response to changes in relative humidity. *Proc Natl Acad Sci U S A*. 2003;100:3461-3466.

38. Opie DB, Goulet EM. *D-Value Measured Using NO2 at 40 % RH and 50 % RH*. 2018. Noxilizer internal report: NR.0078. Maintained at Noxilizer, Inc.

39. Shomali MF, Bernstein JE, Opie DB, Sahay A, Soreide JC, inventors; Eniware, LLC, Noxilizer Inc, assignees. Gas generation module. US patent 2018/0021466. January 25, 2018.

40. Shomali MF, Opie D, Avasthi T, Trilling A. Nitrogen dioxide sterilization in low-resource environments: a feasibility study. *PLoS One*. 2015;10:e0130043.

41. Arnold EV, Doletski BG, Raulli RE, inventors; Noxilizer Inc, assignee. Nitric oxide-releasing molecules. US patent 8,101,589. January 24, 2012.

42. Matsuuchi H, Hirose T, Iwasaki R, et al, inventors; Noxilizer Inc, assignee. High concentration NO$_2$ generating system and method for generating high concentration NO$_2$ using the generating system. US patent 8,580,086. November 12, 2013.

43. Parvulescu VI, Magurenu M, Lukes P. *Plasma Chemistry and Catalysis in Gases and Liquids*. Hoboken, NJ: John Wiley & Sons; 2013.

44. Wang j, Yi H, Zhao S, Gao F, Zhang R, Yang Z. Products yield and energy efficiency of dielectric barrier discharge for no conversion: effect of O$_2$ content, no concentration, and flow rate. *Energy Fuels*. 2017;31:9675-9683.

45. Finlayson-Pitts BJ, Wingen LM, Sumner AL, Syomin D, Ramazan KA. The heterogeneous hydrolysis of NO$_2$ in laboratory systems and in outdoor and indoor atmospheres: an integrated mechanism. *Phys Chem Chem Phys*. 2003;5:223-242.

46. Caulfield JL, Wishnok JS, Tannenbaum SR. Nitric oxide-induced deamination of cytosine and guanine in deoxynucleosides and oligonucleotides. *J Biol Chem*. 1998;273:12689-12695.

47. Knudsen SM, Cermak N, Delgado FF, Setlow B, Setlow P, Manalis SR. Water and small-molecule permeation of dormant *Bacillus subtilis* spores. *J Bacteriol*. 2015;198:168-177.

48. Ewing GE. Ambient thin film water on insulator surfaces. *Chem Rev*. 2006;106(4):1511-1526.

49. Liebe HJ, Wolfe VL, Howe DA. Test of wall coatings for controlled moist air experiments. *Rev Sci Instrum*. 1984;55:1702-1705.

50. Ljungström E, Svensson RE, Lindqvist O. Kinetics of the reaction between nitrogen dioxide and water vapor. *Atmos Environ*. 1987;21: 1529-1539.

51. Finlayson-Pitts BJ. *Heterogeneous NOx Chemistry in Polluted Urban Atmospheres: Implications for the Formation of Particles and Ozone and Control Strategy Development*. https://www.arb.ca.gov/research /apr/past/00-323.pdf. Accessed July 9, 2018.

52. Ramazan KA, Wingen LM, Miller Y, et al. New experimental and theoretical approach to the heterogeneous hydrolysis of NO$_2$: key role of molecular nitric acid and its complexes. *J Phys Chem A*. 2006;110: 6886-6897.

53. Troy DB, Beringer P. *Remington: The Science and Practice of Pharmacy*. 21st ed. Philadelphia, PA: Lippincott Williams & Wilkins; 2006:270.

54. Heider D, Gömann J, Junghann U, Kaiser U. Kill kinetics study of *Bacillus subtilis* spores in ethylene oxide sterilisation processes. *Zentr Steril*. 2002;10:158-167.

55. Deegan RD, Bakajin O, Dupont TF, Huber G, Nagel SR, Witten TA. Capillary flow as the cause of ring stains from dried liquid drops. *Nature*. 1997;389:827.

56. Gillitzer E. Spore news. *Mesa Laboratories Newsletter*. 2012;9(3):1-3.

57. Raguse M, Fiebrandt M, Stapelman K, et al. Improvement of biological indicators by uniformly distributing *Bacillus subtilis* spores in monolayers to evaluate enhanced spore decontamination technologies. *Appl Environ Microbiol*. 2016;82:2031-2038.

58. Shintani H. Important points to attain reproducible sterility assurance. *Biochem Physiol*. 2014;3:135.

59. Shintani H. Current mistaken interpretation of microbiological data on gas plasma sterilization. *Pharm Regul Aff Open Access*. 2015;4:138.

60. Opie DB, Goulet EM. *BI Carrier Material Comparison: Stainless Steel and Quartz Fiber Discs*. 2018 Noxilizer internal report: NR.0079. Maintained at Noxilizer, Inc.

61. Chung S, Barengoltz J, Kern R, Koukol R, Cash H. *The Validation of Vapor Phase Hydrogen Peroxide Microbial Reduction for Planetary Protection and a Proposed Vacuum Process Specification*. Pasadena, CA: Jet Propulsion Laboratory. JPL report D-36113, publication 06-6. https://trs.jpl.nasa.gov/bitstream/handle/2014/40601/06-06.pdf?sequence=1&isAllowed=y. Accessed January 19, 2018.

62. Summer AL, Menke EJ, Dubowski Y, et al. The nature of water on surfaces of laboratory systems and implications for heterogeneous chemistry in the troposphere. *Phys Chem Chem Phys*. 2004;6:604-613.

63. Jones K. *The Chemistry of Nitrogen: Pergamon Texts in Inorganic Chemistry*. Vol 2. Oxford, United Kingdom: Pergamon Press; 1973.

64. Saliba NA, Yang H, Finlayson-Pitts BJ. Reaction of gaseous nitric oxide with nitric acid on silica surfaces in the presence of water at room temperature. *J Phys Chem A*. 2001;105:10339-10346.

65. Ali AA, Coulter JA, Ogle CH, et al. The contribution of N$_2$O$_3$ to the cytotoxicity of the nitric oxide donor DETA/NO: an emerging role for S-nitrosylation. *Biosci Rep*. 2013;33:e00031. doi:10.1042/ BSR20120120.

66. International Organization for Standardization. *ISO 10993-12:2012: Biological Evaluation of Medical Devices—Part 12: Sample Preparation and Reference Materials*. Geneva, Switzerland: International Organization for Standardization; 2012.

67. National Institute for Occupational Safety and Health. *NIOSH Pocket Guide to Chemical Hazards*. Vol 6. 3rd ed. Cincinnati, OH: National Institute for Occupational Safety and Health; 2007. DHHS publication no. 2005-149.

68. *Air Quality Guidelines for Europe*. 2nd ed. Copenhagen, Denmark: WHO Regional Publications, European Series; 2000.

69. *Medical Management Guidelines for Ethylene Oxide ([CH₂]2O)*. Atlanta, GA: Agency for Toxic Substances and Disease Registry; 2014. http://www.atsdr.cdc.gov/MHMI/mmg137.html. Accessed July 10, 2018.

70. *Medical Management Guidelines for Hydrogen Peroxide (H₂O₂)*. Atlanta, GA: Agency for Toxic Substances and Disease Registry; 2014. https://www.atsdr.cdc.gov/MHMI/mmg174.html. Accessed July 10, 2018.

71. National Institutes of Health. *Ozone—Haz-Map Category Details*. Bethesda, MD: US National Library of Medicine; 2017. https://hazmap.nlm.nih.gov/category-details?id=68&table=copytblagents. Accessed July 10, 2018.

72. Ruth JH. Odor thresholds and irritation levels of several chemical substances: a review. *Am Ind Hyg Assoc J*. 1986;47(3):A142-A151.

73. International Agency for Research on Cancer. *Chemical Agents and Related Occupations, Ethylene Oxide*. Lyon, France: International Agency for Research on Cancer; 2012. https://monographs.iarc.fr/ENG/Monographs/vol100F/mono100F-28.pdf. Accessed July 10, 2018.

74. International Agency for Research on Cancer. *Chemical Agents and Related Occupations, Formaldehyde*. Lyon, France: International Agency for Research on Cancer; 2012. https://monographs.iarc.fr/ENG/Monographs/vol100F/mono100F-29.pdf. Accessed July 10, 2018.

75. International Agency for Research on Cancer. *Re-Evaluation of Some Organic Chemicals. Hydrazine and Hydrogen Peroxide*. Lyon, France: International Agency for Research on Cancer; 1999. https://monographs.iarc.fr/ENG/Monographs/vol71/mono71.pdf. Accessed July 10, 2018.

76. Sigwarth V, Stärk A. Effect of carrier materials on the resistance of spores of *Bacillus stearothermophilus* to gaseous hydrogen peroxide. *PDA J Pharm Sci and Technol*. 2003;57:228.

77. *VHP (Vaporized Hydrogen Peroxide) Bio-decontamination Technology*. Hampshire, United Kingdom: STERIS; 2003. STERIS technical data monograph 2003.

78. Jellinek HHG, Yokota R, Itoh Y. Reaction of nitrogen dioxide with nylon 66. *Polym J*. 1973;4:601-606.

79. Jellinek HHG, Chaudhuri AK. Inhibited degradation of nylon 66 in presence of nitrogen dioxide, ozone, air, and near-ultraviolet radiation. *J Polym Sci*. 1972;Part A-1:10.

80. Jellinek HHG, Wang TJY. Reaction of nitrogen dioxide with linear polyurethane. *J Polym Sci*. 1973;11:3227-3242.

81. Davydov E, Gapnova I, Pariiski G, Pokholok T, Zaikon G. Reactivity of polymers on exposure to nitrogen dioxide. *Chem Cheml Technol*. 2010;4:281-290.

82. Goulet EM. *Degradation of Nylon and Delrin as a Function of Humidity and Percent NO₂*. 2008. Noxilizer Test Report 2008; TR.0059.00. Maintained at Noxilizer, Inc.

83. Goulet EM. *Effects of the Noxilizer Process on Urethanes, PVC, Buna, and Delrin*. 2008. Noxilizer Test Report 2008; TR.0065.00. Maintained at Noxilizer, Inc.

84. Ivanova LV, Moiseev YV, Zaikov GE, Ivanov VV. Destruction of Polyacetals in Acid Media. *Russ Chem Bull*. 1970;19:2104-2106.

85. *Safety Assessment of Di(2-ethylhexyl)phthalate (DEHP) Released from PVC Medical Devices*. Rockville, MD: Center for Devices and Radiological Health, US Food and Drug Administration; 2002. http://www.fda.gov/downloads/MedicalDevices/DeviceRegulationandGuidance/GuidanceDocuments/UCM080457.pdf. Accessed July 10, 2018.

86. *DEHP Phthalates in Medical Devices*. London, United Kingdom: Medicines and Healthcare Products Regulatory Agency; 2016. https://www.gov.uk/government/publications/dehp-phthalates-in-medical-devices/dehp-phthalates-in-medical-devices. Accessed July 12, 2018.

87. Yackel EC, Kenyon WO. The oxidation of cellulose by nitrogen dioxide. *J Am Chem Soc*. 1942;64:121-127.

88. Pigman WW, Browning BL, McPherson WH, Calkins CR, Leaf RL. Oxidation of D-galactose and cellulose with nitric acid, nitrous acid and nitrogen oxides. *J Am Chem Soc*. 1949;71:2200-2204.

89. Feldman LA, Hui HK. Compatibility of medical devices and materials with low-temperature hydrogen peroxide gas plasma. *Med Device & Diagn Industry*. 1997;19:57-62.

90. Goulet EM, Kase C, Danko E. NO₂ Sterilization as part of a batch release for clinical trials. Paper presented at: 2016 Parenteral Drug Association (PDA) Annual Meeting; 2016; San Antonio, TX. https://www.noxilizer.com/wp-content/uploads/2018/05/poster-201603-pda-annual-meeting.pdf. Accessed October 28, 2019.

91. Goulet EM. NO₂ gas sterilization and decontamination: keeping pace, from start to finish. Paper presented at: PDA Midwest Sterility Assurance and Risk Mitigation; October 2016; Indianapolis, IN.

92. European Pharmacopoeia. Water for injections. 2017;6.0:0169.

93. Kennedy SR. *Process Definition for Noxilizer Part No. NSC.PRT.0300—Ruler 6.0 316 SSTL*. 2015. Noxilizer Test Report 2015; TR.0315.00. Maintained at Noxilizer, Inc.

94. Kennedy SR. *Supplementary Microbiological Performance Qualification for Noxilizer Part No. NSC.PRT.0300—Ruler 6.0, 316 SSTL*. 2015. Noxilizer Test Report 2015; TR.0320.00. Maintained at Noxilizer, Inc.

95. International Organization for Standardization. *ISO 10993-1:2009: Biological Evaluation of Medical Devices—Part 1: Evaluation and Testing Within a Risk Management Process*. Geneva, Switzerland: International Organization for Standardization; 2009.

96. Kennedy SR. *Biocompatibility, Residuals, and Package Performance Exposures for Noxilizer Part No. NSC.PRT.0300—Ruler 6.0, 316 SSTL*. 2015. Noxilizer Test Report 2015; TR.0321.00. Maintained at Noxilizer, Inc.

97. *Guidance for Industry Sterile Drug Products Produced by Aseptic Processing—Current Good Manufacturing Practice*. Rockville, MD: Center for Devices and Radiological Health, US Food and Drug Administration; 2004. https://www.fda.gov/downloads/Drugs/Guidances/ucm070342.pdf. Accessed July 10, 2018.

Formaldehyde

Allan Bennett and Thomas Pottage

Formaldehyde is a monoaldehyde that exists as a gas freely soluble in water. It can be used both as an aqueous solution (formalin) for disinfection and as a gas for fumigation of indoor spaces and equipment. Apart from its use as a disinfectant, it is used in the preparation of human and veterinary vaccines and the preservation of tissues. Formaldehyde is highly efficacious against a broad range of microorganisms, but its activity is relatively slow acting. Its antimicrobial efficacy is reduced in the presence of organic matter. Formaldehyde vapor has a pungent odor and may cause allergic reactions in some workers; is an irritant of mucous membranes; and, as of 2014, was classified as a carcinogen (category 1B), mutagen (category 2), and sensitizer. For these reasons, it is declining in use as a general liquid disinfectant and as part of formulated disinfectants. However, it is still widely used as a gaseous disinfectant in the microbiological laboratory sector and agricultural sectors, where it can be generated by depolymerizing paraformaldehyde by heating, boiling off formalin and water, or historically by adding formalin to potassium permanganate crystals. It is also used as a tissue preservative and in embalming.[1]

▶ CHEMICAL PROPERTIES

Formaldehyde is the simplest of the aldehydes and is also known as methanal. Its chemical formula is CH_2O. Its chemical properties are summarized in Table 36.1. It is obtained either in a polymeric form, paraformaldehyde ($HO[CH_2O]_nH$), or in a liquid aqueous suspension at ~40% vol/vol stabilized with methanol (10%-15%) to prevent oxidation or polymerization generally referred to as formalin.[2]

▶ MECHANISM OF ACTION

The basic mode of action of formaldehyde as an antimicrobial agent is through the irreversible cross-linking or denaturing of protein and through DNA damage potentially though protein-DNA cross-linking.[3] This prevents the operation of essential cell functions causing loss of viability. Formaldehyde has a broad spectrum of action on microorganisms, and it denatures proteins by alkylation with amino and sulfhydryl groups of proteins and ring nitrogen atoms of purine bases such as guanine.[4] In the inactivation of spores, alkylation of nucleic acids may be more important than changes in protein constituents.[3]

Due to this broad mode of action, formaldehyde is considered to have a very wide range of activity against all types of microorganisms, and the development of resistance is considered limited. Some microorganisms have been found to have increased resistance to formaldehyde due to the expression of formaldehyde dehydrogenase.[5] Formaldehyde is oxidized by formaldehyde dehydrogenase. In these experiments it was found that a glutathione-dependent formaldehyde dehydrogenase that oxidizes formaldehyde[6] was found to be encoded by a gene, which can be transferred between the microorganisms via plasmids, and the mechanisms of resistance can be transferred to unrelated strains of the same bacterial species, such as *Escherichia coli*.[7,8] However, Azachi et al[9] described that formaldehyde dehydrogenase was not the sole reason for increased resistance to formaldehyde in two gram-negative bacteria. It was found that formaldehyde-resistant strains had the addition of a high-molecular-mass protein in the outer membrane, and therefore, formaldehyde resistance is conferred by the structure and composition of the outer membrane.[9] Revival in formaldehyde-treated *Bacillus subtilis* spores was increased by up to 1 log using heat shock for 30 minutes before plating out. It was postulated by Williams and Russell[10] that the heat shock could enhance and/or trigger germination after contact with formaldehyde.

Formaldehyde has been used for the inactivation of viruses in vaccine production for a number of years.[11] Complete inactivation depends on the physical state of

TABLE 36.1	Chemical properties of formaldehyde
EC No.	200-001-8
CAS No.	50-00-0
Molecular Weight	30.03 g/mol
Melting Point	−92°C
Boiling Point	−21°C
Conversion Factor	1 ppm = 1.23 mg/m^3 (20°C, 101.3 kPa)

the particles. There have been reported problems with reactivation of the virus particles when clumped prior to treatment with formalin.[11]

Formaldehyde has reduced activity against agents in organic materials.[12] This was demonstrated by the Cutter incident regarding the ineffective inactivation of live polio virus used in the polio vaccination.[13] Approximately 400 000 people, primarily children, were inoculated with a formaldehyde-inactivated vaccine, of these over 250 either of vaccinees or their contacts were reported with polio infections.[14]

Formaldehyde is ineffective against prions and has been shown in some instances to stabilize them and make them more resistant to other modes of disinfection such as autoclaving and incineration.[15]

▶ APPLICATIONS

Tissue Fixative

Formalin is commonly used as a tissue fixative. Solutions used include phosphate-buffered formalin or formalin-saline at a formalin concentration of 10%.[2]

Soil Disinfection or Sterilization

Chemical decontamination of soil can be carried out in small batches collected from a contaminated site or in in situ by the application of formalin to the soil. Formaldehyde was used to decontaminate a Scottish island that had been contaminated with *Bacillus anthracis* spores through the testing of a biological weapon during the Second World War.[16] A 5% suspension of formaldehyde was sprayed at 50 L/m^2 over the contaminated area after burn off of vegetation. The highest areas of contamination were treated by injection of undiluted formalin (38% formaldehyde) to a depth of 50 mm. Soil sampling showed that the process was effective. The soil type facilitated the process allowing easy absorption of the formaldehyde. This approach may not be suitable for different soil types. It was also costly; approximately 2 million liters of 5% formaldehyde were

applied over a 4-hectare (40 000 m^2) area with further direct treatments with formaldehyde necessary for small pockets of spores.

Embalming

Formaldehyde is the major chemical used to preserve cadavers. Its antimicrobial properties delay the decay processes and thus can preserve tissues without destroying their structural detail, which is essential for anatomical study.[17] The embalming fluid fixes the proteins within the body or parts thereof limiting their ability to become a food source for microorganisms. The embalming fluid is either injected arterially or directly into the body's cavities to displace the bodily fluids. The embalming fluid itself is made up of a mixture containing not only predominantly formalin but also glutaraldehyde and methanol, the concentration of these agents can be varied depending on the area to be injected.

Liquid Disinfection

Forty-percent formaldehyde gas dissolved in water constitutes a 100% solution of formalin; 8% formaldehyde in water is 20% formalin. Depending on its concentration, formaldehyde can be classified as a high-level (8% formaldehyde plus 70% alcohol) or intermediate- to high-level (4%-8% formaldehyde in water) disinfectant.[18] Aqueous formaldehyde in concentrations less than 4% may have limited activity against *Mycobacterium* species, particularly the nontuberculous mycobacteria indigenous to certain potable water supplies.[18] The action of formaldehyde on the protein coat of poliovirus progressively slows down the killing rate by obstructing penetration to the nucleic acid core.[19] As mentioned, 8% formaldehyde in water is considered an intermediate- to high-level disinfectant; combining 8% formaldehyde in 65% to 70% isopropanol yields a compound that is rapidly bactericidal, tuberculocidal, and sporicidal, but the time required for achieving sterility using high numbers of spores as a challenge may be up to 18 hours or longer, depending on the test conditions.[18]

Experiments conducted by Sagripanti and Bonifacino[20] in a comparison of different liquid chemical agents found that an 8% formaldehyde solution at different pH, ranging from 3 to 10, produced less than 90% inactivation of *B subtilis* subspecies *Bacillus globigii* (now *Bacillus atrophaeus*) spores after contact for 30 minutes at 20°C. The sporicidal properties of 8% formaldehyde was increased when the temperature was increased from 20°C to 40°C (at pH 3.2) to >99.9% spore inactivation in 20 minutes. A later set of experiments used 8% formaldehyde, this time at pH 3.4, against a range of vegetative bacteria in liquid suspensions. It was found that with a contact time

TABLE 36.2   Bacterial inactivation using 8% formaldehyde for 30 minutes at 20°C[a]

Bacterium	Log$_{10}$ Reduction (Replicates)
Bacillus cereus	>5.0 (2)
Clostridium perfringens	>6.3 (2)
Escherichia coli	>6.9 (2)
Listeria monocytogenes	>6.1 (1)
Pseudomonas aeruginosa	>6.1 (3)
Salmonella typhimurium	>6.2 (3)
Shigella sonnei	>6.3 (2)
Staphylococcus aureus	>6.5 (3)
Staphylococcus epidermidis	5.9 ± 1.1 (3)
Vibrio cholerae	>6.4 (2)
Vibrio parahaemolyticus	>6.2 (2)
Vibrio vulnificus	>6.3 (2)
Yersinia enterocolitica	>6.8 (2)

[a]Data from Sagripanti et al.[21]

of 30 minutes, formaldehyde was able to reduce the recoverable numbers of bacteria to below the detection limit in all cases except *Staphylococcus epidermidis*[21] (Table 36.2).

Alasri et al[22] investigated the minimum sporicidal concentration of formaldehyde to produce a 5 log reduction of *Bacillus* spores (three species of *B subtilis* and one species of *Bacillus amyloliquefaciens*) over a range of exposure periods. Formaldehyde concentrations of 7500 ppm (0.75 %) were required to inactivate spores (5 log reduction) of one wild type *B subtilis* species and *B amyloliquefaciens* within 5 minutes, with a lower formaldehyde concentration (3750 ppm) required for inactivation within a 7-hour period. The concentration of 3750 ppm was also found to inactivate the other *B subtilis* wild-type spores over the range of times investigated from 5 minutes up to 7 hours. Spores of a *B subtilis*–type strain (ATCC 6633) were found to be the least resistant to formaldehyde, being inactivated by 3750 ppm within 5 minutes decreasing to 1875 ppm for 7 hours.[22]

A far lower concentration of formaldehyde, 0.02%, was found to be able to inactivate *E coli*. Conversely, sporicidal activity of 4% (pH 8.0) formaldehyde against *B anthracis* spores was slower, >2 hours for a 10^4 reduction, than 1% and 2% glutaraldehyde treatment for 30 and 15 minutes, respectively, under the same conditions.[23]

Formaldehyde solutions have been demonstrated to be tuberculocidal by Rubbo et al.[23] A concentration of 4% was shown to inactivate 10^4 colony-forming units of *Mycobacterium tuberculosis* within 5 minutes in liquid suspension.[23]

Möller et al[24] have shown that a 2% solution of formaldehyde was effective against vaccinia, adenovirus, and murine norovirus at 25°C. However, long exposure times of 6 hours were required for the enveloped vaccinia virus, and inactivation took days at a lower temperature of 4°C.

Because it is not corrosive to equipment associated with hemodialysis systems, formaldehyde has been used in a concentration of 4% to disinfect dialysis systems and disposable hemodialyzers that are reused in the same patient. In both instances, however, the problem of residual formaldehyde constitutes a potential health hazard to dialysis patients, and hemodialysis systems and hemodialyzers must be thoroughly rinsed free of residual formaldehyde prior to use.[25]

Liquid formaldehyde has also been used to control outbreaks of parasites, such as the ectoparasite *Ichthyophthirius multifiliis*, in aquaculture systems. It was found in these studies not to harm the fish at the concentrations used, but the safety issues to workers using it and environmental discharge have led to alternative agents to be identified and investigated.[26,27]

Gaseous Formaldehyde

Formaldehyde has been used for over 100 years as a gaseous disinfectant in a number of industries. It is an effective and economic way of reducing microbial contamination of buildings and laboratories. Formaldehyde can be vaporized from formalin suspension or from paraformaldehyde, held for an exposure time, and then vented.[28,29] It is at its most effective at temperatures over 18°C and relative humidity values of over 85%.[28] Lach[30] reports that the efficacy of gaseous formaldehyde is caused by the formation of a condensing layer of aqueous formaldehyde over the entire surface area of the space to be disinfected. Spiner and Hoffmann[31] completed studies investigating the effect of relative humidity on formaldehyde disinfection and found that higher relative humidity (at 75% and 100%) provided the quickest kills of the *B subtilis* spores presented on cloth and glass surfaces. Data on the effectiveness of formaldehyde gaseous disinfection against a wide range of microorganisms can be hard to find. The source for most efficacy data is Nordgren[32] who found that formaldehyde fumigation was effective within 1 hour against a range of microorganisms including coliforms staphylococci and mycobacteria. He found that if organisms were suspended in organic soils such as blood or sputum, the exposure period should be increased to 24 hours. The use of higher temperatures of up to 55°C increased antimicrobial action. These studies were carried out using glass tubes as carriers.[32] Later studies carried out in the United Kingdom tested the efficacy of formaldehyde against a variety of organisms such as staphylococci, *B subtilis* spores, *M tuberculosis*, and smallpox dried onto threads.[28] They found that formaldehyde was effective within 2 hours in inactivating 10^4 *M tuberculosis* on a thread and against smallpox in crusts. It was also effective against micrococci in gelatin and other soils, although a study completed by Grossgebauer et al[33] found there was incomplete inactivation of vaccinia virus in scabs when exposed to 10 g of formaldehyde per cubic meter for 24 hours. They postulated that the slow diffusion of formaldehyde was the reason for the incomplete inactivation of the viral particles within the scabs.[33]

More recent studies (Rogers et al[34] and Beswick et al[35]) show formaldehyde fumigation to be effective against a wide range of pathogenic agents including bacterial spores, mycobacteria, and viruses. Rogers et al[34] demonstrated that a commercial formaldehyde system (Certek Model #1414RH formaldehyde gas generator/neutralizer) was effective (>6 log reductions) at inactivating *B anthracis* spores, *Geobacillus stearothermophilus* spores, and *B atrophaeus* spores dried onto various materials (carpet, wood, etc.) when used at 10.5 g paraformaldehyde per cubic meter (<8500 ppm theoretical but <1400 ppm measured peak) for 10 hours. The commercial system heated and depolymerized paraformaldehyde-containing pills and used nebulizers filled with water to increase the relative humidity within the exposure chamber. Beswick et al[35] used a far lower level of formaldehyde in their study at 600 ppm (0.75 g/m³), which is lower than generally used in practice yet still showed high efficacy against *Clostridium difficile* spores (5.73 log reductions) and *Mycobacterium fortuitum* (6.25) but lower efficacy against vaccinia virus (2.43) (potentially due to organic matter from the cell culture solution used) and *G stearothermophilus* spores (2.9). Interestingly, Beswick et al[35] also found that formaldehyde was able to give a greater inactivation of *M fortuitum* and vaccinia virus in liquid spills as opposed to dried inoculations, with an inactivation less in liquid spills compared to dried inoculations for *C difficile*. Ide[36] also reported that formaldehyde gas exposure was effective against liquid suspensions of avian viruses in plastic 96-well microtiter plates (0.3 mL per well). Formalin (37%) was vaporized at 40 mL/min from a commercial insecticide fogger to deliver 1220 mL per chamber (30-min delivery), giving a concentration of 36 mL/m³ at a temperature between 20°C and 22°C. The viruses were completely inactivated after one cycle, including infectious bursal agent, adenovirus, infectious bronchitis virus, and poxvirus. Interestingly, two cycles were required for Newcastle disease virus and reovirus possibly due to the high titers used in these studies.[36]

There are many ways of generating gaseous formaldehyde. In the United Kingdom, the method generally recommended for rooms is to boil off 100 mL formalin and 900 mL water in kettles per 28.3 m³ (1.42 g/m³)[28] and leave overnight, although a higher amount of formalin is recommended when absorbent materials are present. This creates a very wet environment with visible condensation and puddles forming on floors but is generally

found to be effective against spore indicators. This would suggest that condensation could aid the disinfection process, such as helping to penetrate into dried spills to contact organisms that would usually remain uncontacted by drier systems. In the United States, for laboratory uses, paraformaldehyde is vaporized from paraformaldehyde in a skillet at a concentration 1.0 mg/L,[37] although earlier papers suggested 0.3 g/ft³.[29,38] It is typical in such processes that water is boiled off at the same time to increase the relative humidity within the area. For smaller areas, such as a laboratory biosafety cabinets, higher levels tend to be used. The UK standard for a safety cabinet suggests 60 mL formalin and 60 mL water per cubic meter, but a recent publication suggests that this can be lowered considerably to 4.2 and 4.2 mL/m³ of formalin and water, respectively.[39] In the United States, exposure to formaldehyde gas at a concentration of 1 mg/L at 75% relative humidity and 23.9°C (75°F) is recommended for safety cabinets, whereas Munro et al[40] suggested a concentration of 10.5 g/m³ at a relative humidity of 65% and a minimum temperature of 28°C was effective against the bacillus Calmette-Guérin vaccine strain, *B subtilis* spores, and poliovirus. Ackland et al[41] showed that 0.3 g/m³ was effective against spores at 20°C for 6 hours exposure using the UK formalin method. Another method suggested for areas without electrical supply is referred to as "bombing," where potassium permanganate is added to formalin and the reaction creates sufficient heat to vaporize the formaldehyde. This is generally not recommended on grounds of safety and efficacy concerns because it can be uncontrollable.[28]

Cross and Lach[42] assessed the effectiveness of the controlled exposure to formaldehyde in inactivating spores of *B atrophaeus* on filter membranes and obtained D-values for a range of relative humidity values and formaldehyde concentrations. At a humidity of 98%, D-values from 9 minutes for 400 mg/m³ to 373 minutes at 55 mg/m³. Lach[30] also carried out a comparison of a range of conventional formaldehyde fumigation methods. They found that, when double the concentration of the UK method was used in which 63.6 mL water and 7.07 mL formalin were vaporized per cubic meter (theoretical concentration 2.83 g/m³) and held for 18 hours, this gave a 9 log reduction, whereas a 3-hour exposure gave between 6 and >9 log reductions. At far higher concentrations (10.6 g/m³), when produced by reaction with permanganate and formalin, only a 4 to 5 $\log_{10}$ reduction was achieved.[30] Formaldehyde concentration in the air was measured through all fumigation processes. For the double UK method, a range of 89 to 347 mg/m³ was detected in the air, with peak levels of 190 to 580 mg/m³. This demonstrates that most of the formaldehyde was present in condensing layers on room surfaces along with water. This suggests that formaldehyde fumigation is at its most effective when the amount of water vaporized is enough to allow this condensing layer to form.

If the amount of water vaporized is too low, then the condensation layer is not formed. If it is too high, then the formaldehyde concentration in the condensing layer may not be as rapidly sporicidal. However, Casella and Schmidt-Lorenz[43] reported significantly lower D-values during formaldehyde fumigation without condensation for *B atrophaeus* (DSM 675) but not with *Streptococcus faecium* (ATCC 6057) and *Staphylococcus aureus* (ATCC 6538). In this study, condensation was caused by keeping the coupons at a lower temperature with a relative humidity of 90%.[43]

Paraformaldehyde fumigation was used successfully in combination with and following traditional liquid disinfection procedures as part of the remediation of buildings contaminated with *B anthracis* spores during the contamination incident at two mailing machines at the US Department of Justice Mail Facility in 2002.[44]

Measurement of Formaldehyde Gas

Formaldehyde concentration in the air can be measured using a number of tests. Standard methods for occupational exposure include passive sampling methods such as Occupational Safety and Health Administration (OSHA) Method No. 1007 (OSHA 2005) and the Health and Safety Executive - Methods for the Determination of Hazardous Substances (HSE-MDHS) 102 method (2010) as well as active sampling methods including The National Institute for Occupational Safety (NIOSH) Method (2016), L'Institut National de la Recherche Scientifique (INRS) Metropol 001/V01(2005), Association Francaise de Normalisation (AFNOR NFX) 43-264 (2002), NIOSH Method 2541, OSHA 52 (1989), and NIOSH Method 3500. More details on the specification of these methods are reviewed by Bolt et al.[45]

Handheld electronic meters are also available that are often used to ensure there are no leaks of formaldehyde from areas being fumigated, to ensure areas are safe to enter after the completion of the fumigation process, and as a safety control during the use of formaldehyde gas sterilizers. Formaldehyde concentrations can also be measured using Dräger tube-type systems. These systems often have a limited detection range and are used for safety reasons to ensure that levels outside the fumigated area are within threshold limit values.

Low-Temperature Steam Formaldehyde

Low-temperature steam with formaldehyde is commonly used in Scandinavian countries, in other parts of Europe, and South America as a sterilization process. The requirements of such sterilization processes are defined in the Europe and International Standard ISO 14180 *Sterilizers for medical purposes—low temperature steam and formaldehyde sterilizers—requirements and testing.*[46] Such steam

formaldehyde processes are not typically used in other countries such as the United States, United Kingdom, France, Russia, China, and Australia. Despite comparable toxicological concerns, the earlier selection of formaldehyde over ethylene oxide in some parts of the world was based on local familiarity with formaldehyde,[32] an ability to detect the odor of formaldehyde in low concentrations, nonflammability compared with 100% ethylene oxide, availability, and lower cost. Practices similar to those used with modern ethylene oxide sterilization equipment such as equipment design improvements, installation practices, reliable worker exposure/area monitoring technology, process improvements, and educational programs also have minimized safety concerns about formaldehyde use overtime.

Aldehydes are primarily surface-sterilizing agents, and the cross-linking of extraneous materials can limit penetration to the target microorganisms. Aldehyde-alkylating agents such as formaldehyde do not exhibit permeation capabilities necessary to sterilize occluded locations sealed within plastic materials, unless assisted by equipment and process design capabilities as for other sterilization methods (eg, exposure under controlled vacuum conditions). There can be difficulty in sterilizing certain types of porous materials as a result of polymer (such as paraformaldehyde) formation inhibiting further sterilant access. The relatively low concentrations of formaldehyde used typically range from 6 to 50 mg/L. In the case of formaldehyde, low concentrations are used to minimize its condensation and formation of a variety of polymers on materials processed, the sterilizing chamber, and associated equipment piping.[47] Because of low sterilant concentrations required to prevent such complications, processing conditions must be well controlled so that depleted molecules as a percentage of the total sterilant do not affect the efficacy of a sterilization process.

Formalin must be vaporized carefully because the water vaporizes more readily and solid formaldehyde polymers can be left behind. Formaldehyde is also supplied from paraformaldehyde, which releases formaldehyde on heating. The sterilizing temperature is greater than 65°C and typically is performed between 70°C and 80°C to minimize the formation of various solid polymers in the sterilizing chamber and on materials processed. The processing temperature(s) and humidity required are typically higher than range of temperatures commonly used with ethylene oxide (35°C-60°C at 30%-70% relative humidity). Phillips and Warshowsky[48] reported that bacterial spores were 2 to 15 times as resistant toward formaldehyde as were vegetative bacteria, exhibiting a ratio much less than is the case with many other types of disinfectants. Formaldehyde decomposes into carbon dioxide and water vapor, the formaldehyde concentration in an enclosed space decreases by about 2 mg/L/h.[49] Therefore, like air in a steam sterilization process, carbon dioxide can inhibit replenishment of formaldehyde sterilant inside geometric configurations such as lumens and tubing.

Reliable formaldehyde sterilization requires precise temperature and relative humidity control between 75% and 100% relative humidity, with limited steam condensation. This is difficult to achieve in practice. Precise process temperature and humidity control are required to prevent condensation of steam into water. Formaldehyde vapor rapidly dissolves into solution, depleting the environment of formaldehyde, producing an aqueous solution. Formaldehyde exhibits limited biocidal properties at 80°C, with up to 8 to 10 mg/L aqueous solution compared with the effective biocidal combination of vapor (or gas) phase formaldehyde and steam.[50] Experiences in the Scandinavian countries during the 1980s resulted in recommended simultaneous use of *B subtilis* var. *niger* and *G stearothermophilus* spores to evaluate the delivery of the needed humidity and formaldehyde concentration.[50] Other concepts included the use of organisms occluded in water-soluble crystals or organic material, which does not allow the test organisms to be exposed to formaldehyde until a minimum humidity level is attained.

In more recent innovations for formaldehyde sterilization processes, the formalin concentration has been reduced from about 37% (wt/vol) with methanol as a stabilizer, as used in conventional cycles, to about 2% (wt/vol in water to deliver a lower concentration of formaldehyde during the conditioning and sterilization phases. The data presented indicated having sterilization efficacy in lumens at temperatures as low as 45°C with minimal formation of paraformaldehyde.[51]

▶ FORMALDEHYDE NEUTRALIZATION

Because formaldehyde is a hazardous chemical, it is considered to be necessary in some countries to neutralize formaldehyde prior to ventilation of a disinfected area. Residual paraformaldehyde will be present on the surfaces of the exposure chamber after fumigation; without neutralization this can present a safety issue to the user when cleaning residues.[52,53] Neutralization can be done in a number of ways.

Neutralization Using Ammonium Carbonate or Bicarbonate or Ammonia

After the end of fumigation, ammonia can be generated such as from ammonium bicarbonate or carbonate release in the area or prior to release.[54] Ammonia reacts with the formaldehyde to form methenamine and water as follows:

$$6CH_2O + 4NH_3 \rightarrow C_6H_{12}N_4 + 6H_2O$$

Luftman[54] provided the following ratio for neutralization of 1.58 g ammonium bicarbonate to 1 g of paraformaldehyde calculated from theory and demonstrated by experiment; however, care should be taken using this formula because the lower levels of formaldehyde or ammonia remaining may still exceed threshold limit values.

Carbon Filtration

Activated carbon filters have been used in order to remove formaldehyde and other volatile organic compounds from indoor environments and after fumigation of laboratories or safety cabinets. The formaldehyde chemically reacts with the activated carbon and is adsorbed irreversibly. Although this can be effective, care has to be taken to avoid saturation of the carbon filter leading to breakthrough of active formaldehyde.

Oxidative Columns

Air containing formaldehyde can be pulled through devices containing oxidative chemicals such as potassium permanganate that will oxidize formaldehyde into CO_2 and water. Although these columns can cause significant reductions in concentrations, they are unlikely to reduce concentrations to safe levels.

▶ SAFETY

Formaldehyde is a carcinogenic compound and an irritant. It is a hazardous chemical agent and has been the subject of increasing regulatory scrutiny, such as under the requirements of Article 2(b) of Directive 98/24/EC and the scope of this legislation. Formaldehyde is also a carcinogen for humans in accordance with Article 2(a) and (b) of Directive 2004/37/EC and therefore restricts its use under such legislation. Ackland et al[41] demonstrated that when concentrations of more than 2 g/m^3 were used, paraformaldehyde polymerization was found on surfaces and may pose a safety risk to users. To ensure that staff or people in neighboring areas are not exposed to formaldehyde, the area to be fumigated must be sealed and held at a negative pressure, or an exclusion area should be created and patrolled by staff with formaldehyde monitors. If personnel need to enter an area under fumigation or above the exposure limit, they must wear positive pressure respiratory protective equipment fitted with appropriate filters. In some countries, the use of self-contained breathing apparatus is required.

The occupational exposure limits for formaldehyde vary from country to country (Table 36.3).

TABLE 36.3 Occupational exposure limits for formaldehyde[a,b]

Country	TWA (8 h)		STEL (15 min)	
	ppm	mg/m^3	ppm	mg/m^3
Australia	1	1.2	1	2.5
Canada	Not available	Not available	1	2.5
China	Not available	Not available	Not available	0.5
France	0.5	Not available	1	2.5
Germany	0.3	0.37	0.6	0.74
Japan	0.1	0.12	Not available	Not available
Netherlands	Not available	0.15	Not available	0.5
Spain	Not available	Not available	0.3	0.37
Sweden	0.3	0.37	0.6	0.74
Europe (SCOEL)	0.3	0.37	0.6	0.74
United Kingdom	2	2.5	2	2.5
United States	0.1	Not available	0.3	Not available

[a]Listed are the time-weighted averages (TWA) for an 8-hour shift and the short-term exposure limit (STEL) (15 min) in various countries. The Scientific Committee on Occupational Exposure Limits (SCOEL) value is a consensus value agreed by the authors of the review.

[b]Based on Bolt et al.[45]

REFERENCES

1. Dreyfus W. Review of formaldehyde fumigation. *Am J Public Health (N Y)*. 1914;4(11):1046-1049.
2. Cheney JE, Collins CH. Formaldehyde disinfection in laboratories: limitations and hazards. *Br J Biochem Sci*. 1995;52:195-201.
3. Loshon CA, Genest PC, Setlow B, Setlow P. Formaldehyde kills spores of *Bacillus subtilis* by DNA damage and small, acid-soluble spore proteins of the alpha/beta-type protect spores against this DNA damage. *J Appl Microbiol*. 1999;87(1):8-14.
4. Habeeb AJ, Hiramoto R. Reaction of proteins with glutaraldehyde. *Arch Biochem Biophys*. 1968;126(1):16-26.
5. Kaulfers PM, Marquardt A. Demonstration of formaldehyde dehydrogenase activity in formaldehyde-resistant Enterobacteriaceae. *FEMS Microbiol Lett*. 1991;63(2-3):335-338.
6. Kümmerle N, Feucht HH, Kaulfers PM. Plasmid-mediated formaldehyde resistance in *Escherichia coli*: characterization of resistance gene. *Antimicrob Agents Chemother*. 1996;40(10):2276-2279.
7. Kaulfers PM, Karch H, Laufs R. Plasmid-mediated formaldehyde resistance in *Serratia marcescens* and *Escherichia coli*: alterations in the cell surface. *Zentralbl Bakteriol Mikrobiol Hyg A*. 1987;266(1-2):239-248.
8. Dorsey CW, Actis LA. Analysis of pVU3695, a plasmid encoding glutathione-dependent formaldehyde dehydrogenase activity and formaldehyde resistance in the *Escherichia coli* VU3695 clinical strain. *Plasmid*. 2004;51(2):116-126.
9. Azachi M, Henis Y, Shapira R, Oren A. The role of the outer membrane in formaldehyde tolerance in *Escherichia coli* VU3695 and *Halomonas* sp. MAC. *Microbiology*. 1996;142(pt 5):1249-1254.
10. Williams ND, Russell AD. Revival of biocide-treated spores of *Bacillus subtilis*. *J Appl Bacteriol*. 1993;75(1):69-75.
11. Kim KS, Sharp DG. Influence of the physical state of formalinized vaccinia virus particles on surviving plaque titer: evidence for multiplicity reactivation. *J Immunol*. 1967;99(6):1221-1225.
12. The Committee on Formaldehyde Disinfection. Disinfection of fabrics with gaseous formaldehyde. *J Hyg*. 1958;56(4):488-515.
13. Fitzpatrick M. The Cutter incident: how America's first polio vaccine led to a growing vaccine crisis. *J R Soc Med*. 2006;99(3):156.
14. Nathanson N, Langmuir AD. The cutter incident. Poliomyelitis following formaldehyde-inactivated poliovirus vaccination in the United States during the spring of 1955. I. Background. *Am J Hyg*. 1963;78:16-18.
15. Brown P, Liberski PP, Wolff A, Gajdusek DC. Resistance of scrapie infectivity to steam autoclaving after formaldehyde fixation and limited survival after ashing at 360 degrees C: practical and theoretical implications. *J Infect Dis*. 1990;161(3):467-472.
16. Manchee RJ, Broster MG, Stagg AJ, Hibbs SE. Formaldehyde solution effectively inactivates spores of *Bacillus anthracis* on the Scottish Island of Gruinard. *Appl Environ Microbiol*. 1994;60:4167-4171.
17. Brenner E. Human body preservation—old and new techniques. *J Anat*. 2014;224(3):316-344.
18. Spaulding E. Chemical disinfection of medical and surgical materials. In: Lawrence C, ed. *Disinfection, Sterilization, and Preservation*. Philadelphia, PA: Lea & Febiger; 1968:517-531.
19. Gard S. Theoretical considerations in the inactivation of viruses by chemical means. *Ann N Y Acad Sci*. 1960;83:638-648.
20. Sagripanti JL, Bonifacino A. Comparative sporicidal effects of liquid chemical agents. *Appl Environ Microbiol*. 1996;62(2):545-551.
21. Sagripanti JL, Eklund CA, Trost PA, et al. Comparative sensitivity of 13 species of pathogenic bacteria to seven chemical germicides. *Am J Infect Control*. 1997;25(4):335-339.
22. Alasri A, Valverde M, Roques C, Michel G, Cabassud C, Aptel P. Sporocidal properties of peracetic acid and hydrogen peroxide, alone and in combination, in comparison with chlorine and formaldehyde for ultrafiltration membrane disinfection. *Can J Microbiol*. 1993;39(1):52-60.
23. Rubbo SD, Gardner JF, Webb RL. Biocidal activities of glutaraldehyde and related compounds. *J Appl Bacteriol*. 1967;30(1):78-87.
24. Möller L, Schünadel L, Nitsche A, Schwebke I, Hanisch M, Laue M. Evaluation of virus inactivation by formaldehyde to enhance biosafety of diagnostic electron microscopy. *Viruses*. 2015;7(2):666-679.

25. Rutala WA, Weber DJ. *Guideline for Disinfection and Sterilization in Healthcare Facilities, 2008*. Atlanta, GA: US Department of Health and Human Services; 2008.

26. Pedersen L-F, Pedersen PB, Sortjaer O. Temperature-dependent and surface specific formaldehyde degradation in submerged biofilters. *Aqua Engin*. 2007;36(2):127-136.

27. Pedersen L-F, Pedersen PB, Nielsen JL, Nielsen PH. Peracetic acid degradation and effects on nitrification in recirculating aquaculture systems. *Aquaculture*. 2009;296(3-4):246-254.

28. Darlow H. The practical aspects of formaldehyde fumigation. *Mon Bull Minist Health*. 1958;17:270-273.

29. Taylor LA, Barbeito MS, Gremillion GG. Paraformaldehyde for surface sterilization and detoxification. *Appl Microbiol*. 1969;17(4):614-618.

30. Lach VH. A study of conventional formaldehyde fumigation methods. *J Appl Bacteriol*. 1990;68(5):471-477.

31. Spiner DR, Hoffmann RK. Effect of relative humidity on formaldehyde decontamination. *Appl Microbiol*. 1971;22(6):1138-1140.

32. Nordgren G. Investigations on the sterilization efficacy of gaseous formaldehyde. *Acta Pathol Microbiol Scand*. 1939;40:165.

33. Grossgebauer K, Spicher G, Peters J, Kuwert E, Pohle HD, Kerner H. Experiments on terminal disinfection by formaldehyde vapor in the case of smallpox. *J Clin Microbiol*. 1975;2(6):516-519.

34. Rogers JV, Choi YW, Richter WR, et al. Formaldehyde gas inactivation of *Bacillus anthracis*, *Bacillus subtilis*, and *Geobacillus stearothermophilus* spores on indoor surface materials. *J Appl Microbiol*. 2007;103(4):1104-1112.

35. Beswick AJ, Farrant J, Makison C, et al. Comparison of multiple systems for laboratory whole room fumigation. *Appl Biosaf*. 2011;16(3):139-157.

36. Ide PR. The sensitivity of some avian viruses to formaldehyde fumigation. *Can J Comp Med*. 1979;43(2):211-216.

37. National Research Council. *Reopening Public Facilities after a Biological Attack: A Decision Making Framework*. Washington, DC: National Academic Press; 2005.

38. Standard NI. *Biosafety Cabinetry: Design, Construction, Performance, and Field Certification*. Ann Arbor, MI: NSF International; 2014.

39. Ngabo D, Pottage T, Bennett AM, Parks SR. Cabinet decontamination using formaldehyde. *Appl Biosaf*. 2017;22(2):60-67.

40. Munro K, Lanser J, Flower R. A comparative method to validate formaldehyde decontamination of biological safety cabinets. *Appl Environ Microbiol*. 1999;65:873-876.

41. Ackland NR, Hinton MR, Denmeade KR. Controlled formaldehyde fumigation system. *Appl Environ Microbiol*. 1980;39:480-487.

42. Cross GL, Lach VH. The effects of controlled exposure to formaldehyde vapour on spores of *Bacillus globigii* NCTC 10073. *J Appl Bacteriol*. 1990;68(5):461-469.

43. Casella ML, Schmidt-Lorenz W. Disinfection with gaseous formaldehyde. First part: bactericidal and sporicidal effectiveness of formaldehyde with and without formation of a condensing layer. *Zentralbl Hyg Umweltmed*. 1989;188(1-2):144-165.

44. Canter DA, Gunning D, Rodgers P, O'Connor L, Traunero C, Kempter CJ. Remediation of *Bacillus anthracis* contamination in the U.S. Department of Justice mail facility. *Biosecur Bioterror*. 2005;3(2):119-127.

45. Bolt HM, Johanson G, Nielsen GD, Papameletiou D, Klein KL. *SCOEL/REC/125 Formaldehyde. Recommendation from the Scientific Committee on Occupational Exposure Limits*. Luxembourg, Luxembourg: Publications Office of the European Union; 2016.

46. Kanemitsu K, Kunishima H, Imasaka T, et al. Evaluation of a low-temperature steam and formaldehyde sterilizer. *J Hosp Infect*. 2003;55(1):47-52.

47. Hoxey EV. Low temperature steam formaldehyde. In: Morrisey RE, Prokopenko YI, eds. *Sterilization of Medical Products*. Vol 5. Morin-Heights, Quebec, Canada: Polyscience Publications; 1991:359-364.

48. Phillips CR, Warshowsky B. Chemical disinfectants. *Annu Rev Microbiol*. 1958;12:525-550.

49. Phillips CR. Gaseous sterilization. In: Reddish GF, ed. *Antiseptics, Disinfectants, Fungicides, and Physical Sterilization*. Philadelphia, PA: Lea & Febiger; 1954:638-654.

50. Hoxey EV. Gaseous sterilization. In: Fraise AP, Maillard J-Y, Sattar SA, eds. *Russell, Hugo & Ayliffe's: Principles and Practice of Disinfection, Preservation, and Sterilization*. 2nd ed. Oxford, United Kingdom: Blackwell Science; 1992:567-572.

51. Joslyn LJ. Gaseous chemical sterilization. In: Block SS, ed. *Disinfection, Sterilization, and Preservation*. 5th ed. Philadelphia, PA: Lippincott Williams & Wilkins; 2001:1481.

52. Gibson GL, Johnston HP, Turkington VE. Residual formaldehyde after low-temperature steam and formaldehyde sterilization. *J Clin Pathol*. 1968;21(6):771-775.

53. Kanemitsu K, Kunishima H, Saga T, et al. Residual formaldehyde on plastic materials and medical equipment following low-temperature steam and formaldehyde sterilization. *J Hosp Infect*. 2005;59(4):361-364.

54. Luftman HS. Neutralization of formaldehyde gas by ammonium bicarbonate and ammonium carbonate. *Appl Biosaf*. 2005;10(2):101-106.

CHAPTER

37

Prevention of Infection From Food and Water

Christon J. Hurst and Gerald McDonnell

The subject of this chapter is microbial contaminants found either in food or in water, and the chapter primarily addresses microbial contaminants that infect humans. Before considering this topic, it is important for us to reflect on the broader issue of foodborne and waterborne disease. Many types of diseases have been associated with the consumption of food.[1] Diseases also are associated with either ingestion or other types of exposure to water.[2] These food-associated and water-associated diseases may be either acute or chronic. It is important to note that in the modern world today, many of the diseases associated with contaminants present in food or water are often caused by chemicals and are not specifically related to microbial contamination. Despite the disease hazards represented by chemical contaminants, the causative agents of foodborne and waterborne disease outbreaks continue to be frequently microbiological in nature. This is highlighted from the review of the top causes of death in the world today, which varies depending if you live in a high- or low-income country; in high-income countries, the major causes are ischemic heart disease, stroke, and dementia, whereas in low-income countries, communicable disease remains prevalent causes such as diarrheal diseases that are typically associated with food or water contamination.[3] But even in high-income countries, outbreaks of infection and even death linked to such contaminants remain a frequent occurrence. The causes of such microbiological-associated diseases may represent either microbially produced toxins or infectious agents.

In general, foodborne disease outbreaks tend to be smaller but more numerous than waterborne disease outbreaks. Whereas it is true that in some cases, water is considered a food item because it is ingested, this chapter generally keeps with the more traditional custom of considering waterborne disease transmission as independent of food. There are notable connections between the subjects of foodborne and waterborne diseases in that food items can be contaminated by water. These connections

between waterborne and foodborne diseases are noted within the chapter. The acquisition of infection from food items almost always is associated with ingestion of food. Usually, the only rare exceptions to this rule result when a microbial aerosol created during food handling is inhaled and causes a respiratory infection. Infections can be acquired from water by many different routes aside from ingestion, and these waterborne routes are described within the chapter. It is important to recognize that the associated microbial contaminants cause both individual and clusters of disease cases, even in the absence of recognized community-wide outbreaks. Both foodborne and waterborne infectious diseases represent substantial economic costs to society, not only in terms of medical treatment expenses but also the expense resulting from lost human productivity and even premature human death.

Most environmentally transmitted infections of humans seem to result from encountering pathogens that were contributed to the environment by other humans or animals. Therefore, we can prevent the transmission of these infections if we successfully prevent initial contamination of that food or water. This represents the aim of contamination-prevention programs such as crop and watershed protection, food and water disinfection (or commonly referred to as *sanitation*), the use of protective food packaging, and the use of closed containers or plumbing to transport potable water; however, additional environmentally associated illnesses result from microorganisms that are natural environmental inhabitants and many of these defy efforts at blocking the source of contamination. Included in the category of infectious agents that represent natural environmental inhabitants are numerous bacterial organisms such as *Listeria monocytogenes*, a soil organism that can cause meningitis if ingested; *Legionella pneumophila*, a water organism that can cause pneumonia if inhaled in a droplet aerosol; and *Vibrio vulnificus*, which can cause septicemia if it is present in bivalve mollusks that are ingested. *Vibrio cholerae* represents a particularly interesting bacteria because it naturally resides in warm waters on the chitinous shell of crustaceans; we can acquire infections caused by these bacteria either by ingesting macrocrustaceans such as crabs as a food item or if we inadvertently ingest microcrustaceans contained in drinking water. The outcome of ingesting *V cholerae* by either of these processes leads to a diarrheal illness that can be transmitted by sewage; thus, infectious agents that might have been acquired from a food can lead to waterborne infection. Natural environmental microorganisms can cause other noninfectious illnesses associated with food items. Examples of bacterial species that cause such noninfectious illnesses are *Clostridium botulinum*, whose toxin causes nerve paralysis, and *Clostridium perfringens*, which, although normally associated with causing gas gangrene in deep wounds, will produce a toxin that can cause gastroenteritis when consumed.

A disease-causing microbe is less likely to be transmitted by an environmental route that exposes the organism to conditions under which it cannot easily survive; thus, infectious agents that are likely to have the greatest success at being transmitted in foods or water will logically have to be organisms that have evolved abilities to survive and even grow in food or water despite the natural or artificial (eg, preservative) methods employed to prepare them for consumption. We can use this general knowledge to our advantage by exposing the food or water to various treatment processes that impose conditions that will diminish the existing level of many types of pathogens and will help to prevent the growth of any infectious organisms that remain.

▶ INTRODUCTION TO FOODBORNE INFECTIOUS DISEASES

Microbially contaminated foods represent a major source of human illness, and although these are often related to bacteria, they can include other pathogens including a large number of viral and protozoal diseases. Unlike chemical contaminants, some categories of microbial contaminants may be capable of replicating within the food, which can increase the disease hazard associated with the contaminated foods over the course of time. Indeed, *thermal abuse*, a term used to describe food that has been held at temperatures high enough to enable the growth of contaminating pathogenic bacteria or fungi, often has been associated with enteritis. Thermal abuse of foods usually is not implicated in protozoan- or viral-induced illnesses because protozoa that cause human enteric illnesses usually will not grow in stored foods and the human enteric viruses cannot grow in foods because viruses require viable animal host cells in which to replicate. The causative microbial contaminants found in food may have been acquired either

from the environment or during the subsequent steps involved with food processing, packaging, and handling that occur prior to consumption.

Sources of Microbial Contaminants in Food

Microbial contamination of foods can occur within the environment before the food is harvested. Foods contaminated by water in this way include crustaceans and bivalve mollusks in which they live and vegetables contaminated by having been either irrigated with wastewater or fertilized with solids from wastewater. Foods also can be contaminated in the environment by processes that are not directly associated with contaminated water, with examples including *Salmonella* species (the bacterial agents associated with salmonellosis that may be acquired from ingesting eggs) and *Campylobacter* species (bacteria that cause campylobacteriosis, which may be acquired from both poultry and dairy products). Foods also can become contaminated with microorganisms at many different steps between the time of harvesting and eventual consumption. Some contamination is intentional, with certain bacteria and fungi deliberately added to food so that through their associated metabolic processes, these microorganisms will impart desired characteristics to the food. These characteristics include modifications of food coloration, texture, aroma, and taste. As an example, the gases released by respiration of yeasts cause bread to rise. Yeasts can ferment sugars to produce ethanol, which is a desired component of many beverages. Bacteria in the same beverages then can convert the ethanol and other compounds to acetic acid, thereby producing vinegar. Usually, it is the unintentional contamination of foods with microorganisms that is of public health concern. This contamination may result in spoilage of the food, production of microbial toxins, and infections of humans or animals that consume the food. It is the last of these categories of microorganisms—the unintentional contaminants—that will be addressed in the following text. Many of the individual foodborne pathogenic microorganisms are characteristically associated with specific types of foods (Table 37.1). These include not only many different categories of microorganisms (bacteria, protozoa, and viruses) but also some of the smaller types of microbial worms (metazoans such as cestodes and nematodes). These characteristic associations tend to represent contamination acquired either prior to harvesting or during processing operations performed before the food is marketed. Noncharacteristic associations between microorganisms and foods also have been noticed, and these tend to represent contamination that is acquired during the course of food handling after marketing. Some examples of these associations are *Salmonella* in orange juice,[4] *Giardia* on raw sliced vegetables[5] or in salads,[6]

TABLE 37.1	Examples of characteristic associations between foods and infectious diseases[a]	
Food	**Disease**	**Causative Microorganism**
Crops (vegetables)	Bacterial	
	Enteric fever	*Salmonella*
	Enteritis	*Vibrio*
	Viral	
	Hepatitis	*Hepatovirus*
Salads	Bacterial	
	Enteritis	*Shigella*
	Enteritis	*Escherichia*
	Viral	
	Enteritis	*Calicivirus*
Dairy products	Bacterial	
	Enteritis	*Campylobacter*
	Febrile syndrome	*Brucella*
	Meningitis	*Listeria*
Eggs (avian)	Bacterial	
	Enteric fever	*Salmonella*
	Enteritis	*Campylobacter*
Eggs (marine reptiles)	Bacterial	
	Enteritis	*Vibrio*
Fish (sold raw)	Metazoan	
	Worm infestation	*Spirometra*
Poultry (sold raw)	Bacterial	
	Enteric fever	*Salmonella*
	Enteritis	*Campylobacter*
(sold in processed, precooked, prepackaged form)	Bacterial	
	Meningitis	*Listeria*
Red meats (sold raw)	Bacterial	
	Enteritis	*Escherichia*
	Febrile syndrome	*Francisella tularensis*
	Protozoan	*Giardia*
	Metazoan	*Cryptosporidium*
	Worm infestation	*Taenia, Trichinella*
(sold in processed, precooked, prepackaged form)	Bacterial	
	Meningitis	*Listeria*
Shellfish (crustacean)	Bacterial	
	Enteritis	*Vibrio*
Shellfish (bivalve molluskan)	Bacterial	
	Enteritis	*Vibrio*
	Viral	
	Gastroenteritis	*Calicivirus*
	Hepatitis	*Hepatovirus*
Ice	Viral	
	Gastroenteritis	*Calicivirus*

[a]These characteristic associations generally represent microbial contamination that occurs either before harvesting or when food is processed prior to marketing. Many other diseases, such as those associated with *Staphylococcus* and *Clostridium*, are not listed in this table because they generally represent intoxications rather than infections.

Streptococcus in macaroni and cheese,[7] and *Calicivirus* with freshly cut fruit.[8]

Contamination Acquired From the Environment Prior to Harvesting

As suggested in the preceding discussion, microbial contamination can occur before harvesting, which also represents the first link in the chain of food production. As indicated, some of these microbial contaminants are hazardous because they infect consumers, but other microbes are primarily hazardous because of the toxins they produce. The predominant bacterial organisms associated with foodborne infectious disease seem to be *Salmonella*, *Shigella*, and *Campylobacter* species. *Salmonella* tends to be associated with both meat and eggs from poultry when those items are sold raw, and this is due to the fact that members of the genus *Salmonella* represent natural intestinal and cloacal microflora for avians. *Salmonella* also represent some risk for raw meat and eggs from terrestrial and freshwater reptiles because this genus of bacteria likewise colonizes the intestines and cloaca of those reptiles. In comparison, the bacterial contamination associated with raw eggs from marine turtles is of the genus *Vibrio*, which ecologically serves the marine environment in a role similar to that of *Salmonella's* role in the terrestrial environments. *Campylobacter* seems to be associated with milk and likewise with poultry sold raw. The association of *Vibrio* with crustaceans and bivalve mollusks (such as mussels, clams, oysters, and scallops) represents natural microflora. Unfortunately, the natural colonization of the chitinous shells of crustaceans by *Vibrio* species can cause illness following ingestion if the crustaceans are not adequately cooked prior to ingestion. There is also some evidence that *Vibrio* species may be naturally present within the interior of the crustaceans. The association with *Vibrio* species as contaminants in bivalve mollusks presumably results from the mollusks having ingested these naturally present aquatic bacteria during the course of filter feeding.[9] In fact, during the course of filter feeding, bivalve mollusks can become contaminated with any enteric pathogens present in the shellfish-growing waters, including bacteria, protozoans, and viruses.[9] *Salmonella*, *Pseudomonas*, and *Aeromonas* species can be detected in bivalve mollusks, although it is not certain whether many of these contaminants are acquired prior to harvesting or during processing and handling. Disease problems with *Escherichia*, including the shiga-toxin strains of *Escherichia coli* O157:H7 strain, tend to be associated with ground beef sold raw.[10] Interestingly, it is the strains of *E coli* associated with cattle that cause illness in humans, although at the same time, those humans presumably would find their intestines to be naturally colonized by nonpathogenic human-associated strains of *E coli*.

The predominant viruses associated with foodborne diseases are hepatitis A virus, which is the sole member of the *Hepatovirus* genus, and particularly *Calicivirus*, a genus most often represented by noroviruses or Norwalk and Norwalk-like viruses. These viruses are often associated with illnesses acquired from ingesting bivalve mollusks, where they are accumulated from water during the natural filter-feeding process used by the bivalve mollusks. *Caliciviruses* also may be associated with ice, an association that likely results from using virally contaminated water to produce the ice, and are commonly transmitted by the fecal-oral route (eg, known as a winter-vomiting bug). The Centers for Disease Control and Prevention estimates worldwide that noroviruses are responsible for 1 in 5 case of acute gastroenteritis and is the most common cause of diarrhea and vomiting associated with outbreaks of disease.[11] Helminths, such as *Taenia* and *Trichinella*, usually are associated with meat from terrestrial mammals sold either raw or inadequately cooked and represent a disease-related infestation of the animals being slaughtered for food. Helminths of the genus *Spirometra* have a parallel association with fish. These bacterial, viral, and helminth contamination problems are characteristic associations.

The food-associated microorganisms listed earlier in this section cause illness by infecting the consumer. Some other microbial contaminants are notable for producing toxins that, when the food is ingested, cause diseases that represent intoxications.[12] Dinoflagellate toxins can be accumulated by fish and shellfish prior to harvesting. Additional examples of environmentally acquired microbial toxins in foods are fungal toxins, such as aflatoxins, caused by the growth of fungi on plant materials either prior to harvesting or during storage.

Contamination Acquired During Processing and Production Prior to Marketing

Many foods are processed prior to marketing. In some cases, this can involve procedures as simple as washing and sorting, followed by packaging. Of course, processing can involve far more complex operations, including the addition of multiple ingredients from different sources and cooking. Each one of the steps involved, and each one of the ingredients added, represents an opportunity for microbial contamination. Contaminants can come from food contact surfaces, including processing equipment such as vats and plumbing. Biofilms are particular sources of microbial pathogens in these situations that are both actively growing in and associated with the biofilm; their resilience to cleaning and disinfection strategies is discussed further in chapter 67. Other sources of contamination are water used in washing operations, aerosols that can fall into the food as it is being processed and packaged, and the packaging material itself. Cross-contamination can occur between subsequently processed lots of raw ingredients. Cross-contamination also can occur between raw and cooked products if these come into contact with one another either directly or through the use of common processing or packaging equipment. Assuring adequate disinfection at the processing step is particularly important in light of the fact that some microbial contaminants such as bacteria and fungi can grow in foods following packaging, and the distribution and marketing process for some foods may involve long periods during which that growth could occur. A few common examples of food items contaminated during processing are bacterial contaminations of meat, frozen fresh foods, and dairy products. Outbreaks of infection due to bacterial genus such as *Listeria* are frequently reported and linked with foodborne illness.[13] *Listeria* are often associated with milk and other dairy products and is also associated with processed products containing red meat or poultry (such as sausages and luncheon meats) when these meat products are sold in a precooked, prepackaged form. *Listeria* are considered to be sourced from soil and animals and have been shown to be sourced from unsanitary factory production or food-handling practices. The presence of *Shigella* in food items presumably represents direct contact of the food with human feces or with the contaminated hands of workers, which can occur either prior to harvesting, during harvesting, or during processing prior to marketing.[14]

Legal regulations were established to protect the quality of food products, perhaps the most important of which are regulations pertaining to the applications of risk assessment during the food preparation process, such as Hazard Analysis and Critical Control Point (HACCP) and associated controls such as disinfection (in food-associated applications often referred to as *sanitation*) practices. These help in controlling microbial quality not only of the basic material used in a food but also of additives as simple as potable water. Preventing microbial contamination requires close attention to sanitation practices. Good sanitation can result in food products that have a greater health safety level and may increase the shelf life of the product.[15]

Contamination Acquired During Handling and Preparation Following Marketing

Handlers involved in the preparation of food represent a major source of contaminants. Again, the largest factor involved is one of proper sanitation and aseptic practices. The infectious microbial contaminants associated with improper handling during food preparation tend to represent microorganisms that are present in the feces of infected persons and for which the transmission route involves ingestion of fecally contaminated materials.[16] An example of bacterial disease caused by enteric microorganisms introduced during handling and preparation is with *Salmonella typhi* in a reconstituted beverage[4] or with viruses such as noroviruses.[17] These situations can be difficult to control due to the levels of microorganisms produced in different body excretions during illness (eg, 10^5-10^7 colony-forming units [CFUs] *Salmonella* per gram

of feces or up to 10^6 CFU *Staphylococcus* per milliliter of saliva) as well as in asymptomatic individuals (eg, approximately 10^9 hepatitis A virions per gram feces in patients before symptoms of infection are seen).[16] Handlers have even been reported to contaminate food through contact with infected wounds, resulting in outbreaks of diseases that normally are not considered to be enteric. An example of this route of bacterial contamination is an outbreak of streptococcus pharyngitis attributed to prepared macaroni and cheese.[7]

Examples of enteric protozoan contamination of foods that occurred during handling and preparation are *Giardia* in raw sliced vegetables,[5,18] in a pasta salad,[6] and from various grocery foods handled by asymptomatic carriers.[19] Protozoan contamination of vegetables in one of those two outbreaks,[5,18] and of the pasta salad, presumably represented cross-contamination contributed by water that had been used to prepare the food. The common-source giardiasis study[18] represents a particularly interesting example of how microbial contaminants can be transferred from one type of contaminated material to another, creating a cycle of contamination. In that outbreak of giardiasis, it appears that raw food initially became contaminated by washing in tap water, after which the contaminated food was chopped on a cutting board. Other foods appear to have become contaminated when they were later prepared on that same cutting board, which was never adequately washed. Adequate washing of the cutting board to remove contaminating microorganisms physically, or disinfection of the cutting board, would have broken the cycle of contamination. Overall, water contamination is still the most prevalent source of protozoa associated with outbreaks, but food-borne contamination and outbreaks with *Giardia*, usually associated with food handlers, is estimated to be approximately 15% of cases.[20] Examples of enteric viral contamination that may have originated during handling are represented by *Calicivirus* associated with freshly cut fruit[8] and multiple enteric viruses (rotavirus, sapovirus, and norovirus) due to fecal contamination of salad.[21]

Whereas the pathogenic organisms listed in Table 37.1 represent prevalent examples of infectious hazards (in which case, the whole organism itself is considered the pathogen), there also exist characteristic hazards from organisms that are pathogenic by virtue of the toxins they produce. Bacterial toxins can result from the growth of microorganisms on improperly stored foods, and these intoxications usually do not represent an infectious disease. Nevertheless, intoxications of this type are sufficiently notable in a number of bacterial examples. For example, *Staphylococcus* food poisoning is among the top three causes of foodborne illness.[22] *Bacillus cereus* strains can survive cooking temperatures due to the production of spores but if given the opportunity (eg, in cooked rice held at temperature ranging from 10°C to 50°C) can produce toxins such as cereulide that can withstand any subsequent heating and cause nausea/vomiting on ingestion.[23]

Other toxins produced by these strains can lead to more delayed symptoms, particularly diarrhea. *C botulinum* can cause disease by different mechanisms. During the growth of this organism in foods, it produces a toxin that, when ingested, results in a more immediate intoxication. This organism normally cannot grow within the human intestines beyond the age of infancy; however, growth of *C botulinum* within the intestines of infants can result in the intoxication known as *infant botulism*. Fungi can also produce a number of toxins in association with grain or nuts that have been stored incorrectly. The most notable fungal toxins associated with foods are the aflatoxins, such as the aflatoxins B_1 and B_2 produced by *Aspergillus flavus*.[24] These toxins can lead to acute (eg, hepatic necrosis) and chronic (particularly cancer) diseases. Viruses cannot produce toxins, and generally, it is presumed that foodborne pathogenic protozoa do not produce toxins.

It should also be recognized that the predominating types of contaminating microorganisms may change during the chain of events between the time of harvesting and final cooking prior to consumption. Using fish as an example, at the time of harvesting, the predominant bacterial and fungal contaminants will be environmental organisms, many of which will prefer to grow at refrigeration temperatures. During processing by humans, human enteric microflora might be added, and these would prefer to grow at 35°C to 40°C.

Preventing Foodborne Disease Transmission

Preserving the microbiological quality of foods is a subject that can be divided into three principal components. The first component is using protective containers and coverings, including protective packaging, to serve as physical barriers to preserve the existing quality of food items. The second of component is reducing the existing level of pathogenic microbial contaminants both in the food substance and in packaging materials, preferably while limiting the addition of newly introduced microbial contaminants during the course of these treatments. The third component is preventing subsequent growth of the remaining microorganisms before the food can be consumed.

Use of Physical Barriers to Preserve the Existing Quality of Food Items

The use of physical barriers can begin prior to harvesting. Examples of this early application occur with several different types of fruit. For example, plastic bags are wrapped around the individual bunches of bananas during their growth period when they still are on tree. Likewise, in some Asian countries, paper bags are wrapped around individual fruits, such as apples and pears, while they still are growing on the trees. This protection by bagging primarily serves to protect the appearance of the fruit product against damage caused by insects. Similar efforts, directed against microbial rotting, occur when plastic sheeting is placed on the soil surface underneath strawberry plants to keep the fruit from coming into direct contact with the soil. Microbiological quality can be addressed at the time of harvest, when tarpaulins are placed on the ground underneath trees that bear fruits such as olives. Those fruits then are harvested by being shaken from the trees, after which the fruits are collected by gathering the tarpaulins. Many types of food then are protected in bulk using cardboard or plastic containers to transport the food items to processing sites and from the processing sites to markets where the food is to be sold. Other examples of protective packaging used to protect food items against contamination during the interval between food processing and marketing include metal cans, plastic or glass jugs and jars, cardboard boxes, paper wrapping, and plastic bags or plastic sheeting.

Reducing the Levels of Existing Microbial Contaminants

Reducing the existing level of microbial contaminants in food and in the materials used for packaging can be accomplished by many different approaches during the processing that occurs prior to marketing. The simplest of these is washing or washing-disinfecting both the food and packaging materials with water that contains chemical disinfection agents such as chlorine, chlorine compounds, or hydrogen peroxide.

Pathogenic microorganisms that shellfish acquire from the environment during their natural filter feeding can be purged prior to marketing by either relaying or depuration. Relaying involves moving the shellfish to environmental waters known to be uncontaminated. Depuration involves placing the shellfish into an artificial environment of flowing, usually recirculated, water that may be disinfected by a process such as ultraviolet irradiation. In both instances, the shellfish then are kept in the clean water for a time adequate for them to expel their load of microbial contaminants.

All organisms can be destroyed by the application of sufficient heat, one of the oldest methods of disinfecting foods. Applying heat until the food reaches an adequately high temperature and maintaining that temperature for an appropriate period are the most effective methods for reducing the level of microorganisms in foods. *Pasteurization* is the term used to describe the application of heat for a specific period to destroy pathogenic bacteria, demonstrated scientifically by Louis Pasteur in the treatment of beer and wine. Today, this is normally performed when the products are being processed prior to marketing. Pasteurization is often used to treat dairy products. *Retorting* is another heating technique used in food processing. Retorting commonly is used in canning operations, during which externally applied heat generates steam pressure inside sealed containers of food. This process simulates the practice of autoclaving that is used in laboratory sterilization operations. The sensitivity of various groups of microorganisms to the effects of heating varies tremendously (see chapter 11). This is a particular problem in the control of *Bacillus* and *Clostridium* species, two genera of bacteria that produce endospores. Whereas the vegetative cells of these bacteria can be killed easily by heating, their spores are relatively resistant to the effects of heating. After cooked food is allowed to cool, any spores that survived the heat treatment can germinate into new vegetative bacterial cells that subsequently may grow in the food. Because of this resistance, the spore-producing organism *C perfringens* is one of the most prevalent causes of food poisoning in the United States (along with *Salmonella*, *Staphylococcus aureus*, and *Campylobacter*) and is particularly associated with contaminated meats.[25]

Adequately cooking food prior to consumption, performed either during processing before marketing or by the individual consumer, can be effective in reducing foodborne illness. Cooking can be done with externally applied heat or with microwave radiation (as indirect source of heating; see chapter 10). An example of the value of cooking is represented in the control of enteric fever caused by bacteria of the genus *Salmonella*, which is often associated with the consumption of raw or inadequately cooked chicken eggs.[26] In fact, the extent to which eggs are cooked prior to consumption has been found to be associated statistically with the likelihood of acquiring that illness, known as *salmonellosis*. Outbreaks of bacterial disease also are associated with meat and meat products that have been inadequately cooked before consumption, as demonstrated by contamination of raw beef by *E coli* fecal bacteria from cattle. Consumption of undercooked beef contaminated with at least one bovine strain of *E coli*, designated strain O157:H7, can cause enteritis, which in some childhood cases may progress to a fatal hemolytic uremic syndrome.[27] Interestingly, this *E coli* problem is not associated with eating intact cuts of beef because the bacterial contamination is only on the external surface of the meat and can be quickly killed when the surface is heated during frying or grilling of the meat. Instead, this problem of *E coli* contamination occurs with ingestion of beef that has been ground before being cooked. The grinding process inadvertently internalizes the surface microbial contaminants, making it important that even the interior of the ground meat then be cooked thoroughly before that meat is ingested. Consumption of inadequately cooked crustacean shellfish is one of the characteristic associations for foodborne enteritis (cholera and hemolytic diarrhea) caused by various members of the bacterial genus *Vibrio*. Consumption of raw or inadequately cooked bivalve molluskan shellfish characteristically is associated with viral hepatitis and gastroenteritis.

Alternative techniques for destroying pathogenic microorganisms in food include freezing, irradiation, dehydration, and chemical addition. Freezing can be effective for destroying protozoans, although it cannot be considered protective against viruses and bacteria. Gamma irradiation is used during the processing of some foods, both as a microbial reduction and/or sterilization process.[28] Examples include herbs/spices, fruits, vegetables, meats, and shellfish. Other types of radiations, including ultraviolet and electron beams, may have beneficial roles by reducing the levels of contaminating microorganisms in foods during processing. The major drawbacks of some of these approaches can be cost and negative effects on tastes/flavors. Some microorganisms can be destroyed by drying, but the role of drying is more important from the standpoint of its effectiveness at preventing microbial growth. Drying reduces the water activity in foods, a natural preservation method, and is achieved either by vaporization of liquid water or by freeze-drying, which involves the sublimation of ice from frozen foods. Chemical supplements also can be effective at destroying microbial contaminants. These supplements are numerous and include such common natural additives as salt and sugar (eg, in pickling), which act by changing osmolarity and reducing water activity, and the application of smoke, which can contain a complex mixture of chemicals. Enzymes, such as lysozyme and lactoperoxidase, are sometimes added to food because of their antimicrobial or preservative potentials. Other examples include the use of bacteriocins and bacteriophages, essential soil, organic acids (propionic acid, lactic acid, and citric acid), chlorine, carbon dioxide (as a preservative), peracetic acid or hydrogen peroxide, and ozone.[29] Other innovative methods that have been shown to reduce microbial levels include biocide-impregnated packaging (eg, with organic acids), vacuum packaging, high-pressure treatment (eg, 400-600 MPa at room temperature), pulsed electric fields, and pulsed light treatments.[29]

Preventing the Growth of Harmful Microbial Contaminants

Bacteria, fungi, and perhaps algae are groups of pathogenic microbial contaminants whose environmental needs are often sufficiently simple that they can potentially replicate within stored food's condition. Microbial pathogens that, for the most part, cannot replicate in food are protozoa, helminths, and viruses. Water activity, temperature, and the presence of competing microorganisms are factors that play a major role in regulating the growth of microorganisms in food. Other factors, which are slightly less important but still significant in terms of regulating the ability of microorganisms to grow in foods, include pH, the presence of inhibiting chemicals, and the availability of suitable electron acceptors to support metabolic processes.

Control of water activity is probably the oldest technique known for preventing the growth of microorganisms in foods, and it can effectively be accomplished by many different approaches. Of these, drying is the simplest technique for long-term storage of foods, and it will inhibit the growth of all microorganisms below a critical moisture level. Drying offers the benefit that the food can be stored either at ambient temperature or, for longer storage, under refrigeration. Drying is commercially important for preserving many whole, uncooked materials, such as meats, fruits, and vegetables. Drying is also used for preserving many powdered foods, such as eggs, milk, and other assorted dairy products; flour and flour-based products, such as pasta and cereals; and sugar and sugar-containing products, such as flavored beverage mixes. Entire prepackaged dried meals are available to use in settings that necessitate lightweight transportation and extended storage. Drying, followed by maintaining adequate dryness, can protect the microbiological quality of food for decades; however, drying will not prevent the chemical oxidation of food, which, over the course of time, can render some foods unpalatable. Other means for controlling microbial growth through the reduction of water activity include increasing the level of highly soluble compounds such as salt and sugar. This approach may not be effective for as long as drying because some bacteria can grow in salt at low moisture levels and fungi can grow in highly sugared foods including corn syrups.

Temperature control is an old and a reliable technique that can be accomplished by maintaining foods under refrigeration to reduce the growth rate of microbial contaminants. Freezing, which inhibits all growth and severely reduces the rate of chemical oxidation, potentially can preserve food for centuries. Unfortunately, maintaining food in a frozen condition is costly, and freezing can produce undesirable changes in the texture of some foods. Storage of food at temperatures above freezing has contributed to the knowledge that temperature has a clear impact on microbial growth rates. This relationship has proved itself to be well suited to the use of mathematical modeling, with microbial growth a function of time and temperature. Storing foods at warm temperatures that allow the uncontrolled growth of microbial pathogens is termed *thermal abuse* and represents a major cause of illness. Time and salinity also constitute an important relationship in terms of microbial growth, as does the combination of temperature and pH.

Numerous types of supplements can be added to foods to inhibit the growth of undesired microorganisms. The list of chemical supplements includes solid compounds, such as salt and sugar, that reduce water activity, as discussed already; acidulants, such as acetic acid, citric acid, and lactic acid, which lower the pH; nitrite, which may have its effect through inhibiting heme-based microbial enzymes; and gases, such as carbon dioxide and nitrogen, which largely are inert and act by displacing oxygen.

Carbon dioxide, in addition to displacing oxygen from packaging, also can act as an acidulant when solubilized into aqueous liquids and, when solubilized under pressure, has a powerful inhibitory effect on microbial growth. Other gases used for their antimicrobial effects include ozone, sulfur dioxide (which may be added in the form of sulfites), epoxides, and chlorine. Table 37.2 lists examples of chemicals that are commonly used as food preservatives.

Beneficial (as opposed to harmful) microorganisms often may be allowed to remain in foods and sometimes are added intentionally. Those microorganisms deemed beneficial often are identified as such based on their metabolic activities, such as respiration and fermentation, performed within a food item. Metabolic processes for which the electron donor and acceptor exist on different molecules are referred to as *respiration* and, by definition, can occur either aerobically or anaerobically. In the case of aerobic microbial growth, the metabolism is respiration and the electron acceptor is usually oxygen. Production of lactic acid, a key flavor component in some dairy items, can occur during incomplete aerobic respiration and sometimes indicates that the amount of oxygen available is insufficient to support normal aerobic respiration. Other inorganic and organic molecules serve as electron

TABLE 37.2 Examples of chemicals commonly used as food preservatives[a]

Reducers of water activity	Salicylic acid
Salt	Sorbic acid
Sugar	Succinic acid
Enzymes	Tartaric acid
Lysozyme	Gases
Lactoperoxidase	Carbon dioxide
Acidulants	Chlorine
Acetic acid	Epoxides
Dehydroacetic acid	Nitrogen
Halogenacetic acids	Ozone
Adipic acid	Sulfur dioxide
Ascorbic acid	Others
Benzoic acid	Nisin
Boric acid	Ethanol
Citric acid	Hydrogen peroxide
Formic acid	Nitrates
Hydrochloric acid	Nitrites
Lactic acid	Phosphates
Phosphoric acid	Plant oils
Propionic acid	Smoke

[a]From Hurst.[30]

acceptors during the growth of microorganisms under anaerobic conditions. *Fermentation*, a common microbial process often used in food production, is, by definition, a metabolic process wherein both the electron donor and receptor exist on the same molecule. An example of anaerobic fermentation is the microbial food production process by which yeast generates ethanol. Subsequent bacterial aerobic respiration can convert that ethanol to acetic acid, turning wine to vinegar.

Many, indeed possibly most, bacteria and fungi produce and release antimicrobial compounds that are antagonistic to the growth of other microorganisms. This is a common occurrence in microbial ecology and represents evolutionarily developed mechanisms that favor the ability of organisms to compete for available nutrients. Some of these antimicrobial compounds have been developed commercially as antibiotics and antimicrobial peptides (eg, nisin).[31] Others include siderophores that act by binding iron, which is essential for organisms to grow, and bacteriocins, which produce cell death. One of the newer developments in food microbiology is research on the application of microbial competition as a means of preserving the healthful quality of foods, a process termed *biopreservation*.[31] The goal of biopreservation is to seed nonpathogenic strains of bacteria such as *Lactobacillus* into food and to allow the seeded organisms to grow, thereby inhibiting subsequent growth of pathogenic organisms such as *Listeria*.

▶ INTRODUCTION TO WATERBORNE INFECTIOUS DISEASES

Ingestion of contaminated water is perhaps the most notable route by which humans acquire waterborne disease and is the route emphasized in this chapter. Nevertheless, we must not lose sight of the fact that we also acquire infections from water through many other different routes. These other routes include both recreational and occupational activities performed in contaminated water, aerosolization of water in different situations, and the ingestion of foods or other materials that have been contaminated by microorganisms present in water. Table 37.3 lists examples of the numerous types of infectious disease that can be acquired by the various water-associated transmission routes. This section of the chapter is intended to help explain both the sources of and the important aspects about the ecology of these microorganisms.

Sources of Microbial Contaminants in Water

The existence of waterborne infectious disease outbreaks provides evidence that the source waters were contaminated. The microorganisms that cause these waterborne infections originate from numerous reservoirs, the list of which includes humans, domesticated animals, wild animals, and microbes that naturally inhabit the water.

Pathogenic Microorganisms That Are Natural Residents of Water

The environment itself can serve as a reservoir of many types of microorganisms that are pathogenic to humans.[32] These will include various types of bacteria, fungi, protozoa, algae, and associated viruses. The types and levels of these contaminants will also vary depending on the various natural and industrial chemical contaminants present in the water, as highlighted recently with large-scale algae blooms in the Great Lakes in the United States and other areas around the world with associated toxic syndromes.[33] Interestingly, both *L pneumophila* and *V cholerae* seem to exist as natural organisms in water, with *L pneumophila* often residing within free-living amoebae and *V cholerae* existing on the shells of crustaceans, where it presumably degrades the chitinous shells. The natural association of *V cholerae* with the shells of crustaceans may be one of the reasons why cholera can exist as an endemic focus even in areas that do not experience outbreaks of the disease in humans. The ability of various types of bacteria and viruses to survive and even thrive in protozoa, particularly *Acanthamoeba* species, has been an area of further investigations.[34] This may be important due to the ability of these microorganisms, including bacterial pathogens such as *Mycobacterium* species, *Legionella*, *Pseudomonas*, and *Vibrio*, to survive and even multiply both in the vegetative and dormant (cyst) forms of these protozoa, with the cyst forms providing an indirect survival method in the presence of chemical disinfectants.[34] These act in many ways like microbiological Trojan horses and as sources of microbial pathogens.

Animal Reservoirs of Microbial Contaminants

Other animals, besides humans, can contribute fecal microbial contaminants to water. Vertebrate animals can be an important source of microbial contaminants in surface water through two different paths. The first is fecal material and urine that animals deposit directly into the water. The second represents microorganisms in fecal material and urine that are deposited on the land and subsequently washed into surface waters by overland runoff. These problems with bacterial contaminants can come from warm-blooded animals, such as mammals and birds, as well as from cold-blooded animals, such as fish and lizards. The most notable waterborne bacterial diseases of humans that may originate from such animal reservoirs include campylosis, caused by *Campylobacter* and possibly contributed by beavers, migratory birds, muskrats, and other rodents, and leptospirosis caused by *Leptospirillum*

TABLE 37.3   Examples of diseases transmitted by environmental water routes

Exposure Route	Disease	Causative Microorganism(s)
Recreation or aquatic occupation	Bacterial	
	Enteritis	*Vibrio cholerae* (causes cholera)
	Nephritis	*Leptospira interrogans*
	Metazoan	
	Worm infestation	*Schistosoma*
	Protozoan	
	Encephalitis	*Naegleria*
	Enteritis	*Entamoeba histolytica* (causes amebic dysentery)
	Viral	
	Encephalitis	*Enterovirus*
	Gastroenteritis	*Astrovirus, Calicivirus, Coronavirus, Rotavirus*
	Meningitis	*Enterovirus*
	Pharyngoconjunctival fever	*Mastadenovirus*
Domestic use	Bacterial	
	Enteric fever	*Salmonella* (especially *Salmonella* ser Typhi, which causes typhoid fever)
	Enteritis	*Campylobacter, Shigella* (causes bacterial dysentery), *V cholerae* (causes cholera)
	Febrile syndrome	*Francisella tularensis*
	Protozoan	
	Enteritis	*Cryptosporidium parvum, E histolytica, Giardia lamblia*
	Viral	
	Encephalitis	*Enterovirus*
	Gastroenteritis	*Astrovirus, Calicivirus, Coronavirus, Rotavirus*
	Hepatitis	*Calicivirus, Hepatovirus*
	Meningitis	*Enterovirus*
Ice	Viral	
	Gastroenteritis	*Calicivirus*
Shellfish (crustacean)	Bacterial	
	Enteritis	*Vibrio*
Shellfish (bivalve molluskan)	Bacterial	
	Enteritis	*Vibrio*
	Viral	
	Gastroenteritis	*Calicivirus*
	Hepatitis	*Hepatovirus*
Crops (vegetables)	Bacterial	
	Enteric fever	*Salmonella*
	Enteritis	*Vibrio*
	Viral	
	Hepatitis	*Hepatovirus*
Aerosols	Bacterial	
	Pneumonic fever	*Legionella pneumophila*

contributed by livestock.[35] The fact that some protozoans can infect both humans and animals implies that wild animals living in a watershed area also can contribute this category of contaminating microorganisms to the water, thereby leading to human waterborne disease. The protozoa responsible for causing giardiasis (genus *Giardia*) and cryptosporidiosis (genus *Cryptosporidium*) in humans are also capable of cross infecting a variety of animals, including beavers and livestock, with a result that these animals may serve as reservoirs of the diseases and transmit them to humans by surface waters. Rotaviruses, which cause waterborne gastroenteritis, can also cross infect humans and a variety of animals, including cattle and poultry. This suggests that infected livestock and poultry could be reservoirs of waterborne viral gastroenteritis and that the causative microorganisms could enter the water either as fecal waste from feedlots or as waste from slaughterhouses.

Human Reservoirs of Microbial Contaminants

Humans constitute one of the most obvious sources of microbial contaminants in water. Humans carry microorganisms both on and within our bodies and leave a trail of these microorganisms behind us. The organisms that cause intestinal illnesses are of greatest concern caused by ingestion of water. These organisms are naturally present in feces and tend to be transmitted by the fecal-oral route, meaning that infection is acquired either through oral contact with or ingestion of contaminated materials. Humans can become infected by these organisms from sources other than water, such as food (as discussed earlier). The excretion of these organisms in human fecal wastes represents a reservoir in the cycle of waterborne disease transmission. These organisms exist as contaminants in domestic wastewater, a factor that holds true for all categories of microorganisms, including bacteria, protozoa, and viruses. Aside from the microorganisms that are shed in human fecal material, animals such as rats, which dwell in sewerage collection systems, will additionally contribute contaminants directly to the wastewater. Wastewater and the pathogens it can contain are often simply disposed of by direct discharge into surface waters, injection into groundwater, and application onto land surfaces. Microbial contaminants placed on the land surface are not assured of remaining on the land because surface-applied wastewater can percolate into the groundwater and runoff as surface water. Humans subsequently may encounter these pathogens either by contact with, or consumption of, contaminated surface waters and groundwaters. Discharge of wastewater into the environment then results in microbial contamination of environmental waters that may subsequently be used as sources of potable water. Drinking water from these sources thereby completes the cycle of infection, from humans to water and back to humans.

Recreational activities in sewage-polluted water is another way humans become ill from microorganisms in water; however, such illnesses are often acquired even from water that has no known sewage input, suggesting that it was humans themselves who contaminated the water during the course of recreational activities. Humans may contribute microbial contaminants directly to water through fecal shedding during the course of recreational activities in natural wading and swimming areas as well as in artificial swimming pools and spas. Because of surface water runoff, human recreational activities performed on beaches and in the watershed areas immediately surrounding a body of water may indirectly contribute fecal contamination to the water. Protozoan contaminants contributed in this way include the causative agents of cryptosporidiosis and giardiasis, as examples. Viral contaminants contributed to water during recreational activities include causative agents of gastroenteritis and pharyngoconjunctival fever.

Disease Transmission by Environmental Water Routes

Water serves as the vehicle for a large proportion of environmentally transmitted disease. The most obvious means by which infections are acquired from water is by ingestion of the water, which can result in both endemic as well as epidemic disease. Although outbreaks of epidemic disease draw the most notoriety, endemic disease is perhaps more insidious. Consumption of microbially contaminated water can lead to bacterial illnesses such as typhoid (caused by members of the genus *Salmonella*), cholera (caused by the species *V cholerae*), and tularemia (caused by the species *Francisella tularensis*); protozoan illnesses, among which are cryptosporidiosis (caused by members of the genus *Cryptosporidium*) and giardiasis (caused by members of the genus *Giardia*); and a variety of viral illnesses, including gastroenteritis and hepatitis (caused by members of the genera *Calicivirus*, *Hepatovirus*, and *Rotavirus*). Infection with the hepatitis E virus is particularly onerous because it has been associated with a high incidence of death in pregnant women.[36] Of the four diseases that can cause the greatest risk of suffering and death in underdeveloped parts of the world—cholera, hepatitis, malaria, and typhoid—malaria is the only one that is not transmitted by ingestion of water. A list of some of the microbial illnesses acquired by consumption of contaminated water, along with the names of the causative microorganisms, is presented in Table 37.3.

Public health emphasis often is placed on diseases associated with the ingestion of water because this route of transmission has resulted in large outbreaks. It is important to remember that ingesting water is not the only way in which we acquire diseases that are transmitted by contaminated water. Diseases can also be acquired from occupational or recreational activities performed in water as well as from the consumption of water-contaminated shellfish and food crops. Inhalation of aerosols represents yet another, and perhaps underrecognized, route of exposure to microbial contaminants contained in wastewater. Liquid (droplet) aerosols are generated during the processes of wastewater aeration and the spray application of wastewater sludge suspensions onto land. Aerosols generated during wastewater treatment may serve as a source of disease in wastewater workers; however, aerosols generated during community wastewater treatment processes probably do not serve as a major source of disease for members of the general population because many microorganisms were found to die readily in droplet aerosols.[37] This will vary depending on the microorganism and aerosolization method.[38]

The ability of microbial contaminants to survive after they enter water is a major issue in sources of waterborne infectious disease. Microbial contaminants that are released into water will often die if they are unable to replicate in that environment. The results of mathematical analyses have revealed that water temperature is a major factor affecting the survival of microorganisms in water, with survival increasing at lower temperatures. Other important factors, at least from the standpoint of viruses, are the amount of nutrients available in the water that could support the growth of bacterial organisms, generally exhibiting a detrimental effect on viral survival; water hardness, generally having a beneficial effect on viral survival, perhaps because it relates to enhancing the ability of the viruses to adsorb to particulates in the water; and the level of turbidity in the water, with higher turbidity likewise generally being beneficial to survival, presumably by providing those particulates.

Interconnected Flow of Water and Its Microbial Contaminants

Microbial contaminants are not necessarily stationary within the environment. Another major issue is the transport of microbial contaminants, which will occur naturally during water flow. As water flows, microorganisms may be conveyed over long distances, far from visible sources of contamination. Wastewater contaminants applied to the land surface may be carried into surface waters by runoff. Microorganisms contained in wastewater that is applied to the land surface for irrigation of crops or for groundwater recharge may be carried into groundwater by both vertical and horizontal infiltration. Once in the groundwater, natural flow can carry these microbial contaminants into surface waters and they can emerge onto the land surface via springs. Surface waters can dramatically return to the land surface during floods. Flooding also brings attendant concern about mosquito-transmitted illnesses (including malaria) because flooding increases water surface area, which in turn supports the life cycle of mosquitos.

Diseases Acquired From Microbially Contaminated Surface Water

Participation in either occupational or recreational surface water activities frequently is associated with the acquisition of infectious disease. The general symptoms experienced by ill swimmers and occupational aquatic workers include respiratory, gastrointestinal, eye, skin, and allergic ailments. Specific examples of diseases acquired by human activities in water include the bacterial disease leptospirosis and the viral diseases gastroenteritis and pharyngoconjunctival fever.

The domestic use of contaminated water clearly results in disease transmission. The goal of preventing these diseases is the reason for practicing drinking-water treatment at community levels; however, it is possible to find microbial contaminants associated with tap water even when the water lines feeding the taps apparently are free of the suspect organism. The formation of biofilms is an important consideration in many of these cases (see chapter 67). The most commonly suspected mode of transmission associated with domestic water use is through ingestion of the contaminated water. Bacterial diseases acquired in this way include campylosis, cholera, typhoid, and tularemia. Viral diseases acquired from drinking water include diarrhea, hepatitis, and poliomyelitis. Recently, the most notable protozoan disease acquired by the ingestion of water is cryptosporidiosis. Another interesting route by which diseases can be acquired from tap water is using contaminated water when washing wounds. There may also be some concern about microorganisms contained in droplet aerosols inhaled during showering.

Ingestion of shellfish harvested from waters that have been contaminated by discharged wastewater represents another means through which people acquire microbial illnesses, from polluted water. Crustaceans may accumulate pathogenic microorganisms from the environment and then potentially pass these organisms to humans who consume the crustaceans. Mollusks are divided into two categories. The first are *bivalves*, such as oysters and hard-shelled clams. The second group is *gastropods*, such as conch. Human pathogenic viruses, such as the hepatitis A virus (genus *Hepatovirus*) and the Norwalk virus (genus *Calicivirus*), can be detected in bivalve mollusks, and the ingestion of contaminated bivalves has caused outbreaks not only of viral disease but also of bacterial diseases such as cholera. It is presumed that the bivalve mollusks accumulate these microbial contaminants during their natural process of filter feeding. Gastropod mollusks do not filter feed and thus would not be expected to accumulate pathogens by this mechanism.

Diseases Acquired From Land That Has Been Microbially Contaminated by Water

Wastewater sometimes is used for the irrigation of vegetable crops. As mentioned earlier, this practice presents a health hazard because it may contaminate crops with potentially pathogenic microorganisms that have been shed in feces. Human consumption of crops that were irrigated with raw wastewater has been implicated in the spread of cholera. Particulate aerosols may be generated from wastewater sludges that have been applied onto land surfaces either for the purpose of composting that sludge or for final sludge disposal. These aerosols present a pathogenic hazard because they can contain both bacterial and fungal contaminants and they may be transported by the wind.

Diseases Acquired From Microbially Contaminated Groundwater

It is often thought that groundwater is intrinsically pristine and pure, but groundwater can be typically contaminated with various chemicals and microorganisms that are pathogenic for humans as a result of movement of microorganisms in association with the underground flow of water. The result can be the contamination of wells and springs by pathogens originating from the contents of septic tanks, privies, and leaking sewage lines. Domestic use of contaminated groundwater results in outbreaks of the bacterial illness such as cholera. Ingestion of contaminated groundwater also has resulted in outbreaks of the protozoan illnesses cryptosporidiosis and giardiasis and the viral illnesses gastroenteritis and hepatitis. A heavy reliance is often placed on the use of groundwater for crop

irrigation, and this reliance might result in the microbial contamination of crops.

Preventing Waterborne Disease Transmission

Waterborne microbial infections are an important cause of morbidity and mortality in human populations.[39] Outbreaks of human disease associated with the consumption of untreated drinking water probably have occurred for as long as humans have existed. There are several means by which waterborne disease transmission can be prevented. Among these are two categories of infection-control practices. The first category represents establishment of physical barriers to prevent contamination of the water used for recreation or as the source of drinking water. The second category consists of water disinfection treatments, as listed in Table 37.4.

Disinfection of drinking water, defined as the removal or destruction of pathogenic microorganisms, is a practice that can be performed either at the municipal level with formal treatment facilities or at individual and household levels. Disinfection of drinking water on an individual or household basis can be accomplished by boiling water; distilling water; or adding chemicals such as chlorine, ozone, chlorine dioxide, bromine, and iodine to water. Disinfection is also performed on wastewaters to protect the quality of receiving waters. The historically high death

TABLE 37.4 Examples of treatments used for disinfection of water

Category of Water Being Treated	Nature of Process	Process or Compound
Drinking water	Physical removal	Coagulation-flocculation, filtration, sedimentation
	Denaturation	Heat
	Chemical oxidation	Bromine, chlorine and chlorine compounds (chloramines), chlorine dioxide, iodine, ozone
	Metabolic inhibition	Heavy metal ions
	Atomic bond (including DNA) disruption	Electromagnetic radiation (ultraviolet, gamma)
Recreational water	Physical removal	Filtration
	Chemical oxidation	Bromine, chlorine and chlorine compounds (chloramines), chlorine dioxide, iodine, ozone
	Metabolic inhibition	Heavy metal ions
Wastewater	Physical removal	Coagulation-flocculation, filtration, sedimentation
	Denaturation	Heat
	Chemical oxidation	Bromine, chlorine and chlorine compounds (chloramines), ozone
	Atomic bond disruption	Electromagnetic radiation (ultraviolet, gamma)
	Particle bombardment	Electron beam
	Biological	Digestion, retention ponds (lagoons), artificial wetlands

rates associated with cholera, and both epidemic as well as endemic typhoid, helped drive the development of municipal and private drinking water treatment utilities that provide a measure of protection for the communities they serve. Unfortunately, the use of community drinking water treatment facilities does not guarantee against waterborne disease outbreaks. There are three major reasons for this situation. First, the types of treatment used can vary from one region to another. Second, the many available treatment processes differ regarding their capacity for physically removing or disinfecting various categories of microorganisms, a fact that led to the development of treatment facilities that use a series of stepwise treatment processes. And third, even when multistep treatment processes are used, their operation is not always optimal or reliable.

Inadequate treatment, or outright failures in municipal drinking water treatment operations, can lead to microbial contaminants entering the drinking water distribution system. Bacterial diseases spread by this route include, of course, the notorious agents associated with typhoid and cholera. Outbreaks of cholera often take the form of massive, wide-ranging epidemics, termed *pandemics*, which have caused fear in human populations since at least 1817 when they became more defined. A recent American pandemic alone, which occurred during 1991 and 1992, resulted in an estimated 350,000 cases of illness and nearly 4,000 deaths. Larger scale outbreaks continue to be periodically reported and particularly in areas such as Asia and Africa.[40] The disease cholera and its causal organism *V cholerae* continues to be a concern.[41] Examples of disease outbreaks that presumably resulted from inadequate municipal treatment of drinking water even in modern facilities include those of enteritis caused by the protozoans *Cryptosporidium* and *Giardia*.[20,42] Viruses also can enter the water-distribution system in this way and result in human illnesses, among which are gastroenteritis, which has been associated with rotaviruses and Norwalk virus. These can often lead to larger outbreak reports.[43] Microbial contamination can occur following treatment due to cross-connections with wastewater plumbing or seepage into piping and storage tanks. Such posttreatment contamination can lead to disease outbreaks. Contamination can even occur from water taps fed by apparently uncontaminated water supplies, possibly representing microbial colonization of the taps. It has been estimated that ingesting microbial contaminants in tap water, from a distribution system served by fully operational conventional treatment plants, may have caused 35% of the gastrointestinal illnesses reported among drinkers of tap water.[44,45] The sources used for providing drinking water and the techniques used for making that potable have recently been reviewed in detail.[45]

Not all community-distribution water supplies are treated. Often, this represents either a matter of cost or an avoidance of disinfected water because of taste preference. At other times, it may result from an assumption that water from streams, wells, or springs is intrinsically pure and can be consumed without treatment. Even when treated drinking water is available through community distribution systems, people still may prefer to drink water obtained from untreated sources such as springs or wells, thinking that these represent water that somehow is more pure and healthful than the treated water. This assumption often is not valid because water from such sources can be contaminated with pathogenic microorganisms, and their consumption results in outbreaks of waterborne disease. The popular alternative of consuming bottled or otherwise packaged water may not be much better from a health standpoint because commercial bottled water can also contain pathogens.

Although the two bacterial illnesses, cholera and typhoid, were the driving force behind the development of formal drinking water treatment utilities during the middle and end of the 19th century, we are still faced with the fact that these microorganisms consumed in conventionally treated drinking water still may account for 35% of the gastrointestinal illnesses among consumers, even in some developed countries. It is because of these disease risks that many governments have developed ongoing surveillance programs for waterborne disease.[39]

REFERENCES

1. Matthews KR, Montville TJ, Kniel KE. *Food Microbiology: An Introduction*. 4th ed. Washington, DC: ASM Press; 2017.
2. Bitton G. *Microbiology of Drinking Water: Production and Distribution*. Hoboken, NJ: John Wiley & Sons; 2014.
3. World Health Organization. *Global Health Estimates 2016 Summa Tables: Deaths by Cause, Age, Sex, by Country and by Region, 2000-2016*. Geneva, Switzerland: World Health Organization; 2018.
4. Birkhead GS, Morse DL, Levine WC, et al. Typhoid fever at a resort hotel in New York: a large outbreak with an unusual vehicle. *J Infect Dis*. 1993;167(5):1228-1232.
5. Mintz ED, Hudson-Wragg M, Mshar P, Cartter ML, Hadler JL. Foodborne giardiasis in a corporate office setting. *J Infect Dis*. 1993;167(1):250-253.
6. Petersen LR, Cartter ML, Hadler JL. A food-borne outbreak of *Giardia lamblia*. *J Infect Dis*. 1988;157(4):846-848.
7. Farley TA, Wilson SA, Mahoney F, Kelso KY, Johnson DR, Kaplan EL. Direct inoculation of food as the cause of an outbreak of group A streptococcal pharyngitis. *J Infect Dis*. 1993;167(5):1232-1235.
8. Herwaldt BL, Lew JF, Moe CL, et al. Characterization of a variant strain of Norwalk virus from a food-borne outbreak of gastroenteritis on a cruise ship in Hawaii. *J Clin Microbiol*. 1994;32(4):861-866.
9. Zannella C, Mosca F, Mariani F, et al. Microbial diseases of bivalve mollusks: infections, immunology and antimicrobial defense. *Mar Drugs*. 2017;15(16):E182.
10. Rangel JM, Sparling PH, Crowe C, Griffin PM, Swerdlow DL. Epidemiology of *Escherichia coli* O157:H7 outbreaks, United States, 1982-2002. *Emerg Infect Dis*. 2005;11(4):603-609.
11. Centers for Disease Control and Prevention. Norovirus. Centers for Disease Control and Prevention Web site. https://www.cdc.gov/norovirus. Updated June 2018. Accessed April 15, 2019.
12. Martinović T, Andjelković U, Gajdošik MŠ, Rešetar D, Josić D. Foodborne pathogens and their toxins. *J Proteomics*. 2016;147:226-235.

13. Ramaswamy V, Cresence VM, Rejitha JS, et al. *Listeria*—review of epidemiology and pathogenesis. *J Microbiol Immunol Infect.* 2007;40(1):4-13.

14. Torres AG. Current aspects of *Shigella* pathogenesis. *Rev Latinoam Microbiol.* 2004;46(3-4):89-97.

15. Cramer MM. *Food Plant Sanitation: Design, Maintenance, and Good Manufacturing Practices.* 2nd ed. Boca Raton, FL: CRC Press; 2016.

16. Todd EC, Greig JD, Bartleson CA, Michaels BS. Outbreaks where food workers have been implicated in the spread of foodborne disease. Part 5. Sources of contamination and pathogen excretion from infected persons. *J Food Prot.* 2008;71(12):2582-2595.

17. Rumble C, Addiman S, Balasegaram S, et al. Role of food handlers in norovirus outbreaks in London and South East England, 2013 to 2015. *J Food Prot.* 2017;80(2):257-264.

18. Grabowski DJ, Tiggs KJ, Senke HW, et al. Common-source outbreak of giardiasis—New Mexico. *MMWR Morb Mortal Wkly Rep.* 1989;38(23):405-407.

19. Figgatt M, Mergen K, Kimelstein D, et al. Giardiasis outbreak associated with asymptomatic food handlers in New York state, 2015. *J Food Prot.* 2017;12:837-841.

20. Adam EA, Yoder JS, Gould LH, Hlavsa MC, Gargano JW. Giardiasis outbreaks in the United States, 1971-2011. *Epidemiol Infect.* 2016;144(13):2790-2801.

21. Gallimore C, Pipkin C, Shrimpton H, et al. Detection of multiple enteric virus strains within a foodborne outbreak of gastroenteritis: an indication of the source of contamination. *Epidemiol Infect.* 2005;133(1):41-47.

22. Hennekinne JA, De Buyser ML, Dragacci S. *Staphylococcus aureus* and its food poisoning toxins: characterization and outbreak investigation. *FEMS Microbiol Rev.* 2012;36(4):815-836.

23. Schoeni JL, Wong AC. *Bacillus cereus* food poisoning and its toxins. *J Food Prot.* 2005;68(3):636-648.

24. Kowalska A, Walkiewicz K, Kozieł P, Muc-Wierzgoń M. Aflatoxins: characteristics and impact on human health. *Postepy Hig Med Dosw (Online).* 2017;71:315-327.

25. Centers for Disease Control and Prevention. Foodborne illnesses and germs. Centers for Disease Control and Prevention Web site. https://www.cdc.gov/foodsafety/foodborne-germs.html. Accessed April 4, 2019.

26. Whiley H, Ross K. *Salmonella* and eggs: from production to plate. *Int J Environ Res Public Health.* 2015;12(3):2543-2556.

27. Lawrie RA, Ledward DA. *Lawrie's Meat Science.* 7th ed. Cambridge, United Kingdom: CRC Press; 2006.

28. Huang M, Zhang M, Bhandari B. Recent development in the application of alternative sterilization technologies to prepared dishes: a review. *Crit Rev Food Sci Nutr.* 2019;59(7):1188-1196.

29. Sohaib M, Anjum FM, Arshad MS, Rahman UU. Postharvest intervention technologies for safety enhancement of meat and meat based products; a critical review. *J Food Sci Technol.* 2016;53(1):19-30.

30. Hurst CJ. Preventing foodborne infectious disease. In: Hurst CJ, ed. *Modeling Disease Transmission and Its Prevention by Disinfection.* Cambridge, United Kingdom: Cambridge University Press; 1996:193-212.

31. Singh VP. Recent approaches in food bio-preservation—a review. *Open Vet J.* 2018;8(1):104-111.

32. Cabral JP. Water microbiology. Bacterial pathogens and water. *Int J Environ Res Public Health.* 2010;7(10):3657-3703.

33. Berdalet E, Fleming LE, Gowen R, et al. Marine harmful algal blooms, human health and wellbeing: challenges and opportunities in the 21st century. *J Mar Biol Assoc U.K.* 2015;2015:1-62. doi:10.1017/S0025315415001733.

34. Thomas V, McDonnell G, Denyer SP, Maillard JY. Free-living amoebae and their intracellular pathogenic microorganisms: risks for water quality. *FEMS Microbiol Rev.* 2010;34(3):231-259.

35. Hurst CJ. *The Connections Between Ecology and Infectious Disease.* Cham, Switzerland: Springer; 2018.

36. Hakim MS, Wang W, Bramer WM, et al. The global burden of hepatitis E outbreaks: a systematic review. *Liver Int.* 2017;37(1):19-31.

37. Hurst CJ, Murphy PA. The transmission and prevention of infectious disease. In: Hurst CJ, ed. *Modeling Disease Transmission and Its Prevention by Disinfection.* Cambridge, United Kingdom: Cambridge University Press; 1996:3-54.

38. Haddrell AE, Thomas RJ. Aerobiology: experimental considerations, observations, and future tools. *Appl Environ Microbiol.* 2017;83(17):e00809-17.

39. World Health Organization. *Guidelines for Drinking-Water Quality.* 4th ed. Geneva, Switzerland: World Health Organization; 2017.

40. Davies HG, Bowman C, Luby SP. Cholera—management and prevention. *J Infect.* 2017;74(suppl 1):S66-S73.

41. Hurst CJ. Briefly summarizing our understanding of *Vibrio cholerae* and the disease cholera. In: Hurst CJ, ed. *The Structure and Function of Aquatic Microbial Communities: Advances in Environmental Microbiology.* Vol 7. Cham, Switzerland: Springer; 2019:173-184.

42. Chalmers RM, Robinson G, Elwin K, Elson R. Analysis of the *Cryptosporidium* spp. and gp60 subtypes linked to human outbreaks of cryptosporidiosis in England and Wales, 2009 to 2017. *Parasit Vectors.* 2019;12(1):95.

43. Zhang L, Li X, Wu R, et al. A gastroenteritis outbreak associated with drinking water in a college in northwest China. *J Water Health.* 2018;16(4):508-515.

44. Hurst CJ. Understanding and estimating the risk of waterborne infectious disease associated with drinking water. In: Hurst CJ, ed. *The Connections Between Ecology and Infectious Disease: Advances in Environmental Microbiology.* Vol 5. Cham, Switzerland: Springer; 2018:59-114.

45. Hurst CJ. Options for providing microbiologically safe drinking water. In: Hurst CJ, ed. *The Structure and Function of Aquatic Microbial Communities: Advances in Environmental Microbiology.* Vol 7. Cham, Switzerland: Springer; 2019:185-260.

Preservation of Industrial Products and Processes

Tony A. Rook

Many waterborne industrial products, and the processes used to manufacture these products, can be susceptible to microbial contamination if adequate microbial control strategies are not employed. These products and processes have become increasingly more susceptible to microbial spoilage mainly due to the increasing use of environmentally favorable raw materials.[1-3] The development of more sustainable formulations has also seen the replacement of volatile organic compounds with water as raw materials and the incorporation of natural and/or bio-based raw materials.[4-6] The consequences of microbial spoilage can lead to irreparable damage to industrial products because of changes of viscosity, generation of offensive odors (malodors), gas formation resulting in potential container deformation due to excessive pressure buildup, product changes such as discoloration, or gelling of product and enzyme production resulting in instability of product formulation.[7] In addition, the service life of many industrial products may be shortened due to the activities of microbial defacement, such as visible growth of on the surface of materials leading to loss in aesthetic qualities of the product and loss of mechanical integrity due to biodeterioration of the material that may lead to blistering, delamination, or otherwise disfigurement of the products.[8] Within industrial products and processes, there are four main focus areas to consider when employing preservation strategies: manufacturing hygiene, wet-state preservation, finished article dry preservation, and functional fluid preservation.

▶ MANUFACTURING HYGIENE OF INDUSTRIAL PROCESSES

Effective manufacturing hygiene programs for industrial processes require an understanding of the necessity of microbial control practices to be integral to the process.[9-12] Manufacturing environments for waterborne industrial products are complex engineered built environments that can offer many opportunities for microbial contamination to persist if not otherwise mitigated through a systematic approach to microbial control. A successful industrial manufacturing hygiene program consists of the following major components:

- Risk assessment of the manufacturing process, facility, and equipment from a microbial control perspective
- Continuous monitoring of the process with microbiological and analytical methods
- Management and handling of raw materials to prevent microbial contamination
- Effective cleaning and disinfection (or sanitization) of the manufacturing process
- Microbiological testing of finished products
- Establishment of effective preservation of finished products
- Documentation of program, processes, and metrics

Manufacturing Process Equipment Design

The design of the manufacturing process and equipment employed to produce industrial products is an important consideration.[13-15] The equipment chosen for the manufacture of water-based industrial products such as paints, inks, polymers, paper, leather, textiles, and functional fluids should consider a design that is easy to clean and accessible for routine inspections. The built environment of an industrial product manufacturing facility may consist of raw material storage tanks, pumps, filtration units, production tanks, flexible hoses, transfer manifolds, heat exchangers, transfer piping, pigging systems, and filling lines. Integral to these production processes are water delivery systems for production and/or cleaning of the plant environment.

Raw material holding tanks ideally should be accessible for routine monitoring and scheduled (or unscheduled) cleaning. One important consideration for a good sanitary tank design is a domed interior ceiling that reduces the likelihood of product buildup. The venting of the tanks should be accomplished by incorporating a 180-degree pipe facing downward to discourage the ingress of exterior contamination. Additionally, a filtration unit can be applied to the venting pipe to further reduce the chances of contamination to be introduced.[16] Filtration units can either consist of a high efficiency particulate air (HEPA) filter or be designed as a wet air filtration unit, which consists of a small holding vessel containing liquid to entrap airborne particles. If water is used as the liquid for particle entrapment, then it should be treated with a biocide and routinely changed to prevent this filter from becoming the source of contamination.

Production equipment design should be chosen to minimize buildup of product or water within the process.

Pumps, pipes, and filter units should allow for easy draining. Whenever possible, the production process lines should be sloped to allow for easy draining.[17,18] The pumps and filter units chosen should be designed to minimize any stagnant fluid within the process when not in use. Many production processes incorporate the use of filter bag units. These units should be designed to be bottom exiting to allow for the filter housing to drain completely of fluid between production campaigns.

During the engineering design of a new manufacturing facility or during the review of an existing facility, the ability to effectively clean the process should be considered.[19] Consideration should be given to minimize the overall complexity of the process to aide in the ability to clean, disinfect, and fully drain the production process in place. Table 38.1 provides a summary of best practices for facility design of industrial manufacturing processes.[20]

TABLE 38.1 Important considerations for facility design of industrial manufacturing processes

Area of Manufacturing Process	Best Practices to Support Good Plant Hygiene
Floors	Use an easily cleanable material (eg, cementitious epoxy) with minimal point drains; avoid the use of extensive trench drains and materials, which degrade easily or are difficult to clean.
Ceilings	Install a drop ceiling with easily cleanable coatings (eg, PVC coating) and schedule maintenance for cleaning; avoid overhead utilities that create areas to trap dirt (eg, HVAC ducts, water lines).
Valves	Use sanitary valves that are easily cleanable (eg, butterfly valves); avoid valve designs, which are difficult to clean-in-place (eg, ball valves).
Pumps	Use sanitary pumps that are cleanable/drainable in place (eg, rotary lobe PD pumps); if possible, avoid the use of pumps, which are difficult to clean/drain (eg, diaphragm pumps) or incorporate routine maintenance to clean/drain and sanitized pumps.
Piping	Minimize connections, use orbital welds or sanitary tri-clamp connections, and maintain a slope to facilitate effective draining of piping lines; avoid the use of rough welds or threaded connections (when possible) and avoid improperly sloped sections, which don't drain properly.
Hoses	Ensure hoses are smooth bore with sanitary (eg, tri-clamp) fittings and store in a manner to facilitate drainage (eg, vertically or upside down "u"); avoid the use of internally reinforced hoses with threaded connections and avoid leaving hoses with liquid material trapped inside.
In-process filters	Use bottom-exiting filters to promote drainage and self-cleaning filters if possible; avoid any filters that retain fluid (eg, side-exiting filters) or filters that cannot be easily removed for cleaning and maintenance.
Tanks	Use tanks with domed lids (keep closed) and bottoms sloped to drain; avoid the use of tanks with flat top/bottoms (if possible) or incorporate routine inspection, cleaning, and maintenance of tank interiors and limit any unnecessary ports or penetrations into the tanks.
Sample ports	Use ports that can be cleaned/drained/disinfected and appropriately located; avoid maintaining any unused or unnecessary sample ports.
Materials of construction	Employ easily cleanable materials with smooth surface finish (eg, 316 L SS, Ra <0.8 μm); avoid using materials, which are difficult to clean (eg, most plastics and rough metals).
Personnel	Ensure proper gowning and personal protective equipment, all individuals should have up-to-date training including awareness and importance of microbial control.

Abbreviations: HVAC, heating ventilation and air conditioning; PD, positive displacement; PVC, polyvinyl chloride.

Continuous Monitoring of Production Process and Products

A central component to an effective microbial control program is the implementation of a continuous monitoring program of the manufacturing environment and the products manufactured by the process. A continuous monitoring program should consist of evaluation of the microbial condition of process equipment and manufacturing environment, raw materials, and finished products.[21] Within the manufacturing process, locations that may provide an early indication of the microbial condition of the process should be selected to be evaluated in a routine basis for the presence of microbial contamination.[22-25] These locations may be considered critical control points because determining the microbial conditions of these locations can provide an estimated understanding of the overall control of microbial contamination within the entire production process. Critical control points should be selected throughout the process and be relatively easy to access to ensure continuous monitoring of the process will take place. Some common locations within industrial product manufacturing systems include bulk tank lids and side walls, flexible transfer hoses, pump inlet/outlet, filtration unit housings, intermediate and process tank sidewalls, fill bowls, and fill heads (Figure 38.1). In addition to directly sampling process equipment, the routine sampling of representative raw materials should determine the microbial status of these materials.[26] Special attention should be focused on waterborne raw materials that are transported and stored within bulk storage tanks as well as raw materials known to potentially contain high numbers of microorganisms, such as specific dry raw materials.

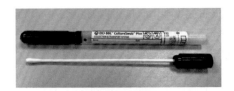
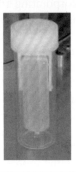

FIGURE 38.2   An example of a common microbiological sampling/transport swab and a test dip slide. For a color version of this art, please consult the eBook.

Assessment of microbial contamination within critical control points are commonly carried out through surface sampling using a sterile transport swab[26] (Figure 38.2). Ideally, the swab should contain a media, such as Aimes Gel, to minimize microbial cell death during transport. If the system is known to contain residual equipment disinfectants during the sampling process, the transport media should also contain a component known to neutralize commonly used agents. The swabs are transported to a laboratory to be evaluated by streaking onto a solid microbiological media known to support the growth of microorganisms commonly known to cause spoilage

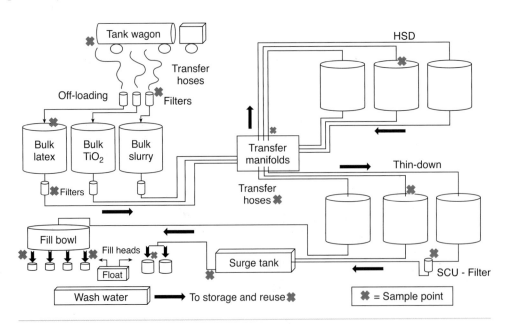

FIGURE 38.1   General layout of an industrial manufacturing facility for paint production, showing examples of critical control points. HSD, high speed dispersion; SCU, self cleaning filter; TiO₂, titanium dioxide.

within the process or products. Alternatively, facilities may choose to employ the use of dip slides.[27] These sampling devices consist of a plastic paddle attached to the inside of a screw top (see Figure 38.2). Typically, the paddles contain a bacterial growth media on one side and a fungal growth media on the other side. The manufacturing operator should be trained to open the twist-off lid without touching the inside of neither the container nor the media and dip the paddle into a raw material, process fluid or finished product. The paddle is then placed back into the sterile container and typically incubated at room temperature. After a specified incubation time, microbial growth can be more easily detected using chromogenic media to induce a color change upon growth. Processes for measuring the presence of microbial contamination consist of traditional microbiological growth media and/or several rapid microbiological methods.[28,29]

▶ PROCESS WATER CONTROLS

Process water within industrial manufacturing processes of waterborne products can be a primary source of bacterial contamination within the process, within the raw material storage, and ultimately within the final products manufactured. Therefore, the manufacturing facilities should ensure measures have been taken to periodically monitor process water for bacterial contamination, consider adding treatments to reduce the incoming microbiological load of the water, and employ sanitary designs of the engineered water systems to increase the likelihood for effective disinfection of these systems.[30-32]

It is critical for any waterborne industrial process to implement a program to sample and monitor the bacterial contamination of the incoming process water. Employment of aseptic sampling techniques for collection of the water is critical to ensure that the data generated is truly representative of current condition of the process water.[33] Sample points within the process should be selected where water samples can be taken that are truly representative of the process water. Some locations to be considered are water lines at point of entry into the manufacturing facility; water lines at the receiving area for raw materials being stored in bulk storage tanks; water lines entering the process, such as an in-process mixing tanks; and water lines at the filling lines. Consideration should be given to how the water is being used within the process and emphasis on water directly impacting the manufacturing for process or being used in the manufacturing of the final products. For instance, special attention should be focused on water that is being directly added to any process tank as a product raw material. Any water being used to clean or rinse the process equipment should also ensure low microbiological content because this water may ultimately be the source of bacterial biofilms within the process that ultimately may lead to quality issues within the final product.[34]

Engineering of a process water system should consider sanitary design both within the material of construction and the overall functioning of the water systems. If possible, water systems should be designed to be compatible with disinfection treatments that may be employed to control the microbiological load within the incoming water. Areas within the water process with little to no flow should be avoided. If these areas are unavoidable due to the design and function of the process, consideration should be taken to consider adding a flowing circulation within the process. An additional area of consideration within an engineered process water system are any flexible hoses that are attached to the water process lines for process equipment rinsing and our addition to production batches. It has been well documented that flexible hoses can be a location for microbiological contamination.[9,15,20,21,33] Consideration should be given to implement a program for removal of the flexible hoses for routine disinfection followed by hanging of the hoses for draining and drying between uses. Allowing the hoses to remain attached to the process and filled with water can create a stagnant zone that increases the opportunity for microbial growth to occur.

Some key factors should be considered when selecting a microbicidal treatment for any water system within an industrial manufacturing process. A critical and often overlooked criteria for determining a treatment process for process water lines is the type of microorganisms that are known to be present within the incoming water itself or known to be resident within the water process equipment of the system. This information can provide critical information regarding the potential presence of aggressive biofilm formers that may require rigorous water treatment for full control.[35,36] This information will also allow the measurement of effectiveness to control these specific microorganisms during the validation of the water treatment system. Another important factor to consider when selecting a disinfection process is the nonmicrobiological (or chemical) quality of incoming water including the residual levels of disinfectant from municipal treatment (if applicable), water hardness, pH, and turbidity of the water. These factors may influence the choice and efficacy of the water treatment process selected.

Treatments of process water can be divided into two major categories: chemical or physical treatments. The chemical treatments of process water can further be divided into two major categories: oxidizing or nonoxidizing chemistries. Physical treatment programs may consist of applying heat to intermediate water storage tanks, where periodic heat treatment of temperature at 180°F (82°C) or higher can be applied through a recirculation loop. Alternatively, water may be treated using physical filtration to remove both gross contamination as well as microbiological contamination with the incoming water. The most commonly used filtration methods include reverse osmosis, membrane filtration, and ultraviolet (UV) filtration.

Reverse osmosis filtration systems should include scheduled maintenance to periodically disinfect the filters. Membrane filter systems should be maintained and evaluated to ensure the membranes remain integral and undamaged during the use life. Filter membranes with larger pores sizes of 5 to 10 μm are commonly installed to remove gross contamination to be filtered out upstream of the terminal (eg, 0.45 μm) filters membranes intended to remove microbial contamination. This design protects and extends the effective life of the downstream filters. The UV disinfection can be applied to treat industrial process water (see chapter 9); however, there are several factors that should be considered for successful implementation. The factors that impact the effectiveness of a UV disinfection system are water turbidity, light intensity, and resident time within the treatment unit. These factors should be measured over the life of the system to ensure the system is effective for microbicidal activity. Additional consideration should be given to the placement of the UV system within the manufacturing process. Installing a single UV filtration unit at a single point where the process water first enters the production plant may not always be the best choice, especially when installing systems within existing manufacturing process with a known history of microbial contamination of process water. In this instance, the UV system may help knock down any incoming microbiological load but will not do anything for the microorganisms that are already resident within the water distribution systems of the plant. Another consideration is to install UV treatment units at the point of water addition to the process, for example, directly prior to point of addition at the processing tanks. This may become cost restrictive for larger manufacturing processes but may be a good choice for smaller processes.

Process water can be treated with oxidizing microbicides such as halogenated chemicals (including chlorine or bromine) or nonhalogenated oxidizing chemicals such as ozone (see chapters 15, 17, 18, and 33). Addition of chlorinated disinfectants to process water creates a mixture of hypochlorous acid and hypochlorite ions with the disinfecting properties being contributed by the hypochlorous acid (see chapter 15). Because stability of hypochlorous acid is pH dependent, chlorinated microbicides such as sodium hypochlorite are most effective when the process water pH is between 6.0 and 7.5 and will quickly lose any meaningful efficacy at pH levels above 8.0. Any residual organic matter present within the process water will react with chlorinated biocide treatments; therefore, higher chlorine concentrations will be required within process that contain higher organic content.

Chlorine dioxide (ClO_2) can effectively be used as a chemical water treatment at much lower concentrations than other chlorinated microbicides (see chapter 27). Systems commonly used within industrial processes generate on-site ClO_2 gas, which can be directly added to a process water stream. This can be accomplished by either mixing a strong chlorine solution with sodium chlorite or by mixing hydrochloric acid with a mixture of hypochlorite and sodium chlorite solutions. Safety precautions should be considered during installation because ClO_2 gas can be explosive. The benefits of ClO_2 treatment is that the active ingredient remains more effective at higher pH ranges than traditional chlorinated biocide choices and is not as highly reactive to residual organic content within process water.

Process water can also be treated with brominated microbicides and are becoming more popular within processes with higher pH because active ingredient of hypobromous acid maintains its biocidal properties across a broader pH range than chlorinated treatments (see chapter 15). Typically, a mixture of hypobromous acid and hydrochloric acid with sodium chloride are prepared through the hydrolysis of either an activated bromide salt or bromine chloride.[37] An additional advantage of using brominated treatment process is that any bromamines generated during the treatment are generally considered to be more environmentally favorable than the chloramines generated during chlorinated treatments.

Ozone is a strong oxidizing agent that can effectively be employed to control incoming microbial contamination of industrial process water (see chapter 33). Systems using ozone as the active biocidal ingredient to treat process water require commitment to install capital equipment to generate ozone on-site. Important factors to consider when implementing an ozone treatment process are pH, temperature, and organic content within the process water because each of these factors impacts on stability of the ozone within the treatment system. One main benefit of using an ozonation system is lower potential of corrosivity than traditional chlorinated treatment systems.

▶ PRESERVATION OF RAW MATERIALS

It is critical to ensure raw materials being received, stored, and used to manufacture waterborne industrial products, such as paints, coatings, and inks, are controlled for unacceptable levels of microbial content that may lead to spoilage events within the process and within the final products. A program should be established to sample and evaluate incoming raw materials as well as raw materials maintained under bulk storage conditions on a continuous frequency to ensure the materials are within good microbiological quality. Raw materials used to manufacture industrial products are not required to be sterile; however, effective wet-state preservation strategies often provide effective control of microorganisms that may lead to product spoilage.[7,38,39] The current industry guidance suggests the upper limit for a microbial content specification should be no more than 1000 colony-forming units (CFUs)/mL within aqueous solutions and suspensions, and no more than 1000 CFUs/g for anhydrous raw materials.[40]

The manufacturing process design can contribute to contamination of waterborne raw materials that are stored in bulk vessels. The production process lines used to off-load bulk raw materials from tanker wagons or railcars should not contain any dead-legs where stagnant raw material may remain as a source of contamination within the delivery lines. The flexible hoses used for off-loading of raw materials are commonly a source of microbial contamination (as discussed earlier), which can contribute to contamination of an entire bulk tank. Systems should be considered that allow for the flexible hoses to be cleaned and disinfected on a regulatory basis and are stored in a manner to facilitate draining and drying of the hoses between uses. The bulk storage tanks themselves can contribute to contamination of the raw material being stored within the tanks. A critical area of a bulk tank that should be monitored is the interior ceiling. The condensation cycle within the tank may deposit raw material and degrade any preservative within the material leading to a potential source of contamination, which may be deposited back into the raw material within the tank upon subsequent condensation cycling.[41] Because the majority of preservatives used within industrial products today do not have a high enough vapor pressure to provide any significant protection of the headspace of a bulk raw material tank, this portion of the process has become an area where alternate strategies are required to provide microbial control. Other important areas to consider within the headspace of the bulk tank where raw material build up can occur is on the side walls of a bulk tank and the shaft of the mixing blades within the tanks. A program should be considered to periodically empty the bulk tanks of the raw material content, physically remove any buildup within the tank through a combination of physical and/or chemical cleaning methods, and then disinfection of the interior surfaces of the bulk tank.

It is critical to ensure aqueous-based raw materials include an effective preservative, which can control the growth of microorganisms known to cause spoilage issues within the raw material or the subsequent finished product.[41,42] Any contamination of raw materials above specified levels can increase the likelihood of quality defects, such as off-odor, discoloration, or viscosity drift within the raw material, and may lead to issues within the performance of the finished product.[43] It is important to consider the handling of raw materials that are susceptible to microbial contamination throughout the supply chain. Many raw materials such as polymer or latex dispersions, emulsions, and pigment slurries may have increased susceptibility due to the extent of handling and time frame within storage prior to being used in the manufacture of a finished product.[7,41,44-46] Raw materials are often manufactured and placed in bulk storage at the raw material manufacturing site until being transferred to a transport vessel. This storage period may significantly vary depending on the current market for the specific raw material.

During transfer to a transport vessel, such as a tote, tank wagon, or railcar, the raw material is pumped through a filling line process being exposed to potential microbial insults within the equipment. The transport vessels may then be transferred to a depot or delivered directly to the manufacturer of finished products. Raw materials that are placed within a depot may further be exposed to environmental pressures such as elevated temperatures, which may reduce the level of preservation within the material. Once the materials are received at the finished product manufacturing sites, the materials are off-loaded by pumping out of the transport vessels through flexible hoses, delivery lines, and/or filtration equipment before being placed into bulk storage. During the off-loading process and storage within bulk containers, the raw materials are once again exposed to potential microbial insults from microorganisms that may persist within the product equipment. Exposure to such microorganisms within a dedicated production process can be especially challenging because they have become accustomed to growth on the very same ingredients that are being delivered and may have acquired an increased level of tolerance to the preservatives within the formulations.

The continuous monitoring of the bulk raw materials for microbial contamination will allow for a plan to quickly remediate high levels through the addition of a biocidal process to reduce the contamination population within the material. One of the most commonly employed biocides for remediation of contaminated waterborne raw materials of industrial products is 2,2-dibromo-3-nitrilopropionamide (DBNPA) due to its very fast-acting activity (Figure 38.3). The DBNPA can break down into inactive decomposition components through either interaction with nucleophilic substances, UV radiation via light, or through a pH-dependent hydrolysis mechanism (Figure 38.4).[47] The hydrolyzed degradation of DBNPA proceeds through decarboxylation to dibromoacetonitrile, whereas the nucleophilic and UV degradation pathway proceeds through debromination to cyanoacetamide. The microbicidal rate of DBNPA is very rapid within materials such as latex or paints; however, the impact of the alkaline pH ranges and/or high processes high temperatures should be considered because these factors can significantly impact the degradation rate of DBNPA (Figure 38.5).[47] Other rapid-acting biocides for consideration include peracetic acid, hydrogen peroxide, glutaraldehyde, and sodium hypochlorite. It is important to consider compatibility of any biocide

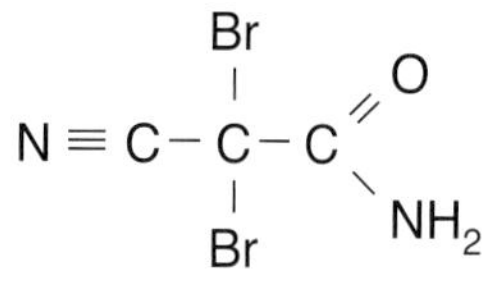

FIGURE 38.3 Molecular structure of 2,2-dibromo-3-nitrilopropionamide (DBNPA).

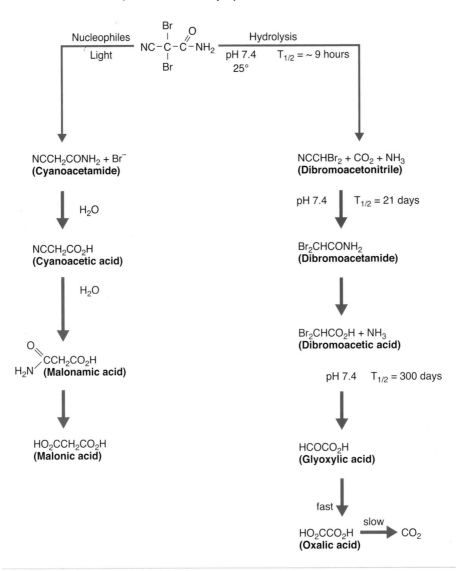

FIGURE 38.4   Decomposition pathway of 2,2-dibromo-3-nitrilopropionamide (DBNPA).

with the raw material matrix that is being treated. Finally, during the remediation of a contaminated raw material, it is important to consider the addition of a long-term preservative appropriate for the raw material to ensure a regrowth of the contamination does not occur within the bulk material (Table 38.2).

PRESERVATION OF FINISHED PRODUCTS

Because industrial products have driven toward more sustainable formulation choices, the proper selection and evaluation of finished product preservation has been increasingly critical to ensure product integrity throughout the service life of the product.[5] Many modern industrial

products are formulated with raw materials that have increased the potential for susceptibility to product spoilage.[39] A major driver toward increased susceptibility to microbial attack has been the trend to replace organic solvents, commonly referred to as volatile organic compounds with water as the main solvent.[3,48-51] Along with water becoming a major component of many environmentally favorable formulations, other components that may provide nutrients to support microbial growth include surfactants, dispersants, rheology modifiers, enzymes, and other naturally occurring additives.[38] For many industrial products, the principal objective is to protect against microbial growth within the wet-state of the product. But for some industrial products such as paints and coatings, plastics, rubbers, leathers, and other building materials, the protection of microbial attack within the dry-state of the

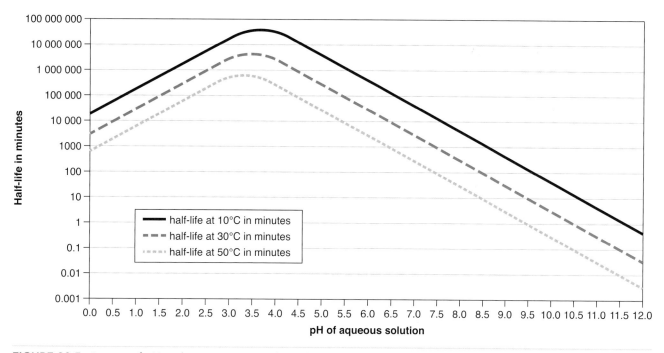

FIGURE 38.5 Impact of pH and temperature on degradation rate of 2,2-dibromo-3-nitrilopropionamide (DBNPA).

product is just as, and often, more critical for the service life of the products.[52-55]

The consequences of ineffective material protection due to microbial degradation within the wet-state of industrial products can result in loss of product integrity due to instability of formulated chemical properties, such as pH or viscosity.[56-59] Additionally, as a result of microbial spoilage, products may exhibit discoloration, generation of offensive malodors, and increased pressure within a container's headspace due to microbial metabolism producing gas that may compromise the integrity of the product's container. Most circumstances of microbial spoilage within the wet-state are the result of contamination due to either bacteria or yeast; however, biodegradation of products within the dry-state are mainly due to fungal and algal attack resulting in offensive appearance and decreased integrity over the service life of the products.

Building Materials

Building materials include a wide variety of product types used within the construction industry including wood, drywall (or gypsum board), asphalt shingles and other roofing materials, siding, thermal insulation, and wallpaper.[60,61] Additional product mixtures used within the construction industry include caulks, grouts, sealants, joint compound, or other construction adhesives. Effective preservation of building materials is necessary to prevent premature failures, which may compromise the integrity of the constructions these materials are used within.

For many building products, prevention of microbial-induced biodegradation not only extends the useful service life of installed product but also reduces the amount of building product waste due to product failures.

Paints and Coatings

Modern-day paints and coatings formulations have substituted historical organic solvents that may have provided some inherent properties to resist microbial ingress, with water as being the essential solvent used both within the formulated product and within many raw materials.[47,49] Many raw materials used to manufacturing paints and coatings are also susceptible to microbial attack if otherwise left unprotected. These raw materials may include polymer or latex emulsions, thickening agents, dispersants, surfactants, wetting agents, and defoamers.[38,41,43-45] All these raw materials contain nutrients that may support microbial growth. Increasingly, production facility hygiene programs have played an important role to attaining microbial control within both the products and processes employed to manufacture these products.[9,12,13,19,33] But effective preservation strategies continue to play a central role to raw material storage and handling, manufacturing of paint formulations with environmentally sustainable properties, and storage throughout the entire supply chain to ensure high-quality products are delivered to customers to meet their performance expectations of the product.[50] Preservatives used to ensure both the wet-state stability of the paints and the dry-film integrity are essential to

TABLE 38.2   Commonly used preservatives in industrial products

Preservative Category	Active Ingredient of Preservative	Microbicidal Spectrum of Activity	Intended Application (Wet-state, Dry-state)
Aldehydes	1,5-pentanediol (glutaraldehyde)	Bacteria, fungi	Wet-state
Carbamates	3-Idoopropynylbutylcarbamate (IPBC)	Fungi	Dry-state
	Methyl benzimidazol-2-ylcarbamate, carbendazim (BCM)	Fungi	Dry-state
Formaldehyde-releasing compounds	1-(3-chloroallyl)-3,5,7-triaza-1-azoniaadamantane chloride (CTAC)	Bacteria	Wet-state
	4,4-dimethyloxazolidine (DMO)	Bacteria	Wet-state
	1,3-dimethylol-5,5-dimethylhydantoin (DMDMH)	Bacteria	Wet-state
Heterocyclic N,S Compounds	1,2-benzisothiazolin-3-one (BIT)	Bacteria	Wet-state
	Mixture of 5-chloro-2-methyl-4-isothiazolin-3-one and 2-methyl-4-isothiazolin-3-one (CMIT/MIT)	Bacteria, fungi	Wet-state
	2-methyl-4-isothiazolin-3-one (MIT)	Bacteria	Wet-state
	2-n-octyl-4-isothiazolin-3-one (OIT)	Fungi	Dry-state
	4,5-dichloro-2-octylisothiazol-3(2H)-one (DCOIT)	Fungi, algae	Dry-state
Halogenated compounds	2-bromo-2-nitropropane-1,3-diol (bronopol, BNPD)	Bacteria	Wet-state
	2,2-dibromo-3-nitrilopropionamide (DBNPA)	Bacteria, fungi	Wet-state
Quaternary ammonium compounds (QAC)	Tetrakishydroxymethyl phosphonium sulfate (THPS)	Bacteria, fungi	Wet-state
	Di-n-decyl-dimethylammonium chloride (DDAC)	Bacteria, fungi	Wet-state
	N-alkyl(C_8-C_{18})-N, N-dimethyl-N-benzylammonium chloride (ADBAC)	Bacteria, fungi	Wet-state
Oxidizing agents	Chlorine dioxide (ClO_2)	Bacteria, fungi	Wet-state
	Sodium hypochlorite	Bacteria, fungi	Wet-state
	Hypobromous acid	Bacteria, fungi	Wet-state
Cyclic thiohydroxamic acid	Zinc pyrithione (ZPT): zinc bis-(2-thioxopyridin-1(2H)-olate)	Fungi	Dry-state
Azoles	Thiabendazole (TBZ): 2-thiazol-4-yl-1H-benzoimidazole	Fungi	Dry-state
	Tebuconazole: (RS)-1-(4-chlorophenyl)-4,4-dimethyl-3-(1H-1,2,4-triazol-1-ylmethyl)-pentan-3-ol; 1:1 ratio of RS enantiomers	Fungi	Dry-state
	Propiconazole: (2RS, 4RS; 2SR, 4SR)-1-[2-(2,4-dichlorophenyl)-4-propyl-1,3-dioxolan-2-yl]-1H-1,2,4-triazole; mixture of 4 biocidal stereoisomers	Fungi	Dry-state
Algicides	Diuron: 3-(3,4-dichlorophenyl)-1,1-dimethylurea	Algae	Dry-state
	Isoproturon: 3-(4-isopropylphenyl)-1,1-dimethylurea	Algae	Dry-state
	Terbutryn: 2-tert-butylamino-4-ethylamino-6-methyl-thio-1,3,5-triazine	Algae	Dry-state

formulating coating products today. Wet-state preservative efficacy testing (commonly referred to as challenge testing) of paints consists of repeated inoculations of microorganisms known to be relevant to spoilage of finished products followed by incubation and recovery to demonstrate the preservative package is capable of adequate protection against spoilage of the finished product.[62-65] Several standard methods have also been developed to evaluate the performance of preservatives within the wet-state, such as ASTM D2574-16, IBRG PDG16-007.3, and IBRG P16-001.2.[66-68] Evaluation of dry film preservation efficacy testing consists of exposure of dry paint films to either fungal or algal microorganisms, which are known to cause defacement of dry paint films. Standard methods have also been developed to evaluate the performance of dry film preservation with mildewcide and/or algaecides, such as ASTM D3273-16, ASTM D3274-09, ASTM D3456, ASTM D5590, and ASTM D5589-09.[69-73]

Wood

As a naturally occurring material, wood is prone to microbial attack leading to biodeterioration and biodegradation of the material (see chapter 69).[74] Most commonly, fungal attack of the cellulosic portion occurs through three major types of attack: white rot, brown rot, and soft rot.[75] The remaining portion of the wood are modified lignin with weakened structural integrity. Other portions of the wood that may be susceptible to microbial attack by cellulolytic bacteria are resins, gums, dyes, tannic acids, waxes, and fats.[76] Finally, many woods may be left susceptible to attack by insects that can impart considerable destructive damage if otherwise left unprotected.[77,78]

Different types of wood inherently have differing levels of ability to naturally resist biodeterioration, with sapwoods commonly being known to be highly susceptible to microbial attack that can reduce the durability of the wood. Using agents for preservation of woods that are susceptible to biodeterioration has permitted these widely available wood species to be broadly used for a variety of end-users where extended service life is critical.[75,79,80] Protection of wood products with preservatives allows for use not only within the construction of buildings but also across several products, such as telephone poles, bridges, wharves and marine pilings, and railroad crossties. These applications support the infrastructure of critical industries, such as the communication industry where transmission of electricity and phone lines are supported by utility poles and transportation industries, such as highway, railroad, and marine transportation where critical infrastructure is dependent on well-preserved wood pilings and crossties.

Pulp and Paper Plastics

The use of preservatives within the pulp and paper industries are important to control a number of defects that may occur within the product and/or process due to unsuppressed microbial growth.[74,81-83] These include unwanted deposits on finished paper products (commonly referred to as "foxing"), accumulation of slime deposits within the manufacturing process, reduced strength of fibers, pH drift, odors due to microbial metabolites, microbial-induced corrosion of the production machinery, degradation of additives used within the manufacturing of paper products, such as starches, polymers, and other filler ingredients.[34,84-86] Preservatives play a key role to ensure levels of microorganisms are controlled to prevent unwanted issues within the process equipment, the raw materials, and the significant volume of water required to manufacture paper products through modern-day continuous processes. A wide variety of industrial products are dependent on the pulp and paper industry to provide materials that have maintained their integrity and provide the characteristics expected by their customers. Some of these products include corrugated cardboard, paper bags, paper towels and tissue, printing and writing paper, magazine, and newsprint. A number of standardized methods have been established by ASTM International, including ASTM E1839-13, ASTM E723-13, and ASTM E875-15.[87-89] Within the Technical Association of the Pulp & Paper Industry (TAPPI), a Microbiology and Microbial Technology Committee of the Research Development Division have established a number of standardized methods, including TAPPI T228: OM 85, TAPPI T449: OM 90, TAPPI T487: PM 85, and TAPPI T631: OM 89.[90-93]

Leathers and Suede Products

Leather and suede products are important to many industries such as footwear, furniture, automotive, garment, and gloves. Because the basic raw materials for leather products are animal hides and skins, biodeterioration may occur during the harvesting, processing, storage, and use of leather products. The process of preparing leather for commercial or industrial goods involves three major steps: hide preparation (commonly referred to as "beamhouse" processes), tanning of the leathers, and post-tanning finishing processes. Preservatives are critical within many of these steps to ensure biodeterioration of the hide or skin does not occur either by bacterial or fungal colonization of the skin and/or process.[94] During the initial preparation steps, the skins are soaked in aqueous solutions to allow for rehydration of water lost during storage. This step is also intended to remove any soil from the skin, such as any blood, dirt, salt, or other soluble material present. The soaking water is highly susceptible to microbial spoilage and therefore, to ensure the skins quality is maintained for the other portions of the process, preservatives are commonly added to control bacterial growth.[95]

During the later stages of hide preparation is a step referred to as pickling, being an acidification step intended to stop the enzymatic activity of the bating process that immediately precedes the pickling step. Preservatives are often incorporated during the pickling step to control both bacterial and fungal contamination that may occur.[96] The tanning process introduces tannins into the skin that may be vegetable, mineral, or synthetic based. The skins and tanning worts used during this process are also susceptible to deterioration mainly by molds due to the acidic nature of the materials. Finally, during the drying stages of the leathering process, the skins are susceptible to microbial attack due to temperatures, humidity levels, and time required to achieve the desired drying. If effective preservation strategies are not employed, rapid microbial contamination can occur with irreparable damage to the leather product.

Metalworking Fluids

During industrial metal machining and grinding operations, metalworking fluids (MWFs) are used to cool and lubricate the metal tools, dies, and the products being created. The use of MWFs during machining processes is also intended to remove fine metal chips being cut away during the production process. For operations where the main function of these fluids is for cooling metal parts, the major constituent of the MWF is water with a lesser portion made up of lubricating additives and those intended to prevent corrosion. These formulations are widely known to be susceptible to microbial attack by both aerobic and anaerobic bacteria as well as fungi.[97-104] The metalworking process recycles the MWF within the machining equipment, which can often be open to the environment and therefore susceptible to environmental contamination.[105-109] The use of preservatives is important to extend the useful performance period of these fluids and protect the equipment for plugging and microbial-induced corrosion.[110-112] Evaluation of the preservatives within MWFs and other water-containing hydraulic fluids can be accomplished using standardized test methods such as ASTM E2275-14, ASTM E979-09, or ASTM E2169-17.[113-115] The addition of preservatives during the process may be triggered by operators' perception of spoilage through detection of odor caused by hydrogen sulfide or ammonia odors. In addition to the detection of fouling odors, the formation of slime within the process, and alterations in pH may impact the overall performance, such as loss of lubricating and/or cooling capabilities, of the MWF within the metalworking operations. Implementation of a microbial monitoring and preservative dosing program can extend the useful life of both the MWF and equipment employed within this industrial process.

Petroleum and Fuels

There are some industrial products where the use of preservatives would be surprising to those people who have not been trained within the industry. Such products are petroleum and fuels. Preservatives are integral to the supply, distribution, storage, and use of many fuels including aviation, diesel, biodiesel, marine, gasoline, and kerosene.[74,116,117] Petroleum products require the addition of preservatives within a variety of product types that can vary from small portions of an aqueous phase to an oil-in-water emulsion. Additionally, many fuel additive products require protection from microbial degradation of both raw materials and finished products. Preservatives can be added throughout the supply chain of fuels, but this is particularly important during production and storage for extending periods of time.

Assessment of preservative effectiveness within liquid fuels can be accomplished using standardized test methods, including ASTM E1259-18,[118] and the methods for evaluation of fuels and fuel systems for microbial contamination include ASTM D6974-16, ASTM D6469-17, and ASTM D7464-14.[119-121]

The infrastructure that supports the fuel industry is critical to ensuring the uninterrupted energy supply that modern-day society has become dependent on. Microbial contamination within these processes poses a risk through biologically mediated corrosion. As with many industrial processes and products, it is very difficult to fully control microbiological ingress into the production and storage processes because these are not sterile environments. It is therefore important to responsibly use preservatives to ensure these products do not become spoiled and unusable.[116,122,123] In the case of fuels, the consequences of microbial spoilage can include product thickening, haziness, condensate or other particulate formation in fuels, reduced service life of associated engines parts and/or fuel filters, microbial-induced corrosion of storage tanks and biodegradation of tank coatings, sludge formation, and increase of sulfur content within fuels.[117] Mechanical issues may arise due to microbial fouling of systems, such as clogging of valves, injectors, and filters. The presence of microbial contamination may also produce biological-derived biosurfactants that may interfere with water separation processes during production and lower the quality of the final product. Microbiological monitoring, routine cleaning, and periodic disinfection of fuel production processes are important in maintaining microbial control within these products and processes.

Oil and Gas Recovery

Preservatives play a critical role to ensure the recovery of oil and gas.[124,125] Microbial contamination can lead to severe problems including equipment failure due to microbial-induced corrosion, souring of reservoirs, generation of hydrogen sulfide due to anaerobic sulfate-reducing bacterial contamination, plugging of equipment due to extensive microbial biofilm formation, and the loss of heat exchange efficiency within processes.[126-130] The various stages of operating an oil and gas recovery process initially involves drilling and preparing the well for production, which is then followed by construction of the recovery facilities and finally the actual production of oil and gas recovered from the well.[131] At each of these stages, preservative products play an important role to protect against spoilage of recovered product, limitation of hazardous generation of hydrogen sulfides, and protection of manufacturing equipment from microbial-induced corrosion.[132-135]

COMMONLY USED PRESERVATIVES FOR THE PROTECTION OF INDUSTRIAL PRODUCTS

The category of industrial products is a wide and varied group of products that directly contribute to the infrastructure and commerce of modern society. A common thread within these products is the necessity use of preservatives within either the wet-state to ensure raw material stability and shelf life of waterborne finished product or within the dry-state to ensure the service life of these products are meaningful for their intended applications. Preservatives for protection of industrial products are included within the following chemical types: aldehydes and acetal/aldehyde-releasing compounds, halogenated compounds, acids and acid esters, amides, azoles, carbamates, dibenzamidines, formaldehyde-releasing compounds, haloalkylthio compounds, organometallic compounds, oxidizing agents, phenolics, pyridine-derived compounds, surface active agents, and various other preservatives not within these chemical categories. Table 38.2 provides an abbreviated summary of the some of the most important preservatives for the protection of materials intended for industrial products.[10,56-59]

REGULATIONS OF ANTIMICROBIALS AS MATERIAL PROTECTION PRESERVATIVES

Antimicrobials for the use of material preservation are regulated globally through several agencies with the intention to provide a thorough review process for ensuring the effectiveness and safety of the products. For example, within the United States, antimicrobials are a category of pesticides regulated by the US Environmental Protection Agency (EPA) under the Federal Insecticide, Fungicide, and Rodenticide Act (FIFRA), 7 USC §135 et. Seq.[136] An antimicrobial pesticide is defined under FIFRA as "a substance intended to disinfect, sanitize or otherwise mitigate the growth of microorganisms, or to protect inanimate objects, industrial processes, surfaces, water or other chemical substances from contamination, fouling or deterioration caused by microorganisms."[136] Antimicrobial pesticides can be viewed as falling into two broad categories:

1. Those intended to control pathogenic microorganisms on inanimate objects, known as "public health pesticides"
2. Those intended to be used in areas essential to the economic health of an industrialized society, including extending the in-use life of manufactured goods and other products, protecting equipment used in industrial processing and manufacturing systems, and preserving energy efficiency in numerous systems and operations, known as "non-public health" pesticides

Pursuant to FIFRA, pesticide products are rigorously reviewed and assessed by the EPA prior to registration. Registrations are issued only for specific uses and applications. Public health pesticides also require EPA review of efficacy data generated under good laboratory practice conditions to substantiate the claims as part of the registration process.[137] It is important to understand that industrial products using antimicrobial pesticides for material preservation do not require the finished products to obtain registrations. Instead, these products are permitted to make limited claims regarding the products' use of material preservations for the purposes of protecting the product (or article) itself. This is commonly referred to as the treated articles exemption.[138]

Antimicrobial pesticides are used as preservatives in a wide range of finished goods to protect them from microbial contaminants that spoil, decrease in-use service life, and compromise product integrity.[8] Products using antimicrobial pesticides for the purpose of material protection are exempt from any requirements to obtain a registration for the finished product itself but must ensure the antimicrobial pesticides label provides instructions for the application within the preserved finished product. Typically, antimicrobial pesticides used as material preservatives are present at low levels in the final goods (less than 1.0% of the total formulation) but are critical because they help preserve the finished product, decrease energy and natural resource consumption, and waste generation by extending the useful life of the finished goods. Overall, this leads to significant economic sustainability and societal benefits.

REFERENCES

1. Geis P, Rook T. Microbiological quality of consumer products. *Happi.* 2011;48:82-87.
2. Tirodkar RB, Menon RB. Microbial spoilage of water-borne paints. *J Colour Soc.* 1983:10-15.
3. Linder W, Horacek GL. *How Microbicides Will Contribute to Further Substantial Reduction of Emissions From Coatings.* Chicago, IL: Federation of Societies for Coating Technologies; 2008.
4. Browne BA, Geis P, Rook T. Conventional vs. natural preservatives. *Happi.* 2012;5:69-74.
5. Kähkönen E. Compliant tools for the future: how can increasingly biodegradable products be preserved? Paper presented at: European Coatings Conference: Novel Biocide Technology IV; September 17-18, 2009; Berlin, Germany.
6. Ravikumari HR, Rao SS, Karigar CS. Biodegradation of paints: a current status. *Indian J Sci Technol.* 2012;5:1977-1987.
7. Gillatt J. The biodeterioration of polymer emulsions and its prevention with biocides. *Int Biodeterioration.* 1990;26:205-216.
8. American Chemistry Council Biocide Panel. *Benefits of Antimicrobial Pesticides in Public-Health and Industrial Uses.* Washington, DC: American Chemistry Council Biocide; 2010.
9. Ogden D. Industrial plant hygiene, cost savings, preservation and life after the BPD. *Surf Coatings Int.* 2006;89:306-309.
10. Sauer F. Coatings preservation. In: Sauer F, ed. *Microbiocides in Coatings.* Hanover, Germany: Vincentz Network; 2017:37-87.
11. Gillatt J. Preservation of paints in the wet-state. In: Karsa DR, Ashworth D, eds. *Industrial Biocides: Selection and Application.* Cambridge, United Kingdom: Royal Society of Chemistry; 2002:65-83.

12. Briggs MA. *Emulsion Paint Preservation, Factory Practice and Hygiene.* Teddington, United Kingdom: Paint Research Association; 1980. Paint Research Association technical report TR18178.

13. Wedderburn DL. Hygiene in the manufacturing plant and its effect on the preservation of emulsions. *J Soc Cosmet Chemists.* 1965;16:395-403.

14. Bilgili SF. Sanitary hygienic processing design. *World Poult Sci J.* 2006; 62:115-122.

15. Mulhall R, Schmidt E, Brannan DK. Microbial environment of the manufacturing plant. In: Brannan DK, ed. *Cosmetic Microbiology: A Practical Handbook.* Washington, DC: CRC Press; 1997:69-91.

16. Felo M. Design considerations and best practices for tank vent filtration. Pharma Manufacturing Web site. https://www.pharmamanufacturing .com/articles/2011/149/. Accessed July 6, 2019.

17. Chemseal Inc. Hygienic Piping Design Guidelinespiping design guidelines. Chemseal Inc Web site. https://www.chemsealinc.net/content /FreeGuide.pdf. Accessed July 6, 2019.

18. Folkmar JA, Boye BBJ, Boye-Møller AR, et al. *Design of Piping Systems for Food Processing Industry—With a Focus on Hygiene.* Denmark, Europe: Danish Competence Center for Stainless Steel Industry; 2006.

19. Harry RG. Cleanliness, hygiene and microbiological control in manufacture. In: Harry RG, ed. *Harry's Cosmeticology.* Aylesbury, England: Leonard Hill Books; 1973:877-897.

20. Domsic J, Lowenstein M, van Komen J, et al. Manufacturing with microbial control in mind (part II). *Happi.* 2017:98-102.

21. Browne BA, van Komen J, Domsic J, et al. Manufacturing with microbial control in mind (part I). *Happi.* 2017;4:72-78.

22. *Guideline on Test Methods for Environmental Monitoring for Aseptic Dispensing Facilities.* 2nd ed. Scotland, United Kingdom: A Working Group of the Scottish Quality Assurance Specialist Interest Group; 2004.

23. Kohn FS. Report: quality management program for environmental monitoring. Novatek International Web site. https://ntint.com /quality-management-program-for-environmental-monitoring -part-1. Accessed July 6, 2019.

24. Sandle T. Environmental monitoring: a practical approach. In: Friedman BA, Ginsbury K, Lowery SA, et al, eds. *Environmental Monitoring Volume 1: Establishing the Program.* Bethesda, MD: DHI Publishing; 2017:23-48.

25. Friedman BA. Environmental monitoring and the microbial control strategy. In: Friedman BA, Ginsbury K, Lowery SA, et al, eds. *Environmental Monitoring Volume 1: Establishing the Program.* Bethesda, MD: DHI Publishing; 2017:127-144.

26. ASTM International. ASTM D5588-97 (2017): standard test method for determination of microbial condition of paint, paint raw materials, and plant areas. ASTM International Web site. https://www.astm.org /Standards/D5588.htm. Accessed July 6, 2019.

27. Chem-Aqua. *Using and Interpreting Dip Slides.* Irving, TX: Chem-Aqua; 2018. Technical Bulletin 2-001 Cooling Systems.

28. Moldenhauer J. Overview of rapid microbiological methods. In: Zourob M, Elwary S, Turner A, eds. *Principles of Bacterial Detection: Biosensors, Recognition Receptors and Microsystems.* New York, NY: Springer; 2008:49-79.

29. Miller MJ, ed. *Encyclopedia of Rapid Microbiological Methods.* Vols 1-3. Bethesda, MD: PDA/DHI; 2015.

30. Suez Water Technologies & Solutions. *Handbook of Industrial Water Treatment.* Paris, France: Suez Water Technologies & Solutions; 2019. https:// www.suezwatertechnologies.com/handbook/handbook-industrial -water-treatment. Accessed July 6, 2019.

31. Samco Technologies. *An Introduction to Industrial Water Treatment Systems.* Buffalo, NY: Samco Technologies; 2019.

32. Royal Haskoning DHV. *Industrial Water Treatment.* Amersfoort, Netherlands: Royal Haskoning DHV; 2019

33. Ogden D. Industrial plant hygiene. *Polym Paint Colour J.* 2010;1:18-22.

34. Johnsrud SC. Biotechnology for solving slime problems in the pulp and paper industry. In: Scheper T, ed. *Advances in Biochemical Engineering/ Biotechnology.* Vol 57. Berlin, Germany: Springer; 1997:311-328.

35. Donlan RM. Biofilm control in industrial water systems: approaching an old problem in new ways. In: Evans LV, ed. *Biofilms: Recent Advances in Their Study and Control.* Amsterdam, Netherlands: Hardward Academic Publishers; 2000:345-373.

36. McBain AJ, Gilbert P. Biofilms: adverse economic impacts and their avoidance. In: Karsa DR, Ashworth D, eds. *Industrial Biocides: Selection and Application.* Cambridge, MA: Royal Society of Chemistry; 2002:41-51.

37. McCoy WF. A new environmentally sensible chlorine alternative. In: Karsa DR, Ashworth D, eds. *Industrial Biocides: Selection and Application.* Cambridge, MA: Royal Society of Chemistry; 2002:52-62.

38. Tothill IE, Seal KJ. Biodeterioration of waterborne paint cellulose thickeners. *Int Biodeterior Biodegradation.* 1993;31:241-254.

39. Jakubolwski JA, Simpson SL, Gyuris J. Microbiological spoilage of latex emulsions: causes and prevention. *J Coating Technol.* 1982;54:39-44.

40. Consumer Specialty Products Association. *Microbiology Quality of Raw Material General Guidelines.* Washington, DC: Consumer Specialty Products Association; 2014.

41. Gillatt JW. The microbial spoilage of polymer dispersions and its prevention. In: Paulus W, ed. *Directory of Microbicides for the Protection of Materials: A Handbook.* Dordrecht, Netherlands: Springer; 2005:219-249.

42. International Biodeterioration Research Group. Tier 1 polymer dispersions method, IBRG PDG16001.2. International Biodeterioration Research Group Web site. http://ibrg.org/methods.aspx. Accessed July 6, 2019.

43. Poulse S, Hansen SL, Kofoed MVW, et al, eds. *Reducing Biocide Concentrations for Preservation of Water-Based Paints.* Copenhagen, Denmark: Danish Environmental Protection Agency; 2018.

44. Woods WB. Prevention of the microbial spoilage of latex paint. *J Water Borne Coatings.* 1982;111:2-4.

45. Cresswell MA, Holland K. Preservation of aqueous-based synthetic polymer emulsions and adhesive formulations. In: Morpeth FF, eds. *Preservation of Surfactant Formulations.* Dordrecht, Netherlands: Springer; 1995:212-261.

46. Bhattacharya A. *Microbial Degradation of Water-Based Pigments.* Montvale, NJ: Rodman Media. https://www.pcimag.com/articles /99317-microbial-degradation-of-water-based-pigments. Accessed July 6, 2019.

47. Dow Chemical. *Dowicil QK-20 Antimicrobial: A Fast-Acting, Broad Spectrum Biocide for Treating Raw Materials, Processing Water, and Contaminated Products.* Midland, MI: Dow Chemical; 2000. Form no. 253-01184-0100X/GW.

48. Counquer L. VOC and the biocide industry. *Eur Coatings J.* 1993; 7:592-597.

49. Kähkönen E, Nordström K, Suominen M. A challenge for biocides. *Eur Coatings J.* 2007;7-8:28.

50. Betancur J. The rise of water-based formulations: addressing microbial contamination challenges in the paint and coatings market. Paint & Coatings Industry Web site. https://www.pcimag.com/articles /105619-the-rise-of-water-based-formulations. Accessed July 6, 2019.

51. Agosta M. Biocides update: preservation is key. Coatings World Web site. https://www.coatingsworld.com/issues/2002-09/view_features /biocides-update-preservation-is-key. Accessed July 6, 2019.

52. Linder W. Surface coatings. In: Paulus W, ed. *Directory of Microbicides for the Protection of Materials: A Handbook.* Dordrecht, Netherlands: Springer; 2005:347-375.

53. Gobakken LR, Høibø OA, Solheim H. Mould growth on paints with different surface structures when applied on wood claddings exposed outdoors. *Int Biodeterior Biodegradation.* 2010;64:339-345.

54. Shirakawa MA, Gaylarde CC, Gaylarde PM, John V, Gambale W. Fungal colonization and succession on newly painted buildings and the effect of biocide. *FEMS Microbiol Ecol.* 2002;39:165-173.

55. Linder W, Horacek GL. Efficacy requirements for microbial resistant coatings. *J Coating Technol.* 2007;3:34-40.

56. Falkiewicz-Dulik M, Janda K, Wypych G, eds. *Handbook of Biodegradation, Biodeterioration, and Biostabilization.* 2nd ed. Toronto, Canada: ChemTec Publishing; 2015.

57. Rossmoore HW, ed. *Handbook of Biocide and Preservative Use.* Glasgow, Scotland: Blackie Academic & Professional; 1995.

58. Karsa DR, Ashworth D, eds. *Industrial Biocides: Selection and Application.* Cambridge, United Kingdom: Royal Society of Chemistry; 2002.

59. Paulus W, ed. *Directory of Microbicides for the Protection of Materials.* Dordrecht, Netherlands: Springer; 2005.

60. Menetrez MY, Foarde KK, Webber TD, Dean TR, Betancourt DA. Mold growth on gypsum wallboard—a research summary. In: Proceedings from Indoor Environmental Quality: Problems, Research and Solutions; July 17-19, 2006; Pittsburgh, PA.

61. D'Orazio M. Materials prone to mould growth. In: Pacheco-Torgal F, Jalali S, Fucic A, eds. *Toxicity of Building Materials.* Cambridge, United Kingdom: Woodhead Publishing; 2012:334-350.

62. Winkowski K. Efficacy of in-can preservatives. *Eur Coatings J.* 2001; 1-2:87-91.

63. Lunenburg-Duindam J, Linder W. In-can preservation of emulsion paints. *Eur Coatings J.* 2000;3:66-73.

64. Obidi OF, Aboaba OO, Mankajuola MS, Nwachukwu SC. Microbial evaluation and deterioration of paints and paint-products. *J Environ Biol.* 2009;30:835-840.

65. Ananth V, Rook T, Shaw D, et al. Preservative efficacy testing. *Happi.* 2015;4:74-78.

66. ASTM International. ASTM D2574-16: standard test method for the resistance of emulsion paints in container to attack by microorganisms. ASTM International Web site. http://www.astm.org/standards /D2574.htm. Accessed July 6, 2019.

67. International Biodeterioration Research Group. Tier 1 Basic efficacy method for biocidal active substances used to preserve aqueous-based products, IBRG PDG16-007.3. International Biodeterioration Research Group Web site. http://ibrg.org/methods.aspx. Accessed July 6, 2019.

68. International Biodeterioration Research Group. Tier 1 Wet state paint method, IBRG P16-001.2. International Biodeterioration Research Group Web site. http://ibrg.org/methods.aspx. Accessed July 6, 2019.

69. ASTM International. ASTM D3273-16: standard test method for resistance to growth of mold on the surface of interior coatings in an environmental chamber. ASTM International Web site. https://www .astm.org/Standards/D3273.htm. Accessed July 6, 2019.

70. ASTM International. ASTM D3274-09 (2017): standard test method for evaluating degree of surface disfigurement of paint films by fungal or algal growth, or soil and dirt accumulation. ASTM International Web site. Accessed July 6, 2019.

71. ASTM International. ASTM D3456-18: standard practice for determining by exterior exposure tests the susceptibility of paint films to microbiological attack. ASTM International Web site. https://www.astm.org /Standards/D3456.htm. Accessed July 6, 2019.

72. ASTM International. ASTM D5590: standard test method for determining the resistance of paint films and related coatings to fungal defacement by accelerated four-week agar plate assay. ASTM International Web site. https://www.astm.org/Standards/D5590.htm. Accessed July 6, 2019.

73. ASTM International. ASTM D5589-09 (2013): standard test method for determining the resistance of paint films and related coatings to algal defacement. ASTM International Web site. https://www.astm.org /Standards/D5589.htm. Accessed July 6, 2019.

74. Biodegradation, biodeterioration, and biostabilization of industrial products. In: Falkiewicz-Dulik M, Janda K, Wypych G, eds. *Handbook of Biodegradation, Biodeterioration, and Biostabilization.* 2nd ed. Toronto, Canada: ChemTec Publishing; 2015:99-375.

75. Leightley L. Biocides used in wood preservation. In: Rossmoore HW, ed. *Handbook of Biocide and Preservative Use.* Glasgow, Scotland: Blackie Academic & Professional; 1995:283-314.

76. Alves da Silva C, Monteiro MBB, Brazolin S, et al. Biodeterioration of brazilwood *Caesalpinia echinata* Lam. (Leguminosae—Caesalpinioideae) by rot fungi and termites. *Int Biodeterioration and Biodegradation.* 2007; 60:285-292.

77. Muñoz GR, Gete AR, Regueiro MG. Sawing yield in oak (*Quercus robur*) wood affected by insect damage. *Int Biodeterior Biodegradation.* 2014;86:102-107.

78. Eaton RA, Hale MDC, eds. *Wood: Decay, Pests and Protection.* London, New York: Chapman & Hall; 1993.

79. Nicholas DD, ed. *Wood Deterioration and Its Prevention by Preservative Treatments.* New York, NY: Syracuse University Press; 1973. *Degradation and Protection of Wood*; vol 1.

80. Richardson BA, ed. *Wood Preservation.* Lancaster, PA: Construction Press; 1978.

81. Eagon RG. Paper, pulp and good grade paper. In: Rossmoore HW, ed. *Handbook of Biocide and Preservative Use.* Glasgow, Scotland: Blackie Academic & Professional; 1995:83-132.

82. Corbel C. Pulp & paper. In: Paulus W, ed. *Directory of Microbicides for the Protection of Materials.* Dordrecht, Netherlands: Springer; 2005:377-409.

83. Simpson P. Biocides in the pulp & paper industry: an overview. In: Karsa DR, Ashworth D, eds. *Industrial Biocides: Selection and Application.* Cambridge, United Kingdom: Royal Society of Chemistry; 2002:17-22.

84. Raaska L, Sillanpää J, Sjöberg AM, Suihko ML. Potential microbiological hazards in the production of refined paper products for food applications. *J Ind Microbiol Biotechnol.* 2002;28:225-231.

85. Choi S. Foxing on paper: a literature review. *J Am Inst Conserv.* 2007;46:137-152.

86. Arai H. Foxing caused by fungi: a 25 year study. *Int Biodeterioration and Biodegradation.* 2000;46:181-188.

87. ASTM International. ASTM E1839-13: standard test method for efficacy of slimicides for the paper industry—bacterial and fungal slime. ASTM International Web site. https://www.astm.org/Standards/E1839 .htm. Accessed July 6, 2019.

88. ASTM International. ASTM E723-13: standard practice for evaluation of antimicrobials as preservatives for aqueous-based products used in the paper industry (bacterial spoilage). ASTM International Web site. https://www.astm.org/Standards/E723.htm. Accessed July 6, 2019.

89. ASTM International. ASTM E875-15: standard practice for evaluation of fungal control agents as preservatives for aqueous-based products used in the paper industry. ASTM International Web site. https://www .astm.org/Standards/E875.htm. Accessed July 6, 2019.

90. Technical Association of the Pulp & Paper Industry. *T228: OM 85 Microbiologial Examination of the Pulp in Sheet Form.* https://www .tappi.org. Accessed July 6, 2019.

91. Technical Association of the Pulp & Paper Industry. *T449: OM 90 Bacteriological Examination of Paper and Paperboard.* https://www.tappi .org. Accessed July 6, 2019.

92. Technical Association of the Pulp & Paper Industry. *T487: PM 85 Fungus Resistance of Paper and Paperboard.* https://www.tappi.org. Accessed July 6, 2019.

93. Technical Association of the Pulp & Paper Industry. *T631: OM 89 Microbiological Examination of Process Water and Slush Pulp.* https://www .tappi.org. Accessed July 6, 2019.

94. Hauber C. Microbicide applications in the leather industry. In: Paulus W, ed. *Directory of Microbicides for the Protection of Materials.* Dordrecht, Netherlands: Springer; 2005:317-324.

95. Falkiewicz-Dulik M. Leather and leather products. In: Falkiewicz-Dulik M, Janda K, Wypych G, eds. *Handbook of Biodegradation, Biodeterioration, and Biostabilization.* 2nd ed. Toronto, Canada: ChemTec Publishing; 2015:133-237.

96. Rother HJ. Microorganisms: the scourge of the leather industry. *World Leather.* 1995;5:48-50.

97. Passman FJ. Microbiology of metalworking fluids. In: Byers JP, ed. *Metalworking Fluids.* 3rd ed. Boca Raton, FL: CRC Press; 2017.

98. Saha R, Donofrio RS. The microbiology of metalworking fluids. *Appl Microbiol Biotechnol.* 2012;94:1119-1130.

99. Koch T. Microbiology of metalworking fluids. In: Mang T, ed. *Encyclopedia of Lubricants and Lubrication.* Berlin, Germany: Springer; 2014:1169-1172.

100. Dilger S, Fluri A, Sonntag HG. Bacterial contamination of preserved and non-preserved metal working fluids. *Int J Hyg Environ Health.* 2005;208:467-476.

101. Thompson IP, van der Gast CJ. The microbiology of metal working fluids. In: Timmis KN, ed. *Handbook of Hydrocarbon and Lipid Microbiology.* Berlin, Germany: Springer; 2010:2369-2376.

102. Lloyd G, Lloyd GI, Schofield J. Enteric bacteria in cutting oil emulsion. *Tribol Int.* 1975;8:27-29.

103. Mattsby-Baltzer I, Sandin M, Ahlström B, et al. Microbial growth and accumulation in industrial metal-working fluids. *Appl Environ Microbiol.* 1989;55:2681-2689.

104. van der Gast CJ, Knowles CJ, Wright MA, Thompson IP. Identification and characterisation of bacterial populations of an in-use metal-working fluid by phenotypic and genotypic methodology. *Int Biodeterior Biodegradation*. 2001;47:113-123.

105. Rossmoore HW. Microbial degradation of water-based metalworking fluids. In: Moo-Young M, ed. *Comprehensive Biotechnology: The Principles, Applications and Regulations of Biotechnology in Industry, Agriculture and Medicine*. New York, NY: Pergamon Press; 1989:249-269.

106. Foxall-VanAken S, Brown JA Jr, Young W, Salmeen I, McClure T, Napier S Jr, Olsen RH. Common components of industrial metal-working fluids as sources of carbon for bacterial growth. *Appl Environ Microbiol*. 1986;51:1165-1169.

107. Rossmoore HW. *Microbiological Causes of Cutting Fluid Deterioration*. New York, NY: American Society of Mechanical Engineers; 1974. Technical paper MR 74-169.

108. Murat JB, Grenouillet F, Reboux G, et al. Factors influencing the microbial composition of metalworking fluids and potential implications for machine operator's lung. *Appl Environmental Microbiol*. 2012;78:34-41.

109. Trafny EA. Microorganisms in metalworking fluids: current issues in research and management. *Int J Occup Med Environ Health*. 2013;26:4-15.

110. Wright MA. The application of biocides in metal working fluids. In: Karsa DR, Ashworth D, eds. *Industrial Biocides: Selection and Application*. Cambridge, United Kingdom: Royal Society of Chemistry; 2002:111-118.

111. Marchand G, Lavoie J, Racine L, et al. Evaluation of bacterial contamination and control methods in soluble metalworking fluids. *J Occup Environ Hyg*. 2010;7:358-366.

112. Rossmoore HW. Biocides for metalworking lubricants hydraulic fluids. In: Rossmoore HW, ed. *Handbook of Biocide and Preservative Use*. Glasgow, Scotland: Blackie Academic & Professional; 1995:133-184.

113. ASTM International. ASTM E2275-14: standard practice for evaluating water-miscible metalworking fluid bioresistance and antimicrobial pesticide performance. ASTM International Web site. https://www.astm.org/Standards/E2275.htm. Accessed July 6, 2019.

114. ASTM International. ASTM E979-09 (2015): standard practice for evaluation of antimicrobial agents as preservatives for invert emulsion and other water containing hydraulic fluids. ASTM International Web site. https://www.astm.org/Standards/E979.htm. Accessed July 6, 2019.

115. ASTM International. ASTM E2169-17: standard practice for selecting antimicrobial pesticides for use in water-miscible metalworking fluids. ASTM International Web site. https://www.astm.org/Standards/E2169.htm. Accessed July 6, 2019.

116. Hill EC. Fuels biocides. In: Rossmoore HW, ed. *Handbook of Biocide and Preservative Use*. Glasgow, Scotland: Blackie Academic & Professional; 1995:207-237.

117. Robbins JA, Levy R. A review of the microbiological degradation of fuel. In: Paulus W, ed. *Directory of Microbicides for the Protection of Materials*. Dordrecht, Netherlands: Springer; 2005:177-201.

118. ASTM International. ASTM E1259-18: standard practice for evaluation of antimicrobials in liquid fuels boiling below 390 °C. ASTM International Web site. https://www.astm.org/Standards/E1259.htm. Accessed July 6, 2019.

119. ASTM International. ASTM D6974-16: standard practice for enumeration of viable bacteria and fungi in liquid fuels—filtration and culture procedures. ASTM International Web site. https://www.astm.org/Standards/D6974.htm. Accessed July 6, 2019.

120. ASTM International. ASTM D6479-17: standard guide for microbial contamination in fuels and fuel systems. ASTM International Web site. https://www.astm.org/Standards/D6469.htm. Accessed July 6, 2019.

121. ASTM International. ASTM D7464-14: standard practice for manual sampling of liquid fuels, associated materials and fuel system components for microbiological testing. ASTM International Web site. https://www.astm.org/Standards/D7464.htm. Accessed July 6, 2019.

122. London SA. *Microbiological Evaluation of Aviation Fuel Storage, Dispensing and Aircraft Systems*. Springfield, VA: National Technical Information Service; 1974. Final report no. AMRL-TR-74-144.

123. Pivnick H. *The Nutrition and Factors Affecting the Growth of Bacteria in Soluble Oils* [dissertation]. East Lansing, MI: Michigan State College; 1952.

124. Herbert BN. Biocides in oilfield operations. In: Rossmoore HW, ed. *Handbook of Biocide and Preservative Use*. Glasgow, Scotland: Blackie Academic & Professional; 1995:185-206.

125. McIlwaine DB. Oilfield application for biocides. In: Paulus W, ed. *Directory of Microbicides for the Protection of Materials*. Dordrecht, Netherlands: Springer; 2005:157-175.

126. National Association of Corrosion Engineers International. *Microbiologically Influenced Corrosion and Biofouling in Oilfield Equipment, TPC 3*. Houston, TX: NACE; 1990.

127. Youssef N, Elshahed MS, McInerney MJ. Microbial processes in oil fields: culprits, problems, and opportunities. In: Laskin AI, Sariaslani S, Gadd GM, eds. *Advances in Applied Microbiology*. Vol 66. Burlington, MA: Academic Press; 2009:141-251.

128. Sunde E, Torsvik T. Microbial control of hydrogen sulfide production in oil reservoirs. In: Ollivier B, Magot M, eds. *Petroleum Microbiology*. Washington, DC: ASM; 2005:201-213.

129. Vance I, Thrasher DR. Reservoir souring: Mechanisms and prevention. In: Ollivier B, Magot M, eds. *Petroleum Microbiology*. Washington, DC: ASM; 2005:123-142.

130. Jack TR, Wardlaw SN, Costerton JW. Microbial plugging in enhanced oil recovery. In: Donaldson EC, Chilingarian GV, Yen TF, eds. *Development in Petroleum Science, Microbial Enhanced Oil Recovery*. New York: Elsevier, 1989, Vol 22: 125-149.

131. Lake LW, ed. *Petroleum Engineering Handbook*. Richardson, TX: Society of Petroleum Engineers; 2007.

132. Sianawati E, Yin B, Williams T, et al. Microbial control management for oil and gas recovery operation. Paper presented at: SPE Kuwait Oil and Gas Show and Conference, Society of Petroleum Engineers; October 8, 2013; Kuwait City, Kuwait. doi:10.2118/167366-MS.

133. Javaherdashti R. *Microbiologically Influenced Corrosion: An Engineering Insight*. Switzerland, Europe: Springer; 2017.

134. Little BJ, Lee JS. *Microbiologically Influenced Corrosion*. Hoboken, NJ: Wiley; 2007.

135. Little BJ, Mansfeld FB, Arps PJ, et al. Microbiologically influenced corrosion. In: Bard AJ, Stratmann M, Gileadi E, Urbakh M, eds. *Encyclopedia of Electrochemistry, Thermodynamics and Electrified Interfaces*. Hoboken, NJ: Wiley; 2007:662-685.

136. US Environmental Protection Agency. Federal Insecticide, Fungicide, and Rodenticide Act, FIFRA § 2(mm)(1)(A); 7 U.S.C. §136(mm)(1)(A) (1996).

137. US Environmental Protection Agency. 40 CFR §158.2220(a)(2) (1996).

138. US Environmental Protection Agency. *PRN 2000-1: Applicability of the Treated Articles Exemption to Antimicrobial Pesticides*. Washington, DC: US Environmental Protection Agency; 2000.

Preservation of Pharmaceutical Dosage Forms

Patrick J. Crowley and David P. Elder

Shelf lives of medications are invariably measured in years, and product usage can be intermittent in some cases. Removing/replacing a product closure during use, a common practice with multidose aqueous liquid products, can inadvertently introduce microbial contaminants. Proliferation of microbes that are present in input materials or introduced during product manufacture or use can also lead to contaminated product, such risks being inflated in products containing ingredients that support microbial growth. The inclusion of a suitable microbicide in products that are aqueous in nature mitigates such risks. However, choosing a preservative is not a simple task. The diversity of the organisms mandated for preservative efficacy testing, the differing regulatory requirements, and seemingly progressive narrowing of choice of suitable preservatives, along with the lack of new preservatives present formidable challenges in dosage form design and preservation. Such challenges and possibilities for their resolution are discussed in this chapter.

◗ BACKGROUND AND CURRENT STATUS

Historically, the risks of microbial contamination in products were manifold. Many active components as well as excipients such as suspending agents were derived from plant or other vegetable sources: They were animal extracts in some cases. Methods of purification were often rudimentary or nonexistent. Preparations of agents such as extracts and tinctures for medicinal use were usually alcohol based, which probably helped limit microbial contamination. The advent of therapeutic agents prepared by chemical synthesis provided opportunities for purification by crystallization and contributed to purer drug substances and excipients. Good Manufacturing Practice (GMP) requirements and associated standards and testing that are now common have also greatly

reduced possibilities for microbial contamination. These, along with tests and controls for microbial contamination in source drugs and excipients, provide reasonable assurance of the microbial cleanliness of the final manufactured product. Focus has therefore shifted to protecting against microbial contamination in pharmaceutical products that are aqueous in composition and not manufactured as single-dose sterile preparations. Nevertheless, product recalls due to microbial contamination are becoming increasingly prevalent and concern both sterile (parenteral) and nonsterile dosage forms.[1] Regulatory agencies are accordingly devoting increased resource and attention to the microbial quality of excipients, drug substances, and drug products. Lack of sterility in purportedly sterile products is a prime concern. Fungal and bacterial contamination of ostensibly sterile products prepared in a compounding pharmacy has caused deaths and illness on administration to patients, being attributable to using nonsterile ingredients and noncompliance with GMP standards.[2]

The excipients and active ingredients used in pharmaceutical products must meet pharmacopoeial limits for microbial quality. Most are not microbe free and, although products may be manufactured and packaged in appropriately clean facilities using controlled operating procedures, microbial growth is possible during subsequent product storage. Inadvertent contamination of multidose liquid products during patient use can also lead to microbial growth and risk to the patient. Hence, it is necessary to include a preservative in products that are not manufactured as sterile unless another product component or mixture of components provide an antimicrobial effect that meets pharmacopoeial standards.

Products manufactured as sterile and contained in single-dose presentations do not require a preservative. Examples are not only single-dose parenteral products but may also include single-dose products for ophthalmic instillation. Sterile products in multidose containers must contain a preservative or components that provide the requisite antimicrobial effects.

Risk assessment tools are described in various compendia and industry documents to help identify potential sources of microbial contamination in nonsterile drug products. These guidelines include

- International Council for Harmonisation Quality Risk Management Q9 (ICH Q9)[3]
- Fault Tree Analysis (FTA)[4]
- Failure Mode and Effect Analysis (FMEA)[5]
- Hazard Analysis Critical Control Point (HACCP)[6]

▶ REGULATORY AND PHARMACOPOEIAL REQUIREMENTS

The US Food and Drug Administration (FDA) requires that all ingredients used in a licensed product must meet pharmacopoeial standards for purity and quality. Any preservative used shall be sufficiently safe so that the amount present in the recommended dose of the product will not be harmful to the recipient. It is also essential that the impact of preservatives on other product quality attributes is considered in dosage form design. The US Code of Federal Regulations (CFR §610.15[a]) directs that "preservatives be examined in the context of the overall product, including the recommended dose, and the requirement that patient safety is not compromised at the level included." The European Medicines Agency (EMA) has comparable guidelines for product components, preservatives, and antioxidants and adopts a similar approach when reviewing, assessing, and approving their inclusion in medicinal products.[7] The EMA also states that the choice of a preservative is supported by the following justifications:

- why the material (preservative) is included
- proof of its effectiveness
- the method and standards for its control in the product
- labeling details on the product
- relevant safety information

If the product is contained in a multidose container and does not contain a preservative because it is intended for single use only, is self-preserving, or is an oil-based formulation, the applicant may justify the absence of preservative(s). The EMA indicates that this requirement emphasizes the risk associated with using nonpreserved materials and highlights the absence of a preservative. The original intent was to stress the need for risk/balance in decision making, bearing in mind that preservatives (being biocidal) can be considered as "toxic" and pose a safety risk in some situations or in vulnerable populations, such as pediatrics or the elderly. It is also feasible that nonpreserved formulations, intended for single use but which might be used in a multidose fashion in certain situations, can pose risks of microbial contamination and

affect patient safety. Subsequently, EMA broadened the guidance to include all excipients in a product.[8]

Products available in multidose presentations, being vulnerable to contamination during use, may benefit from the presence of a preservative. Examples include

- Orally dosed aqueous multidose products. These may be formulated as solutions or suspensions at the outset or are constituted as aqueous liquids at time of dispensing with limited in-use periods in the liquid state.
- Multidose parenteral products such as vaccines for mass immunization programs. Some may be constituted at time of use. Multidose parenterals may also be used to dose patients in health care settings.
- Multidose ophthalmic medications
- Topical products that are aqueous based (creams, lotions etc) for application to the skin and mucosal tissues
- Other aqueous products such as aqueous based liquid metered dose inhalers or nebulized medications that are delivered to regions such as nasal passages, the oro-laryngeal space, the pleural region by inhalation, or to wounds/skin abrasions

The demographics of some users of liquid and semisolid medications (elderly and pediatrics), the cumbersome operations that are sometimes associated with administration or application, and the diversity of microbes in the dosing or application environment can lead to microbes being transferred to the medication during use. Growth during subsequent product storage, particularly when use is only occasional, can compromise quality. Preservation is necessary to prevent such microbial growth and risk to the patient.

Single-dose parenteral products have become increasingly prominent, aided by the advent of technologies, materials, and therapeutic agents that are dosed less frequently, possibly even just once (eg, novel immunotherapeutic agents or vaccines for infectious conditions). Engineered systems are also being developed that make it possible to use multidose presentations that can prevent product contamination during use. Such systems usually incorporate sophisticated technologies, manufacturing operations, and complex packaging. These can inflate costs and be expensive or impractical for operations such as mass vaccination programs. Products in single-dose forms such as sachets for oral dosage can be cumbersome when administering or constituting as liquids; spillage can compromise dose accuracy. Consequently, multidose products are unlikely to be replaced, wholesale in the foreseeable future, and their preservation will remain a prominent requirement in dosage form design.

A preservative may not be required in a product that possesses intrinsic antimicrobial activity. Examples include products containing high levels of sucrose or of polyols such as glycerol or propylene glycol that provide high osmotic pressure or reduced water activity, or products that contain an active ingredient with anti-infective properties, present in solution at levels conferring the requisite preservative activity. In some cases, such an ingredient might not provide the full antimicrobial spectrum for preservation. For example, a preservative with antifungal activity might be required in a medication containing a broad-spectrum antibacterial that has no or limited antifungal activity.

Transdermal patch systems delivering a fixed dose of drug to or through the skin can be considered single dose and, as such, might not seem to warrant a preservative if manufactured such that the system is microbe free. However, if the delivery system is aqueous, microbial growth could occur throughout the application period, where delivery/application is prolonged and the skin is rich in microorganisms. The limited number of transdermal medications including transmucosal patches that are available in the United States are, with three exceptions, preservative-free. However, the preservative-free products have nonaqueous vehicles, whereas the systems that are aqueous contain preservatives. In essence, a single-dose product of this nature does not necessarily obviate the need for a preservative where inclusion may be warranted. There has been much interest in using low-level electric current (iontophoresis) to provide prolonged transdermal delivery of medications, the technique being facilitated by the availability of microsized power (battery) units. Such presentations are single dose but may warrant the inclusion of a preservative. Drug delivery incorporating an ionizable preservative could pose complications such that the presence of preservative may affect drug delivery, or the ionizable preservative might be transported to or beyond dermal barriers causing inflammation, irritancy, or other unwanted effects. Such possibilities warrant consideration during dosage form design.

▶ PERFORMANCE STANDARDS FOR ANTIMICROBIAL QUALITY

Preservative Performance Standards

The diversity of microbes that could be present in a nonsterile product or in the environment during dosing or application requires a preservative system that possesses broad-spectrum antimicrobial activity. Compendial test methods and requirements reflect this, requiring that activity be demonstrated against defined strains of gram-positive (*Staphylococcus aureus*) and gram-negative (*Pseudomonas aeruginosa*) bacteria as well as *Candida* and *Aspergillus*, a yeast and mold respectively. The British Pharmacopoeia (BP) and European Pharmacopoeia (Ph. Eur.) recommend that these test organisms be supplemented where appropriate by additional strains/species. Examples are defined strains of *Escherichia coli* in liquid oral preparations and *Zygosaccharomyces rouxii* in liquid

oral preparations containing high concentrations of sugar. The United States Pharmacopeia (USP) also requires that efficacy be shown against *E coli*. Antiviral activity is not a requirement in any pharmacopoeia.

The pharmacopoeial requirements can be broadly summarized as requiring that the preservative provides a biocidal effect (following deliberate inoculation of the product) during the early incubation period (reduced microorganism counts) and a biostatic effect at later time intervals. Standards reflect the product type, the most stringent concerning parenteral and ophthalmic products. Specific requirements are also provided in the USP for oral antacid products. Liquid antacid products such as those containing aluminum hydroxide and magnesium and calcium hydroxides are difficult to preserve due to their capability to adsorb preservatives such as sodium benzoate and aminobenzoate esters. The relatively high pH of some such products can also cause hydrolysis of aminobenzoates.[9-11] The less stringent requirements in the USP for preservation of antacids reflect such challenges. Other pharmacopoeias do not make allowances for antacid-containing products.

Test methods and performance standards for determining the antimicrobial capabilities of preservatives in pharmaceutical products are detailed in current USP, Ph. Eur., BP, and Japanese Pharmacopoieas (JP). At the time of writing, the International Pharmacopoeia does not contain testing methods nor performance requirements but states that these are defined by the relevant national authority. The requirements of the BP are harmonized with and identical to those in the Ph. Eur. All pharmacopoeial monographs caution that a preservative must not be used as a substitute for GMP.

Protocols to determine antimicrobial effectiveness involve inoculation of defined concentrations of a range of cultured microorganisms to samples of the test product which is then stored at 20°C to 25°C (representing ambient conditions). Microbial counts are performed at times that are product specific over a maximum of 28 days to provide a measure of microbial kill or growth inhibition over time. The performance standards for different products in the various pharmacopoeias are summarized in Table 39.1.

Ph. Eur. stipulates that bactericidal activity be demonstrated over the first 14 days of the incubation period: Fungicidal requirements are slightly less stringent. The USP standards are less demanding, requiring a fungistatic rather than fungicidal effect, while the bactericidal requirements are also less stringent. Such differences can complicate dosage form design programs, particularly with novel therapeutic agents. Developing a single formulation for all regions where the product is to be made available reduces the complexity of dosage form design and clinical evaluation programs. If the dosage form used in pivotal clinical evaluation programs becomes the commercial product, the risks of biological or clinical nonequivalence

TABLE 39.1	Summary of pharmacopoeial preservative efficacy test requirements

Pharmacopoeia	Product Type (Aqueous)	Organisms	Criteria[a]	Log₁₀ Reduction (Minimum)					
				6 h	24 h	48 h	7 d	14 d	28 d
Ph. Eur./BP	Parenteral and ophthalmic	Bacteria	A	2	3				No recovery
			B		1		3		No increase from previous reading
		Fungi	A				2		
			B					1	
	Oral, oromucosal, and rectal	Bacteria						3	No increase from previous reading
		Fungi						1	
	Ear, nasal, cutaneous (topical), and inhalation products	Bacteria	A			2	3		No increase from previous reading
			B					3	
		Fungi	A					2	
			B					1	
USP/JP[b]	Parenteral and ophthalmic	Bacteria					1	3	No increase
		Fungi		No increase from initial					
	Oral, other than antacids	Bacteria						1	No increase
		Fungi		No increase from initial					
	Antacids	Bacteria		No increase from initial					
		Fungi							
	Topical, nonsterile nasal	Bacteria						2	No increase
		Fungi		No increase from initial					

Abbreviations: BP, British Pharmacopoeia; JP, Japanese Pharmacopeia; Ph. Eur., European Pharmacopoeia; USP, United States Pharmacopeia.

[a]A criteria are the recommended performance standards. B criteria may be acceptable, where higher preservative levels might risk adverse reactions. Use of B criteria must be justified.

[b]The JP does not contain requirements for antacid products.

are reduced. This is an important consideration where a conventional bioequivalence study is not possible or is complex, such as with topical or ophthalmic presentations. Regulatory agencies invariably defer to local/national compendial standards when reviewing information in an application for a new product approval. Products developed to meet USP preservative standards might not meet the more stringent Ph. Eur. performance requirements. A higher preservative inclusion level might be required for a product to be used in Europe than for a product formulated to USP standards. Conversely, if a product were to be developed to meet Ph. Eur. standards, it could be considered to be at variance with the generally accepted requirement that preservative levels be minimal so as to reduce possibilities for adverse reactions. Such differing compendial standards could require that two formulations with differing preservative levels be developed, adding complexity to the development program and postapproval supply chain management. There is no evidence that the less stringent USP requirements leads to poorly preserved products.

A useful summary of other subtle differences in pharmacopoeial requirements is provided elsewhere.[12]

An additional inconsistency in test and performance protocols can concern the formulation of antibacterial products, for instance β-lactam antibiotics. Most of these have limited stability in aqueous solution or suspension. Oral formulations for pediatric dosage are accordingly constituted as multidose liquids prior to use. Such liquid products have limited use periods, being constrained by the time that the product in the liquid state retains acceptable drug content, usually 7 to 14 days. Such limitations are usually acceptable because most pediatric infections are cleared within this time frame. But pharmacopoeial standards require that preservative efficacy be sustained over 28 days, a longer period than the dosing interval. Degradation products generated by β-lactam antibiotics can cause product pH to change over the 28-day test period, possibly affecting preservative efficacy. Buffering agents to stabilize pH cannot always be incorporated in such products because of catalytic effects on drug degradation or adverse effects on taste.[13] pH drift over the 14- to 28-day period could reduce the efficacy of the preservative. A requirement that preservative efficacy be sustained for 28 days when product usage time is shorter is difficult to defend. Some oral antibacterial preparations may also require refrigerated storage following constitution as liquids. Microbial growth or inhibition under such conditions may differ from that under pharmacopoeial test conditions (20°C-25°C) and not reflect in-use performance or labeling requirements.

In essence, there are inconsistencies in pharmacopoeial requirements for preservative performance. In practice, it may be impossible to define testing protocols and requirements applicable to every product form but some of the aforementioned anomalies could merit case-by-case decision making by regulatory assessors when reviewing product approval applications.

Preservative Screening

The compendial tests for preservative efficacy are labor-intensive, complex, and time-consuming. Duration of incubation is 28 days, and culture preparation and microbial counts during and postincubation along with data analysis all contribute to significant resource requirements and prolonged testing cycle times. It may also be necessary, based on findings during dosage form design, to change the preservative or adjust its content to meet

requirements. This can necessitate sequential tests that can delay a product development program. It may be prudent therefore to employ faster screening techniques at the outset such as determination of minimum preservative concentrations that inhibit or kill the test microorganisms in relevant media and testing conditions.[14,15] Such tests are used in antimicrobial research and in preservative evaluation programs in other disciplines to determine biocidal and biostatic effects. They can usually be completed in a matter of days and, provided that methodology such as culture media and test conditions are appropriate for the organism and formulation, the findings could increase the probability of subsequent success using compendial tests.

Other Considerations

Microbial contamination in a pharmaceutical product can emanate from materials, processes, and other operations listed in Figure 39.1. Such diversity and complexity can mean that a product that otherwise meets compendial preservative efficacy requirements may not be fully protected from contamination and microbial proliferation. To avoid such possibilities, potential contamination from sources such as materials, processes, containers, etc should be proactively considered during dosage form and process design so that particularly troublesome microbes can be identified and controlled appropriately. Such microorganisms may differ from those employed in compendial tests

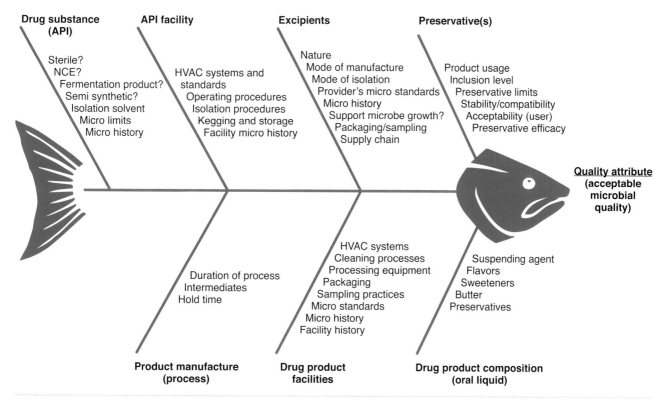

FIGURE 39.1 Fishbone diagram for assuring microbial quality of a preserved product. Abbreviations: API, active pharmaceutical ingredient; HVAC, heating, ventilation, and air conditioning; NCE, novel chemical entity.

and are termed *objectionable* in that their presence in a product can cause illness or product degradation. Parenteral products that were contaminated in this way caused fatalities attributable to contamination with microorganisms such as *Aspergillus fumigatus* and *Exserohilum rostratum* in the United States,[16] whereas *Bacillus cereus*–contaminated total nutrient product caused three fatalities in the United Kingdom.[17]

An objectionable organism has been identified as[18]

- A microorganism that, due to its numbers and pathogenicity, can cause infection, allergic response, or toxemia in patients receiving the product
- A microorganism that can adversely affect the appearance, physicochemical attributes, or therapeutic effect of a nonsterile product

Possibilities for contamination by microorganisms such as *Burkholderia cepacia* and *B cereus* elicit close attention from regulatory agencies, particularly the FDA in the light of their prominence in recalled and other contaminated products. The FDA and other regulatory agencies submit that it is the responsibility of the pharmaceutical manufacturer to show that any microorganisms that may be present in nonsterile medicinal products do not pose a safety risk.[18] The FDA has a well-established record of enforcing product recalls because of objectionable organisms. During the 8-year period, 1998-2006, nearly 90% of microbial-related recalls for nonsterile dosage

forms were attributable to such contamination.[18-20] Numbers approaching 75% were recorded over the period 2004-2011.[1]

Figure 39.2 outlines an approach to managing issues related to objectionable microorganisms. A more comprehensive decision tree is provided in a report by the Parenteral Drug Association (PDA).[20] The issue facing manufacturers is complex. Some level of microbial presence in materials used in nonsterile drug products is inevitable. Microbial limits for such input materials are accordingly included in pharmacopoeial monographs because input materials are not required to be sterile. A control strategy can accordingly be considered as being within the remit of GMP procedures for controlling less desirable organisms, that is, opportunistic pathogens that do not typically cause infections in the normal, healthy population.[1] However, exclusion of objectionable organisms from nonsterile products can be complex, being viewed as an undefined, critical quality attribute. There are no mandated tests nor limits at this time, and control strategies can be difficult to define. The PDA conducted a benchmarking survey to establish the scope of the issue. Respondents indicated that industry has no consistent practices to determine whether a nonspecified microorganism, isolated from a nonsterile product formulation is truly objectionable.[21] The PDA has also published guidance seeking to define risk management associated with manufacture and storage of nonsterile oral products.

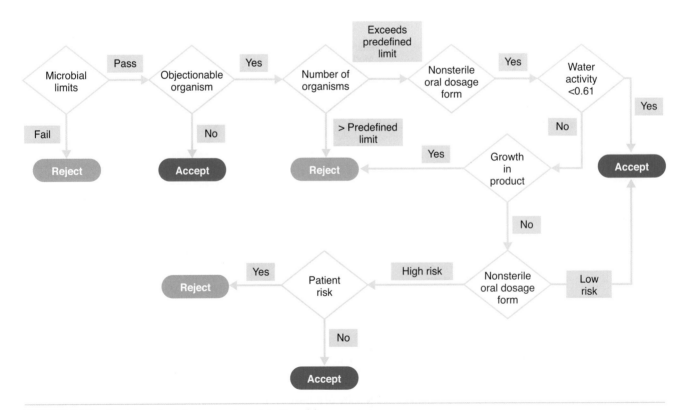

FIGURE 39.2   Decision chart for managing objectionable organisms.

Suggestions are made on how to identify microbes that engender significant concern on the part of regulatory agencies.[21] The PDA report does not list specific objectionable organisms because this could cause undue focus on specific microbes at the expense of an overarching, comprehensive review by the manufacturer. Instead, microbes commonly involved in product contamination/recalls are highlighted along with common opportunistic pathogens. Waterborne opportunistic pathogens, particularly *Pseudomonas* species and related organisms such as *Burkholderia* are most frequently cited in product recalls.[1] Many do not grow well under defined compendial test conditions and, are not readily identifiable and can complicate test findings. Alternative detection techniques can be used if similar or superior methodologies are shown to be appropriate for any suspect microorganisms.[22,23] Compliance with GMP processing requirements is also likely to constrain the presence of problem organisms. Examples of potentially objectionable organisms are provided in Table 39.2.[18,24] Microorganisms associated with the greatest number of major health care–associated outbreaks of infection (linked with nonsterile dosage forms) in rank order were *B cepacia* > *P aeruginosa* > *Serratia marcescens* > *Ralstonia mannitolilytica* > *B cereus* > *Klebsiella pneumoniae* > *Enterobacter cloacae* > *Serratia liquefaciens* > *Paecilomyces lilacinus* > *Enterobacter* species.

TABLE 39.2	Examples of objectionable organisms[a]
Bacteria	**Reported Sources**
Aerobacter species	Counterfeit herbal and medicinal products
Bacillus species	Counterfeit herbal and medicinal products
Brucella species	Hospitals
Burkholderia cepacia	Hospitals, recalled products
Campylobacter jejuni	Hospitals, recalled products
Clostridium botulism	Hospitals, recalled products
Corynebacterium diphtheriae	Hospitals
Enterobacter species	Counterfeit herbal and medicinal products
Escherichia coli	Hospitals
Klebsiella species	Contaminated nonsterile products
Legionella species	Emerging pathogen in hospital setting
Micrococcus species	Contaminated nonsterile products
Mycoplasma species	Emerging pathogen in hospital setting
Proteus species	Contaminated nonsterile products
Pseudomonas species	Hospitals, recalled products
Salmonella species	Hospitals, recalled products
Staphylococcus species	Hospitals, recalled products
Streptococcus species	Hospitals, recalled products
Yeasts/Molds	
Absidia species	Counterfeit herbal/medicinal products
Aspergillus	Recalled products and counterfeit herbal/medicinal products
Candida albicans	Hospitals and counterfeit medicinal/herbal products
Colletotrichum dermatium	Counterfeit herbal/medicinal products
Mucor	Counterfeit herbal/medicinal products
Penicillium species	Product recalls and counterfeit herbal/medicinal products
Pneumocystis jirovoci	Emerging pathogen in hospital setting
Rhizopus	Counterfeit herbal/medicinal products
Verticillium	Counterfeit herbal/medicinal products

[a]Additional examples can be found in Sutton[18] and US Food and Drug Administration.[25]

In contrast, the objectionable organisms that were involved in the greatest number of product recalls were *B cepacia* > unspecified fungal organisms > *B cereus* > *P aeruginosa* > *Elizabethkingia meningoseptica* > *Enterobacter gergoviae* > *Pseudomonas putida* > *Pseudomonas* species > *Salmonella* species. There was particular focus on *B cepacia* and *B cereus* in such reports. *B cepacia* is an opportunistic waterborne pathogen typically infecting immunocompromised people such as cystic fibrosis sufferers. There is accumulating evidence that it is a common contaminant in cosmetics, disinfectants, and in preserved multiuse pharmaceuticals.[26] A review of 16 representative product recalls identified *B cepacia* as the causative organism.[25,26] The primary causes of contamination were cited as

- Poor design of water systems (eg, the system did not prevent stagnant water formation) that can rapidly lead to biofilm formation
- Poor control of water systems (eg, failure to validate operations and processes, lack of scheduled repair and maintenance programs, and improper sanitization procedures)
- Inappropriate quality of water (eg, use of potable water to clean and/or rinse equipment)
- Inadequate cleaning and cleaning procedures (eg, inadequate equipment drying times, inadequate sterilization of finished product, inappropriate storage of intermediates, and inappropriate time/temperature/relative humidity controls)
- Inadequate testing and inappropriate specifications (eg, incomplete or incorrect antimicrobial effectiveness testing, use of contaminated input materials, and inadequate microbiological analysis)
- Inadequate environmental validation of equipment handling processes or product contact surfaces

The prominence of *B cepacia* may be attributable to its prevalence in water and other environments, resistance to many common preservatives, adept biofilm formation, and possession of several efflux pump and other mechanisms. Some strains can even grow in distilled water in the temperature range 12°C to 48°C, highlighting the resilience and adaptability of this organism.[26-30]

The FDA has long had concerns regarding *B cepacia* contamination in pharmaceutical products. The agency recognizes that there are currently no reliable methodologies for its identification in multiuse products but states that "pharmaceutical companies bear the responsibility to monitor their components, processes, and products to prevent contamination of objectionable organisms." The FDA cautions that manufacturers should not be overly reliant on preservatives for such control but use validated in-process controls such as effective cleaning, disinfection, and drying of pharmaceutical manufacturing equipment as part of GMP-related practices. This is aligned with FDA policy that preservatives should not be surrogates for poor GMPs. Overall, the hazards presented by organisms such as *B cepacia* can be summarized as

- Potential to cause infections in some patient populations[25,26]
- Resistance to chemical preservatives and capability to readily share this resistance factor[29]
- Detection difficulties when using conventional microbiological techniques[30]
- Ability to grow in hostile low-nutrient conditions[28,29]

The many possibilities for contamination, the challenges associated with detection, and the resilience of *B cepacia* suggest that a risk-based assessment is preferable for determining the probability of this opportunistic pathogen being present in a medicinal product rather than a compendial "test and limit" approach. Factors germane to such a risk assessment could include

- the route and method of product use
- the patient population (eg, children, immunocompromised patients)
- the type of product and its propensity to support microbial growth

B cereus is a gram-positive aerobic, facultative anaerobic spore-forming bacterium, claimed to be one of the more prevalent spore-forming microbes in soil, dust, sediments, food, and plants.[30] Consequently, it can be consumed in diet and is normally present in human intestinal flora. Its toxicity is closely related to production of tissue-destructive toxins. The *Bacillus* group comprises several closely related bacterial species (eg, *B cereus sensu stricto*, *Bacillus anthracis*, *Bacillus thuringiensis*, *Bacillus mycoides*, *Bacillus pseudomycoides*, *Bacillus weihenstephanensis*, and *Bacillus cytotoxicus*).[34-36] Such heterogeneity may contribute to the technical difficulties associated with their identification, but these could be mitigated using specific media (eg, rapid agar-AES chemunex [BACARA™] or Brilliance™ *B cereus* agar [BBCA™]).[22,23] In addition to association with food poisoning and eye infections, these organisms are also linked with clinical conditions such as anthrax-like progressive pneumonia, sepsis, and central nervous system (CNS) infections, predominantly in immunosuppressed patients and neonates. They are also associated with postsurgical wound infections especially when catheters are used.[31-34] *B cereus* is the spore-forming bacterium most often associated with contaminated nonsterile materials.[35] Contaminated alcohol swabs used in a surgical center in the United States lead to several fatalities.[36] *B cereus* contamination can be caused by inadequacies associated with:[37]

- inadequate cleaning and disinfection procedures
- inadequate controls for air-handling systems
- inadequate microbial controls for input materials
- inadequate contamination control strategies such as deficient environmental monitoring programs

The FDA has indicated that accepting a level of spore-forming microbes as part of the standard environmental flora was a deficiency in such cases, implying that these organisms be totally absent rather than adopting a risk-based assessment process to their presence.[38]

Pitt et al[39] stated that little if any information is available in the literature concerning *B cereus* infections in any body site that could be linked with use of personal care products. The authors conclude that

- Low levels of *B cereus* spores may occasionally be present in near-eye cosmetics and that these products have been used by consumers for many years
- Exposure to *B cereus* is more likely to occur through other routes (eg, dust-borne contamination) due to its ubiquity and the resistance of its spores
- The organism has also been recovered from the eyes of healthy individuals
- Although there may be a potential hazard, the risk of severe eye infections consequent to exposure through contaminated near-eye cosmetics is judged to be vanishingly small

In cases where nonsterile oral products have been microbiologically tested in a clinical setting and shown to be contaminated (eg, with *Bacillus*, *Klebsiella*, or *Candida* species), the cause has been attributable to poor handling of the pharmaceutical products during dispensing or repackaging, rather than GMP inadequacies.[40] *B cereus* has also been linked with contamination of sterile-labeled products in aseptic manufactured products. It was the causative agent in 23 cases of sepsis in babies (including 3 fatalities) being administered intravenous total parenteral nutrition in the United Kingdom during 2013-2014. The source of the strain identified in 19 patients was subsequently traced to environmental samples from the aseptic area on the day of product manufacture. Investigations by the Medicines and Healthcare Products Regulatory Agency (MHRA) found no evidence to suggest that individual ingredients, product components, or materials caused the contamination. Airborne contamination was considered to be the source of the outbreak. The recalled supplies were found to be contaminated with *B cereus*.[17]

The question has been posed whether *B cereus* warrants categorization as an objectionable microorganism.[1,18] For sterile products, the answer was an unequivocal "yes" (as with any microbe), but nonsterile oral products may require a more nuanced attitude. Regarding the related question of it being a significant concern, responses to its presence in a pharmaceutical manufacturing environment may depend on its ubiquity. Opinions have been advanced to the effect that the issue resides with the class as a whole (ie, *Bacillus* species rather than constraining it to *B cereus*).[18] However, *B cereus* is one of the more virulent members of the class. The high resistance of spore-forming bacteria such as *Bacillus* species

and *Clostridium* species to cleaning, disinfection, and drying makes it difficult to eradicate them from a manufacturing environment. Facility design, personnel practices, and compliance as well as cleaning and disinfection procedures must necessarily take account of such challenges.[20] In summary, meeting compendial requirements for preservative efficacy does not necessarily guarantee that microbial contamination and growth will not occur. Product and facility-based risk assessment programs allied to GMP practices, along with validating and securing the supply chain, can all contribute to maintaining microbial cleanliness of the pharmaceutical product.

So-called hurdle technology can be a useful means of developing and implementing what might seem to be daunting risk mitigation programs.[41,42] The tool was originally developed for preservation of spoilable foodstuffs, but it can be equally applicable to pharmaceutical products. Identifying the factors that optimize microbial proliferation (pH, temperature, presence of water, oxygen concentration, nutrient levels, etc) can suggest approaches for impeding microbial growth by creating nonoptimal microbial proliferation conditions ("hurdles") to contribute to microcidal or microstatic environments in materials handling, storage, formulation, product manufacture, packaging, etc and an effective control strategy. Possibilities might include

- Adjust product pH to more acidic or basic regions to attenuate microbial growth.
- Raise temperature during processing or reduce during transit and/or storage.
- Reduce water content/activity in the product by including humectants such as polyols or nonaqueous solvents such as propylene glycol.
- Reduce oxygen concentration during manufacture or replace by nitrogen in product headspace, and otherwise minimized during transport and storage by suitable packaging.
- Include a preservative, possibly more than one or increase its concentration.

It may not always be feasible to implement each and every one of the above possibilities. Product and process-related considerations can decree otherwise. Nevertheless, the concept of hurdle technology merits exploration as a contributor to product preservation.

▶ FACTORS INFLUENCING PRESERVATIVE CHOICE

The prime requirement for preservative performance is to provide the requisite antimicrobial activity for product preservation. There are also usually additional, product-specific considerations that need to be incorporated in the target product profile for dosage form design. A program to design a preservation system for a specific product should take account of the physicochemical properties of the preservative, of the drug substance, and of other product components (excipients) as well as the mode of product manufacture, dosage, and use. Preservatives permitted in pharmaceuticals and foodstuffs can be constrained by specific attribute requirements of the pharmaceutical product and its mode of use/administration (Table 39.3). Properties associated with the preservative such as irritancy (topical, oral, parenteral, ophthalmic), odor, and taste (oral liquid, inhalation, intranasal products)

TABLE 39.3 Allowable preservatives in food and pharmaceuticals in the European Community[a]

E Number	Name	Food	Pharmaceutical
E200	Sorbic acid	Yes	Yes
E202	Potassium sorbate	Yes	Yes
E203	Calcium sorbate	Yes	Limited—less soluble than other salts
E210	Benzoic acid	Yes	Yes
E211	Sodium benzoate	Yes	Yes
E212	Potassium benzoate	Yes	Yes
E213	Calcium benzoate	Yes	Limited—less soluble than other salts
E214	Ethyl p-hydroxybenzoate	Yes	Yes
E215	Sodium ethyl p-hydroxybenzoate	Yes	Yes
E218	Methyl p-hydroxybenzoate	Yes	Yes
E219	Sodium methyl p-hydroxybenzoate	Yes	Yes
E220	Sulfur dioxide	Yes	No—toxicity considerations
E221	Sodium sulfite	Yes	No—toxicity considerations
E222	Sodium hydrogen sulfite	Yes	No—toxicity considerations
E223	Sodium metabisulfite	Yes	No—toxicity considerations
E224	Potassium metabisulfite	Yes	No—toxicity considerations
E226	Calcium sulfite	Yes	No—toxicity considerations
E227	Calcium hydrogen sulfite	Yes	No—toxicity considerations
E228	Potassium hydrogen sulfite	Yes	No—toxicity considerations
E234	Nisin	Yes	No—toxicity considerations
E235	Natamycin	Yes	No—toxicity considerations
E239	Hexamethylene tetramine	Yes	No—toxicity considerations
E242	Dimethyl dicarbonate	Yes	No—toxicity considerations
E243	Ethyl lauroyl arginate	Yes	No
E249	Potassium nitrite	Yes	No—toxicity considerations
E250	Sodium nitrite	Yes	No—toxicity considerations
E251	Sodium nitrate	Yes	No—toxicity considerations
E252	Potassium nitrate	Yes	No—toxicity considerations
E280	Propionic acid	Yes	Yes
E281	Sodium propionate	Yes	Yes
E282	Calcium propionate	Yes	Limited—less soluble than other salts
E283	Potassium propionate	Yes	Yes
E284	Boric acid	Yes	Yes
E285	Sodium tetraborate; borax	Yes	No
E1105	Lysozyme	Yes	No

[a]From EU-approved additives and E numbers: https//www.food.gov.uk/business-guidance/eu-approved-additives-and-e-numbers.[43]

can influence user acceptability, compliance, and consequently product efficacy. A thorough awareness of relevant properties of potential preservatives along with those of the active ingredient and the other product components can avoid much iterative trial and error studies that could otherwise prolong a development program. The compendial standards for antimicrobial effectiveness that were summarized earlier are demanding. For instance, few, if any, therapeutic anti-infectives have both antibacterial and antifungal activity. Yet, a preservative is required to be effective against a diversity of microbes. A target product profile to guide preservative selection might accordingly comprise the following:

- It meets compendial (pharmacopoeial) preservative performance standards.
- Preservative is effective over the product pH range.
- Preservative is effective at the lower limit for preservative content in the product specification.
- Solubility of the preservative (in the appropriate phase if relevant) is not affected by other product components or by conditions encountered during product manufacture, storage, transport, or use that compromise preservative efficacy.
- Preservative is physically and chemically compatible with the other product components.
- Preservative does not adversely affect product-specific quality attributes such as taste, odor, irritation, etc at the inclusion level in the product.
- Effect is sustained throughout product lifetime, including use.

Requirements such as safety and lack of pharmacologic effects at the levels employed, being self-evident, are not listed in the preceding text.

Some textbooks and promotional literature recommend specific inclusion levels or ranges for preservatives. Such information, although useful on occasion, should also be treated with caution. Preservative efficacy can be influenced by components that are included to confer other attributes to the product. Choice of preservative can also be product specific, taking account of preservative properties such as

- Aqueous solubility and pH-solubility profile
- Dissociation constant and partition coefficient (where relevant)
- Product-specific organoleptic properties that may include odor, taste, irritancy, or inflammation
- Compatibility with formulation and packaging components
- Chemical and physical stability in the product

Aqueous Solubility

The properties of the active ingredient may require that a buffer or other pH-modifying agent be included

TABLE 39.4 Aqueous solubility values of *p*-aminobenzoic acid esters (parabens) and product inclusion levels

Ester Type	Solubility (mg/mL at 20°C-25°C)	Usual Inclusion Level (mg/mL)
Methyl	2.50	1-2.5
Ethyl	0.80	1-2.5
Propyl	0.46	1-2.5
Butyl	0.20	1-4

in the formulation. The preservative system needs to be soluble over the pH range engendered by such material. Rate of preservative dissolution should also be rapid within any defined pH range if the product is constituted as a liquid prior to use. Preservative solubility should also not be so temperature dependent that fluctuations during product manufacture, transport, and storage/use could cause precipitation. Such requirements may not be onerous for most commonly used preservatives, with low inclusion levels being helpful in such respects. Exceptions can include the aminobenzoate esters (parabens). These have aqueous solubility values that are close to the inclusion levels required for microbial inhibition (Table 39.4). Modest levels of acceptable nonaqueous solvents such as propylene glycol and glycerol can sometimes be included to enhance preservative solubility; they may also contribute to antimicrobial efficacy. Combinations of preservatives may also be used to ensure that inclusion levels are lower than their saturation solubilities in the product.

Rates of dissolution of aminobenzoate esters can be slow, making them potentially unsuitable for products that are manufactured as solids and constituted as liquids at time of use. Incorporation of these preservatives in conventional liquid products during product manufacture may be facilitated by raising the temperature to increase dissolution, but there can be a risk of preservative loss due to volatilization or due to precipitation when the liquid cools. Low-temperature excursions during product storage or transport may also cause precipitation of preservative when inclusion levels are near saturation solubility. Appropriate travel tests or temperature cycling studies may help identify such potential risks.

Solubility of ionizable preservatives can be influenced by pH. Benzoic acid is essentially in un-ionized form at pH 2, with aqueous solubility being in the region of 3.5 mg/mL at 25°C. Sodium benzoate, in contrast, is highly soluble at neutral pH (630 mg/mL at 25°C). Similar solubility relationships are apparent for the other acids listed in Table 39.5.

Dissociation Constant and Partition Coefficient

Benzoic, sorbic, and propionic acids are most effective at low pH, reflecting their un-ionized states (see Table 39.5). Higher inclusion levels are required where product pH is greater. Some oral liquid formulations containing sodium benzoate contain citrate or other buffers to provide the requisite pH for antimicrobial activity and possibly also to ensure acceptable stability of the active ingredient. Nondissociated forms of preservatives favor hydrophobic environments in biphasic oil/water-based emulsion-type systems rather than the aqueous (hydrophilic) phase. Hence, there is less preservative in the aqueous phase where its presence is required for efficacy. Preservative inclusion levels need to reflect such partitioning tendencies.

Preservative disposition can also be influenced by the nature of the oil phase in biphasic preparations.[44] Cream-based topical products or oral emulsion systems containing a vegetable oil are generally more difficult to preserve than those containing a mineral oil because of the higher oil/water partition coefficients of vegetable oils (Table 39.6). Such partitioning behaviors in cream/lotion (aqueous based) formulations mean that an analytical method to determine total preservative content in a product can provide spurious information on preservation capability. In such cases, analytical methods need to be designed to determine preservative levels in the aqueous phase. Oil/water partitioning rates can also be gradual, so it may be prudent to explore time-related effects on partitioning during dosage form design and product stability studies. Partition coefficients can also be temperature dependent, so there is potential for formulations, stored under different conditions to exhibit what could be spurious or conflicting results if tested for preservative efficacy. It may sometimes be possible to provide a more favorable environment for preservative distribution by including acceptable nonaqueous water-miscible liquids such as propylene glycol or glycerol to confer a measure of "hydrophobicity" in the aqueous phase and enhance preservative disposition.

TABLE 39.6 Oil/water partition coefficients for preservatives and some nonaqueous liquids[a]

Preservative	Oil	Partition Coefficient
Methyl paraben	Almond oil	7.5
	Mineral oil	0.1
	Isopropyl myristate	18
	Diethyl adipate	200
Ethyl paraben		26
Propyl paraben	Soya bean oil	87
Butyl paraben		280
Benzoic acid		6.1
Sorbic acid	Almond oil	3.3
	Mineral oil	0.21
Phenol	Arachis oil	5
	Mineral oil	0.07

[a]From McElroy J. https://www.slideshow.net/JimMcElroy/antimicrobial-presentaton-overview-for-formulation-and-process-scientists.

Organoleptic Considerations

Properties such as palatability (taste/bitterness), irritancy, inflammation, and possibly odor, while not affecting antimicrobial activity *per se*, can influence user acceptability and compliance and, by default, the effectiveness of the medication. Such attributes need to be considered in the context of, the preservative properties, including inclusion level, site and mode of administration or application, and possibly duration of treatment (product use). Information in chemical databases on agents used as preservatives invariably concern neat (undiluted) materials. Undesirable properties like irritancy, odor, or bitterness may not be manifest at concentrations used for product preservation. It may be advisable, in cases where

TABLE 39.5 Ionization (pKa), pH, and partition coefficients (Log P) of organic acid preservatives

| Property | Organic Acid (pKa) | | |
	Benzoic Acid (4.19)	Sorbic Acid (4.76)	Propionic Acid (4.88)
pH	% Un-ionized		
2	99.4	99.8	99.9
3	94.1	98.3	98.7
4	61.3	85.2	88.4
5	13.70	36.5	43.50
5.5	4.78	15.4	19.23
6	1.56	5.4	7.04
6.5	0.50	1.8	2.34
7	0.16	0.6	0.76
Octanol/ Water Partition Coefficient (Log P)	1.87	0.33	0.76

a potential preservative is listed as a known irritant, that a suitable preclinical test be used to determine whether this attribute would present concerns at the product inclusion level. Similar considerations apply to other organoleptic properties.

Children usually find liquid medications easier to swallow than solid units. However, an orally dosed liquid product that is bitter tasting may not be acceptable to pediatric patients or to some adults if dosage is chronic. Bitterness may also be an issue with oral inhalation products and nasal sprays due to the presence of a limited numbers of taste buds in the pharynx and nasopharynx. Preservatives such as benzyl alcohol are listed as bitter, but inclusion levels for preservation may be lower than the bitterness threshold. It may also be possible to attenuate a bitter or similar undesirable taste by including an excipient that elevates the bitterness threshold of the bitter-tasting material. Sucrose can be particularly effective in this respect, but inclusion levels may need to be high. Other saccharides are generally less useful. A flavoring agent such as aspartame may be helpful in some cases.

The freedom from bitterness of sodium benzoate may account for its wide use in pediatric antibacterial formulations constituted as liquids on dispensing. Its good aqueous solubility and rapid dissolution rate are also helpful for ready constitution. Some antibacterials such as β-lactams require mildly acidic environments for acceptable drug stability in the liquid state. The presence of citrate in many products containing sodium benzoate suggests that it is included to provide a favorable pH environment for antimicrobial efficacy as well as acceptable drug stability in the constituted state.

Irritancy or Inflammation

Irritancy can be problematic with parenteral, topical, intranasal, and ophthalmic products and where product is applied to damaged skin or other sensitive tissues. Benzalkonium chloride has been reported as irritant to ocular tissues; yet, it is the most widely used preservative in ophthalmic products. This suggests that irritancy may be less of an issue at the low inclusion levels in such products (0.003%-0.01%). Concerns have also been expressed that prolonged use in ocular may be detrimental to ocular tissue.[48] Such disquiet may become more prominent as prolonged life spans has lead to conditions such as glaucoma becoming more prominent and require chronic use of ophthalmic medications.

Another quaternary ammonium compound, benzododecinium bromide, is present at an inclusion level of 0.012% in an ophthalmic gel available in the United States. It is listed as a serious eye and skin irritant in chemical databases, but irritancy may not be manifest or prominent at the low inclusion levels required for preservation.

▶ PRESERVATIVE SELECTION PROGRAMS

Selecting a preservative system can be relatively straightforward for some products where the required product attributes may be aligned with preservative performance requirements. Others may warrant a comprehensive program because the antimicrobial activity of a preservative can depend on its inclusion level, the environment engendered by the other product components, and the disposition of the preservative in complex formulations such as emulsion-based creams, lotions, multilamellar lipid-based systems, etc. Furthermore, a preservative may provide acceptable antimicrobial efficacy but adversely affect other product quality attributes. Hence, designing a preservation system can be complex.

Product pH

Product pH may be determined or mandated by considerations such as drug solubility, stability, its partition coefficient, or organoleptic properties. A low-solubility form of the drug or a product pH range conferring low solubility may be effective at masking a bitter taste of an orally dosed drug. Conversely, it may be necessary to control product pH to assure adequate drug solubility for a parenterally administered product. Preservative selection must reflect such considerations. Table 39.7 lists pH effects on the ionization and inclusion level requirements of benzoic acid/sodium benzoate for adequate preservation.[46] Relationships such as these may complicate preservative selection if the required higher inclusion levels were to impart a bitter or other unpleasant attribute to the product.

pH change during product shelf life/use can impact preservative efficacy if degree of ionization is affected. Such change might be caused by modest (but acceptable) drug degradation altering pH or possibly by alkali extracted from glass bottle containers. Minor pH changes may not be detrimental to drug stability but could change the degree of preservative ionization and alter antimicrobial performance.

		Concentration for Preservation	
pH	% Un-ionized	%	mg/mL
5	13.70	0.5	5
5.8	2.45	1.5	15
6.5	0.50	2.5	25

TABLE 39.7 pH, ionization, and preservative efficacy of benzoic acid/sodium benzoate[a]

[a]Adapted from Bean.[46] Copyright © 1961. With permission.

Combinations of Preservatives

The wide range of potential microbial contaminants and the diversity of the test organisms to be inhibited can make it difficult to find a single preservative with the requisite broad-spectrum activity that also meets other product attribute requirements. A preservative might meet requirements for activity against some test microbes but not perform adequately against others. An additional preservative, possibly possessing a different mechanism of action or antimicrobial spectrum, may help provide the requisite cover. A combination may also help reduce inclusion levels where a preservative has an undesirable characteristic such as irritancy, odor, or taste or where the level required for efficacy is close to its saturation solubility in the vehicle. Consequently, many products contain more than one preservative.

The solubilities of aminobenzoate preservatives decrease as their molecular masses increase. Their saturation solubility values are also close to the levels required for microbial inhibition (see Table 39.4). Combinations of esters are accordingly used in many oral and topical products to enable lower inclusion levels that pose less risk of precipitation. Sodium benzoate or potassium sorbate is combined with aminobenzoate esters in a number of oral and topical products.[47] Aminobenzoate esters are particularly effective against fungi and gram-positive bacteria but less so against gram-negative bacteria such as *Pseudomonas*. Antipseudomonal activity can be enhanced by combination with benzyl alcohol, ethylenediaminetetraacetic acid (EDTA), or phenylethanol.[48] The aromatic alcohols, benzyl alcohol, and phenylethyl alcohol can enhance the activities of BKC and chlorhexidine against *P aeruginosa*.[49]

The outer surfaces of bacterial cells are negatively charged and stabilized by divalent cations. The chelating agent EDTA binds to and disrupts such sites on microbial cell wall membranes by complex formation with the divalent cations, thereby enhancing the effect of cationic preservatives.[50] Other chelating agents such as citrates can have a similar effect. Benzalkonium chloride is widely used in ophthalmic products but can have irritant and inflammatory effects on ocular tissue, particularly when treatment is long term. Combination with EDTA can enable its concentration to be reduced to alleviate such effects. Coformulation with chlorhexidine or other biguanides can also enhance efficacy of BKC against gram-negative bacteria.[51] Dose-related bronchoconstriction has been reported when BKC is used in nebulizer solutions so use is discouraged in such products.[52,53]

Excipients included in a product for other purposes may also contribute to antimicrobial efficacy. Propylene glycol, glycerol, and ethanol may be used as solvents, emollients, or penetration enhancers in liquid oral and topical formulations. Inclusion levels for such purposes are invariably insufficient for preservation but may broaden the antimicrobial spectrum or help reduce the inclusion level of the formal preservative. Propylene glycol can have a preservative effect as a 10% aqueous solution. It also enhances the antibacterial efficacy (and solubility) of para-aminobenzoate preservatives, being present in several liquid oral pharmaceutical products containing aminobenzoates. Glycerol is also present in several aminobenzoate-containing orally dosed products.[47]

Sucrose and other polyols can be included in oral liquid products as sweetening agents or as lyophilization aids in parenteral products. Sucrose evinces a strong antimicrobial effect at concentrations exceeding 85% but can be a microbial nutrient at lower concentrations. The level required for preservative efficacy probably renders its use as the sole preservative impractical in most cases.

The flavoring agent vanillin and its ethyl analogue possess some antimicrobial activity, being generally more effective as antifungals. Optimum effect is seen at approximately pH 6, although the pH effect is slight.[54] Vanillins are widely used in the food industry and as flavors in solid oral dosage forms that may be chewed or dispersed in water, but there are no reports of use in liquid pharmaceutical products. Combinations of essential oil extracts from frankincense and myrrh have been used as preservatives in some cultures for many centuries, being listed in pharaonic pharmacopoeias, reportedly possessing additive and synergistic antimicrobial effects against pseudomonads.[55] The possible variable quality of natural products (with respect to the active components) may require that the molecular structures of any preserving components be identified and possibly isolated/synthesized if such materials (or their components) were to be adopted for product preservation.

Other Considerations

Preservatives chosen for inclusion in the product need to fulfill the compendial requirements for antimicrobial efficacy discussed earlier. It may also be prudent to determine whether the preservative system is also effective against other microbes such as the objectionable organisms discussed earlier that may be potential product contaminants because of association with the facility, the process, or the product component materials.

▶ RETENTION OF PRESERVATIVE EFFICACY

Preservative efficacy can be compromised during manufacture, shelf life, and use. Possibilities include

- Chemical degradation of the preservative with levels in solution falling below those required to sustain efficacy
- Physical losses due to phenomena such as volatility of the preservative, adsorption on to other product components, or possibly polymorphic transformations that reduce preservative solubility

Preservative Chemical Structure Changes

Preservatives can be considered analogous to drug substances in that they possess functional groups necessary for biological (antimicrobial) activity and to enable their metabolism, transformation, and excretion after ingestion or application. Such properties can also render them susceptible to transformation, facilitated by the aqueous *milieu* in preserved products. Parabens preservatives are particularly susceptible to base-catalyzed ester hydrolysis at higher pH, degrading by classic pseudo-first-order kinetics, shorter chain analogues such as methylparaben being least stable. Their stabilities in solution are not markedly influenced by pH up to about pH 6.5, but degradation rates can be significant at about pH 7.5 and above.[56] The predictable and well-characterized degradation kinetics of these agents may make it feasible to conduct scientifically relevant, accelerated (high temperature) stability studies in prototype products to predict long-term preservative stability. The formulation scientist may then have the information to implement and justify the inclusion of an overage of preservative to compensate for degradation or other losses during product manufacture or storage.

Sorbic acid can be a very good preservative but is relatively unstable in semisolid and liquid preparations. It is also incompatible with bases, oxidizing and reducing agents.[57] Modes of its degradation are complex. Autooxidation generates acetaldehyde and β-carboxyacreloin end products and numerous other volatile aldehydes such as malonaldehyde, acrolein, crotonaldehyde as well as related furans (2-methylfuran, 2-acetyl-5-methylfuran, 2,5-dimethylfuran). These, in turn, may promote aldehyde-type interactions with other formulation components, including the drug substance or another preservative (if present). Sorbic acid can be stabilized by phenolic antioxidants such as 0.02% wt/wt propyl gallate.[58]

Other preservatives that are susceptible to degradation by strong oxidizing agents include phenylethanol, EDTA, thiomerosal, and the antioxidants, propyl gallate and butylated hydroxyanisole (BHA). Interaction between BHA, peroxides, and permanganates might even cause spontaneous combustion under certain conditions. It would be rare for strong oxidizing agents to be present in a medicinal product, but benzoyl peroxide is included in topical formulations to treat acne.

Preservative-excipient interactions may involve polymeric excipients used as suspending agents, viscosity enhancers, or other physical stabilizers. The polyethylene derivatives, polyethylene glycol, and polysorbate 80 can interact with aminobenzoate esters.[59] Cationic preservatives such as BKC are, unsurprisingly, incompatible with anionic surfactants or with suspending agents such as sodium carboxymethylcellulose, sodium alginate, and bentonite.[60] Nonionic surfactants can compromise the activities of benzyl alcohol[61] and phenoxyethanol.[62]

Preservative-excipient interactions may not necessarily be caused by excipients *per se* but by low-level residues or impurities from excipient manufacture or that are formed during their storage or transport. Povidone (polyvinylpyrrolidone), crospovidone, polyethylene glycol, and polysorbates can contain residual peroxides.[63] Levels may be low, but high excipient-preservative ratios in a product could cause significant interaction. Possibilities for such interactions merit exploration in preformulation and early formulation studies to help guide preservative selection. Such studies may not always be fully predictive; interactions may take time to be manifest, or the levels of reactive residues may vary in the materials being tested and complicate assessment programs. Nevertheless, such investigations are good risk assessment and mitigation practice.

Potential consequences of preservative-excipient interactions can be 2-fold; the functionality of excipient or preservative can be compromised or, if a significant level of interaction product is generated, there may be patient-associated effects, such as irritancy. Table 39.8 lists potential residues that may be associated with common excipients. Interactions may not necessarily involve conventional chemical transformations but more subtle phenomena such as hydrogen bonding, aggregation, or complex formation. The overall preservative content, determined by chemical analysis, may not change, but the preservative may not be fully available in its active form, so its efficacy is reduced. Monitoring preservative efficacy regularly during stability studies is advisable, to mitigate such risk. Analytical techniques to monitor preservative content in stability testing programs need to be designed to determine levels in solution in liquid formulations or in the aqueous phase in complex biphasic or multiphase systems because the preservative needs to be in aqueous solution to evince an antimicrobial effect.

TABLE 39.8 Residues and impurities that may be present in common pharmaceutical excipients[a]

Excipient	Impurity/Residue
Povidone, crospovidone	Peroxides
Polysorbates	Peroxides
Fixed oils, lipids	Antioxidants
Lactose	Aldehydes, reducing sugars
Benzyl alcohol	Benzaldehyde
Polyethylene glycol	Aldehydes, peroxides, organic acids
Microcrystalline cellulose	Lignin, hemicelluloses, water
Starch	Formaldehyde

[a]Data from Crowley and Martini.[63]

Some preservatives can form ion pairs or in situ salts with drug substances. The β-blocker, timolol, is used to treat glaucoma and forms an ion pair with sorbic acid. This has been proposed as a mechanism for enhancing its ocular bioavailability, but the impact on preservative efficacy has not been reported.[64] Some preservatives can form cocrystals with drug substances. Behaviors such as these may possibly have positive effects, but unanticipated cocrystal formation would typically be expected to remove free preservative from the aqueous phase in liquid oral or cream/lotion products, reducing the antimicrobial effect. Many approaches used to form cocrystals are akin to those employed during manufacture of semisolid and suspension formulations such as high energy mixing and homogenization. Preservatives such as alcohols, phenols, and carboxylic acids also have the appropriate synthons to act as effective coformers. Examples include nalidixic acid forming cocrystals with phenolic coformers[65] and fluoxetine forming cocrystals with benzoic acid.[66] Even preservatives that do not possess obvious synthons may act as good coformers. Methylparaben has been reported as forming cocrystals with β-lactam antibiotics.[67] The examples summarized in Table 39.8 do not represent the totality of excipient-related interactions but illustrate the wide range of possibilities. Interactions can be specific to the individual preservative, drug, excipient and product environment.

Physical Losses

Many drugs are isolated in salt form to facilitate solubility in aqueous media. If the active moiety of the preservative carries a negative charge, interaction with a positively charged drug could reduce solubility of both components, depress levels in solution and affect preservative activity or biopharmaceutical performance. The physical and chemical properties of antacids that are inorganic salts make their preservation a challenge. Long-established antacids such as aluminum hydroxide, magnesium/calcium hydroxide, or magnesium trisilicate or a combination of these can compromise preservative efficacy by adsorbing preservatives such as the aminobenzoates, sodium benzoate, chlorhexidine, and sorbic acid.[9-11] Such behaviors, together with the relatively high pH of some antacid products, make them difficult to preserve and reflect the lower USP acceptance criteria for antacid products (see Table 39.1). Adsorption by packaging components, excipients and even processing equipment (eg, metal) can also deplete preservative content (Table 39.9)

Sublimation

The para-aminobenzoate esters,[73-76] benzoic acid, and the liquid preservatives benzyl alcohol,[65] phenoxyethanol,[62] can sublime or volatilize. This can cause losses

TABLE 39.9	Preservatives susceptible to adsorption by excipients or packaging materials	
Preservative	**Adsorbent (Substrate)**	**Reference**
Benzalkonium chloride	Hypromellose	68
	Filter membranes	69
Benzoic acid	Kaolin	70
Benzyl alcohol	Polyethylene, natural rubber	61
Chlorobutanol	Polyethylene, rubber stoppers, bentonite, magnesium trisilicate	71
Chlorhexidine	Negatively charged polymeric excipients (eg, sodium carboxymethylcellulose, sodium alginate)	72
p-Aminobenzoate esters	Magnesium trisilicate, ion exchange resins, some plastics	73, 74, 75, 76
Phenoxyethanol	PVC, cellulose-based excipients	62
Phenylmercuric salts	Some suspending agents, rubber stoppers, polyethylene, polypropylene	77
Sorbic acid/sorbates	Polypropylene, PVC, polyethylene	57
Thimerosal	Polyethylene, rubber, metals, quaternary ammonium compounds	78

Abbreviation: PVC, polyvinyl chloride.

during processing if heating or vacuum (lyophilisation) are used, or during product shelf life (long-term storage) due to diffusion of vaporized preservative through or adsorption plastic components of syringes, or elastomeric closures. An overage and appropriate end-of-shelf life limits may need to be considered to compensate for such losses, with limits validated to provide assurance that preservative efficacy is maintained throughout product life.

Precipitation

Precipitation of the preservative from solution during manufacture, transport, or storage reduces antimicrobial efficacy. Reported incidents usually concern ionic interactions, particularly with polyvalent cations. Examples include

- Sorbic acid[57] and chlorhexidine[72] can be "salted out" by calcium ions.
- Chlorhexidine[72] can interact with magnesium ions.
- Phenylmercuric nitrate can be precipitated by aluminum ions.[77]
- EDTA can be precipitated by polyvalent cations.[79]

Container/Closure Interactions

Plastic or elastomeric materials used to fabricate containers and closures for pharmaceutical products invariably contain additives such as antistatic agents, lubricants, plasticizers, antioxidants, and stabilizers.[80] Some of these might be leached from containers during product storage, then encountering and interacting with product components, including preservatives. The literature is generally bereft of examples, and levels that are leached may be low but possibilities are worth considering as part of a risk assessment strategy. Reported examples include

- Plasticizers in polyvinyl chloride (PVC) can interact with phenolic preservatives.[81]
- Mercurial preservatives can be absorbed from solution by rubber vial closures, polythene, and other plastic materials.[77,78]
- Solutions of sorbic acid are rapidly degraded in aqueous solutions stored in polythene or polypropylene containers unless an antioxidant is included.[57]

In essence, preservative efficacy in a product can be compromised in several ways. Possibilities for drug/excipient/preservative interactions can sometimes be apparent by considering the molecular makeup and physicochemical properties of preservative and other product components (including primary packaging materials). Well-designed preformulation and early formulation studies can provide valuable insights on interaction potential, mitigating the risk of findings during subsequent programs that might require additional work, possibly product reformulation and delayed project progression. The potential and possibilities for reduced antimicrobial efficacy in complex multiphase systems has engendered efforts to devise *in silico* approaches to predict the impact of product formulation components on preservative activity. The influence of partition coefficients, binding constants (surfactants and polymers), and oil-water ratios have been investigated but with limited success. The favored approach remains optimizing the preservation system and inclusion levels by laboratory investigations and other established conventional programs.

▶ SAFETY OF PRESERVATIVES

Preservatives that inhibit microbial viability and proliferation possess functional groups harmful to living cells. Hence, they may also pose a risk to humans. The EMA Committee for Medicinal Products for Human Use (CHMP) requirement states that inclusion in a medicinal product needs justification that the concentration used should be at the lowest feasible level.

The EMA has recently updated labeling requirements for common excipients, including preservatives based on assessment of their safety profiles, with special focus on pediatric safety.[82] The EMA also regulates the inclusion and allowable levels of preservatives in food. Some, but not all, food preservatives are used in medicinal products but not necessarily *vice versa*, largely because food products are consumed orally, whereas medicines can have wider modes of administration. A list of allowable preservatives is provided in Table 39.3. Food preservatives such as sulfites, nitrites, and nitrates are considered unsuitable for medicinal products. Equally, some preservatives used in vaccines, such as phenols and organomercurials, are considered too toxic as food additives.

The safety of a preservative needs to be considered in the context of product type, mode and frequency of use (short term or chronic), site of administration, and preservative inclusion level. Many oral liquid products are dosed to children and even neonates, mandating that particular attention be paid to preservatives in products dosed to these groups. Prior use in a particular product or product type may not necessarily justify inclusion in a new product or for a new indication. Preservation of ophthalmic products exemplifies such complexities. Prolonged life spans have resulted in glaucoma and other chronic ocular conditions becoming increasingly prominent. Treatment usually requires long-term use of multidose eye drops or gels. Historically, thimerosal was widely used in such products, but use is now discouraged due to concerns of side effects from chronic dosage. BKC is a frequently used preservative in ophthalmic products, often combined with EDTA to enhance activity against *Pseudomonas* species and to enable BKC inclusion levels to be reduced.[48] However, BKC can be irritant with regular use so adherence can be poor. It has also been asserted that chronic use causes ocular damage.[83] Consequently, there is much interest in preservative-free systems. A number of container types are available, such as pump dispensers and squeeze bottles using valves or other systems to prevent contamination during use. The FDA has recently approved the first preservative-free ophthalmic product.[84]

The EMA has stated that preservative-free ophthalmic formulations should be considered whenever possible for use in pediatrics and particularly in neonates.[85] However, based on a review of the available safety data, a general recommendation not to use preservatives in eye preparations is not supported by the available data. Furthermore, the cost of single-dose presentations is 5 to 10 times greater than for multiuse systems. Single-dose systems are not always easy to dose from a patient or carer perspective, usually because of the lack of sufficient suppleness of plastic containers. Serrated edges on an opened container have the potential to irritate or damage patients' eyes, particularly when hand-eye coordination is poor in elderly patients. Drop size, and hence dose, can be variable being highly dependent on the size of the aperture created on opening.[86,87] Such challenges exemplify the complexities associated with providing preservative-free presentations, particularly for long-term use. In essence, use of preservative-free ophthalmic products is not without hazard. Developing a novel preservative for use in ophthalmic products that are dosed chronically can be daunting. Chronic use demands complex long-term safety studies on a novel material possessing some degree of cytotoxicity to be an effective antimicrobial. Some specific safety considerations for common preservatives used in pharmaceutical presentations are discussed in the following text.

Aminobenzoic Acid Esters (Parabens/Aminobenzoates)

The aminobenzoates have generated much attention, particularly because of potential estrogenic effects especially in neonates and more generally in pediatrics. A reflection paper prepared by the EMA concluded that methyl paraben is not linked with estrogenic effects on male or female reproductive organs in immature juvenile rodents or in embryo-fetal development studies.[88] Concentrations up to 0.2% wt/vol, equating to a maximum intake of 140 mg/d were deemed safe, irrespective of the age of the pediatric subgroup. The situation for

propyl paraben is less clear but, based on its effects on female reproductive organs, a conservative no observed effect level (NOEL) of 100 mg/kg/d was assigned. This equates to an equally conservative permitted daily exposure (PDE) value of 2 mg/kg/d. There is no clear-cut position with respect to ethyl paraben. However, it is evident from the EMA position paper that estrogenic effects are related to the length of the ester alkyl group. A risk mitigation strategy might avoid propyl paraben in pediatric products, possibly by using combinations of methyl and ethyl paraben if they provide acceptable antimicrobial efficacy.

Benzalkonium Chloride

BKC evinces significant regulatory unease when used in multidose products for ocular, nasal, or pulmonary use. Its safety profile in oral products is relatively benign, being neither genotoxic, carcinogenic nor exhibiting reproductive toxicity. No significant differences in adverse safety profiles between adults and pediatrics are manifest, where such data are available. However, a number of reports state that prolonged use may cause ocular irritation and impairment. It was accordingly suggested that, for patients requiring decades-long treatment of opthalmic medications, preservative-free products or combinations of two or more preservatives be used.[89] Reliable and unambiguous evidence for BKC-related toxicity was not apparent from a review of various clinical investigations, and lower safety limits for the general population have not been suggested. EMA guidelines state that BKC is a topical irritant in cosmetic products and may cause skin reactions. It may also cause bronchospasm in inhaled products and inclusion levels are limited to 10 mcg per delivered dose. EMA guidelines also state that BKC may cause eye irritation and discoloration of contact lenses and that users should remove lenses prior to application of the medication and wait at least 15 minutes before insertion in the eye.[90]

Benzoic Acid/Sodium Benzoate

Sodium benzoate is widely used to preserve liquid oral presentations for administration to pediatrics and neonates. Its acceptable taste and ready dissolution (where products are constituted as liquids prior to use) support such usage. The primary safety issue concerns its capacity to displace bilirubin from albumin, leading to bilirubinemia. This can be a concern in pre- and full-term neonates where metabolic enzymes are not fully mature and can lead to accumulation of benzoic acid. Neonatal, unconjugated hyperbilirubinemia is common in newborn infants, although it is usually benign. Such possibilities can exist with oral, parenteral, and topical preparations as percutaneous absorption of benzoic acid can be significant, particularly in neonates. The risk of developing hyperbilirubinemia in neonates is also possible with benzyl alcohol because benzoic acid is a metabolite of benzyl alcohol. Coadministration of medicinal products containing these excipients could lead to benzoic acid accumulation.

The Scientific Committee of Consumer Products (SCCP) of the EMA discussed potential safety issues related to benzoates contained in pediatric and neonatal medications, specifically with respect to pre- and full-term neonates with immature metabolic systems.[91] The SCCP defined an acceptable daily intake (ADI) for benzoic acid and its salts as 0 to 5 mg/kg/d, a value aligned with that in an earlier World Health Organization (WHO) report.[92] Current EU labeling requirements state that benzoates may induce jaundice (yellowing of skin/eyes) in newborn babies when administered orally, parenterally or topically and may be irritant when applied topically.[93]

Benzyl Alcohol

The Scientific Committee on Food (SFC) of the European Commission reviewed animal safety data for benzyl alcohol and allocated an ADI of 0 to 5 mg/kg/d.[94] This is supported by an earlier US Environmental Protection Agency (EPA) review.[95] A subchronic oral reference dose of 1 mg/kg/d for adults was derived based on the no-observed-adverse-effect-level (NOAEL) of 200 mg/kg/d from a 13-week rat study. A chronic oral reference dose of 0.3 mg/kg/d for adults was derived from a lowest-observed-adverse-effect level (LOAEL) of 200 mg/kg value obtained from a 2-year carcinogenicity study in rodents. There are no animal safety data for parenteral or topical use for this excipient. However, oral absorption is such (virtually 100%) that oral dose recommendations can be considered relevant to other routes of administration. A short-term study in juvenile rats established a NOAEL of 300 mg/kg/d, being similar to the NOAEL in adults.[96] No long-term effects were reported from the juvenile animal toxicity studies.

The prime concern with benzyl alcohol concerns its potential for accumulation in pre- and full-term neonates due to immature metabolic enzymes. Intravenous administration equivalent to 100 to 200 mg/kg/d has been associated with gasping syndrome in preterm newborn infants suffering from metabolic acidosis, the majority being fatal.[97,98] Current EU labeling stipulates that benzyl alcohol not be present in products for administration to premature infants or neonates and that exposure exceeding 90 mg/kg/d may cause fatal toxic and allergic reactions in infants and children up to age 3 years.[99]

Ethanol

Ethanol is a well-established CNS depressant. Mild to moderate exposure in adults can result in euphoria, ataxia, sedation, aggressive behavior, nausea, and vomiting. Higher exposure can cause respiratory depression and failure as well as cardiovascular toxicities, including congestive heart failure and severe myocardial depression. Uncertainties exist concerning alcohol tolerance as a function of age due to differences in metabolic maturation in children as well as the impact of differing levels of ethanol over different times. Most of the literature concerns acute exposure and consequent poisoning. Symptoms of ethanol intoxication are more severe in children than in adults.[100,101]

Cutaneous absorption of ethanol can also be significant in neonates due to the newborn child's immature skin: This can cause significant local reactions as well as systemic exposure and associated toxicity.[102] Ethanol is also a known reproductive and developmental toxic agent and can cause genetic defects, probably ascribable to its principal metabolite, acetaldehyde. The effects of long-term exposure, even at very low levels, on the health and development of pediatrics is not known.[103] However, the prevalence of fetal alcohol syndrome (FAS) and fetal alcohol effects (FAE) in children clearly demonstrates the adverse effect potential of chronic alcohol exposure, particularly on neurologic and cognitive developmental processes.[104,105] Ethanol is also a human oral carcinogen.[106,107] Its presence in adult medicinal products is now discouraged due to concerns relating to interactions with other medicines, alcohol-related diseases, the effects on motor skills (eg, driving), and issues with addiction, pregnancy, and breastfeeding.[108] Current labeling requirements for ethanol are extensive and focused on three exposure levels, namely ≥75, 6 to <75, and 1 to <6 mg/kg/d.[109,110] Surprisingly, there appear to be no regulatory requirements concerning use in chronic and short-term medications dosed to adults.

Phenolic Agents

Phenol is used in a variety of products such as mouthwashes, throat lozenges, and throat sprays. It is also used as a preservative in FDA-approved vaccines for pneumococci (Pneumovax 23®), typhoid (Typhim Vi®), and smallpox (ACAM2000®) infections. Each of these vaccines contains 0.25% phenol.[48] Reports on side effects attributable to phenol are fairly rare, probably a reflection of the low inclusion levels typically used. The total daily intake (TDI) limit for phenol was reduced by the European Food Safety Authority (EFSA) in 2013 from 1.5 mg/kg/d to 0.5 mg/kg/d (equivalent to 0.5 mg/kg/d for a 50-kg adult) based on findings from new safety studies.[111]

The relative cytotoxicity of commonly used preservatives in vaccines has been assessed using a cell-based assay.[112] Phenol was found to be the safest, the rank order being phenol < 2-phenoxyethanol < benzethonium chloride < thimerosal. The observed relative toxicity indices were also assessed using the ratio; human/bacterial cells, providing values of 2-phenoxyethanol (4.6-fold) < phenol (12.2-fold) < thimerosal (>330-fold). The authors commented that, with the exception of 2-phenoxyethanol, the required concentrations to induce significant antimicrobial efficacy (pharmacopoeial requirements) were significantly higher than those routinely included in USA-licensed vaccine/biological preparations. The implication is that clinical safety considerations outweigh antimicrobial efficacy considerations when developing such products (ie, risk/benefit considerations apply). The authors further commented that none of the preservatives in vaccine/biological products can be considered ideal in terms of providing optimal antimicrobial efficacy along with minimal mammalian toxicity. They recommended that future vaccines/biologics products be sterile and single dose, eliminating the need for preservatives and unnecessary risk to patients. It may be unrealistic to impose such a strategy in the light of the complexities associated with the development and manufacture of vaccines/biologics. Organizations developing products, including biosimilars or multivalent influenza vaccines, such as those targeted to new strains of *Haemophilus influenzae*, could be reluctant to diverge from using phenol-containing products because of uncertainties concerning potential impact on efficacy and safety of such modified products.

Chlorocresol is less toxic than phenol but can be irritating to skin, eyes, and mucous membranes. It cannot be used in intrathecal, intracisternal, or peridural injections. It is used as a cosmetic preservative in skin care and suntan formulations and as an indirect food additive in the United States.[113] Chlorocresol is approved for use as a preservative by the EMA at concentrations of up to 0.2% but can be used at other concentrations for non-preservative functions. It is banned from topical products that may contact mucous membranes. Chlorocresol showed no evidence of mutagenicity in Ames tests, but there was an increase in SOS-DNA repair synthesis in *E coli*. Acute, short-term, and subchronic tests in animals indicated that there were no dose-related toxicity events other than a reduction in body weight gain. A chronic oral (with food) study in rats showed kidney damage in high-dose male groups and increases in pituitary adenomas in mid- and high-dose female groups. Aqueous solutions (0.05%) caused ocular irritation in rabbits. Additionally, there was some evidence of dermal irritation and sensitization in animal studies. Aqueous solutions containing 2% chlorocresol (20 mg/ml) caused skin irritation. Volunteer predictive patch tests using 0.5% chlorocresol were negative but provocative patch tests yielded positive responses in some sensitive individuals.

Other animal in vitro data are not available. Missing information includes

- The maximum concentration for safe use in cosmetics
- Ultraviolet (UV) absorption (photosensitization where an ingredient absorbs in the UVA or UVB region)
- Dermal developmental toxicity information
- Findings from mutagenicity studies using a mammalian rather than an in vitro test system. A 2-year dermal carcinogenicity study is required in the event of a positive outcome in a mutagenesis study

Overall, the lack of such information means that the safety of chlorocresol in topical/cosmetic formulations is not fully supported.

Chloroxylenol is used in cosmetic products at concentrations up to 5.0%. It is readily absorbed through skin and from the gastrointestinal tract, and postabsorption, it binds readily to plasma proteins. Both free and conjugated chloroxylenol is found in urine. Formulations containing up to 1.0% were reported to be nonsensitizing and essentially nonirritating to human skin, but there was a small incidence (≤1%) of skin sensitization at 1.0% inclusion level. It is nonmutagenic in the Ames test (± S9 activation). A 0.1% aqueous chloroxylenol solution was nonirritant to rabbit skin. Carcinogenicity and teratogenicity studies have not been reported.[114] Chloroxylenol is generally considered to be less irritating than chlorocresol and safe when used as a preservative in cosmetic products. Surprisingly, it does not seem to be included in any prescription products in the United States.

Hexachlorophene usage has declined because of concerns over neurotoxicity.

▶ AIDS TO PRESERVATION

Preservative selection and efficacy can be constrained by a combination of compendial performance requirements, attributes of the preservative, or the pharmaceutical product and by patient requirements. In such cases, it may be feasible to include other materials in the dosage form, which while possessing limited antimicrobial effects can contribute to the overall preservative efficacy in the product.

Water Activity

An aqueous environment is a prerequisite for microbial survival and growth. Microbial viability can be reduced and preservative effects enhanced by reducing the water activity of the product. Water activity (A_w) is defined as the following ratio:

$$A_w = P/P_0$$

where P is the water vapor pressure in a material or product and P_0 is the vapor pressure of pure water at the same temperature. The term has essentially the same meaning as equilibrium relative humidity (ERH), a concept widely used in dosage form design, processing, and packaging of solid pharmaceutical products with ERH values being expressed in percentage rather than fractional terms (ERH = A_w × 100). Reducing water activity is widely used to preserve food products, usually by including sugars, salt, or by freezing.[115] The same strategy can be used with aqueous pharmaceutical products because potentially contaminating organisms can be similar to those in food products.

Bacteria are generally inhibited at A_w <0.9. Some molds require that water activity not exceed A_w <0.8 for inhibition, whereas some yeasts require values as low as A_w <0.6 (Table 39.10). Microbial proliferation is not usual where A_w <0.6 and products with such values are usually considered to be nonaqueous. Table 39.11 lists aqueous solution concentrations of various materials that provide an A_w 0.85.[116] Such high concentrations are probably impractical for many products due to effects on other product attributes. Furthermore, reductions in water activity become progressively less as the level of the

TABLE 39.10	Minimum water activity values required to support growth of a selection of bacteria, molds, and yeasts[a]

Organism	Minimum Water Activity (A_w) Requirement for Growth
Pseudomonas aeruginosa	0.97
Bacillus cereus	0.95
Bacillus subtilis	0.91
Clostridium botulinum type A	0.95
Clostridium perfringens	0.95
Escherichia coli	0.95
Lactobacillus viridescens	0.95
Salmonella species	0.95
Staphylococcus aureus	0.86
Rhizopus nigricans	0.93
Mucor plumbeus	0.92
Rhodotorula mucilaginosa	0.92
Saccharomyces cerevisiae	0.92
Paecilomyces variotii	0.9
Penicillium chrysogenum	0.84
Aspergillus fumigatus	0.82
Zygosaccharomyces rouxii	0.62
Xeromyces bisporus	0.61

[a]USP 38: 1178-1179 <1112>.[116]

TABLE 39.11	Aqueous solution concentration requirements to attain a water activity value of 0.85 at 25°C[a]

Material	Inclusion Level (%)
Propylene glycol	40.0
Glycerol	43.0
Glucose	58.0
Sucrose	67.0
Sorbitol	59.5
Urea	39.7
Xylose	54.0

[a]Adapted from US Pharmacopeia 35.[116]

activity-lowering agent is increased; the relationship is not linear.[117] Water activity is also temperature dependent and can be influenced by storage environment or transport conditions. Such limitations dictate that in many cases, reducing water activity needs to be considered as one component of the overall strategy to aid preservation. Instruments to measure water activity are widely available. Testing is nondestructive and readily applicable to programs for product preservation.

Other Materials

Buckley et al[118] considered the safety and antimicrobial efficacies of materials that are not normally considered as preservatives, using the challenge organisms *Aspergillus brasiliensis* and *P aeruginosa*. They also conducted a hazard assessment, supplemented by *in silico* computational modeling to determine effects in man and any environmental impact. The antioxidant, octyl gallate, exhibited superior antimicrobial efficacy and comparable or lower hazard ratings. The report concluded that octyl gallate could serve an effective preservative in conjunction with other microbicides. Identifying an antimicrobial effect can be straightforward, but using *in silico* tools to predict human safety is a greater challenge. Octyl gallate would need to be assessed either alone or more typically or as a formulation component using a battery of *in vitro* and *in vivo* safety studies to support its long-term safety.

▶ HERBAL PRODUCTS

Herbal products can pose high risks of microbial contamination due to their tendency to have higher bioburdens than chemically derived agents. Spores and mycotoxins may be present, being difficult to eliminate. Herbal medicinal products can also be contaminated with numerous types/species of bacteria, yeasts, fungi, and molds. Levels of viable microorganisms and spore-forming bacteria and fungi in source materials should be determined and limited in accordance with pharmacopoeial requirements. Testing for the presence of pathogens such as *Shigella*, *Campylobacter*, and *Listeria* species is prudent, with acceptance criteria (where required) that are based on the outcomes of appropriate microbial risk assessments.[119]

Microbial limits also need to be established for herbal products presented as multidose oral liquids and other aqueous-based products (eg, cream-based topicals). Standards to maintain the product's microbial quality throughout shelf life and use are identical to those for conventional pharmaceutical products. It may be necessary to supplement testing protocols with additional challenge organisms based on the microbial risk assessment of product, process, and starting materials.

▶ PARENTERAL DOSAGE FORMS

Preservation of multidose parenteral products is vital because the introduction of microorganisms by the parenteral route can have extremely serious consequences, particularly for immunocompromised patients. Thimerosal (or thiomersal) is the most widely used preservative in centrally authorized human vaccines within the EU, principally for influenza pandemic vaccines. Alternative preservatives have been registered nationally or via mutual recognition practices for other human vaccines. Phenol has been used in vaccines for typhus (Typherix®, Typhim Vi®) and vaccines for pneumococcal infections (Pneumovax II®), whereas phenoxyethanol is used in diphtheria/tetanus/pertussis/polio vaccines (Tetravac®, Pediacel®, Revaxis®, Repevax®).

There has been much comment on possibilities for replacement (on safety grounds) of thimerosal in vaccines. Only a small number of vaccines in the United States now contain this preservative. At the same time, it is generally accepted that existing epidemiologic data do not support any causal relationship between thiomersal-containing vaccines and autism or other pediatric developmental disorders. Available evidence supports the conclusion that all currently licensed vaccines containing thimerosal have been proven to be safe under the applicable regulatory framework. Substituting thimerosal with a putatively less toxic alternative has the potential to change vaccine safety, effectiveness, and quality.

The complexity of the active ingredient(s) in vaccine and other biologically derived products and the shortcomings of some of the analytical techniques for characterization of biological constructs make preservative removal or replacement a risky proposition. Uncertainties associated with effects on processing, stability, and particularly the safety and efficacy of the immunizing or other biologically active component(s) are such that comprehensive safety and efficacy information would need to be generated to support any change. The FDA stipulates that a wide-ranging reformulation/evaluation program is required to establish the safety and effectiveness of a product containing a replacement preservative, or a nonpreserved vaccine.[120] EMA and WHO positions are concordant with those expounded by the FDA.[121,122] In essence, the risk inherent in any replacement strategy needs to be mitigated by relevant safety and efficacy investigations and other nonclinical studies. Replacing an established, efficacious preservative with an unproven alternative might increase the risk/benefit ratio rather than decrease it. Quaternary ammonium compounds and phenylmercuric nitrate are rarely if ever used in parenteral products.[123]

Significant efforts are being devoted to total removal of preservatives in vaccines, primarily by using single-dose preservative-free presentations. Some multidose vaccines do not contain preservatives, for example, influenza vaccines (Celvapan® and Vepacel®). These must be used within 3 hours of broaching. By contrast, influenza vaccines containing preservative (Pandemrix and Focetria) can be used for up to 24 hours, postbroaching.

The inclusion of preservatives in parenteral products has steadily declined. Reductions may be due to the increasing availability of single-dose self-administration systems and of single-dose products such as biopharmaceuticals, monoclonal antibody, and other immunotherapeutic presentations, most being provided in single-dose sterile form. Treatments with some of these novel agents may not require regular dosage as dosage intervals can be relatively long, or treatments may comprise single-dose administration. However, manufacture and shipping and storage of single-dose products can be expensive and particularly burdensome in remote regions due to the greater unit numbers. Consequently, multidose presentations are likely to continue to be required for vaccines and some other types of parenteral products for the foreseeable future.

Biopharmaceuticals

Biopharmaceutical products of earlier vintage, being largely replacement or therapeutic proteins, usually contained preservatives. Phenol, *m*-cresol, thimerosal, and benzyl alcohol were usually used in such now-mature products.[124] Biopharmaceutical therapeutic agents developed in recent years are mostly monoclonal antibodies, many based on immunotherapeutic concepts. They are invariably provided in single-dose vials or prefilled syringes and do not contain preservatives. Virtually all such agents contain Polysorbate 80 (or Polysorbate 20 in a few cases) to attenuate aggregation (and associated safety concerns) during product manufacture, reconstitution, and administration. Polysorbate is without peer as an antiaggregant and no suitable replacement has been identified to date. However, polysorbates and other polyethylene glycol–based nonionic surfactants can compromise the activities of many preservatives.[59,124]

Conversely, *m*-cresol can cause precipitation of polysorbates.[125] If future biologically-derived products are to warrant multidose presentations, there may be formidable challenges associated with their preservation.

Macromolecular therapeutic agents can also be adversely affected by preservatives. Benzyl alcohol causes aggregation of recombinant human interferon (rhIFN), recombinant human granulocyte colony-stimulating factor (rhGCSF), recombinant human interleukin-1 receptor antagonist (rhIL1ra) and it can also accelerate the aggregation of partially unfolded proteins.[126-128] Interactions have also been reported between aminobenzoate esters and macromolecules.[129] Instructions on some biopharmaceutical products stipulate that diluent for their constitution should not contain preservative(s) because of the potential for protein/preservative interactions. If future biologically-derived products warrant multidose presentations, there may be formidable challenges associated with their preservation.

Preservatives for multidose insulin preparations must be chosen carefully. Insulin zinc suspensions cannot contain phenol because it destroys the crystallinity of the insulin, so mixtures of aminobenzoate esters are usually used. In contrast, neutral protamine insulin requires the presence of phenol or meta-phenol to form and preserve the crystal form that provides the long-acting effect.

Vaccines

Vaccines for preventing infections usually contain phenol, *m*-cresol, phenoxyethanol, or thimerosal.[50,123] Inclusion is largely based on historical experience with earlier versions of such vaccines. However, regulatory agencies do not necessarily consider prior use as supporting inclusion in other parenteral products.

▶ PACKAGING

Pharmaceutical products may be packaged in glass or plastic containers that are fabricated using polymeric materials. Seals or caps may be metallic, plastic, or, in the case of multidose parenterals in glass vials, rubber closures to facilitate dose withdrawal and resealing. The potential impact of such packaging on preservatives and their efficacy can be summarized as

- Preservatives that are volatile may gradually diffuse through "plastic" container walls or vial closures during long-term storage, depleting levels so possibly compromising preservative efficacy.
- Virtually all plastic containers and elastomers contain additives to confer rigidity, flexibility, and polymer stability or to facilitate container manufacture.[80] Preservatives may interact with such additives, preservative efficacy or the container closure system compromised. Such effects and their consequences may only become

apparent during prolonged product storage. Fortunately, many can be anticipated by carefully designed preformulation or other early investigative studies. Such diligence minimizes the possibilities for late-breaking issues requiring reformulation and delaying program progression. It is also important that appropriate change control and notification systems are agreed, both internally and with suppliers of containers/plastic/elastomeric components as it is not unusual for processes and the input components for such materials to be unilaterally altered by the Provider.

▶ FUTURE TRENDS

Views are sometimes expressed that multidose liquid formulations requiring preservation be discouraged in favor of alternatives such as solid dosage forms: These could consist of single-dose granules in sachets or bulk granules designed to be converted to liquid prior to use. This is based on the assumption that granules are frequently intermediates in the manufacture of medicinal products for adults (eg, tablets or capsules) and can be seamlessly adopted as pediatric products. However, such intermediate granules may not be optimal with respect to patient usage or acceptability. A major challenge can be lack of palatability (particularly for pediatric presentations) requiring that the drug be coated, or a complex be formed to prevent drug from dissolving in the buccal cavity and displaying poor taste, or by using some other taste-masking technique. Moreover, from an efficacy perspective, the patient must swallow the entire dose (ie, all the granules). Granule-based products are often difficult to disperse prior to dosing, unlike a bespoke suspension product, and cause suboptimal dosing. The flow properties of such granule-based products can also be suboptimal for filling into single-dose receptacles such as sachets. Patient adherence/compliance is often linked with the ease of use of products. A patient or caregiver may have to constitute such a product (convert to liquid) and dose 3 times daily for 7 days (eg, in treating a bacterial infection), in essence, performing 21-unit operations if the product is in single-dose form. A bespoke suspension or solution product is more convenient and less prone to constitution and administration errors.

The inclusion of preservatives in medicinal products as well as in cosmetics, foods, and beverages has been controversial at times, mostly but not exclusively in developed countries. Objections range from concerns about autism development in vaccinated children (worldwide) to allegations of conspiracies for male sterilization during polio vaccination programs in West Africa. Little if any scientific evidence is available to substantiate these and other concerns and, in the later-referenced case, a subsequent polio epidemic claimed nearly 800 victims. It is also the case that less well-developed global regions are those most in need of medications. The lack of clean water, facilities for hygienic practices, and the preponderance of infectious diseases all inflate the risk of product contamination, particularly during use. Including a preservative can be considered good practice in such cases. It is unlikely therefore that the practice of including a preservative in relevant pharmaceutical products will cease in the foreseeable future. At the same time, the potential exists for the identification of novel preservatives providing more options, particularly for products for treating chronic conditions that are becoming more prominent in aging populations and where current preservatives may have undesirable long-term effects.

To conclude, the possibilities and constraints for product preservation need to be considered at an early stage in dosage form design to obviate risk of delays to the program. If the program concerns a novel drug or mode of delivery, the clinical evaluation studies should ideally use product containing the preservative intended for inclusion in the commercial product, selection being based on the criteria and evaluation programs discussed in this document. In essence, the preservation system needs to be included and evaluated as part of preclinical and early clinical programs to forestall patient-related issues (such as irritancy or irritation) being encountered in clinical trials that might a change to the preservative. Otherwise, programs are likely to be delayed by the need for reformulation and possibly additional clinical testing. It is also important that product-related strategies such as single or multidose presentations and topical dosage form type (cream/ointment) are considered and defined at the outset of a product development program. There may be uncertainties at such an early stage, but considerations can lead to useful contributions to the construction of a target product quality profile and associated risk mitigation and management systems for product development programs.

REFERENCES

1. Sutton S, Jiminez L. A review of reported recalls involving microbiological control 2004-2011 with emphasis on FDA considerations of "objectionable organisms." American Pharmaceutical Review Web site. https://www.americanpharmaceuticalreview.com/Featured-Articles/38382-A-Review-of-Reported-Recalls-Involving-Microbiological-Control-2004-2011-with-Emphasis-on-FDA-Considerations-of-Objectionable-Organisms. Accessed July 2019.
2. Barlas S. FDA devotes new resources to upgrading generic drug safety: but in some instances, the industry is pushing back. *P T*. 2014;39:353-364.
3. International Council for Harmonisation. ICH harmonised tripartite guideline: quality risk management Q9. International Council for Harmonisation Web site. https://www.ich.org/fileadmin/Public_Web_Site/ICH_Products/Guidelines/Quality/Q9/Step4/Q9_Guideline.pdf. Accessed July 9, 2019.
4. Ericcson A. *Fault Tree Analysis Primer*. Charleston, NC: CreateSpace Inc; 2011.
5. ASQ Service Quality Division. Failure modes and effect analysis (FMEA). ASQ Service Quality Division Web site. http://asqservicequality.org/glossary/failure-modes-and-effects-analysis-fmea. Accessed July 9, 2019.
6. US Food and Drug Administration. Hazard analysis critical control point (HACCP). US Food and Drug Administration Web site. https://www.fda.gov/Food/GuidanceRegulation/HACCP. Accessed July 9, 2019.
7. European Medicines Agency. Note for guidance on inclusion of antioxidants and antimicrobial preservatives in medicinal products. EMEA/CPMP/CVMP/111/95/2003. European Medicines Agency Website.https://www.ema.europa.eu/en/documents/scientific-guideline/note-guidance-inclusion-antioxidants-antimicrobial-preservatives-medicinal-products_en.pdf. Accessed July 9, 2019.
8. European Medicines Agency. Guideline on excipients in the dossier for application for marketing authorisation of a medicinal product. EMEA/CHMP/QWP 396591/2006. European Medicines Agency Web site. https://www.ema.europa.eu/en/documents/scientific-guideline/guideline-excipients-dossier-application-marketing-authorisation-medicinal-product-revision-2_en.pdf. Accessed July 9, 2019.
9. Allwood MC. The adsorption of esters of *p*-hydroxybenzoic acid by magnesium trisilicate. *Int J Pharm*. 1982;11:101-107.
10. Schmidt PC, Benke K. The adsorption and stability of preservatives in antacid suspensions 1. Determination and influence on adsorption. *Pharm Acta Helv*. 1988;63:117-127.
11. Schmidt PC, Benke K. The adsorption and stability of preservatives in antacid suspensions. 2. Stability and reaction kinetics. *Pharm Acta Helv*. 1988;63:188-196.
12. Moser CL, Meyer BK. Comparison of compendial antimicrobial effectiveness tests: a review. *AAPS Pharm Sci Tech*. 2011;12:222-226.
13. Haginaki J, Nakagawa T, Uno T. Stability of clavulanic acid in aqueous solution. *Chem Pharm Bull*. 1981;29:3334-3341.
14. Stanojevic D, Comic L, Stefanovic O, Solujic-Sukdolac S. Antimicrobial effects of sodium benzoate, sodium nitrite and potassium sorbate and their synergistic action *in vitro*. *Bulg J Ag Sci*. 2009;15:307-311.
15. Wiegland I, Hilpert K, Hancock EW. Agar and broth dilution methods to determine the minimal inhibitory concentration (MIC) of antimicrobial substances. *Nat Protoc*. 2008;3:163-175.
16. Levitz SM. Compounding drugs contaminated with fungi: a recipe for disaster. *Emerg Microb Infect*. 2012;1(11):e41. https://www.ncbi.nlm.nih.gov/pmc/articles/PMC3634134/. Accessed July 9, 2019.
17. Public Health England. *Bacillus cereus* infections: 1 July 2014 [press release]. London, United Kingdom: Public Health England. https://www.gov.uk/government/news/bacillus-cereus-infections-1-july-2014. Accessed July 9, 2019.
18. Sutton S. What is an "objectionable organism"? American Pharmaceutical Review Web site. http://www.americanpharmaceuticalreview.com/Featured-Articles/122201-What-is-an-Objectionable-Organism-Objectionable-Organisms-The-Shifting-Perspective/. Accessed July 2019.
19. US Food and Drug Administration. Enforcement home page. https://google2.fda.gov/search?q=enforcement+page&client=FDAgov&site=FDAgov&lr=&proxystylesheet=FDAgov&required fields=-archive%3AYes&output=xml_no_dtd&getfields=*. Accessed July 9, 2019.
20. Parenteral Drug Association. 2013 PDA objectionable microorganisms for nonsterile pharmaceutical, consumer health, medical devices, dietary supplement and cosmetic products. Parenteral Drug Association Web site. https://store.pda.org/TableOfContents/45003_TOC.pdf. Accessed July 9, 2019.
21. Parenteral Drug Association. Exclusion of objectionable microorganisms from nonsterile pharmaceuticals, medical devices, and cosmetics. Parenteral Drug Association Web site. https://store.pda.org/TableOfContents/TR67_TOC.pdf. Accessed July 9, 2019.
22. US Food and Drug Administration. Microbiological methods for cosmetics. US Food and Drug Administration Web site. https://www.fda.gov/Food/FoodScienceResearch/LaboratoryMethods/ucm073598.htm. Accessed July 9, 2019.
23. Microchem Laboratory. PCPC (formerly CTFA) test methods for cosmetics. Microchem Laboratory Web site. http://microchemlab.com/test/pcpc-formerly-ctfa-test-methods-cosmetics. Accessed July 9, 2019.

24. US Food and Drug Administration. Bad bug book: handbook of food-borne pathogenic microorganisms and natural toxins. US Food and Drug Administration Web site. https://www.fda.gov/downloads/food/food borneillnesscontaminants/ucm297627.pdf. Accessed July 9, 2019.

25. Jimenez L. Microbial diversity in pharmaceutical product recalls and environments. *PDA J Pharm Sci Technol.* 2007;61(5):383-399.

26. Torbeck L, Raccasi D, Guilfoyle DE, Friedman RL, Hussong D. *Burkholderia cepacia*: this decision is overdue. *PDA J Pharm Sci Technol.* 2011;65:535-543.

27. Anwar H, Dasgupta MK, Costerton JW. Testing the susceptibility in biofilms to antibacterial agents. *Antimicrob Agents Chemother.* 1990;34:2043-2046.

28. Carson L, Favero MS, Bond WW, Petersen NJ. Morphological, biochemical, and growth characteristics of *Pseudomonas cepacia* from distilled water. *Appl Microbiol.* 1973;25(3):476-483.

29. Cundell T. Excluding *Burkholderia cepacia* complex from aqueous, non-sterile drug products. American Pharmaceutical Review Web site. https://www.americanpharmaceuticalreview.com/Featured-Articles /358427-Excluding-i-Burkholderia-cepacia-i-complex-from -Aqueous-Non-Sterile-Drug-Products/. Accessed July 9, 2019.

30. Ribeiro NF, Heath CH, Kierath J, Rea S, Duncan-Smith M, Wood FM. Burn wounds infected by contaminated water: case reports, review of the literature, and recommendations for treatment. *Burns.* 2009;36(1):9-22.

31. Jensen GB, Hansen BM, Eilenberg JJ, Mahillon J. The hidden lifestyles of *Bacillus cereus* and relatives. *Environ Microbiol.* 2003;5:631-640.

32. Turnbull PCB, Kramer JM. Intestinal carriage of *Bacillus cereus*: faecal isolation studies in three population groups. *J Hyg (Lond).* 1985;95:629-638.

33. Bottone EJ. *Bacillus cereus*, a volatile human pathogen. *Clin Microbiol Rev.* 2010;23(2):382-398.

34. Guinebretière MH, Auger S, Galleron N, et al. *Bacillus cytotoxicus* sp. nov. is a novel thermotolerant species of the *Bacillus cereus* group occasionally associated with food poisoning. *Int J Syst Evol Microbiol.* 2013;63:31-40.

35. Sandle T. The risk of *Bacillus cereus* to pharmaceutical manufacturing. American Pharmaceutical Review Web site. http://www.american pharmaceuticalreview.com/Featured-Articles/169507-The-Risk -of-em-Bacillus-cereus-em-to-Pharmaceutical-Manufacturing/. Accessed July 9, 2019.

36. Centers for Disease Control and Prevention. Notes from the field: contamination of alcohol prep pads with *Bacillus cereus* group and *Bacillus* species—Colorado, 2010. Centers for Disease Control and Prevention Web site. https://www.cdc.gov/mmwr/preview/mmwrhtml /mm6011a5.htm. Accessed July 9, 2019.

37. US Food and Drug Administration. Warning letter. Zeppessis Reprocessing, LCC. 09/08/13. US Food and Drug Administration Web site. https://www.fda.gov/ICECI/EnforcementActions/WarningLetters /ucm365433.htm. Accessed July 9, 2019.

38. https://www.fda.gov/ICECI/EnforcementActions/Warning Letters/2013/ucm365433.htm.

39. Pitt TL, McClure J, Parker MD, Amézquita A, McClure PJ. *Bacillus cereus* in personal care products: risk to consumers. *Inst Cosmet Sci.* 2015;37:165-174.

40. Mugoyela V, Mwambete KD. Microbial contamination of nonsterile pharmaceuticals in public hospital settings. *Ther Clin Risk Manag.* 2010;6:443-448.

41. Leistner L. Hurdle technology and energy savings. In: Downey WK, ed. *Food Quality and Nutrition.* London, United Kingdom: Applied Sciences; 1978:553-557.

42. Leistner L. Shelf-stable products and intermediate moisture foods. In: Rockland LB, Beuchat LR, eds. *Water Activity: Theory and Applications to Food.* New York, NY: Marcel Dekker; 1987:295-328.

43. Food Standards Agency. EU approved additives and E numbers. Food Standards Agency Web site. https://www.food.gov.uk/business-guidance /eu-approved-additives-and-e-numbers. Accessed July 9, 2019.

44. McElroy J. Antimicrobial preservation overview for formulators and process scientists. SlideShare Web site. https://www.slideshow.net /JimMcElroy/antimicrobial-presentation-overview-for-formulation -and process scientists. Accessed July 9, 2019.

45. Baudouin C, Labbé A, Liang H, Pauly A, Badouin FB. Preservatives in eyedrops: the good, the bad and the ugly. *Prog Retinal Eye Res.* 2010;29:312-334.

46. Bean H. pH, ionisation and inhibitory levels for benzoic acid. In: Davis H, ed. *Bentley's Textbook of Pharmaceutics.* 7th ed. London, United Kingdom: Bailliere, Tindall and Cox; 1961:995-1013.

47. US Food and Drug Administration. Drugs@FDA: FDA approved drug products. US Food and Drug Administration Web site. https:// www.accessdata.fda.gov/scripts/cder/daf/. Accessed July 9, 2019.

48. Aalto TR, Firman MC, Rigler NE. *p*-hydroxybenzoic acid esters as preservatives. 1. Uses, antibacterial and antifungal studies, properties and determination. *J Am Pharm Assoc Am Pharm Assoc.* 1953;42:449-457.

49. Richards RME, McBride RJ. Enhancement of benzalkonium chloride and chlorhexidine against *Pseudomonas aeruginosa* by aromatic alcohols. *J Pharm Sci.* 1973;62:2035-2037.

50. Hart JR. Chelating agents as preservative potentiators. In: *Cosmetic and Drug Preservation.* New York, NY: Marcel Dekker; 1984:323-327.

51. Richards RME, McBride RJ. Phenylethanol enhancement of preservatives used in ophthalmic presentations. *J Pharm Pharmacol.* 1971;23:141S-146S.

52. Worthington L. Bronchoconstriction due to benzalkonium chloride in nebuliser solutions. *Can J Hosp Pharm.* 1989;42:165-166.

53. European Medicines Agency. Benzalkonium chloride used as an excipient: report published in support of the 'Questions and answers on benzalkonium chloride used as an excipient in medicinal products for human use' (EMA/CHMP/495737/2013). European Medicines Agency Web site. https://www.ema.europa.eu/en/documents/report /benzalkonium-chloride-used-excipient-report-published-support -questions-answers-benzalkonium_en.pdf. Accessed July 9, 2019.

54. Ngarmsak M, Delaquis P, Toivonen P, Ngarmsak T, Ooraikul B, Mazza G. Antimicrobial activity of vanillin against spoilage microorganisms in stored fresh fruit mangoes. *J Food Prot.* 2006;69:1724-1727.

55. deRapper S, Van Vuuren SF, Kamatou GP, Viljoen AM, Dagne E. The additive and synergistic antimicrobial effects of select frankincense and myrrh oils—a combination for the pharaonic pharmacopeia. *Lett Appl Microbiol.* 2012;54:352-358.

56. Blaug SM, Grant DE. Kinetics of degradation of the parabens. *J Soc Cosm Chem.* 1974;25:495-506.

57. Cook W, Quinn ME, Shesky PJ. Sorbic acid monograph. In: Rowe R, Shesky PJ, Quinn ME, eds. *Handbook of Pharmaceutical Excipients.* 6th ed. London, United Kingdom: Pharmaceutical Press; 2009:672-675.

58. Yarramaraju S, Akurathi V, Wolfs K, Van Schepdael A, Hoogmartens J, Adams E. Investigation of sorbic acid volatile degradation products in pharmaceutical formulations using static headspace gas chromatography. *J Pharm Biomed Anal.* 2007;44:456-463.

59. Patel NK, Foss NE. Interaction of some pharmaceuticals with macromolecules. I. Effect of temperature on the binding of parabens and phenols by polysorbate 80 and polyethylene glycol 4000. *J Pharm Sci.* 1964;53:94-97.

60. Elder DP, Crowley PJ. Antimicrobial preservatives: choosing a preservative. American Pharmaceutical Review Web site. http://www .americanpharmaceuticalreview.com. Accessed October 28, 2019.

61. Cahill E. Benzyl alcohol monograph. In: Rowe R, Shesky PJ, Quinn ME, eds. *Handbook of Pharmaceutical Excipients.* 6th ed. London, United Kingdom: Pharmaceutical Press; 2009:64-66.

62. Owen SC. Phenoxyethanol monograph. In: Rowe R, Shesky PJ, Quinn ME, eds. *Handbook of Pharmaceutical Excipients.* 6th ed. London, United Kingdom: Pharmaceutical Press; 2009:488-489.

63. Crowley P, Martini LG. Drug-excipient interactions. *Pharm Technol.* 2001;13:26-34.

64. Higashiyama M, Inada IK, Ohtori A, Kakehi K. NMR analysis of ion pair formation between timolol and sorbic acid in ophthalmic preparations. *J Pharm Biomed Anal.* 2007;43:1335-1342.

65. Gangavaram S, Raghavender S, Sanphui P, et al. Polymorphs and co-crystals of nalidixic acid. *Cryst Grow Design*. 2012;12:4963-4971.

66. Childs SL, Chyall L, Dunlap J, et al. Crystal engineering approach to forming cocrystals of amine hydrochlorides with organic acids. Molecular complexes of fluoxetine hydrochloride with benzoic, succinic, and fumaric acids. *J Am Chem Soc*. 2004;126:13335-13342. doi:10.1021/ja048114o.

67. Amos JG, Indelicato JM, Passini CE, Reutzel SM, inventors; Eli Lilly and Co, assignee. Bicyclic beta-lactam/parabens complexes. US patent 5,412,094. May 2, 1995.

68. Richards RME. Effect of hypromellose on the antibacterial activity of benzalkonium chloride. *J Pharm Pharmacol*. 1976;28:264.

69. Bin T, Kulshreshtha AK, al-Shakhshir R, Hem SL. Adsorption of benzalkonium chloride by filter membranes: mechanisms and effect of formulation and processing parameters. *Pharm Dev Technol*. 1999;4(2):151-165.

70. Clarke CD, Armstrong NA. Influence of pH on the adsorption of benzoic acid by kaolin. *Pharm J*. 1972;209:44-45.

71. Hanson BA. Chlorobutanol monograph. In: Rowe R, Shesky PJ, Quinn ME, eds. *Handbook of Pharmaceutical Excipients*. 6th ed. London, United Kingdom: Pharmaceutical Press; 2009:166-168.

72. Peltonen L. Chlorhexidine monograph. In: Rowe R, Shesky PJ, Quinn ME, eds. *Handbook of Pharmaceutical Excipients*. 6th ed. London, United Kingdom: Pharmaceutical Press; 2009:161-166.

73. Haley S. Methylparaben monograph. In: Rowe R, Shesky PJ, Quinn ME, eds. *Handbook of Pharmaceutical Excipients*. 6th ed. London, United Kingdom: Pharmaceutical Press; 2009:441-445.

74. Johnson R, Steer R. Butylparaben monograph. In: Rowe R, Shesky PJ, Quinn ME, eds. *Handbook of Pharmaceutical Excipients*. 6th ed. London, United Kingdom: Pharmaceutical Press; 2009:78-81.

75. Haley S. Propylparaben monograph. In: Rowe R, Shesky PJ, Quinn ME, eds. *Handbook of Pharmaceutical Excipients*. 6th ed. London, United Kingdom: Pharmaceutical Press; 2009:596-598.

76. Sandler N. Ethylparaben monograph. In: Rowe R, Shesky PJ, Quinn ME, eds. *Handbook of Pharmaceutical Excipients*. 6th ed. London, United Kingdom: Pharmaceutical Press; 2009:270-272.

77. Matthews BR. Phenylmercuric nitrate monograph. In: Rowe R, Shesky PJ, Quinn ME, eds. *Handbook of Pharmaceutical Excipients*. 6th ed. London, United Kingdom: Pharmaceutical Press; 2009:496-499.

78. Weller PJ. Thimerosal monograph. In: Rowe R, Shesky PJ, Quinn ME, eds. *Handbook of Pharmaceutical Excipients*. 6th ed. London, United Kingdom: Pharmaceutical Press; 2009:736-739.

79. Owen SC. Edetic acid monograph. In: Rowe R, Shesky PJ, Quinn ME, eds. *Handbook of Pharmaceutical Excipients*. 6th ed. London, United Kingdom: Pharmaceutical Press; 2009:247-250.

80. 3.2.2. Plastic containers and closures for pharmaceutical use. Scribd Web site. https://www.scribd.com/document/150657654/3-2-2-Plastic-Containers-and-Closures-for-Pharmaceutical-Use. Accessed July 9, 2019.

81. McCarthy TJ. Storage studies of preservative solutions in commonly used plastic containers. *Cosmet Perfum*. 1973;88:41-42.

82. European Medicines Agency. Annex to the European Commission guideline on 'Excipients in the labelling and package leaflet of medicinal products for human use' (SANTE-2017-11668): excipients and information for the package leaflet. European Medicines Agency Web site. https://www.ema.europa.eu/en/documents/scientific-guideline/annex-european-commission-guideline-excipients-labelling-package-leaflet-medicinal-products-human_en.pdf. Accessed July 9, 2019.

83. Okahara A, Kawazu K. Local toxicity of benzalkonium chloride in ophthalmic solutions following repeated applications. *J Toxicol Sci*. 2013;38:531-537.

84. Waknine Y, Barclay L. FDA approvals: first preservative-free prostaglandin eye drops for glaucoma. Medscape Web site. http://www.medscape.org/viewarticle/759229. Accessed July 9, 2019.

85. Kozaerwicz P. Preservatives: are they safe? European Medicines Agency Web site. https://www.ema.europa.eu/en/documents/presentation/presentation-preservatives-are-they-safe_en.pdf. Accessed July 9, 2019.

86. Loeffler M, Hornblass A. Hazards of unit dose artificial tear preparations. *Arch Ophthalmol*. 1990;108:639-640.

87. Van Santvliet L, Sam T, Ludwig A. Packaging of ophthalmic solutions—influence on stability, sterility, eye drop instillation and patient compliance. *Eur J Pharm Biopharm*. 1996;42:375-384.

88. European Medicines Agency. Reflection paper on the use of methyl- and propylparaben as excipients in human medicinal products for oral use. EMA/CHMP/SWP/272921/2012. European Medicines Agency Web site. https://www.ema.europa.eu/en/documents/scientific-guideline/reflection-paper-use-methyl-propylparaben-excipients-human-medicinal-products-oral-use_en.pdf. Accessed July 9, 2019.

89. European Medicines Agency. Questions and answers on benzalkonium chloride in the context of the revision of the guideline on 'Excipients in the label and package leaflet of medicinal products for human use' (CPMP/463/00). European Medicines Agency Web site. https://www.ema.europa.eu/en/documents/scientific-guideline/questions-answers-benzalkonium-chloride-context-revision-guideline-excipients-label-package-leaflet_en.pdf. Accessed July 9, 2019.

90. European Medicines Agency. EMEA Public statement on antimicrobial preservatives in ophthalmic preparations for human use. EMEA/622721/2009. European Medicines Agency Web site. https://www.ema.europa.eu/en/documents/presentation/presentation-preservatives-are-they-safe_en.pdf. Accessed July 9, 2019.

91. Scientific Committee on Consumer Products. Opinion on benzoic acid and sodium benzoate. European Commission Web site. https://ec.europa.eu/health/ph_risk/committees/04_sccp/docs/sccp_o_015.pdf. Accessed July 9, 2019.

92. World Health Organization. Joint FAO/WHO Expert Committee on Food Additives (JECFA) publications. World Health Organization Web site. https://www.who.int/foodsafety/publications/jecfa/en/. Accessed July 9, 2019.

93. European Medicines Agency. Questions and answers on benzoic acid and benzoates in the context of the revision of the guideline on 'Excipients in the label and package leaflet of medicinal products for human use' (CPMP/463/00). European Medicines Agency Web site. Accessed July 9, 2019.

94. European Commission. Opinion of the Scientific Committee on Food on benzyl alcohol. European Commission Web site. https://ec.europa.eu/food/sites/food/files/safety/docs/fs_food-improvement-agents_flavourings-out138.pdf. Accessed July 9, 2019.

95. US Environmental Protection Agency. Health and environmental effects document for benzyl alcohol. US Environmental Protection Agency Web site. https://nepis.epa.gov/Exe/tiff2png.cgi/900G0J00.PNG?-r+65+-g+3+D%3A%5CZYFILES%5CINDEX%20DATA%5C86THRU90%5CTIFF%5C00001494%5C900G0J00.TIF. Accessed July 9, 2019.

96. European Medicines Agency. Questions and answers on benzyl alcohol used as an excipient in medicinal products for human use. European Medicines Agency Web site. https://www.ema.europa.eu/en/documents/scientific-guideline/questions-answers-benzyl-alcohol-used-excipient-medicinal-products-human-use_en.pdf. Accessed July 9, 2019.

97. Gershanik J, Boecler B, Ensley H, McCloskey S, George W. The gasping syndrome and benzyl alcohol poisoning. *N Engl J Med*. 1982;307:1384-1388.

98. Brown WR, Buist NR, Gipson HT, Huston RK, Kennaway NG. Fatal benzyl alcohol poisoning in a neonatal intensive care unit. *Lancet*. 1982;1:1250.

99. European Medicines Agency. Questions and Answers on benzyl alcohol in the context of the revision of the guideline on 'Excipients in the label and package leaflet of medicinal products for human use' (CPMP/463/00). European Medicines Agency Web site. https://www.ema.europa.eu/en/documents/scientific-guideline/questions-answers-benzyl-alcohol-context-revision-guideline-excipients-label-package-leaflet_en.pdf. Accessed July 9, 2019.

100. Milsap RL, Jusko WJ. Pharmacokinetics in the infant. *Environ Health Perspect*. 1994;102(suppl 11):107-110.

101. Brothers E. Pediatric ethanol toxicity. Medscape Web site. http://emedicine.medscape.com/article/1010220-overview. Accessed July 9, 2019.
102. Mancini AJ. Skin. *Pediatrics.* 2004;113:1114-1119. https://pediatrics.aappublications.org/content/pediatrics/113/Supplement_3/1114.full.pdf. Accessed July 9, 2019.
103. Simon HK, Cox JM, Sucov A, Linakis JG. Serum ethanol clearance in intoxicated children and adolescents presenting to the ED. *Acad Emerg Med.* 1994;1:520-524.
104. Spohr HL, Willms J, Steinhausen HC. Prenatal alcohol exposure and long-term developmental consequences. *Lancet.* 1993;341:907-910.
105. Coles CD. Prenatal alcohol exposure and human development In: Miller MW, ed. *Development of the Central Nervous System. Effects of Alcohol and Opiates.* New York, NY: Wiley-Liss Inc; 1992:9-36.
106. Testino G. The burden of cancer attributable to alcohol consumption. *Maedica (Buchar).* 2011;6(4):313-320.
107. National Toxicology Program. NTP technical report on toxicology and carcinogenesis. Studies of urethane, ethanol, and urethane/ethanol (Urethane, CAS No. 51-79-6; Ethanol, CAS No. 64-17-5). National Toxicology Program Web site. https://ntp.niehs.nih.gov/ntp/htdocs/lt_rpts/tr510.pdf. Accessed July 9, 2019.
108. Association des Centres Antipoison et de Toxicovigilance. *The Recommendations on the Ethanol Threshold in Oral Liquid Preparations Administered to Children.* Paris, France: Association des Centres Antipoison et de Toxicovigilance; 2006. http://www.centresantipoison.net/cctv/rapport_ethanol_cctv_2006.pdf. Accessed July 9, 2019.
109. US Food and Drug Administration. Over-the-counter drug products intended for oral ingestion that contain alcohol. US Food and Drug Administration Web site. https://www.accessdata.fda.gov/scripts/cdrh/cfdocs/cfCFR/CFRSearch.cfm?CFRPart=328&showFR=1. Accessed July 9, 2019.
110. European Medicines Agency. Questions and answers on ethanol in the context of the revision of the guideline on 'Excipients in the Label and Package Leaflet of Medicinal Products for Human Use'. European Medicines Agency Web site. https://www.ema.europa.eu/en/documents/scientific-guideline/questions-answers-ethanol-context-revision-guideline-excipients-label-package-leaflet-medicinal_en.pdf. Accessed July 2018.
111. European Food Safety Authority. Scientific opinion on the toxicological evaluation of phenol. *EFSA J.* 2013;11(4):3189. https://efsa.onlinelibrary.wiley.com/doi/epdf/10.2903/j.efsa.2013.3189.
112. Geier DA, Jordan SK, Geier MR. The relative toxicity of compounds used as preservatives in vaccines and biologics. *Med Sci Monit.* 2010;16:21-27.
113. International Journal of Toxicology. Final report on the safety assessment of *p*-chloro-*m*-cresol. *Int J Toxicol.* 1997;16:235-268.
114. CIR Expert Report. Final report on the safety assessment of chloroxylenol. *J Am Coll Toxicol.* 1985;4:147-169.
115. Fontana AJ. Water activity's role in food safety and quality. *Food Safety Magazine.* February/March 2001. https://www.foodsafetymagazine.com/magazine-archive1/februarymarch-2001-water-activitye28099s-role-in-food-safety-and-quality. Accessed July 9, 2019.
116. United States Pharmacopeia. *USP 35 <1112> Application of Water Activity Determination to Nonsterile Pharmaceutical Products.* Rockville, MD: United States Pharmacopeial Convention; 2012.
117. Chirife J, Fontana CF, Benmergui EA. The prediction of water activity in aqueous solutions in connection with intermediate moisture foods. *J Food Technol.* 1980;15:59-70.
118. Buckley HL, Hart-Cooper WM, Kim JH, et al. Design and testing of safer, more effective preservatives for consumer products. *ACS Sustainable Chem Eng.* 2017;5:4320-4433.
119. European Medicines Agency. Reflection paper on microbiological aspects of herbal medicinal products and traditional herbal medicinal products. European Medicines Agency Web site. https://www.ema.europa.eu/en/documents/scientific-guideline/reflection-paper-microbiological-aspects-herbal-medicinal-products-traditional-herbal-medicinal_en.pdf. Accessed July 9, 2019.
120. Ball R. Substituting thimerosal preservative used in vaccines: FDA perspective. World Health Organization Web site. https://www.who.int/immunization/sage/meetings/2012/april/USFDA_perspective_thimerosal_alternatives.pdf. Accessed July 9, 2019.
121. European Medicines Agency. EMA public statement on thiomersal in vaccines for human use: recent evidence supports safety of thiomersal-containing vaccines. European Medicines Agency Web site. https://www.ema.europa.eu/en/documents/scientific-guideline/emea-public-statement-thiomersal-vaccines-human-use-recent-evidence-supports-safety-thimersal_en.pdf. Accessed July 9, 2019.
122. World Health Organization. Statement on thimerosal. World Health Organization Website. https://www.who.int/vaccine_safety/committee/topics/thiomersal/statement_jul2006/en. Accessed July 9, 2019.
123. Meyer BK, Binghua AN, Shi L. Antimicrobial preservative use in parenteral products: past and present. *J Pharm Sci.* 2007;96:3155-3165.
124. Blaug SM, Ahsan SS. Interaction of parabens with nonionic macromolecules. *J Pharm Sci.* 1961;50(5):441-443.
125. Shi S, Chen Z, Rizzo JM, et al. A highly sensitive method for the quantitation of polysorbates 20 and 80 to study the compatibility between polysorbates and *m*-cresol in peptide formulations. *J Anal Bioanal Tech.* 2015;6:1-8.
126. Zhang Y, Roy S, Jones LS, et al. Mechanism for benzyl alcohol-induced aggregation of recombinant human interleukin-1 receptor antagonist in aqueous solution. *J Pharm Sci.* 2004;93:3076-3089.
127. Thirumangalathu R, Krishnan S, Brems DN, Randolph TW, Carpenter JF. Effects of pH, temperature, and sucrose on benzyl alcohol-induced aggregation of recombinant human granulocyte colony stimulating factor. *J Pharm Sci.* 2006;95:1480-1497.
128. Roy S, Jung R, Kerwin BA, Randolph TW, Carpenter JF. Effects of benzyl alcohol on aggregation of recombinant human interleukin-1-receptor antagonist in reconstituted lyophilized formulations. *J Pharm Sci.* 2005;94:382-396.
129. Patel NK, Kostenbauder HB. Interaction of preservatives with macromolecules 1. Binding of parahydroxybenzoate esters by polyoxyethylene 20 sorbitan monooleate. *J Am Pharm Assoc.* 1958;47:289-293.

CHAPTER 40

Cosmetic Preservatives and Preservation

Philip A. Geis

Archaeologic evidence indicates that humans have been painting their bodies for nearly a half-million years,[1] progressing from sharpened reocher sticks presumed to be used for coloring the bodies of *Homo erectus* to modern cosmetics of such technical and esthetic sophistication. Although early cosmetic use of lead and antimony may have inadvertently served a preservative function, the realization of microbiological risk and need for preservation was largely a mid-20th century realization. The concept of microbiological quality and effective preservation developed early for foods but less rapidly for cosmetics. Despite the early 20th century introduction of parabens[2] and to a limited extent formaldehyde and benzoic acid,[3] and the 1938 US Food Drug and Cosmetic Act, cosmetic preservation as a focused technical effort across the industry did not evolve until the latter half of the last century. Published reports that exposed the poor state of cosmetic and drug microbiological quality were compelling to its development. A US Food and Drug administration (FDA) study of products sold in New York found 25% to be contaminated with various bacteria and fungi.[4] Other studies found similar levels of contaminated drug and cosmetics products in Europe.[5,6] Preservation and preservative testing became important and necessary elements of cosmetic research and development addressing risks of contamination during manufacturing and preservative systems and protocols for their evaluation.[7-10] By contrast, preservative testing developed to address pharmaceutical contamination focused on contaminants encountered in clinical practice.[11,12] An additional concern for microbiological safety of cosmetics was identified by Ahearn et al who reported eye infections, some resulting in blindness, traced to contaminated mascara.[13-15] The same products were shown to be free of contamination before use; however, consumer practices of moistening the mascara brush with tap water and spittle resulted in microbial growth on the brush and in the product. Minor corneal abrasion resulting from misuse of the brush, implanted *Pseudomonas aeruginosa* in a manner that resulted in serious ocular infection, blinding some women. The realization of in-use risk further compelled attention to preservative stability and efficacy through the life of the product.[16] Dr. Ahearn's investigation had been funded by the FDA, and the serious nature of these reports compelled the agency to propose rulemaking to establish regulations for the development of preservative efficacy standards for eye-area products.[17]

Through the following decade, the cosmetic industry organized as the Cosmetic, Toiletry and Fragrance Association (now the Personal Care Products Council or PCPC), developed and broadly implemented industry guidelines and methodologies to control microbiological risks. With the introduction of good manufacturing practices (GMPs), new preservatives and data-driven qualification of preservatives systems, microbiological concerns, recalls and risks of contamination diminished profoundly.[18] Through the remainder of the 20th century, the cosmetic industry focused on maintaining this high level of microbiological quality by the reapplication of a few, very effective combinations of preservatives including esters of parabens, formaldehyde releasers (FAs), isothiazolinone, organic alcohols and acids and the adjunct ethylene diamine tetraacetic acid (EDTA).[7,19] At the turn of the century, Darbre[20] published a troubling report that implied a connection between parabens and breast cancer, a phenomenon that lab and others continued to explore into the 21st century. Although this connection was and continues to be significantly criticized by the scientific community[21] and has not been accepted by the FDA,[22] it provoked closer scrutiny of parabens. The European Union later banned paraben esters of limited use primarily due to lack of current safety data.[23] As these molecules are commodities and the primary paraben was not affected, no supplier chose to invest data development. The overall safety assessment of parabens continues to support their safe use in cosmetics.[24-26]

However, growing consumer desire for alternative and natural products[27] was unfavorable to all traditional preservatives, but most critical of parabens drove application of alternatives.[28,29] The preservative methyl isothiazolinone was introduced as a replacement,[28] but its rapid and extensive adoption apparently proved problematic as it drove an unacceptable level of sensitization among consumers.[30,31] Although major companies have maintained traditional cosmetic preservative combinations,[32] preservation diversified in the hands of some formulators to include more complex combination of less effective chemicals, some of which were largely new, as well as several "natural" preservatives and "preservative-free" packaging innovations.[28,29,33,34] Unfortunately, these alternative preservative systems have, in some cases, driven cosmetic recalls due to microbial contamination at levels not seen for many decades. FDA reported over 70 cosmetic-specific cosmetic products recalled for microbial contamination in 2017.[35] All associated natural or alternative preservative systems, the greatest level this writer recalls in his 40-year career. The following sections will address the rationale for preservative use, the scope of preservation, preservatives and preservation elements, and the methods and risk assessments used by the cosmetic industry to ensure consumer safety.

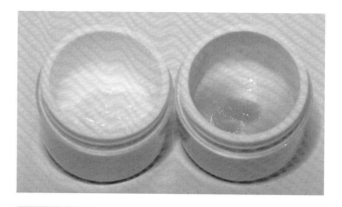

FIGURE 40.1 Example of a cosmetic product as made (left) and contaminated (right). Photo courtesy of halenia.net.

▶ RATIONALE FOR PRESERVATIVE USE

The rationale or objective of cosmetic preservation and preservative use is to establish and maintain microbiological quality. Whereas some degree of preservation is required in nonsterile manufacturing, GMPs are intended to mitigate spoilage risk in this context. The primary objective of the cosmetic preservative is to protect the consumer during product use. Consequences for failure to serve this objective include loss of product functionality and esthetics, regulatory intervention and most importantly compromised consumer safety.

For esthetics and functionality, the classic consumer perception of a contaminated cosmetic is an unsightly mold on the surface of a cream in an open jar. Other visual signals of contamination include discoloration for example by microbial pigments such as prodigiosin from *Serratia marcescens* and pyoverdine from *P aeruginosa*.[36] Manifest as general yellow to muddy brown product discoloration or localized, for example, as a red ring on the surface of a white liquid hand soap contaminated with *S marcescens*; more substantial contamination or extended incubation time is typically required to render these effects obvious (Figure 40.1).

If the consumer investigated further, the consumer would certainly find compromise in other attributes of the products such as odor and changes in product perfume. A common culprit of mold-spoilage odor is 1-Octen-3-ol,[37] and bacteria that contaminate cosmetics can produce

hydrogen sulfide, indole, and skatole.[38] The thresholds of detection of these volatile organic compounds are at parts per billion levels,[39] and ironically some serve as perfume components themselves. The perception of moldy or fecal odor is a critical fault for a cosmetic. In addition, fungal and bacterial contamination can physically comprise product stability with sediment production and breaking of emulsions.[40] Despite these potential manifestations, microbial contamination more often presents no discernable effect, denying the consumer a signal that the product being used may offer a safety risk.

Human safety is clearly the most significant driver for preservation. Whereas topical application at high titers of bacteria representative of cosmetic contaminants may result in transient skin irritation and even infection,[41] consumers with some degree of physical impairment and immunocompromised are at greater risk and the subjects of greatest concern. Historically, cutaneous anthrax infections have been attributed to the use of contaminated shaving implements that allow exposure of abraded skin.[42] Use of contaminated (*Burkholderia cepacia*) moisturizing body milk in an intensive care unit resulted in bacteremia and urinary and respiratory infections.[43] Similarly, multiple publications have reported respiratory infection traced to the use of *B cepacia*-contaminated mouthwash products in hospital intensive care units.[44,45] As described earlier, Ahearn et al[13] reported very serious eye infection with exposure of scratched ocular surface to contaminated mascara. Serious as these were, fatal infections infection from contaminated cosmetics also have been reported. Use of a baby shampoo contaminated with *S marcescens* in a hospital children's ward reportedly resulted in 15 infections in 11 children, 1 of whom died.[46] Shampoo contaminated with *P aeruginosa* was used in cancer hospital salon where patients, in anticipation of chemotherapy-related alopecia, had their heads shampooed and then shaven. Serious infections traced to the contaminated shampoo developed during chemotherapy and one of these proved fatal.[47] Whereas, compromised patients' defenses were associated with each these, it is important to consider that more than 25% of the US population may be considered "immunocompromised" and other transient factors such as broken skin and existing pathologies further elevates that number.[48]

Based on concerns for product safety, regulatory bodies around the world monitor cosmetic product quality including the FDA, Health Canada, Australia's Therapeutic Goods Administration, and the European Commission. Microbiological contamination is considered a significant risk, and product recalls are considered an appropriate response. Although recalls of cosmetics are historically infrequent, microbiological contamination is by far the primary rationale for any such action regarding cosmetics. In considering microbiological quality, it is recognized that cosmetics are not expected to be sterile, but detectable microbes should be very few and should not include "objectionable microorganisms."[49] An exclusive list of specific objectionable microorganisms of concern is difficult if not impossible to assemble as gross contamination with any microorganism could compromise product integrity and safety. In practice, those present at any level that would be considered unacceptable includes pathogenic microbes such as *Staphylococcus aureus*, *P aeruginosa*, and gram-negative bacteria as a group, as well as fungi such as *Candida albicans*, both due to their pathogenicity and potential adaptation to preservatives and growth in products.[7,49]

Microbial contaminants of cosmetics and related products compose a very wide range of mesophilic bacteria and fungi (Table 40.1). This includes some significant pathogens including historical reports of anthrax from shaving brushes[41] and modern reports from developing countries of *Corynebacterium diphtheria* from decongestant sprays[55] and *Salmonella* and *Shigella* species in shampoos.[56,57] Contamination with such frank pathogens is associated with cosmetics manufactured in the developing world. The challenge to the cosmetic microbiologist is to establish a preservative system in context of GMPs and appropriate packaging to mitigate this diverse microbiological risk in the context of global and cultural uses/misuses as well as nonsterile manufacturing environments.

▶ PRESERVATIVES

Although some historic cosmetics included ingredients of antimicrobial potential, purposeful preservation of cosmetics began in the 20th century with several new and very effective preservatives introduced in the 1960s and 1970s, many of which were based on formaldehyde release (Table 40.2).[7,58] Especially in combination with parabens, these formaldehyde-releasing preservatives became widely used for effective preservation and remain in common usage.[7,59] Chloromethyl isothiazolinone (CMIT) was introduced in the late 1970s and expanded in the following decade to become the primary global preservative in rinse-off products—shampoos, conditioners, body washes, and hand soaps.[7,60] Its minor component methyl isothiazolinone (MIT) was introduced in the 1990s.

TABLE 40.1	Common microbiological contaminants of cosmetics and related materials[a]		
Gram-Negative Bacteria	*Pseudomonas aeruginosa* *Burkholderia cepacia* *Burkholderia pickettii* *Stenotrophomonas maltophilia* *Acinetobacter* species *Moraxella* species *Escherichia coli* *Klebsiella pneumoniae* *Klebsiella oxytoca*		*Serratia marcescens* *Aeromonas* species *Salmonella* species *Proteus* species *Raoultella planticola* *Rhizobium radiobacter* *Achromobacter xylosoxidans* *Pantoea agglomerans* *Citrobacter freundii*
Gram-Positive Bacteria	*Staphylococcus aureus* *Staphylococcus epidermidis* *Staphylococcus warneri* *Streptococcus* species *Propionibacterium* species		*Corynebacterium diphtheriae* *Clostridium tetani* *Clostridium perfringens* *Bacillus* species *Bacillus anthracis* (historic)
Fungi	*Candida albicans* *Candida lipolytica* *Saccharomyces cerevisiae* *Rhodotorula* species *Aureobasidium pullulans*		*Paecilomyces variotii* *Aspergillus fumigatus* *Aspergillus niger* *Scopulariopsis* species *Penicillium* species

[a]Data from Geis,[7] Sutton and Jimenez,[50] Chervenak et al,[51] International Standards Organization,[52] Personal Care Products Council,[53] and Schnittger.[54]

TABLE 40.2	Historical review of preservatives used in cosmetics
Date	**Preservative**
1900	Sodium benzoate/benzoic, phenol, cresol
1920s	Parabens, formaldehyde
1940s	Alcohols, sorbic acid
1950s	Phenoxyethanol
1960s	Imidazolidinyl urea (Germall), DMDM hydantoin (Glydant), bromo nitropropane diol (bronopol)
1970s	Hexamethylenetetramine chloroallyl chloride (quaternium-15)
1980s	Diazolidinyl urea (Germall II), chloromethyl isothiazolinone (Kathon-CG), chlorphenesin
1990s	Methyl isothiazolinone (Neolone), expansion of preservative blends
2000s	Glycols (caprylyl glycol), ethylhexyl glycerine, "natural preservatives," pressure to remove parabens
2010s	Expansion of "natural' preservatives, ethylhexyl glycerine, methyl isothiazolinone limitations

Abbreviation: DMDM hydantoin, dimethyl dimethylol hydantoin.

As reported previously, 21st century concerns for preservatives drove considerable interest in parabens replacements, especially in leave-on products. Many formulators chose MIT and to a lesser extent phenoxyethanol as paraben replacements[28,29]; however, reports of skin sensitization to MIT provoked a ban of its use in this application. The growth of consumer interest in natural, organic, parabens-free, and formaldehyde-free free products after the turn of the century have driven much greater diversity into cosmetic preservative use.[32]

Although the mechanism(s) by which the commonly used preservatives exert antimicrobial effect are not well researched, the practical factors associated with their effective applications has been learned through empirical testing of innumerable product development cycles. (Table 40.3).

TABLE 40.3	Application considerations for commonly used cosmetic preservatives				
Preservative	**Primary Application**	**Suggested Active Application Range**	**pH Range**	**Primary Efficacy**	**Efficacy Constraints**
Parabens	Emulsion/leave on	2000-8000 ppm (as total paraben)	3-8	Gram-positive bacteria, Fungi	Nonionic surfactants Polysorbates
Formaldehyde releasers	General	1000-2500 ppm	3-8	Bacteria	Some perfume, amines, protein hydrolysates, amino acids
CMIT	Rinse off	3-7.5 ppm	3-7	Bacteria	Amines, reducing/oxidizing agents
MIT	Rinse off	50-100 ppm	Broad	Bacteria	Reducing/oxidizing agents
Organic acids	Leave on	2000-5000 ppm	6 or less	Gram-positive bacteria, fungi	Nonionic surfactants, formaldehyde
Organic alcohols	General	2000-8000 ppm	Broad	Bacteria, fungi	Oxidation, nonionic surfactants
Long-chain 1,2 glycols	Leave on	1%-5%	Broad	Bacteria	

Abbreviations: CMIT, chloromethyl isothiazolinone; MIT, methyl isothiazolinone.

Parabens

These are esters of p-hydroxybenzoic acid include methyl-, ethyl-, propyl-, isopropyl-, and benzyl- parabens, with methyl parabens as the most commonly used cosmetic preservative. Parabens are most often used in combination to preserve emulsion-based leave-on and fine and color cosmetics at total concentrations 1000 to 8000 ppm.[7,32,61,62] Longer chain parabens have been reported to be more effective but are used at lesser levels due to their decreasing solubility.[32] Parabens are effective across a broad pH range from 3 to 8 and are most effective versus gram-positive bacteria and fungi, especially with the longer chain parabens for the latter.[32,61] Less effective against gram-negative bacteria, they are commonly used in combination with FAs or phenoxyethanol to extend efficacy to these bacteria.[61] During formulation, they are typically added to the heated water preemulsion or via solution in other ingredients such as propylene glycol.[32] As preservatives are most effective in the water phase of emulsions, it is essential for antimicrobial efficacy that aqueous preservative levels are maximized in the formulation. Parabens possess significant lipid solubility and, if formulated poorly, will partition into emulsion oil phase and with loss of product preservative efficacy.[63,64] Parabens undergo hydrolysis in weak alkaline and strongly acidic solutions, and antimicrobial efficacy decreases above pH 8 due to the formation of the phenolate anion.[32] They also physically interact with cyclodextrins and nonionic surfactants such as polysorbates with mitigation of efficacy.[32,61,65] In the presence of sugars and polyols, parabens (especially methyl paraben) may undergo transesterification and some tubing materials may absorb parabens.[66,67]

Formaldehyde-Releasing Preservatives

Direct preservation with formaldehyde preservation was phased out in the latter half of the 20th century and replaced with the so-called FAs. First marketed in the 1960s and 1970s and continuing in frequent application,[32] FAs imidazolidinyl urea, dimethyl dimethylol hydantoin (DMDM hydantoin), and diazolidinyl urea are used at concentrations from 1000 to 3000 ppm.[32,61,68-70] These are effective by the slow release of a low level of formaldehyde,[71] although some have attributed additional efficacy to the parent molecule itself.[72] Effective across a broad pH range, they are used in both leave-on and rinse-off products as well as color cosmetics.[7] Most effective versus bacteria especially gram-negative bacteria, FAs are often used in combination with parabens or organic acids that address yeast and mold contamination risk establishing "broad spectrum" efficacy (see Table 40.3).[61] Due to heat sensitivity, FAs should be formulated at temperatures less than 70°C.[32] Interaction with perfume components, some

protein hydrolysates, amino acids, and sunscreen actives can limit efficacy.[7,32,73,74] In formulation, they should be incorporated in the water phase[58] as addition to lipid phase will result in their precipitation, and addition to finished product may not achieve adequate distribution.

Isothiazolinones

First marketed in the late 1970s, CMIT rapidly became the primary preservative for rinse-off products—shampoos, conditioners, body washes, and hand soaps.[7,60] It is not used in leave-on products such as creams and lotions due to concerns for skin sensitization.[75] At typical usage levels of 5 to 7 ppm, CMIT is primarily effective versus bacteria in products of acidic and neutral pH. The molecule is unstable at alkaline pH especially in the presence of secondary amines.[58,63,76] Although rinse-off surfactant-based products are less prone to fungal contamination, CMIT is typically used with an additional preservative such as benzoic acid (see Table 40.3).[7] As a raw-material ingredient, CMIT is stabilized in a magnesium salt solution, dilution in deionized water without immediate product formulation should be avoided due to stability concerns.[76] The molecule is unstable in the presence of reducing and oxidizing agents and pyrithione zinc and should be formulated at temperatures less than 50°C.[58,61,76] Efficacy may be diminished in the presence of some protein hydrolysates.[58]

Commercially, CMIT includes an ineffective level of MIT. As discussed earlier, the late 1990s saw MI introduced as a stand-alone preservative at use levels up to approximately 100 ppm and found rapid acceptance as a parabens-replacement in leave-on products (see Table 40.3). Unfortunately, significant sensitization issues in this application developed in the early 21st century resulting in regulatory and marketing restraints in its use.

Organic Acids

These are some of the oldest cosmetic preservatives and include benzoic, sorbic, and dehydroacetic acids. As antimicrobial activity is associated with the protonated molecule, these organic acids are primarily effective at pH less than or approximating their pKa (see Table 40.3).[58] However, benzoic acid efficacy has been observed at higher pH in some surfactant-based, rinse-off products. Used at concentrations from 2000 to 8000 ppm, they are primarily effective versus gram-positive bacteria and fungi and are typically combined with FAs, CMIT, or phenoxyethanol to address gram-negative bacterial contamination risk (see Table 40.3).[61] Organic acids can serve as substrate for microbial metabolism and therefore should be used at appropriate levels and pH and in combination with preservatives such as benzyl alcohol, FAs, or isothiazolinone.[58,61,77,78]

Sorbic acid stability is compromised in the presence of some amino acids[79,80] and isothiazolinones.[81] Dehydroacetic acid stability is accelerated in the presence of free formaldehyde, and the insoluble salt formed with magnesium (eg, from combination with commercial CMIT) will compromise stability and efficacy.[81,82] Organic acids can be absorbed by some flexible tubing materials.[83,84] Due to poor solubility at formulation pH, organic acids are typically formulated into the water phase as sodium or potassium salts with product pH subsequently adjusted to establish appropriate efficacy.[58]

Organic Alcohols

These include ethyl, phenoxyethyl, and benzyl alcohols. Ethanol is a cosmetic ingredient that brings substantial preservative capacity to appropriate products. Although concentrations of about 20% and greater are considered necessary for effective preservation,[61] lower levels may have limited effect when combined with other preservatives. Phenoxyethanol is a very commonly used preservative and has found significant use both with parabens and as parabens replacement.[58] At concentrations of 2000 to 8000 ppm, PE is primarily effective versus bacteria, importantly, gram-negative bacteria, and is often combined with preservatives targeting fungi (see Table 40.3).[58] Benzyl alcohol is similarly effective although less so versus gram-negative bacteria and is often formulated with antioxidants such as tocopherol to address potential oxidation.[58] Although not so much at parabens, some have reported loss of organic alcohol efficacy due to partitioning into the lipid phase of emulsions.[85] Organic alcohols can be subject to bacterial degradation, especially if used as sole preservatives and at low levels,[58,86] and are at risk to absorption by some packaging materials.[83,84]

Glycols

Whereas short-chain glycols such as propylene glycol can affect antimicrobial efficacy via modulation of water activity, concentrations beyond typical preservation levels are required. However, longer chain 1,2-glycols show efficacy in addition to any modulation of water activity. Hexylene and caprylyl glycols are effectively used as cosmetic preservatives at concentrations 5000 to 10 000 ppm.[58,87,88] Primarily effective against bacteria, glycols and are often used in preservative combinations (see Table 40.3).[58,89]

Chlorphenesin

This preservative should not be confused with chlorphenesin carbamate, a muscle relaxant. Reportedly effective versus fungi at 1000 to 3000 ppm, chlorphenesin is effectively incorporated in heated aqueous phase in products of pH range 5 to 7.[61] It is primarily effective versus fungi and used in combination with preservatives that are effective versus bacteria (see Table 40.3).[90]

Ethylhexyl Glycerine

A 21st century introduction, this preservative can be considered a multifunctional ingredient as it allegedly establishes skin-feel benefits.[91] As a stand-alone preservative, it has little to no activity but reportedly confers broad-spectrum efficacy in combination with phenoxyethanol and caprylyl glycol.[92,93]

"Natural" Preservatives

Growth of the "natural," organic cosmetic niche provoked significant interest in unconventional preservatives. Preservatives claimed to be natural include natural sourcing of conventional preservatives such as some alcohols and organic acids as well as plant extracts, products of fermentation (eg, leuconostoc radish ferment), essential oils, and enzyme preparations including glucose oxidase.[28,29,33,94-96] Application has been limited by a number of factors. Ingredient costs are substantially greater, and, unlike conventional preservatives, efficacy may not be consistent between product applications sometimes requiring multiple preservative reformulations to achieve necessary efficacy in development. Some preparations have been reported to be adulterated with synthetic disinfectants and preservatives, most notable in this regard is grapefruit seed extract.[97-99] Plant extracts and essential oils are complex and variable mixtures typically consisting of hundreds of components.[100] The qualitative and quantitative chemical dynamics conferring effective preservation of such mixtures in formulated products are very poorly understood. As the composition of such natural mixtures will vary greatly between batches,[100] and such natural materials can also be contaminated with pesticides,[101] substantial analytical and microbiological qualification is required to assure efficacy on a batch basis in each product application.

▶ PRESERVATIVE APPLICATIONS

The diversity of preservative application has evolved substantially. Despite this, the most recent summary of cosmetic preservative used as reported to the FDA (Table 40.4) shows that the parabens remain the most commonly used. Phenoxyethanol, driven by parabens-replacement application, is in substantial application. Whereas MIT shows substantial use in the year addressed, sensitization concerns discussed have certainly diminished application

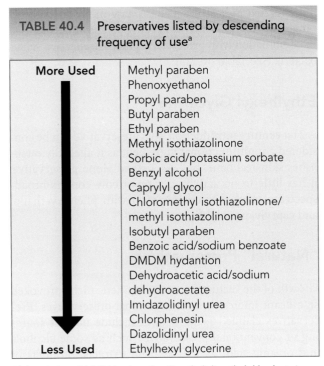

TABLE 40.4   Preservatives listed by descending frequency of use[a]

More Used	
↓	Methyl paraben
	Phenoxyethanol
	Propyl paraben
	Butyl paraben
	Ethyl paraben
	Methyl isothiazolinone
	Sorbic acid/potassium sorbate
	Benzyl alcohol
	Caprylyl glycol
	Chloromethyl isothiazolinone/ methyl isothiazolinone
	Isobutyl paraben
	Benzoic acid/sodium benzoate
	DMDM hydantion
	Dehydroacetic acid/sodium dehydroacetate
	Imidazolidinyl urea
	Chlorphenesin
	Diazolidinyl urea
Less Used	Ethylhexyl glycerine

Abbreviation: DMDM hydantoin, dimethyl dimethylol hydantoin.

[a]Reprinted with permission from Steinberg.[32]

in subsequent years. Organic acids and benzyl alcohol have significant use, largely as copreservatives. Despite concerns, formaldehyde-releasing preservatives continue significant usage.

Preservative Systems

In application, individual preservatives are very rarely used a sole protective agents. Although all possess antimicrobial potential to address the broad range of target organisms, efficacy associated with levels used and effective in cosmetics has their effective application focused on specific groups of microbial contaminants. Therefore, they are used in combination with other preservatives that complement their efficacies to address the wide range of microbiological risks anticipated—grampositive and gram-negative bacteria as well as mycelial and yeast-like fungi.[7,58,61] Table 40.5 lists examples of preservative systems established in major brands. It is significant to note the types of preservatives systems used in specific products categories. Whereas parabens with FAs or phenoxyethanol are often used in leave-on emulsions such as creams and lotions, CMIT with organic acids are commonly found in rinse-off products such as hand and body washes, shampoos and conditioners. Many preservative combinations have been reported to establish "synergy" in preservation, a claim often found invalid when examined in an appropriate statistical consideration.[102]

Preservative Adjuncts

Formula components and characteristics can magnify preservative efficacy. Limitation of water activity (a measure of unbound water available for microbial metabolism and growth) can mitigate the potential for microbial growth in products.[58,103] Gram-negative bacteria generally are the most frequent microbial contaminants of cosmetic products and are also the most sensitive to reduced water activity. Water activity mitigation as the sole preservative mechanism in aqueous products is typically not practical for most cosmetic products but can serve as an adjunct preservative factor.[103] Chelators, especially EDTA, are also very effective as preservative adjuncts. In addition to the anticipated sequestration of divalent cations necessary for microbial stability and metabolism, EDTA also destabilizes microbial capsules and biofilm, allowing better exposure of the cell to preservatives.[58,61,104-106] Other less-used chelators include hinokitiol, phytic acid, and gluconolactone. The antimicrobial efficacy of pyrithione compounds is based in part on chelation capabilities of the molecule although the general resistance of gram-negative bacteria limits their practical application.[58]

Packaging as Preservative

Direct and indirect product packaging is a functional part of the preservative system as well as a target for preservation. In its basic form, product package serves as a physical means preventing incursion from the external, contaminated world and functions with the product chemical preservative to maintain quality.[61] The product package also serves as the dispensing mechanism and establishes a significant risk-control parameter in that role.[107,108,127] For example, cosmetic packaging with large openings offer hand and air-sourced microbes contamination opportunity that, with sufficient time and exposure, can result in microbiological failure.[107,108] Similarly, the screw-off cap of a shampoo used and stored in the shower offers opportunity of tap water ingress. As tap water routinely includes gram-negative bacteria, notably *P aeruginosa*[109] or other pseudomonads, the resulting diluted product is at significant microbiological risk. Risks of this nature can be mitigated to some extent by increasingly robust preservative systems[110] but are better addressed with dispensing mechanisms that reduce exposure to external microbial challenge and product compromise. Brannan and Dille[107] demonstrated that closure system protection of contained product correlated to contamination in use. Pump dispensers further mitigate risk if designed in a manner that prevents "suck back" of external microbes with dispensed product.[108] Packaging has been developed that prevents contamination during use and has been proposed as to serve lower preservative or even preservative-free product formulations,[34] a concept the aerosol products represent in its most effective application.[61,111]

TABLE 40.5	Examples of cosmetic preservative systems of major marketed cosmetics
Product Type	**Preservative System**
Shampoo	CMIT/MIT, benzoic acid, EDTA CMIT/MIT, EDTA Benzoic acid, benzyl alcohol, hexylene glycol Sodium benzoate, benzyl alcohol, phenoxyethanol, leuconostoc ferment filtrate, potassium sorbate, hexylene glycol
Conditioner	CMIT/MIT, benzyl alcohol, EDTA DMDM hydantoin, EDTA CMIT/MIT, IPBC, EDTA CMIT/MIT, DMDM hydantoin, EDTA
Body wash	CMIT/MIT, iodopropyl carbamate, EDTA CMIT/MIT, benzoic acid, EDTA (two such systems) DMDM hydantoin, EDTA (two such systems)
Cream/lotion	Phenoxyethanol, ethylhexyl glycerine DMDM hydantoin, methyl paraben, EDTA methyl paraben, ethyl paraben, propyl paraben, benzyl alcohol, EDTA Diazolidinyl urea, methyl paraben, propyl paraben, EDTA DMDM hydantoin, methyl paraben, iodopropynyl butylcarbamate, EDTA
Mascara	Methyl paraben, propyl paraben, benzyl alcohol Methyl paraben, propyl paraben, phenoxyethanol Methyl paraben, ethyl paraben, propyl paraben, capryloyl glycine, phenoxyethanol, EDTA Caprylyl glycol, dehydroacetic acid, EDTA Phenoxyethanol, methyl paraben, propyl paraben Caprylyl glycol, ethylhexyl glycerol, phenoxyethanol
Eye cream	Phenoxyethanol, sorbic acid, butyl paraben, ethyl paraben, isobutyl paraben, methyl paraben, propyl paraben, sodium benzoate Phenoxyethanol, dehydroacetic acid, EDTA, denatured alcohol Caprylyl glycol, hexylene glycol, Na bisulfite, butylene glycol, phenoxyethanol, EDTA
Pressed powder	Sodium dehydroacetic acid, methyl paraben, propyl paraben Phenoxyethanol, methyl paraben, ethyl paraben, propyl paraben Caprylyl glycol, hexylene glycol; phenoxyethanol, potassium sorbate Sorbic acid, methyl paraben, propyl paraben, butyl paraben, EDTA Ethylhexyl glycerine, sodium dehydroacetic acid

Abbreviations: CMIT, chloromethyl isothiazolinone; DMDM hydantoin, dimethyl dimethyol hydantoin; EDTA, ethylene diamine tetraacetic acid; MIT, methyl isothiazolinone.

▶ PRESERVATIVE RESISTANCE

In this discussion, preservative resistance describes the phenomenon by which the survival and growth of a microbe, typically a product contaminant, is not controlled by a nominally effective concentration of cosmetic preservative. The mechanisms by which cosmetic preservative resistance are considered to occur include alteration of the target site reducing interaction with the preservative, reduction of preservative concentration at the active site and inactivation of the preservative.[112]

Resistance by alteration of target site has only rarely been described as the basis for resistance to preservatives and similar biocides. Triclosan resistance has been attributed to several factors, including mutation of a specific bacterial fatty acid biosynthetic enzyme functional in gram-negative and gram-positive bacteria including mycobacteria, efflux, and other mechanisms.[113] Periame et al[114] described similar resistance-associated phenomena in *Enterobacter gergoviae* including over expression of some protein and membrane alteration that may be related to active site.

Reduction of preservative concentration at the active site has been observed by both active and passive means.[117,120] Efflux as a central mechanism has been shown to be functional for adaptive resistance to a broad range of preservatives in *B cepacia* and *E gergoviae*, two common cosmetic contaminants.[115,116] Davin-Regli et al[116] proposed that the relatively frequent isolation of *E gergoviae* from paraben-preserved cosmetics is directly attributable to the activity of efflux-based resistance. It has long been established that biofilms mechanically reduce preservative concentration access to target microorganisms.[117] Although some would see biofilm as functional in preservative tolerance, allowing survival in the presence of the preservative rather than active resistant growth, the extracellular polysaccharide biofilm matrix of resistance microbes has been shown to include other means of conferring resistance including efflux pumps.[118]

Inactivation, most commonly by metabolic destruction, has been reported for many preservatives. Sondossi et al[119] demonstrated production of formaldehyde dehydrogenase as the basis for resistance to formaldehyde and formaldehyde-releasing preservatives by several microbial contaminants. Similarly, parabens degradation has been demonstrated as a resistance mechanism for both *Pseudomonas* and *Enterobacter* species.[66,116] As noted earlier, organic alcohols and acids can be metabolized by many cosmetic contaminants.[58,85]

Whereas each of the earlier mechanisms has been shown to be uniquely effective for preservative resistance, it is common to find multiple mechanisms in contaminating microorganisms. This is especially true for gram-negative bacteria and most problematically for *B cepacia*.[117,118] Based on records of product recall, the most frequent contaminants of cosmetics are pure cultures of gram-negative bacteria, especially the species *B cepacia* and *P aeruginosa*.[50,121] These products often included preservatives presumed to be at effective concentrations. Where not intrinsic, resistance is presumed to be the result in many cases of exposure of product to resident manufacturing microbes, especially in process water systems. This diluted product allows selection and adaptation progressively from dilute to the full-strength product preservative system. Dynamics of preservatives and microbial contaminants may establish a threshold of concentration of resistance, such that greater concentrations may still provide increased protection against resistance. The common use of preservative in complementary combinations may mitigate risk of resistance,[51] presumably by burdening the contaminating microorganism with necessity to establish multiple mechanisms of resistance. Resistant microorganisms are very difficult to eradicate from manufacturing facilities, causing ongoing quality and economic issues. Although very little information is available regarding in-use contamination, the microbiology of consumer contaminants is much more diverse,[7] apparently reflecting the complexity of unique product usage and effective inoculation and incubation dynamics established by individual consumers.

▶ PRESERVATIVE TESTING

For cosmetic preservatives, specific "in vitro" inhibitory and microbicidal concentrations (minimal inhibitory concentration [MIC] and minimal bactericidal concentration [MBC]) are not very useful. However, "in vivo" preservative challenge testing in product of concern is the central actionable element of risk assessment. Also known as antimicrobial effectiveness testing (AET) and preservative efficacy testing (PET), the prototype for such testing is USP <51>.[12] Designed in the mid-20th century,[11] USP <51> uses three bacterial and two fungal microbial isolates from the American Type Culture Collection (ATCC) collection: *Staphylococcus aureus* ATCC 6538, *Pseudomonas aeruginosa* ATCC 9027, *Escherichia coli* ATCC 8739, *Candida albicans* ATCC 10231, and *Aspergillus brasiliensis* ATCC 16404. The bacteria and yeast-like fungus are clinical isolates dating 60 to 80 years from submission to ATCC. The *A brasiliensis* isolate was recovered from blueberries and submitted in the late 1960s. Efficacy against these has been the benchmark for preserved products (especially drugs) for many decades as considered in microbiological risk assessment for contamination during the use of the product. USP <51> is proscriptive in the preparation of inocula, inoculation of products, validation of recovery of remaining viable microbes, and importantly success criteria based on the rate and extent of kill.[11] Such criteria are specified by product type, and that for "topically used products" is most relevant to cosmetic products. USP <51> methodology, sometimes with modified efficacy standards, has been reapplied globally, most recently by the International Standards Organization.[52]

In the 1960s, the cosmetic industry organized under the then Cosmetic Toiletry and Fragrance Association (CTFA, now Personal Care Products Council or PCPC) and developed industry quality standards. Its microbiology committee adopted the basic USP <51> method and expanded it to include additional isolates, especially those relevant to cosmetic contamination including *B cepacia*, *Staphylococcus epidermidis*, *E gergoviae*, and *S marcescens*.[52] Such microbial contaminants offer a challenge that addresses both consumer contamination and inevitable microbial risks associated with nonsterile manufacturing (see Table 40.1). Compendial tests for preservative efficacy such as those described earlier are offered by many commercial testing laboratories, but most major cosmetic manufacturers evaluate preservative systems using "in-house" testing protocols. Such tests are proprietary and therefore not reported in the literature but historical data and personal observations find their use of microbes described in USP <51> as well as unique isolates from consumer returns and manufacturing contamination events. Preservative efficacy as evaluated by such testing may be further "validated" to consumer use. An example can be found in Brannan et al,[110] where products of graduated preservative efficacy established by formulation and confirmed by differing preservative capacity as judged by preservative efficacy tests were placed in consumer use and tested for contamination on completion of the use test. Success criteria in laboratory testing of preserved product were calibrated to the level of preservation found to resist contamination in consumer use. Although reportedly rare, PET data may lose significance in context of unique formula parameters such as water-in-silicone oil emulsions.[54,122] For these, in-use testing is essential to establish an effective risk assessment. Manufacturers also establish empirical, pragmatic validation of preservative systems to manufacturing GMPs, recognizing the practical level of preservative efficacy in PET needed to protect product made in controlled manufacturing systems. Preservative testing protocols, especially USP <51>, are necessary but may not represent all global consumer risks and may not be sufficient alone during microbiological risk assessments.

▶ CONCLUSION

Cosmetic preservation is often considered an arcane and complex effort. The cosmetic microbiologist must organize a subset of the few approved preservatives available commercially in a manner that establishes protection against a profoundly wide range of potential contaminants and within ranges that do not assault the consumer through product contact with skin and intimate surfaces. Each preservation effort is made unique by the complexities of formulation, manufacturing, packaging, and personal and cultural variation in product application. Successful preservation is accomplished in a manner effective in controlling gram-negative and gram-positive bacteria and fungi. Rather than a single preservative, systems (eg, see Table 40.5) of two or more preservatives combined with an adjunct (especially a chelator) are most effective in ensuring efficacy and minimizing opportunity for resistance development with this range of microorganisms. Unfortunately, even a well-designed preservative system by itself is not sufficient to ensure microbiological quality as dramatized by reports of contamination of disinfectants and even 70% ethanol[123,124] of much greater antimicrobial efficacy than preserved cosmetics. Efficacy nominally confirmed in PET in 28 days may fail to achieve the microbicidal effects of a disinfectant at use dilution established in less than 10 minutes. Microbiological safety in practice is therefore critically associated with effective manufacturing GMPs and packaging for consumers that limit both microbial types, numbers and exposure, as cosmetic preservatives systems are not capable of overcoming all conditions of microbiological-compromised manufacturing and consumer use, and reasonably foreseeable misuse that extend from product adulteration and community sharing to use well beyond the intended preservative system life.[125,126]

Appropriate risk assessment and mitigation can address development and manufacturing risks as well as foreseeable consumer use. Preservation occupies a central role in this risk assessment. Necessary but not sufficient to establish product quality, it demands effective manufacturing hygiene as it cannot completely mitigate all manufacturing and lifetime risks. Similarly, microbiological risks established by packaging can be somewhat but not entirely mitigated by preservation. Microbiological quality in production and use is a function of these combined factors.

REFERENCES

1. Curry JC, Brannan DK, Geis PA. History of cosmetic microbiology. In: Geis PA, ed. *Cosmetic Microbiology: A Practical Approach*. 2nd ed. New York, NY: Taylor & Francis; 2006:3-18.
2. Schubel K, Manger J. Ein beitrag zur pharmakologie einiger para-oxybenzoesaureester: das schicksal im organismus und die toxizitat. *Naunyn Schmiedebergs Arch Exp Pathol Pharmakol*. 1929;146:208-222. As cited in Lueck E. Antimicrobial Food Additives. New York, NY: Springer Verlag; 1980.
3. Held D. The preserving action of benzoic acid. *Arch Hyg*. 1915;84:289. As cited in Lueck E. *Antimicrobial Food Additives*. New York, NY: Springer; 1980.
4. Dunnigan AP, Evans JR. Report of a special survey: microbiological contamination of topical drugs and cosmetics. *TGA Cosmet J*. 1970;2:39-41.
5. Kallings LO, Ringertz O, Silverstolpe L. Microbiological contamination of medical preparations. *Acta Pharm Suec*. 1996;3:219-228.
6. Smart R, Spooner DF. Microbiological spoilage in pharmaceuticals and cosmetics. *J Soc Cosmet Chem*. 1972;23:721-737.
7. Geis PA. Preservation strategies. In: Geis PA, ed. *Cosmetic Microbiology: A Practical Approach*. New York, NY: Taylor & Francis; 2006:163-180.
8. Olsen SW. The application of microbiology to cosmetic testing. *J Soc Cosmet Chem*. 1967;18:191-198.
9. Owen EM. A method for the evaluation of preservative systems in cosmetic formulations. *Soap Chem Spec*. 1969;45:54.
10. Flawn PC, Malcolm SA, Woodroffe RCS. Assessment of the preservative capacity of shampoos. *J Soc Cosmet Chem*. 1973;24:229-238.
11. Sutton SV, Porter D. Development of the antimicrobial effectiveness test as USP chapter<51>. *PDA J Pharm Sci Technol*. 2002;56:300-311.
12. United States Pharmacopeial Convention. <51>Antimicrobial effectiveness test. In: *The United States Pharmacopeia*. 41st Revision. Rockville, MD: United States Pharmacopeial Convention; 2017.
13. Ahearn DG, Sanghvi J, Haller GJ. Mascara contamination: in use and laboratory studies. *J Soc Cosmet Chem*. 1978;29:127-131.
14. Wilson LA, Julian AJ, Ahearn DG. The survival and growth of microorganisms in mascara during use. *Am J Ophthalmol*. 1975;79:596-601.
15. Wilson LA, Ahearn DG. Pseudomonas-induced corneal ulcers associated with contaminated eye mascaras. *Am J Ophthalmol*. 1977;84:112-119.
16. Bhadauria R, Ahearn DG. Loss of effectiveness of preservative systems of mascaras with age. *Appl Env Microbiol*. 1980;39:665-667.
17. US Food and Drug Administration. FDA draft monograph regulation—FDA questions adequacy of preservation of eye area cosmetics. *Fed Regist*. 1977. To be codified at 42 CFR § 54837.
18. US Food and Drug Administration. *FDA Guide to Inspections of Cosmetic Product Manufacturers*. Silver Spring, MD: US Food and Drug Administration; 1995. http://academy.gmp-compliance.org/guidemgr/files/1-2-22.pdf. Accessed October 18, 2019.
19. Steinberg D. Frequency of use of preservatives 2001. *Cosmet Toilet*. 2002;117(4):41-44.
20. Darbre PD. Underarm cosmetics are a cause of breast cancer. *Eur J Cancer Prev*. 2001;10:389-394.

21. Golden R, Gandy J, Vollmer G. A review of the endocrine activity of parabens and implications for potential risks to human health. *Crit Rev Toxicol.* 2005;35:435-458.

22. Nohynek GJ, Borgert CJ, Dietrich D, Rozman KK. Endocrine disruption: fact or urban legend? *Toxicol Lett.* 2013;223:295-305.

23. European Commission. Consumers: commission improves safety of cosmetics. European Commission Web site. http://europa.eu/rapid/press-release_IP-14-1051_en.htm. Published 2014. Accessed October 18, 2019.

24. Centers for Disease Control and Prevention. National Biomonitoring Program: parabens fact sheet. Centers for Disease Control and Prevention Web site. https://www.cdc.gov/biomonitoring/Parabens_FactSheet.html. Accessed October 18, 2019.

25. US Food and Drug Administration. Cosmetics safety Q&A: parabens. US Food and Drug Administration Web site. https://www.fda.gov/Cosmetics/ResourcesForYou/Consumers/ucm397393.htm. Accessed October 18, 2019.

26. Cosmetic Ingredient Review. *Safety Assessment of Parabens as Used in Cosmetics.* Washington, DC: Cosmetic Ingredient Review; 2017. http://www.cir-safety.org/sites/default/files/paraben_web.pdf. Published 2017. Accessed October 18, 2019.

27. Kim S, Seock YK. Impacts of health and environmental consciousness on young female consumers' attitude towards and purchase of natural beauty products. *Int J Cons Stud.* 2009;33:627-638.

28. Janichen J. Reliable and safe replacement of parabens is possible. *Cosmet Sci Technol.* 2013:39.

29. Flanagan J. Preserving cosmetics with natural preservatives and preserving natural cosmetics. In Naya D, Lambros K, eds. *Formulating, Packaging, and Marketing of Natural Cosmetic Product.* Hoboken, NJ: John Wiley & Sons; 2011:169-178.

30. Aerts O, Baeck M, Constandt L, et al. The dramatic increase in the rate of methylisothiazoline contact allergy in Belgium: a multicentre study. *Contact Dermatitis.* 2014;71:41-48.

31. Giménez-Arnau AM. Opinion of the Scientific Committee on Consumer Safety (SCCS)—opinion on the safety of the use of methylisothiazolinone (MI)(P94), in cosmetic products (sensitisation only). *Regul Toxicol Pharmacol.* 2016;76:211-212.

32. Steinberg D. Frequency of preservative use through 2014. *Cosmet Toilet.* 2014;131:56-62.

33. Dweck AC. Natural preservatives. *Cosmet Toilet.* 2013;118:45-50.

34. Devlieghere F, De Loy-Hendrickx A, Rademaker M, et al. A new protocol for evaluating the efficacy of some dispensing systems of a packaging in the microbial protection of water-based preservative-free cosmetic products. *Int J Cosmet Sci.* 2015;37:627-635.

35. US Food and Drug Administration. Enforcement reports. US Food and Drug Administration. https://www.fda.gov/safety/recalls/enforcement reports/default.htm. Accessed October 18, 2019.

36. Moss M. Bacterial pigments. *Microbiologist.* 2002;3:10-12.

37. Schnürer J, Olsson J, Börjesson T. Fungal volatiles as indicators of food and feeds spoilage. *Fungal Genet Biol.* 1999;27:209-217.

38. Stotzky G, Schenck S. Volatile organic compounds and microorganisms. *CRC Crit Rev Microbiol.* 1976:4:333-382.

39. Leffingwell & Associates. Odor & flavor detection thresholds in water (in parts per billion). Leffingwell & Associates Web site. http://www.leffingwell.com/odorthre.htm. Accessed October 18, 2019.

40. Rabenstein A, Koch T, Remesch M, Brinksmeier E, Kuever J. Microbial degradation of water miscible metal working fluids. *Int Biodet Biodeg.* 2009;63:1023-1029.

41. Leyden JJ, Stewart R, Kligman AM. Experimental inoculation of *Pseudomonas aeruginosa* and *Pseudomonas cepacia* on human skin. *J Soc Cosmet Chem.* 1980;31:19-28.

42. Szablewski CM, Hendricks K, Bower WA, Shadomy SV, Hupert N. Anthrax cases associated with animal-hair shaving brushes. *Emerg Infect Dis.* 2017;23:806-808.

43. Álvarez-Lerma F, Maull E, Terradas R, et al. Moisturizing body milk as a reservoir of *Burkholderia cepacia*: outbreak of nosocomial infection in a multidisciplinary intensive care unit. *Crit Care.* 2008;12:R10.

44. Matrician L, Ange G, Burns S, et al. Outbreak of nosocomial *Burkholderia cepacia* infection and colonization associated with intrinsically contaminated mouthwash. *Infect Contr Hosp Epidemiol.* 2000;21:739-741.

45. Molina-Cabrillana J, Bolaños-Rivero M, Alvarez-León EE, et al. Intrinsically contaminated alcohol-free mouthwash implicated in a nosocomial outbreak of *Burkholderia cepacia* colonization and infection. *Infect Control Hosp Epidemiol.* 2006;27:1281-1282.

46. Madani TA, Alsaedi S, James L, et al. *Serratia marcescens*-contaminated baby shampoo causing an outbreak among newborns at King Abdulaziz University Hospital, Jeddah, Saudi Arabia. *J Hosp Infect.* 2011;78:16-19.

47. Fainstein V, Andres N, Umphrey J, Hopfer R. Hair clipping: another hazard for granulocytopenic patients? *J Infect Dis.* 1988;158:655-656.

48. Gerba CP, Rose JB, Haas CN. Sensitive populations: who is at the greatest risk? *Int J Food Microbiol.* 1996;30:113-123.

49. US Food and Drug Administration. Chapter 23. microbiological methods for cosmetics. In: *Bacteriological Analytical Manual.* Silver Spring, MD: US Food and Drug Administration; 2017. https://www.fda.gov/Food/FoodScienceResearch/LaboratoryMethods/ucm565586.htm. Accessed October 18, 2019.

50. Sutton S, Jimenez L. A review of reported recalls involving microbiological control 2004-2011 with emphasis on FDA considerations of objectionable organisms. *Am Pharm Rev.* 2012;15(1):42-57.

51. Chervenak M, Eachus A, Henry B. Biocide resolves bacterial hygiene. *European Coatings J.* 2004;1-2:26-34.

52. International Standards Organization. ISO 11930. 2112. *Cosmetics—Microbiology—Evaluation of the Antimicrobial Protection of a Cosmetic Product.* Geneva, Switzerland: International Standards Organization; 2012.

53. Personal Care Products Council. CTFA M-3 determination of preservative adequacy of water miscible cosmetics. In Krowka JF, Jonas BA, eds. *CTFA Technical Guidelines.* Washington, DC: Personal Care Products Council; 2016:209-216.

54. Schnittger S, Sabourin J, King D. Preservation of water-in-silicone emulsions. *J Cosmet Sci.* 2002;3:78-80.

55. Braide W, Nwosu IL, Offor-Emenike IU, et al. Microbial quality of some topical pharmaceutical products sold in Aba, Abia state, Nigeria. *Int J Pharmacol Ther.* 2012;2:26-37.

56. Al-Mijalli SH. Isolation of human pathogenic bacteria from baby shampoo and their susceptibility to common antibiotics in Riyadh, Saudi Arabia. Paper presented at: International Conference on Medical Sciences and Chemical Engineering; August 28-29, 2013; Penang, Malaysia.

57. Razooki RA, Saeed EN, Hamza H. A study on cosmetic products marketed in Iraq: microbiological aspect. *Iraqi J Pharm Sci.* 2017;18:20-25.

58. Steinberg DC. *Preservatives for Cosmetics.* 2nd ed. Carol Stream, IL: Allured Publishing Corporation; 1996.

59. Richardson EL. Preservatives frequency of use in cosmetic formula as disclosed to the FDA. *Cosmet Toilet.* 1977;92;85-87.

60. Siegert W. Microbiological quality management for the production of cosmetics and detergents. *SOFW J.* 2012;138:30-38.

61. Geis PA, ed. *Cosmetic Microbiology: A Practical Approach.* 2nd ed. New York, NY: Taylor & Francis; 2006.

62. Haag T, Loncrini DF. Esters of para-hydroxybenzoic acid. *Cosmet Sci Technol Ser.* 1984;1:63-77.

63. Patel NK, Romanowski JM. Heterogeneous systems. II. Influence of partitioning and molecular interactions on in vitro biologic activity of preservatives in emulsions. *J Pharm Sci.* 1970;59:372-376.

64. Parker MS, Barnes M, Bradley TJ. The use of the Coulter Counter to detect the inactivation of preservatives by a non-ionic surface-active agent. *J Pharm Pharmacol.* 1966;18:103S-106S.

65. Chin YP, Mohamad S, Abas MR. Removal of parabens from aqueous solution using β-cyclodextrin cross-linked polymer. *Int J Mol Sci.* 2010;11:3459-3471.

66. Hensel A, Leisenheimer S, Müller A, et al. Transesterification reactions of parabens (alkyl 4-hydroxybenzoates) with polyols in aqueous solution. *J Pharm Sci.* 1995;84:115-118.

67. Bahal SM, Romansky JM. Sorption of parabens by flexible tubings. *Pharm Dev Technol.* 2001;6:431-440.

68. Rosen M. Glydant and MDMH as cosmetic preservatives. In: Kabara J, ed. *Cosmetic and Drug Preservation: Principles and Practice.* New York, NY: Marcel Dekker; 1984:160-190.

69. Rosen WE, Berke PA. Germall 115: a safe and effective preservative. In: Kabara J, ed. *Cosmetic and Drug Preservation: Principles and Practice.* New York, NY: Marcel Dekker. 1984:191-205.

70. Berke PA, Rosen WE. Germall II. A new broad spectrum cosmetic preservative. *Cosmet Toilet.* 1982;97:49-50.

71. McDonnell G, Russell AD. Antiseptics and disinfectants: activity, action, and resistance. *Clin Microbiol Rev.* 1999;12:147-179.

72. Kireche M, Peiffer JL, Antonios D, et al. Evidence for chemical and cellular reactivities of the formaldehyde releaser bronopol, independent of formaldehyde release. *Chem Res Toxicol.* 2011;24:2115-2128.

73. Tome D, Naulet N. Carbon 13 nuclear magnetic resonance studies on formaldehyde reactions with polyfunctional amino-acids. *Int J Pept Protein Res.* 1981;17:501-507.

74. Rassat F, Gonzenbach H, Pittet GH. Use of sunscreen and vitamins in daily-use cosmetics. *Drug Cosmet Ind.* 1997:16-20.

75. Heid SE, Kanti A, McNamee PM, et al. Consumer safety considerations of cosmetic preservation. In: Geis PA, ed. *Cosmetic Microbiology: A Practical Handbook.* New York, NY: Marcel Dekker; 1997:193-214.

76. Law AB, Moss JN, Lashen ES. Kathon C-G: a new single component, broad spectrum preservative for cosmetics and toiletries. In: Karaba JJ, ed. *Cosmetic and Drug Preservation: Principles and Practice.* New York, NY: Marcel Dekker; 1984:29-141.

77. Bazire A, Diab F, Jebbar M, Harras D. Influence of high salinity on biofilm formation and benzoate assimilation by *Pseudomonas aeruginosa*. *J Ind Microbiol Biotechnol.* 2007;34:5-8.

78. Karandikar R, Badri A, Phale PS. Biochemical characterization of inducible "reductase" component of benzoate dioxygenase and phthalate isomer dioxygenases from *Pseudomonas aeruginosa* strain PP4. *Appl Biochem Biotechnol.* 2015;177:318-333.

79. Arya SS, Thakur BR. Degradation products of sorbic acid in aqueous solutions. *Food Chem.* 1988;29:41-49.

80. Arya SS. Stability of sorbic acid in aqueous solutions. *J Agric Food Chem.* 1980;28:1246-1249.

81. Bennassi CA, Semenzato A, Lucchiari M, Bettero A. Dehydroacetic acid sodium salt stability in cosmetic preservative mixtures. *Int J Cosmet Sci.* 1988;10:29-32.

82. Melnick D, Luckmann FH, Gooding CM. Sorbic acid as fungistatic agent for foods. *J Food Sci.* 1954;19:44-58.

83. Bahal SM, Romansky JM. Sorption of benzoic acid, sorbic acid, benzyl alcohol, and benzalkonium chloride by flexible tubing. *Pharm Dev Technol.* 2002;7:49-58.

84. McCarthy TJ. Storage studies of preservative solutions in commonly used plastic containers. *Cosmet Perf.* 1973;88:41-42.

85. Puschmann J, Herbig ME, Müller-Goymann CC. Correlation of antimicrobial effects of phenoxyethanol with its free concentration in the water phase of o/w-emulsion gels. *Eur J Pharm Biopharm.* 2018;131:152-161.

86. Horiuchi K, Morimoto K, Ohta T, Suemitsu R. Biotransformation of benzyl alcohol by *Pseudomonas cepacia. Biosci Biotech Biochem.* 1993;57:1346-1347.

87. Kinnunen T, Koskela M. Antibacterial and antifungal properties of propylene glycol, hexylene glycol, and 1, 3-butylene glycol in vitro. *Acta Derm Venereol.* 1991;71:148-150.

88. Ziosi P, Manfredini S, Vandini A, et al. Caprylyl glycol/phenethyl alcohol blend for alternative preservation of cosmetics. *Cosmet Toilet.* 2013;128:538-551.

89. Roden K. A rational approach to the preservative conundrum: preservatives. *S African Pharma Cosmet Rev.* 2015;42:20-22.

90. Shin KH, Kwack IY, Lee SW, et al. Effects of polyols on antimicrobial and preservative efficacy in cosmetics. *J Soc Cosmet Sci Korea.* 2007;33:111-115.

91. Leschke M. Ethylhexylglycerin for improved skin feel. *SOFW J.* 2010; 136:10.

92. Leschke M, Wustermann S. A reliable alternative for traditional preservative systems. *SOFW J.* 2007;132:2-4.

93. Lawan K, Kanlayavattanakul M, Lourith N. Antimicrobial efficacy of caprylyl glycol and ethylhexylglycerine in emulsion. *J Health Res.* 2009;23:1-3

94. Isaiah S, Karthikeyan S. Challenges for formulating natural cosmetics: comparative physiochemical studies on natural and synthetic made shampoo. *Int J Pharm Bio Sci.* 2015;6(1):1269-1274.

95. Tonoyan L, Fleming GT, Mc Cay PH, Friel R, O'Flaherty V. Antibacterial potential of an antimicrobial agent inspired by peroxidase-catalyzed systems. *Front Microbiol.* 2017;2:680-695.

96. Carvalho IT, Estevinho BN, Santos L. Application of microencapsulated essential oils in cosmetic and personal healthcare products—a review. *Int J Cosmet Sci.* 2016;38:109-119.

97. Takeoka GR, Dao LT, Wong RY, Harden LA. Identification of benzalkonium chloride in commercial grapefruit seed extracts. *J Agric Food Chem.* 2005;53:7630-7636.

98. van der Waal JW. Grapefruit seed extracts as organic post-harvest agents: precious lessons on efficacy and compliance. *Organic Agric.* 2015;5:53-62.

99. Li J, Chaytor JL, Findlay B, McMullen LM, Smith DC, Vederas JC. Identification of didecyldimethylammonium salts and salicylic acid as antimicrobial compounds in commercial fermented radish kimchi. *J Agric Food Chem.* 2015;63:3053-3058.

100. De Groot AC, Schmidt E. *Essential Oils: Contact Allergy and Chemical Composition.* Boca Raton, FL: CRC Press; 2017.

101. Saitta M, Di Bella G, Salvo, F, Lo Curto S, Dugo G. Organochlorine pesticide residues in Italian citrus essential oils, 1991-1996. *J Agric Food Chem.* 2000;48:797-801.

102. Lambert RJ, Johnston MD, Hanlon GW, Denyer SP. Theory of antimicrobial combinations: biocide mixtures—synergy or addition? *J Appl Microbiol.* 2003;94:747-759.

103. Kerdudo A, Fontaine-Vive F, Dingas A, Faure C, Fernandez X. Optimization of cosmetic preservation: water activity reduction. *Int J Cosmet Sci.* 2015;37:31-40.

104. Brown MR. Survival of *Pseudomonas aeruginosa* in fluorescein solution. Preservative action of PMN and EDTA. *J Pharma Sci.* 1968;57:389-392.

105. Beloin C, Renar S, Ghigo JM, Lebeaux D. Novel approaches to combat bacterial biofilms. *Curr Opin Pharmacol.* 2014;18:61-68.

106. Holbein BE, Mira de Orduña R. Effect of trace iron levels and iron withdrawal by chelation on the growth of *Candida albicans* and *Candida vini. FEMS Microbiol Lett.* 2010;307:19-24

107. Brannan DK, Dille JC. Type of closure prevents microbial contamination of cosmetics during consumer use. *Appl Environ Microbiol.* 1990;56:1476-1479.

108. Brannan DK. The role of packaging in product preservation. *Cosm Sci Technol Ser.* 1997:227-242.

109. van der Kooij D, Oranje JP, Hijnen WA. Growth of *Pseudomonas aeruginosa* in tap water in relation to utilization of substrates at concentrations of a few micrograms per liter. *Appl Environ Microbiol.* 1982;44:1086-1095.

110. Brannan DK, Dille JC, Kaufman DJ. Correlation of in vitro challenge testing with consumer use testing for cosmetic products. *Appl Environ Microbiol.* 1987;53:1827-1832.

111. Ibrahim YKE, Sonntag HG. Effect of formulation pH and storage temperatures on the preservative efficacy of some gases used as propellants in cosmetic aerosols. *J Appl Microbiol.* 1993;74:200-209.

112. Chapman JS. Antimicrobial mechanisms of selected preservatives and the bacterial response. In: Geis PA, ed. *Cosmetic Microbiology: A Practical Approach.* 2nd ed. New York, NY: Taylor & Francis; 2006: 181-192.

113. Schweizer HP. Triclosan: a widely used biocide and its link to antibiotics. *FEMS Microbiol Lett.* 2001;202:1-7.

114. Périamé M, Pagès JM, Davin-Regli A. *Enterobacter gergoviae* adaptation to preservatives commonly used in cosmetic industry. *Int J Cosmet Sci.* 2014;36:386-395.

115. Rushton L, Sass A, Baldwin A, Dowson CG, Donoghue D, Mahen-thiralingam E. Key role for efflux in the preservative susceptibility and adaptive resistance of *Burkholderia cepacia* complex bacteria. *Antimicrob Agents Chemother.* 2013;57:2972-2980.

116. Davin-Regli A, Chollet R, Bredin J, Chevalier J, Lepine F, Pagès JM. *Enterobacter gergoviae* and the prevalence of efflux in parabens resistance. *J Antimicrob Chemother.* 2006;57:757-760.

117. Mah TFC, O'Toole GA. Mechanisms of biofilm resistance to antimicrobial agents. *Trends Microbiol.* 2001;9:34-39.

118. De Kievit TR, Parkins MD, Gillis RJ, et al. Multidrug efflux pumps: expression patterns and contribution to antibiotic resistance in *Pseudomonas aeruginosa* biofilms. *Antimicrob Agents Chemother.* 2001;45:1761-1770.

119. Sondossi M, Rossmoore HW, Wireman JW. Observations of resistance and cross-resistance to formaldehyde and a formaldehyde condensate biocide in *Pseudomonas aeruginosa*. *Int Biodeterior.* 1985;21:105-106.

120. Rhodes KA, Schweizer HP. Antibiotic resistance in *Burkholderia* species. *Drug Resist Updat.* 2016;28:82-90.

121. Jimenez L, Kulko E, Barron E, Flannery T. *Burkholderia cepacia*: a problem that does not go away! *EC Microbiol.* 2015;2:205-210.

122. Geis PA. Antimicrobial efficacy testing in risk assessment. In: McCullough K, Moldenhaur J, eds. *Microbial Risks and Investigations.* Scottsdale, AZ: Davis Healthcare International; 2015:171-198.

123. Nasser RM, Rahi AC, Haddad MF, Daoud Z, Irani-Hakime N, Almawi WY. Outbreak of *Burkholderia cepacia* bacteremia traced to contaminated hospital water used for dilution of an alcohol skin antiseptic. *Infect Contr Hosp Epidemiol.* 2004:25:231-239.

124. Weber DJ, Rutala WA, Sickbert-Bennett EE. Outbreaks associated with contaminated antiseptics and disinfectants. *Antimicrob Agents Chemother.* 2007;51:4217-4224.

125. Dadashi L, Dehghanzadeh R. Investigating incidence of bacterial and fungal contamination in shared cosmetic kits available in the women beauty salons. *Health Promo Perspect.* 2016;6:159-163.

126. Giacomel CB, Dartora G, Dienfethaeler HS, Haas SE. Investigation on the use of expired make-up and microbiological contamination of mascaras. *Int J Cosmet Sci.* 2013;35:375-380.

127. Schaffner DW, Jensen D, Gerba CP, Shumaker D, Arbogast JW. Influence of soap characteristics and food service facility type on the degree of bacterial contamination of open, refillable bulk soaps. *J Food Prot.* 2018;81:218-225.

Sterile Packaging

Thierry Wagner, Dan B. Floyd, Michael H. Scholla, and Jane E. Severin

In 1668, Francesco Redi, an Italian physician and biologist, published a book entitled *Experiments on the Generation of Insects* challenging the theory of "spontaneous generation" of maggots from dead flesh or, in a more general way, of putrefying matter.[1] Under the theory of spontaneous generation, the widely held belief at the time, microorganisms were formed without reproduction from parents. Redi prepared jars with raw meat, some he left open and others he covered with corks or with "very fine Naples veil" to avoid flies entering the jars to deposit their larvae. Maggots only appeared in uncovered jars. Redi's experiments were a cornerstone of the scientific work that allowed Louis Pasteur, Joseph Lister, Robert Koch, and others to understand the true nature of microorganisms. But what was also remarkable, Redi conducted probably the first scientific experiments with containers covered with a porous lid and he worked with a control, in this case with uncovered jars, to prove his hypothesis, an innovative concept at the time. The veil used was a barrier to flies, and allowed air to enter, important to counter the arguments of those believing that air was required for life to develop. The veil was probably not a good microbial barrier, but by challenging the theory of spontaneous generation, the concept of protection for preservation became possible. It took however two additional centuries to finally root out this ancient theory.

In 1745-1748, John Needham, a Scottish clergyman and naturalist, showed that broth still shows microbial growth when conserved in a hermetically sealed container after being boiled, although the boiling should have destroyed all forms of life. Critics pointed out that he may have recontaminated the broth during transfer to the container.[1] Another Italian, Lazzaro Spallanzani at the University of Reggio Emilia, repeated these experiments during 1765-1767 in sealed glass flasks using a special procedure to avoid recontamination. Spallanzani concluded that the elements at the source of putrefaction could be killed by sufficiently long boiling. He also proposed that these elements can move through air and the hermetic sealing protects from recontamination. He even showed that the liquid could not be preserved in flasks with an integrity issue. His opponents claimed that his hermetically sealed flasks did not allow air to enter, which was believed at the time to be an essential requirement (ER) for life.[1] But it was Louis Pasteur who finally gave the mortal blow to the theory of spontaneous generation with his famous swan neck flask experiments during the period of 1859-1865 (see Figure 2.2, chapter 2). His flasks had a thin and long tub neck shaped like the neck of a swan. Air could enter, but particulates would not get into the flask as they settled somewhere in the S-shaped neck of the flask. Pasteur filled the flasks with a meat broth, sterilized them through boiling, and could demonstrate preservation of these liquids for weeks or months unless the bulb was tilted such that some liquid could reach the bottom of the S-shaped neck where particulates with microorganisms had settled. Microorganisms would also develop when the neck was broken off such that the surrounding air could enter freely into the flask. With his experiments, Pasteur demonstrated that a torturous path could be an effective barrier to microorganisms, a concept still in use today. He also showed the limitations of the swan neck tortuous path. When the flasks were violently shaken such that air would rush in, then it was possible of observe microbial growth. He even demonstrated that the air of Paris was more contaminated than mountain air at 850 m or even 2000 m above sea level (see Vallery-Radot[1]).

In the 19th century, Louis Pasteur, Robert Koch, Joseph Lister, and many others set the basis for moving into modern medicine with the increasing knowledge of microbiology. Sterilization at the point of use with carbolic acid and heat was the first approach without any preservation means. As packaging emerged to preserve the microbiological state, it was mainly based on metal or glass containers. During the 19th century, a lot of research focused on the preservation of foods.

François Nicolas Appert[2] invented the process of food bottling and was awarded by Napoleon in 1810 who was keen to have a method to preserve the food for his armies. The effective and simple method was widely adopted in a short time span. Preservation was first done in glass bottles and later in tin cans invented by Peter Durand. The process of bottling was further improved by Dr Rudolf Rempel who filed a patent in 1892 to close and vent sterilization containers. His patent was the basis for Johann Carl Weck to create the company Weck GmbH, which still marketing their Weck preservation bottles today.[3]

The limitations of boiling for sterilization became quickly apparent. It took until 1879 for the first autoclave for medical purposes to be introduced by Charles Chamberland in Paris, although Denis Papin had already developed a precursor in 1679. Using this equipment, Pasteur demonstrated that steam sterilization was particularly effective to kill microorganisms. Steam sterilization presented a problem that any packaging had to be porous to allow the steam to reach the packaged devices. In 1890, Curt Schimmelbusch[4] filed a patent for sterilization containers, the so-called Schimmelbusch drum (Figure 41.1), and he recommended the steam sterilization of wound dressings in his famous book published in 1892 with the support of Prof Dr E. von Bergmann. Schimmelbusch[4] described the preservation of sterilized wound care products in sterilization drums as well as preservation of surgical catgut ligatures in special containers. The same year, Aesculap (in Germany) created the first rigid sterilization containers responding to the needs of military hospitals. Originally, they were equipped with valves or sliding vents replaced in the 1930s with reusable filters.

As medicine continued to make progress internationally, Fred Kilmer, pharmacist in New Brunswick, New Jersey, saw the potential of offering ready-made packaged sterile dressings, which he described in 1897 in an article entitled "Modern Surgical Dressings."[5] The sterile glass jars were filled aseptically under well-controlled conditions and become the key product for the success of Johnson & Johnson. At the beginning of the 20th century, sterile packaging was still very basic, for example,

Charles E. Parker[6] specified packaging in his catgut ligature and suture patent of June 3, 1902, as follows: "wrapping or container of paper or similar material which is permeable to sterilizing fluids, but will exclude dust or any solid carrier of infection." Parker's description included all the essentials, but engineered microbial barrier materials were not yet available. He included a drawing, which showed an object wrapped in plain paper. The development of the prefilled syringe, combining primary packaging and drug delivery mechanism is an equally fascinating story. Johann Sigismund Elsholtz was one of the first to investigate ways of intravenous (IV) injection in 1667. Literature[7,8] lists several inventors for the syringe working independently in the middle of the 19th century, namely, Alexander Wood (1817-1884), a Scottish physician, and Charles Gabriel Pravaz (1791-1853), a French surgeon. Robert Koch came up with a sterilizable syringe in 1888 and Becton, Dickinson and Company introduced the disposable syringe.[7] In 1939, Erhard[9] of E.R. Squibb and Sons, filed a patent for a "hypodermic unit," which led to the development of the famous "morphine syrette" adopted by the US army during World War II. The design was simple and battlefield compatible; it consisted of a toothpaste-like squeezable metal container with a seal that was pierced by a wire in the attached hypodermic needle before the medication could be administered into the patient. In first aid kits, the syrette was protected with a hard fireboard tube. This innovative device combined the delivery system, packaging, and protection for extreme situations with simplicity and great usability to allow for administration in adverse and difficult conditions.

In the 1940s, the US military commissioned Drs Charles A Phillips and Saul Kaye to develop an efficient biological decontamination process.[10] Their work at Fort Detrick, Maryland, on ethylene oxide (EO) established the scientific foundations for the introduction of EO as a gaseous sterilant. The EO sterilization, also in addition to the use of radiation, enabled the introduction of sterile medical devices made of materials that were not compatible with the high temperatures of steam sterilization. More and more single-use disposable medical devices emerged, and with that the need for appropriate packaging. Fabrics and medical paper were the most used material initially, joined by film packaging and later by DuPont™ Tyvek® in 1972.

Sterile packaging over the many years of its history has developed into an extremely diverse sector covering medical devices, combination products, and pharmaceuticals, addressing professional health care users as well as patients in a variety of situations such as home health, health care facilities, and military applications. The complexity of sterile packaging has grown with the emergence of sophisticated devices, sensitive drug products, new sterilization modalities, and aseptic processing technologies as well as with the development of sophisticated clinical procedures. Packaging continues to evolve with the

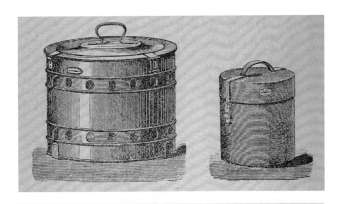

FIGURE 41.1   Schimmelbusch drum.

introduction of new drug delivery and device technology, to enable productivity improvements, the adoption of new materials and manufacturing technologies, the inclusion of active elements to control atmosphere, and the integration of microchips for smart functions, and to address changing regulatory requirements. But the fundamental aspects, discovered by the pioneers, are still true today.

▶ INTENDED USE, FUNCTIONS, AND REQUIREMENTS FOR STERILE PACKAGING

There are a broad range of sterile packaging types to package devices, combination products, or drugs. Before reviewing these in detail, it is worthwhile considering the intended use, typical functions, and key requirements for sterile packaging.

Sterilization Compatibility

The preferred and the lowest risk method to provide a sterile health care product is to package first and then sterilize the contents in the package (referred to as terminal sterilization). For drugs or devices that cannot be sterilized, aseptic processing is another option (see chapter 58). But even in this case, the various components including the packaging should be sterilized before filling the drug or device packaging operation. Packaging needs to allow for and must be compatible with the selected sterilization process(es). As an example, gaseous sterilization modalities require porous packaging for penetration of the gaseous sterilizing agent and evacuation of any residues. Packaging materials need to be able to withstand the specific sterilization process being applied in a way that the properties of the material stay within required limits and there are no chemical or other reactions that could lead to detrimental impacts on the product (safety and efficacy) or limited stability and performance of the packaging over the shelf life.

Package Integrity, Microbial, and Other Barrier Functionalities

The ability to exclude microbial contamination from the packaged product is a key feature of sterile packaging for the maintenance of sterility after sterilization or aseptic processing until the point of use. For preservation of sterile contents, packaging needs to maintain integrity over the shelf life and through the challenges of transportation and handling. In many cases, packaging must also shield the product from environmental impacts such as from oxygen or humidity while maintaining a set atmosphere inside. Porous materials for gaseous sterilization modalities should allow air to enter and exit while retaining

particulates and airborne microorganisms. Air will pass typically through the porous structure of the sheet in a meandering pattern around fibers or filaments, representing a tortuous path with given microbial barrier properties, a concept originally demonstrated as effective by Pasteur. Porous materials are also used to allow packaging to adapt to changes in atmospheric pressure, important for large packages, or if transportation includes airfreight and significant changes in altitude.

The packaging, that is in direct contact with the product, is identified as primary packaging in pharmaceutical applications, whereas the medical device industry has introduced the terminology of sterile barrier system to identify the minimum package that minimizes the risk of ingress of microorganisms and allows aseptic presentation of the sterile contents at the point of use.[11] The sterile barrier system is considered an essential accessory to a sterile device.

Protection of the Product and Its Sterile Barrier System

Packaging must protect the health care product from physical hazards, like shocks, vibration, compression of transport, distribution, and storage as well as from any harmful environmental elements like ultraviolet (UV) light, electromagnetic fields, temperature, or chemical products. To cope with these adverse conditions, packaging systems are often composed of various protective packaging layers, or secondary and tertiary packaging, including means for transportation like pallets or containers. If packaging alone cannot guarantee the protection, special conditions must be maintained like a temperature-controlled supply chain (cool or cold chains).

Biocompatibility Aspects and Interactions With the Health Care Product

Packaging can be in direct contact with a health care product, or during use, it may even come into contact with the patient. Biocompatibility, toxicity aspects, chemical compatibilities, potential leachables, and the risks of adverse impacts on the health care product from such interactions need to be understood. Leachables are chemical entities from materials in direct or even in indirect contact with the product that migrate to the product and as such contaminate it. Leachables could come from plastics and their antioxidants; from residual catalyst respective impurities; or from glass, metals, or any packaging materials. Further sources include printing inks used for labeling, label adhesives, paperboard, and cardboard boxes used for protection and from products used to treat pallets (eg, preservatives; see chapter 69). Leachables can lead to effectiveness alterations of a drug product, inactivate active ingredients, or react with ingredients to form new chemical compounds that have further undesirable secondary effects. Packaging constructs could also bind components of a drug product to change it. Packaging is considered compatible with a health care product if its safety and intended use is not compromised and in case of a drug product if its efficacy is within required limits.[12-15]

Packaging Usability

At the point of product use, packaging will be opened, removed, or the product will be dispensed, administered, or used. There are several functions and requirements for product usability that can impact packaging:

- Identification of the product
- Reading the information on the label, cautions, use-by-date information, required storage conditions, etc
- Opening the package
- Aseptically removing the sterile health care product or administering the drug
- Aseptically handling components in an aseptic filling process

All aspects in the list earlier may have an impact on patient safety. Labels help with identification not only of the product but also design features like transparent web materials or windows in cardboard box allow for visual identification of the product. Label readability is important to support health care personnel that must deal with an increasing complexity under often stressful conditions. The use of symbols is preferred to increase label readability and to eliminate the need for multiple languages of internationally distributed products.

The packaging design must allow for appropriate aseptic technique to remove the sterile device to minimize the risk of cross-contamination and infection. Aseptic presentation after opening is ideally performed by two people, one to open the packaging and the other to remove the product from the package without contact with unsterile areas (Figure 41.2).

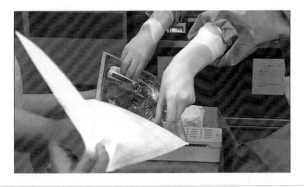

FIGURE 41.2 Aseptic presentation.

Aseptic presentation is defined as "transfer of the sterile contents from their sterile barrier system using conditions and procedures that minimize the risk of microbial contamination."[13] Often, health care acts are only performed by a single health care practitioner and packaging designs need to account for these specific situations. Regulations and standards put increasing focus on usability evaluation of the device, including its packaging, to minimize the risk of adverse events with the patient and to produce evidence that the design allows for easy handling and is safe.

Packaging Sustainability

Finally, empty packaging must be discarded properly, avoiding harm to the environment and to users, like unintended sticks from needles, and increasingly prepared for recycling and fed into the appropriate channels. Many jurisdictions have set ambitious goals to improve recycling rates moving to a more circular economy and packaging designs will have to adapt to optimize reuse and recycling possibilities.[14]

▶ STERILE PACKAGING TYPES, MATERIALS, AND DESIGN

Sterile Packaging Types

There are numerous materials, styles, and formats used for medical packaging. To meet the needs of more and more complex products especially for combination products, there are new combinations of package styles and materials emerging every year. Combination products in these cases refer to a combination of a drug and device; a biological product and a device; a drug and biological product; or a drug, device, and biological product. These can pose a new challenge in the design of packaging and impact on sterilization requirements. Table 41.1 illustrates typical package formats for some common product types and characteristics.

Common Materials—Medical Device Packaging

Medical device packaging must primarily allow its contents to be sterilized and it must then maintain sterility until the time of use. There are exceptions to this, for example, a manufacturer may market a nonsterile device, such as many types of adhesive bandages. Packaging types include bags, overwraps, pouches, trays, fin-seal wrappers, form-fill-seal containers, and clamshells. The packages are made of a variety of materials; porous, nonporous, rigid,

TABLE 41.1	Types of sterile medical packaging formats					
Product Characteristic/ Package Formats	Preformed Rigid Tray With Die Cut Lid	Premade Pouches and Bags	Flexible Peel Pouch	Header Bag	Form Fill Seal	Four-Side Sealing
Hard/rigid product	✓					
Soft product			✓			
Heavy/bulky product	✓			✓		
Dressings/wound care			✓			✓
Surgeon's gloves						✓
Syringes			✓			
Tubing			✓			
Airways			✓			
Kits	✓			✓		
Gowns and drapes				✓		
General medical devices			✓		✓	
Hospital use		✓				

flexible, high barrier, etc. Figure 41.3 shows the typical packaging used for sterile contact lenses.

Medical Grade Paper

Medical grade paper is used primarily for two-dimensional flexible pouches or lidstocks sealed to flexible, rigid, or semirigid trays. It is selected typically because it is porous, which is necessary for sterilization by EO or steam.

FIGURE 41.3 Medical device package thermoformed rigid plastic tray with foil lid/contact lens case. For a color version of this art, please consult the eBook. (https://www.istock.com/yoyochow23.)

Porosity levels of paper structures vary widely. They are made of fibers that can generate particles when the package is opened, which can compromise sterility or lead to other complications following surgical use. Fiber generation, as an example, can be minimized by reinforcing the paper with a polymer. The reinforcement is intended to improve strength and to provide a clean peel, which is critical for medical device packages. Such paper treatments can influence material porosity levels compared to the original substrate, but the levels remain acceptable for use for a medical device package. Paper does require, in most cases, the addition of heat seal coating to one side of the material for sealing to a film web or tray.[15]

DuPont™ Tyvek®

A DuPont brand, DuPont™ Tyvek® is marketed as an alternative to medical grade paper. It is made of virgin high-density polyethylene (HDPE). The unique manufacturing process results in long, spun filaments, randomly laid and bonded into sheet form by heat and pressure. DuPont™ Tyvek® is unique because it provides a superior microbial barrier due to a tortuous path (Figure 41.4) created in its manufacturing process and it is also very breathable. A more breathable or porous material can reduce cycle times for sterilization, which can result in improved operational efficiencies. Unlike paper, the clean peeling characteristic is not dependent on additional treatments.

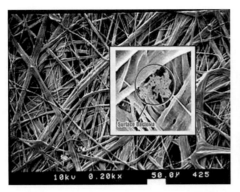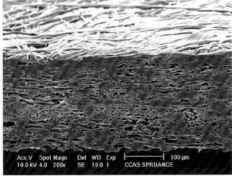

FIGURE 41.4 DuPont™ Tyvek® material. Top view with surface bacteria unable to penetrate (200×) and side view (200×) Illustration of the "tortuous path." (Copyright © 2019 DuPont. DuPont™ and Tyvek® are trademarks or registered trademarks of E.I. DuPont de Nemours and Company or its affiliates. All rights reserved.)

DuPont™ Tyvek® can be sealed to flexible webs and trays with or without the addition of a heat seal coating. DuPont™ Tyvek® also has superior physical strength and more resistance to tearing and puncturing.[16]

Aluminum

Aluminum can be in a foil form or vacuum deposited on films known as metallization. Aluminum is an excellent barrier against light, oxygen, and moisture. These properties are typically critical for the packaging of many types of combination products. When aluminum is the barrier layer in a lamination, it requires a heat-seal layer for sealing because aluminum does not seal. Also, aluminum is typically sandwiched between protective layers to eliminate any possible chemical reactivity and to minimize flex cracking. It is important to consider material thickness because aluminum is susceptible to the formation of pinholes. Pinholes are inherent due to the manufacturing process and are more prevalent in thinner materials.[15]

Plastic

Commonly used plastics for medical device packaging include polyethylene (low-density polyethylene [LDPE], HDPE), polystyrene (PS), high-impact PS, polypropylene (PP), polyvinyl chloride, polyvinylidene chloride (PVDC), polyethylene terephthalate glycol-modified (PETG), and polyester in addition to blends of materials. Plastics are used in flexible, semirigid, and rigid structures, as monolayers, laminations, or coextrusions of more than one material.

Plastics offer numerous characteristics and properties, such as a broad range of opacity, barrier properties, forming properties, sealability, strength, elongation, etc. It is important to thoroughly understand product requirements prior to selecting a plastic material for medical device packaging. Plastic films are compatible

with sterilization methods that don't require porosity (eg, electron beam and irradiation). Sterilization methods that require the ingress and egress of a gas, such as EO, do require material porosity. DuPont™ Tyvek® or medical grade paper are typically used in these cases. The porous material can be one or both sides of a flexible pouch, a lid for a semirigid or rigid tray, or a smaller area can be included as a strip or patch on a film pouch or lid. The adequacy of the reduced porous area for sterilization efficacy must be proven. See Figure 41.5, a nonporous foil pouch with a strip of porous material to allow for gas sterilization.[17]

Flexible Packaging Laminating

Laminating is the process in which two or more flexible packaging webs are joined together using a bonding agent. These webs are composed of films, papers, or

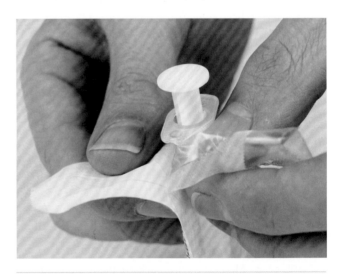

FIGURE 41.5 Flexible pouch containing syringe.
For a color version of this art, please consult the eBook.
(https://www.istock.com/TomekD76.)

aluminum foils.[15] To bond the webs, an adhesive is applied to the less absorbent substrate web, which is then pressed against the second web. This results in a two-layer laminate. Depending on required properties, a laminated structure can consist of several layers. Flexible packaging laminates provide mechanical product protection with excellent strength and tear resistance. They can provide excellent barrier properties to external elements such as light, moisture, and gases while also protecting the loss of product qualities such as freshness, aroma, etc. The laminate structure also provides a sealable layer to produce the finished package.[17]

Coextruded Material

Coextrusion is the process of pressing two or more materials through the same extrusion die to produce a single material structure. When multiple plastics are combined, the result can yield properties different from those of a single material. Very thin layers of resin that cannot be made into a film alone can be layered through coextrusion. Several characteristics can be combined in a single film such as heat resistance, heat sealing capabilities, rigidity, flexibility, cold resistance, and easy-peel capabilities.[17]

Adhesives and Coatings

A medical device package must have a continuous, uninterrupted seal of adequate strength to maintain the integrity of the package. Most medical device packaging heat seals are designed to be peelable. A permanent seal, not intended to be opened for product use, is applied less frequently, for example, the bottom (base) seal of a flexible pouch. The challenge for heat seal designs is that the seal strength must be acceptable for the user to easily open yet strong enough to maintain package integrity through distribution. The user concerns include both the strength of the seal as well as the seal, when opened, providing a clean peel. A clean peel means that upon opening the seal does not generate particulates or fiber fragments that might compromise patient safety.

The processing variables critical for heat sealing are pressure (the force that a tool applies to the materials to make a seal), temperature of both the top and bottom tools, and dwell time or machine speed, which is the amount of time the tool is in contact with the materials to be sealed. It is important that these inputs be balanced to provide the optimum seal and manufacturing efficiency.[17,18]

Inks

Packaging labeling, graphics design, and print are not typically used as a marketing tool as in the consumer industries. There are regulatory requirements concerning ink migration, direct contact, solvents used, etc, that must be met to use an ink for a medical device package. The label content and package printing are primarily for product identification, storage instructions, instructions for use, expiration dating, and lot numbering. Another feature ink can provide is the ability to visually detect if an event occurred with color changing inks. Two common examples are inks that change colors after sterilization providing a visual indicator the package has been sterilized, or temperature extreme indicator inks that indicate any unusual conditions (eg, climate extremes) the product may have been exposed to during distribution.[15,18]

Common Materials—Pharmaceutical Packaging

Glass

The glass used in packaging pharmaceuticals falls into four categories, depending on the chemical constitution of the glass and its ability to resist deterioration. Type I, II, and III glasses are intended for parenteral products, and type IV or NP (non parenteral) is intended for other products. Each type is tested for its resistance to water attack. The degree of attack is determined by the amount of alkali released from the glass under specified test conditions. Obviously, leaching of alkali from the glass into a pharmaceutical solution or preparation could lead to negative effects such as affecting the pH and subsequently the stability of the product.

There are four types of glass:

- Type I (neutral or borosilicate glass)
- Type II (treated soda lime glass)
- Type III (soda lime glass)
- Type IV or NP (general purpose soda lime glass)

Type I glass is the least reactive using higher ingredients and processing cost. It is used for more sensitive pharmaceutical products such as parenteral or blood products. Most ampules and vials are made of type I glass. Type II glass has high chemical resistance but less than type I; therefore, ingredient and processing costs are also less. Many products can be packaged in type II glass; some exceptions include blood products and liquid pharmaceuticals with a pH less than 7.

Examples of the types of products packaged with glass are

- Type I—ampules or vials containing liquid injectables of any pH, blood and related products, and aerosol product
- Type II—injectables of pH <7
- Type III—nonliquid injectables
- Type IV or NP—dry powders for parenteral use (to be reconstituted before use); bottles and jars for tablets, capsules, oral solids, and other solids for reconstitution; oral liquids (solutions, suspensions, emulsions); nasal and eardrops; and droppers

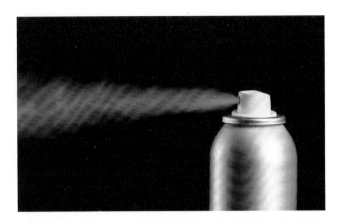

FIGURE 41.6   Metal aerosol container. For a color version of this art, please consult the eBook. (https://www.istock.com/mehmetdinler.)

Metals

Metal containers are used for nonparenteral pharmaceutical products. Metals can be strong, opaque, typically not impacted by temperature extremes, shatterproof, and impermeable to moisture, gases, odors, light, or bacteria. It is the ideal packaging material for pressurized containers (Figure 41.6). Examples include tubes, blisters, cans, aerosol, and gas cylinders. Aluminum is a common choice for both primary and secondary packaging for pharmaceutical products. It is relatively light, yet very strong. It provides a barrier to light and chemicals and is usually impermeable. Thin aluminum is used when a flexible foil is a component of a laminated packaging material such as collapsible tubes for semisolid preparations.[15,19]

Elastomers (Rubber)

Container closures (or seals) are a critical component for container closure systems. The closure, which is typically crimped in place, on the container with a metal ring, and the vial form the primary package for many types of pharmaceutical products, both wet and dry (Figure 41.7).

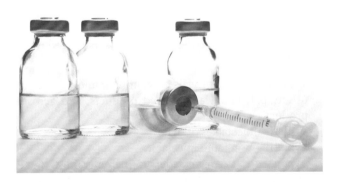

FIGURE 41.7   Elastomeric stoppers vial. For a color version of this art, please consult the eBook. (http://www.istock.com/NikiLitov.)

The closures are commonly referred to as "stoppers" or "bungs" and are typically made from elastomeric materials or also referred to as rubber. An elastomeric material is a material that resumes its original shape when a deforming force is removed, also referred to as viscoelasticity. For example, following the withdrawal with a sterile needle, from a vial, of a dose of the product for administration, an elastomeric closure can reclose after the needle is removed. This characteristic prevents contamination of the contents from the outside and from the closure itself. Less elastomeric closure materials can result in "coring." Coring is when a piece of the stopper is pushed or breaks free due to the needle insertion and can result in the contamination of the vial contents. Low permeability to moisture, vapors, and gases; chemical resistance; and resistance to aging conditions are other important characteristics of a closure. Rubber, an elastomeric material, is an excellent material used to form closures such as stoppers or bungs for vials or gaskets in aerosol cans. Natural rubbers are common for multiple-use closures for injectable products. They do not stand up well to multiple autoclave cycles. The most critical aspect of using components made of natural rubber, including closures, is the possible release of allergenic latex proteins into the container contents or to the user from handling the product. It has compelled manufacturers to seek for less problematic materials that offer the same positive characteristics of natural rubber. Isoprene rubber products provide the flexibility and strength of natural rubber without any of its disadvantages, such as odor, fragmentation coring, and allergic reactions. Some examples of the material usage are for glass or plastic infusion bottles, IV bags, vials, syringe plungers, and insulin pens. Synthetic materials are produced under controlled conditions and are free of the impurities and lot-to-lot variations that are inherent in natural materials, including natural rubber. These materials are often compatible with EO, γ radiation, and steam sterilization. Other common synthetic rubbers currently used for pharmaceutical packaging are butyl, bromobutyl, chlorobutyl, silicon, neoprene, and nitrile. There are many advantages and disadvantages to consider for all elastomeric materials. It is important to thoroughly understand the requirements for the product before selecting a closure material.[15,20-22]

Plastic

Many pharmaceuticals are packaged in plastic materials. Some examples include plastic bags for IV fluids, plastic ointment tubes, plastic film–protected suppositories, plastic tablet, and capsule bottles. There are a vast number of different plastic materials and blends with a range of molecular weights, each with different properties and characteristics. Plastic materials are generally strong, lightweight, reasonably inert, and chemical resistant and can be designed from various polymers for select applications. At certain stages of the manufacturing process, many plastics can be formed, cast, molded, or polymerized into a designed shape or form. There are two classes of plastics: thermoplastics and thermosets. The primary physical difference is that thermoplastics can be remelted back into a liquid, where thermoset plastics always remain in a permanent solid state.

Thermoset plastics contain polymers that cross-link together during the curing process to form an irreversible chemical bond. The cross-linking process eliminates the risk of the product remelting when heat is applied, making thermosets ideal for high-heat applications such as electronics and appliances. Thermoset plastics significantly improve the material's mechanical properties, providing enhanced chemical resistance, heat resistance, and structural integrity. Thermoset plastics are often used for sealed products due to their resistance to deformation. Thermoplastics pellets soften when heated and become more fluid as additional heat is applied. The curing process is completely reversible as no chemical bonding takes place. This characteristic allows thermoplastics to be remolded and recycled without negatively affecting the material's physical properties. There are multiple thermoplastic resins that offer various performance benefits, but most materials commonly offer high strength, shrink resistance, and easy bendability. Depending on the resin types, they can be used for low-stress applications such as plastic bags or higher stress mechanical parts. Some properties of LDPE include ease of processing, moderate barrier to moisture, strength/toughness, flexibility, and ease of sealing. A common application is squeeze bottles used for nasal and eye drops. The HDPE is less permeable to gases and more resistant to oils, chemicals, and solvents. Some properties include stiffness, strength/toughness, and resistance to chemicals. It is widely used in bottles for solid dosage forms. The PP has good resistance to cracking when flexed and good resistance to heat sterilization methods. It is a colorless, odorless thermoplastic material with excellent tensile properties even at high temperature and excellent resistance to strong acids and alkalis.

The PS provides versatility, insulation, and clarity. The PS is used for jars for ointments and creams with low water content. Styrofoam, made from PS, is used for insulation and a cushion material for product protection. The PVC provides versatility, ease of blending, strength/toughness, resistance to grease/oil, resistance to chemicals, and clarity. It is commonly used as a rigid packaging material and main component of intravenous (IV) solution bags. The addition of elastomers to the resin can improve impact resistance. The PVDC provides excellent barrier properties against moisture, water vapor, UV light, aroma, inorganic acids, alkalis, salt solutions, soluble acids, hydrocarbons, detergent base materials, emulsifying agents, and wetting agents. Material coating weight can be customized depending on the barrier requirements of the product. The PVDC is very transparent, which can improve the aesthetics of the product. The PETG has outstanding thermoforming characteristics for applications that require deep draws with precise molding details. It has strong structural integrity and is typically not brittle. The PETG is a common material for thermoformed rigid trays for medical devices that require tray design elements to protect the product. All plastics can contain other substances, such as residues from the polymerization process, plasticizers, stabilizers, antioxidants, pigments, and lubricants.[15,17-19]

Desiccants

Desiccant systems are often included in packaging systems to help protect the product from moisture damage and to help extend product shelf life. There are numerous choices and configurations.

Desiccant canisters are rigid cylindrical, small containers filled with clay, silica gel, or another desiccant material. They are the most commonly used desiccant product for pharmaceutical products. The purpose of the canister is to absorb moisture. Activated carbon, which controls odor, can also be carried in a canister. The canister is commonly used in bottles containing tablets or capsules, such as vitamins, nutraceuticals, and other health or pharmaceutical products. It is important that the canister be designed and produced to be leakproof. They also must comply with regulatory standards governing direct contact with food or drugs.

Desiccant capsules are also rigid and can be molded into a wide range of shapes and sizes to meet different requirements. For example, flat capsules can be placed into blister packages, whereas others can be integrated into packaging closures. These capsules have a distinctive shape and can be made in multiple colors and with different printing options. This clearly distinguishes them from tablets and pills, so they are not accidentally digested.

Desiccant packets are small packs containing desiccant materials of clay, silica gel, or molecular sieve. Like desiccant canisters and capsules, their purpose is to prevent moisture damage. Desiccant packets are used in a wide range of industries, including pharmaceutical. The amount of desiccant needed for an application depends on the chemical and physical composition of the product and container and the volume of the container. Desiccant tubes and stoppers containing a desiccant such as silica gel are sturdy containers made of a combination of HDPE and LDPE. Their purpose is to protect a wide range of pharmaceutical products from moisture and breakage; everything from diagnostic test trips to effervescent tablets or pills.[18,19]

Sterile Packaging Design Considerations

The general functions of packaging are to protect the product and the environment, provide a method of product containment, protect the product as it moves through the supply chain, and to communicate with the user. The paramount feature of a sterile barrier package is to prevent microbial ingress. This barrier must be maintained until the point of product use. Other points to consider when selecting packaging materials or designing a medical package are

- The degree of physical and mechanical protection the product may require. The product must be protected from physical hazards such as shock, vibration, and compression that it may encounter during normal supply chain transportation, handling, and storage.
- Light sensitivity. When applicable for the product type, the package must protect, as needed, from harmful environmental elements like UV light, X-ray, and electromagnetic fields.
- Temperature sensitive products. The product may need to be protected and shipped under controlled thermal conditions.
- Control of the permeation of gases or water vapor. The product may require packaging with superior barrier characteristics or to protect the environment from the product.
- Minimization of contamination, chemical, and/or environmental
- Adequate microbial barrier to prevent microbial ingress over the product life
- Package and product compatibility, including biocompatibility/toxicological considerations
- The type of product identification, coding, and symbology required
- Compatibility with printing and labeling methods
- The facilitation of opening the package and aseptic transfer or presentation of the product at the point of use

- Disposal of the packaging materials
- Conformity with applicable standards
- Identification of the product
- Labeling with instructions for use, cautions, warnings, expiry dating, any required storage conditions
- Material compatibility with the sterilization method

Tables 41.2 and 41.3 provide guidelines on material compatibility with the various sterilization processes based on the Sterile Barrier Association[23] guidance documentation.

When considering all aspects of package usability, including labeling, it is important to consider the context of the use of a package. It often is used in extremely fast-paced and stressful conditions, such as an emergency department. In such an environment, it is important for product identification and information be easy to read and understand. In addition to providing a sterile barrier, all of the other considerations for the design of a medical package also may affect patient safety. Usability evaluations are of increasing importance for medical packaging in addition of the device itself. These evaluations provide evidence that the package design allows for safe and easy handling.

Overall, there are many factors which must be considered when designing a packaging system for a medical device, pharmaceutical or biological, or a combination product. It is important to consider each and assign measurable requirements, such as permeation rates for a film. Once the requirements definition is established, package design and material selection can commence. Following the establishment of the packaging system, it is important

| TABLE 41.2 | Sterilization compatibility porous materials (Copyright © Sterile Barrier Association) |

Materials With Gas and Steam Permeability	Permeability Sufficient for Steam and Gaseous Sterilization Methods	Steam at Least a Part of the Packaging Needs to Be Permeable to Steam	EO/Form at Least a Part of the Packaging Needs to Be Permeable to Gas	Hydrogen Peroxide (Plasma) Natural Fiber-Based Materials Are Incompatible	Gamma/ E-Beam or Beta radiation Impermeable Material May Be Used	Dry Heat (Maximum Temperature) Impermeable Material May Be Used
Medical grade paper	✓	✓	✓	No	✓	✓ (160°C)
Flush spunbond nonwoven materials of polyethylene	✓	✓ (maximum temperature = 127°C) Not suitable for hospitals	✓	✓	✓	No
Wet laid nonwovens (pulp and plastic fibers)	✓	✓	✓	No	✓	No
Spunbond meltblown spunbond (SMS) nonwoven materials of polypropylene	✓	✓	✓	✓	No	No

Abbreviations: E-beam, electron beam; EO, ethylene oxide.

TABLE 41.3 Sterilization compatibility films and composite materials (Copyright © Sterile Barrier Association)

Films and Composite Films	Steam at Least a Part of the Packaging Needs to Be Permeable to Steam	EO/Form at Least a Part of the Packaging Needs to Be Permeable to Gas	Hydrogen Peroxide (Plasma) Natural Fiber-Based Materials Are Incompatible	Gamma/ E-Beam or Beta Radiation Impermeable Material May Be Used	Dry Heat (Maximum Temperature) Impermeable Material May Be Used
Laminated films, widely used for the manufacture of prefabricated sterile barrier systems (pouches, reels), impermeable					
PET/PP films (polyethylene terephthalate/ polypropylene)	✓	✓	✓	No	No
PET/PE films (PET/polyethylene)	No	✓	✓	✓	No
Film components, blister materials, high-barrier composites, impermeable					
Aluminum laminates and composites (ie, high-barrier materials)	✓	✓	See suppliers' specification.	✓	✓
APET film (amorphous polyethylene terephthalate)	No	✓	See suppliers' specification.	✓	No
EP (ethylene propylene copolymer)	See suppliers' specification.	✓	See suppliers' specification.	See suppliers' specification.	See suppliers' specification.
HDPE film (high-density polyethylene)	✓ (121°C)	✓	See suppliers' specification.	✓	No
LDPE film (low-density polyethylene)	No	✓	✓	✓	No
PA film (component) (polyamide)	✓	✓	✓	✓	✓
PE film (component) (polyethylene)	No	✓	✓	✓	No
PP film (component) (polypropylene)	✓	✓	✓	No	No
PET film (component) (polyethylene terephthalate)	✓	✓	✓	✓	✓
PETG (PETG-foam, PETG-PE) film (PET glycol)	No	✓	See suppliers' specification.	✓	No
PS film (polystyrene)	No	✓	See suppliers' specification.	✓	No
HIPS film (high-impact polystyrene)	No	✓	See suppliers' specification.	✓	No
PC film (polycarbonate)	✓	✓	See suppliers' specification.	✓	✓
PVC film (poly vinyl chloride)	No	✓	See suppliers' specification.	No	No
TPU film (thermoplastic polyurethane)	No	✓	See suppliers' specification.	✓	✓

Abbreviations: E-beam, electron beam; EO, ethylene oxide.

to evaluate, produce evidence, and document that requirements set forth have successfully been met. Formal design controls must be applied as well as formal validation processes as described in the next chapter.

THE EVOLUTION OF REGULATIONS AND STANDARDS

In 1938, the United States introduced the Federal Food, Drug, and Cosmetic Act to better regulate product claims and safety requirements. This regulation required new drugs to be tested and to submit the results in a new drug application for market approval. The act also included requirements for labeling and the Federal Trade Commission had to oversee all drug advertising. At the end of 1950s, a specific drug and device branch was formed. In 1976, the US Food and Drug Administration (FDA) got the authority to authorize devices in a premarket review process based on a risk classification scheme.[24] In 1978, the good manufacturing practices (GMPs) for medical devices were introduced to be replaced in 1997 by the quality system regulation (QSR), which is still effective today. When the QSR was introduced, there was still little standardization of how manufacturers evaluated their medical packaging to ensure maintenance of sterility until the point of use. Discussions started early in the 1990s and a monograph on medical packaging was published in 1993 via Health Industry Manufacturers Association (known today as AdvaMed).[25] This document contained most of the fundamentals that are today in international standards on medical packaging. The International Organization for Standardization (ISO) technical committee (TC) 198/working group (WG) 7 met first in 1991 and started in work 1992 to develop a standard for medical packaging, ISO 11607, that was first published in 1997.[26]

The Food and Drug Administration Modernization Act of 1997 introduced a process to facilitate the recognition of national and international medical device consensus standards. Although the regulations mention packaging in many cases, the key requirements are documented in consensus standards as we will see later. The FDA has a long history of promoting standards. The 1995 National Technology Transfer and Advancement Act created a legal basis for federal agencies to get involved with consensus standards development. Today, the Center for Devices and Radiological Health also has 380 individuals participating in more than 600 national and international standards committees across 29 Standards Developing Organizations. The 21st Century Cures Act of 2016 introduced a more formal FDA standards recognition process to further consolidate their approach to standards. The ISO 11607 is the FDA-recognized standard for medical packaging and ISO TC 198/WG 7 has seen continuous participation by agency representatives.

The European Union (EU) introduced its first medical device directive in 1990 for active implantable devices (90/385/European Economic Community[EEC][27]). This directive, as well as all those adopted later, are based on the "new approach" where the law describes high level ERs that must be complied with and where "harmonized" standards can be used to fulfill the requirements of the law. For these directives, the EU Commission issues a mandate (a standardization request) to European Committee for Standardization (CEN), the European standard development organization, to develop standards that will be listed in the EU Official Journal as "harmonized" standards. Authorities and notified bodies must recognize harmonized standards that provide presumption of conformity with the law. The EU adopted the Medical Device Directive (MDD) 93/42/EEC[28] in 1993. The working group CEN TC 102/WG 4 was created to develop European medical packaging standards to be harmonized, but progress was difficult with the parallel standardization activities within ISO. The CEN was working on a suite of standards that included a horizontal standard (EN 868-1[29]) as well as several vertical standards to address specific performance requirements of typical packaging materials used in medical packaging (EN 868 parts 2-10[30-38]). On the other side, the ISO working group developed a single standard addressing the required performance attributes of medical packaging but without specific acceptance criteria.

Experts from both ISO TC 198 and CEN TC 102 met in Ottawa, Ontario, Canada in 1993, and agreed on a resolution for ISO to develop one standard (ISO 11607) and CEN to develop an independent separate series of standards (EN 868 series). After publication of these standards, the next revision would be the time to harmonize the ISO and CEN documents. The resolution outlining this strategy was approved in ISO and CEN and EN 868-1[29] and ISO 11607 were then both published in 1997.[26]

The ISO 11607 was published as a revised version in 2003[39] with notes highlighting the requirements in EN 868-1.[29] This was the basis to merge EN 868-1[29] and ISO 11607 into ISO 11607: 2006 parts 1 and 2.[40,41] A separate standard (ISO 11607-2[41]) was created for process validation as EN 868-1 did not include this important validation aspect at the time.

European directives require the adoption of a national EU member state law complying with the requirements of the directive as a minimum. This approach may result in subtle differences between requirements in member states because there is some freedom on how to transpose the directives, but it was the process to move toward a single market for all EU member states. The recent medical device regulation (MDR),[42] adopted in 2017 by the European Council and the European Parliament, entered into force in all EU member states on the 26th of May 2017 without the need for national transposition legislation. The MDR confirmed the concept of harmonized standards, but the EU Commission introduced a formal process to harmonize standards with increased scrutiny as well as new requirements to be met by those standards. The formal review process, with the newly introduced harmonized standards' consultants to assess such standards during development and prior to publication clearly raises the bar for all harmonized standards.

The European MDR[42] takes a product life cycle (PLC) approach to medical device management covering all the steps from development, clinical evaluation, certification, and postmarket management. Although the former medical device directive (MDD)[28] focused more on the CE certification, the MDR PLC approach requires data gathered during postmarket management to be used to improve the risk management, instructions for use and labeling, clinical evaluation, and identify options to improve the usability, performance, and safety of the device. This impacts sterile packaging as a key accessory of sterile devices. The regulation puts more focus on sterile packaging in key areas. In addition to all the general requirement, there are three general safety and performance requirements (GSPR) in Annex I of the MDR that are highly relevant for sterile packaging:

- In GSPR 11.1, device design and manufacturing processes should "eliminate, or reduce as far as possible, the risk of infection to patients." It further requires that the design allows for "easy and safe handling" and to "prevent microbial contamination of the device." The new requirements are much more explicit, and it is obvious that this requirement requires an assessment of the usability of device including its packaging.
- In GSPR 11.4, the devices delivered in a sterile state . . . "remain sterile, under the storage and transport conditions specified by the manufacturer until that packaging is opened at the point of use." It further requires to "ensure that the integrity of that packaging is clearly evident to the final user" which is a new requirement. The maintenance of sterility has always been a key requirement for packaging, but the specification to the "point of use" adds an additional complexity.
- In GSPR 11.5, devices labeled as sterile are "processed, manufactured, packaged and sterilised by means of appropriate, validated methods." Traditionally, the focus was only on the validation of sterilization processes but now explicitly mentions packaging.

Standards like EN ISO 11607, which are currently harmonized with the previous MDD, need to be reharmonized with the MDR to meet the amended GSPR. At the end of 2018, a revised version of EN ISO 11607 was submitted for review by the harmonization consultants of the EU Commission and remains to be finalized at this time this chapter was prepared. It can be expected, though, that this process may lead to further changes to ISO 11607 in the future, with its latest revision published in February 2019.[13,43]

The essential principles of the MDD and the more evolved GSPR of the MDR are aligned with the essential principles as published by the International Medical Device Regulators Forum (IMDRF).[44] The principles are also published in ISO 16142-1.[45] The objective of these principles is to create the basis for country regulations that build on standards that are recognized to provide conformity with these principles. Such standards can be national, but the idea is that they will evolve over time toward international standards to remove barriers for international trade. The regulations of many countries like Australia, India, Russia, and the Association of Southeast Asian Nations countries like Malaysia, Singapore, Thailand, Vietnam, etc, are all based on the IMDRF essential principles and standards. Other countries such as China, Japan, and Korea have also adopted many of the key sterilization standards and the packaging standard ISO 11607 as national standards.

Quality Management Over the Packaging Life Cycle

The historic evolution of product quality went from *quality control*, where products were tested or inspected to comply with approved specification to *quality assurance* where more focus was put on manufacturing processes by requesting compliance with GMPs to *quality systems* that introduced a design control process taking a quality-by-design approach as well as introducing other essential quality processes. The latest development takes a total PLC approach to fully integrate clinical studies and postmarket follow-up and to close the loop when adverse events occur that require improvements to the design, the instructions for use, or the product claims.

The 1997 FDA QSR[46] was a major regulatory development. The QSR introduced requirements for design controls, materials and supplier controls, production and process controls, records, documents, change controls, etc.[47,48] The QSR included also important requirements for packaging. Packaging is included in the scope (§820.1), packaging and the labeling are specified as one of the design outputs (§820.3), clause §820.120 requires establishing and maintaining procedures to control labeling activities, and clause §820.130 requires device packaging and shipping containers to be "designed and constructed to protect the device from alteration or damage during the customary conditions of processing, storage, handling, and distribution." And finally, packaging and labeling specifications, including methods and processes used, must be documented in the device master record (§820.181).

In 1996, ISO introduced a specific quality management systems standard for medical devices, ISO 13485, which is now available in its 2016 version[49] supported with guide to help with implementation.[50] Whereas the 1996 version of ISO 13485 was applied in conjunction with the application of ISO 9001, to specify the "quality system requirements for the design/development and, when relevant, installation and servicing of medical devices", the 2016 version has evolved into an independent quality standard applicable to the entire life cycle of the device considering regulatory requirements from design and development, documentation, through clinical evaluation, to postmarket follow-up, etc.

Included was the concept of continuous improvement for the medical device (and its accessories) based on market feedback, whereas earlier versions only focused on the efficiency of the quality system.

Requirements for packaging have evolved recognizing the need for preservation of the product, to considering the risks of transport, storage, and distribution and addressing specifically the requirements of sterilization, maintenance of sterility of sterilized products, and related validations. What is true for the product is also true for packaging; quality cannot be reliably confirmed by testing the product and can only be truly and sustainably achieved through a quality-by-design approach. Implementation of effective product design controls including for packaging is ever more relevant and important.

Labeling

Packaging plays an important role as a carrier of labeling. Labeling includes instructions for use of the health care product and information that allows proper identification of the product and provides details regarding its technical description. Clause §820.120 of the US QSR requires "establishing and maintaining procedures to control labeling activities", whereas ISO 13485:2016[49] requires "implementation of defined operations for labelling and packaging." Labeling controls is not only a regulatory requirement, but a good business practice because labeling errors are the primary source of product recalls. From a packaging point of view, it is important that inks and adhesives used or labeling supports do not have adverse effects on the medical devices. Labeling must be compatible with the sterilization process and remain legible until at least the use-by-date of the device.

Current Medical Packaging Standards

As described earlier, standards have developed over the last decades and despite their voluntary nature, they have become unavoidable especially for medical devices. Even in pharmaceutical applications, standards are increasingly taking over areas that pharmacopoeia monographs and GMPs used to address. This section summarizes the requirements of ISO 11607-1 and ISO 11607-2, as republished in 2019 in their latest revised versions.[13,43]

Principles of Packaging Validation

Validation is a key and essential activity for achieving and maintaining sterility because sterility cannot be verified without destructive and technically limited tests. It is essential to make the difference between validation, defined as "confirmation, through the provision of objective evidence that the requirements for a specific intended use or application have been fulfilled" and verification, defined

as "confirmation, through the provision of objective evidence that specified requirements have been fulfilled."[9,51,52] Although it may be theoretically possible for some types of packaging to verify each unit in terms of integrity with a nondestructive test method, the accuracy and sensitivity of such verification will be far from perfect. Even if integrity verification after manufacturing reaches a high degree of accuracy and ability to detect the smallest defects, this activity does not provide full evidence to support the maintenance of integrity (respectively maintenance of sterility) through the hazards of distribution, storage, and handling, which is part of the intended use of the product. Verification of integrity by the user can only be done visually and will be even less reliable. It is best practice that users verify integrity of packaging to eliminate breaches that are evident; however, the user cannot be left with the burden to make the selection between packaging that made it through the transportation hazards and those that experienced a loss of integrity. Especially in emergency situations or faced with more and more demands, health care workers may only glance at packaging if at all. It is obvious that integrity cannot be verified reliably, and what cannot be verified needs to be validated considering the intended use or application of a product. Based on this, it is logical that ISO 13485:2016[49] requires sterile packaging to be validated. The ISO 11607-1[13,53] provides the basis for sterile packaging validation and the fundamental principle to use integrity testing instead of sterility testing as integrity tests are significantly easier to perform and more reliable. When developing a product or a packaging through a systematic controlled design process, it is important to make sure that design outputs can be verified and respectively validated.

The 1997 FDA design control guidance[54] provided guidance and a framework on how to develop and implement design controls including those for packaging. It was developed with contributions from the Global Harmonization Task Force, which included members from Canada, Japan, EU, Australia, and the United States. As such, it represented the state of the art of design controls thinking at the time, and it is still valid today. It states the following on packaging:

> Validation should also address product packaging and labeling. These components of the design may have significant human factors implications, and may affect product performance in unexpected ways . . . Validation should include simulation of the expected environmental conditions, such as temperature, humidity, shock and vibration, corrosive atmospheres, etc. For some classes of device, the environmental stresses encountered during shipment and installation far exceed those encountered during actual use, and should be addressed during validation.

It is interesting to note that this already addressed the human factors implications, which has received more attention in the latest revision of ISO 11607-1 for packaging[13] and for devices in general with the recent publication of ISO 62366-1:2015.[55] The 2019 version of ISO 11607-1[13] states that "packaging systems that meet the requirements of design, usability, performance testing and stability testing shall be considered validated if the sterile barrier system conforms with ISO 11607-2." This statement provides a summary of all aspects that must be included into a validation including usability.

Performance Testing

One of the key functions of packaging is to protect the device and the sterile barrier system through the hazards of storage, distribution, and transport. For maintenance of sterility, it is necessary that the sterile barrier system maintains integrity until the point of use and no breaches of integrity occur. The anticipated storage, handling, and distribution are key design inputs for the design. Distribution locally in a region, transnationally, or even via intercontinental shipments means that packaging may be exposed to very different hazards that have to be in considered. Quality management systems[49] require that the planned storage, handling, and distribution are considered and that procedures for preserving the conformity of the product are documented. The ISO 11607-1 requires that based on the storage, handling, and distribution environment, the worst case packaging system is exposed to a simulated distribution tests typically according to American Society for Testing and Materials (ASTM) D4169[56] or International Safe Transit Association guidelines.[57] The packaging system will also be exposed to environmental challenges. The objective of these tests is to produce evidence that the packaging system is capable to protect the sterile barrier system and the product and that integrity is maintained. It is the manufacturer's responsibility, when applicable, to review changes in the distribution environment and to determine if revalidation may be required. The EU MDR[42] now insists to maintain sterility until the point of use. Although performance testing has focused mainly on shipping units in the past, it will be important to consider handling of unit boxes in a health care facility environment after protective cartons for several unit boxes are removed.

Stability Testing

Maintenance of sterility must also be ensured over any stated shelf life. The objective of stability testing is to produce evidence that the sterile barrier system will maintain integrity until a stated expiry date. The ISO 11607-1[13] requires this evidence to be generated via real-time aging, products can be released to market based on accelerated aging studies and pending the availability of real-time aging data. Accelerated aging is well accepted in the industry to evaluate if materials and their seals and closures are sufficiently stable over time and do not lose their physical properties due to oxidation or other chemical reactions that could have a negative impact. The main focus of ISO 11607 is to make

sure that integrity is maintained over time. It is also important to assess if aseptic presentation is not impaired due to changes in seal strength or fiber tear issues during peeling, for example. Accelerated aging is based on the fact that rates of chemical reactions typically double with every temperature increase of 10°C. This dependence was expressed by Arrhenius in 1889.[58] The practice of calculating appropriate accelerated aging temperatures for sterile barrier system packaging is documented in ASTM F1980.[59] The higher the temperature, the shorter the accelerated aging time; however, at higher temperatures, the relationship gets less precise so that a maximum accelerated aging temperature of 50°C to 56°C is typically recommended. It may be required to age at even lower temperatures if the device is temperature sensitive and aged with the packaging. For many materials, humidity has little to no impact, but for some, the low humidity in aging ovens may lead to an underestimate of materials hydrolysis in real-life conditions.[60]

Evaluation of Aseptic Presentation

The ability to aseptically present a sterile medical device is a key feature of packaging. Practices have improved over time with the health care community focused on the importance of minimizing or eliminating microbial contamination and the risk of health care–acquired infections (HAIs). With the emergence of good hospital hygiene practices and the emergence of potent antibiotics in the beginning of the 20th century, HAIs were considered under control. But by the end of the 20th century, the incidence of antibiotic-resistant bacteria became alarming, and there was a growing renewed interest to further mitigate contamination risks. Recent data published for Europe, for example, suggested that the problem cannot be underestimated with "the estimated burden of infections with antibiotic-resistant bacteria in the EU and EEA was similar to the cumulative burden of influenza, tuberculosis, and HIV, was notably diverse across countries, and has increased between 2007 and 2015."[61] Based on ISO 11607-1:2019,[13] manufacturers are now required to conduct a formal evaluation of aseptic presentation for their sterile packaging applications. This can be done by usability evaluations of the medical device including its packaging following ISO International Electrotechnical Commission (IEC) 62366-1:2015.[55] The purpose is to demonstrate that the sterile barrier system can be opened without contaminating the sterile contents and the contents can be presented aseptically, in other words risks of microbial contamination are mitigated to an acceptable level.[62]

Packaging Assembly, Closure, or Sealing Process Validation

The packaging assembly processes, including the placement of the content in the packaging and the closure or sealing operations, will impact the integrity of the final package. These processes need to be of high reliability and capability even under worst conditions. The validation must include an installation qualification (IQ), operational qualification (OQ), and a performance qualification (PQ). The objectives of IQ are to make sure that the process equipment is properly installed and adheres to the approved specification. During OQ, the focus is to determine that the installed equipment operates within the predetermined limits in accordance with its operational procedures.[63] During OQ, the sealing process window and the process specification are developed and confirmed. The process specification includes process parameters, controls, settings, alarms, and monitoring of process variables necessary to produce a product meeting the specification. And finally, during PQ, it must be demonstrated that the process has a high capability considering all potential sources of variability and anticipated conditions. These will typically include replicates to demonstrate consistency, such as three lots of materials, different operators, and production runs after change over procedures or during different seasons.

Inspection and Control

Implementation of adequate inspections and controls is a last fundamental step to maintain a packaging process in a state of validation. Regular seal strength measurements and integrity tests are important measures to maintain the process in that state of control. Incoming quality inspections of materials and preformed sterile barrier systems as well as supplier audits are essential steps of supplier controls.

Change Management and Revalidations

Supplier agreements should include change notification agreements and any changes need to be thoroughly investigated to determine the potential impact on the validation status. The ISO 11607, QSRs, and ISO 13485 require the implementation of a change control procedure to review the impact of changes in materials, design, device, distribution channels, sterilization processes, or anything that could negatively impact the maintenance of sterility, the stability of the packaging over the shelf life, the packaging performance, or the aseptic presentation. Revalidation protocols must be established to validate such changes before implementation to maintain a high degree of safety for the patient. Depending on the changes, the revalidation steps can focus only on those aspects that are potentially impacted. Any rationales must be documented in the change control files.[64]

Application of Packaging Validation Principles in Health Care Facilities

Validation is a key regulatory requirement and a necessity to ensure sterility up to the point of use. And yet, many health care facilities consider validation and design as an activity to be done exclusively by medical device manufacturers, although they perform similar activities

in their central services (reprocessing and sterilization) departments. Health care users normally have no or limited possibility to perform data intensive validation efforts, but the same essential principles apply. Validations will be typically based on packaging manufacturers labeling and provided compliance and conformity certificates. The final sealing or closure process needs to be validated to demonstrate that the process is capable. The selection of appropriate packaging solutions is a design activity that needs to consider various design inputs and that must be based on a risk-based decision process. The packaging solutions used in health care facility sterilization department are normally very standardized so that health care users can build their validation efforts on data received from their suppliers. Often this data is not available so that health care facilities usually adopt an "event-related" shelf life for sterility defined as being sterilized until the packaging is opened or otherwise compromised within a relatively short date of expiration. They may also use validation services offered by service providers or by the suppliers themselves. A revision process has been initiated in 2018 for ISO technical specification (TS) 16775 *Packaging for Terminally Sterilized Medical Devices—Guidance on the Application of ISO 11607-1 and ISO 11607-2"* with an extensive annex on the application in health care facilities.[65]

▶ TEST METHOD CONSIDERATIONS

Test Method Overview

To demonstrate that the integrity of the package can be maintained throughout the useful life of the product, there must be appropriate means to test it. Unfortunately, a single test does not exist that can adequately assess the entire package. Testing only the packaging seals does not detect pinholes or abrasions in other areas of the package. Conversely, testing only the materials themselves for microbial barrier, strength, or puncture resistance will not detect channels in the seals. A glass vial with an elastomeric stopper must be tested much differently than a porous pouch. The manufacturer is therefore left to determine and justify an appropriate combination of tests for their specific device and packaging situation. Just as there are a myriad of different tests, there are also dozens of different standards and guidance documents that the user must be familiar with. The most recognized standard for packaging validation is the harmonized international standard, EN ISO 11607 parts 1 and 2.[53,66-68] Some countries can have their own national standards. There are also regional specific standards such as the European EN 868 series parts 2 to 10,[29-38] which include numerous test methods and proposed acceptance criteria. The ASTM standards outline many test methods and are used globally in over 140 countries. They are arguably the most widely followed packaging testing standards.

The ISO 11607-1 Annex B[13] and ASTM F2097-16[69] contain an informative list of the most commonly used test methods and guidance for medical device packaging, although this is not an exhaustive list. United States Pharmacopeia (USP) <1207>[70] defines package integrity for nonporous packages for pharmaceutical products. Pharmaceutical products are most often packaged in nonporous packaging to prevent leakage of the product out, in the case of liquid drug products, and to keep environmental contaminants, such as oxygen or water, away from products that could adversely be affected by exposure to these substances. To determine the adequacy of any package, various tests must be performed from at least three categories: strength, integrity, and microbial barrier. Some of the most commonly used tests are discussed in this section.

Strength Testing

Most packaging is made by joining two materials to form a seal at the interface (with G_c representing the intrinsic adhesion at the interface of the two materials in Figure 41.8) of the two materials. The same material may be joined to itself, as is the case with an all film pouch, or two dissimilar materials as is the case with a thermoformed tray with a DuPont™ Tyvek® lid.

For joining dissimilar materials, some type of adhesive is normally applied to at least one of the materials. Two types of seals exist: weld seals that are not meant to be opened or peelable seals that provide a means to access the contents aseptically. The integrity of the seals is critical in the maintenance of sterility. The seal must be made with enough force to stay intact during the rigors of sterilization, transportation, and handling but must also allow ease of opening and aseptic presentation for the end user. It is not desirable to have a seal so easy to open that the end user has doubts about the integrity of the seals. Conversely, it should not be difficult to open that the end user has trouble accessing the device in an aseptic manner. The true adhesion of the surfaces, or the force holding the two surfaces together (see F in Figure 41.8), is difficult to measure accurately. The most common tests to determine the strength properties are seal strength, burst testing, and creep testing.

Seal strength, which more appropriately should be named "peel strength", is determined by measuring the force that it takes to pull the seal apart with a tensile machine (Figure 41.8). The peel force measured is the combination of the intrinsic adhesive force and the force required to deform the material. The most common method of measuring the seal strength is ASTM F88[71] or EN 868-5.[38] The test involves cutting a specified width of package either 15 mm (ASTM or EN) or 25 mm (ASTM) wide. The cut is made 90 degrees perpendicular to the seal and placing the material on either side of the seal in the grips of a tensile strength machine (Figure 41.9).

The material is either oriented with the "tail" unsupported (ASTM F88 technique A), supported at 90 degrees (ASTM F88 technique B) or supported at 180 degrees with an alignment plate (ASTM F88 technique C). The jaws are moved apart at a constant rate and the force required to peel the seal, the average force, and the point of failure is measured and documented. The results can be graphed to represent a seal curve as shown in Figure 41.10.

It is common to exclude 10% at the beginning and 10% at the end of the curve to yield a more reliable curve. The orientation and angle of placing the sample in the machine grips can lead to significant variability. For consistency, it is important to perform the test in the same manner each time. The material that is the most flexible is usually placed in the upper grips and the more rigid material in the lower grips. There is no generally accepted requirement for a minimum seal strength value. Many in the industry have historically relied on a 1 lb-f/in minimum value, but there never has been a regulatory requirement or scientific basis for this value. Others have

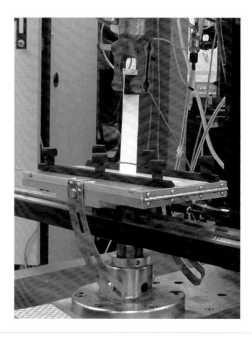

FIGURE 41.9 Seal strength testing using a tensile strength test machine.

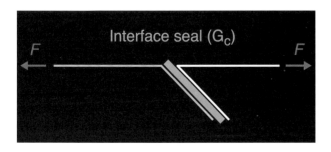

FIGURE 41.8 Illustration of seal interface.

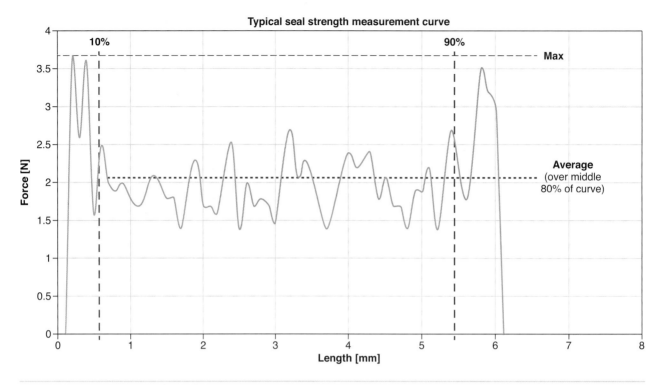

FIGURE 41.10   Example of a seal curve.

used the value proposed by EN 868-5[38], but this standard has been developed for pouches used in healthcare sterilization applications. The manufacturer is responsible for determining an appropriate specification based on their specific product and packaging combination.

A second type of strength test is the burst test. This test involves inflating the package with air until it fails. Burst testing is performed according to ASTM F2054[72] with restraining plates to hold the package or an alternate version ASTM F1140[73] without the use of restraining plates. The use of restraining plates allows most of the stress to be focused on the seals around the outside perimeter of the package while testing unrestrained may put more of the stress on the middle of the package and may not as accurately detect the part of the seal that is weakest.

Also outlined in ASTM F1140, creep testing inflates the package to a pressure below the burst pressure (typically 80% of the burst value) and holds it for either a specified amount of time or until the package fails. These tests can be useful to estimating effects of sterilization processes and transportation, where the packages will undergo varying degrees of pressure differentials. The seal may experience "creep" or start to narrow, essentially opening from the inside due to the higher internal pressure expanding the package when subjected to vacuum in a steam, gas, or other sterilization process. Both the depth of the vacuum as well as the rate of attainment can affect seal integrity. Seal creep can also be possible with the change in pressure associated with air transport or even by truck at higher altitudes, especially with nonporous packaging. Porous packaging must

have sufficiently breathable area to equilibrate the pressure differential. Labels placed over areas of the breathable surface can potentially contribute to seal creep. Another factor that can lead to narrowing of the seals or seal creep is the device weight placing stress against the seal.

Integrity Testing

In the ASTM terminology standard,[74] package integrity is defined as the physical capability of a given package to protect its contents with the desired level of protection over a defined period of service, including as a barrier to physical, microbiological, and/or chemical challenge. Pharmaceutical products such as drugs contained in nonporous packaging such as glass or blow-filled plastic ampules, vials with screw cap or elastomeric closures, autoinjectors, and syringes must be protected from not only microbial contamination getting in but also of environmental gases and product leakage. These environmental contaminants could also include loss of nitrogen or other inert gases from the container, loss of vacuum, or entry of oxygen, water vapor, or air into product that may be adversely affected by the breach.

The integrity of the package can be tested in a variety of ways. Integrity can be separated into seal integrity and overall package integrity, such as detecting a pinhole in foil pouch. The simplest test for package integrity is visual inspection. Visual inspection based on ASTM F1886[75] looks for channels across the seal where microbiological or environmental contaminants may breach the sterile barrier. According to this standard, channels of 125 μm may be detected reliably at 94% and 75 μm detected at 79%. Types of defects investigated with visual inspection are unsealed areas, nonhomogenous or undersealed areas, oversealed areas, narrow seals (creep or rupture), channels, wrinkles/cracks/fold-overs, and tears and pinholes. The operator must assess the package using controlled lighting conditions of 540 lumens/m^2, and there may be subjectivity and variability based on the operator's level of training and/or experience.

Dye penetration testing across the seal area of porous packaging is a method to determine if channels exist across the seal. Testing based on ASTM F1929[76] allows detection of channels down to 50 μm (Figure 41.11). This test is used on materials with a transparent film side and a porous sheet component. The packages are tested either by injecting a toluidine dye solution into the package to a depth of 3 to 6 mm, edge dipping the outside edge of the seal or using an eye dropper and laying a bead of dye material in the area between the two different materials and looking for channels.

If dye penetrates across the seal area, the package fails. The dye must be in contact for a relatively short duration (ie, 5 s on each side) or the dye may begin to wick into the porous material making the test hard to interpret. If a true channel exists, it is typically detected almost immediately by visual assessment. Folding and bending can cause sheet separation in most porous materials allowing the dye to enter the center of the sheet, and appearing as a channel, when in fact it is a false positive. A reference article published on the topic of sheet separation goes into this topic in more detail.[77]

Testing nonporous packages or flexible barrier material based on ASTM 3039-15[78] also allows detection of channels. Method A involves injection of intact packages with a toluidine dye solution at a volume of 0.25 mL for each 25 mm (1 inch) of seal area and allowing the dye to contact the seal for no more than 5 seconds. If the material has a transparent side the seal edge can be visually examined for the presence of channels. If the material is opaque, it is placed on an absorbent pad, and following the test interval, the pad is examined for staining indicative of a leak. Channels down to 50 μm can be detected with this method. Method B is not for whole packages but is for testing flat nonporous sheets (such as foils and films) can detect leaks down to as small as 10 μm. The flat sheets of material are placed on an absorbent material, placing dye on all areas the top surface and rolling the dye over the surface with a small roller. The absorbent material is then observed for the presence of any stains, which would indicate a leak.

Parenteral Drug Association (PDA) Technical Report No. 27[79] recommends both a physical and a microbial test when evaluating container closure. For nonporous sterile containers such as pharmaceutical vials or ampules, or other containers that can be immersed and withstand pressure changes, containers filled with microbiological media may be immersed into a microbial challenge of an indicator organism. One of the most common microorganisms used is *Brevundimonas diminuta*, a motile bacteria that can be cultured as a very small cell size when grown under certain conditions. The challenge may be performed at ambient pressure or a dynamic test can be performed by subjecting the samples to vacuum or pressure changes to simulate air shipment. Following the challenge, the vials are incubated and then visually examined for growth of the indicator organism to determine if the closure system was breached. Because the test organism is typically aerobic and therefore requires oxygen, it is required to leave a headspace in the media filled containers. This is commonly referred to as a microbial ingress study. The physical counterpart to the microbial ingress test is the dye ingress study. This may also be referred to as tracer liquid. This test is used on products such as containers, vials, autoinjectors, and prefilled syringes to place them in a similar chamber and immersed in a dye solution. A vacuum or series of pressure and vacuum changes may be performed, and the products are either visually examined or analyzed through spectrophotometry for presence of the dye (eg, methylene blue) indicating a leak in the container closure system.

Bubble emission is an integrity test based on either ASTM D3078[80] for packages containing a headspace gas or ASTM F2096[81] for packages that are internally pressurized. The first method submerges the packages in water in a vacuum chamber and a vacuum is pulled. The vacuum creates a lower surrounding pressure and thus a higher pressure inside the package and any headspace gas that leaks out can be visualized as a steady stream of bubbles. The second method involves manual inflation of the packages while submerged and can be performed on both porous or nonporous packages. Porous packaging can be more difficult to analyze as you will see an effervescence of bubbles through the porous material. A steady stream of bubbles is indicative of a leak. These tests mostly will determine only gross leaks.

The tests mentioned earlier are the most common tests historically performed and are considered probabilistic in nature. Probabilistic tests are more error prone,

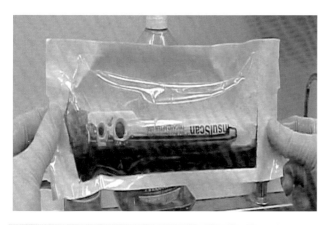

FIGURE 41.11   Dye penetration test.

not as reproducible, have more uncertainties and rely more on human interpretation. More recently developed tests are deterministic. They are less error prone, more quantitative, and are highly sensitive. The USP<1207.1>[82] encourages the use of deterministic test methods such as tracer gas detection, high-voltage leak detection, mass extraction, pressure decay, and vacuum decay. The USP <1207.2>[83] describes each of these methods and lists the corresponding ASTM method where applicable. These methods are commonly performed on nonporous pharmaceutical products such as ampoules and vials and such methods are generally more sensitive than the tests available for porous packaging. Minute leaks can be detected well below the values that could result in microbial ingress and compromise pharmaceutical products.

Microbial Barrier Testing

In the 1990s, various methods to challenge packaging with microorganisms were used. It was thought that a real-world challenge would be the ultimate way to demonstrate adequate integrity of the package and its ability to maintain sterility. Many variations of microbial tests were used including aerosol spore challenge tests, spores in talcum powder, inoculation of test organisms onto swatches of material, and others. At that time, no consensus standards existed. The industry began to move away from these tests due to the lack of sensitivity and inability to validate them consistently. Industry and regulatory bodies began accepting a combination of test methods such as both the seals and microbial barrier properties of the material in lieu of whole package challenges. This led to a decline in the use of these tests. The ASTM F1608[84] was one of the next generation test standards developed and used globally. This microbial aerosol challenge tests for the passage of airborne *Bacillus atrophaeus* spores through swatches of porous packaging material. The organisms passing through the samples are trapped on a membrane filter, enumerated, and a log reduction of the sample in comparison to a control can be calculated. This is useful for comparing materials to each other and is known as microbial barrier ranking. The drawbacks include lengthy incubation, relatively high variability, microbiological waste, and the use of face velocities significantly higher than real world conditions. In 1998, a group of medical packaging companies funded research to develop an improved microbial barrier test. The studies demonstrated that particles behave much like spores and a correlation with filtration theory was shown.[85] This led to the development of ASTM F2638.[86] This test determines the barrier properties of the porous component of the sterile barrier system. It is not used for nonporous samples. Swatches 120 mm in diameter are placed in a housing and the sample is challenged with 1.0 µm PS spheres. Any particles penetrating through the material are counted by

laser particle counters. Multiple face velocities are used to generate a curve of maximum penetration. This can be used to compare different material types. No lengthy incubation time is required, and the face velocities are more representative of those seen during routine package handling. The test was accepted by the FDA in 2013.

Conclusion

There are seemingly countless packaging test methods available, yet not a single test by itself will adequately demonstrate the appropriateness of the package and closures. The combination of tests chosen must consider product requirements, sensitivity of the product to environmental contaminants such as oxygen or moisture, allowable leakage rates, sterilization method and parameters employed, resterilization requirements (if allowed), shipping methods, and end-user requirements to name a few. Prior to testing, samples must undergo a worst-case simulation of what could happen to the package in real life situations. This involves sterilization, accelerated, and real-time aging to determine if the package deteriorates over time as well as a systematic series of distribution tests and environmental challenges to simulate the rigors of shipping and handling. An appropriate combination of strength, integrity, and microbial barrier tests can help ensure a robust package that meets the essential requirements of packaging to include sterilization, provide physical protection, maintain sterility up to the point of use, and allow for aseptic presentation.

▶ THE FUTURE OF STERILE PACKAGING

Although the fundamentals of the maintenance of sterility will never change, packaging has and continues to evolve. The drive for efficiency improvements and cost reductions will continue, but with a more regulatory focus, a healthy balance is emerging as the safety of the patient must continue to be the first priority. Products become increasingly complex and packaging engineers must cope with new requirements. The focus on optimizing supply chain requirements and traceability will further increase; the software tools to support those will achieve maturity and allow innovative smart packaging solutions to become ubiquitous as the cost of those technologies continues to fall. Packaging design will also become more users centric from a more product centric approach in the past. Furthermore, minimizing the contamination risk during aseptic presentation will only be possible by carefully analyzing the usability (or human factors) of packaging and product designs and supplemented by targeted training of users.

The biggest challenge may be sustainability needs to find the right answers to enable a more circular economy and optimize recycling of packaging. This will only be possible by carefully selecting materials and combinations thereof that can be easily recycled and optimizing recycling processes. These may be further influenced by additional regulatory requirements in the future. State of the art packaging solutions overall enable and are fundamental to modern health care.

REFERENCES

1. Vallery-Radot R. *Louis Pasteur: His Life and Labours*. Hamilton EEP, trans. New York, NY: Appleton; 1886.
2. Appert N. *The Art of Preserving All Kinds of Animal and Vegetable Substances for Several Years. A Work Pub by Order of the French Minister of the Interior on the Report of the Board of Arts and Manufactures*. London, United Kingdom: Black, Parry and Kingsbury; 1811.
3. J. Weck GmbH u. Co. KG. Die Geschichte der Firma WECK. J. Weck GmbH u. Co. KG Web site. http://www.weck.de/docs/Geschichte_WECK.pdf. Accessed January 1, 2019.
4. Schimmelbusch C. *Anleitung zur aseptischen Wundbehandlung*. Berlin, Germany: August Hirschwald; 1892.
5. Kilmer FB. Modern surgical dressings. *Am J Pharm*. 1897;69:15.
6. Parker CE, inventor. Catgut ligature and suture and method of preparing same. US patent 701,501. June 3, 1902.
7. Akers MJ. *Sterile Drug Products: Formulation, Packaging, Manufacturing, and Quality*. New York, NY: Informa Healthcare; 2010.
8. Nema S, Ludwig JD, eds. *Pharmaceutical Dosage Forms: Parenteral Medications. Volume 1: Formulation and Packaging*. 3rd ed. New York, NY: Informa Healthcare; 2010.
9. Erhard W, inventor; ER Squibb and Sons, LLC, assignee. Hypodermic unit. US patent 2,219,301. October 29, 1940.
10. Gaughran ERL, Kereluk K, eds. Sterilization of medical products. Paper presented at: Kilmer Conference Proceedings; December 1976; East Windsor, NJ.
11. International Organization for Standardization. *ISO 11607-1:2006/ Amd 1:2014: Packaging for Terminally Sterilized Medical Devices— Part 1: Requirements for Materials, Sterile Barrier Systems and Packaging Systems*. Geneva, Switzerland: International Organization for Standardization; 2014.
12. Jenke D. *Compatibility of Pharmaceutical Products and Contact Materials: Safety Considerations Associated With Extractables and Leachables*. Hoboken, NJ: Wiley; 2009.
13. International Organization for Standardization. *ISO 11607-1:2019: Packaging for Terminally Sterilized Medical Devices—Part 1: Requirements for Materials, Sterile Barrier Systems and Packaging Systems*. Geneva, Switzerland: International Organization for Standardization; 2019.
14. European Commission. 2018 Circular economy package. European Commission Web site. http://ec.europa.eu/environment/circular-economy/index_en.htm. Accessed February 18, 2018.
15. Bakker M. *The Wiley Encyclopedia of Packaging Technology*. New York, NY: Wiley; 1986.
16. DuPont Medical and Pharmaceutical Protection. *DuPont Technical Reference Guide for Medical and Pharmaceutical Packaging*. Midland, MI: DuPont Medical and Pharmaceutical Protection; 2017. http://www.dupont.com/content/dam/dupont/products-and-services/packaging-materials-and-solutions/medical-and-pharmaceutical-packaging-materials/documents/DPT_MPP_Technical_Reference_Guide.pdf. Accessed November 3, 2019.
17. Hernandez RJ, Selke SEM, Culter JD. *Plastics Packaging: Properties, Processing, Applications, and Regulations*. Vol 1. Cincinnati, Ohio: Hanser Gardner; 2000.
18. O'Brien JD, Sherman M. *Medical Device Packaging Handbook*. 2nd ed. New York, NY: Marcel Dekker; 1998.
19. US Food and Drug Administration. *Guidance for Industry—Container Closure Systems for Packaging Human Drugs and Biologics—Chemistry, Manufacturing, and Controls Documentation*. Silver Spring, MD: US Food and Drug Administration; 1999.
20. United States Pharmacopoeia. *USP <381> Elastomeric Closures for Injections, General Chapter*. Bethesda, MD: United States Pharmacopeia; 2011.
21. Sandle T. Closures for pharmaceutical preparations: a review of design and test considerations. *BioPharm Int*. 2012;25(12):32-36.
22. United States Pharmacopoeia. *USP <797> Pharmaceutical Compounding Sterile Preparations*. Bethesda, MD: United States Pharmacopeia; 2016.
23. Sterile Barrier Association. Compatibility of materials used for sterile barrier systems with sterilisation processes. Sterile Barrier Association Web site. http://www.sterilebarrier.org/media/71547/Sterilisation-compatibility-August-2017.pdf. Accessed September 1, 2018.
24. Fiedler BA, ed. *Managing Medical Devices Within a Regulatory Framework*. Amsterdam, Netherlands: Elsevier; 2016.
25. Spitzley J, Larsen C, Liebler BL. *HIMA Reference on Sterile Packaging*. Washington, DC: Health Industry Manufacturers Association; 1993.
26. International Organization for Standardization. *ISO 11607:1997: Packaging for Terminally Sterilized Medical Devices (Now Withdrawn)*. Geneva, Switzerland: International Organization for Standardization; 1997.
27. European Union. Council directive of 20 June 1990 on the approximation of the laws of the member states relating to active implantable medical devices (90/385/EEC). *Off J Eur*. 1990;L189:1-35.
28. European Union. Council directive 93/42/EEC of 14 June 1993 concerning medical devices. *Off J Eur*. 1993;L169:1-43.
29. European Committee for Standardization. *EN 868-1:1997: Packaging Materials and Systems for Medical Devices Which Are to Be Sterilize— Part 1. General Requirements and Test Methods*. Brussels, Belgium: European Committee for Standardization; 1997.
30. European Committee for Standardization. *EN 868. Packaging for Terminally Sterilized Medical Devices—Part 2: Sterilization Wrap— Requirements and Test Methods*. Brussels, Belgium: European Committee for Standardization; 2017.
31. European Committee for Standardization. *EN 868. Packaging for Terminally Sterilized Medical Devices—Part 3: Paper for Use in the Manufacture of Paper Bags (Specified in EN 868-4) and in the Manufacture of Pouches and Reels (Specified in EN 868-5)—Requirements and Test Methods*. Brussels, Belgium: European Committee for Standardization; 2017.
32. European Committee for Standardization. *EN 868. Packaging for Terminally Sterilized Medical Devices—Part 4: Paper Bags—Requirements and Test Methods*. Brussels, Belgium: European Committee for Standardization; 2017.
33. European Committee for Standardization. *EN 868. Packaging for Terminally Sterilized Medical Devices—Part 6: Paper for Low-Temperature Sterilization Processes—Requirements and Test Methods*. Brussels, Belgium: European Committee for Standardization; 2017.
34. European Committee for Standardization. *EN 868. Packaging for Terminally Sterilized Medical Devices—Part 7: Adhesive Coated Paper for Low-Temperature Sterilization Processes—Requirements and Test Methods*. Brussels, Belgium: European Committee for Standardization; 2017.
35. European Committee for Standardization. *EN 868. Packaging for Terminally Sterilized Medical Devices—Part 8: Re-Usable Sterilization Containers for Steam Sterilizers Conforming to EN 285—Requirements and Test Methods*. Brussels, Belgium: European Committee for Standardization; 2018.
36. European Committee for Standardization. *EN 868. Packaging for Terminally Sterilized Medical Devices—Part 9: Uncoated Nonwoven Materials of Polyolefins—Requirements and Test Methods*. Brussels, Belgium: European Committee for Standardization; 2018.
37. European Committee for Standardization. *EN 868. Packaging for Terminally Sterilized Medical Devices—Part 10: Adhesive Coated Nonwoven Materials of Polyolefins—Requirements and Test Methods*. Brussels, Belgium: European Committee for Standardization; 2018.

38. European Committee for Standardization. *EN 868. Packaging for Terminally Sterilized Medical Devices—Part 5: Sealable Pouches and Reels of Porous Materials and Plastic Film Construction—Requirements and Test Methods.* Brussels, Belgium: European Committee for Standardization; 2018.

39. International Organization for Standardization. *ISO 11607:2003: Packaging for Terminally Sterilized Medical Devices (Now Withdrawn).* Geneva, Switzerland: International Organization for Standardization; 2003.

40. International Organization for Standardization. *ISO 11607-1:2006: Packaging for Terminally Sterilized Medical Devices—Part 1: Requirements for Materials, Sterile Barrier Systems and Packaging Systems.* Geneva, Switzerland: International Organization for Standardization; 2006.

41. International Organization for Standardization. *ISO 11607-2:2006: Packaging for Terminally Sterilized Medical Devices—Part 2: Validation Requirements for Forming, Sealing and Assembly Processes.* Geneva, Switzerland: International Organization for Standardization; 2006.

42. European Union. Regulation (EU) 2017/745 of the European Parliament and of the Council of 5 April 2017 on medical devices, amending Directive 2001/83/EC, Regulation (EC) No 178/2002 and Regulation (EC) No 1223/2009 and repealing Council Directives 90/385/EEC and 93/42/EEC. *Off J Eur.* 2017;L117:1-175.

43. International Organization for Standardization. *ISO 11607-2:2019: Packaging for Terminally Sterilized Medical Devices—Part 2: Validation Requirements for Forming, Sealing and Assembly Processes.* Geneva, Switzerland: International Organization for Standardization; 2019.

44. International Medical Device Regulators Forum. *IMDRF GRRP WG/N47 FINAL: 2018—Essential Principles of Safety and Performance of Medical Devices and IVD Medical Devices.* Ottawa, Canada: International Medical Device Regulators Forum; 2018.

45. International Organization for Standardization. *ISO 16142-1: Medical devices—Recognized Essential Principles of Safety and Performance of Medical Devices—Part 1: General Essential Principles and Additional Specific Essential Principles for All Non-IVD Medical Devices and Guidance on the Selection of Standards.* Geneva, Switzerland: International Organization for Standardization; 2016.

46. US Food and Drug Administration. *Part 820—Quality System Regulation.* Electronic Code of Federal Regulation Web site. http://www.ecfr.gov/cgi-bin/text-idx?SID=39df3a74818e54ae1ca405f599ac630f&mc=true&node=pt21.8.820&rgn=div5.

47. Trautman KA. *The FDA and Worldwide Quality System Requirements Guide Book for Medical Devices.* Milwaukee, WI: ASQC Quality Press; 1997.

48. Daniel A, Kimmelman E, Trautman KA. *The FDA and Worldwide Quality System Requirements Guidebook For Medical Devices.* 2nd ed. Milwaukee, WI: ASQ Quality Press; 2008.

49. International Organization for Standardization. *ISO 13485:2016: Medical Devices—Quality Management Systems—Requirements for Regulatory Purposes.* Geneva, Switzerland: International Organization for Standardization; 2016.

50. International Organization for Standardization. *ISO 13485:2016: Medical Devices—A Practical Guide.* Geneva, Switzerland: International Organization for Standardization; 2017.

51. International Organization for Standardization. *ISO 9000:2015: Quality Management Systems—Fundamentals and Vocabulary.* Geneva, Switzerland: International Organization for Standardization; 2015.

52. International Organization for Standardization. *ISO 9001:2015: Quality Management Systems—Requirements.* Geneva, Switzerland: International Organization for Standardization; 2015.

53. European Committee for Standardization. *EN ISO 11607-1:2017/Amd 1:2014: Packaging for Terminally Sterilized Medical Devices—Part 1: Requirements for Materials, Sterile Barrier Systems and Packaging Systems.* Brussels, Belgium: European Committee for Standardization; 2017.

54. US Food and Drug Administration. *Design Control Guidance for Medical Device Manufacturers.* Silver Spring, MD: US Food and Drug Administration; 1997.

55. International Electrotechnical Commission. *IEC 62366-1:2015: Medical Devices—Part 1: Application of Usability Engineering to Medical Devices.* Geneva, Switzerland: International Electrotechnical Commission; 2015.

56. American Society for Testing and Materials International. *D4169-09: Standard Practice for Performance Testing of Shipping Containers and Systems.* West Conshohocken, PA: American Society for Testing and Materials International; 2009.

57. International Safe Transit Association. *Guidelines for Selecting and Using ISTA® Test Procedures & Projects.* East Lansing, MI: International Safe Transit Association; 2012.

58. Arrhenius S. *Über die Dissociationswärme und den Einfluss der Temperatur auf den Dissociationsgrad der Elektrolyte.* Leipzig, Germany: Wilhelm Engelmann; 1889.

59. American Society for Testing and Materials International. *F1980-16: Standard Guide for Accelerated Aging of Sterile Barrier Systems for Medical Devices.* West Conshohocken, PA: American Society for Testing and Materials International; 2016.

60. Sterilization Packaging Manufacturers Council. *Sterile Packaging: The Facts of Shelf Life in Medical Device Developments.* Annapolis, MD: Sterilization Packaging Manufacturers Council; 2006.

61. Cassini A, Högberg LD, Plachouras D, et al; and Burden of AMR Collaborative Group. Attributable deaths and disability-adjusted life-years caused by infections with antibiotic-resistant bacteria in the EU and the European Economic Area in 2015: a population-level modelling analysis. *Lancet Infect Dis.* 2019;19:56-66.

62. European Committee for Standardization. *EN ISO 14971:2012: Medical Devices—Application of Risk Management to Medical Devices.* Brussels, Belgium: European Committee for Standardization; 2012.

63. International Organization for Standardization. *ISO 11607-2:2006/Amd 1:2014: Packaging for Terminally Sterilized Medical Devices—Part 2: Validation Requirements for Forming, Sealing and Assembly Processes.* Geneva, Switzerland: International Organization for Standardization; 2014.

64. Wagner T, Scholla MH. Sterile barrier systems: managing changes and revalidations. *J Validation Technol.* 2013;19(3). http://www.ivtnetwork.com/article/sterile-barrier-systems-managing-changes-and-revalidations. Accessed November 3, 2019.

65. International Organization for Standardization. *ISO/TS 16775: Packaging for Terminally Sterilized Medical Devices—Guidance on the Application of ISO 11607-1 and ISO 11607-2.* Geneva, Switzerland: International Organization for Standardization; 2014.

66. European Committee for Standardization. *EN ISO 11607-1:2009/Amd 1:2014: Packaging for Terminally Sterilized Medical Devices—Part 1: Requirements for Materials, Sterile Barrier Systems and Packaging Systems.* Brussels, Belgium: European Committee for Standardization; 2014.

67. European Committee for Standardization. *EN ISO 11607-2:2006/Amd 1:2014: Packaging for Terminally Sterilized Medical Devices—Part 2: Validation Requirements For Forming, Sealing And Assembly Processes.* Brussels, Belgium: European Committee for Standardization; 2014.

68. European Committee for Standardization. *EN ISO 11607-2:2006: Packaging for Terminally Sterilized Medical Devices—Part 2: Validation Requirements for Forming, Sealing and Assembly Processes.* Brussels, Belgium: European Committee for Standardization; 2006.

69. American Society for Testing and Materials International. *F2097-16: Standard Guide for Design and Evaluation of Primary Flexible Packaging for Medical Products.* West Conshohocken, PA: American Society for Testing and Materials International; 2016.

70. United States Pharmacopeia. *USP <1207> Sterile Product Packaging—Integrity Evaluation.* Bethesda, MD: United States Pharmacopeia; 2015.

71. American Society for Testing and Materials International. *ASTM F88/F88M-15: Standard Test Method for Seal Strength of Flexible Barrier Materials.* West Conshohocken, PA: American Society for Testing and Materials International; 2015.

72. American Society for Testing and Materials International. *F2054/F2054M-13: Standard Test Method for Burst Testing of Flexible Package Seals Using Internal Air Pressurization Within Restraining Plates.* West Conshohocken, PA: American Society for Testing and Materials International; 2013.

73. American Society for Testing and Materials International. *ASTM F1140/F1140M-13: Standard Test Methods for Internal Pressurization Failure Resistance of Unrestrained Packages.* West Conshohocken, PA: American Society for Testing and Materials International; 2013.

74. American Society for Testing and Materials International. *ASTM F17-18a: Standard Terminology Relating to Primary Barrier Packaging.* West Conshohocken, PA: American Society for Testing and Materials International; 2018.

75. American Society for Testing and Materials International. *F1886/F1886M-16: Standard Test Method for Determining Integrity of Seals for Flexible Packaging by Visual Inspection.* West Conshohocken, PA: American Society for Testing and Materials International; 2016.

76. American Society for Testing and Materials International. *ASTM F1929-15: Standard Test Method for Detecting Seal Leaks in Porous Medical Packaging by Dye Penetration.* West Conshohocken, PA: American Society for Testing and Materials International; 2015.

77. Larsen CL. Porous sterile barrier integrity testing: failure anomalies. *Medical Device & Diagnostic Industry Magazine.* January 1, 2006. https://www.mddionline.com/porous-sterile-barrier-integrity-testing-failure-anomalies. Accessed November 3, 2019.

78. American Society for Testing and Materials International. *ASTM F3039-15: Dye Penetration—Nonporous Packaging.* West Conshohocken, PA: American Society for Testing and Materials International; 2015.

79. Parenteral Drug Association. PDA Technical Report No. 27 (TR 27) pharmaceutical package integrity. *PDA J Pharm Sci Technol.* 1998; 52(suppl 2):49.

80. American Society for Testing and Materials International. *ASTM D3078-02(2013): Standard Test Method for Determination of Leaks in Flexible Packaging by Bubble Emission.* West Conshohocken, PA: American Society for Testing and Materials International; 2013.

81. American Society for Testing and Materials International. *F2096-11: Standard Test Method for Detecting Gross Leaks in Packaging by Internal Pressurization (Bubble Test).* West Conshohocken, PA: American Society for Testing and Materials International; 2011.

82. United States Pharmacopoeia. *USP <1207.1> Package Integrity and Test Method Selection.* Bethesda, MD: United States Pharmacopeia; 2016.

83. United States Pharmacopoeia. *USP <1207.2> Package Integrity Leak Test Technologies.* Bethesda, MD: United States Pharmacopeia; 2016.

84. American Society for Testing and Materials International. *ASTM F1608-16: Standard Test Method for Microbial Ranking of Porous Packaging Materials (Exposure Chamber Method).* West Conshohocken, PA: American Society for Testing and Materials International; 2016.

85. Sinclair CS, Tallentire A. Definition of a correlation between microbiological and physical particulate barrier performances for porous medical packaging materials. *PDA J Pharm Sci Technol.* 2002; 56(1):11-19.

86. American Society for Testing and Materials International. *ASTM F2638-18: Standard Test Method for Using Aerosol Filtration for Measuring the Performance of Porous Packaging Materials as a Surrogate Microbial Barrier.* West Conshohocken, PA: American Society for Testing and Materials International; 2018.

CHAPTER

42

Hand Hygiene

Günter Kampf

▶ TYPES OF HAND FLORA AND RELEVANCE FOR INFECTION CONTROL

The effects of antiseptics applied to intact skin varies depending on the location of the skin (eg, in moist or drier skin areas, or in skin with a higher or lower density of sebaceous glands). In this review, the focus is on the hands. Three types of hand flora are distinguished since 1938: the resident flora, the transient flora, and the infectious flora.[1,2]

Resident Hand Flora

Inhabitants of the resident hand flora are typically found on the epidermal surface and especially under the superficial cells of the stratum corneum.[3] The species are not considered to be pathogens on intact skin, but in sterile body cavities or on damaged skin, they may cause infections.[4] The resident skin flora protects the skin from the adhesion of transient pathogenic species (colonization resistance) by exhibiting a microbial antagonism and competition in the dermal ecosystem.[5]

Staphylococcus epidermidis can almost always be found on hands.[6-8] The rate of oxacillin resistance can be as high as 64.3%.[6] *Staphylococcus hominis, Staphylococcus warneri*, and other coagulase-negative staphylococci[9,10] as well as propionibacteria, corynebacteria, dermabacteria, and micrococci can also be found as permanent skin inhabitants.[11,12] *Malassezia* (previously known as *Pityrosporum*) has been described as a fungus to reside on human skin.[13] Viruses, however, are not considered permanent skin inhabitants.

The total colony count of resident flora on both hands has been described to be between 3.9×10^4 and 4.6×10^6 in health care workers.[1,14-16] The highest density with approximately 60 000 CFUs/cm^2 is found in the subungual spaces; other areas on the hand have lower counts with 90 to 850 CFUs/cm^2.[17]

Transient Hand Flora

The transient flora describes microorganisms which can only be transiently found on the skin (eg, after contact with patients, animals, or food). Typical transient species on health care workers hands are summarized in Table 42.1. Overall, gram-negative bacteria species are less frequently found on health care workers hands. The density of bacterial transient hand flora increases with the duration of patient care on average by 6 CFUs/min.[19]

Infectious Flora

In addition, the infectious flora can be described as species such as *Staphylococcus aureus* or β-hemolytic streptococci, which are frequently isolated from skin infections, such as from abscesses, whitlows, paronychia, or infected eczema.[20]

Relevance for Infection Control

Hand hygiene is considered to be a key element for prevention of health care–associated infections. In one particular study, it was shown that increasing the compliance in hand hygiene from 48% to 66% over 4 years reduced the rate of health care–associated infection from 16.9% to 9.9%.[21] As a consequence, indications for hand hygiene were harmonized, initially called "five moments of hand hygiene." These included recommendations of hand hygiene before touching a patient, before clean and aseptic procedures, after contact with body fluids, after touching a patient, and after touching patient surroundings.[22] Another consequence

TABLE 42.1 Frequency of nosocomial pathogens detected on health care workers' hands (range)[a]

Species	Colonization Rates on Health care Workers' Hands (Range)
Staphylococcus aureus	2.5%-85.4%
MRSA	0%-16.7%
VRE	0%-41%
Acinetobacter baumannii	1.5%-16.1%
Enterobacter aerogenes	2.9%-13.3%
Enterobacter agglomerans	12.9%-34.4%
Enterobacter cloacae	0.7%-10.6%
Escherichia coli	0.7%-3.2%
Klebsiella pneumoniae	0%-75%
Klebsiella oxytoca	2.2%-10.6%
Pseudomonas aeruginosa	1.0%-25.0%
Serratia marcescens	1.0%-16.7%
Proteus mirabilis	0.7%-4.0%
Clostridium difficile	0%-62.5%
Candida albicans	2.1%-23.0%
Candida parapsilosis	13.1%-53.8%

Abbreviations: MRSA, methicillin-resistant *S aureus*; VRE, vancomycin-resistant Enterococcus species.

[a]From Kampf.[18] Reprinted with permission from Günter Kampf, MD.

was to establish different types of multimodal campaigns to improve compliance among health care workers.[23]

The World Health Organization (WHO) alliance for patient safety has started the first global campaign on patient safety on October 13, 2005 ("clean care is safer care").[24] Promoting hand hygiene has been considered a key element in the campaign.[25] The goal is to implement national strategies for improving hand hygiene in all countries.[26] In 2009, the first global guideline on hand hygiene was published by the WHO.[27] As of January 2018, 139 member states have formally committed themselves to reduce the rate of nosocomial infections in their country, to report their results, and to learn from each other. In 2015, two alcohol-based hand rubs were added to the WHO list of essential medicines: one based on 80% (vol/vol) ethanol and one based on 75% (vol/vol) iso-propanol.[28] The increase of antimicrobial, specifically antibiotic resistance worldwide, makes targeted hand hygiene even more important to prevent transmission in health care facilities.[29]

▶ SIMPLE HAND WASH

Originally, the washing of the hands had a primarily symbolic meaning in rituals of the great world religions (eg, before a prayer). Hands were also washed when they had to be cleaned, although often to remove gross materials from the hands rather than to reduce the impact of microbial transmission (eg, after a meal because cutlery to eat was not always available in antiquity). In the Middle Ages, the washing of hands became more and more important for infection control and prevention.[30] Today, simple hand washing is still the method of choice for keeping hands clean at home and in other situations; however, in patient care, it should be an exception.

Definition

A simple hand wash describes a rinse-off procedure with water with the aim of cleaning hands. Plain liquid or bar soap may be used during washing, particularly in the removal of soils. Soaps used for a simple hand wash do not contain active, antimicrobial ingredients. That is why the effect is physical removal, both on the reduction of soil and on the reduction of microorganisms.

Typical Applications

A simple hand wash is usually carried out on visibly soiled hands with the aim of cleaning them. Four different types of soiling can be distinguished (Table 42.2). In health care, one can expect mainly a slight or medium grade of

TABLE 42.2 Types of soils and proposals for suitable cleaning agents[a]

Grade of Contamination	Kind of Soil	Area of Application	Cleanser
Slight	Not available	Office, administration	Liquid soap
Medium	Not available	Shops, garages, farming, gardening	Skin cleanser with scrubber
Severe	Oils, greases, carbon black, graphite, metallic dust, lubricants	Mining, heavy industry, mechanical engineering	Skin cleanser with scrubber (and solvent)
Special	Paints, lacquers, resins, adhesives	Paint shops, printing offices	Special hand cleansers

[a]Reprinted by permission from Klotz et al.[31] Copyright © 2003 Springer-Verlag.

TABLE 42.3   Mean $\log_{10}$ reduction of different bacterial spores by washing hands with plain soap and water

Species	Duration	Mean $\log_{10}$ Reduction	Reference
Clostridium difficile	10 s	2.0-2.4	Bettin et al[35]
	20 s	2.1	Nerandzic et al[36]
Bacillus subtilis	20 s	2.0	Nerandzic et al[36]
Bacillus atrophaeus	10 s	2.2	Weber et al[37]
	20 s	2.1	Nerandzic et al[36]
	30 s	2.2	Weber et al[37]
	60 s	2.2	Weber et al[37]
Bacillus thuringiensis	20 s	2.2	Nerandzic et al[36]
Bacillus stearothermophilus	15 s	2.0	Hübner et al[38]

Reprinted with permission from Lineaweaver et al.[39]

contamination so that washing hands with water and soap should be sufficient.

Another reason is the proven or suspected contamination of hands with bacterial spores such as *Clostridium difficile* in health care settings or *Bacillus anthracis* in bioterrorism. Infections caused by *C difficile* are among the four most common types of health care–associated infections[32] which were transmitted in the hospital in 70% of all cases.[33] In 2001, letters were sent in the United States, contaminated with spores of *B anthracis*. A total of 22 anthrax infections were observed, 11 of them with pulmonary anthrax and 11 with dermal anthrax.[34] Bacterial spores can be reduced by a simple hand wash by approximately 2 $\log_{10}$, irrespective of the duration of washing (Table 42.3). In case of suspected or proven contamination of the hands with *C difficile*, it is advisable to perform the hand wash after a hand disinfection because patients colonized with *C difficile* are co-colonized with vegetative bacteria pathogens, such as 55.8% with vancomycin-resistant enterococci (VRE)[40] and in 31% with extended spectrum β-lactamase (ESBL) enterobacteriaceae.[41] Patients with a *C difficile* infection carry ESBL enterobacteriaceae in 62% of cases.[41]

Bar soap has no place in health care[42] because it is basically always contaminated and may be a reservoir for pathogens such as *Pseudomonas aeruginosa* or *Klebsiella pneumoniae*.[43] Liquid soap is first choice, although it often does not show an increase in the overall microbial reduction on clean hands in a 20-second hand wash (0.3 $\log_{10}$ difference), as shown with *Enterobacter aerogenes*.[44] On hands soiled with meat, however, the hand wash with liquid soap was more effective by 1.1 $\log_{10}$.[44] Liquid soaps may, themselves, be occasionally contaminated due to poor preservation activity (see chapter 6) (eg, with *Pseudomonas cepacia*,[45,46] *P aeruginosa*,[46-49] *Escherichia coli*,[47] *E aerogenes*,[47] *K pneumoniae*,[46,47,50] *Enterobacter cloacae*,[46,47] *Serratia marcescens*,[47,51] *Klebsiella oxytoca*,[47]

Citrobacter species,[50] *Pseudomonas putidas*,[46] or *Pseudomonas luteola*[46]). In case of a soap dispenser contamination, biofilm is likely to be found inside the dispenser design[52] so that a simple rinse of the dispenser is not an effective way of decontamination.[45]

A procedure of hand washing was recommended by the WHO to be done using specific steps of hand movement, being first described in 1978[53] based on data with insufficient hand coverage.[54,55] Recent data obtained with *C difficile* suggest that the effect on spore removal is significantly better using a structured compared to an unstructured hand washing technique (1.7 versus 1.3 $\log_{10}$ reduction).[56] A similar finding was described in contact lenses washing studies. A multistep hand washing for 34 seconds transferred less lipids to the contact lenses compared to an 11-second unstructured hand washing.[57] In clinical practice, however, the duration of a hand wash is typically between 7 and 10 seconds.[58]

The applied volume of soap in clinical practice is variable and has been described in a study of 47 nursing staff and 10 other persons to be between 0.4 and 9 mL per hand wash.[59]

The fastest drying of hands can be achieved with cotton or paper towels with 4% to 10% or water remaining on the hands after 10-second drying.[60,61] Hot air dryers have actually worse drying effects[60] and can even distribute microorganisms in the air within a radius of 1 m.[62] Finally, air driers can irritate the skin and cause skin dryness, roughness, and redness over time.[61]

Test Methods and Efficacy Requirements

The effect is 2-fold, reduction of soil and microorganisms. There are currently no specific methods used to measure the reduction of soil or microorganisms for simple

TABLE 42.4 Mean $\log_{10}$ reduction of different bacterial species by washing hands with plain soap and water

Species	Duration	Mean $\log_{10}$ Reduction	Reference
Escherichia coli	10 s	0.5	Ansari et al[70]
	15 s	0.6-1.7	Ojajärvi[71] and Mahl[72]
	30 s	1.4-3.0	Ayliffe et al,[53] Lowbury and Lilly,[68] Lowbury et al,[73] and Ayliffe et al[74]
	1 min	2.6-3.2	Kampf and Ostermeyer,[75] Mittermayer and Rotter,[76] Rotter and Koller,[77] Rotter and Koller,[78] and Messager et al[79]
	2 min	3.3	Mittermayer and Rotter[76]
Pseudomonas aeruginosa	30 s	2.0-3.0	Lowbury et al[73]
Acinetobacter baumannii	30 s	2.0-3.8	Cardoso et al[80]
Serratia marcescens	10 s	1.9	Sickbert-Bennett et al[81]
	15 s	1.7	Mahl[72]
	30 s	2.3	Nicoletti et al[82]
	30 s	2.0	Kim et al[83]
Klebsiella species	20 s	1.7	Casewell and Phillips[84]
Enterobacter aerogenes	20 s	1.7	Jensen et al[44]
Micrococcus species	30 s	1.5	Nicoletti et al[82]
Staphylococcus aureus	30 s	0.5-3.0	Ayliffe et al,[53] Lowbury et al,[73] and Lilly and Lowbury[85]
MRSA	20 s	1.4	Huang et al[86]
	30 s	1.4-1.9	Guilhermetti et al[87]
Staphylococcus saprophyticus	30 s	2.5	Ayliffe et al[53]

Abbreviation: MRSA, methicillin-resistant *S aureus*.

hand washing, including no specific efficacy requirements (definition of a minimum to qualify as an effective soap). Nevertheless, some studies describe the effect of a simple hand wash on reducing microorganisms.

Efficacy on Resident Hand Flora

A simple hand wash reduces the resident hand flora only marginally with mean $\log_{10}$ reductions of 0.32 after 30 seconds,[63] −0.05 after 2 minutes,[64] 0.62 after 3 minutes,[65] and between 0.3 and 0.4 after 5 minutes.[66-69] The volume of applied soap (1 or 3 mL) does not make a difference.[59]

Efficacy on Transient Hand Flora

The effect on the transient bacterial flora is better (Table 42.4). A hand wash of 30 seconds or longer usually reduced transient bacteria by about 2 $\log_{10}$. A higher contamination resulted in a lower efficacy as shown with *Acinetobacter baumannii* (2.0 versus 3.8 $\log_{10}$)[80] or methicillin-resistant *S aureus* (MRSA) (1.4 versus 1.9 log).[87] Viruses can also be reduced by hand washing (Table 42.5), but $\log_{10}$ reductions with feline calicivirus (FCV) and rotavirus were quite low.

Side Effects

The overall dermal tolerance of hand washing is rather poor.[97] An analysis of 1932 skin evaluations revealed that washing hands with soap and water is a risk for dry and irritated skin.[98] Frequent hand washing (>10 times per day) is a relevant risk for irritated skin with a relative risk of 1.55.[99] The composition of the soap can have a significant impact on the dermal tolerance and the cleaning efficacy.[31,100] Reducing the frequency of hand washing and increasing the use of alcohol-based hand rubs can significantly reduce skin redness (21.7% versus 11.0%) and

TABLE 42.5 Mean $\log_{10}$ reduction of different viruses by washing hands with or without plain soap and water measured as reduction of viral infectivity in cell culture assays

Species	Duration	Mean Log$_{10}$ Reduction	Reference
Rotavirus	10 s	0.7-1.2	Ansari et al[70]
	30 s	1.2	Bellamy et al[88]
Poliovirus	30 s	2.1	Davies et al[89]
	1 min	1.0-1.1	Steinmann et al[90]
	5 min	2.1	Steinmann et al[90]
	5 min	Ca. 3	Schürmann and Eggers[91]
Feline calicivirus	30 s	1.4	Kramer et al[92]
	30 s	0.3	Lages et al[93]
	30 s	1.2	Gehrke et al[94]
	2 min	0.4	Lages et al[93]
Murine norovirus	30 s	1.7	Paulmann et al[95]
	30 s	2.9	Steinmann et al[96]

itchiness (15.8% versus 7.1%) as shown on health care workers from seven intensive care units (ICUs).[101] A direct comparison of hand washing or hand rubbing over 8 days among 52 nurses showed a significantly worse skin condition and a significantly higher degree of skin damage in the hand washing group.[102]

Only few studies are available to describe the risk of allergies. Specific preservatives such as quaternium-15 (a formaldehyde-releasing agent) or methyldibromoglutaronitrile have been described as allergens, but more relevant are probably fragrances used in soaps.[103,104]

◗ HYGIENIC HAND WASH

Washing hands with an antiseptic agent was introduced in human medicine in 1847 when Ignaz Semmelweis performed hand washes with chlorinated lime in a basin.[105] The first washing lotions contained two active ingredients such as chlorhexidine and cetrimide.[106] Today, chlorhexidine or octenidine are commonly used. Many other microbicides have also been traditionally used in such hand washes. But, regular use of antimicrobial soaps in countries with low incomes did not show reduced infection rates compared to the use of plain soaps.[107] Triclosan and 18 other substances that have been used are now banned by the US Food and Drug Administration (FDA) in 2016[108] as an active ingredient in consumer antimicrobial soaps because of a lack of direct clinical benefit (ie, a reduction of infection), risks of toxic reactions including hormonal effects, environmental concerns, and the risk of triggering bacterial cross-resistance to antibiotics by sublethal concentrations.[109]

Definition

A hygienic hand wash (FDA: health care personnel hand wash) describes a rinse-off procedure with water with the aim of cleaning hands and to have an antimicrobial effect at the same time. Liquid soaps based on biocidal agents such as 4% chlorhexidine or 1% octenidine may be used during washing. The overall effect is 2-fold: a physical one removing soil and microorganisms and a chemical one killing bacteria and yeasts to some extent during the application.

Typical Applications

In patient care, there is rarely an indication to perform a hygienic hand wash because clean hands should be routinely treated with alcohol-based hand rubs when an indication for hand hygiene occurs. The WHO recommends that health care facilities using alcohol-based hand rubs should not provide health care workers antimicrobials soaps.[110] Preparing or handling food, however, is a different scenario because hands may often be soiled and contaminated so that a combined procedure with cleaning the hands and having some antimicrobial activity can be valuable.

It is recommended by WHO to perform the hygienic hand wash with a six-step procedure.[110] If the six-step procedure provides an additional benefit (eg, more reduction of soil, stronger antimicrobial efficacy) compared to other washing procedures is unknown. A 30-second application time is usually required to exhibit a bactericidal and yeasticidal activity. Transient flora such as *E coli* (EN 1499) or *S marcescens* (ASTM E1174) is usually reduced by 2 to 3 $\log_{10}$ steps within 30 to 60 seconds, depending on the specific product tested. The efficacy is often reported to be remarkably lower compared to alcohol-based hand rubs (approximately 4-5 $\log_{10}$).

Test Methods and Efficacy Requirements

In Europe, the spectrum of antimicrobial activity of products used in human medicine must include bactericidal activity according to EN 13727 and yeasticidal activity according to EN 13624.[111] The same spectrum of antimicrobial activity is required in the United States, although the number of bacterial species to be investigated to determine bactericidal activity is much higher with at least 20 species compared to 4 species in EN 13727.[112] In veterinary medicine, the products must be at least bactericidal according to EN 13727.[111] Hygienic hand wash products used in food, industrial, domestic and institutional areas have in Europe no specific minimum spectrum of antimicrobial activity. Tests are available to demonstrate bactericidal (EN 1276) and yeasticidal (EN 1650) activity.[111]

In Europe, the in vivo efficacy of hygienic hand wash products is evaluated according to EN 1499 for all fields of application.[113] In the United States, it was determined for many years according to the test method described in the Tentative Final Monograph for Healthcare Antiseptic Products published in 1994[112] similar to ASTM E1174.[114] In 2015, the FDA has proposed a new test method for hand scrub products with a single application and defined new efficacy requirements.[115] The methods are summarized in Table 42.6. Although hygienic hand wash products have to show superiority compared to a negative control according to EN 1499 (relative requirement, similar to clinical trials), they are required to show at least a 2.5 $\log_{10}$ reduction according to the FDA proposed rules (absolute requirement).

Side Effects

The skin compatibility of antimicrobial soaps used for hygienic hand wash is often reported to be poor especially when used frequently. This is mainly explained by the types of detergents used in the formulation. In addition, adding chlorhexidine or octenidine to the product formulation can influence dermal tolerance and affect the irritation potential of a final formulation.[97] The potential for allergic reactions is described below (side effects, surgical hand rubbing, page 871).

TABLE 42.6	Overview on critical test parameter of EN 1499, ASTM E1174, and the proposed FDA rules for antiseptic hand wash products		
Parameter	**EN 1499 (2013)[113]**	**ASTM E1174 (2013)[114]**	**Proposal by FDA (2015)[115]**
Number of subjects	12-15 subjects	"Sufficient number"	A sample size large enough to show statistically significant differences to the vehicle control
Baseline count on hands	Mean $\log_{10}$ baseline count at least 5.0	Not specified	Not specified
Number of applications	Single application of product and reference soap	Ten applications	Single application
Sampling times	Immediately after hand treatment	Within 1 min after hand washes 1 and 10	Within 5 min after hand wash
Neutralizer	Required in sampling and dilution fluid, optional in agar plates	Required in the sampling and dilution fluid	All recovery media (ie, sampling solution, dilution fluid, plating media); demonstration of neutralizer validation
Sampling method	Finger tips in broth	Whole hand by glove juice method	Whole hand by glove juice method
Study design	Crossover	Uncontrolled trial	Crossover
Type of control(s)	Negative control: 5 mL of unmedicated kalisoap with water for 1 min	No controls required	Vehicle control to show the contribution of the active ingredient (test product should be superior) Active control to validate the study conduct (active control should meet the appropriate log reduction criteria)
Efficacy requirements	Superiority to negative control	Not specified	≥2.5 $\log_{10}$ on each hand after a single application

Abbreviations: ASTM, American Society for Testing and Materials; FDA, US Food and Drug Administration.

▶ HYGIENIC HAND DISINFECTION

The term *hygienic hand disinfection* was introduced by Wilhelm Speck in 1905, who described procedures for hand decontamination with alcohol-based solutions so that neither the user nor the environment of canalization were contaminated during use ("hygienic").[116] In the 1960s, alcohol-based hand rubs containing emollients were offered for the first time in central Europe[117] in order to reduce skin dryness when used frequently.[118,119]

Definition

Hygienic hand disinfection (FDA: health care personnel hand rub) describes a leave-on procedure with an alcohol-based hand rub, gel, or foam. It should be performed in the following clinical situations: before touching a patient, before clean and aseptic procedures, after contact with body fluids, after touching a patient, after touching patient surroundings, and after glove removal.[22] The formulations are typically based on ethanol, iso-propanol, n-propanol, or a combination of these alcohols. The overall concentration of alcohol(s) is often between 60% and 95% with a trend to better antimicrobial efficacy with higher alcohol concentrations.[120] The antimicrobial efficacy of lower alcohol concentrations may theoretically be increased by retarding the evaporation time of the alcohol (ie, by adding specific excipients to a formulation). But so far, published data indicate that alcohol-based gels or lotions tend to be often less effective compared to alcohol-based solutions. The WHO has described hand rubs–based ethanol at 80% (vol/vol) or iso-propanol at 75% (vol/vol) as essential medicines,[28] although they are not found to meet European efficacy requirements when applied with 3 mL for 30 seconds.[121]

Typical Applications

Alcohol-based hand rubs are usually applied to clean and dry hands. During an application time of 30 seconds, the product is distributed all over both hands to ensure complete hand coverage. The WHO recommends to apply a specific rub-in technique with six steps similar to the one used for testing the efficacy according to EN 1500.[122] In clinical practice, however, hand coverage is often incomplete. In a study with 546 students, 55.1% of hands were incompletely covered with even 7.1% incomplete coverage on the palmar side where complete coverage is easy to accomplish.[123] Treatment gaps are typically found on the thumb and the index finger.[124] The recommended six steps are rarely done in clinical practice. In South Korea, 2174 hand disinfections were observed. In only 7.4%, all six steps were done as recommended.[125] Similar results were reported from Switzerland with 8.5% of 2480 hand disinfections being performed with all six steps.[126] Alternatives such as the "responsible technique" (individual technique with feedback) yield better hand coverage.[127] It is particularly important to cover the thumb and the finger tips (Figure 42.1). A good rub-in technique and professional experience are relevant factors that can have a significant impact on the efficacy of the hand disinfection.[124] That is why education and feedback are important to optimize personal practices.[129] The presence of soil may not significantly reduce the efficacy of certain alcohol-based hand rubs,[130] depending on the level and type of soil, but overall, the soil will not be removed during a hand disinfection.

Test Methods and Efficacy Requirements

In Europe, the spectrum of antimicrobial activity must include bactericidal activity according to EN 13727 and yeasticidal activity according to EN 13624. The same spectrum of antimicrobial activity is required in the United States, although the number of bacterial species to be investigated to determine bactericidal activity is much higher with at least 20 species compared to 4 species in EN 13727.[112] A mycobactericidal or virucidal activity is optional.[111] In veterinary medicine, the products must be at least bactericidal according to EN 13727.[111]

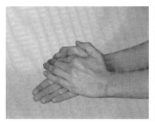 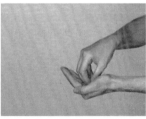 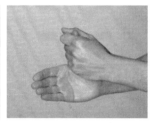

FIGURE 42.1 Steps of a clinically relevant rub-in technique; covering all surfaces of the hand, rotational rubbing of fingertips, and rubbing of both thumbs. For a color version of this art, please consult the eBook. Copyright © Aktion Saubere Hände, Charité University Medicine, Berlin, Germany.[128]

Hygienic hand rub products used in food, industrial, domestic, and institutional areas in Europe have no specific minimum spectrum of antimicrobial activity. Tests are available to demonstrate bactericidal (EN 1276) and yeasticidal (EN 1650) activity.[111]

In Europe, the in vivo efficacy of hygienic hand rub products is evaluated according to EN 1500.[122] In the United States, this was determined for many years according to the test method described in the Tentative Final Monograph for Healthcare Antiseptic Products published in 1994[112] and similar to ASTM E1174, which was designed for hand wash testing. In 2010, a new ASTM test method (ASTM E2755) was developed and published for alcohol-based hand rubs.[131] In 2015, the FDA has proposed a new test method for hand rub products with a single application and defined new efficacy requirements.[115] These are summarized in Table 42.7. It is noteworthy that the FDA proposal from 2015 suggests a minimum $\log_{10}$ reduction for a single hand rub application of 2.5, whereas the reference procedure of EN 1500 (positive control) usually results in a 4.6 $\log_{10}$ reduction and the reference hand wash procedure with unmedicated soap of EN 1499

(negative control) results in a 2.8 $\log_{10}$ reduction[75,132] suggesting that the FDA requirement for a hand rub procedure may be rather low.

Side Effects

Typical hand rubs contain, in addition to the active ingredients, emollients with the aim to reduce skin dryness and irritation.[119] The proportion of emollients in a product can be up to 1.45%.[121] Such commercially available hand rubs are usually well tolerated on intact skin in comparison to aqueous alcohol solutions.[133] Skin barrier, skin hydration, and dermal sebum content are usually not changed even when hand rubs are used frequently.[134,135] The irritation potential of most hand rubs is low[98,136-138] even on skin of subjects with an atopic predisposition.[139] But differences of the local tolerance between hand rubs may be found when used intensively.[140] The risk for dermal sensitization of hand rubs is very low.[136,137] Some gels have been described to increase skin hydration to some extent.[135,137,141,142]

The dermal tolerance may be worse for alcohol-based hand rubs with a virucidal activity because they may

TABLE 42.7 Overview on critical test parameter of EN 1500, ASTM E2755, and the proposed FDA rules for alcohol-based hand rub products

Parameter	EN 1500 (2013)[122]	ASTM E2755 (2010)[131]	Proposal by FDA (2015)[115]
Number of subjects	18-22 subjects	"Sufficient number"	A sample size large enough to show statistically significant differences to the vehicle control
Baseline count on hands	Mean baseline count at least 5.0	≥8.0 $\log_{10}$ CFUs per hand	Not specified
Number of applications	Single application of product and reference alcohol	Single application; up to 11 applications are possible	Single application
Sampling times	Immediately after hand treatment	Within 1 min after product application	Within 5 min after hand rub
Neutralizer	Required in sampling and dilution fluid, optional in agar plates	Required in the sampling and dilution fluid	All recovery media (ie, sampling solution, dilution fluid, plating media); demonstration of neutralizer validation
Sampling method	Finger tips in broth	Whole hand by glove juice method	Whole hand by glove juice method
Study design	Crossover	Uncontrolled trial	Crossover
Type of control(s)	Positive control: 2 × 3 mL of iso-propanol (60%, vol/vol) for 1 min	No controls required	Vehicle control to show the contribution of the active ingredient (test product should be superior) Active control to validate the study conduct (active control should meet the appropriate log reduction criteria)
Efficacy requirements	Noninferiority to positive control	Not specified	≥2.5 $\log_{10}$ on each hand after a single application

Abbreviations: ASTM, American Society for Testing and Materials; CFUs, colony-forming units; FDA, Food and Drug Administration.

contain substances like propan-1,2-diol (10%) in combination with butan-1,3-diol (10%), phosphoric acid (0.45%-0.7%), citric acid (0.5%), or hydrochloric acid (0.1%-0.3%).[92,143] One study shows that virucidal formulations with phosphoric acid have a worse dermal tolerance.[144] The results are supported by postmarketing surveillance data for a virucidal hand rub.[145]

Do Hand Rubs Reveal a Persistent Efficacy?

The WHO provides the following definition of persistent activity: the prolonged or extended antimicrobial activity that prevents the growth or survival of microorganisms after application of a given antiseptic. It is also called residual, sustained, or remnant activity. Both substantive and nonsubstantive active ingredients can show a persistent effect significantly inhibiting the growth of microorganisms after application. According to the WHO guideline on hand hygiene published in 2009, persistent activity is not necessary for hygienic hand rub products.[27]

Alcohols alone are not expected to demonstrate persistent activity because they do not remain in the skin over time. A persistent effect may be expected by the inclusion of other nonvolatile biocidal ingredients such as chlorhexidine or triclosan. Sound evidence to support a persistent activity of specific hand rub products is currently missing.

Nevertheless, a persistent efficacy has been claimed for a hand rub based on 70% iso-propanol and 0.5% chlorhexidine within 60 minutes[146,147] because it apparently reduced a bacterial contamination on hands after use of the hand rub. But the effect is doubtful. First, an effect within 60 minutes has no real clinical relevance as pathogens may have been transmitted already from these hands. Second, residual activity in the samples was not neutralized as current standards require,[148] suggesting false-positive results.[149] Third, chlorhexidine needs some water on the skin to be able to have some persistent activity within 15 minutes.[150] Other alcohol-based hand rubs contain 4% chlorhexidine, 0.2% mecetronium etilsulfate, or 0.5% triclosan as nonvolatile active ingredient. In a study with some of these products, all had no persistent efficacy on dry hands after 30 or 60 minutes when used for hygienic hand disinfection.[151] In Germany, alcohol-based hand rubs with an additional antimicrobial persistent agent are not recommended in health care because the efficacy is not better but the risks increase (acquired bacterial resistance, skin irritation, allergy).[152]

▶ SURGICAL HAND SCRUBBING

The use of antimicrobial soaps for surgical scrubbing was first mentioned in the middle of the last century: in 1949 using hexachlorophene,[153] in 1960 using povidone-iodine,[73] and in 1973 using chlorhexidine.[147] Currently, soaps based on chlorhexidine or povidone-iodine are mainly used for this purpose.[154] It has been common practice for decades in numerous Anglo-American countries[155] but is becoming less popular and often replaced by surgical hand rubbing.[156] The main reasons are the faster efficacy, the broader spectrum of antimicrobial activity, and the lack of risk of recontaminating hands by the final rinse with water.[156] In central-European German-speaking countries, for example, surgical hand scrubbing is rarely done and not recommended.[157]

Definition

Surgical hand scrubbing is the application of an antimicrobial soap (eg, based on 4% chlorhexidine) with water to the hands and forearms before surgery ("rinse-off procedure").[110] In Europe, the procedure is called "surgical hand wash."[112]

Typical Applications

The first step is rinsing the hands and forearms with water, followed by distributing the necessary soap volume and scrubbing it in to hands and forearms, followed by rinsing off all remaining soap with tap water and drying hands. The necessary volume of the antiseptic soap and the application procedure depends on the selected product.

Antimicrobial soaps based on 4% chlorhexidine are usually recommended with a total volume of 10 mL for surgical hand scrubbing.[158] The total application time is typically 6 minutes. Other application times have been evaluated, but this will vary depending on the label claims. Using the scrub product for 10 minutes revealed a similar efficacy compared to a 5-minute application, both during short surgical procedures with a duration up to 90 minutes and during longer operations with a duration >90 minutes.[159] Comparable products based on povidone-iodine are usually recommended with volumes between 6 and 10 mL with a total application time between 5 and 6 minutes.[158]

Brushes were used traditionally for a surgical hand scrubbing[160,161] until increasing skin irritations among the users lead to investigations without brushes showing similar efficacy.[162,163] Using a brush was not found to increase the overall efficacy significantly among volunteers[164,165] or health care workers[166] but could increase skin irritation significantly especially in winter time.[167] That is why the use of brushes is not recommended during surgical hand scrubbing.[110,152] Observational data from surgical theaters, however, show that brushes are still used in clinical practice, for example, in Scotland in 69% for the first operation of a day[168] or in Turkey in 16.8% for treating the fingernails.[169] Education and training for not using a brush remains an important target.

Nail picks are quite often used especially since the FDA declared the use of nail picks to be standard part of the surgical hand scrubbing procedure in 1994,[112] even if hands are clean. An additional effect on the efficacy, however, cannot be expected.[164,166] The WHO still recommends nail picks for visibly soiled hands to clean the subungual spaces[110] based on a study published in 1938.[1]

Surgical hand scrubbing requires using quite large amounts of tap water. The total volume per application has been described to be between 5.0 and 20.2 L.[170-172] Clean tap water is not easily available in many countries, so that for this reason, the practice of surgical hand scrubbing should be reviewed critically in those situations.

Test Methods and Efficacy Requirements

In Europe, the spectrum of antimicrobial activity must include bactericidal activity according to EN 13727 and yeasticidal activity according to EN 13624. The same spectrum of antimicrobial activity is required in the United States, although the number of bacterial species to be investigated to determine bactericidal activity is much higher with at least 20 species compared to 4 species in EN 13727.[112] In veterinary medicine, the products must be at least bactericidal according to EN 13727.[111]

In Europe, the in vivo efficacy of surgical hand scrub products is evaluated according to EN 12791.[173] In the United States, a test method described in the Tentative Final Monograph for Healthcare Antiseptic Products published in 1994[112] was used similar to ASTM E1115.[174] In 2015, the FDA has proposed a new test method for hand scrub products with a single application and defined new efficacy requirements.[115] These are summarized in Table 42.8.

Whereas a surgical hand scrub product has to show noninferiority to a positive control according to EN 12791 (relative requirement, similar to clinical trials), it has to show at least a 2 $\log_{10}$ reduction according to the FDA proposed rules (absolute requirement). In addition, bacterial counts should not exceed baseline after 6 hours according to the FDA proposed rules.

TABLE 42.8   Overview on critical test parameter of EN 12791, ASTM E1115, and the proposed FDA rules for surgical hand rub and hand scrub products

Parameter	EN 12791 (2015)[173]	ASTM E1115 (2011)[174]	Proposal by FDA (2015)[116]
Number of subjects	23-26 subjects	"Sufficient number"	A sample size large enough to show statistically significant differences to the vehicle control
Baseline count	Mean $\log_{10}$ baseline count at least 3.5	At least 1.0×10^5 bacteria from each hand	Not specified Criteria from 1994: at least 1.5×10^5 bacteria from both hands
Number of applications	Single application of product and reference alcohol	Single application; in order to show a cumulative effect 11 additional applications are optional	Single application
Sampling times	0 and 3 h	0 and 6 h	0 and 6 h
Neutralizer	Required in sampling and dilution fluid, optional in agar plates	Required in sampling fluid, optional in dilution fluid and agar plates	All recovery media (ie, sampling solution, dilution fluid, plating media); demonstration of neutralizer validation
Sampling method	Fingertips in broth	Whole hand by glove juice method	Whole hand by glove juice method
Study design	Crossover	Uncontrolled trial	Crossover
Type of control(s)	Positive control: n-propanol 60% (vol/vol) for 3 min	Not required	Vehicle control to show the contribution of the active ingredient (test product should be superior) Active control to validate the study conduct (active control should meet the appropriate log reduction criteria)
Efficacy requirements	Noninferiority to positive control after 0 and 3 h	Not specified	$\geq 2 \log_{10}$ on each hand after a single application; does not exceed baseline at 6 h; superiority to the vehicle control

Abbreviations: ASTM, American Society for Testing and Materials; FDA, Food and Drug Administration.

Side Effects

A survey in Scotland in 1984 among 623 surgical theater staff revealed that 37.2% had visible skin irritation. The skin damage was so severe in 5% of the health care workers that a dermatologist was consulted.[162] In Canada, 26% of 184 surgical theater staff had skin damage on hands which was explained by the type of antiseptic soap used.[175] Detergents remaining on the skin and kept under gloves for hours can significantly increase skin irritation.[176] That is why final rinsing should be done carefully.

Type IV allergies to chlorhexidine are not rare. A survey among 307 physicians in Japan revealed that 7.5% claim to be allergic. A patch test, however, was not done to confirm a potential allergy.[177] In Australia, at least four confirmed cases of allergic contact dermatitis among health care workers were reported. As possible sources, 7 products for hand hygiene and 11 other products were identified. In a second step, 549 health care worker were patch tested with 10 of them (1.8%) showing a clinically relevant skin reaction.[178] Another study from Australia showed that among 276 health care workers with an allergic contact dermatitis, chlorhexidine was the causative agent in 2.2%.[179] In Thailand, 5% of 92 health care workers were found to be allergic to chlorhexidine.[180]

Type I allergies can also be found with chlorhexidine. The risk is usually underestimated by health care workers.[181] Repeated contact may result in sensitization[182] and finally in severe allergic reactions.[183] A type I allergy may present as an allergic contact dermatitis, as urticaria or an anaphylactic shock,[181,184,185] which may even develop after topical application.[186,187] The FDA has published a warning in 2016 because the frequency of severe allergic reactions to chlorhexidine has increased.[188]

Do Surgical Scrubs Reveal a Persistent Efficacy?

In 2009, WHO recommended the use of suitable antimicrobial soaps, preferably with a product ensuring sustained activity.[27] In 2016, however, WHO changed the recommendation to "suitable antimicrobial soap" due to a lack of evidence that products with chlorhexidine were more effective in directly reducing the risk of surgical site infections.[189] A persistent activity may be demonstrated by sampling a site several hours after application and demonstrating bacterial antimicrobial effectiveness when compared with a baseline level.[189] One study complies with the new FDA and ASTM E1115 requirements on neutralization and allows determining if such an effect can be found after a single application of a surgical scrub product based on 4% chlorhexidine and applied with 2×5 mL over 2×3 minutes.[191] Mean bacterial counts were still $1.2 \log_{10}$ below baseline similar to the application of 60% n-propanol over 3 minutes. A long-term efficacy

(or persistent) according to EN 12791 has so far never been described for surgical scrub products (superiority to the reference procedure).

▶ SURGICAL HAND RUBBING

Surgeons hands were described in 1886 as "an object which is most difficult to disinfect."[192] In 1888, Fürbringer[193] postulated four essential criteria for a successful surgical hand disinfection: (1) reliable efficacy, (2) time saving, (3) gentle to the skin, and (4) cheap. These criteria are still valid today.

Definition

The application of an alcohol-based hand rub ("surgical hand rubbing") is another option for preoperative hand preparation as defined by WHO[110] and FDA[115] and is a "leave-on procedure." In Europe, the procedure is called "surgical hand disinfection."[111] The products are usually based on ethanol, iso-propanol, n-propanol, or a combination of these. Commercially available products contain emollients to reduce skin dryness. Some products contain, in addition, nonvolatile active ingredients such as chlorhexidine with the aim to achieve persistent antimicrobial activity (see page 872). Surgical hand rubbing is carried out in human medicine as well as veterinary medicine.[194] It is indicated before surgery, before contact with sterile medical devices or materials, and before other medical interventions with the same level of asepsis as in surgery.[110,152] In addition, it is recommended before donning sterile gloves when aseptic procedures are to be performed in clean room areas.[195]

The aim of surgical hand rubbing is to eliminate the transient flora from the hands of the surgical team and to reduce the resident hand flora to a minimum.[156] The contaminated glove juice or sweat which develops under the sterile surgical glove during an operation may cause surgical site infections by glove perforation[196] so that the overall number of microorganisms inside the surgical glove shall be reduced as much as possible.[189]

Typical Application

History

The surgical hand rubbing procedure has changed substantially over the last 120 years based on new evidence.[197] Traditionally, it has a washing period and a hand rubbing or disinfection period. In 1888 in Germany, a washing period of 10 minutes was described, followed by the application of ethanol to remove lipids and finished with the application of a mercury chloride solution.[198] For decades, the washing period was recommended with 5 to

7 minutes, often using hot water, soap, and a brush.[199-201] Occupational dermatology would reject this type of washing today.[202] Even washing for 15 minutes was not effective in significantly reducing the resident microbial load on hands.[199] Using sand for washing had no additional effect.[199] Hand washing was reduced in Germany to 3 minutes in 1972[203] and to 1 minute in 2000.[204]

The hand rubbing period was initially considered less important and lasted usually between 3 and 7 minutes.[201,205,206] In 1939, alcohol in a reusable basin should not be used too long or by too many persons.[201] In 2005, an application time of 1.5 minutes was found for one hand rub to be equally effective to the 3-minute application time; a 1-minute application, however, failed the efficacy EN 12791 requirements.[207]

Washing Period

The surgical theater should always be entered with clean hands. Visibly clean hands do not need to be washed.[110] Nevertheless, WHO recommends washing hands and forearms before the first operation of the day.[189] The main reason is to reduce the load of bacterial spores. Routine hand washing before applying the surgical hand rub product for any following operations is not recommended.[189] A specific duration of the hand washing has not been recommended. Maximum reduction of bacterial spores (approximately 2 $\log_{10}$) is usually achieved within 10 seconds of thoroughly washing both hands. Longer hand washing had no additional effect.[37] Brushes have been used traditionally[203] but should not be used anymore during the hand washing[110] because it damages the skin[208] and may even increase the bacterial density on the skin.[209,210] When hands are washed for 1 minute, skin hydration increases significantly for up to 10 minutes.[38] When the hand rub is applied immediately after the hand washing, skin hydration is at a maximum and can impair the efficacy of the hand rub to some extent.[211] Similar results were obtained by Rotter and Koller in 1990.[212] It is, therefore, advisable to wash hands before entering the theater block so that hands can dry before the surgical hand rubbing protocol is started. A hand wash should always be finished with thoroughly drying hands and forearms.

Hand Rubbing Period

Commercially available hand rubs are usually applied for 1.5 minutes to hands and forearms. As many aliquots as necessary should be applied to ensure that the treated skin remains wet for the total application time. The effect usually lasts for approximately 6 hours. Some manufacturers in the United States have recommended small volumes for the entire surgical hand rubbing procedure (eg, 6 or even 4 mL).[213] This recommendation is supported by efficacy data according to the national test methods. Proposing specific volumes irrespective of hand size, however, is critical. First, data

| TABLE 42.9 | Mean $\log_{10}$ reduction (three-hour values) by the three-minute reference procedure of EN 12791 according to hand size (shown as glove size) and the applied volume[a] |

Glove Size	Applied Volume for Three-Minute Surgical Hand Disinfection Reference Procedure				P Value[b]
	All Volumes	6 mL	9 mL	12 mL	
7	2.25	1.73[c]	2.20	3.23[c]	0.021
7.5	2.03	1.32[c]	2.14[c]	2.21	0.025
8	2.18	1.27[c]	2.47[c]	2.10	0.013
8.5	2.37	NA	2.51	2.05	0.502
9	1.03	NA	1.50	0.79	0.461

[a]From Kampf and Ostermeyer.[213] http://creativecommons.org/licenses/by/2.0.

[b]ANOVA, comparison between three volumes.

[c]Pairwise comparison with significant difference.

Abbreviations: NA, not available.

obtained with the EN 12791 reference procedure showed that 200 subjects required variable volumes. In 73% of all applications, 9 mL were necessary to keep hands wet for 3 minutes; in 24%, it was 12 mL; and in 3%, it was 6 mL.[207] Second, large hands require larger volumes for surgical hand rubbing and may not be sufficiently covered with a standard smaller volume like 4 mL. An evaluation of the necessary volume for a 3-minute surgical hand rubbing revealed that 6 mL were consistently not enough on large hands with a glove size of 8.5 or 9.[213] Interestingly, larger antiseptic volumes had only a small effect on large hands (Table 42.9).

Based on these data, a general recommendation of a small volume such as 4 mL for all hand sizes may not always be effective. This assumption is supported by a report with an increase of surgical site infections from 1.3 to 2.9 per 100 operations. Overall, 77 cases were identified: 29 after colon or small bowel surgery, 21 after vascular surgery, 16 after open orthopedic surgery, and 11 after mastectomies. It was found by observation that the surgical hand rub based on 61% ethanol and 1% chlorhexidine (recommended by the manufacturer with 6 mL) was not correctly applied suggesting that the applied volume in real life was even smaller.[214]

An analysis of the microbial population kinetics on hands after the 3-minute reference treatment of EN 12791 shows that the reference alcohol alone (n-propanol 60%, vol/vol) keeps the microbial density below baseline for at least 6 hours (Figure 42.2).[215,216]

Sweating under the surgical glove has been shown to speed up recolonization. When the dry inner surface of a

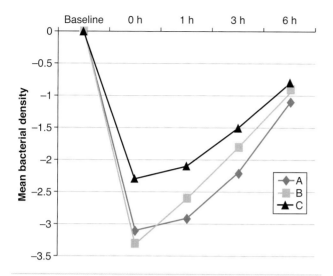

FIGURE 42.2 Mean log$_{10}$ reduction of microbial hand flora after performing the EN 12791 reference treatment (*n*-propanol 60%, vol/vol, applied for 3 min); three data sets (A, B, C) from two studies with 24 subjects.[215,216]

surgical glove revealed approximately 20 CFUs *S aureus* after 2 hours, it was between 500 and 1000 CFUs after 30 minutes following sweating under the glove.[217] The use of a brush during the application of the hand rub is not recommended, although some studies indicate that the immediate effect can be increased by 0.4 log$_{10}$ (*n*-propanol 60%, vol/vol), 0.7 log$_{10}$ (iso-propanol 60%, vol/vol), or even 1.0 log$_{10}$ (ethanol 80%, vol/vol) when a brush is used gently for 30-second treatment under the nails. After 3 hours, however, the effect was not significant anymore.[38] Similar results have been described earlier in 1988.[218]

For consecutive surgical hand rubbing procedures, it was found that the baseline count before the second application is only 2.2 log$_{10}$ compared to 4.4 log$_{10}$ before the first application and a simulated 3-hour surgical procedure. With a lower baseline count, it is possible to achieve the same efficacy with a propanol-based hand rub in 30 seconds, 1 minute, and the recommended 1.5 minute.[219] Whether hands were washed or not before the second surgical hand rubbing had no significant influence on the overall efficacy.[220,221] These findings may be relevant in emergency surgery when every minute counts and a short surgical hand rubbing is all that can be done (eg, in aortic aneurysm).

The majority of studies indicate that surgical hand rubbing procedures are more effective compared to surgical hand scrubbing procedures.[157,189] A comparative study with three hand scrubs and two hand rubs all applied for 3 minutes showed that the hand rubs fulfilled the prEN 12791 efficacy requirements, whereas two surgical scrubs failed them.[222] Another study with a scrub based on 4% chlorhexidine, 70% (vol/vol) iso-propanol, and 85% (vol/vol) ethanol also showed a better efficacy for the

alcohols.[223] Studies with other methods found that the efficacy of surgical hand rubs was at least as good or better compared to surgical scrubs based on chlorhexidine[224-231] or povidone-iodine.[232-234] In clinical practice, the overall results are similar with a better efficacy of surgical hand rubs compared to surgical scrubs.[235,236]

Test Methods and Efficacy Requirements

In Europe, the spectrum of antimicrobial activity must include bactericidal activity according to EN 13727 and yeasticidal activity according to EN 13624. The same spectrum of antimicrobial activity is required in the United States, although the number of bacterial species to be investigated to determine bactericidal activity is much higher with at least 20 species compared to 4 species in EN 13727.[112] In veterinary medicine, the products must be at least bactericidal according to EN 13727.[111]

In Europe, the in vivo efficacy of alcohol-based hand rubs for surgical hand disinfection is evaluated according to EN 12791.[173] In the United States, a test method described in the Tentative Final Monograph for Healthcare Antiseptic Products published in 1994 was recommended, although the method was designed for hand scrub products and not for hand rub products.[112] In 2015, the FDA has proposed a test method for hand rub products and defined efficacy requirements.[115] These are summarized in Table 42.8.

A surgical hand rub product has to show noninferiority compared to a positive control according to EN 12791 (relative requirement, similar to clinical trials), and it has to demonstrate at least a 2 log$_{10}$ reduction according to the FDA proposed rules (absolute requirement). In addition, bacterial counts should not exceed baseline after 6 hours. An example shows that a hand rub based on 61% ethanol has been described to have a 1.1 log$_{10}$ reduction and would have failed the proposed FDA requirement. After 6 hours, bacterial counts were still 0.5 log$_{10}$ below baseline so that this requirement would have been met.[231]

Side Effects

Skin irritation caused by surgical hand rub products is rare. Using alcohol-based hand rubs for surgical hand rubbing is usually well tolerated by the skin, especially in comparison to surgical scrub products. After 6 or 24 applications of a surgical hand rub based on 61% ethanol and 1% chlorhexidine, skin dryness and redness were significantly lower compared to using surgical scrub product based on 4% chlorhexidine.[237] Similar results were reported from 20 surgeons in the United States[236] and 400 users in a surgical theater in Mexico.[238] In France, a propanol-based surgical hand rub applied for 5 minutes yielded significantly less skin dryness and skin irritation among 77 surgeons in comparison to surgical scrub products also applied for 5 minutes.[155]

Type IV allergies to ingredients of surgical hand rub products are extremely rare. In a study on 1828 health care workers in five university hospitals in Germany, a total of 50 were identified by medical history and a clinical evaluation with a possibility of a type IV allergy to the alcohol-based hand rub. None of the health care workers had a positive allergic reaction in occlusive patch tests using ethanol (80%), n-propanol (60%), or iso-propanol (70%).[239] In 2011, a total of 44 patients with a positive patch test result to iso-propanol were reported from 1450. Four of the 44 cases were considered to be occupational with 3 of them being nurses. But, there were doubts if the positive patch test results prove an allergy in the study because iso-propanol was used at 100%, although it is recommended for patch tests at 10%.[240] Case reports with a proven type IV allergy to iso-propanol exist but are extremely rare.[241-244] Type IV allergies have also been described to the emollient lanolin alcohol in 1.7% of 276 health care workers[179] or to the preservative diazolidinyl urea in a gel as a case report.[179]

Do Surgical Hand Rubs Reveal a Persistent Efficacy?

In 2009, WHO recommended the use of suitable alcohol-based hand rub, preferably with a product ensuring sustained activity.[27] In 2016, however, WHO changed the recommendation to "suitable alcohol-based hand rub" due to a lack of evidence that products with additional biocidal agents such as chlorhexidine were more effective in directly reducing the risk of surgical site infections.[189]

A persistent efficacy is traditionally only expected from alcohol-based hand rubs containing an additional nonvolatile active ingredient. In the scientific literature, chlorhexidine is mostly mentioned as such an ingredient[245] (eg, at 0.5% or 1% in combination with iso-propanol or ethanol). Another ingredient in this category is mecetronium etilsulfate, which is typically used at 0.2% in combination with n-propanol and iso-propanol. Hand rubs are also available containing 0.1% octenidine or 0.1% polyhexanide.

In 2002, the Centers for Disease Control and Prevention (CDC) guideline on hand hygiene provided a definition of "persistent activity." It is the prolonged or extended antimicrobial activity that prevents or inhibits the proliferation or survival of microorganisms after application of the product. This activity may be demonstrated by sampling a site several minutes or hours after application and demonstrating bacterial antimicrobial effectiveness when compared with a baseline level.[190] Bacterial load on hands has been compared to baseline levels after application of n-propanol (60%, vol/vol) for up to 6 hours

(reference alcohol for surgical hand disinfection in EN 12791). This alcohol alone applied for 3 minutes kept the bacterial load approximately 1 $\log_{10}$ below baseline for 6 hours.[215,216] All hand rubs fulfilling the EN 12791 efficacy requirement are likely to have a "persistent activity" based on the CDC definition of 2002. No additional active ingredients would be necessary. There is, however, another way to look at a potential superior efficacy for hand rubs with additional active ingredients.

EN 12791 allows determining a "long-term efficacy," which is often described as persistent efficacy. According to this norm, a hand rub has a long-term efficacy when the antimicrobial efficacy under the sterile surgical glove is significantly better after 3 hours ($P < .01$) compared to the reference alcohol (n-propanol, 60%, vol/vol) without any nonvolatile active ingredients.[173,246] A literature review on persistent efficacy in surgical hand rubs published in 2017 showed interesting results.[247] Two different hand rubs with 0.5% or 1% chlorhexidine did not have a long-term efficacy. Hand rubs with 0.2% mecetronium etilsulfate did not have a long-term efficacy when used as recommended for 1.5 minutes as shown by 14 published data sets. The lack of persistent efficacy for mecetronium etilsulfate were supported by a controlled trial with identical formulations with and without the ingredient,[248] similar to a vehicle control suggested by the FDA to demonstrate a superior efficacy of the formulation with an additional active ingredient.[115] One study according to the FDA test methods published in 1994, however, demonstrated a significantly better efficacy at all nine sampling times for the combination of 61% and 1% chlorhexidine compared to 61% ethanol alone.[231] The study has two major limitations. First, the concentration of ethanol is quite low compared to international standards (usually ≥80%) so that it is rather easy to demonstrate a significant additional effect by 1% chlorhexidine. Second, the sampling fluid did not contain any neutralizing agents so that false-positive results for the ethanol-chlorhexidine combination are likely.[149,249] Today, ASTM 1115 and the FDA require neutralization in the sampling fluid to obtain valid efficacy data.[115,174] Overall, there is currently solid evidence available to demonstrate that additional nonvolatile ingredients have very little if any additional efficacy benefit.

The WHO recommendation on the prevention of surgical site infection published in 2016 has, therefore, clearly postulated that a surgical hand rub should be "suitable." A persistent efficacy is not required and is not easily achieved when it must be shown with a lower incidence of surgical site infections.[189] In Germany, the addition of active ingredients with an expected persistent effect is regarded with caution by the Commission for Hospital Hygiene and Infection Prevention at the Robert Koch Institute because the risk-benefit ratio is not clear.[152] Chlorhexidine has been described with an increasing risk of acquired bacterial resistance[250] including cross-resistance to antibiotics and the increasing risk for anaphylactic reactions.[188] The risk of a mild skin irritation has been described which is plausible for a detergent-like molecule.[251] Current evidence suggests that substances, such as chlorhexidine, mecetronium etilsulfate, octenidine, or polyhexanide are dispensible in alcohol-based products for surgical hand rubbing because of the additional effect is more than doubtful, and some clinically relevant risks have been described. These aspects should be taken into consideration whenever alcohol-based hand rubs with any of these agents are preferred with the expectation to have persistent efficacy.

REFERENCES

1. Price PB. The bacteriology of normal skin: a new quantitative test applied to a study of the bacterial flora and the disinfectant action of mechanical cleansing. *J Infect Dis.* 1938;63:301-318.
2. Rotter M. Hygiene der hände. *Zeitschrift für die gesamte Hygiene.* 1990;36(2):77-79.
3. Montes LF, Wilborn WH. Location of bacterial skin flora. *Br J Dermatol.* 1969;81(suppl 1):23-26.
4. Lark RL, VanderHyde K, Deeb GM, Dietrich S, Massey JP, Chenoweth C. An outbreak of coagulase-negative staphylococcal surgical-site infections following aortic valve replacement. *Infect Control Hosp Epidemiol.* 2001;22(10):618-623.
5. Sullivan A, Edlund C, Nord CE. Effect of microbial agents on the ecological balance of human microflora. *Lancet Infect Dis.* 2001;1(2):101-114.
6. Lee YL, Cesario T, Lee R, et al. Colonization by *Staphylococcus* species resistant to methicillin or quinolone on hands of medical personnel in a skilled-nursing facility. *Am J Infect Control.* 1994;22(6):346-351.
7. Rayan GM, Flournoy DJ. Microbiologic flora of human fingernails. *J Hand Surg Am.* 1987;12(4):605-607.
8. Slight PH, Weber JM, Campos JM, Plotkin SA. Oxacillin-resistant coagulase-negative staphylococcal carriage rates in neonatal intensive care nurses and non-patient care hospital personnel. *Am J Infect Control.* 1987;15(1):29-32.
9. Aiello AE, Cimiotti J, Della-Latta P, Larson EL. A comparison of the bacteria found on the hands of "homemakers" and neonatal intensive care unit nurses. *J Hosp Infect.* 2003;54(4):310-315.
10. Cimiotti JP, Haas JP, Della-Latta P, Wu F, Saiman L, Larson EL. Prevalence and clinical relevance of *Staphylococcus warneri* in the neonatal intensive care unit. *Infect Control Hosp Epidemiol.* 2007;28(3):326-330. doi:10.1086/511998.
11. Evans CA, Smith WM, Johnston EA, Giblett ER. Bacterial flora of the normal human skin. *J Invest Dermatol.* 1950;15:305-324.
12. Aly R, Maibach HI. Aerobic microbial flora of intertrigenous skin. *Appl Environ Microbiol.* 1977;33(1):97-100.
13. Elsner P. Antimicrobials and the skin physiological and pathological flora. *Curr Probl Dermatol.* 2006;33:35-41. doi:10.1159/000093929.
14. Larson E. Effects of handwashing agent, handwashing frequency, and clinical area on hand flora. *Am J Infect Control.* 1984;12:76-82.
15. Larson EL, Hughes CA, Pyrak JD, Sparks SM, Cagatay EU, Bartkus JM. Changes in bacterial flora associated with skin damage on hands of health care personnel. *Am J Infect Control.* 1998;26:513-521.
16. Maki DG. Control of colonization and transmission of pathogenic bacteria in the hospital. *Ann Intern Med.* 1978;89(5, pt 2 suppl):777-780.
17. McGinley KJ, Larson EL, Leyden JJ. Composition and density of microflora in the subungual space of the hand. *J Clin Microbiol.* 1988;26(5):950-953.
18. Kampf G. Die epidemiologische Bedeutung der Hände. In: Kampf G, ed. *Kompendium Händehygiene.* Wiesbaden, Germany: mhp-Verlag; 2017:1-33.
19. Pittet D, Dharan S, Touveneau S, Sauvan V, Perneger TV. Bacterial contamination of the hands of hospital staff during routine patient care. *Arch Intern Med.* 1999;159(8):821-826.
20. McDonald LS, Bavaro MF, Hofmeister EP, Kroonen LT. Hand infections. *J Hand Surg Am.* 2011;36(8):1403-1412. doi:10.1016/j.jhsa.2011.05.035.
21. Pittet D, Hugonnet S, Harbarth S, et al. Effectiveness of a hospital-wide programme to improve compliance with hand hygiene. Infection Control Programme. *Lancet.* 2000;356:1307-1312.
22. Sax H, Allegranzi B, Uçay I, Larson E, Boyce J, Pittet D. 'My five moments for hand hygiene': a user-centred design approach to understand, train, monitor and report hand hygiene. *J Hosp Infect.* 2007;67(1):9-21.
23. Pittet D. Improving adherence to hand hygiene practice: a multidisciplinary approach. *Emerg Infect Dis.* 2001;7(2):234-240.
24. Pittet D, Donaldson L. Clean care is safer care: a worldwide priority. *Lancet.* 2005;366(9493):1246-1247. doi:10.1016/S0140-6736(05)67506-X.
25. Pittet D, Allegranzi B, Storr J, Donaldson L. 'Clean care is safer care': the global patient safety challenge 2005-2006. *Int J Infect Dis.* 2006;10(6):419-424. doi:10.1016/j.ijid.2006.06.001.
26. Pittet D, Donaldson L. Clean care is safer care: the first global challenge of the WHO World Alliance for Patient Safety. *Am J Infect Control.* 2005;33(8):476-479. doi:10.1016/j.ajic.2005.08.001.
27. World Health Organization. *Guide to Implementation: A Guide to the Implementation of the WHO Multimodal Hand Hygiene Improvement Strategy.* Geneva, Switzerland: World Health Organization; 2009. https://www.who.int/gpsc/5may/Guide_to_Implementation.pdf. Accessed May 28, 2019.
28. World Health Organization. *20th WHO Model List of Essential Medicines.* Geneva, Switzerland: World Health Organization; 2017. https://apps.who.int/iris/bitstream/handle/10665/273826/EML-20-eng.pdf. Accessed May 28, 2019.
29. World Health Organization. Hand hygiene a key defence in Europe's fight against antibiotic resistance. World Health Organization Web site. Updated April 5, 2017. http://www.euro.who.int/en/health-topics/Health-systems/health-workforce/news/news/2017/05/hand-hygiene-a-key-defence-in-europes-fight-against-antibiotic-resistance. Accessed May 28, 2019.
30. Bifulco M, Capunzo M, Marasco M, Pisanti S. The basis of the modern medical hygiene in the medieval Medical School of Salerno. *J Matern Fetal Neonatal Med.* 2015;28(14):1691-1693. doi:10.3109/14767058.2014.964681.
31. Klotz A, Veeger M, Röcher W. Skin cleansers for occupational use: testing the skin compatibility of different formulations. *Int Arch Occup Environ Health.* 2003;76(5):367-373. doi:10.1007/s00420-002-0427-0.
32. Behnke M, Hansen S, Leistner R, et al. Nosocomial infection and antibiotic use: a second national prevalence study in Germany. *Dtsch Arztebl Int.* 2013;110(38):627-633. doi:10.3238/arztebl.2013.0627.
33. Geffers C, Gastmeier P. Nosocomial infections and multidrug-resistant organisms in Germany: epidemiological data from KISS (the Hospital Infection Surveillance System). *Dtsch Arztebl Int.* 2011;108(6):87-93. doi:10.3238/arztebl.2011.0087.
34. National Research Council. *Review of the Scientific Approaches Used during the FBI's Investigation of the 2001 Anthrax Letters.* Washington, DC: National Academies Press; 2011.
35. Bettin K, Clabots C, Mathie P, Willard K, Gerding DN. Effectiveness of liquid soap vs. chlorhexidine gluconate for the removal of *Clostridium difficile* from bare hands and gloved hands. *Infect Control Hosp Epidemiol.* 1994;15(11):697-702.
36. Nerandzic MM, Rackaityte E, Jury LA, Eckart K, Donskey CJ. Novel strategies for enhanced removal of persistent *Bacillus anthracis* surrogates and *Clostridium difficile* spores from skin. *PLoS One.* 2013;8(7):e68706. doi:10.1371/journal.pone.0068706.
37. Weber DJ, Sickbert-Bennett E, Gergen MF, Rutala WA. Efficacy of selected hand hygiene agents used to remove *Bacillus atrophaeus* (a surrogate of *Bacillus anthracis*) from contaminated hands. *JAMA.* 2003;289(10):1274-1277.
38. Hübner NO, Kampf G, Löffler H, Kramer A. Effect of a 1 min hand wash on the bactericidal efficacy of consecutive surgical hand disinfection with standard alcohols and on skin hydration. *Int J Hyg Environ Health.* 2006;209(3):285-291.

39. Lineaweaver W, McMorris S, Soucy D, Howard R. Cellular and bacterial toxicities of topical antimicrobials. *Plast Reconstr Surg.* 1985;75(3):394-396.

40. Fujitani S, George WL, Morgan MA, Nichols S, Murthy AR. Implications for vancomycin-resistant Enterococcus colonization associated with *Clostridium difficile* infections. *Am J Infect Control.* 2011;39(3):188-193. doi:10.1016/j.ajic.2010.10.024.

41. Vervoort J, Gazin M, Kazma M, et al. High rates of intestinal colonisation with fluoroquinolone-resistant ESBL-harbouring Enterobacteriaceae in hospitalised patients with antibiotic-associated diarrhoea. *Eur J Clin Microbiol Infect Dis.* 2014;33(12):2215-2221. doi:10.1007/s10096-014-2193-9.

42. Kabara JJ, Brady MB. Contamination of bar soaps under "in-use" conditions. *J Environ Pathol Toxicol Oncol.* 1984;5(4-5):1-14.

43. Afolabi BA, Oduyebo OO, Ogunsola FT. Bacterial flora of commonly used soaps in three hospitals in Nigeria. *East Afr Med J.* 2007;84(10):489-495.

44. Jensen DA, Danyluk MD, Harris LJ, Schaffner DW. Quantifying the effect of hand wash duration, soap use, ground beef debris, and drying methods on the removal of *Enterobacter aerogenes* on hands. *J Food Prot.* 2015;78(4):685-690. doi:10.4315/0362-028X.JFP-14-245.

45. Graf W, Kersch D, Scherzer G. Microbial contamination of liquid-soap wall dispensers with one-way bottles. *Zentralbl Bakteriol Mikrobiol Hyg B.* 1988;186(2):166-179.

46. Caetano JA, Lima MA, Di Ciero Miranda M, Serufo JC, Ponte PR. Identification of bacterial contamination in liquid soap for hospital use. *Rev Esc Enferm USP.* 2011;45(1):153-160.

47. Aktas E, Taspinar E, Alay D, Ögedey ED, Külah C, Cömert F. Extrinsic contamination of liquid soap with various gram-negative bacteria in a hospital in Turkey. *Infect Control Hosp Epidemiol.* 2010;31(11):1199-1201. doi:10.1086/657077.

48. Yapicioglu H, Gokmen TG, Yildizdas D, et al. *Pseudomonas aeruginosa* infections due to electronic faucets in a neonatal intensive care unit. *J Paediatr Child Health.* doi:10.1111/j.1440-1754.2011.02248.x.

49. Blanc DS, Gomes Magalhaes B, Abdelbary M, et al. Hand soap contamination by *Pseudomonas aeruginosa* in a tertiary care hospital: no evidence of impact on patients. *J Hosp Infect.* 2016;93(1):63-67. doi:10.1016/j.jhin.2016.02.010.

50. Biswal M, Prasad A, Dhaliwal N, Gupta AK, Taneja N. Increase in hospital purchase of hand hygiene products: the importance of focusing on the right product. *Am J Infect Control.* 2015;43(7):765-766. doi:10.1016/j.ajic.2015.02.031.

51. Sartor C, Jacomo V, Duvivier C, Tissot-Dupont H, Sambuc R, Drancourt M. Nosocomial *Serratia marcescens* infections associated with extrinsic contamination of a liquid nonmedicated soap. *Infect Control Hosp Epidemiol.* 2000;21(3):196-199.

52. Lorenz LA, Ramsay BD, Goeres DM, Fields MW, Zapka CA, Macinga DR. Evaluation and remediation of bulk soap dispensers for biofilm. *Biofouling.* 2012;28(1):99-109. doi:10.1080/08927014.2011.653637.

53. Ayliffe GAJ, Babb JR, Quoraishi AH. A test for 'hygienic' hand disinfection. *J Clin Pathol.* 1978;31:923-928.

54. Taylor LJ. An evaluation of handwashing techniques—1. *Nurs Times.* 1978;74:54-55.

55. Taylor LJ. An evaluation of handwashing techniques—2. *Nurs Times.* 1978;74:108-111.

56. Deschênes P, Chano F, Dionne LL, Pittet D, Longtin Y. Efficacy of the World Health Organization—recommended handwashing technique and a modified washing technique to remove *Clostridium difficile* from hands. *Am J Infect Control.* 2017;45(8):844-848. doi:10.1016/j.ajic.2017.04.001.

57. Campbell D, Mann A, Hunt O, Santos LJ. The significance of hand wash compliance on the transfer of dermal lipids in contact lens wear. *Cont Lens Anterior Eye.* 2012;35(2):71-76. doi:10.1016/j.clae.2011.11.004.

58. Kampf G. Die einfache Händewaschung. In: Kampf G, ed. *Kompendium Händehygiene.* Wiesbaden, Germany: mhp-Verlag; 2017:78-91.

59. Larson EL, Eke PI, Wilder MP, Laughon BE. Quantity of soap as a variable in handwashing. *Infect Control.* 1987;8(9):371-375.

60. Patrick DR, Findon G, Miller TE. Residual moisture determines the level of touch-contact-associated bacterial transfer following hand washing. *Epidemiol Infect.* 1997;119(3):319-325.

61. Huang C, Ma W, Stack S. The hygienic efficacy of different hand-drying methods: a review of the evidence. *Mayo Clin Proc.* 2012;87(8):791-798. doi:10.1016/j.mayocp.2012.02.019.

62. Ngeow YF, Ong HW, Tan P. Dispersal of bacteria by an electric air hand dryer. *Malays J Pathol.* 1989;11:53-56.

63. de Almeida e Borges LF, Silva BL, Gontijo Filho PP. Hand washing: changes in the skin flora. *Am J Infect Control.* 2007;35(6):417-420. doi:10.1016/j.ajic.2006.07.012.

64. Babb JR, Davies JG, Ayliffe GAJ. A test procedure for evaluating surgical hand disinfection. *J Hosp Infect.* 1991;18(suppl B):41-49.

65. Crémieux A, Reverdy ME, Pons JL, et al. Standardized method for evaluation of hand disinfection by surgical scrub formulations. *Appl Environ Microbiol.* 1989;55(11):2944-2948.

66. Heeg P, Oßwald W, Schwenzer N. Wirksamkeitsvergleich von desinfektionsverfahren zur chirurgischen händedesinfektion unter experimentellen und klinischen bedingungen. *Hygiene + Medizin.* 1986;11:107-110.

67. Larson EL, Butz AM, Gullette DL, Laughon BA. Alcohol for surgical scrubbing? *Infect Control Hosp Epidemiol.* 1990;11(3):139-143.

68. Lowbury EJL, Lilly HA. Disinfection of the hands of surgeons and nurses. *Br Med J.* 1960;1:1445-1450.

69. Rotter M, Koller W, Wewalka G. Eignung von chlorhexidinglukonat- und PVP-iod-haltigen präparationen zur händedesinfektion. *Hygiene + Medizin.* 1981;6:425-430.

70. Ansari SA, Sattar SA, Springthorpe VS, Wells GA, Tostowaryk W. In vivo protocol for testing efficacy of hand-washing agents against viruses and bacteria: experiments with rotavirus and *Escherichia coli.* *Appl Environ Microbiol.* 1989;55(12):3113-3118.

71. Ojajärvi J. Effectiveness of hand washing and disinfection methods in removing transient bacteria after patient nursing. *J Hyg (Lond).* 1980;85:193-203.

72. Mahl MC. New method for determination of efficacy of health care personnel hand wash products. *J Clin Microbiol.* 1989;27(10):2295-2299.

73. Lowbury EJL, Lilly HA, Bull JP. Disinfection of hands: removal of transient organisms. *Br J Med.* 1964;2:230-233.

74. Ayliffe GAJ, Babb JR, Davies JG, Lilly HA. Hand disinfection: a comparison of various agents in laboratory and ward studies. *J Hosp Infect.* 1988;11:226-2243.

75. Kampf G, Ostermeyer C. Intra-laboratory reproducibility of the hand hygiene reference procedures of EN 1499 (hygienic hand wash) and EN 1500 (hygienic hand disinfection). *J Hosp Infect.* 2002;52(3):219-224.

76. Mittermayer H, Rotter M. Vergleich der wirkung von wasser, einigen detergentien und äthylalkohol auf die transiente flora der haut. *Zentralbl Bakteriol.* 1975;160:163-172.

77. Rotter ML, Koller W. A European test for the evaluation of the efficacy of procedures for the antiseptic handwash. *Hygiene + Medizin.* 1991;16:4-12.

78. Rotter ML, Koller W. Test models for hygienic handrub and hygienic handwash: the effects of two different contamination and sampling techniques. *J Hosp Infect.* 1992;20:163-171.

79. Messager S, Hammer KA, Carson CF, Riley TV. Effectiveness of hand-cleansing formulations containing tea tree oil assessed ex vivo on human skin and in vivo with volunteers using European standard EN 1499. *J Hosp Infect.* 2005;59(3):220-228. doi:10.1016/j.jhin.2004.06.032.

80. Cardoso CL, Pereira HH, Zequim JC, Guilhermetti M. Effectiveness of hand-cleansing agents for removing *Acinetobacter baumannii* strain from contaminated hands. *Am J Infect Control.* 1999;27:327-331.

81. Sickbert-Bennett EE, Weber DJ, Gergen-Teague MF, Sobsey MD, Samsa GP, Rutala WA. Comparative efficacy of hand hygiene agents in the reduction of bacteria and viruses. *Am J Infect Control.* 2005;33(2):67-77.

82. Nicoletti G, Boghossian V, Borland R. Hygienic hand disinfection: a comparative study with chlorhexidine detergents and soap. *J Hosp Infect.* 1990;15:323-337.

83. Kim SA, Moon H, Lee K, Rhee MS. Bactericidal effects of triclosan in soap both in vitro and in vivo. *J Antimicrob Chemother.* 2015;70(12):3345-3352. doi:10.1093/jac/dkv275.

84. Casewell M, Phillips I. Hands as route of transmission for Klebsiella species. *Br Med J.* 1977;2:1315-1317.

85. Lilly HA, Lowbury EJL. Transient skin flora: their removal by cleansing or disinfection in relation to their mode of deposition. *J Clin Pathol.* 1978;31:919-922.

86. Huang Y, Oie S, Kamiya A. Comparative effectiveness of hand-cleansing agents for removing methicillin-resistant *Staphylococcus aureus* from experimentally contaminated fingertips. *Am J Infect Control.* 1994;22(4):224-227.

87. Guilhermetti M, Hernandes SE, Fukushigue Y, Garcia LB, Cardoso CL. Effectiveness of hand-cleansing agents for removing methicillin-resistant *Staphylococcus aureus* from contaminated hands. *Infect Control Hosp Epidemiol.* 2001;22(2):105-108.

88. Bellamy K, Alcock R, Babb JR, Davies JG, Ayliffe GA. A test for the assessment of 'hygienic' hand disinfection using rotavirus. *J Hosp Infect.* 1993;24:201-210.

89. Davies JG, Babb JR, Bradley CR, Ayliffe GAJ. Preliminary study of test methods to assess the virucidal activity of skin disinfectants using poliovirus and bacteriophages. *J Hosp Infect.* 1993;25:125-131.

90. Steinmann J, Nehrkorn R, Meyer A, Becker K. Two in-vivo protocols for testing virucidal efficacy of handwashing and hand disinfection. *Zentralbl Hyg Umweltmed.* 1995;196:425-436.

91. Schürmann W, Eggers HJ. An experimental study on the epidemiology of enteroviruses: water and soap washing of poliovirus 1—contaminated hands, its effectiveness and kinetics. *Med Microbiol Immunol.* 1985;174(5):221-236.

92. Kramer A, Galabov AS, Sattar SA, et al. Virucidal activity of a new hand disinfectant with reduced ethanol content: comparison with other alcohol-based formulations. *J Hosp Infect.* 2006;62(1):98-106.

93. Lages SLS, Ramakrishnan MA, Goyal SM. In-vivo efficacy of hand sanitisers against feline calicivirus: a surrogate for norovirus. *J Hosp Infect.* 2008;68(2):159-163.

94. Gehrke C, Steinmann J, Goroncy-Bermes P. Inactivation of feline calicivirus, a surrogate of norovirus (formerly Norwalk-like viruses), by different types of alcohol in vitro and in vivo. *J Hosp Infect.* 2004;56(1):49-55.

95. Paulmann D, Steinmann J, Becker B, Bischoff B, Steinmann E, Steinmann J. Virucidal activity of different alcohols against murine norovirus, a surrogate of human norovirus. *J Hosp Infect.* 2011;79(4):378-379.

96. Steinmann J, Paulmann D, Becker B, Bischoff B, Steinmann E, Steinmann J. Comparison of virucidal activity of alcohol-based hand sanitizers versus antimicrobial hand soaps in vitro and in vivo. *J Hosp Infect.* 2012;82(4):277-280. doi:10.1016/j.jhin.2012.08.005.

97. Larson E, Girard R, Pessoa-Silva CL, Boyce J, Donaldson L, Pittet D. Skin reactions related to hand hygiene and selection of hand hygiene products. *Am J Infect Control.* 2006;34(10):627-635. doi:10.1016/j.ajic.2006.05.289.

98. Chamorey E, Marcy PY, Dandine M, et al. A prospective multicenter study evaluating skin tolerance to standard hand hygiene techniques. *Am J Infect Control.* 2011;39(1):6-13. doi:10.1016/j.ajic.2010.03.021.

99. Callahan A, Baron E, Fekedulegn D, et al. Winter season, frequent hand washing, and irritant patch test reactions to detergents are associated with hand dermatitis in health care workers. *Dermatitis.* 2013;24(4):170-175. doi:10.1097/DER.0b013e318290c57f.

100. Girard R, Carré E, Pires-Cronenberger S, et al. Field test comparison of two dermal tolerance assessment methods of hand hygiene products. *J Hosp Infect.* 2008;69(2):181-185. doi:10.1016/j.jhin.2008.03.016.

101. Souweine B, Lautrette A, Aumeran C, et al. Comparison of acceptability, skin tolerance, and compliance between handwashing and alcohol-based handrub in ICUs: results of a multicentric study. *Intensive Care Med.* 2009;35(7):1216-1224. doi:10.1007/s00134-009-1485-5.

102. Winnefeld M, Richard MA, Drancourt M, Grobb JJ. Skin tolerance and effectiveness of two hand decontamination procedures in everyday hospital use. *Br J Dermatol.* 2000;143:546-550.

103. Suneja T, Belsito DV. Occupational dermatoses in health care workers evaluated for suspected allergic contact dermatitis. *Contact Dermatitis.* 2008;58(5):285-290. doi:10.1111/j.1600-0536.2007.01315.x.

104. Clayton TH, Wilkinson SM. Contact dermatoses in healthcare workers: reduction in type I latex allergy in a UK centre. *Clin Exp Dermatol.* 2005;30(3):221-225. doi:10.1111/j.1365-2230.2005.01768.x.

105. Ataman AD, Vatanoğlu-Lutz EE, Yildirim G. Medicine in stamps—Ignaz Semmelweis and puerperal fever. *J Turk Ger Gynecol Assoc.* 2013;14(1):35-39. doi:10.5152/jtgga.2013.08.

106. Hall R. Chlorhexidine/cetrimide mixture for washing hands. *Lancet.* 1961;278(7207):876-877.

107. de Witt Huberts J, Greenland K, Schmidt WP, Curtis V. Exploring the potential of antimicrobial hand hygiene products in reducing the infectious burden in low-income countries: an integrative review. *Am J Infect Control.* 2016;44(7):764-771. doi:10.1016/j.ajic.2016.01.045.

108. Food and Drug Administration, Department of Health and Human Services. Safety and effectiveness of consumer antiseptics; topical antimicrobial drug products for over-the-counter human use. Final rule. *Fed Regist.* 2016;81(172):61106-61130.

109. McNamara PJ, Levy SB. Triclosan: an instructive tale. *Antimicrob Agents Chemother.* 2016;60(12):7015-7016. doi:10.1128/aac.02105-16.

110. World Health Organization. *WHO Guidelines on Hand Hygiene in Health Care: First Global Patient Safety Challenge: Clean Care Is Safer Care.* Geneva, Switzerland: World Health Organization; 2009.

111. Comité Européen de Normalisation. *EN 14885:2015. Chemical Disinfectants and Antiseptics. Application of European Standards for Chemical Disinfectants and Antiseptics.* Brussels, Belgium: Comité Européen de Normalisation; 2015.

112. Tentative final monograph for health care antiseptic products; proposed rule. *Fed Regist.* 1994;59(116):31401-31452.

113. Comité Européen de Normalisation. *EN 1499:2013. Chemical Disinfectants and Antiseptics. Hygienic Hand Wash. Test Method and Requirement (Phase 2/Step 2).* Brussels, *Belgium*: Comité Européen de Normalisation; 2013.

114. American Society for Testing and Materials International. *ASTM E 1174 - 06. Standard Test Method for Evaluation of the Effectiveness of Health Care Personnel Handwash Formulations.* West Conshohocken, PA: American Society for Testing and Materials; 2006.

115. Department of Health and Human Services, Food and Drug Administration. Safety and effectiveness of healthcare antiseptics; topical antimicrobial drug products for over-the-counter human use; proposed amendment of the tentative final monograph; reopening of administrative record. *Fed Regist.* 2015;80(84):25166-25205.

116. Speck A. Hygienische händedesinfektion. *Zeitschrift für Hygiene.* 1905;50:502-578.

117. Kalmár P, Meyer-Rohn J. Experiences with a new hand disinfectant. *Chirurg.* 1968;39(5):231-236.

118. Rotter ML, Koller W, Neumann R. The influence of cosmetic additives on the acceptability of alcohol-based hand disinfectants. *J Hosp Infect.* 1991;18(suppl B):57-63.

119. Kampf G, Wigger-Alberti W, Schoder V, Wilhelm KP. Emollients in a propanol-based hand rub can significantly decrease irritant contact dermatitis. *Contact Dermatitis.* 2005;53:344-349.

120. Kramer A, Rudolph P, Kampf G, Pittet D. Limited efficacy of alcohol-based hand gels. *Lancet.* 2002;359:1489-1490.

121. Suchomel M, Kundi M, Pittet D, Weinlich M, Rotter ML. Testing of the World Health Organization recommended formulations in their application as hygienic hand rubs and proposals for increased efficacy. *Am J Infect Control.* 2011;40(4):328-331.

122. Comité Européen de Normalisation. *EN 1500:2013. Chemical Disinfectants and Antiseptics. Hygienic Hand Disinfection. Test Method and Requirement (Phase 2, Step 2).* Brussels, Belgium: Comité Européen de Normalisation; 2013.

123. Škodova M, Gimeno-Benítez A, Martínez-Redondo E, Morán-Cortés JF, Jiménez-Romano R, Gimeno-Ortiz A. Hand hygiene technique quality evaluation in nursing and medicine students of two

academic courses. *Rev Lat Am Enfermagem*. 2015;23(4):708-717. doi:10.1590/0104-1169.0459.2607.

124. Widmer AF, Dangel M. Alcohol-based handrub: evaluation of technique and microbiological efficacy with international infection control professionals. *Infect Control Hosp Epidemiol*. 2004;25(3):207-209.

125. Park HY, Kim SK, Lim YJ, et al. Assessment of the appropriateness of hand surface coverage for health care workers according to World Health Organization hand hygiene guidelines. *Am J Infect Control*. 2014;42(5):559-561. doi:10.1016/j.ajic.2013.12.014.

126. Tschudin-Sutter S, Sepulcri D, Dangel M, Schuhmacher H, Widmer AF. Compliance with the World Health Organization hand hygiene technique: a prospective observational study. *Infect Control Hosp Epidemiol*. 2015;36(4):482-483. doi:10.1017/ice.2014.82.

127. Kampf G, Reichel M, Feil Y, Eggerstedt S, Kaulfers PM. Influence of rub-in technique on required application time and hand coverage in hygienic hand disinfection. *BMC Infect Dis*. 2008;8:149.

128. Aktion Saubere Hände. Berlin, Germany: Charité University Medicine.

129. Widmer AF, Conzelmann M, Tomic M, Frei R, Stranden AM. Introducing alcohol-based hand rub for hand hygiene: the critical need for training. *Infect Control Hosp Epidemiol*. 2007;28(1):50-54.

130. Pickering AJ, Davis J, Boehm AB. Efficacy of alcohol-based hand sanitizer on hands soiled with dirt and cooking oil. *J Water Health*. 2011;9(3):429-433. doi:10.2166/wh.2011.138.

131. ASTM International. *ASTM E2755-10: Standard Test Method for Determining the Bacteria-Eliminating Effectiveness of Hand Sanitizer Formulations Using Hands of Adults*. West Conshohocken, PA: ASTM International; 2010.

132. Kampf G, Ostermeyer C. Inter-laboratory reproducibility of the hand disinfection reference procedure EN 1500. *J Hosp Infect*. 2003;53(4):304-306.

133. Hartmann RS, Pietsch H, Sauermann G, Neubert R. Untersuchung zur hautverträglichkeit von alkoholischen händedesinfektionsmitteln. *Dermatosen*. 1994;42:241-245.

134. Kramer A, Bernig T, Kampf G. Clinical double-blind trial on the dermal tolerance and user acceptability of six alcohol-based hand disinfectants for hygienic hand disinfection. *J Hosp Infect*. 2002;51(2):114-120.

135. Houben E, de Paepe K, Rogiers V. Skin condition associated with intensive use of alcoholic gels for hand disinfection: a combination of biophysical and sensorial data. *Contact Dermatitis*. 2006;54:261-267.

136. Kampf G, Muscatiello M. Dermal tolerance of Sterillium, a propanol-based hand rub. *J Hosp Infect*. 2003;55(4):295-298.

137. Kampf G, Muscatiello M, Häntschel D, Rudolf M. Dermal tolerance and effect on skin hydration of a new ethanol-based hand gel. *J Hosp Infect*. 2002;52(4):297-301.

138. Girard R, Bousquet E, Carré E, et al. Tolerance and acceptability of 14 surgical and hygienic alcohol-based hand rubs. *J Hosp Infect*. 2006;63(3):281-288.

139. Kampf G, Wigger-Alberti W, Wilhelm KP. Do atopics tolerate alcohol-based hand rubs? A prospective, controlled, randomized double-blind clinical trial. *Acta Derm Venereol*. 2006;86(2):140-143.

140. Pittet D, Allegranzi B, Sax H, Chraiti MN, Griffiths W, Richet H; and World Health Organization Global Patient Safety Challenge Alcohol-Based Handrub Task Force. Double-blind, randomized, crossover trial of 3 hand rub formulations: fast-track evaluation of tolerability and acceptability. *Infect Control Hosp Epidemiol*. 2007;28(12):1344-1351. doi:10.1086/523272.

141. Kampf G, Muscatiello M, Segger D. Dermal tolerance and effect on skin hydration of an improved ethanol-based hand gel. *Int J Infect Control*. 2009;5:1-6.doi:10.3396/ijic.V5i1.003.09.

142. Traore O, Hugonnet S, Lübbe J, Griffiths W, Pittet D. Liquid versus gel handrub formulation: a prospective intervention study. *Crit Care*. 2007;11(3):R52. doi:10.1186/cc5906.

143. Harada YU, Lekcharoensuk P, Furuta T, Taniguchi T. Inactivation of foot-and-mouth disease virus by commercially available disinfectants and cleaners. *Biocontrol Sci*. 2015;20(3):205-208. doi:10.4265/bio.20.205.

144. Conrad A, Grotejohann B, Schmoor C, Cosic D, Dettenkofer M. Safety and tolerability of virucidal hand rubs: a randomized, double-blind, cross-over trial with healthy volunteers. *Antimicrob Resist Infect Control*. 2015;4:37. doi:10.1186/s13756-015-0079-y.

145. Kampf G, Reichel M. Gehäufte hautirritationen durch ein viruzides händedesinfektionsmittel mit hohem phosphorsäuregehalt. *ASU*. 2010;45(9):546-547.

146. Wade JJ, Casewell MW. The evaluation of residual antimicrobial activity on hands and its clinical relevance. *J Hosp Infect*. 1991;18(suppl B):23-28.

147. Lowbury EJL, Lilly HA. Use of 4% chlorhexidine detergent solution (Hibiscrub) and other methods of skin disinfection. *Br Med J*. 1973;1:510-515.

148. Casewell MW, Law MM, Desai N. A laboratory model for testing agents for hygienic hand disinfection: handwashing and chlorhexidine for the removal of klebsiella. *J Hosp Infect*. 1988;12(3):163-175.

149. Kampf G. What is left to justify the use of chlorhexidine in hand hygiene? *J Hosp Infect*. 2008;70(suppl 1):27-34.

150. Rutter JD, Angiulo K, Macinga DR. Measuring residual activity of topical antimicrobials: is the residual activity of chlorhexidine an artefact of laboratory methods? *J Hosp Infect*. 2014;88(2):113-115. doi:10.1016/j.jhin.2014.06.010.

151. López-Gigosos RM, Mariscal-López E, Gutierrez-Bedmar M, García-Rodriguez A, Mariscal A. Evaluation of antimicrobial persistent activity of alcohol-based hand antiseptics against bacterial contamination. *Eur J Clin Microbiol Infect Dis*. 2017;36(7):1197-2203. doi:10.1007/s10096-017-2908-9.

152. Empfehlung der Kommission für Krankenhaushygiene und Infektionsprävention (KRINKO) beim Robert Koch-Institut (RKI). Händehygiene in einrichtungen des gesundheitswesens. *Bundesgesundheitsbl*. 2016;59(9):1189-1220.

153. Nungester WJ, Thilby RL, Vial AB. Evaluation of hexachlorophene and detergents as substitutes for the surgical scrub; a biological technique. *Surg Gynecol Obstet*. 1949;88(5):639-642.

154. Jarral OA, McCormack DJ, Ibrahim S, Shipolini AR. Should surgeons scrub with chlorhexidine or iodine prior to surgery? *Interact Cardiovasc Thorac Surg*. 2011;12(6):1017-1021. doi:10.1510/icvts.2010.259796.

155. Parienti JJ, Thibon P, Heller R, et al. Hand-rubbing with an aqueous alcoholic solution vs traditional surgical hand-scrubbing and 30-day surgical site infection rates: a randomized equivalence study. *JAMA*. 2002;288(6):722-727.

156. Widmer AF, Rotter M, Voss A, et al. Surgical hand preparation: state-of-the-art. *J Hosp Infect*. 2010;74(2):112-122.

157. Widmer AF. Surgical hand hygiene: scrub or rub? *J Hosp Infect*. 2013;83(suppl 1):S35-S39.

158. Tavolacci MP, Pitrou I, Merle V, Haghighat S, Thillard D, Czernichow P. Surgical hand rubbing compared with surgical hand scrubbing: comparison of efficacy and costs. *J Hosp Infect*. 2006;63(1):55-59. doi:10.1016/j.jhin.2005.11.012.

159. O'Farrell DA, Kenny G, O'Sullivan M, Nicholson P, Stephens M, Hone R. Evaluation of the optimal hand-scrub duration prior to total hip arthroplasty. *J Hosp Infect*. 1994;26:93-98.

160. Ginsberg F. Scrub brushes and nail files essential to aseptic technic. *Mod Hosp*. 1960;94:130.

161. McBride ME, Duncan WC, Knox JM. An evaluation of surgical scrub brushes. *Surg Gynecol Obstet*. 1973;137(6):934-936.

162. Mitchell KG, Rawluk DJ. Skin reactions related to surgical scrub-up: results of a Scottish survey. *Br J Surg*. 1984;71(3):223-224.

163. Galle PC, Homesley HD, Rhyne AL. Reassessment of the surgical scrub. *Surg Gynecol Obstet*. 1978;147(2):215-218.

164. Okgün Alcan A, Demir Korkmaz F. Comparison of the efficiency of nail pick and brush used for nail cleaning during surgical scrub on reducing bacterial counts. *Am J Infect Control*. 2012;40(9):826-829. doi:10.1016/j.ajic.2011.10.021.

165. Loeb MB, Wilcox L, Smaill F, Walter S, Duff Z. A randomized trial of surgical scrubbing with a brush compared with antiseptic soap alone. *Am J Infect Control*. 1997;25:11-15.

166. Tanner J, Khan D, Walsh S, Chernova J, Lamont S, Laurent T. Brushes and picks used on nails during the surgical scrub to reduce bacteria: a randomised trial. *J Hosp Infect.* 2009;71(3):234-238. doi:10.1016/j.jhin.2008.11.023.

167. Kikuchi-Numagami K, Saishu T, Fukaya M, Kanazawa E, Tagami H. Irritancy of scrubbing up for surgery with or without a brush. *Acta Derm Venereol.* 1999;79(3):230-232.

168. Ezzat A, Safdar MM, Ahmed I. Are we following the WHO recommendations for surgical scrubbing? *Scott Med J.* 2014;59(4):214-219. doi:10.1177/0036933014554885.

169. Umit UM, Sina M, Ferhat Y, Yasemin P, Meltem K, Ozdemir AA. Surgeon behavior and knowledge on hand scrub and skin antisepsis in the operating room. *J Surg Educ.* 2014;71(2):241-245. doi:10.1016/j.jsurg.2013.08.003.

170. Petterwood J, Shridhar V. Water conservation in surgery: a comparison of two surgical scrub techniques demonstrating the amount of water saved using a 'taps on/taps off' technique. *Aust J Rural Health.* 2009;17(4):214-217. doi:10.1111/j.1440-1584.2009.01074.x.

171. Ahmed A. Surgical hand scrub: lots of water wasted. *Ann Afr Med.* 2007;6(1):31-33.

172. Somner JE, Stone N, Koukkoulli A, Scott KM, Field AR, Zygmunt J. Surgical scrubbing: can we clean up our carbon footprints by washing our hands? *J Hosp Infect.* 2008;70(3):212-215.

173. Comité Européen de Normalisation. *EN 12791:2005. Chemical Disinfectants and Antiseptics. Surgical Hand Disinfection. Test Method and Requirement (Phase 2, Step 2).* Brussels, Belgium: Comité Européen de Normalisation; 2005.

174. American Society for Testing and Materials International. *ASTM E 1115 - 11. Standard Test Method for Evaluation of Surgical Hand Scrub Formulations.* West Conshohocken, PA: American Society for Testing and Materials; 2011.

175. Holness DL, Tarlo SM, Sussman G, Nethercott JR. Exposure characteristics and cutaneous problems in operating room staff. *Contact Dermatitis.* 1995;32(6):352-358.

176. Antonov D, Kleesz P, Elsner P, Schliemann S. Impact of glove occlusion on cumulative skin irritation with or without hand cleanser-comparison in an experimental repeated irritation model. *Contact Dermatitis.* 2013;68(5):293-299. doi:10.1111/cod.12028.

177. Sato K, Kusaka Y, Suganuma N, Nagasawa S, Deguchi Y. Occupational allergy in medical doctors. *J Occup Health.* 2004;46(2):165-170.

178. Toholka R, Nixon R. Allergic contact dermatitis to chlorhexidine. *Australas J Dermatol.* 2013;54(4):303-306. doi:10.1111/ajd.12087.

179. Higgins CL, Palmer AM, Cahill JL, Nixon RL. Occupational skin disease among Australian healthcare workers: a retrospective analysis from an occupational dermatology clinic, 1993-2014. *Contact Dermatitis.* 2016;75(4):213-222. doi:10.1111/cod.12616.

180. Apisarnthanarak A, Mundy LM. High incidence of chlorhexidine-induced rash among Thai health care workers. *Clin Infect Dis.* 2011;53(8):848-849. doi:10.1093/cid/cir518.

181. Wittczak T, Dudek W, Walusiak-Skorupa J, Świerczyńska-Machura D, Pałczyński C. Chlorhexidine—still an underestimated allergic hazard for health care professionals. *Occup Med (Lond).* 2013;63(4):301-305. doi:10.1093/occmed/kqt035.

182. Liippo J, Kousa P, Lammintausta K. The relevance of chlorhexidine contact allergy. *Contact Dermatitis.* 2011;64(4):229-234. doi:10.1111/j.1600-0536.2010.01851.x.

183. Beaudouin E, Kanny G, Morisset M, et al. Immediate hypersensitivity to chlorhexidine: literature review. *Eur Ann Allergy Clin Immunol.* 2004;36(4):123-126.

184. Hong CC, Wang SM, Nather A, Tan JH, Tay SH, Poon KH. Chlorhexidine anaphylaxis masquerading as septic shock. *Int Arch Allergy Immunol.* 2015;167(1):16-20. doi:10.1159/000431358.

185. Odedra KM, Farooque S. Chlorhexidine: an unrecognised cause of anaphylaxis. *Postgrad Med J.* 2014;90(1070):709-714. doi:10.1136/postgradmedj-2013-132291.

186. Ohtoshi T, Yamauchi N, Tadokoro K, et al. IgE antibody-mediated shock reaction caused by topical application of chlorhexidine. *Clin Allergy.* 1986;16(2):155-161.

187. Vu M, Rajgopal Bala H, Cahill J, Toholka R, Nixon R. Immediate hypersensitivity to chlorhexidine. *Australas J Dermatol.* 2018;59(1):55-56. doi:10.1111/ajd.12674.

188. US Food and Drug Administration. FDA drug safety communication: FDA warns about rare but serious allergic reactions with the skin antiseptic chlorhexidine gluconate. 2017. https://www.fda.gov/Drugs/DrugSafety/ucm530975.htm. Accessed May 28, 2019.

189. World Health Organization. *Global Guidelines for the Prevention of Surgical Site Infections.* Geneva, Switzerland: World Health Organization; 2016.

190. Boyce JM, Pittet D. Guideline for hand hygiene in health-care settings. Recommendations of the healthcare infection control practices advisory committee and the HICPAC/SHEA/APIC/IDSA hand hygiene task force. *MMWR Recomm Rep.* 2002;51:1-45.

191. Kampf G, Reichel M, Hollingsworth A, Bashir M. Efficacy of surgical hand scrub products based on chlorhexidine is largely overestimated without neutralizing agents in the sampling fluid. *Am J Infect Control.* 2013;41(1):e1-e5. doi:10.1016/j.ajic.2012.07.018.

192. Schlich T. Asepsis and bacteriology: a realignment of surgery and laboratory science. *Med Hist.* 2012;56(3):308-334. doi:10.1017/mdh.2012.22.

193. Fürbringer P. *Untersuchungen und Vorschriften über die Desinfektion der Hände des Arztes nebst Bemerkungen über den Bakteriologischen Charakter des Nagelschmutzes.* Wiesbaden, Germany: J. F. Bergmann; 1888.

194. Verwilghen DR, Mainil J, Mastrocicco E, et al. Surgical hand antisepsis in veterinary practice: evaluation of soap scrubs and alcohol based rub techniques. *Vet J.* 2011;190(3):372-377. doi:10.1016/j.tvjl.2010.12.020.

195. Herbig S, Kaiser V, Maurer J, Taylor L, Thiesen J, Krämer I. ADKA-leitlinie: aseptische herstellung und prüfung applikationsfertiger parenteralia. *Krankenhauspharmazie.* 2013;34(2):93-106.

196. Misteli H, Weber WP, Reck S, et al. Surgical glove perforation and the risk of surgical site infection. *Arch Surg.* 2009;144(6):553-558.

197. Kampf G, Voss A, Widmer AF. Die chirurgische händedesinfektion zwischen tradition und fortschritt. *Hygiene + Medizin.* 2006;31(7-8):316-321.

198. Fürbringer P. Zur desinfection der hände des arztes. *Dtsch Med Wochenschr.* 1888;48:985-987.

199. Reinicke EA. Bakteriologische untersuchungen über die desinfektion der hände. *Zentralbl Gynäkol.* 1894;47:1189-1199.

200. Kampf G, Kramer A, Rotter M, Widmer AF. Optimierung der chirurgischen händedesinfektion. *Zentralbl Chir.* 2006;131(4):322-326.

201. Price PB. Ethyl alcohol as a germicide. *Arch Surg.* 1939;38:528-542.

202. Kampf G, Löffler H. Prevention of irritant contact dermatitis among health care workers by using evidence-based hand hygiene practices: a review. *Ind Health.* 2007;45(5):645-652.

203. Nonnemann HC, Kisseih G. Untersuchungen verschiedener händewaschmethoden im chirurgischen operationssaal. *Chirurg.* 1972;43:484-487.

204. Händehygiene. *Bundesgesundheitsblatt.* 2000;43(3):230-233.

205. Ahlfeld F. Die desinfection des fingers und der hand vor geburtshülflichen untersuchungen und eingriffen. *Dtsch Med Wochenschr.* 1895;51:851-855.

206. Hingst V, Juditzki I, Heeg P, Sonntag HG. Evaluation of the efficacy of surgical hand disinfection following a reduced application time of 3 instead of 5 min. *J Hosp Infect.* 1992;20:79-86.

207. Kampf G, Ostermeyer C, Heeg P. Surgical hand disinfection with a propanol-based hand rub: equivalence of shorter application times. *J Hosp Infect.* 2005;59(4):304-310.

208. Decker LA, Gross A, Miller FC, Read JA, Cutright DE, Devine J. A rapid method for the presurgical cleansing of hands. *Obstet Gynecol.* 1978;51(1):115-117.

209. Blech MF, Hartemann P, Paquin JL. Activity of non antiseptic soaps and ethanol for hand disinfection. *Zentralbl Bakteriol Mikrobiol Hyg B.* 1985;181:496-512.

210. Dineen P. An evaluation of the duration of the surgical scrub. *Surg Gynecol Obstet.* 1969;129:1181-1184.

211. Hübner NO, Kampf G, Kamp P, Kohlmann T, Kramer A. Does a preceding hand wash and drying time after surgical hand disinfection influence the efficacy of a propanol-based hand rub? *BMC Microbiol.* 2006;6:57.

212. Rotter ML, Koller W. Surgical hand disinfection: effect of sequential use of two chlorhexidine preparations. *J Hosp Infect*. 1990;16:161-166.

213. Kampf G, Ostermeyer C. Small volumes of n-propanol (60%) applied for 3 minutes may be ineffective for surgical hand disinfection. *Antimicrob Resist Infect Control*. 2014;3:15. doi:10.1186/2047-2994-3-15.

214. Haessler S, Connelly NR, Kanter G, et al. A surgical site infection cluster: the process and outcome of an investigation—the impact of an alcohol-based surgical antisepsis product and human behavior. *Anesth Analg*. 2010;110(4):1044-1048.

215. Rotter ML, Kampf G, Suchomel M, Kundi M. Population kinetics of the skin flora on gloved hands following surgical hand disinfection with 3 propanol-based hand rubs: a prospective, randomized, double-blind trial. *Infect Control Hosp Epidemiol*. 2007;28(3):346-350.

216. Rotter ML, Kampf G, Suchomel M, Kundi M. Long-term effect of a 1.5 minute surgical hand rub with a propanol-based product on the resident hand flora. *J Hosp Infect*. 2007;66(1):84-85.

217. Devenish EA, Miles AA. Control of *Staphylococcus aureus* in an operating-theatre. *Lancet*. 1939;233(6037):1088-1094. doi:10.1016/S0140-6736(00)60700-6.

218. Heeg P, Ulmer R, Schwenzer N. Verbessern händewaschen und verwendung der handbürste das ergebnis der chirurgischen händedesinfektion? *Hygiene + Medizin*. 1988;13:270-272.

219. Kampf G, Ostermeyer C, Kohlmann T. Bacterial population kinetics on hands during 2 consecutive surgical hand disinfection procedures. *Am J Infect Control*. 2008;36(5):369-374.

220. Kampf G, Ostermeyer C. A 1-minute hand wash does not impair the efficacy of a propanol-based hand rub in two consecutive surgical hand disinfection procedures. *Eur J Clin Microbiol Infect Dis*. 2009;28(11):1357-1362.

221. Rehork B, Rüden H. Investigations into the efficacy of different procedures for surgical hand disinfection between consecutive operations. *J Hosp Infect*. 1991;19:115-127.

222. Marchetti MG, Kampf G, Finzi G, Salvatorelli G. Evaluation of the bactericidal effect of five products for surgical hand disinfection according to prEN 12054 and prEN 12791. *J Hosp Infect*. 2003;54(1):63-67.

223. Rotter M, Kundi M, Suchomel M, et al. Reproducibility and workability of the European test standard EN 12791 regarding the effectiveness of surgical hand antiseptics: a randomized, multicenter trial. *Infect Control Hosp Epidemiol*. 2006;27(9):935-939.

224. Macinga DR, Edmonds SL, Campbell E, McCormack RR. Comparative efficacy of alcohol-based surgical scrubs: the importance of formulation. *AORN J*. 2014;100(6):641-650. doi:10.1016/j.aorn.2014.03.013.

225. Hobson DW, Woller W, Anderson L, Guthery E. Development and evaluation of a new alcohol-based surgical hand scrub formulation with persistant antimicrobial characteristics and brushless application. *Am J Infect Control*. 1998;26(10):507-512.

226. Reverdy ME, Martra A, Fleurette J. Effectiveness of 9 soaps and/or antiseptics on hand flora after surgical-type washing. *Pathol Biol (Paris)*. 1984;32(5 Pt 2):591-595.

227. Bryce EA, Spence D, Roberts FJ. An in-use evaluation of an alcohol-based pre-surgical hand disinfectant. *Infect Control Hosp Epidemiol*. 2001;22(10):635-639.

228. Chen CF, Han CL, Kan CP, Chen SG, Hung PW. Effect of surgical site infections with waterless and traditional hand scrubbing protocols on bacterial growth. *Am J Infect Control*. 2012;40(4):e15-e17. doi:10.1016/j.ajic.2011.09.008.

229. Burch TM, Stanger B, Mizuguchi KA, Zurakowski D, Reid SD. Is alcohol-based hand disinfection equivalent to surgical scrub before placing a central venous catheter? *Anesth Analg*. 2012;114(3):622-625. doi:10.1213/ANE.0b013e31824083b8.

230. Weight CJ, Lee MC, Palmer JS. Avagard hand antisepsis vs. traditional scrub in 3600 pediatric urologic procedures. *Urology*. 2010;76(1):15-17. doi:10.1016/j.urology.2010.01.017.

231. Mulberry G, Snyder AT, Heilman J, Pyrek J, Stahl J. Evaluation of a waterless, scrubless chlorhexidine gluconate/ethanol surgical scrub for antimicrobial efficacy. *Am J Infect Control*. 2001;29(12):377-382.

232. Choi JS. Evaluation of a waterless, scrubless chlorhexidine gluconate/ethanol surgical scrub and povidone-iodine for antimicrobial efficacy. *Taehan Kanho Hakhoe chi*. 2008;38(1):39-44.

233. Lai KW, Foo TL, Low W, Naidu G. Surgical hand antisepsis—a pilot study comparing povidone-iodine hand scrub and alcohol-based chlorhexidine gluconate hand rub. *Ann Acad Med Singapore*. 2012;41(1):12-16.

234. Grabsch EA, Mitchell DJ, Hooper J, Turnidge JD. In-use efficacy of a chlorhexidine in alcohol surgical rub: a comparative study. *ANZ J Surg*. 2004;74(9):769-772. doi:10.1111/j.1445-1433.2004.03154.x.

235. Pietsch H. Hand antiseptics: rubs versus scrubs, alcoholic solutions versus alcoholic gels. *J Hosp Infect*. 2001;48(suppl A):S33-S36.

236. Larson EL, Aiello AE, Heilman JM, et al. Comparison of different regimes for surgical hand preparation. *AORN J*. 2001;73:412-420.

237. Grove GL, Zerweck CR, Heilman JM, Pyrek JD. Methods for evaluating changes in skin condition due to the effects of antimicrobial hand cleaners: two studies comparing a new waterless chlorhexidine gluconate/ethanol-emollient antiseptic preparation with a conventional water-applied product. *Am J Infect Control*. 2001;29:361-369.

238. Vergara-Fernández O, Morales-Olivera JM, Ponce-de-León-Rosales S, et al. Surgical team satisfaction levels between two preoperative hand-washing methods. *Rev Invest Clin*. 2010;62(6):532-537.

239. Stutz N, Becker D, Jappe U, et al. Nurses' perceptions of the benefits and adverse effects of hand disinfection: alcohol-based hand rubs vs. hygienic handwashing: a multicentre questionnaire study with additional patch testing by the German Contact Dermatitis Research Group. *Br J Dermatol*. 2009;160(3):565-572.

240. Löffler H, Kampf G, Lachenmeier D, Diepgen TL, John SM. Allergic or irritant contact dermatitis after patch testing with alcohol—that is the point. *Contact Dermatitis*. 2012;67(6):386-387. doi:10.1111/cod.12003.

241. García-Gavín J, Pérez-Pérez L, Zulaica A. Hand eczema due to hygiene and antisepsis products: not only an irritative etiology. *Actas Dermosifiliogr*. 2012;103(9):845-846. doi:10.1016/j.ad.2012.06.002.

242. Ludwig E, Hausen BM. Sensitivity to isopropyl alcohol. *Contact Dermatitis*. 1977;3(5):240-244.

243. Kwon JA, Lee MS, Kim MY, Park YM, Kim HO, Kim CW. Allergic contact dermatitis from dodecyldiaminoethyl-glycine and isopropyl alcohol in a commercial disinfectant swab. *Contact Dermatitis*. 2003;48(6):339-340.

244. Vujevich J, Zirwas M. Delayed hypersensitivity to isopropyl alcohol. *Contact Dermatitis*. 2007;56(5):287. doi:10.1111/j.1600-0536.2006.00983.x.

245. Rotter ML. Hand washing and hand disinfection. In: Mayhall CG, ed. *Hospital Epidemiology and Infection Control*. 2nd ed. Philadelphia, PA: Lippincott Williams & Wilkins; 1999:1339-1355.

246. Comité Européen de Normalisation. *EN 12791:2015. Chemical Disinfectants and Antiseptics. Surgical Hand Disinfection. Test Method and Requirement (Phase 2, Step 2)*. Brussels, Belgium: Comité Européen de Normalisation; 2015.

247. Kampf G, Kramer A, Suchomel M. Lack of sustained efficacy for alcohol-based surgical hand rubs containing "residual active ingredients" according to EN 12791. *J Hosp Infect*. 2017;95(2):163-168.

248. Kampf G. Lack of antimicrobial efficacy of mecetronium etilsulfate in propanol-based hand rubs for surgical hand disinfection. *J Hosp Infect*. 2017;96(2):189-191.

249. Kampf G, Shaffer M, Hunte C. Insufficient neutralization in testing a chlorhexidine-containing ethanol-based hand rub can result in a false positive efficacy assessment. *BMC Infect Dis*. 2005;5:48.

250. Kampf G. Acquired resistance to chlorhexidine—is it time to establish an 'antiseptic stewardship' initiative? *J Hosp Infect*. 2016;94(3):213-227.

251. Slotosch CM, Kampf G, Löffler H. Effects of disinfectants and detergents on skin irritation. *Contact Dermatitis*. 2007;57:235-241.

Surgical Antisepsis

Gerald McDonnell

Surgical antisepsis is the application of microbicidal or microbistatic antimicrobial chemicals to skin, mucosa, and wounds to reduce the risk of infection. Antimicrobials have been used, at least since Pharaonic times, in the form of natural products or chemicals to care for wounds and to prevent miasma or contagia causing putrefaction and death.[1] Ignaz Semmelweis[2] and Joseph Lister[3] are considered the fathers of modern antisepsis because of their development of the early principles of antiseptic technique before the new science of bacteriology had evolved. Semmelweis,[2] in his treatise on childbed fever, observed a significantly higher rate of postpartum infections among women whose childbirth was managed by physicians compared with those managed by midwives. He recognized the relationship between puerperal infections and physicians' frequent practice of performing autopsies prior to providing obstetric care and childbirth. Following the implementation of simple hand washing, he demonstrated a decrease in the infection rate from 9.9% to approximately 2%. In 1867, Joseph Lister[3] published a technique of surgical preparation with carboxylic acid spray applied to the patient's skin, all instruments, and gauze, which also led to a dramatic decrease in the postoperative infection rate. Subsequently, the early bacteriologists, beginning with Robert Koch, studied the bacteria of the skin, suggested the possible contribution of these bacteria to the infection of wounds, and studied their reduction or elimination with antimicrobial agents. Price,[4] in his classic study of 1938, first proposed that skin bacteria could be considered as two sorts: transients and residents. He demonstrated the effect of hand washing and surgical scrubbing on the removal of skin flora and first showed that viable skin cannot be truly sterilized. Skin flora was studied by many investigators using various techniques as well as more detailed analysis on the various microbiomes that can exist on healthy and compromised skin.[5-12]

The major premise of surgical antisepsis is the removal or reduction of normal flora by the topical application of antimicrobial substances to the skin before a surgical procedure. With preoperative scrubbing and patient skin preparation, one hopes to reduce both transient and resident flora to the greatest extent and to maintain this state for the duration of the surgical procedure. Despite confident statements that skin disinfection can be achieved, considerable numbers of resident bacteria are found to survive antiseptic treatment in the deeper layers of the skin.[13] Early studies suggested that despite best attempts using widely accepted antiseptic agents, the number of skin bacteria cannot be lowered below a certain level.[14]

▶ SKIN AND SKIN FLORA

It is well established that skin flora plays an essential role in the development of wound infection.[7,10,15-17] Because an important function of the skin is to serve as a barrier against infection, antiseptic treatment should not be toxic or damaging to the skin,[18] cause skin reactions,[19,20] or interfere with the normal protective function of the skin.[16,17] Indirect effects such as removal of skin lipids, interference with the "acid mantle," and excessive drying may result in damage to skin, especially in frequent users of antiseptics such as surgeons and nurses.[16] As assessed by using objective physiologic parameters by Larson et al,[21,23] frequent hand washing can cause some damage to the stratum corneum. Such physiologic studies are needed for all antiseptics in addition to assessing efficacy, toxicity, absorption, and inactivation.[24-26]

The skin is a multilayered surface with irregular pits, ridges, and creases covered by cornified epithelial cells that are loosely attached to the deeper cell layers; thus, the skin provides a nesting place for bacterial flora and is also a potential source of airborne particles carrying microorganisms.[27] The surface is interrupted by the openings of sweat glands and pilosebaceous units. Because sweat is essentially sterile, slightly acidic, and flows continually, it keeps the sweat ducts clean of bacteria. In contrast, the ducts of sebaceous glands contain fatty and proteinaceous materials as well as cells, cell detritus, and salts that can serve as nutrients for a number of organisms composing the resident flora. The fat covers the epidermal surface and makes it water repellent. Its composition changes with age and thereby affects the type and quantity of normal flora. Normal flora also differs on various parts of the body surface, depending on the distribution of the skin secretory glands and their activity; the type, size, and density of hair; bacterial adherence; and antimicrobial antagonism.[6-9] In addition, certain regions of the body, such as the groin and the paragenital area of women, have extremely high bacterial counts (up to 10^7 colony-forming units [CFUs]/mL stripping solution).[28] Others confirmed Price's work from 1938 that the resident flora is concentrated mainly around and under fingernails.[4,29] Unfortunately, whereas it has been established that the subungual space is a significant reservoir of bacteria,[30] the routine surgical scrub is often ineffective at reducing the subungual counts to acceptable levels.[31] Recognizing the subungual space as a good indicator of the efficacy of personnel hand washes and surgical scrubs, new methods were developed for testing antiseptics by assessing the fluid obtained from artificially contaminated hands after scrubbing the subungual space.[32]

Many of these earlier studies have been verified in the detailed, molecular analysis of the microbiome on various parts of the skin and the role of resident and transient bacteria as part of a healthy population in comparison to a diseased or unhealthy skin state.[33,34] These studies have verified that the microbial population can highly diverse and variable depending on the person, regional anatomy, environmental factors, and various host factors (eg, immune system, personal hygiene, and genetic factors). The range of microorganisms present is now known to be wider than first observed in traditional microbiological culture methods.[7-9] The most commonly isolated bacteria included gram-positive, coagulase-negative staphylococci (eg, *Staphylococcus epidermidis*), *Micrococcus*, and Actinobacteria (eg, *Corynebacterium* and *Propionibacterium* species). Modern molecular techniques allow for the identification of a wider range of bacteria. Skin and mucous membrane bacteria are found to be in four major phyla: Actinobacteria (gram-positive bacteria such as *Propionibacterium*), Firmicutes (gram-positive bacteria such as *Staphylococcus*, *Bacillus*, and *Clostridium*), Bacteroidetes (gram-negative bacteria such as *Bacteroides*), and Proteobacteria (gram-negative bacteria such as *Escherichia coli* and *Pseudomonas*). The proportions of each of these can vary depending on the area of the skin or mucous membranes. For example, areas with increased moisture can lead to greater proportions of bacteria that grow well under humid conditions, such as gram-negative rods and *Staphylococcus aureus*, and areas with increased presence of sebaceous glands (eg, the face) see a greater proportion of lipophilic bacteria (eg, *Propionibacterium*)

due to the production of sebum in these areas. In addition to bacteria, other members of the skin flora can include a wide range of resident and transient microorganisms such as fungi, arthropods, and viruses. Of particular note are *Malassezia* species of fungi and *Demodex* arthropods (mites) are often considered as resident skin flora.[33,34]

Despite the differentiation of transient and resident flora, both types of flora play important roles in the development of health care–acquired infection (HAI). Many transient bacteria are loosely attached to the lipoidal components of the skin and are generally considered easy to remove using mechanical means. Resident flora, on the other hand, is much more difficult to completely remove and are relatively stable in terms of the density and types of organisms; however, the simple historical notion that transient bacteria are bad and resident flora are harmless can no longer be supported. Researchers demonstrated during the *S aureus* epidemic in the 1950s and 1960s that this pathogen may become part of the resident flora and may even be disbursed in large quantities by shedders.[24] Gram-negative bacteria also may lodge persistently, especially in damaged or moist skin.[35] Gram-negative bacteria recovered from nurses' hands after five consecutive hand washings with nonmedicated bar soap and tap water suggests that these organisms, found independently of patient contact, should be considered *nontransient* (or transitional) flora.[36] Regarding skin carriage of gram-negative bacteria, especially in the axilla, groin, and toe webs, it has been emphasized that each patient may carry his or her own environment.[9,10] In addition, the skin flora of personnel from different hospital services (eg, dermatology and oncology) can differ in both its composition and its antimicrobial susceptibility.[37] Dermatology personnel showed *S aureus* more frequently, whereas oncology personnel had a significantly higher carriage of gram-negative bacteria, yeast, and multiple antibiotic-resistant *Corynebacterium*. The isolates from nurses were found to be generally more resistant to many antibiotics, and two-thirds of the oncology nurses had methicillin-resistant staphylococci. These results support more recent studies with skin flora, where the microbial flora can vary depending on environmental factors (such as working locations). Furthermore, it should be reemphasized that there is wide variation in log differences in the density of bacteria across various sites of the body, with relatively low counts on the palm and much higher counts at other sites, such as the axilla and forehead.[6-10]

▶ MUCOSA AND WOUNDS

Whereas antisepsis can be more or less successful on unbroken skin, its use on exposed or visceral mucosa, open wounds, and burns is more problematic. Side effects that result from increased absorption of the antimicrobial chemical by the tissue and by the reduction of its activity by blood, exudates, and tissue result in less efficacious antiseptic regimens. Prevention of surgical infection and therapy of local infection are still considered achievable more effectively with systemic antibiotics.[15,38] Although there are many agents that can be specifically applied to wound and burn injuries to decrease infection, it should be emphasized that the primary therapy for prevention of infection in these settings is early mechanical or surgical debridement in association with early skin grafting of burn injuries. Antimicrobial agents, including antiseptics and antibiotics, should only be used in accordance with manufacturers' label claims, and these can vary regionally. But despite the emphasis on the appropriate use of prophylactic antibiotics to reduce the risk of surgical site infections (SSIs), the parallel use of different antiseptics is recommended to include preoperative bathing (with antimicrobial soaps or antiseptic agents), use of 2% mupirocin ointment in the nares (for decolonization of methicillin-resistant S aureus [MRSA] carriers), surgical site preparation (with an emphasis on the use of alcohols or alcohol/chlorhexidine combinations), surgical hand preparation (uses of antimicrobial soaps or alcohol hand rubs prior to glove donning), and triclosan-containing sutures.[15,38]

▶ SURGEONS AND ANTISEPSIS

Since Lister's[3] work, surgeons have been aware that wound infections can be prevented by the topical use of antimicrobial chemicals. Because bacteriologists could demonstrate that bacteria on the skin of surgeons or patients could cause wound infections, hand washing and preoperative surgical scrubbing became part of the system of aseptic surgery introduced since 1882 by Trendelenburg, von Bergmann, and Schimmelbusch in Germany and

by Halsted in the United States. Antisepsis and asepsis contributed to the rapid development of surgery, and the advent of antibiotics promised further expansion of the surgical horizons. Despite these advances, the rates of SSIs remain a concern and vary internationally. The SSIs are defined as infections of the incision or organ or space that occur after surgery[15] and usually occurring within 30 days of an operative procedure.[38] They can be further subdivided into infections that are limited to the skin and subcutaneous tissue at the site of incision (*superficial incisional*), including deep soft tissue (eg, muscle and fascia) at the surgical site (*deep incisional*), and/or any other part of the anatomy that was accessed during the procedure (*organ or space* SSIs). The SSIs can also be associated with infections that are associated with deep incisional or organ/space infections that occur within 1 year if implant is left in place. The surgical wound can also be classified into four major types that are also associated with increased infection risk due to the level of damage associated at the wound and other factors (Table 43.1).[38] The SSIs remain one of the most common HAIs, estimated to comprise 31% of all infections among hospitalized patients. Between 2006 and 2009, SSIs complicated an estimated 1.9% of surgical procedures in the United States. The Centers for Disease Control and Prevention (CDC) HAI prevalence survey found there were an estimated 157 500 SSIs associated with inpatient surgeries in 2011.[15] The SSIs alone can cause serious injury or death at significant cost to patients, families, and health care organizations. A systematic review of the literature on SSI from 1998 to 2014 found the estimated average cost of an SSI ranged between $10 433 and $25 546, which equates to approximately $13 300 to $35 400 in 2019 costs.[15,44] In addition, infection remains a further limiting factor of surgical success in certain patients (eg, the obese, diabetics, trauma patients). But, as highlighted earlier,

TABLE 43.1 Surgical wound classification

Class	Wound Infection Rate[a]	Definition
Class I/clean	0.2%-2.9%	An operative wound in which infection or inflammation is not encountered; aseptic technique is maintained; and the respiratory, gastrointestinal, genital, or urinary tract is not entered
Class II/clean-contaminated	0.9%-3.9%	An operative wound in which the respiratory, gastrointestinal, biliary, genital, or urinary tracts is entered under controlled conditions without unusual contamination or when a minor break in aseptic technique occurs
Class III/contaminated	1.3%-8.5%	Open, fresh, accidental wounds. In addition, operations with major breaks in sterile technique or gross spillage from the gastrointestinal tract and incisions in which acute, nonpurulent inflammation are encountered
Class IV/dirty	2.1%-48%	Old wounds with devitalized tissue and those that involve existing clinical infection or perforated viscera

[a]Rates are estimated and can vary depending on the reports in the literature. (Based on Berríos-Torres et al,[15] World Health Organization,[38] Reichman and Greenberg,[39] Onyekwelu et al,[40] Ortega et al,[41] Rosenthal et al,[42] and Cruse.[43])

infections cannot always be controlled by antibiotics alone and are becoming a greater risk with the continuing development of antibiotic-resistant gram-positive (eg, MRSA, vancomycin-resistant *Enterococcus* [VRE], and various types of mycobacteria) and gram-negative (eg, carbapenem-resistant Enterobacteriaceae) bacteria. Fortunately, the surgical community has retained antisepsis and various usages of biocides as an important component of surgical technique as well as continuing to identify alternatives to antibiotic dependence.[15,38,45] Guidelines for the prevention of surgical wound infections in the United States[15] and internationally[38] address the continuing need for appropriate surgical antisepsis.

Staff selecting an antiseptic must be familiar with the spectrum of activity and limitations, appropriate use, potential side effects, risk of failures, potential contamination, cost-effectiveness, and, last but not least, the art to motivate people to use these agents correctly.[17,46-49] An initial recommendation of the CDC[50] that hand washing with plain soap suffices for routine use in hospitals was accepted but with some reservations. The data in laboratory and clinical studies could often be variable, depending on the product formulation, test methods used, and comparisons to controls. The overall evidence of the benefit of antimicrobial soaps in many settings continues to be of some debate. For example, the US Food and Drug Administration (FDA) issued a final ruling in 2016 that over-the-counter (OTC) consumer antiseptic wash products containing certain active ingredients (eg, triclosan and triclocarban) can no longer be marketed due to safety and effectiveness concerns in comparison to regular soap and water but at that time deferred ruling on other biocides such as benzalkonium chloride and chloroxylenol (PCMX).[51] Similarly, for health care antiseptics, such as health care personnel hand washes, health care personnel hand rubs, surgical hand scrubs, surgical hand rubs, and patient antiseptic skin preparations, a range of biocides (particularly including triclosan) could no longer be generally recognized as safe for health care antiseptic use. In addition, they deferred ruling on a further six types of widely used biocides in antiseptic use (benzalkonium chloride, benzethonium chloride, chloroxylenol, alcohol, isopropyl alcohol, and povidone-iodine). Some widely used biocides such as chlorhexidine have a unique situation as they are currently ineligible for evaluation under the FDA's OTC drug review for use as a health care antiseptic and therefore continue to require approval under a new drug application to the FDA prior to marketing.

But overall, the use of antiseptics (or skin/hand disinfectants) in health care environments continues to be supported by consensus and evidence-based guidelines internationally.[15,17,38,52] But the recommendations have changed depending on the evidence, such as with the emphasis on the use of alcohol-based antiseptics (hand rubs) over antimicrobial soaps (hand washes) than in the past (particularly in the United States, where initial use of various hand rubs was initially low in comparison to other areas such as in Europe; see chapters 19 and 42). These guidelines provide a detailed review of the evidence to support these recommendations and in summary include

- For general health care hand hygiene, hand washing with water and soap (that may or may not contain antimicrobials) is recommended when the hands are visibly soiled. In other cases, alcohol-based antiseptics/hand disinfectants or washing with antimicrobial soap and water are recommended in many clinical situations such as before direct patient contact, prior or following glove use etc.
- For surgical hand antisepsis or hand disinfection, alcohol-based antiseptics/hand disinfectants or washing with antimicrobial soap and water are recommended prior to glove donning. Some guidelines specifically recommend the use of products that have some persistent activity on the skin following application, such as in the case of chlorhexidine-containing soaps or alcohol hand rubs (see chapter 22).
- Patient showering or bathing prior to surgery with either nonantimicrobial or antimicrobial soap or an alternative antimicrobial agent. The most commonly used biocide for the application is chlorhexidine (eg, in soaps or washcloth impregnated products) but also other biocides such as triclosan and chloroxylenol.
- Presurgical, intraoperative skin preparation with alcohol-based antiseptics, which may or may not include chlorhexidine. Other widely used biocides include chlorhexidine and iodine (eg, iodophor) products, but alcohols are generally found to be more effective.

Intraoperative irrigation of tissues with an aqueous iodophor solution under restrictive situations, such as of deep or subcutaneous tissues, or in certain situations before wound closure of clean or clean-contaminated wounds.

In addition, it is clear that such products should meet the required efficacy, safety, and registration requirements (as applicable) for the countries in which they are marketed in (eg, under the FDA requirements[26] or the European Union Biocidal Product Regulation[53] and associated efficacy test standards) (see chapters 61, 62, and 63). These products should also be specifically used in compliance to manufacturer's instructions and labeled claims.

▶ ANTISEPTICS USED IN SURGERY

In this chapter, we use the definitions proposed by the FDA OTC Antimicrobial Panel II[54] and finalized in 2017 for the use classification of health care antiseptics.[26] These are considered drug products that are generally intended for use by health care professionals in a hospital setting or other health care situations outside the hospital. They can include washes that are designed to be applied with water (eg, health care personnel hand washes and surgical hand scrubs) or rubs (or leave-on products) that are applied and not rinsed off after use (eg, health care personnel hand rubs, surgical hand rubs, and patient antiseptic skin preparations). Overall these include

- Health care personnel hand washes or hand rubs: antiseptic-containing preparation designed for frequent use; they reduce the number of transient microorganisms on intact skin to an initial baseline level after adequate applications (eg, with hand washes by washing, rinsing, and drying); they are considered broad-spectrum, fast acting, and, if possible, persistent. Note that persistence refers prolonged activity of the applied product that assures antimicrobial activity during the interval between washings and is considered an important for a safe and effective health care personnel hand wash (as well as other products in the following text).
- Surgical hand scrubs or rubs: an antiseptic-containing preparation that significantly reduces the number of microorganisms on intact skin; it is broad-spectrum, fast acting, and persistent.

Patient antiseptic skin preparations (ie, patient preoperative and preinjection skin preparations): fast-acting, broad-spectrum, and persistent antiseptic containing preparation that significantly reduces the number of microorganisms on intact skin. Examples include products used for patient preoperative or preinjection skin preparations.

The antimicrobial ingredients of such preparations were initially placed by the FDA[54] in three categories: *category I*, generally recognized as safe and effective and not misbranded; *category II*, not generally recognized as safe and effective or misbranded; and *category III*, available data insufficient to classify as safe and effective, and further testing is required. These have now been replaced with products defined as being under monograph conditions (ie, previously considered category I) and nonmonograph conditions (referring to the original categories II and III products). First aid antiseptics are considered separately under a separate monograph.[55] These regulatory requirements led to many restrictions on the range of biocides that may be used in these products as well as the continuing requirements for new drug applications for the specific use of certain types of biocides (as discussed earlier). Equally in Europe, the range of antimicrobials are restricted based on the environmental safety, antimicrobial effectiveness, and toxicity requirements defined for these types of products.[53,56] For detailed information on the chemical, antimicrobial, and toxic properties of each active component, the reader is referred to the respective chapter of this book.

Alcohols

Alcohols are effective antiseptic agents with a broad spectrum of activity (see chapter 19). Isopropyl alcohol is known to be effective against bacteria, mycobacteria, fungi, and large or lipid-containing viruses (eg, human

immunodeficiency virus [HIV] and hepatitis B virus [HBV]) but is significantly less effective against hydrophilic viruses (eg, rotavirus or parvoviruses) in the use of dilutions of 60% to 95%. Ethyl alcohol has a similar spectrum of activity, with similar restrictions on efficacy against hydrophilic viruses (see chapters 19 and 42).[57] Alcohols are now well established as offering the most rapid and reliable reduction of microbial counts on skin for personnel hand rubbing, surgical scrub, and patient preoperative skin preparations (see chapters 16, 20, 21, 42, and 49). One of the concerns regarding the use of alcohol preparations is the flammability and potential for burn injury in the operating room,[58] although when they are used appropriately, there is little risk of such injury.[16,17,59]

The benefit of alcohol preparations containing emollient and refatting additives that retard evaporation and in combination with other antimicrobial chemicals have been reported in multiple studies (see chapter 42).[60] Other opportunities include the optimized concentration of alcohols in these formulations and application times.[61] The call for more effective and rapidly acting antiseptics has increased the interest of health care workers in alcohol antiseptics and has stimulated the industry to offer such preparations with and without the addition of an additional antimicrobial chemical, such as chlorhexidine gluconate.

Chlorhexidine

Chlorhexidine gluconate replaced hexachlorophene as an active ingredient for surgical antiseptics in the 1970s. In wash formulations that can typically range from 0.5% to 4% detergent preparation, it has a broad antimicrobial spectrum, but it is less active against gram-negative than gram-positive bacteria, it is not active against mycobacteria (see chapter 22), it is moderately active against fungi, and it is generally active against enveloped viruses (but no nonenveloped viruses). Although not as rapidly acting as alcohol, chlorhexidine gluconate is well accepted as a surgical antiseptic, with residual activity caused by its strong affinity for the skin and little interference by blood. In addition to wash products, it is also marketed at lower concentrations (eg, 0.1%-0.5%) in alcohols, thereby combining the rapid effect of alcohol with the residual effect of chlorhexidine as well as in impregnated dressing (eg, used for application to the skin prior to and during the insertion of vascular devices through the skin). Chlorhexidine is considered relatively safe but has been associated with isolated episodes of hypersensitivity, including anaphylactic shock (see chapter 22).[62,63]

Iodine

Tincture of iodine has been used in surgery since its introduction by Grossich in Fiume in 1908 for preoperative skin preparation (see chapter 16).[64] The old-fashioned tincture (7% iodine and 5% potassium iodide in 85% ethyl alcohol) was much too strong and caused considerable skin burns.[65] Examples of more modern iodine tinctures include solutions or tinctures containing 2 ± 0.2 g iodine and 2.1 to 2.6 g sodium iodide in 100 mL purified water or in 44% to 50% ethyl alcohol. Both preparations are considered reasonably safe and rapidly acting with a broad antimicrobial spectrum, but the solution has overall been found to be inferior to the tincture in clinical use.[65] One percent or 2% iodine with an equal amount of potassium iodide in 70% ethyl alcohol was considered as the most effective in reducing skin flora.[65] Due to previous risks of skin burns, these products were often recommended in the past to be removed from the operative site immediately on drying with 70% alcohol to prevent skin burns. This also applied to the use of tincture of iodine in other applications such as before punctures to obtain blood, body fluids, or tissue specimens. The problem of local toxicity has limited the use of tincture of iodine or aqueous iodine in recent years, mainly because of the arrival of alternative iodophor preparations. Iodophors are complexes of iodine with carriers such as the nonsurfactant compound polyvinylpyrrolidone (povidone or PVP) or the surfactant compound poloxamer that slowly release free iodine and thereby reduce staining and local toxicity while retaining the broad antimicrobial activity of iodine (see chapter 16). An "iodine flux" between the deeper layers of the skin and the skin surface has been claimed in the past to allow several hours of residual bactericidal activity after the initial scrub, but these effects are not consider as effective as in chlorhexidine applications.[16,17]

Initially, iodophors were used widely on skin, mucosa, wounds, burns, and even in body cavities, and an elevation of blood iodine levels was noted.[54] Although safety and efficacy reports in the literature do vary, overall the use of iodophors in these applications are considered to have a favorable risk/benefit profile and including in acute and chronic wound treatments.[66] Iodophors, most commonly povidone- or poloxamer-iodine, are used in concentrations of 0.75% to 2.0% available iodine (0.75-2 mg free iodine/L). Their activity is relatively slow, and the presence of organic materials can neutralize the free iodine (see chapter 16). Studies following the surprising finding of contamination of povidone-iodine with *Pseudomonas cepacia* showed that the ratio of free to bound iodine increases with dilution.[67,68] Other reports suggested that *P cepacia* was protected in these formulations in a biofilm, likely to be sourced during the manufacturing of the product.[69] Example of a low-iodine hand soap (eg, 0.05% complexed iodine) have been patented and developed and shown to be effective as personnel hand washing products, but these has not seen widespread use in clinical practice.[70]

Phenol Derivatives

Substituted phenols were discussed extensively by the FDA OTC Antimicrobial Panels (FDA[71]) and are widely used an antiseptic antimicrobials.[46,51,54,71] For health care

use (including patient skin preparation, in health care personal hand washes/hand rubs, and surgical preparations), these have predominantly included triclosan, para-chloro-*meta*-xylenol (chloroxylenol or PCMX), and in the past hexachlorophene (see chapter 42).[51] Hexachlorophene at 0.1% to 3% in various formulations was widely used as an antiseptic from the 1950s up to the early 1970s, when reports of toxicity eventually led to the restrictive use of this biocide under prescription.[17,72] Similar to other bisphenols, like triclosan, it had good bactericidal activity against gram-positive bacteria (particular those associated with the skin microbiome) but less activity against gram-negative bacteria and fungi (which could be improved by formulation effects such as in combination with chelating agents). This led to an increased interest in alternative biocides such as triclosan, another bisphenol used in concentrations of 0.5% to 4%. Triclosan became one of the widely used antimicrobials in both consumer and health care applications, due to its spectrum of antimicrobial activity, persistent activity on the skin, and was considered relatively nontoxic. The widespread use of triclosan led to concerns over its benefit over the use of nonantimicrobial soaps (particularly in the consumer area) and more recently the banning or restrictive use of triclosan in antiseptic applications, such as by the FDA in 2016.[26,51] These included risk-benefits discussion on the benefits of the broad use of antimicrobial in the general public, increased reports of toxic reactions including hormonal effects, environmental concerns due to the persistence of the biocide and risks to aquatic life, and, finally, reports on the development of increased resistance in bacteria and cross-resistance to antibiotics.[51] Although these reports continue to be the subject of debate,[73,74] the use of triclosan in both consumer and health care antiseptic applications has significantly reduced and have more focused on particular applications such as the use in antimicrobial sutures that have shown clinical benefit.[15,38,75]

The decreased used of triclosan for surgical applications has been in parallel with an increased (or renewed) interest in the use of chloroxylenol, a halophenol.[51] Similar to other antiseptic phenolics, chloroxylenol (in the 0.5% to 4% concentration range) is very dependent on formulation effects to optimize antimicrobial activity, intrinsically having greater activity against gram-positive bacteria than gram-negative bacteria (such as *Pseudomonas* species) or fungi.[17,51] It can also demonstrate persistent activity on the skin, a particular benefit on surgical antiseptic applications. Studies on the potential or resistance or biocide tolerance development with chloroxylenol do not appear to show the same risks as with triclosan.[74,76] At this time, the FDA has delayed final rulemaking on the safety and efficacy of chloroxylenol in consumer and health care antiseptic use.[26,51]

A further phenol derivative that is widely used as an antiseptic is salicylic acid, in particular for the treatment of acne due to being an exfoliant and demonstrating bactericidal/fungicidal activity. Typical concentrations used in these applications range from 0.5% to 6%, in skin washes and as ointments/skin paints.[51] Other applications include their use for the topical treatment of warts and psoriasis, but they are not generally used for surgical applications.

In general, it can be important to understand the length of surgical operation when deciding on the agents for skin preparation. Some studies have reported a direct relationship between the length of operation and risk for infection.[77,78] Alcohol has the most rapid onset but is limited as a single agent by its lack of residual activity but can be combined with other antimicrobials (such as chlorhexidine as described earlier). Iodine/iodophors have minimal residual activity, and some residual activity has been reported with triclosan and chloroxylenol. The excellent residual effect of chlorhexidine may be advantageous in prolonged procedures.[15,17,38,51]

▶ PERSONNEL HAND WASHING WITH ANTISEPTIC PREPARATIONS

For more than 140 years, it has been known that infectious agents can be carried on hands.[79] Whether acquired from corpses, patients, unclean dressings, or contaminated instruments and surfaces, they can survive as transient flora on the skin for some time, and some may become part of the "nontransient" flora.[24,35,36] Hand washing has been accepted for many decades as the most effective way to interrupt the chain of transmission of infection from one person to another. The guidelines for the hand washing and hand antisepsis have evolved over the years since the publication of widely used evidence-based guidelines such as the 1985 CDC *Guidelines for Handwashing and Hospital Environment Control*.[80] These include changes in the recommendations in the types and methods of hand antisepsis.[17,52] It is practical to consider that the use of soap (antimicrobial or nonantimicrobial) and water is preferred when the hands are visible soiled (such as with blood or other body fluids), but for routine use that convenient use of antimicrobial (usually alcohol-based) hand rubs (that are often preferred) or antimicrobial soap and water can be used. The guidelines specify situations when the use of antiseptic hand rubs or hand washes should be used, to include before and after direct contact with a patient, prior to donning gloves before specific patient procedures (such as catheter insertion), and on contacting patient fluids or inanimate surfaces in close vicinity to a patient (even if not visibly soiled). The methods of handling are equally important to observe. Although deferring to manufacturer's instructions, the guidelines recommend steps in the use of hand rubs and hand washes, such as prewetting the hands before applying soap, washing for at least 15 seconds, followed by rinsing and drying.[17,52] In many clinical situations, washing with plain soap has been recommended for some time unless otherwise indicated.[80] Unfortunately, such guidelines were often interpreted to mean that antiseptic hand wash agents were to be replaced in all hospital areas with nonmedicated soap. Routine hand washing practices in hospitals already were often less than optimal in frequency, length and technique of washing, and quantity of soap used.[81-86] Thus, the removal of antimicrobial soaps with residual activity may have had a negative effect on infection control in some institutions. Several studies demonstrated that hand washing with antiseptic soaps can reduce HAIs.[70,87-90] Therefore, the guidelines continue to recommend the appropriate use of antiseptics in higher risks situations, including in surgical wards to minimize or eliminate the transient flora acquired from infected patients and reduce the resident flora, which may include gram-positive and gram-negative bacteria.[17,52] Hand washing frequency and technique are dependent on many factors such as the motivation of personnel, the selection of an acceptable hand washing agent, and the availability of either sinks for hand washing or dispensers for waterless preparations.[17,52,90] Alcohol-based hand rinses are highly efficacious, and such products are recommended as a health care personnel hand wash, particularly when a sink and running water are inaccessible.[17,52] Senior clinicians and nurses play important roles both as decision makers and as role models for their associates.

When selecting an antimicrobial preparation for personnel hand washing, a number of points should be considered. These include efficacy of removing and killing microorganisms (in accordance with label claims), rapidity of antimicrobial action, persistent (residual) activity or substantivity, ease of use, and lack of skin irritation. Other issues include input from employees regarding the use of the product (eg, feel and fragrance, to improve compliance), cross-reactivity potential (eg, with gloves), and use of dispenser systems (eg, dispensing of defined product volumes).

Using a standardized 15-second hand washing technique, in many cases, antimicrobial soaps may not show significant increases over plain soap, such as with chlorhexidine gluconate preparations.[85] But such reports can vary depending on the test methods used and specific product formulation under investigation. Plain soaps also vary considerable in microbial removal from the skin and can also be associated with negative effects such as irritation, increased in bacterial levels, and as sources of pathogens due to contamination.[17] But antimicrobial hand washes such as those containing chlorhexidine, over repeated washes, because of the persistent activity of the biocide, can show a significantly higher reduction of skin flora than nonantimicrobial soaps. In most cases, comparisons of higher concentrations of chlorhexidine (eg, 4% in comparison to 1% or 2% formulations) demonstrate greater antimicrobial activity, but this can also vary depending on the formulation.[17] Chlorhexidine gluconate

(0.5%) in 70% isopropyl alcohol also was compared with 7.5% povidone-iodine surgical scrub in a 15-second personnel hand wash after artificial contamination.[91] The alcoholic preparation produced significantly lower counts with substantive (residual) effect after 24 washes over 8 hours. A similar study comparing alcohol-based hand rinses with 4% chlorhexidine gluconate and plain soap showed that alcohol rinses caused the most rapid, immediate reduction of skin flora, but chlorhexidine resulted in more persistent reduction.[23] Based on subjective measures of product acceptability, chlorhexidine gluconate was the mildest and most preferred preparation in these studies.

Alcohol-containing hand rubs are often preferred and not just due to their convenience in use, as not requiring water (see chapters 19 and 42). Many studies of antimicrobial detergent/soap-based preparations were performed using 1- to 2-minute exposure to the active agent. Using the Vienna test method, as an example, a 3 log reduction of bacteria from artificially contaminated fingertips was obtained after a 2-minute wash with povidone-iodine and after a 1-minute wash with chlorhexidine gluconate.[92] In comparison, a 1-minute rubbing with 60% isopropanol resulted in a more than 4 log reduction. Using the same test method, in a comparison of 14 hand washing, alcoholic preparations showed the highest log reduction, followed by chlorhexidine and povidone-iodine, with chlorhexidine showing the best residual activity after 10 applications.[93] From these studies, alcohol preparations were the fastest acting because of mildness and persistent activity, chlorhexidine soap is the most acceptable for frequent washes, chlorhexidine alcohol combines the rapidity of alcohol with the persistence of chlorhexidine, and povidone-iodine requires at least a 2-minute wash to develop its activity fully. Older studies did reports that antimicrobial hand washes containing PCMX[94,95] or triclosan[93] were overall less effective than chlorhexidine- and iodophor-based products, and the rapidity of their antimicrobial action was considered intermediate.[96] But formulations of these biocides have improved overall efficacy and compliance to standardized test method requirements.[46,97]

Because of universal precautions, health care workers are required to wear gloves during patient contact if contamination with blood or body fluids could occur. The present recommendation is removal of gloves and hand washing after each contact.[17,52] The reuse of gloves by washing following use is not recommended. There are conflicting reports exist regarding the efficacy of disinfecting the gloved hand.[98-100] It may be expected that the use of different soaps in removing bacteria from gloved hands can reduce microbial levels.[99] But in other studies, such as in a controlled, experimental trial with artificially contaminated gloves, showed after treatment with a 10-second wash with nonmedicated soap, a 60% isopropanol commercial preparation, or 4% chlorhexidine gluconate were not consistently cleaned, and the internal hands of the study persons were cross-contaminated with

the test organisms after removal of the gloves after the use of nonmedicated soap.[98] These authors concluded that it may not be prudent to wash and reuse gloves between patients. A further practical consideration is the potential for damage to the gloves from the use of antiseptics and water on the gloves, which can lead to a loss of glove integrity and the potential for the leaching of glove-based chemicals due to damage that can lead to issues such as irritation.[17]

▶ SURGICAL SCRUB

The preoperative antiseptic preparation of the surgeon's hands and forearms has been accepted as an effective infection control measure since the late 1800s. Price[4] performed the first scientifically sound study to show the effect of surgical scrubbing on the skin flora. Despite his and numerous subsequent studies, the technique and length of time required for the most effective surgical scrub are still being discussed, and no single procedure is accepted by all surgeons. Overall, as products can vary in formulation and concentration of biocides, it is important to follow approved (or regulatory cleared) instructions for use to ensure optimum antimicrobial activity. In general, the recommended surgical scrub procedures require that surgeons and nurses first remove any jewelry (eg, rings and watches), clean under the fingernails with water, and then antiseptic use (preferably with a biocide that presents with persistent activity such as chlorhexidine) in accordance with manufacturer's instructions.[17,52] For hand washes, this includes washing the hands and forearms thoroughly with an antimicrobial soap, followed by rinsing and drying prior to donning gloves. For hand rubs, it is recommended that the hands are first washed with a nonantimicrobial soap, rinsed, and dried, and then the alcohol solution is applied and rubbed into the hands and forearms; the hands should be allowed to dry before donning gloves. The volume of antiseptic used can vary depending on the size of the hands/forearms being treated, and there is no need to require extended contact times for antisepsis over those typically recommended by the manufacturer (2-6 min, in general). After the scrub, the prepared areas are covered with a sterile gown and sterile gloves, adhering to the concept of asepsis by establishing an effective barrier between personnel and the patient's surgical wound.[101]

In the past 20 years, numerous alterations of the "classic" scrub procedures were proposed and accepted. Bristle brushes were replaced by disposable plastic brushes, sponges were impregnated with an antiseptic, antiseptic agents were changed, the time of scrubbing was shortened, and recently the need for brushing itself was no longer recommended due to no direct benefit in reduce microbial levels and potential of damage to the skin.[17,52,102,103] For example, a "classic" 10-minute two-brush scrub using an iodophor surgical scrub preparation was compared to a 5-minute no-brush scrub using another iodophor and a 3-minute no-brush with plain soap, drying with a sterile towel, and subsequent application of an ethanol-hexachlorophene foam; the shorter no-brush scrubs were as effective as the two-brush technique.[104] The lack of any benefit for using a brush or even a sponge has been particularly highlighted in studies than compared soap-based products to alcohol-based hand rubs, such as in studies comparing application of a 61% alcohol/1% chlorhexidine gluconate formulation being more effective at reducing levels on the skin compared to using a 4% chlorhexidine soap-based formulation with brushing.[103] Other researches have suggested the use of alternative, mechanical-based devices as methods for surgical hand preparation. An example was a 90-second jet washing method that was found to be more effective than a 10-minute scrub[105] as well as many other patent devices that include other types of antimicrobials (eg, hydrogen peroxide or ultraviolet [UV] light),[106,107] but such devices have not been commercially successful.[105]

Antiseptic scrubbing compounds other than alcohols have been shown to be more effective than soap and water, and many also have persistent and accumulative effects.[17,108-110] Hexachlorophene, used previously as a 3% antiseptic soap, was replaced as a surgical scrub in the early 1970s, as discussed earlier.[111] Iodophors and, later, chlorhexidine gluconate became the antiseptics of choice for surgical scrubbing. A 6-minute scrub with a widely used 4% chlorhexidine gluconate detergent preparation (Hibiclens®) was demonstrated many years ago to be effective at removing transient flora from the artificially infected hand and showed good activity and long-term (residual) activity against the resident flora.[112,113] Generally, this preparation was established to be more effective than 0.75% povidone-iodine and 3% hexachlorophene soaps used at that time. This report confirmed earlier findings in England, where 4% chlorhexidine had been introduced several years before it was available in the United States. Chlorhexidine gluconate has also been shown to reduce bacterial skin counts faster, to a greater degree, and more persistently.[114] Generally, chlorhexidine gluconate has been found to be less affected by blood than povidone-iodine.[114] Despite many experimental studies suggesting distinct advantages of certain preparations, the relative impact of these scrub agents on the postoperative infection rate remains an area of debate, but they are widely respected as being important in reducing the levels of bacteria under gloves during surgical use and thereby reducing the risk of infection from these sources.[17,52]

It was initially established in the 1960s that a 2-minute standard hand wash using 0.5% chlorhexidine in 70% ethanol reduced more of the resident skin flora than a 2-minute wash with an antiseptic detergent. But more recent investigations (summarized in chapters 22 and 49) have firmly established the benefits of alcohol-based hand rubs in surgical hand preparation and particularly when incorporating other biocides with persistent activity such as chlorhexidine. Despite their widespread use in Europe and other parts of the world for these applications, up to recently in the United States iodophors and chlorhexidine gluconate soaps were still the preferred agents for surgical scrubbing. Alcohol preparations, such as those with 0.5% chlorhexidine, are now used more frequently and not only in emergency medicine but also in operating rooms, especially by people with skin irritation caused by detergent-based antiseptics. Generally, alcohol preparations are well accepted by the user, but their acceptance depends greatly on the emollients and other ingredients added to alcohol formulations and when not excluded due to personnel (eg, religious) reasons and their refatting capability.[17,21-23,115]

The time required for scrubbing with nonalcoholic agents has historically been reported to be between 5 and 10 minutes for the classic scrubbing procedure[4,116] with the use of modern antimicrobial agents. But more recent studies that examined several different antiseptic preparations, such as chlorhexidine, suggested that scrubbing durations as short as 3 minutes may be as beneficial as longer classic scrub durations.[17,52] Overall, the optimal duration of the surgical scrub and the agent of choice will depend on the manufacturer's instructions, and these should be established based on the conducting standardized in vivo efficacy tests in comparison to controls.[26,117] The current guidelines recommend at least a 2- to 6-minute scrub depending on the labeling of the scrub preparations, and that there is little to no benefit to apply longer scrub times that were traditionally used.[17,52]

Other factors such as the use of artificial nails, nail length, the use of nail polish, and the wearing of jewelry in the operating theater have been discussed as factors potentially contributing to the development of infection. These are generally regarded as being bad practices, even though sufficient data may not be available to confirm the independent relationship between these factors and postoperative infection rates.[17,52,101]

Antiseptic principles for the conduct of surgical procedures have been recognized since the time of Lister. Although much appears to be ritualistic, closer examination of the practice of surgery led to recognized ways to increase and decrease the risk of infection in the surgical wound. Virtually all surgical procedures begin with the preparation of the staff's skin at the site of surgery as a first step in reducing the risk in a "sterile" surgical field and before donning sterile gloves. The bacteria of the skin that remain or proliferate after a surgical scrub are at risk of colonizing the incision (in particular during a breach of the gloves) and effect a postoperative wound infection. The three primary tenets of the surgical scrub include removal of debris, maximal killing of both transient and resident bacteria, and essentially abiding by the general principle to "do no harm."

▶ PREOPERATIVE PREPARATION OF PATIENTS' SKIN

As discussed earlier, the skin is contaminated with a variety of microorganisms that can be both resident or transient parts of the many types of microbiomes that can exist on various parts of the skin and mucous membranes. It is also clear that many surgical sites infections are caused by the patient's own, endogenous microorganisms, and particularly is cases with *S aureus* and coagulase-negative staphylococci.[39,118] Therefore, the control of the cross-contamination of the surgical incision area and development of infection by growth of a microorganism is a key goal in the guidelines to prevent SSIs.[15,38] These include the correct preoperative use of prophylactic antibiotics and antiseptic treatment of the skin prior to surgical incision. It is impossible to practically sterilize the skin and indeed likely that every surgical site is a (or is at risk of) contamination from endogenous skin flora. But reducing the levels and types of microorganisms on the skin at these incision areas is good practice.[15,38,101]

There is no one way to prepare the skin surface for an operation. Lister's carbolic acid was the first of many agents used to reduce the risk of infection for the patient. For many years, the traditional recommendation had been a 5-minute scrub with an antimicrobial detergent (or 1-minute alcohol wash) to remove skin debris as well as to defat the skin, exposing the bacteria within hair follicles. Application of an antiseptic solution (usually povidone-iodine or chlorhexidine) was then undertaken as the final preparation of the skin before draping.[15,38] This approach led to excellent clinical results of wound infections of 1% to 2% in clean cases during the 1970s, when compared to other practices.[43] In more recent years, the use of alcohol-based antiseptics that may or may not include other biocides like chlorhexidine and iodophors has been recommended in most international, evidence-based guidance's to reduce the risks of SSIs[15,38]; however, there are some exceptions, for example, when the use of alcohol is contraindicated such as on mucous membranes and in the ear, or when a risk of pooling can lead to a fire risk during the procedure. In these latter cases, the use of chlorhexidine is preferred in comparison to other biocides such as iodophors,[15] but this may vary depending the antiseptic product claims and regulatory clearances. The preoperative skin preparation methods, types of antimicrobials used, and duration of skin preparation continue to be a matter of some debate and investigation. Other impacts include the removal of hair from the skin, antiseptic lavage of wounds, the use of antimicrobial drapes, preoperative bathing with antiseptics, the use of antimicrobial sutures, and advanced antimicrobial wound dressing.[15,38]

Overall, the guidelines internationally have gained consensus on the evidence to support the following practices to reduce the risk of SSIs.[15,38,101]

- It is logical to remove gross debris from the skin surface and any associated crevices prior to surgery.[119,120] Patient showering or bathing prior to surgery is recommended with either nonantimicrobial or antimicrobial soap or an alternative antimicrobial agent. The evidence would suggest the overall benefit is to reduce the level of resident and transient microorganisms on the skin, but the overall benefit of the use of antimicrobials remains of some debate.[38,120,121] The mostly commonly used and studied antimicrobial for this purpose is chlorhexidine (in various types of antiseptic products such as soaps or washcloth impregnated products), but others include triclosan and chloroxylenol.

- Further preoperative skin preparation or nasal decolonization in patients known to have nasal carriage of *S aureus*. This will typically include the use of a 2% mupirocin ointment in intranasal applications (eg, two times daily for 5 days) and may (or may not) also include preoperative bathing with a chlorhexidine-containing antiseptic. This is particularly recommended in patients preparing for cardiothoracic and orthopedic surgery but may also be appropriate for other surgeries.[38]

- Aesthetics were often the reason for traditional preoperative removal of hair from the operative site, but this practice is now discouraged. Hair removal is not considered necessary prior to incision, unless it may specifically interfere during the surgical procedure.[122] If hair removal is required, shaving is not recommended and methods such as clipping or the use of depilatory (hair removal) products should be used. These will overall reduce the risks of skin damage, when used appropriately.

- Presurgical, intraoperative skin preparation with alcohol-based antiseptics, which may or may not include chlorhexidine. Other widely used biocides include chlorhexidine and iodine (eg, iodophor) products, but alcohols are generally found to be more effective. Overall, no one type of preoperative skin preparation has been shown consistently to reduce SSI rates, despite studies that show differences in their safety and effectiveness.[121] But overall, the selection of a product will depend on the needs of the surgical procedure on the patient (eg, the location on the body) and the surgical staff. Products should be chosen and used in accordance with the manufacturer's labeling. In the United States, for example, this will include clearance by the FDA in compliance to antiseptic requirements.[26,54] The guidelines also highlight the importance of the safe and effective use of any antiseptic used, including any contraindications, storage, and disposal requirements.

- In general, it is not recommended to apply antimicrobial agents (eg, antiseptic or antibiotic ointments, solutions, or powders) to the surgical wound. Although the intraoperative irrigation of tissues with an aqueous iodophor solution under restrictive situations has been recommended, such as of deep or subcutaneous tissues, or in certain situations before wound closure of clean or clean-contaminated wounds.[15,38]

- Equally, the use of advanced, including antimicrobial, wound dressings are not generally recommended over standard dressings that use dry absorbent materials. Advanced dressings are defined by the World Health Organization (WHO) as types of material dressing that promote wound healing by maintaining a moist environment in the wound during the healing process.[38] These dressings are based on materials such as semipermeable membranes, hydrocolloids, and alginates but can also include antimicrobials such as polyhexamethylene biguanides (PMHB) and silver (eg, in nanoparticles; see chapter 74). The benefits of these dressing can vary in efficacy (for wound healing and reducing SSIs), costs, and potential harms.[38,123,124] Overall, the guidelines suggest that there is not enough evidence on the risk benefits of using these materials, and they are therefore not generally recommended to be used to reduce SSIs.[15,38]
- At this time, the use of other technologies are not generally recommended, due to a lack of evidence to support a reduction in SSI rates.[15,38,101,125,126] Examples are the use of plastic adhesive drapes with or without antimicrobial properties (such as iodine-based drapes),[127] although some guidance do recommend the use of adhesive drapes that contain iodophors due to more recent evidence.[120,128] The use of these materials in accordance with manufacturer's instructions is important to ensure effectiveness and reduce the impact of negative factors (such as bacterial growth under the dressing). It is important to note these are different to sterile drapes that are generally recommended as good practice to prevent contact during surgery with various environmental surfaces and surrounding equipment in the patient vicinity.[38,120] Another example is skin sealants that are presterile liquids (eg, cyanoacrylate-based sealants) designed to form a film when applied to the skin after skin antisepsis. Depending on the formulation, they may allow for moisture/air penetration but also claim to cause the immobilize microorganisms on the skin surface to retard their penetration into the wound. Some reports have also suggested an antimicrobial effect during this process.[125,126] Following incision, the sealant remains in place to provide an additional antimicrobial effect at the wound site and then dissolves away over time. There is also the potential benefit of the incorporation of defined antimicrobials, such as chlorhexidine, into such sealant to improve efficacy claims.

Antimicrobial sutures are also used to reduce the risk of skin/wound infection postclosure. The most widely used by far to date are triclosan-containing sutures (in various forms), and moderate date is available to support their use to reduce SSIs.[19,38]

OTHER FACTORS IN REDUCING SURGICAL SITE INFECTIONS

Although outside the scope of this chapter, the guidelines also highlight the importance of other best practices in reducing SSIs,[15,38] including

- Appropriate antibiotic prophylaxis, although the guidelines do vary on recommendations regarding the use of antibiotics directly in the wound or applied during surgery to implantable device surfaces
- Perioperative glycemic control
- Maintaining normothermia
- The optimal skin preparation for the conduct of a surgical procedure has not yet evolved. The general theme remains to reduce the level of microorganisms residing on the skin of the patient with the expectation that there will be fewer bacteria to contaminate the wound and to produce postoperative infections. To the extent that a procedure is entirely clean of endogenous contaminating organisms, this is a laudable, although not quite achievable, goal.

Surgical wound infections are often the result of many diverse factors. Even with similar skin preparations, different procedures have varied infection rates (Tables 43.1 and 43.2).[15,38-43] Some of these variables, in addition to those discussed earlier, can be controlled by the surgical staff, whereas others cannot. These include:

- Prolonged preoperative hospitalization increases the resultant risks of wound infection for various reasons.[78,129] Earlier reports demonstrated that 1 day, 1 week, and more than 2 weeks of preoperative stays resulted in an infection rate of 1.2%, 2.1%, and 3.4%, respectively.[129] The relative risk of postoperative wound infection was subsequently reported to be 1.74 (95% CI, 1.13-2.69) for patients with a preoperative stay beyond 3 weeks.[78]
- A direct relation exists between the length of operating time and the infection rate, with the clean rate roughly doubling for every hour of operating time.[78] This phenomenon may be the consequence of proliferating bacteria within the wound and on the skin surface and increased injury to the wound (eg, desiccation, electrocautery, and retraction pressure) associated with longer procedures. In addition, distant-site infections at the time of surgery significantly increase the risk of postoperative wound infection.[78]
- It has been difficult to prove that contamination from dust and environment is implicated when the operating theater conforms to standard association guidelines.[38,130] But the impact of levels of associated air/surface contamination, the absence of these best practices, and outbreak situations continue to support the role of controlled, filtered, laminar-flow air in operating rooms in reducing SSI risks.[130,131] This is an area of continued debate[132] but generally less movement and traffic within the area and room maintenance (eg, periodic cleaning) are equally important.[130,133,134]

TABLE 43.2 Summary of infections following 100 or more operations[a]

Operative Procedure	National Research Council			Foothills Hospital		
	No. of Wounds	Infections		No. of Wounds	Infections	
		No.	%		No.	%
General surgery						
Radical mastectomy	227	43	18.9	—	—	—
Modified radical mastectomy	—	—	—	383	16	4.2
Appendectomy	551	63	11.4	1148	73	6.4
Cholecystectomy	756	52	6.9	1330	26	2.0
Inguinal hernia	1312	25	1.9	1857	9	0.5
Thyroidectomy	406	9	2.2	254	3	1.2
Nephrectomy	127	22	17.3	130	8	6.1
Orthopedics						
Bone biopsy and excision of bone lesion	109	6	5.5	372	10	2.7
Cardiovascular-thoracic						
Exploratory thoracotomy (with or without biopsy)	137	8	5.8	54	3	5.6
Lobectomy segmental resection	131	9	6.9	145	8	5.5

[a]Based on an older study,[43] but note that the rates of infection can vary from facility to facility and country to country.[42]

- Patient factors are also important to consider. Extremes in age,[135] coincident remote site of infection,[80] malnutrition,[129,136] diabetes,[136,137] use of nicotine,[136] and obesity[136,137] all have been associated with an increased risk of wound infections for some time.[15,38] In addition, intraoperative hypothermia is now strongly associated with increased risk of postoperative infection, with the guidelines recommending the use of warming device to maintain normal body temperature.[15,38] It is important to recognize these factors to minimize risk and to maximize effort to prevent surgical wound infections.

A final consideration is surveillance. As far back as the 1970s, it was established that the risks of wound infections decreased over a period during which dissemination of information occurred.[43,138] In this respect, surveillance can be defined as an ongoing collection, analysis, interpretation, and evaluation of SSI case, including the reporting of this data (to include infection control and surgical staff). Surveillance of SSI rates are now recommended as an essential part of the WHO guidelines to reduce SSIs as well as being mandatory (eg, in the United Kingdom) or voluntary in different countries.[38,139]

The prevention of infection in the surgical wound is an important goal. No single factor may be isolated and given sole credit or blame for the result. Certainly, spontaneous generation of bacteria in wounds does not occur, and it is incumbent on the operating team to keep the inoculum in the wound to an absolute minimum, to minimize the trauma inflicted on the wound, and to promote the speedy repair of necessarily produced injuries.

▶ ROLE OF ANTISEPTICS IN SURGICAL WOUNDS

The aim of treatment of injured tissue (whether by trauma or surgical procedure) is to provide optimal conditions for healing. It has long been recognized that infection or high tissue burden of bacteria will interfere with the biologic process of healing. To this end, wound disinfectants or antiseptics of a variety of types have been widely used by physicians and surgeons with the purpose of counteracting the detrimental effect of wound contamination and infection. As noted previously, the commonly used antiseptics are potent agents and have the capacity to injure not only the infectious organisms but also viable human tissue. This balance in the favor of the human tissue is an important consideration confronting the practicing clinician.

Historical Perspective

In the pre-antibiotic era, the complication of wound infection was disastrous with significant morbidity and mortality. After the lessons learned by Semmelweis,[2] Lister,[3] and many others that demonstrated the beneficial effect of antiseptics and disinfectants, much clinical attention was given to the careful and judicious application of antiseptics to the surgical wound. During the First World War, two schools of wound treatment arose: the *psychological school*, which concentrated on aiding the body to clear infection, and the *antiseptic school*, which attempted to kill microbes in a wound with a chemical agent. The 1919 Hunterian Lecture before the Royal College of Surgeons was given by Alexander Fleming[140] and entitled "The Action of Chemical and Physiological Antiseptics in a Septic Wound" (Figure 43.1). During this discourse, the point was repetitively made that when wounds were analyzed, antiseptics of that era (eg, carbolic acid, mercuric chloride, iodine, sodium hypochlorite, Lysol, flavine, chloramine-T, hydrogen peroxide) used in the manner of the time did not give a significant reduction in microbial burden. Conversely, wounds often were made more susceptible to microbial proliferation. It was hypothesized to be the consequence of the nonspecific effect of toxic chemicals on biologic tissues (unlike many antibiotics, antiseptics are generally not able to discriminate bacteria from viable or dead tissue), and the physical properties of wounds prevented contact between antiseptics and bacteria.

To this day, the debate remains even as many have been responsive to developing newer types of antiseptics or applications with different delivery systems. Many advocates urge practitioners to use these agents not only for disinfection of keratinized surfaces (skin, oropharynx, and vagina) but also in epithelial or serosal surfaces (bladder, bowel, and peritoneum) and directly in wounds (surgical wounds, pressure ulcers). Some of the information on this subject is reviewed further in the following text, but the reader is also encouraged to follow the various different evidence-based guidelines worldwide to determine when and if this is appropriate.[15,38,130]

Experimental Studies

The use of in vitro experiments to draw conclusions about the clinical environment is fraught with assumptions. The usual experiment to demonstrate antimicrobial activity consists of placing bacteria (or other test microorganisms), broth, and a test antiseptic in a single test situation and quantitating the number of viable organisms after

THE ACTION OF CHEMICAL AND PHYSIOLOGICAL ANTISEPTICS IN A SEPTIC WOUND.

The Hunterian Lecture delivered before the Royal College of Surgeons of England on February 12, 1919.

By ALEXANDER FLEMING, London.

Since the war began, much attention has been directed to the treatment of suppurating wounds, for in the earlier years—1914–15–16—practically all the gunshot wounds became infected, and even in 1918 nearly all the wounds which were left open for more than a week became grossly infected with pyogenic cocci and other organisms.

Prior to the war, the surgeon gave most of his attention to aseptic methods, his great object being to exclude microbes from the wound. The question of how to deal with the bacteria after they were in possession was a problem of much less interest to him. I can remember in the days when I was first admitted to the surgical wards as a dresser, there were always a certain number of septic wounds which we were instructed to dress with this or that antiseptic, which stood in jars around the fire, and which we were told possessed great virtue as destroyers of microbes in the wound. These antiseptics were chiefly carbolic acid, mercury salts, and boric acid. The wounds were religiously dressed once or twice a day with these lotions, and although it was obvious that the antiseptic did not kill all the microbes in the wound, we were always told that it would kill many of them, and so the condition would be better than if no antiseptic were used. We were not then in a position to criticize this view.

At the beginning of the war in 1914, all the old antiseptics were used in military hospitals, in just such a manner as when I started surgery. Carbolic acid, perchloride or biniodide of mercury, boric acid, and hydrogen peroxide were poured into septic wounds once or twice a day, either singly or in mixtures of two or more, according to the fancy of the medical officer.

FIGURE 43.1 Fleming's[140] 1919 lecture on antiseptics in septic wounds.

a defined period (see chapters 61-63). These can readily demonstrate that many agents (eg, povidone-iodine, Dakin's solution, hydrogen peroxide, chlorhexidine) are effective at clinically relevant concentrations in effecting antimicrobial activity (especially against many of the common causes of SSIs discussed previously); however, missing from these studies are the usual controls for what is typically present in clinical wounds, large amounts of amorphous tissues. Even Fleming[140] in 1919 added tissue to such tests under in vitro conditions and found that bacterial killing capacity was abrogated. The effectiveness of antiseptic solutions on bacteria in the open healing wound is uncertain from many studies in the literature. One can surmise that efficacy can be reduced drastically by inactivating the antiseptic by the wound material but equally can be effective depending on variables such as the antimicrobial concentration and method or timing of application. The benefit of reducing microbial levels or even temporarily reducing the growth of such contaminants in the wound can allow for a greater opportunity for the body's immune system to deal with the rest and overall the risk of SSI development.

Antiseptics are nonspecific in their interaction with living organisms, and normal mammalian cells can be expected to be injured by antiseptic application. To evaluate these disinfectants, a bactericide/leukocide ratio was proposed in 1958.[141] Of 15 compounds analyzed, only three had less toxicity to phagocytes than to bacteria. Additionally, although fibroblasts survive in antibiotics, antiseptics (1% povidone-iodine, 0.25% acetic acid,

0.5% sodium hypochlorite, and 3% hydrogen peroxide) produce 100% cell death after 24 hours of in vitro exposure (Table 43.3).[142,143] Impaired function of polymorphonuclear leukocytes, cytotoxicity to neoplastic tumor lines, and injury to endothelial cells have been reported with antiseptic use.[142-144]

In vitro assays of cytotoxicity should draw criticism similar to that expressed for bacterial efficacy testing in vitro. Antiseptics applied to wounds with large amounts of necrotic debris (fresh) would in all likelihood leave less of an injurious effect on viable host cells than antiseptics placed in a fresh surgical wound. In vivo studies using experimental animal wounds have proved valuable in delineating the effect of antiseptics on the healing process, although alternatives to these types of tests (including clinical studies) are preferred. For example, an investigation of the use of a quaternary ammonium compound (cetylpyridinium) on an acute surgically created wound demonstrated intravascular hemolysis, intravascular disruption of granulocytes, fibrin deposition on vascular endothelium, and tissue edema.[145] Although other agents produced variable results, there was an overall deleterious effect by antiseptics on the host cells of the *acute* surgical wound.

To evaluate the healing wound, an ear chamber model in rabbits was used to compare the use of a calcium hypochlorite antiseptic with 0.3% available chlorine with povidone-iodine (5% and 1%), hydrogen peroxide, chloramine-T (1% = 0.24% available chlorine), and chlorhexidine gluconate (0.05%).[146] After approximately

TABLE 43.3 Toxicity of antimicrobial agents to fibroblasts in comparison with antibacterial activity[a]

Agent	% Fibroblast Survival (24 h)	Bacterial % Survival (24 h)
Povidone-iodine		
0.01%	0	0
0.001%	105 ± 6	0
Sodium hypochlorite		
0.05%	0	0
0.005	97 ± 6	0
0.0005	107 ± 12	71 ± 5
Hydrogen peroxide		
3.0%	0	0
0.3%	0	103 ± 5
0.03%	41 ± 7	105 ± 8
Acetic acid		
0.25%	0	78 ± 3
0.025%	74 ± 7	97 ± 2

[a]Data from Lineweaver et al.[143]

4 weeks, all the agents tested caused adverse effects, but the hypochlorite antiseptics caused blood flow in the capillary of the granulation tissue to cease. Moreover, a delay in production of collagen was demonstrated when chloramine-T was applied to an experimental wound.[147] It has been suggested that a physician should not put anything into a wound that could not safely be put in one's eye. Thus, the corneal toxicity of some commonly used skin antiseptics comparing tincture of iodine, Hibiclens (4% chlorhexidine and detergent), pHisoHex (3% hexachlorophene and detergent), Lavacol (70% ethanol), 7.5% povidone-iodine scrub (with detergent), and 10% povidone-iodine solution was performed in rabbits.[148] With all products except 10% povidone-iodine solution, marked corneal epithelialization, conjunctival chemosis, and edema occurred (these effects were reversible within a week). At the same time, advances in the topical treatment of eye infections, in particular with resilient microorganisms such as *Acanthamoeba*, do show that the right balance between the application of an antiseptic formulation (including biocides such as PVPI, biguanides, and hydrogen peroxide) to meet antimicrobial efficacy and tissue toxicity is possible.[149-151]

Many of these studies suggested that the uncontrolled or off-labeled application of antiseptic solutions to open wounds is a risky procedure. In a study of experimental peritonitis, it was demonstrated that lethality was *increased* after the instillation of povidone-iodine.[152] The balance between reducing bacterial numbers and injuring host mammalian cells is tenuous. On theoretic grounds, many antiseptic solutions have little advantage over topical high-dose antibiotics, which have minimal toxicity to mammalian cells. But there is an opportunity to balance these requirements with appropriate formulations and labeled (regulatory cleared or approved) products for various wound applications.[15,38,153]

Clinical Studies

Since the time of Lister,[3] physicians have put antiseptics onto wounds with the putative intent of "sterilizing" the wound and improving healing. Both the clinician and the patient invest much energy in the process. Clinical studies that demonstrate benefits, risks, or efficacy have often provided inconclusive evidence, and these will be expected to vary based on the product type (not just based on the presence or absence of a certain type of biocide), application method, and many complicating patient factors; consequently, multiple conflicting reports regarding the use of topical antiseptic agents in surgical wounds remain.[15,38,130,154,155]

An earlier review on topical therapy of pressure ulcers from 1900 to 1974 found that although improved healing often was asserted, rarely was the claim supported by results that were controlled.[156] Overall, the conclusion

was that no specific antiseptic agent used was shown to be useful for pressure ulcers. Povidone-iodine used as treatment for chronic pressure ulcers was shown to be no more effective in reducing wound bacterial numbers than physiologic saline[157] and is still recommended as a benefit over saline for wound irrigation, particularly in clean and clean-contaminated wounds.[38,154] Topical silver sulfadiazine (1%), as another example, was also found to be effective in the reduction of pressure-ulcer bacteria, as it has been in the prevention of burn-wound infection. The use of silver for various wound applications continues to be a matter of some debate, including efficacy and toxicity concerns (see chapter 25).

The role of antiseptics in the contaminated wound has been open to much discussion.[15,38,155] Because the contaminating inoculum is often polymicrobial and can consist of unknown types and resistant forms of bacteria, antiseptics have been used to decrease their numbers and, by analogy, the risk of wound infection. Some studies show benefit from instillation of antiseptics into surgical wounds when used appropriately. Intraperitoneal taurolin (an agent that degrades to formaldehyde) was shown to be nontoxic and to improve survival rates.[158] In patients undergoing abdominal surgery, intraparietal povidone-iodine resulted in a reduction of wound infections from 24% to 9%.[159] A study to compare topical antiseptic (5% available iodine), aerosol (12% povidone-iodine), and topical polyantibiotic aerosolized powder (neomycin, bacitracin, and polymyxin B) during appendectomy also was performed.[160] The beneficial effect in the reduction of wound infections for povidone-iodine treatment to 8% ($P < .025$) and polyantibiotic to 9.3% ($P < .06$) was found when compared with controls with an infection rate of 16%. Intraperitoneal application of low-molecular-weight povidone-iodine solution also reduced wound infections and intra-abdominal infectious complications when compared with saline lavage in 75 patients.[161] In contrast, others reported that full-strength povidone-iodine does not reduce the incidence of wound infection in patients undergoing head and neck surgery and, in fact, may increase the risk.[162] In a series of 294 pediatric surgery patients, treatment of an appendectomy wound with 5% povidone-iodine aerosol *increased* the wound infection rate (19% versus 8% in controls).[163] When the concentration of povidone-iodine was reduced to 1%, the increased wound infection rate diminished. Such studies highlight the importance of using antiseptics in accordance with manufacturer's instructions and ensuring that such products or applications are supported by clinical evidence. Furthermore, these studies strongly support the notion that the cytotoxicity demonstrated in the laboratory carries over to the clinic. If an agent is applied to a wound that is more toxic to host-reparative processes than bacteria, the outcome can favor nonhealing and infection risk.

Other studies give equivocal results. In a small study, saline lavage was compared with the use of specific chlorhexidine gluconate and povidone-iodine products.[164]

The incidence of postoperative fever, wound infection, and duration of hospital stay were unaffected by lavage grouping, and all deaths were due to either coexistent disease or the severity of presenting disease. Others demonstrated no difference in wound infection rates in acute appendicitis when comparing metronidazole with either povidone-iodine or ampicillin.[165] The clinical experience serves many functions, but it can leave enough vagaries and uncertainties to allow individual opinion to persist with literature to support essentially any position on the use of antiseptics in wounds.

When examined in the light of in vitro studies and in vivo animal experiments, it can be concluded that the application of antiseptic solutions to surgical wounds is a risky procedure. There is a high likelihood that injury to the host cells (phagocytes, fibroblasts, endothelial cells) will be more prevalent than eradication of bacteria or fungi. The geography of wounds and the contact with biologic material resulting in inactivation of antiseptics make this probable. The consequence of this series of events is the *increased* likelihood that a deleterious effect (ie, delayed healing or wound infection) will occur. The maxim "never put anything in a wound which you wouldn't place in your eye" continues to be sound. There continues to be an opportunity for the successful use of antiseptics in wound situations to reduce SSI when supported with adequate safety and efficacy data as well as regulatory approval but any off-label use of such products should be discouraged.

Use of Antiseptics to Prepare Contaminated Surgical Sites

Antiseptic solutions have proved utility in the preparation of thick keratinized surfaces for operative manipulation and have serious drawbacks when applied to injured wounds, no matter how contaminated with bacteria. It is often desirable to diminish the bacterial numbers in either mucosal-lined viscera or squamous cell-lined oropharynx and vagina/perineum.[166] The "instant bowel prep," as first popularized by Jones et al,[167] was performed with the instillation of povidone-iodine into an isolated bowel segment.[168] Experimentally, this proved to decrease the numbers of luminal bacteria dramatically; however, experimental models demonstrated that bowel wall–associated organisms were minimally affected. Although used clinically with good results,[169] there has been little information to suggest that intracolonic antiseptic is superior to the administration of systemic antibiotics. Most modern guidelines either recommend the use of oral antibiotics or not at all for such applications to impact SSI rates.[38] There is a worry that large amounts of iodine could lead to toxicity, although this is controversial.[170] The use of oral hydrogen peroxide or povidone-iodine has been tried to decrease oral colonization of pathogens and

to improve hygiene.[171] Its efficacy is not known, but the toxic potential is probably minimal if the agent used in small quantities. The overall same conclusions have been reported in the use of antiseptics for intracavity lavage and wound irrigation in the prevention of SSIs.[172]

Antiseptic solutions can play an important role in surgery in preparation of patient and surgeon. The benefits are numerous, and microbial killing is rapid and covers many types of microorganisms. Rarely are normally sensitive microorganisms and particularly pathogens capable of developing high-level resistance to antiseptics, unlike with antibiotics and bacteria.[46] But all this comes with a cost, and that typically resides in the toxicity to mammalian cells or damage to the exposed tissue. Loss of cellular integrity and increased susceptibility to wound nonhealing are the detrimental side effects. It is the correct balance of these effects that can provide the optimum benefit in reducing SSIs.

▶ CONCLUSION

Since the introduction of antisepsis by Semmelweis[2] and Lister,[3] outcomes after surgical procedures have been improved dramatically. Whereas the techniques of antisepsis continue to evolve, current practices effectively minimize postoperative SSIs. Despite these advances, surgical antisepsis is only an adjunct to appropriate and prompt management of surgical diseases, careful surgical technique, and the limitation of multiple other factors that may contribute to wound infections.

▶ ACKNOWLEDGMENT

The chapter has been updated based on the previous fifth edition and owes substantially to the contributions of Traves D. Crabtree, Shawn J. Pelletier, and Timothy L. Pruett at the Department of Surgery, University of Virginia Health Sciences Center, Charlottesville, Virginia.

REFERENCES

1. Craig CP. Preparation of the skin for surgery. *Todays OR Nurse.* 1986;8:17-20.
2. Semmelweis IP. The etiology, concept and prevention of childbed fever, 1861. *Am J Obstet Gynecol.* 1995;172:236-237.
3. Lister J. The antiseptic system on a new method of treating compound fracture, abscess, etc. *Lancet.* 1867;1:326,357,387,507.
4. Price PB. The bacteriology of normal skin: a new quantitative test applied to a study of the bacterial flora and the disinfectant action of mechanical cleansing. *J Infect Dis.* 1938;63:301-318.
5. Larson E. Handwashing and skin. Physiologic and bacteriologic aspects. *Infect Control.* 1985;6:14-23.
6. Aly R, Maibach HI. *Clinical Skin Microbiology.* Springfield, IL: Charles C. Thomas; 1978.
7. Aly R, Maibach H. Factors controlling skin bacterial flora. In: Maibach HI, Aly R, eds. *Skin Microbiology: Relevance to Clinical Infection.* New York, NY: Springer; 1981:29-39.

8. Noble WC, Somerville DA. *Microbiology of Human Skin*. Philadelphia, PA: WB Saunders; 1974:316-319.

9. Noble WC. *Microbiology of Human Skin*. London, United Kingdom: Lloyd-Luke Medical Books; 1981.

10. Noble WC. Microbiology of special sites in relation to infection. In: Maibach HI, ed. *Microbiology: Relevance to Clinical Infection*. New York, NY: Springer; 1981:40-44.

11. Sanchez DA, Nosanchuk JD, Friedman AJ. The skin microbiome: is there a role in the pathogenesis of atopic dermatitis and psoriasis? *J Drugs Dermatol*. 2015;14:127-130.

12. Dréno B, Araviiskaia E, Berardesca E, et al. Microbiome in healthy skin, update for dermatologists. *J Eur Acad Dermatol Venereol*. 2016;30:2038-2047.

13. Selwyn S, Ellis H. Skin bacteria and skin disinfection reconsidered. *Br Med J*. 1972;1:136-140.

14. Lilly HA, Lowbury EJ, Wilkins MD. Limits to progressive reduction of resident skin bacteria by disinfection. *J Clin Pathol*. 1979;32:382-385.

15. Berríos-Torres SI, Umscheid CA, Bratzler DW, et al. Centers for Disease Control and Prevention guideline for the prevention of surgical site infection, 2017. *JAMA Surg*. 2017;152:784-791.

16. Larson EL. APIC guideline for handwashing and hand antisepsis in health care settings. *Am J Infect Control*. 1995;23:251-269.

17. Boyce JM, Pittet D; for Healthcare Infection Control Practices Advisory Committee, Society for Healthcare Epidemiology of America, Association for Professionals in Infection Control, Infectious Diseases Society of America, Hand Hygiene Task Force. Guideline for hand hygiene in health-care settings: recommendations of the Healthcare Infection Control Practices Advisory Committee and the HICPAC/SHEA/APIC/IDSA Hand Hygiene Task Force. *Infect Control Hosp Epidemiol*. 2002;23:S3-S40.

18. Kramer A, Weuffen W, Adrain V. Toxic risks by the use of disinfectants on skin. *Hyg und Med*. 1987;12:134-142.

19. Roberts DL, Summerly R, Byrne JP. Contact dermatitis due to the constituents of Hibiscrub. *Contact Dermatitis*. 1981;7:326-328.

20. Mitchell KG, Rawluk DJ. Skin reactions related to surgical scrub-up: results of a Scottish survey. *Br J Surg*. 1984;71:223-224.

21. Larson E, Leyden JJ, McGinley KJ, Grove GL, Talbot GH. Physiologic and microbiologic changes in skin related to frequent handwashing. *Infect Control*. 1986;7:59-63.

22. Larson E, McGinley KJ, Grove GL, Leyden JJ, Talbot GH. Physiologic, microbiologic, and seasonal effects of handwashing on the skin of health care personnel. *Am J Infect Control*. 1986;14:51-59.

23. Larson EL, Eke PI, Laughon BE. Efficacy of alcohol-based hand rinses under frequent-use conditions. *Antimicrob Agents Chemother*. 1986;30:542-544.

24. Lowbury EJL. Topical antimicrobials: perspective and issues. In: Maibach HI, Aly R, eds. *Skin Microbiology: Relevance to Clinical Infection*. New York, NY: Springer; 1981:158-168.

25. Allegranzi B, Pittet D. Hand hygiene. In: Fraise AP, Maillaurd JY, Sattar SA. *Principles and Practice of Disinfection, Preservation, and Sterilization*. 5th ed. Chichester, United Kingdom: Wiley-Blackwell; 2013:418-444.

26. Safety and effectiveness of health care antiseptics; topical antimicrobial drug products for over-the-counter human use. *Fed Regist*. 2017;82(242):60474-60503. To be codified at 21 CFR §310.

27. Meers PD, Yeo GA. Shedding of bacteria and skin squames after handwashing. *J Hyg (Lond)*. 1978;81:99-105.

28. Vorherr H, Ulrich JA, Messer RH, Hurwitz EB. Antimicrobial effect of chlorhexidine on bacteria of groin, perineum, and vagina. *J Reprod Med*. 1980;24:153-157.

29. Hann JB. The source of the "resident" flora. *Hand*. 1973;5:247-252.

30. McGinley KJ, Larson EL, Leyden JJ. Composition and density of microflora in the subungual space of the hand. *J Clin Microbiol*. 1988;26:950-953.

31. Gross A, Cutright DE, D'Alessandro SM. Effect of surgical scrub on microbial population under the fingernails. *Am J Surg*. 1979;138:463-467.

32. Mahl MC. New method for determination of efficacy of health care personnel hand wash products. *J Clin Microbiol*. 1989;27:2295-2299.

33. Byrd AL, Belkaid Y, Segre JA. The human skin microbiome. *Nat Rev Microbiol*. 2018;16:143-155.

34. Grice EA, Segre JA. The skin microbiome. *Nat Rev Microbiol*. 2011;9:244-253.

35. Larson EL. Persistent carriage of gram-negative bacteria on hands. *Am J Infect Control*. 1981;9:112-119.

36. Guenthner SH, Hendley JO, Wenzel RP. Gram-negative bacilli as nontransient flora on the hands of hospital personnel. *J Clin Microbiol*. 1987;25:488-490.

37. Horn WA, Larson EL, McGinley KJ, Leyden JJ. Microbial flora on the hands of health care personnel: differences in composition and antibacterial resistance. *Infect Control Hosp Epidemiol*. 1988;9:189-193.

38. World Health Organization. *Global Guidelines on the Prevention of Surgical Site Infection*. Geneva, Switzerland: World Health Organization; 2018.

39. Reichman DE, Greenberg JA. Reducing surgical site infections: a review. *Rev Obstet Gynecol*. 2009;2:212-221.

40. Onyekwelu I, Yakkanti R, Protzer, L, Pinkston CM, Tucker C, Seligson D. Surgical wound classification and surgical site infections in the orthopaedic patient. *J Am Acad Orthop Surg Glob Res Rev*. 2017;1:e022.

41. Ortega G, Rhee DS, Papandria DJ, et al. An evaluation of surgical site infections by wound classification system using the ACS-NSQIP. *J Surg Res*. 2012;174:33-38.

42. Rosenthal VD, Richtmann R, Singh S, et al; for International Nosocomial Infection Control Consortiuma. Surgical site infections, International Nosocomial Infection Control Consortium (INICC) report, data summary of 30 countries, 2005-2010. *Infect Control Hosp Epidemiol*. 2013;34:597-604.

43. Cruse PJ. Incidence of wound infection on the surgical services. *Surg Clin North Am*. 1975;55:1269-1275.

44. Anderson DV, Podgorny K, Berríos-Torres SI, et al. Strategies to prevent surgical site infections in acute care hospitals: 2014 update. *Infect Control Hosp Epidemiol*. 2014;35:605-627.

45. Ploegmakers IB, Olde Daminik SW, Breukink SO. Alternatives to antibiotics for prevention of surgical infection. *Br J Surg*. 2017;104:e24-e33.

46. McDonnell G. *Antisepsis, Disinfection, and Sterilization: Types, Action, and Resistance*. 2nd ed. Washington, DC: ASM Press; 2017.

47. Favero MS, Bond WW. Sterilization, disinfection, and antisepsis in the hospital. In: Balows A, Hausler W, eds. *Manual of Clinical Microbiology*. 5th ed. Washington, DC: ASM Press. 1991:183-200.

48. Richter A, Chaberny IF, Surikow A, Schock B. Hygiene in medical education—increasing patient safety through the implementation of practical training in infection prevention. *GMS J Med Educ*. 2019;36:Doc15.

49. World Health Organization. *Patient Safety Curriculum Guide*. Geneva, Switzerland: World Health Organization; 2011.

50. Garner JS. CDC guideline for prevention of surgical wound infections, 1985. Supersedes guideline for prevention of surgical wound infections published in 1982. (Originally published in November 1985). Revised. *Infect Control*. 1986;7:193-200.

51. Safety and effectiveness of consumer antiseptics; topical antimicrobial drug products for over-the-counter human use. *Fed Regist*. 2016;81(172):61106-61130. To be codified at 21 CFR §310.

52. World Health Organization. *Guidelines on Hand Hygiene in Health Care*. Geneva, Switzerland: World Health Organization; 2009.

53. European Chemicals Agency. *Guidance on the Biocidal Products Regulation: Volume V, Guidance on Active Micro-organisms and Biocidal Products. Version 2.1*. Helsinki, Finland: European Chemicals Agency; 2017. ECHA-17-G-06-EN.

54. Topical antimicrobial drug products for over-the-counter human use: tentative final monograph for health-care antiseptic drug products—proposed rule. *Fed Regist*. 1994;59:31441-31452. To be codified at 21 CFR §333 and 369.

55. Topical antimicrobial drug products for over-the-counter human use; tentative final monograph for first aid antiseptic drug products. *Fed Regist*. 1991;56:33644-33702.

56. Sheldon AT. Assessing the efficacy of professional healthcare antiseptics: a regulatory perspective. In: *Principles and Practice of Disinfection, Preservation and Sterilization*. 5th ed. Chichester, United Kingdom: Wiley-Blackwell; 2013:247-254.

57. Klein M, Deforest A. Antiviral action of germicides. *Soap and Chemical Specialties*. 1963;39:70-72,95-97.

58. Rocos B, Donaldson LJ. Alcohol skin preparation causes surgical fires. *Ann R Coll Surg Engl*. 2012;94(2):87-89.

59. Hardin W. Handwashing and patient skin preparation. In: Malangoli M, ed. *Critical Issues in Operating Room Management*. Philadelphia, PA: Lippincott-Raven; 1997:133-149.

60. Spaulding EH. Alcohol as a surgical disinfectant. *AORN J*. 1964;2:67-71.

61. Suchomel M, Kundi M, Pittet D, Weinlich M, Rotter ML. Testing of the World Health Organization recommended formulations in their application as hygienic hand rubs and proposals for increased efficacy. *Am J Infect Control*. 2012;40:328-331.

62. Fujita S, Sumita S, Kawana S, Iwasaki H, Namiki A. Two cases of anaphylactic shock induced by chlorhexidine [in Japanese]. *Masui*. 1997;46:1118-1121.

63. Krautheim AB, Jermann TH, Bircher AJ. Chlorhexidine anaphylaxis: case report and review of the literature. *Contact Dermatitis*. 2004;50:113-116.

64. Muller R. *Medizinische Mikrobiologie*. Munich, Germany: Urban & Schwarzenberg; 1950:57-65.

65. Altemeier WA. Surgical antiseptics. In: Block SS, ed. *Disinfection, Sterilization, and Preservation*. 3rd ed. Philadelphia, PA: Lea & Febiger; 1983:493-504.

66. Bigliardi PL, Alsagoff SAL, El-Kafrawi HY, Pyon JK, Wa CTC, Villa MA. Povidone iodine in wound healing: a review of current concepts and practices. *Int J Surg*. 2017;44:260-268.

67. Berkelman RL, Lewin S, Allen JR, et al. Pseudobacteremia attributed to contamination of povidone-iodine with *Pseudomonas cepacia*. *Ann Intern Med*. 1981;95:32-36.

68. Berkelman RL, Holland BW, Anderson RL. Increased bactericidal activity of dilute preparations of povidone-iodine solutions. *J Clin Microbiol*. 1982;15:635-639.

69. Anderson RL, Vess RW, Carr JH, Bond WW, Panlilio AL, Favero MS. Investigations of intrinsic *Pseudomonas cepacia* contamination in commercially manufactured povidone-iodine. *Infect Control Hosp Epidemiol*. 1991;12:297-302.

70. Onesko KM, Wienke EC. The analysis of the impact of a mild, low-iodine, lotion soap on the reduction of nosocomial methicillin-resistant *Staphylococcus aureus*: a new opportunity for surveillance by objectives. *Infect Control*. 1987;8:284-288.

71. OTC topical antimicrobial products: over-the-counter drugs generally recognized as safe, effective, and not misbranded. *Fed Regist*. 1978;43:1210-1249. To be codified at 21 CFR §333.

72. Shuman RM, Leech RW, Alvord EC Jr. Neurotoxicity of hexachlorophene in humans. II. A clinicopathological study of 46 premature infants. *Arch Neurol*. 1975;32:320-325.

73. Lee JD, Lee JY, Kwack SJ, et al. Risk assessment of triclosan, a cosmetic preservative. *Toxicol Res*. 2019;35:137-154.

74. Scientific Committee on Emerging and Newly Identified Health Risks. *Assessment of the Antibiotic Resistance Effects of Biocides*. Brussels, Belgium: European Commission; 2009. Accessed April 15, 2019.

75. Leaper D, Wilson P, Assadian O, et al. The role of antimicrobial sutures in preventing surgical site infection. *Ann R Coll Surg Engl*. 2017;99:439-443.

76. Lear JC, Maillard J-Y, Dettmar PW, Goddard PA, Russell AD. Chloroxylenol and triclosan-tolerant bacteria from industrial sources—susceptibility to antibiotics and other biocides. *Int Biodeter Biodegrad*. 2006;57:51-56.

77. Bruun JN. Post-operative wound infection. Predisposing factors and the effect of a reduction in the dissemination of staphylococci. *Acta Med Scand Suppl*. 1970;514:3-89.

78. Velasco E, Thuler LC, Martins CA, Dias LM, Conalves VM. Risk factors for infectious complications after abdominal surgery for malignant disease. *Am J Infect Control*. 1996;24:1-6.

79. Hebra E. Most important experiences about the etiology of puerperal fevers epidemic in birth institutions. *Z Gesellschaft KK Artze Wien*. 1848;2:242-244.

80. Garner JS, Favero MS. CDC guideline for handwashing and hospital environmental control, 1985. *Infect Control*. 1986;7:231-243.

81. Albert RK, Condie F. Hand-washing patterns in medical intensive-care units. *N Engl J Med*. 1981;304:1465-1466.

82. Larson E, Killien M. Factors influencing handwashing behavior of patient care personnel. *Am J Infect Control*. 1982;10:93-99.

83. Larson E, Lusk E. Evaluating handwashing technique. *J Adv Nurs*. 1985;10:547-552.

84. Larson E. Effects of handwashing agent, handwashing frequency, and clinical area on hand flora. *Am J Infect Control*. 1984;12:76-82.

85. Larson EL, Eke PI, Wilder MP, Laughon BE. Quantity of soap as a variable in handwashing. *Infect Control*. 1987;8:371-375.

86. Donowitz LG. Handwashing technique in a pediatric intensive care unit. *Am J Dis Child*. 1987;141:683-685.

87. Maki DG, Hecht J. Antiseptic-containing handwashing agents reduce nosocomial infections: a prospective study. Paper presented at: 28th Intersociety Conference on Antimicrobial Agents and Chemotherapy of American Society of Microbiology; September 1982; Miami Beach, FL.

88. Massanari RM, Hierholzer WJ. A crossover comparison of antiseptic soaps on nosocomial infection rates in intensive care units. *Am J Infect Control*. 1984;12:247-248.

89. Tyzack R. The management of methicillin-resistant *Staphylococcus aureus* in a major hospital. *J Hosp Infect*. 1985;6(suppl A):195-199.

90. Rigby R, Pegram A, Woodward S. Hand decontamination in clinical practice: a review of the evidence. *Br J Nurs*. 2017;26:448-451.

91. Ulrich JA. Clinical study comparing Hibistat (0.5% chlorhexidine gluconate in 70% isopropyl alcohol) and Betadine surgical scrub (7.5% povidone-iodine) for efficacy against experimental contamination of human skin. *Curr Ther Res*. 1982;31:27-30.

92. Rotter M, Koller W, Wewalka G. Povidone-iodine and chlorhexidine gluconate-containing detergents for disinfection of hands. *J Hosp Infect*. 1980;1:149-158.

93. Ayliffe GA, Babb JR, Davies JG, Lilly HA. Hand disinfection: a comparison of various agents in laboratory and ward studies. *J Hosp Infect*. 1988;11:226-243.

94. Davies J, Babb JR, Ayliffe GA, Wilkins MD. Disinfection of the skin of the abdomen. *Br J Surg*. 1978;65:855-858.

95. Sheena AZ, Stiles ME. Efficacy of germicidal handwashing agents in hygienic hand disinfection. *J Food Prot*. 1982;45:713-720.

96. Larson E, Mayur K, Laughon BA. Influence of two handwashing frequencies on reduction in colonizing flora with three handwashing products used by health care personnel. *Am J Infect Control*. 1988;17:83-88.

97. Messager S, Goddard PA, Dettmar PW, Maillard JY. Comparison of two in vivo and two ex vivo tests to assess the antibacterial activity of several antiseptics. *J Hosp Infect*. 2004;58:115-121.

98. Doebbeling BN, Pfaller MA, Houston AK, Wenzel RP. Removal of nosocomial pathogens from the contaminated glove. Implications for glove reuse and handwashing. *Ann Intern Med*. 1988;109:394-398.

99. Gobetti JP, Cerminaro M, Shipman C Jr. Hand asepsis: the efficacy of different soaps in the removal of bacteria from sterile, gloved hands. *J Am Dent Assoc*. 1986;113:291-292.

100. Newsom SW, Rowland C. Application of the hygienic hand-disinfection test to the gloved hand. *J Hosp Infect*. 1989;14:245-247.

101. Association of periOperative Registered Nurses. *2019 Guidelines for Perioperative Practice*. Denver, CO: Association of periOperative Registered Nurses; 2019.

102. Kikuchi-Numagami K, Saishu T, Fukaya M, Kanazawa E, Tagami H. Irritancy of scrubbing up for surgery with or without a brush. *Acta Derm Venereol.* 1999;79:230-232.

103. Mulberry G, Snyder AT, Heilman J, Pyrek J, Stahl J. Evaluation of a waterless, scrubless chlorhexidine gluconate/ethanol surgical scrub for antimicrobial efficacy. *Am J Infect Control.* 2001;29:377-382.

104. Galle PC, Homesley HD, Rhyne AL. Reassessment of the surgical scrub. *Surg Gynecol Obstet.* 1978;147:215-218.

105. Decker LA, Gross A, Miller FC, Read JA, Cutright DE, Devine J. A rapid method for the presurgical cleansing of hands. *Obstet Gynecol.* 1978;51:115-117.

106. Sias RM, Sias HE, Foster M, Stewart T, inventors; TOMI ENVIRONMENTAL SOLUTIONS Inc, assignee. Apparatus and method for cleaning particulate matter and chemical contaminants from a hand. US patent 6,706,243. March 16, 2004.

107. Gordon EI, inventor; Germgard Lighting LLC, assignee. Hand sanitizer/sterilizer. US patent 8,142,713. March 27, 2012.

108. Lilly HA, Lowbury EJ. Disinfection of the skin: an assessment of some new preparations. *Br Med J.* 1971;3:674-676.

109. Lowbury EJL. Special problems in hospital antisepsis. In: Russell AD, Hugo WB, Ayliffe GAJ, eds. *Principles and Practice of Disinfection, Preservation, and Sterilization.* Oxford, United Kingdom: Blackwell Scientific Publications; 1982:262-284.

110. Ayliffe GA. Surgical scrub and skin disinfection. *Infect Control.* 1984;5:23-27.

111. Hexachlorophene, as a component of drug and cosmetic products. *Fed Regist.* 1972;37:160-164. To be codified at 21 CFR §250.

112. Peterson AF, Rosenberg A, Alatary SD. Comparative evaluation of surgical scrub preparations. *Surg Gynecol Obstet.* 1978;146:63-65.

113. Wade JJ, Casewell MW. The evaluation of residual antimicrobial activity on hands and its clinical relevance. *J Hosp Infect.* 1991;18(suppl B):23-28.

114. Aly R, Maibach H. Comparative evaluation of chlorhexidine gluconate (Hibiclens) and povidone-iodine (E-Z Scrub) sponge/brushes for pre-surgical hand scrubbing. *Curr Ther Res.* 1983;34:740-745.

115. Larson E, Talbot GH. An approach for selection of health care personnel handwashing agents. *Infect Control.* 1986;7:419-424.

116. Laufman H. The operating room. In: Bennett JV, Brachman PS, eds. *Hospital Infections.* 2nd ed. Boston, MA: Little, Brown; 1986:315-324.

117. Comité Européen de Normalisation. *EN 14885:2018: Chemical Disinfectants and Antiseptics. Application of European Standards for Chemical Disinfectants and Antiseptics.* Brussels, Belgium: Comité Européen de Normalisation; 2018.

118. Hidron AI, Edwards JR, Patel J, Horan TC, Sievert DM, Pollock DA, Fridkin SK; for National Healthcare Safety Network Team, Participating National Healthcare Safety Network Facilities. NHSN annual update: antimicrobial-resistant pathogens associated with healthcare-associated infections: annual summary of data reported to the National Healthcare Safety Network at the Centers for Disease Control and Prevention, 2006-2007. *Infect Control Hosp Epidemiol.* 2008;29(11):996-1011.

119. Association of periOperative Registered Nurses. Recommended practices for skin preparation of patients. *AORN J.* 1996;64:813-816.

120. Association of periOperative Registered Nurses. Patient skin antisepsis. In: *Guidelines for Perioperative Practice.* 2018 ed. Denver, CO: Association of periOperative Registered Nurses; 2018.

121. Webster J, Osborne S. Preoperative bathing or showering with skin antiseptics to prevent surgical site infection. *Cochrane Database Syst Rev.* 2012;(9):CD004985.

122. Tanner J, Norrie P, Melen K. Preoperative hair removal to reduce surgical site infection. *Cochrane Database Syst Rev.* 2011;(11):CD004122.

123. Dumville JC, Gray TA, Walter CJ, Sharp CA, Page T. Dressings for the prevention of surgical site infection. *Cochrane Database Syst Rev.* 2014;(9):CD003091.

124. Dickinson Jennings C, Culver Clark R, Baker JW. A prospective, randomized controlled trial comparing 3 dressing types following sternotomy. *Ostomy Wound Manage.* 2015;61(5):42-49.

125. Wood C, Phillips C. Cyanoacrylate microbial sealants for skin preparation prior to surgery. *Cochrane Database Syst Rev.* 2016;(5):CD008062.

126. Prince D, Kohan K, Solanki K, et al. Immobilization and death of bacteria by Flora Seal® microbial sealant. *Internat J Pharma Sci Invent.* 2017;6:45-49.

127. Webster J, Alghamdi A. Use of plastic adhesive drapes during surgery for preventing surgical site infection. *Cochrane Database Syst Rev.* 2015;(4):CD006353.

128. Rezapoor M, Tan TL, Maltenfort MG, Parvizi J. Incise draping reduces the rate of contamination of the surgical site during hip surgery: a prospective, randomized trial. *J Arthroplasty.* 2018;33:1891-1895.

129. Cruse PJ, Foord R. A five-year prospective study of 23,649 surgical wounds. *Arch Surg.* 1973;107:206-210.

130. Association of periOperative Registered Nurses. *Guidelines for Perioperative Practice.* 2018 ed. Denver, CO: Association of periOperative Registered Nurses; 2018.

131. Erichsen Andersson A, Petzold M, Bergh I, Karlsson J, Eriksson BI, Nilsson K. Comparison between mixed and laminar airflow systems in operating rooms and the influence of human factors: experiences from a Swedish orthopedic center. *Am J Infect Control.* 2014;42(6):665-669.

132. McHugh SM, Hill AD, Humphreys H. Laminar airflow and the prevention of surgical site infection. More harm than good? *Surgeon.* 2015;13:52-58.

133. Pryor F, Messmer PR. The effect of traffic patterns in the OR on surgical site infections. *AORN J.* 1998;68:649-660.

134. Parvizi J, Barnes S, Shohat N, Edmiston CE Jr. Environment of care: is it time to reassess microbial contamination of the operating room air as a risk factor for surgical site infection in total joint arthroplasty? *Am J Infect Control.* 2017;45:1267-1272.

135. Beitsch P, Balch C. Operative morbidity and risk factor assessment in melanoma patients undergoing inguinal lymph node dissection. *Am J Surg.* 1992;164:462-466.

136. Nagachinta T, Stephens M, Reitz B, Polk BF. Risk factors for surgical-wound infection following cardiac surgery. *J Infect Dis.* 1987;156:967-973.

137. Slaughter MS, Olson MM, Lee JT Jr, Ward HB. A fifteen-year wound surveillance study after coronary artery bypass. *Ann Thorac Surg.* 1993;56:1063-1068.

138. Haley RW, Quade D, Freeman HE, Bennett JV. The SENIC project. Study on the efficacy of nosocomial infection control (SENIC project). Summary of study design. *Am J Epidemiol.* 1980;111:472-485.

139. Centers for Disease Control and Prevention. *Surgical Site Infection (SSI) event.* Centers for Disease Control and Prevention Web site. https://www.cdc.gov/nhsn/pdfs/pscmanual/9pscssicurrent.pdf. Published January 2019. Accessed April 15, 2019.

140. Fleming A. The action of chemical and physiological antiseptics in a septic wound. *Brit J Surg.* 1919;7:99-129.

141. Greenberg L, Ingalls JW. Bactericide/leukocide ratio: a technique for the evaluation of disinfectants. *J Am Pharm Assoc Am Pharm Assoc.* 1958;47:531-533.

142. Lineaweaver W, Howard R, Soucy D, et al. Topical antimicrobial toxicity. *Arch Surg.* 1985;120:267-270.

143. Lineaweaver W, McMorris S, Soucy D, Howard R. Cellular and bacterial toxicities of topical antimicrobials. *Plast Reconstr Surg.* 1985;75:394-396.

144. Blenkharn JI. The differential cytotoxicity of antiseptic agents. *J Pharm Pharmacol.* 1987;39:477-479.

145. Brånemark PI, Ekholm R. Tissue injury caused by wound disinfectants. *J Bone Joint Surg Am.* 1967;49:48-62.

146. Brennan SS, Leaper DJ. The effect of antiseptics on the healing wound: a study using the rabbit ear chamber. *Br J Surg.* 1985;72:780-782.

147. Brennan SS, Foster ME, Leaper DJ. Antiseptic toxicity in wounds healing by secondary intention. *J Hosp Infect.* 1986;8:263-267.

148. MacRae SM, Brown B, Edelhauser HF. The corneal toxicity of presurgical skin antiseptics. *Am J Ophthalmol.* 1984;97:221-232.

149. Carrijo-Carvalho LC, Sant'ana VP, Foronda AS, de Freitas D, de Souza Carvalho FR. Therapeutic agents and biocides for ocular infections

by free-living amoebae of *Acanthamoeba* genus. *Surv Ophthalmol.* 2017;62:203-218.

150. Grzybowski A, Kuklo P, Pieczynski J, Beiko G. A review of preoperative manoeuvres for prophylaxis of endophthalmitis in intraocular surgery: topical application of antibiotics, disinfectants, or both? *Curr Opin Ophthalmol.* 2016;27:9-23.

151. Gili NJ, Noren T, Törnquist E, Crafoord S, Bäckman A. Preoperative preparation of eye with chlorhexidine solution significantly reduces bacterial load prior to 23-gauge vitrectomy in Swedish health care. *BMC Ophthalmol.* 2018;18:167.

152. Ahrenholz DH, Simmons RL. Povidone-iodine in peritonitis. I. Adverse effects of local instillation in experimental *E, coli* peritonitis. *J Surg Res.* 1979;26:458-463.

153. Slaviero L, Avruscio G, Vindigni V, Tocco-Tussardi I. Antiseptics for burns: a review of the evidence. *Ann Burns Fire Disasters.* 2018;31:198-203.

154. Mangram AJ, Horan TC, Pearson ML, Silver LC, Jarvis WR. Guideline for prevention of surgical site infection, 1999. Hospital Infection Control Practices Advisory Committee. *Infect Control Hosp Epidemiol.* 1999;20:250-280.

155. Fry DE. Prevention of infection at the surgical site. *Surg Infect (Larchmt).* 2017;18:377-378.

156. Morgan JE. Topical therapy of pressure ulcers. *Surg Gynecol Obstet.* 1975;141:945-947.

157. Kucan JO, Robson MC, Heggers JP, Ko F. Comparison of silver sulfadiazine, povidone-iodine and physiologic saline in the treatment of chronic pressure ulcers. *J Am Geriatr Soc.* 1981;29:232-235.

158. Browne MK, MacKenzie M, Doyle PJ. C controlled trial of taurolin in established bacterial peritonitis. *Surg Gynecol Obstet.* 1978;146:721-724.

159. Gilmore OJ, Sanderson PJ. Prophylactic interparietal povidone-iodine in abdominal surgery. *Br J Surg.* 1975;62:792-799.

160. Gilmore OJ, Martin TD. Aetiology and prevention of wound infection in appendicectomy. *Br J Surg.* 1974;61:281-287.

161. Sindelar WF, Brower ST, Merkel AB, Takesue EI. Randomised trial of intraperitoneal irrigation with low molecular weight povidone-iodine solution to reduce intra-abdominal infectious complications. *J Hosp Infect.* 1985;6(suppl A):103-114.

162. Becker GD. Identification and management of the patient at high risk for wound infection. *Head Neck Surg.* 1986;8:205-210.

163. Viljanto J. Disinfection of surgical wounds without inhibition of normal wound healing. *Arch Surg.* 1980;115:253-256.

164. Vallance S, Waldron R. Antiseptic vs. saline lavage in purulent and faecal peritonitis. *J Hosp Infect.* 1985;6(suppl A):87-91.

165. Parker MC, Mathams A. Systemic metronidazole combined with either topical povidone-iodine or ampicillin in acute appendicitis. *J Hosp Infect.* 1985;6(suppl A):97-101.

166. Byatt ME, Henderson A. Preoperative sterilization of the perineum: a comparison of six antiseptics. *J Clin Pathol.* 1973;26:921-924.

167. Jones FE, DeCosse JJ, Condon RE. Evaluation of "instant" preparation of the colon with povidone-iodine. *Ann Surg.* 1976;184:74-79.

168. Rotstein OD, Wells CL, Pruett TL, et al. Reevaluation of the "instant" colon preparation with povidone-iodine. *Surgical Forum.* 1985;36:70-71.

169. Hay JM, Boussougant Y, Roverselli D, Regnard JF, Meyrignac P, Lacaine F. The use of povidone-iodine enema as pre-operative preparation for colorectal surgery: bacteriological study. *J Hosp Infect.* 1985;6(suppl A):115-116.

170. Glöbel B, Glöbel H, Andres C. The risk of hyperthyroidism following an increase in the supply of iodine. *J Hosp Infect.* 1985;6(suppl A):201-204.

171. Brun-Buisson C, Legrand R, Rauss A, et al. Intestinal decontamination for control of nosocomial multiresistant gram-negative bacilli. Study of an outbreak in an intensive care unit. *Ann Intern Med.* 1989;110:873-881.

172. Norman G, Atkinson RA, Smith TA, et al. Intracavity lavage and wound irrigation for prevention of surgical site infection. *Cochrane Database Syst Rev.* 2017;(10):CD012234.

Infection Prevention for Skin and Burns

Gerald McDonnell

This chapter is divided into two parts. The first deals with infections located in or originating from the skin, and the second deals with burn wound management insofar as the prevention of microbial colonization or infection is concerned. The role of antisepsis for the prevention and/or treatment of specific skin infections may not be considered as being as prominent as in the prophylaxis of burn wound infections. Other chapters have considered antisepsis of the skin for hand hygiene (see chapter 42), surgical site and associated wound infection prevention (see chapter 43), and in oral and mucous membrane applications (see chapter 45).

▶ PREVENTION OF SKIN INFECTIONS

Skin infections can be generally classified as being primary or secondary. Primary infections generally occur on normal, intact skin and are typically caused by a single type of microorganism.[1,2] Examples include impetigo, cellulitis, and folliculitis. Secondary infections are associated with a preexisting diseased or damaged skin, with examples such as intertrigo (inflammation caused by skin-to-skin friction) or a wound infection. For the prevention and treatment of skin infections, antisepsis typically contributes in very specific circumstances, and the use of antiseptics is often only one among other measures. To analyze the role of antisepsis, it may be useful to list some examples of skin infections and conditions originating from the skin that are common or can have severe consequences:

- Cutaneous abscesses (including impetigo)
- Cellulitis and related skin infections
- Wound infections, including puncture wound, animal and human bites, decubitus ulcers, and surgical sites (but not burn wounds)
- Tetanus, particularly neonatal tetanus

Cutaneous Abscesses

Together with impetigo, a pathologic skin condition related to abscesses and often found in children, the immunocompromised and in other populations living under conditions of poor hygiene, skin abscesses are among the most common soft tissue infections. The pathogenesis of the various types of abscesses (eg, furuncles, carbuncles, recurrent furunculosis, superficial and bullous impetigo) and their etiologic agents are considered in detail by other authors.[1-3] But overall, the most frequent of these are bacteria such as *Staphylococcus aureus,* group A streptococci (with nephritogenic strains causing special problems), and anaerobic bacteria, either in pure culture or mixed with coliforms, especially in the perineal region. Because general preventive measures against these primary skin infection conditions usually cannot be taken, apart from good hygiene practices, only therapy of already manifest infections is required (or possible), usually by incision and drainage or—under certain conditions—with antibiotics. In some of these cases, such as during or following drainage, antiseptics can be used to reduce the microbial load around the infection/intervention area to provide an advantage to the immune system in resolving the infection, reduce the risk of cross-infection to other areas of the skin, or to reduce the risk of secondary infections. Any example is the use of hydrogen peroxide for this that can aid in cleaning the wounded area and reducing the microbial load. Prevention of recurrent furuncles (or boils) has often been achieved by eradication of staphylococcal nasal carriage in the patient with mupirocin or chlorhexidine digluconate (CHG) or oral antibiotics such as clindamycin.[4] But the successful use of antiseptics in these situations, as for antibiotics, can be variable depending on the patient/treatment.

Antisepsis has a place in the prevention of impetigo, which is a contagious condition. Although until the 1980s, mercurochrome, an organic mercury compound, was regarded as the antiseptic of choice for this purpose, its use, at least for large skin surface areas, is discouraged today because of toxicologic considerations.[5] Instead, aqueous or detergent-containing preparations of CHG, povidone-iodine, or mupirocin are most commonly used. Topical (localized) or in more severe cases oral or parenteral antibiotics are also used.[1,6]

Cellulitis and Related Skin Infections

This condition represents a superficial, erythematous inflammation of the skin that must be distinguished from infections of deeper tissues such as subcutaneous fat, fascia, and muscle. Sometimes, these tissues may be affected by extension of a superficial cellulitis. Underlying disorders such as diabetes mellitus, preceding trauma, other skin infections (eg, varicella), lymphedema of the legs, genetic disposition such as in familial Mediterranean fever, skin lesions, and defects in cellular or humoral immunity are also known risk factors for cellulitis.[1-3]

The most frequent forms and causes for cellulitis are as follows:

- Streptococcal infections are most often due to group A streptococci, such as erysipelas, an inflammatory process characterized by sharply demarcated margins (occasionally also due to group G streptococci). Phlegmonous processes sometimes lead to streptococcal toxic shock syndrome or extend to deeper soft tissue areas and cause necrotizing fasciitis or myositis, which can be life-threatening. Group B streptococcal cellulitis is not infrequently encountered in the elderly, those with diabetes or an underlying malignant process, and those with immunodeficiency.
- Staphylococcal cellulitis often cannot be distinguished clinically from streptococcal cellulitis and can, indeed, occur in conjunction with it. This has, of course, consequences for the choice of antibiotics.
- Erysipeloid is a cellulitis that also has well-defined margins. It is caused by *Erysipelothrix rhusiopathiae*, an animal pathogen, and therefore is located mostly on the fingers or hands of people handling raw meat or fish. In contrast to erysipelas, fever is not a common symptom.
- Other etiologic agents of cellulitis include *Haemophilus influenzae*, which causes blue-red to purple-red skin inflammation with indistinct margins. *Pseudomonas aeruginosa* can cause various dermatologic manifestations including ecthyma gangrenosum, nodules, abscesses, vesicles, and cellulitis, some of which may also occur in healthy users of poorly maintained whirlpools and hydrotherapy tanks or erysipelas-like lesions in immunocompromised hosts with systemic infection. Some saltwater-specific bacteria such as *Vibrio vulnificus* and other vibrios can cause various mild to severe skin infections that may lead to necrotizing infections of deeper

soft tissues and septicemia, both of which may be fatal in immunocompromised patients. Enterobacteriaceae, alone or in combination with anaerobic bacteria, play an important role in perineal cellulitis affecting the perirectal and perivulvar area or the scrotum. Clostridial cellulitis due to the gas gangrene/edema group of clostridial species occurs only under conditions of anaerobiosis, such as in areas with devitalized or hypoperfused tissue. *Corynebacterium diphtheriae* can cause cutaneous and wound infection, especially in humid tropical areas with poor hygiene. These infections are characterized by skin lesions that, in their final status, appear as oval, well-demarcated ulcers with a gray membrane at the base. The preventive measure of choice is immunization with diphtheria toxoid.

An analysis of these infections with respect to prevention reveals that treatment of underlying disorders in the host, whenever possible, and reducing external risk factors such as contaminated bathing water, whirlpools, and hydrotherapy devices, are probably the most effective prophylactic measures achievable. Antiseptic measures can play a supportive, although very limited role in the treatment of superficial skin lesions.

Wound Infections (Excluding Burn Wounds)

Puncture wounds may create local infection problems if they originate from contaminated sharps such as butcher's knives or pointed objects such as nails and thorns. For example, puncture wounds occur most commonly in children's feet during warm weather.[7,8] Other risks come from deliberate puncture wounds such as in tattooing and intravenous drug use. These wounds can lead to cellulitis, soft tissue infection, osteomyelitis, and tetanus. Although a wide range of microorganisms can be associated with these infections (due to the nature/source of the trauma), *Streptococcus* species, *P aeruginosa*, and *S aureus* are often cited as the most frequent causative agents.[8,9] More severe infections can result with bacteria such as atypical *Mycobacterium* and *Clostridium tetani* (tetanus).

Prevention of infection and treatment of the fresh wound consists of cleaning with an iodophor or alcohol antiseptic, surgical intervention for search and removal of any residual foreign body, and tetanus prophylaxis. In fresh (<6 h) wounds, antibiotic prophylaxis is not routinely indicated, unless the patient is at a higher risk for infection (eg, diabetics or when the wound is found to be infected).

The management of bite wounds is very similar and has also been extensively reviewed elsewhere.[10-12] With respect to frequency and severity of infections after bites, some facts have been established that may help to prevent complications. Dog bites account for the majority (approximately 70% to 80%) of animal bite wounds, and it is estimated that 10% to 20% of them become infected, although this may range as high as 50% in some situation.[10,13] There is some evidence that the rates of infection are lower with human bites than with dog bites, but the cat bites can be much higher.[13] Due to increases in tourism worldwide and exchange or exotic animals as pets, many cases of infection (in some cases serious) linked to other animal bites, for example with bats that are often associated with outbreaks of Ebola and coronaviruses.[14,15] Equally, our knowledge of the risks associated with tick-borne infections has increased in the last 10 years (eg, with Lyme disease and *Borrelia burgdorferi*).[16] But in general, the main causative organisms of bite wound infections are *Pasteurella*, α-hemolytic streptococci, various *Staphylococcus* species, *Enterococcus*, *Neisseria*, and *Corynebacterium*, independent of the source animal.[10,12,13,15] In bites of cats and cat-like predatory animals, the incidence of infection can greater than 50% and may involve not only skin and soft tissues but also bones and joints. The *Pasteurella multocida* is the pathogen most frequently isolated ($>$50%). A wide range of other bacteria have also been identified, especially anaerobes such as *Propionibacterium* and *Fusobacterium*. Although trivial wounds do not require antibiotic prophylaxis, this is recommended for more severe wounds, especially if hands and joints are involved or if a high risk of infection is suspected.[10,11,13,15] Clearly, antibiotics would not be effective in high-risk cases for virus infection (eg, with bats and animals suspected to have rabies). In any case, wound irrigation with soap/water, a saline solution or an antiseptic such as with alcohol, CHG or Povidone-Iodine (PVPI), debridement (if applicable), and tetanus prophylaxis are often used. Depending on the epidemiologic situation, rabies prophylaxis must be considered, especially as many countries no longer have recommended rabies vaccination due to low risks of infection in those countries, but this will not apply when travelling outside of those countries. Although these initial steps can be effective, subsequent signs of infection in the wound (such as swelling, redness, and pain) are indicative of the need for further intervention.

Infections after occlusion bites (when teeth break into the skin) and clenched-fist injuries, as happen when a person's fist strikes another person's teeth, are distinguished on the basis of their outcome and causative agents. Occlusion bites are most often infected by *S aureus, Eikenella corrodens, H influenzae,* and oral anaerobic bacteria, whereas the most serious clenched-fist injuries are usually infected by anaerobic bacteria, some of them producing β-lactamase, and by *E corrodens* (25%). In addition to the previously mentioned measures, antibiotic prophylaxis is necessary to prevent deep-space infection, septic arthritis, and osteomyelitis; patients with clenched-fist injuries require hospitalization and the attention of a hand surgeon.

Although antisepsis is not a key issue in the prevention of bite wound infections, some authorities have advocated treatment of fresh bite wounds with a solution of 0,1% benzalkonium chloride or with 56% to 70% ethanol instead of or in addition to the usual cleansing procedure with soap or detergent and water or only with saline.[17-19] Recommended preparations have also included a combination formulation of povidone-iodine and ethanol (Betaseptic®) and 0.1% to 0.2% polyhexanide, a polyhexamethylene bisguanidine for all kinds of traumatogenic wounds.[19,20]

Decubital ulcers are skin ulcerations caused by prolonged pressure resulting in ischemic necrosis of the skin and underlying soft tissue. They are common in patients who, for various reasons, are not mobile enough to allow their pressurized body parts to recover from local ischemia. Malnutrition, incontinence, and low concentration of serum albumin may aggravate the condition. Complications arising from these skin lesions are cellulitis, soft tissue necrosis, osteomyelitis in adjacent bones, and systemic infection. The infectious flora is usually a mixed flora of aerobic and anaerobic bacteria, but differentiation between colonization and infection may be difficult. Bacteria most commonly isolated are staphylococci, streptococci, enterobacteria, and a range of anaerobic species.

The most important preventive measure is to remove the pressure from the affected skin area by special mattresses and beds ranging from egg-crate foam and automatic mattresses to turning or fluidized beds. Physiotherapy and massage increase local perfusion. High-calorie nutritional preparations and parenteral amino acid mixtures supplement protein loss from permanent wound secretion. Administration of antibiotics is considered necessary only when signs of tissue or systemic infection occur. Surgical debridement may be necessary in some cases, followed by plastic surgery. The role of antisepsis is limited to the attempt to delay heavy bacterial colonization of the wound. Aqueous povidone-iodine solutions or ointments are most commonly applied. In some countries, tetrachlorodecaoxide (Oxoferin®) was also used for many years for both prevention and eradication of bacterial colonization and, because of its stimulating effect on epithelial granulation, as a preparation for the base of ulcers for skin transplantation.[21] Other examples include the use of advanced, including biocide-impregnated dressings such as those containing silver, CHG, and polyhexamethylene biguanides (see chapters 73 and 74).[22] Although the benefits of many of dressings or topical treatments in these cases can range considerably, advances in the development of optimum biocide delivery, effectiveness, and novel application are areas of recent research, in particular as alternatives to combat emerging antibiotic resistance trends.[23]

Since the onset of surgery, the surgical wound has always been recognized as a site of increased infection risk (see chapter 43). The pathogenesis, epidemiology, and prevention of surgical site infection (SSI) and the factors determining these risks have been well studied since Joseph Lister, at the latest, but exhaustively so during the 40 years to enable surgeons to apply continuously improving surgical techniques without jeopardizing the results of their work. Excellent guidelines and recommendations for prevention of SSI have been published,[24,25] that have continued to build on previous versions.[26] In addition, the Centers for Disease Control and Prevention (CDC) had developed a system of standardized surveillance criteria for defining SSI[27] that have been widely used. According to this CDC system, SSIs are classified into superficial incisional, deep incisional, and organ/space infections. Similar classification systems are used worldwide but can vary from country to country.[25] Surveillance of SSI rates are recommended as an essential part of the World Health Organization (WHO) guidelines to reduce SSIs, as well as being mandatory (eg, in the United Kingdom) or voluntary in different countries.[25,28,29]

The literature on this subject cannot be reviewed in full here and is further considered in chapter 43. But a few facts should be recalled and explained to define the role of antisepsis within the range of other preventive measures or factors influencing infection risk. SSIs are the most common of reported health care-acquired infections, are a major cause of morbidity and mortality, and a significant cost burden.[25,30] In the United States alone, it is estimated that approximately 2% of surgical procedures are associated with an SSI, and these rates can range for facility to facility and country to country. According to various sources,[25,31,32] the most frequent causative agents of SSI are bacteria including *S aureus* (approximately 30%), coagulase-negative staphylococci (approximately 12%), *Escherichia coli* (approximately 9%), *Enterococcus faecalis* (6%), *P aeruginosa* (approximately 5%), *Enterobacter* species (4%), and *Klebsiella* species (4%). Other bacteria and fungi (especially *Candida albicans*) are also frequently implicated. It is generally accepted that the main source of this flora is the patient.[24,25,33] Apart from specific carrier dispersers (such as those carrying *S aureus* in the nares), surgical personnel are regarded as a less important source if the rules of good surgical practice are adhered to.[34]

Among the risk factors associated with SSI are patient-related (ie, patient characteristics), procedure-related ones (ie, operative characteristics), and postoperative characteristics (see chapter 43). Examples of the former are patient age, nasal carriage of *S aureus*, underlying diseases and pathologic conditions such as obesity and diabetes, presence of infection at other sites, malnutrition and glucose levels, the length of the preoperative hospital stay, and others.[24,25] Examples of operative characteristics include type of procedure, such as orthopedic, breast, or heart surgery, with or without implanted foreign material; duration of the surgical procedure, whether it is an emergency or elective operation; hair removal; blood transfusion; and antibiotic prophylaxis.[24-26,33]

The risk for development of an infection can be affected by the quality of the surgical technique (which is often difficult to assess objectively) and by the degree of microbial contamination of the surgical site during the operation. Based on the latter, the National Academy of Sciences and the National Research Council[35] developed a widely accepted classification of surgical wounds that is used worldwide,[24,25] stratifying them into four major categories:

- *Clean* sites are those in which no inflammation is encountered and in which areas with a physiologic microbial colonization, such as the respiratory, alimentary, genital, and urinary tracts, are not entered.
- *Clean-contaminated sites* are colonized by a natural flora and are entered under controlled conditions and without unusual contamination. Typical operative sites include the biliary tract, appendix, vagina, and oropharynx, provided no evidence of infection or major break in technique is encountered.
- *Contaminated* surgical sites include open, fresh accidental wounds or operations with major breaks in sterile technique or gross spillage from the gastrointestinal tract. Typical surgical sites are those entering the urinary tract with infected urine or the biliary tract with infected bile, and surgical sites with acute, nonpurulent inflammation.
- *Dirty and infected* sites include old traumatic wounds with residual devitalized tissue, foreign bodies, or fecal contamination, and sites where a perforated viscus or pus is encountered during the operation.

There is a clear correlation between the class of surgical wound and the postoperative infection rate,[24,25,32,36-38] which ranges for the four classes between 0.2% to 2.9%, 0.9% to 3.9%, 1.3% to 8.5%, and 2.1% to 48%, respectively (see chapter 43). Among all these risk factors, the patient's own colonizing and, even more, the infecting microflora play an important role, as does the flora of the environment surgical team.[25] This has been considered in attempts to minimize the infection risk by including relevant recommendations for the management of both infected patients or staff members and for antiseptic measures to reduce the level of colonizing microbial flora that might reach the surgical site (chapter 43).

The latest guidelines for the prevention of SSI[24,25] provide recommendations that are categorized based on existing scientific data, theoretic rationale, and applicability. For example, the CDC category IA and IB recommendations are regarded as effective by experts in the fields of surgery, infectious diseases, and infection control based on the quality of scientific evidence suggesting net clinical benefits. Category II recommendations have, based on the review committee, less supporting scientific data than for category I in the balance between clinical benefits and harms. For some practices, no recommendation is given because the available scientific evidence is not considered sufficient, or there is lack of consensus as to their efficacy.[25] But the subjectivity of some of these recommendations is highlighted in a comparison between international recommendations based on the same data review.[24,25] Examples include the use of antimicrobial sutures and the benefit/harms balance of the identification of underlying conditions and/or infections. Others seem to make practical sense, such as the identification of personnel with potentially transmissible infection (eg, such as the carriage of *S aureus* in the nares) should be identified or encouraged to report the condition, and policies should be developed that allow work restrictions and require clearance to resume work after an illness that required work exclusion.

For antiseptic measures at the incisional site or the team's hands, there are many data on the antimicrobial efficacy of various agents on the skin (see chapters 42 and 43), but the clinical effects of optimum preoperative skin antisepsis on the risk of SSI remain the subject of debate. Nevertheless, use of an appropriate antiseptic agent is recommended for preparation of the incision site, which has been previously washed and cleaned to remove gross contamination.[24,25] Overall, the guidelines highlight the use of alcohol-based antiseptics that may or may not include CHG for presurgical, intraoperative skin preparation (see chapter 43). Other widely used biocides include CHG and iodine (eg, iodophor) products, but alcohols are generally found to be more effective. No one type of preoperative skin preparation has been shown consistently to reduce SSI rates, despite studies that shows differences in their safety and effectiveness.[39] But overall, the selection of a product will depend on the needs of the surgical procedure on the patient (eg, the location on the body) and the surgical staff. The timing and method of application depends on the specific and approved labeled claims of the preoperative skin preparation product.

Likewise, the recommendations for hand antisepsis of the surgical team are recommended using an appropriate antiseptic, despite the subsequent use of surgical, sterile gloves.[24,25] The recommended surgical scrub procedures require that staff first remove any jewelry (eg, rings and watches), clean under the fingernails with water, and then apply an appropriate antiseptic (preferably with a biocide that presents with persistent activity such as CHG) in accordance with manufacturer's instructions.[40,41] For hand washes, this includes washing the hands and forearms thoroughly with an antimicrobial soap, followed by rinsing and drying prior to donning gloves. For hand rubs, it is recommended that the hands are first washed with a nonantimicrobial soap, rinsed, and dried and then applying the alcohol solution to hands and rubbing into the hands and forearms; the hands should be allowed to dry before donning gloves. Antiseptics should be used as recommended by the manufacturer (2-6 minutes, in general), with no need for arbitrary extended contact time recommendations that were often cited in the past.[26] It is equally important to follow aseptic practices following hand washing/scrubbing in gowning (including donning of sterile gloves) and subsequent surgical practices to reduce cross-contamination risks.[34]

For skin and hand antisepsis, only a few groups of chemical agents are suitable, some of them only in combination with alcohols:

- Alcohols
- Iodine/iodophors
- CHG
- Some phenolic compounds, such as parachloro-metaxylenol (PCMX or chloroxylenol), biphenylol (2-phenylphenol), and others
- Triclosan

Of these, alcohols are by far the fastest acting and most efficacious.[24,25,40-43] Almost exclusively, the short-chain, aliphatic alcohols—ethanol, isopropanol, and in Europe, *n*-propanol—are used for skin and hand antisepsis (see chapters 19 and 42). They have excellent activity against bacteria, fungi, and enveloped viruses. Against nonenveloped viruses such as enteroviruses, including picornavirus and hepatitis A virus, their activity is less pronounced and limited to high concentrations (>90% volume per volume [vol/vol]) of ethanol.[44,45] Antimicrobial activity against these viruses is often considered less important because viruses are not members of the resident skin flora and are not typically cited as become sources of SSIs but may in some cases be associated with cross-infection in particular for blood-borne pathogens.[46] In addition, alcohols are not effective against bacterial spores and instances of alcohol contamination with spore-forming pathogens or the carriage of spores in health care worker hands have been reported,[47] suggesting the use of products that are known to be free of spores or the use of the physical removal of spores (by washing) have been recommended. Alcohols are also flammable, and this may be a disadvantage for their use in the operating room and requires special considerations for storage.[34] Furthermore, the surgical team must ensure that no alcohol residues are left on the skin and under the patient to avoid burns when a thermocautery is used, and to prevent postoperative skin necrosis at the contact surface when the patient is left lying in a pool of alcohol.

There is a clear association between the alcohol species and antimicrobial efficacy, with *n*-propanol being the most active, followed by isopropanol and ethanol (see chapters 19 and 42).[42,43] The activity also depends on the concentration. The strongest and fastest action is seen with *n*-propanol and isopropanol at concentrations of 100%, and with ethanol at concentrations of 85% to 95% vol/vol. The traditional belief that the best activity of ethanol is achieved at 77% vol/vol is true only for dry bacteria,[42,48] and this will also depend on the formulation of the alcohol product (see chapter 19). Skin bacteria are never considered dry. To be effective in the discussed areas of application, alcohol concentrations (here, always vol/vol) should typically not fall below 60% with *n*-propanol, 80% with isopropanol, and 90% with ethanol. This opinion is based on the observation[49] that the efficacy of isopropanol against the resident skin flora of hands is comparable with that of *n*-propanol 60. At 70%, the bacterial reduction was considered significantly less. Likewise, with ethanol 85%, it was shown that even this high concentration was significantly less effective than 80%, although significantly more effective than isopropanol at 70%.[50] Only at 95% was the activity of ethanol comparable with that of *n*-propanol 60%, but these results may depend not only on the specific alcohol concentration but also the overall formulation and demonstrated effectiveness of the specific antiseptic. It must be admitted, that the antimicrobial activity of *n*-propanol 60% was arbitrarily chosen as a reference for a European Standard,[51] and there are no data to prove its clinical superiority in terms of a reduced rate of SSI.

In Table 44.1, the antibacterial efficacy of *n*-propanol 60% vol/vol is demonstrated for preoperative incision site antisepsis. Biopsy and cylinder scrub samplings were taken before the alcohol had been swabbed for exactly 1 minute onto the abdominal skin of recently deceased patients. After this procedure, samples were taken again at both points of time immediately and after complete drying, which extended the total disinfection time to 2 to 3 minutes.[52] It can be seen that bacterial reduction by the alcohol is significantly associated with the disinfection time and that the antiseptic effect on anaerobic bacterial flora is less pronounced when the biopsy method is used, which samples the deeper anaerobic flora more effectively. This difference was not considered significant.

From very sebaceous areas such as scalp and forehead, the deep-lying skin flora is much more difficult to reduce. Sixty percent vol/vol *n*-propanol achieved a 2.1 log reduction of aerobic flora on the skin surface but only a 1.4 log reduction at depth, and propionibacteria were specifically reduced only by 0.6 log.[53] The corresponding values for isopropanol 60% vol/vol were 0.8, 0.4, and 0.5 log, respectively. With a 4-minute rub of ethanol 77% vol/vol on the

(sebum-free) palm a reduction in aerobic flora of 2.3 log was reported but only 1.3 log on the forehead.[54] This problem was also originally reported by Christiansen,[55] who initially developed the German Society of Hygiene and Microbiology guidelines for testing skin antiseptics in sebum-rich and in other skin areas.

Table 44.2 provides a summary of different alcohols according to their efficacy as surgical hand scrubs/disinfectants at various concentrations and times of application. These results were obtained by comparable methods to the European norm, EN 12791.[66] They demonstrate that not only the alcohol species and its concentration but also the application time are determining factors for the efficacy of surgical scrubs, even if this could not be shown in all trials by some authors.[67] Furthermore, the data indicate that the immediate antibacterial effect of these alcohols is good enough to keep bacterial release under the glove low for at least 3 hours. This is explained by the slow regrowth of the skin flora, as observed with combination alcohol products such as with CHG.[24,25] According to EN 12791, the immediate effect of a product for surgical hand disinfection used for 3 to 5 minutes must not be significantly less than that of the reference (ie, *n*-propanol 60% vol/vol within 3 minutes), a test for a 3-hour sustained effect is required only if there is an explicit claim about this effect (see chapter 42). In this case, the mean bacterial reduction caused by the product must be significantly stronger than that of the reference scrub after 3 hours on the gloved hand.

Alcohols are used either alone or in combination with one of the other chemicals listed previously, mainly to confer sustained activity, which they lack, but also to increase the antimicrobial effect. But overall impact of such combined products continues to be an area of debate (see chapters 19 and 42).[24,25] As an example, when ethanol 77% vol/vol was used for skin antisepsis in combination with 1.5% iodine, a bacterial reduction of 2.3 log on a sebum-free and of 1.3 log on a sebum-rich environment was achieved in only 45 seconds,[68] whereas with ethanol alone, 4 minutes was needed. In combination with 0.5% CHG, the respective reductions were 2.2 and 0.9 log for the same period of application. For surgical scrubs, it has also been shown that the combination of 70% isopropanol with 0.5% CHG causes significant sustained (3 h) effects on the gloved hand regardless of the application time. A 5-minute application achieved, for example, an immediate 2.5 log reduction, but a sustained effect of 2.7 log,[60] and a 2-minute application caused corresponding effects of 0.7 and 1.4 log.[61] With respect to the strong immediate and the resulting sustained effects of alcohols alone (if valid), it must be questioned whether a real sustained effect is needed for the surgical scrub if a product meets the requirement of EN 12791 regarding the immediate effect (see chapters 42 and 43).

In the past, surgical scrubs based on iodine (PVPI) and CHG were traditionally preferred in North America, and alcohols were not as widely used, often due to being more drying on the skin and leading to decreased compliance in use. In contrast, alcohols were well accepted

TABLE 44.1	Results of skin antisepsis with rubbing *n*-propanol 60% vol/vol onto abdominal skin for exactly 1 minute versus 2 to 3 minutes (until dry)[a]

Sampling Method	Culture	Mean (*N* = 12) Log Reduction After Disinfection (min)	
		1	2-3
Biopsy	Aerobic	1.3[b]	1.7
	Anaerobic	0.9[b]	1.5
Cylinder scrub	Aerobic	1.4[b]	1.7
	Anaerobic	1.2[b]	1.8

Abbreviation: vol/vol, volume per volume.

[a]From Semradova et al.[52]

[b]All *p* < .05.

TABLE 44.2	Effect of surgical hand rub with alcohols on the release of autochthonous flora from clean hands				
Alcohol	**Concentration[a] (%)**	**Time (min)**	**Mean Log Reduction**		**References**
			Immediate	Sustained (3 h)	
n-Propanol	60	5	2.9	1.6	Rotter et al[56]
		5	2.7	NA	Heeg et al[57]
		5	2.5	1.8	Rotter and Koller[58]
		5	2.3	1.6	Rotter and Koller[59]
		3	3.2	1.8	Rotter et al (unpublished data, 2001)
		3	2.8	NA	Rotter et al[50]
		3	2.4	1.0	Rotter et al[49]
		3	2.0	1.0	Rotter and Koller[59]
		1	1.1	0.5	Rotter and Koller[59]
Isopropanol	90	3	2.4	1.4	Rotter et al[49]
	80	3	2.3	1.2	Rotter et al[49]
	70	5	2.4	2.1	Wewalka et al[60]
		5	2.1	1.0	Rotter and Koller[59]
		3	2.0	0.7	Rotter et al[49]
		3	1.7	NA	Rotter et al (unpublished data, 2001)
		3	1.5	0.8	Rotter and Koller[59]
		2	1.2	0.8	Lowbury et al[61]
		1	0.7	0.2	Rotter and Koller[59]
		1	0.8	NA	Aly and Maybach[62]
	60	5	1.7	1.0	Rotter et al[63]
Ethanol	95	2	2.1	NA	Lilly et al[64]
	90	3	3.2	2.2	Rotter and Lhotsky (unpublished data, 2001)
	85	3	2.3	NA	Rotter et al[50]
	80	2	1.5	NA	Altemeier[65]
	70	2	1.0	0.6	Lowbury et al[61]

Abbreviation: NA, not available.

[a]Volume per volume (vol/vol).

as surgical scrubs in the German-speaking countries, and in the Scandinavian countries. Hospital personnel were advised to replace soap and other detergents with alcohol preparations containing suitable emollients to take advantage of the faster antimicrobial action of alcohols without creating skin problems that were often reported with the frequent use of soap and water-based scrubbing action for extended exposure times.[69] The beneficial effect of appropriate emollients has been demonstrated,[70] and there is consensus that alcohols without such additives should not be used for frequent hand rubs (see chapters 19 and 42).

Despite its wide antimicrobial spectrum, elemental iodine used as an (alcoholic) tincture or as an aqueous solution of potassium iodine (Lugol solution) has virtually been replaced by preparations containing iodine complexed with polymers such as polyvinylpyrrolidone (ie, povidone), polyether glycols, or polyoxyethanol derivatives (see chapter 16). These preparations do not cause skin burns, do not need to be removed on skin application (to prevent excessive irritation), and are much better accepted. Their strongest antimicrobial effect occurs with dilute rather than concentrated solutions,[71,72] and in some cases, these solutions have been found to be contaminated with pseudomonad biofilms (see chapter 16).[73,74] Like many biocides at lower concentrations, they can be inactivated by organic matter (including blood); 1 g of hemoglobin was estimated to inactivate 58 mg of iodine.[75]

The antimicrobial spectrum of iodophors is wide, including even bacterial spores at certain concentrations, although not practically at concentrations typically used in antiseptics (see chapter 16).[40,41,76] Although the latter activity may be useful for long-term preparation of the incision site, it is much too slow to make use of it in the surgical scrub.[77] Without special precautions such as addition of potassium iodide, the antimicrobial efficacy of iodophors decreases during storage (see chapter 16).

Up to recently, for preoperative preparation of skin and mucus membranes, iodophors were among the most widely used antiseptics (but now with a preference being for the use of alcohols or alcohol/CHG combinations in such applications). Their antibacterial effect is rapid, although not considered as fast and strong as that of alcohols-based product formulations currently in widespread use, and they exert hardly any sustained effect if used on the skin.[70] Table 44.3 gives an example of the efficacy on skin flora of an aqueous solution of povidone-iodine with approximately 1% available iodine, compared with that of *n*-propanol 60% vol/vol, both of which were rubbed for 1 minute onto the abdominal skin of recently deceased patients. Independent of the sampling method (biopsy or cylinder scrub), the bacterial reduction achieved with the alcohol proved significantly stronger.

When used for the surgical scrub, the antimicrobial efficacy of an aqueous solution of povidone-iodine is comparable with that of isopropanol 60% vol/vol, producing, after a hand rub of 5 minutes, a bacterial reduction of 1.7 to 1.9 log. This was significantly less efficacious than a hand rub with *n*-propanol 60%, which results in mean log reductions of 2.3 to 2.9 (see Table 44.2).[56] Many detergent-based preparations of povidone-iodine are considered even less active but can vary depending on their formulation (see chapter 16). A 15-minute hand wash with povidone-iodine liquid soap reduces the release of skin flora only by 0.9 to 1.1 log (Table 44.4), although this is significantly better than the results with unmedicated soap, which was found to have reductions of approximately 0.4 log in the studies reported (see Table 44.4). On the skin of the hands, a sustained activity was hardly demonstrable, as would be expected for the type of biocide activity (see Table 44.4).[70]

The bisbiguanide compound CHG is more commonly used for antisepsis of the skin and hands as a digluconate salt, but the acetate has also been used (see chapter 22). Formulations of CHG can vary considerably in antimicrobial activity on the skin and not just based on the concentration of CHG in the product. For example, washing of hands for 2 to 6 minutes with a detergent preparation of CHG caused bacterial reductions of 0.8 to 1.2 log in comparison to other antiseptics (see Table 44.4). A sustained effect after 3 hours under surgical gloves is demonstrable (see Table 44.4) and is considered one of the particular benefits of this biocide in skin or wound applications (see chapters 22 and 43).[85] The CHG can also be used for reducing the load of bacteria on the skin in prewashing prior to surgery[24,25,86,87] and for the prevention of catheter-related skin and bloodstream infections (see chapter 22). In an early study comparing a 2% aqueous CHG with 70% (vol/vol) isopropanol and an aqueous solution of povidone-iodine in preventing insertion site infection and catheter-related septicemia,[88] CHG prevented both local infection (2.3%) and bacteremia (0.5%) significantly more effectively than isopropanol (7.1% and 2.3%, respectively) or povidone-iodine (9.3% and 2.6%, respectively).

Both groups of agents, iodophors and CHG (as well as soap and water), are also used for preoperative bathing or showering of patients prior to surgery.[24,25] There is good evidence that the skin flora and rate of wound contamination are reduced by two preoperative antiseptic baths or showers; however, a reduction of the SSI rate with or without the use of specific antiseptics has not always been shown convincingly.[24,25]

For preoperative antisepsis of both the patient's skin and the surgical team's hands, other chemical agents such as triclosan, phenolics, and cationic and amphoteric compounds have been used,[41,42] but to date, none of them has proved to be superior to the use of alcohols, iodophors, or CHG preparations mentioned previously (see Table 44.4).

TABLE 44.3	Results of skin antisepsis with rubbing either *n*-propanol 60% vol/vol or aqueous povidone-iodine (1% wt/wt) onto abdominal skin for 1 minute[a]

| Sampling Method | Mean (*N* = 12) Log Reduction | |
	n-Propanol	Povidone-Iodine
Biopsy	1.4	0.7[b]
Cylinder scrub	1.4	0.6[b]

Abbreviations: vol/vol, volume per volume; wt/wt, weight per weight.

[a]From Semradova et al.[52]

[b]All *p* < .05.

Tetanus

Tetanus is an infectious disease is caused by exotoxins (particularly tetanospasmin, a neurotoxin) produced at the site of wound entry by the anaerobic, spore-forming bacterium *C tetani*. The bacteria are widely distributed and commonly found in soil, dust and mature, the source of which is the gut of plant-eating animals. Therefore, those working in agricultural areas are at a higher risk and are frequently found to have *C tetani* spores on their skin. Infection is commonly associated with puncture wounds with contaminated objects but can also be linked to existing wound contamination (eg, umbilical cord stump postdelivery in neonates, poor aseptic practices on circumcision, and skin/mucous membrane damage).[89] Disease is initiated by introduction of the bacterial spores of the organism into the area of injury, and

TABLE 44.4 Effect of surgical hand wash on the release of resident flora from clean hands

Agent	Concentration[a] (%)	Time (min)	Mean Log Reduction		References
			Immediate	Sustained (3 h)	
Unmedicated soap		5	0.4	−0.1	Rotter et al[56]
		5	0.4	NA	Heeg et al[57]
		5	0.4	0.0	Larson et al[78]
Povidone-iodine liquid soap	0.8	5	1.1	0.3	Larson et al[78]
		5	1.0	NA	Heeg et al[57]
		5	1.0	0.2	Rotter et al[63]
		5	0.9	0.2	Rotter et al[63]
		2	0.5	NA	Lilly and Lowbury[79]
Chlorhexidine liquid soaps	4.0	6	1.2	NA	Furuhashi and Miamae[80]
		5	0.9	0.9	Rotter et al[56]
		5	0.9	0.6	Larson et al[78]
		3	1.2	1.4	Holloway[81]
		3	0.8	1.0	Rotter et al[56]
		3	0.8	0.8	Rotter et al[63]
		2	1.0	1.2	Babb et al[82]
		2	0.9	1.6	Lowbury et al[83]
		5 × 3	1.6	0.2	Bendig[84]
Zephirol	0.1	2	0.4	NA	Altemeier[65]
		2	0.3	NA	Lilly and Lowbury[79]
Cetrimide	1.0	2	0.4	NA	Lilly and Lowbury[79]
Chloro-cresol	0.3	2	0.4	NA	Lilly and Lowbury[79]
Triclosan	1.0	5	0.6	0.5	Larson[78]
	2.0	5 × 3	0.8	1.1	Bendig[84]

Abbreviation: NA, not available.

[a]Weight per volume (wt/vol).

particularly deeper into the skin where low-oxygen (anaerobic) conditions allow for germination and growth of the bacteria, with subsequent toxin production. The toxin can enter the blood/lymphatic system and be carried to the central nervous system, where the toxin interferes with neurotransmission. After an incubation period that can range from 3 to 21 days, tonic muscle spasms and hyperreflexia occur. There are three forms of tetanus based on clinical manifestations, local, cephalic, and general tetanus. The rarer forms (local or cephalic) show muscle effects localized to the site of infection, such as the wound site or facial features respectively. But at least 80% of cases are general tetanus, classically showing "lock-jaw," with muscle stiffness to the neck and jaw, but also other effects including fever, muscle spasms, seizures, and headache. Since the 1920s, based on pioneering work by Ramon on toxin inactivation using formaldehyde and the development of tetanus toxoid by Descombey,[89,90] tetanus is

preventable by immunization with and used during treatment of the disease with tetanus toxoid–containing vaccines These are now recommended in routine immunization programs by the WHO and others globally, and in high-risks areas of population (eg, neonates).[91] These guidelines have dramatically reduced the rates of tetanus reported worldwide.[92] In 2015, estimates of mortality due to tetanus suggest approximately 56,700 deaths, with about 35% reported in neonates (especially in South Asia and Sub-Saharan Africa).[92] These rates have been significantly reduced, with approximately 90% reduction in neonates alone from previous estimates in 1990. For neonates, the infection risks remain high because of unhygienic conditions and unsafe umbilical care practices at delivery, such as unsafe practices such as covering the umbilical wound with cow dung.[93]

Overall, the emphasis on infection prevention and control with tetanus is vaccination (both for pre- and postexposure prophylaxis). But, there continues to be debate on the benefits of other preventative measures, including the use of antiseptics following wounds or in high-risk situations with neonates.[94] It continues to be good practice to ensure all wounds are cleaned, in particular to remove necrotic tissue and the presence of any foreign bodies.[95] Necrotic tissue and foreign material should be removed. With neonates, proper cord care during the first days of life is recommended by several institutions, such as the WHO and United Nations Children's Fund. But overall, the impact of the use of antiseptics specifically is not known and may be considered low due to the lack of substantial efficacy against bacterial spores with most antiseptics; however, the impact of reducing the microbial load by cleaning and preventing the outgrowth of bacterial spores may have an impact. For example, in a randomized trial, daily application of triple dye, povidone-iodine ointment, silver sulfadiazine, or bacitracin ointment to the umbilical stump produced no significant differences in the incidence of colonization with any organism,[96] but povidone-iodine ointment was preferred because of cleanliness, ease of use, and excellent tolerance. But overall, the evidence would suggest that the use of antiseptics may have a benefit, particularly in developing countries as part of best practices in infection prevention.[97] Similarly, antibiotic prophylaxis is not considered beneficial in managing associated wounds, with emphasis placed on immunization strategies.[95]

▶ PREVENTION OF COLONIZATION AND INFECTION OF BURN WOUNDS

Although the survival of patients with burn wounds has increased considerably since the early 1970s,[33] infections are still the most common cause of death in burn patients, with the most frequent sites of infection being the burn wound and the lungs.[98,99] Mortality continues to be directly related to the extent of body surface area injured and the age of patient. For children and young adults with 59% of body surface area injured, the mortality rate was reported to be less than 20%, whereas for 70-year-old patients with the same extent of injury, it was 70%.[100,101] The proportion of deaths related to burn wound infection was estimated to be approximately 86%[102] but can range depending on the country and other patient factors.

The high infection risk of burn wounds is easily understood when the following facts related to pathogenesis are considered. The thermal lesion represents an open wound comprising avascular, necrotic tissue, which combined with serum proteins, provides a rich culture medium for microorganisms. In addition, general and local immunosuppression together with impaired function of neutrophils as a consequence of the thermal injury favors the multiplication of colonizing microbial flora. This can be followed by microbial invasion of neighboring viable tissue and other sources of microorganisms, particularly antibiotic-resistance bacteria that are often more prevalent in health care facilities.[99,102,103] The most frequently encountered pathogens are bacteria and yeasts, similar to those reported for wound infections discussed previously, including *S aureus* (26%), *P aeruginosa* (21%), enterococci (12%), *Enterobacter* (9%), *E coli* (8%), and *Candida* (5%).[104,105] Increasing reports of infections with multidrug-resistant bacteria, as in all health care acquired infections but particularly in high-risk patients, is a concern such as with strains of methicillin-resistant *S aureus*, *P aeruginosa* and other pseudomonads, *Acinetobacter baumannii*, *Stenotrophomonas maltophilia*, and carbapenem-resistant Enterobacteriaceae.[105,106] Also, early burn wound infections are predominantly caused by gram-positive cocci from the endogenous flora; gram-negative bacteria and fungi are typically found in the wound later, such as 4 to 10 days after injury.[102,105,107,108] Yeasts (*Candida* species) and filamentous fungi can also cause common infectious complications.[107] Common fungi are *Aspergillus* species, Zygomycetes such as *Mucor* and *Rhizopus* species, *Geotrichum* species, and *Fusarium* species. Viral infections, although less common are reported. Herpes simplex is the most important viral cause of infection in burned patients, followed by cytomegalovirus. Both viruses, which are usually reactivated, may produce symptomatic or asymptomatic infection.[102,109]

The diagnosis of burn infection requires a distinction to be made from mere microbial colonization and can be difficult to define.[110,111] The only reliable method to do this traditionally has been by biopsy of the wound, with the specimen containing viable tissue adjacent to the eschar. Definite evidence of infection is attained only by the histopathologic proof of microbial tissue invasion, although less than 10^5 colony-forming units (CFUs)/g tissue, as determined by quantitative culture, has been used as an indication of the absence of infection with high probability.[112] Specimens containing 10^5 to 10^8 CFUs/g cannot be interpreted without histopathologic analysis, and those with more than 10^8 CFUs/g tissue are usually considered to be infected.

Early studies on the epidemiology of burn wound infection identified the patients' burn wound and their gastrointestinal tract as the most important reservoirs of microorganisms.[33,102,105] Carriers among the hospital personnel can act as a source of burn wound infection, but their role is limited when routine precautions are taken.[33] Hydrotherapy equipment (at one stage widely used for treating burn patients for purposes such as reducing microbial load and patient comfort) was identified as one of the most important inanimate reservoirs and as a source of serious infections.[113,114] Pathogens can be transmitted to the burn wound by the hands of the medical personnel, by fecal contamination, by *air* (eg, staphylococci), by hydrotherapy, and, in patients with more than 50% injured body surface area, possibly by bacterial translocation from the patient's gut through the (now permeable) gut mucosa into the mesenteric lymph system, blood circulation, and, finally, to the wound.[102,105,115] Risk factors for microbial colonization and/or infection of the burn wound can include the age of the patient,[100] the size of the wound,[100,115] duration of hospitalization,[99] resistance of microorganisms to topical antimicrobial agents,[33,34] and resistance to systemically administered antibiotics,[102,105] although they are assumed not to reach therapeutic concentrations in the eschar.

The prevention of burn wound infection must aim at both reducing the infection susceptibility of the wound and limiting the extent of microbial colonization by preventing the transmission of pathogens to the wound and reducing their numbers in the wound. To achieve these goals, the following strategies have proven successful, although the role of each individual measure alone is not always clear and continue to be debated[103,105]:

- Reduction of infection susceptibility by interventions such as early excision of necrotic tissue and closure of the burn wound with grafts. Early excision and closure of the burn wound is a generally accepted treatment method thought to improve local defense and greatly reduce the incidence of invasive burn wound sepsis, despite much debate.[33,103,105,107,116] It has been argued that several studies showing apparent reductions of infection were not sufficiently controlled and that during the introduction of early excision and wound closure, many aspects of burn wound care were also improved at same time as a typical bundle approach to infection prevention.[102]
- An understanding and monitoring of the antibiotic sensitivity of bacteria associated with infection in the burn.[117]
- Prevention of microbial transmission by best practices including barrier nursing techniques, use of protected environment (including isolation of high-risk patients known to be infected with multidrug-resistant bacteria), hand hygiene practices and correct sterile glove use, strict environmental cleaning/disinfection practices in particular for "high-touch" surfaces in close proximity to the patient, and correct use and handling of any associated invasive devices (including catheters).
- Reduction in the presence of colonizing microbial flora. The use of systemic antibiotics is particularly controversial, due to the limit of penetration to the site of infection but may play a role in preventing the further dissemination of bacteria systematically[103,105] or as established a best practice in the reduction of infection during surgical intervention (see chapter 43). The application of topical antimicrobials, including antibiotics or biocides, is often preferred.

Prevention of Microbial Transmission

Barrier nursing is well established as best practice in patient nursing and to reduce the incidence of burn wound sepsis.[99,103,118] Hand washing and hand disinfection and the use of gloves and patient-assigned aprons have been proven to lower the frequency of cross-contamination.[119]

Because the antimicrobial activity of alcoholic hand rubs is often preferred to that of soap and water or antimicrobial soaps, a suitable dispenser for alcoholic rub preparations should be provided conveniently (eg, next to each bed) to increase compliance (see chapters 19 and 42). But hand washing itself will not be effective if not combined with correct aseptic technique prior to patient contact, particularly on skin, materials or environmental surfaces that can be contaminated.[120] This logic applies in the use of sterile gloves, such as during dressing changes.

Because all surfaces and objects in the direct environment of the patient should be considered contaminated,[102,103] they must be cleaned and disinfected to reduce the risk of microbial transmission to the wound. Noncritical items such as stethoscopes, blood pressure cuffs, and thermometers should be used only on the same patient for the duration of his or her stay, and/or routinely cleaned and disinfected (see chapter 47). Mattresses are also recommended to be disinfected and covered after each patient; outbreaks related to mattresses have been reported.[121,122]

To prevent cross-contamination by hydrotherapy equipment and treatment, special barrier techniques must be used, and the equipment has to be adequately disinfected after each patient.[103,113,114,123] In addition, the water in hydrotherapy tanks may transfer the patient's own fecal or other flora to the burn wound; therefore, the addition of disinfectants such as chlorine-releasing agents has been used to reduce microbial loads. Sodium hypochlorite (see chapter 15), at concentrations of 120 to 780 mg/L, proved to be effective in eliminating all bacteria from the tank water and reducing bacterial numbers on burned and unburned skin (10- to 100-fold), but a number of adverse effects were experienced by patients and health care personnel.[124] Other biocides have been used or recommended for this application including chloramine-T, povidone-iodine, and CHG.[125,126] But in these cases, care should be taken to only use such products in accordance with their labeled claims because they can lead to other negative impacts including bacterial overgrowth and toxicity. Overall, the use of hydrotherapy baths is seen as a higher risk than alternatives such as showering.

Use of a Protected Environment

Whether an individual patient room, which has been reported to allow the use of barrier techniques most effectively,[127] is necessary is still a matter for discussion. At any rate, protected environments include patient isolators or rooms with unidirectional ventilation supplying sterile air, and personnel required to wear sterile gloves, gowns, caps, and masks. Although in theory, this environment protects the patient from cross-contamination, this has never been convincingly shown.[128,129] Furthermore, it cannot prevent colonization of the burn wound with the patient's own gastrointestinal flora. Furthermore, sufficiently controlled studies are still needed, the results of which could justify the high financial investments and running costs of such units as well as the psychic disturbances in patients confined to such units for prolonged periods.

Intestinal Tract Decontamination

Selective microbial reduction (referred to as "decontamination") of the gastrointestinal tract has been suggested to reduce the risk of endogenous and autoinfection from the patient's own gut. The idea is to remove potential pathogens from the gastrointestinal tract using oral, nonabsorbable antibiotics that do not attack the main part of the anaerobic bacterial flora, which physiologically confers a kind of local colonization resistance. Several studies have produced conflicting results, and in the only randomized—although small—trial, no evidence was found for decreased or delayed colonization of the burn wound by enteric bacteria, but severe side effects prompted discontinuation of the treatment in 9 of the 27 patients.[130] From the available data, it was concluded that selective gastrointestinal microbial reduction is still of unproven to reduce the risk of burn wound sepsis and that possible side effects of this prophylactic measure are not well defined.[102] Despite this, a recent review of clinical studies on the mortality, incidence of infection, and its adverse effects in burn patients concluded an overall beneficial effect of these practices, but this remains controversial.[131]

Reduction of Colonizing Microflora

Antimicrobial agents are widely used to diminish colonization and growth of microorganisms on the surface of the burn wound, thereby reducing the risk of invasion into living tissue. Both systemic and topical antimicrobials have been used, but topical antimicrobials are preferred.[103,105] The systemic administration of antibiotics is limited by two facts: (1) at therapeutic doses the antibiotic concentrations in the avascular eschar often remain below the minimum inhibitory concentration of the colonizing microflora; and (2) under the preceding condition, selection of resistant strains among the colonizing flora is virtually unavoidable during continued, long-term use of the same antibiotic.[132] Therefore, the prophylactic use of systemic antibiotics should be limited to clear indications, such as perioperative prophylaxis before surgical intervention to reduce the risk of bacterial dissemination due to manipulation of the colonized burn wound (see chapter 43).[99,103,105] Furthermore, the microbial flora colonizing the burn wound should be monitored by culturing swabs, and the results of antimicrobial susceptibility tests should guide the choice of antibiotics. Burn wound biopsies for histopathologic examination and quantitative

cultures may be necessary for detection and effective therapy of superinfected burn wounds.

Topical administration of antimicrobials can help ensure that higher concentrations in the wound and on its surface. This can aid in inhibiting multiplication and even reducing the number of colonizing microflora. In general, antibiotics that are used for systemic administration should not be used topically and especially off-label use. Instead, certain antibiotics (eg, sulfonamides) and antiseptics (eg, silver sulfadiazine) are used. The most prominent antiseptics used are based on silver sulfadiazine, mafenide acetate, and silver nitrate.[99] Other biocides used include povidone-iodine and CHG (Table 44.5). Applications methods include the direct use of the biocide in the wound (using creams, ointments, or liquid rinses) of the indirect use as integrated in wound dressings.

The most commonly used antiseptic for burn applications has been silver sulfadiazine, is essentially the combination of two antimicrobials, silver and a sulfonamide. It is typically used in cream formulations (at approximately 1%) and demonstrates broad-spectrum bactericidal (against gram-negative and gram-positive bacteria) and yeasticidal activity.[133] But increased tolerance to silver has been described due to multiple mechanisms, such as efflux and exclusion, and including plasmid-borne resistance mechanisms (*sil* genes for silver as well as other antibiotic-resistance genes) in gram-negative (*Salmonella, Pseudomonas,* and *Acinetobacter*) and gram-positive bacteria (*S aureus*).[133,134] These mechanisms are often effective in render bacteria resistant to the antimicrobial levels of silver used in impregnated dressings. The precise mechanism of action of silver sulfadiazine is not known and not very well studied, but it is particularly focused on the cell wall/membrane. The proposed polymeric structure of six silver atoms bonding to six sulfadiazine molecules via the nitrogens of pyrimidine rings allows for release of silver over time as the main mechanisms of action (see chapter 25), but there also appears to be a synergistic action with sulfadiazine.[133,135] In contrast, the mode of action of silver alone has been well studied.[133,136] Silver is particularly active as the cell surface (wall/membrane) to affect the structure and function of proteins by binding to sulfhydryl, amino, and carboxyl groups of amino acids. This can lead to an overall distribution of wall/membrane functions, including increased permeability.

Silver sulfadiazine (1%) cream has a long history of use for burn treatment, with few side effects, but penetration into the wound is considered low.[137] A typical side effect of sulfonamides, crystalluria, has been rarely reported. It is often used as a comparative in the investigation of alternative biocide usage in clinical trials.[99,138] As mentioned previously, the development of bacterial resistance is common and can lead to clinical failure and may require changing to another antimicrobial.

TABLE 44.5   Characteristics of common topical antimicrobial agents for prevention of burn wound infections

Antimicrobial Agent	Formulation Example	Advantages	Side Effects and Disadvantages
Silver sulfadiazine (Flamazine®, Silvadene®)	1% in water-soluble cream	Broad antimicrobial spectrum, mediocre penetration into wound, fewest side effects of the three most used agents	Allergy to sulfonamides; crystalluria (rare); methemoglobinemia, leukopenia (transient and mild); resistance common
Mafenide acetate (Sulfamylon®, Napaltan®)	10% in water-soluble cream or 5% in aqueous solution soaks	Broad antimicrobial spectrum; very good penetration into wound; resistance uncommon	Application may be painful; allergic reactions; hyperchloremic acidosis
Silver nitrate	0.5% in aqueous solution soaks	Broad antimicrobial spectrum	Poor penetration into wound; hyponatremia; hypochloremia; methemoglobinemia; frequent changing of soaks necessary
Povidone-iodine	10% in aqueous solution or water-soluble cream	Broad antimicrobial spectrum; good penetration into wound; antimycotic activity	High absorption of iodine associated with effects on the function of the thyroid gland
Chlorhexidine	0.1% in combination with 0.5% silver nitrate in creams	Often more convenient to use than silver nitrate soaks; persistence on the skin	As for silver nitrate but can also be associated with irritancy or sensitivity in some patients

Another sulfonamide, initially developed for treatment of large wound areas, is mafenide acetate (Sulfamylon®), the acetate of 4-aminomethylbenzol-sulfonamide. Its broad antimicrobial spectrum and excellent penetration of eschar have made it an indispensable first-line agent in the local prevention and therapy of burn wound infections. Mafenide acetate (10%) cream has to be applied at least twice daily because the concentration of the sulfonamide decreases considerably within 8 to 12 hours. Compresses soaked with 5% mafenide acetate have been recommended to be changed every 3 to 4 hours.[107] Bacterial resistance is also known but uncommon. Some side effects are worrisome and should be carefully monitored. For example, application of the cream is often accompanied by a (transient) burning sensation, and, in addition to allergic reactions, hyperchloremic acidosis may be observed in patients with a large wound surface area.[139]

Silver nitrate, a classic antiseptic, has a broad antimicrobial spectrum (see chapter 25). It is used at a concentration of 0.5% in aqueous solutions that are administered with soaked compresses. The agent does not penetrate the eschar. Side effects such as hyponatremia, hypochloremia, and methemoglobinemia may occur. Development of resistance has also been observed, as discussed earlier. It has been recommended to delay the development of resistance by regularly alternating the use of the aforementioned topical antimicrobials[99] or change to alternative (but not necessarily more efficacious) agents such as povidone-iodine preparations, polyhexanide, sodium hypochlorite, merbromin (a considered weak antiseptics containing mercury) or those containing low concentrations of CHG alone or in combination with silver nitrate.[102,105,138] Other

alternatives include natural products such as honey and aloe vera that also had some benefits over nonantimicrobial treatments,[138] with honey being now well established for its benefits in wound healing.[139] Overall, these agents are useful alternatives but have not to date replaced the classic antimicrobials.[20,99,140,141]

As previously mentioned, many of these biocides are used not only for wound cleaning and application but also in combination with dressings that can have multiple benefits in addition to reduce the risks of microbial multiplication. Examples include exudate management, wound healing, and cross-contamination prevention. These dressings are composed of alginate and/or polyurethane that are coated with biocides, particularly silver.[20,99] More advanced dressings include vacuum (or negative pressure)-assisted closure dressings that typically consist of a foam or gauze material (that can be impregnated with biocides such as silver) that are applied to the wound and covered with an adhesive covering to allow for a seal around the wounded area.[99,142] The adhesive cover is connected to a drain line and to a vacuum pump to allow for the application of a negative pressure on the wound (in the 25-200 mm Hg range, either continuously or periodically). Modifications of these systems can also be used in combination with the use of liquid biocide formulation to reduce microbial load. But microbial levels are also claimed to be kept low by cleaning (removal of fluid) and retaining the wound clean, including microorganism removal; there may also some benefit in reducing the ability of aerobes to grow due to the lower availability of oxygen but equally an increased risk in the growth of facultative or strict anaerobes.

▶ ACKNOWLEDGMENT

The chapter has been updated based on the previous 5th edition and owes substantially to the contributions of Manfred L. Rotter (retired): Institute of Hygiene, University of Vienna, Vienna, Austria A-1095; Department of Clinical Microbiology, General Hospital (Medical School), Vienna, Austria A-1095.

REFERENCES

1. Moffarah AS, Al Mohajer M, Hurwitz BL, Armstrong DG. Skin and soft tissue infections. *Microbiol Spectr.* 2016;4(4). doi: 10.1128/microbiolspec .DMIH2-0014-2015.
2. Aly R. Microbial infections of skin and nails. In: Baron S, ed. *Medical Microbiology*. 4th ed. Galveston, TX: University of Texas Medical Branch at Galveston; 1996: chap 98.
3. Kang S, Amagai M, Bruckner AL, et al. *Fitzpatrick's Dermatology*. 9th ed. New York, NY: McGraw-Hill Education; 2019.
4. Ibler KS, Kromann CB. Recurrent furunculosis—challenges and management: a review. *Clin Cosmet Investig Dermatol.* 2014;7:59-64.
5. Breuninger H, Bruck JC, Bühler M, et al. Klinische und hygienische Aspekte der Wundbehandlung. *Hyg Med.* 1990;15:298-306.
6. Williamson DA, Carter GP, Howden BP. Current and emerging topical antibacterials and antiseptics: agents, action, and resistance patterns. *Clin Microbiol Rev.* 2017;30:827-860.
7. Fitzgerald RH Jr, Cowan JD. Puncture wounds of the foot. *Orthop Clin North Am.* 1975;6:965-972.
8. Eidelman M, Bialik V, Miller Y, Kassis I. Plantar puncture wounds in children: analysis of 80 hospitalized patients and late sequelae. *Isr Med Assoc J.* 2003;5:268-271.
9. Raz R, Miron D. Oral ciprofloxacin for treatment of infection following nail puncture wounds of the foot. *Clin Infect Dis.* 1995;21:194-195.
10. Goldstein EJC. Bite wounds and infection. *Clin Infect Dis.* 1992;14:633-638.
11. Goldstein EJC. Bites. In: Mandell GL, Bennett JE, Dolin R, eds. *Mandell, Douglas, and Bennett's Principles and Practice of Infectious Diseases.* 4th ed. New York, NY: Churchill Livingstone; 1995:2765-2769.
12. Loder RT. The demographics of dog bites in the United States. *Heliyon.* 2019;5:e01360.
13. Bula-Rudas FJ, Olcott JL. Human and animal bites. *Pediatr Rev.* 2018;39:490-500.
14. Han HJ, Wen HL, Zhou CM, et al. Bats as reservoirs of severe emerging infectious diseases. *Virus Res.* 2015;205:1-6.
15. Abrahamian FM, Goldstein EJC. Microbiology of animal bite wound infections. *Clin Microbiol Rev.* 2011;24:231-246.
16. Cardenas-de la Garza JA, De la Cruz-Valadez E, Ocampo-Candiani J, Welsh O. Clinical spectrum of Lyme disease. *Eur J Clin Microbiol Infect Dis.* 2019;38:201-208.
17. Kramer A, Heeg P, Harke H-P, et al. Wundantiseptik. In: Kramer A, Groeschel D, Heeg P, et al, eds. *Klinische Antiseptik.* Berlin, Germany: Springer; 1993:163-191.
18. Magnussen CR. Skin and soft tissue infections. In: Reese RE, Betts RF, eds. *A Practical Approach to Infectious Diseases*, 4th ed. Boston, MA: Little, Brown; 1996:96-132.
19. Kramer A, Assadian O, Frank M, Bender C, Hinz P. Prevention of post-operative infections after surgical treatment of bite wounds. *GMS Krankenhhyg Interdiszip.* 2010;5:Doc12.
20. Kramer A. Antiseptika and Händedesinfektionsmittel. In: Korting HC, Sterry W, eds. *Therapeutische Verfahren in der Dermatologie: Dermatika und Kosmetika.* Berlin, Germany: Blackwell Scientific; 2000.
21. Zenker W, Thiede A, Dommes M, Ullmann U. Die Wirksamkeit von Tetrachlorodecaoxid zur Behandlung komplizierter Wundheilungsstörungen. *Chirurg.* 1986;57:334-339.

22. Dumville JC, Gray TA, Walter CJ, Sharp CA, Page T. Dressings for the prevention of surgical site infection. *Cochrane Database Syst Rev.* 2014;(9):CD003091.
23. Mulani MS, Kamble EE, Kumkar SN, Tawre MS, Pardesi AR. Emerging strategies to combat ESKAPE pathogens in the era of antimicrobial resistance: a review. *Front Microbiol.* 2019;10:539.
24. Berríos-Torres SI, Umscheid CA, Bratzler DW, et al; for Healthcare Infection Control Practices Advisory Committee. Centers for Disease Control and Prevention guideline for the prevention of surgical site infection, 2017. *JAMA Surg.* 2017;152:784-791.
25. World Health Organization. *Global Guidelines on the Prevention of Surgical Site Infection.* Geneva, Switzerland: World Health Organization; 2018.
26. Mangram AJ, Horan TC, Pearson ML, Silver LC, Jarvis WR. Guideline for prevention of surgical site infection, 1999. Hospital Infection Control Practices Advisory Committee. *Infect Control Hosp Epidemiol.* 1999;20:247-280.
27. Horan TC, Gaynes RP, Martone WJ, Jarvis WR, Emori TG. CDC definitions of nosocomial surgical site infections, 1992: a modification of CDC definitions of surgical wound infections. *Infect Control Hosp Epidemiol.* 1992;13:606-608.
28. Centers for Disease Control and Prevention. Surgical site infection (SSI) event. https://www.cdc.gov/nhsn/pdfs/pscmanual/9pscssicurrent .pdf. Published January 2019. Accessed April 15, 2019.
29. Bruce J, Russell EM, Mollison J, Krukowski ZH. The quality of measurement of surgical wound infection as the basis for monitoring: a systematic review. *J Hosp Infect.* 2001;49(2):99-108.
30. Harbarth S, Sax H, Gastmeier P. The preventable proportion of nosocomial infections: an overview of published reports. *J Hosp Infect.* 2003;54(4):258-266, 321.
31. Sievert DM, Ricks P, Edwards JR, Schneider A, Patel J, Srinivasan A, et al; for National Healthcare Safety Network (NHSN) Team and Participating NHSN Facilities. Antimicrobial-resistant pathogens associated with healthcare-associated infections: summary of data reported to the National Healthcare Safety Network at the Centers for Disease Control and Prevention, 2009-2010. *Infect Control Hosp Epidemiol.* 2013;34(1):1-14.
32. Rosenthal VD, Richtmann R, Singh S, et al; for International Nosocomial Infection Control Consortium. Surgical site infections, International Nosocomial Infection Control Consortium (INICC) report, data summary of 30 countries, 2005-2010. *Infect Control Hosp Epidemiol.* 2013;34:597-604.
33. Kluytmans J. Surgical infections including burns. In: Wenzel RP, ed. *Prevention and control of nosocomial infections.* 3rd ed. Baltimore, MD: Williams & Wilkins; 1997:841-865.
34. Association of periOperative Registered Nurses. *AORN's Guidelines for Perioperative Practice.* Denver, CO: Association of periOperative Registered Nurses; 2019.
35. Berard F, Gandon J. Postoperative wound infections: the influence of ultraviolet radiation of the operating room and of various other factors. *Ann Surg.* 1964;160(suppl 2):1-192.
36. Reichman DE, Greenberg JA. Reducing surgical site infections: a review. *Rev Obstet Gynecol.* 2009;2:212-221.
37. Onyekwelu I, Yakkanti R, Protzer L, Pinkston CM, Tucker C, Seligson D. Surgical wound classification and surgical site infections in the orthopaedic patient. *J Am Acad Orthop Surg Glob Res Rev.* 2017;1:e022.
38. Ortega G, Rhee DS, Papandria DJ, et al. An evaluation of surgical site infections by wound classification system using the ACS-NSQIP. *J Surg Res.* 2012;174:33-38.
39. Webster J, Osborne S. Preoperative bathing or showering with skin antiseptics to prevent surgical site infection. *Cochrane Database Syst Rev.* 2012;(9):CD004985.
40. Boyce JM, Pittet D. Guideline for hand hygiene in health-care settings. *Infect Control Hosp Epidemiol.* 2002;23:S3-S40.
41. World Health Organization. *Guidelines on Hand Hygiene in Health Care.* Geneva, Switzerland: World Health Organization; 2009.

42. Rotter ML. Alcohols for antisepsis of hands and skin. In: Ascenzi JM, ed. *Handbook of Disinfectants and Antiseptics*. New York, NY: Marcel Dekker; 1996:177-233.

43. Rotter ML. Hand washing, hand disinfection, and skin disinfection. In: Wenzel RP, ed. *Prevention and Control of Nosocomial Infections*. 3rd ed. Baltimore, MD: William & Wilkins; 1997:691-709.

44. Sattar SA, Jacobsen H, Springthorpe VS, Cusack TM, Rubino JR. Chemical disinfection to interrupt transfer of rhinovirus type 14 from environmental surfaces to hands. *Appl Environ Microbiol*. 1993;59: 1579-1585.

45. Klein M, Deforest A. Antiviral action of germicides. *Soap Chem Spec*. 1963;39:70-72,95-97.

46. Danzmann L, Gastmeier P, Schwab F, Vonberg RP. Health care workers causing large nosocomial outbreaks: a systematic review. *BMC Infect Dis*. 2013;13:98.

47. Sasahara T, Ae R, Watanabe M, et al. Contamination of healthcare workers' hands with bacterial spores. *J Infect Chemother*. 2016;22:521-525.

48. Larson EL, Morton HE. Alcohols. In: Block SS, ed. *Disinfection, Sterilization, and Preservation*. 4th ed. Philadelphia, PA: Lea & Febiger; 1991:191-203.

49. Rotter ML, Simpson RA, Koller W. Surgical hand disinfection with alcohols at various concentrations: parallel experiments using the new proposed European standards method. *Infect Control Hosp Epidemiol*. 1998;19:778-781.

50. Rotter ML, Stoklasek B, Koller W, et al. Surgical hand disinfection: intralaboratory reproducibility and reliability of the model described by prEN 12791. Paper presented at: The 26th Biannual Meeting of the Austrian Society of Hygiene, Microbiology, and Preventive Medicine; May 26-28, 1998; Millstatt, Austria.

51. European Committee for Standardization. *EN 1500:2013. Chemical Disinfectants and Antiseptics. Hygienic Hand Disinfection. Test Method and Requirement (Phase 2, Step 2)*. Brussels, Belgium: European Committee for Standardization; 2013.

52. Semradova S, Ulrich W, Kundi M, et al. Systematische Untersuchungen zur Prüfung von Hautdesinfektionsmitteln: Wirkung von n-Propanol und wässriger PVP-Jod-Lösung an der Leichenhaut. Paper presented at: The 13th DOSCH-Symposium for Sterilization, Disinfection, Hospital Cleaning of the Austrian Society for Hygiene, Microbiology, and Preventive Medicine; May 18-19, 1995; Vienna, Austria.

53. Hartmann AA, Pietsch C, Elsner P, et al. Antibacterial efficacy of Fabry's tinctura on the resident flora of the skin at the forehead. Study of bacterial population dynamics in stratum corneum and infundibulum after single and repeated applications. *Zentralbl Bakteriol Mikrobiol Hyg B*. 1986;182:499-514.

54. Evans CA, Mattern KL. The bacterial flora of the antecubital fossa: the efficacy of alcohol disinfection on this site, the palm and the forehead. *J Invest Dermatol*. 1980;75:140-143.

55. Christiansen B, Höller CH, Gundermann KO. Vorschlag einer neuen quantitativen Methode zur Prüfung der Eignung von Präparaten zur prä- und postoperativen Hautdesinfektion. *Hyg Med*. 1984;9:471-473.

56. Rotter ML, Koller W, Wewalka G. Eignung von Chlorhexidinglukonat- und PVP-Jod-haltigen Präparationen zur Händesinfektion. *Hyg Med*. 1981;6:425-430.

57. Heeg P, Oszwald W, Schwenzer N. Wirksamkeitsvergleich in Desinfektionsverfahren zur chirurgischen Händesdesinfektion unter experimentellen und klinischen Bedingungen. *Hyg Med*. 1986;11:107-110.

58. Rotter ML, Koller W. Sequential use of chlorhexidine detergent and alcohol for surgical hand disinfection. Poster presented at: The 2nd International Conference of the Hospital Infection Society; September 2-6, 1990; London, United Kingdom. Poster no. 0073.

59. Rotter ML, Koller W. Surgical hand disinfection: the influence of time on the effectiveness. Paper presented at: The 24th Biannual Meeting of the Austrian Society of Hygiene, Microbiology, and Preventive Medicine. May 17-19, 1994; Salzburg, Austria.

60. Wewalka G, Rotter M, Koller W. Wirksamkeit verschiedener Mittel zur Chirurgischen Händesinfektion und zur präoperativen Hautdesinfektion. In: Porpaczy P, ed. *10 Jahre Ludwig Boltzmann Institut zur Erforschung der Infektionenund Geschwülste des Harntrakts*. Wien, Austria: H. Egermann; 1980:9-15.

61. Lowbury EJ, Lilly HA, Ayliffe GA. Preoperative disinfection of surgeons hands: use of alcoholic solutions and effects of gloves on skin flora. *BMJ*. 1974;4:369-372.

62. Aly R, Maybach HI. Comparative study on the antimicrobial effect of 0.5% chlorhexidine gluconate and 70% isopropyl alcohol on the normal flora of hands. *Appl Environ Microbiol*. 1979;37:610-613.

63. Rotter ML, Koller W, Wewalka G. Povidone-iodine and chlorhexidine gluconate-containing detergent for disinfection of hands. *J Hosp Infect*. 1980;1:149-158.

64. Lilly HA, Lowbury EJ, Wilkins D. Detergents compared with each other and with antiseptics as skin "degerming" agents. *J Hyg (Lond)*. 1979;82:89-93.

65. Altemeier WA. Surgical antisepsis. In: Block SS, ed. *Disinfection, Sterilization, and Preservation*. 2nd ed. Philadelphia, PA: Lea & Febiger; 1977:641-653.

66. European Committee for Standardization. *EN 12791:2005. Chemical Disinfectants and Antiseptics. Surgical Hand Disinfection. Test Method and Requirement (Phase 2, Step 2)*. Brussels, Belgium: European Committee for Standardization; 2005.

67. Hingst V, Juditzki I, Heeg P, Sonntag HG. Evaluation of the efficacy of surgical hand disinfection following a reduced application time of 3 instead of 5 min. *J Hosp Infect*. 1992;20:79-86.

68. Selwyn S, Ellis H. Skin bacteria and skin disinfection reconsidered. *Br Med J*. 1972;1:136-140.

69. Kristiansen BE, Johnsen RL. Preoperativ handdesinfeksjon. *Tidsskr Nor Laegeforen*. 1994;114:3463-3465.

70. Koller W, Rotter M, Gottardi W, et al. Langzeitwirkung eines PVP-Jodpräparates bei der Händedesinfektion. *Hyg Med*. 1991;16:111-114.

71. Berkelman RL, Holland BW, Anderson RL. Increased bactericidal activity of dilute preparations of povidone-iodine solutions. *J Clin Microbiol*. 1982;15:635-639.

72. Birnbach DJ, Stein DJ, Murray O, Thys DM, Sordillo EM. Povidone iodine and skin disinfection before initiation of epidural anesthesia. *Anesthesiology*. 1998;88:668-672.

73. Craven DE, Moody B, Connolly BS, Kollisch NR, Stottmeier KD, McCabe WR. Pseudobacteremia caused by povidone-iodine solution contaminated with *Pseudomonas cepacia*. *N Engl J Med*. 1981;305:621-623.

74. Panlilio AL, Beck-Sague CM, Siegel JD, et al. Infections and pseudoinfections due to povidone-iodine solution contaminated with *Pseudomonas cepacia*. *Clin Infect Dis*. 1992;14:1078-1083.

75. Lacey RW. Antibacterial activity of povidone iodine towards non-sporing bacteria. *J Appl Bacteriol*. 1979;46:443-449.

76. Reybrouck G. Handwashing and hand disinfection. *J Hosp Infect*. 1986;8:5-23.

77. Lowbury EJL, Lilly HA, Bull JP. Disinfection of hands: removal of transient organisms. *BMJ*. 1964;2:230-233.

78. Larson EL, Butz AM, Gullette DL, Laughon BA. Alcohol for surgical scrubbing? *Infect Control Hosp Epidemiol*. 1990;11:139-143.

79. Lilly HA, Lowbury EJL. Disinfection of the skin: an assessment of some new preparations. *BMJ*. 1971;3:674-676.

80. Furuhashi M, Miamae T. Effect of preoperative hand scrubbing and influence of pinholes appearing in surgical rubber gloves during operation. *Bull Tokyo Med Dent Univ*. 1979;26:73-80.

81. Holloway PM, Platt JH, Reybrouck G, Lilly HA, Mehtar S, Drabu Y. A multi-centre evaluation of two chlorhexidine-containing formulations for surgical hand disinfection. *J Hosp Infect*. 1990;16:151-159.

82. Babb JR, Davies JG, Ayliffe GA. A test procedure for evaluating surgical hand disinfection. *J Hosp Infect*. 1991;18(suppl B):41-49.

83. Lowbury EJL, Lilly HA, Bull JP. Disinfection of hands: removal of resident bacteria. *BMJ*. 1963;1:1251-1256.

84. Bendig JW. Surgical hand disinfection: comparison of 4% chlorhexidine detergent solution and 2% triclosan detergent solution. *J Hosp Infect*. 1990;15:143-148.

85. Peterson AF, Rosenberg A, Alatary SD. Comparative evaluation of surgical scrub preparations. *Surg Gynecol Obstet*. 1978;146:63-65.

86. Kaiser AB, Kernodle DE, Barg NL, Petracek MR. Influence of preoperative showers on staphylococcal skin colonisation: a comparative trial of antiseptic skin cleansers. *Ann Thorac Surg.* 1988;45:35-38.

87. Brandberg A, Holm J, Hammarsten J, et al. Postoperative wound disinfection by shower bath with chlorhexidine soap. In: Newsom SWB, Caldwell ADS, eds. *Problems in the Control of Hospital Infection.* London, United Kingdom: RSM/Academic Press; 1980:71-75. Royal Society of Medicine International Congress and Symposium Series, No. 23.

88. Maki DG, Ringer M, Alvarado CJ. Prospective randomized trial of povidone iodine, alcohol and chlorhexidine for prevention of infection associated with central venous or arterial catheters. *Lancet.* 1991;338:339-343.

89. Atkinson W. *Tetanus Epidemiology and Prevention of Vaccine-Preventable Diseases.* 12th ed. Washington, DC: Public Health Foundation: 2012: 291-300.

90. Hopkins A, Lahiri T, Salerno R, Heath B. Diphtheria, tetanus, and pertussis: recommendation for vaccine use and other preventive measures. *MMWR Recomm Rep.* 1991;40:1-28.

91. World Health Organization. The "high-risk" approach: the WHO-recommended strategy to accelerate elimination of neonatal tetanus. *Wkly Epidemiol Rec.* 1996;71:33-36.

92. Kyu HH, Mumford JE, Stanaway JD, et al. Mortality from tetanus between 1990 and 2015: findings from the Global Burden of Disease study 2015. *BMC Public Health.* 2017;17:179.

93. Bennett J, Macia J, Traverso H, Banoagha S, Malooly C, Boring J. Protective effects of topical antimicrobials against neonatal tetanus. *Int J Epidemiol.* 1997;26:897-903.

94. Bennett JV, Schooley M, Traverso H, Agha SB, Boring J. Bundling, a newly identified risk factor for neonatal tetanus: implications for global control. *Int J Epidemiol.* 1996;25:879-884.

95. Centers for Disease Control and Prevention. The pink book: epidemiology and prevention of vaccine-preventable diseases. Tetanus. Centers for Disease Control and Prevention Web site. https://www.cdc.gov/vaccines/pubs/pinkbook/tetanus.html. Accessed May 16, 2018.

96. Gladstone IM, Clapper L, Thorp JW, Wright DI. Randomized study of six umbilical cord care regimens. Comparing length of attachment, microbial control, and satisfaction. *Clin Pediatr (Phila).* 1988;27:127-129.

97. Mullany LC, Darmstadt GL, Tielsch JM. Role of antimicrobial applications to the umbilical cord in neonates to prevent bacterial colonization and infection: a review of the evidence. *Pediatr Infect Dis J.* 2003;22:996-1002.

98. Mooney DP, Gamelli RL. Sepsis following thermal injury. *Compr Ther.* 1989;15:22-29.

99. Coban YK. Infection control in severely burned patients. *World J Crit Care Med.* 2012;1:94-101.

100. Tomkins RG, Burke JF. Infections in burn wound. In: Bennett JV, Brachman PS, eds. *Hospital Infections.* 3rd ed. Boston, MA: Little, Brown; 1992.

101. Peng YZ, Yuan ZQ. Standardized definitions and diagnostic criteria for infection in burn patients. *Zhonghua Shao Shang Za Zhi.* 2007;23:404-405.

102. Mayhall CG. Nosocomial burn wound infections. In: Mayhall CG, ed. *Hospital Epidemiology and Infection Control.* Baltimore, MD: Williams & Wilkins; 1996:225-236.

103. International Society for Burn Injury. Practice guidelines for burn care. *Burns.* 2016;42:953-1021.

104. Schaberg DR, Culver DH, Gaynes RP. Major trends in the microbial etiology of nosocomial infection. *Am J Med.* 1991;91(3B):72S-75S.

105. Lachiewicz AM, Hauck CG, Weber DJ, Cairns BA, van Duin D. Bacterial infections after burn injuries: impact of multidrug resistance. *Clin Infect Dis.* 2017;65:2130-2136.

106. Kanamori H, Parobek CM, Juliano JJ, et al. A prolonged outbreak of KPC-3-producing *Enterobacter cloacae* and *Klebsiella pneumoniae* driven by multiple mechanisms of resistance transmission at a large academic burn center. *Antimicrob Agents Chemother.* 2017;61: e01516-16.

107. Pruitt BA Jr, McManus AT, Kim SH, Goodwin CW. Burn wound infections: current status. *World J Surg.* 1998;22:135-145.

108. Dodd D, Stutman HR. Current issues in burn wound infections. *Adv Pediatr Infect Dis.* 1991;6:137-162.

109. Park KC, Han WS. Viral skin infections: diagnosis and treatment considerations. *Drugs.* 2002;62:479-490.

110. Pruitt BA Jr. The diagnosis and treatment of infection in the burn patient. *Burns Incl Therm Inj.* 1984;11:79-91.

111. Greenhaigh DG, Saffie JR, Holmes JH IV, et al; for American Burn Association Consensus Conference on Burn Sepsis and Infection Group. American Burn Association Consensus Conference to define sepsis and infection in burns. *J Burn Care Res.* 2007:28:776-790.

112. McManus AT, Kim SH, McManus WF, Mason AD Jr, Pruitt BA Jr. Comparison of quantitative microbiology and histopathology in divided burn-wound biopsy specimens. *Arch Surg.* 1987;122:74-76.

113. Tredget EE, Shankowsky HA, Joffe AM, et al. Epidemiology of infections with *Pseudomonas aeruginosa* in burn patients: the role of hydrotherapy. *Clin Infect Dis.* 1992;15:941-949.

114. Embil JM, McLeod JA, Al-Barrak AM, et al. An outbreak of methicillin resistant *Staphylococcus aureus* on a burn unit: potential role of contaminated hydrotherapy equipment. *Burns.* 2001;27:681-688.

115. Fleming RY, Zeigler ST, Walton MA, Herndon DN, Heggers JP. Influence of burn size on the incidence of contamination of burn wounds by fecal organisms. *J Burn Care Rehabil.* 1991;12:510-515.

116. Sheridan RL, Tompkins RG, Burke JF. Management of burn wounds with prompt excision and immediate closure. *J Intensive Care Med.* 1994;9:6-17.

117. Girerd-Genessay I, Bénet T, Vanhems P. Multidrug-resistant bacterial outbreaks in burn units: a synthesis of the literature according to the ORION statement. *J Burn Care Res.* 2016;37:172-180.

118. McManus AT, McManus WF, Mason AD Jr, Aitcheson AR, Pruitt BA Jr. Microbial colonization in a new intensive care burn unit: a prospective cohort study. *Arch Surg.* 1985;120:217-223.

119. Lee JJ, Marvin JA, Heimbach DM, Grube BJ, Engrav LH.. Infection control in a burn center. *J Burn Care Rehabil.* 1990;11:575-580.

120. Cobrado L, Silva-Dias A, Azevedo MM, Rodrigues AG. High-touch surfaces: microbial neighbours at hand. *Eur J Clin Microbiol Infect Dis.* 2017;36:2053-2062.

121. Fujita K, Lilly HA, Kidson A, Ayliffe GA. Gentamicin-resistant *Pseudomonas aeruginosa* infection from mattresses in a burns unit. *Br Med J (Clin Res Ed).* 1981;283:219-220.

122. Sherertz RJ, Sullivan ML. An outbreak with *Acinetobacter calcoaceticus* in burn patients: contamination of patients' mattresses. *J Infect Dis.* 1985;151:252-258.

123. Linnemann CC Jr. Nosocomial infections associated with physical therapy, including hydrotherapy. In: Mayhall CG, ed. *Hospital Epidemiology and Infection Control.* Baltimore, MD: Williams & Wilkins; 1996:725-730.

124. Cardany CR, Rodeheaver GT, Horowitz JH, Kenney JG, Edlich RF. Influence of hydrotherapy and antiseptic agents on burn wound bacterial contamination. *J Burn Care Rehabil.* 1985;6:230-232.

125. Steve L, Goodhart P, Alexander J. Hydrotherapy burn treatment: use of chloramine-T against resistant microorganisms. *Arch Phys Med Rehabil.* 1979;60:301-303.

126. Thomson PD, Bowden ML, McDonald K, Smith DJ Jr, Prasad JK. A survey of burn hydrotherapy in the United States. *J Burn Care Rehabil.* 1990;11:151-155.

127. Shirani KZ, McManus AT, Vaughn GM, McManus WF, Pruitt BA Jr, Mason AD Jr. Effects of environment on infection in burn patients. *Arch Surg.* 1986;121:31-36.

128. Sehulster L, Chinn RY; for Centers for Disease Control and Prevention, Healthcare Infection Control Practices Advisory Committee. Guidelines for environmental infection control in health-care facilities. Recommendations of CDC and the Healthcare Infection Control Practices Advisory Committee (HICPAC). *MMWR Recomm Rep.* 2003;52:1-42.

129. Garner JS. Guideline for isolation precautions in hospitals. *Infect Control Hosp Epidemiol.* 1996;17:53-80.

130. Deutsch DH, Miller SF, Finley RK Jr. The use of intestinal antibiotics to delay or prevent infections in patients with burns. *J Burn Care Rehabil.* 1990;11:436-442.

131. Rubio-Regidor M, Martín-Pellicer A, Silvestri L, van Saene HKF, Lorente JA, de la Cal MA. Digestive decontamination in burn patients: a systematic review of randomized clinical trials and observational studies. *Burns.* 2018;44:16-23.

132. Mayhall CG, Polk RE, Haynes BW. Infections in burned patients. *Infect Control.* 1983;4:454-459.

133. McDonnell GE. *Antisepsis, Disinfection, and Sterilization.* 2nd ed. Washington, DC: ASM Press; 2017.

134. Finley PJ, Norton R, Austin C, Mitchell A, Zank S, Durham P. Unprecedented silver resistance in clinically isolated Enterobacteriaceae: major implications for burn and wound management. *Antimicrob Agents Chemother.* 2015;59:4734-4741.

135. Fox CL Jr. Topical therapy and the development of silver sulfadiazine. *Surg Gynecol Obstet.* 1983;157:82-88.

136. Fox CL Jr, Modak SM. Mechanism of silver sulfadiazine action on burn wound infections. *Antimicrob Agents Chemother.* 1974;5: 582-588.

137. Monafo WW, Freedman B. Topical therapy for burns. *Surg Clin North Am.* 1987;67:133-145.

138. Norman G, Christie J, Liu Z, et al. Antiseptics for burns. *Cochrane Database Syst Rev.* 2017;(7):CD011821.

139. Molan P, Rhodes T. Honey: a biologic wound dressing. *Wounds.* 2015;27:141-151.

140. Yurt RW. Burns. In: Mandell GL, Bennett JE, Dolin R, eds. *Mandell, Douglas, and Bennett's Principles and Practice of Infectious Diseases.* 4th ed. New York, NY: Churchill Livingstone; 1995:2761-2765.

141. Brown TP, Cancio LC, McManus AT, Mason AD Jr. Survival benefit conferred by topical antimicrobial preparations in burn patients: a historical perspective. *J Trauma.* 2004;56:863-866.

142. Anghel EL, Kim PJ. Negative-pressure wound therapy: a comprehensive review of the evidence. *Plast Reconstr Surg.* 2016;138:129S-137S.

Oral and Mucous Membrane Treatments

Prerna Gopal and Lipika Gopal Chugh

The oral cavity is rightly referred to as the mirror of the body. It plays an important role in digestion, respiration, speech, and innate immune responses. It constitutes a complex environment of hard and soft tissues with constantly changing microflora, from predentate to dentate to the postdentate period. The typical oral flora comprises a diverse population of eubacteria, fungi, archaea, mycoplasma, and protozoa. A healthy oral flora follows a cross-feeding model and lives in harmony until an underlying disease or modifiable factor brings about dysbiosis leading to oral infections. These infections can be local bacterial, viral, or fungal, as well as manifestation of systemic diseases. The oral cavity is an integral part of the human body. Any change in the oral cavity mirrors the disturbances in general systemic health of the individual. Several systemic diseases have oral manifestations and sometimes even appear first and foremost in the oral cavity. For example, Koplik spots (bluish white spots on the buccal mucosa) is an early diagnostic clue for measles.[1,2] Autoimmune diseases like systemic lupus erythematosus, rheumatoid arthritis also can manifest as erosive lesions on the buccal mucosa in conjunction with systemic manifestations.

In order to understand the complexity of the oral cavity, a brief introduction to oral histology and immunology is provided in this chapter. The most commonly occurring oral and mucous membrane conditions and their treatments are also briefly discussed. Oral hard tissue and mucosal lesions are multifactorial and can be from a variety of bacterial, viral, or fungal habitats, including contaminated instruments. The first part of the chapter discusses oral histology, immunology, and microbiology within the scope of the chapter. The second part focusses on the lesions and oral mucous membrane treatments.

ORAL HISTOLOGY

The hard tissues of the oral cavity include the bones of the maxilla and mandible, hard palate, and teeth (occupying almost 20% of the total surface of the mouth) (Figure 45.1).

The entire oral cavity is lined by a wet mucous membrane consisting of an epithelium and connective tissue named as the lamina propria. Based on the histology of the tissue, the mucosa is divided into three types[3]:

1. Masticatory: stratified squamous keratinized epithelium covering the gingiva and the hard palate. The lamina propria is tightly bound to the underlying bone, is immovable, and helps withstand the masticatory pressure.
2. Lining: stratified squamous nonkeratinized epithelium lining the lips, cheeks, in the vestibules, floor of the mouth, alveolar processes, ventral surface of tongue and soft palate. The lamina propria is not tightly bound to bone and is designed for protection and mobility.
3. Specialized: This specialized masticatory mucosa containing papillae and taste buds lines the dorsal surface of tongue.

The tooth proper consists of enamel, dentin, and pulp. Enamel is 96% inorganic composing of hydroxyapatite crystals and is acellular. This nonvital and insensitive tissue cannot be repaired or regenerated but allows ion exchange between the enamel and saliva. Dentin forms the bulk of the tooth and supports the enamel. It is highly mineralized and made up of odontoblasts, harbors open nerve endings, and is capable of regeneration and/or repair (sclerotic or secondary dentin). Pulp is a specialized connective tissue present in a chamber underlying the dentin. It consists of collagen, noncollagenous protein, glycoproteins, enzymes, growth factors, and phospholipids.

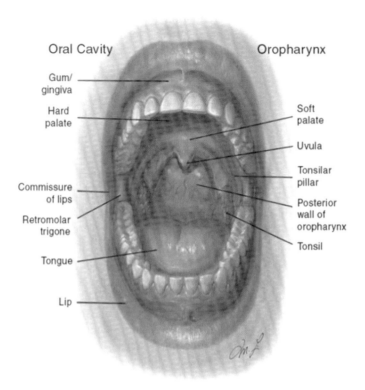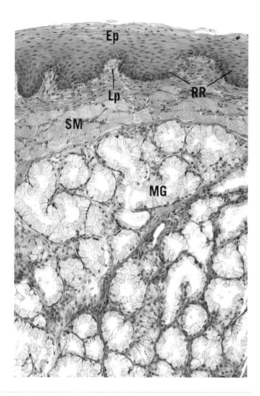

FIGURE 45.1 Anatomy of the oral cavity (left). Histologic section of the oral surface (soft palate; right). The top surface is lined by a stratified squamous nonkeratinized epithelium (Ep) that interdigitates with the lamina propria (Lp) by the formation of rete ridges (RR). It is a movable structure, supported by the presence of skeletal muscle (SM) fibers, below which are numerous mucous glands (MG) that deliver secretory products into the oral cavity.

The other supporting structures of the tooth include alveolar bone, periodontal ligament, and the cementum. Cementum covers the root dentin, and periodontal ligament fibers help anchor the tooth to the alveolar bone of maxilla and mandible.

▶ ORAL INNATE IMMUNE RESPONSES

The different habitats in human oral cavity, hard and soft tissues shedding, and nonshedding surfaces can harbor over 600 known diverse bacterial species.[4] Despite the anatomical complexity and diversity of oral microorganisms, the oral cavity's innate immune response helps maintain the integrity of oral epithelium.[5] The various innate immune factors present include the following:

- Oral mucosa: The stratified squamous epithelium acts as a mechanical barrier to oral microorganisms.[6] A rapid oral epithelial turnover rate helps limit the attachment of bacteria to the mucosa.[7] Moreover, several studies have shown the ability of oral keratinocytes to distinguish between commensal and pathogenic microorganisms by mediating the production of immunoinflammatory responses by their dendritic cells[5,8,9] as well as a wide range of cytokines like interleukin IL-1β,

tumor necrosis factor-alpha, granulocyte-macrophage colony stimulating factor, etc.[10]
- Odontoblasts: They represent the first line of defense on the tooth surface. Studies have shown that gram-positive and gram-negative bacteria can activate the toll-like receptors TLR2 and TLR4.[11,12] The upregulation of these factors can lead to the secretion of several antimicrobial agents, proinflammatory cytokines, and chemokines.[13] Odontoblasts also secrete broad-spectrum antimicrobial agents like β-defensins that are effective against oral bacteria.[14]
- Gingival crevicular fluid (GCF): GCF is composed mainly of serum components and organic molecules, such as albumins, globulins, lipoproteins, and cellular components. The concentration of immune cells present in GCF is higher than the peripheral blood with polymorphonuclear neutrophils being the most predominant.[15]
- Saliva: A versatile clear fluid consisting of organic and inorganic components that continuously bathes the oral cavity. An adult secretes an average ∼1 to 1.5 L of saliva per day, 90% of which is secreted by the major salivary glands (parotid, submandibular, and sublingual glands).[16,17] The remaining 10% is contributed by the minor salivary glands. Saliva plays an important

role in both innate and acquired immunity. Proteins like lactoferrin (that binds iron), lysozyme (that can break down bacterial cell wall structures), histatins (inhibiting the growth of *Candida albicans*), and lactoperoxidase act as general antimicrobial enzymes. Other proteins like salivary amylase, cystatins, proline-rich proteins, mucins, peroxidases, and statherin are also primarily involved in innate immunity.[18]

Salivary immunoglobulin IgA aggregates oral cariogenic bacteria like *Streptococcus mutans* and prevents its attachment on the tooth surface. Constituents like bicarbonates, phosphates, and urea help maintain the pH of the oral cavity, whereas calcium, phosphate, and various proteins can modulate demineralization and remineralization of enamel.

In the human body, the oral cavity and the gastrointestinal tract are the only two dynamic microenvironments, where the attachment of microflora is site specific and the bacterial load changes over time depending on the time of the day, diet intake, and overall health status. Microorganisms from the oral cavity have been shown to cause a number of oral infectious diseases, including caries (tooth decay), periodontitis (gum disease), endodontic (root canal) infections, alveolar osteitis (dry socket), and tonsillitis. Moreover, when oral bacteria enters systemic circulation, they can cause conditions like cardiovascular disease,[19] stroke,[20] preterm low-birth-weight babies,[21] diabetes,[22] and pneumonia.[4]

DYNAMICS OF THE HUMAN ORAL MICROBIOME

At birth, a neonate's oral cavity is exposed to diverse microorganisms of the outside world and the establishment of the oral microflora begins. The initial microbial colonization depends on the type of delivery (vaginal or cesarean), diet (breastfed or formula-fed), and contact with parents and medical staff. Within the first 24 hours, gram-positive cocci such as *Streptococcus* and *Staphylococcus* species are the most common organisms. As the first tooth (lower central incisors at the age of 6-9 months) erupts in the oral cavity, the cariogenic bacteria *S mutans* is found to have the greatest affinity to the nonshedding tooth surface and fights for a niche on the tooth.[23] The diversity of bacteria and their interdependencies for nutrition and niche leads to a complex consortium of microorganisms known as a biofilm. The biofilm continues to grow and harbor organisms like streptococci, *Actinomyces*, *Haemophilus*, *Neisseria*, *Fusobacterium*, and *Prevotella*. Children's oral microbiota can vary throughout the development of teeth, mixed or permanent dentition, diet and lifestyle changes, and hormonal changes associated with growth and puberty. The progression and maturation of biofilms can continue until adulthood. Different bacterial species within the biofilm interact by various cell signaling mechanisms and contribute to ecologic

stability by differentiation and maturation of the host mucosa and immune system. Normal resident microflora can keep pathogenic bacteria out by maintaining basic pH around the tooth surface, thereby preventing the invasion and growth of pathogens. Saliva and GCF provide nutrients (salivary amylase breaks down starch) for microbial growth and also contain (lactoferrin, lactoperoxidase, mucins, cystatins, etc) antimicrobial activities, thereby stabilizing the microbial community.

DEVELOPMENT OF DENTAL PLAQUE AND COMMON BACTERIAL INFECTIONS

Tooth surface is never dry (in physiologic conditions) and gets covered by a thin proteinaceous layer called the acquired enamel pellicle (AEP).[24] This 100 to 1000 nm thick film is attached to the enamel surface due to selective physical forces and plays an important role in determining the fate of an oral microbiome.[25] Selective oral streptococci have the ability to attach to this pellicle as initial colonizers and occupy sites at the tooth surface and selective oral sites such as the tongue and buccal epithelium.[26] Once established, these colonizers provide attachment sites for secondary and tertiary colonizers leading to a complex ecosystem of symbiotic microbial communities—the dental biofilm known as "plaque." The communities stabilize and live with a simple cross-feeding model in harmony with the host until the balance is tipped off leading to dysbiosis. The modifiable factor of dysbiosis can range from being a change in the salivary flow, lifestyle changes (like inclusion of more sugar in the diet), poor oral hygiene, or an underlying disease. Dysbiosis leads to a shift in the microflora, such as from aerobic to anaerobic and aciduric bacteria. The predominance of aciduric bacteria around the tooth surface causes the dissolution of mineral salts from enamel leading to one of the most common dental diseases of the world—dental caries. Based on the location and depth of lesion, the dental caries can be on the enamel, root, or reach deep into the pulp. Enamel and dentin caries is caused by *S mutans* and *Lactobacillus* species. Initial enamel caries is referred to as "white spot lesions" and can be reversed if the bacterial growth is arrested and symbiosis of oral microorganisms is achieved. But if the carious lesion reaches deeper tissues, it can even lead to irreversible pulpitis rendering the tooth nonvital. Because bacteria are site specific, certain bacteria like *Aggregatibacter actinomycetemcomitans*, *Porphyromonas gingivalis*, and *Prevotella intermedia*, etc, can target the supporting structures of the tooth leading to periodontitis and gingivitis.[27] Periodontal disease is a chronic bacterial infection characterized by persistent inflammation, connective tissue breakdown, and alveolar bone destruction. With advancing gingivitis and periodontitis, *Actinomyces* and other anaerobic species can

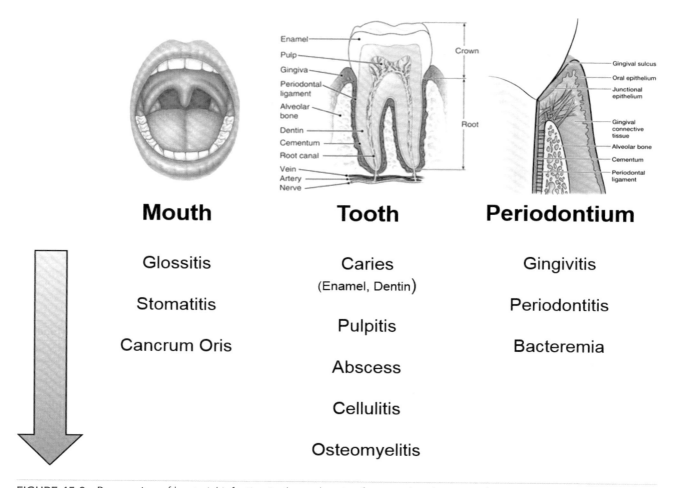

FIGURE 45.2 Progression of bacterial infection in the oral cavity: from tooth to bone, on the periodontium, and other tissues of the mouth such as the tongue.

gain entry to the exposed root surfaces causing root caries. As long as bacteria are present on the hard tissue and do not enter the systemic circulation, the best mode of treatment is to excavate the carious lesion with a suitable dental bur and restore the structure and function of the tooth by restorations like the use of an amalgam or composite. In cases of extensive decay extending to the pulp, root canal treatment or extraction is required.

In cases of gingivitis and periodontitis, excessive microbial load and the oral epithelium's innate immune responses can lead to inflammation and tissue breakdown. Hence, supragingival and subgingival debridement of the tissue (such as scaling and root planing) targeted toward the reduction of plaque and microflora can help revert disease states to health. Untreated pulpal or periodontal pathology may progress to the neighboring soft tissues, causing cellulitis and osteomyelitis if bone is infected. The host's local defense factors, regional anatomy, microbial load, and bacterial virulence will determine the extent of the damage. Because dental diseases are multifactorial, the presence of bacteria and the host tissue response along with predisposing factors like immunocompromised state, malnutrition,

smoking, and poor oral hygiene can lead to severe destructive orofacial lesions like cancrum oris. Figure 45.2 shows the progression of bacterial infections in the mouth.

For dental-related infections, the advantage of reducing microbial load by caries excavation and scaling and root planing should be utilized before resorting to antibiotics. In today's era of increased antibiotic resistance and improved culture sensitivity testing, the identification of the associated bacteria is of utmost importance. Dentist should be encouraged to prescribe antibiotics only if necessary. Patient compliance, nutrition support, and medical care including analgesics, antipyretics, and anti-inflammatory drugs constitute the proper management of every infection.

▶ MANAGEMENT OF ORAL BACTERIAL INFECTIONS

The overall goal of managing bacterial infections is to reduce the microbial burden and eliminate the modifying factors that lead to the dysbiosis of oral microflora.

Depending on the severity of infection and presence of local factors, the treatment will range from a minor change in brushing habits or type of brush/toothpaste to mechanical debridement of factors by a dental professional. Figure 45.3 shows an example of pre- and postscaling leading to reduction in the local factors and inflammation. Table 45.1 summarizes the various treatment options for common bacterial infections of the oral cavity.

▶ BIOCIDES IN PREVENTION AND DISINFECTION

Oral health can be maintained at home with mechanical and chemical methods, lifestyle changes (if need be), and regular visit to the dentist.[28] The mechanical methods include tooth brushing and flossing. Some of the various factors affecting mechanical method include the type of brush (manual versus powered; soft, medium, hard bristled), frequency of brushing, brushing technique, type of toothpaste, and the type of floss.[29-31] Poor patient compliance is a major factor in reducing the effectiveness of mechanical plaque control. Hence, chemical methods, mouthrinses, and chewing gums are based as an adjunct to tooth brushing and flossing. Several clinical studies have been conducted on the efficacy of mouthrinses as an antiplaque agent.[32] Based on the studies, an ideal mouthrinse should be tolerated well by the hard and soft tissues (pH regulated) and maintain bacterial homeostasis, thereby reducing dental plaque and caries occurrence. Most of the available mouthrinses contain a biocide, which according to the European commission, is defined as "an active chemical molecule to control the growth of or kill bacteria in a biocidal product."[33]

Biocides range from naturally occurring to synthetic compounds and are used in various personal care products due to their broad-spectrum antimicrobial activity.[34] Systemic antibiotics and biocide differ in their mode of action, availability, and susceptibility to resistance. Direct biocide delivery and availability in the form of mouthrinses, skin ointments, gels, etc, will limit systemic side effects, if any, and their multiple target sites on microorganisms make them less susceptible to the development of resistance.[35] Moreover, higher concentrations of biocides than that required to inhibit microorganisms also contribute to their effectiveness, lack of resistance development, and concerns on the development of opportunistic flora. Combination of biocides in oral health care have been shown to reduce certain adverse effects like staining or irritation while maintaining the positive effect of antibacterial properties intact. For instance, a combination of chlorhexidine (CHX) + hydrogen peroxide (H_2O_2) is superior to CHX alone, and it minimizes extrinsic tooth discoloration (especially in pits and fissures) without affecting the plaque-inhibiting efficacy of CHX. Other examples include the use of 5% to 10% of polyvinylpyrrolidone (PVP) with 0.06% CHX (for slow release overtime) to reduce the staining of tongue and teeth compared to when 0.06% CHX is used alone[36] and a combination of CHX and sodium hypochlorite (NaOCl) has been suggested to demonstrate enhanced antibacterial activity.[37]

More recent advances have been made in the field of dental materials where antimicrobial agents are added to the increase the longevity of the restoration and help reduce the microbial load. Most of the studies indicate antimicrobial effect in laboratory studies, and more evidence is required clinically.[38] But meta-analysis of a 6-month clinical trial on mouthrinses with CHX, essential oils, or cetylpyridinium chloride (CPC) concluded that essential oils and CHX are superior to CPC in their antiplaque and anti-gingivitis potential.[38] Their effects are maximized when used as an adjunctive therapy with toothbrushing.[39,40] Multiple clinical studies ranging from a period of 6 months to 3 years show the antiplaque and antigingivitis effect of biocides used worldwide.

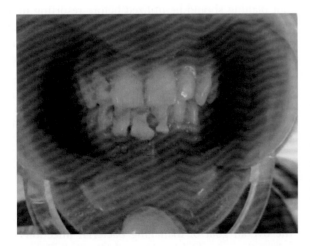
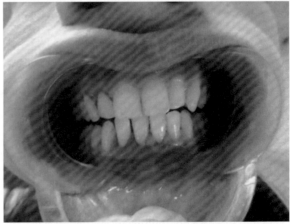

FIGURE 45.3 Pre- (left) and postscaling (right) and root planing. Removal of plaque depicts the underlying inflammation and bleeding of gingiva that heals in 2 weeks with proper oral hygiene maintenance.

TABLE 45.1 Summary of treatment options for most common bacterial infections of the oral cavity

Infection	Appearance	Most Commonly Associated Microorganisms	Treatment
Enamel and dentin caries	Brown or black spots on enamel/dentin, sensitivity to hot/cold (dentin caries)	*Streptococcus mutans* *Lactobacillus*	• Caries excavation and restoration • Erbium family of lasers (erbium-doped yttrium aluminum garnet [ErYAG]) treatment
Pulpitis—reversible and irreversible	Tooth sensitivity, pain and swelling	*Enterococcus faecalis*	• Reversible: deep caries excavation, pulp capping and restoration • Irreversible: root canal and restoration with crown • Post and core • Extraction
Root caries		*Actinomyces*	• Restoration
Gingivitis	Gingival bleeding, suppuration, recession	*Fusobacterium nucleatum* *Bacteroides* species	• Scaling and root planing • Curettage • Soft tissue graft • Gingival augmentation • Proper oral hygiene maintenance
Periodontitis	Pocket formation, tooth mobility	*Treponema denticola* *Porphyromonas gingivalis* *Aggregatibacter actinomycetemcomitans*	• Scaling and root planing • Curettage • Chlorhexidine mouthwash • Oral hygiene maintenance
Dentoalveolar abscess	Painful swelling Trismus (difficulty in opening mouth)	Facultative anaerobic bacteria	• Incision and drainage of abscess • Management of the associated tooth pathology • Antibiotics if required
Cellulitis and osteomyelitis	pain, trismus, warm erythematous swelling of the face	Aerobic and anaerobic *Streptococci*, *Peptostreptococci*, *Prevotella*, *Fusobacterium*, and *Bacteroides*	• Incision and drainage of abscess • Antibiotics • Palliative medical care
Glossitis and stomatitis	Inflammation of tongue	Polymicrobial, fungi, viral	• Oral hygiene maintenance • Removal of causative agent
Cancrum oris	Painful ulceration of gingiva/buccal mucosa Sequestration of bone and nearby tissues	Anaerobic bacteria (fusiform bacilli)	• Antibiotics • Tissue debridement • Medical care

▶ VIRAL INFECTIONS IN THE ORAL CAVITY

The oral cavity encounters a wide range of DNA and RNA viruses.[41] Viruses can gain entry in the mouth via the food we eat, the water we drink, and through the air we breathe.[42] With the advent of modern detection technology, viruses can be easily identified and accounted for the ulcerogenic and tumorigenic growth in the oral cavity. Some viral infections can manifest in the oral environment before their systemic counterparts (eg, oral mucosal vesicles with varicella zoster virus, oral tumors with human papillomavirus (HPV), and Koplik spots with rubeola). Hence, dentist can play a major role in the early detection of some threatening infections and tumors of the mouth.

The major oral manifestations of a viral infection are oral ulcers, oral tumors, oral infectious diseases, and periodontitis.[43] Oral ulceration involves a breach in epithelium, covered by white to yellow pseudomembranes, and surrounded by an inflammatory halo. Major viruses associated with oral ulcers are herpes simplex virus 1 and 2; varicella/herpes zoster; herpangina; hand, foot, and mouth disease viruses; and verrucous carcinoma-associated viruses. Conditions like stress, infection, or any immunocompromised state can activate a latent virus leading to recurrent ulceration like aphthous ulcers (commonly known a canker sores). Viral infections with predisposing factors of age, sex, genetic susceptibility, alcohol, tobacco chewing, and sexual behavior can lead to oral tumors such as oral squamous cell carcinoma (with HPV), Kaposi sarcoma (with HHV 8), and

Burkitts lymphoma (with Epstein-Barr virus EBV).[44] Acute infections of the salivary gland (sialadenitis), xerostomia, and oral lichen planus are a few of the pathoses commonly associated with hepatitis C and HPV infections. Prodromal symptoms like fever, malaise, lymphadenopathy, and predisposition to other viral and bacterial infections can be secondary to an active viral infection.

Most of the viral infections are self-limiting and resolve themselves in healthy individuals; however, to help accelerate healing of oral lesions, antiviral drugs like acyclovir can be prescribed. Analgesics, anesthetic gel, and nonsteroidal anti-inflammatory drugs can be applied to virus-associated ulcers. Oral mouthrinses and local biocide applications such as those listed in Table 45.2 can also be used to treat infections and help improve overall oral hygiene.

The management of oral tumors involves a multidisciplinary approach with the efforts of dental surgeons, radiation oncologists, chemotherapy oncologists, and nutritionists. Based on the size of the lesion and extent of metastasis, the treatment might range from surgical excision of the tumor to extensive head and neck chemotherapy and radiation. More recent advances in cancer treatment include gene therapy, monoclonal antibody therapy, tumor growth factors, and targeted therapy. The Food and Drug Administration (FDA)-approved drug cetuximab (Erbitux®) has been successful in shrinking oral cancers when given along with radiation.[53,54] But, radiation and chemotherapy can decrease patient salivary flow leading to poor oral hygiene and growth of other opportunistic bacterial and fungal infections. Therefore, changes in the dietary habits, exclusion of sugar and starch with the administration of lozenges, or artificial saliva is often recommended.

In recent times, HPV is the most common sexually transmitted virus[55] and appears to be more fatal than HIV. The HPV can be transmitted by engaging in orogenital sex with multiple sex partners.[56] It is postulated that young adults engage in oral sex more frequently than vaginal sex due to increased awareness of HIV transmission, leading to potential increased HPV transmission. There are various types of HPV viruses associated with cervical cancer in women and are also associated with anogenital, penile, and oral cancers. The HPV is commonly linked with head and neck cancers (specifically those of the tonsils and the base of the tongue) in relatively young individuals with no history of smoking or tobacco chewing.[57,58] The HPV-16 and HPV-18 are considered to be the most commonly associated with oropharyngeal squamous cell carcinoma (OSCC). These cancers exhibit relatively high mortality rates as they are detected fairly late due to asymptomatic growth of the lesion that goes unnoticed by the patient. The World Health Organization (WHO) recommends vaccination against HPV 16 and HPV 18 to reduce the occurrence of oropharyngeal carcinoma.[13,59] Lesions detected later require radical head and neck dissection, postoperative radiotherapy,

and/or chemotherapy. The various other HPV-associated infections include[60]

1. Verruca vulgaris: "common wart" can be present on any part of the mouth or body
2. Oral lichen planus: an autoimmune disorder linked with HPV 7 and 8
3. Verrucous carcinoma: variant of OSCC linked with HPV 2 and 6
4. Focal epithelial hyperplasia: Heck disease: HPV 13 and 32
5. Condyloma acuminatum: HPV 6 and 11

There are two widely used HPV vaccines available: Gardasil® and Cervarix®. Both can protect against the strains of HPV that cause the most prominent cervical cancers (HPV 16 and 18). Dentists play a major role in educating the patient regarding the risk and transmission of the disease. Moreover, a thorough examination of the head and neck area for unusual swelling/lump must be conducted at regular intervals at the dental office. The medical history, knowledge of patient's sexual behavior, and oral examination are the connecting dots to an early diagnosis of OSCC.

The other common viral infections and associated treatments are summarized in Table 45.3.

▶ FUNGAL INFECTIONS OF THE ORAL CAVITY

Fungi are eukaryotes and the most important fungi to dentistry are *Candida*. *Candida* species are considered inhabitants of the normal oral and gastrointestinal flora.[63] They are predominantly present on the dorsum surface of the tongue, followed by palate and buccal mucosa.[64] On an average, the concentration of *Candida* in saliva is approximately 300 to 500 cells/mL,[65] and their presence is benign until a disruption in the local oral environment causes their overgrowth leading to oral candidiasis. The disrupting factor can include reduced salivary flow due to drug therapy or radiation, poor oral hygiene, and removable or fixed dentures.[66,67] Xerostomia or reduced salivary flow leads to reduced intrinsic antifungal properties of salivary components such as lactoferrin, lysozyme, histatins, and immunoglobulins. Nutritional deficiency of iron, folate, vitamin B$_{12}$, systemic conditions like diabetes mellitus, hypothyroidism, Sjögren syndrome, and HIV infection (AIDS) are also contributing factors to the occurrence of candidiasis. The various *Candida* species associated include *C albicans*, *Candida tropicalis*, *Candida krusei*, *Candida parapsilosis*, *Candida dubliniensis*, *Candida glabrata*, and *Candida lusitaniae*. *C albicans* is the most commonly associated causative agent of oral candidiasis.

Pseudomembranous/erythematous candidiasis is commonly known as oral thrush. This is observed more in immunocompromised patients, patients on corticosteroids or broad-spectrum antibiotics.[68] This is observed as a

TABLE 45.2 Various chemical agents (biocides) available for prevention and disinfection of the oral cavity, including their classification, activity, dosage, and disadvantages

Biocide	Class	Activity	Dosage	Disadvantage
Chlorhexidine (CHX)	Biguanide	• Bactericidal • Bacteriostatic • Also used as sub-gingival irrigant and preprocedural rinse[45]	• 0.12%-0.2% • 30-60 s	• Brown/black discoloration of teeth, mucosa, and restoration • Increased roughness of restoration • Development of tolerance in some microbial strains[46]
Cetylpyridinium chloride	Amphiphilic quaternary compound	Reduces bacterial adhesion to tooth surfaces by binding to negatively charged bacterial cells	Long-term therapy effective (6 mo)	Dose-dependent dental staining (less than CHX)
Essential oils	Thymol, eucalyptol, menthol, methyl salicylate	• Antimicrobial • Anti-inflammatory		• Strong taste • Tissue irritant[47]
Ethanol, isopropanol	Alcohol	• Used as a solvent	0%-27%	• Contraindicated in children • Associated with carcinogenesis
Triclosan	Bisphenol	• Antibacterial • Anti fungal (eg, *Candida*)	0.2-6.2 µg/mL	• Health risks[48] • Bioaccumulation[34]
Octenidine	Biguanide	• Antiseptic • Interferes with microbial coaggregration	0.1%	• Unpleasant taste • High staining potential than CHX[49]
Polyvinylpyrrolidone (PVP) complexes	Hydrophilic polymer that releases CHX	PVP + CHX	5%-10%	• Few studies done • Slow release of CHX[36]
Hyaluronic acid (HA)	Nonsulfated glycosaminoglycan	• Anti-inflammatory • Bacteriostatic • Antioxidant	• 0.2% gel • Spray	• Further research required[50]
Delmopinol hydrochloride	Cationic agent	Interferes with dental biofilm formation by altering attachment and acid formation	0.2%[51]	Unknown
Natural compounds[52]	Variety of formulated products that contain various natural plant extracts such as from green team, peppermint, and other oil extracts	• Antibacterial • Anti-inflammatory claims • Anti-oxidant	Varies from product to product	Ulceration and burning sensation
Fluoride compounds	NaF 0.05% SnF$_2$ 0.2%	Remineralization potential	0.05%-0.2%	• Dental stains • Unstable compound in mouthrinses versus dentifrices
Dilute sodium hypochlorite	NaOCl	• Antimicrobial, root canal irrigant • Tooth whitening	0.25%	Sensitive to tissues and mucous membrane
Hydrogen peroxide	H$_2$O$_2$	• Antiseptic • Stain removal	3%	Redness or irritation of mucous membrane

TABLE 45.3   Common oral viral infections and treatments

Virus	Disease	Oral Lesions	Treatment and Prevention
Herpes simplex virus 1 (HSV 1) and 2 (HSV 2)—deoxyribonucleic acid (DNA) virus	Recurrent herpeti-form ulcerations called cold sores Herpes labialis, primary herpetic gingivostomatitis	Ulcers on lips, mucosa characterized by burning/itching sensation before appearance of vesicles Mostly seen in children Accompanied by fever and malaise	• Antiviral treatment[61,62] • Acyclovir: 200-400 mg × 5 times a day • Analgesics, nonsteroidal anti-inflammatory drugs (NSAIDs), lavage, hydration. • 5% topical acyclovir for herpes labialis
Varicella zoster virus—DNA virus Herpes Zoster	Children—chicken pox Adults—shingles	Oral lesions—mucosal vesicles precedes skin lesions Vesicular development distributed along the second division of trigeminal nerve	• Vaccination available • Palliative medical care-analgesics, hydration • Aspirin contraindicated. (Reye syndrome)
Epstein-Barr virus Human herpes virus 8	Infectious mononucleosis	Petechiae on hard and soft palate Necrotizing ulcerative gingivitis	• Self-limiting • NSAIDs
Cytomegalovirus	Fatal in immu-nocompromised patients and neonates	Ulceration—present with coinfections of HSV/human immunodeficiency virus Enamel hypoplasia, discoloration of teeth	• Intravenous ganciclovir
Enterovirus Herpangina Acute lymphonodular pharyngitis Hand, foot and mouth syndrome	Vesicular eruption	Vesicles (2-4 mm) in the posterior areas of mouth—tonsillar pillars, soft palate Yellow to dark pink nodules in area of oropharynx Intraoral lesions on palate, tongue, and buccal mucosa	Supportive care and over the counter pain medications Self-limiting and clears up in 7-10 d
Rubeola	Measles	Koplik spots—red macular lesions with a blue white center on oral mucosa	• Vaccination available: measles, mumps, and rubella (MMR) vaccine in 2 doses • Rest, fluids, antipyretic
Paramyxovirus	Mumps	Bilateral swelling of the parotid gland Swelling and pain begin from the ear and extend to the mandible	• Vaccination available: MMR vaccine in 2 doses • Palliative care
Human papillomavirus	Oral squamous cell carcinoma Verruca vulgaris Condyloma acuminatum	Small, white, exophytic, and pedunculated growth on hard and soft palate, uvula and vermillion border of lips Nodular lesion on lips, gingiva, and hard palate Multiple pink nodules on labial mucosa, soft palate, and lingual frenum	Surgical excision with scalpel or laser ablation
Human immunodeficiency virus	Immunocompromised oral and general health	Oral candidiasis, oral hairy leukoplakia, Kaposi sarcoma, periodontal disease	Highly active antiretroviral therapy Palliative care Good oral hygiene maintenance

TABLE 45.4	Other common oral fungal infections and treatments		
Fungi	**Disease**	**Oral Lesions**	**Treatment and Prevention**
Aspergillus	Aspergillosis—in immunocompromised patients	Marginal gingiva and gingival sulcus are portal of entry of spores; painful gingival ulcerations and mucosal soft tissue swelling with gray hue	Multidisciplinary treatment involving antifungal agents with surgical debridement and reduction of immunosuppression
Cryptococcus neoformans	Cryptococcosis	Oral mucosal ulcers nodules; granulomas on gingiva, palate, and tooth socket after extraction	Antifungal therapies—intravenous amphotericin B, oral flucytosine, and oral fluconazole
Histoplasma capsulatum	Histoplasmosis	Ulcerative or nodular lesion on oral mucous membrane—tongue, palate, or lips; ulcers with raised and rolled borders, covered by a yellow or greyish membrane	Usually self-resolving Itraconazole—antifungal for 3-12 mo for worse symptoms
Zygomycetes spp	Zygomycosis	Necrotic palatal ulcer with well-defined borders that appear either white or black	Amphotericin B, hyperbaric oxygen therapy in combination with antifungal and surgical therapies
Coccidioides immitis	Coccidioidomycosis (valley fever)	Ulcerated granulomatous nodules	Oral triazole antifungals, usually self-resolving. Follow up every 3-6 mo.
Geotrichum candidum	Geotrichosis	Oral lesions very similar to pseudomembranous candidiasis—white plaques with erythematous background	Nystatin or Gentian violet 1%

thick white plaque on the tongue, buccal mucosa, and hard palate. The plaques consist of necrotic material, debris, desquamated epithelial cells, and fungal hyphae and are usually asymptomatic. Pseudomembranous candidiasis with localized erythema and burning sensation is called erythematous candidiasis.[69] Denture stomatitis, associated with ill-fitting dentures and/or poor oral hygiene can lead to the development of similar lesions,[70] characterized by erythema and burning sensations at the fitting surface of the prosthesis. Median rhomboid glossitis is localized to the posterior surface of the tongue and presents as an erythematous, rhomboidal area of atrophic papillae on the dorsal tongue.[68] Finally, angular cheilitis is a chronic inflammatory lesion characterized by a bilateral crusting, erythema at the angle of the mouth. This is most frequently seen in elderly patient with a loss of vertical dimension leading to pooling of saliva at the labial fissure that favors candidal growth.[68] Because candidiasis is multifactorial, identification of the underlying cause is the key to proper management. Hence, nutritional deficiencies, salivary flow rate and composition, denture adequacy, and patient oral/dental hygiene status should be identified. For pseudomembranous types, topical azole or polyene antifungal agents are often directly applied to the lesion. Nystatin oral suspension (100 000 U/mL) four times daily for 7 to 14 days and/or systemic antifungal agents like ketoconazole, flucanozole, and amphotericin B can be administered for widespread cases. For denture stomatitis, patients should be advised to practice proper oral and denture hygiene measures. Dentures should be not be worn at night and be

placed in a cleaning solution. Antifungal agents can also be applied to the base of the denture for site-directed antifungal action. Amphotericin B lozenges (10 mg) or suspension (100 mg/mL) can also be considered.

Other fungal infections of oral cavity are summarized in Table 45.4.

▶ HABIT-ASSOCIATED ORAL MUCOSAL LESIONS

Smoking in the form of cigarettes and tobacco chewing, certain medicines, and faulty restorations can have a major effect on the teeth and oral mucosa. Tobacco use in any form affects the oral epithelium, resulting in changes to the tissues ranging from a mild increase in pigmentation to a premalignant thickening of the oral epithelium. It increases the risk of periodontal disease and can also irritate minor salivary glands. Smoking-associated oral lesions are mentioned in the following text.

In 1978, oral leukoplakia was defined by the WHO as a "white patch or plaque that cannot be characterized clinically or pathologically as any other disease."[71] It is associated with use of tobacco in smoke and smokeless form. Leukoplakia can affect any part of the oral cavity. Depending on the form and use of tobacco, the most common sites are hard palate (reverse cigar smoking) and the buccal mucosa (betel nut placement and chewing).[72] Leukoplakia can present as homogenous white patches usually asymptomatic in nature or nonhomogenous irregular, flat, nodules with red and white nonuniform patches. These are classified as premalignant lesions. Smoker's palate (or nicotinic stomatitis) presents as painless papules on the hard palate in response to heat produced by smoking a pipe or cigar. The smoke causes irritation of the minor salivary gland ducts, and the tiny papules represent the dilated orifice of the glands.[73] Oral submucous fibrosis is a premalignant condition caused by betel nut chewing. The copper and arecoline from these nuts can produce blanching of the oral mucosa leading to hypovascularity and fibrosis. The other symptoms include staining of teeth and gums, trismus, and thick and rubbery appearance of lips.[74]

Acetylsalicylic acid (aspirin) is used by patients sometimes to manage tooth pain. When the tablet is placed in the mucobuccal fold adjacent to the painful tooth for a prolonged period of time, it can cause white keratotic lesion known as aspirin burn.[75] Aspirin reduces the pH of the oral environment, and the acids bind with the epithelial and tissue proteins can lead to denaturation and coagulative necrosis.[76,77]

Frictional keratosis present as reactive white lesions caused by prolonged irritation and/or regular friction of the mucous membrane. They appear as white patches due to extra epithelial cell turnover on the tongue, cheek, or the buccal mucosa (linea alba—the white line on the buccal mucosa adjacent to the line of occlusion). The etiology can be a constant irritation from ill-fitting dentures/restoration, habitual tongue/cheek biting, broken/maligned teeth, stress-induced grinding of teeth at night (bruxism), etc. Acute trauma can cause ulcers, whereas chronic mild trauma may lead to hyperkeratosis.[78]

The management of such lesions, first and foremost, is habit cessation, removal of the causative agent (tobacco, smoking, aspirin, and faulty restoration) to prevent further damage to the oral mucosa. Analgesics like Triamcinolone 0.1% ointment in Orabase® and tretinoin 0.05% gel can be applied to alleviate pain. Bite guards, in cases of bruxism or grinding of teeth, should be worn at night. For severe cases when the lesions are malignant, chemoprevention, surgical removal with lasers, cryotherapy, and regular observation can also be advised. As always, early diagnosis by thorough dental examination and history is vital.

▶ DENTIST-INDUCED COMPLICATIONS

Dentist use chemicals like silver nitrate, dental varnishes, and acid etching materials for restoration of carious tooth, NaOCl, and H_2O_2 for root canal debridement. These chemicals can sometimes leach out to the soft tissue and contribute to the formation of superficial pseudomembranes composed of necrotic surface tissue and an inflammatory exudate. Even commercially available mouthrinses can lead to superficial burn or ulceration with sloughing of the mucosa in certain groups of individuals. In these cases, dentist should be encouraged to

use rubber dams and proper tooth isolation protocols when using certain chemicals in the oral cavity. Dentist should have a good knowledge of the patient's medical and general health (allergies or sensitivity history). Most superficial burns and ulcers will heal in 1 to 2 weeks. For palliative care, an analgesic gel or glycerin can be applied at the lesion. In areas of severe necrosis, tissue debridement, biocide treatment, and antibiotic coverage is sometimes indicated.

Reusable medical instruments can be subdivided into critical, semicritical, and noncritical types depending on the risk of transmitting infection.[79,80] There are many guidance documents (eg, International Standards Organization, Association for the Advancement of Medical Instrumentation, and FDA) available concerning the reprocessing of reusable medical devices (see chapter 47), but reusable dental instruments are often considered separately and often lack such well-defined processing protocols particularly in the United States.[81] The American Dental Association[82] classifies dental instruments based on the same Spaulding classification as follows:

1. Critical instruments: Instruments are those used to penetrate soft tissue or bone, or enter into or contact the bloodstream or other normally sterile tissue. They should be cleaned and sterilized after each use. Examples in dentistry: forceps, scalpels, bone chisels, scalers, and surgical burs.

2. Semicritical instruments are those that do not penetrate soft tissues or bone but contact mucous membranes or nonintact skin, such as mirrors, reusable impression trays, and amalgam condensers. These should also be cleaned and sterilized, although high-level disinfection is often considered as an alternative to sterilization.

3. Noncritical instruments are those that come into contact only with intact skin such as external components of x-ray heads, blood pressure cuffs, and pulse oximeters. They are recommended to be cleaned and disinfected (see chapter 47).

The reprocessing of dental instruments is often found to be inefficient, and devices have been shown to possess residual patient materials, such as bone, saliva, and other debris.[83,84] Dentists have been fortunate, to date, to have low reported numbers and less severe cases of associated infections associated with insufficient reprocessing, in comparison to those compared in other medical areas, such as with the use of flexible endoscopes.[85-87] But, there have been studies showing the direct presence of HIV and HBV viruses on reprocessed dental instruments.[88] Potential outbreaks of infection with dental instrumentation can include lack of adequate cleaning, ineffective sterilization, and cross-contamination from reusable water lines.[89] Moreover, the well-defined connection between oral cavity and systemic infections mandates the reduction in cross-contamination risks with dental instruments.

▶ DENTISTS AS ORAL PHYSICIANS

The oral cavity is an integral and unique part of the human body, where dental practitioners can play a key role in diagnosis of many diseases. Careful examination of the oral cavity may reveal findings indicative of an underlying systemic condition and allow for early diagnosis and treatment. A dentist is taught to examine, diagnose, and treat the oral cavity and related structures with often-limited primary medical care training. With today's dynamic health care reforms, increased life expectancy, and prevalence of many chronic diseases, a greater number of patients avail of dental care and visit dentists at least once or twice a year for routine dental examinations. A thorough dental examination of oral hard and soft tissues, lymph nodes palpitation, medical history questionnaire, and oral cancer screening will go long way in preventative care, such as the asymptomatic swelling on the lower jaw of a patient leading to an early diagnosis of infections such as with HPV. A plethora of research studies have linked oral bacteria with life-threatening conditions like cardiovascular diseases, diabetes, rheumatoid arthritis, inflammatory bowel disease, and even obesity.[19,90] Common oral and systemic links include the following:

- Several dermatologic conditions present with oral mucosal involvement, either concurrent with the skin pathology or sometimes as the only clinical presentation. Examples include hand, foot and mouth disease, varicella zoster, and Koplik spots.
- Blood disorders like thrombocytopenia and leukemia present as gingivitis and prolonged postextraction bleeding.
- Anemic patients present with facial pallor, atrophic glossitis, angular cheilitis, and candidiasis.
- Oral ulceration is a common manifestation of several diseases like autoimmune diseases; metabolic disorders; and viral, bacterial, and fungal infections. Careful inspection of the type of ulcer, its edges and appearance along with medical history can help diagnose the underlying systemic condition. An example is oral ulcerations with diffuse mucosal swelling, cobblestone mucosa, and localized mucogingivitis suggests underlying Crohn disease.
- Severe periodontal inflammation or bleeding with absence of local factors like dental plaque indicates conditions such as diabetes mellitus, HIV infection, and leukemia.
- In patients with gastroesophageal reflux disease, bulimia, or anorexia, dental erosion on the palatal surface of upper anterior teeth is a classical sign.

The dentist clinical goal should be to reestablish the oral flora's symbiotic equilibrium and maintain its natural diversity. In cases of periodontal disease, first line of treatment should include scaling and root planing and use of biocides to reduce the microbial load of the pathogenic bacteria and help the commensals grow to bring a healthy equilibrium back. Use of antibiotics should be discouraged to prevent the development of antibiotic resistance and further complications. Moreover, probiotics with active cultures may be prescribed to help outnumber the presence of pathogens.[91] Emphasis should be placed on the active maintenance of health and educating the patient on healthy lifestyle and diet choices. The traditional and proper guidance on oral hygiene maintenance (brushing twice a day with a soft bristle brush, flossing, and use of mouthwash) should be provided at every dental visit reinforcing the concept of balancing the good and the bad bacteria. Overall, dentists and patients should embrace the concept of balanced oral microbiomes and their connection to oral and systemic health. The dentists of the near future should become "oral physicians"[92] and go the extra step by bridging the gap between oral and systemic infections.

REFERENCES

1. Jiménez Gómez N, Ballester Martínez MA, Alcántara González J, Jaén Olasolo P. Koplik spots as a diagnostic clue in a case of measles. *Med Clin (Barc)*. 2012;139:560.
2. Xavier S, Forgie SE. Koplik spots revisited. *CMAJ*. 2015;187:600.
3. Nanci A. *Ten Cate's Oral Histology: Development, Structure, and Function*. St. Louis, MO: Elsevier Health Sciences; 2007.
4. Dewhirst FE, Chen T, Izard J, et al. The human oral microbiome. *J Bacteriol*. 2010;192:5002-5017.
5. Novak N, Haberstok J, Bieber T, Allam JP. The immune privilege of the oral mucosa. *Trends Mol Med*. 2008;14:191-198.
6. Squier CA, Kremer MJ. Biology of oral mucosa and esophagus. *J Natl Cancer Inst Monogr*. 2001;7-15.
7. Abu Eid R, Sawair F, Landini G, Saku T. Age and the architecture of oral mucosa. *Age (Dordr)*. 2012;34:651-658.
8. Feller L, Altini M, Khammissa RA, Chandran R, Bouckaert M, Lemmer J. Oral mucosal immunity. *Oral Surg Oral Med Oral Pathol Oral Radiol*. 2013;116:576-583.
9. Walker DM. Oral mucosal immunology: an overview. *Ann Acad Med Singapore*. 2004;33:27-30.
10. Okada H, Murakami S. Cytokine expression in periodontal health and disease. *Crit Rev Oral Biol Med*. 1998;9:248-266.
11. Durand SH, Flacher V, Roméas A, et al. Lipoteichoic acid increases TLR and functional chemokine expression while reducing dentin formation in vitro differentiated human odontoblasts. *J Immunol*. 2006;176:2880-2887.
12. Farges JC, Alliot-Licht B, Renard E, et al. Dental pulp defence and repair mechanisms in dental caries. *Mediators Inflamm*. 2015;2015:230251.
13. Turner MD, Nedjai B, Hurst T, Pennington DJ. Cytokines and chemokines: at the crossroads of cell signalling and inflammatory disease. *Biochim Biophys Acta*. 2014;1843:2563-2582.
14. Song W, Shi Y, Xiao M, et al. In vitro bactericidal activity of recombinant human beta-defensin-3 against pathogenic bacterial strains in human tooth root canal. *Int J Antimicrob Agents*. 2009;33:237-243.
15. Barros SP, Williams R, Offenbacher S, Morelli T. Gingival crevicular fluid as a source of biomarkers for periodontitis. *Periodontol 2000*. 2016;70:53-64.
16. Humphrey SP, Williamson RT. A review of saliva: normal composition, flow, and function. *J Prosthet Dent*. 2001;85:162-169.
17. Greabu M, Battino M, Mohora M, et al. Saliva—a diagnostic window to the body, both in health and in disease. *J Med Life*. 2009;2:124-132.

18. Fábián TK, Hermann P, Beck A, Fejérdy P, Fábián G. Salivary defense proteins: their network and role in innate and acquired oral immunity. *Int J Mol Sci.* 2012;13:4295-4320.

19. Leishman SJ, Do HL, Ford PJ. Cardiovascular disease and the role of oral bacteria. *J Oral Microbiol.* 2010;2.

20. Lucchese A. Streptococcus mutans antigen I/II and autoimmunity in cardiovascular diseases. *Autoimmun Rev.* 2017;16:456-460.

21. Cobb CM, Kelly PJ, Williams KB, Babbar S, Angolkar M, Derman RJ. The oral microbiome and adverse pregnancy outcomes. *Int J Womens Health.* 2017;9:551-559.

22. de Groot PF, Belzer C, Aydin Ö, et al. Distinct fecal and oral microbiota composition in human type 1 diabetes, an observational study. *PLoS One.* 2017;12:e0188475.

23. Caufield PW, Cutter GR, Dasanayake AP. Initial acquisition of mutans streptococci by infants: evidence for a discrete window of infectivity. *J Dent Res.* 1993;72:37-45.

24. Lendenmann U, Grogan J, Oppenheim FG. Saliva and dental pellicle—a review. *Adv Dent Res.* 2000;14:22-28.

25. Skjørland KK, Rykke M, Sonju T. Rate of pellicle formation in vivo. *Acta Odontol Scand.* 1995;53:358-362.

26. Jenkinson HF. Beyond the oral microbiome. *Environ Microbiol.* 2011;13:3077-3087.

27. Lovegrove JM. Dental plaque revisited: bacteria associated with periodontal disease. *J N Z Soc Periodontol.* 2004;87:7-21.

28. American Dental Association. Oral health topics: home oral care. American Dental Association Web site. https://www.ada.org/en/member-center/oral-health-topics/home-care. Accessed August 29, 2019.

29. Rosema N, Slot DE, van Palenstein Helderman WH, Wiggelinkhuizen L, Van der Weijden GA. The efficacy of powered toothbrushes following a brushing exercise: a systematic review. *Int J Dent Hyg.* 2016;14:29-41.

30. Slot DE, Wiggelinkhuizen L, Rosema NA, Van der Weijden GA. The efficacy of manual toothbrushes following a brushing exercise: a systematic review. *Int J Dent Hyg.* 2012;10:187-197.

31. Santos AP, Oliveira BH, Nadanovsky P. Effects of low and standard fluoride toothpastes on caries and fluorosis: systematic review and meta-analysis. *Caries Res.* 2013;47:382-390.

32. Sreenivasan P, Gaffar A. Antiplaque biocides and bacterial resistance: a review. *J Clin Periodontol.* 2002;29:965-974.

33. Scientific Committee on Emerging and Newly Identified Health Risks. Effects of biocides on antibiotic resistance; 2009. http://ec.europa.eu/health/scientific_committees/opinions_layman/en/biocides-antibiotic-resistance/l-3/1-definition-antimicrobials.htm. Accessed June 22, 2010.

34. Dhillon GS, Kaur S, Pulicharla R, et al. Triclosan: current status, occurrence, environmental risks and bioaccumulation potential. *Int J Environ Res Public Health.* 2015;12:5657-5684.

35. McDonnell G, Russell AD. Antiseptics and disinfectants: activity, action, and resistance. *Clin Microbiol Rev.* 1999;12:147-179.

36. Claydon N, Addy M, Jackson R, Smith S, Newcombe RG. Studies on the effect of polyvinyl pyrrolidone on the activity of chlorhexidine mouthrinses: plaque and stain. *J Clin Periodontol.* 2001;6:558-564.

37. Mohammadi Z, Shalavi S, Moeintaghavi A, Jafarzadeh H. A review over benefits and drawbacks of combining sodium hypochlorite with other endodontic materials. *Open Dent J.* 2017;11:661-669.

38. Gunsolley JC. A meta-analysis of six-month studies of antiplaque and antigingivitis agents. *J Am Dent Assoc.* 2006;137:1649-1657.

39. Haps S, Slot DE, Berchier CE, Van der Weijden GA. The effect of cetylpyridinium chloride-containing mouth rinses as adjuncts to toothbrushing on plaque and parameters of gingival inflammation: a systematic review. *Int J Dent Hyg.* 2008;6:290-303.

40. Stoeken JE, Paraskevas S, van der Weijden GA. The long-term effect of a mouthrinse containing essential oils on dental plaque and gingivitis: a systematic review. *J Periodontol.* 2007;78:1218-1228.

41. Hairston BR, Bruce AJ, Rogers RS III. Viral diseases of the oral mucosa. *Dermatol Clin.* 2003;21:17-32.

42. Grinde B, Olsen I. The role of viruses in oral disease. *J Oral Microbiol.* 2010;2.

43. Slots J. Oral viral infections of adults. *Periodontol 2000.* 2009;49:60-86.

44. Hillbertz NS, Hirsch JM, Jalouli J, Jalouli MM, Sand L. Viral and molecular aspects of oral cancer. *Anticancer Res.* 2012;32:4201-4212.

45. Löe H. Oral hygiene in the prevention of caries and periodontal disease. *Int Dent J.* 2000;50:129-139.

46. Kulik EM, Waltimo T, Weiger R, et al. Development of resistance of mutans streptococci and *Porphyromonas gingivalis* to chlorhexidine digluconate and amine fluoride/stannous fluoride-containing mouthrinses, in vitro. *Clin Oral Investig.* 2015;19:1547-1553.

47. Richards D. Effect of essential oil mouthwashes on plaque and gingivitis. *Evid Based Dent.* 2017;18:39-40.

48. Dinwiddie MT, Terry PD, Chen J. Recent evidence regarding triclosan and cancer risk. *Int J Environ Res Public Health.* 2014;11:2209-2217.

49. Beiswanger BB, Mallatt ME, Mau MS, Jackson RD, Hennon DK. The clinical effects of a mouthrinse containing 0.1% octenidine. *J Dent Res.* 1990;69:454-457.

50. Casale M, Moffa A, Vella P, et al. Hyaluronic acid: perspectives in dentistry. A systematic review. *Int J Immunopathol Pharmacol.* 2016;29:572-582.

51. Hase JC, Attström R, Edwardsson S, Kelty E, Kisch J. 6-month use of 0.2% delmopinol hydrochloride in comparison with 0.2% chlorhexidine digluconate and placebo. (I). Effect on plaque formation and gingivitis. *J Clin Periodontol.* 1998;25:746-753.

52. Chen Y, Wong RW, McGrath C, Hagg U, Seneviratne CJ. Natural compounds containing mouthrinses in the management of dental plaque and gingivitis: a systematic review. *Clin Oral Investig.* 2014;18:1-16.

53. Specenier P, Vermorken JB. Cetuximab: its unique place in head and neck cancer treatment. *Biologics.* 2013;7:77-90.

54. Hartner L. Chemotherapy for oral cancer. *Dent Clin North Am.* 2018;62:87-97.

55. Rietbergen MM, Leemans CR, Bloemena E, et al. Increasing prevalence rates of HPV attributable oropharyngeal squamous cell carcinomas in the Netherlands as assessed by a validated test algorithm. *Int J Cancer.* 2013;132:1565-1571.

56. Dahlstrom KR, Li G, Tortolero-Luna G, Wei Q, Sturgis EM. Differences in history of sexual behavior between patients with oropharyngeal squamous cell carcinoma and patients with squamous cell carcinoma at other head and neck sites. *Head Neck.* 2011;33:847-855.

57. Chaturvedi AK, Engels EA, Anderson WF, Gillison ML. Incidence trends for human papillomavirus-related and -unrelated oral squamous cell carcinomas in the United States. *J Clin Oncol.* 2008;26:612-619.

58. Centers for Disease Control and Prevention. Human papillomavirus–associated cancers—United States, 2004-2008. *MMWR Morb Mortal Wkly Rep.* 2012;61(15):258-261.

59. Human papillomavirus vaccines: WHO position paper, October 2014-Recommendations. *Vaccine.* 2015;33:4383-4384.

60. Kim S. Human papilloma virus in oral cancer. *J Korean Assoc Oral Maxillofac Surg.* 2016;42:327-336.

61. Slezák R, Buchta V, Förstl M, Prásil P, Sustová Z, Bukac J. Infections of the oral mucosa caused by herpes simplex virus. *Klin Mikrobiol Infekc Lek.* 2009;15:131-137.

62. Glick M. Clinical aspects of recurrent oral herpes simplex virus infection. *Compend Contin Educ Dent.* 2002;23(7 suppl 2):4-8.

63. Gerard R, Sendid B, Colombel JF, Poulain D, Jouault T. An immunological link between Candida albicans colonization and Crohn's disease. *Crit Rev Microbiol.* 2015;41:135-139.

64. Zahir RA, Himratul-Aznita WH. Distribution of Candida in the oral cavity and its differentiation based on the internally transcribed spacer (ITS) regions of rDNA. *Yeast.* 2013;30:13-23.

65. Cannon RD, Chaffin WL. Oral colonization by *Candida albicans. Crit Rev Oral Biol Med.* 1999;10:359-383.

66. Peterson DE. Oral candidiasis. *Clin Geriatr Med.* 1992;8:513-527.

67. Shulman JD, Rivera-Hidalgo F, Beach MM. Risk factors associated with denture stomatitis in the United States. *J Oral Pathol Med.* 2005;34:340-346.

68. Reichart PA, Samaranayake LP, Philipsen HP. Pathology and clinical correlates in oral candidiasis and its variants: a review. *Oral Dis.* 2000;6:85-91.

69. Krishnan PA. Fungal infections of the oral mucosa. *Indian J Dent Res.* 2012;23:650-659.

70. Grimoud AM, Lodter JP, Marty N, et al. Improved oral hygiene and Candida species colonization level in geriatric patients. *Oral Dis.* 2005;11:163-169.

71. Kramer IR, Lucas RB, Pindborg JJ, Sobin LH. Definition of leukoplakia and related lesions: an aid to studies on oral precancer. *Oral Surg Oral Med Oral Pathol.* 1978;46:518-539.

72. Pindborg JJ, Roed-Peterson B, Renstrup G. Role of smoking in floor of the mouth leukoplakias. *J Oral Pathol.* 1972;1:22-29.

73. Andersson G, Vala EK, Curvall M. The influence of cigarette consumption and smoking machine yields of tar and nicotine on the nicotine uptake and oral mucosal lesions in smokers. *J Oral Pathol Med.* 1997;26:117-123.

74. Sharma A, Kumar R, Johar N, Sabir H. Oral submucous fibrosis: an etiological dilemma. *J Exp Ther Oncol.* 2017;12:163-166.

75. Dellinger TM, Livingston HM. Aspirin burn of the oral cavity. *Ann Pharmacother.* 1998;32:1107.

76. Deo SP, Shetty P. Accidental chemical burns of oral mucosa by herbicide. *JNMA J Nepal Med Assoc.* 2012;52:40-42.

77. Gilvetti C, Porter SR, Fedele S. Traumatic chemical oral ulceration: a case report and review of the literature. *Br Dent J.* 2010;208:297-300.

78. Cam K, Santoro A, Lee JB. Oral frictional hyperkeratosis (morsicatio buccarum): an entity to be considered in the differential diagnosis of white oral mucosal lesions. *Skinmed.* 2012;10:114-115.

79. Spaulding EH. Chemical disinfection of medical and surgical materials. In: Lawrence C, Block SS, eds. *Disinfection, Sterilization, and Preservation.* Philadelphia, PA: Lea & Febiger; 1968.

80. Rutala WA, Weber DJ; and Healthcare Infection Control Practices Advisory Committee. *Guideline for Disinfection and Sterilization in Healthcare Facilities, 2008.* Chapel Hill, NC: Centers for Disease Control and Prevention.

81. Alfa MJ, Olson N, DeGagne P, Jackson M. A survey of reprocessing methods, residual viable bioburden, and soil levels in patient-ready endoscopic retrograde choliangiopancreatography duodenoscopes used in Canadian centers. *Infect Control Hosp Epidemiol.* 2002;23:198-206.

82. American Dental Association. Oral health topics: infection control and sterilization. http://www.ada.org/en/member-center/oral-health-topics/infection-control-resources. Accessed September 18, 2019.

83. Vassey M, Budge C, Poolman T, et al. A quantitative assessment of residual protein levels on dental instruments reprocessed by manual, ultrasonic and automated cleaning methods. *Br Dent J.* 2011;210:E14.

84. Smith A, Letters S, Lange A, Perrett D, McHugh S, Bagg J. Residual protein levels on reprocessed dental instruments. *J Hosp Infect.* 2005;61:237-241.

85. Bourvis N, Boelle PY, Cesbron JY, Valleron AJ. Risk assessment of transmission of sporadic Creutzfeldt-Jakob disease in endodontic practice in absence of adequate prion inactivation. *PLoS One.* 2007;2.

86. Walker JT, Dickinson J, Sutton JM, Raven ND, Marsh PD. Cleanability of dental instruments—implications of residual protein and risks from Creutzfeldt-Jakob disease. *Br Dent J.* 2007;203:395-401.

87. Kovaleva J, Peters FT, van der Mei HC, Degener JE. Transmission of infection by flexible gastrointestinal endoscopy and bronchoscopy. *Clin Microbiol Rev.* 2013;26:231-254.

88. Epstein JB, Rea G, Sibau L, Sherlock CH. Rotary dental instruments and the potential risk of transmission of infection: herpes simplex virus. *J Am Dent Assoc.* 1993;124:55-59.

89. The Future Dentist. Classification of instruments. https://nicolasmontagnat.wordpress.com/2016/03/07/2-classification-of-instruments/. Accessed March 3, 2018.

90. Le Bars P, Matamoros S, Montassier E, et al. The oral cavity microbiota: between health, oral disease, and cancers of the aerodigestive tract. *Can J Microbiol.* 2017;63:475-492.

91. Pujia AM, Costacurta M, Fortunato L, et al. The probiotics in dentistry: a narrative review. *Eur Rev Med Pharmacol Sci.* 2017;21:1405-1412.

92. Giddon DB. Should dentists become 'oral physicians'? Yes, dentists should become 'oral physicians.' *J Am Dent Assoc* 2004;135:438-442.

Laundry Hygiene

Dirk P. Bockmühl and Marlitt Honisch

▶ MICROORGANISMS ON TEXTILES

Microbial contaminations on laundry items originate from numerous sources. During the different stages of the utilization cycle of textiles, various microbial species are introduced to the fabric on the one hand and they are being removed, inactivated, or killed on the other (Figure 46.1). This cycle includes the process of wearing or using a textile followed by its reconditioning (ie, sorting, laundering, drying, and storing). Thus, the presence of microorganisms on textiles is closely linked to their way of use: Microbial contaminants on textiles with narrow body contact, such as clothing and towels, are expected to be predominantly members of the human skin and mucosal biota as well as contaminations that result from bodily excretions. Another source of microbial contamination on textiles that is closely related to their use is the environment, including dust, soil, or food. Moreover, the washing machine itself has been shown to be a source of microbial contaminations being of particular importance in the context of laundering (Table 46.1). Although a major proportion of the microbial cells that are present on a used textile will be removed or inactivated during laundering, microbial biofilms colonizing the detergent distribution system of the washing machine can be detached in the washing process and transported with the rinsing water, resulting in a recontamination of the laundry after the main wash cycle. As a result, the microbial load on the textiles might even increase by laundering.[10]

In general, it can be assumed that most of the microorganisms found on clothes do not pose an immediate health risk because everybody is in regular contact with them anyway because they are also part of the human microbiome or the environment. However, there are situations where an increased health risk from laundry must be considered (eg, in the case of an infectious disease present in a household or when immunocompromised people are concerned), which is particularly important in the case of domestic health care as well as for care facilities or hospitals. Other situations in which deficient laundry hygiene might pose a health risk include reinfection by insufficiently decontaminated items and the transmission of infections among household members via cross-contamination (ie, the transfer of microbial cells from contaminated to non-contaminated textiles). Consequently, contaminations of facultative or obligatory pathogenic microorganisms on laundry items should be reduced to a noninfectious level as one measure among others to avoid the transmission of infections.

Besides the risk of infection, microbial contaminations on textiles or in washing machines can also cause aesthetic impairments, such as the generation of malodors on washed textiles or the formation of biofilms in the washing machine. Particularly in the domestic environment, the generation of malodors might be considered as one of the most prominent microbiological problems related to laundry.[11-14]

It can be assumed that there are two major types of typical laundry-associated malodors: acidic, sweat-like odors on the one hand and musty, "wet-and-dirty-dustcloth-like" odors on the other hand.[15] The formation of malodors on washed textiles is thought to be caused by the bacterial metabolization of sweat residues,[16] whereas microorganisms that colonize the washing machine represent another origin of malodor, comprising a musty "wet-cloth-like" odor, which is believed to be associated with the presence of *Moraxella* species.[15] However, *Moraxella* is not one of the bacteria most commonly isolated from biofilms in European washing machines[2,5,17] and might be more relevant in Asia if not being able to form malodorous substances even if present in low numbers. Callewaert et al[3] observed exchange of waterborne microorganisms and skin colonizers on the textile during the laundry process. It seems likely that the

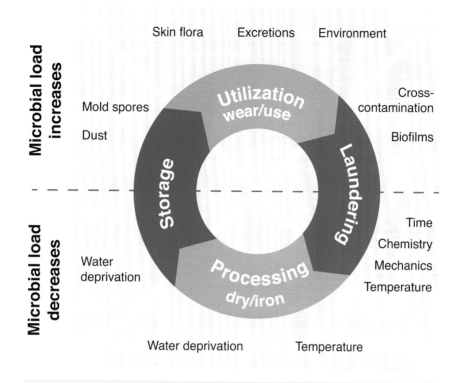

FIGURE 46.1 Utilization cycle of textiles showing the input and removal of microorganisms. Modified after Bockmühl.[1]

formation of laundry-associated malodor is not caused by the presence of one specific species alone but that the mixture of biofilm-forming microorganisms transferred from the washing machine to the fabric and of residual contaminants from the skin remaining on the textile leads to the generation of malodor on the washed textiles. Neither the compounds that are responsible for this type of malodor nor the way these substances are formed are well understood yet. Takeuchi et al[18] proposed C7-branched fatty acids to be mainly responsible for this phenomenon, which remarkably resemble molecules that are present in human sweat after bacterial metabolization. Measures against malodor generation in laundry thus include, in particular, machine care, including the use of high wash temperatures at regular intervals and thorough machine cleaning.

▶ PRINCIPLES OF LAUNDRY HYGIENE—FACTORS INFLUENCING THE HYGIENE EFFICACY

Laundering aims to restore the usable state of textiles by removing malodors and visible dirt and also provide a safe and sanitized textile. Whereas the term *cleaning* mostly refers to the removal of dirt and stains, laundry sanitization and hygiene also includes measures to (1) lower the bioburden (ie, the population

of viable microorganisms on laundry items), (2) prevent cross-contamination (ie, the transfer of microorganisms from one item to the other), and (3) reduce the microbial load in the washing liquor. The reduction of the microbial load on laundry items results from the inactivation or killing of the microorganisms that are attached to the fiber as well as from the detachment and mechanical removal of the microbial cells. Because reducing the infection risk is not the only aim of laundering, especially in the domestic area, laundering can thus be understood as all means that help to make textiles fit for their dedicated purpose.

According to Sinner,[19] the cleaning performance of a washing process is determined by four parameters: chemistry, temperature, time, and mechanical action. Because these factors also affect the antimicrobial performance of the process, their role in laundry hygiene is discussed here. Despite these process parameters, the quality and quantity of contamination (ie, the microbial species and the soil matrix embedding the cells as well as the amount and nature of soil) are some of the additional factors that might affect the antimicrobial efficacy of the laundering process.

Detergents and Additives

When discussing the influencing parameters in laundry according to the Sinner[19] principle, the term *chemistry* can be understood as the action of detergents and laundry additives. Two ingredient categories particularly

TABLE 46.1	Microorganisms present on textiles (tex) and in the washing machine (wm) possibly originating from environment (en) or from human sources (h)			
Classification	**Genus**	**Presence**	**Possible Origin**	**Reference**
Gram-negative bacteria	*Acinetobacter*	tex, wm	en, h	Nix et al,[2] Callewaert et al,[3] Babič et al[4]
	Brevundimonas	tex, wm	en	Nix et al,[2] Callewaert et al,[3] Babič et al[4]
	Citrobacter	tex, wm	h	Gattlen et al,[5] Scott et al[6]
	Enhydrobacter	tex	en	Callewaert et al[3]
	Enterobacteriaceae	tex, wm	h	Nix et al,[2] Gattlen et al,[5] Scott et al,[6] Blaser et al,[7] Smith et al[8]
	Flavobacterium	tex, wm	en	Nix et al,[2] Callewaert et al[3]
	Ochrobactrum	wm	en	Nix et al,[2] Babič et al[4]
	Pseudomonas	tex, wm	en	Nix et al,[2] Callewaert et al,[3] Babič et al,[4] Gattlen et al,[5] Scott et al,[6] Blaser et al,[7] Smith et al[8]
Gram-positive bacteria	*Corynebacterium*	tex	h	Callewaert et al,[3] Robinton and Mood[9]
	Enterococcus	tex	en, h	Scott et al,[6] Smith et al[8]
	Microbacterium	wm	en	Nix et al,[2] Gattlen et al,[5] Babič et al[4]
	Micrococcus	tex, wm	en	Callewaert et al,[3] Babič et al,[4] Robinton and Mood[9]
	Propionibacterium	tex	h	Callewaert et al[3]
	Staphylococcus	tex, wm	h	Callewaert et al,[3] Gattlen et al,[5] Scott et al,[6] Blaser et al,[7] Smith et al,[8] Robinton and Mood[9]
Mould	*Cladosporium*	wm	en	Nix et al,[2] Babič et al[4]
	Fusarium	wm	en	Nix et al,[2] Babič et al[4]
Yeast	*Candida*	tex, wm	h	Nix et al,[2] Babič et al,[4] Blaser et al,[7]
	Rhodotorula	wm	en	Nix et al,[2] Babič et al,[4] Gattlen et al,[5]

determine the antimicrobial performance of detergents: surfactants and bleaching agents. Whereas the main function of surfactants in the laundering process is to provide a basic cleaning efficacy by removing hydrophobic soil, hence also supporting the detachment and the physical removal of microbial cells from the fibers, rather than the inactivation of the microorganisms,[20,21] the main function of bleach in laundering is achieving a discoloration by oxidizing the chromophore groups in the stain molecules. Moreover, bleach oxidizes other organic compounds like odorous substances and reacts with microorganisms, making it the major antimicrobial component in laundry detergents. Today, the most common types of bleach are sodium hypochlorite and activated oxygen bleach (AOB). In Japan, America, Southern Europe, and other regions where traditionally cold water is used for laundering, the use of chlorine bleach is common due to its high activity at temperatures as low as 20°C (68°F), whereas oxygen-based bleach systems have prevailed in Western and Northern Europe. Most of these agents use percarbonate and a bleach activator, such as tetraacetylethylenediamine (TAED), which leads to a strong and permanent release of peracetic acid also at rather low temperatures. For domestic use, liquid and

solid detergent types are available, which, apart from the way of dosage, also differ in their composition. Whereas solid heavy-duty detergents normally contain AOB, exerting a high antimicrobial efficacy in laundry washing processes, liquid detergents do not. The application of AOB in detergents was shown to significantly increase the reduction of the microbial load on textiles.[22] In liquid detergents, surfactants may be considered as the only ingredient mediating the antimicrobial efficacy of a laundering process. However, although surfactants can support the detachment of the microorganisms from the surface, they do not have a microbicidal action per se. Application-oriented experiments suggest that the effect of the detergents on the reduction of microbial loads on textiles largely depends on the type of microorganism. Whereas the reduction of *Staphylococcus aureus* and *Enterococcus hirae* was strongly increased with liquid detergent compared to laundering with water alone, the reduction was not affected in case of *Pseudomonas aeruginosa*, *Candida albicans*, and *Trichophyton mentagrophytes*.[21] It should be mentioned that special products and those used in industrial and institutional laundering may contain other oxidizing agents (eg, hydrogen peroxide or phthalimidoperoxyhexanoic acid [PAP]).

Due to the high degree of dilution in the washing liquor, only a few substances are capable to exert an antimicrobial performance in the washing process. Besides bleach, quaternary ammonium cations (QAC) are the most commonly used substances. However, these compounds are not compatible with anionic surfactants due to their cationic nature. Hence, they are not used in detergents, but primarily in rinse aids, which are applied after the main cycle of the washing process. Two important representatives of this group are benzalkonium chloride (BAC) and didecyldimethylammonium chloride (DDAC). The antimicrobial activity of QACs largely varies between the different groups of microorganisms. Although these substances are highly effective against gram-positive bacteria even in low concentrations (with a minimum inhibitory concentration [MIC] of approximately 10 ppm), the inactivation of fungi or gram-negative bacteria requires significantly higher concentrations.[23]

Although products that contain QACs may enhance the level of hygiene in laundering (in particular with regard to delicate laundry that must not be washed with bleach or hot water), they should be used prudently, as QACs are discussed to promote resistance against biocides and perhaps even against antibiotics.[24,25]

Temperature

The washing temperature affects the reduction of the bioburden on textiles during laundering not only by thermal inactivation of the microorganisms but also by facilitating mechanical removal and accelerating the activation of bleach. Traditionally, hot-temperature washing ($\geq$60°C [140°F]) is regarded as best choice to ensure a certain level of hygiene in laundry and is still widely applied in institutional and industrial laundry. This concept has been questioned because heating the wash liquor requires the largest share of energy in the washing process with hot water, thus making lower wash temperatures an effective means to save energy. Lowering the wash temperature, however, might significantly decrease the antimicrobial performance of the washing process. According to Sinner,[19] decreased wash temperatures can be compensated for by a prolonged wash cycle, providing virtually the same stain removal efficacy and—to a limited extent—also a comparable antimicrobial performance (Figure 46.2). This strategy is often applied in energy-saving programs of modern washing machines. Yet, there are limits to this approach because the effect of a prolonged wash cycle time on the antimicrobial efficacy of laundering processes depends on the washing temperature: For cold temperatures (around 20°C [68°F]), it could be shown that a longer wash cycle time would not further enhance the antimicrobial performance of laundering. However, if high temperatures cannot be chosen, whether due to energy-saving reasons or temperature-sensitive clothing, the impaired

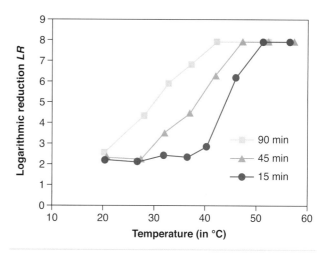

FIGURE 46.2 Effect of temperature and time on logarithmic reduction of *Staphylococcus aureus* by laundering in a domestic drum-type washing machine with bleach-free detergent. Lines are used for visualization only, based on Honisch et al.[26]

antimicrobial efficacy at low wash temperatures can be compensated by increasing the chemical part (eg, by using bleach-containing detergents).[26]

Apart from the technical parameters, the level of reduction that is reached within the washing process also depends on the type of microorganism. Experimental studies suggest that washing temperatures above 50°C (122°F) ensure a high level of hygiene in domestic laundry for a wide range of microorganisms, even without biocidal ingredients.[26-36] At this point, it should be mentioned that the actual temperature inside domestic washing machines does often not reach the selected temperature due to technical reasons because the temperatures are not measured inside the load.

Washing Machines and Programs

In the different regions of the world, three different construction types of household washing machines have prevailed. Whereas mainly horizontal axis washing machines predominate in Europe, vertical axis washing machines are traditionally used in North America and Asia.

There are no data available comparing the antimicrobial effect with regard to different types of washing machines, although it must be assumed that the mechanical effect of the washing machine significantly contributes to the reduction of the microbial load on the textile.[21] Thus, in low-temperature programs with mild, bleach-free detergents, the mechanical action and the associated dilution might be important antimicrobial factors in physically removing the microbial cells from the textile surface. Depending on the test strain, for horizontal-axis drum-type washing machines under these mild conditions, microbial reductions from 0.5 to 4.1 logarithmic units were detected for bacteria.[21,27] It is thus likely that differences in mechanics, which are to be expected due to the different construction types, also have an effect on the contribution of this factor to the reduction of the microbial load.

In context of the antimicrobial efficacy of laundering processes, two types of washing programs of domestic washing machines must be mentioned: hygiene programs and eco-programs. Compared to classical programs, hygiene programs have an extended temperature holding time and more rinsing steps. In energy-saving eco-programs, washing temperatures below the nominal (selected) temperature are applied. In a random sample of washing machines sold in Germany, temperatures of 2°C to 25°C below the chosen nominal temperatures were detected.[37] In those programs, an extended washing time was used to achieve an equivalent cleaning performance as in the reference process of a classical program at the nominal temperature, wherein the energy saving due to the lower washing temperature exceeds the energy expenditure for the extended washing.[38] In general, this principle can also be applied to the antimicrobial performance of a washing process, but compensating for lower washing temperatures by prolonging the washing time can only be achieved to a limited extent.[21,26]

In addition to the adaptation of the classic cleaning factors in the course of washing programs, there are several new technologic approaches by appliance manufacturers to enhance the antimicrobial efficacy of the washing process. Among others, the generation of ozone in the machine during the wash cycle, the use of silver nanoparticles as antimicrobial agent in the main wash cycle and in the final rinse step, and the application of electrostatic atomized water particles, which it is claimed to suppress allergens, bacteria, fungi, and viruses, can be mentioned.

Drying, Ironing, and Storage

The way of treating textiles after laundering (ie, by drying, ironing, and storage) can also be expected to affect the microbial load on the laundry items. Microbial counts that have resisted the washing process can be further reduced during drying under favorable conditions. It could be shown that the chosen drying method (eg, drying in a clothes dryer, drying on a clothes line on the inside, and drying on a clothes line outside) would strongly influence the microbial reduction by the deprivation of water as well as by temperature effects.[39] Data suggest that drying programs at moderate temperatures do not show any antimicrobial benefit compared to drying on the leash (indoors). On the other hand, drying on the leash outside, an additional reduction of the bioburden can be expected by the antimicrobial effect of the ultraviolet (UV) radiation contained in the sunlight. Under poor drying conditions, such as presence in dump rooms, however, a formation of malodors on the washed fabrics might be observed, which

indicates microbial activity.[16,40] Although the specific microbial species might behave very different when it comes to drying, gram-positive bacteria can be considered more resistant to drying than gram-negative bacteria, in general.[16] Ironing is a further step of laundry treatment that can help to reduce the microbial load on the textile. Although there are only few data available, it seems to be obvious that the application of steam during ironing enhances the sanitizing effect of ironing.[41]

During storage of textiles under dry conditions, the remaining microbial load will further decrease during the storage period.[42] However, some potentially harmful species can survive without moisture for a longer period (ie, days to several weeks).[42-45]

▶ METHODS FOR EVALUATING THE ANTIMICROBIAL PERFORMANCE OF LAUNDERING

As mentioned, the reduction of the bioburden on textiles by laundering is based on a combination of removal and inactivation of microbial cells on the fabric. In order to consider this interplay, tests measuring the antimicrobial performance of laundering use contaminated textiles because alternative methods, such as suspension tests, cannot correctly simulate the washing process because the mechanical component of automatic laundering is not taken into account in these procedures.[46]

Laundry disinfection processes using a combination of heat and (antimicrobial) detergents are referred to as chemo-thermal disinfection processes and have, therefore, to be distinguished from purely chemical or purely thermal disinfection approaches. Methods for testing chemo-thermal laundry disinfection are described in the American Society for Testing and Materials (ASTM) standards E2274 and E2406 and the European standard EN 16616. Whereas the ASTM methods use lab-scale devices simulating a vertical- or horizontal-axis machine, the European method is performed in a standard washing machine.

The standards basically assess the antimicrobial efficacy of the process according to the standard by contaminating cotton fabric with suspensions of test microorganisms. The microorganism carriers are then laundered together with ballast textiles and additional organic load, and the remaining microbial count on the carriers and the bacterial count in the wash liquor are determined after the laundering process. The comparison of the microbial load on the textile before and after the disinfection step is used to evaluate the reduction of the microbial load by the process. In addition, the occurrence of cross-contamination is detected on sterilized pieces of cotton test fabrics washed together with the load. The ASTM standards use *Klebsiella pneumoniae*, *S aureus*, and *P aeruginosa* as regular test strains, but other microorganisms may be included as well. For the European standard EN 16616, the intended claim determines the test strains as listed in Table 46.2.

Apart from these standards aiming to evaluate the antimicrobial efficacy of the whole laundering process, there are others that focus on the machine part. These include the International Electrotechnial Commission/Publicly Available Specification IEC/PAS 62958 and National Sanitation Foundation (NSF) Protocol 172 that strive to determine the antimicrobial effect without relying on the chemistry. An

overview of all mentioned standards is shown in Table 46.2. Besides other aspects, they also differ in the selection of test strains and the specified passing criteria. Whereas IEC/PAS 62958 is merely a descriptive test procedure that does not specify criteria for passing, ASTM E2274 and ASTM E2406 distinguish between disinfecting and sanitizing processes.

In addition to the regular application of the described standard procedures, naturally contaminated laundry items have been used to investigate the antimicrobial effectiveness of laundering.[7,10,47] Although these samples

TABLE 46.2 Specifications of standards on testing the antimicrobial efficacy of laundry processes and products

Standard	Field of Application	Test Strains	Passing Criteria
ASTM E 2274	Laundry sanitizers and disinfectants (detergents/additives) for use in traditional top-loading automatic clothes washing operations	*Klebsiella pneumoniae* ATCC 4352, *Staphylococcus aureus* ATCC 6538, *Pseudomonas aeruginosa* ATCC 15442, and other microorganisms as applicable	Not defined
ASTM E 2406	Laundry sanitizers and disinfectants (detergents/additives) for use in front-loading high efficiency automatic clothes washing operations	*K pneumoniae* ATCC 4352, *S aureus* ATCC 6538, *P aeruginosa* ATCC 15442, and other microorganisms as applicable	Not defined
DIN EN 16616	Hospitals, community medical facilities, and dental areas; schools, kindergartens, and nursing homes; other areas requiring hygienic treatment of textiles (eg, food processing facilities, hotels and restaurants, work clothing from special areas, textiles from facilities potentially capable of transmitting infectious diseases)	*P aeruginosa* ATCC 15442, *Escherichia coli* (K12) ATCC 10538, *S aureus* ATCC 6538, *Enterococcus hirae* ATCC 10541 (*Enterococcus faecium* ATCC 6057), *Candida albicans* ATCC 10231 *Aspergillus brasiliensis* ATCC 16404, *Mycobacterium avium* ATCC 15769, *Mycobacterium terrae* ATCC 15755	Bactericidal activity: *LR* ≥7 for *each* carrier with bacteria Yeasticidal activity: mean *LR* ≥6 for carrier with *C albicans* Fungicidal activity (additional): mean *LR* ≥6 for carrier with *A brasiliensis* Tuberculoidal activity (additional): mean *LR* ≥7 for carrier with *M terrae* Mycobactericidal activity (additional): *LR* ≥7 for carrier with *M avium* no cross-contamination, no test organisms in 100 mL washing liquor
IEC/PAS 62958	Clothes washing machines for household use, washing machines for communal use in blocks of flats and in launderettes	*Pseudomonas putida* (ATCC 1172), *S aureus* ATCC 6538, *C albicans* ATCC 10231 or *Pseudomonas fluorescens* ATCC 17397, *Staphylococcus arlettae* ATCC 43957 *Saccharomyces cerevisiae* ATCC 9763	No requirements specified, only descriptive
NSF Protocol 172	Sanitization performance of residential and commercial family-sized clothes washers	*K pneumoniae* ATCC 4352, *S aureus* ATCC 6538, *P aeruginosa* ATCC 15442	Average reduction of triplicate test runs for each test organism must meet 3 log reduction (reduction by 99.9 %).

Abbreviations: ASTM, American Society for Testing and Materials; ATCC, american type culture collection; DIN, deutsches institut für normung; IEC/PAS, international electrotechnial commission/publicly available specifications; LR, log reduction; NSF, national sanitation foundation.

are closer to realistic conditions than artificially contaminated textiles, the use of naturally contaminated textiles has some limitations because the highest detectable reduction of the microbial load depends on the initial contamination. Thus, the upper detection limit with naturally contaminated textiles is often too low to allow for an accurate differentiation of washing processes.

REQUIREMENTS FOR LAUNDRY DISINFECTION IN THE INDUSTRIAL AND INSTITUTIONAL AREA

Preventing the transmission of pathogens is one key element of an effective infection prevention program. Because textiles might serve as vectors for the transmission of pathogens, the processing of potentially contaminated laundry is crucial, resulting in the fact that many national authorities (such as the US Center for Disease Control and Prevention or the German Robert Koch Institut) publish recommendations on the handling of laundry in hospitals or other institutions. Depending on the field of application, clean laundry must either be sterile (in areas with particular high requirements [eg, surgical units]) or of low microbial contamination (in other medical areas). In addition, regular monitoring of the antimicrobial effectiveness of laundering processes is recommended. Additional controls might be necessary in the case of exceedance of guideline limits. These controls include samples of dry and wet laundry items and determining the microbial load on process-related surfaces, hands, air, and water. When handling possibly contaminated laundry in a professional environment, also the provisions of occupational safety and health must be followed in order to prevent possible infections of the employees.[48]

LAUNDRY HYGIENE IN THE DOMESTIC ENVIRONMENT

Unlike in institutional and industrial applications, the required level of hygiene in domestic laundering is mostly not defined and may depend on various factors. On the one hand, the type of laundry item and therefore the expected contamination must be regarded; on the other hand, the specific risk situation of the individual household members must be considered. In everyday life, sterilization of laundry items might not be necessary. Two current trends, however, have to be taken into account in the context of domestic laundry hygiene: First, the number of people with increased hygiene needs will probably increase in future due to the demographic development. Second, there is an ongoing trend to avoid high temperatures during washing, which might result in a change of the microbiological status of the laundry items and the washing machine.[49] Because epidemiologic studies linking the

consumers' washing behavior to the incidence of infections are missing, it is not possible to assess the impact of laundry hygiene on the household members' health based on evidence. Moreover, establishing minimum hygiene performance standards for domestic laundry is a problem because there is a lack of knowledge on the bioburdens of pathogens or resistant strains to be expected on textiles used in the domestic environment. Furthermore, a level of residual contamination after laundering that is considered to be safe has not been defined yet.

Even though it might not be necessary to define requirements for domestic laundry hygiene, it is important to generate a scientific base for assessing the antimicrobial efficacy of domestic laundering products. Additionally, sustainability issues should be taken into account, when setting general recommendations for domestic laundering. These include the environmental impact of high wash temperatures, the use of laundry detergents and additives, water-saving measures, and sewage reduction.

REFERENCES

1. Bockmühl DP. Wäschehygiene bei niedrigen Temperaturen—Erkenntnisse und Herausforderungen. *SOFW J.* 2011;137:2-6.
2. Nix ID, Frontzek A, Bockmühl DP. Characterization of microbial communities in household washing machines. *Tenside Surfactants Deterg.* 2015;52(6):432-440.
3. Callewaert C, Nevel S, Kerckhof F-M, Granitsiotis M, Boon N. Bacterial exchange in household washing machines. *Front Microbiol.* 2015;6:1-11.
4. Babič MN, Zalar P, Ženko B, Schroers HJ, Džeroski S, Gunde-Cimerman N. *Candida* and *Fusarium* species known as opportunistic human pathogens from customer-accessible parts of residential washing machines. *Fungal Biol.* 2015;119(2-3):95-113.
5. Gattlen J, Amberg C, Zinn M, Mauclaire L. Biofilms isolated from washing machines from three continents and their tolerance to a standard detergent. *Biofouling.* 2010;26(8):873-882.
6. Scott E, Bloomfield SF, Barlow CG. An investigation of microbial contamination in the home. *J Hyg (Lond).* 1982;89:279-293.
7. Blaser MJ, Smith PF, Cody HJ, Wang WL, LaForce FM. Killing of fabric-associated bacteria in hospital laundry by low-temperature washing. *J Infect Dis.* 1984;149(1):48-57.
8. Smith JA, Neil KR, Davidson CG, Davidson RW. Effect of water temperature on bacterial killing in laundry. *Infect Control.* 1987;8(5):204-209.
9. Robinton ED, Mood EW. A study of bacterial contaminants of cloth and paper towels. *Am J Public Health Nations Health.* 1968;58(8):1452-1459.
10. Lucassen R, Blümke H, Born L, et al. The washing machine as a source of microbial contamination of domestic laundry—a case study. *Househ Pers Care Today.* 2014;9(5):54-57.
11. Kruschwitz A, Karle A, Schmitz A, Stamminger R. Consumer laundry practices in Germany. *Int J Consum Stud.* 2014;38:265-277.
12. Laitala K, Klepp IG, Boks C. Changing laundry habits in Norway. *Int J Consum Stud.* 2012;36:228-237.
13. Abeliotis K, Candan C, Amberg C, et al. Impact of water hardness on consumers' perception of laundry washing result in five European countries. *Int J Consum Stud.* 2015;39:60-66.
14. Arild A-H, Brusdal R, Tore J, Gunnarsen H, Terpstra PMJ, van Kessel IAC. *An Investigation of Domestic Laundry in Europe—Habits, Hygiene and Technical Performance.* Oslo, Norway: Statens Institutt for Forbruksforskning; 2003.

15. Kubota H, Mitani A, Niwano Y, et al. *Moraxella* species are primarily responsible for generating malodor in laundry. *Appl Environ Microbiol.* 2012;78(9):3317-3324.

16. Munk S, Johansen C, Stahnke LH, Adler-Nissen J. Microbial survival and odor in laundry. *J Surfactants Deterg.* 2001;4(4):385-394.

17. Rehberg L, Frontzek A, Melhus Å, Bockmühl DP. Prevalence of β-lactamase genes in domestic washing machines and dishwashers and the impact of laundering processes on antibiotic resistant bacteria. *J Appl Microbiol.* 2017;123(6):1396-1406.

18. Takeuchi K, Hasegawa Y, Ishida H, Kashiwagi M. Identification of novel malodor compounds in laundry. *Flavour Fragr J.* 2012;27: 89-94.

19. Sinner H. *Über das Waschen mit Haushaltswaschmaschinen.* 2nd ed. Hamburg, Germany: Haus und Heim Verlag; 1960.

20. Brands B, Brinkmann A, Bloomfield S, Bockmühl DP. Microbicidal action of heat, detergents and active oxygen bleach as components of laundry hygiene. *Tenside Surfactants Deterg.* 2016;53(5): 495-501.

21. Honisch M, Brands B, Weide M, Speckmann H, Stamminger R. Antimicrobial efficacy of laundry detergents with regard to time and temperature in domestic washing machines. *Tenside Surfactants Deterg.* 2016;53(6):547-552.

22. Honisch M. Antimicrobial efficacy of laundering processes: a systematic study on the impact of wash temperature, wash cycle time, and detergents. In: Stamminger R, ed. *Schriftenreihe der Haushaltstechnik Bonn 2/17.* Aachen, Germany: Shaker Verlag; 2017:1-83.

23. Fredell DL. Biological properties and applications of cationic surfactants. In: Cross J, Singer EJ, eds. *Cationic Surfactants.* New York, NY: Marcel Dekker; 1994:31-60.

24. Lambert RJW. Comparative analysis of antibiotic and antimicrobial biocide susceptibility data in clinical isolates of methicillin-sensitive *Staphylococcus aureus,* methicillin-resistant *Staphylococcus aureus* and *Pseudomonas aeruginosa* between 1989 and 2000. *J Appl Microbiol.* 2004;97:699-711.

25. Mc Cay PH, Ocampo-Sosa AA, Fleming GTA. Effect of subinhibitory concentrations of benzalkonium chloride on the competitiveness of *Pseudomonas aeruginosa* grown in continuous culture. *Microbiology.* 2010;156:30-38.

26. Honisch M, Stamminger R, Bockmühl DP. Impact of wash cycle time, temperature and detergent formulation on the hygiene effectiveness of domestic laundering. *J Appl Microbiol.* 2014;117(6):1787-1797.

27. Bloomfield SF, Exner M, Signorelli C, Scott EA. *Effectiveness of Laundering Processes Used in Domestic (Home) Settings.* Somerset, United Kingdom: International Scientific Forum on Home Hygiene; 2013.

28. Ossowski B, Duchmann U. Der Einfluß des haushalts- üblichen Waschprozesses auf mykotisch kontaminierte Textilien. *Hautarzt.* 1997;48:397-401.

29. Wiksell JC, Pickett MS, Hartman PA. Survival of microorganisms in laundered polyester-cotton sheeting. *Appl Microbiol.* 1973;25(3): 431-435.

30. Walter WG, Schillinger JE. Bacterial survival in laundered fabrics. *Appl Microbiol.* 1975;29(3):368-373.

31. Lichtenberg W, Girmond F, Niedner R, Schulze I. Hygieneaspekte beim niedrigtemperaturwaschen. *SÖFW J.* 2006;132:28-34.

32. Fijan S, Koren S, Cencic A, Sostar-Turk S. Antimicrobial disinfection effect of a laundering procedure for hospital textiles against various indicator bacteria and fungi using different substrates for simulating human excrements. *Diagn Microbiol Infect Dis.* 2007;57:251-257.

33. Bellante S, Engel A, Hatice T, et al. Hygienische aufbereitung von textilien in privathaushalten—eine studie aus der praxis. *Hyg und Medizin.* 2011;36:300-305.

34. Hammer TR, Mucha H, Hoefer D. Infection risk by dermatophytes during storage and after domestic laundry and their temperature-dependent inactivation. *Mycopathologia.* 2011;171(1):43-49.

35. Linke S, Gemein S, Koch S, Gebel J, Exner M. Orientating investigation of the inactivation of *Staphylococcus aureus* in the laundry process. *Hyg und Medizin.* 2011;36:8-12.

36. Lucassen R, Merettig N, Bockmühl DP. Antimicrobial efficacy of hygiene rinsers under consumer-related conditions. *Tenside Surfactants Deterg.* 2013;50(4):259-262.

37. Stiftung Warentest. 60 Grad? Schön wärs! *Test.* 2013;(6):64-67.

38. Janczak F, Stamminger R, Nickel D, Speckmann D. Energy savings by low temperature washing. *SÖFW J.* 2010;136(4):75-80.

39. Brands B, Honisch M, Wegner S, Bockmühl DP. The effect of drying processes on the microbial load of laundry. *Househ Pers Care Today.* 2016;11(1):24-27.

40. Nagoh Y, Tobe S, Watanabe T, Mukaiyama T. Analysis of odorants produced from indoor drying laundries and effects of enzyme for preventing malodor generation. *Tenside Surfactants Deterg.* 2005;42:7-12.

41. Eckert A, Booten Y, Jarchow M, Lucassen R, Nemitz L, Bockmühl DP. Reduction of microorganisms by ironing. *Househ Pers Care Today.* 2014;9(4):34-35.

42. Bloomfield SF, Exner M, Signorelli C, Nath KJ, Scott EA. *The Infection Risks Associated with Clothing and Household Linens in Home and Everyday Life Settings, and the Role of Laundry.* Somerset, United Kingdom: International Scientific Forum on Home Hygiene; 2011.

43. Neely AN, Maley MP. Survival of enterococci and staphylococci on hospital fabrics and plastics. *J Clin Microbiol.* 2000;38(2):724-726.

44. Neely AN. A survey of gram-negative bacteria survival on hospital fabrics and plastics. *J Burn Care Rehabil.* 2000;21(6):523-527.

45. Traoré O, Springthorpe VS, Sattar SA. A quantitative study of the survival of two species of *Candida* on porous and non-porous environmental surfaces and hands. *J Appl Microbiol.* 2002;92(3):549-555.

46. Block C, ten Bosch C, Hartog B, Lemaire P. Determination of the microbicidal effect of laundry detergents. *Tenside Surfactants Deterg.* 2001;38:140-146.

47. Lakdawala N, Pham J, Shah M, Holton J. Effectiveness of low-temperature domestic laundry on the decontamination of health-care workers' uniforms. *Infect Control Hosp Epidemiol.* 2011;32(11): 1103-1108.

48. Robert Koch Institut. Richtlinie für die Erkennung, Verhütung und Bekämpfung von Krankenhausinfektionen" Bundesgesundheitsblatt, 22 Jg 1979, Nr 10. In: *Richtlinie für Krankenhaushygiene und Infektionsprävention.* München, Germany: Elsevier, Urban & Fischer; 2003:181-183.

49. Corsten H, Roth S, eds. *Bericht Nachhaltigkeit in der Wasch-, Pflege- und Reinigungsmittelbranche in Deutschland 2011–2012.* Wiesbaden, Germany: Gabler Verlag; 2013.

Processing of Reusable Medical Devices

Emily Mitzel

A medical device can include an instrument, apparatus, implement, machine, appliance, implant, reagent for in vitro use, software, material or other similar or related article, intended by the manufacturer to be used, alone or in combination, for medical purpose(s). These can include the diagnosis, prevention, monitoring, treatment or alleviation of disease, compensation for an injury, the investigation, replacement, modification, or support of the anatomy or of a physiological process, for supporting or sustaining life, in the control of conception, for the disinfection or sterilization of medical devices, and providing information by means of examination of specimens derived from the human body.[1] Legally, products that may be medical devices in some jurisdictions but not in others can include disinfection substances, aids for persons with disabilities, devices incorporating animal and/or human tissue, and devices for in vitro fertilization or assisted reproduction technologies. A reusable medical device is a device that has been designated by the device manufacturer as suitable for processing and reuse. As they are used, they can become contaminated, and processing must ensure that the devices are rendered safe for the next patient use. Effective processing can include cleaning, disinfection, inspection and maintenance, and sterilization between patient use and is important to prevent adverse patient effects, particularly health care acquired infections (HAIs). In addition to medical devices, a variety of other surfaces can be contaminated in clinical practice, and these are also be subjected to routine processing to reduce the risks of pathogen transmission. Health care facility environments are known to be sources of pathogens such as methicillin-resistant *Staphylococcus aureus* (MRSA), *Clostridium difficile*, vancomycin-resistant enterococci, and other pathogenic organisms.[2] These organisms have been isolated from surfaces frequently contacted by health care personnel or patient intact skin but regardless can lead to cross-contamination and infection.

The purpose of this chapter is to describe the risk classification of medical and surgical devices, determine the proper steps for processing, supporting validations to be performed to confirm the effectiveness of those steps, and current standards and guidance documents that apply. The types of processing that is appropriate for different device types is considered as well as what a manufacturer needs to do to ensure those processing steps are appropriate.

▶ PROCESSING OF MEDICAL DEVICES

The definition of processing is the steps performed between patient use and the activities to prepare a new or used device for its intended use. A "processor" may be an organization and/or individual with the responsibility for carrying out actions necessary to prepare a new or reusable device for its intended use. Processing devices can range from just cleaning for some noncritical devices or surfaces to a full cycle of cleaning, disinfecting, and terminal sterilization for semicritical and critical devices. These processes are explained in detail later in this chapter. Figure 47.1 shows the typical processing cycle of devices as can occur in a health care facility or center.

The important steps of processing medical devices in a health care facility, depending on their risk criticality, can include

1. Precleaning to prevent soil from drying on devices, making it easier to clean and to ensure safe transport, reducing risk to staff or others that may be at risk of contacting the devices

2. Transport to a central processing area in which devices should be kept moist in a container by adding a towel moistened with water. Appropriate foam-, spray-, or gel-based products may also be used.

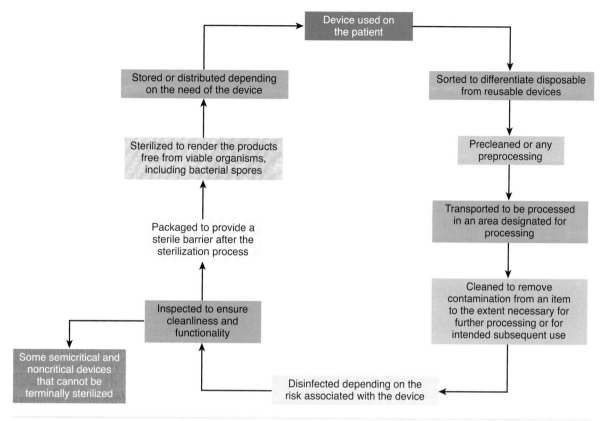

FIGURE 47.1 The typical processing cycle for reusable medical devices. The full cycle is typical for critical (eg, surgical) devices, with acceptable steps indicated for semicritical and noncritical devices.

3. Disassembly, sorting, and cleaning pretreatment that can include rinsing, soaking, and brushing
4. Thorough cleaning by manual or automated methods. This includes thorough rinsing and drying.
5. Disinfection
6. Terminal disinfection or sterilization according to the Spaulding classification (see in the following text) or other specific, local regulatory requirements
   a. Low-, intermediate-, or high-level disinfection using physical (eg, heat) or chemical processes
   b. Sterilization by processes using steam or gases such as vaporized hydrogen peroxide
7. Appropriate packaging of devices for terminal disinfection or sterilization, if applicable
8. Appropriate storage until subsequent use

Cleaning is of particular concern, and there are many factors that affect the efficacy of the cleaning processes. These include the following[3]:

1. Amount and type of soil (contamination on a device following its use) present on the device can affect the effectiveness of cleaning chemicals and sterilants used because they may become diluted or ineffective in the presence of soils.

2. Water quality and temperature as cleaning chemicals are designed to be optimally effective at specific temperatures and water hardness (concentration of calcium and magnesium ions in water) can alter the effectiveness of cleaning.
3. Availability and use of cleaning chemicals, for example, if specific cleaning chemicals recommended to be used are not available, can alternatives be used?
4. It is essential that the staff performing the processing are trained and competent in the use of all equipment, chemicals, and accessories to adequately clean each device (eg, lumens and other hard to access areas, disassembly, and reassembly of items).
5. Rinsing of the devices ensures that no harmful residuals (from soil or the cleaning process) remain on the device that can interfere with subsequent processing or patient use.

One important aspect of processing medical devices is to have a quality management system at the facility responsible for processing. This includes the requirements for

- Documentation and document maintenance for the appropriate time period
- Infection prevention and control

- Education and training
- Risk management
- Personal protective equipment (PPE) requirements specific for each process performed
- Automated washer or washer-disinfector, disinfectant, and sterilizer monitoring (eg, biological and chemical indicator controls) and preventative maintenance procedures
- Key parameter monitoring (eg, temperature, exposure time, concentration) to ensure that the processed device has met the validated process parameters
- Traceability to ensure the ability to track back to a patient from the devices and appropriate processing steps conducted in the event of a device recall or investigation of an adverse patient event

▶ MEDICAL DEVICE PROCESSING GOALS AND RISKS

The main goal of processing medical devices is to ensure devices are safe and effective for the next patient use. The definition of "safe" in this application is not only for the device to be clean and free of harmful microorganisms but also to ensure that there are no toxic substances present or damage that could cause it to malfunction. The goals and risks associated with processing that are important to address include

1. Providing a clean and disinfected or sterile (if appropriate) device for the next patient use to reduce the risk of infection.
2. Ensuring no toxic substances remain on the devices after the processing steps, which may include detergent residuals, disinfectant residuals, water-contaminant residuals (eg, due to poor water chemical quality), or chemical interactions with device materials.
3. Ensuring there is no physical damage of the device due to use, chemical interactions, incorrect cleaning, disinfection or sterilization parameters, or incorrect water quality.
4. Environmental considerations, including reducing wastes, optimal utility utilization, and "green" chemical use

▶ HUMAN FACTORS ISSUES

The incidence of hospital-acquired infections (HAIs) is a concern throughout the world. They have heightened regulatory attention on reusable devices, with impacts on manufacturers and health care users of these devices. Reusable devices must be designed to be cleaned, disinfected, and sterilized, when appropriate, between patient use. Manufacturers are expected to design devices and perform associated validations to ensure that the devices

can be processed at health care facilities and publish clear procedures in their instructions for use (IFU) that are easy for health care personnel to follow. Health care personnel should also carefully follow the manufacturer's instructions. Correct processing of medical devices plays an important role in the prevention of HAIs. Many cases of inappropriate cleaning, disinfection, or sterilization of medical devices have been identified as causes of HAIs or other adverse patient reports. Other concerns such as epidemics and increasing prevalence of antimicrobial resistance has intensified resources and improved practices to strengthen infection prevention strategies in health care facilities.

Human factor safety margins should be built into design and instructions to better manage device safety in the health care setting. Considerations include the complexity of device design, accuracy of validated processing instructions, and the practical use of instructions in health care facilities. Common human factor consideration practices can include[4]

- Processing instructions that are clear, legible, and written in a step-by-step manner (chronological) from the initial processing step through to the terminal processing step and storage requirements
- Instructions written in simple and clear language
- The use of charts, pictures, or diagrams that provide visual aids for processing steps
- Specific instructions for known risk areas due to the design of the device, for example, difficult to clean locations
- Visual inspection procedures following the cleaning processes

The ability to clean a medical device should be considered early in the initial device design and engineering planning. Features that effectively facilitate processing (eg, the design of flushing ports for internal device areas or the ease of device disassembly) should be incorporated when designing a reusable medical device. This has a significant impact on the ability of health care personnel to effectively clean the device, which correlates directly to patient safety. Human factors in medical device processing can be as minor as a simple variation in a cleaning step. For example, health care facility personnel may scrub laterally instead of the recommended circular motion to ensure proper cleaning. Manufacturers may also need to be aware that some health care facilities have elected to develop facility-specific cleaning processes instead of following device manufacturer's validated cleaning instructions that may be unpractical or less efficient.

Health care facility processing personnel must be properly trained to follow manufacturer's written cleaning instructions but then also assessed to show competency in following those instructions. If instructions and department requirements are not followed, the subsequent patient that comes into contact with that device is at risk for developing a HAI or other complication. A notable example of this has been highlighted by outbreaks of HAIs following the use of contaminated flexible endoscopes.[5-9] In a recent safety communication, the US Food and Drug Administration (FDA) noted that "although the complex designs of duodenoscopes improves the efficiency and effectiveness of endoscopic retrograde cholangiopancreatography (ERCP), it causes challenges for cleaning and high-level disinfection. Some parts of the scope may be extremely difficult to access and effective cleaning of all areas of the duodenoscope may not be possible." In addition, a recent FDA engineering assessment and a growing body of literature have identified design issues in duodenoscopes that complicate processing of these devices. For example, one step of the manual cleaning instructions in the device labeling is to brush the elevator area at the patient insertion end of these devices; however, the moving parts of the elevator mechanism contain microscopic crevices that may not be easily reached with a brush. Residual body fluids and organic debris may remain in these crevices after cleaning and disinfection. If these fluids contain microbial contamination, subsequent patients may be at risk of serious infection development.[10]

The ability of health care personnel to be able to practically follow the IFU should be considered. A US FDA guidance recommends in-use testing to verify that medical devices can be adequately cleaned after patient contact in a health care facility.[4,11] First, the contaminants present on the device during patient procedures should be identified and understood. Next, the devices determined to have the greatest cleaning challenges should be subjected to a worst-case contamination challenge. Complex invasive devices that have a clear potential for serious harm resulting from use errors should be particularly considered for human factors. Identification of such risk design can be based on investigation of medical device adverse reports and recall information, such as those in the United States.[12] Human factor data may need to be considered in developing and submitting instructions for processing for regulatory approval, unless the submission does not involve any changes to users, user tasks, user interface, or use environments from those of predicates. These devices can include but may not be limited to[4]

- ablation generators (associated with ablation systems)
- anesthesia machines
- artificial pancreas systems
- autoinjectors
- automated external defibrillators
- duodenoscopes with elevator channels
- gastroenterology-urology endoscopic ultrasound systems with elevator channels
- hemodialysis and peritoneal dialysis systems
- implanted infusion pumps
- Infusion pumps
- insulin delivery systems
- negative-pressure wound therapy intended for use in the home
- robotic catheter manipulation systems
- robotic surgery devices
- ventilators
- ventricular assisted devices

Classroom training for health care personnel can be important to educate personnel on how to appropriately clean, inspect, and further process devices during in-use testing. During this exercise, the manufacturer solicits feedback from the trainees about the ease of use of the processing instructions. This training can aid the manufacturer in understanding how their processing instructions are being interpreted in a health care facility setting. Depending on the feedback, the manufacturers may adjust the processing instructions if any issues with usability are identified.

Overall, human factor analysis related to health care processing of medical devices is a valuable component during product development of medical devices. In-use testing can be a powerful method to ensure health care personnel can appropriately follow and perform all of the processing steps. This is an integral part of ensuring the device can be processed properly between patient use. Manufacturers are recommended to use similar methods, terminology, and document layout to aid health care personnel in the comprehension and adherence to the instructions. The processing instructions for a device should be validated to ensure health care personnel will be able to understand and follow the processes. This can include observing and documenting participants while performing the cleaning and subsequent processing steps as well as asking if the instructions are feasible or at all difficult. This information should be documented, and changes to the instructions should be made if appropriate.

▶ SPAULDING CLASSIFICATION

Dr E. H. Spaulding originally categorized reusable medical devices into four groups: critical, semicritical, noncritical, and nonpatient contacting surfaces.[13] These categories have been essentially accepted worldwide, are endorsed by many regulatory agencies including in the United States by the Centers for Disease Control and Prevention (CDC) and FDA and are commonly used today. These classifications are used to specify what level of disinfection or sterilization is appropriate for the device, depending on the risk to the patient; however, it is important to note that thorough cleaning of the device is typically required prior to any terminal disinfection and sterilization processes.

Critical devices have a substantial risk of transmitting infection if the item is contaminated with microorganisms at the time of use. These are devices that are introduced directly into the body, either into or in contact with the bloodstream or other sterile areas of the body. Examples include needles, scalpels, transfer forceps, cardiac catheters, implants, and the inner surface components of extracorporeal blood-flow devices such as of the heart-lung oxygenator and the blood side of artificial kidneys (hemodialyzers). These items must be, at a minimum, cleaned and then sterilized between patients.

Devices classified as semicritical come in contact with mucous membranes (that can be naturally contaminated with microorganisms) but do not ordinarily penetrate body surfaces. Examples of these devices are many types of flexible fiber-optic endoscopes, endotracheal and aspirator tubes, bronchoscopes, laryngoscopes, respiratory therapy equipment, vaginal specula, and some urinary catheters. These devices are recommended to be cleaned and preferably sterilized, although high-level disinfection is acceptable at a minimum. If sterilization is not an option, treatment with a broad-spectrum chemical disinfectant that labeled with a tuberculocidal claim (a high-level disinfectant) may be used.

Noncritical devices usually come into direct contact with the patient but, in most instances, only with intact skin. Such items include facemasks, blood pressure cuffs, and most neurologic or cardiac diagnostic electrodes. Use of these devices carry a relatively lower risk of transmitting infection directly to patients but can be a source of microbial transmission. These devices are processed by cleaning and may require low- to intermediate-level disinfection.

The category that carries the least risk of disease transmission is nonpatient contacting surfaces. These surfaces potentially contribute to secondary cross-contamination such as by the hands of health care personnel that will subsequently come into contact with patients. Examples of these devices are medical equipment surfaces, such as frequently touched adjustment knobs or handles on hemodialysis machines, instrument carts, or dental units. These devices are often recommended to be processed by cleaning and may also benefit from periodic low- to intermediate-level disinfection. A wide range of disinfectants may therefore be used.

◗ MICROORGANISM RESISTANCE

Microorganisms vary widely in their resistance to physical and chemical disinfection and sterilization methods (see chapter 3). The types of microorganisms that are present on medical items or surgical materials following patient use can have a significant effect on the desired effectiveness of disinfection or sterilization. The most resistant types of microorganisms are generally regarded to be bacterial spores, some of which are significantly more resistant to both chemical and physical stresses than a wide variety of other microorganisms.[14-16] In a broad descending order of relative resistance, considerably below that of bacterial endospores are considered mycobacteria species (eg, *Mycobacterium tuberculosis*). Following that, in descending order of resistance, are small nonlipid viruses, the vegetative and spore forms of fungi, vegetative bacteria, and medium-sized or lipid-containing viruses (Figure 47.2). This hierarchy is useful in determining the appropriate level of disinfection or sterilization process that needs to

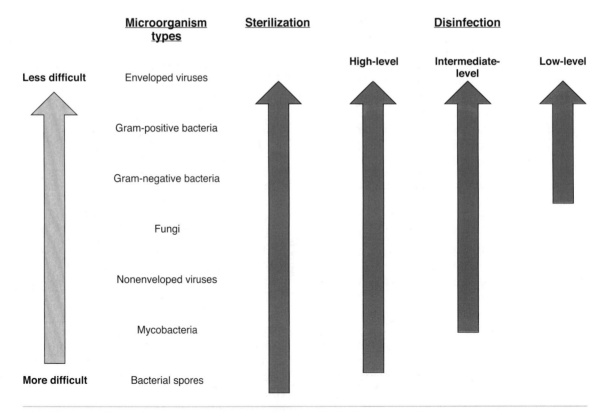

FIGURE 47.2 General resistance of microorganisms to disinfection and sterilization.

TABLE 47.1	Level of disinfection or sterilization appropriate to kill microorganisms
Microorganisms	**Level of Disinfection or Sterilization**
Prions (eg, causative agent in Creutzfeldt-Jakob disease)	Prion processing[a]
Bacterial spores (eg, *Bacillus subtilis, Clostridium difficile*)	Sterilization
Mycobacteria (eg, *Mycobacterium tuberculosis*)	High-level disinfection
Nonlipid or small viruses (eg, poliovirus, rhinovirus) Fungi (eg, *Cryptococcus neoformans, Candida albicans*)	Intermediate-level disinfection
Vegetative bacteria (eg, *Pseudomonas aeruginosa, Escherichia coli, Staphylococcus aureus*) Lipid or medium-sized viruses (eg, herpes simplex, hepatitis B)	Low-level disinfection

[a]Unique processing recommendations (see chapter 68).

occur after the cleaning process and before the next patient use.[17,18] This hierarchy is also important in determining the correct level of terminal disinfection or sterilization recommended to be appropriate (Table 47.1).

Examples of notable pathogens that produce bacterial spores include *Bacillus cereus, Clostridium botulinum*, and *C difficile. M tuberculosis* and nontuberculous mycobacteria are frequently associated with heath case–associated transmission, including cases due to inappropriately cleaned, disinfected, and sterilized device. Examples of fungal pathogens include *Candida albicans* and *Aspergillus fumigatus*. Important pathogenic gram-negative bacteria include *Pseudomonas aeruginosa, Klebsiella pneumoniae*, and *Salmonella* species. *P aeruginosa* is known for its preference for moist environments and its propensity to form biofilms that are difficult to remove or inactivate (see chapter 67). *Salmonella* species are found to be common microorganisms associated with gastrointestinal (GI) endoscopy procedures. Outbreaks with these bacteria are often related to inappropriate use of disinfectants that did not meet the criteria of high-level disinfection. Examples of gram-positive bacteria include *S aureus* and *Streptococcus pyogenes*. Finally, enveloped viruses including key blood-borne pathogens such as HIV and hepatitis B viruses (HBVs).

▶ CLINICAL CONTAMINANTS ON MEDICAL DEVICES

Even though critical and semicritical devices are often considered to present the greatest challenge to cleaning, disinfection, and sterilization with the amount of contaminants

following clinical use and associated patient risks following processing, noncritical devices and surfaces also need to be cleaned and disinfected properly. Clinical contaminants found on medical devices directly relate to the surgical procedure in which they are used or the environment the device or surface is located. Noncritical devices and surfaces can be contaminated with a variety of soils including patient materials and microorganisms, including notable pathogens often associated with outbreaks such as *C difficile*, noroviruses, MSRA, etc. A recent review on the role of the patient environment in the transmission of microorganisms, in particular multidrug-resistant organisms, highlighted that the role of the environment in the acquisition of HAIs are underestimated.[19] New techniques and technologies may be used to reduce these risks such as improving manual chemical disinfection, the use of automated environmental disinfection methods (eg, ultraviolet [UV] and hydrogen peroxide gas), environmental monitoring, molecular detection methods, and self-disinfecting surfaces.[19]

The clinical contaminants that can be present on devices following patient use include organic and inorganic materials. Organic materials include blood, mucus, urine, tissue, carbohydrates, fats, protein, and microorganisms (such as bacteria, virus, and fungi). Inorganic materials can include salts, metals, calcium deposits, and iodine or chlorhexidine (eg, from antiseptics use during surgery). Studies on the biochemical nature of contaminants following surgical use of devices found that the levels of visible contamination can range considerably, as did the quantitative levels of contaminants, including detectable microorganisms.[20] This is important to note that many of these contaminants may inhibit the activity of subsequent disinfection or sterilization processes and, if present following processing, may also lead to toxic reactions in patients or device damage. High levels of total organic carbon (TOC), protein, and hemoglobin were observed on many device types indicating how important processing is between patient use.[19] Overall, the levels of microorganisms on surgically used devices were actually low (<600 detectable colony-forming units [CFUs]).[20] Another study showed that surgical devices used in sterile body cavity procedures have relatively low bioburden levels, averaging about 10^2 per device when compared with devices used in nonsterile body areas (eg, GI endoscopes), which are in the range of 10^5 to 10^9.[21] These results would suggest that the microbial challenge may actually be greater on many of the semicritical devices in comparison to critical devices. In a study that tested 50 surgical instruments obtained from 25 surgical procedures, 30% of the devices resulted in no growth, 14% resulted in 11 to 100 CFUs, and 14% resulted in greater than 100 CFUs.[22] Two devices had higher levels of bacterial growth and both were contaminating with coagulase-negative *Staphylococcus*, a normal part of the skin flora.

Any contaminating soil (such as blood, mucus, or feces) remaining on a device after the cleaning process may contribute to the failure of a disinfection or sterilization process. The clinical soil may prevent penetration to microorganisms and may inactivate disinfectant chemicals such as chlorine, iodine, oxidizing agents, and quaternary ammonium compounds. This effect can be a greater concern when lower concentrations of biocides are used and with low-level disinfectants compared to higher concentrations or more potent, high-level disinfectants. In addition, this factor underscores the necessity and importance of thoroughly cleaning a medical device prior to chemical disinfection or sterilization. An example of this was reported in an outbreak of septicemia caused by a *Serratia* species from a flexible fiber-optic endoscope.[23] This device had been sterilized in an ethylene oxide (EO) gas process but had not been cleaned properly before the sterilization cycle. This testing and other research has shown that even a rigorous cycle capable of killing all microorganisms, including bacterial spores, may not kill even relatively sensitive vegetative bacterial cells if they are protected by extraneous organic material. This observation may also be intimately associated with the number of microorganisms present. Effective cleaning procedures that remove organic soil simultaneously tend to lower the general level of microbial contamination associated with the soil by physical removal alone and increase the effectiveness of the subsequent antimicrobial process.

Because the presence of microbial pathogens are assumed to be present as biohazards on contaminated devices, specialized protective equipment for the eyes, face, head, and extremities (eg, masks, gloves, goggles, face shields, and gowns) are appropriate, particularly during the handling and cleaning of devices prior to an antimicrobial process. Protective clothing, respiratory devices, and protective shields and barriers have been designed to protect the wearer from injury. The PPE is used by health care personnel and others whenever necessary to protect from such hazards and reduce the risks of injury or impairment in the function of any part of the body through absorption, inhalation, or physical contact.

▶ CLEANING METHODS

Cleaning is the first and most important step of processing. The formal definition in regard to processing medical devices is the removal of contaminants to the extent necessary for further processing or for intended use.[1] Cleaning consists of the removal, usually with a detergent-based formulation and water, of clinical soil (eg, blood, protein substances, and other debris) from the surfaces, crevices, serrations, joints, and lumens of a medical device by a manual and/or automated process that prepares the devices for safe handling and/or further processing. The goals of these processes are to remove microbiological and chemical (organic and inorganic materials) contaminants. These processes include the use of various cleaning (detergent-based) chemistries with

water combined with various brushing, flushing, soaking, and rinsing steps. Cleaning can be performed manually, by wiping and immersion in a sink or basin, or by using automated systems such as ultrasonic cleaning systems and automated washers or washer-disinfectors.

For many devices, precleaning moistens and loosens gross clinical soil and makes the subsequent cleaning steps more efficient. This should be performed as soon as possible after devices have been used and most often includes just the use of water. Other chemicals that may be available in surgical or clinical practice (eg, antiseptics and saline solutions) should be avoided due to the potential for device damage and other complications. Close attention to rinsing devices at this stage can reduce the gross clinical soil load in the subsequent cleaning steps. Manual cleaning in many countries is the most widely used method performed to thoroughly clean devices using a variety of methods such as immersion, wiping, brushing, and flushing. If a device is able to go through an automated process, this method is preferred and is often conducted in addition to manual cleaning steps when appropriate. This allows minimal handling of contaminated devices and allows for larger processing capacity. The automated process, such as in washer-disinfectors, combines cleaning with disinfection (and often drying) to allow devices to be safely used or handled for packaging depending on the terminal antimicrobial process applicable. The steps for a manual cleaning may typically include

1. Prerinsing to remove soil
2. Washing with a detergent-based formulation diluted according to manufacturer's recommendations and at the appropriate water temperature
3. Soaking, brushing, and flushing (as applicable for the device type)
4. Rinsing to remove any remnants of soil and cleaning chemistries
5. Manual disinfection and/or drying as appropriate

The steps for a manual cleaning with the use of ultrasonics can include

1. Prerinsing to remove soil
2. Washing with a detergent-based solution diluted according to manufacturer's recommendations and used at the appropriate water temperature
3. Soaking, brushing, and flushing (as applicable for the device type)
4. Cleaning in an ultrasonic washer at a given power frequency (eg, >38 kHz) and time, which will typically be conducted in a detergent-based solution
5. Rinsing to remove any remnants of soil and cleaning chemistries
6. Manual disinfection and/or drying as appropriate

Note that during these cleaning processes, it is important to consider parameters for efficient cleaning, including time, temperature, type(s) of cleaning agent(s), and water quality specifications. The steps for an automated cleaning may include

1. Prerinsing to remove soil
2. Detailed manual washing of certain device features (if appropriate) with a detergent-based solution diluted according to manufacturer's recommendations and at the appropriate water temperature. This may include soaking, brushing, moving, and flushing of device features.
3. Rinsing to remove any remnants of soil and cleaning chemistries
4. Processing in a mechanical washer-disinfector compliant with International Organization for Standardization (ISO) 15883-1 with a defined, validated cycle.[24] The automated cycle may include the following cleaning cycle parameters
   - prewash phase
   - cleaning agent(s) and wash phase(s)
   - rinse and final rinse phases

These parameters also include requirements to meet time, temperature, type(s) of cleaning agent(s), and water quality specifications.

5. Automated washer-disinfectors may also include validated disinfection and drying phases of cycles, such as thermal or chemical disinfection, purging, and hot air drying.

The final results from the cleaning process must result in a visually clean device, a device that meets the appropriate low amounts of organic soil and microbial load, is not cytotoxic, and must be fully functioning for the next patient use or further processing (eg, packaging and sterilization).

Detergents

The determination of the appropriate type of detergent(s) used in the cleaning processes is an important part of the cleaning process. Considerations include appropriate labeling with the detergent product (eg, safe for use on medical devices), material compatibility, tolerance of water quality being used during cleaning, types of processing methods that can be used, temperature and contact times, and even in some cases environmental safety requirements. Currently, there are no specific regulatory requirements to determine the effectiveness or specifications for such detergent formulations. But the characteristics of an ideal cleaning agent can include nonabrasiveness, low foaming, free rinsing, biodegradable, able to rapidly dissolve/disperse various types of soil (lipids, proteins, etc), nontoxic, effective in the presence of varying water quality, have an acceptable shelf life, and be cost effective.[24]

Cleaning chemistries are typically classified by the type of active chemistry present such as acidic, alkaline, and enzymatic (although these can often be combined). Acidic cleaners are commonly more effective at removing mineral (inorganic) deposits and, when appropriately used, can also allow for oxidation to protect certain types of material surfaces, such as stainless steel. Certain types of formulated enzymatic and acidic cleaners are also better for removing certain types of starches, carbonates, and insoluble hydroxides from surfaces. Alkaline cleaners are very effective at breaking down and removing various organic materials such as patient soil components (eg, blood, proteins, hemoglobin). Alkaline cleaners can remove oils, fats, greases, proteins, and an array of other soils. For medical device cleaning, the most widely used cleaning chemistry formulations are enzymatic (which can be alkaline or acidic in formulation), neutral detergent cleaners, and mild to strong alkaline cleaners, or combinations of these. In some cases, combinations of an alkaline cleaner followed by an acidic (or neutralizing) cleaner are used in different phases of a cleaning cycle. Enzymatic detergents often have the benefit of being in the neutral pH range (pH 6-8), with enzymes added to enable soil component breakdown, and classically demonstrate the greatest compatibility on surfaces, depending on the detergent formulation. The different types of enzymes that may be added in these products can include

- Proteases that break down many proteins contained in blood and saliva
- Amylases that target starches and certain carbohydrates
- Lipases that break down certain types of fats and lipids
- Cellulases, which are active against certain types of fibers and may even be useful against certain types of biofilms

Overall, the effectiveness of enzymatic-based detergents depends on the enzymes included, as well as the other components in the formulation (eg, buffers, surfactants), and the correct use in accordance with manufacturer's instructions. Acidic and alkaline-based products, in general, can be equally effective cleaning chemistries, when used correctly but may also be more aggressive on device surfaces over repeated use. Overall, the cleaning abilities and device compatibility profiles can vary considerably based on the individual product formulations.

Lubricants

The benefits of lubrication include easing stiffness, prolonging instrument life, and reducing the risk of rust, tarnish, and corrosion damage. The typical recommendation is to add lubrication to the appropriate device after the cleaning and drying steps (eg, prior to sterilization or clinical use). Lubricants should be used in accordance with their manufacturer's instructions and only on devices requiring lubrication.

Equipment Used in Cleaning

A variety of accessories can be used for manual cleaning. Example of these accessories are brushes of many shapes and sizes that are specified by the size and length or by a part number. Brushes are an integral part of cleaning various types of device crevices, surfaces, and lumens. It is particularly important to use the appropriate-sized brush for cleaning device lumens to ensure cleaning and reduce the risk of damage to the inside of the lumen. ISO 17664 states that the requirements for brushes and all of the accessories required need to be included in the cleaning steps in the IFU.[1] A variety of other cleaning accessories include cloths and sponges as well as specific aids to safely remove certain types of stubborn soils (such as cements and cauterized blood) if present. It is important to note that most manufacturers recommend against the use of accessories such as scouring pads due to potential damage to device surfaces over time.

Ultrasonic cleaning equipment provides a sonication process to aid in the cleaning process while the device is immersed in a low-foaming detergent solution. Sonication is a process using ultrasonic waves, which cause the disruption and removal of soil from surfaces by the effect of cavitation. Cavitation is a process where microbubbles are produced in the presence of sonication and implode on contact with surfaces to dislodge soil from the device surfaces. Because ultrasonic cleaning is especially effective in removing soil and other debris from hard-to-reach areas, it is usually a necessary step for complex devices.[25]

Automated washers and washer-disinfectors are designed to clean and disinfect (when applicable) a large range of devices. These are computerized processes that are programmed for cleaning, disinfection, and most often drying. There are many different types, sizes, and processes available. ISO 15883-1 describes the central design and performance criteria for such equipment, including cleaning, disinfection, and drying requirements.[24]

▶ DISINFECTION METHODS

The next steps after cleaning are appropriate disinfection and/or sterilization. Disinfection may be an intermediary step between cleaning and sterilization to render devices safe for handling during inspection and packaging or it may be the terminal step of processing, depending on the classification and intended use of the device. Disinfection is the process to reduce the number of viable microorganisms to a level specified as being appropriate for a defined purpose. High-level disinfection is a process that is expected to kill all microorganisms but not necessarily large numbers of bacterial spores (see Figure 47.2) and is often recommended during the processing of critical device (prior to packaging and sterilization) or the terminal processing of semicritical devices. Intermediate-level disinfection is a process that is expected to kill most viruses, fungi, vegetative bacteria, and some mycobacteria but not typically fungal or bacterial spores. Low-level disinfection is a process that should inactivate most vegetative bacteria, some viruses, and some fungi but not mycobacteria or fungal and bacterial spores.[26,27] These terms are widely used in certain parts of the world, such as in the United States, but may not be widely used or defined in other areas (see chapter 2).

There are many methods of disinfection depending on the device type, but these can be generally divided into two major types, high-temperature or low-temperature (chemical) disinfection. These methods include manual disinfection by means of soaking, spraying, or wiping with a chemical disinfectant, automated chemical disinfection within a washer-disinfector, or automated thermal disinfection that takes place under controlled temperature conditions in a pasteurizer or washer-disinfector or by immersing the devices into hot water at a specified temperature for a specific amount of time.

In the United States high-level disinfection is the minimum treatment recommended by CDC in guidelines for the processing of semicritical devices.[28,29] The most widely used high-level disinfection process is the use of hot water typically at >70°C. Common chemical high-level disinfectants include a number of glutaraldehyde-, chlorine dioxide-, hydrogen peroxide-, and peracetic acid-based formulations; these are commercially available disinfectants but often require regulatory approval in different countries such as being cleared by FDA in the category of sterilants/disinfectants.

Intermediate-level disinfectants are not necessarily capable of killing bacterial spores, but they do inactivate *Mycobacterium* species, which are significantly more resistant to chemical disinfectants than other vegetative bacteria. These disinfectants are also expected to be effective against fungi including asexual spore forms but not necessarily dried chlamydospores or sexual spores as well as lipid and many nonlipid medium-sized and small viruses. The specific activity of these disinfectants can vary and may require specific antimicrobial test requirements to support label claims in different areas of the world (see chapter 61). Examples of intermediate-level disinfectants can include alcohol-based formulations (eg, containing 70%-90% ethanol or isopropanol), chlorine compounds (free chlorine, ie, hypochlorous acids derived from sodium or calcium hypochlorite, or chlorine dioxide, 500 mg/L, and certain chloramines), and some phenolic or iodophor preparations, depending on the formulation and label claims. The effects of intermediate-level disinfectants can often vary in efficacy against specific microorganisms, for example, alcohol efficacy against nonenveloped viruses (see chapter 19).

Low-level disinfectants cannot be relied on to destroy, within a practical period, bacterial spores, mycobacteria, most fungi, or all small or nonlipid viruses. But these disinfectants may rapidly kill vegetative forms of other types of bacteria and most fungi as well as medium-sized or lipid-containing viruses. Examples of low-level disinfectants are products based on quaternary ammonium compounds, iodophors, or phenolics. They, like other disinfectants, can be marketed in a variety of ways such as concentrates (requiring dilution in water before use), ready-to-use products (not requiring dilution), two-part components (that are activated prior to use), and as saturated wipes. Many of these products, such as those based on quaternary ammonium compounds, may be used for both cleaning and disinfection due to the surfactant activity in aiding the physical removal of microorganisms from surfaces. The antimicrobial activity of these products can be variable, depending on the concentration and/or formulation of the active ingredients. Some iodophor- and phenolic-based disinfectant formulations may be labeled for use for intermediate-level or low-level disinfection depending on the concentrations of the products being used. All disinfection chemicals do not have this capacity, such as the limited capacity of many quaternary ammonium compound–based formulation to meet the tuberculocidal or viricidal criteria of intermediate-level disinfectants.[30] Overall, care should be taken to review and understand the label claims associated with chemical disinfectants to ensure safe and effective use, rather than depending on a list of antimicrobials present.

Chemical disinfection occurs with many types of chemicals and chemical processes. The correct disinfectant to be used depends on the device material, device characteristics, and level of disinfection necessary. It is also important to ensure that the chemicals are labeled for use on medical devices, when applicable, and approved for use in accordance with local regulatory requirements (eg, in the United States, cleared by FDA or US Environmental Protection Agency [EPA] depending on their use and label requirements), and used in accordance with the label claims. In many applications, removal of disinfectant residuals may be required due to toxicity concerns postdisinfection and depending on the subsequent use of the device or equipment. It is also important in these cases that the disinfected surfaces are not recontaminated, such as in the case of using contaminated rinse water.[31-33] The following section provides a brief overview of some of the most widely used disinfectants for device disinfection.

Alcohols

Isopropanol, ethanol, and *n*-propanol are prevalent types of alcohols used for disinfection. Alcohols are not usually used for device disinfection with the exception of noncritical devices or to facilitate drying following high-level disinfection but are often used for surface disinfection of consoles or other areas in health care facilities. Use of alcohols can meet the acceptance criteria for intermediate- and high-level disinfection claims, depending on the associated label claims. Alcohols can be expected to rapidly kill vegetative microorganisms, including *Mycobacterium* species but have little to no activity against certain types of nonenveloped viruses and bacterial spores (see chapter 19).

Aldehydes

Aldehydes include glutaraldehyde and ortho-phthalaldehyde (OPA) formulations that are used frequently for high-level disinfection (see chapter 23). Formaldehyde, in gas form, is also used in certain countries as an area fumigant and as a device sterilization method (see chapter 36). Glutaraldehyde is a saturated dialdehyde that is widely accepted as an overall effective high-level disinfectant and chemical sterilant in formulation. It has a broad antimicrobial range and is generally effective against vegetative bacteria, most *Mycobacterium* species, fungi, and viruses. It is also effective against bacterial spores but generally at longer exposure times depending on the formulation and temperature of application. The OPA formulations are also used for high-level disinfection (HLD) of heat-sensitive semicritical devices and can be used manually and in an automated endoscope reprocessor (AER), depending on the product labeling. These formulations are especially active against mycobacteria, including many glutaraldehyde-tolerant strains of *Mycobacterium* species.

Peroxygens

Hydrogen peroxide, peracetic acid, chlorine dioxide, and ozone are widely used peroxygens for disinfection. Most peroxygens in formulation can provide a high-level disinfection claim with some activity against bacterial spores, but their antimicrobial activity will depend on the formulation and in-use conditions (eg, temperature).[34] Hydrogen peroxide is widely used in both liquid and gas forms for disinfection and sterilization as a broad-spectrum antimicrobial (see chapters 18 and 32). Peracetic acid also demonstrates broad-spectrum activity in both liquid and gas forms. Liquid peracetic acid formulations have been widely used in health care facilities as a biocidal oxidizing agent, are effective biocides even at low temperatures, and can be effective (depending on the formulation/use) in the presence of organic matter (see chapter 18).

Quaternary Ammonium Compounds

Quaternary ammonium compounds (also referred to as "quats") have important advantages as they are commonly used for both cleaning and disinfection due to surfactant abilities (see chapter 21). The microbial activity depends on the chemicals used and typically as a mixture of two or three biocides in formulation with other excipients (see chapter 6). Commonly low-level disinfection claims are associated with such products; however, an intermediate-level disinfection may be claimed depending on the formulation and demonstrated efficacy.

Halogens

The chlorine-containing groups of detergents and disinfectants fall into the category of halogens. Chlorine or chlorine-releasing agents are some of the most widely used chemicals for disinfection. This includes sodium hypochlorite (NaOCl), which is the source of active chlorine in typical household bleach solutions. Chlorine can inactivate all microorganisms, depending on its formulation and concentration (see chapter 15); however, higher concentrations or contact times are required to inactivate spore-forming organisms and other dormant forms. The other widely used halogen is iodine but has had limited applications in device processing (see chapter 16).

Thermal Disinfection

Thermal disinfection, also referred to as pasteurization, is an effective and efficient disinfection method. Temperatures above 70°C in a time/temperature-related process are typically used for medical device processing, and most microorganisms are inactivated under these temperatures except heat-resistant bacterial spores. Time/temperature correlations are of key importance for disinfection efficacy (see chapter 11). As the temperature goes up, the time necessary to facilitate an effective disinfection process goes down similar to the concepts used for steam sterilization (see chapter 28). For example, 90°C for 1 minute or 80°C for 10 minutes are well-accepted high-level disinfection processes.

▶ STERILIZATION—HIGH AND LOW TEMPERATURE

Sterilization is the terminal process that most semicritical and all critical medical devices should go through prior to next patient use. Sterilization provides the highest level of expected microbial inactivation and is a validated process used to render products free from viable microorganisms. In a sterilization process, the nature of microbial inactivation is an expected, exponential function. The survival of a microorganism on a device is expressed in terms of probability. Although this probability of survival can be reduced to a very low number, it can never be statistically reduced to zero (see chapter 5). With device processing, sterilization is typically defined as a process after which the probability of a microorganism surviving on an item is reduced to a low level (typically 10^{-6}). This is referred to as the sterility assurance level (SAL) and this overkill

approach is widely used by medical device manufacturers in the validation of sterilization of reusable medical devices. The heath care facility uses the subsequent validated instructions from the medical device company to sterilize the cleaned devices prior to patient use. But the facility is also responsible to ensure that the equipment used to sterilize reusable devices is appropriate, validated, and maintained appropriately according to the sterilizer manufactured instructions.

The two methods most commonly used to validate and confirm that medical devices are properly sterilized by predefined processes are parametric release and/or by demonstrating direct microbial reduction. Parametric release is the declaration that the product has been sterilized, based on records demonstrating that the process parameters were delivered as expected within specified tolerances. It allows the product to be released based on verified process records (eg, time, temperature, pressure) instead of the approach of waiting for the incubation of exposed biological indicators during the process that were traditionally used in the past.[35] The other validation approach is achieved by using biological indicators containing the most resistant organism to the sterilization process (see chapter 65). This may be performed by directly confirming the kill of $\geq 1.0 \times 10^6$ bacterial spores in a half-cycle or equivalent, thereby confirming that a 12 $\log_{10}$ reduction can be achieved in a full cycle as an overkill cycle validation. This half-cycle approach is typically confirmed during validation studies by performing a minimum of three half-cycles with the test devices, using established sterilization cycle parameters used at health care facilities.

Steam Sterilization

The most widely used method of sterilization in health care facilities is high-temperature steam under pressure (see chapter 28). Steam sterilization is effective against all types of microorganisms, is economical, is easy to monitor, and is a very well-understood process. Prion inactivation can also be achieved at higher temperatures and times depending on the prior cleaning process (see chapter 68). Devices that cannot withstand high temperatures, pressures, or moisture are not able to be sterilized with this method. One of the benefits of steam sterilization is the lack of toxic residuals or the need for residual analysis to ensure no residuals are left onto the device after sterilization; however, this will be dependent on the purity of water being used to generate the steam.[33] Chemical and microbial (eg, endotoxin) residues from the water can be transferred in the steam and remain on device surfaces following the sterilization process.

Commonly used health care facility steam sterilization cycles have three phases: conditioning (eg, by a prevacuum or gravity displacement process), sterilization for

TABLE 47.2 Examples of steam sterilization exposure and drying times used in health care processing[a]

Item	132°C (270°F)	135°C (275°F)	Drying Times
Wrapped instruments	4 min		20-30 min
		3 min	16 min
Textile packs	4 min		5-10 min
		3 min	3 min
Wrapped utensils	4 min		20 min
		3 min	16 min
Unwrapped nonporous items (eg, instruments)	3 min	3 min	NA
Unwrapped nonporous and porous items in a mixed load	4 min	3 min	NA

Abbreviation: NA, not applicable.
[a]Data from Association for the Advancement of Medical Instrumentation.[31]

a defined time/temperature, and drying. Examples of typical sterilization and drying parameters are given in Table 47.2.

Ethylene Oxide Gas and Hydrogen Peroxide Gas Sterilization

Two of the most commonly used types of low-temperature sterilization methods for the processing of reusable devices are processes based on Ethylene Oxide (EO) or vaporized hydrogen peroxide (VHP) gases. Others can include processes based on liquid peracetic acid, gas peracetic acid, ozone, ozone–hydrogen peroxide gas combinations, and formaldehyde gas. These processes are considered in more detail in other chapters.

An EO is an essentially colorless gas that dissolves easily in water, alcohol, and most organic solvents. It is used mainly for industrial sterilization but in some cases is used in health care facilities for sterilization of processed devices between patient use. The EO sterilization processes occur in sterilizer designs typically under vacuum and at temperatures between 30°C and 65°C (86°F and 149°F), EO concentrations ranging from 400 to 1200 mg/L, and with a humidity level at 40% to 80% (see chapter 31). Following the sterilization process, devices often require extended aeration, depending on the device design and materials of construction, to ensure the safe removal of toxic process residuals.

Hydrogen peroxide gas (or "vapor") processes are continually becoming more popular for the sterilization of reprocessed medical devices (see chapter 32). These sterilization processes occur at temperatures between 30°C and 55°C (86°F and 131°F) with a hydrogen peroxide gas concentration

of 2 to 10 mg/L that is produced during the cycle from liquid formulations of 35% to 55% hydrogen peroxide in water. This type of sterilization is good for both metal and nonmetal medical devices at low temperatures. Because defined cycles can typically operate within a dry environment and at low temperatures, it is especially suitable for devices sensitive to heat and moisture. In some processes, the cycle can include the use of plasma generation for various purposes such as degradation of peroxide residuals following gas exposure (eg, the STERRAD® series of sterilizers). These systems have the advantage of safely and rapidly sterilizing medical devices and materials without leaving any significant toxic residues. Hydrogen peroxide is an oxidizing agent that affects sterilization by oxidation of key cellular components (see chapters 18 and 32). Cycle times can vary, depending on the manufacturers' instructions, from 28 minutes to a few hours.

Gas sterilization methods are normally validated under half-cycle process conditions using biological indicators to confirm an effective process in the presence of device loads. Validation to confirm that toxic levels of sterilization residuals are not left on devices after the sterilization processes is often necessary. ISO 10993-7 specifies the allowable limits for residual EO and ethylene chlorohydrin residuals as an example.[32]

▶ WATER QUALITY FOR DEVICE PROCESSING

The quality (or chemical purity) of water used for processing is an important consideration in all stages of medical device processing for many reasons. Unfavorable water quality can have an adverse effect on both the processing procedure and on the appearance of the devices and material(s). Some effects of water quality during device processing are[33]

1. Device malfunction and other effects due to the retention of minerals. Calcium and magnesium salts may cause scaling, lime deposits, or corrosion. Iron, manganese, and copper may cause brownish red deposits or secondary rust. Silicates and silicic acid may cause white-grey colored appearance. Chlorides may cause pitting.
2. Toxic effects or pyrogenic reactions may occur, such as in the presence of excessive levels of copper or if residual levels of endotoxin from bacteria are present.
3. Infections may occur where inorganic salts or other organic deposits inactivate the disinfectant or sterilant and are therefore inefficient or if the final rinse water used following a terminal processing step (eg, after high-level disinfection) contains unacceptable levels of microorganisms.
4. Water contaminants could reduce the effectiveness of detergents used for cleaning leading to ineffective cleaning, disinfection, and sterilization.
5. Steam used for sterilization may compromise product safety due to contaminants in the water leading to product damage or toxicity.

A treatment system used to control the purity of water can often have three key elements: pretreatment processes, principal water treatment processes, and controls during the distribution process. The pretreatment consists of processes such as iron filtration, depth filtration, softening, and carbon filtration. The principal treatment processes generally consists of de-ionization (DI), reverse osmosis (RO), distillation, or a combination of these processes. The distribution system should be designed appropriately to be routinely disinfected by means of chemical treatment, UV light, ozone, heat, or a combination of these processes.

The requirement for water quality used during device processing can be defined locally or regionally. The ANSI AAMI TIR34:2014 describes two categories of water quality in terms of the characteristics that are important for medical device processing and the level of treatment that may be needed as found in Table 47.3.[33] Utility water is water that comes from the tap (or potable water) and may require further treatment to achieve the desired specifications. These treatments may include the removal of excessive levels of water hardness or chlorine that may lead to negative effects.[33] This quality of water is mainly used for the processing steps of flushing, washing, and rinsing following washing. Critical water is water that is extensively treated usually by a multistep treatment process that can include a carbon bed, softening, DI, and RO or distillation to ensure that the microorganisms and the inorganic and organic materials are removed from the water. This water is recommended for final rinsing, thermal disinfection, and steam generation.

Other standards may also specify certain water quality requirements such as ISO 15883-1:2019, which recommends water quality required at each stage of the washer-disinfector process,[24] and EN 285,[36] which provides recommendations for steam purity and quality.

Routine sampling and testing of water must be performed to ensure the appropriate water quality is achieved and maintained over time. Tests for chemical purity include testing such as conductivity, pH, oxidizable substances, total hardness, and dissolved solids. Other testing that should be considered includes the level of bacterial endotoxins and total viable microorganisms.

▶ MAJOR CONSIDERATIONS IN PROCESSING VALIDATIONS

Validation is the confirmation through the provision of objective evidence that the requirements for a specific intended use or application have been fulfilled, including cleaning, disinfection, and sterilization. The first step in a device processing validation is to consider a risk-based scientific rationale that needs to be assessed during processing. These can include the criteria in Figure 47.3.

These design risks can include

1. risk of infection based on intended clinical use (eg, the Spaulding classification)
2. the physical and material design restrictions
3. any potential chemical interactions
4. use life
5. total system design
6. potential of misuse

TABLE 47.3	Recommended levels of water purity used for device processing[a]			
Contaminant	Units	Utility Water (Used for Flushing, Washing, or Rinsing)	Critical Water (Used for Final Rinsing or Steam Generation)	
Hardness	mg/L	<150	<1	
Conductivity (mg/L = ppm)	μS/cm	<500	<10	
pH		6-9	5-7	
Chlorides	mg/L	<250	<1	
Bacteria	CFUs/ mL	NA	<10	<10
Endotoxin	EU/mL	NA	<20	<10

Abbreviation: CFUs, colony-forming units; NA, not applicable.
[a]Data from Association for the Advancement of Medical Instrumentation.[33]

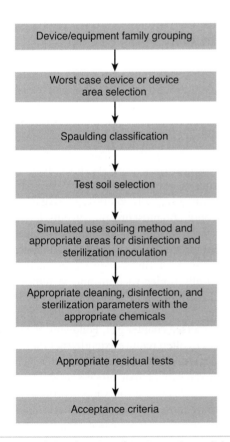

FIGURE 47.3 Considerations for processing validations.

Standards, such as ISO 17664,[1] ISO 17665-3,[37] ANSI/AAMI ST81,[38] and AAMI TIR12,[17] can be used to help establish family groupings and worst-case devices or areas of a device for processing validations. A family grouping is a collection of medical devices based on classification of risk, surgical procedure, design and manufacturing process, and physical attributes. In this respect, ISO 17664 states that "if a manufacturer supplies a number of different medical devices that share common attributes, then validation studies may be performed as a product family.[1] If this approach is taken, the medical device manufacturer shall demonstrate commonality between the different medical devices and the validation studies shall address the worst case attribute(s) of the product family." Similarly, ANSI/AAMI ST81:2004 states that "where the manufacturer supplies a number of different medical devices which share common features and attributes, the validation specified may be performed with respect to these medical devices as a group or family, provided that the manufacturer can demonstrate the commonality of the medical devices and that the tests and assessments address the 'worse case' feature or attribute of the group or family."[38]

There are three main ways to ascertain the family grouping for cleaning validations, as an example

1. Device use: Group families by similar use during the surgical procedures.
2. Material type: Materials can have greater or less affinity for residues and, therefore, should be grouped accordingly.
3. Size and challenge features: Group families of similar size and challenge features.

Examples of family groupings for sterilization validation can include evaluating weight, mass, complexity of devices, volume to vent ratio of trays or containers used to sterilize devices, and the ability of trays including all contained devices to allow proper air removal and penetration of steam or gas. Sterilization validation considerations for device sets and trays include proper air removal and steam flow throughout the tray contents and that holders should have limited contact with device, not block steam penetration, and allow devices to be in unlocked and open positions. Mass should be distributed throughout a tray of devices and devices should not be stacked on top of each other.

▶ CLEANING VALIDATION

According to ISO 17664: 2017,[1] the manufacturer shall validate each process that is identified in the information supplied with the medical device as being suitable. An automated cleaning method is preferred to be validated unless the device cannot go through an automated process. In this case a manual cleaning should be validated.

The automated cleaning validation may include some manual cleaning steps as part of the overall cleaning validation and associated IFU. If the IFU recommends both manual and automated processes, then both processes must be validated as specified. Objective evidence should be available that cleaning will be effective when the devices are processed as directed.

The cleaning methods specified should include all applicable accessories, cleaning chemicals and concentrations, water qualities, chemical residual risks, temperatures, exposure times, and all techniques including rinsing specific to the cleaning process and device type being processed. Prior to the commencement of the cleaning validations, consideration should be given to the impact of repeated clinical use on the device over time. The devices may need to be subjected to simulated use cycles to ensure that they are in a "used" state including the potential for soil accumulation or wear and tear over time. This can be performed by simulated clinical soiling, cleaning, then disinfection or sterilization processes, where appropriate or by using clinically used devices. The appropriate number of cycles is dependent on the device type, clinical use expectations, and associated labeling.

Selecting the test soil and soiling process requires identifying the clinical use of the device. This process should simulate the clinical procedure as close as possible. This will determine the test soil as well as how the specific device is soiled for the validation.[18,39,40] Some questions that arise in this process are

1. How is the device used during the surgical procedure? Does the device only get handled by surgical staff?
2. How long is the surgical procedure?
3. What is the expected time between the surgical procedure and the cleaning?

Examples of soiling of a simple surgical scissor are

1. Handling and actuating the device in a test soil (Figure 47.4)
2. Immersing the tip of the device into a test soil (Figure 47.5)

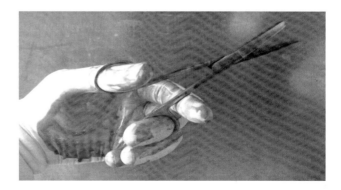

FIGURE 47.4 Picture of handling devices with gloves dipped into test soil. For a color version of this art, please consult the eBook.

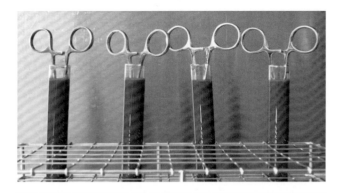

FIGURE 47.5   Picture of soiling of the tip of devices into the test soil. For a color version of this art, please consult the eBook.

Other options to contaminate devices may also be appropriate depending on the clinical use of the device. If the device is used for cauterization, causing blood burning on the device, then the test soil should be heated onto the device. All areas of surgical contamination should be soiled with the test soil during the validation process.

Detergent selection used for cleaning purposes should be conducted depending on what is compatible with the device, what is available where the device will be marketed, and what contaminants will be on the device during the surgical procedure (see Detergent section earlier). Determination of all cleaning supplies must ensure compatibility with the device design and the manufacturer should either supply these to the health care facility or supply the part number(s).

After all cleaning processes have taken place, the first acceptance criteria is to ensure a visibly clean device through direct inspection. This process can be device dependent. The minimum process is conducting the inspection with a naked eye under normal lighting conditions or some enhanced magnification such as 2x to 10x. If the device has a lumen, a borescope may also be used to view the internal areas of the device. If there is any visual soil on the device, the device should be cleaned again. The next process of the validation is the extraction of the device to quantitatively assess the amount of residual soil components such as protein, hemoglobin, and TOC. The extraction method that is used depends on the size and delicacy of the device as well as the residuals that will be tested. Sonication, manual shaking, swabbing, or brushing-flushing of device lumens are the most common methods of extraction. If a device has a lumen or any restricted access areas, those should be flushed during the extraction process. A swabbing method of extraction can be used if the device cannot be fully immersed. All extraction processes must be validated to ensure appropriateness of the method. An extraction efficiency from a positive control device should be performed to ensure it is an appropriate method. This will aid in the estimation of an extraction efficiency.

Common analytes that are recommended to be tested in device extractions include protein, hemoglobin, TOC,

and carbohydrate. Protein residual analysis is the most common and considered the most important residual to be analyzed because most surgical contamination contains proteinaceous substances.[18] If devices come into contact with blood, then hemoglobin may be appropriate for the contamination test soil and residual analysis. The TOC test is very sensitive for many organic materials such as proteins and lipids but is not specific; therefore, if levels of contaminations are detected on the device, their specific identification is unknown. Results must be quantitative.

Cytotoxicity or other specific residual assessments can be used to ensure that no harmful residues remain from the cleaning processes. This includes ensuring that rinsing techniques are sufficient to remove all detergent residuals from the cleaning processes. The presence of cytotoxic residues may be determined by minimal essential media (MEM) testing[18,32] or the ultraviolet/visible (UV/Vis) method to determine any detergent residuals present on the device after the cleaning processes. ISO 10993-5 and USP <87>[42] include recommended test methods and acceptance criteria for the MEM test.[41] The MEM test is a rapid, standardized test that is very sensitive and is an inexpensive way to determine if the materials contain significant quantities of harmful extractables and the effect on cellular components. Results must also be quantitative. The levels of acceptable residuals on a cleaned device is still a matter of some debate but are regionally defined and are becoming more standardized. Examples of guidance on appropriate residuals are summarized in Tables 47.4 and 47.5. Lower levels of protein, for example, are recommended in guidance from the United Kingdom stating 5 µg bovine serum albumin (BSA) equivalent per device side[43] and guidance from Germany stating 3 µg/cm².[44] An attempt to harmonize these criteria is ongoing, such as in the revision of ISO 15883-5 that includes proposed action and alert levels (see Table 47.5).[39]

The results of the MEM test is recommended to be a reactivity grade of ≤2.[32] There are currently no specific acceptance criteria when testing for detergent residual using a UV/Vis method. A proposed acceptance criteria is that the test device extracts be below the detection limit of the test.

TABLE 47.4   Recommended analyte levels in the United States[a]

Analyte	Recommended Level
Protein	≤6.4 µg/cm²
Hemoglobin	≤2.2 µg/cm²
Carbohydrate	≤1.8 µg/cm²
Endotoxin	≤2.2 EU/cm²

[a]Data from Association for the Advancement of Medical Instrumentation.[18]

TABLE 47.5 Recommended analyte levels from ISO 15883-5[a]

Analyte	Alert Level	Action Level
Protein	≤3 μg/cm^2	≤6.4 μg/cm^2
Hemoglobin	≤1.0 μg/cm^2	≤2.2 μg/cm^2
Carbohydrate	NA	≤1.8 μg/cm^2
Endotoxin	≤2.2 EU/cm^2	≤22 EU/cm^2
ATP	≤10 fmoles of ATP/cm^2	≤22 fmoles of ATP/cm^2
TOC	≤6 μg/cm^2	≤12 μg/cm^2

Abbreviations: ATP, adenosine triphosphate; NA, not applicable; TOC, total organic carbon.
[a]The figure taken from International Organization for Standardization.[39] Copyright remains with ISO.

DISINFECTION VALIDATION

A processing disinfection step must be validated if it is specified in the manufacturer's IFU.[1] Examples of disinfection steps include interim thermal disinfection as part of the automated washer-disinfector cycle to reduce contamination on critical devices prior to handling and packaging for sterilization, as the final step of processing devices that are unable to be sterilized (eg, high-level disinfection for semicritical devices), or for other devices/surfaces recommended to be disinfected in accordance to the Spaulding classification. A validated method of automated disinfection is recommended, unless the medical device cannot withstand this process. A validated method of manual disinfection should be specified if automated disinfection is not possible.[1] The level of disinfection that should be used depends in part on the category and nature of the device and the way it is to be used. The criticality of the device determines the level of disinfection necessary (see Figure 47.2 and Table 47.1).

Standards such as ISO 17664 and the ISO 15883 series give specific recommendations such that all accessories, contact times, temperatures, types and concentrations of disinfectants, water quality, chemical residues, and rinsing techniques should be considered (as applicable), as well as specifying correct disinfectant types (eg, chemical or thermal disinfection), any potential toxic residual, materials compatibility, and expected disinfection efficacy.[1,24,39,45]

The requirements for demonstrating disinfection efficacy can vary from region to region. In Europe, this can depend on specific regional requirements, such as in Germany where the recommended thermal disinfection for critical devices during processing is typically 90°C for 5 minutes (or equivalent). In the ISO 15883 series of standards,[24,39,45] thermal disinfection is determined parametrically based on a time-temperature relationship

known as the A_0 (see in the following text). A series of EN test methods define requirements to support chemical disinfectant claims.[26] In the United States, an FDA guidance document on medical washer-disinfectors[27] states acceptance criteria for the demonstration of disinfection, depending on the level:

- Low-level disinfection requires a 6 log$_{10}$ reduction in a mixed population of vegetative organisms including *Pseudomonas aeruginosa*, *Staphylococcus aureus*, *Escherichia coli*, and a representative of the *Klebsiella-Enterobacter* family.
- Intermediate-level disinfection requires a 6 log$_{10}$ reduction of the same mixed population of vegetative organisms to be demonstrated in conjunction with a 3 log$_{10}$ reduction of a thermophilic *Mycobacterium* species.
- High-level disinfection requires a 6 log$_{10}$ reduction of a thermophilic *Mycobacterium* species.

Chemical Disinfection Validation

A method including the inoculation of a known concentration of the specific microorganism(s) onto a surface and evaluating the level of reduction following the disinfection process is used to ensure that chemical disinfection processes are appropriate for the device type. This is necessary even though the disinfectant label claim itself might show appropriate log reduction kill of specified microbial populations in tests with the disinfectant itself (see chapter 61). Neutralization verification is required during disinfection testing to demonstrate that any residual chemical is neutralized and won't allow additional kill or inhibition of the test microorganisms following the indicated exposure time. Accurate microbial population determinations are required to verify the starting inoculation population as well as the appropriate log reduction of the applicable microorganisms over the defined exposure time.

Residuals of chemicals used for disinfection may result in toxic effects in patients due to inadequate rinsing of the devices following chemical disinfectant exposure. Cytotoxicity testing can be performed to ensure the disinfectant is removed from the device following the rinsing steps, if required for the safe use of the device (eg, with semicritical devices).

Thermal Disinfection Validation

Parametric testing is frequently used to ensure the thermal disinfection step, and this can be used for both manual disinfection or in the use of an automated washer-disinfector or disinfector. The main method for validation of thermal disinfection processes is the A_0 concept as outlined in ISO 15883-1.[24] The A_0 of a thermal disinfection process is the equivalent time in seconds at 80°C to produce a given disinfection effect, where the z-value is expected to be 10°C (see chapter 11). The A_0 value recommended to be achieved can depend on intended use of the device.[24] This is based on a time-temperature relationship and the fact that most microbial pathogens are inactivated at temperatures above 65°C to 70°C.[46]

$$A_0 = \Sigma\ 10[(T - 80) / z] \times \Delta t$$

Where:

A_0 is the A value when z is 10°C

t is the chosen time interval, in seconds

T is the temperature in the load, in degrees Celsius

The washer-disinfector standards recommend a minimum A_0 value of 60 for noncritical devices as a terminal disinfection step and an A_0 value of 600 for critical devices to render these devices safe for handling/packaging.[24] An A_0 value of 600 is recognized as the appropriate value for devices that are intended to contact intact mucous membranes or nonintact skin.[46] An A_0 value of 600 is achieved by 100 minutes at 70°C, 10 minutes at 80°C, 1 minute at 90°C, as examples. An A_0 value of 3000 was traditionally recommended in certain countries (such as Germany) as being appropriate to inactivate enveloped viruses such as HBV, hepatitis C virus (HCV), and HIV and should be applied when medical devices may be contaminated with these organisms of concern; this commonly equates to 90°C for 5 minutes.[24] But subsequent evidence would suggest that such virus types are rapidly inactivated at lower temperatures and contact times, which is the basis of the washer-disinfector standard recommendations.[24]

▶ STERILIZATION VALIDATION

Parametric release, particularly in the case of thermal (steam) sterilization, or the use of a microbiological challenge ("overkill") test methods are traditionally used to verify that a sterility assurance level (SAL) of 10^{-6} is achieved in a given sterilization process. This is a typical overkill approach because the specific bioburden associated with critical devices following clinical use, cleaning, and handling is generally unknown or is expected to be low.[20] For example, a half exposure cycle in an established sterilization process is often used to demonstrate $\geq 6\ \log_{10}$ reduction of a representative bacterial spore population to extrapolate to a desired SAL of 10^{-6}. The biological indicators (BIs) are used in these tests that have a known population and resistance.[48] For steam sterilization validations, in addition or as an alternative to BI testing, it is also typical to perform temperature profiling of the device in a typical load during the sterilization cycle as a reliable predictor of sterilization efficacy.

The BI overkill validations are widely used for low- and high-temperature sterilization cycle testing, particularly

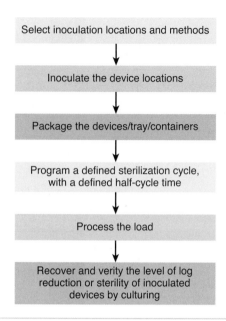

FIGURE 47.6 An example of a sterilization validation approach using 10^6 BIs at a half-cycle sterilization exposure cycle for reusable devices.

in the United States. An example of a validation approach using BIs is shown in Figure 47.6. The BIs that are used for validation must be appropriate for the sterilization modality being used and to be able to be placed in worst-case locations. The choice of test organisms is usually defined based on most resistant organism for the sterilization method should be used for testing.[47] *Geobacillus stearothermophilus* spores are considered the most resistant organism for testing of steam sterilization processes, as well as certain gas-based processes such as hydrogen peroxide–based processes.[49] Similarly, *Bacillus atrophaeus* spores are used as representative resistant organisms to EO.[50] The BI can consist of a variety of materials (or carriers) including the use of sutures, discs or coupons of many materials, diameters, and lengths. The BIs are placed in the most difficult-to-sterilize areas, which include lumens, mated surfaces, cannulas, and heat sink areas. Direct inoculation of the test device(s) with a spore preparation can be used as an alternative, particularly when the use of a BI may interfere with the penetration of the sterilization process to a device location. Important considerations in steam sterilization validations can include the BI spore population and its resistance to steam. During validation, BI population verification should be performed on the lot of BIs being used for testing, and the resistance ($D_{121.1°C}$ or D_{ref}) is referenced from the labeling provided by the BI manufacturer. The true biological challenge for each inoculation site to a steam process in a half-cycle validation should be greater than or equal to 6 F_{bio} (see chapter 11).[17,51] For example, *G stearothermophilus* spore preparations with a population less than 10^6, with a

$D_{121.1°C}$ value of greater than 1 minute can be used to verify a 6 $\log_{10}$ reduction under half-cycle test conditions, as

$$F_{bio} = \log_{10} (BI\ population) \times D_{121.1°C}\ value$$

Example 1:
Spore population $= 1 \times 10^6$
$D_{121.1°C}$ value $= 1.0$ minute
$F_{bio} = \log 10^6 \times 1.0 = 6 \times 1 = 6$

Example 2:
Spore population $= 1 \times 10^4$
$D_{121.1°C}$ value $= 1.5$ minutes
$F_{bio} = \log 10^4 \times 1.5 = 4 \times 1.5 = 6$

After devices are inoculated, they are packaged for sterilization. A variety of systems can be used to include single or multiple devices placed in holding trays, cassettes, and/or caddies and then placed into a flexible or rigid primary packaging system (or sterile barrier system; see chapter 41) for exposure to the sterilization process. Devices can also be placed individually into such packaging systems if desired. Sterile packaging is primarily used to maintain sterility poststerilization. The specific packaging requirements for devices needs to be determined and validated to show that devices in their final packaging configuration are capable of being sterilized under typical health care facility conditions and then recommendations are made in the IFU regarding these parameters. The ISO 11607 series specifies the requirements for materials, sterile barrier systems, and packaging as well as the test methods for validation requirements (see chapter 41). It is important that these materials not only allow for successful sterilization but also maintain sterility of terminally sterilized medical devices until the point of use.[52,53] The types of packaging can depend on the device or device trays or containment systems being used, but overall, they must be compatible with the devices being held and with label claims associated with packaging materials, including the attainment of sterilization. Sterilization pouches, sterilization wraps, and rigid containers come in many shapes, sizes, and materials.

During the validation, the test devices are packaged and placed in the worst-case location of the sterilizer. For steam sterilization this is often referred to as the "cold" spot and is typically over the drain area of the sterilizer. It is important not to place the test devices in a way that would inhibit the cycle process or in a manner contrary to the sterilizer manufacturer instructions. The devices are then processed through a typical half-cycle sterilization exposure. As part of the overkill validation approach, the BIs are recovered, placed into containers of media (or in the case of products, extracted into media to recover spores using a validated method), and then incubated at the required temperature and time (eg, for *G stearothermophilus* spores, at 55°C-60°C for 7 d or as appropriate for the labeling of the BI used). Following incubation,

the samples are then scored for the presence or absence of growth of the indicator organism. As an alternative, the population of the test organism on the BI can be quantified to determine the population reduction.

Steam sterilization considerations during validation can include the device design, weight of the device/load, limiting blind holes or dead-ended lumens, the use of cannulas to allow for sterilant penetration, and ensuring that the sterilant can contact the entire device for the minimum time and temperature requirement. The packaging tray design must allow for adequate sterilant penetration, allow for materials to heat up quickly (in the case of heat-based processes), and remain under the defined conditions for the desired sterilization cycle. A recommended limitation of the overall weight of the tray for steam sterilization is less than 25 lb (11 kg), to meet sterilizer manufacturers' requirements and to reduce handling injuries following sterilization.[31]

A further requirement for steam sterilization is the dry time. Drying is important to ensure the integrity of the microbial barrier properties of the packaging materials. The devices are packaged then exposed to the full sterilization cycle time, including the drying phase. Drying is typically validated by preparing and weighing the packaging before and after the test cycle and by direct inspection for the presence of any moisture on the packaging and internally within the tray and devices following the sterilization cycle. The weight gain of the packaging is then calculated by

$$[(postweight - preweight) / preweight] \times 100 = weight\ gain\ percentage$$

The packaging and devices must pass visual inspection with no moisture observed and the packaging weight gain is recommended not to exceed 3%.[17] Some considerations for minimizing the dry time during validation testing can include location of devices within the load, reducing the mass of the load, minimizing surfaces or positioning of devices that allow water to pool, and considering the ability of the packaging material to allow water to properly drain during the cycle. If needed, extended drying outside of a normal sterilization cycle may be necessary to ensure load or device drying, and this should be described in the processing IFU, if appropriate.

It is important to ensure that the temperature throughout the devices and chamber are appropriate especially for high-temperature sterilization processes. Temperature profiling is performed under full cycle parameters.[51,54] This process allows for the physical validation of cycle effectiveness and identifies sterilizer and/or load cold and hot zones.

Reuse Life of Processed Devices

It is important that the labeling of reusable medical devices defines the expected end of the reuse life for the medical device. Some reusable devices can be designed to only withstand a limited number of processing cycles (eg, 5, 10, or 20), and others can go through thousands of uses and processing cycles. Methods of accomplishing this include

1. A restricted number of processing cycles by determining how many times the device can be used
2. Inspection criteria by specifying what visual attributes of the device show that the device should not be used again
3. Combination of the two above

The IFU should also recommend how to evaluate deterioration of the device(s) during inspection because damage can occur during the clinical use, handling, and/or processing of the devices. These instructions may also include appropriate disposal instructions.[4]

Following sterilization, a defined shelf life of the device should be suggested. In general, sterile packaged devices are considered sterile until an event causes the sterile barrier to be compromised (eg, the packaging is damaged or opened for device use). This is referred to as event-related shelf life. Consideration of the validation of the packaging materials that define the recommended shelf life following sterilization based on the manufacturer's validation is important. Storage requirements may also include humidity, temperature, and airflow specification. If the packaging material is damaged during storage (eg, tearing, wetness) the device cannot be assumed to be sterile and should be processed again.

▶ ENDOSCOPE CHALLENGES

Endoscopic devices deserve further consideration in this chapter as important examples of device with complex designs that are prone to inadequate processing practices.[55] They can be classified as being critical or semicritical devices but also as being temperature resistant or temperature sensitive (Figure 47.7).

Based on their complex design and clinical use, these devices can pose a unique challenge to device processing.[56] Recent reports indicated that physically complex accessories to the endoscopic sets, such as suction valves or biopsy forceps, can also be extremely difficult to clean and process.[57] Inadequate cleaning has been consistently associated with the transmission of a variety of organisms such as *Mycobacterium* species[55] and *Salmonella ser Newport*.[58] Many reusable rigid endoscopes and endoscopic accessories are heat stable and can be steam sterilized, whereas others are not and require high-level disinfection or, preferably, low-temperature sterilization.

The FDA, for example, issued guidance regarding scope processing.[4,59] Documented reports of postendoscopic infection were reviewed and in virtually every case significant departures from contemporary endoscope processing guidelines were reported.[60] After investigating episodes of disease transmission, some have suggested the need for the redesign of certain types of endoscopic devices and associated equipment.[61] This view is also reflected in many processing guidelines, such as from the Association for Professionals in Infection Control and Epidemiology (APIC) on infection control in endoscopy[62] and other related professional guidelines and reviews.[63-73] These guidelines highlight the importance of the following:

- Greater attention to device design for processing, with clear, validated IFU
- Close attention to IFU requirements in health care facilities, particularly cleaning instruction
- The higher risks associated with many of these devices, particularly semicritical upper and lower GI endoscopy devices, due to the potential of high levels of microbial contamination and the levels of microorganisms that can be present even after rigorous cleaning, with a lower margin of error risk with terminal high-level disinfection
- Cross-contamination risks from inappropriate rinse water following chemical disinfection
- Device inspection and maintenance
- The importance of staff training and competency

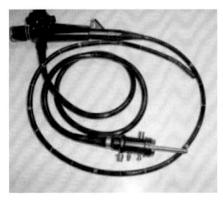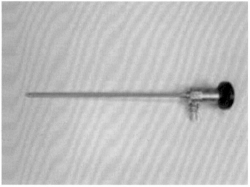

FIGURE 47.7   Examples of a heat-sensitive (flexible) endoscope (left) and a heat-resistant (rigid) endoscope (right).

Overall, endoscope manufacturers, regulatory bodies, and health care facilities are increasingly concerned about the spread of communicable diseases on processed medical devices. For these reasons, many of these guidelines have begun to recommend the routine microbial surveillance of high-level disinfected endoscopes as a periodic quality indication of device safety, in addition to existing quality requirements.[73] Many country-specific guidelines already recommend routine microbiological monitoring in addition to the other processing quality controls. Documents associated with endoscope surveillance include sampling the duodenoscopes.[56,74,75] Microbiological endoscope surveillance can be used as proficiency assessment for health care practices but may not be appropriate as a routine safety assessment for the processing of scopes (unless under outbreak situations for investigation purposes). This is important because health care personnel will need to assess the data, interpret results, and determine if the scope is safe for use or requires additional processing, additional testing, or be quarantined. Many countries have specific endoscope guidance, standards, and publications to reduce the risks of infection from endoscope use.[56,74] Some include the recommendation to perform routine monitoring of the scopes to ensure processing was performed correctly. An important aspect of this testing is the extraction method used to sample the scope. For example, the entire process needs to be optimally done in as aseptic environment with aseptic procedures to prevent cross-contamination. The next important part of the testing is the culturing method that is performed in a laboratory. There are many ways to culture extraction samples but the most typical way is to determine the number of bacterial colonies or "high-concern" microorganisms. The CDC has defined high-concern organisms as those more often associated with disease.[74] Examples include gram-negative bacteria (eg, *E coli*, *K pneumoniae* or other *Enterobacteriaceae*, as well as *P aeruginosa*), *S aureus*, and *Enterococcus*. Low-concern organisms are defined as organisms that are less often associated with disease and their presence could result from the simple cross-contamination of samples during collection or environmental contamination. Examples of low-concern organisms include species of gram-positive bacteria such as coagulase-negative staphylococci (excluding *Staphylococcus lugdunensis*) and diphtheroids that are routinely found on the skin as well as *Bacillus* species routinely found in the air and environment.[74]

▶ STANDARDS FOR PROCESSING REUSABLE MEDICAL DEVICES

When designing a reusable medical device, it is important to consider the standards organizations that write and publish applicable design and processing-associated standards (see chapter 70). These include

- ISO—an independent, nongovernmental international organization. Examples include the washer-disinfector series (ISO 15883 series), various sterilization standards (including the steam sterilization process ISO 17665), and the criteria for processing IFU (ISO 17664).
- Comité Européen De Normalisation (CEN), European Committee for Standardization—is an association that brings together the National Standardization Bodies of European countries. The CEN is officially recognized by the European Union and by the European Free Trade Association (EFTA) as being responsible for developing and defining voluntary standards at European level. Many standards associated with processing are published in combination with ISO, such as EN ISO 17664.
- Country-specific standard organizations—ISO and CEN are composed of representatives from various national standards organizations. The British Standards Institution (BSI), as an example, is the national standards body of the United Kingdom. Many standards associated with processing are published in combination with ISO and CEN, such as BS EN ISO 17664. Similarly, the Deutches Institut für Normung (DIN) is the equivalent German Institute for Standardization and Association Francaise de Normalisation (AFNOR) is the French national organization. Standardization Administration of China (SAC) is the standards organization authorized by the State Council of China to exercise administrative responsibilities by undertaking unified management, supervision, and overall coordination of standardization work in China. Standards Australia is a nongovernment standards development body in Australia. Standards Australia is recognized as Australia's representative on ISO and published standards such as AS/NZ 4187: 2014.

Even though there are many standards and guidance documents available on processing requirements for reusable medical devices (eg, see https://wfhss.com/members), it is important to ensure that labeling, including associated IFU and validations, meet the regulatory requirements of the areas the devices are sold and regulated. Examples of regulatory bodies that govern the processing of medical devices include

- European Parliament, Member States, and designated Notified Bodies under the Medical Device Regulation (EU) 2017/745
- The FDA Center for Devices and Radiological Health (CDRH) that regulates medical device manufacturers marketing in the United States
- EPA—regulates the registration of environmental surface disinfectants
- Therapeutic Good Administration (TGA)—regulates medical devices in Australia
- Health Canada—regulates medical devices in Canada

REFERENCES

1. International Organization for Standardization. *ISO 17664:2017: Processing of Health Care Products—Information to Be Provided by the Medical Device Manufacturer for the Processing of Medical Devices.* Geneva, Switzerland: International Organization for Standardization; 2017.

2. Walker J. *Decontamination in Hospital and Healthcare.* Cambridge, United Kingdom: Woodland; 2013.

3. World Health Organization. *Decontamination and Reprocessing of Medical Devices for Health-Care Facilities.* Geneva, Switzerland: World Health Organization; 2016.

4. US Food and Drug Administration. *Guidance for Industry and FDA Staff—Processing/Reprocessing Medical Devices in Health Care Settings: Validation Methods and Labeling.* Silver Spring, MD: US Food and Drug Administration; 2015.

5. Kovaleva J, Peters FTM, van der Mei HC, Degener JE. Transmission of infection by flexible gastrointestinal endoscopy and bronchoscopy. *Clin Microbiol Rev.* 2013;26:231-254.

6. NBC Universal. UCLA superbug outbreak: how endoscopes got dirty. NBC News Web site. https://www.nbcnews.com/health/health-news/ucla-superbug-outbreak-how-endoscopes-got-dirty-n309146. Published February 20, 2015.

7. NBC Universal. Two more hospitals report 'superbugs' on endoscopes. NBC News Web site. https://www.nbcnews.com/health/health-news/two-more-hospitals-report-superbugs-endoscopes-n317591. Published March 5, 2015.

8. Cohen E, Christensen J. Scope superbug: how long did the FDA know about problem? CNN International Web site. http://www.cnn.com/2015/02/25/health/duodeonoscopes-cleaning-issue/index.html. February 25, 2015.

9. Newmarker C. The deadly superbug outbreak: what it means for you. MDDI Web site. https://www.mddionline.com/deadly-superbug-outbreak-what-it-means-you. Published February 25, 2015.

10. US Food and Drug Administration. Design of endoscopic retrograde cholangiopancreatography (ERCP) duodenoscopes may impede effective cleaning: FDA safety communication. US Food and Drug Administration Web site. https://www.ecri.org/Resources/Superbug/CRE_Alert_022015.pdf. Published February 19, 2015.

11. International Organization for Standardization. *ISO 14971:2012: Medical Devices. Application of Risk Management to Medical Devices.* Geneva, Switzerland: International Organization for Standardization; 2012.

12. European Union. *Regulation (EU) 2017/745 of the European Parliament and of the Council on Medical Devices, of 5 April 2017.* Brussels, Belgium: European Union; 2017

13. Spaulding EH. Role of chemical disinfection in the prevention of nosocomial infections. In: Brachman PS, Eickhoff TC, eds. *Proceedings of the International Conference on Nosocomial Infections, 1970.* Chicago: American Hospital Association; 1971:247-254.

14. Bond WW, Favero MS, Petersen NJ, Marshall JH. Dry-heat inactivation kinetics of naturally occurring spore populations. *Appl Microbiol.* 1970;20:573-578.

15. Bond WW. Disinfection and sterilisation of flexible fiberoptic endoscopes (FEE) and accessories. *Endosc Rev.* 1987;5:55-58.

16. Carson LA, Petersen NJ, Favero MS, Aguero SM. Growth characteristics of atypical mycobacteria in water and their comparative resistance to disinfectants. *Appl Environ Microbiol.* 1978;36:839-846.

17. Association for the Advancement of Medical Instrumentation. *ANSI/AAMI TIR12:2010. Designing, Testing, and Labeling Reusable Medical Devices for Reprocessing in Health Care Facilities: A Guide for Device Manufacturers.* Arlington, VA: Association for the Advancement of Medical Instrumentation; 2010.

18. Association for the Advancement of Medical Instrumentation. *ANSI/ AAMI TIR30:2011. A Compendium of Processes, Materials, Test Methods, and Acceptance Criteria for Cleaning Reusable Medical Devices.* Arlington, VA: Association for the Advancement of Medical Instrumentation; 2011.

19. Chemaly RE, Simmons S, Dale C Jr, et al. The role of healthcare environment in the spread of multidrug-resistant organisms: update on current best practices for containment. *Ther Adv Infect Dis.* 2014;2(3-4):79-90.

20. Cloutman-Green E, Canales M, Zhou Q, Ciric L, Hartley JC, McDonnell G. Biochemical and microbial contamination of surgical devices. *Am J Infect Control.* 2015;43:659-661.

21. Chu NS, Chan-Myers H, Ghazanfari N, Antonoplos P. Levels of naturally occurring microorganisms on surgical instruments after clinical use and after washing. *Am J Infect Control.* 1999;27:315-319.

22. Rutala WA, Gergen MF, Jones JF, Weber DJ. Levels of microbial contamination on surgical instruments. *Am J Infect Control.* 1998;26:143-145.

23. Webb SF, Vall-Spinosa A. Outbreak of *Serratia marcescens* associated with the flexible fiber bronchoscope. *Chest.* 1975;68:703-708.

24. International Organization for Standardization. *ISO 15883-1:2019: Washer-Disinfectors. Part 1: General Requirements, Terms, and Definitions and Tests.* Geneva, Switzerland: International Organization for Standardization; 2019.

25. McDonnell G, Sheard D. *A Practical Guide to Decontamination in Healthcare.* Hoboken, NJ: Wiley-Blackwell; 2012.

26. British Standards Institution. *BS EN 14885:2015. Chemical Disinfectants and Antiseptics—Application of European Standards for Chemical Disinfectants and Antiseptics.* London, United Kingdom: British Standards Institution; 2015.

27. US Food and Drug Administration, Center for Devices and Radiological Health. *Class II Special Controls Guidance Document: Medical Washers and Medical Washer-Disinfectors; Guidance for the Medical Device Industry and FDA Review Staff.* Silver Spring, MD: US Food and Drug; 2002.

28. Garner JS, Favero MS. CDC guideline for handwashing and hospital environmental control, 1985. *Infect Control.* 1986;7:231-243.

29. Rutala WA, Weber DJ. *Guideline for Disinfection and Sterilization in Healthcare Facilities, 2008.* Atlanta, GA: Healthcare Infection Control Practices Advisory Committee, Centers for Disease Control and Prevention; 2008. https://www.cdc.gov/infectioncontrol/guidelines/disinfection/index.html.

30. Klein M, Deforest A. Antiviral action of germicides. *Soap Chem Specifications.* 1963;39:70-72, 95-97.

31. Association for the Advancement of Medical Instrumentation. *ANSI/AAMI ST79:2010. Comprehensive Guide to Steam Sterilization and Sterility Assurance in Health Care Facilities.* Arlington, VA: Association for the Advancement of Medical Instrumentation; 2010.

32. International Organization for Standardization. *ISO 10993-7:2008: Biological Evaluation of Medical Devices. Part 7: Ethylene Oxide Sterilization Residuals.* Geneva, Switzerland: International Organization for Standardization; 2008.

33. Association for the Advancement of Medical Instrumentation. *ANSI/AAMI TIR34:2014. Water for the Reprocessing of Medical Devices.* Arlington, VA: Association for the Advancement of Medical Instrumentation; 2014.

34. Association for the Advancement of Medical Instrumentation. *ANSI/AAMI ST58:2013. Chemical Sterilization and High-Level Disinfection in Health Care Facilities.* Arlington, VA: Association for the Advancement of Medical Instrumentation; 2013.

35. International Organization for Standardization. *ISO 11135:2014: Sterilization of Health Care Products—Ethylene Oxide—Requirements for the Development, Validation and Routine Control of a Sterilization Process for Medical Devices.* Geneva, Switzerland: International Organization for Standardization; 2014.

36. British Standards Institution. *BS EN 285:2015. Sterilization—Steam Sterilizers—Large Sterilizers.* London, United Kingdom: British Standards Institution; 2015.

37. International Organization for Standardization. *ISO 17665-3:2013: Sterilization of Health Care Products. Moist Heat. Part 3: Guidance on the Designation of a Medical Device to a Product Family and Processing Category for Steam Sterilization.* Geneva, Switzerland: International Organization for Standardization; 2013.

38. Association for the Advancement of Medical Instrumentation. *ANSI/AAMI ST81:2004/(R2010). Sterilization of Medical Devices—Information to Be Provided by the Manufacturer for the Processing*

of Resterilizable Medical Devices. Arlington, VA: Association for the Advancement of Medical Instrumentation; 2010.

39. International Organization for Standardization. *ISO 15883-5:2019: Washer-Disinfectors. Part 5: Performance Requirements and Test Method Criteria for Demonstrating Cleaning Efficacy.* Geneva, Switzerland: International Organization for Standardization; in press.

40. American Society for Testing and Materials. *ASTM F3208-18. Standard Guide for Selecting Test Soils for Validation of Cleaning Methods for Reusable Medical Devices.* West Conshohocken, PA: American Society for Testing and Materials; 2018.

41. International Organization for Standardization. *ISO 10993-5:2009: Biological Evaluation of Medical Devices. Part 5: Tests for In Vitro Cytotoxicity.* Geneva, Switzerland: International Organization for Standardization; 2009.

42. United States Pharmacopeia and National Formulary 35. *Official Monograph: Biological Reactivity Tests, In Vitro (USP <87>).* Rockville, MD: United States Pharmacopeial Convention; 2017.

43. UK Department of Health. *Health Technical Memorandum 01-01: Management and Decontamination of Surgical Instruments (Medical Devices) Used in Acute Care.* London, United Kingdom: UK Department of Health; 2016.

44. Deutsche Gesellschaft für Krankenhaushygiene, Deutsche Gesellschaft für Sterilgutversorgung, Arbeitskreis Instrumentenaufbereitung. *Zentral Sterilisation: Guideline Compiled by DGKH, DGSV and AKI for the Validation and Routine Monitoring of Automated Cleaning and Thermal Disinfection Processes for Medical Devices.* 5th ed. Wiesbaden, Germany: mph-Verlag GmbH; 2017.

45. British Standards Institution. *BS EN ISO 15883-2:2009. Washer-Disinfectors. Part 2: Requirements and Tests for Washer-Disinfectors Employing Thermal Disinfection for Surgical Instruments, Anaesthetic Equipment, Bowls, Dishes, Receivers, Utensils, Glassware, etc.* London, United Kingdom: British Standards Institution; 2009.

46. McCormick PJ, Schoene MJ, Dehmler MA, McDonnell G. Moist heat disinfection and revisiting the A_0 concept. *Biomed Instrum Technol.* 2016;50(suppl 3):19-26.

47. Association for the Advancement of Medical Instrumentation. *ANSI/AMI/ISO 11138-3:2006/(R)2010. Sterilization of Health Care Products—Biological Indicators. Part 3: Biological Indicators for Moist Heat Sterilization Processes.* Arlington, VA: Association for the Advancement of Medical Instrumentation; 2010.

48. International Organization for Standardization. *ISO 11138-1:2017: Sterilization of Health Care Products—Biological Indicators. Part 1: General Requirements.* Geneva, Switzerland: International Organization for Standardization; 2017.

49. International Organization for Standardization. *ISO 11138-5:2017: Sterilization of Health Care Products—Biological Indicators. Part 5: Biological Indicators for Low-Temperature Steam and Formaldehyde Sterilization Processes.* Geneva, Switzerland: International Organization for Standardization; 2017.

50. International Organization for Standardization. *ISO 11138-2:2017: Sterilization of Health Care Products—Biological Indicators. Part 2: Biological Indicators for Ethylene Oxide Sterilization Processes.* Geneva, Switzerland: International Standards Organization; 2017.

51. International Organization for Standardization. *ISO 17665-1:2006: Sterilization of Health Care Products. Moist Heat. Part 1: Requirements for the Development, Validation and Routine Control of a Sterilization Process for Medical Devices.* Geneva, Switzerland: International Organization for Standardization; 2006.

52. International Organization for Standardization. *ISO 11607-1:2006: Packaging for Terminally Sterilized Medical Devices. Part 1: Requirements for Materials, Sterile Barrier Systems and Packaging Systems.* Geneva, Switzerland: International Organization for Standardization; 2006.

53. International Organization for Standardization. *ISO 11607-2:2006/ (R)2015: Packaging for Terminally Sterilized Medical Devices. Part 2: Validation Requirements for Forming, Sealing and Assembly Processes.* Geneva, Switzerland: International Organization for Standardization; 2015.

54. Association for the Advancement of Medical Instrumentation. *ANSI/AAMI ST77:2013. Containment Devices for Reusable Medical Device Sterilization.* Arlington, VA: Association for the Advancement of Medical Instrumentation; 2013.

55. US Food and Drug Administration. Additional guidance related to scope reprocessing and complexities due to design. US Food and Drug Administration Web site. https://www.fda.gov/medical-devices /reprocessing-reusable-medical-devices/factors-affecting-quality -reprocessing. Published January 12, 2018.

56. Gastroenterological Nurses College of Australia. *Infection Control in Endoscopy—Microbiological Testing of Gastrointestinal and Respiratory Endoscopes and Automated Flexible Endoscope Processors.* Victoria, Australia: Gastroenterological Nurses College of Australia; 2010.

57. Association for the Advancement of Medical Instrumentation. *ANSI/AAMI ST91:2015. Comprehensive Guide to Flexible and Semi-Rigid Endoscope Processing in Health Care Facilities.* Arlington, VA: Association for the Advancement of Medical Instrumentation; 2015.

58. Wheeler PW, Lancaster D, Kaiser AB. Bronchopulmonary cross-colonization and infection related to mycobacterial contamination of suction valves of bronchoscopes. *J Infect Dis.* 1989;159:954-958.

59. Dwyer DM, Klein EG, Istre GR, Robinson MG, Neumann DA, McCoy GA. *Salmonella newport* infections transmitted by fiberoptic colonoscopy. *Gastrointest Endosc.* 1987;33:84-87.

60. Mitzel E. Comments on "Reprocessing Guidance for Industry and FDA Staff," issued March 17, 2015. US Food and Drug Administration Web site. https:// nelsonmedtechinsights.com/2015/03/20/comments-on-reprocessing-guidance-for-industry-and-fda-staff-issued-march-17-2015/.

61. Spach DH, Silverstein FE, Stamm WE. Transmission of infection by gastrointestinal endoscopy and bronchoscopy. *Ann Intern Med.* 1993;118:117-128.

62. Birnie GG, Quigley EM, Clements GB, Follet EA, Watkinson G. Endoscopic transmission of hepatitis B virus. *Gut.* 1983;24:171-174.

63. Martin MA, Reichelderfer M. APIC guidelines for infection prevention and control in flexible endoscopy. Association for Professionals in Infection Control and Epidemiology, Inc. 1991, 1992, and 1993 APIC Guidelines Committee. *Am J Infect Control.* 1994;22:19-38.

64. Favero MS. Strategies for disinfection and sterilization of endoscopes: the gap between basic principles and actual practice. *Infect Control Hosp Epidemiol.* 1991;12:279-281.

65. Bond WW, Ott BJ, Franke K, McCracken JE. Effective use of liquid chemical germicides on medical devices: instrument design problems. In: Block SS, ed. *Sterilization, Disinfection, and Preservation.* 4th ed. Philadelphia, PA: Lea & Febiger; 1991:1097-1106.

66. American Public Health Association. Public Policy Statement 9417: establishment of clearly defined performance standards for between-patient processing of reusable endoscopic instruments and accessories. *Am J Public Health.* 1995;85:449-450.

67. Favero MS, Pugliese G. Infections transmitted by endoscopy: an international problem. *Am J Infect Control.* 1996;24:343-345.

68. DiMarino AJ, Bond WW. Flexible gastrointestinal endoscopic reprocessing. *Gastrointest Endosc.* 1996;43:522-524.

69. Society of Gastroenterology Nurses and Associates. *Standards for Infection Control and Reprocessing of Flexible Gastrointestinal Endoscopes.* Chicago, IL: Society of Gastroenterology Nurses and Associates; 1997.

70. Bond WW. Endoscope reprocessing: problems and solutions. In: Rutala WA, ed. *Disinfection, Sterilization, and Antisepsis in Health Care.* Washington, DC: Association for Professionals in Infection Control and Epidemiology; 1998:151-163.

71. American Society for Gastrointestinal Endoscopy. Infection control during gastrointestinal endoscopy: guidelines for clinical application. From the ASGE. American Society for Gastrointestinal Endoscopy. *Gastrointest Endosc.* 1999;49:836-841.

72. Petersen BT. Gaining perspective on reprocessing of GI endoscopes. *Gastrointest Endosc.* 1999;50:287-291.

73. Bond WW. Overview of infection control problems: principles in gastrointestinal endoscopy. *Gastrointest Endosc Clin N Am.* 2000;10:199-213.

74. Centers for Disease Control and Prevention. *Interim Duodenoscope Surveillance Protocol Which Included a Sampling Plan and Culture Method.* Atlanta, GA: Centers for Disease Control and Prevention; 2015.

75. Beilenhoff U, Neumann CS, Rey JF, et al. ESGE–ESGENA guideline for quality assurance in reprocessing: microbiological surveillance testing in endoscopy. *Endoscopy.* 2007;39(2):175-181.

Targeted Decontamination of Environmental Surfaces in Everyday Settings

Elizabeth A. Scott, Elizabeth Bruning, and Mohammad Khalid Ijaz

The concept of acquiring infectious agents from contact with contaminated surfaces is age-old and predates the germ theory of disease. The Book of Leviticus in the Old Testament of the Bible cites religious guidelines that apparently were intended not only to limit the acquisition of foodborne parasitic worms but also to limit the spread of infectious agents through contaminated drinking water and environmental surfaces, such as eating utensils and clothing, capable of transmitting infectious agents (pathogens).

In more modern times, concerns about public health issues date back to at least the mid-19th century and to the work of the sanitary reformers, who themselves were the precursors of the public health movement. The history of the development of *hygiene* and cleaning practices in the home dates to approximately the same period.

In recent years, there has been a significant shift in attitudes about microbes in our environment and their association with human health and disease. The revised viewpoints are likely to have a profound effect on *hygiene* policies.[1] On the one hand, infectious diseases, including community-based infections such as respiratory, gastrointestinal, and skin infections, continue to exert a heavy toll on human health and prosperity.[2] The problem is exacerbated by the aging of the population and the associated increase in percentage (approximately 20%) of immunocompromised individuals living in the community, who are often cared for at home.[3] Contrary to predictions made during the mid-20th century, infectious diseases have clearly not been eradicated. Indeed, new infectious agents (eg, Zika virus, severe acute respiratory syndrome coronavirus [SARS-CoV], Middle East respiratory syndrome coronavirus [MERS-CoV], Ebola virus, pandemic influenza strains, *Vibrio cholerae*, *Escherichia coli* 0157, and *Yersinia pestis*) continue to emerge and/or reemerge globally. In addition, the emergence of antibiotic-resistant pathogens (eg, methicillin-resistant *Staphylococcus aureus* [MRSA] and multidrug-resistant *Mycobacterium tuberculosis*) has become, and continues

to represent, a massive global concern. The concern is not only the risk in health care settings but also the risk in the home and general public settings. It is hard to overstate the risk associated with the emergence of such multidrug-resistant pathogens. The government of the United Kingdom has referred to this issue as a *post-antibiotic apocalypse*, which threatens to kill 10 million people globally by 2050.[4]

At the same time, there also is much concern about the rapid rise in allergies (especially asthma and food allergies) and other chronic inflammatory diseases (CID). The *hygiene hypothesis* proposed by Strachan[5] postulated that a lower incidence of early childhood infection (predominantly in first-world countries) might explain the rapid rise of allergic diseases during the 20th century. As discussed in a 2016 review by Bloomfield et al,[6] our current understanding of host-microbiome interactions and immune dysfunction suggests that increases in CID are the combined result of lifestyle, medical, and public health (*hygiene* and sanitation) changes, all of which have deprived humans of exposure to potentially beneficial microbial agents currently described as *old friends* (OF), particularly in early life.[6] These OF microbes are not pathogenic (as argued by Strachan[5]) and include nonharmful species that inhabit the human gastrointestinal tract and our natural environment. Based on these immunologic understandings, Dowling[7] has introduced the concept of *age-appropriate and health-appropriate hygiene practices for home and everyday life*. Such practices include age-appropriate vaccination and exposure to nonharmful microbes that prime the immune system.[8]

It is now widely accepted that the *hygiene hypothesis* of Strachan resulted in the inherently dangerous concept of our being *too clean* that has persisted in the media and in the minds of the public. The general public, as a result, now appears to be confused about the real meaning and value of *hygiene*. This is happening at a time when health agencies worldwide are emphasizing the necessity of basic *hygiene* practices at both the individual and community levels. Most importantly, *hygiene* is now being seen as a key component of strategies to tackle the global problem of antibiotic resistance. It is hoped that by reducing the level of infections, fewer people will need to seek antibiotic treatment, thereby limiting the selective pressure for generating antibiotic-resistant strains of pathogens. A balance in the use of hygiene practices, such as surface decontamination or hand antisepsis, in order to fight pathogens and the restoration of natural microbial diversity is, therefore, thought to be essential for enabling a healthy coexistence with the microbial world (ie, "bidirectional *hygiene*" or "bygiene"), a concept introduced by Al-Ghalith and Knights.[9]

The purpose of this chapter is to take a more holistic look at the risks posed by pathogen-contaminated surfaces, primarily in general living areas such as homes, by (1) taking a closer look at pathogen-contaminated environmental sites and surfaces in home and community settings in order to assess their roles for transmission of infectious agents; (2) exploring the role of human hands in disseminating infectious agents between *common-touch surfaces* (ie, the role of the *air-surface-hands nexus* in the chain of infection); (3) considering the current use of chemical and physical decontamination procedures; and (4) looking toward the future, including new technologies and probiotics, the potential insights to be gained from microbiome studies of the indoor environment, and best approaches for communicating information about *targeted hygiene* and surface decontamination practices in everyday settings.

Globally, the home captures a large cross-section of the human population in terms of age, health, nutritional status, and susceptibility to infectious agents and is, therefore, representative of many other community settings in terms of the necessity for *hygiene* practices. A constant dynamic exists between the home and other settings (day care, work, school, travel, leisure, health care, etc) in terms of the dissemination of infectious agents from infected individuals, contaminated food, and domesticated animals to surfaces and, via the intermediacy of human hands, through the entire cycle of reinfection. In day care settings, young children are immunologically immature and exhibit behaviors that may encourage transmission of infectious agents (eg, poor personal *hygiene* and mouthing of objects). Problems associated with day care staffing and varying educational levels may compound the problem.

In determining the role that surfaces play in the transmission of disease, it is important first to develop a working definition of inanimate surface contamination. The chain of events leading to the occurrence and spread of infectious agents is then discussed. With the recognition that decontamination of environmental surfaces may not be necessary in all situations, the prudent use of effective targeted approaches as a possible means of reducing the burden of infectious agents is described.

The terminology that is commonly used for surface contamination includes the word *fomite* (an environmental surface that might be contaminated and then serve as a vehicle for dissemination of the infectious agent) and terms describing a subclass of fomites, namely *common-touch surfaces* (also referred to as *high frequency–touch surfaces* [HITES] in health care settings).[10] *Common-touch surfaces* include fomites such as door knobs, toilet flush handles, faucet handles, light switches, remote controls, cell phones, and other digital devices. The concern over *common-touch surfaces* reflects the important role that hands play in the dissemination of infectious agents in everyday settings.

To define the risk associated with surface contamination, several factors must be considered. These include (1) the presence of pathogenic contaminants in the environment and their minimum infective doses (MID), (2) the length of time over which such pathogens remain viable and infectious on fomites, and (3) the likelihood of their being transferred from such fomites to a new host. We must also consider the types of *common-touch surfaces* that are most likely to become contaminated in the home. Pathogens travel via well-defined routes from an infected source to another individual. Numerous sampling studies have recorded the presence of both pathogenic bacteria, fungi, parasites, and viruses as well as nonpathogenic microbes on environmental surfaces in home and community settings. Both laboratory and field studies have evaluated the rates of transfer of pathogens via hands and *common-touch surfaces*, as reviewed by Bloomfield et al.[3] These studies demonstrate that the surfaces with the highest risk of transmitting pathogens and which are, therefore, the critical control points in the transmission of infection, are the hands, *common-touch surfaces*, food-contact surfaces, and the cleaning utensils used on these surfaces, as shown in Figure 48.1.

For an infection to result from human contact with a contaminated surface, the following must be in place: (1) the presence of an infectious agent (implying the existence of a source or reservoir for the pathogen), (2) a means or mode of transmission, and (3) the presence of a susceptible host. The greatest risk is associated with hosts characterized as at higher risk for infection (ie, the very young, very old, immunocompromised, malnourished, etc), although potentially any individual may be at risk of acquiring infectious agents from pathogen-contaminated surfaces. The cycle of pathogen contamination of surfaces leading to the reinfection of a new host, and possible approaches for interruption of this cycle, are displayed in Figure 48.2. The overwhelming importance of the human hand in dissemination of pathogens that have been deposited on surfaces is depicted by the placement of the hands at the top of this figure. We return to the theme of the *air-surface-hand nexus* throughout this chapter to emphasize that the surfaces serve as reservoirs for contamination, and the hand and air are primary disseminators for the contamination to other hosts and surfaces.

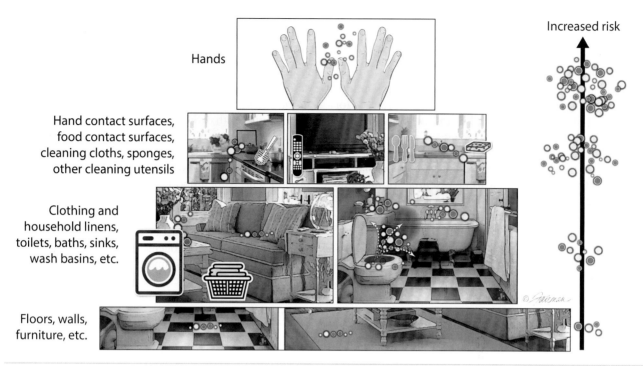

Hands

Hand contact surfaces, food contact surfaces, cleaning cloths, sponges, other cleaning utensils

Clothing and household linens, toilets, baths, sinks, wash basins, etc.

Floors, walls, furniture, etc.

Increased risk

FIGURE 48.1 Ranking of sites and surfaces based on risk of transmission of infection through the intermediacy of the hand. The filled dots and unfilled dots represent pathogenic and nonpathogenic microorganisms, respectively. For a color version of this art, please consult the eBook. Modified from Bloomfield et al.[6] Copyright © 2016 SAGE Publications.

Targeting those *common-touch surfaces* at high risk for pathogen transmission/acquisition by hosts and applying appropriate decontamination practices form the basis for an evidence-based *hygiene* policy known as *targeted hygiene*. *Targeted hygiene* is intended to manage the microbial diversity of environmental surfaces as well as the human microbiome[6] and incorporates the novel concept of *bygiene*.[9]

▶ DISSEMINATION OF PATHOGENS BY ENVIRONMENTAL SURFACES

Common-touch surfaces may become contaminated by pathogens and subsequently serve as reservoirs for transmission of infectious agents through the intermediacy of the human hand.[2,11,12] Knowledge of, and focus of remediation efforts on, such *common-touch surfaces* will have the greatest economic and infectious disease prevention impact. According to the Centers for Disease Control and Prevention,[13] 80% of infectious diseases are transmitted by contaminated hands and, therefore, the human hand is a common denominator in transmission of infectious agents via *common-touch surfaces*. According to this view, high-risk *common-touch surfaces* include door knobs/handles, kitchen counters, toilet flush handles, telephone handsets, personal digital electronic devices, shopping carts, handrail belts for escalators and people movers, toys, contaminated fabrics, automated banking teller machines, currency coins and bills, etc (Figure 48.3). Again, this

figure emphasizes the central role of the human hand in dissemination of infectious agents acquired by handling various common-touch objects.

Pathogens that are most likely to be transmitted from common-touch reservoirs are those that are capable of surviving in the absence of a host under ambient conditions following release from a source of infectious agents. For this reason, pathogens of particular concern include nonenveloped viruses, spore-forming bacteria, fungi, and parasitic ova/(oo)cysts. Although the ambient environment is relatively less conducive for survival of vegetative bacteria and enveloped viruses, these also may be disseminated from *common-touch surfaces*. To better appreciate the risk of pathogen spread via *common-touch surfaces* and the mitigation of such risk, the following need to be considered:

1. Certain pathogens may remain infectious outside of a host for extended periods of time.
2. There is evidence for the recovery of pathogens from environmental surfaces.
3. The transmission of pathogens from contaminated surfaces to human hands has been demonstrated.
4. Targeted use of microbicidal products and hygienic practices may disrupt pathogen transfer from environmental surfaces to human hands.
5. The combination of hygiene practices and education (including knowledge of when, where, and how to apply these practices) can reduce the transmission and thus the risk of infectious diseases in home and community settings.

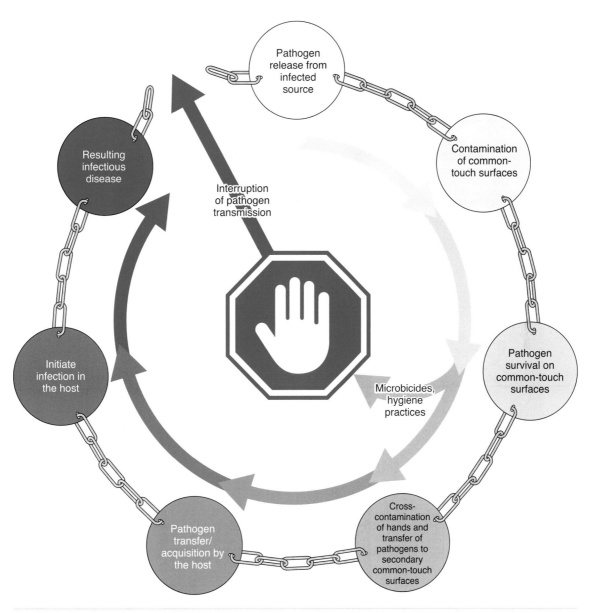

FIGURE 48.2 The cycle of surface contamination, dissemination, and reinfection and possible approaches for interrupting the cycle.

◗ PATHOGENS MAY REMAIN INFECTIOUS ON SURFACES FOR EXTENDED PERIODS OF TIME IN THE ABSENCE OF A HOST

Pathogens such as bacteria, fungi, viruses (especially non-enveloped), and enteric parasitic ova/(oo)cysts have been found to remain infectious for extended periods of time following contamination of environmental surfaces. For instance, nonenveloped viruses including the adenoviruses, astroviruses, picornaviruses (eg, coxsackie virus, hepatitis A virus, poliovirus, and rhinovirus), caliciviruses (eg, norovirus and feline calicivirus), and reoviruses (eg, rotavirus) have been found to survive for up to 3 months on contaminated

environmental surfaces (reviewed by Kramer et al[15] and Boone and Gerba[11]). On the other hand, enveloped viruses, such as the herpesviruses (eg, cytomegalovirus, herpes simplex), paramyxoviruses (eg, Sendai virus, respiratory syncytial virus), orthomyxoviruses (eg, influenza A and B viruses), and coronaviruses (eg, SARS-CoV, MERS-CoV), and blood-borne retroviruses (eg, human immunodeficiency virus) tend to remain infectious on the order of hours or days, rather than months (Table 48.1).[11,14,15,21,29]

Most gram-positive bacteria, such as *Enterococcus species.* (including vancomycin-resistant *enterococcus*), *S aureus* (including MRSA), or *Streptococcus pyogenes*, survive for months on dry surfaces.[15] Many gram-negative bacteria, such as *Acinetobacter species*, *E coli*, *Klebsiella species*, *Pseudomonas aeruginosa*, *Serratia marcescens*, or *Shigella*

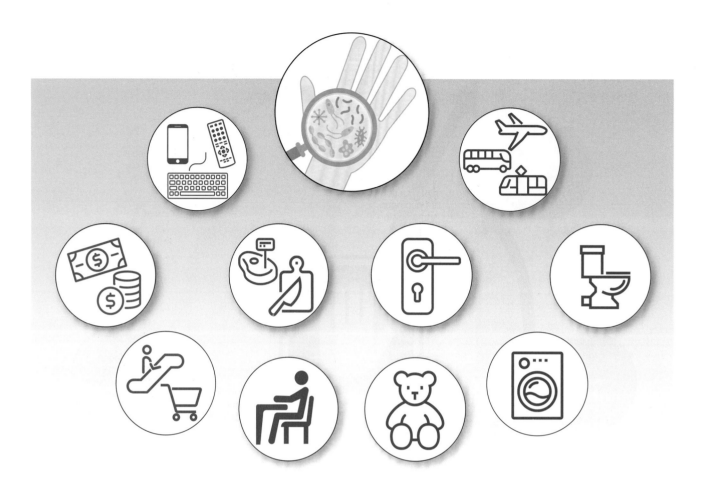

FIGURE 48.3   High-risk *common-touch surfaces* for transmission of pathogens in the home or outside of the home. Adapted from Alum et al.[14] Copyright © 2010 International Society for Infectious Diseases. With permission.

species, can also survive for months.[15] The fungal pathogen *Candida albicans* can survive up to 4 months on surfaces.[15] Enteric parasitic (oo)cysts (*Cryptosporidium*) or (oo)cysts (*Giardia*) and enteric parasitic ova have been found to survive on experimentally contaminated environmental surfaces (both animate and inanimate) for weeks to months (A. Alum et al, unpublished data, August 19, 2011) (see Table 48.1).[30]

In general, it can be assumed that the nonenveloped viruses (hepatitis A, rhinoviruses, noroviruses, and rotaviruses) will survive longer than enveloped viruses. In the case of bacteria, sporeformers (eg, *Clostridium difficile*) will survive the longest, and for parasites, the encysted (*Cryptosporidium* and *Giardia*) forms will survive longer than nonencysted parasites. Vegetative bacteria such as MRSA, *Acinetobacter* species, and *E coli* may also survive for months. Although enveloped viruses (eg, influenza) may survive only for days, the human minimal infective dose for these viruses may be low enough that, for instance, it might take 6 to 9 days for an influenza-contaminated surface to be rendered noninfectious (see Table 48.1).

Surface porosity or roughness, temperature, relative humidity (RH), and presence of organic matter associated with pathogens released from the source are also significant determinants of pathogen survival outside of a host.[11,15,16,21,29-32] Biofilm formation also promotes persistence of bacteria.[33] As a generality, the lower the temperature, the longer the time that the pathogen will remain infectious (see also chapter 67).[15,30,32] The presence of organic matter has been found to provide added stability to infectious agents present on contaminated environmental surfaces.[16,30,32,34]

Indoor air temperature, RH, presence of organic load, and types of environmental surfaces (hard/soft and porous/nonporous) have each been shown to impact the survival of viruses. At room temperature, survival of enveloped viruses such as transmissible gastroenteritis virus and murine hepatitis virus (surrogates for SARS-CoV) on surfaces is greater at relatively low RH (20%),[21] whereas human coronavirus 229E has been reported to persist on six surface materials common to communal and domestic environments for at least 5 days under

TABLE 48.1 Examples for survival of pathogens on fomites in the absence of decontamination and duration of time required to reach a noninfectious state

Pathogen (Reference)	Minimum Infective Dose	Fomite	k_i (Log$_{10}$ Reduction in Titer/d)	Time Needed for 3 Log$_{10}$ Reduction[a]	Time Needed to Get Below MID[b]
Nonenveloped viruses					
Adenovirus 40 (Abad et al[16])	150 TCID$_{50}$	Nonporous	0.264	11 d	14 d
Feline calicivirus (Doultree et al[17])	10-100 particles	Nonporous	0.286	10 d	21 d
Hepatitis A virus (Abad et al[16])	10-100 TCID$_{50}$	Nonporous[c] Porous[d]	0.0667 0.0667	45 d 45 d	90 d 90 d
Rhinovirus 14 (Sattar et al[18])	1-10 TCID$_{50}$	Nonporous	0.526	5.7 d	13 d
Rotavirus p13 (Abad et al[16])	10-100 TCID$_{50}$	Nonporous Porous	0.0667 0.0667	45 d 45 d	90 d 90 d
Enveloped viruses					
Coronavirus 229E (Warnes et al[19])	No data	Nonporous Porous	0.50 1.0	6 d 3 d	No data
Influenza virus (Bean et al[20])	2-790 TCID$_{50}$	Nonporous Porous	0.667 1.00	4.5 d 3.0 d	9 d 6 d
Mouse hepatitis virus (Casanova et al[21])	No data	Nonporous	0.685	4.4 d	No data
Transmissible gastroenteritis virus (Casanova et al[21])	No data	Nonporous	0.896	3.3 d	No data
Bacteria					
Acinetobacter species (Otter and French[22])	No data	Nonporous	0.107	28 d	No data
Campylobacter jejuni (Humphrey et al[23])	500 organisms (Kothary and Babu[24])	Nonporous	6.6	11 h	18 h
Clostridium difficile (Otter and French[22])	No data	Nonporous	0.0238	107 d	No data
Escherichia coli (Wilks et al[25])	>10^5 organisms (Kothary and Babu[24])	Nonporous	0.196	15 d	10 d
Staphylococcus aureus (Otter and French[22])	10^3-10^5 organisms (Otter and French[22])	Nonporous	0.131	23 d	31 d
Fungi					
Candida albicans (Traoré et al[26])	No data	Nonporous Porous	1.0 0.143	3 d 21 d	No data
Parasites					
Ascaris lumbricoides	No data	Nonporous Porous	0.0174 0.0160	172 d 188 d	No data
Cryptosporidium parvum (Alum et al[30])	10 (oo)cysts (Kothary and Babu[24])	Nonporous Porous	0.0769 0.0909	39 d 33 d	78 d 66 d
Entamoeba histolytica	1000 organisms (Health Canada Pathogen Safety Data Sheets[27])	Nonporous Porous	0.107 0.143	28 d 21 d	37 d 28 d

TABLE 48.1	Examples for survival of pathogens on fomites in the absence of decontamination and duration of time required to reach a noninfectious state *(Continued)*				
Pathogen (Reference)	Minimum Infective Dose	Fomite	k_i (Log$_{10}$ Reduction in Titer/d)	Time Needed for 3 Log$_{10}$ Reduction^a	Time Needed to Get Below MID^b
Enterobius vermicularis	No data	Nonporous Porous	0.0938 0.115	32 d 26 d	No data
Giardia muris (Alum et al[30])	10 (oo)cysts (Stachan and Kunstýr[28])	Nonporous Porous	0.100 0.107	30 d 28 d	100 d 93 d

Abbreviations: k_i, inactivation constant; MID, minimum infective dose; TCID$_{50}$, tissue culture infective dose$_{50}$.

^{a}The time in days for 1 log$_{10}$ inactivation = 1 / k_i. For the days required to obtain 3 log$_{10}$ inactivation, multiply the days required for 1 log$_{10}$ inactivation by 3.

^{b}Assumes an initial burden of 10^6 pathogens. The log$_{10}$ reduction needed to achieve a bioburden 1 log$_{10}$ lower than the lowest MID is divided by k_i to arrive at the time required (days).

^{c}Nonporous surfaces include aluminum, stainless steel, and glass.

^{d}Examples of porous surfaces include paper, latex glove, and cloth.

ambient conditions (21°C; RH, 30%-40%).[19] At room temperature, nonenveloped viruses (eg, picornaviruses including poliovirus and murine norovirus [used as a surrogate for human norovirus]) remain infectious longer on surfaces at higher RH,[32,35] with the exception of rotavirus and hepatitis A virus, which survive best at a low to medium RH.[36-38]

▶ RECOVERY OF PATHOGENS FROM NATURALLY CONTAMINATED ENVIRONMENTAL SURFACES

The cycle of infection/reinfection begins with the contamination of a surface with pathogens from a source of infectious agents. This might represent shedding of pathogens from an infected human or domesticated animal through pathophysiologic secretions (feces, respiratory aerosols, oral or urogenital excretions, or blood/serum exudates). Other sources of pathogens include contaminated raw foods and water. Indoor environmental surfaces may become contaminated directly or indirectly, and a continual redistribution of pathogens then may occur at the *air-surface-hand nexus*, leading to a *surface contamination network* of pathogen dissemination.[39] As shown schematically in Figure 48.4, activities such as surface cleaning, flushing of toilets, air movement, and human and domesticated animal activities each may contribute to the distribution and redistribution of infectious agents among various environmental surfaces.

Various types of pathogens have been recovered from naturally (ie, not experimentally) contaminated environmental surfaces. Of special concern in this context are common foodborne pathogens such as *Salmonella*

species, *Campylobacter* species, *S aureus*, *E coli*, *Bacillus cereus*, and *Listeria monocytogenes*.[23,40] The kitchen is a high-risk area due to the possibility of spread of pathogens from contaminated foods to surfaces or from infected food preparers' hands to food or surfaces.[41-43]

The microbiome of sponges and cleaning cloths used in the kitchen has been the subject of recent, albeit controversial, research activity.[44] The controversy is not regarding the role of kitchen sponges and other kitchen cleaning cloths as reservoirs and disseminators of pathogens, which has been well documented in the past[42,45] but rather about the reported population density values for certain pathogens on sponge surfaces proposed by these authors.

The bathroom/restroom is another high-risk area for dissemination of pathogens, due to generation there of oral secretions and enteric excrements. The generation of pathogen-containing aerosols through flushing of toilets has been convincingly demonstrated by Gerba et al[46] in studies using coliform bacteria, bacteriophage MS2, and poliovirus. The pathogen-containing aerosols were found to remain airborne long enough to contaminate surfaces throughout the bathroom. Various enteric viruses have been recovered from 78% of surfaces and 81% of aerosols produced by toilet flushing in office buildings and health care facilities.[47] These results indicate that toilets are an important reservoir of viral contaminants, both in the home as well as in offices and health care settings.

Infants have been found to be a source of secondary infection in dense family units, and careful handling and hygiene around diaper changing is proposed as the primary means of mitigating risk.[48] Ibfelt et al[49] studied the prevalence of pathogenic bacteria and viruses and characterized the most contaminated fomites in a day care center. Coliform bacteria were primarily found in the toilet

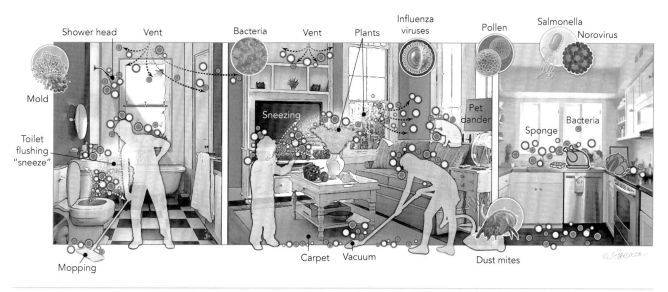

FIGURE 48.4 High-risk sources of airborne pathogens in the home and potential for environmental surface contamination. The filled dots and unfilled dots represent pathogenic and nonpathogenic microorganisms, respectively. For a color version of this art, please consult the eBook.

and kitchen, whereas nasopharyngeal bacteria were found mostly on toys and fabric surfaces in the playroom. Respiratory viruses were detected throughout the day care center, especially on the toys.

A norovirus outbreak on rental vacation houseboats was documented by Jones and coworkers.[50] Various environmental surfaces were sampled, with five of six bathroom samples being found positive for norovirus, two of five kitchen samples being found positive, and three of three doorknob samples being found positive by reverse transcriptase polymerase chain reaction (RT-PCR). The contamination of various *common-touch surfaces* within the houseboat and subsequent dissemination by human hands was suggested to play a role in sustaining the outbreak among passengers during three consecutive rental trips of the same houseboat.

Enteric parasitic ova/(oo)cysts have been recovered from the hands of naturally contaminated Bangladeshi and Indian populations.[51] A total of 972 stool samples were collected from volunteers from the surveyed sites (300 from Kolkata, India, and 672 from Dhaka, Bangladesh). Of these, 38% of the Kolkata samples and 40% of the Dhaka samples were found to be positive for parasitic ova/(oo)cysts. Of corresponding hand wash samples, 14% from stool-positive subjects in Kolkata and 7% from stool-positive subjects in Dhaka were positive for ova/(oo)cysts. *Ascaris lumbricoides* ova and *Giardia lamblia* cysts predominated in hand wash samples from both sites (53% and 31% of positive samples, respectively, in Kolkata, and 47% and 19% of positive samples, respectively, in Dhaka). Genotypic analysis has shown that enteric parasitic ova/(oo)cysts obtained from stool and corresponding hand wash samples from a given subject were found to be identical, consistent with fecal-oral trans-

mission of the infectious agents via hands.[51] The enteric parasitic (oo)cysts and ova have been shown to survive for months on experimentally contaminated environmental surfaces, as described earlier (A. Alum et al, unpublished data, August 19, 2011) (see Table 48.1).[30] This emphasizes the importance of proper hand washing in reducing the parasite burden in low socioeconomic communities.

A discussion of the fomites with potential to disseminate infectious agents would not be complete without consideration of the pathogen load of our modern digital devices (cell phones, laptop computers, etc), automated banking teller machines,[52,53] and conveyances (escalators, people movers, and *common-touch surfaces* within urban transport systems). Each of these, not unexpectedly, has been shown to reflect pathogen deposition by human interaction with these devices or conveyances.[54-57]

TRANSMISSION OF PATHOGENS FROM CONTAMINATED ENVIRONMENTAL SURFACES TO HUMANS

The role of indoor environmental surfaces in dissemination of infectious agents has been reviewed by Barker et al,[58] Kagan et al,[59] and, more recently, Boone and Gerba.[11] Barker and coworkers[58] concluded that "there is growing evidence that person-to-person transmission via the hands and contaminated fomites plays a key role in the spread of viral infections and there is a need for wider understanding of the potential for contaminated surfaces to act as unidentified vectors of pathogens in the transmission cycle."

Kagan et al[59] have reviewed the evidence for transmission within the home of members of the *Enterobacteriaceae* and other bacteria, including *E coli, Klebsiella pneumoniae, Enterobacter cloacae, Bacillus subtilis, P aeruginosa, Salmonella ser Typhimurium, S aureus,* and *Enterobacter aerogenes*. These authors identified the importance of the kitchen, bathroom, and laundry as reservoirs for such bacteria. Sattar and coworkers[60] examined the transfer of *S aureus* from experimentally contaminated fabrics to hands and to other fabrics. Transfer was enhanced from moist versus dry fabrics, and friction was also found to increase transfer from fabric to fingerpads by at least fivefold.

Winther et al[61] found, using RT-PCR, that adults with naturally acquired rhinovirus infections contaminated 35% of environmental surfaces in hotel rooms during overnight occupancy. Rhinovirus RNA was detected on a variety of *common-touch surfaces*, such as light switches, phone buttons, and telephone handsets. Virus-containing mucous experimentally seeded onto *common-touch surfaces* and allowed to dry for 1 to 18 hours was shown to be transferred to the fingers of subjects touching the seeded surfaces. These findings were then replicated in a home setting, where rhinovirus-infected subjects touched pre-identified *common-touch surfaces* (doorknobs, refrigerator door handles, TV remote controls, and bathroom faucets) in their homes within 24 hours of confirmation of their infections by RT-PCR and cell culture–based assay. Of the touched surfaces, 41% were later found to be positive for rhinovirus by RT-PCR. When infectious rhinovirus was seeded onto *common-touch surfaces* and touched by subjects within 1 hour, rhinovirus was detected on 22% of fingertips. Transfer of virus dropped to 3% of fingertips after 24 hours, and no transfer occurred after 48 hours.[62]

More recently, Oristo et al[63] demonstrated the presence of norovirus and adenovirus on environmental surfaces and military conscripts' hands in two Finnish garrisons. The same norovirus genotypes were observed on surfaces and in fecal samples or on hand swabs, suggesting possible transmission of viruses via contaminated surfaces and hands.

Koganti et al[12] demonstrated that bacteriophage MS2 seeded on a hospital floor adjacent to a patient bed was subsequently recovered within 1 day from the patient's hands and footwear and from *common-touch surfaces* within the patient room including bed rails, phone, bed linens, tray tables, furniture, door handle, and as far away as the nursing station computer keyboards and phones.

Yuguo Li's group[39] at the University of Hong Kong have recently identified the existence of a community structure to what they refer to as the *surface contamination network* in an aircraft cabin. Similar to the connectivity that exists between different housing communities, the aisle seatback surfaces become the root surfaces for dissemination of norovirus by hand touch to other surfaces within each subcommunity and eventually throughout the aircraft cabin. This emphasizes again the importance of the human hand in dissemination of pathogens. This study of dissemination of an infectious agent through an aircraft cabin is mentioned because the latter may be used as a model for pathogen dissemination within other crowded indoor settings. This study highlights the importance of the *air-surface-hand nexus* (see Figure 48.4) and the role of the *common-touch surface* network for dissemination of aerosolized pathogens once deposited onto a surface. This model could potentially be applicable to dissemination of pathogens such as influenza, norovirus, MERS-CoV, or SARS-CoV within other crowded settings, such as homes, cruise ships, urban transport systems, day care centers, and schools. This is also suggested by findings that seasonality associated with norovirus outbreaks correlates with the school year in the northern and southern hemisphere.[64]

▶ MICROBICIDAL INTERVENTIONS TO DISRUPT PATHOGEN DISSEMINATION FROM ENVIRONMENTAL SURFACES TO HUMANS

Mitigating the risk of disseminating infectious agents while maintaining the nonpathogenic natural diversity microbiome of such environmental surfaces requires implementation, both at the home and community level, of targeted hygienic measures that can interrupt the infectious cycle through removal or inactivation of pathogens from *common-touch surfaces* (see Figure 48.2).[58,65]

Transfer of norovirus from food preparers' hands to food items is proposed as a dissemination mechanism for this enterovirus from the *Caliciviridae* family.[66] Bidawid et al[67] used feline calicivirus as a surrogate for human norovirus to study this mechanism and to assess the potential for interruption of virus transfer from contaminated hands to food items and vice versa, through use of hand antisepsis (see also chapter 42). Transfer in both directions was observed, with 13% to 46% of available virus being transferred from hands to food and 6% to 14% of available virus being transferred from food items to hands. Significant interruption of transfer was observed using hand hygiene incorporating ethanol-based antisepsis. Similar results were obtained when the picornavirus hepatitis A virus was used as the test pathogen.[68]

The risk of dissemination of foodborne infectious agents during food preparation activities can also be mitigated through use of targeted microbicidal applications. Josephson and coworkers[69] evaluated the pathogens on naturally contaminated *common-touch surfaces* (cutting boards, sponges, countertops, sinks, faucets, refrigerator doors, oven controls, etc) from 10 kitchens pre- and postapplication of a microbicidal kitchen cleaning (MKC) product. Prior to application of MKC products, the sinks and sponges were found to contain fecal coliforms and specific pathogens. Microbicidal products targeted to high-risk surfaces soon after contamination with foods or hands decreased the incidence of contamination significantly. In another study,[70] *common-touch surfaces* in the kitchen surfaces were experimentally contaminated and the microbicidal efficacy of MKC products was assessed. In both studies, pathogen contamination postapplication of MKC products was significantly reduced, compared with the levels on surfaces before product application.

The risk of dissemination of foodborne infectious agents during food preparation activities can also be mitigated through use of microbicidal wipes, as demonstrated by Lopez et al.[71] These authors used Monte Carlo simulation to demonstrate that the use of microbicidal wipes to decontaminate surface areas after chicken preparation could reduce the annual risk of *Campylobacter jejuni* infections 100- to 1000-fold. A recent study performed in a health care setting[72] suggested that frequent use of microbicidal wipes applied to *common-touch surfaces* is more effective in preventing MRSA dissemination than whole-room cleaning. These results imply that for home settings, frequent application of microbicidal products in the form of wipes or surface cleansers to common-touch and especially high-risk surfaces such as kitchen countertops, cutting boards, refrigerator door handles, kitchen cabinet door handles, microwave door handles, stove knobs, faucet handles, and knives should be practiced along with proper hand hygiene when raw foods are handled to avoid foodborne pathogen spread (see Figure 48.1).

Murine norovirus (used as a surrogate for human norovirus) displays markedly faster inactivation (measured in minutes instead of days) on copper surfaces relative to stainless steel (see also chapter 24).[73] Replacement of stainless steel surfaces with copper surfaces in food preparation areas could, therefore, reduce the persistence of foodborne pathogens. The efficacy of an antibacterial dishwashing liquid for reducing the burden of *E coli*, *Salmonella* ser Enteritidis, *S aureus*, and *B cereus* in kitchen sponges with and without organic load was investigated by Kusumaningrum et al.[74] Although the dishwashing liquid (4% wt/wt) was found to be effective in inactivating each of the bacteria when tested in a liquid suspension assay at 3% wt/wt, the dishwashing liquid was relatively ineffective for reducing the burden of bacteria in the kitchen sponge.

A commonly used household microbicidal spray was found[75] to interrupt the transmission of rotavirus to human subjects exposed to experimentally contaminated environmental surfaces. None of the subjects exposed to microbicide-treated surfaces acquired infection, whereas 93% of the subjects exposed to nontreated surfaces acquired rotavirus infection. Sattar et al[76] found that a household microbicidal spray and a sodium hypochlorite

solution diluted to provide 800 ppm of free chlorine were each effective in interrupting the transfer of rhinovirus type 14 from stainless steel disks to the fingerpads of human volunteers. Viral infectivity was reduced $>4 \log_{10}$ by a contact time to the spray of 1 or 10 minutes and no virus was transferred from the treated disks to fingerpads. The sodium hypochlorite solution reduced the infectious virus titer by approximately $3 \log_{10}$ after a contact time of 10 minutes and, again, no virus was transferred from the treated disks to fingerpads.

A modified American Society for Testing and Materials (ASTM) E1838-02 method[77] has been used to assess activity of hand hygiene agents against viruses, bacteria, and fungi.[77-80] This method has also been used to determine the effectiveness of a bar soap for removing soil-transmitted helminth ova from the fingerpads of adult volunteers (M.K.I. and J. Rubino, unpublished data, September 10, 2009). In this pilot study, hand washing with the soap reduced ova from *Ascaris suum* (a surrogate of *A lumbricoides*) by ≥ 3 $\log_{10}$, compared to the baseline control when applied for a 30-second contact time. This confirms that proper hand hygiene may play a significant role in reducing fecal-oral transmission of enteric parasites in humans.

A number of investigators have studied the presence of bacteria on used toothbrushes and the use of microbicidal products to reduce pathogen load. Chlorhexidine gluconate– and sodium hypochlorite–based microbicidal products have been found to be efficacious for decontamination of toothbrushes.[81,82]

The pathogenic and malodourous microbes in contaminated laundry can potentially survive the laundering process (see also chapter 46). Globally, in some health care settings, the recommended laundering process is standardized and includes a combination of high temperature (at least 60°C) and oxidizing agents.[83] Apart from removing visible stains and dirt, such processes also provide hygienically clean textiles by removal/inactivation of malodorous microbial contaminants and pathogens. In the typical domestic setting, however, where energy-conserving machines may use water at $<40°C$, many nonenveloped viruses and fungi are likely to survive the laundry process (reviewed by Bockmühl[83]). Gerba and Kennedy[84] showed that enteric nonenveloped viruses (adenovirus, rotavirus, and hepatitis A virus) added to cotton cloth swatches survived a 20°C to 23°C wash cycle, the rinse cycle, and a 28-minute permanent press (approximately 55°C) drying cycle as commonly practiced in households in the United States. Washing with detergent alone reduced only approximately $2 \log_{10}$ of enteric viruses. Viruses were readily transferred from contaminated laundry to washed laundry. The use of bleach (5.25% sodium hypochlorite) in the wash step reduced a number of infectious viruses by at least $4 \log_{10}$.[84]

To determine if application of hygiene products combined with hygiene education could provide health benefits, a field intervention study was performed in a periurban area (near Cape Town, South Africa). The study assessed the differential effects of hygiene education alone versus hygiene education plus consistent use of hygiene products (soap, a 0.074% benzalkonium chloride–based surface cleaner, and a 4.8% chloroxylenol-based skin antiseptic) on reduction of target illnesses/infections in children.[85] The study investigated subjects in a government housing and in an informal housing community. Within the government housing community, the hygiene education–only group was 2.5 times more likely to experience gastrointestinal illnesses and 4.6 times more likely to experience respiratory illnesses, compared to the education plus hygiene products group. In the informal community where communal taps and latrines were used, subjects with hygiene education only experienced 1.6 times more gastrointestinal illnesses, 4.6 times more respiratory illnesses, and 1.3 times more skin infections compared to the education plus hygiene products group.[85] These results indicate the importance of access both to education and to hygiene products for reducing the likelihood of acquiring infectious agents leading to various infectious diseases. Another example of the importance of hygiene education and product use to manage the risk of acquiring infectious agents and maintenance of the natural vulvovaginal microbiome is in the field of personal intimate hygiene.[86]

Morvai and Szabó[55] reviewed the literature for reports on the potential for dissemination of infections by mobile communication devices and interventions for mitigating this risk. The successful interventions included staff education, hand hygiene, and regular decontamination of mobile communication devices.

These studies demonstrate that microbicidal products can potentially interrupt the transfer of pathogens from contaminated surfaces to human hands and the subsequent dissemination to other hosts and surfaces, possibly through *surface contamination networks*,[39] emphasizing the potential role of proper hygiene practices in interrupting the cycle of infection/reinfection discussed earlier (ie, the concept of the *air-surface-hand nexus*).

◗ CURRENT DECONTAMINATION APPROACHES AND TECHNOLOGIES

"Microbicide" is an older term that has recently been reintroduced[87] to denote pathogen-reducing actives that are chemical in nature. Chemical agents include formulations of quaternary ammonium compounds (QACs), alcohols, aldehydes, phenolics, acids, caustics, and oxidizing agents such as peroxide, sodium hypochlorite, and other halogens. Fu et al[88] surveyed approximately 500 microbicidal products registered with the US Environmental Protection Agency (EPA) for use in households, reporting that five types of active ingredients predominate (Figure 48.5A). The QACs are used in well over half of the microbicidal products, followed in rank by pine oil, alcohol, phenolics, and hypochlorites. A similar survey of the more than 2300 EPA-registered microbicidal products targeted for industrial and institutional use revealed that QACs again were the predominant active (36%), followed in rank by hypochlorites (>18%) (Figure 48.5B).

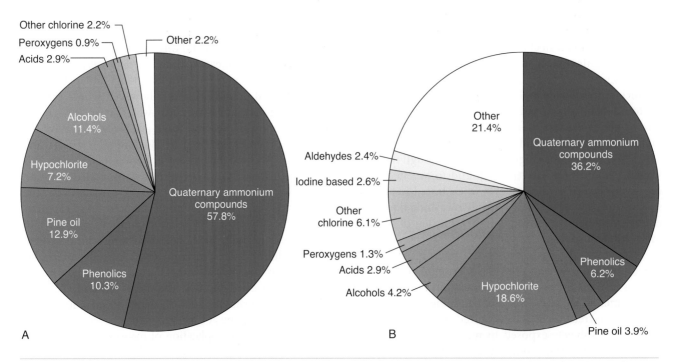

FIGURE 48.5 Distribution of active ingredients in US Environmental Protection Agency–registered microbicidal products intended for household use (A) and industrial and institutional use (B).

It is important to note that all microbicidal products display activity that is dependent on factors such as concentration applied, contact time, temperature, and presence of organic load. Contact time refers to the duration of time that an agent is applied to a pathogen-contaminated surface. Reduction of pathogen load on surfaces during application of a microbicidal product involves both inactivation by the active ingredients as well as removal of pathogens during the wiping off of the microbicide following the contact time. The downside of this fact is that, if the active is not a potent inactivating agent, the pathogens may simply be spread around during the application process.

Air, water, and surface decontamination may also be achieved through use of physical methods such as ultraviolet light (UV) treatment. Water decontamination by means of UV treatment devices to reduce the levels of infectious coliforms is commonly employed within developed countries, especially in rural settings where water wells supply the potable water for daily use. Surface decontamination using UV is more common in industrial/health care settings than in the home, due primarily to safety issues. Air decontamination devices based on physical removal (filtration) and/or UV treatment are available, although again, are not widely used in home settings.[31] A recent study from Dr Sattar's lab (B. Zargar et al, unpublished data, September 10, 2009) demonstrated that decontamination of experimentally aerosolized bacteria prevents microbial contamination of nonporous environmental surfaces by approximately 90%. This suggests that targeting airborne pathogens can reduce the risk of spread of infections to environmental surfaces and subsequent dissemination through the *air-surface-hand nexus*.[89]

The recent emergence of Ebola Makona variant virus (EBOV/Mak) resulted in unprecedented morbidity and mortality as human-to-human spread resulted in extensive virus dissemination across six African nations. Nosocomial transmission of this virus also occurred as patients were evacuated to Europe and the United States. The evaluation of Ebola virus survival on experimentally contaminated environmental surfaces and the study of efficacy of microbicidal products for surface decontamination were, therefore, undertaken in a BL4 laboratory by Cook et al.[90,91] It was reported that despite being an enveloped virus, EBOV/Mak survived for up to 8 days on fomites. Survival was favored on stainless steel (inactivation constant [k_i] is equal to approximately 0.4 log_{10}/day, compared with a k_i of approximately 7.3 log_{10}/day on a cloth gown).[90] Sodium hypochlorite– and ethanol-based microbicidal products demonstrated concentration- and contact time–dependent inactivation of EBOV/Mak suspended in simulated organic load on steel carriers.[90,91] Studies using coliphage MS2 as a surrogate for Ebola virus demonstrated that the addition of microbicidal products (peracetic acid, QAC, or hydrogen peroxide) to contaminated toilet bowls reduced the viral contamination of nearby surfaces after flushing.[92]

Recent studies on personal protective equipment for use with Ebola have demonstrated that liquid stress/saturation during hot humid conditions and wearer perspiration/condensation can impact the ability of masks to exclude the virus and could potentially compromise the protection of mask-wearers. Based on these findings, the use of powered air-purifying respirators has been suggested because these provide air circulation and liquid-impermeable protection.[93]

Evaluation of the comparative efficacies of several microbicidal products against murine norovirus (a surrogate for human norovirus) revealed significant efficacy for formulations based on sodium hypochlorite, oxidizing agents, and for a formulation containing a QAC, alcohol, and aldehyde. This led the authors to recommend these microbicidal products for application on potentially contaminated environmental surfaces or materials with food contact.[94] The efficacy of neutral electrolyzed water at 250 ppm free available chlorine as an environmentally friendly, less corrosive/irritant, alternative to bleach has been evaluated against norovirus-contaminated environmental surfaces.[95] Neutral electrolyzed water applied for a 30-minute contact time reduced the infectious titer of Tulane virus (a norovirus surrogate) by 4.1 log_{10}. For hard-to-reach surfaces, methods for decontamination using microbicidal fogging have been employed. For instance, Montazeri et al[96] reported that hydrogen peroxide (7.5%) delivered by fog achieved >4 log_{10} reduction of infectious feline calicivirus within a 5-minute contact time, thereby meeting the EPA 4 log_{10} reduction required for a claim of norovirucidal activity.[97]

The requisite efficacy of a microbicidal product to be used as a disinfectant, sanitizer, or a virucide is a topic of current interest. Historically, registration and use of microbicidal products in the United States has been based on specific log_{10} inactivation requirements in defined test methods set forth by the EPA (see also chapter 62). For instance, the EPA defines a sanitizer as "a substance, or mixture of substances, that reduces the bacterial population in the inanimate environment by significant numbers, (e.g., 3 log_{10} reduction) or more, but does not destroy or eliminate all bacteria."[98] Note that the emphasis is on bactericidal efficacy, and virucidal efficacy (in particular, against nonenveloped viruses) cannot be assumed from this claim. As mentioned earlier, a registered norovirucide must demonstrate a 4 log_{10} inactivation of a norovirus surrogate.[97] The practical significance of a 3 or 4 log_{10} reduction (ie, 99.9% or 99.99%, respectively) in burden of a pathogen for mitigating risk of pathogen transfer, of course, can only be determined if the initial burden of the pathogen on the surface is known. For instance, it has been reported that approximately 10^{12} rotavirus and approximately 10^{11} norovirus particles are present per gram of stool from infected patients during the acute phase of illness.[99,100] If surfaces in the bathroom are contaminated with only 10^8 virus particles during this phase of infection, a risk of transfer of sufficient infectious viral particles to cause infection (considering the low MID for these viruses—see Table 48.1) might remain for over 100 days in the absence of decontamination of the virus-contaminated surface.

In fact, the initial burden of a pathogen during a contamination event is typically not known; therefore, the safety of a contaminated surface cannot be assured following application of a microbicide. For example, the impact of a 99% (2 $\log_{10}$), 99.9% (3 $\log_{10}$), or 99.99% (4 $\log_{10}$) reduction in titer of an infectious agent depends on the initial pathogen burden, as depicted in Figure 48.6. The risk associated with any remaining pathogen titer following application of a microbicidal product will depend on the MID of the pathogen. This argues that the requirement for efficacy of a microbicidal product based on a fixed $\log_{10}$ (or percentage) reduction may not be appropriate, or, at best, may be misleading to the public.

A new approach being used for determining the necessary $\log_{10}$ reduction to be achieved by a microbicidal product is the use of quantitative microbial risk assessment (QMRA). This approach has, until now, been applied primarily to water treatment systems but is more recently also being applied to environmental surface decontamination. In this case, the QMRA is based on specific dose-response models, determination of aerobic bacteria and specific pathogens on fomites, exposure assessment, and risk characterization.[101] A QMRA analysis performed for seven pathogens, including *E coli*, *E coli* 0157:H7, *L monocytogenes*, norovirus, *Pseudomonas* species, *Salmonella* species, and *S aureus* suggested, for instance, that a reduction in bacterial numbers on a

fomite by 99% (2 $\log_{10}$) might reduce the risk of infection from a single contact to less than 1 in 1 million.

Pathogens within biofilms tend to be much less susceptible to microbicidal products compared to their planktonic counterparts (see also chapter 67).[102,103] For biofilm-forming bacteria, including mycobacteria, it could be argued that the use of a method such as the ASTM E2871-13 method[104] is more appropriate than the methods more typically used for assessing activity of microbicidal products intended for decontamination of environmental surfaces and to support product registrations.

In certain areas of the world (especially India, China, Brazil), the concept of *complementary and alternative medicine* has been practiced in the past, and this practice continues to the present. Natural products, such as therapies derived from neem (*Azadirachta indica*), as an example, are used for a variety of antimicrobial, antifungal, antiviral, and antiparasitic applications.[105] This efficacy also includes activity against foodborne pathogens.[106]

It should be noted that the efficacy of microbicidal products on contaminated environmental surfaces are typically not specific to pathogens. The indoor microbiome of the surfaces, including commensals that might compete with pathogenic microbial agents in a beneficial manner, are likely to be disrupted through nonjudicious use of current microbicidal products. The desirability of managing "healthy"/balanced versus pathogenic microbial populations is discussed in the following text.

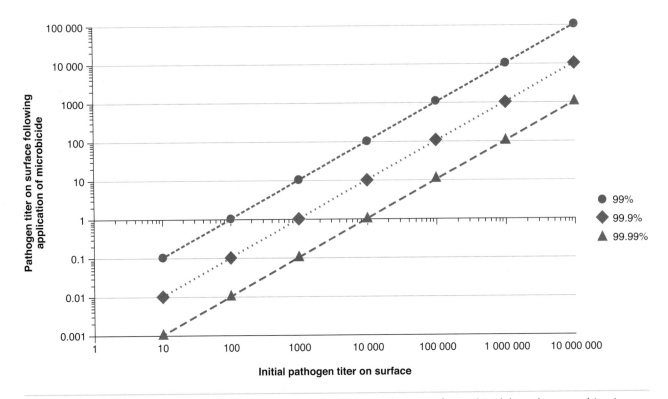

FIGURE 48.6   The pathogen burden (titer) on a surface following application of microbicidal products resulting in various percentage reduction: dependency on the initial pathogen titer.

▶ FUTURE PERSPECTIVES

As mentioned throughout this chapter, the historical approach to pathogen reduction on surfaces has involved attempts to effectively reduce microbes naturally present in those areas. For decades, we have been bombarded with advertisements in the media implying that, for maintaining health, we must eradicate all *germs* from our environments. This approach has not accounted for the possible beneficial impact of nonpathogenic microorganisms in managing a natural diverse versus a dysbiotic indoor microbiome. More recently, it has become clear that establishing, maintaining, and regulating health involves a paradigm shift that goes beyond our antiquated *germ theory* of disease toward a more holistic *microbial theory of health, wellness, and disease prevention.*

As a result of the recent evolution of molecular sequencing techniques and methodologies enabling rapid and less cost-prohibitive study of microbial communities, a wealth of scientific literature on human and indoor microbiomes has been accumulating over the past decade. In addition, there is an increased scrutiny on the indiscriminate use of microbicidal products and the resulting impacts on the environment as well as public concerns about generating microbicide-resistant infectious agents.[4]

Probiotics for maintaining a healthy gastrointestinal microbiome, such as those contained in yogurts and fermented products such as kimchi and more recently kombucha,[107] are well established in the food industry, and the use of such products is becoming more mainstream in personal health care. As an example, recent studies of the oral microbiome have suggested that disruption of the natural diversity of microorganisms (dysbiosis) occurs in periodontal disease.[108] This suggests the possibility of future treatments aimed at tailoring the oral microbiome, rather than simply attempting to eliminate oral microbial populations altogether.

The human skin microbiome of healthy adults is relatively stable and resilient.[109] It is interesting that there appears to be a different skin microbiome associated with populations, such as the Yanomami Amerindians of Venezuela, who have been devoid of contact with individuals from developed countries.[110] The study of such communities suggests that westernization and urbanization has led to a substantial loss in diversity of exposure to the beneficial environmental microorganisms our ancestors were exposed to for centuries and that apparently were essential for appropriate development of our immune systems. Differences in the skin microbiome of individuals living in megacities have been reported by Kim et al.[111] The skin microbiomes were impacted by factors such as environment and socioeconomic status. The outdoor environment and level of physical activity may also contribute to the acquisition of the human microbiome via skin and airways.[6]

On the other hand, the indoor microbiome seems to be more transient.[112] The modern home is not considered a *natural* setting and the composition of the indoor microbiome in such dwellings is not stable, being heavily influenced by the daily activities of the human, domesticated animal, and plant inhabitants as well as external factors, such as pollution and other chemical contributors to our exposome.[113] The types of shelters or habitats in which our ancestors lived in the distant past would have provided continuous exposure to external elements such as dirt, animals, plants, and natural water sources. Exposure to this natural outdoor microbiome has now been reduced. The consequent impact to health is thought to include an increased incidence of asthma and other manifestations of allergies. For instance, children growing up on traditional Amish farms in contact with animals have been shown to be less prone to asthma and other types of allergic reactions.[114] The reduced incidence of allergic reactivity in such children is attributed to the inhalation of air containing bacterial endotoxin (lipopolysaccharide), which is thought to reduce the overall reactivity of the immune system.[114] In support of this, a reduction in development of house dust mite–related asthma induced by an allergic stimulus in mice chronically exposed to bacterial endotoxin has been demonstrated by Schuijs et al.[115] This protection relied on the induction, by endotoxin, of the ubiquitin-modifying enzyme A20 in the lung epithelium of mice. In humans, the level of a variant of A20 correlates with increased susceptibility to asthma and allergy in children growing up on farms. Endotoxin was found to reduce epithelial cell cytokines that activate dendritic cells, thus suppressing type 2 immunity to house dust mites. Loss of A20 function in lung epithelium abolished this protective effect of endotoxin.[115]

These results support the *old friends hypothesis* ("bidirectional hygiene or bygiene" concept) mentioned earlier,[9] which is gaining ground as a viable replacement for the *hygiene hypothesis*[5] that attributed increased allergic reactivity to absence of exposure to pathogens during childhood. The term *old friends* in this context refers to nonpathogenic microbes that are found in the natural environment and help shape the development of our immune systems. The most impactful window of exposure to these OF is postulated to be during early childhood.[6]

A beneficial indoor home microbiome product of the future might make the indoors more like the outdoors. For instance, products containing probiotics, beneficial environmental bacteria, or components of these bacteria might be capable of interacting with the developing immune system in a manner that reduces the types of allergic reactions now being seen in children. This type of product might also provide a constant exposure to such bacteria in order to keep the immune system functioning appropriately. We note the recent introduction into the market of the first type of this product, the probiotic-based cleaning hygiene system (PCHS).[116] The PCHS has been evaluated in a hospital setting and is claimed to provide nonpathogenic bacteria to outcompete pathogens, with the objective of minimizing risk of exposure to nosocomial infections and increasing exposure to a healthy indoor microbiome.

At the time of writing of this chapter, a paucity of studies has been reported in the published literature on such alternative approaches, and the mechanism of action that might best be employed remains to be elucidated. Therefore, regarding products intended to serve this purpose, there currently are more questions than answers, and it will be interesting to watch this field evolve. Future research should be conducted to identify the best mix of probiotics; the appropriate or optimal delivery systems; the safety profiles/considerations; potential for causing or preventing infections; the potential impacts of age (particularly the benefit for young children, infants, newborns, as well as older children/adults); and the potential risks for the immunocompromised, aging, and malnourished populations.

Finally, there is a need to promote greater public understanding of the role of the microbiome in human health and wellness. Shifting this paradigm toward a microbial theory of health, wellness, and disease prevention should not be allowed to undermine the critical role that

targeted personal and surface hygiene practices play in interrupting the dissemination of infectious agents. It is the responsibility of subject matter experts to restore the public understanding of the basic principles of good hygiene practices and the importance of the concept of targeted hygiene as a means of minimizing the dissemination of infectious agents. In devising best practices for informing the public in both developed and developing countries, it will be wise to draw on field studies from developing countries (eg, Cole et al[85]) that have demonstrated the critical importance of hygiene education in addition to the use of appropriate microbicidal "tools." In explaining targeted hygiene to the public with reference to *common-touch surfaces* such as those outlined in Figure 48.7, key questions to consider include the following:

1. What are the key targets for microbicidal product use?
2. When is the right time and place to act?
3. Who is most at risk in home and community settings?
4. Which smart, targeted hygiene interventions can be employed?

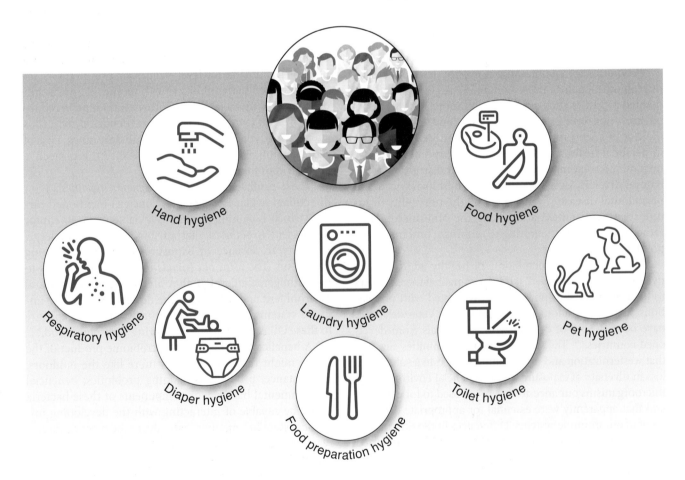

FIGURE 48.7 Public education should highlight the *common-touch surfaces* for practicing targeted hygiene. Practicing hygiene is particularly important during and after activities such as handling food or eating, handling raw foods (such as meat, poultry, fish, eggs, fruits, and vegetables), using the toilet, diapering, contacting blood or body fluids, touching contaminated porous or nonporous surfaces, dressing a wound or administering medications, touching animals, or performing outdoor activities such as gardening.

Focusing on selected behaviors, such as hand washing with soap and clean water, is particularly impactful, and encouraging hand washing at appropriate times before and after high-risk activities can help to significantly reduce the risk of exposure to infectious agents.

◗ CONCLUSIONS

In conclusion, it is time to recognize the paradigm shift from the germ theory of disease to the *microbial theory of health*. This also will require a change in the approaches that we take to manage the indoor microbiome to those that reduce the risk posed by infectious agents, using targeted hygiene and intentional exposure to naturally diverse microbial communities. Interestingly, health care providers have started shifting their emphasis in this direction by promoting critical care microbiome research/applications to treat dysbiosis in intensive care patients, an ambitious but encouraging goal.[117] Recently, a pragmatic use of currently practiced therapeutic agents for treatment/prevention of infectious agents has also been suggested by Rook and coworkers.[118]

Environmental surfaces may serve as reservoirs for infectious agents deposited following shedding from humans or domesticated animals or arising from contaminated raw meats, fruits, and vegetables including pathogen-contaminated air and water. Infectious agents have been found to survive on indoor environmental surfaces for extended periods of time, in many instances remaining for days to months at populations high enough to initiate infection of a new host. *Common-touch surfaces* such as door knobs, toilet flush handles, faucet handles, remote controls, digital devices, and light switches play an important role in dissemination of these infectious agents throughout the indoor space. The cycle of infection and reinfection involves dissemination, primarily through the intermediacy of the human hand, from these *common-touch surfaces* to new surfaces and/or other hosts. This cycle may be interrupted through the timely/judicial use of microbicidal products targeted to decontaminate *common-touch surfaces* following high-risk activities such as using the toilet, preparing food, or handling other *common-touch surfaces*.

An effective strategy for minimizing the risks associated with the deposition of infectious agents on *common-touch surfaces* and the ensuing cycle of infection requires the availability of effective microbicidal products and hygiene practices, including the knowledge of how and when to exercise these practices. The points to be considered in developing targeted surface decontamination practices include (1) the probability of significant pathogen contamination at the surface under consideration, (2) the types of pathogens that are most likely to survive on surfaces and the time periods over which these might remain infectious at levels in excess of the minimum

human infectious dose, (3) the likelihood of pathogen transfer from the contaminated surface to human hands and to other surfaces and hosts, and (4) the susceptibility of the new hosts to acquiring infection.

In considering targeted surface decontamination practices, it is important to select appropriate microbicidal products for each potential application. In making this selection, the spectrum of microbicidal activity, contact time required, presence of organic load, and efficacy should be considered. Efficacy of microbicidal products (ie, the $\log_{10}$ or percentage reduction of pathogens that is required) should be determined on the basis of a QMRA, rather than relying on a set of fixed and somewhat arbitrary requirements. However, for extending application of QMRA to the broad range of human pathogens of concern, further research is needed to provide the necessary data on (1) typical surface pathogen burdens to be expected when a person is ill and excreting the pathogen at the highest rate, (2) the survival and persistence (ie, the k_i) of pathogens on contaminated *common-touch surfaces*, (3) the distribution of pathogens in indoor settings and transfer/acquisition of pathogens during different activities highlighted earlier (*air-surface-hand nexus*), and (4) reduction below the minimum infectious dose for a given pathogen posttargeted application of appropriate microbicidal product.

This chapter attempts to put into perspective the various factors associated with transmission to humans of pathogens from contaminated surfaces in everyday settings and the associated risks to human health. There is much evidence indicating that targeted decontamination can play an important role in prevention and control of the acquisition, through the intermediacy of the hand, of infectious agents from pathogen-contaminated environmental surfaces. Such decontamination may help to minimize the risk of transmission of infectious agents and, at the same time, may preserve a naturally diverse home microbiome. The future brings the exciting possibility for implementation of new technologies for decontaminating everyday settings that are based on our emerging understanding of the complex relationships between humans and microorganisms.

◗ ACKNOWLEDGMENTS

The authors gratefully acknowledge Joseph Rubino, BA, MA (RB Research and Development), for critically reviewing this chapter; Jennifer Fairman, CMI, FAMI (Fairman Studios, LLC), for creating the illustrations; and Dr Raymond W. Nims (RMC Pharmaceutical Solutions, Inc) for editorial support. We are also indebted to Dr Charles P. Gerba (University of Arizona) for insightful discussions and for relating results obtained with the Ebola virus from his laboratory, Dr Yuguo Li (The University of Hong Kong) for sharing the concept of surface contamination networks, Dr Absar Alum (Arizona State University) for providing enteric parasite survival data, Dr Syed A. Sattar (University of Ottawa and CREM Co) for sharing results on the role of indoor air decontamination to reduce contamination of environmental surfaces, and Drs Syed A. Sattar and Jean-Yves Maillard (Cardiff University) for clarifying some of the terminologies used.

REFERENCES

1. Bloomfield S. The hygiene hypothesis: identifying microbial friends and protecting against microbial enemies. *Perspect Public Health.* 2013;133:301-303.

2. Scott E. Community-based infections and the potential role of common touch surfaces as vectors for the transmission of infectious agents in home and community settings. *Am J Infect Control.* 2013;41:1087-1092.

3. Bloomfield SF, Exner M, Nath KJ, Signorelli C, Scott EA. The chain of infection transmission in the home and everyday life settings, and the role of hygiene in reducing the risk of infection. International Scientific Forum on Home Hygiene Web site. https://www.ifh-homehygiene .org/review/chain-infection-transmission-home-and-everyday-life -settings-and-role-hygiene-reducing-risk. Accessed May 30, 2019.

4. Barber S, Swaden-Lewis K, Harker R. Antimicrobial resistance. https://researchbriefings.parliament.uk/ResearchBriefing/Summary /CBP-8141. Published November 15, 2017. Accessed May 30, 2019.

5. Strachan DP. Hay fever, hygiene, and household size. *BMJ.* 1989; 299:1259-1260.

6. Bloomfield SF, Rook GAW, Scott EA, Shanahan F, Stanwell-Smith R, Turner P. Time to abandon the hygiene hypothesis: new perspectives on allergic disease, the human microbiome, infectious disease prevention and the role of targeted hygiene. *Perspect Public Health.* 2016;136:213-224.

7. Dowling D. Developing an approach to consumer hygiene practice and products that can maximize protection from infection and minimize the risk of disrupting our microbial friends. Paper presented at: 3rd Annual Translational Microbiome Conference; April 11-13, 2017; Boston, MA.

8. Dowling DJ, Levy O. Ontogeny of early life immunity. *Trends Immunol.* 2014;35:299-310.

9. Al-Ghalith GA, Knights D. Bygiene: the new paradigm of bidirectional hygiene. *Yale J Biol Med.* 2015;88:359-365.

10. Sattar SA, Maillard JY. The crucial role of wiping in decontamination of high-touch environmental surfaces: review of current status and directions for the future. *Am J Infect Control.* 2013;41:S97-S104.

11. Boone SA, Gerba CP. Significance of fomites in the spread of respiratory and enteric viral disease. *Appl Environ Microbiol.* 2007;73:1687-1696.

12. Koganti S, Alhmidi H, Tomas ME, Cadnum JL, Jencson A, Donskey CJ. Evaluation of hospital floors as a potential source of pathogen dissemination using a nonpathogenic virus as a surrogate marker. *Infect Control Hosp Epidemiol.* 2016;37:1374-1377.

13. Centers for Disease Control and Prevention. Wash your hands. Centers for Disease Control and Prevention Web site. https://www.cdc.gov /cdctv/healthyliving/hygiene/wash-your-hands.html?CDC_AA_ref Val=https%3A%2F%2Fwww.cdc.gov%2Fcdctv%2Fhealthyliving%2F hygiene%2Fhands-together-hygiene.html. Accessed May 30, 2019.

14. Alum A, Rubino JR, Ijaz MK. The global war against intestinal parasites—should we use a holistic approach? *Int J Infect Dis.* 2010;14:e732-e738.

15. Kramer A, Schwebke I, Kampf G. How long do nosocomial pathogens persist on inanimate surfaces? A systematic review. *BMC Infect Dis.* 2006;6:130. doi:10.1186/1471-2334-6-130.

16. Abad FX, Pintó RM, Bosch A. Survival of enteric viruses on environmental fomites. *Appl Environ Microbiol.* 1994;60:3704-3710.

17. Doultree JC, Druce JD, Birch CJ, Bowden DS, Marshall JA. Inactivation of feline calicivirus, a Norwalk virus surrogate. *J Hosp Infect.* 1999;41:51-57.

18. Sattar SA, Karim YG, Springthorpe VS, Johnson-Lussenburg CM. Survival of human rhinovirus type 14 dried onto nonporous inanimate surfaces: effect of relative humidity and suspending medium. *Can J Microbiol.* 1987;33:802-806.

19. Warnes SL, Little ZR, Keevil CW. Human coronavirus 229E remains infectious on common touch surface materials. *mBio.* 2015;6:e01697-15. doi:10.1128/mBio.01697-15.

20. Bean B, Moore BM, Sterner B, Peterson LR, Gerding DN, Balfour HH Jr. Survival of influenza viruses on environmental surfaces. *J Infect Dis.* 1982;146:47-51.

21. Casanova LM, Jeon S, Rutala WA, Weber DJ, Sobsey MD. Effects of air temperature and relative humidity on coronavirus survival on surfaces. *Appl Environ Microbiol.* 2010;76:2712-2717.

22. Otter JA, French GL. Survival of nosocomial bacteria and spores on surfaces and inactivation by hydrogen peroxide vapor. *J Clin Microbiol.* 2009;47:205-207.

23. Humphrey TJ, Martin KW, Slader J, Durham K. *Campylobacter* spp. in the kitchen: spread and persistence. *Symp Ser Soc Appl Microbiol.* 2001;(30):115S-120S.

24. Kothary MH, Babu US. Infective dose of foodborne pathogens in volunteers: a review. *J Food Safety.* 2001;21:49-73.

25. Wilks SA, Michels H, Keevil CW. The survival of *Escherichia coli* O157 on a range of metal surfaces. *Int J Food Microbiol.* 2005;105:445-454.

26. Traoré O, Springthorpe VS, Sattar SA. A quantitative study of the survival of two species of *Candida* on porous and non-porous environmental surfaces and hands. *J Appl Microbiol.* 2002;92:549-555.

27. Health Canada Pathogen safety data sheets. Government of Canada Web site. https://www.canada.ca/en/public-health/services/laboratory -biosafety-biosecurity/pathogen-safety-data-sheets-risk-assessment .html#t. Accessed May 30, 2019.

28. Stachan R, Kunstýr I. Minimal infectious doses and prepatent periods in *Giardia muris*, *Spironucleus muris* and *Tritrichomonas muris*. *Zentralbl Bakteriol Mikrobiol Hyg A.* 1983;256:249-256.

29. van Doremalen N, Bushmaker T, Munster VJ. Stability of Middle East respiratory syndrome coronavirus (MERS-CoV) under different environmental conditions. *Euro Surveill.* 2013;18. doi:10.2807/1560-7917 .ES2013.18.38.20590.

30. Alum A, Absar IM, Asaad H, Rubino J, Ijaz MK. Impact of environmental conditions on the survival of *Cryptosporidium* and *Giardia* on environmental surfaces. *Interdiscip Perspect Infect Dis.* 2014;2014:210385. doi:10.1155/2014/210385.

31. Ijaz MK, Zargar B, Wright KE, Rubino JR, Sattar SA. Generic aspects of the airborne spread of human pathogens indoors and emerging air decontamination technologies. *Am J Infect Control.* 2016;44:S109-S120.

32. Vasickova P, Pavlik I, Verani M, Carducci A. Issues concerning survival of viruses on surfaces. *Food Environ Virol.* 2010;2:24-34.

33. Prakash B, Veeregowda BM, Krishnappa G. Biofilms: a survival strategy of bacteria. *Curr Sci.* 2003;85:1299-1307.

34. Wilde C, Chen Z, Kapes T, et al. Inactivation and disinfection of Zika virus on a nonporous surface. *J Microb Biochem Technol.* 2016;8:422-427.

35. Mormann S, Heißenberg C, Pfannebecker J, Becker B. Tenacity of human norovirus and the surrogates feline calicivirus and murine norovirus during long-term storage on common nonporous food contact surfaces. *J Food Prot.* 2015;78:224-229.

36. Sattar SA, Lloyd-Evans N, Springthorpe VS, Nair RC. Institutional outbreaks of rotavirus diarrhoea: potential role of fomites and environmental surfaces as vehicles for virus transmission. *J Hyg (Lond).* 1986;96:277-289.

37. Mbithi JN, Springthorpe VS, Sattar SA. Effect of relative humidity and air temperature on survival of hepatitis A virus on environmental surfaces. *Appl Environ Microbiol.* 1991;57:1394-1399.

38. Kim SJ, Si J, Lee JE, Ko G. Temperature and humidity influences on inactivation kinetics of enteric viruses on surfaces. *Environ Sci Technol.* 2012;46:13303-13310.

39. Lei H, Li Y, Xiao S, et al. Logistic growth of a surface contamination network and its role in disease spread. *Sci Rep.* 2017;7:14826. doi:10.1038/s41598-017-13840-z.

40. Teixeira P, Silva S, Araújo F, Azeredo J, Oliveira R. Bacterial adhesion to food contacting surfaces. In: Méndez-Vilas A, ed. *Communicating Current Research and Educational Topics and Trends in Applied Microbiology*. Badajoz, Spain: Formatex; 2007:13-20. https://repositorium.sdum.uminho.pt/bitstream/1822/7711/1/Pilar_Teixeira_etal.pdf. Accessed May 30, 2019.

41. Gibson KE, Crandall PG, Ricke SC. Removal and transfer of viruses on food contact surfaces by cleaning cloths. *Appl Environ Microbiol.* 2012;78:3037-3044.

42. Rossi EM, Scapin D, Tondo EC. Survival and transfer of microorganisms from kitchen sponges to surfaces of stainless steel and polyethylene. *J Infect Dev Ctries.* 2013;7:229-234.

43. Tuladhar E, Hazeleger WC, Koopmans M, Zwietering MH, Duizer E, Beumer RR. Transfer of noroviruses between fingers and fomites and food products. *Int J Food Microbiol.* 2013;167:346-352.

44. Cardinale M, Kaiser D, Lueders T, Schnell S, Egert M. Microbiome analysis and confocal microscopy of used kitchen sponges reveal massive colonization by *Acinetobacter, Moraxella* and *Chryseobacterium* species. *Sci Rep.* 2017;7:5791. doi:10.1038/s41598-017-06055-9.

45. Scott E, Bloomfield SF. The survival and transfer of microbial contamination via cloths, hands and utensils. *J Appl Bacteriol.* 1990;68:271-278.

46. Gerba CP, Wallis C, Melnick JL. Microbiological hazards of household toilets: droplet production and the fate of residual organisms. *Appl Microbiol.* 1975;30:229-237.

47. Verani M, Bigazzi R, Carducci A. Viral contamination of aerosol and surfaces through toilet use in health care and other settings. *Am J Infect Control.* 2014;42:758-762.

48. Miura F, Watanabe T, Watanabe K, Takemoto K, Fukushi K. Comparative assessment of primary and secondary infection risks in a norovirus outbreak using a household model simulation. *J Environ Sci (China).* 2016;50:13-20.

49. Ibfelt T, Engelund EH, Permin A, Madsen JS, Schultz AC, Andersen LP. Presence of pathogenic bacteria and viruses in the daycare environment. *J Environ Health.* 2015;78:24-29.

50. Jones EL, Kramer A, Gaither M, Gerpa CP. Role of fomite contamination during an outbreak of norovirus on houseboats. *Int J Environ Health Res.* 2007;17:123-131.

51. Ijaz MK, Talukder KA, Aslam M, et al. Natural contamination of human hands with enteric parasites in Indian subcontinent. *World J Clin Infect Dis.* 2013;3:13-19.

52. Nagajothi J, Duraipandian J, Vigneshwaran S, Kumar P. Study of prevalence of microbial contamination with its antibiotic resistance pattern in automated teller machine in and around Puducherry, India. *Int J Earth Environ Health Sci.* 2015;1:27-31.

53. Onuoha SC, Fatokun K. Bacterial contamination and public health risk associated with the use of banks' automated teller machines (ATMs) in Ebonyi State, Nigeria. *Am J Public Health Res.* 2014;2:46-50.

54. Meadow JF, Altrichter AE, Green JL. Mobile phones carry the personal microbiome of their owners. *PeerJ.* 2014;2:e447. doi:10.7717/peerj.447.

55. Morvai J, Szabó R. The role of mobile communication devices in the spread of infections. *Orv Hetil.* 2015;156:802-807.

56. Bik HM, Maritz JM, Luong A, Shin H, Dominguez-Bello MG, Carlton JM. Microbial community patterns associated with automated teller machine keypads in New York City. *mSPhere.* 2016;1. doi:10.1128/mSphere.00226-16.

57. Hsu T, Joice R, Vallarino J, et al. Urban transit system microbial communities differ by surface type and interaction with humans and the environment. *mSystems.* 2016;1(3). doi:10.1128/mSystems.00018-16.

58. Barker J, Stevens D, Bloomfield SF. Spread and prevention of some common viral infections in community facilities and domestic homes. *J Appl Microbiol.* 2001;91:7-21.

59. Kagan LJ, Aiello AE, Larson E. The role of the home environment in the transmission of infectious diseases. *J Commun Health.* 2002;27:247-267.

60. Sattar SA, Springthorpe S, Mani S, et al. Transfer of bacteria from fabrics to hands and other fabrics: development and application of a quantitative method using *Staphylococcus aureus* as a model. *J Appl Microbiol.* 2001;90:962-970.

61. Winther B, McCue K, Ashe K, Rubino JR, Hendley JO. Environmental contamination with rhinovirus and transfer to fingers of healthy individuals by daily life activity. *J Med Virol.* 2007;79:1606-1610.

62. Winther B, McCue K, Ashe K, Rubino J, Hendley JO. Rhinovirus contamination of surfaces in homes of adults with natural colds: transfer of virus to fingertips during normal daily activities. *J Med Virol.* 2011;83:906-909.

63. Oristo S, Rönnqvist M, Aho M, et al. Contamination by norovirus and adenovirus on environmental surfaces and in hands of conscripts in two Finnish garrisons. *Food Environ Virol.* 2017;9:62-71.

64. Kraut RY, Snedeker KG, Babenko O, Honish L. Influence of school year on seasonality of norovirus outbreaks in developed countries. *Can J Infect Dis Med Microbiol.* 2017;2017:9258140. doi:10.1155/2017/9258140.

65. Bloomfield S, Carling PC, Exner M. A unified framework for developing effective hygiene procedures for hands, environmental surfaces and laundry in healthcare, domestic, food handling and other settings. *GMS Hyg Infect Control.* 2017;12:1-16.

66. Towers S, Chen J, Cruz C, et al. Quantifying the relative effects of environmental and direct transmission of norovirus. *R Soc Open Sci.* 2018;5(3):170602. doi:10.1098/rsos.170602.

67. Bidawid S, Malik N, Adegbunrin O, Sattar SA, Farber JM. Norovirus cross-contamination during food handling and interruption of virus transfer by hand antisepsis: experiments with feline calicivirus as a surrogate. *J Food Prot.* 2004;67:103-109.

68. Bidawid S, Farber JM, Sattar SA. Contamination of foods by food handlers: experiments on hepatitis A virus transfer to food and its interruption. *Appl Environ Microbiol.* 2000;66:2759-2763.

69. Josephson KL, Rubino JR, Pepper IL. Characterization and quantification of bacterial pathogens and indicator organisms in household kitchens with and without the use of a disinfectant cleaner. *J Appl Microbiol.* 1997;83:737-750.

70. Zhao P, Zhao T, Doyle MP, Rubino JR, Meng J. Development of a model for evaluation of microbial cross-contamination in the kitchen. *J Food Prot.* 1998;61:960-963.

71. Lopez GU, Kitajima M, Sherchan SP, et al. Impact of disinfectant wipes on the risk of *Campylobacter jejuni* infection during raw chicken preparation in domestic kitchens. *J Appl Microbiol.* 2015;119:245-252.

72. Lei H, Jones RM, Li Y. Exploring surface cleaning strategies in hospital to prevent contact transmission of methicillin-resistant *Staphylococcus aureus. BMC Infect Dis.* 2017;17:85. doi:10.1186/s12879-016-2120-z.

73. Warnes SL, Summersgill EN, Keevil CW. Inactivation of murine norovirus on a range of copper alloy surfaces is accompanied by loss of capsid integrity. *Appl Environ Microbiol.* 2015;81:1085-1091.

74. Kusumaningrum HD, van Putten MM, Rombouts FM, Beumer RR. Effects of antibacterial dishwashing liquid on foodborne pathogens and competitive microorganisms in kitchen sponges. *J Food Prot.* 2002;65:61-65.

75. Ward RL, Bernstein DI, Knowlton DR, et al. Prevention of surface-to-human transmission of rotaviruses by treatment with disinfectant spray. *J Clin Microbiol.* 1991;29:1991-1996.

76. Sattar SA, Jacobsen H, Springthorpe VS, Cusack TM, Rubino JR. Chemical disinfection to interrupt transfer of rhinovirus type 14 from environmental surfaces to hands. *Appl Environ Microbiol.* 1993;59:1579-1585.

77. Sattar SA, Ansari SA. The fingerpad protocol to assess hygienic hand antiseptics against viruses. *J Virol Methods.* 2002;103:171-181.

78. Liu P, Yuen Y, Hsiao HM, Jaykus LA, Moe C. Effectiveness of liquid soap and hand sanitizer against Norwalk virus on contaminated hands. *Appl Environ Microbiol.* 2010;76:394-399.

79. Larson EL, Cohen B, Baxter KA. Analysis of alcohol-based hand sanitizer delivery systems: efficacy of foam, gel, and wipes against influenza A (H1N1) virus on hands. *Am J Infect Control.* 2012;40:806-809.

80. World Health Organization. *WHO Guidelines on Hand Hygiene in Health Care: First Global Patient Safety Challenge Clean Care Is*

Safer Care. Geneva, Switzerland: World Health Organization. https://apps.who.int/iris/bitstream/handle/10665/44102/9789241597906_eng.pdf;jsessionid=127C400A969C0704C8F801750C61CECC?sequence=1. Accessed May 30, 2019.

81. Mehta A, Sequeira PS, Bhat G. Bacterial contamination and decontamination of toothbrushes after use. *NY State Dent J*. 2007;73:20-22.

82. Naik R, Ahmed Mujib BR, Telagi N, Anil BS, Spoorthi BR. Contaminated tooth brushes-potential threat to oral and general health. *J Family Med Prim Care*. 2015;4:444-448.

83. Bockmühl DP. Laundry hygiene—how to get more than clean. *J Appl Microbiol*. 2017;122:1124-1133.

84. Gerba CP, Kennedy D. Enteric virus survival during household laundering and impact of disinfection with sodium hypochlorite. *Appl Environ Microbiol*. 2007;73:4425-4428.

85. Cole EC, Hawkley M, Rubino JR, et al. Comprehensive family hygiene promotion in peri-urban Cape Town: gastrointestinal and respiratory illness and skin infection reduction in children aged under 5. *S Afr J CH*. 2012;6:109-117.

86. Chen Y, Bruning E, Rubino JR, Eder DE. Role of female intimate hygiene in vulvovaginal health: global hygiene practices and product usage. *Womens Health (Lond)*. 2017;13:58-67.

87. Maillard JY, Bloomfield S, Coelho JR, et al. Does microbicide use in consumer products promote antimicrobial resistance? A critical review and recommendations for a cohesive approach to risk assessment. *Microb Drug Resist*. 2013;19:344-354.

88. Fu E, McCue K, Boesenberg D. Chemical disinfection of hard surfaces—household, industrial and institutional settings. In: Johansson I, Somasundaran P, eds. *Handbook for Cleaning/Decontamination of Surfaces*. Oxford, United Kingdom: Elsevier; 2007:573-593.

89. Sattar SA, Kibbee RJ, Zargar B, Wright KE, Rubino JR, Ijaz MK. Decontamination of indoor air to reduce the risk of airborne infections: studies on survival and inactivation of airborne pathogens using an aerobiology chamber. *Am J Infect Control*. 2016;44:e172-e182.

90. Cook BW, Cutts TA, Nikiforuk AM, et al. Evaluating environmental persistence and disinfection of the Ebola virus Makona variant. *Viruses*. 2015;7:1975-1986.

91. Cook BW, Cutts TA, Nikiforuk AM, Leung A, Kobasa D, Theriault SS. The disinfection characteristics of Ebola virus outbreak variants. *Sci Rep*. 2016;6:38293. doi:10.1038/srep38293.

92. Sassi HP, Reynolds KA, Pepper IL, Gerba CP. Evaluation of hospital-grade disinfectants on viral deposition on surfaces after toilet flushing. *Am J Infect Control*. 2018;46(5):505-511.

93. Nikiforuk AM, Cutts TA, Theriault SS, Cook BW. Challenge of liquid stressed protective materials and environmental persistence of Ebola virus. *Sci Rep*. 2017;7:4388. doi:10.1038/s41598-017-04137-2.

94. Zonta W, Maurov A, Famir F, Thiry E. Comparative virucidal efficacy of seven disinfectants against murine norovirus and feline calicivirus, surrogates of human norovirus. *Food Environ Virol*. 2016;8:1-12.

95. Moorman E, Montazeri N, Jaykus LA. Efficacy of neutral electrolyzed water for inactivation of human norovirus. *Appl Environ Microbiol*. 2017;83. doi: 10.1128/AEM.00653-17.

96. Montazeri N, Manuel C, Moorman E, Khatiwada JR, Williams LL, Jaykus LA. Virucidal activity of fogged chlorine dioxide- and hydrogen peroxide-based disinfectants against human norovirus and its surrogate, *feline calicivirus*, on hard-to-reach surfaces. *Front Microbiol*. 2017;8:1033. doi:10.3389/fmicb.2017.01031.

97. Antimicrobials Division, US Environmental Protection Agency. Confirmatory virucidal effectiveness test using feline calicivirus as surrogate for norovirus. US Environmental Protection Agency Web site. https://www.epa.gov/sites/production/files/2015-09/documents/fcv2_confirm_surf_pcol.pdf. Accessed May 30, 2019.

98. US Environmental Protection Agency. Pesticide registration manual: chapter 4—additional considerations for antimicrobial products. US Environmental Protection Agency Web site. https://www.epa.gov/pesticide-registration/pesticide-registration-manual-chapter-4-additional-considerations. Accessed May 30, 2019.

99. Atmar RL, Opekun AR, Gilger MA, et al. Norwalk virus shedding after experimental human infection. *Emerg Infect Dis*. 2008;14:1553-1557.

100. Cortese MM, Prashar UD. Prevention of rotavirus gastroenteritis among infants and children recommendations of the Advisory Committee on Immunization Practices (ACIP). *MMWR Recomm Rep*. 2009;58(RR02):1-25. https://www.cdc.gov/mmwr/preview/mmwrhtml/rr5802a1.htm. Accessed May 30, 2019.

101. Ryan MO, Haas CN, Gurian PL, Gerba CP, Panzl BM, Rose JB. Application of quantitative microbial risk assessment for selection of microbial reduction targets for hard surface disinfectants. *Am J Infect Control*. 2014;42:1165-1172.

102. Bridier A, Briandet R, Thomas V, Dubois-Brissonnet F. Resistance of bacterial biofilms to disinfectants: a review. *Biofouling*. 2011;27:1017-1032.

103. Vázquez-Sánchez D, Cabo ML, Ibusquiza PS, Herrera JJ. Biofilm-forming ability and resistance to industrial disinfectants of *Staphylococcus aureus* isolated from fishery products. *Food Control*. 2014;39:81-16.

104. ASTM International. E2871-13. Standard test method for evaluating disinfectant efficacy against *Pseudomonas aeruginosa* biofilm grown in CDC biofilm reactor using single tube method. ASTM International Web site. https://www.astm.org/Standards/E2871.htm. Accessed May 30, 2019.

105. Alzohairy MA. Therapeutics role of *Azadirachta indica* (neem) and their active constituent in diseases prevention and treatment. *Evid Based Complement Alternat Med*. 2016;2016:7382506. doi:10.1155/2016/7382506.

106. Mahfuzul Hoque MD, Bari ML, Inatsu Y, Juneja VK, Kawamoto S. Antibacterial activity of guava (*Psidium guajava* L.) and neem (*Azadirachta indica* A. Juss.) extracts against foodborne pathogens and spoilage bacteria. *Foodborne Pathog Dis*. 2007;4:481-488.

107. Kozyrovska NO, Reva OM, Goginyan VB, de Vera JP. Kombucha microbiome as a probiotic: a view from the perspective of post-genomics and synthetic ecology. *Biopolymer Cell*. 2012;28:103-113.

108. Costalonga M, Herzberg MC. The oral microbiome and the immunobiology of periodontal disease and caries. *Immunol Lett*. 2014;162:22-38.

109. Oh J, Byrd AL, Park M, Kong H, Segre J; and NISC Comparative Sequencing Program. Temporal stability of the human skin microbiome. *Cell*. 2016;165:854-866.

110. Clemente JC, Pehrsson EC, Blaser MJ, et al. The microbiome of uncontacted Amerindians. *Sci Adv*. 2015;1:e150018.

111. Kim HJ, Kim H, Kim JJ, et al. Fragile skin microbiomes in megacities are assembled by a predominantly niche-based process. *Sci Adv*. 2018;4:e1701581.

112. Lax S, Smith DP, Hampton-Marcell J, et al. Longitudinal analysis of microbial interaction between humans and the indoor environment. *Science*. 2014;345:1048-1052.

113. Dai D, Prussin AJ II, Marr LC, Vikesland PJ, Edwards MA, Pruden A. Factors shaping the human exposome in the built environment: opportunities for engineering control. *Environ Sci Technol*. 2017;51:7759-7774.

114. Stein MM, Hrusch CL, Gozdz J, et al. Innate immunity and asthma risk in Amish and Hutterite farm children. *New Engl J Med*. 2016;375:411-421.

115. Schuijs MJ, Willart MA, Vergote K, et al. Farm dust and endotoxin protect against allergy through A20 induction in lung epithelial cells. *Science*. 2015;349:1106-1110.

116. Caselli E, D'Accolti M, Vandini A, et al. Impact of a probiotic-based cleaning intervention on the microbiota ecosystem of the hospital surfaces: focus on the resistome remodulation. *PLoS One*. 2016;11(2):e0148857. doi:10.1371/journal.pone.0148857.

117. Kitsios GD, Morowitz MJ, Dickson RP, Huffnagle GB, McVerry BJ, Morris A. Dysbiosis in the intensive care unit: microbiome science coming to the bedside. *J Crit Care*. 2017;38:84-91.

118. Rook G, Bäckhed F, Levin BR, McFall-Ngai MJ, McLean AR. Evolution, human-microbe interactions, and life history plasticity. *Lancet*. 2017;390:521-530.

Basic Principles of Infection Prevention and Control

Charles Edmiston Jr and Gwen Borlaug

Health care–associated infections (HAIs), formerly called nosocomial infections, are infections that sometimes occur among patients receiving medical care. They are associated with the use of invasive medical devices such as central venous catheters (CVC), urinary catheters, and mechanical ventilators and can also occur following surgical and other invasive procedures. The four major HAI types of concern include central line–associated bloodstream infections (CLABSI); catheter-associated urinary tract infections (CAUTI); surgical site infections (SSIs); and ventilator-associated adverse events (VAE), which include ventilator-associated pneumonia (VAP). Exposure to antibiotic agents also puts patients at risk of acquiring *Clostridium difficile* infections (CDI) and infections caused by multidrug-resistant organisms (MDRO) such as methicillin-resistant *Staphylococcus aureus* (MRSA), vancomycin-resistant *Enterococcus* (VRE), and carbapenem-resistant gram-negative bacteria.

The HAIs are associated with increased morbidity, mortality, and higher cost of health care delivery.[1] During the 1960s, hospitals developed infection control programs to conduct HAI surveillance and to implement measures to address these adverse events. By the mid-1970s, the Joint Commission on Accreditation of Healthcare Organizations (JCAHO) included a standard that required hospitals to develop and implement infection control programs as part of the accreditation process. At that time, approximately 30% of HAIs were considered preventable, based on a study conducted by the Centers for Disease Control and Prevention (CDC).[2] Today, because the science of prevention has advanced, we now know much larger proportions of HAIs are preventable than once thought. Furthermore, attitudes among providers, health care quality experts, infection preventionists, and public health officials toward HAIs have changed. Once considered inevitable consequences of providing health care, HAIs are currently viewed as unacceptable and largely preventable outcomes of patient care.

◗ PREVALENCE OF HEALTH CARE–ASSOCIATED INFECTIONS

During 2011, the CDC conducted a multistate point-prevalence survey to estimate the occurrence of HAIs among hospital patients, using the surveillance definitions from the National Healthcare Safety Network (NHSN), the national HAI database maintained by the CDC. The study revealed that approximately 650 000, or 4% of hospital patients, acquired 722 000 HAIs, and 75 000 patients died with an HAI during their hospital stay. The most prevalent types of HAI were non-VAP (157 000) and SSIs (157 000), each of which comprised 22% of the total number of HAIs identified in the survey. *C difficile* was the most prevalent health care–associated pathogen, with approximately 12% of HAIs caused by this organism, compared to 7% of HAIs caused by MRSA.

This study highlights the changing epidemiology of HAIs. Historically, device-associated infections have been the most prevalent type of HAI; however, in this study, they comprised only 25% of HAIs, with CDI, other gastrointestinal infections, and non-VAP comprising half of all reported HAIs. Modern-day health care infection prevention efforts must include strategies to prevent these types of HAIs in addition to the traditional focus on device-associated and invasive procedure–associated infections.[3]

◗ FINANCIAL BURDEN OF HEALTH CARE–ASSOCIATED INFECTIONS

In addition to posing threats to patient safety and favorable patient care outcomes, HAIs exert significant financial burdens on the health care system. A 2009 report estimated that HAIs can add up to $4.5 billion in excess health care costs annually in the United States. This figure does not account for HAIs occurring outside of hospital settings.[4]

TABLE 49.1	Aggregate attributable patient hospital costs by site of infection[a]
Type of HAI	**Range of Cost Estimates (Based on 2007 Consumer Price Index)**
SSI	$11 874-$34 670
CLABSI	$7288-$29 156
VAP	$19 633-$28 508
CAUTI	$862-$1007
CDI	$6408-$9124

Abbreviations: CAUTI, catheter-associated urinary tract infections; CDI, *Clostridium difficile* infections; CLABSI, central line–associated bloodstream infections; HAI, health care–associated infection; SSI, surgical site infection; VAP, ventilator-associated pneumonia.

[a]Data from Scott.[5]

TABLE 49.2	2020 National health care–associated infection prevention plan targets[a]
Measure (Data Sources)	**2020 Target**
CLABSI (NHSN)	50% Reduction in the national SIR[b]
CAUTI (NHSN)	25% Reduction in the national SIR
Invasive MRSA infections (NHSN/EIP)	50% Reduction in the national SIR
Facility onset MRSA (NHSN)	50% Reduction in the national SIR
CDI (NHSN)	30% Reduction in the national SIR
SSI (NHSN)	30% Reduction in the national SIR
CDI hospitalizations (HCUP)	30% Reduction in the national SIR

Abbreviations: CAUTI, catheter-associated urinary tract infections; CDI, *Clostridium difficile* infections; CLABSI, central line–associated bloodstream infections; EIP, emerging infections program; HCUP, health care cost and utilization project; MRSA, methicillin-resistant *Staphylococcus aureus*; NHSN; National Healthcare Safety Network; SIR, standardized infection ratio; SSI, surgical site infection.

[a]Data from US Department of Health and Human Services.[6]

[b]Progress is tracked using the SIR to compare actual health care–associated infection occurrence to predicted occurrence, which is based on risk-adjusted estimates using 2015 national baseline data.

The CDC estimated HAI costs that same year to range from $5.7 to $6.8 billion annually. Cost varied by HAI type, with CAUTI the least costly to treat and SSI and VAP the most costly HAI types to treat (Table 49.1).[5]

▶ A NATIONAL CALL TO ACTION

During the mid-2000s, as health care leaders, public health officials, and political leaders recognized that HAIs continued to be significant patient safety and public health issues, a national collective will to intensify HAI reduction and elimination efforts resulted in a national call to action to eliminate all preventable HAIs through broad application of evidence-based prevention strategies. Congressional leaders called on the US Department of Health and Human Services (HHS) to escalate national HAI prevention efforts, and in response to this directive, HHS convened the Federal Steering Committee for the Prevention of Health Care-Associated Infections to coordinate HAI prevention efforts across federal government agencies. Members of the Steering Committee included clinicians, scientists, and public health officials representing myriad private and government entities.

During 2009, the Steering Committee issued the National Action Plan to Prevent Health Care-Associated Infections: Roadmap to Elimination, which outlined a phased approach to expand HAI prevention beyond acute care facilities. Phase 1 focused on preventing the most prevalent HAIs in hospital settings. Phase 2 focused on reducing HAIs in ambulatory surgery centers (ASCs) and dialysis centers and increasing influenza vaccination among health care personnel. Phase 3 described strategies to address HAIs in long-term care facilities (LTCF). Each phase included goals and metrics for measuring progress toward reaching those goals by December 2013. New targets for HAI reduction have been set for 2020, (Table 49.2) using the 2015 national baseline determined by national data obtained from the NHSN.[6]

The HHS also directed its key agencies involved in HAI prevention—the CDC, the Centers for Medicare & Medicaid Services (CMS), and the Agency for Healthcare Research and Quality (AHRQ)—to sharpen their focus on HAI prevention. During 2009, the CDC Division of Healthcare Quality Promotion began funding state, territorial, and local health departments to build and strengthen HAI prevention activities in their jurisdictions. Using grants provided under the American Recovery and Reinvestment Act, public health agencies were charged with enhancing HAI surveillance and developing collaborative public and private health partnerships to ensure broad implementation of HAI prevention measures across the population at risk. State health departments were strongly encouraged to work with key partners such as hospital associations and quality improvement organizations (QIO) to develop and implement statewide HAI prevention plans.

The CMS created incentives under the Inpatient Prospective Payment System (IPPS), aimed at improving health care quality by providing financial incentives to hospitals, physicians, and other health care providers.[7] The CMS payments to providers were converted during 2008 from a fee-for-service system to value-based purchasing, under which health care institutions are being rewarded for high-quality care and performance improvement with bonus payments. Conversely, penalties can be imposed if health care institutions fail to achieve certain goals, such as preventing certain conditions among patients during their hospital stay. Some of the conditions that are the basis for penalties include selected HAIs.

The role of AHRQ in HAI prevention is to support research leading to evidence-based HAI prevention measures, to create teaching and training tools for health care professionals to improve health care delivery, and to create systems of measuring performance improvement in health care systems. This agency has funded initiatives to bring science into practice using techniques such as the Comprehensive Unit-based Safety Program (CUSP), aimed at reducing CLABSI occurrence among hospitalized patients.

PROGRESS TOWARD HEALTH CARE–ASSOCIATED INFECTION REDUCTION

The CDC 2016 National and State Healthcare-Associated Progress Report revealed that progress was made toward HAI reduction during 2008-2014 (Table 49.3), and during 2014, the national action plan goal for CLABSI reduction was met. Although CAUTI occurrence increased during 2009-2013, progress toward reductions occurred among non–intensive care unit patients, and progress in all settings occurred during 2013-2014. Additionally, SSI following abdominal hysterectomy procedures decreased by 17%, and CDI decreased by 8% from 2011 to 2014. The MRSA bacteremia decreased by 13% from 2011 to 2014.[8]

TABLE 49.3	Progress toward reduction in occurrence of health care–associated infections[a,b]
HAI	**Status of Progress**
CLABSI	50% Reduction during 2008-2014
CAUTI	No change during 2009-2014
SSI following abdominal hysterectomy	17% Reduction during 2008-2014
SSI following colon surgery	2% Reduction during 2008-2014
CDI	8% Reduction during 2011-2014
MRSA bacteremia	13% Reduction during 2011-2014

[a]Progress was tracked using the standardized infection ratio to compare actual health care–associated infection (HAI) occurrence to predicted occurrence, which was based on risk-adjusted estimates using baseline data (2008 for central line–associated bloodstream infections [CLABSI] and surgical site infection [SSI], 2009 for catheter-associated urinary tract infections [CAUTI], and 2011 for *Clostridium difficile* infections [CDI] and methicillin-resistant *Staphylococcus aureus* [MRSA] bacteremia).

[b]Data from Centers for Disease Control and Prevention.[8]

The HAIs are known to occur outside hospital settings but have not been tracked until 2013, when CMS mandated selected HAI reporting among long-term acute care (LTAC) hospitals and inpatient rehabilitation facilities (IRF). During 2013-2014, CLABSI and CAUTI decreased among LTAC patients by 9% and 11%, respectively, and among IRF patients, CAUTI decreased by 14%.

During 2010, the CDC launched its "Winnable Battles" campaign, in which HAIs were deemed one of six public health priorities because they were leading causes of death and disability but were preventable if known effective prevention strategies were broadly implemented across the population at risk. Despite the successes described earlier, the national focus on HAIs and collaborative efforts among health care providers and public health professionals must continue if future HAI goals are to be met, and health care institutions should continue to prioritize HAI reduction as part of their patient safety and health care quality improvement goals. Infection prevention and control professionals in all health care settings should continue to work with internal and external partners to further drive HAI occurrence toward zero preventable infections.

We subsequently describe the basic infection prevention infrastructure and functions necessary to develop and maintain robust and effective HAI prevention and control programs in health care settings.

THE HEALTH CARE INFECTION PREVENTION PROGRAM INFRASTRUCTURE

Hospitals

The CMS requires hospital infection prevention programs to designate at least one individual as the infection control officer, or infection preventionist. Most hospitals employ a nurse, clinical laboratory scientist, microbiologist, or communicable disease epidemiologist to serve as the infection preventionist. Hospitals must demonstrate this individual's qualifications through documentation of training and education, experience, or certification. Certification in Infection Prevention and Control (CIC) is obtained through successfully completing a written examination administered by the Certification Board of Infection Control and Epidemiology (CBIC). Certified infection preventionists must renew their certification every 5 years by successfully completing a computer-based self-assessment test.

The Association for Professionals in Infection Control and Epidemiology (APIC) defines core competencies that all infection preventionists should possess to function within the realm of patient safety science and HAI prevention. These core competencies include the ability to identify infectious disease processes, conduct surveillance and epidemiologic investigations, prevent transmission of infectious agents, support employee and occupational health activities, manage and communicate effectively, provide education, and conduct research.[9] Infection preventionists who can demonstrate advanced skills in the APIC future-oriented domains of technology, infection prevention and control, leadership and program management, and performance improvement and implementation science are eligible to become APIC fellows.

In addition to the infection preventionist, the CMS also requires hospitals to designate a leader responsible for the institution's antibiotic stewardship program. This individual can be a physician, pharmacist, or other hospital staff person responsible for the coordination and oversight of the antibiotic stewardship program.

Although not a CMS requirement, most hospital infection prevention programs include a hospital epidemiologist. This individual is usually an infectious disease physician with training and education in identifying infectious disease outbreaks and understanding the epidemiology of HAIs.[10] The role of the hospital epidemiologist has expanded considerably during the past 20 years, to include emergency preparedness, collaboration with public health professionals, education, occupational health, patient safety, and antibiotic stewardship. These individuals may also function as the medical director for the hospital infection prevention program.

The Joint Commission, as well as many state legislatures, directs hospitals to organize infection control committees to oversee the institution's infection prevention and control program.[11] These committees are typically composed of the infection preventionist; hospital epidemiologist; quality resource director; microbiology laboratory staff; pharmacy representatives; risk management, central processing, and environmental services representatives; infectious disease physicians; and providers and managers representing the various patient care services provided by the institution. The purpose of the committees is to oversee all aspects of the hospital infection prevention program, including surveillance, outbreak investigation, policy and procedure development, and education of hospital staff and patients.[12]

Ambulatory Surgery Center Infection Prevention Program Infrastructure

Following a 2008 outbreak of hepatitis C virus infections at a Las Vegas ASC, it became evident that little was known regarding infection prevention practices in these settings. Thus, the CMS conducted surveys during 2008 among a sample of ASCs using a pilot audit tool focused on assessment of key infection prevention practices such as hand hygiene, injection safety, equipment reprocessing, and environmental cleaning and disinfection.[13] At least one lapse in infection prevention practices was found among most

facilities. As a result, the CMS added infection prevention requirements to the ASC conditions of participation.

The CMS conditions of participation for ASCs include a requirement for the facility to designate a qualified, licensed health care professional with training in infection control to direct the ASC infection prevention program. If the designated infection control professional is not certified in infection control, evidence of training in infection control methods must be provided.

The facility must also demonstrate the existence of an infection control program and adherence to nationally recognized infection control guidelines. The requirements do not specify the amount of time that must be spent on infection prevention activities, but sufficient time should be allowed to direct an effective infection prevention program.

Components of an ASC infection prevention program must include systems to actively identify postprocedure infections, report notifiable conditions to public health agencies, to train personnel regarding infection prevention strategies, and to comply with current standards for prevention practices such as hand hygiene, safe injection practices, and equipment reprocessing.

Long-Term Care Facility Infection Prevention Program Infrastructure

During October 2016, the CMS issued new requirements for participation for LTCF, the first comprehensive update to health and safety standards for these facilities since 1991. The Final Rule, also called the Mega Rule, aims to improve resident safety and quality care through reduction of hospital readmissions and incidence of HAIs.[14]

The LTCF must designate an individual who is trained in infection prevention practices to coordinate the facility's infection prevention program, and antibiotic stewardship programs must be created to develop antibiotic use protocols and systems to monitor antibiotic use. A formal surveillance process to monitor trends in HAI occurrence must also be in place.

▶ SENTINEL ELEMENTS OF AN INFECTION PREVENTION PROGRAM

Well-designed and executed health care infection prevention programs are successful in reducing device-associated infections such as CLABSI, CAUTI, VAP, and SSI and other invasive procedure–associated infections. They are also aimed at protecting patients and health care personnel from acquiring communicable diseases such as influenza and other respiratory virus infections, gastrointestinal illnesses, and infections with health care–associated pathogens such as CDI and MDRO (eg, MRSA, carbapenem-resistant *Enterobacteriaceae*) while receiving or giving health care. Infection prevention program activities can be divided into two main domains: surveillance for HAIs and prevention and control of HAIs.

Surveillance for Health care–Associated Infections

Surveillance is the process of collecting and analyzing data regarding HAIs and other health care–associated events to monitor trends in occurrence and to evaluate the effectiveness of strategies implemented to prevent adverse events and increase positive patient outcomes. Surveillance is the foundation of quality assurance, performance improvement, and prevention activities and is a major activity of the infection preventionist.

Surveillance for all HAIs is not feasible or necessary; thus, infection prevention program activities should include development of annual surveillance plans to prioritize surveillance activities based on the patient populations most at risk of adverse outcomes and that align with the overall quality improvement goals of the institution. Outcomes associated with high-volume and high-risk treatments and procedures should be considered for surveillance.

Surveillance plans must also accommodate federal and state HAI reporting requirements. The CMS value-based purchasing initiative is based in part on submission of selected HAI data to the NHSN, and facilities that fail to complete data entry into that system do not receive full reimbursement from CMS. Most states have also enacted laws requiring hospitals and other health care facilities to report certain HAIs. As of October 2017, 32 states have enacted laws mandating reporting of at least one HAI.[15]

The NHSN is a national HAI database maintained by the CDC and is the central repository of HAI data used to monitor national, state, and individual facility progress toward HAI reduction. It is also the system used to meet federal and state HAI reporting requirements. More than 17 000 health care facilities including acute care hospitals, LTAC hospitals, psychiatric and rehabilitation hospitals, dialysis centers, ASCs, and skilled nursing facilities participate in NHSN, and more facilities will enroll in the future as HAI surveillance expands to additional health care facilities.[16]

To track HAI occurrence over time at the national, state, and individual facility level, a standardized infection ratio (SIR) is used to compare the actual number of HAIs occurring at the state or facility level to the predicted number of infections, a risk-adjusted number calculated from NHSN aggregate data. The SIRs that are significantly higher than 1 indicate HAI occurrence worse than predicted, and SIRs significantly lower than 1 indicate HAI occurrence better than predicted. Because SIRs are based on risk-adjusted data, they have replaced the use

of incidence rates as the preferred method to track and monitor trends in HAI occurrence over time.

Surveillance includes not only detecting outcomes (eg, HAIs) but also measuring compliance with processes implemented to achieve the desired outcome. Examples of HAI prevention processes that are typically measured to maintain or increase compliance include hand hygiene and influenza vaccination of health care personnel. Process measurement should be an integral part of HAI prevention efforts, and both outcomes and process surveillance data should be disseminated to facility staff, managers, and administrators to motivate further quality improvement.

Although surveillance activities are foundational to successfully reducing HAIs, the modern-day infection preventionist is increasingly burdened with surveillance-related tasks in response to reporting mandates and expansion of health care services and size of facilities. A 2015 survey conducted by the APIC determined that approximately 25% of infection preventionists' work time is spent conducting surveillance, more than any other single task. This means that less time is available for participating in HAI prevention activities.[17] Fortunately, technologic solutions such as installation of electronic medical records systems and development of automated surveillance algorithms have enhanced the efficiency and reliability of surveillance methods. These technologic trends are expected to continue to evolve and further enhance automated surveillance in the future.[18]

Prevention of Health Care–Associated Infections

Knowledge gained through HAI surveillance, outbreak investigations, and laboratory research has contributed to the dramatic evolution of HAI prevention science since the inception of infection control programs during the 1970s. Organizations such as the APIC and the CDC have developed evidence-based prevention guidelines based on that knowledge to improve patient safety by reducing HAI occurrence.

The Healthcare Infection Control Practices Advisory Committee (HICPAC) is a federal advisory committee that assists the CDC in the development of strategies to prevent device-associated infections and procedure-associated infections; reduce the prevalence of MDRO; prevent transmission of infectious agents among patients and health care personnel; and promote best practices in disinfection and sterilization, environmental infection control, and employee health. These evidence-based strategies are compiled into systematically reviewed guidelines containing multiple recommendations that should be practiced by all health care facilities to prevent HAI occurrence. The recommendations are categorized according to the strength of scientific evidence supporting the strategy or regulatory requirements (Table 49.4).[19]

| | TABLE 49.4 | Healthcare Infection Control Practices Advisory Committee categorization scheme for strength of evidence of recommendations[a] |

Rank	Description
Category 1A	A strong recommendation supported by high- to moderate-quality evidence suggesting net clinical benefits or harms
Category 1B	A strong recommendation supported by low-quality evidence suggesting net clinical benefits or harms or an accepted practice supported by low- to very low-quality evidence
Category 1C	A strong recommendation required by state or federal regulation
Category 2	A weak recommendation supported by any quality evidence suggesting a trade-off between clinical benefits and harms
No recommendation/ unresolved issue	An issue for which there is low- to very low-quality evidence with uncertain trade-offs between the benefits and harms or no published evidence on outcomes deemed critical to weighing the risks and benefits of a given intervention

[a]Data from Centers for Disease Control and Prevention.[19]

Health care–Associated Infection Prevention Guidelines

Guidelines for preventing device-associated infections include the 2009 Guideline for Prevention of Catheter-Associated Urinary Tract Infections, which includes recommendations for appropriate urinary catheter use, proper techniques for catheter insertion and maintenance, and meaningful surveillance for CAUTI. Two key strategies include limiting use of urinary catheters to only the recommended indications and removing them as soon as possible.

Guidelines for the Prevention of Intravascular Catheter-Related Infections were developed during 2011 and updated in 2017. The use of maximal sterile barrier precautions during insertion and site dressing regimens are emphasized in these guidelines. The 2017 update recommends use of chlorhexidine-impregnated dressings with a US Food and Drug Administration (FDA)-cleared label specifying a clinical indication for reducing catheter-related bloodstream infections to protect the insertion site of short-term, nontunneled CVC.

Procedure-associated HAI prevention guidelines include the US Public Health Service Guideline for Reducing Human Immunodeficiency Virus, Hepatitis B Virus, and Hepatitis C Virus Transmission Through Organ Transplantation (2013) and the 2017 Guideline for Prevention of Surgical Site Infections. Both documents are aimed at increasing the probabilities of good surgical outcomes and preventing potentially catastrophic surgery-related events. Because SSIs are currently the most prevalent HAI type in the United States, and because SSI prevention is relatively more complex compared to prevention of other HAIs, a separate section of this chapter has been devoted to this topic.

Patients in acute care and LTAC facilities and residents of LTCF are at risk of acquiring infections or becoming colonized with MDRO such as MRSA, VRE, and various gram-negative bacteria such as carbapenem-resistant *Enterobacteriaceae* and multidrug-resistant *Pseudomonas* and *Acinetobacter*. In the CDC document, Management of Multidrug-Resistant Organisms in Healthcare Settings (2006), MDRO are defined as microorganisms that are resistant to one or more classes of antimicrobial agents. Historically, most MDRO organisms have been bacteria, but multidrug-resistant fungi, specifically *Candida auris*, emerged during 2013 in the United States, posing a significant patient safety threat.

Because MDRO are transmitted among facilities as patients and residents are transferred, a regional approach to MDRO prevention is recommended. In this way, hospitals and LTCF can work together to standardize the management of patients infected or colonized with MDRO according to state and local public health recommendations and to ensure effective intra- and interfacility communications so that appropriate infection prevention measures are promptly implemented upon admission.

In addition to reducing the prevalence of MDRO through infection prevention strategies, health care organizations are required by accreditation organizations and public health agencies to implement antibiotic stewardship programs to reduce the overuse and inappropriate use of antimicrobial agents. Recommended elements of an effective antibiotic stewardship program include collection of data regarding institutional antibiotic use, leadership support, prescriber education, and pharmacy expertise to implement policies that support optimal antibiotic use.[20] Infection preventionists can support antibiotic stewardship programs by conducting data collection and analysis to monitor trends and progress toward improved antibiotic use.

◗ BREAKING THE CHAIN OF INFECTION

Transmission of infectious agents in health care settings occurs when susceptible hosts (patients, health care personnel) are exposed to an infectious source (other patients, visitors, health care personnel, the environment, medical devices and equipment) and the infectious agent enters the body of the susceptible host through a portal of entry (open skin, eyes, nose, mouth). Organisms can be transmitted via contact, droplet, or airborne modes of transmission from the source to a susceptible host. These components form the "chain of infection," or the series of steps that occur as infectious diseases are transmitted in health care settings and in the community. Multiple strategies are implemented in the health care setting to break the chain of infection and thereby prevent transmission of infectious agents. For example, standard and transmission-based precautions interrupt the modes of transmission, environmental cleaning and disinfection and disinfection and sterilization of medical devices eliminate sources of infection, and vaccination of patients and health care personnel reduces host susceptibility.

Preventing Modes of Transmission of Infectious Agents and Protecting Portals of Entry

Infectious agents are transmitted from infectious sources to susceptible hosts via three main modes of transmission—contact, droplet, and airborne transmission.

Contact transmission is the most common means by which infectious agents are transmitted and occurs either directly or indirectly. Direct contact transmission occurs when an individual has direct contact with an infectious person, whereas indirect contact transmission involves the transfer of infectious agents via an intermediary contaminated object, surface, or person. Patient to patient transmission of infectious agents from the hands of health care personnel is an example of indirect contact transmission. Examples of diseases transmitted by direct or indirect contact transmission include *S aureus* infections, *C difficile* infections, and viral infections caused by respiratory syncytial virus or herpes simplex virus.

Droplet transmission is the transfer of infectious agents via respiratory droplets that travel directly from the respiratory tract of infected individuals to mucosal surfaces of susceptible hosts. Respiratory droplets are generated through coughing, sneezing, and talking or during procedures such as suctioning, intubation, and cardiopulmonary resuscitation. Influenza virus, adenovirus, *Mycoplasma pneumoniae*, and the severe acute respiratory syndrome (SARS) virus are transmitted by droplet transmission.

Airborne transmission occurs when airborne droplet nuclei or small aerosol particles containing infectious agents are carried by air currents over large distances, and the contaminated air is inhaled by a susceptible host. Airborne transmission is the least common mode of transmission, with few diseases transmitted in this way. Tuberculosis, measles, and chickenpox are transmitted by airborne transmission.

Strategies to prevent infectious disease transmission by blocking modes of transmission include hand hygiene practices, standard precautions, and transmission-based precautions.[21]

Hand hygiene is one of the most important measures to prevent transmission of infectious diseases in health care settings. During 1975, the CDC issued written guidelines regarding hand washing practices that were to be followed by all health care personnel. The recommendations directed staff to wash hands with soap and water for 1 to 2 minutes before and after patient contact. At that time, the use of waterless antiseptic agents such as alcohol-based hand rubs (ABHR) was recommended only when sinks were not readily available. However, the promulgation of the 2002 CDC Guideline for Hand Hygiene in Healthcare Settings marked a paradigm shift in hand hygiene practices in health care settings because the prevailing evidence supported preferential use of ABHR in the clinical setting. Hand washing with soap and water is now indicated only when hands are visibly soiled or when caring for patients infected with *C difficile*. Otherwise, health care personnel are to use ABHR instead of soap and water because a greater log reduction of transient organisms on the hands is achieved with use of the ABHR than with soap and water (0.6-1.1 $\log_{10}$ versus 3.5 $\log_{10}$, respectively). The ABHR are also more convenient to use, require less time to use, and maintain skin integrity more effectively than soap and water. Hand hygiene is so key to protecting patients and health care personnel against infectious diseases that ongoing monitoring for compliance and methods to maintain high levels of compliance must be incorporated into all infection prevention programs in all health care settings.

Standard precautions are based on the premise that all blood and body fluids are potentially infectious, and thus, this infection prevention strategy must be practiced on all patients. In addition to hand hygiene, standard precautions include health care personnel use of personal protective equipment such as gloves, gowns, masks, and eye protection when contact with blood, body fluids, mucous membranes, or nonintact skin is anticipated. Standard precautions also include safe injection practices, respiratory hygiene, and specific infection control measures for special lumbar puncture procedures.

Safe injection practices entail the use of a new syringe and needle for every injection and the use of single dose vials whenever possible. Bags or bottles of intravenous solutions must not be used as common sources for multiple patients.[22]

Respiratory hygiene includes placing tissues, ABHR, and masks in common areas for patients and visitors to use to prevent transmission of respiratory illnesses. Covering coughs and sneezes to prevent droplet spread should be encouraged through posting of signs at entrances, elevators, and other strategic locations. Visitors with symptoms of respiratory illness should be discouraged from entering the facility, if possible.[21]

Following reports of bacterial meningitis associated with myelogram and other spinal procedures, recommendations for special precautions during procedures involving placement of catheters or injection of materials into the spinal or epidural space were added to standard precautions practices. Individuals performing such procedures should wear a face mask during the procedure to help prevent transmission of oropharyngeal flora.[21]

Transmission-based precautions are practiced when the infectious agent is known or is presumed to be the cause of illness in a patient. These include contact, droplet, and airborne precautions.

Contact precautions are used for patients infected or colonized with organisms that are transmitted by direct or indirect contact. The practice of contact precautions includes placing patients in private rooms and requiring all health care personnel entering the room to wear gowns and gloves. Patient care items, medical equipment, and all other items located in the room should be cleaned and disinfected before removing from the room or, if disposable, should be discarded in the room. Movement of patients outside the room should occur only when medically necessary.[21]

Patients known or suspected to have infectious respiratory illnesses are placed in droplet precautions. If possible, patients should be placed in private rooms. Health care personnel should wear surgical masks upon entry to the room, and if patients leave the room, they should wear a surgical mask if able and observe respiratory hygiene measures.[21]

Airborne precautions are used to manage patients with infections transmitted by the airborne route and necessitate placement in an airborne infection isolation room (AIIR), a specially engineered room that provides negative air flow relative to the corridor, specified air exchanges per hour, and exhaustion of air to the outside environment. Health care personnel entering the room must wear certified, fit-tested N95 respirators to prevent inhalation of tiny infectious droplet nuclei. If facilities do not have AIIR rooms, patients should be masked and placed in a private room until they are transported to a facility with an AIIR.[21]

Eliminating or Reducing Infectious Sources

Environmental infection control, disinfection and sterilization of medical devices and surgical equipment, and implementation of policies to address ill health care personnel and visitors are methods of breaking the chain of infection at the point of the infectious source.

Environmental infection control has become more important as the immunocompromised patient population grows. Most environmental sources of infection involve opportunistic pathogens (eg, *Aspergillus*, *Legionella*) that are seldom problematic for the immunocompetent host but can be catastrophic to medically fragile patients. A comprehensive environmental infection control program can, however, greatly mitigate risk to these susceptible patient populations by addressing water and air sources of infection, reducing contamination of surfaces and items in the immediate patient care area, and implementing measures to contain potentially infectious sources during construction and renovation projects.

Strategies to eliminate water sources of infection include routine cleaning and disinfecting sinks and wash basins, avoiding placement of decorative fountains in patient care areas, implementing water maintenance measures to minimize growth of *Legionella* and other opportunistic pathogens, and maintaining constant recirculation in hot water distribution systems.[23]

Standards for design, construction, and maintenance of air handling systems can be found in the American Institute of Architects guidelines for health care facilities and in most state or local construction regulations and codes. Institution policies should include proper installation and maintenance of heating, ventilation, and air-conditioning filters and monitoring of areas with special ventilation requirements (eg, AIIR, procedure rooms, operating rooms) for the appropriate air exchanges, filtration rates, and pressure differentials. Temperature and humidity should also be maintained within recommended parameters. Prior to construction or renovation projects, infection prevention staff should conduct an infection control risk assessment to determine the necessary risk mitigation strategies that must be implemented during the project.

Cleaning and disinfecting the patient care environment, including surfaces and noncritical medical equipment and patient care items, is also an important step to reduce sources of infection for patients and health care personnel. Environmental service staff play a critical role in protecting patients from HAI and should be trained and educated regarding the proper use of disinfectant agents to ensure products are being diluted, applied, and in contact with the item to be disinfected according to manufacturer's instructions.[23]

Laundry and linens have rarely been identified as a source of patient infections because washing and drying at recommended temperatures and chemical applications during the laundry process will remove pathogen from gowns, linens, towels, and bedding. However, an outbreak of fungal infections at a children's hospital during 2008-2009 was associated with linens that were likely contaminated following the laundry process, presumably from being stored in dusty, dirty, or humid bins.[24] Laundry facilities and equipment, even if located off-site, should be inspected by infection prevention staff to ensure laundry processes occur according to recommendations, and environmental rounds conducted in the institution should include assessment of laundry storage to ensure linens, bedding, gowns, and towels do not become contaminated during storage.

Disinfection and sterilization of medical devices and surgical equipment represent another crucial means of breaking the chain of infection through elimination of infectious sources. Millions of surgical and invasive medical procedures are performed each year in the United States and involve use of complex medical devices and equipment that must be adequately cleaned and disinfected or sterilized to safely use on multiple patients. A detailed description of sterile processing procedures is included in the "Prevention of Surgical Site Infections" section of this chapter.

Policies that discourage visitors with signs and symptoms of infectious illnesses from entering the facility are also methods that help reduce patient exposure to infectious sources. Signs that direct visitors to refrain from entering while ill should be posted to help protect patients, but if emergent circumstances necessitate patient contact, ill persons should be provided the appropriate personal protective equipment (eg, gowns, gloves, masks) to help prevent infectious disease transmission.

To reduce risk of infectious disease transmission, health care personnel should not work while experiencing symptoms of infection, yet many continue to work and treat patients while ill. A 2014 survey of physicians and advanced practice clinicians working at a children's hospital revealed that 83% reported working while sick at least once during the past year, even though 95% of respondents believed that working while sick put their patients at risk.[25] Health care facilities should develop human resource policies and create cultures of patient safety that support exclusion from work while ill.

Immunization of Susceptible Hosts

Even when infectious agents are transmitted from a source to a portal of entry of an individual via an effective mode of transmission, infection will not occur if the exposed individual is immune to the infectious agent. Immunization of patients and health care personnel is a long-recognized and effective way to prevent transmission of vaccine-preventable diseases such as measles, mumps, pertussis, hepatitis B virus infection, and influenza among patients and their health care providers. The Advisory Committee on Immunization Practices[26] publishes recommendations for health care personnel vaccination, and most states have enacted laws mandating vaccination of health care personnel against certain diseases, predominately hepatitis B virus infection, influenza, pertussis, pneumococcal disease, and chickenpox.[27] The CMS conditions of participation include offering influenza and pneumococcal vaccine to hospitalized patients, and hospitals, ASCs, dialysis centers,

and IRF must report their health care personnel influenza vaccination rates to CMS using the NHSN. Health care employee health programs that ensure best practices and compliance with state vaccination mandates are important components of infection prevention programs.

▶ PREVENTION OF SURGICAL SITE INFECTIONS

During 2017, the CDC published Guideline for the Prevention of Surgical Site Infections, which was composed of two sections. The Core section addresses six specific content areas: antimicrobial prophylaxis, nonparenteral antimicrobial prophylaxis, glycemic control, normothermia, oxygenation, and antiseptic prophylaxis. The second section, Prosthetic Joint Arthroplasty, addresses blood transfusion, systemic immunosuppressive therapy, intra-articular corticosteroid injection, anticoagulation, orthopedic space suits, postoperative antimicrobial prophylaxis, and use of drains and biofilms. However, several shortcomings in the evidence-based literature limited the number of class 1 recommendation, which have proven to be problematic in efforts to prevent SSIs.[28] Two additional SSI prevention guidelines have been published as supplements to the CDC recommendations, the American College of Surgeons and Surgical Infection Society: Surgical Site Infection Guidelines and the Wisconsin Division of Public Health Supplemental Guidance for the Prevention of Surgical Site Infections: An Evidence-Based Perspective.[29,30] A synopsis of selective components of the SSI prevention guidelines for all three recommendations is reviewed in Table 49.5. A fourth guideline regarding SSI prevention was published during 2016 by the World Health Organization (see Table 49.5). Although this guideline is quite instructive, its primary focus is for underdeveloped countries.[31]

The fundamental strategy for preventing an SSI involves reducing the vulnerability of the surgical wound to intraoperative contamination. This can be accomplished by selective evidence-based practices such as skin antisepsis or use of innovative wound protection sleeves, limiting the risk of wound contamination. Other adjunctive strategies involve appropriate perioperative antibiotics or enhancing the immune integrity of the surgical wound itself through the process of normothermia, glycemic control, and smoking cessation.[28-31]

An SSI can occur through one or more of these interrelated risk factors: (1) microbial-related factors that center primarily around bacterial virulence and antimicrobial resistance; (2) host-related factors that may present as multiple comorbidities such as obesity, diabetes, and history of corticosteroid therapy; (3) intraoperative risk factors that include perioperative team factors, operative technique, organizational and management factors, and the operating room environment; (4) and finally,

TABLE 49.5   Comparative summary of selective components of WHO, proposed CDC, ACS, and Wisconsin SSI prevention guidelines

Intervention	WHO Guidelines[31]	CDC Guidelines[28]	ACS Guidelines[29]	Wisconsin SSI Prevention[30]
Normothermia	Maintain normothermia.	Maintain normothermia.	Maintain normothermia.	Maintain normothermia—FAW reduces incidence of SSI.
Wound irrigation	No recommendation	Intraoperative irrigation recommended—povidone-iodine	No recommendation	Intraoperative irrigation recommended—CHG
Antimicrobial prophylaxis	Short duration	Short duration	Short duration	Short duration—follow ASHP weight-based dosing
Glycemic control	Recommended	Recommended—no recommendation for HbA_{1c}	Highly beneficial	Highly beneficial HbA_{1c} ≤7.0
Perioperative oxygenation	Recommended	Administer increased Fio_2 during surgery after extubation, immediate postoperative period	Recommended	Recommended—strongest evidence in colorectal surgery
Preadmission showers	Advise patients to bathe or shower with soap.	Advise patients to bathe or shower with soap or antiseptic agent—at least night before surgery.	Advise patients to bathe/shower with CHG.	Two standardized shower/cleansing with 4% or 2% CHG night before, morning of surgery
Antimicrobial sutures	Use antimicrobial sutures independent of type of surgery.	Consider use of triclosan-coated sutures for prevention of SSI.	Recommendation for clean and clean-contaminated abdominal procedures	The use of triclosan sutures represents 1a clinical evidence.

Abbreviations: ACS, American College of Surgeons; ASHP, American Society of Health-System Pharmacists; CDC, Centers for Disease Control and Prevention; CHG, chlorhexidine gluconate; FAW, forced-air warming; Fio_2, fraction of inspired oxygen; HbA_{1c}, glycated hemoglobin; SSI, surgical site infection; WHO, World Health Organization.

postoperative care–related factors such as inadequate postoperative wound management can adversely impact outcome once the patient leaves the operating room.

Effective SSI risk reduction should be viewed as a three-pronged approach, mitigating risk in the preadmission, perioperative, intraoperative, and postoperative periods. In the preadmission period, a minimum of two (night before, morning of surgery) showers/cleansings using a standardized process with 4% chlorhexidine gluconate (CHG) or 2% CHG-impregnated cloths has been shown to be an effective risk reduction strategy.[32] Although the surface of the skin can never be rendered sterile, use of a standardized evidence-based antiseptic preadmission shower will result in several log reduction of typical gram-positive and gram-negative surgical wound pathogens, including drug-resistant strains such as MRSA.[32-34] Multiple randomized controlled trials (RCTs) have documented that intensive smoking cessation 4 weeks prior to surgery leads to a significant reduction in postoperative complications, such as wound dehiscence and poor wound healing.[35]

Embracing an effective preoperative smoking cessation program results in improved angiogenesis, which is necessary for postoperative wound healing and potentially diminishing anastomotic leaks following colon surgery.

Intraoperative contamination leading to a postoperative SSI can occur by a variety of mechanisms, including[32-34,36]

- Dispersion of microbial aerosols within the vicinity of the surgical wound during the intraoperative period—excessive room traffic can increase the microbial burden in room air
- Deviation from recommended environmental conditions such as reduced air changes or excessive humidity
- Contamination of the wound bed by endogenous host flora originating from the sebaceous glands at the time of surgical incision
- Insertion of a contaminated biomedical device or use of surgical instruments that have been inadequately cleaned or sterilized

- Contamination of the fascial or subcuticular tissues by the hands of surgical team members following bowel manipulation/resection
- Contamination following any inadvertent break in aseptic technique by a member of the surgical team
- Failure to adequately irrigate the surgical wound prior to closure
- Contamination of the intraoperative irrigation fluid
- Poor communication among members of the surgical team
- Failure to deliver the correct weight-based antimicrobial prophylaxis or failure to redose the patient during surgical procedures lasting greater than 3 hours

Clinical practices in nursing, medicine, and surgery have evolved from the dogmatic to evidence-based practices based on well-designed laboratory, prospective cohort clinical studies, case-controlled studies, RCT, systematic reviews, and meta-analyses. Peer-reviewed publications from several surgical disciplines have documented the benefit of combining selective evidence-based practices to form what is identified as a comprehensive "surgical care bundle" (SCB) for reducing the risk of SSIs. However, implementation of a well-founded and well-thought-out SCB requires continuous monitoring to ensure compliance to the bundled intervention because poor compliance will diminish the interventional benefit of this valuable risk reduction strategy.[37-44]

Sterile Processing Department

The sterile processing department (SPD) is defined as a service within the hospital in which medical/surgical supplies and equipment, both sterile and, are cleaned, prepared, processed, stored, and issued for patient care. The effectiveness of an SPD department relies on expert execution of processes, facility design, resources (including equipment and personnel), education and training, quality control, and documentation of processes. There are professional guidelines directing the protocols for this area, including the Association of periOperative Registered Nurses (AORN) and the Association for the Advancement of Medical Instrumentation (AAMI).[45-49] The SPD leadership should have access to these guidelines, be familiar with their contents, and be able to speak to any policies for all elements of decontamination, disinfection, sterilization, and storage as performed within SPD.

All SPD staff should have easy access to the manufacturer's written instructions for use (IFU) for every instrument that is processed as well as for the machines, products, solutions, and chemicals that are used. Indeed, the importance of these documents cannot be overstated. When any questions arise, these documents should be consulted to ensure compliance. The IFU should be followed and if they are not followed, a risk assessment should be completed to justify this practice.

The major areas of the SPD are decontamination, assembly/packaging, sterilization, and sterile storage. These areas are considered restricted and attire and covering of all head and facial hair are required. In addition, jewelry on the hands and wrists are prohibited. Ideally, these areas should be separated either into rooms or via physical barriers. This may not, however, be possible in all facilities. The most crucial area to separate is the decontamination area. The decontamination area is considered "dirty," whereas the rest of the areas are considered "clean." Separating the dirty area decreases the chances for cross-contamination. The directional flow of items through SPD should be from contaminated to increasingly more clean.

The surfaces in the department (including countertops, cabinets, floors, doors, walls, and ceilings) should be smooth, made of cleanable materials, and durable enough to withstand frequent use and abuse. Lighting should be adequate to facilitate the attention to detail required for instrument reprocessing. Hand hygiene stations, including soap and water washing and waterless alcohol-based hand sanitizer, should be readily available throughout the department. All personnel should comply with the facility's hand hygiene policies.

American National Standards Institute (ANSI), American Society of Heating, Refrigerating, and Air-Conditioning Engineers (ASHRAE), and the American Society for Healthcare Engineering (ASHE) Standard 170-2013 provide guidance regarding heating, ventilation, and air-conditioning parameters, including temperature and humidity in the various areas within the SPD. Facilities Guideline Institute (FGI) 2014 Guidelines for Design and Construction of Hospitals and Outpatient Facilities provide standards to be used when constructing or completing major renovations.[50,51] The AAMI and AORN guidelines provide clinical practice recommendations.[45,49]

As instruments enter the SPD, additional pretreatment (or other methods to ensure bioburden remains moist) is advisable if the instruments will not be immediately cleaned. All hinged instruments must be open for the pretreatment. At the beginning of processing, instruments should be separated based on cleaning method (hand wash/delicate, etc). Instruments should be disassembled as much as possible, and jointed instruments should be opened. It is important to ensure that the solution used for presoaking and cleaning is approved by the device or instrument manufacturer. In addition, the solution manufacturer's requirements should be followed, including dilution, temperature, and contact time. If an automatic dilution device is used, it should be routinely verified and calibrated. The solution should be clean before use and may require changing after every use. Thorough rinsing after presoaking and cleaning is also necessary to ensure removal of all solutions.

Any brushes that are used should be designed for that specific purpose. Instruments that require brushing (such as those with lumens) will have instructions on how to obtain the correct size and type of brush. It is critical to obtain the correct brush for each item and for SPD personnel to be able to speak to the process of determining which brush to use. Brushes should be checked for visible soil and damage after each use, and reusable brushes should be reprocessed and dried for storage. If ultrasonic cleaning is used, it is important to ensure that gross soil is removed prior to placing instruments in the machine. The cleaning solution that is used should be labeled for ultrasonic use and it should be changed after each load. As always, the manufacturer's recommendations must be followed for proper loading of instruments and items, for daily cleaning of the machine, performance verification, and degassing of the machine.

When automated washers are used, it should be as the last step of the cleaning process in decontamination. Manufacturer's IFU must be followed, including how to load items (avoidance of overloading is critical) and how to maintain all working parts of the equipment, including any connectors. In addition, staff must be able to speak to selecting the correct washing cycle. Reusable containers, such as rigid container systems and transportation carts, should be inspected for damage, including breaks in gaskets and malfunctioning latching mechanisms. Processing of rigid containers (for cleaning and disinfection) and transport carts should follow manufacturer's IFU. In general, filters and filter holders, valves, and interior baskets should be removed and processed separately.

Items are typically rinsed in critical water (although each manufacturer's IFU should be consulted). Critical water is defined as having been extensively treated, so it can be used during the final rinsing stage or steam sterilization. Items should be inspected for damage at the end of the manual cleaning process. Instrument lubricants should be applied at this time.

Verification of cleaning starts with a visual inspection for any visible soil. Magnifiers can assist with this process. Additional verification methods, such as adenosine triphosphate (ATP) testing or microbiological sampling, may be used. If used, the processes for testing should be approved by the facility and rigorously followed. Verification of cleaning also includes monitoring of the parameters of the cleaning process. For example, automated washers and ultrasonic machines often provide a digital readout or printout; when they do, these records should be reviewed to ensure all parameters are met. In addition, the documentation should be maintained. There are a variety of additional verification methods, such as use of coupons contaminated with proteins, which should only be used with facility-approved testing procedures. In addition, all mechanical equipment should be properly maintained according to manufacturers' IFU, along with documentation of routine, preventive, and other types of maintenance. After nonroutine maintenance, cleaning verification should be completed prior to use.

Critical items that enter sterile tissue or the vascular system must be sterile and are packaged to ensure they stay sterile during storage. Examples of items that require sterilization include surgical instruments and ultrasound probes used in sterile body cavities. There are three common sterilization processes:

- Heat: Steam sterilization is the preferred method.
- Gas: Items that are heat sensitive are typically sterilized by ethylene oxide or hydrogen peroxide vapor.
- Chemical: The same chemicals used in high-level disinfection can render an item sterile, but the contact time is much longer (3-12 h). The disadvantage of the chemical sterilization process is that items cannot be wrapped to maintain sterility (and must be rinsed).

Monitoring the Sterilization Process

Three different types of monitoring are used to monitor the sterilization process. These monitors are used in a variety of ways and places and will be evaluated by sterilization personnel at the end of the process as well as by any health care workers who open the item at the point of use. If there is concern about any process monitor, the item should not be used, management should be notified, and an investigation should be undertaken to remedy any problems. The first type of monitor is a physical monitor. Physical monitors include a sterilizer's time, temperature, and pressure. The sterilizer will produce this information, usually via printout or electronic display. The staff member that is operating the sterilizer is required to verify that the information shows that necessary parameters are met and to maintain documentation.

The second type of monitoring is a chemical indicator. There are six types of chemical indicators. Type 1 is a process indicator, which is found on the outside of individual containers or packs and gives a visual indication that an item has been exposed to the sterilization process. The Bowie-Dick is an example of a type 2 indicator, which tests for air leaks, adequate air removal, and steam penetration in steam sterilization. Bowie-Dick tests should be run daily for all steam sterilizers. Types 3 and 4 only test some of the process variables and have little use in health care. Type 5, also referred to as an integrating indicator, is designed to react to all of the critical process variables. Type 6 is an emulating indicator and it reacts to all critical process variables for specific sterilization processes.

A type 5 or 6 chemical indicator should be placed inside each container or pack of the cycle (many times, multiple indicators are placed in packages, depending on the manufacturer's IFU) and evaluated by the staff member who opens the item at the point of use. These indicators are specific to the sterilization cycle and should be selected based on the cycle required for the items being sterilized. A type 5 or 6 indicator will also be placed within a process control device that is evaluated at the end of the sterilization load (prior to releasing the items for use).

The final type of monitoring is a biological indicator. Biological indicators are composed of very hearty bacterial spores and provide clear indication that the sterilization cycle was adequate to kill organisms. The biological indicator is placed within a process control device and incubated after the sterilization cycle is complete. After the manufacturer's recommended incubation time has passed, the indicator is evaluated for growth (ie, to indicate whether the sterilization process has succeeded or failed). Biologicals should be run daily or weekly depending on facility's policy and with every sterilization load that contains an implant. When used for implant loads, the biological incubation should be completed prior to use of the implant on a patient.

High-Level Disinfection

The process of high-level disinfection involves the elimination of all microorganisms (mycobacteria, fungi, viruses, and bacteria) in or on a device, with the exception of high numbers of bacterial spores. Devices processed by high-level disinfection include such heat-sensitive, semicritical items including endoscopes (gastrointestinal, bronchoscopes, and laryngoscopes), laryngoscope blades, endocavitary probes (rectal and vaginal), and respiratory therapy and anesthesia equipment.[50,51] The SPD staff may be responsible for performing high-level disinfection on medical devices used in hospital or outpatient clinics, emergency rooms, OB/GYN clinics, operating rooms, special procedure rooms, and endoscopy suites. High-level disinfection can involve heat, pasteurization (65°C-77°C for 30 minutes), or, more typically, chemical disinfection.[47] Table 49.6 identifies common disinfectants used for high-level disinfection along with the estimated kill times.

TABLE 49.6	Common disinfectants used for high-level disinfection along with the estimated kill times[a]
Method	**Duration**
>2% Glutaraldehyde (GLUT)	20-45 min
0.55% ortho-Phthalaldehyde (OPA)	12 min
1.12% GLUT/1.93% phenol	20 min
7.5% Hydrogen peroxide (HP)	30 min
7.35% HP/0.23% peracetic acid (PA)	15 min
1.0% HP/0.08% PA	25 min
400-500 ppm chlorine	10 min
2.0% HP	8 min
3.4% GLUT/26% isopropanol	10 min

[a]Data from Rutala and Weber.[47]

Although these chemical disinfectants have proven to be effective for high-level disinfection, several of the selective agents have been documented to cause skin, eye, and respiratory irritation; contact dermatitis; and anaphylactic irritation in bladder cancer patients. All require the use of personal protective equipment (long-sleeved impervious gown, protective eyewear, mask, gloves, and cap). Personal protective equipment is also worn to protect the health care worker from blood and body fluids. The determination of level of disinfection or sterilization required for any instrument is determined by the Spaulding classification. The Spaulding classification is a classification scheme using the degree of risk of infection, and the intended use of the object, to determine how items should be reprocessed. There are three levels to the Spaulding classification:

- Critical: Items that enter sterile tissue must be sterilized.
- Semicritical: Items that contact mucous membranes require at least high-level disinfection.
- Noncritical: Items that come in contact with intact skin require low-level disinfection.

▶ FINAL CONSIDERATIONS

Implementation of an effective infection control and prevention program requires a multidisciplinary effort, one that embraces health care professionals, quality engineers, health care administrators, and public health professionals. The historic perspective that once viewed healthcare-associated infections as inevitable consequences of the care process was shortsighted, due in a great part to our failure to recognize the tremendous number of infections that occurred yearly in US health care institutions. The recognition of the role of evidence-based practices as a pathway to improving patient outcome is reflected in the current WHO, CDC, American College of Surgeons (ACS), and Wisconsin supplemental SSI prevention guidelines.[28-31] However, evidence-based medicine is a moving target, and sentinel improvements in infection control and prevention practices should be frequently updated to address not only the complexity of the health care process but also the challenges that must be faced in caring for patients with substantial comorbid risk factors.

REFERENCES

1. Zimlichman E, Henderson D, Tamir O, et al. Health care-associated infections: a meta-analysis of costs and financial impact on the US health care system. *JAMA Intern Med.* 2013;173(22):2039-2046.
2. Haley R, Quade D, Freeman H, et al. Special issue: the SENIC project. *Am J Epidemiol.* 1980;111(5):465-653.
3. Magill S, Edwards J, Bamberg W, et al; for Emerging Infections Program Healthcare-Associated Infections and Antimicrobial Use Prevalence Survey Team. Multistate point-prevalence survey of health care-associated infections. *N Engl J Med.* 2014;370(13):1198-1208.
4. Reed D, Kemmerly SA. Infection control and prevention: a review of hospital-acquired infections and the economic implications. *Ochsner J.* 2009;9(1):27-31.

5. Scott RD. The direct medical costs of healthcare-associated infections in U.S. hospitals and the benefits of prevention. Centers for Disease Control and Prevention Web site. https://www.cdc.gov/hai/pdfs/hai/scott_costpaper.pdf. Accessed October 16, 2017.

6. US Department of Health and Human Services. National action plan to prevent health care-associated infections: roadmap to elimination. Office of Disease Promotion and Prevention Web site. https://health.gov/hcq/prevent-hai-measures.asp. Accessed October 30, 2017.

7. James J. Health policy brief: pay-for-performance. *Health Aff.* 2012. doi:10.1377.hpb20121011.

8. Centers for Disease Control and Prevention. 2016 National and state healthcare-associated infections progress report. Centers for Disease Control and Prevention Web site. https://www.cdc.gov/hai/surveillance/progress-report/index.html. Accessed October 17, 2017.

9. Murphy D, Hanchett M, Olmsted R, et al. Competency in infection prevention: a conceptual approach to guide current and future practice. *Am J Infect Control.* 2012;40(4):296-303.

10. Bryant KA. The role of the hospital epidemiologist. In: Bearman G, Munoz-Price S, Morgan D, Murthy R, eds. *Infection Prevention: New Perspectives and Controversies.* Cham, Switzerland: Springer; 2018:181-186. doi:10.1007/978-3-319-60980-5_19.

11. Hoffmann K. Developing an infection control program. *Infection Control Today.* December 1, 2000. https://www.infectioncontroltoday.com/articles/2000/12/developing-an-infection-control-program.aspx. Accessed November 4, 2017.

12. Lee F, Lind N. The infection control committee. *Infection Control Today.* June 1, 2000. https://www.infectioncontroltoday.com/articles/2000/06/the-infection-control-committee.aspx. Accessed November 4, 2017.

13. Schaefer M, Jhung M, Dahl M, et al. Infection control assessment of ambulatory surgical centers. *JAMA.* 2010;303(22):2273-2279.

14. Centers for Medicare & Medicaid Services. Medicare and Medicaid programs; reform of requirements for long-term care facilities. Final rule. *Fed Regist.* 2016;81(192):68688-68872.

15. Association for Professionals in Infection Control and Epidemiology. Interactive legislative map. Association for Professionals in Infection Control and Epidemiology Web site. http://cqrcengage.com/apic/home. Accessed October 30, 2017.

16. Centers for Disease Control and Prevention. National Healthcare Safety Network. Centers for Disease Control and Prevention Web site. https://www.cdc.gov/nhsn/about-nhsn/index.html. Accessed November 2, 2017.

17. Landers T, Davis J, Crist K, Malik C. APIC MegaSurvey: methodology and overview. *Am J Infect Control.* 2017;45(6):584-588.

18. Sips ME, Bonten MJM, van Mourik MSM. Automated surveillance of healthcare-associated infections: state of the art. *Curr Opin Infect Dis.* 2017;30(4):425-431. doi:10.1097/QCO.0000000000000376.

19. Centers for Disease Control and Prevention. Healthcare Infection Control Practices Advisory Committee infection control guideline library. Centers for Disease Control and Prevention Web site. https://www.cdc.gov/infectioncontrol/guidelines/index.html. Accessed November 2, 2017.

20. Centers for Disease Control and Prevention. Core elements of hospital antibiotic stewardship programs. Centers for Disease Control and Prevention Web site. https://www.cdc.gov/antibiotic-use/healthcare/implementation/core-elements.html. Accessed December 22, 2017.

21. Centers for Disease Control and Prevention. Guideline for isolation precautions: preventing transmission of infectious agents in healthcare settings (2007). Centers for Disease Control and Prevention Web site. https://www.cdc.gov/infectioncontrol/guidelines/isolation/index.html. Accessed November 2, 2017.

22. Dolan SA, Arias KM, Felizardo G, et al. APIC position paper: safe injection, infusion, and medication vial practices in health care. *Am J Infect Control.* 2016;44(7):750-757.

23. Centers for Disease Control and Prevention. Guidelines for environmental infection control in health-care facilities. Centers for Disease Control and Prevention Web site. https://www.cdc.gov/infectioncontrol/pdf/guidelines/environmental-guidelines.pdf. Accessed November 2, 2017.

24. Duffy J, Harris J, Gade L, et al. Mucormycosis outbreak associated with hospital linens. *Pediatr Infect Dis J.* 2014;33(5):472-476. doi:10.1097/INF.0000000000000261.

25. Szymczak J, Smathers S, Hoegg C, Klieger S, Coffin S, Sammons J. Reasons why physicians and advanced practice clinicians work while sick: a mixed-methods analysis. *JAMA Pediatr.* 2015;169(9):815-821. doi:10.1001/jamapediatrics.2015.0684.

26. Advisory Committee on Immunization Practices. Immunization of health-care personnel: recommendations of the Advisory Committee on Immunization Practices (ACIP). *MMWR Recomm Rep.* 2011;60(RR-7):1-45.

27. Centers for Disease Control and Prevention. Public health law: vaccination laws. Centers for Disease Control and Prevention Web site. https://www.cdc.gov/phlp/publications/topic/vaccinationlaws/html. Accessed November 3, 2017.

28. Berríos-Torres SI, Umscheid CA, Bratzler DW, et al; for Healthcare Infection Control Practices Advisory Committee. Centers for Disease Control and Prevention guideline for the prevention of surgical site infection, 2017. *JAMA Surg.* 2017;152(8):784-791.

29. Ban KA, Minei JP, Laronga C, et al. American College of Surgeons and Surgical Infection Society: surgical site infection guidelines, 2016 update. *J Am Coll Surg.* 2017;224(1):59-74.

30. Wisconsin Division of Public Health Services. Supplemental guidance for the prevention of surgical site infections: an evidence-based perspective. Wisconsin Department of Health Services Web site. https://www.dhs.wisconsin.gov/publications/p01715.pdf. Accessed December 12, 2017.

31. World Health Organization. Global guidelines for the prevention of surgical site infections. World Health Organization Web site. http://apps.who.int/iris/bitstream/10665/250680/1/9789241549882-eng.pdf?ua=1. Accessed December 12, 2017.

32. Anderson DJ, Podgorny K, Berríos-Torres SI, et al. Strategies to prevent surgical site infections in acute care hospitals: 2014 update. *Infect Control Hosp Epidemiol.* 2014;35(6):605-627.

33. Edmiston CE Jr, Lee CJ, Krepel CJ, et al. Evidence for a standardized preadmission showering regimen to achieve maximal antiseptic skin surface concentrations of chlorhexidine gluconate, 4%, in surgical patients. *JAMA Surg.* 2015;150(11):1027-1033.

34. Edmiston CE, Krepel CJ, Spencer MP, et al. Preadmission application of 2% chlorhexidine gluconate (CHG): enhancing patient compliance while maximizing skin surface concentrations. *Infect Control Hosp Epidemiol.* 2016;37(3):254-259.

35. Thomsen T, Tønnesen H, Møller AM. Effect of preoperative smoking cessation interventions on postoperative complications and smoking cessation. *Br J Surg.* 2009;96(5):451-461.

36. Edmiston CE Jr, Seabrook GR, Cambria RA, et al. Molecular epidemiology of microbial contamination in the operating room environment: is there a risk for infection? *Surgery.* 2005;138(4):573-582.

37. Waits SA, Fritze D, Banerjee M, et al. Developing an argument for bundled interventions to reduce surgical site infection in colorectal surgery. *Surgery.* 2014;155(4):602-606.

38. Tanner J, Padley W, Assadian O, Leaper D, Kiernan M, Edmiston C. Do surgical care bundles reduce the risk of surgical site infections in patients undergoing colorectal surgery? A systematic review and cohort meta-analysis of 8,515 patients. *Surgery.* 2015;158(1):66-77.

39. Keenan JE, Speicher PJ, Thacker JK, Walter M, Kuchibhatla M, Mantyh CR. The preventive surgical site infection bundle in colorectal surgery: an effective approach to surgical site infection reduction and health care cost savings. *JAMA Surg.* 2014;149(10):1045-1052.

40. Johnson MP, Kim SJ, Langstraat CL, et al. Using bundled interventions to reduce surgical site infection after major gynecologic cancer surgery. *Obstet Gynecol.* 2016;127(6):1135-1144.

41. van der Slegt J, van der Laan L, Veen EJ, Hendriks Y, Romme J, Kluytmans J. Implementation of a bundle of care to reduce surgical site infections in patients undergoing vascular surgery. *PLoS One.* 2013;8(8):e71566.

42. Schweizer ML, Chiang HY, Septimus E, et al. Association of a bundled intervention with surgical site infections among patients undergoing cardiac, hip, or knee surgery. *JAMA.* 2015;313(21):2162-2171.

43. Featherall J, Miller JA, Bennett EE, et al. Implementation of an infection prevention bundle to reduce surgical site infections and cost following spine surgery. *JAMA Surg.* 2016;151(10):988-990.

44. Leaper DJ, Tanner J, Kiernan M, Assadian O, Edmiston CE Jr. Surgical site infection: poor compliance with guidelines and care bundles. *Int Wound J.* 2015;12(3):357-362.

45. American National Standards Institute/Association for the Advancement of Medical Instrumentation. Comprehensive guide to steam sterilization and sterility assurance in health care facilities. Association for the Advancement of Medical Instrumentation Web site. https://standards.aami.org/higherlogic/ws/public/download/11091/Public%20review%20CDV-2%20ST79.pdf. Accessed December 12, 2017.

46. American National Standards Institute/Association for the Advancement of Medical Instrumentation. Chemical sterilization and high-level disinfection in health care facilities. Association for the Advancement of Medical Instrumentation Web site. http://my.aami.org/aamiresources/previewfiles/ST58_1308_preview.pdf. Accessed December 12, 2017.

47. Rutala WA, Weber DJ; and Healthcare Infection Control Practices Advisory Committee. Guidelines for disinfection and sterilization in healthcare facilities, 2008. Centers for Disease Control and Prevention Web site. https://www.cdc.gov/infectioncontrol/pdf/guidelines/disinfection-guidelines.pdf. Accessed December 12, 2017.

48. Association of periOperative Registered Nurses. Guideline for cleaning and care of surgical instruments. Association of periOperative Registered Nurses Web site. http://www.aornstandards.org/content/1/SEC36.extract. Accessed December 12, 2017.

49. Association of periOperative Registered Nurses. Guideline for sterilization. Association of periOperative Registered Nurses Web site. https://www.aorn.org/guidelines/guideline-implementation-topics/sterilization-and-disinfection. Accessed December 12, 2017.

50. Rousseau CP. ANSI/ASHRAE/ASHE Standard 170-2013: ventilation of health care facilities. American Health Care Association Web site. http://www.ahcaseminar.com/AHCA%202015%20PDF%20For%20Flash%20Drives/Mechanical%20Engineering%20Sessions/1.%20Updates%20to%20ANSI_ASHRAE_ASHE%20Standard%20170-2013%20.pdf. Accessed December 12, 2017.

51. Facilities Guideline Institute. 2014 Guidelines for Design and Construction of Hospitals and Outpatient Facilities. American Hospital Association Web site. https://ams.aha.org/eweb/DynamicPage.aspx?WebCode=ProdDetailAdd&ivd_prc_prd_key=8d03858d-980b-4a66-9d68-71dabd5fca14. Accessed December 12, 2017.

Disinfection and Sterilization of Living and Scaffold Tissue Engineered Medical Products

Kelvin G.M. Brockbank and Alyce Linthurst Jones

The use of human allogeneic tissues, such as arteries, bone, heart valves, skin, tendon, veins, and organs in medicine has become standard practice. Allogenic refers to biological material from the same species with a different genetic composition, with an allograft being biological material intended for transplantation into another individual of the same species. In contrast, autologous is related to self (or belonging to the same organism), where autografts are biological material intended for implantation into the individual from whom they were recovered. Finally, xenografts are from nonhuman animal source and implanted into a human recipient. Although clinical demand for organs and tissues continues to grow, the supply of these valuable human resources is a limiting factor. The United Network for Organ Sharing reported over 33 000 organ transplants in 2016, which represents a 20% increase since 2011.[1] The American Association of Tissue Banks (AATB) estimates that there are more than 39 000 deceased tissue donors annually in the United States and more than 3.2 million tissue grafts (allografts) are implanted annually[2]; however, there remains over 113 500 people in the United States alone waiting on the organ transplant list and the number of people awaiting tissue grafts is not maintained. As a result, the development of scaffolds and living engineered constructs has become an important discipline in biomedical science. Many tissue engineered products are under development, including wound covering and repair systems, orthopedic tissue repair systems, encapsulated tissues, cardiovascular products, and organs on a chip. Tissue engineering in this context refers to the development, design, and implantation of devices consisting of materials and living cells to replace defective or diseased organs and tissues. The long-term goal of tissue engineering is essentially to being able to replace or repair virtually every tissue and organ system. Four examples of marketed living engineered tissue products are Apligraf® (Organogenesis, Inc, Canton, MA) for wound repair, Carticel™ (Genzyme Tissue Repair, Inc, Cambridge, MA) for

articular cartilage repair, DeNovo® NT Natural Tissue Graft by Zimmer Biomet (Warsaw, IN) (particulate, juvenile human cartilage for the repair of articular cartilage damage), and ViviGen® Bone Matrix (LifeNet Health, Virginia Beach, VA) for new bone regeneration (cryopreserved, viable cortical cancellous bone matrix, and demineralized bone). Two of these engineered tissues are co-formulated with a cellular component of either an allogeneic material with different genetic composition within the same species (Apligraf®) or autologous material (Carticel™) along with one or more natural or synthetic biomaterials. Apligraf® is a bilayered human skin equivalent consisting of an epidermal layer made of human keratinocytes (the cells forming the keratinized epidermal layer of skin) and a dermal layer made of human fibroblasts (the most commonly found cell in connective tissues and are responsible for the synthesis of collagen, extracellular matrix, and can differentiate into a variety of cells types), in a bovine collagen matrix. Carticel™ is an implant consisting of concentrated autologous human chondrocytes (differentiated cells found in all types of cartilage) in culture medium that is injected beneath a periosteal flap into an articular cartilage defect.[3] DeNovo® NT is a minimally manipulated tissue product, regulated as a 361 human cells, tissues, and cellular and tissue-based product (HCT/P) by the US Food and Drug Administration (FDA) and not a medical device or biologic. It purports its efficacy in repairing articulating joints based on a large density of chondrocytes due to the donors being juveniles.[4] Additionally, there are many tissue engineered products that are regulated as 361 HCT/Ps under the US 21 CFR Part 1271 and do not require premarket approval prior to commercial availability. Some examples are live bone products (Osteocel®, Trinity Evolution®, and ViviGen®) used to stimulate new bone formation through osteoconduction (support new bone formation by providing an environment in which preexisting osteoid cells capable of synthesizing and secreting components essential to the formation lead to growth of new host bone), osteoinduction (the ability of a substance to stimulate cells to differentiate along some osteoprogenitor pathway resulting in those capable of synthesizing and secreting components essential to the formation of bone), and osteogenic (the presence of cells capable of synthesizing and secreting components essential to the formation of bone) properties of the bone in orthopedic, spine applications, and trauma repair. Decellularized dermis is another tissue engineered product requiring no premarket approval in the United States (AlloDerm®, DermaMatrix®, DermACELL®, FlexHD®, and AlloMax™) for breast augmentation postmastectomy, burns, soft tissue augmentation, and wounds. The FDA held a panel meeting for the General and Plastic Surgery Devices on March 25 to 26, 2019, indicating that premarket approval may be required in the future for decellularized dermis indicated for breast reconstruction because its homologous use for this indication is in question.[5]

▶ REGULATION OF HUMAN TISSUES

Human tissues are regulated in the United States by the FDA in the Center for Biologics Evaluation and Research. This jurisdiction and the regulations are outlined in 21 CFR Part 1271 and were promulgated May 25, 2005.[6] These products may have different or similar regulatory pathways in other parts of the world. For instance, in Canada, some tissues are similarly regulated, where tissue bank are assigned a Human Cells, Tissues and Organs number to include in their labeling[7] and in other stances, like cryopreserved heart valves, they are considered class IV medical devices. In the European Union, tissues only require registration, but some member states can require additional information above and beyond the European Union Tissue and Cells Directives.[8] Germany and India are special cases where human tissues are regulated as drugs, which can be exceptionally complex in compliance given how different drugs are from human tissues in that there is no active pharmaceutical ingredient in tissues.

The US regulations are often referred to as *Good Tissue Practices* (GTPs). FDA has issued many guidance documents to provide its current thinking on the implementation of 21 CFR 1271 across such topics as donor screening and eligibility,[9] minimal manipulation, homologous use, use of donor screening tests, current GTPs, small entity compliance guide, and validation.[10] Allografts that are regulated as 361 HCT/Ps are deemed to be

1. Minimally manipulated, for homologous use.
2. The manufacture of the HCT/Ps does not involve the combination of cells or tissues with another article, except for water, crystalloids, or a sterilizing, preserving, or storage.
3. The HCT/P does not have a systemic effect and is not dependent on the metabolic activity of living cells for its primary function.

4. The HCT/P has a systemic effect or is dependent on the metabolic activity of living cells for its primary function and (1) is for autologous use, (2) is for allogeneic use in a first-degree or second-degree blood relative, or (3) is for reproductive use.

These products are regulated under section 361 of the US Public Health Services Act as 361 HCT/Ps. If the tissue does not meet all four of these definitions, then it is either regulated in the United States as a device or a biologic; however, the tissues are still subject to the rules and regulations outlined in 21 CFR 1271. To further elaborate on two key definitions, minimal manipulation and homologous use, the FDA has further defined these two attributes.[11] Minimal manipulation is (1) for structural tissue, processing that does not alter the original relevant characteristics of the tissue relating to the tissue's utility for reconstruction, repair, or replacement, and (2) for cells or nonstructural tissues, processing that does not alter the relevant biological characteristics of cells or tissues, as defined in 21 CFR 1271.3. Homologous use means the repair, reconstruction, replacement, or supplementation of a recipient's cells or tissues with an HCT/P that performs the same basic function or functions in the recipient as in the donor, 21 CFR 1271.3. Therefore, Center for Biologics Evaluation and Research regulates products whose primary mode of action is the result of its cellular component, such as cultured cartilage cells where the cells are expanded in culture, whereas a product whose primary mode of action is structural in nature, such as a decellularized heart valve, is regulated by the Centers for Devices and Radiological Health.

The safety standards for tissue engineered products are driven by their regulatory status; however, one unifying theme for human tissues, regardless if regulated as a 361 HCT/P, a medical device, or a biologic, is that they do not introduce, transmit, or communicable diseases. Therefore, products without viable cells are often terminally sterilized using a validated sterilization dose via electron beam or γ irradiation (see chapter 29).[12] Grafts with viable cells cannot be irradiated without killing the constituent cells via formation of free radicals and/or direct damage to the DNA that is unable to be repaired (see chapter 5). For example, the typical cumulative dose of irradiation for a breast cancer patient is 50 Gy, and a typical absorbed dose for tissue being terminally sterilized is 15 kGy or 15 000 Gy; thus, mammalian cells that absorb this much irradiation are likely to be necrotic and proinflammatory once implanted as a result of the lethality of the terminal sterilization dose. Often allografts are irradiated on dry ice to minimize free radical damage from free water in the product, thereby overcoming many of the limitations reported in older literature (1970s-1990s) of the loss of functionality or early failure because the tissues were γ irradiated at 25 kGy (2.5 Mrad) at ambient temperatures. In addition to irradiation in the presence of dry ice, there are other strategies that may be employed.

The traditional terminal sterilization requirement of a sterility assurance level (SAL) of 10^{-6} is giving way to less-stringent SALs as a compromise to achieve a sterility claim for regenerative medicine products but at a dose or treatment process that does not negatively impact the product for its intended surgical purpose (see chapter 5). The difference between SALs is in the theoretical probability of a viable microorganism, such as in 1 in a 1000 for an SAL 10^{-3} versus 1 in a million for an SAL 10^{-6}. Guidance documents such as International Organization for Standardization (ISO)/TS 19930 and, specific for radiation processes, AAMI TIR 76 provide some instructions for alternatives.[13,14] The AAMI TIR 76 provides instruction supplementary to the radiation sterilization standard ISO 11137 for additional options for VD_{max} doses and charts to achieve alternative SALs (10^{-5}, 10^{-4}, 10^{-3}, and 10^{-2}) using lower doses of irradiation.[12] The radiation validation method 1 (see chapter 29) can also be used to achieve alternative SALs to 10^{-6} like 10^{-3}, but at this time, this approach requires minimally 139 samples (30 bioburden, 100 verification dose, 6 for method suitability testing to validate the test of sterility, and 3 for bioburden recovery efficiency test to determine the correction factor to be applied to bioburden count) to execute verses 29 for the VD_{max} protocols (10 bioburden, 10 test of sterility, and the balance of 9 for the aforementioned test method validations). To achieve the lowest possible dose at a desired SAL, method 2B can be used; however, it requires around 300 samples to execute the validation as described in AAMI TIR 37.[15] To determine the optimal validation strategy and SAL, knowledge of the maximum absorbed dose the product can withstand through functional testing such as biomechanical integrity or other appropriate functional testing is important. The range between the minimum absorbed dose, maximum absorbed dose, dose uniformity ratio, and the correction factor to a reference location in the carrier must be considered because commercial irradiators generally require a 35% spread between the minimum and maximum specified delivered doses (minimum or maximum dose location in the product payload container multiplied by the reference to minimum ratio or reference to maximum ratio). Many considerations for terminal irradiation of allografts are further discussed in guidances such as AAMI TIR 37.[15] The other option for nonviable and viable grafts is end point microbiological testing of the lot that conforms to the United States Pharmacopeia (USP) chapter 71 or 21 CFR Part 610.12 to demonstrate no bacterial growth after a 14-day incubation period in appropriate media.[16,17] But it is important to note that USP <71> microbiological testing is intended to be an adjunct to a validated process demonstrated not to introduce bioburden and to reproducibly disinfect the graft. One significant difference between processed tissue-based products and pharmaceuticals is that the tissue entering the process is not sterile, whereas pharmaceutical components are typically sterile and need only be aseptically combined without cross-contamination. USP <71> testing generally involves testing 10% of the lot aerobically and 10% of the lot anaerobically. There are strategies that involve incubating the same sample at 25°C to 30°C for 3 to 5 days and then moving the sample to 35°C for the remaining 9 days on test (see chapter 64). Samples can be assessed through direct immersion into nutrient media or rinsates, filtered and the filter placed on agar or nutrient media for 14 days. The final result from USP <71> testing is often mistakenly referred to as demonstrating an SAL of 1×10^{-3}, but this is incorrect. It is only appropriate to use SAL in the context of products that have been terminally sterilized by a validated method in the final packaging and not handled until needed for implantation. USP <71> can provide the probability of a nonsterile unit, which is generally 10^{-3} (1 in 1000), and not to be confused with a SAL 10^{-3} because it is typically arrived upon by conducting an aseptic fill validation and not having a positivity rate of more than 1 in 1000. This level of performance for aseptic tissues is highly unlikely—only 1 in 1000 donors found to be culture-positive during end point microbiological testing.

To provide additional guidance to the allograft tissue community, the AATB has established standards and guidance documents that provide minimum performance requirements for all aspects of tissue banking activities.[18,19] These standards and guidance documents include requirements for donor suitability, handling of transplantable human tissue, and a guidance document focused on microbial surveillance testing of donor tissue and environmental monitoring of dedicated recovery suites as well as processing clean rooms.[19] The intent is to ensure allograft tissue recipients receive disease and contaminant-free implants and optimal clinical performance of transplanted tissues.

Regardless of whether the transplantable material is a US 361 HCT/P allograft, 351 HCT/P allograft, or a tissue engineered medical device, recipient safety must be ensured by starting with the administration of strict donor screening criteria along with stringent quality control measures that encompass the entire tissue preparation protocol and highly controlled environments, such as an ISO 14644-1 class 7 cleanroom or cleaner that are designed for unidirectional flow from clean to dirty to minimize cross-contamination.[20] The gowning of processing technicians has advanced from gowns, gloves, and surgical masks to surgical togas and contained head gear with fans to reduce skin contaminants from entering into the sterile field.[21] Various tools and aseptic training techniques can be used to reduce cross-contamination risks in these areas (see chapter 58). Overall, approaches involve employing the essential requirements in ISO 13485 for quality management systems and ISO 14871 for risk management to ensure that high-quality and microbiologically safe grafts are accomplished and brought to market with the risk to the patient as low as reasonably practicable and thus the risk-benefit ratio being in the patients' favor.[22,23]

◗ ENGINEERED TISSUE GRAFTS

There is no current need for modification from existing best clinical practices in the autologous situation, in which cells or tissues are removed from a patient and transplanted back into the same patient in a single surgical procedure. The FDA recently issued guidance on this subject.[24] If the autologous cells or tissues are banked, transported, or processed with other donor cells or tissues, then there exist opportunities for the introduction of transmissible disease. When this additional manipulation occurs, good manufacturing practices and GTPs should be implemented and it becomes necessary to screen for infectious agents (21 CFR 1271 Subpart C: Donor Eligibility).[6] For example, in the case of the Carticel™ process, in which biopsies of healthy cartilage are used as a source of chondrocytes, the biopsies are minced, washed, and cultured with cell culture medium containing antibiotics. As prescribed in USP <71>, method suitability testing, previously referred to a bacteriostasis/fungistasis (B/F) testing, must be performed prior to using a nutrient growth-based culture method to confirm the culture negative status of the lot for at least detectable bacteria/fungi (see chapter 64). To confirm that the test method will not result in a false-negative result at low numbers of bacterial colony forming units (CFUs), tissue products processed at the maximum residuals of antimicrobials (maximum concentration, maximum exposure time, and minimum rinses) are placed into nutrient media and inoculated with 10 to 100 CFUs of typical human flora and assessed for growth within five day of inoculation.[16] The turbidity of the test grafts must closely approximate the turbidity of the positive control flasks that contain no tissue but were inoculated with the same number of CFUs. Other methods such as filtration of the final solution are also appropriate; however, the time the tissue is incubated prior to the fluid being tested should be validated with a dwell time study to ensure if there were microorganisms present, they would be removed from the tissue into the fluid during the extraction period. A microbiologist should be consulted to ensure proper conductance of these studies. Incorrect performance of method suitability testing could give in false-negative culture results and the potential for disease transmission in the recipient.

Tissue Grafts and Prevention of Infectious Agent Transmission

All tissues, whether they be allografts, autografts, and/or engineered grafts, should be delivered to patients with the highest possible assurance that they are free of pathogens. The most effective and common methods for the prevention of infectious agent transmission are thorough donor screening, donor serological testing for relevant viruses, donor tissue microbiological testing, and adherence to sterile techniques during procurement, transport, pro-

cessing, and terminal sterilization if applicable. There are six pillars to ensure tissue safety (1) medical suitability determination through a detailed medical history, physical examination, and detailed social history; (2) serology testing for viral diseases such as human immunodeficiency virus (HIV), hepatitis B, hepatitis C, and the bacterial disease syphilis; (3) microbiological testing of recovered tissues prior to disinfection; (4) validated processing to clean and disinfect tissues; (5) validated end point microbiological testing or a validated terminal sterilization process; and (6) validated packaging to maintain the sterile barrier for the shelf life of the graft.

In United States, the first step in confirming eligibility of a potential donor is to obtain authorization for organ and/or tissue donation from the donor's legal next of kin. This is the case even if a potential donor has registered as an organ and tissue donor with the Department of Motor Vehicles, Donate Life State Registry, various health applications (eg, on mobile phones), or legal agreements such as advanced directives. Alternatively, authorization may be obtained via telephone on a recorded line and documented as such in the donor record. Once authorization for donation is obtained, the donor must be screened to minimize the potential for disease transmission as a result of health status, travel, social influences such as drug and alcohol, or sexual orientation. The AATB, for example, has developed a standardized process for its member banks to use, the *Uniform Donor Risk Assessment Interview* (DRAI) that ensures compliance with FDA's requirements.[25] Some AATB member banks add additional questions to the DRAI to aid medical directors in making medical suitability determinations. These determinations are living documents and account for emerging infectious diseases such as Zika virus. The DRAI consists of flowcharts, guidance documents, and questionnaires to assess medical history, behavioral history, travel history, and social history. The DRAI also covers a range of age groups, newborns, donors younger than 12 years, and those 12 years or older. This age range accounts for maternal contribution to the disease/health status of the child and in the instance of children younger than 12 years there are differences in hemodilution (explained in the following text) calculations due to their size. The DRAI is completed by a knowledgeable historian such as a family member or partner and assessed in conjunction with the donor's medical records. The next step in assessing medical suitability is a physical examination of the donor by the recovery teams prior to recovery as detailed in Appendix III of the AATB standards.[18] Some of the elements of this are, but not limited to, conclusive identification of the donor and authorization for donation, documentation of trauma, nonmedical needle punctures, presence of jaundice, presence of infection in tissue recovery areas, skin lesions, enlarged lymph nodes, enlarged liver, genital and anal lesions, tattoos, and piercing. The next critical element in determining donor suitability is serological testing for viral load using FDA-approved/cleared test kits for use on cadaveric samples by laboratories that are registered with the FDA as a tissue establishment to perform infectious disease testing and that hold a current Clinical Laboratory Improvement Amendments certification. Prior to testing, the donor record is reviewed for evidence of hemodilution, which if present would result in the donor's blood being significantly diluted (>2 L) by blood donor products, colloids, or crystalloids within 48 hours of asystole. Getting an accurate assessment of viral load in the donor under such conditions is impossible with current technology, and thus, the donor tissue is discarded. It would be difficult to demonstrate freedom from relevant communicable virus with deference to the window period where virus is present in the blood below the detection limit of the nucleic acid test (NAT), which is maximally 60 days for hepatitis C. But once the specimen is determined to be suitable, the following tests shall be performed:

1. Antibodies to the HIV, type 1 and type 2 (anti-HIV-1 and anti-HIV-2)
2. NAT for HIV-1
3. Hepatitis B surface antigen
4. NAT for the hepatitis B virus
5. Total antibodies to hepatitis B core antigen (anti-HBc—total, meaning immunoglobulin G and M)
6. Antibodies to the hepatitis C virus (anti-HCV)
7. NAT for hepatitis C virus
8. Tests for syphilis (a nontreponemal or treponemal-specific assay may be performed)

All tissue from donors who test repeatedly reactive on a required screening test shall be quarantined and shall not be used for transplantation.

The next step in reducing the risk of disease transmission is determination of the microorganisms on the tissue postrecovery, prior to the use of an antimicrobial or other solution that could obscure a positive result, false negative. Theoretically, other than skin, the tissue should be sterile; however, surface contamination can and does occur during recovery in spite of detailed and thorough disinfection of the donor skin and aseptic practices employed during donor recovery (Appendix IV, AATB Standards[18]). These risks become greater in the recovery of animal tissues (eg, in an abattoir), as compared to a surgical suite. The AATB maintains a list of objectionable microorganisms "considered to be pathogenic, highly virulent microorganisms that shall result in tissue discard unless treated with a disinfection or sterilization process validated to eliminate the infectivity of such organisms." Those organisms include *Clostridium* species, fungi (yeasts and molds), and *Streptococcus pyogenes* (group A streptococci). Some tissue types have additional specific high-risk microorganisms as well, such as with cardiovascular tissues.[26] Additionally, each member bank can develop a list of additional organisms that their medical directors and laboratory professionals find to be objectionable in spite of the

bank's validated cleaning, disinfection, and possible terminal sterilization validations. The development of such a list should take the cleaning and disinfection reagents, concentration, contact time, and temperature into account as well as the susceptibility of the organisms to method of terminal sterilization and pathogenicity should there be survivors detected. The FDA and AATB require all processing and sterilization activities to be validated through the demonstration of documented, objective evidence. Terminal sterilization validations are verified minimally on an annual basis per applicable ISO standard to ensure the susceptibility of the remaining organisms to the mode of sterilization has not changed.

Many tissue processors have proprietary or in-licensed cleaning and disinfection processes to help ensure the safety of the allografts distributed for implantation. One of the most widely used is the Allowash® technology that was developed by Lloyd Wolfinbarger, PhD, at LifeNet Health Inc (Virginia Beach, VA) and was protected by multiple US patents. Given the interest of allograft safety in the United States, this process was further out-licensed to other tissue banks. The Allowash® process had demonstrated superior cleaning and bactericidal/virucidal capabilities, which was of the upmost concern in at the height of the HIV epidemic in the 1980s and 1990s. The process involves 3% hydrogen peroxide, nonionic detergents, antibiotics, isopropanol combined with centrifugation, ultrasonics, and elevated temperatures to provide the desired cleaning, disinfection, and adventitious agent removal. Another major cleaning and disinfection process developed to address the threat of disease transmission and improve throughput efficacy with the hope of donor pooling was the BioCleanse® process, developed by RTI Surgical Holdings Inc (Marquette, MI).[27]

Ultimately, in these cases, the initial goal of donor pooling was not realized due to FDA requirements (defined in 21 CFR 1271.220) that prohibit the pooling of donor tissues.[6] The rationale for this was if a pathogen does get through screening, serology, processing, and/or terminal sterilization by limiting each processing event to one donor, the harm to recipients is finite and limited by the number of grafts one donor can produce that range anywhere from 1 to in excess of 500 if demineralized particle bone for dental implants are considered. These regulations represent the state of science at the time they were developed, the 1990s, and may not properly consider the many technological advances in disease detection, treatment, and efficacy of terminal sterilization processes; however, they have prevented the spread of disease as the result implantation of allograft tissues.

The next step in providing microbiologically safe tissues is terminal sterilization that can be achieved through several methods. The use of physical or chemical inactivating methods has been supported by laboratory data and clinical experience.[28-31] Despite this, the primary means of terminal sterilization today uses low dose, <20 kGy/2.0 Mrad, electron beam irradiation or γ irradiation at dry ice temperatures to reduce free radical formation and prevent damaging the tissues (see chapter 29). The international standards, ISO 11137 and associated standards in that series, define the minimum requirement for the definition, validation, and maintenance of radiation sterilization methods.[12] There are at least two mechanisms by which ionizing radiation is effective (see chapter 5).[32] First, it causes lethal strand breaks in the nucleic acids of the infecting microorganism rendering it incapable of proliferation or infectivity. Secondarily, irradiation induces several sublethal chemical alterations through free radicals and their propagation in an aqueous, room temperature environment that collectively become lethal. The required dose of γ radiation to achieve sterility varies with the number and types (radiosensitivity) of microorganisms (bioburden) present on the tissue and may also be impacted by the temperature at which sterilization is performed (see chapter 29). As discussed previously, an SAL of 10^{-6} is the typical validation target for such processes, but alternative SALs may be acceptable. Because absolute sterility is not achievable, it is determined through mathematical probability of a single organism surviving based on the collective D_{10} (dose of irradiation to cause a 90% decrease the number of viable microorganisms on a graft) value for a diverse population of organisms. The ISO 11137 standard refers to this concept as "population C."

It may be suggested that freedom from viral contamination cannot be assumed under validated SAL conditions with radiation because this has been particularly demonstrated with bacteria and to a much lesser extent with viruses. Some viruses may have higher D_{10} values than do bacteria,[33] but also bacteria themselves can range in radiation sensitivity (see chapter 29). The reduction of viruses is also considered a mathematical probability; however, the kinetics of kill (as with other microorganisms) can vary relative to the antimicrobial agents and the substrate involved and thus do not lend themselves as readily demonstrable as the mathematical modeling that occurred with bacteria and fungi (as the basis in ISO 11137).[12] As an example, there is an international standard defining requirements for viral inactivation/removal validation,

ICH Q5A (R1).[34] The first step is to identify the relevant viruses or model viruses to test and then identify those steps in the tissue processing regime to test keeping in mind solutions with the same mode of kill, for example, oxidation, may not have their levels of log kill combined because the virus may become recalcitrant to solutions with the same mechanisms of action. The ideal outcome is a 6 $\log_{10}$ reduction above, which is expected on the incoming tissues achieved through two to three different steps. Minimally, regulatory agencies prefer to see at least 4 logs of kill/removal for each relevant virus. For human tissues, the relevant viruses/model viruses represent a variety of DNA and RNA viruses, as listed in Table 50.1.

Briefly, after the appropriate method, validations for toxicity and ensuring the method of inactivation can be stopped (neutralized) to get an accurate log kill (see chapter 61), the tissue is seeded with a known amount of virus, exposed to one step in the process, and the amount of virus remaining on the tissue and solution are determined through plaque formation assays with susceptible cell lines. Ideally, this is repeated over multiple time points to determine the consistency of the inactivation kinetics and whether or not it is first order. With respect to kill by γ irradiation, many researchers have tried to determine the amount of radiation lethal to HIV. Results have been equivocal and range from 10 to 40 kGy.[32,35,36] Given the structure of HIV, it is not considered to be highly resistant to inactivation (see chapter 3). The γ radiation doses greater than 25 kGy have been recommended to inactivate most other viruses, including those of similar structure and nucleic acid type to HIV; therefore, procedures have been developed that incorporate multiple antiviral treatment methods in order to produce the optimum possibility of a disease-free graft. It should be recalled that bacterial and viral safety are part of a continuum starting with donor screening, medical, behavioral, and social history as well as bacteriological/fungal testing of the recovered tissues and viral testing of the donor plasma and serum. During chemical treatments, each viral inactivation step will not only depend on the chemical type and exposure process conditions (including concentration, time, and temperature) but may also involve physical removal through centrifugation, ultrasonic cavitation, or

TABLE 50.1 Examples of relevant model viruses used in demonstrate viricidal efficacy in tissues

Test Virus	Virus Family	Nucleic Acid (Size, nm)	Enveloped
Bovine viral diarrhea virus	Flaviviridae (eg, hepatitis C)	RNA	Yes
Hepatitis A virus	Picornaviridae	RNA	No
HIV-1	Retroviridae (eg, HIV)	RNA	Yes
Pseudorabies virus	Herpesviridae	DNA	Yes
Porcine parvovirus	Parvoviridae	DNA	No

Abbreviation: HIV, human immunodeficiency virus.

other mechanical means. If there are multiple steps that inactivate by the same mechanism, such as oxidation, only the kill from one of the oxidation steps can be counted toward total kill per the ICH guidance. The reason for this, despite its limitations, is the suggestion that viruses can become recalcitrant to kill from the same mechanism of action in subsequent steps and thus cannot be reliably counted on to result in the presumed kill. This approach is considered very conservative.

In the past, a particular emphasis was placed on the risks of HIV,[37] but fortunately, there have been relatively few documented cases of HIV transmission by allograft transplant. The majority of these cases, which included both organs and tissues, occurred prior to the availability of the currently used HIV blood tests and the implementation of donor social history screening in 1985. Studies have reviewed the blood, tissues, and organs implicated in HIV transmission and are still relevant 25 years later because there have been no reported transmissions since these in the mid-1980s.[38,39] The most publicized case of allograft HIV transmission, and the case most relevant for this overview, was a case in which the HIV-antibody test was negative at the time of donation.[31] Six years after death of the donor, the donor was shown to have been HIV-positive by polymerase chain reaction tests. Three recipients of vascular organs and three fresh-frozen bone and tendon recipients from this donor were found to be infected with HIV. In contrast, 34 recipients of relatively avascular structures, including fascia lata, tendons, ligaments, dura mater, corneas, and highly processed bone did not become infected with HIV. A variety of other infectious organisms have been transmitted by allogeneic tissue transplantation, including bacterial infections, viruses (hepatitis, cytomegalovirus, herpes simplex, and rabies), fungal infections, and parasites.[38,39] Special consideration may also be given to the risks associated with prion contamination in certain high-risk tissues, given reports of tissue transplantation transmission of prion diseases.[40] But, as the screening of donors' behavioral, medical, and social history have become more robust and standardized in the last 25 years as well as the use of detection methods, the risks of disease transmission have been significantly reduced. Additionally, with more banks terminally sterilizing their allografts, the risk of viral and bacterial disease transmission has also been significantly reduced. Those grafts, not able to undergo terminal sterilization that are assessed for their culture positive status, have also seen significant improvement in testing methods and validation of those test methodologies using USP <71> method suitability testing, ensuring a significant reduction in false negatives due to processing reagent residuals that can mask bacterial growth. Also, the banks have undertaken and completed characterizations and validations of the tissue cleaning and disinfection processes used for the various tissue types, viable and nonviable produced. It is to their benefit to maximize the donor gift, reducing the amount of tissue

that is discarded, and reduce the risk of disease transmission. Thus, there is multifactorial motivation to ensure the safety of the allografts produced.

The final aspect to ensuring allograft safety is that the packaging will maintain a sterile/aseptic barrier for the shelf life of the graft. Many considerations go into choosing packaging that exceeds the scope of this chapter (see chapter 41). Overall, selection and pretreatment of packaging materials, validating sealing parameters, and ensuring packaging can withstand any applicable terminal sterilization, effects of freezing (if applicable), and confirming that there is no negative interaction between the graft or any preservation agents are essential examples. There are several standards and guidances to help navigate these elements as well as details on appropriate packaging validation requirements. For example, the AATB has a guidance on executing packaging validations[41] and the international packaging standards.[42] Even though the title of the international standard indicates requirements for terminally sterilized products, most of the information is also applicable to aseptically manufactured products.

▶ HEART VALVES AND OTHER VIABLE ALLOGRAFTS

The most commonly employed viable allografts involving disinfectant treatments are aortic and pulmonary heart valves. There is a growing use of viable bone void filler allografts that contain one or more cell types such as osteocytes, mesenchymal stem cells, and adipose combined with demineralized cortical bone and corticocancellous bone chips to collectively provide an osteogenic, osteoinductive, and osteoconductive product, respectively. The processing, particularly of the live bone component, and testing of these grafts for their culture negative status is similar to that of heart valves. In the United States, as discussed, all tissue donors must fall within the AATB standards, but it is further stipulated that heart valve donors shall meet additional criteria in order to reduce the risks of infectious disease transmission. These additional criteria are the following:

1. There shall be no history of bacterial endocarditis, rheumatic fever, or semilunar valvular disease, or a cardiomyopathy of viral or idiopathic etiology.
2. Any history of previous cardiac surgery, closed chest massage, penetrating cardiac injury, or other potentially deleterious cardiac intervention shall be evaluated on a case-by-case basis.
3. In the case of suspected sudden infant death syndrome, an autopsy should be performed, and results reviewed to confirm the cause of death.

Donor tissues for transplantation are obtained aseptically in an operating room or, alternatively, at autopsy in a clean fashion. The donor is usually prepared in a manner similar to preparing the incision site of a patient for surgery, for example, with 2% chlorhexidine gluconate, povidone-iodine, and/or 70% isopropanol (see chapter 43). Surgical techniques for the recovery of hearts for valve procurement in an autopsy setting have been presented.[43] In order to provide a culture negative allograft for transplantation, identification and elimination of any potential contaminants are required. Antibiotics, despite their limitations in their spectrum of activity to bacteria, have been traditionally used. The AATB standards dictate that "processing shall include an antibiotic disinfection period followed by rinsing, packaging, and cryopreservation" and that "disinfection of cardiovascular tissue shall be accomplished via a time-specific antibiotic incubation."[18,19] The effectiveness of allograft disinfection by incubation in low-concentration, broad-spectrum antibiotics was reported.[44,45] Skin was also treated with gentamicin[44] or combinations of penicillin and streptomycin.[46,47] Others reported better results with combinations of ceftazidime, ampicillin, and amphotericin.[48] Reduction in antibiotic concentrations also improved the viability of refrigerated stored skin (Figure 50.1).[47] Antibiotic selection also varies depending on the type of tissue to be treated. For example, a patented method of cryopreserving saphenous vein grafts used imipenem as the antibiotic of choice.[49]

In addition to surgical techniques and recipient variables, the most crucial aspects influencing posttransplant allograft valve function are the methods of aseptic procurement, antibiotic treatment, and storage of donor heart valves. There have been five eras, beginning in the 1950s, related to the development and advancement of these critical factors. It is important to review the history of allografts in order to gain perspective on the current state-of-the-art and future trends. At the present, allograft heart valves have become commonly used for right ventricular outflow tract reconstructions in children and adults. They have also become the first choice of many surgeons for complex left ventricular outflow reconstructions, par-

ticularly valve or root replacements for bacterial endocarditis that has dramatically increased over the last 5 years in parallel with the opioid epidemic in the United States. In 2017, the American Association for Thoracic Surgery issued a consensus on surgical treatment of infective endocarditis recommending the use of allograft heart valves in this patient population due to excellent inherent risk of infection and supporting clinical data.[50]

Fresh Viable Grafts

During the first era, fresh aseptic procurement was performed, with transplantation occurring within hours or a few days.[51,52] In the 1950s, animal studies that simulated the transplantation of fresh human aortic allograft valves into the descending thoracic aorta were reported.[53] This work was later supported by others in studies using aortic valve allografts for surgical treatment of native aortic and mitral valve insufficiency.[51,52,54-58] In 1962, the initial clinical procedures utilizing aortic valve allografts for valve replacement were nearly simultaneously reported with excellent results.[59,60] Consequently, because allografts became more popular, supply of viable grafts for transplantation became a problem. This shortfall led to further experimentation designed to improve sterilization and storage techniques. Radiation and chemical methods of sterilization (utilizing β-propiolactone and ethylene oxide) had been described in the early 1950s[61-64] but were not generally used.

Experimental Disinfection/Sterilization and Storage Techniques

Beginning in the 1960s, a second era saw clean procurement combined with further experimentation in disinfection/sterilization and storage.[56,65-73] Limited donor availability led to preservation attempts to thereby lengthen storage time and enable the establishment of heart valve banks. Storage techniques included freeze drying and flash freezing (submersion in liquid nitrogen) followed by frozen storage at −70°C. In 1977, a 6-year review reported that flash freezing resulted in poor clinical results and laboratory evidence of altered biomaterial properties.[71] Similar poor results were reported with frozen irradiated valves.[69] These valves demonstrated an increased failure rate after 5 years *in vivo*. Additional concerns about transmission of infection led to aggressive disinfection or sterilization techniques, including highly concentrated antibiotic incubation, irradiation, and chemical pretreatment. Although all of these methods were capable of increasing valve availability, allograft valve durability was significantly reduced and subsequently caused disenchantment with the transplantation of allograft valves. As early as 1966,[65] radiation methods were described for heart valve sterilization. Pretreatment with γ radiation or β-propiolactone

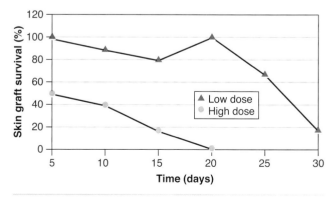

FIGURE 50.1 Refrigerated human skin graft cell survival during exposure to high- and low-dose antibiotics (penicillin G and streptomycin). From Cram et al.[47]

markedly diminished the *in vivo* durability of valves.[56-58] The use of radiation was subsequently confirmed by others as having deleterious effects on valve performance and was completely abandoned.[72] At that time, recognizing the damaging effects of these sterilization techniques, it was suggested that the use of fresh valve grafts was clinically superior.

Antibiotic-Treated Refrigerated Grafts

The third and longest era emerged from the above period of experimentation. In several studies, aseptic allograft procurement was combined with antibiotic treatment during 4°C storage, in various culture media and salt solutions, for up to 6 weeks. These relatively gentle techniques improved valve durability and, ultimately, patient survival.[74,75-82] The Stanford group demonstrated actuarial estimates of freedom from all modes of valve failure of 83 ± 4% at 5 years, 62 ± 6% at 10 years, and 43 ± 7% at 15 years[81]; 92 ± 3% of patients were free from endocarditis at 8 years after operation. Freedom from reoperation was 88 ± 4% at 5 years, 67 ± 6% at 10 years, and 45 ± 7% at 15 years. The Harefield group substantiated these findings by demonstrating actuarial patient survival rates of 87% at 5 years and 81% at 8 years.[83-87] Ten- to 13-year follow-up of their aortic valve replacements demonstrated 71.6% freedom from valve failure at 10 years. Studies on allograft valves culminated in the demonstration of 50% valve survival at 12 years and 23 ± 6% valve survival at 15 years.[88] Patient survival was 75% at 15 years. In New Zealand, an actuarial survival of 77% at 5 years, 57% at 10 years, and 38% at 14 years was demonstrated.[73] Thus, allograft valves studies produced results, which were either comparable or better than those seen with prosthetic valves. Furthermore, statistics on patient survival were even better than those for valve durability. This was due to the typically noncatastrophic failure mode of allograft valves, which permitted valve deterioration to be detected by the patient's cardiologist before the situation became life-threatening. The only problem encountered with antibiotic-treated, refrigerated storage has been the relatively short shelf life of the stored allografts. Although commonly used after 6 weeks of storage, 4°C-stored allograft valves were clearly more durable *in vivo* when storage was limited to no more than 3 weeks. Several other studies have demonstrated that valves stored for less than 3 weeks retain significant levels of cell viability.[89,90]

Cryopreserved Grafts

The fourth era was characterized by an aseptic procurement combined with a short period between donor death and valve procurement (less than 24 hours), gentle antibiotic treatment, and cryopreservation with liquid nitrogen storage. Cryopreservation of allograft

heart valves started in the 1970s in response to the short shelf life of antibiotic-treated, refrigerated allograft heart valves. Studies showed that one of two approaches ensured the viability of the valve and generated the best clinical results. First, the current method wherein the valves received antibiotic treatment followed by short-term refrigerated storage.[85,91,92] The second effective technique was antibiotic treatment followed by long-term cryopreserved storage.[93,94] Long-term function of allograft heart valves generally correlates with the level of cell viability in the heart valve leaflets at the time of transplantation. Others provided evidence of a direct correlation of cell viability with *in vivo* function.[91,95,96]

It has been suggested that hearts recovered from multi-organ donors are essentially microbiologically sterile and, with correct aseptic technique on procurement and handling, may be immediately transplanted or cryopreserved without antibiotic treatment[97]; however, more recent studies have documented that a significant percentage (32%-53%) of donor heart valves or intact hearts in these conditions have yielded positive bacterial cultures.[98] It is difficult to determine if such infections were endogenous or exogenous in source (see chapter 43), but it is still current state of the industry that all allograft heart valves are subjected to antibiotic treatment and robust microbiological end point testing to ensure the culture negative status of the graft.

Many different antibiotic mixtures for treatment of tissues for transplantation have been used with varying degrees of success. Indicators of effectiveness, documented in many studies over the years, include cellular viability, host in-growth rate, treatment efficiency, and valve survival rates.[71,82,99-104] Various formulas using penicillin, gentamicin, kanamycin, azlocillin, metronidazole, flucloxacillin, streptomycin, ticarcillin, methicillin, chloramphenicol, colistimethate, neomycin, erythromycin, and nystatin have been tried by several investigators but were often reported to be unsatisfactory for a variety of reasons. Many reported a decrease in cellular viability.[105,106] Other documented molecular cross-linkages with collagen and mucopolysaccharides, which inhibited host ingrowth into the disinfected valve leaflets.[100,101,107,108] A modified version of the antibiotic treatment regimen with cefoxitin, lincomycin, polymyxin B, and vancomycin added to a sterile-filtered RPMI 1640 tissue culture medium was commonly used in the United States to disinfect allograft heart valves.[45] Banks have looked at the incoming flora on the tissue and reformulated their cocktails to address those organisms and included such antibiotics as gentamicin, vancomycin, ciprofloxacin, meropenem, rifampin, and anidulafungin. Some of the frequent organisms seen are *Streptococcus viridians*, *Staphylococcus* coagulase negative, *Lactobacillus* species, *Veillonella* species, group B streptococci, *Enterococcus faecalis*, and *Clostridium* species. Various nutrient media have also been used, including modified Hank's solution, TCM 199, Eagle's

TABLE 50.2	Antibiotic cocktails employed for heart valves		
Antibiotics	**Nutrient Media**	**References**	
Cefoxitin, lincomycin, polymyxin B, vancomycin, +/− amphotericin	RPMI 1640 and TCM 199	Strickett et al,[45] Barratt-Boyes et al,[73] Lange and Hopkins,[98] McNally et al[111]	
Colistimethate, gentamicin, kanamycin, lincomycin	TCM 199	Angell et al[104]	
Streptomycin, penicillin	Eagle's MEM	O'Brien et al[93]	
Gentamycin, methicillin, nystatin, erythromycin, streptomycin	Modified Hank's balanced salts	Lockey et al[75]	
Cefoxitin, ticarcillin, neomycin, polymyxin, Mycostatin	RPMI 1640 and fetal calf serum	Gonzalez-Lavin et al[97], Gonzalez-Lavin et al[112]	
Penicillin, streptomycin, amphotericin B	RPMI 1640	Kirklin et al[113]	
Gentamycin, azlocillin, flucloxacillin, metronidazole, amphotericin B	RPMI 1640 and human serum	Yankah and Hetzer[114]	

Abbreviations: MEM, Minimum Essential Medium.

MEM, and RPMI 1640 in conjunction with various antibiotic cocktails.[45,91,104,109,110] Although many different antibiotics in various tissue culture media have been employed (Table 50.2), all are employed at relative low doses with varying incubation times at either 4°C or 37°C. Care should be taken to optimize the antibiotic concentrations and conditions to minimize loss of heart valve leaflet cells (Figure 50.2).

The antibiotic solutions developed for the antiseptic treatment of heart valves were originally formulated to ensure preservation after weeks of storage at 4°C. But it was soon shown that antibiotics are more effective at

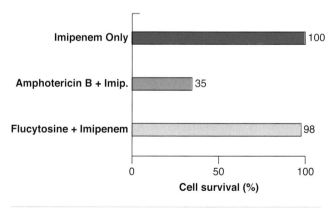

FIGURE 50.2 An example of studies with antibiotics and fungicides (flucytosine and amphotericin) for tissue treatment. Canine saphenous veins were incubated in antibiotic solutions, cryopreserved, thawed, and the endothelial cells removed by an enzyme digestion technique. The endothelial cells were cultured using a limiting dilution assay. The data are expressed as the number of clonogenic endothelial cells in percent of untreated controls. The amphotericin B treatment was statistically different ($P > .05$) compared to the untreated controls. From Schmehl et al.[115]

physiological temperatures (approximately 37°C) than at refrigerator temperatures.[106] In fact, there is little evidence that antibiotics even provide significant bactericidal action at 4°C because most function through interference with temperature-dependent processes of nucleic acid synthesis or the bacterial cell wall. It is possible that the effectiveness of some of the 4°C antibiotic treatment protocols can be credited to antibiotic binding during low-temperature incubation and that upon subsequent rewarming, the antibiotic action is effective. Nevertheless, and regardless of the mechanism, most allograft heart valve programs advocate the use of antibiotics, although the disinfection processes vary.[116] Antibiotic treatment is an effective and necessary component in the processing of allografts for transplantation. All antibiotics should be reconstituted with sterile fluids per the manufacturer's instructions and premixed with a HEPES-buffered nutrient medium, such as Dulbecco's Modified Minimal Eagle's Medium (DMEM), RPMI 1640, or MEM, to maintain the pH within normal physiological ranges for mammalian cells.

The treatment stage of processing begins once the pulmonary and aortic valves are fully dissected from the donated heart. The dissected valves are placed in sterile containers and a quantity of antibiotic solution is added to completely cover the tissue. The tissues are then incubated under immersion at 37°C for up to 24 hours. Protocol efficacy may be enhanced, such as by continuous, gentle agitation of the container during the antibiotic exposure period. Following incubation, the heart valves are removed from the antibiotic solution, rinsed with tissue culture medium and packaged aseptically in a cryosolution, such as containing 10% dimethylsulfoxide and 10% fetal calf serum from a bovine spongiform encephalopathy–free certified herd for subsequent cryopreservation and storage in liquid nitrogen, below −120°C.

Antibiotic treatment of heart valves has been reported to cause some changes in cell morphology,[105] inhibition of cell ingrowth,[108] and reduction of heart valve leaflet cell viability.[106] The utilization of the fungicide amphotericin B in antibiotic formulas was reported to reduce porcine heart valve leaflet cell viability to zero after 12 hours of exposure at 4°C.[117] Overall, there is an opportunity to further optimize alternative antibiotic and even microbicide treatment processes.

Decellularized Heart Valves

Decellularized heart valves hold the promise of tissue engineering, providing a biologic, biocompatible, hemodynamically optimized valve that will not sensitize the recipient to the donor HLA profile but develop within a child born with congenital heart anomalies. This is quite the challenge to sufficiently decellularize the myocardial skirt and conduit wall while not stripping the delicate leaflets of collagen and proteoglycans.[118] There are numerous reports in the literature that describe a variety of approaches.[119] As examples, a German approach has been to use trypsin and endonuclease, a Brazilian approach uses the anionic denaturing detergent sodium dodecyl sulfate, and American approaches include the use of water with protease inhibitors and endonuclease (CryoLife), or the anionic nondenaturing detergent sodium lauroyl sarcosinate and recombinant endonuclease (LifeNet Health, nonvalved grafts only). Insufficiently decellularizing the tissue can lead to catastrophic failures because the partially decellularized valve is more antigenic than a cryopreserved one. At this time, CryoLife (http://www.cryolife.com) has the only decellularized heart pulmonary valve cleared by the FDA, and this is also claimed to reduced sensitization potential. It was announced in 2019 that the FDA would act on the recommendation of the 2014 panel meeting on more-than-minimally manipulated allograft heart valves and upregulate them from class II to class III medical devices. One common theme of all of these valves is they are still aseptically processed and are not terminally sterilized and thus rely on USP <71> microbiological testing to determine if they have been adequately disinfected. In recent years, there has been an increased need for human valves because the opioid epidemic has increased the incidence of bacterial endocarditis and allograft valves are uniquely indicated for use in infected fields because human tissues tend to be resistant to bacterial colonization.[120]

▶ FUTURE PERSPECTIVES

Since the original writing of this chapter, most tissues that do not have active cells are terminally sterilized using γ or E-beam radiation to an SAL of 10^{-6} to 10^{-3} (see chapter 29). Those grafts that do not have cells and are released for implantation based on USP <71> testing are often irradiated

preprocessing due to the microorganisms detected on recovery cultures. As much of the emphasis in regenerative medicine is now on cellular products, there is a need for optimizing disinfection and aseptic technique for the future. It is also of interest to note that there has not been a death associated with allograft tissue transmitting bacterial disease since 2001.[121] Thus, the focus within the tissue banking industry is on nanofibers, bioprinting, cellular therapeutics, and novel regenerative medicine solutions. Additionally, the tissue banks have developed compendia of clinical evidence with their proprietary processing regimes and use these data with hospital value analysis committees, so changing processing methods for these grafts generally does not have a safety, clinical, or business benefit at this time. But novel disinfectants and sterilizing methodologies are needed to maximize the impact of these new aforementioned technologies that may not be able to withstand traditional sterilization methodologies even at the lowest doses, so the donor gift is maximized.

REFERENCES

1. United Network for Organ Sharing. Increasing the number of transplants in the United States: 2016 in review. United Network for Organ Sharing Web site. https://unos.org/about/annual-report/2016-annual-report/. Accessed November 20, 2019.
2. American Association of Tissue Banks. National Tissue Recovery through Utilization Survey. American Association of Tissue Banks Web site. https://www.aatb.org/about-us/tissue-bank-surveys. Accessed November 20, 2019.
3. Brittberg M, Lindahl A, Nilsson A, Ohlsson C, Isaksson O, Peterson L. Treatment of deep cartilage defects in the knee with autologous chondrocyte transplantation. *N Engl J Med*. 1994;331:889-895.
4. Coetzee JC, Giza E, Schon LC, et al. Treatment of osteochondral lesions of the talus with particulated juvenile cartilage. *Foot Ankle Int*. 2013;34:1205-1211.
5. US Food and Drug Administration. March 25-26, 2019: General and Plastic Surgery Devices Panel of the Medical Devices Advisory Committee meeting announcement. US Food and Drug Administration Web site. https://www.fda.gov/advisory-committees/advisory-committee-calendar/march-25-26-2019-general-and-plastic-surgery-devices-panel-medical-devices-advisory-committee. Accessed November 20, 2019.
6. US Food and Drug Administration. Part 1271: human cells, tissues, and cellular and tissue-based products. 21 CFR. https://www.accessdata.fda.gov/scripts/cdrh/cfdocs/cfCFR/CFRSearch.cfm?CFRPart=1271. Accessed November 20, 2019.
7. Government of Canada. Human cells, tissues and organs (CTO) for transplantation establishment registration application form (FRM-0171). Government of Canada Web site. https://www.canada.ca/en/health-canada/services/drugs-health-products/compliance-enforcement/establishment-licences/human-cells-tissues-organs-transplantation-registration-application-form-0171.html. Accessed November 20, 2019.
8. European Commission. Blood, tissues, cells and organs. European Commission Web site. https://ec.europa.eu/health/blood_tissues_organs/tissues_en. Accessed November 20, 2019.
9. US Food and Drug Administration. Eligibility determination for donors of human cells, tissues, and cellular and tissue-based products: guidance for industry. US Food and Drug Administration Web site. https://www.fda.gov/BiologicsBloodVaccines/GuidanceComplianceRegulatoryInformation/Guidances/Tissue/default.htm. Accessed November 20, 2019.

10. US Food and Drug Administration. Search for FDA guidance documents. US Food and Drug Administration Web site. https://www.fda.gov/regulatory-information/search-fda-guidance-documents. Accessed November 20, 2019.

11. US Food and Drug Administration. Regulatory considerations for human cells, tissues, and cellular and tissue-based products: minimal manipulation and homologous use. US Food and Drug Administration Web site. https://www.fda.gov/media/124138/download. Accessed November 20, 2019.

12. International Organization for Standardization. *ISO 11137-1:2006: Sterilization of Health Care Products—Radiation—Part 1: Requirements for Development, Validation and Routine Control of a Sterilization Process for Medical Devices.* Geneva, Switzerland: International Organization for Standardization; 2006.

13. International Organization for Standardization. *ISO/TS 19930:2017: Guidance on Aspects of a Risk-Based Approach to Assuring Sterility of Terminally Sterilized, Single-Use Health Care Product That Is Unable to Withstand Processing to Achieve Maximally a Sterility Assurance Level of 10^{-6}.* Geneva, Switzerland: International Organization for Standardization; 2017.

14. Kowalski JB. Setting standards: extending the VD_{max} approach: AAMI TIR76 and its web-based calculation tool. *Biomed Instrum Tech.* 2019;53:232-236.

15. Association for the Advancement of Medical Instrumentation. *AAMI TIR37:2013: Sterilization of Health Care Products-Radiation-Guidance on Sterilization of Biologics and Tissue-Based Products.* Arlington, VA: Association for the Advancement of Medical Instrumentation; 2013.

16. United States Pharmacopeia. *USP <71>. Sterility Testing.* Rockville, MD: United States Pharmacopeial Convention; 2012.

17. US Food and Drug Administration. General biological products standards: sterility. 21 CFR §610.12. https://www.accessdata.fda.gov/scripts/cdrh/cfdocs/cfcfr/CFRSearch.cfm?fr=610.12. Accessed November 20, 2019.

18. American Association of Tissue Banks. *Standards for Tissue Banking.* 14th ed. McLean, VA; American Association of Tissue Banks; 2016.

19. American Association of Tissue Banks. *Guidance Document: Microbiological Process Validation & Surveillance Program [No. 5, version 2, July 18, 2016].* McLean, VA; American Association of Tissue Banks; 2016.

20. International Organization for Standardization. *ISO 14644-1:2015: Cleanrooms and Associated Controlled Environments—Part 1: Classification of Air Cleanliness by Particle Concentration.* Geneva, Switzerland: International Organization for Standardization; 2015.

21. Stryker. Stryker SurgiCool™ personal protection hood. Stryker Web site. http://www.strykermeded.com/media/1083/surgicool-brochure.pdf. Accessed November 20, 2019.

22. International Organization for Standardization. *ISO 13485:2016: Medical Devices—Quality Management Systems—Requirements for Regulatory Purposes.* Geneva, Switzerland: International Organization for Standardization; 2016.

23. International Organization for Standardization. *ISO 14971:2019: Medical Devices—Application of Risk Management to Medical Devices.* Geneva, Switzerland: International Organization for Standardization; 2019.

24. US Food and Drug Administration. Same surgical procedure exception under 21 CFR 1271.15(b): questions and answers regarding the scope of the exception. US Food and Drug Administration Web site. https://www.fda.gov/regulatory-information/search-fda-guidance-documents/same-surgical-procedure-exception-under-21-cfr-127115b-questions-and-answers-regarding-scope. Accessed November 20, 2019.

25. American Association of Tissue Banks. What is the Uniform DRAI? American Association of Tissue Banks Web site. https://www.aatb.org/?q=standards/uniform-drai. Accessed November 20, 2019.

26. Hansen-Suss P, Ribeiro V, Cieslinski J, Kraft L, Tuon F. Experimental procedures for decontamination and microbiological testing in cardiovascular tissue banks. *Exp Biol Med (Maywood).* 2018;243:1286-1301.

27. Mills CR, Wironen JF, Hanstke S, inventors; RTI Surgical Inc, assignee. Cyclic implant perfusion, cleaning and passivation process and implant produced thereby. US patent 8,142,991. March 27, 2012.

28. Feinstone S, Mihalik K, Kamimura T, Alter HJ, London WT, Purcell RH. Inactivation of hepatitis B virus and non-A, non-B hepatitis by chloroform. *Infect Immun.* 1983;41:816-821.

29. Spire B, Barré-Sinoussi F, Montagnier L, Chermann JC. Inactivation of lymphadenopathy associated virus by chemical disinfectants. *Lancet.* 1984;2:899-901.

30. Spire B, Dormont D, Barré-Sinoussi F, Montagnier L, Chermann JC. Inactivation of lymphadenopathy-associated virus by heat, gamma rays, and ultraviolet light. *Lancet.* 1985;1:188-189.

31. Simonds RJ, Holmberg SD, Hurwitz RL, et al. Transmission of human immunodeficiency virus type 1 from a seronegative organ and tissue donor. *N Engl J Med.* 1992;326:726-732.

32. Tomford W. Transmission of disease through transplantation of musculoskeletal allografts. *J Bone Joint Surg Am.* 1995;77:1742-1754.

33. Sullivan R, Fassolitis AC, Larkin EP, Read RB Jr, Peeler JT. Inactivation of thirty viruses by gamma radiation. *Appl Microbiol.* 1971;22:61-65.

34. European Medicines Agency. *ICH Q5A (R1) Quality of Biotechnological Products: Viral Safety Evaluation of Biotechnology Products Derived From Cell Lines of Human or Animal Origin.* Amsterdam, Netherlands: European Medicines Agency; 1997.

35. Campbell DG, Li P. Sterilization of HIV with irradiation: relevance to infected bone allografts. *Aust N Z J Surg.* 1999;69:517-521.

36. Campbell DG, Li P, Stephenson AJ, Oakeshott RD. Sterilization of HIV by gamma irradiation. A bone allograft model. *Int Orthop.* 1994;18:172-176.

37. Patijn GA, Strengers PF, Harvey M, Persijn G. Prevention of transmission of HIV by organ and tissue transplantation. HIV testing protocol and a proposal for recommendations concerning donor selection. *Transpl Int.* 1993;6:165-172.

38. Eastlund T. Infectious disease transmission through cell, tissue, and organ transplantation: reducing the risk through donor selection. *Cell Transplant.* 1995;4:455-477.

39. Eastlund T. Infectious disease transmission through tissue transplantation. Reducing the risk through donor selection. *Transplant Coordination.* 1991;1:23-30.

40. Bonda DJ, Manjila S, Mehndiratta P, et al. Human prion diseases: surgical lessons learned from iatrogenic prion transmission. *Neurosurg Focus.* 2016;41(1):E10.

41. American Association of Tissue Banks. Guidance document: qualification of packaging and validation of shipping/transport procedures. American Association of Tissue Banks Web site. https://www.aatb.org/sites/default/files/sites/default/files/private/AATB%20Guidance%20Doucment%20No.%209%20final%2010.23.17%5B1%5D.pdf. Accessed November 20, 2019.

42. International Organization for Standardization. *ISO 11607-1:2019: Packaging for Terminally Sterilized Medical Devices—Part 1: Requirements for Materials, Sterile Barrier Systems and Packaging Systems.* Geneva, Switzerland: International Organization for Standardization; 2019.

43. Kirklin JW, Barratt-Boyes BG, eds. *Cardiac Surgery.* New York, NY: Wiley; 1986:421.

44. Ross DN, Martelli V, Wain WH. Allograft and autograft valves used for aortic valve replacement. In: Ionescu MI, ed. *Tissue Heart Valves.* Boston, United Kingdom: Butterworth; 1979:127-172.

45. Strickett MG, Barratt-Boyes BG, MacCulloch D. Disinfection of human heart valve allografts with antibiotics in low concentration. *Pathology.* 1983;15:457-462.

46. Raju S, Grogan JB. Effect of storage on skin allograft survival. *Arch Surg.* 1969;99:100-102.

47. Cram AE, Domayer M, Shelby J. Human skin storage techniques: a study utilizing a nude mouse recipient. *J Trauma.* 1983;23:924-926.

48. Csönge L, Pellet S, Szenes A, István J. Antibiotics in the preservation of allograft and xenograft skin. *Burns.* 1995;21(2):102-105.

49. McNally RT, McCaa C, Brockbank KGM, Heacox AE, Bank HL, inventors; Medical University of South Carolina, assignee. Method for cryopreserving blood vessels. US patent 5,145,769. September 8, 1992.

50. Pettersson GB, Coselli JS, Hussain ST, et al; for American Association for Thoracic Surgery. 2016 The American Association for Thoracic Surgery (AATS) consensus guidelines: surgical treatment of infective endocarditis: executive summary. *J Thorac Cardiovasc Surg.* 2017;153:1241.e29-1258.e29.

51. Murray G. Homologous aortic-valve-segment transplants as surgical treatment for aortic and mitral insufficiency. *Angiology.* 1956;7:466-471.

52. Murray G. Aortic valve transplants. *Angiology.* 1960;11:99-102.

53. Lam CR, Aram HH, Munnell ER. An experimental study of aortic valve homografts. *Surg Gynecol Obstet.* 1952;94:129-135.

54. Kerwin AG, Lenkei SC, Wilson DR. Aortic-valve homograft in the treatment of aortic insufficiency. Report of nine cases, with one followed for six years. *N Engl J Med.* 1962;266:852-857.

55. Heimbecker RO. Durability of fresh homograft. *Ann Thorac Surg.* 1986;42:602-603.

56. Heimbecker RO. The homograft cardiac valve. In: Marendino KA, ed. *Prosthetic Valves for Cardiac Surgery.* Springfield, IL: Charles C. Thomas; 1961:157-159.

57. Heimbecker RO. Whither the homograft valve? *Ann Thorac Surg.* 1970;9:487-488.

58. Heimbecker RO, Aldridge HE, Lemire G. The durability and fate of aortic valve grafts. *J Cardiovasc Surg.* 1968;9:511-517.

59. Barratt-Boyes BG. Homograft aortic valve replacement in aortic incompetence and stenosis. *Thorax.* 1964;19(2):131-150.

60. Ross DN. Homograft replacement of the aortic valve. *Lancet.* 1962;2:487.

61. Meeker IA Jr, Gross RE. Sterilization of frozen arterial grafts by high-voltage cathode-ray irradiation. *Surgery.* 1951;30:19-28.

62. LoGrippo GA, Overhulse PR, Szilagyi DC, Hartman FW. Procedure for sterilization of arterial homografts with beta-propiolactone. *Lab Invest.* 1955;4:217-231.

63. Sutherland TW, Williamson GM, Zinnemann K, Shucksmith HS. Graft sterilization; a bacteriological and histological study of the relative merits of ethylene oxide and beta-propiolactone as tissue sterilizing agents, with special reference to arterial grafts. *Br Med J.* 1958;1:734-736.

64. Scott HW Jr, Collins HA, Foster JH. Clinical experience with arterial homografts sterilized with ethylene oxide and preserved by the freeze-dry method. *J Tn State Med Assoc.* 1955;48:435-445.

65. Hudson R. Pathology of the human aortic valve homograft. *Brit Heart J.* 1966;228:291.

66. Malm JR, Bowman FO Jr, Harris PD, Kovalick ATW. An evaluation of aortic valve homografts sterilized by electron beam energy. *J Thorac Cardiovasc Surg.* 1967;54:471-477.

67. Smith J. The pathology of human aortic valve homografts. *Thorax.* 1967;22:114-138.

68. Beach PM Jr, Bowman FO Jr, Kaiser GA, Malm JR. Frozen irradiated aortic valve homografts. Long-term evaluation. *NY State J Med.* 1973;73:651-654.

69. Merin G, McGoon DC. Reoperation after insertion of aortic homograft as a right ventricular outflow tract. *Ann Thorac Surg.* 1973;16:122-126.

70. Parker R, Nandakumaran K, Al-Janabi N, Ross DN. Elasticity of frozen aortic valve homografts. *Cardiovasc Res.* 1977;11:156-159.

71. Barratt-Boyes BG, Roche AHG, Whitlock RML. Six year review of results of freehand aortic valve replacement using an antibiotic sterilized homograft valve. *Circulation.* 1977;55:353-361.

72. Wain WH, Greco R, Ignegeri A, Bodnar E, Ross DN. 15 Years experience with 615 homograft and autograft aortic valve replacements. *Int J Artif Organs.* 1980;3(3):169-172.

73. Barratt-Boyes BG, Roche AHG, Subramanyan R, Pemberton JR, Whitlock RM. Long-term follow-up of patients with the antibiotic-sterilized aortic homograft valve inserted freehand in the aortic position. *Circulation.* 1987;75:768-777.

74. Kosek J, Iben A, Shumway N, Angell W. Morphology of fresh heart valve homografts. *Surgery.* 1969;66:269-274.

75. Lockey E, Ai-Janabi N, Gonzales-Lavin L, Ross DN. A method of sterilizing and preserving fresh allograft heart valves. *Thorax.* 1972;27:398-400.

76. Anderson ET, Hancock EW. Long-term follow-up of aortic valve replacement with the fresh aortic homograft. *J Thorac Cardiovasc Surg.* 1976;72:150-156.

77. Barratt-Boyes BG. Cardiothoracic surgery in the antipodes: including a report of a randomized trial of medical and surgical treatment of asymptomatic patients with severe coronary artery disease; a long-term follow-up of both fresh and antibiotic-treated homograft valves; and some observations on glutaraldehyde-preserved valve tissue. *J Thorac Cardiovasc Surg.* 1979;78:804-822.

78. Thomson R, Yacoub M, Ahmed M, Somerville W, Towers M. The use of "fresh" unstented homograft valves for replacement of the aortic valve. Analysis of 8 years' experience. *J Thorac Cardiovasc Surg.* 1980;79:896-903.

79. Saravalli OA, Somerville J, Jefferson KE. Calcification of aortic homografts used for reconstruction of the right ventricular outflow tract. *J Thorac Cardiovasc Surg.* 1980;80:909-920.

80. Penta A, Qureshi S, Radley-Smith R, Yacoub MH. Patient status 10 or more years after 'fresh' homograft replacement of the aortic valve. *Circulation.* 1984;70:I182-I186.

81. Miller DC, Shumway NE. "Fresh" aortic allografts: long-term results with free-hand aortic valve replacement. *J Cardiac Surg.* 1987;2:185-191.

82. Stelzer P, Elkins RC. Pulmonary autograft: an American experience. *J Card Surg.* 1987;2:429-433.

83. Ross DN, Yacoub MH. Homograft replacement of the aortic valve. A critical review. *Prog Cardiovasc Dis.* 1969;11:275-293.

84. Thompson R, Yacoub M, Ahmed M, Seabra-Gomes R, Rickards A, Towers M. Influence of preoperative left ventricular function on results of homograft replacement of the aortic valve for aortic stenosis. *Am J Cardiol.* 1979;43(5):929-938.

85. Al-Yanabi N, Ross D. Enhanced viability of fresh aortic homografts stored in nutrient medium. *Cardiovasc Res.* 1973;7:817-822.

86. Sabolinski ML, Alvarez O, Auletta M, Mulder G, Parenteau NL. Cultured skin as a 'smart material' for healing wounds: experience in venous ulcers. *Biomaterials.* 1996;17:311-320.

87. Thompson R, Ahmed M, Seabra-Gomes R, et al. Influence of preoperative left ventricular function on results of homograft replacement of the aortic valve for aortic regurgitation. *J Thorac Cardiovasc Surg.* 1979;77(3):411-421.

88. Ross DN. Application of homografts in clinical surgery. *J Card Surg.* 1987;2(suppl 1):175-183.

89. Mochtar B, van der Kamp A, Roza-de Jongh E, Nauta J. Cell survival in canine aortic heart valves stored in nutrient medium. *Cardiovasc Res.* 1984;18:497-501.

90. Brockbank KGM, Carpenter JF, Dawson PE. Effects of storage temperature on viable bioprosthetic heart valves. *Cryobiology.* 1992;29:537-542.

91. Kirklin JW, Blackstone EH, Maehara T, et al. Intermediate-term fate of cryopreserved allograft and xenograft valved conduits. *Ann Thorac Surg.* 1987;44:598-606.

92. Okita Y, Franciosi G, Matsuki O, Robles A, Ross DN. Early and late results of aortic root replacement with antibiotic-sterilized aortic homograft. *J Thorac Cardiovasc Surg.* 1988;95:696-704.

93. O'Brien MF, Stafford EG, Gardner MA, Pohlner PG, McGiffin DC. A comparison of aortic valve replacement with viable cryopreserved and fresh allograft valves, with a note on chromosomal studies. *J Thorac Cardiovasc Surg.* 1987;94:812-823.

94. McGiffin DC, O'Brien MF, Stafford EG, Gardner MA, Polner PG. Long-term results of the viable cryopreserved allograft aortic valve: continuing evidence for superior valve durability. *J Card Surg.* 1988;3:289-296.

95. Stark J. Do we really correct congenital heart defects? *J Thorac Cardiovasc Surg.* 1989;97:1-19.

96. O'Brien MF, Johnston N, Stafford G, et al. A study of the cells in the explanted viable cryopreserved allograft valve. *J Cardiac Surg.* 1988;3(suppl):279-287.

97. Gonzalez-Lavin L, McGrath L, Alvarez M, Graf D. Antibiotic sterilisation in the preparation of homovital homograft valves: is it necessary? In: Yankah AC, Hetzer R, Miller DC, Ross DN, Somerville J, Yacoub MH, eds. *Cardiac Valve Allografts 1962-1987*. New York, NY: Springer; 1987:17-21.

98. Lange PL, Hopkins RA. Allograft valve banking: techniques and technology. In: Hopkins RA, ed. *Cardiac Reconstructions With Allograft Valves*. New York, NY: Springer; 1989:37-63.

99. Yacoub M, Kittle CF. Sterilization of valve homografts by antibiotic solutions. *Circulation*. 1970;41(suppl 5):II29-II32.

100. Gavin JB, Herdson PB, Monro JL, Barratt-Boyes BG. Pathology of antibiotic-treated human heart valve allografts. *Thorax*. 1973;28:473-481.

101. Gavin JB, Barratt-Boyes BG, Hitchcock GC, Herdson PB. Histopathology of 'fresh' human aortic valve allografts. *Thorax*. 1973;28:482-487.

102. Waterworth PM, Lockey E, Berry EM, Pearce HM. A critical investigation into the antibiotic sterilization of heart valve homografts. *Thorax*. 1974;29:432-436.

103. Wain WH, Pearce HM, Riddell RW, Ross DN. A re-evaluation of antibiotic sterilisation of heart valve allografts. *Thorax*. 1977;32:740-742.

104. Angell WW, Angell JD, Oury JH, Lamberti JJ, Grehl TM. Long-term follow-up of viable frozen aortic homografts. A viable homograft valve bank. *J Thorac Cardiovasc Surg*. 1987;93:815-822.

105. Girinath MR, Gavin JB, Strickett MG, Barratt-Boyes BG. The effects of antibiotics and storage on the viability and ultrastructure of fibroblasts in canine heart valves prepared for grafting. *Aust N Z J Surg*. 1974;44:170-172.

106. Angell JD, Christopher BS, Hawtrey O, Angell WW. A fresh, viable human heart valve bank: sterilization, sterility testing, and cryogenic preservation. *Transplant Proc*. 1976;8(2 suppl 1):139-147.

107. Armiger LC, Gavin JB, Barratt-Boyes BG. Histological assessment of orthotopic aortic valve leaflet allografts: its role in selecting graft pre-treatment. *Pathology*. 1983;15:67-73.

108. Gavin JB, Monro JL. The pathology of pulmonary and aortic valve allografts used as mitral valve replacements in dogs. *Pathology*. 1974;6:119-127.

109. Watts LK, Duffy P, Field RB, Stafford EG, O'Brien MF. Establishment of a viable homograft cardiac valve bank: a rapid method of determining homograft viability. *Ann Thorac Surg*. 1976;21:230-236.

110. Karp RB. The use of free-hand unstented aortic valve allografts for replacement of the aortic valve. *J Card Surg*. 1986;1:23-32.

111. McNally RT, Heacox A, Brockbank KGM, Bank HL, inventors; CryoLife Inc, assignee. Method for cryopreserving heart valves. US patent 4,890,457. January 2, 1990.

112. Gonzalez-Lavin L, Bianchi J, Graf D, Amini S, Gordon CI. Homograft valve calcification: evidence for an immunological influence. In: Yankah AC, Hetzer R, Miller DC, Ross DN, Somerville J, Yacoub MH, eds. *Cardiac Valve Allografts 1962-1987*. New York, NY: Springer; 1987:69-74.

113. Kirklin JK, Kirklin JW, Pacifico JAD, Phillips S. Cryopreservation of aortic valve homografts. In: Yankah AC, Hetzer R, Miller DC, Ross DN, Somerville J, Yacoub MH, eds. *Cardiac Valve Allografts 1962-1987*. New York, NY: Springer; 1987:35-36.

114. Yankah AC, Hetzer JR. Procurement and viability of cardiac valve allografts. In: Yankah AC, Hetzer R, Miller DC, Ross DN, Somerville J, Yacoub MH, eds. *Cardiac Valve Allografts 1962-1987*. New York, NY: Springer; 1987:23-26.

115. Schmehl MA, Bank HL, Brockbank KGM. Effects of antibiotics on the endothelium of fresh and cryopreserved canine saphenous veins. *Cryobiology*. 1993;30:164-171.

116. Germain M, Strong DM, Dowling G, et al. Disinfection of human cardiac valve allografts in tissue banking: systematic review report. *Cell Tissue Bank*. 2016;17:593-601.

117. Hu J-F, Gilmer L, Hopkins R, Wolfinbarger L Jr. Effects of antibiotics on cellular viability in porcine heart valve tissue. *Cardiovasc Res*. 1989;23:960-964.

118. Nachlas A, Li S, Davis ME. Developing a clinically relevant tissue engineered heart valve—a review of current approaches. *Adv Healthc Mater*. 2017;6(24);201700918.

119. Naso F, Gandaglia A. Different approaches to heart valve decellularization: a comprehensive overview of the past 30 years. *Xenotransplantation*. 2018;25(1).

120. Pettersson GB, Hussain ST. Current AATS guidelines on surgical treatment of infective endocarditis. *Ann Cardiothorac Surg*. 2019;8:630-644.

121. Centers for Disease Control and Prevention. Update: allograft-associated bacterial infections—United States, 2002. Centers for Disease Control and Prevention Web site. https://www.cdc.gov/mmwr/preview/mmwrhtml/mm5110a2.htm. Accessed November 20, 2019.

Sterilization, Disinfection, and Asepsis in Dentistry

Chris H. Miller and Charles John Palenik

◗ CROSS-CONTAMINATION IN DENTISTRY

The practice of dentistry spans a wide variety of oral treatments, ranging from the simple polishing of a restoration (filling) to complex and extensive surgery of the osseous and soft orofacial tissues. Standard procedures of sterilization, disinfection, and asepsis must be applied to all types of dental care to reduce the chances of cross-contamination that may lead to serious infectious diseases. The main source of potential pathogenic microbes in dental facilities is the patients' mouths. Cross-contamination is the spread of microorganisms from one person to another, and there are three main pathways by which this may occur in dentistry: (1) patient to dental personnel, (2) dental personnel to patient, and (3) patient to patient.[1] These pathways involve one or more of the four major modes by which microorganisms may be shared between individuals: (1) *direct contact* (touching oral surfaces and fluids), (2) *droplet infection* (airborne contamination with larger droplets of aerosols or spatter of oral and respiratory fluids), (3) *indirect contact* (contact with contaminated instruments, needles, environmental surfaces or hands), (4) *airborne* (spread of smaller particles of respiratory fluids such as droplet nuclei through the air). In the dental setting, microbes can enter the body through (1) needlesticks and instrument punctures and cuts; (2) invisible breaks or cuts in the skin; (3) mucous membranes of the mouth, nose, eyes; (4) through open lesions; (5) inhalation; and (6) ingestion. Thus, the pathways for cross-contamination in dentistry involve numerous possible combinations of modes of microbe spread and entrance into the body, all of which must be addressed in a dental infection prevention program.

Cross-contamination from patient to the dental team mainly involves microorganisms present in the patient's mouth in saliva, blood, gingival crevice fluid, plaque, subgingival debris, or open lesions. The dental team may be exposed to these microbes through all three routes of spread by directly touching any oral surface; through dental aerosols and body fluid spatter; and by contact with previously contaminated instruments, surfaces, and supplies. In the absence of adequate protective measures, the dental team is exposed to the risk of infection by oral microorganisms and blood-borne pathogens present in the patients' mouths. For example, the incidence of hepatitis B among dentists (before the hepatitis B vaccine became available) was approximately two to six times greater than that of the general population.[2] Similar increases were noted among other health care professionals who also had frequent exposures to human blood and body fluids that may harbor the hepatitis B virus (HBV).

The risk of exposure to blood-borne and other pathogens for all health care workers (HCWs) and patients and the need for prevention have been recognized by the Centers for Disease Control and Prevention (CDC)[3] and by professional health care organizations, including the American Dental Association (ADA)[4] and the Organization for Safety and Asepsis Procedures (OSAP).[5] In 1991, the Occupational Safety and Health Administration (OSHA) of the US Department of Labor promulgated the blood-borne pathogens standard that requires employers to protect employees from exposure to human body fluids such as blood and saliva. Similar best practices and regulations are applicable internationally. Guidelines and specific local, state, and federal regulations now exist requiring all health care facilities to practice specific sterilization, disinfection, cleaning, and aseptic techniques.

Cross-contamination from a member of the dental team to the patient is a relatively rare event in dentistry that might involve the hands or respiratory fluids of dental personnel. This pathway of disease spread has been documented with case reports of dentist-to-patient transmission of hepatitis B.[2] Because these carrier dentists did not routinely wear gloves during care of the patient, it is assumed that the blood-borne virus periodically contaminated their hands as a result of blood or serum leaking through small cuts or abrasions. The virus was then apparently transferred to patients through a break in their oral mucosa during intraoral care. Instances of apparent occupational spread of the human immunodeficiency virus (HIV) from an infected dentist[6] and physician[7] to patients have been reported.

Cross-contamination from one patient to another patient may occur by indirect routes through contaminated instruments, surfaces, equipment, or the hands of dental personnel. This pathway, involving improperly washed hands of a dental hygienist, has been documented in the spread of herpes simplex virus from a herpes labialis lesion of one patient to the mouths of several other patients, resulting in herpes gingivostomatitis.[8] In another incident, the CDC confirmed that hepatitis B was spread from one patient to another on the same day in 2001 in an oral surgery practice.[9] The source patient was an asymptomatic carrier of the HBV and did not tell anyone in the office she was a carrier. After, she has some teeth extracted the same oral surgeon, and staff extracted seven teeth from another patient (a 61-year-old female) who later developed hepatitis B. Molecular epidemiology techniques determined that the same virus caused hepatitis B in both women. Fourteen of 15 employees in the practice showed evidence of hepatitis B vaccination, and none had a history of the disease. Several of the patients seen after the source patient that week tested positive for hepatitis B immunity. Although the transmission was clearly documented, no clear-cut mode of viral spread was identified. The spread was likely limited to one patient due to the high incidence of hepatitis B immunity in the staff and several patients.

Two other routes of microbe spread involving dentistry are (1) dental office to community (eg, improper containment of contaminated medical waste during transport or sending a contaminated dental impression to a dental laboratory) and (2) community to dental office (eg, contaminated municipal water being used in patient care). A report from England in 1987 describes how two cancer patients acquired oral infections with *Pseudomonas aeruginosa* from dental unit water.[10] In 2015, 20 children ages 3 to 11 who received pulpotomies (removal of tooth pulps) in a pediatric dental practice in Georgia, developed oral infections with *Mycobacterium abscessus*.[11] All required hospitalization with granulomatous swellings of the face or neck. *M abscessus* (an opportunistic microbe commonly present in domestic water supplies) was isolated from the water exiting all seven dental units in the practice and the isolates were indistinguishable from those isolated from the children. The water samples from the dental units had a total microbial count averaging 93,333 colony-forming units (CFUs) per milliliter well above the CDC-recommended

maximum of 500 CFUs/mL (the drinking water standard indicated by the US Environmental Protection Agency [EPA]). One CFU is considered as one or a small number of bacterial cells.

The two main approaches to control cross-contamination involve reducing the dose of microorganisms that might be shared between patients and the dental team and increasing the resistance of the dental team through immunization against specific diseases. The infection control procedures in these approaches can be categorized into the eight major areas discussed in this chapter. These are (1) personal protective equipment (PPE), (2) reusable instrument processing, (3) surface and equipment asepsis, (4) aseptic techniques, (5) laboratory asepsis, (6) radiographic asepsis, (7) safe handling of dental waste, and (8) immunization.

◗ PERSONAL PROTECTIVE EQUIPMENT

Prevention of Contamination

The three basic steps in the development of an infectious disease are (1) contamination (a portion of the body is exposed to microorganisms), (2) infection (the microorganisms survive and grow on or in the body), and (3) disease (growth of the microorganisms causes damage to our body).[12]

Preventing or reducing contamination interferes with the initial step in the development of an infectious disease. It is always best to prevent contamination (when possible) than to rely totally on the body's resistance to a given disease agent. One of the important approaches in attempts to accomplish this is the use of approved PPE, such as gloves, protective eyewear, masks, face shields, and protective clothing, to prevent or reduce exposure to potentially infectious materials. Many blood-borne pathogens prevention standards indicate that PPE is to be provided by an employer to any employee who may have potential for exposure to human body fluids at work. Also, the employer must maintain, clean, launder, and properly dispose of soiled PPE and provide alternatives (eg, latex-free gloves) when necessary (eg, Occupational Safety and Health Administration, US Department of Labor[13]).

Gloves

Gloves not only protect the hands of dental personnel from direct or indirect contact with patients' saliva and blood but also protect the patient from contamination with microorganisms on the hands of dental personnel.

Gloves must be worn by the dental team where there is the potential to have direct contact with blood, saliva, other potentially infectious body fluids, mucous membranes, and nonintact skin, and when handling items or surfaces soiled with blood or other potentially infectious materials (OPIM).[3,13] Disposable gloves must be replaced when torn or punctured or when their ability to function as a barrier is compromised. A fresh pair of gloves is to be used for each patient. Thus, gloves must not be washed or disinfected for reuse on another patient. In restricted conditions, heavy utility gloves may be cleaned and disinfected for reuse if the integrity of the glove is not compromised, but they should be discarded if they are cracked, peeling, discolored, torn, punctured, or exhibit other signs of deterioration.

Because the use of powder on medical gloves presents numerous risks to patients and HCWs, including inflammation, granulomas, and respiratory allergic reactions, the US Food and Drug Administration (FDA) has banned the sale of powdered surgeon's gloves and powdered examination gloves.[14] This rule became effective January 2017 and includes powdered latex and nonlatex gloves.

Sterile surgeon's gloves are to be worn when performing oral surgical procedures.[3] The sterile latex surgeon's gloves offer the best fit, with half-sizes and right and left thumb orientation. Nonsterile latex, nitrile, and vinyl examination gloves are adequate for nonsurgical intraoral procedures. Heavy utility gloves should be worn during operatory cleanup when disinfecting surfaces, handling other chemicals, and handling contaminated instruments (eg, during cleaning). Heat-resistant gloves should be worn when working with heat-based sterilizers.

Reactions to Gloves

One study of dental and other HCWs reported that 19% had some type of reaction to gloving and 3.8% reported having a latex allergy.[15] Another study involving testing of dental workers for latex allergy indicated that 6.2% were positive.[16] Reports for the general population range from 0.12% to 6%.[17,18]

There are three types of reactions to gloves: irritant contact dermatitis, allergic contact dermatitis, and latex allergy.[19] Irritant contact dermatitis is the most common and results from a nonimmunologic irritation of the skin from chemicals in the gloves or powder. Allergic contact dermatitis is an immunologic reaction to one of the many nonlatex chemicals in gloves. This reaction is the same in those sensitive to the poison ivy plant. Latex allergy is an immunoglobulin E (IgE)-mediated immunologic response to the protein allergens in latex. Latex allergy may not only result in skin reactions of hives, redness, burning, or itching but may also involve respiratory symptoms with difficulty breathing and, more rarely, anaphylactic shock. The protein allergens involved are not only present in the latex glove material but are also absorbed into cornstarch powder from the glove. During donning and removing of powdered gloves, the powder becomes airborne and can be widely distributed through a health care facility.

If inhaled, it may cause respiratory symptoms in the allergic and possibly enhance sensitization to latex proteins in others. Thus, as mentioned earlier, FDA has instituted a ban on powdered gloves to help reduce these potential reactions.

In the United States, both sterile surgeon's and nonsterile patient examination gloves are medical devices regulated by the FDA.[20] Accepted quality levels with respect to inherent perforations are actually 4.0% and 2.5% (maximum percentage of gloves with defects) for examination and sterile surgeon's gloves, respectively.

Gloving and Personal Protection

Small cuts and abrasions on the hands and fingers may serve as a route through which pathogenic microorganisms enter the body. A study of 26 second-semester senior dental students who did not routinely wear gloves at chairside revealed a total of 101 areas of trauma (cuts and abrasions) on their hands.[21] Twelve percent of these areas became painful on swabbing with alcohol, suggesting an open epidermis. Of interest was that a few additional alcohol-induced painful responses were detected in visually intact areas between the fingernail and peripheral epidermis, including the subungual area. This indicates that even a close visual inspection of the hands may not detect areas that could serve as a portal of entry for microorganisms into the body.

Wearing gloves provides a physical barrier over such portals of entry for pathogenic organisms from the saliva or blood of dental patients. The lack of routine gloving may have been a major contributing factor to the once alarmingly high occurrence of hepatitis B among dental personnel.[2] Like hepatitis B, herpetic whitlow (herpes simplex infection of the hands) is also an occupational disease of dental personnel.[22-24] Gloving prevents the occurrence of herpes simplex infections on the fingers acquired through direct contact with lesions or contaminated saliva.

Another personal protection aspect of wearing gloves involves providing a barrier against contact with contaminated inanimate objects or with irritating chemicals used in the office. For example, office staff responsible for post-treatment operatory cleanup or use of disinfecting or sterilizing solutions should wear heavy, chemical-resistant utility gloves. This reduces chances of accidental instrument puncture or direct contact with agents that may cause skin irritations or allergic reactions.

Hand Hygiene and Gloving for Protection of Patients

Besides offering personal protection to members of the dental team, gloves also provide an important measure of protection to patients. Hands have long been known to be one of the most important sources of nosocomial infection, and hand hygiene is generally considered the single most important procedure for preventing such infections.[25-27] There are two approaches to hand hygiene. Hand washing with plain or antimicrobial soap suspends dirt and microbes that are removed by thorough rising with water. When hands are not visibly soiled an alcohol hand rub can be used.[3,28] Hand hygiene facilities are recommended to include liquid soaps in no-touch dispensers, no-touch faucets, and disposable paper towels.

Although proper hand hygiene can remove/kill the transient skin flora, which is the most important in disease spread, no hand washing procedure sterilizes the skin, not even properly performed surgical scrubs with antiseptic agents.[29,30] Thus, sterile gloving is used to prevent transmission of organisms not removed by hand washing. Surgical hand scrubbing is a standard procedure, but hand hygiene should also be performed before routine nonsterile gloving to reduce the number of skin microbes that can multiply under the gloves and cause skin irritation. Hands also need to be washed after removing gloves to remove perspiration, materials that may have come through glove defects/punctures/tears, and microbes that may have multiplied beneath the gloves. Recognized antiseptic hand washing agents that have residual activity on the skin (long-lasting effect) include biocides such as chlorhexidine gluconate or parachlorometaxylenol.[31]

Ungloved hands of dental personnel become contaminated with potentially infectious materials from patients' mouths. Blood impaction under the fingernails does occur, and this material may be retained for several days after treating a patient.[21] This occult (concealed) blood could serve as a source of infection for subsequent patients through a leaching process. Routine gloving prevents blood or saliva impaction in those parts of the hands that are difficult to clean, such as under the fingernail or areas of dermatitis.

Microorganisms that might be present in the blood periodically contaminate the hands and fingers as a result of blood or serum leaking through small cuts or abrasions. This process may be enhanced if the site of the cut or abrasion is kept moist, as when performing barehanded dentistry. This seems to be a likely route of HBV and other pathogen transmission from carrier dentists to their patients.

The eight reported instances of HBV transmission from dental personnel to patients resulted in numerous cases of the disease.[2,32,33] Most of the implicated dental personnel acquired subclinical infections and became chronic carriers of the virus; none had worn gloves, and some had skin lesions or dermatitis on their hands. Although intact gloves would protect patients from this route of disease transmission, other routes of disease transmission from carrier dental personnel to patients clearly do exist.

The report of an outbreak of herpes simplex virus type I gingivostomatitis in a dental hygiene practice also offers a vivid line of evidence for the role of contaminated hands in disease transmission.[8] A hygienist with dermatitis on her ungloved hands contracted a herpes infection on her hands after treating a patient with active herpes labialis. Before vesicles developed in the areas of chronic dermatitis on her hands, she unknowingly transmitted the virus to other patients, resulting in gingivostomatitis in 20 of 46 patients treated over the next few days with ungloved hands. When the herpes vesicles appeared on her hands she began to wear gloves, and this prevented further spread of the virus.

Surgical Masks

Surgical masks covering the mouth and nose were originally developed for the protection of the patient from respiratory organisms of health care personnel. This is an important reason to use surgical masks in dentistry, but equally important in dentistry is that surgical masks help protect the dental staff from the patient's microorganisms. They reduce the number of infectious particles that may enter the mouth or nose while the staff person performs techniques that generate dental spatter (the larger particles of oral fluids). Respirators (eg, N95 respirator) are needed to protect against inhalation of the smaller aerosol-type particle that cause airborne infections (eg, the causative agents of tuberculosis, measles, and severe acute respiratory syndrome [SARS]). Patients with many high-risk infections may need to be treated in specialized facilities. Respirators are not part of the normal PPE needed in dental offices. Masks made of glass fiber or synthetic fiber mats are more efficient in filtering bacteria than gauze or paper masks.[34]

For FDA clearance, mask manufacturers are required to submit performance data that includes fluid resistance, particulate filtration efficiency, bacterial filtration efficiency, differential pressure (degree to which the passage of air is impeded through the mask material and flammability).[35] Surgical masks are available that claim at least a 99% bacterial filtration efficiency against particles that are 3 to 5 μm in diameter, as determined by the modified Greene and Vesley method.[36] The filterability of any mask is destroyed if the mask does not fit well, however; this permits excessive contaminated air to leak around the edges of the mask.[37] A key feature of a mask is that it must be comfortable to wear, and the mask should fit snugly over the bridge of the nose to reduce fogging of the protective eyewear from exhaled air.

Masks are single-use disposable items and should not be reused with another patient and should be changed when wet.

Protective Eyewear

Protective eyewear can reduce the chance of physical and microbial injury to the eyes.[38] Microorganisms may contact the eye by aerosol spray or droplet deposition.

Tooth or restorative material expelled from the mouth also may be contaminated with potentially pathogenic microorganisms.

Usually, the eye eliminates transient infections, but if the contamination is heavy, if a highly virulent organism is involved, or if physical damage accompanies the contamination, serious disease may result. Of particular concern is a herpesvirus infection of the eye that may recur and produce increasing ocular damage. Hepatitis B infection may also develop after initial contamination of the eye with the virus.[39,40]

Review of a report of 10 cases of ocular injuries sustained in dental offices demonstrates a compelling need for protective eyewear for both patients and dental personnel.[41] The cases included impalement of a patient's eye by an excavator, corneal abrasions in patients from an exploding anesthetic carpule or a piece of acrylic denture tooth, subconjunctival hemorrhage after a dentist hit a patient's eye with his or her thumb, corneal abrasions and hemorrhage in dental assistants' eyes by projectiles emitted from patients' mouths during operative procedures, and damage to an assistant after splashing varnish into his or her eyes while working in the laboratory.

Protective eyewear should be worn at chairside, in the laboratory, in darkrooms, in the use of chemical disinfectants, and in the sterilization area when mixing and using chemicals. The OSHA blood-borne pathogens standard as well as the CDC require protective eyewear to have side shields.[3,13]

Face Shields

Plastic face shields have become more popular for use at chairside during procedures that generate salivary droplets. Face shields protect the skin, eyes, and mucous membranes of the mouth and nose from potentially infectious droplets but offer little protection from inhalation of aerosols. Thus, masks need to be worn beneath face shields.

Protective Clothing

Dental procedures generate salivary droplets, particularly during the use of handpieces, ultrasonic scalers, and air/water syringes. Protective clothing should be worn to protect underlying work clothes, street clothes, undergarments, and skin.[3,13] Protective clothing worn at work should be changed before leaving for home, and this clothing is not to be taken home for laundering. Disposable gowns are available for use at chairside or reusable protective clothing may be worn. A laundry service may be used for reusable clothing or laundering may be performed in the office with a washer and dryer. As a related precaution, work shoes should be kept at work or at least out of reach of small children at home because at work the shoes are constantly in contact with salivary spatter that rapidly settles to the floor.

Donning and Doffing PPE

The CDC recommends the following sequence for putting on and removing PPE to avoid unnecessary spread of contaminants.[42] For donning (1) protective clothing, (2) mask, (3) protective eyewear, and (4) gloves. For doffing: (1) gloves, (2) protective eyewear, and (3) gown, and (4) mask.

▶ INSTRUMENT REPROCESSING

The goal of instrument reprocessing is to prevent transfer of infectious agents to patients from contaminated dental hand instruments and handpieces and, at the same time, to protect the staff who must handle these items. The steps in this process involve instrument transport, presoaking, cleaning, packaging, sterilization, monitoring, storage, and distribution, as summarized in Table 51.1. Heavy utility gloves, protective clothing, a mask, and protective eyeglasses should be worn during the cleaning and disinfection of instrument processing to help protect against sharps injuries, direct contact with contaminated surfaces, and splashing of chemicals or contaminated fluids. Following thermal disinfection, devices are considered safe for handling, but critical and semicritical devices are required to be sterilized prior to patient use. Processing dental handpieces is described at the end of this section.

The central processing area should be divided physically or, at a minimum spatially, into distinct areas for (1) receiving, cleaning, and decontamination; (2) preparation and packaging; (3) sterilization; and (4) storage.[3] This helps prevent the intermingling of contaminated with sterile instruments. The responsibility for reprocessing dental instruments needs to be assigned to personnel with the appropriate training, and the manufacturers' instructions for reprocessing instruments/equipment are to be readily available, ideally in or near the reprocessing area.[3]

Instrument Transport

Contaminated instruments should be transported to the processing area in a manner that minimizes the risk of exposure to people and the environment. This includes the use of covered, rigid, leak-proof containers or carts that are appropriately marked with biohazard symbols. The containers used for these sharp contaminated instruments must not permit a person to reach into them without being able to see the instruments. It is considered best practice to not allow soil to dry on devices prior to cleaning, but if this occurs, then instrument presoaking is recommended prior to cleaning (see in the following text). This may be achieved such as cleaning solution,

TABLE 51.1	Critical dental instrument reprocessing
1. Transport	Separate and dispose all single-use devices and materials. Transport contaminated reusable instruments to a defined decontamination area so that exposure of staff and the environment are minimized. It is best practice not to allow soil to dry on devices prior to cleaning.
2. Presoak and rinse	If used (eg, if soil has dried on devices), submerge in pH neutral to mild alkaline detergent in accordance with manufacturer's instructions.
3. Clean, rinse, and dry	Carefully remove gross soil using a cleaning solution in compliance to manufacturer's instructions, ensuring cleaning of any restricted access device features (eg, brushing of lumens, articulating moving parts). Ultrasonic cleaning systems may be used and devices may also be cleaned and/or disinfected in a washer or washer-disinfector.
4. Inspection and maintenance	Dry devices using a drying over or lint-free materials. Inspect devices to ensure they are clean and undamaged. Lubricate any devices in accordance to manufacturer's instructions.
5. Package	Include any applicable biological or chemical indicators to test for steam sterilization. Package in an approved sterilization wrap, bags, pouches, or rigid containters.
6. Sterilize and monitor	Steam sterilization is preferred, unless the devices are heat sensitive. Ensure to check all indicators used to test the sterilization process, including mechanical gauges or monitors (eg, temperature and pressure). Ensure packaging is dry prior to storage. Record results of monitoring.
7. Store or distribute	Sterilized cassettes or packages are ready for storage or use at chairside. Store in a dry place in a manner that does not allow for accidental damage of the packaging material.

transportation gel or foam, or water. The containers or carts used during transport (where applicable) need to be decontaminated (cleaning and disinfected with an environmental surface disinfectant) between each use and should be indicated as "contaminated" or "sterile."

Instrument Presoaking

If saliva and blood on instruments are allowed to dry, the cleaning process becomes more difficult. This occurrence is not uncommon because seldom, is it possible in a busy practice to clean instruments immediately after use. Thus, contaminated instruments can be presoaked in a pH neutral to mild alkaline detergent solution (which may or may not include enzymes) until time is available for full cleaning. The manufacturer's instructions for use (IFU) need to be followed, including not only those provided with the instruments but also the cleaning chemistries or other equipment used for reprocessing. This process also is referred to as instrument *holding* and is most effective when it begins immediately after the patient is dismissed. This step in instrument processing prevents drying of blood and saliva and actually begins the cleaning process. Some enzyme- or alkaline-based detergents designed to break down proteins may facilitate this process, but such detergents should be labeled for use on medical or dental instrumentation. The use of environmental disinfectants (eg, bleach solutions), saline or antiseptic formulations (eg, chlorhexidine- or iodine-based soaps) are not appropriate and can even damage devices. Instruments should

not be presoaked for more than a few hours, for the longer the instruments remain wet, the greater the chances for corrosion of stainless steel and other metals, as well as the risk of bacterial growth.

If ultrasonic cleaning is used, gross contamination should be manually removed, and the contaminated instruments then placed in the ultrasonic cleaning basket or the cassettes in a cassette rack, and the basket or rack placed in the presoak solution. This reduces the direct handling of the contaminated instruments. If the clinician uses "plastic-type" instrument cassettes that retain the instruments during use at chairside and during ultrasonic cleaning, the manufacturer of the cassettes should be consulted as to which type of presoak solution will not damage the cassette. After the presoak period, the instruments should be carefully rinsed under running tap water with minimal splashing.

Instrument Cleaning

One approach to instrument cleaning is hand washing, which includes manual cleaning of exposed and restricted access parts of the devices. It is particularly important to ensure that any restricted access device features are manually cleaned (eg, brushing of lumens, articulating moving parts). However, hand scrubbing is directly contrary to one of the dogmas of infection prevention—reduce direct contact with contaminated surfaces as much as possible. Hand scrubbing increases such contact and involves the added danger of handling sharp and pointed objects.[43]

If an item must be hand scrubbed, then heavy-duty utility gloves, mask, protective eyewear, and clinic attire must be worn and spattering must be avoided by scrubbing the item while it is submerged under water using a long-handled brush.

Approved automated cleaning (or cleaning-disinfection) equipment should also be considered.[3] Ultrasonic cleaning or using an instrument washer or washer/disinfector is effective and generally much safer than hand scrubbing. It is, however, important to understand the limitations of such equipment depending on their IFU. For example, gross soiling should be removed prior to ultrasonics and lumens (or other device restricted access features) may not be adequately cleaning by such equipment. Several brands of ultrasonic cleaners are available in a variety of sizes.[1] A metal cleaning basket or cassette rack and a lid over the tank always should be used, and the IFU followed for optimal results. An ultrasonic cleaning detergent solution should be used that is specifically recommended for use with medical/dental instruments in sonic cleaners.

For ultrasonic cleaning, the rinsed instruments contained in the cleaning basket are submerged into the cleaning solution. The basket suspends the instrument in the tank. Loose instruments should not be placed on the bottom of the tank because this usually results in less effective cleaning. Place the lid on the bath and operate the unit in accordance with manufacturer-validated instructions (eg, for 6 to 10 min or until no visible debris remains). Note that the efficiency of ultrasonic cleaning will depend on the equipment device, ultrasonic energy, and cleaning detergent solution. If the instruments are to be in cassettes, it may be recommended to increase cleaning time to 15 minutes.[44] Cleaning time in these cases is not time lost because other tasks can be performed during this process. After cleaning, thoroughly rinse the instruments while they are still in the cleaning basket or cassette rack to remove dislodged debris, microorganisms, and residual cleaning solution.

Instrument washers that automatically clean and rinse instruments and cassettes are becoming more popular in group practices and large clinics. They operate somewhat like a home dishwasher but are much more sophisticated and are specifically designed for processing medical/dental instruments. Washer-disinfectors may also be used and are recommended to be compliant to International Organization for Standardization (ISO) 15883-1.[45] These typically have separate phases to validated cycles to include cleaning, thermal disinfection (to render devices safe for handling), and drying. It is important that such equipment is calibrated and maintained in accordance with manufacturer's instructions.

Cleaned instruments should be visually inspected for cleanliness and carefully dried before packaging and sterilization.[3] If nonstainless steel instruments are to be sterilized in a steam autoclave, a rust inhibitor (dip or spray) such as sodium nitrite should only be applied to the instruments after cleaning if recommended by the device manufacturer. Other instrument maintenance recommendations may be appropriate at this time, such as handpiece lubrication. Only approved lubricants should be used that are compatible with subsequent steam sterilization.

Ultrasonic cleaners, instrument washers, and washer-disinfectors may be excellent for cleaning but are not sterilizers. Thus, the cleaned and rinsed instruments (but not thermally disinfected) are still considered biohazardous and must be handled only while wearing protective gloves. The used cleaning solution in ultrasonic cleaning tanks is also contaminated.[46] Use of the ultrasonic cleaning basket or cassette rack with handles avoids excessive contact with this solution, and rinsing after cleaning reduces this contamination on the instruments. The ultrasonic cleaning solution should be changed periodically, some suggest every use, by someone wearing gloves, protective clothing, eyewear, and a mask. At the end of the day, the ultrasonic cleaner tank should be cleaned, disinfected (eg, using alcohol), rinsed (if appropriate for the disinfectant type), and dried.

Note that the quality of water use during reprocessing can also be an important consideration due to the potential presence of chemical, microorganisms, and other contaminants in water. Tap water, for example, may be suitable for cleaning, but a higher purity of water is generally recommended for final rinsing and, for example, in the generation of steam for sterilization. Guidelines from the Association for the Advancement of Medical Instrumentation (AAMI), such as AAMI TIR34, can provide useful discussions on the impact and safety requirements for water used during device reprocessing.[47]

Packaging

Wrapped Instruments

Packaging cleaned instruments in an appropriate microbial barrier material before sterilization will help protect the instruments from recontamination after removal from the sterilizer. The instruments may be packaged in functional sets and then opened when required for patient use at chairside, or they may be packaged individually or in smaller groups and then distributed at chairside on sterile or disposable trays intended for use at chairside.

A variety of packaging materials are available for this purpose including peel pouches of plastic or paper, sterilization wraps (including woven or unwoven materials), and sterile rigid containers. In choosing the appropriate packaging material, they should be designed and labeled for use for the type of sterilization process and used in accordance to the manufacturer's claims. Packaging materials should be compliant to the appropriate standards, such as ISO 11607[48,49] and may need to be cleared for such uses in certain countries (as in the United States by the FDA).[3,50] Some types of materials may not be appropriate in certain cases, such as thin material bags through which pointed instruments may protrude. "See-through" bags and pouches facilitate instrument identification. One type is provided as a clear tubing of different widths on a roll that is cut and heat sealed. These are available for steam or dry-heat sterilization, and self-sealing paper/"plastic" pouches are also available for use in the steam autoclave or chemical gas sterilizers.[1] Sterilization paper wrap may be used for dry-heat processes as long as protrusion of sharp instruments is prevented. Each package to be sterilized should be labeled with the sterilizer used, the cycle or load number, and the date of sterilization. Use a writing device that does not run or fade during sterilization, and do not penetrate the packaging material with the writing device. Some permanent markers can be used on the plastic of paper/plastic pouched. Labels can be used on other types of packaging material.

Instruments in Trays or Cassettes

One option in this approach involves using a cassette that retains the instruments at chairside and during ultrasonic cleaning, rinsing, and subsequent sterilization.[44] This maintains the instruments in functional sets and minimizes potentially dangerous handling of the contaminated instruments during the cleaning or distribution process. After ultrasonic cleaning and rinsing, sterilizable supply items may be added to the cassette, and the cassette is wrapped, sterilized, and stored or used immediately.

The other option in this approach involves placing the cleaned instruments in one of several types of sterilizable trays.[1] Some types of solid metal trays with lids, that are designed and labeled to provide a sterile barrier, need no additional wrapping and can be used in standard dry-heat sterilization. However, their suitability as sterilization containers needs to be confirmed by proper sterilization monitoring using chemical and biological indicators as described later. "Plastic-type" or metal trays for steam or chemical vapor sterilization must have no lids or be perforated to permit penetration of the steam or chemical vapors. These trays, like cassettes, must be wrapped in an appropriate sterile barrier material before sterilization.

The use of sterilizable trays requires sterilizers with adequate chamber size to accommodate the trays. Larger size office sterilizers are available.

Unwrapped Instruments (Special Circumstances Only)

This approach should be used only in special circumstances, such as when one or a very small number of instruments are needed quickly on an emergency basis, and a short-time, high-temperature steam autoclave cycle is to be used. This is sometimes referred to as flash or immediate-use sterilization. This involves sterilizing previously cleaned and unpackaged instruments that will be used immediately after sterilization, if they do not become contaminated with blood or saliva from hands, surfaces, or aerosols before use. An aseptic protocol must be established for handling these instruments after sterilization, during conveyance from sterilizer to chairside. For example, this might include using sterile tongs to place the instruments in sterile bags for transport. It is recommended that these procedures are only used under emergency situations.

Sterilization Versus Disinfection

Sterilization is defined as a validated process that kills all microorganisms, as verified by demonstrating the kill of highly resistant bacterial spores. Sterilization is the highest level of microbial kill. If a process can be routinely shown to kill bacterial spores, then it is correctly assumed that the process can kill all other microorganisms, yielding sterilization. Disinfection is considered a less lethal form of microbial killing, usually involving the use of heat (eg, hot water) or a liquid disinfectant at room temperature. Disinfection can be achieved at different levels depending on the process or product claims (see chapter 2). Disinfection processes are directed at pathogenic microorganisms and are considered less lethal than sterilization. Unfortunately, the level of killing that does occur with liquid disinfectants in particular cannot be easily verified during actual use. On the other hand, the level of killing that occurs in a heat-based sterilizer can be monitored parametrically (eg, based on temperature, pressure, and time monitoring) and/or the routine use of chemical and biological indicators. Thus, the safest approach to preventing disease transmission by contaminated instruments is to sterilize them rather than disinfecting them.

All items used in the mouth must be cleaned, packaged, and sterilized before they are reused on another patient. For example, the CDC recommendations for infection prevention in dentistry indicate that surgical and other instruments used to penetrate soft tissue or bone and those that do not penetrate soft tissues or bone but contact oral tissues should be heat sterilized routinely between uses using steam under pressure (autoclave), dry heat, or chemical vapor.[3,51]

The only exceptions are disposable items that are used with only one patient and items that can be covered with a barrier that prevents contamination, such as light-curing devices and some camera lens probes and x-ray sensors. In these latter cases, equipment can be periodically disinfected using an approved environmental disinfectant.

Sterilization Processes

Sterilization equipment should be approved for use and used in accordance with equipment manufacturers requirements.[3] In dentistry, the three most commonly used forms of heat sterilization of instruments in the United States are (1) steam sterilizers (also known as autoclaves), (2) unsaturated chemical vapor sterilizers, and (3) dry heat. A fourth form of sporicidal disinfection in the United States involves submerging items in a liquid sterilant (eg, properly prepared glutaraldehyde or hydrogen peroxide solutions) often for extended contact times (eg, 3-10 h) followed by rinsing to remove toxic residuals; however, this method cannot be verified by spore testing and should be reserved for plastic and other items that are incompatible in the heat systems. Alternative low-temperature gaseous sterilization processes (such as those based on ethylene oxide or hydrogen peroxide gas) may be used as alternatives. The use of ethylene oxide gas sterilizers are reliable methods of low-temperature sterilization that can be verified with spore testing but requires special safety and postprocess aeration time (to remove toxic residuals). This method is primarily used in hospitals, some universities, and industry however, with only minimal use in dental offices. These low-temperature processes are described in more details in other chapters (see chapters 31 and 32).

Microorganisms are rapidly killed after they come in direct contact with a heat-sterilizing agent (steam, chemical vapor, air) that is at the proper temperature. Thus, time, temperature, and exposure are the minimum three key factors. The actual surfaces of the instruments must be exposed to the agent for the appropriate time, and the sterilizing agent must be at an appropriate temperature. Anything that interferes with exposure or temperature may prevent the sterilization or extend the time required for sterilization.[52] This will include trapped air (prevent steam or chemical penetration) or the presence of residual soil (due to inadequate cleaning or rinsing). An example is that device packages need to be loaded in sterilizers loosely and in accordance with device manufacturer's instructions so as not to impede contact with the sterilizing agent.

A comparison of the three heat-sterilization methods appears in Table 51.2. Each of the three methods, when performed properly, yields sterilization. Special care must be taken to follow the sterilizer manufacturer's IFU. Moreover, the manufacturer's IFU for the type of

TABLE 51.2 Comparison of heat-sterilization methods with small office sterilizers

Method	Sterilizing Conditions[a]	Advantages	Precautions	Spore Testing
Steam autoclave	15-30 min at 121°C (250°F) or 3.5-10 min at 132°C (270°F)	Time efficient Good penetration	Some materials can corrode or be damaged. Items can be wet after normal cycle and require extended drying afterward. Do not use nonvented, closed containers. May damage plastic and rubber items Use of hard water may leave deposits (white spotting).	*Geobacillus stearothermophilus* strips or vented vials
Unsaturated chemical vapor	20 min at 132°C (270°F)	Time efficient Less corrosion risk Items typically dry after cycle.	Must use special solution Ventilation must be adequate. Predry instruments. May damage plastic and rubber items Do not use closed, nonvented containers. May not be appropriate for handpieces[b] Devices must be compatible with the heat/chemical process. Do not use absorptive materials.	*G stearothermophilus* strips
Dry heat (oven type)	60-120 min at 160°C (320°F)	No corrosion Items dry after cycle. Closed containers may be used.[c]	May damage plastic and rubber items Predry instruments. Long cycle time May not be appropriate for handpieces[b]	*Bacillus atrophaeus* strips
Dry heat (rapid heat transfer)	12 min at 190°C (375°F)	No corrosion Items dry after cycle. Time efficient	May damage plastic and rubber items Predry instruments. May not be appropriate for handpieces[b]	*B atrophaeus* strips

[a]These cycle times are representative; they do not include warm-up times, and they may vary with the brand of sterilizer. Some sterilizers will include drying phase, whereas others will not. Follow the sterilizer manufacturer's directions for using the sterilizer, sterilizing conditions, and confirming kill by spore testing.

[b]Check with handpiece manufacturer.

[c]Use spore tests to confirm appropriate kill in closed containers.

wrapping material to use must be followed, and the sterilizing process should be routinely monitored, as described later.

Steam Autoclave

Steam autoclaves are the most popular sterilizers in dental settings. A variety of models are available and should be approved for use.[1] Minimal features to look for are a temperature gauge independent of the pressure, an automatic timer that begins once the sterilizing temperature has been reached, and a print-out that documents the sterilizing conditions. Local recommendations for the use of steam sterilizers in dental facilities have been made such as in the United States by the AAMI ST79:2017,[53] and in the United Kingdom by Health Technical Memorandum 01-05:2013.[54] There are also local (eg, AAMI,[55] American National Standards Institute[56]) and international standards[57] describing the requirements for equipment and sterilization processes, respectively. Follow the manufacturer IFU for proper sterilization. Be sure to dry the packages either during or following sterilization to avoid damage to the packaging material when handling and to avoid wicking, the drawing through of microbes from the outside of paper packaging.

Unsaturated Chemical Vapor Sterilizer

The unsaturated chemical vapor sterilizer is a noncorrosive form of sterilization because of the low level of water present during the cycle. The sterilizing agent is mainly heated alcohol-formaldehyde vapor that is generated from the special solution added to the sterilizer for each cycle. Instruments need to be dry before sterilizing and compatible with the process. This keeps the presence of water at a minimum, so the noncorrosive environment can be maintained. Further information about the unsaturated chemical vapor sterilizer is available.[58,59]

Dry-Heat Oven

More and more dry-heat ovens are being used in dental offices to sterilize items as alternatives to steam autoclave. Smaller models are available through dental and scientific supply companies. The instruments must be dry before sterilizing. Care should be taken during use of the dry-heat sterilizer not to open the door until the entire cycle is completed. Opening the door reduces the chamber temperature and requires that the sterilizing cycle be started again.

An example of a new type of dry-heat sterilizer is called a rapid heat-transfer unit, with claims of sterilization after 12 minutes at a chamber temperature of 190°C (375°F) with wrapped instruments. Further information about dry-heat sterilizers is available (see chapter 28 and AAMI[60]). There is also an international standard for the requirements for dry-heat sterilization.[61]

Sterilization Monitoring

Monitoring the sterilization process is one of the few standard quality-assessment procedures available in infection control. The three forms of monitoring can include

1. Mechanical monitoring: observation of read-outs, dials, and/or gauges (monitors sterilizer functioning such as time, temperature, pressure)
2. Biological monitoring: spore-based biological indicator testing, a main guarantee of sterilization
3. Chemical monitoring: color or physical change chemical indicators that monitor exposure to sterilizing agents or conditions

Proper monitoring typically can involve all three forms and includes keeping records of the results.[58] At least weekly biological monitoring (spore testing) of the use and functioning of dental office sterilizers is recommended by the CDC.[3] Some states in the United States also require that dental sterilizers be spore tested at least weekly. Spore testing should also be performed at certain times in addition to routine testing (Table 51.3). AAMI guidelines recommend that biological monitoring should be performed at least weekly but preferably every day that a sterilizer is used.[53]

Biological indicators (spore strip or vial) should always be placed inside packages, bags, or trays next to the instruments themselves just before placing the items into the sterilizer. Sterilization monitoring services that function through the mail are available at a few dental schools and from some companies.[63] Most of these services can test steam autoclaves, unsaturated chemical vapor sterilizers, dry-heat sterilizers, and ethylene oxide sterilizers. Some also provide infection control newsletters, certificates of participation, and an available contact person to answer questions about infection control. The necessary supplies and instructions are sent, and the processed biological indicators are mailed back to the service for culturing, analysis, and return of a testing report. Although a mail-in spore testing service requires a delay in culturing the biological indicators, a study has shown that immediate and delayed culturing of biological indicators yields comparable results in relation to detection of sterilization failures.[64] Alternatively, steam autoclaves can be tested in the office with purchase of spore vials and an appropriate 56°C incubator for culturing. In-office testing of other types of sterilizers is more difficult.[58] Modern self-contained and rapid read-out biological indicators can be easily incubated and evaluated on site.

The CDC recommends monitoring each sterilizer load with mechanical and chemical indicators (CIs).[3] Mechanical monitoring consists of observing the gauges on the sterilizer and checking the timer to make sure the unit appears to be working properly. The CIs are generally recommended to be placed inside each package to be sterilized. If that internal indicator is not visible from the outside of the package, a second CI is to be placed

TABLE 51.3   Spore testing of small office sterilizers[a]

When	Why
At least once per week	To verify proper use and functioning
Whenever a new type of packaging material or tray is used	To ensure that the sterilizing agent is getting inside to the surface of the instruments
After training new sterilization personnel	To verify proper use of sterilizer
During initial use of a new sterilizer	To ensure unfamiliar operation instructions are being followed
First run after repair of a sterilizer	To ensure sterilizer is functioning properly
With every implantable device and hold until results are known	Extra precautions for items implanted in tissue
After any other change in sterilization procedure	To ensure change does not interfere with sterilization

[a]Spore (biological indicator) testing is recommended in many countries, including the United States. Alternative classifications of chemical indicators (such as class 5 or 6, in accordance to International Organization for Standardization [ISO] 11140-1 requirements)[62] may be appropriate alternatives in other countries.

on the outside. Chemical monitoring of dental office sterilizers involves use of color change or other indicators (eg, autoclave tape, special markings on bags, strips, and packets). These CIs, which can range in labeling and sensitivity (eg, from class 1 to Class 6 CIs in accordance with ISO 11140-1:2014),[62] are available for most types of sterilizers and give immediate indication that the items have at least been exposed to the sterilizing agent or to defined sterilizing conditions.

If mechanical, chemical, or biological monitoring indicates failure, the instruments/equipment need to be recleaned, repackaged, and resterilized. Failures should be investigated to determine root cause such as sterilizer malfunction or overloading of the sterilizer chamber.

Instrument Storage

Placing the instruments in drawers at chairside is not recommended because the drawers are likely to be contaminated from previous instrument retrieval with saliva-coated fingers. A drawer distribution system of unwrapped instruments at chairside carries a great potential for cross-contamination.

Because of the need for rapid instrument recirculation in most dental settings, storage of instruments is usually not a problem. Some items that are used less frequently must be stored; however, and this relates to the question of what is the shelf life of sterilized instruments.

Unwrapped instruments have no shelf life. They are susceptible to contamination immediately after being removed from the sterilizer or disinfecting solution. The shelf life of sterile, wrapped instruments, or instruments in completely closed containers depends on the integrity of the wrap or container. If the wrap or container is not opened, punctured, or torn and remains sealed and dry, then internal sterility should be maintained indefinitely. Thus, shelf life

is event related rather than time related. Each instrument package must be carefully inspected before being opened for use to help ensure that integrity of the packaging has been maintained during storage and distribution. Care should be taken when handling sterilized packs so the wrapping material is not torn. If packs or trays are stored, the storage area should be dry, out of direct sunlight, away from heat sources, and free of dust (eg, in a closed cabinet).[53,58] Sterile instruments must be kept completely separated from nonsterilized instruments so there is no chance of intermingling. This is one of the advantages of using an external CI to readily identify packages or trays that have been processed through the sterilizer.

Handpiece Reprocessing

High-speed dental handpieces, slow-speed handpieces, motors, reusable prophy angles, contra angles, and nose cones should be cleaned, packaged, and heat sterilized (unless indicated as thermos sensitive) between patients.[3] Patient saliva, blood, and other oral debris may enter the internal portions of handpieces and their attachments during use.[65-70] Unless these internal portions are properly decontaminated, these materials may be spewed out into the mouth of the next patient. Adequate cleaning followed by heat sterilization, in accordance to manufacturers validated IFU, addresses both the external and internal portions of handpieces and their attachments.[71] Different manufacturers of handpieces have different recommendations for how to clean, lubricate, and sterilize their handpieces. The specific manufacturer directions need to be followed. Most, for example, cannot be ultrasonically cleaned. Most can be sterilized in the steam autoclave, but few can be sterilized in the dry-heat sterilizer or unsaturated chemical vapor sterilizer.[58,72,73]

▶ SURFACE AND EQUIPMENT ASEPSIS

Surface Contamination

Dental operatory surfaces can become heavily contaminated during care of patients.[74-75] Use of handpieces, ultrasonic scalers, and air/water syringes generate salivary aerosols and spatter containing microorganisms.[34,76] The smaller aerosol particles may remain airborne for some time, enhancing the possibility of inhaling microorganisms.[77] The larger spatter droplets hit the skin, lips, and mucous membranes of the nose and eyes or settle rapidly and contaminate nearby operatory surfaces. These surfaces are also contaminated by touching with saliva/blood-coated fingers during care of patients. Although no evidence indicates dental aerosol spread of hepatitis B surface antigen (HBsAg) from HBsAg-positive patients,[78] other studies have shown that a variety of inanimate environmental surfaces can become contaminated with HBV particles.[79,80] Investigators have theorized that HBV contamination of surfaces may explain instances of disease transmission in the absence of overt percutaneous or mucous membrane exposures.[79,81] This hypothesis is strengthened by the finding that HBV in human plasma can remain infective (under laboratory conditions) for at least 1 week in the dry state at a room temperature of 25°C.[82] It is likely that similar or more environmentally tolerant microorganisms can pose at least similar risks.[77]

Thus, operatory surfaces and equipment that are contaminated by touching or by salivary droplets may serve as a potential source of indirect spread of disease agents.

Approaches to Surface Care and Protection

Reducing the spread of disease agents through contaminated operatory surfaces and equipment involves the following general approaches (Figure 51.1)[83]:

1. Differentiate between clinical contact surfaces (surfaces that may be touched or contaminated with salivary droplets during an appointment) and housekeeping surfaces (eg, floor sinks, walls).
2. Cover the clinical contact surfaces, especially those that are difficult to clean and disinfect (chair buttons, control switches, air/water syringe buttons, hoses, light handles).
3. Clean and disinfect uncovered surfaces that become contaminated.

Surface Covers

The most effective and efficient way to prevent cross-contamination by operatory surfaces is to cover them with disposable plastic wrap, plastic sheets or tubing,

Order of Preference

S = Sterilization C = Covering D = Disinfection

1. Head rest — C, D
2. Chair arm rest/controls — C, D
3. Light handles — S, C, D
4. Hand piece connectors — C, D
5. Table surface — C, D
6. Instruments — S

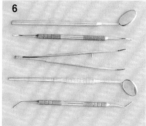
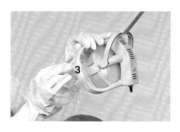
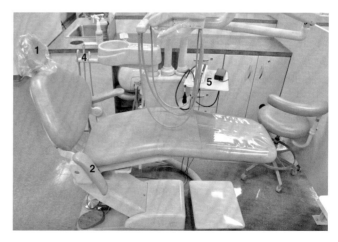

FIGURE 51.1 Surface components of a dental operatory and their aseptic care. Data from Crawford.[83]

plastic-backed paper, or other material impervious to moisture and replace with fresh covers between each patient.[83,84] It is not necessary to disinfect a properly covered surface between patients unless the cover fails or the surface is accidentally contaminated during cover removal.

Surface Cleaning

Uncovered contaminated surfaces must be precleaned and then disinfected.[85] Because the presence of blood on uncleaned surfaces can reduce or impair environmental disinfectant activity,[85] it is important to follow the CDC guideline to perform thorough cleaning before final disinfection.[3] It is best to use a disinfectant in the initial cleaning step (eg, the use of QAC-based disinfectants, which provide cleaning activity combined with low-level disinfection; chapter 21), and this, along with the wearing of heavy-duty gloves, provides protection during cleaning and reduces the chances of spreading contamination to adjacent surfaces during the process.[86] It is also prudent to wear protective eyewear during the mixing, handling, and use of any chemical solution.

Surface Disinfection

There are two approaches to cleaning and disinfecting.[87] One is the *spray-wipe-spray* technique. The spray and wipe is the cleaning step, and the second spray is the disinfection step. For the cleaning step, the surface is thoroughly sprayed with the disinfectant and vigorously wiped (spray-wipe). For the disinfecting step the disinfectant is thoroughly sprayed on the surface and allowed to remain wet for the longest contact time recommended by the disinfectant manufacturer. The second approach is the *wipe-discard-wipe* techniques using a disinfectant towelette. Preclean the surface with a towelette (or disinfectant-impregnated wipe) and discard the towelette. For disinfection, wipe the surface with a second towelette allowing the surface to remain wet for the contact time recommended by the disinfectant manufacturer.

For disinfection of precleaned surfaces, the disinfectant should be applied and allowed to remain in contact with the surface for the maximum contact time indicated on the disinfectant label. The chemical nature and properties of liquid disinfectants and sterilants are described elsewhere in this book. Chemicals used for surface disinfection in the dental operatory should be specific for use on surfaces and should be registered for such applications (such as in the United States with EPA or in compliance to European Norms requirements in the European Union).[88] In general, it is recommended that such disinfectants should be intermediate-level to include bactericidal and tuberculocidal activity, and killing highly resistant hydrophilic viruses or viruses of intermediate resistance.[86] Disinfectant formulations based on phenolics, chlorine-based solutions,

iodophors, and combinations of alcohol and quaternary ammonium compounds are typically considered to be effective against the relatively low levels of microbes left on dental equipment and surfaces after cleaning.[89-92] A variety of these surface disinfectants are available but can vary widely in antimicrobial activity (see chapter 5).[1]

▶ ASEPTIC TECHNIQUE

Disposable Items

More and more disposable items are becoming available for use in dental care. From the point of view of infection prevention, a disposable item (defined as an item to be used only on one patient and then discarded) has major advantages in preventing disease transmission. Disposal of the item after use on one patient prevents transfer of microbes to another patient. The best known example is the sterile disposable needle. Others include saliva ejector tips, high-volume evacuation tips, air/water syringe tips, impression trays, prophy cups, prophy angles, brushes, surgical and examination gloves, bib/napkin holders, some dental instruments, and surface barriers. It is important that such items are handled correctly, using aseptic technique in preparing for use and during their use to prevent accidental cross-contamination.

Disposable needles always should be used, and they should be discarded properly after use on a single patient. Other disposable items should be used whenever possible, but their cost should be compared with that of using the nondisposable or reusable item. The frequency of item use and the labor costs and any supplies required to properly prepare (clean, package, and sterilize) the reusable item for the next patient should be taken into consideration. Once a disposable item rather than a reusable item has been chosen, the clinician should not try to save money and reuse the disposable item. Disposable, single-use items for patient care are not designed for reuse, except under specifically validated and approved procedures (see chapter 55). In fact, the FDA states that the user is liable for any problem that may develop from reuse of an item manufactured as disposable. Disposable patient care items are often difficult or impossible to clean properly and are frequently damaged by cleaning agents or sterilization procedures. Risks include transmission of infection, toxicity, and device damage (eg, leading to breakage during use).

Packaging, Storage, and Dispensing

Aseptic storage and dispensing of supplies and instruments can be difficult to manage. The goal is to protect these items from contamination. Packaging of instruments in covered trays or sterilization bags or wraps in preparation for and during sterilization, prevents their subsequent contamination during storage, as described earlier. Packaging or dispensing instruments on trays or in drawers after sterilization permits contamination before use on the next patient. Consider for example the handling of packaged materials stored under inappropriate conditions and then the subsequent difficulty in aseptically removing the instruments in preparation for use. Storing previously sterilized or disinfected, unprotected instruments in a drawer at chairside results in contamination every time the drawer is opened and saliva-coated fingers are used to retrieve an instrument. Instruments should be cleaned, arranged in functional sets for use on a single patient, then packaged and sterilized.

Some manufacturers of dental supply items are beginning to package these items in unit doses for use on a single patient; however, many items are still bulk packaged, a method that increases the chances of contaminating many items in the package when the practitioner attempts to retrieve just one with saliva-coated fingers. The solution is to repackage in unit doses or devise an aseptic technique using sterile forceps to retrieve a unit dose from the bulk package. If supplies must be stored near chairside, their contamination from dental aerosols and spatter can be prevented by storing them behind the patient or in drawers. Supply containers or drawer handles that are touched during care of patients must be covered or cleaned and disinfected between patients.

Limiting Surface Contamination

Strictly speaking, if an operatory surface is not contaminated during care of patients, then that surface need not be disinfected between patients. Surfaces that are visually soiled (eg, with blood) often get the greatest attention, but at the same time, microbial contaminated surfaces can appear visually clean but can present a transmission risk. Overall, the fewer surfaces that must be disinfected between patients, the less time required for operatory cleanup, but obvious exposed areas in the patient zone should be considered for disinfection or barrier protection between patients. Contamination may occur by dental aerosols or spatter and by touching with saliva/blood-coated fingers or contact with contaminated items. Gloves used for care of patients are contaminated, and that contamination is transferred to any surface touched by those gloves (eg, switches, pens, charts, doorknobs, telephones, drawer knobs, cabinet handles, supply containers, unit surfaces, chairbacks).

Every effort must be made to dispense *all* items needed at chairside before the patient is seated. This includes placement of disposable surface covers as described earlier. The practitioner should touch as few surfaces as possible with saliva/blood-coated fingers during care of

patients. If possible, an uninvolved person should retrieve items needed unexpectedly. Disposable plastic sheets or inexpensive plastic overlay (food handlers) gloves should be available to protect an uncovered surface that must be touched.

Preprocedure Mouthrinse

The application of an approved antiseptic agent to skin (see chapter 43) or mucous membranes (see chapter 45) before surgery or needle injection has been practiced for many years. The objective of this procedure is to reduce the number of microbes at the surgical or needle injection site and to reduce the risk of the entry of surface microbes into underlying tissues, which may cause bacteremias, septicemias, or surgical site infections.[31] These procedures reduce the chances of an autogenous infection (one caused by a person's own microbes). The principle of these procedures is applied to reducing the spread of oral microbes to others. Rinsing with an antiseptic mouthrinse has long been known to reduce the number of oral microbes available for spread through aerosols, spatter, or direct contact.[93] More recent studies have shown that preprocedure mouthrinsing with agents containing chlorhexidine gluconate or certain phenolic substances can reduce the number of oral microbes in saliva and reduce the number expelled from the mouth during dental procedures.[94-96]

Reduction of Contaminated Dental Aerosols

Use of the rubber (or dental) dam during dental procedures that generate salivary aerosols and spatter reduces the number of oral bacteria that are sprayed into the environment.[76,97] These are single-use thin sheets of plastic or rubber used to isolate the localized operative site (eg, a single or multiple teeth) from the rest of the mouth. The reduction in bacterial counts with use of the rubber dam can approach 100%, depending on the type and site of the intraoral procedure and the environmental site of microbial sampling. The use of high-volume evacuation during operative procedures also reduces the production of both spatter and aerosols, but without simultaneous use of the rubber dam, this still permits the generation of considerable contamination.[76] The saliva ejector also removes saliva from the mouth so that less fluid will be available to generate aerosols and spatter. However, patients should not close their mouths around the saliva ejector to expectorate. In about 20% of the cases, research has shown that previously suctioned fluids may be retracted toward the patients' mouths.[98] Some disposable ejector tips have a small hole in the side that relieves the pressure when the tip is closed off.

Cough Etiquette

The CDC recommends procedures to limit the spread of respiratory droplets from patients in waiting rooms and other areas.[3] These include using posters depicting cough etiquette, providing a box of facial tissues, a no-touch waste container, an alcohol hand rub in reception areas, and offering a mask to those with respiratory symptoms. Those with specific symptoms of infection are encouraged to sit as far away as possible from others in the area.

Safe Injection Practices

The CDC has several recommendations related to preventing cross-contamination from injection devices.[3,51] They include

- Prepare injections using aseptic techniques.
- Disinfect the rubber septum on a medication vial with alcohol before piercing.
- Do not use needles or syringes for more than one patient.
- Use single-dose vials for parenteral medications whenever possible.
- Do not use single-dose medication vials, ampules, or bags for more than one patient.
- Medication containers are always entered with a new needle and syringe even when obtaining doses for the same patient.
- Do not combine leftover contents form medication vials.

Dental Unit Water Asepsis

The insides of dental units, with their small-bore waterlines and frequent periods of water stagnation, are conducive to microbial attachment and growth in the waterlines. This growth that forms on the inside walls of the tubing is called biofilm (see chapter 67)[99] and is much like the biofilm that forms on teeth, referred to as dental plaque. Dental unit waterline biofilm is a potential source of high levels of microbes (particular gram-negative bacteria and atypical mycobacteria) present in dental unit water that exits the dental unit through high-speed handpieces, the air/water syringe, and ultrasonic scalers. The municipal water (tap water) entering the dental unit may typically contain 15 to 50 CFUs of bacteria/mL As this water passes over the biofilm in the dental unit waterlines, it becomes highly contaminated and commonly exits the dental unit at levels ranging from a few thousand to a few hundred thousand CFUs/mL and may reach as high as 1 million CFUs/mL. Reviews of studies demonstrating such contamination are available.[67,100,101] Although this water contains the typical waterborne bacteria, these frequently include species of *Pseudomonas* and mycobacteria (opportunistic pathogens) and sometimes *Legionella*

TABLE 51.4	Approaches to improve the microbial quality of dental unit water
1. Use a water delivery system other than the dental unit. • Sterile water and sterile water delivery system • Separate water reservoir and sterilizable lines
2. Use the dental unit water delivery system but improve the quality of the incoming water. • Add an antimicrobial agent to the treatment water. • Treat incoming water with ultraviolet light. • Use high-quality water in a separate water reservoir.
3. Use the dental unit water delivery system, but prevent or control biofilm formation in the waterlines. • Heat or chemically treat the water.

(which may cause a type of pneumonia called Legionnaires' disease).[102,103] There are reports of disease transmission from dental unit water as mentioned earlier. However, there is currently no evidence for the occurrence of any widespread public health problem from exposure to dental unit water. The CDC[3] indicates that dental facilities should do the following:

- Use water that meets local regulatory standards for drinking water (ie, EPA recommend less than 500 CFUs/mL of heterotrophic water bacteria and the absence of *Legionella* or coliforms).
- Consult with the dental unit manufacturer for appropriate methods and equipment to maintain the quality of dental water.
- Follow recommendations for monitoring water quality provided by the manufacturer of the dental unit or waterline treatment product.
- Use sterile saline or sterile water as a coolant/irrigant when performing surgical, invasive procedures.

Some current approaches to improve the microbial quality of dental unit water and to achieve the 500 CFUs/mL goal are described in Table 51.4.

▶ LABORATORY ASEPSIS

Any instrument or piece of equipment used in the oral cavity or any orally soiled prosthetic device or impression is a potential source of cross-infection. All patients must be considered capable of transmitting highly infectious diseases, in accordance with universal precautions. The same procedures and materials must be used in all cases.[104,105]

If contaminated items were to enter the laboratory environment, infectious materials could be spread to prostheses and appliances of other patients. Unsuspecting laboratory personnel also could be placed at increased risk for cross-infection.[3,104]

Two factors are of greatest importance. These are the use of proper methods and materials for handling and decontaminating soiled items and the establishment of a coordinated infection control program between dental offices and commercial dental laboratories.

Protective Barriers

All items coming from the oral cavity must be sterilized or disinfected before entering the dental laboratory or before being returned to patients. Procedures vary depending on the type(s) of material(s) involved. Use of PPE is required because both infectious materials and potentially hazardous materials/chemicals can be present.

Receiving Areas

A specific area should be identified where all materials being sent to the in-house or commercial laboratories initially can be placed. Running water, a sink, and hand washing facilities are required. Prostheses, appliances, and impressions need to be properly disinfected prior to entering the receiving area. Use of water-resistant protective covers (eg, plastic sheeting or impervious paper) and regular chemical surface disinfection are required. Frequency of barrier changes and disinfection is based on the number of items coming through the area.[104]

Microbially Soiled Prostheses and Impressions

Prostheses coming from the oral cavity are potential sources of infection. Most prostheses and appliances cannot undergo standard heat sterilization. Instead, such items must be disinfected by immersion after a thorough cleaning. The best way to decontaminate soiled prostheses is through chairside disinfection immediately after removal. Disinfection should include use of an EPA-registered disinfectant having at least an intermediate level of activity (an actual tuberculocidal claim) prior to handling in the laboratory. Consult manufacturer recommendations concerning disinfectant-prostheses/appliance (and impression) compatibility.[104]

Gloves, protective eyewear, and some type of clinical gown must be worn when handling orally soiled prostheses until they have been properly decontaminated. Such personal protective barriers limit exposure to both infectious body fluids as well as hazardous materials, such as disinfectants.[3,104,105]

Some prostheses or appliances are soiled to an extent that a simple rinse followed by disinfection will not remove all adherent debris. More extensive cleaning, or even, scrubbing may be required. First, the prosthetic device is rinsed with tap water and shook dry. The most effective (and safest) procedure is to place the item into a glass or plastic beaker or a "zippered" plastic bag containing an appropriate ultrasonic detergent solution. Make sure the beaker is off the cleaner's floor or suspend the plastic bag from the cleaner's lid. Best cleaning typically occurs in the middle of the cleaning solution bath, but this can vary depending on the equipment design. After at least 15 minutes, the prosthetic device is removed and rinsed well using good quality tap water.[47] Some recalcitrant items may need hand scrubbing or air-powered blasting. The item is then ready for disinfection.[104,105] It is important to remember that rinsing of the items may be required following disinfection to remove toxic residuals and the water used for rinsing should be of adequate quality not to recontaminate the item.

The same procedure is used when a prosthesis or appliance comes back from a commercial dental laboratory. The properly disinfected and rinsed prosthesis then can be delivered to the patient (but not stored long term) in bag containing a mouthrinse solution. Because of a chance of adverse reaction by patient or office staff, prostheses and appliances should never be sent out or returned in a disinfecting solution.[104,105]

Dental Impressions

Dental impressions easily become contaminated with patient blood and saliva. Transfer of oral microorganisms onto and into impressions is well-documented. Movement of these organisms into dental casts while setting has been demonstrated. Some microbes have been shown to remain viable within gypsum cast materials for up to 7 days.[106] Improper handling of orally soiled impressions, therefore, offers a definite opportunity for cross-infection.

Personal protective barriers must be in place until the impression is properly decontaminated. This minimizes the chances of an exposure to patient fluids as well the hazardous chemicals used. After removal, impressions are rinsed gently under tap water and shook to eliminate adhering water droplets. Rinsed impressions are then placed into a well-sealed glass or plastic beaker or a zippered plastic bag containing an appropriate disinfecting solution.[86,107] Consultant product manufacturers for advice. Contact should not be prolonged. Impressions are removed following the recommended disinfectant exposure time, rinsed again, and shaken, after which the impressions are ready for pouring.[104]

Some types of impressions are sensitive to extended contact with disinfectant solutions and even water. In such cases, the impression is often completely sprayed with a disinfectant and wrapped in a paper towel moistened with the same disinfectant. Consultant product manufacturers for advice. Spraying is probably not as effective as immersion because coverage of all surfaces cannot be ensured. Also, spraying releases disinfectant as an aerosol into the environment. After following the recommended disinfectant exposure time, the impression is ready to be rinsed and poured up.[86,105,107]

Other Laboratory Activities

Laboratory work should be done only on prostheses, appliances, or impressions that have been properly disinfected. Bringing untreated items into the laboratory increases the chances of cross-infections.

Dental lathes are used to perform a variety of procedures on laboratory materials, including grinding and polishing. Protective eyewear must be in place whenever using a dental lathe. The poly(methyl methacrylate) (eg, Plexiglas) shield should be down and the unit's vacuum system activated. Lathe attachments, such as rag wheels, stones, burs, and bands should either be disposable or, if reusable, cleaned and sterilized between uses. For each case, a new pan liner and pumice must be used. It is best when polishing to use as many disposable attachments as possible and to "unit dose" the polishing materials (eg, rouge) used.[86,105,107]

Intermediate and Completed Cases

Complete and partial dentures often undergo an intermediate step called the wax try-in stage. Sometimes, fixed prostheses are also sent back to the office for fitness checks. After examination, these materials are returned to the dental laboratory for final processing.

It is best that these items be disinfected before placement in the patient and again before being returned to the dental laboratory. The same processes described for microbial soiled prostheses and impressions should be used.

Appliances and prostheses being returned to the patient for final placement are not free of microbial contamination. Today, many dental laboratories disinfect these items before they are sent back. The dental office is responsible for providing disinfected prostheses to the patient. If the office is confident that the laboratory has properly disinfected the item, then their responsibility is met. If not, then the office must perform the disinfection.[104,105]

▶ RADIOGRAPHIC ASEPSIS

Proper infection prevention practices for dental radiology use most of the materials and procedures used during restorative dental treatments. The overall goals are to minimize exposure of dental personnel to patient body fluids, prevent cross-infections in patients, and protect the community from regulated dental waste.[104,105]

The use of effective PPE, such as gloves, clinic gowns, and protective eyewear, is central to the protection of employees. Such barriers also protect patients from exposure to employee body fluids. Protective of both dental personnel and patients is the routine cleaning and sterilization of reusable instruments and equipment and the proper disinfection of orally soiled environmental surfaces. The use of protective environmental barriers, such as disposable plastic sheets or bags, is also an effective procedure.[104,105]

Dental radiology also involves occupational exposure to hazardous materials. Involved personnel must be familiar with the chemical and radiological hazards involved. Correct hazardous materials management is based on continuous employee training and minimizing the chances of exposure. The goal of a properly constructed and maintained written office hazard communication (HazCom) program is better assure that employees and employers are familiar with workplace hazards and how to protect themselves.[104]

All materials and processes must be used in conjunction with a well-written office infection prevention and control as well as HazCom office manuals. Establishing written procedures is very valuable; however, employees must be aware of the manual's tenets, be provided regular training sessions, and show competence in their use. Any effective and efficient office safety and health program must also have a consistent monitoring element.

Unit, Film, and Patient Preparation

The radiographic process offers the possibility of employee contact with patient body fluids. Both disposable and reusable items can become contaminated. Taking radiographs is a clinical procedure that requires the wearing of PPE, such as gloves, clinic gowns, and protective eyewear. These barriers protect against fluid contact as well as exposure to the hazardous chemicals used to develop radiographic films.[104]

Many of the materials used to take radiographs are single-use disposable items. Almost all reusable instruments and pieces of equipment can be cleaned and sterilized by heat between patient uses. The few heat-sensitive materials (eg, some plastic items) can be treated after cleaning by immersion in a full-strength disinfectant solution labeled for such use carefully following manufacturer's IFU.

Environmental surface disinfection and the use of surface covers are essential elements of radiographic asepsis. All surfaces soiled must either be covered or properly disinfected. Covered surfaces do not need to be disinfected after the barriers have been removed. In some situations, it is more efficient to use plastic drapes, bags, covers, or tubing on the radiograph unit (tube, head, arm, and cone), the chair headrest, and control panel.[104,105,107]

Taking Radiographs

Clean gloves (almost any type will work) are worn when unexposed films are placed onto a clean paper towel. Films should be arranged in the order of use. Exposed films are then rinsed and placed into a plastic cup.

For a number of years, films have been sold already covered with a removable plastic (eg, FDA-cleared barrier) pouch. Also, pouches are available that can be placed onto films before exposure. Proper opening of the pouch releases an exposed, yet unsoiled film. These films can then be handled with bare hands. This also eliminates potential contact of glove powder with the films. Tests indicate that when correctly placed, film covers do not allow penetration of fluids, nor do they interfere with the quality of the exposed film.[104,105,107]

Taking radiographs also includes the use of environmental and personal barriers and proper disinfection. Offices need to determine the best combination of barriers and disinfection to use. However, several switches and dials are often involved and these are best covered while being used. The unit cone can be covered or readily disinfected. Some items used intraorally should be sterilized by heat.

Digital radiographic sensors and associated computer hardware are used in place of x-ray films. The digital system generates an electronic image onto a computer screen where it can be manipulated, stored, and transmitted. Most of these systems cannot be heat sterilized or chemically disinfected. The only alternative to use some type of disposable plastic cover to protect the sensor. Some systems are wireless. Local regulatory-cleared barriers should always be used as covers. Consult sensor manufacturers for advice.[104]

In the Darkroom

Some offices have a darkroom for the development of radiographic films. Ideally, exposed films can be released from their protective pouches and carefully collected in a plastic cup or within a folded paper towel and transported directly into the darkroom while avoiding touching environmental surfaces. The films packets can then be opened onto new clean paper towel or plastic sheet using a new pair of gloves. If care is taken, the result is a film that is not contaminated (fewer artifacts). Films can then be developed manually or placed into an automatic processor. Again, the use of protective pouches decreases further the chances of film or practitioner exposure.[104,105]

All items to be discarded are collected and placed into the regular office waste system. Because none of the items is considered regulated medical waste, they do not require special handling, storage, and neutralization processes. Hands must be washed immediately after removal of gloves.[104,105]

Using Daylight Loaders

Potential problems can arise with the use of daylight loaders attached to automatic processors or with "portable darkrooms" that contain small beakers or cups of developing solutions. These units have portals that allow the entrance of hands and arms with a maximum exclusion of light. This is accomplished using cloth or rubber sleeves or cuffs. Because such units have a limited amount of operational space, the chances of cross-contamination are significant. Once contaminated, the sleeves or cuffs are extremely difficult to disinfect.[104,105]

The best way to use daylight loaders aseptically is to insert only properly disinfected or unsoiled film packets (eg, previously pouched films). Films can then be unwrapped and processed automatically or, in some cases, by hand. Manual processing requires the use of gloves to protect against the film developing chemicals.

❯ DENTAL WASTE

Effective and efficient waste management programs are complex due to numerous regulations, differing guidelines, evolving technologies, increasing numbers and diversity of health care settings, and the threat of emerging diseases.[108]

Dental Waste Management Programs

Proper waste management is an essential part of a dental practice's written exposure control plan. Components of the plan should include assignment of risk, types of waste, regulated medical waste, isolation schemes, handling, storage, neutralization, training, and community relations.[109]

Assignment of Risk

Many countries will have specific guidelines or regulations addressing dental waste management, and example is the 2003 CDC Guidelines for Infection Control in Dental Health-Care Settings updated in 2016.[3] This guidance makes two general recommendations—offices must develop a medical waste management program that which follows federal and local regulations and offices must ensure that dental workers who handle and dispose of regulated medical waste are appropriately trained and informed of possible health and safety hazards.[3,109]

Dental waste has differing levels of associated risk, depending on host susceptibility, waste type (ie, hollow vs solid sharps), level/type of contamination (presence of pathogens and pathogen virulence), contamination source and exposure route (eg, portal of entry, direct versus indirect). Proper waste management helps protect practitioners, patients, the surrounding population, and the local environment.[3,108,109]

Types of Waste

The terms *hospital waste*, *biohazardous waste*, *biomedical waste*, *red bag waste*, *medical waste*, and *infectious waste* often are used synonymously (Table 51.5). Hospital waste, dental office waste, or household waste refer to the total discarded solid waste generated by all sources within a given facility.[3,108,109,113]

Studies have compared microbial load and diversity in residential waste versus waste from multiple types of health care settings. Health care waste can have a greater variety of microorganisms than domestic waste, whereas those from households usually are more heavily contaminated.[3,108] Despite that, there is no epidemiological evidence that most medical/dental waste is any more infectious than residential waste. Except for a relatively limited number of items, most soiled items in dental offices are general medical waste and can be disposed of with ordinary waste (via regular waste streams). Examples include used gloves, masks, gowns, lightly soiled gauze or cotton rolls, and environmental barriers (eg, plastic sheets or bags) used to cover equipment during treatment. Although any item that has had contact with blood, exudates, or secretions might be a greater infectious risk, treating all such waste as infectious is neither necessary nor practical.[3,109,110]

Infectious waste is a small subset (estimated to be 3%-10% in hospitals and 1%-2% in dental offices) of the total discarded. Infectious waste is that part of medical/dental waste that has been shown through controlled studies capable of transmitting an infectious disease. Infectious medical/dental waste is also known as regulated waste (as regulated by some governmental agency) because certain segregation, storage, and disposal procedures must be followed.[3,108-111]

Regulated Medical Waste

Waste generated in dental offices must deal with two types of waste-regulated medical waste and nonregulated medical waste.[3,109] In the United States, for example, OSHA defines regulated waste as "liquid or semi-liquid blood or other potentially infectious materials; contaminated items that would release blood or other potentially infectious materials in a liquid or semi-liquid state if compressed; items that are caked with dried blood or other potentially infectious materials (OPIM) and are capable of releasing these materials during handling; contaminated sharps; and pathological and microbiological wastes containing OPIM." OPIM in dentistry include saliva.[13]

Handling, Isolation, Storage, Neutralization, and Disposal

For dental offices, there are five basic types of regulated medical waste. These require special isolation, handling, storage, and disposal methods because they have been shown capable of transmitting infectious diseases (Table 51.6).

Regulated waste must be placed into appropriately designed containers, usually biohazard bags or sharps containers/boxes, which are labeled or color coded. Usually, these are red, yellow, or orange and have biohazard symbols attached. Such containers should be impervious, rigid, puncture resistant, leakproof on the sides and bottom, and closable. Ideally, segregation and storage should occur as close as possible to the point of origin with a minimum of transport. Segregation increases patient and practitioner safety and prevents contamination of nonregulated waste.[3,13,108-110,114]

TABLE 51.5	Types of waste defined[a]
Type	**Definition**
Contaminated waste	Items that have had contact with blood or other body secretions
Hazardous waste	Waste posing a risk or peril in human beings or the environment
Infectious waste	Waste capable of causing an infectious disease
Regulated medical waste	Infectious medical waste that requires special handling, neutralization, and disposal
Medical waste	Any solid waste generated in the diagnosis, treatment, or immunization of human beings or animals in research pertaining thereto, or the production or testing of biologicals (does not include hazardous waste or household waste; only a small percentage of medical waste is infectious and needs to be regulated)[b]
Toxic waste	Waste capable of having a poisonous effect

[a]Modified from Centers for Disease Control and Prevention,[3] Miller,[109] Palenik,[110] Krisiunas,[111] Rutala and Mayhall.[112]

[b]Examples of solid waste include discarded solids, liquids, semiliquids, or contained gaseous materials.

TABLE 51.6	OSHA regulated waste[a]
Waste	**Dental Example**
Liquid or semiliquid blood or other potentially infectious material (OPIM)	Liquid blood or saliva
Contaminated items that would release blood or OPIM in a liquid or semiliquid state if compressed	Cotton 2 × 2 squares and rolls saturated with blood or saliva
Items that are caked with blood or OPIM capable of releasing these materials during handling	Cotton 2 × 2 squares and rolls saturated/caked with blood or saliva
Contaminated sharps	Used needles, scalpel blades, orthodontic wires, broken instruments, burs, or endodontic files/rasps
Pathological or microbiological wastes containing blood and saliva	Biopsy specimens, excised tissue, extracted teeth not returned to the patient

[a]Modified from references Centers for Disease Control and Prevention[3]; Occupational Safety and Health Administration, US Department of Labor[13]; Miller[109]; Palenik[110]; Rutala and Mayhall.[112]

Safe collection, handling, and storage of regulated medical waste are essential. Written procedures will help. Workers must be informed of possible occupational hazards and trained in appropriate handling, storage, and disposal methods.[3,109,110]

Regulated waste must be stored in a properly ventilated, secured area, which patients cannot readily see. Generally, waste should not be stored for more than 30 days. Waste containers must be designed to prevent the development of offensive odors.[3,109,110]

In most locations, blood in a liquid or semiliquid form, even when mixed with other fluids such as saliva, can be poured or evacuated into the office waste water system (sanitary sewers of septic tanks). Proper PPE must be worn when pouring. Sink traps and evacuation lines should be thoroughly rinsed at least daily and treated with an effective, environmentally compatible disinfectant (nonbleach) or evacuation cleaner. A final water rinse should follow. There are a limited number of locations that regulate types and amounts of body fluids discharged into the environment. It is important to check with local, state, or country-specific water quality agencies.[3,109,110]

Many areas allow in-house treatment of regulated medical/dental waste. An easy and effective procedure is moist heat sterilization (autoclaving). However, sterilizer cycles should be validated for such treatments and performance must be biologically monitored on a regular basis.[3,109,110] Sharps containers left open should be placed into the sterilizer in an upright position (avoiding spilling contents). The containers should be only three-fourths full and are often recommended to be exposed through two consecutive sterilizer treatment cycles. In-house treated regulated waste items then can be added to the nonregulated office waste. These items should be labeled as "treated medical waste" and with other information as required by local laws. All treated waste should be well packaged.[3,109,110]

Pathologic waste is potentially infectious and, thus, regulated medical waste. Teeth without amalgam restorations and other tissues can be placed directly into a biohazard bag or a sharps container. Where allowed, these wastes can then be heat sterilized using and approved sterilizer cycle for that purpose. Teeth with amalgams could release mercury vapor during sterilization, therefore, they should be disinfected at room temperature (ideally, immersion for 30 minutes in a fresh solution of a tuberculocidal disinfectant held within a sealed container). Treated teeth can then be rinsed with water and are ready for disposal or return to pediatric patients.[3,109,110]

Items heavily soiled (even saturated) with blood/saliva can be placed into sharps containers. However, it may be easier to store them in small biohazard bags until treated or disposed. Used anesthetic cartridges should be placed into sharps containers.[3,109,110]

Some areas require that regulated medical waste be removed, neutralized, and disposed of by a locally approved (eg, EPA) commercial waste hauling service. Even though a service is hired, the office still retains ultimate responsibility for its regulated medical waste.[3,108-110]

Employee Training

Training of employees concerning all stages/steps of the regulated medical waste management process is needed. Training should include infectious waste definitions, handling procedures, appropriate PPE, hand hygiene, labeling/coding of infectious waste, and postexposure management.[3,108-110]

Community Relations and Training

All treated waste should be well packaged. This protects practitioners, patients, and the public from exposure to infectious materials and to facilitate proper handling, storage, treatment, and disposal. When it comes to regulated medical waste, "out of sight is out of mind."[3,108-110,113]

An effective and efficient office waste management plan addresses each step in the process, from acquiring materials that will become waste, collection, isolation, storage, transportation, treatment (neutralization), and final disposal. Informed and training workers perform better and in a safer manner. If the plan is not in writing then, it does not exist.[3,108-110]

Amalgam Separators

Amalgam separators can greatly reduce the discharge of mercury-containing amalgam into publicly owned treatment works (POTWs) and are practical, affordable, and readily available. Separators are designed to remove solids from dental office wastewater. The process removes amalgam particles through centrifugation, sedimentation, filtration, or a combination of methods. Almost all separators sold today rely on sedimentation because of its effectiveness and operational simplicity. The mercury collected by separators can be recycled.[115,116] The EPA has promulgated a standard under the Clean Water Act to reduce discharges of mercury from dental offices into municipal sewage treatment plants known as POTWs. The rule requires affected dental offices to use amalgam separators and the best

management practices for amalgam waste management issued by the ADA.[115,117]

The US dental industry consists of an estimated 133,000 offices. It is thought that 40% of offices to the rule have already installed amalgam separators. The rule applies to any location where the dentistry practiced discharges wastewater into a POTW. It does not apply to mobile units or offices where the practice of dentistry consists only of the following dental specialties: oral pathology, oral and maxillofacial radiology, oral and maxillofacial surgery, orthodontics, periodontics or prosthodontics. Approximately, 80% of US dentists are generalists.[115,116]

Dental offices that discharge into POTWs that do not place or remove amalgam need only submit a one-time certification. Dental offices that place or replace amalgam must operate and maintain an amalgam separator and must not discharge scrap amalgam down a drain and use certain kinds of line cleaners. Bleach and chlorine-containing cleaners as well as acids can lead to the dissolution of solid mercury in chairside traps and vacuum lines. Cleaners should have a pH between 6 and 8. In the United States, these offices must also submit a One-Time Compliance Report.[115-118]

In addition to separators and traps, the Final Rule indicates the need to use the ADA best management practices for amalgam waste handling and disposal plus regular inspections and cleaning of traps and use of appropriate commercial waste services to recycle and/or dispose of collected amalgam (Table 51.7).

TABLE 51.7 Americal Dental Association best management practices for amalgam waste[a]

Do	Don't
Do stock a variety of precapsulated alloy capsules.	**Do not** use bulk mercury.
Do recycle used disposable amalgam capsules.	**Do not** place used disposable amalgam capsules into biohazard containers.
Do salvage, store, and recycle noncontact (scrap) amalgam.	**Do not** place noncontact (scrap) amalgam into biohazard containers, infectious waste containers (sharps containers or red bags), or the regular garbage.
Do salvage, store, and recycle contact amalgam pieces from restorations after removal.	**Do not** place contact amalgam into biohazard containers, infectious waste containers (sharps containers or red bags), or the regular garbage.
Do use chair-side traps, vacuum pump filters, and amalgam separators to retain amalgam and recycle their contents regularly.	**Do not** rinse instruments or devices containing amalgam over drains or sinks.
Do recycle extracted teeth containing amalgam restorations. Ask your recycler if they require disinfection of such teeth.	**Do not** dispose of extracted teeth containing amalgam restorations into biohazard containers, infectious waste containers (sharps containers or red bags), or the regular garbage.
Do recycle amalgam as much as possible.	**Do not** flush amalgam waste down drain or the toilet.
Do use line cleaners that minimize dissolution of amalgam (pH 6-8).	**Do not** use acid or bleach or other chlorine-containing cleaners to flush wastewater lines.

[a]Modified from American Dental Association.[117] Copyright © 2012 American Dental Association. All rights reserved. Reprinted with permission.

Collected materials can be recycled. It is important to hire a reputable service, one that follows all applicable federal and state laws and has adequate indemnification for their actions.[115] The hope is that the application of such rules will ensure dental amalgam waste is captured before entering the waste stream. Ideally, such materials can be properly recycled.

▶ IMMUNIZATIONS FOR DENTAL PERSONNEL

Dental personnel are exposed daily in their offices, clinics, and laboratories to a variety of communicable diseases. Personal physical barriers, such as gowns, gloves, masks, and protective eyewear, help prevent many cross-infections; however, immunization, when available, is the best method for preventing infectious diseases. Maintenance of immunity is an essential component of any effective infection prevention program. Dental personnel must be made aware of their risk for cross-infection and those diseases that can be prevented by immunization.

It is known that compliance with a vaccination scheme is greatest when the program is mandatory, rather than voluntary. It is also known that when the employer pays for vaccinations, compliance is markedly higher than if the employees must pay all or a significant portion of their immunization costs.

The CDC, for example, recommends routine immunization to prevent 17 vaccine-preventable diseases that occur in infants, children, adolescents, or adults. Of these, 5 are commonly recommended for HCW, including dental professionals.[119,120]

The five recommended vaccines, HCW immune status factors and recommendations are presented in Table 51.8. Also, meningococcal vaccine is recommended for HCW routinely exposed to isolates of *Neisseria meningitidis* and involves 1 dose.

HBV is spread through skin punctures or mucosal contact with infectious fluids, including blood and saliva, exposure to patient open wounds and needlesticks. HBV under some conditions can survive outside humans and remain infectious for at least 7 days. Between 2% and 6% of infected adults develop chronic infections, which can lead

TABLE 51.8	Centers for Disease Control and Prevention recommended vaccines for health care worker[a]
Vaccine Applications	**Situations and Recommendations**
Hepatitis B (HB)	If you do not have documented evidence of a complete hepatitis vaccine series or if you do not have an up-to-date blood test that shows you are immune to hepatitis B (eg, no serologic evidence of immunity or prior vaccination), then you should (1) get the 3-dose series (dose no.1 now, no. 2 in 1 month, and no. 3 approximately 5 months after no. 2) and (2) get anti-HBs serologic screening 1-2 months after dose no. 3.
Flu (influenza)	Get 1 dose of influenza vaccine annually.
Measles, mumps, and rubella (MMR)	If you were born in 1957 or later and have not had the MMR vaccine or if you do not have an up-to-date blood test that shows you are immune to measles or mumps (eg, no serologic evidence of immunity or prior vaccination), get 2 doses of MMR (1 dose now and the second dose at least 28 days later). If you were born in 1957 or later and have not had the MMR vaccine or if you do not have an up-to-date blood test that shows you are immune to rubella, only 1 dose of MMR is recommended. However, you may end up receiving 2 doses because the rubella component is in the combination vaccine with measles and mumps. Although birth before 1957 generally is considered acceptable evidence of MMR immunity, 2 doses of MMR vaccine should be considered for unvaccinated HCP born before 1957 who do not have laboratory evidence of disease or immunity to measles and/or mumps. Those born before 1957 should visit https://www.cdc.gov/vaccines/hcp/acip-recs/vacc-specific/mmr.html.
Varicella (chickenpox)	If you have not had chickenpox (varicella), if you have not received the varicella vaccine or if you do not have an up-to-date blood test that shows you are immune to varicella (eg, no serologic evidence of immunity or prior vaccination), get 2 doses of varicella vaccine, 4 weeks apart.
Tetanus, diphtheria, and pertussis (Tdap)	Get a one-time dose of Tdap as soon as possible if you have not received Tdap previously (regardless of when a previous dose of Td was received). Get Td boosters every 10 years, thereafter. Pregnant HCW need to get a dose of Tdap during each pregnancy.

Abbreviations: HCP, health care personnel; HCW, health care workers.

[a]Modified from references Centers for Disease Control and Prevention.[120,121]

to cirrhosis and liver cancer. After three properly spaced intramuscular doses of hepatitis B vaccine, more than 90% of healthy adults develop adequate antibody responses.[121]

Available data show that vaccine-induced antibody levels decline with time. However, immune memory remains intact for more than 20 years following immunization. Those with declining antibody levels are still protected against significant HBV infection (eg, clinical disease, HBsAg antigenemia, or significant elevation of liver enzymes). Exposure to HBV results in an anamnestic anti-HBsAg response that prevents clinically significant HBV infection. Chronic HBV infection has only rarely been documented among vaccine responders. The need for booster doses after longer intervals will continue to be assessed as additional information becomes available.[121,122]

Influenza is a serious disease that can lead to hospitalization and sometimes even death, especially among the very young and the elderly. Influenza vaccinations are recommended each year. The seasonal flu vaccine protects against the influenza viruses that research indicated will be most common during the upcoming season. Infected HCWs can spread influenza to their patients, coworkers, and families.[121,122]

If not already immune to measles, mumps, or rubella, HCW should be vaccinated. Even mild or undetectable rubella disease during pregnancy can cause fetal anomalies. Measles can cause encephalitis, whereas mumps can cause swelling of the salivary glands and testicles. Measles, mumps, and rubella (MMR) vaccination is >90% effective against measles and rubella and 80% or more effective against mumps after 2 doses.[121,122]

Varicella (or specifically the varicella-zoster virus, which causes chickenpox or shingles) can be transmitted in hospitals by patients, staff, and visitors. If not already immune based on a prior infection or vaccination, immunization is recommended.

Initially, most individuals receive a single dose of tetanus, diphtheria, and pertussis (Tdap) vaccine (tetanus, diphtheria, and pertussis) and then a booster of Td vaccine every 10 years. An HCW lacking Tdap vaccination that have direct patient contact and/or have been injured are recommended to have a Tdap dose.[121,122]

Immunization is a key component of a dental practice's infection control program, which is a system of, procedures and practices that when successfully implemented, will minimize the risk of transmission of pathogenic microorganisms. The goal is to prevent health care-associated infections in patients and injuries and illnesses among HCW, including dental practitioners.

REFERENCES

1. Miller CH. Infection control strategies for the dental office. In: Ciancio SG, ed. *Dental Therapeutics*. 3rd ed. Chicago, IL: American Dental Association; 2003:551-566.
2. Cottone JA. Hepatitis B virus infection in the dental profession. *J Am Dent Assoc*. 1985;110:617-621.
3. Centers for Disease Control and Prevention. *Summary of Infection Prevention Practices in Dental Settings: Basic Expectations for Safe Care*. Atlanta, GA: Centers for Disease Control and Prevention; 2016.
4. American Dental Association. American Dental Association statement on infection control in dental settings. American Dental Association Web site. http://www.ada.org/en/press-room/news-releases/2017-archives/august/statement-on-infection-control. Accessed December 12, 2017.
5. Eklund KJ, Bednarsh H, Haaland CO. *OSHA and CDC Guidelines: Combining Safety with Infection Control and Prevention for Dentistry*. 5th ed. Atlanta, GA: Organization for Safety, Asepsis and Prevention; 2017.
6. Ciesielski C, Marianos D, Ou CY, et al. Transmission of human immunodeficiency virus in a dental practice. *Ann Intern Med*. 1992;116:798-805.
7. Lot F, Séguier JC, Fégueux S, et al. Probable transmission of HIV from an orthopedic surgeon to a patient in France. *Ann Intern Med*. 1999;130:1-6.
8. Manzella JP, McConville JH, Valenti W, Menegus MA, Swierkosz EM, Arens M. An outbreak of herpes simplex virus type I gingivostomatitis in a dental hygiene practice. *JAMA*. 1984;252:2019-2022.
9. Redd JT, Baumbach J, Kohn W, Nainan O, Khristova M, Williams I. Patient-to-patient transmission of hepatitis B virus associated with oral surgery. *J Infect Dis*. 2007;195:1311-1314.
10. Martin MV. The significance of the bacterial contamination of dental unit water systems. *Brit Dent J*. 1987;163:152-154.
11. Peralta G, Tobin-D'Angelo M, Parham A, et al. Notes from the field. *Mycobacterium abscessus* infections among patients of a pediatric practice—Georgia, 2015. *MMWR Morb Mortal Wkly Rep*. 2016;65:355-356.
12. Miller CH, Cottone JA. The basic principles of infectious diseases as related to dental practice. *Dent Clin North Am*. 1993;37:1-20.
13. Occupational Safety and Health Administration, US Department of Labor. Occupational exposure to blood-borne pathogens; final rule. *Fed Regist*. 1991;56(64):175-164. To be codified at 29 CFR §1910.1030.
14. US Food and Drug Administration. Banned devices; powdered surgeon's gloves, powdered patient examination gloves, and absorbable powder for lubricating a surgeon's glove. Federal Register Web site. https://www.federalregister.gov/d/2016-30382/page-91723. Accessed December 12, 2017.
15. Hill JG, Grimwood RE, Hermesch CB, Marks JG Jr. Prevalence of occupationally related hand dermatitis in dental workers. *J Am Dent Assoc*. 1998;129:212-217.
16. Hamann CP, Turjanmaa K, Rietschel R, et al. Natural rubber latex hypersensitivity: incidence and prevalence of type I allergy in the dental profession. *J Am Dent Assoc*. 1998;129:43-53.
17. National Institute of Occupational Health and Safety. *Preventing Allergic Reactions to Natural Rubber Latex in the Workplace*. Cincinnati, OH: National Institute of Occupational Health and Safety; 1997. Publication no. 97-100.
18. Turjanmaa K, Makinen-Kiljunen S, Reunala T, et al. Natural rubber latex allergy: the European experience. In: Fink JN, ed. *Immunology and Allergy Clinics of North America: Latex Allergy*. Philadelphia, PA: WB Saunders; 1995:71-88.
19. Miller CH, ed. Personal protective equipment. In: *Infection Control and Management of Hazardous Materials for the Dental Team*. 6th ed. St. Louis, MO: Elsevier; 2018:107-119.
20. US Food and Drug Administration. Medical devices; patient examination glove; revocation of exemptions from the premarket notification procedures and the current good manufacturing practice regulations. *Fed Regist*. 1989;54:1602-1604. To be codified at 21 CFR §880.
21. Allen AL, Organ RJ. Occult blood accumulation under the fingernails: a mechanism for the spread of blood-borne infections. *J Am Dent Assoc*. 1982;105:455-459.
22. Merchant V. Herpes simplex virus infection: an occupational hazard in dental practice. *J Mich Dent Assoc*. 1982;64:199-203.
23. Palenik CJ, Miller CH. Occupational herpetic whitlow. *J Indiana Dent Assoc*. 1982;61:25-27.

24. Rowe NH, Heine CS, Kowalski CJ. Herpetic whitlow: an occupational disease of practicing dentists. *J Am Dent Assoc* 1982;105:471-473.

25. Larson EL. APIC guideline for handwashing and hand antisepsis in health care settings. *Am J Infect Control.* 1995;23:251-269.

26. Palenik CJ, Miller CH. Handwashing. *Dent Asepsis Rev.* 1981;2(3):1-2.

27. Steere AC, Mallison GF. Handwashing practices for the prevention of nosocomial infections. *Ann Intern Med.* 1975;83:683-690.

28. Miller CH, ed. Hand hygiene. In: *Infection Control and Management of Hazardous Materials for the Dental Team.* 6th ed. St. Louis, MO: Elsevier; 2018:94-100.

29. Crawford JJ, Parker WD, Parker NH. Asepsis in periodontal surgery [abstract 177]. *J Dent Res.* 1974;53:99.

30. Gross A, Cutright D, D'Alessandro SM. Effect of surgical scrub on microbial population under the fingernails. *Am J Surg.* 1979;138: 463-467.

31. Miller CH, Byrne BE. Topical antiseptics. In: Ciancio SG, ed. *Dental Therapeutics.* 3rd ed. Chicago, IL: American Dental Association; 2003:189-199.

32. Kane MA, Lettau LA. Transmission of HBV from dental personnel to patients. *J Am Dent Assoc.* 1985;110:634-636.

33. Centers for Disease Control and Prevention. Hepatitis B among dental patient—Indiana. *MMWR Morb Mortal Wkly Rep.* 1985;34:73-74.

34. Micik RE, Miller RL, Leong AC. Studies on dental aerobiology. 3. Efficacy of surgical masks in protecting dental personnel from airborne bacterial particles. *J Dent Res.* 1971;50:626-630.

35. US Food and Drug Administration. Guidance for industry and FDA staff: surgical masks—premarket notification [510(k)] submissions; guidance for industry and FDA, 2004. US Food and Drug Administration Web site. https://www.fda.gov/medicaldevices/device regulationandguidance/guidancedocuments/ucm072549.htm. Updated 2015. Accessed December 12, 2017.

36. Greene VW, Vesley D. Method for evaluating surgical masks. *J Bacteriol.* 1962;83:663-667.

37. Pippin DJ, Verderame RA, Weber KK. Efficacy of face masks in preventing inhalation of airborne contaminants. *J Oral Maxillofac Surg.* 1987;45:319-323.

38. Palenik CJ. Eye protection for the entire dental office. *J Indiana Dent Assoc.* 1981;60:23-25.

39. Bond WW, Peterson NJ, Favero MS. Transmission of a type B viral hepatitis via eye inoculation of a chimpanzee. *J Clin Microbiol.* 1982;15:533-534.

40. Kew MC. Possible transmission of serum (Australia-antigen-positive) hepatitis via the conjunctiva. *Infect Immun.* 1973;7:823-824.

41. Hales RH. Ocular injuries sustained in the dental office. *Am J Ophthalmol* 1970;70:221-223.

42. Centers for Disease Control and Prevention. Guidance for the Selection and use of personal protective equipment (PPE) in healthcare settings, 2016. Centers for Disease Control and Prevention Web site. https://www.cdc.gov/hai/pdfs/ppe/PPEslides6-29-04.pdf. Accessed December 12, 2017.

43. Palenik CJ, Miller CH. Use of the ultrasonic cleaner in the dental office. *J Indiana Dent Assoc.* 1980;59:11-12.

44. Miller CH, Hardwick LM. Ultrasonic cleaning of dental instruments in cassettes. *Gen Dent.* 1988;36:31-36.

45. International Organization for Standardization. *ISO 15883-1:2006: Washer-Disinfectors—Part 1: General Requirements, Terms and Definitions and Tests.* Geneva, Switzerland: International Organization for Standardization; 2006. https://www.iso.org/standard/41076.html. Accessed September 23, 2019.

46. Miller CH, Riggen SD, Sheldrake MA, Neeb JM. Presence of microorganisms in used ultrasonic cleaning solutions. *Am J Dent.* 1993;6:27-31.

47. Association for the Advancement of Medical Instrumentation. *AAMI TIR34:2014/(R)2017. Water for Reprocessing of Medical Devices.* Arlington, VA: Association for the Advancement of Medical Instrumentation; 2017. http://my.aami.org/store/SearchResults .aspx?searchterm=Water+for+reprocessing&searchoption=L. Accessed September 23, 2019.

48. International Organization for Standardization. *ISO 11607-1:2006: Packaging for Terminally Sterilized Medical Devices—Part 1: Requirements for Materials, Sterile Barrier Systems and Packaging Systems.* Geneva, Switzerland: International Organization for Standardization; 2006. https://www.iso.org/standard/38712.html. Accessed September 23, 2019.

49. International Organization for Standardization. *ISO 11607-2:2006: Packaging for Terminally Sterilized Medical Devices—Part 2: Validation Requirements for Forming, Sealing and Assembly Processes.* Geneva, Switzerland: International Organization for Standardization; 2006. https://www.iso.org/standard/38713.html. Accessed September 23, 2019.

50. US Food and Drug Administration. Medical devices: premarket notification 510(k). US Food and Drug Administration Web site. https:// www.fda.gov/medicaldevices/deviceregulationandguidance/howto marketyourdevice/premarketsubmissions/premarketnotification510k /default.htm. Accessed September 23, 2019.

51. Centers for Disease Control and Prevention. Guidelines for infection control in dental health-care settings—2003. *Morb Mortal Wkly Rep.* 2003;52(RR-17):3.

52. Miller CH, Sheldrake MA. Sterilization beneath rings on dental instruments. *Am J Dent.* 1991;4:291-293.

53. Association for the Advancement of Medical Instrumentation. *ANSI/ AAMI ST79:2017. Comprehensive Guide to Steam Sterilization and Sterility Assurance in Health Care Facilities.* Arlington, VA: Association for the Advancement of Medical Instrumentation; 2017. http:// my.aami.org/store/detail.aspx?id=ST79. Accessed September 23, 2019.

54. UK Department of Health and Social Care. *Decontamination. Health Technical Memorandum 01-05: Decontamination in Primary Care Dental Practices.* Richmond, United Kingdom: UK Department of Health and Social Care; 2013. https://www.gov.uk/government/uploads /system/uploads/attachment_data/file/170689/HTM_01-05_2013.pdf. Accessed September 23, 2019.

55. Association for the Advancement of Medical Instrumentation. *ANSI/AAMI ST8:2013. Hospital Steam Sterilizers.* Arlington, VA: Association for the Advancement of Medical Instrumentation; 2013. http://my.aami.org/store/SearchResults.aspx?searchterm=hospital +steam+sterilizers&searchoption=ALL. Accessed September 23, 2019.

56. American National Standards Institute. Sterilization. Steam sterilizers, large sterilizers (British Standard). BS EN 285:2015. American National Standards Institute Web site. https://webstore.ansi.org/RecordDetail .aspx?sku=BS+EN+285%3a2015. Accessed September 26, 2019.

57. International Organization for Standardization. *ISO 17665-1:2006: Sterilization of Health Care Products—Moist Heat—Part 1: Requirements for the Development, Validation and Routine Control of a Sterilization Process for Medical Devices.* Geneva, Switzerland: International Organization for Standardization; 2006. https://www.iso.org /standard/43187.html. Accessed September 26, 2019.

58. Miller CH, ed. Instrument processing. In: *Infection Control and Management of Hazardous Materials for the Dental Team.* 6th ed. St. Louis, MO: Elsevier; 2018:120-151.

59. Association for the Advancement of Medical Instrumentation. *ANSI/ AAMI ST58:2013. Chemical Sterilization and High Level Disinfection in Health Care Facilities.* Arlington, VA: Association for the Advancement of Medical Instrumentation; 2013. http://my.aami.org/store /SearchResults.aspx?searchterm=Chemical+sterilization&search option=ALL. Accessed September 26, 2019.

60. Association for the Advancement of Medical Instrumentation. *ANSI/ AAMI ST40:2004/(R)2018. Table-Top Dry Heat (Heated Air) Sterilization and Sterility Assurance in Health Care Facilities.* Arlington, VA: Association for the Advancement of Medical Instrumentation; 2018. http://my.aami.org/store/detail.aspx?id=ST40-PDF. Accessed September 26, 2019.

61. International Organization for Standardization. *ISO 20857:2010: Sterilization of Health Care Products—Dry Heat—Requirements for the Development, Validation and Routine Control of a Sterilization Process for Medical Devices.* Geneva, Switzerland: International Organization for Standardization; 2010. https://www.iso.org/standard /39778.html. Accessed September 26, 2019.

62. International Organization for Standardization. *ISO 11140-1:2014: Sterilization of Health Care Products—Chemical Indicators—Part 1: General Requirements*. Geneva, Switzerland: International Organization for Standardization; 2014. https://www.iso.org/standard/55080.html. Accessed September 26, 2019.

63. American Dental Association. Biological indicators for verifying sterilization. *J Am Dent Assoc*. 1988;117:653-654.

64. Miller CH, Sheldrake MA. The ability of biological indicators to detect sterilization failures. *Am J Dent*. 1994;7:95-97.

65. Lewis DL, Arens M, Appleton SS, et al. Cross-contamination potential with dental equipment. *Lancet*. 1992;340:1252-1254.

66. Lewis DL, Boe RK. Cross-infection risks associated with current procedures for using high-speed dental handpieces. *J Clin Microbiol*. 1992;30:401-406.

67. Miller CH. Microbes in dental unit water. *J Calif Dent Assoc*. 1996;24:47-52.

68. Miller CH, Waskow JR, Riggen SD, et al. Justification for heat sterilization of slow-speed handpiece motors between patients [abstract 3182]. *J Dent Res*. 1996;75:415.

69. Chin JR, Miller CH, Palenik CJ. Internal contamination of air-driven low-speed handpieces and attached prophy angles. *J Am Dent Assoc*. 2006;137:1275-1280.

70. Herd S, Chin JR, Palenik CJ, Ofner S. The in vivo contamination of air-driven low-speed handpieces with prophylaxis angles. *J Am Dent Assoc*. 2007;138:1360-1365.

71. Miller CH. Cleaning, sterilization, and disinfection: basics of microbial killing for infection control. *J Am Dent Assoc*. 1993;124:48-56.

72. Young JM, Cottone JA. Dental handpieces: maintenance and sterilization. In: Cottone JA, Terezhalmy GT, Molinari JA, eds. *Practical Infection Control in Dentistry*. 2nd ed. Baltimore, MD: Lippincott Williams & Wilkins; 1996:176-189.

73. Kolstad RA. How well does the chemiclave sterilize handpieces? *J Am Dent Assoc*. 1998;129:985-991.

74. Edmunds LM, Rawlinson A. The effect of cleaning on blood contamination in the dental surgery following periodontal procedures. *Aust Dent J*. 1998;43:349-353.

75. McColl E, Bagg J, Winning S. The detection of blood on dental surgery surfaces and equipment following dental hygiene treatment. *Br Dent J*. 1994;176:65-67.

76. Cochran MA, Miller CH, Sheldrake MA. The efficacy of the rubber dam as a barrier to the spread of microorganisms during dental treatment. *J Am Dent Assoc*. 1989;119:141-144.

77. Jones RM, Brosseau LM. Aerosol transmission of infectious disease. *J Occup Environ Med*. 2015;57(5):501-508.

78. Petersen NJ, Bond WW, Favero MS. Air sampling for hepatitis B surface antigen in a dental operatory. *J Am Dent Assoc*. 1979; 99:465-467.

79. Bond WW, Petersen NJ, Favero MS. Viral hepatitis B: aspects of environmental control. *Health Lab Sci*. 1977;14:235-252.

80. Lauer JL, VanDrunen NA, Washburn JW, Balfour HH Jr. Transmission of hepatitis B virus in clinical laboratory areas. *J Infect Dis*. 1979;140:513-516.

81. Francis DP, Maynard JE. The transmission and outcome of hepatitis A, B, and non-A, non-B: a review. *Epidemiol Rev*. 1979;1:17-31.

82. Bond WW, Favero MS, Petersen NJ, Gravelle CR, Ebert JW, Maynard JE. Survival of hepatitis B virus after drying and storage for one week. *Lancet*. 1981;1:550-551.

83. Crawford JJ. *Clinical Asepsis in Dentistry*. Mesquite, TX: Oral Medicine Press; 1987:27-35.

84. Miller CH, Palenik CJ. Surface disinfection. *Dent Asepsis Rev*. 1988;9:1-2.

85. Molinari JA, Gleason MJ, Cottone JA, Barrett ED. Cleaning and disinfectant properties of dental surface disinfectants. *J Am Dent Assoc*. 1988;117:179-182.

86. Miller CH, ed. Surface and equipment asepsis. In: *Infection Control and Management of Hazardous Materials for the Dental Team*. 6th ed. St. Louis, MO: Elsevier; 2018:142-154.

87. Molinari JA, Harte JA. How to choose and use environmental surface disinfectants. In: Molinari JA, Harte JA, eds. *Cottone's Practical Infection Control in Dentistry*. 3rd ed. Baltimore, MD: Lippincott Williams & Wilkins; 2010:185-193.

88. American National Standards Institute. Chemical disinfectants and antiseptics. EN 14885: 2015. Application of European Standards for chemical disinfectants and antiseptics (British Standard). American National Standards Institute web site. https://webstore.ansi.org/RecordDetail.aspx?sku=BS+EN+14885%3a2015. Accessed September 26, 2019.

89. Bond WW, Favero MS, Petersen NJ, Ebert JW. Inactivation of hepatitis B virus by intermediate-to-high level disinfectant chemicals. *J Clin Microbiol*. 1983;18:535-538.

90. Martin LS, McDougal JS, Loskoski SL. Disinfection and inactivation of the human T lymphotrophic virus type III/lymphadenopathy-associated virus. *J Infect Dis*. 1985;152:400-403.

91. Molinari JA, Harte JA. Environmental surface infection control: Disposable barriers and chemical disinfection. In: Molinari JA, Harte JA, eds. *Cottone's Practical Infection Control in Dentistry*. 3rd ed. Baltimore, MD: Lippincott Williams & Wilkins; 2010:171-184.

92. Rutala WA. APIC guideline for selection and use of disinfectants. 1994, 1995, and 1996 APIC Guidelines Committee. Association for Professionals in Infection Control and Epidemiology, Inc. *Am J Infect Control*. 1996;24:313-342.

93. Litsky BY, Mascis JD, Litsky W. Use of an antimicrobial mouthwash to minimize the bacterial aerosol contaminations generated by the high-speed drill. *Oral Surg Oral Med Oral Pathol*. 1970;29:25-30.

94. Fine DH, Furgang D, Korik I, Olshan A, Barnett ML, Vincent JW. Reduction of viable bacteria in dental aerosols by preprocedural rinsing with an antiseptic mouthrinse. *Am J Dent*. 1993;6:219-221.

95. Veksler AE, Kayrouz GA, Newman MG. Reduction of salivary bacteria by pre-procedural rinses with chlorhexidine 0.12%. *J Periodontol*. 1991;62:649-651.

96. Bin-Shuwaish MS. Effects and effectiveness of cavity disinfectants in operative dentistry: a literature review. *J Contemp Dent Pract*. 2016;17(10):867-879.

97. Stevens RE Jr. Preliminary study—air contamination with microorganisms during use of air turbine handpieces. *J Am Dent Assoc*. 1963;66:237-239.

98. Watson CM, Whitehouse RL. Possibility of cross-contamination between dental patients by means of the saliva ejector. *J Am Dent Assoc*. 1993;124:77-80.

99. Costerton JW, Lewandowski Z, Caldwell DE, Korber DR, Lappin-Scott HM. Microbial biofilms. *Annu Rev Microbiol*. 1995;49:711-745.

100. Garg SK, Mittal S, Kaur P. Dental unit waterline management: historical perspectives and current trends. *J Investig Clin Dent*. 2012;3(4):247-252.

101. Barbeau J, Gauthier C, Payment P. Biofilms, infectious agents, and dental unit waterlines: a review. *Can J Microbiol*. 1998;44:1019-1028.

102. Atlas RM, Williams JF, Huntington MK. Legionella contamination of dental-unit waters. *Appl Environ Microbiol*. 1995;61:1208-1211.

103. Miller CH, ed. Dental unit water asepsis and air quality. In: *Infection Control and Management of Hazardous Materials for the Dental Team*. 6th ed. St. Louis, MO: Elsevier; 2018:155-164.

104. Miller CH, ed. Laboratory and radiographic asepsis. In: *Infection Control and Management of Hazardous Materials for the Dental Team*. 6th ed. St. Louis, MO: Elsevier; 2018:170-175.

105. Palenik CJ. Laboratory and radiographic asepsis. In: Miller CH, Palenik CJ, eds. *Infection Control and Management of Hazardous Materials for the Dental Team*. 2nd ed. St. Louis, MO: Mosby; 1998:210-221.

106. Huizing KL, Palenik CJ, Setcos JC, et al. Method of evaluating the antimicrobial abilities of disinfectant-containing gypsum products. *QDT Yearbook*. 1994;17:172-176.

107. Molinari JA, Harte, JA. Dental services. APIC Text Web site. http://text.apic.org/toc/infection-prevention-for-practice-settings-and-service-specific-patient-care-areas/dental-services. Accessed September 26, 2019.

108. Pate WJ. Waste management. In: Grota PG ed. *APIC Text on Infection Control and Epidemiology*. Washington, DC: Association for Professionals in Infection Control and Epidemiology; 2014:chap 13.

109. Miller CH, ed. Waste management. *Infection Control and Management of Hazardous Materials for the Dental Team*. 6th ed. St. Louis, MO: Elsevier; 2018:176-180.

110. Palenik CJ. Managing regulated waste in dental environments. *Dent Today*. 2004;23:62-63.

111. Krisiunas, E. Healthcare waste management. In: Friedman C, ed. *IFIC Basic Concepts of Infection Control*. 3rd ed. Craigavon, Northern Ireland: International Federation for Infection Control; 2016:chap 24.

112. Rutala WA, Mayhall CG. Medical waste. *Infect Control Hosp Epidemiol*. 1992;13:38-48.

113. Miller CH. No wasted effort. *Dent Prod Rep*. 2007;41:130-134.

114. Gordon JG, Denys GA. Infectious wastes: efficient and effective management. In: Block SS, ed. *Disinfection, Sterilization and Preservation*. 5th ed. Philadelphia, PA: Lippincott Williams & Wilkins; 2001:1139-1157.

115. US Environmental Protection Agency. Effluent limitations guidelines and standards for the dental category. *Fed Regist*. 2017;82(113)27154-27178. To be codified at 40 CFR §441.

116. US Environmental Protection Agency. *Technical and Economic Development Document for the Final Effluent Limitations Guidelines and Standards for the Dental Category, EPA-821-R-16-005*. Washington, DC: US Environmental Protection Agency, Office of Water; 2016.

117. American Dental Association. *Oral Health Topics—Amalgam Separators and Waste Best Management*. Washington, DC: American Dental Association; 2007. http://www.ada.org/en/member-center/oral-health-topics/amalgam-separators. Accessed December 2017.

118. Vadeven, J, McGinnis S. An assessment of mercury in the form of amalgam in dental wastewater in the United States. *Water Air Soil Pollut*. 2005;164(1-4):349-366.

119. Advisory Committee on Immunization Practices, Centers for Disease Control and Prevention. Immunization of health-care personnel: recommendations of the Advisory Committee on Immunization Practices (ACIP). *MMWR Recomm Rep*. 2011;60(RR-7):1-45.

120. Centers for Disease Control and Prevention. Recommended vaccines for healthcare workers. Centers for Disease Control and Prevention Web site. https://www.cdc.gov/vaccines/adults/rec-vac/hcw.html. Accessed February 13, 2018.

121. Centers for Disease Control and Prevention. Healthcare personnel: are your vaccinations up-to-date. Centers for Disease Control and Prevention Web site. https://www.cdc.gov/vaccines/pubs/downloads/f_hcp_color_print.pdf. Accessed February 13, 2018.

122. Hamborsky J, Kroger A, Wolfe S, eds. *Epidemiology and Prevention of Vaccine-Preventable Diseases*. 13th ed. Washington, DC: Public Health Foundation; 2015.

Disinfection and Biosecurity in the Prevention and Control of Disease in Veterinary Medicine

Patrick J. Quinn, Bryan K. Markey, Finola C. Leonard, and Eamonn S. FitzPatrick

Strategies for limiting the impact of infectious diseases on animal populations are often determined by the nature of the infectious agents responsible for disease production, the importance of the diseases produced on animal and human health, and the range of measures available to animal owners for the control and prevention of such diseases. Although there have been major advances in the development of chemotherapeutic drugs including antimicrobial compounds and anthelmintics as well as in the use of effective veterinary vaccines, infections caused by pathogenic microorganisms still constitute major obstacles to increased productivity, particularly in intensively reared animal populations. Among food-producing animals, infectious diseases may result in increased mortality, decreased production of meat, milk, or eggs and reproductive failure. The cost of chemotherapy is an additional expense for animal owners. In recent decades, increased reliance on intensive livestock production has resulted from increasing demands for food of animal origin and declining profit margins for producers. Although reliable data documenting losses attributable to disease in animals are difficult to determine, global estimates indicate average losses of more than 20%.[1] The mortality rate associated with infectious diseases is strongly influenced by the species and ages of animals involved, by husbandry methods used, and by the measures employed to limit transmission of pathogenic microorganisms on the farm or in the production unit.

Characteristics of infectious agents, their modes of transmission, and both management and environmental factors influence the outcome of an encounter between a susceptible host and a virulent pathogenic microorganism. In some instances, a number of infectious agents either in combination or acting sequentially may cause well-recognized "complex" diseases, particularly affecting the respiratory tract. Such disease conditions may not be amenable to control through chemoprophylaxis, chemotherapy or vaccination, and other control measures relating to the animals' immediate environment may be required to minimize adverse environmental conditions that predispose animals to opportunistic infections. For exotic infectious diseases of major economic importance in domestic animals, control measures include accurate identification of animals, control of their movement within a herd, flock or country, isolation followed by testing and where necessary, slaughter of infected animals. Contaminated buildings, equipment, and transport vehicles should be thoroughly disinfected to minimize transfer of pathogens to other locations. When dealing with endemic infectious diseases within a country, chemotherapy, chemoprophylaxis, and vaccination may be supplemented with appropriate disinfection and sterilization programs. Control measures applied to particular infectious diseases are determined by their status within a farm or country, their economic importance, and their public health significance.

▶ TRANSMISSION OF INFECTIOUS AGENTS

Contamination of the environment, including buildings, equipment, transport vehicles, vegetation, water and soil, is an important consequence of outbreaks of many infectious diseases. Such contamination can occur on farms or in other locations where animals are reared or assembled for sales, shows, or sporting events. In association with outbreaks of many infectious diseases such as those that cause abortions in horses, cattle and sheep, extensive environmental contamination can occur as animals are aborting and subsequently from contamination of aborted fetuses and fetal fluids. Scavenger animals, transport vehicles, footwear and clothing of farm workers can amplify the extent of microbial contamination before effective control measures are implemented. Salmonellosis, brucellosis, and leptospirosis as well as parvovirus, herpesvirus, and rotavirus infections are examples of diseases in which extensive environmental contamination occurs. Depending on their predilection sites in the host animal's body, pathogenic microorganisms may be shed in secretions, fluids, excretions and animal products such as meat, eggs, and offal (Figure 52.1). For some infectious agents, aerosol transmission is an important mode of transfer among susceptible animals. Avian chlamydiosis, caused by *Chlamydia psittaci*, occurs in a wide range of both wild and domestic species. The organism, which is present in respiratory discharges and feces of infected birds, is usually acquired by inhalation or ingestion. In addition to its importance in avian species, *C psittaci* is recognized as a cause of sporadic disease in the human population, often with respiratory symptoms.

Some infectious agents can survive for long periods outside the animal's body, thereby facilitating prolonged exposure of healthy animals to sources of infection. Mycobacteria, coccidial oocysts, parvoviruses, and bacterial endospores are particularly able to survive for long periods in animal products, in the environment, in feces, soil and water, in animal buildings, and on pasture. Apart from clinically affected animals, carrier animals that appear clinically normal may shed microbial pathogens intermittently if stressed by transportation over long distances, by adverse housing conditions, or by severe climate changes.

The role of animal feeds in disease transmission became an issue of international importance following the unexpected appearance of bovine spongiform encephalopathy (BSE) in British cattle. The extreme resistance of the agent of BSE to thermal and chemical inactivation renders recycling food of animal origin, especially if derived from ruminants, an undesirable practice.

Insect vectors have an important role in the dissemination of infectious agents, especially viral pathogens. Wildlife reservoirs of infectious agents, both mammals and birds, often limit the efficacy of disease control measures and, in some instances, render them ineffective.

SURVIVAL OF INFECTIOUS AGENTS IN THE ENVIRONMENT

Microbial pathogens shed in the excretions, secretions, or body fluids of infected animals may contaminate farm buildings, transport vehicles, soil, water, pasture, food, and fomites. There is considerable variation in the survival times of animal pathogens in the environment, which, for *Mycoplasma* species and some viruses, may be days, unlike bacterial endospores, which may survive for decades in soil (Figure 52.2). For more labile pathogens, duration of survival is influenced by the number of infectious agents excreted by an infected animal, the availability of nutrients, competition from other microorganisms in the same environment, and other microenvironmental factors such as the type and amount of organic material present, temperature, pH, humidity, and exposure to ultraviolet (UV) light. Although accurate information relating to pathogen survival in the environment is available for some infectious agents,[2-4] in many instances, the persistence of pathogens in soil, water, and animal waste is of uncertain duration. Infectious agents that are capable of prolonged survival in the environment include mycobacteria, coccidial oocysts, parvoviruses, bacterial endospores, and prions.

Lability is a feature of mycoplasmas, many enveloped viruses, and spirochetes, and these microbial pathogens usually have short survival times outside the animal body. In contrast, pathogenic mycobacteria, parvoviruses, and coccidial oocysts, because of their stability in the environment, remain viable in feces, soil, or contaminated buildings for many months and in favorable microenvironmental conditions for more than 1 year. Prions and bacterial endospores exhibit exceptional resistance to environmental factors and can survive for many years in soil.

Although the resistance of prions to physical and chemical inactivation has been well documented, the duration of their survival in the environment has been rarely reported. Scrapie-infected hamster brain homogenates mixed with soil and packed in perforated petri dishes retained infectivity for more than 3 years when buried in soil at ground level.[5] This important report raises serious questions about the safety of burying the carcasses of sheep that had scrapie or bovine carcasses from animals with BSE. It also raises questions about the possibility of residual infectivity on pasture, which has been grazed by animals with transmissible spongiform encephalopathies (TSEs).

PRINCIPLES OF DISEASE CONTROL

The control measures applicable to a particular infectious disease are determined by its status in the country, its public health significance, and its importance internationally. Diseases that are endemic within a country may be confined to domestic animals or may be present in and transmitted from wildlife reservoirs. National governments implement control and eradication programs for infectious diseases in accordance with the importance of the diseases for the animal population, their public health importance, and their impact on national and international trade. Ultimately, the success of a disease control program is determined by the feasibility of the procedure, the reliability of the diagnostic tests, reservoirs of infection, and the national resources available for the implementation of the eradication program. Examples of the particular methods appropriate for the prevention, treatment, and control of particular infectious agents are presented in Table 52.1.

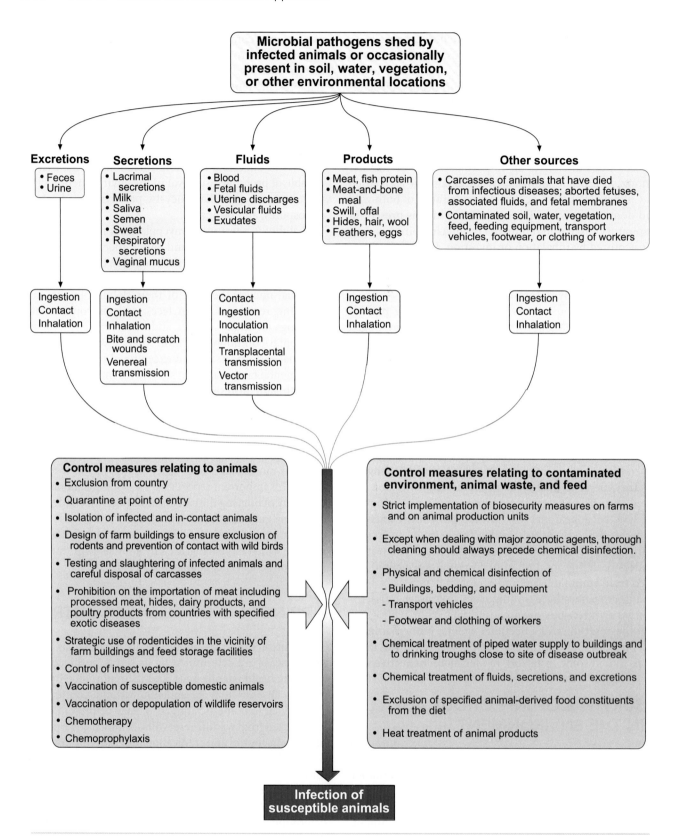

FIGURE 52.1   Modes of transmission of infectious agents from infected to susceptible animals and relevant control measures.

Infectious agents	**Survival times**

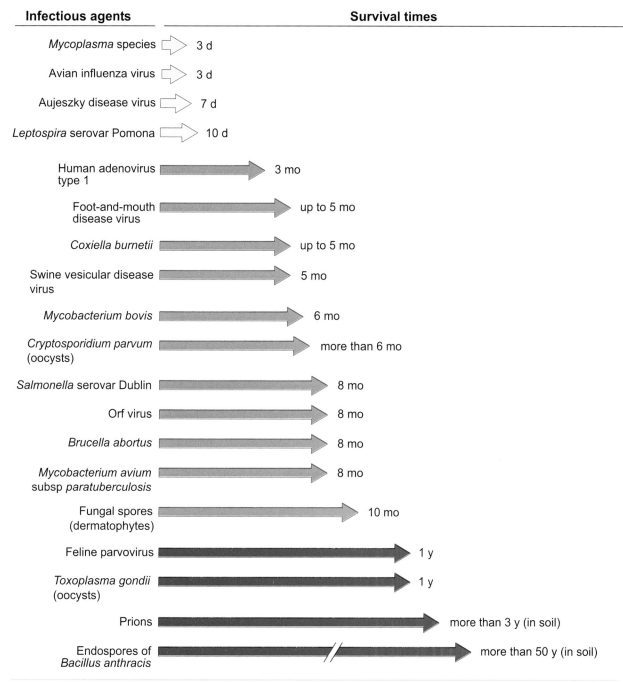

Infectious agents	Survival times
Mycoplasma species	3 d
Avian influenza virus	3 d
Aujeszky disease virus	7 d
Leptospira serovar Pomona	10 d
Human adenovirus type 1	3 mo
Foot-and-mouth disease virus	up to 5 mo
Coxiella burnetii	up to 5 mo
Swine vesicular disease virus	5 mo
Mycobacterium bovis	6 mo
Cryptosporidium parvum (oocysts)	more than 6 mo
Salmonella serovar Dublin	8 mo
Orf virus	8 mo
Brucella abortus	8 mo
Mycobacterium avium subsp *paratuberculosis*	8 mo
Fungal spores (dermatophytes)	10 mo
Feline parvovirus	1 y
Toxoplasma gondii (oocysts)	1 y
Prions	more than 3 y (in soil)
Endospores of *Bacillus anthracis*	more than 50 y (in soil)

FIGURE 52.2 Survival times of microbial pathogens in the environment at ambient temperature. The duration of survival is influenced by the number of infectious agents shed in the environment and by microenvironmental factors including the availability of nutrients, competition from other microorganisms in the same location, prevailing temperature, pH, humidity, and exposure to ultraviolet light.

Biosecurity

The term *biosecurity* includes a range of measures designed to limit or prevent exposure of domestic animals on a farm or in a production unit to pathogenic microorganisms from sources outside the premises, referred to as bioexclusion. Appropriate measures for establishment of a closed herd or flock are illustrated in Figure 52.3. Biocontainment refers to procedures for preventing or limiting the spread of infectious diseases among animals on a farm, in kennels, in poultry production units, or wherever animals are housed or reared in close contact with each other. Infectious agents can be transmitted to healthy animals by purchase of infected animals, through contaminated feed,

TABLE 52.1   Methods for the prevention, treatment, and control of particular infectious agents

Infectious Agent	Disease/Hosts	Methods[a]					Comments
		Movement Restriction[b]	Vector Control	Chemotherapy	Disinfection	Vaccination	
African swine fever virus	African swine fever/pigs	++	++	–	++	–	Soft ticks of the genus *Ornithodoros* are vectors of the virus.
Bacillus anthracis	Anthrax/many species	+	–	+	++	++	Endospores survive for many years in soil; vaccination is permitted where disease is endemic.
Clostridium tetani	Tetanus/many species	–	–	+	±	++	Endospores of *C tetani* are widely distributed in soil and in feces of animals.
Foot-and-mouth disease virus	Foot-and-mouth disease/many species	++	–	–	++	+	Vaccination is permitted where disease is endemic. Vaccinal strain must match field strain, and duration of protection is limited.
Histoplasma capsulatum	Histoplasmosis/many species	–	–	+	+	–	Soilborne fungus that causes opportunistic infections
Microsporum canis	Ringworm/many species	+	–	+	+	+	*M canis* is transmitted by direct and indirect contact.
Streptococcus equi	Strangles/horses	+	–	+	++	±	Efficacy of vaccines uncertain

[a]++, effective method; +, effective under defined conditions; ±, of questionable value; –, not applicable.

[b]Exclusion from a country, quarantine, or restriction of movement on affected farm.

by vectors, and from environmental sources. An effective biosecurity program has many components, all aimed at ensuring that the risks of healthy animals acquiring infection are minimized (Table 52.2). Design considerations for farms engaged in the implementation of biocontainment policies are illustrated in Figure 52.4.

A number of well-defined measures can be used for the prevention and control of infectious diseases within a country or in a region of a country. These include exclusion of suspect animals, quarantine at point of entry, and isolation and slaughter of infected animals if an exotic disease is confirmed by clinical or laboratory tests. If infectious diseases are endemic in a country, control measures include vaccination, chemotherapy, and chemoprophylaxis. Effective control measures relating to the environment, animal waste, and animal products are central to the success of a disease eradication program. These include

- Chemical disinfection of
  - buildings, bedding, and equipment
  - transport vehicles
  - footwear and clothing of workers
- Chemical treatment of water supply, following disinfection of building
- Chemical treatment of fluids, excretions, secretions
- Heat treatment of milk and milk products; mandatory boiling of waste food if swill feeding to pigs is permitted

The forms and amount of animal waste generated on a farm are determined by the number and species of animals present, building design, and the type of material used as bedding for large animals or as poultry litter.

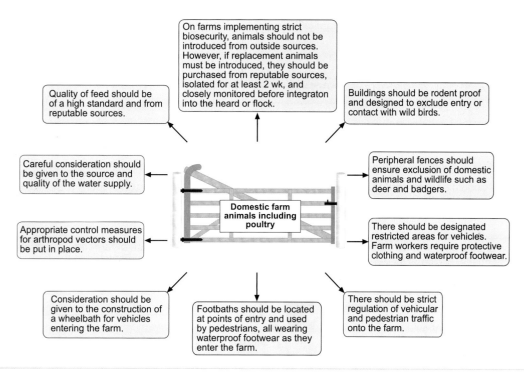

FIGURE 52.3 Bioexclusion measures appropriate for establishment and maintenance of a closed herd or flock and farm policies aimed at minimizing the risk of introducing specific infectious agents to such animal populations.

TABLE 52.2	Components of a biosecurity program for farm animals, including poultry	
Component	**Considerations**	**Comments**
Animals	Replacement animals should be purchased from reputable sources.	Newly purchased animals should be isolated for at least 2 wk and closely monitored.
Feed	Source and quality of feed requires close attention.	Feed can become contaminated by wild birds and rodents during storage.
Water supply	Water quality is influenced by source, climatic factors, and local environmental influences.	Drinkers within buildings or water troughs for grazing animals can become contaminated with feces or urine containing microbial pathogens.
Environment of animals	Building design should incorporate features that promote animal health and facilitate cleaning and disinfection.	Improper building design, inadequate ventilation, and insufficient floor space can predispose animals to stressful conditions.
Vehicular and pedestrian traffic	Delivery vehicles should be visibly clean, and drivers should be advised at point of entry on the control measures that apply. Staff, service personnel, and others visiting the farm should wear protective clothing and use footbaths provided.	Particular care is required with vehicles used for transportation of animals, slurry tankers, and vehicles used for disposal of used bedding or poultry litter.
Equipment used on farms	Sharing of farm equipment such as trailers used for transportation of animals should be avoided.	Any equipment used for cleaning farm buildings or spreading animal waste should not be borrowed or loaned.
Animal waste	Liquid animal waste is usually stored in slurry tanks; solid waste may be composted on the farm or removed at frequent intervals for dispersal on arable land.	An interval of up to 2 mo should elapse between the application of slurry to pasture and commencement of grazing.
Rodents, wild birds, wildlife	Rodents can act as reservoirs of a number of microbial pathogens; wild birds can transmit avian influenza to commercial poultry flocks; a number of wildlife species can transmit infectious agents to grazing animals.	Where feasible, buildings should be rodent proof; wild birds should not have access to poultry houses or to feed mills where poultry feed is prepared or stored.
Cleaning and disinfection	Effective cleaning followed by thorough disinfection is essential for the elimination of microbial pathogens from farm buildings.	Cleaning can reduce the number of microbial pathogens in a building, but chemical disinfection is required to inactivate residual microbial pathogens.

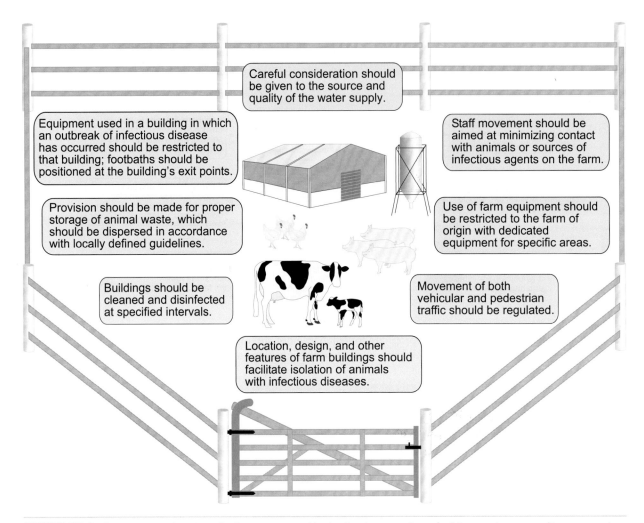

FIGURE 52.4 Design considerations for farms engaged in the implementation of a biocontainment policy appropriate for the prevention or control of outbreaks of infectious disease in farm animals, including poultry.

For buildings with slatted floors, animal waste is stored in slurry tanks. These tanks should be constructed to high specifications and have ample capacity to avoid overflowing of contents. Slurry spreading is usually restricted to defined times of the year when ground conditions are suitable for slurry tankers and when the risk of runoff is low. An interval of at least 2 months should elapse between the application of slurry to pasture and the commencement of grazing. A longer interval between the application of slurry and the commencement of grazing may be required if enteric pathogens such as *Salmonella* species or pathogenic acid-fast bacteria are likely to be present in the slurry.

Straw used for bedding animals and litter from poultry houses should be composted for at least 2 months at a site remote from farm buildings before spreading on land used for tillage. Composting should take place on a site where runoff is minimized by location and by the design of the holding facility. Alternatively, the bedding material can be removed at regular intervals and dispersed on arable land. If an infectious disease has occurred on the farm from

which the bedding material derived, composting should be carried out for at least 2 months before dispersal of the material on arable land.

▶ SELECTION AND USE OF DISINFECTANTS

Control of infectious diseases at farm level requires procedures that are practical, realistic, and cost-effective. Although a number of potentially useful physical methods for disinfection such as dry heat, moist heat, ionization radiation, UV light, and mechanical methods may be used for disinfection in many situations, chemical disinfection procedures usually find wider application than physical methods in clinical facilities and at farm level. By employing specific physical dispersal methods for chemical disinfectants, enhanced distribution and greater reliability in surface decontamination can be achieved.

A number of new chemical formulations, many based on combinations of antimicrobial compounds that have been in continual use for decades, are gaining acceptance as effective disinfectants for infectious diseases of animals. Combinations of antimicrobial compounds that have received favorable evaluation in published reports include quaternary ammonium compounds (QACs) combined with glutaraldehyde (a proprietary disinfectant), accelerated hydrogen peroxide (containing a reduced concentration of hydrogen peroxide supplemented with acids, surfactants, wetting agents, and chelating agents), and hydrogen peroxide combined with silver nitrate. Characteristics of an ideal chemical disinfectant include

- Broad antimicrobial spectrum with effective activity against vegetative bacteria (including mycobacteria), bacterial endospores, fungal spores, enveloped and nonenveloped viruses, oocysts of pathogenic protozoa, and prions
- Absence of irritancy, toxicity, teratogenicity, mutagenicity, and carcinogenicity for personnel implementing disinfection programs and also for animals occupying buildings where the chemical disinfectant will be used
- Stability, with a long shelf life at ambient temperatures
- Effectiveness against bacteria in biofilms or pathogenic microorganisms dried on surfaces
- Compatibility with a wide range of chemicals including acids, alkalis, and anionic and cationic compounds
- Retention of antimicrobial activity in the presence of organic matter
- Solubility in water to the concentration required for effective antimicrobial activity
- Absence of corrosiveness or chemical interactions with metallic fittings, plastic, rubber, or synthetic structural materials
- Absence of tainting or toxicity following application to surfaces or equipment in dairies, meat, plants, or food processing areas
- Moderately priced and readily available
- Nonpolluting for groundwater or air, nontoxic for aquatic species and biodegradable

It is evident that no currently available antimicrobial compounds possess all of these attributes. With further refinements, chemical disinfectants with enhanced antimicrobial and fewer undesirable characteristics are emerging. Disinfection has become a central part of disease control strategies in the dairy industry, in the poultry industry, and in pig production. Teat dipping is an integral component of mastitis control programs for dairy cattle and routine cleaning, and terminal disinfection has become a standard procedure for the prevention of infectious diseases in pigs and poultry. Regardless of the species of animal involved or the intensity of production, disinfection should play a central role in the prevention and control of infectious diseases in farm animals or captive animals.

The relative susceptibility of pathogenic microorganisms to chemical disinfectants is illustrated in Figure 52.5.

Marked differences in susceptibility occur among infectious agents, and consequently, selection of disinfectants for a disinfection program should be based on the particular infectious agents likely to be present and the spectrum of activity of the disinfectant selected. A clinical history of animals on the farm, laboratory reports, and other sources of relevant information can assist in the selection of a suitable chemical disinfectant for a particular farm. Ultimately, the choice of a disinfectant for a particular purpose should take into account its spectrum of activity, efficacy, susceptibility to inactivation by organic or inorganic materials, compatibility with surface materials or other chemicals such as detergents, toxicity for personnel and animals, contact time required, optimal temperatures, residual activity, corrosiveness and effect on the environment, and cost. Infectious agents also exhibit variation in their susceptibility to moist heat (Figure 52.6).

The Influence of Structural and Other Features of Microbial Pathogens on Disinfectant Efficacy

The great structural, biochemical, and metabolic diversity exhibited by bacterial, fungal, protozoal, and viral pathogens partially accounts for the wide variation in their patterns of resistance or susceptibility to chemical disinfectants. The presence of lipopolysaccharide (LPS) in the cell walls of gram-negative bacteria is associated with their intrinsic resistance to particular disinfectants. Mycobacterial resistance to disinfectants is linked to the hydrophobic nature of cell wall mycolic acids, which act as permeability barriers to hydrophilic disinfectants. The six-layered structure of bacterial endospores, the presence of dipicolinic acid in their cores, and their metabolically inactive state contribute to their exceptional resistance to chemical disinfectants and also to adverse environmental conditions. Fungal species etiologically implicated in human and animal infections share many common features in the structure of their cell walls, which are composed primarily of carbohydrates such as α-glucan polymers, chitin, mannans, and proteins. Composition, porosity, and thickness of fungal cell walls are features that may limit uptake of chemical disinfectants. As fungal cells age, their relative porosity decreases, probably due to increased cell wall thickness.

Viruses with lipid envelopes are susceptible to inactivation by lipophilic-type disinfectants, but nonenveloped viruses are resistant to the action of lipophilic disinfectants and demonstrate higher resistance to heat. Unlike conventional infectious agents, prions are resistant to many chemical compounds that readily inactivate pathogenic microorganisms. The basis of this exceptional resistance is not well understood but may

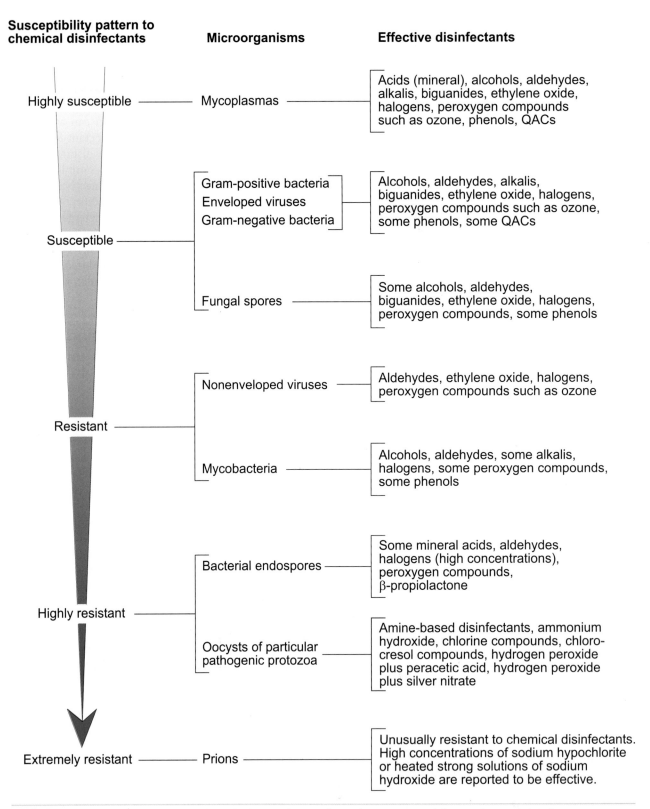

FIGURE 52.5   Microorganisms broadly ranked according to their relative susceptibility to chemical disinfectants. The effectiveness of disinfectants is influenced by many factors, including their composition and concentration, the presence of organic matter or other interfering substances, and the temperature at which they are used. Abbreviation: QACs, quaternary ammonium compounds.

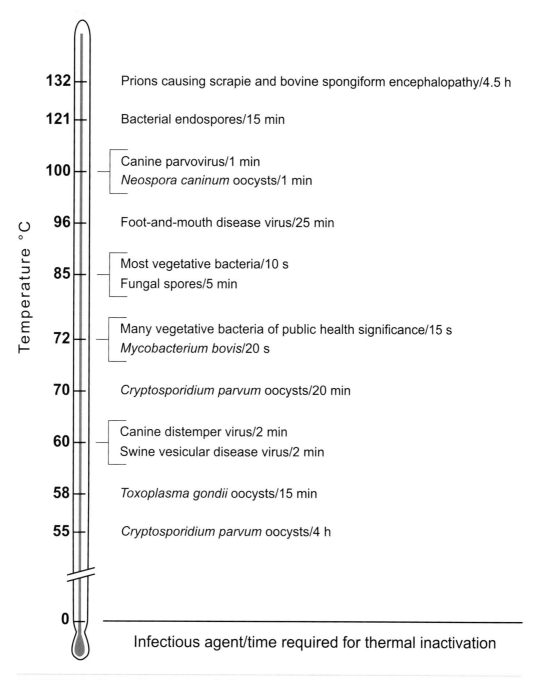

Temperature °C

132 — Prions causing scrapie and bovine spongiform encephalopathy/4.5 h

121 — Bacterial endospores/15 min

100 — Canine parvovirus/1 min
       Neospora caninum oocysts/1 min

96 — Foot-and-mouth disease virus/25 min

85 — Most vegetative bacteria/10 s
      Fungal spores/5 min

72 — Many vegetative bacteria of public health significance/15 s
      Mycobacterium bovis/20 s

70 — *Cryptosporidium parvum* oocysts/20 min

60 — Canine distemper virus/2 min
      Swine vesicular disease virus/2 min

58 — *Toxoplasma gondii* oocysts/15 min

55 — *Cryptosporidium parvum* oocysts/4 h

0 — Infectious agent/time required for thermal inactivation

FIGURE 52.6   Thermal inactivation of infectious agents by moist heat. The number of infectious agents initially present and sensitivity of the detection system used to determine survival or inactivation may alter the reliability of the results.

relate to the chemical composition of prions, which are described as being composed of altered or denatured protein.

The oocysts of a number of protozoal parasites such as *Cryptosporidium parvum* are particularly resistant to most chemical disinfectants but are more sensitive to the effects of heat. The resistance of these oocysts to chemical inactivation is attributed to the inability of many chemical disinfectants to penetrate the rigid bilayer of

acid-fast lipids in the oocyst wall and the inner layer of oocyst wall proteins. Structural and other features of particular infectious agents are presented in Figure 52.7. Distinguishing structural features of four pathogenic fungi are presented in Figure 52.8. Although a substantial amount of biochemical detail relating to fungal cell walls is available, much of this information cannot be readily illustrated in diagrammatic representations of these fungal agents.

Microorganisms	Structural, biochemical, or other features that influence susceptibility or resistance to chemical disinfectants	Relative susceptibility to chemical disinfectants	Suitable disinfectants
Mycoplasmas	Devoid of cell wall, peptidoglycan not synthesized, flexible, triple-layered outer membrane, unusual "fried egg" colonies formed, as illustrated	Highly susceptible	Acids (mineral), alcohols, aldehydes, alkalis, biguanides, ethylene oxide, halogens, peroxygen compounds, phenols, QACs
Gram-positive bacteria	Because of their high content of peptidoglycan, relatively large molecules such as disinfectants can readily move through their cell walls; the cytoplasmic membrane, a lipid-protein bilayer, acts as a selective barrier.	Susceptible	Alcohols, aldehydes, alkalis, biguanides, halogens, peroxygen compounds, some phenols, QACs
Gram-negative bacteria	The cell walls of these bacteria contain lipopolysaccharide in their outer membranes. The cytoplasmic membrane, composed of lipoprotein, may contribute to the intrinsic resistance of these bacteria. *Pseudomonas aeruginosa, Burkholderia cepacia,* and *Proteus* species may exhibit resistance to particular disinfectants.	Susceptible	Some alcohols, aldehydes, biguanides, ethylene oxide, halogens, peroxygen compounds, some phenols, some QACs

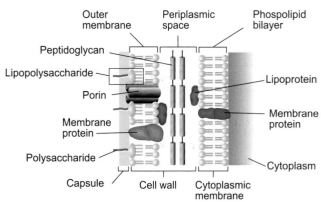

FIGURE 52.7 Structural, biochemical, and other features of bacteria, bacterial endospores, pathogenic fungi, pathogenic mycobacteria, protozoal oocysts, viruses, and prions, which may influence and, in some instances, determine their resistance to chemical disinfectants. Abbreviation: QACs, quaternary ammonium compounds.

Microorganisms	Structural, biochemical, or other features that influence susceptibility or resistance to chemical disinfectants	Relative susceptibility to chemical disinfectants	Suitable disinfectants
Proteobacteria *Coxiella burnetii*	An atypical obligate intracellular bacterial pathogen, *C burnetii* forms small intracellular resistant endospore-like forms. Although resistant to many disinfectants, the basis of this resistance, which has not been determined, is attributed to metabolic dormancy.	Resistant	Ethyl alcohol (70%), chloroform (5%), specific QAC-type disinfectant combined with detergent
Bacterial endospores	A typical bacterial endospore has six layers: an exosporium, an outer coat composed mainly of protein, an inner coat composed mainly of protein, a cortex rich in peptidoglycan, a core wall, and an inner membrane surrounding the core containing the cell genome. The core contains dipicolinic acid, a chelating agent, and small acid-soluble DNA-binding proteins that protect DNA from thermal and ultraviolet radiation. Endospores, which are produced inside the bacterial cell, exhibit species variation in size and shape. Structural and biochemical features, along with their metabolically inactive state, contribute to the exceptional resistance of endospores to chemical disinfectants and to adverse environmental conditions.	Highly resistant	Some mineral acids, aldehydes, halogens (high concentrations), peroxygen compounds, ethylene oxide

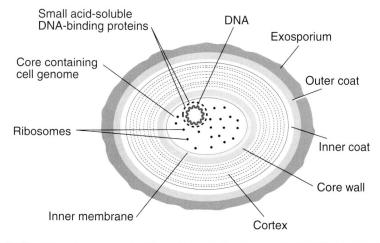

FIGURE 52.7 *Continued*

Microorganisms	Structural, biochemical, or other features that influence susceptibility or resistance to chemical disinfectants	Relative susceptibility to chemical disinfectants	Suitable disinfectants
Pathogenic mycobacteria	Mycobacterial resistance to disinfectants is linked to the cell wall composition of these bacteria. The outer surface of mycobacteria is composed of medium-chain and short-chain lipids and glycolipids, forming a hydrophobic layer of mycolic acids. Porin channels in their cell walls may allow diffusion of some hydrophilic disinfectants, but the permeability barrier associated with the hydrophobic cell walls of these acid-fast bacteria limits penetration by hydrophilic disinfectants, which may not be able to exert a mycobactericidal effect.	Resistant	Alcohols, aldehydes, some alkalis, halogens, peroxygen compounds, some phenols
Pathogenic fungi	Fungal species associated with infections in humans and animals represent a number of very diverse groups in the kingdom Fungi. Despite this diversity, fungi share many common features, especially in the structure of their cell walls, which are composed primarily of carbohydrates such as α-glucan polymers, chitin, mannans, and proteins, as illustrated in Figure. 52.8. The fungal cell membrane is rich in ergosterol, which is the target of many antifungal drugs. Fungal pathogens are more resistant to chemical disinfectants than non-sporulating bacteria.	Susceptible	Aldehydes, halogens, biguanides, ethylene oxide, peroxygen compounds, halogenated phenols, some QACs

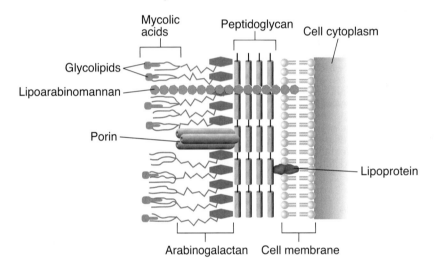

FIGURE 52.7 *Continued*

Microorganisms	Structural, biochemical, or other features that influence susceptibility or resistance to chemical disinfectants	Relative susceptibility to chemical disinfectants	Suitable disinfectants
Enveloped viruses	Viruses with lipid envelopes are susceptible to inactivation by lipophilic-type disinfectants. Both lipid content and virion size influence viral susceptibility to disinfectants.	Susceptible	Alcohols, aldehydes, alkalis, some mineral acids, biguanides, ethylene oxide, halogens, some QACs

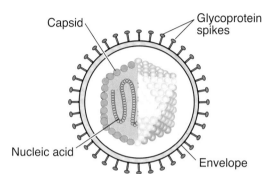

Nonenveloped viruses	Unlike enveloped viruses, nonenveloped viruses are resistant to the action of lipophilic disinfectants, and broad-spectrum disinfectants are required for their inactivation. Effective disinfectants may induce conformational changes in capsid proteins or attach to capsid receptors; they may induce alterations in nucleic acid, capsid proteins, virus-encoded enzymes, or sulfhydryl groups in viral proteins.	Resistant	Aldehydes, ethylene oxide, β-propiolactone, halogens, ozone, peracetic acid

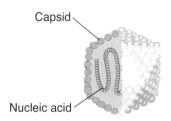

FIGURE 52.7 *Continued*

Microorganisms	Structural, biochemical, or other features that influence susceptibility or resistance to chemical disinfectants	Relative susceptibility to chemical disinfectants	Suitable disinfectants
Protozoal oocysts	The oocysts of *Cryptosporidium parvum*, a zoonotic, intestinal protozoan parasite, cause enteric disease in many species of domestic animals and also in humans. Because the oocysts are resistant to chlorine-based compounds used to treat drinking water, periodic outbreaks of cryptosporidiosis are reported in the human population in many countries. These oocysts are resistant to most chemical disinfectants that are effective against bacterial and viral pathogens. Although the basis of resistance of the oocysts to chemical inactivation is not explained, it is attributed to the inability of many chemical disinfectants to penetrate the rigid bilayer of acid-fast lipids in the oocyst cell wall and the inner layer of oocyst wall proteins.	Highly resistant	Amine-based disinfectants, ozone, ammonium hydroxide, formol saline, hydrogen peroxide plus peracetic acid, hydrogen peroxide plus silver nitrate, specific phenolic compounds such as *p*-chloro-*m*-cresol
Prions	Unlike conventional infectious agents, prions are resistant to the majority of chemical compounds that inactivate bacteria, bacterial endospores, fungi, viruses, and protozoal oocysts. The basis of this exceptional resistance, which is not well understood, may relate to the fact that prions are altered proteins that resist further chemical degradation, especially when attached to walls of containers or dried on metal surfaces.	Extremely resistant	High concentrations of sodium hypochlorite or heated strong solutions of sodium hydroxide are reported to be effective.

FIGURE 52.7   *Continued*

▶ CHARACTERISTICS OF CHEMICAL DISINFECTANTS USED IN VETERINARY MEDICINE

Table 52.3 provides a summary of the different properties and spectra of action of the main disinfectant chemical groups.

Acids

Low concentrations of organic acids such as citric acid and acetic acid are nonirritating; mineral acids such as hydrochloric acid and sulfuric acid are corrosive and hazardous for workers. At pH values below 3, acids exert a bactericidal effect. Mineral acids are used as cleaning agents in food processing and for removing lime scale, milk stone, and other alkaline deposits in pipes, milking machines, and on surfaces. Organic acids are used as preservatives in food and in pharmaceutical products.

Both organic and mineral acids can inactivate the virus of foot-and-mouth disease. Hydrochloric acid at a 2.5% concentration, has been used for inactivation of the endospores of *Bacillus anthracis* on skins and hides.

Alcohols

Two forms of alcohol, ethyl alcohol and isopropyl alcohol, are widely used as disinfectants. They are relatively nontoxic, nontainting, colorless, and evaporate quickly without leaving a residue. Their solvent activity can damage rubber and some plastic material. Because they are flammable at concentrations recommended for disinfection, they should not be used close to naked flames.

When used at appropriate concentrations on intact skin, alcohols provide a rapid and effective reduction in the microbial skin population. This characteristic accounts for their extensive use in hand rinses and other preparations used for minimizing the transmission of flora acquired from infected patients in clinical environments.

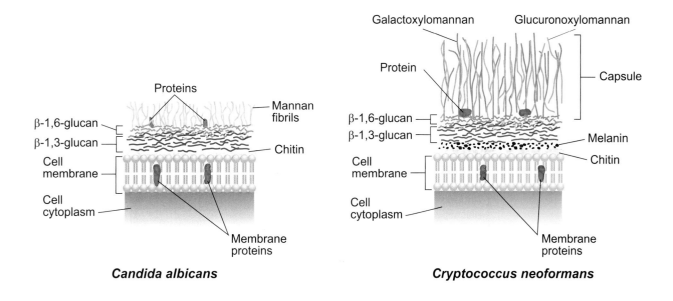

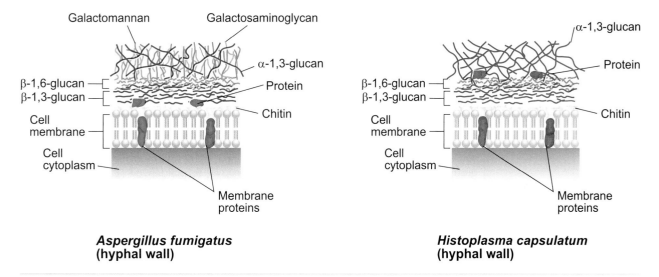

FIGURE 52.8 Structural features of the cell walls of four fungal species: two yeasts, *Candida albicans* and *Cryptococcus neoformans*; the saprobic mold, *Aspergillus fumigatus*; and the dimorphic fungus, *Histoplasma capsulatum*. Based on Erwig and Gow[6] and Brown et al.[7]

TABLE 52.3   General characteristics and antimicrobial spectrum of disinfectants commonly used in veterinary medicine[a]

| Disinfectant Group | Examples | Modes of Action | Characteristics | | Undesirable Interactions With Other Chemicals, Inherent Toxicity, and Risks Associated With Their Use | Substances or Environmental Conditions That Adversely Affect Disinfectant Activity |
			Positive Features	Negative Features		
Acids	Acetic acid, citric acid, hydrochloric acid	Antimicrobial activity is related to hydrogen ion concentration, precipitation of protein, and nucleic acid disruption.	Organic acids inactivate viruses of foot-and-mouth disease; strong mineral acids inactivate the endospores of *Bacillus anthracis*	Mineral acids are corrosive and hazardous for workers.	Because mineral acids are hazardous for workers, protective clothing is required; should not be mixed with alkaline solutions	Activity may be neutralized by alkaline solutions and can be reduced by hard water; organic matter reduces effectiveness.
Alcohols	Ethyl alcohol, isopropyl alcohol	Denature proteins and are lipid solvents	Inexpensive, nontoxic, non-tainting, fast acting	Some rubber and plastic materials may be damaged; highly flammable, not sporicidal	Highly flammable	Organic matter dried on surfaces reduces effectiveness.
Aldehydes	Formaldehyde, glutaraldehyde	React with sulfhydryl and amino groups in cell walls and cell membranes of microorganisms; denature nucleic acids by alkylation	Highly reactive chemicals with wide spectrum of activity	Irritating vapor and pungent odor; toxic for humans and animals; mutagens and potential carcinogens	Because of the toxicity of formaldehyde vapor, breathing apparatus should be mandatory for workers in confined spaces.	Effectiveness reduced by organic matter, some soaps, and hard water; glutaraldehyde activity affected by pH of environment; efficiency is best above pH 7.
Alkalis	Sodium hydroxide, ammonium hydroxide	Hydroxyl ions at high pH values exert antimicrobial activity and denature lipids.	Sodium carbonate often used to raise pH of industrial cleaners; heated sodium hydroxide used for inactivation of prions	Corrosive for metals; caustic alkaline solutions hazardous for workers; protective clothing required	Sodium hydroxide forms caustic solutions; protective clothing required for workers; should not be added to acid solutions	Activity influenced by pH of environment; may be neutralized by low pH values; organic matter reduces effectiveness.

(continued)

TABLE 52.3 General characteristics and antimicrobial spectrum of disinfectants commonly used in veterinary medicine[a] *(Continued)*

Disinfectant Group	Examples	Modes of Action	Characteristics		Undesirable Interactions With Other Chemicals, Inherent Toxicity, And Risks Associated With Their Use	Substances or Environmental Conditions That Adversely Affect Disinfectant Activity
			Positive Features	Negative Features		
Biguanides	Chlorhexidine gluconate, alexidine	These cationic compounds alter bacterial cell wall osmotic equilibrium by binding to negatively charged groups on cell membranes but without causing cell wall lysis.	Broad spectrum of activity against bacteria; relatively nontoxic; longer persistence on skin than many other chemical compounds	Activity is pH-dependent (5-8); soaps and anionic compounds inhibit activity; toxic for aquatic species	These cationic compounds are toxic for fish and should not be released into the environment.	Inactivated by anionic soaps/detergents, cotton, cork, and organic matter; optimal pH range 5-8
Chlorine compounds	Sodium hypochlorite, chlorine dioxide	Oxidation of peptide links and denaturation of proteins; damage to viral nucleic acids	Broad spectrum; inexpensive; chlorine-releasing compounds are potent virucides and require short contact time.	Organic matter and alkaline substances inhibit chlorine compounds; due to their instability, freshly prepared solutions should be used.	Addition of acids can release chlorine gas, which is toxic; chlorine-releasing agents used in association with formaldehyde produce bis(chloromethyl) ether, a potent carcinogen.	Organic matter rapidly reduces effectiveness; soaps and detergents can have an inhibitory effect; an alkaline pH inhibits their antimicrobial activity; should be stored in opaque containers due to instability in light
Iodine compounds	Iodophors, povidone-iodine, tincture of iodine	Denature proteins and interfere with microbial enzyme systems; interact preferentially with thiol groups in proteins of the cytoplasmic membrane	Broad spectrum, stable during storage, relatively nontoxic; short contact time required; widely used in food industry	Environmental pH highly influences their activity; may cause skin irritation; activity is reduced by organic matter.	Optimal pH is in the neutral or acid range; stable in acid solutions	Inactivated by organic matter

TABLE 52.3   General characteristics and antimicrobial spectrum of disinfectants commonly used in veterinary medicine[a] *(Continued)*

Disinfectant Group	Examples	Modes of Action	Characteristics		Undesirable Interactions With Other Chemicals, Inherent Toxicity, And Risks Associated With Their Use	Substances or Environmental Conditions That Adversely Affect Disinfectant Activity
			Positive Features	Negative Features		
Peroxygen compounds	Hydrogen peroxide, peracetic acid	Denature microbial proteins and lipids; act as oxidizing agents, producing free hydroxyl radicals that interact with lipids, proteins, and DNA	Fast acting; low toxicity; wide antimicrobial spectrum; some commercial preparations of hydrogen peroxide may have enhanced activity.	Some cause metal corrosion; high concentrations can be hazardous.	At room temperature, higher concentrations can be hazardous and in air (as vapor) can cause respiratory distress.	Hydrogen peroxide loses its potency when heated; antimicrobial activity inhibited by the presence of degrading enzymes (eg, catalase and reducing agents); effect of organic matter usually moderate
Phenolic compounds	Ortho-phenylphenol, chloroxylenol	Low concentrations act on cell membrane inactivating cellular enzymes; high concentrations act as protoplasmic poisons disrupting the cell wall and precipitating cell proteins.	Effective bactericidal compounds in the presence of organic matter; stable during storage	Toxic for some animals, particularly cats; unsuitable for surfaces in contract with food due to tainting; disposal restrictions apply; strong odors	Denature and coagulate protein and are general protoplasmic poisons; toxic for humans and animals, especially cats and pigs	Most active at neutral or slightly alkaline pH values; oils or fats reduce their activity.
Quaternary ammonium compounds (QACs)	Benzalkonium chloride, cetrimide	By binding to phospholipids and proteins in the cell membrane and inactivating enzyme systems, these surface-active agents disrupt cell membrane activity.	Relatively nontoxic; effective at high temperatures and high pH values; stable during storage	Limited antimicrobial spectrum; organic matter, soaps, and detergents inhibit activity; some gram-negative bacteria are resistant; moderately expensive	Toxic for fish; should not be discharged into streams or ponds; turkeys reported to be sensitive to low levels of QACs; exposure to QACs impaired reproductive health in mice.	Organic matter, anionic detergents, soaps, and material such as cotton and gauze pads reduce their microbicidal activity; optimal pH range neutral or slightly alkaline

[a]Note that characteristics can vary depending on the formulation and labeling on specific disinfectant products.

Alcohols denature protein and are lipid solvents. The most effective concentration of ethyl alcohol is approximately 70%. In the presence of organic matter, the antimicrobial activity of alcohols can be limited. The antimicrobial spectrum of alcohols includes gram-positive and gram-negative bacteria, acid-fast bacteria, *Coxiella burnetii*, some fungi, and many enveloped viruses. They are not sporicidal.

Aldehydes

As a group, aldehydes are highly reactive chemicals with a wide antimicrobial spectrum. Three aldehydes are used as disinfectants: formaldehyde, glutaraldehyde, and ortho-phthalaldehyde. A number of chemical disinfectants including aldehydes, ethylene oxide (EO), and β-propiolactone are alkylating agents: they inactivate enzymes and other proteins with labile hydrogen atoms such as sulfhydryl groups. Aldehydes react readily with amino, carboxyl, sulfhydryl, and hydroxyl groups on proteins, causing irreversible changes in protein structure. Some aldehydes react with amino groups on purine and pyrimidine bases in nucleic acids and with peptidoglycan.

Formaldehyde is a monoaldehyde that occurs as a gas, which is freely soluble in water. Formaldehyde solution, formalin, is an aqueous solution containing up to 38% formaldehyde with methyl alcohol added to prevent polymerization. Vapor-phase formaldehyde can be used for fumigation of sealed buildings. The vapor can be produced by evaporation of formalin, by the addition of formalin to potassium permanganate crystals, or by heating paraformaldehyde. The antimicrobial spectrum of formaldehyde is wide. It is effective against vegetative bacteria including mycobacteria, endospores, fungi, and viruses, but it acts more slowly than glutaraldehyde. In addition to its use as a disinfectant, formaldehyde is used in the preparation of veterinary vaccines and also in footbaths to prevent or treat foot lameness in cattle and sheep. Even at low concentrations, the irritating vapor and pungent odor of formaldehyde is evident. The use of formaldehyde as a broad-spectrum antimicrobial agent is declining due to its known toxicity and potential carcinogenicity. Chlorine-releasing agents should not be used in association with formaldehyde because bis(chloromethyl) ether, a potent carcinogen, is produced by the reaction of formaldehyde with hydrochloric acid, sodium hypochlorite, or other chlorine-releasing compounds.

Glutaraldehyde, a dialdehyde, is usually supplied commercially as a 2%, 25%, or 50% acidic solution. Although stable at acid pH, it is more active at values close to pH 8. It has high microbicidal activity against vegetative bacteria, bacterial endospores, fungal spores, and viruses. It is noncorrosive and usually does not damage rubber or plastic components. Glutaraldehyde is reported to have a marked inhibitory effect on bacteria within biofilms by penetrating and inhibiting bacterial activity and by

contributing to bacterial detachment from the biofilm. This dialdehyde is widely used for high-level disinfection of thermosensitive medical equipment such as endoscopes and anesthetic equipment at various concentrations and exposure times depending on the formulation. Even at low levels, glutaraldehyde vapor is irritating for the eyes and mucous membranes. Concerns about the risks of exposure to glutaraldehyde have resulted in a marked decline in its use as a broad-spectrum disinfectant.

Ortho-phthalaldehyde, an aromatic aldehyde, has some characteristics in common with glutaraldehyde. It is bactericidal and virucidal, but its sporicidal activity is much less than that of glutaraldehyde. This chemical is stable over a wide pH range, has a mild odor, and is less irritating to mucous membranes than glutaraldehyde. Absence of corrosiveness and compatibility with most rubber and plastic components is another positive feature of this disinfectant.

Alkalis

The antimicrobial activity of alkalis is related to hydroxyl ion concentration. Alkalis are frequently used to increase the pH of many industrial sanitizers and cleaners and are sometimes used as cleaning and disinfecting solutions in their own right. Sodium hydroxide, potassium hydroxide, and sodium carbonate (washing soda) are the alkalis most often employed for cleaning the surfaces of buildings and transport vehicles. Calcium oxide (lime) has been used as a traditional disinfectant in agricultural locations for decades, and calcium hydroxide (slaked lime) is sometimes used for whitewashing building surfaces following an outbreak of an infectious disease. At high concentrations, these chemicals have effective microbicidal properties. Caustic alkaline solutions inactivate many viruses including foot-and-mouth disease virus, adenoviruses, and swine vesicular disease virus. A pH value above 12 may be required for inactivation of pathogens such as *Mycobacterium bovis*. Although sodium carbonate at a 4% concentration is used primarily as a cleaning agent, it is particularly effective against foot-and-mouth disease virus. At concentrations over 5%, sodium hydroxide has a wide antimicrobial spectrum including bacterial endospores. Prions, which are resistant to most decontaminating procedures, are inactivated by treatments including 2 M sodium hydroxide at 121°C for 30 minutes. Both sodium hydroxide and potassium hydroxide are corrosive for metals and hazardous for workers. All workers using strong alkaline solutions should be informed of their caustic nature and should wear eye protection, rubber gloves, and protective clothing.

Endospores of *B anthracis* have the ability to persist in the environment for decades, even under adverse environmental conditions. Outbreaks of anthrax are often associated with alkaline soil. Formerly, lime was used as a disinfectant when carcasses of animals, which had died of anthrax, were being buried. Current scientific observations indicate that lime, rather than acting as a disinfectant for endospores of *B anthracis*, may actually prolong their survival.[8]

Ammonium hydroxide, described as a weak base, under some conditions, has been shown to inactivate coccidial oocysts that are resistant to the majority of standard chemical disinfectants. Strong solutions of ammonium hydroxide emit intense pungent fumes.

Biguanides

This group of cationic compounds includes chlorhexidine, alexidine, and some polymeric forms. Biguanides are widely used as aqueous solutions for hand washing and preoperative skin preparation. Because biguanides are cationic, their activity is greatly reduced by certain soaps and other anionic compounds. The most important member of this group, chlorhexidine, is available as dihydrochloride, diacetate, and gluconate. Chlorhexidine gluconate (CHG), which is water-soluble, is the form most commonly used. It binds to the negatively charged bacterial cell wall, altering the bacterial cell osmotic equilibrium.[9] At low concentrations, this membrane-active agent inhibits membrane enzymes and promotes leakage of cellular constituents. When the concentration is increased, cytoplasmic constituents are coagulated and a bactericidal effect is observed. The optimal pH range for chlorhexidine is 5.5 to 8. Absence of toxicity is an important feature of biguanides.

Chlorhexidine has a wide antibacterial spectrum, which includes gram-positive and many gram-negative bacteria. It has limited antifungal activity. Some gram-negative bacteria such as *Proteus* species and *Pseudomonas* species may be highly resistant to this disinfectant, and, in addition, it is neither mycobactericidal nor sporicidal. Although it may be active against some enveloped viruses, the antiviral activity of chlorhexidine is variable, and it cannot be recommended as an effective antiviral disinfectant. Chlorhexidine-alcohol solutions are particularly effective as topical disinfectants: They combine the antibacterial rapidity of alcohol with the persistence of chlorhexidine at the site of application. Because it has longer residual activity on teat skin than many other disinfectants, chlorhexidine is often used in teat dips for mastitis control programs in dairy herds. The antimicrobial activity of chlorhexidine is reduced by the presence of organic matter. Because biguanides may be toxic for aquatic species, care should be taken when disposing of chlorhexidine solutions.

Gas Phase Sterilizing Agents

A number of chemical disinfectants with broad-spectrum antimicrobial activity are used for sterilizing medical devices that are heat sensitive. Ethylene oxide, formaldehyde and hydrogen peroxide (including some systems that use gas plasma as part of these processes) are among the vapor-phase disinfectant systems used for sterilizing heat-sensitive equipment. Some of these technologies are also used for area fumigation, such as hydrogen peroxide and formaldehyde.

At room temperature, EO is a colorless gas with a faint odor and an irritating effect on eyes and mucous membranes. It is soluble in water and a range of organic solvents. EO is toxic and can be flammable, and when present in the air at a concentration exceeding 3%, it forms an explosive mixture. This safety problem can be reduced by mixing EO with carbon dioxide or other suitable noninflammable gases. EO is generally not corrosive for metals and decomposes spontaneously into methane, ethane, and carbon dioxide. As an alkylating agent, EO reacts with amino, carboxyl, sulfhydryl, and hydroxyl groups, leading to denaturation of microbial proteins including enzymes and also nucleic acids. It is a highly effective antimicrobial agent with bactericidal, fungicidal, virucidal, and sporicidal activity. It does not inactivate prions. A desirable feature of the gas is its ability to penetrate a variety of materials including large packages, bundles of cloth, and certain plastics. Inactivation of microorganisms, however, takes place slowly. The antimicrobial activity of EO is influenced by relative humidity, temperature, gas concentration, contact time, and the presence of water vapor. Organic residues and salt crystals interfere with the activity of EO. Since the 1990s, EO has been listed as a mutagen and a human carcinogen, and consequently, there has been a decline in its use as a vapor-phase disinfectant. An additional concern relates to the potential risks arising from release of this alkylating agent into the environment in the immediate vicinity of establishments employing EO for low-temperature sterilization of equipment. Hydrogen peroxide gas (or vapor) processes are realistic alternatives to EO for sterilization of heat-labile equipment.

Halogens

Chlorine and iodine compounds are widely used in veterinary medicine for their antimicrobial activity. These compounds have wide antimicrobial spectra, are usually inexpensive, have low toxicity, and are convenient disinfectants in health care facilities, for agriculture buildings, food-processing units, and for veterinary facilities.

Chlorine Compounds

The antimicrobial activity of chlorine preparations is determined by the amount of available chlorine in solution. The stability of free available chlorine in solution is strongly influenced by chlorine concentration, pH, the presence of organic matter, and exposure to light. Chlorine-releasing compounds include sodium hypochlorite and *N*-chloro compounds, also referred to as organic chlorides. Chloramine-T, halazone, sodium dichloroisocyanurate, and potassium dichloroisocyanurate are examples of organic chlorine compounds. The antimicrobial activity of these compounds is reported to be slower than that of hypochlorites, but some of these organic chloride compounds are less susceptible to inactivation by organic matter than sodium hypochlorite. Chlorine dioxide, which is a gas at room temperature, is being increasingly used for chlorination of potable water, also in swimming pools and for treatment of wastewater. This gas, which is soluble in water, forming a stable solution in the dark, decomposes slowly when exposed to light. At concentrations above 10% in air, chlorine dioxide is unstable and explosive. However, it is an effective antimicrobial compound and nonflammable and not explosive at concentrations used for sterilization. Chlorine dioxide has a broad antimicrobial spectrum. It is bactericidal, fungicidal, virucidal, and sporicidal and reported to be capable of inactivating prions. The sterilizing capability of chlorine dioxide is reported to be equivalent to EO. The antimicrobial activity of chlorine and its compounds is due to the formation of hypochlorous acid, which forms when free chlorine is added to water. Hypochlorites and chloramines undergo hydrolysis when added to water, leading to the formation of hypochlorous acid. This acid releases nascent oxygen, a powerful oxidizing agent. Chlorine compounds combine directly with bacterial cytoplasmic proteins and with viral capsid proteins. Sodium hypochlorite and other chlorine compounds are most effective at pH values below 7, and their antimicrobial activity is inversely proportional to the pH of the environment in which they are used. As diluted chlorine disinfectants lose their potency, fresh solutions should be prepared for use. Hypochlorites are among the most widely used disinfectants. Sodium hypochlorite is fast acting, nonstaining, and inexpensive. Its use in veterinary medicine, however, is limited by its corrosiveness, its inactivation by organic matter, and its relative instability.

Chlorine-releasing compounds are potent virucides. Chlorination, a standard treatment for preventing the spread of waterborne infectious diseases, is generally considered a safe procedure. Household bleach, which usually contains high concentrations of sodium hypochlorite, is used at suitable dilutions in dairies, food-processing plants, and for general disinfection of equipment and farm buildings. Health risks associated with the use of chlorine compounds appear to be limited. Detection of trihalomethanes in chlorinated water has raised concerns about the safety of this form of treatment of public water supplies because trihalomethanes are reported to be carcinogenic in laboratory animals. Currently, few alternative treatment methods for rendering public water supplies safe for human consumption are available. Advantages of chlorine compounds over other disinfectants include low toxicity at effective concentrations, wide antimicrobial spectra, ease of use, and relatively low cost.

Iodine Compounds

The antimicrobial activity of iodine has been recognized since the 1830s. As halogens, iodine and chlorine share some common characteristics: both are effective antimicrobial agents. Although less chemically reactive than chlorine compounds, iodine compounds are effective antimicrobials that are more active in the presence of organic matter than chlorine compounds. The antimicrobial activity of iodine is greater at acid pH than alkaline pH.

Elemental iodine, a bluish-black crystalline substance with a metallic luster, is only slightly soluble in water. Despite its low solubility, iodine was formerly used for its antimicrobial activity as an aqueous solution. Iodine is readily soluble in ethyl alcohol and in aqueous solutions of potassium iodide and sodium iodide. When dissolved in ethyl alcohol (tincture of iodine), high levels of free iodine are obtained. Disadvantages of using iodine solutions include instability, staining of skin and fabrics, toxicity, and skin irritation. Inorganic iodine has been largely replaced by iodophors in which iodine is complexed with surface-active compounds or polymers that allow both increased solubility and sustained release of free iodine. In iodophors, the iodine is bound to a carrier of high-molecular-weight as micellar aggregates. When complexed, free iodine levels are limited and the disadvantages of using aqueous or alcoholic solutions are avoided. An iodophor in which iodine is complexed with polyvinylpyrrolidone, referred to as povidone-iodine, is a commonly used disinfectant. When an iodophor is diluted with water, dispersion of the micellar aggregates of iodine occurs leading to slow release of iodine. The amount of free iodine in iodophor solutions depends on the concentration used and, paradoxically, more concentrated solutions have less antimicrobial activity than diluted solutions. Within defined limits, as the degree of dilution increases, the bactericidal activity increases. The increased antimicrobial activity results from the higher level of free iodine in dilute solutions. For maximum antimicrobial effect, iodophor solutions should be diluted in accordance with the manufacturers' instruction. Iodophors retain much of their activity in the presence of organic matter and are effective at both low and high temperatures.

When used at appropriate dilutions and at pH values below 5, iodophors have a broad range of antimicrobial activity. They are bactericidal, fungicidal, and virucidal. It has been suggested that the amino acids tyrosine and histidine in the viral capsid are specific targets of iodine. These disinfectants are reported to react with sulfhydryl groups. Some nonenveloped viruses are less sensitive than enveloped viruses to iodophors. It has been observed that when using iodophors, prolonged contact times are required to inactivate certain fungal species and bacterial endospores. With endospores, the spore coat and cortex are the sites affected. Reports of prolonged survival of *Pseudomonas aeruginosa* and *Burkholderia cepacia* in povidone-iodine solution have been attributed to the protection of these bacteria by the presence of organic matter and inorganic material or by biofilm formation on the items being treated. Addition of alcohol improves the antimicrobial activity of iodophors. In some countries, alcoholic solutions of iodophors are widely used for disinfection of hands and sites prior to surgical procedures. Acidic iodophor solutions are used as sanitizers in the food industry. When employed as disinfectants in dairy plants, the pH of iodophors is kept acidic by the addition of phosphoric acid to ensure the removal of dried milk residues. Effective postmilking teat dipping is an important control measure for contagious mastitis in dairy cattle, and iodophors are among the common teat dips used for this purpose.

Heavy Metals and Their Derivatives

The salts of mercury, lead, zinc, silver, and copper have been used for their antimicrobial activity in farming, horticulture, and in human and veterinary medicine for many years. The ability of extremely low levels of certain metals such as copper and silver to exert a marked inhibitory effect on bacteria, algae, and fungi has been observed for centuries. The antimicrobial and antifungal activity of heavy metal derivatives such as copper salts is attributed to their ability to inhibit enzymatic activity in microbial membranes and within the cytoplasm, by binding to sulfhydryl groups. The virucidal action of copper salts is attributed to their binding to thiol groups of protein molecules and also to their strong affinity for DNA.[10] Three footbath treatment methods were evaluated for their ability to control digital dermatitis in dairy cows.[11] Formalin (5% solution), a commercial footbath product (5% solution), and copper sulfate (10% solution) were used in the study. The results indicated that the commercial product performed better than formalin, and there was no therapeutic difference between copper sulfate and the commercial product. In a Norwegian study of infectious foot diseases of dairy cattle, a number of treatment methods were evaluated.[12] Automatic stationary flushing with water alone had no beneficial effect on interdigital dermatitis or heel horn erosion. The claw horn of cows walking through a disinfectant containing 7% copper sulfate became harder, and the claw horn of cows that had their hind feet flushed with water became softer, compared with control animals. In the European Union (EU), the possible environmental impact of copper sulfate has been a cause of concern in recent years. Despite these concerns, few chemical compounds of comparable potency to copper sulfate for use in footbaths for cattle are currently available. To minimize the risks arising from the use of copper sulfate in footbaths, used solutions should be mixed with the contents of slurry tanks and subsequently dispersed widely on arable land. The algicidal activity of copper sulfate has been used to prevent algal growth on open bodies of water and pools. A number of copper compounds are used as preservatives in wood, paper, and paint industries.

Interference with sulfhydryl groups has been proposed as the likely method of interference by silver compounds with bacterial and fungal enzyme systems. Binding to nucleic acids has also been reported. Aqueous solutions of silver nitrate, which are bactericidal, have been used to prevent infection of burn wounds in human patients. The antibacterial effect of silver-releasing surgical dressings has been documented. Sand coated with silver has been used in filters for water purification, and silver-coated charcoal has been used for similar purposes. The virucidal activity of silver compounds against a range of enveloped and nonenveloped viruses has been described. Although the mode of action has not been explained, alteration of capsid proteins was proposed as the likely method of inactivation. Many published reports have confirmed the resistance of the fecal oocysts of *C parvum* to chemical disinfectants. Treatment of these oocysts with hydrogen peroxide combined with silver nitrate at a concentration of 3% completely eliminated oocyst infectivity for mice after exposure for 30 minutes.[13]

β-Propiolactone

This alkylating compound has a wide antimicrobial spectrum. It is bactericidal, fungicidal, sporicidal, and virucidal. The antimicrobial activity of β-propiolactone depends on its concentration and on relative humidity and temperature. It can be a highly effective gaseous sporicidal disinfectant. Demonstrable changes induced in viruses by β-propiolactone include structural alterations and modifications of viral capsids.[14] This compound has been widely used for the production of inactivated viral vaccines. Health hazards associated with the use of β-propiolactone include skin lesions and eye irritation following direct exposure. The suspected carcinogenic activity of β-propiolactone has limited its use as a disinfectant in veterinary medicine.

Peroxygen Compounds

Broad antimicrobial spectra, safety for personnel engaged in disinfection programs, and absence of residual toxicity are dominant considerations in the selection and use of many chemical compounds for inactivation of infectious agents in human and veterinary medicine. Oxidizing agents, which include hydrogen peroxide, peracetic acid, ozone, and a number of peroxygen-based disinfectants, are antimicrobial compounds, which fulfill many of these requirements. Their wide antimicrobial spectra, low toxicity, and spontaneous breakdown into harmless products are attractive attributes of these strongly oxidizing agents. A number of published reports, however, indicate that some peroxygen compounds including peroxymonosulfates are ineffective as mycobactericidal agents. The characteristics of individual compounds determine their usefulness as disinfectants in veterinary medicine.

Hydrogen peroxide is a clear, colorless liquid, which is commercially available in concentrations ranging from 3% to 90%. It is a nonpolluting compound that rapidly degrades into water and oxygen. Because hydrogen peroxide solutions are unstable, benzoic acid or other suitable substances are added as stabilizers. This oxidizing agent is bactericidal, fungicidal, and virucidal depending on its concentration and how it is delivered (as a liquid, liquid formulation, or gas/vapor). There is a limited number of publications dealing with the virucidal activity of hydrogen peroxide. Under some conditions, the liquid disinfectant inactivates herpes viruses and rhinoviruses but not poliovirus.[10] Virucidal and cysticidal activity have been shown with gas-based processes in particular.[15] Hydrogen peroxide is an effective sporicidal agent, and its activity is enhanced by increased concentrations and elevated temperatures. In common with some other peroxygen compounds, the activity of hydrogen peroxide can vary against mycobacteria depending on the concentration, formulation, and delivery method. The presence of catalase and peroxidases in some bacteria can increase their tolerance to low levels of hydrogen peroxide. The antimicrobial activity of hydrogen peroxide is attributable to the formation of free hydroxyl radicals, which interact with lipids, proteins, and nucleic acids.[16] Hydrogen peroxide vapor has been developed as an effective method for environmental decontamination. Two types are used: a noncondensing hydrogen peroxide vapor system and a condensing method. Both systems have proven effective against bacterial endospores and other infectious agents. The virucidal activity of a condensing hydrogen peroxide vapor system was evaluated against feline calicivirus, human adenovirus type 1, transmissible gastroenteritis, coronavirus of pigs, avian influenza virus, and swine influenza virus.[17] The system proved virucidal for all the viruses included in the trial. Of note is that gas peroxide systems have been shown to neutralize the infectivity of prions.[18] When an electromagnetic field is applied to a solution of hydrogen peroxide under appropriate conditions, the disinfectant becomes a gas plasma, a highly efficient disinfectant system with sporicidal activity. The term *accelerated hydrogen peroxide* is used to describe proprietary disinfectants containing reduced concentrations of hydrogen peroxide supplemented with compounds used in industrial cleaners such as surfactants, wetting agents, acids, and chelating agents. Disinfectants containing these compounds are reported to have a wide antimicrobial spectrum with short contact times. Undesirable features of these disinfectants include their reactions with brass, copper and aluminium, and some surgical instruments.

Peracetic acid, a colorless liquid with a pungent odor, is a strong oxidizing agent. It is miscible with water, has greater lipid solubility, and has more potent antimicrobial activity than hydrogen peroxide. This oxidizing agent decomposes into water, acetic acid, and oxygen. It is rapidly lethal for a wide range of infectious agents including bacteria and their spores, fungi, algae, and viruses. It is virucidal for a wide range of viruses including picornaviruses, adenoviruses, coxsackie viruses, and herpes viruses.[10] Even at low temperatures and in the presence of organic matter, peracetic acid is mycobactericidal and sporicidal. It oxidizes sulfhydryl and amino groups and induces structural changes in nucleic acids. Because of its wide antimicrobial spectrum, it is used as a cold sterilizing agent for thermolabile medical devices. Peracetic acid can corrode steel, copper, and other metals, and it can also damage natural and synthetic rubber. Stainless steel, glass, and plastics are generally more resistant. Therefore, the formulation of the biocide is important to consider in optimizing antimicrobial efficacy while limiting surface damage. On account of its strong antimicrobial action at low temperatures and absence of residues, peracetic acid has been widely used in food processing and beverage industries. At concentrations close to 60%, peracetic acid can be explosive at room temperature. Exposure to peracetic acid vapor has an irritating effect on the eyes and respiratory tract. More serious health care risks may possibly arise from prolonged exposure to peracetic acid because it has been implicated in tumor development in mice and has been referred to as a carcinogen.

Ozone, an allotropic form of oxygen, is a blue-colored gas at ambient temperatures with strong oxidizing properties. It is bactericidal, mycobactericidal, sporicidal, and virucidal. The primary viral changes caused by ozone appear to be structural damage to the viral capsids followed by inactivation of viral nucleic acid. The sporicidal activity of ozone is attributed to changes induced in the outer spore coat layers. Ozone is sometimes used for disinfection of the air and water, being described as having the highest oxidation potential among most chemicals used in water treatment. The inactivation of infectious prion protein by ozone has been investigated.[19] The efficacy of ozone inactivation of scrapie prion protein (PrP^{Sc}) was both pH and temperature dependent. The results were a preliminary indication that ozone was effective for prion inactivation in ozone-demand-free water; the findings suggested that ozone could be used for inactivation of infectious prion protein in prion-contaminated water and in wastewater.

Novel Developments Using Hydrogen Peroxide

Traditional systems for cleaning and disinfecting large surface areas require an experienced workforce and proper supervision to ensure thorough cleaning and effective application of disinfectant. Hydrogen peroxide vapor, a novel automated decontamination system that requires minimal human involvement, has been introduced for environmental decontamination to improve the efficacy of disinfection.[16] Other advantages of this system over alternative vapor-phase methods are low toxicity and absence of toxic residues. Two types of hydrogen peroxide vapor systems are available: a noncondensing vaporized hydrogen peroxide system and a condensing hydrogen peroxide vapor system.[17] Condensing systems require the injection of hydrogen peroxide until the air in the enclosed space becomes saturated with hydrogen peroxide and the vapor begins to condense on surfaces. Noncondensing systems dry the vapor stream as it is returned to the generator. Both systems have been evaluated using bacterial endospores and other infectious agents, and published reports confirm their effectiveness.

The virucidal efficacy of hydrogen peroxide vapor was evaluated using feline calicivirus, human adenovirus type 1, transmissible gastroenteritis coronavirus of pigs, avian influenza virus, and swine influenza virus.[17] The viruses were dried on stainless steel discs and exposed to hydrogen peroxide vapor using a condensing hydrogen peroxide vapor system. All viruses were inactivated by the hydrogen peroxide vapor, indicating the suitability of this system for decontamination of virus-contaminated surfaces.

Phenolic Compounds

More than 150 years ago, phenol was recognized as a substance with antimicrobial activity. It has the distinction of being one of the first chemicals used as an antiseptic in surgical procedures. Phenol was also the standard disinfectant with which other chemical compounds with potential antimicrobial activity were compared in a procedure known as the phenol-coefficient technique. In former times, most of the phenolic compounds used for the manufacture of disinfectants were obtained from tar, hence the use of the term *coal-tar disinfectants*. Tar itself, a by-product of the destructive distillation of coal, contains a number of products. Fractionation of tar yields phenols, organic bases, and neutral products. The temperature employed for fractionation determines the range of products produced and their biological activity. A progressive increase in desirable biological properties of coal-tar phenols is observed with increasing boiling point, but this is accompanied by decreased solubility in water. Many phenolic compounds are now synthesized. In addition to a wide range of coal-tar phenols, non-coal-tar phenols such as ortho-phenylphenol are also available. Simple and substituted phenols constitute a vast group of chemicals, but their antimicrobial activity cannot be related directly to their chemical structures. Phenolic compounds range from phenol and cresylic acid to a collection of high-boiling point tar acids. Because of differences in formulation, generalizations relating to the antimicrobial activity of particular phenolic disinfectants are not justified. The antimicrobial activity and the toxicity of individual phenolic disinfectants depend on the exact formulation and concentration of each active constituent in the preparation. By binding to amino acid residues and displacing

water molecules, phenols denature protein. Conformational changes in membrane proteins result in cytoplasmic membrane damage, leading to leakage of intracellular components. Some phenolic compounds also react with thiol groups, causing metabolic disturbance.

At recommended concentrations, phenolic compounds are typically bactericidal, fungicidal, and virucidal. Ortho-phenylphenol and some coal-tar fractions are particularly effective against mycobacteria, but bisphenols are not mycobactericidal. When halogenated, phenols and cresols have antifungal activity. As a group, phenolic compounds are not sporicidal, and their effectiveness against viruses is formulation dependent. They are usually effective against enveloped viruses, but their activity against nonenveloped viruses may be unpredictable. Due to the great diversity of phenolic compounds available and the wide variation in their formulations, this group of disinfectants cannot be recommended as reliable virucidal agents.

Phenolic compounds are usually moderately priced and not seriously inhibited by the presence of organic matter. Contact with the skin should be avoided because of the irritation and depigmentation produced by some of these compounds. As cats and pigs are particularly susceptible to the toxic effects of phenolic disinfectants, all treated surfaces should be thoroughly rinsed before the reintroduction of animals. Phenolic compounds often impart a tarry odor and leave a residual film on surfaces, which can cause tainting of food and agricultural products. Accordingly, these disinfectants should not be used in meat plants, dairies, or food storage areas. They are unsuitable for disinfecting surfaces or containers that come into direct contact with food for human consumption. Disinfectant solutions containing phenolic compounds are potentially toxic for workers, domestic animals, wildlife, and aquatic species. In circumstances where substantial amounts of these disinfectants are used in farm buildings, runoff should not be discharged directly into ponds, lakes, or streams. Fluid containing phenolic compounds should be collected in slurry tanks or other suitable holding areas and spread on arable land remote from watercourses.

Quaternary Ammonium Compounds

The QACs are cationic and have surface-active properties, but they are incompatible with a wide range of chemical agents including organic matter and anionic detergents. They are most effective at neutral or slightly alkaline pH values, depending on the specific compound. These disinfectants are reported to exert their antimicrobial action by reacting with anionic lipids in the cytoplasmic membrane and with the outer membrane of gram-negative bacteria. Reactions with lipid and protein components of the cytoplasmic membrane lead to its disruption, inactivation of associated enzymes, and denaturation of cell proteins. Succeeding generations of QACs, each reported to have improved antimicrobial qualities, have become available.[20] Currently, the seventh generation of these cationic disinfectants, composed of bis-quaternary ammonium chlorides and polymeric ammonium chlorides, is available with claims of enhanced efficacy and less toxicity. Because of changes that have occurred in successive generations of QACs, objective comments on the antimicrobial spectra, efficacy, and toxicity of current formulations are difficult to determine from independent sources. Assertions in promotional literature that these disinfectants offer broad-spectrum efficacy require experimental confirmation and claims of absence of toxicity for these new generation compounds are often not supported by recent published information.[21]

Reports on earlier generations of QACs as a group indicated a limited antimicrobial spectrum with greater activity against gram-positive than gram-negative bacteria. Some gram-negative bacteria such as *Pseudomonas* species and *Serratia marcescens* survived and even grew in certain disinfectant formulations. These cationic compounds were neither sporicidal nor mycobactericidal. Although some of these compounds had activity against enveloped viruses, nonenveloped viruses were resistant and, consequently, they could not be recommended as reliable virucides.

Earlier generations of these cationic compounds were inactivated by soaps, detergents, proteins, organic matter, and fibrous material. Newer generations are reported to be less affected by organic matter and anionic compounds. In comparison to other disinfectants, QACs are moderately expensive.

Because they are nonstaining, odorless, and usually noncorrosive, these disinfectants are used extensively in food processing industries. They are also used for disinfecting farming equipment and have been included in sheep dips for controlling microorganisms associated with fleece problems. They are often used for combined cleaning and disinfecting applications, due to their detergent nature.

Although generally described as nontoxic disinfectants, some species of animals are sensitive to low levels of QACs. Turkeys are reported to be sensitive to these cationic compounds, and exposure to low levels of these disinfectants has resulted in high mortality in turkeys. Because these chemical disinfectants are toxic for fish, they should not be discharged into rivers, streams, ponds, or lakes. Decreased reproductive performance in laboratory mice coincided with the introduction of a disinfectant containing both alkyl dimethyl benzyl ammonium chloride and didecyl dimethyl ammonium chloride.[21] The QACs were detected in caging material over a period of several months following discontinuation of disinfectant use. Breeding pairs exposed for 6 months to this disinfectant exhibited decreases in fertility and fecundity, increased time to first litter, longer pregnancy intervals, fewer offspring per litter, and fewer pregnancies. In addition, there was a significant increase in morbidity in near-term dams. The results of these experiments indicated that exposure to a common QAC mixture significantly impaired reproductive health in mice.

Products containing QACs are widely used in health care institutions, in domestic activities, and for a number of industrial products. The presence of these chemicals in wastewater and their accumulation in sludge and sediment has been reported in many countries.[22] The toxicity of these compounds for many aquatic species combined with their documented toxicity for some avian and mammalian species calls for a greater awareness on the part of health professionals, the agricultural community, and others using these chemicals, of their undesirable environmental impact if discharged into wastewater.

Recent Developments That Have Improved Disinfection Choice and Efficacy

Formerly, disinfection in veterinary medicine relied on individual chemical compounds for the planning and implementation of disinfection programs. Companies engaged in the provision of disinfection services selected particular chemical compounds that were best suited for the prevailing conditions on the farm or the clinical facility being serviced. In recent years, pharmaceutical companies engaged in the manufacture of chemical disinfectants have embarked on the provision of combinations of chemical disinfectants rather than individual compounds. Many of these recently developed chemical combinations have been in response to the need for disinfectants effective against resistant pathogenic microorganisms such as the fecal oocysts of pathogenic protozoa or for the inactivation of prions. In addition to a wider choice of chemical compounds, novel developments for decontamination of surfaces such as hydrogen peroxide vapor and the introduction of gas plasma for sterilization have become available for inactivation of infectious agents. These developments have expanded the choice of chemical disinfectant available for the veterinary profession and for the farming community. Improvements in physical methods for surface decontamination with chemical compounds have increased the reliability of disinfection at farm level and in veterinary establishments. Finally, improvements in formulation technology based around the development of unique mixtures of chemicals are resulting in improved product performance.

▶ PRACTICAL ASPECTS OF DISINFECTION

Environment of Domestic Animals

The immediate environment of farm animals can have a positive or negative influence on their health status. Farm buildings, farmyards, paddocks, and other grazing areas can be designed to promote animal health. Conversely, improper building design, inadequate ventilation, and insufficient floor space for the animal population can predispose to stressful environmental conditions for intensively reared animals. Apart from farm buildings, animals, especially young animals, may acquire infectious agents from their immediate environment at pasture. Dusty paddocks and heavily grazed pastures can lead to a buildup of *Rhodococcus equi*, which can cause suppurative bronchopneumonia in foals up to 4 months of age. Rough pastures offer cover for many tick species such as *Ixodes ricinus*. The acquisition of tick-borne diseases such as louping ill and tick-borne fever is usually associated with animals grazing rough pasture.

Cleaning of Farm Buildings

In farm buildings, the survival time of many infectious agents outside the host is extended by the presence of organic material. Removal of all forms of organic matter—feces, urine, exudates, blood, bedding, food, and dust—is essential before disinfection proceeds. If carried out in a competent manner, cleaning alone can substantially reduce the number of actual or potential pathogens in a building, thereby decreasing the risk of a heavy challenge to animals in that environment. It has been estimated that cleaning alone may remove over 90% of bacteria from some surfaces.[23]

Organic matter in the form of dried feces or exudates may shield pathogenic microorganisms from direct contact with disinfectants. In addition, the antimicrobial activity of many disinfectants especially halogens and also some QACs is adversely affected by the presence of organic material. With the exception of buildings that have housed animals with major zoonotic diseases such as anthrax, effective cleaning should always precede disinfection. Particular care is required when personnel carrying out cleaning and disinfection are entering premises contaminated with suspected exotic pathogens or where notifiable diseases have been confirmed. All personnel should wear protective clothing and rubber boots and, where necessary, gloves, face masks, goggles, and headwear.

When routine cleaning is being carried out, personnel should be made aware of the importance of removing all traces of organic material before disinfection commences. Cleaning should begin with the removal of all gross organic matter, including bedding, feces, feed, and dust, immediately after removal of animals. Equipment which can be removed should be brushed and soaked in detergent prior to disinfection. The organic matter removed from the building may be composted, burned, or buried, depending on the level of risk and disease status of the unit. Brushing, scraping, and sweeping form part of dry cleaning, which is followed by wet cleaning. Soaking before washing requires a reliable water supply and suitable equipment. If the water source for soaking and cleaning is from an adjacent river, pond, or well, it may be necessary to confirm its freedom from high levels of pathogenic microorganisms or toxic substances. Electrical equipment used for power hosing should be well maintained and fitted with fuses of appropriate ratings. If electrical appliances installed in the building cannot be conveniently removed, they should be covered with waterproof material and cleaned and disinfected manually at a later stage. Before washing commences, the electricity supply to the building should be disconnected and an alternative supply from an adjacent building should be used to supply power for electrical equipment used for washing. Cables carrying electrical power for washing equipment should be fitted with earth leakage circuit breakers. The building and its contents should be soaked for up to 3 hours before washing commences. Pressure washing should begin at surfaces at higher levels and move down to the walls and floor. Care should be taken to adjust the pressure of the equipment to avoid aerosol generation with the risk of spreading pathogens to surfaces already cleaned. Good lighting is required to ensure that surfaces are visibly clean. Hot water with cleaning agents such as sodium carbonate or trisodium phosphate can facilitate removal of caked material and grease.

Footbaths

Microbial pathogens shed in feces or urine can be transferred on contaminated footwear to many different locations on a farm including buildings and transport vehicles. If placed in appropriate locations and maintained properly, footbaths can limit the risk of pathogen transfer on footwear of farm workers or farm visitors. Unless all personnel visiting the farm or working on the farm wear waterproof footwear and use footbaths, this method of preventing transmission of infectious agents will not be successful. Suggested dimensions for a footbath are indicated in Figure 52.9. Disinfectants suitable for footbath use include phenols, iodophors, and particularly surface-active compounds, such as fifth-generation QACs, potassium peroxymonosulfate, and occasionally formalin. If a specific infectious agent is identified as the cause of an outbreak of disease, a disinfectant known to be effective against that agent should be used in all footbaths on the farm.

Disinfectants in footbaths should be changed frequently, and the date of change should be displayed on the container. A designated member of staff who has an understanding of the preparation of accurate dilutions should be assigned to footbath maintenance. If used constantly on a large farm or unit, the disinfectant should be changed daily or more frequently if there is evidence of gross contamination. On smaller farms, replacement of disinfectant at intervals of 3 days may be adequate. If gross soiling of footwear is unavoidable, a second footbath with diluted

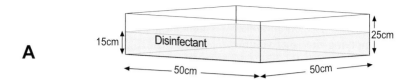

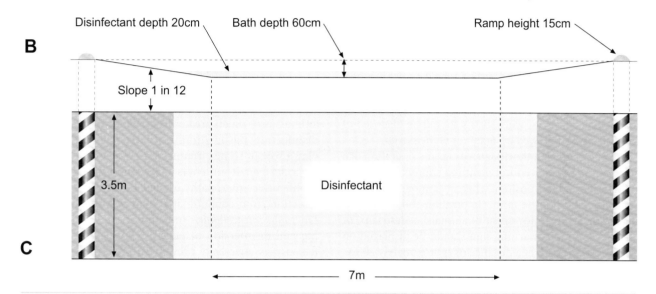

FIGURE 52.9 Suggested dimensions for a footbath (A) for personnel. On premises where footbaths are used, waterproof footwear should be mandatory for all staff and visitors. Elevation (B) and plan (C) for a wheel bath, with suggested dimensions. The design of a wheel bath should ensure immersion of the entire wheel surface in disinfectant.

detergent and a brush should be placed alongside the footbath with disinfectant for washing footwear before immersion in disinfectant.

Brief immersion of footwear in a footbath cannot be considered satisfactory as a disease control measure. Immersion of clean footwear to a depth of 15 cm in an effective disinfectant for at least 1 minute is a minimum requirement. Footbaths, located at suitable entry points to a farm or building, should be protected from flooding by surface water or rainfall. Antifreeze compatible with the disinfectant may be added in frosty weather. Alternatively, footbaths may be moved indoors close to entry points to avoid freezing.

Wheel Baths

Vehicles that visit a number of farms in succession may be considered as creating a potential risk of transferring infectious agents on the body of the vehicle or on its wheels. Consequently, wheel baths are sometimes installed at farm entrances as part of a disease control program.

The design, construction, and use of wheel baths should ensure that there is adequate contact with disinfectant for a sufficient time to ensure destruction of infectious agents on the surface of the wheels. The site for construction of a wheel bath should be carefully selected to minimize the risk of flooding, contamination by surface water, or subsidence. In countries with severe freezing conditions during winter months, wheel baths may be inoperable at freezing temperatures. A plan and elevation for a wheel bath with suggested dimensions is shown in Figure 52.9. The dimensions of the bath should ensure accommodation of the largest vehicles entering the farm. The tyres of the largest wheel entering the bath should be completely immersed in disinfectant in one complete revolution. Wheel baths should be built to high specifications, should be waterproof, and free from structural defects. Valves or openings that might allow accidental pollution of watercourses should not form part of the design. The capacity of the bath should allow for heavy rainfall without the risk of disinfectant overflow. A depth gauge could be incorporated into the design to indicate dilution or evaporation of disinfectant.

In addition to the cost of construction of a wheel bath, there are additional associated expenses. A vacuum tanker (slurry tanker) for filling and emptying the large volume of disinfectant is essential. For the wheel bath shown in Figure 52.9, a volume of approximately 6600 L of diluted disinfectant is required. The type of disinfectant selected and the interval between changing require careful consideration. Iodophor disinfectants are relatively stable with a broad antimicrobial spectrum and are more environmentally safe than phenolic disinfectants and more stable than hypochlorite based compounds. Particular surface-active compounds such as fifth-generation QACs are reported to exert improved antimicrobial activity over those formerly used, and these compounds may be suitable for use in wheel baths. If wheels have caked organic matter or grease on their surfaces, a wheel bath exerts minimal antimicrobial activity. Used disinfectant from wheel baths should be disposed of into slurry tanks followed by agitation of the slurry.

In some countries, the design, siting, and operation of a wheel bath may require local planning approval. The bath should be located in a position where it cannot be bypassed by vehicles entering the farm. Its position should not interfere with the free movement of animals, pedestrians, or cyclists. A luminous warning sign should be displayed on either side of the bath at a distance of approximately 20 m.

Compared with other possible sources of infectious agents, wheels of vehicles are unlikely to feature in disease transmission. Vehicles used for transporting animals, however, require special consideration. The contents of such vehicles, including animals and their secretions and excretions, animal feed, clothing and footwear of drivers and their assistants, pose a much greater threat to healthy animals than the vehicle's wheels. Installation and maintenance of a wheel bath is an expensive undertaking, which may impart a false sense of security to those involved in the transportation of animals and to those visiting the premises. The possible contribution of wheel baths to disease control measures is difficult to assess and must be balanced against the high initial expenditure associated with their construction and routine maintenance costs.

▶ THE ROLE OF DISINFECTION IN CONTROL OF BACTERIAL DISEASE IN ANIMALS

The importance of environmental contamination and indirect transmission of an infectious agent differs depending on the bacterium, environmental conditions, and the physiologic status of the host. As a result, the importance of the role of cleaning and disinfection in control of bacterial disease will vary depending on the disease in question and it is essential to understand this when designing a disease control program. *Salmonella* serotypes may persist for many months in the environment,[24] but Hill et al[25] found that cleaning and disinfection practices have little impact on *Salmonella* prevalence in finishing pigs if any of the pigs entering cleaned pens are high or "super" shedders of salmonella. In such situations, the authors suggest that separation of pigs with strict adherence to an all-in, all-out policy is of much greater importance than adherence to good cleaning practices. However, correct use of footbaths and other internal biosecurity practices have a role in such segregation.

M bovis is a resistant organism that can survive for long periods in the environment. However, acquisition of infection by the oral route from a contaminated environment in the case of tuberculosis in cattle requires significantly higher numbers of organisms than when infection occurs through aerosol infection, and the latter is considered the most important route of natural infection.[26,27] Thus, control of *M bovis* infection in cattle by removal of infected animals is of much greater importance than cleaning and disinfecting the environment, although the latter may play a role in some circumstances. In contrast, maintaining a clean environment is highly important in controlling proliferative enteropathy of pigs. Indirect transmission of infection from contaminated pens was demonstrated for *Lawsonia intracellularis* infection in pigs, whereas cleaning and disinfection of pens previously occupied by infected pigs effectively prevented further transmission to subsequent batches of pigs.[28] Recurrence of anthrax after many years of absence in a region may be due to survival of *B anthracis* endospores in the environment and confirms the importance of destruction of such endospores in control of this disease. Although hygiene and inactivation of bacterial pathogens is an important part of control of bacterial disease in animals, they are only one aspect of disease prevention, and their limitations must be recognized. The efficacy of individual compounds against bacteria, bacterial endospores, and *C burnetii* is summarized in Table 52.4.

Bacterial Endospores

Bacterial endospores are much more resistant to adverse environmental conditions, heat, and chemical disinfectants than their corresponding vegetative cells. The ability of certain bacteria such as clostridia and *B anthracis* to form spores confers on them unique attributes such as prolonged survival under adverse conditions and resistance to chemical disinfectants. Thermal resistance is a common characteristic of many endospores, and temperatures exceeding 100°C are usually required for their inactivation. Although disinfectants such as alcohols, biguanides, phenols, and QACs may be sporostatic, they are not sporicidal.

Diseases of animals caused by spore-forming bacteria are of considerable importance. Clostridia, a group of anaerobic, spore-forming bacteria whose habitat is soil, cause many fatal diseases in animals such as tetanus,

TABLE 52.4 A guide to the typical antibacterial spectrum of chemical disinfectants[a]

Disinfectant Class[b]	Gram-positive	Gram-negative	Mycobacteria	Endospores	Coxiella burnetii
Acids (mineral)	++	+	−	±[c]	ND
Alcohols	++	++	++	−	++
Aldehydes	++	++	+	++	+[d]
Alkalis	++	++	+	+	
Biguanides	++	+	−	−	+
Halogens					
Chlorine compounds	++	++	+	+	+
Iodine compounds	++	++	+	+	ND
Peroxygen compounds					
Hydrogen peroxide	++	++	±	+[d]	+[d]
Peracetic acid	++	++	+[e]	++	+[f]
Phenol[g]	++	++	+	−	+
QACs	++	+	±[h]	−	+[i]

Abbreviations: ++, highly effective; +, effective; ±, limited activity; −, no activity; ND, no data; QACs, quaternary ammonium compounds.

[a]This can vary depending on the product formulation, label claims, application conditions, and other factors. Based on the following sources: Bocian et al,[29] Boothe,[30] Bruins and Dyer,[31] Dagher et al,[32] de Jong,[33] Elkholy et al,[34] Holton et al,[35] Jeffrey,[36] Lemarié and Hosgood,[37] Malloch and Stoker,[38] McDonnell and Russell,[39] Russell,[40] Russell et al,[41] Scott and Williams,[42] and Widmer and Frei.[43]

[b]The activity of complex disinfectants may vary in accordance with their formulation and the data presented relate to use under ideal conditions.

[c]Hydrochloric acid is sporicidal under some conditions.

[d]High concentrations required.

[e]Efficacy is dependent on formulation of the product, with some products being highly effective.

[f]A peroxymonosulfate-based product was effective in the presence of high soiling in a Dutch study.[33]

[g]Individual phenolic compounds may vary in their antimicrobial spectrum.

[h]A novel QAC-based compound had limited activity against some mycobacterial species.[29,34]

[i]Some QACs are reported to be effective.

botulism, colitis, and malignant edema. Because of their widespread distribution in soil and the sporadic nature of the diseases that clostridia cause, vaccination rather than disinfection is the preferred method for the prevention of clostridial diseases in animals. However, cleaning and disinfection to reduce environmental contamination with endospores has a role in the control of *Clostridium difficile* infections in equine hospitals.[44]

Bacillus anthracis

B anthracis produces endospores of high resistance, and serious environmental contamination may follow if the carcass of an animal that died of anthrax is inadvertently subjected to postmortem examination.

Methods for the control of anthrax including disinfection methods and strategies for decontamination of the environment following outbreaks of anthrax in domestic animals and wildlife are reviewed in the World Health Organization (WHO) document on anthrax in animals and humans.[45] Animals acquire infection from spores in the environment, and although much is still unknown about the epidemiology of disease including the dose required to initiate infection, removal or inactivation of spores in the environment is an essential part of control and prevention of disease in animals. Vegetative bacteria within the carcasses of animals that have died from anthrax do not survive putrefaction within days, but spores that form in serosanguineous discharges from the carcass can remain viable for many decades. The preferred method of carcass disposal is by incineration, and different methods are described in the annexes to the WHO document.[45] Where incineration is not possible, decontamination has been described using formalin.

Gruinard Island, off the northwest coast of Scotland, was heavily contaminated with the endospores of *B anthracis* during biological weapons trials in 1942 and 1943. Forty years later, after an extensive survey that revealed that contamination was confined to the top 8 cm of soil, decontamination of the island was planned.[46] A solution of 5% formaldehyde in seawater, applied by surface spraying, was shown to be the most effective disinfection procedure. Large-scale decontamination of affected areas of the island was carried out. Isolated pockets of surviving endospores, which were located after extensive sampling, received further treatment with formaldehyde solution. A flock of 40 Cheviot sheep were placed on the island and allowed to graze there for 5 months. No cases of anthrax occurred in the sheep flock placed on the island after decontamination of the soil with formaldehyde.

Guidelines issued by the WHO for dealing with carcasses of animals that have died from anthrax recommend treatment of carcasses and the environment with 10% formalin, including mixing with undiluted formalin to a final concentration of 10% for decontamination of slurry.[45] For full efficacy of formalin solutions, the temperature should be at least 15°C. Previously, lime (calcium oxide) was recommended for use as a disinfectant for control of anthrax, but, because calcium is an important constituent of the spore coat and has been shown to play an essential role in its resistance, use of lime may, in fact, be contraindicated.[8,45] Other disinfectants with sporicidal activity include alkaline glutaraldehyde, hydrogen peroxide, and peracetic acid. Hypochlorites are also sporicidal but are rapidly inactivated by organic matter and are therefore of limited value in agricultural settings.

The sporicidal effect of peracetic acid on endospores of *B anthracis* in soil was investigated by Hussaini and Ruby.[47] Treatment with 3% peracetic acid for 10 minutes at 4°C proved effective. The efficacy of a chlorine-releasing compound, peracetic acid, formaldehyde, glutaraldehyde, and other disinfectants against the endospores of *B anthracis* was studied by Lensing and Oei.[48] The chlorine-releasing compound (2400 ppm available chlorine) and 0.25% peracetic acid had a significant sporicidal effect after 30 minutes at 20°C in the presence of 4% horse serum. Formaldehyde at a 4% concentration and 2% glutaraldehyde were sporicidal after 2 hours under the same test conditions.

An additional factor that should be considered when testing the sporicidal effect of disinfectants and highlighted by March et al[49] is the effect of heat shock. Exposure of spores to a high temperature (80°C for 20 minutes) after disinfection may aid the revival of injured spores. Testing for the effect of heat shock should be carried out to ensure the efficacy of a disinfectant is accurately determined and not overestimated. March et al[49] demonstrated a significant interaction between the effect of heat shock, disinfectant product, and spore-producing bacterial species. These results clearly showed that the effects of a particular product on the spores of one species may not be easily extrapolated to another bacterial species; each species should be tested independently.

Mycobacteria

Tuberculosis is still a major disease in humans and animals, especially in developing countries. Before the introduction of programs for the elimination of *M bovis* infection in cattle, zoonotic infection with this pathogen was a common cause of tuberculosis in humans. Milk pasteurization and tuberculin testing have led to a progressive decrease in human disease acquired from cattle in many developed countries. In developing countries, however, inadequate monitoring of tuberculosis in cattle and the absence of control measures expose human populations to constant sources of infection in milk from tuberculous animals and from occupational exposure to aerosols containing *M bovis*.[50] The proportion of tuberculosis cases in humans attributable to *M bovis* was estimated at 1.4% in the United States, 17% in Ethiopia, and 28% in Mexico among certain population subgroups.[51] Mycobacteria shed by infected animals have the ability to survive for long periods in the environment, particularly in dark or shaded locations such as poorly maintained and infrequently cleaned buildings, sales yards, or transport vehicles. Survival times differ depending on soil conditions and temperature, with low temperatures apparently favoring survival.[52] Mycobacteria, a diverse group of acid-fast bacteria, are, in general, more resistant to chemical disinfection than other vegetative bacteria. Heat is one of the most effective methods of inactivating mycobacteria. The resistance of mycobacteria to chemical disinfectants, which is considered intermediate between those of vegetative bacteria and endospores, is attributed to the unusually high lipid content of their cell wall, which renders them highly hydrophobic.[53] As a consequence, hydrophilic antibacterial agents are unable to penetrate the cell wall in sufficiently high concentrations to exert a deleterious effect and, accordingly, comparatively few chemical compounds are mycobactericidal. In addition, variation in the resistance pattern of some mycobacterial strains has been observed. Although the activity of chemical disinfectants against *Mycobacterium tuberculosis* has been actively investigated,[54-57] only a limited number of reports relating to the chemical inactivation of *M bovis* have been published. Standardization of mycobactericidal testing of disinfectants has proved difficult, and a number of modifications to established procedures have been proposed.[56,58-60] Factors influencing antimycobacterial activity of disinfectants, mechanisms of mycobacterial inactivation by biocides, and mycobacterial resistance to disinfectants[61] have been comprehensively reviewed by Russell[53] and McDonnell.[62]

There are few recent studies examining the efficacy of disinfectants against *M bovis* specifically, with most recent publications reporting research investigating inactivation of nontuberculous mycobacteria (NTM) by both standard disinfectant agents and novel products in human hospital and environmental settings. The importance of NTM is increasing because of the growing numbers of immuno-compromised human patients, although disease also occurs in immunocompetent people.[63] Increasing numbers of immunosuppressed small animal patients are treated in companion animal practice also.[64] In addition, occasional cases of *M bovis* infection in dogs and cats, including nosocomial infections, are reported.[65,66] Control programs for *M bovis* in cattle rely principally on detection and removal of infected cattle and reservoir hosts, but farmers also implement measures relating to biosecurity including cleaning and disinfection.[67,68] Thus, inactivation of mycobacteria remains an important consideration in veterinary medicine. Statutory bodies responsible for the control of mycobacterial infection in farm animals in many countries publish lists of approved disinfectants for use during outbreaks of disease, including tuberculosis (eg, Department for Environment, Food and Rural Affairs[69]).

The most effective disinfectants against mycobacteria include aldehyde, phenolic, and peracetic acid-based preparations, although efficacy can differ depending on the species of *Mycobacterium* in question. The mycobactericidal activity of phenol and a phenolic disinfectant containing ortho-phenylphenol was tested against five strains of *M bovis* suspended in cows' milk.[70] The phenolic disinfectant at a 1:8 dilution and phenol diluted 1:32 killed each of the five strains of *M bovis* after exposure for 6 hours at 23°C.

Ten formulations that included 5% phenol, sodium hypochlorite at two concentrations (10 000 and 6000 ppm available chlorine), sodium dichloroisocyanurate (6000 ppm), 70% ethyl alcohol, a QAC (0.04% dimethylbenzylammonium chloride), two iodophors (1% titratable iodine and 0.008% titratable iodine), CHG (4%), and a number of glutaraldehyde-based disinfectants at a 2% concentration were tested for their mycobactericidal activities against *M tuberculosis* using a minimum contact time of 1 minute in suspension tests and carrier tests with sputum added as organic matter.[71] The QAC, CHG, and the iodophor (with 0.008% titratable iodine) were ineffective in all tests. Ethyl alcohol at a 70% concentration was effective against *M tuberculosis* only in suspension tests and in the absence of sputum. Povidone-iodine (1% titratable iodine) was less effective against mycobacteria dried on surfaces than in suspension, and its activity was further reduced by the presence of sputum. A higher concentration of available chlorine in sodium hypochlorite than in sodium dichloroisocyanurate was required to achieve an effective level of disinfection against *M tuberculosis*. Phenol, at a 5% concentration, was effective under all test conditions. The glutaraldehyde-based disinfectants, which were tested at contact times of 10 and 30 minutes, were mycobactericidal even in the presence of dried sputum.

Fourteen disinfectants, including glutaraldehyde, halogens, hydrogen peroxide, ethyl alcohol, a phenolic formulation, and QACs, were tested for their mycobactericidal activity.[72] Three disinfectants, chlorine dioxide, 0.8% hydrogen peroxide plus 0.06% peracetic acid, and an iodophor completely inactivated both *M tuberculosis* and *M bovis*. Alkaline glutaraldehyde at a 2% concentration, a phenolic compound, and a chlorine disinfectant were highly effective against *M tuberculosis* but less effective against *M bovis*. Hydrogen peroxide at a concentration of 6% appeared to be highly effective against *M bovis* but ineffective against *M tuberculosis*. Conversely, 70% ethyl alcohol was mycobactericidal for *M tuberculosis* but ineffective for *M bovis*. The unexpected findings with 6% hydrogen peroxide and 70% ethyl alcohol are inconsistent with other published reports, yet the authors offered no explanation for these surprising results.

The effects of a range of biocides that included QACs, a phenolic disinfectant (chlorocresol), esters of para-4-hydroxybenzoic acid, chlorhexidine diacetate, and glutaraldehyde on the growth and viability of *M tuberculosis*, *M bovis*, *Mycobacterium avium-intracellulare*, *Mycobacterium fortuitum*, and *Mycobacterium phlei* were studied by Broadley et al.[73] The *M phlei* was the most sensitive of the test strains, and the strain of *M avium-intracellulare* was the most resistant. Chlorhexidine diacetate, QACs, the phenolic disinfectant, and esters of para-4-hydroxybenzoic acid were inhibitory but not lethal for *M avium-intracellulare*, whereas glutaraldehyde at a 2% concentration was mycobactericidal for all strains. A peroxygen-based disinfectant (Virkon®), at concentrations of 2%, 3%, and 4%, was tested against *M tuberculosis* and *M avium-intracellulare* using contact times of 30 to 120 minutes.[74] No reduction in the numbers of viable *M tuberculosis* was evident after treatment with a 4% concentration for 60 minutes, and this disinfectant did not exhibit a satisfactory mycobactericidal activity even after a contact time of 2 hours.

The feasibility of a combined carrier test for disinfectants using a mixture of five types of organisms, including *M bovis* bacillus Calmette-Guerin (BCG), was investigated by Best et al.[75] Contact times ranging from 1 minute to 3 hours were used. Of 11 products tested, 2% alkaline glutaraldehyde, 0.6% sodium hypochlorite, 0.4% of a QAC containing 23% hydrochloric acid, 70% ethyl alcohol, and povidone-iodine (1% available iodine) were effective against *M bovis*. A 3% solution of peroxygen compounds, 1.5% CHG, 0.06% QAC, a 0.03% phenolic compound, and 3% hydrogen peroxide were not mycobactericidal.

Treatment of fresh clinical isolates of *M tuberculosis* and *M avium-intracellulare* in the presence or absence of organic matter, with 2% glutaraldehyde, 6% QAC, 0.2% peracetic acid, and 5% organic beta-ene for up to 60 minutes inactivated both mycobacterial species.[55] Although all the disinfectants had comparable mycobactericidal activity, *M avium-intracellulare* appeared to be more resistant to short-term chemical disinfection than *M tuberculosis*.

An iodine-containing compound (0.034% iodine) was less effective, allowing some survival of mycobacteria. A beta-ene compound at a concentration of 5% and a peroxygen disinfectant (Virkon®) at a 1% concentration totally lacked mycobactericidal activity.

The mycobactericidal activity of a disinfectant containing acetic acid, peracetic acid, and hydrogen peroxide (Nu-Cidex®) against *M tuberculosis*, *M bovis*, and *Mycobacterium avium* after contact times of 5, 10, 30, and 60 minutes was investigated by Holton et al.[35] This disinfectant was rapidly mycobactericidal even against drug-resistant isolates of *M tuberculosis* in both suspension tests and surface tests. No survival of mycobacteria was detected after exposure for 5 minutes. A newer formulation of peracetic acid is now available, which involves the synthesis of peracetic acid through reaction of tetraacetylethylenediamine (TAED) and a peroxy compound such as perborate, percarbonate, or persulfate. This method yields "Bioxy" compounds that are solid rather than liquid and have several advantages because they are stable in storage, are safe to handle, and odorless.[32] A 5% aqueous solution of Bioxy reduced *M bovis* levels by 3.93 log within 10 minutes.[32]

The activity of three disinfectants, 2% alkaline glutaraldehyde, a QAC containing 15.3% isopropyl alcohol, and 0.55% sodium hypochlorite solution, against five *M bovis* BCG suspensions was evaluated.[76] A 20-minute exposure time was required to achieve a 6 log reduction with 2% glutaraldehyde. The QAC achieved a 6 log reduction in less than 20 minutes, whereas the sodium hypochlorite solution required more than 4 hours to achieve the same reduction. Culture variability among the five *M bovis* suspensions contributed to the wide variation observed with individual disinfectants, especially with the hypochlorite solution.

Glutaraldehyde and ortho-phthalaldehyde disinfectants are frequently used for inactivation of NTM, although De Groote et al[77] reported resistance of some clinical isolates of *Mycobacterium abscessus* subsp *abscessus* to these compounds. The presence of NTM, specifically *M avium*, in water systems is also of increasing concern in both hospital and community settings.[78] *M avium* is considered a natural inhabitant of drinking water and plumbing systems, and its resistance to disinfectants is compounded by its ability to form biofilm, survive the warm temperatures in hot water systems, and grow in amoebas. Hsu et al[79] found that installation of a chlorine dioxide disinfection unit in a hospital water system reduced NTM in both hot and cold water systems.

Brucella abortus

Brucellae, obligate intracellular pathogens of animals and humans, can survive for long intervals in the environment. They usually enter the host through the alimentary tract, conjunctival mucosa, respiratory tract, or skin, and,

although many species of animals are susceptible to these bacteria, individual *Brucella* species exhibit host preference.[80] Among non–spore-forming bacteria, brucellae are unique in their resistance to environmental conditions.

The survival of *Brucella abortus* outside the host has been investigated by many workers. Dried fetal membranes of cattle retained infectivity for 120 days, and, in moist soil, culture suspensions remained viable for 66 days.[81] In liquid manure, *B abortus*, shed by cattle that had aborted, survived for at least 8 months in high numbers.[82] Infected animals shed extremely high numbers of organisms in aborted fetuses and associated fluids, of the order of 10^9 or 10^{10} colony-forming units (CFUs)/g of fluid. Thus, isolation of aborting animals and cleaning and disinfection of premises are important components of disease control measures.

Brucellae are susceptible to most commonly used disinfectants,[83] but activity is reduced in the presence of organic matter.[84] CHG gave a 5 log reduction in *B abortus* numbers in 60 seconds at room temperature.[85] The initial concentration of organisms was not specified, and no organic matter was added to the test system. The *in vitro* activity of povidone-iodine against *B abortus* (strain 19) was evaluated by Mansi and Lakin.[86] The brucellae were killed within 30 seconds by the iodophor at full strength or diluted 1/10 and within 2 minutes by a 1/25 dilution.

When cattle slurry containing *B abortus* was treated with 0.1% xylene, brucellae were recovered from the slurry at 14 days but not at 21 days.[87] However, the recommendations of the WHO are that if xylene is added to, for example, liquid slurry, to increase destruction of brucellae, material should be stored for at least 6 months before it can be considered safe for disposal.[88] Seven disinfectants, which included representatives of phenolic, halogen, QACs, and aldehyde compounds, were evaluated for their activity against high concentrations of *B abortus* in the presence and absence of organic matter.[84] At 1% and 0.5% concentrations, these disinfectants performed well in the absence of organic matter. The addition of organic matter, in the form of bovine serum, had a marked inhibitory effect on the bactericidal activity of most of the disinfectants apart from 1% formalin, which proved consistently reliable in the presence of organic matter.

▶ THE ROLE OF DISINFECTION IN CONTROL OF FUNGAL DISEASE IN ANIMALS

Diseases caused by pathogenic fungi can be conveniently categorized according to the sites of fungal lesions as superficial mycoses, subcutaneous mycoses, and systemic mycoses. In superficial mycoses, lesions are confined to the epidermis, other keratinized structures, and mucous membranes. Subcutaneous mycoses are confined to subcutaneous tissues, whereas systemic mycoses affect the respiratory and digestive tracts and sometimes other organ systems. Fungal species associated with infections in humans and animals represent a number of very different groups in the kingdom Fungi. Despite this diversity, fungi share many common features, especially in the structure of their cell walls. Currently, there is limited published information on the basis for the susceptibility or resistance of fungal pathogens to chemical disinfectants.

Many fungal species, some of which are zoonotic, cause disease in domestic animals. Infection with *Microsporum canis*, an important pathogen of dogs and cats, can result in extensive environmental contamination. A number of dimorphic fungi such as *Histoplasma capsulatum* and *Sporothrix schenckii* are associated with disease in animals and humans. In addition to their role in disease production, several fungal species contribute to food spoilage, contamination of stored animal feed, and damage to growing crops, fabrics, timber fittings, and other susceptible materials. The shape and strength of the fungal cell is maintained by the cell wall, which also provides structural integrity and protection against adverse environmental influences.

Based on detailed studies of a number of pathogenic fungi, the cell wall has been shown to be composed primarily of chitin, glucans, mannans, and glycoproteins. The cell walls of many fungal species have some common features and some distinguishing features.[6,7,89] Structural features of the cell walls of four fungal species are illustrated in Figure 52.8.

The cell wall of the yeast *Candida albicans*, an opportunistic fungal pathogen, is composed mainly of β-1,3-glucans, β-1,6-glucans (glucose polymers), chitin (an *N*-acetylglucosamine polymer), and mannoproteins.[90] Up to 60% of the cell wall biomass is composed of β-glucans. Mannoproteins account for up to 40% of the cell wall biomass, and, although it represents a small percentage of the cell wall biomass, chitin is a vital component of fungal cell walls. Unlike *C albicans*, the cell wall of the yeast *Cryptococcus neoformans* is surrounded by a thick capsule of galactoxylomannan and glucuronoxylomannan. A layer of melanin is interposed between the chitin layer and the β-1,3-glucan layer.[6]

The hyphae of the saprobic mold, *Aspergillus fumigatus*, have similar features to *C albicans* in their inner layers, whereas outer layers contain galactosaminoglycan, galactomannan, and α-1,3-glucan. The hyphae of the dimorphic fungus *H capsulatum* have an outer layer containing α-1,3-glucan over the β-1,6-glucan and β-1,3-glucan layers.

The fungal cell membrane, which is rich in ergosterol, is the target of many antifungal drugs such as azoles and polyene antibiotics. Composition, porosity, and thickness of fungal cell walls have been mentioned as features that influence the resistance of pathogenic fungi to chemical disinfectants. Molds are reported to be more resistant than yeasts to chemical disinfectants, and both fungal forms are more resistant to disinfectants than nonsporulating bacteria. Fungal spores are more susceptible to disinfectants than bacterial endospores. A number of *Aspergillus* species, particularly *A fumigatus*, cause clinical infections in animals. Toxins produced by *Aspergillus flavus* in stored food cause aflatoxicosis. The *in vitro* susceptibility of 18 *Aspergillus* species isolated from veterinary hospital surfaces in Brazil were tested against four disinfectants.[91] Nine isolates of *A fumigatus*, seven of *A flavus*, and two of *Aspergillus niger* were used in the study. One halogen disinfectant, sodium hypochlorite, a QAC, benzalkonium chloride, a chlorhexidine compound, and a chlorophenol derivative were evaluated for their fungicidal activity. Apart from sodium hypochlorite, the other disinfectants were effective against all isolates at the concentrations used. Sodium hypochlorite was ineffective against a number of *Aspergillus* isolates used in the study.

Areas of a concrete floor deliberately contaminated with *M canis*–infected hair were treated with household bleach, three aqueous chlorhexidine solutions, a number of phenolic compounds, a QAC, and an enilconazole environmental spray.[92] Water served as a negative control, and 1% formalin was used as a positive control. Only undiluted bleach and 1% formalin inactivated all of the fungal spores with one application. The authors concluded that many products recommended for surface disinfection have minimal efficiency against *M canis*–infected hair.

Twelve disinfectants that included chlorine-releasing compounds, ethyl alcohol, chloroxylenol, and glutaraldehyde were evaluated for their ability to kill *M canis* in naturally infected feline hair.[93] Hypochlorite, benzalkonium chloride, and glutaraldehyde-based compounds were the most effective disinfectants. Phenolic compounds, ethyl alcohol, and anionic detergents were inadequate.

Five disinfectants, sodium hypochlorite, enilconazole, accelerated hydrogen peroxide, potassium peroxymonosulfate, and calcium hypochlorite, were tested against two fungal pathogens, *M canis* and *Trichophyton erinacei*.[94] The *M canis* isolate was obtained from an infected kitten, and the *T erinacei* isolate was obtained from infected hedgehogs. Enilconazole, sodium hypochlorite, accelerated hydrogen peroxide, and 2% potassium peroxymonosulfate inhibited growth of both fungal pathogens. Calcium hypochlorite showed no antifungal activity. Enilconazole at a 1/100 dilution, sodium hypochlorite at a 1/100 dilution, accelerated hydrogen peroxide at a 1/16 dilution, and 2% potassium peroxymonosulfate were recommended for decontamination of kennels contaminated with dermatophytes.

Accelerated hydrogen peroxide, a proprietary disinfectant sold as concentrates or ready-to-use products, contains a reduced concentration of hydrogen peroxide supplemented with surfactants, wetting agents, and chelating agents. The antifungal efficacy of disinfectants containing accelerated hydrogen peroxide against conidial arthrospores and isolated infective spores of *M canis* and *Trichophyton* species was evaluated.[95] The authors concluded that accelerated hydrogen peroxide products were suitable for decontamination of surfaces following thorough mechanical cleaning in association with a detergent. They also proposed that these products may be suitable alternatives to sodium hypochlorite for decontaminating homes where *M canis*–infected animals are being treated. The fungicidal efficacy of eight commercial disinfectants against *M canis* and *Trichophyton* species was evaluated using infective spores on an experimentally contaminated gauze sponge.[96] The disinfectants selected included sodium hypochlorite, two QACs, lactic acid, hydrogen peroxide, an ethoxylated alcohol mixture, and potassium peroxymonosulfate. Using a contact time of 10 minutes, all of the disinfectants tested were fungicidal for the two fungal pathogens used.

The inhibitory effect of 4% sodium hypochlorite and 6.6% chlorhexidine digluconate on clinical isolates of *S schenckii* was investigated using broth microdilution, agar diffusion, and direct exposure techniques.[97] After 20 minutes in the direct exposure test, sodium hypochlorite performed better than chlorhexidine digluconate, which showed little antifungal activity. The results demonstrated that sodium hypochlorite had a greater antifungal activity against *S schenckii* than chlorhexidine digluconate in the presence and absence of organic matter.

The antifungal activities of chemical disinfectants against a saprobic mold, dermatophytes, and a dimorphic fungus are presented in Table 52.5. The lack of consistency evident in different publications relating to the antifungal activity of chemical disinfectants may be due in part to differences in the experimental methods used and also to the variety of chemical compounds selected by some workers.

THE ROLE OF DISINFECTION IN CONTROL OF VIRAL DISEASE IN ANIMALS

Viruses are a unique class of infectious agents that differ in many respects from other infectious microorganisms such as bacteria and fungi. They replicate but it is a matter of some debate whether they can be considered as being alive. For certain viruses, the nucleic acid alone is capable of initiating infection and disruption of the viral envelope or capsid may not be sufficient to inactivate a virion. As a result, viruses present several unique challenges in terms of disinfection. In addition to the chemical composition of a disinfectant and environmental factors such as the presence of organic matter, temperature, and relative humidity, the physicochemical nature of the virus being targeted greatly influences the outcome of a specific disinfection procedure. Attempts have been made to group viruses according to those physicochemical properties thought to influence resistance to disinfectants. Noll and Younger[98] proposed a classification system based on the lipophilic properties of viruses. Subsequently, Klein and Deforest[99]

TABLE 52.5   The antifungal activity of chemical disinfectants against a saprobic mold, dermatophytes, and a dimorphic fungus[a]

Disinfectants	Fungal Species[b]			
	Aspergillus Species	*Microsporum canis*	*Trichophyton* Species	*Sporothrix schenckii*
Alcohols		±	±	
Accelerated hydrogen peroxide		+	+	
Biguanides	+	±		±
Calcium hypochlorite		−		
Enilconazole		+	+	
Formalin		++		
Glutaraldehyde		++		
Potassium peroxymonosulfate		+	+	
Phenolic compounds	+	±		
QACs	+	+	+	
Sodium hypochlorite	±	++	+	++

Abbreviation: QACs, quaternary ammonium compounds.

[a]Compiled from published scientific papers cited in the text.

[b]++, highly effective; +, effective; ±, limited activity; −, no activity.

proposed that the lipid content and size of a virus were useful indicators of the susceptibility of a virus to particular disinfectants. Three categories were proposed by these workers: viruses that possess lipoprotein envelopes (lipophilic) and are highly susceptible to many disinfectants, small nonenveloped viruses (hydrophilic) that are resistant to lipophilic disinfectants, and nonenveloped viruses that are capable of adsorbing some lipids (capsomeric lipophilicity) and are intermediate in their pattern of susceptibility to disinfectants. Prince et al[100] expanded the Klein and Deforest scheme to include viroids and prions, resulting in six groups of viruses/prions ranked according to susceptibility to chemical disinfectants (Table 52.6).

Specific data on susceptibility to chemical disinfectants have been generated for a limited number of viral species. Where such data are not available, predictions about the susceptibility of a specific virus to a particular disinfectant based on a related virus (often, a virus in the same family) and the general rankings of Prince et al[100] are generally considered to be broadly valid and frequently relied on. However, it is evident that in some instances, even closely related viruses may differ substantially in their susceptibility to disinfectants. For example, although foot-and-mouth disease virus and swine vesicular disease virus are both picornaviruses, they have different susceptibility to low pH values.[102,103] Foot-and-mouth disease virus is unstable at pH values below 6.5, whereas swine vesicular disease virus is stable at low pH values. In addition, it is often inferred that if efficacy for a particular disinfectant is demonstrated against a "more resistant" virus, then it must be effective against a "less resistant" virus. This idea of "high level" and "low level" disinfectants is inherent in classification systems for patient care items such as that of Spaulding,[104] which are designed to

aid health care workers in choosing the most appropriate level of cleaning, disinfection, or sterilization required to render surfaces, particularly those of medical and surgical devices, safe. Again, this is considered a reasonable and pragmatic approach but is only a guide.[105] In many instances, the studies on which susceptibility rankings are based have been carried out *in vitro*, in "clean" laboratory environments. An overreliance on such guides has been called into question.[106] Certain lipophilic viruses may have a particularly high affinity for organic material containing proteins or mucopolysaccharides that may interfere with the action of a disinfectant. Therefore, in nature, some viruses may behave in a more "resistant" manner than expected. Unfortunately, the number of studies carried out on such viruses under field conditions is even more limited in number than *in vitro* studies.

A limited number of scientific studies evaluating the ability of different disinfectants to inactivate viruses of veterinary importance have been published. Information available on the activity of disinfectants against some viruses is summarized in Table 52.7. Most published studies have reported on the virucidal activity of disinfectants under laboratory conditions only, and the efficacy of many disinfectants under field conditions can only be inferred from these publications. Some studies have evaluated particular commercial products containing a number of active compounds with different modes of action, giving additive or sometimes synergistic effects. Soaps or detergents are frequently combined with a particular disinfectant. It is important to carefully read the claims made by a manufacturer for the activity of a particular disinfectant preparation. Regulatory authorities recognize that products, which ostensibly contain similar active chemicals, often differ in terms of the range of components used in their formulation and in the process of manufacture. Bodies such as the US Environmental Protection Agency insist on statistically valid antimicrobial testing against a range of marker organisms for each product approved. Conditions and tests used to determine virucidal activity vary in accordance with the virus used and the experimental design, rendering decisions on applicability to various field situations difficult to determine. The efficacy of a disinfectant against a test virus is usually measured in terms of the degree of reduced infectivity for tissue culture, chick embryos, or susceptible animals. The sensitivity of different test systems varies, depending on the ability of a specific virus to infect the host cells and the method of demonstrating virus survival. Many disinfectants are toxic for cells, and further procedures such as dialysis or chemical neutralization may be required to remove disinfectant activity, procedures that may influence the test result. After their release from cells, viruses frequently remain clumped or associated with cellular debris. There is also a tendency for individual virions to adhere to particulate matter and surfaces. The resulting aggregations may contain a matrix of organic molecules

TABLE 52.6	Viruses and prions grouped according to their susceptibility to chemical disinfectants from most susceptible (group A) to most resistant (group F)[a]
Group	**Virus/Prion**
A	Lipophilic viruses
B	Nonenveloped viruses capable of adsorbing some lipids (eg, adenoviruses, rotaviruses, papillomaviruses)
C[b]	Picornaviruses
D	Parvoviruses
E	Viroids
F	Prions

[a]Based on Prince and Prince.[101]

[b]Members of the family *Caliciviridae*, in particular noroviruses, are considered to be intermediate between picornaviruses and parvoviruses.

TABLE 52.7   A guide to the antiviral spectrum of disinfectants against viruses of veterinary importance[a]

Viruses	Acids	Alkalis	Alcohols	Aldehydes	Biguanides	Halogens		Phenolic Compounds	Peroxygen Compounds	QACs
						Chlorine	Iodine			
Ruminant viruses										
Infectious bovine rhinotracheitis virus[107,108]	+	nt	nt	±	nt	+	+	V	+	nt
Bovine viral diarrhea virus[107]	nt	nt	nt	+	nt	+	±	±	+	nt
Parainfluenza virus type 3[107,108]	±	nt	nt	+	nt	+	+	±	+	nt
Orf virus[107,109]	nt	nt	−	+	nt	+	±	+	+	±
Bovine rotavirus[110,111]	nt	nt	+	+	nt	+	nt	+	nt	+
Foot-and-mouth disease virus[102]	+	+	nt	nt	nt	+	nt	±	nt	nt
Porcine viruses										
Aujeszky's disease virus[112]	nt	+	+	+	+	+	+	+	nt	+
Transmissible gastroenteritis virus[107,112]	−	+	+	+	+	+	+	V	+	+
Porcine adenovirus[113]	nt	+	+	+	−	+	±	+	nt	±
Swine vesicular disease virus[103]	−	+	nt	+	−	+	±	−	nt	nt
Porcine enterovirus[107,108,113]	−	+	+	+	−	+	±	−	+	−
Porcine circovirus type 2[114-116]	nt	+	−	+	−	+	−	V	+	V
Porcine rotavirus[117]	nt	nt	nt	+	nt	nt	nt	+	+	nt
Equine viruses										
Equine infectious anemia virus[118]	nt	+	+	+	+	+	+	+	nt	nt
Equine rotavirus[119]	nt	nt	nt	+	nt	+	+	nt	+	±

(continued)

TABLE 52.7   A guide to the antiviral spectrum of disinfectants against viruses of veterinary importance[a]
(Continued)

Viruses	Acids	Alkalis	Alcohols	Aldehydes	Biguanides	Halogens — Chlorine	Halogens — Iodine	Phenolic Compounds	Peroxygen Compounds	QACs
Canine viruses										
Canine coronavirus[120]	nt	nt	+	+	−	+	+	+	nt	+
Canine distemper virus[121,122]	nt	nt	+	+	nt	+	+	+	nt	+
Canine adenovirus[122-124]	nt	+	±	+	nt	V	V	V	nt	±
Canine parvovirus[120,122,125]	nt	+	−	+	−	+	+	−	nt	−
Feline viruses										
Feline viral rhinotracheitis virus[126]	nt	nt	+	+	+	+	+	+	nt	+
Feline calicivirus[126,127]	+	nt	±	+	−	+	±	+	+	−
Feline panleukopenia virus[126]	nt	nt	−	+	−	+	±	−	+	−
Poultry viruses										
Newcastle disease virus[123,128]	nt	+	+	+	nt	+	+	V	+	V
Avian metapneumovirus[128]	nt	nt	+	+	nt	−	nt	+	+	+
Avian influenza virus[128]	nt	nt	nt	+	nt	−	nt	+	+	−

Abbreviations: QACs, quaternary ammonium compounds; nt, not tested (in the specific publication cited); +, effective; −, ineffective; ±, limited efficacy; V, variable (published data inconsistent).

[a]Note that efficacy can vary depending on the biocide formulation, concentration, exposure time, and other factors.

and inorganic salts from body fluids, cellular debris associated with shed viruses, and large numbers of virions. Such structures provide physical protection from disinfectants as well as reacting chemically with and inactivating many disinfectants. As a result, virions in the center of cellular aggregations may retain infectivity.[129,130] The repeated use of disinfectants such as alcohols or aldehydes, which act as fixatives, may result in the buildup of organic material on surfaces, shielding viruses from disinfectant activity. Temperature and time of contact may also influence the activity of a disinfectant. In general, the higher the temperature and the longer the contact time, the more effective the disinfection program. In summary, there is a dynamic interaction between virus (physical properties, concentration, aggregation), disinfectant (chemical properties, exposure time), and the environment (organic material, relative humidity, temperature) that may determine the effectiveness of a disinfection program. The selection of a chemical disinfectant must not only be based on knowledge of the spectrum and mode of action of the active compound(s) in the preparation but must also take into consideration a variety of other factors operating in a particular situation.

In addition, the toxicity of the disinfectant for the animal, the personnel, and more generally to the environment should also influence the decision making. It is not simply a matter of choosing the most effective disinfectant but rather the most appropriate disinfectant for a particular set of circumstances.

Ruminant Viruses

Nine disinfectants were evaluated by Evans et al[107] for their activity against several viruses of veterinary importance, including infectious bovine rhinotracheitis virus. Glutaraldehyde, Lysol™, sodium hypochlorite, a commercial iodophor, peracetic acid, and citric acid were all found to be effective. Slavin[108] found a number of phenolic compounds and sodium hypochlorite effective against infectious bovine rhinotracheitis virus. Bovine viral diarrhea virus, also an enveloped virus, was inactivated by glutaraldehyde, formalin, Lysol™, sodium hypochlorite, and peracetic acid. The virus was partially sensitive to an iodophor.[107] In the same study, orf virus was sensitive to glutaraldehyde, formalin, Lysol™, sodium hypochlorite, an iodophor, phenol, and peracetic acid. Gallina and Scagliarini[109] found that sodium hypochlorite and certain products containing QACs were effective against orf virus, whereas 70% ethanol was ineffective and the presence of organic material greatly inhibited the action of sodium hypochlorite. Parainfluenza virus type 3 was sensitive to glutaraldehyde, formalin, phenolic compounds, sodium hypochlorite, a commercial iodophor, and peracetic acid.[107,108]

In one study, foot-and-mouth disease virus was rapidly inactivated in the presence of acid or alkali.[102] In the same study, sodium hypochlorite was also shown to be effective provided organic matter was not present, and a number of phenolic compounds were found to inactivate the virus slowly. Formaldehyde, phenol, sodium hypochlorite, alcohol, and a commercial product containing a QAC, amphoteric salts, and propylene glycol were effective against bovine rotavirus.[110,111] Snodgrass and Herring[131] reported that a commercial iodophor, Lysol™, and formol-saline had activity against an ovine rotavirus in intestinal contents after a 2-hour contact period. Under the same conditions, the performance of sodium hypochlorite was unsatisfactory. A bovine adenovirus isolate was sensitive to glutaraldehyde, sodium hypochlorite, a commercial iodophor, and peracetic acid.[107]

Porcine Viruses

Transmissible gastroenteritis virus, an enveloped coronavirus, was sensitive to aldehydes, sodium hypochlorite, iodine-containing compounds, certain phenolic compounds, ethanol, sodium hydroxide, QACs, and peracetic acid.[107,112] Aujeszky disease virus, which is also enveloped, was sensitive to a wide range of disinfectants, including aldehydes, sodium hypochlorite, iodine-containing compounds, phenolic compounds, ethanol, sodium hydroxide, and QACs.[112] In contrast, in the same study, the small nonenveloped virions of porcine parvovirus were sensitive only to aldehydes, sodium hypochlorite, and sodium hydroxide. Porcine enterovirus type 1, a picornavirus responsible for Teschen/Talfan disease, was sensitive to a narrow range of disinfectants, including aldehydes, sodium hypochlorite, ethanol, sodium hydroxide, and peracetic acid.[107,113] Another picornavirus, swine vesicular disease virus, which is similar to human coxsackievirus B5, was sensitive to formaldehyde, sodium hypochlorite, and sodium hydroxide.[103] The QACs did not inactivate swine vesicular disease virus, but, when combined with 0.1% sodium hydroxide, did inactivate the virus.[132] A porcine adenovirus isolate was shown to be susceptible to formaldehyde, sodium hypochlorite, ethanol, sodium hydroxide, and a commercial phenolic preparation.[113] Blackwell[133] reported that vesicular exanthema of swine virus, a calicivirus, was inactivated by sodium hypochlorite, sodium hydroxide, citric acid, and phenol. Stone and Hess[134] evaluated 10 commercially available disinfectants under conditions of low and high pH for their ability to inactivate African swine fever virus. A phenolic compound containing ortho-phenylphenol was the most effective agent. Sodium hypochlorite and a number of phenolic compounds were effective against the rhabdovirus, vesicular stomatitis virus.[135] Porcine circovirus type 2 was shown to be sensitive to sodium hypochlorite, sodium hydroxide, and peroxygen compounds.[114-116] Iodine, chlorhexidine, and ethanol were ineffective, whereas phenolic compounds and QACs gave variable results. Peroxygen compounds and a glutaraldehyde-based disinfectant inactivated porcine rotavirus.[117] Two phenolic disinfectants based on 4-chloro-3-methylphenol differed in their activity against the rotavirus, and it was concluded that this was due to other chemical components in the products used.

Equine Viruses

Equine infectious anemia virus, a retrovirus, was tested for sensitivity to 12 disinfectants, including aldehydes, halogen compounds, phenolic compounds, sodium hydroxide, and ethanol.[118] The virus was inactivated by all the disinfectants used. Glutaraldehyde, halogen-based, and peroxygen compounds were all effective against equine rotavirus.[119]

Canine Viruses

Saknimit et al[120] showed that canine coronavirus was susceptible to a wide range of compounds. Canine distemper virus was sensitive to formalin, halogen compounds, alcohols, cresol soap, and QACs.[121] In contrast, canine parvovirus was sensitive only to aldehydes, halogen compounds, and sodium hydroxide.[120,125,136] Mahnel and Herlyn[123] reported that halogen compounds and sodium hydroxide were effective even at low temperatures against canine adenovirus 1, the cause of infectious canine hepatitis. Sanekata et al[122] compared chlorine dioxide and sodium hypochlorite against a range of canine viruses. Both of these halogen compounds were effective against canine distemper, canine adenovirus 2, and canine parvovirus. However, the antiviral activity of chlorine dioxide was estimated to be about 10 times greater than that of sodium hypochlorite.

Feline Viruses

Commercial disinfectants, representing all the main classes of disinfectants, were evaluated for their virucidal activity against common feline viruses by Scott.[126] Of 35 products tested against feline calicivirus, only 11 products, including sodium hypochlorite, aldehydes, and a number of phenolic compounds, were effective. Only 3 of 27 products tested against feline panleukopenia virus, sodium hypochlorite, and two different aldehydes were effective. All of the 22 products tested against feline rhinotracheitis virus were effective. Sodium hypochlorite solution (0.175%) was considered to be the most effective and practical broad-spectrum disinfectant for the feline viruses tested. There has been renewed interest in feline calicivirus in recent years given its use as a surrogate virus for human norovirus, on account of the absence of a cell culture system for the latter virus.[122,127,137,138]

Poultry Viruses

Five commercial phenolic disinfectants evaluated for their activity against Newcastle disease virus were shown to be effective.[139] Mahnel and Herlyn[123] reported that formalin, sodium hydroxide, and halogen compounds were active against Newcastle disease virus, whereas phenol had a minimal effect. A proprietary iodophor was reported to be active against infectious bronchitis virus by Jordan and Nassar.[140] The activity of eight commercial disinfectants against budgerigar fledgling disease polyomavirus was evaluated by Ritchie et al.[141] Sodium hypochlorite, stabilized chlorine dioxide, ethanol, and a phenolic compound were effective. Patnayak et al[128] examined the efficacy of nine commercially available disinfectants against Newcastle disease virus, avian influenza virus, and avian metapneumovirus. Phenolic compounds, potassium peroxymonosulfate, and glutaraldehyde were effective against all three viruses. The QACs were effective against avian metapneumovirus. Sodium hypochlorite was effective against Newcastle disease virus but was not as effective against avian influenza virus and avian metapneumovirus.

▶ THE ROLE OF DISINFECTION IN CONTROL OF PROTOZOAL DISEASE IN ANIMALS

The oocysts of two protozoan parasites, *C parvum* and *Toxoplasma gondii*, which cause disease in animals and humans, are widely distributed in the environment and transmitted by the fecal-oral route. Fecal oocysts of pathogenic protozoa are much more resistant to chemical disinfectants than bacteria, fungi, or viruses.[142-144]

Contamination of food, water, or equipment with the fecal oocysts of *C parvum* has caused major outbreaks of cryptosporidiosis, sometimes in urban populations, involving public water supplies. Clinical features of disease in humans include diarrhea and abdominal pain. The parasite invades intestinal epithelial cells, and subsequently, oocysts are excreted in the feces for several weeks. In a moist environment, oocysts may remain infective for 6 months or longer.[145] A major outbreak of waterborne cryptosporidiosis was reported among residents of Milwaukee in 1993 in which more than 400 000 people were estimated to have acquired infection.[146] This massive outbreak of disease was caused by oocysts of *C parvum* that passed through the filtration system of the city's water treatment plants. Their small size (5.0-5.5 μm), the large number shed by an infected human or animal, and their resistance to chemical inactivation by chlorine-based disinfectants may account for the frequency and importance of this protozoan parasite in outbreaks of waterborne disease in the human population. In addition to its frequent association with waterborne disease in humans, *C parvum* is also an important cause of enteric disease in farm animals, especially in newborn ruminants.

Fecal oocysts of *T gondii* share some common characteristics with those of *C parvum* in their resistance to chemical disinfectants and in their ability to withstand adverse environmental conditions. In other respects, however, these two protozoan parasites have little in common. The definitive hosts of *T gondii* are cats that usually acquire infection by eating infected rodents, birds, or meat from infected farm animals, especially sheep. Fecal oocysts shed in cat feces are another possible source of infection for cats, grazing animals, and humans. When fecal oocysts are ingested by susceptible animals, they form cysts in muscle or other tissues, which may remain viable for the animal's lifetime. For humans, infection with *T gondii* is primarily from cat feces or from soil contaminated with fecal oocysts and from ingestion of undercooked meat with tissue cysts, especially mutton. If a pregnant woman acquires a primary infection with *T gondii*, there may be a risk of congenital toxoplasmosis in her baby.

Monoclonal antibodies or mass spectrometry were employed to investigate structural components of the oocyst walls of *T gondii* and *C parvum*.[147] Structural components of *T gondii* include β-1,3-linked glucose; acid-fast lipids are present in both *T gondii* and *C parvum*. Oocyst walls of *Toxoplasma* have two distinct layers with β-1,3 glucan in the inner layer, resembling that of fungi, and with acid-fast lipids in the outer layer as occur with mycobacteria. The oocyst walls of *Cryptosporidium* have a fibrillar glycocalyx, a rigid bilayer of acid-fast lipids, an inner layer of oocyst wall proteins, and tethers that have a globular appearance when disrupted. The oocyst walls of *T gondii* and *C parvum* contain O-glycans, and oocyst wall proteins are the most abundant proteins in the cryptosporidial wall. Oocysts of *Toxoplasma* and *Eimeria* also contain wall proteins.

The activities of chemical disinfectants against the oocysts of *C parvum*, *T gondii*, *Neospora caninum*, and *Eimeria tenella* are presented in Table 52.8.

Cryptosporidium parvum

Important structural components of the oocyst wall include acid-fast lipids, an inner layer containing oocyst wall proteins, and an abundance of O-glycans.[147] Numerous published reports confirm the exceptional resistance of the fecal oocysts of *C parvum* to chemical disinfectants. Although the basis of this resistance has not been determined, the inability of chemical compounds to penetrate the thick-walled oocyst has been proposed as the reason for this intrinsic resistance.[13] Oocysts of *C parvum* suspended in aqueous solutions of sodium hypochlorite at 21°C survived exposure to a range of concentrations up to 5.25% for more than 120 minutes.[148] Treatment with a commercial disinfectant composed of 25% chlorocresol at a concentration of 4% for up to 120 minutes significantly inhibited *Cryptosporidium* development.[149] Two commercial peroxygen-based disinfectants containing hydrogen peroxide combined with either peracetic acid or silver nitrate were evaluated for their ability to inactivate *C parvum* oocysts.[13] Treatment with hydrogen peroxide combined with silver nitrate at a concentration of 3% completely eliminated oocyst infectivity for mice after 30 minutes exposure. The combination of hydrogen peroxide with peracetic acid used at a concentration of

TABLE 52.8   A guide to the activity of chemical disinfectants against the oocysts of selected pathogenic protozoa of human and veterinary importance[a]

Disinfectant	Pathogenic Protozoa[b]			
	Cryptosporidium parvum	Eimeria species	Neospora caninum	Toxoplasma gondii
Alcohols			−	−
Aldehydes	−		−	−
Amine-based disinfectants	++			
Ammonia	−	++	−	
Biguanides				−
Halogens				
Chlorine compounds	±		++	−
Iodine compounds			−	
Peroxygen compounds				
Hydrogen peroxide plus peracetic acid	++			
Hydrogen peroxide plus silver nitrate	++			
Potassium peroxymonosulfate				−
Ozone				−
Phenolic compounds				
Phenol				−
p-chloro-*m*-cresol	++			
Chlorinated phenols		++		
Quaternary ammonium compounds				−
Sodium hydroxide				−

[a]Compiled from published scientific papers cited in the text.

[b]++, highly effective; ±, limited activity; −, no activity.

5% required 120 minutes to inactivate *C parvum* oocysts. An integrated field study in which calves were treated with halofuginone lactate and calf pens were disinfected with *p*-chloro-*m*-cresol controlled cryptosporidiosis completely for the first 2 weeks after birth.[150]

The effect of an amine-based disinfectant on the infectivity of *C parvum* oocysts was investigated using oocysts suspended in water and treated with a 2% and 3% concentration of the disinfectant for 2 hours.[151] The infectivity of the treated oocysts was assessed using neonatal mice. At a concentration of 3%, infectivity of the oocysts was completely eliminated. Treatment of oocysts with two commercial disinfectants containing *p*-chloro-*m*-cresol (Neopredisan® 135-1 and Aldecoc® TGE) at a 4% concentration for 2 hours consistently inactivated more than 99.5% of oocysts.[144] The susceptibility of *C parvum* to heat inactivation was investigated using cell cultures.[149] Heating oocysts at 55°C for 4 hours resulted in a complete loss of infectivity for cell cultures. In another study, heating oocysts at 70°C for 20 minutes resulted in complete inactivation of oocysts.[152]

Prevention and control of cryptosporidiosis in animals requires treatment of infected animals with effective cryptosporicidal drugs and intensive cleaning to reduce oocyst numbers on contaminated building surfaces followed by physical or chemical inactivation of residual oocysts. Reducing the number of oocysts ingested by susceptible animals may lessen the severity of infection and allow the development of active immunity to infection. The environment of calves at birth should be clean, and each animal should have an optimal intake of colostrum. For the first 2 weeks of life, calves should be reared separately and with strict attention to equipment used for feeding to avoid mechanical transmission of oocysts. From a disease transmission perspective, the prevention of contact with other calves may be desirable, but from an animal welfare consideration and in many countries in order to comply with legislation, contact with at least one other calf is required. Calves, which develop diarrhea, should be isolated immediately from healthy calves and remain isolated until clinical signs of illness are no longer evident.

In the event of an outbreak of cryptosporidiosis, oral therapy with halofuginone lactate combined with thorough cleaning of contaminated buildings and disinfection with *p*-chloro-*m*-cresol disinfectant may decrease oocyst shedding and lessen the severity of enteric disease.[150] Drugs that have been used for treating cryptosporidiosis in animals include halofuginone, nitazoxanide, and azithromycin.[153] Thermal inactivation of *C parvum* oocysts offers an effective method for decontaminating buildings, equipment, and transport vehicles following an outbreak of cryptosporidiosis. Appropriate facilities, however, are required to maintain water at the correct temperature for the requisite time to ensure oocyst inactivation.

In the absence of an effective vaccine, the availability of a range of chemical compounds with documented activity against the oocysts of *C parvum* is an important resource that can be employed as part of a strategic program for the control of cryptosporidiosis in animals, thereby decreasing the risk of environmental contamination and associated human infection by this protozoan parasite, often a consequence of fecal contamination of public water supplies.

A newly developed *in vitro* germ carrier assay system to assess disinfectant efficacy of chemical disinfectants against *C parvum* has been described.[152] Oocysts of *C parvum* on stainless steel discs were incubated in chemical disinfectants for 2 hours, rinsed to remove disinfectants, and recovered oocysts were transferred to human ileocecal adenocarcinoma cell monolayers. After 48 hours, genomic DNA was extracted and quantified by real-time polymerase chain reaction (PCR) assay, targeting the *hsp* gene to estimate parasite reproduction. Inactivation rates obtained by suspension tests and germ carrier tests were comparable, and the authors propose that both the suspension assay and germ carrier assay be used if products are being tested against oocysts of *C parvum*. They also propose a threshold of 99.5% inactivation for *in vitro* evaluation of disinfectants, using *C parvum* as a model organism, in comparison with the *E tenella* animal infection assay.

Toxoplasma gondii

Some of the components present in the oocyst walls of *T gondii* resemble those present in fungi and in mycobacteria. The inner layer of the oocyst wall contains β-1,3-glucan, and the outer layer contains acid-fast lipids. The oocyst wall contains sugar polymers composed of β-1,3-glucan, acid-fast lipids, glucanase, and other proteins together with an abundance of O-glycans.[147]

Oocysts of *T gondii* were completely inactivated by heating at 58°C for 15 minutes.[154] Sporulated oocysts of *T gondii* treated with 95% and 75% ethyl alcohol, 100% methyl alcohol, and 10% formalin for up to 24 hours retained infectivity for mice. Treatment with CHG in 70% ethyl alcohol, sodium dichloroisocyanurate, and a peroxygen compound failed to inactivate the oocysts.[155]

Physical and chemical methods for inactivating oocysts of *T gondii* in water have been evaluated. Pulsed UV radiation of oocysts with doses as low as 40 mJ/cm² resulted in inactivation, and continuous UV radiation with doses as low as 45 mJ/cm² also resulted in inactivation.[142] This method of inactivation, however, was not 100% reliable, and the results suggested that a minimum UV exposure dose of 1000 mJ/cm² for water treatment may be required to increase the probability of consistent and complete oocyst inactivation.

Sodium hypochlorite and ozone were used to assess their ability to inactivate oocysts of *T gondii* in water.[143] Oocysts were exposed to 100 mg/L of chlorine for 30 minutes or for 2, 4, 8, 16, and 24 hours and to 6 mg/L of ozone for 1, 2, 4, 8, and 12 minutes. The results of chemical exposure of the oocysts to sodium hypochlorite or ozone indicated that neither treatment effectively inactivated the oocysts of *T gondii* in water.

Neospora caninum

The oocyst-forming coccidian parasite *N caninum*, which affects a wide range of host species, is an important cause of abortions in cattle. Dogs, wolves, and coyotes are definitive hosts of this parasite, and they shed fecal oocysts that infect intermediate hosts, especially ruminants. *Neospora* oocysts survive in soil and water for prolonged periods and also in decomposed canine feces. The viability of sporulated oocysts of *N caninum* after exposure to different physical and chemical treatments has been investigated.[156] Sporulated oocysts were treated with absolute ethyl alcohol for 1 hour, 20°C for 6 hours, 4°C for 6 hours, 60°C for 1 minute, 100°C for 1 minute, 10% formaldehyde for 1 hour, 10% ammonia for 1 hour, 2% iodine for 1 hour, 10% sodium hypochlorite for 1 hour, and 70% ethyl alcohol for 1 hour. All chemical treatments were carried out at 37°C. Heating at 100°C for 1 minute and treating with 10% sodium hypochlorite for 1 hour were the only methods that effectively inactivated all oocysts of *N caninum*.

Eimeria tenella

The ability of two phenolic disinfectants and ammonia to kill sporulated oocysts of *E tenella* was investigated by Williams.[157] One phenolic compound, a coal-tar phenol, was effective at a concentration of 0.8%, whereas the other containing coal-tar and chlorinated phenols was effective at 0.4% concentration. Ammonia at a concentration of approximately 0.5% was the most effective agent against sporulated oocysts of *E tenella*.

▶ THE ROLE OF DISINFECTION IN CONTROL OF PRION DISEASE IN ANIMALS

A group of fatal neurologic diseases of mammals, including humans (Table 52.9), which share several unusual features, are termed TSEs. Their incubation period in mammals is prolonged, ranging from 2 months to more than 20 years. Although frequently lasting months or years, the clinical course is always progressive and invariably fatal. The histopathologic changes in the brain associated with each of these diseases are characteristic and include a reactive astrocytosis and vacuolation of neurons. In 1982, Prusiner[158] introduced the term *prion* to distinguish the novel pathogens responsible for these

TABLE 52.9	Transmissible spongiform encephalopathies of importance that affect humans and animals
Disease	**Affected Host(s)**
Scrapie	Sheep, goats
Bovine spongiform encephalopathy (BSE)	Cattle
Chronic wasting disease (CWD)	Elk, mule deer, white-tailed deer, moose
Transmissible mink encephalopathy[a]	Mink
Feline spongiform encephalopathy[a]	Cats
Ungulate spongiform encephalopathy[a]	Nyala, oryx, greater kudu
Kuru	Humans
Creutzfeldt-Jakob disease (CJD)	Humans
Variant Creutzfeldt-Jakob disease[a] (vCJD)	Humans, linked to BSE
Gerstmann-Straussler syndrome	Humans
Fatal familial insomnia	Humans

[a]Incorporation of ruminant tissues containing scrapie prion protein (PrP^{Sc}) in foodstuffs is considered to have been the cause of vCJD, feline spongiform encephalopathy, transmissible mink encephalopathy, and ungulate spongiform encephalopathy.

diseases from viruses and viroids. He defined prions as "small proteinaceous infectious particles that resist inactivation by procedures which modify nucleic acids." It is now widely accepted that prions do not contain nucleic acid and therefore are at odds with all other known infectious agents. Prions have also been described in fungi. In 2013, Zhang et al[159] successfully generated an infectious prion *de novo* using recombinant prion protein expressed in bacteria.

Cellular prion protein (PrP^C) is a normal sialoglycoprotein encoded by a chromosomal gene and found in association with the cell membrane of mammalian and avian cells, particularly neurons. A disease-associated isoform of PrP termed PrP^{Sc} (named after scrapie, the prototypic prion disease) is derived from PrP^C and accumulates in the brains of affected humans and animals. The two proteins are chemically identical but differ in tertiary structure in that PrP^{Sc} has a significantly higher ratio of β sheets compared with PrP^C. A posttranslational modification is responsible for the conformational misfolding of PrP^C into PrP^{Sc}. Prion replication proceeds at a much faster rate when a PrP^{Sc} nucleus or "seed" provides the template for this misfolding. This self-propagating process is known as nucleation-dependent polymerization.

Predisposition to TSE is significantly influenced by the genome of the host. Certain polymorphisms of the prion protein (*PrP*) gene are strongly associated with the incidence of TSEs. The primary PrP^C amino acid sequence determines both the susceptibility of the molecule to misfold and the range of PrP^{Sc} conformations with which it is able to interact ("species barrier"). Three different manifestations of prion diseases are described[160]:

- *Acquired "slow" infection.* Kuru is a slowly progressive disease transmitted by cannibalism practiced by the Fore people, inhabiting the Eastern Highlands of Papua New Guinea. A number of cases of Creutzfeldt-Jakob disease (CJD) have been associated with the use of human cadaver tissues or extracts such as corneal transplants and human growth hormone. The epidemic of BSE in Britain is believed to have resulted from changes in rendering practices permitting the survival of prions, possibly derived from scrapie-infected sheep, in meat-and-bone meal.[161] The agent of BSE is transmissible to humans and is responsible for the appearance of a new variant form of CJD (vCJD) in humans.[162] There is evidence that prions are shed into the environment by sheep suffering from scrapie and by deer suffering from chronic wasting disease (CWD) and that prions are taken up by and bind to plants thus completing the cycle of infection in such herbivores.[163]
- *Sporadic disease.* Most sporadic CJD (sCJD) cases occur in a sporadic manner in the human population at a rate of approximately 1 case per million people each year. These cases are thought to arise from a somatic mutation in the gene controlling PrP production or spontaneous conversion of PrP^C into PrP^{Sc}.
- *Familial genetic disorder.* Familial CJD, Gerstmann-Straussler syndrome (GSS), and fatal familial insomnia are all associated with germline mutations in the *PrP* gene.

The disease-associated prion PrP^{Sc} has traditionally referred to a PrP molecule that is resistant to proteinase K (PK) digestion (designated $rPrP^{Sc}$). However, several disease-related forms of PrP, including PK-sensitive isoforms of PrP^{Sc} (referred to as $sPrP^{Sc}$), have been demonstrated[164,165] and shown to make up a significant fraction of PrP^{Sc} in sCJD and GSS.[166] The role of $sPrP^{Sc}$ in disease is unclear, but the concentration of these protease-sensitive isoforms has been shown to correlate with the progression rate of disease.[167] Furthermore, it appears that PrP^{Sc}, as originally defined by its relative protease resistance and detergent insolubility, constitutes only a small proportion of total disease-related PrP isoforms present in infectious brain material.[168] The studies described here involving brain tissue do not distinguish between these different isoforms, but it is assumed that the remarkable resistance of prions to inactivation is due to the PK-resistant isoform. The resistance of prions to inactivation by heating, exposure to chemicals, and irradiation has been summarized in Quinn et al.[169]

Physical and chemical methods of inactivation of prions have been reviewed by Taylor[170,171] and McDonnell.[172]

Extensive research has been carried out into physical methods of inactivating the agents of BSE and scrapie because of the need for safe disposal of carcasses and the possibility that meat-and-bone meal may act as a source of infection.[173,174] Resistance of these agents to normal methods of inactivation of viruses resulted in exposure of several thousand sheep to the scrapie agent in a louping ill vaccine prepared from formalin-treated suspensions of brain, spinal cord, and spleen.[175] In fact, the treatment of prions with alcohols or aldehydes that fix proteins may help to protect these agents from inactivation and enhance their thermostability. There are differences in the thermostability of different strains of prions obtained by serial passage in laboratory animals,[176] and both BSE and vCJD prions are considered to be more thermostable than other prions.[177,178] In addition, Giles et al[179] highlighted differences in resistance between cattle and mouse-passaged BSE prions. They concluded that inactivation procedures must be validated using the prion strain for which they were intended. Dry heat is not as effective as moist heat in reducing the infectivity titer of prions. Brown et al[180] ashed scrapie-infected brain samples at 600°C but failed to fully inactivate the prion, whereas incineration at 1000°C was successful.[181]

Variables such as type of tissue preparation, exposure time, and temperature frequently differ from study to study. Equivocal results are sometimes reported. Ideally, the conditions used in decontamination studies should mimic the most adverse natural circumstances. It has been shown that prion infectivity binds avidly to steel surfaces.[182,183] A standardized testing method involves the contamination of stainless steel wires with high titers of TSE-infected brain homogenates, allowing the material to dry on the surface before decontamination treatment and the determination of residual infectivity using a mouse bioassay that may require more than 500 days. This greatly increases the cost and time required to carry out these inactivation trials.

Prions are usually unaffected by acidic pH changes but are susceptible to treatment with particular alkalis. Exposure of CJD agent to 1N hydrochloric acid for 60 minutes resulted in little loss of infectivity.[184] The inclusion of a formic acid step in formaldehyde fixation of brain tissue has been shown dramatically to reduce the infectivity of scrapie, BSE, and CJD agents without significantly affecting the quality of histologic sections.[185,186] The effectiveness of formic acid is most likely due to its fixation effect on proteins preventing the release of the prion protein. Brown et al[184] found that exposure of scrapie-infected brain material to 1N sodium hydroxide for 1 hour resulted in loss of infectivity. However, Taylor et al[187] demonstrated significant residual infectivity in brain material containing the scrapie agent after exposure to 1 or 2 mol/L sodium hydroxide for 1 or 2 hours; it is important to note that these studies were conducted in the presence of significant amounts of interfering brain material. Neither autoclaving nor exposure to sodium hydroxide can be relied on alone to completely inactivate prions in brain material. Taguchi et al[188] found that treatment with 1N sodium hydroxide for 60 minutes followed by autoclaving at 121°C for 30 minutes was capable of completely inactivating the agent of CJD in mouse brain homogenates. Taylor et al[189] showed no infectivity in mouse brain infected with the scrapie agent after subjecting the material to gravity displacement autoclaving at 121°C for 30 minutes in the presence of 2 mol/L sodium hydroxide. Taylor et al[190] reported that a particularly thermostable strain of BSE could be inactivated by boiling in 1 mol/L sodium hydroxide for 1 minute. Murphy et al[191] confirmed the effectiveness of alkaline hydrolysis for inactivating scrapie-positive mouse brains using KOH treatment at 150°C and a pressure of 4.14 bars. One of the most widely used methods for the reprocessing of reusable medical devices, steam sterilization at 134°C for 18 minutes, gave equivocal results in contaminated surface studies, whereas immersion in 1N sodium hydroxide or in 2.5% sodium hypochlorite for 1 hour were both consistently effective.[192]

Organic solvents, including acetone,[193] ethanol,[194] chloroform,[195] and commercial formulations involving hexane, heptane, perchlorethylene, or petroleum[196] have little effect on prion infectivity. Similarly, alkylating agents such as formalin,[197,198] glutaraldehyde,[194] β-propiolactone,[199] acetylethylenimine,[200] and EO[201] are considered ineffective for the inactivation of prions.

Halogen compounds, particularly sodium hypochlorite at high concentrations, are active against prions. Brown et al[184] found 2.5% sodium hypochlorite (25 000 ppm available chlorine) capable of inactivating scrapie-infected brain material after exposure for 1 hour. Exposure to hypochlorite containing 10 000 ppm of available chlorine for 30 minutes reduced the infectivity titer for two mouse-passaged strains of scrapie by 10^4 to 10^5, leading to the recommendation that 2% hypochlorite should be used for the decontamination of surfaces.[176] The corrosive nature of such strong concentrations of hypochlorite prompted investigations with the less corrosive chlorine-releasing compound, sodium dichloroisocyanurate.[187] Homogenates of BSE-infected bovine brain were treated with sodium hypochlorite and sodium dichloroisocyanurate containing up to 16 500 ppm available chlorine for up to 2 hours. Although the sodium hypochlorite solutions were fully effective, none of the dichloroisocyanurate solutions produced complete inactivation under the test conditions. At the end of the exposure periods, it was found that the residual available chlorine in the sodium dichloroisocyanurate samples was 3.5 times greater than in the sodium hypochlorite samples, indicating inhibition of the release of free chlorine from sodium dichloroisocyanurate. Iodine at a 2% concentration (wt/vol) gave only a modest reduction in the infectivity of scrapie-infected brain homogenates.[197]

The treatment of prion-infected brain homogenates with 4% phenol[195] was not effective, but unusually, a proprietary phenolic disinfectant was[176,197] only partially effective. Oxidizing agents such as chlorine dioxide at a concentration

of 50 ppm and 3% (vol/vol) hydrogen peroxide only partly inactivated the scrapie agent after exposure for 24 hours[197]; hydrogen peroxide in gas form was reported to be effective, even under room fumigation conditions.[18,192] Although 2% peracetic acid was effective against the scrapie agent in intact brain tissue, concentrations of up to 19% were ineffective with supernatants of homogenized brain.[202]

A number of other compounds, including sodium metaperiodate,[203] potassium permanganate,[204] and urea,[203] have been reported to be highly effective against prions, but other studies have found only low to moderate activity against TSE agents.[184,197]

The work of Chesney et al[205] suggested that the oxidant peroxymonosulfate may be useful in decontaminating instruments and soil. However, they did not confirm reductions in infectivity using a mouse bioassay. Ding et al[206] used the protein misfolding cyclic amplification (PMCA) assay to evaluate the effect of ozone on scrapie strain 263K and concluded that ozone may be effective for inactivating prions in water and wastewater.

Interest has also focused on the use of proteolytic methods for prion decontamination.[207] Jackson et al[208] showed that a sodium dodecyl sulfate (SDS), pK, and pronase three-stage procedure significantly reduced prion infectivity. Beekes et al[209] demonstrated the effectiveness of a combination of 0.2% SDS and 0.3% sodium hydroxide in 20% n-propanol in decontaminating steel wires contaminated with brain material containing scrapie strain 263K.

The extreme resistance of prions requires cautious extrapolation from in vitro studies to practical applications. Most published studies have involved brain tissue. The presence of animal tissue, particularly when dried on glass or metal surfaces, has been shown in autoclave studies to dramatically increase the resistance of prions. Organic matter may hinder decontamination of surfaces of equipment and benches in a similar manner. The possibility of transmission of animal prions to humans necessitates a rigorous examination of decontamination procedures in the laboratory. Uncertainties regarding the ability of rendering processes to fully inactivate prions resulted in the EU banning the feeding of ruminant-derived protein to ruminants in 1994 (Commission Decision 94/381/EC). Since April 1997, in the EU, a temperature of at least 133°C for 20 minutes at an absolute pressure of three bars is required for the disposal of infected BSE carcasses (Commission Decision 96/449/EC). Studies have shown that autoclaving according to these guidelines is generally effective but does not destroy prion infectivity in all instances.[207,208] Even if more efficient rendering procedures are developed and scientifically validated to ensure the reliable destruction of prions in ruminant-derived protein, it is unlikely that these decisions will be revoked in the future, given the disastrous impact of BSE on the British beef trade and the occurrence of new-variant CJD in humans.

Similarities between the pathogenesis of TSEs and several age-related noninfectious neurodegenerative diseases has led to suggestions to redefine prions as "proteinaceous nucleating particles."[210] This expands the prion concept to encompass other proteopathic diseases, such as Alzheimer disease, Parkinson disease, and Huntington disease, which lack an infectious origin.[211] Others feel that this is a step too far and prefer the term *prionoid* to distinguish these nontransmissible (at least under natural conditions) neurodegenerative conditions.[212] In any case, this debate has added renewed impetus to the design and implementation of decontaminating protocols for human surgical equipment and materials. The safest option is to use disposable materials and new equipment, but this is not always practical or affordable. Instruments and other materials subject to reuse should be kept moist from time of exposure to subsequent decontamination and cleaning. The removal of adherent particles through mechanical cleaning will enhance the decontamination process but must be carried out in a manner that safeguards personnel. The WHO[213] developed infection control guidelines for TSEs. For the sterilization of heat-resistant surgical instruments following contact with high-risk tissues (brain, spinal cord, eyes) to ensure that they are fully decontaminated for prions, the guidelines recommend immersion in 1N sodium hydroxide and heating in a gravity displacement autoclave at 121°C for 30 minutes or alternatively immersion in 1N sodium hydroxide or sodium hypochlorite (20 000 ppm available chlorine) for 1 hour. The instruments can then be cleaned and autoclaved as usual. The use of sodium hydroxide is considered to be preferable to sodium hypochlorite because it is much less corrosive for surgical instruments. However, such high concentrations of sodium hydroxide or sodium hypochlorite are not suitable for use on various pieces of medical equipment such as endoscopes. Lehmann et al[214] investigated the effect of copper and hydrogen peroxide (Fenton reaction) for 30 minutes on brain homogenate (263K scrapie strain) dried onto stainless steel wires and demonstrated full decontamination. Fichet et al[18] found that a gaseous hydrogen peroxide sterilization process was effective against the scrapie 263K strain, whereas liquid hydrogen peroxide was not. A mildly acidic, electrochemically activated hypochlorous acid formulation was shown by Hughson et al[215] to pose no apparent hazard to either users or surfaces and successfully eliminated hamster-adapted scrapie infectivity in brain homogenates.

▶ APPLIED ASPECTS OF DISINFECTION

Disinfection and Disease Prevention in Pig Production

Pig farming is an intensive industry in many countries with high numbers of animals kept indoors in large groups. If facilities and husbandry practices are suboptimal, this system of production can lead to problems with infectious disease. Although the carrier pig is highly important in the transmission of many of the most prevalent infections in the pig industry, environmental contamination remains a significant source of infection on many units. Accordingly, cleaning and disinfection is an integral part of internal and external biosecurity procedures and disease control measures in pig production.

Because antimicrobial resistance (AMR) in bacterial pathogens impacts more widely on human and veterinary medicine, there is increasing pressure from bodies such as the WHO, the World Organisation for Animal Health (OIE), and many other national and international scientific groups to reduce antimicrobial use in animal production. Reduced reliance on prophylactic and therapeutic use of antimicrobial drugs in animal production and in the intensive pig and poultry industries in particular requires alterative measures such as increased biosecurity, strategic vaccination use, and improved hygiene practices. Postma et al[216] reported that it was possible to reduce antimicrobial use by 52% in pigs from birth to slaughter on 61 Flemish herds by improving hygiene and increasing the use of vaccines and anthelminthic treatments. However, not all proposed measures were adopted. Thus, although farmers may acknowledge the importance of biosecurity and hygiene measures, they may be slow to implement such measures. In the study by Postma et al,[216] measures that required increased labor and possible reductions in stocking density such as leaving facilities vacant after cleaning and disinfection or always cleaning the loading area after use were implemented by less than half of those given such advice. In addition, even where cleaning and disinfection are carried out on farms and considered effective by the farmer, residual contamination may remain in some locations. Mannion et al[217] reported that *Enterobacteriaceae* counts were significantly reduced on finisher pig pen floors in 14 farms following cleaning and disinfection procedures by the farmer, but feeding troughs within the pens remained highly contaminated. Luyckx et al[218] found that although feeding troughs of nursery pens were clean, drinking nipples were highly contaminated postcleaning and disinfection.

A number of studies have examined efficacy of different disinfectants in the intensive production systems, in both experimental and on-farm settings. McLaren et al[219] carried out extensive studies on the efficacy of several Department of Environment, Food and Rural Affairs (DEFRA)-approved disinfectants for inactivating *Salmonella* serotypes in the poultry industry. Chlorocresol-based disinfectants were highly effective at eliminating *Salmonella* in the presence of feces, whereas the formaldehyde-based products were effective in the dry environment but less so in the wet model. A chlorocresol-based disinfectant (Interkokask®) was also effective when tested in the lairage of a pig abattoir where it reduced levels of *Enterobacteriaceae* below the limit of detection.[220] In an experimental study examining the efficacy of six commercial disinfectants against porcine rotavirus in the presence and absence of organic matter, a phenolic product (Bi-OO-cyst®) was the only compound that was effective in the presence of high levels of organic matter.[117] Another phenolic product, BioPhen™, although not significantly affected by the presence of organic matter, was much less effective against rotavirus than Bi-OO-cyst®. These results illustrate the variability in efficacy of different commercial products, although the principal chemical components may be chemically similar. Other compounds tested by Chandler-Bostock and Mellits[117] including peracetic acid (Vanodox®), glutaraldehyde (GPC8®), and peroxygen-based (peroxymonosulfate, Virkon S®) products inactivated rotavirus only when organic matter contamination levels were low. However, when used to prevent transmission of *L intracellularis* to uninfected pigs, Virkon S® was effective if used after cold-water pressure washing to remove fecal matter.[28]

Gosling et al[221] conducted an extensive study of the efficacy of 15 different disinfectants under conditions simulating those present on pig farms, including the presence of fecal material and biofilm. Incompatibility with detergents or other cleaning agents was also examined. Glutaraldehyde/formaldehyde, peracetic acid, and iodine-based products showed reduced efficacy when used following alkaline detergents, whereas the chlorocresol-based product, Interkokask®, was not inhibited by any of the detergents tested. Interkokask® was also highly effective in the presence of biofilm, as was one of the glutaraldehyde/formaldehyde products (Intercid®) and an iodine-based product (Virophor®). Gosling et al[221] also examined the efficacy of different products under conditions simulating boot dips and surfaces. Differences in efficacy were detected depending on whether a product was used in a boot dip or to disinfect surfaces in a pig unit. This finding highlights the importance of considering the proposed conditions of use of a product when selecting a disinfectant and that one disinfectant may not be suitable for all purposes on a unit.

Hancox et al[222] examined the effect of drying duration following disinfection on total aerobic counts and *Enterobacteriaceae* levels. Results showed that although bacterial counts were reduced following drying for 24 hours, further reductions in counts did not occur when metal surfaces or stock board (recycled plastic product) were left to dry for more than 24 hours after cleaning and disinfection. Addition of a drying interval did not reduce counts on cleaned and disinfected concrete surfaces.

Martelli et al[223] found that intensive cleaning and disinfection of pens by trained contractors was effective in reducing *Salmonella* contamination at slaughter of finisher pigs introduced into cleaned pens. However, these authors emphasized that because of the high level of *Salmonella* carriage in pigs, good cleaning and disinfection practices form only one of a number of measures that should be used to reduce *Salmonella* levels on pig farms.

New approaches to disinfection of pig units include use of activated water or acidified water. However, few peer-reviewed publications evaluating these methods have been published. Slightly acidic electrolyzed water (SAEW) is generated by electrolysis of dilute salt solution; it has pH of 5.0 to 6.5 and contains a high concentration of hypochlorous acid (HOCl, approximately 95%) and the hypochlorite ion (ClO, approximately 5%). Hao et al[224] investigated the effectiveness of SAEW for inactivating microorganisms on the surfaces of pig units and compared it to the efficacy of another oxidizing agent, trichloroisocyanurate, and to povidone-iodine disinfectant. They found that SAEW had comparable efficacy to the trichloroisocyanurate product and performed better than the povidone-iodine disinfectant, and they concluded that SAEW had potential for use in the pig industry. Luyckx et al[225] examined another novel approach to disinfection of pig nursery units based on the principle of competitive exclusion and using a commercial probiotic product. They found that it was less effective than conventional methods of cleaning and disinfection.

Disinfection and Disease Prevention in Poultry Production

Prevention and control of infectious diseases in poultry rely on high standards of hygiene, effective flock management, vaccination, chemoprophylaxis, and disinfection. Vaccination for specific infectious diseases has become a routine and effective measure for the prevention of many infectious diseases of poultry. Chemoprophylaxis for coccidiosis is an established practice in most poultry units with high stocking densities. Although vaccination and medication are effective for a number of infectious diseases, many pathogens of poultry are not amenable to control by these means, and consequently, disinfection is an integral part of disease control programs.

The objective of poultry house disinfection is the elimination of pathogens, especially those of economic or public health importance. Disinfection is routinely recommended after depopulation and before restocking takes place. If carried out in a competent manner, disinfection of a poultry unit can be relied on to reduce the risk of infectious diseases and thereby, enhance production. It can also contribute to disease control measures aimed at reducing the risk of flock infections with pathogens of public health importance, which can be transmitted through poultry meat and eggs. Complete disinfection of a large poultry farm, which is time-consuming and expensive, requires thorough planning, careful selection of disinfectants, and appropriate application methods to ensure success. Attention to detail in the design of the program ensures cost-effectiveness, feasibility, and reliability. Critical evaluation of flock records, a detailed knowledge of building design and quality, the management system, vaccination policy, and the biosecurity measures in place should be assessed before implementation of a disinfection program. Selection of a disinfectant, preparation for disinfection, and the application methods require careful consideration and approval by management and personnel implementing the disinfection program. Factors influencing the choice of disinfectant include its spectrum of activity, dilution rate, cost, application rate, activity in the presence of organic material, and safety for workers. Inclusion of detergents during the cleaning program and optimal contact time and prevailing temperature should also be considered. Because disinfectants are not equally effective against all poultry pathogens, selection of a chemical compound with activity against the infectious agent causing disease in the flock is a requirement for success. Pest control should feature prominently in decisions relating to disinfection. Cleaning and vector control should commence immediately after birds are removed from each building. Vector control measures should be initiated while the building is still warm because ectoparasites tend to retreat from building surfaces into less accessible spaces as the temperature drops. Ectoparasites, rodents, and insect vectors require special control measures relating to design, quality, and age of the building. Rats sometimes shed leptospires in their urine and can transmit these virulent pathogens to domestic mammals and also to humans. In many poultry units, mice may harbor *Salmonella* ser Enteritidis, and accordingly, rodent control measures should feature prominently in building cleaning and preparation.[226] Rats and mice are often attracted to farm buildings because they provide shelter in cold weather and because of the abundance of food available in such buildings. Farm buildings, especially food storage facilities, should be designed to exclude rodents. Feed bins should be rodent proof, and feed spillages should be cleared up promptly to lessen the attraction of rodents and wild birds to farm buildings. Strategic use of rodenticides should form part of a rodent control program. The availability of grain and shelter often attracts wild birds to farmyards and farm buildings. Migratory waterfowl can transmit avian influenza and Newcastle disease to commercial poultry flocks. Native species of wild birds can transmit microbial pathogens such as *Salmonella* species, *Yersinia* species, and *Mycoplasma* species to poultry flocks. All poultry house openings, including ventilation shafts, should be covered with wire mesh to exclude wild birds.

When feasible, cleaning and disinfection should be carried out in all buildings in a poultry enterprise in a coordinated manner to minimize the risk of recontamination of buildings already cleaned and disinfected. Cleaning protocols in broiler houses, which were preceded by overnight soaking with water, resulted in a greater reduction in total aerobic flora than protocols that omitted the overnight presoaking.[227] In addition, soaking of broiler houses resulted in lower water consumption and a reduction in

working time during high pressure cleaning. Drinkers, drain holes, and floor cracks were identified as critical locations for cleaning in broiler houses. Troughs, drinkers, and inaccessible corners require particular attention in routine cleaning procedures. A final rinse of all surfaces with cold water at low pressure is recommended. The building should be allowed to dry overnight before application of disinfectant. Tanks supplying drinking water should be emptied, cleaned, and if necessary disinfected with sodium hypochlorite.

Hatcheries

Egg contamination with bacterial pathogens contributes to poor hatchability and high mortality shortly after hatching is likely to occur. The degree of contamination usually reflects the prevailing hygiene standards of the poultry unit. In some circumstances, up to 20% mortality can occur within days of hatching.[228] Newly hatched chicks are susceptible to many microbial pathogens, and they often acquire infectious agents from debris in incubators. Brooder pneumonia caused by a buildup of spores of *A fumigatus* in incubators can be prevented by strict hygiene standards and fumigation of incubators.

Methods that can be used to reduce egg contamination before hatching include the application of disinfectants by wiping, spraying, or dipping. Fumigation with formaldehyde, treatment with iodophors, fumigation with ozone, and dipping in hydrogen peroxide solution are among the methods that have been used to reduce egg contamination before hatching.[229]

Treatment and Disposal of Waste

After depopulation of the premises, buildings and equipment should be prepared for the arrival of a new batch of birds. There should be strict adherence to hygiene standards in the cleaning and disinfection of each unit. Litter, manure, and other waste material from poultry houses should be stored at a site remote from buildings occupied by birds and composted for up to 2 months before dispersal on arable land. Composting should take place on a site where runoff is minimized by location and design of the holding facility. Alternatively, the material can be removed at regular intervals and, if climatic and environmental factors permit, spread on a suitable site on arable land. If an endemic, infectious disease has occurred on the farm from which the bedding derived, all material should be composted in heaps, sprayed with an appropriate disinfectant, and covered with plastic sheeting to prevent wind dispersal. Identification of an exotic poultry disease on a farm warrants special measures, and all waste material from the farm should be either burned or buried on the farm involved.

Two experimental models, one wet and the other dry, were used to evaluate the efficacy of commonly used disinfectants against *Salmonella* Enteritidis or *Salmonella* ser Typhimurium.[219] In the wet model, a slurry of poultry feces inoculated with *Salmonella* species was treated with disinfectants. In the dry model, *Salmonella*-inoculated poultry feces, which were air-dried onto wooden dowels, were immersed in disinfectants. Chlorocresol-based disinfectants provided consistently high rates of *Salmonella* inactivation in both wet and dry tests. Formaldehyde-containing disinfectants displayed high efficacy in the dry test but were less effective in the wet test. The efficacy of glutaraldehyde without formaldehyde varied between products. The QACs, amphoteric surfactants, iodine preparations, peroxygen compounds, and a substituted phenol blend were only moderately effective. Some disinfectants when used at recommended concentration showed almost no activity against *Salmonella* in dried feces when compared with water alone.

The effects of time, temperature, and organic matter on the efficacy of four commonly used disinfectants against *Staphylococcus aureus* and *Salmonella* Typhimurium were evaluated under simulated field conditions.[230] A QAC, a phenolic disinfectant, a chlorhexidine compound, and a binary ammonium-based solution were used in the studies. In the first study, spanning a range of temperatures and time, all disinfectants tested were effective. In the second study, the addition of sterile chicken litter had an inhibitory effect on the four classes of disinfectants against *Salmonella* Typhimurium. The phenolic compound retained its efficacy against *S aureus*. In the third study, the bactericidal activities of freshly prepared and 30-week-old disinfectants in the presence of organic matter were compared. The presence of organic matter significantly reduced the efficacy of the 30-week-old QAC and the phenolic disinfectant against *Salmonella* Typhimurium. The fresh QAC and the binary compound achieved a greater inactivation of *S aureus* than the 30-week-old quaternary disinfectants.

Nine commercially available disinfectants were evaluated for their virucidal activity against avian metapneumovirus, avian influenza virus, and Newcastle disease virus.[128] The disinfectants used included phenolic compounds, QACs, glutaraldehyde, sodium hypochlorite, peroxyacetic acid, and potassium peroxymonosulfate. Phenolic compounds and glutaraldehyde were found to be the most effective disinfectants against all three viruses. The QACs were effective against avian metapneumovirus but not against the other two viruses.

Swab samples from 50 turkey houses, which had housed *Salmonella*-positive flocks, were collected following cleaning and disinfection.[231] A minimum of 45 swab samples from different surfaces we collected per house and cultured in selective enrichment media for detection of *Salmonella*. The houses in the study were grouped into four categories according to the disinfectants that had been used in each house. The disinfectants used were as follows: phenol-based products, disinfectants containing a mixture of formaldehyde, glutaraldehyde, and QAC, products containing glutaraldehyde, QAC, and phosphoric acid, and products containing hydrogen peroxide and peracetic acid. Following cleaning and disinfection, 68% of houses tested positive for *Salmonella*. Products containing a mixture of formaldehyde, glutaraldehyde, and QAC performed significantly better than products containing hydrogen peroxide and peracetic acid. Houses disinfected with phenol-based products were given an intermediate rating as were houses disinfected with glutaraldehyde, QAC, and phosphoric acid.

Five pathogenic viruses, namely high-pathogenic avian influenza virus H7N1, low-pathogenic avian influenza virus H5N3, bovine parainfluenza virus type 3, feline coronavirus, and feline calicivirus, used as models of important avian pathogens were incorporated into untreated hatchery waste for treatment with ammonia.[232] Bacteriophage MS2 was also monitored as a stable indicator in the hatchery waste. The spiked hatchery waste was treated with different concentrations of ammonia at different temperatures. Feline coronavirus was the most sensitive virus, and the high-pathogenic avian influenza virus was the most resistant virus. The results indicated that ammonia treatment, at the concentrations and temperatures specified, was an efficient method for inactivating enveloped and nonenveloped viruses in hatchery waste. Damage to viral DNA was proposed as the method of viral inactivation. To ensure inactivation of viruses in hatchery waste by ammonia, treatment must take place in a closed container.

The ability of the agricultural herbicide referred to as metam sodium to inactivate low-pathogenic avian influenza virus (an enveloped virus) and infectious bursal disease virus (a nonenveloped virus) was investigated.[233] Treatment with the appropriate concentration of metam sodium for 1 hour inactivated both the enveloped virus and the nonenveloped virus in chicken litter. In the presence of moisture, metam sodium forms a gas, methyl isothiocyanate, which can penetrate litter and act as a fumigant. Methyl isothiocyanate is reported to interact with amino acids, and its ability to inactivate infectious agents is attributed to alteration of protein structures in pathogenic microorganisms.

Animal Waste

Many pathogenic microorganisms are shed in the feces of infected mammals and avian species. *Salmonella* species, *M bovis*, *M avium* subsp *paratuberculosis*, *M avium* complex, *B anthracis*, and *Clostridium tetani* are among the more important bacterial pathogens, which may be shed in animal feces. Porcine parvovirus, bovine viral diarrhea virus, and rotaviruses may be shed in large numbers in feces of infected animals. Fecal oocysts of *C parvum*, *Eimeria* species, and other coccidial oocysts may be shed in feces. Although not shed in feces, *B abortus* and serovars of *Leptospira interrogans* may be present in animal excretions and contaminate liquid manure or stored slurry.

The form and amount of animal waste generated on a farm are determined by the number and species of animals present, building design, and the type of material used for bedding large animals or as poultry litter. In buildings with slatted floors, animal waste is stored in slurry tanks. These tanks should be constructed to high specifications and have ample capacity to ensure that overflowing of contents does not occur. Slurry spreading is usually restricted to defined times of the year when ground conditions are suitable for slurry tankers and when the risk of runoff is low. In many European countries, slurry spreading is restricted by government regulations to specified times of the year. An interval of at least 2 months should elapse between the application of slurry to pasture and the commencement of grazing. If enteric pathogens such as *Salmonella* species or pathogenic acid-fast bacteria are likely to be present in slurry, a longer interval between the application of slurry and the commencement of grazing may be required.

Farmyard manure, typically a mixture of feces, urine, and bedding was formerly stacked adjacent to animal dwellings or stored in purpose-built pits and allowed to compost for long intervals. Composted manure generates temperatures capable of inactivating most pathogens contained in animal excretions. In many European countries, food-producing animals are reared intensively during the winter months on slatted floors and fed, housed, and managed in a system that results in the production of large volumes of slurry. Unlike composted manure, slurry, with its low content of solids, high water content, and alkaline pH, often favors the prolonged survival of microbial pathogens.[234,235] Many months may be required for the natural inactivation of viruses in slurry.[235]

B abortus can survive for more than 8 months in cattle slurry.[82] Methods used for slurry spreading often generate aerosols, which may be potentially hazardous for humans or livestock in close proximity. Spreading of slurry during stormy weather may result in drifting of aerosols with the risk of contamination of adjacent land and watercourses.

In many countries, regulations stipulate a minimum storage period for contaminated animal slurry and specify how land application should be carried out. Long-term storage, if appropriate, or physical, biological, or chemical treatment of slurry may be employed to reduce the risk of infectious agents being spread by contaminated animal waste. Physical methods that have been used include gamma irradiation and heat treatment. Temperatures between 65°C and 100°C for at least 30 minutes have been recommended. Biological treatment methods that have been employed include anaerobic digestion.[236] Chemical disinfection of slurry is a difficult procedure that requires careful planning, accurate estimation of the volume to be

treated, and the availability of appropriate chemical compounds. Where vigorous and sustained agitation of slurry is necessary, specialized equipment may be required. After an outbreak of a notifiable disease, chemical treatment of slurry to ensure inactivation of the pathogens present may be specified in regional or national legislation.

Although the choice of disinfectant is invariably determined by the infectious agents present, aldehydes, acids, oxidizing agents, and alkalis, including ammonium hydroxide, are potentially useful for chemical treatment of slurry.

Formalin, a 35% to 37% solution of formaldehyde in water, has a broad spectrum of activity and can be used at a rate of 25 to 40 L/m^3.[234] At temperatures below 10°C, formalin has little antimicrobial activity. Because of its irritant nature and toxic activity, special care is required when large volumes of formalin are used. An advantage of formalin is that its activity is minimally affected by environmental pH and organic matter. At 20°C, up to 4 days should be allowed for inactivation of pathogens in treated slurry, and at lower temperatures, a longer time may be required. The exceptional resistance of fecal oocysts of pathogenic protozoa such as those of *C parvum* to many chemical disinfectants, including aldehydes, emphasizes the importance of the careful selection of chemical compounds for inactivation of microbial pathogens in slurry.

Peracetic acid, a very strong oxidizing agent, can be used at low ambient temperatures, but because of the large amounts of foam produced, it is not widely used. This chemical can be used at a rate of 25 to 40 L/m^3 with a contact time of 4 hours.

Slaked lime (calcium hydroxide) is sometimes used for treating animal waste, including slurry. When used as a 40% solution, it should be added to slurry at a rate of 40 to 60 L/m^3 with a contact time of at least 4 days.[234] Its activity is minimally influenced by ambient temperature. Advantages of lime treatment include the low cost involved and ease of disposal of treated slurry. However, thorough mixing, which is labor-intensive, may be required and this may take several days. A pH value between 11 and 12 is usually required to ensure inactivation of pathogens treated with alkalis.

Ammonium hydroxide has been used to raise the pH of slurry for inactivation of pathogens. It has the advantage of being a by-product of slurry and, accordingly, increases the fertilization capacity of slurry applied to land. It is readily mixed with animal waste and when used at a 1% concentration in cattle slurry, it will raise the pH to a value above 10.

Sodium hydroxide (caustic soda) used as a 50% solution can be added to slurry at a rate of 16 to 30 L/m^3.[234] An exposure time of 4 days is recommended, and treatment can be carried out at temperatures between 0°C and 10°C. When treated in this manner, the pH of slurry usually rises to a value close to 13. Sodium hydroxide is corrosive for metals, and because it is hazardous for personnel, protective clothing, rubber gloves, and safety glasses should be worn when working with this chemical.

Certain guidelines should be observed in the storage and spreading of slurry. When possible, slurry should be stored for at least 60 days before being spread on pasture. Ideally, slurry should be spread on arable land and plowed into the soil. Following application to pasture, a period of at least 60 days should elapse before the pasture is grazed.

If chemical treatment of slurry is required following an outbreak of a notifiable disease, it is essential that storage tanks should not be full to allow for the addition of chemicals. Thorough mixing must take place to ensure dispersal of the added chemical, which should be introduced to the tank at several points. An aqueous solution of a chemical is preferable to a powdered or granular preparation. Vigorous agitation of slurry for several hours should precede the addition of the selected chemical, and high-performance agitation equipment is required to ensure thorough mixing. Agitation should continue as the chemical is being added and for at least 6 hours afterward. During the treatment period, no new slurry should be added to the tank and stirring should continue for at least 2 hours.

The possible environmental impact of chemically treated slurry should be considered, and dispersal on dry land used for tillage, remote from watercourses, is the preferred choice. If chemically treated slurry has been thoroughly mixed and stored for more than 4 days, damage to vegetation in particular and the environment in general is considered unlikely.

Toxicologic Hazards Associated With Slurry Agitation and Slurry Dispersal

All personnel engaged in slurry agitation or in the addition of chemical disinfectants to slurry prior to the spreading of this form of animal waste on farmland should be informed by supervisory staff of the toxicity of gases produced by slurry decomposition during storage. Toxic gases produced include hydrogen sulfide, carbon dioxide, ammonia, and methane. These gases are released from slurry tanks during slurry agitation immediately before spreading or during the vigorous and sustained agitation required if chemical disinfection of slurry is required following an outbreak of a notifiable disease in animals on the farm.

Hydrogen sulfide, which is slightly heavier than air, accumulates in low-lying, poorly ventilated spaces such as slurry tanks. It has a characteristic "rotten-egg" odor, which can be detected at low concentrations. This toxic gas inactivates mitochondrial cytochrome oxidase, resulting in failure of oxidative metabolism and causing histotoxic hypoxia. All animals should be moved from buildings with slatted floors before slurry agitation commences. Personnel in the vicinity should vacate the buildings and

should not return to the well-ventilated buildings involved for several hours after agitation is completed.

Teat Disinfection in Mastitis Prevention

Despite advances in disease control through development of recommended milking practices, chemotherapy, and disinfection, mastitis remains one of the most common diseases of dairy cattle. It is also of major economic importance because of the resulting decrease in milk production, the cost of treatment, loss of milk sales, and the cost of preventive measures, including teat disinfection, use of internal teat sealants, and dry cow therapy. Additional losses may result from the time required for treatment of affected animals and the cost of culling and replacement of cattle of high genetic potential due to the development of mastitis-related problems.

The usual route of entry of microorganisms that cause intramammary infection in dairy cattle is the teat duct. Transfer of pathogens during milking may be related to the milking cluster, udder cloths, and the milkers' hands. Measures aimed at decreasing the microbial population on teat skin decrease the probability of intramammary infections. Acquisition of infection from contaminated environments also occurs and thus maintenance of good hygiene standards in housing and animal handling areas is of the utmost importance.

S aureus, *Streptococcus agalactiae*, and *Streptococcus dysgalactiae* are the bacteria commonly transmitted through milking machines or during the milking procedure. Other bacteria more widely distributed in the environment, such as *Escherichia coli*, *Streptococcus uberis*, and *Pseudomonas* species, may contaminate the teats between milkings. However, the distinction between "contagious" and "environmental" pathogens is now accepted to be less clear than previously thought, and, for example, some *E coli* isolates appear to cause persistent infections in the mammary gland and some *S aureus* are spread in a more "environmental" manner rather than directly from cow to cow.[237] Disinfection is an important aspect of disease prevention in the dairy industry, and many disinfectants have been developed for preventing the spread of bacteria that cause mastitis. Strategies for the control of mastitis include the proper use of milking machines that are functioning optimally, the application of premilking and postmilking teat disinfectants, treatment of clinical mastitis during lactation, use of internal teat sealants and selective antibiotic therapy at drying off, and culling of chronically infected cows unresponsive to standard treatment.

Disinfectants that are of benefit to the dairy farmer and acceptable to the consumer should meet certain criteria. They should have residual activity after application to the teat skin. They should be nonirritating and nontoxic and should promote healing of lesions on teats. They should remain active in the presence of organic matter such as milk and should not be absorbed into the tissues or leave undesirable residues in milk. Many teat disinfectants are expensive, therefore, cost-effectiveness should be considered. Few commercial disinfectants fulfill all of the criteria sought by farmers and required by consumers.

Teat disinfectants may be applied as dips or as sprays using manual or automated systems. When automated systems are used, it is essential to ensure that they operate correctly. Edmondson[238] described the spread of *S aureus* mastitis in a 135-cow dairy herd because the automatic teat spray missed the outside of the teats. Reintroduction of manual teat dipping in the herd solved the problem.

Most teat disinfectants are based on a limited range of chemicals, including chlorine-releasing compounds, iodophors, QACs, and CHG. Preparations containing other constituents, including natural germicides, have been used to minimize residues and avoid teat irritation. In addition, some products, so-called barrier teat disinfectants, contain components that form a film on the teat that effectively prolong the protection provided by the chemical disinfectant and seal the teat against bacteria.[239] The usefulness of teat disinfectant chemicals has been established using negative control trials over many years, with the result that postmilking teat disinfection is recommended as a standard effective method for reducing the incidence of new intramammary infections by contagious pathogens. It is also recognized, however, that postmilking teat disinfection does not control mastitis pathogens acquired mainly from environmental sources such as *S uberis* and coliform bacteria.[240]

Standard methods for testing the efficacy of teat disinfectants have been developed over a number of years.[241] These methods describe protocols for animal selection, experimental challenge including bacterial culture methods, recording, analysis, and reporting of results. It is noteworthy that negative control trials are now deemed unethical and that positive control trials are standard for evaluation of product efficacy in many countries including EU member states.[242]

There are ample experimental data supporting the use of products as teat disinfectants including products containing iodophors, chlorous acid, chlorine compounds, and chlorhexidine. A document produced by the National Mastitis Council was updated annually until 2009 and provides comprehensive information on teat disinfectants.[243] Using an excised teat assay, 57 teat dip formulations were tested for their germicidal activity against *S aureus*, *S agalactiae*, and *E coli*.[244] Four teat dips containing 4% sodium hypochlorite and three containing glutaraldehyde were effective against the three bacterial pathogens. Formulations containing 1% to 0.5% iodine were not consistently effective against the three test organisms, and teat dips containing 0.5% chlorhexidine also showed inconsistency in their antimicrobial activity. However, although these types of data provide useful preliminary information, excised teat assays are no longer

recommended for product testing because they demonstrate only bactericidal activity and not efficacy of teat disinfectants *in vivo*.[245] For *in vivo* negative control trials, the National Mastitis Council has defined a 40% reduction in new intramammary infections as the minimum a product must achieve before it can be declared effective.[241] Based on these criteria, most of the products tested in the research studies published during the 1990s and summarized below can be considered effective.

An *in vivo* study using controlled experimental challenge infection evaluated two iodophor teat germicides with low iodine concentration against *S aureus* and *S agalactiae*.[246] New intramammary infections with *S aureus* and *S agalactiae* were reduced by 80.7% and 56.6%, respectively, by one iodophor at a concentration of 0.1%.

Three developmental postmilking teat dip formulations containing CHG were evaluated against *S aureus* and *S agalactiae* in sequential experimental exposure trials.[247] Two additional commercial CHG teat dip products were evaluated in natural exposure trials by the same workers. Under conditions of experimental challenge, the developmental formulations were effective against *S aureus* but did not significantly reduce the incidence of new intramammary infections by *S agalactiae*. In the natural exposure trials with negative controls, a 0.35% chlorhexidine teat sanitizer had an efficacy of 88.7% against *S aureus* and 51.4% against *S agalactiae*. The 0.5% chlorhexidine product reduced *S aureus* and *S agalactiae* intramammary infections by 86% and 56%, respectively.

Two postmilking teat dips, one containing chlorous acid with lactic acid as activator and the other chlorous acid with mandelic acid as activator, were tested for their efficacy against experimental challenge by *S aureus* and *S agalactiae*.[248] The teat dip activated with mandelic acid significantly reduced new intramammary infections due to *S aureus* by 68.7% and infections due to *S agalactiae* by 56.4%. The teat dip activated with lactic acid significantly reduced new intramammary infections due to *S aureus* by 69.3% but did not significantly reduce new *S agalactiae* intramammary infections. Neither teat dip affected teat skin condition.

Two teat dip formulations containing sodium dichloroisocyanurate, which released hypochlorous acid as active ingredient, were tested for their efficacy against new *S aureus* and *S agalactiae* intramammary infections using an experimental challenge model[249] and reduced new infection rates by between 65% and 74%, depending on product and pathogen.

A natural exposure trial of 12 months' duration was carried out in a commercial herd of 125 lactating cows to compare the efficacy of an experimental barrier teat dip containing 0.55% CHG with that of a 1% iodophor for preventing new intramammary infections and clinical mastitis.[250] After milking, teats of half the cows were dipped in the experimental barrier product and teats of the other half of the herd were dipped in the 1% iodophor product. Quarters where postmilking teat disinfection with the experimental barrier product was carried out had fewer new intramammary infections caused by *E coli*, coagulase-negative staphylococci, or gram-positive bacilli than quarters where postmilking teat disinfection with the 1% iodophor was used.

Under conditions of experimental challenge, two test germicides applied postmilking, one containing 0.5% CHG and the other an iodophor containing 1% iodine, reduced new intramammary infections caused by *S aureus* and *S agalactiae*.[251] New intramammary infections caused by *S aureus* were reduced by 73.2% with 0.5% chlorhexidine and by 75.6% with the iodophor. The chlorhexidine and iodophor products reduced new intramammary infections caused by *S agalactiae* by 53.9% and 53.5%, respectively. No overall differences in the condition of teat skin or teat ends before or after the trial were evident in control quarters or in quarters treated with either product.

A comparison of the efficacy of postmilking teat disinfection with 4% benzyl alcohol and a 1% iodophor in the prevention of new intramammary infections in lactating cows was carried out by Erskine et al.[252] Five dairy herds participated in a split-herd study to compare the efficacy of the two teat dips. The 1% iodophor teat dip was more effective in the prevention of new intramammary infections caused by *S aureus* and *Corynebacterium bovis* than 4% benzyl alcohol. The rate of new intramammary infections for other pathogens did not differ between the groups.

The effect of two postmilking teat dip barrier products, one containing lactic acid, sodium chloride, and iodine and the other a commercial iodophor teat dip, on colonization by *S aureus* of teat skin after experimental challenge, was investigated.[253] The experiments were carried out during cold, windy conditions with mean daily temperatures close to 0°C. *S aureus* counts tended to be higher on teat skin and in milk from treated teats than control teats. The results from the trial suggested that iodine-based teat disinfectants could negatively interact with chapped teat skin and retard healing during harsh weather.

Three postmilking teat dips were tested for their efficacy against *S aureus* and *S agalactiae* in two separate studies using experimental challenge procedures.[254] The first study evaluated a barrier teat dip product containing chlorous acid–chlorine dioxide as the germicidal agent. The second study evaluated a sodium chlorite product with a barrier component as well as sodium chlorite without a barrier component. The chlorous acid–chlorine dioxide teat dip reduced new intramammary infections caused by *S aureus* by 91.5% and reduced new intramammary infection caused by *S agalactiae* by 71.7%. The barrier dip containing sodium chlorite reduced new intramammary infections caused by *S aureus* and *S agalactiae* by 41% and 0%, respectively. The nonbarrier dip containing sodium chlorite reduced new intramammary infections caused by *S aureus* by 65.6% and new intramammary infections caused by *S agalactiae* by 39.1%.

Recent trials investigating the efficacy of teat disinfection mainly use a positive control design, consider new product types, and address concerns such as residues in milk and effects on biofilm-producing and antimicrobial-resistant organisms. The criterion for establishing efficacy in a positive control trial is that the test product should be at least as effective as a control product that is known to reduce new intramammary infections by 70%.[241] Lago et al[239] investigated a novel glycolic acid-based product using approximately 300 cows in a split-herd natural exposure design. The novel product was compared with a recognized iodine-based disinfectant (positive control). They concluded that the new product was effective because it showed a relative improvement of 17% in reducing new infections compared to the control product. Infections were mostly by coagulase-negative staphylococci and streptococci other than *S agalactiae*. Another natural exposure study investigating a glycolic acid-based product also concluded that the product had equivalent efficacy to a proven iodine-based commercial teat disinfectant.[255] Comparable efficacy was demonstrated for a new hydrogen peroxide–based product versus an established commercial product also based on hydrogen peroxide in an experimental study by Leslie et al.[256] There was no significant difference between the products in the number of new infections by either *S aureus* or *S agalactiae*, and teat skin condition was significantly improved with the new formulation. Martins et al[257] investigated two iodine-based products, one of which had barrier properties and high free iodine levels, in a natural exposure study in two commercial dairy herds. The barrier product with high free iodine content reduced the probability of the cows acquiring a new clinical mastitis infection by 46% compared with the nonbarrier product.

Scientifically reviewed studies employing accepted National Mastitis Council protocols to test the efficacy of unconventional novel teat disinfectants are not yet published. However, some initial studies suggest that teat disinfectants based on cultures of lactobacilli or antimicrobial peptides may be beneficial. Yu et al[258] investigated the effect of a probiotic lactobacilli-based product on somatic cell count (SCC) and bacterial community types in milk collected from a small group of 11 cows over time. They showed a decrease in SCC and a relative reduction in numbers of mastitis-causing bacteria over the course of the trial. Another report indicated that a bacteriocin, Hyicin 4244, was able to prevent biofilm formation by planktonic staphylococcal organisms isolated from bovine mastitis and could also penetrate and kill staphylococci within biofilm during *in vitro* studies.[259]

Programs designed to reduce subclinical mastitis and bulk milk SCCs have been moderately successful. Such programs, which include postmilking teat disinfection, can contribute to a decrease in the prevalence of subclinical mastitis in many herds. However, although postmilking teat disinfection is accepted as part of standard practice for mastitis control, the effectiveness of premilking teat disinfection is not as conclusive. Trials designed to investigate the effect of premilking teat dipping on mastitis caused by environmental pathogens were carried out in nine matched pairs of dairy herds over 24 weeks during the winter housing period.[260] In one group of herds, normal udder preparation was adhered to throughout the trial and an iodophor teat dip was used after milking. In the other nine herds, preparation of all teats at all milking sessions included dipping with an iodine disinfectant (0.25% available iodine) that was left to act for 30 seconds. Each teat was then wiped with a paper towel before cluster attachment. No differences in the overall rate of mastitis or in the incidence of mastitis between the trial groups was evident. Premilking teat dipping appeared to have no effect on total bacterial cell count, milk cell count, or iodine content of bulk tank milk. Oliver et al[261] compared predipping with a 0.25% iodine premilking teat disinfectant to a negative control using a split-udder experimental design in a natural exposure study. All teats were dipped after milking with the same teat dip. New intramammary infections caused by gram-negative bacteria were significantly lower in quarters where premilking and postmilking teat disinfection was applied. Premilking and postmilking teat disinfection was no more successful against *S aureus* and *C bovis* than postmilking teat dipping alone. Williamson et al[262] found no benefit of premilking teat disinfection with a chloramine-T product in a study of three New Zealand dairy herds. The environmental pathogen, *S uberis*, is the most common cause of mastitis in New Zealand and was also the most common pathogen in the three study herds, but differences in new intramammary infection rates were not detected between groups treated with both pre- and postmilking teat disinfection compared to groups treated postmilking only. Another study in five pasture-based herds in Australia found similar results, with no significant differences in new infection rates or cases of clinical mastitis detected between groups receiving premilking teat disinfectant and control groups.[263] However, significantly fewer cases of clinical mastitis were recorded in cows given premilking disinfectant in one of the five study herds where teat soiling was observed, and the authors suggested that premilking teat disinfection may be worthwhile in wet weather if teats are obviously soiled. An additional role for premilking disinfectants is in the reduction of contamination of milk with environmental spoilage organisms that may affect milk processing, including cheese making. Predipping with a commercial detergent and emollient mixture significantly reduced anaerobic spore-forming bacteria on teat skin and in milk in a study by Bava et al.[264] Predipping may be particularly important where cows are fed on ensiled forages or where certain types of bedding materials that contain high levels of endospores are used.

In addition to teat disinfection, environmental hygiene and disinfection of milking parlor equipment is important in mastitis control. Automatic cluster disinfection is employed between every cow in many milking systems. Depending on the disinfectant used, however, this practice may have implications for the liner material. Baxter[265] suggests the usual interval of 2500 milkings between liner changes may have to be reduced by approximately one-third if disinfectants such as peracetic acid are used for flushing clusters between cows. Replacing steam disinfection of an automatic milking system with peracetic acid disinfection was part of a number of measures used to successfully control *S aureus* mastitis in a small dairy herd.[266] Biofilm formation by mastitis-causing organisms is not only associated with persistent infections in the udder[267] but also contributes to problems with environmental contamination. Control of persistent problems with mastitis due to *Pseudomonas* species using disinfection of milking equipment by SAEW was described by Kawai et al.[268] *Pseudomonas* species were isolated not only from mastitis cases but also from hoses, teat liners, and the inside walls of the water tank. Previous use of sodium hypochlorite had failed to remove contamination by *Pseudomonas* species of the milking equipment and milking parlor environment, and the authors suggested that the production of biofilm by the organisms contributed to the problem. Following introduction of the use of SAEW, environmental contamination by *Pseudomonas* species was no longer detected and intramammary infections decreased from approximately 10% of cows to 1%.

Disinfection in Veterinary Hospitals

Recognition of the importance of formal infection control protocols and practices in veterinary hospitals is increasing, and the use of disinfectants is a basic component of such practices. Although much of the information available for human hospitals can be extrapolated for use in the veterinary setting, there are major differences that must be accounted for including higher levels of fecal material, hair and dust, conduct of procedures on floors, and greater sharing of equipment than occurs in human premises. Cleaning and disinfection protocols should be developed in accordance with the species of animal being treated, the principal pathogens being targeted, and the structural features and purpose of the veterinary facility. Hygiene protocols may differ depending on whether a loose box is to be cleaned following a case of *C difficile* diarrhea in a horse or if a kennel area is to be cleaned and disinfected following cases of methicillin-resistant *Staphylococcus pseudintermedius* (MRSP) infection in dogs.

The practice of veterinary medicine has changed in recent decades with an increase in the number of specialized secondary and tertiary referral practices. Such practices frequently deal with animals that have received some treatment previously, often involving antimicrobial use, and as a result, AMR is a particular issue. There are increasing numbers of patients, especially in companion animal practice, which are being treated for chronic illnesses, immunosuppressive conditions, or have received surgical implants. As in human medicine, such patients are at particular risk of acquiring infection with multidrug resistant organisms, and effective infection control procedures are essential to minimize this risk. Some of the organisms causing nosocomial infections in veterinary hospitals are similar to those causing problems in human hospitals, with gram-negative multidrug resistant bacteria of increasing concern in both human and animal medicine.[269] Methicillin-resistant *S aureus* (MRSA) infections are a concern in companion animal hospitals, including equine hospitals, but for dogs and cats, infections with MRSP are possibly of even greater significance.[270,271] Other infectious agents that require control in a small animal veterinary hospital setting include pathogens that cause canine and feline respiratory disease, parvoviruses, and dermatophytes.[272] Apart from MRSA and multidrug resistant gram-negative organisms, pathogens such as *C difficile*, *Salmonella* serotypes, equine influenza virus, rotavirus, and equine herpesviruses 1 and 4 may cause nosocomial infections in equine hospitals.

Infection control in veterinary as well as in human hospitals is multifaceted. Control policies should be clearly defined, comprise written protocols, and be overseen by an individual or individuals with responsibility for the area. Some of the many relevant topics for inclusion are biosecurity and implementation of screening for specific pathogens such as MRSA, procedures for determining whether animals should be admitted to an isolation area, operation of isolation areas, hand hygiene, cleaning and disinfection protocols, surveillance of infections, and monitoring of compliance with protocols.[272] Good hand hygiene practices are well recognized as the cornerstone in controlling hospital acquired infections, but it is acknowledged that in addition to clean hands, equipment and the environment must be clean if the number of infections is to be reduced.[273] Defined cleaning and disinfection protocols are central to this objective. The choice of disinfectant to be used depends on the target pathogens, the surface to be disinfected, toxicity to the user, cost, and other considerations. Although there are relatively few publications detailing the use of specific disinfectants in the control of nosocomial infections in veterinary hospitals, some data are available.

Grönthal et al[271] described the eventual control of a large outbreak of MRSP infections in a veterinary teaching hospital by implementation of a suite of control measures including enhanced cleaning and disinfection procedures. Increased use of alcohol-based hand sanitizers and disinfection with a peroxymonosulfate-based product were specifically mentioned. Bergström et al[274] reported an outbreak of MRSA in an equine teaching hospital and outlined the extensive measures required to control the

outbreak. Specific cleaning and disinfectant products were not described, but it was noted that expenditure on gloves and disinfectants doubled following the implementation of new infection control protocols. Controls implemented during an outbreak of salmonellosis in an equine hospital included steam cleaning, scrubbing surfaces with bleach, and subsequent disinfection with a phenolic product.[275] Ward et al[276] also described the monitoring and control of a *Salmonella* outbreak in an equine hospital. Steam cleaning and disinfection with ammonium chloride and peroxymonosulfate-based products were used successfully in this instance. An outbreak of virulent feline calicivirus infection in a small animal hospital was contained by closure of the hospital for 3 weeks, steam cleaning, and disinfection with a solution of 9.6% hypochlorite diluted 1:30 in water.[277] Eleraky et al[278] tested four disinfectants against feline calicivirus and feline parvovirus *in vitro* and noted that, although chlorine dioxide and potassium peroxymonosulfate were fully effective against these two viruses, the QAC and a grapefruit extract tested had no effect on feline calicivirus.

Fungal spores can persist for prolonged periods in the environment, and contamination with dermatophyte spores may be a concern in veterinary hospitals and animal shelters. However, acquisition of infection by pets from the environment alone, in the absence of direct animal contact, is extremely rare.[279] Although dermatophytes were cultured from 23 of 401 sites monitored in a small animal veterinary teaching hospital over a period of a year, outbreaks of ringworm were not recorded.[280] Nevertheless, environmental decontamination is important, primarily to prevent contamination of the skin and hair of animals under treatment, subsequent false-positive culture results, and unnecessary prolongation of therapy. Cleaning alone can be highly effective in reducing fungal contamination of a premises as well as controlled humidity and wetness within an area. Shampooing of carpets twice with a commercial detergent or hot water treatment using a machine that extracts the water following application is effective. Machine washing of clothes without disinfectant is also successful in removing fungal spores.[279] Disinfectants such as sodium hypochlorite and accelerated hydrogen peroxide compounds are among a number of effective antifungal disinfectants (see Table 52.5).

Methods employed for the application of disinfectants in a veterinary hospital may vary and use of fogging, misting, or spraying may be particularly useful in large animal hospitals. Cold fogging (low-temperature aerosolization) was investigated by Dunowska et al[281] using artificial contamination of surfaces with *S aureus* and *Salmonella* Typhimurium in a large animal hospital. Fogging with a 1% solution of a potassium peroxymonosulfate disinfectant reduced counts of the test organisms by between 1 and 5 log with the exception of counts on a wooden desk where counts were reduced by only 0.02 log. The authors suggested that fogging would be a useful adjunct to cleaning and disinfection protocols particularly for inaccessible areas. Best results were obtained on horizontal nonporous surfaces; activity in the presence of biofilm was not examined. A study by Saklou et al[282] using a 2% solution of peroxymonosulfate disinfectant applied as a directed mist onto vertical smooth surfaces showed much lower reductions of only 0.2 to 1 log. However, the authors used a small volume of disinfectant solution (35 mL/m^2) and suggested that larger volumes and a higher concentration (4%) would have greater effect as demonstrated in a previously published study.[283] Overall, results of these studies suggest that care must be taken of the concentration and volume of product used, in addition to the type of surface to be treated, when disinfecting veterinary premises with fogging or misting. Steam disinfection is another possible choice and was shown to be effective when tested on stainless steel and concrete surfaces in a veterinary hospital.[284] Rapid action, ability to reach inaccessible areas, and lack of toxicity are some of the advantages of using steam. However, steam may not disinfect some surfaces such as rubber effectively and because of the high temperature used, this method is unsuitable for use on some plastic and other materials.[284] Traverse and Aceto[273] suggest that hydrogen peroxide vapor systems may be suited to occasional use in veterinary settings. These systems are effective against a wide range of pathogens, but cost and long room turnaround times are disadvantages.[285]

The use of disinfectant footbaths has been covered elsewhere, but some researchers have specifically examined their usefulness in veterinary hospitals. Footbaths or foot mats containing a potassium peroxymonosulfate product reduced counts on contaminated footwear to a limited extent, by approximately 1 to 1.5 log, in studies by Amass et al[286] and Dunowska et al[281] when footwear was immersed for approximately 2 seconds. Hornig et al[287] tested four disinfectant products using a protocol that involved standing on a foot mat for 3 seconds. They recorded reductions of up to 0.26 log for the potassium peroxymonosulfate and quaternary ammonium products tested and suggested that disinfectant foot mats could be useful adjunct measures in infection control in large animal hospitals. However, when Stockton et al[288] examined the effects of different footwear and disinfection protocols on the number of bacteria recovered from floors in an equine hospital, they could not find consistent differences between treatments.

Specialized equipment such as endoscopes used in veterinary and human hospitals can be difficult to decontaminate due to problems with cleaning including lack of attention to detail on cleaning/disinfection protocols and the potential for biofilm formation.[289] Protocols for reprocessing endoscopes have been developed in human medicine and are also suitable in a veterinary setting. These usually comprise vigorous cleaning of all surfaces (including internal lumens) with a detergent-based cleaning agent, flushing with water and air, followed by soaking in disinfectant. Thorough rinsing with the appropriate quantity of water and drying after disinfection are critical, and drying needs to be performed using pressurized air.[290] Sometimes, additional sterilization using an EO or hydrogen peroxide gas system is employed, where there is evidence of failure of the normal reprocessing procedures.[291] Hydrogen peroxide gas sterilization, if available, is suitable for some endoscope sterilization and is safer and more rapidly acting than EO.[105]

Other equipment such as mobile (cell) phones, stethoscopes, computer keyboards, and other "high hand-touch" surfaces may be possible reservoirs of nosocomial pathogens and must be included when developing cleaning and disinfection protocols for use in animal hospitals.[273] These surfaces require frequent disinfection, and alcohol-based disinfectant wipes are often used for this purpose. Bender et al[292] showed that wiping of computer keyboards with 70% isopropyl alcohol wipes improved cleanliness as measured by a luminometer and significantly reduced recovery of staphylococci. It is important to consider which pathogens may be contaminating surfaces when selecting a disinfection method. Although alcohol wipes are widely used, they are not sporicidal and thus would not be effective for disinfection of hand-touch surfaces during an outbreak of *C difficile* or similar infections in an equine hospital.

Monitoring the effectiveness of cleaning and disinfection practices can be a useful component of infection control in veterinary hospitals. Most published studies report the use of microbiological monitoring, which may include determination of total bacterial counts and/or detection of specific pathogens or indicator organisms. Regular monitoring is required because, in the absence of baseline data, results of sporadic testing are usually difficult to interpret meaningfully. Other methods for environmental monitoring such as use of adenosine triphosphate (ATP) bioluminescence or fluorescence tagging systems may be employed. Weese et al[293] used a small hand-held UV light source to detect whether a fluorescent dye, previously applied to over 500 different sites in a veterinary teaching hospital, was removed, indicating adequate cleaning. The authors concluded this was a cheap, practical, and effective method of monitoring compliance with cleaning protocols. The ATP bioluminescence meters measure the concentration of ATP as relative light units (RLU) in organic material and living cells. Monitoring of cleaning practices using these systems is widely used in the food industry and increasingly in human hospitals. The method is easy, and results are available directly, although there is an initial cost in buying the meter and associated ongoing costs for the swabs used. Ongoing compliance with cleaning protocols in a small animal veterinary hospital can be monitored using this system. In addition, such systems can be used to assess cleaning in situations where there is a high risk of cross-contamination, and it is essential to ensure cleaning is adequate as, for example, postdischarge of an animal with a multidrug resistant pathogen.

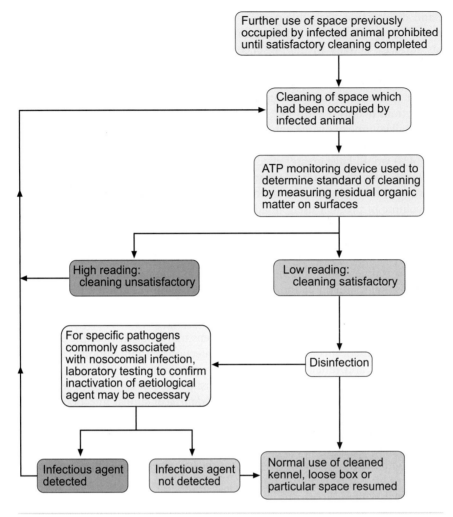

FIGURE 52.10 Evaluation of the effectiveness of cleaning in a hospital space previously occupied by an animal with a confirmed transmissible infectious disease. For particular infectious agents that may be resistant to many commonly used disinfectants or are often associated with nosocomial infection, elimination of the pathogen may require laboratory confirmation. Abbreviation: ATP, adenosine triphosphate.

Other cleaning indicators include the use of various protein or hemoglobin swabbing methods. Figure 52.10 illustrates a possible scheme for the monitoring of the effectiveness of cleaning of hospital areas. A low reading obtained following swabbing of a cleaned space indicates adequate cleaning; disinfection and resumption of use of the area can proceed. If a reading above the set threshold is obtained, further cleaning of the space must be carried out. Threshold values are set for individual premises by repeated monitoring of selected areas during a pilot program. Analysis of these data allows infection control personnel to select appropriate threshold values. Values may differ depending on area, for example, the threshold value for a floor may be set at a higher level than for hand-touch surfaces. The ATP bioluminescence meters are probably most useful in a small animal setting; their use in large animal hospitals is likely to be restricted to cleaner areas such as surgery suites or particular treatment areas.

Disease Control on Stud Farms

An all-in and all-out husbandry policy combined with appropriate cleaning and disinfection of buildings is extremely effective for limiting transmission of pathogens from one group of animals to succeeding groups. As a result, it has become an integral part of modern husbandry practices for the intensive farming of pigs and poultry. It is also appropriate on larger stud farms where the careful design and separation of yards or buildings facilitate such an approach. However, large yards, broodmare barns, and smaller enterprises are generally not managed in such a manner and complete depopulation along with the discarding of all stored feed and bedding may not be realistic or feasible. As a result, there are certain considerations regarding disinfection of equine facilities on stud farms that are worthy of individual attention. A review of the role of disinfection in the control of equine infectious disease is provided by Dwyer.[294] In addition, codes of practice for the equine industry in dealing with infectious diseases are available in many countries, for example those of the Horserace Betting Levy Board (https://codes.hblb.org.uk), the Irish Thoroughbred Breeders' Association (http://www.itba.info/wp-content/uploads/2013/07/Codes-of-Practice-2018-_.pdf), the National Trainers Federation (https://www.racehorsetrainers.org/publications/pdfs/cop.pdf), and the American Association of Equine Practitioners (https://aaep.org/guidelines/infectious-disease-control).

Equine Pathogens

Some pathogens are labile and easily removed from the environment by cleaning and inactivated by disinfection (Table 52.10). However, because some infectious agents are highly contagious and may be shed by carrier animals, exclusion from the farm or premises is the preferred method for controlling such pathogenic agents. Equine influenza virus is an example of a viral pathogen the risk of transmission of which can be minimized by reducing movement of horses on or off the premises and by quarantining all newly arrived horses. Younger horses returning from large gatherings such as race meetings or showjumping competitions are often the source of viral pathogens for animals on the farm. Because influenza A virus is labile and does not survive well in the environment, efforts should concentrate on preventing animals at the acute stage of the disease from entering the farm. Another labile virus, equine arteritis virus, is typically introduced by horses incubating the infection or more importantly by carrier stallions. Serologic screening of breeding animals is essential for identification of suspect animals.

TABLE 52.10 Bacterial and viral pathogens frequently encountered on stud farms

Pathogen	Type	Disease(s)	Comments
Rotavirus	Nonenveloped reovirus	Diarrhea in foals	Relatively resistant, requiring disinfectants effective in the presence of organic matter
Equine herpesvirus 1 and 4	Enveloped viruses	Herpesvirus abortion, respiratory disease, neurologic disease	Labile, easily destroyed by disinfectants, but latently infected horses continue to pose a risk to susceptible animals
Salmonella enterica, various serotypes	Gram-negative bacteria	Salmonellosis, diarrhea, septicemia	Carriers can be a source of ongoing shedding of salmonellae in feces. Cleaning and disinfection of buildings and equipment are essential measures for limiting transmission; important zoonosis
Rhodococcus equi	Gram-positive bacterium	Suppurative bronchopneumonia of young foals	Present in the soil on affected farms
Clostridium species such as *Clostridium perfringens*, *Clostridium difficile*, and *Clostridium tetani*	Gram-positive endospore-producing bacteria	Diarrhea, tetanus	Present in the intestinal tract and soil. Clostridial endospores are resistant to many chemical disinfectants.
Klebsiella species, *Enterobacter* species	Gram-negative bacteria	Metritis, septicemia	Disinfection is usually effective once organic matter is removed but commonly found in the equine environment.
Escherichia coli	Gram-negative bacterium	Wide range of opportunistic infections including diarrhea, metritis, septicemia	Disinfection is usually effective once organic matter is removed but part of gut flora and commonly found in the equine environment. Pathogenicity varies according to strain and virulence factors.
Actinobacillus equuli	Gram-negative bacterium	Septicemia in neonates (sleepy foal disease)	Carried in intestinal and reproductive tracts of dam; present in equine environment
Streptococcus equi	Gram-positive bacterium	Strangles	Highly contagious, acute outbreaks following introduction. Cleaning and disinfection are important control measures. However, a chronic, convalescent carrier state can develop in some animals with persistence of the bacterium in the guttural pouch and intermittent shedding occurring over months or years. Such animals may appear clinically normal.

In contrast with labile viruses, many other potential pathogens such as *Klebsiella* species are carried by normal horses and others such as *R equi* or *Clostridium* species may be present in the environment of susceptible animals. Often, such pathogens require the presence of predisposing factors to establish infection and induce disease. In the case of alpha herpesvirus infections, the ongoing concern is the introduction or presence of latently infected animals that may shed virus without evidence of clinical signs. Cleaning and disinfection programs can be very effective for containing environmental contamination in a single stable or perhaps in a small yard following an acute episode of disease such as a herpesvirus abortion or an outbreak of salmonellosis[295,296] but are of limited benefit in circumstances where carrier animals, for example, subclinical carriers of salmonella or *Streptococcus equi*, are present in the horse population or where infectious agents are widely distributed in feces and in soil on the farm or where infection is carried by vectors such as rodents or birds. The management of horses in separate groups such as broodmares, mares and foals, and yearlings without new introductions or contact with other groups can be a helpful disease control strategy.

Environment

A range of surfaces may be present in the equine environment. Porous, rough materials such as raw wood or concrete are more difficult to clean effectively and disinfect than smooth, nonporous materials such as stainless steel, glass, and enamel-painted surfaces. Raw wood should be varnished with marine-quality varnish or painted with polyurethane to give an impervious, smooth finish. Concrete block should be sealed with a good-quality enamel paint. Surface coverings should be maintained and kept in good condition. Flooring may be more problematic, varying from soil to expensive poured rubber with sealed perimeters to prevent material seeping underneath. Commonly, a poured cement floor topped with bedding materials such as wood shavings, moss peat, shredded paper, and straw for the horse's comfort is used. Such bedding material is very difficult to disinfect but usually can be removed and composted. Dirt floors cannot be disinfected, and the only solution may be the removal of the top 20 to 30 cm and replacement with fresh material. Removable objects such as feed buckets, water containers, and hay mangers should be removed to facilitate cleaning and disinfection of both the stable and its contents. Consideration should also be given to cleaning and disinfecting any equipment that a horse has been in contact with including veterinary equipment, dental equipment, trailers, horse vans, halters, brushes, combs, bridles, and saddles. Ideally, other items such as smaller objects are not shared but used exclusively in association with a particular animal. Following an outbreak of salmonellosis in a large animal veterinary teaching

hospital, Ewart et al[297] conducted an evaluation of the effect of several disinfectants on recovery of salmonella from various surface materials. They found that sodium hypochlorite was the most effective disinfectant on the largest number of surfaces tested but emphasized that removal of all organic material was an essential first step. Hancox et al[222] also found that surface type affected the effectiveness of disinfection when they evaluated the interaction between different bacterial groups and surface materials using a peroxygen compound.

It is unrealistic to disinfect a paddock occupied by animals shedding salmonellae or excreting *R equi*. Manual removal of manure and chain harrowing may help to reduce fecal contamination. Resting the pasture for several weeks may deplete the microbial pathogens, but some microorganisms such as salmonellae are capable of surviving for several months in damp, shaded soil.

Choice of Disinfectant on a Stud Farm

Because there is no ideal disinfectant, selection of a particular chemical compound must relate efficacy to safety. Some disinfectants such as aldehydes are effective but highly toxic for workers and for animals. The presence of residual organic material has a marked inhibitory effect on disinfectants such as sodium hypochlorite. The choice of disinfection should be related to the pathogenic organisms likely to be present and the environment in which it is to be used. Many commercial disinfectants in current use contain mixtures of chemical compounds, and consumers should rely on independent assessment of their efficacy before selecting these commercial products. Purchasers should avoid arbitrary blending of chemical disinfectants because of the possibility of chemical reactions leading to reduction in disinfectant activity or generation of toxic gases.

Disinfection and Biosecurity for Zoologic Gardens and for Wildlife Parks

This section is concerned with collections of nondomesticated, typically exotic species (although not exclusively), open to the public in zoos and wildlife parks. Although there may be areas of common interest with establishments such as wildlife rehabilitation centers, veterinary hospitals catering for wildlife species, crocodile farms, and aviaries, such topics are not specifically covered in this section.

Some animal species being cared for in zoos may be rare, valuable species threatened with extinction. The diverse range of exotic species encountered in zoologic collections presents many challenges for veterinary personnel dealing with issues related to biosecurity. The fungal disease chytridiomycosis, which was first reported in large outbreaks in Australia in recent years, has resulted in high mortality in frogs through the formation of skin lesions that interfere with their ability to respire through their skin. This disease has resulted in dramatic amphibian population declines in California, Central America, and in regions of South America. Consequently, it is essential that fungal pathogens etiologically implicated in this devastating disease are excluded from collections of susceptible species and are not inadvertently introduced into regions currently free of this disease.[298] Disease control measures for animals in zoos may apply to fish, amphibians, reptiles, avian species, and mammals. In addition to their roles in education of those who visit zoos, many aspire to become centers of animal conservation and breeding. To achieve this objective, their standard of animal husbandry for diverse species must include consideration of environmental temperature control, nutrition, and patterns of behavior related to animal breeding. Failure to provide suitable surroundings and appropriate diets could have a direct impact on animal welfare relating to their interactions with members of homologous species such as chimp bands or avian flight patterns in confined spaces. Because of the unique requirements of some species and the wide range of infectious agents to which they may be susceptible, exclusion of pathogenic microorganisms may be difficult to achieve. Textbooks such as *Fowler's Zoo and Wild Animal Medicine*[299] provide a useful introduction to many of the infectious agents, which may be encountered in exotic species. The risk of visitors to zoos acquiring a disease of animal origin is an important consideration as zoonotic agents can be easily acquired in such surroundings. Transmission of infectious agents from humans to animals should be clearly understood and a "One Health" approach relating the ease of transmission of infectious agents from humans to animals and from animals to humans is a principle that has wide application in biology and public health aspects of disease transmission. This "One Health" policy should identify basic rules for staff caring for animals and visitors to premises housing exotic species of animals. Information relating to control of infectious diseases in zoologic collections is available on the Internet, which provides extensive sources of scientific data relevant to animals kept in zoologic collections and also on wildlife species. There are a number of excellent, readily available publications that specialize in this area. Both the American Association of Zoo Veterinarians (AAZV) and the European Association of Zoo and Wildlife Veterinarians (EAZWV) have produced very useful publications on infectious diseases that threaten zoologic collections, the *Infectious Disease of Concern to Captive and Free Ranging Animals in North America*[300] and the *Transmissible Diseases Handbook*,[301] respectively. In particular, the chapter by Kiupel et al[301] on "Guidelines for Cleaning and Disinfection in Zoological Gardens" in the EAZWV publication has proven to be a very useful reference source. In addition, the Zoo and Aquarium

Association (ZAA) of Australia and New Zealand have, in collaboration with the Australian Government and others, produced the *National Zoo Biosecurity Manual*.[302] These publications are a reflection of the excellent tradition of sharing specialist knowledge between individuals and institutions involved in the care of zoo animals. There is also a significant amount of legislation, enacted in many countries, that regulates zoologic collections. This legislation tends to be largely concerned with animal welfare and the disease risks associated with animal/human interaction. The National Association of State Public Health Veterinarians[303] has produced a compendium of measures for prevention of disease associated with animals in public settings. According to AAZV guidelines, a preventive medicine program should be in place in every zoo.[304] Such programs should include strictly enforced quarantine protocols, infectious disease screening, vermin control, immunization schedules, and parasite surveillance. Zoos and fauna parks are included within the remit of the Australian Veterinary Emergency Plan (AUSVETPLAN), which is a coordinated national response plan for the control and where possible eradication of exotic diseases known as emergency animal diseases (EAD). As a result, an *Enterprise Manual: Zoos*[305] has been produced by the Australian government.

Appropriate sanitary and disinfection practices are essential for the prevention, control, and containment of infectious diseases in zoos or wildlife parks. Nursery facilities for young captive animals are of particular importance, and both feeding utensils and animal accommodation require high hygiene standards.[306] The two practices complement one another greatly, disinfection cannot be expected to compensate for poor hygienic practices. In any case, a clean environment is also an attractive and necessary feature in a public venue. This section aims to provide some guiding principles and to highlight some unique features with regard to cleaning and disinfection programs in zoologic collections. However, each individual zoo needs to develop its own detailed and specific protocols that will take into account the range of animal species as well as diverse accommodation types and building designs. The disease control procedures need to be practical and to become an integral part of routine husbandry practices in the zoo. Where a specific infectious disease has occurred, then detailed information regarding the transmission routes, environmental stability, and effective disinfectants is required. The individual fact sheets in the *Transmissible Diseases Handbook* (http://www.eazwv.org/page/inf_handbook) and in the AAZV *Infectious Disease Manual*[300] provide disease-specific information about prevention and control. The psittacosis guidelines provided by National Association of State Public Health Veterinarians should be consulted in the case of infected birds.[307] In addition, the National Association of State Public Health Veterinarians have published a compendium of measures for prevention of rabies.[308]

Disinfection is most effective for diseases acquired by indirect contact. For example, disinfection of facilities was a key component in the successful eradication of *Shigella flexneri* from primates at the National Zoological Collection in Washington, DC.[309] However, disinfection will not prevent the risk of insect-borne or vermin-associated infections such as West Nile virus and leptospirosis, respectively. Additionally, it will not eliminate risks associated with the introduction of animals or personnel harboring infections such as tuberculosis or food sources containing salmonellae. In recent years, the threat of avian influenza introduction by contact with native wild birds such as pigeons or ducks attracted to water features and supplemental feed has become a concern.[310] Therefore, routes of entry, spread within, and possible dispersal outside the confines of the zoo must be considered when developing a comprehensive and effective disease control program. Routes of entry will include introduction of new animals, free-ranging species such as birds, rodents, and feral dogs/cats, feedstuffs, water sources, vehicles, zoo personnel, visitors, bedding, semen, and embryos. Spread within a zoologic gardens could be facilitated by movement of personnel, the public, feeding utensils, tools, vehicles, vermin, and flies. Possible modes of dispersal of infection beyond the zoo include exchange of animals between zoos, personnel (in particular where there is contact with pets/farm animals outside of working hours or where neonatal animals are brought home for hand rearing), removal of waste, free-ranging animals such as birds, rodents, and feral dogs/cats, vehicles, effluent, dead animals sent for disposal or postmortem examination, sick animals removed to veterinary hospitals for specialist treatment, and visitors to the premises. An effective cleaning and disinfection plan can mitigate some of the risks posed. For example, vehicles can be properly decontaminated, but the public is unlikely to accept the imposition of a cleaning and disinfection regime or the use of personal protective equipment. As a result, a strict cleaning and disinfection regime incorporated into daily routines becomes a mandatory measure. Every building and facility should have a tailored program that is revised at frequent intervals, following the occurrence of an infectious disease or prior to introducing new animals into the facility. Sanitation procedures and their proper implementation comprise several components including thorough scrubbing and power hosing, training of personnel, proper food storage, handling and distribution, removal of uneaten food, timely removal of animal waste and bedding, selection of suitable cleaning agents, and assessment of water quality. The disinfection process is the last step in a cleaning and disinfection program. It aims to eliminate pathogens and minimize the microbial load to very low levels. Lists of evaluated disinfectants are available from bodies such as the DEFRA and the German Veterinary Medical Society. The number of chemical disinfectant products has increased in recent years. Traditionally,

zoos have opted for broad-spectrum disinfectant such as ortho-phenylphenol while using QAC for routine sanitization and sodium hypochlorite in clean areas free of organic material.[306] It is important to consider the possible toxicity or caustic nature of many disinfectants. Consequently, animals should be removed from their quarters to permit a proper cleaning and disinfection program to be implemented and to protect the animals from any toxic effects. Once completed and after a suitable exposure time, the facilities need to be rinsed and ventilated before animals are allowed to return.

The Association of Zoos and Aquariums (AZA) has accreditation standards that insist on staff training on the risks of zoonotic disease. Since 2005, the National Association of State Public Health Veterinarians and the Centers for Disease Control and Prevention (CDC) have published a Compendium of Measures to Prevent Disease Associated With Animals in Public Settings. The compendium highlights published cases (Table 52.11) and is largely aimed at managing health risks to the public associated with animal contact at agricultural fairs and open farms. However, the measures are also applicable to petting zoos and zoologic gardens that include a pet's corner or facilitate human interaction with animals such as handling snakes, stroking rabbits, pony rides, and similar activities. A suspect case of rabies in a bear cub in a petting zoo that involved the CDC tracing 200 visitors from across 10 US states and from Australia[314] is illustrative of the significant challenge when dealing with the risk of human infection following animal contact. Such animal attractions are particularly appealing to children. However, the risk of serious illness is particularly high in children under the age of 5 years. Some of this vulnerability is due to their immature immune system, whereas other aspects relate to behavior such a placing small items in the mouth, sucking of thumbs or soothers, and a general lack of awareness of danger. One approach to reduce the risk is to adequately separate animals and humans. Good facility design can greatly help to ensure that the public does not have contact with animals or their wastes by using double barriers, restricted areas, locked doors/gates, and signage. However, there are significant educational and psychological benefits from having contact with animals and the associated risks need to be managed. Eliminating all risk associated with animal contact is not possible, but it is feasible to minimize risks. As a rule, contact with animals should only take place in controlled settings where measures are in place to reduce the potential for disease transmission.

Hand washing is one of the most important disease prevention methods, but it must be facilitated by the presence of sufficient numbers of suitable stations. Ensuring compliance with hand washing advice and the insistence on the correct procedure can be an issue. During investigation of an outbreak of *E coli* O157:H7 in Canadian children following a visit to a petting zoo, it was found that running water for washing hands was not available,

TABLE 52.11	Examples of zoonotic disease incidents in zoos (including petting zoos)			
Disease	**Pathogen**	**Animal Species Involved**	**Comments**	**Reference**
Salmonellosis	*Salmonella ser* Enteritidis	Komodo dragon	Associated with touching a wooden barrier around a temporary exhibit	Friedman et al[311]
Enteritis	Shiga toxin–producing *Escherichia coli* O157:H7	Goat	Inadequate hand washing facilities at a petting zoo	David et al[312]
Enteritis	Shiga toxin–producing *E coli* O157:H7	Sheep and goats	Large outbreak (155 cases)	Warshawsky et al[313]
Rabies	Rabies virus	Bear	Handling of a bear cub that died following acute neurologic signs; initial diagnostic tests were positive but could not be confirmed.	Centers for Disease Control and Prevention[314]
Ringworm	*Microsporum canis*	Tiger	Hand rearing of a tiger cub	Scott[315]
Cowpox	Orthopoxvirus similar to cowpox virus	*Felidae* species and anteaters	Zoo attendant affected	Marennikova et al[316]
Monkeypox	Monkeypox virus	Prairie dogs	Prairie dogs housed by pet distributor alongside wild African rodents; 70 people exposed, 9 clinical cases	Kile et al[317]
Fish tank granuloma	*Mycobacterium marinum*	Fish species	Human cases associated with cleaning out fish tanks	Gray et al[318] and Lewis et al[319]
Tuberculosis	*Mycobacterium tuberculosis*	Elephant	12 elephant handlers affected	Michalak et al[320]
Tuberculosis	*Mycobacterium bovis*	Rhinoceros and monkeys	7 animal handlers exposed	Stetter et al[321]
Tuberculosis	*M tuberculosis*	Elephant, rhinoceros, and Rocky Mountain goat	Staff exposure in a large city zoo	Oh et al[322]
Tuberculosis	*Mycobacterium pinnipedii*	Sea lions	Several animal keepers infected	Kiers et al[323]
B virus infection	Macacine herpesvirus 1	Rhesus macaque monkey	Worker at a primate center splashed in the eye, fatal encephalomyelitis	Centers for Disease Control and Prevention[324]
Ornithosis	*Chlamydia psittaci*	Avian species	Pneumonia in a staff member at Copenhagen zoo	Christensen et al[325]
Shigellosis	*Shigella flexneri*	Barbary macaque, orangutan	Animal keeper developed dysentery.	Lederer et al[326]

signs recommending hand washing were absent, and hand sanitizers were placed at a level too high for most of the children to reach.[312] Education has a very important part to play in highlighting potential risks to the public and encouraging correct and timely hand washing. There is evidence that people who are knowledgeable about potential risks are less likely to become ill in these circumstances.[327] Washing with soap and water is considered optimal. Alcohol-based (60%-70% alcohol) hand sanitizers are considered to be the next best thing, but washing with soap and water should always be encouraged to take

place as soon as possible after leaving the animal housing area. Poor design of facilities can lead to visitor congestion and less compliance with hand hygiene advice.

Enteric bacteria and parasites are considered to pose the highest risk of human disease following human-animal interaction in public settings.[328] In one US study,[329] the percentage causes of the total number of enteric illnesses attributable to animal contact were estimated to be *Campylobacter* species (42%), nontyphoidal *Salmonella enterica* (29%), *Cryptosporidium* species (26%), non-O157 Shiga toxin–producing *E coli* (STEC) strains (2%), and

STEC O157:H7 (1%). Many of these pathogens have a low infectious dose and may be carried by clinically healthy animals. The primary route of infection is fecal-oral, and transmission can occur following contact with contaminated skin, feathers, fur, scales, and saliva, which can harbor these microorganisms. Contaminated surfaces such as barriers and contact with animal bedding or floor surfaces can also facilitate transmission. The removal of animals with diarrhea or that show signs of illness from areas of public contact is a sensible precautionary measure. However, animals may shed pathogens intermittently and show few, if any, signs and yet manage to significantly contaminate the environment with pathogens such as *Salmonella*. Some animal species that are considered to be of higher risk in terms of transmission include amphibians, reptiles, and birds. Shedding of certain pathogens such as *C psittaci* and salmonellae are known to increase because of stress induced by overcrowding, confinement, handling, transport, and commingling. In certain circumstances, diseases such as psittacosis can give rise to significant mortality.[330] Amphibians and reptiles are known to frequently carry and shed salmonella. A large outbreak of *Salmonella* Enteritidis in visitors to Denver Zoological Gardens was found to be associated with touching a temporary wooden barrier around a Komodo dragon exhibit.[311] Interestingly, children who washed their hands after visiting the exhibit were significantly less likely to become ill. Good hand hygiene practices are essential in reducing disease risks following human-animal interactions, and legislation may be used to enforce the provision of suitable sanitation stations.[331] Compliance by the public with hand hygiene advice needs to be encouraged through active interventions such as good quality signage combined with personnel offering hand disinfectant solution and verbal reminders by personnel to visitors to clean their hands before leaving the animal display area.[332]

▶ FACTORS THAT MAY CONTRIBUTE TO FAILURE OF A DISINFECTION PROGRAM

Designing and implementing a successful disinfection program require effective cleaning of all surfaces by an experienced workforce, the careful selection of a disinfectant suitable for the circumstances in which it is being used, and an awareness of the pathogenic microorganisms likely to be present. Thorough cleaning of all surfaces before application of disinfection is essential for the inactivation of infectious agents because the antimicrobial activity of many chemical compounds is seriously impaired by residual organic material such as feces, blood, exudates, food, and bedding. Even moderate amounts of organic matter interfere with the activity of halogen disinfectants, particularly sodium hypochlorite, whereas phenolic disinfectants retain much of their activity in similar

circumstances. For optimal activity, disinfectants should be used at the correct concentration and allowed sufficient contact time with the surfaces or equipment being treated. Failure of a disinfection program may result from human factors such as delegation of cleaning to an inexperienced workforce, disinfection factors including selection of an unsuitable chemical compound for the pathogens present, environmental factors, particularly the presence of organic material on surfaces or equipment, and the presence of large numbers of resistant infectious agents such as coccidial oocysts, pathogenic mycobacteria, or bacterial endospores (Table 52.12). Disinfection is but one component of a properly designed biosecurity program, and any deficiencies that occur in these disease-exclusion measures can permit the reintroduction of infectious agents into buildings or facilities already cleared of pathogenic microorganisms by chemical disinfection.

Microbial Resistance to Disinfection

Disinfectants are used extensively for limiting the spread of bacterial and viral pathogens where animals are reared and where food of animal origin is prepared for human consumption. Chemical compounds with antimicrobial activity are also used for dealing with surfaces or equipment contaminated with fungal or protozoal pathogens. The continuous use of chemical disinfectants as part of a biosecurity program in veterinary medicine and for other purposes in agriculture and also in human medicine could potentially lead to the emergence of bacterial resistance to these important antimicrobial compounds. If used under suboptimal conditions, bacteria treated with disinfectants may survive the treatment. Conditions that can contribute to such developments include incorrect dilution, the presence of residual organic material, or the incorrect application of the disinfection to surfaces or equipment. Although resistance to disinfectants is less common among bacteria than antibiotic resistance, different veterinary pathogens including *E coli*, *Campylobacter* species, *Listeria* species, staphylococci, and *Pseudomonas* species have demonstrated resistance to different classes of disinfectants.[333,334]

A number of resistance mechanisms to disinfectants are used by bacteria, and many of these overlap with the mechanisms that facilitate antibiotic resistance.[169] These include target site modification, alteration in cell permeability, active efflux of disinfectant from the bacterial cell, and resistance associated with bacterial populations within biofilms. Disinfectants against which bacterial resistance has been demonstrated include formaldehyde, glutaraldehyde, chlorhexidine, triclosan, and QAC. The majority of bacterial species with demonstrable resistance to disinfectants are gram-negative but, in addition, *S aureus* and some *Mycobacterium* species exhibit resistance to chemical disinfectants. Intrinsic bacterial resistance is a feature of many gram-negative bacteria

TABLE 52.12	Factors that may adversely affect the outcome of a disinfection program or contribute to its failure			
Human Factors	**Disinfectant Factors**	**Environmental Factors**	**Nature, Number, and Resistance of the Infectious Agents Present**	**Comments**
Inexperienced workforce Inadequate supervision of cleaning staff Protective clothing, footwear, and associated items not provided for workers Disinfectant selected inappropriate for the infectious agents likely to be present and not prepared in accordance with the manufacturers' recommended concentration	Selected disinfectant ineffective against the pathogens present Too dilute to be effective Insufficient contact time allowed Temperature too low for optimal activity Relative humidity too low for gaseous disinfectants Loss of potency due to improper storage such as warm and bright conditions, storage for an extended period following dilution or use after its expiry date	Residual organic matter due to inadequate cleaning Improper application of disinfectant to surfaces, equipment, or transport vehicles Lack of contact with infectious agents due to nature of surfaces Inactivation of quaternary ammonium compounds and biguanides by residual soaps and detergents Inadequate treatment of water supply to contaminated buildings	The presence of large numbers of specific infectious agents such as coccidial oocysts, bacterial endospores, pathogenic mycobacteria, or parvoviruses, which are resistant to many chemical disinfectants, requires the careful selection of suitable disinfectants to ensure their inactivation.	Because the antimicrobial activity of disinfectants does not persist, infectious agents can be reintroduced into buildings or equipment by carrier animals, fomites, rodents, wild birds, transport vehicles, or on the footwear or clothing of personnel.

such as members of the *Enterobacteriaceae* and among *Pseudomonas* species. Structural components of the outer cell membranes of these bacteria are a barrier to the entry of some disinfectants. Gram-positive endospore-forming bacteria possess an intrinsic resistance to many disinfectants. The multilayered endospore structure provides an effective physical barrier to many potentially deleterious influences such as heat, UV light, dehydration, and chemical disinfectants, treatments, which would effectively inactivate vegetative bacterial cells.

Efflux pumps are membrane-associated proteins that eliminate a range of structurally dissimilar toxic compounds from the cytoplasm of bacterial cells. Five classes of efflux pumps, which are widely distributed among bacteria, are described.[169] In gram-positive bacteria, genes encoding efflux pumps are frequently located on plasmids. Among gram-negative bacteria, transporters are located on plasmids or in some instances on chromosomes. Bacteria resistant to various classes of disinfectants can exhibit cross-resistance to some important antibiotics used for treatment of animals.

Many bacterial populations are associated with surfaces and grow as a biofilm rather than as planktonic cells. The resistance of such microorganisms to disinfectants is frequently associated with biofilm formation. In both natural and engineered ecosystems, bacteria, some potentially pathogenic, can grow as biofilms. Bacterial biofilms constitute the prevalent way of growing for many bacteria, and this form of existence affords a greater tolerance to antimicrobial compounds than occurs with planktonic bacteria.[335] The term *biofilm* is used to describe a bacterial population enclosed in a self-produced polymer matrix adhering to each other or to inert surfaces or to viable structures such as tissue cells. Formerly, much experimental research relating to biofilms was carried out on single-strain biofilms. Natural biofilms, however, are typically composed of multiple species of bacteria, and the presence of different bacterial species renders the structure and function of such biofilms difficult to interpret.[336] Growth as a biofilm is considered to have a protective role for the enclosed bacteria, which promotes survival in unfavorable environments.

Biofilm formation involves a number of sequential steps.[337] Bacterial cells in the biofilm are held together by an extracellular matrix composed mainly of exopolysaccharide, proteins, lipids, and nucleic acid. Formation of a biofilm occurs in response to extracellular signals deriving from the initiating bacteria and from environmental sources. For biofilm formation, bacteria must attach to a surface and special bacterial components are required for adhesion. Following attachment to a surface, the bacteria autoaggregate into microcolonies. Subsequently, the bacteria produce exopolysaccharide matrix that surrounds and binds the microbial population, resulting in the formation of complex three-dimensional structures. A final stage in the process is detachment and dispersal of bacteria from the biofilm and colonization of new surfaces by the released bacteria. The composition of biofilm matrices varies according to the bacterial species present and environmental conditions. One matrix exopolysaccharide, a polymer of β-1,6-N-acetyl-D-glucosamine, is produced by *E coli*, *S aureus*, *Yersinia pestis*, and *Actinobacillus* species.

Benefits for the enclosed bacteria deriving from biofilms include resistance to chemical disinfectants, antibiotics, and host immune defences.[335]

Biofilms found in natural and industrial environments are resistant to bacteriophages, amoebas, and chemical disinfectants. Interference with the ability of disinfectants to penetrate biofilms may be a factor that contributes to the resistance of bacteria in biofilms to disinfectants.[336] Numerous studies confirm that multispecies biofilms are generally more resistant to the antibacterial effect of disinfectants than monospecies biofilms.

Pathogenic bacteria of veterinary importance, which are capable of forming biofilms, include *Actinobacillus pleuropneumonia*, *Trueperella pyogenes*, *B anthracis*, *Brucella melitensis*, *Clostridium perfringens*, strains of *E coli*, *Leptospira* species, *Mycobacterium* species, *Yersinia* species, *Salmonella* species, and *Staphylococcus* species. There are indications that biofilm formation by pathogenic bacteria may promote their survival in the environment and in the host. A point of particular importance associated with biofilms is that bacterial interactions in spatially organized biofilms can promote bacterial tolerance to chemical disinfectants. An additional concern relates to the possibility that pathogen persistence is favored by the protection afforded by resident flora.[335]

◗ CONCLUSION

Prevention and control methods appropriate for infectious diseases are determined by their status in the country, public health significance, and importance internationally. Implementation of control measures is ultimately determined by the country's financial resources and the expertise of those with responsibility for planning and implementing the eradication or control program at a regional or national level. The success of a disease control program is determined by the feasibility of the procedure, the reliability of the diagnostic tests, reservoirs of infection, and the national resources available for implementation of the eradication program. A number of well-defined measures can be used for the prevention and control of infectious diseases within a country or in a region of a country. These include, exclusion of suspect animals, quarantine at point of entry and isolation and slaughter of infected animals if an exotic disease is confirmed by clinical or laboratory tests. If infectious diseases are endemic in a country, control measures include vaccination, chemotherapy, and chemoprophylaxis. Effective control measures relating to the environment, animal waste, and animal products are central to the success of a disease eradication program. These include chemical decontamination of buildings, equipment, transport vehicles, footwear, and clothing. Effective cleaning followed by thorough disinfection is essential for the elimination of microbial pathogens from farm buildings, transport vehicles, and equipment. Successful integration of an effective disinfection program

into a disease control plan requires the application of relevant scientific knowledge on the part of those designing and implementing control measures. An understanding of the fundamental concepts relating to transmission of infectious agents and the role of chemical compounds in the inactivation of pathogenic microorganisms provides essential information for personnel engaged in the planning and implementation of disinfection programs. Staff involved in the cleaning of buildings, equipment, or transport vehicles should, ideally, have experience in this area. Alternatively, they should be instructed on the procedures involved and their work should be closely supervised.

On farms or animal production units, which have effective disease control policies as part of management structures, biosecurity should feature prominently. Biosecurity incorporates a series of measures that combine practical decisions such as those relating to purchase of replacement animals, disposal of animal waste, and design of cleaning and disinfection programs. If properly implemented, biosecurity should minimize the risks of disease transmission among animals on the farm and reduce risks of acquiring disease from external sources such as rodents, wildlife, and migrating birds.

Although chemical disinfectants are extensively used for preventing the transmission of infectious diseases in animals, they also have a central role in the prevention of zoonotic diseases. When environmental contamination of animal origin contributes to the spread of pathogenic microorganisms, disinfectants can interrupt and sometimes prevent the spread of zoonotic agents. *C parvum*, a zoonotic protozoan parasite that can cause enteric disease in a wide range of young ruminants, also infects humans. Infective oocysts, shed in feces in large numbers, are resistant to environmental conditions and also to commonly used disinfectants. In addition to foodborne transmission, waterborne transmission can occur. Outbreaks of cryptosporidiosis have been associated with contamination of public water supplies in a number of countries. Because the fecal oocysts are resistant to conventional chemical agents added to drinking water, including chlorine, water supplies are periodically contaminated with these resistant oocysts. In a number of outbreaks of waterborne cryptosporidiosis in the human population, water contamination by ruminant feces was the suspected cause of the disease outbreaks. In recent years, chemical disinfectants that can inactivate the fecal oocysts of *C parvum* have been developed. These compounds offer the possibility of reducing environmental contamination in buildings housing young susceptible ruminants and also of decreasing the widespread dissemination of oocysts due to fecal dispersion, which can contribute to contamination of public water supplies. A number of fungal diseases of animals are transmissible to humans. Dermatophytes, fungal pathogens, which cause ringworm in domestic animals, are readily acquired from infected animals. In cattle, *Trichophyton verrucosum* can be transmitted to humans by contact with the superficial lesions produced by this fungal pathogen. Ringworm in dogs and cats caused by *M canis* infects humans, especially children. Extensive environmental contamination with the arthrospores of *M canis* can occur in buildings occupied by infected animals. Disinfection is an effective means of dealing with environmental contamination caused by the arthrospores of *M canis*.

Disinfection is but one component of the measures that form part of a biosecurity program for control and prevention of infectious diseases in animal populations. Its effectiveness is influenced by the mode of spread of infectious agents, the nature of the pathogen involved, and the thoroughness of the disinfection program itself. Removal of all traces of organic matter from contaminated surfaces followed by the application of a chemical compound known to be effective against the infectious agents likely to be present are essential for the successful implementation of a disinfection program. Because no single chemical disinfectant has characteristics that render it suitable for every purpose and circumstance where it may be required, at farm level, in food processing, or in veterinary hospitals, the selection and use of disinfectants for particular purposes and environmental conditions requires a clear understanding of their antimicrobial spectra and their limitations. Disinfectants such as aldehydes have a wide antimicrobial spectrum, whereas other chemical compounds such as biguanides are limited in their antimicrobial activity. Cost, availability, stability, inactivation by organic matter, and toxicity are features that influence the selection, safety, and general use of many chemical compounds on the farm, in food processing industries, or for specific aspects of disease control programs. For particular chemical compounds with known toxicity for wildlife, fish, or other aquatic species, there should be strict adherence to the manufacturer's disposal instructions. Because disinfectant solutions containing phenolic compounds are potentially toxic for workers, domestic animals, wildlife, and aquatic species, runoff from buildings where these chemicals have been used should not be discharged directly into streams, rivers, or lakes. Where possible, wastewater containing disinfectants should be discharged into slurry tanks, liquid holding tanks, or composting sites to allow for dilution, inactivation, or degradation before land application.

A number of realistic alternatives to routine and unnecessary use of toxic chemical disinfectants may be feasible. Improved animal management systems that incorporate building designs which promote animal welfare, could decrease reliance on chemical disinfectants. Hot water or steam cleaning of surfaces or equipment with the inclusion of suitable detergent if required can inactivate vegetative bacteria, fungi, mycobacteria, and enveloped viruses. In many instances, however, chemical disinfectants are indispensable for the successful implementation of disease eradication programs. To ensure success, the selection, use, application, and limitations of these compounds should be understood by those implementing such programs. With careful selection, accurate dilution and judicious use of disinfectants, tissue residues, food tainting, and environmental pollution can be readily avoided while still ensuring destruction of microbial pathogens of zoonotic and veterinary importance.

ACKNOWLEDGMENTS

The facilities and support provided by the librarian, Carmel Norris, and the staff of the Veterinary Library, University College Dublin are acknowledged with gratitude. The constructive criticism of the authors' colleagues is also acknowledged.

REFERENCES

1. World Organisation for Animal Health. Feeding the world better by controlling animal diseases. World Organisation for Animal Health Web site. http://www.oie.int/for-the-media/editorials/detail/article/feeding-the-world-better-by-controlling-animal-diseases/. Accessed May 23, 2018.
2. Wray C. Survival and spread of pathogenic bacteria of veterinary importance within the environment. *Vet Bull.* 1975;45:543-550.
3. Pirtle EC, Beran GW. Virus survival in the environment. *Rev Sci Tech.* 1991;10:733-748.
4. Scanlon MP, Quinn PJ. The survival of *Mycobacterium bovis* in sterilized cattle slurry and its relevance to the persistence of this pathogen in the environment. *Ir Vet J.* 2000;53:412-415.
5. Brown P, Gajdusek DC. Survival of scrapie virus after 3 years' internment. *Lancet.* 1991;337:269-270.
6. Erwig LP, Gow NA. Interactions of fungal pathogens with phagocytes. *Nat Rev Microbiol.* 2016;14:163-176.
7. Brown L, Wolf JM, Prados-Rosales R, Casadevall A. Through the wall: extracellular vesicles in Gram-positive bacteria, mycobacteria and fungi. *Nat Rev Microbiol.* 2015;13:620-630.
8. Himsworth CG. The danger of lime use in agricultural anthrax disinfection procedures: the potential role of calcium in the preservation of anthrax spores. *Can Vet J.* 2008;49:1208-1210.
9. Milstone AM, Passaretti CL, Perl TM. Chlorhexidine: expanding the armamentarium for infection control and prevention. *Clin Infect Dis.* 2008;46:274-281.
10. Maillard JY, Russell AD. Viricidal action and mechanisms of action of biocides. *Sci Prog.* 1997;80:287-315.
11. Teixeira AG, Machado VS, Caixeta LS, Pereira RV, Bicalho RC. Efficacy of formalin, copper sulfate, and a commercial footbath product in the control of digital dermatitis. *J Dairy Sci.* 2010;93:3628-3634.
12. Fjeldaas T, Knappe-Poindecker M, Bøe KE, Larssen RB. Water footbath, automatic flushing, and disinfection to improve the health of bovine feet. *J Dairy Sci.* 2014;97:2835-2846.
13. Quilez J, Sanchez-Acedo C, Avendaño C, del Cacho E, Lopez-Bernard F. Efficacy of two peroxygen-based disinfectants for inactivation of *Cryptosporidium parvum* oocysts. *Appl Environ Microbiol.* 2005;71:2479-2483.
14. Fan C, Ye X, Ku Z, et al. Beta-propiolactone inactivation of coxsackievirus A16 induces structural alteration and surface modification of viral capsids. *J Virol.* 2017;91:e00038-17.
15. Zonta W, Mauroy A, Farnir F, Thiry E. Virucidal efficacy of a hydrogen peroxide nebulization against murine norovirus and feline calicivirus, two surrogates of human norovirus. *Food Environ Virol.* 2016;8:275-282.
16. Linley E, Denyer SP, McDonnell G, Simons C, Maillard JY. Use of hydrogen peroxide as a biocide: new consideration of its mechanisms of biocidal action. *J Antimicrob Chemother.* 2012;67:1589-1596.

17. Goyal SM, Chander Y, Yezli S, Otter JA. Evaluating the virucidal efficacy of hydrogen peroxide vapour. *J Hosp Infect*. 2014;86:255-259.

18. Fichet G, Antloga K, Comoy E, Deslys JP, McDonnell G. Prion inactivation using a new gaseous hydrogen peroxide sterilization process. *J Hosp Infect*. 2007;67:278-286.

19. Ding N, Neumann NF, Price LM, et al. Kinetics of ozone inactivation of infectious prion protein. *Appl Environ Microbiol*. 2013;79: 2721-2730.

20. Gerba CP. Quaternary ammonium biocides: efficacy in application. *Appl Environ Microbiol*. 2015;81:464-469.

21. Melin VE, Potineni H, Hunt P, et al. Exposure to common quaternary ammonium disinfectants decreases fertility in mice. *Reprod Toxicol*. 2014;50:163-170.

22. Zhang C, Cui F, Zeng GM, et al. Quaternary ammonium compounds (QACs): a review on occurrence, fate and toxicity in the environment. *Sci Total Environ*. 2015;518-519:352-362.

23. Fotheringham VJ. Disinfection of livestock production premises. *Rev Sci Tech*. 1995;14:191-205.

24. Carrique-Mas JJ, Breslin M, Snow L, McLaren I, Sayers AR, Davies RH. Persistence and clearance of different *Salmonella* serovars in buildings housing laying hens. *Epidemiol Infect*. 2009;137:837-846.

25. Hill AA, Simons RL, Swart AN, Kelly L, Hald T, Snary EL. Assessing the effectiveness of on-farm and abattoir interventions in reducing pig meat-borne salmonellosis within E.U. member states: salmonella in pigs intervention analysis. *Risk Anal*. 2016;36:546-560.

26. Neill SD, Bryson DG, Pollock JM. Pathogenesis of tuberculosis in cattle. *Tuberculosis*. 2001;81:79-86.

27. Pollock JM, Rodgers JD, Welsh MD, McNair J. Pathogenesis of bovine tuberculosis: the role of experimental models of infection. *Vet Microbiol*. 2006;112:141-150.

28. Collins AM, Fell SA, Barchia IM. Cleaning and disinfection with Virkon S significantly reduces *Lawsonia intracellularis* survival and transmission to naive pigs. *J Swine Health Prod*. 2013;21:144-147.

29. Bocian E, Grzybowska W, Tyski S. Evaluation of mycobactericidal activity of selected chemical disinfectants and antiseptics according to European standards. *Med Sci Monit*. 2014;20:666-673.

30. Boothe HW. Antiseptics and disinfectants. *Vet Clin North Am Small Anim Pract*. 1998;28:233-248.

31. Bruins G, Dyer JA. Environmental considerations of disinfectants used in agriculture. *Rev Sci Tech*. 1995;14:81-94.

32. Dagher D, Ungar K, Robison R, Dagher F. The wide spectrum high biocidal potency of Bioxy formulation when dissolved in water at different concentrations. *PLoS One*. 2017;12:e0172224.

33. de Jong R. *Determination of Veterinary Bactericidal Activity of Virkon-S Against Coxiella burnetii in High Soiling Conditions*. Lelystad, Netherlands: Central Veterinary Institute; 2011. Report no. 11/CVI0408/JOR/sn.

34. Elkholy YS, Hegab AS, Ismail DK, Hassan RM. Evaluation of a novel commercial quaternary ammonium compound for eradication of mycobacteria, HCV, and HBV in Egypt. *J Microbiol*. 2016;54(1): 39-43.

35. Holton J, Shetty N, McDonald V. Efficacy of "Nu-Cidex" (0.35% peracetic acid) against mycobacteria and cryptosporidia. *J Hosp Infect*. 1995;31:235-237.

36. Jeffrey DJ. Chemicals used as disinfectants: active ingredients and enhancing additives. *Rev Sci Tech*. 1995;14:57-74.

37. Lemarié RJ, Hosgood G. Antiseptics and disinfectants in small animal practice. *Compend Contin Educ Pract Vet*. 1995;17:1339-1350.

38. Malloch RA, Stoker MG. Studies on the susceptibility of *Rickettsia burnetii* to chemical disinfectants, and on techniques for detection small numbers of viable organisms. *J Hyg (Lond)*. 1952;50:502-514.

39. McDonnell G, Russell AD. Antiseptics and disinfectants: activity action and resistance. *Clin Microbiol Rev*. 1999;12:147-179.

40. Russell AD. Microbial susceptibility and resistance to chemical and physical agents. In: Collier L, Balows A, Sussman M, eds. *Tapley and Wilson's Microbiology and Microbial Diseases*. Vol 2. 9th ed. London, United Kingdom: Arnold; 1998:149-184.

41. Russell A, Hugo W, Ayliffe G. *Principles and Practice of Disinfection, Preservation, and Sterilization*. 3rd ed. Oxford, United Kingdom: Blackwell Science.

42. Scott GH, Williams JC. Susceptibility of *Coxiella burnetii* to chemical disinfectants. *Ann N Y Acad Sci*. 1990;590:291-296.

43. Widmer AF, Frei R. Decontamination, disinfection, and sterilization. In: Murray PR, Barron EJ, Pfaller MA, et al, eds. *Manual of Clinical Microbiology*. Washington, DC: ASM Press; 1999:138-164.

44. Båverud V. *Clostridium difficile* diarrhea: infection control in horses. *Vet Clin North Am Equine Pract*. 2004;20:615-630.

45. World Organisation for Animal Health, World Health Organization, Food and Agriculture Organization of the United Nations. *Anthrax in Humans and Animals*. 4th ed. Geneva, Switzerland: World Health Organization; 2008.

46. Manchee RJ, Broster MG, Stagg AJ, Hibbs SE. Formaldehyde solution effectively inactivates spores of *Bacillus anthracis* on Scottish island of Gruinard. *Appl Environ Microbiol*. 1994;60:4167-4171.

47. Hussaini SN, Ruby KR. Sporicidal activity of peracetic acid against *Bacillus anthracis* spores. *Vet Rec*. 1976;98:257-259.

48. Lensing HH, Oei HL. A study of the efficacy of disinfectants against anthrax spores. *Tijdschr Diergeneeskd*. 1984;109:557-563.

49. March JK, Pratt MD, Lowe CW, et al. The differential effects of heat-shocking on the viability of spores from *Bacillus anthracis*, *Bacillus subtilis*, and *Clostridium sporogenes* after treatment with peracetic acid- and glutaraldehyde-based disinfectants. *Microbiologyopen*. 2015;4:764-773.

50. Müller B, Dürr S, Alonso S, et al. Zoonotic *Mycobacterium bovis*–induced tuberculosis in humans. *Emerg Infect Dis*. 2013;19:899-908.

51. Olea-Popelka F, Muwonge A, Perera A, et al. Zoonotic tuberculosis in human beings caused by *Mycobacterium bovis*—a call for action. *Lancet Infect Dis*. 2017;17:e21-e25.

52. Barbier E, Rochelet M, Gal L, Boschiroli ML, Hartmann A. Impact of temperature and soil type on *Mycobacterium bovis* survival in the environment. *PLoS One*. 2017;12(4):e0176315.

53. Russell AD. Activity of biocides against mycobacteria. *Soc Appl Bacteriol Symp Ser*. 1996;25:87S-101S.

54. Collins FM, Montalbine V. Mycobactericidal activity of glutaraldehyde solutions. *J Clin Microbiol*. 1976;4:408-412.

55. Holton J, Nye P, McDonald V. Efficacy of selected disinfectants against mycobacteria and cryptosporidia. *J Hosp Infect*. 1994;27:105-115.

56. Sattar SA, Best M, Springthorpe VS, Sanani G. Mycobactericidal testing of disinfectants: an update. *J Hosp Infect*. 1995;30(suppl): 372-382.

57. van Klingeren B, Pullen W. Comparative testing of disinfectants against *Mycobacterium tuberculosis* and *Mycobacterium terrae* in a quantitative suspension test. *J Hosp Infect*. 1987;10:292-298.

58. Ascenzi JM. Standardization of tuberculocidal testing of disinfectants. *J Hosp Infect*. 1991;18(suppl A):256-263.

59. Ascenzi JM, Ezzell RJ, Wendt TM. A more accurate method for measurement of tuberculocidal activity of disinfectants. *Appl Environ Microbiol*. 1987;53:2189-2192.

60. Lind A, Lundholm M, Pedersen G, Sundaeus V, Wåhlén P. A carrier method for the assessment of the effectiveness of disinfectants against *Mycobacterium tuberculosis*. *J Hosp Infect*. 1986;7:60-67.

61. Fisher CW, Fiorello A, Shaffer D, Jackson M, McDonnell G. Aldehyde-resistant mycobacteria associated with the use of endoscope reprocessing systems. *Am J Infect Control*. 2012;40:880-882.

62. McDonnell GE. *Antisepsis, Disinfection, and Sterilization: Types, Action, and Resistance*. 2nd ed. Washington, DC: ASM Press; 2017.

63. Whiley H, Keegan A, Giglio S, Bentham R. *Mycobacterium avium* complex—the role of potable water in disease transmission: *Mycobacterium avium* complex in potable water. *J Appl Microbiol*. 2012;113:223-232.

64. Weese JS. Infection control in veterinary practice; the time is now. *J Small Anim Pract*. 2011;52:507-508.

65. Murray A, Dineen A, Kelly P, et al. Nosocomial spread of *Mycobacterium bovis* in domestic cats. *J Feline Med Surg*. 2015;17:173-180.

66. Roberts T, O'Connor C, Nuñez-Garcia J, de la Rua-Domenech R, Smith NH. Unusual cluster of *Mycobacterium bovis* infection in cats. *Vec Rec*. 2014;174:326.

67. More SJ, Radunz B, Glanville RJ. Lessons learned during the successful eradication of bovine tuberculosis from Australia. *Vec Rec*. 2015;177:224-232.

68. O'Hagan MJ, Matthews DI, Laird C, McDowell SW. Herd-level risk factors for bovine tuberculosis and adoption of related biosecurity measures in Northern Ireland: a case-control study. *Vet J*. 2016;213: 26-32.

69. Department for Environment, Food and Rural Affairs. List of approved disinfectants for use in England, Scotland and Wales. http://disinfectants.defra.gov.uk/DisinfectantsExternal/Default.aspx?Module=ApprovalsList_SI. Accessed May 24, 2018.

70. Richards WD, Thoen CO. Chemical destruction of *Mycobacterium bovis* in milk. *J Food Prot*. 1979;42:55-57.

71. Best M, Sattar SA, Springthorpe VS, Kennedy ME. Efficacies of selected disinfectants against *Mycobacterium tuberculosis*. *J Clin Microbiol*. 1990;28:2234-2239.

72. Rutala WA, Cole EC, Wannamaker NS, Weber DJ. Inactivation of *Mycobacterium tuberculosis* and *Mycobacterium bovis* by 14 hospital disinfectants. *Am J Med*. 1991;91:267S-271S.

73. Broadley SJ, Jenkins PA, Furr JR, Russell AD. Anti-mycobacterial activity of biocides. *Lett Appl Microbiol*. 1991;13:118-122.

74. Broadley SJ, Furr JR, Jenkins PA, Russell AD. Antimycobacterial activity of "Virkon." *J Hosp Infect*. 1993;23:189-197.

75. Best M, Springthorpe VS, Sattar SA. Feasibility of a combined carrier test for disinfectants: studies with a mixture of five types of microorganisms. *Am J Infect Control*. 1994;22:152-162.

76. Robison RA, Osguthorpe RJ, Carroll SJ, Leavitt RW, Schaalje GB, Ascenzi JM. Culture variability associated with the U.S. Environmental Protection Agency tuberculocidal activity test method. *Appl Environ Microbiol*. 1996;62:2681-2686.

77. De Groote MA, Gibbs S, de Moura VC, et al. Analysis of a panel of rapidly growing mycobacteria for resistance to aldehyde-based disinfectants. *Am J Infect Control*. 2014;42:932-934.

78. Falkinham J. Common features of opportunistic premise plumbing pathogens. *Int J Environ Res Public Health*. 2015;12:4533-4545.

79. Hsu MS, Wu MY, Huang YT, Liao CH. Efficacy of chlorine dioxide disinfection to non-fermentative Gram-negative bacilli and non-tuberculous mycobacteria in a hospital water system. *J Hosp Infect*. 2016;93:22-28.

80. Corbel M, MacMillan A. Brucellosis. In: Collier L, Balows A, Sussman M, eds. *Topley and Wilson's Microbiology and Microbial Infections*. 9th ed. London, United Kingdom: Arnold; 1998:819-847.

81. Jones G. The epidemiology of bovine brucellosis. *State Vet J*. 1976; 31:7-17.

82. Verger JM. Prevalence and survival of *Brucella* species in manures. In: Walton JR, White EG, eds. *Communicable Diseases Resulting From Storage, Handling, Transport and Landspreading of Manures*. Luxembourg: Commission of the European Communities; 1982: 157-160.

83. Scott Williams Consulting. *Persistence of Disease Agents in Carcases and Animal Products*. Canberra, Australia: Animal Health Australia; 2003.

84. Quinn PJ. An investigation of the activity of selected disinfectants against *Brucella abortus*. *Ir Vet J*. 1984;38:86-94.

85. Hall R. The activity of chlorhexidine gluconate against *Brucella abortus*. *Vet Rec*. 1979;105:305-306.

86. Mansi W, Lakin C. In vitro activity of povidone-iodine using *Brucella abortus* (strain 19) as the test organism. *Vet Rec*. 1968;82:444.

87. Plommet M, Plommet A. Destruction par le xylène de diverses bacteries pathogènes dans le lisier de bovins. *Ann Rech Vet*. 1974;5:213-221.

88. Corbel MJ. *Brucellosis in Humans and Animals*. Geneva, Switzerland: World Health Organization; 2006.

89. Bowman SM, Free SJ. The structure and synthesis of the fungal cell wall. *Bioessays*. 2006;28:799-808.

90. Ene IV, Walker LA, Schiavone M, et al. Cell wall remodeling enzymes modulate fungal cell wall elasticity and osmotic stress resistance. *MBio*. 2015;6(4):e00986.

91. Mattei AS, Madrid IM, Santin R, Schuch LF, Meireles MC. In vitro activity of disinfectants against *Aspergillus* spp. *Braz J Microbiol*. 2013;44:481-484.

92. DeBoer DJ, Moriello KA, Cairns R. Clinical update on feline dermatophytosis: part II. *Compend Contin Educ Pract Vet*. 1995;17:1471-1480.

93. Rycroft AN, McLay C. Disinfectants in the control of small animal ringworm due to *Microsporum canis*. *Vet Rec*. 1991;129(11):239-241.

94. Moriello KA. Kennel disinfectants for *Microsporum canis* and *Trichophyton* sp. *Vet Med Int*. 2015;2015:853937.

95. Moriello KA, Hondzo H. Efficacy of disinfectants containing accelerated hydrogen peroxide against conidial arthrospores and isolated infective spores of *Microsporum canis* and *Trichophyton* sp. *Vet Dermatol*. 2014;25:191-194.

96. Moriello KA, Kunder D, Hondzo H. Efficacy of eight commercial disinfectants against *Microsporum canis* and *Trichophyton* spp. infective spores on an experimentally contaminated textile surface. *Vet Dermatol*. 2013;24:621-623.

97. Madrid IM, Mattei AS, Santin R, dos Reis Gomes A, Cleff MB, Meireles MC. Inhibitory effect of sodium hypochlorite and chlorhexidine digluconate in clinical isolates of *Sporothrix schenckii*. *Mycoses*. 2012;55:281-285.

98. Noll H, Younger JS. Virus-lipid interactions: the mechanism of adsorption of lipophilic viruses to water insoluble polar lipids. *Virology*. 1959;8:319-343.

99. Klein M, Deforest A. Principles of viral inactivation. In: Block SS, ed. *Disinfection, Sterilization, and Preservation*. 3rd ed. Philadelphia, PA: Lea & Febiger; 1983:422-434.

100. Prince HN, Prince DL, Prince RN. Principles of viral control and transmission. In: Block SS, ed. *Disinfection, Sterilization, and Preservation*. 4th ed. Philadelphia, PA: Lea & Febiger; 1991:411-444.

101. Prince HN, Prince DL. Principles of viral control and transmission. In: Block SS, ed. *Disinfection, Sterilization, and Preservation*. 5th ed. Philadelphia, PA: Lippincott Williams & Wilkins; 2001:543-571.

102. Sellers RF. The inactivation of foot-and-mouth disease virus by chemicals and disinfectants. *Vet Rec*. 1968;83:504-506.

103. Blackwell JH, Graves JH, McKercher PD. Chemical inactivation of swine vesicular disease virus. *Br Vet J*. 1975;131:317-322.

104. Spaulding EH. Chemical disinfection and antisepsis in the hospital. *J Hosp Res*. 1957;9:5-31.

105. Weese JS. Cleaning and disinfection of patient care items, in relation to small animals. *Vet Clin North Am Small Anim Pract*. 2015;45:331-342.

106. McDonnell G, Burke P. Disinfection: is it time to reconsider Spaulding? *J Hosp Inf*. 2011;78:163-170.

107. Evans DH, Stuart P, Roberts DH. Disinfection of animal viruses. *Br Vet J*. 1977;133:356-359.

108. Slavin G. A reproducible surface contamination method for disinfectant tests. *Br Vet J*. 1973;129:13-18.

109. Gallina L, Scagliarini A. Virucidal efficacy of common disinfectants against orf virus. *Vet Rec*. 2010;166:725.

110. Ferrari M, Gualandi GL, Minelli MF. A study on the sensitivity of bovine rotavirus to some chemical agents. *Microbiologica*. 1986;9: 147-150.

111. Kurtz JB, Lee TW, Parsons AJ. The action of alcohols on rotavirus, astrovirus, and enterovirus. *J Hosp Infect*. 1980;1:321-325.

112. Brown TT. Laboratory evaluation of selected disinfectants as virucidal agents against porcine parvovirus, pseudorabies virus, and transmissible gastroenteritis virus. *Am J Vet Res*. 1981;42:1033-1036.

113. Derbyshire JB, Arkell S. The activity of some chemical disinfectants against Talfan virus and porcine adenovirus type 2. *Br Vet J*. 1971;127:137-142.

114. Martin H, Le Potier MF, Maris P. Virucidal efficacy of nine commercial disinfectants against porcine circovirus type 2. *Vet J*. 2008;77:388-393.

115. Kim HB, Lyoo KS, Joo HS. Efficacy of different disinfectants in vitro against porcine circovirus type 2. *Vet Rec*. 2009;164:599-600.

116. Royer RL, Nawagitgul P, Halbur PG, Prem SP. Susceptibility of procine circovirus type 2 to commercial and laboratory disinfectants. *J Swine Health Prod.* 2001;9:281-284.

117. Chandler-Bostock R, Mellits KH. Efficacy of disinfectants against procine rotavirus in the presence and absence of organic matter. *Lett Appl Microbiol.* 2015;61:538-543.

118. Shen DT, Crawford TB, Gorham JR, McGuire TC. Inactivation of equine infectious anaemia virus by chemical disinfectants. *Am J Vet Res.* 1977;38:1217-1219.

119. Nemoto M, Bannai H, Tsujimura K, Yamanaka T, Kondo T. Virucidal effect of commercially available disinfectants on equine group A rotavirus. *J Vet Med Sci.* 2014;76:1061-1063.

120. Saknimit M, Inatsuki I, Sugiyama Y, Yagakami K. Virucidal efficacy of physicochemical treatments against coronaviruses and parvoviruses of laboratory animals. *Exp Anim.* 1988;37:341-345.

121. Watanabe Y, Miyata H, Sato H. Inactivation of laboratory animal RNA-viruses by physicochemical treatment. *Exp Anim.* 1989;38:305-311.

122. Sanekata T, Fukuda T, Miura T, et al. Evaluation of the antiviral activity of chlorine dioxide and sodium hypochlorite against feline calicivirus, human influenza virus, measles virus, canine distemper virus, human herpesvirus, human adenovirus, canine adenovirus and canine parvovirus. *Biocontrol Sci.* 2010;15:45-49.

123. Mahnel H, Herlyn M. Stabilität von Teschen-, HCC-, ND-, und Vacciniavirus gegenüber 5 desinfektions wirkstoffen. *Zentralbl Veterinarmed B.* 1976;23:403-411.

124. Nomura Y, Ohita C, Shirahata T, et al. Virucidal effect of disinfectants on several animal viruses. *Research Bulletin of Obihiro University.* 1991;17:103-107.

125. McGavin D. Inactivation of canine parvovirus by disinfectants and heat. *J Small Anim Pract.* 1987;28:523-535.

126. Scott FW. Virucidal disinfectants and feline viruses. *Am J Vet Res.* 1980;41:410-414.

127. Zonta W, Mauroy A, Farnir F, Thiry E. Comparative virucidal efficacy of seven disinfectants against murine norovirus and feline calicivirus, surrogates of human norovirus. *Food Environ Virol.* 2016;8:1-12.

128. Patnayak DP, Prasad AM, Malik YS, Ramakrishnan MA, Goyal SM. Efficacy of disinfectants and hand sanitizers against avian respiratory viruses. *Avian Dis.* 2008;52:199-202.

129. Springthorpe VS, Sattar SA. Chemical disinfection of virus-contaminated surfaces. In: Straub CP, ed. *Critical Reviews in Environmental Control.* Vol 20. Boca Raton, FL: CRC Press; 1990:169-229.

130. Thurman RB, Gerba CP. Molecular mechanisms of viral inactivation by water disinfectants. *Adv Appl Microbiol.* 1988;33:75-105.

131. Snodgrass DR, Herring AJ. The action of disinfectants on lamb rotavirus. *Vet Rec.* 1977;101:81.

132. Shirai J, Kanno T, Inoue T, Mitsubayashi S, Seki R. Effects of quaternary ammonium compounds with 0.1% sodium hydroxide on swine vesicular disease virus. *J Vet Med Sci.* 1997;59:323-328.

133. Blackwell JH. Comparative resistance of San Miguel sea lion virus and vesicular exanthema of swine virus to chemical disinfectants. *Res Vet Sci.* 1978;25:25-28.

134. Stone SS, Hess WR. Effects of some disinfectants on African swine fever virus. *Appl Microbiol.* 1973;25:115-122.

135. Wright HS. Test method for determining the viricidal activity of disinfectants against vesicular stomatitis virus. *Appl Microbiol.* 1970;19:92-95.

136. Kennedy MA, Mellon VS, Caldwell G, Potgieter LN. Virucidal efficacy of the newer quaternary ammonium compounds. *J Am Anim Hosp Assoc.* 1995;31:254-258.

137. Cromeans T, Park GW, Constantini V, et al. Comprehensive comparison of cultivable norovirus surrogates in response to different inactivation and disinfection treatments. *Appl Environ Microbiol.* 2014;80:5743-5751.

138. Morino H, Fukuda T, Miura T, Lee C, Shibata T, Sanekata T. Inactivation of feline calicivirus, a norovirus surrogate, by chlorine dioxide gas. *Biocontrol Sci.* 2009;14:147-153.

139. Wright HS. Virucidal activity of commercial disinfectants against velogenic viscerotropic Newcastle disease virus. *Avian Dis.* 1974;18:526-530.

140. Jordan FT, Nassar TJ. The survival of infectious bronchitis (IB) virus in an iodophor disinfectant and the influence of certain components. *J Appl Bacteriol.* 1973;36:335-341.

141. Ritchie BW, Pritchard N, Pesti D, et al. Susceptibility of avian polyomavirus to inactivation. *J Avian Med Surg.* 1993;7:193-195.

142. Wainwright KE, Lagunas-Solar M, Miller MA, et al. Physical inactivation of *Toxoplasma gondii* oocysts in water. *Appl Environ Microbiol.* 2007;73:5663-5666.

143. Wainwright KE, Miller MA, Barr BC, et al. Chemical inactivation of *Toxoplasma gondii* oocysts in water. *J Parasitol.* 2007;93:925-931.

144. Shahiduzzaman M, Dyachenko V, Keidel J, Schmäschke R, Daugschies A. Combination of cell culture and quantitative PCR (cc-qPCR) to assess disinfectants efficacy on *Cryptosporidium* oocysts under standardized conditions. *Vet Parasitol.* 2010;167:43-49.

145. Heymann DL, ed. *Control of Communicable Diseases Manual.* Washington, DC: American Public Health Association; 2015:614-617.

146. MacKenzie WR, Hoxie NJ, Proctor ME, et al. A massive outbreak in Milwaukee of cryptosporidium infection transmitted through the public water supply. *N Engl J Med.* 1994;331:161-167.

147. Samuelson J, Bushkin GG, Chatterjee A, Robbins PW. Strategies to discover the structural components of cyst and oocyst walls. *Eukaryotic Cell.* 2013;12:1578-1587.

148. Fayer R. Effect of sodium hypochlorite exposure on infectivity of *Cryptosporidium parvum* oocysts for neonatal BALB/c mice. *Appl Environ Microbiol.* 1995;61:844-846.

149. Najdrowski M, Joachim A, Daugschies S. An improved *in vitro* infection model for viability testing of *Cryptosporidium parvum* oocysts. *Vet Parasitol.* 2007;150:150-154.

150. Keidel J, Daugschies A. Integration of halofuginone lactate treatment and disinfection with p-chloro-m-cresol to control natural cryptosporidiosis in calves. *Vet Parasitol.* 2013;196:321-326.

151. Naciri M, Mancassola R, Fort G, Danneels B, Verhaeghe J. Efficacy of amine-based Keno™Cox on the infectivity of *Cryptosporidium parvum* oocysts. *Vet Parasitol.* 2011;179:43-49.

152. Dresely I, Daugschies A, Lendner M. Establishment of a germ carrier assay to assess disinfectant efficacy against oocysts of coccidian parasites. *Parasitol Res.* 2015;114:273-281.

153. Shahiduzzaman M, Daugschies A. Therapy and prevention of cryptosporidiosis in animals. *Vet Parasitol.* 2012;188:203-214.

154. Kuticic V, Wikerhauser T. Studies on the effects of various treatments on the viability of *Toxoplasma gondii* tissue cysts and oocysts. *Curr Top Microbiol Immunol.* 1996;219:261-265.

155. Kuticic V, Wikerhauser T. Effects of three disinfectants on the viability of *Toxoplasma gondii* oocysts. *Periodicum Biologorum.* 1993;95:345-346.

156. Alves Neto AF, Bandini LA, Nishi SM, et al. Viability of sporulated oocysts of *Neospora caninum* after exposure to different physical and chemical treatments. *J Parasitol.* 2011;97:135-139.

157. Williams RB. Laboratory tests of phenolic disinfectants as oocysticides against the chicken coccidium *Eimeria tenella. Vet Rec.* 1997;141:447-448.

158. Prusiner SB. Novel proteinaceous infectious particles cause scrapie. *Science.* 1982;216:136-144.

159. Zhang Z, Zhang Y, Wang F, et al. De novo generation of infectious prions with bacterially expressed recombinant prion protein. *FASEB J.* 2013;27:4768-4775.

160. Prusiner SB. Prion diseases and the BSE crisis. *Science.* 1997;278:245-251.

161. Wilesmith JW. Epidemiology of bovine spongiform encephalopathy and related diseases. *Arch Virol.* 1993;7:245-254.

162. Will RG, Ironside JW, Zeidler M, et al. A new variant of Creutzfeldt–Jakob disease in the UK. *Lancet.* 1996;347:921-925.

163. Pritzkow S, Morales R, Moda F, et al. Grass plants bind, retain, uptake and transport infectious prions. *Cell Rep.* 2015;11:1168-1175.

164. Cronier S, Gros N, Tattum MH, et al. Detection and characterization of proteinase K-sensitive disease-related prion protein with thermolysin. *Biochem J.* 2008;416:297-305.

165. Safar J, Wille H, Itri V, et al. Eight prion strains have PrP^{Sc} molecules with different conformations. *Nat Med.* 1998;4:1157-1165.

166. Das AS, Zou WQ. Prions: beyond a single protein. *Clin Microbiol Rev.* 2016;29:633-658.

167. Kim C, Haldiman T, Cohen Y, et al. Protease-sensitive conformers in broad spectrum of distinct PrPSc structures in sporadic Creutzfeldt-Jakob disease are indicator of progression rate. *PLoS Pathog.* 2011;7:e1002242.

168. Sandberg MK, Al-Doujaily H, Sharps B, et al. Prion neuropathology follows the accumulation of alternate prion protein isoforms after infective titre has peaked. *Nat Commun.* 2014;5:4347.

169. Quinn PJ, Markey BK, Leonard FC, FitzPatrick ES, Fanning S, Hartigan PJ. *Veterinary Microbiology and Microbial Disease.* 2nd ed. Oxford, United Kingdom: Wiley-Blackwell; 2011.

170. Taylor DM. Transmissible degenerative encephalopathies: inactivation of the unconventional causal agents. In: Russell AD, Hugo WB, Ayliffe GM, eds. *Principles and Practice of Disinfection, Preservation, and Sterilization.* 3rd ed. Oxford, United Kingdom: Blackwell Science; 1999:222-236.

171. Taylor DM. Inactivation of transmissible degenerative encephalopathy agents: a review. *Vet J.* 2000;159:10-17.

172. McDonnell G. Transmissible spongiform encephalopathies and decontamination. In: Fraise A, Maillard J, Sattar S, eds. *Russell, Hugo and Ayliffe's: Principles and Practice of Disinfection, Preservation and Sterilization.* 5th ed. Chichester, United Kingdom: Wiley-Blackwell; 2013:208-228.

173. Taylor DM, Woodgate SL, Atkinson MJ. Inactivation of the bovine spongiform encephalopathy agent by rendering procedures. *Vet Rec.* 1995;137:605-610.

174. Taylor DM, Woodgate SL, Fleetwood AJ, Cawthorne RJ. Effect of rendering procedures on the scrapie agent. *Vet Rec.* 1997;141:643-649.

175. Greig JR. Scrapie in sheep. *J Comp Pathol.* 1950;60:263-266.

176. Kimberlin RH, Walker CA, Millson GC, et al. Disinfection studies with two strains of mouse-passaged scrapie agent. Guidelines for Creutzfeldt-Jakob and related agents. *J Neurol Sci.* 1983;59:355-369.

177. Fernie K, Hamilton S, Somerville RA. Limited efficacy of steam sterilization to inactivate vCJD infectivity. *J Hosp Infect.* 2012;80:46-51.

178. Schreuder BE, Geertsma RE, van Keulen LJ, et al. Studies on the efficacy of hyperbaric rendering procedures in inactivating bovine spongiform encephalopathy (BSE) and scrapie agents. *Vet Rec.* 1998;142:474-480.

179. Giles K, Glidden DV, Beckwith R, et al. Resistance of bovine spongiform encephalopathy (BSE) prions to inactivation. *PLoS Pathog.* 2008;4:e1000206.

180. Brown P, Rau EH, Johnson BK, Bacote AE, Gibbs CJ Jr, Gajdusek DC. New studies on the heat resistance of hamster-adapted scrapie agent: threshold survival after ashing at 600°C suggests inorganic template of replication. *Proc Natl Acad Sci U S A.* 2000;97:3418-3421.

181. Brown P, Rau EH, Lemieux P, Johnson BK, Bacote AE, Gajdusek DC. Infectivity studies of both ash and air emissions from simulated incineration of scrapie contaminated tissues. *Environ Sci Technol.* 2004;38:6155-6160.

182. Flechsig E, Hegyi I, Enari M, Schwarz P, Collinge J, Weissman C. Transmission of scrapie by steel-surface bound prions. *Mol Med.* 2001;7:679-684.

183. Fichet G, Comoy E, Duval C, et al. Novel methods for disinfection of prion-contaminated medical devices. *Lancet.* 2004;364:521-526.

184. Brown P, Rohwer RG, Gajdusek DC. Newer data on the inactivation of scrapie virus or Creutzfeldt-Jakob disease virus in brain tissue. *J Infect Dis.* 1986;153:1145-1148.

185. Brown P, Wolff A, Gajdusek DC. A simple and effective method for inactivating virus infectivity in formalin-fixed tissue samples from patients with Creutzfeldt-Jakob disease. *Neurology.* 1990;40:887-890.

186. Taylor DM, Brown JM, Fernie K, McConnell I. The effect of formic acid on BSE and scrapie infectivity in fixed and unfixed brain-tissue. *Vet Microbiol.* 1997;58:167-174.

187. Taylor DM, Fraser H, McConnell I, et al. Decontamination studies with the agents of bovine spongiform encephalopathy and scrapie. *Arch Virol.* 1994;139:313-326.

188. Taguchi F, Tamai Y, Uchida K, et al. Proposal for a procedure for complete inactivation of the Creutzfeldt-Jakob disease agent. *Arch Virol.* 1991;119:297-301.

189. Taylor DM, Fernie K, McConnell I. Inactivation of the 22A strain of scrapie agent by autoclaving in sodium hydroxide. *Vet Microbiol.* 1997;58:87-91.

190. Taylor DM, Fernie K, Steele PJ. Boiling in sodium hydroxide inactivates mouse-passaged BSE agent. Paper presented at: The 53rd Scientific Meeting of Association of Veterinary Teachers and Research Workers; March 1999; Scarborough, United Kingdom.

191. Murphy RG, Scanga JA, Powers BE, et al. Alkaline hydrolysis of mouse-adapted scrapie for inactivation and disposal of prion-positive material. *J Anim Sci.* 2009;87:1787-1793.

192. McDonnell G, Dehen C, Perrin A, et al. Cleaning, disinfection and sterilization of surface prion contamination. *J Hosp Infect.* 2013;85:268-273.

193. Hunter GD, Millson GC. Further experiments on the comparative potency of tissue extracts from mice infected with scrapie. *Res Vet Sci.* 1964;5:149-153.

194. Dickinson AG, Taylor DM. Resistance of scrapie agent to decontamination. *N Engl J Med.* 1978;229:1413-1414.

195. Dickinson AG. Scrapie in sheep and goats. In: Kimberlin RH, ed. *Slow Virus Diseases of Animals and Man.* Amsterdam, Netherlands: North-Holland; 1976:209-241.

196. Taylor DM, Fernie K, McConnell I, Ferguson CE, Steele PJ. Solvent extraction as an adjunct to rendering: the effect on BSE and scrapie agents of hot solvents followed by dry heat and steam. *Vet Rec.* 1998;143:6-9.

197. Brown P, Rohwer RG, Green EM, Gajdusek DC. Effect of chemicals, heat, and histopathologic processing on high-infectivity hamster-adapted scrapie virus. *J Infect Dis.* 1982;145:683-687.

198. Fraser H, Bruce ME, Chree A, McConnell I, Wells GA. Transmission of bovine spongiform encephalopathy and scrapie to mice. *J Gen Virol.* 1992;73:1891-1897.

199. Haig DA, Clarke MC. The effect of beta-propiolactone on the scrapie agent. *J Gen Virol.* 1968;3:281-283.

200. Stamp JT, Brotherston JC, Zlotnik I, Mackay JM, Smith W. Further studies on scrapie. *J Comp Pathol.* 1959;69:268-280.

201. Brown P, Gibbs CJ, Amyx HL, et al. Chemical disinfection of Creutzfeldt-Jakob disease virus. *N Engl J Med.* 1982;306:1279-1282

202. Taylor DM. Resistance of the ME7 scrapie agent to peracetic acid. *Vet Microbiol.* 1991;27:19-24.

203. Hunter GD, Gibbons RA, Kimberlin RH, Millson GC. Further studies of the infectivity and stability of extracts and homogenates derived from scrapie affected mouse brains. *J Comp Pathol.* 1969;79:101-108.

204. Adams DH, Field EJ, Joyce G. Periodate: an inhibitor of the scrapie agent? *Res Vet Sci.* 1972;13:195-198.

205. Chesney A, Booth C, Lietz CB, Li L, Pedersen JA. Peroxymonosulfate rapidly inactivates the disease-associated prion protein. *Environ Sci Technol.* 2016;50:7095-7105.

206. Ding N, Neumann NF, Price L, et al. Inactivation of template-directed misfolding of infectious prion protein by ozone. *Appl Environ Microbiol.* 2012;78:613-620.

207. Edgeworth JA, Sicilia A, Linehan J, Brandner S, Jaxckson GS, Collinge J. A standardized comparison of commercially available prion decontamination reagents using the standard steel-binding assay. *J Gen Virol.* 2011;92:718-726.

208. Jackson GS, McKintosh E, Flechsig E, et al. An enzyme-detergent method for effective prion decontamination of surgical steel. *J Gen Virol.* 2005;86:869-878.

209. Beekes M, Lemmer K, Thomzig A, Joncic M, Tintelnot K, Mielke M. Fast, broad-range disinfection of bacteria, fungi, viruses and prions. *J Gen Virol.* 2010;91:580-589.

210. Walker LC, Jucker M. Neurodegenerative diseases: expanding the prion concept. *Annu Rev Neurosci.* 2015;38:87-103.

211. Prusiner SB. Biology and genetics of prions causing neurodegeneration. *Annu Rev Neurosci.* 2013;47:601-623.

212. Ashe KH, Aguzzi A. Prions, prionoids and pathogenic proteins in Alzheimer disease. *Prion.* 2013;7:55-59.

213. World Health Organization. WHO infection control guidelines for transmissible spongiform encephalopathies. Report of a WHO consultation, Geneva, Switzerland, 23-26 March 1999. World Health Organization Web site. https://apps.who.int/iris/bitstream/handle/10665/66707/WHO_CDS_CSR_APH_2000.3.pdf;jsessionid=28B736D5EC23BD9A432FB8802C08FF9C?sequence=1. Accessed July 5, 2019.

214. Lehmann S, Pastore M, Rogez-Kruz C, et al. New hospital disinfection processes for both conventional and prion infectious agents compatible with thermosensitive medical equipment. *J Hosp Infect.* 2009;72:342-350.

215. Hughson AG, Race B, Kraus A, et al. Inactivation of prions and amyloid seeds with hypochlorous acid. *PLoS Pathog.* 2016;12:e1005914.

216. Postma M, Vanderhaeghen W, Sarrazin S, Maes D, Dewulf J. Reducing antimicrobial usage in pig production without jeopardizing production parameters. *Zoonoses Public Health.* 2017;64:63-74.

217. Mannion C, Leonard FC, Lynch PB, Egan J. Efficacy of cleaning and disinfection on pig farms in Ireland. *Vec Rec.* 2007;161:371-375.

218. Luyckx K, Millet S, Van Weyenberg S, et al. A 10-day vacancy period after cleaning and disinfection has no effect on the bacterial load in pig nursery units. *BMC Vet Res.* 2016;12:236.

219. McLaren I, Wales A, Breslin M, Davies R. Evaluation of commonly-used farm disinfectants in wet and dry models of *Salmonella* farm contamination. *Avian Pathol.* 2011;40:33-42.

220. Walia K, Argüello H, Lynch H, et al. The efficacy of different cleaning and disinfection procedures to reduce *Salmonella* and *Enterobacteriaceae* in the lairage environment of a pig abattoir. *Int J Food Microbiol.* 2017;246:64-71.

221. Gosling RJ, Mawhinney I, Vaughan K, Davies RH, Smith RP. Efficacy of disinfectants and detergents intended for a pig farm environment where *Salmonella* is present. *Vet Microbiol.* 2017;204:46-53.

222. Hancox LR, Le Bon M, Dodd CE, Mellits KH. Inclusion of detergent in a cleaning regime and effect on microbial load in livestock housing. *Vet Rec.* 2013;173:167.

223. Martelli F, Lambert M, Butt P, et al. Evaluation of an enhanced cleaning and disinfection protocol in *Salmonella* contaminated pig holdings in the United Kingdom. *PLoS One.* 2017;12:e0178897.

224. Hao XX, Li BM, Zhang Q, et al. Disinfection effectiveness of slightly acidic electrolysed water in swine barns. *J Appl Microbiol.* 2013;115:703-710.

225. Luyckx K, Millet S, Van Weyenberg S, et al. Comparison of competitive exclusion with classical cleaning and disinfection on bacterial load in pig nursery units. *BMC Vet Res.* 2016;12:189.

226. Davies RH, Wray C. Observations on disinfection regimens used on *Salmonella enteritidis* infected poultry units. *Poult Sci.* 1995;74:638-647.

227. Luyckx KY, Van Weyenberg S, Dewulf J, et al. On-farm comparisons of different cleaning protocols in broiler houses. *Poult Sci.* 2015;94:1986-1993.

228. Willinghan EM, Sander JE, Thayer SG, Wilson JL. Investigation of bacterial resistance to hatchery disinfectants. *Avian Dis.* 1996;40:510-515.

229. Quinn PJ, Markey BK. Disinfection and disease prevention in veterinary medicine. In: Block SS, ed. *Disinfection, Sterilization, and Preservation.* 5th ed. Philadelphia, PA: Lippincott Williams & Wilkins; 2001:1069-1103.

230. Stringfellow K, Anderson P, Caldwell D, et al. Evaluation of disinfectants commonly used by the commercial poultry industry under simulated field conditions. *Poult Sci.* 2009;88:1151-1155.

231. Mueller-Doblies D, Carrique-Mas JJ, Sayers AR, Davies RH. A comparison of the efficacy of different disinfection methods in eliminating *Salmonella* contamination from turkey houses. *J Appl Microbiol.* 2010;109:471-479.

232. Emmoth E, Ottoson J, Albihn A, Belák S, Vinnerås B. Ammonia disinfection of hatchery waste for elimination of single-stranded RNA viruses. *Appl Environ Microbiol.* 2011;77:3960-3966.

233. Gay L, Mundt E. Testing of a new disinfectant process for poultry viruses. *Avian Dis.* 2010;54:763-767.

234. Haas B, Ahl R, Böhm R, Strauch D. Inactivation of viruses in liquid manure. *Rev Sci Tech.* 1995;14:435-445.

235. Turner C, Burton CH. The inactivation of viruses in pig slurries: a review. *Bioresour Technol.* 1997;61:9-20.

236. Kearney TE, Larkin MJ, Levett PN. The effect of slurry storage and anaerobic digestion on survival of pathogenic bacteria. *J Appl Bacteriol.* 1993;74:86-93.

237. Zadoks RN, Middleton JR, McDougall S, Katholm J, Schukken YH. Molecular epidemiology of mastitis pathogens of dairy cattle and comparative relevance to humans. *J Mammary Gland Biol Neoplasia.* 2011;16:357-372.

238. Edmondson PW. Raised herd somatic cell count due to *Staphylococcus aureus* following the failure of an automatic teat spraying system. *Vet Rec.* 2012;170:287.

239. Lago A, Bruno DR, Lopez-Benavides M, Leibowitz S. Short communication: efficacy of glycolic acid-based and iodine-based postmilking barrier teat disinfectants for prevention of new intramammary infections in dairy cattle. *J Dairy Sci.* 2016;99:7467-7472.

240. Pankey JW, Drechsler PA. Evolution of udder hygiene. Premilking teat sanitation. *Vet Clin North Am Food Anim Pract.* 1993;9:519-530.

241. Schukken YH, Rauch BJ, Morelli J. Defining standardized protocols for determining the efficacy of a postmilking teat disinfectant following experimental exposure of teats to mastitis pathogens. *J Dairy Sci.* 2013;96:2694-2704.

242. European Medicines Agency. Guideline on the conduct of efficacy studies for intramammary products for use in cattle. European Medicines Agency Web site http://www.ema.europa.eu/docs/en_GB/document_library/Scientific_guideline/2017/01/WC500220206.pdf. Accessed July 5, 2019.

243. National Mastitis Council. Summary of peer-reviewed publication on efficacy of premilking and postmilking teat disinfectants published since 1980. Paper presented at: 52nd National Mastitis Council Annual Meeting; January 27-29, 2013; San Diego, CA.

244. Murdough PA, Pankey JW. Evaluation of 57 teat sanitizers using excised cow teats. *J Dairy Sci.* 1993;76:2033-2038.

245. Middleton JR, Saeman A, Fox LK, Lombard J, Hogan JS, Smith KL. The National Mastitis Council: a global organization for mastitis control and milk quality, 50 years and beyond. *J Mammary Gland Biol Neoplasia.* 2014;19:241-251.

246. Boddie RL, Nickerson SC, Adkinson RW. Evaluation of teat germicides of low iodine concentrations for prevention of bovine mastitis by *Staphylococcus aureus* and *Streptococcus agalactiae*. *Prev Vet Med.* 1993;16:111-117.

247. Drechsler PA, O'Neil JK, Murdough PA, Lafayette AR, Wildman EE, Pankey JW. Efficacy evaluations on five chlorhexidine teat dip formulations. *J Dairy Sci.* 1993;76:2783-2788.

248. Boddie RL, Nickerson SC, Kemp GK. Efficacy of two barrier teat dips containing chlorous acid germicides against experimental challenge with *Staphylococcus aureus* and *Streptococcus agalactiae*. *J Dairy Sci.* 1994;77:3192-3197.

249. Boddie RL, Nickerson SC. Efficacy of teat dips containing a hypochlorous acid germicide against experimental challenge with *Staphylococcus aureus* and *Streptococcus agalactiae*. *J Dairy Sci.* 1996;79:1683-1688.

250. Hogan JS, Smith KL, Todhunter DA, Schoenberger PS. Efficacy of a barrier teat dip containing .55% chlorhexidine for prevention of bovine mastitis. *J Dairy Sci.* 1995;78:2502-2506.

251. Boddie RL, Nickerson SC, Adkinson RW. Efficacies of teat germicides containing 0.5% chlorhexidine and 1% iodine during experimental challenge with *Staphylococcus aureus* and *Streptococcus agalactiae*. *J Dairy Sci.* 1997;80:2809-2814.

252. Erskine RJ, Sears PM, Bartlett PC, Gage CR. Efficacy of postmilking disinfection with benzyl alcohol versus Iodophor in the prevention of new intramammary infections in lactating cows. *J Dairy Sci.* 1998;81:116-120.

253. Fox LK, Burmeister JE. Barrier teat dip application during cold, windy conditions: *Staphylococcus aureus* colonization and teat skin health. *Dairy Food Environ Sanitation.* 1998;18:732-734.

254. Boddie RL, Nickerson SC, Adkinson RW. Germicidal activity of a chlorous acid-chlorine dioxide teat dip and a sodium chlorite teat dip during experimental challenge with *Staphylococcus aureus* and *Streptococcus agalactiae. J Dairy Sci.* 1998;81:2293-2298.

255. Godden SM, Royster E, Knauer W, et al. Randomized noninferiority study evaluating the efficacy of a postmilking teat disinfectant for the prevention of naturally occurring intramammary infections. *J Dairy Sci.* 2016;99:3675-3687.

256. Leslie KE, Vernooy E, Bashiri A, Dingwell RT. Efficacy of two hydrogen peroxide teat disinfectants against *Staphylococcus aureus* and *Streptococcus agalactiae. J Dairy Sci.* 2006;89:3696-3701.

257. Martins CMMR, Pinheiro ESC, Gentilini M, Benavides ML, Santos MV. Efficacy of a high free iodine barrier teat disinfectant for the prevention of naturally occurring new intramammary infections and clinical mastitis in dairy cows. *J Dairy Sci.* 2017;100:3930-3939.

258. Yu J, Ren Y, Xi X, Huang W, Zhang H. A novel lactobacilli-based teat disinfectant for improving bacterial communities in the milks of cow teats with subclinical mastitis. *Front Microbiol.* 2017;8:1782.

259. Duarte AF, Ceotto-Vigoder H, Barrias ES, Souto-Padrón TCBS, Nes IF, Bastos MD. Hyicin 4244, the first sactibiotic described in staphylococci, exhibits an anti-staphylococcal biofilm activity. *Int J Antimicrob Agents.* 2018;51:349-356.

260. Hillerton JE, Shearn MF, Teverson RM, Langridge S, Booth JM. Effect of pre-milking teat dipping on clinical mastitis on dairy farms in England. *J Dairy Res.* 1993;60:31-41.

261. Oliver SP, Lewis MJ, Ingle TL. Gillespie BE, Matthews KR. Prevention of bovine mastitis by a premilking teat disinfectant containing chlorous acid and chlorine dioxide. *J Dairy Sci.* 1993;76:287-292.

262. Williamson JH, Lacy-Hulbert SJ. Effect of disinfecting teats postmilking or pre- and post-milking on intramammary infection and somatic cell count. *N Z Vet J.* 2013;61:262-268.

263. Morton JM, Penry JF, Malmo J, Mein GA. Premilking teat disinfection: is it worthwhile in pasture-grazed dairy herds? *J Dairy Sci.* 2014;97:7525-7537.

264. Bava L, Colombini S, Zucali M, et al. Efficient milking hygiene reduces bacterial spore contamination in milk. *J Dairy Res.* 2017;84:322-328.

265. Baxter K. Mastitis control in practice. Paper presented at: British Mastitis Conference; November, 2015; Worcester, United Kingdom.

266. Ruf J, Johler S, Merz A, Stalder U, Hässig M. Success of interventions in mastitis problems with *Staphylococcus aureus* after the introduction of an automatic milking system. *Schweiz Arch Tierheilkd.* 2015;157:153-156.

267. Gomes F, Saavedra MJ, Henriques M. Bovine mastitis disease/pathogenicity: evidence of the potential role of microbial biofilms. *Pathog Dis.* 2016;74(3).

268. Kawai K, Shinozuka Y, Uchida I, et al. Control of *Pseudomonas* mastitis on a large dairy farm by using slightly acidic electrolyzed water. *Anim Sci J.* 2017;88:1601-1605.

269. Walther B, Tedin K, Lübke-Becker A. Multidrug-resistant opportunistic pathogens challenging veterinary infection control. *Vet Microbiol.* 2017;200:71-78.

270. Pires Dos Santos T, Damborg P, Moodley A, Guardabassi L. Systematic review on global epidemiology of methicillin-resistant *Staphylococcus pseudintermedius*: inference of population structure from multilocus sequence typing data. *Front Microbiol.* 2016;7:1599.

271. Grönthal T, Moodley A, Nykäsenoja S, et al. Large outbreak caused by methicillin resistant *Staphylococcus pseudintermedius* ST71 in a Finnish veterinary teaching hospital—from outbreak control to outbreak prevention. *PLoS One.* 2014;9:e110084.

272. Stull JW, Weese JS. Hospital-associated infections in small animal practice. *Vet Clin North Am Small Anim Pract.* 2015;45:217-233.

273. Traverse M, Aceto H. Environmental cleaning and disinfection. *Vet Clin North Am Small Anim Pract.* 2015;45:299-330.

274. Bergström K, Nyman G, Widgren S, Johnston C, Grönlund-Andersson U, Ransjö U. Infection prevention and control interventions in the first outbreak of methicillin-resistant *Staphylococcus aureus* infections in an equine hospital in Sweden. *Acta Vet Scand.* 2012;54:14.

275. Schott HC, Ewart SL, Walker RD, et al. An outbreak of salmonellosis among horses at a veterinary teaching hospital. *J Am Vet Med Assoc.* 2001;218:1152-1159

276. Ward MP, Brady TH, Couëtil LL, Liljebjelke K, Maurer JJ, Wu CC. Investigation and control of an outbreak of salmonellosis caused by multidrug-resistant *Salmonella typhimurium* in a population of hospitalized horses. *Vet Microbiol.* 2005;107:233-240.

277. Reynolds BS, Poulet H, Pingret JL, et al. A nosocomial outbreak of feline calicivirus associated virulent systemic disease in France. *J Feline Med Surg.* 2009;11:633-644.

278. Eleraky NZ, Potgieter LND, Kennedy MA. Virucidal efficacy of four new disinfectants. *J Am Anim Hosp Assoc.* 2002;38:231-234.

279. Moriello KA, Coyner K, Paterson S, Mignon B. Diagnosis and treatment of dermatophytosis in dogs and cats: clinical consensus guidelines of the World Association for Veterinary Dermatology. *Vet Dermatol.* 2017;28:266-e68.

280. Oldenhoff W, Moriello KA. One year surveillance of the isolation of pathogenic dermatophyte spores from risk areas in a veterinary medical teaching hospital. *Vet Dermatol.* 2013;24:474-475.

281. Dunowska M, Morley PS, Hyatt DR. The effect of Virkon S fogging on survival of *Salmonella enterica* and *Staphylococcus aureus* on surfaces in a veterinary teaching hospital. *Vet Microbiol.* 2005;105:281-289.

282. Saklou NT, Burgess BA, Van Metre DC, Hornig KJ, Morley PS, Byers SR. Comparison of disinfectant efficacy when using high-volume directed mist application of accelerated hydrogen peroxide and peroxymonosulfate disinfectants in a large animal hospital. *Equine Vet J.* 2016;48:485-489.

283. Patterson G, Morley PS, Blehm KD, Lee DE, Dunowska M. Efficacy of directed misting application of a peroxygen disinfectant for environmental decontamination of a veterinary hospital. *J Am Vet Med Assoc.* 2005;227:597-602.

284. Wood CL, Tanner BD, Higgins LA, Dennis JS, Luempert LG. Effectiveness of a steam cleaning unit for disinfection in a veterinary hospital. *Am J Vet Res.* 2014;75:1083-1088.

285. Boyce JM. Modern technologies for improving cleaning and disinfection of environmental surfaces in hospitals. *Antimicrob Resist Infect Control.* 2016;5:10.

286. Amass SF, Arighi M, Kinyon JM, Hoffman LJ, Schneider JL, Draper DK. Effectiveness of using a mat filled with a peroxygen disinfectant to minimize shoe sole contamination in a veterinary hospital. *J Am Vet Med Assoc.* 2006;228:1391-1396.

287. Hornig KJ, Burgess BA, Saklou NT, et al. Evaluation of the efficacy of disinfectant footmats for the reduction of bacterial contamination on footwear in a large animal veterinary hospital. *J Vet Intern Med.* 2016;30:1882-1886.

288. Stockton KA, Morley PS, Hyatt DR, et al. Evaluation of the effects of footwear hygiene protocols on nonspecific bacterial contamination of floor surfaces in an equine hospital. *J Am Vet Med Assoc.* 2006;228:1068-1073.

289. Kovaleva J, Peters FT, van der Mei HC, Degener JE. Transmission of infection by flexible gastrointestinal endoscopy and bronchoscopy. *Clin Microbiol Rev.* 2013;26:231-254.

290. Portner JA, Johnson JA. Guidelines for reducing pathogens in veterinary hospitals: hospital design and special considerations. *Compend Contin Educ Vet.* 2010;32:E1-E8.

291. Naryzhny I, Silas D, Chi K. Impact of ethylene oxide gas sterilization of duodenoscopes after a carbapenem-resistant *Enterobacteriaceae* outbreak. *Gastrointest Endosc.* 2016;84:259-262.

292. Bender JB, Schiffman E, Hiber L, Gerads L, Olsen K. Recovery of staphylococci from computer keyboards in a veterinary medical centre and the effect of routine cleaning. *Vet Rec.* 2012;170:414.

293. Weese JS, Lowe T, Walker M. Use of fluorescent tagging for assessment of environmental cleaning and disinfection in a veterinary hospital. *Vet Rec.* 2012;171:217.

294. Dwyer RM. Environmental disinfection to control equine infectious diseases. *Vet Clin North Am Equine Pract.* 2004;20:531-542.

295. Hartmann F, Callan R, McGuirk S, West S. Control of an outbreak of salmonellosis caused by drug-resistant *Salmonella anatum* in horses at a veterinary hospital and measures to prevent future infections. *J Am Vet Med Assoc.* 1996;209:629-631.

296. Alinovi C, Ward M, Couetil L, Wu C. Detection of *Salmonella* organisms and assessment of a protocol for removal of contamination in horse stalls at a veterinary teaching hospital. *J Am Vet Med Assoc.* 2003;223:1640-1644.

297. Ewart S, Schott HC, Robison RL, Dwyer RM, Eberhart SW, Walker RD. Identification of sources of *Salmonella* organisms in a veterinary teaching hospital and evaluation of the effects of disinfectants on detection of *Salmonella* organisms on surface materials. *J Am Vet Med Assoc.* 2001;218:1145-1151.

298. Peel AJ, Hartley M, Cunningham AA. Qualitative risk analysis of introducing *Batrachochytrium dendrobatidis* to the UK through the importation of live amphibians. *Dis Aquat Organ.* 2012;98: 95-112.

299. Miller RE, Fowler ME, eds. *Fowler's Zoo and Wild Animal Medicine.* Vol 8. St. Louis, MO: Elsevier Saunders; 2015.

300. Gamble KC, Clancy MM, eds. *Infectious Diseases of Concern to Captive and Free Ranging Animals in North America.* 2nd ed. Yulee, FL: Infectious Disease Committee, American Association of Zoo Veterinarians; 2013. http://www.aazv.org/?page=IDM2013. Accessed July 5, 2019.

301. Kiupel M, Mecklem R, Hunsinger B, Marschang RE. Guidelines for cleaning and disinfection in zoological gardens. In: *Transmissible Diseases Handbook.* European Association of Zoo and Wildlife Veterinarians; 2010:chap 8. http://www.eazwv.org/page/inf_handbook. Accessed July 5, 2019.

302. Reiss A, Woods R, eds. *National Zoo Biosecurity Manual.* Canberra, Australia: Commonwealth of Australia; 2011.

303. National Association of State Public Health Veterinarians Animal Contact Compendium Committee. Compendium of measures to prevent disease associated with animals in public setting, 2013. *J Am Vet Med Assoc.* 2013;243:1270-1288.

304. Carpenter N, Chinnadurai S, Helmick K, et al. *Guidelines for Zoo and Aquarium Veterinary Medical Programs and Veterinary Hospitals.* 6th ed. Yulee, FL: American Association of Zoo Veterinarians; 2016. https://www.aazv.org/resource/resmgr/files/aazvveterinaryguidelines2016.pdf. Accessed July 5, 2019.

305. Animal Health Australia. *Enterprise Manual: Zoos (Version 3.0). Australian Veterinary Emergency Plan (AUSVETPLAN).* 3rd ed. Canberra, Australia: Agriculture Ministers' Forum; 2014. https://www.animalhealthaustralia.com.au. Accessed July 5, 2019.

306. Heuschele WP. Use of disinfectants in zoos and game parks. *Rev Sci Tech.* 1995;14:447-454.

307. Smith KA, Campbell CT, Murphy J, Stobierski M, Tengelsen LA. Compendium of measures to control *Chlamydophila psittaci* infection among humans (psittacosis) and pet birds (avian chlamydiosis), 2010 National Association of State Public Health Veterinarians (NASPHV). *J Exot Pet Med.* 2011;20:32-45.

308. Brown CM, Slavinski S, Ettestad P, Sidwa TJ, Sorhage FE. Compendium of animal rabies prevention and control. *J Am Vet Med Assoc.* 2016;248:505-517.

309. Banish LD, Sims R, Bush M, Sack D, Montali RJ. Clearance of *Shigella flexneri* carriers in a zoological collection of primates. *J Am Vet Med Assoc.* 1993;203:133-136.

310. Redrobe SP. Avian influenza H5N1: a review of the current situation and relevance to zoos. *International Zoo Yearbook.* 2007;41:96-109.

311. Friedman CR, Torigian C, Shillam PJ, et al. An outbreak of salmonellosis among children attending a reptile exhibit at a zoo. *J Pediatr.* 1998;132:802-807.

312. David S, MacDougall L, Louie K, et al. Petting zoo-associated *Escherichia coli* O157:H7—secondary transmission, asymptomatic infection, and prolonged shedding in the classroom. *Can Commun Dis Rep.* 2004;30:173-180.

313. Warshawsky B, Gutmanis I, Henry B, et al. Outbreak of *Escherichia coli* O157:H7 related to animal contact at a petting zoo. *Can J Infect Dis.* 2002;13:175-181.

314. Centers for Disease Control and Prevention. Public health response to a potentially rabid bear cub—Iowa, 1999. *MMWR.* 1999;48:971-973.

315. Scott WA. Ringworm outbreak. *Vet Rec.* 1986;118:342.

316. Marennikova SS, Maltseva NN, Korneeva VI, Geranina N. Outbreak of pox disease among *Carnivora (Felidae)* and *Edentata. J Infect Dis.* 1977;135:358-366.

317. Kile JC, Fleischauer AT, Kuehnert MJ, et al. Transmission of monkeypox among persons exposed to infected prairie dogs in Indiana in 2003. *Arch Pediatr Adolesc Med.* 2005;159:1022-1025.

318. Gray SF, Smith RS, Reynolds N, Williams E. Fish tank granuloma. *BMJ.* 1990;300:1069-1070.

319. Lewis FMT, Marsh BJ, von Reyn CF. Fish tank exposure and cutaneous infections due to *Mycobacterium marinum*: tuberculin skin testing, treatment and prevention. *Clin Infect Dis.* 2003;37:390-397.

320. Michalak K, Austin C, Diesel S, Bacon J, Zimmerman P, Maslow J. *Mycobacterium tuberculosis* infection as a zoonotic disease: transmission between humans and elephants. *Emerg Infect Dis.* 1998;4: 283-287.

321. Stetter M, Mikota S, Gutter A, et al. Epizootic of *Mycobacterium bovis* in a zoological park. *J Am Vet Med Assoc.* 1995;207:1618-1621.

322. Oh P, Granich R, Scott J, et al. Human exposure following *Mycobacterium tuberculosis* infection of multiple animal species in a metropolitan zoo. *Emerg Infect Dis.* 2002;8:1290-1293.

323. Kiers A, Klarenbeek A, Mendelts B, Van Soolingen D, Koeter G. Transmission of *Mycobacterium pinnipedii* to humans in a zoo with marine mammals. *Int J Tuberc Lung Dis.* 2008;12:1469-1473.

324. Centers for Disease Control and Prevention. Fatal cercopithecine herpesvirus 1 (B virus) infection following a mucocutaneous exposure and interim recommendations for worker protection. *MMWR Morb Mortal Wkly Rep.* 1998;47:1073-1076.

325. Christensen AL, Jarlov JO, Ingeberg S. The risk of ornithosis among the staff of Copenhagen zoo. *Ugeskr Laeger.* 1990;152:818-820.

326. Lederer I, Much P, Allerberger F, Voracek T, Vielgrader H. Outbreak of shigellosis in the Vienna Zoo affecting human and non-human primates. *Int J Infect Dis.* 2005;9:290-291.

327. Goode B, O'Reilly C, Dunn J, et al. Outbreak of *Escherichia coli* O157:H7 infections after petting zoo visits, North Carolina State Fair, October-November 2004. *Arch Pediatr Adolesc Med.* 2009;163: 42-48.

328. LeJeune JT, Davis MA. Outbreaks of zoonotic enteric disease associated with animal exhibits. *J Am Vet Med Assoc.* 2004;224: 1440-1445.

329. Hale CR, Scallan E, Cronquist AB, et al. Estimates of enteric illness attributable to contact with animals and their environments in the United States. *Clin Infect Dis.* 2012;54(suppl 5):S472-S479.

330. Ornelas-Eusebio E, Sánchez-Godoy FD, Chávez-Maya F, De la Garza-García JA, Hernández-Castro R, García-Espinosa G. First identification of *Chlamydia psittaci* in the acute illness and death of endemic and endangered psittacine birds in Mexico. *Avian Dis.* 2016;60: 540-544.

331. Hoss A, Basler C, Stevenson L, Gambino-Shirley K, Robyn MP, Nicholas M. State laws requiring hand sanitation stations at animal contact exhibits—United States, March-April 2016. *MMWR Morb Mortal Wkly Rep.* 2017;66:16-18.

332. Anderson MEC, Weese JS. Video observation of hand hygiene practices at a petting zoo and the impact of hand hygiene interventions. *Epidemiol Infect.* 2012;140:182-190.

333. Randall LP, Ridley AM, Cooles SW, et al. Prevalence of multiple antibiotic resistance in 443 *Campylobacter* spp. isolated from humans and animals. *J Antimicrob Chemother.* 2003;52:507-510.

334. Brenwald NP, Fraise AP. Triclosan resistance in methicillin-resistant *Staphylococcus aureus* (MRSA). *J Hosp Infect.* 2003;55:141-144.

335. Sanchez-Vizuete P, Orgaz B, Aymerich S, Le Coq D, Briandet R. Pathogens protection against the action of disinfectants in multispecies biofilms. *Front Microbiol.* 2015;6:1-12.

336. Bridier A, Briandet R, Thomas V, Dubois-Brissonnet F. Resistance of bacterial biofilms to disinfectants: a review. *Biofouling.* 2011;27: 1017-1032.

337. Jacques M, Aragon V, Tremblay YDN. Biofilm formation in bacterial pathogens of veterinary importance. *Anim Health Res Rev.* 2010;11:97-121.

Disinfection of Contact Lenses

Manal M. Gabriel and Donald G. Ahearn

Soft contact lenses and rigid gas-permeable lenses have provided a practical and safe alternative for eyeglasses. Successful contact lens wear (enhanced vision without irritation) can be achieved during many physical activities unsuitable for glasses. Advanced technologies in biocompatible lens materials, particularly silicone hydrogels, and lens solutions underlie the significant worldwide increases in all types of lens wear over the past two decades. Convenience and comfort have been stimulating factors for increased contact lens wear, but curative usage (eg, treatment of myopia and controlled provision of ocular medications to the cornea) offers further advances.

Contact lens wear in North America is highest in the United States and estimated at near 41 million users.[1,2] In Europe, the United Kingdom, Germany, France, Russia, and Italy are estimated, in decreasing order, to include near 100 million users. Brazil, China, and Japan, in the Asia-Pacific region, are leading markets for increased use of contact lenses.

A contact lens placed on the eye is a foreign body that could adversely affect tear flow, its composition, and evaporation. Furthermore, specific lens types may differentially absorb or/adsorb tear components, such as lysozyme, mucin, and lipids, and be impacted by interactions with host ocular tissues and their microbiota. These may also affect the disinfectant efficacy of some multipurpose contact lens solutions.[3-6] In essence, individual ocular homeostasis may be altered to varying extents following lens insertion and the discrete alterations may not be readily observable in the "asymptomatic eye of the wearer."[7,8] Therefore, for avoidance of possible adverse events, successful contact lens wear requires good hygienic practices by the user as guided by clinicians and the manufacturers of these products.

Anoxia (lack of oxygen) damage to cornea tissue as a risk factor for infections (despite being rare) was a primary concern in early conventional soft hydroxyethyl-methacrylate (HEMA) lens wear. This concern, in part, and the quest for development of more biocompatible extended wear (EW) lens materials has stimulated a shift from HEMA type lenses to soft higher oxygen diffusion silicone modalities.[9-11] The further shift from HEMA lenses and soft silicone EW modalities to mostly daily silicone disposables would theoretically reduce unhygienic lens manipulation and storage[12,13]; however, the incidence of rare infection and vision loss associated with contact lens wear, at least with bacteria, have not been detected to change overall with the current shift in wear to select higher oxygen diffusion silicone lens types.[11]

▶ LENS TYPES

Rigid gas permeable (RGP or GP) contact lenses (copolymers of polymerizable silicone acrylates or fluorosilicone acrylates, and the latter cross-linked with polymerizable hydrophobic-hydrolyzable silicone monomers) have largely replaced polymethyl methacrylate (PMMA) hard lenses. RGP lenses offer clear vision, excellent oxygen diffusion, and durability with ease for cleaning and disinfection. The lenses may be customized for the individual eye shape and worn with comfort; after reasonable adaptation to use, RGPs have increasing applications in orthokeratology, particularly controlling myopia progression.

Conventional hydrogel (soft) lenses first were composed of homopolymers of cross-linked chains of poly(2-hydroxyethylmethacrylate) (pHEMA) with various concentrations of absorbed water. Addition of N-vinylpyrrolidone (NVP) or methacrylic acid (MA) increased hydrophilic properties and related oxygen diffusion.[14,15] The polymer type and organization of ionic groups on the hydrogel surface interact with water content and affect the deposition of proteins, lipids, and microorganisms on the lens surface.[14,16,17] The backbone chains of the polymers commonly have hydroxyl ($-OH$), carboxylic ($-COOH$), esoteric ($-COOCH3$), or etheric ($-COCH3$) functional groups. Hydroxyl or polar groups provide the hydrophilicity required for the increased water-swelling activity.

TABLE 53.1 Original US Food and Drug Administration groups of hydrogen lenses

Group 1 Low Water (<50% H₂O) Nonionic Polymers	Group 2 High Water (>50% H₂O) Nonionic Polymers	Group 3 Low Water (<50% H₂O) Ionic Polymers	Group 4 High Water (>50% H₂O) Ionic Polymers
Nelfilcon A&B (45%)	Lidofilcon B (79%)	Droxifilcon A (47%)	Perfilcon (71%)
Tefilcon (38%)	Surfilcon (74%)	Bufilcon A (45%)	Etaflcon A (58%)
Polymacon (38%)	Lidofilcon A (70%)	Ocufilcon (44%)	Bufilcon A (55%)
Tetrafilcon A (43%)		Deltafilcon A (43%)	Ocufilcon C (55%)
Crofilcon (38%)	Omafilcon A (59%)	Phemfilcon A (38%)	Phemfilcon A (55%)
Isofilcon (36%)			Methafilcon (55%)
Mafilcon (33%)			Vifilcon A (55%)
			Ocufilcon B (53%)

The US Food and Drug Administration (FDA) grouped traditional hydrogel lenses into four major divisions on the basis of ionic charge and water content (Table 53.1). Lenses with nonionic polymers (groups 1 and, particularly, 2) allow more lipid deposition from the tears than hydrogel lenses with ionic radicals (groups 3 and 4). Jones et al[14] indicated that high lipid accumulation may be associated with group 2 lenses because of their content, NVP. Group 4 material (ionic, high water content) is more attractive to protein because of the negative charge that methacrylic acid gives to the material. These first groupings served as a guide for probable physical-chemical compatibilities of traditional lens types with their care solutions.

Early silicone hydrogel lenses (such as lotrafilcon and balafilcon, initially grouped in 1 and 3, respectively) and subsequent innovative silicone formulations have deviated in their physical-chemical interaction from the patterns recognized for the above four traditional hydrogel groups. Goals for extending wear time and comfort while addressing potential adverse hypoxia and modulus stresses have guided the shift of soft lens compositions to include mobile siloxy groups of silicone complexed with varied conventional components.[17] Also, current silicone soft lenses have gone through several generations of development and modifications in surface properties and treatments and intrabinding of wetting agents.[18] Formulation changes among various silicone lens types may differentially alter interactions with host comfort, microorganisms, and solutions.[3,5,19] The overall groupings with silicone lenses as discrete types are expected to facilitate the determination of compatibilities with cleaning and disinfection regimens by lens type. A fifth group has been proposed for inclusion of silicone hydrogels and was under evaluation.[20]

Hutter et al[20] proposed a system for silicone hydrogel lens materials that further subdivides group 5 into five subgroups. Group 5-A: low-water content, nonionic, and surface-treated lenses; group 5-B1: low-water content, nonionic, nonsurface treated, and hydrophilic monomer-containing lenses; group 5-B2: low-water content, nonionic, nonsurface treated and semi-interpenetrating network-containing lenses; group 5-C: high-water content and nonionic lenses; and group 5-D: ionic materials, both low-water and high-water content lenses. However, International Organization for Standardization (ISO) 18369-1: 2017 classified group 5 differently as 5A ionic subgroup, 5B high-water subgroup (≥50%), and 5C low-water subgroup, which contains <50%. Representative contact lenses for the five groups are described in Table 53.2.

▶ CLEANING AND DISINFECTANT SOLUTIONS

The selection of chemicals for the cleaning and disinfection of contact lenses requires a compromise between toxicity of the chemicals to the eye and activity against the more

TABLE 53.2 ISO 18369-1:2017 classification for group 5 silicone lenses[a]

5A[b] Ionic Subgroup	5B[c] High-Water Subgroup (≥50%)	5C[d] Low-Water Subgroup (<50%)
Balafilcon A (36%)	Efrofilcon A (74%)	Lotrafilcon A (24%) Lotrafilcon B (33%) Comfilcon A (48%) Senofilcon A (38%)

[a]From International Organization for Standardization.[21]

[b]A subgroup of group 5 that contains monomers or oligomers, which are ionic at pH 6 to 8.

[c]A subgroup of group 5 that contains 50% water or more and no ionic monomer or oligomer at pH 6 to 8.

[d]A subgroup of group 5 that contains less than 50% water and no ionic monomer or oligomer at pH 6 to 8.

common ocular pathogens. The cleaning step itself can reduce significantly (several logs) the microbial bioburden on a lens.[22] Daily cleaners are typically a combination of nonionic or amphoteric surfactants (nonirritating to the eye compared with cationic and anionic surfactants) combined with preservatives and frequently with chelating agents such as ethylenediaminetetraacetic acid (EDTA). Some alcohol-based cleaning formulations (that include approximately 20% isopropyl alcohol) effectively clean and can have some disinfection activity for hard lenses, but because of their toxicity to the eye, they must be thoroughly rinsed from the lens before insertion. Weekly cleaners typically contain proteolytic enzymes (eg, subtilisin-A, stabilized papain, porcine pancreatin) that are designed to remove tear proteins from the hydrogel surface. In combination with daily cleaning, including disinfection with hydrogen peroxide (H_2O_2), protein deposits and the risk of microbial biofilm formation on hydrogel lenses are reduced with a weekly cleaning regimen. Unit-dose preservative-free saline (15-mL vials) and multidose preservative-free saline also are commercially available for rinsing and for use with heat disinfection units, respectively. Borate buffer in conjunction with certain contact lens care solutions might be essential for optimal preservation (Table 53.3).

TABLE 53.3   Contact lens care solutions

Solutions	Preservatives	Chelators	Surfactants	pH	Buffer	Regimen	Storage
Single Disinfection							
Peroxide system 1	3% hydrogen peroxide	None	Pluronic 17R4	6.2	Phosphate	Rinse only (6 h soak).	7 d
Peroxide system 2	3% hydrogen peroxide	None	HPMC	NA	Phosphate	Rinse only (6 h soak).	7 d
MPS 1	PQ	EDTA	None	7.5	Phosphate	Rub/rinse (6 h soak).	30 d
MPS 1	PHMB 0.0001%	EDTA	Pluronic F127	7.2	Sodium phosphate	Rinse only (4 h soak).	30 d
MPS 2	PHMB 0.0001%	EDTA	Polaxemer 237	7.2	Sodium phosphate	Rub/rinse (6 h soak).	30 d
MPS 3	PHMB 0.0001%	EDTA	Poloxamine hydranate	7.3	Boric acid; sodium borate	Rub/rinse (4 h soak).	30 d
MPS 4	PHMB 0.00005%	EDTA	Poloxamine	7.3	Boric acid; sodium borate	Rub/rinse (4 h soak).	30 d
Dual Disinfection							
MPS 5	PHMB 0.00013% PQ-1 0.0001%	EDTA	Hyaluronan; poloxamine	7.5	Boric acid; sodium citrate	Rub/rinse (4 h soak).	30 d
MPS 6	PQ-1 0.0001% MAPD 0.0005%	EDTA	Tetronic 1304	7.8	Boric acid; sodium citrate	Rub/rinse (6 h soak).	30 d
MPS 7	PQ-1 0.0001% MAPD 0.0005%	None	Tetronic 1304; nonanoyl ethylenediaminetriacetic acid	7.8	Boric acid; sodium citrate	Rub/rinse (6 h soak).	30 d
MPS 8	PQ-1 0.0001% MAPD 0.0006%	EDTA	Tetronic 1304; EOBO-41*-polyoxyethylene-polyoxybutylene	7.8	Boric acid; sodium citrate	Rub/rinse (6 h soak).	30 d
MPS 8	PQ-1 0.0003% Alex 0.00016%	EDTA	Tetronic 904	7.8	Boric acid; sodium borate; sodium citrate	Rub/rinse (6 h soak).	30 d
Triple Disinfection							
MPS 9	PHMB 0.00005% PQ-1 0.00015% and Alex 0.0002%	EDTA	Poloxamine; poloxamer 181; diglycine	NA	Sodium citrate; boric acid; sodium borate	Rub/rinse (4 h soak).	30 d

Abbreviations: Alex, alexidine; EDTA, ethylenediaminetetraacetic acid; HPMC, Hydroxypropyl methylcelluose; MAPD, myristamidopropyl dimethylamine; MPS, multipurpose solutions; NA, not available; PHMB, polyhexamethylene biguanide; PQ, polyquaternium.

The antimicrobial components in current representative multipurpose solutions (MPS) and oxidizing solutions that have addressed FDA and ISO guidelines are listed in Table 53.3. The primary preservative concentrations individually are below standard minimal inhibitory concentrations for most contaminants. However, the presence of unique and proprietary combinations of poloxamers, chelators, and often borates complex in the formulations to provide the overall enhanced antimicrobial and concordant properties of different preservatives. Not all solutions are suitable for all lenses, usages and hygienic approaches or lack thereof. [6,23-25] The prominent active agents used in contact lens disinfectant formulations are considered in the following text, the structures are shown in Table 53.4.

Hydrogen Peroxide

The H_2O_2 was the first "nonthermal" system used for the disinfection of contact lenses. The antimicrobial action of H_2O_2 is particularly based on its dissociated peroxide ion state that is a transitory phase during its decomposition into water and oxygen (see chapter 18). The highly reactive hydroxyl radical oxidizes has been shown to have effects associated with cell membrane lipids, proteins, and DNA. Disinfection solutions are typically at 3.0% concentrations; levels of 1.0% are usually sufficient to eradicate 10^6 suspended cells per milliliter of the typical cells of the typical challenge vegetative bacteria within 10 minutes, but with certain fungi and their associated spores, the 3.0 % concentration

TABLE 53.4	Disinfectants and their structures
Disinfectants	**Structure**
Hydrogen peroxide	
Quaternary ammonium compounds	
Polyquaternium 1 (Polyquad-1)	
Myristamidopropyl dimethylamine (MAPD)	
Polyhexamethylene biguanides (PHMB)	
Chlorhexidine	
Alexidine	
Thimerosal	
Sorbic acid and potassium sorbate	$CH_3-CH=CH-CH=CH-COOH$

may require exposures longer than an hour.[26,27] When the protozoa *Acanthamoeba* is the contaminating organism, up to 4 hours of exposure to 3.0% H_2O_2 may be necessary for acceptable disinfection, particularly due to the presence of cyst-forms.[28] The strong biocidal activity of H_2O_2 combined with its oxidizing-cleaning power and nontoxic decomposition products accounts for its successful application as a disinfectant for contact lenses.

The 3.0% H_2O_2 solution, however, is directly toxic to the eye, and it must be neutralized before a lens can be inserted. Whether the neutralization is by platinum disk, catalase, or sodium pyruvate, the end result is a nonpreserved rinsing solution that is subject to contamination. Microorganisms that may contaminate this solution may produce a biofilm within the lens case or on a stored lens. Cells and associated biofilm can be present on the plastic contact lens case, including the cap area, and in some of these cases may not be directly exposed to subsequent disinfection. Even with direct exposure during disinfection, the cells in the biofilm may survive further the disinfection regimens. The addition of fresh H_2O_2 will kill most cells in the planktonic state, but cells present in a progressively expanding biofilm in the case, particularly if the substratum is neutralizing, can increase the potential for survival and infection, particularly if disinfected lenses are stored in the case in neutralized H_2O_2 for several days and then placed on the eye. This same problem exists with lenses disinfected with heat, ultraviolet, or chemicals if the holding solution is insufficiently preserved during the required storage time. Although H_2O_2 when properly employed may be an efficacious disinfectant for contact lenses, it may cause transient alteration of lens parameters, fading of certain tinted lenses, and requires extended neutralization times for certain lens materials.

Povidone-Iodine

Aqueous povidone-iodine 5% to 10% (see chapter 16) is employed as a surfactant disinfectant prior to corneal surgery with minor toxicity concerns. Commercially available contact lens solutions have exhibited broad antimicrobial properties including the cysts of amoeba.[29-32]

Quaternary Ammonium Compounds

In most ocular medications, including antibiotic preparations, quaternary ammonium compounds (QACs) such as benzalkonium chloride (BAK) are used as preservatives (see chapter 21). The QAC molecule (as a type of surfactant) has a hydrophilic head and a lipophilic tail that may range from C8 to C30 branch length disinfectant or preservative BAK preparations containing at least 20% of the C14•H29 homologue and 40% of the C12•H25 homologue.

The polar portion of the molecule is cationic and readily adsorbed to bacterial/fungal cell walls from which

the tail portion is inserted (intercalation) into the phospholipid bilayer of the cell membrane. The degree of intercalation is affected by the numbers of C in the tail chain and the cell wall/membrane composition of the target species. BAK preparations may vary somewhat in antimicrobial activity because of homologue differences, but 100 to 200 μg/mL of most preparations in solution cause cell lysis of gram-positive and gram-negative bacteria and fungi. At these concentrations, BAK is used exclusively in contact lens solutions for PMMA and RGP lenses; at least 10-fold dilution of these concentrations is used in solutions for hydrogel lenses. EDTA, a chelating agent with some synergistic potential, is present at concentrations of 0.1% to 0.25% in lens solutions with BAK. Levels of BAK of 1.0 μg/mL may be toxic to cornea tissues[33]; low concentrations of BAK may absorb to certain lenses and accumulate to toxic levels (see chapter 21).

Polyquaternium-1 (Polyquad)

Polyquaternium-1 is a straight-chained molecule of repeating 4C groups randomly terminated with triethanolamine.

The compound is nonfoaming and relatively nontoxic. Solutions formulated and preserved with this biocide have been employed successfully when used meticulously in a complete regimen of cleaning, disinfection, and storage[34]; however, it has been reported that microbicidal activity against certain fungi and strains of *Serratia marcescens* in laboratory test was relatively low.[35,36]

Myristamidopropyl Dimethylamine

Myristamidopropyl dimethylamine (MAPD) has a broad activity against bacteria and fungi (membrane leakage). Codling et al[37] and others[6,38] have demonstrated enhanced activity of MAPD and Polyquad formulated in combination.

Polyhexamethylene Biguanides

May[39] reviewed the use of polyhexamethylene biguanides (PHMB) as in preservative, sanitizer, and disinfectant formulations in various food, water, and clinical applications, including contact lens disinfection systems.[40,41] PHMB is a complex of polymeric biguanides with an average polymer length of 5(n) and molecular weight of 3000.[42,43]

The specific proportion of short to long polymer lengths enhances antimicrobial activity against bacteria, fungi, and amoebae, as does their formulation in a borate buffer with nonionic surfactants. Concentrations of PHMB in all contact lens solutions (because of toxicity) are typically found to be below minimal biocidal concentrations found for challenge microorganisms in laboratory procedures. For example, a minimum biocidal concentration of PHMB for 10^6 to 10^7 cells of *Pseudomonas aeruginosa* in water with a 1-hour exposure could range from about 20 to 500 μg/mL. Formulations with PHMB may vary in their polymer mixtures in different manufactured lots. The type of poloxamer or nonionic surfactants used as emulsifiers and the presence of chelating agents such as EDTA may have a significant effect on the antimicrobial efficacy of the final formulation.[44]

Polyquad and PHMB have been formulated into MPS that allow for a simple one-step cleaning, disinfection, and storage process. This one-step procedure resulted in greater compliance, which appeared to be associated with reduced incidence of infections.[37,38,45]

Chlorhexidine

The chemical properties of chlorhexidine and its mode of antimicrobial activity were reviewed extensively by Denton[46] (see chapter 22). This cationic bisbiguanide at concentrations of >0.05% (500 μg/mL) is used extensively as a skin disinfectant. At sublethal concentrations, the compound causes cell membrane damage and ion leakage; at lethal concentrations, proteins in the cytoplasm are coagulated. The native compound is poorly soluble in water; thus, the water-soluble gluconate salt is used in contact lens solutions.

Because of the previously mentioned hypersensitivity reactions and toxicity for ocular tissues, contact lens solutions do not typically contain more than 0.006% of the gluconate salt. At these concentrations, inocula of 10^6 cells of *P aeruginosa* and *Staphylococcus epidermidis* were reduced by more than 1 log within 1 minute, whereas more than 3 minutes were required for a log reduction of *S marcescens* and from 8 minutes to 24 minutes for *Candida albicans* and *Aspergillus fumigatus*.[47] Chlorhexidine formulations with borate salts have greater antimicrobial activity than chlorhexidine solutions in phosphate buffers (PBS).[48-50] Isolates of *S marcescens* may adapt to growth in the latter type formulations, and these adapted cells show increased resistance to BAK and other preservatives.[49] Chlorhexidine has demonstrated therapeutic value in the treatment of *Acanthamoeba* keratitis (AK)[51] and is used in the cleaning and disinfection of rigid lenses.

Alexidine

Like chlorhexidine, alexidine (1,1′-hexamethylene-bis [5-(2-ethylhexyl)biguanide]) is a cationic preservative with broad antimicrobial properties for vegetative bacteria, fungi, and amoeba.[52] Both compounds are recognized oral and skin disinfectants (see chapter 22). Alexidine, however, has wider applications as a copreservative in formulations compatible with a broader diversity of current contact lens materials.[53-58]

Chlorhexidine and alexidine are structurally similar hydrophobic-lipophilic molecules that bind to lipopolysaccharides and lipoteichoic acids affecting cell membrane integrities that can culminate in cell lysis. Alexidine differs from chlorhexidine in possessing ethylhexyl end groups. Modes and rates of membrane disruption by alexidine vary with cell type and for amoeba and fungi may involve downregulation of mitochondrial-protein tyrosine phosphatase.[54,58-62] Alexidine is used in approved concentration of 0.00045%, 0.0002%, and 0.00016% in various contact lens solutions.

Thimerosal

Thimerosal is an organomercurial compound (ethylmercury thiosalicylate) with a broad antimicrobial spectrum but is most effective when used in combination with other preservatives. Penley et al[63] found that 10^6 cells of *S marcescens*, but not 10^3 cells, introduced into saline preserved with 400 μg/mL remained viable for 24 hours.

A combination of chlorhexidine (50 μg/mL) and thimerosal (10 μg/mL) produced efficacious D-values for *S marcescens* (0.22 min) and species of *Aspergillus* (90 min), *Candida* (0.67-15 min), and *Fusarium* (3.0-4.7 min) relatively similar to those of H_2O_2 in a comparison with other preservatives.[64] All these challenge organisms were considered resistant types compared with isolates of *Pseudomonas* and *Staphylococcus*. Gandhi et al[49] and Parment el al[65] found that *S marcescens* grew in certain chlorhexidine- and BAK-preserved solutions; there is no report of growth of *S marcescens* in lens solutions preserved both with thimerosal and chlorhexidine. Unfortunately, thimerosal and chlorhexidine have been associated with rare unacceptable incidents of ocular hypersensitivity reactions.[66,67] Nevertheless, thimerosal serves as a preservative in limited types of multidose preparations and worldwide topical-ocular formulations with noted activity against certain fungi.[68]

Chlorine

Tablets of sodium dichloroisocyanurate when dissolved in water are used to release approximately 3 μg/mL chlorine, as a strong oxidizing agent that rapidly inactivate planktonic bacteria via hypochlorous acid and the hypochlorite ion (see chapter 15). These highly reactive chlorine solutions are neutralized rapidly by residual cleaner and organic material and are typically unsuitable for other than short periods of lens storage.

Alcohols

Benzyl alcohol as a disinfection agent for hard and RGP lenses and isopropyl alcohol (propan-2-ol) in a surfactant-based cleaning formulation are examples of the use of alcohols in current contact lens systems. May et al[69] found that cells of *S marcescens* in the planktonic state and cells of *S marcescens* and *P aeruginosa* adhered to lenses survived in an RGP cleaning-disinfecting and storage solutions containing 0.1% benzyl alcohol. Challenge inocula introduced into the alcohol solution were not recoverable within 1 minute. The mode of action is primarily through protein coagulation and dissolution of the cell membrane. The isopropyl cleaning solution is toxic to the cornea, and unless lenses are rinsed thoroughly, their insertion causes immediate eye irritation.

Sorbic Acid and Potassium Sorbate

Sorbic acid and its salt, potassium sorbate, are used as preservatives in cleaning solutions and preserved salines, offering protection mainly as fungistatic agents.

The observed activity against bacteria decreases as the pH increases above pH 6.5 (see chapter 12). The unsaturated carboxylic acid is effective in contact lens solutions only in combination with borate buffers or H_2O_2.

▶ MICROBIAL KERATITIS

Contact lens–related keratitis can be divided into three categories: (1) infectious keratitis with positive cultures; (2) infectious keratitis with negative cultures; and (3) sterile infiltrates, which may result from corneal, hypoxia, or immune-mediated hypersensitivity reactions.[70] Changes in the local environment of the eye (eg, pH, corneal hydration, carbon dioxide, and lactic acid production) associated with interactions of hydrogel contact lenses and microbial populations may induce corneal infiltration. It is difficult in many cases to distinguish a slowly developing infectious infiltration from a sterile infiltration. Stein et al[71] observed that most (70%) sterile infiltrates and some (35%) infectious infiltrates are less than 1.0 mm in diameter.

The true "sterility" of the cornea mucosa may be questioned by several 16S rRNA gene sequencing studies that demonstrated significant differences in the diversity and abundance of certain bacteria in comparison to traditional culture techniques.[72-74] These reports seem in general agreement that any commensal component of the cornea mucosa (eg, *Delftia*) that may not present by routine culture procedures are in low abundance relative to other mucosal tissues of the individual. The relative abundance of the prominent genera in these studies did shift in some instances with contact lens wear.[74,75] Commensals in ocular tissue have been projected to elicit protective immune responses for extant microbiota.[76] The observed alterations of the ocular/mucosal-commensal microbiome from contact lens wear have not been associated with rare contact lens–associated microbial keratitis (CLMK).

Recent approaches in discerning what factors are the greater risks related to microbial keratitis in lens wear have centered on contaminated lens storage cases and poor lens hygiene practices (over time found with nearly all contact lens users).[68] The contact lens may serve as a fomite or, in some cases, a vector in transporting potentially pathogenic microorganisms from a contaminated contact lens case to the eye resulting in rare CLMK.[23,77]

Incidence

A CLMK is a rare infection that occurs at an overall incidence of about 1 to 4 per 10 000 contact lens wearers per year.[78-81]

Epidemiological studies by Morgan et al[82] reported a higher incidence of severe keratitis among those who wear hydrogel lenses while sleeping, but the risk for severe keratitis was 5 times lower for silicone hydrogels versus conventional hydrogels.

Dart et al[83] indicated that the severity, but not the incidence of CLMK, was reduced with use of daily disposable (DD) silicone hydrogel lenses versus other daily wear (DW) reusable silicone hydrogel modalities. Presumably, use of DD under optimal circumstances (eg, no napping or finger manipulation during wear) would negate the need for contact lens cleaning, disinfection, and storage. DD use carried a somewhat higher risk for any form of CLMK. Dart et al[83] suggest that exposure of the lens to a contaminated lens case was possibly less important than lens wear stressors such as tear film stagnation or reduced corneal epithelial cell turnover. The data also suggested a brand association risk. A similar study in Australia, however, did not detect any increased incidence of CLMK with DD use or differences in risk with lens type from previous reports.[81] The above surveys and adjunct laboratory studies that supported an overall rare incidence of CLMK were inclusive of several overlapping outbreaks of contact lens–associated *Fusarium* and AK.[84-87]

Demographics for lens wear in 39 countries surveyed during 5 consecutive years (2006-2010) indicated a near 80% soft daily lens wear modality. The EW modalities decreased over this study from about 12% to 8%.[88] Various lens wear modalities noted for different countries and environments shifted with time and ranged in use from less than 1.0% to near 30%.[88] Data tabulated at the Centers for Disease Control and Prevention for 2010-2015 noting instances of adverse lens events were highest for soft DW at 57%, soft EW at 35%, and 3% to 4% for soft DD, RGP, and decorative types.[1]

Consensus opinions noted that overnight wear presented the highest risk factor for CLMK with poor storage case hygiene (eg, evaporation, topping-off, or reuse of solution) as an additional overriding risk factor. Maintaining low rates of CLMK for specific geographies has been challenged by outbreaks emanating from microbial outbreaks of ill-defined etiology.

Overall, the minimum risk for CLMK seemed associated with soft silicone hydrogel DD wear, but an unknown degree of this regimen may have involved sporadic disinfection and storage of lenses.[24,34,77,89-92] Regardless of the actual circumstance of (inappropriate) handling and geographic-environmental influences, all DD soft contact lens wear, whether with high oxygen-permeable silicone or conventional HEMA lenses, seem to bear a risk for CLMK approximating that of other DW modalities.[80,93]

Contamination of Contact Lens Cases

Essentially, all contact lens users at one time or another are inserting lenses on the eye from contaminated storage contact lens cases. New cases with fresh solutions inappropriately handled may have high levels of *Pseudomonas*, *Serratia*, or *Acinetobacter* within 1 to 2 days of use without any immediate association of ocular events. Surveys indicating above 50% incidences of microbe-contaminated cases among contact lens users are not unusual.[68]

When isolated and tested, pseudomonads, in particular from contaminated contact lens cases, mostly prove susceptible to the manufacturers' recommended contact lens disinfection regime and to routine challenge tests with planktonic inocula. Monitored cleaning and disinfection regimens with various solutions and lenses have demonstrated that contamination of cases can be significantly reduced.[34,89] Noncompliance with manufacturers' recommendations for hand washing, cleaning, and disinfection of lenses and storage cases seem to be major causative factors in case contaminations. It needs to be recognized that multiple microbes, particularly strains of *P aeruginosa* from the aerosol environment of a bathroom or shower for example, may bind within seconds of contact to certain lenses or lens case surfaces and exhibit increased resistance to a routine disinfectant regimen. Within only minutes to a few hours, these attached and adhered cells may be expected to develop biofilms with survivable cells following standard exposures to various MPS.[34,77,94,95] A variety of protocols have been recommended for cleaning and disinfecting contact lens cases with various MPS that include wiping, air-drying, and so on and avoidance of water and topping-off of solutions.[68,96,97]

Bacterial Keratitis

Bacteria such as *S epidermidis* (part of the normal eye biota and the most common microorganism isolated from used contact lens paraphernalia) and various fungi, amoeba, and viruses may be associated with slowly developing corneal infiltrates.

The two most common gram-negative bacteria causing contact lens–associated keratitis are *P aeruginosa* and *S marcescens*. Neither of these bacteria are normal eye biota, but both are ubiquitous in the environment. These bacteria colonize water systems in swimming pools, hot tubs, and bathroom sinks and showers. Because of this ubiquity in nature, their presence in lens cases of asymptomatic contact lens users is not uncommon.[98] The more serious and rapidly progressive keratitis is caused by *P aeruginosa*. *P aeruginosa* is often associated with contamination of saline solutions or neutralized disinfectant solutions during storage,[99,100] whereas *S marcescens* is more readily established as a contaminant in preserved solutions.[49,100]

The microbiota of the conjunctiva and corneal surfaces of asymptomatic contact lens wearers may differ in species diversity and densities from those identified with asymptomatic noncontact users.[72,98,101] The differences may be transient and lack clear correlation with infections. Ocular microbiota associated with contact lens users because of normal handling probably reflect greater numbers of finger and eyelid microbiota than seen with noncontact lens users.[102,103]

Fungal Keratitis

Historically, and particularly in agriculture regions, fungal keratitis in uncompromised patient eyes is caused by molds representative of the genera *Aspergillus*, *Curvularia*, and *Fusarium*. The ocular infections are associated with the traumatic implantation of soil or vegetation that serves as fomites for viable mold propagules. With a few exceptions, the overall reported incidence of such infections relative to bacterial keratitis remains rare and tend to be associated with males. In some geographic regions with probable seasonal influence, fungi may be a prominent cause of infectious keratitis irrespective of contact lens wear.[104,105] Increasingly, over the past 30 years, however, contact lens wear inclusive of females has been recognized as a risk factor for rare infections by environmental molds.[106-113] Kredics et al[114] summarized the global involvement of near 70 different etiological agents of fungal keratitis stressing the significance and need for molecular identifications in selecting antifungal drugs.

Fungal conidia from the extant environs may be entrapped on the corneal surface by a contact lens. Also, certain soft contact lenses, both silicone and conventional (HEMA) types, may be invaded by fungi while being worn but apparently most often during storage in a lens case.[3,35,47,106,115-119]

A rare outbreak of several hundred infections of *Fusarium* keratitis during 2004-2006 was associated statistically with the use of an MPS seemingly incompatible with certain poor hygiene stresses during use and uptake of preservative in the solution by some lenses.[6,56,84,85,120-122] Bullock and colleagues[123] in a series of reports theorized a single point-source temperature event, and, later, temperature-increased absorption of the preservative (alexidine) by the MPS container bottle as possible factors in the outbreak. These studies used surrogate MPS formulations and bottles, the original products no longer being available. Unopened containers of the outbreak, MPS collected from localities of infection, had demonstrated antifusaria and antibacteria capacities sufficient to meet normal antimicrobial challenge requirements but insufficient in regard to the fusaria under multi-environmental stress factors of use.[3,24,124] Short et al[125,126] identified two new unique molecular species in the *Fusarium solani* complex (*Fusarium petroliphilum* and *Fusarium keratoplasticum*) as major adventitious pathogens associated with shower drains of patients in the outbreak. Isolates of the complex from patients and their contact lenses also were identified with a proclivity for producing biofilms with chlamydospores on lens cases and penetrating lenses.[3,118] The *F solani* complex is noted for involvement with water systems and human infections.[127,128] Following withdrawal of the MPS from the market in 2006, the overall incidence and geography of fusaria keratitis returned to their near prior status but overall fungal keratitis tended to increase.[112,113,122]

Walther et al[113] verified gene sequencing involvement of the *F solani* complex (FSSC-1) in 13 out of 15 cases of infections. Eighteen of 22 patients studied were females with use of soft contact lenses as a risk factor. There were no associations of infections with specific lens disinfection regimen in these studies (2007-2016). The MPS implicated in the 2004-2006 outbreaks was not involved as it had been withdrawn from the market.

Acanthamoeba Keratitis

Acanthamoeba keratitis (AK is caused by free-living amoeba broadly distributed in indoor and outdoor environments where they actively propagate in damp environments.[52,129-131] About 20 species have been described in the genus with cyst morphology as a base for group divisions; isolates identified as *Acanthamoeba castellanii* and *Acanthamoeba polyphaga* were prime species associated with rare CLMK.[30,132,133] A molecular basis in development (analysis of 18S rDNA gene typing) has indicated about 20 genotypes and a disconnect between classic and molecular species.[134,135] An AK infection may be initiated by invasion of microtraumatized corneal tissue by the feeding trophozoite stage (mostly T4 genotype) and, if a rare disease stage is attained, a slowly developed corneal ulcer that is recalcitrant to treatment. The dormant resistant cyst stage of the amoeba may be induced in the host tissues and could result in recurrent disease states.[136-138] *Acanthamoeba* have been associated with rare skin lesions and grave granulomatous encephalitis of immunocompromised.[139,140] Following the availability of contact lens wear to the general public in the 1970s, AK has been increasingly associated with contact lens wear (85%-95%) and exposures to extant water.[130,132,141] The persistence of the dormant stage with inappropriate lens hygiene is of major concern (Figure 53.1). The overall incidence of AK varies with water quality (eg, well water, tap water, flood water,

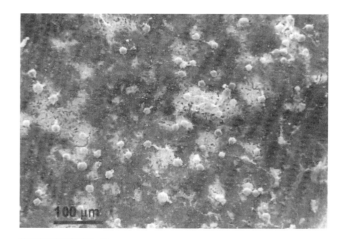

FIGURE 53.1 Cysts of *Acanthamoeba castellanii* in the bottom of a lens case from patient with amoebic keratitis. Viable amoeba and the fungus *Exophiala spinifera* were recovered from the case after more than 9 mo of dry storage.

grey water from roof reservoirs, and geography) and has been estimated at about 17 to 70 per million contact lens users per year.[86,131,134,141,142]

Increased AK in the Chicago, Illinois, area beginning in the early 2000s and peaking in 2007 was statistically associated with the use of an MPS separate from that involved with the *Fusarium* outbreak. The AK was independently associated with 35 of 38 patients using the MPS; however, nearly 39% of the AK patients never used the MPS. Topping-off and water exposures were noted.[143] Shortly after recall of the MPS, the numbers of AK decreased but not to the preoutbreak levels.[86,87,143]

The FK and AK outbreaks overlapped in time and to some extent geography but were deemed independent events. Dual infections independent of the implicated MPS have occurred.[144,145] Potentially, such infections are more prevalent because both eukaryotic organisms may present similar diagnostic difficulties and syndromes that in early stages may be resolved with similar therapies.[137,141,146,147]

Epidemiological Considerations: Indoor (Built) Environments

Select genotypes of the *A castellanii-A polyphaga* complex and fusaria complexes may co-colonize biofilms in filters and sumps of swimming pools, spas, tap water, and particularly in drains in residential, hospital, and industrial buildings.[87,125-128,134,148-151] Drains are subject to rapid temperature changes, periodic toxic chemicals and desiccation, conditions that may induce cells of fusaria to differentiate to chlamydoconidia, and those of amoeba to cyst-like stages.[118,152-155]

Acanthamoeba is noted for the intracellular harboring of *Legionella* and other human pathogens both in its feeding trophozoite- and dormant-resistant stages.[156-158]

Lateral gene transfer between genotypes of the *A castellanii* complex and various pathogenic fungi may underlie their virulence capacities.[159-161] The T4 group included isolates with intron clusters close relatives to those of fungi.[151,162]

Acanthamoeba spp are voracious feeders of microbiota in general and may be cannibalistic within the genus. They phagocytize conidia and other morphotypes of various fungi including ascospores and chlamydospores of *Fusarium*. The propagules may be lysed supporting trophozoite growth or they may harbor some fungal propagule for ill-defined periods with or without internal fungal propagation prior to their expulsion or the lysis of the trophozoite.

Cateau et al[163] examined coculture of trophozoites of *A castellanii* with conidia of *F oxysporum* in filtered tap water as well as effects of the tap water-amoeba supernatant on *F oxysporum*. Trophozoites and their supernatant-enhanced recovery of colony-forming units (CFUs) of *F oxysporum* on Sabouraud dextrose agar after 48 hour and 72 hour, respectively. Conidia germination was enhanced. The numbers of viable amoeba in coculture remained constant at 24 hour and 48 hour when compared with controls without conidia.[163] Conidia of the *F solani* genotypes of the *A castellanii-A polyphaga* complex and fusaria complexes may co-colonize. *F oxysporum* complexes internalized by trophozoites may germinate and exit amoeba. Cocultures established in nutrient-deficient PBS may demonstrate enhancement of hyphal development with conidia production versus conidia germination in PBS without amoeba.[163,164] Dependent on strains of fusaria and amoeba and test conditions (eg, volume of PBS, inocula ratios), some encystment may be observed.

Mutualistic cosurvival in PBS of trophozoites of *A castellanii* with internalized conidia of *F solani* engulfed from growing hyphal elements after 8 days is shown in Figure 53.2.

Cateau et al[163] proposed "the simultaneous presence of free-living amoeba and *F oxysporum* in the same environments can therefore lead to an increase in the fungal population." Such coexistence could provide conditions for lateral gene transfer and virulence enhancement between the fusaria and amoeba complexes.[162]

Keratitis among contact lens wearers caused by *Acanthamoeba* and *Fusarium* are infrequent relative to rare bacterial keratitis associated with lens wear. The sporadic or chronic occurrence of adventitious pathogens of the genera *Fusarium* and *Acanthamoeba* in water systems of a given building may be expected. The sparsity of reports on their concurrence in individual samples suggests a low cohabitation incidence or in situ monitoring procedures, which perhaps are tangent for such an observation. The concurrence of these microbes in extant damp ecosystems would be expected.

The demographics for the built environment itself (water system, central heating and air-conditioning, geography-climate) may affect the integrity of components

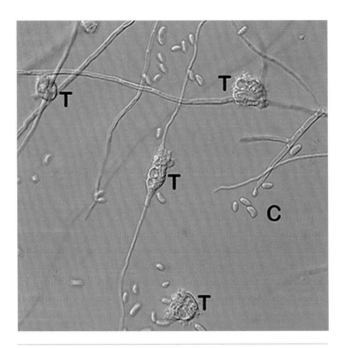

FIGURE 53.2 The replication-survivor relationships between *Acanthamoeba castellanii* and *Fusarium solani* hyphal strands without observable cyst or chlamydospore formation occurred under oligotrophic-like conditions over 8-10 d in two separate experiments. C, conidiophore of *Fusarium solani* complex with apical microconidium; T, trophozoites with phagocytized microconidia.

of a contact lens regimen facilitating contamination of the case with one or both organisms. Individual wearer stress factors from poor hygienic practices, perhaps even subtle dry-eye inflammation linked to ergonomics of the "digital screen area" could trigger rare tissue invasion.[165,166]

An epidemiological scheme for *Acanthamoeba* and *Fusarium* keratitis (AK-FK) is proposed in Figure 53.3.

▶ DISINFECTION SYSTEMS

Various electrically powered units for cleaning and disinfection of contact lenses, for example, standard wave and ultrasound devices,[167] integrated ultraviolet light units,[168] and heat devices, have been developed. A standard wave system (designed only for cleaning) removed mascara that had been applied to hydrogel and PMMA lenses, whereas some mascara remained on high-water content and RGP lenses after ultrasound treatment. Standard wave had no appreciable effect on the viability of microbes used in a lens challenge procedure, whereas ultrasound device was ineffective against fungi.[167] Admoni et al[168] reported that an integrated ultraviolet light cleaning and disinfection system was effective on lens when challenged with microorganisms. This same unit was not associated with any severe eye complications in clinical trials among 76 contact lens wearers who used the unit for up to 3 months. The major difficulty appeared to be malfunction of the unit.

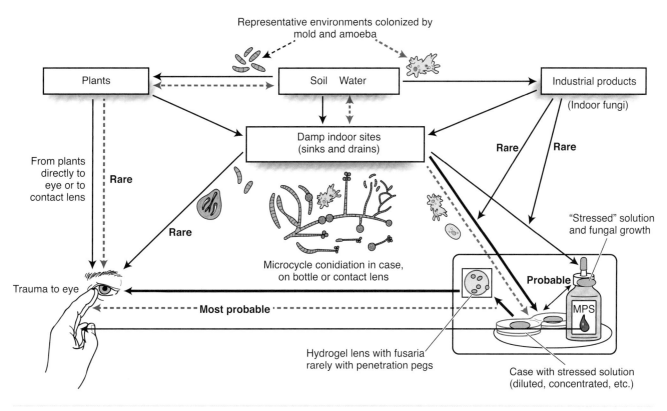

FIGURE 53.3 Environmental life cycle of *Acanthamoeba* and *Fusarium*.

Only heat, the first FDA approved system for disinfection of hydrogel lenses, has had successful and broad commercial application. Heating at 80°C for at least 10 minutes will kill most bacteria, fungi, and amoebae associated with ocular disease and contact lens wear (see chapter 11). Nevertheless, heat disinfection in the United States is decreasing in use. Disadvantages of the use of heat include discoloration and reduction in optical properties of certain types of lenses, inducement of deposits that cause eye irritation, and the need for a power source. Storage of heat-disinfected lenses in nonpreserved saline was a major cause of gram-negative bacterial keratitis during the 1980s. Miller[169] reviewed in detail the chemical composition uses and manufacturers of contact lens disinfectants.

A BAK at concentrations of 30 to 100 µg/mL provided for disinfection of PMMA and certain RGP lenses, but the adsorption of the BAK to soft lenses resulted in progressive eye irritation. Concentrations as low as 1.0 µg/mL of BAK induced growth arrest and apoptotic cell death in a continuous human conjunctival cell line.[33] Similarly, thimerosal, an antimicrobial first used in combination with chlorhexidine in early soft contact lens disinfection systems, gave broad-spectrum antimicrobial activity but induced delayed hypersensitivity in some wearers.[66] In certain Asian markets, concern remains over several serious hypersensitivities to chlorhexidine following release of the disinfectant from central venous catheters.[170] Such possible associations of anaphylactic shock with release

from catheters of chlorhexidine into the bloodstream have not been noted in the United States.[171]

LABORATORY DETERMINATIONS OF EFFICACY

Since 1990, contact lens care products, such as cleaners, chemical disinfection products, conditioning solutions, lubricating or rewetting solutions, saline solutions, and heat-disinfection units (with the exception of contact lens cases and cleaning accessories), have been grouped by the FDA as class II devices. Class II devices are governed by both general and special controls. General controls involve regulations on manufacturing practices, quality assurance of composition, labeling, records, submission of premarket notification, and so forth. Special controls for contact lens care products include the promulgation of performance standards for assurance of the safety and effectiveness of the device. Evidence must be presented that any new product demonstrates a substantial equivalence to similar or "generic" legally marketed devices.

In May 1997, the FDA released a premarket notification (510k) guidance document for industry for the evaluation of contact lens care products. Topics addressed in the guidelines include sterilization, manufacturing chemistry, toxicology, clinical evaluations, labeling, and microbiology. Microbiology data are required for all "in-eye" contact lens solutions, such as lubricating drops.

The guidelines advise that these types of products should not be packaged in bottle sizes that exceed 30 mL and that their formulations should be antimicrobial. A synopsis of the FDA recommended microbial challenge procedures for substantiating the microbial efficacy of various eye-care products is presented herein.

Multidose Preserved Contact Lens Products

Contact lens products such as artificial tears (10-mL volumes, three separate lots) are challenged with separate inoculum (10^5 to 10^6 cells in Dulbecco's phosphate-buffered saline without calcium chloride or magnesium chloride [DPBS] or with 0.05% wt/vol Tween 80 [DPBST]) of *Pseudomonas aeruginosa* NCIMB 8626, ATCC 9027; *Staphylococcus aureus* NCTC 10788, ATCC 6538; *Escherichia coli* NCIB 8245, ATCC 8739; *C albicans* ATCC 10231; *Aspergillus niger* IMI 149007, ATCC 16404.

The challenge inocula of bacteria, after steps for appropriate neutralization for preservative carryover, should be reduced by at least a mean value of 3.0 log by 7 and 14 days of incubation of the product at 20°C to 25°C. The product is rechallenged at day 14, and a similar 3.0 log reduction should be seen at day 28. The numbers of recoverable fungi should be within ±0.5 log of the initial inoculum at 14 days and also after the rechallenge at day 28. The products should be able to maintain this level of efficacy throughout their indicated shelf-life.

Bacteriostasis Test

Multidose saline products that do not contain conventional preservatives but do contain bacteriostatic agents, such as borates, EDTA, or potassium sorbate, should have a discard date. The discard date is based on results of a challenge test similar to that for multidose preserved products. The product label should indicate that the product be discarded within a specified time after its initial opening. The specified time should be within the period before an increase in the number of any of the challenge organisms in the bacteriostasis test.

▶ FDA AND ISO DISINFECTION GUIDELINES

Heat

The disinfection systems for contact lenses vary with the type of lens and its particular chemical composition. Microbiological data for heat disinfection units are not generally required for contact lenses, provided the temperature and cycle time of the unit are at least maintained at 80°C for 10 minutes. Heat disinfection is highly effective against most contact lens–associated microorganism, including trophozoites of *Acanthamoeba*,[172,173] but it adversely affects the physical properties of most high-water content lenses and RGP lenses and requires a power source. For these reasons, cold disinfection procedures prevail currently.

Chemical Disinfection

Stand-alone Procedures

Disinfecting products for contact lenses should show efficacy by at least one of two procedures. The *stand-alone procedure* according to ISO 14729 consists of an individual challenge by five microorganisms of three batches of product (chemical disinfecting solution),[174] with each batch challenged with a separate inoculum preparation of each organism. The challenge microorganisms are to include *P aeruginosa* ATCC 9027, *S aureus* ATCC 6538, *S marcescens* ATCC 13880, *C albicans* ATCC 10231, and *F solani* ATCC 36031. The freshly prepared inocula of each bacterium and yeast should give final challenge concentrations of 10^5 to 10^6 CFUs/mL of sample volume (inoculum volume not to exceed 1.0% of the sample volume). At 25%, 50%, 75%, and 100% of the minimum recommended disinfection time for the product, and, in addition, at not less than 4 times the minimum recommended disinfection time for yeast and molds, 1.0 mL of product should be processed for recoverable microorganisms. If overnight disinfection is recommended, recoveries should be processed after 8 hours.

All samples should be processed with validated conditions for neutralizing possible preservative carryover. The number of bacteria recovered per milliliter should be reduced by a mean value of not less than 3.0 log within the minimum recommended disinfection time. There should be a reduction in numbers of yeasts and molds of not less than 1.0 log within the minimum recommended disinfection time with no increase in densities within at least 4 times the minimum disinfection time. Multipurpose disinfecting solutions currently marketed are used in regimen that include "rub and rinse" protocol.[68,96]

Regimen Procedure

Disinfection products that fail to pass the stand-alone protocol but demonstrate a minimum reduction per bacterium of at least 1 log, a combined mean reduction of all bacteria of not less than 5.0 log, and stasis for the yeast and mold (±0.5 log) within the recommended disinfection period may be evaluated by a regimen test procedure (ISO 14729).[174] This procedure is prescribed for multifunctional disinfection regimens, which may include cleaning, rinsing, and soaking of a lens. The test procedures should be developed to include all steps in product labeling and patient instructions. A minimum of three lots of product should be tested. Each lot should be challenged with a separate inoculum preparation of each challenge organism. Challenge organisms include *P aeruginosa* ATCC 9027, *S aureus* ATCC 6538, *S marcescens* ATCC 13880, *C albicans* ATCC 10231, and *F solani* ATCC 36031. All regimen items, including cases, lenses, cleaning devices, solutions, and other items, should be new and unused. If the test product or regimen is compared with a predicate device, data for the predicate device should be included in the evaluation (eg, an H_2O_2 system compared with an approved H_2O_2 system). Separate inocula of each challenge organism (1×10^7 to 10^8 CFUs/ml) (three separate preparations for each organism, each used in separate challenges) are prepared in heat-inactivated bovine serum containing 10^8 heat-killed cells of *S cerevisiae*. The challenge inocula of 0.01 mL to give a final concentration of 10^5 to 10^6 cells is applied to both sides of the test lens. The test lenses (eight per lot of test product per microbial species tested) should be representative of those for which the product is intended. If the product is to be qualified for all hydrophilic lenses, representatives of groups 1 and 4 and the new group 5 of silicone lenses should be used (ISO 14729).[174] For hydrophobic lenses, four silicone-acrylate and four fluorosilicone-acrylate lenses are used. This procedure overall involves the testing of at least 120 lenses each for qualifying regimens for soft or RGP lenses. The inoculated lenses are held in a petri dish for 5 to 10 minutes at 20°C to 25°C and then processed identically as described in the manufacturer's consumer instructions, including all specified cleaning, rinsing, and soaking steps. If the regimen is compared with a predicate device, the procedures should be performed in similar fashion to those for the predicate device. Any deviations from the predicate protocol should be addressed in the manufacturer's instructions to consumers.

After the regimen is completed, test lenses with any surviving microorganisms should be transferred into an appropriate neutralizing solution. This solution, with the test lenses, is filtered through a membrane filter, and both lenses and membranes are transferred each to separate agar media.

No more than 10 CFUs per each lens-membrane combination should be recovered per challenge microorganism. Alternatively, the average number of surviving microorganisms on the last lens and filter should be essentially the same as numbers obtained with a predicate device (ie, within ≤0.5 log).

Few published studies have applied the FDA guidelines of 1997 to currently approved contact lens materials. All current materials and systems presumably would pass the microbiology laboratory criteria, particularly when "rinse and rub" procedures that remove up to several logs of inoculum from lenses are involved. Nevertheless, hydrogel lenses of wearers using any of the approved systems may become contaminated with bacteria, with

noncompliance with the manufacturer's regimen a major contributing factor.[23,68,96,175,176] The increasing use of multipurpose solutions has been suggested to be accompanied by a decrease in grave pseudomonads infections, however, an increasing incidence of minor inflammatory events.[73,93,177,178] The exact causes of these changes whether due to noncompliance, improper fit, dry eye syndrome, or combination of these are yet to be resolved.

Disinfection Effectiveness in the Presence of the Lens Case and the Lens—ISO 18259

This methodology—antimicrobial efficacy endpoint methodology to determine compatibility of contact lens solutions, lens cases, and hydrogel lenses for disinfection (AEEMC)[179]—provides a process for evaluating compatibility of solutions with specific lens and lens case materials with time in the presence of challenge organisms and organic soil. For practical purposes, this does not apply to oxidative systems.

New lenses and new lens cases with no preconditioning are to be used unless otherwise justified. A variety of lenses and case(s) recommended for use with the test solution are included in the protocol, for example, group 1, group 4, and representative silicone hydrogel materials. Log reductions for all five challenge organisms specified in ISO 14729 are for all exposure times. Preliminary applications of this protocol indicate that the commercially available disinfecting solutions antimicrobial efficacy varies depending on challenge organism, types and presence of contact lenses, and MPS biocide system, thus highlighting the importance of evaluating MPS for compatibility with lenses and lens cases. Some silicone hydrogel or soft hydrophilic contact lens materials interact with PHMB when soaked in commercially available MPS.[6,180] The study found that after soaking with lenses, the PHMB concentrations in the remaining solution as measured using high performance liquid chromatography were reduced. These lowered PHMB concentrations were associated with a decrease in antimicrobial efficacy against *S aureus*.[181] Another study reported by Clavet et al[24] demonstrated that PHMB uptake by contact lenses over time can reduce its concentration in the formulation and subsequently reduce the fungicidal activity of the MPS against *F solani*.

Method for Evaluating *Acanthamoeba* Encystment by Contact Lens Care Products—ISO 19045-1

This standard specifies a method[182] for evaluating the potential of products for contact lens disinfection to induce trophozoites of *Acanthamoeba* to form immature or mature cysts. This method excludes the evaluation of oxidative systems that require a special lens case for use. After exposure to test solutions, trophozoites are treated with detergent (for lysis) and calcofluor white staining that provide for microscopic observations of cysts. Earlier studies with nonstandard conditions indicated that various MPS in comparative tests differed significantly in cyst induction and under conditions of MPS evaporation.[183]

During recent decades, the incidence of infection keratitis, the spectrum of their etiological agents, and their association with contact lens wear have remained similar.[93,184,185]

The global contact lens market become somewhat stable with a near 50% turnover ratio between new and experienced wearers, with discomfort seemingly related to the dry eye syndrome and meibomian gland disorders.[186] Poor hygiene and noncompliance, however, seems to persist with contact lens wear. Appropriate disinfection is essential for fungi and amoeba that may threaten grave infections.[6,187] Future contact lens wear, however, is anticipated to expand with extension in the Asian countries and more personalized diversity in contact lens types and regime including therapeutic usage.

REFERENCES

1. Cope JR, Collier SA, Srinivasan K, et al. Contact lens-related corneal infections—United States, 2005–2015. *MMWR Morb Mortal Wkly Rep*. 2016;65(32):817-820.

2. Cope JR, Collier SA, Nethercut H, Jones JM, Yates K, Yoder JS. Risk behaviors for contact lens-related eye infections among adults and adolescents—United Sates, 2016. *MMWR Morb Mortal Wkly Rep*. 2017;66(32):841-845.

3. Zhang S, Ahearn DG, Noble-Wang J, et al. Growth and survival of *Fusarium solani-F. oxysporum* complex on stressed multipurpose contact lens care solution films on plastic surfaces in situ and in vitro. *Cornea*. 2006;25(10):1210-1216.

4. Zhao Z, Wei X, Aliwarga Y, Carnt NA, Garrett Q, Willcox MD. Proteomic analysis of protein deposits on worn daily wear silicone hydrogel contact lenses. *Mol Vis*. 2008;14:2016-2024.

5. Nash WL, Gabriel MM. Ex vivo analysis of cholesterol deposition for commercially available silicone hydrogel contact lenses using a fluorometric enzymatic assay. *Eye Contact Lens*. 2014;40(5):277-282.

6. Gabriel MM, McAnally C, Bartell J. Antimicrobial efficacy of multipurpose disinfecting solutions in the presence of contact lenses and lens cases. *Eye Contact Lens*. 2016;44(2):125-131.

7. Situ P, Simpson TL, Fonn D, Jones LW. Conjunctival and corneal pneumatic sensitivity is associated with signs and symptoms of ocular dryness. *Invest Ophthalmol Vis Sci*. 2008;49(7):2971-2976.

8. Efron N, Morgan PB. Rethinking contact lens aftercare. *Clin Exp Optom*. 2017;100(5):411-431.

9. Tighe B. Silicone hydrogels: structure, properties and behavior. In: Sweeney DF, ed. *Silicone Hydrogels: Continuous-Wear Contact Lenses*. 2nd ed. Edinburgh, United Kingdom: Butterworth-Heinemann; 2004:1-27.

10. Jones L. Hydrogel contact lens materials: dead and buried or about to give rise again? Contact Lens Update Web site. https://contactlensupdate .com/2013/10/07/hydrogel-contact-lens-materials-dead-and-buried -or-about-to-rise-again/. Accessed October 7, 2013.

11. Stapleton F, Keay L, Edwards K, Holden B. The epidemiology of microbial keratitis with silicone hydrogel contact lenses. *Eye Contact Lens*. 2013;39(1):79-85.

12. Morgan P, Woods CA, Tranoudis IG, et al. International contact lens prescribing in 2015. Our 15th annual report in CLS provides information about 23,000 fits in 34 markets. *Contact Lens Spectr*. 2016;31:24-29.

13. Nichols JJ. Contact lenses 2016. A status quo remains for much of the contact lens industry. *Contact Lens Spectr*. 2017;32:22-25,27,29,55.

14. Jones L, Evans K, Sariri R, Franklin V, Tighe B. Lipid and protein deposition of N-Vinyl pyrrolidone-containing group II and group IV frequent replacement contact lenses. *CLAO J*. 1997;23:122-126.

15. LaPorte RJ, ed. Common hydrophilic polymers. In: *Hydrophilic Polymer Coatings for Medical Devices: Structure/Properties, Development, Manufacture and Applications*. Lancaster, PA: Technomic; 1997:57-80.

16. Cook AD, Sagers RD, Pitt WG. Bacterial adhesion to protein-coated hydrogels. *J Biomater Appl*. 1993;8:72-89.

17. Tighe B. A decade of silicone hydrogel development: surface properties, mechanical properties, and ocular compatibility. *Eye Contact Lens*. 2013;39(1):4-12.

18. Jones L, Subbaraman LN, Rogers R, Dumbleton KA. Surface treatment, wetting and modulus of silicone hydrogels. *Optician*. 2006;232(6067):28-34.

19. Beattie TK, Tomlinson A, Seal DV. Surface treatment or material characteristic: the reason for the high level of *Acanthamoeba* attachment to silicone hydrogel contact lenses. *Eye Contact Lens*. 2003;29(suppl 1):S40-S43.

20. Hutter JC, Green JG, Eydelman MB. Proposed silicone hydrogel contact lens grouping system for lens care product compatibility testing. *Eye Contact Lens*. 2012;38(6):358-362.

21. International Organization for Standardization. *Ophthalmic Optics—Contact Lenses—Part 1: Vocabulary, Classification System and Recommendations for Labeling Specifications*. Geneva, Switzerland: International Organization for Standardization; 2017.

22. Houlsby RD, Ghajar M, Chavez G. Microbiological evaluation of soft contact lens disinfecting solutions. *J Am Optom Assoc*. 1984;55:205-211.

23. Ahearn DG, Gabriel MM. Disinfection of contact lenses. In: Block SS, ed. *Disinfection, Sterilization, and Preservation*. 5th ed. Baltimore, MD: Lippincott Williams & Wilkins; 2001:1105-1114.

24. Clavet CR, Chaput MP, Silverman MD, et al. Impact of contact lens materials on multipurpose contact lens solution disinfection activity against *Fusarium solani*. *Eye Contact Lens*. 2012;38:379-384.

25. Tilia D, Lazon de la Jara P, Weng R, Willcox MD. Short-term clinical comparison of two dual-disinfection multipurpose disinfecting solutions. *Eye Contact Lens*. 2014;40:7-11.

26. Penley CA, Llabrés C, Wilson LA, Ahearn D. Efficacy of hydrogen peroxide disinfection systems for soft contact lenses contaminated with fungi. *CLAO J*. 1985;11:65-68.

27. Lowe R, Brennan NA. Hydrogen peroxide disinfection of hydrogel contact lenses: an overview. *Clin Exp Optom*. 1987;70:190-197.

28. Davies DJG, Anthony Y, Meakin BJ, Kilvington S, Anger CB. Evaluation of the anti-acanthamoebal activity of five contact lens disinfectants. *Int Contact Lens Clin*. 1990;17:14-21.

29. Gottardi W. Iodine and iodine compounds. In: Block SS, ed. *Disinfection, Sterilization, and Preservation*. 5th ed. Baltimore, MD: Lippincott Williams & Wilkins: 2001:159-183.

30. Kilvington S, Gray T, Dart J, et al. *Acanthamoeba* keratitis: the role of domestic tap water contamination in the United Kingdom. *Invest Ophthalmol Vis Sci*. 2004;45:165-169.

31. Yanai R, Yamada N, Ueda K, et al. Evaluation of povidone-iodine as a disinfectant solution for contact lenses: antimicrobial activity and cytotoxicity for corneal epithelial cells. *Cont Lens Anterior Eye*. 2006;29:85-91.

32. Martin-Navarro CM, Lorenzo-Morales J, López-Arencibia A, Valladares B, Piñero JE. *Acanthamoeba* spp.: efficacy of Bioclen FR One Step, a povidone-iodine based system for the disinfection of contact lenses. *Exp Parasitol*. 2010;126:109-112.

33. De Saint Jean M, Brignole MF, Bringuier AF, Bauchet A, Feldmann G, Baudouin C. Effects of benzalkonium chloride on growth and survival of Chang conjunctival cells. *Invest Ophthalmol Vis Sci*. 1999;40:619-630.

34. Wilson LA, Sawant AD, Ahearn DG. Comparative efficacies of soft contact lens disinfectant solutions against microbial films in lens cases. *Arch Ophthalmol*. 1991;109:1155-1157.

35. Richardson LE, Begly CG, Keck GK. Comparative efficacies of soft contact lens disinfection systems against a fungal contaminant. *J Am Optom Assoc.* 1993;64:210-214.

36. Lever AM, Miller MJ. Comparative antimicrobial efficacy of multi-purpose lens care solutions using the FDA's revised guidance document for industry: stand-alone primary criteria. *CLAO J.* 1999;25:52-56.

37. Codling CE, Maillard JY, Russell AD. Aspects of the antimicrobial mechanisms of action of a polyquaternium and an amidoamine. *J Antimicrob Chemother.* 2003;51:1153-1158.

38. Codling CE, Hann AC, Maillard JY, Russell AD. An investigation into the antimicrobial mechanisms of action of two contact lens biocides using electron microscopy. *Cont Lens Anterior Eye.* 2005;28:163-168.

39. May OW. Polymeric antimicrobial agents. In: Block SS, ed. *Disinfection, Sterilization, and Preservation.* 4th ed. Philadelphia, PA: Lea & Febiger; 1991:322-333.

40. Mashat BH. Polyhexamethylene biguanide hydrochloride: features and applications. *Br J Environ Sci.* 2017;4(1):40-55.

41. Place LW, Gulcius-Lagoy SM, Lum JS. Preparation and characterization of PHMB-based multifunctional microcapsules. *Colloids Surf A.* 2017;530:76-84.

42. Gilbert P, Pemberton D, Wilkinson DE. Barrier properties of the gram-negative cell envelope towards high molecular weight polyhexamethylene biguanides. *J App Bacteriol.* 1990;69:585-592.

43. Gilbert P, Pemberton D, Wilkinson DE. Synergism within polyhexamethylene biguanide biocide formulations. *J Appl Bacteriol.* 1990;69:593-598.

44. Portolés M, Leong F-L, Refojo MF. Inhibition of *Pseudomonas aeruginosa* adherence to hydrophilic contact lenses with poloxamers [poly(oxyethylene)/poly(oxypropylene) block copolymers]. *Invest Ophthalmol Vis Sci.* 1992;33(suppl):1292.

45. Stevenson RNW, Seal DV. Has the introduction of multi-purpose solutions contributed to a reduced incidence of *Acanthamoeba keratitis* in contact lens wearers? A review. *Cont Lens Anterior Eye.* 1998;21:89-92.

46. Denton GW. Chlorhexidine. In: Block SS, ed. *Disinfection, Sterilization, and Preservation,* 4th ed. Philadelphia, PA: Lea & Febiger; 1991:274-289.

47. Shih KL, Raad MK, Hu JC, et al. Disinfecting activities of non-peroxide soft contact lens cold disinfection solutions. *CLAO J.* 1991;17:165-168.

48. Houlsby RD, Ghajar M, Chavez L. Antimicrobial activity of borate-buffered solutions. *Antimicrob Agents Chemother.* 1986;29:803-806.

49. Gandhi PA, Sawant AD, Wilson LA, et al. Adaptation and growth of *Serratia marcescens* in contact lens disinfectant solutions containing chlorhexidine gluconate. *Appl Environ Microbiol.* 1993;59:183-188.

50. Ogunbiyi L, Smith FX, Reidhammer TM, inventors; Bausch and Lomb Inc, assignee. Disinfecting and preserving systems and methods of use. US patent 4,758,595. July 19, 1988

51. Seal D, Hay J, Kirkness C, et al. Successful medical therapy of *Acanthamoeba* keratitis with topical chlorhexidine and propamidine. *Eye (Lond).* 1996;10:413-421.

52. Llyod D. Encystment in *Acanthamoeba castellanii*: a review. *Exp Parasitol.* 2014;145(suppl):S20-S27.

53. Borazjani RN, Kilvington K. Efficacy of multipurpose solutions against *Acanthamoeba* species. *Cont Lens Anterior Eye.* 2005;28(4):169-175.

54. Alizadeh H, Neelam S, Cavanagh D. Amoebicidal activities of Alexidine against 3 pathogenic strains of *Acanthamoeba. Eye Contact Lens.* 2009;35(1):1-5.

55. Kilvington S, Huang L, Kao E, Powell C. Development of a new contact lens multipurpose solution: comparative analysis of microbiological, biological and clinical performance. *J Optom.* 2010;3(3):134-142.

56. Green AJ, Phillips KS, Hitchins VM, et al. Material properties that predict preservative for silicone hydrogel contact lenses. *Eye Contact Lens.* 2012;38(6):350-357.

57. Bausch & Lomb. *renu* advanced multi-purpose solution brings you innovations in lens care. Bausch & Lomb Web site. https://www.renu.com/why-renu. Accessed August 2019.

58. McDonnnell G, Russell AD. Antiseptics and disinfectants: activity, action, and resistance. *Clin Microbiol Rev.* 1999;12:147-179.

59. Khunkitti W, Lloyd D, Furr JR, Russell AD. Aspects of the mechanisms of action of biguanides on trophozoites and cysts of *Acanthamoeba castellanii. J Appl Microbiol.* 119;82:107-114.

60. Chawner JA, Gilbert P. A comparative study of the bactericidal and growth inhibitory activities or the bisbiguanides alexidine and chlorhexidine. *J Appl Bacteriol.* 1989;66:243-252.

61. Zorko M, Jerala RJ. Alexidine and chlorhexidine bind to lipopolysaccharides and lipoteichoic acid prevent cell activation by antibiotics. *J Antimicrob Chemother.* 2008;62:730-737.

62. Niemi NM, Lanning NU, Westrate LM, MacKeigan JP. Down regulation of the mitochondrial phosphatase PTPMT 1 is sufficient to promote cancer cell death. *PLoS One.* 2013;8(1):e53803.

63. Penley CA, Schlitzer RL, Ahearn DG, Wilson LA. Laboratory evaluation of chemical disinfection of soft contact lenses. *Contact Intraocul Lens Med J.* 1981;7:101-110.

64. Penley CA, Ahearn DG, Wilson LA. Inhibition of fungi by soft lens solutions as determined by FDA-recommended tests. *Dev Ind Microbiol.* 1983;24:369-375.

65. Parment PA, Colucci B, Nystrom B. The efficacy of soft contact lens disinfection solutions against *Serratia marcescens* and *Pseudomonas aeruginosa. Acta Ophthalmol Scand.* 1996;74:235-237.

66. Wilson LA, McNatt J, Reitschel R. Delayed hypersensitivity to thimerosal in soft contact lens wearers. *Ophthalmology.* 1981;88:804-809.

67. Wright P, Mackie I. Preservative-related problems in soft contact lens wearers. *Trans Ophthalmol Soc UK.* 1982;102:3-6.

68. Wu YT, Willcox M, Zhu H, Stapleton F. Contact lens hygiene compliance and lens case contamination: a review. *Cont Lens Anterior Eye.* 2015;38:307-316.

69. May LL, Gabriel MM, Simmons RB, Wilson LA, Ahearn DG. Resistance of adhered bacteria to rigid gas permeable contact lens solutions. *CLAO J.* 1995;21:242-246.

70. Mertz PH, Bouchard CS, Mathers WD, Goldman J, Shields WJ, Cavanagh HD. Corneal infiltrates associated with disposable extended wear soft contact lenses: a report of nine cases. *CLAO J.* 1990;16:269-272.

71. Stein M, Clinch TE, Cohen EJ, et al. Infected vs sterile corneal infiltrates in contact lens wearers. *Am J Ophthalmol.* 1988;105:632-636.

72. Shin H, Price K, Albert L, Dodick J, Park L, Dominguez-Bello MG. Changes in the eye microbiota associated with contact lens wearing. *MBio.* 2016;7(2):e00198.

73. Zhang H, Zhao F, Hutchinson DS, et al. Conjunctival microbiome changes associated with soft contact lens and orthokeratology lens wearing. *Invest Ophthalmol Vis Sci.* 2017;58:128-136.

74. Ozkan J, Nielsen S, Diez-Vives C, Coroneo M, Thomas T, Willcox M. Temporal stability and composition of the ocular surface microbiome. *Sci Rep.* 2017;7:9880.

75. Wiley L, Bridge DR, Wiley LA, Odom JV, Elliott T, Olson JC. Bacterial biofilm diversity in contact lens-related disease: emerging role of *Achromobacter, Stenotrophomonas,* and *Delftia. Invest Ophthalmol Vis Sci.* 2012;53:3896-3905.

76. Lu L, Liu J. Human microbiota and ophthalmic disease. *Yale J Bio Med.* 2016;89:325-330.

77. Mayo MS, Schlitzer RL, Ward MA, Wilson LA, Ahearn DG. Association of *Pseudomonas* and *Serratia* corneal ulcers with use of contaminated solutions. *J Clin Microbiol.* 1987;25:1398-1400.

78. Poggio EC, Glynn RJ, Schein OD, et al. The incidence of ulcerative keratitis among users of daily-wear and extended-wear soft contact lenses. *N Engl J Med.* 1989;321:779-783.

79. Schein OD, Glynn RJ, Poggio EC, Seddon JM, Kenyon KR. The relative risk of ulcerative keratitis among users of daily-wear and extended-wear soft contact lenses. A case-control study. *Microbial Keratitis Study Group. N Engl J Med.* 1989;321:773-778.

80. Schein OD, McNally JJ, Katz J, et al. The incidence of microbial keratitis among wearers of a 30-day silicone hydrogel extended-wear contact lens. *Ophthalmology.* 2005;112:2172-2179.

81. Stapleton F, Keay L, Edwards K. The incidence of contact lens-related microbial keratitis in Australia. *Ophthalmology.* 2008;115(10):1655-1662.

82. Morgan PB, Efron N, Hill EA, Raynor MK, Whiting MA, Tullo AB. Incidence of keratitis of varying severity among contact lens wearers. *Br J Ophthalmol.* 2005;89:430-436.

83. Dart JK, Radford CF, Minassian D, Verma S, Stapleton F. Risk factors for microbial keratitis with contemporary contact lenses: a case-control study. *Ophthalmology.* 2008;115(10):1647-1654.

84. Chang DC, Grant GB, O'Donnell K, et al. Multistate outbreak of *Fusarium* keratitis associated with use of a contact lens solution. *JAMA.* 2006;296:953-963.

85. Khor WB, Aung T, Saw SM, et al. An outbreak of *Fusarium* keratitis associated with contact lens wear in Singapore. *JAMA.* 2006;295:2867-2873.

86. Verani JR, Lorick SA, Yoder SJ, et al. National outbreak of *Acanthamoeba* keratitis associated with use of a contact lens solution, United States. *Emerg Infect Dis.* 2009;15:1236-1242.

87. Tu EY, Joslin CE. Recent outbreaks of atypical contact lens-related keratitis: what have we learned? *Am J Ophthalmol.* 2010;150:602-608.e2.

88. Efron N. *Contact Lens Complications.* 3rd ed. Edinburgh, United Kingdom: Elsevier; 2012.

89. Wilson LA, Sawant AD, Simmons RB, Ahearn DG. Microbial contamination of contact lens storage cases and solutions. *Am J Ophthalmol.* 1990;110:193-198.

90. Borazjani RN, Levy B, Ahearn DG. Relative primary adhesion of *Pseudomonas aeruginosa, Serratia marcescens* and *Staphylococcus aureus* to HEMA-type contact lenses and an extended wear silicone hydrogel contact lens of high oxygen permeability. *Cont Lens Anterior Eye.* 2004;27:3-8.

91. Amos CF, George MD. Clinical and laboratory testing of a silver-impregnated lens case. *Cont Lens Anterior Eye.* 2006;29:247-255.

92. Eydelman MB, Tarver ME, Kiang T, Alexander KY, Hutter JC. The Food and Drug Administration's role in establishing and maintaining safeguards for contact lenses and contact lens care products. *Eye Contact Lens.* 2012;38(6):346-349.

93. Stapleton F, Carnt N. Contact lens-related microbial keratitis: how have epidemiology and genetics helped us with pathogenesis and prophylaxis? *Eye.* 2012;26:185-193.

94. Miller MJ, Wilson LA, Ahearn DG. Effects of protein, mucin, and human tears on adherence of *Pseudomonas aeruginosa* to hydrophilic contact lenses. *J Clin Microbiol.* 1988;26:513-517.

95. Szczotka-Flynn L, Ahearn DG, Barr J, et al. History, evolution, and evolving standards of contact lens care. Moderator: *Cont Lens Anterior Eye.* 2013;36(suppl 1):S4-S8.

96. Vijay AJ, Willcox M, Zhu H, Stapleton F. Contact lens storage case hygiene practice and storage case contamination. *Eye Contact Lens.* 2015;41(2):91-97.

97. Boost M, Lai S, Ma C, Cho P. Do multipurpose contact lens disinfecting solutions work effectively against non-FDA/ISO recommended strains of bacteria and fungi? *Ophthalmic Physiol Opt.* 2010;30(1):12-19.

98. Ahanotu EN, Ahearn DG. Association of *Pseudomonas aeruginosa* and *Serratia marcescens* with extended-wear soft contact lenses in asymptomatic patients. *CLAO J.* 2002;28(3):157-159.

99. Cokington CD, Hyndiuk RA. Bacterial keratitis. In: Tabbara KF, Hyndiuk RA, eds. *Infections of the Eye.* 2nd ed. Boston, MA: Little, Brown and Company; 1996:328-348.

100. Parment PA. The role of *Serratia marcescens* in soft contact lens associated ocular infections. A review. *Acta Ophthalmol Scand.* 1997;75:67-71.

101. Willcox MD. Characterization of the normal microbiota of the ocular surface. *Exp Eye Res.* 2013;117:99-105.

102. Mowrey-McKee MF, Monnat K, Sampson HJ, et al. Microbial contamination of hydrophilic contact lenses. Part I: quantitation of microbes on patient worn-and-handled lenses. *CLAO J.* 1992;18:87-91.

103. Mowrey-McKee MF, Sampson HJ, Proskin HM. Microbial contamination of hydrophilic contact lenses. Part II: quantitation of microbes after patient handling and after aseptic removal from the eye. *CLAO J.* 1992;18:240-244.

104. Chowdhary A, Singh K. Spectrum of fungal keratitis in North India. *Cornea.* 2005;24(1):8-15.

105. Ansari Z, Miller D, Galor A. Current thoughts in fungal keratitis: diagnosis and treatment. *Curr Fungal Infect Rep.* 2013;7(3):209-218.

106. Wilson LA, Ahearn DG. Association of fungi with extended-wear soft contact lenses. *Am J Ophthalmol.* 1986;101:434-436.

107. Rosa RH, Miller D, Alfonso EC. The changing spectrum of fungal keratitis in South Florida. *Ophthalmology.* 1994;101:1005-1013.

108. Thomas PA. Fungal infections of the cornea. *Eye.* 2003;17(8):852-862.

109. Alfonso E, Miller D, Cantu-Dibildox J, O'brien TP, Schein OD. Fungal keratitis associated with non-therapeutic soft contact lenses. *Am J Ophthalmol.* 2006;142:154-155.

110. Pouyeh B, Galor A, Miller D, et al. New horizons in one of ophthalmology's challenges: fungal keratitis. *Exp Rev Ophthalmol.* 2011;6(11):529-540.

111. Collier SA, Gronostaj MP, MacGurn AK, et al. Estimated burden of keratitis—United States, 2010. *MMWR Morb Mortal Wkly Rep.* 2014;63(45):1027-1030.

112. Ong HS, Fung SSM, Macleod D, Dart JKG, Tuft SJ, Burton MJ. Altered patterns of fungal keratitis at a London ophthalmic referral hospital: an eight-year retrospective observational study. *Am J Ophthalmol.* 2016;168:227-236.

113. Walther G, Stasch S, Kaeger K, et al. *Fusarium* keratitis in Germany. *J Clin Microbiol.* 2017;55(10):2983-2995.

114. Kredics L, Narendran V, Shobana CS, Vágvölgyi C, Manikandan P. Filamentous fungal infections of the cornea: a global overview of epidemiology and drug sensitivity. *Mycoses.* 2015;58(4):243-260.

115. Simmons RB, Buffington JR, Ward M, Wilson LA, Ahearn DG. Morphology and ultrastructure of fungi in extended-wear soft contact lenses. *J Clin Microbiol.* 1986;24:21-25.

116. Buffington JR, Simmons RB, Wilson LA, et al. Effect of polymer differences on fungal penetration of hydrogel lenses. *J Ind Microbiol.* 1988;3:29-32.

117. Ahearn DG, Simmons RB, Zhang S, et al. Attachment to and penetration of conventional and silicone hydrogel contact lenses by *Fusarium solani* and *Ulocladium* sp. in vitro. *Cornea.* 2007;26:831-839.

118. Ahearn DG, Zhang S, Stulting RD, et al. *Fusarium* keratitis and contact lens wear: facts and speculations. *Med Mycol.* 2008;46:397-410.

119. Ahearn DG, Zhang S, Stulting RD, et al. Relative in vitro rates of attachment and penetration of hydrogel soft contact lenses by haplotypes of *Fusarium. Cornea.* 2009;28:447-450.

120. Saw SM, Ooi P-L, Tan DTH, et al. Risk factors for contact lens-related *Fusarium* keratitis: a case-control study in Singapore. *Arch Ophthalmol.* 2007;125:611-617.

121. Ma SK, So K, Chung PH, Tsang HF, Chuang SK. A multi-country outbreak of fungal keratitis associated with a brand of contact lens solution: the Hong Kong experience. *Int J Infect Dis.* 2009;13:443-448.

122. Gower EW, Keay LJ, Oechsler RA, et al. Trends in fungal keratitis in the United States, 2001 to 2007. *Ophthalmology.* 2010;117:2263-2267.

123. Bullock JD, Warwar RE, Elder B, Khamis HJ. Microbiological investigations of ReNu plastic bottles and the 2004 to 2006 ReNu with MoistureLoc-related worldwide *Fusarium* keratitis event. *Eye Contact Lens.* 2016;42(3):147-152.

124. Ramani R, Chaturvedi V. Evaluations of shorter exposures of contact lens cleaning solutions against *Fusarium oxysporum* species complex and *Fusarium solani* species complex to simulate inappropriate usage. *Antimicrob Agents Chemother.* 2011;55:2265-2275.

125. Short DPG, O'Donnell K, Zhang N, Juba JH, Geiser DM. Widespread occurrence of diverse human pathogenic types of the fungus *Fusarium* detected in plumbing drains. *J Clin Microbiol.* 2011;49:4264-4272.

126. Short DPG, O'Donnell K, Thrane U, et al. Phylogenetic relationships among members of the *Fusarium solani* species complex in human infections and the descriptions of *F. keratoplasticum* sp. nov. and *F. petroliphilum* stat. nov. *Fungal Genet Biol.* 2013;53:59-70.

127. Anaissie EJ, Kuchar RT, Rex JH, et al. Fusariosis associated with pathogenic *Fusarium* species colonization of a hospital water system: a new paradigm for the epidemiology of opportunistic mold infections. *Clin Infect Dis.* 2001;33:1871-1878.

128. Mehl HL, Epstein L. Sewage and community shower drains are environmental reservoirs of *Fusarium solani* species complex group 1, a human and plant pathogen. *Environ Microbiol.* 2008;10:219-227.

129. Marciano-Cabral F, Cabral G. *Acanthamoeba* spp. as agents of disease in humans. *Clin Microbiol Rev.* 2003;16(2):273-307.

130. Cateau E, Delafont V, Hechard Y, Rodier MH. Free-living amoebae: what part do they play in healthcare-associated infections? *J Hosp Infect.* 2014;87:131-140.

131. Walochnik J, Scheikl U, Haller-Schober EM. Twenty years of *Acanthamoeba* diagnostics in Austria. *J Eukaryot Microbiol.* 2015;62:3-11.

132. Ahearn DG, Gabriel MM. Contact lenses, disinfectants, and *Acanthamoeba* keratitis. *Adv Appl Microbiol.* 1997;43:35-56.

133. Tu EY, Joslin CE, Sugar L, Shoff ME, Booton GC. Prognostic factors affecting visual outcome in *Acanthamoeba* keratitis. *Ophthalmology.* 2008;115:1998-2003.

134. Booton GC, Rogerson A, Bonilla TD, et al. Molecular and physiological evaluation of subtropical environmental isolates of *Acanthamoeba* spp., causal agent of *Acanthamoeba* keratitis. *J Eukaryot Microbiol.* 2004;51:192-200.

135. Fuerst PA, Booton GC, Crary M. Phylogenetic analysis and the evolution of the 18S rRNA gene typing system of *Acanthamoeba. J Eukaryot Microbiol.* 2015;62(1):69-84.

136. Mathers WD, Nelson SE, Lane JL, Wilson ME, Allen RC, Folberg R. Confirmation of confocal microscopy diagnosis of *Acanthamoeba* keratitis using polymerase chain reaction analysis. *Arch Ophthalmol.* 2000;118:178-183.

137. Mathers WD. Use of higher medication concentrations in the treatment of *Acanthamoeba* keratitis. *Arch Ophthalmol.* 2006;124(6):923.

138. Carnt N, Stapleton F. Strategies for the prevention of contact lens-related *Acanthamoeba* keratitis: a review. *Ophthalmic Physiol Opt.* 2016;36(2):77-92.

139. Martinez AJ, Visvesvara GS. Free-living, amphizoic and opportunistic amoebas. *Brain Pathol.* 1997;7(1):583-598.

140. Walochnik J, Aichelburg A, Assadian O, et al. Granulomatous amoebic encephalitis caused by *Acanthamoeba* amoebae of genotype T2 in a human immunodeficiency virus-negative patient. *J Clin Microbiol.* 2008;46(1):338-340.

141. Seal DV. *Acanthamoeba* keratitis update—incidence, molecular epidemiology and new drugs for treatment. *Eye (Lond).* 2003;17(8):893-905.

142. Joslin CE, Tu EY, McMahon TT, Passaro DJ, Stayner LT, Sugar J. Epidemiological characteristics of a Chicago-area *Acanthamoeba* keratitis outbreak. *Am J Ophthalmol.* 2006;142(2):212-217.

143. Joslin CE, Tu EY, Shoff ME, et al. The association of contact lens solution use and *Acanthamoeba keratitis. Am J Ophthalmol.* 2007;144(2):169-180.

144. O'Brart DPS, Gavin EA. Contact-lens associated simultaneous *Fusarium* and *Acanthamoeba* keratitis treated with therapeutic penetrating keratoplasty. *J Clinic Exp Ophthalmol.* 2011;2:171.

145. Babu K, Murthy KR. Combined fungal and *Acanthamoeba* keratitis: diagnosis by in vivo confocal microscopy. *Eye (Lond)* 2007;21:271-272.

146. Gupta S, Shrivastava RM, Tandon R, Gogia V, Agarwal P, Satpathy G. Role of voriconazole in combined *Acanthamoeba* and fungal corneal ulcer. *Cont Lens Anterior Eye.* 2011;34:287-289.

147. Iovieno A, Gore DM, Carnt N, Dart JK. *Acanthamoeba* sclerokeratitis: epidemiology, clinical features, and treatment outcomes. *Ophthalmology.* 2014;121:2340-2347.

148. Boost M, Cho P, Lai S, Sun WM. Detection of *Acanthamoeba* in tap water and contact lens cases using polymerase chain reaction. *Optom Vis Sci.* 2008;85:526-530.

149. Trzyna WC, Mbugua MW, Rogerson A. *Acanthamoeba* in the domestic water supply of Huntington, West Virginia, U.S.A. *Acta Protozool.* 2010;49:9-15.

150. Stockman U, Wright CJ, Visvesvara GS, Fields BS, Beach MJ. Prevalence of *Acanthamoeba* spp. and other free-living amoebae in household water, Ohio, USA—1990-1992. *Parasitol Res.* 2011;108:621-627.

151. Corsaro D, Köhsler M, Montalbano FM, et al. Update on *Acanthamoeba* jacobsi genotype T15, including full-length 18S rDNA molecular phylogeny. *Parasitol Res.* 2017;116(4):1273-1284.

152. Coulon C, Collignon A, McDonnell G, Thomas V. Resistance of *Acanthamoeba* cysts to disinfection treatments used in health care settings. *J Clin Microbiol.* 2010;48:2689-2697.

153. Ahearn DG, Zhang S, Stulting RD, et al. In vitro interactions of *Fusarium* and *Acanthamoeba* with drying residues of multipurpose contact lens solutions. *Invest Ophthalmol Vis Sci.* 2011;52:1793-1799.

154. Ahearn DG, Simmons RB, Ward MA, Stulting RD. Potential resistant morphotypes of *Acanthamoeba castellanii* expressed in multipurpose contact lens disinfection systems. *Eye Contact Lens.* 2012;38:400-405.

155. Son H, Lee J, Lee YW. Mannitol induces the conversion of conidia to chlamydospore-like structures that confer enhanced tolerance to heat, drought, and UV in *Gibberella zeae. Microbiol Res.* 2012;167:608-615.

156. Fritsche TR, Gautom RK, Seyedirashti S, Bergeron DL, Lindquist TD. Occurrence of bacterial endosymbionts in *Acanthamoeba* spp. Isolated from corneal and environmental specimens and contact lenses. *J Clin Microbiol.* 1993;31:1122-1126.

157. Cirillo JD, Falkow S, Tomkins LS. Growth of *Legionella pneumophila* in *Acanthamoeba castellanii* enhances invasion. *Infect Immun.* 1994;62:3254-3261.

158. Choi SE, Cho MK, Ahn SC, et al. Endosymbionts of *Acanthamoeba* isolated from domestic tap water in Korea. *Korean J Parasitol.* 2009;47(4):337-344.

159. Steenbergen JN, Shuman HA, Casadevall A. *Cryptococcus neoformans* interactions with amoebae suggest an explanation for its virulence and intracellular pathogenic strategy in macrophages. *Proc Natl Acad Sci U S A.* 2001;98:15245-15250.

160. Thomas V, McDonnell G, Denyer SP, Maillard JY. Free-living amoebae and their intracellular pathogenic microorganisms: risks for water quality. *FEMS Microbiol Rev.* 2010;34(3):231-259.

161. Derengowski LS, Paes HC, Albuquerque P, et al. The transcriptional response of *Cryptococcus neoformans* to ingestion by *Acanthamoeba castellanii* and macrophages provides insights into the evolutionary adaptation to the mammalian host. *Eukaryot Cell.* 2013;12(5):761-774.

162. Clarke M, Lohan AJ, Liu B, et al. Genome of *Acanthamoeba castellanii* highlights extensive lateral gene transfer and early evolution of tyrosine kinase signaling. *Genome Biol.* 2013;14:R11.

163. Cateau E, Hechard Y, Fernandez B, et al. Free living amoebae could enhance *Fusarium oxysporum* growth. *Fungal Ecol.* 2014;8:12-17.

164. Nunes TET, Brazil NT, Fuentefria AM, Rott MB. *Acanthamoeba* and *Fusarium* interactions: A possible problem in keratitis. *Acta Trop.* 2016;157:102-107.

165. Chalmers RL, Young G, Kern J, Napier L, Hunt C. Soft contact lens-related symptoms in North America and the United Kingdom. *Optom Vis Sci.* 2016;93:836-847.

166. Nichols JJ. The impact of dry eye on modern contact lens wearers. *Contact Lens Spectrum.* 2017;32(36):38-40.

167. Efron N, Lowe R, Vallas V, et al. Clinical efficacy of standing wave and ultrasound for cleaning and disinfecting contact lenses. *Intl Contact Lens Clin.* 1991;18:24-29.

168. Admoni MM, Bartolomei A, Qureshi MN, Bottone EJ, Asbell PA. Disinfection efficacy in an integrated ultraviolet light contact lens care system. *CLAO J.* 1994;20:246-248.

169. Miller MJ. Contact lens disinfectants. In: Ascenzi JM, ed. *Handbook of Disinfectants and Antiseptics.* New York, NY: Marcel Dekker; 1995:83-109.

170. Terazawa E, Shimonaka H, Nagase K, Masue T, Dohi S. Severe anaphylactic reaction due to a chlorhexidine-impregnated central venous catheter. *Anesthesiology.* 1998;89:1296-1298.

171. Veenstra DL, Saint S, Saha S, Lumley T, Sullivan SD. Efficacy of antiseptic-impregnated central venous catheters in preventing catheter-related bloodstream infection. *JAMA.* 1999;281:261-267.

172. Connor CG, Blocker Y, Pitts DG. *Acanthamoeba culbertsoni* and contact lens disinfection systems. *Optom Vis Sci.* 1989;66:690-693.

173. Kilvington S. Moist-heat disinfection of *Acanthamoeba* cysts. *Rev Infect Dis.* 1991;13(suppl 5):S418.

174. International Organization for Standardization. *Ophthalmic Optics—Contact Lens Care Products—Microbiological Requirements and Test Methods for Products and Regimens for Hygienic Management of Contact Lenses.* Geneva, Switzerland: International Organization for Standardization; 2001.

175. Stone JH, Gabriel MM, Ahearn DG. Adherence of *Pseudomonas aeruginosa* to inanimate polymers including biomaterials. *J Ind Microbiol Biotechnol.* 1999;23:713-717.

176. Ky W, Scherick K, Stenson S. Clinical survey of lens care in contact lens patients. *CLAO J.* 1998;24:216-219.

177. Forster RK. The management of infectious keratitis as we approach the 21st century. *CLAO J.* 1998;24:175-180.

178. Stern GA. Contact lens associated bacterial keratitis: past, present, and future. *CLAO J.* 1998;24:52-56.

179. International Organization for Standardization. *Ophthalmic Optics—Contact Lens Care Products—Method to Assess Contact Lens Care Products with Contact Lenses in Lens Case, Challenged with Bacterial and Fungal Organisms.* Geneva, Switzerland: International Organization for Standardization; 2014.

180. Rosenthal RA, Dassanayake NL, Schlitzer RL, Schlech BA, Meadows DL, Stone RP. Biocide uptake in contact lenses and loss of fungicidal activity during storage of contact lenses. *Eye Contact Lens.* 2006;32(6):262-266.

181. Shoff ME, Lucas AD, Brown JN, Hitchins VM, Eydelman MB. The effects of contact lens materials on a multipurpose contact lens solution disinfection activity against *Staphylococcus aureus*. *Eye Contact Lens.* 2012;38:368-373.

182. International Organization for Standardization. *Ophthalmic Optics—Contact Lens Care Products—Method for Evaluating* Acanthamoeba *Encystment by Contact Lens Care Products.* Geneva, Switzerland: International Organization for Standardization; 2015.

183. Kilvington S, Heaselgrave W, Lally JM, Ambrus K, Powell H. Encystment of *Acanthamoeba* during incubation in multipurpose contact lens disinfectant solutions and experimental formulations. *Eye Contact Lens.* 2008;34(3):133-139.

184. Bennett L, Hugo YH, Tai S, et al. Contact lens versus non-contact lens-related corneal ulcers at an academic center. *Eye Contact Lens.* 2018;00:1-5. doi: 10.1097/ICL.0000000000000568.

185. Kowalski RP, Nayyar SV, Romanowski EG, et al. The prevalence of bacteria, fungi, viruses, and *Acanthamoeba* from 3,004 cases of keratitis, endophthalmitis, and conjunctivitis. *Eye Contact Lens.* 2019;00:1-4. doi: 10.1097/ICL.0000000000000642.

186. Pucker AD, Jones-Jordan LA, Marx S, et al. Clinical factors associated with contact lens dropout. *Contact lens and Anterior eye.* 2019; 42(3):318-324.

187. Gabriel MM, McAnally C, Bartell J, et al. Biocidal efficacy of a hydrogen peroxide lens care solution incorporating a novel wetting agent. *Eye Contact Lens.* 2019;45:164-170.

Infectious Waste Management, Treatment, and Disposal

Lawrence G. Doucet

In the modern era, for well over 200 years, medical waste management and disposal were of minor concern to most hospitals and health care facilities. Medical waste was essentially not covered in any particular regulations, and ample, low cost disposal options were readily available. Except for pathologic waste, such as body parts, almost all medical wastes were routinely disposed in local municipal landfills, with no special treatment, and with minimal concerns for segregation or special handling. Over this entire period, there were no documented or reported epidemics or public health impacts associated with medical waste disposal practices. However, that all changed dramatically in the early 1980s shortly after the Centers for Disease Control and Prevention (CDC) released its first report about the disease now known as AIDS, which led to rampant fears of a possible worldwide epidemic. At the time of CDC's first AIDS report, little was known about what caused the disease or how it was spread which fostered confusion, consternation, and great concern among health care providers about how best to protect against transmission of the disease. The supposition among many experts, regulators, and most of the general public was that just about any waste generated at hospitals and other health care facilities was a likely source of the AIDS pathogen contamination and posed substantial threats to anyone that could be possibly exposed to it. Such suppositions, in turn, led to overreactions and panic-based decisions that sparked the promulgation of increasingly stringent infectious waste regulations, tremendous increases in "infectious waste" generation rates, launching of the commercial infectious waste disposal industry, and the development and promotion of countless alternative medical waste treatment technologies.

This chapter provides an overview of infectious waste regulations and standards with a particular focus on the United States as well as the basis and background of their development and promulgation. It also provides a general overview of recommended policies and procedures for managing

infectious waste as well currently available systems and technologies for infectious waste treatment and disposal.

◗ INFECTIOUS OR MEDICAL WASTE GENERATORS

Health care institutions are obviously the predominant generators of infectious or medical waste. These are categorized by the North American Industry Classification System (NAICS) under the sector entitled *Health Care and Social Assistance*, and facilities in the health care industry are identified under NAICS Code 62. This code comprises four subsectors that include ambulatory health care services, hospitals, nursing and residential care facilities, and social assistance. The facilities included within each of these subsectors and respective NAICS code numbers are shown on Table 54.1.

In addition to health care facilities, other generators or sources of infectious or medical waste include academic, industrial, and governmental research laboratories; microbiological production facilities; biotechnology and pharmaceutical laboratory; and production facilities. Veterinary facilities including veterinarians' offices, veterinary hospitals, and animal pharmaceutical research and production facilities are also generators. The following is a list of known and potential sources of medical waste:

- Hospitals, medical centers, and polyclinics
- Clinics, diagnostic facilities, dialysis centers, and other specialized outpatient treatment facilities
- Primary health centers, rural health stations, basic health units, or health posts
- Maternity centers or birthing facilities
- Physicians' offices
- Dental clinics and offices
- Medical laboratories, biomedical laboratories, research centers, and biotechnology laboratories

- Blood banks, blood collection centers, and blood transfusion centers
- Nursing homes for the elderly and long-term residential care facilities
- Facilities and hospices for the chronically and terminally ill
- Pharmacies and dispensaries, drug stores, and pharmaceutical manufacturing facilities
- Alternative medicine treatment facilities such as acupuncture centers
- Veterinary hospitals, veterinarians' clinics, and veterinary offices
- Animal research and testing centers and animal quarantine stations
- Home health care settings

- Emergency service facilities including ambulance stations, paramedic units, and rescue operations
- Coroners' or medical examiners' facilities, forensic pathology or autopsy laboratories, and crime laboratories
- Drug addiction rehabilitation centers
- Funeral homes and mortuaries
- Tattoo and cosmetic ear piercing establishments
- Health and quarantine stations in airports, ports, and immigration/customs facilities
- First-aid positions
- Health facilities, infirmaries, clinics, or health stations in colleges and universities, children's schools and summer camps, military establishments, police stations, prisons, and commercial or industrial establishments

According to a 2012 United Nations study,[1] hospitals in the United States alone comprise only about 1% of the number of health-related facilities but account for more than 70% of total medical waste generation. Doctors' offices, nursing homes, clinics, and medical laboratories collectively make up about 36% of the health-related facilities and generated about 22% of total medical waste. The study also indicated that this is typical in most countries whereby larger health care facilities generate the large majority of medical waste, even though they account for a small percentage of health care establishments, whereas small health centers, clinics, primary health stations, doctors' offices, etc, comprise the majority of health care facilities but generate a much smaller portion of the medical waste stream.

TABLE 54.1	Health care industry classifications Code 62 for the North American Industry Classification System (NAICS) under the Health Care and Social Assistance sector

NAICS Sectors	NAICS Nos.
Ambulatory health care services subsector	**NAICS 621**
Offices of physicians	NAICS 6211
Offices of dentists	NAICS 6212
Offices of other health practitioners	NAICS 6213
Outpatient care centers	NAICS 6214
Medical and diagnostic laboratories	NAICS 6215
Home health care services	NAICS 6216
Other ambulatory health care services	NAICS 6219
Hospitals subsector	**NAICS 622**
General medical and surgical hospitals	NAICS 6221
Psychiatric and substance abuse hospitals	NAICS 6222
Specialty hospitals	NAICS 6223
Nursing and residential care facilities subsector	**NAICS 623**
Nursing care facilities	NAICS 6231
Mental retardation, mental health, and substance abuse facilities	NAICS 6232
Community care facilities for the elderly	NAICS 6233
Social assistance subsector	**NAICS 624**
Individual and family services	NAICS 6241
Community food and housing and emergency and other relief services	NAICS 6242
Vocational rehabilitation services	NAICS 6243
Child day care services	NAICS 6244

INFECTIOUS OR MEDICAL WASTE TERMS AND DEFINITIONS

The definition or meaning of the term *infectious waste* has been debated for decades, and there is no universally accepted definition. More than a dozen different terms, such as *medical waste*, *biohazardous waste*, *hospital waste*, *red bag waste*, *pathologic waste*, and others are typically used interchangeably with or in place of the term *infectious waste* in scientific and medical literature, regulations and standards, guidance manuals, and in press reports and journals. There are distinct technical differences in the meanings of these terms, but they essentially refer to the same type of waste. However, as discussed in the following text, because only a small fraction of so-called infectious waste generated at hospitals and other health care facilities is actually or potentially infectious or capable of causing or transmitting an infectious disease, the term *medical waste* is used herein to refer to all health care waste that is collectively managed or typically considered as being potentially infectious, and the term *infectious waste* is intended to refer only to waste that is actually or potentially infectious.

Discussions or analysis involving waste management, treatment, or disposal, which is collectively termed herein as waste management, should always begin with the establishment of clear definitions or at least a good understanding of the waste itself. In fact, failure to properly identify or correctly describe a particular waste stream and its characteristics in the course of making waste management decisions could result in any number of problems ranging from general misunderstandings and confusion to unexpected compliance difficulties or the procurement of an inadequate waste treatment system.

This may seem obvious and easily done, but it is not typically the case. Terms commonly used to identify waste types and categories are sometimes a bit vague and could have multiple meanings. For example, there are about 20 synonyms for the term *waste*, including *trash*, *refuse*, *garbage*, *rubbish*, *debris*, and so on, that are often used indiscriminately and interchangeably when referring to a waste, but the composition and characteristics applicable to these terms could be different under different scenarios. For example, the term *garbage* technically only means animal or vegetable waste from food service or kitchen activities, which is quite different from trash or rubbish typically

originating from such activities as warehousing operations and office buildings. As another example, the term *solid waste* would normally be assumed to mean waste having a solid form or state, but the US Environmental Protection Agency (EPA) regulations define "solid waste" to include sludges from wastewater treatment plants, which, by most definitions and in most all cases, is far from being a solid.

The term *infectious waste* is a prime example of a waste type or category where clarification and specificity are often needed to avoid potential problems. This is particularly important to prevent misunderstandings about potential risks for a particular waste stream that impact decisions on its management and disposal. As an example, usage of terms like *infectious* or *biohazardous waste* by local newspaper reports when referring to waste generated at any particular hospital or health care facility could readily lead to unwarranted fears within the local community as well as unjustifiable opposition by environmental activist groups of a proposed medical waste treatment, transport, or disposal of project. Examples of various synonyms typically used for infectious or medical waste are summarized in Table 54.2.

TABLE 54.2 Typical infectious waste synonyms

Terms	Comments
Biohazardous waste	Used primarily because "infectious waste" was included in the EPA's *draft* hazardous waste regulations
Biological waste	More applicable to activities in clinical, research, or pathology laboratories involving cells, tissues, organs, or other organisms
Biomedical waste	General term combining terms for biological- and medical-type waste; does not necessarily mean infectious or potentially infectious but commonly assumed to be so
Clinical waste	More applicable to activities in clinical, research, or pathology laboratories; is also a common term used for describing "infectious waste" in a number of countries
Contaminated waste	Disposed items that have contacted blood or body fluids regardless of whether such blood or body fluids are contaminated by a pathogen
Health care waste	Used to describe or identify *all* waste generated from a health care facility whereby potentially infectious waste is typically only a small fraction
Hospital waste	Used to describe or identify *all* waste generated from a hospital whereby potentially infectious waste is typically only a small fraction of total hospital waste
Infectious medical waste (IMW)	Common regulatory term to define waste that must be managed and disposed as being potentially infectious; does not technically apply to any other health care waste
Medical waste	Defined by the EPA as waste generated at health care facilities such as hospitals, doctors' offices, etc, that has the *potential* to be contaminate by blood or body fluids
Pathologic waste	Comprises recognizable body parts, tissues, organs, animal carcasses; also termed anatomical waste; may or may not be infectious or potentially infectious
Red bag waste	Color-coded bags typically used in the United States to collect and contain regulated or *potentially* infectious waste. For most health care facilities, most of the waste in such bags is not contaminated or potentially infectious. It should be noted that yellow-colored bags are used to collect potentially infectious waste in many other countries.
Regulated medical waste (RMW)	Waste specifically designated or defined as being potentially infectious according to regulatory definitions

Abbreviation: EPA, US Environmental Protection Agency.

Regardless of origin or composition, any waste that is identified or designated as being infectious is almost always understood and assumed to have been contaminated by an infectious agent and therefore readily capable of causing or transmitting an infectious disease. However, the fact is that a very high percentage of waste generated from hospitals and other health care facilities is *not* infectious and poses virtually no threat of transmitting an infectious disease. Instead, only a small fraction of health care waste is even considered potentially infectious and only under very specific conditions.

Technically and scientifically, infectious waste comprises disposed items or materials that have been contaminated by a pathogenic microorganism, or etiologic agent, or pathogen, such as bacteria, viruses, parasites, or fungi, having sufficient virulence and in sufficient quantity that it is capable of causing infectious disease in healthy humans. The primary means or source for such contamination is direct contact in some manner with contaminated blood or body fluids during medical procedures or diagnostic activities. Accordingly, medical waste is either infectious if pathogenically contaminated or it is not infectious if not so contaminated. However, this distinction is often not clear because it is typically problematic if not impossible to know with certainty whether blood or body fluids released or exposed in connection with most health care–related activities is in fact infectious or contaminated with a pathogen. Likewise, it is not possible to know whether any particular waste or disposed item has been in contact with blood or body fluids that are not readily discernible or that are possibly too small to be visibly detected. Therefore, prudent practice is that any and all waste or disposed items having been in contact with or exposed to blood and/or body fluids be managed as "potentially infectious waste," and this is the basis of most medical waste regulations and standards. In addition, practice at most health care facilities and most medical waste regulations standards also identify specific health care procedures, areas, and activities where there is a high likelihood that waste and disposed items generated therein have contacted blood and/or body fluids and, accordingly, need to be managed as being potentially infectious.

CDC Medical Waste Definitions

Decisions by most health care facilities to manage any and all waste that may have contacted blood or body fluids as being potentially infectious originated from interpretations of CDC's 1983 guidance commonly known as *Universal Precautions*.[2] These guidelines were published shortly after CDC's initial reports about AIDS and subsequent concerns that just about all health care waste was likely to be contaminated by the HIV and that such waste posed unacceptable risks to patients and public health.

Universal Precautions guidelines were originally interpreted by most health care facilities as meaning anything whatsoever that came into contact with any patient or staff person should be considered and managed as potentially infectious. This interpretation had far-reaching consequences because countless health care facilities suddenly began considering just about all waste as being potentially infectious thereby greatly increasing medical waste generation rates nationwide. At that time in the United States, not only was there insufficient on-site or off-site capacity for treating such waste but also many municipal waste disposal firms abruptly refused to pick up or dispose of any waste from hospitals, including trash, cardboard, and recyclables, because of fears that it was possibly contaminated with HIV.

In light of continued uncertainties and confusion about HIV and its transmission as well as increasing problems associated with health care waste management and disposal, CDC undertook efforts to clarify the meaning and intent of the universal precautions in the 1985 publication *Guideline for Handwashing and Hospital Environmental Control*.[3] This identified four specific health care waste categories as having "sufficient potential risk of causing infection during handling and disposal and for which some precautions are prudent since precise definition of infective waste that is based on the quantity and type of etiologic agents present is virtually impossible." The listed categories are

- **Microbiology laboratory waste** such as microbiological cultures and stocks of microorganisms including specimen containers; slides and cover slips; and disposable gloves, aprons, and laboratory coats
- **Pathology and anatomical waste** such as from surgery and autopsy including body parts, soiled dressings, sponges, drainage sets, underpads, and surgical gloves
- **Blood and blood products** including blood specimens and body fluid specimens
- **Contaminated sharps** including used needles, scalpel blades, and broken glass

EPA Medical Waste Definitions

The US Congress enacted the Solid Waste Disposal Act of 1965 (SWDA) to promote improved waste management technologies and standards for reducing pollutants in municipal waste disposal programs, but it did not address medical waste in any manner. The Resource Conservation and Recovery Act of 1976 (RCRA) amended the SWDA and gave the EPA authority to regulate hazardous waste. Initial drafts of EPA's hazardous waste regulations included the term *infectious characteristic* as a descriptor for waste to be regulated as hazardous, but EPA's final Hazardous Waste Regulations in 1980 neither listed infectious waste as a hazardous waste nor included "infectiousness" as one of the characteristics for identifying a waste as being hazardous. However, in anticipation that infectious waste would eventually be identified as hazardous waste, the EPA published the *Draft Manual for Infectious Waste Management*[4] in 1982 and the *EPA Guide for Infectious Waste Management*[5] in 1986.

During the summers of 1987 and 1988, there were numerous reported incidents of needles and other medical waste washing up on beaches and shorelines of the United States along the eastern seaboard and Great Lakes that caused a national sensation and great public concern. These incidents led to congressional enactment of the Medical Waste Tracking Act (MWTA) of 1988.[6] The MWTA was only a 2-year program that ran from June 1989 through June 1991, and it only applied to four states (New York, New Jersey, Connecticut, and Rhode Island as well as Puerto Rico). Its primary objectives were to gather information about medical waste management, to evaluate various medical waste treatment technologies, and to provide a model for states and other federal agencies to use in developing their own medical waste programs.

The MWTA adopted the definitions and descriptions that were included in the EPA's 1986 *Guide for Infectious Waste Management*.[5] It defined medical waste as "any solid waste that is generated in the diagnosis, treatment, immunization or autopsy of human beings or animals, in research pertaining thereto, in the preparation of human or animal remains for interment or cremation, or in the production or testing of biologicals" and it included the following categories:

1. **Cultures and stocks of infectious agents** and associated biologicals including cultures from medical and pathologic laboratories; cultures and stocks of infectious agents from research and industrial laboratories; wastes from the production of biologicals; discarded live and attenuated vaccines except for residue in emptied containers; and culture dishes, assemblies, and devices used to conduct diagnostic tests or to transfer, inoculate, and mix cultures
2. **Pathologic wastes** including tissues, organs, body parts, and body fluids that are removed during surgery or autopsy
3. **Waste human blood and blood products** including serum, plasma, and other blood components
4. **Contaminated sharps that have been used** in patient care or in medical research or industrial laboratories including hypodermic needles, syringes, pipettes, broken glass, and scalpel blades
5. **Contaminated animal carcasses, body parts, and animal bedding** that were exposed to infectious agents during research, production of biologicals, or testing of pharmaceuticals
6. **Waste from surgery or autopsy** that was in contact with infectious agents including soiled dressings, sponges, drapes, underpads, and surgical gloves
7. **Laboratory waste** from medical, pathologic, or pharmaceutical laboratories that were in contact with infectious agents

8. **Dialysis waste** that was in contact with blood of patients undergoing hemodialysis including contaminated disposal equipment and supplies
9. **Discarded medical equipment and parts** that were in contact with infectious agents
10. **Isolation waste** including biological waste and discarded materials contaminated with blood, excretion, exudates, or secretion from humans or animal who are isolate to protect others from communicable diseases

US State Medical Waste Definitions

Incidents leading up to enactment of the MWTA as well as the fact that the EPA appeared to have no intentions of enacting more permanent medical waste regulations after the 2-year program ended prompted most US states to enact their own medical regulations. To date, all states in the United States have enacted medical waste regulations, and the regulations and requirements among each state vary widely with particular differences in the terminology and definitions of the waste being regulated. Many states adopted definitions and categories identical to those in the MWTA, whereas others established relatively unique definitions and identifiers of medical waste types, categories, and sources. As an example, some states define medical waste strictly in accordance with its degree of contamination, that is, whether it has only been in contact with blood or body fluids or whether it is saturated or grossly contaminated with blood or body fluids.

Most state environmental protection agencies are primarily responsible for developing and enforcing medical waste management regulations, but the department of health is the agency primarily responsible for medical waste management in some states. In several states, both agencies have responsibility for medical waste management, with the department of health typically responsible for on-site management and the environmental protection agency responsible for off-site transportation and disposal. In addition to definitions and designations, most states also specify requirements for medical waste containerization, labeling, storage, transportation, treatment, and disposal. They also specify procedures for permitting, operating, and testing medical waste treatment systems and equipment inclusive of requirements for training and certifying medical waste treatment system operators and for recording and reporting operating parameters of medical waste treatment systems.

▶ MEDICAL WASTE MANAGEMENT REGULATIONS AND STANDARDS

Agencies that have enacted regulations and standards applicable to medical waste management in the United States are the EPA, the CDC, the Occupational Safety and

Health Administration (OSHA), and the US Department of Transportation (DOT). Each of these has its own congressional mandate that serves to direct or focus the approach that each adopts with respect to implementing its regulations and standards, but their collective goal is to protect the environment, public health, and workers including practices and procedures involving the management and disposal of infectious or medical waste. These are discussed in the following text.

EPA Regulations

The EPA has not had congressional authority to regulate medical waste management since expiration of the MWTA in 1991. However, the EPA strives to serve as a resource for medical waste management information and to work with or help support state health departments and environmental agencies in matters involving environmental protection as related to off-site medical waste disposal.

The EPA has authority to regulate two specific medical waste treatment technologies, namely, medical waste incinerators and treatment technologies using chemicals for disinfection or sterilization. The EPA regulates medical waste incinerators pursuant to the Clean Air Act (CAA) amendments of 1990 under regulations entitled Hospital, Medical, and Infectious Waste Incinerators (HMIWI). The HMIWI regulations, which were promulgated in 1997 (40 CFR §60 Subparts Ce and Ec) and amended in 2009 (40 CFR §62, Subpart HHH), establish highly stringent emissions standards for nine different air pollutants along with requirements for incinerator system operations, compliance testing, monitoring and reporting, and the training and certification of incinerator system operators and supervisors.[7,8]

The EPA regulates medical waste treatment technologies that use antimicrobial chemicals proclaimed to reduce the infectiousness of waste under the authority of the US Federal Insecticide, Fungicide, and Rodenticide Act (FIFRA). Companies making such claims are required to register their product or technology under FIFRA through the EPA's Office of Prevention, Pesticides, and Toxic Substances (OPPTS) Antimicrobial Division.

OSHA Regulations

Congress established OSHA as an agency of the United States Department of Labor under the Occupational Safety and Health Act of 1970 with a mandate to "assure safe and healthful working conditions for working men and women by setting and enforcing standards and by providing training, outreach, education, and assistance." The OSHA regulations cover most private-sector employers and their workers as well as some public-sector employers and their workers in all states and certain territories either through federal OSHA or through an OSHA-approved state plan. Currently, 22 US states or territories have OSHA-approved state programs.

The OSHA regulations generally cover hazards associated with specific workplace activities, conditions, or practices, and they include certain aspects of medical waste management designed to protect health care workers and other employees against possible injury and risks of infection under the Bloodborne Pathogen Standard of 1991.[9] This standard includes specific requirements covering the management of contaminated sharps, the containerization and labeling of medical waste, employee training, hazard communications, and hepatitis B virus (HBV) vaccinations. Although medical waste management operations are not identified as a specific OSHA workplace activity with its own activity-specific regulations, workers involved with such operations are protected against workplace injury under the OSHA General Duty Clause (Section 5[a][1]). The General Duty Clause states that employers are required to provide their employees a workplace that is "free from recognized hazards that are causing or are likely to cause death or serious physical harm."

DOT Regulations

The DOT regulates the transportation of medical waste as an "infectious substance" (49 CFR Parts 171-180), particularly under Subchapter C, "Hazardous Materials Regulations" (HMR), which includes information on various hazardous materials and pertinent requirements for their packaging and their shipment by rail, air, vessel, and public highway. The HMR applies to any material the DOT determines is "capable of posing an unreasonable risk to health, safety, and property when transported in commerce." The DOT regulations adopted the definitions for medical waste that were included in the MWTA.[10]

The DOT regulations primarily apply to medical waste transporters rather than medical waste generators. However, the DOT regulations include specific requirements for the packaging, labeling, and manifesting of medical waste that is transported off-site via public highways for treatment or disposal. Such requirements include mandatory Hazardous Materials Training for all managers and employees who prepare, assist, or who are responsible for the packaging and loading of hazardous materials, including medical waste, for off-site transport. Such training is also required for anyone who signs hazardous or medical waste transport manifest papers.

International Regulations and Standards

There are no international regulations or standards exclusively covering medical waste management, treatment, or disposal. However, two international agreements or treaties have been established and signed by a number of participating countries that are designed to reduce the transboundary movement of hazardous waste, including those designated as "biohazardous," between countries. The particular focus of these agreements is to prevent the transfer of hazardous waste from developed to less developed countries. One treaty, the *Basel Convention on the Control of Transboundary Movements of Hazardous Wastes and Their Disposal* (typically known as the Basel Convention), became effective in 1992. The other treaty, the *Bamako Convention on the Ban on the Import into Africa and the Control of Transboundary Movement and Management of Hazardous Wastes within Africa* (typically known as the Bamako Convention), was negotiated by 12 African nations in 1991 and became effective in 1998 because of reported failures of the Basel Convention to prohibit trade or imports of hazardous waste to less developed African countries.

It is believed that most developed countries have medical waste regulations in place that are comparable in many respects to those enacted in the United States. Such regulations vary widely in terms of content and specific requirements, and most are a component of or included within a country's hazardous waste regulations whereby medical waste is defined as a type of hazardous waste. On the other hand, most developing countries have no such regulations in place and have no legal policies or standards in place for managing and disposing of medical waste in a safe, sanitary manner that will not endanger the environment or public health. Additionally, a high percentage of developing countries lack proper sanitary landfills such that medical waste is typically disposed at dump sites that not only are regularly scavenged by people for goods but also are sources of ground and drinking water contamination. As a means to help deal with such disposal problems, health care facilities in some developing countries use incinerators for on-site medical waste disposal, but such incinerators are typically of an inferior quality that operate poorly, at best, and tend to have exceedingly high air pollutant emissions during operations. International organizations, such as the United States Agency for International Development (USAID), typically attempt to work with or assist developing countries to help correct such problems whenever possible, but doing so tends to be exceptionally difficult if not insurmountable.

Medical Waste Management Guidelines and Resources

Medical Waste Management Association

The Medical Waste Management Association (MWMA) is a nonprofit trade group in the United States for the medical waste disposal industry that was formed in July 2016. The stated goal of the association is to "promote operating standards, research, education and regulatory advocacy for organizations that transport, process, store or dispose of biological and medical waste." The

MWMA is reportedly open to membership from health care professionals responsible for medical waste disposal and compliance.

Clinical and Laboratory Standards Institute

The Clinical and Laboratory Standards Institute (CLSI), which was formerly called National Committee for Clinical Laboratory Standards (NCCLS), is a volunteer-driven, membership-supported, nonprofit, standards development organization. Its stated goal is to "promote the development and use of voluntary laboratory consensus standards and guidelines within the healthcare community," and its stated mission is to develop clinical and laboratory practices and promote their use worldwide. CLSI guidance with respect to the management, treatment, and disposal of medical waste, chemical waste, multihazardous waste, and other waste is included in the publication entitled *Clinical Laboratory Waste Management—Approved Guideline.*[11]

Healthcare Infection Control Practices Advisory Committee

The Healthcare Infection Control Practices Advisory Committee (HICPAC) is a federal advisory organization chartered to provide advice and guidance to the CDC on infection control practices and strategies for surveillance, prevention, and control of health care–associated infections, antimicrobial resistance, and related events. The HICPAC has posted a number of medical waste management guidelines on their Web site. Of note is a 2003 HICPAC publication entitled *Guidelines for Environmental Infection Control in Health-Care Facilities.*[12] This publication reported "no epidemiologic evidence suggests that most of the solid- or liquid wastes from hospitals, other healthcare facilities, or clinical/research laboratories is any more infective than residential waste." It also reported that "no epidemiologic evidence suggests that traditional waste-disposal practices of health-care facilities whereby clinical and microbiological wastes were decontaminated on site before leaving the facility have caused disease in either the health-care setting or the general community." These statements and other similar reported findings are considered very significant because they provide a documented basis for assuaging persistent, exaggerated fears and anxieties that abound about medical waste and its disposal.

Health Care Facility Accreditation Organizations

In order for US hospitals, health care facilities, and similar organizations to receive federal payments from Medicare or Medicaid programs, they must obtain accreditation or certification of compliance with certain health and safety requirements that are set forth in federal regulations. Such accreditation is achieved on the basis of surveys conducted by a state agency on behalf of the federal government or by a national accrediting organization such as The Joint Commission. The Joint Commission, which was formerly named The Joint Commission on Accreditation of Healthcare Organizations (JCAHO) and prior to that The Joint Commission on Accreditation of Hospitals (JCAH), accredits upward of 90% of hospitals throughout the US. Until relatively recently, The Joint Commission was widely considered as the only viable or acceptable accreditation organization, but several competitive accreditation organizations have become increasingly popular options including the Healthcare Facilities Accreditation Program (HFAP) and Det Norske Veritas Healthcare, Inc. (DNV).

The Joint Commission and the other accreditation organizations have standards in place for assessing health care facility performance in numerous areas and functions including compliance with environmental, safety, and health standards that encompass the management of medical and hazardous waste and materials. An example is The Joint Commission's *Environment of Care Standard 3.10.9* under Element of Performance 3—Implementation of Hazardous Material and Hazardous Waste Program.[13] Accordingly, most health care facilities are mandated not only to comply with all applicable medical waste regulations but also, consistent with accreditation standards, to implement, monitor, and continually improve on a comprehensive waste management program that ensures continued compliance.

International Guidelines

As discussed earlier, a number of developed countries and many developing countries have no medical waste management and disposal regulations in place as well as no regulatory or legislative authority or structure to enforce medical waste management and disposal policies or practices. However, many at least reference or avail themselves of guidelines published by the World Health Organization (WHO) such as *Safe Management of Wastes from Health-Care Activities.*[14] Also, whenever USAID becomes involved with medical waste management and related environmental issues in various developing countries, the guidance document *Sector Environmental Guidelines: Healthcare Waste* is typically referenced and applied to the extent possible.[15]

▶ MEDICAL WASTE GENERATION RATES

Medical waste generation rates, or the quantities of medical waste generated as a percentage of total waste, vary widely among health care facilities not only in relation to the different types of health care facilities but also in relation to health care facilities of the same type. In addition, medical waste generation rates often vary widely among the same types of facilities that are within the same organization or ownership. Generation rates appear to be independent of such factors as facility location, facility size, off-site disposal costs or charge rates, or labor and utility rates. As an example, one study involving a comparative analysis of medical waste management programs at 129 different hospitals across the United States involving a total of about 43 000 beds and a combined waste generation rate of about 240 million lb (109 million kg) per year of waste found medical waste generation rates to range from less than 5% to as high as about 93% of the total solid waste generated with the average being about 15% of total waste.[16]

The fundamental reason for the wide variations of medical waste generation rates for different types of health care facilities, such as between hospitals and dentist offices, is quite obvious. However, the reasons for wide variations among similar types of hospitals are not so obvious because they are typically due to relatively unique, site-specific factors, as well as consequential analysis of different options for dealing with such factors. The most significant factors can be broken into four categories as follows:

1. Applicable medical waste regulations
2. Facility-specific waste management policies and procedures
3. Administrative oversight of waste management activities
4. Off-site disposal availability and costs

These are discussed in further detail in the following text.

Applicable Medical Waste Regulations

Site-specific medical waste generation rates are most influenced by applicable state and local regulations. Health care facilities in areas or states having regulations with relatively vague or generalized medical waste definitions and/or nonspecific requirements for identifying and managing waste are likely to have substantially lower rates as compared to facilities in locations having more extensive, detailed definitions and more restrictive management requirements. For example, medical waste generation rates for those facilities in states that adopted the CDC's 1985 Universal Precaution waste guidelines, whereby only microbiology laboratory waste, pathology waste, blood and blood products, and contaminated sharps are to be managed as potentially infectious, are likely to have as much as a 5 to 10 times *lower* medical waste generation rate in comparison to those facilities in states that adopted the 1989 MWTA guidance document, whereby 10 different waste types and categories are required to be managed as potentially infectious.

Another regulatory-related factor that often impacts facility-specific waste generation rates is how a particular regulatory agency or individuals within an agency chooses to interpret and subsequently enforce certain sections of the regulations. For example, some agencies or regulators stipulate that *all* waste generated in surgery areas and emergency rooms should be considered potentially infectious, whereas others stipulate that only those items obviously contaminated with blood or body fluids should be considered potentially infectious.

Facility-Specific Waste Management Policies and Procedures

It is essential that health care facilities develop and implement policies and procedures as part of a formal medical waste management program with the objective of attaining and ensuring continued compliance with applicable medical waste regulations. However, such programs vary widely among facilities with respect to content and levels of detail. At one end of the spectrum are those facilities having minimal, poorly written, and outdated policies and procedures with unclear and undesignated responsibilities concerning program implementation and oversight, and at the other end of the spectrum are those facilities having detailed, frequently updated, and widely communicated policies and procedures in place along with clear, designated responsibilities. Differences in the content and quality of such programs tend to correlate directly with varying medical waste generation rates.

At most health care facilities, prevailing medical waste generation rates are the result of site-specific analysis of waste management program options involving varying degrees of infectious waste segregation with particular consideration of disposal options combined with comparative risks and costs. Many facilities have chosen to undertake extraordinary efforts to minimize the quantity of medical waste to be managed and disposed as potentially infectious due to high costs for its off-site disposal; however, many other facilities have chosen to implement a much more conservative approach because increasingly stringent medical waste segregation proportionally increases the likelihood of segregation errors, involving the intermixing or commingling of medical waste with general waste or trash. Such commingling not only poses health and safety risks to employees and the general public but also increases risks of regulatory compliance violations, fines, and adverse publicity.

Administrative Oversight of Waste Management Activities

Regardless of the quality and content of any particular waste management program or the details of its respective policies and procedures, it is of diminished value if not properly implemented. For example, a health care facility may have developed a robust waste management programs, but it is of no value if never instituted. Likewise, problems, inefficiencies, regulatory violations, and injuries to waste handling personnel and others are likely if these policies and procedures are not properly communicated to waste management personnel. Similar concerns apply if such personnel are not properly trained in implementing program requirements and/or if administrative and supervisory monitoring and oversight are not provided or are inadequate to ensure continued, facility-wide adherence to the program.

Off-site Disposal Availability and Costs

Another factor impacting medical waste generation rates for many health care facilities is the availability and proximity of off-site treatment and disposal locations. Those facilities in relatively remote locations or in areas for which medical waste needs to be transported long distances for treatment and disposal usually have much higher unit costs or rates for medical waste disposal as compared to facilities where suitable treatment facilities or disposal site are relatively closer and, accordingly, such facilities typically strive to minimize their medical waste generation rates.

▶ MEDICAL WASTE MANAGEMENT

Medical waste management generally encompasses all measures, steps, policies, and procedures involved from points of generation through ultimate disposal. Specific components of a medical waste management program or plan include the following:

- Waste minimization, segregation, and containment
- Collection and containerization
- Waste pickup and transport
- Interim storage
- Treatment and disposal

Waste Minimization

A fundamental element of a sound and strategic waste management program is to reduce, to the extent possible, the quantity or volume of materials, items, products, and the like to be managed and disposed as waste. This process is termed waste minimization, and it is achieved by procedures that include source reduction, reuse, recycling, and similar measures. In addition to the benefits of reducing the quantity of waste to be managed and disposed, waste minimization measures can reduce occupational and environmental risk exposures as well as treatment and disposal costs.

Typical waste minimization techniques include source reduction, waste segregation, and containment, and they are discussed in the following text.

Source reduction involves the minimization of materials or items to be managed and disposed at their points of origin, thereby reducing the volume of waste, and such measures should be considered a high priority when establishing, implementing, and administering a health care waste management program. It also involves the elimination of hazardous materials to the extent possible through the substitution of products such as feedstocks, laboratory chemicals, and cleaning agents to those being less hazardous. It similarly involves the elimination of hazardous materials via implementation or changes of technologies or processes such as using non–mercury-containing devices instead of mercury thermometers or mercury switches. However, product and material minimization and substitution measures do not technically apply to medical waste except possibly with respect to changes in treatment, diagnostic, or clinical procedures that result in reduced waste generation with less chance of contamination or blood and body fluid contact.

Substantial waste minimization is also typically achieved by improved materials management practices that include such practices as the implementation of inventory controls to minimize the accumulation of expired or outdated products as well as the consumption of all contents within product containers, especially those having chemical and pharmaceutical products, prior to disposal. Preferential purchasing controls, such as the selection of products, supplies, and materials that have less packaging materials as well as the purchasing of products in bulk quantities, also serve to substantially minimize waste generation rates. The use of products and items having less packaging is particularly pertinent to medical waste management programs because it is typical in a number of health care activities, particularly those involving surgical and emergency procedures, for product packaging to be disposed in infectious waste containers regardless of whether it has been contaminated.

Another waste minimization technique is the utilization of reusable products and materials rather than those requiring disposal after single use (see chapters 47 and 55). Examples include reusable drapes and gowns in surgery suites, reusable dishware and utensils in cafeterias and dining areas, and reusable items in patient rooms such as bedpans, water pitchers, and the like. However, the risks and costs associated with the safe reprocessing of such items for reuse should be duly considered. Finally, substantial waste minimization is achieved by recycling programs that involve the segregation, recovery, and recycling of waste stream components and constituents for reuse, resale, or return. Almost all recycling efforts apply to components in the general waste stream such as paper, corrugated boxes, glassware, plastics, aluminum cans, and the like. Contaminated or potentially infectious waste items are almost never recovered and recycled due to infection prevention measures or regulatory requirements.

Waste Segregation and Containment

After all feasible, practical measures have been implemented to minimize waste generation to the extent possible, the next key element of a comprehensive waste management program is to institute reliable and effective waste segregation procedures. Waste segregation basically involves the implementation of measures to ensure that different waste stream types and components are kept separated and not intermixed or commingled with each other. A common problem for health care facilities is the intermixing of potentially infectious waste with general-type waste. This results from the inadvertent depositing of potentially or apparently infectious waste into general waste collection containers, but it also occurs when medical waste containers, such as boxes or bags, are placed or loaded alongside containers of general waste either within storage areas or in waste transport bins or containers. Whenever intermixing (termed comingling) occurs, the general waste portion typically becomes designated as being potentially infectious. The typical consequence of such commingling is a substantial increase in the quantity of medical waste to be managed and disposed as being potentially infectious which thereby also increases waste disposal costs and associated occupational, safety, health and environmental risks.

Typical waste segregation techniques involve the use of color-coded waste containers (bags, boxes, or collection bins) having special identification labels as well as the use of containers meeting certain criteria for the specific waste being contained. Specific requirements for such containment are included in the medical waste regulations of most US states as well as in sections of the OSHA and the DOT regulations. Red-colored containers are used almost exclusively for the collection of potentially infectious waste in the United States and a number of other countries. Yellow-colored containers are often used for collecting medical waste in many countries such as Canada, Great Britain, and South Africa, but yellow-colored containers are used almost exclusively in the United States for the collection of chemotherapy-type waste which is basically medical waste that has been in contact with chemotherapy drugs during oncology treatment procedures.

In addition to color coding, special labels or symbols are also often used or applied to waste containers as well as entryways to areas or locations in which such waste is being stored, handled, or treated. Requirements and details for such labeling are typically included in medical waste management regulations. Figure 54.1 shows the biohazard symbol that is used internationally to indicate containers, rooms, materials, equipment, and other locations and items that are actually or potentially contaminated with an infectious agent. This symbol is universally required to be placed on infectious waste containers either as an imprint on the container itself or as a

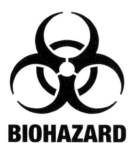 

BIOHAZARD

FIGURE 54.1   Universal or international biohazard symbols. These are used internationally to identify the actual or potential presence of an infectious agent or material. The symbol may be black, fluorescent orange, or orange-red with a contrasting background.

separate adhesive-backed label. The symbol may be black, fluorescent orange, or orange-red, and the background color is optional so long as there is sufficient contrast to ensure that the biohazard symbol is clearly discernible.

Waste collection containers should not only be color-coded/labeled, but they must also be designed to be able to fully contain the collected waste securely and without breakage, spillage, leakage, or rupture. This is particularly important for the containment of potentially infectious waste, especially contaminated sharps, as well as other wastes having hazardous properties or characteristics that could endanger workers and waste handling personnel, public health, or the environment. State and federal medical waste regulations, including sections of the OSHA and DOT regulations, as well as the regulations in a number of developing countries include specific requirements and criteria for medical waste containers such as minimum thickness, degree of puncture resistance, leak resistance, break resistance, and testing standards for strength.

On-site Waste Management and Handling

The next steps in a comprehensive waste management program involve the collection, or pickup, of waste containers from points of generation and their transport either to an interim on-site storage location, or to an on-site treatment and disposal system, or to a vehicle for off-site transport and disposal.

Efficient and effective waste collection and transport procedures require proper, well-designed planning to ensure that wastes do not overaccumulate at points of generation but are collected frequently and in a manner safe for transport. Typical requirements for a well-managed waste collection program include the following:

- Waste containers should not be overfilled but limited to a maximum of about three-fourths of container capacity. Overfilled containers increase the risks of waste

spillage and worker exposures to potentially infectious, hazardous, or dangerous items.
- Waste containers should not be picked up and transported unless they have been closed or sealed correctly and tightly.
- Waste containers that are damaged, leaking, split open, or subject to breakage should not be picked up and transported. Such waste should be repackaged or the damaged container placed within another sound container.

There are two categories of health care waste transport: internal (on-site) transport and external (off-site) transport. On-site refers to the transport of waste from points of generation to interim storage areas and/or to a central storage area for eventual treatment and disposal. Off-site transport involves transport from any on-site storage area to an off-site facility or location for disposal. Both categories of waste transport also require proper, well-designed planning to ensure that wastes are managed and disposed safely and without imposing unacceptable risks of harm or injury. Basic or typical requirements for a well-managed on-site waste transport program include the following:

- Waste collection and transport should best take place during low activity times whenever possible.
- Regular transport routes and collection times should be standardized to minimize potential problems. Specific transport routes should be planned to minimize possible exposures to staff, patients, and the public; that is, the transport of loaded waste carts through public spaces, patient care areas, and other clean areas should be avoided or minimized to the extent possible.
- Cross-contamination or commingling of transported waste items and containers must be avoided.
- Waste transport carts, such as wheeled bins and trolleys, should be specifically sized and designed for the type and volume of waste to be transported, and they should not be used for any other purpose.
- Carts used for transporting medical waste should be prominently labeled with an international biohazard symbol and possibly color coded.
- Carts used for transporting medical waste should either be frequently cleaned and disinfected or lined with a disposable plastic liner for containing potential spills and leaks from damaged or improperly closed waste containers.

Collected health care wastes are typically transported either to interim on-site waste storage areas or to a centralized waste storage area for eventual treatment and/or disposal. Interim storage areas or rooms are usually places within departments or floors of a health care facility where waste is temporarily stored before being brought to a central storage area. Such area are typically termed "dirty" or "soiled" utility rooms that are typically also used for storing cleaning equipment, dirty linen, and supplies. Central storage is the place within a health care facility where waste is brought for safe retention until it is either treated on-site or collected for off-site transport and disposal. Basic or typical requirements for on-site waste storage areas or rooms include the following:

- Storage areas should be capable of ensuring complete and continued separation of general waste from medical waste and other special or hazardous wastes.
- Access doors to waste storage areas should be lockable and adequately secured at all times to prevent entry of unauthorized persons.
- Storage areas should be protected from the sun, rain, or snow, and they should be designed and protected to prevent access by animals, insects, vermin, and birds.
- Waste storage areas should have good lighting and at least passive air ventilation.
- Waste storage areas should not be situated near fresh food storage or food preparation areas.
- Waste storage areas or rooms should be kept neat and clean at all times, and spills and debris should be cleaned and disinfected promptly and thoroughly.
- Waste containers or carts should be stored or stacked within storage areas in an unobtrusive, orderly manner to prevent accidental spillage or exposures. Aisle ways should be kept clear and unobstructed.
- Waste storage areas should have conspicuously posted door signage that clearly identifies the type and nature of wastes stored within. Medical waste storage area doors or entryways should be labeled with the term *Medical Waste*, *Infectious Waste*, or *Biohazardous*, along with the international biohazard symbol.

Off-site Transportation of Medical Waste

Health care facilities and other generators are fully responsible for the proper, safe containment and correct labeling of waste collected and transported off-site for treatment and disposal. Packaging and labeling must comply with all applicable regulations and standards governing the transport of the specific wastes to be transported, including, in the United States, the DOT regulations pertaining to medical waste. Additionally, transported packaging must be secured in a manner that will prevent any adverse risks or dangers to anyone during its handling and vehicular loading for off-site transport as well as during its transport and unloading for eventual treatment and disposal.

The regulations of most US states and a number of countries include specific standards and requirements applicable to firms or individuals that pickup medical waste for off-site transport and disposal. A particular requirement is that medical waste transporters be officially permitted and certified for doing so and that health care facilities must only use such transporters. In addition, the regulations of many states and the DOT require that

shipping papers or manifests be prepared and signed by the medical waste transporter, the facility from which the waste is picked up for transport, and the facility at which the waste is delivered and disposed. The DOT regulations also specify that anyone signing such manifests must attend a formal, approved hazardous material training course or program.

▶ MEDICAL WASTE TREATMENT AND DISPOSAL

Two fundamental medical waste disposal options are available to health care facilities; namely, off-site treatment and disposal and on-site treatment in combination with off-site disposal. The option of using a commercial or third-party vendor for off-site transport, treatment, and disposal of medical waste is essentially available to all health care facilities, but the costs or affordability of this option vary widely. As discussed earlier, off-site disposal rates for small health care facilities in remote locations whereby their medical waste needs to be picked up and transported over long distances are much greater than the rates charged to larger facilities having relatively short transport distances to an approved treatment facility.

Medical Waste Treatment Terminology

The term *waste processing* is often used interchangeably with the term *waste treatment*, but they are different. Waste processing involves the application of physical, chemical, mechanical, thermal, or other processes or combinations of processes to change the characteristics, composition, or nature of a waste or waste stream for a particular purpose including the preparation of waste for introduction into a particular waste treatment technology or device. Waste processing systems and equipment typically include such components as shredders, granulators, compactors, dryers, separators, and solidifiers for such purposes as weight or volume reduction, size reduction, disfigurement, blending, resource recovery and recycling, secondary processing, and/or the conversion of waste to a fuel for firing or burning in conventional boilers and furnaces. On the other hand, waste treatment systems are typically understood to comprise equipment used to render or convert wastes that are considered or regulated as being infectious, hazardous, toxic, radiologic, pathologic, physically dangerous, and/or potentially harmful to a residue that is considered safe and suitable for general landfill disposal. For simplicity and clarity, the term *waste treatment* is used herein to refer to systems or technologies that process and/or treat waste.

The terms *disinfection* and *sterilization* are also used interchangeably, particularly in the descriptive, technical, and promotional literature for most alternative medical waste treatment technologies, but they also have different meanings (see chapter 2). Although both of these terms refer to antimicrobial processes, disinfection is the process of eliminating or reducing *harmful* microorganisms from objects and surfaces, but sterilization is the process of killing *all* microorganisms including viruses and bacterial spores. Only a few treatment technologies are able to provide sterilization, such as high-temperature incineration, but other treatment technologies provide a sufficiently high level of disinfection as to be considered acceptable for medical waste treatment in accordance with the regulations of most states.

Evolution of Medical Waste Treatment

Up until about the mid-1990s, on-site incineration and steam sterilization (autoclaving) were widely considered the only viable, proven treatment technologies suitable for medical waste. Relatively few facilities used autoclaves for medical waste treatment, and most were of limited capacity and installed at smaller facilities. Between about the late 1980s and the early 2000s, a series of events and associated federal regulations spurred the rapid development and promotion of literally hundreds of different, nonincineration-type medical waste treatment technologies. However, despite encouraging market projections and high motivations combined with the development of claimed reliable, effective, efficient, and cost-effective, nonincineration technologies, virtually of all of the technologies introduced during that period were unsuccessful and are no longer available. Today, much as was the situation before the mid-1990s, incineration and autoclaving are still widely considered the only proven medical waste treatment technologies.

It is useful to consider a brief summary of the key historical events and trends in the United States relative to the evolution of medical waste treatment technologies from the 1960s through today. This is intended to provide context and insights for a better understanding of the recommendations presented in this chapter with particular respect to evaluating and selecting technologies for site-specific applications. The SWDA identified hospital waste as a "significant component of the municipal solid waste stream" and designated it as being "potentially hazardous." This marked the first time that hospitals and other medical waste generators had to be concerned with more than just pathologic waste disposal and whether other waste stream components should be considered potentially hazardous thereby requiring special treatment and disposal. The OPEC oil embargos in the 1970s created drastic fuel oil shortages throughout the United States and drove energy prices to very high levels. These embargos resulted in medical waste incinerators with energy recovery systems, or waste heat boilers, becoming a cost-effective way for health care facilities to offset increasing fuel costs, and this situation greatly increased the number of on-site medical waste incinerator systems nationwide.

As discussed earlier, public fears about a possible national AIDS epidemic in the early 1980s led many to consider all waste from hospitals and health care facilities to be a serious health threat. The CDC's response to this situation resulted in the publication of the *Universal Precautions* guidelines, the interpretation of which motivated facilities to institute exceptionally conservative waste segregation policies that resulted in as much as a 10-fold increase in infectious waste generation rates nationwide. At about the same time, solid waste transport and disposal firms in many areas of the country refused to handle any waste from hospitals, and the off-site medical waste disposal industry was only in its infancy; this caused a serious problem for most health care facilities not having on-site incineration capabilities. These circumstances further increased the desirability of on-site medical waste incinerator systems and essentially ignited interest in alternative treatment technologies.

The exceedingly stringent air pollutant emissions standards and other onerous requirements imposed by the EPA's HMIWI regulations of 1997 resulted in an estimated 95% closure or shutdown of the medical waste incinerator systems in operation at the time by about 2000 due to very high compliance costs and other difficulties. The closure of most medical waste incinerator systems, combined with growing opposition against incineration by environmental activist groups and increasing medical waste volumes, spawned an exceptionally rapid growth and interest in alternative, nonincineration treatment technologies. By 1991, as many as 18 different alternative treatment technologies were reportedly under development or available, and the number rose to as many as 45 by 1997.[17,18] However, by about 2001, the growth rate went into a steep decline with very few new technologies being introduced and with less than a dozen or so of the alternative treatment technology vendors still in business. It is estimated that well over 200 different nonincineration treatment technologies were developed or promoted by different firms between about 1987 and about 2001, and possibly as many as 50 or more different technologies were developed and promoted since that time through today. Failures at promoting and advancing these alternative technologies were due to a combination of overly optimistic economic forecasts of demands, overestimates of medical waste volumes nationwide, increased competitiveness of the off-site medical waste disposal industry, improved medical waste segregation efficiencies at most facilities, and an oversaturation of offerings in a market with somewhat limited opportunities.

Medical Waste Treatment Technologies

There are only a few viable, proven, effective, and environmentally sound technologies for treating medical waste available today. They include incineration, autoclaving, and possibly pyrolysis. There may be other specialized or unique treatment technologies available having demonstrated successful performance on specific applications in some parts of the world, but it is recommend that before such technologies be considered viable or possibly suitable for any site-specific applications that they first be thoroughly evaluated using criteria as recommended and discussed in the following text in this chapter.

Incinerator Systems

Incineration is a high-temperature combustion process that is long proven suitable for destroying virtually all types and forms of waste. A properly designed, controlled, and operated incinerator system readily converts medical waste and almost all other types of waste generated at health care facilities to an inert, sterile, nonhazardous, unrecognizable ash residue that is safe for disposal in a general or municipal landfill. Incinerator systems typically reduce the weight and volume of medical waste by upward of 95% or more, and they provide the opportunity to recover useful energy from the waste in the form of steam via heat recovery boilers.

The most widely used incineration technology or type for medical waste disposal is commonly termed controlled air incineration. Controlled air incinerators are also called modular incinerators, starved air incinerators, and two-stage incinerators. This technology was originally developed in the early 1970s to comply with emission standards imposed by the newly enacted CAA

without the need for installing air pollution control (APC) devices, and not long thereafter, countless controlled air–type incinerators were installed at health care facilities throughout the United States. As discussed earlier, the EPA's HMIWI regulations resulted in the closure of nearly all medical waste incinerator systems in the United States by about 2000, and it is estimated that less than a dozen medical waste incinerator systems are still in operation in the United States with most of them located at commercial, off-site treatment facilities.

Controlled air–type incinerators are so-called because of the way air for combustion is introduced and controlled during burning process. They are composed of a primary combustion chamber (PCC) into which waste is loaded and typically burned under air-deficient, or starved-air, conditions. This process minimizes particulate entrainment and carryover but causes volatile gases and smoke to be generated and carried into a secondary combustion chamber (SCC). In the SCC, excess combustion air is introduced along with auxiliary fuel firing to combust the volatile gases and any entrained organic particulate matter discharged from the PCC. The PCCs are typically controlled to operate in the range of 1400°F to 1600°F (760°C-871°C), and SCCs are typically controlled to operate in the range of 1800°F to 2000°F (982°C-1093°C). Figure 54.2 includes a schematic diagram for a controlled air–type incinerator system.

Incinerator systems for medical waste disposal are being offered throughout the world by several manufacturers (Figure 54.3). Such systems vary widely in

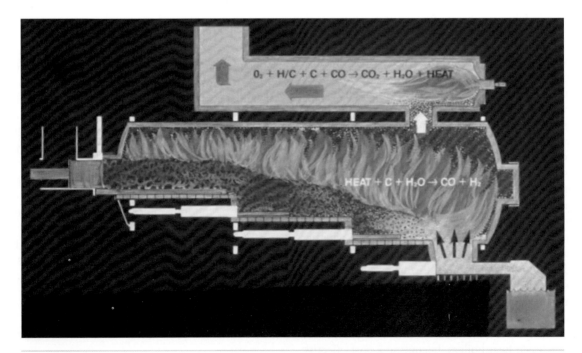

FIGURE 54.2 Internal schematic of a controlled air incinerator system. Schematic shows a waste loader on the left charging waste into the lower primary combustion chamber, with a secondary combustion chamber above and a wet quench type ash removal system on the lower right. For a color version of this art, please consult the eBook. Courtesy of Consutech Systems, LLC.

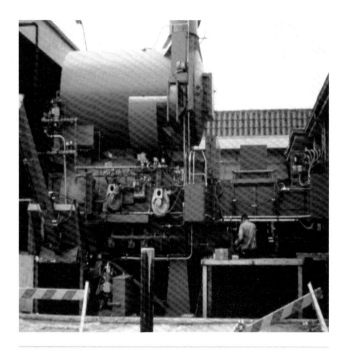

FIGURE 54.3 Example of a medical waste incinerator system. This controlled air–type incineration system was designed to burn up to 1000 lb/hr (455 kg/hr) of medical waste. The waste loader system is on the right and ash removal system on right. For a color version of this art, please consult the eBook.

construction quality, degree of controls and instrumentation, sufficiency of auxiliary components (such as burners and blowers), type and quality of waste loading, and ash removal systems and equipment. Medical waste incinerator system need not necessarily be of a conventional controlled air–type, but there are basic, minimum standards or criteria that are applicable to any waste combustion system and should be considered mandatory for any type of incinerator system. These include the following:

- Incinerator combustion chambers must be sized on the basis of well-established engineering criteria, such as volumetric heat release rate standards, for the specific type of waste to be incinerated at a specific hourly burning rate. Failure to do so results in the procurement of a system having insufficient burning capacity, excessive smoke or pollutant emissions, extensive maintenance and repair problems, and a low degree of online reliability.
- Chambers must be lined with a sufficient thickness of high-quality, high-temperature refractory selected specifically for incinerator system operations. This should be backed by high-temperature insulation to ensure long-term operations without major equipment damage as well as to provide sufficiently low outer casing temperatures to prevent burn injuries to operating personnel.
- Chambers must be equipped with auxiliary fuel burners for waste ignition, preheating, and automatically maintaining proper, elevated operating temperatures

at all times. The burners should be automatically and independently controlled for each chamber, equipped with independent, dedicated air supply blowers, and equipped with all necessary safeguard devices and management systems.

- Chambers must be equipped with an independent, properly sized combustion air supply system comprising a blower, air supply ductwork, air injection nozzles, and means of automatic control based on burning rates and operating temperatures.
- Means or a mechanism should be provided to ensure safe and controlled loading or charging of waste into the PCC that will both minimize the release or exfiltration of hot gases or flames from the chamber as well as the infiltration of excessive ambient air into the chamber during loading and burning.
- Means or a mechanism should be provided to enable the safe removal and handling of ash residues from the PCC without endangerment to operating personnel, excessive dust proliferation, or the potential of uncontrolled fires from glowing ash embers.
- Instrumentation and devices should be provided to enable the continuous monitoring of combustion conditions, such as temperatures and draft, in all chambers at all times.

As discussed, all existing and new medical waste incinerator system in the United States are required to comply with the highly stringent pollutant emission standards specified in the EPA's HMIWI regulations, and such compliance requires the installation of high-efficiency and highly sophisticated APC systems and equipment. The most commonly used and proven APC systems comprise high-pressure drop, wet scrubbers complete with quench chambers for cooling flue gases from the SCC to saturation temperature levels, condenser/absorbers for acid gas removal, and venturi sections for particulate removal. They also include separator sections for removing entrained water droplets; induced draft fans for pulling flue gases through the APC system; heat exchangers system for subcooling flue gases below their adiabatic saturation level; caustic feed systems for acid gas removal and controlling pH levels; and associated circulation pumps, piping, valves, and fittings. Carbon bed adsorbers and cartridge filter units may also be needed to enable new medical waste incinerators to meet the pollutant emission standards in EPA's HMIWI regulations.

Steam Autoclave Systems and Equipment

Steam autoclaving is a thermal process that uses pressurized, saturated steam injection within an insulated pressure vessel for inactivating infectious agents or pathogenic microorganisms (see chapter 28). Autoclaves are typically operated at temperatures in excess of 250°F (121°C), with pressures of 15 psi (103 kPa), and with typical operating cycle times ranging from 30 to 60 minutes. Autoclaves used for off-site, commercial medical waste disposal are typically operated at a higher temperature of 275°F (135°C) and at pressures in the range of 60 to 75 psi (412-515 kPa).

Autoclaving is suitable for treating most types and compositions of medical waste. However, it is not considered suitable or acceptable for treating pathologic waste, such as gross anatomical wastes and body parts, or waste containing bulk quantities of blood and body fluids. Also, autoclaving should never be used for treating disposed pharmaceuticals, chemotherapy waste, radioactive waste, or hazardous wastes and chemicals, particularly those which could be volatilized or vaporized when heated. Furthermore, autoclaving alone may not always be considered an acceptable treatment technology for some types of waste, such as human or animal tissues contaminated with high levels of prions (associated with diseases such as Creutzfeldt-Jakob disease [CJD] or bovine spongiform encephalopathy [BSE]; see chapter 68).

Autoclaving effectiveness or efficiency is a direct function of steam temperatures, the ability of the steam to directly contact pathogenic microorganisms within loaded waste, and the duration of steam contact. Factors that influence treatment efficiencies include the type, composition, and density of the waste as well as the means for waste containment or packaging within the treatment vessel or chamber. As an example, autoclaving is considered unsuitable for treating waste containing high percentages of bulk fluids or pathologic remains because of difficulties in heating such fluids to temperature levels sufficient to achieve an acceptable degree of disinfection. Also, if waste items are not packaged within bags, containers, or carts that enable or allow steam penetration to directly contact waste therein, disinfection efficiencies will likely be low and unacceptable. As such, effective waste autoclaving requires either the use of autoclavable bags, or bags that melt and enable steam penetration during treatment, or the opening of each bag and container prior to treatment. Furthermore, if waste carts are used to hold waste containers as part of the autoclave process, the carts need to have openings or perforations to facilitate steam contact with the waste contained therein.

There are two basic types of autoclave systems; namely gravity displacement and prevacuum autoclaves (see chapter 28). With gravity displacement–type systems, steam is admitted at the top or the sides of the treatment chamber, and because the steam is lighter than air, it forces air out the bottom of the chamber through a drain vent. The time needed for steam penetration into waste loads is prolonged for gravity displacement systems because of incomplete air elimination. On the other hand, prevacuum-type systems are fitted with a vacuum pump or steam eductor to ensure air is removed from the treatment chamber to the extent possible before steam is admitted (Figure 54.4).

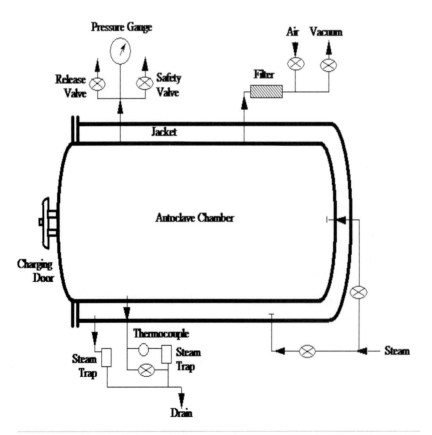

FIGURE 54.4 Schematic of a prevacuum-type autoclave for waste disposal.
From: UNDP GEF Global Healthcare Waste Project.

The advantage of creating a prevacuum is that there is nearly instantaneous steam penetration into waste loads, thereby maximizing treatment efficiencies while minimizing treatment times.

Autoclaves are batch-processing systems, where waste to be treated is loaded into the treatment chamber in individual batches to undergo a process cycle. A typical process cycle includes closure of the chamber door and initiation of the process from a control panel, steam injection for a gravity-type system or air evacuation followed by steam injection for a prevacuum-type system, steady-state steam contact time for a selected duration, exhausting of steam and condensate from the chamber, and opening of the chamber door for removal of treated waste residue containers or carts. The size of the autoclave treatment chamber dictates the volume of waste that can be loaded for each batch and, therefore, the quantity of waste that can be treated over any particular time period. Accordingly, autoclaves are sized and designed on the basis of facility-specific needs ranging from systems suitable for treating small waste volumes and batches to very large waste volumes of upward of 5000 lb (2268 kg) per batch as used at commercial, off-site treatment facilities (Figure 54.5). Because most autoclaved waste remains recognizable after treatment and because sharps within the waste stream remain as potential puncture hazards, it may be necessary to consider processing the autoclaved waste residues within a shredder or granulator to render it unrecognizable and safe for general handling and landfill disposal. A number of state regulatory agencies, in fact, require postshredding of autoclaved waste prior to its off-site transport and disposal.

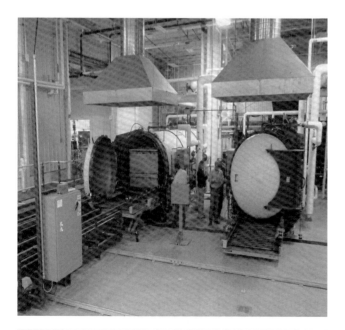

FIGURE 54.5 High-volume, high-pressure, and high-temperature commercial autoclave facility processing up to 50 tons of waste per day. For a color version of this art, please consult the eBook. Courtesy of Bondtech Corporation.

Most, if not all, state regulatory agencies specify requirements and procedures for using biological, mechanical, and chemical indicators for monitoring autoclave system performance efficiencies. Biological indicators, or spore test samples, are often considered reliable and acceptable performance monitors, but because spore tests are typically only done weekly with the results not immediately available, mechanical and chemical monitoring are also typically required. Biological indicators provide for direct monitoring assessments of autoclave system effectiveness via analysis of the kill rate, or log reduction, of known, high-resistant microorganisms that are typically bacterial spores with a defined resistance. On a periodic basis, biological indicators are placed within randomly selected, recognizable waste loads as spore strips or within self-contained vials for a treatment cycle of operation. Afterward, the indicator samples are collected and analyzed via an incubator to determine the extent of kill (typically presence/absence of growth in comparison to positive controls). State requirements for an acceptable kill levels vary, but a 4 log reduction in the concentration of *Geobacillus stearothermophilus* spores, as the most resistant to moist heat, is the most widely accepted standard for autoclave system operations.

Chemical indicators involve the use of heat-sensitive chemicals that change shape or color when exposed to specific high temperatures (see chapter 65). Examples include chemical indicator tapes, strips, or tabs as well as special markings on waste containers or packaging materials. Chemical indicator results are obtainable immediately following an autoclave treatment cycle and therefore can provide more timely information about the operating process parameters than a spore test. The CDC recommends placing or affixing a chemical indicator either inside or outside of every waste container depending on visibility. The color change of chemical indicator can provide direct indication of whether an acceptable operating temperature was achieved; however, such color change may not indicate whether the waste or the contents of a particular waste container was heated for an appropriate length of time or at the proper pressure to assure acceptable effectiveness. It may also verify that the outside of a waste container reached a sufficiently high temperature, but it would not reflect temperature levels achieved inside the container during operations.

Mechanical indicators basically include computer displays, or printouts, and written, recorded documentation of autoclave system operating pressures, temperatures, and exposure times. Most state agencies and the CDC specify or recommend that such conditions be recorded at all times during autoclave system operations with typical recorders be strip charts or computerized data acquisition systems.

Nonconventional Medical Waste Treatment

The organization Health Care Without Harm (HCWH) published a report in 2001 entitled *Non-Incineration Medical Waste Treatment Technologies* that included discussions and overviews of nonincineration treatment technologies that were being offered or promoted at the time by 49 different vendors or manufacturers.[19] It included descriptions for the following treatment technology categories:

- Nineteen different "low-heat thermal processes" or technologies using steam, microwaves, dry heat, and electrical resistance in combination with an array of mechanical processing methods
- Two different "medium-heat thermal processes" or technologies using polymerization and depolymerization
- Fifteen different "high-heat thermal processes" or technologies using pyrolysis, plasma pyrolysis, superheated steam, and laser beams
- Ten different "chemical processes" or technologies using sodium hypochlorite, chlorine dioxide, ozone, peracetic acid, and other disinfection chemicals in combination with various methods for shredding or granulating waste to be treated
- Two different "irradiation processes" or technologies using electron beams and cobalt 60 as sources of ionizing radiation
- One "biological process" using microorganisms

As discussed earlier, apart from conventional, steam autoclave systems, and possibly a few others, none of technologies described in the 2001 report are commercially available. The regulatory agencies in a number of states maintain and frequently update a listing of what have been deemed "approved" alternative, nonincineration, medical waste treatment technologies. As examples, the current approved list for the California Department of Public Health includes 30 treatment technologies, West Virginia Department of Health and Human Resources includes 22 technologies, and the approved list for the New York State Department of Environmental Conservation includes 14 technologies. Such lists could be considered potential resources when evaluating any particular treatment technology; however, the problem with these and similar lists is that almost all of the listed technologies have never been installed or proven successful on an actual, full-scale application and almost all of them are no longer commercially available. Most technologies are only included on such lists because, at some time, vendors or developers submitted documentation to respective state agencies for approval, regardless of being actually installed or made operational.

Pyrolysis Treatment Technologies

One of the few, nonconventional-, nonincineration-type medical waste technologies that appear to remain potentially viable is pyrolysis. The 2001 HCWH report listed more than a dozen different pyrolysis-type technologies, none of which are known to be in operation or commercially available, but some of these continue to be

developed and promoted for medical waste treatment applications. The main reason for this is that the EPA specifically excluded pyrolysis technologies from meeting the requirements in the HMIWI regulations for medical waste incinerator systems.

Whereas incineration is a combustion or high-temperature oxidation process, pyrolysis involves heating to high temperatures using indirect heating sources or selective fuel-firing in the absence of oxygen. Pyrolysis, which is also termed destructive distillation or thermal decomposition, has long been used in a number of industrial applications, such as coal gasification, carbon black manufacturing, and coke manufacturing for the steel industry. Pyrolysis technologies have also been used in various solid waste processing applications over the years including the conversion of municipal solid waste to a type of low-grade fuel oil or a fuel gas for firing in conventional boilers. Pyrolytic-type technologies, typically termed gasification systems, have further been used to produce what are known as biofuels from disposed organics such as wood waste and agricultural by-products.

Pyrolysis-type medical waste treatment systems are similar to and have the same basic components as conventional incinerator systems. For example, they have a primary chamber into which waste is loaded for treatment, a secondary chamber such as an afterburner or similar device for combusting or cleaning volatile gases discharged from the primary chamber, and means for adding and controlling heat input for processing or treatment. Due to the inherent nature of their operations, pyrolysis systems present a number of challenging problems when treating wastes that are difficult to overcome and which likely limited their widespread use. The more significant problems or difficulties include the following:

- The need for special handling and the further processing of solid residues remaining in the primary or pyrolytic chamber after each cycle of operation. Unless waste to be pyrolyzed is shredded or granulated beforehand, treated residues are recognizable, not disfigured, and not destroyed because no combustion takes place and, additionally, its volume is only slightly reduced because carbonaceous solids are not burned.
- The need for specialized APC equipment combined with the burning of large quantities of natural gas in an afterburner in order to remove or clean dense concentrations of volatile gases and organic pollutants released from waste components, such as plastics and chemicals, when they are heated
- The need to closely control and strictly limit any ambient air infiltration into the pyrolyzing chamber during operations that restricts such systems to batch-type operations, comparable to autoclave operations, and to smaller throughput rates or capacities in comparison to comparably sized incinerator systems

▶ EVALUATING AND SELECTING MEDICAL WASTE TREATMENT TECHNOLOGIES

Seven fundamental criteria are recommended for consideration and comparative analyses in the process evaluating and selecting the most viable and cost-effective technology for a site-specific application. It should be relatively easy to apply a weight rating to each of the criteria based on site-specific considerations and then to derive a total numerical rating value for each alternative as a metrical means of determining or deciding that which is best. These criteria are discussed in the following text:

1. **Demonstrated performance criteria**

   This is paramount for evaluating or comparing either different treatment technologies or different vendors of a preferred type of technology. It essentially focuses on the overall viability and degree of demonstrated success of any particular technology or technology variation. For example, technologies that are still under development with no full-scale operational systems in place should be rated or ranked much lower than those technologies having long-term demonstrated successful installations at multiple facilities or locations. Key factors under this criterion can include the following:

   - The status or viability of the technology or process; that is, is it conceptual, under development, or proven in full-scale operation?
   - The number of full-scale operational systems in place and their respective capacities or process rates
   - Years of successful performance of full-scale operational systems based on discussions with independent reference contacts at those facilities at which operational system are in place

2. **Technical and performance criteria**

   This comprises assessments of the suitability of any particular technology for satisfying site-specific or user-specific medical waste treatment requirements including considerations of processing capacity, degree of destruction or disinfection, and ease of operation without the need for specialized handling or waste segregation. As an example, technologies that can process large volumes of medical waste at a high hourly capacity and without requiring repackaging or special handling should be rated or ranked higher than those technologies having a small capacity with a need for the waste to be loaded in small batches. Key factors under this criterion can include the following:

   - Process throughput capacity on an hourly and daily basis
   - Waste type or component exclusions or limitations
   - Waste container size limitations
   - Weight reductions or increases of treated waste residues
   - Volume reductions or increases of treated waste residues
   - Degree of destruction, disfigurement, or recognizability of treated waste residues
   - Degree of disinfection or sterilization and suitability for meeting applicable regulatory requirements
   - Process and operational complexity

3. **Vendor qualification criteria**

   This comprises assessments of the ability and resources of the treatment technology vendor or supplier to provide support services for system installation and commissioning as well as during continued operations over the long term. For example, larger vendors that have been in business for many years in manufacturing and servicing waste treatment systems may be ranked higher than vendors having limited resources, a small support staff, and without a track record of successful installations. Key factors can include the following:

   - Years in business, both overall and in manufacturing the specific technology
   - Financial stability
   - Staffing and levels of expertise
   - Ability and staffing expertise to provide support services such as responses to problems, emergency repairs, scheduled maintenance, spare parts, etc

4. **Environmental and permitting criteria**

   This includes assessments of the ability of any particular technology to comply with all applicable, site-specific environmental regulations and requirements inclusive of its acceptability or approval by the environmental agency in the state or region in which the technology is to be installed. It may also include the public perceptions and the potential of public opposition to the technology. Key factors include the following:

   - Air pollutant emissions from stacks and vents, their potential impacts on the surrounding environment and public health, and the possible need to install APC equipment to meet applicable emission standards
   - Liquid effluent discharges and contaminants, or pollutants, and the possible need to install wastewater treatment equipment to meet applicable discharge or pretreatment standards
   - Characteristics and components of treated waste residue and their acceptability for off-site disposal
   - Degree of difficulty and demonstrated success in obtaining approvals, acceptance, and permits from applicable environmental and regulatory agencies
   - Public perceptions and acceptability

5. **Occupational safety and health criteria**

   This considers the ability of facility personnel or staff to operate, maintain, and service any particular technology without unacceptable or exceptionally high safety and health risks or exposures as well as the possible need for any special personnel protection measures. Depending on the type of technology, risks can include potential exposures to high temperatures or flames, toxic or corrosive chemicals, toxic fumes or vapors, and/or poorly protected moving parts and components. Factors to consider can include the types and degree of risk (including protective measures) during normal, routine system operations, and during scheduled or unscheduled maintenance and repair.

6. **Facility and infrastructure requirement criteria**

   This considers utility services and connections and necessary site or general construction work required. It also includes considerations of space requirements, such as the overall area needed for the treatment equipment, the staging of waste to be delivered and stored for treatment, and the containment and interim storage of treated residues destined for off-site disposal. It can also include any special building or general construction requirements for dealing with potential operational issues such as excessive vibrations, high noise levels, high temperatures, odors, and the uncontrolled release of chemicals and fumes. Key factors include the following:

   - Overall space area and clear elevation requirements
   - Special general construction requirements, such as foundations, structural supports, and equipment pads
   - Utility requirements such as fuel, steam, electrical power, ventilation air, blowdown water drainage. This should include peak demand levels and normal levels during steady-state operations.
   - Special heating, ventilation, exhaust, and/or air conditioning requirements

7. **Economic assessment criteria**

   This includes budgetary cost estimates and preliminary economic analysis, or life cycle costing, of treatment technologies that are deemed to be potentially viable or suitable for a particular application. Life cycle costing based on processing the quantities of medical waste to be treated should provide a reliable means for a good economic comparison. Economic assessments can include the following:

   - Estimated total capital cost requirements inclusive of system and equipment procurement and installation, site and general construction work, utility supply and connections, startup and commissioning, permitting, compliance testing, etc
   - Estimated total annual costs inclusive of operating labor, utility usage, consumables such as chemicals or special containers, maintenance and repair, treated waste residue disposal, annual testing and certifications, and the handling and disposal of any excluded waste items
   - Life cycle costing analyses including annualized costs, unit costs, and return on investment (ROI) comparisons to other technologies under consideration or being evaluated

REFERENCES

1. United Nations Environment Programme. *Compendium of Technologies for Treatment/Destruction of Healthcare Waste*. Osaka, Japan: United Nations Environment Programme; 2012.
2. Centers for Disease Control and Prevention. *CDC Guideline for Isolation Precautions in Hospitals*. Atlanta, GA: Centers for Disease Control and Prevention; 1983. Health & Human Services Publication No. 83-8314.
3. Centers for Disease Control and Prevention. *Guideline for Handwashing and Hospital Environmental Control*. Atlanta, GA: Centers for Disease Control and Prevention; 1985.
4. Environmental Protection Agency. *Draft Manual for Infectious Waste Management. SW-957*. Washington, DC: Environmental Protection Agency, Office of Solid Waste and Emergency Response; 1982.
5. Environmental Protection Agency. *EPA Guide for Infectious Waste Management. EPA/530-SW-86-014*. Washington, DC: Environmental Protection Agency, Office of Solid Waste and Emergency Response; 1986.
6. Environmental Protection Agency. Standards for the tracking and management of medical waste. 1989. Codified as 40 CFR Part 259.
7. Environmental Protection Agency. Standards of performance for new stationary sources and emission guidelines for existing sources: hospital/medical/infectious waste incinerators; final rule. 1997. Codified as Title 40 CFR Part 60 & Subpart Ce—Standards of Performance for New Stationary Sources; Subpart Ec—Standards of performance for hospital/medical/infectious waste incinerators for which construction commenced after June 20, 1996.
8. Environmental Protection Agency. Federal plan requirements for hospital/medical/infectious waste incinerators constructed on or before December 1, 2008, and standards of performance for new stationary sources: hospital/medical/infectious waste incinerators: final rule. 2013. Codified as 40 CFR Parts 60 and 62, Subpart HHH.
9. Occupational Safety and Health Administration. Bloodborne pathogens. 1991. Codified as Title 49 CFR Part 1910.1030.
10. Department of Transportation. Hazardous materials regulations. 1996. Codified as 49 CFR Parts 171-180: Subparts 172 & 173—Infectious Substances & Regulated Medical Waste.
11. Gile TJ, Cook CR, Glotzer JM, et al. *GPO5-A3 Clinical Laboratory Waste Management—Approved Guideline*. 3rd ed. Wayne, PA: Clinical and Laboratory Standards Institute; 2011.
12. Centers for Disease Control and Prevention, Healthcare Infection Control Practices Advisory Committee. *Guidelines for Environmental Infection Control in Health-Care Facilities*. Atlanta, GA: Centers for Disease Control; 2003.
13. The Joint Commission. *Guide to JCAHO Environment of Care Standard 3.10.9*. Oakbrook Terrace, IL: The Joint Commission; 2005.
14. Prüss A, Giroult E, Rushbrook P. *Safe Management of Wastes from Health-Care Activities*. 2nd ed. Geneva, Switzerland: World Health Organization; 2014.
15. United States Agency for International Development. *Sector Environmental Guidelines—Healthcare Waste*. Washington, DC: United States Agency for International Development. Contract No. GS-10F-01055, 2003 & 2015.
16. Doucet L. *Calculating True Biomedical Waste Generation Rates*. Chicago, IL: American Society for Healthcare Environmental Services; 1992. Professional Development Series No. 057018.
17. Doucet L. *Medical Waste Management: Regulatory & Technical Background Report*. Palo Alto, CA: Electric Power Research Institute. EPRI TR-100978, Project 2662-1B; 1992.
18. Doucet L. *Evaluating & Selecting the Best Medical Waste Treatment and Disposal Alternatives*. Chicago, IL: American Society for Healthcare Engineering; 2001. Professional Development Series No. 197110.
19. Health Care Without Harm. *Non-Incineration Medical Waste Treatment Technologies*. Reston, VA: Health Care Without Harm; 2001.

CHAPTER 55

Reprocessing and Remanufacturing of Single-Use Medical Devices

D. J. Vukelich

Worldwide reuse of single-use devices (SUDs) is commonplace. However, historically, regulatory requirements applied to SUD reuse have not been consistent. Because SUDs most often do not come with reprocessing instructions, the reprocessing of SUDs has varied from facility to facility, region to region, and country to country. In 2000, the US Food and Drug Administration (FDA) began to regulate the reuse of SUDs as a medical device manufacturing activity, subject to the same requirements applicable to any other medical device manufacturer. Globally, other nations have begun taking similar regulatory steps, subjecting SUD reuse to medical device manufacturing regulations. The impact of such regulations has generally been the consolidation of SUD reprocessing into a limited number of regulated firms, subject to medical device regulatory agency oversight (eg, FDA).[1] Where regulated, health care facilities have generally ceased reprocessing SUDs in-house or in the hospital's central sterile departments alongside reusable devices; instead, they rely on commercial firms to conduct the reprocessing according to medical device manufacturing standards. The impact of regulation has also been to narrow the scope of SUDs commonly reprocessed to only those for which reprocessors can demonstrate to regulatory authorities that the devices are as safe and as effective as original equipment. Furthermore, the subset of SUDs that are reprocessed is practically limited to those products that are expensive and common enough to make it financially worthwhile to commercial reprocessors. From the patient or health care provider's perspective, where regulated, this means that reprocessed SUDs are subject to all the same safety and efficacy standards applicable to any other medical device.

The objective of this chapter is to provide historical perspectives on SUD reprocessing, the circumstances that led to its growth, the types of devices commonly reprocessed, and a discussion of the SUD label. Most importantly, this chapter provides an overview of the regulatory requirements for organizations that reprocessors SUDs including hospitals, commercial reprocessor, and/or medical device manufacturers. As part of this, the chapter addresses emerging international regulatory trends applicable to SUD reprocessing.

DEFINITIONS

Single-use medical devices are those designated or intended by the manufacturer for use on one patient during a single procedure.[2] The manufacturer does not intend for SUDs to be further processed and used again. This contrasts with **reusable medical devices** that are designated or intended by the manufacturer as suitable for processing and reuse. Medical devices intended for reuse are sold to hospitals and health care providers with processing/reprocessing instructions. **Processing** is the activity to prepare a new or used health care product for its intended use. Processing may include various steps such as cleaning, disinfection, and sterilization.[3] Most SUDs do not come with processing/reprocessing instructions, as the manufacturer does not intend for the device to be reused (see chapter 47). In this chapter, *reprocess* may be used interchangeably with *process*; both, in the context of this chapter, refer to any reuse of an SUD. **Remanufacturing**, with regard to SUDs, is a term increasingly used outside the United States to differentiate regulated SUD reprocessing in hospital reprocessing centers.

LABELING

Because SUDs are not intended by the original manufacturer to be reprocessed, no discussion of SUD reprocessing would be appropriate without a discussion of labeling. After all, why would health care institutions want to reprocess devices clearly labeled as disposable or for single use? It is important to understand the regulatory implications of device labeling. As noted, regulatory requirements, including FDA requirements,[4] place the responsibility on the manufacturer to correctly label a device based on the intended use. A US Government Accountability Office (GAO) report succinctly addressed the usage of a single-use label as follows:

> The decision to label a device as single-use or reusable rests with the manufacturer. If a manufacturer intends to label a device as reusable, it must provide data demonstrating to FDA's satisfaction that the device can be cleaned and sterilized without impairing its function. Thus, a device may be labeled as single-use because the manufacturer believes that it cannot be safely and reliably used more than once, or because the manufacturer chooses not to conduct the studies needed to demonstrate that the device can be labeled as reusable.[5]

In contrast to labeling a device for single use, which requires no cleaning validation or other reprocessing instructions, medical device manufacturers desiring to market a device as reusable must have sufficient data to demonstrate that the device can be reused and that the validated processing instructions will consistently render a device appropriate for use (eg, cleaned, disinfected, and/or sterilized; see chapter 47). Thus, there is a strong regulatory incentive to label devices as single use because the regulatory burden is lower than labeling a device as reusable.

Prior to the 1980s, most medical devices were made of durable reusable materials such as metal, rubber, or glass. These were considered relatively easy to clean. With the advent of new plastic materials, less regulatory demands for SUDs, developments of sterilization technologies (eg, ethylene oxide optimization and the use of oxidizing agents), growing device intricacy, and the threat of iatrogenic HIV transmission in the early 1980s, the demand and use of disposable devices increased. Health care facilities found disposable devices to be convenient and safe and thus the beginning of a greater "throwaway" mentality. The pendulum began to swing back in the 1990s with managed care capping procedural costs, greater financial pressures, and a concern over the environmental implications in relying on disposable medical devices. It was at this time that hospitals began to consider the reuse of some SUDs.[6] In addition to these financial and environmental pressures, health care facility skepticism of original equipment manufacturer (OEM) use of the single-use label grew, contributing to greater SUD reprocessing. In 2000, the first GAO report about SUD reprocessing found that some manufacturers had "contributed to the sense that compliance with the single-use label is not always necessary." The GAO identified a manufacturer of pulse oximeter sensors that provided health care facilities with "remanufactured" sensors at a reduced price if the hospitals returned their

used, single-use sensors to the company. This recycling of devices by the manufacturer, who itself had originally labeled the devices as single use, contributed to the sense among health care professionals that the single-use label was primarily for marketing purposes. Hospital skepticism of the single-use label was summarized in the 2000 GAO report, suggesting that health care personnel distrusted single-use labeling with some devices because of issues such as the FDA not being able to require manufacturers to support the designation of a device as single use and the perception that there was an economic incentive to market SUDs that could be reusable.[5]

Third-party or commercial SUD reprocessors emerged in the late 1990s. The competitive effect of their lower cost offerings placed greater attention on disposable medical devices, prices, and environmental impact (or sustainability). One article at the time estimated that if 1% to 2% of disposable medical devices were reprocessed/reused in the United States at that time, the health care savings could be approximately a billion dollars every year.[7] Thus, many factors including economic, regulatory, and marketing considerations contributed to growing reprocessing of SUDs.

▶ DEVICE TYPES

There are three main categories of SUDs commonly reprocessed in the United States: operating room (OR) instruments, noninvasive devices, and cardiovascular products. In the category of OR instruments, prices have escalated for hospitals for such devices including laparoscopic and electrosurgical instruments. Commercial reprocessors have offered reprocessed versions of these instruments including trocars, ultrasonic scalpels, graspers, and forceps, among others. Noninvasive devices include sequential compression sleeves and cuffs, tourniquet cuffs, bed alarms, and pulse oximetry sensors. Cardiovascular products include electrophysiology and ultrasonic cardiac catheters and associated instruments. Internationally, a greater range of SUD types have been subjected to routine processing and in many cases under unregulated controls or insufficient risk considerations. But such uncontrolled processing has heightened attention to the importance of meticulous process controls and safety considerations.[8-10]

▶ REPROCESSING AND REGULATION

Before 1995, there were no federal regulations for the reprocessing of SUDs in the United States and no known regulations in other countries. The Joint Commission on Accreditation of Healthcare Organizations at that time maintained that SUDs should not be reprocessed unless the OEM had provided written instructions. Despite this, in one 1986 survey, the Institute of Health Policy

Analysis reported that 82% of US hospitals reused devices marked as disposable.[6] As is much the case internationally, the full extent of SUD reprocessing by US hospitals in the 1980s and 1990s was not fully known. Not until 2000 did federal US regulations apply to SUD reuse and did a clearer picture of the extent of SUD reprocessing emerge.

Commercial SUD reprocessors, distinct from health care facilities that may reprocess devices, were subject to FDA oversight in the United States. Since at least 1998, the FDA considered third-party or commercial reprocessors of SUDs to be medical device manufacturers. Manufacturers could market a device for one more single use from a raw material that was previously used if the device met the same specifications described in the original clearance.[11] The FDA did inspect commercial reprocessors in accordance with the quality system regulation (QSR).[12] But, as noted, FDA did not assert any regulation against hospitals, surgical centers, or other entities that reprocessed SUDs, or did it assert the agency's premarket controls against SUD reprocessing, regardless of where it took place. Beginning in 2000, pursuant to the Federal Food, Drug, and Cosmetic Act (FDCA), FDA began requiring all SUD reprocessors to comply with all device manufacturing requirements that apply to OEMs[2] as well as some additional requirements added later that apply only to SUD reprocessors.[13] They issued guidance in 2000 outlining its enforcement priorities as it phased in new requirements. The implications of this move are multifold. First, this is the first known medical device regulatory authority to assert that the reuse of SUDs is a manufacturing activity and therefore subject to medical device manufacturing requirements. For reasons outlined in the following text, this not only put SUD reprocessors on a level regulatory footing with other device manufacturers but also put in motion a model regulatory approach to SUD reprocessing. Second, for the first time, FDA was asserting its regulatory authority over hospitals. Traditionally, as FDA only has jurisdiction to regulate device manufacturing, most FDA enforcement was against manufacturers at traditional manufacturing operations. Now, despite some protest from American hospitals and their trade associations, FDA would inspect and stop US hospitals from reusing SUDs if not meeting specific requirements. Third, by asserting it had authority over all SUD reprocessing, the FDA essentially forced a consolidation of all US SUD reprocessing into a handful of regulated firms. Hospitals, after a few high-profile warning letters,[14,15] ceased to reprocess SUDs in-house and began to depend on FDA-regulated commercial firms. Of note, the scope of FDA's 2000 guidance did exclude permanently implantable pacemakers, opened but unused SUDs, health care facilities that are not hospitals, and reprocessing of hemodialyzers. Since 2000, FDA has not acted to terminate the exemption for these four exclusions. As a result, medical device manufacturers, third-party, or commercial reprocessors and hospitals are all subject to the same FDA requirements when it comes to reprocessing SUDs.[2]

Since the issuance of FDA's 2000 guidance, the agency has required SUD reprocessors, like OEMs, to comply with the agency's establishment registration and medical device listing, medical device reporting, medical device tracking, reports of corrections and removals, the QSR, and labeling requirements.[2] Including in this, like all devices, reprocessed devices are subject to premarket review by FDA, unless the agency has, by regulation, declared the device to be exempt from premarket requirements. Unless exempt, FDA class I and class II reprocessed devices are required to have cleared premarket notification submissions ("510(k)s").[16] In the 18 years since the introduction of FDA regulation of SUD reprocessing, over 250 FDA clearances have been issued for reprocessed SUDs, overwhelmingly to third-party or commercial firms. Only four instances exist where ownership of clearances belong to hospitals, but those hospitals are not registered or listed with the FDA to reprocess.[17] It is unclear why these hospitals acquired a clearance to reprocess these devices if they lack the establishment registration and listing to do so.

As noted, the FDA requires that reusable devices come with validated reprocessing instructions (see chapter 47). Devices intended for single use do not require such data. Any subsequent reuse of an SUD, by a hospital, reprocessor, or manufacturer, is done absent FDA review or inspection of any validated reprocessing instruction. In its move to regulate SUD reprocessing, FDA put in place a mechanism by which to obtain validated reprocessing protocols from any entity wishing to reprocess an SUD. It is the reprocessor (now the manufacturer) that has the burden to demonstrate to the FDA that a reprocessing validation has taken place and that the new, reprocessed SUD will be as safe and as effective as the predicate medical device. Since 2002, FDA has required this validation data of SUD reprocessors on a premarket basis, meaning the reprocessed product is not marketable for sale until such time as the agency has reviewed and cleared the data, in conjunction with all others submitted as part of the premarket filing.[16] Specifically, reprocessors are, in many cases, required to include validation data for cleaning and sterilization and functional performance to show that the reprocessed device remains substantially equivalent after the maximum number of times the device is intended to be reprocessed.[13]

In 2017, FDA increased its requirements of OEMs marketing reusable devices with its *Reprocessing Medical Devices in Health Care Settings: Validation Methods and Labeling* guidance.[18] In the guidance appendix E, FDA outlined those devices for which it expects validated reprocessing instructions data to be submitted on a premarket basis, meaning, to be inspected by the agency as part of the review for new such products. Historically, the agency had only sought to inspect to ensure manufacturers had such data, on a postmarket basis. This long-anticipated guidance addressed recent attention given to the problems associated with inadequate hospital reprocessing or inadequate manufacturer reprocessing instructions with *reusable* devices. This begins to level the regulatory requirements for all reprocessed devices, single use or reusable. Since 2002, SUD reprocessors had, in many cases, to include in their premarket submissions greater data packages than OEMs have traditionally been required to submit for reusable devices.[13]

Also pursuant to provisions added to the FDCA in 2002 by the Medical Device User Fee and Modernization Act (MDUFMA), FDA withdrew the exemptions from the premarket notification requirement for a significant number of previously exempt reprocessed devices, although the original devices remain exempt from premarket review.[13] Title III of MDUFMA amended the FDCA.[19] The law required FDA to identify critical and semicritical 510(k)-exempt devices for which the exemptions should be terminated when the devices are reprocessed, in order to provide a reasonable assurance of the safety and effectiveness of these devices.[19] For devices that lost exemption from premarket notification, reprocessors had to submit a 510(k) within 15 months of FDA's publication of a notice terminating the exemption, or the device in question could no longer be legally marketed.[19]

The FDA's regulation of SUD reprocessing can arguably be regarded as a success story and a potential guide to other agencies internationally. All reprocessed SUDs in the United States are subject to medical device manufacturer requirements, ensuring the same levels of safety and efficacy. The intent of regulation has been to stop the unvalidated reprocessing of SUDs and ensure that it is only done under regulated circumstances. Patients and health care providers can therefore depend on reprocessed SUDs meeting these same standards. Device manufacturers and reprocessors are held to the same requirements, ensuring a consistent regulatory approach. With this strong regulatory framework in place, US SUD reprocessing has been legitimized, takes place in an open and transparent market, and can provide a competitive market advantage.

▶ SUSTAINABILITY CONSIDERATIONS

An additional hospital consideration for using SUD reprocessing is the financial and economic sustainability that reprocessing may offer. In addition to the cost savings per device, reprocessing allows hospitals to lower their environmental footprint by reducing the number of devices they consume and therefore dispose of, reducing the cost associated with both waste and waste removal.

The Emergency Care Research Institute (ECRI), a nonprofit organization dedicated to bringing the discipline of applied scientific research to discover which medical procedures, devices, drugs, and processes are best practice, has weighed in on SUD reprocessing. The ECRI reported

that the use of reprocessed medical devices had become commonplace; the use of reprocessed SUDs was a cost-effective practice, reduced medical waste, and without increasing risk to patient safety.[20] Large health systems have reported saving many millions of dollars annually and diverting many hundreds of tons of medical waste by using reprocessed SUDs.

▶ INTERNATIONAL REGULATION

The reuse of SUDs is common in international hospitals. In many cases (particularly in Africa and Asia), uncontrolled reuse of such devices is relatively common, if not the norm.[21] Whereas FDA's regulatory framework for SUD reprocessing is perhaps the longest standing in the world, Germany also began regulation of SUD reprocessing beginning in 2002 under the German Medical Devices Law and the Medical Devices Operator Ordinance.

Germany

The German regulatory framework does not distinguish between the reprocessing of reusable and single-use medical devices. The guidelines, therefore, allow for SUD reprocessing if conformance with certain standards is achieved. The German Medical Devices Law and the Medical Devices Operator Ordinance regulate the reprocessing of medical devices and in doing so refer to the mutual recommendation by the Kommission für Krankenhaushygiene und Infektionsprävention (KRINKO) and the Federal Institute for Drugs and Medical Devices (BfArM) for the reprocessing of medical devices. As a result, the KRINKO requirements must be observed.[22] Institutions that want to reprocess single-use medical devices must adopt and implement a quality management system according to DIN EN ISO 13485.[23] Compliance with the quality management requirements is monitored annually by Notified Bodies that have been accredited by the Central Authority of the states (Länder) for Health Protection for Medicinal Products and Medical Devices (ZLG).

European Union

In April 2017, after nearly 5 years of negotiations at council and in parliament, the European Union (EU) adopted a comprehensive new EU-wide medical device regulation (MDR). With it, the EU adopted manufacturer standards for SUD reprocessors and remanufacturers, much akin to the FDA approach. Prior to that, the EU did not have a single policy regarding the reprocessing of SUDs. Previously in 1993, with the publication of the previous Medical Device Directive, the issue of medical device reprocessing was identified as requiring additional clarification and the European Commission was instructed to submit a report on the issue by 2010.[24] In short, after a lengthy deliberative process between the European Commission, Council, and Parliament, on March 7, 2017 a final agreement was reached and resulted in the final regulation, published in the *Official Journal of the European Union* on May 5, 2017. The regulation treats SUD reprocessing as *manufacturing*.[25]

With the adoption of this new regulation, the EU is poised to take on the same trajectory as the United States in curtailing unvalidated SUD reprocessing and allowing regulated, commercial firms. This regulatory position allows commercial reprocessors to legitimize their products by demonstrating their devices are safe and meet the same requirements as original equipment. However, unlike the uniform application of FDA regulations in the United States, a provision in the EU regulation requires the European member states to allow or disallow such products within their own borders. This means, that in addition to reprocessor compliance with the regulation, each European member state must also adopt a law or regulation explicitly allowing reprocessed products within their borders.[26]

Already, the United Kingdom took regulatory action consistent with the new MDR paradigm in June 2016. In it, the Medicines & Healthcare products Regulatory Agency (MHRA) adopted the term SUD "remanufacturing" to describe regulated SUD reuse as distinct from SUD reprocessing or what typically happens in hospitals. In short, MHRA advises hospitals *not* to reprocess SUDs in-house but opens the door to allowing regulated, remanufactured SUDs to the British market.[26] Similarly, in April 2014, the Portuguese Secretary of State Health published in the *Official Gazette* the conditions and requirements applicable to the reprocessing of SUDs. The National Authority of Medicines and Medicinal Products is empowered to regulate SUD reprocessing and to require, among other things, that reprocessed SUDs meet the essential requirements established in Annex I of Decree-Law No. 145/2009 or the Medical Device Directive.[27]

Other member states, such as Spain[28] and France,[29] discouraged or prohibited SUD reprocessing. Most member states in Europe do not have similar national regulations regarding SUD reprocessing, as of now. With full implementation of the EU regulation by late 2019 or early 2020, more member states are expected to assess their position on SUD reprocessing.

Australia/New Zealand

Australia enacted regulations regarding the reprocessing (or remanufacturing) of SUDs in 2003. Like the United States, in Australia, all reprocessors (third-party, hospital, and OEM) must conform to medical device manufacturer requirements as regulated by the Therapeutic Goods

Administration (TGA).[30,31] Prior to implementation of these requirements, hospital reprocessing of SUDs was common. Also, it is believed that due to the costs and high technical standards required to meet the TGA's conformity assessment requirements, hospitals have ceased reprocessing SUDs in-house. In New Zealand, the regulator Medsafe requires either compliance with the US 510(k), CE approval, or a listing with the Australian TGA for the sale of medical devices within the country. Besides a notification procedure, no further regulatory approval was required.[21]

Canada

Historically, Health Canada asserted that it did not have the legal authority to regulate the reprocessing of SUDs. The Canadian *Food and Drugs Act* and Canadian *Medical Device Regulations* do not address the way in which health care facilities use, maintain, or sterilize medical devices *after* sale. This changed in 2014. The agency released a letter in July 2014 to all provincial and territorial Ministers of Health indicating that the agency would, henceforth, apply the existing regulations to all incoming applications for reprocessed SUDs. In that same letter, Health Canada announced that it had issued, for the first time, a license to an SUD reprocessor.[32]

In February 2015, the agency issued a notice to all stakeholders confirming that Health Canada would have the authority under the existing Food and Drugs Act and Medical Devices Regulations to require commercially reprocessed devices to meet appropriate standards for safety, effectiveness, and labeling. Furthermore, the agency gave an 18-month time frame by which companies that reprocessed and distributed medical devices originally labeled as single use in Canada would now have to meet the same requirements as manufacturers of new devices. This meant meeting requirements including quality system management, investigating and handling complaints, conducting recalls, reporting incidents or changes to license applications, etc. The requirements apply to commercial reprocessors in or outside of Canada.[33]

The SUD reprocessing in Canada had historically been left to the territorial and provincial health ministries and hospital boards, and in-hospital reprocessing continues to remain a provincial and territorial responsibility. The large provinces have adopted similar positions, essentially requiring any hospital that wishes to reprocess critical SUDs to do so through an FDA-regulated vendor. Examples include the following:

- British Columbia issued a policy to its health authorities stating that by January 1, 2008, all health authorities must have eliminated the reprocessing and reuse of critical contact SUDs, unless they have been reprocessed by a licensed third-party reprocessor that was certified by a national regulatory authority such as

Health Canada or the FDA.[34] A 2011 policy required that critical and semicritical devices labeled as single use shall not be reprocessed and reused unless the reprocessing is done by a licensed reprocessor.[35]

- Manitoba does not permit hospitals to reuse SUDs in-house but does permit hospitals to contract with an FDA-regulated vendor, among other requirements.[35]
- Since 2005, the Northwest Territories have prohibited reprocessing. Specifically, the Northwest Territories Department of Health and Social Services revised its *Hospital and Health Care Facility Standards Regulations* to require that a disposable device intended to be used on a patient should only be used on that patient for one procedure and not used with another patient.[35]
- In 2013, Public Health Ontario released its third edition document developed by its Provincial Infectious Diseases Advisory Committee (PIDAC) advising that critical and semicritical SUDs must not be reprocessed and reused, unless the reprocessing is done by a licensed reprocessor.[36]
- In 2013, Saskatchewan Health affirmed a policy outlining requirements for hospitals that reprocess SUDs. Consistent with the earlier policies of other provinces, Saskatchewan requires, among other things, that hospitals outsource to an FDA-regulated vendor.[34]

Japan

In June 2017, Japan released guidance making the reuse of SUDs subject to manufacturing requirements.[37]

South Africa

In December 2016, South Africa's Department of Health issued long-awaited regulations for medical devices, pursuant to Section 35 of the Medicines and Related Substances Act 101 of 1965 as amended by Act 59 of 2002. In it, the reprocessing, refurbishment, repair, relabeling, or repackaging of medical devices is defined as a manufacturing activity and therefore subject to the regulation's requirements. The SUD reprocessors must, like all other device manufacturers, comply with the regulation's requirements, including obtaining an establishment license and registration for each of the products marketed in the country. Furthermore, according to the labeling requirements for medical devices in part 22, reprocessors must include the name of the reprocessor and identify the device as being reprocessed.[38]

There are no known regulations for SUD reprocessing in the rest of Africa. The lack of resources, including medical devices and distribution channels, is often used to justify the reuse of SUDs in much of Africa. This includes the reuse of syringes and needles that have not been sterilized, and even rubber gloves.[21]

Israel

Israel does not have regulations in place specifically to the reprocessing of SUDs, but as a general matter, medical devices must be registered with the Ministry of Health (MOH) before they can be sold in the country. If a product is approved by the FDA, it will generally be registered by the MOH with no further testing requirements and, therefore, may be lawfully marketed in the country. Consistent with this policy, FDA-cleared reprocessed devices have been registered with MOH and are actively imported into this country.[39,40]

REFERENCES

1. Williamson RB, Yamane K, Byer M, et al. *Reprocessed Single-Use Medical Devices: FDA Oversight Has Increased, and Available Information Does Not Indicate That Use Presents an Elevated Health Risk.* Washington, DC: US Government Accountability Office; 2008. Report No. GAO-08-147.
2. Center for Devices and Radiological Health. *Guidance for Industry and for FDA Staff: Enforcement Priorities for Single-Use Devices Reprocessed by Third Parties and Hospitals.* Rockville, MD: Center for Devices and Radiological Health; 2000.
3. International Organization for Standardization. *ISO 17664: 2017: Processing of Health Care Products—Information to Be Provided by the Medical Device Manufacturer for the Processing of Medical Devices.* Geneva, Switzerland: International Organization for Standardization; 2017.
4. General Labeling Provisions, 21 CFR §801. Revised April 1, 2012.
5. Scanion W, Bradley E, Crosse M, Gahart M, Johnson J, Weldon S. *Single-Use Medical Devices: Little Available Evidence of Harm from Reuse, but Oversight Warranted.* Washington, DC: US Government Accountability Office; 2000. Report No. GAO/HeHS-00-123.
6. Dunn D. Reprocessing single-use devices—the ethical dilemma. *AORN J.* 2002;75:989-999.
7. Selvey D. Medical device reprocessing: is it good for your organization? Infection Control Today Web site. https://www.infectioncontroltoday.com/environmental-hygiene/medical-device-reprocessing. Accessed August 27, 2019.
8. Kapoor A, Vora A, Nataraj G, Mishra S, Kerkar P, Manjunath CN. Guidance on reuse of cardio-vascular catheters and devices in India: a consensus document. *Indian Heart J.* 2017;69:357-363.
9. Larose E. Legal implications of single-use medical device reprocessing. *Healthc Q.* 2013;16:48-52.
10. Shuman EK, Chenoweth CE. Reuse of medical devices: implications for infection control. *Infect Dis Clin North Am.* 2012;26:165-172.
11. Burlington DB. *Letter to: N Singer.* Washington, DC: US Food and Drug Administration; 1998.
12. Plaisier MK. *Letter to: TJ Bliley, Jr.* Washington, DC: US Food and Drug Administration; 2000.
13. Office of Device Evaluation. *Guidance for Industry and FDA Staff: Medical Device User Fee and Modernization Act of 2002, Validation Data in Premarket Notification Submissions (510(k)s) for Reprocessed Single-Use Medical Devices.* Rockville, MD: Center for Devices and Radiological Health; 2004.
14. Chappell M. *Warning Letter. Letter to: JE Crumpler.* Bowie, TX: US Food and Drug Administration; 2003.
15. Frappalo PJ. *Warning Letter. Letter to: GR Angle.* Tucson, AZ: US Food and Drug Administration; 2002.
16. Federal Food, Drug, and Cosmetic Act, 21 USC §360k (2012).
17. US Food and Drug Administration. Establishment registration & device listing. US Food and Drug Administration Web site. https://www.fda.gov/industry/fda-basics-industry/registration-and-listing. Accessed August 27, 2019.

18. US Food and Drug Administration. *Guidance for Industry and Food and Drug Administration Staff. Reprocessing Medical Devices in Health Care Settings: Validation Methods and Labeling.* Rockville, MD: Center for Devices and Radiological Health; 2015.

19. Pub L No. 107-250, 116 Stat 1588.

20. Emergency Care Research Institute. Use of reprocessed single-use medical devices. *Healthc Risk Control.* 2015;3:1-13.

21. Popp W, Rasslan O, Unahalekhaka A, et al. What is the use? An international look at reuse of single-use medical devices. *Int J Hyg Environ Health.* 2010;213:302-307.

22. Medizinprodukte A, Arzneimittel B. Hygiene requirements for the reprocessing of medical devices. Recommendation of the Commission for Hospital Hygiene and Infection Prevention (KRINKO) at the Robert Koch Institute (RKI) and the Federal Institute for Drugs and Medical Devices (BfArM) [in German]. *Bundesgesundheitsblatt Gesundheitsforschung Gesundheitsschutz.* 2012;55:1244-1310.

23. International Organization for Standardization. *ISO 13485: 2016: Medical Devices—Quality Management Systems—Requirements for Regulatory Purposes.* Geneva, Switzerland: International Organization for Standardization; 2016.

24. European Commission. Council Directive 93/42/EEC of 14 June 1993 concerning medical devices. European Commission Web site. https://eur-lex.europa.eu/legal-content/EN/TXT/PDF/?uri=CELEX :32017R0745. Accessed August 27, 2019.

25. European Commission. Regulation (EU) 2017/745 of the European Parliament and of the Council of 5 April 2017 on medical devices, amending Directive 2001/83/EC, Regulation (EC) No 178/2002 and Regulation (EC) No 1223/2009 and repealing Council Directives 90/385/EEC and 93/42/EEC. European Commission Web site. https://eur-lex.europa.eu/legal-content/EN/TXT/PDF/?uri=CELEX :32017R0745. Accessed August 27, 2019.

26. Medicines & Healthcare products Regulatory Agency. *Single-Use Medical Devices: UK Guidance on Re-Manufacturing.* London, United Kingdom: Medicines & Healthcare products Regulatory Agency; 2016.

27. National Authority of Medicines and Medicinal Products Health, IP. *Decision Paper No. 939/2014 Which Is Pursuant to Paragraph 9 of Order No. 7021/2013.* Lisbon, Portugal: National Authority of Medicines and Medicinal Products Health, IP; 2013.

28. Ministry of Health and Consumption. *Royal Decree 414/1996 of March 1, Regulating Medical Devices. BOE. No. 99. 14670-14702.* Madrid, Spain: Ministry of Health and Consumption; 2007.

29. Ministry of Social Affairs. *Circulaire DGS/DH No 51 on the Use of Sterile Medical Devices for Use in Public and Private Health Facilities.* Paris, France: Ministry of Social Affairs; 1994.

30. Therapeutic Goods Administration. *Statement by the TGA on Regulations for Sterilisation of Single Use Devices.* Symonston, Australia: Department of Health, Australian Government; 2003.

31. Parliament of Australia. *The Regulatory Standards for the Approval of Medical Devices in Australia.* Canberra, Australia: Parliament of Australia; 2011.

32. Sabourin BJ. *Re: Medical Device License. Letter to: Provincial and Territorial Ministries of Health.* Ottawa, Canada: Health Canada; 2014.

33. Medical Devices Bureau. *Notice to Stakeholders—Health Canada's Regulatory Approach to Commercial Reprocessing of Medical Devices Originally Labelled for Single-Use.* Ottawa, Canada: Health Canada; 2015.

34. Cowling T, de Léséleuc L. *Reprocessing of Single-Use Medical Devices: a 2015 Update. (Environmental Scan; Issue 48).* Ottawa, Canada: Canadian Agency for Drugs and Technologies in Health; 2015.

35. BC Health Authorities. *Best Practice Guidelines for Cleaning, Disinfection and Sterilization of Critical and Semi-Critical Medical Devices.* Surrey, United Kingdom: BC Health Authorities; 2011.

36. Public Health Ontario. *Best Practices for Cleaning, Disinfection and Sterilization of Medical Equipment/Devices in All Health Care Settings.* Ottawa, Canada: Provincial Infectious Diseases Advisory Committee on Infection Prevention and Control; 2013.

37. Ministry of Health, Labour and Welfare, Ministry of Health, and Physicians, Department of Monitoring Guidance, Drug Administration. *Remanufacturing Single-Use Medical Equipment and Medicine for In Vitro Diagnosis. No. 12(0731).* United Kingdom, Ministry of Health, Labour and Welfare, Ministry of Health; 2017.

38. South Africa Department of Health. *Medicines and Related Substances Act, 1965 (Act No. 101 of 1965) Regulations Relating to Medical Devices and In Vitro Diagnostic Medical Devices (IVDs). Staatskoerant No. 40480(1515) 61-93.* South Africa, South Africa Department of Health; 2016.

39. Israel Ministry of Health. *Reuse of Single-Use Medical Devices.* Jerusalem, Israel: Israel Ministry of Health; 2005.

40. US Department of Commerce. *Global Import Regulations for Pre-Owned (Used and Refurbished) Medical Devices.* Washington, DC: US Department of Commerce; 2005.

Food- and Waterborne Microorganisms

Gerald McDonnell

Food- and waterborne infective microorganisms constitute a diverse group that includes viruses, bacteria, algae, protozoa, fungi, and helminths. These agents can cause acute, chronic, or latent infections with incubation periods of a few hours, days, or even weeks; severity ranges from mild, transient, to fatal episodes. The illness may be manifested by preformed toxins or by the invading pathogens or both. The organism may be free living and saprophytic in nature or fastidious, multiplying only in the host. The agent may show single host specificity, or it may infect hosts of different species. The organism may be highly susceptible to physical-chemical agents, or it may form highly resistant spores. The pathogens may be highly aerobic, or they may show extreme oxygen sensitivity and be anaerobic. Some of these agents may cause local intestinal infections, whereas others cause septicemia. Some pathogens have the potential to cause explosive epidemics, and others only localized outbreaks; however, all these pathogens use food and water as a common vehicle and the gastrointestinal tract as a common route of infection.

▶ CHANGING PATTERN OF INFECTIONS

Food and water have been the most common sources of infectious diseases because the gastrointestinal tract offers pathogens a more direct access to the interior of the host. The pathogenic microorganisms often use food and water both as a vehicle and as a growth medium. Ingestion of contaminated food and water has been the cause of serious outbreaks, large epidemics, or waves of pandemics of diseases. One of the pathogens that have caused ravaging epidemics with high fatality rates is the etiologic agent of cholera, *Vibrio cholerae*. A brief historical perspective of this typical food- and water-infective pathogen is interesting. *Cholera*, as the term was used in Hippocratic writings 2400 years ago, represented sporadic gastrointestinal derangements of diverse origin.[1] Since the late 19th century, cholera has designated the illness caused by *V cholerae*. The illness represents most significantly an altered disease pattern resulting from industrialization without sanitation practices.[2] In seven pandemics, each starting from 1817, 1829, 1852, 1863, 1881, 1889, and 1961, respectively, it has claimed millions of lives in several countries. Transmission of cholera through water was discovered during the study known as "the cause of Broad street pump."[3] The victims used well water that had been contaminated by drainage. The epidemic was arrested by removal of the handle of the pump located on Broad Street, and sand filtration of water was effective in containing the cholera epidemic in Altona, Germany, at the end of the 19th century. The original biotype of *V cholerae* has been replaced by the El Tor strain in most parts of the world.[4]

During the first half of the 20th century, pathogens such as *Salmonella* ser Typhimurium, *V cholerae*, *Shigella* species, *Brucella* species, *Streptococcus pyogenes*, *Clostridium botulinum*, *Entamoeba histolytica*, and viruses such as polio viruses were known as primary foodborne and waterborne pathogens. Most recent and notable examples include outbreaks with *Escherichia coli* (including the shiga-toxin producing strains, such as the serogroup O157),[5] *Listeria*,[6] *Campylobacter*,[7] and norovirus.[8] Indeed, recent reports from the United States suggested that the top 5 pathogens associated with foodborne outbreaks were norovirus, *Salmonella*, *Clostridium perfringens*, *E coli*, and *Campylobacter* species.[9] Many of these are equally associated with waterborne sources, particularly *Cryptosporidium*, norovirus, *Giardia*, *Campylobacter*, and rotavirus.[10] These and many other pathogens still cause widespread illnesses in developing countries. For foodborne illness, the World Health Organization has estimated that the global burden of such diseases is significant and particularly in developing countries, with the main pathogens being norovirus and *Campylobacter*

TABLE 56.1 The most common causes worldwide of food- and waterborne outbreaks

Microorganism Type	Examples
Viruses	Hepatitis A virus Norovirus
Bacteria	*Bacillus cereus* *Brucella* species *Campylobacter* species *Clostridium* species *Escherichia coli* *Listeria* species *Mycobacterium bovis* *Salmonella* species *Shigella* species *Staphylococcus aureus* *Vibrio cholerae*
Protozoa	*Cryptosporidium* species *Giardia* species
Helminths	*Ascaris* species *Echinococcus* species *Fasciola* species *Taenia solium* *Toxoplasma gondii* *Trichinella* species
Toxins	Aflatoxin

species leading to diarrheal diseases.[11] Others included *Salmonella* species, *Taenia solium*, hepatitis A virus, and from fungal sources of aflatoxins. Examples of some of the more notable causes of food- and waterborne microbiological risks associated with outbreaks are summarized in Table 56.1.

Salmonella ser Typhi (leading to typhoid fever) and *Salmonella* ser Paratyphi (paratyphoid fever) continue to be leading causes of morbidity and mortality worldwide, despite the availability of a vaccine for at least typhoid fever and available antibiotic therapies.[12] These rates are further exasperated by increased reports of antibiotic resistance.[13] Incident rates vary from region to region, being particularly high in African, Latin American, and other developing countries. *S* Typhi was encountered in probably one of the largest recorded epidemics of typhoid fever in recent history, resulting from contaminated well water in Sangli, India, during 1975 through 1976.[14] Another similarly large typhoid epidemic (10 766 cases) was reported in Dushanbe, Tajikistan, as a result of contaminated municipal water supply.[15] Recent estimates worldwide suggest at least 27 million cases of typhoid and some 200 000 deaths annually, particularly in African and Asian countries,[16] although outbreaks are also frequently reported in other countries that are considered to have better controls on food and water sources.[17] *V cholerae* infections are estimated to occur in 3 to 5 million cases, and responsible for 100 000

to 120 000 deaths annually.[18] Reports and outbreaks continue to be endemic in certain regions of the world seasonally, including in parts of the Americas, Africa, and Asia. Large outbreaks are also frequently reported.[19] Other examples include larger outbreak with *Shigella* species in bacillary dysentery in Nigeria,[20] in India,[21] and more recent concerns with antibiotic-resistant strains such as in China.[22] High incidence of brucellosis, one of the most common causes of zoonotic disease reported worldwide, was once consider high in countries such as Argentina, Peru, Iran, Laos, Spain, Malta, and Italy,[23] but the implementation of control measures in developing countries have led to some success but remains of concern.[24] Of the viruses, in the last 10 years, the rates of reported norovirus and rotavirus outbreaks have become very common, particularly seasonally (autumn/winter) with common sources being food, water, and associated outbreak due to dissemination by infected patients (eg, due to vomitus and diarrhea).[8,25,26] Tables 56.2, 56.3, and 56.4 present lists of specific food- and waterborne microorganisms

TABLE 56.2 Food- and water-infective bacteria[a]

Produce Toxins in Food
Bacillus cereus
Clostridium botulinum
Escherichia coli
Staphylococcus aureus
Produce Infection
Aeromonas hydrophila
Brucella abortus, Brucella suis, Brucella melitensis
Campylobacter jejuni, Campylobacter coli, Campylobacter fetus
Clostridium botulinum
Clostridium perfringens
Escherichia coli
Klebsiella pneumoniae
Legionella pneumophila
Listeria monocytogenes
Mycobacterium bovis
Plesiomonas shigelloides
Salmonella species
Shigella sonnei, Shigella dysenteriae, Shigella flexneri
Streptococcus pyogenes (Group A)
Vibrio cholerae, Vibrio mimicus, Vibrio vulnificus, Vibrio parahaemolyticus
Yersinia enterocolitica, Yersinia pseudotuberculosis

[a]From Madden et al.[27]

TABLE 56.3 Food- and water-infective viruses[a]
Adenoviruses
Astroviruses
Caliciviruses, noroviruses (or Norwalk viruses)
Coronaviruses
Cytomegaloviruses
Enteroviruses: coxsackie, ECHO, polio, and hepatitis A
Hepatitis E virus
Norwalk-like viruses
Papovaviruses
Parvoviruses
Rotaviruses

Abbreviation: ECHO, enteric cytopathogenic human orphan.

[a]From European Food Safety Authority.[28]

pertaining to bacteria, viruses, and parasites, respectively. Each of these classes of microbes includes several genera and species of infective agents. Mention should be made that there are more than 45 types of parasites, and a number of toxin-producing fungi and algae that should also be considered as concerning food- and water-infective microorganisms. Harmful algal blooms in water bodies (and associated drinking water contamination with cyanobacterial toxins) have been associated with human, fish, and animal toxicity, such as in the Great Lakes in the United States.[29] Parasitic infections are endemic and widespread in developing countries, with pathogens such as *Cryptosporidium* and *Giardia* frequently associated with outbreaks.[30-32]

In many countries, different patterns of food- and waterborne infections are often considered as "emerging" because of previously little-noticed or newly discovered pathogens.[33] The increasing incidence of many of these pathogens becomes more evident in developed countries because our mechanisms of diagnosis and detection have improved and in the era of modern infection prevention strategies or controls leading to the declining incidence of previously recognized pathogens and emergence of new pathogens. Examples may include the following:

- Antibiotic-resistant bacteria including various strains of carbapenem-resistant Enterobacteriaceae, including *Klebsiella*, *E coli*, and *Pseudomonas* species that are associated with a high mortality rate[34]
- Bacterial pathogens with newly identified virulence factors, such as Shiga toxin-producing *E coli* O157: H7[35]
- Viral pathogens, such as rotaviruses and noroviruses.[8,25,26] Further examples include other nonenveloped viruses such as sapovirus, adenoviruses, coxsackievirus, mamastrovirus, and torovirus.[36]

- Transmissible spongiform encephalopathies (TSEs), particularly scrapie, bovine spongiform encephalopathy (BSE), and chronic wasting disease (CWD) (see chapter 68)[37,38]
- Sources of even low levels of fungal and algal toxins that have been linked to acute and chronic health effects[39,40]

Many previously recognized pathogens, such as *Staphylococcus aureus*, *E histolytica*, *Shigella*, and *Cryptosporidium* species are also often included as the emerging pathogens because they either maintain a significant incidence or are sporadically encountered even in developed countries. Therefore, at present, the term *emerging* should be assigned to the incidence of the pathogens under apparently improved sanitary conditions or have been newly identified. These are further considered in the next section.

RECOGNITION OF EMERGING PATHOGENS

Numerous related or unrelated factors have been responsible for the recognition of emerging pathogens. An emerging pathogen may be a new agent, a pathogen jumping the species barrier, a reemerging or reappearing known pathogenic agent of the past, or a pathogen showing a sudden and noteworthy increase in otherwise uneventful or low incidence of infection. Some of the pathogens, such as *Legionella pneumophila*, rotavirus, or noroviruses (often referred to as Norwalk or Norwalk-like agents), are relatively newer examples, whereas others, such as *Giardia lamblia*, have been known for centuries. The increased detection of psychrotrophic *Listeria monocytogenes* or *Yersinia enterocolitica* could be linked to certain practices in the modern food industry, such as longer storage of products at refrigeration temperature. Emergence of *L pneumophila* and atypical *Mycobacterium* species (eg, *Mycobacterium chelonae*, *Mycobacterium avium*, and *Mycobacterium chimaera*) have been associated with piped cold- and hot-water systems. Higher incidences of latent and otherwise uneventful infections, such as with the parasites *Isospora belli*, *Cryptosporidium* species, or *Sarcocystis* species have been associated with the increased population of immunocompromised persons in health care systems worldwide (eg, during cancer chemotherapy or associated with viral infections such as AIDS). Regardless of the factors associated with recognition of the emerging pathogens, their emergence has been marked by outbreaks that are often cited in the popular media. Outbreaks associated with food contamination or cross-contamination are frequent examples. Although improvement have been made to reduce the risks of waterborne outbreaks due to better standards and guidance to control chemical and microbiological quality worldwide,[41] outbreaks are still commonly reported.

TABLE 56.4   Common food- and water-infective protozoa and helminths

Source	Agent	Comments
Amoeba		
Fecal contamination of food and water	*Entamoeba histolytica*	Human pathogen; incubation period is variable, from a few days to several weeks. Invasion of colonic tissue results in acute diarrhea, abdominal pain, and bloody mucoid stools. Complication of lung, brain, or liver in severe cases
Recreational water (swimming)	*Naegleria fowleri*	Free living; found in soil, fresh water, sewage, and sludge; more common in lakes used for cooling water; causes amebic meningoencephalitis
Recreational water (swimming)	*Acanthamoeba culbertsoni, Acanthamoeba castellanii, Acanthamoeba polyphaga, Acanthamoeba astronyx*	Free living; found in soil, fresh water, brackish water, and sea water; causes chronic granulomatous amebic encephalitis that may be fatal. May cause eye infections, immunocompromised individuals may get infection by inhalation of cysts from soil
Flagellates		
Community water and raw vegetables	*Giardia lamblia*	Both warm- and cold-blooded animals serve as carriers; does not multiply outside the body Causes diarrhea, flatulence, cramps, nausea, anorexia, and fatigue and acute and chronic infection in asymptomatic persons
Oral-fecal contamination of food and water	*Dientamoeba fragilis*	Flagellate without flagella and cyst form. Infection is associated with *Enterobius* (pinworm infection). Probably uses *Enterobius* eggs to bypass stomach acidity. Illness results in diarrhea, nausea, and vomiting.
Ciliates		
Food and water contaminated with pig feces	*Balantidium coli*	More common in tropics; largest protozoan parasite. Both cyst and trophozoite. Symptoms include nausea, vomiting, and watery diarrhea. Both acute and chronic infections and colonic ulcers are observed.
Coccidia		
Fecal contamination of food and water by carnivorous host	*Isospora belli*	Inhabits mucosa of small intestine. Intracellular parasite; can produce severe intestinal disease with diarrhea, nausea, and fever. Disease may persist for months or years. Fatal in immunocompromised persons
Fecal contamination of food and water	*Cryptosporidium parvum*	Infects brush border of intestinal epithelium, infects other organs in immunocompromised individuals; causes profuse and watery diarrhea, epigastric pain, and nausea that is prolonged in immunocompromised persons
Fecal contamination of food and water	*Cyclospora cayetanensis*	Watery diarrhea, mild-to-severe nausea, anorexia, abdominal cramping, fatigue, and weight loss; diarrhea can be intermittent and protracted. Persons with no previous immunity and very young children are likely to exhibit symptoms.
Fecal contamination of food water	*Sarcocystis hominis, Sarcocystis suihominis*	Intestinal mucosa as the primary site of infection
Fecal contamination of cats and undercooked meat of intermediate hosts	*Toxoplasma gondii*	Causes acute and chronic infections; disease may resemble mononucleosis. Congenital infection may involve CNS and ocular abnormalities and may be fatal. Reactivated in immunocompromised individuals, resulting in encephalitis, pneumonitis, and myocarditis. Cats serve as primary host. Frequency of infection can be as high as 80% in regions of France to as low as 1% in the United States.

TABLE 56.4 Common food- and water-infective protozoa and helminths *(Continued)*

Source	Agent	Comments
Helminths	Nematodes (tissue)	
Undercooked raw pork, bear meat	*Trichinella spiralis*	Develop in mucosa of small intestine. Nonspecific gastroenteritis, fever eosinophilia, and myositis
Ingestion of animal livers or food contaminated with eggs from soil	*Capillaria hepatica*	Develops in liver parenchyma
Food contaminated with dog feces	*Toxocara canis*	Hyper-eosinophilia, hepatomegaly, fever, and pneumonitis
Consumption of raw fish dishes: sushi, sashimi, and ceviche	*Anisakis* species	Anisakiasis, abdominal pain, vomiting, eosinophilic granuloma
	Phocanema species	
	Terranova species	
Raw or undercooked shrimp, crabs, large edible snails; improperly washed lettuce, fruits, and strawberries	*Angiostrongylus cantonensis*	Lungworms inhabiting pulmonary artery of rats and passed on to slugs and snails. Causes human eosinophilic meningitis or meningoencephalitis. Observed in Hawaii, Thailand, Indonesia, and other southeast Asian countries and Cuba. Worms migrate to brain, spinal cord, and eye, giving prolonged severe headache and other CNS complications.
Nematodes (intestinal)		
Fecal contamination of food and water	*Enterobius vermicularis*	Infections associated with gastrointestinal tract. Human pinworm. Primarily infects children; eggs survive for prolonged periods in feces.
	Ascaris lumbricoides	Human large roundworm found in cecum
	Trichuris trichiura	Human whipworm common in moist, warm regions
Raw and poorly cooked fish	*Capillaria philippinensis*	Parasite of fish-eating birds and fish. Common in Philippines, Thailand, and areas around South China Sea
Cestodes (tissue)		
Poorly cooked fish or the use of frog and snake poultices	*Spirometra mansoni*	Parasites of cats, dogs, wild canids, and wild felids; common in China, Japan, Korea, and Vietnam
	Spirometra mansonoides	Common in United States
Food contaminated by dog feces	*Taenia multiceps*	Parasite of dogs, cats, and fishes. Human infection through dog feces
Consumption of undercooked meat	*Echinococcus granulosis*	Domestic and wild canids as primary host. Common in sheep and cattle raising areas.
		Forms hydatid cysts and CNS complications
	Echinococcus multilocularis	Develops invasive cysts in liver. Common in Europe, Japan, North and South America, Australia, and New Zealand
	Echinococcus vogeli	Primarily found in Latin America. Bush dogs and large rodents are primary hosts. Develops invasive cysts in liver
Cestodes (intestinal)		
Undercooked fish	*Diphyllobothrium latum*	Fish tapeworm found in cold, clear lakes of United States, Canada, Russia, Japan, and Europe
Beef	*Taenia saginata*	Cattle tapeworm
Pork	*Taenia solium*	Pig tapeworm. Most prevalent in Latin America, India, China, Africa, and Europe. Can cause severe CNS and eye infections

(continued)

TABLE 56.4 Common food- and water-infective protozoa and helminths *(Continued)*

Source	Agent	Comments
Grains and cereals	*Hymenolepis nana*	Mice are primary host; grains- and cereal-infecting beetles are secondary host.
Food contaminated with dog and cat feces	*Dipylidium caninum*	Dogs and cats are primary hosts; children are most susceptible.
Trematodes		
Consumption of under-cooked water vegetables like water chestnut and water caltrop and watercress	*Fasciolopsis buski*	Largest and most pathogenic intestinal fluke. Common in China, India, Indonesia, Thailand, Taiwan, and Vietnam
Water vegetables such as watercress	*Fasciola hepatica*	Worldwide occurrence
Undercooked and pickled fish	*Clonorchis sinensis*	Parasite found in bile duct of humans, cats, and dogs
Poorly cooked crustaceans	*Paragonimus westermani*	Parasite of dogs, cats, and wild animals

Abbreviation: CNS, central nervous system.

Noteworthy Outbreaks and Events

G lamblia is probably one of the earliest recognized pathogens, discovered or observed by Antonie van Leeuwenhoek in 1681.[42] It was recognized as an important pathogen during one of the largest laboratory-confirmed outbreaks in Rome, New York, during 1974 through 1975, with an estimated 4000 to 5000 cases.[43] In the United States alone, giardiasis continues to be one of the leading causes of human enteric disease. *G intestinalis* is now estimated to cause approximately 1.2 million reported cases of infection, with an estimated number of 242 reported outbreaks associated with at least 41 000 people affected and about 3581 hospitalizations yearly.[44] The infectious dose is considered low, at an estimated level of 10 cysts, noting than an infected individual can release billions of cysts per day and over many months of active and latent infection. The dormant, or cyst forms have known higher resistance levels to inactivation by chemical disinfectants (see chapter 3, including chlorine concentrations traditionally used for water disinfection; see chapter 37) and are therefore more robust under environmental conditions. Reports in outbreaks, which may be due to improvement in diagnosis and reporting in the United States, had actively increased from 1996 to 2001 but since that time have been stable or even decreased. The majority (approximately 75%) of these outbreaks were sources to contaminated drinking water, with the remaining sources being from recreational water (approximately 16%) and zoonotic or human-to-human transmission particularly through food. A greater emphasis on preventative measures, such as filtration or different chemical disinfection applications to control drinking water and as emphasis on good hygiene practices on handling of animals and food clearly have an impact of reducing the potential for outbreaks. But it may be suggested that

the emphasis in recent years has turned to another protozoal source of outbreaks, *Cryptosporidium* species. From 2009 to 2017, again in the United States, active surveillance and reporting had identified over 444 outbreaks of infection, with an estimated impact on at least 7465; overall, it was estimated during this time to have been a 135 increase per year of outbreaks.[30] The source of the outbreaks in most of these cases was due to recreational water, but cases associated with human-to-human and zoonotic transmission have also been reported and similar to *Giardia* outbreak cases. Large outbreaks have also been reported in drinking water,[45] highlighting limitations in chemical and filtration disinfection practices due to the lack of controls and tolerance of *Cryptosporidium* oocysts that are even more resistant to chemical inactivation compared to investigations with *Giardia* cysts.[46,47] The rates of such protozoal infections are likely to be higher in other parts of the world but are often not reported or investigated. There is also a risk in many of these cases that protozoa may be the source of other bacterial and viral infection associated with water and food contamination due to the ability of many protozoa to maintain or even allow the active growth of other pathogens within their vegetative and dormant forms of their respective life cycles (see chapter 3).[48]

There continues to be attention on various gram-negative bacteria associated with water- and foodborne outbreaks, such as those associated with *Salmonella* species such as *Salmonella enteritidis* and *S* Typhi that were probably some of the earliest bacteria identified to be associated with foodborne infections.[49,50] The importance of these and other nontyphoidal salmonellae even in the countries with well-established controls was realized after the largest milk-borne outbreak of *S* Typhi in Illinois, United States, in 1985 resulted in 16 000 cases.[51] Other larger outbreaks include a toasted oatmeal cereal product was an unlikely source of multistate outbreaks of *Salmonella agona* infections, with 209 cases in 11 states in the United States,[52] and with *Salmonella* species infections linked to backyard poultry in 768 people (approximately 30% hospitalized and two deaths) across 48 states.[53]

The most prominent causes of bacterial gastrointestinal infections in the United States is still considered to be *Campylobacter jejuni*, with an estimated 1.3 million illnesses each year in the United States.[54] These are often associated with contamination poultry, water, or other products such as unpasteurized milk. The magnitude of these infections was realized only after improved isolation procedures were developed during the early 1980s[55] and now including part or whole genome sequencing.[56] *Y enterocolitica* was recognized as an emerging pathogen after an epidemic in New York state, which was marked by several unnecessary appendectomies[57] and a multistate outbreak in Arkansas, Tennessee, and Mississippi that involved several thousand cases.[58] *Y enterocolitica* and other species are frequently linked to pigs and other environmental sources.[59,60] The pathogenic potential of the gram-positive bacteria *L monocytogenes* was initially observed after the epidemics in Germany,[61] Canada,[62] and the United States.[63] In 1998, several cases of illnesses caused by a strain of *L monocytogenes*, serotype 4b, were reported in 11 states, associated with the consumption of hot dogs and deli meat.[64] Some of these epidemics involved several hundred cases and were marked by high mortality rates linked to contaminated foods, with recent examples including from salads[65] and apples.[6] The widespread nature of *Vibrio parahaemolyticus* infection became evident after its first isolation in Japan in 1950.[66] The pathogen accounted for 40% to 50% of bacterial gastroenteritis cases in Japan[67] and is commonly associated with the consumption of seafood.[68,69] *C perfringens*, long known to be the causative agent of gas gangrene, was associated with food poisoning during the early 1960s.[70] The ability of this bacterium to survive in food due to spore formation and subsequently sporulate in the intestines results in poisoning from the production of various toxins.[71] *C perfringens* infections are in the top three causes of bacterial foodborne illness, along with *Salmonella* and *Campylobacter* species in the United States.[72] Similar spore-forming bacteria such as *C botulinum* (types A, B, and E) have been known as the classic toxin-producing bacterium in canned foods.[73] They can produce various neurotoxins (8 types, designated A-H) that can enter the body following digestion, but it is known that the toxins can be neutralized by heat treatment (eg, at 85°C for 5 min). During the 1960s, the ability of different *C botulinum* strains to grow and produce toxin under refrigeration conditions was recognized.[74] In addition to direct ingestion of the toxin, the bacterium also can multiply in the gastrointestinal tract and activity product toxin overtime. Outbreaks are most often associated with canned foods,[75] but others have included contaminated honey

in infants.[76,77] This pathogen has also been incriminated in botulism attributed to contaminated rainwater in rural Australia.[78] *Aeromonas hydrophila* was first described as an enteropathogen in 1955,[79] and since then, it has been associated with gastrointestinal infections.[80,81] Its ubiquitous nature and enhanced virulence for immunocompromised persons make it an important member of the emerging pathogens both in food and water sources.[81]

E coli was previously considered as a nonpathogenic inhabitant of the human and animal intestine; however, pathogenic strains were found to account for the largest number of diarrheal infections in developing countries and in the young associated with contaminated food or water.[82,83] In many cases, *E coli* strains can be harmless or may cause mild disease associated with short-lived diarrhea, but some strains can lead to more severe cases of disease associated with toxin production including vomiting, abdominal pain, and severe diarrhea. Virulent strains can also lead to other complications such as urinary tract and bloodstream infections.[83,84] A particularly virulent strain, referred to as coli-hemorrhagic or Shiga toxin-producing *E coli* O157:H7 (STEC), was isolated during rapidly spreading outbreaks of hemorrhagic colitis in Canada[85] and in the United States.[86,87] Since that time, a variety of pathogenic *E coli* and their virulence determinants have been described.[83] These have been classified into different pathotypes such as enteropathogenic, STEC (including enterohemorrhagic strains), enteroinvasive, enteroaggregative, diffusely adherent, enterotoxigenic, adherent invasive *E coli*. The presence of various virulent factors includes toxins, adhesins, and invasins in these and other *E coli* strains are further exasperated by the increasing development of multiantibiotic-resistant strains; antibiotic resistance has been well described with antibiotics that have been traditionally used for many years in humans and animals (eg, penicillin and ampicillin), but in more recent years, there has been an alarming increase in reports of multidrug resistance to include newer antibiotics such as cephalosporins and fluoroquinolones.[83,84] Environmental detection of and outbreaks with these strains are frequently reported and often due to their difficulty in treating patients and persistence of the infection leading to greater rates of morbidity and mortality.[88-90] Most of these virulent factors, including antibiotic-resistant genes, are associated with mobile genetic elements such as transposons and plasmids. These are of further concern because they can be transferred from one strain to another and even between different gram-negative bacteria species. The impact of this can be highlighted by the growing incident rates of the detection of carbapenem-resistant strains of Enterobacteriaceae, such as in *Klebsiella*, *Pseudomonas*, and *E coli*.[91] The rates of infection with these pathogens in patients that are immunocompromised (eg, health care–acquired infections) is a major threat given that treatment options in these patients are limited. Many of these outbreaks are associated with water sources, such as from sinks and drains,[92,93] as well as associated with food contamination.[90,94]

L pneumophila is an example of fairly recent member of the emerging pathogens from water sources. Numerous outbreaks of infections of *L pneumophila* since 1977 give testimony to its virulence potential and the link to various water sources.[95,96] The initial discovery of *L pneumophila* in an outbreak of respiratory illness associated with the American Legion convention in Philadelphia was unusual and widely publicized.[97] The etiologic agent turned out to be a gram-negative bacterium, not a rickettsia-like agent as indicated by isolation procedures and the nature of illness. Since then, *L pneumophila* was found to have been associated with past outbreaks of unknown cause[98] and often found to be persistent in water systems despite remediation (including waterline disinfection) attempts.[96]

Increasing reports of outbreaks due to atypical mycobacteria have been linked to the persistence of many of these strains in water sources and, in some cases, unusual tolerance profiles to disinfectants. These infections are often difficult to treat due to the intrinsic (or acquired) resistance to antibiotics in these isolates. Examples include outbreaks (or pseudo-outbreaks) associated with ice machines (*Mycobacterium fortuitum*[99]), *M chimaera* infections following cardiac surgery and sources to heater-cooler units,[100] *Mycobacterium massiliense* outbreaks associated with resistance to aldehyde-based disinfectants, antibiotic resistance and increased virulence,[101,102] *M avium* outbreak from contaminated pork meat.[103] Atypical (or nontuberculous) mycobacteria are found to be ubiquitous in the environment and widely detected in water sources, although they do require specific attention to culturing methods (media, growth temperatures, and extended incubation times) to allow for their detection. Interestingly, the ability of bacteria such as *Legionella* and mycobacteria to enter and survive within protozoa is used a method to detect fastidious strains (using protozoa essentially as a cell culture method) and as a mechanism of resistance (or persistence) to water disinfection due to their survival in the dormant (cyst/oocyst) forms of these microorganisms (see chapter 3).[104]

Overall, many outbreaks associated with food and water will be further exasperated by our ability to travel more widely and rapidly than in previous times. Examples include the speed at which strains of bacteria or viruses can transfer from one, isolated area of the world to other. Probably the most noteworthy example of this in recent years is the Spanish flu that peaked in 1918-1919.[105] Although it is unsure where exactly the source of the outbreak was, in recent years, the H1N1 virus was found to have genes of avian origin. Estimates of infection rates was approximately 500 million people, which at the time was about one-third of the world's population, and about one-tenth of those infected died (although it is generally believed that many died due to complications of virus infection, such as secondary bacterial infections). Recent cases

or concerns on pandemics include severe acute respiratory syndrome, Middle East respiratory syndrome, viral hemorrhagic fevers (eg, Ebola or Marburg viruses), and antibiotic-resistant bacteria. Food and water sources, as well as being mechanisms of transmission, will continue to be of concern.[106]

It is clear that a wider range of infection or outbreaks can occur in individuals or groups that are immune or otherwise compromised, as highlighted earlier in hospitalized patients. This will include populations that are younger, older, or with underlying infections that affect the immune system (such as acquired immunodeficiency syndrome [AIDS]) or open the body to a greater risk of infection (eg, during surgery or in damaged skin; see chapters 43 and 44) or following cancer therapy. In may be that as we see increases in populations (especially those concentrated in urban areas), longevity, obesity or poor eating habits, use of more common or invasive medical treatment, and different types of pharmaceutical treatment (eg, depression of the immune system in case of psoriasis or inflammatory bowel disease), that we will continue to identify unique or emerging pathogens. Earlier examples include *M avium* serovars that had caused enteritis, bacteremia, or granulomata in the liver and bone marrow in patients with AIDS.[106] A large percentage of these population (20%-80%) were found to be infected by *Toxoplasma gondii* through fecal contamination or by consumption of undercooked meat.[107] This normally uneventful infection is reactivated in AIDS or transplantation patients to give rise to encephalitis, pneumonitis, and myocarditis. Similarly, *I belli*, *Sarcocystis* species, and *Cryptosporidium* species are known to cause severe and often fatal infections in immunocompromised persons.[108] Large outbreaks of protozoan infections in healthy population resulted from the survival of *Cryptosporidium* cysts in chlorinated water. One massive outbreak of *Cryptosporidium* infection originated from contaminated municipal water supply in Wisconsin and another from recreational water fountain in Minnesota.[45,109] Cyclosporiasis outbreaks are frequently reported due to contaminated foods such with the consumption of raspberries and snap peas imported to the United States and Canada.[110-112] Approximately 370 clinically defined cases of cyclosporiasis were reported from eight states (California, Florida, Maryland, Nebraska, Nevada, New York, Rhode Island, and Texas) and one province in Canada (Ontario). In addition, approximately 220 clinically defined cases were reported among persons on a cruise ship that departed from Florida. *Microsporidia* and *Blastocystis* are further intestinal protozoa associated with infections in the immunocompromised.[113] Other bacterial and protozoal pathogens associated with food and waterborne outbreaks emerge from time to time as summarized in Tables 56.1, 56.2, and 56.4, but as diagnostic methods have and continue to improve, it is likely that further emerging pathogens will continue to be identified in outbreaks.

As highlighted earlier, many types of viruses are associated such as hepatitis A and emerging pathogens including hepatitis E, sapovirus, adenoviruses, coxsackievirus, mamastrovirus, and torovirus (see Table 56.3).[36] But special consideration is given to rotavirus and norovirus as recent leading causes of viral outbreaks.[8,25,26] Rotaviruses are one of the leading causes of diarrheal diseases in the United States. The most common species associated with infection is rotavirus A, but there are at least 8 other species that can infect humans, animals, and birds (norovirus B to I). Infection is usually associated with severe diarrhea, vomiting, and abdominal pain. In the past, infection was often associated with severe illness and high rates of death, but overall, these rates have been reduced with prevention methods (vaccination) and management of disease (eg, oral rehydration therapy). These viruses have been recognized as a major cause of viral diarrhea in infants and young children, acquired by the fecal-oral route. Outbreaks associated with food[114,115] and water[10,116] are now frequently reported in both children and adults. Noroviruses (Norwalk or Norwalk-like viruses), which are also small, nonenveloped viruses, are now the more prevalent causes of gastroenteritis associated with food and water contamination in the United States and other countries.[10,117] In the United States alone, out of 31 major pathogens, norovirus was the top cause of illness at 58%, followed by major bacterial sources such as *Salmonella* (11%), *Clostridium* (10%), and *Campylobacter* (9%); however, *Salmonella* remained the leading cause of death (at 28%) and norovirus was at 11%.[72] In 1989 a major outbreak of 900 cases of gastroenteritis was reported in north central Arizona traced to contaminated well water.[118] Outbreaks are now frequently reported with food,[119,120] often associated with nonsymptomatic food handlers, and with water (including ice).[121,122] It is interesting to note, in a review of drinking water-associated outbreaks during 2000 and 2014 affecting large numbers of consumers, that norovirus and rotavirus, as well as the protozoal pathogens *Cryptosporidium* and *Giardia* species, were prevalent and that these pathogens are associated with higher levels of resistance to disinfection and water preservation methods (see chapter 3).[123]

Finally, one of the most notable causes of foodborne disease has to be the transmission of BSE (commonly known as mad cow disease) in cattle and the association to a variant form of Creutzfeldt-Jakob disease (vCJD) in humans. These diseases are examples of TSEs or generally known as prion diseases. These are progressive, neurodegenerative diseases that are associated with the deterioration of mental and physical effects in humans and animals and culminate in death. Although the incubation times can be long, once these effects are diagnosed the progression of the disease can be rapid, with patients dying within a year. Prions are unique as both infectious and transmissible agents because they are proposed to be composed exclusively of proteins (see chapter 3 and 68).[124] The protein associated with these diseases is known as PrP (in its

normal form, PrP[c]), a glycoprotein associated with the cell membrane of human/animal cells including the neurons as various neural tissues such as the brain and spinal cord. The exact function of the protein in normal cells is not known but is known to be associated with functions such as copper trafficking and/or oxidative stress.[125] But during the disease progression, the secondary/tertiary structure of PrP[c] is converted to an abnormal, protease-resistant form of the protein (PrP[res]). This form cannot be fully degraded by normal cellular processes and therefore accumulates to eventually lead to cell death and transmission to other neighboring cells. As the disease progresses, further neurons are destroyed, and this eventually leads to the interruption of normal neural tissue structure and function that eventually culminates in death. Prion diseases are generally rare diseases in humans (eg, the classic form of CJD being the most prevalent at rates approximately 1.4 cases in a million population worldwide),[124] although some animal forms of these diseases are considered more prevalent (eg, the rates of scrapie in sheep is difficult to estimate but has been reported to be as low as 0.3% and as high at 35%).[126] But the sudden outbreak of BSE in the United Kingdom (and to a less extent in some other countries such as Ireland, France, and Switzerland) was associated with the disease in approximately 200 000 confirmed cases, that was first identified in the United Kingdom in 1986, peaked in 1991-1993, and has subsequently declined but are still reported yearly.[127] It is considered that the outbreak was sourced from the contamination (that was speculated to have been sourced from sheep with scrapie) of meat and bone meal that had been rendered (by grinding and heat treatment) of waste meat and bone from animals.[128] This outbreak was further exasperated by the emergence of a new form of CJD (variant or vCJD) that occurred in humans at the same time, which has been linked to the consumption of contaminated meat.[129,130] By 2019, 178 deaths (peaking at 28 in 2000) from vCJD have been confirmed as being likely caused during the outbreak in the United Kingdom alone, with cases being reported in other countries such as in France, Ireland, United States, and Spain.[131] No new cases had been identified in the United Kingdom since 2016 (when one case was reported), but there remains much speculation about the potential for a further wave of cases in the future.[132] In addition to BSE and vCJD, there remains much speculation about the potential of transmission of other TSEs, particularly scrapie and CWD. In the United States, for example, CWD is a concern in deer and elk populations, but there is a continued debate on the transmissibility of this disease to humans by contaminated meat.[133]

A whole new spectrum of emerging pathogens ranging from viruses to protozoa and prions has been observed during foodborne and waterborne outbreaks of infections. The emergence of new infectious diseases has been associated with changes taking place during human evolution. Multiple, sometimes similar, factors were responsible for these outbreaks, but greater diagnostic methods and attention to investigating and reporting such outbreaks will continue to highlight the risks of food- and waterborne infections.

Causative and Recognition Factors of Outbreaks Caused by Emerging Pathogens

Awareness of Inadequacy of Legislative Guidelines on Sanitation in the Food Industry

Automation of large-scale food-processing facilities has resulted in the reduction of contamination of food as a result of manual handling. The practices of pasteurization and refrigeration and the use of disinfectant (sanitizers) during processing, transportation, and storage have increased shelf life and improved organoleptic properties of food products. Early legislative guidelines on sanitation were directed toward control of infections caused by previously recognized pathogens. These measures also resulted indirectly in the production of desired organoleptic quality of food through the control of mesophilic spoilage and pathogenic microorganisms. Thus, desired organoleptic properties and microbiological safety became synonymous in the food industry; the microbiological aspect apparently became secondary as long as the organoleptic quality of food product was maintained. This brought about certain degree of consumer complacency with regard to safe handling of food and other food safety precautions. The practice of using outdated but organoleptically acceptable pasteurized milk that had been returned from supermarket shelves for the preparation of ice cream and other frozen dairy products presented an underlying danger of contamination by psychrotrophic pathogens such as L monocytogenes. The ability of L monocytogenes to multiply at refrigeration temperatures in stored dairy products, hot dogs, and delicatessen meats resulted in large outbreaks of infection.[63,64] Listeria is also found to be ubiquitous in the environment and persist in food processing environments.[134] Factors such as the operation of the processing facilities for extended periods, poor sanitation of hard-to-reach dead spaces (eg, in water or product pipelines), and difficult-to-clean intricate mechanical parts (eg, fillers) may result in an ill-defined loss of microbiologic quality. Mechanical parts also result in cross-contamination with pathogens. Defeathering rubber fingers were found to spread C jejuni in poultry processing plants.[135] Similarly, Salmonella species were spread by cross-contamination in a cattle-slaughtering plant.[136] Overall attention to process design, sanitization practices, and environmental monitoring are all important to control Listeria as well as other bacterial pathogens.[137]

Production of larger quantities of food requires pooling of small batches, such as in the comingling of milk.

Thus, a single contaminated source can spread pathogens to the bulk quantity. Past legislative guidelines for monitoring pathogens in these situations were not often adequate or are difficult to implement because of a lack of time, techniques, economic resources, or some other factors.[138] Increasing incidence of foodborne and waterborne infections and exposure in the mass media resulted in awareness and acknowledgment of the importance of legislative guidelines to implement safety procedures for food and water. This awareness was followed by many governments to introduce food safety initiatives, such as in the United States with the US Food and Drug Administration Food Safety Modernization Act both for the food sourced from the United States or imported.[139] Implementation of new initiatives and guidelines certainly will help to reduce the future incidence of emerging infections. For example, in the case of BSE, similar initiatives worldwide have probably helped to halt the risk of transmission of infection by preventing recycling of ruminant food animal parts as an animal feed additive.[140]

Age, Packaging, and Distribution

Compromise, abuse, or ignorance of the temperature factor in food storage can lead to growth of pathogens in food. Storage temperature a few degrees above 4°C to 5°C can permit the growth of many pathogens such as L monocytogenes, Y enterocolitica, A hydrophila, C botulinum, Salmonella species, S aureus, C perfringens, Bacillus cereus, and V parahaemolyticus.[141-143] Many of these pathogens, such as Listeria, Yersinia, and Aeromonas species, can grow even at proper refrigeration temperatures.[141] A hydrophila increased from 10^3 to 10^8/mL in 14 days at 4°C,[144] and the generation time of L monocytogenes in dairy food was reported to be 1.2 to 1.7 days at 4°C.[145] With better transportation facilities, food processed in a single plant has been distributed to larger sections of population over wide geographic areas. Large outbreaks of salmonellosis, listeriosis, and yersiniosis have been traced to single food-processing facilities.[52,58,63,146,147] This can include many cases of international outbreaks, such as with brie cheese produced in one factory in France caused outbreaks of E coli-associated illness in multiple states in the United States.[148]

The center of hot food can remain at 50°F (approximately 10°C) for 24 hours even when stored in a refrigerator, thus resulting in optimal growth temperatures for some pathogens in contaminated food.[149] Pathogens can also survive on the surface of refrigerated packages, as potential sources of cross-contamination on handling and opening prior to food contact.[150] One of the largest epidemics of enteritis due to Y enterocolitica resulted from contamination of the external surfaces of fresh milk cartons. The cartons in turn were contaminated by milk crates previously used to transfer outdated products to a pig farm. The crates were contaminated by runoff from the pig pens during heavy rains.[151,152]

Increasing Number of Immunocompromised Individuals

As mentioned earlier, the population of immunocompromised persons appears to be increasing in the era of modern medicine. Less virulent and opportunistic microorganisms often produce severe illnesses in these persons, and virulent pathogens may cause fatal infections.[63,113,153,154] Some of the factors that cause immunosuppression are (1) human immunodeficiency virus infection; (2) inherited diseases; (3) aging; (4) premature birth; (5) radiation or chemotherapy treatment; (6) immunosuppressive treatment for transplantation, autoimmune disease, and malignancy; (7) malnutrition; (8) pregnancy; (9) severe trauma and burn; (10) other concurrent infections; and (11) malignancy.[113,155,156] Thus, increasing numbers of persons are becoming immunosuppressed and more susceptible to infections, including from water and food sources.

Use of Antibiotics and Drugs

The use of antibiotics, either in animal feed or for therapy, can alter the pattern of foodborne infections. Antibiotics in animal feed have been well-associated with emergence of drug-resistant strains in foodborne salmonellosis and other bacteria.[157,158] The use of antibiotics as growth promoters in food animals has led to the appearance of multidrug-resistant pathogenic strains.[158-160] Early examples include S Typhi strains, first associated with the consumption of beef, became an important emerging pathogen with broad spectrum to ampicillin, chloramphenicol, streptomycin, sulfonamides, and tetracycline, and poultry-associated quinolone-resistant C jejuni.

Therapeutic use of antibiotics, as well as other factors that can lead to intestinal dysbiosis such as stress and diet, are contributing factors to chronic diseases and appears to enhance the infectious process in persons undergoing treatment.[161] As an example, antibiotic-resistant Salmonella newport has been reported to cause serious illness among persons taking antimicrobials. Intestinal flora also may initiate infection when shifted out of balance during therapy. Clostridium difficile, a normal intestinal inhabitant and a common soil and water bacterium, is associated with diarrhea and pseudomembranous colitis, particularly in health care–acquired infections.[162] There has been an increase in reports of more aggressive C difficile infections and particularly in patient that are taking certain classes of antibiotics, such as clindamycin and fluoroquinolones.[163] As a spore-forming organism, it may be better able to survive the oral antibiotic treatments that will reduce other bacterial flora in the gut but also be able to spread and survive easier in the environment. But there has also been an increase in the antibiotic resistance profile of C difficile strains that will make infections harder to treat, thereby increasing morbidity

and mortality rates.[164] C difficile transmission, as well as other spore-forming pathogens, can be associated with lower oral infectious doses due to their innate resistance to the acidic stomach environment on ingestion. Gastric acidity (pH 2.5) is one of the natural defenses of the host against infection from food- and water-infective microorganisms.[165] Although oral infectious doses can be hard to quantify, there is a direct correlation between acid resistance and infectious dose. For example, the infectious dose of more acid-sensitive V cholerae is approximately 10^9 in comparison to lower doses of Salmonella species (10^5) and Shigella flexneri (10^2) being more acid tolerant, respectively.[166] Therefore, it may be expected that more resistant forms of microorganisms such as nonenveloped viruses (rotaviruses and noroviruses), bacterial spores, and protozoal (oo)cysts will be associated with lower infectious doses and therefore higher risks in food, water, and environmental transmission when present (see chapter 3). Earlier studies reported that illness-inducing oral doses of V cholerae ranged between 10^3 to 10^4 and 10^8 to 10^{11} cells under buffered and unbuffered conditions, respectively,[167] highlighting that not only the intrinsic resistance of the microorganism is important but also their association with various food sources. For example, Salmonella was shown to be protected from the effects of acidic inactivation when present in food with high protein and fats (eg, in egg whites), which may dramatically reduce the infection dose from the 10^5 range to as low as 10^1 to 10^2.[168] Equally, when L monocytogenes was exposed to mild acid treatment, it developed greater acid resistance and therefore virulence.[169] Despite this, normal stomach acid was reported to protect against infections due to L monocytogenes, whereas reduced gastric acid levels due to antacid and cimetidine therapy was associated with increased Listeria infections.[170,171] Reduced gastric acidity also enhanced pathogenesis in Salmonella infections.[172] These results indicated that altering gastric acidity by increasing use of antacids and other drugs may result in exposure to infections that otherwise could be naturally prevented. Thus, the widespread use of antibiotics and other drugs can alter the course of infection by foodborne and waterborne infective microorganisms.

Travel and Tourism

Movement of populations has been associated with the spread of infections since antiquity. Darius' campaigns against the Greeks (492 BC) and the British campaign in Gallipoli in 1915 over the same ground suffered because of food- and water-infective microorganisms.[173] Modern transportation facilities have increased the exposure of susceptible populations to foodborne and waterborne infections by many orders of magnitude. Tourism and increased traveling populations resulting from military movements, political refugees, pilgrimages, and international business bring exposure to foodborne and waterborne infective pathogens endemic in certain areas. It has been estimated that up to 70% of tourists traveling each year are likely to acquire traveler's diarrhea, depending on the destination.[174,175] Infections are predominantly identified as bacterial, with the most common pathogen being *E coli* but also *C jejuni*, *Salmonella* and *Shigella*, although this may be due to limitation in attempts to diagnose root cause due to other pathogens such as viruses and protozoa. *Giardia* is the most frequently identified protozoa in cases, and emerging pathogens have included *Aeromonas*, *Plesiomonas*, and *Bacteroides fragilis*, as well as viral pathogens discussed previously such as rotavirus and norovirus.[175]

Intercontinental travel or tourism often involves confinement in planes or cruise ships. Limitations of space, water, toilet facilities, mass catering, and improper storage temperatures can create hazardous conditions with respect to microbiologic safety. Food prepared in flight kitchens is often stored for prolonged periods at temperatures conducive for the growth of pathogens. *S aureus* and *Salmonella* species have been encountered in foodborne infection outbreaks on international flights.[176,177] Foodborne outbreaks of gastroenteritis caused by *Salmonella* species, enteropathogenic *E coli*, *V parahaemolyticus*, *Shigella* species, *Trichinella spiralis*, and *S aureus* have been reported on cruise ships.[176,178] Reports of viral (especially due to norovirus) outbreaks in these situations are also frequently reported,[179] including in the popular press. Travelers may acquire local culinary habits and consume raw food dishes such as sushi and sashimi, which are often more likely to be contaminated with pathogens than are cooked dishes.

Developments in Detection Methods

Newer and more sensitive detection methods have resulted in associating previously unknown or unsuspected pathogens with gastroenteritis outbreaks. Earlier, the use of new isolation media led to realization of the widespread nature of *C jejuni* infections.[180] Nonenveloped virus infections (eg, norovirus or Norwalk agent) were first associated with gastroenteritis through the use of electron microscopy.[181] Improvement in detection methods reduced the time required for the isolation and identification of *L monocytogenes*.[182] The application of fluorescent and immunofluorescent methods expedited identification of intestinal parasites.[183] Improvements in isolation of sublethally injured bacteria in processed food also resulted in increased frequency of isolating pathogens.[184] Further modern techniques, including molecular and immunologic identification, and direct visualization by endoscopy are now widely used and allow for the more rapid diagnosis of pathogens, which can impact the choice of optimal treatment including the use of antimicrobials.[185,186]

Role of Modern Communications Media

Instant communication through radio, television, and newspapers often has alarmed the general population about outbreaks of illness from foodborne and waterborne infective agents. Thus, modern communications media played an important role in educating people about the emergence of new pathogens. Public interest about illness caused by emerging pathogens such as *Salmonella*, *Campylobacter*, *Listeria*, and norovirus could be compared with that of agents of cholera and typhoid in the early 20th century.[187-189] But public interest in the impact of infection prevention practices, such as handwashing, environmental disinfection, quarantine of subjects with active infection, correct handling/cooking of food, vaccination, and boiling of drinking water in high-risk areas has also had an impact in reducing potential infections (see chapter 48).[190]

▶ FACTORS THAT INFLUENCE INFECTIONS THROUGH FOOD AND WATER

Contamination with, survival, and growth of pathogens in food and water primarily determine the course of the infectious process. Some of the factors that determine the survival and growth are pH, water activity, and resistance to antimicrobial processes (used for preservation, disinfection, and sterilization), temperature, osmotic pressure, and salt content as well as the ability of the pathogens to form resistant, dormant forms such as (oo)cysts or spores. These factors were discussed individually in great detail by others and have changed little since the previous version of this chapter.[191,192] Some other parameters that determine the probability of infection are the nature and source of food and water, processing and handling, association of the pathogens with particulate matter, soil (organic or inorganic), or sediment, and environmental interaction with other microorganisms. The number of infecting organisms is also an important factor in determining the infectious process. Some virulent pathogens can initiate infections in lower numbers, whereas others require much larger doses to cause illness (Table 56.5).[193-198] Host resistance also should be considered as an important aspect in determining the outcome of the infectious process. Evidence suggests that, besides immunologic heterogeneity of the human population, chemical composition of food can influence the infective dose by protective mechanisms and by increasing virulence due to stressful environments.[198,199] For example, high-lipid foods can encapsulate and protect pathogens from the lethal action of gastric acidity; the dispersing action of bile salts can subsequently release the encapsulated pathogens in the duodenum. In addition, stressful environments (such as in the presence of growth inhibitors

TABLE 56.5	Estimated number of pathogens associated with oral ingestion of foods suggested to produce illness[a,b]
Organism	**Number**
Bacillus cereus	>10^5/g of food
Campylobacter jejuni	5×10^2-10^6
Clostridium perfringens	10^6-10^9 or ≥10^5/g of food
Escherichia coli	10^6-10^{10}
E coli O157:H7	0.3-15/g of food
Giardia lamblia	10^1-10^2
Hepatitis virus	10^3
Norovirus (Norwalk)	10^1
Salmonella species	1-10^1
Shigella species	10^1-10^2
Staphylococcus aureus	≥10^5/g of food
Streptococcus faecalis	10^9-10^{10}
Vibrio cholerae	10^6-10^{11}
Vibrio parahaemolyticus	10^3-10^7 or ≥10^5/g of food
Yersinia enterocolitica	10^9

[a]From Bryan,[193] National Research Council,[194] Banwart,[195] Rendtorff,[196] Doyle et al,[197] and D'Aoust.[198]

[b]These estimates can vary depending on the contaminated food types, subject health, strain of microorganisms (and associated virulence factors), etc.

such as food pH or residual chlorine in water, high or low temperatures, etc) can lead to changes in bacterial/fungal gene expression to increase their tolerance to inactivation and survival, leading to changes in virulence factors such as bacterial adhesion, toxin or other chemical production, capsule production, etc.[199]

Nature and Source of Food and Water

The sources of water, food, and food products are often important factors in determining the type and number of infecting pathogens. In an earlier review of worldwide medical and engineering literature, it was concluded that disease such as typhoid fever, infectious hepatitis, fascioliasis, and cholera are more frequently associated by foods such as vegetables, fish, shrimp, and shellfish contaminated by sewage or irrigation water in agricultural or aquacultural practices.[200] Infected food and farm animals were particularly responsible for diseases such as tuberculosis, brucellosis, salmonellosis, and parasitic infection in developing countries.[177] Milk and associated products are common sources of pathogens and reported occurrence of emerging pathogens such as L monocytogenes,

Y enterocolitica, C jejuni, enteropathogenic E coli, and S Typhi in milk and milk products in the United States.[201] Poultry, eggs, and beef have been common sources of Campylobacter and Salmonella infections.[135,202] Water is a common source of gram-negative bacteria, as well as viruses and protozoa due to fecal contamination. Droppings by nocturnal roosting gulls in winter on a water storage reservoir, supplying water to Glasgow, Scotland, resulted in deterioration of water quality.[203] Contamination of water by bird feces corresponded with the appearance of E coli and salmonellae in untreated water and on three occasions in treated water samples. Outbreaks of norovirus are commonly reported due to cross-contamination from food handlers, presumably due to fecal carriers and in many cases from asymptomatic individuals[204,205]; these and similar bacterial outbreaks highlight the importance of simple hygiene practices in food preparation and handling, such as hand washing, lessons that have been learned many times over from modern epidemiology.[206] Thermal pollution of man-made lakes as well as that of rivers used for cooling electrical power plants has resulted in increased numbers of pathogenic Naegleria fowleri in water[207]; the use of water from these sources either for recreational or drinking purposes presents a danger of infection by N fowleri, which can cause fatal human primary amebic meningoencephalitis.

Processing and Handling

Food can become contaminated during processing and handling. The level of pathogens in contaminated food may increase, depending on processing and handling practices. In decreasing order of frequency, the first 10 most important factors that result in foodborne infections were improper cooling (44%), delay of 12 hours or longer between preparation and consumption of food (23%), food handlers as carriers of pathogens (18%), mixing of uncooked and cooked food or ingredients (16%), inadequate processing (16%), improper hot holding (14%), inadequate reheating (11%), unsafe sources (10%), cross-contamination (5%), and improper cleaning (5%).[148] These risks, most often associated with mistakes made during food handling, have not changed much over the years.[208]

For example, eight outbreaks of foodborne infections resulting from the consumption of meat and meat products were examined.[209] Undercooking, improper cooling of cooked food, unsanitary handling practices, ingestion of raw products, a delay of 24 hours or longer between preparation and consumption, food handlers as carriers of pathogens, and improper thawing of raw food were important factors that contributed to 46%, 34%, 16%, 15%, 13%, 12%, and 10% of outbreaks, respectively. The restaurants, care institutions, and small food businesses were most often the suspected locations in which food became contaminated.[210] Overall, the top five causes of foodborne infection outbreaks are as follows:

- Improper handling of higher risk foods at hot or cold temperatures
- Inadequate cooking temperatures/times
- Contamination from dirty equipment used in food preparation
- Hygiene or health concerns in food handlers
- Foods from higher risk or nonapproved sources

Interaction of Pathogens With Other Environmental Microorganisms

In some cases, the interaction between pathogens and nonpathogenic environmental microorganisms can determine the survival and virulence of pathogens in food and water. *Flavobacterium breve*, a common environmental water bacterium, probably supports the growth of *Legionella pneumophila* in sediments on taps, sinks, and other water distribution systems by providing L-cysteine to the fastidious pathogen.[211] Microorganisms interact more efficiently in sediments because of proximity to each other. The transfer of antibiotic resistance between *E coli* strains was shown in marine sediments[212] and subsequently for a wider range of Enterobacteriaceae in many other environmental sources such as in biofilms or microbiomes.[213,214] Protozoa present in the environment, particularly associated with water or biofilms, can support the growth of bacterial and viral pathogens. *L pneumophila* was found to multiply intracellularly in an amoeba and two ciliates,[215] a phenomenon that is now widely shown for many other types of pathogens that are associated with food/water outbreaks such as *E coli*, *Vibrio*, *Pseudomonas*, *Listeria*, *Shigella*, and *Campylobacter*.[104] On the other hand, brachiopods (marine invertebrates) removed *E coli* from a wastewater pond.[216]

Association of Pathogens With Sediment and Soil

Water-infective pathogens have been found concentrated on sediment particles, as compared with being found in the body of water. For example, the concentration of *V parahaemolyticus* was 436/100 g of sediment compared with 36/100 mL of seawater near Alexandria, Egypt.[217] Similarly, the concentration of enteroviruses in sediment was 10 times higher than that in water.[218] Compared with poliovirus I and ECHO virus 1, hepatitis A virus was less readily adsorbed to soils,[219] which probably explains in part the cause of some outbreaks of hepatitis A infections resulting from drinking groundwater.[220] Enteroviruses have been found at 67 m and up to an aquifer depth of 18 m from a subsurface leaching pool.[221] Various factors such as sediment type, pH, electric charge, and moisture content of the soil can determine adsorption of pathogens on the sediments.[222] Increased concentration of pathogens in the sediment accounted for increased risk of infection for young bathers in shallow waters of wading pools.[223]

Virulence Factors

Microbial toxins are important determinants of bacterial, fungal, and algal virulence. Some of the toxins produced by these organisms are presented in Tables 56.6, 56.7, and 56.8. Table 56.9 also gives a brief outline of the symptoms and illness caused by some important pathogens. Besides toxin production, the ability of food- and water-infective microorganisms to cause illness depends on their survival under the hostile conditions present in the gastrointestinal tract. Gastric acidity, digestive enzymes, bile salts, peristalsis, osmolarity, and high temperatures may inhibit some pathogens. Successful pathogens not only survive but even use the unfavorable environment to their advantage. The enteroviruses, *Giardia* cysts, and *Dientamoeba fragilis* all survive gastric acidity. *G lamblia* probably uses gastric acidity for triggering excystation into the trophozoite form for growth in the small intestine.[229] The trophozoite form of *D fragilis* apparently escapes gastric acidity by hiding inside *Enterobius* eggs.[108] *Helicobacter pylori* has been associated with peptic and other intestinal ulcers.[230,231] They resist gastric acidity by first burrowing into the stomach mucus lining, bind to epithelial cells, and a number of resistance mechanisms such as the production of urease to breakdown urea into ammonia that allows for local neutralization of acids around the bacteria.[232]

To colonize, the pathogens must be able to attach to a suitable site in the intestinal tract. Therefore, the ability to attach is also a virulence-determining factor, such as by the expression of adhesins.[233] The distribution of receptors to which pathogens attach on the host cells may influence tissue tropism and thus may determine the expression of certain virulence characteristics such as neurovirulence of poliovirus.[234] Studies of coxsackieviruses suggest that pathogens that exhibit a wider host range may show specificity to more than one receptor.[235] Parasites use physical processes for attachment, for example, ventral disc of *G lamblia*. Bacterial and viral pathogens attach by means of chemical moieties and adhesins to the receptor sites on the host cells. In the case of pathogenic *Y enterocolitica*, the adhesins are always expressed on the surface of the cells, whereas in *S* Typhi and *Salmonella choleraesuis*, they are induced by trypsin- and neuraminidase-sensitive structures on the epithelial cells.[233] In the case of *Vibrio* species, the pilus needed for attachment is synthesized in response to environmental signals such as pH, temperature, and osmolarity.[236]

Invasion of the host cells is an integral part of active pathogenesis. The pathogens are endocytosed and

TABLE 56.6	Examples of bacterial pathogens and their toxins	
Organism	**Toxin/Virulence Determinant**	**Comment/Effect/Activity**
Aeromonas hydrophila	Beta hemolysin	Cytotoxic activity
	Cytotonic enterotoxin	Intestinal fluid secretion
	Aerolysin	Attacks glycophorin; forms pore in cell membranes
	Invasive factors	
	Adhesins	
Bacillus cereus	Enterotoxin	Increased intestinal permeability, diarrhea, tissue necrosis, vomiting
	Emetic toxin	
	Edema factor	
	Lethal toxin	
	Hemolysin	
Campylobacter jejuni	Enterotoxin	Acts through cyclic AMP-mediated adenylate cyclase
	Cytotoxin	Cell toxicity
	Motility due to spiral shape and flagellum	Facilitates movement through viscous mucin layer toward intestinal wall
	Chemotaxis	For mucin and L-fucose
	Adhesins: outer membrane protein, lipopolysaccharide, and microcalyx material	Attachment to cell receptors: specific for L-fucose, D-mannose, and D-fucose
Clostridium botulinum A, B, E, F	Neurotoxin	Respiratory paralysis; inhibits release of acetylcholine
	Neurotoxins A-G	Zinc-metalloprotease; target: VAMP/synaptobrevin, SNAP-25 syntaxin
	C2 and C3 toxin	ADP-ribosyltransferase; target: monomeric G-actin, Rho-G protein
Clostridium perfringens	Enterotoxin	Spore-coat protein alters transport of fluid and glucose: causes tissue damage and inhibits metabolic process
	Gamma and beta toxins	Lethal activity
	Delta toxin (B and C strains)	Lethal activity, hemolysis
	Theta toxin	Lethal activity, hemolysis, and necrotizing activity
	Kappa toxin	Collagenase
	Lambda toxin (B, E, and D strains)	Protease
	Mu toxin	Hyaluronidase
	Nu toxin	Deoxyribonuclease
	Alpha toxin	Phospholipase C, lysis of cell membrane, intravascular hemolysis
	Beta and iota toxins	Increased capillary permeability
	Epsilon toxin	Prototoxin converted by trypsin; increased vascular permeability leading to tissue necrosis
	Perfringolysin O	Pore former
	Sialidase	

(continued)

TABLE 56.6   Examples of bacterial pathogens and their toxins *(Continued)*

Organism	Toxin/Virulence Determinant	Comment/Effect/Activity
Escherichia coli	Heat-labile toxin	Cyclic AMP-mediated fluid loss; ADP-ribosyltransferase; target: G-proteins
	Heat-stable toxin	Cyclic GMP-mediated fluid loss by disrupting intracellular signaling pathways (e.g., by binding to and activating guanylate cyclase)
	Cell-associated toxin	
	Cytotoxin	
	Colonization factors: CFA/I, CFA/II, CFA/III	Colonization in human intestine
	Pill adhesins type 1	Mannose-specific
	Pyelonephritis-associated pili (PAP)	α Gal (1-4) β Gal-specific
	S pill	Sialic acid-specific
	Afimbrial adhesin	Specific for squamous and transitional epithelial cells
	Cytotoxic necrotizing factor	
Listeria monocytogenes	Listeriolysin O	Pore-forming protein, facilitates entry of the pathogen into cytoplasm from endocytic vacuole
	Oxygen radicals	Survival in macrophages
	Internalin A & B	Internalization of bacteria into eukaryotic cell
	ActA	Actin-based movement to invade adjacent cell
	Lecithinase	Lysis of the vacuole
Salmonella species	Enterotoxin (cell associated)	Probably fluid loss
	Delayed permeability factor	Cyclic AMP-mediated fluid loss
	Cytotoxin	Inhibition of host protein synthesis
	Mannose-resistant hemagglutinin	
Shigella species	Exotoxin	Inhibition of host protein synthesis, cytotoxic, and neurotoxic activity
	N-glycosidase	Target: 28S rRNA
	Hemolysin	Invasion of cytoplasm by lysis of endocytic vacuole
	Active metabolism	Required for invasion
	Cell-associated invasive factors	
	Aerobactin	
	Lipopolysaccharide with 0 antigen	
Staphylococcus aureus	Enterotoxins (A, B, C, D, E, F)	Emetic; superantigen target: T-cell receptor and major histocompatibility complex II
	Hemolysins (α, β, γ, δ)	Hemolytic
	Hemolysin α	Lethal and dermonecrotic
	Hemolysin δ	Enteric hemolytic
	Exfoliative toxin (AB)	Exfoliation; superantigen (and serine protease); target: T-cell receptor and major histocompatibility complex II
	Fibronectin-binding protein	Attachment to epithelial cells
	Hyaluronidase	Invasive factor
	Coagulase	Plasma coagulation
	Staphylokinase	Fibrinolytic
	Leucocidin	Lethal to leucocytes

TABLE 56.6 Examples of bacterial pathogens and their toxins *(Continued)*

Organism	Toxin/Virulence Determinant	Comment/Effect/Activity
Vibrio cholerae	Cholera toxin	Cyclic AMP-mediated fluid loss
	Al	Acts on adenylate cyclase system
	A2	Facilitates entry of toxin into the cell
	B (5 subunits)	Bind to cell receptors
	Invasive and adhesin factors	Pilus synthesized in response to pH, temperature, and osmolarity
	Flagellum	Facilitates colonization
Yersinia enterocolitica	Invasion factors	Ca^{+2} dependent and expressed at 37°C
	V (protein)	
	W (lipoprotein) outer membrane protein	
	Autoagglutination	
	Heat-stable (ST) toxin	Mediates guanylate cyclase system
	Ail	Outer membrane protein associated with attachment and invasion

Abbreviations: ADP, adenosine diphosphate; AMP, adenosine monophosphate; CFA, colonization factor antigen; GMP, guanosine monophosphate; VAMP, vesicle associated membrane protein.

TABLE 56.7 Food poisoning by microalgae and dinoflagellate toxins[a]

Organisms	Toxin	Comment
Gambierdiscus toxicus, Prorocentrum concavum, Prorocentrum lima, Prorocentrum hoffmannianum, Prorocentrum mexicana, Ostreopsis lenticularis, Orthogonius siamensis, blue-green algae (*Trichodesmium erythraeum* Ehrenberg)	Ciguatera finfish poisoning (CFP): ciguatoxin, maitotoxin, scaritoxin etc, poorly characterized	Ciguatera poisoning through reef- or bottom-feeding fishes: barracuda, grouper, red snapper, and sea bass
Dinoflagellates (*Gymnodinium catenatum, Alexandrium* species), *Gonyaulax catenella, Gonyaulax tamarensis*	Paralytic shellfish poisoning (PSP): saxitoxins neosaxitoxins (≥18 carbamate, decarbamoyl, and sulfocarbamoyl derivatives)	PSP through clams, mussels, cockles, and scallops. Cosmopolitan (Northwest, Northeast, and Florida)
Gymnodinium breve, Gymnodinium species, *Ptychodiscus brevis*	Neurotoxic shellfish poisoning (NSP): more than nine polyether brevetoxins and derivatives	Neurotoxic shellfish poisoning associated with red tide; subtropical/warm temperate Gulf coast, eastern Florida, and North Carolina
Dinophysis fortii, Dinophysis acuminata, Prorocentrum lima	Diarrhetic shellfish poisoning (DSP): okadaic acid, dinophysis toxins, pectenotoxins, yessotoxins, and derivatives	Cold and warm temperate Atlantic, Pacific, and Indo-Pacific (Canada, Northeast)

[a]From Taylor[224] and Burkholder.[225]

TABLE 56.8   Examples of fungal toxins found in food products[a]

Organism	Toxin	Food Product
Aspergillus flavus, Aspergillus parasiticus	Aflatoxins	Wheat, corn, soybean, flour, bread, barley, cornmeal, peanut, cheese, hops, moldy meats
Alternaria species	Alternariol, altenuisol, alternuene, tenuazonic acid	Processed tomato products, pecans
Penicillium citrinin, Penicillium implicatum, Penicillium chrzaszczi, Penicillium citreosulfuratum, Penicillium lividum, Penicillium phaeojanthinellum, Penicillium viridicatum, Aspergillus terreus, Aspergillus candidus, Aspergillus niveus	Citrinin	Cereal grains, barley, rice
Claviceps purpurea	Ergot alkaloids	Cereal grains, forage grasses
Aspergillus flavus, Aspergillus oryzae, Aspergillus tamarii, Aspergillus glaucus	Kojic acid	Foods stored in homes
Penicillium brevicompactum, Penicillium roqueforti, Penicillium viridicatum, Penicillium brunneum	Mycophenolic acid	Cheese
Aspergillus nidulans	Nidulin	Corn
Aspergillus ochraceus, Aspergillus melleus, Aspergillus sulphureus, Penicillium viridicatum	Ochratoxins	Corn, wheat, oats, barley, and green coffee
Aspergillus clavatus, Aspergillus giganteus, Aspergillus terreu, Penicillium patulum, Penicillium griseofulvum, Penicillium claviforme, Penicillium expansum, Penicillium novae-zelandiae, Penicillium melinii, Penicillium leucopus, Penicillium equinum, Gymnoascus species	Patulin	Apple products
Penicillium viridicatum, Trichophyton megnini, Trichophyton rubrum, Trichophyton violaceum	Xanthomegnin	Stored grains
Penicillium rubrum	Rubratoxins	Feedstuff
Aspergillus versicolor, Aspergillus favus, Aspergillus nidulans, Penicillium luteum, Bipolaris species	Sterigmatocystins	Feed wheat, coffee, cheese
Fusarium species, *Myrothecium* species, *Trichothecium* species	Trichothecenes	Corn, wheat, mixed feed
Gibberella zeae	Zearalenone	Corn, moldy hay, feed

[a]From Bullerman[226] and Stoloff.[227]

internalized by the epithelial cells in response to either constitutive or induced invasion factors present on the surface of the microorganisms.[237,238] Both *Shigella* species and *L monocytogenes*, respectively, produce hemolysin and listeriolysin to lyse intracellular membrane vacuole and enter the cell cytoplasm. *Salmonella* species can use fused vacuoles to traverse the cell barrier.[239] Both *Y enterocolitica* and *Shigella* species use temperature-dependent (37°C) expression of the virulence factors.[240,241] The expression of virulence factors to environmental signals is an important characteristic of some emerging pathogens.

Host range is also an important aspect of virulence. Wide host range is another feature of some emerging pathogens. Host-adapted pathogens such as *S* Typhi, *V cholerae*, or polioviruses cannot maintain their infective cycle through animals used for food. Pathogens with a wide host range, on the other hand, can maintain a continuous chain of growth from humans to animals and thus

have greater infective potential. *S* Typhi, *L monocytogenes*, and *C jejuni* can be transmitted from species to species with increasing numbers.

Intoxication of food by bacteria, fungi, and algae are also important virulence-determining factors of foodborne and waterborne pathogens. Accumulation of histamine-like metabolites during growth on scombroid fishes, such as tuna or mackerel, may be considered an aspect of pathogenicity of *Proteus morganii, Klebsiella pneumoniae,* and *C perfringens.*

▶ CONTROL OF FOOD- AND WATER-INFECTIVE MICROORGANISMS

Control of food- and water-infective microorganisms has been a challenging problem for microbiologists as well as for public health scientists since a greater understanding

TABLE 56.9   Food- and waterborne pathogens: illness and symptoms[a]

Associated Organism or Toxin	Onset Time	Predominant Symptoms
Staphylococcus aureus and its enterotoxins	1-6 h, mean 2-4 h	Nausea, vomiting, retching, diarrhea, abdominal pain, prostration
Bacillus cereus and its exotoxins	8-16 h (2-4 h emesis possible)	Vomiting, abdominal cramps, diarrhea, nausea
Bacillus anthracis, Brucella melitensis, Brucella abortus, Brucella suis, Coxiella burnetii, Francisella tularensis, Listeria monocytogenes, Mycobacterium tuberculosis, Mycobacterium species, *Pasteurella multocida, Streptobacillus moniliformis, Campylobacter jejuni, Leptospira* species	Varying periods (depends on specific illness)	Fever, chills, head or joint ache, prostration, malaise, swollen lymph nodes, and other specific symptoms of disease in question
Streptococcus pyogenes	12-72 h	Sore throat, fever, nausea, vomiting, rhinorrhea, sometimes a rash
Corynebacterium diphtheriae	2-5 d	Inflamed throat and nose, spreading grayish exudate, fever, chills, sore throat, malaise, difficulty in swallowing, edema of cervical lymph node
Clostridium perfringens, Bacillus cereus, Streptococcus faecalis, Streptococcus faecium	2-36 h, mean 6-12 h	Abdominal cramps, diarrhea, putrefactive diarrhea associated with *C perfringens*, sometimes nausea and vomiting
Salmonella species (including *Salmonella arizonae*), *Shigella,* enteropathogenic *Escherichia coli,* other *Enterobacteriaceae, Vibrio parahaemolyticus, Yersinia enterocolitica, Pseudomonas aeruginosa, Aeromonas hydrophila, Plesiomonas shigelloides, Campylobacter jejuni, Vibrio cholerae* (O1 and non-O1) *Vibrio vulnificus, Vibrio fluvialis*	12-74 h, mean 18-36 h	Abdominal cramps, diarrhea, vomiting, fever, chills, malaise, nausea, headache, possible. Sometimes bloody or mucoid diarrhea, cutaneous lesions associated with *V vulnificus*. *Yersinia enterocolitica* mimics flu and acute appendicitis.
Salmonella ser Typhi	7-28 d, mean 14 d	Malaise, headache, fever, cough, nausea, vomiting, constipation, abdominal pain, chills, rose spots, bloody stools
Clostridium botulinum and its neurotoxins	2 h-6 d, usually 12-36 h	Vertigo, double or blurred vision, loss of reflex to light, difficulty in swallowing, speaking, and breathing, dry mouth, weakness, respiratory paralysis
Histamine (scombroid) (produced by bacteria)	Less than 1 h	Headache, dizziness, nausea, vomiting, peppery taste, burning of throat, facial swelling and flushing, stomach pain, itching of skin
Enteric viruses	3-5 d	Diarrhea, fever, vomiting abdominal pain, respiratory symptoms
Giardia lamblia	1-6 wk	Mucoid diarrhea (fatty stools) abdominal pain, weight loss
Entamoeba histolytica	1 to several weeks	Abdominal pain, diarrhea, constipation, headache, drowsiness, ulcers, variable—often asymptomatic
Toxoplasma gondii	10-13 d	Fever, headache, myalgia, rash
Trichinella spiralis	4-28 d, mean 9 d	Gastroenteritis, fever, edema about eyes, perspiration, muscular pain, chills, prostration, labored breathing

(continued)

TABLE 56.9 Food- and waterborne pathogens: illness and symptoms[a] *(Continued)*

Associated Organism or Toxin	Onset Time	Predominant Symptoms
Taenia saginata, Taenia solium	3-6 mo	Nervousness, insomnia, hunger pains, anorexia, weight loss, abdominal pain, sometimes gastroenteritis
Toxoplasma gondii	10-13 d	Fever, headache, myalgia, rash
Ciguatera finfish poisoning (CFP) toxin	1-6 h	Tingling and numbness, gastroenteritis, dizziness, dry mouth, muscular aches, dilated pupils, blurred vision, paralysis
Paralytic shellfish poisoning (PSP) (saxitoxins)	0.5-2 h	Tingling, burning, numbness, drowsiness, incoherent speech, respiratory paralysis
Neurotoxic shellfish poisoning (NSP) (brevetoxins)	2-5 min to 3-4 h	Reversal of hot and cold sensation, tingling; numbness of lips, tongue and throat: muscle aches, dizziness, diarrhea, vomiting
Diarrhetic shellfish poisoning (DSP) (dinophysis toxin, okadaic acid, pectenotoxin, yessotoxin)	30 min to 2-3 h	Nausea, vomiting, diarrhea, abdominal pain, chills, fever
Amnesic shellfish poisoning (ASP) (domoic acid)	24 h (gastrointestinal) to 48 h (neurologic)	Vomiting, diarrhea, abdominal pain, confusion, memory loss, disorientation, seizure, coma

[a]From US Food and Drug Administration.[228]

of microbiology arose in the 1800s, if not before by serendipitous means. New problems have arisen after the use of newer processing, storage and transportation procedures in the food industry. Several measures, including cleaning, preservation, disinfection (eg, pasteurization), and even sterilization methods, are available to control foodborne and waterborne pathogens. Foodborne and waterborne infective agents are controlled by prevention through the practice of good practices in these areas of cleaning, disinfection, preservation, and personal hygiene. Other measures such as the use of vaccines and anti-infectives such as antibiotics also can be used preventative or active control the pathogens. Prevention of intestinal colonization by pathogens through microbiological, chemical, and genetic methods has potential to control these microorganisms. These include the growing interest in the study, understanding, and use of beneficial or healthy-associated microbiomes of microorganisms in the gut to prevent infections and other chronic diseases such as inflammatory bowel diseases and obesity, and not only associated with intestinal diseases.[242,243]

HAZARD ANALYSIS AND CRITICAL CONTROL POINTS SYSTEM

The system was first introduced to meet the stringent food safety requirement for manned space flights.[244] A preplanned integrated approach to control the pathogens in the food industry and related establishments was recommended by the US National Research Council[194] and was termed the

Hazard Analysis and Critical Control Point (HACCP) system. The HACCP system includes preemptive measures to ensure food safety. It is designed to do the following:

- Identify and assess hazards (*hazard analysis*, or *HA*) associated with growing, harvesting, processing, marketing, preparation, and use of a given raw material or food product that may cause an unacceptable consumer health risk.
- Evaluate, monitor, and control precise steps (*critical control points*, or *CCP*) at which deviation (*loss of control*) from specified criteria (*limits or range of values*) can adversely affect the safety of the food product.

This system is like other risk assessment methodologies or tools (such as failure modes and effects analysis) now widely used in other design, manufacturing, or production systems. The HACCP system identifies and evaluates potential hazards, severity of hazards, likelihood of exposure, and risk of exposure prior to the production of food. Microbiologic, chemical, and physical tests as well as visual observations are used to monitor the CCP. The HACCP system mandates detailed monitoring, record keeping, and verification activities associated with food production, preparation, processing, storage, distribution, and handling by the consumer. This implies that good manufacturing practices are also in place to implement the HACCP system. The HACCP-based system specifies *horizontal* or common safeguards for all food types as well as *vertical* or product-specific safeguards. Because appropriate safeguards are built in at each critical step of food preparation to ensure food safety and quality, the HACCP system does not rely on the earlier procedures of sampling and end-product testing.[194,244,245]

Factors Considered in Hazard Analysis Process

Several factors related to food products, processing plants, and consumer habits are considered during hazard analysis, including the following:

1. Hazards related to food products: (1) microbiological quality of ingredients; (2) influence of intrinsic factors such as pH, acidity, content of fermentable carbohydrate, water activity, salinity, and packaging on growth of microorganisms or toxin production; and (3) microbial population density of pathogens, spore formers, and total microbial count under normal conditions and during storage (before, during, and after preparation) or during handling of food by the consumer

2. Hazards related to plant and processes: (1) efficacy of procedures used during preparation or processing of food to destroy microorganisms or to prevent its recontamination; (2) effect of plant design and equipment for adequate separation of raw material and finished good to prevent cross-contamination, positive air pressure in packaging area, traffic pattern, and temperature control; (3) optimum use of sanitizing chemicals and procedures and verification of efficacy; (4) impact of packaging method, material, labeling, consumer instructions, tamper-evident packaging, and identification of coding for production lot and coding for shelf life; (5) employee health, hygiene, and education; and (6) conditions of storage and transportation between packaging and delivery to the consumer

3. Consumer-dependent hazards: (1) consumer practices: washing hands, cleaning of utensils and food-contact surfaces, maintenance of proper personal hygiene; (2) age and health of the consumer whether elderly, immunocompromised, pregnant, infants, and so forth; and (3) intended use by the consumer: heating, cooking, ready-to-eat, storage temperature, storage with raw foods, treatment of left overs, etc

A well-defined HACCP team consists of members knowledgeable of a food (or indeed water treatment) operation and the specific production steps. With the responsibility of each member clearly defined, the team operates along the following seven guiding principles of the HACCP system[194,244,245]:

1. Hazard analysis: The HA (1) identifies significant (moderate- to high-risk) hazards, (2) assesses the likelihood of occurrence and the severity of hazards, and (3) develops preventive measures to ensure or improve food safety.

2. Identify the CCP in food preparation and storage at which hazard is likely to occur (ie, foodborne hazards arise from unacceptable limits of biologic, chemical, or physical properties of food as a result of the presence of high microbial population density, pathogens, toxins, pesticides, glass, metal debris, or such).

3. Establish critical limits for preventive measures required at each identified CCP: Critical limits of time, temperature, humidity, water content (a_w), pH, titratable acidity, preservatives, salt concentration, available chlorine, and viscosity are most frequently used.

4. Establish procedures to monitor CCP by visual observations, or by monitoring temperature, time, pH, a_w, etc.

5. Establish the corrective action to be taken when monitoring procedure shows that a critical limit had been exceeded. (Such food product must be kept on hold to perform appropriate tests of its safety, and expert opinion should be sought for additional testing or disposition of the product.)

6. Establish effective record keeping procedures that document the HACCP operative system.

7. Establish procedures to verify that the HACCP system is working as stipulated.

Factors that can be considered in microbiologic HA include (1) epidemiologic evidence of food as a vehicle of disease; (2) the ability of pathogens to contaminate, survive, and grow in the food during manufacture, storage, distribution, preservice preparation, and serving; and (3) susceptibility of probable consumers to the infective agent or toxins. Table 56.10 shows the identification and risk rating (severity) of biological hazards that may be associated with food being prepared, processed, stored, served, or sold in food establishments.

Standards, guidelines, and specifications for both pathogens and indicator organisms are considered for evaluating microbiologic criteria during hazard analysis. The presence of pathogens relates directly to the risk, whereas the presence of indicator organisms point to the probable presence of a pathogen or its toxins, improper practices adversely affecting safety or shelf life, or unsuitability of food or an ingredient for its intended use. When detection of pathogens is difficult or otherwise restrictive, assessment of fecal contamination can be determined by the presence of indicator organisms such as *E coli*, *Streptococcus faecalis*, or bacteriophages, which are commonly found in the intestine in large numbers. Sensitive and faster detection of indicator and other organisms can be used to implement disinfection (or sanitization) procedures for the control of pathogens[246]; however, the absence of indicator organisms may not always indicate absence of pathogens. For example, potable water that meets regulatory indicator standards may still be present with pathogens such as enteroviruses.[41]

Some of the hazards or risk factors responsible for foodborne infections in industrialized countries have

TABLE 56.10 Examples of severity rating of biological hazards[a]

Hazards From Infectious Agents		Naturally Present Hazards in Food	
Severe Hazard	**Moderate Hazards: Potentially Extensive Spread**	**Moderate Hazards: Limited Spread**	**Moderate-to-Severe Hazard**
Clostridium botulinum types A, B, E, and F	Listeria monocytogenes	Bacillus cereus	Mycotoxins (eg, aflatoxin) from mold
Shigella dysenteriae	Salmonella species	Campylobacter jejuni	Toxic mushroom species
Salmonella ser Typhimurium; Salmonella ser Paratyphi A, B	Shigella species	Clostridium perfringens	Scombrotoxin (histamine) from protein decomposition
	Enterovirulent Escherichia coli	Staphylococcus aureus	
	Streptococcus pyogenes	Vibrio cholerae, non-O1	Ciguatoxin from marine dinoflagellates
Hepatitis A and E	Rotavirus	Vibrio parahaemolyticus	
Brucella abortus; Brucella suis	Norovirus	Yersinia enterocolitica	Shellfish toxins (from marine dinoflagellates)
	Entamoeba histolytica	Giardia lamblia	
Vibrio cholerae O1	Diphyllobothrium latum	Taenia saginata	Neurotoxic shellfish poison
Vibrio vulnificus	Ascaris lumbricoides		Amnesic shellfish poisoning
Taenia solium	Cryptosporidium parvum		
Trichinella spiralis			

[a]From US Food and Drug Administration.[244]

been discussed earlier in this chapter (processing and handling). Prevention or elimination of these hazards by appropriate measures can result in the prevention of foodborne infections. Table 56.11 shows precautions and practices necessary for the control of foodborne and waterborne pathogens in poor rural areas of developing countries.[41,247]

Physical and Chemical Agents

The application of various preservation, disinfection, and sterilization methods has important applications in controlling the risks associated with food- and water-borne pathogens. These can range from the treatment of raw materials, treatment of foods, prevention of cross-contamination (eg, using surface disinfectants and hand antiseptics), and transport/storage systems. The application of heat (eg, pasteurization) and radiation (ionizing and nonionizing), low-temperature storage, filtration, and desiccation are some of the physical methods used to control pathogens in the food industry (see chapter 37). Irradiation of food for the control of pathogens continues to be highlighted as one of the most versatile technologies that has found some applications (eg, in dried foods such as herbs and spices and animal feeds) but has not been as widely used as initially proposed.[248,249] This can be due to many factors such as perception of radioactive risk (the misconception that radiation of food can render

the food radioactive), practical application in comparison to other heat or chemical methods, costs, and changes in perceptions of the organoleptic properties of the food. The use of chemicals for preservation as well as water/food or associated surface disinfection and sanitation can result in effective control of most of the water- and food-infective microorganisms. Commonly used food plant preservatives and disinfectants/sanitizers such as acids, salts, quaternary ammonium compounds, iodophors, and organic and inorganic hypochlorites are effective against both gram-positive and gram-negative bacteria as well as other pathogens depending on their applications (see chapter 37).[250] Heat, filtration, and chemical methods are also used for water disinfection/sterilization depending on the application. For example, water disinfection and sterilization can be achieved by heating methods (see chapters 11 and 28), such as distillation processes that not only inactivate microorganisms but also can be used to purify water of chemical contamination (eg, for the generation of water for infection). Chemical disinfectants such as chlorine, ozone, bromine, and chlorine dioxide have a broad disinfecting range against viruses, bacteria, and protozoa and continue to be widely used in the disinfection of drinking (potable) or other qualities of water (see chapter 37).[41,190] Filtration of water is not only used for the disinfection or even sterilization of water (see chapter 30) but also is often used as a pretreatment prior to chemical treatment to remove particulate matter and many microorganisms (eg, protozoa) by using sand and

TABLE 56.11	Preventive practices for food- and water-infective microorganisms in poor rural areas of developing countries[a]
Food preparation	
Washing hands with soap and water before food handling	
Avoidance of fecal contamination during food preparation	
Safe preparation of dried or artificial milk	
Short delay between preparation and consumption of food	
Thorough cooking	
Washing fruits and vegetables	
Appropriate storage of leftover foods	
Protection of food from insects and rodents	
Feeding of children	
Breastfeeding and delaying onset of weaning	
Feeding safe supplements in clean bottles or by cups and spoons	
Handling of water	
Use of safe water supply	
Treatment of unsafe water supply	
Boiling water for drinking	
Storage of drinking water in separate and clean containers	
Toilet practices	
Use of toilet and latrines	
Washing hands with soap and water after toilet visits or after handling of human or animal feces	

[a]From World Health Organization.[247]

polymers effectively increasing activity of the subsequent disinfectants. The technologies are considered in further details in other chapters of this book.

Principle of Competitive Exclusion

The use of either microorganisms or chemicals for preventing attachment and subsequent colonization by pathogens in the intestine are comparatively new and upcoming concepts.[242,243] This approach can be used to protect the host from infection by some food- and water-infective pathogens. For example, the prevention of colonization of pathogens such as *C jejuni* in poultry was identified as one of the most important approaches in the control of pathogens in food derived from animals.[251] Since that time, there has been a focus on the investigation of the

impact of microbiomes and the control of microorganism populations in the gut, not only in preventing infection but also in a wide range of other health effects.[242,243] These new ways of things challenge us in the traditional approaches to controlling food- and waterborne infections, particularly in the decreased use of antibiotics will become less widely used as our knowledge increases for the benefit of animal/human health. Other methods such as immunization and the use of genetics for breeding birds, animals, or other sources of food that are resistant to colonization by pathogens also can be considered as further control measures.

The "Nurmi" Concept

Poultry-associated human salmonellosis originates primarily from bacteria colonized in the intestinal tract of chickens. Commercial poultry flocks often become carriers of pathogenic microorganisms.[135,252,253] Non–host-specific salmonellae readily colonize the intestinal tracts of newly hatched chicks and turkey poults on commercial farms. Freshly hatched chicks are more susceptible to *Salmonella* colonization than adult birds. It has been known for some time that more than 50% of freshly hatched chicks could be infected with only 10 cells, whereas by day 14, approximately 90% of birds resist infection with one million cells of S Typhi.[254] Thus, preventing colonization of these bacteria in freshly hatched chicks would be an important method of preventing human salmonellosis.

It was also reported in the 1970s that newly hatched chicks fed a suspension of gut contents of *Salmonella-free* adult birds resisted colonization by *Salmonella infantis*.[255] The inhibition was first evident after 1 to 2 hours of feeding adult gut microflora and does not appear to be related to inhibition of *Salmonella* by volatile fatty acids that reach inhibitory concentration a few days later.[256] This led to the interpretation that inhibition was the result of steric hindrance, that is, the blocking of epithelial attachment sites of *Salmonella* by adult gut microflora.[257] The protection from *Salmonella* colonization was not due to activation of the immune system because chicks immunosuppressed with cyclophosphamide also were protected by gut microflora to the same degree as the controls. Birds receiving adult microflora become resistant to colonization by higher numbers of salmonellae. The treatment reduces the incidence of the carrier state and the number of salmonellae being shed. The birds also show increased resistance to colonization by other pathogens such as *C jejuni*, *C botulinum* type C, *C perfringens*, pathogenic *E coli*, and *Y enterocolitica*.[252] The mechanism can be speculated to involve the saturation of attachment sites by adult microflora on intestinal epithelium, resulting in exclusion and subsequent prevention of colonization by pathogens.

These findings lead to the development of earlier microbiome treatments, such as the commercial product,

PREEMPT, consisting of mixed bacterial culture prepared using gut microflora from adult birds for the practical prevention of *Salmonella* colonization.[258] The culture of 29 bacterial isolates maintained in a continuous-flow (CF3) system was used to feed chicks to prevent *Salmonella* colonization in chick intestines by what is presumed to be competitive exclusion. After the chicks were fed with the culture, their cecal propionic acid concentrations increased and the challenged *Salmonella* population decreased within 1-day posttreatment. Increase of propionic acid in the cecal crop indicated establishment of the adult culture. These results were soon followed by similar reports using probiotics based on lactobacilli isolated from chicken intestines, with the suggestion that the prevention of *Salmonella* colonization could be due partially to the direct competitive inhibition and partially due to the inhibitory chemicals produced by the adult culture.[259,260] These earlier reports lead to the continued interest in probiotics and modern microbiome treatment available or under development today.[261]

Use of Chemical Moieties

Many types of chemical moieties can show potential for use in preventing the first major interaction and attachment of pathogens and the host. Small chemical molecules with high specificity can bind either to the adhesins of the pathogens or to the receptors on the host cells, thereby preventing attachment of pathogens or toxins to host cells.[238,262,263] Of the numerous receptor sites present on the host cell, only a few serve as targets for the attachment of pathogens. Many species of *Enterobacteriaceae* attach by means of adhesins that specifically bind to D-mannose residue on the host cell receptors.[264,265] Cholera toxin and heat-labile (LT) *E coli* toxin bind to the same ganglioside receptors on mammalian cell surface.[263] *S aureus* and *S pyogenes* (group A) use fibronectin, a glycoprotein molecule present on epithelial cell surface, as a receptor for attachment.[266] Lipoteichoic acid present on *S pyogenes* (group A) cells acts as an adhesin to attach to fibronectin molecules.[267]

These specific binding characteristics can be useful in controlling infection processes. A mannose-containing glycoprotein (the Tam-Horsfall protein) produced in the kidney and present in urine binds to type 1 pili of *Enterobacteriaceae*. It may protect the host from bacterial infection of the kidney.[237] N-acetyl-D-galactosamine, L-fucose, D-galactose, L + arabinose, and D + mannose were found to reduce attachment of *S* Typhi to ceca of 1-week-old chicks.[268] L-Fucose inhibited adhesion of *V cholerae* to intestinal brush borders of the adult rabbit in vitro.[269] Fructose and tannin-like material from cranberry juice were reported to interfere in the attachment of *E coli* cells to receptors through type 1 and P pili, respectively.[270] P pili bind specifically to galactose disaccharide present on the host cell receptors. Overall, such interventions may prove to be successful alternatives to the use of drugs and anti-infectives, but they have had little development commercial to date.[271]

Economic Factors

Acceptance and implementation of measures at the national and community levels to control food- and water-infective microorganisms require cost-effectiveness and net benefit from these measures. The economic losses due to illness will vary with the infective agent and will differ from country to country. The estimated annual cost of foodborne infections due to *Salmonella* and *E coli* O157:H7 alone in the United States was estimated in 2010 to be $3.13 billion, with a total cost estimate for all foodborne illness in the $152 billion.[272] The overall costs worldwide can be equally staggering,[11] not to mention similar costs associated with waterborne infection.[41] Maintenance of cleanliness, education of personnel associated with food processing and food service sectors, and the use of chemical sanitizers were reported to be some of the least expensive control measures, whereas irradiation and competitive exclusion were found to be relatively more expensive control measures against human salmonellosis associated with poultry. On a large-scale and long-term basis, the last two measures and similar developments of modern methods of microbial control may prove to be more cost-effective over time, but time will tell. Implementation of more than one single control measure is necessary for success in preventing infections and illnesses due to food- and water-infective microorganisms. Table 56.9 displays an overview of symptoms associated with major food- and waterborne illnesses caused by the infective agents. Each of these symptoms can translate into economic factors considering drug treatment cost, absence from work, hospitalization cost, personal loss, involvement of supportive personnel, burden on community, emotional trauma, and even loss of life. It is hard to put an economic cost on the true impact of morbidity and mortality associated with these associated diseases, especially as in many cases there are preventable. Considering how far we have come in public health in our understanding of the risks associated with water- and foodborne infections, it would seem we remain to learn more in reducing these rates worldwide.

▶ ACKNOWLEDGMENTS

This chapter was updated from a previous excellent review by J. A. Lopes and S.S. Block.

REFERENCES

1. van Heyningen WE, Seal JR. *Cholera: The American Scientific Experience, 1947-1980.* Boulder, CO: Westview Press; 1983.
2. Fenner F. Sociocultural change and environmental diseases. In: Stanley NF, Joske RA, eds. *Changing Disease Pattern and Human Behaviour.* New York, NY: Academic Press; 1980:8-25.
3. Snow J, York J. *Report on the Cholera Outbreak in the Parish of St. James, Westminster, During the Autumn.* London, United Kingdom: Churchill; 1855.

4. Kaper JB, Morris JG, Levine MM. Cholera. *Clin Microbiol Rev.* 1995;8:48-86.

5. Smith JL, Fratamico PM, Gunther NW IV. Shiga toxin-producing *Escherichia coli. Adv Appl Microbiol.* 2014;86:145-197.

6. Angelo KM, Conrad AR, Saupe A, et al. Multistate outbreak of *Listeria monocytogenes* infections linked to whole apples used in commercially produced, prepackaged caramel apples: United States, 2014-2015. *Epidemiol Infect.* 2017;145:848-856.

7. Kang CR, Bang JH, Cho SI. *Campylobacter jejuni* foodborne infection associated with cross-contamination: outbreak in Seoul in 2017. *Infect Chemother.* 2019;51:21-27.

8. Morgan M, Watts V, Allen D, et al. Challenges of investigating a large food-borne norovirus outbreak across all branches of a restaurant group in the United Kingdom, October 2016. *Euro Surveill.* 2019;24:18.

9. Centers for Disease Control and Prevention. *Surveillance for Foodborne Disease Outbreaks United States, 2016: Annual Report.* Atlanta, GA: US Department of Health and Human Services, Centers for Disease Control and Prevention; 2018.

10. Moreira NA, Bondelind M. Safe drinking water and waterborne outbreaks. *J Water Health.* 2017;15:83-96.

11. World Health Organization. *WHO Estimates of the Global Burden of Foodborne Diseases: Foodborne Disease Burden Epidemiology Reference Group 2007-2015.* Geneva, Switzerland: World Health Organization; 2015.

12. Buckle GC, Walker CL, Black RE. Typhoid fever and paratyphoid fever: systematic review to estimate global morbidity and mortality for 2010. *J Glob Health.* 2012;2:010401.

13. Zaki SA, Karande S. Multidrug-resistant typhoid fever: a review. *J Infect Dev Ctries.* 2011;5:324-337.

14. Sathe PV, Karandikav VN, Gupte MD, et al. Investigation report of an epidemic of fever. *Int J Epidemiol.* 1983;12:215-219.

15. Centers for Disease Control and Prevention. Epidemic typhoid fever—Dushanbe, Tajikistan, 1997. *MMWR Morbid Mortal Wkly Rep.* 1998;47:752-756.

16. Dougan G, Baker S. *Salmonella enterica* serovar Typhi and the pathogenesis of typhoid fever. *Annu Rev Microbiol.* 2014;68:317-336.

17. Loharikar A, Newton A, Rowley P, et al. Typhoid fever outbreak associated with frozen mamey pulp imported from Guatemala to the western United States, 2010. *Clin Infect Dis.* 2012;55:61-66.

18. World Health Organization. *Global Report for Research on Infectious Diseases of Poverty.* Geneva, Switzerland: World Health Organization; 2012.

19. Conner JG, Teschler JK, Jones CJ, Yildiz FH. Staying alive: *Vibrio cholerae* cycle of environmental survival, transmission, and dissemination. *Microbiol Spectr.* 2016;4. doi:10.1128/microbiolspec.VMBF-0015-2015.

20. Umoh JU, Adesiyun AA, Adekeye JO, Nadarajah M. Epidemiological features of an outbreak of gastroenteritis/cholera in Kastina, Northern Nigeria. *J Hyg (Lond).* 1983;91:101-111.

21. Kapadia CR, Bhat P, Baker SJ, Mathan VI. A common source epidemic of mixed bacterial diarrhea with secondary transmission. *Am J Epidemiol.* 1984;120:743-749.

22. Shen H, Chen J, Xu Y, et al. An outbreak of shigellosis in a Children Welfare Institute caused by a multiple-antibiotic-resistant strain of *Shigella flexneri* 2a. *J Infect Public Health.* 2017;10:814-818.

23. Thimm BM. *Brucellosis: Distribution in Man, Domestic and Wild Animals.* New York, NY: Springer; 1982.

24. Zhang N, Huang D, Wu W, et al. Animal brucellosis control or eradication programs worldwide: a systematic review of experiences and lessons learned. *Prev Vet Med.* 2018;160:105-115.

25. Hall AJ, Vinjé J, Lopman B, et al. Updated norovirus outbreak management and disease prevention guidelines. *MMWR Recomm Rep.* 2011;60:1-15.

26. Sadiq A, Bostan N, Yinda KC, Naseem S, Sattar S. Rotavirus: genetics, pathogenesis and vaccine advances. *Rev Med Virol.* 2018;28:e2003.

27. Madden JM, McCardell BA, Archer DL. Virulence assessment of food borne microbes. In: Pierson MD, Stern NJ, eds. *Food-Borne Microorganisms and Their Toxins: Developing Methodology.* New York, NY: Marcel Dekker; 1986:291-315.

28. European Food Safety Authority. Update on the present knowledge on the occurrence and control of foodborne viruses. *EFSA J.* 2011;9:2190.

29. Bláha L, Babica P, Maršálek B. Toxins produced in cyanobacterial water blooms—toxicity and risks. *Interdiscip Toxicol.* 2009;2(2):36-41.

30. Gharpure R, Perez A, Miller AD, Wikswo ME, Silver R, Hlavsa MC. Cryptosporidiosis outbreaks—United States, 2009-2017. *MMWR Morb Mortal Wkly Rep.* 2019;68:568-572.

31. Ryan U, Hijjawi N, Xiao L. Foodborne cryptosporidiosis. *Int J Parasitol.* 2018;48:1-12.

32. Budu-Amoako E, Greenwood SJ, Dixon BR, Barkema HW, McClure JT. Foodborne illness associated with *Cryptosporidium* and *Giardia* from livestock. *J Food Prot.* 2011;74:1944-1955.

33. Foster EM. A half century of food microbiology and a glimpse at the years ahead. *Dairy Food Sanit.* 1988;8:586-592.

34. Mathys DA, Mollenkopf DF, Feicht SM, et al. Carbapenemase-producing Enterobacteriaceae and *Aeromonas* spp. present in wastewater treatment plant effluent and nearby surface waters in the US. *PLoS One.* 2019;14(6):e0218650.

35. Lim JY, Yoon JW, Hovde CJ. A brief overview of *Escherichia coli* O157:H7 and its plasmid O157. *J Microbiol Biotechnol.* 2010;20:5-14.

36. Rodríguez-Lázaro D, Cook N, Ruggeri FM, et al. Virus hazards from food, water and other contaminated environments. *FEMS Microbiol Rev.* 2012;36:786-814.

37. Asher DM, Gregori L. Human transmissible spongiform encephalopathies: historic view. *Handb Clin Neurol.* 2018;153:1-17.

38. European Food Safety Authority. The European Union summary report on surveillance for the presence of transmissible spongiform encephalopathies (TSEs) in 2017. *EFSA J.* 2018;16:5492.

39. Miller TR, Beversdorf LJ, Weirich CA, Bartlett SL. Cyanobacterial toxins of the laurentian great lakes, their toxicological effects, and numerical limits in drinking water. *Mar Drugs.* 2017;15:E160.

40. Lee HJ, Ryu D. Worldwide occurrence of mycotoxins in cereals and cereal-derived food products: public health perspectives of their co-occurrence. *J Agric Food Chem.* 2017;65:7034-7051.

41. World Health Organization. *Guidelines for Drinking-Water Quality, Incorporating the First Addendum.* 4th ed. Geneva, Switzerland: World Health Organization; 2017.

42. Dobell C. The discovery of intestinal protozoa of man. *Proc R Soc Med.* 1920;13:1-15.

43. Shaw PK, Brodsky RE, Lyman DO, et al. A community wide outbreak of giardiasis with evidence of transmission by a municipal water supply. *Ann Intern Med.* 1977;87:426-432.

44. Adam EA, Yoder JS, Gould LH, Hlavsa MC, Gargano JW. Giardiasis outbreaks in the United States, 1971-2011. *Epidemiol Infect.* 2016;144:2790-2801.

45. MacKenzie WR, Hoxie NJ, Proctor ME, et al. A massive outbreak in Milwaukee of *Cryptosporidium* infection transmitted through the public water supply. *N Engl J Med.* 1994;331:161-167.

46. Betancourt WQ, Rose JB. Drinking water treatment processes for removal of *Cryptosporidium* and *Giardia. Vet Parasitol.* 2004;126:219-234.

47. Barbee SL, Weber DJ, Sobsey MD, Rutala WA. Inactivation of *Cryptosporidium parvum* oocyst infectivity by disinfection and sterilization processes. *Gastrointest Endosc.* 1999;49:605-611.

48. Harb OS, Gao LY, Abu Kwaik Y. From protozoa to mammalian cells: a new paradigm in the life cycle of intracellular bacterial pathogens. *Environ Microbiol.* 2000;2:251-265.

49. Gärtner A. Über die Fleischvergiftung in Frankenhausen a. K. und dea Erreger derselben. *Cor. Bl. d. allg. aärztl. Ver. v. Thuäringen, Weimar.* 1888;XVII:573-600.

50. de Nobele J. Du Séro-diagnostic dans les affections gastro-intestinales d'origine alimentaire. *Ann Soc Med Gand.* 1898;77:281-306.

51. Ryan CA, Nickels MR, Hargrett NT, et al. Massive outbreak of antimicrobial-resistant salmonellosis traced to pasteurized milk. *JAMA.* 1987;258:3269-3274.

52. Centers for Disease Control and Prevention. Multistate outbreak of *Salmonella* serotype Agona infections linked to toasted oats cereal—United States, April-May, 1998. *MMWR Morb Mortal Wkly Rep.* 1998a;47:462-464.

53. Centers for Disease Control and Prevention. Outbreaks of *Salmonella* infections linked to backyard poultry. Centers for Disease Control and Prevention Web site. https://www.cdc.gov/salmonella/backyardpoultry-05-19/index.html. Accessed July 25, 2019.

54. Centers for Disease Control and Prevention. Surveillance for foodborne disease outbreaks—United States, 2009-2010. *Morb Mortal Wkly Rep*. 2013;62:41-47.

55. Blaser MJ. *Campylobacter jejuni* and food. *Food Technol*. 1982;36:69-92.

56. Oakeson KF, Wagner JM, Rohrwasser A, Atkinson-Dunn R. Whole-genome sequencing and bioinformatic analysis of isolates from foodborne illness outbreaks of *Campylobacter jejuni* and *Salmonella enterica*. *J Clin Microbiol*. 2018;56:e00161-18.

57. Black RE, Jackson RJ, Tsai T, et al. Epidemic *Yersinia enterocolitica* infection due to contaminated chocolate milk. *N Engl J Med*. 1978;298:76-79.

58. Lofgren JP, Koningsberg C, Rendtorff R, et al. Multistate outbreak of yersiniosis. *MMWR Morb Mortal Wkly Rep*. 1982;31:505-506.

59. Marder EP, Griffin PM, Cieslak PR, et al. Preliminary incidence and trends of infections with pathogens transmitted commonly through food—foodborne diseases active surveillance network, 10 U.S. sites, 2006-2017. *MMWR Morb Mortal Wkly Rep*. 2018;67:324-328.

60. Le Guern AS, Martin L, Savin C, Carniel E. Yersiniosis in France: overview and potential sources of infection. *Int J Infect Dis*. 2016;46:1-7.

61. Ortel S. Bakteriologische serologische and epidemiologische untersuchungen warhend einer Listeriose-epidemie. *Deutshe Gesundheitswes*. 1968;16:753-759.

62. Schlech WF III, Lavigne PM, Bostolussi RA, et al. Epidemic listeriosis—evidence for transmission by food. *N Engl J Med*. 1983;308:203-206.

63. James SM, Fannin SL, Agee BA, et al. Listeriosis outbreak associated with Mexican-style cheese—California. *MMWR Morb Mortal Wkly Rep*. 1985;34:357-359.

64. Centers for Disease Control and Prevention. Multistate outbreak of listeriosis—United States, 1998. *MMWR Morb Mortal Wkly Rep*. 1998;47:1085-1086.

65. Self JL, Conrad A, Stroika S, et al. Multistate outbreak of listeriosis associated with packaged leafy green salads, United States and Canada, 2015-2016. *Emerg Infect Dis*. 2019;25:1461-1468.

66. Fujino T, Okuno Y, Nakada D, et al. On bacteriological examination of Shirasu-food poisoning. *J Jpn Assoc Infect Dis*. 1951;25:11-12.

67. Sakazaki R, Shimada T. Vibrio species as causative agents of food-borne infection. In: Robinson RK, ed. *Development in Food Microbiology—2*. New York, NY: Elsevier; 1982:123-151.

68. Taylor M, Cheng J, Sharma D, et al. Outbreak of *Vibrio parahaemolyticus* associated with consumption of raw oysters in Canada, 2015. *Foodborne Pathog Dis*. 2018;15:554-559.

69. Su YC, Liu C. *Vibrio parahaemolyticus*: a concern of seafood safety. *Food Microbiol*. 2007;24:549-58.

70. Hall HE, Angelotti R, Lewis KH, Foter MJ. Characteristics of *Clostridium perfringens* strains associated with food and food-borne disease. *J Bacteriol*. 1963;85:1094-1103.

71. Li J, Paredes-Sabja D, Sarker MR, McClane BA. *Clostridium perfringens* sporulation and sporulation-associated toxin production. *Microbiol Spectr*. 2016;4. doi:10.1128/microbiolspec.TBS-0022-2015.

72. Scallan E, Hoekstra RM, Angulo FJ, et al. Foodborne illness acquired in the United States—major pathogens. *Emerg Infect Dis*. 2011;17:7-15.

73. Palma NZ, da Cruz M, Fagundes V, Pires L. Foodborne botulism: neglected diagnosis. *Eur J Case Rep Intern Med*. 2019;6:001122.

74. Cann DC, Wilson BB, Hobbs G, Shewan JM, Johannsen A. The incidence of *Clostridium botulinum* type E in fish and bottom deposits in the North Sea and off the coast of Scandinavia. *J Appl Bacteriol*. 1965;28:426-430.

75. Bergeron G, Latash J, Da Costa-Carter CA, et al. Notes from the field: botulism outbreak associated with home-canned peas—New York City, 2018. *MMWR Morb Mortal Wkly Rep*. 2019;68:251-252.

76. Midura TF, Arnon SS. Infant botulism. Identification of *Clostridium botulinum* and its toxins in faeces. *Lancet*. 1976;2:934-935.

77. Pickett J, Berg B, Chaplin E, Brunstetter-Shafer MA. Syndrome of botulism in infancy: clinical and electrophysiologic study. *N Engl J Med*. 1976;295:770-772.

78. Sugiyama H, Sofos JN. Botulism. In: Robinson RK, ed. *Developments in Food Microbiology*. New York, NY: Elsevier; 1982:77-120.

79. Caselitz FH. Ein neues Bacterium der Gaming: Vibrio muller, Vibrio jamaicensis. *Z Tropenmed Parasitol*. 1955;6:52.

80. Altwegg M, Geiss HK. Aeromonas as human pathogen. *Crit Rev Microbiol*. 1989;16:253-286.

81. Janda JM, Abbott SL. The genus *Aeromonas*: taxonomy, pathogenicity, and infection. *Clin Microbiol Rev*. 2010;23:35-73.

82. Kornacki J, Marth EH. Foodborne illness caused by *Escherichia coli*: a review. *J Food Prot*. 1982;45:1051-1067.

83. Croxen MA, Law RL, Scholz R, Keeney KM, Wlodarska M, Finlay BB. Recent advances in understanding enteric pathogenic *Escherichia coli*. *Clin Microbiol Rev*. 2013;26:822-880.

84. Vila J, Sáez-López E, Johnson JR, et al. *Escherichia coli*: an old friend with new tidings. *FEMS Microbiol Rev*. 2016;40:437-463.

85. Stewart PJ, Desormeaux W, Chene J. Hemorrhagic colitis in a home for the aged—Ontario. *Can Dis Wkly Rep*. 1983;9:29.

86. Taylor WR, Schell WL, Wells JG, et al. A foodborne outbreak of enterotoxigenic *Escherichia coli* diarrhea. *N Engl J Med*. 1982;306:1093-1095.

87. Ryan CA, Tauxe RV, Hosek GW, et al. *Escherichia coli* O157:H7 diarrhea in a nursing home: clinical, epidemiological, and pathological findings. *J Infect Dis*. 1986;154:631-638.

88. Frank C, Werber D, Cramer JP, et al. Epidemic profile of Shiga-toxin-producing *Escherichia coli* O104:H4 outbreak in Germany. *N Engl J Med*. 2011;365:1771-1780.

89. Yang SC, Lin CH, Aljuffali IA, Fang JY. Current pathogenic *Escherichia coli* foodborne outbreak cases and therapy development. *Arch Microbiol*. 2017;199:811-825.

90. Canizalez-Roman A, Flores-Villaseñor HM, Gonzalez-Nuñez E, et al. Surveillance of diarrheagenic *Escherichia coli* strains isolated from diarrhea cases from children, adults and elderly at northwest of Mexico. *Front Microbiol*. 2016;7:1924.

91. Iovleva A, Doi Y. Carbapenem-resistant *Enterobacteriaceae*. *Clin Lab Med*. 2017;37:303-315.

92. Kizny Gordon AE, Mathers AJ, Cheong EYL, et al. The hospital water environment as a reservoir for carbapenem-resistant organisms causing hospital-acquired infections—a systematic review of the literature. *Clin Infect Dis*. 2017;64:1435-1444.

93. Kotsanas D, Wijesooriya WR, Korman TM, et al. "Down the drain": carbapenem-resistant bacteria in intensive care unit patients and handwashing sinks. *Med J Aust*. 2013;198:267-269.

94. Pattabiraman V, Katz LS, Chen JC, McCullough AE, Trees E. Genome wide characterization of enterotoxigenic *Escherichia coli* serogroup O6 isolates from multiple outbreaks and sporadic infections from 1975-2016. *PLoS One*. 2018;13:e0208735.

95. Meyer RD. *Legionella* infections: a review of five years of research. *Rev Infect Dis*. 1983;5:258-278.

96. Mouchtouri VA, Rudge JW. Legionnaires' disease in hotels and passenger ships: a systematic review of evidence, sources, and contributing factors. *J Travel Med*. 2015;22:325-337.

97. McDade JE, Shepard CC, Fracier DW, Tsai TR, Redus MA, Dowdle WR. Legionnaires' disease: isolation of a bacterium and demonstration of its role in other respiratory disease. *N Engl J Med*. 1977;297:1197-1203.

98. Sharrar RG. Prior outbreaks of legionellosis. In: Katz SM, ed. *Legionellosis*. New York, NY: CRC Press; 1985:12-18.

99. Labombardi VJ, O'brien AM, Kislak JW. Pseudo-outbreak of *Mycobacterium fortuitum* due to contaminated ice machines. *Am J Infect Control*. 2002;30:184-186.

100. van Ingen J, Kohl TA, Kranzer K, et al. Global outbreak of severe *Mycobacterium chimaera* disease after cardiac surgery: a molecular epidemiological study. *Lancet Infect Dis*. 2017;17:1033-1041.

101. Duarte RS, Lourenço MC, Fonseca Lde S, et al. Epidemic of postsurgical infections caused by *Mycobacterium massiliense*. *J Clin Microbiol*. 2009;47:2149-2155.

102. Shang S, Gibbs S, Henao-Tamayo M, et al. Increased virulence of an epidemic strain of *Mycobacterium massiliense* in mice. *PLoS One*. 2011;6:e24726.

103. Pérez de Val B, Grau-Roma L, Segalés J, Domingo M, Vidal E. Mycobacteriosis outbreak caused by *Mycobacterium avium subsp.* avium detected through meat inspection in five porcine fattening farms. *Vet Rec.* 2014;174:96.

104. Thomas V, McDonnell G, Denyer SP, Maillard JY. Free-living amoebae and their intracellular pathogenic microorganisms: risks for water quality. *FEMS Microbiol Rev.* 2010;34:231-259.

105. Morens DM, Taubenberger JK, Harvey HA, Memoli MJ. The 1918 influenza pandemic: lessons for 2009 and the future. *Crit Care Med.* 2010;38:e10-e20.

106. Young LS, Inderlied BC, Berlin OG, Gottlieb MS. Mycobacterial infections in AIDS patients, with an emphasis on *Mycobacterium avium* complex. *Rev Infect Dis.* 1986;8:1024-1033.

107. Korgstad DJ, Visvesvara GS, Walls KW, et al. Blood and tissue protozoa. In: Lennette EH, Balows A, Hausler WJ, Shadomy HJ, eds. *Manual of Clinical Microbiology.* 4th ed. Washington, DC: American Society for Microbiology; 1985:612-630.

108. Melvin DM, Healy GR. Intestinal and urogenital protozoa. In: Lennette EH, Balows A, Hausler WJ, et al, eds. *Manual of Clinical Microbiology.* 4th ed. Washington, DC: American Society for Microbiology; 1985:631-650.

109. Centers for Disease Control and Prevention. Outbreak of cryptosporidiosis associated with a water sprinkler fountain—Minnesota, 1997. *MMWR Morb Mortal Wkly Rep.* 1998;47:856-860.

110. Centers for Disease Control and Prevention. Update: outbreaks of Cyclosporiasis—United States and Canada, 1997. *MMWR Morb Mortal Wkly Rep.* 1997;46:521-523.

111. Herwaldt BL, Ackers ML. *Cyclospora* working group: an outbreak in 1996 of cyclosporiasis associated with imported raspberries. *N Engl J Med.* 1997;336:1548-1556.

112. Whitfield Y, Johnson K, Hanson H, Huneault D. 2015 Outbreak of cyclosporiasis linked to the consumption of imported sugar snap peas in Ontario, Canada. *J Food Prot.* 2017;80:1666-1669.

113. Marcos LA, Gotuzzo E. Intestinal protozoan infections in the immunocompromised host. *Curr Opin Infect Dis.* 2013;26:295-301.

114. Chia G, Ho HJ, Ng CG, et al. An unusual outbreak of rotavirus G8P[8] gastroenteritis in adults in an urban community, Singapore, 2016. *J Clin Virol.* 2018;105:57-63.

115. Pacilli M, Cortese MM, Smith S, et al. Outbreak of gastroenteritis in adults due to rotavirus genotype G12P[8]. *Clin Infect Dis.* 2015;6:e20-e25.

116. Rebato ND, de Los Reyes VCD, Sucaldito MNL, Marin GR. Is your drinking-water safe? A rotavirus outbreak linked to water refilling stations in the Philippines, 2016. *Western Pac Surveill Response J.* 2019;10:1-5.

117. Rushton SP, Sanderson RA, Reid WDK, et al. Transmission routes of rare seasonal diseases: the case of norovirus infections. *Philos Trans R Soc Lond B Biol Sci.* 2019;374:20180267.

118. Lawson HW, Braun MM, Glass RIM, et al. Waterborne outbreak of Norwalk virus gastroenteritis at a southwest US resort: role of geological formations in contamination of well water. *Lancet.* 1991;337:1200-1204.

119. Verhoef L, Hewitt J, Barclay L, et al. Norovirus genotype profiles associated with foodborne transmission, 1999-2012. *Emerg Infect Dis.* 2015;21:592-599.

120. Monini M, Ostanello F, Vignolo E, et al. Occurrence of two Norovirus outbreaks in the same cafeteria in one week. *New Microbiol.* 2019;42.

121. Blanco A, Guix S, Fuster N, et al. Norovirus in bottled water associated with gastroenteritis outbreak, Spain, 2016. *Emerg Infect Dis.* 2017;23:1531-1534.

122. Cheng HY, Hung MN, Chen WC, et al. Ice-associated norovirus outbreak predominantly caused by GII.17 in Taiwan, 2015. *BMC Public Health.* 2017;17:870.

123. Coker RJ, Hunter BM, Rudge JW, Liverani M, Hanvoravongchai P. Emerging infectious diseases in southeast Asia: regional challenges to control. *Lancet.* 2011;377:599-609.

124. Scheckel C, Aguzzi A. Prions, prionoids and protein misfolding disorders. *Nat Rev Genet.* 2018;19:405-418.

125. Wulf MA, Senatore A, Aguzzi A. The biological function of the cellular prion protein: an update. *BMC Biol.* 2017;15:34.

126. Hoinville LJ. A review of the epidemiology of scrapie in sheep. *Rev Sci Tech.* 1996;15:827-852.

127. Casalone C, Hope J. Atypical and classic bovine spongiform encephalopathy. *Handb Clin Neurol.* 2018;153:121-134.

128. Taylor DM, Woodgate SL. Bovine spongiform encephalopathy: the causal role of ruminant-derived protein in cattle diets. *Rev Sci Tech.* 1997;16:187-198.

129. Will RG, Ironside JW, Zeidler M, et al. A new variant of Creutzfeldt-Jakob disease in the UK. *Lancet.* 1996;347:921-925.

130. Bruce ME, Will RG, Ironside JW, et al. Transmissions to mice indicate that 'new variant' CJD is caused by the BSE agent. *Nature.* 1997;389:498-501.

131. European Creutzfeldt-Jakob Disease Surveillance Network. *Variant CJD Cases Worldwide.* Solna, Sweden: European Centre for Disease Prevention and Control; 2019. https://www.cjd.ed.ac.uk/sites/default/files/worldfigs.pdf. Accessed August 15, 2019.

132. Mok T, Jaunmuktane Z, Joiner S, et al. Variant Creutzfeldt-Jakob disease in a patient with heterozygosity at PRNP Codon 129. *N Engl J Med.* 2017;376:292-294.

133. Waddell L, Greig J, Mascarenhas M, Otten A, Corrin T, Hierlihy K. Current evidence on the transmissibility of chronic wasting disease prions to humans—a systematic review. *Transbound Emerg Dis.* 2018;65:37-49.

134. Ferreira V, Wiedmann M, Teixeira P, Stasiewicz MJ. *Listeria monocytogenes* persistence in food-associated environments: epidemiology, strain characteristics, and implications for public health. *J Food Prot.* 2014;77:150-170.

135. Genigeorgis C, Hassuneh M, Collins P. *Campylobacter jejuni* infection on poultry farms and its effect on poultry meat contamination during slaughter. *J Food Prot.* 1986;49:895-903.

136. Stolle A. Spreading of salmonellas during cattle slaughtering. *J Appl Bacteriol.* 1981;50:239-245.

137. Malley TJ, Butts J, Wiedmann M. Seek and destroy process: *Listeria monocytogenes* process controls in the ready-to-eat meat and poultry industry. *J Food Prot.* 2015;78:436-445.

138. National Research Council. Current status of microbiological criteria and legislative bases. In: Subcommittee on Microbiological Criteria for Foods and Food Ingredients, ed. *An Evaluation of the Role of Microbiological Criteria for Foods and Food Ingredients.* Washington, DC: National Academy Press; 1985:152-173.

139. US Food and Drug Administration. FSMA rules & guidance for industry. US Food and Drug Administration Web site. https://www.fda.gov/food/food-safety-modernization-act-fsma/fsma-rules-guidance-industry. Accessed August 15, 2019.

140. Willesmith JW. *Manual on Bovine Spongiform Encephalopathy. Food and Agriculture Organization of the United Nations.* Rome, Italy: Food and Agriculture Organization of the United Nations; 1998. http://www.fao.org/livestock/agap/frg/feedsafety/special/fao-bse.htm. Accessed August 15, 2019.

141. Jackson V, Blair IS, McDowell DA, Kennedy J. The incidence of significant foodborne pathogens in domestic refrigerators. *Food Control.* 2007;18:346-351.

142. Corlett DA. Refrigerated foods and use of Hazard Analysis and Critical Control Point principles. *Food Technol.* 1989;43:91-94.

143. Palumbo SA. Is refrigeration enough to restrain foodborne pathogens? *J Food Prot.* 1986;49:1003-1009.

144. Palumbo SA, Morgan DR, Buchanan RL. The influence of temperature, NaCl, and pH on the growth of *Aeromonas hydrophila. J Food Sci.* 1985;50:1417-1421.

145. Rosenow M, Marth EH. Growth patterns of *Listeria monocytogenes* in skim, whole, and chocolate milk and whipping cream at 4, 8, 13, 21, and 35°C. *J Food Prot.* 1987;50:452-459.

146. Health Protection Bureau. Salmonellosis associated with cheese consumption—Canada. *MMWR Morb Mortal Wkly Rep.* 1985;33:387.

147. Centers for Disease Control and Prevention. Milk-borne salmonellosis—Illinois. *MMWR Morb Mortal Wkly Rep.* 1985;34:200.

148. Bryan FL. Risks of practices, procedures and processes that lead to outbreaks of foodborne diseases. *J Food Prot.* 1988;51:663-673.

149. Smith M, Fancher W, Blumberg R, et al. Turkey associated salmonellosis at an elementary school—Georgia. *MMWR Morb Mortal Wkly Rep*. 1985;34:707-708.

150. Stanfield JT, Wilson CR, Andrews WH, Jackson GJ. Potential role of refrigerated milk packaging in the transmission of listeriosis and salmonellosis. *J Food Prot*. 1987;50:730-732.

151. Schiemann DA. *Yersinia enterocolitica* in milk and dairy products. *J Dairy Sci*. 1987;70:383-391.

152. Tacket CO, Narain JP, Sattin R, et al. A multistate outbreak of infections caused by *Yersinia enterocolitica* transmitted by pasteurized milk. *JAMA*. 1984;251:483-486.

153. Johnson RW. Microbial food safety. *Dairy Food Sanitization*. 1987;7:174-176.

154. Sperber SJ, Schleupner CJ. Salmonellosis during infection with human immunodeficiency virus. *Rev Infect Dis*. 1987;9:925-934.

155. Lederberg J, Shope RE, Oaks SC Jr, et al. Factors of emergence. In: *Emerging Infections: Microbial Threats to Health in the United States*. Washington, DC: National Academy Press; 1992;2:34-112.

156. Lockhart SR, Guarner J. Emerging and reemerging fungal infections. *Semin Diagn Pathol*. 2019;36:177-181.

157. Holmberg SD, Osterholm MT, Senger ICA, Cohen ML. Drug-resistant *Salmonella* from animals fed antimicrobials. *N Engl J Med*. 1984;311:617-622.

158. Morehead MS, Scarbrough C. Emergence of global antibiotic resistance. *Prim Care*. 2018;45:467-484.

159. Glynn MK, Bopp C, Dewitt W, Dabney P, Mokhtar M, Angulo FJ. Emergence of multi-drug resistant *Salmonella enterica* serotype typhimurium DT104 infections on the United States. *N Engl J Med*. 1998;338:1333-1338.

160. Smith KE, Besser JM, Hedberg CW, et al. Quinolone-resistant *Campylobacter jejuni* infections in Minnesota, 1992-1998. *N Engl J Med*. 1999;340:1525-1532.

161. Hawrelak JA, Myers SP. The causes of intestinal dysbiosis: a review. *Altern Med Rev*. 2004;9:180-197.

162. Abt MC, McKenney PT, Pamer EG. *Clostridium difficile* colitis: pathogenesis and host defence. *Nat Rev Microbiol*. 2016;14:609-620.

163. Spigaglia P, Mastrantonio P, Barbanti F. Antibiotic resistances of *Clostridium difficile*. *Adv Exp Med Biol*. 2018;1050:137-159.

164. Brown KA, Khanafer N, Daneman N, Fismana DN. Meta-analysis of antibiotics and the risk of community-associated *Clostridium difficile* infection. *Antimicrob Agents Chemother*. 2013;57:2326-2332.

165. Peterson WL, Mackowiak PA, Barnett CC, Marling-Cason M, Haley ML. The human gastric bactericidal barrier: mechanisms of action, relative antibacterial activity, and dietary influences. *J Infect Dis*. 1989;159:979-983.

166. Blaser MJ, Newman LS. A review of human Salmonellosis. I. Infective dose. *Rev Infect Dis*. 1982;4:1096-1106.

167. Hornick RB, Music SI, Wenzel R, et al. The Broad Street pump revisited: response of volunteers to ingested cholera vibrios. *Bull NY Acad Med*. 1971;47:1181-1191.

168. Waterman SR, Small PLC. Acid-sensitive enteric pathogens are protected from killing under extremely acidic conditions of pH 2.5 when they are inoculated onto certain solid food sources. *Appl Environ Microbiol*. 1998;64:3882-3886.

169. Conte MP, Petrone G, Di Biase AM, Ammendolia MG, Superti F, Seganti L. Acid tolerance in *Listeria monocytogenes* influences invasiveness of enterocyte-like cells and macrophage-like cells. *Microb Pathog*. 2000;29:137-144.

170. Ho JL, Shands KN, Friedland G, Eckind P, Fraser DW. An outbreak of type 4b *Listeria monocytogenes* infection involving patients from eight Boston hospitals. *Arch Intern Med*. 1986;146:520-524.

171. Vázquez-Boland JA, Kuhn M, Berche P, et al. *Listeria* pathogenesis and molecular virulence determinants. *Clin Microbiol Rev*. 2001;14:584-640.

172. Gionella RA, Broitman SA, Zamcheck N. Salmonella enteritis. I. Role of reduced gastric secretions in pathogenesis. *Am J Dig Dis*. 1971;16:1000-1006.

173. Pearson RD, Hewlett EL. Amebiasis in travellers. In: Ravdin JI, ed. *Amebiasis*. New York, NY: John Wiley & Sons; 1988:556-562.

174. Fernandes HVJ, Houle SKD, Johal A, Riddle MS. Travelers' diarrhea: clinical practice guidelines for pharmacists. *Can Pharm J (Ott)*. 2019;152:241-250.

175. Connor BA. Travelers' diarrhea. Centers for Disease Control and Prevention Web site. https://wwwnc.cdc.gov/travel/yellowbook/2018/the-pre-travel-consultation/travelers-diarrhea. Accessed August 15, 2019.

176. Jackson Tartakow L, Vorperian JH, eds. Gastrointestinal illness aboard cruise ships and aircraft. In: *Food-Borne and Water-Borne Diseases*. Westpoint, CT: AVI Publishing; 1980:259-264.

177. Todd ECD. Impact of spoilage and foodborne diseases on national and international economies. *Int J Food Microbiol*. 1987;4:83-100.

178. Rooney RM, Cramer EH, Mantha S, et al. A review of outbreaks of foodborne disease associated with passenger ships: evidence for risk management. *Public Health Rep*. 2004;119:427-434.

179. Bert F, Scaioli G, Gualano MR, et al. Norovirus outbreaks on commercial cruise ships: a systematic review and new targets for the public health agenda. *Food Environ Virol*. 2014;6:67-74.

180. Dekeyser P, Gossuln-Detrain M, Butzler JP, Sternon J. Acute enteritis due to related vibrio: first positive stool cultures. *J Infect Dis*. 1972;125:390-392.

181. Kapikian AZ, Wyatt RG, Dolin R, Thornhill TS, Kalica AR, Chanock RM. Visualization by immune electron microscopy of a 27-nm particle associated with acute infectious nonbacterial gastroenteritis. *J Virol*. 1972;10:1075-1088.

182. Lovett J. Isolation and enumeration of *Listeria monocytogenes*. *Food Technol*. 1988;42:172-175.

183. Gallard L, Bueno H. Advances in laboratory diagnosis of intestinal parasites. *Am Clin Lab*. 1989;8:18-19.

184. Ray B. Impact of bacterial injury and repair in food microbiology: its past, present, and future. *J Food Prot*. 1986;49:651-655.

185. Verweij JJ, Stensvold CR. Molecular testing for clinical diagnosis and epidemiological investigations of intestinal parasitic infections. *Clin Microbiol Rev*. 2014;27(2):371-418.

186. Clark B, McKendrick M. A review of viral gastroenteritis. *Curr Opin Infect Dis*. 2004;17:461-469.

187. Martelle S, Tschirhart D. Ailment is infectious, can be dangerous. *The Detroit News*. October 15, 1988:22.

188. Kendall D. One in three chickens contaminated, USDA sarns. *The Detroit News*. July 1, 1989:20.

189. Prentice T, Wood N, Ford R. Health chief warns of new food danger. *The Times*. February 11, 1989:3.

190. Centers for Disease Control and Prevention. Water, sanitation & environmentally-related hygiene. Centers for Disease Control and Prevention Web site. https://www.cdc.gov/healthywater/hygiene/index.html. Accessed August 15, 2019.

191. Silliker JH, Elliot RP, Baird-Parker AC, et al. *Microbial Ecology of Foods: Factors Affecting Life and Death of Organisms*. Vol 1. New York, NY: Academic Press; 1980.

192. Troller JA. Water relations of foodborne bacterial pathogens—an updated review. *J Food Prot*. 1986;49:656-670.

193. Bryan FL. Factors that contribute to outbreaks of foodborne diseases. *J Food Prot*. 1978;41:816-827.

194. National Research Council. Selection of pathogens as components of microbiological criteria. In: *An Evaluation of the Role of Microbiological Criteria for Foods and Food Ingredients*. Washington, DC: National Academy Press; 1985:72-103.

195. Banwart GJ. *Basic Food Microbiology*. New York, NY: AVI Publishing; 1981.

196. Rendtorff RC. The experimental transmission of human intestinal protozoa parasites. II. *Giardia lamblia* cysts given in capsules. *Am J Hyg*. 1954;59:209-270.

197. Doyle MP, Zhao T, Ming J, et al. *Escherichia coli* O157:H7. In: Doyle MP, Beuchat LR, Montville TJ, eds. *Food Microbiology—Fundamentals and Frontiers*. Washington, DC: ASM Press; 1997:177-191.

198. D'Aoust JY. *Salmonella* species. In: Doyle MP, Beuchat LR, Montville TJ, eds. *Food Microbiology—Fundamentals and Frontiers*. Washington, DC: ASM Press; 1997:129-158.

199. Horn N, Bhunia AK. Food-associated stress primes foodborne pathogens for the gastrointestinal phase of infection. *Front Microbiol.* 2018;9:1962.

200. Bryan FL. Diseases transmitted by foods contaminated by waste water. *J Food Prot.* 1977;40:45-56.

201. Vasavada PC. Pathogenic bacteria in milk—a review. *J Dairy Sci.* 1988;71:2809-2816.

202. Centers for Disease Control and Prevention. Update: *Salmonella enteritidis* infections in the Northeastern United States. *MMWR Morb Mortal Wkly Rep.* 1987;36:204-205.

203. Benton C, Khan F, Monaghan P, Richards WN, Shedden CB. The contamination of a major water supply by gulls (*Larus* spp.). *Water Res.* 1983;17:789-798.

204. Guix S, Pintó RM, Bosch A. Final consumer options to control and prevent foodborne norovirus infections. *Viruses.* 2019;11:E333.

205. Iturriza-Gomara M, O'Brien SJ. Foodborne viral infections. *Curr Opin Infect Dis.* 2016;29:495-501.

206. Todd EC, Greig JD, Michaels BS, Bartleson CA, Smith D, Holah J. Outbreaks where food workers have been implicated in the spread of foodborne disease. Part 11. Use of antiseptics and sanitizers in community settings and issues of hand hygiene compliance in health care and food industries. *J Food Prot.* 2010;73:2306-2320.

207. Tyndall RL, Ironside KS, Metler PS, Tan EL, Hazen TC, Fliermans CB. Effect of thermal additions on the density distribution of thermophilic amoebae and pathogenic *Naegleria fowleri* in a newly created cooling lake. *Appl Environ Microbiol.* 1989;55:722-732.

208. Kasowski EJ, Gackstetter GD, Sharp TW. Foodborne illness: new developments concerning an old problem. *Curr Gastroenterol Rep.* 2002;4:308-318.

209. Genigeorgis C. Problems associated with perishable processed meats. *Food Technol.* 1986;40:140-154.

210. Beckers HJ. Incidence of foodborne diseases in The Netherlands: annual summary 1982 and an overview from 1979 to 1982. *J Food Prot.* 1988;51:327-354.

211. Wadowsky RM, Yee RB. Satellite growth of *Legionella pneumophila* with an environmental isolate of *Flavobacterium breve. Appl Environ Microbiol.* 1983;46:1447-1449.

212. Stewart KR, Kodistschek L. Drug-resistance transfer in *Escherichia coli* in New York Bight Sediment. *Mar Pollut Bull.* 1980;11:130-133.

213. Maheshwari M, Ahmad I, Althubiani AS. Multidrug resistance and transferability of blaCTX-M among extended-spectrum β-lactamase-producing enteric bacteria in biofilm. *J Glob Antimicrob Resist.* 2016;6:142-149.

214. Mo SS, Sunde M, Ilag HK, Langsrud S, Heir E. Transfer potential of plasmids conferring extended-spectrum-cephalosporin resistance in *Escherichia coli* from poultry. *Appl Environ Microbiol.* 2017;83:e00654-17.

215. Barbaree JM, Fields JM, Feeley JC, Gorman GW, Martin WT. Isolation of protozoa from water associated with legionellosis outbreak and demonstration of intracellular multiplication of *Legionella pneumophila. Appl Environ Microbiol.* 1986;51:422-424.

216. Seaman MT, Gophen M, Cavari BZ, Azoulay B. *Brachionus calyciflorus* Pallas as an agent for removal of *E. coli* in sewage ponds. *Hydrobiologia.* 1986;135:55-60.

217. El-Sahn MA, El-Banna AA, El-Tabbey Shehata AM. Occurrence of *Vibrio parahaemolyticus* in selected marine invertebrates, sediment, and seawater around Alexandria, Egypt. *Can J Microbiol.* 1982;28:1261-1264.

218. Lewis GD, Austin FJ, Loutit MW. Enteroviruses of human origin and faecal coliforms in riverwater and sediments downstream from a sewage outfall in Taieri River, Otago. *J Mar Res.* 1986;20:101-105.

219. Sobsey MD, Shields PA, Hauchman FH, Hazard R, Caton L. Survival and transport of hepatitis A virus in soils, groundwater, and wastewater. *Water Sci Technol.* 1986;18:97-106.

220. Bowen GS, McCarty MA. Hepatitis A associated with a hardware store water fountain and contaminated well in Lancaster County, Pennsylvania, 1980. *Am J Epidemiol.* 1983;117:695-705.

221. Vaughn JM, Landry EF, Thomas MZ. Entrainment of viruses from septic tank leach fields through a shallow, sandy, soil aquifer. *Appl Environ Microbiol.* 1983;45:1474-1480.

222. Hassard F, Gwyther CL, Farkas K, et al. Abundance and distribution of enteric bacteria and viruses in coastal and estuarine sediments—a review. *Front Microbiol.* 2016;7:1692.

223. Vasconcelos GJ, Anthony NC. Microbiological quality of recreational waters in the Pacific northwest. *J Water Pollut Control.* 1985;57:366-377.

224. Taylor SL. Marine toxins of microbial origin. *Food Technol.* 1988;42:94-98.

225. Burkholder JM. Implications of harmful microalgae and heterotrophic dinoflagellates in management of sustainable marine fisheries. *Ecol Appl.* 1998;8:537-562.

226. Bullerman LB. Mycotoxins and food safety. *Food Technol.* 1986;40:59-66.

227. Stoloff L. Toxigenic fungi. In: Speck M, ed. *Compendium of Methods for the Microbiological Examination of Foods.* Washington, DC: American Public Health Association; 1954:557-572.

228. US Food and Drug Administration. *Foodborne Pathogenic Microorganisms & Natural Toxins Handbook: Onset, Duration, and Symptoms of Foodborne Illness.* Giza, Egypt: US Food and Drug Administration, Center for Food Safety and Applied Nutrition; 1998.

229. Bingham AK, Meyer EA. Giardia excystation can be induced in vitro in acidic solutions. *Nature.* 1979;277:301-302.

230. Marshall BJ, Warren JR. Unidentified curved bacilli in the stomach of patients with gastritis and peptic ulceration. *Lancet.* 1984;323:1311-1315.

231. Goodwin CS, McConnell W, McCullough RK, et al. Transfer of *Campylobacter pylori* and *Campylobacter mustelae* to *Helicobacter* gen. nov. as *Helicobacter pylori*, comb. nov. and *Helicobacter mustelae* comb. nov. respectively. *Int J Syst Bacteriol.* 1989;39:397-405.

232. Sachs G, Weeks DL, Wen Y, Marcus EA, Scott DR, Melchers K. Acid acclimation by *Helicobacter pylori. Physiology.* 2005;20:429-438.

233. Klemm P, Schembri MA. Bacterial adhesins: function and structure. *Int J Med Microbiol.* 2000;290:27-35.

234. Racaniello VR, Mendelsohn CL, Morrison M, et al. Molecular genetics of cellular receptors for polio-virus. In: Brinton MA, Heinz FX, eds. *New Aspects of Positive-Strand RNA Viruses.* Washington, DC: American Society for Microbiology; 1990:278-294.

235. Hsu KL, Paglini S, Alstein B, et al. Identification of a second cellular receptor for a coxsackievirus B3 variant, CB3-RD. In: Brinton MA, Heinz FX, eds. *New Aspects of Positive-Strand RNA Viruses.* Washington, DC: American Society for Microbiology; 1990:271-277.

236. Miller JF, Mekalanos JJ, Falkow S. Coordinate regulation and sensory transduction in the control of bacterial virulence. *Science.* 1989;243:916-921.

237. Finlay BB, Falkow S. Common themes in microbial pathogenicity. *Microbiol Rev.* 1989;53:210-230.

238. Finlay BB, Heffron F, Falkow S. Epithelial cell surfaces induce *Salmonella* proteins required for bacterial adherence and invasion. *Science.* 1989;243:940-943.

239. Fields PL, Groisman EA, Heffron E. A *Salmonella* locus that controls resistance to microbial proteins from phagocytic cells. *Science.* 1989;243:1059-1061.

240. Portnoy DA, Moseley SL, Falkow S. Characterization of plasmids and plasmid-associated determinants of *Yersinia enterocolitica* pathogenesis. *Infect Immun.* 1981;31:775-782.

241. Maurelli AT, Blackmon B, Curtiss R III. Temperature-dependent expression of virulence genes in *Shigella* species. *Infect Immun.* 1984;43:195-201.

242. Gargiullo L, Del Chierico F, D'Argenio P, Putignani L. Gut microbiota modulation for multidrug-resistant organism decolonization: present and future perspectives. *Front Microbiol.* 2019;10:1704.

243. Gentile CL, Weir TL. The gut microbiota at the intersection of diet and human health. *Science.* 2018;362:776-780.

244. US Food and Drug Administration. *HACCP Guidelines.* Washington, DC: US Department of Health and Human Services Public Health Service, US Food and Drug Administration; 1997.

245. Food and Agriculture Organization, World Health Organization. HACCP principles and practice: teacher's handbook; 1999. World Health Organization Web site. https://www.who.int/foodsafety/publications/haccp-principles/en/. Accessed August 15, 2019.

246. Fung F, Wang HS, Menon S. Food safety in the 21st century. *Biomed J.* 2018;41:88-95.

247. World Health Organization. *The Role of Food Safety in Health and Development. Report of a Joint FAO/WHO Expert Committee on Food Safety.* Geneva, Switzerland: World Health Organization; 1984. World technical report series 705.

248. Urbain WM. Food irradiation: the past fifty years as prologue to tomorrow. *Food Technol.* 1989;43:76:76-92.

249. Taub IA. Radiation pasteurization and sterilization of food. *Stud Phys Theor Chem.* 2001;87:705-737.

250. Doyle MP, Diez-Gonzalez F, Hill C. *Food Microbiology: Fundamentals and Frontiers.* 5th ed. Washington, DC: ASM Press; 2019.

251. Stern NJ, Meinersmann RJ. Potentials for colonization control of *Campylobacter jejuni* in the chickens. *J Food Prot.* 1989;52:427-430.

252. Mead GC, Impey CS. The present status of the Nurmi concept for reducing carriage of food-poisoning salmonellae and other pathogens in live poultry. In: Smulders FJM, ed. *Elimination of Pathogenic Organisms From Meat and Poultry.* Amsterdam, Netherlands: Elsevier; 1987:57-77.

253. Beery JT, Hugdahl MB, Doyle MR Colonization of gastrointestinal tracts of chicks by *Campylobacter jejuni. Appl Environ Microbiol.* 1988;54:2365-2370.

254. Milner KC, Shaffer ME. Bacteriologic studies of experimental *Salmonella* infection in chicks. *J Infect Dis.* 1952;90:81-96.

255. Nurmi E, Rantala M. New aspects of *Salmonella* infection in broiler production. *Nature.* 1973;241:210-211.

256. Seuna E. Sensitivity of young chickens to *Salmonella typhimurium* var. Copenhagen and *S. infantis* infection and the preventive effect of cultured intestinal microflora. *Avian Dis.* 1979;23:392-400.

257. Snoeyenbos GH, Weinack OM, Soerjadi AS. Our current understanding of the role of native microflora in limiting some bacterial pathogens of chickens and turkeys. In: *Australian Veterinary Poultry Association and International Union of Immunological Societies. Proceedings No. 66: Disease Prevention and Control in Poultry Production.* Sydney, Australia: Australian Veterinary Poultry Association and International Union of Immunological Societies; 1983:45-51.

258. Hume ME, Corner DE, Nisbet DJ, DeLoach JR. Early *Salmonella* challenge time and reduction in chick cecal colonization following treatment with a characterized competitive exclusion culture. *J Food Prot.* 1998;61:673-676.

259. Gusils G, Pérez Chaia A, González S, Oliver G. Lactobacilli isolated from chicken intestines: potential use as probiotics. *J Food Prot.* 1999;62:252-256.

260. Ashenafi M, Busse M. Inhibitory effect of *Lactobacillus plantarum* on *Salmonella infantis, Enterobacter aerogenes* and *Escherichia coli* during tempeh fermentation. *J Food Prot.* 1989;52:169-172.

261. Markowiak P, Śliżewska K. Effects of probiotics, prebiotics, and synbiotics on human health. *Nutrients.* 2017;9: E1021.

262. Paulson JC. Interaction of animal viruses with cell surface receptors. In: Conn PM, ed. *The Receptors.* Vol 2. New York, NY: Academic Press; 1985:131-219.

263. Eidels L, Proia RL, Hart DA. Membrane receptors for bacterial toxins. *Microbiol Rev.* 1983;4:596-620.

264. Clegg S, Gerlach GF. Enterobacterial fimbriae. *J Bacteriol.* 1987;169: 934-938.

265. Eisenstein BI. Type I fimbriae of *Escherichia coli*: genetic regulation, morphogenesis, and role in pathogenesis. *Rev Infect Dis.* 1988;10(suppl 2):341-344.

266. Proctor RA. The staphylococcal fibronectin receptor: evidence for its importance in invasive infection. *Rev Infect Dis.* 1987;9:335-340.

267. Courtney HS, Stanislawski L, Ofek I, Simpson WA, Hasty DL, Beachey EH. Localization of a lipoteichoic acid binding site to a 24-kilodalton NH2-terminal fragment of fibronectin. *Rev Infect Dis.* 1988;10:360-362.

268. McHan F, Cox NA, Blankenship LC, Bailey JS. In vitro attachment of *Salmonella typhimurium* to chick ceca exposed to selected carbohydrates. *Avian Dis.* 1989;33:340-344.

269. Jones GW, Freter R. Adhesion properties of *Vibrio cholerae*: nature of the interaction with isolated rabbit brush border membranes and human erythrocytes. *Infect Immun.* 1976;14:240-245.

270. Fox JL. Bacterial lectins and the cranberry factor. *ASM News.* 1989;55:657.

271. Ofek I, Hasty DL, Sharon N. Anti-adhesion therapy of bacterial diseases: prospects and problems. *FEMS Immunol Med Microbiol.* 2003;38:181-191.

272. US Department of Agriculture. Cost estimates of foodborne illnesses. US Department of Agriculture Web site. https://www.ers.usda.gov/data-products/cost-estimates-of-cost-estimates-of-foodborne-illnesses/. Accessed August 15, 2019.

CHAPTER
57

Groundwater Purification

Nicholas P. Cheremisinoff and Chris Brown

Water purification is the process by which undesired chemical compounds, organic and inorganic materials, as well as biological contaminants are removed from water. There are multiple processes that serve this purpose. Selection and costs depend on the type and nature of contaminants, the extent of contamination, the cleanup or purification levels that are defined or established from statutory standards, and the intended use of the purified water. A major purpose of water purification is to provide potable drinking water. Water purification is also intended to meet the needs of medical, pharmacological, chemical, and industrial applications for clean and potable water as well as agricultural use. Purification reduces the concentration of contaminants such as suspended particles, parasites, bacteria, algae, viruses, fungi, as well as chemical constituents introduced from manufacturing operations that are often the result of spills and other unintentional releases to ground and surface water sources.

Water purification operations are implemented on scales spanning from the large (eg, for an entire city) to the small (eg, for individual households). Most communities rely on natural bodies of water as intake sources for water purification and for day-to-day use. In general, these resources can be classified as groundwater or surface water and include underground aquifers, creeks, streams, rivers, and lakes. Oceans and saltwater seas have also been used as alternative water sources for drinking and domestic use. This chapter provides an overview of water purification technologies that are commonly applied in industrial settings and remedial activities. Available technologies must be carefully assessed in terms of their suitability for an intended application. Although the processes can be classified generically, many purification applications require unique engineering solutions to meet water quality targets.[1]

GROUNDWATER CONTAMINATION RISK

When groundwater has been adversely impacted, a variety of sciences, strategies, technologies, and actions are needed to assess human and ecological risks from contamination. The first step in assessing impacts requires an environmental site assessment. The goal of an environmental site assessment is to identify recognized environmental conditions, referring to the presence of any hazardous or petroleum substances on a property under conditions that indicate release into the ground, groundwater, or surface water.[2]

In the United States, as an example, the control and prevention of the entry of hazardous substances into the environment is the objective of several acts of congress. Rules regulating various aspects of hazardous waste can be attributed to the Toxic Substances Control Act; Clean Water Act; Clean Air Act; Federal Insecticide, Fungicide, and Rodenticide Act; Safe Drinking Water Act; Resource Conservation and Recovery Act (RCRA); and the Comprehensive Environmental Response, Compensation, and Liability Act (CERCLA). The RCRA and CERCLA are the two that are most often associated with environmental site assessments. Many, if not most, state agencies publish risk-based cleanup criteria for industrial sites and recognize "mixing zone" concepts that allow stable contaminated plumes to attenuate in place so long as surface water and drinking water resources are protected. The ASTM International has also developed a risk-based corrective action standard for chlorinated solvents that is similar to the standard developed for fuel.[3]

The nature and extent of a site's groundwater contamination must be defined in part with a conceptual model. The investigator needs to develop a useful conceptual site model or update an existing one and determine what human or ecological receptors may be at risk and how to limit their exposure to the contamination. An accurate conceptual site model is critical to evaluating the true risk of contamination as well as the possibilities and limitations of site remediation strategies. A complete model should include a visual representation of contaminant source and release information, site geology and hydrology, contaminant distribution, fate and transport parameters, and risk assessment features such as current and future land use and potential exposure pathways and receptors. The conceptual site model should be developed as a part of the site investigation or feasibility study phase of site remediation. Many interim remedial systems have been installed and are operating without a well-defined model, oftentimes leading to major cost overruns or inability to achieve cleanup goals within reasonable time periods. Some remedial systems were designed based on an initial model that requires updating based on recent operations and monitoring data. Changes in land use, or changes in the enforcement of institutional controls, can also alter the exposure and risk assumptions of the model. It is important to recognize that the conceptual site model is intended to be a dynamic representation of site conditions based on a continual influx of information from the site. The following are important elements of a conceptual site model.

Source and Release Information

The model should include a description of the source of contamination and what is known about the timing and quantity of the release. Most site characterizations begin by locating areas where chemical contaminants were originally released to the subsurface. In many cases, the distinct source of contamination is known to be a former underground storage tank, disposal pit, a leaking pipeline, a spill, etc; however, many industrial source areas are dispersed and sometimes difficult to delineate. For example, oil/water separators and sanitary and storm sewers have historically received chlorinated solvents from process operations or various plant maintenance shops. At such sites, it may be impossible to pinpoint the exact source of contamination.

The timing and amount of chemical contaminants released are equally difficult to estimate. Historical records on chemical uses are sometimes difficult to obtain, and if they exist are generally found in Phase I Installation Restoration Program documents developed in the United States in the early 1980s. Many sites as examples used chlorinated solvents like trichloroethylene (TCE), which was used for decades at some operations before it was phased out in the early 1980s. Such chemicals may not have been widely used at a facility for nearly 20 to 30 years. This fact is important when evaluating the fate and transport of chlorinated solvents or any chemical contaminant and is especially important when estimating

degradation rates based on the breakdown products of certain chemicals like the chlorinated solvents.

Geological and Hydrogeological Characterization

The model must include a complete description of the site geology and hydrogeology. The descriptions should include the following at a minimum:

- A general description of site geology including major soil strata that are impacted by or influence the migration of contaminants. Strata thickness, lateral extent, continuity and depositional features should be described.
- Physical and chemical properties of subsurface materials such as sieve analysis, bulk density, porosity, and total organic carbon
- Geological or man-made features, which may provide preferential migration of chemicals, dense nonaqueous phase liquids (DNAPLs), solvent vapors, or dissolved contaminants
- Depth to groundwater, seasonal variations, recharge, and discharge information including interactions with surface waters
- Ranges of hydraulic gradients (horizontal and vertical)
- Ranges of hydraulic properties (eg, hydraulic conductivity, storage coefficient, effective porosity, seepage velocity)
- Geochemical properties influencing the natural biodegradation of the chemical contaminants

This may need to be updated to reflect current estimates of these properties based on site remediation experience. For example, the hydraulic properties of an aquifer can be more accurately estimated after a groundwater extraction system has operated several months. On sites where natural attenuation has been selected as the groundwater remedy, tracking the movement (or stability) of the contaminant plume provides essential information that can be introduced into an updated model.

Contaminant Distribution, Transport, and Fate

The model should include a summary of the chemical, physical, and biodegradation properties of key contaminants of concern and describe their distribution, movement, and fate in the subsurface environment. Descriptions should include the following:

- Chemical and physical properties of the chemical contaminants that impact subsurface transport (eg, partitioning coefficients, solubility, vapor pressure, Henry's law, density, viscosity)
- Estimates of the phase distribution of each contaminant in the saturated and unsaturated zone

- Temporal trends in contaminant concentrations in each phase
- Geochemical evidence of contaminant natural attenuation processes (destructive and nondestructive)

Geochemistry Impacting Natural Biodegradation

Under certain conditions, geochemical parameters may favor natural biodegradation of some chemicals. Examples of these can be found with chlorinated solvents. Geochemical indicators such as dissolved oxygen, nitrate, iron, manganese, sulfate, methane, and hydrogen ion concentrations should be reported in the conceptual site model. In the case of groundwater contamination caused by chlorinated solvents, the relative distribution of primary solvents such as tetrachloroethene (PCE) and TCE and daughter products such as 1,2-dichloroethane (DCE) and vinyl chloride should be documented in relation to the geochemical profile of the site.

Risk-Based Cleanup Goals and Screening Level Evaluations

Important considerations for defining risk-based goals are the following:

- Determining the risk-based screening levels that are appropriate for a contaminated site
- Developing site-specific cleanup goals based on realistic exposure scenarios at the site
- Estimating the average exposure concentration as opposed to the maximum concentration at the site

Once a conceptual site model has been devised, defining the source of chemical contamination, potential pathways, and potential receptors, the task of defining risk-based cleanup objectives may begin. This can be approached as a two-step process involving the following actions:

- First, an initial comparison of potential exposure concentrations to conservative industrial screening levels for each contaminant of concern can be made. For sites with potential discharges to surface water bodies, a comparison to ecological screening levels may be deemed appropriate.
- Second, any contaminant exceeding conservative screening levels can be evaluated using more realistic, site-specific exposure assumptions to determine if an unacceptable human health or ecological risk could or potentially exist.

A two-step approach provides flexibility to replace potentially conservative, nonsite-specific exposure assumptions with site-specific information while still providing the same level of human health and environmental

resource protection. The investigator is likely to encounter increasingly complex levels of data collection and risk along the process. The evaluation will need to be performed in order to establish the type and magnitude of remediation required to reduce or eliminate unacceptable risks at a particular site. This may be accomplished by replacing nonsite-specific (ie, default) assumptions about how chemicals behave in the environment and how receptors may be exposed, with site-specific data and assumptions that are more representative of actual site conditions and realistic exposure pathways for human and ecological receptors.

A screening level evaluation provides a means of identifying whether a particular chemical warrants additional risk evaluation. Screening levels are conservative (health protective), generic cleanup criteria that define the residual amount of a contaminant that can remain onsite and not present an unacceptable risk to potential receptors. For sites with the potential for discharge to surface waters, ecological screening levels are appropriate. Industrial screening levels for human receptors are generally based on reasonable maximum exposure assumptions and can be either health protective or designed to mitigate nuisances associated with chemical contamination (eg, taste and odor). In order to select (or develop) appropriate screening levels, information about the current and potential future land and groundwater uses at/or down-gradient from the affected site must be thoroughly documented in the conceptual site model. It is common practice to consider screening levels for industrial land use scenarios over prolonged periods of say 25 years and by taking into consideration exposure to all contaminated media. Many published industrial screening levels assume ingestion of onsite groundwater by a specific receptor group (eg, industrial onsite workers). Such assumptions may or may not be realistic; however, such conservative screening levels may be appropriate if groundwater use cannot be absolutely controlled through pumping restrictions or pump and treat strategies.

Once the appropriate land use category has been defined, the types of exposure pathways to be considered in the screening evaluation should be defined. An essential step in defining appropriate screening levels is determining the risk target level. Acceptable target risk ranges for carcinogens (eg, chlorinated solvent contamination and in particular vinyl chloride) fall between 10^{-6} and 10^{-4}.[1] The risk ranges are equivalent to an added lifetime cancer risk of 1 in 1 000 000 to 1 in 10 000 for people exposed to site contamination. Screening levels for carcinogens typically are based on an extremely protective 10^{-6} target risk level that is referred to as a *de minimis* risk level, meaning that a 1 in 1 000 000 risk level is so small as to be of negligible concern. A 10^{-6} target risk level should be considered health protective, given that the "normal background level" of cancer in the general population is about 1 in 3 persons (30%-35%). The US Environmental Protection Agency (EPA) reports that for carcinogens, a 10^{-6} target risk level for individual chemicals and pathways generally will lead to cumulative risks within the 10^{-4} to 10^{-6} risk range for the combinations of chemicals typically found at contaminated sites.[4] In addition to potential human receptors, a screening level evaluation should consider potential ecological receptors and other environmental resources that could be impacted by site contaminants.[5]

Once applicable screening levels are identified, the evaluation process consists of comparing representative exposure-point concentrations from recent site sampling events to applicable screening levels. It is important to use the most recent site contamination data. It is good practice to evaluate the two most recent sampling events and a comparison of maximum detected site concentrations to applicable screening levels. The use of statistically averaged site concentrations may be appropriate at some sites.

▶ DENSE NONAQUEOUS PHASE LIQUIDS

The DNAPLs are liquids that are only slightly soluble in water and therefore exist in the subsurface as a separate fluid phase immiscible with both water and air. Common types include wood treating oils such as creosote, transformer and insulating oils containing polychlorinated biphenyls, coal tar, and chlorinated solvents such as TCE and PCE with other, less frequently encountered being mercury and certain crude oils. Most DNAPL products are toxic and some compounds are highly mobile in the subsurface and groundwater. Unlike light nonaqueous phase liquids such as gasoline and heating oil (products that are less dense than water), DNAPLs are denser than water

and have the ability to migrate to significant depths below the water table. There they slowly dissolve into flowing groundwater, giving rise to aqueous phase plumes. Releases of DNAPLs at the ground surface can result in long-term contamination of both the unsaturated and saturated zones at a site. Although DNAPLs have been produced and heavily used in industry since the beginning of the 20th century, their importance as soil and groundwater contaminants was not recognized or understood until the 1980s. This lack of recognition was partly due to the fact that the analytical methods and tools required to detect low concentrations of organic compounds in groundwater were not widely available or used until relatively recently.

Essentially, all DNAPLs can be characterized by their density, viscosity, interfacial tension with water, component composition, solubility in water, vapor pressure, and wettability. When a DNAPL is released at the ground surface, it will migrate both vertically and laterally in the subsurface (Figure 57.1). The amount of residual DNAPL retained by a typical porous medium such as silt, sand, and gravel may range between 5% and 20% of the available pore space.

Remedial strategies and technologies are selected by taking into consideration the effectiveness, practicability, durability, and likely costs and benefits of the various remediation options. The EPA seeks to ensure that within this framework, the most sustainable approach to remediation is selected. The area of contamination that is the focus of remediation may vary from site to site but typically involves one or both of the following:

- A DNAPL present within the source zone along with the associated aqueous and sorbed phase contamination in the source zone. If unsaturated media is involved, vapor phase contamination may also be addressed.

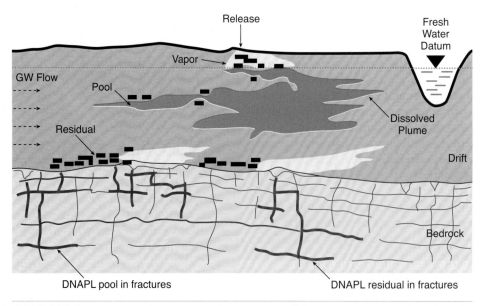

FIGURE 57.1 Conceptual illustration of a migration of dense nonaqueous phase liquid (DNAPL) released to ground surface. Abbreviation: GW, ground water.

- Aqueous phase contamination present downstream of the DNAPL source zone. This will typically have sorbed phase contamination (on the soil or aquifer materials) associated with it and may include vapor phase contamination in unsaturated media.

GROUNDWATER REMEDIATION STRATEGIES FOR CHLORINATED CHEMICALS

The selection of effective remediation strategies is often not straightforward due to the nature of chlorinated compound contamination. Site soil conditions can limit the selection of a treatment process. Process-limiting characteristics such as pH or moisture content may sometimes be adjusted. In other cases, a treatment technology may be eliminated based on the soil classification (eg, particle-size distribution) or other soil characteristics. Soils are inherently variable in their physical and chemical characteristics. Usually, the variability is much greater vertically than horizontally, resulting from the variability in the processes that originally formed the soils. The soil variability, in turn, will result in variability in the distribution of water and contaminants and in the ease with which they can be transported within, and removed from, the soil at a particular site. The following are common treatment technologies.

Soil Excavation, Treatment, and Disposal

If a discrete source zone containing DNAPL is identified and isolated, then a possible remediation strategy is the excavation of contaminated soil. Soil excavation methods are well established; after soil containing DNAPL has been removed from a source zone, it may be properly disposed, or treated—strategies include disposal in hazardous waste landfills, biodegradation cells, thermal desorption, chemical oxidation. Soils contaminated with chlorinated solvents generally cannot be disposed of in landfills unless they can be shown to be nontoxic based on the Toxic Characteristic Leaching Procedure.

Successful contaminant source removal/excavation starts with the collection of a sufficient number of soil/sediment samples to adequately characterize the extent of the contaminant source area, including variations in lithologies. A variety of equipment has been used to excavate contaminated soil or remove contaminated media. Typical machinery includes backhoes and track hoes for soil excavations and storage tank removals. Small track hoes are used inside buildings to excavate contaminated soils inside a building. Vacuum trucks are used to excavate contaminated soil, remove contaminated sediments from soakage pits and cleanout contaminated sludge and wastewater from septic tanks. Vacuum trucks can be used for shallow excavations under building floor slabs where access is limited. At some sites where remediation is performed indoors, a portion of the floor slab is cut out at contaminant source areas and the vacuum truck is parked near the facility, where the vacuum hose can access the excavation via the service door. Contaminated soil is removed down to the water table and then the excavation is backfilled with grout or sand and the floor slab restored.

Soil Vapor Extraction

Soil vapor extraction (SVE) strategies were developed to remove volatile contaminants from unsaturated soils. The SVE is a frequently used remedial strategy in situations where excavation is not feasible due to the presence of physical obstructions (eg, buildings, utilities, trees, etc), or where the extent of soil contamination is extensive. The SVE systems can be very effective at minimizing indoor vapor intrusion by keeping the contaminated soil vapors closer to the source area. The technology involves the application of a vacuum to slotted pipes in the vadose zone to draw air through contaminated material. The air flow volatilizes contaminants from the DNAPL, soil, and aqueous phases. The goal of most SVE operations at DNAPL sites is to remove sufficient contaminant mass so that water percolating through the vadose zone will no longer dissolve contaminants and transport them to the water table at concentrations exceeding regulatory limits. An SVE is capable of achieving the goal in relatively homogeneous, coarse-grained soils where air can rapidly move through the contaminant zone. An SVE is not as effective in mobilizing contaminants from the capillary fringe or in fine-grained or very moist strata. Slow diffusion of contaminants from residual DNAPL entrapped in these zones limit restoration rates.

Enhanced Methods of Soil Vapor Extraction

Multiphase extraction refers to remediation strategies that incorporate combinations of groundwater pumping, DNAPL removal, and SVE using a single well to extract both liquid and vapor. Depending on the site, the depth at which SVE can be applied is increased by lowering the water table with groundwater extraction. At sites with mobile DNAPL, a low rate of groundwater pumping can be applied to lower the water table while applying SVE to enhance liquid migration toward the well and to remove volatiles from the expanded unsaturated zone. The multiphase extraction strategy is applicable at sites with permeable soils, where the majority of the DNAPL is trapped within the upper 10 ft (3.05 m) of the aquifer. Multiphase extraction is less successful at sites with low-permeability soils because dewatering at the well may not result in a significant reduction in the water saturation level of the soil. In this case, the air permeability of the soil will not be improved by application of simple dewatering.

Another strategy is applying thermal enhancements to SVE system. In situ heating methods that have received attention are aimed at reducing soil moisture and thereby enhancing SVE effectiveness by extending SVE influence into shallow aquifers. In situ heating strategies offer potential to increase the permeability of silt and clay soils and increase the removal efficiency of SVE. Steam injection combined with vacuum extraction may also be considered an approach to remove volatile DNAPL from the vadose and shallow groundwater zones. When high pressure "dry" steam is injected into contaminated soil, volatile chemicals with boiling points lower than that of water are vaporized. The SVE wells are then used to remove the resulting vapor. This process has been applied at smaller sites with relatively uniform permeable soils but may not be as effective in layered soils. Other methods use resistive or radio frequency heating for increasing soil temperatures and volatilizing DNAPL residuals. The most promising of the resistive heating technologies is a six-phase system, which uses metal and graphite electrodes to set up an alternating electrical current in the soil.[6] This strategy is limited to sites with soil moisture levels above 10% because water is required to conduct the electricity and to create resistive heating. Resistive heating can reach a maximum temperature of 100°C, which boils away the groundwater and can volatilize residual DNAPLs. Once volatilized, volatile organic compounds are removed by a concurrently operating SVE system. Radio frequency heating is a process that uses electrodes placed in the subsurface to deliver radio frequency energy that excite molecular motion and induce heating (in the same way that microwave ovens heat food). Radio frequency heating has the potential to heat soil to temperatures in excess of 200°C and can be used to volatilize higher boiling point compounds such as mixtures of jet fuel and solvents. The SVE wells are then used to remove the resulting vapor.[7]

In situ Air Sparging

In situ air sparging is the process of injecting air into the saturated zone with the objective of stripping the contaminants from the dissolved phase and transferring these compounds to a vapor phase. The strategy competes with conventional baseline technologies of pump-and-treat and pump-and-treat combined with SVE. Vertical well air sparging and in well recirculation technologies have been implemented at a number of sites.

An air sparge network consists of sparge points designed to deliver air to a specific zone of contaminated groundwater. Air compressors deliver contaminant-free air under pressure to the target zones. The vapor migrates upward from the saturated zone to the unsaturated zone. The vapor phase is then vented through the unsaturated zone to the atmosphere and typically uses an SVE in the unsaturated zone to more effectively control, treat, and remove the vapor plume from the unsaturated zone.

Volatile, semivolatile, and nonvolatile organic contaminants in dissolved, free-phase, sorbed, and vapor phases can be treated using air sparging. Air sparging is applicable for the treatment of less volatile and/or tightly sorbed chemicals that could not be remediated using vapor extraction alone. Contaminants affected by the volatilization and biodegradation processes of air sparging include various fuels (eg, gasoline, diesel, jet fuel), oils and greases, and the chlorinated solvents (PCE, TCE, DCE, etc). Some commercially available systems (eg, BioSparge®) employs an ozone generator with the air sparging technique to extend the capabilities of the technology to chlorinated phenols (pentachlorophenol [PCP]), alcohols, ketones, and other industrial solvents. The injected ozone breaks the chlorine bonds, facilitating biodegradation of the resulting compounds.

Enhanced Biodegradation

Combinations of anaerobic and aerobic biological degradation represent a strategy that is theoretically capable of completely degrading chlorinated solvents to harmless by-products.[1] The strategy has been primarily applied to the dissolved phase of chlorinated solvent plumes. A promising biotechnology for DNAPL removal is enhanced reductive dechlorination. Under highly anaerobic conditions, chlorinated solvents such as PCE, TCE, and DCE are used as electron acceptors by subsurface bacteria. In this process, chlorine atoms are sequentially removed from the chlorinated solvent molecule.

Natural attenuation processes refer to biodegradation, dispersion, sorption, and volatilization, all of which affect the fate and transport of chlorinated solvents in all hydrological systems. When these processes are shown to be capable of attaining site-specific remediation objectives in a time period that is reasonable compared to other strategies, they may be selected alone or in combination with other more active remedies as the preferred remedial strategy. The EPA defines monitored natural attenuation as the reliance on natural attenuation processes (within a controlled and monitored cleanup approach) to achieve site-specific remedial objectives within a time frame that is reasonable compared to other methods.[8] Natural attenuation processes include biodegradation, dispersion, dilution, sorption, volatilization, and chemical or biological stabilization, transformation, or destruction of contaminants. Such processes are typically used in conjunction with other active remediation measures or as a follow-up these that have already been implemented.

In-Well Aeration and Recirculation

In-well aeration is a strategy that involves injecting air into a well with the intended purposes of

- stripping volatile organics from groundwater that enters the well
- adding oxygen to the groundwater
- displacement and recirculation of groundwater outside of the well

The first two (stripping of volatiles and addition of oxygen) are almost certain to occur at any site; however, the recirculation of groundwater outside of the well has not been consistently proven in sandy aquifers, and most will not occur in low-permeability soils. The shortfall of this strategy is the limited influence that oxygen addition or volatiles stripping will have outside of the well. The strategy has a limited radius of influence, and as such, large number of recirculation wells may be needed to contain a plume; an inordinate number of wells would be required for total plume remediation. Geochemical changes inside of the recirculation well have led to fouling and high costs.

Reactive and Permeable Walls

A strategy of improving the uniformity of groundwater treatment is to install a semipermeable barrier that can either physically or biologically remove contaminants as groundwater passes through an in situ treatment wall. In situ treatment walls may be effective for preventing plumes from discharging to a drainage ditch or migrating off of a site. Several types of physical, chemical, and biological treatment can be completed using semipermeable barriers. Barrier wall technologies are best suited for sites where the plume is not stable and is migrating off-site or toward receptors. This strategy is more effective in shallow aquifers and can become unworkable and costly as the thickness of the aquifer increases.

Volatile chlorinated solvent contamination can be physically removed from shallow groundwater by creating an air sparging curtain of closely spaced sparge wells or by placing a horizontal sparge well in a gravel-filled trench that intercepts groundwater flow. By using a gravel-filled trench, some of the short-circuiting problems common to air sparging can be eliminated. The removal of dilute concentrations of chlorinated compounds can generally be completed without an SVE collection system. Zero-valent iron barrier walls are currently being applied for the reductive dechlorination of chlorinated solvent plumes. This approach has been applied at many sites and is achieving contaminant destruction with only minimal geochemical fouling.[9] Initial installation costs for zero-valent iron barrier walls can be high for sites with rapid groundwater movement because of the residence time required for complete dechlorination of vinyl chloride. This technology can achieve complete remediation in with just a few feet of iron wall where biological treatment can require hundreds of feet.

Biologically induced reductive dechlorination can also occur in an engineered, semipermeable barrier wall. A variety of organic material can be placed in a trench creating a flow-through bioreactor where reductive dechlorination can take place.

▶ MEMBRANE TECHNOLOGIES FOR MINERAL IONS AND NATURAL CONTAMINANTS

Ground water contains mineral ions. These ions slowly dissolve from soil particles, sediments, and rocks as the water travels along mineral surfaces in the pores or fractures of the unsaturated zone and the aquifer. These are referred to as dissolved solids. Some dissolved solids may have originated in the precipitation water or river water that recharges the aquifer. Dissolved solids in any water can be divided into three groups: major constituents, minor constituents, and trace. The total mass of dissolved constituents is referred to as the total dissolved solids (TDS) concentration. All of the dissolved solids are either positively charged ions (cations) or negatively charged ions (anions). The total negative charge of the anions equals the total positive charge of the cations. A high TDS value means that there are more cations and anions in the water than a sample with low TDS. With more ions in the water, the water's electrical conductivity increases. A measurement of water's electrical conductivity provides an indirect measurement of its TDS concentration. At a high TDS concentration, water becomes saline. Water with a TDS above 500 mg/L is not recommended for use as drinking water (eg, in the United States known as EPA's secondary drinking water guidelines[10] or equivalent World Health Organization guidelines[11]). Water with a TDS above 1500 to 2600 mg/L (electrical conductivity [EC] greater than 2.25-4 mmho/cm) is generally considered problematic for irrigation use on crops with low or medium salt tolerance.

Except for natural organic matter originating from top soils, all naturally occurring dissolved solids are *inorganic* constituents, such as minerals, nutrients, and trace elements, including trace metals. Concentrations are measured in milligrams per liter (mg/L) or micrograms per liter (μg/L). Also used to measure concentration are the units parts per billion (ppb) and parts per million (ppm), where 1 ppb ≈ 1 μg/L and 1 ppm ≈ 1 mg/L. Salinity as TDS in units of mg/L can be estimated by assuming 65% of the electrical conductivity value in μS/cm or in μmho/cm. For example, 65 mg/L ≈ 100 μmho/cm or 650 mg/L ≈ 1 mmho/cm. Generally, trace elements occur in such low concentrations that they are not a threat to human health. Many of the trace elements are considered essential for the human metabolism. Water from springs and wells with certain levels of trace elements has long been considered a remedy for ailments. Popular health spas usually are located near such areas. High concentrations of trace metals can also be found in ground water near contaminated sources; however, these may pose potential health threats. Some trace constituents that are associated with industrial pollution, such as arsenic and chromium, may also occur in completely pristine ground water at concentrations that are high enough to make that water unsuitable as drinking water.

Microbial matter is also a natural constituent of ground water. Just as microbes are ubiquitous in the environment, they are common in the subsurface, including ground water. Hydrogeologists increasingly rely on these, for instance, for subsurface bioremediation of contaminated ground water.

Secondary Drinking Water Standards

The United States has National Secondary Drinking Water Regulations (NSDWRs known as secondary standards).[10] These are nonmandatory water quality standards that have been set for 15 contaminants. The EPA does not enforce these secondary maximum contaminant levels. They are established as guidelines to assist public water systems in managing their drinking water for aesthetic considerations, such as taste, color, and odor. These contaminants are not considered to present a risk to human health at these levels. Public water systems may test for these standards on a voluntary basis; however, states generally choose to adopt these as enforceable standards. The EPA reports that if these contaminants are present in water at levels above the standards, the contaminants may cause the water to appear cloudy or colored or to taste or smell bad. This may cause people to stop using water from their public water system even though the water may be safe to drink. Secondary standards are set to give public water systems guidance on removing these chemicals to levels that are below what most people will find to be noticeable.

There are several problems related to secondary contaminants. These problems can be grouped into three categories.

- Aesthetic effects—undesirable tastes or odors, color, and foaming
- Cosmetic effects—effects which do not damage the body but are still undesirable such as skin discoloration, tooth discoloration and pitting
- Technical effects—damage to water equipment or reduced effectiveness of treatment for other contaminants including corrosivity, scaling, and sedimentation

Examples of secondary US federal and specific California standards are summarized in Table 57.1.

TABLE 57.1 US Environmental Protection Agency (EPA) Secondary Drinking Water Standards for inorganics (Federal[a] and California[b])[c]

Contaminant	Maximum Contamination Levels (MCL; mg/L)	
	EPA	California
Inorganics		
Aluminum	0.05-0.2[d]	1 (0.2)[d]
Antimony	0.006	0.006
Arsenic	0.01	0.01
Asbestos	7 MFL[e]	7 MFL[e]
Barium	2	1
Beryllium	0.004	0.004
Cadmium	0.005	0.005
Chromium	0.1	0.05
Copper	1.3[f]	1.3[f]
Cyanide	0.2	0.15
Fluoride	2[d]	2
Lead	0.015[f]	0.015[f]
Mercury	0.002	0.002
Nickel	Remanded	0.1
Nitrate	(As N) 10	(As NO$_3$) 45
Nitrite (as N)	1	1
Total Nitrate/ nitrite (as N)	10	10
Perchlorate	NA	0.006
Selenium	0.05	0.05
Thallium	0.002	0.002

[a]From US Environmental Protection Agency.[10]

[b]From California Water Boards.[12]

[c]Further standards are provided for other contaminants such as radionuclides, volatile organic compounds (VOCs), and disinfection by-products.

[d]Secondary MCL.

[e]MFL = million fibers per liter, with fiber length >10 μm.

[f]Regulatory action level; if system exceeds, it must take certain actions such as additional monitoring, corrosion control studies and treatment, and for lead, a public education program; replaces MCL.

Water Treatment Membrane Technologies

Membrane technologies are considered the most suitable for treating the types of water discussed. A membrane or, more properly, a semipermeable membrane, is a thin layer of material capable of separating substances when a driving force is applied across the membrane. Once considered a technology restricted to desalination, membrane processes are increasingly employed for removal of bacteria and other microorganisms, particulate material, and natural organic material, which can impart color, tastes, and odors to the water and react with disinfectants to form disinfection by-products. As advancements are made in membrane production and module design, capital and operating costs continue to decline. The pressure-driven membrane processes include reverse osmosis (RO), nanofiltration (NF), microfiltration (MF), and ultrafiltration (UF). Another technology worth noting but not discussed here is electrodialysis reversal (ED/EDR). For water with high TDS (TDS >3000 mg/L), ED/EDR or RO may be less costly than the other technologies. As a rough guide, the following provides a summary of the suitability of each technology in terms of contaminant removal type:

- RO—most suitable for salts and low molecular weight (MW) organics
- NF—suitable for organics with MW >400 (daltons); hardness ions
- MF—particles >0.2 μm
- UF—organics with MW >10 000; viruses and colloids
- ED/EDR—most suitable for salts

Note that selection of a membrane technology must take into consideration factors such as membrane pore size, molecular weight cutoff (MWCO), and the applied pressure needed when comparing different membrane systems. The parameter MWCO should be regarded as a measure of membrane pore dimensions because it is a specification used by membrane suppliers to describe a membrane's retention capabilities.

Reverse Osmosis

Osmosis is a natural phenomenon in which a solvent (water) passes through a semipermeable barrier from the side with lower solute concentration to the higher solute concentration side (Figure 57.2). In this case, water flow continues until the chemical potential equilibrium of the solvent is established (Figure 57.2A). At equilibrium, the pressure difference between the two sides of the membrane is equal to the osmotic pressure of the solution. To reverse the flow of water, a pressure difference greater than the osmotic pressure difference is applied (Figure 57.2B). The result is the separation of water from the solution occurs as pure water flows from the high concentration side to the low concentration side. This phenomenon is termed *reverse osmosis* (it has also been referred to as hyperfiltration).

An RO membrane acts as the semipermeable barrier to flow in the RO process, which permits selective passage of a particular species (the solvent, water) while partially or completely retaining other species (solutes).

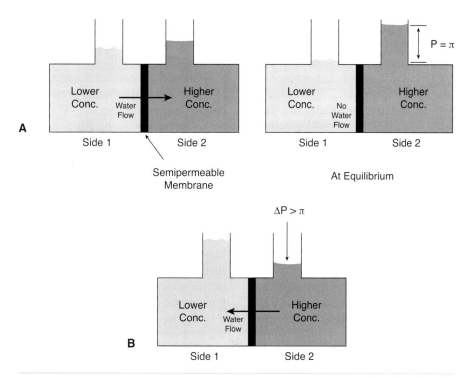

FIGURE 57.2 The basic concept of reverse osmosis. **A** shows the normal process of osmosis, reaching as equilibrium, and **B** the reverse osmosis process. π is the osmotic pressure, and P is pressure.

Chemical potential gradients across the membrane provide the driving forces for solute and solvent transport across the membrane: $-\Delta\mu_s$, the solute chemical potential gradient, is usually expressed in terms of concentration; and $-\Delta\mu_w$, the water chemical potential gradient, is usually expressed in terms of pressure difference across the membrane.[1] Advantages that make it particularly attractive for dilute aqueous wastewater treatment include the following:

- Simple to design and operate. They have low maintenance requirements and are modular in nature, making expansion of systems straightforward.
- Both inorganic and organic pollutants can be removed simultaneously.
- Allow recovery/recycle of waste process streams with no effect on the material being recovered
- Often require less energy and offer lower capital and operating costs than many conventional treatment systems
- Can reduce the volume of waste streams so that these can be treated more efficiently and cost-effectively by other processes such as incineration
- RO systems can replace or be used in conjunction with other treatment processes such as oxidation, adsorption, stripping, or biological treatment (as well as other technologies) to produce a high-quality product water that can be reused or discharged.

Typical industrial applications for RO processes include the treatment of organic containing wastewaters; wastewaters from electroplating and metal finishing operations; pulp and paper effluent streams; mining and petrochemical waste stream; textile manufacturing effluents; generation of high-purity water systems for medical device and pharmaceutical manufacturing processes; and wastes from food processing industries, radioactive wastewater, municipal wastewater, and contaminated groundwater. The ability of RO membranes to remove both inorganic and organic compounds has made the technology attractive for the treatment of contaminated drinking water supplies. The RO processes can simultaneously remove hardness, color, many kinds of bacteria and viruses, and organic contaminants such as agricultural chemicals and trihalomethane precursors.

The RO membrane separations are governed by the properties of the membrane used in the process. These properties depend on the chemical nature of the membrane material that is almost always a polymer as well as its physical structure. Properties for the ideal RO membrane include that it is resistant to chemical and microbial attack, mechanically and structurally stable over long operating periods, and have the desired separation characteristics for each particular system. Few membranes satisfy all these criteria and so compromises must be made to select the best RO membrane available for each application. The RO membranes fall into two categories: asymmetric membranes containing one polymer, and thin-film, composite membranes consisting of two or more polymer layers. Asymmetric RO membranes have a very thin, permselective skin layer supported on a more porous sublayer of the same polymer. The dense skin layer determines the fluxes and selectivities of these membranes, whereas the porous sublayer serves only as a mechanical support for the skin layer and has little effect on the membrane separation properties. Because the skin layer is very thin (from 0.1 to 1 μm), the membrane resistance to water transport (which is proportional to the dense skin thickness) is much lower and, consequently, water fluxes much higher than those through comparable symmetric membranes. Examples of asymmetric membranes include cellulose acetate membranes and linear aromatic polyamide membranes. Among the most widely used thin-film, composite membranes are cross-linked aromatic polyamide on a polysulfone support layer.

Although RO membranes have been formed and tested with a wide range of different materials and preparation techniques, the cellulosic polymers, linear and cross-linked aromatic polyamide, and aryl-alkyl polyetherurea are considered the most important RO membrane materials. Asymmetric cellulose acetate membranes continue to be widely used despite disadvantages such as a narrow pH operating range (pH 4.5-7.5) because it is subject to hydrolysis, susceptibility to biological attack, compaction (mechanical compression) at high pressures that results in reduced water flux, and low upper temperature limits (approximately 35°C). Polyamide and polyurea composite membranes display higher water fluxes and salt and organic rejections, can withstand higher temperature and larger pH variations (pH 4-11), and are more immune to biological attack and compaction. These membranes tend to be less chlorine resistant and more susceptible to oxidation compared to cellulose acetate membranes. They also tend to be more expensive.

Cellulose acetate membranes have often been used in seawater desalination. Although strongly limited in index of pH, the advantages are low material costs and resistance to chlorine, which is used in feed water to inhibit biological fouling. Cellulose acetate membranes have a relatively short operating life and suffer pressure compaction (ie, deterioration of permeate water flow because of creep buckling of the membrane material at high pressure and high temperature). Polyamide and thin-film composite membranes generally have higher water fluxes and higher salt rejections than cellulose acetate membranes. These types of membranes are subject to chlorine attack. If chlorine is added to feed water to control biological growth, the feed water must be dechlorinated before entering the membrane modules.

The RO membranes are commercially available in a variety of configurations. Two of the commercially successful configurations are the spiral-wound module and hollow-fiber module (Figure 57.3). In both

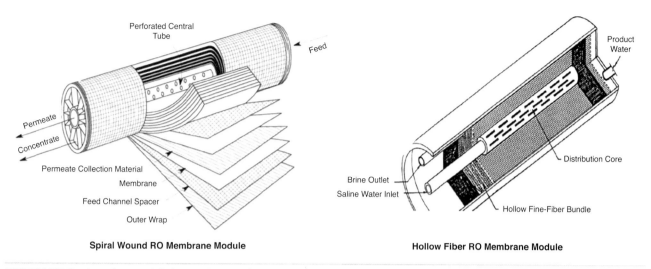

Perforated Central Tube

Feed

Permeate

Concentrate

Permeate Collection Material

Membrane

Feed Channel Spacer

Outer Wrap

Spiral Wound RO Membrane Module

Product Water

Distribution Core

Brine Outlet

Saline Water Inlet

Hollow Fine-Fiber Bundle

Hollow Fiber RO Membrane Module

FIGURE 57.3   Spiral-wound (**left**) and hollow-fiber (**right**) reverse osmosis (RO) membrane modules.

configurations, module elements are serially connected in pressure vessels (up to seven in spiral-wound modules and up to two in hollow-fiber modules). A spiral-wound module element consists of two membrane sheets supported by a grooved or porous support sheet. The support sheet provides the pressure support for the membrane sheets as well as providing the flow path for the product water. Each sheet is sealed along three of its edges, and the fourth edge is attached to a central product discharge tube. A plastic spacer sheet is located on each side of the membrane assembly sheets to provide the flow channels for the feed flow. The entire assembly is spirally wrapped around the central discharge tube forming a compact RO module element. The recovery ratio (permeate flow rate divided by the feed flow rate) of spiral-wound module elements is very low, permitting up to seven elements to be arranged in a single module enabling a higher overall recovery ratio. Spiral-wound membranes have a simple design and relatively high resistance to fouling, operating at pressures as high as 69 bars and recovery ratios up to 45%. Hollow-fiber membranes are made of hairlike fibers, which are united in bundles and arranged in pressure vessels. Typical configurations of hollow-fiber modules are U-tube bundles, which resemble shell and tube heat exchangers. The feed is introduced along a central tube and flows radially outward on the outside of the fibers. The pure water permeates the fiber membranes and flows axially along the inside of the fibers to a header at the end of the bundle. Hollow fibers can withstand pressures as high as 82.7 bar and have high recovery ratios up to 55%.

Basic individual components in an RO system are the high-pressure feed pump and the RO membranes (Figure 57.4). These components are essential and require careful selection and application for an efficient operation. Other important components include pretreatment of the inlet water and equipment for final modifications

and cleanup of treated water. Overall, there are typically four major components to a system.

- Pretreatment section, where the feed water is pretreated to be compatible with the membranes by removing suspended solids, pH adjustment, and the incorporation of a threshold inhibitor to control scaling caused by constituents such as calcium sulfate
- Pressurization section, where the pump raises the pressure of the pretreated feed water to an operating pressure appropriate for the membrane and the salinity of the feed water
- Separation section, where the permeable membranes inhibit the passage of dissolved salts while permitting the desalinated product water to pass through. The saline feed is pumped into a closed vessel where it is pressurized against the membrane. As a portion of the water passes through the membrane, the salt content in the remaining brine increases. At the same time, a portion of this brine is discharged without passing through the membrane.
- Stabilization section, where the product water from the membrane assembly requires a final pH adjustment and degasification before being transferred to the distribution system for use. The product stream may pass through an aeration column in which the pH is elevated from a value of about 5 to close to 7. Oftentimes, this water is discharged to a storage cistern for later use.

Nanofiltration

The NF is often referred to as using "loose" RO membranes. These membranes typically have much higher water fluxes at low pressures compared to traditional RO membranes. The NF membranes are usually charged with carboxylic groups, sulfonic groups, etc, and, as a result, ion repulsion (known as Donnan exclusion) is the major

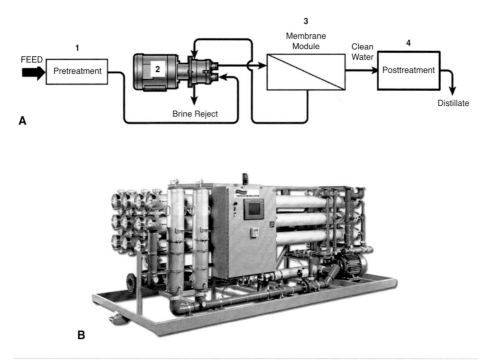

FIGURE 57.4 Basic schematic of an reverse osmosis (RO) system showing the major system components (**top**) and example of a skid-mounted RO unit for water treatment (**bottom**).

factor in determining salt rejection; that is, more highly charged ions such as SO_4^{2-} are more highly rejected than monovalent ions such as Cl^- by a negatively charged NF membrane. This is essentially a membrane process that rejects solutes approximately 1 nanometer (10 angstroms) in size with molecular weights above 200. Because they feature pore sizes larger than RO membranes, these membranes remove organic compounds and selected salts at lower pressures than RO systems. Such systems are a lower pressure version of RO where the purity of product water is not as critical as with pharmaceutical grade water as an example, or the level of dissolved solids to be removed is less than what typically is encountered in brackish water or seawater.

The NF membranes have good rejections of organic compounds with molecular weights above 200 to 500. The most important NF membranes are composite membranes made by interfacial polymerization; aromatic polypiperazine is an example of a one type of NF membrane. The NF systems function similarly to RO, but these are generally targeted to remove only divalent and larger ions. It is therefore sometimes referred to as "selective reverse osmosis." Monovalent ions such as sodium and chloride will pass through a membrane, thus many of the uses of this technology involve desalting of the process stream. An example is the production of lactose from cheese whey; the NF process is designed to concentrate the lactose molecules while passing salts, a procedure

that purifies and concentrates the lactose stream. In water treatment, NF membranes are used for hardness removal (in place of water softeners), pesticide elimination, and color reduction. The NF can also be used to reclaim spent sodium hydroxide (NaOH) solutions. In this case, the permeate (filtrate) stream is purified NaOH, allowing reuse many times over. While RO systems are capable of removing the smallest of solute molecules, in the range of 0.0001 μm in diameter and smaller, NF removes molecules in the 0.001 μm range. The technology is applied where the high salt rejection of RO is not necessary. Like RO, NF also is capable of removing bacteria and viruses as well as organic-related color without generating undesirable chlorinated hydrocarbons and THMs. The NF is used to remove pesticides and other organic contaminants from surface and ground waters to help insure the safety of public drinking water supplies.

Because NF systems operate on lower pressure than RO, energy costs are lower than for a comparable RO treatment system. This makes NF well suited for the treatment of well water or water from surface supplies such as rivers or lakes. NF is also an osmotic pressure–dependent process, but due to the passage of monovalent ions, the net osmotic driving force required is less than RO. Operating pressures are lower and filtration rates are higher. The NF membranes typically operate in the range of 100 to 600 psi (7-42 bars). An important distinction between RO and NF to bear in mind is that while an RO membrane will typically remove 98% to 99% of monovalent ions, such as chlorides or sodium, an NF membrane typically removes 50% to 90%, depending on the material and manufacture of the membrane. Because of its ability to effectively remove di- and trivalent ions, NF is frequently used to remove hardness from water while leaving the TDS content much less affected than would RO. The NF is often used to filter water with low amounts of TDS, to remove organic matter, and soften water. The NF membranes are less likely to foul or scale and require less pretreatment than RO. Sometimes, it is even used as pretreatment to RO. The NF can be employed in a variety of water and wastewater treatment industries for the cost-effective removal of ions and organic substances. Besides water treatment, NF is employed in the manufacturing process for pharmaceuticals, dairy products, textiles, and bakeries.

Microfiltration

The MF is a membrane separation process that relies on membranes with a pore size of approximately 0.03 to 10 μm, an MWCO of greater than 100 000 Da, and a relatively low feedwater operating pressure of approximately 15 to 60 psi (100-400 kPa). Examples of materials removed include sand, silt, clays, protozoa-like *Giardia lamblia* and *Cryptosporidium* (vegetative or oocyst/cyst forms), algae, and some bacterial species. It is not considered to be an absolute barrier to viruses; however, when used in combination with chemical and physical removal disinfection, MF is recognized to control these microorganisms in water. This is noteworthy because by physically removing pathogens, membrane filtration can significantly reduce the need for chemical addition, such as chlorination. Another application for the technology is for removal of natural or synthetic organic matter to reduce fouling potential. In its normal operation, it removes little or no organic matter; however, when pretreatment is applied, increased removal of organic material as well as a retardation of membrane fouling can be achieved. Other applications include as a pretreatment to RO or NF to reduce fouling potential.

The MF membranes are described by suppliers as capable of providing absolute removal of particulate contaminants from a feed stream by separation based on retention of contaminants on a membrane surface. The technology is generally described as the "loosest" of the membrane processes, and as a consequence of its large pore size, it is used primarily for removing particles and microbes and can be operated under ultralow pressure conditions.

With simple configurations, the process involves pre-screening raw water and pumping it under pressure onto a membrane. In comparison to conventional water clarification processes, where coagulants and other chemicals are added to the water before filtration, there are few pretreatment requirements for hollow-fiber systems when

particles and microorganisms are the target contaminants. Prefilters must be employed to remove large particles that may plug the inlet to the fibers within the membrane module. More complex pretreatment strategies are employed either to reduce fouling or enhance the removal of viruses and dissolved organic matter. In such cases, pretreatment by adding coagulants or powdered activated carbon (PAC) has been used. In some cases, the cake layer built up on the membrane during the water production cycle can remove organic materials. As with RO, it may be necessary to adjust the feedwater pH by chemical dosing prior to membrane filtration in order to maintain the pH within the recommended operating range for the membrane material employed. Note that pH adjustment is not required for scaling control because these membranes do not remove uncomplexed dissolved ions.

Commercially available membrane geometries employed are spiral wound, tubular, and hollow capillary fiber. Spiral-wound configurations are not preferred due to the flat-sheet nature of the membrane, which presents difficulties in keeping the membrane surface clean. Unlike spiral-wound membranes, hollow-fiber and tubular configurations allow the membrane to be backwashed. There are two methods for maintaining or re-establishing permeate flux after the membranes are fouled:

- Membrane backwashing. To prevent the continuous accumulation of solids on the membrane surface, the membrane is backwashed. Unlike backwashing for conventional media filtration, the backwashing cycle takes only a few minutes. Both liquid and gas backwashing are used with this technology. For most systems, backwashing is fully automatic. If backwashing is incapable of restoring the flux, then membranes must be chemically cleaned. The variables that should be considered in cleaning membranes include frequency and duration of cleaning, chemicals and their concentrations, cleaning and rinse volumes, temperature of cleaning, recovery and reuse of cleaning chemicals, neutralization and disposal of cleaning chemicals.
- Membrane pretreatment. Also known as feedwater pretreatment, this is employed to improve the level of removal of various natural water constituents. It is also used to increase or maintain transmembrane flux rates and/or to retard fouling. The two most common types of pretreatment are coagulant and PAC addition.

Ultrafiltration

The UF involves the pressure-driven separation of materials from water using a membrane pore size of approximately 0.002 to 0.1 μm, an MWCO of approximately 10 000 to 100 000 Da, and an operating pressure of approximately 30 to 100 psi (200-700 kPa). It can remove all microbiological species removed by MF (partial removal of bacteria) as well as some viruses (but not an absolute barrier to viruses) and humic materials. The UF allows most ionic inorganic species to pass through the membrane and retains discrete particulate matter and nonionic and ionic organic species. It is a single process that removes many water-soluble organic materials as well as microbiological contaminants. Because all membranes are capable of effectively straining protozoa, bacteria, and most viruses from water, the process offers a disinfected filtered product with little load on any posttreatment sterilization method, such as ultraviolet radiation, ozone treatment, or even chlorination. Disinfection can provide a second barrier to contamination. Major advantages of low-pressure UF membrane processes compared with conventional clarification and disinfection (postchlorination) processes include the following:

- No need for chemicals (coagulants, flocculants, disinfectants, pH adjustment)
- Size-exclusion filtration as opposed to media depth filtration
- Good and constant quality of the treated water in terms of particle and microbial removal
- Compact plant
- Simple automation

Unlike RO, the pretreatment requirement for UF is normally quite low. Due to the chemical and hydrolytic stability of membrane materials, some of the pretreatment steps essential for RO membranes, such as adjustment of pH or chlorine concentration levels, do not apply. But it may be necessary to adjust the pH to decrease the solubility of a solute in the feed so that it may be filtered out. The UF is best suited for the removal of suspended and dissolved macromolecular solids from fluids. Modules are designed to accept feedwaters that carry high loads of solids. Because of the many uses for membranes, pilot studies are normally conducted to test how suitable a given stream is for filtration process. Water containing dissolved or chelated iron and manganese ions require treatment by an adequate oxidation process in order to precipitate these ions prior to filtration. The same applies to all membrane processes. This is recommended to avoid precipitation of iron and manganese in the membrane, or even worse, on the permeate side of the membrane (membrane fouling during the backwash procedure). Preoxidation processes include aeration, pH adjustment to a value greater than eight, or addition of strong oxidants, such as chlorine, chlorine dioxide, ozone, or potassium permanganate. Natural organic matter is of importance in potential fouling of the membranes and, consequently, in permeate flux that can be used under normal operating conditions. The use of PAC or coagulants to pretreat the water to remove these constituents is recommended, which also decreases the surface of membrane needed.

The UF membranes are supplied in one of two forms: tubular or flat sheet. Package plants, skid-mounted standard units that allow significant cost savings, are usually employed for plants treating less than 1.5 mgd (million gallons per day). The primary skid-mounted system components may include an autocleaning prefilter, raw water pump, recirculation pump, backwash pump, chlorine dosing pump for the backwash water, air compressor (valve actuation), chlorine tank, chemical tank (detergent), programmable logical controller with program and security sensor (high pressure, low level, etc). Full-scale plant operations have several subcategories.

- Raw water intake and pressure pumps
- Pretreatment, which includes prescreening, prefiltration, and pH adjustment (if required) or any of the needed pretreatments
- UF units
- Chemical cleaning station, backwash station (which uses chlorinated product water), chlorine station, conditioner/preservative station
- Line for discharging or treatment of backwash water

Operation and performance are influenced by raw water quality variations. Turbidity as well as total organic carbon of the raw water are water quality parameters of major significance that drive operation mode and membrane flux for UF plants.

Secondary Wastes

Membrane technologies generate secondary wastes that can pose a challenge depending on country or region-specific requirements. Conventional treatment processes can generate roughly 5% to 10% of the influent water as waste. In contrast, membrane processes produce waste streams amounting to as much as 15% of the total treated water volume. These wastes are highly concentrated. Disposal methods include deep well injection, dilution and spray irrigation, or disposal in the municipal sewer. These alternatives are usually necessary for NF wastes, which usually contain concentrated organic and inorganic compounds. Regardless of the type of membrane, disposal must be carefully considered in decisions about the use of membrane technology. Applicable local discharge regulations must be carefully considered.

Selection Criteria

Membrane selection for a given application can be complicated because of the many choices among new types of membranes, applications, and site-specific conditions. Bench and pilot tests are generally recommended to minimize the risks and uncertainties and to accurately assess cost impacts. Membrane classification standards vary considerably from one filter supplier to another. What one supplier markets as a UF product, another manufacturer calls an NF system. It is best to examine pore size, MWCO, and the applied pressure needed when

TABLE 57.2 Suitability of membrane technologies and selection criteria

Technology	Ease of Operation	Pretreatment and Other Requirements	Secondary Waste Generation	Limitations
Reverse osmosis (RO)	Intermediate: increases with pre-/posttreatment and membrane cleaning needs	May require conventional or other pretreatment for surface water to protect membrane surfaces: may include turbidity or Fe/Mn removal; stabilization to prevent scaling; reduction of dissolved solids or hardness; pH adjustment	Briny waste. High volume, for example, 25%-50%; may be toxic to some species	Bypassing of water (to provide blended/stabilized distributed water) cannot be practiced at risk of increasing microbial concentrations in finished water. Post-disinfection required under regulation is recommended as a safety measure and for residual maintenance. Other post-treatments may include degassing of CO_2 or H_2S and pH adjustment.
Nanofiltration	Intermediate: increases with pre-/posttreatment and membrane cleaning needs	Very high quality or pretreatment required (eg, micro- or ultrafiltration to reduce fouling/extend cleaning intervals). See also RO pretreatments.	Concentrated waste: 5%-20% volume	Disinfection required under some regulations and recommended as a safety measure or for residual protection
Microfiltration	Basic: increases with pre-/posttreatment and membrane cleaning needs	High quality or pretreatment required. TOC rejection generally low, so if disinfection by-product precursors are a concern, nanofiltration may be preferable.	Low-volume waste may include sand, silt, clay, cysts, and algae.	Additional chemical or thermal disinfection required for viral control
Ultrafiltration	Basic: increases with pre-/posttreatment and membrane cleaning needs	High quality or pretreatment required (eg, microfiltration). TOC rejection generally low, so if disinfection by-product precursors are a concern, nanofiltration may be preferable.	Concentrated waste: 5%-20% volume. Waste may include sand, silt, clays, cysts, algae, viruses, and humic material.	Additional chemical or thermal disinfection required for viral control

Abbreviation: TOC, total organic carbon.

comparing different membrane systems. The MWCO is widely regarded as a measure of membrane pore dimensions and is a specification used by membrane suppliers to describe a membrane's retention capabilities. Table 57.2 provides some general comparisons among the membrane technologies that may assist in initial screening for selection.

▶ ION EXCHANGE

Ion exchange processes are reversible chemical reactions for removing dissolved ions from solution and replacing them with other similarly charged ions. They have little to no impact on microbial contamination. In water treatment, it is primarily used for softening where calcium and magnesium ions are removed from water; however, it is being used more frequently for the removal of other dissolved ionic species. In a cation exchange process, positively charged ions on the surface of a resin are exchanged with positively charged ions available on the resin surface, typically sodium. Water softening is the most widely used cation exchange process. Similarly, in anion exchange, negatively charged ions are exchanged with negatively charged ions on the resin surface, typically chloride. Contaminants such as nitrate, fluoride, sulfate, and arsenic, as well as others, can all be removed by anion exchange. The exchange medium consists of a solid phase of naturally occurring materials (zeolites) or a synthetic resin having a mobile ion attached to an immobile functional acid or base group.

Both anion and cation resins are produced from the same basic organic polymers, but they differ in the functional group attached to the resin. The mobile ions are exchanged with solute ions having a stronger affinity to the functional group (eg, calcium ion replaces sodium ion or sulfate ion replaces chloride ion). When the capacity of the resin is exhausted, it is necessary to regenerate the resin using a saturated solution to restore the capacity of the resin and return the resin to its initial condition. Brine, or sodium chloride solution, is most the commonly used regenerant, although others, such as strong acids (hydrochloric acid, sulfuric acid) or strong bases (NaOH) may also be used.

Chelating Agents

Chelating resins behave similarly to weak acid cation resins but exhibit a high degree of selectivity for heavy metal cations. Chelating resins are analogous to chelating compounds found in metal finishing wastewater; that is, they tend to form stable complexes with the heavy metals. In fact, the functional group used in these resins is an EDTAa (ethylenediaminetetraacetic acid) compound. The resin structure in the sodium form is expressed as R-EDTA-Na.

The high degree of selectivity for heavy metals permits separation of these ionic compounds from solutions containing high background levels of calcium, magnesium, and sodium ions. A chelating resin exhibits greater selectivity for heavy metals in its sodium form than in its hydrogen form. Regeneration properties are similar to those of a weak acid resin; the chelating resin can be converted to the hydrogen form with slightly greater than stoichiometric doses of acid because of the fortunate tendency of the heavy metal complex to become less stable under low pH conditions. Potential applications of the chelating resin include polishing to lower the heavy metal concentration in the effluent from a hydroxide treatment process or directly removing toxic heavy metal cations from wastewaters containing a high concentration of nontoxic, multivalent cations.

Batch and Column Exchange Systems

Ion exchange processing can be accomplished by either a batch method or a column method. In batch mode, the resin and solution are mixed in a batch tank, the exchange is allowed to come to equilibrium, on which the resin is separated from solution. The degree to which the exchange takes place is limited by the preference the resin exhibits for the ion in solution. Consequently, the use of the resins exchange capacity will be limited unless the selectivity for the ion in solution is far greater than for the exchangeable

ion attached to the resin. Because batch regeneration of the resin is chemically inefficient, batch processing by ion exchange has limited potential for application. Passing a solution through a column containing a bed of exchange resin is analogous to treating the solution in an infinite series of batch tanks.

Process Configurations

Industrial applications of ion exchange use fixed-bed column systems (Figure 57.5). Column designs are intended to

- Contain and support the ion exchange resin
- Uniformly distribute the service and regeneration flow through the resin bed
- Provide space to fluidize the resin during backwash
- Include the piping, valves, and instruments needed to regulate flow of feed, regenerant, and backwash solutions

Once the feed solution is processed to the extent that the resin becomes exhausted and cannot accomplish any further ion exchange, the resin is regenerated. In a normal column operation, for a cation system being converted first to the hydrogen then to the sodium form, regeneration employs the following steps:

- Backwashing. The column is backwashed to remove suspended solids collected by the bed during the service cycle and to eliminate channels that may have formed during this cycle. The backwash flow fluidizes the bed thereby releasing trapped particulate matter. Backflushing also serves to reorient the resin particles according to size. During the backwash cycle, the larger, denser particles tend to accumulate at the base and the particle size decreases moving up the column. This distribution yields a good hydraulic flow pattern and resistance to fouling by suspended solids.
- The resin bed is brought in contact with the regenerant solution. In the case of the cation resin, acid elutes the collected ions and converts the bed to the hydrogen form. A slow water rinse then removes any residual acid.
- The bed is brought in contact with an NaOH solution to convert the resin to the sodium form. Again, a slow water rinse is used to remove residual caustic. The slow rinse pushes the last of the regenerant through the column.
- The resin bed is subjected to a fast rinse that removes the last traces of the regenerant solution and ensures good flow characteristics.
- The column is then returned to service.

Regeneration of a fixed-bed column usually requires between 1 and 2 hours. Frequency depends on the volume of resin in the exchange columns and the quantity of heavy metals and other ionized compounds in the wastewater. Columns are designed to operate as either

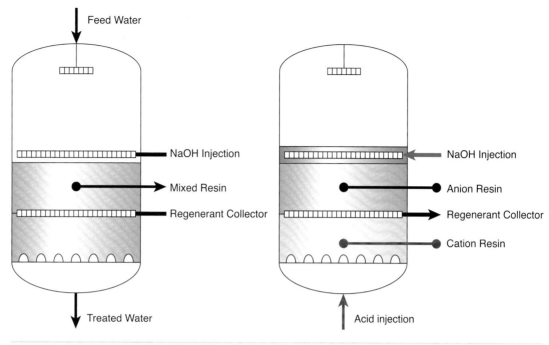

FIGURE 57.5 Ion exchange resin columns.

cocurrent or countercurrent regeneration. In cocurrent mode, both feed and regenerant solutions make contact with the resin in a downflow mode. These units are the less expensive of the two in terms of initial equipment cost. On the other hand, cocurrent flow uses regenerant chemicals less efficiently than countercurrent flow; they have higher leakage concentrations (the concentration of the feed solution ion being removed in the column effluent) and cannot achieve as high a product concentration in the regenerant.

▶ ACKNOWLEDGMENTS

This chapter has used some materials from a previous publication, Cheremisinoff NP. *Groundwater Remediation: A Practical Guide for Environmental Engineers and Scientists.* Beverly, MA: Scrivener; 2017, by permission.

REFERENCES

1. Cheremisinoff NP. *Groundwater Remediation: A Practical Guide for Environmental Engineers and Scientists.* Beverly, MA: Scrivener; 2017.
2. ASTM International. *ASTM E 1527-97: Standard Practice for Environmental Site Assessments: Phase 1 Environmental Site Assessment Process.* West Conshohocken, PA: ASTM International; 2000.
3. ASTM International. *ASTM E2081-00(2015): Standard Guide for Risk-Based Corrective Action.* West Conshohocken, PA: ASTM International; 2015.
4. US Environmental Protection Agency. *Water Quality Criteria Summary.* Washington, DC: US Environmental Protection Agency; 1991.
5. US Environmental Protection Agency. *Soil Screening Guidance: Technical Background Document.* Washington, DC: US Environmental Protection Agency; 1996.
6. US Environmental Protection Agency. *Cost and Performance Report: Six-Phase Heating at a Former Manufacturing Facility Skokie, Illinois.* Washington, DC: US Environmental Protection Agency; 1999.
7. US Environmental Protection Agency. *Groundwater Cleanup: Overview of Operating Experience at 28 Sites.* Washington, DC: US Environmental Protection Agency; 1999.
8. US Environmental Protection Agency. *Use of Monitored Natural Attenuation at Superfund, RCRA Corrective Action, and Underground Storage Tank Sites.* Washington, DC: US Environmental Protection Agency; 1999.
9. US Environmental Protection Agency. *Field Applications of In Situ Remediation Technologies: Permeable Reactive Barriers.* Washington, DC: US Environmental Protection Agency; 2002.
10. US Environmental Protection Agency. Drinking water regulations and contaminants. US Environmental Protection Agency Web site. https://www.epa.gov/dwregdev/drinking-water-regulations-and-contaminants. Accessed May 21, 2019.
11. World Health Organization. *Recommendations.* 3rd ed. Geneva, Switzerland: World Health Organization; 2008. *Guidelines for Drinking-Water Quality: Incorporating First and Second Addenda;* vol 1.
12. California Water Boards. California drinking water-related laws. California Water Boards Web site. https://www.waterboards.ca.gov/drinking_water/certlic/drinkingwater/Lawbook.html. Accessed May 21, 2019.

Aseptic Processing and Facilities for the Control of Microbial Contamination

James E. Akers Jr

From the earliest days of parenteral administration of health care products, there have been active ingredients that could not withstand a sterilization process, or in the parlance of the pharmaceutical industry, could not be terminally sterilized. Historically, these products were sufficiently heat labile, and moist heat, the principal method for end-product sterilization, could not be used.[1] Advancements in sterilization technology, such as the discovery that radiation could be used to sterilize some heat labile products safely, increased the use of terminal processing. Currently, the majority of sterile parenteral preparations are still not able to withstand traditional sterilization in their final container. Surveys done in the 1990s reported that more than 80% of all sterile preparations were aseptically manufactured without terminal sterilization.[2] Since those surveys were conducted, there has been an increasing prevalence of biological products that are incompatible with terminal sterilization technologies.

It is a widely held view in the health care industry that no manufacturing process is as technically challenging to accomplish and maintain as the aseptic processing production of sterile drug products. Aseptic manufacturing of sterile products without terminal sterilization requires the complex melding of several skills and technologies.[3] These technologies typically include sterilization of all product contact packaging components and product contact manufacturing equipment. The most challenging technological requirement is an environment that can be designed and operated in a manner that renders it as free of contaminating microorganisms as possible. The challenges and risks of aseptic processing have been well described and have resulted in complex regulatory compliance requirements and standards.[4-8]

The recent emergence of new types of health care products derived from biotechnology has imposed an even more difficult process control challenge than that of traditional aseptic processing. In research and development as well as production, some biotechnology processes, such as genetic therapy, require not only that the product is sterile but also that potentially hazardous materials such as virus vectors are absent. Aseptic process controls with simultaneous containment of process generated hazards requires exacting process and facility design as well as operational controls.

Facilities used solely for the control of product microbiological quality do not require the same level of critical activities as those used for aseptic processing. In these types of operations, the systematic control of microbial contamination need not approach perfection, but instead, it must be good enough to protect adequately the process or product contained within the clean environment (see chapter 60). Whereas these facilities may be less technically demanding than those built for aseptic processing, they nevertheless require careful consideration regarding design and operation.

ASEPTIC PROCESSING

The term *aseptic processing* has been widely used in the health care industry to describe the manufacturing of sterile products without the benefit of terminal sterilization. In the science of microbiology, the word aseptic means the absence of microbial contaminant capable of causing sepsis. Literally, the most concise description of aseptic is "without infection." Thus, aseptic has a meaning that is quite distinct from that of sterility, where aseptic implies the elimination of all organisms having the ability to reproduce. In the health care field, the essential meaning of sterility is that any microorganisms in or on a material must be nonviable.

It is not surprising that there has been a heated debate for decades regarding the labeling of products that cannot be terminally sterilized. Some industry scientists have held that aseptically manufactured products could not accurately be labeled sterile.[1] In spite of the firmly held opinions on both sides of this issue, the word *sterile* continues to be used to describe both products manufactured aseptically and using terminal sterilization. The regulatory application of the word *sterile* is not, it must be emphasized, a mere semantic distinction. Aseptic processing does not kill microorganisms, rather it functions to separate microorganisms from the product and prevent them from entering the product from the surrounding environment. Some microorganisms such as viruses are not always filterable and therefore may not be separable from the product stream. A further complication is that aseptic processing relies on environmental controls to prevent microorganisms from entering product containers, and attaining definitive proof of sterility in this aspect of manufacturing is dubious. So dubious in fact that it may be considered technically impossible both analytically and statistically.

Terminally sterilized products are considered different regarding patient risk than those manufactured aseptically. This difference is attributed to the capability of terminal sterilization to inactivate microorganisms with an exceptionally high rate of success. Nevertheless, regulatory requirements make it necessary for industry to apply the label *sterile* to both terminally sterilized and aseptically processed products. At the same time, government regulators, industry experts, and standard setters acknowledge that the two methods for the manufacture of products labeled sterile are not entirely equivalent.

The microbiological analytical tools currently available lack the ability to distinguish between a product free of any viable organism and one that contains no potential infectivity. Even if assessment tools of the requisite limit of detection and sensitivity did exist, it would not be possible to assert with absolute certainty that an aseptic product was always sterile. There are organisms that are known pathogens, but others are opportunistic pathogens that can cause disease rarely and only in a subset of patients. Given the fact that many product recipients are to one extent or another unwell, or even immunocompromised, it is difficult to ascribe complete harmlessness to any organism. The pharmacological and chemical characteristics of products further complicate risk assessment. Many products are either inherently antimicrobial or contain antimicrobials in the form of preservatives (see chapters 39 and 40). Furthermore, there is no method given in the current international regulations or guidelines applicable to aseptic manufacturing for assessing the effect the product or its preservative system has on reducing the risk of microbial contamination. Although we do not formally consider the antimicrobial factors possessed by a product in any comprehensive way, the antimicrobial effect might reduce the risk of patient infection.

The only means currently used for directly evaluating the capability of an aseptic process is the process simulation or media fill test. This test is the filling and subsequent incubation of actual product containers with microbiological media under realistic simulated production conditions. The object of the media fill or process simulation test is to assess the ability of the process to manufacture uncontaminated (aseptic) product. The media fill test has been required in industrial aseptic manufacturing for about 40 years.[9] Because the media fill test is used universally in industry, there exists an understanding of the facility and process conditions resulting in low rates of contamination.

Microbiological assessment of the facility environment, known as environmental monitoring (EM) is given critical importance by many practitioners and many regulatory authorities (see chapter 60). The principle technical limitation of EM is that it is only an indirect measurement of microbiological controls. The EM provides a means of assessing facility hygiene in general terms rather than a specific assessment of sterility assurance. The EM is not a suitable method for accurately determining patient risk.[10] The value of EM is that it allows us to understand the factors in facility design and operation that consistently result in low microbiological and particulate contamination.

The antimicrobial effect produced by any preservative system present or by the nature of the product itself is by convention not considered in determining a patient safety factor for an aseptically filled product. The inherent antimicrobial factor(s) possessed by the formulation can abate hazards associated with microbial contamination. This risk abatement is excluded from the determination of contamination rate tabulated from media fill testing. It is possible in every case to estimate the antimicrobial effect of a formulation. This is a critical element of what is broadly known as product characterization that should not be excluded from patient risk analysis. The exclusion of antimicrobial risk abatement factors that are part of many product formulations when considering sterility assurance is unfortunate. We do not possess a means for objective quantitative assessment of the attribute of "sterility" in aseptic processing, and the substitution of nonquantitative subjective or even intuitive factors should be discouraged.[11]

The aseptic manufacture of products requires not only the ability to use a variety of contamination control technologies in concert with one another but also a high level of engineering, supervisory, and risk-assessment skills. Our forebearers in the health care industry were both wise and intellectually honest when they used the word *aseptic* to describe parenteral products that could not withstand terminal sterilization. It is challenging, even with 21st century technology, to manufacture products in a clean, aseptic environment. But we have learned from industrial aseptic processing experience that it is possible in the current state of practice to manufacture products that provide superb patient safety.[12,13]

Although the safety of products can be extremely high, aseptic processing manufacturing methods, at the current state of the art, can lack precision and sensitive safety assessment tools. The sterility test has been required for product-release testing for sterile products for decades (see chapter 64); however, this test lacks the sensitivity to prove reliably that a product is pathogen or microbe free.[14] Process simulation tests or media fills are important tools for proving process capability, and these tests have quite rightly taken on increasing importance over the years. It is important to know that the broad-spectrum microbiological medium typically used for these studies is not able to recover or grow all types of microbes that could be present in a product. Although the media fill is the most comprehensive evaluative tool available in aseptic processing, it is both statistically and microbiologically limited. Finally, the EM program, although it is useful for assessing background contamination in the manufacturing environment, does not directly assess the product. Additionally, we must recognize that any microbial test that relies on humans to conduct the test can and most likely will yield false-positive results.

The best approach to the aseptic manufacture of health care products is a strong proactive one focused on contamination control and prevention rather than on measurement. Once the limitations of measurement-based strategies are acknowledged, the importance of proper design and operation of the aseptic environment and the process becomes clear. It can be stated accurately that the most important element in aseptic product safety is a process and environmental design that eliminates the potential for hazards. Fortunately, a great deal is known about the factors that introduce hazards into an aseptic process. It has been widely acknowledged since at least the late 1970s that the major causes of microbiological contamination in an aseptic processing clean room are the human beings working in those areas. In fact, human operators represent nearly all the contamination risk in aseptic manufacturing and are the only potential vector for pathogenic organisms in a clean room. Therefore, an obvious and generally quite successful approach to contamination control in the clean room is simply the elimination of personnel.[15] Fortuitously, advanced automated equipment has provided the health care industry with an outstanding means of contamination control.[16]

It is also well accepted that contamination hazards are reduced by reducing the length of time sterile objects are exposed to the environment during aseptic manufacture.[4,17] Therefore, equipment that can operate at high throughput smoothly and without human intervention is far safer than equipment that requires numerous interventions (or is manual) and operates at a low speed. For these reasons, equipment selection is an important factor in reducing hazards, which relate entirely to controlling contamination. High-speed, reliable, automated equipment that requires little human intervention for assembly, running adjustments, in-process maintenance, component charging, or quality-control sampling is far

safer than equipment that is less able to run without operator intervention.[18] Thus, equipment selection is an important factor in controlling contamination.

Another vital factor in reducing hazards associated with microbial contamination in aseptic manufacturing environments is the separation of hazards from the critical zone[19] of the process that area within the aseptic environment where product, containers, and closures are brought together and assembled aseptically. It follows, given that operators are the most significant risk factor, anything that can be done to separate the operators from the critical zone will be an important control measure. In the 1970s, this separation typically was achieved primarily by the placement of flexible polyvinyl chloride (PVC) sheets. These sheets or curtains were an easily defeated barrier but nevertheless provided at least a psychological reinforcement of need for operators to keep their distance from the critical zone. A barrier in this case refers to any device that limits opportunity for human-derived or production-associated contamination to affect the quality of a product. Unfortunately, most process equipment available during that era required consistent and, in some cases, extensive human intervention. By the 1980s, equipment speed and reliability had increased to the point that less permeable fixed barriers could be used. Equipment manufacturers began to offer equipment that was enclosed in typically clear, solid polycarbonate panels. Equipment with these enclosures is still widely used in human scale clean rooms. Although these solid enclosures are less permeable than PVC sheets, the panels typically are mounted on hinges, which allows operator access for adjustment, maintenance, or sampling. As sophistication and automation of the equipment increased, light barriers or interlocks were added to stop moving parts when the panels were opened. In the mid-1980s, isolation technology was first used in the health care industry.[20] Isolators can be defined as self-contained clean facilities and offer optimal control of human contamination because human operators work outside the clean zone. Isolators had been widely used in other industries since the 1960s, but they were used more for the containment of poisonous or otherwise hazardous materials than for the control of microbial contamination. Scientists and engineers recognized that a technology that was well suited to keeping contamination in, if properly employed, could be equally good at keeping microbial contamination out.

The devices the pharmaceutical industry calls isolators have been very widely adopted in the production of aseptic foods and beverages, where they are known as aseptic chambers. In the aseptic food and beverage industry, aseptic chambers have become universal in their application. These aseptic chambers often operate at throughput rates in the range of 600 to 1300 units per minute, so not only is the environment effectively controlled but the length of time that each unit produced is exposed to the environment is also extremely short.[21] Isolators and the entire field of isolation technology (aseptic chambers) have evolved considerably since their introduction to aseptic manufacturing industries and now represent the pinnacle of aseptic processing safety. Isolators, automation, robotics, and sensor technology will continue to advance, assuring a future in which human involvement in aseptic processing is limited to process supervision and review of processing data. The less complete barrier production operations sometimes called open restricted access barrier systems (RABS), which accommodate the possibility of human intervention, will in this author's view become extinct along with all other manned clean rooms. The most likely trajectory for aseptic processing is the implementation of complete automation, where the nature of the enclosure will need to allow access during maintenance and changeover only, and never during routine aseptic operations. There is a species of separative technology used on the pharmaceutical and biopharmaceutical industries that is very similar to the aseptic chamber or isolator in performance. These are the so-called closed RABS systems, which are kept closed in operation and do not accommodate any direct human interventions during aseptic manufacturing. These closed systems were built to circumvent the decontamination processes generally required by regulatory agencies for isolator systems or aseptic barriers. In this author's view, both closed and open RABs will face extinction because automation technology will render them unnecessary. Evidence of this can be found in the aseptic food and beverage industry where a RABS alternative has not evolved and human scale or manned clean rooms are already extinct.[21]

PLANNING A FACILITY

Facility Design Attributes

The first step in a facility planning exercise should be a detailed analysis of microbial hazards as they apply to the production process. A formal, documented method of hazard analysis is the most effective method for identifying and assessing hazards and can be extremely useful in determining what level of controls should be applied for each step in the manufacturing process. Hazard analysis critical control point (HACCP) planning is widely used to assess risks to a process, and environmental- or facility-related hazards should be included as components of a thorough HACCP program. The HACCP planning is a general regulatory requirement in food manufacturing and is being applied more broadly in health care manufacturing processes as well. An HACCP team for an aseptic process may overlap in membership with a facility planning team. The HACCP methods and program organization are beyond the scope of this chapter; however, the reader is urged to research these methods independently.[22]

There are other risk management systems that may be applied that suggest other statistical or computation means for conducting risk assessment. These include systems that consider intervention risk or use elements of a failure mode effect analysis approach. In the author's view, risk analysis systems reliant on EM data alone as a metric are inherently suspect. This is because EM results in well controlled aseptic processing manufacturing environments typically show the absence of viable microorganisms. It is necessary to consider that the absence of growth, or zero (0), in microbiological plate cultivation methods has no clear meaning beyond the obvious conclusion that nothing grew (see chapter 64). It is not uncommon for a finding of no growth to be interpreted as a "sterile" outcome. This is analytically incorrect as it assumes that any organism that might be present would grow in the medium/media and growth conditions used in testing. It is well known that the efficiency of this type of testing for detection and quantitation is limited.[23]

Facilities that require human scale clean rooms for aseptic processing are often expensive to build and to operate. At the same time, manned clean room facilities for less than fully aseptic levels of control contamination can be relatively simple and contain only minimal environmental control features. In facilities where separative technologies are employed, such as with isolation technology, a simpler surrounding clean room environment can suffice. Facilities also may need to be designed to protect the worker from hazards associated with pathogenic organisms or chemical contaminants used for research, development, or manufacturing. Depending on the nature of the process, these facilities also may be required to protect the manufacturing process and the product from contamination with other microorganisms. Facilities that must provide both chemical and/or biological containment for the operator or environmental protection as well as microbial control for process hazard reduction, impose unique design constraints. Those that require a blend of hazardous material containment and microbiological control are among the costliest to install, test, and operate. But if isolators can be used, a combination of aseptic safety and containment of hazards can be accomplished optimally and at with minimal cost implications.

Facilities can be designed and built to accomplish varying degrees of control or containment, depending on the process and a variety of regulatory requirements. Thorough, rigorous planning is absolutely necessary to ensure that the best cost-to-performance ratio is achieved.[24] Among the critical issues to be addressed in the design of a facility are

- Process layout
- Personnel access and personnel load
- Location of the manufacturing process within a multipurpose building
- Relationship, if any, with other work areas within the building

- Relationships and the potential effect on other operations located on the same property or group of buildings
- Current regulatory requirements including
  - Product regulatory requirements (eg, US Food and Drug Administration)
  - Environmental/civil engineering issues, including sewage discharge, safety, emergency planning
  - Occupational health and safety and others as applicable (eg, radiation safety, live organism control)
  - Likely changes in regulations or the need to comply with international regulations (It is vital to consider in any new facility the potential for increasing stringency in regulatory requirements as they evolve over time.)
  - Flexibility of design if the facility is converted to other uses or if other processes are likely to be added in the future
  - Emergency management

Facility Classification

Over the years, ventilation supply air quality classifications have evolved for facilities designed to control contamination. Probably the first official classification scheme to be used on a broad industrial scale was the US Federal Standard 209 entitled *Airborne Particulate Cleanliness Classes in Cleanrooms and Clean Zones*.[25] This standard described the general design and particulate air quality performance requirements for facilities commonly called clean rooms. It emerged in the early 1970s with the iteration designated FS209B and remained the gold standard of classification until the global adoption of International Organization for Standardization (ISO) 14644 in 1999.[26,27] The final iteration of FS209 (designated version E), even though was retired with the adaptation of ISO 14644, can still be read and referenced to the original clean room classification standard at the present time.

Technically, FS209E was a legal requirement only for organizations doing work for the United States government. Thus, FS209E was officially allied to products,

manufactured in classified clean rooms or clean zones, that were purchased by the United States. In broad practice, FS209E became by far the most important general reference in the classification of clean rooms in its time. Many of the clean room operational parameters delineated initially in FS209 have become general design and control specifications that have been captured in one way or another in a variety of industrial and regulatory guidelines. The British, French, German, and Japanese governments, as well as others, also introduced clean room performance standards. The European Union (EU, then European Economic Community) incorporated a classification scheme in their good manufacturing practices document first issued in 1989. Although EU Annex 1 has been revised several times since its clean room grades were introduced and is currently under revision again, the fundamental requirements assigned to each grade have not changed.[8] Tables 58.1 and 58.2 show internationally referenced room classification schemes commonly used in aseptic processing. Although these standards differ in units of measure and in some cases particulate size specified for classification, experience has proven that these clean room standards generally resulted in demonstrably equivalent levels of facility performance.

Historically, facilities that complied with the requirements of one standard would not comply with others because of differences is compliance testing and differences in the statistics applied to test results. This situation has been improved by the harmonization of most of the world on the classification requirements given in ISO 14644-1, which first issued in 2001 and revised in 2015.[27] Although minor differences remain, the international requirements for clean room classification are in the case of particulate air quality now mostly reconcilable if not precisely harmonized. At the present time, there is effectively only one international standard (ISO 14644) for clean room classification, although the current version of EU Annex 1 is nearly but not fully harmonized with this consensus international standard. There are two major issues thwarting full harmonization; the first is the EU Annex 1 requirement for testing 5 μm particles and the second is

TABLE 58.1 ISO 14644-1 classification standards for clean rooms[a]

Class Number	Particle Size and Limits (Particles/m³)				
	0.1 μm	0.2 μm	0.3 μm	0.5 μm	1.0 μm
Class 5	100 000	23 700	10 200	3520	832
Class 6	1 000 000	237 000	102 000	35 200	8320
Class 7	—	—	—	352 000	83 200
Class 8	—	—	—	3 520 000	832 000

[a]Classes 5, 6, and 7 are those used for aseptic processing, whereas International Organization for Standardization (ISO) 8 may be used for controlled areas outside the aseptic processing area. Class 5 is used for the critical zone of aseptic processing, where aseptically manufactured products are assembled and placed in their primary package. Particle numbers for each class and particulate size are per cubic meter.

TABLE 58.2 European Good Manufacturing Practice Annex 1 microbiological monitoring limits

Grade	Maximum Permitted Number of Particles Equal to or Greater Than 0.5 μm		
	At Rest Equal to or Greater Than 0.5 μm/m³	**In Operation** Equal to or Greater Than 0.5 μm/m³	**ISO Classification In Operation/at Rest**
A	3520	3520	5/5
B	3520	352 000	5/7
C	352 000	3 520 000	7/8
D	3 520 000	Not defined	8

Abbreviation: ISO, International Organization for Standardization.

the insistence on microbiological conditions for classification. Neither of these requirements are logical from either the analytical or the statistical perspectives. Fortunately, these remaining issues awaiting full harmonization have very little impact on the design or operation of most clean rooms.

The ISO class 5 (or EU grade A) clean room is used for aseptic processing or other activities requiring the lowest concentration of microorganisms per unit volume of room air. The areas surrounding an ISO class 5 suite are generally class ISO class 6 or 7 or grade B/C. In many modern aseptic facilities, the entire room in which aseptic filling, sealing, or assembly is done is ISO class 5 throughout. This obviates the need for an ISO class 6 or 7 surrounding space and makes the entire room ISO class 5 rather than restricting that classification to only the critical space in which product is filled, sealed, or assembled. The ISO class 7 rooms also may be used as stand-alone suites for operations that require excellent control of microbial contamination but for which ISO class 5 conditions are not required. Examples of processes often conducted in ISO class 7 rooms are product purification, compounding, and moderately critical testing and research laboratory operations. ISO class 8 facilities are used for operations that require greater control than can be achieved in a standard building environment. ISO class 8 environments are used

for laboratories and manufacturing facilities in which the microbial hazards to the operation are minor. See Tables 58.3 and 58.4 for microbial contamination levels or rates recommended by the EU and the current United States Pharmacopeia (USP) for the commonly used facility classifications.[28]

Common Characteristics of Clean Room Facilities

Conditioning of Air

Experience has shown that control of heat and humidity can be an important factor in the control of microbial contamination. Therefore, the control of excessive temperature and humidity conditions is an essential design element in classified clean rooms designed to reduce hazards from microbial contamination. Moisture levels, particularly when levels are reached that approach the dew point, can result in colonization by microorganisms. Cooler areas within the filters themselves are particularly dangerous in this regard because they can provide a cool, damp supporting matrix that is conducive to mold growth. Additionally, temperature and humidity levels that result in discomfort for human operators result

TABLE 58.3 Total particulate air classification limits and microbiological monitoring levels[a]

Clean Area Classification (0.5 μm Particles/ft³)	ISO Designation	≥0.5 μm Particles/m³	Microbiological Active Air Action Levels (CFUs/m³)	Microbiological Settling Plates Action Levels (diam = 90 mm; CFUs/4 h)
100	5	3520	1	1
1000	6	35 200	7	3
10 000	7	352 000	10	5
100 000	8	3 520 000	100	50

Abbreviations: CFUs, colony-forming units; diam, diameter; ISO, International Organization for Standardization.

[a]From US Food and Drug Administration[6] and International Organization for Standardization.[27]

TABLE 58.4 United States Pharmacopeia microbiological monitoring incident rate recommendations for aseptic processing[a,b]

Grade	Active Air Sample	Settle Plate (9 cm) 4-h exposure	Contact Plate or Swab	Glove or Garment
Isolator or closed restricted access barrier system (International Organization for Standardization [ISO] 5 or better)	<0.1%	<0.1%	<0.1%	<0.1%
ISO 5	<1%	<1%	<1%	<1%
ISO 6	<3%	<3%	<3%	<3%
ISO 7	<5%	<5%	<5%	<5%
ISO 8	<10%	<10%	<10%	<10%

[a]From United States Pharmacopeia.[28]

[b]Values applicable to full aseptic gowning requirements only.

in poor control of contamination. Uncomfortable and sometimes perspiring operators are prone to making undesirable movements, such as wiping the brow or fanning. Any heat or humidity condition that results in perspiration for operators is a concern in contamination control. Perspiration can result in higher levels of contamination on human skin and can compromise the filtration effects of clean room clothing.

To obviate the hazards associated with heat and humidity, clean room air is typically maintained at a somewhat cooler and drier condition than homes or offices. Target temperatures of 68°C or even lower are common, and humidity targets of 50% ± 10% are routinely specified.[29,30] It is important to consider that the clean room operator often may wear two or more layers of clothes and outer garments, and if any skin at all is left exposed, it is usually only a small patch of skin around the face mask. Therefore, attempting to economize on either capital investment or operating costs to maintain appropriate temperature and humidity levels in a facility can seriously compromise contamination control. For aseptic processing facilities, there should be no compromise in temperature and humidity control, even in areas that are relatively distant from the most critical processing areas. It may be possible to liberalize temperature and humidity control requirements for some less critical processes, but this should be carefully reviewed using HACCP or similar hazard analysis techniques.

Air Filtration

Air filtration is an essential element in the design of ventilation systems used in facilities designed to control contamination. The most commonly used grade of filter used in classified facilities is the high-efficiency particulate air filter, or HEPA filter. The HEPA filters are depth-type filters that work to a not less than 99.95%

(H13 rating) efficiency rating or a 99.995% (H14 rating) level of efficiency. The H13 and H14 filters are often referenced to as "three 9" or "four 9" HEPA filters. In practice for aseptic processing application, both H13 and H14 filters have proven suitable for use, and experience has shown no discernible difference in contamination control performance.

The HEPA filters have proven extremely effective at the removal of airborne microbial contamination from facility air supply systems. Other types of filters are occasionally used in facilities designed to control microbial contamination. Some users have specified ultra-low particulate air filters, or ULPA filters. The ULPA filters are rated at an efficiency range of 99.9995%. The ULPA filters often are used in clean rooms that must be operated at exceedingly low levels of nonviable particulate contamination (eg, electronics manufacturing); however, there is little evidence to indicate that ULPA filters do a measurably better job of reducing airborne microbial contamination than HEPA filters.[31]

The HEPA filters remain the most commonly used for efficient filtering of airborne microbial control applications, both in conventional human-scale clean rooms and in isolator systems. There has been some interest in the use of sterilizing grade membrane filters in isolators. Membrane filters, typically of a 0.2-μ nominal pore rating are commonly used to remove microbial contamination from liquids or in venting applications. These filters are also used to sterilize compressed gases and rarely used in microbially controlled environments. Membrane filters are typically not used in human-scale conventional clean rooms because they impose a limited airflow rate. It has generally been considered impractical to use membrane filters in areas where high airflow rates, and therefore high volumes, are required, although in small isolator enclosures, this drawback may be minimized. There is no experimental reason to consider that membranes of "sterilizing grade" filters would afford any contamination control advantage at all under these situations.

Air Movement and Dilution of Contamination

For many years, the movement or "pattern" of airflow in a microbially controlled environment has been considered a critical design element. Much has been written in both design and operation guidance documents and in some regulations regarding laminar airflow. It is widely believed that airflow sweeps both viable and nonviable contamination away from critical work zones. It is important to note that little actual scientific data exist on the effects of airflow in a broad general sense on contamination control. The work of Ljungqvist and Reinmüller[32] showed that the ability of filtered air to limit the effects of contamination on a critical zone is quite real and can be demonstrated empirically. These investigators and others pointed out that laminar airflow (ie, an airstream moving in the same direction and at the same rate without turbulence) does not exist in "real-world" facilities. Rather, the best that can be hoped for is unidirectional airflow in which turbulence exists but where the overall mass of airflow is in the same general direction. It cannot be easily demonstrated that airstreams actually wash or sweep all contamination away from critical work zones. It is more likely that zones bathed with high flow rates of filtered air bar to some extent the entry of contamination. Of equal or even greater effect may be the ability of high flow rates of clean air to dilute microbial contamination and by so doing reduce the probability of such contamination adversely affecting the facility or the process being conducted.

In considering the beneficial effects of relatively large volumes of clean, filtered air in reducing contamination risk, it is important to examine the potential sources of contamination within a controlled facility. There is agreement among microbiologists and engineers that the human operator poses the greatest hazard to the control of microorganisms within the manufacturing environment.[33] In fact, in many environments, the human operator represents the only hazard to the environment. It then follows that the human operator population and load are critical factors that must be considered in the design of an air supply system for any clean environment.[34] In quite simple terms, the greater the number of operators, the greater the risk of human-contributed microorganisms to the process within a facility. It also follows that the closer these operators approach areas in which the product is exposed to the possibility of microbial contamination, the greater the risk to the process (Figure 58.1). Therefore, the highest airflow rates are typically used in the most critical zones of the process. In isolators or other devices that limit the risk from human operators, airflow rates become far less critical. As noted in the discussion of air filtration, in general, the same grades of filters are used in all types of clean rooms and isolators; therefore, airflow is the

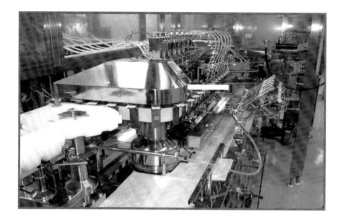

FIGURE 58.1 A high speed vial filling stoppering machine installed in a conventional clean room. Courtesy of Shibuya Co, Kanazawa, Ishikawa, Japan.

design characteristic that differs among clean rooms of different control classifications. Rooms designed to provide a higher level of control use much higher flow rates and therefore must be provided with a higher volume air supply system. This, of course, means that higher blower capacity and, in most cases, more filter area are required to achieve the required airflow.

Other Air Movement Characteristics

Direction of Flow

Air supplies are commonly oriented to provide air that moves in a vertical pattern. Air in this case approaches the work surface from above. This is the so-called vertical laminar airflow, which is widely specified in the health care manufacturing industry. Laminar airflow is a condition in which airflow is at a uniform velocity along streamlines. Laminar flow is the complete absence of turbulence, and although the term is used widely in clean room design and control, in practice, it does not actually exist. Of course, as previously mentioned, this air is not truly laminar flow, but at best, it is unidirectional. It is important to note that in practice, the requirement for unidirectional, or as it is commonly but incorrectly called, laminar airflow, is applied only to clean rooms classified at ISO class 5 (EU class A) level or higher. Orienting a room with vertical flow is advantageous from the standpoints of space utilization and convenience of maintenance. In this design, the air-handling systems can be located between the floors of a building and the filter systems mounted at or in the ceiling.[34]

In the case of vertical airflow, the airstream is actually moving perpendicular to the work surface. Therefore, the air strikes horizontal surfaces of equipment and can deflect in rather unpredictable ways against this work surface. It is hoped that the air will flow relatively smoothly over equipment and sweep contamination away, but the effectiveness of airflow in this regard is quite difficult to predict. In some research facilities, testing laboratories, and occasionally in health care product manufacturing, horizontal airflow is used. In horizontal airflow, the air moves across the work area and toward the human operator. Although this orientation appears to have a theoretical advantage in terms of control of human-borne contamination, it requires that all operators be stationed on the same side of a work surface. This is generally easily done in research and testing settings, but it can be difficult to accomplish in a production environment.

Regardless of airflow orientation, it is important to optimize airflow to ensure that the flow is as efficient as possible in protecting the most critical work areas within the facility. Studies conducted by ventilation engineers demonstrated that the low-density particulate contamination (both viable and nonviable) in a clean facility are affected little by gravity. It has long been a generally accepted notion that contamination in clean rooms follows streamlines or, in other words, is transported by convection along with the stream of airflow. If we can ignore the contribution of gravity, two other factors could affect the movement of contaminants: turbulence, in which the airstreams mix and move the particles by turbulent diffusion or, in the absence of turbulence, could diffuse by Brownian motion. It also has been suggested that electrostatic attraction may be a significant factor in particle movement in clean rooms, but presently, this is generally not considered in facility design for the control of microbial contamination.[35]

The wakes and vortices created by fixed equipment are constant; however, the movement of operators is not predictable. Therefore, the disruptions to airflow caused by operators working in clean facilities are of the utmost concern. A method has been developed to assist users in optimizing and testing the effectiveness of airflow.[36] This method consists of two steps, the first of which is a visualization of airflow under mock operational conditions using conventional smoke generators. The second step is to determine a risk factor, which is an evaluation of the ability of the airflow to reduce the likelihood of contamination in the critical zone. This is accomplished by measuring airborne particulate levels within the critical zone while generating particulate matter in the surrounding ambient environment. During this test, operators are working within the environment and equipment is in full operation. It is suggested that the movements of operators be somewhat exaggerated compared with their normal operations because this will give a more accurate reading of the robustness of the facility design. It was demonstrated experimentally that if the risk factor is less than 10^{-4} (0.01%), the probability of microbial contamination within the critical work zone is low; however, if the risk factor is greater than 10^{-4}, some remedial action is required. This remediation could include equipment

orientation, barrier curtain placement, reduction in personnel movement, or modification to the airflow.

Over the last 20 years, airflow visualization by smoke studies has become a heavily emphasized activity in aseptic processing clean rooms. Such smoke studies are subject to video recording for review by the clean room operator and to be shown to regulatory inspectors as required. But the metrics for determination of smoke study success are not easily defined, which results in subjective evaluation principles.

Airflow Volume

The amount of HEPA filtered air flowing through a clean room facility has long been considered an important design consideration. The volume of air flowing into a room is a function of the velocity of air (flow rate) through the filters. The flow rate through the filters for ISO class 5 environments is quite frequently specified at 90 ft/min or approximately 0.45 m/s as measured about 30 cm from the filter face, which is in most cases the air entry point. This rate, or as it is commonly known velocity, is typically the controlling factor regarding the total airflow volume for a facility and hence the air-exchange rate and its recommendation dates to US Federal Standard 209B.[25] Air velocity was a mandatory specification in this standard; in subsequent versions, stipulations regarding air velocity were dropped. The authors realized that airflow rate and volume requirements are extremely dependent on the purpose for which the facility will be used. For example, for aseptically dispensed medicines or medical device manufacturing, high flow rates may be desirable, particularly if there are large number of operators stationed in a facility, making a high dilution rate desirable. In a germ-free animal research facility, high airflow rates may cause desiccation resulting in discomfort to animals. Also, in facilities where both containment of dangerous substances and maintenance of high levels of contamination control are required, high flow rates may be contraindicated. Therefore, it can be suggested that the air velocity in clean facilities should not be standardized. It is still common in the health care industry for air velocities in the range of 0.45 m/s to be specified. Over the years, many clean rooms have been designed to this specification, and the level of performance attained has been excellent.[32]

Over the last decade, there has been increasing emphasis placed on measuring air velocity at the level of the work table or just above the work surface. The result has been air velocity requirements historically expected at the air entry point being expected or demanded at or slightly above the work surface. This practice has not been proven beneficial. The actual height of the work surface is typically a variable rather than a constant, and this complicates accurate measure. Also, boundaries such as walls and barriers provide resistance to air velocity, which result in unavoidable slowing of air movement diminishing uniformity. An upshot of this requirement has been the increase in air velocity at the room entry point to achieve a 0.45 μm air velocity (or greater) at the work surface. This can depend on air return baffle settings that result in high air flow rates through a room and therefore a greater number of air changes per hour. This results in higher energy consumption that runs contrary to the desire to reduce carbon emissions. High air flow rates beyond those achieved at customary flow rates of 0.45 m/s at or slightly below the filter face are often considered sufficient. The use of automation to reduce operator contamination potential would be a far more effective way to reduce microbiological risk, than an increase in air flow.

The traditional 90 ft/min or 0.45 m/s specifications are best considered arbitrary recommendations rather than as hard and fast standards. Air velocity increases or undo emphasis on uniformity across the room are generally expected at the historical velocity tolerances of about ±20%. Also, in aseptic chambers or isolator enclosures where the bioload from personnel is low or zero, much lower air velocities compared to those used in clean rooms have been used successfully. Total airflow, and thus the number of air changes per hour, relates both to the air velocity across each filter and the number of filters installed. In some ISO class 5 clean rooms, it will be necessary to have as much filter area in the ceiling of the room (assuming vertical airflow) as possible. In facilities where the need for ISO class 5 quality air is limited to a discrete area within a room, the air supply volume will be proportionately less. Therefore, rooms may be entirely ISO class 5 (EU class A), or they may be some combination of ISO class 5/6 (EU A/B) or ISO class 5 space surrounded by ISO class 7. Rooms that are totally ISO class 5, of course, typically have a higher total airflow per unit of room volume and therefore more air exchanges per hour. Rooms used for critical operations may have anywhere from 100 air changes per hour up 700 or more depending on total air flow through the room. Generally, ISO class 5 facilities rarely have fewer than 20 air changes per hour, with a typical target of 30 to 50 air changes per hour. ISO class 7 rooms typically have 50 to more than 100 air exchanges per hour, although more or less could be provided, depending on the nature of the work to be done in the facility.

Recirculation of Air

In most clean room facilities, about 80% of the air is recirculated from the return ducts back through the filters and into the room, and 20% of the air is fresh. Fresh air is conditioned and prefiltered prior to routing to the principal (or final) room air-filtration system. The introduction of fresh air is required to ensure that a buildup of carbon dioxide in breathing air does not occur. In some operations, particularly those in which powders or dangerous materials are handled, it may be desirable to use 100% fresh air. These issues are not significant from a medicines or medical device regulatory perspective but rather are economic and occupational safety issues.

Pressure Differentials

It is standard practice in clean room operations to have zones of operation. Generally, classification of individual clean rooms within a facility and the criticality of activities define these zones. The most critical areas, that is those with the most stringent level of classification, should operate at the highest relative pressure. It is common for clean facilities to have two or three zones of operation. Typically, the pressure differentials between adjacent zones are in the range of 10 to 15 Pa, although lower and higher differentials are possible, depending on process requirements.

Facilities designed to control the dissemination of hazardous substances typically are run at a negative pressure relative to the surrounding area. Where aseptic processing is conducted, microbial control must take precedence in the design over containment. In aseptic operations in which containment is required, buffer rooms or air locks may represent the most effective design approach. An air lock is a clean room design feature typically used to transfer materials into or out of clean room suites; it prevents the flow of air from a lower classified or unclassified zone into an area of higher air quality.

Ingress and Egress of Personnel

Because human operators have a great capacity for contributing contamination to a clean environment, the method by which workers don protective clothing is vital to the control of microbial contamination. Modern clean rooms typically are equipped with a three-stage gowning facility in which the operator changes from plant clothing into sterile, full-coverage, clean room apparel.[1] Aseptic processing facilities and other clean room housing critical or relatively critical activities typically have three-stage gowning suites. All three stages are provided with their own air supply system, and the air quality increases from one stage to the next. Generally, the last stage of the gowning operation is classified at the same level as the most critical zone in the suite of clean rooms served by the gowning suite. Accordingly, the pressure is highest in the final stage of gowning and lowest at the entry point into the gowning suite. The second state of gowning is controlled at a pressure that falls in between the other two stages. In some facilities, an air shower is installed between the last stage of gowning and the clean room facility.

Great care should be given to designing the gowning rooms and to laying out the clothing storage and supply areas. The design should consider the number of staff members that will be using the facility and allow sufficient room for movement during the gowning process.

Clothing and supplies should be easy to access and should require a minimum of difficult movement. The doors between the gowning rooms as well as the main entry door into the gowning suit and the door between the third gowning stage and the main portion of the clean facility should be provided with interlocks. There must never be more than one of these doors open at any given point in time. Wherever possible, a separate exit air lock should be provided for personnel egress. The exit air-lock doors always should be interlocked and alarmed. This air lock also can be used to move used equipment and waste out of the clean facility. In some facilities, it may be appropriate to use this same air lock for the introduction of materials into the clean room; however, in critical operations, it is best to provide a separate air lock, preferably with its own filtered air supply for the introduction of materials.

Cleaning and Disinfection of the Facility

Large clean room suites typically are subjected to sanitation or disinfection on a frequent and regularly scheduled basis.[37] The selection of wall finishes, flooring, glazing, sealing materials, and ceilings that are resistant to the antimicrobial agents and cleaning materials used is imperative. The reader is referred to other chapters in this book that specifically describe typical antimicrobial agents used and for specific guidance in the selection and testing of these substances. In critical ISO class 5 zones used for aseptic processing or other activities demanding tight control over microbial contamination, sporicidal agents are strongly recommended.

The design of the air ducts supplying the facility should allow for frequent inspection and cleaning. Strategically located hatches allowing access for visual inspection of the ducts is strongly recommended. In many critical applications, the ducts and filters are also subjected to treatment with antimicrobial agents. Historically, formaldehyde vapor has been the most common agent for treating ducts and filters. Recently, vaporized hydrogen peroxide (VHP) and chlorine dioxide (CD) have been used for this purpose.[38,39]

Enhanced Clean Devices and Separative Technologies

Since the mid-1980s, there has been a dramatic increase in the use of advanced enhanced clean devices of various types to control microbial and particulate contamination (Figure 58.2). The terms *enhanced clean devices* and *separative technologies* are terms coined by ISO technical committee 209 working group 7 to describe various types of equipment used to improve the performance of contamination control facility. This category of equipment

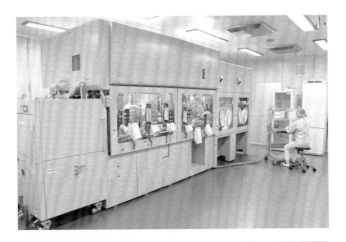

FIGURE 58.2 A fully automated isolator system used for aseptic processing of cytotherapy products or regenerative medicines. An incubator can be seen on the left of the main isolators and a transfer pass box may be seen on the right. These modules or others as required can be connected to the main isolator system by docking ports, which can be decontaminated as required. Courtesy of Shibuya Co, Kanazawa, Ishikawa, Japan.

ranges from rather simple barrier equipped flow cabinets or hoods to isolators, which are as close to fully closed clean work environments as current technology allows.

All enhanced clean devices have one important feature in common, and that is a much higher level of separation between workers and the process than is possible in a conventional human-scale clean room. Isolators have become widely used in health care manufacturing and product testing. During the last 30 years, isolators have replaced scores of conventional clean room facilities for sterility testing, and many isolators have been validated and approved for the manufacturing and containment of hazardous substances.

Key Features of Isolators

The advantages that isolators have over conventional clean rooms in terms of contamination control are related to four key performance attributes. First, a true isolator must not exchange air with any environment in which human operators' work, except after that air has been treated by filters to remove contamination (Figure 58.3). Second, all manipulations performed by humans on materials within an isolator must be conducted remotely. In practice, this means that all manipulations are done using gloves mounted on flexible sleeve assemblies or using body suits mounted into the wall of the isolator. Third, the isolator—including all enclosure surfaces, equipment, and manipulation devices—must be disinfected[40] such that the entire enclosure is rendered essentially free of microorganisms. Fourth, conventional air locks or transfer hatches are not used to transfer materials into the isolator; instead, special

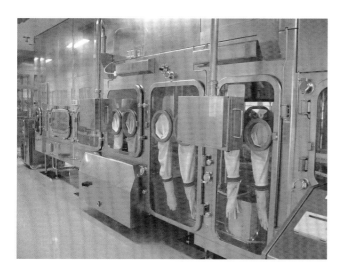

FIGURE 58.3 An isolator network enclosed aseptic vaccine production line capable of 400 containers per minute. This photograph shows the aseptic filing and stopper placement sections of the network. The system uses robots, which can be decontaminated in situ along with the isolator network. Robots are used for parts loading of sterilized stoppers and placement operations. The system operates with minimal need for operator involvement. Courtesy of Shibuya Co, Kanazawa, Ishikawa, Japan.

rapid transfer ports (RTPs) are used, which greatly reduce the risk of environmental contamination entering the isolator on materials RTPs are specialized transfer devices used to make connections between isolators or between adjacent zones in a clean room. Examples of equipment docked to isolators using disinfection-capable transfer ports can be seen in Figure 58.2.

Types of Isolators

There are two general types of isolators. A closed isolator is an enclosure that has no direct opening to the external environment. The air supply for the closed isolator is filtered through an HEPA or better grade filter and a filter of at least HEPA quality protects the air exhaust as well. Closed isolators are extremely useful for batch production operations and laboratory work, such as product testing or research. A useful attribute of the closed isolator is their ability to provide simultaneously a high level of sterility assurance and containment of hazardous materials.[22]

The second type of isolator is an air-sealed or open isolator. An air-sealed isolator, as the name implies, relies on air overpressure rather than a physical seal to maintain its integrity. These isolators are useful for continuous production operations, such as continuous container filling. Management and control of the air system are essential because these function as isolators only as long as an effective air seal is maintained.

Materials of Construction

Isolators may be fabricated out of sturdy, flexible thermoplastic materials, PVC being the most common material. These flexible wall isolators have the advantage of being light, relatively portable, and easy to assemble. Their flexible design also affords them some ergonomic benefits because the walls can flex to accommodate human movement. They have the disadvantages of being structurally limited and cannot be easily fit with a unidirectional air supply system. The PVC is also less than perfect optically and typically becoming more opaque over time. In addition, flexible wall isolators can be physically difficult to clean because of the movement of the walls and concerns regarding abrasion and chemical compatibility.

Rigid wall isolators are fabricated out of steel, the 300 series of stainless steels being the most commonly selected. Isolators always incorporate glazing materials to provide a suitable view of the work area within the enclosure. Glass, acrylic, and polycarbonate are the most common glazing materials. Rigid wall isolators are able to support large, complex air supply systems and can readily be configured to provide unidirectional airflow. They are relatively easy to clean and generally are more resistant to harsh chemicals than flexible walled isolators. Rigid wall isolators are more difficult to use for applications requiring portability, such as transfer of materials, because they can be heavy, even for rather small enclosure volumes.

Isolator Air Supply Systems

Isolator air supply systems can be extremely simple but, in some installations, have been nearly as complex as those for conventional clean rooms. The air supply system for flexible wall isolators are generally simple and consists only of an inlet filter, exhaust filter, and a blower. Conditioning and dehumidification of the air are generally not required. The flexible wall isolator simply uses the room air from the surrounding facility as makeup air.

Rigid wall isolators also can have a simple air supply system if turbulent or mixing airflow is specified. If unidirectional airflow is required, however, the air supply system is typically of a recirculating design similar to those used in conventional clean rooms. It is not uncommon for a large, rigid wall isolator to be equipped with some air conditioning and dehumidification capability.

Airflow velocity and air exchange rate can be much lower in an isolator than in a conventional clean room. The isolator enclosure is much smaller, and typically the air entry point is far closer to the work surface than in a human scale clean room.[41] Also, the contamination load in an isolator is much less due to the absence of human operators and the improved protection against environmental contamination provided by an isolator. Thus, the air volume needed to dilution of contamination is not nearly as high as would be needed in a large clean room.

In practice, air velocities of 0.1 m/s have proven satisfactory. Correspondingly, high air exchange rates, such as the several hundred an hour typical in conventional clean rooms are not required in isolators. Simpler air supply systems have numerous advantages, including reduced cost, simple maintenance, more efficient decontamination, and easier cleaning and inspection.

Isolator Air Quality Standards

In terms of particulate air quality, isolators equipped with HEPA filters will readily meet ISO class 5, or EU class A, standards. It is important to note that these particulate air standards do not require unidirectional airflow patterns. The level of microbial contamination control provided by an isolator is much higher than the human-scale clean room. In fact, the consensus is that a target value of zero contamination is reasonable. USP <1116> suggests that isolators should produce contamination control rates at least 10-fold lower than manned clean rooms.[28]

Material Transfer Systems (Rapid Transfer Systems)

A number of material transfer systems have been successfully used with isolators. The RTPs are available from a large number of manufacturers. These systems originated in the nuclear industry during the 1960s and have proven reliable in both containment and sterility assurance applications. Currently, some manufacturers are further enhancing the microbiological safety of RTPs by offering systems that are fully sterilizable. Standard clean room transfer hatches or air locks never should be used with isolators unless these hatches can be reproducibly and quantitatively decontaminated prior to use. Numerous transfer hatch or tunnel devices have been used successfully in conjunction with isolators. A gaseous disinfectant agent may treat materials on a batch or continuous basis, or they may be treated by ultraviolet light. It is critical that the surface of any material taken into the isolator enclosure be free of microbial contamination.

Disinfection (or Biodecontamination) of Isolators

One of the key advantages of isolators is the ability to develop and validate a rigorous and fully reproducible method for disinfection of both the enclosure and its contents. Isolator disinfection (or fumigation) methods are most commonly based on vapor or gaseous antimicrobial agents. The VHP is currently the most commonly used method; given careful attention to temperature and vapor concentration, this method has worked well. The CD has also been used successfully, and atomized liquid hydrogen peroxide has been used in the disinfection of aseptic chambers (isolators) used in the aseptic manufacture of extended shelf-life beverages or food products. These methods have all but replaced the use of traditional methods that used formaldehyde fumigation or liquid disinfectants.[21] These gaseous methods can be evaluated using biological indicators, which are distributed throughout the enclosure, to provide a quantitative assessment of effectiveness. A suitable resistant spore population from a *Bacillus* or *Geobacillus* species is used as the indicator organism. Although requirements may vary depending on the application, process, and regulatory requirements, in general, a 3 to 6 spore log reduction will result in an isolator environment that is suitably decontaminated for the aseptic processing of medicines, biologicals, and medical devices.[42]

▶ CONCLUSION

A wide range of facilities and equipment to provide a suitable microbially controlled environment is available to the user than ever before. Given the near universal agreement that the control of human-borne contamination is the most critical factor in the control of microbial cross-contamination, it comes as no surprise that automation and isolation have moved to the forefront of facility and equipment design objectives. Although there are many complexities involved in the control of environmental microorganisms, if the user can focus on control and dilution of human-borne microbial contamination, it will be possible to employ better methods to control these hazards both in the design of facilities and in the day-to-day operation. It is impossible to cover all the critical issues in facility design in a summary chapter such as this; however, if the reader keeps the basic principles discussed here in mind, a sufficient understanding of this subject can be attained to explore this topic in greater depth in the numerous books and trade publications that cover this important subject.

REFERENCES

1. Agalloco J, Akers J, Madsen R. Aseptic processing: a review of current industry practice. *Pharm Tech*. 2004;28(10):126-129.

2. Akers J, Agalloco J, Carleton F, Korczynski M. A review of current technology in parenteral manufacturing. *J Parenter Sci Technol*. 1988;42(2):53-56.

3. Akers J. Environmental monitoring and control: proposed standards, current practices, and future directions. *PDA J Pharm Sci Technol*. 1997;51(1):36-47.

4. Akers JE, Agalloco JP. A revised aseptic risk assessment and mitigation methodology. *Pharm Tech*. 2017;41(11):32-39.

5. Akers J, Agalloco J. Clean rooms, RABS, and isolators: validation and monitoring in the diverse world of aseptic processing. *American Pharm Rev*. 2011;14(4). https://www.americanpharmaceuticalreview.com/Featured-Articles/36878-Clean-Rooms-RABS-and-Isolators-Validation-and-Monitoring-in-the-Diverse-World-of-Aseptic-Processing/. Accessed May 27, 2019.

6. US Food and Drug Administration. *Guideline for Industry on Sterile Drug Products Produced by Aseptic Processing—Current Good Manufacturing Practice*. Silver Spring, MD: US Food and Drug Administration; 2004.

7. ICH Expert Working Group. *ICH Harmonised Tripartite Guideline: Quality Risk Management Q9*. Geneva, Switzerland: International Conference on Harmonisation; 2005. https://www.ich.org/fileadmin/Public_Web_Site/ICH_Products/Guidelines/Quality/Q9/Step4/Q9_Guideline.pdf. Accessed May 27, 2019.

8. Sandle T. New guidance for sterile products manufacture is coming: review of EU GMP Annex 1. Institute of Validation Technology Web site. http://www.ivtnetwork.com/article/new-guidance-sterile-products-manufacture-coming-review-eu-gmp-annex-1. Accessed May 27, 2019.

9. Parenteral Drug Association. Process simulation testing for aseptically filled products. *PDA J Pharm Sci Technol.* 1996;50(suppl 1):S1-S16.

10. Akers J, Agalloco J. Environmental monitoring: myths and misapplications. *PDA J Pharm Sci Technol.* 2001;55(3):176-184.

11. Akers J. Technological advances in microbial contamination control. In: Prince R, ed. *Microbiology in Pharmaceutical Manufacturing*. Bethesda, MD: Parenteral Drug Association; 2001:125-145.

12. Bryce DM. Tests for the sterility of pharmaceutical preparations: the design and interpretation of sterility tests. *J Pharm Pharmacol.* 1956;8(8):561-572.

13. Hughes JB, Hellmann JJ, Ricketts TH, Bohannan BJ. Counting the uncountable: statistical approaches to estimating microbial diversity. *Appl Environ Microbiol.* 2000;67(10):4399-4406.

14. Sutton SVW. The sterility tests. In: Moldenauer J, ed. *Rapid Sterility Testing*. Bethesda, MD: Parenteral Drug Association; 2011:7-18.

15. Meyer D. Design and engineering of isolators. In: Akers J, Agalloco J, eds. *Advanced Aseptic Processing Technologies*. London, United Kingdom: Informa Healthcare; 2010:65-75.

16. Akers J, Tanimoto K, Kawata M. Highly automated isolator-based vaccine filling—a case study. In: Akers J, Agalloco J, eds. *Advanced Aseptic Processing Technologies*. London, United Kingdom: Informa Healthcare; 2010:395-403.

17. Whyte W, Agricola K, Derks M. Airborne particulate deposition in cleanrooms: deposition mechanisms. *Clean Air Containment Rev.* 2015;24:4-9.

18. Katayama H, Toga A, Tokunaga Y, Katoh S. Proposal for a new categorization of aseptic processing facilities based on risk assessment scores. *PDA J Pharm Sci Technol.* 2008;62(4):235-243.

19. US Food and Drug Administration. *Guideline on Sterile Drug Products Produced by Aseptic Processing*. Silver Spring. MD: US Food and Drug Administration; 1987.

20. Wagner CM, Akers JE. *Isolator Technology: Applications in the Pharmaceutical and Biotechnology Industries*. Buffalo Grove, IL: Interpharm Press; 1995.

21. Akers JE, Izumi Y. Technological advancements in aseptic processing and the elimination of contamination risk. In: Akers J, Agalloco J, eds. *Advanced Aseptic Processing Technologies*. London, United Kingdom: Informa Healthcare; 2010:404-410.

22. Pierson MD, Corlett DA. *HACCP Principles and Application*. New York, NY: Van Nostrand Reinhold; 1992.

23. Tomasiewicz DM, Hotchkiss DK, Reinbold GW, Read RB Jr, Hartman PA. The most suitable number of colonies on plates for counting. *J Food Prot.* 1980;43(4):282-286.

24. De Vecchi F. Validation of environmental control systems. In: Agalloco J, Carleton F, eds. *Validation of Pharmaceutical Products—Sterile Products*. New York, NY: Marcel Dekker; 1998:217-259.

25. Institute of Environmental Sciences and Technology. *Federal Standard 209E. Airborne Particulate Cleanliness Classes in Cleanrooms and Clean Zones*. Mt. Prospect, IL: Institute of Environmental Sciences and Technology; 1992.

26. International Organization for Standardization. *ISO 14644-7:2015: Cleanrooms and Associated Controlled Environments—Part 7: Separative Devices (Clean Air Hoods, Gloveboxes, Isolators and Mini-Environments)*. Geneva, Switzerland: International Organization for Standardization; 2015.

27. International Organization for Standardization. *ISO 14644-1:2015: Cleanrooms and Associated Controlled Environments—Part 1: Classification of Air Cleanliness by Particle Concentration*. Geneva, Switzerland: International Organization for Standardization; 2015.

28. United States Pharmacopeia. *National Formulary (USP_NF) 41 General Chapter <1116> Microbiological Control and Monitoring of Aseptic Processing Environments*. Bethesda, MD: United States Pharmacopeia; 2018.

29. Cole JC. *Pharmaceutical Production Facilities—Design and Applications*. Chichester, United Kingdom: Ellis Norwood; 1990.

30. Institute of Environmental Sciences and Technology. *Compendium of Standards, Practices, Methods and Similar Documents Relating to Contamination Control. CC009/IESCC009.2*. Mt. Prospect, IL: Institute of Environmental Sciences and Technology; 1995.

31. International Organization for Standardization. *ISO 29464-1:2017: High Efficiency Filters and Filter Media*. Geneva, Switzerland: International Organization for Standardization; 2017.

32. Ljungqvist B, Reinmüller B. Interaction between air movements and the dispersion of contaminants: clean zones with unidirectional air flow. *J Parenter Sci Technol.* 1993;47(2):60-69.

33. Ljungqvist B, Reinmüller B. Microbiological assessment in clean zones for aseptic production. *J R3 Nordic.* 1994;3:7-10,27-28.

34. Whyte, W. *Cleanroom Design*. 2nd ed. Chichester, United Kingdom: John Wiley & Sons; 1999.

35. Sandle T. Distribution of particles within the clean room: a review of contamination control considerations. Institute of Validation Technology Web site. http://www.ivtnetwork.com/article/distribution-particles-within-cleanroom-review-contamination-control-considerations. Accessed May 27, 2019.

36. Ljungqvist B, Reinmüller B. Supplementary microbiological assessment test with the air of particle challenge test and visualization technique. In: Proceedings from the 11th International Symposium on Contamination Control; September 21-25; 1995; London, United Kingdom.

37. Agalloco J, Akers J. Current practices in the validation of aseptic processing—1992. *J Parenter Sci Technol.* 1993;47(suppl 1):S1-S21.

38. Kokubo M, Inoue T, Akers J. Resistance of common environmental spores of the genus *Bacillus* to vapor hydrogen peroxide. *PDA J Pharm Sci Technol.* 1998;52(5):228-231.

39. Sintim-Damoa K. Other gaseous sterilization methods. In: Morrissey R, Phillips G, eds. *Sterilization Technology—A Practical Guide for Manufacturers and Users of Health Care Products*. New York, NY: Van Nostrand Reinhold; 1992:335-347.

40. Parenteral Drug Association. *Design and Validation of Isolator Systems for Manufacturing and Testing of Sterile Health Care Products*. Bethesda, MD: Parenteral Drug Association; 2001. Technical report no. 34.

41. Akers JE, Agalloco J. Environmental monitoring of advanced aseptic processing technology. In: Akers J, Agalloco J, eds. *Advanced Aseptic Processing Technologies*. London, United Kingdom: Informa Healthcare; 2010:267-275.

42. Akers JE, Agalloco J. Decontamination of advanced aseptic processing environments. In: Akers J, Agalloco J, eds. *Advanced Aseptic Processing Technologies*. London, United Kingdom: Informa Healthcare; 2010:276-288.

Safe Handling of Biological Agents in the Laboratory

Alan J. Beswick, Brian Crook, and Catherine Makison Booth

Working with biological agents in the laboratory environment may involve the handling of microorganisms, cell cultures, or human endoparasites, including those that have been genetically modified, which may cause infection, allergy, toxicity, or other negative impact to human and/or animal health or the environment. Not all biological agents are hazardous by nature, but those that are harmful are often referred to as biohazards. When working in laboratories, the protection of test materials and sample integrity are important considerations, but these are secondary to the safety of personnel who may regularly be required to work with potentially infectious material. Risk assessment, management, and control are therefore important to laboratory biosafety to protect laboratory personnel and the wider community against inadvertent exposures and release of hazardous biological agents. This chapter has been prepared from authoritative information sources, including those from North America and Europe, in order to provide material that is internationally relevant for laboratory workers.

Four risk or hazard groups are often used to categorize biological agents based on several key factors associated with their inherent characteristics. These are

- ability to cause disease
- severity of disease
- likelihood of spreading to the wider community
- availability of prophylaxis or treatment

These groups are then often associated with an equivalent biosafety level (BSL; also known as containment level). Each BSL (ranging from levels 1 to 4) has a specific set of facility and operational requirements that must be complied with before work with the associated biological agents can be started. Most routine microbiological analytical work is undertaken in laboratories operated at BSL-2. Although biological agents handled at BSL-2 can cause disease, these typically present a low-to-moderate risk to employees and are unlikely to spread to the wider community because effective treatment or prophylaxis is available.[1,2] Examples of these include common bacteria such as *Staphylococcus aureus*, *Mycobacterium fortuitum*, and *Acinetobacter baumannii* as well as viruses such as respiratory syncytial virus and norovirus. Fungal isolates such as *Aspergillus fumigatus* and *Microsporum* species also fall into this category. Many other examples exist and are listed by most national regulatory bodies as well as by international agencies.[3-7]

Work with biological agents may also be undertaken in facilities such as pharmaceutical production or with more hazardous pathogens in higher containment (BSL-3 or BSL-4) laboratories. Procedures and room design in these areas should reflect the nature of the activities undertaken. In some countries, regulations will specify the controls required, usually supported by codes of practice and guidance. These will typically allow for a broad range of clinical, diagnostic, and research work with biological agents.

In addition to identifying the hazards associated with the biological agents, other factors are important to ensure that work can take place within any laboratory setting safely and efficiently. These include effective health and safety management, including local risk assessment to identify what measures are needed to eliminate or control risk, implementation of these control measures, the competency of the staff to undertake the work, robust operational and safety procedures, and the fitness for purpose of the laboratory space itself (work surfaces, equipment, freedom of movement, appropriate waste disposal procedures, etc).

▶ RISK ASSESSMENT

A hazard is something that has the potential to cause harm and a risk is the likelihood that somebody could be harmed by the hazard, together with an indication of how serious the harm could be. For example, in a microbiology laboratory, workers may be at risk of adverse health consequences from exposure to microorganisms. The risk to workers will increase if the *likelihood* of exposure increases, which will depend on the activities being performed. The risk will also increase if the *severity* of the health consequences increases, which will be dependent on the type and number of microorganisms being handled. It is important to note that there may also be a risk of harm to people who do not work in the laboratory.

The aim of a risk assessment is to decide whether appropriate control measures are in place to eliminate or effectively control risks, or to determine whether more are required. The first step in assessing risk from biological agents in the laboratory is to identify and characterize the hazard(s) (ie, sources of harm), the nature of that harm, who might be affected, and how they may be harmed (ie, what they are doing and what could happen to cause harm).

Therefore, it is necessary to identify

- What biological agents will be used
- The activities or procedures to be undertaken, including whether sharps are used, and the potential for causing an exposure, for example, to generate aerosols or splash
- The potential health consequences to both laboratory personnel and others who could be exposed

An estimation of risk can then be made. This will include consideration of both the severity of the hazard and the likelihood of harm, taking into account the control measures in place (or those planned for new activities). Having estimated the risk, the next stage of the risk assessment is to determine whether appropriate control measures are in place so that work can proceed or whether additional or different, more effective control measures are needed. Risk evaluation criteria will need to conform to national and local requirements.

Characterizing Biohazards

When making a biological risk assessment, the hazards relate directly to the biological agents to be handled. The risk associated with a biological agent will be dependent on several key factors including

- the likelihood of infection if exposed
- severity of disease (morbidity or mortality)
- infectious dose
- route(s) of transmission (natural versus laboratory; see in the following text)
- communicability/R_0 (basic reproduction rate—used to measure the transmission potential of a disease)
- epidemiology (exotic or endemic)
- effective prophylaxis and treatments (availability, practical, appropriate)
- susceptibility of local population (naive)

Other factors that should be considered can include

- environmental robustness (persistence outside of host/culture conditions) of the biological agent
- natural host range (ie, coming across agents in laboratory not normally encountered), such as rabies being

exotic in United Kingdom but endemic in mainland Europe and multi-drug-resistant tuberculosis (MDR TB) considered a greater risk pathology in laboratories at an inner city compared to a rural location
- zoonosis
- history of laboratory-acquired infection
- susceptibility of staff working in the laboratory (immunocompromised)
- symptoms (possibility of asymptomatic disease)
- shedding (likelihood and type)
- official control (is the agent on a national notifiable disease database, subject to human, plant, animal, or other regulations)
- the concentration and volume of the biological agent to be handled

Routes of Transmission and Exposure

Biological agents usually have a certain route of entry into the body, although in some cases, infection can occur via multiple routes. *Bacillus anthracis* (the causative agent of anthrax), for example, is infectious via inhalation, percutaneous entry, or ingestion. It is important to note that natural routes of transmission and pathogenicity can differ from those associated with laboratory-acquired infection. This could be due to the use of high concentrations and high volumes of fluids, the generation of splashes and aerosols, use of sharps, and working with infected animals. In addition, the disease may also present itself differently if there has been an unconventional route of transmission. The nature of microorganisms being handled in the laboratory may vary, but one of the determining factors for an increased likelihood of microbiological exposure is when they are present at high titers as a result of their intensive propagation.

Using the inadvertent spillage of a bacterial culture as an example, the numbers of microorganisms involved will depend on the natural growth rate and age of the culture under laboratory growth conditions. A bacterial culture in late exponential growth typically has between 10^6 and 10^9 colony-forming units per millilitre (or milliliter) (CFUs)/mL,[8] whereas cell concentration techniques may increase this to between 10^{10} and 10^{11} CFUs/mL. Viral particles can be similarly propagated and concentrated, for example, by filtration and centrifugation, to achieve high viral levels, usually measured as plaque-forming units per millilitre (or milliliter) (PFUs/mL) or ID_{50}. Although less commonly used, fungal cultures for pathogen testing (eg, *Coccidioides immitis*[9]) produce stock suspensions of between 10^7 and 10^8 spores/mL. Therefore, there is the potential for significant exposure to microorganisms even when small volumes of cultures are being handled.

The main routes of infection in the laboratory are discussed in the following sections.

Percutaneous

Within the laboratory, routes of percutaneous transmission can include

- sharps injury such as needles, broken glass, scalpel blades
- splashing of the mucous membranes of the eye, nose, or mouth
- contamination of unprotected skin lesions, for example, eczema
- animal bites or scratches
- presence of a vector, for example, biting or piercing insects

Blood-borne viruses (BBVs) are transmitted in contaminated blood or other body fluids following entry into the body of a susceptible person. The rate of viral transmission is dependent on the level of exposure to the virus, the type of virus, and the immune status of the exposed person. The BBVs are generally not thought to be transmitted via the respiratory route, although this possibility cannot be dismissed entirely if, under laboratory conditions such as in high-titer in vitro cultures, BBVs are present in concentrations far exceeding that found in normal body fluids. In the laboratory setting, BBVs are mainly transmitted by direct exposure to infected blood or other body fluids contaminated with infected blood, most likely via sharps injury.

Because most microbiology laboratory work involves handling cultures in aqueous suspension, splashing onto the mucous membranes is a real and feasible route of exposure and potential transmission through laboratory incidents, resulting from loss of primary containment. Aerosols may be created by, for example, spills or dropped and broken flasks.[10] The loss of primary containment in these situations is likely to be in the form of material derived from a splash (see in the following text) and subsequently transferred on to other surfaces by the hands of workers.[11-13]

Damage to the skin barrier such as cuts, abrasions, or lesions caused by ongoing dermatological conditions can leave a person generally more susceptible to percutaneous transmission of infection. Consequently, it is important that laboratory workers are aware of any skin conditions, including broken or punctured skin and allergies, prior to handling biological agents or potentially contaminated materials, and take any additional precautions necessary to avoid exposure.

Contact

Direct contact with microbiologically contaminated objects or surfaces (fomites) can readily result in

- ingestion of microorganisms, typically after pick up and hand-to-mouth transfer
- their contact with mucus membranes
- contact with the skin (commonly through broken skin but can occur via contact with intact skin)

The transfer of microorganisms, or other hazardous substances, via surfaces and objects is a well-known exposure route and has been particularly well studied in the health care settings. In poorly controlled work environments, there is a risk of cross-contamination from hazardous materials on surfaces and inadvertent transfer, for example, via gloved or unprotected hands.[12] Human factors are also a significant factor. Even in a laboratory setting where the risks of hand to face contact are stressed, those contacts may still be made. In a study of 93 laboratory workers at BSL-2, 67 (72%) touched their face at least once, with contact to the nose being most common (44.9% of contacts), followed by contact with the forehead (36.9%), cheek/chin (12.5%), mouth (4.0%), and eye (1.7%).[14] Another potential contact exposure scenario is while cleaning up a spill, warranting additional protection. The prevention of worker exposure via contact is therefore dependent on the effective use of primary containment, good laboratory technique and, where required, the decontamination of affected surfaces and equipment. Any intervention in the laboratory setting is also likely to include a disinfection step. The diligence of the operator and appropriateness of any products used for cleaning and disinfection are therefore critical to effective worker protection from surface contamination.

Airborne

The airborne route of exposure is commonly implicated in occupational exposures to all types of hazards including chemicals, nonbiological particulates, and bioaerosols. It is also an exposure that can be readily controlled in the laboratory setting using good laboratory techniques and effective engineering solutions, especially ventilation controls. Failure to do this can result in inhalation of infectious aerosols, conjunctival exposure, inhalation of infectious aerosols followed by swallowing/ingestion (eg, with norovirus), and droplet exposure.

Pottage et al[11] examined the potential for routine microbiological techniques, such as serial dilution and pipetting, to be transmission routes by the generation of bioaerosols or splashing. Test activities, undertaken by staff with a range of experience and training, showed that aerosol and splash contamination was produced by all users, even those highly trained and experienced but that a correctly operating biological safety cabinet (BSC) will contain these aerosols. More experienced operators did not necessarily generate fewer aerosols, but those trained to work at BSL-3 did, suggesting that good microbiological technique was important. When preparing serial dilutions, those not trained at BSL-3 generated significantly more aerosols on average by over seven times. The study also showed that splash contamination on gloves and surfaces could potentially be spread within and outside the laboratory, emphasizing the importance of effective personal protective equipment (PPE) and hygiene controls.

Working with animals, both large and small, may involve handling pathogenic microorganisms, and the animal's physical activity may be the source of infectious bioaerosols. The containment of contaminated materials, such as fecal or urine-contaminated bedding, may be challenging under such circumstances. One study used a mouse parvovirus (MPV) model to assess the potential transfer from rodent housing containment to surrounding surfaces.[15] The chosen virus represented the possible cross-contamination routes for other harmful viruses. The study found little evidence of significant deposition of the virus onto transfer surfaces, such as gloves and work surfaces outside of contained rodent storage cages. Even the positive pressure in ventilated cages did not result in animal room floor contamination, a suspected bioaerosol route of transfer, despite exhaust air escaping from the cage-top lip prior to high-efficiency particulate air (HEPA) filtration. However, soiled animal bedding and its handling by laboratory personnel was implicated in bioaerosol generation.

Infectious Dose and Environmental Robustness

The ability of a pathogen to cause infection requires its contact with susceptible host receptors (a combination of routes of transmission and exposure, as mentioned earlier) in a sufficient quantity, that is, at an infectious dose. Data on infectious dose for the wide range of human pathogens are limited. However, some notable examples illustrate the importance of taking this into consideration. *Escherichia coli* is an ubiquitous bacterium. Most *E coli* strains can cause minor infection via the oral route (hand-to-mouth transfer) but require a high dose to do so; therefore, it is safe to work with them in a general-purpose microbiology laboratory (BSL-2) using routine laboratory precautions. Disabled strains are commonly used tools in laboratory work, especially in genetic and molecular biology modifications and because of this attenuation, they are of minimal hazard (equivalent of BSL-1). However, verocytotoxigenic strains of *E coli*, such as O157, are zoonotic agents that can cause severe infection in humans at a very low infectious dose, estimated at just tens or hundreds of cells.[16,17] This *E coli* serotype therefore requires laboratory handling using enhanced precautions (equivalent to BSL-3) that minimize exposure.

Where data on infectious dose are available, it is important to factor this into the biohazard assessment in developing a risk assessment. In addition to evidence from research papers, public and occupational health Web sites also provide a valuable source of data on infectious dose of human pathogens (eg, European Centre for Disease Prevention and Control,[18] World Organisation for Animal Health,[19] Public Health Agency of Canada,[20] Health

and Safety Executive,[21] Public Health England,[22] Centers for Disease Control and Prevention,[23] World Health Organization[24]). However, such data must be used with caution because it is typically based on infectious dose derived from natural routes of transmission. In the laboratory, much higher titers of pathogens may be handled in culture and laboratory activities and, as described in the following text, this may create different potential routes of transmission. For example, although some vector-borne pathogens are most likely to be transmitted in the laboratory when handling infected mosquitoes or ticks, percutaneous injury from contaminated sharps may mimic the vector-borne route. These laboratory-specific routes of transmission must be taken into consideration.

Environmental robustness, that is, persistence of a pathogen outside its host, or outside of ideal culture conditions, is a further factor in assessing biohazard. At the one extreme, some enveloped viruses are more sensitive to ambient humidity and pH and quickly lose viability on surfaces or in aerosols,[25] whereas at the other extreme, spore-forming bacteria have been shown to survive in the wider environment for decades.[26]

▸ EXAMPLES OF LABORATORY ACTIVITIES AND INHERENT RISK

Laboratory work covers a broad range of procedures. This section describes how these procedures translate into laboratory activities and how these activities correlate with the risk of exposure to biological agents. The inherent hazard is the natural level of hazard associated with the agent being handled. The work carried out using the agent, eg, amount, titre used or procedures undertaken, will in turn influence any handling risk associated with the hazard.

Procedures that are less likely to result in exposure to biological agents include those that use low volumes and at low titer, such as molecular testing and use of diagnostics kits. For example, polymerase chain reaction (PCR) assays are unlikely to lead to significant exposure because of the preliminary steps in the process to lyse cells and extract nucleic acid, thus eliminating viable pathogens. Procedures that confer an increased likelihood of exposure include those that introduce energy into handling microbial cultures, for example, aspirating and ejecting liquids with pipettes, vortex mixing, or centrifuging. It should be noted that the potential for exposure via vortex mixing or centrifugation can and should be reduced with the use of sealed vessels and rotors. Procedures that present the greatest likelihood of exposure are those associated with handling high volumes with high titers of infectious agents in less contained conditions, including infected human or animal tissues. Figure 59.1 illustrates the relationship between examples of different types of laboratory procedure and the related likelihood of exposure to the hazard (the infectious agent) associated with the material/activity.

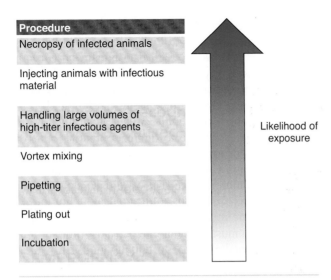

Procedure

Necropsy of infected animals

Injecting animals with infectious material

Handling large volumes of high-titer infectious agents

Vortex mixing

Pipetting

Plating out

Incubation

Likelihood of exposure

FIGURE 59.1   Increasing likelihood of exposure versus common laboratory procedures.

Estimating the Risks

To estimate the risks associated with the handling of microorganisms, the following need to be considered: consequence of release, consequence of exposure, likelihood of exposure, what could go wrong, and how likely it would be to go wrong.

Consequence of Release

The consequence of release (loss of containment in the laboratory) may immediately impact the operator directly involved, coworkers in neighboring laboratories, or others in the immediate vicinity. If loss of containment spreads beyond the laboratory environment, it may have implications for the nearby community or the wider environment (including farmed, domestic, or wild animal populations). As an example, foot-and-mouth disease (FMD) virus causes minimal harm to humans but seriously affects some farm animals. A nationwide outbreak of FMD in 2001 was estimated to cost the UK economy £8 billion, and another outbreak in 2007, although limited to eight farms, was estimated to cost the government department responding to it an estimated £47 million and the British livestock industry £100 million.[27] The overall impact, in terms of health and economics, will be dependent on the key factors associated with the biological agent, such as infectious dose and method of dissemination. It is important to note that the likelihood of acquiring infection in the event of exposure may differ between laboratory personnel and the community, for example, laboratory staff might have been vaccinated lowering their risk of infection.

Considerations in determining the consequences if the biological agent was released can include

- impact/consequence
- environmental survival
- natural distribution (of the agent in the country)
- novelty (new or emerging biological agent, eg, pandemic influenza)
- country preparedness (public health context)
- epidemiology (endemic, exotic)

In cases where the consequences of the release can be significant, the characteristics of the biological agent (as previously noted) that may also be important to consider can include the overall impact to populations (eg, FMD on livestock), survival for long periods in the environment (eg, *B anthracis*), being a new or emerging pathogen, exotic epidemiology (nonendemic), and minimal country preparedness.

Consequence of Exposure

Several countries collect information on the nature of laboratory-acquired incidents (LAIs) and any reported operator infection as well as the wider impact. In addition, the American Biological Safety Association (ABSA) has developed a database of reported LAIs.[28] The main exposure risks associated with working in this environment are therefore well identified, with some of these reports extending back many years. Some key examples are presented in the following text and provide an international insight into LAIs that help to put in perspective the biological agents implicated in these exposures and how they occurred. Most are based on human error, rather than failure of engineering controls.

The laboratory environment is no different from any other workplace in that there is the potential for incidents to occur, including due to human error. Where it does differ from many workplaces is the higher potential for those incidents to lead to exposure to infectious agents. The consequence of such exposures could be the potential for an LAI, or an actual infection, where the outcome could be fatal depending on the nature of the agent. From early in the development of laboratory-based work, incidents leading to serious infections and fatalities have underpinned the development and improvement of biosafety procedures. However, although improvements may have diminished such problems, they are not eradicated. Table 59.1 provides details of recent historical case reports of LAIs, the agents responsible, and underlying causes, providing useful evidence on the underlying causes of these exposures.

In addition to individual case reports and some surveys as described earlier, wider ranging summaries and surveys have previously been published but, with information dating back to the 1970s[42] or the late 1990s,[43] it is

TABLE 59.1 Summary of reported laboratory-acquired incidents, agents responsible, and underlying causes

Infectious Agent	Case Details	Underlying Causes	Reference
Escherichia coli 0157:H7	Review: 28 case reports in 1982-2007 showing 167 potential exposures and 71 LAI	18 (11%) due to laboratory accidents, 147 (88%) due to aerosolization during routine identification work	Tuttle et al[17]
Brucella (Turkey)	Survey: 38 of 667 laboratory workers with history of infection	Risk factors for infection were being male, a lack of compliance with personal protective equipment, and biosafety cabinets	Ergönül et al[29]
Brucella (Spain)	Survey: of 628 respondents, 75 (43 microbiologists and 32 technicians; 11.9%) infected	Major break in biosafety measures identified in 60 cases (80%)	Bouza et al[30]
Dengue virus	Case report: 1 laboratory worker	Possible bite during laboratory procedure infecting mosquito colony with virus	Britton et al[31]
Ebola virus	Case report: 1 virologist (no infection)	Needlestick injury while inoculating mouse	Kortepeter et al[32]
Genetically modified organism (GMO) incidents	Survey: 139 reported occupational exposures resulting in 14 reported LAI	See separate summary in Table 59.3.	Campbell[33]
Neisseria meningitidis	Survey: 16 cases (8 fatal) worldwide 1985-2001 probably associated with laboratory work	Isolate manipulation with engineered or personal protection	Sejvar et al[34]
Sabiá virus	Case report: 1 researcher	Working alone in BSL-3, cleaned up leakage from bottle into centrifuge after centrifugation. Underestimated problem, wore inadequate PPE, and did not report incident until symptoms occurred.	Barry et al[35]
SARS virus	Two student laboratory workers	Unknown	Fleck[36]
SARS virus	Case report: 1 laboratory worker	Unfamiliar with work at BSL-3. Working with West Nile virus but cell cultures cross-contaminated with SARS; inadequate training, supervision, or use of PPE	Lim et al[37]
Vaccinia virus	Case report: 1 laboratory worker	Needlestick injury while inoculating mouse	Hsu et al[38]
Vibrio species	Case report: 1 microbiology student	Cleanup of spillage of culture from flask; infected despite wearing gloves and gown	Huhulescu et al[39]
Yersinia pestis	Case fatality report: 1 researcher	Unknown route of transmission; attenuated strain but case was high susceptibility due to underlying health problems	Ritger et al[40]
Various	Survey	See Table 59.2.	Willemarck et al[41]

Abbreviations: BSL, biosafety level; LAI, laboratory-acquired incident; PPE, personal protective equipment; SARS, severe acute respiratory syndrome.

TABLE 59.2   Summary of recent laboratory-acquired incidents worldwide, agent responsible, and number of cases[a]

Infectious Agent	Biosafety Level	Number of LAI Cases (%)
Salmonella	2	130 (42)
Brucella	3	123 (40)
Neisseria meningitidis	2	11 (4)
Vaccinia virus	2	11 (4)
Francisella tularensis	3	6 (2)
Filovirus (Ebola, Marburg)	4	5 (2)
Escherichia coli O157:H7	3	4 (1)
Mycobacterium	2-3	4 (1)
Staphylococcus aureus	2	3 (1)
Bacillus anthracis and *Bacillus cereus*	2-3	2 (1)
Burkholderia pseudomallei and *Burkholderia mallei*	3	2 (1)
Clostridium difficile	2	2 (1)
Chlamydia psittaci	3	1 (<1)
Cowpox virus	2	1 (<1)
Dengue virus	3	1 (<1)
Leptospira	2	1 (<1)
SARS	3	1 (<1)
Shigella sonnei	2	1 (<1)

Abbreviations: LAI, laboratory-acquired incident; SARS, severe acute respiratory syndrome.

[a]Data from Willemarck et al.[41]

questionable how relevant they are to current laboratory practices. However, Willemarck et al[41] sourced 57 more recent surveys and reports and selected 47 for further review, with a total of 309 LAIs included. These are summarized in Table 59.2 and offer a useful focus on the known infectious microorganisms most associated with LAI.

One survey reviewed laboratory exposures to genetically modified organisms (GMOs) that had infectious outcomes.[33] Out of 139 reported exposures, 14 LAIs were reported. The most frequent agents associated with these incidents, summarized in Table 59.3, largely reflect the most frequently used GMOs. Of these, Vaccinia virus was responsible for 10 of the 14 LAIs, the others being adenovirus, *E coli*, *Shigella flexneri* (one LAI from two exposure incidents), and *Neisseria meningitidis* (one LAI from one exposure incidents).

Table 59.4 summarizes the 14 reported LAIs associated with GMOs and the underlying causes attributed to the infections, which were most often associated with needlestick injuries.

Several countries have established reporting mechanisms that capture LAI occurrences. For example, in Great

TABLE 59.3   Summary of genetically modified biological agents most frequently reported in association with occupational exposures[a]

Agent	Occupational Exposures	LAI Reported
Lentivirus	21	0
Vaccinia virus	19	10
Adenovirus	15	1
Toxoplasma gondii	9	0
Escherichia coli	7	1
HIV-1	6	0
Shigella flexneri	2	1

Abbreviations: HIV, human immunodeficiency virus; LAI, laboratory-acquired incident.

[a]Reprinted with permission from Campbell.[33] Copyright © 2015 SAGE Publications.

TABLE 59.4 Summary of occupational exposures to genetically modified organisms and failures leading to infection[a]

Agent	Incident	Underlying Cause
Vaccinia virus	Fomite transfer; touched eye and ear with contaminated gloved hand	Failures in administrative controls,[b] engineering controls,[c] and PPE use
	Needlestick	Failures in administrative controls and PPE use
	Needlestick	Failures in administrative controls, engineering controls, and PPE use
	Needlestick	Failures in administrative controls and engineering controls
	Needlestick	Failures in engineering controls, PPE use, and, possibly, administrative controls
	Needlestick	Possibly failures in administrative controls
	Needlestick	Failures in engineering controls
	Needlestick	Possibly failures in engineering controls and PPE use
	Broken glass	No underlying failures identified
	Droplet or splash	Failures in administrative controls and engineering controls
Shigella flexneri	Not identified	No underlying failures identified
Escherichia coli O157:H7	Not identified	Failures in administrative controls, possibly in engineering controls, safe working practices, and PPE use
Neisseria meningitidis	Fomite transfer (improper disposal of contaminated gloves)	Failures in administrative controls and engineering controls
Adenovirus type 5	Not identified	Possibly failures in administrative controls, engineering controls, safe working practices, and PPE use

Abbreviation: PPE, personal protective equipment.

[a]Based on and reprinted with permission from Campbell.[33] Copyright © 2015 SAGE Publications.

[b]Administrative controls include training and protocols.

[c]Engineering controls include biological safety cabinets or similar, sharps safety devices, autoclaves, high-efficiency particulate air–filtered animal cage racks, sealed centrifuge cups, and so on. Failures proposed to be due to improper use of these controls.

Britain, there is a legal requirement set by Parliament and enforced by the Health and Safety Executive (HSE) for health and safety at workplaces, requiring employers to report work-related incidents under the Reporting of Injuries, Diseases and Dangerous Occurrences Regulations (RIDDOR). "Dangerous occurrences" cover near misses, and therefore, the legislation covers incidents in laboratories handling biological agents both causing infection and the potential to cause infection. Examples include breaches of containment; samples being handled at the wrong BSL, or on open benches when they should have

been handled in BSCs; spillages or leakages; needlestick injuries; and animal bites.

Canada recently introduced a similar legal requirement, administered by the Public Health Agency of Canada, to notify laboratory incidents involving a biological agent. Results from the first year of data were reported, yielding 46 exposure incidents, exposing an estimated 100 people, with three suspected and one confirmed case of LAI.[44] The most common occurrences leading to an incident were 15 cases attributed to failures in procedure and 14 to sharps incidents, whereas issues related to PPE failures and to animal handling incidents accounted for a further 8 and 7 incidents, respectively. Spills, equipment malfunction, and loss of containment together accounted for a further 8 incidents.

In summary, whereas historical data helped to shape biosafety procedures, more recent evidence shows the need, when working with biological agents in laboratories, to identify hazards, routes of transmission, and high-risk activities and apply suitable and proportionate controls.

The consequence of infection will be dependent on the key factors associated with the biological agent noted earlier. Where the consequence of the resulting infection is high, characteristics of the biological agent would include high morbidity or mortality and may also be associated with a combination of the following:

- low infectious dose
- high communicability
- airborne route of transmission
- no preventive or therapeutic treatment available
- history of laboratory-acquired infection
- exotic epidemiology (nonendemic)
- highly susceptible population (eg, immunocompromised, naive)

Likelihood of Exposure

Although pathogenic biological agents are intrinsically hazardous, they only pose a risk to laboratory personnel when they are manipulated. Procedures need to be risk assessed prior to use to consider the severity of the hazard and the likelihood of harm. Considering these consequences, together with the potential for release and therefore the likelihood of exposure, will determine the level of risk. It is important to consider the transmission route(s) and infectious dose of biological agents when assessing the risks associated with the procedures to be carried out. For example, procedures that confer high likelihood of exposure include the handling of sharps (with the opportunity for percutaneous injury), working with large volumes and concentrations of infectious material, infecting animals, and necropsy where infection is suspected.

Errors, Failures, and their Likelihood

Although this will have been considered when identifying hazards, considering the consequences of release/infection and the likelihood of exposure, it is important to consider what could go wrong, the likelihood that this would occur, and subsequently lead to an exposure event or release. Considerations should include the potential for splashes and spills, breakages (eg, glassware), inadvertent aerosol generation, equipment failure, system failure (eg, liquid waste treatment failure), and power failure.

▶ DETERMINING AND APPLYING CONTROL MEASURES

There are risks associated with undertaking every procedure with biological agents in the laboratory. The ability to identify hazards and to estimate and control the risks will depend on the nature of the work. For example, in research laboratories undertaking work with known pathogens, the hazards are known and therefore the risks are more clearly defined and specific controls can be applied. By comparison, in laboratories where specific pathogens may not be known, such as in clinical testing laboratories, universal precautions may be more appropriate. Assessing those risks will determine whether appropriate control measures are in place for the work to go ahead or whether additional or different control measures are required in line with national legislation or requirements.

Appropriate and proportionate control measures need to be determined and implemented to reduce the risk. The greater the consequence of release or infection from a biological agent and the higher the likelihood of exposure from the procedure, the greater the overall risk and therefore the higher the level of control required. Control measures, as described in the following text, are typically tiered in the order in which they should be considered. They may also be categorized as engineering control, personal protection, decontamination, and waste management. To this may be added elimination or substitution.

Elimination or Substitution

The ultimate control is not to work with a hazardous substance or material, but in the context of work in a microbiology laboratory, this is not often feasible. However, for some work such as performance testing, it may be appropriate to use a less hazardous surrogate agent, so long as it is validated to ensure it behaves in a sufficiently similar way to the more hazardous pathogen. For example, the pathogen *B anthracis* is often substituted for other *Bacillus* species for biocidal testing purposes, including *Bacillus thuringiensis* and *Bacillus atrophaeus* strains.[45] Similar situations are the use of nonpathogenic strains of mycobacteria as surrogates for *Mycobacterium tuberculosis* and other pathogenic species (eg, using *Mycobacterium terrae*) and alternatives to using polio virus in disinfectant efficacy testing (see chapters 62 and 63).

Engineering Controls

Suitably designed and implemented engineering controls provide effective protection against exposure of laboratory personnel to pathogens and against breaches leading to wider environmental exposure. Such controls include

- Robust building structure of the laboratory to prevent release in case of microbial aerosols being generated or to contain chemicals if undertaking laboratory disinfection by fumigation. This includes well-fitting doors and windows, also avoiding such features as suspended ceilings and voids as often found in offices.
- Laboratory design features to enhance cleaning and surface disinfection, such as impervious bench tops, walls and floors, simplifying design to avoid areas where contamination can be trapped
- For work with higher hazard pathogens, it may be appropriate to operate laboratories under negative air pressure to further contain any potential airborne hazards (see earlier discussion), possibly including the use of HEPA filtration on air mechanically extracted from such facilities. Different countries may have their own guidance and regulation related to this, although often, these identify common control requirements.
- For work with higher hazard pathogens, it may also be appropriate to have in place buffer zones such as lobbies or other laboratories to segregate public spaces or general work areas from higher hazard activities.
- When working with higher hazard pathogens and with high-titer cultures of other microorganisms, especially where handling procedures could generate an aerosol, it may be appropriate to work within the additional containment of a BSC.

A BSC is a ventilated enclosure intended to offer protection to the user and the environment from infected and hazardous biological material. They combine airflow and filtration to contain airborne droplets and particles, thus preventing their escape and exposure of workers and the local environment. All exhaust air discharged to atmosphere from a BSC must be HEPA filtered, usually ducted to outside the laboratory through at least a single HEPA,

although in some circumstances, it is feasible to discharge air into the laboratory through at least two exhaust HEPA filters, in line. The BSCs are the safety critical workhorses of most microbiology laboratories and, if operated and used correctly, provide full protection for the operator when handling pathogens.[46] They are categorized according to their design and function as class I, II, or III. It is worth noting that these classifications do not necessarily correspond to BSL classifications.

Class I BSCs have an aperture at the front through which the operator works (Figure 59.2). They provide operator protection by maintaining an inward flow of air through the same aperture, past the operator, and over the work surface in a single pass to the exit duct. As incoming air is unfiltered, this type of BSC is designed to prioritize operator protection but is not designed to offer protection to material being handled. Class I BSCs are suitable for work with all categories of biological agent except BSL-4.

Class II BSCs also have a working aperture at the front, but they provide protection to both the operator and the materials being handled as the inward airflow is diverted beneath the work surface and is HEPA filtered prior to circulation within the work area (see Figure 59.2). The downward airflow onto the work surface also minimizes the possibility of cross-contamination within the cabinet. Although modern class II BSCs offer similar operator protection to a class I BSCs, the latter are less affected by external factors (movement of the operator, others passing close by, drafts from opening doors) and internal flow rates (including large pieces of equipment inside the BSC) than class II. Users should consider the needs of the work and be aware of the limitations of the equipment before selection. Class II BSCs are suitable for work with all categories of biological agent except BSL-4.

Class III BSCs are totally enclosed and provide maximum protection for the operator, the work, and the environment (see Figure 59.2). All inward and exhaust air is HEPA filtered and access to the work area is provided

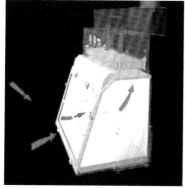 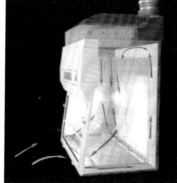 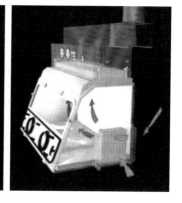

FIGURE 59.2 Schematic diagram of typical class I, II, and III biological safety cabinets (BSCs) (from left to right, respectively) showing air flow. Red arrows denote "dirty" unfiltered air; blue arrows denote "clean" filtered air. For a color version of this art, please consult the eBook.

via the use of full arm-length gloves or gauntlets that are sealed to ports in the front. Usually, they incorporate a side-mounted "pass-box" for aseptic transfer of material in and out of the BSC, or, where more than one BSC is linked together, for transfer from one to the other. Use of class III BSCs is usually restricted to work with BSL-4 biological agents or within enhanced BSL-3 facilities (BSL-3$^+$).

Flexible film isolators (FFI) function by the same principle as class III BSCs, but rather than a rigid cabinet, are usually made from robust plastic material supported by a metal frame. The FFI are sometimes used for animal handling work, where they may incorporate an upper body half-suit in which the operator works. Often stand-alone, with air exhausted through double HEPA filters, they can provide a low-cost and portable option for work with high-hazard pathogens in resource-limited circumstances.[47] However, because of the material from which they are constructed, regular examination is necessary to ensure no damage could lead to breaches and air leaks. In both class III BSCs and FFI, this includes regular examination of the gloves or gauntlets, these being the most safety-critical and probably the most vulnerable components of the units.

Personal Protection

A PPE appropriate for laboratory work usually involves laboratory coats, although for some work, surgical gowns or coveralls may be a convenient alternative. Any garment used, which can be disposable or reusable, should provide adequate cover to protect the wearer's clothing underneath and for the same reason be made from material that is sufficiently impervious to prevent liquid penetration. In some instances, it may be worth considering additional protection such as waterproof aprons or sleeves for specific tasks. Suitable means of decontamination of reusable garments prior to laundering may need to be considered or appropriate means of safe disposal of single-use items.

Hand protection in the laboratory, where appropriate, is usually achieved by wearing disposable surgical gloves, although for some tasks, more robust gloves may be necessary instead or as an extra layer. For work with higher hazard pathogens, use of a double layer of gloves enables the wearer to remove the outer pair if contaminated while still retaining skin protection by the inner pair. It is important to ensure that disposable surgical gloves have been product tested to provide the required protection, as depicted with the labeling provided. Recent changes to BS ISO 374-5:2016 (Protective Gloves Against Dangerous Chemicals and Micro-Organisms—Part 5: Terminology and Performance Requirements for Micro-Organisms Risks[48]) mean that gloves offering protection against viruses, as well as bacteria and fungi, must pass an additional penetration test as described in ISO 16604:2004 (Clothing for Protection Against Contact With Blood and Body Fluids—Determination of Resistance of Protective Clothing Materials to Penetration by Blood-borne Pathogens—Test Method Using Phi-X 174 Bacteriophage[49]). In addition to the marking and pictograms on the product labeling that shows the protection afforded by the gloves, those providing protection against viruses also have the word "VIRUS" next to the pictograms.

It is also important to ensure that gloves are removed in such a way as to prevent cross-contamination, for example, by the pinch-at-the-wrist removal method (see guidance and video at Health and Safety Executive)[50] and that they are safely discarded. Disposable gloves made from latex are still widely used in laboratories and health care settings worldwide, but these may result in allergic reactions and dermatitis due to the presence of natural rubber latex proteins. If used, single-use latex gloves should therefore be low-protein and powder-free, manufactured to an applicable standard such as BS EN 420:2003 + A1:2009 (Protective Gloves. General Requirements and Test Methods[51]) or equivalent to reduce the likelihood of skin reaction. If possible, for regular glove wearers such as laboratory workers, alternative disposable gloves should be sought (eg, those made from nitrile), which offer equivalent levels of approved protection with a reduced likelihood of adverse skin reaction.

Other PPE, often as optional equipment specific to certain tasks, includes disposable overshoes, eye protection such as safety spectacles, goggles or visors, and face masks or respirators. Personal respiratory protection should be unnecessary in the laboratory under normal conditions where BSCs provide protection from airborne transmission but may be used when dealing with emergency situations such as cleaning up a major spill or if work is undertaken outside of normal containment conditions.

▶ DECONTAMINATION AND WASTE MANAGEMENT

In the typical laboratory, decontamination and waste management is routinely achieved by a combination of liquid disinfectants and steam sterilization (autoclaving), in some instances supplemented by incineration.

Liquid disinfectants are used to wipe down potentially contaminated work surfaces, to decontaminate equipment or reusable laboratory ware or to inactivate spills during cleanup. Gordon et al[52] describe how surface decontamination using a liquid disinfectant is often the simplest approach and is ideal for day-to-day cleaning. However, they also state that when large areas and complex equipment require disinfecting, fumigants (eg, formaldehyde gas or hydrogen peroxide gas) are often a better choice for areas that are sealable and able to be so treated. In these situations, the authors believe that liquid disinfectant wipe-down techniques can be time-consuming and difficult to standardize. It is important to ensure that any disinfectants used, whether applied wet or in airborne form, are validated against the agents typically being handled in the laboratory, and are used at least at the concentration and for the minimum contact time against, which they have been validated. Another important factor to consider when choosing the appropriate disinfectant is the potential for some (if not all) disinfectants to have reduced activity in the presence of organic matter, which may include some laboratory reagents such as liquid culture nutrient supplements. For disinfectants with active ingredients that decay with time, it is important that fresh solutions are regularly prepared and old stock disposed of to ensure effectiveness is maintained. Another important factor is dilution. Many disinfectants require appropriate dilution before use, but any further dilution caused by the addition of liquid waste must be considered during use; otherwise, the product may be over diluted and this will affect its efficacy.

Meszaros et al[53] describe other limitations of disinfectants, including a lack of efficacy and control when using wet disinfectants. This study describes how a wide variety of liquid-based detergents and disinfectants, including alcohols, quaternary ammonium compounds, and phenol-based formulations, can vary considerably in their antimicrobial activity. The authors explain how formulations may be termed bactericidal, virucidal, and fungicidal but that some have limited to no activity against more resistant microorganisms, including *Mycobacterium* species and bacterial spores. They emphasized that some liquid-based formulations demonstrate good efficacy against even these more resistant microorganisms, with the use of oxidizing agents and aldehyde-based formulations of particular importance. The most common chemicals used include sodium hypochlorite, chlorine dioxide, hydrogen peroxide, peracetic acid, or combinations of these.

The use of steam sterilization, usually by autoclaving, exposes materials to a combination of elevated temperature (steam under high pressure) and is the most reliable method of treating potentially contaminated waste material prior to disposal or for suitably robust reusable items. However, laboratory autoclaves need to be operated correctly and within validated parameters to achieve complete and reliable kill. This will include consideration to the load type (eg, liquid versus solid waste), weight, and density (see chapter 28). Well-documented autoclave operating conditions can achieve complete kill with almost all biological agents, the exception being prions that require specific consideration, such as supplementary sodium hydroxide treatment (see chapter 68). The autoclave system typically includes a prevacuum or similar conditioning step to remove air and ensure the steam and heat penetrate to the center of densely packed loads and achieve the necessary temperature for the right length of time. It is therefore important for autoclave bags and any rigid waste containers to be at least partially open inside the load to allow air removal and steam penetration. The whole autoclave process can be validated by the use of temperature probes or thermocouples as well as by the use of biological indicators such as bacterial spore strips (see chapter 65). Autoclaves need to be tested, maintained, and serviced regularly to ensure the preset parameters continue to be met.

Incineration is mainly used as an adjunct to autoclaving, not only providing additional assurance but also having the advantage of complete destruction/reduction of laboratory waste, therefore removing the possibility of identifiable laboratory waste ending up in landfill sites (see chapter 54). The most frequent use is for sharps (needles, scalpel blades, glass slides, etc) disposal via robust, sealable single-use containers. It is important that these containers are not damaged or overfilled and only used for disposal of appropriate items. Sharps containers must conform to international quality and safety requirements, for example, compliance with ISO 23907:2012 for single-use sharps containers (at the time of writing being under review and to be replaced by ISO 23907-1:2019).[54,55]

Management of laboratory waste potentially containing pathogens includes a validated means of inactivation as described in the earlier discussion. It is also important to consider segregation (clean from contaminated materials, contaminated materials from personnel) and containment, for example, secure bagging and boxing of waste during handling and transfer of waste from the laboratory bench to the autoclave. In any busy microbiology laboratory, it is important to have a dedicated area for safely holding waste briefly, prior to its prompt processing and disposal. This should ideally be separate from the busy work/analytical area of the laboratory and away from areas where clean and sterile items are stored or processed.

◗ MONITORING THE EFFECTIVENESS OF CONTROL MEASURES

It is recommended that critical equipment, such as sterilizers and BSCs, are qualified prior to use to include demonstrated installation, operational, and performance qualification testing (IQ, OQ, and PQ, respectively). This will ensure that the equipment is installed and operates correctly in accordance with manufacturer's instructions as well as meeting the needs for the desired laboratory use. Routine monitoring of these control measures will include checks such as

- visual assessment of equipment for wear or damage
- in-use tests such as safety alarms on BSCs
- periodic performance tests
- statutory or risk assessment-based servicing and testing of equipment

The frequency of these checks will be based on a combination of factors including the inherent biohazard of the procedures being undertaken, the inherent likelihood of exposure associated with the procedures, the age and general state of repair of the equipment/facility. In some instances, there is a legal requirement to test some safety critical equipment within a minimum period, for example, the statutory annual testing of BSCs or of pressure vessel equipment such as autoclaves. However, based on a risk assessment of the work being done and the agents handled, it may be appropriate to conduct some of these tests more frequently. All the above should be supported by protocols on how to perform the checks, if done in-house, and a mechanism for corrective action if the control measure is found to be less than fully effective.

▶ EMERGENCY CONTROL MEASURES

In addition to routine control measures being put in place to reduce risk, consideration should be given to procedures required in case an exposure or release event occurs or other emergencies. Considerations should include

- how splashes and spills should be handled
- how personnel should be managed if exposure occurs
- how equipment will be maintained and decontaminated in the event of contamination or failure
- how to deal with emergencies such as power failure or fire that could result in a release event
- training of personnel
- local/regional preparedness in the event of release

Written protocols and procedures should be in place that specifically relate to the laboratory environment to which they are applied. Laboratory personnel should be sufficiently familiar with emergency responses to enact them swiftly and minimize potential exposure or breach of containment. Following personnel training, practicing emergency scenarios can be beneficial. Support materials, such as spill kits, should be kept close to hand in higher risk areas. Emergency alarms should be tested regularly. It is important that information and lessons learned from incidents and emergencies, including near misses, are used to review and revise procedures to reduce the likelihood of these event recurring.

▶ TRAINING, COMPETENCY, AND THE DEVELOPMENT AND USE OF GOOD MICROBIOLOGICAL PRACTICES

Well-trained personnel, working to established procedures, underpin the principles of working safely with biological agents in the laboratory. Staff should be selected for their competency in being able to conduct laboratory work not only in terms of techniques but also in their ability to work safely to protect themselves and not endanger others. Appropriate training should be given to

achieve and continue to develop this competency. This is especially important if moving into new areas of work, to include handling of higher risk pathogens, producing larger scale batches (eg, flask to fermenter), increased complexity, animal work, and so on.

Documented procedures are a key component of laboratory work, including staff training and competency and safe working procedures. Developing, documenting, and following good microbiological practices not only provide quality assurance, for example, by ensuring aseptic technique but also control potentially harmful exposure to biological agents. The use of these practices is of key importance to prevent exposure of the laboratory worker to biological agents, accidental release of biological agents outside the laboratory facility, contamination of the laboratory, and cross-contamination of samples.

Written codes of practice and standard operating procedures (SOPs) for safe ways of working should cover all work being undertaken, including the use and maintenance of equipment, storage of samples, transport of samples, inactivation and decontamination, and plans for contingency and emergency operations.

In developing and documenting good microbiology procedures, it is important to include laboratory workers in the process to ensure that the procedures put in place are practical, sensible, achievable, and compatible with the facilities and equipment available. It is then also important to ensure that personnel follow practices and that they report any changes that could warrant a review of procedures. A program of refresher training may also be beneficial, with the level and frequency of training proportionate to the complexity and hazardous nature of the work being done. This will not only maintain good practice but will also assist the process of reviewing procedures by highlighting any necessary changes or possible improvements.

REFERENCES

1. Advisory Committee on Dangerous Pathogens. The management and operation of microbiological containment laboratories. Health and Safety Executive Web site. www.hse.gov.uk/biosafety/management-containment-labs.pdf. Accessed May 31, 2019.
2. Advisory Committee on Dangerous Pathogens. Biological agents: managing the risks in laboratories and healthcare premises. Health and Safety Executive Web site. www.hse.gov.uk/aboutus/meetings/committees/acdp/.../acdp88p6.pdf. Accessed May 31, 2019.
3. World Health Organization. Laboratory biosafety manual: third edition. World Health Organization Web site. http://www.who.int/ihr/publications/WHO_CDS_CSR_LYO_2004_11/en/. Accessed May 31, 2019.
4. Centers for Disease Control and Prevention. Biosafety in microbiological and biomedical laboratories (BMBL) 5th edition. Centers for Disease Control and Prevention Web site. https://www.cdc.gov/biosafety/publications/bmbl5/. Accessed May 31, 2019.
5. European Agency for Safety and Health at Work. Directive 2000/54/EC—biological agents at work. European Agency for Safety and Health at Work Web site. https://osha.europa.eu/en/legislation/directives/exposure-to-biological-agents/77. Accessed May 31, 2019.

6. Advisory Committee on Dangerous Pathogens. Approved list of biological agents. Health and Safety Executive Web site. www.hse.gov.uk/pubns/misc208.pdf. Accessed May 31, 2019.

7. Canadian biosafety handbook, second edition. Canada.ca Web site. https://www.canada.ca/en/public-health/services/canadian-biosafety-standards-guidelines/handbook-second-edition.html. Accessed May 31, 2019.

8. Maier RM, Pepper IL, Gerba CP. *Environmental Microbiology*. 2nd ed. Burlington, MA: Academic Press; 2009.

9. Vogler AJ, Nottingham R, Parise KL, Keim P, Barker BM. Effective disinfectants for *Coccidioides immitis* and *C. posadasii*. *Appl Biosafety*. 2015;20(3):154-158.

10. Bennett A, Parks S. Microbial aerosol generation during laboratory accidents and subsequent risk assessment. *J Appl Microbiol*. 2006;100:658-663.

11. Pottage T, Jhutty A, Parks SR, Walker JT, Bennet AM. Quantification of microbial aerosol generation during standard laboratory procedures. *Appl Biosafety*. 2014;19:124-131.

12. Fleury-Souverain S, Mattiuzzo M, Mehl F, et al. Evaluation of chemical contamination of surfaces during the preparation of chemotherapies in 24 hospital pharmacies. *Eur J Hosp Pharm*. 2015;22:333-341.

13. Wen Z, Yang W, Li N, et al. Assessment of the risk of infectious aerosols leaking to the environment from BSL-3 laboratory HEPA air filtration systems using model bacterial aerosols. *Particuology*. 2014;13:82-87.

14. Johnston JD, Eggett D, Johnson MJ, Reading JC. The influence of risk perception on biosafety level-2 laboratory workers' hand-to-face contact behaviors. *J Occup Environ Hyg*. 2014;11(9):625-632.

15. Compton SR, Paturzo FX, Smith PC, Macy JD. Transmission of mouse parvovirus by fomites. *J Am Assoc Lab Anim Sci*. 2012;51(6):7757-7780.

16. Bolton FJ, Crozier L, Williamson JK. Isolation of *Escherichia coli* O157 from raw meat products. *Lett Appl Microbiol*. 1996;23:317-321.

17. Tuttle J, Gomez T, Doyle MP, et al. Lessons from a large outbreak of *Escherichia coli* O157:H7 infections: insights into the infectious dose and method of widespread contamination of hamburger patties. *Epidemiol Infect*. 1999;122:185-192.

18. European Centre for Disease Prevention and Control. Infectious diseases and public health A-Z. European Centre for Disease Prevention and Control Web site. https://ecdc.europa.eu/en/infectious-diseases-public-health. Accessed May 31, 2019.

19. World Organisation for Animal Health. Technical disease cards. World Organisation for Animal Health Web site. http://www.oie.int/en/animal-health-in-the-world/technical-disease-cards/. Accessed May 31, 2019.

20. Public Health Agency of Canada. Pathogen safety data sheets. Canada.ca Web site. https://www.canada.ca/en/public-health/services/laboratory-biosafety-biosecurity/pathogen-safety-data-sheets-risk-assessment.html. Accessed May 31, 2019.

21. Health and Safety Executive. Biosafety and microbiological containment. Health and Safety Executive Web site. http://www.hse.gov.uk/biosafety/index.htm. Accessed May 31, 2019.

22. Public Health England. Infectious diseases. GOV.UK Web site. https://www.gov.uk/topic/health-protection/infectious-diseases. Accessed May 31, 2019.

23. Centers for Disease Control and Prevention. Diseases and Conditions. Centers for Disease Control and Prevention Web site. https://www.cdc.gov/DiseasesConditions/. Accessed May 31, 2019.

24. World Health Organization. Health topics. World Health Organization Web site. http://www.who.int/topics/en/. Accessed May 31, 2019.

25. Yang W, Marr LC. Mechanisms by which ambient humidity may affect viruses in aerosols *Appl Environ Microbiol*. 2012;78(19):6781-6788.

26. Setlow P. Mechanisms which contribute to the long-term survival of spores of *Bacillus* species. *Soc Appl Bacteriol Symp Ser*. 1994;23:49S-60S.

27. Department for Environment, Food and Rural Affairs. Foot and mouth disease 2007: a review and lessons learned. GOV.UK Web site. https://www.gov.uk/government/publications/foot-and-mouth-disease-2007-a-review-and-lessons-learned. Accessed May 31, 2019.

28. American Biological Safety Association. Laboratory-acquired infection (LAI) database search tips. American Biological Safety Association Web site. https://my.absa.org/LAI. Accessed May 31, 2019.

29. Ergönül O, Celikbaş A, Tezeren D, Güvener E, Dokuzoğuz B. Analysis of risk factors for laboratory-acquired *Brucella* infections. *J Hosp Infect*. 2004;56:223-237.

30. Bouza E, Sánchez-Carrillo C, Hernangómez S, González MJ. Laboratory-acquired brucellosis: a Spanish national survey. *J Hosp Infect*. 2005;61:80-83.

31. Britton S, van den Hurk AF, Simmons RJ, et al. Laboratory-acquired dengue virus infection—a case report. *PLoS Negl Trop Dis*. 2011;5:e1324.

32. Kortepeter MG, Martin JW, Rusnak JM, et al. Managing potential laboratory exposure to Ebola virus by using a patient biocontainment care unit. *Emerg Infect Dis*. 2008;14(6):881-887.

33. Campbell MJ. Characterizing accidents, exposures, and laboratory-acquired infections reported to the National Institutes of Health's Office of Biotechnology Activities (NIH/OBA) division under the NIH Guidelines for Work with Recombinant DNA materials from 1976–2010. *Appl Biosafety*. 2015;20:12-26.

34. Sejvar JJ, Johnson D, Popovic T, et al. Assessing the risk of laboratory-acquired meningococcal disease. *J Clin Microbiol*. 2005;43:4811-4814.

35. Barry M, Russi M, Armstrong L, et al. Brief report: treatment of a laboratory-acquired Sabiá virus infection. *N Engl J Med*. 1995;333:294-296.

36. Fleck F. SARS outbreak over, but concerns for lab safety remain. *Bull World Health Organ*. 2004;82(6):470.

37. Lim PL, Kurup A, Gopalakrishna G, et al. Laboratory-acquired severe acute respiratory syndrome. *N Engl J Med*. 2004;350:1740-1745.

38. Hsu CH, Farland J, Winters T, et al. Laboratory-acquired vaccinia virus infection in a recently immunized person—Massachusetts, 2013. *MMWR Morb Mortal Wkly Rep*. 2015;64(16):435-438.

39. Huhulescu S, Leitner E, Feierl G, Allerberger F. Laboratory-acquired *Vibrio cholerae* O1 infection in Austria, 2008. *Clin Microbiol Infect*. 2010;16:1303-1304.

40. Ritger K, Black S, Weaver K, et al. Fatal laboratory-acquired infection with an attenuated *Yersinia pestis* strain—Chicago, Illinois, 2009. *MMWR Morb Mortal Wkly Rep*. 2011;60(7):201-205.

41. Willemarck N, van Vaerenbergh B, Descamps E, et al. Laboratory-acquired infections in Belgium (2007–2012): an online survey. ResearchGate Web site. https://www.researchgate.net/publication/291331348_Laboratory-Acquired_Infections_in_Belgium_2007-2012_An_online_survey. Accessed May 31, 2019.

42. Pike RM. Laboratory-associated infections: summary and analysis of 3921 cases. *Health Lab Sci*. 1976;13:105-114.

43. Sewell DL. Laboratory acquired infections. *Clin Microbiol Newsl*. 2000;22:73-77.

44. Bienek A, Heisz M, Su M. Surveillance of laboratory exposures to human pathogens and toxins: Canada 2016. *Can Commun Dis Rep*. 2017;43:228-235.

45. Bishop AH, Stapleton HL. Aerosol and surface deposition characteristics of two surrogates for *Bacillus anthracis* spores. *Appl Environ Microbiol*. 2016;82:6682-6690.

46. British Standards Institute. *Biotechnology. Performance Criteria for Microbiological Safety Cabinets*. London, United Kingdom: British Standards Institute; 2000.

47. Bennett A, Parks S, Pottage T. Containment and Ebola in an outbreak setting. *Clean Air and Containment Review*. 2015;24:24-26.

48. Swedish Standards Institute. *ISO 374-5:2016: Protective Gloves Against Dangerous Chemicals and Micro-Organisms—Part 5: Terminology and Performance Requirements for Micro-Organisms Risks*. Stockholm, Sweden: Swedish Standards Institute; 2016.

49. International Organization for Standardization. *ISO 16604:2004: Clothing for Protection Against Contact With Blood and Body Fluids—Determination of Resistance of Protective Clothing Materials to Penetration by Blood-borne Pathogens—Test Method Using Phi-X 174 Bacteriophage*. Geneva, Switzerland: International Organization for Standardization; 2004.

50. Health and Safety Executive. Removing single-use gloves without contaminating your hands. Health and Safety Executive Web site. http://www.hse.gov.uk/skin/videos/gloves/removegloves.htm. Accessed August 21, 2018.

51. International Organization for Standardization. *BS EN 420:2003+A1: 2009: Protective Gloves. General Requirements and Test Methods*. Geneva, Switzerland: International Organization for Standardization. 2003.

52. Gordon D, Carruthers BA, Theriault S. Gaseous decontamination methods in high-containment laboratories. *Appl Biosafety*. 2012;17:31-39.

53. Meszaros JE, Antloga K, Justi C, Plesnicher C, McDonnell G. Area fumigation with hydrogen peroxide vapor. *Appl Biosafety*. 2005;10: 91-100.

54. International Organization for Standardization. *ISO 23907:2012: Sharps Injury Protection—Requirements and Test Methods—Sharps Containers*. Geneva, Switzerland: International Organization for Standardization; 2012.

55. International Organization for Standardization. *ISO 23907-1:2019: Sharps Injury Protection—Requirements and Test Methods—Part 1: Single-Use Sharps Containers*. Geneva, Switzerland: International Organization for Standardization; 2019.

CHAPTER 60

Control and Monitoring of Microbiological Quality in Nonsterile Manufacturing Facilities

Amy Jo Karren

In the health care industry, there is minimal guidance and, in fact, standards do not exist for establishing a microbiological monitoring program in a nonsterile environment. As a result, there are inconsistent practices, and in some cases, inadequate monitoring programs exist. There is a regulatory expectation that an environmental monitoring program is established that includes the monitoring of the microbial burden in the manufacturing area. This requirement applies to nonsterile, terminally sterilized, and aseptically manufactured products. Although the required state of control will vary depending on the product being manufactured, the requirement for microbiological environmental monitoring is universal across all health care manufacturing.

In the manufacturing of health care products, manufacturing controls provide assurance that the process is in a state of control and is the appropriate for the protection of product. A comprehensive environmental control and monitoring program typically includes the control and monitoring of air, water, and compressed gases (including compressed air). Microbiological monitoring provides a means to assess the current state of cleanliness and the stability of the cleanliness over time. During the course of the manufacturing process, the microbiological challenge on the environment will change due to the activity level of personnel, materials, components, packaging, etc. Throughout the year, seasonal changes may also impact the potential microbial burden on the environmental control systems depending on the geographical location. The culmination of these and other environmental stresses can impact the ability of the manufacturing control systems to maintain the required level of cleanliness, therefore establishing a robust sampling plan, based on risk, is prudent so that excursions or loss of control can be quickly identified, contained, and remediated.

For the purposes of microbial control, the controlled environment (a defined zone in which sources of viable and nonviable particulates are controlled by specified means)

does not necessarily have to meet the requirements as defined by International Organization for Standardization (ISO) 14644-1.[1] Particles (or particulates) are minute pieces of matter with defined physical boundaries and, for purposes of classification of air cleanliness, they fall within a cumulative distribution that is based on a lower limit size in the range from 0.1 to 5 μm. Viable particulates are those that consist of, or support, one or more viable microorganisms. In addition, the ISO standard does not specify the level of environmental control that is required in a manufacturing area. There are no regulatory requirements defining the level of environmental control to be used for the manufacture of nonsterile health care products based product classification. The only exception is that the People's Republic of China requires ISO-classified cleanrooms for the manufacture of all types of nonsterile products. A cleanroom is a room within which the number of airborne particles is controlled and classified and which is designed, constructed, and operated in a manner to control the introduction, generation, and retention of particles inside the room.[1] Additionally, the ISO 14644 standards address particle counts and do not discern between viable and nonviable particles. It is recognized that the levels of microorganisms and particulates are not necessarily directly related, but it is understood that particles could carry microorganisms and are frequently associated with particles of 10 to 20 μm in size.[2,3] To provide some guidance, the international pharmaceutical community has recommended minimal cleanroom classification according to the following scheme[4]:

- ISO 5: Aseptic processing zone, sterile product, and/or packaging component is exposed.
- ISO 7: Area immediately surrounding the aseptic processing zone (ISO 6 may be employed but is neither required nor recommended.)
- ISO 8: Nonsterile manufacturing, manufacturing area for terminally sterilized products

A classification in this case describes a method of assessing the level of cleanliness against a specification for a cleanroom, clean zone, controlled zone, or a defined location therein. Levels are expressed in terms of an ISO class, which represents maximum allowable concentrations of contaminants in a unit volume of air.[1] A contaminant is any particulate, molecular, nonparticulate, and biological entity that can adversely affect the product or process. The decision on the level of control and cleanroom classification required for the manufacturing process is made by the manufacturer, with the approval of the regulatory or advisory body. The majority of terminally sterilized products are not manufactured using an aseptic process, so the presence of microorganisms in the environment is expected. The sampling strategies and responses to excursions in a nonsterile manufacturing environment should be significantly different than an aseptic process (see chapter 58). The program should be representative of the risk to the process and product. For nonsterile products and environments, the emphasis should be placed on the long-term trends including any seasonal variations, if applicable, rather than individual events.

▶ RISK ASSESSMENT

The risk assessment for environmental control of the product is typically a separate activity performed prior to conducting the risk assessment for the environmental monitoring program. Both assessments are critical and provide complimentary information.

Environmental Control Risk

An appropriate and practical environmental control program requires an in-depth analysis of the manufacturing process to determine the impact of the environment on the product.[5,6] A risk assessment to determine the potential for the production environment to affect product quality, including the presence of viable and nonviable particles, should be performed to determine the level of control that is needed to assure product quality.[7,8] The program should be designed to monitor selected environmental control parameters in order to detect adverse conditions and be an integral part of the quality management system.[9] The advantage to performing a thorough risk assessment is that the level of control required, and in turn, the investment for maintenance of that control can be established based on risk to the product and not on the expectation for absolute environmental control. If an appropriate environmental control risk assessment is not conducted, the facilities and environmental controls in manufacturing environment may be over- or underengineered. By performing a risk assessment, the level of environmental control implemented can be addressed with a pragmatic approach and appropriate for the product to be manufactured.

Environmental Monitoring Program Risk

Once the environmental control risk for the product is established, the environmental monitoring program can use this information. Microbial levels in controlled environments are not typically uniform (normally distributed) in a given area or over time. Because of this, during the initial risk assessment of the manufacturing area, it is important to establish and document a rationale when selecting the criteria for the monitoring program. To design a comprehensive environmental monitoring program, the following should be included in the assessment[10]:

- Requirement for product microbial quality (eg, nonsterile, terminally sterilized, aseptically processed)
- Requirements of applicable standards and regulations (eg, ISO 14644)
- The product sterilization claim, if applicable (eg, sterile, sterile fluid path, sterile contents)
- The validated method for terminal sterilization, if applicable (eg, moist heat, radiation, ethylene oxide, dry heat)
- Environmental control parameters that should be monitored, as deemed critical for patient safety (eg, particulates, microbial levels and types)
- Factors that might affect the environmental control (eg, number of personnel, raw material flow, relative humidity, disinfectant and method of application, seasonal changes)
- Particulate and microbial monitoring method selection (eg, passive or active air sampling, surface sampling method)
- Monitoring of water (eg, microbial, bacterial endotoxin, pH, total organic carbon, conductivity)
- Monitoring of compressed air or gasses (eg, microbial, moisture, particulates)
- Sampling plans (eg, number of sites sampled and frequency)
- Microbial characterization (eg, Gram staining, colony morphology, phenotypic identification, genotypic identification)
- Alert and action levels (eg, data required to set levels, statistical model, frequency of reassessment)
- Trending requirements (eg, frequency, method of analysis, microbial characterization)
- Process for handling excursions (eg, investigation procedure and documentation, evaluation of risk of an undetected excursion over time)

Maintenance of Risk Assessment

A review of the environmental monitoring risk assessment should be performed periodically as it might indicate that the parameters for the routine monitoring need to be adjusted. Additionally, there should be established requirements when there are planned or unplanned interruptions to a controlled environment. The monitoring program should define the activities required to demonstrate that the controlled environment has returned to a qualified state, including demonstration of acceptable data following the interruption.

ENVIRONMENTAL MONITORING PROGRAM CONSIDERATIONS

Particulate and microbial contamination is not usually uniformly distributed throughout a controlled environment and will fluctuate over time. Individual monitoring events and the derived data represent only a single point in time and may not reflect overall environmental conditions that are evident only by trending. The controlled environment and the respective monitoring results are influenced by a wide variety of factors and reflect the state of control at the time of sampling. Significance should be placed on trends and consistency of results rather than individual data points. The trending of the data over time provides evidence of a continued state of control of the environment. While alert and action levels should be established, the impact of an excursion (in well-controlled process) may not correlate with an increase in the product bioburden. Common factors that can influence the controlled environment include facility design, cleaning and disinfection processes, personnel, and monitoring methods.

Facility Design

Design factors such as air flow pattern, the number of air exchanges, differential pressures, materials of construction, traffic flow, doorways, and equipment placement all have the potential to impact the controlled environment. The initial design and construction of the cleanroom should use materials of construction that reduce the potential for particle shedding and facilitate cleaning. The layout of the room should consider the movement of the product and the personnel throughout the area to minimize disruption in the air flow. Equipment should be placed appropriately, to work effectively with the location of air returns and vents to ensure the air flow pattern is effective at maintaining the controlled environment.

Water or excessive moisture in the area can promote microbial growth as well as geographical areas with high humidity. The use or presence of water in a controlled environment elevates the microbial contamination risk, therefore, highlights the need for control measures and monitoring in the area of use.

The occupancy level of the area should also be a consideration in the design and control of the environment. At-rest monitoring data provides useful information related to facility design and performance, but operational conditions create greater stresses on the environmental controls. The occupancy of the room should be considered during qualification of the area, so that when routine monitoring is employed, the impact of the occupancy level is understood. At-rest sampling is useful to determine if there are changes to the baseline environment, such as after a major cleaning or maintenance events, but should not be used for routine monitoring. The facility design, layout, and occupancy should influence the selection of the sampling sites. Areas that have a greater potential for turbulent air (eg, doorways or equipment) or particle shedding (eg, equipment or known materials) or the presence of water should be considered in the sample site selection.

Cleaning and Disinfection Processes

There are many processes that facilitate microbiological control that should be considered when establishing and maintaining a controlled environment. One critical element of the overall control process is cleaning and disinfection of the room, equipment, and materials brought into the room. The effectiveness of the cleaning methods and frequency of cleaning can have a direct impact on level of control and resulting monitoring data. The disinfectants used should be effective for the expected microbial challenge in the area and associated risk to the product from specific types of organisms. The type of disinfectant, concentration used, application method, surface type, temperature, and contact time should all be considered when establishing a cleaning and disinfection program.[11] The cleaning frequency should be adequate to maintain the required level of cleanliness. When performing microbial monitoring, consideration should be given to the residues from cleaners and disinfectants. There is potential that residues may influence the results of the monitoring. To overcome potential inhibition, media that contains neutralizers should be used in surface sampling to ensure accurate microbial monitoring results.

Personal gowning requirements are also critical to control the number and types of particulates from skin and clothing that may be introduced into the controlled environment. These (gloves, gowns, etc) may be sourced as sterile, single-use items but may also be reused and, in the latter case, are required to be periodically laundered (cleaned and disinfected) to reduce contamination risks. ISO 14644-5 provides considerations for a gowning process, based on the criticality of the associated environment.[11] Additionally, raw materials and equipment may introduce microorganisms if not prepared or cleaned, as appropriate, prior to entering into the controlled environment. The following items are typically not recommended for entry into the cleanroom: cardboard, exposed paper, pallets, and unsealed wood. Items of this nature can be significant sources of microorganisms, are difficult to adequately clean or disinfect, and have a high potential to shed particles.

Personnel

Data indicate that people are the greatest contributors to microbial contamination in the cleanroom.[12] The number of people and the behaviors in the cleanroom can influence the ability to control the environment. The majority of microorganisms related to personnel originate from skin and clothing. Proper gowning procedures provide measures to minimize the transfer of microorganisms from personnel into the controlled environment. Personnel also have the potential to add microorganisms to the environment by sneezing, coughing, talking, and touching surfaces with exposed hands. The process of hand washing, hand sanitization, and the use of gloves can reduce the transfer of microorganisms by touch. Practices such as use of cell phones, use of cosmetics, exposed body piercing, ear buds, or exposed wires should be avoided. There should also be no eating, drinking, or the consumption of chewing gum, lozenges, etc, in the cleanroom. No hair, beards or mustaches, jewelry, or clothing should be exposed with the use of proper gowning practices.

The training of personnel on acceptable behavior in the controlled environment can have a significant impact on microbial control. An example of training for behavior is teaching personnel that even the speed of their movements can impact the environment, whereas rapid movements can generate higher levels of particulates than deliberate and methodical movements. If there is an understanding of the criticality of proper behavior and the need for compliance to procedures to iterate and influence personnel, there is generally compliance. Personnel need to know that what they do impacts product quality and the patients we all serve. Established procedures and training for proper hygiene, gowning, and behaviors are required.

Monitoring Methods

Microbial monitoring results can be highly variable due to the methods used for measurement. Sources of variation might include the sampling technique, sample volume or duration of exposure, timing of sampling during routine manufacturing, distribution of microorganisms in the environment, and the methods used to culture and quantify the microorganisms. The microbial sampling methods used for routine monitoring should be the same sampling methods used during qualification of the controlled environment. If the sampling method is changed, an evaluation of the change should take into consideration the following impact to the routine monitoring:

- Applicability of established alert and action levels (eg, relationship with historical data)
- Ability to detect similar microflora (eg, fastidious or vegetative organisms)

- Ability to neutralize potential disinfectant residuals
- Ability to detect organisms at a similar frequency (eg, impact of active versus passive sampling methods)

In controlled environments, the potential microbiological contamination is most often from human skin, human mucosal membranes, sources of water, and soil. The types of microbiological media and incubation conditions selected should be appropriate for the types of microorganisms present in the environment, with additional consideration regarding the ability to detect organisms that are a known risk to the product. A nonselective growth media, such as Soybean Casein Digest agar, incubated for greater than 3 days at 30°C to 35°C is generally acceptable to detect most heterotrophic environmental organisms. For the culturing of fungal isolates, a selective media that promotes the cultivation of fungi and suppresses aerobic bacterial growth, such as Sabouraud Dextrose agar or Potato Dextrose agar, is appropriate. The incubation conditions for fungal plates are generally greater than 5 days at 20°C to 25°C. The standard for product bioburden testing, ISO 11737-1, is a good source of information on appropriate media and incubation conditions for cultivation of environmental isolates.[13]

Methods for viable sampling are not equivalent. For example, when sampling air, the data generated from a sieve impactor sampler is not equivalent to that of a settling plate. The impactor provides data based on a volume of air sampled, whereas the settling plate results represent the time of exposure. This is true also for methods for viable surface sampling. Changes in culture media and incubation conditions may also impact the detection of the organisms. If the established method for monitoring or the media used in the test system changes, the alert and action levels of the sampling sites must be reassessed and, if appropriate, trend data must be reestablished.

The timing of sampling in the manufacturing area can also influence the data. Periods of time such as shift change or when there is the high level of activity in the controlled environment tend to be worst case for monitoring results. Conversely, monitoring during an at-rest state may falsely provide confidence in the effectiveness of the controls. The time of the monitoring should be understood and defined so that the monitoring provides relevant and consistent data to demonstrate the state of control. Facilities with no history should perform more extensive qualification testing at a greater frequency (eg, daily, weekly, monthly) when establishing the environmental monitoring program. Once baseline testing has been completed, routine monitoring with a reduced sampling plan might be appropriate. The sampling site selection, frequency, and method of monitoring should be designed to provide long-term historical data regarding the microbiological characterization and to provide early indication of changes to the environment.

▶ SAMPLING PLANS

For medical device manufacturing, as an example, most classifications of cleanrooms are monitored for microbiological (bacteria/fungi) levels to meet the expectation of good manufacturing practices. The extent of the monitoring and the associated sampling plan should be defined by the associated risk to the product. No single sampling plan is appropriate for all environments. Sampling plans may be tailored to the level of control required for the manufacturing process with additional consideration for the defined cleanroom classification for the associated environment. Risk assessment tools such as Failure Mode and Effects Analysis and Hazard Analysis and Critical Control Points are useful when determining sampling plan requirements.[14]

Sampling plans should consider not only the potential process and product risk but also any subsequent processes such as cleaning and/or sterilization intended for the manufactured product, if applicable. A product that will be terminally sterilized based on a validation with an overkill method may not require the level of control as one based on product bioburden.[13] Conversely, if the product requires maintenance of a controlled or low bioburden level to demonstrate compliance to the validated sterilization parameters, a more extensive sampling plan may be warranted. The common elements when defining a sampling plan are sample site selection, frequency, the number of sampling sites, and the sampling method.

Sample Site Selection

The sample site locations should be made based on product exposure to the controlled environment. It is common to see sample sites defined by sampling grids, especially for airborne particulate testing.[15] Locations where product are directly exposed to the environment should be considered more critical.[5] When performing microbial monitoring, consider the product exposure location, even when a grid based system is employed. Viable microbial sampling should be performed on locations that provide data to evaluate the microbial risk to the product. The sample should be taken in areas or from the work surfaces where the product has been, or is exposed to the controlled environment, for the longest or most significant amount of time (Table 60.1). A sample taken from a table leg does not provide as much value as a sample from table top surface that has the potential for direct product contact.

Selection of sampling locations should also take into consideration that the sampling process itself should not cause product contamination. It may not be practical to select a site at the most critical location, due to an increased risk of possible direct product contact. If this risk is likely, sampling may be conducted after the risk to product exposure is removed, or another logical location

TABLE 60.1	Examples of sampling sites
System	**Site**
Room air	Proximal to product work area
Surface (equipment)	Control panels, access points, product contact areas
Surface (facility)	Handles, tables, walls, floors
Operators	Finger glove impressions, gowns
Water	Point of use
Compressed air	Point of use site in the system farthest away from compressor and/or on each distribution leg of system

selected. Microbial sampling site selection should provide meaningful data to evaluate the risk of the product, not just to monitor a location on the grid.

Frequency

The sampling frequency should provide a good understanding of the effectiveness of environmental controls over time as well as the ability to detect change due to potential or planned changes in the manufacturing environment. The goal is to select monitoring frequencies that can identify potential system deficiencies. Sampling frequencies for aseptic processing areas are defined in regulatory guidance for aseptic processing and are therefore not addressed in this chapter (see chapter 58). The sampling frequency selected must adequately detect changes in manufacturing environmental conditions, for example, major manufacturing process and/or personnel changes and seasonal variations (if applicable). Consideration of product risk may also impact the sampling frequency selected. For example, products validated using a bioburden-dependent sterilization approach, such as with radiation, might warrant more frequent sampling than those products sterilized using a conservative or overkill approach.[10] It is common to see an increased frequency during the initial implementation of a controlled environment (ie, daily or weekly), then a reduction as the trends indicate stability of the environment (ie, monthly or quarterly). Any change in frequency should be justified with a risk-based assessment of the product and monitoring data. The sampling plan should address conditions under which additional sampling might be necessary, such as product or process changes, construction or excursions, as well as address when it is appropriate to return to the routine sampling plan.

Environmental monitoring data represents a finite point in time. When establishing sampling frequencies, consideration should be given to the design and capability of the environment to maintain control over time. Based on the environmental control risk assessment, if there is a need for rigorous control of the environment, monitoring frequency should be increased to ensure that the required control is maintained.

Number of Sampling Sites

As with other elements of the sampling plan, potential risk to product should be a factor when determining the number of samples that will be taken at a given location. One option is to use a grid-based sampling plan for airborne particulate qualifications of cleanrooms and associated controlled environments. Another option is to monitor identified critical control points in the environment and manufacturing process. The number of locations sampled during routine microbial monitoring should be based on the level of control required in the controlled manufacturing environment and the associated product risk. Typically, more sampling sites will provide increased confidence in detecting changes in the overall environment.

▶ SAMPLING METHODS

Results can vary significantly among different monitoring methods; therefore, it is important to define the method of sampling in the sampling plan. Because of this variability, any changes to the method of sampling require a reassessment of the alert and action levels of sampling sites and, if appropriate, reestablishment of trending. Sampling should occur when the controlled environment is in operation so that it is representative of the conditions present during routine manufacturing. Samples taken when the controlled environment is at rest can be used to demonstrate the continued effectiveness of the cleaning and disinfection as well as the condition of the air supplied to the environment. Routine fungal monitoring may not be necessary depending on outcome of the qualification of the environment and risk assessment; however, fungal monitoring should be considered to monitor the effectiveness of construction cleanup or movement of large equipment into the controlled environment, due to the heightened potential risk of the presence of fastidious fungal organisms.

Table 60.2 provides a summary of the air and surface environmental methods and the associated common environmental monitoring methods (note, this list is not all inclusive).

Airborne Particulate Monitoring

The data derived from airborne particulate monitoring defines the classification of the associated controlled environment (see ISO 14644-1) based on the level of airborne

TABLE 60.2 Examples of common air and surface monitoring methods

Characteristic	Monitoring Method(s)
Air (particulates)	Refer to Annex B of ISO 14644-1 for airborne particulate instruments and testing requirements.[a]
Air (microbial)	Slit impactors Sieve impactors Centrifugal impactors Settling plates Water/broth impingement
Surface (microbial)	Contact plates/flexible films Swabs Surface rinses

Abbreviation: ISO, International Organization for Standardization.

[a]From International Organization for Standardization.[1]

particulate control. Nonclassified areas or controlled environments, can also apply air particulate data to characterize the level of control in the area. Nonviable particulate counts use precise, calibrated instruments and therefore have less variation than methods used for microbial monitoring. Annex B of ISO 14644-1 specifies requirements for airborne particulate instruments and testing.

Air Microbial Monitoring

Airborne microbial monitoring methods vary based on the sampling method, device, rate, and duration of sampling. These variables can influence the airborne microbial monitoring results. Common airborne microbial monitoring methods are settling plates and various types of impaction or impingement samplers. A brief description for each air microbial sampling method is described in Table 60.3.

Surface Microbial Monitoring

The method used for surface microbial monitoring methods should consider the configuration of the surface to be monitored. Contact plates are the most common method for surface monitoring and are appropriate for flat surfaces (eg, tables, walls, floors). Swabs should be considered when the surface is irregular and contact plates are not suitable (eg, equipment). Rinses are for the large surfaces that are difficult to be monitored by other methods (eg, interior surfaces of tanks). Surface sampling media generally contains neutralizers to address the potential of inhibitory residues from disinfectants that are expected on the surface to be tested. A brief description for each surface microbial method is described in Table 60.4.

TABLE 60.3	Air microbial sampling methods
Sampler	**Description of Method**
Slit impactor	Air is drawn through a slit in a dome by a vacuum onto an agar plate (typically 150 mm in diameter) that is slowly rotating. The rotation of the plate provides additional monitoring information in that it indicates when a microorganism was recovered during the sampling period. The air flow (vacuum) and speed of the rotation of the agar plate can be adjusted to control the volume of air sampled and the duration of the sampling.
Sieve impactor	Sieve impactor samplers use vacuum to draw air at a calibrated flow rate through a perforated plate containing holes of equal size across the surface of the plate. The viable particles are impacted onto a surface below the perforated plate, which is typically an agar plate. The air flow rate can be adjusted. Dependent on the air flow rate, the duration of the sampling is set to achieve the desired air sample volume. An advantage of sieve impactors is the ability to perform sampling on different medium. Selective/differential agar or membrane filters may be used to detect different types of contamination, including fungal or fastidious organisms.
Centrifugal impactors	Centrifugal samplers draw air into the sampler by means of an impeller rotating at a measured rate of speed. The impeller creates a centrifugal force that directs the air outwardly and creates a central vacuum. Particles are thrown out of the airstream and onto a solid media surface. The volume of air measured can be extrapolated by the duration of the sampling. A disadvantage to centrifugal impactors is the sourcing of the media strips and the inability to perform selective agar plating.
Settling plates	Media plates are placed open at the sampling location in the controlled environment for a defined period of time (typically 1-4 h) and then closed for incubation and enumeration. The air volume to which the plate was exposed is unknown; therefore, results are interpreted as an exposure time. Factors such as media dehydration during extended exposures (eg, >4 h for static air or >30 min for dynamic air flow such as laminar flow conditions) can negatively impact the results. An advantage to the use of settling plates is that general and selective media can be used simply by exposing multiple plates in the same location. A disadvantage to settling plates is they must be put in a location that will not be disturbed during the duration of the sampling time.
Impingement	Air sampling by impingement involves using a sterile impingement device containing a defined liquid medium, typically sterile water. A known volume of air is bubbled through the impinger containing liquid medium. The flow rate of the air entering the impinger is regulated to determine the volume of air sampled, based on duration of the sampling. Following the impinging process, the liquid media is plated to quantify the organisms present. Note: Impingement is not as common as other methods for viable air monitoring due to the multiple steps and complexity of the monitoring process.

▶ WATER MONITORING

As with microbiological monitoring of nonsterile environments, there is minimal guidance on the quality of water that can and should be used in the manufacturing of nonsterile products; however, most regulatory bodies require the evaluation of water quality. United States Pharmacopeia (USP) monographs for water provide defined types of water and their associated requirements, but often, the water used in the manufacturing of nonsterile product may not need to be held to USP standards. But if the water is to be used as an ingredient in a pharmaceutical product, water used must meet the minimal classification of USP Purified Water, as defined by the associated USP monograph for USP Purified Water.[17] Because there is minimal guidance on the microbial control of the water to be used, as part of the risk assessment for environmental control, the water quality attributes used in the manufacturing process should be defined, controlled, and monitored.

Water used in a manufacturing process poses potential microbial risk for both the product and the environment. First, there is an increased risk for microbial proliferation in the manufacturing environment due to the presence of water. Low levels of microorganisms can flourish in a wet or moist environment. Additionally, there is risk to the product contributed by direct or indirect contact with the water. Water may be a component of coatings, used during extrusion, or used in product cleaning steps. Water has the potential to transfer viable microorganisms to the product as well as the additional risk of increased bacterial endotoxins (see chapter 66). Bacterial endotoxin, which is a component of the cell walls of Gram-negative bacteria, is clinically relevant pyrogenic substance.[18] Because Gram-negative bacteria are typically found in water, the control and monitoring of water for bacterial endotoxin should be performed when endotoxin levels might adversely affect product quality or safety.

Monitoring of the total viable microbial count is performed to demonstrate the water is maintained at

TABLE 60.4 Surface microbial sampling methods

Sampler	Description of Method
Contact plates/ flexible films	Contact plates are filled with agar media to form a convex surface that is pressed against the test surface. Alternately, agar media can be applied to a flexible film and used in a similar way to the contact plate. This method provides direct transfer of potential microbial contamination to the agar media. This method may not be suitable for irregular surfaces where it is difficult to make contact with the entire surface. The media employed typically contains neutralizers such as lecithin and Polysorbate 80 (Tween®80) to facilitate neutralization of disinfectant residues that may be on surfaces that are tested. Results are reported as the number of colonies detected on the area of the contact plate.
Swabs	Sterile swabs made from materials such as cotton, rayon, Dacron™, or calcium alginate are wetted with a transfer medium and a defined surface area is swabbed. Alternately, a defined surface area is wetted and a swab is used to sample the wetted area, facilitating the absorption of microorganisms onto the swab. The swab is then tested for microbial levels qualitatively by placing it in liquid growth media or quantitatively by extracting the swab and plating the extract. Qualitative testing is reported as growth or no growth. Quantitative testing is reported as the number of colonies detected in the area swabbed, which requires an extrapolation of the result of the plating accounting for the amount of extraction liquid plated. It is not recommended to transfer the exposed swab directly onto agar media by streaking the media with the swab. When performing quantitative analysis for critical environments, the efficacy of swabbing method for the detection of organisms should be evaluated to ensure recovery of organisms.[a]
Surface rinses	The surface rinse technique involves rinsing the surface with a known volume of a liquid rinse solution. Sterile water is often used as the rinse solution. Following the rinsing of the surface, the rinse is collected and plated. Membrane filtration is typically used to plate the rinse solution. The results are reported as the number of colonies detected in the rinse solution, which is then extrapolated to the surface sampled using the known volume of the liquid rinse solution.

[a]From Dalamso et al.[16]

appropriate levels to minimize microbial contamination of product. When determining the frequency of monitoring, consider both the level of microbial control provided by the water purification system and criticality of the process step. Microbial controls for water used in a manufacturing environment should, at a minimum, include the following:

- Qualification of the water system, including initial qualification and criteria for requalification after a significant change. It is recommended to have defined intervals for requalification of the system to address any small incremental changes that may have impacted the system.
- Maintenance and disinfection (or sanitization) procedures, including frequency. If biofilms are allowed to form in a water system they can be very difficult to remove. Disinfection and monitoring frequencies should be established to minimize the likelihood of biofilm formation.
- Established procedures on appropriate use of water for cleaning/disinfection
- Established procedures for use of water in quench tanks, sonicators, water baths, extrusion processes, etc. The duration the water is to be used, as well as the procedure for cleaning and maintenance of the equipment, should be defined in the procedures.
- Defined alert and/or action levels for microbial counts and bacterial endotoxin levels, if applicable
- Procedures for routine monitoring, including defined sampling points and procedures for collection, storage, transportation and testing of water

The sampling plan for the monitoring of the water, including the sample sites and frequency should be derived from the qualification of the water system. The methods for the microbial analysis of water are also highly variable as well as quite controversial when debated among industry water experts. Historically, the microbial analysis of water has been performed on low-nutrient media, according to methods prescribed by the Standard Methods for the Examination of Water and Wastewater.[19] This method is designed for the detection of microorganisms, commonly found in water. Due to the nature of the organisms in water typically being slow growers, longer incubation times are required. Conversely, recent guidance provided in USP <1231>, *Water for Pharmaceutical Purposes,*[17] recommends comparative cultivation studies using the native microbiome of the water system to determine the appropriate media and incubation parameters to use for the microbial analysis of water samples. The reason for this recommendation is that the decision to use culturing conditions requiring longer incubation periods to recover higher counts should be balanced with the timeliness of the results. The USP <1231> states "the detection of marginally higher counts at the expense of a significantly longer incubation period may not be the best approach for monitoring water systems, particularly when the slow growers are not new species but the same as those recovered within shorter incubation times." When looking for contaminants, the use of nonselective growth media, such as plate count agar, is generally acceptable. Incubation performed at the time and temperatures used for the detection of aerobic bacteria in environmental air and surface samples are generally used.

COMPRESSED GAS (AIR) MONITORING

Equipment that is used in the manufacture of health care products in a controlled environment may require a source of compressed gas (air) for proper function. Additionally, compressed gas or air may be used directly on the product, such as for drying or curing. The use of compressed air and gasses may adversely affect the product and environmental conditions, if not controlled. Whereas compressed air can be a potential source of particulate and microbial contamination, dependent on the design of the system. The quality of compressed gasses and air should meet or be better than the quality of the air in the controlled environment.

The most common control measure employed on compressed air systems is the use of air filters to control the amount of particulates that could be introduced into the controlled environment. Air filters may be in-line and/or at the point of use. Additionally, a mechanism for reducing the moisture and hydrocarbon content of the compressed air is recommended. The desiccation system should have proper drainage to prevent moisture buildup in the system, which can lead to potential microbial proliferation.

Microbial monitoring of the compressed air or gasses is typically performed similar to the monitoring of air by impaction. This can be accomplished by reducing the pressure of the air in the system to facilitate sampling or by using an air flow regulator to control the flow into the sampler.[20] Monitoring sample site selection and frequency should be based on the design and qualification of the system.

MICROBIAL CHARACTERIZATION

A valuable but often overlooked part of an environmental monitoring program is microbial characterization. Understanding the "normal" types of organisms found in the controlled environment aids in effective microbial excursion investigations as well as can be beneficial to detect shifts in microbial flora. The criticality of the data should drive the level of characterization performed. Start with observing the colony morphology of the isolates to see the diversity of the growth on the sample. Then perform a simple Gram stain on similar morphologic isolates, to determine the cellular morphology to identify potential sources of the contamination. As the need for additional data increases, as recommended for excursion investigations, elevate to microbial identification to genus and species. Typical microbial characterization methods include colony morphology, cellular morphology, staining properties, selective culturing, and microbial identification to genus and species level via phenotypic or genotypic systems. Methods for microbial characterization are summarized in Table 60.5.

TABLE 60.5   Microbial characterization methods

Characterization	Description of Method
Colony morphology	A description of the colony morphology is somewhat subjective and includes color, shape, size, texture, margin, elevation, and other physically observable characteristics of the colony. This information alone is not conducive to trending but can be used to distinguish between bacterial and mold isolates and to initially determine if the colonies on a plate are likely the same microorganism.
Cellular morphology and staining	Cellular morphology techniques such as a wet mount, Gram stain, and spore stains are often used to characterize microorganisms. The benefit to these methods is that they require minimal equipment and time and can provide valuable information regarding the general characteristics of the microorganisms and potential sources. Characterization of fungi (ie, mold and yeast) via a physical description and a wet mount can be sufficient for the majority of isolates.
Selective culturing/ differential media	Media and/or growth conditions that inhibit the growth of particular microorganisms, select for certain organisms, or that assist in differentiating some microorganisms from others (eg, color) are a method for characterization of isolates. A selective method for detection of spore-forming bacteria is to heat shock a liquid sample. Heat shocking essentially eliminates vegetative organisms, so when plated the only the surviving spores are detected.
Microbial identification systems	Various phenotypic and genotypic methods may be used to identify the isolate to genus and species. To facilitate investigations, identification at least to genus can be helpful in identifying the potential source of the microbiological contamination.

TABLE 60.6	Common isolates from controlled environments[21]
Characteristic	**Typical Sources**
Gram-positive cocci	Humans, such as the skin
Gram-positive rods Gram-variable rods Spores	Soil, plants, air, humans
Gram-negative rods	Water
Yeast	Soil, plants
Mold	Soil, plants, air

Common characterization of isolates (Gram stains and cellular morphology) from controlled environments and their typical sources are summarized in Table 60.6.[21]

▶ TRENDING RESULTS

Environmental monitoring processes generate a significant amount of data over time. In order to effectively use the data to demonstrate control, the data must be managed and trended. The use of control charts or graphs provides an efficient way to review data and detect events or trends. Trending allows for detection of short- and long-term drifts from historical performance and can be capable of indicating the potential for an excursion before the observed values achieve statistical significance. Short-term trending (eg, monthly or quarterly) helps to identify individual excursions. Long-term trending (eg, yearly) documents the overall state of control as well as identifies the typical variability of results and potential seasonal impacts, if applicable.[22] The identification of adverse trends should lead to corrective action or remediation, prior to loss of control that could potentially impact the product quality or safety.

▶ ALERT AND ACTION LEVELS

Establishing levels for selected environmental parameters is a necessary to assess the state of control. The use of levels provides a mechanism to determine when corrective actions should be undertaken to return the environment to an acceptable state of environmental control. Alert and action levels must be meaningful and intended to detect changes in the environment that might slowly drift over time. Alert and action levels can also indicate a potential loss of environmental control. An action level is defined as a level set by the user in the context of controlled environments, which, when exceeded, requires immediate action.[23] An alert level is also set by the user, giving early warning of a drift from normal conditions,

which, when exceeded, should result in increased attention in the process.[23]

A two-tiered system allows for the appropriate response when a trend is observed. The established alert level provides an early warning of a drift from normal conditions, which, when exceeded, should result in increased attention in the process. The established action level indicates a potential loss of control and requires immediate action.

Although there are numerous methods to establish alert and action levels, the recommended approach is to use historical data and apply a statistical model. Use of historical data reflects actual performance of the environment control parameter being measured over time. The choice of the statistical model should be based on composition of the data set. It is often difficult to establish levels based on statistical models when the numbers are low and not variable. Because of this, it is highly probable that the established levels may need to be subjective and should be relevant to the risk to the product. It is recommended that you document the rationale for the established levels, so that thought process behind the method used for establishing the levels is understood and can be adjusted when changes occur. Additional guidance on the application of approaches used for establishing alert and action levels in the pharmaceutical industry can be found in Parenteral Drug Association Technical Report No. 13.[4]

Controlled environments that have been newly established may require temporary alert and action levels arbitrarily set based on environments with similar designs and controls or similar manufacturing operations. Once sufficient data is generated, the levels should be reassessed. Alert and action levels should be reviewed periodically to determine if they are still appropriate. At a minimum, an annual review is suggested.[24]

▶ CONCLUSION

In the health care industry, where there is minimal guidance related to the microbial control and monitoring of manufacturing environments, a comprehensive environmental control and monitoring program should be established, as required by regulatory and notified bodies. The program should be defined by an evaluation of risk to the product that then leads to establishment of the appropriate monitoring practices to be employed, based on the extent of the control needed. Using the information presented in this chapter can result in a compliant environmental monitoring program that demonstrates microbial quality in the non-sterile manufacturing facility. Although it is impossible to cover all the factors in detail for an effective environmental control and monitoring program in a single chapter, this chapter is intended to provide a basic understanding of the subject and to research this topic in greater depth in the numerous publications on environmental control.

REFERENCES

1. International Organization for Standardization. *ISO 14644-1:2015: Cleanrooms and Associated Controlled Environments—Part 1: Classification of Air Cleanliness by Particle Concentration.* Geneva, Switzerland: International Organization for Standardization; 2015.

2. United States Pharmacopeia and National Formulary. *<1116> Microbiological Control and Monitoring of Aseptic Processing Environments.* Rockville, MD: United States Pharmacopeial Convention; 2019. https://online.uspnf.com/uspnf/document/GUID-B9A1739F-E171-4E11-A0C7-E43A318EA17F_1_en-US. Accessed May 13, 2019.

3. Ljungqvist B, Reinmüller B. Airborne viable particles and total number of airborne particles: comparative studies of active air sampling. *PDA J Sci Technol.* 2000;54:112-116.

4. Parenteral Drug Association. *Fundamentals of an Environmental Monitoring Program: Technical Report No. 13 (Revised).* Bethesda, MD: Parenteral Drug Association; 2014.

5. Institute of Environmental Sciences and Technology. *IEST-RP-CC023.2 Microorganisms in Cleanrooms.* Schaumburg, IL: Institute of Environmental Sciences and Technology; January 2008.

6. International Organization for Standardization. *ISO 14971:2007: Medical Devices—Application of Risk Management to Medical Devices.* Geneva, Switzerland: International Organization for Standardization; 2007.

7. US Food and Drug Administration. *Guidance for Industry: Sterile Drug Products Produced by Aseptic Processing—Current Good Manufacturing Practice.* Silver Spring, MD; 2004.

8. US Food and Drug Administration. Quality system regulation. 21 CFR Part 820. accessdata.fda.gov/scripts/cdrh/cfdocs/cfcfr/CFRsearch.cfm?CFRPart=820. Accessed January 02, 2020.

9. International Organization for Standardization. *ISO 14698-1:2003: Cleanrooms and Associated Controlled Environments—Biocontamination Control—Part 1: General Principles and Methods.* Geneva, Switzerland: International Organization for Standardization; 2003.

10. Association for the Advancement of Medical Instrumentation. *AAMI TIR52:2014: Environmental Monitoring for Terminally Sterilized Healthcare Products.* Arlington, VA: Association for the Advancement of Medical Instrumentation; 2014.

11. International Organization for Standardization. *ISO 14644-5:2015: Cleanrooms and Associated Controlled Environments—Part 5: Operations. Annex F.5.3.* Geneva, Switzerland: International Organization for Standardization; 2015.

12. Favero M, Puleo JR, Marshall J, Oxborrow G. Comparative levels and types of microbial contamination detected in industrial clean rooms. *Appl Microbiol.* 1966;14:539-551.

13. International Organization for Standardization. *ISO 11737-1:2018: Sterilization of Health Care Products—Microbiological Methods—Part 1: Determination of a Population of Microorganisms on Products.* Geneva, Switzerland: International Organization for Standardization; 2018.

14. International Organization for Standardization. *ISO 14644-5:2015: Cleanrooms and Associated Controlled Environments—Part 5: Operations. Annex A.2.1.* Geneva, Switzerland: International Organization for Standardization; 2015.

15. Institute of Environmental Sciences and Technology. *IEST-RP-CC006: Testing Cleanrooms.* Schaumburg, IL: Institute of Environmental Sciences and Technology; August 2004.

16. Dalamso G, Bini M, Paroni R, Ferrari M. Qualification of high-recovery, flocked swabs as compared to traditional rayon swabs for microbiological environmental monitoring of surfaces. *PDA J Pharm Sci Technol.* 2008;62(3):191-199.

17. United States Pharmacopeia and National Formulary. *<1231> Water for Pharmaceutical Purposes.* Rockville, MD: United States Pharmacopeial Convention; 2019. https://online.uspnf.com/uspnf/document/GUID-07416921-813B-43A7-A494-F190E610AD6F_6_en-US. Accessed May 13, 2019.

18. Association for the Advancement of Medical Instrumentation. *ANSI/AAMI ST72:2011 (R2016): Bacterial Endotoxins—Test Methods, Routine Monitoring, and Alternatives to Batch Testing.* Arlington, VA: Association for the Advancement of Medical Instrumentation; 2011.

19. Rice EW, Baird RB, Eaton AD, eds. *Standard Methods for the Examination of Water and Wastewater.* 23rd ed. Washington, DC: American Public Health Association, American Water Works Association, Water Environment Federation; 2017.

20. Pina R. Testing compressed air lines for microbiological contamination. Biocompare Web site. https://www.biocompare.com/Application-Notes/43423-Testing-Compressed-Air-Lines-For-Microbiological-Contamination/. Accessed May 11, 2019.

21. Sandle T. A review of cleanroom microflora: types, trends, and patterns. *PDA J Pharm Sci Technol.* 2011;65(4):392-403.

22. Moldenhauer J. *Environmental Monitoring: A Comprehensive Handbook.* Vol 2. Bethesda, MD: Parenteral Drug Association; 2005.

23. International Organization for Standardization. *ISO 14644-7:2004: Cleanrooms and Associated Controlled Environments—Part 7: Separative Devices (Clean Air Hoods, Gloveboxes, Isolators and Mini-Environments).* Geneva, Switzerland: International Organization for Standardization; 2004.

24. Winters M, Patch E, Wangsgard W, Bushar H, Ferry A. Establishing bioburden alert and action levels. MDDI/Qmed Web site. https://www.mddionline.com/establishing-bioburden-alert-and-action-levels. Accessed May 11, 2019.

CHAPTER

61

Disinfectant Efficacy Testing

Dan Klein

Disinfectant test methods vary considerably depending on their scope and applicability and can be difficult to generalize (see chapter 5). Disinfectant testing is not solely to advance registration efforts or market new disinfectant products but also applicable when choosing and verifying the use of a disinfectant for a given application, understanding the strengths and limitations of a disinfectant formulation or process, or even when studying characteristics of microbial populations. Understanding the characteristics of a disinfectant's ability to kill microbes is key to creating safe and effective products and surfaces, and efficacy testing is vital for anyone seeking to better understand how microbial threats, whether infection or contamination, can be mitigated through the appropriate use of disinfection. Many methods exist for the characterization of the antimicrobial properties of disinfectants, but like many test methods, inaccurate information can be much more harmful than no information at all. Proper methodology selection for testing disinfectants and diligent application of that methodology is key.

Microbiology is often referred to as art as well as a science. Millions of living creatures rarely act alike, or in perfect order, regardless of their complexity or the status of their place on the phylogenetic tree. Diversity and unpredictability are especially evident in disinfectant testing, where the goal can be to determine the ability of a disinfectant to eradicate low to high numbers (eg, millions) of individual organisms. During these studies of the destruction of microorganisms, variables, some obvious and some extremely subtle, can dramatically impact the test results and the accuracy of a scientific evaluation. This challenge exists for all types of tests and for all classes of microorganisms, although different systems can show different impact. The three main types of disinfectant testing can be classified as regulatory testing, research/development testing, and validation testing. Although controls and documentation can vary depending on the use of the data, the challenges and potential for variability remain the same regardless of application.

Because of inherent variability, in combination with microscopic nature of the test system, it is essential for an experimenter to ensure strict adherence and consideration of all controllable parameters. Many of these controls have been standardized, including confirmation of effective neutralization (stopping antimicrobial action at given time), effective enumeration of population counts, and selection of growth and recovery mechanisms. Others are more elusive and include unseen variables that must be addressed to increase the chances of an accurate results. These types of proper controls, safeguards, and best practices exist for all disinfectant testing, including those designed for research purposes or to meet European, United States, or other regulatory standards (see chapters 62, 63, and 70). In this chapter, important factors affecting antimicrobial test methods will be addressed.

Antimicrobial testing can take multiple forms including the following:

- Simple studies designed to generally evaluate the effectiveness of an active ingredient at different concentrations, such as minimum inhibitory concentration (MIC) studies
- Studies to evaluate the effectiveness of a disinfectant formulation over time, including time kill suspension studies
- More complex studies designed to simulate real-world conditions using different surface types and conditions such as those required by the US Environmental Protection Agency (EPA) and outlined as standardized test methods such as the AOAC International standards or compiled by other similar industry consensus groups

Regardless of the complexity of the study or the anticipated use of the data, there are many key components that must be realized and properly controlled.

▶ KEY CONSIDERATIONS

Usually one of the most important considerations during any test method is adequate neutralization. Some methods, such as an MIC test that just determines the concentration of a microbicide to inhibit the growth of microorganisms, are not time dependent. But these types of tests have limited application, except for the examination of preservation systems (see chapters 37-40). Most other antimicrobial efficacy tests look at the ability of a disinfectant to kill microorganisms over time. Whether defining the amount of time required to kill a specified population of a certain microorganism or determining the time required to destroy a single $\log_{10}$ of a microbial population (eg, to determine the D-value), the importance of stopping a disinfectant's activity at the proper contact time cannot be overstated. Failure to properly neutralize a sample can cause overestimation of activity and a gross mischaracterization of the potency of a product, active ingredient, or formula.

Neutralization in efficacy testing is simply the quenching of antimicrobial activity of a disinfectant at a specified time point. This is typically accomplished through chemical neutralization, although filtration (separation of the microorganisms from the disinfectant) and other methods (eg, rapid cooling in heat processes) can be used. Chemical neutralization is the addition of a single quenching agent (or combination of agents) to the study that inactivates the antimicrobial being tested. When chemical neutralization is selected, the two variables to consider are the ability of the neutralizer to immediately stop the antimicrobial activity upon addition to the test system and to not have a deleterious or toxic effect on the microorganisms being tested. For the first, there are many references to neutralizers to consider based on active class.[1,2] Common chemical neutralizers use lecithin, TWEEN®, reducing agents, or simple dilution. Examples include both prepared media such as Letheen broth or Dey and Engley neutralizing broth as well as other media supplemented with additional TWEEN®, lecithin, or other specific ingredients to address a particular chemistry. These include chemical (eg, sodium thiosulphate, a reducing agent) or enzymatic (catalase) neutralizers used for oxidizing agents such as hydrogen peroxide. With a complicated formula, often the efficacy of an active is not solely related to just the defined active ingredient alone (see chapter 6). Neutralization effectiveness testing must be incorporated using the final formula and the microorganism(s) being tested. A neutralization effectiveness test such as ASTM E1054, *Standard Test Methods for Evaluation of Inactivators of Antimicrobial Agents*, provides great detail on how to perform the evaluation and what the acceptance criteria should look like,

but this can grow increasingly complicated during the research of multiple disinfectants or formulations or the evaluation of a single product with multiple microorganisms.[3] A basic overview of the ASTM test includes adding the active product to the neutralizing solution at the proper test ratios, then inoculating this neutralized mixture with a microbial challenge and determining whether any disinfectant activity still persists when compared to a control, such as using an isotonic buffer in place of the active material. The microbial challenge must be at a low enough titer that even a small amount of residual activity is detected. It is of no value to challenge a neutralization system with relatively high levels (eg, 1.5×10^7 colony-forming units [CFUs]) of bacteria because there may be sufficient residual activity to kill a half a million bacteria and not have the sensitivity to detect this when comparing diluted plate counts (eg, detecting 1.0×10^7 CFUs). The strain of microorganism tested can also be important and is another key consideration. A neutralized product may have a small amount of residual active or excipients that do not impact a particular microorganism, for example, the gram-negative bacteria *Pseudomonas aeruginosa*, but might inhibit another bacteria such as *Staphylococcus aureus*. When testing multiple microorganisms or strains of similar species, it is sufficient to choose the most sensitive strains to a particular active as long as the experimenter understands that there remains some risk inherent in any scientific assumption. For example, it would not be required to confirm the neutralization of 15 different *Burkholderia cepacia* strains, when one or two would suffice, but it shouldn't be assumed that neutralization will be complete for other *Pseudomonas* species, gram-positive bacteria, or even harder to kill microorganisms such as filamentous fungi or spores. It is typically safe to assume that the ability to neutralize a product at a higher concentration will ensure adequate neutralization for more dilute forms; however, even slight changes in a formula or a product, other than dilution, can impact the activity of the system and neutralization may need to be periodically confirmed during disinfectant formulation optimization.

In the absence of a good neutralization process and control, it will not be possible to understand whether the antimicrobial reaction has stopped at the desired time. The test article simply keeps killing as further microbial handling (eg, dilutions) is performed and will likely also continue to kill or inhibit growth of the microorganism during culturing. Occasionally, microbiological indications of inefficient neutralization can be detected on close inspection, such as a nondilutional plate series. This is when the serially diluted plates do not have counts that correspond in a serial manner. For example, with bacterial culturing, a 10^{-1} plate with no colonies followed by a 10^{-2} plate with 100 and a 10^{-3} plate with 10 will give an instant signal that antimicrobial activity was still present in the first plate and subsequent dilution finally stopped this. Although ensuring that neutralizing ingredients are present in the recovery agar as well as in a neutralizing broth will help, any indication of a neutralization issue should be investigated. When a neutralization problem is noted, either through a control or a failed test, alternatives must be considered. These include the use of a different neutralizer, the use of greater neutralizer volumes (and potential change in limits of detection), or the use of neutralization through filtration. Filtration can be a powerful tool when chemical neutralization is improbable. It is possible to pass the antimicrobial chemicals through an inert filter while trapping viable microorganisms that can be subsequently rinsed and plated. Other creative solutions are certainly possible when finding and confirming neutralizers, and neutralization should be at the forefront of factors to consider in order to ensure antimicrobial tests are reliable.

Whether qualitative or quantitative, the number of microorganisms in the initial challenge is a key piece of information to understand. Although it seems basic to have a good enumeration of your starting point, there are challenges. Most microbiologists investigating bacteria and fungi use plate counts to enumerate colonies and assume that each colony arose from a single cell. With this information, the number of survivors can be determined. Microbiologists will understand that colonies form from CFUs that can contain single or small groups of cells, and therefore, quantitation can only be an estimate. Bacteria like to clump and they like to associate. Proper vortexing, sonication, and accurate volume usage during serial dilution can mitigate this effect, but the imperfections in the test system must be understood. Vortex speed and duration can be important, and sonication intensity as well as the position and composition of the tubes being sonicated can matter.[4] Also, something as basic as ensuring 10-fold serial dilutions can make a difference and often go unnoticed. Tenfold serial dilutions are typically done by adding 1 to 9 mL diluent (or equivalent) repeatedly until the bacterial numbers are low enough to count. If errors occur during media preparation and the volumes are not exact, miscalculations can magnify and give dramatically inaccurate counts. Just a half of a milliliter less diluent than projected can result in baseline counts that are many cells away from the actual number after these compounding effects are considered.

Growth media selection in the preparation of a challenge inoculum is another overlooked variable. Although the number of passes a culture undergoes may result in some genetic drift, it is the final incubation conditions that can really impact results. There is much discussion, appropriately, over the phase of growth and incubation time. An actively growing culture at 6 hours may be more vulnerable to the uptake of some antimicrobial agents than a dormant or dying culture that is 35 hours old. There is also a dramatic impact in the preparation of a test culture on solid agar-based media or in liquid broth conditions. Solid agar cultures can be generally more difficult to kill than their liquid equivalents (D.A.K., unpublished data, December 2007). It is not just the nature of

the media but also the ingredients and constituents of the media that matter. Microorganisms will naturally uptake different growth elements depending on the medium to which they are subjected. This can occur regardless of the total titer achieved, impacting the susceptibility of the isolate. Examples of these effects can be seen in experiments using the AOAC International use-dilution method and a marketed disinfectant at a shortened contact time with *S aureus*.[4] The only variable studied was the change in the media used to cultivate the challenge microorganism. As can be seen in Figure 61.1, the two medias selected produced nearly identical carrier populations. But when these carriers were tested in a qualitative (growth or no growth) disinfectant assay, the experimental outcome was dramatically different (Table 61.1). This difference would cause the test product to fail this EPA-required method with tryptic soy broth and pass with nutrient broth.

When discussing neutralization, it was noted that care should be taken in the selection of species to test for adequate neutralization. When cultivating a microorganism for disinfectant evaluations, the particular strain of a species can also matter. Variability can exist even in those cases where identical culture conditions are used. Notorious for this intraspecies heterogeneity is the spore-forming organism, *Bacillus cereus* (Figure 61.2). Comparisons of three different strains classified as the same species showed dramatically different disinfectant efficacy results (D.A.K., unpublished data, December 2007).

The variability between strains (or isolates), species, and genus of microorganisms is well described for bacteria and fungi but also in comparisons of virus types.[5] Variability has been particularly reported in comparison between standardized, type culture strains, and more recent environmental isolates. Therefore, a challenge microorganism should be carefully selected that is representative of the goals of the experiment, whether it is for regulatory registration, research, or validation purposes.

▶ METHOD CONSIDERATIONS

Once a microorganism is selected, neutralization confirmed, and the protocol is established for enumeration and growth, there are many different types of methods to which these principles can be applied. Earlier, three tiers of disinfectant tests were referenced. These include studies to characterize active ingredients, simple studies to test formulations, and tests using critical surface materials that are used to predict product performance in the real world. Further, new methods continue to emerge as new microbial knowledge is uncovered and threats determined, such as bioreactor testing and evolving visualization studies.

The first, and simplest, approaches are tests designed to generally screen an active ingredient to determine its ability to kill certain microorganisms. This type of testing can take several forms. One such approach is the MIC or the

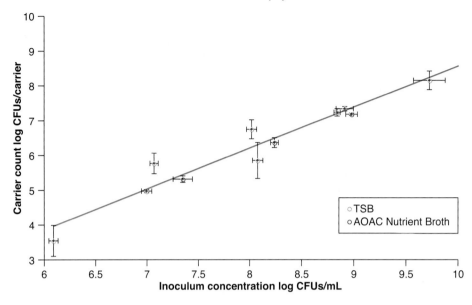

FIGURE 61.1   Comparison of carrier inoculation enumeration from bacterial cultures prepared in two types of growth media (tryptic soy broth [TSB] and AOAC International nutrient broth). Abbreviation: CFUs, colony-forming units.

modification that creates the minimum bactericidal concentration (MBC) test. Although the MIC is much more common in antibiotic testing than disinfectant testing, there is value in using this method for other antimicrobials because of the ease of testing and the ability to screen multiple concentrations, actives, and microorganisms. This method does not apply well to formulated products because the dilution can dramatically impact the ability of the formulation's excipients to work together. The MIC test will typically use a multi-well plate with increasing dilutions of the active that are then each inoculated with a standard test culture. Following incubation, the concentration that inhibits the challenge microorganism is considered the MIC. Note that in these tests, growth culture media will be present, which will limit the availability of the antimicrobial to act on the test microorganism and thereby overestimating the true MIC; this is particularly important with certain types of reactive microbicides such as iodine and hydrogen peroxide. By modifying this test to check the viability of the test microorganism from the

MIC, it is easy to determine the MBC to differentiate preservative (microbiostatic) and microbicidal (kill) activity. Although the information is limited, MIC/MBC analysis can be a good first step when screening multiple actives.

When testing disinfectant formulations, not just specific microbicides alone, the workhorse of disinfectant testing remains the time kill study. Known by multiple names, including D-value, time kill kinetic test, or kill time test, this method is both simple and informative. These tests study the effect of a disinfectant against a microorganism (or population of microorganisms) over time. A typical liquid disinfectant time kill study uses a test tube, filled with disinfectant, that is then inoculated with the challenge microorganism. After the appropriate exposure periods or times, samples are removed, neutralized, and the number of survivors determined. This method is adaptable to an extensive number and classes of microorganisms and can be modified quickly and easily. The selection of time points is important to get an accurate understanding of the kill kinetics of a formulation (and/or associated process

TABLE 61.1   AOAC International use-dilution method results comparing the efficacy of a disinfectant with carriers inoculated with *Staphylococcus aureus* cultures prepared in two different growth media

Growth Medium	No. of Positive Carriers	Total No. of Carriers Tested
TSB	25	90
AOAC nutrient broth	4	90

Abbreviation: TSB, tryptic soy broth.

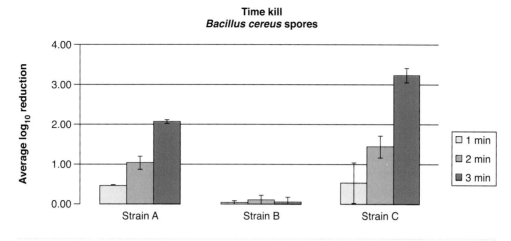

FIGURE 61.2 Disinfection efficacy against different strains of *Bacillus cereus* spores.

conditions such as temperature) and care must be taken to fully understand and report the variables. The problem with such disinfectant tests is that hard surface antimicrobials are often too effective to be characterized in such a method even when using short contact times such as 15, 30, and 60 seconds. Clearly, the value of a time kill suspension study is contingent on the microorganism selected. While vegetative microorganism may be rapidly killed in chemical disinfectant suspension, fungi such as *Aspergillus* species, mycobacteria, or bacterial spores can often survive for an extended time in many broad-spectrum disinfectants. Table 61.2 outlines a guide for the relative hierarchy of susceptibility for different classes of microorganisms,

although this can vary depending on the antimicrobial or disinfectant process under test.[6]

The time kill method, when applicable, does offer flexibility in design and can be used to understand the impact of time and get a good understanding of the differences in antimicrobial activity in formulations, exposure conditions, or microorganism susceptibility. As an example with a liquid inoculum, the test can typically use 10 mL of disinfectant to which 100 μL of a challenge inoculum is added. The volume of product or culture can vary as long as the volume of the inoculum is not great enough to influence the dynamics of the formulation. This ratio should be 100:1 or greater depending on test conditions.

TABLE 61.2 The relative hierarchy of microbial susceptibility to inactivation

	Microorganism	Examples
More Resistant	Prions	Scrapie, Creutzfeldt-Jacob disease, chronic wasting disease
	Bacterial spores	*Bacillus, Geobacillus, Clostridium*
	Protozoal oocysts	*Cryptosporidium*
	Helminth eggs	*Ascaris, Enterobius*
	Mycobacteria	*Mycobacterium tuberculosis, Mycobacterium terrae, Mycobacterium chelonae*
	Small, nonenveloped viruses	Poliovirus, parvoviruses, papillomaviruses
	Protozoal cysts	*Giardia, Acanthamoeba*
	Fungal spores	*Aspergillus, Penicillium*
	Gram-negative bacteria	*Pseudomonas, Providencia, Escherichia*
	Vegetative fungi and algae	*Aspergillus, Trichophyton, Candida, Chlamydomonas*
	Vegetative helminths and protozoa	*Ascaris, Cryptosporidium, Giardia*
	Large, nonenveloped viruses	Adenoviruses, rotaviruses
	Gram-positive bacteria	*Staphylococcus, Streptococcus, Enterococcus*
Less Resistant	Enveloped viruses	HIV, hepatitis B virus, herpes simplex virus

After adding the microorganism to the disinfectant, aliquots (typically 1 mL) are removed and neutralized at the exact contact times to be tested. It is important that the experimenter adds the product/microorganism mixture to the neutralization tube, often 9 mL for a 1:10 dilution, at the exact contact time to stop the reaction. This can make short contact times difficult as the sample must be fully mixed when inoculated before drawing an exposed sample. Fifteen seconds is routine, but times as short as 5 seconds are possible with two analysts. The selection of contact times should be carefully considered, and it must be understood that the time kill method is the easiest challenge that a disinfectant can face, so care must be taken when interpreting results. After neutralizing the sample, aliquots are serially diluted, CFUs (or equivalent) remaining are enumerated and $\log_{10}$ reductions are calculated from a baseline count in which a buffer is substituted for the test article. Time kills can also be modified into extended contact studies to look at preservative systems intended to control, not necessarily quickly eradicate, a microbial population. These tests to determine a preservative's effectiveness face the same challenges as a time kill with short contact times but may use time points of days or weeks instead of minutes or seconds.

Although efficient and easy to conduct, time kills have limitations both in the inability to test highly effective disinfectants but also in their lack of correlation to real-world applications. For many applications, bacteria are not typically found in a uniform suspension of liquid. Because of this, the vast majority of efficacy tests require a method using an inoculated surface. This surface can be any material, from steel to carpet, but often uses a hard surface as a representative real-world situation. Hard surface testing uses bacteria dried to a material of interest to which a disinfectant is added, and efficacy determined. Although conceptually very simple, there are an infinite number of variables at play and results can be much more variable than observed with a time kill method or MIC test. Many of the standard hard surface disinfectant tests have been in use for decades. The phenol coefficient method, which remains the predecessor of the standard bactericidal hard surface methods still in use today, was first established in 1953 by Stuart et al.[7] By 1954, the accuracy of the results obtained by the testing was already being questioned.[8] Hard surface tests are truly infinite in their potential design. Like suspension studies, hard surface testing can be used for testing a variety of microorganisms. It is the inclusion of a surface material that can truly create some new challenges and drive additional variability. Microorganisms on a surface are typically harder to kill than those in suspension. Further, the characteristics of the surface type as well as the porosity or potential imperfections in the surface can drive variability. In many standard methods, glass or stainless steel coupons are used; however, even different grades or finishes of stainless steel can impact test results.[9] Hard surface

methods are frequently used to validate the use of disinfectants in some critical environments. This testing will use isolated microorganisms and can include specific surfaces, such as from a pharmaceutical cleanroom or other controlled areas. The need to test specific surfaces can also directly impact the methodology selected for an antimicrobial evaluation.

The most straightforward hard surface tests include tests with a qualitative endpoint. Methods such as the use-dilution test and other methods within the disinfectant testing section of AOAC International use penicylinders that are coated with bacteria, placed in disinfectant, and then placed in media to ascertain whether any microorganisms survived the treatment.[4] In these tests, a stainless steel or porcelain penicylinder is soaked in a broth culture of the challenge microorganism. These penicylinders are 10 mm long with an 8-mm outer diameter and a 6-mm inner diameter (Figure 61.3). After a period of soaking in the culture media, the carriers are put on edge in a petri dish matted with filter paper and allowed to dry. The dried carriers are then added, one at a time, to a tube of disinfectant. Following the desired contact time, these carriers are removed and placed into a neutralizing broth, incubated, and then scored for growth at the end of the incubation period. Typically performed in sets of 10 or more, this testing is very labor intensive but as a qualitative test gives little information beyond the positive or negative test result. Although the concept is simple, this qualitative method is extremely technique sensitive. If the contaminated carrier is allowed to touch the sides of the tube containing the disinfectant upon insertion, it can easily be reinoculated during retrieval and removal. A carrier with no microorganisms remaining after disinfection will then potentially be a false positive as the penicylinder reacquires the challenge bacteria. The fact that a single surviving microorganism can cause a positive result is one of the greatest challenges of this and other qualitative hard surface tests. In addition to a false positive from reinoculation, small imperfections within the carrier surface can also easily result in an adverse result. For AOAC International tuberculocidal and sporicidal testing, porcelain penicylinders are used. These are notorious for suffering small imperfections that can easily harbor the challenge microorganism and potentially shield or protect it from the action of the disinfectant and are very hard to see visually (see Figure 61.3). Even variables as subtle as what previous disinfectant was tested can have an impact when the penicylinders are reused. If a protein cross-linking disinfectant was used, this fixative could potentially mitigate imperfections and make for an easier challenge that what is intended.

Overall qualitative methods compare poorly to methods with a quantitative endpoint. Industry and academic groups are frequently investigating new and improved methodology. Hard surface methods are incredibly difficult to replace or improve because many small changes

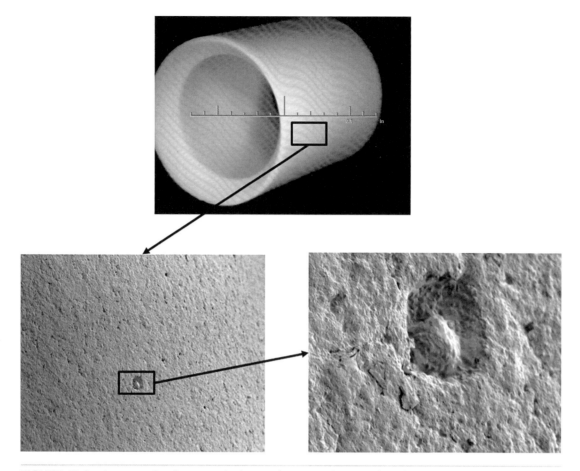

FIGURE 61.3 An example of a penicylinder used as a simulated surface for disinfectant efficacy, showing magnification at 65× and 500×.

can have unanticipated results. There are biases in every test method, and understanding those biases is important if one wants to best characterize their test article. Efforts continue to develop new and improved methods, but these can literally take decades before data is established and analyzed and consensus is reached. One example is the development of the Quantitated Carrier Test at the Centre for Research on Environmental Microbiology at the University of Ottawa.[10] This method uses a small stainless steel disc, onto which a spot inoculum of the challenge microorganism is dried and then covered in disinfectant. After the desired contact time, the disinfectant is neutralized by the addition of neutralizing broth and the number of surviving microorganisms is enumerated. In addition to estimating a quantitative log reduction value that can provide key information about the disinfectants mode of action and kill kinetics, this method reduces the transfer and manipulation of the carrier that is required in some of the qualitative tests. By performing inoculation, disinfectant treatment, and neutralization of this quantitative test within a single test vessel, the possibility of inadvertently producing a false positive is eliminated. Despite obvious improvements, any new method can quickly draw

debate, and this method continues to evolve over the last several decades. With each new investigation into method improvements, whether minor or major efforts, more is learned and incremental improvements and understanding continue to grow.

Still, no method is perfect nor universal nor will it ever be. Although liquid disinfectant testing comprises the bulk of evaluations for most indications, other dosage forms are critically important in many areas. These alternative types of applications, including sprays and wipes, have many of the same seen and unseen variables that can impact experimental outcomes as well as new challenges related to their dosage form. Testing disinfectant towelettes and wipes present some unique challenges. Simply testing the disinfectant expressed from the wipe can provide some information but will not fully characterize the efficacy of the wipe in a typical intended application. Factors including the size of the wipe, the amount of product per wipe, the wipe material, the mechanical action, and the physical force while using the wipe will impact the test results. Different wipe materials have different absorption characteristics and can react differently based on the microorganisms present. Some wipes may simply push the microorganisms to another location, whereas others may absorb them into their matrix. Wiping pressure is also a logical variable to consider. It seems reasonable that the use of a great amount of force would produce different experimental outcomes than light pressure addressing a surface. Efforts have been made over the years to standardize the force application with variable results.[11] Regardless, the experimenter needs to understand and harmonize each variable to any extent possible. Spray products should also be tested in their final dosage form, that is, as a spray and not solely as a liquid. Product dispersion, droplet size, and spray volume can dramatically affect disinfection. It is also important to ensure a consistent and representative spray each time a trigger or other mechanism is actuated during product usage. Although spray products are extremely useful for many applications, their testing does add another layer of complexity that should be controlled.

Many other hard surface methods have evolved based on the microorganism to be tested or the environment in which a product will be used (see chapters 62 and 63). Some methods use a porous surface to present a greater challenge to disinfectants and mirror some real-world situations. Although most disinfectants target hard, nonporous surfaces, microorganism can exist equally well on other surface types and methods must adapt. Laundry, carpet, textiles, wood, and building materials may need to be specifically tested to determine the ability to disinfect or sanitize these surfaces. One such worst case, porous surface, includes the suture loop requirements for AOAC International sporicidal testing.[12]

Another example of modifying antimicrobial test methods for multiple surfaces with different characteristics is the validation of disinfectants per United States Pharmacopeia (USP) criteria to meet US Food and Drug Administration (FDA) regulatory requirements. For this application, pharmaceutical and other FDA regulated manufacturers must validate the performance of their disinfectant for repeatable and effective use in their facility. This testing uses surfaces of construction found in critical areas such as a cleanroom and must also use microorganisms of potential concern in that environment. Only after a disinfectant is validated for an application can its use be endorsed for the regulated process. Similar test methods that simulate the actual use conditions for the antiseptic or disinfectant are intrinsic in the development of antimicrobial test methods in the European Union (see chapter 63). Other examples include standardized tests specifically used to study the efficacy of antiseptics on the skin (see chapters 42 and 43).

Not only are methods needed for different surfaces but also for simulating a microorganism's true environmental conditions. A perfect example is the associated growth of microorganisms in a biofilm matrix (see chapter 67). Biofilms will form anywhere there is a nonsterile interface of a liquid and a surface and exhibit phenotypic and genotypic differences associated with the collective ability of microorganisms to grow in an associated mass. The characteristics that allow microorganisms in biofilms to survive under harsh environmental conditions create a challenge for disinfection. Bacteria do not want to be washed away, whether on a stone in a stream or a valve in the heart. Therefore, to survive, cells will attach to a surface, often where nutrients are present, and secrete an exopolymeric substance to facilitate adhesion and the incorporation of other microorganisms within the mass. Although biofilms have been present since the evolution of microorganisms and the descriptions in the literature date back to 1936, testing biofilm for disinfectant activity is a relatively new process.[13] Despite this, much progress has been made in recent years to grow and test the destruction of different biofilms.[14] In biofilm testing, there are multiple ways to grow biofilms, but fewer consensus tests that outline how to test the activity of disinfectants against them. When growing biofilms, one can usually classify based on flow conditions and sheer force. The tougher the growth conditions, that is, the faster the flow of liquid trying to wash away the microorganisms, the more tenacious the biofilm becomes and the harder it is to disinfect. Although any biofilm modeling system can be employed based on the conditions in the real world that you are trying to mimic, the variability in biofilm testing can be significantly higher than the variability in all other disinfectant test methods. This is because of the associated growth of biofilms and the extreme difficulty in disaggregating and enumerating the CFUs.[15] Every biofilm growth method is created differently and attempts to standardize them to create a consensus standard that can be used for regulatory or validation testing has been difficult. The primary standard method for growing a high sheer biofilm for disinfectant testing is the Centers for Disease Control and Prevention rotating disk reactor. This method uses high sheer conditions and laminar flow with a dilute media containing organisms passing over coupons that are held in rotating reactor arms.[16] The coupons, fully coated with biofilm, can then be removed and placed into disinfectant for testing via the ASTM single-tube method or other applicable test.[17]

▶ OTHER CONSIDERATIONS

Correlating laboratory studies to field research is always difficult and no standard method will ever suffice. One will not likely encounter perfectly planktonic, well-fed microorganisms under typical environmental conditions. Neither will one expect to encounter 10^8 dried microorganisms onto a hard surface in a typical clean room, health care, or critical manufacturing setting. There are many considerations when correlating to real-world conditions including organic materials, uneven surfaces, temperature ranges, and an infinite number of other challenges. These challenges exist regardless of industrial or clinical application, and it can be a particular challenge in those situations with a regulatory requirement for validation testing. In the United States, the FDA requires manufacturers of products classified as drugs to perform testing on materials that represent their critical manufacturing areas using similar conditions and microorganisms of concern in that environment. These validation tests can be very difficult to design and conduct. Conceptually, it is quite simple, where sections of steel that match those in an isolation chamber can be used, inoculated with a spore species that is known to be present or persists in the room, and test a sporicidal disinfectant with this challenge. But in real life, a multitude of variables can come into play.

Whereas validation studies are difficult to correlate, other hard surface disinfectant studies become even more challenging, if not impossible. In a controlled environment, such as a pharmaceutical clean room, it is possible to identify each material of construction and even a good estimation of the microorganisms present. In less controlled or variable environment, whether a hospital room, food processing plant, or home bathroom, it is not feasible. There are literally an infinite number of combinations between surface type, materials present, existing microorganisms, and environmental conditions. Scientists do their best to simulate such real-world conditions, but with each guess or change comes additional variability.

In any study, the test conditions as well as the product composition can be varied in order to get a better understanding of how the product will work in the field. Although all studies must consider those obvious variables such as neutralization, population controls, growth and recovery methods, individual experiments also have a myriad of potential variables to consider and can impact the results depending on the test system employed, with the impact of these factors often not as straightforward as expected. Such variables can include the addition of an organic/inorganic load, a modification of the diluent used in the study as well as product concentration, contact time, and temperature. One example is the use of an organic load within a disinfectant study. The EPA mandates a relatively low challenge when adding organic material; these are reasonable levels for many applications because this level of soil will be visible on a surface but may not match many other applications where disinfectants are expected to be effective under gross soil conditions (such as in animal husbandry; see chapter 52). The EPA requirement for a one-step cleaner/disinfectant is 5% soil (eg, blood serum or the presence of a challenge protein suspension such as bovine serum albumin) added to the inoculum that constitutes a small volume relative to the disinfectant used in the test. Even at 5%, it can make a difference for some microbicides. The choice of organic load can also make a difference as soils such as fetal bovine serum, horse serum, or calf serum can have distinct differences in their effect on the outcome as the chemical composition and protein content of an organic challenge must be considered by the

types of antimicrobial.[18] Other organic and inorganic materials are often added to disinfectant experiments in different ways depending on product application, and their selection should be based what may be encountered under use conditions as well as to meet regulatory requirements. Standardization efforts continue to seek new and more appropriate interfering substances.[19]

Another factor that should be considered is the diluent to prepare concentrated disinfectants. Although ready-to-use disinfectants are very common, there are many concentrated products that must be prepared in a diluent, typically water, prior to use. Water hardness (essentially the measure of the amount of calcium and magnesium salts in the water) is a common consideration because it is known to interfere with disinfectant efficacy. Hard water is frequently used to better mimic the actual preparation conditions in the real world, but water hardness values can vary. Four hundred–ppm hardness is a de facto standard as a worst-case test condition, although those values are much higher than typically found in most of the developed world.[20] Product concentration may be as simple as following the label instructions for preparing a disinfectant; however, when testing disinfectants it is important to understand the impact of concentration in the study. Although more active is typically more effective, this is not always the case as some actives, such as alcohols, have a threshold of activity that requires some water to be present (see chapter 19). Finished products will also have detailed formulation specifics in which the active and excipients in the product are optimized to work at a specific concentration and less dilute samples may exhibit a significant drop in efficacy. The influence of formulation effects on chemical antimicrobials cannot be underestimated, even in products with similar or different concentrations of the same microbicides (see chapter 6).

Clearly, contact time is also an obvious and important test variable. The methodology selected can dramatically affect the speed at which a disinfectant can (or should) effectively reduce a microbial population. Antimicrobial activity may be expected to be much quicker in a suspension study with planktonic bacteria that what would be observed on a hard surface or with a biofilm. When evaluating the impact time on a disinfectant's efficacy, it is important to remember that very few disinfectants have perfectly linear kill kinetics in which the rate of kill is a straight line (or sometimes biphasic lines) when plotting log reduction versus time (see chapter 7). Although this may occur with steam and other sterilization processes making it easier to calculate a sterility assurance level, it rarely happens with liquid disinfectants. Depending on the quantity and the bioavailability of the active material, it is very possible to see rapid initial kill followed by a long tailing effect that requires significantly more time to reach a complete kill endpoint. The analysis of the kinetics of such kill curves can be useful in understanding and optimizing the disinfection formation and/or process (Figure 61.4).

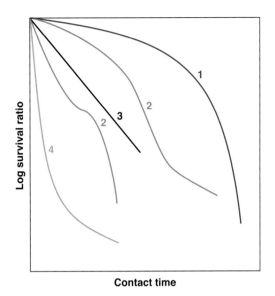

FIGURE 61.4 Examples of the differences in disinfection survival curves. Line 3 shows a linear response, which is often shown for sterilization process but is less commonly described for disinfection processes. Many of these curves may indicate the presence of test microorganisms in a population that range in resistance levels to the disinfectant. Similarly, in the case of line 1, it may take a longer initial time for the disinfectant to penetrate into the test microorganisms to have an antimicrobial effects, or for line 2 where a subpopulation of microorganisms are harder to inactivate.

Contact temperature is often overlooked as most hard surface disinfectant testing specifies "room temperature" as the standard most likely to mirror actual in use conditions. Many, if not most, disinfectants are dramatically affected by testing in cold temperatures with a significant drop in efficacy noted when tested around refrigeration temperatures as a result of thermodynamics. Even subtle changes in "room temperature" can make a difference as some formulations may be more active at 22°C than they might be at 18°C. Clearly, when evaluating disinfectants in more extreme cases, such as the use in cold room applications, the impact on efficacy can be dramatic. Temperature, along with humidity, can also impact the challenge organism when dried onto a hard surface. If the culture is insufficiently dried, the challenge will become less as the liquid suspension creates a time kill effect, whereas an overly dried culture will quickly lose viability and skew the numbers the other way. This is very organism specific, with parallel controls and direct observation being recommended.

As discussed earlier, the test microorganism can be an important variable and consideration for efficacy testing. For example, with fungal or mycobacterial testing, where the challenge cells tend to clump, proper maceration and separation (including filtration as necessary to remove mycelial matting) is important to ensure a standardized test. For virus testing, the introduction of a compatible cell line for enumeration of the surviving plaque-forming units, the viral equivalents of the CFUs, can add a new concern as cytopathic effect on these cells can be achieved independently of the viral load if the product or product excipients maintain residual toxicity. Similar considerations apply for the testing of protozoa and helminths.

Whereas it is imperative to understand the potential impact of both unseen as well as more obvious variables when testing disinfectants, basic design of experiments is a final consideration that must be well thought out to reduce the possibility of confounding or confusing results and the potential mischaracterization of activity. Biocidal data tends to be more variable than other scientific disciplines, especially when evaluating disinfectants that have an efficacy profile that demonstrates neither very high or very low activity.[21] It is essential that each individual study includes sufficient replicates within the study. Duplicate or triplicate plating may offer little added benefit relative to the amount of effort required, but within reason, more replicates is often considered beneficial with newer products or applications. If possible, testing disinfectants repeatedly on different test days and with different challenge populations can provide even more clarity. Despite the strength of the data, interpretation of the results should always be made with care. Many microbiologists accept that results within 0.5 log$_{10}$ of each other are equivalent. Although this can be difficult to explain to analytical or engineering counterparts, the diversity of the populations and the challenges of their enumeration can afford only a certain degree of precision (see chapter 64). Still, a properly controlled and designed study will show trends in the data to allow for significant conclusions to be made. When testing any method, the selection of time points, proper use of parallel controls, and the complete understanding of the test system should be carefully considered in order to prevent wasted time, effort, and misinterpretation. Although not as bad as getting misinformation from testing, getting no information at all can be frustrating and time-consuming.

It is easy to focus on method selection as the only key variable to consider. That, coupled with a well-thought out design of experiments, seems to be enough to get the answers needed from a microbiological disinfectant experiment whether intended for research, validation, or registration. But microbiology remains unique is still a dynamic field of investigation. We are truly in the early days of microbial exploration, and many factors that influence test outcomes are still ambiguous in their nature and our understanding. As in the study of any heterogeneous populations, all possible steps must be taken to enable a true evaluation of a disinfectant product's efficacy. Therefore, it is important to control what can be tested and understand what cannot. Failure to do so can produce the wrong conclusions. Making the wrong conclusions with infectious or contaminating microorganisms can have dramatic consequences.

REFERENCES

1. Russell AD, Ahonkhai I, Rogers DT. Microbiological applications of the inactivation of antibiotics and other antimicrobial agents. *J Appl Bacteriol.* 1979;46:207-245.

2. Sutton SVW. Neutralizer evaluations as control experiments for antimicrobial efficacy tests. In: Ascenzi JM, ed. *Handbook of Disinfectants and Antiseptics.* New York, NY: Marcel Dekker; 1996:43-62.

3. ASTM International. *ASTM E1054-08:2013. Standard Test Methods for Evaluation of Inactivators of Antimicrobial Agents.* West Conshohocken, PA: ASTM International; 2013.

4. AOAC International. Use-dilution methods. In: *AOAC Official Methods of Analysis of the Association of Official Analytical Elements.* 15th ed. Arlington, VA: AOAC International; 1990:chap 6.

5. Eterpi M, McDonnell G, Thomas V. Disinfection efficacy against parvoviruses compared with reference viruses. *J Hosp Infect.* 2009;73: 64-70.

6. McDonnell G. *Antisepsis, Disinfection, and Sterilization: Types, Action, and Resistance.* 2nd ed. Washington, DC: ASM Press; 2017.

7. Stuart L, Ortenzio LF, Friedl JL. Use dilution confirmation tests for results secured by phenol coefficient methods. *J Assoc Offic Agr Chemists.* 1953;36:466-480.

8. Litchfield J, Ordal, Z. *A Study of the Stuart Method for the Evaluation of Germicides.* Urbana, IL: Department of Food Technology, University of Illinois, Urbana; 1954.

9. Black E, Owens K, Staub R, et al. Evaluation of AISI Type 304 stainless steel as a suitable surface material for evaluating the efficacy of peracetic acid-based disinfectants against *Clostridium difficile* spores. *PLoS ONE.* 2017;12(10).

10. Springthorpe VS, Sattar SA. Carrier tests to assess microbicidal activities of chemical disinfectants for use on medical devices and environmental surfaces. *J AOAC Int.* 2005;88:182-201.

11. Sattar SA. Decontamination of high-touch environmental surfaces in healthcare: quantitative assessment of disinfectant pre-soaked wipes. *Int J Infect Dis.* 2016;45:285.

12. AOAC International. Sporicidal activity of disinfectants. In: *Official Methods of Analysis.* 21st ed. Gaithersburg, MD: AOAC International; 2013:chap 6.

13. Zobell CE, Anderson DQ. Observations on the multiplication of bacteria in different volumes of stored sea water and the influence of oxygen tension and solid surfaces. *Biol Bull.* 1936;71:324-342.

14. Buckingham-Meyer K, Goeres DM, Hamilton MA. Comparative evaluation of biofilm efficacy tests. *J Microbiol Methods.* 2007;70:236-244.

15. Hamilton MA, Buckingham-Meyer K, Goeres DM. Checking the validity of the harvesting and disaggregation steps in laboratory tests of surface disinfectants. *J AOAC Int.* 2009;92:1755-1762.

16. ASTM International. *ASTM E2196-17: Standard Test Method for Quantification of* Pseudomonas aeruginosa *Biofilm Grown with Medium Shear and Continuous Flow Using Rotating Disk Reactor.* West Conshohocken, PA: ASTM International; 2017.

17. ASTM International. *E2871-19: Standard Test Method for Determining Disinfectant Efficacy Against Biofilm Grown in CDC Reactor Using Single Tube Method.* West Conshohocken, PA: ASTM International; 2019.

18. Gélinas P, Goulet J. Neutralization of the activity of eight disinfectants by organic matter. *J Appl Bacteriol.* 1983;54:243-247.

19. Meyer B, Morin VN, Rödger HJ, Holah J, Bird C. Do European Standard Disinfectant tests truly simulate in-use microbial and organic soiling conditions on food preparation surfaces. *J Appl Microbiol.* 2010;108:1344-1351.

20. Kaiser H. The importance of water quality on the reprocessing and steam sterilization of surgical instruments. *Infect Control Today.* 2000;4:54-58.

21. Parker A, Hamilton M, Goeres D. Reproducibility of antimicrobial test methods. *Sci Rep.* 2018;8:12531.

Standard Microbiological Methods for Antimicrobial Products in North America

Scott Steinagel and Elaine Black

Products used for the reduction and elimination of microorganisms, known broadly as antimicrobial products, have become part of our daily lives. They are used across the health care, food production, food service, and hospitality industries as well as in private households across the globe.[1-5] In order to measure the effectiveness of new and existing antimicrobial products, a set of repeatable and reproducible standard methods must exist. Standard test methods are vital, science-based, regulatory, and research tools that help ensure antimicrobial products perform as expected.[6-8] Standard microbiological methods are modeled on typical use conditions for the products being tested, and for this reason, a range of methods exists to mimic immersion, spray, wipe, and other product applications.[7,8] Other use conditions that can affect the efficacy or performance of a product can be incorporated and, in some cases, altered depending on the nature of the product and its intended use. Conditions such as product diluent (water hardness level) and the presence of interfering substances (eg, organic soil), which model bodily fluids or environmental soils, are often part of standard methods.[6,9]

The basic premise of an antimicrobial test method is the exposure of a test microorganism (such as vegetative bacteria, bacterial spores, fungal spores, or viruses) to the test product for a defined period of time (contact time), neutralization of the biocidal activity, and subsequent determination of efficacy (enumeration of survivors).[6-8] Standard microbial test methods in North America are generally developed, adapted, and maintained by standard setting bodies such as AOAC International (formerly Association of Official Analytical Chemists) and ASTM International (formerly American Society for Testing and Materials). The membership of these organizations include academic, industrial, and governmental stakeholders. Methods are developed, tested, or improved through collaborative trials involving multiple stakeholder laboratories and are reviewed and voted on by members of these bodies.

The following chapter describes many, although not necessarily all, of the test methods used by producers of antimicrobial products to substantiate efficacy and product label claims of typical antimicrobial products. All information is current at time of publication but is subject to change. The opinions expressed in this chapter are those of the authors and not of the agencies referenced. The information within should not be used in lieu of the most current regulatory guidance or consultation with the relevant regulatory authority.

▶ ANTIMICROBIAL JURISDICTION IN NORTH AMERICA

In the United States, the Federal Insecticide, Fungicide, and Rodenticide Act (FIFRA) establishes the authority of the US Environmental Protection Agency (EPA) over the registration, labeling, sale, distribution, and use of pesticidal products.[10] The FIFRA's definition of a "pest" includes but is not exclusive to any fungus, bacterium, virus, or other microorganism that is injurious to health or the environment. The act defines a "pesticide" as "any substance or mixture of substances intended for preventing, destroying, repelling, or mitigating any pest." By definition, the word *pesticide* is a misnomer because it includes modes of action that are not technically "cidal." In the United States, disinfectants, sanitizers, and sporicides are regarded as pesticides for regulatory purposes. Some antimicrobials, however, do not fall under the jurisdiction of the EPA. Under the Federal Food Drug and Cosmetics Act,[11] the US Food and Drug Administration (FDA) has authority over high-level disinfectants (HLDs) and sterilants used for critical and semicritical medical devices and for food additives, including but not limited to antimicrobials used as processing aids and food additives used for the reduction of pathogenic bacteria in food. Consequently, EPA and FDA have dual jurisdiction over antimicrobials for the treatment of raw agricultural products and for the treatment of process water in food processing facilities.

In Canada, antimicrobial products are regulated mainly by Health Canada's Pest Management Regulatory Agency (PMRA) or the Natural and Nonprescription Health Products Directorate (NNHPD). Other agencies or directorates are involved for specific product types and are discussed elsewhere in the chapter. Through the Food and Drugs Act, NNHPD is the regulatory body responsible for disinfectants used on environmental surfaces or inanimate objects.[12] These products are referred to as "disinfectant drugs" by NNHPD and require a drug identification number (DIN). The PMRA, however, is given authority over some antimicrobial products such as soft surface sanitizers, laundry antimicrobials, bacteriostatic surface treatments, and nonfood contact sanitizers without disinfection claims through the Pest Control Products Act.[13] Canada and the United States are closely aligned with respect to efficacy standards and require data be generated by many of the same methods. With the exception of some minor nomenclature differences, the contents of this chapter reflect the typical methods needed for registration of pesticides/antimicrobial agents used on inanimate surfaces under both EPA and Health Canada jurisdictions. This chapter does not necessarily reference every standard test method that can be used and excludes those antimicrobials used as food tissue treatments and antiseptics.

Antimicrobial Product Efficacy Guidelines in North America

In order to assess the safety and effectiveness or efficacy of antimicrobial products, the EPA has published a series of testing guidelines that serve as testing recommendations. The 810 series Product Performance Test Guidelines describe the testing requirements used to substantiate the efficacy of antimicrobial products that bear public health claims—claims against organisms that pose threat to human health, on inanimate or environmental surfaces.[14] A series of documents authored by Health Canada are Canada's equivalent to the 810 series[15-18] and cover disinfectant drugs, disinfectant sanitizers, and HLDs/sterilants for critical and semicritical medical devices. The FDA testing requirements for HLDs used for medical devices can be found in the Guidance for Industry and FDA Reviewers: Content and Format of Premarket Notification [510(k)] Submissions for Liquid Chemical Sterilants/High Level Disinfectants.[19]

Within these guidance documents, antimicrobial products can be classified as follows:

- Sanitizer—a substance, or mixture of substances, that reduces the bacterial population on environmental surfaces and inanimate objects by significant numbers (eg, a minimum of 3 $\log_{10}$ reduction) due to the antimicrobial action

of the active ingredient(s) but which does not destroy or eliminate all bacteria

- Disinfectant-sanitizer (Canada only)—a chemical product represented for use as a sanitizer on hard nonporous environmental surfaces and inanimate objects which is also represented for use as a hard surface disinfectant
- Disinfectant—a substance, or mixture of substances, capable of destroying or irreversibly inactivating pathogenic (disease causing) and potentially pathogenic (opportunistic) microorganisms (eg, bacteria, fungi, and viruses) but not necessarily bacterial spores, present on environmental surfaces and inanimate objects due to the antimicrobial action of the active ingredient(s)
- Sporicide—a substance, or mixture of substances, capable of destroying or irreversibly inactivating bacterial spores present on environmental surfaces and inanimate objects
- HLD—a substance, or mixture of substances, capable of destroying or irreversibly inactivating all microbial pathogens, but not necessarily large numbers of bacterial spores
- Sterilant—a substance, or mixture of substances, capable of destroying or irreversibly inactivating all forms of microbial life present on inanimate objects, including all forms of vegetative bacteria, bacterial spores, fungi, fungal spores, and viruses

◗ EFFICACY TEST METHOD TERMINOLOGY

Efficacy claims for pesticides are substantiated in the laboratory by standardized test methods. The methods can be classified as either qualitative or quantitative test methods and as suspension-based or carrier-based test methods.[8]

Qualitative test methods—Qualitative test methods provide results classified by the presence or absence of the microorganism following treatment rather than a numerical count of survivors (eg, colony-forming units [CFUs] or plaque-forming units). In qualitative methods, a series of coupons used to represent the intended treatment surface, called "carriers," are inoculated with the test system or a suspension of the microorganism is treated with the antimicrobial product. The treated carrier or a sample of the treated suspension is then transferred to a neutralizing growth medium, incubated, and examined for presence or absence of the test system as indicated by turbidity or other visual end point. This positive/negative end point is the hallmark of a qualitative method. Although these methods have a qualitative end point, the advent of more advanced statistical methods and extensive replication has allowed for "semiquantitative" conclusions to be made in some methods.[20]

Quantitative test methods—Quantitative test methods provide quantifiable results that allow for the calculation of $\log_{10}$ or percentage reductions following treatment. In these methods, an inoculated and subsequently treated coupon or treated suspension of the test system is neutralized and quantitatively assayed for survivors using standard enumeration techniques (eg, standard plate count for bacteria/fungi or cell culture recovery of viruses). The survivors are enumerated as compared to an analogous untreated control and microorganism reductions can be calculated.

Suspension-based test methods—In a suspension-based test method, a sample of test system is introduced directly into the antimicrobial solution and contact with the antimicrobial begins immediately. A sample of the test system/antimicrobial solution mixture is removed and is neutralized once the desired contact time has been reached. Survivors may then be enumerated as compared to an analogous untreated control suspension. Alternatively, assessments of survival following treatment may be made qualitatively. These methods do not rely on the specific use of a treatment surface material, or carrier, and instead involve direct treatment of the test system with the antimicrobial.

Carrier-based test methods—In a carrier-based test method, the test system is first placed onto a coupon or carrier intended to represent the surface to be treated. The test system is then dried to the carrier surface. The coupon is then introduced to or treated by the antimicrobial product. Carrier-based test methods differ from suspension-based test methods in that the antimicrobial product must penetrate a dried organism or virus film to inactivate the test system. The treated surface is then neutralized once the desired contact time has been reached. The neutralized material can either be evaluated quantitatively or qualitatively to evaluate the efficacy of the treatment procedure.

In addition to the mechanism of action process followed in the test method (suspension versus carrier), some key use conditions must also be considered when developing antimicrobial products and evaluating their efficacy. These include contact time and temperature, the intended diluent for concentrated antimicrobial products, and the organic burden (soiling) that might be present under claimed use conditions. For spray products, the spray time and distance traveled by the chemistry can impact efficacy. For towelette products, the folding and wiping procedure can impact efficacy. The following provides more detail regarding intended diluent and organic soiling.

Intended diluent (hard water)—Antimicrobial products can be produced in the form of ready-to-use products or concentrated liquids/solids for dilution in water at the use site. In North America, concentrated antimicrobials to be diluted in water are required to be tested under conditions that demonstrate efficacy in the presence of the water type listed on the label such as hard water.[14] Synthetic hard water introduces minerals into the diluted product including magnesium and calcium. This inorganic burden may interfere with the activity of the product, particularly those actives sensitive to cationic binding.[21] As such, efficacy testing should be conducted in the presence of hard water to confirm the efficacy of the product in use. Two routinely used efficacy test methods give instruction on the preparation of synthetic hard water for use in testing.[22,23]

Organic burden—In North America, disinfectants may be identified as one-step cleaner disinfectants or one-step cleaner sanitizers, which provide efficacy claims in the presence of light to moderate levels of organic burden.[14] This is an important consideration because organic burden can have a negative impact on the activity of various chemicals, particularly those sensitive to the presence of protein.[9] Because of this, an organic soil load should be included in testing to simulate these use conditions in order to substantiate one-step cleaner-disinfectant/sanitizer claims. For many methods, this involves the introduction of a minimum 5% organic soil such as blood serum into the test system prior to treatment. In other methods, as in the case for efficacy claims against *Clostridium difficile* spores, a three-part soil load including bovine serum albumin, yeast extract, and mucin is required to simulate the environment these spores are likely to be found.[24] Once substantiated, these one-step treatment claims provide labor-saving value to the end user of these products by limiting the effort required to effectively disinfect or sanitize surfaces or materials. It should be noted that in all cases where heavy soil is present, the use directions must require precleaning prior to antimicrobial product treatment.

▶ SANITIZERS

The term *sanitizer* is not a globally used term but is widely used in North America.[14] Generally speaking, sanitizers have lower levels of efficacy than disinfectants and are used in areas where complete kill of microorganisms is not necessary or the bioburden in these use sites is lower. There are many types of sanitizer treatments including food contact and nonfood contact sanitization of hard surfaces, soft surface sanitization, toilet sanitization, laundry sanitization, carpet sanitization, and residual hard surface sanitization. Sanitizers play an important role in protecting public health as well as protecting the safety of the food supply in North America.

Classification of Sanitizers

In North America, hard surface sanitizers can be broken into two main categories: food contact surface sanitizers and nonfood contact surface sanitizers.

Food Contact Surface Sanitizers

Food manufacturing/food service industries rely heavily on food contact sanitizers to prevent foodborne illness and spoilage/quality issues in foods. Food contact sanitizers are used to treat the surfaces which food may come into contact and require a higher bactericidal performance than those required by nonfood contact sanitizers. Food contact sanitizers are most often used as part of a broader sanitation process that includes a cleaning step to remove visible soil from the surface.[25] Proper cleaning is essential to remove any soils that may protect microorganisms or neutralize the activity of the sanitizer. The selection of a sanitizer can be based on a number of factors other than efficacy that include cost, stability, safety, and material compatibility.[25]

In 2015, the US Food Safety Modernization Act established a number of rules related to the production and transportation of human and animal food.[26] In the final rule on current good manufacturing and risk-based preventative controls, the FDA requires that food manufacturers adhere to controls that prevent hazards in the US food system including sanitation controls to ensure a facility is maintained in sanitary condition.[27] The US Federal Food Code outlines model guidance on food safety sanitation that can be uniformly adopted for restaurants and food retail establishments. The Food Code includes detailed practices for the use of food contact sanitizers.[28] These laws and guidance underline the importance of sanitizers for maintenance of a safe food supply. Although FDA and the United States Department of Agriculture (USDA) regulate the production of food in the United States, sanitizers used in the food industry are classified as pesticides and are therefore regulated under FIFRA. Standard test methods for the measurement of the efficacy of sanitizers incorporate test organisms that are representative of those found on surfaces to be sanitized.[29]

Food contact sanitizers come in direct contact with the food we eat, are classified as Indirect Food Additives in the United States, and are regulated under 21 Code of Federal Regulations (CFR) 178.1010 because they are reasonably expected to become incorporated into food through contact with treated processing equipment or utensils. Sanitizers must therefore be shown to be safe prior to their use .[30] A manufacturer of a sanitizer must provide assurance to the governing regulatory body that the product does no harm to the public by estimating the sanitizer residue following use and establishment of the probable daily intake of the substance.

In Canada, food contact sanitizers are assessed by Health Canada's Bureau of Chemical Safety (BCS) and the Food Directorate. The BCS determines whether or not the level of sanitizer product residues that could remain on the surface of food is acceptable in terms of human safety and Health Canada BCS issues a No Objection Letter for these products. This allows a registrant to add a "no rinse required" statement to the label, and the product can remain on the surface prior to actual food contact, saving time and labor in processing environments. This "no rinse" paradigm is not accepted globally, making these use directions very North America-centric.

Sanitizer uses include (1) use in public eating establishments to sanitize eating utensils, (2) use on processing equipment and utensils in dairy plants, and (3) use on processing equipment and utensils in other (ie, nondairy) food-processing plants.[31] The storage, dispensing, and use of sanitizers are often strictly controlled by the food processing company following internal Sanitation Standard Operating Procedures (SSOPs), which follow EPA labeling on concentration and contact time.[25] Food contact surface sanitizers used in food service and private homes are often used on food preparation areas such as counter tops and on eating utensils in manual and machine dishwashing systems. Application of sanitizers in these use sites rely heavily on the EPA label and use instructions.

For the purpose of efficacy testing, food contact surface sanitizers are further broken into halide and nonhalide product types. Halide chemical products include those formulated with iodophors, mixed halides, and chlorine-bearing chemicals.[29] Nonhalide products include but are not limited to quaternary ammonium compounds, acids, and peroxygens.

Nonfood Contact Surface Sanitizers

Nonfood contact surface sanitizers are products used on surfaces that will not come into contact with foods or beverages. These sanitizers have a lower hurdle for kill and allow for longer contact times, which is indicative of the less critical nature of their use compared to food contact surface sanitizers. Nonfood contact sanitizers are used routinely on floors, walls, and other hard surfaces not directly used for food production.

Hard-Surface Sanitizer Test Methods

The EPA Product Performance Test Guidelines Office of Chemical Safety and Pollution Prevention (OCSPP) 810.2300 describes the efficacy data requirements and testing recommendations for sanitizers used on hard surfaces.[29] According to the Guideline, the following sanitizer classifications exist:

- Food contact surface sanitizers (halide based)
- Food contact surface sanitizers (nonhalide based)
- Nonfood contact surface sanitizers

Halide-Based Food Contact Sanitizers: AOAC Chlorine (Available) in Disinfectants (955.16)

The AOAC Chlorine (Available) in Disinfectants describes a qualitative, suspension-based test method used to evaluate the germicidal properties of halide-based antimicrobial products.[32] In this method, 10 mL of the sanitizing product, diluted to its use-solution in AOAC hard water, if applicable, is inoculated with 50 μL of the test organism suspension. The solution is mixed and allowed to stand for 1 minute. After mixing, a 10 μL loopful of the suspension is transferred to 10 mL of neutralizing growth medium. Thirty seconds later, the same tube of sanitizing product is inoculated with 50 μL of test organism again. One minute later, the suspension is mixed and 10 μL is transferred (subcultured) to a second tube containing 10 mL of neutralizing growth medium. The inoculation and subculturing procedure is repeated until 10 tubes of growth medium have been subcultured. The test procedure is repeated for three known and verified concentrations of available chlorine (50 parts per million [ppm], 100 ppm, and 200 ppm) to be used as reference solutions. The subculture tubes are incubated and subsequently examined for the presence or absence of test organism growth as determined by the presence or absence of turbidity. The number of consecutive tubes showing growth for the sanitizing product is compared to the number of consecutive tubes showing growth for the three available chlorine reference solutions, allowing the analyst to compare the germicidal efficacy of the test product to the three concentrations of available chlorine. Refer to Table 62.1 for the test organisms and performance standard associated with this method.

Nonhalide-Based Food Contact Sanitizers: AOAC Germicidal and Detergent Sanitizing Action of Disinfectants (960.09)

The AOAC Germicidal and Detergent Sanitizing Action of Disinfectants method describes a quantitative, suspension-based test method used to evaluate the germicidal properties of nonhalide-based food contact sanitizers.[22] In this method, the sanitizer is diluted to its use-solution in AOAC synthetic hard water, if applicable, and a 99-mL sample of the prepared sanitizer solution is equilibrated to 25°C. A standardized suspension of the test organism is prepared, and a 1-mL sample of the organism is added to the sanitizer solution. The solution is mixed and the organism is exposed to the sanitizer for 30 seconds. After exposure, a 1-mL sample is removed and transferred to 9 mL of a neutralizer medium. The neutralized

TABLE 62.1 Sanitizer efficacy data requirements

Product Type	Test Methods	Test Organisms	Evaluation of Success
Halide-based food contact sanitizers (water-soluble powders/liquids)	AOAC Chlorine (Available) in Disinfectants (955.16)	*Staphylococcus aureus* (ATCC 6538) or *Salmonella enterica* (ATCC 6539)	Test results should demonstrate product concentrations equivalent to 50, 100, or 200 ppm of available chlorine.
Nonhalide-based food contact sanitizers (water-soluble powders/liquids)	AOAC Germicidal and Detergent Sanitizing Action of Disinfectants (960.09)	*S aureus* (ATCC 6538) and *Escherichia coli* (ATCC 11229) The control counts must demonstrate 7.0-8.0 logs.	A 99.999% reduction in the number of each test organism within 30 s
Nonfood contact sanitizers[a]	ASTM Standard Test Method for Efficacy of Sanitizers Recommended for Inanimate, Hard, Nonporous, Nonfood Contact Surfaces (E1153)	*S aureus* (ATCC 6538) and *Klebsiella pneumoniae* (ATCC 4352) or *Klebsiella* (formerly *Enterobacter*) *aerogenes* (ATCC 13048) The control counts for the organisms listed earlier must demonstrate a minimum average of 7.5×10^5 CFUs per carrier.	A 99.9% reduction over parallel control counts within 5 minutes
Laundry sanitizers (in wash)	ASTM E2274 or ASTM E2406 (for high efficiency)	*S aureus* (ATCC 6538)[b] *K pneumoniae* (ATCC 4352)[b] *Pseudomonas aeruginosa* (ATCC 15442)[b] A minimum of 1×10^4 CFUs per carrier and 1×10^4 CFUs per mL must be recovered on the control carriers and in the wash water control, respectively.	A minimum 99.9% (3 $\log_{10}$) reduction in bacteria over the control count for both the treated swatches and treatment solution wash water

Abbreviations: AOAC, Association of Official Analytical Chemists; ATCC, American Type Culture Collection; CFUs, colony-forming units; ppm, parts per million.

[a]This method may also be used to support laundry presoak sanitizing treatment claims. A 5% organic soil load must be included in the organism suspension.

[b]For broad-spectrum laundry sanitizers, test *S aureus* and *K pneumoniae*. For laundry sanitizers used in health care facilities, test *S aureus*, *K pneumoniae*, and *P aeruginosa*.

contents are mixed and enumerated by plating onto an appropriate agar. Following incubation, the surviving bacteria are enumerated and bacterial reduction is calculated as compared to the starting population of bacteria used in the test. The method includes sterility controls and a numbers control intended to enumerate the population of organism added to the sanitizer as well as a confirmation that the neutralizer used was suitable. The performance standard for the method can be found in Table 62.1.

ASTM Standard Test Method for Efficacy of Sanitizers Recommended for Inanimate, Hard, Nonporous Nonfood Contact Surfaces (E1153)

The ASTM Method E1153 describes a carrier-based, quantitative test method used to evaluate the efficacy of nonfood contact sanitizers.[33] In this method, glass, stainless steel, or other appropriate surface material 25 mm $\times$ 25 mm coupons are inoculated with 10 to 30 μL of test organism. The carriers are placed in an incubator to dry and are sequentially treated with 5 mL of the sanitizer at its use-solution. After the contact time ($\leq$5 min), the treated carriers are neutralized with 20 mL of neutralizer. The neutralized carriers are mixed and enumerated by plating onto an appropriate agar. Following incubation, the surviving bacteria are enumerated and the bacterial reduction is calculated compared to a control treatment. The method includes controls to enumerate the number of viable organisms present on the carriers (carrier counts) as well as a confirmation that the neutralizer used was suitable for the sanitizer. The performance requirements for the method can be found in Table 62.1.

▶ DISINFECTANTS

In the United States, disinfectants are regarded as products that provide a high level of public health protection when used according to label instructions. In health care environments, disinfectants are extremely important in making and keeping surfaces safe in the clinical environment by killing bacteria, viruses, and fungi. They reduce the likelihood of microbial cross-contamination from inanimate objects like bedrails and equipment to patients and staff, thus reducing the spread of infection in hospitals.[4] Disinfectants are similarly used in workplaces, hotels, and homes to reduce the spread of infectious agents. Disinfectants are most commonly applied by mopping, wiping, or spraying onto a hard surface but can, in some cases, be fogged, misted, or applied as a foam.

Classification of Disinfectants

The EPA Product Performance Test Guideline OCSPP 810.2200 describes the efficacy data requirements and testing recommendations for disinfectants used on hard surfaces.[34] According to the guideline, the following disinfectant classifications exist:

- Limited-spectrum (bactericidal) disinfectants
- Broad-spectrum (bactericidal) disinfectants
- Hospital or health care (bactericidal) disinfectants
- Fungicidal disinfectants
- Virucidal disinfectants
- Tuberculocidal disinfectants

Limited-Spectrum Disinfectants

Limited-spectrum disinfectants are classified as possessing disinfection efficacy against either the model gram-positive bacterium, *Staphylococcus aureus* American Type Culture Collection (ATCC) 6538, or the model gram-negative bacterium, *Salmonella enterica* ATCC 10708. Any additional bactericidal claims that can be made must match the gram stain type (positive or negative) base claim. Virucidal, fungicidal, and tuberculocidal claims cannot be made for limited-spectrum disinfectants.

Broad-Spectrum Disinfectants

Broad-spectrum disinfectants are classified as possessing disinfection efficacy against both gram-positive and gram-negative bacteria and thus must demonstrate efficacy against both *S aureus* ATCC 6538 and *S enterica* ATCC 10708 or *Pseudomonas aeruginosa* ATCC 15442. Additional bactericidal, virucidal, fungicidal, and tuberculocidal claims can be made, where substantiated.

Hospital or Health Care Disinfectants

Health care disinfectants used in hospitals, clinics, dental offices, nursing homes, or any other health care–related facility are classified as possessing disinfection efficacy against both gram-positive bacterium, *S aureus* ATCC 6538, and a clinically significant and difficult to kill gram-negative bacterium, *P aeruginosa* ATCC 15442. Additional bactericidal, virucidal, fungicidal, and tuberculocidal claims can be made, where substantiated.

Fungicidal Disinfectants

Broad-spectrum or hospital disinfectants may possess claims against pathogenic fungi to be classified as a fungicidal disinfectant. Disinfectant efficacy must be demonstrated against a clinically relevant fungus: *Trichophyton interdigitale* ATCC 9533 (formerly known as *Trichophyton mentagrophytes*), the fungus associated with athlete's foot. Once efficacy against *T interdigitale* is established, claims against fungi can be made. For example, mildewcidal disinfectant claims can be made where efficacy is demonstrated against *Aspergillus niger*, a mildew-causing black mold.

Virucidal Disinfectants

Broad-spectrum or hospital disinfectants may possess claims against viruses and be classified as virucidal disinfectants. Efficacy must be demonstrated against each virus listed on the label unless an acceptable surrogate for the virus exists. For example, label claims against hepatitis B virus, hepatitis C virus, and norovirus can be substantiated by testing the surrogate viruses duck hepatitis B virus, bovine viral diarrhea virus, and Feline calicivirus, respectively, because the human viral strains are not conducive to laboratory testing.

Tuberculocidal Disinfectants

Broad-spectrum or hospital disinfectants may possess tuberculocidal disinfection claims. To substantiate such claims, the EPA recommends disinfectant efficacy be demonstrated against *Mycobacterium bovis*-bacille Calmette-Guérin (BCG), a bovine surrogate for *Mycobacterium tuberculosis*, the causative strain of human tuberculosis (TB).

In addition to fungicidal, virucidal, or tuberculocidal claims, the following additional claims are permitted for hospital disinfectants:

- "Kills bacteria in biofilms"
  Liquid- or spray-based hospital disinfectants may be eligible for public health biofilm claims if a 6 $\log_{10}$ reduction can be achieved against pure biofilms composed of *S aureus* and *P aeruginosa*.[35]
- "Kills or inactivates *C difficile* spores"
  Liquid-, spray-, or wipe-based hospital disinfectants may be eligible for this claim if a 6 $\log_{10}$ reduction can be achieved against spores of *C difficile*.[24]

Disinfectant Test Methods

A variety of disinfectant test methods are recommended by the EPA and Health Canada to evaluate the efficacy of a disinfectant claim.[17,34] A summary of these methods, their applicability, and associated performance standards can be found in Tables 62.2 and 62.3.

AOAC Use-Dilution Method (964.02, 955.14, 955.15)

The AOAC Use-Dilution method[36-38] describes a carrier-based, qualitative test method used to evaluate water-soluble and liquid disinfectants commonly used in mop and bucket applications. In this method, stainless steel penicillin cups ("penicylinders") are inoculated by immersion in a suspension of the test organism. The carriers are then removed, dried, and sequentially immersed in 10 mL of the disinfectant at its use-dilution for the prescribed contact time ($\leq$10 min) and temperature. After the contact time, the carriers are transferred

to a neutralizing growth medium, incubated, and examined for growth as indicated by the presence or absence of turbidity. The number of negative carriers (no turbidity) is counted to determine if efficacy was achieved. The method includes controls to enumerate the number of viable organisms present on the carriers (carrier counts) as well as a confirmation that the neutralizer used was suitable for the disinfectant. This method can be used to evaluate disinfectant performance against bacteria and fungi, and the performance standard for the method can be found in Table 62.2.

AOAC Germicidal Spray Products as Disinfectants (961.02)

The AOAC Germicidal Spray Products as Disinfectants method describes a carrier-based, qualitative test method used to evaluate disinfectants applied by spray application.[39] In this method, glass microscope slides are inoculated with 10 μL of test organism. The carriers are dried, sequentially treated by the spray disinfectant, and exposed for the prescribed contact time ($\leq$10 min). After the contact time, the carriers are transferred to a neutralizing growth medium, incubated, and examined for growth as indicated by the presence or absence of turbidity. The number of negative carriers (no turbidity) is counted to determine if efficacy was achieved. The method includes controls to enumerate the number of viable organisms present on the carriers (carrier counts) as well as a confirmation that the neutralizer used was suitable for the disinfectant. This method can be used to evaluate disinfectant performance against bacteria and fungi. The performance standard for the method can be found in Table 62.2.

AOAC Germicidal Spray Products as Disinfectants Modified for Wipes (961.02)

The AOAC Germicidal Spray Products as Disinfectants method can be modified to describe a carrier-based, qualitative test method used to evaluate disinfectants applied in the form of presaturated wipes or towelettes.[39] This modified procedure is also described in ASTM Method E2362: Standard Practice for Evaluation of Pre-saturated or Impregnated Towelettes for Hard Surface Disinfection.[40] In these methods, glass microscope slides are inoculated with 10 μL of test organism. The carriers are dried and sequentially wiped by the disinfectant, providing for simulated mechanical action. Typically, 10 coupons are wiped by a single towelette, rotating the towelette between carriers to expose an unused surface. The treated carriers are held for the prescribed contact time ($\leq$10 min), and after contact, transferred to a neutralizing growth medium. The neutralized carriers are incubated and examined for growth as indicated by the presence or absence of turbidity. The number of negative carriers is counted to determine if efficacy was achieved. The method includes

TABLE 62.2	Bacterial disinfection efficacy requirements		
Product Type	**Test Methods**	**Test Organisms**	**Evaluation of Success**
Water-soluble powder/liquid disinfectants	AOAC Use-Dilution Method (955.14, 955.15, 964.02)[a]	*Staphylococcus aureus* (ATCC 6538)[b] *Salmonella enterica* (ATCC 10708)[b] *Pseudomonas aeruginosa* (ATCC 15442)[b] The control counts must demonstrate an average log density of 6.0-7.0 for *S aureus* and *P aeruginosa* and 5.0-6.0 for *S enterica*.	*S aureus*: At least 57/60 carriers are negative for growth. *S enterica*: At least 59/60 carriers are negative for growth. *P aeruginosa*: At least 54/60 carriers are negative for growth. *Additional bacteria*: 10/10 carriers are negative for growth.
Spray disinfectants	AOAC Germicidal Spray Products as Disinfectants (961.02)	*S aureus* (ATCC 6538)[b] *S enterica* (ATCC 10708)[b] *P aeruginosa* (ATCC 15442)[b] The control counts must demonstrate an average log density of 5.0-6.5 for *S aureus* and *P aeruginosa* and 4.0-5.5 for *S enterica*.	At least 59/60 carriers are negative for growth. *Additional bacteria*: 10/10 carriers are negative for growth.
Towelette disinfectants	AOAC Germicidal Spray Products as Disinfectants (961.02) modified for wipes or ASTM E2362 Standard Practice for Evaluation of Pre-saturated or Impregnated Towelettes for Hard Surface Disinfection		
Laundry disinfectants (in wash)	ASTM E2274 or ASTM E2406 (for high efficiency)	*S aureus* (ATCC 6538)[c] *Klebsiella pneumoniae* (ATCC 4352)[c] *P aeruginosa* (ATCC 15442)[c] A minimum of 1×10^4 CFUs per carrier and 1×10^4 CFUs/mL must be recovered on the control carriers and in the wash water control, respectively.	No growth is observed on each of 9 swatches and in the wash water.

Abbreviations: AOAC, Association of Official Analytical Chemists; ASTM International, American Society for Testing and Materials International; ATCC, American Type Culture Collection; CFUs, colony-forming units.

[a]These methods may also be used to support laundry presoak disinfecting treatment claims. A 5% organic soil load must be included in the organism suspension.

[b]For limited-spectrum disinfectants, test *S aureus* or *S enterica*. For broad-spectrum disinfectants, test *S aureus* and *S enterica* or *P aeruginosa*. For hospital or health care disinfectants, test *S aureus* and *P aeruginosa*.

[c]For broad-spectrum laundry disinfectants, test *S aureus* and *K pneumoniae*. For laundry disinfectants used in health care facilities, test *S aureus*, *K pneumoniae*, and *P aeruginosa*.

controls to enumerate the number of viable organisms present on the carriers (carrier counts) as well as a confirmation that the neutralizer used was suitable for the disinfectant. This method can be used to evaluate disinfectant performance against bacteria and fungi and the performance standard for the method can be found in Table 62.2.

AOAC Fungicidal Activity Test (955.17)

The AOAC Fungicidal Activity Test describes a qualitative, suspension method for evaluating the fungicidal efficacy of a water-soluble powders or liquid disinfectants against *T interdigitale*.[41] The method is a qualitative, suspension-based method and involves inoculating 5 mL of

disinfectant with a 0.5-mL sample of fungal spores (fungal conidia) at 20°C. After 5 minutes, 10 minutes, and 15 minutes of exposure, a 10 μL loopful of the mixture is transferred to tubes of neutralizing growth medium. The tubes are incubated and examined for growth of the fungus after each time point. The method includes controls to enumerate the concentration of the spore (conidial) suspension used in testing as well as a confirmation that the neutralizer used was suitable for the disinfectant. The performance standard for the method can be found in Table 62.3. It should be noted that the method may only be used to support a 10-minute label claim. As an alternative, the AOAC Use-Dilution or AOAC Germicidal Spray Products methods can be modified to evaluate liquid-based, spray-based, or wipe-based disinfectants against *T interdigitale*.

TABLE 62.3 Additional disinfectant-associated efficacy requirements

Claim Type	Product Type	Test Methods	Test Organism or Virus	Evaluation of Success
Fungicidal disinfectants[a]	Water-soluble powder/liquid disinfectants	AOAC Fungicidal Activity Test (955.17) or AOAC Use-Dilution Method modified for fungi	*Trichophyton interdigitale* (ATCC 9533) For the AOAC Fungicidal Activity method, the titer must demonstrate 5×10^6-5×10^7 CFUs/mL. For the AOAC Use-Dilution, AOAC Germicidal Spray Products as Disinfectants, and ASTM E2362 methods, the control counts must demonstrate an average log density of 4.0-5.0.	For the AOAC Fungicidal Test, all fungal spores should be killed at 10 and 15 min to support a 10-min label claim. For the Use-Dilution or Germicidal Spray/Wipes test methods, all carriers are negative for growth (10/10).
	Spray disinfectants	AOAC Germicidal Spray Products as Disinfectants (961.02)		
	Towelette disinfectants	AOAC Germicidal Spray Products as Disinfectants (961.02) modified for wipes or ASTM E2362 Standard Practice for Evaluation of Pre-saturated or Impregnated Towelettes for Hard Surface Disinfection		
Virucidal disinfectants[a]	Water-soluble powder/liquid disinfectants	Standard Test Method to Assess Virucidal Activity of Chemicals Intended for Disinfection (ASTM E1053)	Each virus claimed on the label or approved surrogate[b] A minimum recoverable virus end point titer of 4.80 $\log_{10}$ must be achieved.	A minimum 3 $\log_{10}$ reduction of the virus past neutralization and cytotoxicity, if present, must be shown.
	Spray disinfectants			
	Towelette disinfectants			
Tuberculocidal disinfectants[a]	Water-soluble powder/liquid disinfectants	AOAC Tuberculocidal Activity of Disinfectants (965.12) or Quantitative Tuberculocidal Activity Test (Ascenzi) for glutaraldehyde products	*Mycobacterium bovis*-BCG For the AOAC Tuberculocidal Activity method, the control carrier counts must demonstrate an average log of 4.0-6.0. For the Quantitative Tuberculocidal Activity test, the organism titer must demonstrate 1×10^7-1×10^8 CFUs/mL	Ten of 10 carriers are negative for growth in all three subculture media types. or At least a 4.0 $\log_{10}$ reduction is achieved for each replicate at the stated contact time.
	Spray disinfectants	AOAC Germicidal Spray Products Test modified for tuberculocidal activity		Ten of 10 carriers are negative for growth in all three subculture media types.
	Towelette disinfectants	Modified Germicidal Spray Test or ASTM E2362 Standard Practice for Evaluation of Pre-saturated or Impregnated Towelettes for Hard Surface Disinfection modified for tuberculocidal activity		Ten of 10 carriers are negative for growth in all three subculture media types.
Kills bacteria in biofilms[c]	Water-soluble powder/liquid disinfectants	EPA Microbiology Laboratory Branch (MLB) SOP MB-19, "Growing a Biofilm Using the CDC Biofilm Reactor" and EPA MLB SOP MB-20, "Single Tube Method for Determining the Efficacy of Disinfectants Against Bacterial Biofilms"	*Staphylococcus aureus* (ATCC 6538) and *Pseudomonas aeruginosa* (ATCC 15442) The control counts must demonstrate a mean $\log_{10}$ density of 7.5-9.0 for *S aureus* and 8.0-9.5 for *P aeruginosa*.	A minimum 6 $\log_{10}$ reduction of viable bacteria in biofilm is achieved.
	Spray disinfectants			

TABLE 62.3	Additional disinfectant-associated efficacy requirements *(Continued)*			
Claim Type	**Product Type**	**Test Methods**	**Test Organism or Virus**	**Evaluation of Success**
Kills or inactivates *Clostridium difficile* spores[c]	Water-soluble powder/liquid disinfectants	EPA MLB SOP MB-28, "Production and Storage of Spores of *C difficile* for Use in the Efficacy Evaluation of Antimicrobial Agents" and EPA MLB SOP MB-31, "Procedure for the OECD Quantitative Method for Testing Antimicrobial Products against Spores of *C difficile* on Inanimate, Hard Nonporous Surfaces"	*C difficile* (ATCC 43598) The control carrier counts must demonstrate an average $\log_{10}$ of 6.0-7.0.	A minimum mean 6 $\log_{10}$ reduction in viable spores is achieved.
	Spray disinfectants			
	Towelette disinfectants (liquid expressed from the wipes)			

Abbreviations: AOAC, Association of Official Analytical Chemists; ASTM International, American Society for Testing and Materials International; ATCC, American Type Culture Collection; BCG, bacille Calmette-Guérin; CFUs, colony-forming units; EPA, Environmental Protection Agency; MB, Microbiology Branch; MLB, Microbiology Laboratory Branch; OECD, Organisation for Economic Co-operation and Development.; SOP, Standard Operating Procedure.

[a]The product must also have a broad-spectrum or hospital disinfectant label claim.

[b]For label claims against hepatitis B virus, hepatitis C virus, and norovirus, the duck hepatitis B virus, bovine viral diarrhea virus, and Feline calicivirus, respectively, are considered acceptable surrogates by EPA for testing.

[c]The product must also have hospital disinfectant label claim.

Standard Test Method to Assess Virucidal Activity of Chemicals Intended for Disinfection (ASTM E1053)

This method describes a quantitative, carrier-based method used to assess the virucidal activity of disinfectants.[42] In this method, a 0.2 mL aliquot of a virus suspension is dried onto the surface of a glass Petri dish. The disinfectant is applied to the dish either by transferring a 2-mL aliquot of the disinfectant (mopping applications) or by spraying or wiping the disinfectant in a manner consistent with its use conditions. After treatment, the prescribed contact time is observed ($\leq$10 min). After exposure, the treated virus film is scraped from the dish, collected, and neutralized. Neutralization is commonly achieved by passing the suspension through a gel filtration column or by using a chemical neutralizer. The neutralized suspension is serially diluted and aliquots of the dilutions are transferred to four or more cell culture wells containing a cell monolayer appropriate for the virus. The cell cultures are incubated and examined for cytopathic effect (CPE), a structural change of the host cells that occurs when the infective virus is present. The method includes a neutralization control used to confirm the effectiveness of the neutralizer or neutralization technique used for the disinfectant. Additionally, a cytotoxicity control is included to assess the potentially toxic effects of the neutralized contents on the host cell to distinguish the effects of cytotoxicity from CPE. A virus recovery control

is also conducted using an inert solution in place of the disinfectant to enumerate the level of infective units recovered after drying and a $\log_{10}$ reduction associated with treatment is determined. The performance standard for the method can be found in Table 62.3.

AOAC Tuberculocidal Activity of Disinfectants (965.12)

The AOAC Tuberculocidal Activity of Disinfectants method describes a qualitative, carrier-based test method used to evaluate the tuberculocidal activity of water-soluble powders or liquid disinfectants, excluding glutaraldehyde-based formulations.[43] In this method, porcelain penicylinders are inoculated by immersion into a suspension of *M bovis*-BCG. The carriers are dried and sequentially immersed in 10 mL of the disinfectant at its use-dilution for the prescribed contact time ($\leq$10 min) at 20°C. After the contact time, the carriers are transferred to a neutralizing medium and then to one of three growth media used to recover *M bovis* survivors. Additionally, 2-mL aliquots of the neutralized carrier suspension are added to two additional growth media used to recover *M bovis*. The three sets of subculture media are incubated for up to 90 days and examined for visible growth of the test organism. The number of negative tubes is counted to determine if efficacy was achieved. The method includes controls to enumerate the number of viable organisms present on the carriers (carrier counts) as well as a confirmation that the neutralizer and subculture media used were suitable. The performance standard for the method can be found in Table 62.3. This method can also be adapted to support testing of spray-based and wipe-based disinfectants.

Quantitative Tuberculocidal Activity Test (Ascenzi method)

The Quantitative Tuberculocidal Activity Test describes a quantitative, suspension-based test method used to assess the tuberculocidal activity of specific disinfectants.[44] Based on the EPA's "Data Call-in Notice for Tuberculocidal Effectiveness for All Antimicrobial Pesticides with Tuberculocidal Claims," dated June 13, 1986,[45] EPA strongly recommends using the AOAC Tuberculocidal Activity of Disinfectants method to evaluate all disinfectants except glutaraldehyde-based products. For these products, the Quantitative Tuberculocidal Activity Test should be used.[46] In this method, a suspension of *M bovis*-BCG is inoculated into the disinfectant prepared at its use-solution. The suspension is mixed and allowed to stand for the desired contact time(s). At each contact time, an aliquot is removed, neutralized, and quantitatively assayed for survivors by filtration recovery technique. Quadruplicate replicates are typically evaluated for each batch of disinfectant. The average survivors found in the four test replicates is determined for each contact time as compared to an untreated control run. The EPA requires a minimum 4 log reduction at the contact time stated. Claims are granted in 5-minute increments for this test method, and verification testing in a second lab or with a second set of staff may be required for certain active ingredients such as products formulated solely with quaternary ammonium compounds as the active. Refer to Table 62.3 for more information on the performance standard.

Biofilm Test Methods

Based on guidance published in 2017, the EPA recommends the use of two methods to evaluate hospital disinfectants claiming to kill bacteria present in biofilms.[35] The first method, EPA Microbiology Laboratory Branch (MLB) SOP MB-19, "Growing a Biofilm using the CDC Biofilm Reactor," prescribes a method for growing a biofilm of *P aeruginosa* ATCC 15442 and *S aureus* ATCC 6538.[47] This method derives from ASTM Method E2562: Standard Method for Quantification of *Pseudomonas aeruginosa* Biofilm Grown with High Shear and Continuous Flow using CDC Biofilm Reactor.[48] In this method, a Centers for Disease Control and Prevention (CDC) reactor is assembled, which includes a carboy of nutrient broth, a continuously stirred reactor tank with sterile coupons affixed to rods and a waste carboy. The test organism is inoculated into the reactor and allowed to grow for a

period of time (eg, 24 h). A continuous flow of nutrients with waste collection is then initiated, and the reactor is allowed to mix to simulate high shear flow for a period of time (eg, 24 h). After the growth period has ended, the rods are removed, planktonic bacteria are rinsed away, and the biofilm-coated coupons, produced under high shear flow conditions, can be used in the efficacy phase of testing.

With biofilm-coated coupons prepared, the EPA recommends biofilm efficacy for hospital disinfectants be substantiated by using the EPA MLB SOP MB-20, "Single Tube Method for Determining the Efficacy of Disinfectants against Bacterial Biofilms."[49] This method derives from ASTM Method E2871: Standard Test Method for Evaluating Disinfectant Efficacy against *Pseudomonas aeruginosa* Biofilm Grown in CDC Reactor Using Single Tube method.[50] In this procedure, a series of five biofilm-coated coupons are individually immersed in 4 mL of the disinfectant prepared at its use-solution. The coupons are exposed for the prescribed contact time ($\leq$10 min). Once the contact time has elapsed, an aliquot of neutralizer is added to each tube. The neutralized carriers are sequentially vortex-mixed and sonicated to remove and disaggregate surviving bacteria from the biofilm-inoculated carrier surface. The neutralized material is then serially diluted and recovered by filtration techniques to enumerate survivors. A $\log_{10}$ reduction is determined as compared to control coupons. The method includes controls to enumerate the number of viable organisms present on untreated carriers (control coupons) as well as a confirmation that the neutralizer used was suitable for the disinfectant. The performance standard for the method can be found in Table 62.3.

Clostridium difficile Test Methods

Based on guidance published in 2018, the EPA recommends the use of two methods to evaluate hospital disinfectants claiming to kill spores of *C difficile*.[24] The first method, EPA MLB SOP MB-28, "Production and Storage of Spores of *Clostridium difficile* for Use in the Efficacy Evaluation of Antimicrobial Agents,"[51] describes the procedures used to propagate, purify, assess robustness, and store spores of *C difficile* ATCC 43598. This method has been adapted from ASTM Method E2839: Standard Test Method for Production of *Clostridium difficile* Spores for Use in Efficacy Evaluation of Antimicrobial Agents.[52] Briefly, spores of *C difficile* are grown under anaerobic conditions on CDC anaerobic blood agar for 10 days. The spores are collected from the agar surface in a phosphate buffer solution containing polysorbate 80, washed several times, and purified using a nonionic, density-gradient medium. The purified spores are evaluated for titer and chemical resistance to sodium hypochlorite, are adjusted in concentration, and are frozen at $\leq$−70°C for up to 90 days.

Once the *C difficile* spores have been prepared, hospital-grade disinfectants can be evaluated for efficacy against *C difficile* using the following method: EPA MLB SOP MB-31, "Procedure for the OECD Quantitative Method for Testing Antimicrobial Products against Spores of *Clostridium difficile* on Inanimate, Hard Nonporous Surfaces."[53] This method has been adapted from the method described in the Organisation for Economic Co-operation and Development (OECD) Guidance Document on Quantitative Methods for Evaluating the Activity of Microbicides Used on Hard Non-porous Surfaces, dated June 21, 2013.[23] In this method, brushed discs made of either 430 or 304 type stainless steel, depending on the active ingredient, are inoculated with a 10-μL aliquot of the spores that have been mixed with a three-part soil load including bovine serum albumin, yeast extract, and mucin. The spores are then dried onto the surface under vacuum desiccation. A set of 10 inoculated disks are treated by placing 50 μL of the disinfectant at its use-dilution over the inoculated surface. The coupons are exposed for the prescribed contact time (≤10 min) and a 10-mL aliquot of neutralizer is added to the treatment vial containing the coupon. The coupons are vortex mixed to elute surviving spores from the surface, and the neutralized material is assayed for survivors by filtration technique onto agar appropriate for the recovery of *C difficile*. After 120 hours of anaerobic incubation, a log_{10} reduction is determined for the treated coupons as compared to control coupons. The method includes controls to enumerate the number of viable spores present on untreated carriers (control coupons) as well as a confirmation that the neutralizer used was suitable for the disinfectant. A control to assess the resistance of the spores to sodium hypochlorite is also included. For towelette products, additional wetness testing may be required. The performance standard for the method can be found in Table 62.3.

◗ HIGH-LEVEL DISINFECTANTS, SPORICIDES, STERILANTS, AND DECONTAMINANTS

Sterilants are used to eliminate vegetative bacteria, bacterial spores, fungi, fungal spores, and viruses on hard, nonporous surfaces. In the United States, those used in the medical field on critical and semicritical medical devices and are regulated by the FDA[19] and are referred to as HLDs or liquid chemical sterilants. Those used on environmental surfaces may be referred to as sporicides or sterilants and are regulated by the EPA. Sporicides or sterilants used for the disinfection of manufacturing, filling, and packaging equipment in the food industry and for the aseptic packaging of low-acid food are also regulated by the EPA.[54] Products shown to be effective in eliminating spores of *Bacillus anthracis* are classified by the EPA as decontaminants.[54]

In Canada, a recent notice of the reclassification of HLDs and sterilants used only on medical devices was released by Health Canada. As of March 16, 2018, these products are regulated under the Medical Devices Bureau as Class II Medical Devices and will no longer be regulated as drugs under the Food and Drugs Act.[55]

Sporicide/Sterilant/High-Level Disinfectant Test Methods

Efficacy claims for sporicidal and sterilant pesticides are described in EPA Product Performance Test Guideline OCSPP 810.2100.[54] Testing requirements for HLDs used for medical devices are regulated by the FDA and can be found in the Guidance for Industry and FDA Reviewers: Content and Format of Premarket Notification [510(k)] Submissions for Liquid Chemical Sterilants/High-Level Disinfectants.[19]

AOAC Sporicidal Activity of Disinfectants (966.04)

The AOAC Sporicidal Activity of Disinfectants method describes a carrier-based, qualitative test method used to evaluate water-soluble powders, liquid sterilants/sporicides, or gases used to treat hard and soft environmental surfaces for the mitigation of bacterial spores.[56] In this method, porcelain penicillin cups ("penicylinders") and suture loops, silk or polyester depending on the active ingredient tested, are individually inoculated by immersion into spore suspensions of *Bacillus subtilis* and *Clostridium sporogenes*. The carriers are then dried under vacuum desiccation and are sequentially immersed in sets of five into 10 mL of the sterilant/sporicide at its use-dilution for the prescribed contact time. After the contact time, the carriers are transferred to a series of neutralizing growth media, incubated, and examined for growth as indicated by the presence or absence of turbidity. The number of negative carriers is counted to determine if efficacy was achieved. The method includes controls to enumerate the number of viable spores present on the carriers (carrier counts), a control to evaluate the resistance of the spores used in the study after exposure to hydrochloric acid, and a confirmation that the neutralizing medium used was suitable for the sterilant/sporicide. A total of three batches of product are evaluated against each spore-forming organism on each carrier type. Sets of 60 carriers are evaluated for a total of 720 treated test carriers. Depending on the nature of the final claim, for example, base sterilant claim, sporicidal claim or additional/supplemental spore former claim, batch, carrier number, and carrier material requirements differ.[54] For a sterilant or sporicide to be effective, complete kill must be shown on all test carriers. In addition, verification testing by a second lab or second set of staff must demonstrate complete kill on one batch of product tested against 30 carriers per organism per carrier type. The method can be adapted for commercial sterilants used for aseptic packaging of low acid food by using stainless steel penicylinders as the carrier type in testing, the required test conditions specified for this type of use in 810.2100, and for some antimicrobial products, including a third spore-forming bacterium, *Bacillus cereus* to the test plan.[54]

Liquid Chemical Sterilants/High Level Disinfectants

The Guidance for Industry and FDA Reviewers: Content and Format of Premarket Notification [510(k)] Submissions for Liquid Chemical Sterilants/High Level Disinfectants describes a variety of testing requirements that must be satisfied to market a liquid chemical sterilant/HLD for use on reusable, heat-sensitive critical and semicritical medical devices.[19] As it relates to microbiological laboratory testing, one requirement to market an HLD is microbiological potency testing. These potency tests are conducted at the minimum effective concentration to establish a broad spectrum of microbicidal activity of the HLD and may be modified to accommodate manual versus automated reprocessing treatments. Furthermore, testing to ensure the efficacy of reusable HLDs must be confirmed through simulated reuse tests.[19,57] The list of efficacy tests is as follows:

- AOAC Sporicidal Activity of Disinfectants (966.04): *B subtilis* and *C sporogenes* tested against both carrier types (porcelain penicylinders and suture loops) against three batches of the HLD and 60 carriers/batch/strain/carrier type. Additionally, one lot is repeated under independent test conditions against both spore-forming bacteria and both carrier types at 30 carriers/strain/carrier type. All test carriers must be negative for growth to demonstrate efficacy.[56]
- A quantitative modification of AOAC Tuberculocidal Activity of Disinfectants (965.12) or Quantitative Tuberculocidal Activity Test (Ascenzi method) for which two batches of the HLD are shown to kill 10^6 CFUs of an appropriate mycobacterium species (eg, *M bovis* or *Mycobacterium terrae*) within the prescribed contact time[43]
- AOAC Fungicidal Activity Test (955.17) for which one batch of the HLD shows complete kill against *T interdigitale* ATCC 9533[41]
- AOAC Use-Dilution Method (964.02, 955.14, 955.15) for which one batch of the HLD shows efficacy against *S enterica* ATCC 10708, *S aureus* ATCC 6538, and *P aeruginosa* ATCC 15442 as described in Table 62.1[36-38]
- Standard Test Method to Assess Virucidal Activity of Chemicals Intended for Disinfection (ASTM E1053) for which one batch of the HLD shows efficacy for the claimed virus(es) as described in Table 62.2[42]

▶ OTHER ANTIMICROBIAL CLAIMS AND ASSOCIATED TEST METHODS

Although sporicidal, disinfectant, and sanitizer claims are the most common antimicrobial claims in North America, other claims do exist. For example, according to EPA Test Guidance 810.2400, ASTM Method E1153 can be modified to evaluate nonfood contact sanitizing efficacy on fabric or textile materials.[33,58] In addition, laundry products intended to reduce or eliminate bacteria from household or commercial linens can be assessed using various test methods depending on the level of kill required. These types of products are particularly important in the health care environment where outbreaks of bacterial illness have been linked to improperly laundered sheets.[59,60] This section describes some of these claims and their associated test methods. Test methods used to assess the microbiostatic nature of nonpublic health products are also discussed.

Laundry Treatments and Additives With Antimicrobial Activity

Product performance guidelines for evaluating disinfectants and sanitizers used on fabrics or textiles is described by the EPA in the 810.2400 test guideline.[58] For example, antimicrobial products that bear label recommendations for use in the treatment of laundry (as a presoak treatment or in household and commercial laundering) provide various levels of efficacy including disinfection and sanitization. The effectiveness of disinfecting presoak treatments can be evaluated using the AOAC Use-Dilution Method, incorporating a 5% organic soil load, as described previously.[36-38] According to the EPA, the effectiveness of sanitizing presoak treatments can be evaluated using the ASTM Test Method for Efficacy of Sanitizers Recommended for Nonfood Contact Surfaces (E1153), incorporating a 5% organic soil load, as described previously.[33] The effectiveness of laundry disinfectants and sanitizers used during laundering cycles can be tested using the following methods.

Test Methods for Laundry Disinfectants and Sanitizers

ASTM Standard Test Method for Evaluation of Laundry Sanitizers and Disinfectants (E2274)

Describes a carrier-based, quantitative test method used to evaluate the efficacy of laundry sanitizers and laundry disinfectants.[61] In this method, swatches of fabric are inoculated with the test organism. The carriers are dried and placed inside a spindle that has been wrapped with sterile fabric used to simulate a fabric-loaded laundry machine. The spindle containing the inoculated carrier swatches is then placed into a canister containing the sanitizer or disinfectant. The canisters are spun to simulate the laundry cycle for the desired contact time. After the contact time, the carrier swatches are removed from the spindle and transferred to 10 mL of neutralizing medium. For disinfectant claims, the neutralized swatches are incubated and examined for the presence or absence of growth as demonstrated by turbidity. For sanitizer claims, the neutralized swatch carriers are mixed and serially diluted, plating samples onto an agar medium. For both claims, the treatment solution, representing the wash water, is also evaluated for the presence of the test organism. For disinfection claims, the number of negative carriers is used to evaluate efficacy. For sanitizer claims, the level of $\log_{10}$ reduction achieved is used to evaluate efficacy. The method includes controls to enumerate the number of viable organisms present on the swatch carriers (carrier counts) as well as a confirmation that the neutralizer used was suitable for the disinfectant. A modification of this test method, ASTM E2406: Standard Test Method for Evaluation of Laundry Sanitizers and Disinfectants for Use in High Efficiency Washing Operations[62] can be used to evaluate the efficacy of disinfectants and sanitizers in high-efficiency laundering operations. The performance standard for sanitization claims can be found in Table 62.1, and the performance standard for disinfection claims can be found in Table 62.2.

Microbiostatic Agents

Microbiostatic agents are antimicrobial compounds that inhibit the growth of microorganisms (such as bacteria, fungi, or algae). These agents are generally broken down into categories that describe the target organism type (eg, a bacteriostat inhibits the growth of bacteria, an algistat inhibits the growth of algae, a fungistat inhibits the growth of yeast and fungi, and a mildewstat inhibits growth of mildew). These lower levels of efficacy are not considered suitable for use in areas where public health is a concern. Instead, microbiostatic claims are generally deemed acceptable only for products explicitly recommended for the control of microorganisms of aesthetic significance (eg, spoilage bacteria, nonpathogenic fungi, odor-causing bacteria, protection of product integrity) and are therefore considered to be nonpublic health claims.[10] The EPA's "Pesticide Assessment Guidelines—subdivision G: Product Performance" describes test methods that may be used to support various nonpublic health claims related to algistat or mildewstat claims, whereas various ASTM International and American Association of Textile Chemists and Colorists (AATCC) methods exist to support the testing of bacteriostatic claims.[63]

Control of Bacteria on Textiles

Although considered nonpublic health claims, fabrics or textiles treated or impregnated with bacteriostatic agents can only make claims that have been substantiated with

appropriate data. A variety of standardized test methods exist to substantiate these claims. One method described by AATCC is AATCC 100: Assessment of Antibacterial Finishes on Textiles method.[64] The AATCC 100 describes a quantitative, carrier-based method in which a stack of treated swatches is inoculated with the organism of interest. The stack is held in a sealed container for a period of time (eg, 24 h), neutralized, and assayed for surviving bacteria by serial dilution and plating. An inoculated stack of untreated swatches is similarly inoculated, held, neutralized, and assayed for survivors. A percentage and/or $\log_{10}$ reduction is calculated to assess the effectiveness of the antibacterial finish. Typically, regulatory agencies seek at least a minimum 90% or 1 $\log_{10}$ reduction of both gram-positive and gram-negative bacteria for an effective treatment.

Control of Bacteria on Hard Surfaces

Hard surfaces such as rigid or flexible plastics impregnated or treated with bacteriostatic agents can be evaluated for efficacy using a variety of methods including the following.

The ASTM E2180: Standard Test Method for Determining the Activity of Incorporated Antimicrobial Agents in Polymeric or Hydrophobic Materials describes a quantitative, carrier-based method that can be used to evaluate the effectiveness of bacteriostatic agents in hydrophobic materials like vinyl pool liners, shower curtains, or other materials treated with material-bound antimicrobial agents.[65] The use of an agar slurry assists with overcoming the hydrophobic nature of these materials. In this method, a standardized bacterial culture is incorporated into a molten agar slurry. The agar slurry is inoculated over the surface of the treated material, and a prescribed contact time is monitored (eg, 24 h). The treated material is then neutralized, and surviving bacteria are enumerated. Similar untreated materials are inoculated, exposed, and evaluated for survivors by serial dilution and plating techniques. Percentage and/or $\log_{10}$ reduction are determined by comparing survivors from the treated surface to the untreated surface to assess the efficacy of the bacteriostatic agent. Typically, regulatory agencies seek at least a minimum 90% or 1 $\log_{10}$ reduction of both gram-positive and gram-negative bacteria for an effective treatment.

The ASTM E2149: Test Method for Determining the Antimicrobial Activity of Antimicrobial Agents Under Dynamic Contact Conditions describes a quantitative, carrier-based method that can be used to evaluate the effectiveness of nonleaching, surface bound bacteriostatic under dynamic conditions.[66] This method helps to overcome challenges associated with maintaining contact of the test organism with various flexible materials. In the method, a standardized bacterial culture is prepared and enumerated by serial dilution and plating (time zero inoculum). Next, a measured mass (eg, 1 g) of the treated material is placed into a flask containing 50 mL of the standardized culture of bacteria. The flask is placed onto a wrist-action shaker for a specified contact time to create dynamic interaction of the surface-bound antimicrobial agent with the bacterial culture. After the contact time (eg, 1 h), a sample of the bacterial culture is removed and enumerated by serial dilution and plating. Similarly, an untreated sample is placed into a flask containing 50 mL of inoculum, exposed for the contact time, and enumerated. After incubation, surviving bacteria are calculated for the time zero inoculum, treated sample(s), and the untreated sample(s). Percentage and/or $\log_{10}$ reductions are determined for the treated sample by comparison to either the time zero inoculum control or the untreated sample results. Typically, regulatory agencies seek at least a minimum of 90% or 1 $\log_{10}$ reduction of both gram-positive and gram-negative bacteria for an effective treatment.

Control of Mold and Mildew on Textiles

The EPA's Pesticide Assessment Guidelines—subdivision G: Product Performance sections 93-15 and 93-30(I) item 1 describe a fabric mildew fungistatic test method intended to support claims for control of mildew on fabric.[63] In this method, strips of cotton fabric are treated with a sterile growth medium and dried. Ten test strips of fabric are then treated with the test fungistatic product and are allowed to dry. The strips of treated fabric are sprayed with a mold spore (conidia) suspension containing a mixture of *Aspergillus niger* and *Penicillium variabile*, suspended in bottles containing water, and incubated. A set of 10 identical, untreated control fabric strips are inoculated with the test fungi and incubated alongside the treated samples. The treated and control fabric strips are incubated and evaluated weekly for fungal growth. A product dosage is considered an acceptable mildewstat for a specific period of time when all treated test fabric strips are shown to be free of fungal growth after 7, 14, 21, or 28 days, as claimed. The control fabric strips are used to confirm validity of the study, requiring at least 50% coverage of mold after 7 days of incubation.

Control of Mold and Mildew on Hard Surfaces

The EPA's Pesticide Assessment Guidelines—subdivision G: Product Performance sections 93-15 and 93-30(I) item 2 describes a hard-surface mildew fungistatic test method, supporting claims for control, prevention, or inhibition of mildew-causing fungi on various hard surfaces.[63] In this method, 10 sterile, glazed ceramic tiles (or other materials such as plastic, porcelain, glass, or metal) are treated with the fungistatic product and allowed to dry. The treated tiles are then sprayed with a spore (conidia) suspension of *A niger* and dried. The treated, inoculated tiles are transferred to sterile water agar plates incubated in a humidified environment. A set of 10 identical, untreated control tiles are inoculated with the test fungi and incubated alongside the test. Following 1 week of incubation, the treated and control tiles are evaluated for fungal growth. A product dosage is considered acceptable when all treated tiles are

shown to be free of fungal growth. The control tiles are used to confirm validity of the study, requiring at least 50% coverage of mold after incubation.

▶ THE FUTURE OF EFFICACY TEST METHODS

Many of the efficacy test methods used today are decades old and are based on classical microbiology methods. The most commonly used methods undergo continuous improvement through the processes of standard setting bodies such as ASTM International or through stakeholder engagement with regulatory agencies. In recent years, new methods have and continue to be developed; examples are the methods described earlier for determining the efficacy of disinfectants against biofilms.[35] In the United States, the EPA encourages registrants to develop protocols for testing the efficacy of new or unusual product applications. These methods have the potential of becoming standard methods if the method has significant public health or economic benefit to stakeholders.

Overall, antimicrobial methods have not been standardized or harmonized across the globe. This means that the development of a "universal" or "global" disinfectant is difficult and expensive, owing to the fact that disinfectant manufacturers have to abide by regulations, standard test methods, and performance criteria that vary across multiple geographic regions in order to have a truly global product. A substantial amount of effort is currently underway in the development of a globally harmonized method that has the potential to alleviate these problems. The OECD, for example, is working to release a method for evaluating hard surface disinfectants for bacteria, TB, virus, and fungi.[23] The success of this project could have the potential to set a global standard of disinfection (a common log reduction) and the development of a mutually acceptable efficacy data set across many of countries worldwide. If countries insist on maintaining unique test conditions and/or performance standards, the global acceptance of such a method will be limited. It should be noted that a version of this OECD method is currently used in both the United States and Canada, in a limited capacity, for the evaluation of disinfectants with activity against *C difficile*[17,24,54] and *Candida auris*.[67] Continuous improvement and harmonization efforts help ensure that the antimicrobial products available on the market are performing as expected, giving us confidence in tackling important food safety and public health issues today and in the future.

REFERENCES

1. Rutala WA, Weber DJ; and Healthcare Infection Control Practices Advisory Committee. *Guideline for Disinfection and Sterilization in Healthcare Facilities, 2008*. Atlanta, GA: Centers for Disease Control and Prevention; 2008.

2. Dancer SJ. Controlling hospital-acquired infection: focus on the role of the environment and new technologies for decontamination. *Clin Microbiol Rev.* 2014;27(4):665-690.

3. Rutala WA, Barbee SL, Aguiar NC, Sobsey MD, Weber DJ. Antimicrobial activity of home disinfectants and natural products against potential human pathogens. *Infect Control Hosp Epidemiol.* 2000;21(1):33-38.

4. Rutala WA, Weber DJ. Disinfection and sterilization in health care facilities: an overview and current issues. *Infect Dis Clin North Am.* 2016;30(3):609-637. doi:10.1016/j.idc.2016.04.002.

5. World Health Organization. *Infection Prevention and Control of Epidemic-and Pandemic Prone Acute Respiratory Infections in Health Care.* Geneva, Switzerland: World Health Organization; 2014.

6. Chick H, Martin CJ. The principles involved in the standardisation of disinfectants and the influence of organic matter upon germicidal value. *J Hyg.* 1908;8:654-697.

7. Humphreys PN. Testing standards for sporicides. *J Hosp Infect.* 2011;77(3):193-198.

8. Tomasino SF. Development and assessment of disinfectant efficacy test methods for regulatory purposes. *Am J Infect Control.* 2013;41(suppl 5): S72-S76.

9. Guan J, Chan M, Brooks BW, Rohonczy L. Influence of temperature and organic load on chemical disinfection of *Geobacillus stearothermophilus* spores, a surrogate for *Bacillus anthracis. Can J Vet Res.* 2013;77(2):100-104.

10. US Environmental Protection Agency. Federal Insecticide, Fungicide, and Rodenticide Act (1910).

11. US Food and Drug Administration. Federal Food, Drug, and Cosmetic Act, USC §21 (1938).

12. Canada. Food and drug regulations. Section C.01A.001 (2019).

13. Canada. Pest control products regulations, SOR/2006-124 (section1) (2016).

14. US Environmental Protection Agency. *Product Performance Test Guidelines OCSPP 810.2000: General Considerations for Testing Public Health Antimicrobial Pesticides.* Washington, DC: US Environmental Protection Agency; 2018.

15. Health Canada. *Guidance Document—Disinfectant Drugs (2018).* Ontario, Canada: Health Canada; 2018.

16. Health Canada. *Guidance Document—Management of Disinfectant Drug Applications.* Ontario, Canada: Health Canada; 2018.

17. Health Canada. *Guidance Document—Efficacy Requirements for Hard Surface Disinfectant Drugs.* Ontario, Canada: Health Canada; 2014.

18. Health Canada. *Guidance Document—Safety and Effectiveness Requirements for High-Level Disinfectants and Sterilants for Use on Reusable Semi-Critical and Critical Medical Devices (2018).* Ontario, Canada: Health Canada; 2018.

19. US Food and Drug Administration. *Guidance for Industry and FDA Reviewers: Content and Format of Premarket Notification [510(k)] Submissions for Liquid Chemical Sterilants/High Level Disinfectants.* Silver Spring, MD: US Food and Drug Administration; 2000.

20. Parker AE, Hamilton MA, Tomasino SF. A statistical model for assessing performance standards for quantitative and semiquantitative disinfectant test methods. *J AOAC Int.* 2014;97(1):58-67.

21. Kravitz E, Stedman RL. Retention of disinfectant activity in the presence of hardware. *Appl Microbiol.* 1957;5:34-35.

22. Association of Official Analytical Chemists International. *Germicidal Detergent Sanitizing Action of Disinfectants Test.* Rockville, MD: Association of Official Analytical Chemists International; 2013.

23. Organisation for Economic Co-operation and Development. *Guidance Document on Quantitative Methods for Evaluating the Activity of Microbicides Used on Hard Non-Porous Surfaces.* Paris, France: Organisation for Economic Co-operation and Development; 2013.

24. US Environmental Protection Agency. *Methods and Guidance for Testing the Efficacy of Antimicrobial Products Against Spores of Clostridium difficile on Hard Non-Porous Surfaces.* Washington, DC: US Environmental Protection Agency; 2018.

25. Marriott N. Sanitation and the food industry. In: *Principles of Food Sanitation.* 5th ed. New York, NY: Aspen Publishers; 2006:165-189.

26. US Food and Drug Administration. Food Safety Modernization Act, USC §302 (2011).

27. US Food and Drug Administration. Sanitary operations. Current good manufacturing practice, hazard analysis, and risk-based preventive controls for human food, 21 CFR §117.35 (2017).

28. US Food and Drug Administration. *Cleaning Agents and Sanitizers in Food Code.* 9th ed. Silver Spring, MD: US Food and Drug Administration; 2017.

29. US Environmental Protection Agency. *Product Performance Test Guidelines OCSPP 810.2300: Sanitizers for Use on Hard Surfaces— Efficacy Data Recommendations.* Washington, DC: US Environmental Protection Agency; 2012.

30. US Food and Drug Administration. Indirect food additives: adjuvants, production aids and sanitizers, CFR §178.1010. (2017).

31. US Food and Drug Administration. Sanitizing Solutions: Chemistry Guidelines for Food Additive Petitions. Silver Spring, MD: US Food and Drug Administration; 1986.

32. Association of Official Analytical Chemists International. *AOAC Chlorine (Available) in Disinfectants.* Rockville, MD: Association of Official Analytical Chemists International; 1955.

33. American Society for Testing and Materials International. *Method E1153: Standard Test Method for Efficacy of Sanitizers Recommended for Inanimate, Hard, Nonporous Non-food Contact Surfaces.* West Conshohocken, PA: American Society for Testing and Materials International; 2014.

34. US Environmental Protection Agency. *Product Performance Test Guidelines OCSPP 810.2200: Disinfectants for Use on Environmental Surfaces, Guidance for Efficacy Testing.* Washington, DC: US Environmental Protection Agency; 2018.

35. US Environmental Protection Agency. *Methods and Guidance for Testing the Efficacy of Antimicrobials Against Biofilm Bacteria on Hard, Non-Porous Surfaces.* Washington, DC: US Environmental Protection Agency; 2017.

36. Association of Official Analytical Chemists International. *Testing Disinfectants Against* Pseudomonas aeruginosa *Use-Dilution Method. Official Method 964.02.* Rockville, MD: Association of Official Analytical Chemists International; 2013.

37. Association of Official Analytical Chemists International. *Testing Disinfectants Against* Salmonella enterica *Use-Dilution Method. Official Method 955.14.* Rockville, MD: Association of Official Analytical Chemists International; 2013.

38. Association of Official Analytical Chemists International. T*esting Disinfectants Against* Staphylococcus aureus *Use-Dilution Method. Official Method 955.15.* Rockville, MD: Association of Official Analytical Chemists International; 2013.

39. Association of Official Analytical Chemists International. *Germicidal Spray Products as Disinfectants. Official Method 961.02.* Rockville, MD: Association of Official Analytical Chemists International; 2012.

40. American Society for Testing and Materials International. *Method E2362: Standard Practice for Evaluation of Pre-Saturated or Impregnated Towelettes for Hard Surface Disinfection.* West Conshohocken, PA: American Society for Testing and Materials International; 2015.

41. Association of Official Analytical Chemists International. F*ungicidal Activity of Disinfectants. Official Method 955.17.* Rockville, MD: Association of Official Analytical Chemists International; 1955.

42. American Society for Testing and Materials International. *Method E1053: Standard Test Method to Assess Virucidal Activity of Chemicals Intended for Disinfection.* West Conshohocken, PA: American Society for Testing and Materials International; 2011.

43. Association of Official Analytical Chemists International. *Tuberculosis Activity of Disinfectants. Official Method 965.12.* Rockville, MD: Association of Official Analytical Chemists International; 2012.

44. Ascenzi JM, Ezzell RJ, Wendt TM. A more accurate method for measurement of tuberculocidal activity of disinfectants. *Appl Environ Microbiol.* 1987;53:2189-2192.

45. US Environmental Protection Agency. *Data Call-in Notice for Tuberculocidal Effectiveness Data for All Antimicrobial Pesticides with Tuberculocidal Claims.* Washington, DC: US Environmental Protection Agency; 1986.

46. US Environmental Protection Agency. *MLB SOP MB-16: Standard Operating Procedure for Quantitative Suspension Test Method for Determining Tuberculocidal Efficacy of Disinfectants Against* Mycobacterium bovis (BCG). Washington, DC: US Environmental Protection Agency; 2014.

47. US Environmental Protection Agency. *MLB SOP MB-19: Growing a Biofilm Using the CDC Biofilm Reactor.* Washington, DC: US Environmental Protection Agency; 2017.

48. American Society for Testing and Materials International. *Method E2562: Standard Method for Quantification of* Pseudomonas aeruginosa *Biofilm Grown with High Shear and Continuous Flow Using CDC Biofilm Reactor.* West Conshohocken, PA: American Society for Testing and Materials International; 2017.

49. US Environmental Protection Agency. *MLB SOP MB-20: Single Tube Method for Determining the Efficacy of Disinfectants Against Bacterial Biofilm.* Washington, DC: US Environmental Protection Agency; 2017.

50. American Society for Testing and Materials International. *Method E2871: Standard Test Method for Evaluating Disinfectant Efficacy Against* Pseudomonas aeruginosa B*iofilm Grown in CDC Reactor Using Single Tube Method.* West Conshohocken, PA: American Society for Testing and Materials International; 2013.

51. US Environmental Protection Agency. *MLP SOP MB-28: Production and Storage of Spores of* Clostridium difficile *for Use in the Efficacy Evaluation of Antimicrobial Agents.* Washington, DC: US Environmental Protection Agency; 2018.

52. American Society for Testing and Materials International. *Method E2839: Standard Test Method for Production of* Clostridium difficile *Spores for Use in Efficacy Evaluation of Antimicrobial Agents.* West Conshohocken, PA: American Society for Testing and Materials International; 2011.

53. US Environmental Protection Agency. *MLB SOP MB-31: Procedure for the OECD Quantitative Method for Testing Antimicrobial Products Against Spores of* Clostridium difficile *on Inanimate, Hard Non-Porous Surfaces.* Washington, DC: US Environmental Protection Agency; 2018.

54. US Environmental Protection Agency. *Product Performance Test Guideline OCSPP 810.2100: Sterilants, Sporicides, and Decontaminants.* Washington, DC: US Environmental Protection Agency; 2018.

55. Health Canada. *Notice: Classification and Licensing of High-level Disinfectants and Sterilants as Medical Devices.* Ontario, Canada: Health Canada; 2018.

56. Association of Official Analytical Chemists International. *Sporicidal Activity of Disinfectants.* Rockville, MD: Association of Official Analytical Chemists International; 2013.

57. US Environmental Protection Agency. *Re-use Test Protocol Specifications, Draft Pesticide Assessment Guidelines 91A.* Washington, DC: US Environmental Protection Agency; 1982.

58. US Environmental Protection Agency. *Product Performance Test Guidelines OCSPP 810.2400: Disinfectants and Sanitizers for use on Fabrics and Textiles—Efficacy Data.* Washington, DC: US Environmental Protection Agency; 2012.

59. Dohmae S, Okubo T, Higuchi W, et al. *Bacillus cereus* nosocomial infection from reused towels in Japan. *J Hosp Infection.* 2008;69: 361-367.

60. Hosein IK, Hoffman PN, Ellam S, et al. Summertime *Bacillus cereus* colonization of hospital newborns traced to contaminated, laundered linen. *J Hosp Infection.* 2013;85:149-154.

61. American Society for Testing and Materials International. *Method E2274: Evaluation of Laundry Sanitizers and Disinfectants.* West Conshohocken, PA: American Society for Testing and Materials International; 2016.

62. American Society for Testing and Materials International. *Method E2406: Standard Test Method for Evaluation of Laundry Sanitizers and Disinfectants for Use in High Efficiency Washing Operations.* West Conshohocken, PA: American Society for Testing and Materials International; 2016.

63. US Environmental Protection Agency. *Pesticide Assessment Guidelines: Subdivision G: Product Performance.* Washington, DC: US Environmental Protection Agency; 1982.

64. American Association of Textile Chemists and Colorists. *Method AATCC-100: Assessment of Antibacterial Finishes on Textile Materials.* Research Triangle Park, NC: American Association of Textile Chemists and Colorists; 2012.

65. American Society for Testing and Materials International. *Method E2180: Standard Test Method for Determining the Activity of Incorporated Antimicrobial Agents in Polymeric or Hydrophobic Materials.* West Conshohocken, PA: American Society for Testing and Materials International; 2017.

66. American Society for Testing and Materials International. *Method E2149: Test Method for Determining the Antimicrobial Activity of Antimicrobial Agents Under Dynamic Contact Conditions.* West Conshohocken, PA: American Society for Testing and Materials International; 2013.

67. US Environment *Methods for Antimicrobial Efficacy Testing.* Washington, DC: US Environmental Protection Agency; 2017.

CHAPTER

63

Antimicrobial Test Methods in the European Union

Lionel Pineau

In Europe, any biocidal product falling under the scope of European Medical Devices Directive (MDD) 93/42/EEC[1] and, in the future, the regulation (EU) 2017/745[2] or under the scope of European Biocides Regulation 528/2012[3] shall be tested according to the test methods developed by Technical Committee 216 of the European Committee for Standardization and listed in the European standard EN 14885.[4] These tests are used to support claims appropriate to their intended application. Other test methods can be used when the models specified in the standards are not sufficient and/or appropriate to demonstrate the product claim (eg, activity against biofilm).

In Europe, three different areas of application are defined for antiseptics and disinfectants:

- Medicine (hospitals, medical facilities and dental institutions, laundries and kitchens supplying products directly for the patient)
- Veterinary area
- Food, industrial, domestic, and institutional areas (processing, distribution, and retailing of food of animal or vegetable origin)

For each area, EN 14885 specifies European standards to which products should conform to support their claims for microbicidal activity (Tables 63.1 to 63.3). This standard is also intended to enable users of the product to understand the antimicrobial efficacy information provided by the manufacturer and assist competent bodies in assessing claims made by the manufacturer. Even if this approach could be considered comparable to what is done in other countries or regions to register a chemical disinfectant, the definitions, methods used, and performance requirements are different. The most important differences concern the nature and definition of the products intended to be tested. In some countries like in United States[33] or in Australia,[34] some chemicals can be used to sterilize critical medical devices (eg, products labeled as sterilants), whereas in Europe, the terms *sterility*, *sterile*,

sterilization, or *sterilant* are not defined in this series of European disinfectant testing standards and a disinfectant cannot be regarded as a sterilant; sterilization requirements are defined in other European (EN) and/or International Organization for Standardization (ISO) standards (chapter 70).

▶ TEST CATEGORIES

In the EN chemical disinfection standards, four categories of tests are described:

- Phase 1 tests: quantitative suspension tests to demonstrate that an active substance or a product under development presents bactericidal, fungicidal, or sporicidal activity in fixed conditions (obligatory test conditions) without considering the use conditions specified by the manufacturer. In that case, the contact time and the temperature to be tested are fixed (see Table 63.4).
- Phase 2, step 1 tests: quantitative suspension tests to establish that a product has bactericidal, fungicidal, sporicidal, or virucidal activity simulating practical conditions. Tests shall be performed first in obligatory tests conditions, and some additional test conditions are permitted.
- Phase 2, step 2 tests: quantitative tests equivalent to phase 2 step 1 tests but performed against microorganisms dried on test surfaces (with obligatory and additional test conditions)
- Phase 3 tests: field tests under practical use conditions. Validated methodology for this type of test is not yet available.

Phase 1 and 2 tests are conducted to establish the broad spectrum of microbial activity of the disinfectant. They can be comparable to potency tests because they are described in the United States requirements such as the U.S. Food and Drug Administration (FDA) 510(k)

TABLE 63.1   Medical area—standard test methods to be used to substantiate claims for products (as of May, 2019)

Activity Claims	Phase/Step	Type and/or Purpose of Product							
		Hygienic Hand Rub	Hygienic Hand Wash	Surgical Hand Rub and Surgical Hand Wash	Surface Disinfection		Instrument Disinfection	Textile Disinfection	Water Disinfectant
					Mechanical Action				
					Without	With			
Bactericidal	2.1		EN 13727[5]		EN 13727[5]		EN 13727[5]	*	**
	2.2	EN 1500[6]	EN 1499[7]	EN 12791[8]	EN 13697[9]	EN 16615[10]	EN 14561[11]	EN 16616[12]	**
Yeasticidal	2.1		EN 13624[13]		EN 13624[13]		EN 13624[13]	***	**
	2.2	**	**		EN 13697[9]	EN 16615[10]	EN 14562[14]	EN 16616[12]	**
Fungicidal	2.1		**		EN 13624[13]		EN 13624[13]	*	**
	2.2		**		EN 13697[9]	*	EN 14562[14]	EN 16616[12]	**
Tuberculocidal	2.1	EN 14348[15]	EN 14348[15]	**	EN 14348[15]	*	EN 14348[15]	EN 14348[15]	**
	2.2		**		*	*	EN 14563[16]	EN 16616[12]	**
Mycobactericidal	2.1	EN 14348[15]	EN 14348[15]	**	EN 14348[15]		EN 14348[15]	EN 14348[15]	**
	2.2		**		*	*	EN 14563[16]	EN 16616[12]	**
Virucidal	2.1	EN 14476[17]	EN 14476[17]	**	EN 14476[17]		EN 14476[17]	EN 14476[17]	**
	2.2	*	*	**	***	***	*	***	**
Sporicidal	2.1		**		***	***	***	*	**
	2.2		**		***	*	*	**	**
Legionella	2.1		**			**	**	**	EN 13623[18]

Abbreviations: *, no work items are yet approved; **, no intention to develop a test; ***, work item approved.

TABLE 63.2 Veterinary area—standard test methods to be used to substantiate claims for products (as of May 2019)

Activity Claims	Phase/Step	Type and/or Purpose of Product				
		Surface Disinfection		Teat Disinfection	Immersion of Contaminated Objects High-Level Soiling	Hygienic Hand Rub Hygienic Hand Wash Surgical Hand Rub and Surgical Hand Wash
		Mechanical Action				
		Without	With			
Bactericidal	2.1	EN 1656[19]	*	EN 1656[19]	EN 1656[19]	EN 13727[5]
	2.2[a]	EN 14349[20]	*	**	EN 14349[20]	EN 1499[7] or EN 1500[6] or EN 12791[8]
	2.2[b]	EN 16437[21]	NA	**	**	**
Yeasticidal	2.1	EN 1657[22]	*	**	EN 1657[22]	**
	2.2[a]	EN 16438[23]	NA	**	EN 16438[23]	**
	2.2[b]	*	*	**	**	**
Fungicidal	2.1	EN 1657[22]	*	**	EN 1657[22]	EN 13624[13]
	2.2[a]	EN 16438[23]	NA	**	EN 16438[23]	**
	2.2[b]	*	*	**	**	**
Mycobactericidal	2.1	EN 14204[24]	*	**	EN 14204[24]	**
	2.2[a]	*	*	**	*	**
	2.2[b]	*	NA	**	**	**
Virucidal	2.1	EN 14675[25]	*	**	EN 14675[25]	EN 14476[17]
	2.2[a]	*	*	**	*	**
	2.2[b]	*	NA	**	**	**
Sporicidal	2.1	*	*	**	*	**
	2.2[a]	*	*	**	*	**
	2.2[b]	*	*	**	**	**

Abbreviations: *, no work items are yet approved, but relevant standards may become available in the future; **, no intention to develop a test; NA, not available.

[a]Nonporous surfaces.

[b]Porous surfaces.

guidance document for liquid chemical sterilants and high-level disinfectant.[33] Phase 3 tests are field trials performed to establish the performance of a product under actual use conditions. They correspond to simulated use tests or in use tests described in US and Australian regulations.[33,34]

▶ PRINCIPLES OF THE EUROPEAN TESTS

- Most of the European standards used to evaluate the biocidal activities of disinfectants at this time are quantitative suspension or carrier tests. A defined number of viable bacteria (in suspension or dried on a surface) are exposed to the disinfectant, and the activity of the

product is evaluated by comparing the number of viable bacteria remaining in the suspension or on the surface with the number of bacteria initially inoculated.
- Phase 1 tests[30-32]: Eight milliliter of the product to be tested is mixed with 1 mL of the test microorganism suspension and 1 mL of sterile water. After the obligatory contact time, 1 mL of the test mixture is transferred into 9 mL of neutralizer or filtrated through 0.45 μm membrane filter to neutralize/eliminate all chemical residues. After 10 minutes of neutralization (or filtration), 2×1 mL are transferred on agar culture medium (or the filter is placed onto a poured agar plate) and incubated. Results are expressed as decimal logarithm reductions of the number of test organisms.
- Phase 2, step 1 tests[5,6,9,13,15,17-19,22,24-29]: Eight milliliter of the product to be tested is mixed with 1 mL interfering

TABLE 63.3   Food, industrial, domestic and institutional—standard test methods to be used to substantiate claims for products (as of May 2019)

Activity Claims	Phase/ Step	Type and/or Purpose of Product									
		Surface Disinfection	Products Used for "Cleaning in Place"	Hygienic Hand Wash	Hygienic Hand Rub	Wipes	Products for Use in Breweries	Beverage Soft Drink Industry	Products for Use in Dairies	Products Used in Manufacture of Cosmetics	Products Used in the Pharmaceutical Industry
Bactericidal	2.1	EN 1276[26]	EN 1276[26]	EN 1276[26]	EN 1276[26]	EN 1276[26]	EN 1276[26]	EN 1276[26]	EN 1276[26]	EN 1276[26]	EN 1276[26]
	2.2	EN 13697[9]	NA	EN 1499[7]	EN 1500[6]	*	EN 13697[9]	EN 13697[9]	EN 13697[9]	EN 13697[9]	EN 13697[9]
Yeasticidal	2.1	EN 1650[27]	EN 1650[27]	**	**	**	EN 1650[27]	EN 1650[27]	EN 1650[27]	EN 1650[27]	EN 1650[27]
	2.2	EN 13697[9]	NA	**	**	**	EN 13697[9]	EN 13697[9]	EN 13697[9]	EN 13697[9]	EN 13697[9]
Fungicidal	2.1	EN 1650[27]	EN 1650[27]	EN 1650[27]	EN 1650[27]	EN 1650[27]	EN 1650[27]	EN 1650[27]	EN 1650[27]	EN 1650[27]	EN 1650[27]
	2.2[a]	EN 13697[9]	NA	**	**	**	EN 13697[9]	EN 13697[9]	EN 13697[9]	EN 13697[9]	EN 13697[9]
Virucidal	2.1	**	EN 13610[28,a]	**	**	**	**	**	EN 13610[28,a]	**	**
	2.2[a]	*	NA	**	**	**	*	*	**	**	**
Sporicidal	2.1	EN 13704[29]	EN 13704[29]	**	**	**	EN 13704[29]	EN 13704[29]	EN 13704[29]	EN 13704[29]	EN 13704[29]
	2.2[a]	**	NA	**	**	**	*	*	*	**	**

Abbreviations: *, no work items are yet approved, but relevant standards may become available in the future; **, no intention to develop a test; NA, not available.

[a]Bacteriophages.

TABLE 63.4 EN phase 1 chemical disinfectants and antiseptics test methods and requirements

EN Test Method	EN 1040[30]	EN 1275[31]	EN 14347[32]
Antimicrobial Activity	Bactericidal	Fungicidal or yeasticidal	Sporicidal
Test Organisms	*Staphylococcus aureus* ATCC 6538	*Candida albicans* ATCC 10231	*Bacillus subtilis* ATCC 6633
	Pseudomonas aeruginosa ATCC 15442	*Aspergillus niger* ATCC 16404	*Bacillus cereus* ATCC 12826
Temperature (°C)	20°C		
Contact Time (min)	60	60	120
Interfering Substances	None		
Reduction (log)	5	4	4

substances (see following discussion) and 1 mL of the test microorganism suspension. After the obligatory contact time, 1 mL of the test mixture is transferred into 9 mL of neutralizer or filtrated through a 0.45 μm membrane filter to neutralize/eliminate all chemical residues. After 10 minutes of neutralization (or filtration), 2 × 1 mL (or the membrane filter) are transferred on agar culture medium and incubated. Results are expressed as decimal logarithm reductions of the number of test organisms.

Phase 2, step 2 tests[6-8,10-12,14,16,20,21,23]: Fifty microliters of the microorganisms suspension containing interference substances are spread through a 1 cm² area of the carrier. After drying, the inoculated carrier is transferred in a test tube containing the product to be tested (test without mechanical action). After the obligatory contact time, the carrier is transferred into 9 mL of neutralizer. The surface of the carrier is then scraped to aid in microbial recovery, and the number of viable test microorganisms remaining is determined by the pour plate technique. Results are expressed as decimal logarithm reduction of the number of test organisms.

In some cases, where the product is intended to be tested with mechanical action (eg, for medical area applications as defined in EN 16615),[10] the inoculated carrier is treated to simulate the mechanical action, for example, with a wipe previously soaked in the disinfectant solution and the number of viable bacteria remaining on the carrier is determined by swabbing. The swabs are then washed out in the neutralizer and 2 × 1 mL of the mixture transferred onto agar culture medium and incubated. Results are expressed as decimal logarithm reduction of the number of test organisms.

▶ TEST CONDITIONS

Except for phase 3 tests where the product shall be tested according to the instruction provided by the disinfectant manufacturer, all other tests (phases 1 and 2)

are performed under fixed conditions (temperature and contact time) called *obligatory* test conditions. Some additional tests conditions are also described, but they can be slightly different than the recommended use conditions. The obligation to test products under obligatory test conditions is something specific to European standards. For most other standards, such as Association of Official Agricultural Chemists (AOAC) and American Society for Testing and Materials (chapters 61 and 62), the product is tested according to the specific manufacturer's instructions for use and there is often no obligatory test conditions. In European practice, most of the disinfectant manufacturers test products according to European standards under obligatory and additional test conditions; this is used to demonstrate compliance with the specific standards and to demonstrate product activity under recommended use conditions.

Concentration to Be Tested

All European standards required to evaluate the efficacy of the disinfectant at three different concentrations, with a least one active and one nonactive. This requirement is specific to European standard tests, and in other parts of the world, tests are only performed at the concentration recommended by the manufacturer. EN 14885 does not provide any guidance to the disinfectant manufacturer regarding all different aspects that need to be considered regarding the definition of the concentration to be tested. Thus, variables such as stability of both open and closed containers, dilution or accumulation of interfering substances due to the reuse of the same disinfectant solution, variation between batches, and shelf life are not considered during testing. In other regions, such as with the FDA guidance document on high-level disinfectants,[33] all these factors are used to define the disinfectant concentration to be tested.

Interfering Substances

With the exception of phase 1 tests where no interfering substances are required, all antimicrobial efficacy tests include two test conditions:

- *Clean* conditions—conditions representative of surfaces that have received a satisfactory cleaning program and/or are known to contain minimal levels of organic and/or inorganic substances
- *Dirty* conditions—conditions representative of surfaces that are known to or may contain organic and/or inorganic substances. For veterinary area applications, two different dirty conditions are defined: (1) low-level soiling: condition representative of surfaces, regarding the veterinary area, where a level of soiling can be expected, that is equivalent to dirty conditions and (2) high-level soiling: condition representative of surfaces with regard to the veterinary area, where heavy soiling can be expected.

In contrast, as defined in the FDA 510(k) document,[33] all potency tests are to be performed under worst case conditions (including for disinfectants intended to be reused) to include the presence of inorganic (ie, 400 ppm carbonate calcium; $CaCO_3$) and organic (ie, 5% bovine serum albumin or calf serum) loads.

▶ QUANTITATIVE VERSUS SEMIQUANTITATIVE OR QUALITATIVE TESTS

In Europe, standard test methods used to evaluate the antimicrobial efficacy of a disinfectant are quantitative test methods, in contrast to other standardized tests such as many of the AOAC tests used for disinfectant evaluation in United States that are based on a qualitative growth/no-growth method. For example, to demonstrate its activity against *Staphylococcus aureus*, a disinfectant shall:

- Demonstrate at least a 5-decimal log (log_{10}) reduction when tested according to EN 13727[5] and when the initial challenge is between 1.5×10^8 CFUs/mL and 5.0×10^8 CFUs/mL.

Kill all microorganisms on at least 10 carriers inoculated with $\geq 1.0 \times 10^6$ CFUs, when tested according to AOAC 955.15.[35]

The European approach seems to be more appropriate if the objective of the tests is to compare the antimicrobial activity of two different formulations or test conditions (eg, exposure time or concentration). On the opposite side, growth/no-growth tests are considered more sensitive, and according to the number of tests perform, they may provide a much more important safety margin.

▶ ACCURACY/NUMBER OF REPLICATES

In the process of evaluating the activity of disinfectant, European standards are not required to be performed more than in one assay, and this situation may lead to a reduction of the accuracy or reliability of the results. Thus, for EN 13727 as an example, 4 to 6 repetitions are necessary for a precision of ± 1 log_{10} in reduction, and to reduce the lack of precision due to the limited number of replicates performed, the European standard recommends that the laboratory routinely evaluates a reference chemical disinfectant in order to demonstrate accuracy in performing the test. In contrast, with the AOAC tests, multiple replicates (between 10 and 360, depending in the specific test method) have to be tested. Complete inactivation of 10 out of 10 replicates provides a reasonable reliability index in most cases, and killing in 59 of 60 replicates provides a confidence level of 95%.[35,36]

▶ SPECIFIC TEST METHODS

Other European (and/or international, such as ISO) test methods have been developed to cover specific applications where the standard suspension or carrier tests presented earlier cannot be used or are not appropriate to evaluate the antimicrobial efficacy of the disinfectant/disinfection process. Examples of these include:

- For antiseptics, specific skink tests have been developed (eg, EN 1499[7] and EN 1500,[6] where products are tested in practical conditions, specifically on volunteer hands artificially contaminated with *Escherichia coli* K12 NCTC 10538).
- For disinfectants intended to be used in a washer-disinfector, complementary tests based on the evaluation of the disinfection stage using surrogate devices and/or test devices artificially contaminated with a bacterial suspension in the presence of an organic and inorganic load[37,38]
- Specifically, for disinfectants intended to be used for the periodic disinfection of endoscope washer-disinfector water lines, a specific test has been proposed in EN 15883-4 to evaluate the ability of the disinfectant to inactivate bacteria within biofilms.[39]
- Preservative efficacy tests, by challenging preserved products with various test microorganisms (eg, *S aureus*, *Pseudomonas aeruginosa*, *E coli*, *Candida albicans*, and *Aspergillus brasiliensis*) and determining the log reduction over time.[40] The European Pharmacopeia test is essentially harmonized to other international pharmacopeia tests.[41]

Finally, other methods or requirements are defined for the evaluation of the disinfection of critical equipment used in aseptic processes,[42] for sterilization methods (and associated sterilization standards),[43] and in using/testing biological indicators.[44,45]

▶ CONCLUSION

The test program developed by the Technical Committee 216 of the European Committee for Standardization provides an appropriate testing scheme for any biocidal product to support a claim of specific antimicrobial activity. Nevertheless, the major issues for the CEN/TC 216 test methods concern the performance of the tests in practice, especially their statistical reliability and the production of standard test methodologies for phase 3 tests. At this time, the demonstration of phase 1 and 2 test efficacy is widely used to verify the activity of disinfectants, but it is also important to note that these tests have been developed to be a prerequisite to phase 3 tests, defined as field tests under practical use conditions. These tests are yet to be developed; therefore, in higher risk situations, it is considered good practice to verify the practical applications of these labeled antiseptics and disinfectants under their intended use conditions.

REFERENCES

1. European Union. Council Directive 93/42/EEC of 14 June 1993 concerning medical devices. *Off J Eur.* 1993;L169:1-43.
2. European Union. Regulation (EU) 2017/745 of the European Parliament and of the Council of 5 April 2017 on medical devices, amending Directive 2001/83/EC, Regulation (EC) No 178/2002 and Regulation (EC) No 1223/2009 and repealing Council Directives 90/385/EEC and 93/42/EEC. *Off J Eur.* 2017;L117:1. http://data.europa.eu/eli/reg/2017/745/oj. Accessed September 2019.
3. European Parliament and of the Council. European Parliament and Council of Regulation (EU) No 528/2012 of the European Parliament and of the Council of 22 May 2012 concerning the making available on the market and use of biocidal products. *Off J Eur Union.* 2012;167:1-123.
4. European Committee for Standardization. *EN 14885. Chemical Disinfectants and Antiseptics. Application of European Standards for Chemical Disinfectants and Antiseptics.* Brussels, Belgium: European Committee for Standardization; 2018.
5. European Committee for Standardization. *EN 13727. Chemical Disinfectants and Antiseptics. Quantitative Suspension Test for the Evaluation of Bactericidal Activity in the Medical Area. Test Method and Requirements (Phase 2, Step 1).* Brussels, Belgium: European Committee for Standardization; 2012.
6. European Committee for Standardization. *EN 1500. Chemical Disinfectants and Antiseptics. Hygienic Handrub. Test Method and Requirements (Phase 2/Step 2).* Brussels, Belgium: European Committee for Standardization; 2013.
7. European Committee for Standardization. *EN 1499. Chemical Disinfectants and Antiseptics. Hygienic Hand Wash. Test Method and Requirements (Phase 2/Step 2).* Brussels, Belgium: European Committee for Standardization; 2013.
8. European Committee for Standardization. *EN 12791. Chemical Disinfectants and Antiseptics. Surgical Hand Disinfection. Test Method and Requirements (Phase 2, Step 2).* Brussels, Belgium: European Committee for Standardization; 2016.
9. European Committee for Standardization. *EN 13697. Chemical Disinfectants and Antiseptics. Quantitative Non-Porous Surface Test for the Evaluation of Bactericidal and/or Fungicidal Activity of Chemical Disinfectants Used in Food, Industrial, Domestic and Institutional Areas. Test Method and Requirements Without Mechanical Action (Phase 2, Step 1).* Brussels, Belgium: European Committee for Standardization; 2015.
10. European Committee for Standardization. *EN 16615. Chemical Disinfectants and Antiseptics. Quantitative Test Method for the Evaluation of Bactericidal and Yeasticidal Activity on Non-Porous Surfaces With Mechanical Action Employing Wipes in the Medical Area (4-Field Test). Test Method and Requirements (Phase 2, Step 2).* Brussels, Belgium: European Committee for Standardization; 2015.
11. European Committee for Standardization. *EN 14561. Chemical Disinfectants and Antiseptics. Quantitative Carrier Test for the Evaluation of Bactericidal Activity for Instruments Used in the Medical Area. Test Method and Requirements (Phase 2, Step 2).* Brussels, Belgium: European Committee for Standardization; 2006.
12. European Committee for Standardization. *EN 16616. Chemical Disinfectants and Antiseptics. Chemical-Thermal Textile Disinfection. Test Method and Requirements (Phase 2, Step 2).* Brussels, Belgium: European Committee for Standardization; 2015.
13. European Committee for Standardization. *EN 13624. Chemical Disinfectants and Antiseptics. Quantitative Suspension Test for the Evaluation of Fungicidal Activity of Chemical Disinfectants for Instruments Used in the Medical Area. Test Method and Requirements (Phase 2, Step 1).* Brussels, Belgium: European Committee for Standardization; 2013.
14. British Standards Institution. *BS EN 14562:2006. Chemical Disinfectants and Antiseptics. Quantitative Carrier Test for the Evaluation of Fungicidal or Yeasticidal Activity for Instruments Used in the Medical Area. Test Method and Requirements (Phase 2, Step 2).* London, United Kingdom: British Standards Institution; 2006.
15. European Committee for Standardization. *EN 14348. Chemical Disinfectants and Antiseptics. Quantitative Suspension Test for the Evaluation of Mycobactericidal Activity of Chemical Disinfectants in the Medical Area Including Instrument Disinfectants. Test Methods and Requirements (Phase 2, Step 1).* Brussels, Belgium: European Committee for Standardization; 2005.
16. European Committee for Standardization. *EN 14563. Chemical Disinfectants and Antiseptics. Quantitative Carrier Test for the Evaluation of Mycobactericidal or Tuberculocidal Activity Used for Instruments in the Medical Area. Test Method and Requirements (Phase 2, Step 2).* Brussels, Belgium: European Committee for Standardization; 2008.
17. British Standards Institution. *BS EN 14476:2013. Chemical Disinfectants and Antiseptics. Virucidal Quantitative Suspension Test for Chemical Disinfectants and Antiseptics Used in Human Medicine. Test Method and Requirements (Phase 2, Step 1).* London, United Kingdom: British Standards Institution; 2013.
18. European Committee for Standardization. *EN 13623. Chemical Disinfectants and Antiseptics. Quantitative Suspension Test for the Evaluation of Bactericidal Activity Against Legionella of Chemical Disinfectants for Aqueous Systems. Test Method and Requirements (Phase 2, Step 1).* Brussels, Belgium: European Committee for Standardization; 2010.
19. European Committee for Standardization. *EN 1656. Chemical Disinfectants and Antiseptics. Quantitative Suspension Test for the Evaluation of Bactericidal Activity of Chemical Disinfectants and Antiseptics Used in the Veterinary Area. Test Method and Requirements (Phase 2, Step 1).* Brussels, Belgium: European Committee for Standardization; 2009.
20. British Standards Institution. *BS EN 14349:2013. Chemical Disinfectants and Antiseptics. Quantitative Surface Test for the Evaluation of Bactericidal Activity of Chemical Disinfectants and Antiseptics Used in the Veterinary Area on Non-Porous Surfaces Without Mechanical Action. Test Method and Requirements (Phase 2, Step 2).* London, United Kingdom: British Standards Institution; 2013.

21. British Standards Institution. *BS EN 16437:2014. Chemical Disinfectants and Antiseptics Quantitative Surface Test for the Evaluation of Bactericidal Activity of Chemical Disinfectants and Antiseptics Used in Veterinary Area on Porous Surfaces Without Mechanical Action. Test Method and Requirements (Phase 2, Step 2)*. London, United Kingdom: British Standards Institution; 2014.

22. European Committee for Standardization. *EN 1657. Chemical Disinfectants and Antiseptics. Quantitative Suspension Test for the Evaluation of Fungicidal or Yeasticidal Activity of Chemical Disinfectants and Antiseptics Used in the Veterinary Area. Test Method and Requirements (Phase 2, Step 1)*. Brussels, Belgium: European Committee for Standardization; 2019.

23. British Standards Institution. *BS EN 16438:2014. Chemical Disinfectants and Antiseptics. Quantitative Surface Test for the Evaluation of Fungicidal or Yeasticidal Activity of Chemical Disinfectants and Antiseptics Used in the Veterinary Area on Non-Porous Surfaces Without Mechanical Action. Test Method and Requirements (Phase 2, Step 2)*. London, United Kingdom: British Standards Institution; 2014.

24. European Committee for Standardization. *EN 14204. Chemical Disinfectants and Antiseptics. Quantitative Suspension Test for the Evaluation of Mycobactericidal Activity of Chemical Disinfectants and Antiseptics Used in the Veterinary Area. Test Method and Requirements (Phase 2, Step 1)*. Brussels, Belgium: European Committee for Standardization; 2012.

25. British Standards Institution. *BS EN 14675:2015. Chemical Disinfectants and Antiseptics. Quantitative Suspension Test for the Evaluation of Virucidal Activity of Chemical Disinfectants and Antiseptics Used in the Veterinary Area. Test Method and Requirements (Phase 2, Step 1)*. London, United Kingdom: British Standards Institution; 2015.

26. European Committee for Standardization. *EN 1276. Chemical Disinfectants and Antiseptics. Quantitative Suspension Test for the Evaluation of Bactericidal Activity of Chemical Disinfectants and Antiseptics Used in Food, Industrial, Domestic and Institutional Areas. Test Method and Requirements (Phase 2, Step 1)*. Brussels, Belgium: European Committee for Standardization; 2019.

27. European Committee for Standardization. *EN 1650. Chemical Disinfectants and Antiseptics. Quantitative Suspension Test for the Evaluation of Fungicidal or Yeasticidal Activity of Chemical Disinfectants and Antiseptics Used in Food, Industrial, Domestic and Institutional Areas. Test Method and Requirements (Phase 2, Step 1)*. Brussels, Belgium: European Committee for Standardization; 2019.

28. European Committee for Standardization. *EN 13610. Chemical Disinfectants. Quantitative Suspension Test for the Evaluation of Virucidal Activity Against Bacteriophages of Chemical Disinfectants Used in Food and Industrial Areas. Test Method and Requirements (Phase 2, Step 1)*. Brussels, Belgium: European Committee for Standardization; 2002.

29. British Standards Institution. *BS EN 13704:2018. Chemical Disinfectants. Quantitative Suspension Test for the Evaluation of Sporicidal Activity of Chemical Disinfectants Used in Food, Industrial, Domestic and Institutional Areas. Test Method and Requirements (Phase 2, Step 1)*. London, United Kingdom: British Standards Institution; 2018.

30. European Committee for Standardization. *EN 1040. Chemical Disinfectants and Antiseptics. Quantitative Suspension Test for the Evaluation of Basic Bactericidal Activity of Chemical Disinfectants and Antiseptics. Test Method and Requirements (Phase 1)*. Brussels, Belgium: European Committee for Standardization; 2005.

31. European Committee for Standardization. *EN 1275. Chemical Disinfectants and Antiseptics. Quantitative Suspension Test for the Evaluation of Basic Fungicidal or Basic Yeasticidal Activity of Chemical Disinfectants and Antiseptics. Test Method and Requirements (Phase 1)*. Brussels, Belgium: European Committee for Standardization; 2005.

32. European Committee for Standardization. *EN 14347. Chemical Disinfectants and Antiseptics. Basic Sporicidal Activity. Test Method and Requirements (Phase 1, Step 1)*. Brussels, Belgium: European Committee for Standardization; 2005.

33. Content and format of premarket notification [510(k)] submissions for liquid chemical sterilants/high level disinfectants, and user information and training. *Fed Regist*. 2000;65:36325. To be codified at CFR §880.6885.

34. Australian Government Department of Health and Aging, Therapeutics Goods Administration. *Guidelines for the Evaluation of Sterilants and Disinfectants*. Barton, Australia: Commonwealth of Australia; 1998.

35. Association of Official Analytical Chemists. Official method 955.15: testing disinfectants against *Staphylococcus aureus*, use-dilution method. In: Helrich K, ed. *Official Methods of Analysis*. Arlington, VA: Association of Official Analytical Chemists; 1990:136-137.

36. Association of Official Analytical Chemists. Official method 966.04: sporicidal activity of disinfectants: In: Cunniff P, ed. *Official Methods of Analysis*. Arlington, VA: Association of Official Analytical Chemists; 1995:12-13.

37. International Organization for Standardization. *ISO 15883-1:2006: Washer-Disinfectors—Part 1: General Requirements, Terms and Definitions and Tests*. Geneva, Switzerland: International Organization for Standardization; 2006.

38. International Organization for Standardization. *ISO 15883-7:2016: Washer-Disinfectors—Part 7: Requirements and Tests for Washer-Disinfectors Employing Chemical Disinfection for Non-Invasive, Non-Critical Thermolabile Medical Devices and Healthcare Equipment*. Geneva, Switzerland: International Organization for Standardization; 2016.

39. International Organization for Standardization. *ISO 15883-4:2018: Washer-Disinfectors—Part 4: Requirements and Tests for Washer-Disinfectors Employing Chemical Disinfection for Thermolabile Endoscopes*. Geneva, Switzerland: International Organization for Standardization; 2018.

40. European Pharmacopoeia. *EP <5.1.3> Efficacy of Antimicrobial Preservation*. Strasbourg, France: European Pharmacopoeia; 2011.

41. Moser CL, Meyer BK. Comparison of compendial antimicrobial effectiveness tests: a review. *AAPS PharmSciTech*. 2011;12(1): 222-226.

42. International Organization for Standardization. *ISO 13408-1:2008: Aseptic Processing of Health Care Products—Part 1: General Requirements*. Geneva, Switzerland: International Organization for Standardization; 2008.

43. International Organization for Standardization. *ISO 14937:2009: Sterilization of Health Care Products—General Requirements for Characterization of a Sterilizing Agent and the Development, Validation and Routine Control of a Sterilization Process for Medical Devices*. Geneva, Switzerland: International Organization for Standardization; 2009.

44. International Organization for Standardization. *ISO 11138-1:2017: Sterilization of Health Care Products—Biological Indicators—Part 1: General Requirements*. Geneva, Switzerland: International Organization for Standardization; 2017.

45. International Organization for Standardization. *ISO 18472:2018: Sterilization of Health Care Products—Biological and Chemical Indicators—Test Equipment*. Geneva, Switzerland: International Organization for Standardization; 2018.

CHAPTER 64

Bioburden Assessment and Tests for Sterility

Martell Winters and Trabue Bryans

Microbiology is central to all aspects of disinfection, sterilization, and preservation processes, primarily because the overall intent of these processes is to reduce, eliminate, or maintain the level of viable microorganisms. Bioburden estimation and sterility testing are likely the two most common microbiological tests performed in the validation of microbial reduction or prevention processes. These tests are useful tools in understanding the extent of microorganisms on or in a product, either before, during, or after bioburden reduction or prevention steps are applied; as such, the two tests are complimentary.

In standards relating to sterilization, bioburden is defined as the "population of viable microorganisms on or in product and/or sterile barrier system."[1] The bioburden can therefore consist of viable microorganisms found on a solid product, where an extraction process must be performed prior to plating, incubation, and enumeration. International Organization for Standardization (ISO) 11737-1 contains substantial information regarding bioburden testing of product where an extraction of microorganisms from product is required. Bioburden can also consist of viable microorganisms in a liquid sample or a sample that is soluble, where an extraction is not required prior to plating, incubation, and enumeration. Bioburden tests are addressed in ISO 11737-1[1] and pharmacopoeial documents such as United States Pharmacopeia (USP),[2] European Pharmacopoeia (EP),[3] Japanese Pharmacopoeia (JP),[4] etc, in the chapters regarding microbiological examination of nonsterile products (microbial enumeration tests). The pharmacopoeial chapters are not called bioburden tests per se, but the intent and results are the same. The bioburden test is a quantitative test that results in microorganism counts, usually referred to as colony-forming units (CFU). This type of test is appropriate when there is expected to be some quantity of bioburden on or in product (ie, ≥1 CFU for the majority of product units tested).

In standards relating to sterility testing, specifically ISO 11737-2, "sterile" is defined as "free from viable microorganisms" and the primary focus of the standard is on validation of terminally sterilized products.[5] Pharmacopoeial documents also address sterility testing with the primary focus being on validation and release of aseptically produced products.[6] With these tests, the sterile state is difficult to prove with completeness. It is understood that there are limitations to what commonly used microbiological tests can demonstrate due to the inability of growth media to promote replication of every type of microorganism that could be present on or in a product. A sterility test is a qualitative or attribute test and is usually performed by immersing the product in, or adding the product to, a liquid growth medium followed by incubating and scoring as positive or negative for growth. This type of test is appropriate when there is expected to be no bioburden on or in product (ie, <1 CFU for the majority of units tested). Thus, the sterility test is often used to measure the presence/absence of a viable microorganism on a certain number of samples tested.

It is important to determine which test—the bioburden test or the sterility test—should be selected based on the situation. If a bioburden test is performed on product that is sterile, the result might be 0 CFU on the plated aliquot, but this result in a bioburden test is generally not as sensitive as a sterility test due to the extraction processes and/or dilutions that are often included. This means that a bioburden result of 0 CFU carries with it more uncertainty than a negative growth result in a sterility test. Alternatively, if a sterility test is performed on a group of products that likely are known to contain viable microorganisms, the expected result would be that many or all items tested were positive for growth, which usually provides no useful information as to the quantity of microorganisms per product. The focus of this chapter is to provide a review of these two tests, in some cases beyond what is generally known, or what is already contained in standards and guidance documents.

▶ KNOWLEDGEABLE MICROBIOLOGIST

It is difficult to fully explain the need for knowledgeable microbiologists in the field of industrial microbiology. There are many microbiologists who have become testing experts, due to the many hours of time performing tests in their laboratory. This is a critical first step in developing true expertise; however, this kind of experience does not, in and of itself, develop true industrial expertise. Without exposure to other methods, alternate approaches, and regulatory challenges (external to the laboratory), true expertise cannot be gained. Indeed, the term *expert* is used too often by those who have become an expert at one aspect of microbiology in their industry.

True expertise is developed by the additional experience gained outside of the laboratory. Spending time in the manufacturing environment is necessary to help the microbiologist understand all that can transpire in the microbiological world. Microbiology tests performed in a laboratory often could be modified to be more appropriate for a specific product from a specific manufacturer once a better background of the manufacturing process is gathered. Involvement in industry associations, conventions and meetings also helps to develop expertise. There are few things as helpful to building expertise as working together on industry standards or guidance documents, sharing ideas and new technologies in a forum, or giving and observing presentations on the relevant topics.

It seems to be that many industries are losing needed microbiology expertise on the manufacturing side due to microbiology aspects becoming one of many routine assignments that is folded into quality, regulatory, or manufacturing. In some cases, this may be necessary due to the inability to maintain a full-time person devoted to microbiology, especially for smaller manufacturing firms. The disadvantage is that manufacturing (or industrial) microbiology as a discipline is consequently not addressed, unless an outside expert is involved in such cases. This often results in manufacturers relying on laboratory personnel for guidance on performing tests and interpreting data. Many laboratories are willing to provide this assistance, but it is often given based on what is commonly known or done rather than what is best for the specific product/process. Nonetheless, it is best if product manufacturers develop a good relationship with their laboratories, whether they are internal or external. Developing appropriate test methods and correctly interpreting bioburden and sterility test data must be a collaborative effort with the viewpoints of both the laboratory and manufacturing represented.

▶ BIOBURDEN TESTING

Disinfection, sterilization, and preservation processes do not always address all microbial issues that might be present in the production of acceptable product; some degree of control over the product components and manufacturing processes is required to allow the processes to yield consistent results. Bioburden testing is commonly performed on product obtained under standard manufacturing conditions in order to gather information (quantitative and qualitative) on the typical microbial load during or after manufacturing and packaging. Obtaining and trending these data help the manufacturer to demonstrate continued microbial control over an entire process; however, it is important to note that merely performing bioburden testing alone on a limited basis, for example, semiannually, does not constitute a robust bioburden control program.

Bioburden testing of finished product often results in reactive activities, meaning that the bioburden test data are used to determine if the process has been under some semblance of control over a specified time. The bioburden test on finished product is commonly implemented without any preliminary understanding of the contribution of microbial contamination from subprocesses or components during manufacturing. Use of bioburden testing in this manner is considered a single "end-point" test. If the data are acceptable, it is assumed that the entire process is under reasonable control. If the data are not acceptable, it could mean that any of the many upstream components and processes might have changed, or that certain processes—single or multiple—might be out of control. A thorough bioburden control program uses bioburden testing to understand and qualify higher risk components and steps of the overall process. These higher risk components and processes can usually be identified by a knowledgeable microbiologist who is familiar with the pertinent aspects of product manufacturing. The microbiologist establishes a testing scheme and gathers data either to demonstrate that the current practice is acceptable or to identify where attention is needed or corrections are appropriate.

An understanding of bioburden can be used in several situations such as the following:

- Validation and maintenance of sterilization processes
- Routine monitoring to demonstrate control of manufacturing processes
- Monitoring of raw materials, components, or packaging
- Assessment of the efficiency of cleaning or disinfection processes
- Investigation into root cause for bioburden excursions
- Development/maintenance of an overall environmental monitoring program

Bioburden on a finished product is the sum of the microbial contributions from several sources, including raw materials, manufacturing of components, assembly processes, personnel, manufacturing environment, assembly/manufacturing aids (eg, compressed gases, water, lubricants), cleaning processes, and packaging of finished product. To control product bioburden, attention must be

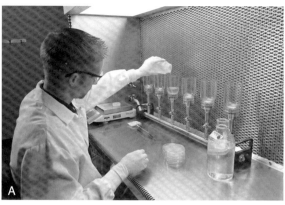 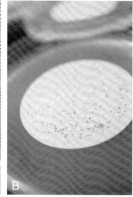 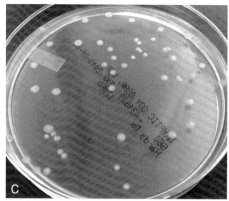

FIGURE 64.1 Examples of a membrane filtration method (A), a membrane filter with colonies (B), and a spread plate with colonies (C). For a color version of this art, please consult the eBook.

given to the microbiological status of these and other relevant sources. Strategic implementation of bioburden testing allows the microbiologist to correct practices or issues before they affect finished product, and to go into full-scale manufacturing with a degree of knowledge that it will be successful. When this approach is taken, the bioburden test of the finished product consequently becomes confirmation of the effort previously completed, rather than a hopeful exercise that will demonstrate control.

Bioburden testing is commonly performed on solid products (eg, plastics and metals) by performing an extraction with a water-based solution, followed by testing all or a portion of the extraction solution using membrane filtration, pour plating, or spread plating. For liquid products, bioburden testing is commonly performed by using membrane filtration, pour plating, or spread plating. When using the membrane filtration method, the membrane through which the liquid has been filtered is placed onto an agar plate or an absorbent pad saturated with liquid medium. After filtration and plating, or pour or spread plating, the agar plates are incubated at a specified temperature for a specified period to obtain visible colonies, followed by counting the colonies (Figure 64.1). Membrane filtration is often a preferred method because it allows for testing a larger volume of extraction solution or product. Pour or spread plating are good methods for bioburden enumeration but are limited by the quantity of solution or product that can be tested per plate. Bioburden testing is commonly performed in an environment to prevent contamination, usually a laminar flow hood in a controlled environment room, but usually not in a cleanroom because that level of control is not necessary.

It is sometimes assumed that bioburden testing will provide results of all types of microorganisms present on or in the product. This is not realistic because there are some types of microorganisms that require specific or unique growth nutrients, conditions, or incubation times to replicate and form a visible colony. For this reason, it is important that a microbiologist who is knowledgeable in

the specific raw materials and manufacturing processes be involved in test development. Based on that information, growth media type(s) and incubation conditions can be selected that are best suited for the various microorganisms expected to be on the product. Most often, this assessment results in selection of media and incubation conditions that are ideal for the majority of bacteria (eg, those from surfaces, humans, and water) and environmental fungi (ie, molds and yeasts). Cultivation and detection of more unique bacteria and fungi, specific viruses, protozoa, etc, is often not practical nor indeed necessary in most situations. Specific applications, such as bioburden testing for allograft tissues and animal serum for human use, might need to consider the detection of certain material-related pathogens.[7]

Change is ever-present in most manufacturing environments. With multiple personnel involved in different aspects of product and processes, and each one of the personnel tasked to improve what is in their control, it is inevitable that change will happen. In many cases, change is for the better, but it must be controlled such that other aspects of the product or process are not inadvertently, negatively impacted. Bioburden tests, along with some degree of microorganism characterization (eg, morphology, selective culturing, Gram stain), are commonly employed as part of the change control process and are effective in understanding if the change has an unintended impact on the process or product.

▶ VALIDATION OF A BIOBURDEN TEST

The validation of a bioburden test, in its strictest interpretation, is not usually necessary if classical microbiological methods are being used. The terms *qualification* or *verification* usually apply, but if bioburden validation is to be considered, as with most microbiological tests, it should be assessed in two different manners. Validation of a bioburden test method is conducted as part of the laboratory's preparation to perform bioburden testing. This type of validation is not specific to a product type but can include several general product types to understand the variability that occurs in the parameters of the overall test method. At this stage, items such as the limits of detection (LOD) and limits of quantification as well as other components of validation such as ruggedness, precision, and accuracy can be addressed. This validation provides the laboratory with valuable information regarding the different parameters of the bioburden test method and the variability that can occur. In microbiology, it is not expected that the variability be as small as might be expected in more precise sciences such as chemistry or physical analysis.

Once a bioburden test method has been validated, and when applying the test for a specific product, the product qualification process becomes the key factor, rather than the traditional components of a complete validation exercise. When addressing a bioburden test for a specific product, topics such as method suitability and recovery efficiency (see the following text) play a larger—and often exclusive—role compared to the other aspects of validation that are addressed in general validation of the test method. In the stage of bioburden qualification, it is usually also determined whether the entire product can be tested, which is called a sample item portion (SIP) of 1.0, or whether it is necessary to test a portion of the product (an SIP of <1.0). Most often, when testing a portion of the product becomes necessary, it is due to the large size of a product or to overcome inhibition of microbial growth in the test system. Whenever possible an SIP of 1.0 should be tested, and only when it is not practicable should an SIP <1.0 be considered. Some approaches (eg, when used in support of testing associated with radiation sterilization) require verification of the appropriateness of the SIP to ensure that the SIP is not too small to accurately represent the entire product, based on the purpose for the test.

Bioburden Method Suitability

Bioburden tests depend on the microorganisms' ability to replicate in the growth conditions provided during incubation; hence, it is critical that the growth conditions allow replication to occur. If microorganisms are not able to replicate, a result of no colonies on an agar plate could be the result of inhibition in the test system rather than an indication of a low or negligible count of bioburden on the product. Until recently, this aspect of qualifying a bioburden test method for a specific product was not well addressed in ISO 11737-1.[1] In contrast, it had been addressed for many years in the pharmacopoeial chapters on testing of nonsterile products.[8] The demonstration of the absence of inhibitory substances in a bioburden test method can be addressed in different ways. The most common is to actively generate data to

TABLE 64.1	Example of bioburden method suitability data	
Sample Number	**Product Extraction Fluid (CFU)[a]**	**Control Fluid (CFU)[a]**
1	60	90
2	51	68
3	71	72
Average	61	77
Percent age difference	61/77 = 0.79 or 79%	

Abbreviation: CFU, colony-forming units.

[a]The product extraction fluids and control fluids were inoculated with a suspension of *Bacillus atrophaeus* at a titer of approximately 8.5×10^1 (85) CFU.

verify that microorganisms can replicate following the performance of the test method on a product. One common option is performing the proposed test method (eg, filtering aliquots of the extraction fluid being proposed to recover the microorganisms from the test device) and then inoculating the filter with known, low numbers of a selected microorganism (or microorganisms) followed by incubation and enumeration. The colony count on the filters through which the product extraction fluid was filtered is then compared to the count on control filters (in the absence of the product extraction fluid) of the same test microorganism suspensions (Table 64.1). Other variations of this approach can also be used, if there is a demonstration of a lack of microbiological inhibition in the test system.

Alternatively, manufacturers who either have data on similar products or who more fully understand their processes can document that there are no inhibitory factors on their products or in associated test methods. This can be a simple exercise for synthetic materials, such as plastic and metal components, where the materials are previously qualified/understood as having no inhibitory factors and where all aspects of component manufacturing, cleaning, assembly, and packaging are generally understood and controlled. If documentation is provided in lieu of performing the test, the manufacturer must document that inhibitory substances are absent on product, such as leachable substances that might come from different polymer or component suppliers.

Bioburden recovery methods that include filtration of either an extraction fluid or filtration of the liquid product are effective methods to help eliminate or reduce inhibitory substances from the test system because the substances can potentially pass through the filter thereby being eliminated or reduced from the test system. Additionally, selection of the correct membrane filter or sufficient rinsing of the filter can minimize association or binding of inhibitory substances to the filter material itself. If filtration and selection of specific membrane filters is not enough to eliminate or reduce inhibition in a test, options such as dilution and the addition of neutralizers into the extraction fluid, rinse fluid, or growth medium are commonly employed (see chapter 61).

Recovery Efficiency

The intent of the recovery efficiency test is to gather data regarding the ability of a bioburden extraction method to remove and culture microorganisms from a product. When the product can be directly tested, such as by filtration of a liquid product or a water-soluble product, the extraction of microorganisms from a surface is not required, so a recovery efficiency test would not be necessary. However, for solid products, the microorganisms need to be removed from the surface for an accurate estimation of the bioburden. This is not a new test because it has been performed for many years in the medical device and pharmaceutical industries. Typically, between 3 and 10 recovery efficiency values are determined for a product and then an average recovery efficiency is calculated, which is used to adjust bioburden data in future testing. But recent changes to the ISO standard merit some discussion on the topic.[1]

There are two commonly used options in performing the recovery efficiency test—the inoculated product technique and the repetitive recovery technique. The inoculated product option is more suitable for products that carry low numbers of naturally occurring bioburden (eg, <100 CFU), and involves inoculating the product with a known number of microorganisms (usually spores) followed by application of the extraction method, plating, incubation, and enumeration. The recovery efficiency is calculated by comparing the number of CFU known to have been inoculated onto the product to the number of CFU that were removed in the single extraction process. The repetitive recovery technique is more suitable for products that carry higher numbers of naturally occurring bioburden (eg, >100 CFU) and involves application of the extraction method multiple times on the same product (using the naturally occurring product bioburden), with each extraction process being followed by plating, incubation, and enumeration. The recovery efficiency is calculated by comparing the number of CFU that were removed in the first extraction process to the number of CFU that were removed in all of the extraction processes combined. Significant information and guidance on recovery efficiency is provided in the ISO standard,[1] Annex C.

Previously, Annex A of ISO 11737-1 stated that for a recovery efficiency less than 50%, one should consider investigation whether the extraction method could be improved to obtain a value greater than 50%. This 50% value was arbitrarily selected, and it resulted in confusion in the industry that led many to believe that recovery efficiencies equal to or greater than 50% were a requirement. Because a requirement of this nature is not scientifically necessary, the 2018 version of the standard no longer contains the <50% recovery efficiency value. Instead, the new ISO 11737-1 standard states that the recovery efficiency value be viewed considering the purpose of the data and that a more important item regarding a set of recovery efficiency data is that the values are relatively consistent with each other and that they are appropriate for the intended use.

It is important in a bioburden test that the extraction method be capable of removing microorganisms in a consistent manner. This consistency is especially important when evaluating bioburden data over time or when the data are being used to establish sterilization processes or criteria for future reference. If this consistency is present, it is less critical whether the average recovery efficiency value is less than or greater than an arbitrary value. The new approach for recovery efficiency in the standards focuses on the use of the data in establishing an acceptable recovery efficiency. Annex C of ISO 11737-1 provides a good discussion of recovery efficiency and some examples of data.[1]

It could be argued that when an extraction is being performed on any product for a bioburden test that a recovery efficiency should be performed, but it should be noted that there are situations where it can be appropriate to not perform a recovery efficiency. For example, bioburden tests being performed on product components as part of routine monitoring of a supplier might not require a recovery efficiency to provide the necessary information, especially when the test is performed in the same manner over time. The intended purpose for the bioburden data is what should determine the need for and/or the use of a recovery efficiency.

▶ BIOBURDEN CHARACTERIZATION

Bioburden characterization is an underused practice in most industries. Where bioburden data are being gathered for health care products, it is often assumed that numerical data is the primary factor for evaluation rather than characterization data. Often, the need for, or the usefulness of, characterization is not fully understood, especially when microbiologists are not involved in the process. Characterization also requires an additional expense without—as it might appear—a direct, immediate correlation to outcome. Lastly, characterization data can be difficult for a nonmicrobiologist to interpret and trend, and therefore, the benefit can be difficult to demonstrate. Characterization should normally occur more frequently in the earlier stages of a manufacturing setting or process, to establish a baseline of the numbers and types of microorganisms present in the normal manufacturing scenario. Following that, characterization is an important key to demonstrating a controlled, stable process and product.

An understanding of the bioburden count alone is sometimes not enough to make an educated decision regarding interpreting microbiological data, assessing the potential impact of the bioburden to the product or process, or understanding the general microbiology of a product or process. Bioburden characterization is a broad term used to describe tests performed on the microorganisms after they have been recovered from the product or process. The most common methods of characterization are selection of specific growth conditions for groups of microorganisms, determination of colony morphology, Gram or other staining methods, and identification to genus and species.

The first step of characterization can include selection of specific growth conditions for groups of microorganisms. In some industries, it is common to employ use of selective or differential media to exhibit growth of specific microorganism types. Although this is considered characterization, it is sometimes too broad to be meaningful, depending on the purpose of the test. Certain types of media (Figure 64.2) or incubation temperatures can result in very specific outcomes. The important issue in using growth conditions as a means of characterization is to understand the desired end points and to ensure that the level of characterization provided meets those end points.

In the health care product industry, it is common to perform bioburden testing using different media and/or temperatures to encourage growth of both aerobic bacteria and fungi (molds and yeasts). This form of characterization helps the manufacturer gain a knowledge of the breakdown of microorganisms that are likely bacteria compared to molds. There is some usefulness in this knowledge, especially for trending bacteria and mold contamination over time. Less overlap and more differentiation will result when a different medium, specific for selection, is used for each microorganism type (eg, tryptic

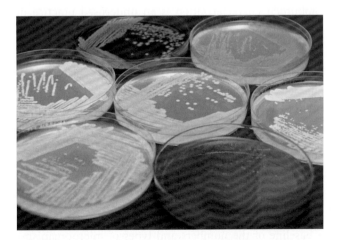

FIGURE 64.2 Different media types with microbial growth. For a color version of this art, please consult the eBook.

soy agar or nutrient agar for bacterial growth and potato dextrose agar or rose bengal agar for fungal growth). For bioburden testing in the health care industry, information regarding characterization to detect the presence of spores and anaerobes can also be considered. Testing for the presence of spores in product or environmental bioburden is sometimes performed in support of moist heat or ethylene oxide (EO) sterilization, where spores are considered more resistant to the process. Typically, spore testing is performed by applying high heat for a short period of time (eg, a heat shock at around 80°C for at least 10 min) to the bioburden extraction fluid to inactive vegetative bacteria, followed by plating and incubation.[9] If testing for aerobic bacteria is also being performed on the same products, it must be understood that spores that grow after heat shocking will generally also grow without the heat shock in the aerobic bacteria test. Thus, although the spore selection test helps to distinguish the percentage of microorganisms that are spores, the spore test results should not automatically be summed with the aerobic bacteria test results, as the total number could likely be overestimated because the spores can be a subset of the aerobic bacteria.

Testing for the presence of anaerobes often results in a similar issue as with spores. Most health care products are composed of different types of synthetic materials, such as plastic and metal, where there is, first, no potential source for strict anaerobes (termed *obligate anaerobes*) and, second, little potential for survival of obligate anaerobes. With these products, an anaerobe test, if not properly conducted, will result in the growth of microorganisms that are facultative rather than obligate anaerobes, meaning that they can also grow in the aerobic bacteria test. Again, summing these two results, without a screening or differentiating step, could result in over estimation of the total bioburden as well as possibly the false assumption that the product contains obligate anaerobes. In the case of tissue or tissue-based products, there is a potential source for obligate anaerobes, therefore anaerobic testing could be warranted. Even in this case, the presence of facultative anaerobes is just as likely as that of strict anaerobes, so an evaluation is recommended prior to summing the results or assuming the presence of obligate anaerobes.

Another means of characterization involves documentation of the colony morphology, which includes visible aspects of the microorganism growth such as colony size, shape, and color (Figure 64.3). Colony morphology by itself is not usually sufficient for making decisions or trending, as there are both Gram-positive and Gram-negative microorganisms that are, for example, of similar size, shape, and pigmentation. Morphology comparisons are useful when looking for a specific microorganism, or for other general activities such as noting predominant colony types. Colony morphology is often accompanied by staining (most commonly a Gram stain) and microscopic inspection (cell morphology), which can prove to be a useful data point.

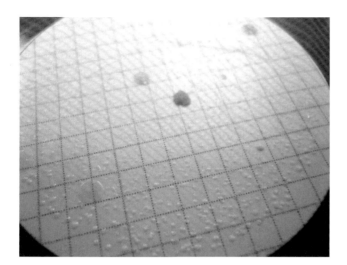

FIGURE 64.3 Example of various colony morphologies on a membrane filter. For a color version of this art, please consult the eBook.

A microbiologist can use colony morphology and Gram stain information, along with an in-depth knowledge of the components and manufacturing processes, to assess potential source(s) of contamination, and, if needed, determine what kinds of mitigating activities can be employed. For example, Gram stains can provide information to assist a microbiologist in understanding whether the microorganisms comprising the product bioburden likely came from water, humans, or the environment.

Microbial identifications to the genus and species level are usually performed as part of investigations, for specific trending purposes, or to characterize predominant microorganisms for a general characterization program. There are many systems available for the specific identification of microorganisms, and it is not the intent of this chapter to go into any detail regarding these systems.[10] These include various types of biochemical, lipid, and genetic identification techniques, where the genetic methods are currently generally considered necessary when establishing critical information that might be reviewed by regulatory bodies.

It should be mentioned that even though a quick search of a microbial genus and species might show that the microorganism in question can originate from a specific source, for example, animals or birds, it should not be assumed that such sources automatically relate to components or are present in the manufacturing area. Microorganisms have a way of populating multiple habitats, and of being spread from one place to another. Truly, they are a perfect example of how "life finds a way." A microbiologist, armed with the genus and species information of a microorganism, is usually able to determine a likely source and, if needed, a potential means of prevention or elimination. For example, bacteria such as the Gram-positive cocci *Staphylococcus epidermidis* and *Staphylococcus hominis* are common bacteria found on human skin, whereas strains of Gram-positive rods such as *Bacillus* species are common dust or surface contaminants (Figure 64.4). Equally, many types of fungi (eg, species of *Aspergillus* and *Penicillium*) can be associated with airborne/dust contamination but may also indicate more serious problems such as water damage. Gram-negative rods, such as strains of *Pseudomonas* and *Escherichia coli*, are often associated with water contamination during the manufacturing process.[11-13]

Examples of Bioburden Characterization

The amount of characterization needed is dependent on the use of the data. The following are a few examples of how much characterization might be necessary in different situations. In a test where a specific microorganism is being investigated, such as an antimicrobial log reduction study, a simple comparison of the colony morphology to that of the control is often enough to accomplish characterization. In these cases, if the stock culture is pure, it is unlikely—in a laboratory with reasonable controls—that a contaminant could be introduced in sufficient numbers, with the same or similar colony morphology, to impact the results of this type of study. In these situations, it is

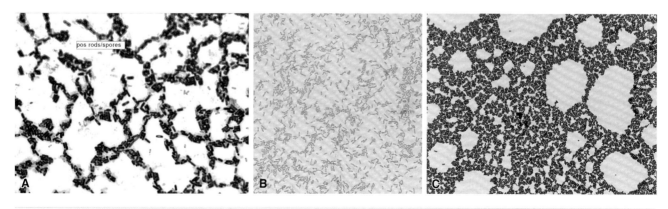

FIGURE 64.4 Examples of gram-positive rods with spores (A), gram-negative rods (B), and gram-positive cocci (C). For a color version of this art, please consult the eBook.

quite common to rely on the colony morphology as proof that the microorganism recovered is the microorganism being studied, rather than having to identify several colonies to genus and species to confirm the identity.

In an investigation into an out of specification result that is high, but not critically so, a Gram stain plus colony morphology can be acceptable to determine the likely source. For example, a high result where all colonies appear the same, and the Gram staining shows Gram-negative rods, it can suggest that the source is water contamination. It is common that water contamination causes high counts composed of a single or only a few microorganism types. Other types of contamination, such as from humans or the environment, will usually result in many types of microorganisms being present, which is usually evident by observing the various types of colonies on the plate.

In an investigation of a result that could be considered a failure of a process, such as a high bioburden count that would raise concerns regarding the acceptability of the product, it is more common to document colony morphology and perform an identification to genus and species. Although this might not provide significantly more information into the source compared to a Gram stain, it is more valuable from a comparison or trending perspective. The frequent appearance of the same genus and species on products or components, or having the same genus and species appear on both a sample and a control, for example, could demonstrate a trend, and be very valuable for investigations. This is a benefit compared to only performing a Gram stain, where there are many microorganisms that could exhibit the same Gram stain result.

It should be noted that the performance of bioburden characterization is only beneficial if a thorough baseline has been established. Characterization that is performed only when results are aberrant is usually of little benefit because there is nothing to which the results can be compared. It is important to be able to distinguish if a microorganism in an investigation is one that has routinely been present but is now present in higher numbers, or if a new type of microorganism has been introduced into the system. A solid baseline of microorganism data is usually established by more frequent monitoring—both of bioburden numbers and bioburden types—in the earlier stages of manufacturing or processing.

Characterization in Support of Sterilization and Aseptic Processing

Another aspect of characterization is in support of a sterilization process, or of aseptic processing of sterile products. All means of providing sterile product can benefit by incorporating some level of microbial characterization. Terminally sterilized products usually do not require as much characterization and overall understanding of the

manufacturing process and product microbiology as does a process such as aseptic processing.

For terminal sterilization, modalities that most often employ an overkill process, such as EO, moist heat, dry heat, and vaporized hydrogen peroxide,[14-17] generally need the least amount of initial bioburden characterization to demonstrate that the manufacturing process is in a state of control prior to conducting validation of the routine sterilization process. Typically, a more basic level of characterization is usually sufficient because these sterilization methods are typically established using worst-case situations and contain the highest level of additional safety for the sterilization process. In these instances, it is usually enough to establish a baseline bioburden characterization and then employ routine bioburden testing. Such testing could include a Gram stain, with occasional identifications to genus and species of predominant microorganisms, especially if the product bioburden is consistent and relatively low. Sometimes, testing for the presence of spores or identifying microorganisms to determine if they are spore-forming is recommended for overkill methods because spores are the types of microorganisms typically used to develop and validate the sterilization process. From a scientific standpoint however, if the product bioburden is moderate to low (eg, less than 1000 CFUs), even if 100% of the microorganisms are spore formers, there is almost no potential that this bioburden would impact the sterilization process based on the extreme high count of spores with a specific resistance that are used to challenge the sterilization process.

Sterilization methods that are validated using a bioburden-based approach, such as is often the approach used for radiation processes,[18] usually require a higher level of microbiological characterization than that required for overkill methods. Bioburden-based sterilization methods rely on both the quantity and the resistance of the microorganisms comprising the product bioburden. Thus, more frequent use of characterization, especially colony morphology paired with Gram stains and/or identifications, is recommended in order to better predict the success of the initial radiation validation and the routine sterilization maintenance. More extensive characterization is especially helpful when determining if a trend exists over time.

Aseptic manufacturing processes[19] rely heavily on bioburden characterization due to the greater inherent risk of not employing a terminal sterilization process. As aseptic processes are initially being established and validated, Gram staining and other identification methods are routinely performed on most or all microorganisms recovered from either the product or surface/air/personnel samples, to facilitate actions that should reduce or eliminate microorganism sources. Generally, it is expected that there are no microorganisms present during any step of the aseptic manufacturing and packaging process. As an aseptic process becomes routine, bioburden characterization is a key component in demonstrating continued control over the process and discovering opportunities for improvement. In the validation of an aseptic process, the data obtained are helpful in identifying at which points of the process it is most beneficial to perform bioburden testing on components or product and also to what level of characterization the recovered microorganisms are subjected. It is common to identify all microorganisms recovered to genus and species and to evaluate them in the context of the cleaning and disinfection validations being employed.

▶ EVALUATION OF BIOBURDEN DATA

Bioburden determination is called many terms, such as plate count, total count, colony count, viable count, mesophilic count, microbial count and heterotrophic plate count. Most of these terms apply to the same essential test where a quantitation is needed of the viable microorganisms on or in a product, but the terms differ in the purpose for the test as well as within the associated industry. Because of the many purposes of a bioburden test, there are consequently many uses of the data and therefore many approaches to evaluating the data. The parameters of the test, the extent of validation and the application of mathematical analyses all depend on the purpose, use, and criticality of the data.

Bioburden data typically vary for health care products, such as medical devices, because the bioburden test is usually performed on product to detect its natural microbial flora and that natural flora is present on the product due to the various materials that make up the product as well as the handling, storage, and processes that occur during manufacturing. Due to these many variables, the expectation for health care products/medical devices is a nonuniform microbial content in both numbers and types from product unit to unit within a batch as well as from batch to batch. Other types of products, such as pharmaceutical formulations, bulk ingredients, and liquid or powder components, will typically have less variation in the bioburden between production units because they are usually composed of fewer components/ingredients, include less handling and manipulations, and have, of necessity, been thoroughly mixed or blended and, in some cases, presterilized to reduce the bioburden prior to entry into aseptic manufacturing. Therefore, the expectation for mixed/blended products is a more uniform microbial content in both numbers and types.

In disciplines such as chemistry and physics, differences between results, such as values in the parts per million level (ppm) or measurements in micrograms, are often considered significant. However, in the discipline of microbiology, much larger differences in results are considered normal. Sometimes, it is said that microbiology is a logarithmic science, meaning that until values differ from each other by a factor of 10, the values can almost be

considered equivalent. Although a log-based approach in assessing significant differences is not always appropriate, the concept is important when identifying data as significantly different.

It must be understood that variation in bioburden counts from product unit to unit is expected and that values such as 15 CFU and 20 CFU, for example, can be considered microbiologically equivalent. In some pharmacopoeia test methods and ISO sterilization-related documents, differences between microbiological values as much as 30% or even 50% are similar enough to be considered equivalent. This concept becomes even more critical when establishing alert and action levels with bioburden data as discussed later in this chapter. In support of this expected variation in bioburden counts, USP <1116> states "growth and recovery in microbiological assays have normal variability in the range of $\pm$ 0.5 $\log_{10}$."[20] It further states "in a practical sense, numerical values that vary by as much as five- to tenfold may not be significantly different."

Viable but Not Culturable Microorganisms

There is another type of bioburden variation that should be considered; it is often called viable but not culturable. The foundation behind this variation is that not all microorganisms need the same nutrients and environment to replicate. Bioburden counts for a specific product type using one agar medium and incubation environment or time can be dramatically different than counts for the same product type using a different medium and/or incubation environment or time. Generally, it is not expected that subtle differences in incubation temperature will have significant effects, such as incubating at 25°C compared to 20°C. Changes such as different agar types and/or longer incubation times are what will sometimes result in significantly different counts. A microbiologist should be able to make an educated decision on agar types and growth environments without having to perform substantial testing using a variety of conditions. The decision will be based on an understanding of the expected types of microbial flora for the types of products being tested and the processes involved.

▶ ENUMERATION METHODS

Plating Method

Bioburden test parameters also vary widely. In general, there are two types of tests: direct plating and most probable number (MPN). Plating is the more common method and involves either (1) incorporating a product extract or a product mixture into molten agar or onto the surface of solidified agar or (2) filtering a liquid product or the extract of a product through a membrane that captures the microorganisms for subsequent plating on growth medium. Both plating methods result in colonies growing in or on the agar or filter. These colonies are called CFU because a colony can be formed from growth of a single cell or from the growth of a cluster of cells. Because of this fact, it should be understood than any count using the term *CFU* will consist of one or more cells originating in each colony, and therefore, the actual cell count is always greater than or equal to the number shown. This translates into a likely underestimation of the bioburden based solely on CFU counts.

Most Probable Number Method

In the MPN method, the actual product and/or dilutions of the non-sterile product are introduced directly into a growth medium followed by incubation. The test samples are scored as positive or negative for growth and results are determined using either MPN tables or a formula. The steps used in performing this test are more related to those used for a sterility test than those for a plated bioburden test because of the immersion and incubation approach rather than extraction, plating, and enumeration. Accurate MPN results rely on uniformity of bioburden on a product; therefore, the natural bioburden uniformity of mixed/blended products or liquids and powders is a good candidate for the MPN technique. It is primarily used for products with low bioburden. The primary advantage of MPN is that an extraction is not performed on the products prior to testing, so there are fewer issues with extracting and capturing microorganisms on or in the product.

The primary disadvantages of the MPN method are that it is not directly quantitative in that colonies are not isolated and counted, and thus, colony characteristics cannot be evaluated until a subculture has been performed of the media after the test is completed. Additionally, if the bioburden count is higher than expected, the MPN results can show all samples are positive for growth, which means that a calculation cannot be performed. Although this method is typically used for product with very low bioburden counts, it can be appropriately applied in situations with higher bioburden, usually facilitated by the appropriate dilution scheme. A few articles have provided detail on this method because it is often misunderstood.[21-23]

Know the Intent

Calculating and reporting bioburden results relies on an understanding of microbiology as well as math. A poor understanding of the purpose of a test, along with an improperly designed test, coupled with subsequent misunderstanding of the nature of the test can lead to confusing, incorrect results or unusable results. The bioburden test must be designed with the intent of the test in mind, in other words, with an understanding of how the data will be used and how that will influence the test method. The intent might be acceptance criteria per a standard, an approximate bioburden number for evaluation of a change, or a less than or equal to result for meeting alert or action levels. Regardless, the test must be designed such that the result can be evaluated considering the purpose for the data.

Limit of Detection

One issue to address with the bioburden test methods that use a plating method is the limit of detection (LOD). If the purpose of a bioburden test is meeting an acceptance criterion of <10 CFU/product, the test cannot be performed by testing dilutions of 1:10 of the product (or product extracts) because this is not sensitive enough. In this instance, one or more colonies detected will result in a count greater than 10 CFU. The product might truly have an average count less than 10 CFU, but it cannot be accurately measured because the LOD is too high. Alternately, if the purpose of a test is to obtain an accurate count for comparison to another product, and the MPN test is used for product with a moderate to high bioburden and if all test units are positive for growth, it could result in, for example, >110 CFU, which reveals very little about the actual count.

Reporting Results

Reporting bioburden counts should always follow the typical rules found in official microbiology standards and guidelines.[1] The rules for colony counts and dilution factors are relatively straightforward, but negative results—zero colony counts—have often been misreported, miscalculated, and misused. For negative results using plating methods, results are always reported as less than the lowest dilution. This means that if a dilution is 1:5, or if one-fifth of the extraction fluid is tested, the results of plates with no colonies is reported as <5 CFU. Consequently, if there is no dilution, that is, the dilution is 1:1 or if the entire volume of extraction fluid is tested, the results are reported as <1 CFU, as 1 CFU is the lowest detection limit.

In considering a result of <5 CFU, one must realize that it means there could be a count of 0, 1, 2, 3, or 4 colonies for that sample. Because the LOD is 5, one cannot know which of those results is correct. In using the data, it cannot be assumed the count is zero due to no colonies being detected because that is a best-case assumption that would be considered falsely representing the data. Depending on the purpose for the data, it is usually expected that one assumes the worst-case, which is 4 or even 5 CFU. This means that when calculating an average using data with less than numbers (eg, <5), it is common to use the LOD as a number (ie, to use 5 for <5).

Some standards mention concerns with use of less than numbers when calculating bioburden averages, in that they might artificially inflate the results.[1] These concerns do not stem from the use of less than values being inappropriate, but because it is often important to design a bioburden test with the lowest LOD possible. It is certainly easier to perform, for example, a spread plate of 0.5 mL compared to performing membrane filtration of a large volume that must be split between two filters, but if the volume of extraction fluid is 200 mL for this example, the LOD of the spread plate becomes very high (ie, 400) and will not be appropriate to demonstrate a state of control for a manufacturing process or trends in the manufacturing process.

It should be noted that bioburden testing is, by its nature, complex and imprecise. For example, as explained earlier, a CFU is either one or more cells, recovery is an average or the worst-case value, and culturing will not recover all microorganisms present; therefore, the bioburden test cannot be assumed or expected to have a level of precision that cannot be achieved or does not apply.

▶ BIOBURDEN SPIKES AND TOO NUMEROUS TO COUNT

On the other end of the spectrum from the issue of LOD and counts that are represented as "less-than" values are bioburden issues such as bioburden spikes and TNTC (too numerous to count) (Figure 64.5). Because bioburden is

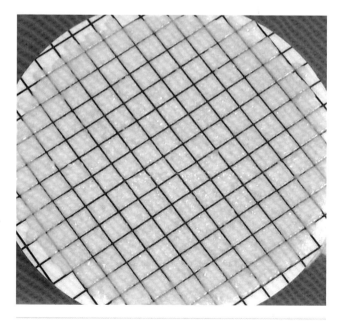

FIGURE 64.5 Example of a too numerous to count result on a membrane filter. For a color version of this art, please consult the eBook.

considered an estimate of the microorganism count on product, it is usually determined on a number of products in a batch or product family and then averaged. When discussing bioburden spikes the focus is on what should happen when the spread of the data is wide or if one specific product sample indicates results that are significantly higher than the rest. A bioburden spike is defined as an individual value that is significantly greater than other bioburden values in a set.

As in calculating and reporting LOD values, one must look at a bioburden spike in light of microbiology, not math alone. For example, in a set of 10 individual product test results, a value of 15 CFUs might seem significantly higher than the other nine counts that are all between 1 and 5 CFUs. This higher value is 3 to 4 times higher than the other counts; however, in the world of bioburden of a health care product or medical device, those differences are commonly seen, are normal data, and would not automatically be considered a spike value (see previous discussion on bioburden variability). But in an example where there is an individual count of 1500 CFUs and the other nine counts are between 100 and 500 CFUs, the high value might be considered a spike, even though it is also about 3 to 4 times the other counts. This is an example of where knowledge of the microbiology of a product and the bioburden distribution from unit to unit and batch to batch is critical.

The issue of TNTC falls into two categories—an anomaly or a contamination. The ISO 11737-1 bioburden standard acknowledges that there will be anomalies in bioburden results, but the expectation is that they should be infrequent.[1] For an unexpected high result or anomaly that cannot be explained through an investigation and is out of line with other results and historical data, it is common practice to simply discard the TNTC results for calculation of an average. But these results might be valid results and should be kept in mind for the future regarding trending. Also, it is wise that the investigation includes an identification of the TNTC microorganism(s) to assist in understanding its potential source, which can include laboratory operations.

The other type of TNTC result is identified as contamination, and it is usually established as such through an investigation where the root cause can be reliably surmised. The test results are noted to be contamination resulting from something related to handling, testing, materials, or other identifiable cause. In this case, the results are considered invalid and a retest is typically warranted. Sometimes, a laboratory will identify a result as TNTC when it might be a single colony, or a low number of colonies, that has spread over the surface of the filter or plate (Figure 64.6). This misinterpretation of results is significant and can result in unnecessary actions at the manufacturing facility. Thus, it is critical that the observation of the plate be interpreted correctly. A knowledgeable microbiologist can often detect the difference, even if all that is available is a good-quality picture of the plate.

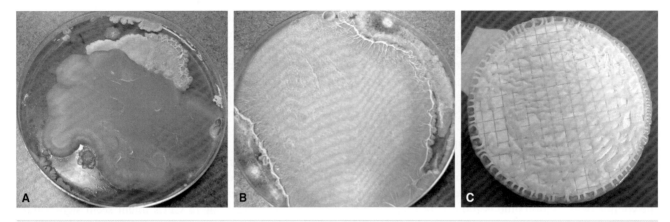

FIGURE 64.6 Examples of spreading colonies on agar plates (A and B) and membrane filters (C). For a color version of this art, please consult the eBook.

Historically, the term *spike* has been used to represent any value that is high compared to the other values in a data set. This general term can have different meanings. One manner of qualifying a value as a spike is if the occurrence is consistent, and the microorganisms are what is normal for that product. "Consistent" means that the occurrence of a high value is not rare, but there is a systematic occurrence of high values across a given number of samples. "Normal" means that the microorganisms that make up the spike are generally the same ones that make up the other samples in that set. These two things indicate that the high value is to be expected to occur periodically on that product and should be considered a real value and not an outlier or a contaminant. An outlier could be considered a high value that is not expected and has not occurred previously on any consistent basis. A contaminant could be considered a high value that does not reflect the microorganisms that were on the product but does reflect something that went awry during the testing or incubation process. In determining whether a value is a spike, there should be enough history of the product's bioburden so that the numbers and types of microorganisms can be evaluated based on the historical data.[24-27]

Establishing Alert and Action Levels

In many applications, there is a recommendation or even a requirement to establish alert and action levels for bioburden of a product, component, or material. This expectation is usually associated with bioburden-based processes such as radiation sterilization[18] or a situation where there is a specified acceptance criterion for the bioburden, such as some pharmacopoeial and nutritional/dietary supplements sections on microbial enumeration tests.[28] Alert and action levels can certainly be established using statistical methods, but the microbiology needs to be taken into consideration as well as the purpose for establishing the levels. Some statistical approaches are not applicable to or are not necessary for bioburden data, mainly because

bioburden varies naturally and often has very high or very low values that do not follow a normal distribution. Alternatively, some statistical approaches are still applicable even though bioburden does not follow a normal distribution. For example, a simple standard deviation calculation can be useful in understanding the dispersion of the bioburden data even though the data might not fit a normal distribution.[1,27] On the subject of statistical approaches associated with bioburden testing, it should also be noted that ISO 11737-1 points out that measurement of uncertainty, precision, and bias usually do not apply in validating a bioburden test method for a specific product.

Setting bioburden levels using pure statistical methods will often result in numbers that are not practical or are too restrictive for the situation. For example, a bioburden alert and action level for a product with low bioburden counts that has been substantiated for radiation sterilization should be different from a bioburden alert and action level for a product that has been qualified for an overkill steam sterilization cycle. In the former, the bioburden is the determining factor for the efficacy of the process and alert and action levels should be established and should be at a level that will be meaningful in detecting changes that could impact the process. In the latter, the bioburden is usually not linked to the efficacy of the process and alert and action levels might be established for general control purposes but may be assigned higher values.

▶ STERILITY TESTING

Although sterility testing—the presence/absence of microbial growth in a sample—could potentially be used in supporting aspects of disinfection and preservation, its main purpose is in support of sterilization processes. In disinfection and preservation, studies are often performed with inoculated solutions or surfaces to determine the log reduction that occurs over time. In these instances, it is possible to perform a sterility test as part of development of the data for the label claim, especially when a sensitive

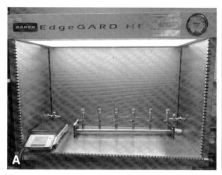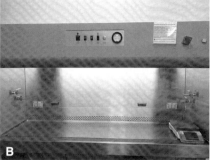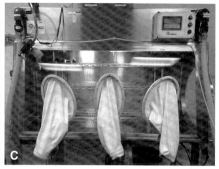

FIGURE 64.7 Examples of a horizontal laminar flow hood (A), a biosafety cabinet (B), and an isolator (C).

test is desired, and a high log reduction is expected, but it is much more common to perform a bioburden test where actual counts will be more applicable. In these instances, the data explain the capability of the full disinfection or preservation process, meaning that the data are generally not used to extrapolate to a longer contact time and more extensive log reduction.

A sterility test for sterilization activities typically is used during development and validation exercises intended to demonstrate the appropriateness of a terminal sterilization process for a specific product. In these instances, the sterility test is applied to products that have undergone a fraction of the intended sterilization process, and the data are subsequently used to extrapolate to a longer exposure time and more extensive log reductions. As will be discussed later, a sterility test should not be performed after exposure to the complete sterilization process because there are no valid scientific data that can be obtained from such studies.[26] A sterility test for aseptic processing activities typically is used as part of a process simulation to demonstrate that the assembly/manufacturing process can be carried out on presterilized components without contaminating the finished product. Although this chapter will deal with aspects of a sterility test that pertain to any given application, the underlying theme regards tests for the sterility of a group of products that have been exposed to a fractional process as part of validation of a sterilization process.

The sterility test is an assay for which, in most cases, there is no readily available automated system. Because of this, the test requires exacting conditions and relies on aseptic technique throughout the process to ensure that the test results reflect the attributes of the test sample versus extraneous contamination associated with the test. There are automated systems for limited applications during the test, such as filtration of liquid products. For most health care products, especially medical devices and tissue-based products/biologics, the test will typically be performed in a laminar flow hood within a cleanroom environment by trained technicians using aseptic technique. Testing can be performed in an isolator to reduce the chances of contamination, but the space limitations of most isolators restricts not only the types of products but also the number of products that can be tested using this technology. Testing of aseptically processed pharmaceutical products, however, is often performed in isolators to obtain the best possible environment to minimize the possibility for contamination during testing (Figure 64.7). Therefore, the type of equipment and conditions used for the sterility test is based on the nature of the test, capability of the testing facility, purpose for the data, and associated risk.

Intent of the Test

A sterility test performed for any purpose involves essentially the same overall technique. It most commonly entails determining the presence of viable microorganisms through incubation of a product in liquid medium to promote growth of microorganism(s) to a detectable level, typically facilitated by visible observation of the medium. Techniques might vary, such as total immersion of a solid item versus membrane filtration of a liquid, but essentially, the test relies on the direct growth of microorganisms. Although the process of performing the overall test method is usually the same, the purpose for performing the test can vary. There is a general distinction between the purposes of the test, which are delineated by two defined terms: the test *for* sterility and the test *of* sterility. Throughout this chapter, the term *sterility test* will be used, except for instances where a distinction needs to be made between these two terms based on the purpose of the test.

The test for sterility is defined in ISO 11737-2 as a test performed to confirm the sterility of products that have been aseptically processed, and can be performed on the entire batch of products in some instances or on a representative number of products in others. It is an appropriate use of the sterility test because it is performed to assist in confirming the claim being made, which is that the products in that batch are sterile. When the entire batch of products is tested for sterility, it is used as part of validation of an aseptic process and typically involves samples from a simulated batch that are tested by filling the container with growth medium rather than product.[19,29] The batch used for this purpose is typically simulated, rather than consisting of actual product, but the test nonetheless does assay the entire run. The sample size of the batch to be tested for sterility can be quite large, such as 1000 units or as many as 10 000 units. When a representative number of products from the batch are tested for sterility, it is intended to verify a previously validated process (eg, pharmacopoeial sterility test).[6] In this instance, it is meant to not be the only criteria for release of the product, but rather, it is one of many controls and monitors that are used to determine the acceptability of the batch for use.

The test of sterility is defined as a test performed in the validation of a sterilization process. It is intended to be performed on products that have received a partial sterilization process, the data then being used to confirm that the sterilization process can be extrapolated using additional processing, to reach a specified sterility assurance level (SAL). This test of sterility can use varying numbers of samples and may depend on the SAL that needs to be determined for a partial sterilization process. In most cases, the number of samples can fall between 10 and 100 product units.[5,30]

Limitations and Uses of the Test

It has long been recognized that the sterility test is limited in its ability to confirm results for which it has been purported to verify.[31] For decades, the sterility test has been employed to confirm the sterility of a batch of products; this can include a batch that has been aseptically processed to achieve and maintain sterility in the finished product or a batch that has been terminally sterilized to a 10^{-6} SAL. In either case, the sterility test used for these purposes does not achieve what the sponsor of the test may be attempting to prove—that the entire batch is sterile to the level claimed. As well-meaning as the original intent or purpose might be, the limits of the sterility test are real, and the scientific community has, for the most part, realized those limitations. There are appropriate and inappropriate applications for the sterility test, and the test is only meaningful for certain applications.

If the intent is to confirm the sterility of a batch of products, this can only be correctly accomplished in one of three ways:

1. Aseptically processed or terminally sterilized product: to perform a sterility test on all product items in the batch (as described earlier)
2. Terminally sterilized product: to perform a sterility test on items that have been processed using a partial sterilization process and then, based on the test results, extrapolate to the extent of the full sterilization process[5,32]

3. Aseptically processed product: to perform a sterility test on a preselected number of products from the batch processed using a previously validated aseptic process

The health care industry has for many years acknowledged that a claim of sterility for a batch is one that cannot be verified by the first, which would involve testing—and consequently destruction—of every product in that batch.[31] Altering the first option to testing of a number of products in the batch will only confirm the sterility of the products tested and, based solely on these results, this information should not be extrapolated to the other products in the batch because they were not tested. In the third option, when a representative number of products from a batch are tested from aseptically processed product, and the aseptic process applied to that batch has been previously validated, the results of the sterility test serve as one of many controls and monitors to confirm that that the previously validated aseptic process has been correctly applied to the production batch. Hence, the proper way of confirming sterility for aseptic processing includes testing of a simulated batch of product at a predetermined frequency (often every 6 months) and does include a test of all samples from a batch to verify that the process is capable of producing a sterile product with a certain degree of confidence.

For confirming that a sterilization process provides a defined SAL, the first option of testing cannot be applied for most SALs (eg, 1 million products for a 10^{-6} SAL), and therefore, the second option of testing from a partial sterilization process, is the only valid means of confirming the SAL claim. Additional uses of the sterility test, such as demonstrating package integrity, confirming sterility due to sterilization or aseptic process deviations, or demonstrating sterility following a catastrophic event, are invalid for proving the purported claim, yet are still often being practiced and/or requested. The remainder of this section discusses the appropriate and inappropriate uses of sterility testing.

The sterility test is still being widely used for inappropriate reasons. As mentioned previously, in order to claim the sterility and/or SAL of a specific batch of fully sterilized products, one cannot select a limited number of samples from that batch and test those samples for sterility. The principle is generally understood throughout the health care product sterilization industry, yet in the broader industry, the practice continues to be performed of testing a limited number of samples from a fully processed batch of product to confirm a claim of sterility. A summary of examples of the inappropriate use of sterility testing to verify a sterile condition can include the following:

- Batch release of a terminally sterilized product
- Investigation into a process deviation
- Catastrophic event, for example, flood or gross contamination
- Package integrity
- Product shelf life

- Environmental monitoring excursion
- Assessment of change, for example, supplier or process
- Confirmation of supplier quality

For the purposes of proving batch sterility, from some of the examples earlier, the number of samples truly needed to confirm an SAL would be between 1000 (for a 10^{-3} SAL) and 1 000 000 (for a 10^{-6} SAL). A typical, yet erroneous, practice is to test a much smaller number, such as 20 or 40 product items, and then use those results to claim that sterility of these samples means all other product in the batch is sterile. For the purposes of proving package integrity or shelf life, the test is inappropriate for the same reasons, plus an additional reason of using an invalid measurement system. The integrity of a package relies on the physical attributes of the package itself and must be verified by actively challenging the seals and materials and not by passively measuring a different attribute of an internal product, the results of which may or may not be affected by inadequate packaging.

In addition to the cited reasons that a sterility test of limited samples cannot verify the sterile claim of a batch of fully sterilized product, there is the overarching issue of the integrity of the sterility test itself. It is extremely difficult to perform the test without some chance of contamination coming into play—either through the environment, materials, or technicians. With the general chance of contamination in a sterility test being between 0.2% and 0.05% even under rigorous aseptic conditions, a positive growth test result always carries with it the question of whether the microorganism(s) arose from the sample itself or as a result of some aspect of the test.

Examples of appropriate uses of sterility tests can include the following:

- Aseptic process validation
- Batch release of a previously validated aseptic process
- Validation approaches for a terminal sterilization process
- In some cases, specific test methods used to validate the efficacy of a disinfection or sterilization product/process[33] (see chapters 61 and 62)

As mentioned, using the sterility test as part of an aseptic process validation is an appropriate use of the test. This is because the entire manufacturing batch is recommended to be tested,[19,34] which then defines an assurance that the process can produce sterile product. This test is called a process simulation, and in most cases, simulated products are used and filled with media (media fill), with the number of samples tested in the thousands. This has long been accepted as a valid way to verify that an aseptic process is capable of reliably and consistently producing sterile product. Often an aseptic process validation is performed on three batches for an aseptic process once, followed by periodic, single-batch requalifications, often every 6 months.

For validation of a terminal sterilization process, the sterility test should only be performed on product from a partial or fractional sterilization exposure. This testing can be used to verify a specific SAL or log reduction for the partial process, and the desired SAL can then be determined by extrapolation for the full process. The validation of terminal sterilization processes can differ in the approaches used to demonstrate sterility as well as the number of samples required,[5,14,17] but the principle is the same: Sterility testing is only performed on partially processed product, with the purpose of proving a known log reduction or SAL associated with that partial process. The full sterilization process does not call for product to be tested because many thousands or millions of product items would have to be tested to verify the desired SAL, which is clearly not appropriate or possible.

An example of how this is properly performed is in the establishment of a radiation sterilization dose (see chapter 29). A radiation dose much lower than the sterilization dose (called a verification dose) is determined based on the product bioburden and taken from a reference table in the applicable standard.[5] The verification dose predicts a 10^{-1} or 10^{-2} SAL, which corresponds to a probability of 1 in 10 or 1 in 100 product items being positive for growth, respectively. After receiving the verification dose, the product items undergo a test of sterility. The purpose of the test of sterility is to verify that the predicted SAL of 10^{-1} or 10^{-2} is met, with the product's naturally occurring bioburden. If the acceptance criteria of the test of sterility are met, the higher radiation dose corresponding to the selected SAL, such as 10^{-6} is confirmed as appropriate for use.

Because there are two different and major uses of the sterility test, there are also two different types of standards that are followed: the pharmacopoeia for aseptically produced products (eg, USP[2], EP[3], JP[4]) and ISO 11737-2 for terminally sterilized products.[30] The primary difference between these test methods is that the pharmacopoeia requires two types of media (soybean-casein digest medium or SCDM and fluid thioglycollate medium) and two incubation temperatures (20°C-25°C and 30°C-35°C, respectively), and ISO defaults to one type of media and one temperature (SCDM at 28°C-32°C). The two media types and temperatures specified in the pharmacopoeia potentially provide greater assurance that the test can recover a broader range of microorganisms that might be present on aseptically prepared products. Also, when a terminal sterilization step is not a direct part of the product manufacturing process, the final product sterility test is expected as a component of product release, making a broader spectrum test method appropriate using two media types and two incubation temperatures. The selection of the single media type in ISO 11737-2 necessitates a rationale that the media type and incubation temperature are appropriate for the microorganisms expected to be present on the product.[30] This rationale is usually based on a microbiological understanding of the raw materials and manufacturing processes as well as bioburden data demonstrating the types of microorganisms that will be found on a product. The incubation time of 14 days is the same in both test requirements.[6,30]

VALIDATION OF STERILITY TESTS

True validation of a test method (meaning evaluation of aspects such as LOD, limit of quantification, linearity, specificity, accuracy, precision, etc) is usually not needed for sterility tests. To borrow a term from the pharmacopoeia,[2-4] sterility tests are considered a compendial method, meaning that they have been sufficiently validated and studied in the industry. If the laboratory can demonstrate that they have properly implemented the method, per the information in standards and including the appropriate controls, they do not have to perform full validation of the test method; a verification is usually appropriate. The same approach is used for sterility tests performed for validation of terminal sterilization.[30]

Verification can include aspects that influence the test system such as media growth promotion, test area certification (eg, cleanroom and/or horizontal/vertical flow hood or isolator), sterilization of instruments, and items specific to individual employees such as training, demonstration of competency, and qualifications. When verification of a sterility test method is addressed (ie, use of a compendial method and demonstrating that the laboratory in question has properly implemented the test), ensuring that the test method can be applied to a specific product becomes an easier task. Generally, it is only necessary to ensure that the product in question does not negatively impact the test system (ie, inhibition of viable microorganisms), which is usually called a suitability test.[6,30]

Sterility Test Method Suitability

Sterility tests are meant to be among the most sensitive of the microbiological tests performed, which makes them critical tests. As with all scientific assays, the test must be shown to be appropriate for the product being tested. This means that the product should not exhibit any effects on the test system that would interfere with the outcome. For the sterility test, the outcome is either no growth of microorganisms or growth of microorganisms. Hence, the appropriateness of the test method for the specific product being assayed, which is essentially the absence of interfering substances and the ability of microorganisms to grow, is demonstrated by performing a method suitability test.

The most well-accepted approach for showing the suitability of the sterility test for a specific product is provided in various national pharmacopoeias that are generally harmonized across the world.[2-4] This test was previously called bacteriostasis/fungistasis for decades, then became known as sterility test validation, and finally was termed the *method suitability test*. The specifics of the suitability test have changed little over this time, with the general technique involving introduction of a low number of representative microorganisms (ie, not more than 100 CFUs, Table 64.2) into the test system, which is the microbiological growth medium containing the product. The desired outcome after incubation is growth of the microorganisms that is visually comparable to the growth of the positive controls, thereby showing no interference in the test system.

Health care products, especially biologics, pharmaceuticals, or tissue-based products, can possess inhibitory or microbicidal substances. Even medical devices can have additives, coatings, or leachable substances that might interfere with microbial growth. For this reason, a sterility test cannot be considered acceptable without a suitability test supporting the validity of the test. Without supporting evidence, a sterility test with results of no growth is suspect and could be considered a false negative. For aseptically processed products, the parameters of the method suitability test as described in the pharmacopoeia[6] provide good assurance that there is no inhibition in the test system. Use of a variety of microorganism types (ie, Gram-positive and Gram-negative bacteria including rod and cocci forms, and yeasts and molds) is a typical

TABLE 64.2	Typical microorganisms used in the method suitability test		
Category	**Gram Stain**	**Microorganism**	**Media Type**
Aerobic bacteria	Gram-positive cocci	*Staphylococcus aureus*	FTM
	Gram-positive rods	*Bacillus subtilis*	TSB
	Gram-negative rods	*Pseudomonas aeruginosa*	FTM
Anaerobic bacterium	Gram-positive rods	*Clostridium sporogenes*	FTM
Yeast	NA	*Candida albicans*	TSB
Mold	NA	*Aspergillus brasiliensis* (*Aspergillus niger*)	TSB

Abbreviations: FTM, fluid thioglycollate medium; NA, not applicable; TSB, tryptic soy broth (soybean-casein digest broth).

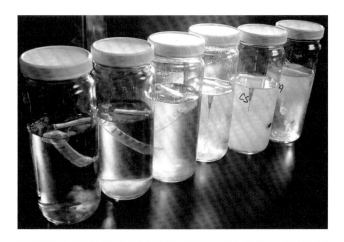

FIGURE 64.8 Method suitability test, showing the presence of growth with product test samples. For a color version of this art, please consult the eBook.

approach to qualifying microbiology tests as being appropriate for a specific product (Figure 64.8).

For terminally sterilized products, the ISO 11737-2 standard does reference the parameters of the pharmacopoeial method suitability test procedure but with some recommended modifications. Because only one media type is called for in the ISO test of sterility, only that media type should be used in the method suitability test along with the recommended microorganisms for that media type. The other modification is regarding the incubation temperature. If the recommended ISO temperature of 28°C to 32°C is used for the sterility test, the method suitability should also be incubated at that temperature. During the development of the ISO sterility test standard, the question arose regarding whether a specific method suitability procedure should be placed into the ISO standard, but it has been determined that the parameters outlined for the pharmacopoeial approach are sufficient, and thus to continue to reference the pharmacopoeia with the applicable modifications.

Neither the ISO nor the pharmacopoeia documents require that method suitability be performed on multiple batches of a product. This is something that should be evaluated on a product-by-product basis. For a simple plastic and/or metal product with little potential process variability from batch to batch, demonstration of method suitability on a single batch might be appropriate. But for a product that includes potentially inhibitory substances as part of the finished product or as part of the manufacturing/assembly process, a determination should be made as to whether testing a single batch is sufficient. After the initial method suitability test is completed, it might be warranted to perform it periodically, usually as part of assessment of change to the product or process. It is not expected or common to perform method suitability on a routine basis; thus, it is worthwhile that in the initial evaluations, sufficient testing is performed to ensure consistently acceptable results.

Variations in the Sterility Test

Sometimes it is necessary, whether the product in question is terminally sterilized or not, to alter the test conditions due to a failing method suitability test. The method suitability test fails when one or more of the test microorganisms does not replicate to demonstrate turbidity (microbial growth) that is comparable to the corresponding positive control. This is usually caused by a substance(s) inherent in or released from the product being tested that inhibits growth of microorganism(s) in the medium and usually indicates that an alteration to the test method is required. One of the most common alterations to overcome inhibitory substances is to test the product in a greater volume of media. Another common option is to alter the media by the addition of neutralizing chemicals to the standard growth medium being used. The additional ingredients are either general neutralizers, such as polysorbate 80 and lecithin, or specific neutralizers for the specific inhibitory substance eliciting microbiostatic activity. It is important to be cautious when adding ingredients into growth media because there might be unintended consequences, such as causing a new type of inhibition. Usually, the new media type, with the additional ingredients included, should be fully qualified for growth promotion with a range of microorganisms to ensure the additive does not inhibit one microorganism type to allow other types to replicate. The additives/neutralizers mentioned in various pharmacopoeias[35] are generally assumed to be acceptable due to their widespread use.

An occasional problem with method suitability is that some product types are intended to be inhibitory, such as an antibiotic-containing product, a naturally inhibitory product such as latex, or products with residual chemicals, preservatives, or disinfectants that are expected parts of the manufacturing process. In these instances, extensive amounts of time and product may need to be expended to obtain acceptable results in the method suitability test. It is for these situations that the phrase in Clause 6.6 of ISO 11737-2[30] says " . . . a system to neutralize, remove, or, if this is not possible, minimize the effect of any such released substance shall be used." It is not expected that every combination of media, media additive(s), temperature, volume, etc, be tested until acceptable results are obtained for every microorganism type. It is expected that a reasonable attempt be made to obtain acceptable results for microorganisms that represent those commonly expected to be present. Although "reasonable attempt" is not defined in the standards, it would make sense that it may include using different media volumes, testing portions of the product in different containers, using different commercially available media types, and adding different neutralizers to the test media, where appropriate. If a reasonable attempt has been made, and one or more of the microorganisms is still not demonstrating consistent, comparable growth, it is appropriate to couple the incubation conditions giving the best results with a well-documented rationale, which can include a risk assessment. The rationale and, if performed, risk assessment, can address variables such as, for example, the amount of sterilization or disinfection being applied (ie, SAL or log reductions), the microorganism type that is demonstrating inhibition, whether the inhibition is complete or partial, and the use of the product on the patient. This type of rationale can vary significantly depending on the industry and use of the product.

There is one aspect of product sterility testing that is usually not variable, the incubation time. It is well accepted that an incubation time of 14 days is sufficient to allow the vast majority of microorganisms time to repair (if needed) or prepare for growth in the lag phase and move into the exponential phase and replicate to the point that the growth is visible in the media. The need for longer incubation times for most products is currently not substantiated. Modifications to the incubation period should only be addressed if there is a specific microorganism known to potentially be present that has definitively demonstrated the need for extended incubation.

Sterility Positive Results

After incubation, the results of a sterility test are determined based on the visual observation of turbidity in the growth media. It should be noted that sterility positive results may not always indicate a sterility failure. The purpose for which the test is being performed will dictate whether sterility positives constitute a sterility failure or acceptable results. Not all microbial growth appears the same in test media. Although sometimes the growth is obvious and evident throughout the media, some microorganisms do not dissociate, and the turbidity is more localized within the test container (see Figure 64.8). Other types of turbidity are not due to microorganism growth but can appear to be so. Some types of products can give the appearance of growth due to particulate matter coming from the product, substances leaching out of the product, or elements of the product itself, such as insoluble powders and viscous liquids.

Sterility positives, or potential sterility positives, should always be subcultured, both to verify that the turbidity is due to microorganism growth and to determine the type of microorganism present. Subculturing is performed in several ways, such as removing a small aliquot (eg, 0.5 mL or a loop full) and streaking onto an agar plate followed by incubation, or transferring a small aliquot (eg, not less than 1 mL) to another container of sterile media, followed by incubation. Verification of growth might also be performed by a simple microscopic examination of the media. It is best to verify growth, if needed, using more than one method due to the criticality of accurately scoring a product as positive or negative for growth.

Identification and Trending of Sterility Positives

As discussed earlier, sterility tests are performed for a variety of reasons. In most cases, the test is intended to provide important information regarding a manufacturing or sterilization process. Thus, it is usually important to identify all microorganisms that grow in sterility tests. Microorganism identifications are beneficial to a microbiologist in understanding likely source(s) and likely ways to reduce or eliminate its presence on/in the product. Trending of microorganisms identified from sterility positives is also a useful tool to help manufacturers understand whether the cause of the positive is a consistent issue or something that might be erratic or changing over time.

Not all sterility positives indicate a problem in manufacturing or sterilization. There are some instances where positives are expected, although usually at low frequencies. Those responsible for requesting and reviewing sterility test information must understand the purpose for which the testing is being performed and the criticality of sterility positives for that purpose. Sometimes, action is required when sterility positives occur, and sometimes, action is not required, based on the purpose for the test.

Investigation of Sterility Positives

It is usually important to perform an investigation of sterility positive results. The investigation might be as simple as identifying the microorganism and adding it to the trending information. During validation, a positive may trigger a detailed investigation to understand the design of the manufacturing process or terminal sterilization process under study. But the investigation might be as serious as halting manufacturing, quarantining product, and reviewing every piece of information related to the manufacture of the product batch. Regardless of the seriousness of the sterility positive, it is always important to start an investigation without any preconceived notions of the outcome. Preconceived notions about the cause of a sterility positive, or a sterility failure, can result in an insufficient investigation and lead to an incorrect root cause. All information available should be gathered and reviewed by a competent microbiologist prior to establishment of a conclusion regarding root cause and potential corrective and/or preventive actions. Important examples of information to review can include the test laboratory methods, controls, and practices during the preparation for, testing of, and incubation of samples, or any unique circumstances that can be identified in the review of the manufacturing processes or handling of products chosen for testing. Other quality indicators in these processes such as environmental monitoring data and sterilization process parameter monitors, when applicable, may provide useful information during such investigations.

RAPID MICROBIOLOGY METHODS FOR BIOBURDEN AND STERILITY TEST METHODS

Rapid microbiology methods (RMM) have different platforms, but the intent is always to detect viable microorganisms in a sample faster than is possible with the traditional methods of growth to the point of observation with the naked eye. Systems are available for both bioburden and sterility testing, although for both, there are some limitations. The systems currently available for sterility testing are either liquid-or filter-based, and the liquid volumes are often small. This means that it may not be possible to place a product into a liquid medium and to assay the sterility test medium while in the container with the product. It is usually required that an aliquot be drawn from the product to assay in the RMM equipment. Examples of RMM systems include adenosine triphosphate (ATP) detection (eg, Celsis Advance®, Growth Direct™, Milliflex®) and flow cytometry (eg, CHEMUNEX®, FACSMicroCount™). There is at least one platform that can perform the analysis on a tube containing the product, but the tube is small and thus the product must also be small (eg, BacT/ALERT®).[10,36,37]

The RMM have been available for many years for both bioburden and sterility tests, but incorporation of these methods into routine use in the sterilization industry has still not happened on a significant level. There is some routine use in other industries (eg, food and cosmetic) as both product release tests and as interim quality control tests. The greatest concern for incorporation of RMM in the eyes of medical device and pharmaceutical manufacturers, especially for release tests, is often cited as regulatory acceptance. This concern might be unfounded, as some regulatory bodies have demonstrated an openness to incorporation of RMM. To assist with RMM use, USP recently initiated a new chapter dedicated to providing guidance for product types that may gain the greatest potential benefit to RMM systems, such as products with a short shelf life.[38]

Another part of the concern for use of RMM might stem from the incorrect notion that the current microbiology test methods are the gold standard or are perfect. Simply because the standard 14-day sterility test is the tried-and-true legacy method, it should not be assumed that it is a perfect method and will be impossible to replicate or improve on in an RMM system. There are issues with the standard sterility test that leave some things to be desired. Scoring of samples as positive or negative is

dependent on a visual observation of growth in the medium, which does not occur until the titer achieves levels of approximately 10^5 or 10^6 CFU/mL. There are some microorganisms that either grow slowly or that only grow to a certain point and then slow or stop their growth due to competition with other microorganisms in the media. Many RMM can detect viable microorganisms at the level of 10^1 to 10^2 CFU/mL, which makes the test not only faster but more sensitive.

There is also a timeliness issue that can be improved with RMM systems. Using the traditional methods for product bioburden, sterility tests, and environmental monitoring, for example, results are obtained after 7 to 14 days at a minimum. Some RMM systems can provide results in a fraction of this time, lessening the risk associated with the lapse of time that occurs between taking the sample and being able to take any necessary actions due to the data obtained. Sometimes there are concerns that the newer methods must be proven to be superior to the traditional methods. This would result in significant validation work if that were the case. Fortunately, it appears that regulatory acceptance is more based on a demonstration that the RMM is not inferior to the traditional method, which is a less stringent requirement. In many cases, the RMM equipment manufacturer has performed significant testing to demonstrate the ability to detect growth of a wide variety of microorganisms and at low numbers. This can lessen the requirement for the users, who might only need to focus on proper implementation of the equipment and test method into their systems and then demonstrate feasibility with each product that is intended to be used.

REFERENCES

1. International Organization for Standardization. *ISO 11737-1:2018: Sterilization of Health Care Products—Microbiological Methods—Part 1: Determination of a Population of Microorganisms on Products.* Geneva, Switzerland: International Organization for Standardization; 2018.
2. United States Pharmacopeia. United States Pharmacopeia Web site. https://www.usp.org.
3. European Pharmacopoeia. European Pharmacopoeia (Ph. Eur.) 9th edition. European Pharmacopoeia Web site. https://www.edqm.eu/en/european-pharmacopoeia-ph-eur-9th-edition.
4. Japanese Pharmacopoeia. Japanese Pharmacopoeia 17th edition. Japanese Pharmacopoeia Web site. https://www.pmda.go.jp/english/rs-sb-std/standards-development/jp/0019.html.
5. International Organization for Standardization. *ISO 11137-2:2013: Sterilization of Health Care Products—Radiation—Part 2: Establishing the Sterilization Dose.* Geneva, Switzerland: International Organization for Standardization; 2013.
6. United States Pharmacopeia. *USP <71> Sterility Tests.* Bethesda, MD: United States Pharmacopeia; USP42-NF37.
7. American Association of Tissue Banks. *Microbiological Process Validation & Surveillance Program.* McLean, VA: American Association of Tissue Banks; 2016.
8. United States Pharmacopeia. *USP <61> Microbiological Examination of Nonsterile Products: Microbial Enumeration Tests.* Bethesda, MD: United States Pharmacopeia; USP42-NF37.

9. United States Pharmacopeia. *USP <55> Biological Indicators—Resistance Performance Tests.* Bethesda, MD: United States Pharmacopeia; USP42-NF37.

10. Lovatt A, Sandle T. *Guide to Bacterial Identification.* Stanstead Abbotts, United Kingdom: Pharmig; 2018.

11. Rintala H, Pitkäranta M, Täubel M. Microbial communities associated with house dust. *Adv Appl Microbiol.* 2012;78:75-120.

12. Barberán A, Dunn RR, Reich BJ, et al. The ecology of microscopic life in household dust. *Proc Biol Sci.* 2015;282:20151139.

13. Ren P, Jankun TM, Leaderer BP. Comparisons of seasonal fungal prevalence in indoor and outdoor air and in house dusts of dwellings in one Northeast American county. *J Expo Anal Environ Epidemiol.* 1999;9:560-568.

14. International Organization for Standardization. *ISO 11135:2014: Sterilization of Health Care Products—Ethylene Oxide—Requirements for Development, Validation and Routine Control of a Sterilization Process for Medical Devices.* Geneva, Switzerland: International Organization for Standardization; 2014.

15. International Organization for Standardization. *ISO 17665-1:2013: Sterilization of Health Care Products—Moist Heat—Part 1 Requirements for the Development, Validation and Routine Control of a Sterilization Process for Medical Devices.* Geneva, Switzerland: International Organization for Standardization; 2013.

16. International Organization for Standardization. *ISO 20857:2015: Sterilization of Health Care Products—Dry Heat—Requirements for the Development, Validation and Routine Control of a Sterilization Process for Medical Devices.* Geneva, Switzerland: International Organization for Standardization; 2015.

17. International Organization for Standardization. *ISO 14937:2009/(R)2013: Sterilization of Health Care Products—General Requirements for Characterization of a Sterilizing Agent and the Development, Validation and Routine Control of a Sterilization Process for Medical Devices.* Geneva, Switzerland: International Organization for Standardization; 2009.

18. International Organization for Standardization. *ISO 11137-1:2006: Sterilization of Health Care Products—Radiation—Part 1: Requirements for Development, Validation and Routine Control of a Sterilization Process for Medical Devices.* Geneva, Switzerland: International Organization for Standardization; 2006.

19. International Organization for Standardization. *ISO 13408-1:2008: Aseptic Processing Of Health Care Products—Part 1: General Requirements.* Geneva, Switzerland: International Organization for Standardization; 2008.

20. United States Pharmacopeia. *USP <1116> Microbiological Control and Monitoring of Aseptic Processing Environments.* Bethesda, MD: United States Pharmacopeia; 2018.

21. Cochran WG. Estimation of bacterial densities by means of the "most probable number." *Biometrics.* 1950;6:105-116.

22. Sutton S. The most probable number and its use in QC microbiology. *J GXP Compliance.* 2010;14(4):28-33.

23. Winters M, Patch E, Shepherd S, Teeples T. Consider the most probable number method for bioburden testing. MDDI Online Web site. https://www.mddionline.com/consider-most-probable-number-method-bioburden-testing. Accessed October 22, 2018.

24. Bryans T. Using bioburden spikes in radiation dose setting. *The Validation Consultant.* 1996;3(1):3-10.

25. Fairand B, Le V, Tumaitis Z. Statistical analysis of spikes in bioburden. *Radiat Phys Chem.* 2012;81:1241-1243.

26. Bryans T, Hansen J. The bioburden estimate: not just math, but microbiology. In: *Industrial Sterilization: Research from the Field.* Arlington, VA: Advancement of Medical Instrumentation; 2013:53-62.

27. Winters M, Patch E, Wangsgard W, Bushar H, Ferry A. Establishing bioburden alert and action levels. MDDI Online Web site. https://www.mddionline.com/establishing-bioburden-alert-and-action-levels. Accessed May 31, 2013.

28. United States Pharmacopeia. *USP <2023> Microbiological Attributes of Nonsterile Nutritional and Dietary Supplements.* Bethesda, MD: United States Pharmacopeia; USP42-NF37.

29. European Commission. *EU Guidelines to Good Manufacturing Practice Medicinal Products for Human and Veterinary Use, Annex 1 Manufacture of Sterile Medicinal Products.* Brussels, Belgium: European Commission; 2008.

30. International Organization for Standardization. *ISO 11737-2:2009: Sterilization of Medical Devices—Microbiological Methods—Part 2: Tests of Sterility Performed in the Definition, Validation and Maintenance of a Sterilization Process.* Geneva, Switzerland: International Organization for Standardization; 2009.

31. Bruch CW. The philosophy of sterilization validation. In: Morrissey RF, Phillips GB, eds. *Sterilization Technology.* New York, NY: Van Nostrand Reinhold; 1993.

32. Daniell E, Bryans T, Darnell K, Hansen J, Hitchins VM, Saavedra M. Product sterility testing . . . to test or not to test? That is the question. *Biomed Instrum Technol.* 2016;50(suppl 3):35-43.

33. US Environmental Protection Agency. *AOAC Sporicidal Activity of Disinfectants Test.* Washington, DC: US Environmental Protection Agency; 2018.

34. US Food and Drug Administration. *Guidance for Industry Sterile Drug Products Produced by Aseptic Processing—Current Good Manufacturing Practice.* Silver Spring, MD: US Food and Drug Administration; 2004.

35. United States Pharmacopeia. *USP <1227> Validation of Microbial Recovery from Pharmacopeial Articles.* Bethesda, MD: United States Pharmacopeia; USP42-NF37.

36. Henriques J, Cardoso C, Vitorino C. Rapid microbiological methods. They are rapid! Are they fast? In: *Research Trends of Microbiology.* Reno, Nevada: MedDocs Publishers; 2019.

37. Moldenhauer J, ed. *Rapid Sterility Testing.* Bethesda, MD: PDA/DHI; 2011.

38. United States Pharmacopeia. *USP <1071> Rapid Sterility Testing of Short-Life Products: A Risk-Based Approach.* Bethesda, MD: United States Pharmacopeia. In press.

Biological Indicators, Chemical Indicators, and Parametric Release

Richard Bancroft

The number of microorganisms can decrease exponentially during exposure to a steady-state disinfection or sterilization process; only by infinite exposure to a defined antimicrobial process can the absence of all viable microorganisms be assured with certainty. At the same time, it is acknowledged that indefinite exposure to the antimicrobial agent is impractical and may have deleterious effects on the device or product being processed, especially when this involves sterilization by heat or irradiation. A compromise must be struck between assuring the sterility of the final device or product and ensuring that the device or product remains fit for purpose. For sterilization processes, as an example, the concept of a sterility assurance level (SAL) can therefore be used to "measure" or define the level of exposure to a sterilization process, with the result expressed in terms of a probability of a surviving microorganism (see chapter 2).[1] Once defined, through validation studies, what process is needed in order to achieve a given disinfected or sterile state, the attributes of this process can then be monitored to ensure that the process is performing to its specification. These attributes may be chemical or physical in nature, and changes in them can alter the process effectiveness; these are known as process variables, with examples including time and temperature. The specified value for a process variable is known as a process parameter. Sterilization processes are particularly defined, or specified, according to their process parameters. Biological and chemical indicators (CIs), as well as physical sensors, are used to ensure that these process parameters are attained and are used both in defining this process specification as well as ensuring the process maintains its specification by means of process monitoring.

▶ BIOLOGICAL INDICATORS

Commercial biological indicators (BIs) are products containing known numbers of disinfectant-resistant or sterilant-resistant microorganisms deposited on a carrier that are often in the form of either metal foil, paper strips, or discs; BIs are also available in a self-contained format (Figure 65.1). These self-contained BIs (SCBIs) consist of the spore-inoculated carrier and a separate sealed container with the microbiological recovery media all packaged together within an ampoule or a container. This packaging also contains a sterilant-permeable filter that allows the SCBI to be used without any disassembly. After processing, the recovery medium is released from its sealed container to allow it to be in contact with the spore-inoculated carrier, and the BI can be incubated as a whole unit. The BIs can also be created by directly inoculating a suspension of microorganisms directly onto or into a product or device. The BIs are often used within a process challenge device (PCD) that is designed to create a defined challenge to the process. For disinfection process monitoring, BIs typically use vegetative microorganisms (see chapter 65); bacterial endospores, or spores, are typically used for sterilization processes because they can be extremely resistant to inactivation. These microorganisms are also selected based on their safety to those using them. Any large numbers of microorganisms should be treated with care to minimize any opportunity for human infection, hence the use of microorganisms that do not require special containment facilities due to being nonpathogenic is always preferred. These reference microorganisms will typically have a resistance to the disinfection or sterilization process that is significantly greater than many common bioburden microorganisms (see chapter 64). The population of the test organism can vary according to the intended application of the BI; for disinfection process monitoring, vegetative microorganisms are used in a range of populations that may be as low as 1×10^3 microorganisms per BI, to much higher. For sterilization process monitoring, the population per BI is typically in the range of 1×10^5 to 5×10^6 bacterial endospores per BI. The BI chosen will provide a challenge to the disinfection or sterilization process through a combination of

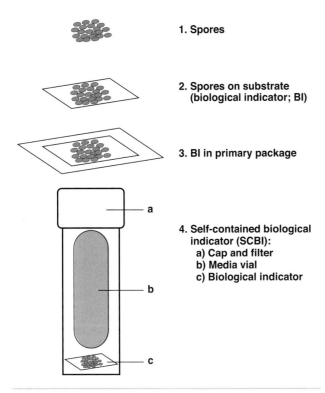

1. **Spores**

2. **Spores on substrate (biological indicator; BI)**

3. **BI in primary package**

4. **Self-contained biological indicator (SCBI):**
   a) Cap and filter
   b) Media vial
   c) Biological indicator

— a

— b

— c

FIGURE 65.1 Components of a biological indicator and self-contained biological indicator.

the microorganism population, and its resistance to the process. For product loads that naturally have either high bioburden or very resistant microorganisms, the reference microorganisms can be used as a basis for understanding and then defining the disinfection or sterilization process.

Microorganisms are inoculated onto the BI carrier and are usually protected from mechanical abrasion or contamination by a disinfectant- or sterilant-permeable package, such as a glassine peel-pouch or similar, allowing the BI to be used either within this packaging or removed and used simply as an inoculated carrier. The BIs containing bacterial spores are typically more stable in use and storage, whereas BIs containing vegetative cells are much more labile and may need to be manufactured and used in a very short time, sometimes as short as a few hours. Commercially available BIs should be carefully stored according to the labeled storage conditions and not used beyond their labeled expiry date.

The carrier onto which the microorganisms are inoculated is usually selected depending on the type of process that the BI will be used to test or monitor. Hard, and largely inert, surfaces like stainless steel and some polymeric substrates have advantages in being robust and largely not interfering with the process they are used within; however, the specific design of these carriers must consider physical protection, during handling and use, of the surface where microorganisms are inoculated. Carriers based on cellulose, such as filter paper, can afford this physical protection but may not be suitable for use in some processes based on fluids such as found in washer-disinfectors and heat-based fluid sterilization processes. In addition, some oxidative chemistries may interact with these cellulosic materials or bind the disinfectant or sterilizing agent such that false-negative results are created.

As mentioned earlier, a BI can be manufactured by directly inoculating an actual device or product with microorganisms. This approach has the advantage that placement of the microorganisms on the device intended to be disinfected or sterilized can be in a location that has been considered to be the most challenging to the process. It can also assess any inherent interactions between the device or product and the microorganism; the resistance of a microorganism to a specific disinfection or sterilization process may be increased or reduced if it is exposed to physicochemical factors on or within the product being processed, such as pharmaceutical actives. This approach does create additional practical consequences; recovery of the microorganism can present challenges, particularly if enumeration of any surviving organisms is necessary because a recovery validation will need to be conducted to ensure that an acceptable microorganism recovery is acceptable. Typically, recovery methods will use either simple elution to remove the microorganisms or a more aggressive method such as abrasion with ballotini beads (small glass beads to aid in mechanical removal) or by ultrasonication (see chapter 64). The intent is to maximize recovery while minimizing potential damage or destruction of the microorganism. If the intent is to simply determine growth or no growth of the microorganism, it may be acceptable to immerse the entire device in recovery media and observe for the presence of growth by turbidity of the media. But there may be practical implications of this approach; examples include if the device is very large, such as a large endoscope, or ensuring that the recovery media is in contact with all parts of the device, including any internal channels or areas. Direct inoculation has other consequences too, such as the need to ensure that aseptic technique is observed throughout, from inoculation to recovery, and that any microorganism detected by growth must be determined to be the reference microorganism that was originally inoculated, and not an environmental contaminant.

The microorganism used in a BI is typically selected based on a prior knowledge of which microorganism is most resistant to a given disinfection or sterilization modality; for example, *Geobacillus stearothermophilus* spores are generally considered to be the most resistant to moist heat sterilization processes. There are of course other considerations for the most suitable microorganism; these may include safety (pathogenic microorganisms are generally avoided unless there are specific justifications why these should be used). Labile organisms may be also unsuitable. Depending on whether the process is a disinfection or sterilization process, as mentioned earlier, the known microbial challenge is usually composed of aerobic bacterial endospores, predominantly *Bacillus* and *Geobacillus* species, although occasionally *Clostridium* species may be used, based on their resistance to a given sterilization process. The BIs are, therefore, characterized by the strain of test organism, the number of colony-forming units per BI, the D-value (decimal reduction value) determined under defined (and specified) conditions, and the Z-value (relating the heat resistance of a microorganism to changes in temperature) (see chapter 2).

The International Organization for Standardization (ISO), based in Geneva, Switzerland, has published a range of product standards for BIs used in sterilization processes. The ISO 11138 series of standards gives prescriptive requirements for a range of BI properties for the different sterilization modalities. General requirements for BIs are given in ISO 11138-1,[2] and specific requirements for BIs are given in ISO 11138-2 for ethylene oxide sterilization,[3] ISO 11138-3 for moist heat sterilization,[4] ISO 11138-4 for dry heat sterilization,[5] and ISO 11138-5 for low-temperature steam and formaldehyde.[6] Recommended reference strains of the microorganisms are as follows:

Steam and other moist heat processes: *G stearothermophilus* spores
Low temperature vaporized hydrogen peroxide processes: *G stearothermophilus* spores
Dry heat processes: *Bacillus atrophaeus* spores
Ethylene oxide sterilization: *B atrophaeus* spores

Note that BIs are not commonly used for ionizing radiation processes, but *Bacillus pumilus* has been used as the reference resistant organism in the past.

The ISO 11138 series of standards also specifies the spore population range, the D-value under defined conditions, the Z-value (where applicable), and standardized labeling requirements, including the lot and expiry date. The resistance of a microorganism to a disinfection or sterilization process is defined as the D-value, which is also sometimes known as the D_{10} value. The D-value is defined as the time or dose required to achieve inactivation of 90% of a population of the test microorganisms, under stated conditions. This 90% inactivation or population reduction is sometimes referred to as a 1 log reduction. The basis for the calculation for D-values is based on microbial inactivation typically following first-order reaction kinetics. When BIs are used for thermal disinfection or sterilization, the Z-value is used to describe the temperature susceptibility of the microorganism; this is more precisely defined as the change in temperature of the thermal disinfection or sterilization process that produces 10 times change in D-value. For example, if the Z-value is 10°C, this means that if the temperature of the process is increased by 10°C, there will be a 10-fold reduction in D-value of that microorganism at that temperature.

INCUBATION OF BIOLOGICAL INDICATORS

Following exposure to the disinfection or sterilization process, BIs must be cultured as soon as possible after the process in suitable media and under appropriate recovery conditions, as specified by the manufacturer. Handling of the BIs must be done aseptically in order to prevent contamination or cross-contamination. In the simplest approach to the use of BIs, they can be immersed in the appropriate recovery media and incubated at the correct temperature for the minimum incubation time, and the result expressed as either the presence of growth or no growth, usually detected by turbidity. A much more complicated approach counts, or enumerates, any surviving organisms, first by removing the microorganisms from the carrier, then serially diluting and plating onto recovery media (agar) plates, before incubation. In order to enumerate a BI, the viable microorganisms must be removed from their carrier, ideally as soon as possible after being exposed to the disinfection or sterilization process, as microorganisms that may have been damaged, but still viable, may not be able to survive without growth media. Removal from the carrier can be carried out using a number of methods that are not damaging to the microorganisms (see chapter 64). These include elution, gentle mechanical abrasion using sterile ballotini beads (small glass beads) in water, or by ultrasonication. The recovery efficacy of this process should be determined as well as the limitation of microbial detection during the recovery and incubation process. Once the microorganisms are in solution, they can be enumerated by plating onto agar plates and incubated. By assuming that each colony that forms originates from a single microorganism, it is possible to then calculate the number of microorganisms that survived the process. It is very difficult to count the colonies that form if there are more than 250 colonies per typical agar plate; because it is not possible to know if there are large numbers of microorganisms surviving from the BI, it is normal practice to serially dilute the extracted sample using sterile water or another diluent. Typically, 1 mL of sample is added to 9 mL of sterile water, thus creating a 10-fold reduction in count per dilution; a number of these dilutions can then be plated onto recovery media for enumeration.

The recovery media can have a significant effect on the performance of the BI as a whole; small changes in the formulation of the recovery medium can have great consequences for the growth of the organism. If no growth occurs, the level of lethality can be calculated to be greater than the logarithm of the population of the BI; in the event of growth occurring, it is sometimes considered necessary to establish whether the growth is derived from the original inoculum or whether it represents accidental contamination during handling or culturing.

During incubation, detection of growth of the reference microorganism can be by a number of methods. The most basic of these is the presence of turbidity (or cloudiness in the media); this may be quite difficult to see in an SCBI format, hence commercially available SCBIs typically include a pH indicator within the recovery media. As microorganism germination and subsequent growth occurs, there is an associated drop in pH as the microorganisms digest the recovery media. This drop in pH causes the pH indicator to change color, hence showing microorganism growth and a positive (ie, growth) result. The incubation time taken to germinate and grow these microorganisms is dependent on many factors, but a 7-day incubation is a standard reference incubation time for normal growth conditions of bacterial spores. Many commercially available BIs have been validated by their manufacturers to have a significantly shorter incubation time than the reference period and can reduce the incubation time to typically around 24 hours. In recent years, other methods of detecting early germination and growth of the reference microorganism have reduced the potential incubation time down to as little as 20 minutes. This has been achieved by adding a nonfluorescent α-glucosidase substrate to the recovery media; as the microorganisms germinate, the substrate is metabolized by the microorganisms, resulting in formation of a fluorescent compound. This fluorescence can be detected using purpose-made incubators that incorporate fluorescent detection capabilities. Other methods for detection of microbial growth are also available.

▶ USE OF BIOLOGICAL INDICATORS

The BIs are used extensively in disinfection and sterilization cycle validation and in routine monitoring of these processes. They integrate all the process variables such as time, temperature, gas or chemical concentration, humidity, etc. In common with CIs (see the following text), because BIs are placed directly in the container or load, they will reflect the actual process conditions in or on the product or load itself, rather than just in the environment in which the container or load has been placed. As mentioned earlier, BIs generally use a bacterial or other microorganism strain that has been specially selected for its high resistance to the given process. Moreover, because the microorganisms on the BIs are likely to present considerably more of a challenge in terms of population and resistance to the process than the expected bioburden of the product, then considerable confidence can be placed in the expected level of process or sterility assurance associated with the process.

Further information for BIs used in sterilization processes employed in the manufacture of sterile medical devices can be obtained from ISO 11138 Part 7 that gives guidance on the use and application of BIs.[7] Use of BIs requires a good appreciation of aseptic technique; the BIs that are recovered after processing need to be aseptically transferred to microbiological recovery media without contamination. Any forceps or tools used to place the BI in position prior to processing must of course be

subsequently sterilized before they are used to remove the processed BIs from within the load or PCD; otherwise, false-positive results may occur due to contamination with the reference organism. These aseptic handling issues are largely mitigated using SCBIs, at the expense of a much larger unit, making the SCBI more difficult to place into inaccessible parts of the load.

The BIs may be used for three main purposes: disinfection/sterilization cycle development, validation, and routine monitoring of processes. During cycle development, the ability of a given process to destroy a challenge from resistant organisms must be assessed. The microorganisms on or within the load can originate from a number of sources, including raw materials, operators, or the production environment itself. Once their resistance has been characterized, test microorganisms can then be used as resistant microbiological reference standards. From purely a sterilization perspective, the term *validation* describes tests on a sterilizer, sterilization process and a given product to determine that the sterilization process operates efficiently and performs repeatedly as expected (other aspects must also be considered, such as device and material compatibility; however, these aspects are outside the scope of this chapter; see chapter 5). Any validation exercise must therefore assess not only the physical performance of the sterilizer but also the sterilization performance of the process on the product. The term *monitoring*, on the other hand, implies the routine control of a process.

The use of BIs in practice depends not only on the regulatory requirements of the country or region in question but also on the efficacy of alternative methods. In some instances, they represent the only practical method of monitoring of some sterilization cycles, whereas in other situations, physical and CI methods offer a much more reliable and efficient alternative. But in practice, careful use of both BIs, CIs, and physical parameter monitoring are all routinely used. On an industrial scale, routine monitoring of moist heat (steam), ethylene oxide, and irradiation sterilization are largely based on physical parameter measurement (and ultimately allows for parametric release, see the following text); however, the use of BIs in routine monitoring is still prevalent, largely because this is a custom and practice, or a regulatory requirement in some parts of the world. Smaller scale or hospital use of ethylene oxide sterilization, for example, would not necessarily have the expensive ethylene oxide concentration monitoring equipment and so would place increased reliance on BIs, in combination with other methods, namely physical parameter and CI monitoring. In some circumstances, BIs may be used as part of the validation program for moist or dry heat sterilization cycles. But they have little use in routine monitoring cycles because the required SAL can be defined in terms of easily and reliably measured physical parameters (see chapter 28). Occasionally, their use may be justified in performance qualification (PQ), when difficulties arise in ensuring adequate contact and penetration of steam in a particular product or load.

With sterilization by irradiation, BIs are regarded to be of little value because the process is defined in terms of a minimum absorbed dose of radiation, best and most reliably measured by dosimeters (see chapter 29). These dosimeters may also be forms of CIs (see the following text); however, they are not defined in the same way as many CIs due to their very specific ad restricted application; these dosimeters are used to calibrate and monitor the dose as an absorbed dose of radiation, usually measured in grays or kilograys (Gy or kGy). Dosimeters are located on or adjacent to the items being irradiated during each load. In some countries, BI use is obligatory for routine monitoring of irradiation sterilization in each batch. During validation work, they may be used for initial characterization of inactivation rates within a given product.

▶ CHEMICAL INDICATORS

The CIs are test systems that indicate, usually by way of a color change, a reaction to one or more predefined disinfection or sterilization process variables, resulting from exposure to that process. This color change is then interpreted by the user, according to the instructions provided by the CI manufacturer. The point of the color change is defined as the endpoint. The CIs are available for many types of disinfection or sterilization process, and specific forms of CIs are available for monitoring of adjunct processes such as washing, which would typically take place in a washer-disinfector, especially in the decontamination of reusable medical devices (Figure 65.2).

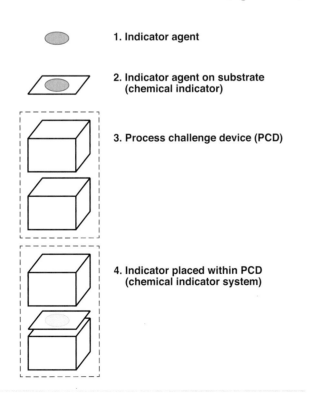

1. Indicator agent

2. Indicator agent on substrate (chemical indicator)

3. Process challenge device (PCD)

4. Indicator placed within PCD (chemical indicator system)

FIGURE 65.2 Components of chemical indicator and process challenge device.

The performance of CIs for sterilization processes are specified by ISO in ISO 11140-1,[8] where they are identified according to the sterilization process that they are designed to be used in, and the type of CI based on their intended application and function (see the following text). Their reliability, stability, and safety must also be considered when choosing which type of CI is best suited to the application. As is the case for any disinfection or sterilization process monitor, CIs should be viewed as one of several complementary indicators of process conditions that include both biological and physical sensors (such as temperature probes). The CIs are typically marked with their lot number and expiry date, together with storage criteria. In all cases, the instructions given by the manufacturer must be followed if the CIs are to function as specified.

ISO 11140-1[8] defines six types of CI for sterilization process monitoring that have different functions, and these must be considered when choosing which to use:

- Type 1 CIs, sometimes referred to as process indicators, are intended for use with individual packs or load components to show that the load component has been exposed to a sterilization process (ie, to show that a load item has been processed, eg, autoclave tape or adhesive labels with an indicator printed onto it). This type of indicator does not indicate that the load has been processed correctly, so are typically used to differentiate between load items that have been sterilized to those that have not been processed.
- Type 2 CIs are designed for use in specific test procedures, such as the Bowie-Dick test.[9] ISO 17665-1[10] requires that a steam penetration test, or Bowie-Dick test, is performed at the commencement of each day (after a warm-up cycle) in all prevacuum steam sterilizers to assess the ability of the sterilizer to penetrate steam into a load of defined resistance (see chapter 28). The Bowie-Dick test consists of a stack of standardized cotton towels and a specific CI placed into the center; if rapid and even steam penetration occurs, an even color change will result. Any air remaining in the center of the towel pack (ie, a steam penetration fault) will be evident by a noncomplete color change of the CI. A Bowie-Dick test should be placed into an otherwise empty chamber because this is the worst case scenario for steam penetration.
- Type 3 CIs will respond only to a single sterilization variable, such as time or temperature. As such, class 3 indicators are not usually considered useful in processes that have two or more critical variables.
- Type 4 CIs are multivariable indicators that will respond to two or more of the variables for the sterilization process for which they are intended. These indicators are designed to be placed within the load to monitor attainment of sterilization critical variables.

- Type 5 CIs are designed to integrate all sterilization variables and to be equivalent to, or exceed, the performance of reference BIs that are specified in the ISO 11138 series. These indicators are designed to be placed within the load to monitor attainment of sterilization critical variables.
- Type 6 CIs, sometimes termed *cycle verification indicators*, are designed to integrate all sterilization variables, with their performance correlated to the actual settings of the sterilization cycle. These CIs are designed to be placed within the load to monitor attainment of sterilization critical variables.

Types 3, 4, 5, and 6 CIs are additionally defined by the CI manufacturer in terms of their performance by stated values (SVs). These SVs effectively define the parameters of each sterilization variable that the CI will respond to; SVs should be carefully considered by the user to ensure that the performance of the indicator is suitable for their intended application. For example, a type 6 indicator may have SVs of 134°C and 3.5 minutes. This means that the indicator will reach its endpoint (point of color change) after 3.5 minutes at 134°C. It therefore stands to reason that this indicator is suited to monitoring a 134°C, 3.5-minute sterilization process. If the same indicator were to be used in a 134°C, 18-minute process, for example, the indicator would be giving much less information about the total process; in this latter case, an indicator with SVs of 134°C and 18 minutes would be more appropriate.

DOSIMETERS USED IN RADIATION STERILIZATION MONITORING

Although rarely referenced as CIs, dosimeters are a specific type of indicator commonly used for validation and routine control of sterilization processes using radiation, such as exposure to ^{60}Co and other forms of ionizing radiation (see chapter 29). One common form of dosimeter is that based on alanine. Alanine dosimeters contain crystalline alanine and a wax binder that allows them to be compressed into a pellet shape and then packaged. The pellet is placed throughout the load to be irradiated. During processing, the alanine within the dosimeter registers the absorbed dose by the formation of alanine-derived free radicals. These free radicals are then analyzed using an electron paramagnetic resonance spectrometer. The dose calculation is then performed, typically within the range of 0.5 to 150 kGy (depending on the design of the dosimeter). Other forms of dosimeter are those based on polymethylmethacrylate (PMMA) and a red or yellow dye, depending on the absorbed dose range that they will be used within (eg, Red 4034 or Amber 3042); these are sometimes referred to as Harwell dosimeters based on their origin (Harwell, near Oxford, United Kingdom, as the site of the UK Atomic Energy Authority).

When these dyes are impregnated into PMMA and then exposed to absorbed radiation doses, the color darkens; this darkening is proportional to the absorbed radiation dose. Dosimeters can then be analyzed using a spectrophotometer.

USE OF CHEMICAL INDICATORS

The CIs have the advantage over other forms of process monitors in that they are very cost-effective and can be easily located within load items to monitor the conditions delivered to what may otherwise be very difficult areas of the load to monitor. Combined with their simple-to-read endpoint, they form a very useful tool for process validation and routine load monitoring. Although CIs have either a qualitative or semiquantitative response (they do not normally give a quantification or numerical value of the variables they have been exposed to), they can easily discriminate between different media such as air and steam in a steam sterilizer; air and steam may exist together at the same temperature during a steam sterilization process, hence will appear to be identical to a physical parameter sensor such as a thermocouple; however, from a microbiological perspective, the difference in lethality between these two media will be very marked and can also be detected by the use of a correctly specified BI.

One disadvantage in using CIs is during the routine monitoring of internal loads of a sterilization process, where the CI result may not be visible to the operator at the completion of the sterilization process due to the positioning of the CI deep within the load and visually inaccessible due to the sterile barrier system in use. This limitation does not apply when CIs are placed within the load in a manner where they can be seen without opening the sterile barrier system, for example, via a sterile packaging peel pouch that has a clear film side to allow viewing of the contents as well as the CI. This limitation also does not apply when the CI is used for sterilization process validation. When the CI is used for routine process monitoring, it is usual for the CI to be placed within a defined commercially available or user-assembled PCD or test pack. The PCD is designed to provide a disinfectant or sterilant penetration challenge and allows the CI to be removed from the PCD and immediately interpreted at the conclusion of the process.

VALIDATION AND ROUTINE CONTROL USING INDICATORS

Validation is the process of objectively assessing and recording that a process delivers its expected outcome. This validation process is typically broken down into installation qualification (IQ), operational qualification (OQ), and PQ. The BI and CIs can be used during both OQ and

PQ tests and can be applied equally to disinfection and sterilization processes; the same general principles apply to both processes.

Regardless of the method of disinfection or sterilization, the specification, construction, installation, and operation of the disinfector or sterilizer are fundamental to disinfection or sterility assurance. Before being taken into routine use, correct functioning of the equipment must be shown, first by a process of IQ, then OQ, and finally by PQ. The responsibility for these tasks is typically different for each stage and usually involves the equipment manufacturer, the installer, and the legal user of the equipment. The IQ involves the demonstration and certification that all parts of the equipment have been correctly installed, all measuring instruments have been correctly calibrated and all other items of equipment comply with their performance specifications. During OQ, it must be demonstrated that, for any given load, the disinfector or sterilizer performs reliably under automatic control, and that disinfection or sterilization conditions are attained within every part of the load. Test and surrogate loads are often used at this stage to show that these conditions are capable of being delivered to defined loads. These tests and loads may contain BIs and/or CIs. The European standard for steam sterilizers, EN 285,[11] for example, gives type and performance test requirements that could be used as part of the OQ stage that include performing a steam penetration test (eg, Bowie-Dick test) that is based on the performance of a CI. The ISO standard for the validation and routine control of steam sterilization, ISO 17665-1,[10] gives specific information for moist heat sterilization validation and process monitoring and makes extensive references to the use of biological and CIs. Further guidance in this area is given in part 2 of this standard, ISO/TS 17665-2.[12] Records of the results of indicator used, together with permanent records of the physical process monitoring, in the form of chart recordings, computer printouts, or electronic data archives, will provide evidence that disinfection or sterilization conditions have been generated in the load.

Tests carried out during OQ and PQ studies will vary according to the method of sterilization used. In the example of a sterilization process employing heat as one of the process variables, heat distribution and penetration studies are undertaken using thermocouples positioned at strategically determined places within the chamber and load. These functional tests, as discussed earlier, prove that the equipment and process are performing to specification. But it must then be shown that these conditions within the chamber are simultaneously provided within the microenvironments throughout the load. One of the limitations of using thermocouples is the difficulty in gaining access to all parts of the load, particularly narrow lumens. The CIs may be more easily placed within devices that may be disassembled, and in cases where even this is not possible, BIs in the form of inoculated microorganisms may be used. Such tests would normally need to be reviewed and if necessary repeated if there is any change in such variables as product type, shape, or size of load. In the case of irradiation sterilization, the penetration of the ionizing radiation within the load is best monitored using an adequate number of dosimeters, again strategically distributed, based on the type of load. Where gas sterilizers are used, the process variables, such as temperature, relative humidity, and gas concentration, are measured by physical sensors within the chamber and/or load and supported by the results of BIs and CIs. Indicators may also be used during routine process monitoring to demonstrate attainment of the critical parameters necessary for sterilization, although use of a BI alone in full-cycle conditions may not solely be capable of demonstrating an SAL of 10^{-6} needed for a declaration of sterility using the overkill method of sterility assurance.[13]

Disinfection and sterilization practices place much greater emphasis on the concept of process assurance, rather than reliance on end-product testing. By understanding the kinetics of microbial inactivation, individual protocols can be designed to destroy a known and previously determined bioburden with a desired level of confidence in the specified process. In other words, by introducing the notion of a required margin of safety, the probability of detecting a viable survivor of a sterilizing process can be assessed on a mathematical scale, known as the sterility assurance level, or SAL, as mentioned earlier. This process will be practically different for disinfection processes as the result is not destruction of all microorganisms, but similar concepts can be applied. As a result, by investing confidence in process validation practices, a system of parametric release can be used for approval of products, as discussed in detail later.

A specific microbial population, exposed to a given process, will have a characteristic response, and the death curve often follows a logarithmic pattern. It will also depend on the resistance of the organism concerned, the physicochemical environment where the treatment takes place, and the lethality of the process itself. If these do not vary, the number of survivors in a known population can be computed after a given period of exposure to the lethal process. Microbial death can be measured in terms of the D-value, as discussed earlier. For a steam sterilization process, if the original population is 10^2 spores and if the D-value is 1 minute at 121°C, then by definition, after 1 minute at 121°C, the population will have been reduced to 10^1 spores. For each additional minute of exposure to the sterilization cycle, a further reduction of 1 log cycle in the population will ensue. Thus, after an 8-minute cycle at 121°C, the population will have been reduced by an estimated total of 8 log cycles, that is, from 10^2 to 10^{-6}. The importance of minimizing bioburden levels in any product prior to disinfection or sterilization is therefore immediately obvious.

The earlier discussion also highlights one of the limitations of using BIs for routine process monitoring, when the overkill approach to sterility assurance is used. In the health care setting, many health care facilities adopt this overkill approach, where sterilization cycles are designed in theory to inactivate considerably larger populations than are likely to be present in actual situations. The advantage of this approach is that knowledge of the bioburden is not necessary, although sensible precautions need to be taken to keep this bioburden as low as reasonably possible. A conservatively high bioburden of 1×10^6 microorganisms per load is assumed. It is also assumed that the bioburden microorganisms have a lower resistance (ie, D-value) than the reference microorganism for the process; in the case of steam sterilization, this is *G stearothermophilus* spores. When considering that loads reprocessed would have been cleaned and often disinfected (in a washer-disinfector) prior to packaging under controlled conditions, it is highly unlikely that both the number and the resistant nature of the reference organism would ever be observed. When validating such processes, the total log reduction of such a resistant test microorganism required is 12, from an initial population of 1×10^6 to an SAL of 1×10^{-6}. As BIs typically do not contain a population of bacterial spores significantly above 1×10^6, to validate this process, it is necessary to halve the cycle exposure time that it is anticipated will be necessary; so if a steam sterilization cycle exposure time is anticipated to be, for example, 134°C for 3 minutes, the validation cycles will be conducted at 134°C for 1.5 minutes. If the microorganisms on the BIs used in these cycles with a population of 1×10^6 are rendered nonviable, it is then known that a half cycle can achieve a 6 $\log_{10}$ reduction. Using simple mathematics, a half cycle achieving a 6 $\log_{10}$ reduction means that a full cycle (in this example, 3 minutes) will achieve a 12 $\log_{10}$ reduction. Applying the assumption of a theoretical starting bioburden of 1×10^6 microorganisms, the 12 $\log_{10}$ cycle will achieve the required SAL of 1×10^{-6}. The same concept can be applied using lower populations of spores to test other fractional sterilization cycle conditions (eg, a 4 $\log_{10}$ reduction at a quarter cycle). The BIs with a population of 1×10^6 spores will only be able to monitor half of this process, hence are not always the most suitable indicator; CIs, however, may be calibrated such that they will reach their endpoint at the full, rather than half-cycle conditions.

There are two components to process validation: selection and then validation of the disinfection or sterilization process. This is followed by routine monitoring of each cycle. Once the disinfection or sterilization process is defined and validated, it must then be monitored using the most appropriate methods available. As highlighted earlier, in practice, there is not one single approach that is adequate to monitor all aspects of a disinfection or sterilization process, so a combined approach, using BIs, CIs, and physical sensors, such as temperature probes, can be used.

PARAMETRIC RELEASE

The method of assuring disinfection or sterility by monitoring the physical conditions of the applicable process and then release of the load or product is termed *parametric release*. It is defined as a declaration that product is disinfected or sterile based on records demonstrating that the process variables were delivered within specified tolerances.[14] Parametric release can be used for product release from many sterilization processes, including steam, ethylene oxide, vaporized hydrogen peroxide, dry heat, and ionizing radiation, where the sterilization variables are understood and can be adequately monitored. If the sterilization variables are not sufficiently understood or cannot be adequately monitored, parametric monitoring is not possible and alternative means of product release are necessary. The same fundamental principles can be applied also to disinfection processes, where the load will be released, of course, as disinfected, rather than sterile.

Parametric release is accepted as the preferential method for the release of sterile products. Products or devices exposed in their final packaging to predetermined, fully validated sterilization using steam, vaporized hydrogen peroxide, ethylene oxide, dry heat, or ionizing radiation may be batch released on the basis of accumulated process data. Through parametric release, the user can provide assurance that the product or device conforms to specification, that is, sterile. By reviewing holistically the upstream manufacturing and preparation of the load, the documentation of successful validation of the sterilization process, together with the process monitoring data of each process and load as well as the outcome of routine equipment checks and tests and evidence of required maintenance activities, the user can make an informed decision that the load has been processed according to the predetermined process specification and can then release the load as sterile.

Parametric release is common practice in the sterile medical device industry for the release of product batches sterilized by many processes, providing that the requirements of applicable sterilization process standards are met. If alternative methods of sterilization are used, other means of product release may be required, depending on the type of device, company practice, or the intended destination of the product. Other methods of load release may be by evidence of nonviable BIs and/or successful sterility tests. When using parametric release, the responsible entity must demonstrate not only sufficient control of the general manufacturing or assembly process (based on both historical and current batch data) but also that the sterilization process is adequately validated and reliably controlled and meets the requirements of the relevant regulations. In particular, standard operating procedures (SOPs) of significance for sterility should be in place to ensure sufficient quality assurance of the starting and packaging materials and the manufacturing environment. The SOPs should also detail the reporting and course of action to be taken for both approval and rejection of devices or product. Regarding sterilization issues, the choice of a sterilization method must be well founded, based on either device manufacturers' reprocessing instructions (eg, with reusable devices; see chapter 47), or knowledge of product stability and information gained during development studies. Qualification of sterilization equipment and validation of the process (eg, heat distribution and sterilizing agent penetration studies for a given load, accompanied by thermometric and/or biological validation) are expected to be demonstrated. Once defined, the sterilization process should be shown to be reproducible and appropriate, based on the appropriate method of sterilization validation. Moreover, specific requirements for parametric release must be met, for example, segregation of sterilized from nonsterile products. This latter point may be addressed both by the use of pass-through (double-ended) sterilizers as well as the use of process CIs that indicate that loads have been exposed to a sterilization process.

In the case of ionizing radiation sterilization, parametric release can be applied to those products exposed to a minimum absorbed dose, such as 25 kGy. But lower doses may be acceptable if justified by low, routinely checked bioburden levels and adequate validation data.[15] Once parametric release has been approved as the releasing mechanism, release or rejection decisions of a batch must then be based on the approved specification.

Regardless of the disinfection or sterilization process, no process can be considered in isolation but must be viewed in the context of good manufacturing practice (GMP), enforced by regulatory agencies around the world, or a quality management system (QMS) such as that detailed in ISO 9001[16] and ISO 13485.[17] A discussion of these GMP or QMS requirements is outside the scope of this chapter, but essentially, they require minimum standards and consistency in manufacture based on a well-developed system of documentation and record-keeping (see chapter 70). Thus, all records associated with the sterilization process itself must be retained for reference purposes, including sterilizer planned preventive maintenance and breakdown records, physical parameter monitoring records, indicator results and experimental data on bioburden and D-values, as well as protocols and their validation. Regulatory agencies and/or notified bodies would expect to scrutinize all appropriate results with BIs and CIs, along with the records of any ancillary processes such as cleaning and microbiological monitoring of associated controlled environmental areas; equipment maintenance and calibration; personnel training and qualification; and control over the packaging, labeling, wrapping, handling, and storage of sterile items.

When parametric release is used, due to the increased reliance on parametric data, it is usual to have process monitoring sensors that are independent of the control function. These independent sensors may be placed in the same location as those that control the process or may be placed in additional locations that have been determined as being representative of the actual loads being processed, through process validation studies. The independent sensors will typically have limiting values (process tolerances) that were determined during validation, and particularly PQ, where knowledge of the relationship of the load to these sensor outputs will be generated. Depending on which sterilization processes are used, an understanding of one variable, such as pressure, can be derived from a different variable, such as sterilizing agent concentration or temperature. The BIs and CIs are often used to supplement the parametric data that is generated. Typically, all sensor results, together with indicator results, should be in specification for the process to be considered in a state of control and that the load can be released.

REFERENCES

1. European Committee for Standardization. *EN 556:2001. Sterilization of Medical Devices. Requirements for Medical Devices to Be Designated "Sterile." Requirements for Terminally Sterilized Medical Devices.* Brussels, Belgium: European Committee for Standardization; 2001.
2. International Organization for Standardization. *ISO 11138-1:2017: Sterilization of Health Care Products—Biological Indicators—Part 1: General Requirements.* Geneva, Switzerland: International Organization for Standardization; 2017.
3. International Organization for Standardization. *ISO 11138-2:2017: Sterilization of Health Care Products—Biological Indicators—Part 2: Biological Indicators for Ethylene Oxide Sterilization Processes.* Geneva, Switzerland: International Organization for Standardization; 2017.
4. International Organization for Standardization. *ISO 11138-3:2017: Sterilization of Health Care Products—Biological Indicators—Part 3: Biological Indicators for Moist Heat Sterilization Processes.* Geneva, Switzerland: International Organization for Standardization; 2017.
5. International Organization for Standardization. *ISO 11138-4:2017: Sterilization of Health Care Products—Biological Indicators—Part 4: Biological Indicators for Dry Heat Sterilization Processes.* Geneva, Switzerland: International Organization for Standardization; 2017.
6. International Organization for Standardization. *ISO 11138-5:2017: Sterilization of Health Care Products—Biological Indicators—Part 5: Biological Indicators for Low-Temperature Steam and Formaldehyde Sterilization Processes.* Geneva, Switzerland: International Organization for Standardization; 2017.
7. International Organization for Standardization. *ISO 11138-7: 2019: Sterilization of Health Care Products—Biological Indicators—Part 7: Guidance for the Selection, Use and Interpretation of Results.* Geneva, Switzerland: International Organization for Standardization; 2019.
8. International Organization for Standardization. *ISO 11140-1:2015: Sterilization of Health Care Products. Chemical Indicators.* Geneva, Switzerland: International Organization for Standardization; 2015.
9. Bowie JH, Kelsey JC, Thompson GR. The Bowie and Dick autoclave tape test. *Lancet.* 1963;1(7281):586-587.
10. International Organization for Standardization. *ISO 17665-1:2006: Sterilization of Health Care Products—Moist Heat—Part 1—Requirements for the Development, Validation, and Routine Control of a Sterilization Process for Medical Devices.* Geneva, Switzerland: International Organization for Standardization; 2006.
11. European Committee for Standardization. *EN 285:2015. Sterilization—Steam Sterilizers—Large Sterilizers.* Brussels, Belgium: European Committee for Standardization; 2015.

12. International Organization for Standardization. *ISO/TS 17665-2:2009: Sterilization of Health Care Products. Moist Heat. Guidance on the Application of ISO 17665-1*. Geneva, Switzerland: International Organization for Standardization; 2009.

13. International Organization for Standardization. *ISO 14937:2009: Sterilization of Health Care Products. General Requirements for Characterization of a Sterilizing Agent and the Development, Validation and Routine Control of a Sterilization Process for Medical Devices*. Geneva, Switzerland: International Organization for Standardization; 2009.

14. International Organization for Standardization. *ISO 11139:2018: Sterilization of Health Care Products—Vocabulary*. Geneva, Switzerland: International Organization for Standardization; 2018.

15. International Organization for Standardization. *ISO 11137-1:2015: Sterilization of Health Care Products. Radiation. Requirements for Development, Validation and Routine Control of a Sterilization Process for Medical Devices*. Geneva, Switzerland: International Organization for Standardization; 2015.

16. International Organization for Standardization. *ISO 9001:2015: Quality Management Systems—Requirements*. Geneva, Switzerland: International Organization for Standardization; 2015.

17. International Organization for Standardization. *ISO 13485:2016: Medical Devices—Quality Management Systems—Requirements for Regulatory Purposes*. Geneva, Switzerland: International Organization for Standardization; 2016.

CHAPTER

66

Bacterial Endotoxin

Kimbrell R. Darnell and Amy Jo Karren

Bacterial endotoxin is a toxic biologic compound of significant medical importance. It is most often broadly characterized as a pyrogen, which describes a substance that acts to elicit fever in a susceptible host. Pyrogens are classified into two groups: microbial-based (sourced from bacteria, fungi, viruses, and their products) and non–microbial-based (eg, drugs, steroids, plasma fractions, or other chemicals). The most significant microbial pyrogens have been found to be endotoxins from gram-negative bacteria. Although gram-positive bacteria, fungi, and viruses can be pyrogenic during infection stages, they do so through a different mechanism and to a lesser degree than gram-negative bacterial endotoxins. Whereas bacterial endotoxins are pyrogenic, the pathologic effects caused by these substances are much more profound than just fever. These effects can include meningitis and a rapid loss of blood pressure such as in the highly and rapidly lethal condition known as septic shock that sometimes occurs in infections with gram-negative bacteria caused by the introduction of bacterial endotoxin into the circulatory system. Endotoxin may also lead to other initially latent effects as immune stimulators when introduced in the body that is the subject of further research.[1,2] Bacterial endotoxin is a component of the outer membrane of gram-negative bacteria (Figure 66.1).

Chemically, bacterial endotoxin is a high-molecular-weight lipopolysaccharide (LPS) typically consisting of three distinct regions (see Figure 66.1). The outermost region is the O-antigen or O-polysaccharide that extends outward from the cell and is attached to a central polysaccharide core. The innermost region, also attached to the core but extending into the cell wall, is a compound called lipid A, which is a disaccharide of glucosamine highly substituted with amide-linked and ester-linked long-chain fatty acids. Lipid A is responsible for most of the biologic reactivity associated with endotoxin.

Bacterial endotoxins are constantly released from gram-negative bacteria into the environment as a result of cell division, damage, or lysis and can pose a biologic threat apart from the intact microorganism if introduced to a susceptible host in sufficient quantity. Extracellular bacterial endotoxin in nature is usually associated with other outer membrane components such as proteins or phospholipids. Endotoxin contamination is difficult to prevent because it is prevalent in the environment, it's chemical stability makes it quite challenging to inactivate, and it's size allows it to easily pass through conventional microbially retentive filters. Due to its chemical stability, bacterial endotoxins are generally not considered to be significantly affected by many sterilization methodologies (with the notable exception of dry heat; see chapter 28) and can therefore persist in or on various medical products or surfaces after they have been rendered "sterile." Thus, bacterial endotoxin represents a clinical hazard if present in sufficient quantity and is introduced into certain areas of the body, particularly the vasculature, the lymphatics, the central nervous system, or the intraocular space. For these reasons, bacterial endotoxin contamination is a primary concern for manufacturers of parenteral pharmaceuticals and certain medical devices that are used to access susceptible anatomical sites.

Conversely, bacterial endotoxin is prevalent in the alimentary canal; therefore, oral dosage forms and medical devices intended for indications in the gastrointestinal tract do not generally pose the same risk of pyrogenicity.

▶ CONTROL OF BACTERIAL ENDOTOXINS

Endotoxin, or LPS, is located in the outer layer of the dual-layered cell wall separated by a thin layer of peptidoglycan that protects gram-negative bacteria from their environment (see Figure 66.1). Because LPS is located on the outer membrane, it possesses several properties that tends to activate a number of host defense mechanisms.

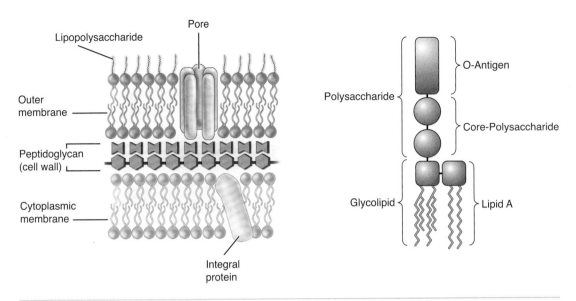

FIGURE 66.1 A representation of the cell wall of gram-negative bacteria (left) and the outer membrane lipopolysaccharide molecule (right). Panel A reprinted with permission from Aschenbrenner and Venable.[3] Figure 39-1.

A single gram-negative bacterial cell wall is estimated to contain approximately 3.5 million LPS molecules occupying about 75% of the cell's outer surface area.[4] The LPS molecules provide several vital functions for the microorganism including structural, physiologic, and transport operations. No gram-negative bacterial species have been found to be able to survive when totally lacking LPS.[5] Bacterial LPS molecules are shed from the cell into the environment through various processes such as multiplication, death, and lysis as well as constant sloughing as outer membrane vesicles (OMV) in a manner analogous to shedding of hair or skin in animals. As these processes take place, the concentration of endotoxin can accumulate and attach to dust particles, raw materials, and/or components that they come into contact with. It is important to note that bacterial endotoxin can come from the direct presence of intact microorganisms or from released, extracellular endotoxin (eg, in water or dust particles) as the source of contamination for health care products. Because gram-negative bacteria are found in virtually every environment on earth, bacterial endotoxin is also equally common in the environment. Given its ubiquity, it is interesting to speculate why endotoxin elicits such an acute response in multicellular animals to its presence in the blood stream. This response is likely due to a type of "early warning system" related to the pathogenicity of many gram-negative species.[6] In fact, a study of bacterial infection in horseshoe crabs led to the discovery of a blood component in this organism that is used as a reagent (*Limulus* amebocyte lysate [LAL]) for the quantitation of bacterial endotoxin. Another reason that significant levels of bacterial endotoxin are often found separate from significant levels of viable microorganisms is the stability of the LPS molecule. Bacterial endotoxin is extremely heat stable and remains active after typical moist heat sterilization and desiccation. They can pass through sterilizing filters that remove whole bacterial cells from liquids such as parenteral solutions. The hydrophobic lipid ends of the molecules are believed to facilitate the adherence to hydrophobic surfaces such as glass or plastic, which are used for many medical devices and container closures for pharmaceutical products.

The production of pharmaceuticals and medical devices, particularly those with a use profile that would require nonpyrogenicity, almost always takes place in a microbiologically controlled environment. Manufacturing operations must be designed to minimize the presence of bacterial endotoxin on the product. They should operate within a state of control and assess for factors that could contribute to the presence of endotoxins (with examples given in Table 66.1). From these examples, it is obvious that processes that expose products to water or other aqueous solutions are generally the highest risk as a source of endotoxins. In fact, dry products that are produced in a controlled environment normally have a significantly lower risk of endotoxin, as do manufacturing steps in which water is not used in the process. Manufacturing processes that involve the use of water (particularly when used at ambient temperatures) are at a higher risk because many vegetative microorganisms typically reproduce in aqueous environments, and some gram-negative bacteria are particularly adept at growing even in purified water with very little available nutrients. Therefore, it is important when seeking to control endotoxins to give primary consideration to exposure to an aqueous environment in all phases of the manufacturing process, including at raw material and other suppliers. Also, natural materials can be a significant source of bacterial endotoxin such as animal or tissue-based products.

TABLE 66.1 Examples of common sources of endotoxins in manufacturing operations

Source	Hazard
Supplied raw materials or components	• Incoming materials contaminated with endotoxin due to suppliers with inadequate microbiological control measures. • Proliferation of microorganisms in raw materials that support growth
Extrusion operations	• Contact with inappropriately treated or controlled water in extrusion troughs
Aqueous washing or finishing processes	• Contact with inappropriately treated water from municipal or purified water system
Drying or curing processes	• Inadequate drying that facilitates the proliferation of microorganisms in the presence of residual water
Aqueous leaching or soaking	• Contact with inappropriately treated water from municipal or purified water system • Prolonged contact with water that facilitates the proliferation of microorganisms
Manual handling	• Shedding of hair or skin bacteria by personnel and transfer to materials during manual manipulations
Product or material storage	• Containers used for transportation or storage during movement between manufacturing areas that are not appropriately cleaned • Product stored in a humid environment that supports the proliferation of microorganisms

Overall, manufacturing processes should be designed and controlled to reduce the risk of potential sources of endotoxins. Considerations for these control measures may include:

1. Supplier quality such as monitoring endotoxin level of incoming raw materials, components, and subassemblies. This also might include supplier certification or attesting to no contact of product with water.
2. Control and monitoring of process water or other process solutions. Control may be demonstrated by microbiologic testing, endotoxin monitoring, or monitoring of control measures such as temperature or chemical disinfectants/preservatives such as chlorine.
3. Monitoring of in-process product at specified control points. This could include product endotoxin testing or manufacturing control parameters such as time or temperature.
4. Regularly scheduled cleaning, disinfection, and maintenance of equipment, particularly those that convey or contain product or aqueous processing materials
5. Microbiologic control of the environment and associated processing materials

Depyrogenation

Another control measure that might be used to eliminate endotoxins is through depyrogenation of materials, equipment, and/or final finished products. Depyrogenation can be accomplished by two primary means: inactivation or removal. Inactivation is accomplished by denaturing or destroying the LPS molecule by chemical or physical means. Due to the inherent chemical stability of LPS, the extent of treatment necessary to achieve inactivation of endotoxin is often severe and often beyond the capability of most health care product to withstand. Chemical inactivation involves treatment to break chemical bonds or bind active sites. Physical inactivation typically involves incineration or dry heat inactivation of LPS at high temperatures. Endotoxin removal can be achieved by several techniques related to the physical characteristics of endotoxin such as size, binding affinity, solubility, and molecular weight. Where possible, manufacturing processes may incorporate design features that can act to mitigate the potential for endotoxins. Some examples of these might include the following:

1. Exposure to dry heat: typically, temperatures greater than 250°C for adequate duration
2. Acid or base hydrolysis
3. Oxidation
4. Distillation, ultrafiltration, reverse osmosis
5. Rinsing

For chemical and physical depyrogenation, it is often very difficult to achieve parameters that provide the necessary effectivity while preserving product activity and/or function. Depyrogenation by dry heat is the most often used method and is widely used in laboratory and manufacturing operations for treatment of heat-tolerant items such as glassware, metal equipment, and some heat-stable chemicals. Depyrogenation by this method is typically accomplished by exposure to temperatures of not less than 250°C for not less than 30 minutes.[7] Validation of such processes is typically required to demonstrate their effectivity.

NONPYROGENIC HEALTH CARE PRODUCTS

Many health care products, both pharmaceuticals and medical devices, are required to be nonpyrogenic. Sterile parenteral drugs and implantable medical devices that contact nonintact tissue during use or that have indirect intravascular, intralymphatic, intrathecal, and intraocular contact are recommended to be nonpyrogenic. The claim of "nonpyrogenic" refers to endotoxin derived from gram-negative bacteria.[8] This requirement can be related to a label claim of "nonpyrogenic," the intended use of the product, or both. The substantiation of a product as being nonpyrogenic is made by demonstrating that the product does not expose the individual on which the product is used to levels of bacterial endotoxin above specific regulatory limits. These limits can vary depending on the product and its intended use. The general regulatory limits for these products are listed in Table 66.2.

TABLE 66.2	Regulatory limits for bacterial endotoxin[a]
Product Contact	**Regulatory Limit (EU = Endotoxin Unit[b])**
Devices—intravascular, intralymphatic	20 EU/device
Devices—intrathecal	2.15 EU/device
Devices—intraocular	2.0 EU/eye
Parenteral drugs—nonintrathecal	5.0 EU/kg
Parenteral drugs—intrathecal	0.2 EU/kg
Parenteral drugs—ophthalmic	0.5 EU/mL
Radiopharmaceuticals	175 EU
Parenteral drug—administered per surface area	100 EU/m³

[a]From International Organization for Standardization,[9] US Food and Drug Administration,[10] American National Standards Institute,[11] US Pharmacopeial Convention,[12] US Food and Drug Administration,[13,14] and US Pharmacopeial Convention.[15,16]

[b]Endotoxins are measured in EU. This is a standard unit of measure for endotoxin activity established relative to the activity contained in 0.2 ng of the US Reference Standard Endotoxin Lot EC-2 (US Pharmacopeia standard reference material).

Endotoxin limits for devices are considered more straight forward as they are generally considered as conservative with a defined endotoxin content per device, no matter the size or intended use, although even more conservative levels as defined for devices for intrathecal or intraocular use.[9,10] But the label claim for devices can vary such as "nonpyrogenic fluid path" in which only the surfaces relevant to the fluid path have patient contact and would therefore only be considered a risk for those parts of the device. Also, devices can contain components or regions that do not have patient contact and are inappropriate to include in product testing such as a device-associated handle or cord. The exemption of any part of a product from evaluation for a "nonpyrogenic" claim should be based on an evaluation of the patient contact profile of the product. Some multiple component device products such as kits or trays can contain components that have applicable patient contact and others that do not. Typically, the "nonpyrogenic" claim only applies to those devices or components that have applicable patient contact.

Pharmaceutical endotoxin limits are also managed based on the patient contact or dosage form; however, the limits are typically based on the product dose administered. The limits for pharmaceuticals are typically expressed as K/M, which is a dose concentration–based approach where

K is the regulatory limit as described in Table 66.2, and
M represents the maximum human dose per kilogram that would be administered in a single bolus or continuously over a single 1-hour period.

For example, the calculation of the endotoxin limit for a nonintrathecal drug administered parenterally at 2 mL/person would be

$$\text{Maximum dose per kg assuming 70 kg}$$
$$\text{body mass} = 2 \text{ mL/70 kg} = 0.0286 \text{ mL/kg}$$

$$\text{Endotoxin limit (K/M)} = [5.0 \text{ EU/kg}] /$$
$$[0.0286 \text{ mL/kg}] = 175 \text{ EU/mL}$$

But the endotoxin limit for a dose of 2 mL/person administered intrathecally would be

$$\text{Maximum dose} = 0.0286 \text{ mL/kg (see above)}$$

$$\text{Endotoxin limit (K/M)} = [0.2 \text{ EU/kg}] /$$
$$[0.0286 \text{ mL/kg}] = 7 \text{ EU/mL}$$

And a topical drug administered based on a defined surface area with a maximum recommended dose of 30 mg/m³ would be

$$\text{Endotoxin limit (K/M)} = [100 \text{ EU/m}^3] /$$
$$[30 \text{ mg/m}^3] = 3.33 \text{ EU/mg}$$

The limits for radiopharmaceuticals are typically expressed as EU/V where

EU is the regulatory limit as described in Table 66.2, and
V is the maximum dose in milliliter. This is a whole-body dose not dose per kilogram.

Therefore, for a radiopharmaceutical with a maximum dose of 7 mL, the endotoxin limit would be 175 EU/7.0 mL, which is 25 EU/mL.

Application of any nonpyrogenic label claim or statement to health care products must be substantiated. This substantiation can be verified by directly testing each finished batch of a product to quantify the endotoxin content. For medical devices, options other than testing each finished batch are considered acceptable, and these options are discussed later in this chapter. The term *pyrogen free* has been historically used in some instances as a label claim; however, such a claim is generally inappropriate because it implies a complete absence of bacterial endotoxin and this cannot be demonstrated empirically due to the detection limits inherent to current test methods.

▶ PRODUCT ENDOTOXIN TESTING AND RELEASE

Bacterial Endotoxins Test

The rabbit pyrogen test was introduced just prior to World War II to test and prevent pyrogenic products from entering the health care system.[17] In this test, rabbits are monitored for a rise in body temperature after injection with a test solution. The LAL test, using a reagent made from amebocytes from the blood of the horseshoe crab, *Limulus polyphemus*, was introduced in 1971 as a potential replacement for the rabbit pyrogen test and is now known as the bacterial endotoxins test (BET).[18,19] The LAL test is an enzymatic reaction that operates in a cascading fashion and has a high sensitivity to gram-negative bacterial endotoxins. First, factor C, an endotoxin-sensitive serine protease zymogen present in the LAL reagent, is activated by endotoxin. This activated factor C then activates factor B, and this converts a proclotting enzyme to clotting enzyme. Finally, the clotting enzyme converts coagulogen to coagulin, and this leads to the formation of a gel. In addition to factor C, LAL reagent might also contain factor G that is activated by (1,3)-β-D-glucans and subsequently converts the proclotting enzyme to a clotting enzyme causing interference with the ability to quantify endotoxin in the presence of these glucans. Endotoxin-specific LAL reagent has been developed by removing factor G or saturating its function.

Because the LAL test is based on an enzymatic reaction, it is influenced by temperature, pH, and it is also interfered with by various compounds such as protease,

protease inhibitors, metal ions, surfactants, chelates, salts, and sugars in sufficient concentrations. Therefore, tests for interfering factors should be performed to check the presence of inhibitors and enhancers of the reaction in sample solution. The effect of the interfering factors can be avoided by the dilution of the sample solution.

The parenteral drug industry and the US Food and Drug Administration (FDA) agreed on a guideline in 1987 to replace the rabbit pyrogen test with the LAL test because this in vitro test was more sensitive, specific, accurate, and cost-effective.[8] The LAL test became the official replacement for most parenteral pharmaceuticals in the United States in 1993, with a sweeping revision of the BET and adoption of product endotoxin limits; the revision of the BET contained more than 650 limits for US Pharmacopeia (USP) articles.[20] Although BET and LAL test are commonly used to describe the method, BET is now the appropriate abbreviation for the test.

For the BET, it was essential to clarify issues of equivalency, safety, endotoxin limits, and regulatory oversight before this new test could be accepted. The FDA's Bureau of Biologics (now the Center for Biologics Evaluation and Research) elected to regulate LAL reagents as an in vitro biologic, due to its potential as a human diagnostic test and as a replacement for the rabbit pyrogen test.[21,22] The LAL reagents were first introduced to the market in 1977, but their use was limited to in-process testing of parenteral pharmaceuticals. A collaborative study between medical device manufacturers and the FDA, supported by the Health Industry Manufacturers Association, established 0.1 ng/mL as the product endotoxin limit for device extracts.[23] This study further verified that the threshold pyrogenic dose of an endotoxin (*Escherichia coli* 055:B5) was approximately 1 ng/kg in rabbits when administered at a dose of 10 mL/kg.

The issue of nonendotoxin pyrogens was a major concern for the pharmaceutical industry. In 1979, a manufacturer of large volume parenterals reported on its experience with LAL testing compared with rabbit pyrogen testing.[24] The study evaluated the results of 143,196 LAL tests and 28,410 rabbit tests performed on intravenous fluids and other health care products. The data concluded the following:

1. All pyrogens detected in the fluids and devices tested were bacterial endotoxins.
2. No unexplained, false-negative results occurred among the LAL tests.
3. Most of the bacterial endotoxin detected by LAL testing was undetected by rabbits because of LAL test's greater sensitivity.
4. The rabbit pyrogen testing often gave equivocal results that were reproducible in the LAL test.

The study had a significant impact on the future of pyrogen testing. The FDA approved the LAL assay (BET) due to concerns with the relative insensitivity and potential unreliability of the rabbit test. Today, the BET is the definitive assay for quantitation of bacterial endotoxin.

There are several documents in the United States that are primarily used for guidance on bacterial endotoxins testing. These include *ANSI/AAMI ST72* Bacterial endotoxins—Test methods, routine monitoring, and alternatives to batch testing[11]; two USP chapters, *USP <85> Bacterial Endotoxin Test,*[20] *USP <161> Medical Device— Bacterial Endotoxin and Pyrogen Test*[12]; and several FDA documents such as *Guidance for Industry: Pyrogen and Endotoxins Testing: Questions and Answers,*[13] *Endotoxin Testing Recommendations for Single-Use Intraocular Ophthalmic Devices,*[10] and *Submission and Review of Sterility Information in Premarket Notification (510(k)) Submissions for Devices Labeled as Sterile.*[14] The FDA also uses quality systems regulations in its enforcement program to require the BET for validating depyrogenation processes and for monitoring water, raw materials, and in-process product.

Various pharmacopeia from developed nations contains BET guidance with similar requirements to the USP. Parts of *USP <85>* have now been harmonized with the *European Pharmacopeia* and the *Japanese Pharmacopeia.*

There are currently three commonly used BET types or techniques. The selection of technique is typically based on several factors such as the capability of the laboratory, the sample throughput requirements, data handling requirements, and the characteristics of the test sample. Current techniques and the methods for each include the following:

1. Gel-clot techniques, which are based on formation of a solid gel. These include the limit test and assay methods.
2. Chromogenic techniques based on the development of color due to cleavage of a synthetic peptide-chromogen complex—kinetic and end point methods.
3. Turbidimetric technique based on development of turbidity due to cleavage of an endogenous substrate—kinetic and end point methods.

Gel-Clot Techniques—Limit Test and Assay Methods

The gel clot methods are typically the simplest of the BET techniques to carry out. These methods require less technical expertise to perform a valid assay and data interpretation/analysis and the equipment needed is minimal, requiring only a properly qualified and maintained water bath or heating block and accessories. The gel-clot test uses equal volumes of test sample diluted to a validated concentration and LAL reagent mixed in a small glass reaction tube. After incubation, individual reaction tubes are carefully removed from the incubating device and slowly inverted 180 degrees. A firm gelatinous clot that remains intact after inversion constitutes a positive test. A tube that does not form a gel or a gel that does not remain intact after inversion is scored as a negative test. The advantages of these tests are that they are typically simpler and less expensive than kinetic methods. They also can have high throughput for products that rarely exceed limit of detection. But the disadvantages are that additional testing is required when limit of detection is exceeded, and these tests are often not as sensitive or precise as kinetic methods.

Chromogenic and Turbidimetric Techniques—End Point and Kinetic Methods

The end point methods are based on the linear relationship between endotoxin concentration and formation of a color (chromogenic) or turbidity measured by optical density at a given wavelength, which is assessed over a relatively short range of standard dilutions. A standard curve is constructed by plotting the optical densities of a series of endotoxin standards prepared in LAL reagent water (LRW) as a function of the endotoxin concentration. Using linear regression analysis, the resulting best-fit standard curve covers an endotoxin range of approximately 1 log, usually 1.0 to 0.1 EU/mL or 0.1 to 0.01 EU/mL. The correlation coefficient is a statistical measure of the scatter of the observed points of the optical density of the standard curve relative to the calculated regression line. Linearity is defined as a correlation coefficient of an absolute value of $r \geq 0.980$. The endotoxin level in an unknown sample is calculated by measuring the optical density of the sample and interpolating the endotoxin concentration from the standard curve. Chromogenic and turbidimetric end point methods are generally performed in microtiter plates and require a heating block, a qualified microplate reader, and software with a statistical package (for linear regression analysis) for the construction of standard curves and analysis of samples. These methods are dependent on good analyst technique, and a knowledge of basic statistics is helpful when analyzing and interpreting data.

The photometric methods, also known as kinetic methods, including the chromogenic and turbidimetric techniques measure the amount of time it takes for a series of standards to achieve a predetermined optical density (turbidimetric) or color intensity (chromogenic), sometimes called the onset or reaction optical density. Quantitation is based on a standard curve constructed by plotting the log of the reaction time (ie, the time it takes for each standard or sample to reach the onset optical density) versus the log of the endotoxin concentration. This log/log plot of the data results in a linear standard curve. The range of the curve for a kinetic method is up to 4 logs as compared to the 1 log curve generated in the end point method. Unless approved alternate regression analyses are used (currently authorized by the FDA only on an individual reagent manufacturer basis), the resulting standard curve is constructed using linear regression analysis across the observed points. A correlation coefficient of the absolute value of r ≥0.980 is the minimum linearity requirement for a kinetic method. As with the end point methods, the endotoxin content of the unknown is calculated by interpolation from the standard curve using the logarithm of the onset time of the sample. The kinetic methods are performed in multiwell plates, glass reaction tubes, or other validated technology. Both methods require suitable, qualified equipment to incubate, read the results and software to carry out a regression analysis to construct a standard curve used to quantify the endotoxin content of test article. A spreadsheet or database application is often used in conjunction with these methods to aid in the analysis and trending of data. The kinetic methods are typically more sensitive and precise than gel-clot methods as well as providing more immediate quantitative capability. But disadvantages include being more expensive to operate and requiring more complex operator skill. Throughput is often not as fast as for gel-clot methods.

Bacterial Endotoxins Test Method Selection and Suitability Testing

The selected BET method must be deemed compatible with the product or product being tested to adequately demonstrate that the product does not cause inhibition, enhancement, or otherwise interfere with the accuracy and sensitivity of the assay. Relative to method suitability, products may be placed into groups or families according to common components or formulations and select a representative product from each group for suitability testing. Historically, method suitability testing for medical devices was required to be performed on three batches of product, using the same sampling plan as determined for routine analysis. Recent changes in guidance now only require a single-method suitability test for medical device product validation to assess interfering factors with the assay (ANSI/AAMI ST72:2019). This change is substantiated by increased knowledge of the ruggedness of the test as well as the data provided by the positive product controls in the kinetic test methods.

For the test method suitability of a BET, a manufacturer may logically divide its products into groups of products according to common components (chemical formulations) and may then choose representative product from each such group.

The product chosen from each group should ideally be

- For polymeric samples such as devices or containers, representative product may be based on size such as the greatest surface area or mass thus contributing the largest potential source of interfering substances.
- For liquids or powders, representative product may be based on chemical content that might present the most inhibitory factors such as pH, divalent ions, or enhancement, such as beta glucans.

Interferences with the BET typically arise from two general sources. The first are factors that acts on the proteins in the LAL-clotting cascade to cause nonspecific interferences; examples of this include nonneutral pH, beta glucans, and serine proteases. The second type of interference acts on the LPS in the purified endotoxin standard used as a control for the BET to change the aggregation state of the purified material causing it to be less reactive. Fortunately, most LAL reagents have enough sensitivity to allow dilution of samples or sample extracts to overcome most interference.

The clotting cascade in LAL reagent may be activated by materials that contain (1,3)-β-D-glucan, a nonpyrogenic polysaccharide typically found in cellulose and yeast cell wall.[25] To avoid a false-positive endotoxin tests, some LAL reagents contain a β-D-glucan blocking agent. These reagents facilitate a valid BET for products that may contain cellulosic products such as depth filters, yeast fermentation, and other sources of LAL reactive materials. Glucans are often suspected if there is an unexpectedly high endotoxin level measured; nonlinear reactions are observed with multiple dilutions, or enhancement is observed in the positive controls of a kinetic BET.

A selected BET method must be qualified or determined to be suitable for its intended use. If the test method or technique is changed, validation or demonstration of continued suitability must be carried out. Suitability testing is based on spiking a product solution or product extract solution with a known amount of a standardized bacterial endotoxin control and determining how accurately the test was able to quantify the spike. The setup for suitability testing for the different BET techniques are noted in Tables 66.3 and 66.4.

Recovery of Endotoxin From a Sample

The BET requires an aqueous sample for the analysis to quantify the amount of endotoxin in or on a test sample. Typically, liquid samples (eg, parenteral drugs, biologics) are tested directly or with dilution. Whereas solid samples, such as medical devices, require an extraction to create an aqueous sample extract for testing. Because of this, the scenario of "recovery of endotoxin" from the test sample has the potential to mean different things dependent on the sample type.

All samples, including liquid samples or extracts of solid samples, employed in the BET should have a positive product control performed during testing. The positive product control is performed by adding a known amount of a standardized endotoxin solution, generally purified LPS, to the sample preparation to determine whether endotoxin can be recovered from the sample matrix without interference from the test sample itself. Low endotoxin recovery indicates that the presence of

TABLE 66.3 Typical setup for suitability testing (inhibition/enhancement) for bacterial endotoxins test gel-clot technique[a]

Solution	Diluent	Endotoxin Spike	Endotoxin Concentration	Number of Replicates
Product positive control series	Sample solution	Prepare 2 λ solution and then 2-fold serial dilutions of initial 2 λ prep	2 λ λ 0.5 λ 0.25 λ	4 4 4 4
Product negative control	Sample solution	None	None	4
Standard control series	LAL reagent water (LRW)	Prepare 2 λ solution and then 2-fold serial dilutions of initial 2 λ prep	2 λ λ 0.5 λ 0.25 λ	2 2 2 2
Negative control	LRW	None	None	2

[a]The test is suitable for the product if
1. The LAL sensitivity (λ) in the product positive control series is within 0.5 λ and 2 λ.
2. Negative controls are nonreactive.
3. The standard control series confirms λ within 0.5 to 2 λ.

a substance in the sample preparation that inhibits the recovery of endotoxin by the BET. Inhibition can be caused by many factors including salts, metals, detergents, and proteins that bind or hide endotoxin from the LAL reagent.[26] Low endotoxin recovery is a phenomenon of concern for the pharmaceutical and biologics industry that has led to many studies to address the issue.[27] It is recognized by industry experts that significant biochemical and physical differences exist between endotoxins found in nature and the purified endotoxin, or LPS, used for reference/control standards. During the gram-negative bacterial cell's normal growth cycle, parts of the cell membrane are pinched off from the growing cell forming extracellular spherical vesicles, OMV. Once released, these OMV float freely in the environment without the same aggregation patterns seen with purified endotoxin. Electron micrographs clearly demonstrate the physical and structural differences between the natural endotoxin OMV and purified LPS in aqueous solution.[28] The hypothesis is that the purified LPS solutions are inappropriate surrogates for natural endotoxin contamination in endotoxin recovery and hold time studies; however, at this time, there is insufficient evidence from observed clinical data or peer reviewed scientific literature that would suggest that low endotoxin recovery poses a patient safety concern when routine testing is performed using LPS as the calibration standard in the BET. Therefore, recovery of a standardized endotoxin solution, either a solution of purified LPS or naturally occurring endotoxin, is maintained and

TABLE 66.4 Typical setup for suitability testing (inhibition/enhancement) for chromogenic and turbidimetric techniques[a]

Solution	Diluent	Endotoxin Spike	Minimum Number of Replicates
Product positive control (PPC)	Sample solution	Middle concentration of the standard curve	2
Sample solution	Sample solution	None	2
Standard control series	LAL reagent water (LRW)	Minimum of three different concentrations	2 per concentration
Negative control	LRW	None	2

[a]For chromogenic or turbidimetric methods, an acceptable suitability test is if the test results confirm the PPC within 50% to 200% of the known added endotoxin concentration.

deemed acceptable as a positive control when performing the BET to demonstrate recovery of endotoxin from the sample matrix.

Extraction efficiency from a solid sample to determine the effectiveness of the sample extraction is a different endotoxin recovery scenario. In contrast to pharmaceuticals, endotoxins must be extracted or flushed from medical devices and then the extract/eluate is tested by the BET. Studies by FDA investigators have demonstrated that extraction of endotoxin from spiked device materials may not achieve complete recovery. Unlike extraction efficiency testing for bioburden testing (see chapter 64), there is no standardized method to evaluate the efficacy of the extraction process for bacterial endotoxin. There are many reasons for this, but the main reason is that purified endotoxin solutions do not adequately mimic endotoxin contamination from natural sources, as noted previously. Additionally, the medium used for extraction must be aqueous, with water being the most common and effective extractant, without additional surfactants or solvents to facilitate the removal of endotoxin. Surfactants and solvents have the potential to interfere with the test system, and the ability to detect endotoxin. It has been demonstrated that surfactants can cause the LPS to form micelles, which in turn may interfere with the detection of the endotoxin by the lysate by hiding the receptor sites for the activation of the enzymatic cascade with the lysate. Solvents have the potential to denature the endotoxin in the sample, therefore resulting in less endotoxin detected than indicated by the true endotoxin burden on the product. Therefore, it is currently advised not to perform extraction efficiency studies on medical devices to demonstrate endotoxin recovery from a sample extraction.[29] Additionally, the established endotoxin limits for devices account for the uncertainty of the extraction process for devices.[8,11] Because the efficiency of the endotoxin recovery is uncertain, a more stringent product endotoxin limit of 20 EU per device was established to account for any potential inefficiency in the extraction method. When this assumption is applied, there is no requirement for performing efficiency testing for each medical device; however, as with pharmaceutical solutions, the validity of the assay must still be demonstrated by use of a spiked endotoxin control.

Sampling Plans

Sampling plans for the BET were first recommended in the FDA's *Guideline on Validation of the Limulus Amebocyte Lysate Test as an End-Product Endotoxin Test for Human and Animal Parenteral Drugs, Biological Products, and Medical Devices* (also known as the "FDA LAL Guideline").[8] This document is still maintained as a primary guidance that describes a minimum sampling regimen for finished products. For pharmaceutical products, the guideline suggests a minimum of three samples from

TABLE 66.5 A suggested sampling plan for medical device bacterial endotoxins test[a]

Batch Size	No. of Samples
<30	2
30-100	3
≥101	3% of batch, up to a maximum of 10

[a]From US Food and Drug Administration[8] and American National Standards Institute.[11]

the beginning, middle, and end of the production batch. Whereas these minimal sampling requirements are not statistically based using confidence levels for the detection of an aberrant result, the beginning/middle/end concept assumes that the most likely points for contamination to occur are at the beginning or end of the manufacturing process, with the median sample being used as a control. For medical devices, a sampling plan (Table 66.5) was also previously defined in the guideline, has been commonly used, and is generally considered to be acceptable. Samples of medical devices are typically pooled during testing.

In most cases, each batch of product is tested using an appropriate number of samples, with not more than 10 samples, taken randomly to represent the quality of the batch. Ten samples are considered the maximum based on the derivation of the established endotoxin limits. Whereas the endotoxin limit for medical devices with intravascular and intralymphatic indications was based on a reduction of the typical 350 EU limit for pharmaceuticals, this limit was reduced to 200 EU to account for potential inefficiency in the extraction method, as noted above. This limit was further reduced to 20 EU based on a maximum amount of endotoxin of 200 EU for the combined extracts from 10 samples. The assumption being that in the worst case, all of the endotoxin in the pooled extract could have come from a single device. Using more than 10 devices in a pooled extraction skews the worst-case scenario and potentially masks endotoxin from a single device that could exceed the pyrogenicity threshold. The sampling plans for endotoxin testing are based on the premise that the manufacturing process is controlled and in compliance with quality system requirements. These include all potential sources of endotoxin risk (raw materials, water, equipment, containers/packaging) have very low endotoxin risk and that the manufacturing process is validated and in a state of control that will minimize variability across the batch.

Selection of Product Units for Testing

Samples selected for end-product testing should be in the finished form. This includes all factors that might affect or contribute to the levels of endotoxin including the container closure or primary sterile barrier system that may normally come into direct contact with the finished product. When the samples are terminally sterilized, sterilization of the samples should also be considered during sample selection. Even though guidance allows for samples to be obtained prior to (pre-) sterilization or after (post-) sterilization, an assessment to the equivalency should be done. Poststerilization samples encompass all of the factors that could affect the product or the endotoxin test. When presterilization samples are selected for testing, it should be determined that the samples represent endotoxin level on the finished product. It is recognized that most modes of sterilization, with the exception of dry heat, do not dramatically impact the endotoxin levels on the finished product, but this conclusion may require further investigation.[25,30,31] For products that support microbial growth (eg, products that contain nonpreserved aqueous liquids or gels), endotoxin levels might increase if there is an increase in bioburden levels on or in the product prior to sterilization. In such cases, poststerilization testing might be necessary to ensure that BET results are representative of the finished product. Presterilization testing is inappropriate for products that support microbial growth. For products that do not support microbial growth, consideration of factors such as the materials, manufacturing processes, historical data (eg, shown by comparative endotoxin testing), etc, should be sufficient to allow for presterilization testing.

Bioburden testing may be performed to determine if a product supports microbial growth, if it is unknown or uncertain. This can be accomplished by bioburden testing multiple time points of samples from the same batch to assess the ability of the product to support growth and hence the suitability of presterilization endotoxin testing. Water activity testing can also assess the capacity of supporting microbial growth for the product.[32]

Identification of Products Requiring Testing and Product Release

Pharmaceutical Products

In the pharmaceutical industry, there is an expectation that the BET is used as a batch release test to ensure the test requirements for product quality in the associated pharmacopeia are met. In general, batch testing is performed on sterile drug products in their finished form. The dosage form, content of the general chapter for BET, and specific test requirements in the associated monographs provide guidance on when testing is required. The drug products that require endotoxin testing include dosage forms for injection or implanted drug products (parenterals) and mucosal drug products used specifically for ophthalmic applications.[15,16]

Individual Medical Devices

Sterile implantable medical devices that contact nonintact tissue during use or medical devices that have direct or indirect intravascular, intralymphatic, intrathecal, and/or intraocular contact are required to have a defined specification and associated evaluation for bacterial endotoxins.[12] Additionally, if the product is labeled as being nonpyrogenic, these must be evaluated and meet the same applicable regulatory requirements for bacterial endotoxin content as products required to be nonpyrogenic due to intended use. Conversely, some implantable medical devices are not required to be evaluated for bacterial endotoxins as the device only contacts intact tissue during use. Examples include implantable medical devices such as ureteral and biliary stents, gastric balloons, hearing aids, breathing strips, Foley catheters, etc. The sampling group for medical devices is generally defined as the production batch.

Medical Device Kits

A kit is defined as a collection of individual health care products in a single sterile barrier system, or a variety of procedure-related health care products. In the testing of multicomponent kits (procedure packs) or sets of individual products within the same sterile barrier system, there are instances where each component may be evaluated individually and other instances where the entire contents may be considered as a single entity. Each individual type of device might have its own product endotoxin limit or the endotoxin limit can be applied to the entire kit. Guidance on how a medical device should be tested and evaluated on an individual basis, if necessary, to support individual claims is provided in Table 66.6.

Product Family and Batch Definition

Product families can be defined in order to further define a batch within the product family. The product families can be established based on an evaluation of products, processes, components, and materials. For routine endotoxin testing for product families, the selection of a single product type from within a product family might be acceptable, using the concept of a representative master product. The designation of product families for endotoxin testing might not necessarily fit the criteria of product families as identified for other purposes, such as a bioburden product family or sterilization equivalence. Each manufacturer should evaluate, analyze, and document the appropriate product family designation based on product components, manufacturing processes, and intended usage.

When performing batch testing for endotoxin, the endotoxin batch may be defined as several similar products with the same endotoxin risk. Caution should be given when defining the batch, whereas what is defined as a "batch" might differ from the definition of a "batch" for other purposes. For example, multiple production batches

TABLE 66.6 Guidance on the selection of product units for testing[a]

Product	Packaging	Item for Testing	Basis for Nonpyrogenic Claim	Rationale
1. One medical device	One sterile barrier system	Individual medical device or applicable patient contact portion	The medical device and its use	The medical device is used in clinical practice as a unit.
2. Components assembled into medical device at the point of use	One or more sterile barrier systems	All components or applicable patient contact portion	The assembled medical device and its use	Components must be combined to assemble the medical device before its use in clinical practice.
3. Number of identical medical device[b]	One sterile barrier system	Individual medical device or applicable patient contact portion	One medical device within the sterile barrier system	Each medical device can be used independently in clinical practice.
4. Procedure-related medical devices[b]	Within a single sterile barrier system	Each type of medical device or applicable patient contact portion	The medical device and its use	Each type of medical device can be used independently in a procedure and can have different product endotoxin limits.
5. Procedure-related medical devices[b]	Medical devices each in a sterile barrier that are combined in secondary packaging.	Each type of medical device or applicable patient contact portion	The medical device and its use	Each type of medical device is used in clinical practice and might have different product endotoxin limits. (The extent of the number of potential devices might not be known; therefore, individual packaged testing is performed.)

[a]From American National Standards Institute.[11]

[b]Manufacturers can choose to test the procedure-related medical devices together to provide a single collective nonpyrogenic claim; however, this is not required. Manufacturers that combine procedure-related medical devices can support nonpyrogenicity by using supplier certification or by performing testing.

that each requires separate endotoxin testing might be sterilized together in the same run or an endotoxin batch may be defined as several similar product types or groupings with the same endotoxin risk. It should be considered that the endotoxin distribution within a batch of samples might not be uniform.

In establishing a sampling group and selecting samples for endotoxin testing, the following factors should be considered:

- Raw materials or components (eg, device containing extruded tubing from the same supplier exposed to the same manufacturing processes and only differing in dimensions)
- Production quantities from a single shift or defined time period (eg, 8 h or 24 h, products with similar endotoxin risks sterilized in the same sterilization load, etc)
- Product produced on specific equipment or in the same manufacturing environment with equivalent endotoxin

risk (eg, all product cleaned or finished in the same immersion bath)
- Product families (eg, different volume or size of the same drug or device)
- Product risk factors (eg, products that undergo the same endotoxin reduction steps, products that have the same endotoxin limits, etc)
- Product produced using the equivalent manufacturing processes (eg, handling, automated versus manual, drying, storage)
- Other logical divisions that contribute, control, or result in consistent end-product endotoxin levels

Alternatives to Batch Testing

Since the recognition and application of ANSI/AAMI ST72 in 2002, the application of alternatives to batch testing has been successfully applied in the medical device industry, allowing manufacturers to assess endotoxin risk and perform in process monitoring and control, in lieu of routine final product batch testing.[33] When developing alternatives to batch testing, the use of the failure mode and effects analysis (FMEA) is an effective assessment tool for risk analysis. Practical examples of this approach to risk analysis have been reported.[34] This approach enables a manufacturer to successfully conduct an analysis of bacterial endotoxin risk during the manufacturing process that may or may not use potentially contaminated process water as a source of endotoxin. An FMEA is not a zero-risk system but is designed to minimize the risk of potential hazards. An FMEA provides supporting documentation toward developing a rationale for alternatives to batch release testing.

As stated, the application of alternatives to batch testing requires a comprehensive risk assessment and corresponding data demonstrating that the manufacturing process is capable of producing product that consistently meets specified endotoxin limits. Such data typically includes testing of a specified number of batches, testing over a specified period of time, testing representative master products, raw materials and components, in-process testing, and verification of manufacturing operational controls (particularly water processes) etc. A review of historical product test data is a key component to determining if a device is an appropriate candidate for alternatives to batch testing.

Specifically, the application of alternatives to batch testing involves several options, including:

- Reduced number of samples (eg, from 10 samples per batch to 3 samples per batch)
- Reduced frequency of testing (eg, from every batch to every nth batch *or* from every batch to one batch per shift or per day)
- Specified combinations of products based on product grouping
- Testing of raw materials and monitoring of risks in the manufacturing process (eg, testing critical components or rinse water)
- Other logical alternatives

In order to apply alternatives to batch testing, specific criteria must be established in the risk assessment. These criteria include identification of key process steps or control points as well as additional risk assessment to demonstrate the process is appropriate for such an approach. The manufacturing process associated with the alternatives to batch testing must have an appropriate manufacturing operation design, validation, and monitoring/controls, as well as periodic review and adjustments made as necessary. Additional guidance on the application of alternatives to batch testing is published.[11]

ALTERNATIVE DETECTION TECHNOLOGIES

In addition to the traditional LAL-based BET, there are several alternative and emerging technologies for the *in-vitro* detection and quantification of bacterial endotoxin. These include recombinant factors C and B.[35] Current LAL reagents are produced from amebocytes that are extracted from the hemolymph of horseshoe crabs. Reagents produced from recombinant factors C and B would still use the same enzymatic cascade as traditional LAL but would not require the use of horseshoe crabs, as an environmental concern. Advances have been made in the development of hand-held instruments intended to provide rapid point of use testing for endotoxin.[36] These technologies are typically LAL reagent based and use miniaturized instrumentation similar to bench top kinetic systems. Another advance is the use of the human cell-based pyrogen test, or the monocyte activation test. Human cell-based pyrogen test is based on immunologic reaction at the cellular level and is a new in vitro method for detecting and quantifying pyrogens through activation of human immune cells such as monocytes and macrophages.[37] This test is designed to evaluate endotoxin-in-mediated pyrogenicity and pyrogenicity mediated by other microbial components corresponding to a febrile response induced by toll-like receptor agonists. This test is nonspecific to bacterial endotoxin and as such is perhaps better suited for evaluation of material-mediated pyrogenicity like the rabbit test discussed earlier in this chapter.

CONCLUSIONS

Limiting bacterial endotoxin contamination of health care products with certain specific types of body contact is critical to patient safety. Bacterial endotoxin testing provides an appropriate mechanism for the detection and quantification of bacterial endotoxin in and on these health care products (pharmaceuticals, biologics, and medical devices). The test assures the product is safe from the risk of pyrogenicity and other systemic effects from the exposure to gram-negative bacterial endotoxin, which is the most significant source of microbial pyrogens. It is critical that manufacturers control and/or mitigate bacteria endotoxins in the manufacturing process to ensure the final products are nonpyrogenic. Routine batch testing is typically performed on the final product; however, with a comprehensive risk assessment, alternatives to batch testing may be applied. Appropriate endotoxin limits should be established for the product.

Products tested by the BET must have method suitability testing performed to ensure that the test method is capable of detecting endotoxin in or on the product. The sample selection for testing should take into consideration guidance provided in various pharmacopeia and other recognized standards for the sampling plan and sample selection, ensuring that the product tested represents the finished product form. For more than 30 years, there has been an accepted use of the BET as a finished product test for endotoxins, in lieu of the rabbit pyrogen test, providing assurance to mitigate patient risk of pyrogenicity from the use of healthcare products.

REFERENCES

1. Zhang C, Tian F, Zhang M, et al. Endotoxin contamination, a potentially important inflammation factor in water and wastewater: a review. *Sci Total Environ*. 2019;681:365-378.
2. Farokhi A, Heederik D, Smit LAM. Respiratory health effects of exposure to low levels of airborne endotoxin—a systematic review. *Environ Health*. 2018;17(1):14.
3. Aschenbrenner DS, Venable SJ. *Drug Therapy in Nursing*. 4th ed. Philadelphia, PA: Wolters Kluwer Health; 2011.
4. Raetz CR, Ulevitch RJ, Wright SD, Sibley CH, Ding A, Nathan CF. Gram-negative endotoxin: an extraordinary lipid with profound effects on signal transduction. *FASEB J*. 1991;5(12):2652-2660.
5. Rietschel ET, Kirikae T, Schade FU, et al. Bacterial endotoxins: molecular relationships of structure to activity and function. *FASEB J*. 1994;18(2):217-225.
6. Kluger MJ. Fever: role of pyrogens and cryogens. *Physiol Rev*. 1991;71(1):93-127.
7. Welch H, Price CW, Chandler VL, Hunter AC. The thermostability of pyrogens and their removal from penicillin. *J Pharm Sci*. 1945;34:114.
8. US Food and Drug Administration. *Guideline on Validation of the Limulus Amebocyte Lysate Test as an End-Product Endotoxin Test for Human and Animal Parenteral Drugs, Biological Products, and Medical Devices*. Washington, DC: US Department of Health and Human Services; 1987.
9. International Organization for Standardization. *ISO 15798:2010: Ophthalmic Implants—Ophthalmic Viscosurgical Devices*. Geneva, Switzerland: International Organization for Standardization; 2010.
10. US Food and Drug Administration. *Endotoxin Testing Recommendations for Single-Use Intraocular Ophthalmic Devices*. Washington, DC: Division of Ophthalmic and Ear, Nose, and Throat Devices; 2015.
11. American National Standards Institute. *ANSI/AAMI ST72:2011(R)2016: Bacterial Endotoxins—Test Methods, Routine Monitoring, and Alternatives to Batch Testing*. New York, NY: American National Standards Institute; 2016. (Approved December 19, 2011. Reaffirmed June 9, 2016.)
12. US Pharmacopeial Convention. *<161> Medical Devices—Bacterial Endotoxin and Pyrogen Tests*. Rockville, MD: United States Pharmacopeial Convention; 2019. USP42-NF37.
13. US Food and Drug Administration. *Pyrogen and Endotoxins Testing: Questions and Answers*. Washington, DC: US Food and Drug Administration. http://www.fda.gov/downloads/drugs/guidancecompliance regulatoryinformation/guidances/ucm310098.pdf. Published June 2012. Accessed January 15, 2020.
14. US Food and Drug Administration. *Submission and Review of Sterility Information in Premarket Notification (510(k)) Submissions for Devices Labeled as Sterile*. Washington, DC: Center for Device and Radiological Health; 2016.
15. US Pharmacopeial Convention. *<1> Injections and Implanted Drug Products (Parenterals)—Product Quality Tests*. Rockville, MD: US Pharmacopeial Convention; 2019. USP42-NF37.
16. US Pharmacopeial Convention. *<4> Mucosal Drug Products—Product Quality Tests*. Rockville, MD: United States Pharmacopeial Convention; 2019. USP42-NF37.
17. McClosky WT, Price CW, Van Winkle W Jr, Welch H, Calvery HO. Results of first U.S.P. collaborative study of pyrogens. *J Pharm Sci*. 1943;32:69-73.
18. Cooper JF, Levin J, Wagner HN. Quantitative comparison of in vitro and in vivo methods for the detection of endotoxin. *J Lab Clin Med*. 1971;78:138-148.
19. Levin J, Bang F. Clottable protein in *Limulus*: its localization and kinetics of its coagulation by endotoxin. *Thromb Diath Haemorrh*. 1968;19:186.
20. US Pharmacopeial Convention. *<85> Bacterial Endotoxins Test*. Rockville, MD: US Pharmacopeial Convention; 2019. USP42-NF37.
21. US Public Health Service. Licensing of Limulus amebocyte lysate. *Fed Regist*. 1997; 40014.
22. Weary M. Pyrogen testing of parenteral products—status report. *J Parenter Sci Technol*. 1984;38:20-23.
23. Health Industry Manufacturers Association. *HIMA Collaborative Study for the Pyrogenicity Evaluation of a Reference Endotoxin by the USP Rabbit Test*. Washington, DC: Health Industry Manufacturers Association; 1969. HIMA Document Series; vol 1, no 7.
24. Mascoli C, Weary M. *Limulus* amebocyte lysate (LAL) test for detecting pyrogens in parenteral injectable products and healthcare products and medical services: advantages to manufacturers and regulatory officials. *J Parenter Drug Assoc*. 1979;33:81-95.
25. Ravikumar M, Hageman DJ, Tomaszewski WH, Chandra GM, Skousen JL, Capadona JR. The effect of residual endotoxin contamination on the neuroinflammatory response to sterilized intracortical microelectrodes. *J Mater Chem B*. 2014;2(17):2517-2529.
26. John Dubzak, CS. The bacterial endotoxins test: a practical guide. In: McCullough KZ, ed. *Resolving Test Interferences*. Bethesda, MD: PDA and River Grove, IL: DHI Publishing; 2011;9:195-214.
27. McCullough, KZ. Current USP perspectives on low endotoxin recovery (LER). American Pharmaceutical Review Web site. https://www .americanpharmaceuticalreview.com/Featured-Articles/190808 -Current-USP-Perspectives-on-Low-Endotoxin-Recovery-LER/. Published July 29, 2016. Accessed January 15, 2020.
28. Brogden KA, Phillips M. The ultrastructural morphology of endotoxins and lipopolysaccharides. *Electron Microsc Rev*. 1988;1:261-277.
29. Bryans TD, Braithwaite C, Broad J, et al. Bacterial endotoxin testing: a report on the methods, background, data, and regulatory history of extraction recovery efficiency. *Biomed Instrum Technol*. 2004;38(1):73-78.
30. Guyomard S. Defining the pyrogenic assurance level (PAL) of irradiated medical devices. *Int J Pharm*. 1987;173-174.
31. Guyomard S, Goury V, Darbord JC. Effects of ionizing radiations on bacterial endotoxins: comparison between gamma radiations and accelerated electrons. *Radiat Phys Chem*. 1988;31(4-6):679-684.
32. Parenteral Drug Association. *PDA Technical Report 67: Exclusion of Objectionable Microorganisms from Nonsterile Pharmaceuticals, Medical Devices, and Cosmetics Technical Report Team*. Bethesda, MD: Parenteral Drug Association; 2014.
33. American National Standards Institute. *ANSI/AAMI ST72:2002: Bacterial Endotoxins—Test Methodologies, Routine Monitoring, and Alternatives to Batch Testing*. New York, NY: American National Standards Institute; 2002.
34. Lee P, Plumlee B, Rymer T, Schwabe R, Hansen J. *Using FMEA to Develop Alternatives to Batch Testing*. Los Angeles, CA: Medical Device and Diagnostic Industry; 2004.
35. Loverock B, Baines A, Burgenson A, Simon B. A recombinant factor C procedure for the detection of gram-negative bacterial endotoxin. *Pharm Forum*. 2010;36(1).
36. Suzuki Y, Suzuki K, Shimamori T, Tsuchiya M, Niehaus A, Lakritz J. Evaluation of a portable test system for assessing endotoxin activity in raw milk. *J Vet Med Sci*. 2016;78(1):49-53.
37. Hartung T, Wendel A. Detection of pyrogens using human whole blood. *In Vitro Toxicol*. 1996;9:353-359.

Biofilm and Biofilm Control

Joey S. Lockhart, Andre G. Buret, and Douglas W. Morck

Microbial biofilms are ubiquitous, naturally occurring aggregates of microorganisms that are among the most successful life forms in the natural world. These unique communities can be composed of bacteria, fungi, and viruses and pose serious medical problems, particularly in the context of chronic infections and especially where medical implants are involved. Biofilms can occur in almost any aqueous or dry[1,2] milieus and therefore are significant, persistent contaminates in most environments. The microorganisms in a biofilm are able to attach to almost any substrate. Examples of this include a rock in a stream, the hull of a ship, suture material or implanted medical device in a host, and the natural growth of intestinal bacteria. Biofilm communities are typically encased in polysaccharide capsules that contain various antigens, components of dead microorganisms (proteins, lipids, nucleic acids), inorganic and organic materials, and host-derived materials such as immune cells and DNA.[3] Observations of biofilm-like structures date back to the 1670s with Antonie van Leeuwenhoek and his observations of dental plaque biofilms; however, the significance of the biofilm mode of growth was not fully appreciated until 1978, when J. William (Bill) Costerton and colleagues[4] published their theories about this sessile form of bacterial growth. The observation that bacteria can and do exist as a community attached to a substrate, encased in a polysaccharide-rich matrix (referred to as glycocalyx by Costerton), was a critical step in the progression of biofilm research. Costerton noted that this was the predominant mode of growth in the vast majority of natural aquatic environments and concluded that these attached communities exhibit significant differences in physiology when compared to their planktonic (or free floating) counterparts.[4] He suggested a phenotypic plasticity in biofilms[5] with mechanisms that enable the bacteria to respond to environmental conditions and improve survival.[6,7]

Prior to the pioneering biofilm research by Costerton, in vitro work performed on bacteria considered the planktonic growth of microorganisms in liquid culture as the "gold standard" for studying bacterial physiology[7] as well as virtually all medical and industrial applications. This is particularly true for the vast majority of research studying the bactericidal activity of various disinfectants, biocides, and antibiotics. Experiments investigating planktonic organisms do not necessarily provide valuable insight into the in situ efficacy of antimicrobial agents; and now, it is clear that in the natural world, microbes are more likely to exist as complex biofilm communities attached to various substrates in the environment.

Following these initial studies, scientists began exploring this distinctly different form of growth. Initial experiments investigating bacterial susceptibility to various antimicrobials immediately demonstrated that biofilm-associated bacteria are significantly more resilient to these treatments. The biofilm mode of growth involves a complex, multispecies microbial community, complete with water channels, which permit the delivery of nutrients throughout the biofilm. These channels help transport and allow bacteria to trap free nutrients for metabolic use. This also aids in the dissemination of communication molecules among species and between individual microbes within the biofilm community.

▶ BIOFILM CHARACTERISTICS

The physical characteristics of a biofilm allow for the development of antibiotic resistance through horizontal gene transfer events and inhibit the diffusion of various biocides into the center of the mature biofilms. This makes biofilms significantly more difficult to eradicate than planktonic organisms, which float freely within culture medium and have been most commonly studied in laboratory settings over the past century. In addition to presenting a physical barrier to disinfectants, microbes in a biofilm exhibit dramatic differences in gene expression compared to their planktonic counterparts[8] resulting in distinct phenotypes.

Biofilms form when planktonic bacteria are able to attach to a surface.[9] Attached bacteria then produce an extracellular matrix typically consisting of polysaccharides, proteins, and DNA,[10] which enables the bacteria to adhere irreversibly to the surface (Figure 67.1).[9,11,12] These extracellular polysaccharides (EPS) are extensively hydrated, can impede diffusion of antimicrobials, and act as a physical barrier to host innate immune cells allowing the bacteria to cause persistent infections.[9,13,14] The physiological generation of EPS is a critical feature of a biofilm and confers numerous advantages to the microorganisms

residing in the biofilm community (Figure 67.2). One major benefit that the EPS layer provides to the community is resistance to desiccation because water stress is an environmental pressure that organisms frequently experience. The active production of EPS molecules makes biofilm bacteria significantly more resilient to desiccation than their planktonic counterparts (see Figure 67.2).[16]

Diffusion of reactive oxidants such as hydrogen peroxide produced by host immune cells, or similar molecules used in disinfection treatments, can be limited and slowed such that the oxidants are inactivated prior to penetrating the outer layer of the biofilm.[17,18] Antimicrobials administered for the treatment of infections can also be

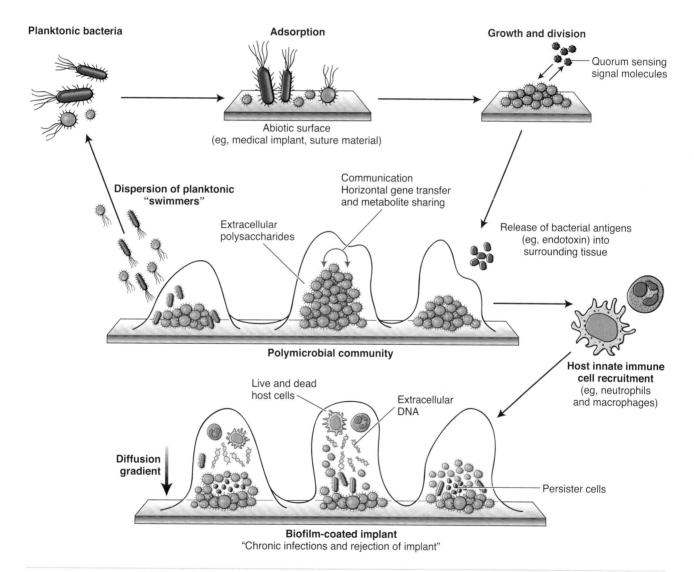

FIGURE 67.1   Biofilm life cycle. Free-floating planktonic bacteria adhere to various abiotic or biotic surfaces. At a certain cell density, bacteria exhibit changes in gene expression and will begin to produce signal molecules such as quorum sensing molecules. This results in the production of a thick extracellular polysaccharide layer around the microbial community, providing protection from host immune cells, desiccation, and an environment conducive to horizontal gene transfer. Planktonic bacteria are periodically released from the community to colonize new locations. Host immune cells such as neutrophils and macrophages are often unable to clear the microbial community and contribute to the structure of the biofilm. Adapted from Harrison et al[11] and Stoodley et al.[12]

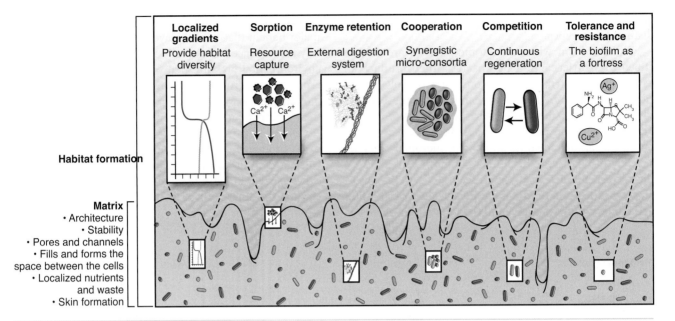

FIGURE 67.2 Properties of mature biofilms. The biofilm mode of growth provides several advantages to the microorganisms living in the community. The production of a hydrated extracellular matrix allows for increased nutrient acquisition and generates localized gradients that result in dramatic differences in nutrient exposure depending on where the organisms are located within the biofilm. This results in differences in growth rates of the microorganisms based on location and leads to the development of bacterial "persister" cells. A similar phenomenon is observed with the diffusion of antimicrobial molecules, and this helps promote the emergence of tolerance and resistance. The close proximity of bacteria to one another also aids in social interactions such as metabolite sharing between different species. Together, these properties make for a much more robust and resilient form of bacterial growth compared with traditional planktonic organisms. Reprinted by permission from Nature: Flemming et al.[15] Copyright © 2016 Springer Nature.

inactivated before they effectively penetrate a biofilm.[19] This diffusion barrier can create an environment that promotes the development of random mutations with the potential of conferring greater antimicrobial resistance to some of the bacteria. Constant low-level exposure to antimicrobial agents in particular can promote increased resistance development within a biofilm. In addition, the physical characteristics and three-dimensional structure of biofilms prevent diffusion of various biocides, and this mode of growth is typically more resistant to biocides than planktonic cells.[14,20] The length of time that biofilms are permitted to grow and generate a more complex EPS enhances this resistance, as mature biofilms show increased tolerance to biocides such as glutaraldehyde.[21] Biofilm-associated microbes experience environmental heterogeneity, meaning that different microniches within the biofilm have different concentrations of nutrients.[15,22] At the center of a biofilm, the oxygen and other nutrient concentrations can be 30 times less than the concentrations at the surface.[23,24] The conditions at the center of the biofilms can even be completely anaerobic in an otherwise aerobic environment.[24] This change in nutrient availability appears to cause cells near the center of the biofilm to exist in a slow-growing state.[9,25] Bacteria growing in this nutrient-restricted state are much less susceptible to antimicrobial agents because the mechanisms of many

antimicrobials target the synthesis of nucleic acids and proteins in growing and dividing cells and minimally affect dormant cells that are not actively and rapidly producing these molecules.[26] The differences in metabolic states of the cells within a biofilm ensure that some bacteria will survive exposure to antimicrobials[9] or other harsh environmental challenging conditions. Channels for water and nutrients are present throughout the entire structure of the biofilm, which help the microbes near the center receive necessary nutrients. Certain populations of planktonic bacteria, known as "swimmers," can tunnel into the biofilm, creating another distinct system of pores that help supply nutrients and oxygen to nutrient-deficient areas.[24,27]

The frequency of mutation in biofilms is significantly higher than in planktonic organisms, leading to the development of antibiotic resistance and other genetic changes more rapidly in biofilms than in planktonic cells.[13] Biofilm-associated bacteria exhibit what is termed a "hypermutable phenotype," creating mutations in the DNA repair pathways leading to the enhanced expression of numerous mutant phenotypes within the community.[13] This seems to be an evolutionary strategy for microbes to survive a variety of unique challenges by rapidly creating a diversity in their genotypes and phenotypes. Biofilm-associated bacteria are more resistant to various environmental stresses such as desiccation, nutrient limitation, toxin actions, oxidative stresses, and heat shock through these mutations, and this hypermutable state can lead to increased antimicrobial resistance opportunities.[13,26,28-31]

All biofilms found in the natural environment are polymicrobial (ie, composed of multiple microbial genera and species) because this provides numerous advantages to the microbes.[32] Multiple species living together exhibit an increased rate of horizontal gene transfer (movement of genes from one bacterium to another), and this, in conjunction with the hypermutable phenotype, allows bacteria living within the biofilm to more efficiently deal with environmental stresses than any single species in planktonic form.[33] Certain types of bacteria are able to promote the growth of other bacterial species when in proximity, such as in coculture. For example, the presence of *Fusobacterium nucleatum* in a culture allows *Porphyromonas gingivalis* to grow under microaerophilic conditions that would otherwise be toxic to monocultures of *P gingivalis*.[34] The process of symbiotic nitrification is another example of metabolite cooperation in biofilms. In this phenomenon, specific bacteria from the genus *Nitrospira* oxidize ammonium to nitrite, which then is oxidized by other members of this genus to nitrate.[35] These observations provide clear evidence for the reasons why bacteria aggregate and form polymicrobial communities that exhibit social interactions such as competition, cooperation, and synergism.

Just like in higher organisms, communication among individual cells is a critical aspect of microbial life in a complex community. All the processes described earlier rely on the exchange of information between microorganisms within a biofilm. Bacteria in biofilms communicate with one another via various signaling molecules in a process initially termed quorum sensing. Waters and Bassler[36] comprehensively review the quorum sensing concept. Disruption of quorum sensing pathways may represent a powerful alternative to traditional antimicrobial treatments. For example, a recent study on aquatic, biofilm-forming species of *Vibrio* demonstrated that intermediates of polyhydroxy butyrates effectively inhibit biofilm formation in a strain-specific fashion by disrupting communication between cells.[37] Such unique strategies may lead to novel mechanisms of inhibiting and killing microbes.

Biofilms are a significant issue in any system that relies on the movement of water or other nutrient-laden liquids through a pipeline, tube, or planar structure. The shear forces in these systems create environments that are conducive toward biofilm development and growth.[31] Biofilms and their associated structures can act as a reservoir for pathogens in various medical devices that require water or other liquids, such as washer-disinfectors, and may result in relatively mild consequences such as water discoloration or, in catastrophic cases, can result in large outbreaks of infectious disease.[38-40] Biofilms present a substantial problem in the water reservoirs and associated liquid delivery systems in surgical and medical equipment

such as those used in eye surgery facilities.[38] One particularly notable pathogen known to be capable of biofilm formation in air conditioner and domestic water supply cooling towers is *Legionella pneumophila*.[40] This particular bacterium can cause serious outbreaks of pneumonia infections or a condition known as legionellosis or Legionnaires' disease. Biofilms of *Legionella* within contaminated cooling towers are one of the earliest reported and major sources of infection in such outbreaks.[40] These outbreaks are particularly severe in immunocompromised populations.[41] New methods to detect bacteria growing in these systems include DNA amplification and next generation DNA sequencing, which have brought biofilms to the attention of researchers particularly in the field of water contamination.[40,42]

Up to 60% of clinical infections treated with antibiotics are estimated to have involved biofilms.[8] Biofilm-associated infections can slowly lead to chronic tissue damage caused by the continual production or overproduction of proinflammatory molecules by frustrated host immune cells such as neutrophils (see Figure 67.1). Inflammation-induced tissue damage occurs in this fashion in conditions such as cystic fibrosis,[43] periodontal disease,[44] and a number of other chronic infectious diseases. In vivo experiments have shown neutrophil migration within biofilms. In some cases, the EPS matrix incorporates damaged and/or dead host immune cells, likely strengthening the barrier to other host immune cells (Figure 67.3).[3] Quiescent biofilms act as nidi of future infection in a host; however, certain toxins (such as endotoxin; see chapter 66) and other bacterial products can be released periodically from mature biofilms that can result in immune responses and inflammation at near and distant locations. Biofilms growing in an environment such as the water reservoirs of medical washing-disinfection equipment can cause postsurgical aseptic inflammation in patients through the release of heat-resistant endotoxins. Such aseptic endotoxin-mediated inflammation events have been implicated in cases of diffuse lamellar keratitis (DLK) in patients undergoing corneal LASIK surgery[38] as well as in outbreaks of toxic anterior segment syndrome (TASS).[45] A combination of mechanical abrasion and biocide application was required to dramatically reduce the incidence of DLK[38] and TASS caused by these biofilm-colonized surfaces.[45]

▶ BIOFILMS AND MEDICAL DEVICES

Biofilms form on a wide variety of medical devices, often resulting in chronic infections that are difficult to treat. Infections surrounding medical implants are a serious therapeutic challenge. The economic effect of such biofilm-associated infections is staggering, with estimates of up to 40 billion US dollars annually in the United States alone.[46] The impact of biofilms in implant infections is reviewed by Costerton et al in 2005.[47]

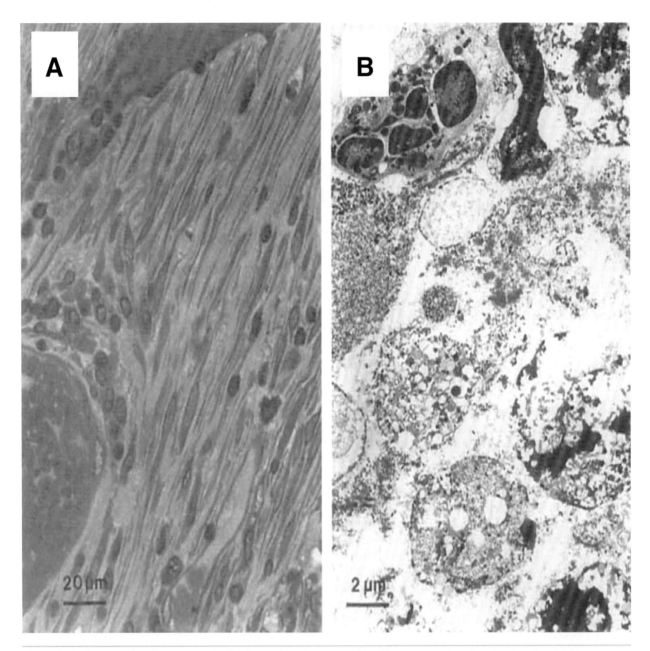

FIGURE 67.3 A, Light photomicrograph of an in vivo–generated biofilm, removed and stained with methylene blue and basic fuchsin and imaged 4 or 28 d after insertion into the peritoneal cavity of a rabbit. The biofilms on the implants were composed of both microbial proteins and host vascularized connective tissue. B, Transmission electron micrograph showing that live and degenerating host immune cells make up a significant proportion of the in vivo biofilm as early as 4 d after biofilm development. Visible in this image are host neutrophils, macrophages, erythrocytes, and a network of fibrin. From Buret et al.[3] Copyright © 1991 John Wiley & Sons, Inc. Reprinted by permission of John Wiley & Sons, Inc.

Biofilms are associated with infections on implanted artificial heart valves, orthopedic joint prostheses, catheters, stents, dental implants, contact lenses, and numerous other artificial substrates placed in or adjacent to host tissue.[48-52] These implant-associated biofilms often result in chronic infections that require multiple treatments and, in severe cases, result in the removal of the afflicted implant.[9,50,53]

Suture material is at high risk of biofilm development from skin-based microorganisms, and this is a significant cause of surgical site infection (SSI)[53] and surgical wound dehiscence. These types of infections are a heavy burden on the medical industry and can account for substantial proportions of the total hospital budget.[54] In a large portion of these infections (up to 30%), clinicians are unable to culture any viable species from the wounds and this may be due to the biofilm mode of growth itself[55] or the involvement of microorganisms that are challenging to culture such as mycobacteria.[56] Similarly, SSIs may involve bacteria that are slow to grow or are not typically scrutinized by medical diagnostic laboratories. Some researchers hypothesize that the slow-growing phenotype makes it more challenging to identify clinically relevant biofilm-associated bacteria because traditional clinical diagnostic approaches do not allow enough time for visible growth on culture plates.[55] Biofilms composed of nontuberculous mycobacteria have also been implicated as causative agents of postsurgical infections, and these are very difficult to treat because many typical antibiotics or antimycobacterial drugs do not eradicate the bacteria.[56]

Using confocal laser scanning microscopy (CLSM) and fluorescent in situ hybridization (FISH) on samples from 15 patients with SSIs associated with biofilm growth on permanent, multifilament sutures, investigators determined that the biofilms on the sutures were all polymicrobial in nature.[53] These biofilms were composed of several microbial taxa, with *Staphylococcus aureus* (and in particular methicillin-resistant *S aureus*) being the most prevalent. An earlier case study demonstrated that a polymicrobial biofilm attached to sutures caused a persistent surgical wound infection in a patient.[57] In these particular cases, which are likely to be more common than the literature suggests, treatments using antibiotics were not successful, and the sutures needed to be removed to eliminate the chronic infections.[53,57] These studies illustrate several complicating issues with biofilm-associated chronic infections. Fortunately, removal of sutures is relatively simple. In other types of biofilm-associated infection, this is not a trivial task (eg, hip and knee joint prostheses or artificial heart valves). As described earlier, treatments with antimicrobials often fail due to lack of diffusion of the antimicrobial into biofilm, the increased incidence of gene transfer (that can convey resistance) within the biofilm as well as the presence of "persister" or metabolically dormant microbial cells in biofilms. The result is increased time spent in health care facilities, making patients even more susceptible to subsequent infections and most particularly when the individual is immunocompromised.

▶ GENERATION OF BIOFILMS IN VITRO

The generation of multiple, equivalent, and uniform biofilms for high-throughput in vitro studies is a significant challenge that microbiologists face. The major issue is reproducibility. There remains controversy among research groups regarding which method of biofilm generation in the laboratory provides the most accurate and realistic representation of biofilms and therefore several different techniques have become widely employed by groups around the globe. The use of a variety of methods creates challenges when reproducing previously published work. Therefore, standardization of experimental design, and perhaps even methods, is crucial in this important field

of microbiological research. The following section briefly describes some of the common methods for biofilm generation in the laboratory, highlighting the advantages and disadvantages of each technique.

Static Systems

Peterson and colleagues[58] review several different methods for the generation of biofilms. Initial experiments investigating biofilm growth relied on static approaches. This method was originally developed to measure adhesion of *S aureus* and has since been used to assess bacterial attachment and associated genes using mutants of several different bacterial species. Many studies have employed the static plate method to assess the effects of various natural and artificial inhibitors on overall biomass and biofilm formation.[59-61] Although this approach is useful for quantifying the initial attachment of bacteria to an abiotic surface, the static method lacks the shear forces necessary for representative mature biofilm development. Additionally, this method does not allow users to supply fresh nutrients to the bacteria in the biofilm. With the limitations of these types of in vitro assays, many researchers advise caution when drawing conclusions and extrapolating results to in vivo and natural biofilms. Results from a study on *Enterococcus faecalis* biofilms (organisms that play a significant role in endocarditis) indicated that biofilms generated using a static method on polystyrene plates were not equivalent to biofilms grown on porcine heart valves.[62] This led the researchers to conclude that *E faecalis* biofilms generated in vitro are not clinically relevant and suggested that these types of studies should be validated using ex vivo approaches prior to publication.[62] Despite such limitations, the static microplate growth method does allow scientists to quantify the biomass of various biofilms and as such, this method is still widely accepted as a tool to assess biofilm growth.[58,63-65] This quick method to assess the total biomass in the wells of microplates using crystal violet is colloquially referred to as the microtiter dish biofilm assay, or O'Toole assay.[66]

Flow Cells and Reactors

Using flow systems has several advantages. There is ample shear force applied to the surface-adhered microbes to stimulate biofilm formation. In addition, a constant supply of growth medium via the flow system provides the organisms with a continuous supply of nutrients. Finally, these systems can be adapted to generate biofilms directly on glass coverslips or slides, allowing for easy fixation and staining. This allows researchers to visualize the biofilms using the various microscopy techniques discussed in the following text in one step.

Costerton and colleagues[67] at the University of Calgary developed one of the first flow reactor systems for monitoring the formation of biofilms in a laboratory setting in 1981. This system was designed to monitor biofilm-associated fouling in industrial settings and was the first platform that allowed researchers to observe relatively undisturbed biofilms due to the presence of removable sampling surfaces.[67] In this fashion, they were able to visualize biofilm growth on the test surfaces with scanning electron microscope (SEM) and bright-field microscopy.[67] This unique approach allowed the authors to conclude that filamentous bacteria are important in biofilm development, particularly at high flow rates, and play a significant role in the loss of energy in these types of tubular systems. This general design has been modified several times since its development, leading to a system now known as the modified Robbins device (MRD) and is commonly used in biofilm research worldwide.

Scientists at the Centers for Disease Control and Prevention (CDC) developed a popular bioreactor that is frequently used today.[68] Further evaluation of this system tested for reproducibility and the results indicated that this system is capable of generating equivalent biofilms; however, researchers need to be cautious when altering parameters such as flow rate to maintain assay validity and reproducibility.[69]

Many studies show that biofilms generated under flow conditions are more representative of real-world natural biofilms[70]; however, other studies indicate that biofilms grown under static conditions behave similarly to those generated with flow systems.[71] For example, Song and colleagues[71] recently demonstrated that dual species biofilms composed of *F nucleatum* and *P gingivalis* did not show statistically significant differences in the physical thickness of biofilm formed when grown in the CDC reactor compared to static plates. Additionally, there was no observable differences in the biocidal activity of chlorhexidine between biofilms generated using the two different methods, but no detailed assessments of microbial physiology were conducted.[71] This result again raises the question of reproducibility between laboratories worldwide because other groups have reported significant differences based on the method of biofilm growth. Recently, high-throughput microfluidic systems have been developed to generate equivalent biofilms without the need for large volumes of media and extensive laboratory space to run equipment such as the CDC reactor.[72] This experimental setup has the powerful advantage of being able to generate realistic, reproducible biofilms and assess antimicrobial efficiency via CLSM in one step.[72] Regardless of what model system is used, standardized, valid, and reproducible assays are required. Biofilm researchers must address this problem going forward. Regulatory agencies such as the United States Environmental Protection Agency have been accepting standardized test methods for biofilm research and associated label claims on products (https://www.epa.gov/pesticides/methods-and-guidance-testing-efficacy-antimicrobials-against-biofilm-bacteria-hard-non). The next section explores one such validated method for assessing the efficacy of antimicrobials on biofilms.

Calgary Biofilm Device

An adaptation to the static method that allows for the application of shear force and the ability to provide fresh nutrients was developed by our group at the University of Calgary in 1999.[73] This approach to in vitro biofilm growth has several advantages and is capable of generating 96 equivalent biofilms on a specialized peg lid that inserts into standard 96-well microplates (Figure 67.4).

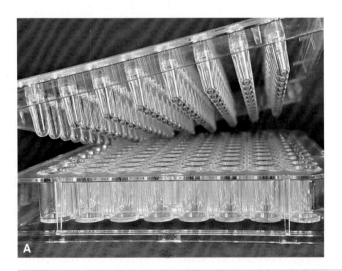
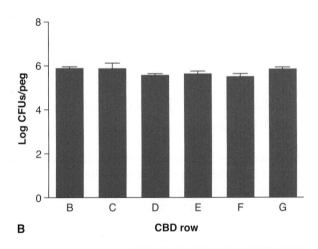

FIGURE 67.4 A, Photograph showing the 96 equivalent pegs of the Calgary Biofilm Device (CBD) and how they fit into the wells of a standard 96-well microplate. B, Equivalent growth of mixed-species biofilms on the pegs of a CBD. *Fusobacterium necrophorum* and *Porphyromonas levii* were mixed in a 1:1 ratio and added to the wells of a 96-well microtiter plate. A CBD peg lid was added and biofilms were grown for 5 d, with fresh medium supplied every 48 h. Four pegs per row were subjected to sonication for 5 min and spot plated for CFUs/peg viable counts. This demonstrates that multiple equivalent biofilms can be generated on the CBD, even with fastidious anaerobic organisms.

Antibiotic and biocide susceptibility testing is easily performed on these 96 equivalent biofilms following a well-designed standard protocol published by Ceri and colleagues[73] that has been accepted as validated methodology for assessing disinfectant efficacy against *P aeruginosa* biofilms (ASTM 2799-11) (ASTM E2799). The minimum biofilm eradication concentration (MBEC) assay, using the Calgary Biofilm Device, is the only microtiter-based assay for assessing biofilm susceptibility to disinfectants currently validated by the American Society for Testing and Materials (ASTM).[74] To generate biofilms for susceptibility testing, standardized suspensions of bacterial cells are inoculated into the wells of a 96-well plate and the peg lid is inserted. The plate is then incubated at the appropriate temperature and placed on a rotary shaker at approximately 120 to 150 rpm; this speed of shaking provides the necessary shear forces for biofilm development. The length of time to generate mature biofilms and appropriate shaking speed depends on the bacterial species of interest. If biofilms are generated over the course of several days (as is often the case with slow-growing bacteria such as anaerobes), the nutrients in the lower wells can be replenished by inoculating a new 96-well plate with growth media and transferring the peg lid with attached biofilms to the fresh media. The frequency of media changes can be altered to optimize biofilm growth on the pegs. Additionally, the pegs can be coated with various solutions such as bovine serum albumin (BSA) or L-lysine to promote bacterial adhesion.[75] Once the biofilms are mature or reach the desired cell density, biofilm antimicrobial resistance or susceptibility is evaluated by submerging the pegs in dilutions of various biocides.[76] Following exposure to the antimicrobials, the biofilms are subjected to sonication to remove the adherent cells and plated to check viable cell counts. This approach has been used in a large number of susceptibility tests focused on biofilms. An additional benefit of this system is that planktonic organisms from the wells of the inoculum plate can also be assessed for antimicrobial resistance or activity, allowing researchers to compare planktonic and biofilm eradication concentrations in a single assay system.[73,75,76] A video describing this assay procedure currently is available through YouTube (*MBEC Assay*, https://www.youtube.com/watch?v=HpBepCYYOJ8). We also have demonstrated that human, or other animal, gut microbiota biofilms may also be grown anaerobically ex vivo using the CBD.[77-79] These CBD-generated biofilms contain the major bacterial classes found in human gut or fecal microbiota, which further underscores the physiological significance of this model system.

Recently, we developed an adaptation of the CBD method where Transwell tissue culture permeable support inserts were used as the substrate for mixed-species biofilm growth.[80] This adaptation allowed growth of multiple equivalent biofilms on the underside of membrane permeable support inserts. Using this approach, researchers can select the appropriate pore size based on their experimental needs and the pores range from 0.1 to 12 μm in diameter. These tissue culture plate inserts are available from a number of commercial retailers including VWR and Corning. The membranes can be composed of various materials, such as polycarbonate, polyester, and polytetrafluoroethylene, depending on the researcher's needs. This approach has additional versatility over the CBD and facilitates investigation of innate immune cell interactions with biofilms.

▶ VISUALIZATION OF BIOFILMS

Several microscopy techniques enable researchers to visualize and characterize biofilm growth. The development of CLSM was a major advancement that allowed researchers to visualize hydrated, living biofilms.[81] Costerton and colleagues[81] used this technique to image biofilms composed of various pathogens such as *Pseudomonas aeruginosa*, *Pseudomonas fluorescens*, and *Vibrio parahaemolyticus*. Since this development, scientists have used the technique to assess parameters such as biofilm depth, distribution and density of cells, and the presence of water channels (with water flowing) throughout the biofilm extracellular architecture.[82-84] The CLSM has been adapted to allow for time-lapse video microscopy to observe interactions of biofilms with host cells.[83] This imaging method also allows researchers to monitor diffusion rates of various nutrients into the biofilm matrix as well as accurately assess the bactericidal activity of various antimicrobials (Figure 67.5).[76,81]

The CLSM techniques can be augmented using fluorescent labels that are specific for bacterial taxa of interest.[85] This approach allows scientists to follow specific types of microorganisms in the biofilm community to investigate parameters such as mutualistic growth and spatial distribution of taxa throughout the biofilm itself.

The FISH is an addition to basic confocal techniques that allows for the specific labeling of various sequences of DNA or RNA in a biofilm[86,87] using complementary sequence probes. This provides the ability to view genes and gene expression within biofilms.

The SEM is another powerful tool to assess the morphology of bacteria present in various biofilms. Once again, Costerton and colleagues[88] were among the first to use this approach in a study of *S aureus* biofilm formation on the surface of a pacemaker lead. The SEM continues to be used to demonstrate biofilm growth on a variety of medical device types. Improper daily care of these devices can lead to serious outbreaks of disease such as DLK and TASS (Figure 67.6).[38]

Prominent advances in the field of metagenomics has allowed researchers to investigate the microbial composition of various biofilm communities through the assessment of gene sequences. Because this type of molecular technique does not rely on the specific cultivation viable bacteria, it provides valuable and more comprehensive information about all types of microorganisms present,[89]

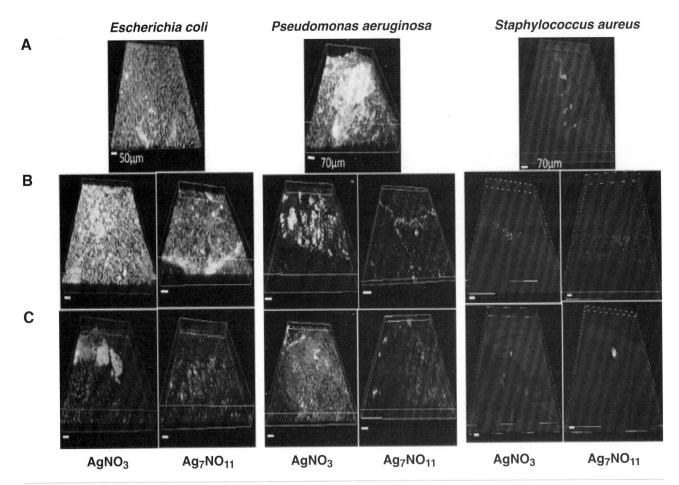

FIGURE 67.5 Confocal laser scanning microscopy (CLSM) investigating the efficacy of silver oxynitrate (Ag$_7$NO$_{11}$) and silver nitrate (AgNO$_3$) at reducing biofilm quantity. The 24-h biofilms of *Escherichia coli*, *Pseudomonas aeruginosa*, and *Staphylococcus aureus* were generated on the pegs of a CBD and subsequently exposed to 0 µM (A), 5 µM (B), and 12.5 µM (C) of AgNO$_3$ or Ag$_7$NO$_{11}$ for 24 h. BacLight Live/Dead staining was used to assess biomass and bacterial viability. Confocal images were taken at 20× magnification using excitation wavelength, 488 nm; emission wavelength, 498 nm for green cells (live); and excitation wavelength, 523 nm; emission wavelength, 617 nm for red cells (dead). All three biofilms were reduced by the metal compound. For a color version of this art, please consult the eBook. From Lemire et al.[76] Reproduced with permission from American Society for Microbiology. Copyright © 2015 American Society for Microbiology.

including those believed to be unculturable. Such tools are now valuable for the investigation of biofilm-associated medical and industrial challenges (Figure 67.7).

▶ PREVENTION, CONTROL, AND ELIMINATION OF BIOFILMS

The previous sections of this chapter have detailed the prevalence of biofilms throughout the natural and medical world and provided details on how the unique physiology of the biofilm structure benefits all the microorganisms in these communities. These complex communities clearly play a significant role in chronic infections, particularly in the context of artificial implants and contamination of materials and surfaces that need to be maintained sterile. The breadth of biofilm impact and importance is still

likely underestimated; however, researchers are beginning to focus on discovering new ways to detect, eradicate, prevent, and improve treatments for biofilms and their associated infections and/or contaminations. As the technique is improved, streamlined metagenomics may provide a practical and valuable tool to monitor development of biofilms in situ and potentially advance our rate of success through early intervention (ie, in advance of biofilm maturation). Despite numerous innovations in the field, biofilms still beleaguer the medical and industrial communities. This slow progress in biofilm science has stemmed from the lack of standardized models to generate biofilms and the challenge of growing biofilms in a laboratory setting that are representative of those in natural settings. In vivo and in situ biofilms contain substantial amounts of host or environmental components, respectively, in addition to the microbe-derived material.[3]

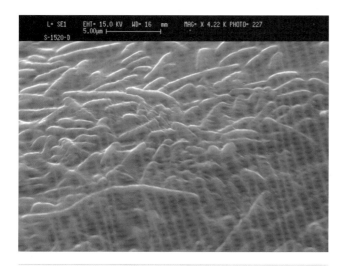

FIGURE 67.6 Scanning electron micrograph of 20-d-old biofilm growth on metal disks in a sterilizer reservoir during an outbreak of diffuse lamellar keratitis (DLK). After treatment with a disinfectant, *Burkholderia pickettii* was able to recolonize the sterilizer reservoir in as few as 7 to 11 d and a considerable biofilm was apparent 20 d after initial disinfection. Reproduced from Holland and Morck,[45] with permission.

Periodontal biofilms stimulate the release of DNA from host neutrophils, and this host DNA is incorporated into the biofilm matrix itself, adding structural stability to the EPS as well as providing an additional diffusion barrier to antimicrobials,[84] and contributes to the hydration of the biofilm. The CBD with an associated MBEC assay is an example of a validated system that can provide users with rapid susceptibility results,[75] but methods will evolve to

better represent the natural phenomenon of biofilm development and persistence.

In industrial settings, a combination of disinfection techniques are employed to ensure the removal of potentially hazardous biofilms. Using only one simple approach, such as the desiccation of stainless steel in the meat industry, allows the bacteria to persist and therefore provides an opportunity to cause serious infections. A recent study demonstrated that biofilms of *Listeria monocytogenes* can survive long-term desiccation practices on stainless steel surfaces for more than 48 days.[90] Therefore, even dried biofilms can pose a serious problem in pathogenic outbreaks. The precise mechanism of biofilm survival in these harsh environmental settings is still unknown, but the presence of metabolically dormant cells likely plays a major role. For these reasons, a combination of disinfection techniques such as the application of appropriate biocides in addition to desiccation is highly recommended, particularly in the food industry.

Biofilm formation is a common problem observed at the fluid-substrate interface in various food-processing settings. This phenomenon even poses an issue in soap dispensers.[91] Even after treatment with high concentrations of sodium hydroxide for 10 minutes, the bacterial biofilms were not fully eradicated, resulting in persistent contamination of the dispenser.[91] Reverse osmosis membranes used in applications such as the production of dairy products also experience a similar circumstance, where biofilms grow at the interface between the membrane and the product.[92] The polysaccharides produced by such biofilms act as a barrier to disinfectants, and this allows for the fouling of the membrane and subsequent

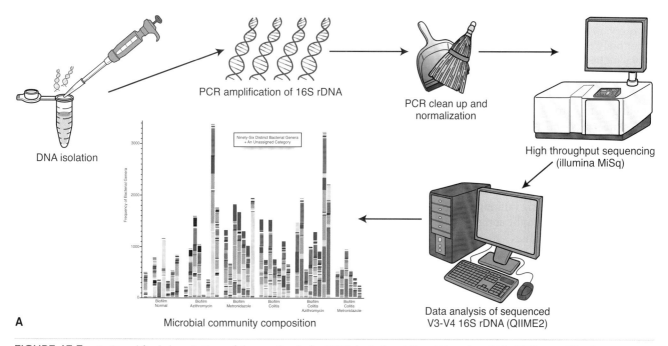

FIGURE 67.7 A, Simplified description of the methods for DNA isolation, V3 to V4 region 16S rDNA amplification, cleaning, high throughput sequencing, and analyzing V3 to V4 16S rDNA from biofilm bacteria. *(Continued)*

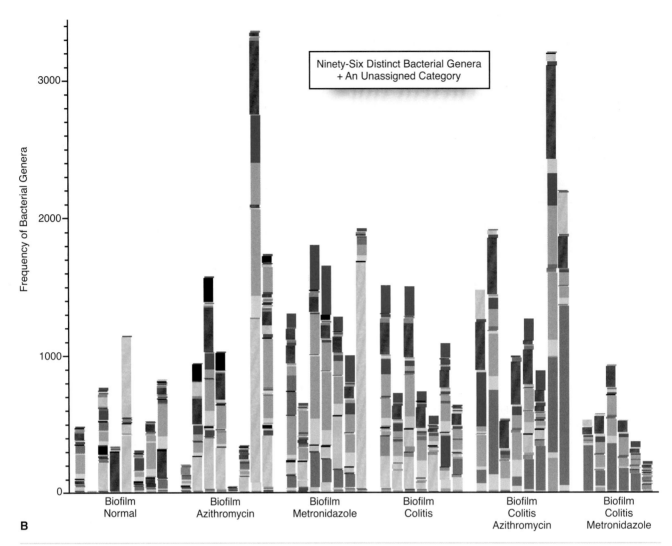

FIGURE 67.7 *(Continued)* B, Example of a genus-level green gene database probed, QIIME2-generated, taxon-stacked bar graph of amplified and sequenced V3 to V4 16S rDNA of colon biofilms from normal mice, normal mice exposed to either oral azithromycin or oral metronidazole, mice with induced colitis, and colitis mice exposed to either oral azithromycin or oral metronidazole. The colored bars represent distinct genera of colon biofilm bacteria. Ninety-six identified genera and substantial unidentifiable genera were observed.

spoiling of the product.[92] Treatment with a combination of disinfectants and even quorum sensing inhibitors is recommended for such surfaces.

Biofouling in oil and gas pipelines due to biofilm formation imparts a huge economic cost on the petroleum industry. These biofilms are typically composed of sulfate-reducing bacteria (among others) and can lead to corrosion, which eventually comprises the integrity of the pipe.[93] Gieg and colleagues[93] review the current strategies to mitigate the issues surrounding these costly biofilms. Various approaches have been used in an attempt to eliminate pipeline biofilms and a combination of mechanical and chemical approaches is the most efficient. One mechanical approach to maintenance and cleaning is termed "pigging" and uses the flow of product in a pipeline to push a physical scraping device termed a "pig" through the pipe to remove biological debris from the internal surface.[94]

Quarini and Shire[94] reviewed this concept. Although this method is effective at removing bulk biological material, the bacteria that produce this debris are often left behind, allowing for the rapid regeneration of biofilm. For this reason, broad-spectrum biocides such as glutaraldehyde, tetrakis hydroxymethyl phosphonium sulfate, and sodium hypochlorite are often used in conjunction with mechanical methods.[95] Certain chemicals used as biocides such as aldehydes also act to fix biomaterials onto surfaces such as pipelines; this can promote further bacterial growth and is another reason why multiple mechanical and chemical approaches are recommended to remove biofilms from any industrial surface.[96] In many of these situations, oxidizing agents (or oxidizing agent-based formulations) such as those based on chlorine, hydrogen peroxide, ozone, and peracetic acid are preferred due to their ability to physically remove and breakdown products, although this can vary depending on the product or application conditions (see chapters 15 and 18).

The most effective way to eliminate the morbidity and costs associated with clinical and industrial biofilms or contaminated equipment is to prevent the initial attachment of the bacteria to the substrate (eg, artificial implant, natural tissue, surgical equipment, and food-processing equipment) or to detect this phenomenon early. As previously discussed, once established as a mature structure, biofilms are very difficult to treat or eradicate; antimicrobials and disinfectants are often ineffective, and residual components of biofilms such as endotoxin (lipopolysaccharides) remain highly biologically active.[38] Persistent contamination and/or chronic infection becomes the typical sequelae. Preventing the adhesion of bacteria is an active field of biofilm research, and several research groups continue to develop a wide variety of antimicrobial coatings for artificial implants as well as alternative materials to construct implants in an attempt to limit biofilm formation.[97] Due to the massive number of examples of diverse methods attempted to limit bacterial adherence on to medical devices, this chapter does not encompass all of the various studies and techniques that have been published to date. Instead, it focuses on a few examples that display significant promise for future applications and some examples where these goals are not met. The material composition of an implant can affect bacterial adherence, as demonstrated decades ago when Lopez-Lopez and colleagues[98] published on the effect of the catheter material on bacterial adherence. The research showed that various biofilm-forming bacteria adhered to polyvinyl chloride and siliconized latex significantly more than to materials such as Teflon.[98] Subsequent research has pursued the ultimate "antibiofilm material" with limited success.

Obviously, the first step when considering implanting a medical device is microbial reduction or elimination via thermal or chemical disinfection or sterilization, but this will not directly prevent the recontamination of the device during insertion into the body or during the continued use within the body. The additional step of impregnating implants such as catheters with antibiotics or microbiocides (eg, chlorhexidine, triclosan, and silver) can significantly reduce the risk of infection in these cases (see chapter 73).[99,100] The inclusion of chemicals that chelate ions essential for microbial growth, such as EDTA, can have some bacteriostatic activity on their own or even increase the efficacy of an antimicrobial. Such chelating agents can act synergistically with antibiotics like minocycline and biocides like triclosan, particularly against gram-negative pathogens.[99] This approach mimics in vivo strategies to limit bacterial growth such as the iron restriction regulated by hepcidin commonly seen in mammals[101] and other animals. The addition of certain enzymes such as DNAses, proteases, or cellulases can help remove the DNA, proteins, and polysaccharides produced

by bacterial biofilms, improving the efficacy of various biocides.[102] Despite such promising studies, there is still controversy regarding the ability of some biocides, such as chlorhexidine, to prevent biofilm colonization over a longer period (greater than 48 h), suggesting that such antimicrobial uses may be most effective[103] in the short term.

Reusable devices such as surgical or medical instruments also provide suitable surfaces for the formation of harmful bacterial biofilms. However, some researchers indicate that if technicians are careful and follow proper decontamination (in particular cleaning) procedures promptly following use of these devices, the risk of biofilm growth and subsequent infection is relatively low.[104] Despite this observation, we highly recommend that proper quality assurance protocols are in place to ensure adequate terminal disinfection or sterility (see chapter 47). One type of reusable medical instrument where biofilm growth poses a significant risk is flexible and rigid endoscopes. The environment within the internal channels or structures of these instruments is perfectly suited for biofilm growth, and therefore, extra caution must be taken when reprocessing them.[105] Special care should be taken in any procedure that requires the use of reusable tools or devices to ensure biofilms are completely removed. Similar to industrial biofilms, this should include a combination of mechanical methods (sonicating, scraping, scrubbing), thermal, and/or chemical disinfectant treatments. Coating presterilized suture material with various antimicrobials limits the amount of bacterial growth following implantation.[106,107] A recent meta-analysis investigating the efficacy of coating sutures with an antimicrobial such as triclosan determined that the strategy is effective in preventing initial attachment of microbes and therefore limits the risk of initial biofilm formation and associated surgical wound infections involving implanted suture material.[106] For intravascular catheters, fewer bacteria have been found to attach to materials such as soft hydrogels of polyethylene glycol dimethacrylate (PEGDMA) compared to stiffer PEGDMA materials.[108] The authors concluded that constructing vascular catheter implants with "softer" materials in combination with traditional antimicrobial coatings would further reduce the risk of contamination, colonization, biofilm formation, and subsequent infection. For infections involving biofilm formation on contact lenses, the incorporation of an organoselenium monomer into the polypropylene contact lens case inhibits bacterial attachment, reduces biofilm formation, and may prevent eye infection involving biofilm formation in inadequately cleaned contact lens cases.[52]

Recently published research on the efficacy of implants coated with a thin film of titanium-copper oxide showed promise in preventing bacterial colonization of prosthetic devices.[109] However, this study only examined the effects in vitro, and the authors recognized that this requires further investigation in an animal model of periprosthetic infection. Many research laboratories are working on projects such as the one described earlier with varying degrees of success. For example, research into the ability of the metal tantalum (tantalium) to prevent bacterial adherence has shown that there were no significant differences in bacterial adhesion or viability between tantalum and titanium materials.[110]

A useful but very challenging model for in vivo evaluation of these approaches is the rabbit model of catheter-associated urinary tract infection.[111-113] This approach allows researchers to investigate the efficacy of different antibiotics on biofilm formation in a living organism, thus providing a more accurate representation of infection compared to the use of in vitro models of biofilm formation. The model requires enormous technical and veterinary input in order to meet the animal welfare requirements of a chronic catheter-related infection and should never be attempted without those expert resources. The intraperitoneal foreign-body infection model using mice is another powerful tool for in vivo evaluation of biofilm interactions with host cells and various antimicrobials.[114,115] Other groups have developed in vivo polymicrobial biofilm wound models to study these types of infections.[116] Lebeaux and colleagues[117] review some other interesting in vivo approaches for studying biofilms, all of which require detailed veterinary input and oversight.

These few examples do not fully represent the breadth of different materials and coatings researchers are investigating to prevent the formation of bacterial biofilms on medical implants, but overall, the results from these studies indicate that scientists are still a great distance from the perfect material that inhibits bacterial adhesion in vivo. Because we are currently unable to fully prevent biofilm formation on contaminated medical implants, work continues on developing effective treatment strategies to eliminate these biofilm infections. It almost goes without stating that very diligent prevention of contamination, such as careful use of aseptic technique, equipment maintenance, and the use of cleaning, disinfection, and sterilization protocols, is essential in any approach for minimizing the adverse effects of biofilms.

Once a biofilm is established on a surface including an implant or surrounding tissues, it is notoriously difficult to eradicate for the reasons discussed earlier in this chapter. The traditional approach of using high doses of potent antibiotics may not be successful in these types of biofilm-related chronic infections. Because of this, researchers around the world are focusing on developing alternative treatments for biofilm-associated infections (often in combination with antibiotics), and these approaches may provide solutions in clinical settings. In the case of SSIs, removal of the biofilm-colonized device is still the recommended course of action in conjunction with the administration of antibiotics.[118] When removal of the afflicted implant is impossible or difficult, new therapies may relieve stress on the patient, personal suffering, and reduce the economic burden of biofilm-associated infections.

Research investigating various metal compounds for their efficacy at preventing and eliminating biofilms has shown some remarkable promise.[76] Lemire et al[76] used the CBD to generate biofilms composed of uropathogenic *Escherichia coli*, fluoroquinolone-resistant *P aeruginosa*, and methicillin-resistant *S aureus*. These were exposed to silver and copper compounds.[76] Silver oxynitrate (Ag_7NO_{11}) exhibited lower MBEC and MBC values than other metal compounds evaluated in this study, indicating Ag_7NO_{11} was more effective at preventing biofilm formation and potentially better at controlling subsequent biofilm-related disease (see Figure 67.5).[76] One caveat to this approach is that these metal compounds remain quite toxic to eukaryotic cells as well as to biofilms; therefore, administration of such antimicrobial agents is likely only viable as a locally applied topical agent or in applications involving more inert surfaces associated with a patient or living animal. Lemire et al[76] proposed the use of this particular compound in silver-impregnated bandages to manage burn wounds and other chronic open wounds that are subject to repeated or constant infection involving biofilm formation. This allows the metal compound to be applied externally to derive maximal antibiofilm effects and it is relatively simple to modify, remove, or replace in these situations.

Certain natural compounds may be effective at preventing biofilm formation. A recent study investigating the efficacy of natural compounds extracted from the marigold flower (*Calendula officinalis*) and sage bush (*Buddleja salviifolia*) suggested that these compounds exhibited antibiofilm properties.[51] The authors proposed the addition of these compounds to contact lenses solutions to assist in preventing biofilm formation on contact lenses and subsequent eye irritation in lens users. The actual efficacy and the mechanisms of action for biofilm inhibition of these compounds are not specified and should be investigated in future studies and before clinical application. There are thousands of other examples of antibiofilm peptides, both naturally occurring and synthetic, and these are the focus of recent reviews.[119-121]

Other novel approaches at developing specific biofilm-eradicating compounds focus on disrupting the bacterial cell-to-cell signaling (ie, quorum sensing) in order to prevent the upregulation and transcription of genes that encode proteins/enzymes involved in the biofilm phenotype. Seghal Kiran and colleagues[37] published research indicating how quorum sensing inhibition can affect the formation of biofilms. Intermediates of polyhydroxy butyrates appear to effectively inhibit biofilm formation by *Vibrio* in a strain-specific fashion through the disruption of quorum sensing and intercellular communication.[37] Another example of this approach includes a recent study that explored the antibiofilm capabilities of an extract from a plant used in traditional Chinese medicine known as *Scutellaria baicalensis* (Baikal skullcap). The compound of interest, baicalin, was effective

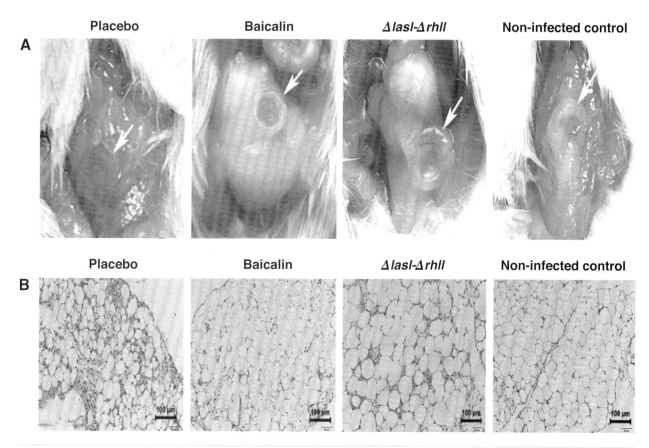

FIGURE 67.8 Gross pathology (A) and histopathologic (B) changes seen in a mouse model of intraperitoneal biofilm infection with *Pseudomonas aeruginosa*. Implants were infected with wild-type *P aeruginosa* (placebo and baicalin treated) or a mutant strain lacking genes essential for proper quorum sensing (ΔlasI-ΔrhlI) and inserted into mice. Treatment with baicalin limited the inflammation observed around these implants, similarly to the mutant strain incapable of quorum sensing when compared with placebo treated mice. A noninfected control showed similar levels of tissue inflammation and immune cell infiltration as the baicalin and the ΔlasI-ΔrhlI exposed-mice. For a color version of this art, please consult the eBook. Reproduced from Luo et al.[115] https://creativecommons.org/licenses/by/4.0/.

at preventing the formation of biofilms by *P aeruginosa* grown in 96-well plates at MICs.[115] The authors assessed the efficacy of baicalin in this part of the study using the crystal violet biomass assay developed by O'Toole, which does not employ shear forces in biofilm development. Baicalin also inhibited the expression of several factors associated with biofilm formation and overall virulence in a dose-dependent fashion.[115] Baicalin targeted and repressed genes that are responsible for the production of several important quorum sensing molecules, including *lasI*, *lasR*, and *rhlI*.[115] The authors further evaluated the effects of baicalin in vivo, employing a mouse model of an intraperitoneal implant infection (Figure 67.8). A silicone implant was preincubated with *P aeruginosa* bacteria to model a biofilm and was surgically inserted into experimental mice. In mice exposed to baicalin, there was a significant decrease in inflammation and inflammatory mediators compared to animals that were not exposed to baicalin. These effects were apparent in the gross pathologic changes in these mice.[115] The authors confirmed these findings with another in vivo model using

Caenorhabditis elegans (roundworms). The *P aeruginosa*–infected *C elegans* worms that were treated with baicalin survived three times longer than untreated worms, suggesting that baicalin limited *P aeruginosa*'s pathogenicity.[115] These observations suggest that baicalin may be an effective intervention for established biofilm-associated infection and may act synergistically when used in combination with traditional antibiotic therapies.

▶ CONCLUSIONS

Future biocide and antimicrobial susceptibility testing needs to consider microbes existing as multispecies biofilms in addition to the nutrient-rich broth culture systems traditionally employed by the majority of laboratories and the developers of drugs as well as cleaning and biocidal technologies. Such an approach is more realistic to what these antimicrobial agents will encounter within practical application. To completely remove biofilm-associated bacteria and their EPS from medical tools, devices, and implants, it is recommended to use a combination of mechanical disruption (eg, sonication, physical scrubbing) and antimicrobials (eg, disinfectants, biocides, and antibiotics). The newer compounds known to disrupt biofilm cell-to-cell communication and/or other biofilm-specific physiological functions (eg, antibiofilm peptides) explored in the final section will also help ensure complete destruction of biofilm. Surfaces colonized by biofilms can cause serious infections in implants, serve as potential sources of contamination of various medical devices, and are a source of toxins. They can also contaminate food processing as well as other critical manufacturing functions in a wide variety of industries.

Despite significant progress in the field of biofilm research, scientists are still searching for the "holy grail" of effective biofilm disinfection and elimination. This goal will vary depending on the application of the technology in various industrial and medical situations. A more complete understanding of biofilm physiology, cell-to-cell communication and signaling, as well as overall biofilm structural morphology, is required. As more research groups focus on this distinct form of bacterial growth and investigate the unique features this phenotype presents, we expect that superior strategies to clean and sterilize biofilm-associated surfaces will be developed. Developing these strategies will be directly dependent on the standardization and validation of biofilm assays such as the MBEC assay to reproducibly assess biofilm form and function. This goal is now within our reach.

REFERENCES

1. Vickery K, Deva A, Jacombs A, Allan J, Valente P, Gosbell IB. Presence of biofilm containing viable multiresistant organisms despite terminal cleaning on clinical surfaces in an intensive care unit. *J Hosp Infect.* 2012;80(1):52-55.

2. Almatroudi A, Gosbell IB, Hu H, et al. *Staphylococcus aureus* dry-surface biofilms are not killed by sodium hypochlorite: implications for infection control. *J Hosp Infect.* 2016;93(3):263-270.

3. Buret A, Ward KH, Olson ME, Costerton JW. An in vivo model to study the pathobiology of infectious biofilms on biomaterial surfaces. *J Biomed Mater Res.* 1991;25(7):865-874.

4. Costerton JW, Geesey GG, Cheng KJ. How bacteria stick. *Sci Am.* 1978;238(1):86-95.

5. Costerton JW, Cheng KJ, Geesey GG, et al. Bacterial biofilms in nature and disease. *Annu Rev Microbiol.* 1987;41(1):435-464.

6. McCowan RP, Cheng KJ, Bailey CB, Costerton JW. Adhesion of bacteria to epithelial cell surfaces within the reticulo-rumen of cattle. *Appl Environ Microbiol.* 1978;35(1):149-155.

7. Lappin-Scott H, Burton S, Stoodley P. Revealing a world of biofilms—the pioneering research of Bill Costerton. *Nat Rev Microbiol.* 2014; 12(11):781-787.

8. Fux CA, Costerton JW, Stewart PS, Stoodley P. Survival strategies of infectious biofilms. *Trends Microbiol.* 2005;13(1):34-40.

9. Costerton JW, Stewart PS, Greenberg EP. Bacterial biofilms: a common cause of persistent infections. *Science.* 1999;284(5418):1318-1322.

10. Singh S, Singh SK, Chowdhury I, Singh R. Understanding the mechanism of bacterial biofilms resistance to antimicrobial agents. *Open Microbiol J.* 2017;11:53-62.

11. Harrison JJ, Turner RJ, Marques LLR, Ceri H. Biofilms: a new understanding of these microbial communities is driving a revolution that may transform the science of microbiology. *Am Sci.* 2005;93:508-515.

12. Stoodley P, Sauer K, Davies DG, Costerton JW. Biofilms as complex differentiated communities. *Annu Rev Microbiol.* 2002;56(1):187-209.

13. Høiby N, Bjarnsholt T, Givskov M, Molin S, Ciofu O. Antibiotic resistance of bacterial biofilms. *Int J Antimicrob Agents.* 2010;35(4):322-332.

14. Campanac C, Pineau L, Payard A, Baziard-Mouysset G, Roques C. Interactions between biocide cationic agents and bacterial biofilms. *Antimicrob Agents Chemother.* 2002;46(5):1469-1474.

15. Flemming H-C, Wingender J, Szewzyk U, Steinberg P, Rice SA, Kjelleberg S. Biofilms: an emergent form of bacterial life. *Nat Rev Microbiol.* 2016;14(9):563-575.

16. Weaver L, Webber JB, Hickson AC, Abraham PM, Close ME. Biofilm resilience to desiccation in groundwater aquifers: a laboratory and field study. *Sci Total Environ.* 2015;514:281-289.

17. Stewart PS. Theoretical aspects of antibiotic diffusion into microbial biofilms. *Antimicrob Agents Chemother.* 1996;40(11):2517-2522.

18. Bylund J, Burgess L-A, Cescutti P, Ernst RK, Speert DP. Exopolysaccharides from *Burkholderia cenocepacia* inhibit neutrophil chemotaxis and scavenge reactive oxygen species. *J Biol Chem.* 2005;281(5): 2526-2532.

19. Dibdin GH, Assinder SJ, Nichols WW, Lambert PA. Mathematical model of beta-lactam penetration into a biofilm of *Pseudomonas aeruginosa* while undergoing simultaneous inactivation by released beta-lactamases. *J Antimicrob Chemother.* 1996;38(5):757-769.

20. Bridier A, Briandet R, Thomas V, Dubois-Brissonnet F. Resistance of bacterial biofilms to disinfectants: a review. *Biofouling.* 2011;27(9): 1017-1032.

21. Vikram A, Bomberger JM, Bibby KJ. Efflux as a glutaraldehyde resistance mechanism in *Pseudomonas fluorescens* and *Pseudomonas aeruginosa* biofilms. *Antimicrob Agents Chemother.* 2015;59(6):3433-3440.

22. Mah TFC, O'Toole GA. Mechanisms of biofilm resistance to antimicrobial agents. *Trends Microbiol.* 2001;9(1):34-39.

23. Davies D. Understanding biofilm resistance to antibacterial agents. *Nat Rev Drug Discov.* 2003;2(2):114-122.

24. de Beer D, Stoodley P, Roe F, Lewandowski Z. Effects of biofilm structures on oxygen distribution and mass transport. *Biotechnol Bioeng.* 1994;43(11):1131-1138.

25. Harrison JJ, Turner RJ, Ceri H. Persister cells, the biofilm matrix and tolerance to metal cations in biofilm and planktonic *Pseudomonas aeruginosa. Environ Microbiol.* 2005;7(7):981-994.

26. Lewis K. Riddle of biofilm resistance. *Antimicrob Agents Chemother.* 2001;45(4):999-1007.

27. Houry A, Gohar M, Deschamps J, et al. Bacterial swimmers that infiltrate and take over the biofilm matrix. *Proc Natl Acad Sci USA.* 2012;109(32):13088-13093.

28. Piercey MJ, Ells TC, Macintosh AJ, Truelstrup Hansen L. Variations in biofilm formation, desiccation resistance and benzalkonium chloride susceptibility among *Listeria monocytogenes* strains isolated in Canada. *Int J Food Microbiol.* 2017;257:254-261.

29. Harrison JJ, Ceri H, Turner RJ. Multimetal resistance and tolerance in microbial biofilms. *Nat Rev Microbiol.* 2007;5(12):928-938.

30. Kuczynska-Wisnik D, Matuszewska E, Laskowska E. *Escherichia coli* heat-shock proteins IbpA and IbpB affect biofilm formation by influencing the level of extracellular indole. *Microbiology.* 2010;156(1):148-157.

31. Olson ME, Ceri H, Morck DW, Buret AG, Read RR. Biofilm bacteria: formation and comparative susceptibility to antibiotics. *Can J Vet Res.* 2002;66(2):86-92.

32. Wolcott R, Costerton JW, Raoult D, Cutler SJ. The polymicrobial nature of biofilm infection. *Clin Microbiol Infect.* 2013;19(2):107-112.

33. Madsen JS, Burmølle M, Hansen LH, Sørensen SJ. The interconnection between biofilm formation and horizontal gene transfer. *FEMS Immunol Med Microbiol.* 2012;65(2):183-195.

34. Diaz PI, Rogers AH, Zilm PS. *Fusobacterium nucleatum* supports the growth of *Porphyromonas gingivalis* in oxygenated and carbon-dioxide-depleted environments. *Microbiology.* 2002;148(2):467-472.

35. Koch H, Lücker S, Albertsen M, et al. Expanded metabolic versatility of ubiquitous nitrite-oxidizing bacteria from the genus *Nitrospira*. *Proc Natl Acad Sci USA*. 2015;112(36):11371-6.

36. Waters CM, Bassler BL. Quorum sensing: cell-to-cell communication in bacteria. *Annu Rev Cell Dev Biol*. 2005;21:319-346.

37. Seghal Kiran G, Priyadharshini S, Dobson ADW, Gnanamani E, Selvin J. Degradation intermediates of polyhydroxy butyrate inhibits phenotypic expression of virulence factors and biofilm formation in luminescent *Vibrio* sp. PUGSK8. *NPJ Biofilms Microbiomes*. 2016;2:16002.

38. Holland SP, Mathias RG, Morck DW, Chiu J, Slade SG. Diffuse lamellar keratitis related to endotoxins released from sterilizer reservoir biofilms. *Ophthalmology*. 2000;107(7):1227-1234.

39. Fish K, Osborn AM, Boxall JB. Biofilm structures (EPS and bacterial communities) in drinking water distribution systems are conditioned by hydraulics and influence discolouration. *Sci Total Environ*. 2017;593-594:571-580.

40. Pereira RPA, Peplies J, Höfle MG, Brettar I. Bacterial community dynamics in a cooling tower with emphasis on pathogenic bacteria and *Legionella* species using universal and genus-specific deep sequencing. *Water Res*. 2017;122:363-376.

41. Fitzhenry R, Weiss D, Cimini D, et al. Legionnaires' disease outbreaks and cooling towers, New York City, New York, USA. *Emerg Infect Dis*. 2017;23(11):1769-1776.

42. Wingender J, Flemming HC. Biofilms in drinking water and their role as reservoir for pathogens. *Int J Hyg Environ Health*. 2011;214(6):417-423.

43. Hassett DJ, Korfhagen TR, Irvin RT, et al. *Pseudomonas aeruginosa* biofilm infections in cystic fibrosis: insights into pathogenic processes and treatment strategies. *Expert Opin Ther Targets*. 2010;14(2):117-130.

44. Cekici A, Kantarci A, Hasturk H, Van Dyke TE. Inflammatory and immune pathways in the pathogenesis of periodontal disease. *Periodontol 2000*. 2014;64(1):57-80.

45. Holland S, Morck D. Autoclave contamination and TASS. *Cataract Refract Surg Today*. 2006:58-60.

46. Neethirajan S, Clond MA, Vogt A. Medical biofilms—nanotechnology approaches. *J Biomed Nanotechnol*. 2014;10(10):2806-2827.

47. Costerton JW, Montanaro L, Arciola CR. Biofilm in implant infections: its production and regulation. *Int J Artif Organs*. 2005;28(11):1062-1068.

48. Cook G, Costerton JW, Darouiche RO. Direct confocal microscopy studies of the bacterial colonization in vitro of a silver-coated heart valve sewing cuff. *Int J Antimicrob Agents*. 2000;13(3):169-173.

49. Fux CA, Quigley M, Worel AM, et al. Biofilm-related infections of cerebrospinal fluid shunts. *Clin Microbiol Infect*. 2006;12(4):331-337.

50. Chan E, Goldstein D, Ceri H, Costerton JW, Morck D, Schultz C. Biofilm development on a post: case report. *Gen Dent*. 2010;58:e184-e186.

51. El-Ganiny AM, Shaker GH, Aboelazm AA, El-Dash HA. Prevention of bacterial biofilm formation on soft contact lenses using natural compounds. *J Ophthalmic Inflamm Infect*. 2017;7(1):11.

52. Tran PL, Huynh E, Pham P, et al. Organoselenium polymer inhibits biofilm formation in polypropylene contact lens case material. *Eye Contact Lens*. 2017;43(2):110-115.

53. Kathju S, Nistico L, Tower I, Lasko L-A, Stoodley P. Bacterial biofilms on implanted suture material are a cause of surgical site infection. *Surg Infect (Larchmt)*. 2014;15(5):592-600.

54. Fry DE. The economic costs of surgical site infection. *Surg Infect (Larchmt)*. 2002;3(suppl 1):S37-S43.

55. Rasnake MS, Dooley DP. Culture-negative surgical site infections. *Surg Infect (Larchmt)*. 2006;7(6):555-565.

56. Ghosh R, Das S, Kela H, De A, Haldar J, Maiti PK. Biofilm colonization of *Mycobacterium* abscessus: new threat in hospital-acquired surgical site infection. *Indian J Tuberc*. 2017;64(3):178-182.

57. Kathju S, Nistico L, Hall-Stoodley L, Post JC, Ehrlich GD, Stoodley P. Chronic surgical site infection due to suture-associated polymicrobial biofilm. *Surg Infect (Larchmt)*. 2009;10(5):457-461.

58. Peterson SB, Irie Y, Borlee BR, et al. Different methods for culturing biofilms in vitro. In: Bjarnsholt T, Jensen P, Moser C, Høiby N, eds. *Biofilm Infections*. New York, NY: Springer; 2011:251-266.

59. Lee J, Bansal T, Jayaraman A, Bentley WE, Wood TK. Enterohemorrhagic *Escherichia coli* biofilms are inhibited by 7-hydroxyindole and stimulated by isatin. *Appl Environ Microbiol*. 2007;73(13):4100-4109.

60. Cady NC, McKean KA, Behnke J, et al. Inhibition of biofilm formation, quorum sensing and infection in *Pseudomonas aeruginosa* by natural products-inspired organosulfur compounds. *PLoS One*. 2012;7(6):e38492.

61. Moreau-Marquis S, O'Toole GA, Stanton BA. Tobramycin and FDA-approved iron chelators eliminate *Pseudomonas aeruginosa* biofilms on cystic fibrosis cells. *Am J Respir Cell Mol Biol*. 2009;41(3):305-313.

62. Leuck A-M, Johnson JR, Dunny GM. A widely used in vitro biofilm assay has questionable clinical significance for enterococcal endocarditis. *PLoS One*. 2014;9(9):e107282.

63. O'Toole GA, Kolter R. Initiation of biofilm formation in *Pseudomonas fluorescens* WCS365 proceeds via multiple, convergent signalling pathways: a genetic analysis. *Mol Microbiol*. 1998;28(3):449-461.

64. Merritt JH, Kadouri DE, O'Toole GA. Growing and analyzing static biofilms. *Curr Protoc Microbiol*. 2005;(1):1B.1.1-1B.1.17.

65. Franklin MJ, Chang C, Akiyama T, Bothner B. New technologies for studying biofilms. *Microbiol Spectr*. 2015;3(4). doi:10.1128/microbiolspec.MB-0016-2014.

66. O'Toole GA. Microtiter dish biofilm formation assay. *J Vis Exp*. 2011;(47). doi:10.3791/2437.

67. McCoy WF, Bryers JD, Robbins J, Costerton JW. Observations of fouling biofilm formation. *Can J Microbiol*. 1981;27(9):910-917.

68. Donlan RM, Piede JA, Heyes CD, et al. Model system for growing and quantifying *Streptococcus pneumoniae* biofilms in situ and in real time. *Appl Environ Microbiol*. 2004;70(8):4980-4988.

69. Goeres DM, Loetterle LR, Hamilton MA, Murga R, Kirby DW, Donlan RM. Statistical assessment of a laboratory method for growing biofilms. *Microbiology*. 2005;151(3):757-762.

70. Thomen P, Robert J, Monmeyran A, Bitbol A-F, Douarche C, Henry N. Bacterial biofilm under flow: first a physical struggle to stay, then a matter of breathing. *PLoS One*. 2017;12(4):e0175197.

71. Song WS, Lee J-K, Park SH, Um H-S, Lee SY, Chang B-S. Comparison of periodontitis-associated oral biofilm formation under dynamic and static conditions. *J Periodontal Implant Sci*. 2017;47(4):219.

72. Nance WC, Dowd SE, Samarian D, et al. A high-throughput microfluidic dental plaque biofilm system to visualize and quantify the effect of antimicrobials. *J Antimicrob Chemother*. 2013;68(11):2550-2560.

73. Ceri H, Olson ME, Stremick C, Read RR, Morck D, Buret A. The Calgary Biofilm Device: new technology for rapid determination of antibiotic susceptibilities of bacterial biofilms. *J Clin Microbiol*. 1999;37(6):1771-1776.

74. Konrat K, Schwebke I, Laue M, et al. The bead assay for biofilms: a quick, easy and robust method for testing disinfectants. *PLoS One*. 2016;11(6):e0157663.

75. Harrison JJ, Stremick CA, Turner RJ, Allan ND, Olson ME, Ceri H. Microtiter susceptibility testing of microbes growing on peg lids: a miniaturized biofilm model for high-throughput screening. *Nat Protoc*. 2010;5(7):1236-1254.

76. Lemire JA, Kalan L, Bradu A, Turner RJ. Silver oxynitrate, an unexplored silver compound with antimicrobial and antibiofilm activity. *Antimicrob Agents Chemother*. 2015;59(7):4031-4039.

77. Sproule-Willoughby KM, Stanton MM, Rioux KP, McKay DM, Buret AG, Ceri H. In vitro anaerobic biofilms of human colonic microbiota. *J Microbiol Methods*. 2010;83(3):296-301.

78. Buret AG. Enteropathogen-induced microbiota biofilm disruptions and post-infectious intestinal inflammatory disorders. *Curr Trop Med Reports*. 2016;3(3):94-101.

79. Beatty JK, Akierman SV, Motta J-P, et al. *Giardia duodenalis* induces pathogenic dysbiosis of human intestinal microbiota biofilms. *Int J Parasitol*. 2017;47(6):311-326.

80. Lockhart JS, Buret AG, Ceri H, Storey DG, Anderson SJ, Morck DW. Mixed species biofilms of *Fusobacterium necrophorum* and *Porphyromonas levii* impair the oxidative response of bovine neutrophils in vitro. *Anaerobe*. 2017;47:157-164.

81. Lawrence JR, Korber DR, Hoyle BD, Costerton JW, Caldwell DE. Optical sectioning of microbial biofilms. *J Bacteriol.* 1991;173(20):6558-6567.

82. Stoodley P, Debeer D, Lewandowski Z. Liquid flow in biofilm systems. *Appl Environ Microbiol.* 1994;60(8):2711-2716.

83. Günther F, Wabnitz GH, Stroh P, et al. Host defence against *Staphylococcus aureus* biofilms infection: phagocytosis of biofilms by polymorphonuclear neutrophils (PMN). *Mol Immunol.* 2009;46(8-9):1805-1813.

84. Hirschfeld J, Dommisch H, Skora P, et al. Neutrophil extracellular trap formation in supragingival biofilms. *Int J Med Microbiol.* 2015;305(4-5): 453-463.

85. Periasamy S, Kolenbrander PE. Mutualistic biofilm communities develop with *Porphyromonas gingivalis* and initial, early, and late colonizers of enamel. *J Bacteriol.* 2009;191(22):6804-6811.

86. Al-Ahmad A, Follo M, Selzer A-C, Hellwig E, Hannig M, Hannig C. Bacterial colonization of enamel *in situ* investigated using fluorescence *in situ* hybridization. *J Med Microbiol.* 2009;58(10):1359-1366.

87. Thurnheer T, Gmür R, Guggenheim B. Multiplex FISH analysis of a six-species bacterial biofilm. *J Microbiol Methods.* 2004;56(1):37-47.

88. Marrie TJ, Nelligan J, Costerton JW. A scanning and transmission electron microscopic study of an infected endocardial pacemaker lead. *Circulation.* 1982;66(6):1339-1341.

89. McLean RJC, Kakirde KS. Enhancing metagenomics investigations of microbial interactions with biofilm technology. *Int J Mol Sci.* 2013; 14(11):22246-22257.

90. Hansen LT, Vogel BF. Desiccation of adhering and biofilm *Listeria monocytogenes* on stainless steel: survival and transfer to salmon products. *Int J Food Microbiol.* 2011;146(1):88-93.

91. Lorenz LA, Ramsay BD, Goeres DM, Fields MW, Zapka CA, Macinga DR. Evaluation and remediation of bulk soap dispensers for biofilm. *Biofouling.* 2012;28(1):99-109.

92. Anand S, Singh D, Avadhanula M, Marka S. Development and control of bacterial biofilms on dairy processing membranes. *Compr Rev Food Sci Food Saf.* 2014;13(1):18-33.

93. Gieg LM, Jack TR, Foght JM. Biological souring and mitigation in oil reservoirs. *Appl Microbiol Biotechnol.* 2011;92(2):263-282.

94. Quarini J, Shire S. A review of fluid-driven pipeline pigs and their applications. *Proc Inst Mech Eng.* 2007;221(1):1-10.

95. Videla HA, Herrera LK. Microbiologically influenced corrosion: looking to the future. *Int Microbiol.* 2005;8(3):169-180.

96. McDonnell GE. *Antisepsis, Disinfection, and Sterilization: Types, Action, and Resistance.* Washington, DC: American Society of Microbiology; 2017.

97. Veerachamy S, Yarlagadda T, Manivasagam G, Yarlagadda PK. Bacterial adherence and biofilm formation on medical implants: a review. *Proc Inst Mech Eng.* 2014;228(10):1083-1099.

98. Lopez-Lopez G, Pascual A, Perea EJ. Effect of plastic catheter material on bacterial adherence and viability. *J Med Microbiol.* 1991;34(6):349-353.

99. Raad I, Hachem R, Tcholakian RK, Sherertz R. Efficacy of minocycline and EDTA lock solution in preventing catheter-related bacteremia, septic phlebitis, and endocarditis in rabbits. *Antimicrob Agents Chemother.* 2002;46(2):327-332.

100. Veenstra DL, Saint S, Saha S, Lumley T, Sullivan SD. Efficacy of antiseptic-impregnated central venous catheters in preventing catheter-related bloodstream infection: a meta-analysis. *JAMA.* 1999; 281(3):261-267.

101. Stefanova D, Raychev A, Arezes J, et al. Endogenous hepcidin and its agonist mediate resistance to selected infections by clearing non–transferrin-bound iron. *Blood.* 2017;130(3):245-257.

102. Stiefel P, Mauerhofer S, Schneider J, Maniura-Weber K, Rosenberg U, Ren Q. Enzymes enhance biofilm removal efficiency of cleaners. *Antimicrob Agents Chemother.* 2016;60(6):3647-3652.

103. Choi YJ, Lim JK, Park JJ, et al. Chlorhexidine and silver sulfadiazine coating on central venous catheters is not sufficient for protection against catheter-related infection: simulation-based laboratory research with clinical validation. *J Int Med Res.* 2017;45(3):1042-1053.

104. Roberts CG. The role of biofilms in reprocessing medical devices. *Am J Infect Control.* 2013;41(5):S77-S80.

105. Aumeran C, Thibert E, Chapelle FA, Hennequin C, Lesens O, Traore O. Assessment on experimental bacterial biofilms and in clinical practice of the efficacy of sampling solutions for microbiological testing of endoscopes. *J Clin Microbiol.* 2012;50(3):938-942.

106. Edmiston CE, Daoud FC, Leaper D. Is there an evidence-based argument for embracing an antimicrobial (triclosan)-coated suture technology to reduce the risk for surgical-site infections? A meta-analysis. *Surgery.* 2013;154(1):89-100.

107. Edmiston CE, Seabrook GR, Goheen MP, et al. Bacterial adherence to surgical sutures: can antibacterial-coated sutures reduce the risk of microbial contamination? *J Am Coll Surg.* 2006;203(4):481-489.

108. Kolewe KW, Peyton SR, Schiffman JD. Fewer bacteria adhere to softer hydrogels. *ACS Appl Mater Interfaces.* 2015;7(35):19562-19569.

109. Norambuena GA, Patel R, Karau M, et al. Antibacterial and biocompatible titanium-copper oxide coating may be a potential strategy to reduce periprosthetic infection: an in vitro study. *Clin Orthop Relat Res.* 2017;475(3):722-732.

110. Harrison PL, Harrison T, Stockley I, Smith TJ. Does tantalum exhibit any intrinsic antimicrobial or antibiofilm properties? *Bone Joint J.* 2017;99-B(9):1153-1156.

111. Morck DW, Olson ME, McKay SG, et al. Therapeutic efficacy of fleroxacin for eliminating catheter-associated urinary tract infection in a rabbit model. *Am J Med.* 1993;94(3A):23S-30S.

112. Morck DW, Olson ME, Read RR, Buret AG, Ceri H. The rabbit model of catheter-associated urinary tract infection. In: Zak O, Sande MA, eds. *Handbook of Animal Models of Infection.* Cambridge, MA: Academic Press; 1999:453-462.

113. Morck DW, Lam K, McKay SG, et al. Comparative evaluation of fleroxacin, ampicillin, trimethoprimsulfamethoxazole, and gentamicin as treatments of catheter-associated urinary tract infection in a rabbit model. *Int J Antimicrob Agents.* 1994;4(suppl 2):S21-S27.

114. Christensen LD, van Gennip M, Jakobsen TH, et al. Synergistic antibacterial efficacy of early combination treatment with tobramycin and quorum-sensing inhibitors against *Pseudomonas aeruginosa* in an intraperitoneal foreign-body infection mouse model. *J Antimicrob Chemother.* 2012;67(5):1198-1206.

115. Luo J, Dong B, Wang K, et al. Baicalin inhibits biofilm formation, attenuates the quorum sensing-controlled virulence and enhances *Pseudomonas aeruginosa* clearance in a mouse peritoneal implant infection model. *PLoS One.* 2017;12(4):e0176883.

116. Dalton T, Dowd SE, Wolcott RD, et al. An *in vivo* polymicrobial biofilm wound infection model to study interspecies interactions. *PLoS One.* 2011;6(11):e27317.

117. Lebeaux D, Chauhan A, Rendueles O, Beloin C. From *in vitro* to *in vivo* models of bacterial biofilm-related infections. *Pathogens.* 2013;2(2):288-356.

118. Turina M, Cheadle WG. Management of established surgical site infections. *Surg Infect (Larchmt).* 2006;7(suppl 3):S33-S41.

119. Pletzer D, Coleman SR, Hancock RE. Anti-biofilm peptides as a new weapon in antimicrobial warfare. *Curr Opin Microbiol.* 2016;33: 35-40.

120. Ribeiro SM, Felício MR, Boas EV, et al. New frontiers for anti-biofilm drug development. *Pharmacol Ther.* 2016;160:133-144.

121. Wang Z, Shen Y, Haapasalo M. Antibiofilm peptides against oral biofilms. *J Oral Microbiol.* 2017;9(1):1327308.

Prions

Kurt Giles, Amanda L. Woerman, and Stanley B. Prusiner

Prions pose unique biosafety challenges. They possess an unusual resistance to inactivation, and quantifying prion infectivity can be time-consuming and expensive. Moreover, guidelines for prion inactivation are often based on limited data from model systems using rodent prions and may not be applicable to the human, bovine, or other natural prions that they are intended to be effective against. To avoid making uninformed and potentially harmful decisions, an understanding of prion pathobiology is required to assess risks related to prions. The difficulties associated with quantifying prion titers have led to the confusing use of the terms *sterilization* and *disinfection* to describe differences in the reduction of prion infectivity titer. However, we prefer the term *inactivation* to imply that the protein conformation can no longer actively template additional refolding of the native protein and, thus, is no longer infective. Although many widely used infection prevention practices can sterilize bacterial and viral contamination under controlled conditions, they typically do not fully inactivate prions. In these circumstances, more stringent prion-specific procedures are required (Figure 68.1).

Prions were initially defined for a group of neurodegenerative diseases, including scrapie in sheep, bovine spongiform encephalopathy (BSE) in cattle, chronic wasting disease (CWD) in deer, and Creutzfeldt-Jakob disease (CJD) in humans. Prototypical prions are unlike any other infectious pathogens, including viruses, because they are composed of an abnormal conformational isoform of a normal cellular protein, termed the prion protein (PrP). The abnormal isoform, designated PrP^{Sc} for *scrapie* isoform of PrP, serves as a template to recruit molecules of the normal, *cellular* isoform (PrP^C) to adopt its misfolded conformation. The PrP prion diseases, therefore, are conditions caused by template-assisted protein misfolding, resulting in PrP^{Sc} accumulation in the brain, which ultimately leads to neuronal dysfunction, degeneration, and death. The term *prion* was derived from a combination of *pro*teinaceous and *in*fectious[1] to differentiate it from nucleic acid–based replication of viruses, bacteria, and fungi. PrP is encoded by the *Prnp* gene (*PRNP* in humans), which is highly conserved in mammals and for which homologs are found in a range of more distant vertebrates including birds, reptiles, and fish.[2] Although the BSE epidemic and the subsequent crisis following the transmission of BSE to people appears to have passed, recent studies showing PrP prion infectivity in skin[3] and evidence that CWD might transmit to people[4] highlight a continuing need to understand prion infection control.

Importantly, the prion concept is not limited to PrP and is now understood to be a much broader biological phenomenon. Some epigenetic inheritance in yeast is transmitted by a prion mechanism in which specific proteins adopt self-templating conformations that may confer selective advantages.[5] More recently, functional mammalian prions have been identified, including cytoplasmic polyadenylation element-binding protein (CPEB), which features in memory,[6,7] and mitochondrial antiviral-signaling protein (MAVS), which contributes to innate immunity.[8] However, the discovery that Aβ, tau, and α-synuclein—the central proteins involved in a range of neurodegenerative diseases including Alzheimer disease (AD) and Parkinson disease (PD)—can become prions[9] has raised new questions about biosafety issues, such as when handling tissue samples from patients with these disorders. Evidence for experimental transmission of prions from non-PrP diseases continues to accumulate. Typically, transmission in cells is first demonstrated, followed by transmission to wild-type or transgenic (Tg) mice, and, subsequently, transmission to nonhuman primates may be tested. Evidence for non-PrP prion transmission to humans is determined epidemiologically. However, with incubation periods potentially spanning decades, it can be difficult to assign direct causality when there is a high incidence of a disease in the aged population (Table 68.1).

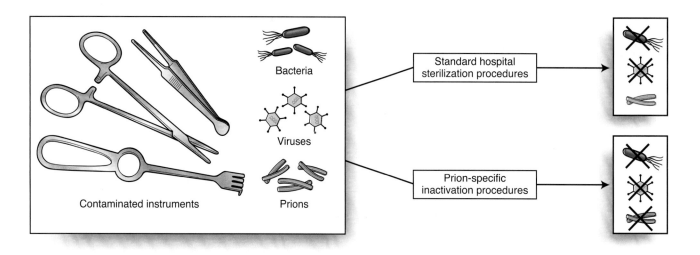

FIGURE 68.1 Prions show an unusual resistance to inactivation. Although standardized hospital sterilization methods used to decontaminate surgical instruments prevent the spread of bacterial or viral infections, these procedures typically do not reduce prion titer sufficiently to mitigate the potential for iatrogenic disease transmission. Instead, specialized cleaning methods are required to inactivate prions before the instruments can be reused.

◗ PrP PRION DISEASE ETIOLOGY AND STRAINS

Of the many distinctive features that separate prion diseases from viral, bacterial, fungal, and parasitic disorders, the most remarkable is that PrP prion diseases are not only acquired but also can manifest as inherited and sporadic disorders. Yet, in all three etiologies, infectious prions are generated in the brain and are composed of PrP^{Sc} molecules with the amino acid sequence encoded by the *Prnp* gene of the affected host. When PrP prions are transmitted to a different host species, there is typically a "transmission barrier," in part related to differences in PrP sequences, resulting in inefficient transmission.[10-12]

TABLE 68.1 Prion diseases, their associated proteins, and observed transmission

Disease	Host	Protein	Cells	Transmission					
				Transgenic Mouse		Nonhuman Primate		Human	
				Neuropathologic Lesions[a]	Lethal	Neuropathologic Lesions[a]	Lethal	Neuropathologic Lesions[a]	Lethal
Scrapie	Sheep	PrP	Yes	+++	Yes	+++	Yes	n.d.	n.d.
BSE	Cow	PrP	Yes	+++	Yes	+++	Yes	+++	Yes
CWD	Deer	PrP	Yes	+++	Yes	++	n.d.	n.d.	n.d.
CJD	Human	PrP	Yes	+++	Yes	+++	Yes	+++	Yes
AD	Human	Aβ	Yes	+++	No	++	No	++	n.d.
		Tau	Yes	++	No	n.d.	n.d.	+	n.d.
PSP	Human	Tau	Yes	+	No	n.d.	n.d.	n.d.	n.d.
CBD	Human	Tau	Yes	++	No	n.d.	n.d.	n.d.	n.d.
CTE	Human	Tau	Yes	n.d.	n.d.	n.d.	n.d.	n.d.	n.d.
MSA	Human	α-synuclein	Yes	+++	Yes	++	No	n.d.	n.d.
PD	Human	α-synuclein	No	+	No	+	No	n.d.	n.d.

Abbreviations: Aβ, β-amyloid; AD, Alzheimer disease; BSE, bovine spongiform encephalopathy; CBD, corticobasal degeneration; CJD, Creutzfeldt-Jakob disease; CTE, chronic traumatic encephalopathy; CWD, chronic wasting disease; MSA; multiple system atrophy; *n.d.*, no data; PD, Parkinson disease; PrP, prion protein; PSP, progressive supranuclear palsy.

[a]Neuropathologic lesion intensity: +, sparse; ++, moderate; +++, robust.

If interspecies transmission does occur, the prions generated in the brain of the host carry the amino acid sequence encoded by the *Prnp* gene of the host species and not the PrP sequence found in the original inoculum. In other words, in interspecies infection, such as from sheep to cattle or from cattle to humans, the prions that replicate in the host brain are not the same as those that initiate replication. In contrast, serial transmission in the same host, in which the inoculum and host PrP sequences match, is generally more rapid and efficient. This scenario is profoundly different from what happens during a viral infection.

Phenotypically distinct strains of prions were first identified following transmission of sheep scrapie to goats.[13] Although this was long used as an argument for the prion containing a nucleic acid, none has ever been found.[14] It was later understood that PrP prion strains represent structurally different conformations of PrP^Sc.[15,16] Yeast prions, which also display this phenomenon, have been important in demonstrating the structural basis of prion strains.[17,18] The strain phenomenon has also been observed for Aβ, tau, and α-synuclein prions,[19-21] which may help explain clinical variability and raises important questions about potential therapeutic specificity.

▶ QUANTIFYING PRION INFECTIVITY

Determining prion inactivation requires quantifiable assays that are ideally rapid and easy to perform. Due to the lack of nucleic acid in prions, quantifying inactivation has been challenging to achieve, with the gold standard still being animal bioassays in wild-type or Tg rodents.

Experimental transmission of sheep scrapie was first demonstrated in the 1930s.[22] Subsequently, both kuru, an acquired human prion disease, and CJD were transmitted to chimpanzees.[23,24] However, the transmission of prions to mice[25] and hamsters[26] greatly accelerated research by providing models with incubation times measured in weeks rather than years. The development of Tg mice expressing PrP from other species, particularly in combination with ablation of endogenous mouse PrP, has provided a range of tools to interrogate prion biology.[27] However, even with these accelerated models, survival time after inoculation is the central metric, which leads to time-consuming and expensive experiments.

A limited number of mouse cell lines have been identified that propagate PrP prions, including N2a,[28] GT1,[29] and CAD5 cells.[30] Interestingly, most of these lines only propagate a subset of mouse-passaged PrP prion strains, the reasons for which are poorly understood. Some success has been achieved by overexpressing heterologous PrP in rabbit RK13 cells,[31] and recent studies have shown infection of some human prions in stem cell–derived astrocytes.[32] However, a scalable cell line for the propagation of the most common strains of human PrP prions is still lacking.

Cell-free replication of PrP prions was first demonstrated by the incorporation of PrP^C into a protease-resistant conformation following incubation with partially denatured PrP^Sc.[33] Subsequent studies using serial sonication, believed to break up PrP prion aggregates, ultimately gave rise to the protein misfolding cyclic amplification (PMCA) assay.[34] Although this method was demonstrated to replicate PrP prion infectivity,[35] the difficulties in generating reproducible results hampered its adoption by many labs. In parallel, assays based on shaking a recombinant PrP substrate led to the development of the real-time quaking-induced conversion (RT-QuIC) assay.[36] Although this is a promising technique for measuring low PrP prion levels, seeding ability in RT-QuIC does not necessarily translate into the replication of PrP prion infectivity, requiring animal bioassays for confirmatory testing.

Experimental models have also been developed for the quantification of Aβ, tau, and α-synuclein prions. Long-term Aβ transmission studies were performed in primates,[37] but the demonstrated transmission of Aβ pathology to Tg mice[38,39] provided experimentally tractable tools. Consistent with the prion hypothesis, distinct Aβ strains are serially passaged with high fidelity in Tg mice.[40-42] However, novel cell lines propagating Aβ prions have only recently been reported.[43] Conversely, although the inoculation models available for studying the tauopathies are less robust than those for Aβ,[44,45] highly sensitive cell models have been used to identify different tau prion strains from various tauopathy patient samples.[20,46]

In contrast to the PrP inoculation model, in which uninoculated animals typically do not have any spontaneous disease, many of the Aβ and tau inoculation models use Tg mice overexpressing the respective human protein, typically with disease-associated mutations. As a result, these mouse lines often exhibit spontaneous disease in older animals. In such cases, there is a "window" between inoculation and spontaneous prion formation that facilitates measuring induced prion propagation. Moreover, these assays typically rely on a neuropathologic readout rather than onset of disease, which can be time-consuming and more difficult to quantify across research groups.

In the five decades since the initial transmission studies of human PrP prions,[23,24] the first new human neurodegenerative disease model to produce a lethal phenotype in an animal model came from a serendipitous discovery. A Tg mouse line, termed TgM83, expresses human α-synuclein with the familial PD–associated mutation A53T. Homozygous TgM83^{+/+} mice develop spontaneous disease beginning at approximately 8 months old, but hemizygous TgM83^{+/−} mice show no signs of disease for at least 20 months.[47] Inoculation of brain homogenate from spontaneously ill TgM83^{+/+} mice, or fibrils of synthetic α-synuclein, into 2- to 4-month-old TgM83$^{+/+}$ mice induced disease onset 3 to 4 months later.[48,49] In an attempt to transmit α-synucleinopathy from PD, we inoculated TgM83$^{+/-}$ mice with brain homogenate from PD patients and from patients who had died from a different α-synucleinopathy, multiple system atrophy (MSA), as a control. To our surprise, whereas the PD samples did not transmit disease to the mice, the MSA samples induced a lethal phenotype approximately 4 months after inoculation.[50] These findings were subsequently confirmed using a much larger cohort of MSA samples from three continents.[51] The MSA strain differs from the spontaneous TgM83$^{+/+}$ strain, exhibiting a shorter incubation period with serial passaging.[51] In contrast to the limitation of cell models for PrP prion diseases, we developed a rapid cell assay for MSA,[52] which correlates well with disease onset in the animal bioassay.[51] This 4-day assay uses human embryonic kidney (HEK) cells that express human α-synuclein with the A53T mutation, conjugated to the yellow fluorescent protein (YFP). Application of exogenous α-synuclein prions induces aggregation of α-synuclein–YFP, which can be automatically identified as puncta by high-content fluorescence microscopy. Importantly, MSA prions propagated in the cell assay also transmitted a lethal disease to TgM83$^{+/-}$ mice following inoculation,[53] which had previously only been demonstrated with CWD and mouse-adapted scrapie strains.

▶ RESISTANCE OF PRIONS TO INACTIVATION

The unusual resistance of PrP prions to inactivation was first identified when formalin-treated sheep's brain and spinal cord, used to immunize animals against the louping-ill virus, resulted in the transmission of scrapie. This was ultimately attributed to the inclusion of tissue from an asymptomatic scrapie-infected sheep in a specific batch of inoculum.[54] Subsequent work showed resistance of PrP prions to heat and chemical denaturants[55,56] and to ultraviolet irradiation.[57]

Resistance to formalin fixation has also been observed for other human prions. MSA brain tissue fixed in formalin for up to 20 years still showed robust α-synuclein prion infectivity in TgM83$^{+/-}$ mice.[58] A similar phenomenon was observed using a Tg mouse model expressing the A30P mutation in human α-synuclein; formalin-fixed tissue from aged animals was able to induce an early onset of neurologic disease when inoculated into young, asymptomatic mice.[59] Likewise, formalin-fixed tissue from AD patients induced robust Aβ-amyloidosis in reporter mice, and, experimentally, formalin fixation only slightly reduced Aβ prion infectivity compared with brain homogenate from frozen tissue.[60] Using an alternative approach, fixed AD patient samples also transmitted tau prions to HEK cells expressing a tau–YFP reporter protein.[61]

▶ ACQUIRED HUMAN PRION DISEASES

Kuru

The first acquired prion disease described was kuru, which was found in the Fore people from the Eastern Highlands of Papua New Guinea. When scientists first became aware of the epidemic in the 1950s, kuru was responsible for more than 200 deaths per year.[62] It was spread by ritualistic mortuary practices, which included consumption of tissue, including brain, from deceased relatives. Following the cessation of this practice beginning in the late 1950s, the number of kuru cases dramatically declined, although rare cases have been observed with incubation periods exceeding 50 years.[63]

Iatrogenic Creutzfeldt-Jakob Disease

Iatrogenic CJD (iCJD) was first identified in the 1970s. In the initial case, the recipient of a corneal transplant from a donor subsequently diagnosed with CJD developed the disease 18 months after surgery.[64] Later, two patients developed CJD approximately 2 years after receiving electroencephalographic (EEG) depth recordings with electrodes that had previously been used on a CJD patient.[65] The suspected iatrogenic transmission was confirmed when the tip of the EEG electrode was implanted into the brain of a chimpanzee, which developed a PrP prion disease 18 months later.[66] Retrospective analysis suggested that neurosurgical procedures performed in the 1950s may have also been responsible for iCJD cases.[67] However, the vast majority of known iCJD cases have come from cadaver-derived growth hormone and dura mater.

In the mid-1980s, young patients who had received injections of human growth hormone (HGH) for hypopituitarism started to develop CJD. Since then, over 220 individuals have succumbed to the disease (Table 68.2).[68] The HGH was purified from batches of thousands of pituitary glands, each batch being processed into multiple lots. Patients treated with HGH often received injections from multiple lots over a period of years. Epidemiologic evidence suggests that multiple independent HGH batches included pituitaries from CJD patients. Some of the hypopituitarism patients who received HGH injections from these contaminated batches later developed iCJD.

A polymorphic residue at position 129 in PrP encodes either methionine (M) or valine (V). Allele distribution differs with ethnicity, but methionine is predominant. In Europeans, the M allele frequency is approximately 60%. However, although MM129 homozygotes make up approximately one-third of the population, they account for more than 70% of sporadic CJD (sCJD) cases. Similarly, valine homozygotes are overrepresented in sCJD, suggesting that MV129 heterozygosity may be protective.[69]

TABLE 68.2	Current status of iatrogenic Creutzfeldt-Jakob disease worldwide	
Tissue Source of Contamination	**No. of Cases**	**Mode of Transmission**
Brain	4	Neurosurgical procedures
Brain	2	Implantation of stereotactic electroencephalography electrode
Eye	2	Corneal transplantation
Dura mater	235	Dura mater transplantation
Pituitary gland	226	Parenteral growth hormone therapy
Pituitary gland	4	Parenteral gonadotropin therapy
Blood	5[a]	Transfusion

[a]Two had preclinical variant Creutzfeldt-Jakob disease.

In iCJD cases that resulted from contaminated HGH, MM129 homozygous individuals are overrepresented in most countries. However, in the United Kingdom, an excess of VV129 homozygotes were observed, suggesting transmission of a different strain.[70] Some heterozygous individuals still developed iCJD, but these patients typically exhibited a longer incubation period.

Over a parallel timespan to the HGH cases, a similar number of iCJD cases occurred following dura mater grafts (see Table 68.2).[68,71] Almost all infections came from a single source that had been distributed worldwide, but the majority of cases occurred in Japan, reflecting the high use of the technique in Japanese medical practice. Due to the very high incidence of the M129 allele in the Japanese population,[72] the influence of genotype is difficult to determine. However, differing clinicopathologic progression in the dura mater cases suggests the possibility that at least two iCJD strains were present in the patients.[73]

Acquired Non-PrP Prion Diseases

The understanding that most, if not all, neurodegenerative disorders are caused by various proteins becoming prions raises the possibility that these diseases may be spread iatrogenically as well. Reanalysis of brain tissue from iCJD patients who received growth hormone or dura mater grafts showed that a number of these brain samples contained Aβ pathology not present in age-matched controls.[74-76] Moreover, Aβ pathology was observed in growth hormone recipients who died from causes other than iCJD.[77] Importantly, Aβ pathology in these cases is typically in the form of cerebral amyloid angiopathy (CAA), which is also the case for Tg mice that have been inoculated with brain extracts from AD patients. A patient who received a cadaver-derived dural graft following removal of a subdural hematoma developed CAA more than four decades later. Genetic testing showed no known mutations or duplications in proteins implicated in familial CAA, leading to the suggestion that this case could represent iatrogenic transmission.[78] Intracellular tau accumulation has also been observed in some iCJD growth hormone recipients, occasionally in the absence of Aβ, suggesting that tau prions may have been transmitted iatrogenically as well.[79]

Although the aforementioned cases reflect the rare instances of patients treated with cadaver-derived material, a recent study identified a link between neurosurgical procedures and the appearance of CAA decades later.[80]

Variant Creutzfeldt-Jakob Disease

The epidemic of BSE arose from industrial cannibalism in which cattle were fed meat and bone meal contaminated with prion-infected cattle and sheep offal as a result of faulty industrial processes, likely starting in the early 1980s.[81] The recycling of infected animals through the food chain meant that by the time BSE was identified, it was endemic throughout the United Kingdom. Ten years after the identification of BSE in cattle, a novel form of CJD appeared in young adults, termed variant CJD (vCJD).[82] In addition to the epidemiologic association, several pieces of experimental evidence linked the BSE and vCJD prion strains. Transmission characteristics and electrophoretic mobility of vCJD were more similar to BSE than to sCJD.[83] Furthermore, multiple BSE and vCJD isolates transmitted to Tg mice expressing bovine PrP with similar incubation periods and resultant neuropathology.[84]

To date, over 200 people have died from vCJD, and all have had a history of exposure to BSE within a country and during a period when the disease was epidemic. Moreover, all of these individuals had the MM129 genotype. However, the most recent case of vCJD, in 2016, occurred in an MV129 heterozygous individual.[85] Whether this portends a new wave of vCJD cases with longer incubation periods remains to be determined. Regardless, the possibility of asymptomatic carriers of vCJD has major public health implications for the blood supply and reuse of surgical instruments. A number of studies have examined archived tonsil and appendix tissue. The largest of these studies suggested that 1 in 2000 people in the United Kingdom may be carriers of vCJD prions.[86]

Because vCJD predominantly affected young adults, individuals with the disease had donated blood. Tragically, three patients died of vCJD 6 to 8 years after receiving whole blood from three different donors who developed clinical symptoms subsequent to donating.[87,88] Two preclinical cases have also been identified: one in an individual who died of a nonneurologic disorder and, notably, had the MV129 genotype, which may have extended the incubation period.[89] A second case was observed in an individual with hemophilia who had received factor VIII prepared from plasma pools known to include donations from vCJD-infected donors.[90]

Recipients of plasma products sourced in the United Kingdom have been notified that they are at a greater risk of vCJD. Interestingly, two patients with a history of extended treatment with fractionated plasma products were recently identified with sCJD; however, a causal link could not be established.[91]

Transmission of Other PrP Prion Strains to Humans

Reports of scrapie in sheep are thought to date from the 18th century, and the lack of evidence for scrapie transmission to humans was the basis for incorrect assumptions that BSE would not transmit to people. CWD in deer was first identified in 1967 and was later understood to be a PrP prion disease.[92] Importantly, CWD has been observed in both wild and captive herds of deer and elk and is contagious within and between herds. From its initial identification in Colorado and Wyoming, CWD has now been reported in 24 US states and two Canadian provinces as well as in South Korea following the importation of infected animals.[93] More recently, CWD was identified in a reindeer in Norway[94] and was subsequently found in moose and red deer as well.[95]

Previously, CWD was shown to transmit to squirrel monkeys but not to macaques, which are more closely related to humans.[96,97] However, early data from ongoing studies of macaques infected orally with CWD showed that these animals are indeed susceptible to infection,[4] raising concerns about the potential for a new human PrP prion disease epidemic.

▶ BIOSAFETY LEVEL CLASSIFICATION

Human PrP prions occupy a somewhat unique position in biological safety classification. Although they are agents that can cause lethal diseases in people and would typically be considered biosafety level (BSL)-3 pathogens, they are generally not thought to be airborne, and respirators are usually not required when experiments are performed in a biosafety cabinet. However, mice exposed to aerosolized prions succumbed to prion disease, albeit with considerably longer incubation periods than occur with intracerebral inoculation.[98] Depending on various national and local regulations, human PrP prions may be considered BSL-2 or BSL-3 agents, depending on the experiments to be performed. BSE prions are likewise considered Risk Group 2 or 3 pathogens because they are transmissible to humans.[99]

All other animal PrP prions are generally considered BSL-2 pathogens. When human prions are passaged in rodents, they have the amino acid sequence of the endogenous PrP (or that of the PrP transgene expressed) and therefore fall in a gray area as to their biosafety status. The "Fukuoka 1" prion strain originated from the transmission to mice of what was likely a case of genetic prion disease.[100] After several subsequent serial passages in additional mice, the resulting prions developed unusual infection characteristics, causing a more rapid disease onset in a Tg mouse line expressing chimeric human/mouse PrP than other mouse-passaged prions. However, the strain failed to cause disease in Tg mice expressing human PrP.[101] Whether these prions are infectious to humans remains unknown, but some laboratories use this strain under BSL-2 conditions. Conversely, human CJD prions transmitted to Tg mice expressing bank vole PrP were still highly infectious in Tg mice expressing human PrP.[102] As a result, experiments using human prions in Tg mice expressing bank vole PrP should be performed under the more stringent BSL-3 conditions where applicable. Unfortunately, few rodent-passaged human prion strains have been validated in Tg mice expressing human PrP. In the absence of evidence to the contrary, these strains should be handled under the same biosafety conditions as human prions to minimize biosafety risks.

The demonstration that proteins involved in other neurodegenerative diseases are transmissible is particularly important for the safety of laboratory and medical workers, who may have direct contact with the most infectious patient tissues, such as brain and possibly cerebrospinal fluid (CSF). Similarly, the production and aggregation of synthetic or recombinant Aβ, tau, and α-synuclein to generate biologically active prions should be considered potential biohazards. We recommend that all such procedures should be handled under BSL-2 conditions at a minimum.

▶ PRION INACTIVATION STUDIES

With the development of the hamster PrP prion model, and the high titers obtained from the brains of these animals, the Sc237 strain, also known as 263K, became a widely used model to quantify prion inactivation. Denaturing detergents, chaotropic agents, and digestion with proteases all reduce infectivity levels but do not completely inactivate prions.[103-105] Instead, more stringent conditions are required to eliminate all detectable infectivity.

Recommended Guidelines

The most widely adopted recommendations for inactivation of prions are based on the World Health Organization (WHO) guidelines arising from a meeting of experts in the field in 1999.[106] These recommendations contain suggestions for reusable instruments based on the probability that an individual has or will develop a prion disease, the likely level of infectivity of the tissue contacted (categorized into high, low, and no detectable infectivity), and how the instruments would be reused. However, this raises a number of practical issues about the potential implementation of these guidelines, such as deciding which of the multiple infection-control protocols to use in each instance based on incomplete information. Moreover, the tissue infectivity distribution tables presented in the WHO guidelines are acknowledged to represent the frequency with which infectivity has been detected rather than data from quantitative bioassays, and the tables are repeatedly updated as more studies are published.[107] The only way to ensure there is no risk of residual infectivity is to destroy the instruments by incineration. When this is not feasible, the Centers for Disease Control and Prevention (CDC) recommends applying one of the three most stringent WHO guidelines:

- Immerse in 1 N sodium hydroxide (NaOH) and heat in a gravity displacement autoclave at 121°C for 30 minutes, rinse in water, and subject to routine sterilization.
- Immerse in 1 N NaOH or sodium hypochlorite (20 000 ppm available chlorine) for 60 minutes, transfer to water and heat in a gravity displacement autoclave at 121°C for 60 minutes, clean, and subject to routine sterilization.
- Immerse in 1 N NaOH or sodium hypochlorite (20 000 ppm available chlorine) for 60 minutes; rinse in water and heat in a gravity displacement autoclave at 121°C, or porous load autoclave at 134°C, for 60 minutes; clean; and subject to routine sterilization.

However, these procedures pose their own safety concerns because the caustic conditions may damage not only the surgical instruments but also the autoclaves themselves in the absence of special precautions.[108]

Noncorrosive Prion Inactivation

The observation that branched polyamine dendrimers diminished prion infectivity in cells, particularly under acidic conditions,[109] led to the study of other denaturants under mildly acidic conditions. Whereas sodium dodecyl sulfate (SDS) at neutral pH had a modest ability to inactivate prions, it was highly effective when combined with acetic acid.[110] Testing inactivation against a range of PrP prion strains using sensitive Tg mouse models for bioassays enabled direct quantification of inactivation with the same treatments. One "acidic SDS" treatment that reduced infectivity of the hamster Sc237 strain by 9 $\log_{10}$ units only reduced infectivity of human CJD prions by less than 4 $\log_{10}$ units, suggesting that human CJD prions can be 100 000 times more difficult to inactivate than the widely

used Sc237 strain (Figure 68.2).[110] Similarly, BSE prions were over 1000-fold more resistant to inactivation than a mouse-passaged BSE strain, termed 301V, that has been widely used as a model for BSE.[111] Unfortunately, few such comprehensive studies have been undertaken. However, these findings strongly argue that prion inactivation procedures must be validated on the specific prion strains they are intended to be used against. Furthermore, these findings show that extrapolating from rodent-passaged prion strains to human prion strains is unreliable.

Inactivation of Surface-Bound Prions

Early prion inactivation studies were generally performed on homogenized PrP prion–infected tissue. To more closely model prions bound to the surfaces of surgical instruments and meat-processing machinery, short sections of stainless-steel wire were incubated in homogenate or briefly inserted into PrP prion–infected brain tissue and then implanted in the brains of reporter mice.[112,113] When equivalent prion inactivation treatments were applied to both brain homogenates and the wires that had been incubated in the homogenates, surface-bound PrP prions were much harder to inactivate.[110,111] Other noncorrosive procedures have been used to inactivate PrP prions, including enzymatic and alkaline cleaners and gaseous hydrogen peroxide.[114-116] However, these have only been validated against rodent-passaged PrP prions, and their efficacy against human or bovine prions is unknown.

Similar models have been used to study Aβ and α-synuclein prions. Stainless-steel wires incubated in brain homogenates from aged Tg amyloid precursor protein (APP) mice generated a robust Aβ-amyloidosis when implanted into the same mouse model.[117] Whereas heating the wires at 95°C for 10 minutes had no effect on the Aβ prions, hydrogen peroxide plasma sterilization (STERRAD S100 long cycle) prevented transmission of amyloid pathology in the APP mice.[117]

Analogously, stainless-steel wires incubated in MSA brain homogenate efficiently produced a lethal phenotype when implanted into TgM83$^{+/-}$ mice.[58] However, efforts to identify methods for inactivating α-synuclein prions have not relied on this bioassay to confirm complete inactivation. Instead, several methods have been used to measure residual protein following exposure of various contaminated surfaces to denaturing reagents. Harsh alkaline treatment, such as with 1 M NaOH or 0.2% SDS and 0.3% NaOH exposure for 1 hour, decreased recoverable α-synuclein from stainless-steel grids by more than 100-fold.[118] Fluorescent labeling of α-synuclein bound to common laboratory surfaces, including plastic, glass, aluminum, and stainless steel, found that NaOH and sodium hypochlorite exposure denatured α-synuclein fibrils on the surfaces but did not solubilize the protein.[119] More recent studies using precise

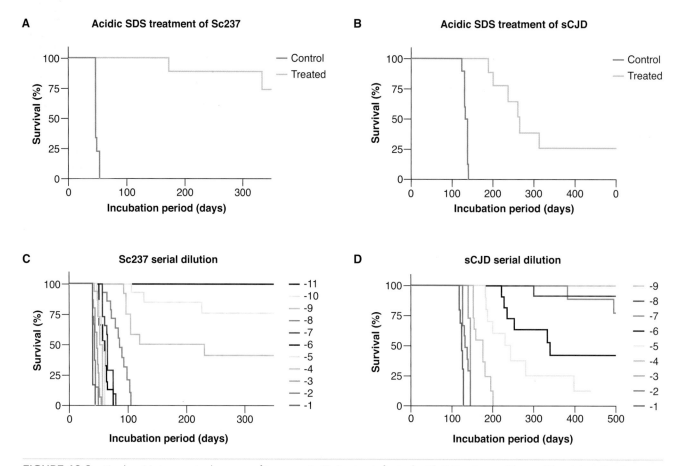

FIGURE 68.2   Kaplan-Meier survival curves of transgenic (Tg) mice infected with PrP prions with or without inactivation treatments. The Sc237 prions assayed in Tg7 mice (A and C), and sporadic Creutzfeldt-Jakob disease (sCJD) prions assayed in Tg22372 mice (B and D). Survival of mice before (dark blue) and after (light blue) incubation with acidic sodium dodecyl sulfate (SDS) (2% SDS, 1% acetic acid) for 30 minutes at 65°C (A and B). Statistical models derived from the serial dilution data (C and D) were used to quantify the difference between control and treatment arms, generating a value for reduction in prion titer. Whereas the treatment produced a 9.0 $\log_{10}$ reduction in infectivity for the hamster Sc237 strain, the same treatment only produced a 3.8 $\log_{10}$ reduction in infectivity for human sCJD prions.

analytical techniques to detect α-synuclein fibrils bound to a stainless-steel surface demonstrated that exposure to 1 N NaOH for 1 hour removes all bound α-synuclein, suggesting that the recommended methods for decontaminating surgical instruments and other surfaces exposed to PrP prions may also be effective for inactivating α-synuclein prions.[120] However, just as inactivation of rodent PrP prion strains is not necessarily a good model for human or bovine prion strains,[110,111] synthetic α-synuclein fibrils do not show the same infectivity characteristics as brain homogenates from MSA patients,[53] so it is unclear whether inactivation of synthetic α-synuclein fibrils is predictive of α-synuclein prions in the human brain.

▶ HANDLING PRIONS IN THE LABORATORY

Individuals entering laboratory space used for prion research should wear the appropriate personal protective equipment, including lab coat and gloves for BSL-2

areas. Eye protection is also advised, and open-toed shoes should be avoided. All procedures using prions that have not been chemically denatured (eg, samples to be run by SDS-polyacrylamide gel electrophoresis [PAGE]) should be carried out within a class II biosafety cabinet. Disposable sleeves and a second pair of gloves should be worn before placing the arms into the cabinet, and gloves should be changed each time the hands are removed from the cabinet. Working in the BSL-3 area requires a full bodysuit, boot or shoe covers, goggles or face shield, and double gloves with the inner pair taped to the bodysuit.

The use of disposable plasticware, which can be discarded as dry waste, is highly recommended. Liquid waste should be treated with NaOH to a final concentration of 1 N for 24 hours before disposal. In BSL-2 areas, solid waste is disposed of as biological waste and sent for incineration. Solid waste from BSL-3 should ideally be autoclaved at 132°C for 4.5 hours before disposal as biological waste. Equipment can be wiped down with 1 N NaOH, followed by 1 N HCl then repeatedly rinsed with water, using pH paper to monitor neutralization.

Because the paraformaldehyde vaporization procedure does not diminish prion titers, biosafety hoods must be decontaminated with 1 N NaOH, followed by 1 N HCl, and rinsed with water. High-efficiency particulate air filters should be autoclaved and incinerated.

▶ CARE OF PATIENTS

In the care of patients dying of human prion disease, the precautions used for patients with acquired immunodeficiency syndrome or hepatitis are adequate. In contrast to these viral illnesses, the human prion diseases are not communicable or contagious. There is no evidence of contact or aerosol transmission of prions from one human to another. However, as outlined earlier, prions are infectious under some circumstances. Noninvasive clinical procedures do not pose a risk to health care workers.[106]

▶ SURGICAL PROCEDURES

Although no well-documented cases of iCJD transmitted from contaminated surgical instruments have been reported for more than 30 years, the potential for such transmission remains a concern for health care facilities. Between 1998 and 2012, 19 incidents of surgeries performed on patients later diagnosed to have CJD were reported to the CDC. These procedures exposed not only operating room personnel to risk but also patients on whom the instruments were reused in subsequent surgeries. The majority of hospitals had multiple sets of instruments and therefore could not determine how many patients were exposed to the instruments used on the index case.[121]

Surgical procedures on patients with a PrP prion disease diagnosis should be minimized. Although there is no documentation of the transmission of prions to humans through droplets of blood or CSF or by exposure to intact skin or gastric and mucosal membranes, the theoretical risk of such occurrences cannot be ruled out definitively. Hospitals should ideally have a CJD policy; in the United Kingdom, this has been a requirement since 2006.[122] Health care workers and the infection control unit should be informed, and a full plan for instrument handling, cleaning, decontamination, and disposal should be implemented. It is recommended that surgeries be scheduled at the end of the day to allow time for the additional decontamination procedures.[106]

Single-use instruments are recommended whenever possible. However, when disposable instruments were introduced for tonsillectomies in the United Kingdom, the increased incidence of hemorrhage resulted in the reinstatement of reusable instruments within a year.[122] Any instruments coming in contact with high-risk tissue should be disposed of or subjected to one of the WHO recommended procedures outlined earlier.

▶ AUTOPSIES

Routine autopsies and the processing of small amounts of formalin-fixed tissues containing human PrP prions require BSL-2 precautions.[123] Historically, human brains have typically either been collected by formalin fixing the whole brain or dividing the hemispheres sagittally, fixing one-half and freezing the other. However, many neurodegenerative diseases are asymmetrical, and for biochemical and infectivity analyses, there is an increasing desire from research groups to have fresh frozen tissue adjacent to identified neuropathologic lesions. We therefore recommend the following procedure: After removing the dura, the olfactory bulbs, brainstem, and cerebellum should be removed. The resulting brain should then be sectioned into 1-cm slabs, with alternating coronal sections being frozen or formalin fixed (Figure 68.3). Sections for freezing should be immediately heat sealed in a heavy-duty plastic bag. The outside of the bag is assumed to be contaminated with prions and other pathogens. With fresh gloves, or with the help of an assistant with uncontaminated gloves,

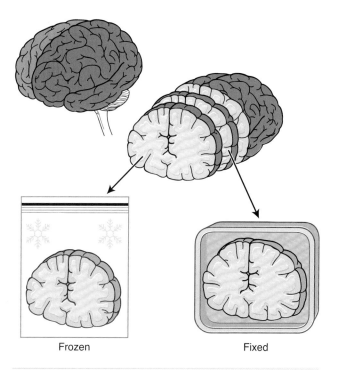

Frozen   Fixed

FIGURE 68.3 Schematic of the recommended procedure for cutting brain sections from prion disease patients. After removing the dura mater, the olfactory bulbs, brainstem, and cerebellum are removed. Then the remaining cerebral hemispheres are sectioned into 1-cm slabs, with alternate slabs being flash frozen or formalin fixed. Given the number of neurodegenerative diseases presenting without bilateral symmetry, previous methods of formalin fixing one cerebral hemisphere and flash freezing the other are becoming less favorable. Instead, to enable biochemical and neuropathologic analysis of adjacent brain regions, alternating sections are increasingly favored among researchers.

the bag containing the specimen should be placed into another plastic bag that does not have a contaminated outer surface. The samples should then be flash frozen on dry ice or placed directly into a −80°C freezer for storage.

The absence of any known effective treatment for prion disease demands caution in the manipulation of tissue from patients with these potentially infectious diseases. The highest concentrations of prions are in the central nervous system and its coverings. Based on data from animal studies, it is possible that high concentrations of prions may also be found in the spleen, thymus, and lymph nodes. The main precaution to be taken when working with prion-infected or contaminated tissue is to avoid puncture of the skin.[124] The prosector should wear cut-resistant gloves if possible. If accidental contamination of the skin occurs, the area should be swabbed with 0.1 N NaOH for 1 minute and then washed with copious amounts of water. Table 68.3 provides guidelines to reduce the risk of skin punctures and contamination from aerosols as well as decontamination of operating room and morgue surfaces and instruments.

Unfixed samples of brain, spinal cord, and other tissues containing human prions should be processed with extreme care at BSL-3. Gross dissection of fixed tissue should only be initiated after adequate formaldehyde fixation (at least 10-14 d), and tissue should be cut on a table covered with an absorbent pad with an impermeable backing. Wherever possible, disposable instruments and plasticware should be used, and decontamination of any instruments should be done following one of the CDC-recommended procedures outlined earlier. Tissue remnants, cutting debris, and contaminated formaldehyde solution should be discarded within a plastic container as infectious hospital waste for eventual incineration. Samples for histologic study should be placed in cassettes labeled "CJD Precautions" and embedded in a disposable embedding mold. In preparing sections, gloves should be worn and disposed of in a biohazard waste receptacle, along with any additional waste collected. The knife stage should be wiped with 1 to 2 N NaOH, and the knife used should be discarded in a biohazard sharps receptacle immediately after use. Slides should be labeled with "CJD Precautions."

▶ SAFETY OF THE BLOOD SUPPLY

The identification of blood transfusion as a source of vCJD led many countries to revisit their donor exclusion policies. However, a risk-benefit analysis must be

---

TABLE 68.3 Autopsies of patients with suspected prion disease: standard precautions

1. Attendance is limited to three staff, including at least one experienced pathologist. One of the staff avoids direct contact with the deceased but assists with handling of instruments and specimen containers.

2. Standard autopsy attire is mandatory. However, a disposable, waterproof gown is worn in place of a cloth gown.
   a. Cut-resistant gloves are worn underneath two pairs of surgical gloves, or chain mail gloves are worn between two pairs of surgical gloves.
   b. Aerosols are mainly created during opening of the skull with a saw. A respirator is required, which can be worn throughout the autopsy; however, when no aerosols are being generated, such as when the brain is being removed or when organ samples are being removed in situ, it is allowable to switch to a surgical mask with a wraparound splash guard transparent visor.

3. To reduce contamination of the autopsy suite:
   a. The autopsy table is covered with an absorbent sheet that has a waterproof backing.
   b. Contaminated instruments are placed on an absorbent pad.
   c. The brain is removed with the head in a plastic bag to reduce aerosol formation.
   d. The brain can be placed into a container with a plastic bag liner for weighing.
   e. The brain is placed onto a cutting board, and after removal of the olfactory bulbs, brainstem, and cerebellum, alternate coronal 1-cm slabs should be flash frozen or formalin fixed.
   f. In most cases of suspected prion disease, the autopsy can be limited to examination of the brain only. In cases requiring a full autopsy, consideration should be given to examining and sampling of thoracic and abdominal organs in situ.

4. Autopsy suite decontamination procedures
   a. Instruments (open box locks and jaws) and saw blades are placed into a large stainless-steel dish and treated by one of the WHO- or CDC-approved decontamination protocols outlined in the text.
   b. The saw is cleaned by repeated wiping with 2 N NaOH solution.
   c. The absorbent table cover and instrument pads, disposable clothing, and so forth are double bagged in appropriate infectious waste bags for incineration.
   d. Any suspected areas of contamination of the autopsy table or room are decontaminated by repeated wetting over 1 h with 2 N NaOH.

Abbreviations: CDC, Centers for Disease Control and Prevention; NaOH, sodium hydroxide; WHO, World Health Organization.

performed by each country before a policy is enacted. In the United States, potential donors are excluded if they have spent 3 months in the United Kingdom between 1980 and 1996, which excludes a small percentage of potential donors. In the United Kingdom, where it is estimated that 1 in 2000 people could be subclinically infected with vCJD,[86] a number of steps have been taken to reduce risk, such as importing plasma from other countries for fractionation to manufacture plasma derivatives and leucodepletion of all blood components. However, the majority of blood components are still derived from UK donors.[125]

▶ ANIMAL TISSUE IN NON-FOODSTUFFS

Following the BSE epidemic, considerable concern erupted in Europe over the safety of not only foodstuffs but also pharmaceutical and biologic products either derived from bovine source materials (active ingredients) or manufactured with bovine raw materials used as reagents in production. In addition, there is concern about products that contain bovine components as excipients in final formulations or as constituents in the ingested product covering (eg, capsule material). The major categories of "at-risk" products include recombinant proteins, vaccines, and gene therapy products produced in cultured cell systems using bovine-derived factors as well as drugs that use tallow or gelatin products as binders. A nonexhaustive list of bovine derivatives in pharmaceuticals is provided in Table 68.4. The pervasiveness of bovine-derived products is remarkable.

A WHO-convened committee recommended that bovine materials not be used in the manufacture of any biological or pharmaceutical products, but when alternatives do not exist, the committee has suggested a series of criteria for risk mitigation. These criteria include sourcing tissues from countries without a record of PrP prion disease and ensuring that high-risk tissues do not contaminate low-risk tissues in processing the carcass and removing the required tissues.[126] However, because the misfolding of prions is a stochastic process, any animal can develop a PrP prion disease in theory. The likelihood of spontaneous PrP prion disease increases with age as the cell mechanisms that clear misfolded proteins begin to break down. Therefore, we believe younger animals should be used to source tissues whenever possible.

TABLE 68.4 Bovine derivatives and their source materials in pharmaceuticals

Active Ingredients		Raw Materials in Manufacturing		Ingested Covering		Excipients	
Bovine Derivative	Bovine Source Material	Bovine Derivative	Bovine Source Material	Bovine Derivative	Bovine Source Material	Bovine Derivative	Bovine Source Material
Aprotinin	Lung	Albumin	Serum	Gelatin	Bone	Gelatin	Bone
Gelatin	Bone/hide	Amicase	Milk (casein)			Lactose	Milk
Glucagon	Pancreas	Brain-heart infusion	Brain and heart			Magnesium stearate	Tallow
Heparin	Intestine	Fetal calf serum	Serum			Polysorbate	Tallow
Insulin	Pancreas	Glycerol	Tallow				
Surfactant	Lung	Liver infusion	Liver				
		Meat extract	Carcass				
		Newborn calf serum	Serum				
		Pepticase	Milk (casein)				
		Peptone	Muscle				
		Polysorbate	Tallow				
		Primatone	Blood/spleen				
		Trypsin	Pancreas				
		Tryptone	Milk				

▶ CONCLUSION

From this review of some of the biosafety issues related to prions, whether transmitted from cattle to humans through BSE-contaminated bovine products or from human to human through CJD-contaminated blood, it is readily apparent that the existing information is insufficient. This situation forces regulatory authorities into the uncomfortable position of having to recommend highly conservative, precautionary measures aimed at precluding a "theoretical risk." Some of these measures are eminently reasonable. Others invite scrutiny and court the danger of provoking medical product shortages while pursuing a theoretical risk.

One of the most frustrating aspects of prion risk assessment and management has been the lack of rapid and sensitive methods for detecting human and animal prions. The need for such methods is imperative if we are to minimize the risk of prion contamination to public health. Animal bioassays have been widely used and have generated much of the data on which we rely, but these bioassays are precluded from routine monitoring because of the prolonged incubation times that are required. Fortunately, a number of advances have been made, including the development of Tg mice that are highly susceptible to bovine[127] and human[128,129] prions with abbreviated incubation periods as well as highly sensitive, conformation-dependent immunoassays that take advantage of the differences between predominantly α-helical PrP^C and the high β-sheet content of PrP^{Sc}.[130] More recently, the cell-free PMCA and RT-QuIC technologies have improved sensitivity to allow detection of PrP^{Sc} in urine,[131] CSF,[132] and blood,[133] offering hope that prion levels will soon be quantifiable using a standardized methodology to mitigate the spread of disease.

▶ ACKNOWLEDGMENTS

The authors acknowledge support from the National Institutes of Health (AG002132), the Brockman Foundation, and the Sherman Fairchild Foundation. We thank Sarah Pyle for figure illustration.

REFERENCES

1. Prusiner SB. Novel proteinaceous infectious particles cause scrapie. *Science*. 1982;216(4542):136-144.
2. Harrison PM, Khachane A, Kumar M. Genomic assessment of the evolution of the prion protein gene family in vertebrates. *Genomics*. 2010;95(5):268-277.
3. Orrú CD, Yuan J, Appleby BS, et al. Prion seeding activity and infectivity in skin samples from patients with sporadic Creutzfeldt-Jakob disease. *Sci Transl Med*. 2017;9(417):eaam7785.
4. Czub S, Schulz-Schaeffer W, Stahl-Hennig C, Beekes M, Schaetzl H, Motzkus D. *Frist evidence of intracranial and peroral transmission of chronic wasting disease (CWD) into cynomolgus macaques: a work in progress*. Paper presented at: Prion 2017; May 25, 2017; Edinburgh, Scotland.
5. Wickner RB. [URE3] as an altered URE2 protein: evidence for a prion analog in *Saccharomyces cerevisiae*. *Science*. 1994;264(5158):566-569.
6. Si K, Lindquist S, Kandel ER. A neuronal isoform of the aplysia CPEB has prion-like properties. *Cell*. 2003;115(7):879-891.
7. Si K, Choi YB, White-Grindley E, Majumdar A, Kandel ER. Aplysia CPEB can form prion-like multimers in sensory neurons that contribute to long-term facilitation. *Cell*. 2010;140(3):421-435.
8. Hou F, Sun L, Zheng H, Skaug B, Jiang QX, Chen ZJ. MAVS forms functional prion-like aggregates to activate and propagate antiviral innate immune response. *Cell*. 2011;146(3):448-461.
9. Prusiner SB. Cell biology. A unifying role for prions in neurodegenerative diseases. *Science*. 2012;336(6088):1511-1513.
10. Pattison IH. Experiments with scrapie with special reference to the nature of the agent and the pathology of the disease. In: Gajdusek DC, Gibbs CJ Jr, Alpers MP, eds. *Slow, Latent and Temperate Virus Infections, NINDB Monograph 2*. Washington, DC: U.S. Government Printing; 1965:249-257.
11. Scott MR, Peretz D, Nguyen HO, Dearmond SJ, Prusiner SB. Transmission barriers for bovine, ovine, and human prions in transgenic mice. *J Virol*. 2005;79(9):5259-5271.
12. Collinge J, Clarke AR. A general model of prion strains and their pathogenicity. *Science*. 2007;318(5852):930-936.
13. Pattison IH, Millson GC. Scrapie produced experimentally in goats with special reference to the clinical syndrome. *J Comp Pathol*. 1961;71:101-109.
14. Safar JG, Kellings K, Serban A, et al. Search for a prion-specific nucleic acid. *J Virol*. 2005;79(16):10796-10806.
15. Bessen RA, Marsh RF. Distinct PrP properties suggest the molecular basis of strain variation in transmissible mink encephalopathy. *J Virol*. 1994;68(12):7859-7868.
16. Telling GC, Parchi P, DeArmond SJ, et al. Evidence for the conformation of the pathologic isoform of the prion protein enciphering and propagating prion diversity. *Science*. 1996;274(5295):2079-2082.
17. Tanaka M, Collins SR, Toyama BH, Weissman JS. The physical basis of how prion conformations determine strain phenotypes. *Nature*. 2006;442(7102):585-589.
18. Toyama BH, Kelly MJ, Gross JD, Weissman JS. The structural basis of yeast prion strain variants. *Nature*. 2007;449(7159):233-237.
19. Lu JX, Qiang W, Yau WM, Schwieters CD, Meredith SC, Tycko R. Molecular structure of β-amyloid fibrils in Alzheimer's disease brain tissue. *Cell*. 2013;154(6):1257-1268.
20. Sanders DW, Kaufman SK, DeVos SL, et al. Distinct tau prion strains propagate in cells and mice and define different tauopathies. *Neuron*. 2014;82(6):1271-1288.
21. Peelaerts W, Bousset L, Van der Perren A, et al. α-Synuclein strains cause distinct synucleinopathies after local and systemic administration. *Nature*. 2015;522(7556):340-344.
22. Cuillé J, Chelle P-L. La maladie dite tremblante du mouton est-elle inoculable? *C R Acad Sci*. 1936;203:1552-1554.
23. Gajdusek DC, Gibbs CJ, Alpers M. Experimental transmission of a kuru-like syndrome to chimpanzees. *Nature*. 1966;209(5025):794-796.
24. Gibbs CJ Jr, Gajdusek DC, Asher DM, et al. Creutzfeldt-Jakob disease (spongiform encephalopathy): transmission to the chimpanzee. *Science*. 1968;161(3839):388-389.
25. Chandler RL. Encephalopathy in mice produced by inoculation with scrapie brain material. *Lancet*. 1961;1(7191):1378-1379.
26. Kimberlin R, Walker C. Characteristics of a short incubation model of scrapie in the golden hamster. *J Gen Virol*. 1977;34(2):295-304.
27. Watts JC, Prusiner SB. Mouse models for studying the formation and propagation of prions. *J Biol Chem*. 2014;289(29):19841-19849.
28. Race RE, Fadness LH, Chesebro B. Characterization of scrapie infection in mouse neuroblastoma cells. *J Gen Virol*. 1987;68(pt 5):1391-1399.
29. Schätzl HM, Laszlo L, Holtzman DM, et al. A hypothalamic neuronal cell line persistently infected with scrapie prions exhibits apoptosis. *J Virol*. 1997;71(11):8821-8831.

30. Mahal SP, Baker CA, Demczyk CA, Smith EW, Julius C, Weissmann C. Prion strain discrimination in cell culture: the cell panel assay. *Proc Natl Acad Sci U S A*. 2007;104(52):20908-20913.

31. Courageot MP, Daude N, Nonno R, et al. A cell line infectible by prion strains from different species. *J Gen Virol*. 2008;89(pt 1):341-347.

32. Krejciova Z, Alibhai J, Zhao C, et al. Human stem cell-derived astrocytes replicate human prions in a *PRNP* genotype-dependent manner. *J Exp Med*. 2017;214(12):3481-3495.

33. Kocisko DA, Come JH, Priola SA, et al. Cell-free formation of protease-resistant prion protein. *Nature*. 1994;370(6489):471-474.

34. Saborio GP, Permanne B, Soto C. Sensitive detection of pathological prion protein by cyclic amplification of protein misfolding. *Nature*. 2001;411(6839):810-813.

35. Castilla J, Saá P, Hetz C, Soto C. In vitro generation of infectious scrapie prions. *Cell*. 2005;121(2):195-206.

36. Wilham JM, Orrú CD, Bessen RA, et al. Rapid end-point quantitation of prion seeding activity with sensitivity comparable to bioassays. *PLoS Pathog*. 2010;6(12):e1001217.

37. Ridley RM, Baker HF, Windle CP, Cummings RM. Very long term studies of the seeding of beta-amyloidosis in primates. *J Neural Transm (Vienna)*. 2006;113(9):1243-1251.

38. Kane MD, Lipinski WJ, Callahan MJ, et al. Evidence for seeding of beta-amyloid by intracerebral infusion of Alzheimer brain extracts in beta-amyloid precursor protein-transgenic mice. *J Neurosci*. 2000;20(10):3606-3611.

39. Meyer-Luehmann M, Coomaraswamy J, Bolmont T, et al. Exogenous induction of cerebral beta-amyloidogenesis is governed by agent and host. *Science*. 2006;313(5794):1781-1784.

40. Heilbronner G, Eisele YS, Langer F, et al. Seeded strain-like transmission of β-amyloid morphotypes in APP transgenic mice. *EMBO Rep*. 2013;14(11):1017-1022.

41. Stöhr J, Condello C, Watts JC, et al. Distinct synthetic Aβ prion strains producing different amyloid deposits in bigenic mice. *Proc Natl Acad Sci U S A*. 2014;111(28):10329-10334.

42. Watts JC, Condello C, Stöhr J, et al. Serial propagation of distinct strains of Aβ prions from Alzheimer's disease patients. *Proc Natl Acad Sci U S A*. 2014;111(28):10323-10328.

43. Olsson TT, Klementieva O, Gouras GK. Prion-like seeding and nucleation of intracellular amyloid-β. *Neurobiol Dis*. 2018;113:1-10.

44. Clavaguera F, Akatsu H, Fraser G, et al. Brain homogenates from human tauopathies induce tau inclusions in mouse brain. *Proc Natl Acad Sci U S A*. 2013;110(23):9535-9540.

45. Kaufman SK, Sanders DW, Thomas TL, et al. Tau prion strains dictate patterns of cell pathology, progression rate, and regional vulnerability in vivo. *Neuron*. 2016;92(4):796-812.

46. Woerman AL, Aoyagi A, Patel S, et al. Tau prions from Alzheimer's disease and chronic traumatic encephalopathy patients propagate in cultured cells. *Proc Natl Acad Sci U S A*. 2016;113(50):E8187-E8196.

47. Giasson BI, Duda JE, Quinn SM, Zhang B, Trojanowski JQ, Lee VM. Neuronal alpha-synucleinopathy with severe movement disorder in mice expressing A53T human alpha-synuclein. *Neuron*. 2002;34(4):521-533.

48. Mougenot AL, Nicot S, Bencsik A, et al. Prion-like acceleration of a synucleinopathy in a transgenic mouse model. *Neurobiol Aging*. 2012;33(9):2225-2228.

49. Luk KC, Kehm VM, Zhang B, O'Brien P, Trojanowski JQ, Lee VM. Intracerebral inoculation of pathological α-synuclein initiates a rapidly progressive neurodegenerative α-synucleinopathy in mice. *J Exp Med*. 2012;209(5):975-986.

50. Watts JC, Giles K, Oehler A, et al. Transmission of multiple system atrophy prions to transgenic mice. *Proc Natl Acad Sci U S A*. 2013;110(48):19555-19560.

51. Prusiner SB, Woerman AL, Mordes DA, et al. Evidence for α-synuclein prions causing multiple system atrophy in humans with parkinsonism. *Proc Natl Acad Sci U S A*. 2015;112(38):E5308-E5317.

52. Woerman AL, Stöhr J, Aoyagi A, et al. Propagation of prions causing synucleinopathies in cultured cells. *Proc Natl Acad Sci U S A*. 2015;112(35):E4949-E4958.

53. Woerman AL, Kazmi SA, Patel S, et al. Familial Parkinson's point mutation abolishes multiple system atrophy prion replication. *Proc Natl Acad Sci U S A*. 2018;115(2):409-414.

54. Gordon WS. Advances in veterinary research. *Vet Rec*. 1946;58(47):516-525.

55. Stamp JT, Brotherston JG, Zlotnik I, Mackay JM, Smith W. Further studies on scrapie. *J Comp Pathol*. 1959;69:268-280.

56. Dickinson AG, Taylor DM. Resistance of scrapie agent to decontamination. *N Engl J Med*. 1978;299(25):1413-1414.

57. Alper T, Cramp WA, Haig DA, Clarke MC. Does the agent of scrapie replicate without nucleic acid? *Nature*. 1967;214(5090):764-766.

58. Woerman AL, Kazmi SA, Patel S, et al. MSA prions exhibit remarkable stability and resistance to inactivation. *Acta Neuropathol*. 2018;135(1):49-63.

59. Schweighauser M, Bacioglu M, Fritschi SK, et al. Formaldehyde-fixed brain tissue from spontaneously ill α-synuclein transgenic mice induces fatal α-synucleinopathy in transgenic hosts. *Acta Neuropathol*. 2015;129(1):157-159.

60. Fritschi SK, Langer F, Kaeser SA, et al. Highly potent soluble amyloid-β seeds in human Alzheimer brain but not cerebrospinal fluid. *Brain*. 2014;137(pt 11):2909-2915.

61. Kaufman SK, Thomas TL, Del Tredici K, Braak H, Diamond MI. Characterization of tau prion seeding activity and strains from formaldehyde-fixed tissue. *Acta Neuropathol Commun*. 2017;5(1):41.

62. Alpers MP. A history of kuru. *P N G Med J*. 2007;50(1-2):10-19.

63. Collinge J, Whitfield J, McKintosh E, et al. Kuru in the 21st century—an acquired human prion disease with very long incubation periods. *Lancet*. 2006;367(9528):2068-2074.

64. Duffy P, Wolf J, Collins G, DeVoe AG, Streeten B, Cowen D. Letter: possible person-to-person transmission of Creutzfeldt-Jakob disease. *N Engl J Med*. 1974;290(12):692-693.

65. Bernoulli C, Siegfried J, Baumgartner G, et al. Danger of accidental person-to-person transmission of Creutzfeldt-Jakob disease by surgery. *Lancet*. 1977;1(8009):478-479.

66. Gibbs CJ Jr, Asher DM, Kobrine A, Amyx HL, Sulima MP, Gajdusek DC. Transmission of Creutzfeldt-Jakob disease to a chimpanzee by electrodes contaminated during neurosurgery. *J Neurol Neurosurg Psychiatry*. 1994;57(6):757-758.

67. Will RG, Matthews WB. Evidence for case-to-case transmission of Creutzfeldt-Jakob disease. *J Neurol Neurosurg Psychiatry*. 1982;45(3):235-238.

68. Brown P, Brandel JP, Sato T, et al. Iatrogenic Creutzfeldt-Jakob disease, final assessment. *Emerg Infect Dis*. 2012;18(6):901-907.

69. Parchi P, Giese A, Capellari S, et al. Classification of sporadic Creutzfeldt-Jakob disease based on molecular and phenotypic analysis of 300 subjects. *Ann Neurol*. 1999;46(2):224-233.

70. Brandel JP, Preece M, Brown P, et al. Distribution of codon 129 genotype in human growth hormone-treated CJD patients in France and the UK. *Lancet*. 2003;362(9378):128-130.

71. Ae R, Hamaguchi T, Nakamura Y, et al. Update: dura mater graft-associated Creutzfeldt-Jakob disease—Japan, 1975-2017. *MMWR Morb Mortal Wkly Rep*. 2018;67(9):274-278.

72. Doh-ura K, Kitamoto T, Sakaki Y, Tateishi J. CJD discrepancy. *Nature*. 1991;353(6347):801-802.

73. Kobayashi A, Matsuura Y, Mohri S, Kitamoto T. Distinct origins of dura mater graft-associated Creutzfeldt-Jakob disease: past and future problems. *Acta Neuropathol Commun*. 2014;2:32.

74. Jaunmuktane Z, Mead S, Ellis M, et al. Evidence for human transmission of amyloid-β pathology and cerebral amyloid angiopathy. *Nature*. 2015;525(7568):247-250.

75. Kovacs GG, Lutz MI, Ricken G, et al. Dura mater is a potential source of Aβ seeds. *Acta Neuropathol*. 2016;131(6):911-923.

76. Cali I, Cohen ML, Haïk S, et al. Iatrogenic Creutzfeldt-Jakob disease with amyloid-β pathology: an international study. *Acta Neuropathol Commun*. 2018;6(1):5.

77. Ritchie DL, Adlard P, Peden AH, et al. Amyloid-β accumulation in the CNS in human growth hormone recipients in the UK. *Acta Neuropathol*. 2017;134:221-240.

78. Hervé D, Porché M, Cabrejo L, et al. Fatal Aβ cerebral amyloid angiopathy 4 decades after a dural graft at the age of 2 years. *Acta Neuropathol.* 2018;135(5):801-803.

79. Duyckaerts C, Sazdovitch V, Ando K, et al. Neuropathology of iatrogenic Creutzfeldt-Jakob disease and immunoassay of French cadaver-sourced growth hormone batches suggest possible transmission of tauopathy and long incubation periods for the transmission of Abeta pathology. *Acta Neuropathol.* 2018;135(20):201-212.

80. Jaunmuktane Z, Quaegebeur A, Taipa R, et al. Evidence of amyloid-β cerebral amyloid angiopathy transmission through neurosurgery. *Acta Neuropathol.* 2018;135(5):671-679.

81. Wilesmith JW, Ryan JB, Atkinson MJ. Bovine spongiform encephalopathy: epidemiological studies on the origin. *Vet Rec.* 1991;128(9):199-203.

82. Will RG, Ironside JW, Zeidler M, et al. A new variant of Creutzfeldt-Jakob disease in the UK. *Lancet.* 1996;347(9006):921-925.

83. Hill AF, Desbruslais M, Joiner S, et al. The same prion strain causes vCJD and BSE. *Nature.* 1997;389(6650):448-450, 526.

84. Scott MR, Will R, Ironside J, et al. Compelling transgenetic evidence for transmission of bovine spongiform encephalopathy prions to humans. *Proc Natl Acad Sci U S A.* 1999;96(26):15137-15142.

85. Mok T, Jaunmuktane Z, Joiner S, et al. Variant Creutzfeldt-Jakob disease in a patient with heterozygosity at *PRNP* codon 129. *N Engl J Med.* 2017;376(3):292-294.

86. Gill ON, Spencer Y, Richard-Loendt A, et al. Prevalent abnormal prion protein in human appendixes after bovine spongiform encephalopathy epizootic: large scale survey. *BMJ.* 2013;347:f5675.

87. Hewitt PE, Llewelyn CA, Mackenzie J, Will RG. Creutzfeldt-Jakob disease and blood transfusion: results of the UK Transfusion Medicine Epidemiological Review study. *Vox Sang.* 2006;91(3):221-230.

88. Agency UKHP. *Health Protection Report: Weekly Report.* London, United Kingdom: Public Health England; 2007.

89. Peden AH, Head MW, Ritchie DL, Bell JE, Ironside JW. Preclinical vCJD after blood transfusion in a PRNP codon 129 heterozygous patient. *Lancet.* 2004;364(9433):527-529.

90. Peden A, McCardle L, Head MW, et al. Variant CJD infection in the spleen of a neurologically asymptomatic UK adult patient with haemophilia. *Haemophilia.* 2010;16(2):296-304.

91. Urwin P, Thanigaikumar K, Ironside JW, et al. Sporadic Creutzfeldt-Jakob disease in 2 plasma product recipients, United Kingdom. *Emerg Infect Dis.* 2017;23(6). doi:10.3201/eid2306.161884.

92. Williams ES, Young S. Chronic wasting disease of captive mule deer: a spongiform encephalopathy. *J Wildl Dis.* 1980;16(1):89-98.

93. Haley NJ, Hoover EA. Chronic wasting disease of cervids: current knowledge and future perspectives. *Annu Rev Anim Biosci.* 2015;3:305-325.

94. Benestad SL, Mitchell G, Simmons M, Ytrehus B, Vikøren T. First case of chronic wasting disease in Europe in a Norwegian free-ranging reindeer. *Vet Res.* 2016;47(1):88.

95. EFSA Panel on Biological Hazards, Ricci A, Allende A, et al. Scientific opinion on chronic wasting disease (II). *EFSA Journal.* 2018;16:5132.

96. Marsh RF, Kincaid AE, Bessen RA, Bartz JC. Interspecies transmission of chronic wasting disease prions to squirrel monkeys (*Saimiri sciureus*). *J Virol.* 2005;79(21):13794-13796.

97. Race B, Meade-White KD, Phillips K, Striebel J, Race R, Chesebro B. Chronic wasting disease agents in nonhuman primates. *Emerg Infect Dis.* 2014;20(5):833-837.

98. Haybaeck J, Heikenwalder M, Klevenz B, et al. Aerosols transmit prions to immunocompetent and immunodeficient mice. *PLoS Pathog.* 2011;7(1):e1001257.

99. Centers for Disease Control and Prevention. *Biosafety in Microbiological and Biomedical Laboratories (BMBL).* Atlanta, GA: US Department of Health and Human Services; 2009.

100. Tateishi J, Ohta M, Koga M, Sato Y, Kuroiwa Y. Transmission of chronic spongiform encephalopathy with kuru plaques from humans to small rodents. *Ann Neurol.* 1979;5(6):581-584.

101. Giles K, Woerman AL, Berry DB, et al. Bioassays and inactivation of prions. In: SB Prusiner, ed. *Prion Biology.* Cold Spring Harbor, NY: Cold Spring Harbor Laboratory Press; 2017:401-416.

102. Watts JC, Giles K, Patel S, et al. Evidence that bank vole PrP is a universal acceptor for prions. *PLoS Pathog.* 2014;10(4):e1003990.

103. Prusiner SB, Groth DF, Cochran SP, Masiarz FR, McKinley MP, Martinez HM. Molecular properties, partial purification, and assay by incubation period measurements of the hamster scrapie agent. *Biochemistry.* 1980;19(21):4883-4891.

104. Prusiner SB, Groth DF, McKinley MP, Cochran SP, Bowman KA, Kasper KC. Thiocyanate and hydroxyl ions inactivate the scrapie agent. *Proc Natl Acad Sci U S A.* 1981;78(7):4606-4610.

105. Prusiner SB, McKinley MP, Groth DF, et al. Scrapie agent contains a hydrophobic protein. *Proc Natl Acad Sci U S A.* 1981;78(11):6675-6679.

106. World Health Organization. *WHO Infection Control Guidelines for Transmissible Spongiform Encephalopathies: Report of a WHO Consultation.* Geneva, Switzerland: World Health Organization; 1999.

107. World Health Organization. *WHO Tables on Tissue Infectivity Distribution in Transmissible Spongiform Encephalopathies.* Geneva, Switzerland: World Health Organization; 2010.

108. Brown SA, Merritt K, Woods TO, Busick DN. Effects on instruments of the World Health Organization—recommended protocols for decontamination after possible exposure to transmissible spongiform encephalopathy-contaminated tissue. *J Biomed Mater Res B Appl Biomater.* 2005;72(1):186-190.

109. Supattapone S, Wille H, Uyechi L, et al. Branched polyamines cure prion-infected neuroblastoma cells. *J Virol.* 2001;75(7):3453-3461.

110. Peretz D, Supattapone S, Giles K, et al. Inactivation of prions by acidic sodium dodecyl sulfate. *J Virol.* 2006;80(1):322-331.

111. Giles K, Glidden DV, Beckwith R, et al. Resistance of bovine spongiform encephalopathy (BSE) prions to inactivation. *PLoS Pathog.* 2008;4(11):e1000206.

112. Flechsig E, Hegyi I, Enari M, Schwarz P, Collinge J, Weissmann C. Transmission of scrapie by steel-surface-bound prions. *Mol Med.* 2001;7(10):679-684.

113. Zobeley E, Flechsig E, Cozzio A, Enari M, Weissmann C. Infectivity of scrapie prions bound to a stainless steel surface. *Mol Med.* 1999;5(4):240-243.

114. Fichet G, Comoy E, Duval C, et al. Novel methods for disinfection of prion-contaminated medical devices. *Lancet.* 2004;364(9433):521-526.

115. Yan ZX, Stitz L, Heeg P, Pfaff E, Roth K. Infectivity of prion protein bound to stainless steel wires: a model for testing decontamination procedures for transmissible spongiform encephalopathies. *Infect Control Hosp Epidemiol.* 2004;25(40):280-283.

116. Fichet G, Comoy E, Dehen C, et al. Investigations of a prion infectivity assay to evaluate methods of decontamination. *J Microbiol Methods.* 2007;70(3):511-518.

117. Eisele YS, Bolmont T, Heikenwalder M, et al. Induction of cerebral beta-amyloidosis: intracerebral versus systemic Abeta inoculation. *Proc Natl Acad Sci U S A.* 2009;106(31):12926-12931.

118. Thomzig A, Wagenführ K, Daus ML, et al. Decontamination of medical devices from pathological amyloid-β-, tau- and α-synuclein aggregates. *Acta Neuropathol Commun.* 2014;2:151.

119. Bousset L, Brundin P, Böckmann A, Meier B, Melki R. An efficient procedure for removal and inactivation of alpha-synuclein assemblies from laboratory materials. *J Parkinsons Dis.* 2016;6(1):143-151.

120. Phan HTM, Bartz JC, Ayers J, et al. Adsorption and decontamination of α-synuclein from medically and environmentally-relevant surfaces. *Colloids Surf B Biointerfaces.* 2018;166:98-107.

121. Belay ED, Blase J, Sehulster LM, Maddox RA, Schonberger LB. Management of neurosurgical instruments and patients exposed to Creutzfeldt-Jakob disease. *Infect Control Hosp Epidemiol.* 2013;34(12):1272-1280.

122. Lumley JS. The impact of Creutzfeldt-Jakob disease on surgical practice. *Ann R Coll Surg Engl.* 2008;90(2):91-94.

123. Ironside JW, Bell JE. The 'high-risk' neuropathological autopsy in AIDS and Creutzfeldt-Jakob disease: principles and practice. *Neuropathol Appl Neurobiol.* 1996;22(5):388-393.

124. Ridley RM, Baker HF. Occupational risk of Creutzfeldt-Jakob disease. *Lancet.* 1993;341(8845):641-642.

125. UK Blood Services Joint Professional Advisory Group. *Position statement: Creutzfeldt-Jakob Disease.* London, UK: Joint United Kingdom (UK) Blood Transfusion and Tissue Transplantation Services Professional Advisory Committee (JPAC); 2015.

126. World Health Organization. *WHO Guidelines on Transmissible Spongiform Encephalopathies in Relation to Biological and Pharmaceutical Products.* Geneva, Switzerland: World Health Organization; 2003.

127. Scott MR, Safar J, Telling G, et al. Identification of a prion protein epitope modulating transmission of bovine spongiform encephalopathy prions to transgenic mice. *Proc Natl Acad Sci U S A.* 1997;94(26):14279-14284.

128. Giles K, Glidden DV, Patel S, et al. Human prion strain selection in transgenic mice. *Ann Neurol.* 2010;68(2):151-161.

129. Korth C, Kaneko K, Groth D, et al. Abbreviated incubation times for human prions in mice expressing a chimeric mouse-human prion protein transgene. *Proc Natl Acad Sci U S A.* 2003;100(8):4784-4789.

130. Safar J, Wille H, Itri V, et al. Eight prion strains have PrP(Sc) molecules with different conformations. *Nat Med.* 1998;4(10):1157-1165.

131. Moda F, Gambetti P, Notari S, et al. Prions in the urine of patients with variant Creutzfeldt-Jakob disease. *N Engl J Med.* 2014;371(6):530-539.

132. McGuire LI, Peden AH, Orrú CD, et al. Real time quaking-induced conversion analysis of cerebrospinal fluid in sporadic Creutzfeldt-Jakob disease. *Ann Neurol.* 2012;72(2):278-285.

133. Concha-Marambio L, Pritzkow S, Moda F, et al. Detection of prions in blood from patients with variant Creutzfeldt-Jakob disease. *Sci Transl Med.* 2016;8(370):370ra183.

Fungal Contamination in the Built Environment: Shipping and Storage

Daniel L. Price and Donald G. Ahearn

▶ INTRODUCTION

Indoor surfaces in the built environment seldom are free of mould propagules from the extant environment. Vegetative and dormant forms of fungi including viable conidia, dormant-resistant chlamydoconidia, and various sexual stages can bind and persist differentially in dust. Select fungi with appropriate dampness can colonize metabolically susceptible surfaces, particularly cellulosic coated gypsum wallboards and ceiling tiles.[1-5] Construction activities, external and internal, can increase airborne fungal densities to objectionable and unhealthy levels.[6-9] Green et al[10] reported the use of a halogen immunoassay (HIA) to document the allergenicity of airborne fungal hyphal fragments and broken spores. The immunoglobulin E (IgE)-based assay documented allergen release from intact germinating conidia as well as the terminal ends of growing hyphal fragments. The data suggested that the total submicron fungal particles could magnify the overall aeroallergen load in the environment beyond that indicated by identifiable spore counts.

Air filters and air duct insulations may support hidden select, reproducing fungal populations contributing to various indoor syndromes (Figure 69.1).[11-14] Water reservoirs and rains in particular may harbor persistent biofilms of aspergilli and fusaria.[15-18] These inherent colonizations, sometimes cryptic within materials as well as on surfaces, can result in indoor air densities significantly distinct in time and composition from those recoverable in the extant airborne mycota.[19,20] Chronic water leaks from plumbing or exterior wall fissures, catastrophic water incursions following floods and storms, and persistent high relative humidity can facilitate fungal growth and metabolism that render the built environment unsuitable for its intended use.[21] Porous structural- or indoor-finishing materials in human habitats inundated with water for over 48 hours, particularly following catastrophic flooding when drying

of materials is impractical, generally are recommended for replacement.[4,22]

Occasionally new, but mostly aged, structures become colonized with fungi without recognized water or construction events. Typically, such colonization can be attributed to the miasma stresses of the structure use and aging (ie, building foundation or envelope integrity issues). In some instances, mostly with new materials, contaminating fungi are not identifiable within the extant geography. The fungus may be from the environment of material processing, sometimes inherent on or within the materials themselves, or from material exposures during shipping and storage.[23,24]

▶ GYPSUM WALLBOARD

Crystalline gypsum ($CaSO_4 \cdot 2H_2O$) bonded between two layers of paper is used worldwide for interior fire-retardant acoustic walls. The product is variable in composition both by design on intended use and the inclusion of inhibitors or nutritive formulations, for example, starch or recycled content.[5,25-27] Products from the same manufacturer may be inhibitory or stimulatory for growth of select fungi varying with the source of raw materials and climatic conditions.[5,28] The paper layers impacted with sufficient moisture support growth and metabolism of fungi, and the core itself may be impacted (eg, after flooding).[25]

The spectrum of fungi capable of growth and metabolism on gypsum wallboards is broad, typically reflecting the adjacent extant environment, and identifiable often with the genera *Aspergillus*, *Alternaria*, *Chaetomium*, *Cladosporium*, *Penicillium*, *Stachybotrys*, and *Ulocladium*.[5,29]

Krause et al[30] demonstrated that commercially available gypsum wallboards, some treated with protective coatings, developed visually detectable mold growth during exposure to bottled water. Untreated wallboard inundated by mold during the exposure appeared devoid of viable

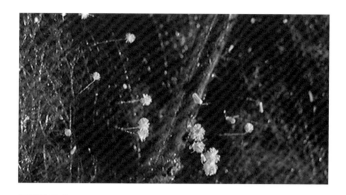

FIGURE 69.1 Emergence of *Aspergillus flavus* growth on the downstream (air leaving) side of a heating, ventilation, and air conditioning (HVAC) filter from a hospital air handling system. For a color version of this art, please consult the eBook.

fungi following cleaning with household chlorine compounds (see chapter 15). The tests were conducted under ambient conditions in a room setting. One end of various uninoculated gypsum board panels was suspended in bottled water to a depth of 1 inch. Various genera such as *Penicillium*, *Cladosporium*, then *Aspergillus*, and later *Ulocladium* were detected sequentially in time at 1 to 6 weeks. Fungi were not observed in ostensibly dry areas about 6 inches above the ascending water stain. *Stachybotrys* was not observed, or was mold observed, on dry control panels maintained in the same room. Several protective coatings delayed fungal development. The extent of growth and splotchy appearance varied among the panels. The source of the fungi in these experiments is problematic. These genera were probably sourced mostly from the extant atmosphere and handling in the test room, but some may have been inherent to the wallboard. Delgado et al[31] reported postprocessing survival and recalcitrance to disinfection chemicals by heat-resistant fungi on paperboard packaging materials. Additional such findings have been mentioned by Rico-Munoz.[32] Menetrez et al[33,34] demonstrated that steam-sterilized coupons of gypsum wallboard, plain and treated with different coatings, supported varied levels of visually detectable growth after inoculation with *Stachybotrys chartarum*. Cleaning and disinfection regimen applied with commercially available products indicated some potential for remediation. The presence of inherent mould among the gypsum boards and the varied coatings may be questioned; it was not part of the study design. Andersen et al[27] examined 13 unused gypsum boards acquired at four different building supply stores that represented three types and two brands. Twelve discs were cut from each panel, submerged with rubbing in 96% ethanol, air-dried, wetted, and stored in sealed Petri dishes at 22°C to 23°C. *Aspergillus hiratsukae* (*Neosartorya*), *Chaetomium globosum*, and *S chartarum* were the most prevalent species observed that developed on all 13, 11, and 7 panels, respectively. The fungi presumably were em-

bedded in the kraft paper surrounding the gypsum core.[27] This was the first report verifying the potential of *A hiratsukae* for colonization of gypsum wallboards and for survival following disinfection procedures. This species at room temperatures (20°C-35°C), in addition to developing conidiophores and conidia similar to those of *Aspergillus fumigatus*, produces cleistothecia encasing asci containing heat-resistant ascospores.[27,35] The maximal temperature for growth on laboratory media such as malt extract is between 45°C and 50°C, but the dormant thermoduric ascospores may survive temperatures above 90°C.[35-37]

The *A hiratsukae* is an emerging pathogen in the fumigati complex, and, as such, its potential colonization of a built environment may be of greater concern for immunocompromised inhabitants in comparison to noxious fungi of lesser or unknown virulence in such as *Avicularia versicolor*, *C globosum*, or *S chartarum*.[38-40]

Lewinska et al[41] used scanning electron microscopy (SEM) and microcomputed tomography to visualize structural changes in gypsum board and plywood samples when exposed to water, *C globosum*, and *S chartarum* over an 8-week period. The *S chartarum* seemed restricted to surface growth on the inoculated paper-layered gypsum wallboard, but inoculated plywood was penetrated into the core. The growth of *Chaetomium* on both substrates was somewhat atypical. Details of the type of gypsum and plywood or presence of potential inhibitory components were not available. Fungal growth was not reported on the uninoculated controls.

Mesophilic fungal isolates identified as *C globosum*, common colonizers in damp buildings, have demonstrated restricted growth, if any, at 37°C to 42°C, although their ascospores may survive exposures at temperatures above 50°C. Such isolates are of possible rare risk for involvement in onychomycosis, otitis, peritonitis, or keratitis, but any associations with invasive mycoses seem unlikely, particularly in noncompromised hosts.[42,43] Some thermotolerant chaetomia capable of growth or survival near 50°C have been recognized as emerging human pathogens in rare infections of competent- and immunocompromised individuals.[42-44] Thermotolerance among these fungi, some of which are yet to demonstrate ascomata, may reside with clusters of chlamydoconidia-like cells.[45,46]

Isolates of the *S chartarum* complex[47] (notorious for toxicity after ingestion) have maximal growth temperatures below 40°C and probably higher survival temperatures if encased in paper, but their capacities for infections remains questioned.[20,26,47,48] The proclivity of this species complex to colonize and metabolize paper coatings of gypsum boards, particularly the inner wall, can result in a hidden source of noxious odors following catastrophic or undetected moisture events. Colonization by the *S chartarum* complex on inner and outer surfaces of interior walls may not be reflected in the detectable airborne mycota because of sluggish conidial release and size versus *Aspergillus* and *Penicillium*.[49] Price and Ahearn[50] earlier noted the development of *S chartarum* on uninoculated

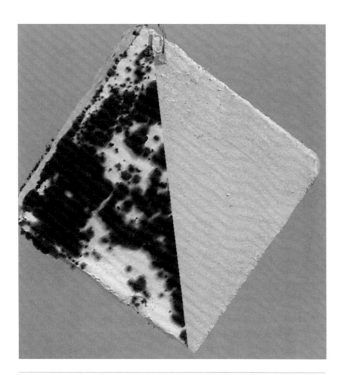

FIGURE 69.2 Gypsum wallboard samples previously colonized by *Stachybotrys chartarum*. Both were disinfected and then coated with preserved paints. Regrowth (shown on the left) on samples with inadequate dry film preservative and minimal regrowth (on the right) after samples were exposed to high relative humidity for 180 d. For a color version of this art, please consult the eBook.

gypsum board controls. Visually detectable fungal colonization on gypsum wallboard is often restricted to untreated surfaces (Figure 69.2).[51]

▶ WOOD

After cutting and milling, the availability of wood sugars on the surface of lumber, coupled with residual or atmospheric moisture, will permit the growth of numerous molds (eg, *Penicillium*, *Paecilomyces*, *Fusarium*). Some will cause a notable blue- or sap-surface staining. Formulations of copper salts combined with azoles, such as tebuconazole and/or thiazolones (octyl isothiazolinones or benzisothiazolinones), are applied often for surface protection, but without moisture control, staining may reoccur from fungi inherent in or on the wood.[52-54]

Iterations of preservative formulations containing azoles (eg, propiconazole), borates, copper salts, alkaline copper quaternary, and copper naphthenate have been incorporated into pressure-treated lumber for above- and in-ground usage.[55-57] These formulations have mostly replaced chromated copper arsenate (CCA) creosote and pentachlorophenol (PCP) for preservation of wood for in-ground dwelling applications. Toxicity concerns (involving chromium and arsenic) and changing

regulatory guidelines, particularly in Europe, spurred the development of the former preservatives. The CCA and PCP have been relegated to be used only for restricted use (ie, railroad crossties, utility poles, and wharf pilings).[56,58,59]

Kiln-dried and pressure-treated lumber and plywood for indoor use, particularly pinewoods, within a single building can encounter a range of ecosystems and stresses. Wood in attics and crawl spaces typically sustain alternating onslaughts from temperatures and humidity. Pine wood in particular, both kiln-dried and pressure-treated, absorbs moisture and can support the growth of species complexes such as *Paecilomyces variotii*.[52,60]

Over 100 countries have agreed that the importation of raw or industrial lumber be in accordance with International Standards for Phytosanitary Measures: Regulation of Wood Packaging Material in International Trade.[61] These standards were adopted to limit the international spread of forest pests, mainly insects, but have been modified to include fungi. Regulations require identification of the protective heat and atmospheric (fumigation) processing applied to the wood product. Lumber and packaging, including pallets and skids, must be identifiable by stamped codes identifying their origin, details of kiln, or other type of heat or protective processing. Wood packaging heat treatment must be at least 30 contiguous minutes for 56°C; kiln exposure should reduce water content to less than 20%. These regulations can vary for the type of wood, even the species, and the intended product use.[24] If appropriate information is unavailable at the port of entry, the shipment may be quarantined.

Heat treatment alters the chemical and structural composition of wood affecting swelling and shrinkage while typically enhancing biological durability against insects and fungi. The capacity to resist fungal decay varies with the type of wood and heat processing conditions. Under optimized conditions, soft and available woods such as pine and poplar may attain antifungal properties akin to hard wood species.[62-64]

Various engineered wood products such as plasticized wallboards and certain plywood varieties may be exempt from inspections because their processing is considered sufficient to prevent a significant role as a fomite for pests. Yet, various plywood types and wood-plastic-composite building materials uninoculated and exposed to moisture in laboratory chambers or in situ conditions in buildings readily develop selective mould populations similar to those associated with gypsum wallboard.[57,65-67]

▶ SHIPPING

The globalization of trade during the past several decades, particularly in the agricultural and pharmaceutical industries, is a recognized factor among microbial concerns (including fungi) for processing, shipping, and storage of product.[24,61,68] Globally, commercial shipping and storage of goods has standardized primarily on the use of pallets bearing products enclosed in metal shipping containers. This format provides a convenient means of multimodal transportation (ie, maritime, rail, road).[69] It is estimated that several billion pallets are in use daily for shipping and storage. Wood comprises the construction of the overwhelming majority of pallets with exceptions for some foods and pharmaceuticals. Rarely are pallet inventories thoroughly inspected for mold contamination.[24]

Finished product and raw material recalls associated with pallet contamination have involved fungal bioconversion of fire-retardant fungicidal treatments (2,4,6-tribromoanisole) or residual chlorophenol-type cleaners to noxious volatiles (2,4,6-trichloroanisole). These volatiles may taint product packaging and final product with a musty odor during shipping and storage.[23,60,70,71] Elevated temperature and relative humidity inside shipping containers provide conditions favorable for mold development on susceptible wooden pallets as well as cardboard and paper packing material.[72,73] Singh et al[72,73] have recorded temperature range shifts near 30°C with highs near 50°C during land/sea and air cargo intermodal container passages within and between Asia and North America. These variable and high temperatures could provide for selective survival of complexes such as *P variotii*.[74] Sporadic climatic cycling of heat, moisture, and dryness may induce microcycle conidiogenesis (ie, rapid, growth-propagation-dispersal-survival stages) from dormant or microcolonization on or inherent in built materials.[52,75] Such rapid life cycles permit perpetuation of select mold in a near imperceptible survival mode to bloom following a chronic or catastrophic moisture event. Potentially, similar scenarios can pertain to wood pallets during shipping.

Vannini et al[53] implicated fungal saprotrophs of mangroves in China as the agents of discoloration of finished wooden kitchen utensils. Seventy pallets, each with 52 packs of 15 boxes per pack, were shipped to warehouse storage in Italy. The packs on the pallets and the boxes in the pack ostensibly were sealed following their manufacturing process and during their container shipping and storage, a total of 54 600 boxes. Discolored utensils noted during retail prompted a microbiological examination using aseptic procedures for examining discolored and apparently acceptable utensils for fungi. Surfaces and inner tissues of utensils were examined, the inner tissues following a surface disinfection process. Surface discoloration of boxes or utensils did not necessarily agree with the demonstration of fungi on inner surfaces. The *P variotii* and the *Penicillium chrysogenum* respectively occurred at high incidences on normal and discolored surfaces of utensils, whereas the *Aspergillus niger* was mainly from discolored regions.[53] Information of any heat treatment or moisture content of the utensils was not available. There was no information on fungi associated with the pallets, but wood boxes containing packs showed fungal growth. The survival and recovery of *P chrysogenum* and *P variotii* in inner layers of the utensils may relate to cryptic dormant ascospores.[74,76]

A somewhat similar episode involved an Asian supplier of composite flooring materials shipped worldwide with packaging that included untreated pallets. Moldy pallets (n >600) were discovered on initial openings of the multimodal cargo containers (n >50); subsequently, no flooring products were released for sale. The tiles were in closed, corrugated cardboard boxes (n >23 000) stacked on pallets and covered with a "shrink wrap" plastic seal. Species of *Aspergillus* (*Eurotium*) and *P variotii* (*Talaromyces*, *Byssochlamys*) were observed in the inner sides of the pallet, particularly the structural runners (Figure 69.3). The decking boards of the pallets appeared

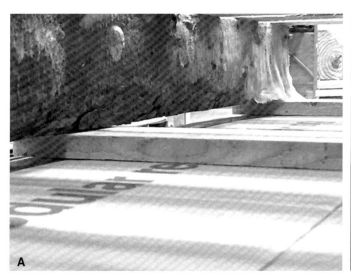
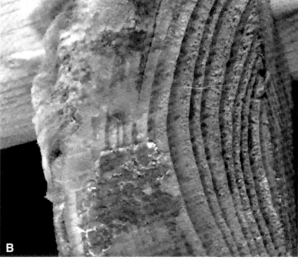

FIGURE 69.3 Fungal growth on pallets used in overseas shipping containers. A, Fungal bloom on interior side of pallet runner. B, Fungal colonization of the cut end of a pallet runner. For a color version of this art, please consult the eBook.

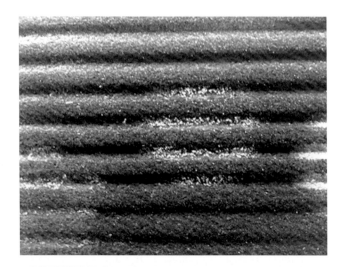

FIGURE 69.4 Colonization of the acoustic layer of a flooring product by *Talaromyces*. The growth developed within a sealed box stacked on a mold-colonized pallet from an overseas cargo container. Presumably, the mold was inherent to the cardboard packing material. For a color version of this art, please consult the eBook.

mostly unaffected. The cardboard liner and paper-based packing materials mostly yielded *Trichoderma* and *Cladosporium*. Deep within ~5% of closed boxes, between adjacent tiles, isolated circular colonies of *Talaromyces* were observed apparently originating from stiffened cardboard within the boxes (Figure 69.4).[77] This event resulted in at least a 6-week disruption of business because of the necessity to identify and quarantine contaminated pallets, open boxes, and visually inspect product for mold colonization, restacking, and storing unaffected product.

▶ SUMMARY

The survival of moulds in building and packaging materials that survive the cyclic temperature and humidity extremes found in cargo containers is to be expected. Nonetheless, if fungal blooms are not observed upon opening of the containers (usually from a pallet association), materials are stored directly in warehouses and at times kept in storage in the cargo container. Potential fungal biodegradation of the indoor structure and finishing materials, particularly organo-celluloses, and their need for preservation are well recognized. Common fungal species complexes from the extant geography are most often involved.

Globalization of trade and associated shipping stresses may be expected to extend fungal diversity not only with susceptible cellulosic products but also to natural rubber products (Figure 69.5)[78] and perhaps synthetic fibers.[79,80] Also, products with recycled content (eg, paper, cardboard, gypsum board) are potential carriers of dormant heat-resistant stages of select moulds and protozoa (see chapter 53).[45,51,81-84]

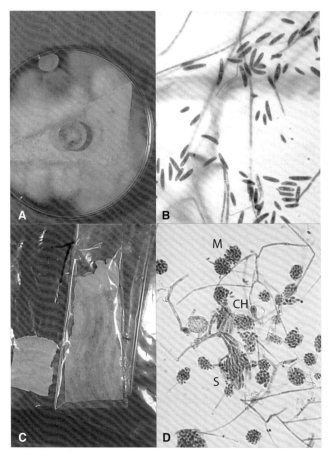

FIGURE 69.5 Recovery of fungi, mainly *Fusarium*, from a rubber mat that had received repeated cleaning/sanitizing treatments. A, Enrichment culture. B, Lacto-phenol cotton blue adhesive tape mount from central region of plate. C, Shower mat section after sanitizing (left side) and postsanitizing (right side) following exposure to high humidity. D, *Fusarium solani* complex with slime clusters of microconidia (M), sporodochium composed of macroconidia (S), and chlamydoconidium (CH). For a color version of this art, please consult the eBook.

Buildings may develop signature microbiomes that reflect the chemical and physical nature of their components with discrete versions expressed from occupant and use stresses.[28,85] Whether native moulds of species complexes such as *S chartarum* and *C globosum* would suppress noxious volatiles or rare pathogenic potentials of alien strains inherent in the imported materials in the recipient, built environment is a consideration.[86,87] Imported susceptible materials should be inspected during storage before release for retail. Renewed emphasis on sustainable building practices along with the specification of more bio-based and recycled content will increase the likelihood of both cryptic and obvious mould colonization of materials associated with transocean cargo. Laminated and corrugated cardboard and other cellulosic packaging components will remain the prime concern.

Current attention therein is focused on quality and environmental control and applications of recycled materials for packaging of food, agricultural, pharmaceutical, and other products. Regulatory enforcements, quarantines, and recalls of unacceptable items in these categories are not uncommon.[24,45,71,84,87-89] Building materials may be unacceptable only to the recipient often after unpacking and/or climatization in storage or after installation.[24] Dormant-resistant stages of some fungi ascospores and amoeba (see chapter 53) embedded in the matrices of built structural materials can remain quiescent over the life time of material use. Ill-defined environmental conditions, possibly associated with fire or flooding, might trigger their emergence.

The protocols for use and need of preservative formulations in materials for the built environment will become increasingly important with expanded world trade. Organic based or naturally derived formulations with broad-spectrum efficacy are desirous, but the need persists that they are durable, substrate bound.

REFERENCES

1. Nielsen KF. *Mould Growth on Building Materials: Secondary Metabolites, Mycotoxins and Biomarkers* [dissertation]. Copenhagen, Denmark: The Mycology Group Technical University of Denmark; 2001.
2. Nielsen KF, Holm G, Uttrup LP, Nielsen PA. Mould growth on building materials under low water activities. Influence of humidity and temperature on fungal growth and secondary metabolism. *Int Biodeterior Biodegradation*. 2004;54:325-336.
3. Institute of Medicine. *Damp Indoor Spaces and Health*. Washington DC: National Academies Press; 2004.
4. WHO Regional Office for Europe. Introduction. In: *WHO Guidelines for Indoor Air Quality: Dampness and Mould*. Copenhagen, Denmark; 2009:61-65.
5. Andersen B, Frisvad JC, Søndergaard I, Rasmussen IS, Larsen LS. Associations between fungal species and water-damaged building materials. *Appl Environ Microbiol*. 2011;77:4180-4188.
6. Burwen DR, Lasker BA, Rao N, Durry E, Padhye AA, Jarvis WR. Invasive aspergillosis outbreak on a hematology-oncology ward. *Infect Control Hosp Epidemiol*. 2001;22(1):45-48.
7. Cooper EE, O'Reilly MA, Guest DI, Dharmage SC. Influence of building construction work on *Aspergillus* infection in a hospital setting. *Infect Control Hosp Epidemiol*. 2003;24(7):472-476.
8. Holý O, Matoušková I, Kubátová A, et al. Monitoring of microscopic filamentous fungi in indoor air of transplant unit. *Cent Eur J Public Health*. 2015;23(4):331-334.
9. Demirel R, Sen B, Kadaifciler D, et al. Indoor airborne fungal pollution in newborn units in Turkey. *Environ Monit Assess*. 2017;189(7):362.
10. Green BJ, Tovey ER, Sercombe JK, Blachere FM, Beezhold DH, Schmechel D. Airborne fungal fragments and allergenicity. *Med Mycol*. 2006;44(suppl 1):S245-S255.
11. Price DL, Simmons RB, Ezeonu IM, Crow SA, Ahearn DG. Colonization of fiberglass insulation used in heating, ventilation and air conditioning systems. *J Ind Microbiol*. 1994;13:154-158.
12. Ezeonu IM, Price DL, Simmons RB, Crow SA, Ahearn DG. Fungal production of volatiles during growth on fiberglass. *Appl Environ Microbiol*. 1994;60(11):4172-4173.
13. Ezeonu IM, Price DL, Crow SA, Ahearn DG. Effects of extracts of fiberglass insulations on the growth of *Aspergillus fumigatus* and *A. versicolor*. *Mycopathologia*. 1995;132:65-69.
14. Simmons RB, Price DL, Noble JA, Crow SA, Ahearn DG. Fungal colonization of air filters from hospitals. *Am Ind Hyg Assoc J*. 1997;58(12):900-904.
15. Anaissie EJ, Kuchar RT, Rex JH, et al. Fusariosis associated with pathogenic *Fusarium* species colonization of a hospital water system: a new paradigm for the epidemiology of opportunistic mold infections. *Clin Infect Dis*. 2001;33:1871-1878.
16. Anaissie EJ, Stratton SL, Dignani MC, et al. Pathogenic molds (including *Aspergillus* species) in hospital water distribution systems: a 3-year prospective study and clinical implications for patients with hematologic malignancies. *Blood*. 2003;101:2542-2546.
17. Mehl HL, Epstein L. Sewage and community shower drains are environmental reservoirs of *Fusarium solani* species complex group 1, a human and plant pathogen. *Environ Microbiol*. 2008;10:219-227.
18. Short DPG, O'Donnell K, Thrane U, et al. Phylogenetic relationships among members of the *Fusarium solani* species complex in human infections and the descriptions of *F. keratoplasticum* sp. nov. and *F. petroliphilum* stat. nov. *Fungal Genet Biol*. 2013;53:59-70.
19. Ahearn DG, Crow SA, Simmons RB, et al. Fungal colonization of fiberglass insulation in the air distribution system of a multi-story office building: VOC production and possible relationship to a sick building syndrome. *J Ind Microbiol*. 1996;16:280-285.
20. Kuhn DM, Ghannoum MA. Indoor mold, toxigenic fungi, and *Stachybotrys chartarum*: infectious disease perspective. *Clin Microbiol Rev*. 2003;16(1):144-172.
21. Straus DC, ed. *Sick Building Syndrome, Advances in Applied Microbiology*. Vol 55. London, United Kingdom: Elsevier Academic Press; 2004.
22. Federal Emergency Management Agency. Cleaning flooded buildings fact sheet (2013). Federal Emergency Management Agency Web site. https://www.fema.gov/. Accessed January 7, 2018.
23. Hill JL, Hocking AD, Whitfield FB. The role of fungi in the production of chloroanisoles in general purpose freight containers. *Food Chem*. 1995;54:161-166.
24. Meissner H, Lemay A, Bertone C, et al. *Evaluation of pathways for exotic plant pest movement into and within the greater Caribbean region*. Washington, DC: United States Department of Agriculture; 2009.
25. Murtoniemi T, Nevalainen A, Hirvonen MR. Effect of plasterboard composition on *Stachybotrys chartarum* growth and biological activity of spores. *Appl Environ Microbiol*. 2003;69:3751-3757.
26. Ahearn DG, Price DL, Simmons RB, et al. Indoor mould and their association with heating, ventilation and air conditioning systems. In: Straus DC, ed. *Sick Building Syndrome, Advances in Applied Microbiology*. Vol 55. San Diego, CA: Elsevier; 2004:113-135.
27. Andersen B, Dosen I, Lewinska AM, Neilsen KF. Pre-contamination of new gypsum wallboard with potentially harmful fungal species. *Indoor Air*. 2017;27(1):6-12.
28. Szulc J, Ruman T, Gutarowska B. Metabolome profiles of moulds on carton-gypsum board and malt extract agar medium obtained using an AuNPET SALDI-ToF-MS method. *Int Biodeterior Biodegradation*. 2017;125:13-23.
29. Gutarowska B. Metabolic activity of moulds as a factor of building materials biodegradation. *Pol J Microbiol*. 2010;59:119-124.
30. Krause M, Geer W, Swenson L, Fallah P, Robbins C. Controlled study of mold growth and cleaning procedure on treated and untreated wet gypsum wallboard in an indoor environment. *J Occup Environ Hyg*. 2006;3:435-441.
31. Delgado DA, de Souza Sant'ana A, Massaguer PR. Occurrence of molds on laminated paperboard for aseptic packaging, selection of the most hydrogen peroxide- and heat-resistant isolates and determination of their thermal death kinetics in sterile distilled water. *World J Microbiol Biotechnol*. 2012;28:2609-2614.
32. Rico-Munoz E. Heat resistant molds in foods and beverages: recent advances on assessment and prevention. *Curr Opin Food Sci*. 2017;17:75-83.
33. Menetrez MY, Foarde KK, Webber TD, Dean TR, Betancourt DA. Testing antimicrobial cleaner efficacy on gypsum wallboard contaminated with *Stachybotrys chartarum*. *Environ Sci Pollut Res Int*. 2007;14(7):523-528.

34. Menetrez MY, Foarde KK, Webber TD, Dean TR, Betancourt DA. Testing antimicrobial paint efficacy on gypsum wallboard contaminated with *Stachybotrys chartarum. J Occup Environ Hyg.* 2008;5(2): 63-66.

35. Berni E, Tranquillini R, Scaramuzza N, Brutti A, Bernini V. Aspergilli with *Neosartorya*-type ascospores: heat resistance and effect of sugar concentration on growth and spoilage incidence in berry products. *Int J Food Microbiol.* 2017;258:81-88.

36. Konstantinos K, Arabatzis M, Bougatsos G, Xanthaki A, Toutouza M, Velegraki A. *Neosartorya hiratsukae* peritonitis through continuous ambulatory peritoneal dialysis. *J Med Microbiol.* 2010;59:862-865.

37. Tranquillini R, Scaramuzza N, Berni E. Occurrence and ecological distribution of heat resistant moulds spores (HRMS) in raw materials used by food industry and thermal characterization of two *Talaromyces* isolates. *Int J Food Microbiol.* 2017;242:116-123.

38. Shivaprakash MR, Jain N, Gupta S, Baghela A, Gupta A, Chakrabarti A. Allergic fungal rhinosinusitis caused by *Neosartorya hiratsukae* from India. *Med Mycol.* 2009;47:317-320.

39. Guarro J, Kallas EG, Godoy P, et al. Cerebral aspergillosis caused by *Neosartorya hiratsukae*, Brazil. *Emerg Infect Dis.* 2002;8:989-991.

40. Frisvad JC, Larsen TO. Extrolites of *Aspergillus fumigatus* and other pathogenic species in *Aspergillus* section fumigati. *Front Microbiol.* 2016;6:1485.

41. Lewinska AM, Hoof JB, Peuhkuri RH, et al. Visualization of the structural changes in plywood and gypsum board during the growth of *Chaetomium globosum* and *Stachybotrys chartarum. J Microbiol Methods.* 2016;129:28-38.

42. Barron MA, Sutton DA, Veve R, et al. Invasive mycotic infections caused by *Chaetomium perlucidum*, a new agent of cerebral phaeohyphomycosis. *J Clin Microbiol.* 2003;41(11):5302-5307.

43. Hubka V, Mencl K, Skorepova M, Lyskova P, Zalabska E. Phaeohyphomycosis and onychomycosis due to *Chaetomium* spp., including the first report of *Chaetomium brasiliense* infection. *Med Mycol.* 2011;49:724-733.

44. Ahmed NE, Abu AS, Idris MO, Elhussein SA. Fungi associated with stored sorghum grains and their effects on grain quality. *Int J Life Sci.* 2016;2:723-729.

45. Ahearn DG, Doyle Stulting R. Fungi associated with drug recalls and rare disease outbreaks. *J Ind Microbiol Biotechnol.* 2014;41:1591-1597.

46. Mohapatra D, Kumar S, Kotwaliwale N, Singh KK. Critical factors responsible for fungi growth in stored food grains and non-chemical approaches for their control. *Int Food Crop Prod.* 2017;108:162-182.

47. Castlebury LA, Rossman AY, Sung GH, Hyten AS, Spatafora JW. Multigene phylogeny reveals new lineage for *Stachybotrys chartarum*, the indoor air fungus. *Mycol Res.* 2004;108:864-872.

48. Centers for Disease Control and Prevention. Facts about *Stachybotrys chartarum* and other molds. Centers for Disease Control and Prevention Web site. https://www.cdc.gov/mold/stachy.htm. Accessed October 20, 2017.

49. Tucker K, Stolze JL, Kennedy AH, Money NP. Biomechanics of conidial dispersal in the toxic mold *Stachybotrys chartarum. Fungal Genet Biol.* 2007;44:641-647.

50. Price DL, Ahearn DG. Sanitation of wallboard colonized with *Stachybotrys chartarum. Curr Microbiol.* 1999;39:21-26.

51. Gaylarde C, Otlewska A, Celikkol-Aydin S, et al. Interactions between fungi of standard paint test method BS3900. *Int Biodeterior Biodegradation.* 2015;104:411-418.

52. Price DL, Drago G, Noble J, Simmons R, Crow S Jr, Ahearn D. Rapid assessment of antimould efficacies of pressure-treated southern pine. *J Ind Microbiol Biotechnol.* 2002;29:368-372.

53. Vannini A, Franceschini S, Vettraino AM. Manufactured wood trade to Europe: a potential uninspected carrier of alien fungi. *Biol Invasions.* 2012;14:1991-1997.

54. Uzunovic A, Dale A, Stirling R, Sidhu A. Effect of fungal preinfection on the efficacy of mold and sapstain control products. *Forest Prod J.* 2013;63(1):31-38.

55. Carll CG, Highley TL. Decay of wood and wood-based products above ground in buildings. *J Test Eval.* 1999;27(2):150-158.

56. Civardi C, Van den Bulcke J, Schubert M, et al. Penetration and effectiveness of micronized copper in refractory wood species. *PLoS One.* 2016;11:e0163124.

57. Kallavus U, Jarv H, Kalamees T, Kurik L. Assessment of durability of environmentally friendly wood-based panels. *Energy Procedia.* 2017;132:207-212.

58. Edlund ML, Nilsson T. Performance of copper and non-copper based wood preservatives in terrestrial microcosms. *Holzforschung.* 1999;53:369-373.

59. Environmental Protection Agency. *Overview of Wood Preservative Chemicals.* Washington, DC: Environmental Protection Agency; 2017.

60. Whitfield FB, Hill JL, Shaw KJ. 2,4,6-Tribromoanisole: a potential cause of mustiness in packaged food. *J Agric Food Chem.* 1997;45:889-893.

61. International Plant Protection Convention. International Standards For Phytosanitary Measures No. 15: Regulation of wood packaging material in international trade. International Plant Protection Convention Web site. https://www.ippc.int/en/publications/640/. Accessed November 22, 2017.

62. Weiland JJ, Guyonnet R. Study of chemical modifications and fungi degradation of thermally modified wood using DRIFT spectroscopy. *Holz als Roh-und Werkstoff.* 2003;61:216-220.

63. Boonstra MJ, van Acker J, Kegel E, Stevens M. Optimisation of a two-stage heat treatment process: durability aspects. *Wood Sci Technol.* 2007;41(1):31-57.

64. Rowell RM, Ibach RE, McSweeny J, Nilsson T. Understanding decay resistance, dimensional stability and strength changes in heat-treated and acetylated wood. *Wood Mat Sci Eng.* 2009;1-2:14-22.

65. Schirp A, Ibach RE, Pendleton DE, Wolcott MP. Biological degradation of wood-plastic composites (WPC) and strategies for improving the resistance of WPC against biological decay. In: Schultz TP, Militz H, Freeman M, Goodell B, Nicholas D, eds. *Development of Commercial Wood Preservatives: Efficacy, Environmental, and Health Issues.* Washington, DC: American Chemical Society; 2008:480-507.

66. Johansson P, Ekstrand-Tobin A, Svensson T, Bok G. Laboratory study to determine the critical moisture level for mould growth on building materials. *Int Biodeterior Biodegradation.* 2012;73:23-32.

67. Barton-Pudlik J, Czaja K, Grzymek M, Lipok J. Evaluation of wood-polyethylene composites biodegradability caused by filamentous fungi. *Int Biodeterior Biodegradation.* 2017;118:10-18.

68. Australian Food & Grocery Council. *Organohalogen Taints in Foods.* Brisbane, Australia: Australian Food & Grocery Council; 2007.

69. Levinson M. *The Box: How the Shipping Container Made the World Smaller and the World Economy Bigger.* Princeton, NJ: Princeton University Press; 2006.

70. Whitfield FB, Shaw KJ, Lambert DE, et al. Freight containers: major sources of chloranisoles and chlorophenols in foodstuff. In: Maarse H, van der Heij DG, eds. *Trends in Flavour Research: Proceedings of the 7th Weurman Flavour Research Symposium.* Amsterdam, Netherlands: Elsevier; 1994:401-407.

71. Sawant P, Callahan W, Clark J, et al. *Detection and Mitigation of 2,4,6-tribromoanisole and 2,4,6-trichloroanisole Taints and Odors in the Pharmaceutical and Consumer Healthcare Industries. Technical Report #55.* Bethesda, MA: Parenteral Drug Association; 2012.

72. Singh SP, Saha K, Singh J, Sandhu APS. Measurement and analysis of vibration and temperature levels in global intermodal container shipments on truck, rail and ship. *Packag Technol Sci.* 2012;25:149-160.

73. Singh SP, Singh J, Saha K. Measurement and analysis of physical and climatic distribution environment for air package shipment. *Packag Technol Sci.* 2015;28:719-731.

74. Houbraken J, Varga J, Rico-Munoz E, Johnson S, Samson RA. Sexual reproduction as the cause of heat resistance in the food spoilage fungus *Byssochlamys spectabilis* (anamorph *Paecilomyces variotii*). *Appl Environ Microbiol.* 2008;74(5):1613-1619.

75. Ahearn DG, Price DL, Simmons RB, Mayo A, Zhang ST, Crow SA Jr. Microcycle conidiation and medusa head conidiophores of aspergilli on indoor construction materials and air filters from hospitals. *Mycologia.* 2007;99:1-6.

76. Böhn J, Hoff B, O'Gorman CM, et al. Sexual reproduction and mating-type-mediated strain development in the penicillin-producing fungus *Penicillium chrysogenum*. *Proc Natl Acad Sci U S A*. 2013;110(4): 1476-1481.

77. Price DL, Ahearn DG, Prestridge BM. Mold contamination of indoor materials for the built environment: shipping, storage, and preservation aspects. Session 4 Biofilms in the built environment. Paper presented at: Montana Biofilm Science & Technology Meeting; July 18-20, 2017; Bozeman, MT.

78. Shamsi S, Chowdury P. Mycoflora associated with rubber sheets and its management by common salt (sodium chloride). *J Asait Soc Bangladesh Sci*. 2014;40(1):79-87.

79. Price DL, Ahearn DG. Activity of an insoluble antimicrobial quaternary amine complex in plastics. *J Ind Microbiol Biotechnol*. 1991;8: 83-90.

80. Friedrich J, Zalar P, Mohoric M, Klun U, Krzan A. Ability of fungi to degrade synthetic polymer nylon-6. *Chemosphere*. 2007;67:2089-2095.

81. Yli-Pirilä T, Kusnetsov J, Haatainen S, et al. Amoebae and other protozoa in material samples from moisture-damaged buildings. *Environ Res*. 2004;96(3):250-256.

82. Yli-Pirila T, Kusnetsov J, Hirvonen MR, Seuri M, Nevalainen A. Survival of amoebae on building materials. *Indoor Air*. 2009;19:113-121.

83. Coombs K, Vesper S, Green BJ, Yermakov M, Reponen T. Fungal microbiomes associated with green and non-green building materials. *Int Biodeterior Biodegradation*. 2017;125:251-257.

84. Potter A, Murray J, Lawson B, Graham S. Trends in product recalls within the agri-food industry: empirical evidence from the USA, UK and the Republic of Ireland. *Trends Food Sci Technol*. 2012;28:77-86.

85. Leung MHY, Lee PKH. The roles of the outdoors and occupants in contributing to a potential pan-microbiome of the built environment: a review. *Microbiome*. 2016;4:21.

86. Došen I, Nielsen KF, Clausen G, Andersen B. Potentially harmful secondary metabolites produced by indoor *Chaetomium* species on artificially and naturally contaminated building materials. *Indoor Air*. 2017;27:34-46.

87. Koster B, Wong B, Straus N, Malloch D. A multi-gene phylogeny for *Stachybotrys* evidences lack of trichodiene synthase (tri5) gene for isolates of one of three intrageneric lineages. *Mycolog Res*. 2009;113:877-886.

88. Nagaich U, Sadhna D. Drug recall: an incubus for pharmaceutical companies and most serious drug recall of history. *Int J Pharm Investig*. 2015;5(1):13-19.

89. Ahearn DG, Stulting RD. Moulds associated with contaminated ocular and injectable drugs: FDA recalls, epidemiology considerations, drug shortages, and aseptic processing. *Med Mycol*. 2018;56(4):389-394.

Regulation of Preservation, Disinfection, and Sterilization Agents, Equipment, and Processes

Eric L. Dewhurst, Helen E. Forsdyke, and Eamonn V. Hoxey

This chapter covers the principles of regulation of the development, manufacture, distribution, and use of processes, agents, and equipment for sterilization, disinfection, and preservation. This chapter discusses the nature of the controls that have been implemented with the intention of ensuring that products are safe, do not harm the environment, and perform as intended. These controls might be implemented through a variety of legal measures depending on the jurisdiction but are often generically described as regulatory requirements. When the term *regulatory requirement* is used, it generally encompasses requirements contained in any applicable law that might, for example, be termed statute, statutory instrument, regulation, ordinance, or directive.

Regulatory requirements often cover two separate aspects of product quality:

- Intrinsic quality—receiving prior approval of the quality, safety, and performance/effectiveness/efficacy before placing on the market
- Extrinsic quality—controlling that products are always manufactured and distributed so as to maintain the intrinsic quality of the approved product

Regulatory requirements, therefore, often cover both the lifecycle of the product and its supply chain; from concept, through development and manufacture, distribution, and monitoring of safety and performance in use to withdrawal at the end of product life. In addition, regulatory requirements can affect different organizations in the supply chain from manufacturers to importers and distributors.

Regulatory requirements can often be statements of principle or description of processes to be applied to obtain approval for products or processes. These are often subject to interpretation and that interpretation can evolve over time. This can be based on experience, developments in science and technology, and changes in the state of the art. The interpretation of regulatory requirements by regulatory authorities in a particular jurisdiction (eg, the US Food and Drug Administration [FDA]) can be thought of as the expression of regulatory expectations. These expectations can go beyond what is actually written in the regulations, for example, the expectations incorporated in what can be described as Current Good Manufacturing Practices (cGMPs or GMPs).[1-3] Regulator positions on such issues are often presented at scientific conferences, in published guidance documents, and on official blogs hosted on regulatory authority websites.

Regulatory requirements can also be supported by voluntary consensus standards, for example, those developed by the International Organization for Standardization (ISO) and adopted by national or regional standards development organizations. Conformance with these standards might be formally recognized as providing a presumption of conformity with regulatory requirements or provide a quicker route through the regulatory approval process. Standards are generally developed in parallel to the regulatory process by consensus of stakeholders, including regulatory authorities. Standards can provide specifications for products or describe methods of test or procedures to demonstrate the effectiveness of a product or process. For medicinal products, many national pharmacopoeias predate medicines legislation. Pharmacopoeias may be integrated into local legislation in which case their contents can become legal public standards. Regulatory requirements and best practice can be supported by recommendations provided by professional societies on how to use products or apply processes in specific applications. Finally, and often overlooked, is the regulatory expectation that a manufacturer adheres to its own procedures.

An example of how cGMP expectations, applicable standards, and regulatory expectations can interact is the expectation within some European authorities that elements of the European Standard EN 285 for large steam sterilizers[4] are applied by pharmaceutical manufacturers when validating sterilization of equipment. EN 285 is itself an equipment standard that includes test methods and acceptance criteria for performance assessment of large steam sterilizers that use vacuum for air removal. The standard specifies the required performance to be achieved against a range of test loads. One measure of the sterilizer's ability to remove air from a test load of cloth material is the equilibration time. This is the time difference between the coolest point of the chamber and the slowest to heat part of the load reaching sterilization temperature. If air removal, and hence steam penetration, is effective, this time difference will be small. EN 285 specifies 30 seconds for the largest sterilizer, when tested with a standard test pack of cloth material. Certain regulatory expectations apply this equilibration time to all production loads. In principle, equilibration time is a valuable measure of air removal effectiveness from any load, but the rigid application of one specification developed for a specific load type can be considered somewhat arbitrary.

It is not practical to cover the regulatory requirements applicable to each and every jurisdiction worldwide, but this chapter focuses on the principles generally included as regulatory requirements and some examples of how these are applied. This chapter describes where key requirements for preservation, disinfection, and sterilization are to be found in the regulatory requirements. It is not intended as an alternative to reference actual regulations, which are subject to change over time.

▶ REGULATORY REGIMES

Antimicrobial agents and their use in methods of disinfection, preservation, and sterilization can be regulated in different ways depending on their application. Examples of regulatory regimes for different applications are summarized in Table 70.1. The regulation of disinfection, preservation, and sterilization generally falls into three main areas depending on the application:

- Health care products—medicinal products, medical devices, and combinations thereof
- Environmental disinfectants or preservatives—biocides, pesticides, or germicides
- Food products—canning, food sterilization, and treatment of ingredients

Sterilizing Agents, Sterilization Processes, Sterilizing Equipment, and Sterile Products

The regulatory requirements for medicinal products apply to sterile pharmaceuticals, including biologics, and would cover the method used to achieve sterility and the validation and routine control of that process. These requirements, including those for biological indicators that may be used in monitoring of sterilization processes

TABLE 70.1 Examples of common regulatory regimes of various applications of disinfection, preservation, and sterilization

Process	Application	Regulatory Regime
Disinfection	Environmental disinfection • Health care facilities • Food handling • Agriculture • Health care product manufacturing	Biocide/germicide/pesticide
	Disinfecting medical devices	Medical device
	Skin disinfection • Antisepsis • Hand disinfection	Medicinal product Biocide
Preservation	Preservation of medicinal products	Medicinal product
	Anti-infective for medical device	Combination product
	Wood preservation	Biocide/pesticide
	Cosmetic preservation	Biocide/pesticide
Sterilization	Sterilizer for medical devices used in health care	Medical device
	Sterilization of medical devices	Medical device
	Sterilization of medicinal product	Medicinal product
	Canning, sterilization of ingredients and foodstuffs	Food

for medicinal products, are generally contained in pharmacopoeia.[5-7] The regulatory requirements for medical devices are applicable for sterile medical devices and cover the methods of sterilization and the validation and routine control of the process to achieve sterility. Medical device regulations also commonly apply to sterilizing equipment used in health care facilities and frequently also encompass ancillary products for monitoring sterilization processes like biological and chemical indicators. The regulatory requirements for food cover processes used for canning and sterilization of food products such as sterilized milk and some sterile baby foods.

Disinfectants, Disinfecting Agents, Disinfection Processes, and Disinfecting Equipment

Environmental disinfectants are usually covered by environmental legislation and might be termed biocides, pesticides, or germicides. Generally, the regulations include disinfectants for use in the health care environment as well as a wide range of other commercial applications. The cGMPs can also apply to the use of disinfectants for environmental control in manufacturing facilities for medicinal products.

Medical device regulations cover disinfectants used specifically on medical devices such as contact lenses or endoscopes. Equipment for disinfection of reusable medical devices, such as anesthetic equipment tubing and facemasks, endoscopes, or bedpans in health care facilities, are also frequently regulated as medical devices.

Specific medicinal product regulations can also typically apply to the variety of antiseptics for human and veterinary use.

Food regulatory regimes cover use of pasteurization to extend the lifetime of perishable foods and preventive treatments to reduce spoilage and application of hygienic practices in food processing.

Preservative and Preservation

Medicinal product regulations cover preservatives incorporated in medicinal products, for example, multiuse ophthalmic preparations. Preservatives in environmental applications, such as treatment of wood, is generally covered by regulatory requirements for environmental disinfectants or pesticides.

Regulation of foods would include preservation by reduction in pH, lowering water content, raising the salt or sugar content, or adding preservatives content. Food safety legislation applies to additives to foods and hygienic practices in food processing.

Regulatory Principles

Health Care Products

Health care products are divided into two principal categories: medicinal products, which might also be described as pharmaceuticals and biologics, and medical devices. The primary distinction is that medicinal products generally have a pharmacologic, metabolic, or immunologic action, whereas medical devices act physically. Where a product combines a physical and a pharmacologic action, for example, a prefilled syringe or a drug-eluting stent, it might be regulated either as a specific category of combination product or under the regime applicable to the principal intended purpose of the product.

It is an essential principle for health care products, and the manufacturing processes used to produce them, that they are designed in a way that eliminates, or reduces as far as possible, the risk of infection to the patient, user, and third parties. In order to achieve this, the product needs to allow ease of handling for its intended use and, where necessary, minimize contamination of the patient by a product or vice versa during use. Packaging systems are intended to prevent deterioration and maintain the level of cleanliness necessary. Products are accompanied by the information needed to use it safely and properly, taking account of the training and knowledge of the potential users.

One approach to reduce the risk of infection to the patient is to provide a product in a sterile state. When a claim of "sterile" is made, a number of regulatory principles can apply. These include that the product is designed and manufactured within the framework of a quality system; is packed in a nonreusable pack to ensure that it is sterile when placed on the market; is manufactured in appropriately controlled environmental conditions; is sterilized by an appropriate, validated method (when applicable); and is labeled "STERILE."

For a terminally sterilized product, a claim that the product is sterile is linked to the delivery of a sterilization process that has been established, validated, and is routinely controlled to predict attainment of a specified maximal sterility assurance level (SAL). Specifying a value for that SAL is a matter for regulatory authorities. It is important to note that

- A product sterilized using a validated process achieving maximally a SAL of 10^{-6} is generally regarded as sterile and is labeled as such.
- Some jurisdictions accept a label claim of sterile for a product for certain defined applications when a sterilization process achieves maximally a SAL of 10^{-3}.
- Regulatory authorities may permit a product processed to achieve maximally a SAL greater than 10^{-6} (eg, 10^{-5}) to be labeled as sterile based on individual analysis of the risk benefit of that particular product if a maximal SAL of 10^{-6} cannot be achieved.
- Generally, a product processed to achieve maximally a SAL greater than 10^{-3}, such as 10^{-2}, is not traditionally

labeled as sterile. There might be individual situations in which such product (such as a cell-based therapy) is appropriate for a specific intended use and has regulatory approval for that use.[8]

When a regulatory body accepts that a maximal SAL greater than 10^{-6} may be used (eg, 10^{-5}) for a product, its consideration will also address how that product should be labeled.[8]

When terminal sterilization is not possible, the manufacture of sterile health care products using aseptic processing is permitted. Aseptic processing requires controls of a number of factors in order designate aseptically processed medical devices as sterile (see chapter 58). These factors relate to controls to and/or records of

a) The manufacturing environment
b) The sterilization of components
c) Associated equipment used during manufacturing
d) The competence of personnel
e) Interventions in the process
f) The performance of process simulations
g) Inspections and tests of finished product

The acceptance limits and actions for occurrence of nonsterile units in process simulations in initial performance qualification and periodic requalification are specified by regulatory authorities or documented in supporting standards or guidance documents. The current expectations are that process simulations should generally not yield any contaminated units.

Medicinal Products

Most regulatory regimes for medicinal products have two separate but related aspects: a marketing authorization (product license) that considers the safety and efficacy of the product and a manufacturing license for each site of manufacture based on continued performance in accordance with GMPs. Part of the approval process is generally a pre-approval inspection (PAI) of the facility that is to make the medicinal product commercially.

Marketing Authorization

The International Council for Harmonisation (ICH) was formed in 1990 by the European Union, Japan, and the United States in order to develop a harmonized format for submissions for marketing authorization of new products. This format is called the Common Technical Document (CTD).[9] It should be noted that the CTD is a common structure for the presentation of data and that data requirements in different jurisdictions can vary. The part of the CTD relevant to sterilization, disinfection, and preservation is module 3, Quality. This section requires details of the active substance and the medicinal product; the method of manufacture and the manufacturing process; and its controls, validation, and

container closure systems. The portion of the submission that details the procedures and methods applied to assure sterility of the product might also be referred to as the chemistry, manufacturing, and controls (CMC) section.

Marketing a medicinal product in the European Union is currently covered by Regulation (EC) No 726/2004.[10] This lays down the procedures within the European Union for the authorization and supervision of medicinal products for human and veterinary use. Applications for market authorization as a medicinal product could be made by a centralized procedure through the European Agency for the Evaluation of Medicinal Products (commonly know by the shortened acronym EMA) or a decentralized procedure through national competent authorities, depending on the nature of the medicinal product and the market strategy of the applicant for market authorization. Applications are prepared in a CTD format. Directive 2001/83/EC, as amended (III Placing on the Market; Chapter 1 Marketing Authorization),[11] details the requirements for making an application for a marketing authorization. Attention is drawn to Article 23 of this directive; this requires that after a marketing authorization has been granted, the marketing authorization holder takes account of technical and scientific progress in methods of manufacture and control and introduces changes that enable their product to be manufactured and checked by "means of generally accepted methods." This indicates that the marketing authorization holder is responsible for keeping processes up to date, whether they are performed in-house or undertaken by a contract manufacturer.

In the United States, drug products are authorized through a New Drug Application (NDA)[12] or, for generics, an Abbreviated New Drug Application (ANDA).[13]

Manufacturing Authorization

In the European Union, Directive 2001/83/EC as amended (IV Manufacture and Importation)[11] details the requirements for holding a manufacturing authorization. Articles 40 to 45 cover the requirements for a manufacturing authorization. Article 47 of this directive requires that the principles and guidelines for GMP are detailed in a separate directive. This is Directive 2003/94/EC,[14] and it contains the current basic requirements for GMP. The GMP is intended to provide assurance that each lot of approved product placed on market is of acceptable quality, safety, and efficacy and meets the marketing authorization commitment. In the European Union GMP, this is described in EudraLex Volume 4,[1] whereas in the United States, it is described in the Code of Federal Regulations (CFR) 210 and 211.[2,3]

Role of Pharmacopoeia

The most influential pharmacopoeias worldwide are those of the United States (USP/NF),[7] Europe (Ph. Eur.),[5] and Japan (JP).[6] The review of the submission for a marketing authorization would consider the requirements in relation to the applicable monographs of the pharmacopoeia. Any submission that did not follow the pharmacopoeia's expectation for sterilization, disinfection, and preservation would be subject to individual review. The pharmacopoeias require medicinal products for parenteral or ophthalmic administration to be provided sterile.

Different pharmacopoeias are arranged in similar formats, although section terminology may differ slightly. Broadly, pharmacopoeias are arranged into general chapters and monographs specific to individual medicinal products. The general chapters contain details of methods of manufacture such as sterilization methods, requirements for product types such as injectables, and test methods applicable to a range of products. These general chapters are informative unless cross-referenced in a product monograph. Pharmacopoeia monographs can contain information on specified excipients, active ingredients, and medicinal products. They might contain definitions and requirements for manufacture, packaging storage, labeling, and testing. The nomenclature for different sections in different pharmacopoeia varies and are presented with key relevant sections indicated in Table 70.2.

US Pharmacopoeia

The USP[7] is arranged in

- General chapters
  - General tests and assays, describing analytical and microbiological test methods
  - General information, describing for example, manufacturing and sterilization methods
- Monographs for official substances (ingredients) and official articles (products)

The general chapters are used to compile into one location information which is applicable to many monographs. Monographs contain requirements such as the product's official name, definition, specification, packaging, and storage requirements where appropriate requirements for sterility and preservation are included.

European Pharmacopoeia

The Ph. Eur.[5] is arranged into

- General chapters containing requirements for test methods, reagents, etc
  - General notices
  - Methods of analysis
  - Materials for containers and containers
  - Reagents
  - General texts
- General monographs containing requirements applicable across any product or product type
- Monographs on specific dosage forms
- Individual monographs containing the requirements for specific medicinal products

The general texts on microbiology contain guidance and requirements on methods of preparation of sterile products. The reference conditions cited for sterilization are

- Aqueous preparations—121°C for 15 minutes
  - The minimum allowable temperature for sterilization is 110°C. Other combinations of conditions are permitted if they give an SAL of 10^{-6} or less.
  - A minimum F_0 (see chapters 11 and 28) of 8 minutes is specified in achieving the SAL of 10^{-6} or less.
- Dry heat—160°C for at least 2 hours
- Irradiation—absorbed dose 25 kGy

For depyrogenation by dry heat, a temperature of 220°C with demonstration of a 3 $\log_{10}$ reduction of heat-resistant endotoxin is specified. Substances that are the subject of an individual monograph are required to comply with the relevant applicable general monographs. It should be noted that the individual monographs do not reference applicable general monographs.

The Japanese Pharmacopoeia

The JP[6] is arranged into

- General rules, containing general notices for preparations and monographs for preparations, specific to preparation types
- General tests, processes, and apparatus giving requirements for tests applicable to a range of products
- Individual monographs containing information on specific products
- General information containing information on methods of sterilization, disinfection, and preservation

Under the general notices for preparations, terminal sterilization is defined as a process performed under the condition where the SAL of 10^{-6} or less is ensured by using suitable biological indicators. Aseptic processing using sterilization by filtration is defined as a "process performed under the condition to give a defined SAL in the clean areas where microbial and particulate levels are adequately maintained by using appropriate techniques." The general notice does not specify which methods should be used preferentially.

The general tests section contains requirements relevant to sterile and preserved products. The section also contains test requirements for primary packaging materials such as glass containers, rubber closures, and plastic containers. The general information section also includes a table indicating which requirements are harmonized with the USP and Ph. Eur. Only the requirements for the sterility test and the bacterial endotoxin test are harmonized.

Role of Standards

There is no formal legislative link between International Standards and regulatory requirements for medicinal products, but they might be referenced as guidance, for

TABLE 70.2 Compilation of relevant topics covered by the European, Japanese, and United States Pharmacopoeia

Topic	European Pharmacopoeia (8th edition, 2013)[5]	Japanese Pharmacopoeia (17th edition, 2016)[6]	United States Pharmacopeia (USP 40, 2017)[7]
General chapters containing requirements for test methods, reagents, etc	2.6.1—Test for Sterility	4.06—Sterility Test	<71> Sterility Tests
	2.6.14—Bacterial Endotoxins	4.01—Bacterial Endotoxins Test	<85> Bacterial Endotoxins Test
			<161> Medical Devices—Bacterial Endotoxin and Pyrogen Tests
		4.04—Pyrogen Test	<151> Pyrogens Test
General monographs containing requirements applicable across any product or product type	5.1—General Texts on Microbiology	G4—Microorganisms	
	5.1.1—Methods of Preparation of Sterile Products	Sterilization and Sterilization Indicators	<1211> Sterilization and Sterility Assurance of Compendial Items
			<1229.1> Steam Sterilization by Direct Contact <1229.2> Moist Heat Sterilization of Aqueous Liquids <1229.4> Sterilizing Filtration of Liquids <1229.7> Gaseous Sterilization <1229.8> Dry Heat Sterilization <1229.10> Radiation Sterilization <1229.11> Vapor Phase Sterilization <1229.12> New Sterilization Methods <1229.13> Sterilization in Place
	5.1.2—Biological Indicators of Sterilization		<1229.5> Biological Indicators for Sterilization
			<55> Biological Indicators—Resistance Performance Tests
			<1229.9> Physicochemical Integrators and Indicators for Sterilization
	5.1.3—Efficacy of Antimicrobial Preservation	Preservatives-Effectiveness Tests	<51> Antimicrobial Effectiveness Testing
	5.1.9—Guidelines for Using the Test for Sterility		
	5.1.10—Guidelines for Using the Test for Bacterial Endotoxins		
			<1229.3> Monitoring of Bioburden
			<1207> Package Integrity Evaluation—Sterile Products
		Parametric Release of Terminally Sterilized Pharmaceutical Products	<1222> Terminally Sterilized Pharmaceutical Products—Parametric Release
		Media Fill (Process Simulations)	

(continued)

TABLE 70.2   Compilation of relevant topics covered by the European, Japanese, and United States Pharmacopoeia *(Continued)*

Topic	European Pharmacopoeia (8th edition, 2013)[5]	Japanese Pharmacopoeia (17th edition, 2016)[6]	United States Pharmacopeia (USP <40> 2017)[7]
		Microbiological Environmental Monitoring Methods of Processing Areas for Sterile Pharmaceutical Products	<1116> Microbiological Control and Monitoring of Aseptic Processing Environments
		Disinfection and Decontamination Methods	
			<1072> Disinfectants and Antiseptics
			<1228> Depyrogenation <1228.1> Dry Heat Depyrogenation <1228.2> Depyrogenation by Filtration <1228.5> Endotoxin Indicators for Depyrogenation
Monographs on specific dosage forms	Parenteral Preparations	(3) Preparations for Injection	
	Eye Preparations	(6) Preparations for Ophthalmic Application	

example, standards on design, construction, and classification of clean rooms (ISO 14644 series)[15] are specifically mentioned in EudraLex Chapter 4, Annex 1.[1]

Standards for the development and routine control of methods of sterilization such as radiation or ethylene oxide which are commonly employed for medical devices but less frequently employed for medicinal products might also be considered as relevant guidance. Some regulators expect certain aspects of standards to apply as cGMPs.

Medical Devices

Generally, the regulation of medical devices is based on a system of risk classification of the device depending on its intended use. Higher risk devices have greater oversight. The extent of oversight can range from self-certification of the lowest risk devices and some form of registration of the manufacturer to premarket review of design and development information including clinical data for the highest risk classes. Additionally, manufacturers of most, if not all classes, of medical devices are required to implement a quality management system. There is a specific international standard, ISO 13485,[16] that specifies requirements for a quality management system for regulatory compliance for medical device organizations. This standard includes requirements for sterile devices in relation to the validation of sterilization and sterile barrier systems.

European Union CE Marking as a Medical Device

The regulatory system for medical devices in the European Union offers a variety of routes for conformity assessment based on the risk classification of the medical device and the strategy for regulatory compliance developed by the manufacturer. The European Union regulations are in the process of transitioning from a series of three directives for active implantable devices,[17] medical devices,[18] and in vitro diagnostic devices[19] that came into force in the 1990s to a Medical Devices Regulation (MDR)[20] and an In Vitro Diagnostic Medical Devices Regulation (IVDR) that entered into force in 2017.[21] The European Union has four levels of medical device classification (I, IIa, IIb, and III) but has specific conformity assessment requirements for some categories of devices within these classifications. For the European Union, third-party review of the aspects related to achieving and maintaining sterility is required irrespective of the classification of the device.

Any device incorporating a medicinal product would be classified as a class III medical device under the most current classification rules (Rule 14 of Annex VII of the MDR[20]). The manufacturer has to prepare and sign a declaration of conformity in order to CE-mark the device and place it on the market. In order to sign such a declaration for a class III device, the manufacturer would require certification from a notified body of review of a design dossier or type test. Both these approaches require the notified body to review the manufacturer's technical documentation. A notified body is an organization designated in the European Union country to assess the conformity of certain types of products as well as a manufacturer's quality management system. The requirements for the technical documentation are set out in Annex II of the MDR and IVDR.

The regulations detail the technical documentation that the manufacturer has to establish and maintain. Aspects of the technical documentation relevant to claims of sterility are

- Design and manufacturing information that includes

    a) Information on design and development stages applied to the device
    b) Information and specifications on the manufacturing processes and their validation
    c) Identification of all sites, including suppliers and subcontractors, where design and manufacturing activities, including sterilization, are performed

- Information for the demonstration of conformity with the general safety and performance requirements that are applicable to the device taking into account its intended purpose together with justification, validation, and verification of the solutions adopted to meet those requirements. The demonstration of conformity includes

    a) The general safety and performance requirements that apply to the device and an explanation as to why others do not apply
    b) The method or methods used to demonstrate conformity with each applicable general safety and performance requirement
    c) The harmonized standards or other solutions applied
    d) The documents providing evidence of conformity with the harmonized standard or other method applied to demonstrate conformity with the general safety and performance requirements

- The general safety and performance requirements that apply in relation to risks of infection. All devices, irrespective of their risk classification, have to meet the general requirements for safety and performance that apply to them. In terms of sterile devices, the applicable requirements are that the device

    a) Is designed, manufactured, and packed in a nonreusable pack and/or according to appropriate procedures to ensure that it is sterile when placed on the market and remains sterile, under the storage and transport conditions laid down, until the protective packaging is damaged or opened
    b) Is manufactured in appropriately controlled environmental conditions
    c) Is manufactured and sterilized by an appropriate, validated method

    d) Is labeled with the word *STERILE* or an accepted symbol indicating sterility
    e) Has packaging and/or labeling that distinguishes between identical or similar product sold in both a sterile and a nonsterile condition

The MDR[20] indicates that devices, systems, or processes that are in conformity with relevant harmonized standards are presumed to be in conformity with those requirements of the regulation covered by those standards. References to standards that are considered to be harmonized are published in the *Official Journal of the European Union*. The list of harmonized standards under the directives for medical devices[17-19] includes standards identifying requirements for terminally sterilized medical devices to be designated sterile, EN 556-1,[22] and the European adoptions of international standards for the development, validation, and routine control of sterilization by the methods of sterilization generally applied for terminal sterilization. It is expected that these same standards will be given the status of harmonized under the MDR.

United States Approval and Clearance of Medical Devices

The US regulation of medical devices also has a system of controls based on classification of devices. The Medical Device Amendments to the Federal Food, Drug and Cosmetic Act[23] created three classifications of medical devices based on the level of risk:

- Class I: low risk, general controls. Generally, these are simple devices considered to present minimal risk to the user. Almost all of these devices are exempt from clearance or approval.
- Class II: moderate risk, special controls. These devices are considered to pose a moderate level of risk to the user. Almost all of these devices require a regulatory submission before they can be legally marketed. As a rule, class II devices require 510(k) submissions.
- Class III: higher risk, such as life-sustaining and implantable devices. These devices are considered to present the highest level of risk to the user. All of these devices require a regulatory submission before they can be legally marketed. As a rule, class III devices require a premarket approval (PMA) submission.

Registration is required regardless of the classification. The extent of regulatory oversight depends on what the manufacturer wishes to claim and whether similar devices have been cleared or approved. Section 510(k) of the Federal Food, Drug and Cosmetic Act[24] requires device manufacturers to register and to notify the FDA of their intent to market a medical device at least 90 days in advance. This is known as premarket notification (PMN) but generally referred to as a 510(k). This allows FDA to determine whether the device is equivalent to a device already placed into one of the three classification categories.

Device manufacturers are required to submit a 510(k) if they intend to introduce a device for the first time or reintroduce a device that will be significantly changed or modified to the extent that its safety or effectiveness could be affected. Such change or modification could relate to the design, material, chemical composition, energy source, manufacturing process, or intended use.

The purpose of a 510(k) submission is to demonstrate that a device is substantially equivalent to a device that has been cleared by the FDA or marketed before 1976 (called a predicate device). The manufacturer compares and contrasts their device with the predicate, explaining why any differences between them should be acceptable. Depending on the type of 510(k), the FDA has either 30 or 90 days to clear the device, ask questions, or reject the application. The FDA does not approve 510(k) submissions, but it clears them. It is therefore not legal to advertise a 510(k)-cleared device as FDA approved. Manufacturers also submit a 510(k) if they alter their device. In general, changes to intended use, contraindications, or basic operation require a new 510(k) clearance. Changes to blood-contacting materials, sterilization method, or performance specifications may also require a new 510(k).

In contrast, a PMA submission is used to demonstrate that a new or modified device is safe and effective. This standard is higher than is required for 510(k) submissions. Human use data from a formal clinical study is almost always required in addition to laboratory studies. The FDA has 180 days to approve, question, or reject the application. Changes to a PMA-approved device may require a PMA supplement or even a new PMA. Manufacturers have far less leeway in modifying PMA devices than they do for changes to 510(k) devices. PMA devices can be advertised as "PMA-approved" or "FDA-approved."

The FDA[25] published guidance specifically for information to be provided in 510(k) submissions for devices labeled as "sterile." The guidance provides expanded information related to advances in sterilization technology. The scope of this guidance includes medical devices that are intended to be labeled sterile as a result of being subjected to industrial terminal sterilization processes based on microbial inactivation and not by microbial exclusion. Consequently, aseptic processing and sterilization by filtration are outside of the scope. This guidance defines three categories of industrial sterilization methods as

- Established A methods for which there is a well-established and extensive history of safe and effective use and extensive literature, including the existence of a dedicated, FDA-recognized consensus standards
- Established B methods for which there is a history of safe and effective use, albeit a relatively shorter one, but without a dedicated, FDA-recognized consensus standard
- Novel methods for which there are inadequate information to conclude that the process is effective, to support a sterile label claim, or to assure that processed devices are safe and effective for patient use

The information that should be included within a 510(k) submission covers five areas:

a) Specific description of the sterilization method, including information on the radiation dose if that method is to be used or residuals information if a chemical sterilizing agent is to be used
b) Description of the validation method used for the proposed sterilization process, citations for all relevant and/or dedicated FDA-recognized consensus standards
c) The SAL achieved
d) Description of the testing performed on the devices, including information on the test method and acceptance criteria
e) Description of the sterile barrier system as well as a simple description of any simulation methods and test methods used to validate package integrity and shelf life claims

Standards for Terminal Sterilization

A European Standard, *EN 556-1. Sterilization of Medical Devices—Requirements for Medical Devices to be Designated "STERILE"—Part 1: Requirements for Terminally Sterilized Medical Devices*,[22] was initially published in 1994 to provide requirements for designating devices as sterile that would be consistent across all methods of terminal sterilization. EN 556-1 was updated in 2001 without changing the core requirement, a corrigendum was issued in 2006, and the standard was subsequently reconfirmed without change. EN 556-1 has been harmonized under the Medical Devices Directive and is expected to be harmonized under the MDR. EN 556-1 has been adopted by countries outside of the European Union, including by Australia, China, Israel, and South Africa. EN 556-1 has a single requirement, that for a terminally sterilized medical device to be designated "STERILE," the probability of there being a viable microorganism present on/in the device is equal to or less than 1×10^{-6}. Compliance with this requirement is demonstrated provision of documentation and records that demonstrate that the devices have been subjected to a validated sterilization process fulfilling this requirement.

Although complying with a harmonized standard such as EN 556-1 provides a presumption of conformity with applicable regulatory requirements, following a harmonized standard is not mandatory. A note in EN 556-1 indicates that permission for acceptance of a probability greater than that specified can be sought through the appropriate regulatory bodies. The note continues by indicating that such permission depends on the individual situation, including consideration of the risk management activities undertaken by the manufacturer of the medical device. The corrigendum to the standard that was issued in 2006 was to update to the note that references the risk management undertaken by the manufacturer of the medical devices. EN 556-1 does not provide any additional guidance on situations where a greater SAL might be accepted or the detailed considerations that would need to be addressed in such circumstances. The ISO TS 19930 was prepared with the intention of providing such guidance.[8]

In contrast in the United States, the AAMI ST 67 standard[26] additionally indicates that there is acceptance of application of a maximal SAL of 10^{-3} for certain devices based on their intended use not coming into contact with breached skin or compromised tissue.

Standards for Validation and Routine Control of Sterilization

There is a portfolio of international standards for the development, validation, and routine control of sterilization of health care products. Similarly, a series of standards has been developed for aseptic processing of health care products. These standards have been adopted by many countries worldwide. For example, the standards have been adopted as European Standards and recognized as providing a presumption of conformity with the regulatory requirements for sterility in the regulations of medical devices. A list of European harmonized standards is available at http://ec.europa.eu/growth/single-market/european-standards/harmonised-standards/medical-devices/.

The US adoptions of the international standards for validation and routine control are also recognized by the FDA. The FDA recommends that applicants use FDA-recognized consensus standards for validation of sterilization processes where available. A current list of these standards is available at http://www.accessdata.fda.gov/scripts/cdrh/cfdocs/cfStandards/search.cfm.

Table 70.3 lists the standards for development, validation, and routine control of sterilization that have been developed or are in development. International standards are subject to regular systematic review and are revised periodically. Refer to www.iso.org for the list of the current editions of the various standards. In addition, the ISO 11607 series[41,42] of international standards provides requirements and guidance for packaging for terminally sterilized health care products.

These standards for development, validation, and routine control are supported by further standards specifying

TABLE 70.3	International standards for development, validation, and routine control of the sterilization and aseptic processing of health care products
Standard Reference	**Standard Title**
ISO 14937 (International Organization for Standardization[27])	Sterilization of Health Care Products—General Requirements for Characterization of a Sterilizing Agent and the Development, Validation and Routine Control of a Sterilization Process for Medical Devices
ISO 11135 (International Organization for Standardization[28])	Sterilization of Health Care Products—Ethylene Oxide—Requirements for Development, Validation and Routine Control of a Sterilization Process for Medical Devices
ISO 11137 series (International Organization for Standardization[29-31])	Sterilization of Health Care Products—Radiation
ISO 17665 series (International Organization for Standardization[32-34])	Sterilization of Health Care Products—Moist Heat
ISO 20857 (International Organization for Standardization[35])	Sterilization of Health Care Products—Dry Heat—Requirements for The Development, Validation and Routine Control of a Sterilization Process for Medical Devices
ISO 25424 (International Organization for Standardization[36])	Sterilization of Medical Devices—Low Temperature Steam and Formaldehyde—Requirements for Development, Validation and Routine Control of a Sterilization Process for Medical Devices
ISO 14160 (International Organization for Standardization[37])	Sterilization of Health Care Products—Liquid Chemical Sterilizing Agents For Single-Use Medical Devices Utilizing Animal Tissues and Their Derivatives—Requirements for Characterization, Development, Validation and Routine Control of a Sterilization Process for Medical Devices
ISO 22441 (International Organization for Standardization[38])	Sterilization of Health Care Products—Low Temperature Vaporized Hydrogen Peroxide—Requirements for the Development, Validation and Routine Control of a Sterilization Process for Medical Devices
ISO 13408 series (International Organization for Standardization[39,40])	Aseptic Processing of Health Care Products

TABLE 70.4 International standards that support the development, validation, and routine control of the sterilization and aseptic processing of health care products

Standard Reference	Standard Title
ISO 11138 series (International Organization for Standardization[43-48])	Sterilization of Health Care Products—Biological Indicators
ISO 14161 (International Organization for Standardization[49])	Sterilization of Health Care Products—Biological Indicators—Guidance for the Selection, Use and Interpretation of Results
ISO 11140 series (International Organization for Standardization[50-53])	Sterilization of Health Care Products—Chemical Indicators
ISO 15882 (International Organization for Standardization[54])	Chemical Indicators—Guidance on the Selection, Use, and Interpretation of Results
ISO 11607 series (International Organization for Standardization[41,42])	Packaging for Terminally Sterilized Medical Devices
ISO 11737 series (International Organization for Standardization[55,56])	Sterilization of Medical Devices—Microbiological Methods

various indicators, packaging materials, and microbiological methods that can be used to implement them. Some of these standards are listed in Table 70.4.

Aseptic Processing and Assurance of Sterility for Medical Devices

The ISO 13408 series of standards[39] specifically addresses aseptic processing and the many requirements associated with that approach to providing sterile product. Although aseptic processing is typically associated with pharmaceutical and biological products, ISO 13408-7 addresses aseptic manufacturing of combination products,[40] products that might use both terminal sterilization and aseptic processing, or similar products that are typically manufactured in small batches. The validation in these cases includes running process simulations that incorporate the largest batch size manufactured. Hence, it must be recognized that the assurance of sterility provided by validation using these lesser batch numbers will not be the same as that provided by traditional 5000 or 10 000 unit runs of the typical pharmaceutical manufacturer.

EN 556-2, Sterilization of Medical Devices—Requirements for Medical Devices to be Designated "STERILE"—Part 2: Requirements for Aseptically Processed Medical Devices,[57] was first published in 2003. This standard parallels EN 556-1 in respect of sterile medical devices that are prepared by aseptic processing. This standard was revised in 2015 to update the references to the European adoption of the ISO 13408 series of standards for aseptic processing. EN 556-2 requires controls of a number of factors in order to designate aseptically processed medical devices as sterile. These factors relate to controls to and/or records of:

- The manufacturing environment
- The sterilization of components

- The competence of personnel
- Interventions in the process
- The performance of process simulations
- Inspections and tests of finished product

The acceptance limits and actions for occurrence of the demonstration of nonsterile units in process simulations in initial performance qualification and periodic requalification are the same as those in ISO 13408-1.[39] Compliance with EN 556-2 is shown by providing documentation and records of the validation and routine control of the aseptic process.[57]

Combination Products

There is an increasing development and introduction to the market of products that combine aspects of medicinal products and medical devices, termed combination products in some jurisdictions. These can be medicinal product supplied with a specific device for delivery to the patient or a device incorporating medicinal substance for improved performance. In the United States, the FDA has established an Office of Combination Products to

a) Serve as a focal point for combination product issues and for medical product classification and assignment issues.
b) Develop guidance and regulations to clarify the regulation of combination products.
c) Classify medical products as drugs, devices, biological products, or combination products and assign them to an FDA center for premarket review and regulation, where their classification or assignment is unclear or in dispute.
d) Ensure timely and effective premarket review of combination products by overseeing the timeliness, alignment of coordination of reviews.

e) Ensure consistent and appropriate postmarket regulation of combination products.

f) Resolve disputes regarding the timeliness of premarket review of combination products.

Combination products are assigned to an FDA center that will have primary jurisdiction for its premarket review and regulation termed the lead center. The assignment is based on the primary mode of action (PMOA) of the combination product. The PMOA is defined as the single mode of action of a combination product that provides the most important therapeutic action of the combination product. If the most important therapeutic action cannot be determined, the assignment of lead center is based on which regulates combination products raising similar types of safety and effectiveness questions or which has the most expertise to evaluate the most significant safety and effectiveness questions raised by the combination product.

There is not a specific category of combination products in European Union regulations; products are categorized as either medicinal products or medical devices depending on their principal mode of action. Products which combine a medicinal product or substance and a medical device are regulated either under the Medical Devices Directive,[18] the MDR,[20] or under the directive for medicinal products.[58] Essentially, if the principal mode of action is physical, for example, a dressing or suture with an antimicrobial coating, this would be classified as a device, but if the principal mode of action is pharmacologic or immunologic, for example, a syringe prefilled with a biopharmaceutical for administration, it would be classified as a medicinal product. The legislative acts for devices and medicinal products are intended to ensure appropriate interaction involving combination products in consultations during premarket assessment and of exchange of information from postmarket oversight.

It is important to be aware that the European Union-MDR,[19] which came into force in May 2017 with a 3-year transition period until full implementation in May 2020, amends the directive on medicinal products in relation to applications for marketing authorization of medicinal products that integrate a medical device element.

Any device that incorporates as an integral part of a substance with an action ancillary to that of the device and, if used separately, would be considered to be a medicinal product, including a medicinal product derived from human blood or human plasma, is assessed and authorized in accordance with the MDR. Such a product would be categorized as a class III device and require review by a notified body designated under the regulation. As part of the process of review to obtain that certificate, this notified body would consult with a competent authority for medicinal products in one of the European Union member states in regard to the safety, quality, and usefulness of any substance considered to be a medicinal product.

A competent authority is an organization within a European Union member state that monitors compliance with the national statutes and regulations and carries out duties on behalf of the government in compliance with European Union law.

▶ STERILIZING EQUIPMENT

Equipment used for sterilization of medical devices within health care facilities are frequently covered by the regulations for medical devices. In both the European Union and the United States, as examples, this is the case. Industrial sterilizing equipment is generally of a larger scale, is often manufactured to an individual specification for a particular application, and is usually out of scope of MDR.

There are a range of standards for sterilizing equipment that provide requirements for safety and performance. Some of these standards are listed in Table 70.5.

▶ ENVIRONMENTAL DISINFECTANTS AND DISINFECTION PROCESSES

Where disinfecting products are regulated as medicinal products (eg, antiseptics for skin preparation), the regulatory requirements previously described for medicinal products can apply, although often specific regulations, monographs, or standards apply to antiseptic products.[72-74] Equally, where disinfecting agents are specifically intended to be used to disinfect medical devices (eg, contact lenses fluids, disinfecting agents for processing flexible endoscopes), they are often regulated as medical devices or accessories to medical devices; in such cases, refer to the previous section on regulation of medical devices. Automated equipment for washing and disinfecting medical devices used in hospitals can be regulated as medical devices in the same way as sterilizing equipment (see earlier). There is a range of international standards for washer-disinfectors listed in Table 70.6.

In the European Union, the Biocidal Products Regulation (BPR)[82] covers products such as preservatives, disinfectants, and rodenticides. It covers the placing on the market of biocidal products used to protect humans, animals, materials, or articles against harmful organisms such as insects, bacteria, or algae. The BPR requires the approval of active substances supplied for use in biocidal products and establishes a list of (1) approved substances and (2) approved suppliers of these substances. Suppliers of the biocidal products containing approved active substances must then obtain an authorization to place each product on the market. The approval of active substances takes place at European Union level, whereas the authorization of the biocidal products is at level of the

TABLE 70.5 Examples of standards containing requirements for sterilizing equipment

Standard Reference	Standard Title
IEC 61010-2-040 (International Electrotechnical Commission[59])	Safety Requirements for Electrical Equipment for Measurement, Control, and Laboratory Use. Part 2-040: Particular Requirements for Sterilizers and Washer-Disinfectors Used to Treat Medical Materials
EN 285 (European Committee for Standardization[4])	Sterilization—Steam Sterilizers—Large Sterilizers
EN 13060 (European Committee for Standardization[60])	Small Steam Sterilizers
ANSI/AAMI ST55 (Association for the Advancement of Medical Instrumentation[61])	Table-Top Steam Sterilizers
ANSI/AAMI ST8 (Association for the Advancement of Medical Instrumentation[62])	Hospital Steam Sterilizers
JIS T 7322 (Japanese Standards Association[63])	Large Steam Sterilizers
JIS T 7324 (Japanese Standards Association[64])	Small Steam Sterilizers
EN 17180 (European Committee for Standardization[65])	Sterilizers for Medical Purposes—Low Temperature Vaporized Hydrogen Peroxide Sterilizers—Requirements and Testing
EN 14180 (European Committee for Standardization[66])	Sterilizers for Medical Purposes—Low Temperature Steam and Formaldehyde Sterilizers—Requirements and Testing
EN 1422 (European Committee for Standardization[67])	Sterilizers for Medical Purposes. Ethylene Oxide Sterilizers. Requirements and Test Methods
JIS T 7323 (Japanese Standards Association[68])	Ethylene Oxide Sterilizers
ANSI/AAMI ST40 (Association for the Advancement of Medical Instrumentation[69])	Table-Top Dry Heat (Heated Air) Sterilization and Sterility Assurance in Health Care Facilities
ANSI/AAMI ST50 (Association for the Advancement of Medical Instrumentation[70])	Dry Heat (Heated Air) Sterilizers
Australian Standard AS 2487 (Standards Australia[71])	Dry Heat Sterilizers

TABLE 70.6 International standards for washer disinfector requirements

Standard Reference	Standard Title
ISO 15883-1 (International Organization for Standardization[75])	Washer-Disinfectors. General Requirements, Terms and Definitions and Tests
ISO 15883-2 (International Organization for Standardization[76])	Washer-Disinfectors. Requirements and Tests for Washer-Disinfectors Employing Thermal Disinfection for Surgical Instruments, Anaesthetic Equipment, Bowls, Dishes, Receivers, Utensils, Glassware, etc
ISO 15883-3 (International Organization for Standardization[77])	Washer-Disinfectors, Part 3: Requirements and Tests for Washer-Disinfectors for Human Waste Containers
ISO 15883-4 (International Organization for Standardization[78])	Washer-Disinfectors—Part 4: Requirements and Tests for Washer-Disinfectors Employing Chemical Disinfection for Thermolabile Endoscopes
ISO TS 15883-5 (International Organization for Standardization[79])	Washer-Disinfectors—Part 5: Test Soils and Methods for Demonstrating Cleaning Efficacy
ISO 15883-6 (International Organization for Standardization[80])	Washer-Disinfectors—Part 6: Requirements and Tests for Washer-Disinfectors Employing Thermal Disinfection for Non-Invasive, Non-Critical Medical Devices and Healthcare Equipment
ISO 15883-7 (International Organization for Standardization[81])	Washer-Disinfectors—Part 7: Requirements and Tests for General Purpose Washer-Disinfectors Employing Chemical Disinfection for Bedframes, Bedside Tables, Transport Carts, Containers, Surgical Tables, Furnishings and Surgical Clogs

individual member countries. Companies can choose between several alternative processes, depending on their product and the number of countries to which they wish to sell it:

a) If the product will be placed only on a single market, authorization from that country is sufficient.
b) If a company wishes to place the product on the market in several countries, it can apply for mutual recognition for the product authorization.
c) A European Union–wide authorization in one go is also available.

The active substances are first assessed by a competent authority in a member country. The results of the assessment are sent to the Biocidal Products Committee at the European Chemicals Agency (ECHA), which prepares an opinion within 270 days. The opinion serves as the basis for the decision on approval which is adopted by the European Commission. The approval of an active substance is granted for a defined period up to 10 years and is renewable.

The BPR also covers products that are protected from the harmful effects of organisms by treatment with, or incorporation of, a biocidal product. These are called treated articles. Examples include paints containing preservative or wood treated to protect it from termites. The BPR requires manufacturers and importers of treated articles to label them if

a) A claim of biocidal properties is made.
b) It is a condition of the approval of the active substance in the biocidal product used to treat the article.

The labels need to be easily understandable and visible for consumers.

There is a large number of European standards that define test methods that can be used for the evaluation of antimicrobial claims on disinfectants and antiseptics[74]

(see chapter 63). These standards define test methods at three different phases of assessment:

a) Assessment of basic activity against different types of microorganism such as vegetative bacteria, spores, or viruses
b) Assessment for different fields of use such as medical, veterinary, or food handling
c) Assessment of specific applications within a field of use such as hand disinfection

Table 70.7 gives some examples of some of the series of European standards at the various levels. There are also other test methods used in other jurisdictions specifically used to demonstrate the antimicrobial activities of antiseptics and disinfectants (eg, as published by AOAC, ASTM, and Organization for Economic Cooperation and Development (OECD); see chapters 62 and 63).

In the United States, the Environmental Protection Agency (EPA) is primarily responsible for regulating pesticides, including disinfectants used on environmental surfaces. But, when such disinfectants are used for high-level disinfection or sporicidal disinfection of medical devices, the FDA is primarily responsible.[87] The Federal Insecticide, Fungicide, and Rodenticide Act (FIFRA)[88] governs the registration, distribution, sale, and use of pesticides and gives the EPA authority to determine which pesticides can be used and how they can be used. A pesticide is defined as any substance or mixture of substances intended for preventing, destroying, repelling, or mitigating any pest, where a pest includes fungus, bacteria, or viruses provided that they are not in a living person or animal. The EPA (in conjunction with other federal and state agencies) evaluates new pesticides and proposed uses, determines if emergency situations warrant temporary approvals of certain pesticides, and periodically reviews current research related to the safety of older pesticides. They also enforce pesticide regulations and provide support to state and regional EPA

TABLE 70.7 Examples of European standards for test methods for the evaluation of disinfectants and antiseptics.

Standard Reference	Standard Title
EN 14885 (European Union[74])	Chemical Disinfectants and Antiseptics—Application of European Standards for Chemical Disinfectants and Antiseptics
EN 1040 (European Committee for Standardization[83])	Chemical Disinfectants and Antiseptics—Quantitative Suspension Test for the Evaluation of Basic Bactericidal Activity of Chemical Disinfectants and Antiseptics—Test Method and Requirements (Phase 1)
EN 14347 (European Committee for Standardization[84])	Chemical Disinfectants and Antiseptics—Basic Sporicidal Activity—Test Method and Requirements (Phase 1)
EN 1499 (European Committee for Standardization[85])	Chemical Disinfectants and Antiseptics—Hygienic Handwash—Test Method and Requirements (Phase 2/Step 2)
EN 1500 (European Committee for Standardization[86])	Chemical Disinfectants and Antiseptics—Hygienic Handrub—Test Method and Requirements (Phase 2/Step 2)

programs designed to protect, certify, and train pesticide applicators. Some pesticides are considered too hazardous for sale to the general public and are designated restricted use pesticides. Only certified applicators can purchase or supervise the application of restricted use pesticides.

The FIFRA requires that all pesticides sold or distributed in the United States are registered. There are four types of registration for pesticide use:

a) Federal registration actions: The EPA can register pesticides in the United States.
b) Experimental use permits (EUPs): The EPA can allow manufacturers of pesticides to field test products under development.
c) Emergency exemptions: In the event of an emergency pest problem, EPA can allow state and federal agencies to permit the use of an unregistered pesticide in a specific area.
d) State-specific registration: In certain circumstances, states can register a new pesticide for general use, or a federally registered product for an additional use, if there is both a demonstrated special local need.

The registration process considers
a) The ingredients of the pesticide
b) Where it is to be used
c) The amount, frequency, and timing of use
d) How it is to be stored and disposed of

Companies submit an application to register a new pesticide active ingredient, new product for an existing pesticide, or add a new use to an existing product. The company provides data from studies that comply with the EPA's testing guidelines. The EPA evaluates the potential for harm to humans, wildlife, fish, and plants, including endangered species and nontarget organisms as well as environmental effects through contamination of surface water or ground water from leaching, runoff, and spray drift. They also evaluate and approve the language that appears on each pesticide label to ensure the directions for use and safety measures are appropriate to any potential risk. Establishments that produce pesticides, active ingredients, or devices and companies or establishments that import into the United States must register and file production reports with EPA.

Preservatives and Preservation

Where preservatives are included as part of the formulation of a medicinal product, for example, in multiple-use ophthalmic preparations, they would be regulated as part of the approval of the medicinal product. There is a recent focus on the safe and effective use of preservatives in such applications, with a particular emphasis on environmental risks and the potential for gram-negative bacteria detection in such products (see chapters 39 and 40). Other preserved industrial products, such as wood preservatives and treated wood, are subject to the requirements of pesticide regulations and specific regulations such as the BPD in Europe. Specific test methods, such as USP <51>,[89] are used to demonstrate the ability of a preserved formulation (medicinal or cosmetic products) to prevent the growth of a bacterial/fungal load (see chapters 39 and 40). See the earlier sections in this chapter for a summary of these regulatory requirements.

Foodstuffs and Ingredients

The GMP concepts have been applied to food processing. As with the production of medicinal products, GMPs addressed personnel, buildings and facilities, plant and grounds, sanitary operations, sanitary facilities and controls, equipment and utensils, production and process controls, and warehousing and distribution. From the early 1990s, GMP for food production has been refined by the principles of Hazard Analysis and Critical Control Point (HACCP). The HACCP is a preventative food safety system in which every step in the manufacture, storage, and distribution of a food product is analyzed for microbiological, physical, and chemical hazards. The HACCP does not replace the concept of GMP but provides a process by which food processors can prioritize and implement GMP. Each food and associated manufacturing processes poses different risks and so each manufacturer needs to address its own situation. The HACCP is based on assessing the risks associated with the product and developing and implementing practices to reduce the risk of unsafe food. The HACCP principles are generally considered and internationally recognized to be a useful tool to control hazards that may occur in food production.

The international standard ISO 22000 outlines Food Safety Management Systems (FSMS) for food businesses along the food chain with focus on enterprises processing or manufacturing food.[90] In addition to this FSMS standard, ISO has produced a number of standards focusing in more detail on specific areas of an FSMS (eg, prerequisites for food manufacturing[91] [ISO 22002-1]; traceability in the feed and food chain[92] [ISO 22005]. A FSMS incorporates the principles of HACCP, GMP, and good hygiene practices.

In the United States, the food processing sector is extensively regulated at both state and federal level. Federal food law applies to all food in considered in interstate commerce where the food or an ingredient of it moved between states. Foods not in interstate commerce are regulated only by state law; however, in practice, most foods fit the definition of being in interstate commerce. There are two federal agencies that provide the regulatory oversight: Food Safety and Inspection Service (FSIS) is the public health agency in the US Department of Agriculture (USDA) for meat and poultry processing and the FDA covers all other food processing businesses. Agencies at state level have an active role in overseeing food processing businesses within their respective states in collaboration with the federal agencies. Food is subject to the laws of the jurisdiction where the food is located, whether the food is being processed there, consumed there, or is merely being moved through the jurisdiction to its final destination. In some situations, FSIS and FDA follow similar practices; in other situations, the practices of these two agencies are quite distinct.

Adulterated or misbranded food cannot be sold. Adulterated food means any food that

a) Contains any substance, food additive, or pesticide chemical residue which may render it injurious to health or unsafe

b) Consists of any filthy, putrid, or decomposed substance

c) Is unfit for food

d) Has been prepared, packed, or held under insanitary conditions whereby it may have become contaminated

e) Is the product of a diseased animal or an animal that died other than by slaughter

f) Its container is composed of any substance which may render the contents injurious to health or has been intentionally irradiated.

Misbranded food means any food that

a) Its labeling or advertising is false or misleading.

b) Is offered for sale under the name of another food

c) Is an imitation of another food but the label does not bear the word *imitation*

d) Its container is made or filled to be misleading.

e) Its label does not provide (1) the name and place of the manufacturer and (2) an accurate statement of the quantity of the contents in terms of weight, measure, or numerical count.

Most food processing involves directly adding ingredients or substances to the food product, contacting the surface of processing equipment or packaging the product. Federal law states that adding anything (directly or indirectly) to food will render the food adulterated, except if the substance is allowed to be added according to an FDA or FSIS regulation. When considering substances that are directly or indirectly added to food, the assessment does not focus solely on the substance; the assessment also focuses on how the substance is used. Substances that can be directly or indirectly added to food are categorized as

- Substances with uses explicitly approved by FDA or USDA prior to September 1958

- Substances with a long history of safe use in food categorized as *generally recognized as safe* (GRAS), such as salt, direct food substances, and indirect food substances (eg, packaging or contact surfaces)

- Food additives—general direct and indirect food additives

- Substances covered by the GRAS notification program and GRAS notice inventory that allows manufacturers

to inform the FDA that a substance is safe and that they intend to use the substance in a food product; the FDA then has an opportunity to accept or to question the assessment of the substance.

- Specifically prohibited substances

Within the broad prohibition of supplying adulterated food is the concept that a food processor conducts the manufacturing process to minimize the risk of adulteration applying HACCP and GMP.

In the European Union, the General Food Law Regulation[93] sets out the general principles and requirements of food law. This regulation is the foundation of food and feed law. It sets out a coherent framework for developing food and feed legislation both at European Union level and in member countries. It covers all stages of food and feed production and distribution. It also sets up an independent agency responsible for scientific advice and support, the European Food Safety Authority (EFSA). The regulation establishes that only safe food and feed can be placed on the European Union market or fed to food-producing animals. It also establishes basic criteria for establishing whether a food or feed is safe. Food cannot be placed on the market if it is (1) injurious to health or (2) unfit for human consumption. Although risk assessment of food and feed is to be primarily based on scientific evidence, societal, economic, ethical, and cultural factors may also be taken into account. The regulation also incorporates the precautionary principle, allowing member countries to take action to protect public health when scientific uncertainty remains about risk. The principle of traceability is extremely important and is to be applied at all stages of the food chain. This includes food and feed business operators keeping records of who supplied the product and who it is subsequently sold to and the requirement of accurate food labeling throughout the food chain. Labeling and packaging must not mislead consumers. The rules apply equally to food being exported from and imported into the European Union. Implementation of a FSMS is fundamental to the legislation.[94]

▶ CONCLUSION

The regulatory requirements that apply to preservation, disinfection, and sterilization vary depending on the product to which they are being applied. Regulations can vary depending on whether the product is considered a health care product (a medicinal product or medical device), environmental biocide use, or a food application. The principles of the regulations are similar, although the detailed requirements and processes and the agency responsible for enforcing the regulatory requirements can differ between jurisdictions. The basis of the various regulatory regimes has a lot of similarities; there are requirements that the agents used for preservation, disinfection, and sterilization are safe and perform as intended and that processes are applied in accordance with principles of management systems, be they quality management systems, FSMS, or cGMPs. The regulatory requirements are often supported by regulatory guidance, voluntary consensus standards, and codes of practice. Similarly, although it was not practical in this chapter to provide detailed explanations of all country or region-specific requirements internationally, the overall requirements are often similar to those described for the United States and the European Union. Substantial efforts at harmonization of technical requirements are underway through organizations such as ICH, the International Medical Device Regulators Forum (IMDRF) and ISO. These efforts are focused on reducing national and regional differences in requirements for products and processes and simplifying requirements for introducing and maintaining products onto the market.

REFERENCES

1. European Commission. EudraLex—volume 4—good manufacturing practice (GMP) guidelines. European Commission Web site. https://ec.europa.eu/health/documents/eudralex/vol-4_en. Accessed June 24, 2019.
2. US Food and Drug Administration. *Current Good Manufacturing Practice in Manufacturing, Processing, Packing or Holding of Drugs: General. Code of Federal Regulations Title 21—Food and Drugs—Chapter 1—Subchapter C—Drugs: General Part 210.* White Oak, MD: US Food and Drug Administration; 2017.
3. US Food and Drug Administration. *Current Good Manufacturing Practice for Finished Pharmaceuticals. Code of Federal Regulations Title 21—Food and Drugs—Chapter 1—Subchapter C—Drugs: General Part 211.* White Oak, MD: US Food and Drug Administration; 2017.
4. European Committee for Standardization. *EN 285. Sterilization—Steam Sterilizers—Large Sterilizers.* Brussels, Belgium: European Committee for Standardization; 2015.
5. European Directorate for the Quality of Medicines. *European Pharmacopoeia.* 8th ed. Strasbourg, France: Council of Europe; 2013.
6. Society of Japanese Pharmacopoeia. *Japanese Pharmacopoeia.* 17th ed. Tokyo, Japan: Society of Japanese Pharmacopoeia; 2016.
7. United States Pharmacopeial Convention. *United States Pharmacopoeia USP 40.* Rockville, MD: United States Pharmacopeial Convention; 2017.
8. International Organization for Standardization. *ISO TS 19930:2017: Guidance on Aspects of a Risk-Based Approach to Assuring Sterility of Terminally Sterilized, Single-Use Health Care Product Including That Unable to Withstand Processing to Achieve Maximally a Sterility Assurance Level of 10-6.* Geneva, Switzerland: International Organization for Standardization; 2017.
9. International Council for Harmonisation of Technical Requirements for Pharmaceuticals for Human Use. M4: The common technical document. International Council for Harmonisation of Technical Requirements for Pharmaceuticals for Human Use Web site. http://www.ich.org/products/ctd.html. Accessed June 24, 2019.
10. European Union. *Regulation (EC) No 726/2004 Community Procedures for the Authorisation and Supervision of Medicinal Products for Human and Veterinary Use and Establishing a European Medicines Agency.* Brussels, Belgium: European Union; 2017
11. European Union. Directive 2001/83/EC of the European Parliament and of the Council of 6 November 2001 on the community code relating to medicinal products for human use. European Union Web site. https://ec.europa.eu/health/sites/health/files/files/eudralex/vol-1/dir_2001_83_consol_2012/dir_2001_83_cons_2012_en.pdf. Accessed June 24, 2019.
12. US Food and Drug Administration. New drug application (NDA). US Food and Drug Administration Web site. https://www.fda.gov/Drugs/DevelopmentApprovalProcess/HowDrugsareDevelopedandApproved/ApprovalApplications/NewDrugApplicationNDA/default.htm. Accessed June 24, 2019.
13. US Food and Drug Administration. Abbreviated new drug application (ANDA). US Food and Drug Administration Web site. https://www.fda.gov/Drugs/DevelopmentApprovalProcess/HowDrugsareDevelopedandApproved/ApprovalApplications/AbbreviatedNewDrugApplicationANDAGenerics/default.htm. Accessed June 24, 2019.
14. European Union. *Directive 2003/94/EC Principles and Guidelines of Good Manufacturing Practice in Respect of Medicinal Products for Human Use and Investigational Medicinal Products for Human Use.* Brussels, Belgium: European Union; 2003.
15. International Organization for Standardization. *ISO 14644 series: Cleanrooms and Associated Controlled Environments.* Geneva, Switzerland: International Organization for Standardization; 2015.
16. International Organization for Standardization. *ISO 13485:2016: Medical Devices—Quality Management Systems—Requirements for Regulatory Purposes.* Geneva, Switzerland: International Organization for Standardization; 2016.
17. European Union. *Active Implantable Medical Devices Directive 90/385/EEC.* Brussels, Belgium: European Union; 1990.
18. European Union. *Medical Devices Directive 93/42/EEC.* Brussels, Belgium: European Union; 1990.
19. European Union. *In Vitro Diagnostic Medical Devices Directive 98/79/EC.* Brussels, Belgium: European Union; 1998.
20. European Union. *Medical Devices Regulation EU 2017/745.* Brussels, Belgium: European Union; 1998.
21. European Union. *In Vitro Diagnostic Medical Devices Regulation EU 2017/746.* Brussels, Belgium: European Union; 1998.
22. European Committee for Standardization. *EN 556-1. Sterilization of Medical Devices—Requirements for Medical Devices to Be Designated "STERILE"—Part 1: Requirements for Terminally Sterilized Medical Devices.* Brussels, Belgium: European Committee for Standardization; 2001.
23. Pub L No. 94-295, 90 Stat 539. https://www.govinfo.gov/content/pkg/STATUTE-90/pdf/STATUTE-90-Pg539.pdf. Accessed June 24, 2019.
24. US Food and Drug Administration. 510(k) clearances. US Food and Drug Administration Web site. https://www.fda.gov/MedicalDevices/ProductsandMedicalProcedures/DeviceApprovalsandClearances/510kClearances/. Accessed June 24, 2019.
25. US Food and Drug Administration. Submission and review of sterility information in premarket notification (510(k)) submissions for devices labeled as sterile. Guidance for industry and Food and Drug Administration staff. US Food and Drug Administration Web site. https://www.fda.gov/media/74445/download. Accessed June 24, 2019.
26. Association for the Advancement of Medical Instrumentation. *ANSI/AAMI ST67. Sterilization of Health Care Products—Requirements and Guidance for Selecting a Sterility Assurance Level (SAL) For Products Labeled "Sterile."* Arlington, VA: Association for the Advancement of Medical Instrumentation; 2011.
27. International Organization for Standardization. *ISO 14937:2009: Sterilization of Health Care Products—General Requirements for Characterization of a Sterilizing Agent and the Development, Validation and Routine Control of a Sterilization Process for Medical Devices.* Geneva, Switzerland: International Organization for Standardization; 2009.
28. International Organization for Standardization. *ISO 11135:2014: Sterilization of Health Care Products—Ethylene Oxide—Requirements for Development, Validation and Routine Control of a Sterilization Process for Medical Devices.* Geneva, Switzerland: International Organization for Standardization; 2014.
29. International Organization for Standardization. *ISO 11137-1:2006: Sterilization of Health Care Products—Radiation—Part 1: Requirements for Development, Validation and Routine Control of a Sterilization Process for Medical Devices.* Geneva, Switzerland: International Organization for Standardization; 2006.
30. International Organization for Standardization. *ISO 11137-2:2013: Sterilization of Health Care Products—Radiation—Part 2: Establishing*

the Sterilization Dose. Geneva, Switzerland: International Organization for Standardization; 2013.

31. International Organization for Standardization. *ISO 11137-2:2017: Sterilization of Health Care Products—Radiation—Part 3: Guidance on Dosimetric Aspects of Development, Validation and Routine Control.* Geneva, Switzerland: International Organization for Standardization; 2017.

32. International Organization for Standardization. *ISO 17665-1:2006: Sterilization of Health Care Products—Moist Heat—Part 1: Requirements for the Development, Validation and Routine Control of a Sterilization Process for Medical Devices.* Geneva, Switzerland: International Organization for Standardization; 2006.

33. International Organization for Standardization. *ISO TS 17665-2:2009: Sterilization of Health Care Products—Moist Heat—Sterilization of Health Care Products. Moist Heat. Guidance on the Application of ISO 17665-1.* Geneva, Switzerland: International Organization for Standardization; 2009.

34. International Organization for Standardization. *ISO 17665-3:2013: Sterilization of Health Care Products—Moist Heat—Sterilization of Health Care Products. Moist Heat. Guidance on the Designation of a Medical Device to a Product Family and Processing Category for Steam Sterilization.* Geneva, Switzerland: International Organization for Standardization; 2013.

35. International Organization for Standardization. *ISO 20857:2010: Sterilization of Health Care Products—Dry Heat—Requirements for the Development, Validation and Routine Control of a Sterilization Process for Medical Devices.* Geneva, Switzerland: International Organization for Standardization; 2010.

36. International Organization for Standardization. *ISO 25424:2009: Sterilization of Medical Devices—Low Temperature Steam and Formaldehyde—Requirements for Development, Validation and Routine Control of a Sterilization Process for Medical Devices.* Geneva, Switzerland: International Organization for Standardization; 2009.

37. International Organization for Standardization. *ISO 14160:2011: Sterilization of Health Care Products—Liquid Chemical Sterilizing Agents for Single-Use Medical Devices Utilizing Animal Tissues and Their Derivatives—Requirements for Characterization, Development, Validation and Routine Control of a Sterilization Process for Medical Devices.* Geneva, Switzerland: International Organization for Standardization; 2011.

38. International Organization for Standardization. *ISO 22441: Sterilization of Health Care Products—Low Temperature Vaporized Hydrogen Peroxide—Requirements for the Development, Validation and Routine Control of a Sterilization Process for Medical Devices.* Geneva, Switzerland: International Organization for Standardization; in press.

39. International Organization for Standardization. *ISO 13408 (all parts): Aseptic Processing of Health Care Products.* Geneva, Switzerland: International Organization for Standardization; 2008.

40. International Organization for Standardization. *ISO 13408-7:2015: Aseptic Processing of Health Care Products. Alternative Processes for Medical Devices and Combination Products.* Geneva, Switzerland: International Organization for Standardization; 2015.

41. International Organization for Standardization. *ISO 11607-1:2006: Packaging for Terminally Sterilized Medical Devices—Part 1: Requirements for Materials, Sterile Barrier Systems and Packaging Systems.* Geneva, Switzerland: International Organization for Standardization; 2006.

42. International Organization for Standardization. *ISO 11607-2:2006: Packaging for Terminally Sterilized Medical Devices—Part 2: Validation Requirements for Forming, Sealing and Assembly Processes.* Geneva, Switzerland: International Organization for Standardization; 2006.

43. International Organization for Standardization. *ISO 11138-1:2017: Sterilization of Health Care Products—Biological Indicators—Part 1: General Requirements.* Geneva, Switzerland: International Organization for Standardization; 2017.

44. International Organization for Standardization. *ISO 11138-2:2017: Sterilization of Health Care Products—Biological Indicators—Part 2: Biological Indicators for Ethylene Oxide Sterilization Processes.* Geneva, Switzerland: International Organization for Standardization; 2017.

45. International Organization for Standardization. *ISO 11138-3:2017: Sterilization of Health Care Products—Biological Indicators—Part 3: Biological Indicators for Moist Heat Sterilization Processes.* Geneva, Switzerland: International Organization for Standardization; 2017.

46. International Organization for Standardization. *ISO 11138-4:2017: Sterilization of Health Care Products—Biological Indicators—Part 6: Biological Indicators for Dry Heat Sterilization Processes.* Geneva, Switzerland: International Organization for Standardization; 2017.

47. International Organization for Standardization. *ISO 11138-5:2017: Sterilization of Health Care Products—Biological Indicators—Part 5: Biological Indicators for Low-Temperature Steam Formaldehyde Sterilization.* Geneva, Switzerland: International Organization for Standardization; 2017.

48. International Organization for Standardization. *ISO 11138-6: Sterilization of Health Care Products—Biological Indicators—Part 6: Biological Indicators for Hydrogen Peroxide Vapour Sterilization Processes.* Geneva, Switzerland: International Organization for Standardization; in press.

49. International Organization for Standardization. *ISO 14161:2009: Sterilization of Health Care Products—Biological Indicators—Guidance for the Selection, Use and Interpretation of Results.* Geneva, Switzerland: International Organization for Standardization; 2009.

50. International Organization for Standardization. *ISO 11140-1:2014: Sterilization of Health Care Products—Chemical Indicators—Part 1: General Requirements.* Geneva, Switzerland: International Organization for Standardization; 2014.

51. International Organization for Standardization. *ISO 11140-3:2009: Sterilization of Health Care Products. Chemical Indicators. Class 2 Indicator Systems for Use in the Bowie and Dick-Type Steam Penetration Test.* Geneva, Switzerland: International Organization for Standardization; 2009.

52. International Organization for Standardization. *ISO 11140-4:2007: Sterilization of Health Care Products. Chemical Indicators. Class 2 Indicators as an Alternative to the Bowie and Dick-Type Test for Detection of Steam Penetration.* Geneva, Switzerland: International Organization for Standardization; 2007.

53. International Organization for Standardization. *ISO 11140-5:2007: Sterilization of Health Care Products. Chemical Indicators. Class 2 Indicators for Bowie and Dick-Type Air Removal Tests.* Geneva, Switzerland: International Organization for Standardization; 2007.

54. International Organization for Standardization. *ISO 15882:2008: Chemical Indicators—Guidance on the Selection, Use, and Interpretation of Results.* Geneva, Switzerland: International Organization for Standardization; 2008.

55. International Organization for Standardization. *ISO 11737-1:2018: Sterilization of Medical Devices. Microbiological Methods. Determination of the Population of Microorganisms on Products.* Geneva, Switzerland: International Organization for Standardization; 2018.

56. International Organization for Standardization. *ISO 11737-2:2009: Sterilization of Medical Devices. Microbiological Methods. Tests of Sterility Performed in the Validation of a Sterilization Process.* Geneva, Switzerland: International Organization for Standardization; 2009.

57. European Committee for Standardization. *EN 556-2. Sterilization of Medical Devices. Requirements for Medical Devices to Be Designated "STERILE." Requirements for Aseptically Processed Medical Devices.* Brussels, Belgium: European Committee for Standardization; 2015.

58. European Union. *Community Code Relating to Medicinal Products for Human Use Directive 2001/83/EC.* Brussels, Belgium: European Union; 2001.

59. International Electrotechnical Commission. *IEC 61010-2-040. Safety Requirements for Electrical Equipment for Measurement, Control, and Laboratory Use. Part 2-040: Particular Requirements for Sterilizers and Washer-Disinfectors Used to Treat Medical Materials.* Geneva, Switzerland: International Electrotechnical Commission; 2015.

60. European Committee for Standardization. *EN 13060. Small Steam Sterilizers.* Brussels, Belgium: European Committee for Standardization; 2014.

61. Association for the Advancement of Medical Instrumentation. *ANSI/ AAMI ST55. Table-Top Steam Sterilizers.* Arlington, VA: Association for the Advancement of Medical Instrumentation; 2016.

62. Association for the Advancement of Medical Instrumentation. *ANSI/ AAMI ST8. Hospital Steam Sterilizers.* Arlington, VA: Association for the Advancement of Medical Instrumentation; 2013.

63. Japanese Standards Association. *JIS T 7322. Large Steam Sterilizers.* Tokyo, Japan: Japanese Standards Association; 2005.

64. Japanese Standards Association. *JIS T 7324. Small Steam Sterilizers.* Tokyo, Japan: Japanese Standards Association; 2005.

65. European Committee for Standardization. *EN 17180. Sterilizers for Medical Purposes—Low Temperature Vaporized Hydrogen Peroxide Sterilizers—Requirements and Testing.* Brussels, Belgium: European Committee for Standardization; in press.

66. European Committee for Standardization. *EN 14180. Sterilizers for Medical Purposes—Low Temperature Steam and Formaldehyde Sterilizers—Requirements and Testing.* Brussels, Belgium: European Committee for Standardization; 2014.

67. European Committee for Standardization. *EN 1422. Sterilizers for Medical Purposes. Ethylene Oxide Sterilizers. Requirements and Test Methods.* Brussels, Belgium: European Committee for Standardization; 2014.

68. Japanese Standards Association. *JIS T 7323. Ethylene Oxide Sterilizers.* Tokyo, Japan: Japanese Standards Association; 2005.

69. Association for the Advancement of Medical Instrumentation. *ANSI/ AAMI ST40. Table-Top Dry Heat (Heated Air) Sterilization and Sterility Assurance in Health Care Facilities.* Arlington, VA: Association for the Advancement of Medical Instrumentation; 2010.

70. Association for the Advancement of Medical Instrumentation. *ANSI/ AAMI ST50. Dry Heat (Heated Air) Sterilizers.* Arlington, VA: Association for the Advancement of Medical Instrumentation; 2010.

71. Standards Australia. *AS 2487. Dry Heat Sterilizers.* Sydney, Australia: Standards Australia; 2002.

72. US Food and Drug Administration. Safety and effectiveness of consumer antiseptics; topical antimicrobial drug products for over-the-counter human use. Federal Register Web site. https://www.federalregister.gov /documents/2016/09/06/2016-21337/safety-and-effectiveness-of -consumer-antiseptics-topical-antimicrobial-drug-products-for. Accessed June 24, 2019.

73. US Food and Drug Administration. Safety and effectiveness of health care antiseptics; topical antimicrobial drug products for over-the-counter human use. Federal Register Web site. https://www.govinfo .gov/content/pkg/FR-2017-12-20/pdf/2017-27317.pdf. Accesses June 24, 2019.

74. European Committee for Standardization. *EN 14885. Chemical Disinfectants and Antiseptics—Application of European Standards for Chemical Disinfectants and Antiseptics.* Brussels, Belgium: European Committee for Standardization; 2015.

75. International Organization for Standardization. *ISO 15883-1:2006: Washer-Disinfectors General Requirements, Terms and Definitions and Tests.* Geneva, Switzerland: International Standards Organization; 2006.

76. International Organization for Standardization. *ISO 15883-2:2009: Washer-Disinfectors. Requirements and Tests for Washer-Disinfectors Employing Thermal Disinfection for Surgical Instruments, Anaesthetic Equipment, Bowls, Dishes, Receivers, Utensils, Glassware, etc.* Geneva, Switzerland: International Organization for Standardization; 2009.

77. International Organization for Standardization. *ISO 15883-3:2009: Washer-Disinfectors, Part 3: Requirements and Tests for Washer-Disinfectors for Human Waste Containers.* Geneva, Switzerland: International Organization for Standardization; 2009.

78. International Organization for Standardization. *ISO 15883-4:2008: Washer-Disinfectors—Part 4: Requirements and Tests for Washer-Disinfectors Employing Chemical Disinfection for Thermolabile Endoscopes.* Geneva, Switzerland: International Organization for Standardization; 2008.

79. International Organization for Standardization. *ISO 15883-5:2005: Washer—Disinfectors—Part 5: Test Soils and Methods for Demonstrating Cleaning Efficacy.* Geneva, Switzerland: International Organization for Standardization; 2005.

80. International Organization for Standardization. *ISO 15883-6:2015: Washer-Disinfectors—Part 6: Requirements and Tests for Washer-Disinfectors Employing Thermal Disinfection for Non-Invasive, Non-Critical Medical Devices and Healthcare Equipment.* Geneva, Switzerland: International Organization for Standardization; 2015.

81. International Organization for Standardization. *ISO 15883-7:2016: Washer-Disinfectors—Part 7: Requirements and Tests for General Purpose Washer-Disinfectors Employing Chemical Disinfection for Bed-frames, Bedside Tables, Transport Carts, Containers, Surgical Tables, Furnishings and Surgical Clogs.* Geneva, Switzerland: International Organization for Standardization; 2016.

82. European Union. *Biocidal Products Regulation EU Regulation 528/2012.* Brussels, Belgium: European Union; 2012.

83. European Committee for Standardization. *EN 1040. Chemical Disinfectants and Antiseptics—Quantitative Suspension Test for the Evaluation of Basic Bactericidal Activity of Chemical Disinfectants and Antiseptics—Test Method and Requirements (Phase 1).* Brussels, Belgium: European Committee for Standardization; 2005.

84. European Committee for Standardization. *EN 14347. Chemical Disinfectants and Antiseptics—Basic Sporicidal Activity—Test Method and Requirements (Phase 1).* Brussels, Belgium: European Committee for Standardization; 2005.

85. European Committee for Standardization. *EN 1499. Chemical Disinfectants and Antiseptics—Hygienic Handwash—Test Method and Requirements (Phase 2/Step 2).* Brussels, Belgium: European Committee for Standardization; 2013.

86. European Committee for Standardization. *EN 1500. Chemical Disinfectants and Antiseptics—Hygienic Handrub—Test Method and Requirements (Phase 2/Step 2).* Brussels, Belgium: European Committee for Standardization; 2013.

87. Association for the Advancement of Medical Instrumentation. *ANSI/ AMI TIR68. Technical Information Report—Low and Intermediate-Level Disinfection in Healthcare Settings for Medical Devices and Patient Care Equipment and Sterile Processing Environmental Surfaces.* Arlington, VA: Association for the Advancement of Medical Instrumentation; 2018.

88. Library of Congress. Act for preventing the manufacture, sale, or transportation of adulterated or misbranded Paris greens, lead arsenates, and other insecticides, and also fungicides, and for regulating traffic therein, and for other purposes. Library of Congress Web site. https://www.loc .gov/law/help/statutes-at-large/61st-congress/session-2/c61s2ch191.pdf. Accessed 24, 2019.

89. United States Pharmacopeial Convention. *USP <51> Antimicrobial Effectiveness Testing.* Rockville, MD: United States Pharmacopeial Convention; 2017.

90. International Organization for Standardization. *ISO 22000:2005: Food Safety Management Systems—Requirements for Any Organization in the Food Chain.* Geneva, Switzerland: International Organization for Standardization; 2005.

91. International Organization for Standardization. *ISO TS 22002-1:2009: Prerequisite Programmes on Food Safety—Part 1: Food Manufacturing.* Geneva, Switzerland: International Organization for Standardization; 2009.

92. International Organization for Standardization. *ISO 22005:2007: Traceability in the Feed and Food Chain—General Principles and Basic Requirements for System Design and Implementation.* Geneva, Switzerland: International Organization for Standardization; 2007.

93. European Union. *The General Principles and Requirements of Food Law, Establishing the European Food Safety Authority and Laying Down Procedures in Matters of Food Safety Regulation (EC) 178/2002.* Brussels, Belgium: European Union; 2002.

94. European Union. *Commission Notice on the Implementation of Food Safety Management Systems Covering Prerequisite Programs (PRPs) and Procedures Based on the HACCP Principles, Including the Facilitation/ Flexibility of the Implementation in Certain Food Businesses.* Brussels, Belgium: European Union; 2016.

Federal Regulation of Liquid Chemical Germicides and Healthcare Sterilization by the US Food and Drug Administration

Elizabeth Claverie-Williams, Steven Elliott, Clarence Murray III, and Elaine Mayhall

Please see eBook for this chapter.

Regulation of Antimicrobial Pesticides by the US Environmental Protection Agency

Stephen F. Tomasino, Tajah L. Blackburn, and Jacqueline L. Hardy

In the United States (US), certain types of antimicrobial agents such as hospital disinfectants used to treat environmental surfaces contaminated with a public health-related pathogen, are pesticides (ie, a substance or mixture of substances intended for preventing, destroying, repelling, or mitigating any pest), and thus are regulated by the US Environmental Protection Agency (EPA). This chapter provides background information about the general considerations associated with the registration of pesticides in the United States with an emphasis on the regulatory requirements for antimicrobial products bearing public health claims. The views expressed in this chapter are those of the authors and do not necessarily reflect the views or policies of the EPA.

▶ REGULATORY FRAMEWORK

The US Federal Insecticide, Fungicide, and Rodenticide Act (FIFRA) provides for federal regulation of the distribution, sale, and use of pesticides.[1] All pesticides distributed or sold in the United States must be registered (ie, licensed) by EPA, unless exempt. The FIFRA's implementing regulations are found in Title 40 of the Code of Federal Regulations (CFR), Parts 150 to 189.[2] Regulations are codified annually in the US CFR. Title 40: Protection of Environment is the section of the CFR that deals with EPA's mission of protecting human health and the environment. Part 152 sets forth procedures, requirements, and criteria concerning the registration of pesticide products under FIFRA §3 (registration of pesticides). The EPA also derives authority to regulate pesticide residues on food items (eg, antimicrobial products intended to be applied to food or material or article that contact food) from provisions in the Federal Food, Drug, and Cosmetic Act (FFDCA).[3] The Food Quality Protection Act (FQPA)[4] amended both FIFRA and FFDCA and broadened the scope of how EPA regulates pesticides. For example, FQPA requires the EPA to make a safety finding when setting maximum residue

levels (tolerances) to consider the special susceptibility of children to pesticides, and to consider aggregate risk from exposure to a pesticide from multiple sources (food, water, residential, and other nonoccupational sources) when assessing tolerances. The FIFRA was further amended by the Pesticide Registration Improvement Act (PRIA) of 2003, which was reauthorized by the Pesticide Registration Improvement Extension Act of 2018.[5] The PRIA establishes pesticide registration fees for some registration actions under which applicants are required to pay a fee and, in exchange, EPA is obligated to perform certain registration functions within defined timeframes.

The following are terms associated with EPA's regulatory authority under FIFRA:

- 40 CFR §152.5. Pests. An organism is declared to be a *pest* under circumstances that make it deleterious to man or the environment, if it is (1) any vertebrate animal other than man; (2) any invertebrate animal, including but not limited to, any insect, other arthropod, nematode, or mollusk such as a slug and snail, but excluding any internal parasite of living man or other living animals; (3) any plant growing where not wanted, including any moss, algae, liverwort, or other plant of any higher order, and any plant part such as a root; or (4) any fungus, bacterium, virus, prion, or other microorganism, except for those on or in living man or other living animals and those on or in processed food or processed animal feed, beverages, drugs (as defined in FFDCA 201(g)(1)), and cosmetics (as defined in FFDCA §201 (i)).
- 40 CFR §152.3. Definitions. In general, the term *pesticide* means any substance or mixture of substances intended for preventing, destroying, repelling, or mitigating any pest. See 40 CFR §152.3 for exclusions.
- 40 CFR §152.3. Definitions. A *pesticide product* means a pesticide in a form (including composition, packaging, and labeling) in which the pesticide is, or is intended to be, distributed or sold. The term includes any

physical apparatus used to deliver or apply the pesticide if distributed or sold with the pesticide.

The EPA's regulation "Data Requirements for Registration," which was issued originally in 40 CFR Part 158, specifies the types of data and information generally required under FIFRA. On October 26, 2007, EPA promulgated final rules establishing updated basic data requirements for conventional, biochemical, and microbial pesticides. On May 8, 2013, EPA published a final rule amending 40 CFR Part 158, to add a subpart setting forth basic data requirements that support an application to register an antimicrobial pesticide product. This final rule, which is codified as 40 CFR Part 158 Subpart W—Antimicrobial Pesticide Data Requirements,[6] contains the basic data requirements specifically applicable to *antimicrobial pesticides* (see the following discussion).

As a useful tool, EPA's Pesticide Registration Manual[7] is intended to provide guidance for companies and individuals who want to have their pesticide products registered by EPA. Chapter 4 of the manual (Additional Considerations for Antimicrobial Products) provides specific information concerning the registration of antimicrobial pesticides.

▶ PESTICIDE REGISTRATION—AN OVERVIEW OF THE PROCESS

Pesticide registration is a scientific, legal, and administrative process through which the EPA examines the ingredients of the pesticide; the particular site or crop where it is to be used; the amount, frequency, and timing of its use; storage and disposal practices; and labeling, to ensure when a product is used according to the label, no unreasonable adverse effects on human health and the environment will occur. The EPA's pesticide review and regulatory activities are conducted by the Office of Pesticide Programs (OPP) within the Office of Chemical Safety and Pollution Prevention (OCSPP).[8] Work related to the registration and regulation of antimicrobial pesticides is handled by the OPP Antimicrobials Division. An application for a registration action, for example, to register a new pesticide active ingredient, new product for an existing pesticidal chemical, or adding a new use to an existing product, is submitted by a company for consideration by EPA. The company seeking to register the pesticide, the applicant, must provide data from studies that comply with EPA data requirements at 40 CFR Part 158 Subpart W. The Antimicrobial Pesticide Use Site Index[9] is used in conjunction with the data tables in the subpart to determine the applicability of data requirements to certain antimicrobial use patterns. Good laboratory practice standards, as defined in 40 CFR Part 160, apply to studies submitted to support the registration of pesticides. The pesticide registration process includes many common requirements applicable to the various types of pesticides, but some requirements are specific to the type of pesticide,

such as the need for product efficacy data for antimicrobial pesticides bearing claims against public health pests.

In evaluating a pesticide registration application for a new active ingredient and/or new use, the EPA assesses a wide variety of potential human health and environmental effects and routes of exposure associated with use of the product to ensure that, when the product is used according to the proposed labeled directions, no unreasonable adverse effects on human health or the environment will occur. Risk assessments are conducted to evaluate the potential for harm to humans, wildlife, fish, and plants, including endangered species and nontarget organisms; contamination of surface water or ground water from leaching, runoff, and spray drift; and potential human risks ranging from short-term toxicity to long-term effects such as cancer and reproductive system disorders. If EPA determines that no unreasonable adverse effects to human health or the environment will result from the sale, distribution, and use of a pesticide product, it may then grant the applicant a license or registration to legally sell and distribute the product in the United States. Once an EPA registration has been granted, then the registrants must also address and comply with any applicable requirements imposed by the states in which they wish to sell or distribute their product.

An applicant who does not wish to register and produce its own unique product may become a supplemental registrant for another company that has already registered a product. This supplemental registration allows the new registrant to market the product under its own company and brand name. If a registrant has a product previously registered with EPA and wishes to make a change to the registration such as change the formulation or labeling text (ie, add, delete, or change formulation components or label precautionary statements, or add or change uses), it must file an application to amend its registered product.

▶ A PESTICIDE PRODUCT LABEL—BASIC PRINCIPLES

All registered products must bear an EPA-approved label on every package. Regulatory requirements for pesticide labels are found in the 40 CFR Part 156. A Label Review Manual[10] issued by EPA provides guidance on pesticide labeling with the goal of improving the quality and consistency of pesticide labels. The EPA reviews pesticide product labels as part of the registration process and must approve all label language before a pesticide can be sold or distributed in the United States. The overall intent of the label is to provide clear directions for use and effective product performance while minimizing risks to human health and the environment. Pesticide product labels provide critical information about how to safely and legally handle, use, and dispose of pesticide products. The label is considered the law and must be followed. In addition, following labeling instructions carefully and precisely is necessary to ensure safe and effective use. Pesticide labels are legally enforceable and all of them carry the statement: "It is a violation of Federal law to use this product in a manner inconsistent with its labeling."

US ENVIRONMENTAL PROTECTION AGENCY REGISTRATION NUMBER

All EPA-registered pesticides bear an EPA registration number on the label. The EPA registration number consists of two groups of numbers separated by a hyphen, for example, EPA Registration Number 12345-12. The first group of numbers refers to the registrant's company identification number and the second group of numbers represents the registrant's product number. Distributors may also sell products with identical formulations and identical efficacy as the primary products. Distributor products frequently use different brand names but can be identified by their three-part EPA Registration Number. The first two parts of the EPA Registration Number match the registrant and their product, whereas the third set of numbers represent the distributor identification number. For example, EPA Registration Number 12345-12-2567 is a distributor product (identified by 2567) with an identical formulation and efficacy to the primary product with the EPA Registration Number 12345-12.

ANTIMICROBIAL PESTICIDE PRODUCTS

Per FIFRA section 2(mm), an *antimicrobial pesticide* is a pesticide that is intended to (1) disinfect, sanitize, reduce, or mitigate growth or development of microbiological organisms or (2) protect inanimate objects, industrial processes or systems, surfaces, water, or other chemical substances from contamination, fouling, or deterioration caused by bacteria, viruses, fungi, protozoa, algae, or slime. In general, antimicrobial pesticides used on inanimate surfaces are subject to FIFRA, whereas antimicrobial substances used in or on living animals or humans are regulated by FDA under FFDCA (eg, human or animal drugs, antiseptics). Furthermore, some antimicrobial products are subject to both FIFRA and FFDCA (ie, dual jurisdiction products) because they involve direct or indirect food uses or use on food contact surfaces. The focus here is on antimicrobial pesticides with claims against public health pathogens intended for use on inanimate environmental surfaces.

Antimicrobial pesticides regulated by EPA contain numerous active ingredients (eg, sodium hypochlorite, quaternary ammonium compounds, hydrogen peroxide) and are marketed in many types of formulations including sprays, towelettes, liquids, concentrated powders, and gases. Many of these products are registered to control

microorganisms infectious to humans on inanimate surfaces, and thus are intended to protect against microorganisms harmful to public health. Per 40 CFR Part 158 Subpart W §158.2204 (a) and (b), antimicrobial pesticide products are considered as either *public health* or *nonpublic health*, depending on the specific claims made on each product's labeling.

- *Public health claim.* In brief, an antimicrobial pesticide is considered to make a *public health claim* if the pesticide product bears a claim to control pest microorganisms that pose a threat to human health and whose presence cannot readily be observed by the user including, but not limited to, microorganisms infectious to man in any area of the inanimate environment. See 40 CFR Part 158 Subpart W §158.2204 (a) for complete definition.
- *Nonpublic health claim.* An antimicrobial pesticide is considered to make a *nonpublic health* claim if the pesticide product bears a claim to control microorganisms of economic or aesthetic significance, where the presence of the microorganism would not normally lead to infection or disease in humans. Examples of nonpublic health claims include, but are not limited to, algaecides, slimicides, preservatives, and products for which a pesticidal claim with respect to odor sources is made.

As noted previously, an Antimicrobial Pesticide Use Site Index has been established to assist applicants for antimicrobial pesticide registration in identifying the data requirements necessary to register a pesticide or to support their product registrations. The index, composed of 12 categories, includes antimicrobial pesticide use sites and general antimicrobial pesticide use patterns to help registrants determine if the uses also require the establishment of a tolerance (maximum residue level for food or feed) or an exemption from the requirement of a tolerance. The Pesticide Use Site Index categories are (1) agricultural premises and equipment; (2) food handling/storage establishments, premises, and equipment; (3) commercial, institutional and industrial premises, and equipment; (4) residential and public access premises; (5) medical premises and equipment; (6) human drinking water systems; (7) materials preservatives; (8) industrial processes and water systems; (9) antifouling coatings; (10) wood preservatives; (11) swimming pools; and (12) aquatic areas.

The following terms are defined in 40 CFR Part 158 Subpart W (§158.2203 Definitions) to describe the most common public health antimicrobial products:

1. Sanitizer—A substance, or mixture of substances, that reduces the bacterial population in the inanimate environment by significant numbers (eg, 3 $\log_{10}$ reduction) but does not destroy or eliminate all bacteria
2. Disinfectant—A substance, or mixture of substances, that destroys or irreversibly inactivates bacteria, fungi, and viruses, but not necessarily bacterial spores, in the

inanimate environment. The EPA registers three types of disinfectants based on the type of efficacy data submitted limited, general (or broad-spectrum), and hospital.

3. Sterilant—A substance, or mixture of substances, that destroys or eliminates all forms of microbial life in the inanimate environment, including all forms of vegetative bacteria, bacterial spores, fungi, fungal spores, and viruses. These products are commonly used in hospitals, laboratories, pharmaceutical clean rooms, and similar environments where sterilization is necessary. The FDA has sole regulatory jurisdiction over liquid chemical sterilants/high-level disinfectants intended for use to process reusable heat-sensitive critical and semicritical medical devices (see 40 CFR §152.6 (a); chapter 71).

4. Fungicide—A substance, or mixture of substances, that destroys fungi (including yeasts) and fungal spores pathogenic to man or other animals in the inanimate environment

5. Tuberculocide—A substance, or mixture of substances, that destroys or irreversibly inactivates tubercule bacilli in the inanimate environment

6. Virucide—A substance, or mixture of substances, that destroys or irreversibly inactivates viruses in the inanimate environment

ANTIMICROBIAL PESTICIDE PRODUCT EFFICACY DATA

In addition to data requirements that apply to all pesticides, all antimicrobial pesticides must have data proving their ability to kill the target pest(s). These data are known as efficacy or product performance data. According to 40 CFR Part 158 Subpart W §158.2220 Product Performance, registrants of public health antimicrobial pesticide products must submit efficacy data to support their application for registration or amendments to add public health claims, whereas registrants of nonpublic health antimicrobial pesticide products are required to generate efficacy data but not required to submit those data to EPA unless requested.

Public health disinfectants are marketed in several formulations including liquids, sprays, and towelettes, and laboratory test methods are in place to accommodate each formulation type. Standard-setting organizations such as AOAC International (AOAC)[11] and ASTM International (ASTM)[12] maintain and publish many of the recommended efficacy test methods. Laboratory testing is conducted to determine the effectiveness of the antimicrobial product to control or kill specific pest organisms when the product is used in accordance with label instructions. In some cases, effectiveness and usefulness of the proposed product is further determined through advanced large-scale laboratory tests, field tests, or simulated-use tests using test methods, which closely approximate actual use and employ typically used application equipment (eg, fumigant sterilants). Guidance documents called the *Series 810—Product Performance Guidelines: Group B*[13] have been developed and posted to assist applicants with current 40 CFR Part 158 Subpart W efficacy data requirements for each category of antimicrobial pesticide products, claims, or patterns of use. The key set of guidance documents about efficacy testing is contained in the Product Performance Test Guideline Series 810.2000 through 810.2700 (Table 72.1). The guidelines generally provide information about the 40 CFR Part 158 Subpart W testing requirements for the effectiveness of antimicrobial pesticides under FIFRA and include information pertaining to the test methodology per product formulation type, performance standards (evaluation of success), specific test organisms, soil load (organic burden) added to the inoculum, water hardness, number of testing batches,

TABLE 72.1 Organization of the OCSPP Test Guideline Series 810 for antimicrobial products[a]	
Product Performance Test Guidelines	**OCSPP Guideline Number**
General Considerations for Testing Public Health Antimicrobial Pesticides—Guidance for Efficacy Testing	810.2000
Sterilants, Sporicides, and Decontaminants—Guidance for Efficacy Testing	810.2100
Disinfectants for Use on Environmental Surfaces—Guidance for Efficacy Testing	810.2200
Sanitizers for Use on Hard Surfaces—Efficacy Data Recommendations	810.2300
Disinfectants and Sanitizers for Use on Fabrics and Textiles—Efficacy Data Recommendations	810.2400
Air Sanitizers—Efficacy Data Recommendations	810.2500
Disinfectants and Sanitizers for Use in Water—Efficacy Data Recommendations	810.2600
Products with Prion-Related Claims	810.2700

Abbreviation: OCSPP, Office of Chemical Safety and Pollution Prevention.

[a]From US Environmental Protection Agency.[14]

and limits for acceptable formulation chemistry. Requirements to develop product efficacy data, including use of standard methods and product performance standards, provide a mechanism to ensure that pesticide products will control the public health pests listed on the label and that unnecessary pesticide exposure to the environment will not occur as a result of the use of ineffective products. Guideline OCSPP 810.2000 (General Considerations for Testing Public Health Antimicrobial Pesticides) provides a directory and overview of the testing guidelines, including pertinent terminology and definitions generally used by the agency regarding different claims and uses of antimicrobial pesticides.

The following are summaries of three of the seven widely used guidelines pertaining to the testing of public health antimicrobial pesticides intended for use on inanimate surfaces:

- Guideline OCSPP 810.2100 (Sterilants, Sporicides, and Decontaminants) addresses efficacy testing for antimicrobial pesticides intended to be used on inanimate, environmental, and food packaging surfaces, which bear label claims for use as a sterilant, sporicide, and decontaminant against *Bacillus anthracis* spores, commercial sterilant for aseptic packaging of low-acid food, and/or disinfectant against *Clostridioides difficile* spores. For products bearing sterilant claims, the guidance recommends the AOAC Sporicidal Activity Method 966.04 and conditions to prove the inactivation of spores of *Bacillus subtilis* and *Clostridium sporogenes* on both hard (test carrier—porcelain penicylinders) and soft (test carrier—silk suture loops) inanimate surfaces.[15] This section also provides testing guidance for products with surface-specific sporicide claims to inactivate spores of *B subtilis* and *C sporogenes*. The guideline provides recommendations for registrants seeking a claim for additional spores such as *B anthracis* (ie, a decontaminant claim) using qualitative methods (AOAC Sporicidal Activity Method 966.04) and quantitative methods such as the AOAC Quantitative Three Step Method[16] or ASTM E2197-11: Standard quantitative disk carrier test method.[17] Efficacy testing for a hospital or health care disinfectant product with a claim to inactivate *C difficile* spores on hard, nonporous, inanimate surfaces is also referenced; separate guidance has been established for applicants seeking a *C difficile* claim.[18]

- Guideline OCSPP 810.2200 (Disinfectants for Use on Environmental Surfaces), addresses efficacy testing for antimicrobial pesticides intended to be used as disinfectants on hard, nonporous surfaces in a variety of product formulation types. Testing guidance for base disinfectant claims is provided for limited, broad-spectrum and hospital-level disinfectants. Per EPA's Pesticide Registration Manual: Chapter 4—Additional Considerations for Antimicrobial Products, and Guideline OCSPP 810.2200 (Disinfectants for Use

on Environmental Surfaces) Table 72.1, the following types of disinfectant claims are

- ○ Limited—A disinfectant that is effective against only a specific major group of microorganisms (such as gram-positive [eg, *Staphylococcus aureus*] or gram-negative [eg, *Salmonella enterica*] bacteria)
- ○ General or broad spectrum—A disinfectant that is effective against both gram-positive and gram-negative bacteria (*S aureus* and *S enterica*). General or broad-spectrum disinfectants have a wide variety of uses in residential, commercial, institutional, and other sites.
- ○ Hospital—A hospital disinfectant is a general or broad-spectrum disinfectant that is also effective against the nosocomial bacterial pathogen *Pseudomonas aeruginosa*. These disinfectants are generally for use in hospitals, clinics, dental offices, or other health care–related facilities.

- The AOAC use-dilution methods[19] are recommended for use to evaluate liquid disinfectants, whereas the AOAC germicidal spray products as disinfectants method[20] is recommended for use in testing spray formulations. The AOAC fungicidal activity of disinfectants test[21] and the AOAC in vitro test for determining tuberculocidal activity[22] are recommended to support fungicidal and tuberculocidal claims, respectively.

- Guideline OCSPP 810.2300 (Sanitizers for Use on Hard Surfaces) provides efficacy data recommendations for sanitizing products such as nonfood contact sanitizers, food contact surface sanitizers (halide and nonhalide products), food contact surface sanitizers such as towelettes, and sanitizers for urinals and toilet bowl water and in-tank sanitizers. The recommended methods include ASTM Method E1153 (Test method for efficacy of sanitizers recommended for inanimate non-food contact surfaces, designation E1153)[23] for the nonfood contact sanitizers and the AOAC Method 960.09 (Germicidal and Detergent Sanitizing Action of Disinfectants)[24] for food contact sanitizers (nonhalide products). *S aureus* and *Klebsiella pneumoniae* are the recommended test microbes used in ASTM E1153, and *Escherichia coli* and *S aureus* are used as test microbes in AOAC Method 960.09.

- Guideline OCSPP 810.2000—General Considerations for Testing Public Health Antimicrobial Pesticides (3) Test Organisms (iii) Additional Microorganisms, covers label claims for additional microbes other than the designated test microorganism(s) permitted, provided that the target microbe is likely to be present in or on the recommended use areas and surfaces, and each claim is supported with appropriate efficacy testing. If efficacy test protocols do not exist for certain microorganisms, the registrant should consult with EPA prior to testing to determine a course of action (eg, use of new or amended protocols). In such cases, the registrant should submit the proposed test protocol to EPA for review and acceptance prior to the study being conducted. Testing guidance for a number of important public health claims currently not included in the 810 Guidelines is available[25] and include claims against biofilm,[26] drug resistant *Candida auris*,[27] and efficacy of copper alloy surfaces.[28]

Information about analytical methods and procedures for pesticides and related guidance can be found on the Pesticide Analytical Methods Web site.[29] In addition to the published standards by AOAC and ASTM, specific standard operating procedures (SOPs) for many of the efficacy test methods are maintained by the EPA Microbiology Laboratory Branch (Environmental Science Center, Fort Meade, Maryland). The primary focus of this branch, under the OPP, is to standardize existing efficacy test methods and to develop and validate methods for new uses and emerging pathogens for antimicrobial products with public health claims. The laboratory is instrumental in advancing the science of antimicrobial product testing and provides technical expertise to standard-setting organizations and various agency stakeholder groups.

The EPA recognizes that novel technologies and claims associated with antimicrobial products may evolve over time and would potentially involve test methods that are not referenced in the guideline series. The EPA updates the guidelines periodically to address such changes; however, the use of new methods may occur prior to guideline updates. In these instances, new methods may be published on the EPA's web page until such time that they can be added to the guidelines. Applicants should consult with the EPA for any method modifications prior to testing.

This chapter has provided a broad summary of the regulatory and scientific requirements for registering pesticides in the US, with an emphasis on antimicrobial pesticides bearing public health claims. Before assembling an application for product registration or an amendment to a product registration, an applicant or registrant should first consider scheduling a pre-application meeting. The preapplication meeting provides an opportunity to discuss and confirm the data and labeling requirements that apply to that application. To schedule a meeting with EPA regarding the registration of antimicrobial pesticides, refer to the OPP Antimicrobials Division Contact List[30] for the Antimicrobial Division Ombudsman or the appropriate product team contact person.

REFERENCES

1. US Environmental Protection Agency. The Federal Insecticide, Fungicide, and Rodenticide Act (2012). Title 7 – Agriculture, Subchapter II, Environmental Pesticide Control. https://www.govinfo.gov/app/collection/uscode/2018/title7/chapter6/subchapterII/Sec.%20136a. 2018.

2. US Environmental Protection Agency. Protection of Environment. 40 CFR parts 150-189. e-CFR Web site. https://www.ecfr.gov/cgi-bin/text-idx?tpl=/ecfrbrowse/Title40/40tab_02.tpl. Accessed October 2019.

3. US Food and Drug Administration. Federal Food, Drug, and Cosmetic Act (FFDCA). US Food and Drug Administration Web site. https://www.fda.gov/regulatoryinformation/lawsenforcedbyfda/federalfooddrugandcosmeticactfdcact/default.htm. Accessed March 2018 .

4. Food Quality Protection Act (FQPA). Pub L No. 104-170, 110 Stat. https://www.gpo.gov/fdsys/pkg/PLAW-104publ170/pdf/PLAW-104publ170.pdf. Accessed August 1996.

5. US Environmental Protection Agency. Pesticide Registration Improvement Extension Act (PRIA 4). 2018. US Environmental Protection Agency Web site. https://www.epa.gov/pria-fees/pria-overview-and-history. Accessed July 2019.

6. US Government Publishing Office. Antimicrobial pesticide data requirements. 40 CFR §158. US Government Publishing Office Web site. https://www.gpo.gov/fdsys/granule/CFR-2014-title40-vol24/CFR-2014-title40-vol24-sec158-2201/content-detail.html. Accessed July 2014.

7. US Environmental Protection Agency. EPA pesticide registration manual. US Environmental Protection Agency Web site. https://www.epa.gov/pesticide-registration/pesticide-registration-manual. Accessed April 2017.

8. US Environmental Protection Agency. About the Office of Chemical Safety and Pollution Prevention (OCSPP). US Environmental Protection Agency Web site. https://www.epa.gov/aboutepa/about-office-chemical-safety-and-pollution-prevention-ocspp. Accessed October 2019.

9. US Environmental Protection Agency. Antimicrobial Pesticide Use Site Index. US Environmental Protection Agency Web site. https://www.epa.gov/pesticide-registration/antimicrobial-pesticide-use-site-index. Accessed October 2016.

10. US Environmental Protection Agency. Label review manual 2018. US Environmental Protection Agency Web site. https://www.epa.gov/pesticide-registration/label-review-manual. Accessed May 2019.

11. AOAC International. *The Official Methods of Analysis of AOAC International*. 21st ed. Rockville, MD: AOAC International; 2019.

12. ASTM International. *Annual Book of ASTM Standards*. West Conshohocken, PA: ASTM International; 2019.

13. US Environmental Protection Agency. Series 810—product performance test guidelines. US Environmental Protection Agency Web site. https://www.epa.gov/test-guidelines-pesticides-and-toxic-substances/series-810-product-performance-test-guidelines. Accessed October 2019.

14. US Environmental Protection Agency. Product performance test guideline, OCSPP 810.2000: general considerations for testing public health antimicrobial pesticides, guidance for efficacy testing. Regulations.gov Web site. https://www.regulations.gov/document?D=EPA-HQ-OPPT-2009-0150-0034. Accessed February 2018.

15. AOAC International. Method 966.04. Sporicidal activity of disinfectants. In: *The Official Methods of Analysis of AOAC International*. 21st ed. Rockville, MD: AOAC International; 2019.

16. AOAC International. Method 2008.05. Quantitative three step method (Efficacy of liquid sporicides against spores of *Bacillus subtilis* on a hard non-porous surface). In: *The Official Methods of Analysis of AOAC International*. 21st ed. Rockville, MD: AOAC International; 2019.

17. ASTM International. Standard quantitative disk carrier test method for determining bactericidal, virucidal, fungicidal, mycobactericidal, and sporicidal activities of chemicals, designation E 2197-11. In: *Annual Book of ASTM Standards*. West Conshohocken, PA: ASTM International; 2019.

18. US Environmental Protection Agency. Methods and guidance for testing the efficacy of antimicrobial products against spores of *Clostridium difficile* on hard non-porous surfaces. US Environmental Protection Agency Web site. https://www.epa.gov/pesticide-registration/methods-and-guidance-testing-efficacy-antimicrobial-products-against-spores. Accessed February 2019.

19. AOAC International. Methods 955.14, 955.15 and 964.02. Use-dilution methods. In: *The Official Methods of Analysis of AOAC International*. 21st ed. Rockville, MD: AOAC International; 2019.

20. AOAC International Method 961.02. Germicidal spray products as disinfectants. In: *The Official Methods of Analysis of AOAC International*. 21st ed. Rockville, MD: AOAC International; 2019.

21. AOAC International. Method 955.17. Fungicidal activity of disinfectants. In: *The Official Methods of Analysis of AOAC International*. 21st ed. Rockville, MD: AOAC International; 2019.

22. AOAC International. Method 965.12. Tuberculocidal activity of disinfectants. In: *The Official Methods of Analysis of AOAC International.* 21st ed. Rockville, MD: AOAC International; 2019.

23. ASTM International. Test method for efficacy of sanitizers recommended for inanimate non-food contact surfaces, designation E1153. In: *Annual Book of ASTM Standards.* West Conshohocken, PA: ASTM International; 2019.

24. AOAC International. Method 960.09. Germicidal and detergent sanitizing action of disinfectants. In: *The Official Methods of Analysis of AOAC International.* 21st ed. Rockville, MD: AOAC International; 2019.

25. US Environmental Protection Agency. Efficacy requirements for antimicrobial pesticides. US Environmental Protection Agency Web site. https://www.epa.gov/pesticide-registration/efficacy-requirements-antimicrobial-pesticides. Accessed August 2019.

26. US Environmental Protection Agency. Methods and guidance for testing the efficacy of antimicrobial products against biofilms on hard, non-porous surfaces. US Environmental Protection Agency Web site. https://www.epa.gov/pesticide-analytical-methods/methods-and-guidance-testing-efficacy-antimicrobial-products-against. Accessed October 2017.

27. US Environmental Protection Agency. Interim guidance for the efficacy evaluation of products for claims against *Candida auris.* US Environmental Protection Agency Web site. https://www.epa.gov/pesticide-registration/interim-guidance-efficacy-evaluation-products-claims-against-candida-auris-0. Accessed May 2017.

28. US Environmental Protection Agency. Updated draft protocol for the evaluation of bactericidal activity of hard, non-porous copper containing surface products. US Environmental Protection Agency Web site. https://www.epa.gov/pesticide-registration/updated-draft-protocol-evaluation-bactericidal-activity-hard-non-porous. Accessed May 2017.

29. US Environmental Protection Agency. Analytical methods and procedures for pesticides. US Environmental Protection Agency Web site. https://www.epa.gov/pesticide-analytical-methods. Accessed April 2019.

30. US Environmental Protection Agency. Contacts in the Office of Pesticide Programs, Antimicrobials Division. US Environmental Protection Agency Web site. https://www.epa.gov/pesticide-contacts/contacts-office-pesticide-programs-antimicrobials-division. Accessed October 2019.

Antimicrobial Surfaces

Nicola J. Irwin, Colin P. McCoy, Matthew P. Wylie, and Sean P. Gorman

Healthcare–associated infections (HAIs) constitute a major challenge for hospitals worldwide and pose a significant risk to patient health. The most recent prevalence surveys report respective HAI incidence rates of 4% and 4.5% in the US and UK health care systems and direct treatments costs of $9.8 billion and $8.1 billion in the United States and Europe, respectively.[1-4] In a recent Scotland-based study, 57.1% of all reported HAIs were attributed to lower respiratory tract infections, urinary tract infections (UTIs), and bloodstream infections, of which 28.0%, 48.7% and 25.0% of these respective infections were associated with the presence of an indwelling device.[1] Indeed, microbial colonization of hospital surfaces, and subsequent cross-contamination of infecting pathogens, is now widely accepted as a predominant source of HAIs.[5] On account of this surface "reservoir" of infection and the increasing prevalence of antibiotic-resistant bacterial strains, there has been widespread implementation of public health guidelines for hygiene control in health care settings over recent years.[6] Poor adherence to these guidelines and the reported inefficiency of cleaning and disinfection procedures to eradicate contamination have fuelled research into the development of materials with inherent antimicrobial properties for use in medical devices and general health care environments to provide an extra layer of protection from fouling pathogens.[7,8]

The focus on the surface results from the preference of bacteria to live as sessile communities, known as biofilms, rather than as free-flowing cells in suspension (see chapter 67). Indeed, many pathogens have been found to persist on surfaces for periods exceeding 5 months at concentrations sufficient for transmission and subsequent establishment of infection.[8] Biofilm development can be broadly categorized in six stages, as illustrated in Figure 73.1. Briefly, this process involves the initial reversible attachment of free-floating planktonic bacteria to a surface, after which the bacterial secretion of extracellular polymeric substances promotes a "gluing" effect at the

cell-substrate interface, leading to irreversible cellular attachment.[9-11] Accumulation of cells and continued secretion of an exopolysaccharide matrix result in formation of a diverse and highly coordinated bacterial community in which cells undergo phenotypic variation and exhibit significant resistance to external and internal stresses, such as shear flow, host defense systems, and, more importantly, antimicrobial agents. The subsequent shedding of surface layers enables dispersal and colonization of distant surfaces, facilitating the spread of infection.[12-14] Eradication of biofilm-associated infections is therefore a major challenge, with some studies highlighting the need for antibiotic concentrations up to 1000-fold higher than those used for treatment of their planktonic counterparts.[15]

In light of the escalating incidence of antibiotic-resistant bacteria, prevention of HAIs is now of paramount importance. The role of antimicrobial surfaces in preventing HAIs stems from their promising ability to inhibit microbial colonization of, for example, medical devices and health care environments such as floors, textiles, bed rails, door handles, and sinks, thereby preventing subsequent biofilm formation and, ultimately, transmission of antimicrobial-resistant pathogens.[7]

An antimicrobial surface has traditionally been described as a surface containing an antimicrobial agent that inhibits survival of microorganisms.[16] This was based on early development of contact-killing surfaces prepared from deposition of, or coating with, an antimicrobial agent such as silver or copper. McLean et al[17] were one of the first groups to show the bactericidal effects of catheter surfaces coated with a silver-copper film against *Staphylococcus aureus*, *Staphylococcus epidermidis*, and *Pseudomonas aeruginosa*. The term has since evolved to include a growing combination of surfaces that prevent bacterial colonization through both lethal and nonlethal mechanisms.[18] As modern health care continues to develop, people are living longer and health care systems are therefore faced with a growing influx of vulnerable

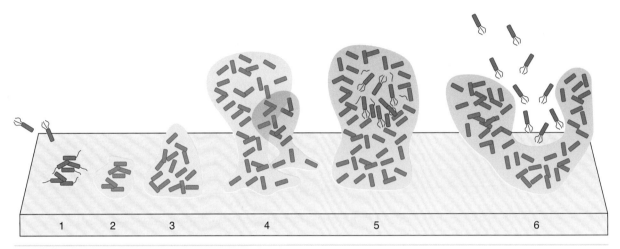

FIGURE 73.1   Illustration of six stages of biofilm development, consisting of reversible attachment (1), irreversible adhesion (2), accumulation and development (3), maturation (4), predetachment assembly (5), and detachment and dispersal of cells (6).

patients requiring treatment or repair of failing physiological functions.[19] The record numbers of hospital admissions coupled with the increasing reliance of medical devices in routine patient care make prevention of surface fouling and transmission of bacteria and other microbes of paramount importance.[20]

This chapter discusses the current development and implementation of antimicrobial surfaces in the manufacture of medical devices and high-touch surfaces as a primary mechanism of addressing the high-priority challenge of HAIs. Many of these concepts may also apply in reducing similar risks in other applications such as industrial, manufacturing, food handling, and public health situations.

▶ ANTIADHERENT SURFACES

Adhesion of bacteria to a material surface is governed by several factors, including characteristics of the adhering bacteria, such as surface charge, hydrophobicity, and the presence of surface appendages, in addition to properties of the surface itself, such as polarity, roughness, surface energy, and porosity.[21,22] Antiadherent surfaces are based on physical or chemical modifications of a material surface to reduce or eliminate the attachment of bacterial cells or other microorganisms.[23]

Superhydrophilic Surfaces

In terms of surface wettability, water contact angles between 54 and 130 degrees have been reported to be favorable for adsorption of bacterial peptidoglycan.[24] Superhydrophilic surfaces are surfaces with a water contact angle below 5 degrees. Their self-cleaning properties are attributed to the pooling and rapid spread of water

droplets, which pick up associated debris as they roll across the surface, as illustrated in Figure 73.2.[25]

Methods to increase surface hydrophilicity include plasma treatment, exposure to ultraviolet radiation, and electrochemical treatments.[26] Reductions in surface contact angles of polycarbonate surfaces from 85 to <5 degrees have been reported on coating with titanium dioxide (TiO_2) and subsequent irradiation by ultraviolet A (UVA) light.[27] In another report, hydrophilization of fibrous polystyrene substrates with air plasma treatment reduced surface contact angles to 0 degree leading to complete wetting of the surface. These superhydrophilic surfaces, with a zeta potential of -40 mV, exhibited significantly greater resistance to adherence of *Escherichia coli* than their comparatively more hydrophobic untreated and fluorinated counterparts due to a combination of electrostatic repulsion and weakened hydrophobic interactions with the gram-negative bacterial membrane lipopolysaccharides.[28] More important, the presence of repulsive surface-bound films of water on superhydrophilic substrates provides an antifouling effect by preventing hydrophobic interactions between adhering macromolecules and the underlying surface.[26]

Superhydrophobic Surfaces

In contrast to superhydrophilic surfaces, a superhydrophobic surface is defined as a surface possessing a water contact angle greater than 150 degrees and typically consists of micro- or nanoscale features inspired by the low-adhesion functionality of leaves of the lotus flower.[28] On contacting a superhydrophobic surface, a water droplet can wet the surface in one of two modes. First, the droplet can fully penetrate the groves, producing a continuous film with a contact angle dictated by physicochemical properties of the liquid-solid interface,

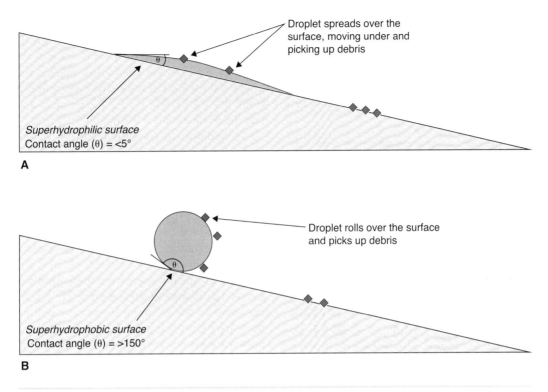

FIGURE 73.2   Illustration of water droplet wetting on self-cleaning (A) and superhydrophobic surfaces (B).

known as the Wenzel state. In the second mode, known as Cassie-Baxter wetting, the water droplet is effectively suspended on a pocket of air trapped between neighboring surface protrusions, with the corresponding contact angle dictated by properties of an additional gas-air interface in addition to the liquid-solid interface present during

Wenzel wetting.[29] Both types of surface wetting are illustrated in Figure 73.3.

In addition to water contact angles above 150 degrees, many self-cleaning superhydrophobic surfaces exhibit low contact angle hysteresis, defined as the difference between the advancing (θ_A) and receding (θ_R) contact angles of a

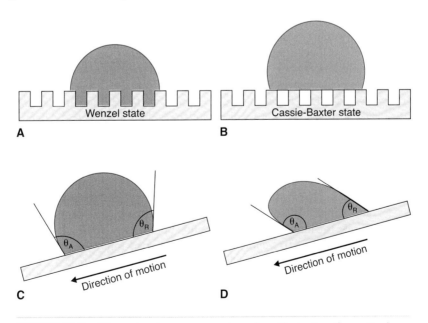

FIGURE 73.3   Water droplets on a rough surface illustrating the wetted Wenzel state (A), the Cassie-Baxter state (B), low-contact angle hysteresis (C), and high-contact angle hysteresis (D).

moving or evaporating water droplet.[30,31] Contact angle hysteresis is directly proportional to the surface retention force exerted on the droplet, and when low, as is typical of most droplets in the Cassie-Baxter state, droplets can roll and slide over the surface with little resistance at low tilt angles, collecting surface debris, and other particulate matter as they pass.[32]

The design and synthesis of self-cleaning superhydrophobic surface analogues mimicking the nonfouling nanoarchitectures of highly water-repellant plant leaves, such as the lotus leaf, has been aided by the parallel investigation of mechanisms responsible for their self-cleaning effects and the associated development of advanced nanofabrication methods, including reactive-ion beam etching, nanoimprint lithography, and laser ablation.[33] By studying the dynamics of droplet impaction on biomimetic hierarchical surfaces fabricated using the *Tobacco mosaic virus*, McCarthy et al[34] have experimentally demonstrated the role of the surface nanoscale features in providing high antiwetting capillary pressures and the distinct, yet complementary, role of surface microstructures in pressure dissipation, thereby impeding transition to a fully wetted state.[35]

Although superhydrophobic surfaces have gained much attention for their self-cleaning properties, particularly regarding their lotus-like ability to remove particulate matter, in light of the escalating incidence of antimicrobial resistance and the toxic properties of many biocides, there has been increasing interest in understanding the potential of these surfaces to resist contamination and therefore help combat HAIs when used in health care environments.[36,37] In studies conducted to date, however, the inherent microbiological resistance of these surfaces have been found to vary widely. For instance, bioinspired highly rough films of silicone elastomer with water contact angles of 165 degrees, prepared via an aerosol-assisted chemical vapor deposition process, achieved modest reductions in adherence of *E coli* and *S aureus* of 38% and 63%, respectively, relative to dip-coated glass controls. Despite a lower overall degree of contact between the elastomer and aqueous bacterial suspensions as a result of the Cassie-Baxter wetting state of the superhydrophobic surface, colonization continued to proceed at the tips of the surface protrusions.[37] In addition, although adhesion of *P aeruginosa* was completely inhibited on two-tier microscale- and nanoscale-patterned superhydrophobic titanium surfaces with water contact angles of 166 degrees, fabricated by laser ablation to mimic the lotus leaf topography, increased colonization of *S aureus* was reported relative to the unmodified smooth surfaces.[38] Indeed, the selective antifouling behavior observed in this study highlights the need for further investigation of the mechanisms controlling bacterial attachment to surfaces to more fully understand factors governing the antiadhesive properties of biomimetic superhydrophobic surfaces. Moreover, the finite sustainability of the Cassie-Baxter state of the

wetting as a result of diffusion of the air pockets into water upon exposure to conditions of high hydrostatic pressure, temperature, humidity, or shear flow limits their potential utility in, for example, nonfouling marine applications or implanted medical devices. The corresponding transition from the metastable Cassie-Baxter state to the Wenzel state leads to complete wetting of the surface.[35,39]

In addition to physical texturing of the surface as a mechanism to engineer superhydrophobic surfaces, functionalization of polyvinyl chloride with low surface energy fluorinated compounds has generated interest for the development of superhydrophobic surfaces inhibiting the early stages of bacterial adhesion and ultimately preventing biofilm formation on medical devices, such as endotracheal tubes.[40] Longevity of the nonfouling properties of superhydrophobic surfaces remains an issue due to masking of the low-energy functionalized surface groups and/or the change in surface structure resulting from attachment of conditioning layers of macromolecules and proteins.[41] One example relates to the heavy surface fouling of roughened superhydrophobic polysiloxane surfaces by macroalgae, bryozoans, and barnacles observed after only 2 months immersion in seawater in contrast to their high resistance to fouling over a 6-month period of exposure to mixed cultures of naturally occurring microfoliant when submerged in tap water.[42] Exposure to shear flow has been reported as an efficacious method of removing surface-adsorbed protein from nanoscale-roughened surfaces; however, this is not a feasible approach in many applications.[43] Therefore, although superhydrophobic surfaces exhibit promising potential for short-term antifouling applications or in situations where periodic resurfacing can be facilitated, further investigation of their antifouling behavior over extended periods is needed to increase longevity of their self-cleaning properties.[42]

Slippery Liquid-Infused Porous Surfaces

A novel self-cleaning surface inspired by the Nepenthes pitcher plant has recently been developed, possessing similar textured features to those of superhydrophobic surfaces. Instead of trapping air within the grooves of the surface, however, the nano- and microstructured features entrap lubricating liquid to create self-healing, slippery liquid-infused porous surfaces (SLIPS).[44,45] These SLIPS demonstrate extreme temperature and pressure stability and superior antiwetting behavior in comparison to their air-entrapped microtextured counterparts.[44] The infused lubricant becomes locked in place through cohesive forces, as illustrated in Figure 73.4.

Stability of SLIPS has been found to be dependent on three key criteria. First, the affinity of the porous substrate to the lubricating liquid must be greater than the affinity of the surface to the liquid to be repelled. Second, the lubricant must be able to infiltrate, wet and robustly adhere

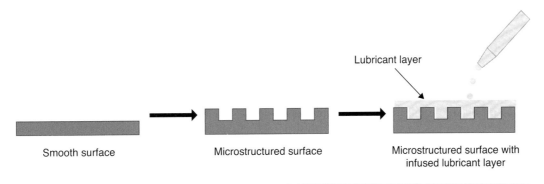

FIGURE 73.4 Illustration of the preparation of slippery liquid-infused porous surfaces (SLIPS) by infusion of a porous or microstructured surface with a chemically inert, low-surface energy lubricant to form a smooth and chemically homogeneous lubricating layer.

to the substrate and, third, the lubricating liquid must be immiscible with the repellant fluids.[46] In contrast to superhydrophobic, lotus leaf–inspired, Cassie-Baxter–type surfaces, which conventionally favor multitiered, hierarchical structures for improved robustness and pressure tolerance, enhanced stability to high-simulated shear and robust nonfouling properties have been observed on uniformly nanostructured SLIPS surfaces. This phenomenon has been attributed to the formation of a stable smooth overcoating of lubricant as a result of the comparatively smaller length scales of the nanotextured structures than the capillary length of the lubricant layer. Even at high spin speeds of 10 000 rpm, where this layer was compressed under gravitational forces to approximately 400 nm, surfaces with nanoscale features approximately 170 nm tall exhibited no signs of deterioration in antiwetting performance.[47]

To date, SLIPS have primarily been investigated for potential application as anti-icing coatings, with only limited assessment of their antibiofouling properties.[47,48] One such study reported the resistance of water-repellent slippery surfaces of microporous poly(butyl methacrylate-co-ethylene glycol dimethacrylate) (BMA-EDMA) infused with a selection of fluorocarbon lubricants, including Krytox 103 and Krytox 100, to attachment of marine microorganisms, namely zoospores of the alga *Ulva linza* and cypris larvae of the barnacle *Balanus amphitrite*.[49] Furthermore, attachment of *P aeruginosa* biofilm was reduced by up to 99.6% on SLIPS prepared from porous Teflon™ membranes with perfluorinated lubricating fluids relative to porous polytetrafluoroethylene (PTFE) membrane controls, based on crystal violet absorbance, following a 7-day challenge period in infected flow cells. Adherence of *S aureus* and *E coli* to the SLIPS was reduced by 97.2% and 96%, respectively, in comparison to PTFE controls over 48 hours under identical flow conditions.[50] Similarly, Li et al[51] demonstrated resistance of BMA-EDMA SLIPS to biofilm formation of various strains of opportunistic *P aeruginosa* for up to 7 days in low-nutrient medium. After a 7-day incubation period, 1.8% and approximately 55% of the surfaces of slippery BMA-EDMA and uncoated glass

controls, respectively, were covered by the *P aeruginosa* PA49 strain.[51] With regard to their potential application in antimicrobial medical devices, Leslie et al[52] have reported antithrombogenic and potent antibiofouling properties of medical tubing modified with SLIPS technology, specifically a tethered liquid perfluorocarbon (TLP) surface. More important, an 8-fold reduction in *P aeruginosa* biofilm formation was reported on TLP-coated loops relative to control tubing after more than 6 weeks incubation in a continuous flow model.[52]

The SLIPS technology undoubtedly holds promising potential for preventing biofilm formation by common bacterial pathogens; however, careful consideration of factors such as the type of lubricant, substrate, durability, and the degree and pattern of surface roughness is required for development of an efficacious SLIPS to prevent contamination while remaining nontoxic to patients.[51]

Antiadherent Strategies Based on Bacterial Targets

Bacterial colonization and subsequent biofilm formation is controlled by a plethora of structural and signaling pathways that have, to date, provided key targets for the action of many conventional antibiotics. On a structural level, bacterial appendages, such as pili and flagella, are important in the anchoring of bacteria to a solid surface, whereas macromolecules, such as enzymes and proteins, are involved in the signaling and regulation of crucial steps during biofilm formation, cell aggregation, swarming, and exopolysaccharide production, in a process of quorum sensing (QS).[53]

A rationale strategy for development of antiadhesive surfaces would therefore involve interference with structural and operational targets of bacteria, for example, by immobilization of inhibitors to facilitate downregulation of key processes involved in bacterial attachment and propagation.[54] Covalent immobilization of virstatin, a small molecule which interferes with the formation of type IV bacterial pili, onto silanized surfaces of silicone was shown to reduce adhesion of *Acinetobacter baumannii* by up to 46% relative to silanized controls after 4 hours incubation.[55] Similarly, covalent attachment of the QS inhibitors, dihydropyrrolones, onto glass substrates reduced adherence of *P aeruginosa* and *S aureus* by up to 97% in comparison to untreated controls. Immobilized dihydropyrrolones could disrupt QS of *P aeruginosa* by interference with the *N*-acyl homoserine lactone–mediated *las* QS system, as demonstrated by the observed repression of a *lasB-gfp* reporter protein of *P aeruginosa* in vitro.[56] This approach has been extended further by combining quorum-quenching and matrix-degrading enzymes into urinary catheter coatings. The enzymes acylase and α-amylase, which degrade bacterial QS molecules and biofilm exopolysaccharides, respectively, were incorporated into multilayer coatings on silicone catheters and challenged with single-species infections of *S aureus* and *P aeruginosa*, and mixed-cultures of *P aeruginosa* and *E coli* in a catheterized bladder model. In dynamic bladder model conditions, coatings with acylase deposited as the outermost layer demonstrated comparatively higher efficacy against clinically relevant gram-negative pathogens, with reductions in biofilm mass of 70%, 50%, and 15%, relative to uncoated controls, after 7 days incubation with *P aeruginosa*, dual-species *P aeruginosa* and *E coli*, and *S aureus* challenges, respectively. In contrast, coatings with amylase as the outermost layer were most active against the gram-positive bacteria, with reductions in biofilm formation of 30% and 10% when infected with *S aureus* and *P aeruginosa*, respectively. Furthermore, after 7 days in an in vivo rabbit model, coatings with acylase as the outermost layer reduced biofilm formation by up to 70% on the balloon portion of the catheter and delayed the spread of biofilm along the inner side of the catheter shaft by 30% in comparison to uncoated silicone controls.[57] These encouraging in vivo results, coupled with the absence of toxicity to human cells in vitro, demonstrate the promising potential of this enzyme-integrated strategy for antifouling medical device coatings.

An increased knowledge and understanding of the bacterial components involved in surface adhesion and regulation of biofilm development, and the associated identification of new molecular targets, is expected to further fuel developments in this area of target-based antifouling surfaces.[58]

Polymer Brushes

Polymer brushes are assemblies of polymer chains tethered at one end to a surface or interface, through covalent attachment or physical adsorption, with sufficient density that the polymer chains stretch away from the surface into the surrounding aqueous medium.[59] Compression of the highly hydrated polymer layer on bacterial approach generates a repulsive osmotic force which, in combination with the reduction in conformational entropy, can significantly reduce particle deposition, bacterial attachment, and resultant surface adhesion, as shown in Figure 73.5.[60]

Polymer chains can be tethered to the surface via the "grafting to" or "grafting from" technique. In the former method, polymerized chains with reactive end-groups, for example, carboxylic, amino, or thiol groups, are attached to a polymer substrate; however, grafting density is limited by the steric barrier generated by previously tethered chains toward the incoming macromolecules. Conversely, in the latter method, polymer chains are grown via surface-initiated polymerization from a substrate functionalized with polymerization initiators, which typically facilitates higher grafting densities and film thicknesses.[59,61]

A common method of producing a polymer brush surface is through a process known as (PEG)ylation, whereby chains of the polymer, PEG, are grafted onto a surface to prevent protein adsorption and cell adhesion.[62] With respect to their antimicrobial abilities, PEGylated surfaces have demonstrated efficacy in delaying biofilm formation of staphylococci and enabling more facile removal of attached biofilm under shear flow.[63]

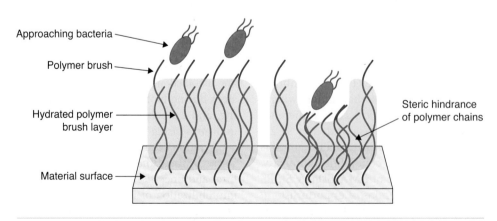

FIGURE 73.5 Hydrated polymer brush surface preventing bacterial adhesion by steric and osmotic repulsion.

Reduced adhesion of *S epidermidis, P aeruginosa, Candida albicans,* and *Candida tropicalis* has been observed on surfaces grafted with PEG chains of molecular weights of 526, 2000, and 9800 Da and corresponding chain lengths of 2.8, 7.5, and 23.7 nm, respectively, relative to pristine glass slides. The effect of molecular weight on adherence was found to be most significant for the smaller bacterial cells than the larger yeast cells, with comparable adhesion of *C albicans* observed between all three brush lengths, and reduced attachment of *S epidermidis* and *P aeruginosa* reported on the longer brushes than on the 2.8 nm brush, as a result of the greater distance of separation from the surface and the corresponding attenuation of the long-range Lifshitz-van der Waals attractions.[64,65] Al-Ani et al[66] have explored the effect of PEG chain grafting density on adherence of proteins, bacteria, and cells by employing different concentrations of the surface initiator, (3-aminopropyl)triethoxysilane, and grafting PEG in solutions of varying salt conditions. The authors observed that adsorption of proteins and human MG63 osteoblast-like and mesenchymal cells was minimal on high polymer density surfaces but increased in a surface- and cell-dependent manner at low and medium grafting densities. With regard to bacterial adherence, attachment of *P aeruginosa* showed a clear relationship with PEG chain density and, accordingly, the high-density PEG layers demonstrated the highest fouling resistance.[66]

In addition to PEG, polymer brush designs based on neutral hydrophilic polymers, including polyacrylamide and poly(2-alkyl-2-oxazoline), have demonstrated promising abilities to resist protein and bacterial adhesion in vitro.[60] Alternatively, zwitterionic polymers, such as poly(2-methacryloyloxyethyl phosphorylcholine), poly(sulfobetaine methacrylate) (PSBMA), poly(*N*4-(2-methacrylamidoethyl) asparagine) (pAspAA), and poly(*N*5-(2-methacrylamidoethyl)glutamine) (pGluAA), have been employed as candidates in the development of nonfouling polymer brush surfaces.[60,67,68] A UV-induced graft polymerization of zwitterionic PSBMA onto hydrophobic microporous polypropylene membranes (MPPMs) at a surface density of 560 $\mu g/cm^2$ enhanced surface hydrophilicity, characterized by a decrease in water contact angle from 145 to 15 degrees. The observed significant reduction in fouling by bovine serum albumin and lysine was attributed to steric repulsion from the hydrated polymer chains on approach of proteins to the surface. Additionally, PSBMA-modified MPPMs completely inhibited adhesion of *E coli, Pseudomonas fluorescens,* and *S aureus* over a 3 hour incubation period.[69]

Current research is aimed at designing bifunctional polymer brush coatings, via the localization of antimicrobial agents onto the polymer chain ends, in an effort to optimize their inherent antiadhesive properties and impart the polymers with lethal activity. For example, the conjugation of an optimized series of antimicrobial peptides (AMPs) to amine-functionalized polymer chains on titanium substrates demonstrated that, despite a possible alteration in the bactericidal mechanism of the AMPs following polymer chain immobilization, broad-spectrum antimicrobial activities were retained. The degree of resistance to bacterial adherence was dependent on the specific conjugated peptide but, in all cases, exceeded that of control copolymer brushes devoid of AMPs, both in vitro and in vivo. Furthermore, the coatings were nontoxic to mammalian cells, compatible with human serum, and displayed antimicrobial properties that could be readily optimized through modification of the copolymer composition and grafting density.[70] Alternatively, a high-efficiency antibacterial surface, demonstrating both antiadherent and microbicidal activities toward *Actinomyces naeslundii* and *E coli,* has been developed through conjugation of the antimicrobial triclosan to zwitterionic PSBMA polymer brushes on a silicone substrate.[71]

Polymer brush surfaces could therefore act as useful "carrier platforms" for antimicrobial agents, with potential benefits of long-term stability, improved biocompatibility of tethered agents, and robustness, in addition to their inherent antiadhesive properties.

▶ ACTIVE STRATEGIES

Active, or bactericidal, surfaces possess the ability to physically or chemically disrupt cells leading to their death, either before or shortly after attachment to the surface.[72]

Antibiotic-Incorporated Surfaces

Many early release-based systems were developed via impregnation of surfaces with antimicrobial agents. These first-generation coatings typically exhibit first- or second-order release kinetics, characterized by an initial burst release of drug followed by a much slower rate of prolonged release. A combination of rifampicin and minocycline in urinary catheter coatings has been found to successfully reduce gram-positive bacteriuria, and, with the addition of chlorhexidine, broad-spectrum coverage against gram-positive and gram-negative bacteria, and fungi, has been reported during short-term implantation of antimicrobial-coated central venous catheters.[73,74] In addition, gentamicin-loaded polymer bone cements have been well described in the literature, and a review of these products has shown their characteristic matrix-style release properties, with a high initial burst release during the first few hours of surface wetting, after which the rate of release significantly declines.[75] Although this release profile is beneficial during the critical first few hours postimplantation, infection-resistance may be required for several weeks or months to facilitate implant-tissue integration as well as providing antimicrobial cover during checkup or resection procedures. Initial attempts to improve the release kinetics of these first-generation coatings typically involved promotion of polymer-antibiotic or antibiotic-antibiotic interactions within polymer matrices to retard release. For example, Piozzi et al[76] loaded a series of acidic and basic polyurethanes with antibiotics containing at least one acidic functional group, including amoxicillin, cefamandole nafate, rifampicin, and vancomycin. Similarly, Ruggeri et al[77] reported synergistic effects of polyurethane-loaded rifampicin and cefamandole nafate against rifampicin-resistant *S aureus* and, moreover, when formulated with the pore-former PEG 10 000, activity was maintained for up to 23 days.

Drawbacks of these first-generation device coatings, mainly related to their suboptimal release kinetics, have limited their widespread application. The burst release of antibiotic, which is followed by a slower and irregular release of drug, can allow bacteria to invade and recolonize a surface, with additional concerns surrounding potential promotion of antibiotic resistance due to prolonged exposure of bacteria to subtherapeutic concentrations. This has recently been observed for gentamicin-loaded bone cements, with some infected orthopedic implants positive for growth of gentamicin-resistant strains.[78] Additionally, many of the release systems suffer from poor overall release, with <10% of loaded antibiotic eventually released from some bone cements, and one study reporting subtherapeutic concentrations of gentamicin in joint aspirates 25 years after the primary total hip arthroplasty procedure.[79,80] These limitations have led to the development of second-generation release coatings with more sophisticated release profiles. Examples include erodible polymer matrices for sustained release of antibiotics and polyelectrolyte multilayers fabricated via layer-by-layer (LbL) deposition techniques for bioresponsive, bacteria-triggered antimicrobial release.[81-83]

Alternatively, the use of cyclic exposure regimens in contrast to conventional coadministration has been shown in recent research to allow continuous exposure to antibiotics with compatible collateral bacterial sensitivities but without the development of resistance.[84] Although this type of release strategy has not yet been reported for nonfouling coatings, polymeric coatings with the ability to sequentially release gentamicin and two growth factors have previously been developed to aid implant integration, and alternating release profiles have been obtained using erodible multilayers or conducting polymers, making collateral sensitivity cycling a potentially feasible strategy for future antimicrobial coatings.[85-87]

Antimicrobial Peptide-Incorporated Surfaces

In addition to the wide variety of loading mechanisms, a diverse range of active agents have been employed, in particular to mitigate the escalating incidence of antimicrobial resistance. In this regard, AMPs (see chapter 26), with their broad-spectrum of activity, including multidrug resistant strains, and reduced risk of promoting bacterial resistance, have gained attention as a potential successor to conventional antibiotics in the treatment and prevention of bacterial infections.[88] AMPs are produced by all living organisms and serve to boost innate immunity as well as provide an immediate lethal response to invading microorganisms.[89] Similar to antibiotics, AMPs have been incorporated into medical device coatings or surfaces to provide antimicrobial cover through sustained release. Incorporation of the positively charged AMP, ponericin G1, into a hydrolytically degradable polyelectrolyte multilayer coating of poly(β-amino ester) and alginic acid was found to completely inhibit attachment of *S aureus* over 2 hour challenge periods due to localized release of active peptide. Furthermore, complexation of the AMPs with the polyanions was postulated to protect mammalian cell lines of NIH 3T3 embryonic murine fibroblasts and human umbilical vein endothelial cells from the cytotoxic effects observed with concentrated solutions of ponericin G1, resulting from interactions of free AMPs with cell membranes.[90]

An alternative mechanism of combatting unwanted cytotoxic effects of AMP-releasing systems involves surface-tethering of AMPs. Because the antibacterial activity of AMPs is attributed to penetration of bacterial membranes, ready accessibility of peptides to their target sites, for example, through use of long spacer molecules, is a critical parameter for effective surface activity.[91] The decreased antimicrobial activity of surface-immobilized AMPs in comparison to their free peptide counterparts observed in some early studies was attributed to steric hindrance from neighboring peptide chains and/or insufficient concentrations of surface-bound AMPs.[92,93] Similarly, Hilpert et al[94] showed a positive correlation between increased concentrations of a series of AMPs tethered to a cellulose surface and their corresponding antimicrobial performance. The orientation of surface-tethered peptides has, in addition, been shown to directly affect their antimicrobial activity. Li et al[95] studied the effect of immobilization of the AMP, MSI-78 (an analogue of the peptide magainin), via the N-terminus or the C-terminus, nMSI-78 and MSI-78n, respectively, on their corresponding structure and behavior. After coupling with alkyne-terminated silane surfaces, the azido-MSI-78 derivatives were observed to form α-helical conformations, however, with different orientations. The nMSI-78 structures adhered in a perpendicular, "standing-up" orientation to the silane surface, whereas the C-terminus tethered peptides ran parallel to the surface in a "lying-down" pose. Although both surface-tethered derivatives killed 100% of adsorbed *S aureus* and *E coli* cells within 60 minutes of exposure, surfaces with the perpendicular nMSI-78 arrangement demonstrated a significantly more rapid response, killing >70% of *E coli* cells within 30 minutes compared to the absence of dead cells observed on the MSI-78n-immobilized surfaces within this same period.[95]

This study therefore provides important insights to inform rational engineering of AMP-tethered surfaces with optimal antibacterial activities.

Metal-Incorporated Surfaces

The use of metals to treat bacterial infections can be dated back to the 16th century when Paracelsus recommended mercurial salts for the treatment of syphilis in place of the more conventionally prescribed botanical medicines.[96] Although largely underresearched during the heights of antibiotic discovery in the mid-1900s, the antibacterial properties of silver and copper have regained interest on account of the reported reductions in efficacy of many conventional antibiotics toward common nosocomial pathogens in combination with the decline in discovery of new antibiotic agents.[97,98] Indeed, the potent antimicrobial activity of these metals against both gram-positive and gram-negative bacteria, and fungi, has been confirmed in numerous studies; however, the cumulative mechanisms of this activity are not completely understood.[99-101] Previous research has shown that their antibacterial activity is likely exerted through the generation of positively charged metal ions that possess an affinity for negatively charged components of microbial cells; this allows for the binding of metal ions to critical structures, such as proteins or DNA, and leads to interference with membrane permeability, interactions with nucleic acids and other components of the cytoplasm, and inactivation of vital enzymes, namely respiratory chain enzymes.[102] Subsequently, cells suffer oxidative stress and/or interruption of key cellular processes. The multifaceted activity of these compounds and their ability to target numerous cellular components make it difficult for bacteria to not only develop resistance to these agents but also to withstand their effects.[98]

Silver has, to date, had a largely controversial role in the prevention of infections related to indwelling devices, such as urinary catheters, intravenous catheters, and endotracheal tubes, based on conflicting findings surrounding the efficacy of silver oxide and silver alloy biomaterial coatings.[17,103-105] A Cochrane Review reported a reduced incidence of asymptomatic bacteriuria with the use of silver alloy catheters for short-term (less than 1 wk) catheterization periods but called for more evidence of their usefulness against symptomatic catheter-associated urinary tract infections (CAUTIs).[106] More important, in a UK multicenter randomized controlled trial by Pickard et al,[107] 12.6% and 12.5% of participants allocated control and silver alloy-coated catheters, respectively, developed symptomatic UTIs, thus providing no support for routine use of these catheters.

A major application of these metals in recent years has been in the fabrication of fomites capable of preventing cross-contamination in hospital wards. Weinstein and

Hota[108] has previously highlighted the significant role played by inanimate objects within hospital environments in contamination and transmission of nosocomial pathogens. In a recent systematic review evaluating the efficacy of numerous antimicrobial surfaces in clinical environments, including bed rails, privacy curtains, and textiles, copper surfaces were found to achieve a median less than 1 log reduction of microbial contamination in a total of seven studies.[109] Two studies have assessed the effect of copper surfaces on two additional outcomes of clinical relevance, including the incidence of HAI and transmission of antibiotic-resistant organisms. The use of copper alloy surfaces on six highly touched items in intensive care units was found to achieve a 58% relative reduction in HAI ($P = .013$) and a 64% relative reduction in transmission of antibiotic-resistant pathogens ($P = .063$) over an 11-month period in a randomized control trial.[110] A 24% reduction in HAIs per 1000 hospitalization days was reported with the use of copper oxide–impregnated textiles, such as bed linen and patient gowns, in comparison to standard materials in a long-term care ward from an uncontrolled before-after study.[111] The poor design, blinding, and randomization of these two studies does, however, limit the quality of this evidence and uncertainty remains regarding the usefulness of copper surfaces in prevention of HAIs or transmission of pathogens.[109]

A comparatively lower number of studies have been conducted to evaluate the efficacy of other noncopper-containing antimicrobial surfaces in clinical settings. Mixed results have been found with the use of organosilane-treated surfaces, with one study reporting a 3 log reduction in microbial contamination and a second study demonstrating no effect from these surfaces.[112,113] With regard to silver, a mean reduction in bacterial adherence of 94.8% was demonstrated on a range of silver-treated items in a single study room compared to comparator untreated products in the control environment of a long-term care facility.[114]

Alternatively, metals such as silver, copper, and zinc oxide in the form of inorganic nanoparticles (NPs) have been found to demonstrate pronounced bactericidal properties at relatively low concentrations as a result of their high surface area to volume ratios, and, as such, nanocomposite materials have emerged as a new generation of nonfouling surfaces.[101,115] These materials may be prepared by plasma-assisted grafting of the antibacterial moieties onto the surface in a two-step process, comprising an initial plasma pretreatment to activate the surface followed by immersion into NP solutions for incorporation of the actives. In addition to inherent properties of the surfaces themselves, including morphology and chemical composition, the efficiency of NP loading and resultant bactericidal activity have been found to be highly dependent on NP properties such as shape, size, and type.[116,117] Several attempts have been made to immobilize antimicrobial NPs onto hydrogel or polymer surfaces for medical device applications.[118-121] Initial approaches have predominately focused on immersion of polymeric materials in concentrated solutions of silver ions, with application of a reducing agent to form metallic NPs, which subsequently deposit on the polymer surface. Maneerung et al[122] were one of the first groups to report this method for the development of silver NP–impregnated bacterial cellulose wound dressings.[112] The NP-impregnated dressings achieved 99.7% and 99.9% reductions in viable counts of *E coli* and *S aureus*, respectively, after 24 hours incubation. In contrast, viable counts for the pure bacterial cellulose dressing increased by 34.6% and 40.7%, respectively.[122] Dubas et al[123] employed a LbL deposition technique to immobilize silver NPs on silk and nylon fibers, with reductions in *S aureus* of 50% and 80% after 24 hours contact with the 20-layer coated nylon and silk, respectively. Furthermore, the development of antimicrobial paints containing silver NPs provides a universal method of instilling wood, glass, metal, and polymer surfaces with antimicrobial properties.[124-126] In addition to silver NPs, NPs of copper or copper oxide, zinc oxide, and selenium have been employed in the development of antimicrobial surfaces over recent years.[127-132]

Despite the promising activities reported to date, toxicological issues and concerns over systemic metal accumulation will have to be addressed before their widespread application in health care environments.[133,134]

▶ STIMULI-RESPONSIVE ANTIMICROBIAL SURFACES

Conventional release-based systems are typically characterized by monotonic and physiologically insensitive release of potentially subtherapeutic levels of bioactive agents, prolonged periods of which may contribute to the serious phenomenon of emerging antibiotic resistance. In an attempt to overcome these limitations, the intrinsic ability of bioresponsive biomaterials to change their mechanical or physicochemical properties in response to a variety of environmental stimuli, including temperature, light, ultrasound, magnetic and electric fields, pH, and enzymes, has recently been exploited in the development of "smart" surfaces.[135,136]

pH-Responsive Surfaces

pH-responsive systems have been engineered to exploit local bacterial-induced acidification and alkalinization processes. The attractiveness of these systems stems from their self-regulating and infection-responsive characteristics, thereby requiring no external control or activation.[137] In the context of HAIs, reference must

be made to the elevation of urine pH typically reported at the onset of CAUTIs by urease-secreting pathogens, for example, *Proteus mirabilis*. This pH elevation, from normal values of approximately pH 6.1 to levels up to pH 8.61, results from the urease-catalyzed hydrolysis of urea to ammonia and has recently been investigated as a trigger for antimicrobial release in the development of contamination-tolerant, drug-eluting urinary catheter coatings.[138-140] In contrast to exploiting infection-induced pH changes to trigger release of active agents, Lu et al[141] have explored the effects of pH-triggered changes in hydrophobicity and charge of poly(2-alkylacrylic acid)s on *S epidermidis* viability in the design of responsive, non-drug-eluting antibacterial polymers. Bactericidal activities of single-component LbL hydrogel thin films of poly(2-ethylacrylic acid), poly(2-*n*-propylacrylic acid) and poly(2-*n*-butylacrylic acid) were switched on upon acidification of the media by bacterial-secreted lactic acid as a result of pH-induced hydrophilic-to-hydrophobic transitions of the coatings.

Temperature-Responsive Surfaces

Recently, surfaces have been developed with biocidal activity that can be triggered in response to changes in temperature. For example, He et al[142] have recently developed thermo-responsive and regenerable antibacterial coatings based on silver NP–loaded copolymers of *N*-isopropylacrylamide (NIPAAm) and sodium acrylate (AANa) with robust bactericidal activity toward *E coli* and *S aureus*. At temperatures below the lower critical solution temperature of poly(NIPAAm) (PNIPAAm), expansion of the polymer network resulted in an increase in surface hydrophilicity and subsequent detachment of dead bacteria from the surface, whereas long-lasting antibacterial properties were achieved by repeated silver NP releasing-reloading cycles of the modified membranes.[142]

Light-Responsive Surfaces

Light has been exploited to eradicate drug-resistant bacteria with no promotion of resistance in the method of photodynamic antimicrobial chemotherapy (PACT), which involves the photoactivation of photosensitizers, in particular porphyrins, to generate reactive oxygen species (ROS), such as hydroxyl radicals and singlet oxygen.[143] Singlet oxygen, in particular, causes irreparable damage to cell walls and membranes of bacteria, fungi, and viruses, ultimately compromising their barrier function and leading to microbial cell death.[144,145] In addition, the majority of the cyclic tetrapyrrole-based macrocycle photosensitizers, including chlorin, porphyrins, and phthalocyanine derivatives, show minimal toxicity in the absence of light, presumably due to their inherent similarity to naturally occurring porphyrins in living tissue.[146]

The use of photosensitizers in PACT to eradicate infections of the skin and mouth has led several groups to investigate the incorporation of photosensitizers into surfaces to confer light-activated antimicrobial properties. McCoy et al[147] were one of the first groups to explore this concept for combatting intraocular lens infections by incorporating the porphyrin, tetrakis(4-N-methylpyridyl) porphyrin (TMPyP), into copolymers of 2-hydroxyethyl methacrylate with methacrylic acid or 2-(diethylamino) ethylmethacrylate. The broad-spectrum efficacy of the TMPyP-incorporated hydrogels was demonstrated by the significant reductions in surface adherence of S epidermidis, S aureus, P aeruginosa, and P mirabilis of up to 99% achieved on exposure to intense white light conditions relative to control copolymers.[147,148]

The phenothiazinium dyes, toluidine blue O (TBO) and methylene blue (MB), are potent photosensitive antimicrobial agents, displaying bactericidal, fungicidal, and spore inactivation properties on irradiation with white or red wavelength light sources due to their efficient generation of singlet oxygen.[149,150] Perni et al[151] reported greater than 4 log reductions in S aureus and E coli on gold NP and TBO- or MB-containing silicone and polyurethane surfaces within 3 minutes exposure to red laser light. The improved performance of dual photosensitizer- and nanogold-containing surfaces in comparison to sole photosensitizer-incorporated surfaces was attributed to the gold NP-induced increase in excited triplet state molecules in addition to the reduced tendency for loss of energy through nonphototoxic fluorescence pathways, thus highlighting the promising potential of photosensitizer-metallic NP complexes for self-sterilizing surfaces.[152,153] In contrast to the previous physical incorporation of photosensitizer molecules, covalent attachment of TBO and MB to modified silicone surfaces was shown to provide similar protection against bacterial adherence, with up to 5 log reductions in surface-localized S epidermidis and E coli reported after 4 minutes exposure to a low-power red laser but, more important, with much lower concentrations of photosensitizer.[154] Covalent attachment of the anthraquinone derivative, 2-(1-bromoethyl)-anthraquinone, to ethylene-acrylic acid films at a surface concentration of 35% wt/wt was demonstrated to reduce Bacillus cereus spore viability by 60% in comparison to inert low-density polyethylene control films when irradiated for 10 minutes with low-power UVA light.[155] Furthermore, broad-spectrum antibacterial activity of cellulosic materials, including paper and cotton fabrics, with covalently grafted porphyrins, has been demonstrated against S aureus and E coli on illumination with visible light. Use of these porphyrin-cellulosic materials in biomedical areas, for example, in antimicrobial patient gowns and bed curtains, offers promising potential for reducing the spread of HAIs.[156,157]

Although the aforementioned approaches have displayed promising antibacterial activity, factors such as the additional cost, ease of solvent recovery, and reproducibility of the photosensitizer-grafting process must be considered before scale-up, transfer, and widespread use of the technology in health care applications.[158] In this regard, an advantage of porphyrin-based photosensitizers is their ability to be used as building blocks for the manufacture of conjugated microporous polymers (CMPs) on account of their structural rigidity and planar geometry. Hynek et al[159] synthesized a series of porphyrin-based CMPs, which generated significant singlet oxygen throughout the polymer. In a similar approach by Wang et al,[160] honeycomb-like porphyrin-based polymer films of Mn(III) meso-tetra(4-sulfonatophenyl)porphine chloride (MnTPPS) dimethyldioctadecylammonium bromide (DODMABr) complexes yielded comparatively higher levels of singlet oxygen than their nonporous MnTPPS-DODMABr film counterparts. Respective reductions in E coli on 60 minutes exposure of the honeycomb films to visible light and dark conditions were 83% and 5%, whereas reductions of 43% and 7% were achieved on 60 minutes incubation of the nonporous thin films under light and in the dark, respectively.[160] This one-step photosensitizer incorporation process provides a convenient and efficient method for the production of active, noneluting, photoresponsive surfaces. Similarly, TBO-incorporated high-density polyethylene (HDpE) films have recently been prepared by a facile hot-melt extrusion process. The observed logarithmic reductions of up to 3.62 and 1.51 in surface adherence of methicillin-resistant S aureus and E coli, respectively, after 2 hours light irradiation in comparison to HDpE dark controls highlight their potential as efficacious antimicrobial materials, or coatings, for medical devices, health care equipment, handrails, counter tops, or finger-plates of hospital doors.

In addition to organic photosensitizers, several metallic substrates have been shown to exhibit photocatalytic activity. One example is TiO_2, which has been widely used in the construction industry for self-cleaning glass and nonfouling paints and concrete. The self-cleaning effect results from a combination of intrinsic superhydrophilic wetting behavior and photocatalytic activity, the latter resulting from UVA light–induced migration of excited electrons to the surface. Subsequent reactions with air or water lead to the production of ROS, such as superoxide and hydroxyl radicals, which can further combine to form hydrogen peroxide or hydroperoxyl.[161] Titanium implants with TiO_2 coatings have demonstrated efficacy in modulating biological responses and reducing surface corrosion to improve long-term stability in vivo.[162] Additionally, Yao et al[163] reported self-cleaning and broad-spectrum antibacterial activity in both dark and illuminated conditions following deposition of silver NPs on TiO_2-coated silicone urinary catheters.

Moreover, the use of fiber-optic cables and lasers to target light extends potential utility of photosensitive surfaces to antimicrobial indwelling medical devices in sites such as the urinary tract and trachea.[164]

ASSESSMENT OF ANTIMICROBIAL SURFACES

Although many of the developed strategies have exhibited promising suppression of surface bacterial colonization, relatively few have been successfully translated into the clinical setting.[165] Factors hindering clinical translation include the complexity of bulk manufacture, poor alignment with industry-standard processing methods, and the resultant high costs.[137] One of the most significant problems concerning the approval and marketing of novel surfaces as antimicrobial relates to the lack of reproducible and reliable performance and safety data obtained from standardized, clinically relevant testing protocols. Current evaluation methods often yield highly variable findings on account of their differing prerequisites, test conditions, and limited configurations.[8]

A common testing protocol used by industry to substantiate marketing claims is International Organization for Standardization (ISO) *22196: Plastics—Measurement of Antibacterial Activity on Plastics and Other Non-Porous Surfaces*. This protocol involves challenging surfaces with infected media and incubating at 37°C and 100% relative humidity for 24 hours after which the surface-adhered bacteria are enumerated. In this test, maximum and direct contact of the bacterial suspension with the antimicrobial surface throughout the period of incubation is ensured by covering inoculated test pieces with plastic film.[166,167] Another widely employed industry-standard test is American Society for Testing and Materials (ASTM) E2149: *Standard Test Method for Determining the Antimicrobial Activity of Antimicrobial Agents Under Dynamic Contact Conditions*. In this protocol, microbial adherence to test surfaces is assessed after a designated period of continuous agitation in inoculum at 37°C.[168] The testing conditions employed in both tests, namely the liquid challenge, high temperatures, and 100% humidity, are not truly representative of those encountered in most clinical settings and, as such, the relevance of performance data generated from these two industry standards to the ultimate efficacy of these surfaces in preventing infection in clinical practice has been questioned.[8]

The importance of the environmental and test conditions employed during testing of antimicrobial surface activity has been highlighted in a recent study by Campos et al.[8] In this study, the authors evaluated the antibacterial activity of two commercially available antimicrobial films and one developmental film, along with a positive (silver) and negative (untreated) control against four nosocomial pathogens using four test protocols: ISO 22196, ASTM E2149, and two novel methods developed by the authors to more closely simulate the clinical environment.

The first of these novel methods was developed to mimic infectious droplets transmitted by, for example, sneezing, coughing, and talking, or produced by systems, such as air conditioning units and nebulizers. Drops of overnight bacterial cultures were placed on the test surfaces and bacterial adherence was measured following 24 hours incubation at room temperature and humidity. A second method involved direct transfer of bacterial strains from infected glass slides to test surfaces by rolling the slides approximately 20 times, with applied pressure, over the test films. Bacteria recovered from the surfaces were enumerated after 24 hours incubation. Regardless of the test method used, the two commercially available silver-containing films exhibited no, or minimal, activity relative to the untreated controls. In contrast, the developmental nanoinorganic particulate-based surfaces displayed significant antibacterial activity when tested by the ISO and ASTM methods, with time- and organism-dependent variations in efficacy reported. When tested by the two novel methods, which employed more clinically relevant conditions of lower temperatures and humidity, minimal and no activity was observed during the transfer and droplet tests, respectively.[8] These varying results highlight the inconsistency of currently available methods and the need for the development of improved, application-specific protocols to more reliably predict clinical performance. Furthermore, the threshold reduction in surface microbial colonization required to prevent HAIs is still not known.[109]

A major aim of an ongoing European Cooperation in Science and Technology action, funded by the EU Framework Programme for Research and Innovation Horizon 2020, is to advance best practice in the selection of optimal testing and characterization methodologies. It has been universally accepted that a "one size fits all" method for testing will not be feasible; therefore, cross-disciplinary efforts between material scientists, microbiologists, clinicians, and industry are required for the production of international standards and guidelines detailing application-specific test conditions, bacterial strains, and reference systems to ultimately facilitate reliable benchmarking and cross-comparison of developed antimicrobial surfaces.[169]

FUTURE DIRECTIONS

Microbial colonization of surfaces remains a serious risk to public health. This chapter discusses some of the ongoing efforts in the development of strategies to combat this global health care challenge, with significant tolerance to bacterial attachment demonstrated by many of the antimicrobial surfaces during short-term challenge periods. Future research should focus on improving longevity of the surface antibacterial and antimicrobial properties to provide tolerance to contamination throughout the period of device usage. Among the various approaches investigated to date, the strategy of "killing-release" offers much promise for the development of antimicrobial surfaces with long-term bactericidal efficacy. Wu et al[170] have reported a highly efficient regenerative surface with both bactericidal and salt-induced bacterial release capabilities based on salt-responsive chitosan-grafted polyzwitterionic brushes of poly(3-(dimethyl (4-vinylbenzyl) ammonium) propyl sulfonate). In addition to the facile fabrication process, the coatings demonstrated the ability to kill >95% of attached *E coli* and *S aureus* cells and, furthermore, approximately 97% of surface-attached bacteria were removed after 10 minutes of gentle shaking in 1.0 M sodium chloride. More important, the retention of the bactericidal efficiency and release rate after four killing-release cycles highlights the promising long-term reusability of this system.[170]

A further area of focus, particularly for indwelling device surfaces, should be deterring attachment not only of bacteria but also of proteins, the adherence of which can mask surface-localized antibacterial moieties.[171] Initial success has been achieved with polymeric impregnation of nitrous oxide (NO) donors, facilitating continuous release of NO from the device surface to give significant antimicrobial activity which is, more important, maintained on adsorption of proteins, such as fibrinogen.[172-174] Furthermore, longevity of the antifouling properties has been enhanced by application of copper wire electrodes or soluble copper complexes, for example, copper(II)-tris(2-pyridylmethyl)amine, within catheter lumen models incorporating a reservoir of inorganic nitrite, allowing periodic electrochemically controlled NO release.[175,176] Moreover, on account of their antithrombotic properties, NO-releasing surfaces represent much promise for dual thrombo- and bacterial-tolerant blood-contacting devices.[177]

In addition to the expanding range of active agents and approaches to reduce susceptibility of surfaces to bacterial colonization, further understanding of the biofilm development process, with complementary investigation of methods to inhibit and disrupt this highly regulated process, is expected to inform the development of enhanced efficiency decontamination procedures for contaminated surfaces. Novel antibiofilm approaches involving application of ultrasonic guided waves, shockwaves, and electrical currents to medical devices have all recently been reported.[178-181] More important, no viable bacteria were detected after 4 days administration of 500 μA direct electrical current (DC) via intraluminally placed platinum electrodes to established biofilms of *S epidermidis* and *S aureus* on peripheral venous catheter surfaces in an in vitro catheter model.[182] This "electricidal" effect has been attributed to DC-generated ROS, which attacks planktonic and biofilm-associated cells, in agreement with previous reports.[183,184] Although contact with human tissue must be avoided due to potential cell lysis or thrombus formation, this approach could offer promise for the treatment of inner catheter lumens and nonindwelling, high-touch devices in health care environments.

In conclusion, significant progress has undoubtedly been made in the development of alternative approaches for the prevention of surface contamination. Interdisciplinary collaborations are crucial to address factors such as cost, complexity of production, and assessment of clinical efficacy, in addition to the longevity of antimicrobial performance, before scale up and clinical translation of highly efficient technologies in "real life" applications, with successful prevention of HAIs or surface-associated contamination risks as the ultimate goal.[117]

REFERENCES

1. Health Protection Scotland. *National Point Prevalence Survey of Healthcare Associated Infection and Antimicrobial Prescribing 2016.* Glasgow, United Kingdom: NHS National Services Scotland; 2017.
2. Magill SS, Edwards JR, Bamberg W, et al; for Emerging Infections Program Healthcare-Associated Infections and Antimicrobial Use Prevalence Survey Team. Multistate point-prevalence survey of health care–associated infections. *N Engl J Med.* 2014;370:1198-1208.
3. Zimlichman E, Henderson D, Tamir O, et al. Health care-associated infections: a meta-analysis of costs and financial impact on the US health care system. *JAMA Intern Med.* 2013;173:2039-2046.
4. European Centre for Disease Prevention and Control. *Annual Epidemiological Report on Communicable Diseases in Europe 2008: Report on the State of Communicable Diseases in the EU and EEA/EFTA Countries.* Stockholm, Sweden: European Centre for Disease Prevention and Control; 2008.
5. Weber DJ, Anderson D, Rutala WA. The role of the surface environment in healthcare-associated infections. *Curr Opin Infect Dis.* 2013;26:338-344.
6. Loveday HP, Wilson JA, Pratt RJ, et al. epic3: national evidence-based guidelines for preventing healthcare-associated infections in NHS hospitals in England. *J Hosp Infect.* 2014;86:S1-S70.
7. Coad BR, Griesser HJ, Peleg AY, Traven A. Anti-infective surface coatings: design and therapeutic promise against device-associated infections. *PLoS Pathog.* 2016;12:e1005598.
8. Campos MD, Zucchi PC, Phung A, et al. The activity of antimicrobial surfaces varies by testing protocol utilized. *PLoS One.* 2016;11: e0160728.
9. Hori K, Matsumoto S. Bacterial adhesion: from mechanism to control. *Biochem Eng J.* 2010;48:424-434.
10. Flemming HC, Wingender J. The biofilm matrix. *Nat Rev Microbiol.* 2010;8:623-633.
11. Renner LD, Weibel DB. Physicochemical regulation of biofilm formation. *MRS Bull.* 2011;36:347-355.
12. Lewis K. Riddle of biofilm resistance. *Antimicrob Agents Chemother.* 2001;45:999-1007.
13. Mah TF, O'Toole GA. Mechanisms of biofilm resistance to antimicrobial agents. *Trends Microbiol.* 2001;9:34-39.
14. Fux CA, Costerton JW, Stewart PS, Stoodley P. Survival strategies of infectious biofilms. *Trends Microbiol.* 2005;13:34-40.
15. Rasmussen TB, Givskov M. Quorum sensing inhibitors: a bargain of effects. *Microbiology.* 2006;152:895-904.
16. Tiller JC. Antimicrobial surfaces. In: Borner HG, Lutz JF, eds. *Bioactive Surfaces.* Berlin, Germany: Springer; 2010:193-217.
17. McLean RJ, Hussain AA, Sayer M, Vincent PJ, Hughes DJ, Smith TJ. Antibacterial activity of multilayer silver-copper surface films on catheter material. *Can J Microbiol.* 1993;39:895-899.
18. Tiller JC, Liao C, Lewis K, Klibanov AM. Designing surfaces that kill bacteria on contact. *Proc Natl Acad Sci U S A.* 2001;98:5981-5985.
19. Kim K, Gollamudi SS, Steinhubl S. Digital technology to enable aging in place. *Exp Gerontol.* 2017;88:25-31.

20. Rechel B, Grundy E, Robine J, et al. Ageing in the European Union. *Lancet.* 2013;381:1312-1322.

21. Katsikogianni M, Missirlis YF. Concise review of mechanisms of bacterial adhesion to biomaterials and of techniques used in estimating bacteria-material interactions. *Eur Cell Mater.* 2004;8:37-57.

22. Song F, Koo H, Ren D. Effects of material properties on bacterial adhesion and biofilm formation. *J Dent Res.* 2015;94:1027-1034.

23. Page K, Wilson M, Parkin IP. Antimicrobial surfaces and their potential in reducing the role of the inanimate environment in the incidence of hospital-acquired infections. *J Mater Chem.* 2009;19:3819-3831.

24. Dou X, Zhang D, Feng C, Jiang L. Bioinspired hierarchical surface structures with tunable wettability for regulating bacteria adhesion. *ACS Nano.* 2015;9:10664-10672.

25. Otitoju TA, Ahmad AL, Ooi BS. Superhydrophilic (superwetting) surfaces: a review on fabrication and application. *J Ind Eng Chem.* 2017;47:19-40.

26. Patel P, Choi CK, Meng DD. Superhydrophilic surfaces for antifogging and antifouling microfluidic devices. *J Assoc Lab Autom.* 2010;15:114-119.

27. Fateh R, Dillert R, Bahnemann D. Preparation and characterization of transparent hydrophilic photocatalytic TiO2/SiO2 thin films on polycarbonate. *Langmuir.* 2013;29:3730-3739.

28. Yuan Y, Hays MP, Hardwidge PR, et al. Surface characteristics influencing bacterial adhesion to polymeric substrates. *RSC Adv.* 2017;7:14254-14261.

29. Wong T, Sun T, Feng L, et al. Interfacial materials with special wettability. *MRS Bull.* 2013;38:366-371.

30. Callies M, Quere D. On water repellency. *Soft Matter.* 2005;1:55-61.

31. Nuraje N, Khan WS, Lei Y, Ceylan M, Asmatulu R. Superhydrophobic electrospun nanofibers. *J Mater Chem A.* 2013;1:1929-1946.

32. Bhushan B, Jung YC, Koch K. Self-cleaning efficiency of artificial superhydrophobic surfaces. *Langmuir.* 2009;25:3240-3248.

33. Ivanova EP, Hasan J, Webb HK, et al. Bactericidal activity of black silicon. *Nat Commun.* 2013;4:2838.

34. McCarthy M, Gerasopoulos K, Enright R, et al. Biotemplated hierarchical surfaces and the role of dual length scales on the repellency of impacting droplets. *Appl Phys Lett.* 2012;100:263701.

35. Kim P, Kreder MJ, Alvarenga J, Aizenberg J. Hierarchical or not? Effect of the length scale and hierarchy of the surface roughness on omniphobicity of lubricant-infused substrates. *Nano Lett.* 2013;13:1793-1799.

36. Simpson JT, Hunter SR, Aytug T. Superhydrophobic materials and coatings: a review. *Rep Prog Phys.* 2015;78:086501.

37. Crick CR, Ismail S, Pratten J, Parkin IP. An investigation into bacterial attachment to an elastomeric superhydrophobic surface prepared via aerosol assisted deposition. *Thin Solid Films.* 2011;519:3722-3727.

38. Fadeeva E, Truong VK, Stiesch M, et al. Bacterial retention on superhydrophobic titanium surfaces fabricated by femtosecond laser ablation. *Langmuir.* 2011;27:3012-3019.

39. Bobji MS, Kumar SV, Asthana A, Govardhan RN. Underwater sustainability of the "Cassie" state of wetting. *Langmuir.* 2009;25:12120-12126.

40. McCoy CP, Cowley JF, Gorman SP, Andrews GP, Jones DS. Reduction of *Staphylococcus aureus* and *Pseudomonas aeruginosa* colonisation on PVC through covalent surface attachment of fluorinated thiols. *J Pharm Pharmacol.* 2009;61:1163-1169.

41. Banerjee I, Pangule RC, Kane RS. Antifouling coatings: recent developments in the design of surfaces that prevent fouling by proteins, bacteria, and marine organisms. *Adv Mater.* 2011;23:690-718.

42. Zhang H, Lamb R, Lewis J. Engineering nanoscale roughness on hydrophobic surface—preliminary assessment of fouling behaviour. *Sci Technol Adv Mater.* 2005;6:236-239.

43. Koc Y, de Mello AJ, McHale G, Newton MI, Roach P, Shirtcliffe NJ. Nano-scale superhydrophobicity: suppression of protein adsorption and promotion of flow-induced detachment. *Lab Chip.* 2008;8:582-586.

44. Guan JH, Wells GG, Xu B, et al. Evaporation of sessile droplets on slippery liquid-infused porous surfaces (SLIPS). *Langmuir.* 2015;31:11781-11789.

45. Bohn HF, Federle W. Insect aquaplaning: *Nepenthes* pitcher plants capture prey with the peristome, a fully wettable water-lubricated anisotropic surface. *Proc Natl Acad Sci U S A.* 2004;101:14138-14143.

46. Wong T, Kang SH, Tang SKY, et al. Bioinspired self-repairing slippery surfaces with pressure-stable omniphobicity. *Nature.* 2011;477:443-447.

47. Kim P, Wong TS, Alvarenga J, Kreder MJ, Adorno-Martinez WE, Aizenberg J. Liquid-infused nanostructured surfaces with extreme anti-ice and anti-frost performance. *ACS Nano.* 2012;6:6569-6577.

48. Wilson PW, Lu W, Xu H, et al. Inhibition of ice nucleation by slippery liquid-infused porous surfaces (SLIPS). *Phys Chem Chem Phys.* 2013;15:581-585.

49. Xiao L, Li J, Mieszkin S, et al. Slippery liquid-infused porous surfaces showing marine antibiofouling properties. *ACS Appl Mater Interfaces.* 2013;5:10074-10080.

50. Epstein AK, Wong T, Belisle RA, Boggs EM, Aizenberg J. Liquid-infused structured surfaces with exceptional anti-biofouling performance. *Proc Natl Acad Sci U S A.* 2012;109:13182-13187.

51. Li J, Kleintschek T, Rieder A, et al. Hydrophobic liquid-infused porous polymer surfaces for antibacterial applications. *ACS Appl Mater Interfaces.* 2013;5:6704-6711.

52. Leslie DC, Waterhouse A, Berthet JB, et al. A bioinspired omniphobic surface coating on medical devices prevents thrombosis and biofouling. *Nat Biotechnol.* 2014;32:1134-1140.

53. Sauer K, Camper AK, Ehrlich GD, Costerton JW, Davies DG. *Pseudomonas aeruginosa* displays multiple phenotypes during development as a biofilm. *J Bacteriol.* 2002;184:1140-1154.

54. Kovacs B, Patko D, Szekacs I, et al. Flagellin based biomimetic coatings: from cell-repellent surfaces to highly adhesive coatings. *Acta Biomater.* 2016;42:66-76.

55. Reffuveille F, Nicol M, Dé E, Thébault P. Design of an anti-adhesive surface by a pilicide strategy. *Colloids Surf B Biointerfaces.* 2016;146:895-901.

56. Ho KK, Chen R, Willcox MD, et al. Quorum sensing inhibitory activities of surface immobilized antibacterial dihydropyrrolones via click chemistry. *Biomaterials.* 2014;35:2336-2345.

57. Ivanova K, Fernandes MM, Francesko A, et al. Quorum-quenching and matrix-degrading enzymes in multilayer coatings synergistically prevent bacterial biofilm formation on urinary catheters. *ACS Appl Mater Interfaces.* 2015;7:27066-27077.

58. Beloin C, Renard S, Ghigo J, Lebeaux D. Novel approaches to combat bacterial biofilms. *Curr Opin Pharmacol.* 2014;18:61-68.

59. Zoppe JO, Ataman NC, Mocny P, Wang J, Moraes J, Klok HA. Surface-initiated controlled radical polymerization: state-of-the-art, opportunities, and challenges in surface and interface engineering with polymer brushes. *Chem Rev.* 2017;117:1105-1318.

60. Hadjesfandiari N, Yu K, Mei Y, et al. Polymer brush-based approaches for the development of infection-resistant surfaces. *J Mater Chem B.* 2014;2:4968-4978.

61. Polanowski P, Halagan K, Pietrasik J, et al. Growth of polymer brushes by "grafting from" via ATRP—Monte Carlo simulations. *Polymer.* 2017;130:267-279.

62. Du H, Chandaroy P, Hui SW. Grafted poly-(ethylene glycol) on lipid surfaces inhibits protein adsorption and cell adhesion. *Biochim Biophys Acta.* 1997;1326:236-248.

63. Nejadnik MR, van der Mei HC, Norde W, Busscher HJ. Bacterial adhesion and growth on a polymer brush-coating. *Biomaterials.* 2008;29:4117-4121.

64. Roosjen A, van der Mei HC, Busscher HJ, et al. Microbial adhesion to poly(ethylene oxide) brushes: influence of polymer chain length and temperature. *Langmuir.* 2004;20:10949-10955.

65. Roosjen A, Kaper HJ, van der Mei HC, Norde W, Busscher HJ. Inhibition of adhesion of yeasts and bacteria by poly(ethylene oxide)-brushes on glass in a parallel plate flow chamber. *Microbiology.* 2003;149:3239-3246.

66. Al-Ani A, Pingle H, P Reynolds N, et al. Tuning the density of poly (ethylene glycol) chains to control mammalian cell and bacterial attachment. *Polymers (Basel).* 2017;9:343.

67. Liu C, Lee J, Small C, Ma J, Elimelech M. Comparison of organic fouling resistance of thin-film composite membranes modified by hydrophilic silica nanoparticles and zwitterionic polymer brushes. *J Membr Sci.* 2017;544:135-142.

68. Li W, Liu Q, Liu L. Antifouling gold surfaces grafted with aspartic acid and glutamic acid based zwitterionic polymer brushes. *Langmuir.* 2014;30:12619-12626.

69. Yang Y, Li Y, Li Q, Wan LS, Xu ZK. Surface hydrophilization of microporous polypropylene membrane by grafting zwitterionic polymer for anti-biofouling. *J Membrane Sci.* 2010;362:255-264.

70. Gao G, Lange D, Hilpert K, et al. The biocompatibility and biofilm resistance of implant coatings based on hydrophilic polymer brushes conjugated with antimicrobial peptides. *Biomaterials.* 2011;32: 3899-3909.

71. Tang Z, Ma C, Wu H, et al. Antiadhesive zwitterionic poly-(sulphobetaine methacrylate) brush coating functionalized with triclosan for high-efficiency antibacterial performance. *Prog Org Coatings.* 2016;97:277-287.

72. Elbourne A, Crawford RJ, Ivanova EP. Nano-structured antimicrobial surfaces: from nature to synthetic analogues. *J Colloid Interface Sci.* 2017;508:603-616.

73. Darouiche RO, Smith JA Jr, Hanna H, et al. Efficacy of antimicrobial-impregnated bladder catheters in reducing catheter-associated bacteriuria: a prospective, randomized, multicenter clinical trial. *Urology.* 1999;54:976-981.

74. Jamal MA, Rosenblatt JS, Hachem RY, et al. Prevention of biofilm colonization by gram-negative bacteria on minocycline-rifampin-impregnated catheters sequentially coated with chlorhexidine. *Antimicrob Agents Chemother.* 2014;58:1179-1182.

75. van de Belt H, Neut D, Uges DRA, et al. Surface roughness, porosity and wettability of gentamicin-loaded bone cements and their antibiotic release. *Biomaterials.* 2000;21:1981-1987.

76. Piozzi A, Francolini I, Occhiaperti L, Di Rosa R, Ruggeri V, Donelli G. Polyurethanes loaded with antibiotics: influence of polymer-antibiotic interactions on in vitro activity against *Staphylococcus epidermidis*. *J Chemother.* 2004;16:446-452.

77. Ruggeri V, Francolini I, Donelli G, Piozzi A. Synthesis, characterization, and in vitro activity of antibiotic releasing polyurethanes to prevent bacterial resistance. *J Biomed Mater Res A.* 2007;81:287-298.

78. Neut D, van de Belt H, Stokroos I, van Horn JR, van der Mei HC, Busscher HJ. Biomaterial-associated infection of gentamicin-loaded PMMA beads in orthopaedic revision surgery. *J Antimicrob Chemother.* 2001;47:885-891.

79. Zilberman M, Elsner JJ. Antibiotic-eluting medical devices for various applications. *J Control Release.* 2008;130:202-215.

80. Webb JCJ, Spencer RF, Lovering AM, Learmouth ID. Very late release of gentamicin from bone cement in total hip arthroplasty (THA). *Orthopaedic Proceedings.* 2005;87-B(suppl I):52.

81. Zhuk I, Jariwala F, Attygalle AB, Wu Y, Libera MR, Sukhishvili SA. Self-defensive layer-by-layer films with bacteria-triggered antibiotic release. *ACS Nano.* 2014;8:7733-7745.

82. Moskowitz JS, Blaisse MR, Samuel RE, et al. The effectiveness of the controlled release of gentamicin from polyelectrolyte multilayers in the treatment of *Staphylococcus aureus* infection in a rabbit bone model. *Biomaterials.* 2010;31:6019-6030.

83. Guillaume O, Garric X, Lavigne J, Van Den Berghe H, Coudane J. Multilayer, degradable coating as a carrier for the sustained release of antibiotics: preparation and antimicrobial efficacy in vitro. *J Control Release.* 2012;162:492-501.

84. Imamovic L, Sommer MO. Use of collateral sensitivity networks to design drug cycling protocols that avoid resistance development. *Sci Transl Med.* 2013;5:204ra132.

85. Strobel C, Bormann N, Kadow-Romacker A, Schmidmaier G, Wildemann B. Sequential release kinetics of two (gentamicin and BMP-2) or three (gentamicin, IGF-I and BMP-2) substances from a one-component polymeric coating on implants. *J Control Release.* 2011;156: 37-45.

86. Jeon JH, Puleo DA. Alternating release of different bioactive molecules from a complexation polymer system. *Biomaterials.* 2008;29: 3591-3598.

87. Valdes-Ramirez G, Windmiller JR, Claussen JC, et al. Multiplexed and switchable release of distinct fluids from microneedle platforms via conducting polymer nanoactuators for potential drug delivery. *Sens Actuators B: Chem.* 2012;161. doi:10.1016/j.snb.2011.11.085.

88. Azzaroni O. Polymer brushes here, there, and everywhere: recent advances in their practical applications and emerging opportunities in multiple research fields. *J Polymer Sci Part A: Polymer Chem.* 2012;50:3225-3258.

89. Hancock RE, Sahl HG. Antimicrobial and host-defense peptides as new anti-infective therapeutic strategies. *Nat Biotechnol.* 2006;24: 1551-1557.

90. Shukla A, Fleming KE, Chuang HF, et al. Controlling the release of peptide antimicrobial agents from surfaces. *Biomaterials.* 2010;31: 2348-2357.

91. Onaizi SA, Leong SSJ. Tethering antimicrobial peptides: current status and potential challenges. *Biotechnol Adv.* 2011;29:67-74.

92. Cho W, Joshi BP, Cho H, Lee KH. Design and synthesis of novel antibacterial peptide-resin conjugates. *Bioorg Med Chem Lett.* 2007;17: 5772-5776.

93. Bagheri M, Beyermann M, Dathe M. Immobilization reduces the activity of surface-bound cationic antimicrobial peptides with no influence upon the activity spectrum. *Antimicrob Agents Chemother.* 2009;53:1132-1141.

94. Hilpert K, Elliott M, Jenssen H, et al. Screening and characterization of surface-tethered cationic peptides for antimicrobial activity. *Chem Biol.* 2009;16:58-69.

95. Li Y, Wei S, Wu J, et al. Effects of peptide immobilization sites on the structure and activity of surface-tethered antimicrobial peptides. *J Phys Chem C.* 2015;119:7146-7155.

96. Borzelleca JF. Paracelsus: herald of modern toxicology. *Toxicol Sci.* 2000;53:2-4.

97. Bazaka K, Jacob MV, Crawford RJ, Ivanova EP. Efficient surface modification of biomaterial to prevent biofilm formation and the attachment of microorganisms. *Appl Microbiol Biotechnol.* 2012;95:299-311.

98. Hobman JL, Crossman LC. Bacterial antimicrobial metal ion resistance. *J Med Microbiol.* 2015;64:471-497.

99. Shih H, Lin YE. Efficacy of copper-silver ionization in controlling biofilm- and plankton-associated waterborne pathogens. *Appl Environ Microbiol.* 2010;76:2032-2035.

100. Grass G, Rensing C, Solioz M. Metallic copper as an antimicrobial surface. *Appl Environ Microbiol.* 2011;77:1541-1547.

101. Araújo EA, Andrade NJ, da Silva LH, et al. Antimicrobial effects of silver nanoparticles against bacterial cells adhered to stainless steel surfaces. *J Food Prot.* 2012;75:701-705.

102. Siddiq DM, Darouiche RO. New strategies to prevent catheter-associated urinary tract infections. *Nat Rev Urol.* 2012;9:305-314.

103. Nandkumar MA, Ranjit M, Pradeep Kumar S, et al. Antimicrobial silver oxide incorporated urinary catheters for infection resistance. *Trends Biomater Artif Org.* 2010;24:156-164.

104. Monteiro DR, Gorup LF, Takamiya AS, Ruvollo-Filho AC, de Camargo ER, Barbosa DB. The growing importance of materials that prevent microbial adhesion: antimicrobial effect of medical devices containing silver. *Int J Antimicrob Agents.* 2009;34:103-110.

105. Tokmaji G, Vermeulen H, Müller MC, Kwakman PH, Schultz MJ, Zaat SA. Silver-coated endotracheal tubes for prevention of ventilator-associated pneumonia in critically ill patients. *Cochrane Database Syst Rev.* 2015;(8):CD009201.

106. Schumm K, Lam TBL. Types of urethral catheters for management of short-term voiding problems in hospitalised adults. *Cochrane Database Syst Rev.* 2008;(2):CD004013.

107. Pickard R, Lam T, MacLennan G, et al. Antimicrobial catheters for reduction of symptomatic urinary tract infection in adults requiring short-term catheterisation in hospital: a multicentre randomised controlled trial. *Lancet.* 2012;380:1927-1935.

108. Weinstein RA, Hota B. Contamination, disinfection, and cross-colonization: are hospital surfaces reservoirs for nosocomial infection? *Clin Infect Dis.* 2004;39:1182-1189.

109. Muller MP, MacDougall C, Lim M; for Ontario Agency for Health Protection and Promotion Public Health Ontario, Provincial Infectious Diseases Advisory Committee on Infection Prevention and Control, Provincial Infectious Diseases Advisory Committee on Infection Prevention and Control. Antimicrobial surfaces to prevent healthcare-associated infections: a systematic review. *J Hosp Infect.* 2016;92:7-13.

110. Salgado CD, Sepkowitz KA, John JF, et al. Copper surfaces reduce the rate of healthcare-acquired infections in the intensive care unit. *Infect Control Hosp Epidemiol.* 2013;34:479-486.

111. Lazary A, Weinberg I, Vatine J, et al. Reduction of healthcare-associated infections in a long-term care brain injury ward by replacing regular linens with biocidal copper oxide impregnated linens. *Int J Infect Dis.* 2014;24:23-29.

112. Tamimi AH, Carlino S, Gerba CP. Long-term efficacy of a self-disinfecting coating in an intensive care unit. *Am J Infect Control.* 2014;42:1178-1181.

113. Boyce JM, Havill NL, Guercia KA, Schweon SJ, Moore BA. Evaluation of two organosilane products for sustained antimicrobial activity on high-touch surfaces in patient rooms. *Am J Infect Control.* 2014;42:326-328.

114. Phillips P, Taylor L, Hastings R. Silver ion antimicrobial technology: decontamination in a nursing home. *Br J Community Nurs.* 2009;14:S25.

115. Chamakura K, Perez-Ballestero R, Luo Z, Bashir S, Liu J. Comparison of bactericidal activities of silver nanoparticles with common chemical disinfectants. *Colloids Surf B Biointerfaces.* 2011;84:88-96.

116. Gorjanc M, Bukosek V, Gorensek M, et al. CF4 plasma and silver functionalized cotton. *Text Res J.* 2010;80:2204-2213.

117. Nikiforov A, Deng X, Xiong Q, et al. Non-thermal plasma technology for the development of antimicrobial surfaces: a review. *J Phys D-Appl Phys.* 2016;49:204002.

118. Sambhy V, MacBride MM, Peterson BR, Sen A. Silver bromide nanoparticle/polymer composites: dual action tunable antimicrobial materials. *J Am Chem Soc.* 2006;128:9798-9808.

119. Ashraf S, Rehman S, Sher F, et al. Synthesis of cellulose-metal nanoparticle composites: development and comparison of different protocols. *Cellulose.* 2014;21:395-405.

120. Qureshi AT, Monroe WT, Lopez MJ, et al. Biocompatible/bioabsorbable silver nanocomposite coatings. *J Appl Polymer Sci.* 2011;120:3042-3053.

121. Travan A, Pelillo C, Donati I, et al. Non-cytotoxic silver nanoparticle-polysaccharide nanocomposites with antimicrobial activity. *Biomacromolecules.* 2009;10:1429-1435.

122. Maneerung T, Tokura S, Rujiravanit R. Impregnation of silver nanoparticles into bacterial cellulose for antimicrobial wound dressing. *Carbohydr Polymers.* 2008;72:43-51.

123. Dubas ST, Kumlangdudsana P, Potiyaraj P. Layer-by-layer deposition of antimicrobial silver nanoparticles on textile fibers. *Colloids Surf A-Physicochem Eng Aspects.* 2006;289:105-109.

124. Kumar A, Vemula PK, Ajayan PM, John G. Silver-nanoparticle-embedded antimicrobial paints based on vegetable oil. *Nat Mater.* 2008;7:236-241.

125. Sahoo PC, Kausar F, Lee JH, et al. Facile fabrication of silver nanoparticle embedded CaCO3 microspheres via microalgae-templated CO2 biomineralization: application in antimicrobial paint development. *RSC Advances.* 2014;4:32562-32569.

126. Szabo T, Mihaly J, Sajo I, et al. One-pot synthesis of gelatin-based, slow-release polymer microparticles containing silver nanoparticles and their application in anti-fouling paint. *Prog Org Coatings.* 2014;77:1226-1232.

127. Cometa S, Iatta R, Ricci MA, et al. Analytical characterization and antimicrobial properties of novel copper nanoparticle-loaded electrosynthesized hydrogel coatings. *J Bioactive Compatible Polymers.* 2013;28:508-522.

128. Thokala N, Kealey C, Kennedy J, Brady DB, Farrell JB. Characterisation of polyamide 11/copper antimicrobial composites for medical device applications. *Mater Sci Eng C Mater Biol Appl.* 2017;78:1179-1186.

129. Palza H, Quijada R, Delgado K. Antimicrobial polymer composites with copper micro- and nanoparticles: effect of particle size and polymer matrix. *J Bioactive Compatible Polymers.* 2015;30:366-380.

130. McGuffie MJ, Hong J, Bahng JH, et al. Zinc oxide nanoparticle suspensions and layer-by-layer coatings inhibit staphylococcal growth. *Nanomedicine.* 2016;12:33-42.

131. Sonkusre P, Singh Cameotra S. Biogenic selenium nanoparticles inhibit *Staphylococcus aureus* adherence on different surfaces. *Colloids Surf B Biointerfaces.* 2015;136:1051-1057.

132. Yip J, Liu L, Wong K, et al. Investigation of antifungal and antibacterial effects of fabric padded with highly stable selenium nanoparticles. *J Appl Polymer Sci.* 2014;131:40728.

133. Yildirimer L, Thanh NTK, Loizidou M, Seifalian AM. Toxicology and clinical potential of nanoparticles. *Nano Today.* 2011;6:585-607.

134. De Giglio E, Cafagna D, Cometa S, et al. An innovative, easily fabricated, silver nanoparticle-based titanium implant coating: development and analytical characterization. *Anal Bioanal Chem.* 2013;405:805-816.

135. Timko BP, Dvir T, Kohane DS. Remotely triggerable drug delivery systems. *Adv Mater.* 2010;22:4925-4943.

136. Manzano M, Vallet-Regi M. Revisiting bioceramics: bone regenerative and local drug delivery systems. *Prog Solid State Chem.* 2012;40:17-30.

137. McCoy CP, Brady C, Cowley J, et al. Triggered drug delivery from biomaterials. *Expert Opin Drug Deliv.* 2010;7:605-616.

138. Stickler DJ, Morris N, Moreno MC, Sabbuba N. Studies on the formation of crystalline bacterial biofilms on urethral catheters. *Eur J Clin Microbiol Infect Dis.* 1998;17:649-652.

139. Irwin NJ, McCoy CP, Jones DS, Gorman SP. Infection-responsive drug delivery from urinary biomaterials controlled by a novel kinetic and thermodynamic approach. *Pharm Res.* 2013;30:857-865.

140. McCoy CP, Irwin NJ, Brady C, et al. An infection-responsive approach to reduce bacterial adhesion in urinary biomaterials. *Mol Pharm.* 2016;13:2817-2822.

141. Lu Y, Wu Y, Liang J, Libera MR, Sukhishvili SA. Self-defensive antibacterial layer-by-layer hydrogel coatings with pH-triggered hydrophobicity. *Biomaterials.* 2015;45:64-71.

142. He M, Wang Q, Zhang J, Zhao W, Zhao C. Substrate independent Ag-nanoparticle loaded hydrogel coating with regenerable bactericidal and thermoresponsive antibacterial properties. *ACS Appl Mater Interfaces.* 2017;9(51):44782-44791.

143. Wainwright M. Photodynamic antimicrobial chemotherapy (PACT). *J Antimicrob Chemother.* 1998;42:13-28.

144. Rajesh S, Koshi E, Philip K, Mohan A. Antimicrobial photodynamic therapy: an overview. *J Indian Soc Periodontol.* 2011;15:323-327.

145. Awad MM, Tovmasyan A, Craik JD, Batinic-Haberle I, Benov LT. Important cellular targets for antimicrobial photodynamic therapy. *Appl Microbiol Biotechnol.* 2016;100:7679-7688.

146. Josefsen LB, Boyle RW. Photodynamic therapy and the development of metal-based photosensitisers. *Met Based Drugs.* 2008;2008:276109.

147. McCoy CP, Craig RA, McGlinchey SM, Carson L, Jones DS, Gorman SP. Surface localisation of photosensitisers on intraocular lens biomaterials for prevention of infectious endophthalmitis and retinal protection. *Biomaterials.* 2012;33:7952-7958.

148. Parsons C, McCoy CP, Gorman SP, et al. Anti-infective photodynamic biomaterials for the prevention of intraocular lens-associated infectious endophthalmitis. *Biomaterials.* 2009;30:597-602.

149. Demidova TN, Hamblin MR. Photodynamic inactivation of *Bacillus* spores, mediated by phenothiazinium dyes. *Appl Environ Microbiol.* 2005;71:6918-6925.

150. Oliveira A, Almeida A, Carvalho CMB, et al. Porphyrin derivatives as photosensitizers for the inactivation of *Bacillus cereus* endospores. *J Appl Microbiol.* 2009;106:1986-1995.

151. Perni S, Prokopovich P, Piccirillo C, et al. Toluidine blue-containing polymers exhibit potent bactericidal activity when irradiated with red laser light. *J Mater Chem.* 2009;9:2715-2723.

152. Perni S, Piccirillo C, Pratten J, et al. The antimicrobial properties of light-activated polymers containing methylene blue and gold nanoparticles. *Biomaterials*. 2009;30:89-93.

153. Noimark S, Dunnill CW, Kay CWM, et al. Incorporation of methylene blue and nanogold into polyvinyl chloride catheters; a new approach for light-activated disinfection of surfaces. *J Mater Chem*. 2012;22: 15388-15396.

154. Piccirillo C, Perni S, Gil-Thomas J, et al. Antimicrobial activity of methylene blue and toluidine blue O covalently bound to a modified silicone polymer surface. *J Mater Chem*. 2009;19:6167-6171.

155. Zerdin K, Horsham MA, Durham R, et al. Photodynamic inactivation of bacterial spores on the surface of a photoactive polymer. *Reactive Functl Polymers*. 2009;69:821-827.

156. Ringot C, Sol V, Barrière M, et al. Triazinyl porphyrin-based photoactive cotton fabrics: preparation, characterization, and antibacterial activity. *Biomacromolecules*. 2011;12:1716-1723.

157. Mbakidi J, Herke K, Alvès S, et al. Synthesis and photobiocidal properties of cationic porphyrin-grafted paper. *Carbohydr Polym*. 2013;91:333-338.

158. McCoy CP, O'Neil EJ, Cowley JF, et al. Photodynamic antimicrobial polymers for infection control. *PLoS One*. 2014;9:e108500.

159. Hynek J, Rathousky J, Demel J, et al. Design of porphyrin-based conjugated microporous polymers with enhanced singlet oxygen productivity. *RSC Advances*. 2016;6:44279-44287.

160. Wang Y, Liu Y, Li G, Hao J. Porphyrin-based honeycomb films and their antibacterial activity. *Langmuir*. 2014;30:6419-6426.

161. Foster HA, Ditta IB, Varghese S, Steele A. Photocatalytic disinfection using titanium dioxide: spectrum and mechanism of antimicrobial activity. *Appl Microbiol Biotechnol*. 2011;90:1847-1868.

162. Sidambe AT. Biocompatibility of advanced manufactured titanium implants—a review. *Materials (Basel)*. 2014;7:8168-8188.

163. Yao Y, Ohko Y, Sekiguchi Y, Fujishima A, Kubota Y. Self-sterilization using silicone catheters coated with Ag and TiO2 nanocomposite thin film. *J Biomed Mater Res B Appl Biomater*. 2008;85:453-460.

164. Timko BP, Kohane DS. Materials to clinical devices: technologies for remotely triggered drug delivery. *Clin Ther*. 2012;34:S25-S35.

165. Ip M, Lui S, Poon V, Lung I, Burd A. Antimicrobial activities of silver dressings: an in vitro comparison. *J Med Microbiol*. 2006;55:59-63.

166. Ando Y, Miyamoto H, Noda I, et al. Calcium phosphate coating containing silver shows high antibacterial activity and low cytotoxicity and inhibits bacterial adhesion. *Mater Sci Eng C-Mater for Biol Appl*. 2010;30:175-180.

167. International Organization for Standardization. *ISO 22196:2007: Plastics—Measurement of Antibacterial Activity on Plastics Surfaces*. Geneva, Switzerland: International Organization for Standardization; 2007.

168. American Society for Testing and Materials. *ASTM E2149-13a. Standard Test Method for Determining the Antimicrobial Activity of Antimicrobial Agents Under Dynamic Contact Conditions*. West Conshohocken, PA: American Society for Testing and Materials; 2013.

169. Gaspar R, Aksu B, Cuine A, et al. Towards a European strategy for medicines research (2014-2020): the EUFEPS position paper on Horizon 2020. *Eur J Pharm Sci*. 2012;47:979-987.

170. Wu B, Zhang L, Huang L, et al. Salt-induced regenerative surface for bacteria killing and release. *Langmuir*. 2017;33:7160-7168.

171. Furno F, Morley KS, Wong B, et al. Silver nanoparticles and polymeric medical devices: a new approach to prevention of infection? *J Antimicrob Chemother*. 2004;54:1019-1024.

172. Ketchum AR, Kappler MP, Wu J, et al. The preparation and characterization of nitric oxide releasing silicone rubber materials impregnated with S-nitroso-tert-dodecyl mercaptan. *J Mater Chem B*. 2016;4:422-430.

173. Nichols SP, Schoenfisch MH. Nitric oxide flux-dependent bacterial adhesion and viability at fibrinogen-coated surfaces. *Biomater Sci*. 2013;1:1151-1159.

174. Handa H, Brisbois EJ, Major TC, et al. In vitro and in vivo study of sustained nitric oxide release coating using diazeniumdiolate-doped poly(vinyl chloride) matrix with poly(lactide-co-glycolide) additive. *J Mater Chem B*. 2013;1:3578-3587.

175. Ren H, Colletta A, Koley D, et al. Thromboresistant/anti-biofilm catheters via electrochemically modulated nitric oxide release. *Bioelectrochemistry*. 2015;104:10-16.

176. Ren H, Wu J, Xi C, et al. Electrochemically modulated nitric oxide (NO) releasing biomedical devices via copper(II)-tri(2-pyridylmethyl) amine mediated reduction of nitrite. *ACS Appl Mater Interfaces*. 2014;6:3779-3783.

177. Brisbois EJ, Davis RP, Jones AM, et al. Reduction in thrombosis and bacterial adhesion with 7 day implantation of S-nitroso-*N*-acetylpenicillamine (SNAP)-doped Elast-eon E2As catheters in sheep. *J Mater Chem B*. 2015;3:1639-1645.

178. Wang H, Teng F, Yang X, et al. Preventing microbial biofilms on catheter tubes using ultrasonic guided waves. *Nature*. 2017;7:616.

179. Gnanadhas DP, Elango M, Janardhanraj S, et al. Successful treatment of biofilm infections using shock waves combined with antibiotic therapy. *Nature*. 2015;5:17440.

180. Chen X, Li X. Extracorporeal shock wave therapy could be a potential adjuvant treatment for orthopaedic implant-associated infections. *J Med Hypotheses Ideas*. 2013;7:54-58.

181. Gomez-Carretero S, Nybom R, Richter-Dahlfors A. Electroenhanced antimicrobial coating based on conjugated polymers with covalently coupled silver nanoparticles prevents *Staphylococcus aureus* biofilm formation. *Adv Healthc Mater*. 2017;6. doi:10.1002/adhm.201700435.

182. Voegele P, Badiola J, Schmidt-Malan SM, et al. Antibiofilm activity of electrical current in a catheter model. *Antimicrob Agents Chemother*. 2015;60:1476-1480.

183. Brinkman CL, Schmidt-Malan SM, Karau MJ, et al. Exposure of bacterial biofilms to electrical current leads to cell death mediated in part by reactive oxygen species. *PLoS One*. 2016;11:e0168595.

184. Schmidt-Malan SM, Karau MJ, Cede J, et al. Antibiofilm activity of low-amperage continuous and intermittent direct electrical current. *Antimicrob Agents Chemother*. 2015;59:4610-4615.

Nanotechnology for Disinfection and Sterilization

David W. Hobson

Naturally occurring mineral, liquid, and organic particles come in a wide range of sizes, shapes, and compositions in the universe, and living things require particles of many types, including particles with dimensions in the nanometer range, nanoparticles (NPs), to support normal biological functions and for survival. In marine, desert, forest, polar, and other free tropospheric environments, natural processes such as secondary aerosol formation, dust storms, and breaking waves are major sources of natural NPs.[1,2] The atmosphere of the earth is so laden with particles, including NPs, that each breath contains roughly 50 million, give or take a few million, particles of 50 nm or less in dimension.[3] The light scattering effects of these particles are largely responsible for the beautiful sunrises and sunsets that we observe.[1,4] In the upper parts of the atmosphere (stratosphere, mesosphere, and thermosphere), meteoritic smoke is also a source of NPs.[5] Regardless of particle size and composition, each different type of NP exhibits distinctive chemical, physical, and optical properties; biotransformation mechanisms; biological deposition; and elimination pathways that are often distinct from the elements that compose the NP and from larger, micron-sized particles of the same composition.[1,2] It is clear then that living with NPs is not exactly new. The NPs that are ever present in our atmosphere such as ocean spray, volcanic ash, airborne soil sediment, and even man-made emissions such as industrial smoke, motor vehicle exhaust, dust and vapor have been around living things for a long time and, in some cases, even since life began on our planet. In fact, many cellular structures and particles with nanometer dimensions are essential for life.[1] Some types of NPs with elemental compositions demonstrate antimicrobial properties such as silver (Ag), gold (Au), copper (Cu), zinc NPs, as well as other nanomaterials of various compositions and molecular structures including NP "functionalized" single-walled carbon nanotubes (SWCNT) and multi-walled carbon nanotubes (MWCNT).[6,7]

The ability to manufacture and engineer nanomaterials, or to control matter at the nanoscale at dimensions between approximately 1 and 100 nm, is termed *nanotechnology* and is a relatively new and rapidly developing and vast technology platform finding application in essentially every area of industry including a growing number of applications in medicine including the development of new, technologically advanced antimicrobial technologies. Some of these new nanotechnological antimicrobial materials have applications in disinfection and sterilization products and processes.[8,9] In the 1 to 100 nm dimensional range, unique phenomena that enable the novel applications occur and represent a technological dimension and tool in our ability to design and develop new products in essentially every area of human endeavor.[10] Nanotechnology encompasses nanoscale science and nanoengineering that involves imaging, measuring, modeling, and manipulating matter at the nanoscale. With the development of current and emerging technology to manipulate matter in the nanoscale and even into the atomic range, humans have arrived at a point where we possess the technological capability to engineer and construct at will essentially any feasible molecular structure using an atomic palette that includes a vast number and variety of natural and synthetic nuclides and an almost unlimited molecular structural potential.[1]

Even though there is great potential to engineer and develop novel nanomaterials, there can be limits to what applications can be commercially successful and at what point a given nanomaterial may pose a potential risk to human, animal, or environmental safety. Therefore, in the application of nanotechnology for disinfection or sterilization, there is a rapidly growing number of engineered nanoproducts in development and commerce that includes effective antimicrobial products that can be safe and others that are of greater concern for potential human, animal, or environmental toxicological effects.[1] Those of greatest concern for safety typically require contact with

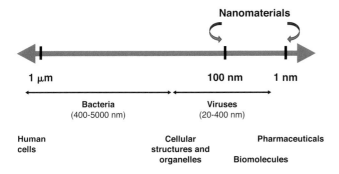

FIGURE 74.1 Nanometer-sized materials dimensions relative to the dimensions of different biological structures and microbes. (Based on Hobson et al.[1])

biological systems that would include uses in antimicrobial technologies as well as pharmaceuticals, medical devices, cosmetics, etc. Conversely, items such as electronics use polymers and coatings (including those that are antimicrobial) applied to metals, glass, and plastics, where the nanomaterial is permanently or very strongly bound to the larger molecular structure or are otherwise not generally available for biological contact, the likelihood of significant toxicological effect, and risk is typically expected to be of lesser concern.[1]

A size-oriented, microbial and cellular (as well as toxicological) dimensional perspective of nanomaterial exposure to biological systems is shown in Figure 74.1. From this figure, it can readily be seen that materials within the critical nanosize range of 1 to 100 nm are also within the size range where cellular structures and biomolecules occur. Therefore, the efficacy and even safety of any given nanomaterial is dependent not only on its chemical composition but also its molecular size and structure.[1] There is increasing toxicological evidence that some types of nanomaterials have both chemical and structural features that could lead to a potential for adverse biological effects.[11] Nanomaterials can be naturally occurring or man-made and are most generally identified as materials having at least one dimension <100 nm.[12] This chapter focuses primarily on the use of man-made, engineered nanomaterials that are products of nanotechnology rather than the effects of naturally occurring nanomaterials.

◗ DESIGN, CHEMISTRY, MOLECULAR STRUCTURE, AND NOMENCLATURE

At the nanometer dimensional level, scientists and engineers endeavor to control individual atoms and molecules to do amazing things. Researchers are employing nanotechnology to advance technology toward solving major challenges in health, energy, agriculture, water quality, materials science, and other areas. Scientists and engineers engaged in the development of nanotechnology

are, for the first time in human history, able to advance nanotechnology by making molecular structures at will to include an almost infinite variety of potential molecules and molecular structures and polymers. Essentially, any reasonably stable, nanomolecular structure and composition is now potentially feasible by design. This advanced materials fabrication capability is translating rapidly into new products in essentially every business sector and so, it should not be surprising that nanotechnology is being used to develop and advance new, safe, and effective sterilization and disinfection products. The use of nanotechnology in these products is especially of interest because it represents a new and potentially useful technology platform to help combat an increasing array of antibiotic-resistant bacteria. So, even in the world of infection prevention as well as the development of novel antimicrobials for other applications, it is imperative that scientists and clinicians working to advance these nanotechnologies have some understanding of their chemistry and structural characteristics and nomenclature in order to stay abreast of technological advances of interest.

The chemistry of nanomaterials covers a broad and increasing landscape and is also diverse. At the simplest level, there are NPs made from pure elements such as NPs of Ag, Au, iron (Fe), silicon, etc. Then, at a slightly higher level of chemical and molecular structural sophistication, there are particles composed of combinations of atoms such as titanium dioxide (TiO_2), Fe oxide, zinc oxide (ZnO), zirconium oxide, etc. For example, zirconium oxide NPs (ZrO_2), like many other elemental NPs, can be fabricated and made available for a variety of applications as nanodots, nanofluids, and nanocrystals. Zirconium oxide NPs are also often doped with yttrium oxide, calcia, or magnesia to impart different antimicrobial properties for a variety of applications including use in dental infection control.[13]

Elemental AgNPs represent the simplest and oldest major use of an engineered NP as an antimicrobial agent that has been used with success since ancient times and into the present in modern antimicrobial products as engineered AgNPs.[14-16] The AgNPs have been shown to possess several mechanisms involved in their bactericidal efficacy. These mechanisms include attachment to the bacterial cell surface and penetration of the bacterial cell membrane, interrupting permeability and disrupting metabolic pathways of the cell.[14,17] In addition, AgNPs can bind to bacterial DNA and prevent its replication and/or through a lethal interaction with bacterial ribosomes.[18,19] The AgNP damage to the structure of the bacterial cell membrane results in leakage and reduces the activity of some membranous enzymes that has been shown to be lethal to *Escherichia coli* bacteria.[20] The AgNPs also typically exhibit greater toxicity to microorganisms and lower toxicity to mammalian cells making them effective and potentially safe antimicrobial candidates that have found their way into commercial antimicrobial products.[21]

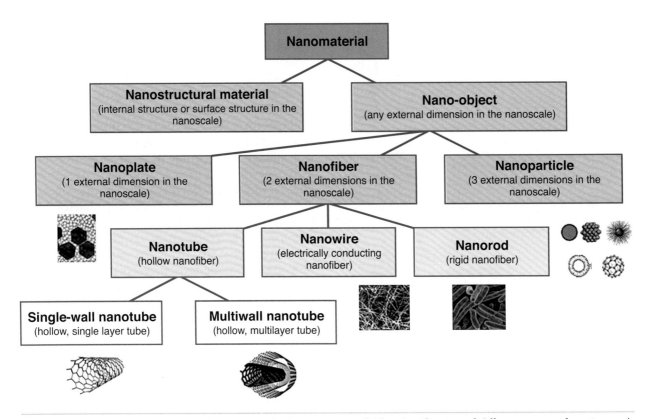

FIGURE 74.2 Nomenclature based on nanoscale dimensions useful for classification of different types of engineered nanomaterials. (Based on Hobson et al.[1])

Combinations or different metals or metals such as Cu, palladium (Pd) and their bimetallic palladium@ copper (Pd@Cu) NPs have been synthesized.[22] The synthesized Cu, Pd, and Pd@Cu NPs were evaluated for antimicrobial activity using specific different microorganism strains that included *Proteus mirabilis*, *Bacillus thuringiensis*, *Shigella flexneri*, *Staphylococcus aureus*, *Klebsiella pneumoniae*, *E coli*, *Pseudomonas aeruginosa*, and *Salmonella* Typhimurium. The antibacterial activities of bimetallic Pd@Cu NPs were found to inhibit the growth of all microorganisms tested at a maximal level of efficacy as compared with the inhibition observed with the standard control antibacterial drug ofloxacin.

Beyond the level at which different atoms are combined into the nanomaterial structure, there are more advanced chemical and polymeric structures such as fullerenes, nanotubes of many types, nanorods, polymer nanocomposites, etc. As an example, polymer nanocomposites consist of a polymer or copolymer having NPs or nanofillers dispersed in a polymer matrix that can be made into different shapes (eg, nanoplatelets, nanofibers, nanospheroids), where at least one dimension is in the range of 1 to 100 nm. Figure 74.2 provides an example of useful nomenclature for classification of most types of nanomaterials based on nanoscale dimensions.

Historically, the technological and commercial advancement of nanotechnology from the first generation to increasingly more complex and potentially profitable next generation nanomedical products has occurred to include the progressive development of four different generations of nanotechnology.[23,24] These began with the first-generation passive nanostructures and then in a time progressive manner the second (active nanostructures), third (nanosystems), and fourth (molecular nanosystems) generations. This concept has been reasonably accurate both in the progression and predicted timeline over the past few decades and is useful in understanding the levels of complexity of nanomedical technologies that have been, are now emerging, and that may emerge in the future from invention, basic research, and into commercial development.

ANTIMICROBIAL MODES OF ACTION OF NANOMATERIALS

Some NP-antimicrobial agents act as potent broad-spectrum antimicrobial agents, disinfection and wound-healing agents, and sustained inhibitors of intracellular pathogens. Like AgNPs, these may employ more than one mechanism in their antimicrobial action. Novel nanomaterials with several antimicrobial properties are not only possible but also likely, and this multiple functionality is beginning to revolutionize clinical medicine and play a significant role in disinfection.[19,25-27] Traditionally, most antimicrobial agents inhibit microbial growth through several mechanisms such as cell wall inhibition and lysis, inhibition of protein synthesis, alteration of cell membranes, inhibition of nucleic acid synthesis, and antimetabolite activity.[28] The NP antimicrobials, on the other hand, have a vast array of possible physiochemical properties with respect to size, shape, surface area, surface energy, charge, crystallinity, agglomeration, aggregation, and chemical composition.[29-31] Although for many NP-antimicrobial materials the precise mechanisms of action are still unknown and are currently under investigation, studies show that NPs often act by causing bacterial cell membrane degradation.[32-35] For example, Li et al[35] found that cell membrane degradation of *S aureus* occurred following exposure to catechin-Cu NPs. Catechin is a crystalline, natural phenol, and antioxidant compound from catechu, the tannic juice or boiled extract of the Mimosa catechu plant (*Acacia catechu* L.). Catechin-Cu NPs were also found to exert different mechanisms of action that resulted in *E coli* cell wall degradation. This is thought to be an indication of potentially different impacts on gram-negative and gram-positive bacteria by these NPs.[35] Similar types of multiple effects have also been observed with CuNPs that exhibit antimicrobial actions, which, in addition to cell membrane damage, include the generation of reactive oxygen species (ROS) and lipid peroxidation.[33]

Other CuNP-antibacterial actions include protein oxidation and DNA degradation within *E coli* cells.[33] Another study by Xie et al[36] showed that ZnO NPs exerted a bactericidal effect by disruption of the cell membrane and oxidative stress in *Campylobacter jejuni*. The NP-antimicrobials such as AgNPs have also been shown to bind to lipopolysaccharides, surface proteins (ie, porin, enzymes, etc), causing microbial cell wall collapse and altering the membrane potential.[36] Similarly, AgNPs have been found to induce efflux of phosphate, reduction of cellular adenosine triphosphate level, interacting with sulfhydryl (or thiol) groups and altering cytoplasmic components as well as inhibiting respiratory enzymes and blocking DNA replication in both gram-negative and gram-positive bacterial pathogens.[36] These studies show that different NPs have very different physiochemical properties and thus exhibit different antimicrobial mechanisms of action.

That the antimicrobial actions of NPs include biocidal destruction of cell membranes, blockage of enzyme pathways, alterations of microbial cell wall, and nucleic materials pathway as well as other, yet to be elucidated modes of action has been observed by many researchers.[37] The NP antimicrobial agents, in general, appear to have excellent potent and low tendency for inducing microbicidal resistance when compared to non–NP-antimicrobial agents.[38] These multiple possible molecular mechanisms by which metal-based NPs have been shown to kill multidrug-resistant (MDR) bacteria via disturbance in respiration, disruption of DNA synthesis, membrane damage, inhibition of cellular growth, etc, have been extensively reviewed.[8,39,40] The microbial toxicity of metal-based NPs

as well as other nanomaterials has been attributed to ROS production such as hydroxyl radicals (•OH), superoxide anions, and hydrogen peroxide (H_2O_2) that inhibit DNA replication as well as amino acid synthesis and damage the bacterial cell membranes via lipid peroxidation, compromising membrane semipermeability and repressing oxidative phosphorylation. The •OH formation has been observed with AgNPs, and H_2O_2 production has been shown with ZnO NPs.[39-42] The TiO_2 NPs have been observed to act via a photocatalytic process.[43] Free Cu^{++} from Cu-containing NPs and Mg halogen (MgX_2)-containing NPs also induce formation of ROS.[33,44]

Different microorganisms have varying sensitivities to metal ions. The Ag and ZnO NPs have been reported to exert antibacterial activity by release of Ag^+ and Zn^{++} that disrupt the cell membrane.[39,42,45] Interaction of Ag^+ with sulfhydryl groups in enzymes and other cellular constituents, making them dysfunctional, is an important antibacterial action of Ag NPs.[8] The Ag^+ also inhibits cell wall synthesis in gram-positive bacteria, Cu^{++} has been shown to interact with amine and carboxyl groups on the surfaces of microbial cells, such as *Bacillus subtilis* and Au NPs have also been shown to act by bacterial membrane disruption.[8,46]

Table 74.1 shows examples the variety of antimicrobial nanomaterials as well as examples of the types of microorganisms that have shown susceptibility and reported mode(s) of action. Many different types of antimicrobial nanomaterials are possible, and their modes of action often involve several molecular targets on and within a variety of microorganisms. This is only snapshot because this list is ever expanding at a rapid pace.

Nanotechnology provides an excellent platform for the development of molecularly targeted nanomaterials. The development of targeted antimicrobial nanomaterials for use in disinfection to include health care applications as well as others shows that nanomaterials of many different types and compositions are possible and that nanomaterials, especially NPs, in general can facilitate:

- Uptake into cells and transcytosis across cells
- Distribution into the blood and lymph circulation to reach potentially sensitive target sites (eg, bone marrow, lymph nodes, spleen, liver, kidneys, and heart)
- Brain entry via nasal nerves (eg, polio virus)
- Recognition and processing by the immune system
- Entry into the cell nucleus
- Skin, inhalation and gastrointestinal absorption
- A growing list of additional antimicrobial processes

In addition to the development of NP-antibacterial technologies, NP-microbicides including those of dendrimer-containing nanoscale microbicides also hold potential safety efficacy against viruses.[59-61] VivaGel® (SPL7013 Gel or astodrimer sodium) is an example of this type of NP use that shows antiviral and antibacterial properties. Several clinical studies have successfully tested

TABLE 74.1 Examples of different types of engineered nanomaterials and their antimicrobial action

NP	Target Microbe(s)	Microbicidal Effects	Source Reference
Ag	*Acinetobacter baumannii, Salmonella typhi, Vibrio cholerae, Bacillus subtilis, Staphylococcus aureus, Escherichia coli, Streptococcus pyogenes, Pseudomonas aeruginosa, Staphylococcus epidermidis, Enterococcus faecalis, Klebsiella pneumoniae, Listeria monocytogenes, Proteus mirabilis, Micrococcus luteus,* hepatitis B virus	ROS generation, lipid peroxidation, inhibition of ETC cytochromes, membrane disintegration, inhibition of cell wall synthesis, increase in membrane permeability, dissipation of proton gradient resulting in lysis, adhesion to cell surface causing lipid and protein damage, ribosome destabilization, intercalation between DNA bases, disruption of biofilms, inhibit virus replication	Lu et al,[19] Dakal et al,[39] Yoon et al[46]
Au	*E coli, S aureus, B subtilis, K pneumoniae*	Loss of membrane potential, disruption of respiratory chain, reduced ATPase activity, decline in subunit of ribosome for tRNA binding, membrane disruption	Shamaila et al,[47] Huo et al[48]
Cu	*B subtilis, E coli*	ROS generation, disorganization of membrane, inhibition of DNA replication Dissipation of cell membrane potential, lipid peroxidation, protein oxidation, DNA degradation	Chatterjee et al,[33] Dakal et al[39]
CdS	*E coli*	Antibiofilm activity	Dhanabalan and Gurunathan[49]
Se	*S aureus, E coli*	Biofilm inhibition	Guisbiers et al[50]
NiO	*S aureus, Streptococcus pneumoniae*	Increase in bacterial cell wall permeability	Khashan et al[51]
MgF₂	*E coli, S aureus*	ROS generation, penetration of cell envelope, lipid peroxidation, biofilm inhibition	Lellouche et al[45]
TiO₂	*E coli, P aeruginosa, S aureus, Enterococcus faecium*	ROS generation, adsorption to cell surface, inhibition of biofilm	Hemeg[8]
ZnO	*S aureus, E coli, P aeruginosa, B subtilis, Stenotrophomonas acidaminiphila, Streptococcus agalactiae,* MRSA	ROS generation, inhibition of biofilm, Zn^{2+} release, enhanced membrane permeability. ROS production, disruption of membrane, adsorption to cell surface, lipids and protein damage, inhibition of microbial biofilm formation	Sirelkhatim et al[42]
YF₂	*E coli, S aureus*	Antibiofilm properties	Lellouche et al[45]
Bi	*Streptococcus mutans*	Inhibition of biofilm	Hernandez-Delgadillo et al[52]
Cu/Zn	*E coli, S aureus,* MRSA	Antioxidant activity	Ashfaq et al[53]
Magnetic FeO	*E coli, S aureus, P aeruginosa, E faecalis*	Inhibition of bacterial biofilms	Liakos et al[54]
Al₂O₃	*E coli*	Cell wall damage, enters cytoplasm	Ansari et al[55]
SiO₂	*E coli, B subtilis, Pseudomonas fluorescens*	Flocculation, membrane disruption	Jiang et al[56]
Chitosan	*E coli, S aureus*	Flocculation, membrane disruption	Qi et al[57]
ZrO₂	*S aureus, E coli, Candida albicans, Aspergillus niger*	Antifungal and antibacterial properties	Gowri et al[58]

Abbreviations: Ag, silver; Al₂O₃, aluminum oxide; ATP, adenosine triphosphate; Au, gold; Bi, bismuth; CdS, cadmium sulfide; Cu, copper; Cu/Zn, copper/zinc; ETC, electron transport chain; FeO, iron oxide; MgF₂, magnesium fluoride; MRSA, methicillin-resistant *S aureus*; NiO, nickel oxide; NP, nanoparticle; ROS, reactive oxygen species; Se, selenium; SiO₂, silicon dioxide; TiO₂, titanium dioxide; tRNA, transfer RNA; Zn^{2+}, zinc ion; ZnO, zinc oxide; ZrO₂, zirconium oxide; YF₂, yttrium fluoride.

the safety and efficacy of VivaGel®, which is formulated as a mucoadhesive gel and delivered vaginally to relieve the signs and symptoms of bacterial vaginosis (BV) and to reduce risk of recurrence of BV in clinical studies. The gel dendrimer is formulated against human immunodeficiency virus (HIV) and herpes simplex virus and has been reported not to interfere with vaginal or rectal physiological pH.[59-62] The microbicide is meant to disrupt and block viral attachment and/or prevent the viral adsorption from targeting cells of the rectum or vagina and is an example of an innovative nanotechnology-enabled product platform being applied to develop safe and effective new antiviral nanoproducts. These include applications to address a variety of sexual and women's health concerns including the treatment and prevention of BV, prevention of sexually transmitted infections, and incorporation into condoms.

Antimicrobial nanomaterials are also being developed with HIV as the target. It has been reported that gp120 of the HIV virus is blocked by the dendrimer microbicide in VivaGel® from attaching to the CD4 receptors of human white blood cells.[59] Similarly, others have reported that a carbosilane dendrimer microbicide is capable of exhibiting anti-HIV activity through targeting principal proteins of HIV in vitro in vaginal epithelial monolayer cells.[63] Other dendrimers such as heparan sulfate-binding peptide have been shown to inhibit human.[60]

Nano-enabled pharmaceuticals that employ nanotechnology in forms such as polymeric NPs, dendrimers, polymer micelles, and solid lipid NPs have been shown to exhibit excellent antimicrobial profiles. Many of these nanomaterials have potent ligand conjugates that improve the pharmacological and therapeutic profile of such drugs to cross cell membranes, internalize, and provide increased and dose-efficient antimicrobial action.[64-66] The enhanced delivery process facilitates the development of NP drugs with multiple functions of carrier, delivery, and antimicrobial capabilities.[64-67] These enhanced delivery attributes are due to their small size (1-100 nm), the vast NP-functionalization ability, and their robust physiochemical properties. These lead to promising new antimicrobial candidates through nanotechnology, even if biodegradability and toxicological challenges must be overcome.[68,69]

▶ DISINFECTION AND MICROBIAL CONTROL

Several natural and engineered nanomaterials, such as Ag, titanium oxide (TiO), ZnO, and carbon nanotubes (CNT) known to have antibacterial properties, are under consideration as disinfecting agents for medical applications and use with water treatment systems.[70,71] For example, the antibacterial efficacy and toxicity of AgNPs is known to depend on their physicochemical properties including size, shape, surface area, surface charge, and surface coatings.[70] Positively charged AgNPs coated by different ionic liquids

with different alkyl chain lengths were evaluated for their antimicrobial activity against *Enterococcus faecalis* as compared to sodium hypochlorite (NaOCl) and chlorhexidine (CHX).[71] They also compared the cytocompatibility of these solutions against L929 mouse fibroblasts. The AgNPs with positive surface charges capped by two different ionic liquids (imidazolium [Im] and pyridinium [Py]) with two alkyl chain lengths (C_{12} and C_{18}) were tested. The results showed that all AgNPs tested had *E faecalis* MIC_{90} values in significantly lower concentrations than CHX and NaOCl. C_{12} Py-coated AgNPs had the lowest MIC_{90} value. The CHX and NaOCl were more toxic on fibroblasts than all tested AgNPs. Im-coated AgNPs exhibited more compatibility with fibroblasts than Py-coated particles, and C_{12} Im-AgNPs showed the greatest cytocompatibility. Variations in alkyl chain length had no effect on the biocompatibility of these AgNPs. It was concluded that Py improved the antibacterial efficacy of AgNPs compared to Im but had a negative effect on cytocompatibility and that alkyl chain length had no effects on AgNP bioactivity.

In addition to using physical techniques to engineer NPs, it is possible to bioengineer (or bio-nano-engineer) antimicrobial NPs economically and in an environmentally friendly manner using biological systems. For example, Halkai et al[72] used cut leaf segments of *Withania somnifera* (ashwagandha) to isolate fungi that were cultured and used to produce AgNPs. Fresh cultures of *Fusarium semitectum* were inoculated in Erlenmeyer flasks containing 100-mL malt glucose yeast peptone broth and incubated at 29°C for 72 hours to grow the biomass, which was harvested and filtered to produce a cell-free fungal filtrate. The filtrate was then mixed with aqueous solution of silver nitrate of 1-mM concentration kept in dark at 29°C for 24 hours for the production of AgNPs, which was monitored by visual observation for color change of the solution. Biosynthesized AgNPs were further characterized using ultraviolet-visible spectrophotometry, transmission electron microscopy, selected area electron diffraction analysis, and Fourier transform infrared spectroscopy. Antibacterial efficacy of the biosynthesized AgNPs was demonstrated with observation of zones of inhibition of ≥17 mm against the periodontal pathogen *Porphyromonas gingivalis*. This research demonstrates that the production of useful, antimicrobial nanomaterials can be accomplished by biotechnology, which may help provide energy efficient, low-cost, renewable, and abundant sources for these nanomaterials.

Protein and peptide NPs of various types are possible and show potentially useful antimicrobial properties with low toxicity.[73,74] For example, antimicrobial peptide (AMP) efficacy against *S aureus* was evaluated by Almaaytah et al.[74] A potent ultrashort AMP named RBRBR was encapsulated into chitosan-based NPs (CS-NPs) using an ionotropic gelation method with an encapsulation efficacy reported for RBRBR into CS-NPs of 51.33% and with a loading capacity of 10.17%. The release kinetics of RBRBR from the nanocarrier exhibited slow release followed by progressive linear release for 14 days. The antibacterial kinetics of RBRBR-CS-NPs was tested against four strains of methicillin-resistant *S aureus* (MRSA) for 4 days, and the RBRBR-CS-NPs exhibited a 3 $\log_{10}$ decrease in the number of colonies when compared to CS-NP and a 5 $\log_{10}$ decrease when compared to controls. The encapsulated peptide NP formulations also were observed to limit the toxicity of the free peptide against both mammalian cells and human erythrocytes and demonstrated up to 98% inhibition of biofilm formation when tested in a commercial biofilm-contaminated device (Innovotech, Edmonton, Canada) with gram-positive *S aureus* (33591) grown at 37°C for 20 hours. The authors concluded that loading RBRBR into CS-NPs could represent an innovative approach to develop delivery systems for achieving potent antimicrobial effects against MDR and biofilm-forming bacteria, with negligible systemic toxicity and reduced synthetic costs, thereby overcoming the obstructions to clinical development of AMPs.

Some antimicrobial NPs act via the photocatalytic production of ROS that inactivate viruses, cleave DNA, and cause disruption of the structural integrity of bacterial cell envelopes resulting in cellular leakage, damaged intracellular integrity, interrupted cellular energy production, and cell death.[75] The NPs used for water disinfection must exhibit potent antimicrobial activity while remaining harmless to humans at antimicrobial exposure concentrations. There are also external factors that may affect the commercial viability of such disinfectants that include the action of salts that promote coagulation and precipitation, the presence of natural organic matter that coats or adsorbs onto NPs and reduces the bioavailability for antimicrobial action, and competing chemical substances that consume ROS.[75] Similarly, the efficacy of NP-containing antimicrobial coatings may also be compromised by the surface deposition of debris (eg, soluble microbial products, inorganic precipitates, or dead cells) that occlude molecular sites for antimicrobial action and then facilitate biofilm formation.[75] The need to retain and recycle NPs to reduce cost and avoid potential health and environmental impacts may also be limitations to commercial viability. Nevertheless, antimicrobial NPs, no matter how they are applied, have the potential to overcome critical challenges associated with traditional chemical water disinfectants such as the generation of free chlorine and/or ozone that can produce harmful disinfection by-products and short-lived antimicrobial activity.

The NP antimicrobials (such as TiO_2) can be used to enhance existing technologies such as ultraviolet inactivation of viruses, solar disinfection of bacteria, and biofouling of filtration membranes.[75] The demand for new antimicrobials to support decentralized or point-of-use water treatment and reuse systems is expected to stimulate further research and commercialization of NPs for water disinfection.[75]

Nanotechnology-enabled materials have potential as low-energy replacements for conventional reverse osmosis membranes in desalination and water reuse applications.[76] Nanoparticulate zeolite coatings, for example, promise a highly selective material that has the chemical, thermal, and mechanical stabilities of conventional ceramic membranes. Nanocomposite membranes, in general, exhibit up to three times greater permeability than current commercial polymeric membranes with no change in salt rejection and can be fabricated with antimicrobial and photoreactive functionalities.[76] Aquaporin (AQP) is an hour glass–shaped protein found in cell membranes with unique water transport properties including molecular transport size restriction of approximately 2.8 angstroms, positively charged amino acid regions that reject the passage of cations, and functional water dipole reorientation to ensure very selective water penetration.

The AQP-based lipid bilayer nanovesicles exhibit nearly 100 times higher water permeability than commercial membranes with near perfect salt rejection. The CNT and graphene-based membranes and self-assembled block copolymer membranes are also capable of forming highly selective structures reminiscent of AQP-based materials.[76]

Nanotechnology has enabled the development of nanoscale oligodynamic disinfection processes using metallic NPs such as Ag, Cu, zinc, titanium, nickel (Ni), and cobalt to engineer a new class of materials capable of killing waterborne disease-causing microbes.[77] These promising nanomaterials have bactericidal and viricidal properties due to their charge capacity, high surface to volume ratios, crystallographic structure, and adeptness to various substrates to increase their contact efficiency. Given the cost and known problems with disinfection by-products of conventional chemical disinfection systems, nanoscale oligodynamic disinfection appears a potentially viable alternative for point of use applications.[77]

Fullerenes are a class of molecular structured nanomaterials that are composed entirely of carbon. They have a size range of 0.65 to 0.7 nm, and their synthesis provided the foundation for carbon-based nanotechnology that has now branched out into a multitude of nanostructures that may include other elements in addition to carbon. The first of these molecules, named Buckminsterfullerene (C_{60} or "Buckyball"), was discovered between 1984 and 1985 and contains 60 carbons in the form of a hollow spherical cage consisting of 12 pentagonal and 20 hexagonal faces.[78] This was named after Buckminster Fuller, an architect of many geodesic dome structures that appear similar to the C_{60} molecular structure. C_{60} is only one example of the entire class of carbon structures now simply called fullerenes discovered in 1985 by Robert Curl, Harold Kroto, and Richard Smalley who were awarded the 1996 Nobel Prize in Chemistry for their work. Many other spherical fullerenes have since been synthesized as well as nonspherical fullerenes that include cylinders (CNTs, which may be single-walled, SWCNT, or multi-walled,

MWCNT tubes) as well as lobed and bowl-like structures. Fullerenes and nanotubes allow an almost infinite variety of functionalities ranging from simple hydroxylation to the grafting of DNA as well as other biomolecules to the carbon structure. The potential for many practical and commercial applications has significantly increased demand for the production of high-quality fullerenes and CNTs.[79] In environmental engineering, fullerenes have received significant interest as a basis for developing new technologies for nanomaterial-enabled oxidation and disinfection, improved membrane functionality, and as adsorbents and biofilm-resistant surfaces.[79] The development of fullerene composite materials for environmental uses (including water purification) includes to strengthen membranes and modify membrane surface chemistry, generate ROS, in situ generation of oxidants to destroy trace organic compounds, inhibit biofilm development, and reduce biofouling. The use of fullerenes in conjunction with UV irradiation is considered as an advanced disinfection process with significant potential for viral inactivation.[79]

The TiO photocatalysts have been widely studied for both solar energy conversion and environmental applications in the past several decades because of their high chemical stability, photoactivity, relatively low cost, and low toxicity.[80] The photocatalytic capability of TiO is limited to only ultraviolet light with a <400-nm wavelength band edge, seriously limiting its solar efficiency. To overcome this limitation, both chemical and physical modifications have been developed to extend the absorption band edge of TiO into the visible-light region of the spectrum. These new TiO visible-light photocatalysts have been further modified by the inclusion of transition metal oxides in addition to TiO and fabricated into NPs, nanoporous fibers, and nanoporous foams. These nanostructured photocatalysts show very fast photocatalytic degradation rates in organics matrices to include bacteria, spores, and virus and have great potential in water disinfection and removal of organic contaminants in water.[80]

Zero-valent Fe and bimetallic NPs such as Ni/Fe and Pd/Fe are effective for the dechlorination of organics (eg, trichloroethylene) but are prone to oxidation when exposed to air.[81] Incorporation of these NPs in a membrane phase minimizes oxidation and simplifies the engineering of nanotechnology-based systems for water treatment.[81] The NPs composed of Fe and combinations with Ni and Pd are synthesized in solution using common microemulsion techniques; they are continuously kept in an organic solvent to inhibit oxidation, until they are transferred to the polymer (eg, cellulose acetate) phase as a polymer dispersion slurry. Flat sheet membranes are made from this polymer dispersion using conventional and scalable phase inversion techniques. These materials show excellent organic degradation rates similar to unsupported NPs. The degradation rate has been observed to depend strongly on the composition of the incorporated NPs. The rate of degradation increased in the order of Fe only, Ni/Fe, and Pd/Fe. For bimetallic NPs, the ratio of secondary metal to Fe also had an effect. For example, an optimum ratio for Ni/Fe was observed at approximately 20 wt% Ni for postcoated particles. Besides the antimicrobial action of the bimetallic NPs, the membrane structure is also a strong absorbent for dissolved organics with a sorption effect that is rapid and decreases only as dechlorination proceeds.[81]

▶ STERILIZATION

Sterilization, when it comes to the products of nanotechnology (NPs as well as other nanomaterials), includes both the procedures needed for the sterilization of the nanoproducts themselves as well as the potential use of some forms of nanotechnology in the improvement sterilization procedures. Several conventionally used methodologies such as filtration, autoclaving, irradiation, as well as treatment with formaldehyde, ethylene oxide, and gas plasma have been implemented for the sterilization of NPs.[82] Although numerous well-established sterilization techniques exist, concerns have been raised regarding the adverse effects that these techniques may have on the physicochemical characteristics of the NPs because changes in these characteristics could potentially affect both the toxicity and the efficacy of the sterilized NPs.

A radiation dose of ≥15 kGy of either γ-irradiation or e-beam irradiation has been shown to be generally effective in the sterilization of poly(butyl cyanoacrylate) NPs that were deliberately contaminated with spore-forming bacteria.[83] However, despite the potential efficacy of this mode of sterilization, various adverse effects have been observed on NPs when irradiation was used for their sterilization.[82] Although effective for the sterilization of uncoated metal NPs, irradiation may not be suitable for the sterilization of coatings to metal NPs and polymeric nanomaterials. Following γ-irradiation, even citrate-stabilized AgNPs were shown to lose their typical polycrystalline structure and form both smaller particulates and larger irregular aggregates.[84] In addition, these γ-irradiated NPs exhibited a 4- to 5-fold increase in their ability to cause platelet aggregation, and therefore, γ-irradiation would not be suitable in the sterilization of these NPs.

Chemical sterilization of nanomaterials using formaldehyde, ethylene oxide, and gas plasma processes also had variable results.[82] Aggregation, impaired resuspension of NPs, and alterations of NP-coating (eg, polyethylene glycol) layers have been observed with chemical sterilization techniques.[85,86]

Sterile filtration has proven to be a reasonable method for the removal of bacterial contamination from NPs, provided that a sufficiently high percentage of NPs can be recovered following filtration.[82] The typical use of 0.2-μm or 0.22-μm filters may not always be possible if the NPs are larger than, or close to, the pore size of the filters because clogging can occur resulting in a decreased.[87,88] It has been observed, for example, that filtration of 200- to 300-nm Poly(D,L-lactide-co-glycolide) (PLGA) nanospheres prepared using the standard emulsion solvent diffusion method resulted in less than 10% of the nanospheres passing through the membrane filter.[89] This problem was circumvented by optimizing the synthesis methodology to produce nanospheres with a particle diameter of 102 to 163 nm, of which 100% to 98% could pass through the membrane filter and successfully pass bacterial sterility tests; however, adjusting the size of the NPs in order to enable them to pass through a membrane filter may not always be feasible or practical.[82,89]

Autoclaving with high-pressurized steam, at a minimum temperature of 121°C, has been used to sterilize a variety of different types of nanomaterials. Selenium NPs have been shown to be essentially unchanged before and after autoclave sterilization.[90] In contrast, autoclaving some types of polymeric NPs (PBLG [PEGylated poly(γ-benzyl-Lglutamate)], PEC [poly(epsilon-caprolactone)], etc) has shown to cause aggregation of the NPs as well as significant size increases.[91,92]

Waterborne health issues continue to grow despite the large number of available solutions. Current sterilization techniques to fight with waterborne diseases struggle to meet the demands on cost, efficiency, and reach. Effective alternatives are pressingly required. Scalable, low-cost, highly efficient, and reusable disinfection or sterilization methods are needed to improve water quality and improve health conditions on a global scale. Prussian blue-coated ferroferric oxide (Fe_3O_4-PB) composites used for water treatment showed that these composites exhibit superior photothermal inactivation of bacteria under solar light irradiation, with nearly complete inactivation of bacterial cells in only 15 minutes.[93] These composites showed excellent bactericidal performance in authentic water matrices. The highly magnetized Fe core of the Fe_3O_4-PB facilitates magnetic separation and recycling. Multiple cycle runs reveal that Fe_3O_4-PB composites have exceptional stability and reusability.

The NPs have been used in many areas of biotechnology including plant tissue sterilization. Green synthesized AgNPs were shown to be effective for the surface sterilization of different Lamiaceae seeds (*Salvia farinacea, Ocimum basilicum, Thymus vulgaris, O basilicum* var purpurascens).[94] Water extracts of dried *Alkanna tinctorum* rhizomes and *Syzygium aromaticum* flowers were used in the bioreduction of Ag ions. The Lamiaceae seeds were exposed to 0-, 1-, 7-, 14-, and 28-day old colloidal solutions of AgNPs, and their effects on germination and surface sterilization were determined. Fresh (0 and 1 day old) colloidal solutions of AgNPs were found very effective for surface sterilization of the seeds (100%). Moreover, they showed no negative effect on both germination and morphology of plantlets. It was shown that AgNPs can be used as a surface sterilization

agent and they have no adverse effects on seed germination and in vitro plantlet growth.

Nanotherapeutics (NTs) are complex systems with multiple components, each of which could be susceptible to the damaging effects of the sterilization procedure in a different way. Sterilization by autoclaving could result in heat-induced chemical and physical changes in NTs, and sterilization by gamma irradiation could induce free radical formation, which could result in immediate chemical changes as well as impact the stability of the product. A suitable battery of tests is required during developmental studies to understand the impact of different modes of sterilization early in the development process. The panel of analytical methods used to evaluate the effects of the process must be appropriate for monitoring the physical and chemical changes to NTs as well as functional changes. In order to accurately assess the impact of sterilization, it is necessary to perform all characterization studies before and after sterilization procedures to confirm effects or lack thereof and to establish a stability program suitable for the detection of chemical degradants that may arise from the sterilization procedure during the shelf life of NTs.

CLINICAL ANTIMICROBIAL AND DISINFECTION APPLICATIONS

The NP-antimicrobial agents can help to eliminate some of the restrictions of conventional antimicrobial agents. The NP-antimicrobial agents have been shown to be clinically useful as potent broad-spectrum antimicrobials, for the sustained inhibition of intracellular pathogens, wound healing antimicrobials, and to impart antimicrobial qualities to various types surfaces and surface coatings. The development of safe and effective NP-antimicrobial agents with multiple functionality is well poised to revolutionize clinical medicine and play a significant role in improving health care practices and alleviating disease.[82] Some examples of emerging clinical applications of antimicrobial nanomaterials in medical products and to help overcome the current problem of microbial resistance are provided in the following text.

Use of Nanomaterials in Medical Products

The antimicrobial properties of NPs were recognized decades ago and have been successfully employed, especially AgNPs, in bandages, as coatings on medical devices, or in suspensions used for wound and burn treatments.[95] Very soon after the initial uses of these NPs, there were concerns of potential toxicity. This concern led to increased scrutiny and investigations related to the safe use of NPs in sunscreens as well as other medical applications; this has established an interest in the research of a new toxicology subdiscipline, nanotoxicology.[96-98]

The earliest intentional use of nanotechnology in medical products involved the use of NPs in the formulation of products such as topical pharmaceuticals and sunscreen formulations.[98-100] This level of nanotechnology development would be considered first-generation nanotechnology.[23] Examples include the use of zinc or titanium NPs to block ultraviolet light in sunscreen formulations, the creation of nanoemulsions of oil in water or water in oil to enhance the solubility and stability of active pharmaceutical agents in various drug products, and the manufacture of nanoparticulate carriers of active pharmaceutical agents with various nanostructures to improve target tissue delivery. This generation of NPs has been foundational to the development and establishment of nanotechnology as a platform for commercial medical product applications and advancements in nanotoxicology.

Bacterial infection is a major concern during the wound healing process. The Ag/silver bromide (AgBr)-loaded mesoporous silica NPs (Ag/AgBr/MSNs) are designed to harvest visible light for rapid disinfection and acceleration of wound healing. The Ag/AgBr nanostructure has a remarkable photocatalysis ability because it can generate electron-hole pairs easily after light absorption. This photocatalytic effect enhances the antibacterial activity by producing ROS.[101] The bacterial killing efficiency of Ag/AgBr/MSNs is 95.62% and 99.99% against S $aureus$ and E $coli$, respectively, within 15 minutes under simulated solar light irradiation due to the generation of ROS. Furthermore, these composites can arrest the bacterial growth and damage the bacterial membrane through electrostatic interaction. The gradual release of Ag^+ not only prevents bacterial infection with good long-term effectiveness but also stimulates the immune function to produce a large number of white blood cells and neutrophils, which favors the promotion of the wound healing process. This platform provides an effective strategy to prevent bacterial infection during wound healing.

Mosselhy et al[102] developed a method for immobilizing small (approximately 5 nm) AgNPs on a silica matrix to form a nanosilver–silica (Ag–SiO$_2$) composite and demonstrated the prolonged antibacterial effects of the composite in vitro. The composite exhibited a rapid initial Ag release after 24 hours and a slower leaching after 48 and 72 hours and was effective against both MRSA) and E $coli$. They also found that UV irradiation was superior to filter sterilization in retaining the antibacterial effects of the composite. Gauze, impregnated with the Ag–SiO$_2$ composite, showed higher antibacterial effects against MRSA and E $coli$ than a commercial Ag-containing dressing, indicating that Ag–SiO$_2$ composites, with prolonged antibacterial effects, are promising technologies with the potential for use in the management and infection control of superficial wounds.

Pagonis et al[103] studied the in vitro effects of PLGA NPs loaded with the photosensitizer methylene blue (MB) and light against E $faecalis$. The bacteria were sensitized in planktonic phase and in experimentally infected root

canals of human extracted teeth with MB-loaded NPs for 10 minutes followed by exposure to red light at a wavelength of 665 nm.[103] The NPs were found to be concentrated mainly on the cell walls of the microorganisms. The synergism of light and MB-loaded NPs led to approximately 2 and 1 log$_{10}$ reduction of colony-forming units in planktonic phase and root canals, respectively. In both cases, mean log$_{10}$ reductions were significantly lower than controls and MB-loaded NPs without light. The utilization of PLGA NPs encapsulated with photoactive drugs appears promising for antimicrobial endodontic treatment.

In recent years, several nanoantimicrobials, that is, nanoscale devices with intrinsic antibacterial activities or capacity for delivering antibiotics, have been developed for the treatment and prevention of bone infections.[104] These nanoantimicrobials can be designed to have controlled and sustained drug release kinetics, surface modifications for bone or bacteria targeting, and increased affinity for biofilms. Given the potential value of these nanoantimicrobials, their clinical application for the treatment of bone infection has been relatively slow and remains an attractive but underserved area of antimicrobial nanomaterial research that is, nevertheless, promising even though the clinical translation of such therapy from bench to bedside is only emerging.[104]

The aforementioned examples of emerging nanomaterial-enabled antimicrobial medical products are just a few of a growing number of products and areas of clinical application. Additional examples of nanotechnology-enabled medical products in development include cancer therapeutics using NPs to improve tumor targeting and localization, radioisotopic NPs (Au, Fe, indium [In], etc), and active pharmaceutical carrying liposomal, polymeric, solid-lipid NPs. Such applications are having an impact on most all aspects of clinical care and is advancing at a rapid pace worldwide.

Use of Nanoparticles to Overcome Microbial Resistance

The use of NPs is among the most promising strategies to overcome microbial drug resistance.[105] The NPs of different types have been developed to combat drug-resistant organisms, including nitric oxide–releasing NPs (NO NPs), chitosan-containing NPs (chitosan NPs), and metal-containing NPs that all use multiple mechanisms simultaneously to combat microbes, thereby making development of resistance to these NPs significantly less unlikely than that experienced with conventional antibiotics. Packaging multiple antimicrobial agents within the same NP also makes development of resistance even more difficult. The NPs can overcome existing drug resistance mechanisms, including decreased uptake and increased efflux of drug from the microbial cell, biofilm formation, and intracellular bacteria. These NPs can target antimicrobial agents to the site of infection, so that higher antimicrobial drug concentrations are delivered to the infected site, thereby overcoming resistance and lowering the potential for toxicity to noninfected tissues.

Antibiotic resistance in *Acinetobacter* species is a serious problem in hospitals around the world. These pathogens are often associated with health care–acquired infections and are associated with high mortality rates in frail or immunocompromised patients. Photodynamic inactivation (PDI) is a noninvasive and safe therapeutic method for such microbial infections.[106,107] Visible light has been shown to be safer than UV for PDI of such pathogens with mammalian cells. ZnO-NPs were used as an antimicrobial agent and a photosensitizer. The ZnO is recognized as safe and has extensive usage in food additives, medical, and cosmetic products. In mammalian cell cultures infected with *Acinetobacter baumannii*, 0.125-mg/mL ZnO-NPs combined with 10.8-J/cm^2 blue light significantly reduced microbial survival; however, it was observed that exposure to ZnO-NPs alone does not affect the viability of *A baumannii*. Irradiation appears to trigger the photocatalytic antimicrobial ability of ZnO-NPs on *A baumannii*. The mechanism of photocatalytic ZnO-NPs treatment appears to occur through bacterial membrane disruptions, and the photocatalytic ZnO-NPs treatment showed high microbial eradication in pathogens, including colistin-resistant and imipenem-resistant *A baumannii* and *K pneumoniae*. Based on these results, the photocatalytic ZnO-NPs treatment could support hygiene control and clinical therapies without antibiotics.

The spread of antibiotic-resistant bacteria through water is a threat to global public health. Das et al[108] studied the effect of Fe-doped ZnO NP (Fe/ZnO NP)-based solar-photocatalytic disinfection (PCD) of multidrug-resistant *E coli* (MDREC). In these studies, Fe/ZnO NPs were synthesized by chemical precipitation technique and, when used as photocatalyst for disinfection, proved to be more effective (time for complete disinfection = 90 min) than ZnO (150 min) and TiO$_2$ (180 min). Lipid peroxidation and potassium ion leakage studies indicated compromise of bacterial cell membranes and electron microscopy and live-dead staining confirmed the detrimental effects on membrane integrity. Investigations indicated that H$_2$O$_2$ was the key species involved in solar-PCD of MDREC by Fe/ZnO NPs. X-ray diffraction and atomic absorption spectroscopy studies showed that the Fe/ZnO NP system remained stable during the photocatalytic process. The Fe/ZnO NP–based solar-PCD process proved successful in the disinfection of real water samples collected from river, pond, and municipal tap. These studies provide important evidence that an Fe/ZnO NP catalyst made from low-cost materials can demonstrate high efficacy under solar photocatalytic conditions may have significant potential for real-world applications to help reduce the spread of bacterial pathogens.

It is clear that the alarming worldwide increase of antibiotic resistance in bacterial pathogens necessitates the development and rapid deployment of new antimicrobial techniques not affected by or lead to resistance development.[109] Light-mediated photocatalytic photoinactivation is only one emerging new technique that uses light to destroy a broad spectrum of pathogens. Most photoinactivation techniques rely on a diverse range of different types of NPs and nanostructures that have dimensions very similar to the wavelength of light that produces antimicrobial photocatalytic inactivation of pathogenic organisms. In contrast, PDI relies on the photochemical production of singlet oxygen from photosensitizing dyes (type II photodynamic pathway) that benefit from formulation in NP-based drug delivery vehicles. Fullerenes are a closed-cage carbon allotrope NP with high absorption coefficients and triplet yield. Their photochemistry is highly dependent on the microenvironment and can be type II in organic solvents and type I (•OH production) in a biological fluid. The TiO$_2$ NPs act as a large band-gap semiconductor that can carry out photo-induced electron transfer under UV-A light and can also produce ROS to kill microbial cells. Some recent PDI studies have shown that significant potentiation of microbial killing can be obtained by the addition of simple inorganic salts such as the nontoxic sodium/potassium iodide, bromide, nitrite, and even the toxic sodium azide in combination with fullerenes and/or TiO$_2$ NPs.[109]

▶ SAFETY CONSIDERATIONS

Because the study of biology does in fact require that we develop an understanding of the practical aspects of exposure to various naturally occurring NPs including smoke, ash, aerosols, and even viruses (which might be viewed as quite elegant NPs), toxicologists have been developing the tools and methods to assess the safety of engineered nanomaterials for over a decade.[1,11,96] Although nanotoxicology is still an emerging subdiscipline of toxicological science, there is a firm fundamental understanding that NPs can have hazard ranges from harmless to profoundly harmful.[1] For example, natural aerosols such as ocean spray, dust, and smoke at natural and atmospheric levels can be generally considered a low hazard (harmless), whereas exposure to the most pathogenic viruses at naturally occurring levels might be considered to be very high hazard (profoundly harmful). It is quite clear that all engineered nanomaterials intended for use as antimicrobials must be evaluated for safety using well-controlled toxicological testing procedures. In addition, if the antimicrobial nanotechnology is to be used in a manner where it will be in intimate contact with humans, the nanomaterial and fully formulated or fabricated product will likely require toxicological testing that adheres to good laboratory practice data standards for the region of the world where its use is to occur and is regulated.

It is already known that the pharmacological properties of some NP-antimicrobial agents may be hampered by potential toxicity.[38,110] The NPs can facilitate the penetration and delivery of antimicrobial agents into biological membranes including microbial cells, thereby enhancing and increasing the biological activities responsible for their antimicrobial efficacy.[28,69] This may also mean that the toxicity of different NP-antimicrobial substances and polymers may exhibit time-dependent toxic exposure response relationships that must be evaluated and taken into account in toxicological testing and risk characterization.[111]

Already some significant issues that require careful consideration in nanotoxicology have been reported. Doak et al[112] observed in their studies of genotoxicity with different nanomaterials that they cannot be treated in the same manner as other chemical compounds in safety assessments because their unique properties can cause unexpected interactions and misleading data. Most nanotoxicity studies (>70%) have been conducted in vitro using a wide variety of models; many of these have not been validated to in vivo toxicological effects or observations. There are very few control or standard reference nanomaterials available for use in the conduct of nanotoxicologic studies, but the degree and methods used in test article characterization in many published studies are substantially variable. In many cases, studies could not be duplicated and scientifically confirmed as state-of-the-art toxicological science would demand. Fortunately, these issues are known, and there is yet no additional toxicological effect shown with a nanomaterial that is unique. Overall, well-controlled, standardized methodologies can usually be adapted for use with nanomaterials to include dose (or exposure) characterizations to establish both the chemical as well as the physical aspects of a given nanomaterial. After decades of study with a growing and vast number of nanomaterials, no pathological effect (nanotoxicosis) unique to these NPs has been observed. Therefore, adverse effects observed with NPs may sometimes include a unique set of findings, but these effects do not appear to be unique to the science of toxicology and existing methods appear adequate to evaluate the safety of emerging nanomaterials.

It has been observed that NPs often are not best characterized by their fundamental material characteristics of size, shape, surface features, and composition but rather by evaluation of the protein corona that coats them following biological introduction. Understanding this for a given NP appears to be of fundamental significance in understanding how NPs and nanomaterials in general interact with different biological systems.[113-116] The corona that coats NPs is a natural process that covers the particle with a combination of "hard" NP-bound protein that is itself then covered with "soft" proteins that are more weakly bound to the outer protein surfaces.[117] These formations appear to be pharmacologically and toxicologically very significant to their biological activity including antimicrobial properties.[73,118,119] Corona proteins may be NP unique, and thousands of different types of proteins may be involved. Important pathophysiological actions such as

immune system recognition, cellular processing, biodistribution, kinetics, elimination, and so on may be affected individually or in combination by corona formation over the surface of an NP.[113,114]

Regulatory agencies such as the US Food and Drug Administration (FDA) and the European Medicines Agency already have some familiarity with the incorporation of nanotechnology in pharmaceutical and medical device products to include antimicrobial use. Both agencies have been continuously learning and improving their ability to understand the unique and potentially beneficial characteristics that the use of nanotechnology may provide to their regulated products. The evaluation of product safety for each nanomaterial-containing product is taken on a case-by-case basis, and it is generally thought that current regulations for medicines and medical devices are sufficiently stringent and comprehensive in scope to cover the theoretical risks associated with nanomaterials. Guidance is in place that requires nanomaterials used in pharmaceutical products be reported and that pharmaceuticals containing nanotechnology be closely evaluated for safety using state-of-the-science risk/benefit principles. The FDA has currently approved or cleared over 100 products that employ nanotechnology as pharmaceuticals and in medical devices.

When used in medical devices for a variety of purposes including antimicrobial surface coatings, the primary toxicological concern is for exposure to unbound nanomaterials. Many devices that employ nanotechnology may not require extensive safety evaluation if it can be established that by design and relevant data the nanomaterial is not bioavailable. In vitro diagnostic tests that employ nanotechnology generally would not require in vivo safety or biocompatibility evaluation. In all cases, the manufacturer is responsible for demonstrating that there is a lack of potential exposure to nanomaterials used in the device. The FDA Draft Guidance for Industry (April 2013) entitled "Use of International Standard ISO-10993, Biological Evaluation of Medical Devices Part 1: Evaluation and Testing" specifically addresses submicron or nanotechnology medical device components. This guidance clearly indicates that considerations for dose characterization and the design and conduct of safety studies will have to take into consideration the unique properties of these materials for all medical device products including those that employ antimicrobial nanomaterials.

▶ CONCLUSION

In conclusion, life depends on and has adapted to the presence of naturally occurring nanostructures and nanomaterials. Modern science and engineering have now developed the ability, termed *nanotechnology*, to make and manufacture nanomaterials in the 1- to 100-nm range for an expanding variety of purposes, including many that involve direct exposure to biological systems and that have antimicrobial properties. Nanotechnology for use in disinfection and sterilization applications is focusing on current problems of antisepsis, sanitation, infection prevention and control, and antimicrobial therapeutics using a wide variety of different of antimicrobial nanotechnologies. Many of these are now demonstrating clear potential for commercial use. There are still hurdles that must be overcome on the path to commercialization of many antimicrobial nanotechnology products. These include ensuring consistent quality in their manufacture, being able to effectively sterilize the product with the nanotechnological properties intact (when applicable) and toxicological testing that must demonstrate sufficient benefit to risk for the intended human or animal use. In order to properly assess risk, the field of nanotoxicology has emerged as a subdiscipline of toxicological science that is needed to support the discovery and development of safe nanotechnology products including those for antimicrobial use.

An understanding of the application of nanotechnology toward the development of novel nanoproducts that can advance current disinfection and sterilization technologies is essential because such products are already entering worldwide markets and are being developed at a rapid pace. This will continue well into the foreseeable future because nanotechnology platforms are not only demonstrating their value as antimicrobials but also ever expanding to include a widening array of structural and compositional possibilities. The benefit of nanotechnology to the development of new antimicrobials has already been demonstrated, but current products are only the beginning for the use of nanotechnology toward solutions to some of the most challenging issues of infection prevention and control.

REFERENCES

1. Hobson DW, Roberts SM, Shvedova AA, Warheit DB, Hinkley GK, Guy RC. Applied nanotoxicology. *Int J Toxicol.* 2016;35(1):5-16.
2. Seinfeld JH, Pandis SN. *Atmospheric Chemistry and Physics, from Air Pollution to Climate Change.* 2nd ed. New York, NY: John Wiley; 2006.
3. Buseck PR, Adachi K. Nanoparticles in the atmosphere. *Elements.* 2008;4:389-394.
4. University of Wisconsin—Madison. What determines sky's colors at sunrise and sunset? ScienceDaily Web site. https://www.sciencedaily.com/releases/2007/11/071108135522.htm. Accessed September 4, 2019.
5. Murphy DM, Thomson DS, Mahoney MJ. In situ measurements of organics, meteoritic material, mercury, and other elements in aerosols at 5 to 19 kilometers. *Science.* 1998;282:1664-1669.
6. Sah U, Sharma K, Chaudhri N, Sankar M, Gopinath P. Antimicrobial photodynamic therapy: single-walled carbon nanotube (SWCNT)-porphyrin conjugate for visible light mediated inactivation of *Staphylococcus aureus. Colloids Surf B Biointerfaces.* 2018;162:108-117.
7. Mohamed NA, Abd El-Ghany NA. Novel aminohydrazide cross-linked chitosan filled with multi-walled carbon nanotubes as antimicrobial agents. *Int J Biol Macromol.* 2018;115:651-662.
8. Hemeg HA. Nanomaterials for alternative antibacterial therapy. *Int J Nanomedicine.* 2017;12:8211-8225.
9. Yah CS, Simate GS. Nanoparticles as potential new generation broad spectrum antimicrobial agents. *Daru.* 2015;23:43.
10. National Nanotechnology Initiative. Nanotechnology 101: definition of nanotechnology. Nano.gov Web site. http://www.nano.gov/. Accessed March 16, 2019.
11. Monteiro-Riviere NA, Tran CL. *Nanotoxicology: Progress Toward Nanomedicine.* 2nd ed. Boca Raton, FL: CRC Press; 2014.
12. Kavoosi F, Modaresi F, Sanaei M, Rezaei Z. Medical and dental applications of nanomedicines. *APMIS.* 2018;126(10):795-803.
13. Fathima JB, Pugazhendhi A, Venis R. Synthesis and characterization of ZrO₂ nanoparticles-antimicrobial activity and their prospective role in dental care. *Microb Pathog.* 2017;110:245-251.
14. Elechiguerra JL, Burt JL, Morones JR, et al. Interaction of silver nanoparticles with HIV-1. *J Nanobiotechnology.* 2005;3:6.
15. Vaidyanathan R, Kalishwaralal K, Gopalram S, Gurunathan S. Nanosilver—the burgeoning therapeutic molecule and its green synthesis. *Biotechnol Adv.* 2009;27(6):924-937.
16. Pal S, Tak YK, Song JM. Does the antibacterial activity of silver nanoparticles depend on the shape of the nanoparticle? A study of the gram-negative bacterium *Escherichia coli. Appl Environ Microbiol.* 2007;73(6):1712-1720.
17. Sharma HS, Hussain S, Schlager J, Ali SF, Sharma A. Influence of nanoparticles on blood-brain barrier permeability and brain edema formation in rats. *Acta Neurochir Suppl.* 2010;106:359-364.
18. Yang W, Shen C, Ji Q, et al. Food storage material silver nanoparticles interfere with DNA replication fidelity and bind with DNA. *Nanotechnology.* 2009;20(8):085102.
19. Lu L, Sun RW, Chen R, et al. Silver nanoparticles inhibit hepatitis B virus replication. *Antivir Ther.* 2008;13(2):253-262.
20. Li WR, Xie XB, Shi QS, Zeng HY, Ou-Yang YS, Chen YB. Antibacterial activity and mechanism of silver nanoparticles on *Escherichia coli. Appl Microbiol Biotechnol.* 2010;85(4):1115-1122.
21. Zhao G, Stevens SE Jr. Multiple parameters for the comprehensive evaluation of the susceptibility of *Escherichia coli* to the silver ion. *Biometals.* 1998;11(1):27-32.
22. Ullah I, Khan K, Sohail M, Ullah K, Ullah A, Shaheen S. Synthesis, structural characterization and catalytic application of citrate-stabilized monometallic and bimetallic palladium@copper nanoparticles in microbial anti-activities. *Int J Nanomedicine.* 2017;12:8735-8747.
23. Roco MC. The US national nanotechnology initiative after 3 years (2001-2003). *J Nanopart Res.* 2004;6:1-10.
24. Roco MC, Bainbridge WS. Societal implications of nanoscience and nanotechnology: maximizing human benefit. *J Nanopart Res.* 2005;7(1):1-13.
25. Muangman P, Chuntrasakul C, Silthram S, et al. Comparison of efficacy of 1% silver sulfadiazine and Acticoat for treatment of partial-thickness burn wounds. *J Med Assoc Thai.* 2006;89(7):953-958.
26. Chen M, Pan X, Wu H, et al. Preparation and anti-bacterial properties of a temperature-sensitive gel containing silver nanoparticles. *Pharmazie.* 2011;66(4):272-277.
27. Podsiadlo P, Paternel S, Rouillard JM, et al. Layer-by-layer assembly of nacre-like nanostructured composites with antimicrobial properties. *Langmuir.* 2005;21(25):11915-11921.
28. Pelczar M, Reid R, Chan ECS. *Microbiologia.* São Paulo, Brazil: McGraw-Hill; 1980.
29. Senior K, Müller S, Schacht VJ, Bunge M. Antimicrobial precious-metal nanoparticles and their use in novel materials. *Recent Pat Food Nutr Agric.* 2012;4(3):200-209.
30. Yah CS. The toxicity of gold nanoparticles in relation to their physiochemical properties. *Biomed Res.* 2013;24(3):400-413.
31. Gatoo MA, Naseem S, Arfat MY, Dar AM, Qasim K, Zubair S. Physicochemical properties of nanomaterials: implication in associated toxic manifestations. *Biomed Res Int.* 2014;2014:498420.
32. Dorotkiewicz-Jach A, Augustyniak D, Olszak T, Drulis-Kawa Z. Modern therapeutic approaches against *Pseudomonas aeruginosa* infections. *Curr Med Chem.* 2015;22(14):1642-1664.
33. Chatterjee AK, Chakraborty R, Basu T. Mechanism of antibacterial activity of copper nanoparticles. *Nanotechnology.* 2014;25(13):135101.

34. Dong Q, Dong A, Morigen. Evaluation of novel antibacterial N-halamine nanoparticles prodrugs towards susceptibility of *Escherichia coli* induced by DksA protein. *Molecules.* 2015;20(4):7292-7308.

35. Li H, Chen Q, Zhao J, Urmila K. Enhancing the antimicrobial activity of natural extraction using the synthetic ultrasmall metal nanoparticles. *Sci Rep.* 2015;5:11033.

36. Xie Y, He Y, Irwin PL, Jin T, Shi X. Antibacterial activity and mechanism of action of zinc oxide nanoparticles against *Campylobacter jejuni. Appl Environ Microbiol.* 2011;77(7):2325-2331.

37. Galdiero S, Falanga A, Vitiello M, Cantisani M, Marra V, Galdiero M. Silver nanoparticles as potential antiviral agents. *Molecules.* 2011;16:8894-8918.

38. Piras AM, Maisetta G, Sandreschi S, et al. Chitosan nanoparticles loaded with the antimicrobial peptide temporin B exert a long-term antibacterial activity in vitro against clinical isolates of *Staphylococcus epidermidis. Front Microbiol.* 2015;6:372.

39. Dakal TC, Kumar A, Majumdar RS, Yadav V. Mechanistic basis of antimicrobial actions of silver nanoparticles. *Front Microbiol.* 2016;7:1831.

40. Durán N, Durán M, de Jesus MB, Seabra AB, Fávaro WJ, Nakazato G. Silver nanoparticles: a new view on mechanistic aspects on antimicrobial activity. *Nanomedicine.* 2016;12(3):789-799.

41. Łysakowska ME, Ciebiada-Adamiec A, Klimek L, Sienkiewicz M. The activity of silver nanoparticles (Axonnite) on clinical and environmental strains of *Acinetobacter* spp. *Burns.* 2015;41(2):364-371.

42. Sirelkhatim A, Mahmud S, Seeni A, et al. Review on zinc oxide nanoparticles: antibacterial activity and toxicity mechanism. *Nanomicro Lett.* 2015;7(3):219-242.

43. Wong MS, Chen CW, Hsieh CC, Hung SC, Sun DS, Chang HH. Antibacterial property of Ag nanoparticle-impregnated N-doped titania films under visible light. *Sci Rep.* 2015;5:11978.

44. Lellouche J, Friedman A, Lahmi R, Gedanken A, Banin E. Antibiofilm surface functionalization of catheters by magnesium fluoride nanoparticles. *Int J Nanomedicine.* 2012;7:1175-1188.

45. Lellouche J, Friedman A, Gedanken A, Banin E. Antibacterial and antibiofilm properties of yttrium fluoride nanoparticles. *Int J Nanomedicine.* 2012;7:5611-5624.

46. Yoon KY, Hoon Byeon J, Park JH, Hwang J. Susceptibility constants of *Escherichia coli* and *Bacillus subtilis* to silver and copper nanoparticles. *Sci Total Environ.* 2007;373(2-3):572-575.

47. Shamaila S, Zafar N, Riaz S, Sharif R, Nazir J, Naseem S. Gold nanoparticles: an efficient antimicrobial agent against enteric bacterial human pathogen. *Nanomaterials (Basel).* 2016;6(4):71. doi:10.3390/nano6040071.

48. Huo S, Jiang Y, Gupta A, et al. Fully zwitterionic nanoparticle antimicrobial agents through tuning of core size and ligand structure. *ACS Nano.* 2016;10(9):8732-8737.

49. Dhanabalan K, Gurunathan K. Microemulsion mediated synthesis and characterization of CdS nanoparticles and its anti-biofilm efficacy against *Escherichia coli* ATCC 25922. *J Nanosci Nanotechnol.* 2015;15(6):4200-4204.

50. Guisbiers G, Wang Q, Khachatryan E, et al. Inhibition of *E. coli* and *S. aureus* with selenium nanoparticles synthesized by pulsed laser ablation in deionized water. *Int J Nanomedicine.* 2016;11:3731-3736.

51. Khashan KS, Sulaiman GM, Abdul Ameer FA, Napolitano G. Synthesis, characterization and antibacterial activity of colloidal NiO nanoparticles. *Pak J Pharm Sci.* 2016;29(2):541-546.

52. Hernandez-Delgadillo R, Velasco-Arias D, Diaz D, et al. Zerovalent bismuth nanoparticles inhibit *Streptococcus mutans* growth and formation of biofilm. *Int J Nanomedicine.* 2012;7:2109-2113.

53. Ashfaq M, Verma N, Khan S. Copper/zinc bimetal nanoparticles-dispersed carbon nanofibers: a novel potential antibiotic material. *Mater Sci Eng C Mater Biol Appl.* 2016;59:938-947.

54. Liakos I, Grumezescu AM, Holban AM. Magnetite nanostructures as novel strategies for anti-infectious therapy. *Molecules.* 2014;19(8):12710-12726.

55. Ansari MA, Khan HM, Khan AA, Cameotra SS, Saquib Q, Musarrat J. Interaction of Al(2)O(3) nanoparticles with *Escherichia coli* and their cell envelope biomolecules. *J Appl Microbiol.* 2014;116(4):772-783.

56. Jiang W, Mashayekhi H, Xing B. Bacterial toxicity comparison between nano- and micro-scaled oxide particles. *Environ Pollut.* 2009;157(5):1619-1625.

57. Qi L, Xu Z, Jiang X, Hu C, Zou X. Preparation and antibacterial activity of chitosan nanoparticles. *Carbohydr Res.* 2004;339(16):2693-2700.

58. Gowri S, Gandhi RR, Sundrarajan M. Structural, optical, antibacterial and antifungal properties of zirconia nanoparticles by biobased protocol. *J Mater Sci Technol.* 2014;30(8):782-790.

59. Rupp R, Rosenthal SL, Stanberry LR. VivaGel (SPL7013 Gel): a candidate dendrimer—microbicide for the prevention of HIV and HSV infection. *Int J Nanomedicine.* 2007;2(4):561-566.

60. Donalisio M, Rusnati M, Cagno V, et al. Inhibition of human respiratory syncytial virus infectivity by a dendrimeric heparan sulfate-binding peptide. *Antimicrob Agents Chemother.* 2012;56(10):5278-5288.

61. McCarthy TD, Karellas P, Henderson SA, et al. Dendrimers as drugs: discovery and preclinical and clinical development of dendrimer-based microbicides for HIV and STI prevention. *Mol Pharm.* 2005;2:312-318.

62. Price CF, Tyssen D, Sonza S, et al. SPL7013 gel (VivaGel®) retains potent HIV-1 and HSV-2 inhibitory activity following vaginal administration in humans. *PLoS One.* 2011;6(9):e24095.

63. Chonco L, Pion M, Vacas E, et al. Carbosilane dendrimer nanotechnology outlines of the broad HIV blocker profile. *J Control Release.* 2012;161(3):949-958.

64. Imbuluzqueta E, Gamazo C, Ariza J, Blanco-Prieto MJ. Drug delivery systems for potential treatment of intracellular bacterial infections. *Front Biosci (Landmark Ed).* 2010;15:397-417.

65. Alizadeh H, Salouti M, Shapouri M. Bactericidal effect of silver nanoparticles on intramacrophage brucella abortus 544. *Jundishapur J Microbiol.* 2014;7:e9039.

66. Upadhyay RK. Drug delivery systems, CNS protection, and the blood brain barrier. *Biomed Res Int.* 2014;2014:869269.

67. Zhang L, Pornpattananangkul D, Hu CMJ, Huang CM. Development of nanoparticles for antimicrobial drug delivery. *Curr Med Chem.* 2010;17:585-594.

68. Yah CS, Simate GS, Iyuke SE. Nanoparticles toxicity and their routes of exposures. *Pak J Pharm Sci.* 2012;25(2):477-491.

69. Simate GS, Yah CS. The use of carbon nanotubes in medical applications—is it a success story? *Occup Med Health Aff.* 2014;2(1):147.

70. Dimapilis EAS, Hsu CS, Mendoza RMO, Lu MC. Review: zinc oxide nanoparticles for water disinfection. *Sustainable Environment Research.* 2018;28:47-56.

71. Abbaszadegan A, Gholami A, Abbaszadegan S, et al. The effects of different ionic liquid coatings and the length of alkyl chain on antimicrobial and cytotoxic properties of silver nanoparticles. *Iran Endod J.* 2017;12(4):481-487.

72. Halkai KR, Mudda JA, Shivanna V, Rathod V, Halkai RS. Biosynthesis, characterization and antibacterial efficacy of silver nanoparticles derived from endophytic fungi against *P. gingivalis. J Clin Diagn Res.* 2017;11(9):ZC92-ZC96.

73. Dutz S, Wojahn S, Gräfe C, Weidner A, Clement JH. Influence of sterilization and preservation procedures on the integrity of serum protein-coated magnetic nanoparticles. *Nanomaterials (Basel).* 2017;7:E453.

74. Almaaytah A, Mohammed GK, Abualhaijaa A, Al-Balas Q. Development of novel ultrashort antimicrobial peptide nanoparticles with potent antimicrobial and antibiofilm activities against multidrug-resistant bacteria. *Drug Des Devel Ther.* 2017;11:3159-3170.

75. Mahendra S, Li Q, Lyon DY, et al. Nanotechnology-enabled water disinfection and microbial control: merits and limitations. In: Street A, Sustich R, Duncan J, Savage N, eds. *Nanotechnology Applications for Clean Water.* 2nd ed. Elsevier; 2014:319-327.

76. Hoek EMV, Pendergast MT, Ghosh AK. Nanotechnology-based membranes for water purification. In: Street A, Sustich R, Duncan J, Savage N, eds. *Nanotechnology Applications for Clean Water.* 2nd ed. Waltham, MA: Elsevier; 2014:133-154.

77. Nameni G, Economy J. Nanometallic particles for oligodynamic microbial disinfection. In: Street A, Sustich R, Duncan J, Savage N, eds. *Nanotechnology Applications for Clean Water*. 2nd ed. Waltham, MA: Elsevier; 2014:283-295.

78. Kroto HW, Heath JR, O'Brien SC, Curl RF, Smalley RE. "C60: Buckminsterfullerene." *Nature*. 1985;318(6042):162-163.

79. Chae SR, Hotze EM, Wiesner MR. Possible applications of fullerene nanomaterials in water treatment and reuse. In: Street A, Sustich R, Duncan J, Savage N, eds. *Nanotechnology Applications for Clean Water*. 2nd ed. Waltham, MA: Elsevier; 2014:329-338.

80. Li Q, Wu P, Shang JK. Nanostructured visible-light photocatalysts for water purification. In: Street A, Sustich R, Duncan J, Savage N, eds. *Nanotechnology Applications for Clean Water*. 2nd ed. Waltham, MA: Elsevier; 2014:297-317.

81. Ritchie SMC. Enhanced dechlorination of trichloroethylene by membrane-supported iron and bimetallic nanoparticles. In: Street A, Sustich R, Duncan J, Savage N, eds. *Nanotechnology Applications for Clean Water*. 2nd ed. Waltham, MA: Elsevier; 2014:351-367.

82. Vetten MA, Yah CS, Singh T, Gulumian M. Challenges facing sterilization and depyrogenation of nanoparticles: effects on structural stability and biomedical applications. *Nanomedicine*. 2014;10(7):1391-1399.

83. Maksimenko O, Pavlov E, Toushov E, et al. Radiation sterilisation of doxorubicin bound to poly(butyl cyanoacrylate) nanoparticles. *Int J Pharm*. 2008;356(1-2):325-332.

84. Zheng J, Clogston JD, Patri AK, Dobrovolskaia MA, McNeil SE. Sterilization of silver nanoparticles using standard gamma irradiation procedure affects particle integrity and biocompatibility. *J Nanomed Nanotechnol*. 2011;2011(suppl 5):001.

85. Franca A, Pelaz B, Moros M, et al. Sterilization matters: consequences of different sterilization techniques on gold nanoparticles. *Small*. 2010;6(1):89-95.

86. Sommerfeld P, Schroeder U, Sabel BA. Sterilization of unloaded polybutylcyanoacrylate nanoparticles. *Int J Pharm*. 1998;164(1):113-118.

87. Memisoglu-Bilensoy E, Hincal AA. Sterile, injectable cyclodextrin nanoparticles: effects of gamma irradiation and autoclaving. *Int J Pharm*. 2006;311(1-2):203-208.

88. Desai N. Challenges in development of nanoparticle-based therapeutics. *AAPS J*. 2012;14(2):282-295.

89. Tsukada Y, Hara K, Bando Y, et al. Particle size control of poly (dl-lactide-co-glycolide) nanospheres for sterile applications. *Int J Pharm*. 2009;370(1-2):196-201.

90. Fesharaki PJ, Nazari P, Shakibaie M, et al. Biosynthesis of selenium nanoparticles using *Klebsiella pneumoniae* and their recovery by a simple sterilization process. *Braz J Microbiol*. 2010;41:461-466.

91. Masson V, Maurin F, Fessi H, Devissaguet JP. Influence of sterilization processes on poly(epsilon-caprolactone) nanospheres. *Biomaterials*. 1997;18(4):327-335.

92. Özcan I, Bouchemal K, Segura-Sánchez F, et al. Effects of sterilization techniques on the PEGylated poly(γ-benzyl-Lglutamate) (PBLG) nanoparticles. *Acta Pharm Sci*. 2009;51:211-218.

93. Jiang T, Wang Y, Li Z, et al. Prussian blue-encapsulated Fe₃O₄ nanoparticles for reusable photothermal sterilization of water. *J Colloid Interface Sci*. 2019;540:354-361.

94. Nartop P. Effects of surface sterilisation with green synthesised silver nanoparticles on Lamiaceae seeds. *IET Nanobiotechnol*. 2018;12(5):663-668.

95. Morones JR, Elechiguerra JL, Camacho A, et al. The bactericidal effect of silver nanoparticles. *Nanotechnology*. 2005;16(10):2346-2353.

96. Oberdörster G, Oberdörster E, Oberdörster J. Nanotoxicology: an emerging discipline evolving from studies of ultrafine particles. *Environ Health Perspect*. 2005;113:823-839.

97. Borm P, Klaessig FC, Landry TD, et al. Research strategies for safety evaluation of nanomaterials, part V: role of dissolution in biological fate and effects of nanoscale particles. *Toxicol Sci*. 2006;90(1):23-32.

98. Nohynek GJ, Lademann J, Ribaud C, Roberts MS. Grey goo on the skin? Nanotechnology, cosmetic and sunscreen safety. *Crit Rev Toxicol*. 2007;37(3):251-277.

99. Alvarez-Román R, Barré G, Guy RH, Fessi H. Biodegradable polymer nanocapsules containing a sunscreen agent: preparation and photoprotection. *Eur J Pharm Biopharm*. 2001;52(2):191-195.

100. Bennat C, Müller-Goymann CC. Skin penetration and stabilization of formulations containing microfine titanium dioxide as physical UV filter. *Int J Cosmet Sci*. 2000;22(4):271-283.

101. Jin C, Liu X, Tan L, et al. Ag/AgBr-loaded mesoporous silica for rapid sterilization and promotion of wound healing. *Biomater Sci*. 2018;6(7):1735-1744.

102. Mosselhy DA, Granbohm H, Hynönen U, et al. Nanosilver-silica composite: prolonged antibacterial effects and bacterial interaction mechanisms for wound dressings. *Nanomaterials (Basel)*. 2017;7:261. doi:10.3390/nano7090261.

103. Pagonis TC, Chen J, Fontana CR, et al. Nanoparticle-based endodontic antimicrobial photodynamic therapy. *J Endod*. 2010;36(2):322-388.

104. Guo P, Xue HY, Wong HL. Therapeutic nanotechnology for bone infection treatment—state of the art. *Curr Drug Deliv*. 2018;15(7):941-952.

105. Pelgrift RY, Friedman AJ. Nanotechnology as a therapeutic tool to combat microbial resistance. *Adv Drug Deliv Rev*. 2013;65(13-14):1803-1815.

106. Ghasemi F, Jalal R.Antimicrobial action of zinc oxide nanoparticles in combination with ciprofloxacin and ceftazidime against multidrug-resistant *Acinetobacter baumannii*. *J Glob Antimicrob Resist*. 2016;6:118-122.

107. Yang MY, Chang KC, Chen LY, et al. Blue light irradiation triggers the antimicrobial potential of ZnO nanoparticles on drug-resistant *Acinetobacter baumannii*. *J Photochem Photobiol B*. 2018;180:235-242.

108. Das S, Sinha S, Das B, et al. Disinfection of multidrug resistant *Escherichia coli* by solar-photocatalysis using Fe-doped ZnO nanoparticles. *Sci Rep*. 2017;7(1):104.

109. Kashef N, Huang YY, Hamblin MR. Advances in antimicrobial photodynamic inactivation at the nanoscale. *Nanophotonics*. 2017;6(5):853-879.

110. Mogharabi M, Abdolahi M, Faramarzi MM. Toxicity of nanomaterials. *Daru*. 2014;22:9.

111. Nuñez-Anita RE, Acosta-Torres LS, Vilar-Pineda J, et al. Toxicology of antimicrobial nanoparticles for prosthetic devices. *Int J Nanomedicine*. 2014;9:3999-4006.

112. Doak SH, Griffiths SM, Manshian B, et al. Confounding experimental considerations in nanogenotoxicology. *Mutagenesis*. 2009;24(4):285-293.

113. Tenzer S, Docter D, Kuharev J, et al. Rapid formation of plasma protein corona critically affects nanoparticle pathophysiology. *Nat Nanotechnol*. 2013;8:772-781.

114. Lee YK, Choi EJ, Webster TJ, Kim SH, Khang D. Effect of the protein corona on nanoparticles for modulating cytotoxicity and immunotoxicity. *Int J Nanomedicine*. 2015;10:97-112.

115. Aggarwal P, Hall JB, McLeland CB, Dobrovolskaia MA, McNeil SE. Nanoparticle interaction with plasma proteins as it relates to particle biodistribution, biocompatibility and therapeutic efficacy. *Adv Drug Deliv Rev*. 2009;61(6):428-437.

116. Karmali PP, Simberg D. Interactions of nanoparticles with plasma proteins: implication on clearance and toxicity of drug delivery systems. *Expert Opin Drug Deliv*. 2011;8(3):343-357.

117. Winzen S, Schoettler S, Baier G, et al. Complementary analysis of the hard and soft protein corona: sample preparation critically effects corona composition. *Nanoscale*. 2015;7:2992-3001.

118. Safi M, Courtois J, Seigneuret M, Conjeaud H, Berret JF. The effects of aggregation and protein corona on the cellular internalization of iron oxide nanoparticles. *Biomaterials*. 2011;32:9353-9363.

119. Lundqvist M, Stigler J, Elia G, Lynch I, Cedervall T, Dawson KA. Nanoparticle size and surface properties determine the protein corona with possible implications for biological impacts. *Proc Natl Acad Sci USA*. 2008;105:14265-14270.

Index

Page numbers in *italics* indicate illustrations; numbers followed by "t" indicate tables.

A

A₀, 16, 953–954
AAMI. *See* Association for the Advancement of Medical Instrumentation
AATB. *See* American Association of Tissue Banks
AATCC. *See* American Association of Textile Chemists and Colorists
AAZV. *See* American Association of Zoo Veterinarians
Abbreviated New Drug Application (ANDA), 1363
Aβ protein, as prion, 1337, 1339, 1341, 1343
ABSA, 1218
Abscesses
   cutaneous, 899–900
   dentoalveolar, 921t
Absolute pore ratings, 637
Absolute temperature, and speed of molecules, 145, *146*
Absorbed dose, 611
Acanthamoeba, 38–39
   contact lens contamination, 69, 1111, 1112, 1113–1116, 1119–1120
   cysts of, 39
   environmental epidemiology of, 1115–1116, *1117*
   food- and water-infective, 1156t
   ozone for, 695
   water contamination by, 773
Acanthamoeba castellanii, 38, 39, *1115*, 1115–1116
Acanthamoeba keratitis, 1112, 1113–1116, *1115*
Acanthamoeba polyphaga, 1115–1116
Accelerated hydrogen peroxide, 1041, 1057, 1067–1058
Acceptable daily exposure (ADE), 160
Accreditation organizations, 1131–1132
Acetic acid, 245, 246t
   peracetic acid and, 370–371
   in veterinary medicine, 1048
Acetylcholine hydroxide, *443*
Acholeplasma laidlawii, 673
Achromobacter guttatus, 457
Acid(s), 121t, 243–251
   common, 245, 246t
   critical limits for microbial growth, 243–245, *244*
   definition of, 243

as disinfectants, factors affecting, 243
in disinfection, 243, 246–247
effects in water, 243, *244*
in food/beverages, 245
modes of action, 248–249, *249*
strong *vs.* weak, 245
tolerance of selected bacteria, 245t
types of, 245
in veterinary medicine, 1048, 1050t
Acid cleaners, 164
Acid-fast mycobacteria, 33
Acidic detergents, for medical devices, 945
Acidic solutions, 243
Acidified water, 1080
Acidophiles, 244, *244*
Acidulants, in food processing, 772, 772t
Acid wash, 163
Acinetobacter
   contact lens contamination, 1114
   heat disinfection for, 228t
   protozoa-associated, 38
   resistance, nanoparticles and, 1414
   resistance to silver, 910
   surface survival time of, 963–964, 965t
Acinetobacter baumannii
   alcohols for, 388
   antiadherent surfaces and, 1392
   burn wound infection, 908
   essential oils for, 272–273
   hand hygiene for, 862, 862t
   health-care acquired infection, 32
   nanoparticles and, 1414
   as objectionable microorganism, 32
   resistance to silver, 552
Acinetobacter calcoaceticus, 526
Acquired enamel pellicle (AEP), 918
Acquired resistance, 34–35, 34t
Acridine(s)
   conventional, 254–255, 255t
   photodynamic, 260–261, 260t
Acridine mepacrine, 254–255
Acridine orange, 260t
Acriflavine, 254–255
Acrolein, 507
Actinobacillus equuli, 1091t
Actinobacteria, in skin flora, 880
Actinomyces, 918–919
Action limits. *See* Alert and action limits

Action spectrum (AS)
   definition of, 179
   of ultraviolet radiation, 179–181, *180*
Activated oxygen bleach (AOB), for laundry, 932
Activated water, 1080
Activation, of bacterial spores, 140–141, *141*
Acute Exposure Guideline Levels for Hazardous Substance (AEGL) values, for peracetic acid, 378, 378t
ADA. *See* American Dental Association
Additive effects, *78*, 78–80, *79*, 120–121
ADE. *See* Acceptance daily exposure
Adenosine triphosphate (ATP), on medical devices, 953t
Adenosine triphosphate (ATP)-binding cassette family, 51
Adenoviruses, 31t
   alcohols for, 389, 390, 392, 396t
   bovine, 1072
   canine, 1071t, 1073
   droplet transmission of, 985
   efficacy studies for, 32
   formaldehyde for, 758
   phenolics for, 424t, 425
   plasma sterilization for, 711–712
   porcine, 1070t, 1072
   resistance of, 27
   surface survival time of, 963, 965t
   ultraviolet radiation for, 179
Adhesion, surfaces reducing or eliminating, 1388–1393
Adhesional forces, 437
Adhesives, for sterile packaging, 841
Adipaldehyde, sporicidal activity of, 512t
Adsorption, 636–637, 648, 654
   of preservatives, 808, 810, 810t
Adulterated food, 1375
Advisory Committee on Immunization Practices, 987
AEGL. *See* Acute Exposure Guideline Levels for Hazardous Substance (AEGL) values, for peracetic acid
AEP. *See* Acquired enamel pellicle
Aeration
   definition of, 16
   in ethylene oxide sterilization, 663–665
   in hydrogen peroxide sterilization, 676–677, 678, 680, *680*